PATIENT CARE SKILLS

Fifth Edition

Mary Alice Duesterhaus Minor, P.T., M.S.
Clinical Assistant Professor of Physical Therapy
Clarkson University
Potsdam, New York

Scott Duesterhaus Minor, P.T., Ph.D.
Associate Dean for Health Science
Associate Professor and Chair
Department of Physical Therapy
Clarkson University
Potsdam, New York

Photography:
Sarah Ruth Minor
Azimuth Incorporated
St. Louis, Missouri and Potsdam, New York

PEARSON

Prentice
Hall

Upper Saddle River, New Jersey 07458

Library of Congress Cataloging-in-Publication Data

Minor, Mary Alice D., (date)
    Patient care skills / Mary Alice Duesterhaus Minor, Scott Duesterhaus Minor.—5th ed.
        p. ;   cm.
    Includes bibliographical references and index.
    ISBN 0-13-111382-8
    1. Transport of sick and wounded. 2. Patients—Positioning.
3. Nursing.
    [DNLM: 1. Nursing Care—methods. 2. Physical Therapy
Techniques. 3. Asepsis—methods. 4. Orthopedic Equipment.
5. Transportation of Patients—methods. WB 460 M666p 2006]
I. Minor, Scott Duesterhaus. II. Title.
    RT87.T72M56 2006
    610.73—dc22

                                                    2005016529

Publisher: Julie Levin Alexander
Assistant to Publisher: Regina Bruno
Executive Editor: Mark Cohen
Associate Editor: Melissa Kerian
Editorial Assistant: Jaquay Felix
Media Editor: John J. Jordan
Director of Production and Manufacturing:
    Bruce Johnson
Managing Production Editor: Patrick Walsh
Production Liaison: Christina Zingone
Production Editor: Jessica Balch, Pine Tree Composition
Manufacturing Manager: Ilene Sanford

Manufacturing Buyer: Pat Brown
Design Coordinator/Cover Designer:
    Christopher Weigand
Director of Marketing: Karen Allman
Channel Marketing Manager: Rachele Strober
Manager of Media Production: Amy Peltier
Media Project Manager: Stephen Hartner
New Media Production: Hector Grillone, Anne
    Lukens, Jody Small, and Kate Stillings, Pearson
    Video Production Services; Red Frog, Inc.
Composition: Pine Tree Composition, Inc.
Printer/Binder: Banta Book Group
Cover Printer: Phoenix Color Corp.

Pearson Education Ltd., *London*
Pearson Education Australia Pty. Limited, *Sydney*
Pearson Education Singapore, Pte. Ltd.
Pearson Education North Asia Ltd., *Hong Kong*
Pearson Education Canada, Ltd., *Toronto*

Pearson Educación de Mexico, S.A. de C.V.
Pearson Education—Japan, *Tokyo*
Pearson Education Malaysia, Pte. Ltd.
Pearson Education, Upper Saddle River, New Jersey

10 9 8 7 6 5 4 3 2 1
ISBN 0-13-111382-8

This book is dedicated to better care for all patients.

CONTENTS

CHAPTER 8 Transfers

CHAPTER 9 Ambulation with Ambulatory Assistive Devices

PREFACE

As the first text of its kind in physical therapy, first published in 1982, it is exciting to see a fifth edition come to fruition 23 years later. It is also extremely exciting to know that this edition is truly a family project. Our daughter, Sarah, born during the first year of publication, has been a photographic subject in previous editions and now is the photographer for the entire text.

We feel extremely fortunate for the continued acceptance of this text. We have worked to meet the responsibility of this faith in our efforts by adding new elements in this fifth edition that build on the strengths of the previous four editions, and by updating information that is changing constantly. We appreciate the faith our colleagues have demonstrated by allowing us to assist them in teaching new generations of physical therapists and physical therapist assistants. We have been fortunate to have received, and we continue to seek, critical commentary and counsel from students and colleagues who have used previous editions of this text and will use this fifth edition. New to this edition is an accompanying CD-ROM providing instructional videos and review questions, an addition to this textbook that has been sought for years and supported by those who have provided critical commentary.

A large number of procedures and variations are included in this manual, although it is not all inclusive. When choosing from among alternative methods or procedures, the most important consideration is to use the safest and most beneficial method for patient and physical therapist. In some cases, this will require modification of previously learned procedures. In all cases, practice will develop safe and efficient performance.

We have found that when teaching these procedures, students can learn both the specifics of the procedures as well as general rules of good body mechanics, patient handling, and safety for patients and physical therapists. Students may require assistance in problem solving when applying procedures in a variety of patient care situations. To assist student learning and problem solving, Suggested Activities and Case Studies have been included.

Each chapter and major section is introduced by a general explanation of the basis for performing the procedures to be described, and by a presentation of general rules or guidelines that are generic to a series of procedures. Wording of instructions in the text are repeated in similar format to enhance generic application when appropriate. Individual rules for specific procedures are associated with each procedure presented. For each procedure presented, step-by-step illustrations are accompanied by brief verbal explanations. Following the sequence of illustrations for a specific procedure decreases the need for extensive text explanations and provides students with a visual reference to determine if the sequence of steps they are performing matches the sequence of steps presented. Each chapter concludes with a series of review questions that provide students an opportunity to test newly acquired knowledge. Review questions can also be used as a study guide by reviewing the questions *before* beginning study of a chapter's content.

Finally, we wish to comment on the terms "patient" and "physical therapist." We have used the term "patient" throughout the text to designate the individual receiving care. This term has been used for its general sense of meaning for consistency throughout the text. We have used the term "physical therapist" throughout the text to designate the individual providing care. This does not mean that only physical therapists can, or will, perform these tasks. We expect that in addition to physical therapists and physical therapist assistants, many health care providers, including home health aides, medical assistants, nurses, nurses' aides, nursing home attendants, occupational therapists, occupational therapy assistants, and orderlies will perform these tasks. Therefore, we hope this text will be useful to the many people receiving and practitioners providing care.

Mary Alice Duesterhaus Minor
Scott Duesterhaus Minor

ACKNOWLEDGMENTS

It is unimaginable to us that any author could create a text and then perform by themselves all the additional tasks required to transform the text into a book and place it before the public. We are aware that this is not possible from our work in creating four previous editions. Each of the four previous editions acknowledge the significant number of people who contributed to each of those editions. With this in mind, we wish to acknowledge those who have contributed significantly to this fifth edition.

We first thank our daughter, Sarah Minor, for the photographic illustrations on which this book depends. We are grateful to Sarah for her critical eye, suggestions, attention to detail, and diligent work in creating the photographic illustrations. We are also grateful to Sarah for willingly putting her education and training as a professional photographer at our disposal.

To Ruth Ann Bosse, Christin Cavoretto, Michelle Deslauriers, Jason Garner, Pradip Grosh, Chuck Gulas, Buddy Heimburger, Nick Heimburger, Kristen Hobgood, Bonnie Hogenkamp, MaryClare Krusing, Chrysta Lloyd, Lewis Mueller, Patty Navarro, Jason Rubel, Abby Schilly, Debbie Schilly, Kathryn Schopmeyer, Joe Shapiro, Tina Shapiro, Sarah Stawizynski, and Michelle Unterberg, we offer thanks and appreciation for their participation in photography sessions. To Gerald Bunker, Heather Caswell, George Fulk, Natalie Gilbert, Justin Hetu, Ellie O'Neill, and King Wilcox, we offer thanks and appreciation for their participation in videography sessions for production of the CD that is an exciting addition to this fifth edition of the text.

We extend our thanks to Joe Neels of Provider Plus Inc. (St. Louis, MO), and Philip Lyons of Orthotic Mobility Systems, Inc. (Kensington, MD), for arranging the loan and use of patient care equipment.

We wish to express our appreciation to Maryville University—St. Louis and Clarkson University for the use of facilities and equipment for photographic and videographic sessions.

We must acknowledge our appreciation to Pearson Education/Prentice Hall personnel who have provided patience, support, and assistance, through an extended period of time during the preparation of this fifth edition. We are grateful to Mark Cohen, Health Professions Editor, and Melissa Kerian, Associate Health Professions Editor, for guiding this project from inception to completion. We are grateful to Jessica Balch of Pine Tree Composition for her work as Production Editor. We are grateful to Christina Zingone, John Jordan, Anne Lukens, Hector Grillone, and Karen Holmes of Pearson Education for their advice, technical savvy, and support for the photographic and videographic aspects of this fifth edition.

Finally, to acknowledge that this is the fifth edition of a successful text, we wish to remember those who contributed to the first four editions. For their participation and contributions to the first two editions, we thank Jim York, photographer, Gary Bergner, Freda Bowden, Mary Edna Harrell, Marvin Levand, Julie Leidecker, and Jennifer McFarland. We thank Cheryl L. Mehalik, Editor, and Sondra Greenfield, Production Editor, for their contributions to the third edition. For their participation and contributions to the fourth edition, we thank Lin Marshall, Editor, Robert Morrison, photographer, Arnie Berger, Deborah Bosse, Jeffrey Bosse, Bettina Brown, Suzanne Cornbleet, Kathleen Dixon, Mustafa Koluman, Janice Loudon, Sarah Minor, and Michael Mueller. For their contributions of facilities and equipment we acknowledge Wichita State University, Maryville University—St. Louis, and Washington University—St. Louis.

REVIEWERS

Marianne Craven, BS, MN
Associate Professor
Department of Nursing
Utah Valley State College
Oren, Utah

Elaine M. Eckel, PT, MA
Program Chair
Physical Therapist Assistant Program
Fayetteville Technical Community College
Fayetteville, North Carolina

Joan E. Edelstein, MA, PT, FISPO
Special Lecturer
Program in Physical Therapy
Columbia University
New York, New York

Eugene D. Hashley, MSEd, PT
Former Director
Physical Therapist Assistant Program
Southeast Missouri State University
Cape Girardeau, Missouri

Rolando Lazaro, PT, DPT, GCS
Assistant Professor
Coordinator, Transitional DPT Program
Department of Physical Therapy
University of the Pacific
Stockton, California

Laura Lee Swisher, PT, PhD
Assistant Professor
School of Physical Therapy
University of South Florida
Tampa, Florida

Robin Ward, PT, MBA
Instructor
Physical Therapist Assistant Program
Linn State Technical College
Linn, Missouri

PROCEDURES

1

PATIENT/CLIENT MANAGEMENT PROCESS

MEDIALINK

A companion CD-ROM, included free with each new copy of this book, supplements the techniques presented in the book. Insert the CD-ROM to watch video clips of patient care skills being demonstrated. This multi-media feature is designed to help you add a new dimension to your learning.

LEARNING OBJECTIVES

Upon completion of this chapter, you will be able to:

1. List and describe the 19 Health Insurance Portability and Accountability Act (HIPAA) identifiers in medical records.
2. Describe the purpose for listing and protecting each patient's 19 HIPAA identifiers.
3. Describe the purposes of an initial interview with the patient.
4. Describe the elements of the Patient/Client Management process presented in the *Guide to Physical Therapist Practice*.[1]
5. Describe the two styles of questions, and when they are used, in an interview.
6. List the areas to be included in an initial interview and provide an overview of the material to be included in each area.
7. List the purposes of documentation in the health care system.
8. Describe two formats of medical records: SOAP[2] note and Patient/Client Management.[3]
9. Describe the sections of the SOAP[2] note format and provide an overview of the material to be included in each section.
10. Describe the elements of the patient/client management[3] note format and provide an overview of the material to be included in each section.
11. Discuss the requirements of proper goal statements.
12. Discuss the requirements of adequate documentation.
13. List the information provided by the medical records audit.

KEY TERMS

Active pathology
Assessment (SOA**P** note)
Audit
Closed-ended question
Database
Diagnosis
Disability
Discharge note
Documentation
Evaluation
Examination
Functional limitations

Health Insurance Portability and Accountability Act (HIPAA)
Identifiers
Impairment
Initial note
Intervention
Interview
Long-term goals (LTGs)
Narrative note
Objective (S**O**AP note)
Open-ended question
Patient/client management note

Plan (SOA**P** note)
Plan of care
Preferred practice pattern
Problem list
Problem-oriented medical record (POMR) method
Prognosis
Progress (interim) notes
Short-term goals (STGs)
SOAP note
Source-oriented method
Subjective (**S**OAP note)

INTRODUCTION

HEALTH INSURANCE PORTABILITY AND ACCOUNTABILITY ACT

In 1996, Federal legislation titled the **Health Insurance Portability and Accountability Act (HIPAA)** was passed. Its effective date of compliance was April, 2002. The purpose of HIPAA is to protect the confidentiality of patient medical records as they are conveyed between health care providers or between health care providers and insurers. The requirements of HIPAA were established because of concern that confidential patient medical information was, on occasion, being handled without appropriate confidentiality, and utilized inappropriately.

Within HIPAA, 18 specific identifiers (the first 18 listed), and 1 general (the last listed) identifier are listed that might allow unauthorized knowledge of a patient's medical information, and thus inappropriate utilization of this knowledge. The 19 identifiers are:

- Name/initials
- Street address, city, county, precinct, zip code, and equivalent geocodes
- All elements of dates (except year) directly related to an individual
- All ages over 89
- Telephone number
- Fax number
- Electronic mail address
- Social security number
- Medical record numbers
- Health plan identification numbers
- Account numbers
- Certificate/license numbers
- Vehicle identifiers and serial numbers, including license plate numbers
- Device identifiers and serial numbers
- Web (Internet) addresses (uniform resource locators [URLs])
- Internet provider (IP) addresses
- Biometric identifiers, including finger and voice prints
- Full face photographic images and any comparable images
- Any other unique identifying number, characteristic, or code (a code is an identifier if the person holding the coded data can re-identify the individual; i.e., if the code is linked to an individual and the person has access to the master list)

This information must not be released without a patient's express written permission. Permission must be requested by each facility with which a patient has a relationship. Facilities are also required to provide each patient with written notification of policies and procedures relating to patient confidentiality under HIPAA regulations and each patient must sign a statement indicating that he or she has been informed of such policies. By protecting any identifiers, confidentiality of patient records is assured. It is vital to follow HIPAA regulations to protect a patient's right to privacy. The same expectations of privacy encompassed by HIPAA regulations should be applied to health care professionals' conversations concerning patients within facility environments, such as discussions in hallways and elevators.

GUIDE TO PHYSICAL THERAPIST PRACTICE

In recent years, the American Physical Therapy Association supported the development of the *Guide to Physical Therapist Practice (Guide)*,[1] an evolving document. Figures 1–1 and 1–3 and Appendices A–F (found at the end of this chapter) are reprinted (with permission) from the *Guide*.[1]

The *Guide* is based, in part, on the disablement model, particularly the four-phased model espoused by Nagi.[2–4] The four phases described by Nagi[2–4] are: (a) active pathology, (b) impairment, (c) functional limitations, and (d) disability.

Active pathology, the first phase, is the interruption of the normal functioning of the body at the cellular level. **Impairment,** the second phase, results when the body cannot compensate or heal itself so that an individual sustains loss of normal function of a system. **Functional limitations,** the third phase, occurs when the loss of a system is sufficient to prevent an individual to perform routine tasks, such as activities of daily living (ADLs), independently and in a timely manner. **Disability,** the fourth phase, occurs when functional limitations prevent an individual from fulfilling his or her life roles, such as parent, employee, or spouse.

In the following discussion, the terms "physical therapist," "physical therapist assistant," and "practitioner" are used. Although this text focuses on physical therapy services, other health professionals may also perform similar tasks.

A **preferred practice pattern** is a description of elements that comprise patient/client management provided by physical therapists. The *Guide*[1] presents five elements by which a preferred practice pattern is defined. Preferred practice patterns are described for each of four categories of conditions within the scope of practice of physical therapists. The four categories within the scope of practice of physical therapists are: (a) musculoskeletal, (b) neuromuscular, (c) cardiovascular/pulmonary, and (d) integumentary. When a preferred practice pattern is followed, physical therapists are guided by results when applying each of the five elements sequentially. The resulting activities comprise the Patient/Client Management process.

The patient/client management process is fundamental to delivery of physical therapy services. The five elements that contribute to identifying and managing a preferred practice pattern are: (a) examination, (b) evaluation, (c) diagnosis, (d) prognosis, and (e) intervention. **Examination** is the process of generating a patient/client history, reviewing all physiologic systems, and applying tests and measures. Upon examination, the physical therapist identifies impairments that produce functional limitations that may limit an individual to such a degree that a temporary or permanent disability occurs. **Evaluation** is the process of making clinical judgments based on the findings from the examination. **Diagnosis** is assignment of a label that states the categorization or classification of the problems identified. **Prognosis** is the determination of the optimal level of improvement and the time necessary to achieve this level. **Plan of care** is a statement that specifies goals, outcomes, and interventions to be provided for a patient's physical therapy care and the timeline for achieving goals and outcomes. **Intervention** is the combination of treatments, communication, education, and other planning that constitute physical therapist and patient/client interaction. A physical therapist's diagnosis is related to the impairments and functional limitations. The diagnosis is selected from the practice pattern or diagnostic category that most closely describes a patient's impairments and functional limitations as presented in the *Guide*.[1] This diagnostic category also indicates the prognosis, plan of care, and directs interventions that allow a patient to achieve expected outcomes. When the examination and evaluation do not result in a physical therapist being able to place a patient in a diagnostic category, it is likely that the patient's active pathology is not within the scope of physical therapy practice and the physical therapist should refer the patient to an appropriate practitioner. Figure 1–1 presents the elements of the Patient/Client Management process leading to optimal outcomes.

DIAGNOSIS
Both the process and the end result of evaluating examination data, which the physical therapist organizes into defined clusters, syndromes, or categories to help determine the prognosis (including the plan of care) and the most appropriate intervention strategies.

PROGNOSIS (Including Plan of Care)
Determination of the level of optimal improvement that may be attained through intervention and the amount of time required to reach that level. The plan of care specifies the interventions to be used and their timing and frequency.

EVALUATION
A dynamic process in which the physical therapist makes clinical judgments based on data gathered during the examination. This process also may identify possible problems that require consultation with or referral to another provider.

INTERVENTION
Purposeful and skilled interaction of the physical therapist with the patient/client and, if appropriate, with other individuals involved in care of the patient/client, using various physical therapy methods and techniques to produce changes in the condition that are consistent with the diagnosis and prognosis. The physical therapist conducts a reexamination to determine changes in patient/client status and to modify or redirect intervention. The decision to reexamine may be based on new clinical findings or on lack of patient/client progress. The process of reexamination also may identify the need for consultation with or referral to another provider.

EXAMINATION
The process of obtaining a history, performing a systems review, and selecting and administering tests and measures to gather data about the patient/client. The initial examination is a comprehensive screening and specific testing process that leads to a diagnostic classification. The examination process also may identify possible problems that require consultation with or referral to another provider.

OUTCOMES
Results of patient/client management, which include the impact of physical therapy interventions in the following domains: pathology/pathophysiology (disease, disorder, or condition); impairments, functional limitations, and disabilities; risk reduction/prevention; health, wellness, and fitness; societal resources; and patient/client satisfaction.

FIGURE 1–1   Elements of Patient/Client Management Leading to Optimal Outcomes. Reprinted with permission from the American Physical Therapy Association.

EXAMINATION

CHART REVIEW

A review of the patient's chart should occur prior to interviewing the patient. When intake history is included in the medical chart, some information for each of the following areas is usually available in the chart: general demographics, current condition or chief complaint, medical/surgical history, general health status, social history, family history, social health habits, previous and present functional status, medications and clinical tests ordered, and results. When the patient is a child, development is also reviewed. The initial chart review must be conducted by a physical therapist. Charts should be reviewed prior to each treatment to determine any relevant changes in patient status or orders. These subsequent reviews should be done by a physical therapist whenever possible, but may be done by a physical therapist assistant. When a chart review is conducted by a physical therapist assistant, the physical therapist must be informed of any significant changes in patient status that affect physical therapy intervention before a physical therapist assistant initiates any intervention.

INTERVIEW

An interview (Figure 1–2) is the next step in the Patient/Client Management process. When conducting an interview, a physical therapist must make sure the patient is comfortable and safe. The physical therapist should ensure that good eye contact can be made with the patient.

Information gathered during a chart review is reviewed with the patient. Specifics of the chief complaint(s) are explored. A survey of all physiologic systems is completed through questioning (see Appendix A). A physical therapist must conduct the initial interview. Brief interviews should be conducted prior to each treatment to determine any relevant changes in patient status. These subsequent brief interviews should be conducted by a physical therapist whenever possible, but may be conducted by a physical therapist assistant. When a follow-up interview is conducted by a physical therapist assistant, the physical therapist must be informed of any significant changes in patient status that may affect physical therapy intervention before a physical therapist assistant initiates any intervention.

A physical therapist/patient relationship usually begins with an initial interview. Experienced physical therapists begin examination of patients as soon as a patient is observed and patients begin to judge health care practitioners when they are first observed and introduced. Dress, body language, and general demeanor convey a message that may be more powerful than a practitioner's words. Health care professionals set the tone for an ongoing patient/practitioner relationship that has a basis of mutual trust.

A physical therapist begins an interview by addressing the patient by his or her proper name and introducing himself or herself using complete name and area of health care he or she represents. The physical therapist should then ask the patient's permission to begin an interview. Two types of questions are used in an interview. **Open-ended questions** allow a patient to tell his or her story in his or her own words. Examples of open-ended questions are: "Tell me about the problem you are having" or "Tell me about your injury." **Closed-ended questions** are used to obtain or confirm specific information. Closed-ended questions, such as "Have you ever had this pain before?," are often answered with a single, or just a few, word(s), such as "Yes," "No," or "Yes, about six months ago."

Questions provide direction for the interview. Interviews begin with open-ended questions to elicit the most information from the patient. During an interview, the

FIGURE 1–2 Physical therapist interviewing a patient.

physical therapist should summarize patient responses periodically. Then, using closed-ended questions, a physical therapist asks the patient if the summary is correct. If the summary is not correct, details must be clarified. Physical therapists also use closed-ended questions to focus discussion and to obtain specific information that a patient may not have thought to include. A physical therapist concludes the interview by asking the patient if there is anything else he or she would like to disclose.

Having a plan and structure for an interview permits a physical therapist to obtain needed information in a reasonable amount of time. Data collection forms (see Appendices B and C) give structure to an interview and assist in collection of data in an organized manner. When data are gathered and entered onto forms during a chart review prior to a patient interview, a physical therapist should ask closed-ended questions to confirm that the data are correct. There may be different forms for inpatients and outpatients. When a patient is encountered in an outpatient setting, the patient can complete a form (see Appendix C) that will provide information about current and prior medical conditions, including family history. During the interview, data on the form are reviewed with the patient. As an interview continues, additional data are elicited to fill in any missing and necessary information.

Once chart review and interview data are collected, information is organized by a physical therapist to determine the tests and measures to be performed (see Appendix D). Figure 1–3 presents types of data that may be generated from a patient/client history.

TESTS AND MEASURES

Upon completion of an interview, tests and measures are selected based upon information retrieved from the chart and elicited from the patient during the interview (see Appendix B). The physical therapist may perform some or all of the selected tests and measures or may delegate performance of specific tests and measures to a physical therapist assistant. These tests and measures generate data used in evaluation.

EVALUATION

Evaluation is the analysis of the data collected during chart review, interview, and application of tests and measures. This analysis is when the physical therapist makes initial clinical judgments with regard to a physical therapist's diagnosis, prognosis, and plan of care. Only a physical therapist may perform these functions.

DIAGNOSIS

The outcome of the evaluation is the physical therapist's diagnosis or recognition that the patient should be referred to a different practitioner. Diagnosis is the assignment of a label that categorizes or classifies a patient's problems. When a categorization or classification of problems is assigned, a specific practice pattern, as presented in the *Guide*,[1] is identified. This function is the responsibility of a physical therapist.

PROGNOSIS

Once categorization or classification of problems is assigned, a specific preferred practice pattern is connected to the diagnosis. From the preferred practice pattern, a physical therapist can provide a prognosis (see Appendix E). This function is the

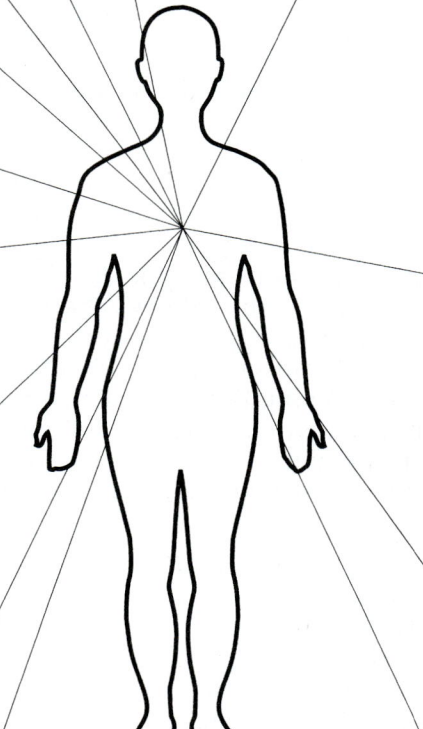

General Demographics
• Age
• Sex
• Race/ethnicity
• Primary language
• Education

Social History
• Cultural beliefs and behaviors
• Family and caregiver resources
• Social interactions, social activities, and support systems

Employment/Work (Job/School/Play)
• Current and prior work (job/school/play), community, and leisure actions, tasks, or activities

Growth and Development
• Developmental history
• Hand dominance

Living Environment
• Devices and equipment (eg, assistive, adaptive, orthotic, protective, supportive, prosthetic)
• Living environment and community characteristics
• Projected discharge destinations

General Health Status (Self-Report, Family Report, Caregiver Report)
• General health perception
• Physical function (eg, mobility, sleep patterns, restricted bed days)
• Psychological function (eg, memory, reasoning ability, depression, anxiety)
• Role function (eg, community, leisure, social, work)
• Social function (eg, social activity, social interaction, social support)

Social/Health Habits (Past and Current)
• Behavioral health risks (eg, smoking, drug abuse)
• Level of physical fitness

Family History
• Familial health risks

Medical/Surgical History
• Cardiovascular
• Endocrine/metabolic
• Gastrointestinal
• Genitourinary
• Gynecological
• Integumentary
• Musculoskeletal
• Neuromuscular
• Obstetrical
• Prior hospitalizations, surgeries, and preexisting medical and other health-related conditions
• Psychological
• Pulmonary

Current Condition(s)/Chief Complaint(s)
• Concerns that led the patient/client to seek the services of a physical therapist
• Concerns or needs of patient/client who requires the services of a physical therapist
• Current therapeutic interventions
• Mechanisms of injury or disease, including date of onset and course of events
• Onset and pattern of symptoms
• Patient/client, family, significant other, and caregiver expectations and goals for the therapeutic intervention
• Patient/client, family, significant other, and caregiver perceptions of patient's/client's emotional response to the current clinical situation
• Previous occurrence of chief complaint(s)
• Prior therapeutic interventions

Functional Status and Activity Level
• Current and prior functional status in self-care and home management, including activities of daily living (ADL) and instrumental activities of daily living (IADL)
• Current and prior functional status in work (job/school/play), community, and leisure actions, tasks, or activities

Medications
• Medications for current condition
• Medications previously taken for current condition
• Medications for other conditions

Other Clinical Tests
• Laboratory and diagnostic tests
• Review of available records (eg, medical, education, surgical)
• Review of other clinical findings (eg, nutrition and hydration)

FIGURE 1–3 Types of Data That May Be Generated from a Patient/Client History. Reprinted with permission from the American Physical Therapy Association.

responsibility of a physical therapist and it is the physical therapist that conveys the prognosis to the patient.

PLAN OF CARE

With establishment of a physical therapist's diagnosis and prognosis, anticipated and expected goals and outcomes are identified. Both the physical therapist and patient contribute to setting goals. Interventions are selected that are appropriate to the diagnosis, prognosis, and goals. A Plan of Care indicates the number of visits, frequency of visits, duration of visits, educational components, equipment to be ordered, and discharge planning (see Appendix F). Designing the Plan of Care is the responsibility of a physical therapist. A physical therapist may delegate appropriate interventions within the Plan of Care to physical therapist assistants.

DOCUMENTATION (MEDICAL RECORDS)

There are many aspects of patient care and a large number of professionals are involved in the care of each patient. Coordination of these aspects and professionals requires a high level of communication among all concerned. A patient's chart serves as the single repository of pertinent facts concerning the patient's history, illness(es), and treatment. Events and actions must be documented and are deemed to have occurred only if documented in the patient's chart.

Documentation is the medico-legal record of patient care provided by all practitioners for a given patient. Documentation that is precise and concise is required for providing appropriate communication and is an essential function of health care professionals. The most important rationale for appropriate documentation is to provide the highest possible level of patient care at all times. With proper documentation, those involved with providing care for the patient and support for the patient's family will know:

1. What has been determined about the patient's condition based upon interviews and tests.
2. Specific problems identified.
3. Goals of treatment.
4. Treatment strategies employed.
5. Patient's response to treatment.
6. Rationale on which goals and treatment are based.

Without proper documentation, initial patient status may not be known, subsequent patient progress may be difficult to monitor, interventions provided may not be known, coordination of patient care may be lost, quality assurance reviews cannot be performed adequately, and reimbursement by third-party payers may be compromised.

Proper documentation provides a valid basis for reflective practice and research. For a physical therapist to review and reflect on his or her practice, he or she requires the data that full and complete documentation provides. Reflecting on one's practice allows a physical therapist to develop as a provider and to ask questions that can be answered within a practice setting. For example, a physical therapist who frequently treats patients with similar diagnoses might ask researchable questions about what interventions seem to promote faster recovery or better long-term outcomes. Without significantly changing what occurs in a treatment environment, a physical therapist can collect data, via routine documentation practices, to answer such questions specific to the treatment environment. When results of this type of inquiry are shared within the profession, the profession's body of knowledge is enhanced.

FORMATS OF MEDICAL RECORDS

There are several major formats of medical records. The **source-oriented method** and the **problem-oriented medical record (POMR) method** are two popular formats. Ideally, all departments within a facility should use the same method of documenting in the medical record. Using a common method within a facility simplifies the process of communication between professionals in different departments. Even if all departments within a facility do not use the same method of record keeping, the formats used need to provide appropriate information in a "user friendly" manner, for both the person providing documentation and for those reviewing the documentation.

In the source-oriented method, a chart is divided into sections for each health profession providing service for a patient (i.e., MD, nursing, PT, etc.). Each discipline provides its documentation in a separate section of the patient's chart. A narrative format is usually used for writing notes in the chart. The source-oriented system segregates patient information by discipline, which may limit the ability to identify patient problems and focus treatment resources on the specific needs of a patient. Documentation of the flow of patient care among professions and the interaction of professional interventions for the benefit of the patient is lost when using the source-oriented format in medical charts.

The POMR system, introduced by Lawrence Weed,[5] was designed to facilitate care provided to patients by organizing each medical record in a standard format. The concept of the POMR initially was received favorably and put into use in medical schools, hospitals, and rehabilitation settings.[6–9]

The POMR is composed of:

1. Database.
2. Problem list.
3. Initial, progress or interim, and discharge notes.

The **database** contains subjective and objective information, including medical, family, and social history, and medical examination and test results. The **problem list** is a list of the patient's problems that are identified from the information contained in the database. Problems may be identified by any professional discipline providing patient care, and may be listed as an abnormal test result, chief complaint, diagnosis, physical finding, physiological finding, or symptom. Notes are a sequential record of decisions, actions, and events describing the course of a patient's treatment by all involved professionals. An **initial note** presents the initial findings and plan of treatment. **Progress (interim) notes** present the progression of treatment, the effects of treatment, and changes in the plan of treatment. A **discharge note** presents the status of the patient's problems and the current course of treatment at the time of patient discharge.

Proper application of the POMR system provides a medical record of each patient that clearly delineates the:

1. Patient's medical history.
2. Medical findings of signs, symptoms, and tests.
3. Patient's problems, based upon an evaluation of signs, symptoms, and test results.
4. Goals of treatment.
5. Methods of treatment.
6. Patient's response to treatment.

When the POMR system is fully implemented, an audit process for peer review and outcome assessment is included. Audit results indicate areas of strengths and weaknesses in patient care rendered, indicating areas for improvement of patient care. The full POMR approach to medical record documentation is seldom used today; however, the format for notes, referred to as the SOAP note format,[5,10] is used.

The Patient/Client Management method of documentation[11] is an outflow of the Physical Therapist Patient/Client Management process. Using the Documentation Template for Physical Therapist Patient/Client Management (in-patient and out-patient) provides a systematic way to generate and record data about a patient. (see Appendices B and C). The information obtained is then summarized into a note for inclusion in the patient's chart/record, as well as for communicating with a referring physician or third-party payers.

When using the Patient/Client Management Note format,[11] a database is initiated upon admission or referral. The database includes identifying information, medical complaints voiced by the patient (symptoms), a brief medical history, and a short review of all physiological systems (signs). The information elicited upon review provides a basis for the initial problem list, determining which health care providers need to be involved in this patient's care and which systems require more extensive medical review.

NOTE FORMATS

Major formats for writing notes include the: (a) **narrative note**, (b) **SOAP note**, and (c) **patient/client management note** formats.

In the narrative format, statements concerning the patient are written in narrative form. Such notes may, or may not, have subheadings to organize information. The organization and flow of information within notes written by different personnel varies, making it difficult to identify where or how specific information is contained within the medical record.

The SOAP note format is the common format used for medical chart notes written by health care providers using the POMR system. SOAP is an acronym containing the SOAP note section headings: (a) **S**ubjective, (b) **O**bjective, (c) **A**ssessment, and (d) **P**lan. Some facilities use the SOAP note format without using the database and problem list sections of the POMR system.

In a SOAP note, a History section often precedes the first "S" section. Others, however, may place this information in the "Subjective" section even though this information is not truly subjective. This section of the note provides background information including identifying information of the patient's name and number, physician names, primary and secondary diagnoses, and date. An example of such content is:

> *Mrs Rita Jones, XXXXX, is a 43-year-old automotive assembly line worker, referred by Dr. Parker. She is 8 weeks post fracture L olecranon process and 10 days post cast removal. First visit today, XX,XX,XX.*

"S" denotes **subjective data.** Relevant data concerning the patient's history that are not verifiable in medical records are considered subjective data. The patient's description of functional problems, pain, and the date of onset are also included as subjective data. Complaints reported by the patient/significant others are considered to be subjective data and are classified as symptoms. The patient's goals of treatment are considered to be subjective data and are included in this section. An example of the Subjective section of a note for a patient with a recently healed fracture is:

> *S. Mrs. Jones' chief complaint is inability to use her left arm for activities of daily living and for work. Patient's goal is to return to previous job.*

"O" denotes **objective data.** Data that are verifiable from medical records are considered objective data. Evaluation and intervention results documented by physical therapists are also included as objective data. Observations by health care personnel and test results are considered objective data and are considered signs. Subheadings are helpful to organize the content of this section. Interventions and patient response(s) to intervention are included in this section. A limitation of the SOAP note format, particularly for an initial note, is the lack of a coherent timeline.

Intervention and responses to intervention provided on a given date are documented in the Objective section before analysis of data in the Analysis section on the same date. An example of the Objective section of a note for a patient with a recently healed fracture is:

O.   *Active ROM: L elbow ext – flex 15–110 degree*
        Passive ROM: L elbow ext – flex 10–115 degree
        Strength: *L elbow ext*   3/5
                          L elbow flex   3+/5
                          L supination   3+/5
                          L pronation   3+/5
                          L wrist (all)   4/5
                          L hand (all)   4/5
                          L shoulder (all)   5/5
        Pain: *L elbow 2/10 in dependent position with no motion.*
                         L elbow 4/10 during passive ROM.
                         L elbow 5/10 during active flexion, supination, pronation.
                         L elbow 7/10 during active extension.

"A" denotes **assessment** or analysis by a physical therapist of the data included in the Subjective and Objective sections. A list of the patient's problems, identified from the Subjective and Objective information, is included in this section. Information contained in this portion of a note may include professional opinion concerning the patient's problems and a discussion of reasoning used as the basis of the plan of care. Hypotheses concerning patient problems listed in the Assessment section must be based on available data that is documented in the Objective section for review by all members of the health care team. A physical therapist's diagnosis and prognosis are included in this section.

In some facilities, goals of treatment are also included in the Assessment section, whereas other facilities include goals in the last section of the note, the Plan section. **Goals** are statements of expected patient capabilities at the end of treatment, when the treatment is successful. These statements of expected outcome are based on the results of the patient evaluation and are written in terms that describe observable and measurable patient behaviors. Goal statements describe what the patient will be able to do when treatment is successful. Goals should be specific, objective, measurable, and related to function. Goals do *not* describe what a physical therapist will do with a patient or the intervention to be provided to a patient.

Long-term goals (LTGs) are statements describing functional capabilities the patient will have upon discharge. **Short-term goals (STGs)** are more discrete activities the patient will have to be able to perform to achieve the functional activities stated as LTGs. There should be a clear progression of goals, indicating that successful achievement of STGs will provide the basis for successful attainment of LTGs.

Goal statements must be complete to be useful. The mnemonic ABCDFT[9] can be used to ensure the inclusion of all components of a goal. A goal is about how a *patient* will perform, *not* what a physical therapist will do. The first component of a goal statement indicates the Audience, "A." The audience of a goal is the patient or patient's family. The second component of a goal is the Behavior, "B," a patient will exhibit. Behaviors are ambulation or dressing. Behavior is described in observable and measurable terms. The third component of a goal is the Conditions, "C." Conditions are distance, type of assistive device used, speed of performance, or other achievements that the patient will demonstrate. The fourth component of a goal is Degree, "D." Degree is how often the patient is expected to perform the behavior under the described conditions. When no specific degree is stated, a patient is expected to perform the behavior under the stated conditions 100% of the time the behavior is required. The fifth component of a goal is a functional behavior, "F." In

STGs, behaviors may not be functional, but the desired behavior must be related to a functional behavior. An STG may be obtaining range of motion (ROM) or strength for the functional behavior of ambulation. It is important to inform others why the described STG is important to attaining the functional behavior of the LTG. The sixth component of the goal is Time, "T." Each goal should include a timeline indicating how long it will take the patient to achieve a specific goal. Time can be stated in terms of number of treatments or days. In *Writing SOAP Notes* (3rd ed.),[11] Kettenbach uses only ABCD of the mnemonic, with Function and Time incorporated within Degree.

An example of the assessment section of a note for a patient with a recently healed fracture is

A.   *Problem 1 – Decreased ROM L elbow*
Problem 2 – Decreased strength L elbow and wrist
Problem 3 – Pain L elbow
Problems 1 through 3 result of recent fracture L olecranon process and casting of L upper extremity.
LTG: The patient is able to use L arm for washing, dressing, and combing hair. Patient will be able to perform pervious job as automotive assembly line worker.
STG: The patient has 5–110 degrees ROM in L elbow to perform job skills in 2 weeks.
The patient has 4/5 muscle strength in all major muscle groups of the L upper extremity to perform job skills in 2 weeks.
The patient is free of pain in L elbow while performing job skills in 5 weeks.

"P" denotes the **plan** to be followed in providing care for a specific patient. Information provided in the Plan section should include:

1. Priority given for treatment of each of the patient's problems.
2. Estimated timetable for meeting the goals for the patient.
3. Enough detail concerning treatment procedures to enable another person to continue treatment.
4. Anticipated duration of each treatment and session.
5. Any actions the physical therapist will take in regard to the patient prior to the next visit.

An example of the plan section of a note for a patient with a recently healed fracture is:

P.   *Priorities: Increase ROM L elbow.*
Increase strength L elbow and wrist muscles.
Decrease in pain expected as ROM and strength return to normal.
Treatment: Cryotherapy prior to and following each exercise session to decrease swelling and pain.
Proprioceptive neuromuscular facilitation (PNF) procedures to increase ROM.
PNF procedures for strengthening exercises in clinic.
Free weight exercises for strengthening in clinic and at-home exercise program.
Schedule: Clinic visits 45 min 3x/wk for 2 weeks followed by 45 min 2x/wk for 2 weeks.
Independent ADL using L arm in 2 weeks.
Return to work in 5 weeks.

Each section of the SOAP note need not be included in every note. Initial notes, however, should include all sections. Only relevant sections are needed for any specific note. Progress notes should include only those sections necessary for indicating changes in patient status (i.e., progress or regression). Discharge notes summarize interventions, progress achieved, and patient profile upon discharge. Thus initial status, final status, and the effectiveness of therapeutic intervention are presented in an organized manner.

The patient/client management note format of documentation is developing in response to the implementation of the Physical Therapy Patient/Client Management Process. This approach has components of both the narrative and SOAP note formats. The elements of the Patient/Client Management process provide the major divisions of the note. Headings are used to enhance the ease of locating specific information (see Appendix F).

The headings for the first division, Examination, are history, systems review, and tests and measures. Each heading can be divided further into subheadings. Subheadings for the History section include those in Figure 1–3 discussed earlier. Systems review is subdivided into (a) cardiovascular/pulmonary, (b) integumentary, (c) musculoskeletal, (d) neuromuscular, (e) communication, (f) affect, (g) cognition, (h) language, and (i) learning style. A systems review directs the selection of test and measures to be conducted. Specific tests and measures within the domain of a physical therapist are used to collect data in the areas of (a) aerobic capacity/endurance; (b) anthropometric characteristics; (c) arousal, attention and cognition; (d) assistive and adaptive devices; (e) circulation; (f) cranial and peripheral nerve integrity; (g) environmental, home, and work barriers; (h) ergonomics and body mechanics; (i) gait, locomotion, and balance; (j) integumentary integrity; (k) joint integrity and mobility; (l) motor function; (m) muscle performance; (n) neruomotor development and sensory integration; (o) orthotic, protective, and supportive devices; (p) pain; (q) posture; (r) prosthetic requirements; (s) range of motion and muscle length; (t) reflex integrity; (u) self-care and home management; (v) sensory integrity; (w) ventilation and respiratory/gas exchange and (x) work, community, and leisure integration or reintegration.

The headings for the second division, Evaluation, in which a physical therapist synthesizes the data collected to determine the patient's problems and the severity of the problem(s), are diagnosis and prognosis. Diagnosis is the physical therapist's diagnosis related to impairments and functional limitations. Specific preferred practice patterns are identified. Situations unique to each patient are taken into consideration as a physical therapist determines a prognosis. A prognosis is the expected outcome a patient will achieve when treated successfully and the amount of time required to achieve the expected outcome. An expected outcome is equivalent to the LTG under the SOAP note format discussed previously. An STG equivalent is referred to as an anticipated outcome. The ABCDFT formula can be used when composing expected outcomes and anticipated outcomes.

The content of the third division, Intervention, includes the interventions and required parameters, frequency of treatment, duration of treatment, plans for obtaining any needed assistive/adaptive devices, coordination with other services, and indication of when reexaminations will be completed. This content is built upon the preceding sections. Expected outcomes give overall direction to the plan of care. Anticipated outcomes establish the progression of the interventions.

REQUIREMENTS FOR ADEQUATE DOCUMENTATION

The primary role of adequate documentation is to enhance communication for medical and legal purposes. Documentation must be precise, concise, legible, and timely. To be **precise**, measurements and test results must be recorded accurately and terminology must be used accurately and appropriately. Only generally accepted abbreviations must be used (see Glossary of Abbreviations). To be **concise**, documentation must be organized effectively, conveying important information in a clear, unfettered fashion. To be **legible**, the method of note entry in a medical record should be one that allows all team members to read the entry of others easily, accurately, and without delay. The increasing adoption of computers as a method of inputting information into the medical record should make the issue of legibility moot and should also assist with the issue of prompt accessibility. **Timeliness** requires that notes be entered into the medical record immediately after the patient is examined or treated, so that subsequent patient care decisions are based upon current information.

An important aspect of medical documentation is the presentation of information in a manner that can be read and interpreted quickly and efficiently. Many facilities recommend outline format, rather than fully formed prose. In many instances, charts or tables can be used to report individual and serial test results. Use of such charts or tables enables communication of large amounts of information quickly and avoids excess use of prose. When prose is used, the rules of proper grammatical usage should be followed. Only relevant information should be included.

AUDIT OF PATIENT CARE

Periodic and consistent evaluation of patient care activities is necessary to measure and analyze the quality of patient care. An **audit** is a systematic review of documentation to examine the efficacy and efficiency of patient care outcomes related to interventions used. Only through the availability of properly completed records can useful audits be performed.

When appropriate and significant data are reported in a consistent format, peer review and quality assurance is facilitated. One question that can be the focus of an audit is to determine if actual patient care outcomes are dependent upon the type of interventions employed. Potential benefits to be gained from performing audits include (a) improved patient care rendered, and (b) improved patient outcomes. A partial list of information that an audit may yield is whether:

1. Individual physical therapists are including pertinent and required information in medical chart notes.
2. Department or individual physical therapist interventions are appropriate for the patients to which the interventions are applied.
3. Changes in department policy or protocols are necessary to improve patient care and patient outcomes.
4. Continuing education is necessary to improve patient care skills.

REVIEW QUESTIONS

1. List the 18 specific HIPAA identifiers.

2. What is the purpose of handling HIPAA identifiers with confidentiality?

3. List the general categories of information found in a medical record.

4. Compare and contrast the source-oriented method and the problem-oriented method of medical record keeping.

5. Describe the three components of a POMR.

6. List the information contained in a patient's medical record using the POMR method.

7. What is the SOAP note format?

8. Define each section of a SOAP note, indicating the information contained in each section.

9. What are the components of the patient/client management process used by physical therapists?

10. What are the areas examined during a chart review?

11. Compare and contrast open-ended and closed-ended questions.

12. Compare LTGs and STGs with each other and with expected outcomes and anticipated outcomes.

13. What are the requirements of adequate documentation?

14. What information can be obtained from an audit?

Suggested Activities

1. Using the following Case Study, identify and redact information that would be covered by HIPAA regulations.

2. Indicate in which component of the SOAP note each of the following statements should be by placing the appropriate letter, S, O, A, or P, before the statement.

_____   ROM: R shoulder flexion: 0–85.

_____   The family reports that the patient frequently falls at night.

_____   TX 2/wk for 3 wks.

_____   The patient will ambulate with a straight cane on all surfaces for functional distances without fatigue within 4 weeks.

_____   Pain 5/10 after treatment.

_____   Patient's pain level ↓ following treatment.

_____   Patient ↑↓12 stairs step over step using the hand rail 4 times.

_____   The patient's ability to assume standing from sitting is impaired because of weakness of both quadricep muscles.

3. Identify the components of the following goal statement by writing the word or phrase in the appropriate space:

Goal statement: The patient will have full left knee extension ROM for ambulation, dressing, and getting in and out of a chair within 2 weeks of daily treatment.

A: _____

B: _____

C: _____

D: _____

F: _____

T: _____

CASE STUDY

Organize the following narrative note into the patient/client management note format:

Edward Jones
415 Main Street
Any City, USA
(555) 212-2222
SSN: 123-45-6789
DOB: 05/08/37
Record: 444-3-45-897

Mr. Ted Jones is a 67-year-old male 2 days post left total knee replacement. Mr. Jones is to be discharged to a skilled nursing care facility in 2 days where he will receive additional therapy. The goal is for Mr. Jones to ambulate independently without an assistive device as a community ambulatory. The physician has indicated that when Mr. Jones has 90 degrees of left knee flexion, good strength of knee flexors and extensors, and can ambulate 200 ft × 4, he can be discharged to his home. Mr. Jones reports pain of 4/10 about the incision. The incision is anterior over the left knee in a proximal distal direction. Some clear discharge is noted at the distal end of the incision. The circumference of the left knee at 2 inches above the tibial tuberosity is 3/4 inch larger than the right.

REFERENCES

1. Guide to Physical Therapist Practice, 2nd ed. *Physical Therapy.* 2001; 81; 1.
2. Nagi S. Some conceptual issues in disability and rehabilitation. In: Sussman M (ed). *Sociology and Rehabilitation.* Washington, DC: American Sociological Association, 1965, 100–113.
3. Nagi S. *Disability and Rehabilitation.* Columbus: Ohio State University Press, 1969.
4. Nagi S. Disability concepts revisited: Implications for prevention. In: Pope A, Tarlov A (eds). *Disability in America: Toward a National Agenda for Prevention.* Washington, DC: Institute of Medicine, National Academy Press, 1991.
5. Weed LL. *Medical Record, Medical Education, and Patient Care.* Chicago: Yearbook Medical Publishers, 1970.
6. Dunsdale SM, Mossman PL, Guleckson G, Jr. et al. The problem-oriented medical record in rehabilitation. *Arch Phys Med Rehabil.* 1970; 51; 488–492.
7. Editorial. Ten reasons why Weed is right. *N Engl J Med.* 1971; 51; 284.
8. Feitelberg SB. *The Problem-Oriented Medical Record System in Physical Therapy.* Self-published. Copyright 1975, revised 1984, 1999.
9. Milhous R. The problem-oriented medical record in rehabilitation management and training. *Arch Phys Med Rehabil.* 1972; 53; 182–185.
10. Kettenback G. *Writing SOAP Notes,* 2nd ed. Philadelphia: F.A. Davis, 1995.
11. Kettenback G. *Writing SOAP Notes,* 3rd ed. Philadelphia: F.A. Davis, 2004.

DOCUMENTATION TEMPLATE FOR
PHYSICAL THERAPIST PATIENT/CLIENT MANAGEMENT
Systems Review

	Not Impaired	Impaired
CARDIOVASCULAR/PULMONARY SYSTEM	☐	☐

Heart rate: _____

Respiratory rate: _____

Blood pressure: _____

Edema: _____

	Not Impaired	Impaired
INTEGUMENTARY SYSTEM	☐	☐

Integrity

Integumentary disruption: _____

Continuity of skin color: _____

Pliability (texture): _____

	Not Impaired	Impaired
MUSCULOSKELETAL SYSTEM		
Gross Symmetry	☐	☐

    Standing: _____

    Sitting: _____

    Activity specific:_____

	Not Impaired	Impaired
Gross Range of Motion	☐	☐
Gross Strength	☐	☐

Other: _____

Height	_____
Weight	_____

	Not Impaired	Impaired
NEUROMUSCULAR SYSTEM		
Gait	☐	☐
Locomotion (includes transfers, sit-to-stand transitions, bed mobility)	☐	☐
Balance	☐	☐
Motor function (motor control, motor learning)	☐	☐

	Not Impaired	Impaired
COMMUNICATION, AFFECT, COGNITION, LEARNING STYLE		
Communication (eg, age-appropriate)	☐	☐
Orientation x 3 (person/place/time)	☐	☐
Emotional/behavioral responses	☐	☐

Learning barriers:
- ☐ None
- ☐ Vision
- ☐ Hearing
- ☐ Unable to read
- ☐ Unable to understand what is read
- ☐ Language/needs interpreter
- ☐ Other: _____

Education needs:
- ☐ Disease process
- ☐ Safety
- ☐ Use of devices/equipment
- ☐ Activities of daily living
- ☐ Exercise program
- ☐ Other: _____

How does patient/client best learn? ☐ Pictures ☐ Reading ☐ Listening ☐ Demonstration ☐ Other: _____

APPENDIX A Documentation Template for Physical Therapist Patient/Client Management: Systems Review. Reprinted with permission from the American Physical Therapy Association.

Systems Review

DOCUMENTATION TEMPLATE FOR
PHYSICAL THERAPIST PATIENT/CLIENT MANAGEMENT
Inpatient Form, Page 1

Today's Date: _____

Patient ID#: _____

IDENTIFICATION INFORMATION

1 Name: _____

a Last _____

b First _____ c MI _____ d Jr/Sr

2 Admission Date: [ ][ ] Month [ ][ ] Day [ ][ ][ ][ ] Year

3 Date of Birth: [ ][ ] Month [ ][ ] Day [ ][ ][ ][ ] Year

4 Sex: a ☐ Male   b ☐ Female

5 Dominant Hand: a ☐ Right   b ☐ Left   c ☐ Unknown

6 Race
a ☐ Asian
b ☐ Native Hawaiian/ Pacific Islander
c ☐ Black
d ☐ White

7 Ethnicity
a ☐ Hispanic or Latino
b ☐ Not Hispanic or Latino

8 Language
a ☐ English understood?
b ☐ Interpreter needed?
c ☐ Primary language: _____

9 Education
a Highest grade completed (Circle one): 1 2 3 4 5 6 7 8 9 10 11 12
b ☐ Some college/technical school
c ☐ College graduate
d ☐ Graduate school/advanced degree

10 Has patient completed an advance directive? a ☐ Yes b ☐ No

11 Referred by: _____

12 Reasons for referral to physical therapy: _____
_____
_____

SOCIAL HISTORY

13 Cultural/Religious
Any customs or religious beliefs or wishes that might affect care?
_____
_____
_____

14 Lives(d) With

	A–Admission	B–Expected at Discharge
a Alone	☐	☐
b Spouse only	☐	☐
c Spouse and other(s)	☐	☐
d Child (not spouse)	☐	☐
e Other relative(s) (not spouse or children)	☐	☐
f Group setting	☐	☐
g Personal care attendant	☐	☐
h Unknown	☐	☐
i Other _____		

15 Available Social Supports (family/friends)
0=No 1=Possibly yes 2=Definitely

	Now	Willing/Able Postdischarge
a Emotional support	☐	☐
b Intermittent physical support with ADLs or IADLs—less than daily	☐	☐
c Intermittent physical support with ADLs or IADLs—daily	☐	☐
d Full-time physical support (as needed) with ADLs or IADLs	☐	☐
e All or most of necessary tranportation	☐	☐

16 Caregiver Status Presence of family member/friend willing and able to assist patient/client? a ☐ Yes   b ☐ No

17 EMPLOYMENT/WORK (Job/School/Play)
a ☐ Working full-time outside of home
b ☐ Working part-time outside of home
c ☐ Working full-time from home
d ☐ Working part-time from home
e ☐ Homemaker f ☐ Student g ☐ Retired h ☐ Unemployed

i Occupation: _____

LIVING ENVIRONMENT

18 Devices and Equipment (eg, cane, glasses, hearing aids, walker)
_____
_____
_____
_____
_____
_____

19 Type of Residence

	A–Admission	B–Expected at Discharge
a Private home	☐	☐
b Private apartment	☐	☐
c Rented room	☐	☐
d Board and care/assisted living/group home	☐	☐
e Homeless (with or without shelter)	☐	☐
f Long-term care facility (nursing home)	☐	☐
g Hospice	☐	☐
h Unknown	☐	☐
i Other _____		

20 Environment

	A–Admission	B–Expected at Discharge
a Stairs, no railing	☐	☐
b Stairs, railing	☐	☐
c Ramps	☐	☐
d Elevator	☐	☐
e Uneven terrain	☐	☐
f Other obstacles: _____		

21 Past Use of Community Services 0=No 1=Unknown 2=Yes

a Day services/programs ☐
b Home health services ☐
c Homemaking services ☐
d Hospice ☐
e Meals on Wheels ☐
f Mental health services ☐
g Respiratory therapy ☐
h Therapies—PT, OT, SLP ☐
i Other (eg, volunteer) ☐
_____

22 GENERAL HEALTH STATUS
a Patient/client rates health as:

☐ Excellent ☐ Good ☐ Fair ☐ Poor

b Major life changes during past year? (1) ☐ Yes (2) ☐ No

[OVER]

APPENDIX B Documentation Template for Physical Therapist/Client Management: Inpatient Form. Reprinted with permission from the American Physical Therapy Association.

23 SOCIAL/HEALTH HABITS (Past and Current)

a Alcohol

(1) How many days per week does patient/client drink beer, wine, or other alcoholic beverages, on average? _____

(2) If one beer, one glass of wine, or one cocktail equals one drink, how many drinks does patient/client have, on an average day? _____

b Smoking

(1) Currently smokes tobacco?

(a) ☐ Yes

1. ☐ Cigarettes # of packs per day _____

2. ☐ Cigars/pipes # per day ____

(b) ☐ No

(2) Smoked in past? (a) ☐ Yes Year quit: ☐☐☐☐

(b) ☐ No

c Exercise

(1) Exercises beyond normal daily activities and chores?

(a) ☐ Yes

Describe the exercise: _____

1. On average, how many days per week does patient/client exercise or do physical activity? _____

2. For how many minutes, on an average day? __

(b) ☐ No

24 FAMILY HISTORY

Condition:	Relationship to Patient/Client:	Age of Onset (if known):
a Heart disease	_____	_____
b Hypertension	_____	_____
c Stroke	_____	_____
d Diabetes	_____	_____
e Cancer	_____	_____
f Other: _____	_____	_____
_____	_____	_____

25 PATIENT/CLIENT MEDICAL/SURGICAL HISTORY: _____

_____

_____

_____

_____

_____

26 FUNCTIONAL STATUS/ACTIVITY LEVEL (Check all that apply.)

a ☐ Difficulty with locomotion/movement:

(1) ☐ bed mobility

(2) ☐ transfers

(3) ☐ gait (walking)

(a) ☐ on level

(b) ☐ on stairs

(c) ☐ on ramps

(d) ☐ on uneven terrain

b ☐ Difficulty with self-care (such as bathing, dressing, eating, toileting)

c ☐ Difficulty with home management (such as household chores, shopping, driving/transportation)

d ☐ Difficulty with community and work activities/integration

(1) ☐ work/school

(2) ☐ recreation or play activity

27 MEDICATIONS (list): _____

_____

_____

_____

_____

_____

_____

_____

_____

_____

_____

28 OTHER CLINICAL TESTS (list):

	Month	Year	Findings
_____	☐☐	☐☐☐☐	_____
_____	☐☐	☐☐☐☐	_____
_____	☐☐	☐☐☐☐	_____
_____	☐☐	☐☐☐☐	_____

APPENDIX B Documentation Template for Physical Therapist/Client Management: Inpatient Form (*cont.*). Reprinted with permission from the American Physical Therapy Association.

Today's Date: _____
Patient ID#: _____

1 Name:

_____
a Last

_____
b First   c MI   d Jr/Sr

2 Street Address: _____

_____
City   State   Zip

3 Date of Birth: Month ☐☐ Day ☐☐ Year ☐☐☐☐

4 Sex: a ☐ Male   b ☐ Female

5 Are you: a ☐ Right-handed   b ☐ Left-handed

6 Type of Insurance: a ☐ Insurer _____
b ☐ Workers' Comp   c ☐ Medicare   d ☐ Self-pay   e ☐ Other

7 Race
a ☐ Asian
b ☐ Native Hawaiian/ Pacific Islander
c ☐ Black
d ☐ White

8 Ethnicity
a ☐ Hispanic or Latino
b ☐ Not Hispanic or Latino

9 Language
a ☐ English understood?
b ☐ Interpreter needed?
c ☐ Language you speak most often:
_____

10 Education
a Highest grade completed (Circle one): 1 2 3 4 5 6 7 8 9 10 11 12
b ☐ Some college / technical school
c ☐ College graduate
d ☐ Graduate school / advanced degree

SOCIAL HISTORY
11 Cultural/Religious
Any customs or religious beliefs or wishes that might affect care?
_____

12 With whom do you live?
a ☐ Alone
b ☐ Spouse only
c ☐ Spouse and other(s)
d ☐ Child (not spouse)
e ☐ Other relative(s) (not spouse or children)
f ☐ Group setting
g ☐ Personal care attendant
h ☐ Other:

13 Have you completed an advance directive?
a ☐ Yes   b ☐ No

14 Who referred you to the physical therapist:
_____

15 Employment/Work (Job/School/Play)
a ☐ Working full-time outside of home
b ☐ Working part-time outside of home
c ☐ Working full-time from home
d ☐ Working part-time from home
e ☐ Homemaker   f ☐ Student   g ☐ Retired   h ☐ Unemployed
i Occupation: _____

LIVING ENVIRONMENT

16 Does your home have:
a ☐ Stairs, no railing
b ☐ Stairs, railing
c ☐ Ramps
d ☐ Elevator
e ☐ Uneven terrain
f ☐ Assistive devices (eg, bathroom): _____
g ☐ Any obstacles: _____

17 Do you use:
a ☐ Cane
b ☐ Walker or rollator
c ☐ Manual wheelchair
d ☐ Motorized wheelchair
e ☐ Glasses, hearing aids
f ☐ Other: _____

18 Where do you live?
a ☐ Private home
b ☐ Private apartment
c ☐ Rented room
d ☐ Board and care / assisted living / group home
e ☐ Homeless (with or without shelter)
f ☐ Long-term care facility (nursing home)
g ☐ Hospice
h ☐ Other: _____

19 GENERAL HEALTH STATUS
a Please rate your health:
(1) ☐ Excellent   (2) ☐ Good   (3) ☐ Fair   (4) ☐ Poor
b Have you had any major life changes during past year? (eg, new baby, job change, death of a family member) (1) ☐ Yes   (2) ☐ No

20 SOCIAL/HEALTH HABITS
a Smoking
(1) Currently smoke tobacco? (a) ☐ Yes   1. ☐ Cigarettes
     # of packs per day __
     2. ☐ Cigars/Pipes
     # per day __
(b) ☐ No
(2) Smoked in past? (a) ☐ Yes Year quit: ☐☐☐☐ (b) ☐ No
b Alcohol
(1) How many days per week do you drink beer, wine, or other alcoholic beverages, on average? ___
(2) If one beer, one glass of wine, or one cocktail equals one drink, how many drinks do you have, on an average day? ___
c Exercise
Do you exercise beyond normal daily activities and chores?
(a) ☐ Yes Describe the exercise: _____
1. On average, how many days per week do you exercise or do physical activity? _____
2. For how many minutes, on an average day? ____
(b) ☐ No

21 FAMILY HISTORY (Indicate whether mother, father, brother/sister, aunt/uncle, or grandmother/grandfather, and age of onset if known)
a Heart disease: _____
b Hypertension: _____
c Stroke: _____
d Diabetes: _____
e Cancer: _____
f Psychological: _____
g Arthritis: _____
h Osteoporosis: _____
i Other: _____

Outpatient History

© American Physical Therapy Association 1999; revised September 2000

APPENDIX C Documentation Template for Physical Therapist Patient/Client Management: Outpatient Form. Reprinted with permission from the American Physical Therapy Association.

22 MEDICAL/SURGICAL HISTORY

a Please check if you have ever had:

(1) ☐ Arthritis
(2) ☐ Broken bones/ fractures
(3) ☐ Osteoporosis
(4) ☐ Blood disorders
(5) ☐ Circulation/vascular problems
(6) ☐ Heart problems
(7) ☐ High blood pressure
(8) ☐ Lung problems
(9) ☐ Stroke
(10) ☐ Diabetes/ high blood sugar
(11) ☐ Low blood sugar/ hypoglycemia
(12) ☐ Head injury

(13) ☐ Multiple sclerosis
(14) ☐ Muscular dystrophy
(15) ☐ Parkinson disease
(16) ☐ Seizures/epilepsy
(17) ☐ Allergies
(18) ☐ Developmental or growth problems
(19) ☐ Thyroid problems
(20) ☐ Cancer
(21) ☐ Infectious disease (eg, tuberculosis, hepatitis)
(22) ☐ Kidney problems
(23) ☐ Repeated infections
(24) ☐ Ulcers/stomach problems
(25) ☐ Skin diseases
(26) ☐ Depression
(27) ☐ Other:_____

b Within the past year, have you had any of the following symptoms? (Check all that apply.)

(1) ☐ Chest pain
(2) ☐ Heart palpitations
(3) ☐ Cough
(4) ☐ Hoarseness
(5) ☐ Shortness of breath
(6) ☐ Dizziness or blackouts
(7) ☐ Coordination problems
(8) ☐ Weakness in arms or legs
(9) ☐ Loss of balance
(10) ☐ Difficulty walking
(11) ☐ Joint pain or swelling
(12) ☐ Pain at night

(13) ☐ Difficulty sleeping
(14) ☐ Loss of appetite
(15) ☐ Nausea/vomiting
(16) ☐ Difficulty swallowing
(17) ☐ Bowel problems
(18) ☐ Weight loss/gain
(19) ☐ Urinary problems
(20) ☐ Fever/chills/sweats
(21) ☐ Headaches
(22) ☐ Hearing problems
(23) ☐ Vision problems
(24) ☐ Other:_____

c Have you ever had surgery? (1) ☐ Yes (2) ☐ No
If yes, please describe, and include dates:

	Month	Year
_____	☐☐	☐☐☐☐
_____	☐☐	☐☐☐☐
_____	☐☐	☐☐☐☐

For men only: d Have you been diagnosed with prostate disease?
(1) ☐ Yes (2) ☐ No

For women only:
Have you been diagnosed with:
e Pelvic inflammatory disease?
  (1) ☐ Yes (2) ☐ No
f Endometriosis?
  (1) ☐ Yes (2) ☐ No
g Trouble with your period?
  (1) ☐ Yes (2) ☐ No

h Complicated pregnancies or deliveries?
  (1) ☐ Yes (2) ☐ No
i Pregnant, or think you might be pregnant?
  (1) ☐ Yes (2) ☐ No
j Other gynecological or obstetrical difficulties?
  (1) ☐ Yes (2) ☐ No
If yes, please describe:
_____

23 CURRENT CONDITION(S)/CHIEF COMPLAINT(S)

a Describe the problem(s) for which you seek physical therapy
_____
_____

	Month	Year
b When did the problem(s) begin (date)?	☐☐	☐☐☐☐

c What happened?_____
_____

d Have you ever had the problem(s) before?
  (1) ☐ Yes
    (a) What did you do for the problem(s)? _____
    _____
    (b) Did the problem(s) get better?
      1. ☐ Yes 2. ☐ No
    (c) About how long did the problem(s) last? _____
  (2) ☐ No

23 Current Condition(s)/Chief Complaint(s) (continued)

e How are you taking care of the problem(s) now? _____

f What makes the problem(s) better? _____

g What makes the problem(s) worse? _____
_____

h What are your goals for physical therapy? _____

i Are you seeing anyone else for the problem(s)? (Check all that apply.)

(1) ☐ Acupuncturist
(2) ☐ Cardiologist
(3) ☐ Chiropractor
(4) ☐ Dentist
(5) ☐ Family practitioner
(6) ☐ Internist
(7) ☐ Massage therapist
(8) ☐ Neurologist
(9) ☐ Obstetrician/gynecologist

(10) ☐ Occupational therapist
(11) ☐ Orthopedist
(12) ☐ Osteopath
(13) ☐ Pediatrician
(14) ☐ Podiatrist
(15) ☐ Primary care physician
(16) ☐ Rheumatologist
Other: _____

24 FUNCTIONAL STATUS/ACTIVITY LEVEL (Check all that apply.)

a ☐ Difficulty with locomotion/movement:
  (1) ☐ bed mobility
  (2) ☐ transfers (such as moving from bed to chair, from bed to commode)
  (3) ☐ gait (walking)
    (a) ☐ on level (c) ☐ on ramps
    (b) ☐ on stairs (d) ☐ on uneven terrain
b ☐ Difficulty with self-care (such as bathing, dressing, eating, toileting)
c ☐ Difficulty with home management (such as household chores, shopping, driving/transportation, care of dependents)
d ☐ Difficulty with community and work activities/integration
  (1) ☐ work/school
  (2) ☐ recreation or play activity

25 MEDICATIONS

a Do you take any prescription medications? (1) ☐ Yes (2) ☐ No
If yes, please list:_____
_____

b Do you take any nonprescription medications? (Check all that apply.)

(1) ☐ Advil/Aleve
(2) ☐ Antacids
(3) ☐ Ibuprofen/ Naproxen
(4) ☐ Antihistamines
(5) ☐ Aspirin

(6) ☐ Decongestants
(7) ☐ Herbal supplements
(8) ☐ Tylenol
(9) ☐ Other: _____
_____

c Have you taken any medications previously for the condition for which you are seeing the physical therapist?
(1) ☐ Yes (2) ☐ No If yes, please list:
_____

26 OTHER CLINICAL TESTS—Within the past year, have you had any of the following tests? (Check all that apply.)

a ☐ Angiogram
b ☐ Arthroscopy
c ☐ Biopsy
d ☐ Blood tests
e ☐ Bone scan
f ☐ Bronchoscopy
g ☐ CT scan
h ☐ Doppler ultrasound
i ☐ Echocardiogram
j ☐ EEG (electroencephalogram)
k ☐ EKG (electrocardiogram)
l ☐ EMG (electromyogram)

m ☐ Mammogram
n ☐ MRI
o ☐ Myelogram
p ☐ NCV (nerve conduction velocity)
q ☐ Pap smear
r ☐ Pulmonary function test
s ☐ Spinal tap
t ☐ Stool tests
u ☐ Stress test (eg, treadmill, bicycle)
v ☐ Urine tests
x ☐ X-rays
y ☐ Other:_____

APPENDIX C Documentation Template for Physical Therapist Patient/Client Management: Outpatient Form (*cont.*). Reprinted with permission from the American Physical Therapy Association.

DOCUMENTATION TEMPLATE FOR
PHYSICAL THERAPIST PATIENT/CLIENT MANAGEMENT
Tests and Measures

KEY TO TESTS AND MEASURES:

1 Aerobic Capacity/Endurance
2 Anthropometric Characteristics
3 Arousal, Attention, and Cognition
4 Assistive and Adaptive Devices
5 Circulation (Arterial, Venous, Lymphatic)
6 Cranial and Peripheral Nerve Integrity
7 Environmental, Home, and Work (Job/School/Play) Barriers
8 Ergonomics and Body Mechanics
9 Gait, Locomotion, and Balance
10 Integumentary Integrity
11 Joint Integrity and Mobility
12 Motor Function (Motor Control and Motor Learning)
13 Muscle Performance (Including Strength, Power, and Endurance)

14 Neuromotor Development and Sensory Integration
15 Orthotic, Protective, and Supportive Devices
16 Pain
17 Posture
18 Prosthetic Requirements
19 Range of Motion (Including Muscle Length)
20 Reflex Integrity
21 Self-Care and Home Management (Including Activities of Daily Living and Instrumental Activities of Daily Living)
22 Sensory Integrity
23 Ventilation and Respiration/Gas Exchange
24 Work (Job/School/Play), Community, and Leisure Integration or Reintegration (Including Instrumental Activities of Daily Living)

NOTES:

Tests and Measures

APPENDIX D   Documentation Template for Physical Therapist Patient/Client Management: Tests and Measures. Reprinted with permission from the American Physical Therapy Association.

DIAGNOSIS:

Musculoskeletal Patterns

☐ A: Primary Prevention/Risk Reduction for Skeletal Demineralization

☐ B: Impaired Posture

☐ C: Impaired Muscle Performance

☐ D: Impaired Joint Mobility, Motor Function, Muscle Performance, and Range of Motion Associated With Connective Tissue Dysfunction

☐ E: Impaired Joint Mobility, Motor Function, Muscle Performance, and Range of Motion Associated With Localized Inflammation

☐ F: Impaired Joint Mobility, Motor Function, Muscle Performance, Range of Motion, and Reflex Integrity Associated With Spinal Disorders

☐ G: Impaired Joint Mobility, Muscle Performance, and Range of Motion Associated With Fracture

☐ H: Impaired Joint Mobility, Motor Function, Muscle Performance, and Range of Motion Associated With Joint Arthroplasty

☐ I: Impaired Joint Mobility, Motor Function, Muscle Performance, and Range of Motion Associated With Bony or Soft Tissue Surgery

☐ J: Impaired Motor Function, Muscle Performance, Range of Motion, Gait, Locomotion, and Balance Associated With Amputation

Neuromuscular Patterns

☐ A: Primary Prevention/Risk Reduction for Loss of Balance and Falling

☐ B: Impaired Neuromotor Development

☐ C: Impaired Motor Function and Sensory Integrity Associated With Nonprogressive Disorders of the Central Nervous System—Congenital Origin or Acquired in Infancy or Childhood

☐ D: Impaired Motor Function and Sensory Integrity Associated With Nonprogressive Disorders of the Central Nervous System—Acquired in Adolescence or Adulthood

☐ E: Impaired Motor Function and Sensory Integrity Associated With Progressive Disorders of the Central Nervous System

☐ F: Impaired Peripheral Nerve Integrity and Muscle Performance Associated With Peripheral Nerve Injury

☐ G: Impaired Motor Function and Sensory Integrity Associated With Acute or Chronic Polyneuropathies

☐ H: Impaired Motor Function, Peripheral Nerve Integrity, and Sensory Integrity Associated With Nonprogressive Disorders of the Spinal Cord

☐ I: Impaired Arousal, Range of Motion, and Motor Control Associated With Coma, Near Coma, or Vegetative State

Cardiovascular/Pulmonary Patterns

☐ A: Primary Prevention/Risk Reduction for Cardiovascular/Pulmonary Disorders

☐ B: Impaired Aerobic Capacity/Endurance Associated With Deconditioning

☐ C: Impaired Ventilation, Respiration/Gas Exchange, and Aerobic Capacity/Endurance Associated With Airway Clearance Dysfunction

☐ D: Impaired Aerobic Capacity/Endurance Associated With Cardiovascular Pump Dysfunction or Failure

☐ E: Impaired Ventilation and Respiration/Gas Exchange Associated With Ventilatory Pump Dysfunction or Failure

☐ F: Impaired Ventilation and Respiration/Gas Exchange Associated With Respiratory Failure

☐ G: Impaired Ventilation, Respiration/Gas Exchange, and Aerobic Capacity/Endurance Associated With Respiratory Failure in the Neonate

☐ H: Impaired Circulation and Anthropometric Dimensions Associated With Lymphatic System Disorders

Integumentary Patterns

☐ A: Primary Prevention/Risk Reduction for Integumentary Disorders

☐ B: Impaired Integumentary Integrity Associated With Superficial Skin Involvement

☐ C: Impaired Integumentary Integrity Associated With Partial-Thickness Skin Involvement and Scar Formation

☐ D: Impaired Integumentary Integrity Associated With Full-Thickness Skin Involvement and Scar Formation

☐ E: Impaired Integumentary Integrity Associated With Skin Involvement Extending Into Fascia, Muscle, or Bone and Scar Formation

PROGNOSIS: _____

_____

_____

_____

_____

_____

_____

_____

_____

_____

Evaluation

APPENDIX E Documentation Template for Physical Therapist Patient/Client Management: Evaluation. Reprinted with permission from the American Physical Therapy Association.

DOCUMENTATION TEMPLATE FOR
PHYSICAL THERAPIST PATIENT/CLIENT MANAGEMENT
Plan of Care

Anticipated Goals: _____

_____

_____

_____

_____

Expected Outcomes: _____

_____

_____

_____

Interventions: _____

Frequency of Visits/Duration of Episode of Care:
_____
_____
_____

Education (including safety, exercise, and disease information): _____

_____

_____

Who was educated? ☐ Patient/client ☐ Family (name and relationship): _____
How did patient/family demonstrate learning:
  ☐ Patient/client verbalizes understanding
  ☐ Family/significant other verbalizes understanding
  ☐ Patient/client demonstrates correctly
  ☐ Demonstration is unsuccessful (describe): _____

_____

_____

Informed Consent:

Does patient/legal guardian agree with plan of care?   ☐ Yes ☐ No

_____
Signature of patient/client or legal guardian

Discharge Plan: _____

_____

_____

_____

_____

_____

_____

_____

_____

_____

© *American Physical Therapy Association 1999; revised September 2000*

Plan of Care

APPENDIX F   Documentation Template for Physical Therapist Patient/Client Management: Plan of Care. Reprinted with permission from the American Physical Therapy Association.

2

PREPARATION FOR PATIENT CARE

LEARNING OBJECTIVES

Upon completion of this chapter, you will be able to:

1. State who is responsible for properly managing the patient care environment.
2. Describe general guidelines for properly managing the patient care environment.
3. Describe correct body mechanics for safety of both the patient and the patient care provider.
4. Describe the physical therapist's, physical therapist assistant's, or other health care provider's position when moving a patient during ROM or guarding a patient during positioning, transfers, and ambulation.
5. Distinguish between instructions and verbal commands by describing the characteristics of instructions and verbal commands.
6. Describe the purposes of proper draping.
7. Describe proper draping techniques.
8. Describe how to transport patients safely via gurney and wheelchair.

MEDIALINK

A companion CD-ROM, included free with each new copy of this book, supplements the techniques presented in the book. Insert the CD-ROM to watch video clips of patient care skills being demonstrated. This multimedia feature is designed to help you add a new dimension to your learning.

KEY TERMS

Body mechanics
Draping
Instructions

Proper posture
Valsalva maneuver
Verbal commands

INTRODUCTION

Fundamental to all patient care are such skills as management of the environment, body mechanics, and communication. Safe implementation of a treatment procedure is best achieved when all components of a procedure are given proper attention. Generally, time taken at the start of a procedure to plan the steps involved and prepare for the procedures will increase the likelihood of safe, efficient, and effective implementation. Safety of the patient and all personnel involved in patient care must be of paramount consideration at all times.

MANAGEMENT OF THE ENVIRONMENT

The patient care environment must be organized for protection of patients and personnel, as well as for efficient use (Figure 2–1). Managing the patient care environment to achieve these goals is a serious responsibility of all personnel. A physical therapist has the responsibility to ensure that all personnel are properly trained in patient care environment management. Although some tasks may be delegated to certain personnel, the user always retains final responsibility for maintaining a safe and efficient environment for patients and personnel.

Preparation for the next treatment to be given in a patient care area begins at the end of the previous treatment. Following use, equipment must be cleaned, if appropriate, and returned to the proper storage area in safe, functioning condition. Used supplies must be disposed of properly. Unused supplies must also be returned to the proper storage area. The person responsible for ordering supplies should be notified in the appropriate manner when consumable supplies are low.

All equipment must be inspected to ensure safe function. A simple examination of equipment before each use helps to ensure patient safety. Malfunctions are to be reported in the appropriate manner to the proper person at the time they occur. Patients can, and should, be taught to inspect their own equipment, such as crutch tips, for wear. Following these guidelines will ensure that supplies and equipment will be available, and function safely, when needed. All personnel will know that equipment and supplies are in the proper place when needed for the plan of care.

Housekeeping requirements must also be considered in management of the environment. The following are examples, and do not cover the entire spectrum of housekeeping requirements. Cleaning of floors, mats, and treatment tables is necessary to provide a clean and safe environment for treatment. Proper cleaning of equipment will prolong its life of safe and effective use. Cleaning should occur on a regular basis and be performed in accordance with facility policies and procedures. Guidelines for, and the basis of, these procedures is outlined by the Centers for Disease Control and Prevention (CDC), and incorporated into facility policies and procedures. Specifics of some of these procedures are covered in Chapter 4, "Aseptic Techniques." All facility personnel, not just Housekeeping/Environmental Services personnel, are responsible for following and implementing policies and procedures correctly. Following these guidelines will ensure that the patient care environment will be safe and clean for use.

Prior to initiating any physical therapy patient interaction, the surrounding area must be readied. For transport, transfer, or intervention, the bed, chair, and surrounding areas must be readied. Treatment tables, mats, chairs, stools, or beds should be prepared before the patient arrives in the treatment area. Supplies necessary in a treatment area include linens and pillows. Additional sheets are used as pull sheets for transfers or for draping. Pillows for patient positioning, comfort, and safety must be within easy reach. Supporting a patient's head while reaching for a misplaced pillow, or leaving a patient in an uncomfortable or unsafe position while equipment is retrieved, is not acceptable patient care. Call bells or patient call buttons must be placed within the patient's reach where patients will be left unattended. Timers, when necessary, must also be available and set properly.

FIGURE 2–1   Preparing a clear patient care environment.

Specific equipment required for implementing a plan of care should be prepared and placed properly prior to beginning work with the patient (Figure 2–2). Having equipment and supplies required for interventions available in the area before intervention begins avoids the possibility of having to leave a patient unguarded or interrupting treatment.

FIGURE 2–2   Equipment and supplies for interventions.

Adequate room must be allowed in a patient care environment for unimpeded movement. Personnel and patients must be able to maneuver in the area without bumping into, or tripping over, equipment. Equipment and furniture not needed during a transport or transfer, such as a mobile stool, should be moved away from the area prior to arrival of the patient in the area. Besides getting in the way, many of these pieces of equipment are not stable and become dangerous when a patient tries to use them as support. When equipment is used in the treatment of a patient, position the equipment and patient to allow easy access for personnel to the patient. Improperly positioned equipment may hamper ability of personnel to provide patient assistance quickly.

PROCEDURE 2-1

BODY MECHANICS

When lifting, lowering, pushing, or pulling, stresses and strains upon the musculoskeletal system are increased. Proper posture and body mechanics are required to limit stress and strain on musculoskeletal structures. **Proper posture** is appropriate alignment of the musculoskeletal system such that the stresses and strains placed on bones, muscles, ligaments, and cartilage are as low as possible. **Body mechanics** requires strength, ROM, and motor control, and uses these elements to maintain proper skeletal alignment during standing and proper skeletal movement during activity. Although the five cardinal rules of correct body mechanics for lifting are titled for lifting only, they apply to any activity in which a person must lift, lower, push, pull, or carry any object or person. By following these rules, a person can maintain balance and decrease the potential for injury. The five cardinal rules are:

1. Keep the load close: The center of mass of the object being lifted/lowered should be kept as close as possible to the body of the person performing the lifting/lowering.

2. Create an appropriate base of support: The base of support of the person performing the lifting/lowering should be as wide (side to side) and long (front to back) as necessary to maintain balance throughout the lifting/lowering activity. If movement beyond the original base of support is required, an appropriately changing base of support must be maintained. While changing a base of support, avoid awkward positions. When movement of feet is required, move in a manner that avoids crossing legs/feet. Use of these strategies decreases the potential for tripping or falling by maintaining an appropriately sized base of support.

3. Use isometric muscle contractions of the trunk (extensor and abdominal muscles): Maintain the trunk in a constant position, preferably erect, during the lifting/lowering activity. Prior to performing the actual lifting/lowering movement, move into position, set trunk position, and then look forward. Setting the trunk and abdominal muscles is performed using isometric contractions and does not permit trunk musculature to extend or flex the trunk actively. Although isometric contractions of trunk musculature are used, avoid performing a Valsalva maneuver. A **Valsalva maneuver** is closing of the glottis during heavy exertion resulting in increased intra-thoracic and intra-abdominal pressure, which can cause a rapid and extreme increase in blood pressure.

4. Lift with the legs: Use the large and strong muscles of the legs to perform the lifting/lowering activity, avoiding active flexion or extension of the trunk.
5. Do not twist: Avoid rotation of the spine as the lifting/lowering activity is performed. When a change of direction is required, movement of the feet should be used to achieve the change of direction.

The initial stance for lifting/lowering requires the feet to be placed in stride and slightly apart. This stance widens the base of support in both the lateral (side to side) and anterior/posterior (front and back) directions, mitigating the effects of shifts in the center of mass during lifting/lowering activities. Centering the load within the base of support, and keeping it close to the base of support, aid stability. In this way, a balanced position can be maintained.

Lifting a person or object from the floor should be initiated from a squatting position. This is the lowest level from which a person or object will need to be lifted. Modifications of these instructions pertaining to lifting from different heights, such as a chair or treatment table, are included in Chapter 8.

The depth of the squat should be sufficient to permit reaching the person or object to be lifted but, if possible, not so deep that the leg muscles are at a disadvantage in regaining the upright position. The person or object is reached by squatting, achieved by flexing the hips and knees, rather than by flexing the trunk. Trunk position should be set or fixed, so muscles maintain this alignment using isometric contractions and do not work to extend the trunk to lift the load during the lifting motion. Creating isometric contractions in the muscles of the trunk prior to lifting can reduce the potential for injury. Being as close as possible to the person or object to be lifted or carried allows the combined center of mass to be maintained within the base of support. When the center of mass is centered within the base of support and near the body's midline, both balance and correct postural alignment are easier to maintain. Lowering a person or object uses the same concepts of posture and alignment as lifting, and the reverse order of steps.

Transfers require movements that move the center of mass away from the center of the base of support. These movements have the potential of causing loss of balance as the combined center of mass moves toward the boundaries of the base of support. Increasing the size of the base of support by setting the feet in stride and slightly apart provides a larger base of support. Proper arrangement of patient and chair, bed, or treatment table can reduce the distance that must be moved during a transfer. Proper environmental management means that the area is free of unnecessary equipment, allowing room for movement and avoiding interference with free movement of the feet. Crossing the legs should be avoided because it decreases the size of the base of support and constrains freedom of foot movement. Specific examples are illustrated in Chapter 8.

When moving large pieces of equipment, such as treadmills or parallel bars, or when guarding a patient during ambulation, the physical therapist, physical therapist assistant, or other health care provider should be positioned behind the equipment or patient, facing in the direction of movement. Positioned this way, the patient's view and path of movement are not obstructed and the view of personnel assisting the patient can then determine a path free from obstruction.

When guarding a patient during ambulation training, a physical therapist, physical therapist assistant, or other health care provider should be positioned with feet in stride, with his or her body at a 45-degree angle slightly to the side and behind the patient. If a patient starts to fall forward, backward, or to either side, this position of the physical therapist allows the patient's center of mass to be pulled toward the physical therapist, and the combined center of mass to be maintained within the base of support with a relatively small shift of the physical therapist's weight, and does not usually require large foot movements. The base of support must be large enough to support such shifts in the center of mass should a patient start to fall. To permit unencumbered weight shifting or foot movements, a physical therapist's feet should not be crossed during ambulation or become entangled with the patient's feet or ambulatory equipment.

In all cases, plan movements and prepare the area to be used prior to implementing any portion of a plan of care. Use of proper body mechanics and safety precautions provides safe and effective patient care. When in doubt about your ability to lift, transfer, or guard a patient or object safely, always obtain appropriate assistance.

INSTRUCTIONS AND VERBAL COMMANDS

To participate effectively during interventions, patients must know what they are to do and when they are to do it. Patients must be able to hear instructions and commands. When a patient cannot hear, or does not understand, spoken words, gestures, and demonstrations may convey necessary meanings. **Instructions** inform a patient of what is to be done and are provided as part of the teaching process for the patient. Instructions may include oral description, visual demonstration, and written description. **Verbal commands** are auditory cues to a patient and are provided during activity performance. Prior to activity performance, it is important to instruct a patient about the verbal commands that will be provided during activity performance.

Instructions must be simple, informative, and in a language and terms the patient can understand. Medical terms should be used only when a patient readily understands medical terminology or when the terms can be explained in a way the patient can understand during patient instruction. When a patient's understanding of English will interfere with safe and effective intervention, providing instructions in a language the patient understands will be necessary. When a physical therapist cannot communicate fluently in the required foreign language, the physical therapist is responsible for securing the services of an interpreter for the patient's benefit. Many facilities maintain lists of personnel who speak specific foreign languages.

A therapist should describe to a patient the general sequence of events that will occur. The patient must also be instructed in what he or she is expected to do. This assists the patient in learning skills for future independent use and increases safety during immediate activity performance. A physical therapist must determine that a patient understands instructions provided before activity performance. Asking a patient,

"Do you understand the instruction?" does not ensure understanding. Having a patient repeat the instructions in proper sequence provides an opportunity for mental rehearsal of the task in addition to indicating an appropriate level of understanding.

Verbal commands focus the patient's attention on specifically desired actions. A command is a cue for a specific action during activity performance. Verbal commands must be clear, brief, specific, properly timed, and spoken in appropriate tone and volume. Tone and volume must vary as a situation requires. Generally, commands spoken in a sharp or loud manner receive quick responses and commands spoken in a soft or low manner elicit slower responses.

Patients may become confused when provided a long series of actions to implement when only one cue is provided. In such situation, each specific action may require a specific verbal command. Verbal commands must be specific to the action desired. For example, counting to three does not direct a patient to perform a specific action. When a patient is to look up, the instruction may be "I will count to three and then say 'look up.' When I say 'look up,' you should look up." The verbal command is "look up," which is a specific command, and does not require translating the word "three" into "look up." In this example, a patient has been provided an instruction that includes the verbal command to be used and the expected response. Commands must be timed for each action to occur in the proper sequence, and at the appropriate time, so the entire activity is completed safely and effectively.

PATIENT PREPARATION

For efficient use of treatment time, patient preparation should be completed prior to transport and treatment. Nursing personnel and transport personnel must be notified of scheduled treatment time and preparation requirements well in advance of scheduled treatment time. Patients should be properly dressed for transfers and treatment to ensure modesty, safety, and effective treatment.

Appropriate draping for modesty, safety, and effective treatment is the right of every patient and the responsibility of all personnel. **Draping** is appropriately covering a patient in a manner that maintains the patient's right to modesty during safe and effective treatment. Draping uses sheets and towels as necessary to achieve the desired effect. Draping (a) protects a patient's modesty; (b) provides warmth; (c) protects wounds, scars, residual limbs, personal clothing, and so forth; and (d) exposes specific body segments for treatment. Edges of sheets and towels should be secured to avoid shifting and resultant inadvertent exposure of a patient. When positioning or transferring a patient, advance planning is required to maintain appropriate draping.

Hospital gowns are designed for ease in dressing and access during nursing care. They may not provide effective draping during movements required for transfers and treatment. Properly securing the ties of a hospital gown may provide some coverage. Mid-length robes or housecoats, or two hospital gowns, with one opening in front and one opening in back, can be used to provide effective draping. Long robes or housecoats interfere with movement and their use as draping should be avoided.

Whenever possible, patients should be dressed in slacks or shorts to provide ease of movement without loss of modesty. Shorts are especially useful if a lower extremity must be observed. If slacks or shorts are loose-fitting, a belt should be worn to prevent them from falling, which would restrict movement and pose a safety hazard. A halter top or bra is useful when a female patient's upper trunk must be observed. Shoes that offer support are required if a patient is to stand, ambulate, or practice transfers. When shoes are worn, socks should be worn for protection, comfort, and sanitation. For patients who are not ambulatory, slippers may be acceptable as they are easier to don and doff as necessary. In all situations, decisions concerning dress must be tempered by the patient's needs, the patient's ability to manipulate clothing, and the requirements of treatment.

Physical therapists treat patients in a variety of settings. In many settings, primarily hospital, but also in nursing homes and some personal homes, patients may present with intravenous (IV) lines, chest tubes, catheters, respirators, cardiac monitors, or combinations of these. When positioning, transferring, or treating patients, care must be taken not to disrupt lines, tubes, or electrodes, as these are vital to patient well-being. If a line, tube, or electrode is disrupted, notify appropriate personnel immediately to obtain assistance. A dislodged chest tube or respirator can be life threatening. Physical therapists must be prepared to react quickly and appropriately.

Lines, tubes, and electrodes limit the amount of movement available to a patient. Prior to moving patients, or having a patient move, physical therapists must check that desired movement will be allowed, or plan in advance to reposition IV containers, catheter bags, oxygen masks, chest tubes, and the like. Repositioning of containers, tubes, lines, and other equipment may require additional equipment or personnel. Do not allow tubes or lines to become tangled, pinched, kinked, stretched, or pulled out from their insertion or attachment site. Any of these occurrences will interrupt proper function, perhaps even be life-threatening. IV drip rates and oxygen flow rates must not be changed without a physician's orders and it is not within the scope of physical therapy practice. IV fluid containers must remain above the level of the patient's heart. Urinary drainage collection bags must remain below the level of the patient's bladder. Proper placement of IV fluid containers and urinary drainage collection bags is necessary to maintain the correct direction of fluid flow.

TRANSPORTING

Transporting patients from one area to another is frequently necessary. A gurney (cart) or wheelchair may be required because of a patient's condition or facility regulations. Patients should be transferred onto/into the required transport device in an appropriate manner, with proper draping maintained throughout transfer and transport. Appropriate transfers in preparation for transporting patients are covered in Chapter 8.

Wheel locks on wheelchairs or gurneys must be locked before initiating transfers. Patient clothing, draping, and medical equipment (IVs, etc.) must be adjusted to avoid problems discussed previously under Patient Preparation, as well as becoming tangled in wheels, or dragged on the floor, during transport. A patient's arms and legs must be within the boundaries of a gurney, or wheelchair to avoid injury during transport. Gurneys may have straps or side rails to keep patients within the confines of the gurney and wheelchairs may have seat belts to keep patients from sliding or falling out of the chair. Such safety devices should be used routinely for patient safety during transport.

Mattresses on gurneys, and cushions on wheelchairs, are used for patient comfort and protection. Additional pillows and padding are positioned for the patient's comfort and protection as necessary. Appropriate patient positioning is covered in Chapter 5.

In some illustrations throughout the text, the physical therapist's position has been altered from the desired position or the physical therapist is absent from the illustration. This was done to provide a clear view of other detail in the illustration.

TRANSPORTING VIA GURNEY

Gurneys have four swivel wheels, making it easier to maneuver the gurney from either end. Locks are located on each wheel. Generally, there are three positions in which the lock can be placed.

With the locking lever in the horizontal position, both swivel and rolling movements are permitted.

When the locking lever is tilted in one direction, swivel movement is locked and rolling motion is permitted. Tilting the locking lever in the other direction locks the wheels completely, prohibiting both swivel and rolling movements. To engage the locking lever, hold the gurney in a stable position and activate the locking lever with your foot.

Gurney side rails raise or swing up to prevent the patient from falling off the gurney. The rails are lowered or swung down for easier transferring.

Gurney rails have a locking mechanism to secure them in the up position.

Gurneys should be pushed from the end at which the patient's head is placed so the patient is moving feet first. The pace of transport should be slow and steady. Quick, jerky movements may upset or nauseate a patient. Control of the gurney must be maintained at all times. Corners must be turned cautiously because of the potential for limited visibility and room for maneuvering. Additional personnel may be needed to maneuver on and off elevators, through doorways, and at blind corners. When necessary, medical equipment, such as IVs, can be attached to a gurney at an appropriate height.

PROCEDURE 2-3

TRANSPORTING VIA WHEELCHAIR

Proper patient positioning in a wheelchair includes having the patient seated well back on the seat, lower extremities placed on the footrests or leg rests, arms resting on armrests or in laps, and available safety straps or seat belts secured. Wheelchairs must be pushed at a slow and steady pace without quick or jerky movements. Control of a wheelchair must be maintained at all times. When necessary, medical equipment, such as IVs, can be attached to the wheelchair at the appropriate height.

The method chosen to ascend and descend curbs depends on the (a) height of the curb, (b) size and weight of the patient and wheelchair, and (c) height and strength of the person transporting the patient. Use of proper body mechanics is necessary to prevent potential injury. When descending an average height curb, the backward method places less stress on a physical therapist. When ascending an average height curb, the forward method places less stress on a physical therapist.

Descending Curb—Backward Method

1. To lower a patient in a wheelchair down a curb, position the wheelchair with the patient facing away from the curb. This positions the larger rear wheels at the edge of the curb to be descended.

2. Facing the wheelchair from behind, the physical therapist steps off the curb backward. Holding onto the wheelchair's push handles, the physical therapist slowly and smoothly rolls the rear wheels of the wheelchair to street level.

3. Securely holding the wheelchair's push handles, and maintaining the wheelchair in a tilted position, the physical therapist continues to roll the wheelchair backward until the front wheels are clear of the curb. The physical therapist slowly lowers the front wheels until all four wheels are securely on the street level.

Descending Curb—Forward Method

1. This method is stressful for a physical therapist, who must maintain a backward tilt of the wheelchair while controlling the roll of the wheelchair's rear wheels over the edge of the curb. There is greater danger of losing control of the wheelchair when using this method. This method is recommended for use only with low curbs.

2. When using the forward method, the wheelchair is positioned with the front of the wheelchair facing the curb. Facing the wheelchair from behind, the physical therapist tilts the wheelchair backward so the front wheels are approximately 8 inches above the ground. The wheelchair is rolled on its rear wheels to the edge of the curb.

3. The rear wheels of the wheelchair are rolled slowly and smoothly off the curb onto the street level. As the wheelchair rolls over the curb, the physical therapist must step forward and bend at the hips and knees to control descent.

4. The therapist then slowly lowers the front wheels until all four wheels are securely on the lower level. The therapist may control the lowering by placing one foot on one anti-tipping bar.

   When a curb is high, a physical therapist may step off the curb while maintaining the wheelchair in a tilted position.

Ascending Curb—Backward Method

This method places more stress on the physical therapist while controlling the roll of the wheelchair over the edge of the curb. This method is recommended only for use with low curbs.

1. To raise a patient in a wheelchair up a curb, position the wheelchair with the patient facing away from the curb. This positions the larger rear wheels at the edge of the curb to be ascended. Facing the wheelchair from behind, the physical therapist tilts the chair backward and steps onto the curb backward. The physical therapist is positioned on the curb with the feet in stride and the hips and knees flexed with the back straight.

   Holding onto the wheelchair's push handles, the physical therapist slowly and smoothly pulls the wheelchair in a tilted orientation up the curb on its rear wheels to sidewalk level.

2. The wheelchair is rolled backward until the front wheels are clearly past the curb and over the sidewalk. The physical therapist then slowly lowers the front wheels until all four wheels are securely on the sidewalk. The physical therapist may place one foot on the anti-tipping bar to control the rate of lowering the wheelchair onto all four wheels.

Ascending Curb—Forward Method

1. To raise a wheelchair with a patient up a curb, position the wheelchair with the patient facing the curb. Facing the wheelchair from behind, the physical therapist tilts the wheelchair backward so that the front wheels are higher than the curb. This can be achieved by the physical therapist assuming a slight squatting position as the push handles are lowered to achieve the tilted orientation.

2. Holding onto the wheelchair's push handles, the physical therapist slowly and smoothly pushes the wheelchair forward until the front wheels are clearly over the sidewalk. The wheelchair is slowly lowered, placing the front wheels on the sidewalk.

3. The physical therapist continues to wheel the wheelchair until the rear wheels contact the curb. The wheelchair is then pushed and lifted so the rear wheels roll up and over the curb. Good body mechanics requires that the arms are held in a steady position and that the legs are straightened during the lifting motion.

Doorways

Most public buildings have automatic doors, both opening and closing, to allow independent access for individuals using ambulation aides. The time an automatic door may take to open or close may vary. Doors with automatic closers may have varying degrees of door closing force. Care should be taken to ensure that patients are instructed to be aware of how automatic doors react and to learn details about specific doors they use frequently.

Assisted Progression Through Doorways

Door Opening Away From Patient

1. To assist a patient in a wheelchair to progress through a doorway opening away from the patient, the physical therapist positions the patient facing away from the door. Using the door handle, the physical therapist releases the latch. The physical therapist walks backward through the doorway pulling the wheelchair backward through the doorway, using his or her back, shoulder, or foot to open and block the door.

2. As the wheelchair passes the doorjamb, the therapist uses one hand to keep the door open and the other hand to steer the wheelchair, turning the wheelchair so that the patient is facing the direction of progression.

3. As the physical therapist, patient, and wheelchair progress through the doorway, the physical therapist may also use his or her shoulder, hip, or foot to continue blocking the door. The door should not be allowed to close and hit the patient or the wheelchair.

Door Opening Toward Patient

1. To assist a patient in a wheelchair to progress through a doorway toward the patient, a physical therapist positions the patient and wheelchair parallel to the door at the latch side of the door. The physical therapist uses one hand to unlatch the door, pulling the door open.

2. The physical therapist opens the door wide enough, sufficient for passage of the wheelchair. Blocking the door open, the physical therapist aligns the patient and wheelchair with the open doorway.

3. Walking forward through the doorway, the physical therapist pushes the wheelchair forward through the doorway, using his or her shoulder, hip, or foot to continue blocking the door. The door should not be allowed to close and hit the patient or the wheelchair.

Independent Progression Through Doorways

Techniques for independent wheelchair ambulation through doorways are determined by the (a) abilities of the patient, (b) direction in which the door opens, (c) direction from which the patient can approach (hinge or latch), and (d) whether or not the door is an automatic opening/closing door.

Door Opening Toward Patient (With Automatic Door Closer)

1. The patient wheels to the latch side of the door and reaches across his or her body for the door handle with the hand toward the hinge side of the door. The patient pulls open the door wider than necessary for progression through the doorway because the door will begin to close prior to the patient completing progression through the door-way.

2. The patient may use the front rigging of the wheelchair and one hand can be used to block open the door. The patient must progress into the doorway quickly to block the closing door. Care must be taken that the closing door does not strike the patient or hit the wheelchair hard enough to cause the patient to lose control of the wheelchair.

3. Patients may pull on the doorjamb to assist propulsion through the doorway. Care must be taken to avoid crushing the patient's fingers between the door and the propulsion wheel as the door is blocked.

*Door Opens Away From Patient
(With Automatic Door Closer)*

1. The patient approaches the door and grasps the door handle.

2. Pushing hard to open the door wide, the patient enters the doorway before the door can close. Care must be taken that the closing door does not strike a patient or hit the wheelchair hard enough to cause a patient to lose control of the wheelchair. Some patients may pull on the doorjamb to assist progression through the doorway, while blocking the closing door with the other hand. Other patients propel their wheelchair in the usual way, or use a combination of pulling on the doorjamb and normal propulsion. The rubber bumper on the footrest closest to the door can also be used to block the closing door.

3. When a patient is nearly through the doorway, the door may be given one more opening push. The patient then propels the wheelchair quickly out of the arc of the closing door. The door is allowed to close behind the patient's wheelchair. Some patients turn their wheelchairs around the latch side of the doorjamb and away from the closing door to quickly move out of the arc of the closing door.

Doors With Automatic Door Openers (Opening Away/Toward Patient)

Several types of activators are available for automatic door openers. A push-plate activator may be located along the path to the door at an appropriate height, or a pressure activator may be located in the floor in front of the door. A motion sensor is another form of activator that may be used. When a door opens toward a patient, patients must make sure to be clear of the arc of the opening door to avoid being struck by the opening door. Doors usually stay open until a patient has progressed completely through the doorway. A patient, however, should not hesitate while progressing through a doorway because the automatic door opener will release after a set amount of time.

WHEELCHAIR WHEELIES

Wheelchair wheelies are performed by balancing on the rear wheels of a wheelchair with the (front) caster wheels in the air. Patients must be able to perform wheelies to ascend and descend curbs independently when no curb ramps/cuts are available. Guarding a patient while a patient learns to perform a wheelie is critical in preventing injury.

1. A physical therapist must be positioned behind, and move with, the wheelchair to guard as patients practice. The physical therapist's hands must be beneath or on the wheelchair push handles, ready to catch the wheelchair if it tilts too far backward.

2. The patient begins a wheelie by grasping the anterior portion of the push rims.

(continued)

3. A quick backward movement of the wheels places the patient's hands in position for the forward thrust that achieves the wheelie position.

4. The quick backward motion of the wheels is immediately followed by a quick forward thrust on both wheel rims. The result of these maneuvers causes the wheelchair to tilt backward, rising onto the rear wheels only.

5. Patients control balancing and moving on the rear wheels by forward and backward movements of the rear wheels.

ELEVATORS

When riding in an elevator, patients should be positioned facing the elevator door, the position most commonly assumed when riding an elevator. When space is sufficient, a patient may enter an elevator forward, and then turn around. When space is limited, patients should enter the elevator backward. Facing forward allows patients to monitor the floor display and have access to the control panel. Exiting facing forward is usually safer.

REVIEW QUESTIONS

1. Who is responsible for ensuring that patient care environments are safe and efficient?

2. Describe the general guidelines for properly managing the patient care environment.

3. List the five rules of proper body mechanics.

4. Describe how to apply the rules of proper body mechanics in each of the following situations:

   a. When transporting a patient on a gurney.
   b. When guarding a patient who is ambulating.
   c. When moving large equipment.

5. Distinguish between instructions and commands, giving examples of each.

6. List the purposes of draping a patient.

7. Describe how to transport a patient in a wheelchair safely.

SUGGESTED ACTIVITIES

1. Demonstrate how to correctly adjust the locking mechanisms on the wheels of a gurney, the railings on a gurney, and the wheel locks on a wheelchair.

2. Demonstrate how to maneuver a gurney and a wheelchair through a doorway, around a corner, and along a hallway properly and safely.

3. Demonstrate how to ascend and descend curbs.

4. Demonstrate how to guard a person performing a wheelie.

5. Perform a wheelie.

6. Discuss experiences in activities 1–5, including:

   a. Perceptions of self when being transported compared to being the person doing the transporting.
   b. Realization of the challenge of moving about the environment while in a wheelchair or on a gurney.

7. Rotate through several stations related to body mechanics. Suggestions for stations include:

   a. Foot placement.
   Place foot marks on the floor indicating foot placement. Make some foot placements correct and some incorrect. Students should perform tasks such as lifting boxes from a wheelchair to a mat table, from a wheelchair to a treatment table, and from a table in front to a table behind. Discuss which foot placements are appropriate and why.
   b. Center of Mass (CoM) centered.
   Carry books in a book bag from the front of the classroom to the rear of the classroom, with the book bag on one shoulder, properly positioned on both shoulders, held in one hand at the side, and held in one hand out in front. Discuss the experiences to determine which are easier and why.

8. Document experiences such as ascending and descending curbs in SOAP note format.

CASE STUDY

You are working in a rehabilitation facility with a patient who has a recent complete cervical spinal cord injury. A power wheelchair has been ordered, but has not yet been delivered, so transport requires family members to maneuver a manual wheelchair. The patient's family wishes to take her to a restaurant in an older section of town. The family has determined that the restaurant is wheelchair accessible. The parking lot, however, is across the street from the restaurant and there are no curb ramps on either side of the street. List and describe the transport activities that might be required. Indicate what you would review with the patient and family prior to their departure for the restaurant.

3

Aseptic Techniques

LEARNING OBJECTIVES

Upon completion of this chapter, you will be able to:

1. Use defined terms correctly.
2. Describe Standard Precautions, including who is responsible for implementation, when to implement, and methods of implementation.
3. Recognize when the guidelines for a sterile field are violated and act appropriately.
4. Demonstrate proper procedure for donning a sterile gown.
5. Demonstrate proper procedure for donning sterile gloves.
6. Demonstrate proper procedure for removal of contaminated gloves.
7. Describe the characteristics of wounds that are evaluated.
8. Describe the purposes, types, materials, and methods of wound dressings.
9. List the five major areas of recommendations for isolation precautions.
10. Describe the five modes of transmission of infectious microorganisms.
11. Describe the implementation of selected procedures of isolation precautions.

MEDIALINK

A companion CD-ROM, included free with each new copy of this book, supplements the techniques presented in the book. Insert the CD-ROM to watch video clips of patient care skills being demonstrated. This multimedia feature is designed to help you add a new dimension to your learning.

KEY TERMS

Airborne precautions
Airborne transmission
Alcohol-based hand rub
Antimicrobial soap
Antiseptic agent
Antiseptic hand rub
Antiseptic handwash
Aseptic technique
Bacterial barrier
Centers for Disease Control and Prevention (CDC)
Cleaning
Cleanliness
Common vehicle transmission
Compression wrap
Contact precautions
Contact transmission
Contaminated
Critical items

Damp-to-damp dressing
Damp-to-dry dressing
Decontaminate hands
Detergent
Direct-contact transmission
Disinfection
Droplet precautions
Droplet transmission
Dry-to-dry dressing
Figure-of-eight wrap
Gauze wrap
Hand antisepsis
Hand hygiene
Handwashing
Hospital Infection Control Practices Advisory Committee (HICPAC)
Indirect-contact transmission
Isolation
Non-critical items

Nosocomial infection
Occlusive dressing
Patient care equipment categories
Plain soap
Recommendations ranking scheme
Rigid dressing
Semi-critical items
Shelf life
Spiral wrap
Standard precautions
Sterile
Sterile field
Sterilization
Surgical hand antisepsis
Transmission-based precautions
Unsterile (non-sterile)
Vectorborne precautions
Waterless antiseptic agent

INTRODUCTION

Although the concepts of cleanliness and aseptic technique in patient care have been in use during the past two centuries, changes in these techniques occur from time to time as the result of research on the prevention of disease transmission. Recent increased emphasis on the importance of prevention of disease transmission and the spread of infection through proper patient care techniques has occurred in part because of the increasing incidence of catastrophic diseases, such as acquired immunodeficiency syndrome (AIDS). The **Centers for Disease Control and Prevention (CDC)** and its **Hospital Infection Control Practices Advisory Committee (HICPAC)**, operating within the Department of Health and Human Services, are responsible for promulgating guidelines related to prevention of disease transmission. These guidelines are updated periodically, and personnel should obtain the most updated information from the infection control officer at their specific institution or directly from the CDC. The Occupational Safety and Health Agency (OSHA), an agency of the federal government, establishes rules and regulations to protect workers in a variety of work environments including workers in health care facilities.

Much of the material in this chapter is from publications in the public domain produced by the CDC,[1-4] which is continually updating recommendations for cleaning, disinfecting, and sterile technique based on an increasing body of scientific knowledge. While the information in this chapter provides a starting point for understanding disease transmission prevention and practices in aseptic techniques, individuals are strongly advised to become familiar with the specific practices of the institution in which they work and to obtain updated information directly from the CDC. Information can be found at the CDC website by entering a key term such as "Isolation Precautions" in the search box, and then downloading the desired information from the Internet.

> Centers for Disease Control and Prevention
> 1600 Clifton Rd, Atlanta, GA 30333
> (404) 639–3311
> (404) 639–3534 / (800) 311–3435 (public inquiries)
> www.cdc.gov

Each institution will use information and protocols specific to that institution. Institution specific information and protocols can be obtained from the appropriate department within the institution.

DEFINITIONS

Definitions are used by the medical community to standardize terminology. Several terms used in this chapter are defined below. Not all definitions related to *Aseptic Techniques* are included.

Alcohol-based hand rub: An alcohol-containing preparation designed for application to the hands for reducing the number of viable microorganisms on the hands. In the United States, such preparations usually contain 60–95% ethanol or isopropanol.

Antimicrobial soap: Soap (i.e., detergent) containing an antiseptic agent.

Antiseptic agent: Antimicrobial substances that are applied to the skin to reduce the number of microbial flora. Examples include alcohols, chlorhexidine, chlorine, hexachlorophene, iodine, chloroxylenol (PCMX), quaternary ammonium compounds, and triclosan.

Antiseptic handwash: Washing hands with water and soap or other detergents containing an antiseptic agent.

Antiseptic hand rub: Applying an antiseptic hand-rub product to all surfaces of the hands to reduce the number of microorganisms present.

Aseptic technique: The methods and procedures used to create and maintain a sterile field.

Bacterial barrier: A barrier that keeps microorganisms from coming in contact with sterile items.

Cleanliness: Three levels of cleanliness—cleaning, disinfection, and sterilization—have been established for equipment use in patient care.

> **Cleaning** is the physical removal of organic material or soil from objects. The process of cleaning is usually performed with water, with or without detergents. Cleaning is the least rigorous of the three levels and is designed to remove microorganisms rather than kill them. Cleaning usually precedes either of the next two levels, disinfection or sterilization.

> **Disinfection** is an intermediate level between cleaning and sterilization. Three levels of disinfection—high, intermediate, and low—have been defined. Disinfection is usually performed using pasteurization or chemical germicides.

> **Sterilization** is the highest level of cleanliness. Sterilization is the destruction of all forms of microbial life by steam under pressure, liquid or gaseous chemicals, or dry heat.

Contaminated: An item, surface, or field is considered to be contaminated whenever it comes in contact with anything that is not sterile.

Decontaminate hands: To reduce bacterial counts on hands by performing antiseptic hand rub or antiseptic hand wash.

Detergent: Detergents (i.e., surfactants) are compounds that possess a cleaning action. They are composed of both hydrophilic and lipophilic parts and can be divided into four groups: anionic, cationic, amphoteric, and nonionic detergents. Although products used for handwashing or antiseptic hand wash in health-care settings represent various types of detergents, the term "soap" is used to refer to such detergents in this guideline.

Hand antisepsis: Refers to either antiseptic hand wash or antiseptic hand rub.

Hand hygiene: A general term that applies to handwashing, antiseptic hand wash, antiseptic hand rub, or surgical hand antisepsis.

Handwashing: Washing hands with plain (i.e., non-antimicrobial) soap and water.

Nosocomial infection: Infection acquired while hospitalized for treatment of other conditions.

Patient care equipment categories: Three categories of patient care equipment—critical, semi-critical, and non-critical[1]—provide a basis for the level of cleanliness deemed necessary.

> **Critical items** are those that are introduced directly into the circulatory system or other normally sterile areas of the body. Surgical instruments, implants, and the blood compartment of a hemodialyzer are examples of critical items.

> **Semi-critical items** are those that are introduced into body cavities not usually considered sterile, and include, but are not limited to, endotracheal tubes and fiberoptic endoscopes. There is less degree of risk of infection associated with semicritical items.

> **Non-critical items** are items that do not touch the patient, or touch the patient in areas that are normally not sterile, such as intact areas of skin. Blood pressure cuffs and crutches are examples of non-critical items.

Plain soap: Detergents that do not contain antimicrobial agents or contain low concentrations of antimicrobial agents that are effective solely as preservatives.

Recommendations ranking scheme: The CDC's Center for Infectious Diseases has established four categories to indicate the scientific support for their recommendations.[3]

> **Category IA:** Strongly recommended for all hospitals, and strongly supported by well-designed experimental or epidemiologic studies.

Category IB: Strongly recommended for all hospitals and reviewed as effective by experts and a consensus of HICPAC, based on strong rationale and suggestive evidence, although definitive scientific studies have not been done.

Category II: Suggested for implementation in many hospitals. Recommendations may be supported or suggested by clinical or epidemiologic studies, a strong theoretical rationale, or definitive studies applicable to some, but not all, hospitals.

No recommendation/unresolved issues: Practices for which insufficient evidence or consensus regarding efficacy exists.

Shelf life: The length of time an unopened sterilized package is considered to remain sterile.

Sterile: An item or environment free from living microorganisms.

Sterile field: An area considered free from living microorganisms.

Standard Precautions: Precautions designed for the care of all patients, particularly hospitalized patients, regardless of their diagnosis or presumed infection status. This is new terminology to replace the term Universal Precautions.

Surgical hand antisepsis: Antiseptic hand wash or antiseptic hand rub performed preoperatively by surgical personnel to eliminate transient, and reduce resident, hand flora. Antiseptic detergent preparations often have persistent antimicrobial activity.

Unsterile (nonsterile): Any item or environment that has not been sterilized, has come into contact with an item that is no longer considered sterile, has entered a field that is not sterile, or has exceeded its shelf life.

Waterless antiseptic agent: An antiseptic agent that does not require use of exogenous water. After applying such an agent, the hands are rubbed together until the agent has dried.

INTRODUCTION TO INFECTION CONTROL

The prevention of disease transmission in hospitals is of major concern.[1] Dramatic changes have occurred in the past 35 years, and the rate at which changes occur has been increasing. For this reason, a brief history of isolation protocols is presented.

One means of preventing disease transmission is placing patients in isolation. **Isolation** is the separation and placement of patients in environments that reduce potential for transmission of infectious microorganisms. The principles followed and the techniques used to prevent disease transmission as part of isolation precautions are generally appropriate for the prevention of disease transmission as part of patient care in general.

When a patient is placed in isolation, signage is posted outside the patient's room, indicating specifically required isolation practices, or a request for visitors to see the patient's nurse prior to entering the patient's room. There are two methods indicating which isolation precautions are to be used. Hospitals choose which method is most appropriate for their facility. In 1970, CDC recommended isolation procedures based on seven categories: Strict Isolation, Respiratory Isolation, Protective Isolation, Enteric Precautions, Wound and Skin Precautions, Discharge Precautions, and Blood Precautions. The precautions recommended for each category were based primarily on the epidemiologic features of the diseases grouped in the category. The diseases were grouped primarily by routes of transmission, and recommended precautions were the minimum believed necessary to prevent transmission of all diseases in a specific category. In 1983, the CDC published new guidelines, which included revision of the original categories, and permitted facilities to use either category-specific guidelines or disease-specific guidelines. Newer CDC guidelines published in 1997 required guidelines to 1) have a basis that is epidemiologically sound, 2) emphasize the importance of all body fluids, secretions, and excretions in the transmission of nosocomial pathogens; 3) contain adequate precautions for infections transmitted by the airborne, droplet, and contact routes of transmission, 4) be simple to understand and use, and 5) use new terms to avoid confusion with existing systems.

Current specific infection control recommendations are contained in *Guidelines for Environmental Infection Control in Health Care Facilities.*[2] Specific infection control recommendations include methods of cleaning and sterilizing whirlpools and other patient contact surfaces, as well as recommendations pertaining to health care provider clothing and jewelry.

ISOLATION PRECAUTIONS IN HOSPITALS[3]

RATIONALE

Transmission of infection requires three elements: 1) a source of infecting microorganisms, 2) a susceptible host, and 3) a means of transmission for the microorganism. Human sources of infecting microorganisms in hospitals may be patients, personnel, or visitors. Included may be persons with acute disease, or persons in the incubation period of a disease, persons who are colonized by an infectious agent but have no apparent disease, or persons who are chronic carriers of an infectious agent. Other sources of infecting microorganisms can be the patient's own endogenous flora, which may be difficult to control, and inanimate environmental objects that have become contaminated, including equipment and medications.

Resistance among persons to pathogenic microorganisms varies greatly. Some may be immune to infection or may be able to resist colonization by an infectious agent. Others exposed to the same agent may establish a commensal relationship with the infecting microorganism and become asymptomatic carriers. Still others may develop clinical disease. Host factors may include, but not be limited to: 1) age, 2) underlying diseases, 3) certain treatments with antimicrobials, corticosteroids, or other immunosuppressive agents, 4) irradiation, and 5) breaks in the first line of defense mechanisms caused by surgical operations, anesthesia, and indwelling catheters, which may render patients more susceptible to infection.

Microorganisms are transmitted in hospitals by several routes, and the same microorganism may be transmitted by more than one route. There are five main routes of transmission: contact, droplet, airborne, common vehicle, and vectorborne. Isolation precautions are designed to prevent transmission of microorganisms by these routes in hospitals. Because agent and host factors are more difficult to control, interruption of transfer of microorganisms is directed primarily at transmission. CDC recommendations are based on this concept.

MODES OF TRANSMISSION

Contact transmission, the most important and frequent mode of nosocomial infection transmission, is divided into two subgroups—direct-contact transmission and indirect-contact transmission. **Direct-contact transmission** involves direct body surface-to-body surface contact, and physical transfer of microorganisms between a susceptible host and an infected or colonized person, such as when turning or transferring a patient, or performing other patient-care activities that require direct personal contact. Direct-contact transmission can also occur when one patient serves as a source of the infectious microorganisms and the other as a susceptible host. **Indirect-contact transmission** involves contact of a susceptible host with a contaminated intermediate object, usually inanimate, such as whirlpool water that is not changed between patient treatments, re-use of self-adhesive electrodes on more than one patient, contaminated hands that are not washed, and gloves that are not changed between patients.

Droplet transmission, theoretically, is a form of contact transmission. The mechanism of transfer of the pathogen, however, is quite distinct from either direct- or indirect-contact transmission. Therefore, droplet transmission is considered a separate route of transmission. Droplets are generated from a source person, primarily during coughing, sneezing, and talking, and during the performance of certain procedures such as suctioning or wound care. Transmission occurs when droplets containing microorganisms generated from the infected person are propelled a short distance through the air and deposited on a host's conjunctivae, nasal mucosa, or mouth. Droplets do not remain suspended in the air, and droplet transmission must not be confused with airborne transmission.

Airborne transmission occurs by two modes of dissemination. The first mode of dissemination is of airborne droplet nuclei, which are small particle residue 5µm or smaller in size. These nuclei are evaporated droplets containing microorganisms that remain suspended in the air for long periods of time. The second mode of dissemination is dust particles containing the infectious agent, dispersed widely by air currents and inhaled by a susceptible host. The distance over which such dissemination may occur is dependent upon environmental factors, thus special air handling and ventilation are required to prevent airborne transmission.

Common vehicle transmission applies to microorganisms transmitted by contaminated items such as food, water, medications, devices, and equipment.

Vectorborne transmission occurs when vectors such as mosquitoes, flies, rats, and other vermin transmit microorganisms; this route of transmission is of less significance in hospitals in the United States than in other regions of the world.

TIERS OF ISOLATION PRECAUTIONS

There are two tiers of isolation precautions. The first, and most important, tier of isolation precautions is **Standard Precautions,** designed for the care of all patients in hospitals, regardless of diagnosis or suspected infection status. Implementation of Standard Precautions is the primary strategy for successful nosocomial infection control. The second tier of precautions is **Transmission-Based Precautions**, based on the concept of avoiding infection by limiting the potential for transmission of microorganisms. Transmission-Based Precautions are designed only for the care of specified patients: patients known, or suspected, to be infected by epidemiologically important pathogens.

Standard Precautions

Standard Precautions synthesize the major features of Universal Precautions and apply them to all patients receiving care in hospitals, regardless of diagnosis or presumed infection status. Standard Precautions apply to 1) blood, 2) all body fluids, secretions, and excretions except sweat, regardless of whether or not they contain visible blood, 3) non-intact skin, and 4) mucous membranes. Standard Precautions are designed to reduce the risk of transmission of microorganisms from both recognized and unrecognized sources of infection in hospitals.

Transmission-Based Precautions

Transmission-Based Precautions are designed for patients documented or suspected to be infected with highly transmissible pathogens for which additional precautions, beyond Standard Precautions, are needed to interrupt transmission in hospitals. There are three types of Transmission-Based Precautions: airborne, droplet, and contact. Combinations of these precautions may be used for diseases that have multiple routes of transmission. Whether used singularly or in combination, they are to be used in addition to Standard Precautions.

RECOMMENDATIONS

When outlining the precautions to be used in isolation the CDC deemed five areas crucial to maintaining isolation precautions in hospitals: 1) administrative controls; 2) standard precautions; 3) airborne precautions; 4) droplet precautions; and 5) contact precautions. Current CDC recommendations for all five areas are at the Category IB level. The recommendations are limited to the topic of isolation. Therefore, they must be supplemented by hospital policies and procedures for other aspects of infection and environment control, occupational health, and administrative and legal issues.

Following are selected isolation precaution recommendations from the CDC.[3]

Administrative Controls

Education.   Develop a system to ensure that hospital patients, personnel, and visitors are educated about use of precautions and their responsibility for adherence to them.

Adherence to Precautions.   Periodically evaluate adherence to precautions and use findings to direct improvements.

Standard Precautions

Use Standard Precautions, or the equivalent, for the care of all patients.

Handwashing.   Hands are to be washed after touching blood, body fluids, secretions, excretions, and contaminated items, whether or not gloves are worn. Hands are to be washed immediately after gloves are removed, between patient contacts, and at other appropriate times to avoid transfer of microorganisms to other patients or environments. Washing hands between tasks and procedures on the same patient to prevent cross-contamination of different body sites may also be necessary.

A plain (non-antimicrobial) soap for routine handwashing is recommended.

An antimicrobial agent or a waterless antiseptic agent is recommended for specific circumstances, such as control of outbreaks or hyperendemic infections.

Gloves.   Clean, non-sterile gloves are adequate when touching blood, body fluids, secretions, excretions, and contaminated items. Clean gloves should be donned just before touching mucous membranes and non-intact skin.

Gloves should be changed between tasks and procedures on the same patient after contact with material that may contain a high concentration of microorganisms.

Gloves should be removed promptly after use, before touching non-contaminated items and environmental surfaces, and before going to another patient.

Hands should be washed immediately after doffing gloves to avoid transfer of microorganisms to other patients or environments.

Mask, Eye Protection, Face Shield.   Mask and eye protection, or a face shield, should be worn to protect mucous membranes of the eyes, nose, and mouth of health care providers during procedures and patient care activities that are likely to generate splashes or sprays of blood, body fluids, secretions, and excretions.

Gown.   A clean, non-sterile gown is adequate to protect skin and to prevent soiling of clothing of health care providers during procedures and patient care activities that are likely to generate splashes or sprays of blood, body fluids, secretions, or excretions. Gowns appropriate for the activity and amount of fluid likely to be encountered should be chosen. Remove soiled gowns promptly and wash hands immediately after removing a gown to avoid transfer of microorganisms to other patients or environments.

Patient Care Equipment.   Handle used patient care equipment soiled with blood, body fluids, secretions, and excretions in a manner that prevents skin and mucous membrane exposure, contamination of clothing, and transfer of microorganisms to other patients and environments. Ensure that reusable equipment is not used for the care of another patient until it has been cleaned and reprocessed appropriately. Ensure that single-use items are discarded properly.

Environmental Control.   Ensure that the hospital has adequate protocols in place and that these protocols are followed for routine care, cleaning, and disinfection of environmental surfaces, beds, bedrails, bedside equipment, and other frequently touched surfaces.

Linen.   Handle, transport, and process used linen soiled with blood, body fluids, secretions, and excretions in a manner that prevents skin and mucous membrane exposures, and contamination of clothing, and that avoids transfer of microorganisms to other patients and environments.

Occupational Health and Bloodborne Pathogens.   Care should be taken to prevent injuries when handling and using needles, scalpels, and other sharp instruments or devices in preparation for, during, and following procedures.

Never recap used needles, manipulate them using both hands, or direct the point of a used needle toward any part of the body. Use a one-handed "scoop" technique or a mechanical device designed for holding a needle sheath. Do not remove used needles from disposable syringes by hand, and do not bend, break, or manipulate used needles by hand.

Used disposable syringes and needles, scalpel blades, and other sharp items must be placed in appropriate puncture-resistant containers, which should be located as close as possible to the area of use. Reusable syringes and needles should be placed in puncture-resistant containers for transport to a reprocessing area.

Mouthpieces, resuscitation bags, or other ventilation devices should be used as an alternative to mouth-to-mouth resuscitation methods in areas where a need for resuscitation is predictable.

Airborne Precautions

Patients known or suspected to be infected with microorganisms transmitted by airborne droplet nuclei (small residue 5µm or smaller in size) of evaporated droplets should be cared for using Airborne Precautions, or the equivalent, in addition to Standard Precautions.

Respiratory Protection.   Respiratory protection (N95 respirator) should be worn when entering the room of a patient with known or suspected infectious pulmonary tuberculosis. Susceptible persons should not enter the room of patients known or suspected to have measles (rubeola) or varicella (chickenpox) if other immune caregivers are available. If susceptible persons must enter the room of a patient known or suspected to have measles or varicella, they also should wear respiratory protection (N95 respirator). Those immune to measles or varicella need not wear respiratory protection.

Patient Transport.   Movement and transport of patients from the room should be limited to essential purposes only. When transport or movement is necessary, minimize patient dispersal of droplet nuclei by placing a surgical mask on the patient, if possible.

Droplet Precautions

For patients known or suspected to be infected with microorganisms transmitted by nonevaporated large-particle droplets (larger than 5µm in size) generated by coughing, sneezing, talking, or the performance of procedures, Droplet Precautions should be used in addition to Standard Precautions.

Mask.   A mask should be worn when working within three feet of the patient. Compliance may be enhanced by requiring a mask to be worn upon entering a patient's room.

Patient Transport.   Movement and transport of patients from the room should be limited to essential purposes only. When transport or movement is necessary, minimize patient dispersal of droplet nuclei by placing a surgical mask on the patient, if possible.

Contact Precautions

Contact Precautions should be used in addition to Standard Precautions for patients known or suspected to be infected with microorganisms that can be transmitted by direct contact or indirect contact with patients, patient care items, or environmental surfaces.

Gloves. Wearing gloves as outlined under *Standard Precautions* is required. Clean, non-sterile gloves should be donned when entering the room. Change gloves during the course of patient care after contact with infective material that may contain high concentrations of microorganisms (fecal material and wound drainage). Remove gloves before leaving a patient's room.

Handwashing. Immediately upon doffing gloves, hands should be washed with an antimicrobial agent or a waterless antiseptic agent. Following glove removal and handwashing, ensure that hands do not touch potentially contaminated environmental surfaces or items in a patient's room.

Gown. A clean, non-sterile gown should be worn upon entering a room if it is anticipated clothing will have substantial contact with the patient, environmental surfaces, or items in the patient's room, or if a patient is incontinent or has diarrhea, an ileostomy, a colostomy, or wound drainage not contained by a dressing. The gown should be removed before leaving the patient's environment. Ensure that clothing does not contact potentially contaminated environmental surfaces after gown removal.

Patient Transport. Movement and transport of patients from the room should be limited to essential purposes only. When transport or movement is necessary, ensure that precautions are maintained to minimize transmission of microorganisms to other persons, environmental surfaces, or equipment.

Patient-Care Equipment. Use of non-critical patient care equipment should be limited to a single patient (or cohort of patients infected or colonized with the specific pathogen requiring precautions) to avoid transmission between patients.

APPAREL

The purposes of apparel have been covered earlier in this chapter. Specific points regarding apparel are presented in this section.

Scrub suits are not sterile. Gowns, whether paper or cloth, should be worn only once, removed properly, and discarded in an appropriate receptacle.

When the use of a mask is indicated, it should be used only once and discarded in an appropriate receptacle. Lowering a mask around the neck and then placing it over the nose and mouth again is the same as reusing a mask and should not be done. Masks should cover both the nose and the mouth.

In most cases, glasses only provide a barrier in front of the eyes. Glasses with side shields provide an additional barrier. When prescription glasses are necessary, shields or goggles should be worn over prescription glasses, providing the best degree of protection. Shields and goggles are usually constructed of clear plastic, providing a barrier in front and on the sides of the eyes.

Non-sterile gloves are worn as a Standard Precaution. Whether using sterile or non-sterile gloves, handwashing is required after gloves are removed. Used gloves should be removed properly and discarded into an appropriate receptacle.

Additional apparel, including caps, beard covers, and shoe covers, must be worn as necessary to maintain clean or sterile fields.

Sterile Field

The primary goal of using aseptic techniques is to prevent infection. One aseptic technique is to provide and maintain a sterile field. A sterile field is most commonly required in an operating room; however, there may also be a necessity for a sterile field in patient care areas other than the operating room for the performance of minor procedures.

There are eight requirements for providing and maintaining a sterile field. The first four requirements concern creation of a sterile field. The remaining four requirements concern maintenance of the sterile field.

Requirement 1

All items used within the boundaries of a sterile field must be sterile. The items must have been properly sterilized and maintained to preserve their sterile state. Once items have been sterilized, they must be used within the allowable shelf life of the item and sterilization process. The expiration date, or end of shelf life, is marked on each sterile package. Certain types of equipment and different types of packaging may affect the shelf life of a sterile package.

Whenever possible, single-use items are preferred. Because single-use items are discarded after use, there is no concern about contamination before they are reused. This does not mean, however, that single-use items cannot become contaminated before the initial use through improper technique or carelessness.

The shelf-life date of a sterile package is not a guarantee that the package is sterile. Packages are only considered to remain sterile when the:

1. Initial packaging was performed properly;
2. Package was stored in a proper manner;
3. Package was not mishandled during distribution; and
4. Shelf-life date has not been exceeded.

Requirement 2

Once a sterile package has been opened, the edges are not considered sterile. Care in opening sterile packages is required to avoid having the edges touch the contents of the package, or having the edges touch the gloved hands or sterile gown. Most sterile packages have enough packaging material around the edges to keep the unsterile edges away from the sterile contents.

Requirement 3

Once donned properly, sterile gowns are considered to be sterile in the front from shoulder level to table top level, including the sleeves. For this reason, the hands must be held above table top level, in front of the body during and after scrubbing, gowning, and gloving.

Requirement 4

In all cases, only the top surface of a table is considered sterile. Sterile drapes cover the top of a surface and descend on all sides of the surface. Such draping may be covering a patient or on an instrument table. Demarcation of sterile surfaces is fairly easy on tables, but more difficult on patients. A guideline to use for demarcation on a patient that is draped is to consider that a surface above the level of the instrument table, or above waist level, whichever is higher, is a sterile surface as long as it is draped properly. Undraped or improperly draped surfaces, or surfaces below the top level of the instrument table or waist, are considered unsterile.

REQUIREMENT 5

Only sterile items and personnel in sterile attire may enter the sterile field or touch items in a sterile area. Personnel considered non-sterile may not touch any item in a sterile area or any item to be placed in a sterile area. Usually, sterile packages are opened by non-sterile personnel and the contents are released into the sterile area without being touched by non-sterile personnel. Transfer of sterile items into a sterile area may also be accomplished by using sterile forceps to hold the item as it is passed into the sterile area. The set of forceps is considered contaminated after a single use, and may not be used again until sterilized properly. Non-sterile personnel may not reach across or into a sterile area.

REQUIREMENT 6

Activity in a sterile area cannot be allowed to render the area unsterile. Personnel in sterile attire should not sit on or lean against unsterile surfaces. Movement within the sterile area must be measured and careful to avoid contact between sterile and unsterile surfaces.

All personnel, sterile or non-sterile, in or around a sterile area must be aware of the boundaries of a sterile area. Any contamination of a sterile area must be pointed out immediately by any personnel present for protection of the patient.

REQUIREMENT 7

Penetration of a sterile covering or barrier is considered to cause contamination of a sterile field. Liquids are the most likely cause of penetration of a sterile barrier. Liquids spilled within a sterile field may cause penetration of a sterile barrier.

A less noticeable but highly potential cause of penetration is air flow. Design of climate control for sterile areas provides for the most purified air possible and a slightly higher gradient of air pressure in the sterile area. Higher air pressure gradient in the sterile area will cause air flow away from the site of potential infection. Climate control systems should also be physically separated from other areas of the institution so that airborne microorganisms picked up in sterile areas do not permeate the atmosphere of the entire institution.

REQUIREMENT 8

Sterile areas and fields should be prepared as close to the time of use as feasible. They should not be left unattended. Sterile fields should not be prepared and then covered for later use. A delay in using equipment or supplies laid out in a sterile field necessitates the preparation of a new sterile field with new sterile equipment and supplies.

When there is doubt about the sterile quality of an area, a field, or an item, it should be considered unsterile. Improper packaging, sterilization processing, storage, or handling can occur without overt signs. Appropriate use of all items in a sterile environment is the responsibility of the user. Only proper judgement, rigid discipline, and appropriate use provides protection for a patient.

HANDWASHING

PROCEDURES

The ideal duration of handwashing is not known. For most activities, a vigorous, brief rubbing together of all surfaces of lathered hands for a minimum of 15 seconds, followed by rinsing under a stream of water is recommended. When hands are visibly soiled, more time may be required for handwashing. The use of antimicrobial products should follow the manufacturer's recommendations, ensuring that all surfaces of the hands and fingers are cleaned.

SCRUBBING

Scrubbing must be performed before entering a sterile field. Scrubbing is a series of specific steps of hand cleaning using nail cleaners, and soap or antimicrobial products.

Prior to beginning the scrubbing procedure, a freshly laundered scrub suit (pants and shirt or gown), scrub cap, and a new mask are donned (Figure 3–1). The scrub suit is fastened completely and properly. All hair must be covered by a scrub cap. Facial hair, when present, must be covered by a mask and beard cover when necessary. The mask is formed to fit tightly but comfortably over the nose and mouth. Eye shields are worn to protect the eyes.

Figure 3–1 Scrub suit and additional apparel.

PROCEDURE 3-1

GOWNING

1. Open the sterile pack containing the gown. The part of the gown facing you as you look at an open sterile pack is the inside, or unsterile side.

2. Grasp the gown firmly and lift it up and away from the sterile field. Move away from the table on which the sterile pack rests, keeping hands above waist height at all times. Shake open the gown so it unfolds. Holding the inside of the gown only, locate the neck and armholes of the gown.

3. Without touching the outside, or sterile side of the gown, work both arms into the sleeves at the same time. Stop when the hands reach the stockinette cuffs.

4. The gown is tied at the back and neck closures by a circulating nurse or other nonsterile personnel.

PROCEDURE 3-2

 GLOVING

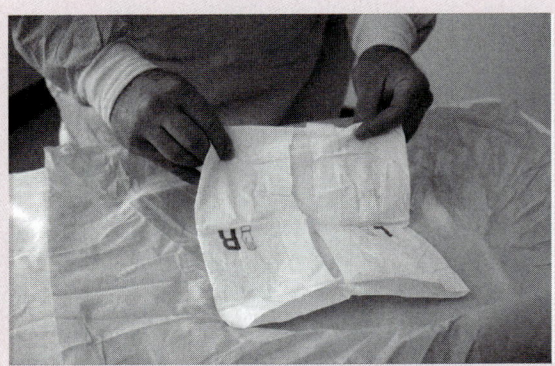

1. A glove pack is opened and the sterile paper enclosure that contains the gloves is placed on a sterile surface with the cuffs toward the person who will be gloving.

2. The sterile portion of a glove pack is opened by grasping the folds of the paper enclosing the gloves.

3. The wrist end of each glove has been turned back on itself, creating a cuff where the inside, or unsterile side, is now outward.

4. Grasping the left glove by its cuff on the non-sterile portion with a bare right hand, the left hand can be worked into the left glove.

5. Once the left glove is in place, it is now a sterile surface. The first two or three fingers of the gloved left hand are now slipped down inside the sterile side of the cuff of the right glove, starting at the palm of the right glove and pointing toward the crease of the cuff at the wrist.

6. The right glove is then lifted using the fingers inside the cuff only. The thumb of the gloved left hand cannot be used to grasp the right hand glove. As the right glove is held by the first two or three fingers on the inside (sterile side) of the cuff, the right hand is worked into the right glove.

7. Once the right hand is gloved, the cuff can be unfolded by pulling the cuff up over the sleeve of the gown and letting the wrist portion of the glove snap into place.

(continued)

8. The fingers of the right hand, now sterile, can now be placed on the inside (sterile side) of the left glove cuff. The left cuff can be unfolded in the same manner as was done for the right glove. If necessary, the gloves can be adjusted on the fingers once both glove cuffs have been properly placed.

9. Once gloved, both hands must remain above waist level or the level of draping that defines the sterile field, whichever is appropriate.

Removal of Contaminated Gloves

When a glove becomes torn or punctured during a sterile procedure, it no longer provides proper protection. Such a glove must be removed and discarded as soon as is feasible, and another sterile glove donned. This may require interruption of a procedure provided that the interruption does not threaten the patient's welfare.

1. Contaminated gloves are removed in a manner that prevents the spread of contaminants. One hand grasps the cuff of the other glove.

2. The glove that has been grasped at the cuff is turned inside out as it is removed.

(continued)

3. The glove that has been removed is compacted into the palm of the hand that still is gloved.

4. The thumb of the ungloved hand is hooked inside the remaining glove and pulls the remaining glove toward the fingers, turning it inside out over the compacted glove.

5. Both gloves are removed with the contaminated sides inward. When removing gloves, the material should not be permitted to snap in order to avoid dislodging material that has accumulated on the gloves. The gloves must be disposed of in an appropriate container, and the hands washed.

WOUND DRESSINGS

The location of a wound can dictate the type of dressing applied or the method of application. Wounds over joints may require rigid dressings to prevent joint motion from disrupting the wound or the dressings may have to be applied in a way that accommodates joint motion. Wounds can require extensive modification of bedding and seating arrangements, so sleeping and sitting activities do not disrupt a dressing or put pressure on a wound.

Underlying pathologic conditions may have an impact on the dressings chosen and the application of dressings. No dressing should ever be applied in a manner that impedes circulation. The existence of peripheral vascular disease is a condition that requires special attention to avoid further impairment of circulation.

When long-term care of a wound is required, care may be provided outside an institutional setting. When non-institutional care is appropriate, a patient or patient's family must be instructed carefully in proper wound care. Whenever possible, simple procedures should be used. Careful evaluation and consideration must be given to the patient's, or family's, ability to understand and carry out specific instructions. A wound site that cannot be seen easily by the patient may not be well cared for by a patient. A physical impairment, such as a stroke, or mental impairment, such as Alzheimer's disease, may prohibit a patient from providing wound care. Supervision must be provided to ensure that proper techniques are followed.

PURPOSE

The purposes of wound dressings are to:

1. Protect physically the site of injury
2. Prevent contamination of a wound
3. Prevent transmission of infection from a wound
4. Promote healing

Many institutions and health care professionals have preferred methods of caring for specific types of wounds, and there is increasing evidence to support several methods. This section presents basic information concerning wound dressings. Information for a specific institution should be sought from the appropriate departments or practitioners within the institution.

EVALUATION

Documentation of wound characteristics is necessary for appropriate selection of dressing materials and protective agents, and for monitoring progress in wound healing. Evaluation of the wound is necessary to determine:

1. The cause of the wound
2. The location, area, and depth of the wound
3. Whether the wound is wet or dry
4. Whether the wound is infected; and if infected, the source, mechanism, and microorganism of infection

Measurement of a wound can be performed using a ruler (Figure 3–2). In addition to regular rulers, there are specialized clear plastic circular rulers. The ruler should not make contact with the wound itself, and should be limited to single patient use. Measurements should include width, length, and depth. Another method of documenting the extent of a wound is by photographing the wound.

FIGURE 3–2   Measuring a wound using a ruler.

TYPES OF DRESSINGS

Five methods of dressing applications generally used for wound management are:

1. Dry to dry
2. Damp to damp
3. Damp to dry
4. Occlusive
5. Rigid

A **dry-to-dry dressing** is the application of a dry absorbent or nonabsorbent dressing to cover the wound. A **damp-to-damp dressing** is the application of a gauze pad moistened with normal saline solution or other similar solution before application. Re-moistening a damp dressing is performed while the dressing remains in place. This prevents the dressing from drying out and becoming embedded in the eschar. The damp-to-damp dressing assists in softening the eschar in preparation for removal. A **damp-to-dry** dressing is the application of a moistened dressing that is allowed to dry before removal. The dressing dries embedded in the eschar, and debrides the wound when the dried, embedded dressing is removed. **Occlusive dressings** are applied to provide a semipermeable barrier to air and moisture penetration. **Rigid dressings** provide physical protection to a wound and the adjacent area.

Choice of materials for, and method of, application of dressings may depend on:

1. The cause of the wound
2. Whether the wound is clean or infected; and if infected, the microorganism causing the infection
3. The type of dressing (damp, dry)
4. The type, if any, of antimicrobial agent to be applied
5. The site, area, and depth of the wound
6. Whether a trained professional, the patient, or the patient's family will be responsible for monitoring and changing the dressing

Identification of the specific microorganism responsible for infection is beneficial in treating any wound. Specific antimicrobial agents may require specific types of dressing materials to ensure that the antimicrobial agent is applied properly to the wound.

When a wound is draining, absorption of exudate can be a consideration requiring a dry dressing. When a wound tends to be dry and the dryness impedes healing, a damp dressing would be required. Limiting exposure to air or maintaining a moist environment within the wound can require an occlusive dressing.

MATERIALS

The size of dressings, whether pre-packaged or constructed, should cover a wound site, plus some portion of healthy tissue on all sides of the wound. In no case should the adhesive portion of a dressing come in contact with a wound.

The most basic dressing is an adhesive strip with a small gauze center, commonly known by the brand name Band-Aid®. These dressings are available from a number of companies in various shapes and sizes. Topical antimicrobial agents may be applied under the gauze portion of this dressing. The adhesive portion of the dressing may be plastic or paper, with a hypoallergenic adhesive that limits skin reaction to the adhesive.

Dressings with non-adhering pads that do not stick to wounds or the exudate from wounds are also available. These dressings, commonly known by the brand name Telfa® pads, are available from a number of companies in various shapes and sizes. These basic dressings are usually best for small wounds, although self-made dressings of the same nature can be constructed in any size when the necessary material is available.

Gauze is the most common material used for dressings, and is available in pads and rolls. Sterile and non-sterile gauze is available in several sizes. If sterile gauze is to be used, proper aseptic handling techniques should be used during opening and application. Dressings constructed from gauze can be used with topical antimicrobial agents under the dressing when required.

Compression wraps are applied to control edema in a limb segment, or to provide some support for a joint. Compression wraps are constructed of an elastic material and are commonly known by the brand name Ace® wrap. Common sizes are 2, 3, 4, 5, and 6-inch widths.

Edges of lacerations can be approximated using thin adhesive strips, commonly known by the brand name Steri-Strips™. The edges of a wound are placed together, and the adhesive strips are placed across the wound. The number of strips required is determined by the open length of the wound.

Tape used to secure a dressing can be cloth adhesive tape or paper tape which has a hypoallergenic adhesive. Tape can be cut to the required length with scissors or torn from the roll. Tape is torn by unrolling the desired amount and firmly grasping the tape between the pad of the thumb and the side of the index finger of each hand, with the hands approximately 1 inch apart. Care should be taken not to roll the edges of the tape over because this makes the tape harder to tear. A quick movement of one hand away from the body and the other hand towards the body will cause the tape to tear between the two hands. Even cloth adhesive tape can be torn in this manner as long as the edges have not been rolled.

PREPARATION

Necessary supplies, such as gauze pads, roll gauze, tape, and topical agents, must be easily accessible during the procedure. Sterile fields, when required, must be prepared appropriately. Protection of the wound from contamination requires the appropriate application of aseptic techniques. Proper preparation for personnel includes handwashing or scrubbing, and masking, gowning, and gloving, when required.

Tape for securing dressings may need to be prepared before starting the application of a dressing because tearing or cutting tape usually takes two hands. The pieces can be hung from the edge of a table, cabinet, or bed frame by sticking only a small portion of one end to the object and letting the remainder of the piece hang free. The pieces should be hung in an accessible place since one hand is usually required to secure the dressing or wrap while tape is applied. When tape is applied circumferentially on a limb segment, the ends should not overlap. Adhesive and paper tape do not have enough elasticity to avoid impairment of circulation if the ends overlap in this situation.

PROCEDURE 3–3

APPLICATION OF DRESSINGS AND WRAPS

Packing a Wound

1. Depending on the depth of a wound, the wound may be packed with gauze, may be required to ensure that deeper layers of a wound heal before surface layers, avoiding development of an unhealed cavity.

2. Once packed, the wound and packing are covered with additional dressing that is secured with tape.

Applying a Gauze Wrap

Gauze pads are secured by tape or a gauze roll. Gauze rolls are applied in a spiral wrap, or in a "figure-of-eight" wrap. To avoid impairing circulation, the amount of pressure applied when using gauze wraps should not be excessive.

1. To apply a **gauze wrap,** lay the portion of the gauze roll that is unwrapping against the limb segment, with the still-rolled gauze away from the limb.

(continued)

2. A **spiral wrap** is applied by wrapping gauze in a continuous manner around the limb segment. The roll of gauze is angled slightly to accommodate for the sloping contour of the limb segment to be wrapped, and to avoid creating a tourniquet. The roll of gauze is unrolled around the limb segment, with each successive wrap overlapping the previous wrap by half. When the wrap is completed, the gauze is secured by tape.

3. Removal of a gauze wrap secured with tape requires careful cutting to avoid injuring patients. Bandage scissors, scissors having one flat arm, are used. The flat arm slides under the wrap and next to the skin, permitting the wrap and tape to be cut without cutting the skin.

Applying a Compression Wrap

Compression wraps may be applied in spiral or figure-of-eight wraps. When applying compression wraps to control edema, a spiral wrap is used, with more pressure applied distally than proximally. This provides for compression on edematous segments without constricting the flow of fluid towards the core of the body for subsequent elimination. When controlling edema, the entire limb segment distal to the proximal edge of the wrap must be covered by the wrap with approximately graded pressure. When applying compression wraps for joint support, a figure-of-eight or spiral wrap may be used. When providing support, a compression wrap is applied with even pressure from distal to proximal. Applying a compression wrap for support does not require the entire limb segment distal to the proximal edge of the wrap to be covered. In no case should a wrap be applied with the proximal pressure greater than the distal pressure.

The technique for applying a compression wrap is the same as for applying a gauze wrap. Frequent examination of compression wraps is necessary to ensure that the amount of compression applied is appropriate and that the wrap remains in place.

A **figure-of-eight wrap** is started in the same manner as a spiral wrap. Rather than a continuous wrap in the same direction, however, the direction of wrapping changes each time the wrap completes one loop of the figure-of-eight. The illustrations for this section demonstrate application of a compression wrap of the ankle.

1. Start with a circumferential anchoring loop around the foot.

2. Wrap from lateral to medial around the ankle.

3. Wrap from lateral to medial around the foot.

(continued)

4. Wrap from lateral to medial around the ankle (second time) with an angle that will permit continuing a spiral wrap up the ankle from distal to proximal. Secure the end of the compression wrap with adhesive tape.

REVIEW QUESTIONS

1. Which federal agency is responsible for developing and issuing guidelines for aseptic techniques and isolation systems?

2. Describe the eight guidelines for providing and maintaining a sterile field.

3. What apparel is necessary for aseptic techniques?

4. What is the most important procedure for preventing transmission of nosocomial infections?

5. List and describe the steps performed during:

   a. Gowning
   b. Gloving
   c. Removal of contaminated gloves

6. List the four purposes of wound dressing.

7. Describe five methods of dressing applications.

8. List five factors affecting selection of wound dressing materials.

9. What are the five main routes of microorganism transmission?

10. Who is responsible for implementing and monitoring isolation procedures?

11. What is the usual level of infection control practiced for contact with all patients?

12. What is the difference between Standard Precautions and Transmission-Based Precautions?

SUGGESTED ACTIVITIES

1. Practice the skills of handwashing, gowning, gloving, wound assessment, and application of wound dressings.

2. Observe other students performing wound dressings using a sterile field and make note of any violation of the guidelines for maintaining a sterile field.

3. Role-play wound assessment and application of dressings.

4. Document wound dressing procedures, including the appropriate portions of a SOAP note.

REFERENCES

1. Department of Health and Human Services. *Part I: Evolution of Isolation Practices.* Centers for Disease Control and Prevention, Hospital Infection Control Practices Advisory Committee, 1997.
2. Schulster L, Chinn RYW. *Guidelines for Environmental Infection Control in Health Care Facilities.* Recommendations of the Centers for Disease Control and Prevention, Healthcare Infection Control Practices Advisory Committee, 2003.
3. Department of Health and Human Services. *Part II: Recommendations for Isolation Precautions in Hospitals.* Centers for Disease Control and Prevention, Hospital Infection Control Practices Advisory Committee, 1997.
4. Boyce JM, Pittet D. *Guideline for Hand Hygiene in Health Care Settings.* Recommendations of the Centers for Disease Control and Prevention, Healthcare Infection Control Practices Advisory Committee and the HICPAC/SHEA/APIC/IDSA Hand Hygiene Task Force, 2002.

4

VITAL SIGNS

LEARNING OBJECTIVES

Upon completion of this chapter, you will be able to:

1. Describe the purposes, methods, and norms for the measurement of vital signs of pulse, blood pressure, respiration, and temperature.
2. Describe the purposes and methods for the subjective measurement of pain levels perceived by a patient.
3. Indicate the sites at which these measurements are usually taken.
4. Correctly and accurately measure pulse, blood pressure, respiration, and temperature.
5. Correctly and accurately measure patient pain levels.
6. Use terms that correctly describe vital sign measurements outside normal ranges.
7. Use terms that correctly describe pain.
8. Identify vital sign measurements that are below, within, or above normal ranges.
9. Correctly and accurately document vital sign measurements.
10. Correctly and accurately document pain measurements.

MEDIALINK

A companion CD-ROM, included free with each new copy of this book, supplements the techniques presented in the book. Insert the CD-ROM to watch video clips of patient care skills being demonstrated. This multimedia feature is designed to help you add a new dimension to your learning.

KEY TERMS

Afebrile	Hyperthermia	Stridor
Auscultation	Hypothermia	Systolic pressure
Basal heart rate	Maximal heart rate	Tachycardia
Blanching	Pain	Target heart rate
Blood pressure	Patency	Temperature
Bradycardia	Pulse	Trophic
Diastolic pressure	Regularity	Visual analog scale
Doppler	Respiratory rate	
Febrile	Resting heart rate	

INTRODUCTION

All personnel providing health care, including physical therapists and physical therapist assistants, should be aware of, and able to perform, objective measurements of physiological functions known as vital signs. Vital signs are used to monitor a patient's status prior to, and at any given time, during patient care. Changes in vital sign measurements indicate physiological responses to treatment. Vital signs consist of heart rate (HR), or pulse (P); blood pressure (BP); respiration (R); and temperature (T).

Although not considered a vital sign, indications of pain levels perceived by a patient are usually measured when vital signs are measured. Pain levels indicated by patients are subjective measurements.

HEART RATE

PURPOSE

Pulse (in beats per minute) is a measurement of heart rate. **Basal heart rate** is the pulse rate measured after an extended period of rest and is one indication of cardiovascular function in the absence of physical stress.

Pulse rate can also be measured before, during, or following an imposed physiological or physical stress arising from physical therapy intervention. Determination of when pulse rate is measured during physical therapy interventions is contingent upon a patient's condition. When measured during rest, pulse rate is called the **resting heart rate**, a measurement of heart rate without imposed stresses. When measured during physical therapy intervention, pulse rate is one measurement of the cardiovascular system's capacity to provide blood flow during imposed physiological or physical stress. When measured after treatment or other exercise, pulse rate is one measure of the cardiovascular system's recovery capability following the imposition of physiological or physical stress.

Measurements of pulse are also used to determine **patency**, which is the openness of the peripheral portion of the cardiovascular system. When used for this purpose, the important measurement is the presence or absence of a pulse at a chosen site. Such measurements of pulse can provide a preliminary indication of arterial occlusion resulting from physical blockage or peripheral vascular insufficiency secondary to disease states, such as diabetes. A lack of patency noted by a physical therapist or physical therapist assistant fits with a known medical diagnosis for a specific patient; the physical therapist will be aware of precautions and contraindications that may affect interventions. This lack of patency must be accurately documented and precautions and contraindications must be reviewed with the physical therapist assistant if interventions are delegated. When a lack of patency is noted that does not fit with a known medical diagnosis for the specific patient, this is a "red flag" that the physical therapist must document and refer immediately to an appropriate health care provider. When such a condition is noted by a physical therapist assistant, the supervising physical therapist and other appropriate health care providers must be notified immediately. Physical therapy interventions should not be implemented with such patients until the medical condition is evaluated and cleared by medical personnel.

Examination for patency of peripheral vessels should be accompanied by observation for **trophic** changes, which are physiological sequelae to decreased circulation, such as loss of hair, dry or flaky skin, and muscle atrophy. Skin temperature changes are often noted in areas of decreased patency. The presence of edema makes the determination of patency difficult. **Blanching** is a noted loss of color of the skin resulting from decreased circulation. Blanching of an extremity is more pronounced and occurs more rapidly when the extremity has decreased circulation. Blanching may be produced by two methods. One method is to raise the extremity above the level of the heart, artificially increasing the difficulty of supplying circulation to the extremity. A second method is to press firmly and briefly on a patient's skin to occlude circulation in the area of pressure. The rate of capillary refill indicates circulatory status in that area.

In addition to patency and rate, pulse regularity and amplitude can provide information concerning cardiovascular status. Measuring pulse rate allows examination of the regularity of the heart beat. **Regularity** refers to the evenness of heart rate. Unless an electrocardiogram (ECG or EKG) is performed, this measure of regularity is subjective. Amplitude of a pulse is rated on a subjective scale of 0–4+. This scale includes the measures of:

0 = absent
1+ = thready, weak
2+ = normal
3+ = strong
4+ = full bounding

A pulse that varies in rate, regularity, or amplitude from normal ranges may be indicative of disease or injury.

METHODS

The most common clinical method of measuring pulse is manual palpation. In addition to manual measures of pulse, there are mechanical devices that may be used. **Auscultation** of the heart, which is monitoring of the heart using a stethoscope, is also used to obtain heart rate. **Doppler** measurements, which use frequency changes during blood flow, are used to examine patency (Figure 4–1).

A pulse oximeter is a device that measures pulse rate and blood oxygen concentrations (Figure 4–2). Results are provided on a digital display. This is an easy method of monitoring pulse rate during activities.

To palpate a pulse manually, the pads of an index and middle finger of one hand are placed over the site where the pulse is to be measured. The pad of the thumb should not be used for palpation when measuring pulse because there is a pulse in the pad of the thumb. If a thumb is used for palpation, one's own pulse may be mistaken for the patient's pulse. Care must be taken not to press too hard while palpating a pulse. Excessive pressure during palpation can obliterate the pulse, impede blood flow, or cause arterial spasm. Obliterating a pulse prevents measurement, and impeding blood flow or causing arterial spasm can be dangerous to a patient. This is especially true when examining distal pulses, which are most commonly palpated when measuring peripheral vascular patency.

FIGURE 4–1 Doppler sonography.

FIGURE 4–2 Pulse oximeter.

Heart rate is measured in beats per minute (bpm). The use of units is advocated to ensure conveying complete information. To obtain a heart rate, a watch or clock that displays time in seconds is used. Once the pulse is palpated, beats are counted within a specified interval of time. The most accurate method is to count beats for a period of 60 seconds. The count is reported without additional calculation.

Alternative methods require less time to monitor the pulse, but require additional calculation. Counting beats for a 10-second time period and multiplying by six, or using a 15-second time period and multiplying by four, are the most common short-cuts used. Using a shorter sampling period may result in a measurement that is less precise. Many times, a whole number of beats does not occur within a shorter period of time. An estimate of a fractional heart rate is not as accurate as an exact count. Irregularities in heart rate are not detected as readily when a shorter sampling period is used. The necessity of additional calculation provides a potential source of error. Sometimes one beat in a time period is missed. In either of these cases, using a shortcut will increase the error, either six-fold or four-fold, respectively.

As an example, an error of one beat during measurements taken over a 60-second period of time and over a 10-second period will provide two very different results. For a patient with an actual heart rate of 72 bpm, missing one beat during the 60-second count produces an error of 1/72 or 1.4%. Using a 10-second count, the same heart rate should yield 12 beats. If one beat is missed during the 10-second count, only 11 beats will be counted. This is multiplied by six, resulting in a calculation of 66 bpm for the same patient, an error of 6/72, or 8.3%. Although shortcut methods are used routinely, and their results are recorded without question, care must be taken to provide an accurate and valid measurement.

There are two methods of timing when counting heart rate. The key factor in counting heart rate is that the number of heart beats within a given time period is counted. The first, or traditional, method starts the time period of counting at a specific time on a clock or watch, and the first heart beat felt after the time period has started is considered beat 1. This is beat 1 because it is the first heart beat within the specified time period. The second method starts the time period of counting when a heart beat is felt and is beat 0. This is beat 0 because it does not occur within the specified time period, but marks the beginning of the specified time period. Whichever method is used will provide an accurate count when attention is paid to the basis for when the interval begins and the number of counts that fall *within* the specified interval.

PROCEDURE 4-1

MEASURING HEART RATE

The radial and carotid arteries are the most commonly used sites for measuring heart rate.

The radial pulse is most easily palpated on the distal volar surface of the wrist just lateral to the tendons of the finger flexors.

The carotid pulse is most easily palpated on the lateral aspect of the neck, just inferior to the angle of the mandible.

Care must be taken to palpate the carotid pulse without reaching across the throat. Palpating the carotid pulse on the side of the neck opposite to where the physical therapist is standing results in the physical therapist placing his or her hand across the patient's throat, providing the potential for compromising the patient's airway. Baroreceptor reflexes produce decreased heart rate and strength of contraction. "Massage" to the carotid artery can elicit this reflex, so care must be taken to be accurate in the placement and type of palpation when measuring a carotid artery pulse.

The site used to obtain a pulse via auscultation is medial to the midclavicular line at the level of the fifth intercostal space.

Common sites for palpation of pulses for determining vacular patency are the brachial, popliteal, posterior tibial, and dorsal pedal pulses. These pulses are usually assessed as present or absent.

(continued)

The pulse in the brachial artery is palpated on the medial aspect of the arm midway down the shaft of the humerus.

The pulse in the femoral artery is palpated in the femoral triangle. Although usually a strong (3+) pulse, the femoral artery lies close to several large muscles, making palpation difficult. Explaining what you are about to do reduces the risk of embarrassing the patient. Palpation that is too firm may cause pain.

Location of the remaining arteries, and avoiding obliteration of the pulse with excessive pressure, can be difficult, even in healthy patients. These pulses are commonly susceptible to degradation of strength in patients with peripheral vascular insufficiency.

The pulse of the popliteal artery is palpated at or just above the knee on the posterior aspect of the leg.

The pulse of the posterior tibial artery is palpated posterior or inferior to the medial malleolus.

The dorsal pedal pulse is palpated on the dorsum of the foot over the cuboid bones.

NORMS

The normal range of heart rate for adults is 60–100 bpm. Resting heart rate in adults can vary greatly, depending on the state of physical conditioning of each individual. Individuals who maintain a high level of physical training may have a resting heart rate between 40 and 60 bpm. Individuals who maintain a moderately sedentary lifestyle may have a resting heart rate between 60 and 85 bpm. A resting heart rate greater than 85 bpm is usually indicative of a state of deconditioning or a medical condition. The normal resting heart rate for infants and young children is between 80 and 100 bpm. A very slow resting heart rate, or **bradycardia**, is a heart rate of less than 60 bpm. A very fast heart rate, or **tachycardia**, is a heart rate greater than 100 bpm. Bradycardia or tachycardia at a resting state may be indicative of disease or side effects of medication. Table 4–1 presents the usual ranges of resting heart rate.

Maximal heart rate is the highest heart rate a person should achieve upon maximal exertion with respect to age and medical condition. The following guidelines for determining maximal heart rate are based on the absence of cardiovascular pathology. Maximal heart rates are calculated for each individual patient based on age. A method of determining maximal heart rate, which does not take into consideration individual patient characteristics, such as weight or cardiovascular or pulmonary disease, is calculated by subtracting the patient's age from 220. For a 43-year-old individual, the maximal heart rate is: 220–43 = 177.

Target heart rate is the heart rate that an individual should achieve during exercise for cardiovascular conditioning with respect to age and medical condition. For a patient without contra-indications, the target heart rate must fall between 60% and 80% of the maximal heart rate. Thus, the formula used to determine a target heart rate for cardiovascular exercise for the 43-year-old person presented earlier is between 106 and 142 bpm.

$(0.60) \times (220\text{–}AGE)$ and $(0.80) \times (220\text{–}AGE)$

$(0.6)(220\text{–}43)$ and $(0.8)(220\text{–}43)$

$(0.6)(177)$ and $(0.8)(177)$

$= 106$ and 142

The target heart rate for a patient with cardiovascular pathology is adjusted by a physician based on clinical findings for the individual patient.

TABLE 4–1	Usual Ranges of Resting Heart Rate
Adult normal range	60–100 bpm
Infant/child normal range	80–100 bpm
Bradycardia	Less than 60 bpm
Tachycardia	Greater than 100 bpm

BLOOD PRESSURE

PURPOSE

Blood pressure is a measure of vascular resistance to blood flow. The primary purposes for measuring blood pressure are to determine vascular resistance to blood flow and the effectiveness of cardiac muscle in pumping blood to overcome vascular resistance. There are two values reported as a measurement of blood pressure. The first value represents **systolic pressure**, which is a measurement of pressure exerted by blood against arterial walls when the heart is contracting. The second value

FIGURE 4–3   Examples of sphygmomanometers.

represents **diastolic pressure**, which is a measure of the pressure exerted by arterial walls against blood when the heart is not contracting.

METHOD

Measurement of blood pressure is performed by auscultation of an artery using a stethoscope while a sphygmomanometer is applied over the artery being auscultated. A sphygmomanometer consists of an air bladder inside a cuff, a device for inflating the bladder, and a device for measuring the pressure in the bladder (Figure 4–3). Blood pressure measurements are actually measurements of the cuff's air bladder pressure. The pressure corresponds to arterial pressure as arterial blood flows, or attempts to flow, past the restrictive cuff.

Blood pressure measurements were originally based on the pressure required to raise a column of mercury in a glass tube. Therefore, blood pressure measurements are stated in millimeters of mercury (mmHg). To avoid potential exposure to mercury, air pressure gauges or electronic devices are now commonly used for measuring blood pressure, but blood pressure measurements continue to be reported in mmHg. Should a mercury sphygmomanometer be used, care must be taken to avoid breaking the glass tube that contains the mercury and to prevent the mercury column from separating. Sphygomomanometers may provide output using a mechanical guage or a digital readout. A stethoscope is used to auscultate the sounds of arterial blood flow through the brachial artery as it passes through the antecubital fossa.

Blood pressure sounds to be monitored are called Korotkoff sounds. Blood pressure readings are reported as the systolic pressure over the diastolic pressure. A systolic pressure of 120 mmHg and a diastolic pressure of 80 mmHg is documented as 120/80 mmHg and verbally reported as "120 over 80." Blood pressure is usually measured in the left arm. Initially, physical therapists should take blood pressure measurements in both arms and subsequently take blood pressure measurements in the arm with the highest reading. Documentation should include the arm in which the measurement was taken.

PROCEDURE 4-2

MEASURING BLOOD PRESSURE

1. Prior to placing the cuff around a patient's left upper arm, the size of the cuff must be considered. Inaccurate readings will be obtained if the wrong size cuff is used. Cuff sizes range from pediatric to large adult. The bladder of a cuff should cover approximately 80% of the circumference of the upper arm and the width should be approximately 40% of the circumference of the upper arm.[1]

2. The blood pressure cuff is placed snugly around the upper arm with the bladder centered over the anterior surface and with the lower border approximately 2–3 cm above the antecubital fossa.
3. The patient's arm is supported, either on a table or by resting on the physical therapist's arm, so the cuff is at the patient's heart level.
4. The inflation bulb and its attaching tube, and the stethoscope and its tubing, must be held so that the tubes do not touch each other. When the respective tubes touch each other, sounds can be distorted.
5. When the patient's arm is supported, the physical therapist locates the brachial artery on the anterior medial surface of the elbow as the artery crosses the antecubital fossa.
6. The pulse is palpated as the bladder is inflated. Note the pressure when the pulse can no longer be palpated.
7. The cuff is deflated.
8. Place the stethoscope drum or bell over the artery and inflate the cuff to about 30 mmHg greater than that noted when the pulse could no longer be palpated. When the cuff is inflated beyond the systolic blood pressure, the artery is totally occluded. Therefore, no sounds of blood flow emanate from the artery.

(continued)

9. Air is evacuated from the cuff by opening the pressure relief valve slowly. The sounds to be monitored are called Korotkoff sounds.

10. As the pressure in the cuff falls to the level of the systolic pressure, blood flows through the artery during systole (contraction phase), but not during diastole (non-contraction phase). The sounds heard through the stethoscope at this cuff pressure are usually described as tapping sounds. Initially, the tapping sound may be difficult to hear as the sounds may be faint or soft and may not occur evenly. As cuff pressure falls, the tapping sounds become more distinct and clear. The tapping nature of the sound is the result of the start of blood flow during systole and the stopping of blood flow during diastole. This occurs because at this level of cuff pressure, arterial flow can only occur during systole. When the first tapping sounds are heard, a pressure reading is noted and represents the value of systolic blood pressure.

11. As more air is evacuated from the cuff, pressure falls toward the diastolic level. When the cuff pressure is at the diastolic pressure level the distinct and clear tapping becomes muffled, and usually disappears after an additional drop of 5 to 10 mmHg. The muffling of sounds occurs because at this level of cuff pressure, blood flows through the brachial artery during both systole and diastole. When the tapping sounds become muffled, the pressure reading is noted. This reading represents the value of diastolic pressure.

12. At this time, the pressure in the cuff can be evacuated rapidly by opening the pressure relief valve completely.

13. The stethoscope and cuff can then be removed from the patient.

Throughout this procedure, care must be taken not to maintain pressure on the artery for more than 2 or 3 minutes without relief. If cuff occlusion occurs for more than 2–3 minutes without relief, the patient may experience symptoms of tingling or numbness, such as when an arm or leg "falls asleep."

SITE

The most common site for measuring blood pressure is the left upper arm. This site corresponds closely to the level of the tricuspid valve of the heart, which is considered the "reference level for pressure measurement." Although body position may change blood pressure, such changes are accurately measured when using the upper arm as the reference.

NORMS

As a reference point for blood pressure, 120/80 mmHg has been considered ideal. New guidelines emphasize a range rather than set numbers. Table 4–2 presents ranges of normal and abnormal blood pressures for an adult.[2] Blood pressure will change with stress, physical activity, and age. Lower levels are considered to indicate the existence of hypotension. Clinical judgments or clinical decision making based on the values presented in Table 4–2 must also include consideration of age and medical status and should take into account all available data concerning patient status. Clinical decision making with respect to the impact of medical status on physical therapy intervention is in the realm of the physical therapist.

TABLE 4–2	Blood Pressure Ranges for Adults	
	Systolic (mmHg)	**Diastolic (mmHg)**
Normal	Less than 120	Less than 80
Prehypertension	120–139	80–89
Stage 1 hypertension	140–159	90–99
Stage 2 hypertension	At or greater than 160	At or greater than 100

Changes from resting blood pressure can result as patients change position or increase activity. Failure of systolic pressure to rise in proportion with increased intensity of activity is a "red flag." A decrease in systolic pressure greater than 10 mm Hg, or a systolic pressure greater than 240 mmHg, indicates a "red flag." An increase greater than 20 mmHg for diastolic pressure during activity also indicates a "red flag." A "red flag" in each of these cases indicates a need to stop activity and examine the patient's cardiac status.

RESPIRATION

PURPOSE

Respiratory rate is the rate of breathing. Each respiratory cycle includes one inspiration and the subsequent expiration. Respiratory rate can be measured and the quality of respiration can be observed.

METHODS

Methods of measuring respiratory rate use auscultation and observation, which may be visual, auditory, or palpation. Unobtrusive visual and auditory observations can be made just prior to, or just after, taking a pulse. In situations where shallow or quiet breathing patterns make visual or auditory observation difficult, auscultation with a stethoscope may improve auditory observation.

Respiratory rate (RR) is measured as the number of breathing cycles per minute. To measure respiratory rate, a watch or clock that displays time in seconds is used. Respiratory cycles are counted for a set period of time. Only complete respiratory cycles, those consisting of both complete inspiratory and expiratory phases, are counted. Measurements may be over a 60-second time period or shorter time periods may be used. The same problems of accuracy noted previously for determining heart rate when using shortcut methods also apply to measurements of respiratory rate. Respiration is measured as cycles per minute but is reported without the use of units. A respiration rate of 12 respirations per minute is reported as 12 RR.

Duration of inspiratory and expiratory phases can also be measured. Depth of inspiration, regularity of inspiration, and use of accessory muscles of respiration can be observed as indicators of the quality of respiration. These measurements are more subjective than rate. Information concerning depth, regularity, and use of accessory muscles should be documented with specific measurements of respiratory rate.

PROCEDURE 4-3

MEASURING RESPIRATORY RATE

Palpation of a patient's thorax will allow a physical therapist to feel the rise and fall of the chest during respiration.

An alternative method of palpation is for a physical therapist to place the dorsum of one hand close to, but not touching or occluding, the patient's mouth and nose. Changes in the direction of air flow during respiration can be felt as slight pressure and temperature changes on the dorsal surface of the hand.

NORMS

Normal resting respiratory rate for adults is approximately 12 breaths per minute. Children normally have a respiratory rate of approximately 20 breaths per minute. The ratio of inspiration time to expiration time within one complete respiratory cycle (I/E ratio) is normally 1 to 2. Resting breathing rates of less than 10 breaths per minute or greater than 20 breaths per minute are considered abnormal. Chronic obstructive lung disease (COPD) may increase the I/E ratio.

A normal breathing pattern should be even, relatively quiet, and have a slight pause between the end of expiration and the initiation of inspiration. Only a very low-level hiss of air movement through the nose or mouth should be evident. Small variations may be noted, depending upon an individual's level of physical training and state of anxiety.

Following periods of exercise, or during respiratory distress, respiration may increase to 40 to 50 breaths per minute for short periods of time. With increased respiratory rates breathing will be more shallow and accessory muscles of respiration around the neck and shoulder region will more likely be involved in breathing patterns. When a patient is in respiratory distress, increased sounds of respiration, termed **stridor**, may be evident.

TEMPERATURE

PURPOSE

Body temperature provides information concerning basal metabolic state, potential presence of infection, and metabolic response to exercise. Physical therapists do not routinely measure a patient's body temperature, but do need to know the methods and norms. Skin temperature provides information concerning circulatory status, potential peripheral nerve injury, and local inflammatory responses. Physical therapists frequently measure skin temperature for these reasons.

METHODS

A variety of devices are available for measuring a patient's temperature (Figure 4–4). Thermometers were originally constructed of a graduated glass tube with a bulb at one end to hold a small quantity of mercury. Increases in temperature cause mercury to expand, and decreases in temperature cause mercury to contract. The degree of expansion or contraction is indicative of specific temperatures. A minimum of three minutes is necessary for a stable reading on a mercury thermometer. After extracting a thermometer from the measurement site, the measurement at the highest level of mercury should be read and recorded as the temperature. Because of the toxic effects of mercury, mercury thermometers should not be used.

Electronic thermometers with disposable probes or probe covers take less time to measure temperature, and have supplanted glass thermometers in many instances. Electronic thermometers are generally used to measure oral temperatures. A tympanic thermometer is used to measure temperature at the ear. Electronic thermometers produce a reading of the temperature, and often make a sound when the maximum temperature is attained. Digital displays of temperature readings will hold the value of the highest temperature until an instrument is reset.

Measurements can be made on the forehead using heat sensitive strips that indicate a temperature range rather than a specific degree. When used on the extremities such strips can also be used to indicate adequacy of peripheral circulation.

When mercury thermometers were used, inspection of the thermometer prior to each use was required to ensure that the mercury in the thermometer had not separated, the mercury in the thermometer had been shaken down to a point below the expected temperature, and the glass that comprised the thermometer was not cracked, split, or chipped, presenting a danger of cuts or mercury leakage.

Reusable thermometers must be cleansed and sterilized between uses. When probes are used, a new probe cover must be used with each patient.

In all situations, patients should remain quiet during the time temperature is being measured. Close supervision of young children and patients with decreased cognition is necessary for safety and to obtain accurate measurements. Temperature measurements may be recorded in degrees Fahrenheit or degrees Celsius and documentation must indicate which temperature scale was used.

SITES

Oral temperature measurements are most commonly used for measurement of body temperature. Traditionally, oral and rectal temperatures are considered the most accurate measures of body temperature. Axillary and tympanic temperature measurements are used primarily for children or when a patient has a medical complication that prevents easy and safe access to the mouth or rectum.

FIGURE 4–4 Examples of devices for measuring temperature.

Oral temperature is taken by placing a thermometer probe under the tongue. The tip of the thermometer probe should be placed as far back as is comfortable for the patient. Probe covers must be changed for each patient.

Palpation of skin temperature is performed using the dorsal surface of the hand. The physical therapist places the dorsum of the hand lightly on the site to be examined and moves the hand slowly from distal to proximal, noting temperature changes throughout the movement. Comparison of one extremity to another, such as left arm to right arm, may provide information concerning differences in temperature.

NORMS

The normal range of body temperature is centered at 98.6°F or 37°C. An individual's temperature will fluctuate throughout a 24-hour period, but these fluctuations should not be more than a few degrees. Depending upon time of day, site of measurement, and level of activity, normal body temperatures vary within general ranges. Therapeutic treatments of heat and cold will cause variations of local site temperatures of several degrees Fahrenheit. Table 4–3 presents temperature ranges for various situations.

Patients with a normal body temperature of 98.6°F are considered to be **afebrile** when oral temperature remains below 100°F (37.8°C). When oral temperature in these patients exceeds 100°F, they are considered to be **febrile. Hyperthermia** is defined as a rectal temperature greater than 106°F (41.1°C). **Hypothermia** is defined as a rectal temperature less than 94°F (34.4°C).

PAIN

Pain is a subjective perception described by patients and thus is difficult to measure. Perceptions of pain are unique to each individual and may depend upon previous experiences, type of injury or disease (laceration, crush, burn, migraine headaches, arthritis, etc.), body part affected, age, time since onset, and ethnic background. There may also be situations in which pain is expressed when an injury or disease does not truly present pain. It is difficult for a physical therapist to determine if malingering is present.

PURPOSE

The purposes of measuring perceptions of pain are to determine (a) diagnosis, (b) prognosis, (c) appropriate interventions, and (d) responses to interventions. Measurements of perceptions of pain that assist in diagnosis seek to determine type of pain (burning, tingling, sharp, dull, etc.), location (specific joint or limb), extent of painful location, intensity, duration, and frequency.

TABLE 4–3	Temperature Ranges for Different Activities				
	Oral			**Rectal**	
Situation	**°F**	**°C**		**°F**	**°C**
Usual normal range	98.6 to 99.5	36.0 to 37.5		96.8 to 99.7	36.0 to 37.6
Morning/Cold weather	95.0 to 96.8	35.0 to 36.0		95.9 to 97.0	35.3 to 36.1
Hard work/Emotion/ A few normal adults/ Many active children	99.7 to 101.0	37.6 to 38.3		99.7 to 101.5	37.6 to 38.6
Hard exercise*				101.2 to 104.0	38.4 to 40.0

*Cannot be measured accurately orally.

METHOD

The most commonly used method of measuring pain is an adaptation of a visual analog scale. A **visual analog scale** is a straight horizontal line with 0 at the left side and 10 at the right side. The left side, 0, represents a complete absence of pain. The right side, 10, represents the worst pain a patient can imagine. Patients are asked to mark on the horizontal line the point that corresponds with their perception of their current pain. The common adaptation of the visual analog scale is that patients are not asked to mark an actual scale, but are asked to provide a number between 0 and 10 that represents where they rank their current perception of pain.

Young children can have difficulty with the concept of ranking pain perceptions. Often a series of faces, from very happy to very unhappy, is used. Children are asked to select the face that represents their perception of pain. This is analogous to selecting a number that represents a perception of pain.

Physical therapists and patients often use body diagrams to document pain. Each site of pain is marked and types of pain are noted by different markings. Intensity may be noted by different colors.

Discussion of more extensive and sophisticated pain scales is beyond the scope of this text.

SITE

Pain may occur in many sites. Every site in which pain is perceived should be documented, including type, intensity, duration, and frequency.

NORMS

Although not universally used, ranges of pain may be listed. One range of pain scoring lists 0 as non existent, 1–3 as minimal, 4–6 as moderate, and 7–10 as severe.

REVIEW QUESTIONS

1. Define pulse rate and list the common sites at which pulse rates are measured.

2. What are the purposes for determining pulse rates and quality of pulses?

3. What are the normal and abnormal ranges of heart rate?

4. Describe how to determine a target heart rate.

5. Define respiratory rate and list the common methods for measuring respiratory rate.

6. What are the normal and abnormal ranges of respiratory rate?

7. Define blood pressure and list the usual site at which blood pressure is measured.

8. What are the normal and abnormal ranges for blood pressure?

9. Define body temperature and list the common sites at which body temperature is measured.

10. What are the normal and abnormal ranges of body temperature?

11. What are the units used when documenting heart rate, respiratory rate, blood pressure, and temperature?

12. What are commonly used methods for measuring pain?

SUGGESTED ACTIVITIES

1. Demonstrate the proper methods to measure pulse, patency, respiratory rate, blood pressure, and temperature.

2. Practice measuring vital signs of classmates in the proper position of sitting or lying quietly.

3. Document results from Activity 2 as the results would be included in the Objective section of a SOAP note.

4. Compare results from Activity 2 to norms to determine if the values obtained are in the normal range.

5. Practice assessing vital signs of classmates before, during, and after activities such as riding a stationary bike, running on a treadmill, or lifting weights.

6. Document results from Activity 5 as the results would be included in the Objective section of a SOAP note.

7. Compare results from Activity 5 to norms to determine if the values obtained are in the normal range.

CASE STUDY

Mr. Stovall is a 47-year-old construction worker. Four days ago he fell from the roof framing of a two-story house currently under construction. His fall was through the unfinished floor/ceiling framing to the first floor, landing on a pile of used lumber with nails. Upon admission to the hospital, Mr. Stovall was diagnosed with two fractured ribs on his right side, a fractured left radius, puncture wounds to his right chest and forearm, a dislocated right shoulder, and a Grade 2 concussion.

A referral for physical therapy services has been forwarded to the Physical Therapy Department.

1. For your first visit, what vital signs would you measure and record?

2. What methods and sites would you use to perform the measurements?

3. What method of measurement of pain perception would you use?

REFERENCES

1. Bickley LS. *Bates' Guide to Physical Examination and History Taking,* 8th ed. Philadelphia: Lippincott Williams & Wilkins, Philadelphia, 2003.
2. National Heart, Lung, and Blood Pressure Institute. *The Seventh Report of the Joint National Committee on Prevention, Detection, Evaluation, and Treatment of High Blood Pressure* (JNC 7), nhlbi.nih.gov/guidelines/hypertension/index.htm.

5

TURNING AND POSITIONING

LEARNING OBJECTIVES

Upon completion of this chapter, you will be able to describe:

1. Goals of proper positioning.
2. How to determine the amount of time a patient can spend in a position.
3. General procedures used to turn and position a patient properly.
4. Specific procedures used to turn a patient to, and to position in, supine, prone, sidelying, and sitting.

KEY TERMS

Long sitting
Orthostatic hypotension
Prone

Sidelying
Supine

INTRODUCTION

Proper positioning is a valuable tool to maintain patient function. Physical therapists and physical therapist assistants often work with other health care professionals to determine the most optimal position(s) for patients. Physical therapists and physical therapist assistants are responsible for positioning patients properly for physical therapy interventions and for function within a patient's environment. For patients who are unable to change position independently, proper positioning is essential for increasing function and preventing complications.

GOALS

The goals of proper positioning are to:

1. Ensure patient comfort.
2. Maintain integumentary integrity by preventing development of pressure sores.
3. Maintain musculoskeletal integrity by preventing deformities.
4. Maintain neuromuscular integrity by preventing pressure on peripheral nerves.

5. Maintain cardiovascular/pulmonary integrity by using changes in position to assist secretion elimination, breathing patterns, and vascular flow.
6. Provide patient access to the environment.
7. Provide proper positioning for specific interventions.

To achieve these goals, patients and environments must be managed properly. Proper positioning includes moving patients into, and out of, desired positions in a safe and effective manner. All health care providers who have contact with a patient have a responsibility to maintain appropriate patient positioning.

TIME IN POSITIONS

The first time a patient is placed in a new position, the patient's skin, particularly over bony protuberances that are pressure sites, should be examined after five to ten minutes and frequently thereafter. Observation over time allows for determination of tolerance for the position. A general rule is initially to reposition a patient at least every two hours to maintain integrity of all four movement systems (integumentary, musculoskeletal, neuromuscular, cardiovascular/pulmonary). Repositioning in less than two hours, even during an initial observation period, may be required for patients who have additional problems, such as poor circulation, fragile skin, decreased sensation, easily compromised peripheral nerves, difficulty breathing or excreting secretions, or inability to move. Establishment of the positioning schedule is the responsibility of a physical therapist, in conjunction with nursing personnel. All health care providers, including physical therapist assistants, have a responsibility to observe and document changes that may require modification of a positioning schedule.

When a patient is repositioned, skin over the area on which the patient was lying should be inspected and observed for color and integrity. Special attention should be paid to areas of skin that cover bony protuberances, such as the greater trochanter or sacrum. Redness of skin should be permitted to resolve before pressure is again placed on that area of skin. When recovery from pressure is delayed, patients should be repositioned more frequently. Excessive or prolonged redness may indicate the occurrence of tissue damage.

When sitting, a patient must relieve pressure in the buttocks and sacrum at least every ten minutes. Sitting push ups, using the arm rests of a chair, leaning first to one side and then to the other, and leaning forward are methods to relieve pressure on the buttocks in the sitting position. Specialized wheelchairs such as tilt-in-space and reclining back are used to relieve pressure areas.

Prolonged periods in one position will affect musculoskeletal structures. Loss of ROM, compromised joint nutrition, decreased joint stress, and loss of strength will occur if changes in position are not required. Loss of ROM may occur in two directions, with tissue (muscle, tendon, ligamentous capsule) shortening on one side and lengthening on the other side of a joint. Musculoskeletal structures respond positively to appropriate stresses of movement. Decreased movement eliminates these stresses and contributes to tissue degeneration and compromised function, such as bone demineralization, loss of sarcomeres, and degeneration of cartilage.

Neuromuscular tissue may be affected by prolonged periods in one position. As with skin, pressure on peripheral nerves will interfere with function. Pain, decreased sensation, and loss of ROM may result. Decreased sensation contributes to integumentary problems discussed previously. Loss of range of motion affects neuromuscular tissue as well as musculoskeletal tissue.

Circulation may be reduced by prolonged periods in one position. Decreased blood flow resulting from pressure on vascular structures may exacerbate integumentary problems, cause pain, and decrease nutrition to all tissues distal to compression. **Orthostatic hypotension,** the inability of the cardiovascular system to adapt to upright postures after prolonged horizontal positioning, can be avoided if changes in position include an upright position in the positioning schedule. Breathing is also easier in an upright position. Moving between a variety of positions aids in a patient's capability to excrete lung secretions.

PROCEDURE 5-1

PREPARING THE ENVIRONMENT

Preparing the environment assists in safe and effective turning and positioning. Preparing the environment means having a clear area for movement and having all necessary supplies, including sheets, pillows, and towels, available within easy reach. A sufficient number of appropriately trained personnel must be available. Following the general procedures reduces the risk of harm to the integumentary, musculoskeltal, neuromuscular, and cardiovascular/pulmonary systems.

1. *Smooth all under sheets, towels, and patient clothing.* Wrinkles in the sheets, blankets, and personal clothing must be avoided because they increase pressure on a small area of skin and cause skin irritation. Such pressure points are uncomfortable for a patient who is unable to move independently.

2. *Pillows, rolled blankets, or towels are used to support body parts and to avoid strain or pressure on ligaments, nerves, and muscles. A sufficient quantity of these items must be available before beginning positioning for safe and efficient positioning.* Pillows or towels are used to provide relief to bony protuberances or areas most susceptible to skin breakdown. Sometimes a sensitive area must be relieved of all pressure but the patient must still be placed in the position. Supporting the body segment just proximal and just distal to, but not under, a sensitive area relieves pressure on the sensitive area. This type of positioning, shown in the photo below, is termed "bridging the gap." To "bridge the gap," pillows or towels are placed close to the involved area, preventing contact of the involved area with the supporting surface. When an area is "bridged," the time in the position should be reduced because pressure may increase at the site of the pillows or towels, thereby compromising circulation.

3. *Ensure that enough clear area exists and equipment is ready for moving patients safely.* A clear area allows all personnel involved in moving and positioning a patient sufficient space to move without impediment, and without bumping into walls, chairs, and other equipment. Beds, gurneys, wheelchairs, and other movable equipment must be locked or secured prior to initiating moving a patient.

(continued)

4. *Ensure that sufficient personnel trained in moving and positioning patients are present.* When turning and positioning patients, patients must be lifted, rather than dragged, across the sheets. Dragging may result in skin irritation, referred to as sheet burn.

5. *Draping should allow appropriate positioning, while maintaining patient modesty and warmth.* Sheets or blankets are used for draping or covering the patient. When covers are tightly tucked at the foot of the bed the ankle is forced into a position of plantar flexion. This should be avoided to reduce the risk of developing contractures.

6. *Whenever possible, patients should participate actively during moving and positioning.* For simple procedures, explanations and directions should be given before initiation of a procedure. Commands are given throughout the procedure. For procedures with many steps, a general explanation is given prior to the start of a procedure. Commands are given prior to each step of the procedure. Additional directions are given as needed. Providing directions and commands as a complex procedure progresses assists patients who may not be able to remember all steps for an entire procedure while concentrating on the first few steps.

Descriptions of turning and positioning procedures presented in this chapter are given as if the patient is unable to assist or is able to assist only minimally. Illustrations in this chapter demonstrate a patient on a treatment table or mat. The same procedures are used when turning or positioning a patient in bed.

SUPINE POSITION

A **supine** position is one in which a person lies on his or her back on a supporting surface. In the supine position, a patient is positioned with shoulders parallel to hips and a straight spine. Many people require a small pillow to support the head for comfort. A pillow can be placed under the knees to relieve strain on the lower back (Figure 5–1). Positioning with a pillow under the knees, however, can lead to decreased hip and knee extension range of motion as a result of prolonged positioning in hip and knee flexion. A pillow placed lengthwise under the legs will reduce knee flexion and relieve pressure on the heels (Figure 5–2).

FIGURE 5–1   Supine position with arm support and a pillow placed crosswise under the knees.

FIGURE 5–2   Supine position with a pillow placed lengthwise under the legs.

PROCEDURE 5-2

TURNING FROM SUPINE TO PRONE

The patient's initial position is supine. The patient is first moved far enough to one side of the treatment table to allow a full turning movement to the prone position without coming too near the opposite edge upon completion of the turning movement. To turn to the left, a patient is first moved to the right side of the treatment table. When segmental movement of the trunk and lower extremities is possible, the patient is moved in stages. When the patient cannot tolerate such movement, more than one person, or specialized beds, will be needed.

To turn a patient from supine to prone, the following steps occur in sequence.

1. Move the upper trunk and head.

2. Move the lower trunk.

3. Move the lower extremities.

(continued)

4. The right lower extremity is crossed over the left lower extremity, with the right ankle resting on top of the left ankle. The patient's left upper extremity is adducted, placing the hand under the left hip, palm against the hip. This positioning of the extremities applies when a patient is being turned to the left, as presented in these figures. In situations where turning is to the right, the positioning movements must be mirror images of these positions.

5. The physical therapist or physical therapist assistant is positioned on the side to which the patient is being turned. When a treatment table is narrow, personnel assisting in turning the patient should stand next to the patient on the side from which the patient is being turned, to prevent the patient from falling while the physical therapist moves from one side of the treatment table to the other. Personnel assisting in turning the patient can help with positioning of pillows and turning the patient.

When a pillow will be under the patient while the patient is in the prone position, position the pillow in the proper orientation before the patient is rolled. The right upper extremity is adducted, placing the hand at the right hip, palm against the hip.

6. When patients have head and neck control, they can assist in turning their head and neck in the direction of the roll as turning is initiated. When patients do not have head and neck control, physical therapists must be aware that a patient's face may be subject to some rubbing on the mattress or mat during turning. When physical therapists are ready to begin the turning movement, they should ask the patient and any assisting personnel if they are ready. Upon receiving an affirmative reply, a preparatory count is given, followed by a specific verbal command as turning is initiated.

    As turning is initiated, the physical therapist's hands are on the patient's back.

7. When a patient reaches the halfway point, gravity can complete the movement, but will do so in an uncontrolled manner. Physical therapists must therefore rotate and reposition their hands as patients reach the midpoint of the turn. The hands are repositioned to the anterior surface of the patient to control the second half of the turning movement.

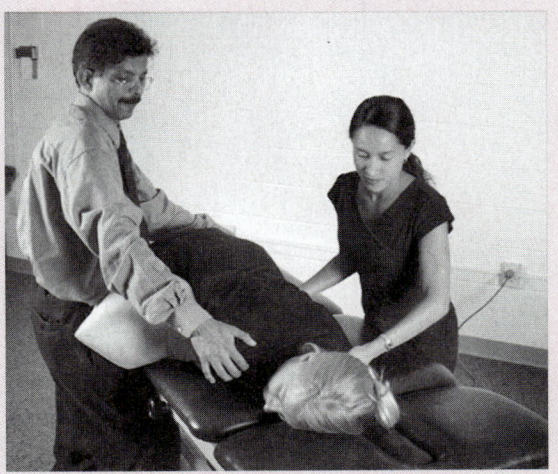

(continued)

8. When a turn is completed, a patient's head and neck are the first body segments to be repositioned. A patient's head is placed in a comfortable position facing the side that will allow best interaction with others and the environment. Positioning the head turned to one side eliminates pressure on the eyes, nose, or mouth, but may increase pressure on the external ear. A small towel may be placed under the temple to relieve pressure on the external ear. In some situations the head may be maintained in the midline, using a small pillow or towel under the forehead to relieve pressure on the eyes, nose, and mouth, and to permit unimpeded respiration.

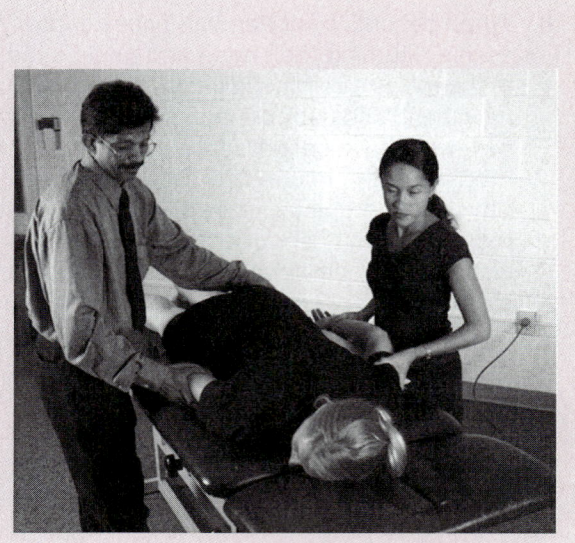

Position of the pillow under the trunk is adjusted as needed. The arms are placed in a position of slight abduction. Finally, the feet are uncrossed if they remained crossed after the turning movement was completed. The lower extremities should be positioned so the feet are approximately six to eight inches apart.

PRONE POSITION

A **prone** position is a position in which a person lies on his or her stomach on a supporting surface. In a prone position, patients are positioned with shoulders parallel to hips and with a straight spine. The head may be turned to either side, or maintained in the midline, as described in the previous section. A patient's upper extremities may be positioned alongside the trunk or alongside the head. For some patients, circulation in the upper extremities may be impaired when they are placed alongside the head. Upper extremities should be positioned alongside the head only when a patient has sensation in the upper extremities and can communicate reliably if a problem arises. When a patient's upper extremities are positioned alongside the head, the physical therapist or physical therapist assistant should question the patient frequently to determine if the patient is experiencing numbness or tingling.

A pillow may be placed lengthwise or crosswise under the trunk to ensure that spinal curvature is not excessive at any segment. A lengthwise position may be more comfortable when patients have limited neck mobility. The lumbar region's lordotic curve is reduced by crosswise positioning of the pillow. Therefore, a crosswise position of a pillow may be more comfortable for patients with low back pain. Patients with tender or large breasts may also be more comfortable with the pillow in a crosswise position, distal to the breasts. A pillow under the lower legs can also be used to avoid positioning the ankles in plantar flexion (Figure 5–3). A patient's feet can be positioned over the end of a treatment table to avoid positioning the ankles in plantar flexion (Figure 5–4). A pillow under the lower legs places the knees in slight flexion, however, and may promote loss of knee extension ROM.

FIGURE 5–3   Prone position with pillows under the trunk and lower legs.

FIGURE 5–4   Prone position with a pillow under the trunk and feet positioned over the end of the treatment table.

PROCEDURE 5-3

TURNING FROM PRONE TO SUPINE

Turning a patient from prone to supine is similar to turning a patient from supine to prone. The patient's initial position is prone. The patient is first moved far enough to one side of the treatment table to allow a full turning movement to the prone position without coming too near the opposite edge upon completion of the turning movement. To turn to the right, a patient is first moved to the left side of the treatment table. When segmental movement of the trunk and lower extremities is possible, the patient is moved in stages. When the patient cannot tolerate such movement, more than one person, or specialized beds, will be needed.

To move a patient from prone to supine, the following steps occur in sequence.

1. Move the upper trunk and head.

2. Move the lower trunk.
3. Move the lower extremities.

4. The patient's hand is placed under the hip with the palm against the body.

5. The physical therapist or physical therapist assistant is again positioned on the side to which the patient is being turned. When a treatment table is narrow, personnel assisting in turning the patient should stand next to the patient on the side from which the patient is being turned to prevent the patient from falling as the physical therapist moves from one side of the treatment table to the other. Personnel assisting in turning the patient can help with positioning of pillows and turning the patient.

   When patients do not have head and neck control, rubbing of the face on the mattress or mat can be avoided by having the patient start by facing away from the physical therapist. Patients with head and neck control can assist by looking up and over their shoulder while being turned toward the physical therapist.

6. The left upper extremity is adducted, placing the hand at the hip, palm against the hip. The physical therapist supports the right upper extremity against the patient's body as the patient is turned.

7. As in turning from supine to prone, physical therapists must control both phases of the turning motion. Initially, physical therapists reach over the patient, placing their hands on the patient's anterior surface.

(continued)

8. When a patient reaches the halfway point, gravity can complete the movement, but will do so in an uncontrolled manner. Physical therapists must therefore rotate and reposition their hands as patients reach the midpoint of the turn. The hands are repositioned to the posterior surface of the patient to control the second half of the turning movement.

9. When a turn is completed, a patient's head and neck are the first body segments to be repositioned. The extremities are then positioned as in the supine position.

PROCEDURE 5-4

TURNING ON A FLOOR MAT

When turning a patient on a floor mat, the same steps and sequence are followed as when turning a patient on a treatment table. Proper body mechanics become more important in preventing injury to a physical therapist or physical therapist assistant when turning a patient on a floor mat.

To turn a patient on a floor mat, the following steps occur in sequence.

1. After a patient is moved to one side of the mat, the physical therapist or physical therapist assistant should be positioned on the side to which the patient will turn. The physical therapist should assume a half-kneeling position, with the "down" knee at the level of the patient's hips and the "up" knee at the level of the patient's shoulders.

2. Using the right hand, the physical therapist places the patient's left hand on the patient's left hip. The physical therapist's left hand is placed on the patient's right shoulder. The physical therapist's hand position must rotate and reposition at the midpoint of the turn, as described for turning on a treatment table.

3. The physical therapist must move out of the patient's way as the turn is completed, allowing the patient to complete the turn without rolling into the physical therapist.

SIDELYING

A **sidelying position** is a position in which a patient is lying on one side. The positions of the upper extremities and lower extremities will vary, depending upon whether the patient's upper trunk is rotated forward or backward while in a sidelying position.

In a sidelying position in which the patient's upper trunk is rotated forward (Figure 5–5), the lowermost upper extremity is slightly flexed at the shoulder so the patient is not lying on the humerus, the uppermost upper extremity is flexed at the shoulder and supported by a pillow, the lowermost lower extremity is relatively extended, and the uppermost lower extremity is flexed at the hip and knee and supported on pillows. The uppermost lower extremity should be support by enough pillows so that it is not lowered into adduction. To avoid excessive pressure on the lowermost lower extremity, the uppermost lower extremity should not lie directly on top of the lowermost lower extremity.

In a sidelying position in which the patient's upper trunk is rotated backward (Figure 5–6), the lowermost upper extremity shoulder girdle is protracted and the shoulder is slightly flexed so the patient is not lying on the humerus, the uppermost upper extremity is extended and supported by pillows behind the patient, the lowermost lower extremity is flexed at the hip and knee, and the uppermost lower extremity is relatively extended and supported on pillows. The uppermost lower extremity should be supported by enough pillows so that it is not lowered into adduction. To avoid excessive pressure on the lowermost lower extremity, the uppermost lower extremity should not lie directly on top of the lowermost lower extremity.

FIGURE 5–5 Sidelying position with upper trunk rotated forward.

FIGURE 5–6 Sidelying position with upper trunk rotated backward.

PROCEDURE 5–5

TURNING FROM SUPINE OR PRONE TO SIDELYING

A patient can be turned to a sidelying position from either the supine or prone positions. The steps in turning a patient from supine to sidelying are similar to those for turning a patient from supine to prone, with the movement stopping when the patient reaches the midpoint of the turn. The patient is then positioned in the chosen one of the two sidelying positions.

The steps in turning a patient from prone to sidelying are similar to those for turning a patient from prone to supine, with the movement stopping when the patient reaches the midpoint of the turn. The patient is then positioned in the chosen one of the two sidelying positions.

PROCEDURE 5–6

MOVING FROM SUPINE TO SITTING

There are various methods for a patient to assume a sitting position with assistance. The method chosen will depend upon a patient's functional abilities, medical problems, and starting position. Whichever method is chosen, patients should not be left unguarded in a sitting position if they cannot maintain the position independently in a safe manner.

Supine to Long Sitting

Long sitting is a position in which a person sits with hips flexed to 90 degrees and knees fully extended on a supporting surface. When patients have sufficient strength, they can assume a long sitting position by doing a sit-up from supine to sitting. To assist a patient in moving from supine to long sitting, the following steps occur in sequence.

1. When minimal assistance is needed, as for patients with generalized weakness, a trapeze bar can be used. In some situations patients can perform a sit-up or use a trapeze bar while a physical therapist or physical therapist assistant provides assistance. A physical therapist can place an arm behind a patient's back to assist the patient in changing position. When a trapeze bar is not available, a physical therapist can stabilize an arm in front of the patient in lieu of a trapeze bar.

(continued)

2. A patient can pull up by pulling on a physical thera-pist's arm. Physical therapists may assist the sit-up movement by placing an arm across a patient's thighs to stabilize the patient's lower extremities.

3. Physical therapists should not move the arm and do the patient's work of pulling up into a sitting position. As necessary, physical therapists should move toward the patient's feet to permit the patient to assume a long sitting position.

Sidelying to Sitting on Side of Table

To assist a patient in moving from sidelying to sitting, the following steps occur in sequence.

1. The patient assumes a sidelying position to the side of the treatment table on which the patient wishes to sit.

    Hips and knees are flexed 60 to 90 degrees and the lower legs are moved over the edge of the treatment table to act as counter-weight to the patient's trunk and upper extremities.

    The physical therapist assists the patient in assuming a sitting position by placing one arm under the patient's thighs to control the rate of lowering the patient's lower extremities and one arm under the patient's shoulder to assist in coming to sitting.

2. With the lower extremities acting as counterweights, the patient uses the upper extremities to push to sitting.

3. The physical therapist assists by controlling lowering of the patient's lower extremities and lifting the upper trunk as necessary.

Supine to Sitting on Side of Table

When patients are dependent upon higher levels of assistance, the physical therapist uses the lower extremities as counterweights and provide additional physical assistance. To move a patient from supine to sitting, the following steps occur in sequence.

1. Starting in supine position, the physical therapist places one arm around the upper trunk at the level of the patient's shoulders and the other arm under the patient's thighs.

2. The physical therapist simultaneously lifts the patient's trunk and lowers the patient's lower extremities over the side of the table.

3. The patient is lifted into a sitting position and pivoted to sitting over the side of the table.

REVIEW QUESTIONS

1. List the goals for proper positioning.

2. State the purposes of proper positioning for the four practice patterns: integumentary, musculoskeletal, neuromuscular, and cardiovascular/pulmonary.

3. Describe how physical therapists determine the proper time a patient can be in a position.

4. Describe how to position a patient properly in the supine, prone, and sidelying positions.

5. Describe how to turn a patient properly from supine to prone, supine to sidelying, sidelying to prone, sideling to supine, and prone to supine.

6. Describe how to assist a patient to sitting from supine.

SUGGESTED ACTIVITIES

1. Demonstrate to students the specific procedures presented.

2. Students should practice specific procedures working in groups of three, role-playing patient, therapist, and assistant.

3. Students should practice performing turning and positioning while other partners role-play diagnoses (see following case studies). The student role-playing the patient can add "character" to the role by employing behaviors such as being cooperative, noncooperative, in pain, hard of hearing, or faint. The "patient" must role-play the diagnosis and character consistently so the students must have researched the diagnosis, signs, and symptoms. The student role-playing the therapist should document the "intervention."

4. Students should monitor vital signs and check for signs of skin irritation as appropriate.

5. Students should practice teaching "family and patients" and other health care providers how to perform turning and positioning. Students should document the intervention.

CASE STUDIES

For the following case study situations, describe and/or demonstrate appropriate turning and positioning procedures. For each procedure or position chosen, provide an appropriate rationale.

1. The patient is a 59-year-old male with right hemiplegia who presents with mild spasticity in both right extremities and expressive aphasia.

2. The patient is a 21-year-old with T12 complete spinal cord injury.

3. The patient is a 12-year-old with moderate spastic cerebral palsy.

4. The patient is a 75-year-old with a fractured right hip status post hip replacement.

6

RANGE OF MOTION EXERCISE

LEARNING OBJECTIVES

Upon completion of this chapter, you will be able to:

1. Describe anatomical position.
2. Define the terms used to describe movements in the anatomical planes.
3. Distinguish between joint range of motion (ROM) and muscle ROM.
4. Indicate when passive ROM (PROM), active assisted ROM (AAROM), or active ROM (AROM) intervention is appropriate.
5. Describe different joint end feels.
6. Describe differences in movement when a patient has normal muscle tone, spasticity, rigidity, and pain.
7. Describe general methods used to perform ROM exercises properly.
8. Describe the benefits of using diagonal patterns of motion.
9. Describe the combining components of motion used in proprioceptive neuromuscular facilitation (PNF) patterns.
10. Describe the specific procedures used to perform ROM exercises in the anatomical planes and diagonal patterns of motion.

KEY TERMS

Abduction
Active assisted range of motion (AAROM)
Active range of motion (AROM)
Adduction
Anatomical planes of movement
Anatomical position
Biarticular
Combining components
Diagonal patterns of movement
End feel
Eversion

Extension
External (lateral) rotation
Flexion
Horizontal abduction
Horizontal adduction
Internal (medial) rotation
Inversion
Joint range of motion
Muscle range of motion
Opposition
Passive range of motion (PROM)
Pronation

Proprioceptive neuromuscular facilitation (PNF)
Protraction
Radial deviation
Range of motion (ROM)
Retraction
Rigidity
Spasticity
Supination
Ulnar deviation
Uniarticular

INTRODUCTION

Range of motion (ROM) is movement of each joint and muscle through its available arc of motion. ROM movements are included in plans of care as interventions to prevent development of contractures, muscle shortening, and tightness in capsules, ligaments, and tendons, all of which can limit mobility. ROM interventions also provide sensory stimulation beneficial to patients.

Joint ROM is moving a joint in all planes of motion appropriate for the specific joint. Limitations of joint ROM may result from bony structure of joint surfaces, internal derangement of joint structures, lack of length of soft tissue (capsule, cartilage, ligament, muscle, skin, tendon) surrounding the joint, or pain. Examples include decreased joint ROM resulting from deterioration of joint surfaces, meniscal tears, ligamentous scarring, or shortness of single joint (**uniarticular**) muscles.

Muscle ROM is lengthening a muscle through its available length for all appropriate joint motions. To lengthen a muscle, joints must be moved in the direction opposite to the shortening action of the specific muscle. This will affect both single joint (uniarticular) and multijoint (**biarticular**) muscles. When a joint is moved through all available ROM, muscle ROM for muscles that cross only that joint (uniarticular muscles) is also achieved. To lengthen muscles that cross more than one joint (biarticular muscles), all joints the biarticular muscles cross must be moved in a manner that achieves full elongation of the biarticular muscles as a final result. An example of decreased muscle ROM occurs when the biceps brachii muscle, a biarticular muscle that flexes the shoulder, flexes the elbow, and supinates the forearm, becomes shortened following prolonged immobilization. To lengthen the biceps brachii muscle to its greatest available length, the shoulder and elbow must be extended and the forearm pronated. These movements may occur simultaneously or in sequence, providing that the end result is having all joint movements at their greatest limit at the same time.

In certain circumstances, a goal of treatment is to allow biarticular muscles to become shortened (not able to be lengthened over all joints at once) to provide a more functional length. Biarticular muscles that cannot be lengthened completely over all joints at the same time will cause these muscles to shorten across one joint when lengthened completely across another joint. This functional use of shortening is called tenodesis action. An example of tenodesis producing function is when shortened long finger flexors cause grasp and release as the wrist is extended and flexed. Patients with quadriplegia use this tenodesis to hold and release utensils, such as a fork, toothbrush, or writing implement.

Physical therapists must differentiate between ROM exercises, which use only the available range of motion, and stretching exercises. Stretching exercises are designed to increase the available range of motion by having an effect on joint structure and soft tissue. Physical therapists determine the appropriate intervention, ROM or stretching. Physical therapist assistants may provide both interventions upon direction by physical therapists.

Joint and muscle range of motion exercises may be performed as passive range of motion (PROM), active assisted range of motion (AAROM), and active range of motion (AROM) exercises. **Passive range of motion** exercise is performed with the patient relaxed and a physical therapist moving the body segment without patient assistance.

Active assisted range of motion is performed by a physical therapist assisting a patient in performing movement. **Active range of motion** exercises are performed independently by a patient, although they may be supervised by a physical therapist to ensure correct performance. Table 6–1 indicates the different types of ROM exercises and the impairments patients may have for which specific types of range of motion exercises are indicated.

TABLE 6–1	Types of Range of Motion and Indications for Use
Type	**Use**
Passive	Paralysis, paresis, weakness, pain, increased muscle tone.
	When active assisted or active would cause excessive cardiopulmonary stress.
	When a patient lacks safe control of movement.
	Maintain joint and soft tissue mobility.
	Maintain joint and tissue nutrition.
	Increase kinesthetic awareness.
Active Assisted	Paresis, weakness, pain, cardiopulmonary problems, abnormal tone.
	Maintain joint and soft tissue mobility.
	Maintain joint and tissue nutrition.
	Increase kinesthetic awareness.
Active	Patient can move correctly without causing undo stress on any body system.
	Maintain joint and soft tissue mobility.
	Maintain joint and tissue nutrition.
	Increase kinesthetic awareness.

The limit of ROM is achieved when a body segment cannot be moved further because of restriction by joint structure or soft tissues, or patient reports of pain. When a limit of motion is reached, the quality of restriction felt by a physical therapist is described as "**end feel.**" End feel may occur based on a number of variables, including joint structure and soft tissue. Normal end feel may vary depending on the reason for nonpathological limitation of further motion. When further motion is limited by bone abutting bone, the end feel is hard and is called bony end feel. An example of a nonpathological bony end feel occurs when complete elbow extension is attained. At this point, movement is halted by contact between the olecranon process of the ulna and the olecranon fossa of the humerus. When further motion is limited by a soft tissue approximation, the end feel is soft. An example of nonpathological soft end feel occurs when elbow flexion is limited by forearm soft tissue approximating the muscle bulk of elbow flexors on the anterior surface of the upper arm. A firm end feel with minimal give is a result of a taut capsule or ligament. This is known as a capsular end feel. An example of nonpathological capsular end feel occurs when a nonpathological knee is stress-tested for varus (adduction) and valgus (abduction) strain. When further motion is limited by pain, there is no tissue limitation to motion and the end feel is described as an empty end feel.

Involuntary muscle contractions or pain can interfere with movement. Patients who have upper motor (central nervous system) lesions, or patients trying to avoid pain, may have involuntary muscle contractions. Muscle tone is altered in upper motor neuron lesions, presenting as spasticity or rigidity. **Spasticity** presents as increased resistance to movement, especially as the velocity of movement is increased. When spasticity is present, a point in the range of motion may be reached where further muscle lengthening is temporarily prevented. If force is maintained, a sudden reduction in tone may occur, and movement through the remaining range of motion is possible. This is referred to as the clasp-knife phenomenon. Spasticity usually occurs in antigravity muscles. **Rigidity** presents as resistance to passive movement that is not affected by movement velocity. Both antigravity and progravity muscles may present with rigidity. In the presence of spasticity or rigidity, slow maintained movement usually permits movement through the complete range of motion without eliciting interference.

METHODS

To assist physical therapists in maintaining proper posture and body mechanics during ROM exercises, a table or bed of appropriate height for the individual therapist should be used. Preparing a treatment area and the use of proper body mechanics is covered in Chapter 2.

Passive ROM exercises during rehabilitation are preferably performed by physical therapists twice each day. Additional exercise times during each day assisted by other personnel or family members can be quite useful. A frequently chosen number of repetitions for each movement is 10; however, fewer repetitions still provide benefits. When a patient can perform active-assisted or active ROM exercises, physical therapists again determine the frequency of treatment periods and the number of repetitions for each movement. Physical therapist assistants, other personnel, or family members may participate or oversee sessions when directed by a physical therapist.

ROM exercises are performed by moving the body segments through each **anatomical plane of motion** separately, or by combining components of motion. **Combining components** of motion occur when more than one plane of joint motion is performed simultaneously. **Diagonal patterns of movement** described by proprioceptive neuromuscular facilitation (PNF) are combining components of motion at one joint as well as all the joints of an extremity. **Proprioceptive neuromuscular facilitation** is a method of exercise that uses combining components of motion for the head/neck/trunk and the extremities and encompasses spiral-diagonal patterns of movement facilitated by proprioceptive inputs.

Physical therapists determine whether anatomical planes of movement or diagonal patterns of movement are used. Physical therapist assistants may provide both interventions upon direction by physical therapists. Anatomical planes of movement allow more specific isolation of joint motions and involved musculature. Full joint motion may be more easily accomplished using anatomical planes of movement, which does not usually occur when using diagonal patterns of movement. Using diagonal patterns of movement simulates functional joint movement more closely than anatomical planes of motion.

Gentle but secure manual contacts are used to provide support when performing range of motion exercises. Hand placement should allow movement of body segments through complete ROM and provide support of all joints with minimal hand repositioning. Velocity of movement should be slow to moderate. Joint ROM exercises should encompass all planes of motion available in a joint. Muscle ROM exercises must result in lengthening biarticular muscles across all joints crossed simultaneously. Even when using anatomical plane movements, multiple joints may be exercised simultaneously. Examples include combinations of hip and knee flexion with ankle dorsiflexion, and hip and knee extension with ankle plantar flexion.

ANATOMICAL PLANES OF MOVEMENT

All motions of the body are described in terms of starting from the anatomical position. The **anatomical position** is described as that position in which a person is standing upright, eyes looking straight ahead, arms at the sides with palms facing forward, and the feet approximately 4 inches apart at the heels with the toes pointing forward (Figures 6–1 and 6–2).

Three anatomical, or cardinal, planes are defined with respect to the anatomical position. The sagittal plane divides the body into two sides—left and right. The midsagittal plane divides the body exactly into left and right halves. Motions of flexion and extension occur in the sagittal plane. The frontal, or coronal, plane divides the body into front and back portions. Motions of abduction and adduction occur in the frontal plane. The only motions of flexion/extension and abduction/adduction that do not occur in their respective planes of motion are motions of the thumb. Thumb flexion and extension occurs in the frontal plane and thumb abduction and adduction occur in the sagittal plane. The transverse plane divides the body into upper and lower portions. All movements of rotation, and horizontal abduction and adduction of the shoulders, occur in the transverse plane.

FIGURE 6–1   Anterior view of anatomical position.

FIGURE 6–2   Lateral view of anatomical position.

The following definitions assume the starting position is the anatomical position.

Flexion: Except for the thumb, flexion is movement in a sagittal plane. For the neck, trunk, upper extremities, and lower extremities except knee and toes, flexion results in approximation of anterior limb segment surfaces. For the knee and toes, flexion results in approximation of the posterior and planter limb segment surfaces respectively. Dorsiflexion, moving the foot and toes upward, is the movement of the ankle considered flexion. Thumb flexion is approximation of the palmer limb segment surfaces and occurs in the frontal plane.

Extension: Except for the thumb, extension is movement in the sagittal plane. For the neck, trunk, upper extremities, and lower extremities other than knee and toes, extension results in anterior limb segment surfaces moving away from each other. For the knee and toes, extension results in posterior and plantar limb segment surfaces moving away from each other, respectively. Plantar flexion, moving the foot and toes downward, is the movement of the ankle considered extension. Thumb extension is moving the palmer limb segment surfaces away from each other and occurs in the frontal plane.

Abduction: Except for the thumb, abduction is movement in the frontal plane and is the result of the limb segment surfaces moving away from the midline of the body. Thumb abduction is movement of the thumb away from the palm of the hand and occurs in the sagittal plane. When the wrist is moved such that the hand moves away from the midline of the body, the movement is labeled *radial deviation*.

Adduction: Except for the thumb, adduction is movement in the frontal plane and is the result of the limb segment surfaces moving toward the midline of the body. Thumb adduction is movement of the thumb into the palm of the hand and occurs in the sagittal plane. When the wrist is moved such that the hand moves toward the midline of the body, the movement is labeled *ulnar deviation*.

Horizontal Abduction: Horizontal abduction is movement of the upper extremity posteriorly when the shoulder has already been abducted to 90° in the frontal plane.

Horizontal Adduction: Horizontal adduction is movement of the upper extremity anteriorly when the shoulder has already been abducted to 90° in the frontal plane.

Protraction: Protraction is multiplanar movement of the scapula around the lateral aspect of the ribs toward the anterior aspect of the thorax. This motion is often termed scapular abduction.

Retraction: Retraction is multiplanar movement of the scapula around the lateral aspect of the ribs as the scapula moves toward the spine. This motion is often termed scapular adduction.

Opposition: Opposition is multiplanar movement of the carpo-metacarpal joint of the thumb that results in approximation of the tip of the thumb and the tip of a finger of the same hand. There is no term that describes the opposite motion.

Internal (medial) rotation: Internal rotation is movement in the transverse plane that results in anterior limb segment surfaces turning inward, toward the midline of the body.

External (lateral) rotation: External rotation is movement in the transverse plane that results in anterior limb segment surfaces turning outward, away from the midline of the body.

Supination: Supination is defined differently for the upper and lower extremities. For the upper extremity, supination of the forearm occurs when the arm is stabilized and the forearm is rotated so that the palm of the hand faces anteriorly. This is a uniplanar movement occurring in the transverse plane. Supination of the forearm is the position of the forearm in the anatomical position. For the lower extremity, supination of the foot occurs when the leg is stabilized and the foot is rotated about the oblique axis of the subtalar and other midfoot joints. This is a triplanar motion that incorporates plantar flexion, forefoot adduction, and inversion of the foot.

Pronation: Pronation is defined differently for the upper and lower extremities. For the upper extremity, pronation of the forearm occurs when the arm is stabilized and the forearm is rotated so that the palm of the hand faces posteriorly. This is a uniplanar movement occurring in the transverse plane. For the lower extremity, pronation of the foot occurs when the leg is stabilized and the foot is rotated about the oblique axis of the subtalar and other mid-foot joints. This is a triplanar motion that incorporates dorsiflexion, forefoot abduction, and eversion of the foot.

Inversion: Inversion is movement of the foot that occurs in the frontal plane about the long axis of the foot. Inversion occurs when the foot is rotated about the long axis of the foot such that the plantar surface of the foot faces toward the midline of the body.

Eversion: Eversion is movement of the foot that occurs in the frontal plane about the long axis of the foot. Eversion occurs when the foot is rotated about the long axis of the foot such that the plantar surface of the foot faces away from the midline of the body.

Confusion exists concerning the use of the terms supination/pronation and inversion/eversion when describing motion at the ankle and foot. The definitions provided earlier are those used by a majority of clinicians in practice. The clinical definitions are based upon the writing of Root and colleagues.[2] Using clinical definitions, supination and pronation are terms describing triplanar movements, of which inversion and eversion are uniplanar components. Anatomists,[3] however, describe these terms of ankle and foot motion in the opposite manner. Under the anatomical definitions, inversion and eversion are terms describing triplanar movement, of which supination and pronation are uniplanar components. In the text, these terms are used in accordance with the clinical definitions presented by Root and colleagues.[2]

DIAGONAL PATTERNS OF MOVEMENT

Two diagonal patterns of movement have been described for the upper and lower extremities.[1,4] Diagonal patterns of movement are achieved by simultaneously combining components of all three cardinal planes of motion and of multiple joints of an extremity. Figure 6–3 illustrates the difference between two successive cardinal planes of motions on the left and the simultaneous combining of three cardinal planes of motion into a diagonal pattern on the right.

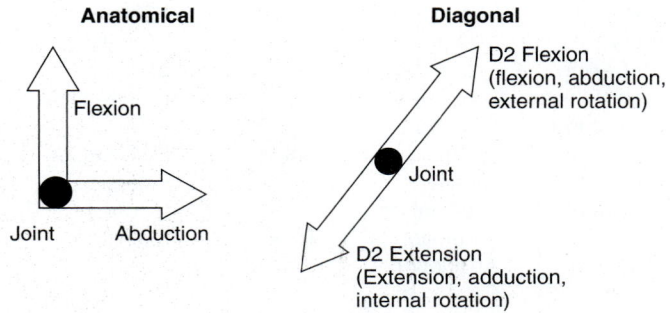

FIGURE 6–3 Anatomical vs. Diagonal Patterns of Movement

Specific diagonal patterns of motion are described by the combination of motions performed by either the shoulder or the hip joints (Figures 6–4 through 6–12). These patterns are modified by varying the position or movement of the elbow or knee, providing the ability to perform both joint ROM and muscle ROM exercises. The two diagonal patterns are commonly referred to as D1 and D2, where "D" stands for diagonal and "1" and "2" refer to specific diagonal patterns.

When combining components of motion are performed, joint movements and muscle lengthening may not occur through as much ROM as when anatomical planes of motion are performed. The mobility, however, that is necessary for function is maintained by use of diagonal patterns. Sensory feedback from movement in diagonal patterns is thought to be closer to the sensory feedback provided by normal active movement than movement in anatomical planes.

Table 6–2 lists the combining components of motion found in the proprioceptive neuromuscular facilitation patterns.

DIRECTIONS

Illustrations in this chapter present ROM performed as passive ROM exercises. Presented are the joint(s) for which the exercise is being performed, the movement, and hand placement of the physical therapist. Where appropriate, precautions have been noted. For procedures specifically involving multijoint muscles, we have listed the muscles involved. Listed are the movements required to *lengthen* muscles, *not* movements produced by the muscles.

The order of presentation will be lower extremity movement in anatomical planes, lower extremity movement in diagonal patterns, upper extremity movement in anatomical planes, upper extremity movement in diagonal patterns, and head/neck/trunk movements.

TABLE 6–2   Combining Components of Motion in PNF Diagonals

Diagonal 1 Upper Extremity			*Diagonal 1 Lower Extremity*		
Segment	**Flexion**	**Extension**	**Segment**	**Flexion**	**Extension**
Scapula	Elevation Abduction Upward rotation	Depression Adduction Downward rotation			
Shoulder	Flexion Adduction External rotation	Extension Abduction Internal rotation	Hip	Flexion Adduction External rotation	Extension Abduction Internal rotation
Elbow	Straight or flexion or extension	Straight or extension or flexion	Knee	Straight or flexion or extension	Straight or extension or flexion
Forearm	Supination	Pronaton			
Wrist	Flexion Radial deviation	Extension Ulnar deviation	Ankle	Dorsiflexion Inversion	Plantar flexion Eversion
Fingers	Flexion Adduction	Extension Abduction	Toes	Extension	Flexion
Thumb	Flexion	Extension			

Diagonal 2 Upper Extremity			*Diagonal 2 Lower Extremity*		
Segment	**Flexion**	**Extension**	**Segment**	**Flexion**	**Extension**
Scapula	Elevation Adduction Upward rotation	Depression Abduction Downward rotation			
Shoulder	Flexion Abduction External rotation	Extension Adduction Internal rotation	Hip	Flexion Abduction Internal rotation	Extension Adduction External rotation
Elbow	Straight or flexion or extension	Straight or extension or flexion	Knee	Straight or flexion or extension	Straight or extension or flexion
Forearm	Supination	Pronation			
Wrist	Extension Radial deviation	Flexion Ulnar deviation	Ankle	Dorsiflexion Eversion	Plantar flexion Inversion
Fingers	Extension Abduction	Flexion Adduction	Toes	Extension	Flexion
Thumb	Extension	Opposition			

FIGURE 6–4 Bilateral upper extremity D1 extension.

FIGURE 6–5 Bilateral upper extremity D1 flexion.

FIGURE 6–6 Bilateral upper extremity D2 extension.

FIGURE 6–7 Bilateral upper extremity D2 flexion.

FIGURE 6–8 Right lower extremity D1 extension with knee extension.

FIGURE 6–9 Right lower extremity D1 flexion with knee flexion.

FIGURE 6–10 Right lower extremity D1 flexion with knee extension.

FIGURE 6–11 Right lower extremity D2 extension with knee flexion.

FIGURE 6–12 Right lower extremity D2 flexion with knee extension.

PROCEDURE 6-1

LOWER EXTREMITY ROM EXERCISES: ANATOMICAL PLANES

Joints:	Hip and knee
Motion:	Extension and flexion
Position:	Supine
Hand Placement:	Heel and posterior knee
Precaution:	Hip motion is complete when pelvic rotation occurs. Anterior pelvic rotation with hip extension, posterior pelvic rotation with hip flexion. Pelvic rotation should not be allowed to occur as hip motion is performed.

Hip and knee extension.

Hip and knee flexion.

Joints:	Hip and knee
Muscles:	Semitendinosus, semimembranosus, biceps femoris
Motions:	Hip flexion with knee extension—Straight leg raise (SLR)
Position:	Supine
Hand Placement:	Heel and posterior knee
Note:	This maneuver lengthens the multijoint muscles of the posterior thigh across both joints at which they act.
Precautions:	The knee must be kept extended. The hip must not be allowed to rotate, adduct, or abduct. The pelvis must not be allowed to rotate posteriorly.

Starting position for straight leg raise (SLR).

Hip flexion with knee extended (SLR).

Joint:	Hip
Motion:	Extension
Position:	Sidelying
Alternative Position:	Prone
Hand Placement:	One hand is placed on the pelvis for stabilization. The other hand and forearm support the patient's lower extremity in the anatomical position.
Note:	The knee is maintained in extension.
Precautions:	The end of hip extension is achieved when the pelvis starts to rotate anteriorly.

Hip extension in sidelying position.

Hip extension in prone position.

Joint:	Hip
Motions:	Abduction and adduction
Position:	Supine
Hand Placement:	Heel and posterior knee
Note:	To perform adduction beyond neutral, the opposite lower extremity is abducted.
Precaution:	Hip flexion, hip rotation, and pelvic motion must be avoided.

Starting position for hip abduction.

End position for hip abduction.

Starting position for hip adduction.

End position for hip adduction.

Joint:	Hip
Muscle:	Tensor facia latae
Motions:	Extension and adduction
Position:	Sidelying
Hand Placement:	One hand stabilizes the pelvis. The other hand and forearm support the leg.
Note:	The tensor fascia latae flexes and abducts the hip and may assist in knee extension. Hip extension, adduction, and knee flexion lengthen this muscle.
Precaution:	Lateral pelvic motion must not be substituted for hip motion.

Starting position for tensor fascia latae lengthening.

End position for tensor fascia latae lengthening.

Joint: Hip
Motions: Internal and external rotation
Position: Sitting
Hand Placement: One hand stabilizes the femur. The other hand grasps the distal leg.

Starting position for hip internal rotation in sitting.

End position for hip internal rotation in sitting.

Starting position for hip external rotation in sitting.

End position for hip external rotation in sitting.

Joint:	Hip
Motions:	Internal and external rotation
Position:	Supine, with hip and knee flexed to 90°
Hand Placement:	Heel and anterior knee
Alternative Placement:	Heel and posterior thigh
Precautions:	Avoid excessive stress on the medial and lateral structures of the knee. Maintain the pelvis flat on the supporting surface.

Starting position for hip internal rotation in supine with hip flexion.

End position for hip internal rotation in supine with hip flexion.

Starting position for hip external rotation in supine with hip flexion.

End position for hip external rotation in supine with hip flexion.

Joint: Hip
Motions: Internal and external rotation
Position: Supine, with hip and knee extended
Hand Placement: Heel and posterior knee.
Precautions: Avoid excessive stress on the medial and lateral structures of the knee. Maintain the pelvis flat on the supporting surface.

Hip rotation in supine with hip extended.

Joint: Knee
Motion: Flexion
Position: Supine with hip flexed to 90°
Hand Placement: Heel and distal femur.

Mid position for knee flexion.

End position for knee flexion.

Joints:	Hip and knee
Muscle:	Rectus femoris
Motion:	Knee flexion with hip extended
Position:	Prone with hip extended
Alternative Position:	Supine with knee at the end of the table
Hand Placement:	One hand is on the posterior thigh or used to stabilize the pelvis. The other hand is on the distal tibia.
Precaution:	The rectus femoris is a hip flexor and knee extensor. Anterior pelvic rotation or hip flexion should not be allowed to occur.

Starting position for rectus femoris range of motion.

End position for rectus femoris range of motion.

Joint:	Ankle (talocrural)
Motion:	Plantar flexion
Position:	Supine
Hand Placement:	Heel and dorsum of foot
Note:	Motion should emphasize movement of the talocrural joint, not midfoot joints.
Precaution:	Force is applied to the heel in the superior direction and not to dorsum of foot.

Starting position for ankle plantar flexion.

End position for ankle plantar flexion.

Joint: Ankle (talocrural)
Motion: Dorsiflexion
Position: Supine with slight knee flexion
Hand Placement: Heel and posterior calf
Note: To move structures of the ankle joint and the one joint soleus muscle, the knee must be flexed such that the gastrocnemius muscle does not limit motion.
Precaution: Force is applied to the heel in the inferior direction, and not to the ball of the foot.

Ankle dorsiflexion.

Joint: Ankle (talocrural)
Muscle: Gastrocnemius
Position: Supine with knee extended
Hand Placement: Heel and leg
Note: To move the gastrocnemius muscle simultaneously across all joints over which it acts, the knee must be kept extended as the ankle is dorsiflexed.
Precaution: Force is applied to the heel in an inferior direction and not to ball of the foot.

Starting position for gastrocnemius range of motion.

End position for gastrocnemius range of motion.

Joint: Foot (intertarsal)
Motions: Inversion and eversion
Position: Supine
Hand Placement: One hand grasps the heel to stabilize the leg. The other hand grasps the forefoot.

Starting position for foot inversion.

End position for foot inversion.

Starting position for foot eversion.

End position for foot eversion.

Joints: Toes (metatarsophalangeal and interphalangeal)
Motions: Extension and flexion
Position: Supine
Hand Placement: One hand stabilizes the foot and leg. The other hand grasps
                     the toes.

Starting position for toe flexion.

End position for toe flexion.

Starting position for toe extension.

End position for toe extension.

PROCEDURE 6–2

LOWER EXTREMITY ROM EXERCISES: DIAGONAL PATTERNS

Pattern: PNF diagonal 1 (D1) extension with knee extended
                                      PNF diagonal 1 (D1) flexion with knee extended

Combining Components
of Motion:
　　D1 extension with knee extended
                                      Hip: extension, abduction, internal rotation
                                      Knee: extended
                                      Ankle and foot: planar flexion, eversion
　　D1 flexion with knee extended
                                      Hip: flexion, adduction, external rotation
                                      Knee: extended
                                      Ankle and foot: dorsiflexion, inversion

Position: Supine
Hand Placement: Heel and posterior thigh
Note: Knee extended (straight) indicates that the knee remains in
                                      complete extension throughout the movement of both pat-
                                      terns. In these patterns motion begins distally, and pro-
                                      gresses proximally, with the motions occuring more or less
                                      simultaneously.

D1 extension with knee extended.

D1 flexion with knee extended.

Pattern: PNF diagonal 1 (D1) extension with knee extension
    PNF diagonal 1 (D1) flexion with knee flexion

Combining Components
of Motion:
    D1 extension with knee extension
        Hip: extension, abduction, internal rotation
        Knee: extension
        Ankle and foot: plantar flexion, eversion
    D1 flexion with knee flexion
        Hip: flexion, adduction, external rotation
        Knee: flexion
        Ankle and foot: dorsiflexion, inversion

Position: Supine
Hand Placement: Heel and posterior thigh
Note: In these patterns motion begins distally, and progresses proximally, with the motions occurring more or less simultaneously.

D1 extension with knee extension.

D1 flexion with knee flexion.

Pattern: PNF diagonal 1 (D1) extension with knee flexion
                      PNF diagonal 1 (D1) flexion with knee extension
Combining Components
of Motion:
    D1 extension with knee flexion
                      Hip: extension, abduction, internal rotation
                      Knee: flexion
                      Ankle and foot: plantar flexion, eversion
    D1 flexion with knee extension
                      Hip: flexion, adduction, external rotation
                      Knee: extension
                      Ankle and foot: dorsiflexion, inversion
Position: Supine
Hand Placement: Heel and posterior thigh
Note: In these patterns motion begins distally, and progresses
                      proximally, with the motions occurring more or less simulta-
                      neously.

D1 extension with knee flexion.

D1 flexion with knee extension.

Pattern: PNF diagonal 2 (D2) extension with knee extended
PNF diagonal 2 (D2) flexion with knee extended

Combining Components
of Motion:

D2 extension with knee extended

Hip: extension, adduction, external rotation
Knee: extended
Ankle and foot: plantar flexion, inversion

D2 flexion with knee extended

Hip: flexion, abduction, internal rotation
Knee: extended
Ankle and foot: dorsiflexion, eversion

Position: Supine

Hand Placement: Heel and posterior thigh

Note: Knee extended indicates that the knee remains in complete extension throughout the movement of both patterns. In these patterns motion begins distally, and progresses proximally, with the motions occurring more or less simultaneously.

Precautions: When performing PNF D2 patterns, the physical therapist must step and move to allow a patient's leg to move through the pattern completely and correctly.

D2 extension with knee extended.

D2 flexion with knee extended.

Pattern: PNF diagonal 2 (D2) extension with knee extension
                                  PNF diagonal 2 (D2) flexion with knee flexion
Combining Components
of Motion:
     D2 extension with knee extension
                                  Hip: extension, adduction, external rotation
                                  Knee: extension
                                  Ankle and foot: plantar flexion, inversion
     D2 flexion with knee flexion
                                  Hip: flexion, abduction, internal rotation
                                  Knee: flexion
                                  Ankle and foot: dorsiflexion, eversion
Position: Supine
Hand Placement: Heel and posterior thigh
Note: In these patterns motion begins distally, and progresses
                                  proximally, with the motions occurring more or less
                                  simultaneously.

D2 extension with knee extension.

D2 flexion with knee flexion.

Pattern: PNF diagonal 2 (D2) extension with knee flexion
                              PNF diagonal 2 (D2) flexion with knee extension
Combining Components
of Motion:
    D2 extension with knee flexion
                              Hip: extension, adduction, external rotation
                              Knee: flexion
                              Ankle and foot: plantar flexion, inversion
    D2 flexion with knee extension
                              Hip: flexion, abduction, internal rotation
                              Knee: extension
                              Ankle and foot: dorsiflexion, eversion
Position: Supine, knee flexed over end of the table
Hand Placement: Heel and posterior thigh
Note: In these patterns motion begins distally, and progresses
                              proximally, with the motions occurring more or less simulta-
                              neously.

D2 extension with knee flexion.

D2 flexion with knee extension.

PROCEDURE 6-3

 UPPER EXTREMITY ROM EXERCISES: ANATOMICAL PLANES

Joint:	Shoulder girdle (scapulothoracic)
Motions:	Protraction (abduction) and retraction (adduction)
	Elevation and depression
	Upward and downward rotation
Position:	Sidelying
Hand Placement:	One hand is placed over the acromion process. The other hand is placed at the inferior angle of the scapula.
Note:	The hand placement for each of the three pairs of motion is the same. The only difference is the direction of force applied to the scapula.

Scapular protraction (abduction).

Scapular retraction (adduction).

Scapular elevation.

Scapular depression.

Scapular upward rotation.

Scapular downward rotation.

Joint:	Shoulder (glenohumeral)
Motion:	Flexion
Position:	Supine
Hand Placement:	One hand supports the arm. The other hand grasps the wrist and hand. Hand placement may need to shift as movement occurs through full flexion.
Precautions:	External rotation must be permitted to avoid impingement.

Beginning shoulder flexion.

Ending shoulder flexion.

Joint:	Shoulder (glenohumeral)
Motion:	Extension
Position:	Sidelying
Alternative position:	Prone
Hand Placement:	One hand supports the arm. The other hand supports the wrist and forearm.
Precaution:	When the end of the range of shoulder extension is reached, shoulder girdle motion will occur.

Beginning shoulder extension.

Ending shoulder extension.

Joint:	Shoulder (glenohumeral)
Motion:	Abduction
Position:	Supine
Hand Placement:	One hand supports the arm and stabilizes shoulder girdle. The other hand grasps the wrist and forearm.
Precautions:	Avoid shoulder flexion and internal rotation during shoulder abduction. External rotation must be permitted to avoid impingement. The physical therapist must move to allow movement through complete range of motion.

Beginning shoulder abduction.

Mid-point of shoulder abduction.

Ending shoulder abduction.

Joint:	Shoulder (glenohumeral)
Motion:	Horizontal adduction
Position:	Supine, shoulder abducted to 90°, and elbow flexed to 90°
Hand Placement:	One hand supports the arm. The other hand grasps the wrist and hand.

Mid-point of shoulder horizontal adduction.   Ending shoulder horizontal adduction.

Joint:	Shoulder (glenohumeral)
Motion:	Internal (medial) rotation
Position:	Supine, shoulder abducted to 90°, elbow flexed to 90°, and the forearm in pronation
Hand Placement:	One hand supports the arm. The other hand grasps the patient's wrist and forearm.
Precaution:	When the end of internal rotation ROM is reached, the shoulder girdle will start to move into protraction. This should not be allowed to occur.

 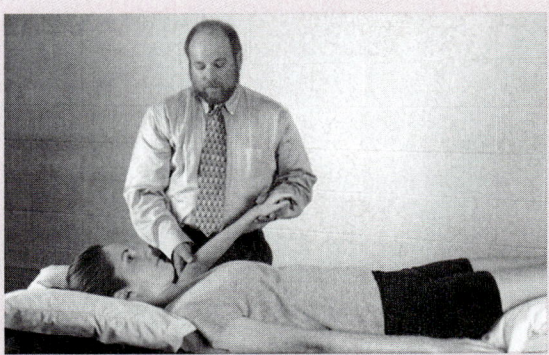

Starting position for shoulder internal rotation.   Shoulder internal rotation.

Joint:	Shoulder (glenohumeral)
Motion:	External (lateral) rotation
Position:	Supine, shoulder abducted to 90°, elbow flexed to 90°, and forearm pronated
Hand Placement:	One hand supports the arm. The other hand grasps the patient's wrist and hand.
Precaution:	When the end of the range of external rotation is reached, the shoulder girdle will start to move into retraction. The patient may also extend the trunk when motion is limited. This should not be allowed to occur.

Starting position for shoulder external rotation.

Shoulder external rotation.

Joints:	Shoulder (glenohumeral) and elbow
Muscle:	Triceps brachii
Motion:	Shoulder and elbow flexion
Position:	Supine
Hand Placement:	One hand supports the arm. The other hand grasps the patient's wrist and hand.
Note:	To move the triceps muscle across both joints over which it acts requires elbow flexion with the shoulder in flexion. This movement is achieved by first flexing the shoulder through its available ROM and then flexing the elbow through its available ROM while shoulder flexion is maintained.

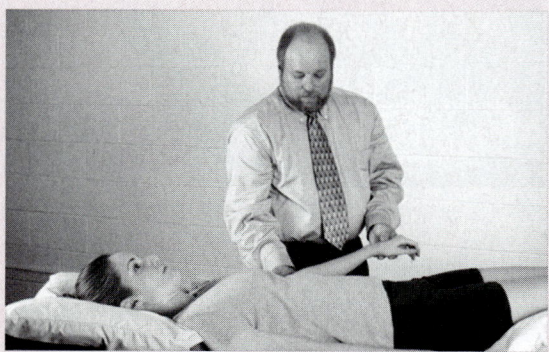

Starting position for shoulder flexion.

Shoulder flexion with elbow flexion.

Joint:	Elbow
Motions:	Flexion and extension
Position:	Supine, upper extremity in anatomical position
Hand Placement:	One hand supports the arm. The other hand grasps the patient's wrist and hand.
Note:	In this illustration, the shoulder is slightly flexed to allow visualization of the elbow.

Elbow extension.　　　　　　　　　　　　　　Elbow flexion.

Joints:	Forearm (radioulnar)
Motions:	Pronation and supination
Position:	Supine, elbow flexed to 90°
Alternative Position:	Sitting
Hand Placement:	One hand stabilizes the arm. The other hand grasps the distal forearm and supports the hand.
Precaution:	This motion occurs in the forearm. Do not apply the force through the wrist by grasping the hand instead of the forearm.

Forearm pronation.　　　　　　　　　　　　　Mid (neutral) position of forearm.

Forearm supination.

Joints: Wrist (radiocarpal and intercarpal)
Motions: Flexion and extension—finger motion is permitted
Position: Supine, elbow flexed, and fingers free to move
Alternative Position: Sitting
Hand Placement: One hand stabilizes the arm and forearm. The other hand grasps the patient's hand.

Wrist flexion.

Mid (neutral) position of wrist.

Wrist extension.

Joints:	Wrist (radiocarpal and intercarpal)
Motions:	Ulnar and radial deviation
Position:	Supine, elbow flexed, and forearm in mid-position
Alternative Position:	Sitting
Hand Placement:	One hand stabilizes the forearm. The other hand grasps the patient's hand.
Note:	The ROM for radial deviation is less than for ulnar deviation.
Precaution:	Avoid wrist flexion and extension, and forearm pronation and supination, while performing ulnar and radial deviation motions.

Ulnar deviation.

Mid (neutral) position of wrist.

Radial deviation.

Joints:	Fingers (metacarpophalangeal and interphalangeal)
Motions:	Flexion and extension
Position:	Supine, elbow flexed to 90°, and wrist in neutral position
Alternative Position:	Sitting
Hand Placement:	One hand stabilizes the forearm and wrist. The other hand grasps the fingers or an individual digit.
Note:	Digits may be moved through the ROM at all joints and in all directions as a group or individually.

Finger flexion.

Neutral position of metacarpophalangeal joints with interphalangeal joint extension.

Finger extension.

Joints:	Elbow, wrist (radiocarpal and intercarpal), and fingers (metacarpophalangeal and interphalangeal)
Muscles:	Flexor digitorum superficialis
	Flexor digitorum profundus
	Palmaris longus
	Extensor digitorum
	Extensor digiti minimi
	Extensor indicis
Motions:	Wrist flexion with finger extension
	Wrist extension with finger extension
	Wrist flexion with finger flexion
	Wrist extension with finger flexion
Position:	Supine, elbow extended, forearm supinated
Alternative Position:	Sitting
Hand Placement:	One hand stabilizes the forearm and wrist. The other hand grasps the hand and fingers.
Note:	These motions move (lengthen) multijoint muscles that cross the joints of the elbow, wrist, and fingers, to the fullest extent possible. Although these muscles cross the elbow joint, the full effect of muscle lengthening can usually be achieved without regard for elbow joint position.
Precaution:	Some patients should not have long finger flexors and extensors moved (lengthened) across all joints simultaneously to permit development of tenodesis action.

Wrist flexion with finger extension.

Wrist extension with finger extension.

Wrist flexion with finger flexion.

Wrist extension with finger flexion.

Joints:	Fingers (metacarpophalangeal)
Motions:	Abduction and adduction
Position:	Supine, elbow flexed to 90°, and wrist in neutral position
Alternative Position:	Sitting
Hand Placement:	One hand supports the hand and fingers and the other hand grasps the finger to be moved through the ROM.
Note:	The middle finger is the reference point for abduction and adduction. Movement of the middle finger in both directions is labeled abduction.

Starting position for finger abduction and adduction.

Finger abduction.

Joints:	Thumb (carpometacarpal) and fifth finger
Motion:	Opposition
Position:	Supine, elbow flexed to 90°, and wrist in anatomical position
Alternative Position:	Sitting
Hand Placement:	One hand grasps the thumb. The other hand grasps the fifth finger.
Note:	To preserve function of the hand, the arches of the hand must be maintained. Opposition of the thumb and fifth finger can contribute to maintaining the arches of the hand.

Beginning opposition.

Opposition of thumb to fifth finger.

Joint:	Thumb (carpometacarpal)
Motions:	Abduction and adduction
Position:	Supine, elbow flexed to 90°, wrist in neutral position, and the thumb extended
Alternative Position:	Sitting
Hand Placement:	One hand grasps the thumb. The other hand grasps the patient's hand.
Note:	Maintaining the "web space" is vital for a functional hand.

Thumb abduction.

Thumb adduction.

Joint:	Thumb (carpometacarpal and metacarpophalangeal)
Motions:	Flexion and extension
Position:	Supine, wrist in neutral position
Alternative Position:	Sitting
Hand Placement:	One hand grasps the thumb. The other hand grasps the patient's hand.

Thumb flexion.

Thumb extension.

PROCEDURE 6–4

UPPER EXTREMITY ROM EXERCISES: DIAGONAL PATTERNS

Pattern:

PNF diagonal 1 (D1) extension with elbow extended
PNF diagonal 1 (D1) flexion with elbow extended

Combining Components
of Motion:

D1 extension with elbow extended
Shoulder: extension, abduction, internal rotation
Elbow: extended
Forearm: pronation
Wrist: extension, ulnar deviation
Digits: extension, abduction

D1 flexion with elbow extended
Shoulder: flexion, adduction, external rotation
Elbow: extended
Forearm: supination
Wrist: flexed, radial deviation
Digits: flexion, adduction

Position:

Supine

Hand Placement:

One hand supports the arm. The other hand grasps the patient's hand. When performing ROM of a patient's left upper extremity, the physical therapist's right hand controls the patient's left wrist and hand.

Note:

Elbow extended indicates that the elbow maintains extension throughout the movement of both patterns. In these patterns motion begins distally, and progresses proximally, with the motions occurring more or less simultaneously.

D1 extension with elbow extended.

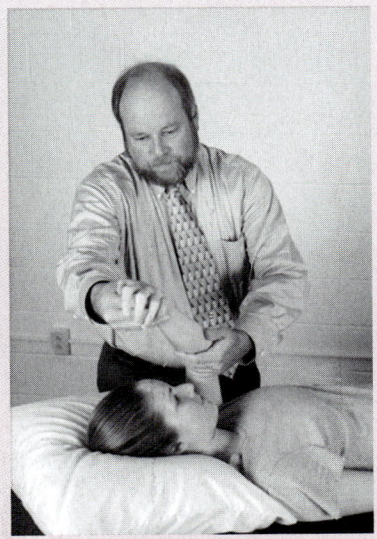

D1 flexion with elbow extended.

Pattern: PNF diagonal 1 (D1) extension with elbow extension
PNF diagonal 1 (D1) flexion with elbow flexion

Combining Components
of Motion:

D1 extension with elbow extension
Shoulder: extension, abduction, internal rotation
Elbow: extension
Forearm: pronation
Wrist: extension, ulnar deviation
Digits: extension, abduction

D1 flexion with elbow flexion
Shoulder: flexion, adduction, external rotation
Elbow: flexion
Forearm: supination
Wrist: flexion, radial deviation
Digits: flexion, adduction

Position: Supine

Hand Placement: One hand supports the arm. The other hand grasps the patient's hand. When performing range of motion of the patient's left upper extremity, the physical therapist's right hand controls the patient's left wrist and hand.

Note: In these patterns motion begins distally, and progresses proximally, with the motions occurring more or less simultaneously.

D1 extension with elbow extension.

D1 flexion with elbow flexion.

Pattern: PNF diagonal 1 (D1) extension with elbow flexion
                                    PNF diagonal 1 (D1) flexion with elbow extension

Combining Components
of Motion:

D1 extension with elbow flexion
                                    Shoulder: extension, abduction, internal rotation
                                    Elbow: flexion
                                    Forearm: pronation
                                    Wrist: extension, ulnar deviation
                                    Digits: extension, abduction

D1 flexion with elbow extension
                                    Shoulder: flexion, adduction, external rotation
                                    Elbow: extension
                                    Forearm: supination
                                    Wrist: flexion, radial deviation
                                    Digits: flexion, adduction

Position: Supine
Hand Placement: One hand supports the arm. The other hand grasps the hand. When
                                    performing ROM of a patient's left upper extremity, the physical thera-
                                    pist's right hand controls the patient's left wrist and hand.

Note: In these patterns motion begins distally, and progresses proximally,
                                    with the motions occuring more or less simultaneously.

D1 extension with elbow flexion.

D1 flexion with elbow extension.

Pattern: PNF diagonal 1 (D1) extension—scapula
                           PNF diagonal 1 (D1) flexion—scapula
Combining Components of Motion:
    D1 extension: Scapula: depression, adduction, downward rotation
    D1 flexion: Scapula: elevation, abduction, upward rotation
Position: Sidelying
Hand Placement: One hand is placed over the scapula. The other hand and forearm
                           support the patient's upper extremity. When performing ROM of the
                           patient's right scapula, the physical therapist's left hand is on the right
                           scapula.
Note: In these patterns, the motion occurs simultaneously.

D1 extension—scapula.

D1 flexion—scapula.

Pattern: PNF diagonal 2 (D2) extension with elbow extended
PNF diagonal 2 (D2) flexion with elbow extended

Combining Components
of Motion:

D2 extension with elbow extended
Shoulder: extension, adduction, internal rotation
Elbow: extended
Forearm: pronation
Wrist: flexion, ulnar deviation
Digits: flexion, adduction
Thumb: opposition

D2 flexion with elbow extended
Shoulder: flexion, abduction, external rotation
Elbow: extended
Forearm: supination
Wrist: extension, radial deviation
Digits: extension, abduction

Position: Supine

Hand Placement: One hand supports the arm. The other hand grasps the patient's hand. When performing ROM of the patient's left upper extremity, the physical therapist's right hand controls the patient's left wrist and hand.

Note: Elbow extended indicates that the elbow maintains complete extension throughout the movement of both patterns. In these patterns motion begins distally, and progresses proximally, with the motions occurring more or less simultaneously.

D2 extension with elbow extended.

D2 flexion with elbow extended.

Pattern: PNF diagonal 2 (D2) extension with elbow extension
                               PNF diagonal 2 (D2) flexion with elbow flexion

Combining Components
of Motion:
      D2 extension with elbow extension
                  Shoulder: extension, adduction, internal rotation
                  Elbow: extension
                  Forearm: pronation
                  Wrist: flexion, ulnar deviation
                  Digits: flexion, adduction
                  Thumb: opposition
      D2 flexion with elbow flexion
                  Shoulder: flexion, abduction, external rotation
                  Elbow: flexion
                  Forearm: supination
                  Wrist: extension, radial deviation
                  Digits: extension, abduction

Position: Supine

Hand Placement: One hand supports the arm. The other hand grasps the patient's
                               hand. When performing ROM of the patient's left upper extremity, the
                               physical therapist's right hand controls the patient's left wrist and
                               hand.

Note: In these patterns motion begins distally, and progresses proximally,
                               with the motions occurring more or less simultaneously.

D2 extension with elbow extension.

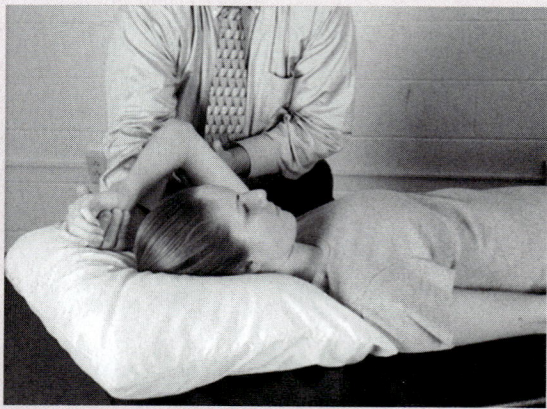

D2 flexion with elbow flexion.

Pattern:	PNF diagonal 2 (D2) extension with elbow flexion
	PNF diagonal 2 (D2) flexion with elbow extension

Combining Components
of Motion:

D2 extension with elbow flexion

Shoulder: extension, adduction, internal rotation
Elbow: flexion
Forearm: pronation
Wrist: flexion, ulnar deviation
Digits: flexion, adduction
Thumb: opposition

D2 flexion with elbow extension

Shoulder: flexion, abduction, external rotation
Elbow: extension
Forearm: supination
Wrist: extension, radial deviation
Digits: extension, abduction

Position:	Supine
Hand Placement:	One hand supports the arm. The other hand grasps the patient's hand. When performing ROM of the patient's left upper extremity, the physical therapist's right hand controls the patient's left wrist and hand.
Note:	In these patterns motion begins distally, and progresses proximally, with the motions occurring more or less simultaneously.

D2 extension with elbow flexion.

D2 flexion with elbow extension.

Pattern:	PNF diagonal 2 (D2) extension—scapula
	PNF diagonal 2 (D2) flexion—scapula
Combining Components of Motion:	
D2 extension	
	Scapula: depression, abduction, downward rotation
D2 flexion	
	Scapula: elevation, adduction, upward rotation
Position:	Sidelying
Hand Placement:	One hand is placed on the scapula. The other hand and forearm are used to support the patient's arm. When performing ROM of the patient's right scapula, the physical therapist's right hand grasps the right scapula.

D2 extension—scapula.

D2 flexion—scapula.

PROCEDURE 6–5

HEAD, NECK, AND TRUNK ROM EXERCISES: ANATOMICAL PLANES

Joints:	Head and neck (atlantooccipital, atlantoaxial, and successive cervical spine joints)
Motions:	Flexion and extension
Position:	Supine
Hand Placement:	One hand grasps each side of the head with the palms above the ears and the fingers spread over the occiput.
Note:	When the treatment table does not have a head support that can be lowered, the patient must lie with his or her head over the end of the table.
Precaution:	The patient's head must be supported carefully. Movement must not be forced. Movement begins with tucking of the chin, rather than jutting the chin forward.

Head and neck (cervical spine) flexion.

Neutral position of head and neck (cervical spine).

Head and neck (cervical spine) extension.

Joints:	Head and neck (atlantooccipital, atlantoaxial, and successive cervical spine joints)
Motions:	Lateral flexion
Position:	Supine
Hand Placement:	One hand grasps each side of the head with the palms above the ears and the fingers spread over the occiput.
Precaution:	The patient's head must be supported carefully. Movement must not be forced. Movement begins with tilting the ear to the shoulder, rather than pushing the head laterally.

Lateral head and neck (cervical spine) flexion to the left.

Neutral position of the head and neck (cervical spine).

Lateral head and neck (cervical spine) flexion to the right.

Joints:	Head and neck (atlantooccipital, atlantoaxial, and successive cervical spine joints)
Motions:	Rotation
Position:	Supine
Hand Placement:	One hand grasps each side of the head with the palms above the ears and the fingers spread over the occiput.
Precaution:	The patient's head must be supported carefully. Movement must not be forced. Movement should not include flexion/extension or lateral flexion.

Head and neck (cervical spine) rotation to the right.

Neutral position of the head and neck (cervical spine).

Head and neck (cervical spine) rotation to the left.

Joint: Lower trunk (lumbar spine) and hip
Motion: Lower trunk rotation
Position: Supine, hips and knees flexed such that the patient's feet are rest-
                    ing flat on the supporting surface close to the buttocks
Hand Placement: One hand grasps the knees. The other hand stabilizes the pelvis.
Alternative Placement: Both hands are placed on the knees.
Precaution: The patient's shoulders remain on the supporting surface as the
                    knees are moved from side to side. When a patient's upper trunk
                    begins to roll, the end point of lower trunk rotation in that direction
                    has been reached.

Lower trunk (lumbar spine) rotation to the left.

Neutral position of the lower trunk (lumbar spine).

Lower trunk (lumbar spine) rotation to the right.

Joint:	Lower trunk (lumbar spine) and hip
Motion:	Lower trunk flexion
Position:	Supine, hips and knees flexed
Hand Placement:	One arm supports the legs on the posterior aspect of the patient's thighs. The other hand supports the patient's feet as the lower trunk (lumbar spine) is flexed.

Starting position for lower trunk (lumbar spine) flexion.

End position for lower trunk (lumbar spine) flexion.

REVIEW QUESTIONS

1. Define passive, active-assisted, and active ROM.

2. How does a physical therapist support body segments during ROM exercises?

3. What are the differences between joint ROM and muscle ROM?

4. Define the different types of end feel and describe the significance of each.

5. Describe differences in movement when a patient has normal muscle tone, spasticity, rigidity, and pain.

6. Compare and contrast anatomical plane motions and diagonal patterns of motion.

7. List the combining components of motion for each of the diagonal patterns.

SUGGESTED ACTIVITIES

1. Demonstrate the specific procedures presented in this chapter.

2. Work in pairs to perform the specific procedures. Rotate partners periodically during practice sessions.

3. Identify the type of end feel for selected motions.

4. Practice ROM exercises for all joints and muscles possible in each position—prone, supine, sidelying and sitting, and on different surfaces—mat on floor, treatment table, bed.

5. Practice performing ROM exercises while a partner role-plays various diagnoses (see Case Studies for suggestions). The student role-playing the patient can add "character" to the role by being cooperative, uncooperative, in pain, hard of hearing, or lacking in ROM to enhance the activity. The "patient" must role-play the diagnoses and character consistently.

6. Practice teaching "family and patients" and other health care providers how to perform ROM exercises.

7. Document "treatments" using the SOAP note format.

CASE STUDIES

Use these case studies to complete Activity #5 above.

1. Patient is a 22-year-old status posttraumatic brain injury and is in a coma.
2. Patient is a 18-year-old with a complete C6 spinal cord injury, presenting with moderate spasticity in the lower extremities.
3. Patient is a 59-year-old former executive with left hemiplegia with mild spasticity in the lower extremity and moderate spasticity in the upper extremity.
4. Patient is a 44-year-old with multiple sclerosis, presenting with moderate spasticity in the lower extremity.
5. Patient is a 70-year-old with advanced Parkinsonism, presenting with moderate to severe rigidity.

6. Patient is a 12-year-old with cerebral palsy, presenting with severe spastic quadriplegia.

REFERENCES

1. Knott M and Voss DE. *Proprioceptive Neuromuscular Facilitation,* 2nd ed. New York: Harper & Row, 1968.
2. Root ML, Orien WP, and Weed JH. *Normal and Abnormal Function of the Foot: Clinical Biomechanics—Volume II.* Los Angeles: Clinical Biomechanics Corporation Publishers, 1977.
3. Warwick R and Williams PL. *Gray's Anatomy,* 37th ed. Philadelphia: WB Saunders, 1989.
4. Sullivan PE, Markos PD, and Minor MAD. *An Integrated Approach to Therapeutic Exercise: Theory and Clinical Application.* Reston, Virginia: Reston Publishing Company, 1982.

7

WHEELCHAIRS

LEARNING OBJECTIVES

Upon completion of this chapter, you will be able to:

1. Identify different components of a wheelchair, including:
   - Anti-tipping components
   - Armrests
   - Front rigging
   - Pelvic positioners
   - Wheels
   - Wheel locks
2. Identify different types of wheelchairs, including:
   - Amputee-frame
   - Fixed frame
   - Folding
   - One-arm drive
   - Reclining-back
   - Standard
   - Tilt-in-space
3. Describe the purpose or function of wheelchair components and types.
4. Describe and demonstrate how wheelchair components and types are manipulated.
5. Describe and demonstrate how to measure an individual to determine correct size and components required for a wheelchair.

KEY TERMS

Armrests
Anti-tipping devices
Caster wheels
Drive wheels
Fixed frame
Folding frame

Footrest
Front rigging
Heel loops
Legrest
One-arm drive

Pelvic positioners
Reclining back
Sacral sitting
Tilt-in-space
Wheel locks

INTRODUCTION

In situations when an individual will use a wheelchair as his or her primary means of mobility, a wheelchair is usually specifically fabricated for that individual. Careful measurement of an individual, and the selection of appropriate components with respect to specific needs, provides the user of a wheelchair with a piece of equipment that allows the individual to function with the most independence and safety possible. Guidelines for selection of a wheelchair design indicate that the wheelchair have a short wheelbase and be as light and narrow as possible. These features make propulsion and maneuvering require less user effort.

Wheelchairs incorporate many common features, but there are a variety of mechanisms that can be selected to meet the needs of each individual. This chapter presents selected components, selected types of wheelchairs, and other mobility devices, and illustrates how to measure a patient for a wheelchair.

WHEELCHAIR COMPONENTS

WHEEL LOCKS

One of the most important safety features on a wheelchair is the wheel lock system (Figure 7–1). **Wheel locks** are devices that stabilize the wheels of a wheelchair *after* the wheelchair has been stopped. Wheel locks usually employ a cam and lever system. In some situations, a slot locking mechanism is used rather than a cam locking mechanism. Previously, wheel locks were referred to as brakes. Some patients understood that to mean that wheel locks functioned as braking devices, such as on an automobile, which is not correct.

FIGURE 7–1   Wheel lock.

A general safety rule is that wheel locks must be engaged whenever an individual is moving into, or out of, a wheelchair. Engaging wheel locks on the rear wheels prevents forward and backward movement of a wheelchair. Wheel locks on front caster wheels minimize side-to-side movement. Although wheel locks are available for front caster wheels, they are not typically placed on wheelchairs. Therefore, slight side-to-side movement of a wheelchair may result as an individual moves into, or out of, a wheelchair when front caster wheels are not secured.

To work properly, wheel locks must make secure contact with tires to prevent movement of the wheels. Effectiveness of wheel locks is reduced if they do not make adequate contact with tires. This may occur when pneumatic tires are not inflated sufficiently, or entire wheel lock mechanisms become loose or slide forward on the wheelchair frame.

The direction of the force needed to engage or release wheel locks can be selected during wheelchair ordering to match a patient's abilities. Wheel locks are usually engaged by pushing a lever on each side forward (Figure 7–2), while pulling the levers backward releases the wheel lock (Figure 7–3). The reverse mechanism, engaging wheel locks by pulling levers backward, and releasing them by pushing levers forward, is an option. A decision as to which method to use is made by a physical therapist and patient, with respect to the patient's strength and balance. The direction of a patient's greatest strength is the direction of movement that should engage the wheel locks.

FIGURE 7–2 Engaging wheel locks.   **FIGURE 7–3**   Releasing wheel locks.

Extensions for wheel lock levers are available (Figure 7–4). Extensions increase the mechanical advantage of a wheel locking mechanism by increasing the length of the wheel lock lever. Increasing the length of the wheel lock lever increases the length of the force arm with respect to the resistance arm of the cam. This increase in mechanical advantage decreases the force required of a patient for engaging or disengaging the wheel lock.

FIGURE 7–4   Wheel lock handle extension.

On some reclining-back wheelchairs, the anterior/posterior dimension of the wheelbase increases when the back is reclined. When the wheelbase is enlarged as the back reclines, the relationship of the wheel lock and the tire is altered, resulting in an ineffective wheel lock because wheel lock contact with the tire is decreased. An additional wheel lock is necessary for these wheelchairs. The additional lock is attached to the back upright of the wheelchair so it is effective when the wheelchair is in the reclined position.

PELVIC POSITIONERS

Pelvic positioners are devices that stabilize a patient's pelvis in the proper position while seated in a wheelchair (Figure 7–5). Pelvic positioners are not intended to be used to prevent a patient from falling out of a wheelchair. Rather, they are part of a positioning system designed to provide proper positioning of a patient in a wheelchair. Pelvic positioners are also not intended to be used as restraints to keep patients from getting out of a wheelchair unexpectedly.

Three mechanisms are used for fastening pelvic positioners: Velcro straps; latching buckles, such as those used for seat belts in airplanes; and push button buckles, such as those used for seat belts in automobiles.

FIGURE 7–5 Pelvic positioner.

CASTER WHEELS

Caster wheels are the small front wheels of a wheelchair. Two basic styles of tire are available—standard solid rubber and pneumatic. Pneumatic tires are filled with air, providing some shock absorption, and thus a smoother ride (Figure 7–6). Pneumatic tires are wider than standard solid rubber tires, making travel easier on soft, or uneven, surfaces such as sand or gravel. Some wheelchair owners use "rollerblade" wheels for front caster wheels (Figure 7–7). Typically these owners are users of ultralight, or sport, wheelchairs. Because of their construction and materials, "rollerblade" wheels are small in size, very durable, and have excellent quality bearings. A tradeoff, however, is that smaller wheels may become caught in sidewalk cracks.

FIGURE 7–6 Pneumatic caster wheels.

FIGURE 7–7 "Rollerblade" caster wheels.

DRIVE (PUSH) WHEELS

Drive wheels are the large rear wheels of a wheelchair, which are used for propulsion. Rear tires may be one of two basic types—standard solid rubber or pneumatic. Pneumatic tires may or may not have tread (Figure 7–8). Treads are used on wheelchairs that are often used outdoors and require more traction than smooth tires provide. Pneumatic tires have been modified to reduce the potential for flat tires.

FIGURE 7–8   Drive wheels—smooth (left), tread (right).

Drive wheels have inner and outer rims. The inner rim is for mounting tires. The outer, or hand, rim is used for propelling the wheelchair. Adaptations of the outer rim, such as projections, are available for use by individuals who do not have sufficient grasp (Figure 7–9). Projections add weight and width to the wheelchair and may make maneuvering in small spaces difficult. Nonslip coatings, rather than projections, are more commonly used on hand rims to assist propulsion when an individual does not have sufficient grasp.

FIGURE 7–9   Drive wheel rim with projections.

Drive wheels come in two types—standard or "mags" (Figure 7–10). Standard wheels are fabricated with multiple steel or aluminum spokes. Spokes are thin and individually adjustable to maintain proper alignment of a wheel. Mag wheels do not use spokes, but usually have eight thicker struts that connect the outer rim to the hub. Mag wheels were named after their fabrication from magnesium, a very strong, lightweight metal. Mag wheels have the material strength to maintain their original alignment, eliminating the need for multiple adjustable spokes. Because of their design and material, maintenance of mag wheels is easier than standard wheels.

FIGURE 7–10 Drive wheels—mag (left), spoke (right).

Drive wheels on some chairs are easily removable (Figures 7–11 and 7–12), making the chair lighter and smaller, increasing the ease of maneuvering the wheelchair into, and out of, a vehicle.

FIGURE 7–11 Releasing quick-release drive wheels.

FIGURE 7–12 Removing quick-release drive wheels.

ARMRESTS

Several configurations of **armrests** are available. Armrests are either full-length or desk-length (Figure 7–13). The height of full-length armrests is the same along the entire length of the armrest. Desk-length armrests have two heights. In a standard set-up, the front portion of the armrest is lower than the rear portion, permitting a wheelchair to be rolled under a table or desk. Most desk-length armrests can be removed and reversed, placing the higher part of the armrest toward the front of the wheelchair. Reversing a desk armrest provides a higher support for patients when pushing to standing or transferring.

FIGURE 7–13 Full-length (left) and desk-length (right) armrests.

Lap trays are available, and can be secured to, or rest on, armrests. Full length armrests offer greater support for lap trays than do desk length armrests.

Both types of armrests have an option for adjustable height with respect to the top of the seat (Figures 7–14 and 7–15). Proper adjustment of armrest height permits the person sitting in the wheelchair to rest his or her forearms on the armrest, with the elbow flexed to approximately 90 degrees.

FIGURE 7–14 Lowered elevating armrest.

FIGURE 7–15 Raised elevating armrest.

Armrests, both full-length and desk-length, can be either removable or fixed. Non-removable armrests usually result in a lighter, and narrower, wheelchair. Removable armrests may be designed so that they wrap around the back uprights of the wheelchair, decreasing wheelchair width (Figure 7–16). When a wrap-around design is used, the posterior upright of the armrest is directly behind the upright of the wheelchair back. Removable armrests often allow easier performance of transfers and permit a patient to sit even closer to a table or desk than desk-length armrests allow.

FIGURE 7–16 Removable wrap-around armrest.

Several types of mechanisms are used to lock armrests in place for patient safety. Both the location and type of armrest locking mechanisms varies. A common type of lock is operated by a lever that is pushed either down or rotated to release the lock (Figures 7–17 and 7–18).

FIGURE 7–17 Removable armrest lock.

FIGURE 7–18 Releasing removable armrest.

Once released, the lever remains in the released position. Thus, only one hand is required to unlock, and then remove, the armrest (Figure 7–19).

FIGURE 7–19 Armrest being removed.

FRONT RIGGING

Front rigging on a wheelchair consists of a footplate attached to either a footrest or an elevating legrest. The purpose of front rigging is to provide support for the lower extremities. Front rigging with a footplate only is called a **footrest**. Front rigging with a footplate and calf pad support is called a **legrest**.

Footplates

A patient's feet rest on footplates. Footplates are available in several sizes to accommodate different size feet. **Heel loops**, constructed of cloth or webbing, attach to footplates and prevent the feet from sliding off the footplates and under the wheelchair (Figure 7–20). Ankle and toe loops, also constructed of cloth or webbing, may also be used to maintain the feet on footplates.

FIGURE 7–20   Heel loop on footrest of front rigging.

Footplates are raised to allow patients to transfer safely in and out of a wheelchair (Figures 7–21 and 7–22). When raising footplates, heel loops must be pushed forward to allow the footplates to be raised completely. Doing this prolongs the life of heel loops by preventing heel loop material from being crushed.

FIGURE 7–21   Footplate in down position.

FIGURE 7–22   Footplate in up position.

Footrests

The distance from seat to footplate for both footrests and legrests can be adjusted to match a patient's lower leg length and to provide proper support for the entire lower extremity. There are several different types of mechanism for making this adjustment. The method illustrated uses a push button release and a clamp to ensure that the desired position is maintained (Figures 7–23 and 7–24).

FIGURE 7–23 Preparing to lengthen front rigging—securing lever and button adjustment.

FIGURE 7–24 Adjusting front rigging length—lengthening while holding button.

Other types of mechanisms use clamps, or tension adjustment screws, located inside the footrest or legrest tube. The adjustment screws for this method of adjustment are accessible from the underside of the footrest or legrest.

Footrests can be fixed or removable. Fixed footrests are usually less expensive and result in a lighter wheelchair. Fixed footrests are part of a unitized construction design in standard wheelchairs. In this design, footplates can be raised but the footrest itself cannot be removed.

Footrests for fixed frame wheelchairs are part of a unitized construction design and cannot be adjusted (Figure 7–25). In this design, footplates are typically bolted to a bar that is positioned so the knees are flexed more than 90 degrees. This results in a shorter overall dimension for the wheelchair. Fixed frame wheelchairs are usually ultra lightweight sport models.

FIGURE 7–25 Fixed frame wheelchair—unitized footrest construction.

Removable footrests typically pivot to the sides of wheelchairs, where they can be removed. Several types of locks are used to secure pivoting footrests (Figure 7–26).

FIGURE 7–26 Preparing to release pivoting footrest.

Pivoting footrests use pivot pins as the center of rotation. To remove a pivoting footrest, the footrest is unlocked or released, pivoted to the side, and then lifted from the pivot pins (Figures 7–27 and 7–28).

FIGURE 7–27 Pushing lever to release pivoting footrest.

FIGURE 7–28 Pivoting footrest.

Elevating Legrests

Elevating legrests are necessary when a patient is unable to flex his or her knee, when a dependent position of the leg contributes to swelling, or with a reclining-back wheelchair. A calf pad support provides a cushion for the calf and support for the leg.

The height of legrest position is adjustable. Legrest height position is maintained by a locking mechanism. The lock is released and activated by a lever. The legrest position is adjusted by releasing the lock with one hand, while raising or lowering the legrest with the other hand (Figures 7–29 and 7–30).

FIGURE 7–29 Preparing to raise elevating legrest by pushing lever.

FIGURE 7–30 Elevating legrest in up position.

To remove an elevating legrest, the calf pad support is pivoted out of the way. The calf pad support must be pivoted before the footplate is raised (Figures 7–31 through 7–33). Failure to use this sequence will not permit the calf pad support to be moved completely out of the way.

Swing-away removable elevating legrests are removed in a similar manner as swing-away removable footrests are removed.

FIGURE 7–31 Calf pad support in down position.

FIGURE 7–32 Calf pad support pivoted to up position.

FIGURE 7–33 Raising footplate with calf pad support in up position.

Anti-Tipping Devices

Anti-tipping devices are small extensions, with or without wheels, attached to the lower horizontal support bar. These devices are used to prevent accidental backward tipping of the wheelchair. Adjustment of anti-tipping devices must permit some tipping of the wheelchair so front casters can roll up and over doorsills, curbs, or other low obstructions.

FIGURE 7–34   Anti-tipping device.

WHEELCHAIR TYPES

Different styles of wheelchairs have been developed to meet specific patient needs. Some styles are minimal modifications of standard wheelchairs. Other styles required extensive re-engineering of basic wheelchair design. Several, but not all, types of specialized wheelchairs are discussed in this section. In addition to manual wheelchairs, motorized wheelchairs and scooters are available.

FOLDING WHEELCHAIR

Wheelchairs that can be folded or collapsed for storage or transport use a similar method for folding (Figures 7–35 and 7–36). Raising footplates, and pulling up on the handles located on either side of the seat will fold most wheelchairs. Do not pull up on the middle of the wheelchair seat upholstery to fold a wheelchair because it will weaken the upholstery and eventually the seat will tear. The wheelchair is unfolded by pushing down on the horizontal bars of the seat.

FIGURE 7–35   Mid-position of folding a wheelchair.

FIGURE 7–36   End position of folding a wheelchair.

STANDARD WHEELCHAIR

A standard wheelchair comes with basic features. This wheelchair is durable and is the standard for facility use. Standard wheelchairs are available in several sizes, to fit patients ranging from pediatric to adult. Seat-to-floor height can be varied, with a lower seat height facilitating propulsion for individuals that propel the wheelchair with their feet (Figure 7–37).

FIGURE 7–37 Seat height—standard (left), low (right)

FIXED FRAME WHEELCHAIR

A **fixed frame** means the wheelchair frame is solid and cannot be folded (Figure 7–38). The front rigging is often part of the frame and not removable. Back height is often lower than a standard wheelchair and many individuals that use fixed frame wheelchairs do not use armrests. Overall frame length in fixed frame wheelchairs is reduced because the front rigging is an integral part of the frame and the front rigging is placed further back on the frame. This improves maneuverability, which is important in small spaces. There are fewer components and the materials used to construct them are lighter than standard wheelchairs. Thus fixed frame wheelchairs are usually ultra lightweight. One disadvantage of the fixed frame is reduced shock absorption because the frame in a unitized design is rigid.

FIGURE 7–38 Unitized, fixed frame, ultralight wheelchair construction.

RECLINING-BACK WHEELCHAIR

Reclining-back wheelchairs are indicated when a patient is unable to sit erect at all, or to sit erect for long periods of time. There are two variations of reclining-back wheelchairs—those that recline completely and those that recline only partially. An extended back is used with both types of reclining-back wheelchairs. An extended back provides support for the upper body when the wheelchair back is in a reclined position. Head support is also required when the back is reclined. Reclining-back wheelchairs usually have elevating legrests, permitting patients to be in a mostly supine position when the back is reclined. A reclining-back wheelchair takes much more space to maneuver when reclined because of the increase in overall length (Figures 7–39 and 7–40).

FIGURE 7–39 Reclining-back wheelchair in upright position.

FIGURE 7–40 Reclining-back wheelchair in reclined position.

There are several types of mechanisms for unlocking and adjusting the angle of inclination of the wheelchair back. To change the wheelchair's back angle, the locking mechanism is released, the angle of the back is adjusted, and the locking mechanism is activated.

A bar across the back of a reclining-back wheelchair provides support and stability. To fold a reclining-back wheelchair, the back support bar must be removed (Figures 7–41 and 7–42). Several different methods of securing the support bar exist. The bar must be released before the wheelchair is folded. A reclining-back wheelchair can then be folded following the same steps used when folding a standard wheelchair.

FIGURE 7–41 Releasing support crossbar to fold reclining-back wheelchair.

FIGURE 7–42 Lowering support crossbar on reclining-back wheelchair.

When a reclining-back wheelchair's back is lowered, the seat-to-back angle widens. As the seat-to-back widens, the wheelbase increases to maintain stability. Traditionally placed wheel locks will not engage the tires in this situation. Therefore, a reclining-back wheelchair typically has two sets of wheel locks. The second set of wheel locks is usually located on the back of the wheelchair to be able to engage the tires and for easy use by an attendant because the individual using a reclining-back wheelchair will not be able to engage the wheel locks during this maneuver.

TILT-IN-SPACE WHEELCHAIR

A variation of a reclining-back wheelchair is a **tilt-in-space** frame (Figures 7–43 through 7–45). A tilt-in-space wheelchair has a fixed seat-to-back angle, even when reclined.

FIGURE 7–43 Tilt-in-space wheelchair in upright position.

FIGURE 7–44 Releasing mechanism to reposition tilt-in-space wheelchair.

FIGURE 7–45 Tilt-in-space wheelchair in a reclined position.

Maintaining this relative seat-to-back angle is useful for individuals that require customized seating systems on their wheelchair. The tilt-in-space frame permits changes of orientation for pressure relief, or for different activities, while maintaining the postural control provided by the customized seating system.

ONE-ARM DRIVE WHEELCHAIR

A patient with only one functional upper extremity may achieve self-propulsion using a one-arm drive wheelchair. One-arm drive wheelchairs have two hand rims on one drive wheel (Figure 7–46). A linking mechanism between the drive wheels provides control for both drive wheels using one upper extremity. With both hand rims on one drive wheel, the two hand rims are used simultaneously to achieve forward or backward propulsion. Applying force to one rim at a time turns the wheelchair.

FIGURE 7–46 One-arm drive wheelchair.

AMPUTEE WHEELCHAIR

An amputee wheelchair frame has the drive wheels set behind the vertical back supports (Figure 7–47). This configuration moves the posterior boundary of the base of support further to the rear. A lower extremity amputation moves the individual's center of mass posteriorly when seated in a wheelchair, necessitating a change in the wheelchair's base of support. If the wheelchair's base of support is not moved posteriorly with respect to the individual, the wheelchair will be less stable and more likely to tip backward.

FIGURE 7–47 Backset drive wheels on frame of amputee wheelchair.

COMPANION WHEELCHAIR

A companion chair, also called a travel chair, is a lightweight wheelchair that does not have drive wheels (Figure 7–48). The rear wheels are the size of caster wheels, so all four wheels are the same size. Smaller wheels, and the use of lightweight components, reduces the weight of a companion chair with respect to a standard wheelchair. A companion pushes the wheelchair. The person using the wheelchair may also be able to propel it using his or her feet.

FIGURE 7–48 Lightweight travel or companion wheelchair.

MOTORIZED WHEELCHAIRS AND SCOOTERS

A variety of motorized or power devices are increasingly available (Figures 7–49 and 7–50). Although expensive, motorized devices offer individuals with minimal or limited functional abilities an opportunity to have independent mobility. There are a large number of choices and complexities in making decisions concerning motorized devices. In addition to determining available components, such as armrests, headrests, and front rigging, the method of power activation must be determined. Given the number of choices, and the complexity involved in making choices for specific patients, a discussion of the types of, and indications for, various methods of power activation and the various configurations of power devices is beyond the scope of this text.

FIGURE 7–49   Standard power wheelchair.

FIGURE 7–50   Power wheelchair with reclining back.

Some motorized wheelchairs also have the capability to use a power mechanism to recline the back of the wheelchair (Figure 7–51). This permits an individual to change position for different activities and provides for pressure relief.

FIGURE 7–51   Power wheelchair with reclining back in reclined position.

Power scooters are an alternative to power wheelchairs for individuals with the ability to ambulate short distances (Figures 7–52 and 7–53).

FIGURE 7–52 Power scooter without armrests.

FIGURE 7–53 Power scooter with armrests.

POWER ASSIST CHAIR

A newer type of wheelchair is a hybrid power-manual wheelchair (Figure 7–54). The individual propels the wheelchair using the drive wheels. The power assist mechanism provides additional propulsion, increasing the duration or distance that may be attained.

FIGURE 7–54 Hybrid power-manual wheelchair.

PROCEDURE 7-1

MEASURING TO DETERMINE WHEELCHAIR SIZE

Selection of the type, size, and components of a wheelchair for an individual depends on a variety of information. Much of this information is determined as a result of the physical therapist/client management process. Some of this information is specific measurement of the individual. Discussion with the patient, caregivers, and determination of the environments in which the device will be used is critical to successful decision making. The decision-making process is the role of a physical therapist. Taking measurements may be delegated to physical therapist assistants.

Wheelchair size is determined by selected measurements of the individual. Care must be taken to use measuring equipment properly and to read a tape measure or ruler accurately. Accurate measurement requires a physical therapist or physical therapist assistant to assume a position that places the tape measure at eye level. The optimal patient position for obtaining accurate measurements is to have the patient sit on a solid flat surface with a solid flat back support. Wood inserts can be used in a wheelchair or straight-back chair to ensure accuracy when measuring. Note that in some of the accompanying photographs, the position of the person performing measurements is altered to allow the tape measure to be seen.

Measuring for Seat Depth

Seat depth is one of the two most important measurements for determining wheelchair size. Proper seat depth provides support for the pelvis and thigh. The front edge of the seat should end two to three inches from the lower leg or knee.

When seat depth is too short, the thighs are not supported properly, which affects weight distribution and comfort adversely. Seat depth that is longer than appropriate may affect circulation or lead to "sacral sitting" by a wheelchair user. **Sacral sitting** occurs when an individual slouches, sliding the buttocks forward and posteriorly tilting the pelvis. Sacral sitting places the posterior aspect of the sacrum on the seat of the chair, resulting in improper postural alignment. This position increases pressure on the posterior aspect of the sacrum and may lead to skin breakdown. In addition, a sacral sitting position is not optimal for efficient propulsion.

One measurement and one calculation are necessary to determine seat depth.

1. When measuring, an individual must sit with proper alignment. Proper alignment requires that the individual's hips and knees be flexed to 90 degrees and his or her back be in contact with the flat back support without a posterior pelvic tilt.
2. The horizontal distance from the flat back support to the posterior aspect of the lower leg is measured parallel to, and at the level of, the solid seat surface.
3. Two or three inches are subtracted from this measurement.
4. The result of this measurement and calculation provides the desired seat depth.

Measuring for Seat Width

Seat width is the other of the two most important measurements for determining wheelchair size. Proper seat width results in properly positioned drive wheels and armrests, resulting in easy and efficient wheelchair use.

When a wheelchair is too wide, an individual may have difficulty reaching the drive wheels for effective propulsion, and may lean to one side or the other to rest on the armrests. When a wheelchair is too narrow, excessive pressure on the lateral aspects of the pelvis and thighs may occur, causing discomfort or skin breakdown. In addition to body width, space for clothing, such as winter coats, prosthetic or orthotic devices when necessary, and ease of movement, must be provided.

One measurement and one calculation are necessary to determine seat width.

1. With the individual sitting in proper alignment on the solid flat seat, the widest aspect of the patient's hips or thighs, whichever is wider, is measured parallel to the solid flat seat.
2. Two inches are added to this measurement.
3. The result of this measurement and calculation provides the desired seat width.

Measuring for Back Height

The amount of back height required depends on how much back support is needed by the individual.

A back height that is too high may restrict an individual's movement. A back height that is not high enough may not provide adequate support. Wheelchair users with adequate sitting balance may choose a lower back height. A lower back height decreases wheelchair weight and improves mobility within the wheelchair. Some wheelchair users also prefer the lower back height for esthetic reasons as it reduces the visual impact of the wheelchair.

One measurement and one calculation are necessary to determine back height.

1. Back height is measured with the individual sitting on the solid flat seat in proper alignment.
2. In most cases, the vertical distance, parallel to the back support, is measured from the top of the seat to the inferior angle of the scapula.
3. The height of the seat cushion to be used must be added to this measurement.
4. The result of this measurement and calculation provides the desired back height.

Measuring for Armrest Height

Proper armrest height promotes proper positioning and alignment. When armrest height is appropriate, and the individual is sitting with proper alignment, an individual's forearms rest comfortably on the armrests. Some individuals may elect not to use armrests if their sitting balance is adequate. Eliminating armrests decreases the weight of the wheelchair; allows the individual to sit close to surfaces such as sinks, desks, and tables; and reduces the visual impact of the wheelchair.

When armrests are at an improper height, an individual will be unable to rest his or her forearms comfortably on the armrests and maintain proper alignment. Improper alignment may cause an individual to be subjected to unequal pressure on the forearms and ischia, and to spinal curvature.

One measurement and one calculation are necessary to determine armrest height.

1. Armrest height is measured with the individual sitting on the solid flat seat in proper alignment, the upper arm held against the chest wall, and the elbow flexed to 90 degrees.
2. The vertical distance between the solid seat surface and the individual's forearm, parallel to the back support, is measured.
3. The height of the seat cushion to be used must be added to this measurement.
4. The result of this measurement and calculation provides the desired armrest height.

Measuring for Seat-to-Footplate Length

Appropriate seat-to-footplate length contributes to proper alignment and support of the lower extremities. When seat-to-footplate length is too great, an individual may sacral sit to rest his or her feet on the footplate. When the length is too short, pressure distribution along the thigh is uneven, forcing excessive weight bearing on the ischia and coccyx. Excessive pressure on the ischia or coccyx may result in skin breakdown.

The seat-to-footplate length is used to determine the type of legrest or footrest selected for the wheelchair, in addition to adjusting the seat-to-footplate length. This measurement is also a factor when considering the seat-to-floor height of a wheelchair. A minimum of two inches between the floor and the under surface of the footplate is necessary to provide clearance over thresholds and other small obstacles. This distance to be measured is from the lowest point of the footplate to the floor. Seat-to-footplate distance and footplate clearance height must be determined in combination with the type of front rigging and wheel size to be chosen.

One measurement and one calculation are necessary to determine seat-to-footplate length.

1. The length of the individual's lower leg and height of the foot are measured from the posterior aspect of the thigh at the popliteal fossa to the sole of the foot at the heel.
2. The height of the seat cushion to be used must be subtracted from this measurement so the total measurement height includes the seat cushion.
3. The result of this measurement and calculation provides the desired seat-to-footplate length.

Measuring for Footplate Size

Footplate size is determined by the size of the patient's foot. Supporting this portion of the foot provides proper support of the lower extremity and assists in preventing development of deformities of the foot and ankle. While a significant portion of the foot must be supported, footrest length should be kept to a minimum to avoid interference with wheelchair maneuverability.

Footplates for the fixed frame ultra lightweight sport wheelchair are often smaller than those used on other frame styles. When footplates on fixed frame wheelchairs are positioned so that the knee is in 90 degrees or more of flexion, more of the forefoot than the hindfoot and heel is on the footplate.

One measurement is necessary to determine footplate size.

1. The portion of the foot that must be supported by a footplate extends from the calcaneus to the heads of the metatarsals.
2. The result of this measurement provides the desired footplate size.

STANDARD WHEELCHAIR SIZES

Table 7–1 provides standard measurements for wheelchairs of different sizes. When a standard-sized wheelchair appropriately fits an individual, the wheelchair is usually less costly and available in a shorter period of time. Custom fabrication, however, has become more commonly used to provide wheelchairs most appropriate for each individual.

TABLE 7–1 Standard Wheelchair Sizes			
Size	Seat Depth (inches)	Seat Width (inches)	Seat Height (inches)
Adult	16.0	18.0	20.00
Narrow adult	16.0	16.0	20.00
Slim adult	16.0	14.0	20.00
Tall adult	17.0	18.0	20.00
Hemi or low seat*			17.50
Pre-school	8.0	10.0	19.50
Tiny tot	11.5	12.0	19.50
Child	11.5	14.0	18.75
Junior	16.0	16.0	18.50

*Hemi or low seat can be any adult-size chair with respect to depth and width.

REVIEW QUESTIONS

1. When are wheel locks used?

2. What are the indications for the following variations of wheelchair components?

   Desk-length armrests
   Full-length armrests
   Adjustable-height armrests
   Elevating legrests
   Footrests

3. How does a tilt-in-space wheelchair differ from a reclining-back wheelchair?

4. How is an amputee wheelchair frame different from a standard frame?

5. Describe how to measure an individual for a wheelchair, including seat width, seat depth, seat height, back height, and armrest height.

6. How do wheelchair cushions affect measurements used to determine wheelchair fit?

7. What are the effects of inappropriate seat depth, seat width, or armrest height on sitting posture?

8. What is the effect of inappropriate footplate-to-seat distance on sitting posture?

9. What are the standard wheelchair sizes?

Suggested Activities

1. Practice as both therapist and patient on a variety of wheelchair components and types.

2. Remove, adjust, and replace all components on the available wheelchairs.

3. Measure available wheelchairs to determine size.

4. Measure several classmates to determine the correct wheelchair size.

5. Review available wheelchairs and discuss which individuals would likely use the wheelchair as it is configured.

6. Practice teaching "patients and family" and other health care providers how to adjust and handle wheelchairs correctly.

7. Document interventions and wheelchair measurements in SOAP note format.

Case Studies

1. An 8-year-old boy with a diagnosis of cerebral palsy presents with spastic quadriplegia. He is nonambulatory and has difficulty adjusting position and maintaining head alignment. Make recommendations for a type of mobility device and components that would be appropriate.

2. A 17-year-old female is 10 weeks post complete T10 spinal cord injury. Prior to her injury she participated on several elite sport teams. She has indicated that she will use a wheelchair rather than ambulate with crutches and orthosis. Indicate the measurements necessary to determine wheelchair size. Recommend the type of mobility device and components that would be appropriate.

3. A 67-year-old male with right hemiplegia following left CVA presents with slight spasticity and minimal voluntary control over both right extremities. Recommend the type of wheelchair and components that would be appropriate.

4. A 46-year-old female with a 20-year history of rheumatoid arthritis has significant involvement of all four extremities. She is able to walk only a few steps and stand for short periods. Recommend the type of mobility device and components that would be appropriate.

8

TRANSFERS

LEARNING OBJECTIVES

Upon completion of this chapter, you will be able to:

1. List transfers, indicating those that are dependent, assisted, or independent.
2. Describe and correctly perform dependent, assisted, and independent transfers.
3. Describe types and levels of assistance used when transferring a patient.

MEDIALINK

A companion CD-ROM, included free with each new copy of this book, supplements the techniques presented in the book. Insert the CD-ROM to watch video clips of patient care skills being demonstrated. This multimedia feature is designed to help you add a new dimension to your learning.

KEY TERMS

Assisted transfers
Close guarding
Contact guarding
Dependent transfers

Gait or transfer belts
Generalizability
Independent transfers
Levels of assistance

Maximum assistance
Minimal assistance
Moderate assistance
Stand-by assistance

INTRODUCTION

The purpose of transfers is to permit patients to function in different environments or use different pieces of equipment. A goal of transfer training is generalizability. **Generalizability** means that some skills learned for one transfer can be used for other transfers. For example, the skills for transferring from a wheelchair to a bed are similar to skills for transferring from a wheelchair to a couch. With modifications of basic transfer skills, transfers into bathtubs, cars, or onto toilets can also be achieved.

The transfer of a patient in or out of a wheelchair, bed, car, or cart may require the maximum assistance of several people, minimal assistance of one person, or no assistance at all. Each patient is examined, or a person knowledgeable about the patient's functional capabilities is interviewed, prior to determining an appropriate method of transfer. Physical therapists evaluate the results of the examination, which includes strength, ROM, pain, cognitive ability, and movement dysfunction to select an appropriate method of transfer that can be performed in a consistent, safe, and efficient manner. During rehabilitation, progression through levels, amounts, and type of assistance may occur.

Patient and physical therapist safety must not be compromised by the selection, or during the performance, of a transfer. Whenever in doubt about the level of assistance necessary to transfer a patient safely, obtain additional assistance. Wheelchairs, carts, or beds must always be stabilized by securing wheel locks, or by other means (i.e., bracing against a wall). Using proper body mechanics reduces the possibility of injury. Before beginning practice of transfers, review material on body mechanics in Chapter 2.

Several systems[1] indicating the level, amount, and type of assistance a patient requires are in current use. Regardless of the system used, documentation of levels, amounts, and types of assistance for each patient is required for safe duplication of transfers.

LEVELS OF TRANSFERS

Independent transfers are those transfers in which a patient consistently performs all aspects of the transfer, including set-up, in a safe manner and without assistance by additional personnel.

Assisted transfers are those transfers in which a patient participates actively, and requires assistance by additional (one or more) personnel. Assisted transfers include, but are not limited to, two-person lift, sliding board transfer, squat pivot, and assisted standing pivot transfer.

Dependent transfers are those transfers in which a patient does not participate actively, or participates only minimally, and additional personnel perform all aspects of the transfer. Dependent transfers include, but are not limited to, sliding transfer from cart to treatment table, three-person carry, dependent standing pivot transfer, and hydraulic lift transfer.

Some transfers may be assisted or independent, depending upon the physical capabilities of a patient. These include, but are not limited to, standing pivot, squat pivot, push-up, sliding board, wheelchair-to-floor, and floor-to-wheelchair transfers.

LEVELS OF ASSISTANCE

Indicating the level and amount of assistance required by a patient during a dependent or assisted transfer provides personnel with information necessary for completing a transfer safely. **Levels of assistance** can be stated as stand-by (supervision), close guarding, contact guarding, minimal, moderate, and maximum assistance. **Stand-by assistance** is indicated for patients who can usually perform the activity without assistance by additional personnel, but do not do so consistently. Examples of stand-by assistance include verbal cues, assistance in problem solving during transfer, or assistance if an emergency arises. In such cases additional personnel are not necessarily in close proximity to the patient. **Close guarding** is indicated for patients who can usually perform the activity without assistance by personnel, but have a greater likelihood for needing physical assistance by additional personnel for support or balance. In such cases additional personnel are in close proximity to the patient, immediately ready to assist the patient. **Contact guarding** is indicated for patients who can usually perform the activity, but have a significant likelihood of requiring physical assistance by additional personnel for support or balance. In such cases additional personnel maintain contact with the patient to be able to provide assistance immediately. **Minimal assistance** is indicated for patients who can perform at least 75% of the activity. **Moderate assistance** is indicated for patients who can perform at least 50% of the activity. **Maximum assistance** is indicated for patients who can perform less than 25% of the activity.

AMOUNT OF ASSISTANCE

When more than one person is required for safe transfers, the number is indicated by adding the number after the level of assistance, such as X2 when two people are required to complete the transfer safely. Therefore, an indication of the level and amount of assistance required when a patient requires moderate assistance of two people during a transfer would be ". . . moderate assist X2 . . . "

TYPE OF ASSISTANCE

Type of assistance is indicated as verbal cuing, balance control, and physical assistance for lifting or supporting. For example, one patient may require minimal assistance for balance control. A second patient may require moderate assistance X2 for lifting. Yet a third patient may require stand-by (supervision) assistance for verbal cuing of instructions.

As a patient improves, the type of transfer may progress from dependent, to assisted, to independent. The amount of assistance may progress from maximum to none as the patient progresses. The type of assistance may progress from the physical therapist doing all the lifting to the physical therapist using only verbal cuing. The goal is for the patient to achieve the maximum level of independent performance of a transfer that is consistent, safe, and efficient.

GENERAL RULES

BODY MECHANICS

Proper attention to body mechanics and the relationship of center of mass and base of support permit physical therapists to maintain the safest position while working with patients. Positioning patients close to a physical therapist's base of support places less stress on the physical therapist's back and upper extremities when physical assistance is required. Such positioning allows a physical therapist's hands to be placed on the appropriate aspect of a patient's anatomy to provide support, such as under the buttocks for lifting, or behind the hips for moving the patient into the physical therapist's base of support. Direct contact with a patient permits a physical therapist's manual contacts to provide input to the patient concerning correct direction of movement, providing a learning tool for a patient to be an active participant during transfers.

GAIT OR TRANSFER BELTS

Gait or transfer belts are belts secured around a patient's waist, providing a secure point of contact and control for a physical therapist. When secured and used properly, gait or transfer belts provide an alternative method to control patient motion during transfers. When direct manual contacts cannot be maintained safely, such as with an extremely large patient, or a patient with wounds or lesions which limit places for contact, a gait or transfer belt provides a method of controlling a patient safely. When a transfer belt is used, patients should be maintained in close proximity to the physical therapist and not at arm's length.

When held at arm's length, a patient is not fully supported and the physical therapist is at greater risk for injury to the back and upper extremity. This occurs because improper use of gait or transfer belts reduces safety for both patients and physical therapists by moving a patient's center of mass away from the physical therapist's base of support. Gait or transfer belts must not become only a handle for maneuvering patients during transfers. Simply pushing, pulling, or lifting on gait or transfer belts alone does not provide specific support needed by patients during transfers. This occurs because improper use of gait or transfer belts does not provide the guidance that manual contacts can to help patients understand the direction of movement required, and to become an active participant in performing a transfer.

In some settings or jurisdictions, gait or transfer belts may be required equipment. Each physical therapist is responsible for determining the administrative and legal requirements of practicing in a specific setting or jurisdiction. Administrative or legal requirements for specific equipment exist in an effort to limit injury or liability. When specific equipment must be used, users must adhere to proper application and use of the equipment.

Preparing the Environment

When preparing the environment for transfers, consideration must be given to the direction in which the patient will move—to the left or right. Generally, when patients have more involvement on one side than the other, transferring toward the stronger side is easier. This direction can be used during initial transfers to ensure success and bolster a patient's confidence. Patients, however, need to be able to transfer to both sides, and transfers should be practiced to both sides. Specific considerations for preparing the environment for each type of transfer will be covered later in this chapter. Additional considerations for preparing an environment can be found in Chapter 2.

Personnel performing transfers should avoid wearing jewelry that can become entangled or scratch patients during patient care. Such jewelry must be removed before patient contact is initiated. For example, watches and rings need to be removed before sliding arms under or around a patient.

Instructions and Verbal Cues

A patient should always be informed about the transfer to be performed, and what he or she is expected to do. Explanations must be provided in a manner understood by patients, using nontechnical terms, and employing a language interpreter if necessary.

Counts and commands are used to synchronize actions of all participants in the transfer. When assistance of more than one person is required for a transfer, the physical therapist at the head of the patient is in charge and is responsible successful completion of the transfer. The physical therapist in charge explains how the transfer will be conducted and indicates the responsibilities of each participant. Counting is used to provide a cue for the ensuing command. This allows all participants to be ready for the command. Specific terms, such as "lift," are used to indicate the command. Commands are the specific action word that participants are to perform when the command term is given. An appropriate count and command is "One, two, three, lift." The word "lift" is a specific indication of the action that is to occur. An inappropriate count and command is "One, two, three." This is inappropriate because the count "three" is not a specific action command. The physical therapist in charge describes the counts and commands that will be given and gives the counts and commands. For example, the sequence of directions and language used by the physical therapist in charge might be:

1. "I will count to three and then give the command to lift."
2. "When I say 'lift,' we will lift."
3. The physical therapist checks visually and verbally to ensure that all assistants and the patient are ready before the transfer is initiated.
4. The physical therapist says "One, two, three, lift."

COMPLETING THE TRANSFER

A transfer is not complete until the patient is safely and securely in the new position. Contact and control of the patient is maintained until the patient is secure in the new position. Appropriate positioning and draping must be completed and necessary equipment placed within usable reach of the patient. The patient must feel secure in his or her new position. Only then is a transfer considered complete.

PROCEDURE 8-1

SLIDING TRANSFER: CART TO TREATMENT TABLE

This transfer can be used to transfer a patient between two treatment tables, a treatment table and cart, or cart and bed. The cart should be positioned parallel to, and against, the treatment table, and secured. The cart should be positioned with the patient's head at the head of the treatment table or cart. In the following illustrations, two treatment tables are used. The first treatment table represents a cart or gurney and will be referred to as a cart. The second treatment table represents a treatment table or bed and will be referred to as a treatment table.

When a patient can perform this transfer with stand-by or minimal assistance, one person may assist by stabilizing the cart, and when necessary, providing minimal verbal or physical assistance.

When a dependent transfer is required, three personnel are needed. A "draw" sheet may be used to move ("draw") the patient from cart to treatment table.

1. A draw sheet is placed under the patient.

2. The portion of the sheet to the patient's sides is rolled and grasped close to the patient. A stronger grip is created when grasping with the forearm supinated.
The physical therapist at the patient's head should be on the side to which the patient is moving. This physical therapist is responsible for coordinating the transfer by instructing the patient and assistants, determining when everyone is ready, and issuing the counts and commands.

3. When patients are unable to control the head and neck, the physical therapist at the patient's head supports the patient's head by placing one arm under the patient's shoulders while cradling the patient's head.

4. When a patient's extraneous movements cannot be controlled during a transfer, or if a patient is agitated, a sheet may be wrapped around the patient to provide control of the patient's extremities.

5. Two people, the physical therapist at the patient's head and the assistant at the lower extremities, stand on the side to which the patient is to be moved and grasp the sheet close to the patient. One assistant stands on the other side and grasps the sheet with one hand at the patient's shoulder and the other hand at the patient's hip. When the two people on the side to which the patient is to be moved are not able to reach across the treatment table to lift the patient, they may kneel on the treatment table.

6. Upon the physical therapist's counts and commands, the patient is lifted and moved part of the way from the cart onto the treatment table.

(continued)

7. Once the patient has been moved part way onto the treatment table, the people on the side to which the patient is being moved remove themselves from the treatment table. The assistant on the side from which the patient is being moved may kneel on the cart to complete the transfer. The transfer is completed by finishing movement of the patient to the treatment table.

PROCEDURE 8–2

THREE-PERSON CARRY

This is a dependent transfer, used to transfer a patient between two treatment tables, a treatment table and cart, or cart and bed. When the two surfaces cannot be arranged parallel to each other, or a sliding transfer is deemed unsafe, a three-person carry is used. As the name of the transfer implies, three people are required to transfer an average size adult.

A cart is positioned and secured at right angles to a treatment table, with the head of the cart at the foot of the table or the foot of the cart at the head of the table. In the following photos, two treatment tables are used. The first treatment table represents a cart or gurney and will be referred to as a cart. The second treatment table represents a treatment table or bed and will be referred to as a treatment table.

1. All three personnel stand on the same side of the cart and are positioned in such a manner that one can support the head and upper trunk, one can support the midsection, and one can support the lower extremities. The strongest person should be at the patient's head or middle position. The tallest person, if strong enough, should be at the patient's head. The physical therapist at the head of the patient is responsible for instructing the patient, determining when everyone is ready, and issuing counts and commands. Personnel stand in stride with their feet slightly apart and knees flexed.

2. Personnel slide their arms under the patient such that their elbows are on the cart and the patient is cradled from head to foot.

(continued)

3. Upon command, the patient is moved to the edge of the cart.

4. By flexing elbows, personnel log-roll the patient onto his side such that he is facing the personnel. The patient is now cradled in the bend of the elbows, bringing the patient's weight closer to the base of support of the personnel.

5. Upon command, personnel stand, lifting the patient from the cart.

6. Upon command, personnel walk backward to pivot 90 degrees.

7. Upon completion of the 90-degree pivot, personnel are aligned parallel to the treatment table.

8. Personnel then move forward in unison to the treatment table.

(continued)

9. Personnel stand in stride at the edge of the treatment table. Upon command, personnel flex their legs until elbows rest on the edge of the treatment table, lowering the patient to the treatment table.

10. The patient is uncradled onto the treatment table, moved to the center of the treatment table, and positioned in proper alignment. Personnel then remove their arms carefully.

HYDRAULIC LIFT

Hydraulic lifts are mechanical devices that provide a method for one person to transfer a dependent patient. Hydraulic lifts have caster wheels for positioning and maneuvering. The following illustrations present a transfer from a treatment table to a wheelchair.

The base of hydraulic lifts can be widened to fit around a wheelchair or other equipment. The base is placed in the narrow position when the patient is being moved to make maneuvering easier. To change the width of the base, the long lever attached to the base is moved from one side to the other (Figures 8–1 and 8–2). This lever is locked by either a slotted mechanism at the bottom of the lever or by a cam locking mechanism that is activated and deactivated by twisting the lever.

FIGURE 8–1   Narrowing the base of a hydraulic lift.

FIGURE 8–2   Widening the base of a hydraulic lift.

A hydraulic release valve (Figure 8–3) on the front of the lift's upright is closed to allow the arm of the hydraulic lift to be raised and opened slowly to allow lowering of the lift arm. After checking that the hydraulic release valve is closed, a physical therapist pumps the handle to raise the arm of the hydraulic lift (Figure 8–4).

FIGURE 8–3 Hydraulic release valve knob for lift arm.

FIGURE 8–4 Hydraulic pump handle.

Patients are supported by a sling, which is attached to a spreader bar on the lift arm, by two chains with hooks (Figure 8–5). Chain lengths must be adjusted to accommodate the height of each patient. The chains are attached to each side of the spreader bar such that each chain is divided into two unequal segments. The shorter segment of each chain is the segment that will be attached to the upper part of the sling, the part that will be supporting the patient's back. The longer segment of each chain is the segment that will be attached to the lower part of the sling, the part that will be supporting the patient's lower extremities. In this way, the patient can be lifted.

FIGURE 8–5 Attaching chains to spreader bar.

Slings are made of a variety of fabrics. Some are one piece and others are two pieces. Slings are positioned so seams are on the outside, away from the patient, to avoid pressure areas. Chain hooks are attached from inside the sling to the outside (Figure 8–6). This reduces the likelihood of patients being injured by the hook.

FIGURE 8–6 Attaching chain hooks to sling.

PROCEDURE 8-3

USING A HYDRAULIC LIFT

1. When a patient is on a cart, treatment table, or bed, slings can be positioned under the patient by rolling the patient onto one side and properly positioning a sling on the treatment table.

2. The patient is rolled onto the sling. If necessary, the patient is then rolled onto her other side to allow proper alignment of the sling under the patient.

3. Once a patient is positioned on the sling, the hydraulic lift is moved into position with the spreader bar suspended across the patient. Both ends of each chain are attached to their respective sides of the sling.

4. With the hydraulic release valve closed, a physical therapist pumps the handle to lift the patient to a safe sitting position.

5. As a patient is lifted above the treatment table, physical therapists place an arm under the patient's lower extremities to remove them from the treatment table.

6. Cradling a patient's lower extremities, physical therapists rotate the lower extremities from over the treatment table and allow the sling to provide full support.

7. Physical therapists may need to steady the patient to prevent excessive sway as the lift, with patient, is maneuvered. The patient is moved to a locked wheelchair. The base is placed in the wide position to fit around the perimeter of the wheelchair.

8. The lift is maneuvered to position a patient directly over the seat of a locked wheelchair.

(continued)

9. The hydraulic release valve is opened slowly to lower the patient into a wheelchair. Seating a patient properly in a wheelchair requires slight pressure in the horizontal plane applied at the knees or thighs. This positions a patient into the wheelchair such that her back is resting firmly against the back of the wheelchair.

10. Once a patient is seated in the wheelchair, the hydraulic release valve is closed to avoid the potential of the lift arm lowering further and striking the patient.

11. After determining that a patient can maintain sitting without assistance, a physical therapist removes the chains from the sling and moves the hydraulic lift away from the patient. The physical therapist must ensure that the spreader bar and chains do not swing and strike a patient as the lift is removed.

12. A one-piece sling is left in place under the patient. Hence, the initial need to position a sling appropriately to avoid pressure from the seams.

13. The wheelchair's pelvic stabilizer is secured and the patient's feet are placed properly on footrests. When a two-piece sling has been used, the upper portion of the sling, which is behind a patient's back, may be removed, while the portion under a patient's thighs remains in place.

PROCEDURE 8-4

TWO-PERSON LIFT

Wheelchair to Floor

The two-person lift transfer is an assisted transfer with maximum assistance of two personnel. This transfer is often used to move a patient between a wheelchair and the floor when the patient has some upper extremity strength and trunk control.

1. Patients participate in this transfer by crossing their upper extremities in front of the trunk. Standing behind the patient, a physical therapist reaches under the patient's upper extremities and grasps the opposite wrists of the patient (left on right and right on left). This prevents patients from abducting upper extremities during the lift. Patients must be able to maintain an upper extremity position of shoulder girdle depression, shoulder extension, adduction, internal rotation, and elbow flexion at approximately 90 degrees to assist in successful completion of the transfer.

2. To prepare for a two-person lift transfer, a wheelchair is positioned close, and parallel, to the surface to which a patient will be transferred. Wheel locks are engaged and the patient's feet are removed from the footrests. The footplates are raised. Footrests are removed from the wheelchair when possible, or swung out of the way. The armrest on the side of the wheelchair to which the patient will be transferred is removed.

3. The physical therapist at the head of the patient places one foot on either side of the drive wheel and leans around the push handle on the side to which the transfer will occur. A second physical therapist faces in the direction of the intended transfer, with feet in stride and hips and knees flexed. This physical therapist places one arm under the thighs and the other arm under the legs. The position of both physical therapists may be modified, depending upon the sizes of patient and physical therapist, and the environment in which the transfer will occur.

4. On command from the physical therapist at the head of the patient, both personnel straighten, lifting the patient to a height, ensuring clearance of all parts of the wheelchair.

5. In unison, the physical therapists step to the side (physical therapist at patient's head) or forward (physical therapist supporting lower extremities), moving away from the wheelchair.

(continued)

6. Both physical therapists squat, using good body mechanics to lower the patient to the floor.

7. Physical therapists continue contact for support until patients are able to maintain a safe and comfortable position.

Floor to Wheelchair

To prepare for a two-person lift transfer, a wheelchair is positioned close, and parallel, to the surface from which a patient will be transferred. Wheel locks are engaged and footplates raised. Footrests are removed from the wheelchair when possible, or swung out of the way. The armrest on the side of the wheelchair closest to the patient is removed.

1. Patients participate in this transfer by crossing their upper extremities in front of the trunk. Squatting behind the patient, a physical therapist reaches under the patient's upper extremities and grasps the opposite wrists of the patient (left on right and right on left). This prevents patients from abducting upper extremities during the lift. Patients must be able to maintain an upper extremity position of shoulder girdle depression, shoulder extension, adduction, internal rotation, and elbow flexion at approximately 90 degrees to assist in successful completion of the transfer.

2. A second physical therapist faces in the direction of the intended transfer, squatting with feet in stride. Although starting in a half-kneeling position may seem easier for the second physical therapist, this necessitates movement into a squatting position, increasing the risk of injury to all participants. This physical therapist places one arm under the thighs and the other arm under the legs. The position of both physical therapists may be modified, depending upon the sizes of patient and physical therapist and the environment in which the transfer will occur.

3. On command from the physical therapist at the head of the patient, the patient is lifted to a height that ensures clearance of all parts of the wheelchair.

(continued)

4. In unison, the physical therapists step to the side (physical therapist at patient's head) or forward (physical therapist supporting lower extremities), moving toward the wheelchair. The physical therapists move until the patient is centered over the seat of the wheelchair. The physical therapist supporting the patient's lower extremities gently pulls the patient's lower extremities away from the back of the wheelchair so the patient will clear the upright of the back of the wheelchair. Once the wheelchair back upright has been cleared, the patient must be pushed toward the back of the wheelchair for the assumption of proper sitting posture.

5. Physical therapists continue contact for support until patients are able to maintain a safe and comfortable position. When the patient is seated in a position she can maintain, the pelvic stabilizer is secured, armrest and footrests are replaced, and the patient's feet are placed on the footrests.

PROCEDURE 8–5

DEPENDENT STANDING PIVOT

The dependent standing pivot transfer is an assisted transfer with maximum assistance of one person. The dependent standing pivot transfer is used for patients who are unable to stand independently, but can bear some weight on their lower extremities. This includes patients with weakness, paresis, or paralysis.

1. To perform a dependent standing pivot transfer, a wheelchair is placed parallel to a treatment table or bed and wheel locks are engaged.

2. The patient's feet are placed on the floor, footplates are raised, and footrests are removed from the wheelchair when possible, or swung out of the way.

3. The armrest nearest the treatment table is removed.

4. To facilitate clearing the wheel, the patient is moved to the front edge of the wheelchair seat.

5. To provide stability for the patient's lower extremities during the transfer, the physical therapist must "block" the patient's lower extremities. Blocking the lower extremities is performed in different ways for different transfers. In this transfer, blocking is achieved by placing the physical therapist's feet and knees outside the patient's feet and knees, with the physical therapist holding the patient's knees between his knees. The physical therapist's foot closest to the treatment table is placed a little behind the other foot, placing the physical therapist's feet in stride. After the patient's lower extremities are blocked, the physical therapist's hands are placed under the patient's buttocks. The physical therapist must create and maintain a static spinal posture throughout this transfer. The position of a physical therapist may be modified, depending upon the sizes of patient and physical therapist and the environment in which the transfer will occur.

(continued)

6. The patient places the upper extremities around the physical therapist's upper back. The purpose of the placement of the patient's arms is to provide control for the patient's upper trunk, and not for the patient to "pull" on the therapist. To avoid injury to the physical therapist, care must be taken that the patient's arms are not placed around the physical therapist's neck, and that the physical therapist maintains static spinal posture throughout the transfer. Improper patient upper extremity placement may also lead to loss of control of the patient during transfer. An alternative position, when a patient cannot place the upper extremities around the physical therapist's upper back, is for a patient to rest the head on one of the physical therapist's shoulders. It is best if the shoulder used is the shoulder on the side of the physical therapist opposite to the direction in which the pivot will occur.

7. To synchronize the effort of the physical therapist and patient, the physical therapist provides counts and commands ("One, two, three, up."). As the physical therapist counts, a rocking motion in time with the counts is initiated to develop momentum. On the command "up," the physical therapist lifts the patient from the wheelchair. The lift is only high enough to clear the wheelchair and the height of the treatment table.

8. The physical therapist pivots toward the treatment table, rotating the patient to the proper position for sitting on the table. The patient is lowered to a sitting position.

9. Physical therapists must continue contact for support until patients are able to maintain a safe and comfortable position.

PROCEDURE 8-6

 SLIDING BOARD

The sliding board transfer is an assisted or independent transfer that may require moderate assistance of two personnel to no assistance at all. The sliding board transfer is used when patients have enough strength to lift most of the weight off the buttocks, sufficient sitting balance to move in a sitting position, but are not able to perform push-up transfers.

When performing a one-person assisted transfer, physical therapists guard a patient by standing in front of the patient and may block the knees to prevent her from sliding off the sliding board. When assistance in lifting is required, physical therapists do so by placing their hands under a patient's buttocks and lifting as the patient performs the push-up. When a patient needs assistance for balance, physical therapists can place their hands on the patient's shoulders. Assistance for lifting or balance is decreased as a patient improves.

1. To perform a sliding board transfer, a wheelchair is positioned parallel, or at a slight angle, to a treatment table or bed, and the wheel locks are engaged. The patient's feet are placed on the floor, footplates are raised, and footrests are removed from the wheelchair when possible, or swung out of the way. The patient moves forward to the front of the wheelchair seat. The armrest on the side nearest the treatment table is removed. In the illustrations presenting the sliding board transfer, assistance is being provided for balance.

2. The patient leans away from the treatment table and a sliding board is placed well under the buttocks. Care must be taken not to pinch the patient between the sliding board and the wheelchair seat.

3. The patient returns to an upright sitting position, with the buttock nearest the treatment table resting on the sliding board.

4. The patient performs the transfer by doing a series of push-ups and slides sideways. Extending the upper extremities, accompanied by shoulder depression, allows patients to lift their body and decrease weight on the sliding board. Reducing body weight on the sliding board permits patients to slide toward the treatment table. A patient may place palms flat on the sliding board, or make a fist and place the outside of the fists on the sliding board to achieve higher lift during push-ups. Wheelchair armrests can be used for the first few push-ups to achieve higher lift. Patients must not grasp the edge of the sliding board as fingers may be pinched as push-ups are performed.

(continued)

5. Repositioning hands, this sequence is repeated until the patient is on the treatment table and only one buttock remains on the sliding board.

6. The patient leans away from the wheelchair to remove the sliding board. Physical therapists must continue contact for support until patients are able to maintain a safe and comfortable position.

The transfer from treatment table to the wheelchair using a sliding board is essentially the same. Follow the steps below.

1. Placing sliding board.

2. Pushing up and sliding.

3. Sliding into wheelchair.

4. Removing sliding board.

PROCEDURE 8-7

PUSH-UP

The push-up transfer is an assisted or independent transfer that may require moderate assistance of two personnel to no assistance at all. The push-up transfer is used when patients have enough strength to lift themselves from the supporting surface and sufficient sitting balance to move in a sitting position. A push-up transfer is performed in a manner similar to a sliding board transfer, except that a push-up transfer does not use a sliding board for support.

To perform a push-up transfer, a wheelchair is positioned parallel, or at a slight angle, to a treatment table or bed, and the wheel locks are engaged. The patient's feet are placed on the floor, footplates are raised, and footrests are removed from the wheelchair when possible, or swung out of the way. The patient moves forward to the front of the wheelchair seat. The armrest on the side nearest the treatment table is removed.

The patient performs the transfer by doing a series of push-ups and moves sideways. Extending the upper extremities, accompanied by shoulder depression, allows patients to lift their body. In the illustrations of a push-up transfer, the physical therapist is blocking the patient's knees to prevent the patient from sliding too far forward and guarding at the patient's shoulders for balance. As a patient's capabilities progress, a push-up transfer may be completed using only one push-up.

1. Pushing up to perform push-up transfer.

2. Lowering from a push-up.

3. Pushing up to treatment table.

4. Lowering onto treatment table.

A push-up transfer from treatment table to a wheelchair is essentially the same. Follow the steps below.

1. Starting to return to wheelchair from treatment table.

2. Midpoint of return to wheelchair from treatment table.

3. Completing return to wheelchair from treatment table.

Physical therapists must continue contact for support until patients are able to maintain a safe and comfortable position.

PROCEDURE 8-8

 ASSIST TO FRONT OF WHEELCHAIR SEAT

A patient must be able to maneuver to the front of a wheelchair seat prior to standing or performing transfers. Sitting on the front of a wheelchair seat allows patients to get their center of mass over their base of support rapidly and easily as they assume standing. When patients are unable to maneuver forward in a wheelchair independently, several methods can be used to assist. As a patient's ability improves, assistance is reduced until the patient is performing the task independently.

To perform these movements, a wheelchair is positioned where desired and the wheel locks are engaged. The patient's feet are placed on the floor, footplates are raised, and footrests are removed from the wheelchair when possible, or swung out of the way.

Side-to-Side Weight Shifting

1. In the side-to-side weight shifting method, physical therapists assist patients to the front of a wheelchair seat by placing one arm around the patient's shoulders from one side and the other arm under the thigh of the opposite lower extremity.
2. The patient's weight is shifted to the side of shoulder support to reduce weight-bearing on the supported thigh and buttock.

3. While the thigh and buttock are unloaded, the patient is assisted in moving the unloaded thigh and buttock forward.

4. The patient's thigh and buttock that have been supported are returned to the wheelchair seat and the patient is returned to an erect sitting position.
5. Physical therapists reverse arm positions and perform the same maneuver to the opposite side. This sequence is repeated from side to side until patients are properly positioned at the front of the wheelchair seat. Physical therapists must continue contact for support until patients are able to maintain a safe and comfortable position.

Pelvic Slide

The pelvic slide method of assisting a patient to the front of a wheelchair seat involves moving a patient's pelvis and upper trunk as separate units. Physical therapists place both hands under a patient's buttocks and assist patients to lift and slide the buttocks to the front of the wheelchair seat.

1. Starting position to slide pelvis forward.

2. Pelvis at front of wheelchair seat.

Physical therapists then place hands behind a patient's shoulders and assist patients in moving their shoulders forward over the pelvis into an erect sitting position. A physical therapist must continue contact for support until patients are able to maintain a safe and comfortable position.

3. Starting position to move shoulders forward.

4. Patient sitting erect with shoulders over pelvis.

Sitting Push-Up

The sitting push-up method of assisting patients to the front of a wheelchair seat requires patients to perform sitting push-ups. Physical therapists may assist by lifting under a patient's buttocks or by guarding at the shoulders. Each time a patient is lowered back to the wheelchair seat, they are lowered closer to the front of the wheelchair seat. Physical therapists must continue contact for support until patients are able to maintain a safe and comfortable position.

1. Starting position to assist sitting push-up.

2. Assisting sitting push-up by lifting.

3. Lowered to front of wheelchair seat.

PROCEDURE 8-9

ASSIST FOR MOVING FROM EDGE OF TREATMENT TABLE

When patients sit on the edge of a treatment table or bed and are unable to move more completely onto the table, physical therapists can assist by using a reversal of the side-to-side weight shifting or push-up maneuvers used to move a patient forward on a wheelchair seat. For the side-to-side weight shifting method, physical therapists assist patients in moving their thighs and buttocks backward onto a treatment table or bed, rather than moving the thighs and buttocks forward to the front of a wheelchair seat.

Physical therapists must guard against patients sliding off the front of the treatment table as the patient's weight is shifted. The maneuver is repeated side to side as needed. These maneuvers can also be used to assist patients in being seated fully against the back of a wheelchair. Physical therapists must continue contact for support until patients are able to maintain a safe and comfortable position.

1. Shifting patient's weight to one side.

2. Moving backward onto treatment table.

3. Shifting patient's weight to opposite side.

PROCEDURE 8–10

 ASSISTED STANDING PIVOT

The assisted standing pivot transfer is an assisted transfer that may require moderate to minimal assistance of one person. The assisted standing pivot transfer is used when patients can sit, stand, pivot, and bear some weight on the lower extremities, but have some weakness, paresis, paralysis, or loss of balance or sensation, which necessitates assistance to transfer safely. This transfer is also used to teach patients to transfer independently. Physical therapists reduce the amount of assistance provided to patients until the highest possible level of independence is achieved.

By varying hand position, physical therapists can vary the amount and type of assistance provided to patients performing this transfer. By placing a hand under the buttocks, physical therapists can assist by lifting as a patient rises to standing.

By placing a hand on the posterolateral aspect of the pelvis, physical therapists can guide as a patient rises to standing. Physical therapists are in a position to control excessive lateral shift of the pelvis and the physical therapist's hand can be moved quickly to the posterior aspect of the pelvis to support patients when necessary.

(continued)

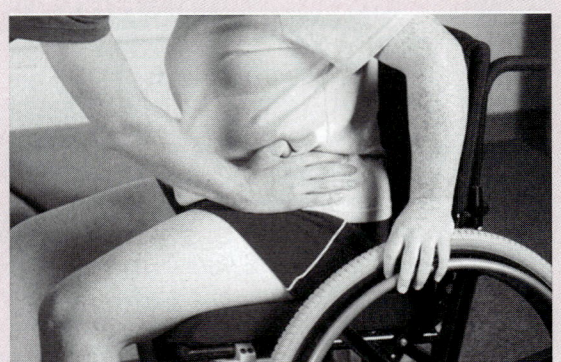

By placing a hand on the anterolateral aspect of the pelvis, physical therapists can guide or resist movement as a patient rises to standing. Resistance may provide facilitation, making the activity easier, and teaches patients to bring the pelvis forward as they rise.

For complete independence, patients must be able to transfer to both sides. When first teaching patients to transfer, moving toward the uninvolved side is easier and safer for many patients because they are moving toward the side in which the lower extremity can provide support. Teaching patients to transfer toward the involved side reinforces a patient's awareness and use of the involved side.

When a physical therapist is unsure of a patient's capability, the patient's uninvolved lower extremity is guarded to ensure support on at least one side during the transfer. Physical therapists always guard the hip and knee on the same side, whether guarding the uninvolved or involved side, by having a knee in contact with the anterolateral aspect of the patient's knee and a hand in contact with the patient's hip.

Guarding the Right Lower Extremity While Transferring to Right

When transferring from a wheelchair to treatment table or bed by pivoting to the right, patients are positioned so the treatment table is to the right during the transfer. The wheelchair is placed parallel, or at a slight angle, to the treatment table and wheel locks are engaged. The patient's feet are placed on the floor, footplates are raised, and footrests are removed from the wheelchair when possible, or swung out of the way. Patients move forward to the front of the wheelchair seat (with assistance when necessary) as described previously.

In this example, the physical therapist is guarding the patient's right knee with his right knee and the patient's right hip with his left hand. This position prevents the patient from collapsing at these joints.

1. The physical therapist's right hand is on the patient's left shoulder to prevent the patient from falling to the left. The physical therapist stands in stride with his right foot medial to the patient's right foot. This position provides a base of support in the direction of transfer and permits both patient and physical therapist to move without tangling feet once the patient is standing. This position also allows the physical therapist to move the patient's foot if the patient does not pivot as the transfer proceeds.

2. The patient positions her feet below the front of the wheelchair seat and initiates standing by leaning forward and pushing to standing using the armrest of the wheelchair.

(continued)

3. The patient pushes to standing using the armrest of the wheelchair. A full upright position, under control, is attained.

4. The patient pivots to the right, toward the treatment table.

5. The patient lowers to the treatment table. If necessary, assistance is provided.

6. A physical therapist must continue contact for support until the patient is able to maintain a safe and comfortable position.

Guarding the Left Lower Extremity While Transferring to Right

When transferring from a wheelchair to treatment table or bed by pivoting to the right, patients are positioned so the treatment table is to the right during the transfer. The wheelchair is placed parallel, or at a slight angle, to the treatment table and wheel locks are engaged. The patient's feet are placed on the floor, footplates are raised, and footrests are removed from the wheelchair when possible, or swung out of the way. Patients move forward to the front of the wheelchair seat (with assistance when necessary) as described previously.

In this example, the physical therapist is guarding the patient's left knee with his right knee, and the patient's left hip with his right hand. This position prevents the patient from collapsing at these joints.

1. The physical therapist's left hand is on the patient's right shoulder to prevent the patient from falling to the right. The physical therapist stands in stride with his right foot lateral to the patient's left foot. This position provides a base of support in the direction of transfer and permits both patient and physical therapist to move without tangling feet once the patient is standing. This position also allows the physical therapist to move the patient's foot if the patient does not pivot as the transfer proceeds.

(continued)

2. The patient positions her feet below the front of the wheelchair seat and initiates standing by leaning forward and pushing to standing using the armrest of the wheelchair.

3. The patient pushes to standing using the armrest of the wheelchair.

4. A full upright position, under control, is attained.

5. The patient pivots to the right, toward the treatment table.

6. The patient lowers to the treatment table. If necessary, assistance is provided. A physical therapist must continue contact for support until the patient is able to maintain a safe and comfortable position.

Wheelchair to Treatment Table: Using a Step Stool

Transferring patients to a high treatment table requires use of a step stool, especially when a patient is short. The position of the wheelchair, guarding techniques, and activity of coming to standing are performed as in an assisted standing pivot transfer. In the following sequence, the patient is demonstrating a transfer to the right, while the physical therapist is guarding the left lower extremity. The guarding position and sequence are performed as in an assisted standing pivot transfer to the right while guarding the left lower extremity, as described in the immediately preceding section.

1. A step stool must be placed close to the physical therapist so the physical therapist can retrieve and position the step stool while guarding the patient.

2. Once the patient has attained a standing position, the stool is placed alongside the treatment table and in front of the patient.

3. Having attained an erect position, the patient places her hand on the treatment table. With her hand on the table, the patient places the foot of her right lower extremity on the stool. The physical therapist guards the left lower extremity to ensure adequate support as the patient lifts and places her foot on the stool. The patient steps onto the stool, lifting and pivoting her body over the stool, and raises her pelvis above the level of the treatment table.

4. The patient then lowers herself to sitting on the treatment table. As described previously, the patient moves completely onto the table. Physical therapists must continue contact for support until patients are able to maintain a safe and comfortable position.

5. To return to a wheelchair from a high treatment table, a stool is not needed. A physical therapist should be prepared to guard either lower extremity as a patient slides from sitting on the treatment table to standing on the floor in a controlled manner.

PROCEDURE 8-11

SQUAT PIVOT TRANSFER

The squat pivot transfer is an assisted transfer that requires minimal assistance of one person. The squat pivot transfer is used when patients can sit, stand, pivot, and bear weight on the lower extremities, but have some weakness, paresis, or loss of balance or sensation, which necessitates assistance to transfer safely.

1. A wheelchair is placed parallel, or at a slight angle, to a treatment table or bed, and wheel locks are engaged. The patient's feet are placed on the floor, footplates are raised, and footrests are removed from the wheelchair when possible, or swung out of the way. Patients move toward the edge of the treatment table (with assistance when necessary) as described previously. A physical therapist sits on a wheeled stool in front of the patient, blocking both of the patient's knees with her knees. The physical therapist's hands are placed on the posterolateral lower thoracic region.

2. The physical therapist assists the patient to perform an anterior pelvic tilt and extension of the upper back, while the patient shifts weight forward onto her feet. This results in the proper position for the patient to rise from the treatment table.

3. Without coming to a complete standing position, the patient raises, pivots toward the wheelchair, and lowers to the treatment table. The patient repeats the sequence until she is seated in the wheelchair.

4. As a patient's capabilities progress, a patient may be able to complete the transfer in one lift and pivot movement.

Raising from treatment table.

Pivoting to wheelchair.

Lowering to sitting in wheelchair.

5. A physical therapist must continue contact for support until patients are able to maintain a safe and comfortable position.

PROCEDURE 8-12

TRANSFERS BETWEEN FLOOR AND WHEELCHAIR

Transfers between a wheelchair and floor are necessary should a patient fall out of a wheelchair, or when patients want to participate in activities on the floor. Occasionally a patient may fall out of, or tip over, a wheelchair.

Dependent One-Person Transfer: Floor to Wheelchair

When an adult patient is unable to transfer from the floor to a wheelchair independently, either a one-person or two-person transfer may be used to get the patient back into the wheelchair. While a two-person lift is desired, because it is safer for patients and personnel, a one-person transfer may be necessary. Safe performance of a one-person transfer depends upon the relative sizes of patients and personnel, the patient's capabilities, and the environment. A physical therapist is responsible for making such a decision and instructing patient and personnel in proper performance.

1. To perform a dependent one-person transfer, a wheelchair is positioned on its back at the patient's feet. A physical therapist places one arm under the patient's lower extremities and the other arm behind the patient's upper back, such that the patient's lower extremities are flexed at the hips and knees.

2. The patient is moved toward the wheelchair seat such that the ankles are placed over the front edge of the wheelchair seat. The physical therapist performs a series of short lifting and sliding maneuvers to move the patient into the wheelchair.

3. When the patient's buttocks are in contact with the wheelchair seat, the physical therapist moves to the patient's head. He then squats to grasp both handles of the wheelchair while cradling the patient's upper trunk on his forearms.

4. The patient and wheelchair are lifted as a unit as the physical therapist moves to a standing position. When a patient is tall, or the back of the wheelchair is low, the physical therapist may grasp one handle of the wheelchair with one hand and support and lift the patient's trunk with the other hand.

Initiating lift.

Midposition of lift.

(continued)

5. As the wheelchair approaches an upright position, the physical therapist shifts one arm to guard the anterior aspect of the patient's upper trunk to prevent her from falling forward.

PROCEDURE 8-13

INDEPENDENT TRANSFER FROM WHEELCHAIR TO FLOOR AND RETURN

Many patients can, and must, learn to move safely from a wheelchair to the floor, and back into the wheelchair. There are several methods for performing this type of transfer. The method of transfer selected depends upon the capabilities of the patient and the environment. A physical therapist, in conjunction with the patient, selects appropriate methods of transfer. The physical therapist must instruct patients to perform the selected transfers in a safe and efficient manner. The transfers selected may begin as assisted transfers (physical or verbal assistance) and then progress to independent transfers. In the following illustrations, patients are performing the transfers with stand-by assistance.

Preparing the Wheelchair

The initial steps for each of these transfers is similar. Wheelchair casters are turned forward, as they would be when a patient is wheeling backward. This increases the base of support of the wheelchair. When casters are not positioned properly, a wheelchair may tip forward as a patient is placed on the front of the wheelchair. After the casters have been turned forward, wheel locks are engaged.

Forward Lowering: Wheelchair to Floor

Forward lowering to the floor and a backward lift into a wheelchair requires the most strength and agility of the methods illustrated.

1. A wheelchair is positioned and locked with caster wheels forward. The patient's feet are placed on the floor, footplates are raised, and footrests are removed from the wheelchair when possible, or swung out of the way. The patient moves to the front of the wheelchair seat and the patient's lower extremities are positioned in front of the patient with knees extended.

(continued)

2. The patient positions one hand on the side, and toward the front, of the wheelchair seat, or the lower portion of a desk armrest. The other hand is placed on the caster or floor. Hand placements depend upon the patient's size, strength, and range of motion. The patient then lowers to the floor.

Positioning upper extremities.

Lowering to floor.

End position on floor.

Backward Lift: Floor to Wheelchair

1. A wheelchair is positioned and locked with caster wheels forward. Footplates are raised and footrests are removed from the wheelchair when possible, or swung out of the way. The patient assumes a long sitting position with her back toward, and close to, the front of the wheelchair. One hand is placed on the side, and toward the front, of the wheelchair seat. The other hand is placed on the caster or floor. Hand placements depend upon the patient's size, strength, and ROM.

2. The patient pushes up by extending the upper extremities and depressing the shoulder girdles.

Starting to lift into wheelchair.

Midposition of lift into wheelchair.

(continued)

3. As the patient's buttocks reach the wheelchair seat, the patient supports on the upper extremity on the wheelchair seat. The hand on the wheelchair seat may stay in place or be moved quickly to the armrest. The other hand is then moved quickly from the caster or floor to the wheelchair seat or lower part of the armrest.

Preparing to move upper extremity from caster to armrest.

Repositioned arms for movement onto wheelchair seat.

4. Again using both upper extremities, the patient moves well back onto the wheelchair seat.

5. The transfer is completed by attaching footrests, positioning feet on footplates, and positioning properly in a sitting position.

Backward Lift Using a Step Stool: Floor to Wheelchair

When a patient is unable to perform an independent floor to wheelchair transfer, a step stool may be used. The reverse of this sequence may be used initially to teach a patient to move from the wheelchair to the floor.

1. A wheelchair is positioned and locked with caster wheels forward. Footplates are raised and footrests are removed from the wheelchair when possible, or swung out of the way. A step stool is placed in front of the wheelchair. The patient assumes a long sitting position with her back toward, and close to, the step stool. Both hands are placed on the step stool.

2. Extending her upper extremities while using scapular depression, the patient pushes upward to lift herself onto the step stool.

Initiating push-up onto step stool.

Completing push-up onto step stool.

(continued)

3. Sitting on the step stool, the patient places both hands on the sides and toward the front of the wheelchair seat, or the lower part of desk armrests, when available. Hand placements depend upon the patient's size, strength, and ROM.

4. Performing another push-up, the patient lifts herself onto the front of the wheelchair seat.

5. The patient then moves her hands to the highest part of the armrests. Using the armrests, the patient performs another push-up to lift herself further onto the wheelchair seat.

6. Using one hand for support, the patient uses the other hand to position one lower extremity such that the foot rests on the step stool. This maneuver is repeated for the other lower extremity.

7. The patient then adjusts her position in the wheelchair until she is sitting erect, well back on the wheelchair seat. The wheelchair is wheeled backward away from the step stool. Footrests and footplates can then be positioned properly and the patient's feet placed on the footplates.

Turn Around: Wheelchair to Floor

1. A wheelchair is positioned and locked with caster wheels forward. Footplates are raised and footrests are removed from the wheelchair when possible, or swung out of the way. The patient moves to the front of the wheelchair seat and turns partially onto one hip.

(continued)

2. The patient moves her right hand behind her to grasp the left side of the seat. Her left hand is moved across the front of her body to grasp the right side of the seat.

3. Extending her upper extremities while depressing her shoulder girdles, the patient lifts herself and turns to face the back of the wheelchair. She then lowers herself to a kneeling position on the floor in front of the wheelchair.

4. From the kneeling position, the patient moves hands-knees position and then may assume a side-sitting position.

Moving to hands-knees position.

Hands-knees position.

Side-sitting position.

Turn Around: Floor to Wheelchair

1. A wheelchair is positioned and locked with caster wheels forward. Footplates are raised and footrests are removed from the wheelchair when possible, or swung out of the way. The patient assumes a hands-knees position in front of the wheelchair.

2. The patient places one hand on the side, and toward the front of, the wheelchair seat, and the other hand on the caster wheel. She then pushes into a kneeling position.

3. The patient moves her hand from the caster wheel to the side, and toward the front of the wheelchair seat, or on the lower part of a desk armrest when available. She is now kneeling in front of the wheelchair.

4. Pushing from the wheelchair seat or lower part of the armrest, the patient lifts herself, starts to turn, and then rests on one hip.

5. The patient repositions her hands onto the appropriate sides of the wheelchair seat, or armrests, and completes the turn.

6. The patient can then position herself properly in the wheelchair.

Forward to Hands-Knees Via Kneeling: Wheelchair to Floor

1. A wheelchair is positioned and locked with caster wheels forward. Footplates are raised and footrests are removed from the wheelchair when possible, or swung out of the way. The patient moves forward to the front of the wheelchair seat and places her feet on the floor under the front of the wheelchair seat.

2. Grasping the lower portion of desk armrests, when available, or the sides of the wheelchair seat, the patient lowers herself to a kneeling position.

3. Holding the lower portion of a desk armrest with one hand, the patient reaches forward to the floor with the other hand.

4. When the patient's upper extremity that is reaching to the floor is in a position to support her, the other hand is moved to the floor.

5. The transfer is completed by movement into a hands-knees position. From the hands-knees position, the patient may assume a side-sitting position.

Forward to Hands-Knees: Wheelchair to Floor

1. A wheelchair is positioned and locked with caster wheels forward. Footplates are raised and footrests are removed from the wheelchair when possible, or swung out of the way. The patient moves forward to the front of the wheelchair seat and places her feet on the floor under the front of the wheelchair seat.

2. The patient reaches to the floor with both upper extremities as she moves from the wheelchair seat, creating forward momentum.

3. With the patient's upper extremities supporting her, momentum shifts weight onto the upper extremities and she assumes a hands-knees position on the floor.

REVIEW QUESTIONS

1. Differentiate between dependent, assisted, and independent transfers.

2. What are the purposes of verbal commands during transfers?

3. Describe the sequences for performing the following transfers:

    Sliding transfer
    Three-person carry
    Hydraulic lift
    Two-person lift
    Dependent standing pivot
    Sliding board
    Push-up
    Assist to front edge of chair (three methods)
    Assist onto treatment table
    Assist standing pivot (three methods)
    Independent one-person transfer from floor to wheelchair
    Independent transfer from wheelchair to floor and return (seven methods)

SUGGESTED ACTIVITIES

1. Demonstrate transfer procedures shown in this chapter.

2. Practice transfers working in groups of 2 to 4 people, with each student participating as a patient, lead therapist, and assistant.

3. Practice transfers with partners role-playing the patient. Students should role-play patients with different diagnoses such as CVA (right or left hemiplegia), spinal cord injury (quadriplegia or paraplegia), multiple sclerosis, cerebral palsy, or Parkinson's disease. Students role-playing patients can add "character" to enhance the activity by being cooperative or noncooperative, in pain, hard of hearing, apprehensive, faint, flaccid, or spastic. Students playing the role of a patient must role-play the diagnosis and character consistently.

4. Practice teaching transfers to "patients and family" and other health care providers.

5. Document treatment using the SOAP note format.

CASE STUDIES

For the following case studies, develop a progression of transfers appropriate for progressing a patient from dependent to independent (as much as feasible) transfer status. Note transfer methods, amount, and type of assistance.

1. The patient is a 23-year-old female with a diagnosis of multiple sclerosis. She was independent in all ADLs and ambulated with a cane for balance until 2 weeks ago. At that time, she experienced an exacerbation that has left her totally dependent in all transfers and unable to ambulate. She becomes faint when moved from supine to sitting, or sitting to standing, too quickly. She is expected to recover most of her prior level of independence.

2. The patient is a 63-year-old male with left CVA onset 20 hours ago, presenting with right hemiplegia and global aphasia (both receptive and expressive aphasia). The cause was a blood clot. Because he received immediate medical treatment, recovery is anticipated to be nearly complete. At present, he is dependent in all ADLs, including transfers and ambulation.

3. The patient is a 18-year-old male who sustained a complete T12-L1 spinal cord lesion in a motorcycle accident 2 weeks ago. Following surgery, he is wearing a thoraco-lumbar-sacral orthosis (TLSO). He has medical clearance to begin transfer training while wearing his TLSO.

4. The patient is a 23-year-old female with cerebral palsy presenting with spastic quadriplegia. While living with her parents, her father lifted her for all transfers. Following her recent college graduation, she is living in a group home for the first time. She ambulates by using a power wheelchair. The staff of the group home requests assistance in selecting appropriate transfers. The staff would like a program to assist her in becoming an active participant in her transfers. Would the transfer method selected be different if she was 5 feet tall weighing 250 pounds versus 5 feet tall weighing 96 pounds?

5. The patient is a 49-year-old female with severe rheumatoid arthritis. She is 5 feet 3 inches tall and weighs 175 pounds. Transfers are currently accomplished using a pneumatic lift. She ambulates by using a power wheelchair. Because her arthritis is in remission at this time, she would like to learn to transfer without the pneumatic lift so she can get out in the community more.

REFERENCE

1. O'Sullivan SB and Schmitz TJ. *Physical Rehabilitation Assessment and Treatment,* 4th ed., chapter 11. Philadelphia: F.A. Davis, 2001.

9

AMBULATION WITH AMBULATORY ASSISTIVE DEVICES

LEARNING OBJECTIVES

Upon completion of this chapter, you will be able to:

1. List indications for use of ambulatory assistive devices for ambulation.
2. Describe and discuss the uses of parallel bars during gait training.
3. Describe and discuss the use of the tilt table during gait training.
4. List and discuss the causes of fatigue during gait training and methods to reduce the effects of fatigue.
5. Discuss the effect of patient concentration on gait training.
6. Describe the use of a scale to teach weight-bearing limits.
7. Describe methods of instruction appropriate for gait training.
8. List activities that a patient must master to be independent in ambulation with an assistive device.
9. List assistive device selection in sequence from those providing most stability to least stability.
10. List assistive device selection in sequence from those requiring the most coordination to least coordination.
11. List evaluations used to determine appropriate ambulatory assistive devices for different patients and pathologies.
12. List contraindications to the use of ambulatory assistive devices when appropriate.
13. Adjust the height of ambulatory assistive devices properly.
14. Describe various styles of walkers, crutches, and canes.
15. Describe and demonstrate common gait patterns used with ambulatory assistive devices.
16. Describe and demonstrate how to guard a patient properly when using ambulatory assistive devices during ambulation on level surfaces, stairs, and curbs; the assumption of sitting from standing and standing from sitting; moving through doorways; falling without injury; and resumption of ambulation after falling.
17. Instruct a patient in the proper method of using various ambulatory assistive devices to perform different gait patterns on level surfaces, stairs, and curbs; moving through doorways; the assumption of sitting from standing and standing from sitting; falling without injury; and resumption of ambulation after falling.

MEDIALINK

A companion CD-ROM, included free with each new copy of this book, supplements the techniques presented in the book. Insert the CD-ROM to watch video clips of patient care skills being demonstrated. This multimedia feature is designed to help you add a new dimension to your learning.

KEY TERMS

Ambulatory assistive devices	Gait pattern	Supervision guarding
Close guarding	Non-weight bearing (NWB)	Toe touch weight bearing (TTWB)
Contact guarding	Partial weight bearing (PWB)	Weight bearing
Full weight bearing (FWB)	Standby guarding	Weight bearing as tolerated (WBAT)

INTRODUCTION

Ambulatory assistive devices are mechanical devices that provide external support for the musculoskeletal system. The ambulatory assistive devices included in this chapter are parallel bars, crutches, canes, and walkers, but not orthotic or prosthetic devices, wheelchairs, or scooters. The ambulatory assistive devices included in this chapter permit some patients with impairments who could not otherwise ambulate to ambulate safely. Three major indications for using ambulatory assistive devices for gait are:

1. Structural deformity, amputation, injury, or disease resulting in decreased ability to bear weight through the lower extremities
2. Muscle weakness or paralysis of the trunk or lower extremities
3. Inadequate balance

Ambulatory assistive devices increase a patient's base of support and provide additional support during ambulation. Increasing a patient's base of support creates a larger area within which the patient's center of gravity can shift without loss of balance. Additional support improves balance control and supports or redistributes weight-bearing during ambulation.

TEACHING TIPS

TRAINING ENVIRONMENT

Initial gait training should occur in an environment that is as free of distractions as possible. Physical therapists should select and monitor the environment to ensure patient safety. Patient rooms or physical therapy departments are usually less distracting than public corridors. When more complex environments are needed to challenge a patient, public corridors can be used for gait training.

PARALLEL BARS

Gait training with ambulatory assistive devices often begins at the parallel bars. Parallel bars provide maximum stability, while requiring the least amount of coordination from patients. Patients can become accustomed to upright posture and learn a gait pattern in the relative safety of parallel bars. Ambulatory assistive devices can be fitted while a patient stands in parallel bars (Figure 9–1). When appropriate, a patient can practice standing or a gait pattern while waiting as physical therapists adjust ambulatory assistive devices, providing efficient use of treatment time.

FIGURE 9–1 Fitting crutches at the parallel bars.

Initial use of ambulatory assistive devices can be in or alongside parallel bars. Patients are reassured by readily available stability provided by parallel bars. A patient may, however, become too dependent on parallel bars. Physical therapists must progress patients to ambulation with ambulatory assistive devices other than parallel bars as rapidly as is safely possible.

Fatigue

Fatigue may occur during gait training as a result of:

1. Performing an activity that has not been performed for a while
2. Using ambulatory assistive devices during ambulation
3. Greater concentration levels while learning a new gait pattern with an assistive device
4. Physiological responses to the stresses of injury or illness

These factors can cause the patient to fatigue rapidly. Frequent rest periods may be necessary during initial gait training sessions. Several short sessions of gait training, rather than one long session, may decrease the effects of fatigue.

Patient Concentration

When first using ambulatory assistive devices, a patient's need to concentrate can be very high. During initial gait training sessions, patients require greater concentration to learn a gait pattern properly. Patients often look at their feet and ambulatory assistive devices as they learn gait patterns because visual input of foot and assistive device location with respect to their body is necessary for coordination and safety. Because patients are paying attention to foot and assistive device position, physical therapists must ensure safety by reducing distraction from other objects and activities in the immediate area.

High levels of concentration exhibited by patients during gait training may interfere with their ability to respond to other inputs, such as conversation. Patients may stop walking to answer questions. Conversation with and around a patient not directly related to gait training should be avoided during initial gait training. Later, however, such additional inputs can be used to test the degree to which patients have mastered use of ambulatory assistive devices and new gait patterns. When gait has again become an automatic activity, patients will be able to respond to questions and attend to other activity in the environment while maintaining appropriate gait patterns. As gait becomes automatic, patients usually start to look around as they ambulate. At this time patients can take over the responsibility of monitoring the environment for themselves, and more complex and distracting environments can be used for gait training.

Weight Bearing

When a patient with a restriction of weight bearing is instructed in gait, bathroom scales can be useful. Placing one lower extremity on a scale can demonstrate different levels of weight bearing and the attendant sensation (Figure 9–2).

FIGURE 9–2   Using one scale to measure weight bearing.

FIGURE 9–3   Using two scales to measure weight bearing.

When using this method, the lower extremity not placed on the scale must be placed on a solid surface. In some cases, two scales may be used, with one lower extremity placed on each scale (Figure 9–3).

Levels of weight-bearing will be discussed later in this chapter when choosing a gait pattern is discussed.

METHODS OF INSTRUCTION

Physical therapists will not always be available to instruct patients in how to perform tasks outside of a rehabilitation setting. Therefore, patients must be assisted in learning how to solve problems on their own when using ambulatory assistive devices. Physical therapists may challenge patients by presenting novel situations and asking patients how they might proceed in the new situation, prior to a patient attempting to maneuver in the new situation as a teaching method. This method may be indicative of a patient's level of independence prior to discharge.

Before a patient begins ambulating, the physical therapist must describe and demonstrate proper use of the chosen assistive device and gait pattern. Demonstration is the primary method of instruction. Verbal descriptions reinforce demonstration and must be simple. Observing other patients who are using ambulatory assistive devices *correctly* may also be a useful method of instruction.

Physical therapists must select specific activities to be mastered in sequence. Ambulation using a chosen gait pattern on level surfaces should be well advanced before gait training in other environments, such as on stairs or in busy corridors, is initiated. A patient's learning capabilities must be balanced with imposed time constraints of treatment sessions or hospital discharge, without compromising patient health and safety.

CONTENT OF INSTRUCTION

Patients must learn to use the chosen assistive device to move out of and into a chair. Initial instruction will most likely be related to using chairs with armrests.

Subsequent instruction for using chairs without armrests, low or soft sofas and chairs, toilets, and car seats, is also necessary. Patients must be taught to sit in a controlled manner, rather than collapsing into a sitting position.

Initial training in the performance of the chosen gait pattern is on level surfaces. When patients can perform safely on a level surface, instruction in the use of stairs, curbs, ramps, elevators, doors, and uneven surfaces, is provided, as well as instruction in how to fall safely. Patients should be taught to ascend and descend stairs on the appropriate side. In the United States, this is the patient's right side when facing the stairs.

Uneven surfaces may present specific problems for patients. Gravel, grass, broken sidewalks and paving, and curb cuts may require additional instruction and practice. Patients should be cautioned to avoid small throw rugs that may slip or become entangled with their feet or ambulatory assistive devices. Wet or highly polished floors can be slippery and should also be avoided whenever possible. When ambulating on icy, wet, or highly polished surfaces, smaller movements and shorter step lengths should be used. Taking shorter steps applies forces placed on ambulatory assistive devices more directly downward, which is more stable and avoids horizontal forces that may cause ambulatory assistive devices to slip.

Patients must be instructed to check that ambulatory assistive devices are in safe working condition. Rubber tips will not grip the floor properly if they become worn excessively or dirt fills the grooves. Wing nuts on crutches often loosen with use and should be checked regularly to ensure they are tightened appropriately.

CHOOSING AN ASSISTIVE DEVICE

A variety of ambulatory assistive devices is available. Some devices provide more stability and support than others. Some devices require more coordination to use. As abilities increase, patients may change from a device that provides relatively greater stability and support to one that provides relatively less stability and support. Other patients may continue to use the same device throughout the entire time an ambulatory assistive device is required. Patients with progressive disorders change from devices that provide relatively less stability and support to devices that provide relatively greater stability and support as their illness progresses.

Different ambulatory assistive devices require the use of different muscle groups. Physical therapists must examine each patient's capabilities to determine which ambulatory assistive device is to be used. Interventions that develop and increase each patient's capabilities must be instituted to ensure that selected ambulatory assistive devices can be used safely and efficiently. Time to improve a patient's capabilities is often limited in hospital environments. This may limit selection of ambulatory assistive devices and may limit a patient's ability to master all necessary skills prior to discharge.

The following list of ambulatory assistive devices is ordered from those providing the most stability and support to those providing the least stability and support.

1. Parallel bars
2. Walker
3. Axillary crutches
4. Forearm (Lofstrand) crutches
5. Two canes
6. One cane

The following list of ambulatory assistive devices is ordered from those requiring the least coordination by a patient to those requiring the most coordination by a patient.

1. Parallel bars
2. Walker
3. One cane
4. Two canes
5. Axillary crutches
6. Forearm (Lofstrand) crutches

Some patients may use one crutch as an intermediate step between two crutches and one cane, or instead of one cane.

When selecting an ambulatory assistive device, physical therapists must choose one that will provide the necessary support and that the patient can easily manipulate. The choice of an ambulatory assistive device is based a patient's impairments and an examination and evaluation of a patient's strength, range of motion, balance, stability, coordination, and general condition. For example, a patient with a fractured lower extremity who must be non-weight bearing may use either crutches or a walker, depending on the results of examination and evaluation. Crutches may be used when necessary strength, stability, and coordination are present. Another patient with the same fracture may require the use of a walker because of poor stability, coordination, or a medically debilitating condition.

A platform for the forearm can be attached to walkers or crutches for patients who are unable to bear weight through their hand, wrist, or forearm, or who have poor grasp (Figure 9–4).

Ambulatory assistive devices come in several sizes—tall, standard, junior, and child. Most ambulatory assistive devices are adjustable within a given range, and there is usually some overlap of adjustment between sizes. Some ambulatory assistive devices have ranges of height marked on them by the manufacturer. These markings are estimates only. Accurate measurement must be performed and confirmed by the physical therapist for each individual patient.

FIGURE 9–4 Walker with forearm platforms.

WALKERS

Walkers provide a relatively greater degree of stability and are generally easy to use. Walkers are chosen for patients with generalized weakness, debilitating conditions, a need to reduce weight bearing on one or both lower extremities, relatively poor balance and coordination, or an inability to use crutches. This may mean that walkers are used more often with elderly patients.

Walkers may, however, be cumbersome. A collapsible walker would be used with patients who will ambulate in the community (Figure 9–5). A collapsible walker is easier to transport in a car and place out of the way in public places, such as movies and restaurants, than is a non-collapsible walker.

(a)

(b)

(c)

FIGURE 9–5 The sides of a collapsible walker fold flat to allow for easier storage and transporting.

Walkers are usually made of aluminum and are adjustable in height. To adjust the height of a walker, the walker is inverted (Figure 9–6). Each leg has a push button lock with a telescoping leg (Figure 9–7). All legs must be adjusted to the same height.

FIGURE 9–6 Walker inverted for height adjustment.

FIGURE 9–7 Push button for height adjustment on walker.

Wheeled walkers are available with either two or four wheels (Figure 9–8). Walkers with four wheels should have a brake that is activated during weight bearing on the walker to ensure stability.

FIGURE 9–8 Four-wheeled walker with brake (left) and two-wheeled walker (right).

A stair climbing walker is available for patients who must use stairs frequently. This walker has an additional pair of handgrips on the rear legs, used when the patient is on the stairs. These handgrips increase the anterior/posterior dimension of the walker, increasing difficulty of maneuvering in small areas. A stair climbing walker in use is shown on pp. 304–308.

Other special walkers are available. A walker with a trunk support is used for patients who have adequate reciprocal lower extremity movements but lack adequate trunk support. These walkers are called ring walkers. Ring walkers are larger than standard walkers in all three dimensions and are not collapsible. An adduction board may be added to a ring walker. Adduction boards are suspended from the frame of the walker to prevent a patient's lower extremities from adducting during the swing phase of gait. Although cumbersome, for some patients an adduction board may be the difference between walking and not walking.

A reciprocal walker is designed with joints that permit each side of the walker to be advanced independently. A reciprocal walker is used when a patient lacks strength or balance to lift a walker completely to advance the walker during gait.

A reverse walker, with or without wheels, is often used by children. Patients stand in the walker with their back to the cross bar. The reverse walker is designed to encourage erect posture. Figure 9–4 shows a reverse walker.

AXILLARY CRUTCHES

Axillary crutches provide a moderate degree of stability and are slightly more difficult to use than walkers. Axillary crutches are generally chosen for patients with weakness of one or both lower extremities, a need to reduce weight bearing on one or both lower extremities, or need some support of the trunk.

Axillary crutches were traditionally made of wood but now may be made of wood or aluminum. Wing nuts and bolts are used to adjust crutch length and handgrip height of wooden crutches. Push button locks and telescoping legs may be used on some aluminum crutches. Alternative designs may be found among the many styles and constructions of axillary crutches (Figure 9–9).

FIGURE 9–9   A variety of aluminum and wooden axillary crutches.

FOREARM (LOFSTRAND) CRUTCHES

Forearm (Lofstrand) crutches (Figure 9–10) are slightly more difficult to use than axillary crutches but provide more ease of movement. The cuff of forearm crutches permits a patient to use his hand for manipulating the environment without dropping the crutch. Forearm crutches are recommended for patients with the same problems as would require axillary crutches, with the exception of decreased trunk stability. Patients who will need crutches permanently or for long periods of time, may find forearm crutches more desirable because they are lighter and more maneuverable than axillary crutches.

FIGURE 9–10 Patient using forearm (Lofstrand) crutches.

CANES

Canes provide limited stability and weight bearing capability. Generally they are made of aluminum or wood. Aluminum canes are adjustable using push button locks and telescoping legs. Wooden canes can be adjusted by cutting them to length, which limits their adjustability. Canes are generally chosen for patients with slight weakness of the lower extremities, who need slight weight reduction because of pain, or who need assistance with balance while ambulating.

When using one cane to limit weight bearing on one lower extremity, the cane is initially used in the hand on the side opposite the involved lower extremity. This placement provides a second point of support, which increases the base of support on the uninvolved side. Increasing the base of support on the uninvolved side permits a patient to shift weight to the uninvolved side during stance on the involved lower extremity. When weight bearing on the involved lower extremity is permitted, the cane may be used on the involved side, which increases the base of support on that side. Increasing the base of support on the involved side encourages weight shifting onto the involved lower extremity. Depending upon the severity of a patient's problem, either one or two canes may be required. Two canes are used primarily for bilateral involvement, or for assistance with balance.

Several styles of canes are available (Figure 9–11). The standard cane has a handgrip, shaft, and a single tip. The most common shape of a standard cane has a curved end for the handgrip. This cane style is often referred to as a "J" cane. Another design has an offset shaft and a straight end for the handgrip. This shape allows forces applied to the handle to be directly over the tip.

FIGURE 9–11   A variety of standard canes.

A variation of the standard cane is a quad cane, so named because it has four feet (Figure 9–12). Quad canes are available with two base sizes, large and small. The design of a quad cane makes it stable. Quad canes are constructed of aluminum, using a telescoping upper shaft for height adjustment. Offset shaft/handgrip design is available for both quad cane sizes. The outer legs of quad cane bases are angled outward from the base to a greater degree than the inner legs to increase the base of support provided. During use, the wider angled legs are placed away from the patient to avoid interference with a patient's feet during gait. Bases on quad canes can be rotated so the same cane can be used on either the right or left side, maintaining appropriate outward orientation of the larger legs with respect to handgrip orientation.

Patients can let go of a quad cane without concern that it will fall or slide to the floor as standard canes do. A disadvantage of large base quad canes is that the larger base does not permit it to be placed on a standard stair tread unless turned sideways.

FIGURE 9–12 Small base quad cane (left) and large base quad cane (right)

Handgrip designs, particularly for the offset cane, are available in varied shapes and textures to make grasp easier. The variety of handgrip designs are used for both standard and quad canes.

In a variation from standard crutches and canes, a "foot" is attached to the shaft with a moveable joint (Figure 9–13). The foot is a flat metal plate with a skid resistant surface and the "ankle" pivots. As the patient ambulates, the shaft "rolls" over the fixed foot (Figure 9–14).

FIGURE 9–13 Footpad canes and crutches.

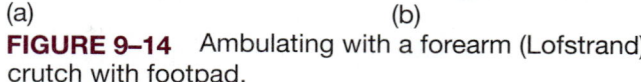

(a)　　　　　　　　　　　　　　　(b)

FIGURE 9–14 Ambulating with a forearm (Lofstrand) crutch with footpad.

CHOOSING A GAIT PATTERN

A **gait pattern** is defined as a selected sequence of movements for the ambulatory assistive device(s) and lower extremities. Five gait patterns are commonly used. The gait patterns described in this section are described for forward progression. These patterns, however, are also used for turning and backward progression. A change in the direction of placement of ambulatory assistive devices and lower extremities is necessary when turning or performing backward progression. Choosing a gait pattern is dependent upon several variables. Among these variables are medical condition, strength, range of motion, balance, and weight bearing status.

WEIGHT BEARING STATUS

Weight bearing is the amount of weight that can be borne on a lower extremity during standing or ambulation. The amount of weight bearing permitted is dependent on the patient's pathology, impairment, and medical management. When ambulating with ambulatory assistive devices, lifting of the body to decrease weight bearing is achieved by shoulder depression and elbow extension.

The amount of weight bearing on a lower extremity can vary from full weight bearing to non-weight bearing. The amount of weight bearing is controlled by the extent to which ambulatory assistive devices are used for weight bearing. There are five commonly used terms to describe weight bearing:

Non-weight bearing (NWB): The involved lower extremity is not to be weight bearing and is usually not permitted to touch the ground.

Toe touch weight bearing (TTWB): The patient can rest the foot of the involved lower extremity on the ground for balance but not for weight bearing.

Partial weight bearing (PWB): A limited amount of weight bearing, such as five pounds, is permitted for the involved lower extremity. When a specific weight is not provided, minimal weight bearing should be permitted on the involved lower extremity until a specific amount is confirmed by the referring physician.

Weight bearing as tolerated (WBAT): The patient determines the amount of weight bearing that will occur on the involved lower extremity. The amount of weight bearing permitted may vary from minimal to full, depending upon the tolerance of the patient.

Full weight bearing (FWB): The patient is permitted full weight bearing on the involved lower extremity. Ambulatory assistive devices are not used to decrease weight bearing but may be used for assistance with balance.

TWO-POINT GAIT PATTERN

A two-point gait pattern is used when two ambulatory assistive devices, such as two canes or two crutches, are required. This gait pattern is used with patients with impairments such as muscle weakness, pain, or decreased balance.

One ambulatory assistive device and the opposite lower extremity are lifted and moved forward simultaneously. When the ambulatory assistive device and lower extremity have been placed on the ground, the patient's weight is shifted to these supports. The other ambulatory assistive device and its opposite lower extremity are then moved forward. This two-part sequence is repeated. Each combination of one ambulatory assistive device and the opposite lower extremity is considered "one point." A complete cycle includes "two points," thus the name two-point gait pattern.

FOUR-POINT GAIT PATTERN

A four-point gait pattern is often described as a deliberate two-point gait pattern. This gait pattern is used when two ambulatory assistive devices, such as two canes or two crutches, are required. A four-point gait pattern is used with patients with the same types of impairments as a two-point gait pattern, but for whom the impairments are more severe. A four-point gait pattern may also be used as a starting point to teach a patient the pairing of the opposite upper and lower extremities before graduating to using the two-point gait pattern.

One ambulatory assistive device is moved forward and placed on the floor, followed by the opposite lower extremity. The other ambulatory assistive device is moved forward and placed on the floor, followed by its opposite lower extremity. Each time an ambulatory assistive device or lower extremity is lifted to be moved forward, weight bearing is shifted to the three supports remaining in contact with the floor. This four-part sequence is repeated. A complete cycle includes "four points."

THREE-POINT GAIT PATTERN

A three-point gait pattern is used by patients with impairments of one lower extremity, such as a fracture, muscle weakness, pain, or injury/surgery requiring decreased weight bearing. The levels of weight bearing described earlier may be used by patients ambulating with a three-point gait pattern. This gait pattern requires two crutches, two canes, or a walker. The example that follows assumes the use of two crutches. The use of two canes follows the same pattern. The use of a walker requires that the walker be advanced as a unit, mimicking the simultaneous advancement of two crutches or two canes.

As patients initially learn this gait pattern, both crutches are moved forward and placed on the floor. The involved lower extremity is moved forward between the two crutches such that the ball of the foot is even with the crutch tips. After the involved lower extremity is moved forward, weight bearing is shifted to the upper extremities, and involved lower extremity if permitted by weight bearing status. The uninvolved lower extremity is then moved forward past the crutches. Weight bearing is then shifted to the uninvolved lower extremity in preparation for the next forward movement of the crutches and involved lower extremity. This three-part sequence is repeated. Thus, a complete cycle includes "three points."

As patients become more confident, the crutches and involved lower extremity are moved forward simultaneously. The shifting of weight bearing and movement of the uninvolved lower extremity follow as before.

Initially, patients may advance the uninvolved lower extremity forward only to the involved lower extremity and crutches. Patients should be encouraged to step beyond the placement of the involved lower extremity and crutches for a faster and more normal gait pattern.

SWING-TO GAIT PATTERN

A swing-to gait pattern requires the use of two crutches or a walker. This gait pattern is used for patients with impairments of the lower extremities such as muscle weakness, paresis, paralysis, or decreased weight bearing on one lower extremity. The levels of weight bearing described earlier may be used by patients ambulating with a swing-to gait pattern. The example that follows assumes the use of two crutches.

The patient moves both crutches forward simultaneously and places the tips on the floor. Weight bearing is shifted onto the crutches. Both lower extremities are moved forward simultaneously to the same point as the crutches were advanced, and placed on the floor. Weight bearing is shifted to one or both lower extremities, as allowed by weight bearing status, for support so the crutches can be advanced again. This two-part sequence is repeated. Each cycle requires that the lower extremities "swing to" the same point as the ambulatory assistive devices were advanced, thus the name "swing-to" gait pattern.

SWING-THROUGH GAIT PATTERN

A swing-through gait pattern requires the use of two crutches. This gait pattern is used for patients with the same impairments as would use the swing-to gait pattern, such as muscle weakness, paresis, paralysis, or decreased weight bearing on one lower extremity. The levels of weight bearing described earlier may be used by patients ambulating with a swing-through gait pattern.

The patient moves both crutches forward simultaneously and places the tips on the floor. Weight bearing is shifted onto the crutches. Both lower extremities swing forward simultaneously beyond the crutch tips. Weight bearing is shifted to one or both lower extremities, as allowed by weight bearing status, for support so the crutches can be advanced again. This two-part sequence is repeated. Each cycle requires that the lower extremities "swing through" the crutches, thus the name "swing-through" gait pattern.

PROCEDURE 9–1

 GUARDING

Guarding is the process of protecting the patient from excessive weight bearing, loss of balance, or falling. Proper guarding requires use of a gait belt. Guarding by holding onto the patient's belt may be uncomfortable for the patient because the narrow belt or belt buckle can bind or pinch the patient. Holding clothing is not appropriate because clothing may tear and does not fit firmly enough to provide control during guarding. A gait belt should fit snugly around the patient's waist. Handles for the physical therapist to grasp the gait belt may or may not be present. The gait belt should be held with the forearm supinated for a stronger grip. Initially the physical therapist grasps the gait belt with one hand and the other hand is placed on the patient's trunk over the shoulder girdle on the side to which the physical therapist is standing.

In and Out of a Wheelchair

When the patient arises from or sits in a chair, the physical therapist stands in stride, to one side and slightly behind the patient. This permits the physical therapist to move with the patient without blocking the patient's movement. In some instances the physical therapist may stand in front of the patient, as for an assisted standing pivot transfer. Standing in front of the patient permits the physical therapist to provide physical assistance, and moves the patient into the physical therapist's base of support.

Level Surfaces

When the patient ambulates, the physical therapist stands in stride behind and slightly to one side of the patient. As the physical therapist grasps the gait belt with a supinated forearm, the other hand is placed over the patient's shoulder girdle, not on the upper extremity. If a hand is placed on the patient's upper extremity, it may interfere with free motion needed to control ambulatory assistive devices.

In all situations, the physical therapist must be positioned in a way that permits the physical therapist to move as the patient moves. This is extremely important because the physical therapist's position must not interfere with the patient's movement. The physical therapist must be alert to the patient's position and movements and to obstacles in the environment.

During initial gait training the physical therapist stands close to the patient to provide increased support and control. As the patient ambulates, the physical therapist moves with the patient. The physical therapist's "outside" foot moves when the ambulatory assistive device on that side is moved. The physical therapist's "outside" foot is the foot most lateral to the patient. The physical therapist's "inside" foot is moved when the patient's foot on the side the physical therapist is guarding is moved. The physical therapist's "inside" foot is the foot directly behind the patient. Such coordination of physical therapist and patient movements allows the physical therapist to move smoothly without kicking or tripping the patient and without interfering with ambulatory assistive devices.

When the physical therapist has both hands on the patient and is behind the patient and ambulatory assistive device, this is described as **close guarding**.

As the patient's ambulation skills improve, the physical therapist removes the hand from the shoulder girdle, stands more to the side of the patient, and continues to grasp the gait belt. This is described as **contact guarding.** As the patient ambulates with this level of guarding, the physical therapist's "inside" foot moves with the ambulatory assistive device. The physical therapist's "outside" foot moves with the patient's lower extremity.

Eventually, the physical therapist walks near the patient without contact or holding the gait belt. This is described as **supervision,** or stand-by, **guarding.**

Falling

If a patient starts to fall, the physical therapist must decide whether to maintain the patient in an upright position, or to permit a controlled lowering to the floor in a manner that will prevent injury to patient or physical therapist. Physical therapists must be alert to a patient's movements at all times, and be able to react quickly to prevent or control a fall.

During early stages of gait training, patients usually lean away from weight bearing on an involved lower extremity because they fear pain or further injury if they put too much weight on the involved lower extremity. This is another reason physical therapists initially guard a patient on the uninvolved or less involved side. By guarding on a patient's uninvolved side, the physical therapist is on the side to which patients are already leaning as they avoid excessive weight bearing on an involved lower extremity. This positioning, and the tendency of patients to lean in this direction, places physical therapists in the best position to pull a patient into the physical therapist's base of support, reducing the risk of increased weight bearing on an involved lower extremity.

(continued)

Pulling the patient into the physical therapist's base of support is the safer method for both patient and physical therapist of preventing a fall. The physical therapist is able to control the patient more completely when the patient's weight is pulled into the physical therapist's base of support. If the patient starts to fall, the physical therapist is better able to provide support and protection of an involved lower extremity by shifting the patient's weight onto the uninvolved lower extremity. This combination of measures is best achieved by guarding a patient on the uninvolved side. For this reason, initial gait training usually begins with the physical therapist guarding the patient on the uninvolved side.

As the patient's capabilities improve, the physical therapist guards on the patient's involved side, encouraging upright posture and appropriate use of the involved lower extremity.

Ascending/Descending Stairs

The physical therapist is positioned below the patient when guarding as the patient ascends and descends stairs. The physical therapist grasps the patient's gait belt with one hand and a handrail with the other hand. Holding a handrail provides the physical therapist with a point of stability to halt a fall. The physical therapist stands in stride on the stairs, placing his or her feet on different stair treads. A stride position enables the physical therapist to shift weight and position as the patient moves, permitting the physical therapist to shift the patient's weight into the physical therapist's base of support should the patient begin to fall.

Occasionally a second person is needed to guard a patient learning to ascend and descend stairs. The second person stands in stride on the stairs above the patient, and also holds the gait belt and handrail.

PROCEDURE 9-2

ASSUMPTION OF STANDING AND SITTING

Preparing the Wheelchair

When assuming standing from a wheelchair or assuming sitting in a wheelchair, the wheelchair is placed against a stable surface, such as a wall or heavy table if possible, and wheel locks are engaged. The footplates are raised and the footrests are removed and placed out of the way of the therapist or patient.

Positioning the Patient

To ease the assumption of a standing position, the patient moves to sitting at the front edge of the seat, as shown in Chapter 8. Both feet are placed flat on the floor below the front edge of the seat. In this position the patient's knees are flexed to approximately 110 degrees and ankles are in slight dorsiflexion. The patient's center of mass can be brought over the base of support quickly from this position as the patient assumes standing. The feet may be placed side by side or in a short stride position. Using a stride position increases the patient's anterior/posterior base of support. When moving to standing with the feet in stride, the foot of the uninvolved lower extremity is placed slightly behind the involved lower extremity. This allows the patient to use the uninvolved lower extremity efficiently for rising to standing. Having the patient place the hands on armrests also increases the base of support, and provides initial assistance to push to a standing position.

Assumption of Standing

1. To assume a standing position, the patient must lean forward to shift the center of mass over the feet and extend the knees and hips to rise from the seat.

2. Initially, the patient pushes directly downward on the armrests. Pushing at an angle creates a horizontal component of the pushing force vector that does not assist the patient to rise and may also propel the patient horizontally and thus off balance.

Ambulatory assistive devices must be accessible to patients when they are sitting in a chair and after the assumption of standing. Initially, ambulatory assistive devices may not be used during the assumption of standing. During initial learning, both hands are placed on the armrests of the chair to assist with pushing to standing. In such cases, the ambulatory assistive devices must be accessible to the physical therapist, who hands them to the patient once standing has been achieved. When using ambulatory assistive devices to assume standing, one of the patient's hands may be placed on the ambulatory assistive devices and the other hand may be placed on the armrest. Whichever hand position is used, the movement to assume standing should be a controlled continuous motion.

Assumption of Sitting

1. To assume a sitting position after walking, the patient must approach the front edge of a chair and then turn away from the chair. When performing this maneuver, the patient may initially feel more confident turning toward the uninvolved side. This occurs because the patient is turning into his/her strength. The patient must, however, be able to turn in both directions, toward the involved and uninvolved sides. As the patient approaches a chair, he or she must ensure that the chair is secure, and if the chair is a wheelchair, that the footrests are out of the way.

2. With the patient standing close to the front edge of the seat and facing away from the chair, the patient's center of mass can be maintained over the base of support during the assumption of sitting. Feet may be placed side by side or placed in a short stride position. Using a stride position increases a patient's base of support. When moving to sitting with the feet in stride, the foot of the uninvolved lower extremity is slightly farther back then the foot of the involved lower extremity. Having patients reach for and use armrests while lowering to the seat also increases a patient's base of support and provides assistance to control the latter stages of lowering.

   Initially, ambulatory assistive devices may not be used for the assumption of sitting. In such cases, ambulatory assistive devices, such as crutches and canes, but not walkers, can be handed to the physical therapist before a patient begins to lower to sitting. Both of the patient's hands then use the armrests of the chair to assist with controlled lowering to sitting. When using ambulatory assistive devices during assumption of sitting, one of the patient's hands, usually the hand on the side of the involved lower extremity, is placed on the assistive device. The other hand is placed on the armrest. The patient then assumes sitting in a controlled manner.

PROCEDURE 9–3

ASCENDING AND DESCENDING STAIRS

Generally, patients ascend and descend stairs on their right side when facing the stairs. When ascending or descending stairs, the patient places the tips of the ambulatory assistive device one-half to two-thirds of the way forward onto the stair tread, in the direction the patient is facing. When two ambulatory assistive devices are used, they are placed far enough apart to allow room for the patient to move between them. When a stair rail is available, the patient should use it for greater stability. When the patient is using two ambulatory assistive devices, both can be placed in one hand to free the other hand for use on the stair rail. When only one upper extremity can be used, the ambulatory assistive device can be held in the hand on the stair rail. If the right upper extremity is unable to be used, patients may use the assistive device only or ascend and descend on the left side when facing the stairs.

When first learning to ascend and descend stairs, patients usually use a step-to gait pattern. As a patient's condition permits, the patient may progress to a step-over-step gait pattern to ascend and descend stairs.

Ascending Stairs

1. When ascending stairs, the uninvolved lower extremity is moved to the next higher stair first because it must lift the body. To do so, weight is shifted to the ambulatory assistive devices, and as permitted to the involved lower extremity, allowing movement of the uninvolved lower extremity.
2. Once the uninvolved lower extremity has been appropriately placed on the next stair, weight is shifted to the uninvolved lower extremity. The uninvolved lower extremity is extended to lift the body.
3. The involved lower extremity and the ambulatory assistive devices are advanced to the same stair at the same time the body is lifted.
4. An alternative is to move the involved lower extremity to the same stair as the uninvolved lower extremity, followed by the ambulatory assistive devices.

Descending Stairs

1. When descending stairs, ambulatory assistive devices are moved to the next lower stair first to provide support for the involved lower extremity.
2. Weight is shifted to the uninvolved lower extremity, permitting the ambulatory assistive devices and involved lower extremity to be lowered to the next lower stair.
3. The uninvolved lower extremity lowers the body until the ambulatory assistive devices and the involved lower extremity are on the next lower stair.
4. An alternative is to lower the ambulatory assistive devices first, followed by the involved lower extremity once the ambulatory assistive devices are in place. Weight is shifted to the ambulatory assistive devices and involved lower extremity when appropriate. The uninvolved lower extremity is than moved down to the same stair.

CURBS

The sequence for ascending and descending curbs is the same as the sequence for ascending and descending stairs. Only ambulatory assistive devices are available for support when ascending and descending curbs because of the absence of handrails.

MOVING THROUGH DOORWAYS

There are many combinations of extremity involvement and doorway configurations. A patient may have one or two functional upper extremities and the impairment of the patient's lower extremities may involve one or both. Doors may open toward or away from the patient, they may be hinged on the left or right, the space around the door available for maneuvering may be ample or limited, and doors may or may not have automatic openers or closers. Each combination of factors will require modifications to the general method of ambulating through doorways. Patient safety must not be compromised regardless of patient level of function and physical configuration of the environment.

Often balance is a major concern. Patients may be required to lean in all directions, moving their center of mass with respect to their base of support while pushing or pulling on doors. Another concern is the danger of a door with an automatic closer striking a patient as it closes. Should a door strike a patient, the patient may lose balance control, resulting in more weight bearing on the involved lower extremity than is permitted, or falling. To avoid an automatic closing door from striking a patient, such doors should be opened wider than the minimal width for a patient to progress through the doorway. This allows the patient time to progress through the doorway before the automatic closing door impedes progress. An alternative technique is to use the tips of ambulatory assistive devices as temporary door stops while progressing through these doorways. Some patients rush to move through such doorways. Rushing can also be hazardous as a patient may not be able to control the ambulatory assistive devices or maintain balance when moving at a faster pace.

The physical therapist's position for guarding the patient during movement through doorways is the same position as for guarding during ambulation. Recognizing that shorter steps and abrupt turns may be required, the physical therapist must be prepared to move with the patient, avoiding interference with the patient's freedom of movement or the arc of movement of a door. During initial gait training through doorways, the physical therapist may need to control opening and closing of the door to protect the patient.

When a door does not have an automatic closer, the door does not have to be opened greater than the width of the patient to prevent the door from closing forcefully on a patient before progress through the doorway is completed. Rapid movement of ambulatory assistive devices to block the door is not necessary. Doors that do not have automatic closers require that the patient turn and close the door after moving through the doorway.

In the sections on ambulation through doorways presented later in this chapter, text and photographs depict independent ambulation. This method was used so a physical therapist does not obscure the desired photographic views of the patient.

TILT TABLE

Some patients must be re-acclimated to upright posture in a safe manner before sitting, standing, or ambulation can be initiated. This is usually necessitated by the existence of orthostatic hypotension in patients who have been in bed for extended periods. Accommodation by the cardiovascular system may be necessary to avoid dizziness or fainting as these patients assume an upright posture. Tilt tables are a safe method to provide maximum support for such patients. Support is provided while the patient is raised slowly to an upright position by the tilt table, leaving the physical therapist free to control the tilt table and monitor the patient. Abdominal binders and elastic wraps or elastic hose on the lower extremities may be used to assist veinous return. Use of lower extremity muscles, such as isometric contractions, often called "muscle setting" exercises, or active range of motion exercises also assists veinous return.

Vital signs are measured, as presented in Chapter 4, before, during, and after the process of raising patients to an upright posture (Figure 9–15). Patients should be lowered when they report feeling faint. A patient who is lowered after feeling faint must be monitored until vital signs return to normal and the patient no longer reports feeling faint. Medical assistance must be obtained when necessary.

FIGURE 9–15 Measuring vital signs before raising tilt table.

Straps are used to secure patients on a tilt table (Figure 9–16). A variety of styles of straps are available. A bar extends along each side of the tilt table surface. Straps used to secure the patient on the tilt table are attached to the bar on one side of the table.

Straps are passed over the patient and secured around the bar on the other side. The location of the straps across the patient depends on the patient's condition. When upper trunk stability is required, a chest strap leaving the upper extremities free is used. A strap over the pelvis stabilizes the lower trunk. A strap at kneel level is used when the patient cannot maintain knee extension.

FIGURE 9–16 Securing patient on a tilt table.

The angle of tilt is adjusted to a position the patient can tolerate safely. Changes in the position of the table should be performed slowly and steadily. Greater degrees of tilt may be assumed as the patient's cardiovascular system adjusts to the demands of an upright posture. For many patients a full upright position provides a sensation of falling forward; therefore, this position is usually avoided.

Patients with non-weight bearing status on one lower extremity can be placed on a tilt table. A lift can be placed under the foot of the uninvolved lower extremity, preventing the involved lower extremity from reaching the supporting surface (Figure 9–17). Thus, the involved lower extremity is non-weight bearing.

FIGURE 9–17 A lift under the uninvolved (right) lower extremity avoids weight bearing on the involved (left) lower extremity.

When an exercise program for one lower extremity is to be implemented, the strap across the knees can be loosened or placed only around the opposite lower extremity. This permits the physical therapist to implement the patient's lower extremity exercise program. Upper extremity and trunk exercises can also be performed on the tilt table (Figure 9–18).

FIGURE 9–18 Exercising on a tilt table.

A tilt table may also be used when patients have restrictions on sitting, or the amount of hip flexion allowed. When individuals move from sitting to standing, the hips ordinarily flex more than 90 degrees. Following total hip replacement, patients are restricted to no more than 90 degrees of hip flexion. For patients unable to assume standing from sitting while maintaining hip precautions, a tilt table can be used to rise to a standing position. Patients can be fitted with ambulatory assistive devices while on a tilt table (Figure 9–19) and "walk," with guarding, off the tilt table for ambulation training.

FIGURE 9–19 Adjusting crutch height while patient is on a tilt table.

WALKERS

FITTING

To measure a walker for proper height adjustment, the patient stands upright with shoulder girdle relaxed within the walker with the crossbar in front. The top of the handgrips should be approximately at the level of the patient's ulnar styloid processes when the upper extremities are relaxed at the side (Figure 9–20). This fitting can be done in a set of parallel bars. When the patient grasps the handgrips with shoulder girdles level and relaxed, the elbows are flexed approximately 20–30 degrees (Figure 9–21).

FIGURE 9–20 Checking handgrip height when fitting a walker.

FIGURE 9–21 Checking elbow flexion angle when fitting a walker.

PROCEDURE 9-4

IN AND OUT OF A WHEELCHAIR WITH A WALKER

Two methods of getting in and out of a wheelchair will be described. In both methods, a wheelchair is prepared and the patient positioned in the manner presented earlier in this chapter under *Assumption of Standing and Sitting.* Reversing wheelchair desk armrests so the higher portion is at the front of the wheelchair will assist patients in pushing to standing and lowering to sitting. A physical therapist is positioned in the manner described earlier in this chapter under *Guarding.*

Assuming Standing Using a Walker

Wheelchair wheel locks are engaged and footrests are moved out of the way. The patient is positioned at the front edge of the seat, with his/her feet in stride or side by side. A physical therapist is positioned in stride, behind and to one side of the patient. The physical therapist grasps the patient's gait belt with one hand. The other hand may be on the patient's shoulder girdle if necessary. If a hand is placed on the patient's shoulder girdle, it should not interfere with a patient's ability to move smoothly using the upper extremity.

1. The patient's hand on the uninvolved side grasps and pushes down on the crossbar of the walker. The patient's hand on the involved side is placed on the armrest of the wheelchair. This ensures that the patient is moving into his/her strength.

2. The patient pushes to standing.

(continued)

3. The patient moves the hand on the involved side from the armrest of the wheelchair and grasps the handgrip of the walker.

4. The patient moves the hand on the uninvolved side from the crossbar to grasp the other handgrip. The patient is now correctly positioned in the walker to begin ambulation.

Force exerted on the crossbar of a walker must be exerted directly downward to avoid tipping the walker.

If force is not exerted directly downward when a patient's hand is placed on the crossbar of a walker, the walker tips forward.

The patient's hand on the uninvolved side may be placed on the walker's handgrip instead of crossbar. There are two disadvantages of this method. First, a walker's handgrip is higher than the crossbar. This location of the handgrip may make pushing directly downward more difficult for a patient. Second, the handgrip is at the very outside of the walker's base of support. Slight deviation from pushing directly downward will cause the walker to tip sideways.

(continued)

Assuming Sitting Using a Walker

1. Wheelchair wheel locks are engaged and footrests are moved out of the way. To sit, the patient is positioned facing away from the wheelchair at the front edge of the wheelchair seat, close enough so that the front edge of wheelchair seat is felt against the back of the lower extremities. The patient's feet can be positioned either in stride or side by side. Positioned in stride, behind and to one side of the patient, the physical therapist grasps the patient's gait belt and shoulder girdle.

2. The patient grasps the middle of the crossbar with the hand on the involved side.

3. The patient reaches backward and grasps the armrest with the hand on the uninvolved side.

4. The patient lowers in a controlled manner to a sitting position.

5. The patient moves the hand from the crossbar to the armrest and adjust the sitting position in the wheelchair.

(continued)

Assuming Standing Using Both Armrests

1. Wheelchair wheel locks are engaged and footrests are moved out of the way. The patients is positioned at the front edge of the seat with the feet in stride or side by side. Positioned in stride, behind and to one side of the patient, the physical therapist grasps the patient's gait belt and shoulder girdle. Sitting on the front edge of the seat, the patient places both hands on the armrests.

2. Using the armrests, the patient pushes to standing.

3. The patient shifts weight completely over the feet. The hand on the uninvolved side is moved first from the wheelchair armrest to the handgrip of the walker.

4. Once the hand on the uninvolved side is properly positioned, the patient moves the hand on the involved side from the wheelchair armrest to the handgrip of the walker.

Assuming Sitting Using Both Armrests

1. Wheelchair wheel locks are engaged and footrests are moved out of the way. To sit, the patient is positioned facing away from the wheelchair at the front edge of the wheelchair seat, close enough so that the front edge of wheelchair seat is felt against the back of the lower extremities. The patient's feet are positioned in stride or side by side. Positioned in stride, behind and to one side of the patient, the physical therapist grasps the patient's gait belt and shoulder girdle.

   The patient retains a grasp on the handgrip of the walker with the hand on the involved side, while reaching back with the hand on the uninvolved side to grasp the wheelchair armrest.

2. After grasping the armrest with the hand on the uninvolved side, the patient moves the hand on the involved side from the handgrip of the walker and grasps the other wheelchair armrest.

3. The patient then lowers to a sitting position in a controlled manner.

4. Once seated, the patient adjusts the sitting position.

PROCEDURE 9–5

 AMBULATING WITH A WALKER

When ambulating with a walker, lifting of the patient's body to decrease weight bearing is achieved by shoulder depression and elbow extension. The patient moves a walker by picking it up, moving it a stride length forward, and placing it on the floor. Walkers should be lifted and set down so that all four legs clear or contact the floor simultaneously.

Some patients will "rock" the walker, lifting and setting down two legs and rocking onto the other two legs. Rocking the walker reduces the base of support and stability a walker provides when used properly. *Rocking the walker should be discouraged.*

The patient's leading lower extremity should *not* be placed beyond the crossbar. Doing so prevents appropriate weight shifting over this lower extremity. When stepping beyond the crossbar occurs, the base of support and stability provided by a walker are compromised.

Three-Point Gait Pattern

Partial to Full Weight Bearing

1. For close guarding, the physical therapist is positioned in stride, behind and to one side of the patient, grasping the patient's gait belt and shoulder girdle. To ambulate using the three-point gait pattern, the patient stands centered within the walker. The walker is lifted and advanced forward. All four legs of the walker are lifted from or lowered to the floor simultaneously. As the patient moves the walker, the physical therapist advances the outside foot.

2. The patient advances the involved lower extremity, moving it into the base of support and stability of the walker.

(continued)

3. Supporting weight as necessary to achieve the desired weight bearing status, the patient bears weight through the upper extremities as she advances the uninvolved lower extremity. The patient may step to or slightly beyond the involved foot, but not beyond the crossbar. Equal step lengths should be encouraged. The physical therapist advances the inside foot to move with a patient. The total sequence is repeated for continued progression.

Non-Weight Bearing

For close guarding, the physical therapist is positioned in stride, behind and to one side of the patient, grasping the patient's gait belt and shoulder girdle. To ambulate using the three-point gait pattern non-weight bearing on the involved lower extremity, the patient stands centered within the walker. The involved lower extremity is not rested on the floor. The involved lower extremity may be held by the patient with the knee extended and the foot in front or it may be held with the knee flexed and the foot behind the patient. The uninvolved lower extremity and both upper extremities provide support.

1. The walker is lifted and advanced forward. All four legs of a walker are lifted from or lowered to the floor simultaneously. As the patient moves the walker, the physical therapist advances the outside foot.

2. Supporting weight as necessary to achieve non-weight bearing status, the patient steps into the walker with the uninvolved lower extremity. The physical therapist advances the inside foot to move with the patient. The total sequence is repeated for continued progression.

Swing-To Gait Pattern

1. For close guarding, the physical therapist is positioned in stride, behind and to one side of a patient, grasping the patient's gait belt and shoulder girdle. To ambulate using a swing-to gait pattern, the patient stands centered within the walker. The walker is lifted and advanced forward. All four legs of a walker are lifted from or lowered to the floor simultaneously. As the patient moves the walker, the physical therapist advances the outside foot.

2. Bearing weight through the upper extremities, the patient lifts the body. The patient then lets the body swing forward ("swing-to") into the walker. The physical therapist moves the inside foot as the patient swings forward.

3. The patient lowers at the end of the swing and bears weight on the lower extremities. The sequence is repeated for continued progression.

PROCEDURE 9–6

AMBULATING ON STAIRS WITH A WALKER

Ambulation on the stairs using a walker can be accomplished with a standard walker or with a stair-climbing walker. When the patient must negotiate stairs frequently, a stair-climbing walker should be considered.

Stair-Climbing Walker

Ascending Stairs

1. For close guarding, the physical therapist is positioned in stride, behind and to one side of the patient, grasping the patient's gait belt and shoulder girdle. The patient stands facing up the stairs with the walker in the usual position for ambulation.

2. A stair-climbing walker is first turned so the crossbar is to the side of the patient.

3. It is turned again so the crossbar is behind the patient.

4. The two legs of the stair-climbing walker closest to the stairs are placed on the first stair.

5. Grasping the handgrips, the patient can support weight on the upper extremities. The physical therapist places one hand on the stair rail and the other on the patient's gait belt. Supporting weight on the upper extremities, the patient advances the uninvolved lower extremity up onto the same stair as the forwardmost legs of the walker.

(continued)

6. Extending the uninvolved lower extremity the patient lifts the body and places the involved lower extremity on the same stair as the uninvolved lower extremity. Guarding becomes more difficult for the physical therapist because placement of the walker may prevent the physical therapist from maintaining a position close behind the patient.

7. The walker is lifted and advanced to the next stair. At this time the physical therapist can again move to a closer position behind the patient. The sequence is repeated to ascend the remaining stairs.

Descending Stairs

1. To descend stairs using a stair-climbing walker, the patient stands facing down the stairs. The walker is positioned with the crossbar of the walker in front of the patient. The patient grasps the handgrips and positions the walker so the forwardmost legs are on the lower stair. Positioned in stride in front of the patient, the physical therapist grasps the patient's gait belt and handrail.

2. Supporting weight on the upper extremities, the patient lowers the involved lower extremity down to the same stair as the front legs of the walker by flexing the uninvolved lower extremity.

(continued)

3. Continuing to support weight with the upper extremities on the walker, the patient lowers the uninvolved lower extremity down to the same stair as the walker's front legs.

4. The sequence is repeated until the patient finishes descending the stairs. When the patient has completed descending the stairs and reaches the landing or floor level, she grasps the handgrips of the walker and positions the walker for ambulation.

Standard Walker

Although it is not the most stable device on stairs, a standard walker can be used to ambulate on stairs.

Ascending Stairs

1. To ascend stairs using a standard walker, the patient stands facing up the stairs with the walker in the usual position for ambulation. The patient turns the walker sideways so the crossbar is on the side of the patient away from the handrail. The patient's hand closest to the walker is placed on the forwardmost handgrip of the walker. The patient's other hand grasps the handrail. Positioned in stride behind the patient, the physical therapist grasps the patient's gait belt and handrail. The patient places the two forwardmost legs of the walker on the first stair.

2. Supporting weight on the upper extremities, the patient advances the uninvolved lower extremity up onto the same stair as the forwardmost legs of the walker.

(continued)

3. Extending the uninvolved lower extremity, the patient lifts the body and places the involved lower extremity on the same stair as the uninvolved lower extremity.

4. The walker is advanced and the sequence is repeated to ascend the remaining stairs.

Descending Stairs

1. To descend stairs using a standard walker, the patient stands facing down the stairs. The walker is turned sideways so the crossbar is on the side of the patient away from the handrail. The patient's hand closest to the walker is placed on the rearmost handgrip of the walker. The patient's other hand grasps the handrail. Positioned in stride in front of the patient, the physical therapist grasps the patient's gait belt and the handrail.

2. Supporting weight on the upper extremities, the patient lowers the involved lower extremity down to the same stair as the forwardmost legs of the walker by flexing the uninvolved lower extremity.

(continued)

3. Continuing to support weight with the upper extremities on the walker, the patient lowers the uninvolved lower extremity down to the same stair as the walker's forwardmost legs.

4. The walker is advanced and the sequence is repeated until the patient completes descending the stairs. When the patient reaches the landing or floor level, she places the walker in front and grasps both handgrips.

PROCEDURE 9-7

 AMBULATING THROUGH DOORWAYS WITH A WALKER

Door Opens Toward Patient

1. The patient approaches the latch edge of the door, standing outside the arc through which the opening door will move. The patient shifts the weight to the side of the walker away from the hand that will be placed on the door handle. The unweighted hand is then placed on the door handle.

2. Using a pulling motion, the door is opened wider than the width of the patient. This is necessary because the door will start to close automatically before the patient can progress through the doorway. The door must be blocked from closing by the walker to allow the patient time to progress through the doorway.

(continued)

3. The hand used to open the door is returned quickly to the walker. The walker is lifted and moved forward into the doorway. All four legs of the walker are placed on the floor with the two legs closest to the door serving as door stops. Using this method, the closing door hits the walker's legs, not the patient.

4. Once the walker has absorbed the contact of a closing door, the patient can step into the walker to advance through the doorway.

5. The patient may have to push the door further open during transit through the doorway to allow a walker to be moved.

6. The patient should wait until the walker's legs have absorbed the contact of the closing door before moving forward. Once the patient has moved completely through the doorway, the door closes behind the patient.

Door Opens Away From Patient

1. When a door with an automatic door closer opens away from a patient, the patient should approach the door and shift the weight to the side of the walker away from the hand that is closest to the door handle. The unweighted hand is then placed on the door handle.

2. Using a pushing motion, the door is opened wider than the width of the patient. The hand used to open the door is returned quickly to the walker. The walker is lifted and moved forward into the doorway. All four legs of the walker are placed on the floor with the two legs closest to the door serve as door stops. Using this method, the closing door hits the walker's legs, not the patient. Once a walker has absorbed the contact of a closing door, the patient can step into the walker to advance through the doorway.

3. Using a walker's legs as doorstops, the patient progresses through the doorway. The patient may have to push a door further open during transit through the doorway to allow a walker to be moved. Whenever this is done, the patient should wait until the walker's legs have absorbed the contact of the closing door before moving forward. Once the patient has moved completely through the doorway, the door closes behind the patient.

AXILLARY CRUTCHES

FITTING

Axillary crutches are fitted with the patient standing and shoulder girdles relaxed. Proper adjustment requires appropriate posture because of the potential for injury. When crutches are too long or when a patient rests on the tops of the crutches, injury to nerves and blockage of blood vessels in the axillae can occur. Patients may report pain or tingling in the upper extremities, and muscle weakness or paralysis may occur.

The first adjustment is the overall length of the crutch (Figure 9–22). Crutch tips are positioned on the floor, approximately 6 inches away from the toes at a 45-degree angle anterior and lateral to the small toe. With the patient's shoulder girdles in a relaxed position, the physical therapist should be able to put two or three fingers between the patient's axillae and the top of the crutch on each side. When axillary pads are to be used on crutches, they should be in place during fitting. In some styles of crutches, nuts and bolts should not be tightened completely until all adjustments are completed.

Handgrip height is adjusted after overall length of the crutch is determined (Figure 9–23). The top of the handgrip should be approximately at the level of the top of the patient's ulnar styloid process when the upper extremities are in a relaxed position at the patient's side. When the patient grasps the handgrips with shoulder girdles level and relaxed, elbows are flexed approximately 20–30 degrees.

FIGURE 9–22 Checking overall height of axillary crutches.

FIGURE 9–23 Checking handgrip height for axillary crutches.

When all length and handgrip adjustments are made, all nuts, bolts, and button locks should be checked to ensure that they are tightened or fully positioned to maintain crutch integrity during ambulation.

PROCEDURE 9-8

IN AND OUT OF A WHEELCHAIR WITH AXILLARY CRUTCHES

Assuming Standing—Physical Therapist on Involved Side

1. Wheelchair wheel locks are engaged and footrests are moved out of the way. Crutches are placed within reach of the physical therapist or patient before the patient starts to stand.

   As the patient moves to the front edge of the seat, the physical therapist may need to support the involved lower extremity the first few times a patient assumes standing.

2. To provide assistance, the physical therapist squats on the involved side of the patient while supporting the involved lower extremity.

   When the patient is unable to flex the knee of the involved lower extremity, an elevating legrest is used for support during sitting. The legrest must be removed or lowered and pivoted to the side before the patient's involved lower extremity is lowered to the floor.

3. The physical therapist supports the involved lower extremity with one hand and arm while the legrest is removed with the other hand. The involved lower extremity is lowered carefully to the floor before the patient attempts to stand.

(continued)

4. Both crutches are placed together in front of and slightly lateral to the patient's foot on the uninvolved side. The patient grasps both crutch handgrips with the hand on the uninvolved side while grasping the wheelchair armrest on the involved side. Positioned in stride to one side of the patient, the physical therapist grasps the patient's gait belt and shoulder girdle.

5. The patient assumes standing using the upper extremities and extending the uninvolved lower extremity. The involved lower extremity must be maintained within the desired weight bearing status.

6. Once a standing position has been assumed, the physical therapist ensures the patient is stable and able to maintain an upright posture. One at a time crutches are positioned properly under the axillae. The patient reaches across the body with the hand on the involved side for a crutch.

7. The crutch that was retrieved by the hand on the involved side is positioned under the axillae first.

8. The crutch that remains in the hand on the uninvolved side is positioned second. The patient is ready to ambulate.

Assuming Sitting—Physical Therapist on Involved Side

1. Wheelchair wheel locks are engaged and footrests are moved out of the way. To sit, the patient is positioned facing away from the wheelchair at the front edge of a wheelchair seat, close enough so that the front edge of wheelchair seat is felt against the back of the lower extremities.
2. The patient's feet can be positioned either in stride or side by side. Positioned in stride, behind and to one side of a patient, the physical therapist grasps the patient's gait belt and shoulder girdle.

3. The crutch on the patient's involved side is removed from the axilla and held by the handgrip only. The crutch on the uninvolved side is removed from the axilla and passed to the hand on the involved side. Both crutches are held by the handgrips. They are placed in front of and slightly lateral to the patient's foot on the involved side.

4. Reaching back with the hand on the uninvolved side, the patient grasps the wheelchair armrest.

5. Using support from the handgrip and armrest, the patient lowers to sitting.

6. Setting crutches aside, the patient grasps both armrests and moves completely into the seat. Physical therapists may or may not need to assist with an involved lower extremity. When necessary, a patient's involved lower extremity is placed on the elevating legrest.

Assuming Standing—Therapist on Uninvolved Side

When the patient can control the involved lower extremity, the physical therapist assists the patient to standing from the patient's uninvolved side.

1. Wheelchair wheel locks are engaged and footrests moved out of the way. The patient is positioned at the front edge of the wheelchair seat. Positioned in stride, behind and to one side of a patient, the physical therapist grasps the patient's gait belt and shoulder girdle.
2. Crutches are placed together to the front and side of the uninvolved foot. The patient grasps the handgrips of both crutches in one hand. The patient's other hand is placed on the wheelchair armrest.

3. The patient pushes to standing using the armrest and the handgrips for support.

4. When the patient has assumed a standing position, the physical therapist should ensure that the patient can control his/her balance. Releasing the grasp on the armrest, the patient reaches for one crutch.

5. One at a time, crutches are positioned properly under the axillae. The crutch on the involved side is positioned first.

6. The crutch on the uninvolved side is positioned second. The patient is then ready to ambulate.

Assuming Sitting—Physical Therapist on Uninvolved Side

1. Wheelchair wheel locks are engaged and footrests are moved out of the way. To sit, the patient is positioned facing away from the wheelchair at the front edge of a wheelchair seat, close enough so that the front edge of wheelchair seat is felt against the back of the lower extremities. The patient's feet can be positioned either in stride or side by side. Positioned in stride, behind and to one side of the patient, the physical therapist grasps the patient's gait belt and shoulder girdle.

2. The crutch on the patient's involved side is removed from the axilla and held by the handgrip only. The crutch on the uninvolved side is removed from the axilla and passed to the hand on the involved side.

3. Both crutches are held by the handgrips on the patient's involved side. The patient reaches back and grasps the wheelchair armrest with the hand on the uninvolved side.

4. Using support from the handgrips and wheelchair armrest, the patient lowers to sitting.
5. Setting crutches aside, the patient grasps both wheelchair armrests and maneuvers completely into the wheelchair seat.

PROCEDURE 9-9

 AMBULATING ON LEVEL SURFACES WITH AXILLARY CRUTCHES

Three-Point Gait Pattern

Partial to Full Weight Bearing

When ambulating with crutches, lifting of the body to decrease weight bearing is achieved by shoulder depression and elbow extension. The patient must also adduct the upper extremities to keep crutches in place under the axillae.

1. The physical therapist is positioned in stride, behind and to one side of the patient, grasping the patient's gait belt. When close guarding is required, the physical therapist maintains contact with the patient's shoulder girdle in addition to the gait belt. In the starting position the patient stands with crutches approximately 6 inches away from the toes at a 45-degree angle anterior and lateral to the small toe. The patient's feet are side by side.
2. To ambulate, both crutches are advanced simultaneously the same distance. The physical therapist advances the outside foot either at the same time or immediately after crutches are advanced.

3. The patient advances the involved lower extremity so the ball of the foot is approximately even with the crutch tips. As the patient improves, she may move crutches and involved lower extremity at the same time, permitting a faster gait.

(continued)

4. Using upper extremities and involved lower extremity weight-bearing as permitted to support body weight, the patient advances the uninvolved lower extremity beyond the crutches. Initially, the patient may "step to" the involved lower extremity, rather than "step through." Stepping through is a normal gait pattern and should be encouraged. The physical therapist advances the inside foot as the patient moves the uninvolved lower extremity closest to him. The sequence is repeated for continued progression.

Non-Weight Bearing

1. The physical therapist is positioned in stride, behind and to one side of the patient, grasping the patient's gait belt. When close guarding is required, the physical therapist maintains contact with the patient's shoulder girdle in addition to the gait belt. In the starting position the patient stands with crutches approximately 6 inches away from the toes at a 45-degree angle anterior and lateral to the small toe. The patient's feet are side by side. The involved lower extremity is not on the floor. Generally, patients hold the involved lower extremity in front when the knee cannot be flexed and behind when the knee can be flexed.

2. To ambulate, both crutches and the involved lower extremity are advanced simultaneously the same distance. The physical therapist advances the outside foot at the same time or immediately after crutches are advanced.

3. Using the upper extremities to support all body weight, the patient advances the uninvolved lower extremity beyond the crutches. Initially, the patient may "step to" the involved lower extremity, rather than "step through." Stepping through is a normal gait pattern and should be encouraged. The physical therapist advances the inside foot as the patient moves the uninvolved lower extremity. The sequence is repeated for continued progression.

(continued)

Four-Point Gait Pattern

1. The physical therapist is positioned in stride, behind and to one side of a patient, grasping the patient's gait belt. In the starting position the patient stands with crutches approximately 6 inches away from the toes at a 45-degree angle anterior and lateral to the small toe. The patient's feet are side by side. To ambulate, the patient advances one crutch. The physical therapist advances the outside foot when the crutch closest to the physical therapist is advanced.

2. The patient then advances the opposite lower extremity so the ball of the foot is approximately even with the tip of the crutch. The physical therapist advances his inside foot when the patient advances the lower extremity closest to the physical therapist.

3. The patient shifts weight to the crutch and lower extremity just advanced, then advances the remaining crutch beyond the other crutch.

4. The patient advances the remaining lower extremity so the ball of the foot is approximately even with the tip of the crutch just advanced. The patient shifts weight to the crutch and lower extremity just advanced. The sequence is repeated for continued progression.

Two-Point Gait Pattern

1. The physical therapist is positioned in stride, behind and to one side of a patient, grasping the patient's gait belt. In the starting position the patient stands with crutches approximately 6 inches away from the toes at a 45-degree angle anterior and lateral to the small toe. The patient's feet are side by side. To ambulate, the patient advances one crutch and the opposite lower extremity simultaneously, placing the ball of the foot approximately even with the tip of the crutch. The patient shifts weight onto this crutch and lower extremity as the physical therapist advances the inside foot.

2. The patient advances the remaining crutch and lower extremity together beyond the first crutch and lower extremity in a normal stride length. The patient shifts weight onto the just advanced crutch and lower extremity as the physical therapist advances the outside foot. The sequence is repeated for continued progression.

Falling

Patients must be taught how to control a fall, as falls may occur during ambulation training or after discharge. When the patient starts to fall, the physical therapist must decide whether to prevent the fall or to permit a controlled fall in a manner that will prevent injury to the patient or physical therapist. The physical therapist must be alert to the patient's movements at all times and be able to react quickly to prevent or control a fall. Proper guarding and attention focused on the patient is required at all times.

1. The physical therapist prevents a fall by using the biomechanical advantages of standing in stride, behind and slightly to the side of a patient. By standing in stride, the physical therapist is able to shift weight onto the back foot and pull the patient into the base of support.

2. When the physical therapist cannot prevent a fall, the fall must be controlled. The patient is instructed to let the crutches fall to the sides, away from the area in which the patient will land, avoiding injury from landing on the crutches. The physical therapist steps forward in a stride position to widen the base of support as the rate at which the patient falls is slowed.

3. Patients can catch themselves on outstretched upper extremities, making sure that the elbows flex slightly to absorb impact. If the elbow is not flexed, injury to the patient's upper extremities may occur.

4. The physical therapist continues lowering the patient to the floor slowly and the patient turns onto the side of the uninvolved lower extremity to avoid additional injury to the involved lower extremity.

5. Turning from the side of the uninvolved lower extremity into a long sitting position, the patient is then in a position to get up from the floor.

   The method used to rise from the floor depends on the patient's initial problem and any additional injury the fall may have caused. When the patient is unsure of the ability to arise after having fallen, assistance should be summoned. Usually the patient can move on the floor to a sitting position near a chair or couch. Using furniture for stability and assistance, the patient can usually assume standing again. Methods of moving from the floor to a sitting position in a chair are described in Chapter 8, "Independent Transfer From Wheelchair to Floor and Return."

PROCEDURE 9-10

AMBULATING ON STAIRS WITH AXILLARY CRUTCHES

Holding the Crutches

Ambulation on stairs can be performed using two crutches without the use of a handrail. Use of a handrail, however, provides stability and thus is an added safety factor. When using a handrail, it takes the place of the crutch on one side. There are several methods of holding crutches when using a handrail. Whichever method of holding crutches is used, the sequence of movements for the lower extremities and ambulatory assistive devices is the same.

There are three common methods of holding crutches while ambulating on stairs.

The first method of holding two crutches while using a handrail is to place both crutches together under the upper extremity on the side opposite the handrail.

The second method of holding two crutches while using a handrail is to hold the crutch on the side of the handrail in the hand that grasps the handrail. This crutch is held by one of its uprights, parallel to the handrail. The crutch on the side opposite the handrail is used in the usual manner.

The third method of holding two crutches while using a handrail is to hold the handrail with one hand. The hand on the side opposite the handrail holds both crutches, one in the usual manner and the other by one of its uprights perpendicular to the first crutch.

Ascending Using a Handrail

1. To ascend stairs using any of the methods of holding crutches, the patient stands facing up the stairs. Positioned in stride behind the patient, the physical therapist grasps the patient's gait belt and the handrail. For the method illustrated in this section, the patient places both crutches under the upper extremity on the side opposite the handrail and grasps the handrail with the other hand.

2. The patient places the uninvolved lower extremity on the next higher stair while the body weight is supported by the upper extremities.

(continued)

3. Weight is shifted to the uninvolved lower extremity on the next higher stair. Extending the uninvolved lower extremity, the patient lifts up to the next higher stair. The crutches and involved lower extremity are advanced to the same stair at the same time.

   Crutches must be placed midway on the stair tread, and placed far enough from the handrail, or far enough from each other when no handrail is used, to permit patients to move through the crutches to the next stair. Proper crutch placement on stairs provides stability and space for patients to maneuver.

4. The physical therapist ascends with the patient. This sequence is repeated to ascend an entire flight of stairs.

Descending Using a Handrail

1. To descend stairs using any of the methods of holding crutches, the patient stands facing down the stairs. Positioned in stride in front of the patient, the physical therapist grasps the patient's gait belt and the handrail. For the method illustrated in this section, the patient places both crutches under the upper extremity on the side opposite the handrails, and grasps the handrail with the other hand.

2. Maintaining support using the uninvolved lower extremity and the hand on the handrail, crutches are placed securely on the next lower stair. Crutches must be placed midway on the stair tread, and placed far enough from the handrail, or far enough from each other when no handrail is used, to permit the patient to move through the crutches to the next stair. Proper crutch placement on stairs provides stability and space for the patient to maneuver.

3. With the body supported by the upper extremities and the uninvolved lower extremity, the involved lower extremity is moved to the same stair as the crutches.

(continued)

4. Bearing weight on the upper extremities and on the involved lower extremity if weight-bearing is permitted, the uninvolved lower extremity is moved to the same stair as the crutches and involved lower extremity. The physical therapist descends with the patient.
5. This sequence is repeated to descend an entire flight of stairs.

Ascending and Descending Stairs Without Using a Handrail

To ascend or descend stairs without using a handrail, crutches are retained in the same position used for ambulating on level surfaces. Rather than using a handrail for support on one side, patients use one crutch on each side for support. Physical therapist position, and the sequence of moving the crutches and lower extremities remains the same as for ascending stairs using a handrail, and descending stairs using a handrail. Physical therapists hold the handrail, when available, for stability, whether a patient is using a handrail or not.

Ascending stairs without using a handrail.

Descending stairs without using a handrail.

PROCEDURE 9-11

 AMBULATING THROUGH DOORWAYS WITH AXILLARY CRUTCHES

Door With Automatic Door Closer
Door Opens Toward Patient

1. The patient approaches the latch edge of the door, standing outside the arc through which the opening door will move. The patient shifts weight onto the crutch on the side away from the hand that will be placed on the door handle. The unweighted hand is then placed on the door handle. Preferably, weight is shifted to the side closest to the door handle and the hand farthest from the door handle is used to pull open the door. Using the hand farthest from the door permits a patient to open a door wider than using the hand closest to the door.

2. Using a pulling motion, the door is opened wider than the width of the patient. This is necessary because a door will start to close automatically before patients can progress through the doorway.

(continued)

3. The hand used to open the door is quickly returned to the crutch. To block automatic closing of the door, the patient turns into the doorway and places the tip of the crutch closest to the door on the floor in the path of the door. This acts as a door stop, permitting the patient to progress through the doorway without being struck by the closing door.

4. Continuing to use the tip of the crutch or shoulder as a door stop, the patient ambulates through the doorway using the appropriate gait pattern.

5. As the patient moves through the doorway, the door may have to be pushed open again. The crutch tip used as a door stop is placed progressively closer to the hinge edge of the door. The physical therapist and patient must be aware that as a crutch tip gets closer to the hinge edge of the door, it becomes more difficult to hold open the door.
6. Once the patient has moved completely through the doorway, the door closes behind the patient.

Door Opens Away From Patient

1. The patient faces the door and shifts weight onto the crutch away from the hand that is closest to the door handle. Using the hand closest to the door permits a patient to open a door wider than using the hand farthest from the door. The unweighted hand is then placed on the door handle.

2. Using a pushing motion, the door is opened wider than the width of the patient. Opening the door wider than the width of a patient is necessary because the door will start to close automatically before a patient can move through the doorway. Automatic closing of the door must be blocked by the tip of the crutch closest to the door, permitting patients time to progress through the doorway. The hand used to open the door is quickly returned to the crutch. The crutch closest to the door is then advanced into the doorway to act as a door stop.

3. As the patient moves through the doorway, the door may have to be pushed open again. Continuing to use the tip of the crutch or shoulder as a door stop, the patient ambulates through the doorway using the appropriate gait pattern.

4. Once a patient has moved completely through the doorway, the door closes behind the patient.

Door Without Automatic Door Closer

When a door does not have an automatic closer, the initial rapid movement to place a crutch tip on the ground as a doorstop is not necessary. Extra wide opening of a door is also not necessary. Crutch movement can be performed more slowly, and placement of a crutch tip as a doorstop between a door and a patient is not required. Patients must turn to close the door because the door will not close automatically.

FOREARM (LOFSTRAND) CRUTCHES

Forearm crutches can be used by patients with the same impairments and with the same gait patterns as patients that use axillary crutches. When ambulating with forearm crutches, lifting of the body to decrease weight bearing is achieved by shoulder depression and elbow extension. The illustrations in this section present the use of forearm crutches for a patient with paraplegia. Patients with paraplegia have paralysis of the musculature of the lower extremities and usually some weakness of trunk muscles. Patients with paraplegia lack sufficient lower extremity and lower trunk muscle strength to support themselves in an upright posture. To overcome this lack of strength, a greater degree of upper trunk and upper extremity strength is required. Ambulation for patients with paraplegia requires upper body movement to control paretic or paralyzed lower extremities.

Patients with paraplegia usually use a swing-to or swing-through gait pattern. They will use bilateral knee-ankle-foot orthoses (KAFOs). KAFOs lock at the knee and ankle joints, maintaining the patient's knees in extension and ankles in slight dorsiflexion during ambulation. Initially, the patient may use a swing-to gait pattern. As ability improves, the patient may progress to the swing-through pattern. The swing-through gait pattern is more efficient, permitting the patient to move more quickly.

FITTING

Setting the length of forearm crutches determines handgrip height. Forearm crutches are positioned with the crutch tip on the floor, approximately 6 inches away from the toes at a 45-dgree angle anterior and lateral to the small toe. Handgrips are level with the ulnar styloid processes when the upper extremities are relaxed at the side (Figure 9–24).

When handgrips are held with the shoulders relaxed, the elbows should be in 20 to 30 degrees of flexion. Forearm cuff height is adjusted after crutch length has been adjusted. Cuff height should be adjusted to a point as high as possible on the forearm without interfering with elbow flexion. Cuff width should be tight enough to stay on the upper extremity when a handgrip is released, but loose enough not to bind. Cuff width is adjusted by squeezing the cuff together, or spreading it apart (Figure 9–25).

FIGURE 9–24 Measuring forearm crutch length.

FIGURE 9–25 Ensuring proper elbow flexion and cuff tightness.

PROCEDURE 9–12

IN AND OUT OF A WHEELCHAIR WITH FOREARM CRUTCHES

Two methods, the turn-around method and the power method, may be used to assume standing using forearm crutches and KAFOs. The turn-around method requires less strength than the power method.

1. Wheelchair wheels are locked and footrests moved out of the way. The patient is positioned at the front edge of the seat. Positioned in stride, behind and to one side of the patient, the physical therapist grasps the patient's gait belt and shoulder.
2. One forearm crutch is placed on either side of the wheelchair. Crutches must be supported securely enough so they will not fall as the patient moves, yet be accessible to the patient.

3. The patient moves forward on the seat of the wheelchair and secures the knee locks of their KAFOs in knee extension.

Assuming Standing Using the Turn-Around Method

For this method, the physical therapist initially assumes the proper position on the side from which the patient will turn. In the illustrations for this section, this is on the patient's right side. The physical therapist must be prepared to move with the patient so as not to inhibit the patient's fluid motion. Initially, the physical therapist may assist by lifting or guiding the patient.

1. When the patient turns to the left, she begins by hooking the medial upright of the right orthosis over the medial upright of the left orthosis. This aids in placement of the lower extremities as the patient stands. The patient then turns onto the left side. As the patient turns, she reaches behind with the left hand to grasp the right armrest, and in front with the right hand to grasp the left armrest.

2. Using the upper extremities, the patient pushes to standing, completing the turn to assume a standing position facing the wheelchair.

3. Using the armrests for support, the patient performs a push-up, lifting the body to position the lower extremities. Feet must be positioned so the patient is centered in front of the wheelchair at a distance that will permit support with one upper extremity as the crutches are retrieved.

4. The patient shifts weight to one side and grasps and positions the forearm crutch on the side that has been un-weighted.

5. Shifting weight onto one forearm crutch, the patient grasps the second forearm crutch and places it properly.

(continued)

6. Using both crutches for support, the patient pushes to a fully upright position, shoulders behind hips to maintain hip extension. This posture is called a "C" curve.

Assuming Sitting Using the Turn-Around Method

1. Wheelchair wheel locks are engaged and footrests moved out of the way. Positioned in stride, slightly behind and to the side to which the patient will turn, the physical therapist grasps the patient's gait belt and shoulder. The physical therapists must be prepared to move as the patient moves to avoid interfering with the patient's fluid motion. Initially, the physical therapist may guide or control the rate at which the patient turns and lowers into the seat.

2. To assume sitting using the turn-around method, the patient approaches and faces the wheelchair with the crutches placed on either side of the wheelchair.

3. Shifting weight onto one forearm crutch, the patient removes the other forearm crutch. The crutch that has been removed is placed against the wheelchair.

4. The patient then grasps the armrest with the free hand and shifts weight onto the upper extremity that is grasping the armrest. The patient then removes the remaining crutch and places it against the wheelchair.

5. The patient is then able to grasp the remaining armrest.

(continued)

6. Turning, the patient then lowers into the wheelchair.

7. Repositioning upper extremities, the patient adjusts the position in the wheelchair. Knee locks on the KAFOs are released. Once KAFO knee locks are released, the patient replaces the wheelchair footrests and assumes a proper sitting position.

Assuming Standing Using the Power Method

1. Wheelchair wheel locks are engaged and footrests moved out of the way. The patient is positioned toward the front edge of the seat. Positioned in stride, behind and to one side of the patient, the physical therapist grasps the patient's gait belt and shoulder. The physical therapist must be prepared to move as the patient moves to avoid interfering with the patient's fluid motion.

2. With knee locks of the KAFOs secured, the patient grasps one crutch in each hand. The tips of the crutches are placed on the floor even with the hips in the anterior/posterior direction, one on each side of the wheelchair.

3. Pushing on the crutches, the patient extends the upper extremities and depresses the shoulders, producing a quick thrusting movement to propel the body upward and forward into a standing position.

4. The patient must move the crutches forward quickly to halt the forward momentum. Placing the crutches slightly ahead and to the side of the toes, the patient assumes a "C" curve. The physical therapist can assist the patient into a "C" curve position by pushing forward on the gait belt and pulling backward on the patient's shoulder.

(continued)

Assuming Sitting Using the Power Method

1. Wheelchair wheel locks are engaged and footrests moved out of the way. Positioned in stride, slightly behind and to the side, the physical therapist grasps the patient's gait belt and shoulder. The physical therapist must be prepared to move as the patient moves to avoid interfering with the patient's fluid motion.

2. To sit, the patient stands facing away from the wheelchair with the feet approximately 12–18 inches in front of the front edge of the seat. The position of the feet must permit the patient to end up sitting securely in the seat as she lowers while the knee locks of KAFOs are locked.

3. Moving the shoulders anterior to the hips, the patient flexes at the hips into a "jack-knife" position. The patient starts falling backward, initiating lowering into the wheel-chair.

4. As the patient sits, the crutches are lifted. After the patient is seated, knee locks on the KAFOs are released. Once the KAFOs have been unlocked, the patient can replace the footrests and assume a proper sitting position.

PROCEDURE 9-13

AMBULATING ON LEVEL GROUND WITH FOREARM CRUTCHES

Swing-To Gait Pattern

1. Positioned in stride, slightly behind and to the side, the physical therapist grasps the patient's gait belt and shoulder. The physical therapist must be prepared to move as the patient moves to avoid interfering with the patient's fluid motion.

   In the starting position, the patient's hips are maintained in extension by keeping shoulders posterior to hips, in the "C" curve posture. The physical therapist can assist maintaining a "C" curve by pushing forward with the hand on the gait belt while pulling backward with the hand on the patient's shoulder.

2. To initiate the swing-to gait pattern, the patient advances the crutches one stride length beyond the patient's toes. The physical therapist advances the outside foot.

3. Pushing down on the crutches, the patients extends the upper extremities and depresses the shoulders. At the same time, the trunk is flexed to lift the feet off the ground. The physical therapist may assist by lifting with the hand on the gait belt.

(continued)

4. With the feet off the ground and trunk flexed, gravity will swing the patient's lower extremities forward. As the lower extremities swing forward, the patient begins to extend the neck and trunk to regain a "C" curve. With the feet placed on the floor between the crutches, momentum continues to move the patient's hips anterior to the shoulders. As the patient swings forward, the physical therapist steps forward with the inside foot. The physical therapist may assist a patient to regain a "C" curve by pushing forward with the hand on the gait belt and pulling backward with the hand on the patient's shoulder. Once a "C" curve is regained, the crutches are advanced. The sequence is repeated for continued progression.

Swing-Through Gait Pattern

A swing-through gait pattern is essentially the same as a swing-to gait pattern. The difference is that during the swing phase of the swing-through gait pattern, the patient swings beyond the crutches and lands anterior to the crutch tips.

1. In the starting position for a swing-through gait pattern, the patient is in a "C" curve, with crutch tips beyond the toes. The role and position of the physical therapist is the same as for a swing-to gait pattern.

2. Pushing down on the crutches, the patient extends the upper extremities and depresses the shoulders. At the same time, the trunk is flexed to lift the feet off the ground. The physical therapist may assist by lifting with the hand on the gait belt.

3. With the feet off the ground and trunk flexed, gravity will swing the patient's lower extremities forward. As the lower extremities swing forward, the patient extends the neck and trunk to regain a "C" curve.

4. The patient lands with the feet anterior to the crutches. As the patient swings forward, the therapist steps forward with the inside foot.

(continued)

5. Because of momentum generated by a larger swing, the crutches must be advanced quickly to prevent the patient from falling. As the crutches are advanced, the physical therapist steps forward with the outside foot.

Falling

The patient must be taught how to control a fall, as falls may occur during ambulation training or after discharge. When the patient starts to fall, the physical therapist must decide whether to prevent the fall or to permit a controlled fall in a manner that will prevent injury to the patient or physical therapist. The physical therapist must be alert to the patient's movements at all times and be able to react quickly to prevent or control a fall. Proper guarding and attention focused on the patient is required at all times.

Patients with paraplegia tend to fall when they lose their "C" curve or when momentum into the "C" curve is interrupted, causing them to "jackknife." The most effective method of preventing falls in these situations is for a physical therapist to assist the patient in regaining the "C" curve. This is achieved by pulling the patient's shoulders backward while pushing forward with the hand on the gait belt.

1. When the physical therapist cannot prevent a fall, she must control the fall. The patient is instructed to let crutches fall to the sides, away from the area in which the patient will land, to avoid injury from landing on the crutches. The physical therapist steps forward in a stride position to widen the base of support while slowing the rate at which the patient falls.

2. The patient catches herself on outstretched hands, keeping the elbows flexed to absorb the impact. If elbows are not flexed, injury to the patient's upper extremities may occur.

3. The physical therapist continues to lower the patient to the floor slowly.

Assuming Standing from the Floor

To assume standing from the floor independently is a difficult maneuver for patients using KAFOs and forearm crutches. The most practical method is to move along the floor to a chair or other sturdy object and use the object as support to rise from the floor. Methods of moving from the floor to a sitting position in a chair are described in the Chapter 8 section, "Independent Transfer from Wheelchair to Floor and Return."

1. To assume standing directly from a prone position on the floor, the patient must first retrieve and position the crutches.

2. Grasping one crutch, the patient places it upright with the tip of the crutch on the floor. The patient places the other hand on the other crutch or on the floor at the level of the shoulder.

(continued)

The following sequence of movements must be performed quickly, without pauses.

3. Pushing with the hand on the floor and pulling with the hand on the crutch, the patient raises the trunk. Positioned in stride, slightly behind and to the side, the physical therapist grasps the patient's gait belt and shoulder. The physical therapist may assist by lifting with the hand on the gait belt.

4. With weight shifted onto the upper extremity that is on the floor, the patient pushes down on the handgrip and floor to assume a "jackknife" position. During initial training, the physical therapist assists by lifting on the gait belt. The physical therapist may also need to block the patient's feet to prevent them from sliding posteriorly. After shifting weight onto the upright crutch, the patient grasps the handgrip of the remaining crutch.

5. The second crutch is positioned upright with the tip on the floor in line with the tip of the first crutch.

6. The patient then uses both crutches to push through an upright position, into a "C" curve. The crutches are properly positioned, one at a time. The patients is then ready to ambulate.

Adjusting first forearm crutch.

Adjusting second forearm crutch.

Ready to ambulate.

Doorways

Patients using forearm crutches maneuver through doorways in the same manner as do patients using axillary crutches.

PROCEDURE 9-14

AMBULATING ON STAIRS WITH FOREARM CRUTCHES

There are two basic methods for patients using KAFOs and forearm crutches to ambulate on stairs, the forward method and the backward method. In both methods, the patient may use a handrail and one crutch, or two crutches. In both methods, the physical therapist is positioned in stride on the stairs below the patient and grasps the patient's gait belt and the handrail. Initially, gait training on stairs may require assistance by two people to ensure patient safety.

Ascending—Forward Method

1. To ascend stairs using the forward method, the patient starts in a "C" curve position facing up the stairs. The feet and crutch tips are parallel with the base of the stair.

2. The same motion used to initiate ambulation on level surfaces is used to initiate ambulation on stairs. Flexing the neck and upper trunk, the patient extends the upper extremities and depresses the shoulders to lift the body. As the patient's feet are lifted from the ground, gravity swings the lower extremities forward onto the next higher stair. The physical therapist may assist by lifting on the gait belt as the patient raises the body.

3. The patient then extends the neck and trunk to regain a "C" curve and places the lower extremities onto the next higher stair. The physical therapist may assist the patient in regaining a "C" curve by pushing forward on the gait belt.

4. Crutches are advanced to the same stair as the feet. The sequence is repeated to ascend an entire flight of stairs.

Descending—Forward Method

1. To descend stairs using the forward method, the patient starts in a "C" curve position facing down the stairs. The feet and crutch tips are parallel with the base of the stair.

(continued)

2. The same motion used to initiate ambulation on level surfaces is used to initiate ambulation on stairs. Flexing the neck and upper trunk, the patient extends the upper extremities and depresses the shoulders to lift the body. The physical therapist may assist by lifting on the gait belt as the patient raises the body. As the patient's feet are lifted from the ground, gravity swings the lower extremities forward over the next lower stair.

3. As the lower extremities swing over the stair, the patient uses the upper extremities to lower in a controlled manner onto the next lower stair.

   Extending the neck and trunk, the patient regain a "C" curve and places the lower extremities on the next lower stair. The physical therapist may assist the patient in regaining a "C" curve by pulling forward on the gait belt.

4. Crutches are advanced onto the same stair as the lower extremities. Patients often descend two steps at a time. The sequence is repeated to descend an entire flight of stairs.

Ascending—Backward Method

1. To ascend stairs using the backward method, the patient starts in a "C" curve position facing away from the stairs. The feet and crutch tips are parallel with the base of the stair. During initial training, two physical therapists may be positioned on the stairs, one above the patient and one below the patient.

2. The same motion used to initiate ambulation on level surfaces is used to initiate ambulation on stairs. Flexing the neck and upper trunk, the patient extends the upper extremities and depresses the shoulders to lift the body. The physical therapist positioned on the stairs above the patient may assist by lifting and pulling back. The physical therapist positioned below the patient pushes on the gait belt as the patient raises the body. When the physical therapist exerts force into the abdominal area to assist patient positioning, care must be taken to avoid injuring the patient.

3. As the patient lifts into a "jackknife" position, backward momentum of the lower extremities moves the patient up and over the higher stair. The patient uses the upper extremities to lower onto the next higher stair.

(continued)

4. Once the patient's lower extremities are on the next higher stair, the patient permits the pelvis to move forward. As this movement occurs, the patient extends the neck and trunk to regain a "C" curve, while moving the crutches onto the same stair as the lower extremities. The physical therapist positioned below the patient may assist the patient in regaining a "C" curve by pulling forward on the gait belt. The sequence is repeated to ascend an entire flight of stairs.

Descending—Backward Method

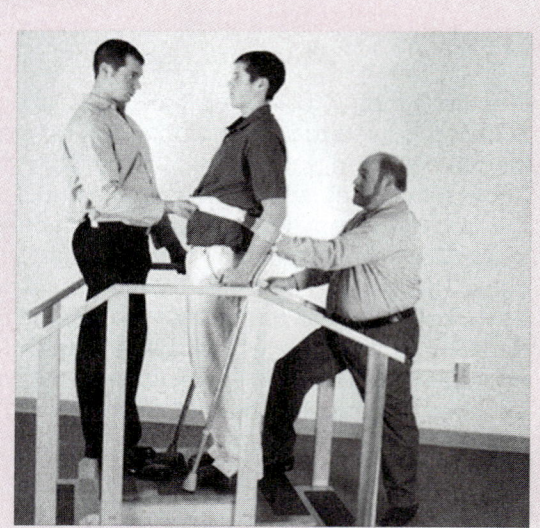

1. To descend stairs using the backward method, the patient starts in a "C" curve position facing up the stairs. The feet and crutch tips are parallel with the base of the stair. During initial training, two physical therapists may be positioned on the stairs, one above the patient and one below the patient.

2. The same motion used to initiate ambulation on level surfaces is used to initiate ambulation on stairs. Flexing the neck and upper trunk, the patient extends the upper extremities and depresses the shoulders to lift the body. The physical therapist positioned on the stairs above the patient may assist by pushing on the gait belt and assisting the lowering. The physical therapist positioned on the stairs below the patient may assist by lifting on the gait belt as the patient raises the body.

3. As the patient lifts into a "jackknife" position, the backward momentum of the lower extremities moves the patient over the next lower stair. Once the lower extremities are over the stair, the patient uses the upper extremities to lower in a controlled manner onto the next lower stair.

4. After the lower extremities are on the next lower stair, the patient extends the neck and trunk to regain a "C" curve. This movement allows the hips to remain in extension. Crutches are then moved onto the same stair as the lower extremities. The physical therapist positioned on the stairs above the patient may assist by pulling on the gait belt to assist the patient in assuming a "C" curve. The physical therapist positioned on the stairs below the patient may assist by pushing on the gait belt.
5. The sequence is repeated to descend an entire flight of stairs.

CANES

FITTING

Canes are fitted with the patient standing and shoulders relaxed. The cane is positioned upright, with the tip on the floor alongside the small toe. With the cane in this position, the top of the cane is adjusted to be at the level of the patient's ulnar styloid process (Figure 9–26). This permits 20 to 30 degrees of elbow flexion when the cane is held in the patient's hand (Figure 9–27). When used properly, forces on a cane should be exerted directly downward.

FIGURE 9–26 Measuring cane height.

FIGURE 9–27 Ensuring proper elbow flexion.

When using a quad cane, the longer legs of the cane are positioned facing away from the patient's lower extremity (Figure 9–28). This reduces the risk of the patient's foot becoming entangled in the legs of the quad cane. Quad canes are measured and used in the same manner as standard canes.

FIGURE 9–28 Proper positioning of a quad cane for ambulation.

PROCEDURE 9-15

IN AND OUT OF A WHEELCHAIR WITH ONE CANE

1. Wheelchair wheel locks are engaged and footrests moved out of the way. The patient is positioned at the front edge of the seat, with the feet in stride or side by side. Positioned in stride, behind and to one side of a patient the physical therapist grasps the patient's gait belt and shoulder.

2. The quad cane is positioned alongside the foot on the side on which it will be held. The patient may place both hands on the respective armrests or place one hand on the cane and one on the armrest to push to standing. When the patient has only one functional upper extremity, that upper extremity is used on the armrest to push to standing. Once the patient is standing, the cane is grasped.

3. The patient pushes to standing, making sure to be erect and balanced. The patient is then ready to ambulate.

Assuming Sitting—Quad Cane and Armrests

1. Wheelchair wheel locks are engaged and footrests moved out of the way. To sit, the patient is positioned at the front edge of the wheelchair seat, facing away from the wheelchair, so the front edge of the wheelchair seat is felt against the back of the lower extremities. The patient's feet are positioned in stride or side by side. Positioned in stride, behind and to one side of a patient, the physical therapist grasps the patient's gait belt and shoulder. The patient reaches for the armrest with one hand while maintaining a grasp on the cane with the other hand.

2. While grasping the armrest and the cane, the patient lowers in a controlled manner onto the seat.

   The patient moves completely onto the seat and positions appropriately.

Assuming Standing—Quad Cane Only

The patient with sufficient strength and balance may assume standing using a quad cane instead of the armrest for support.

1. Wheelchair wheel locks are engaged and footrests moved out of the way. The patient is positioned at the front edge of the seat, with the feet in stride or side by side. Positioned in stride, behind and to one side of a patient, the physical therapist grasps the patient's gait belt and shoulder.

2. The quad cane is positioned alongside the foot on the side on which it will be held. One hand is placed on the quad cane. When the patient has only one functional upper extremity, that upper extremity is used on the quad cane to push to standing. The patient must push directly downward to prevent the cane from tipping.

3. The patient leans forward to initiate standing by pushing downward on the quad cane.

4. The patient must be erect and balanced before initiating ambulation.

Assuming Sitting—Quad Cane Only

1. Wheelchair wheel locks are engaged and footrests moved out of the way. To sit, the patient is positioned at the front edge of the wheelchair seat, facing away from the wheelchair, so the front edge of the wheelchair seat is felt against the back of the lower extremities. The patient's feet are positioned in stride or side by side. Positioned in stride, behind and to one side of a patient, the physical therapist grasps the patient's gait belt.

2. While grasping the quad cane, the patient lowers in a controlled manner onto the seat.

3. The physical therapist continues to guard the patient until safely seated and appropriately positioned.

Assuming Standing—Standard Cane and Two Armrests

1. Wheelchair wheel locks are engaged and footrests moved out of the way. The patient is positioned at the front edge of the seat with the feet in stride or side by side. Positioned in stride, behind and to one side of a patient, the physical therapist grasps the patient's gait belt and shoulder.
2. When using a standard cane, both hands are placed on their respective armrests. Canes are grasped in the same hand as will be used for ambulation. Thus, the patient must grasp both the cane and armrest at the same time with this hand. In the illustrations for this section, the patient is demonstrating the use of two functional upper extremities.

3. Pushing downward on both armrests, the patient pushes to standing.

4. Once standing, the patient releases the grasp on the armrests, stands erect, and positions the cane. The patient is then ready to ambulate

Assuming Sitting—Standard Cane and Two Armrests

1. Wheelchair wheel locks are engaged and footrests moved out of the way. To sit, patients are positioned at the front edge of the wheelchair seat, facing away from the wheelchair, so the front edge of the wheelchair seat is felt against the back of the lower extremities. The patient's feet are positioned in stride or side by side. Positioned in stride, behind and to one side of a patient, the physical therapist grasps the patient's gait belt and shoulder.

2. The patient grasps both armrests. This may be performed with both hands simultaneously or the hands may be moved one at a time. The cane remains grasped in the same hand in which it was used for ambulation. Both cane and armrest are held together by the hand that grasps the cane.

3. The patient lowers in a controlled manner onto the seat. Setting the cane aside, the patient moves completely onto the seat and positions themselves appropriately.

Assuming Standing—Standard Cane and One Armrest

1. Wheelchair wheel locks are engaged and footrests moved out of the way. The patient is positioned at the front edge of the seat, with the feet in stride or side by side. Positioned in stride, behind and to one side of the patient, the therapist grasps the patient's gait belt and shoulder.
2. The cane is positioned alongside the foot on the side on which it will be held. One hand is placed on the armrest and the other hand is placed on the cane. The patient must push directly downward on the cane to prevent the cane from tipping. When the patient has only one functional upper extremity, that upper extremity is used on the cane to push to standing. In the illustrations for this section, the patient is demonstrating the use of two functional upper extremities.

3. The patient then pushes to standing.

4. Once standing and balanced, the patient releases the grasp on the armrest and stands erect. The patient is then ready to ambulate.

Assuming Sitting—Standard Cane and One Armrest

1. Wheelchair wheel locks are engaged and footrests moved out of the way. To sit, the patient is positioned at the front edge of the wheelchair seat, facing away from the wheelchair, so the front edge of the wheelchair seat is felt against the back of the lower extremities. The patient's feet are positioned in stride or side by side. Positioned in stride, behind and to one side of a patient, the physical therapist grasps the patient's gait belt and shoulder.

2. While continuing to use the cane, the patient reaches back and grasps the armrest with the opposite hand.

3. The patient then lowers in a controlled manner onto the seat. Setting the cane aside, the patient moves completely into the seat and positions appropriately.

PROCEDURE 9–16

AMBULATING ON LEVEL SURFACES WITH ONE CANE

The gait pattern and sequence when using one standard cane or one quad cane are the same. To decrease weight-bearing on an involved lower extremity, the cane is used on the uninvolved side. This allows a minimal reduction of weight-bearing on the involved lower extremity.

1. Positioned in stride, behind and to one side of a patient, the physical therapist grasps the patient's gait belt and shoulder. The patient's feet are side by side, with the cane next to the small toe.

2. The cane is advanced first, approximately one stride length ahead. When the physical therapist is guarding on the side opposite the cane, she steps forward with the outside foot.

(continued)

3. The patient advances the lower extremity on the side opposite the cane up to the cane. When the physical therapist is guarding on the side opposite the cane, she steps forward with the inside foot.

4. The patient advances the lower extremity on the same side as the cane. Initially, the patient may only step to the other lower extremity and cane. The patient should, however, be encouraged to step beyond the other lower extremity and cane. This encourages the patient to develop a normal gait pattern.

5. The sequence is repeated for continued progression. The patient should remain erect during this progression and avoid leaning onto the cane.

6. As patients improve, they may move the cane and involved lower extremity at the same time, permitting a faster pace of gait. As patients are able, they may use the cane on the involved side, moving the cane and involved lower extremity simultaneously. Using a cane on the involved side encourages weight-bearing on the involved lower extremity.

PROCEDURE 9-17

AMBULATING ON STAIRS WITH ONE CANE

Holding the Cane

Initially, the patient should be taught to use a handrail for increased stability. Patients who use a cane on the left side continues to grasp the cane with the left hand and grasp the handrail with the right hand. Patients who use a cane in the right hand must do one of three things: 1) continue to use the cane in the right hand and not use the handrail, 2) switch the cane to the left hand and grasp the handrail with the right hand, or 3) grasp both the handrail and cane with the right hand. Patients with a functional right upper extremity only must: 1) either continue to use the cane without using the handrail, or 2) grasp both the handrail and cane with the right hand.

There are two methods for grasping both the cane and handrail in one hand. Note that the method is the same whether the patient uses one cane or two.

In one method the cane is held at mid-shaft, parallel to the handrail.

In the second method, the cane is held at mid-shaft, remaining in a vertical position.

A quad cane's base may be larger than a stair tread.

Turning a quad cane sideways permits all four legs to be supported on the stair.

Ascending Using a Cane and Handrail

In the illustrations for this section, the patient demonstrates the use of two functional upper extremities, permitting use of the cane in the left hand while grasping the handrail with the right hand.

1. Positioned in stride behind the patient, the physical therapist grasps the patient's gait belt and the handrail. To ascend stairs, the patient stands facing up the stairs with the feet and cane parallel to the base of the first stair.

2. The uninvolved lower extremity is moved to the next higher stair and weight is shifted onto this extremity.

3. The patient extends the uninvolved lower extremity, lifting the body. The involved lower extremity is placed on the same stair as the uninvolved lower extremity. The cane is advanced to the same stair as the lower extremities and placed securely on the stair tread. As the patient's balance and strength improve, the cane and involved lower extremity may be moved simultaneously.
4. The sequence is repeated to ascend the remaining stairs.

Descending Using a Cane and Handrail

In the illustrations for this section, the patient demonstrates the use of two functional upper extremities, permitting the use of the cane in the left hand while grasping the handrail with right hand.

1. Positioned in stride and in front of the patient, the physical therapist grasps the patient's gait belt and the handrail. To descend stairs, the patient stands facing down the stairs, with the feet and cane parallel to the stair.

2. The cane is lowered to the next lower stair and placed securely on the stair tread. The patient lowers the involved lower extremity to the next lower stair by flexing the uninvolved lower extremity. As the patient's balance and strength improve, the patient may move the cane and involved lower extremity simultaneously.

3. Weight is shifted to the involved lower extremity and cane and the uninvolved lower extremity is lowered to the same stair as the cane and involved lower extremity.
4. The sequence is repeated to descend the remaining stairs.

Ascending Using One Cane

When not using a handrail, the gait pattern for ascending stairs with one cane is similar to that used when both a cane and handrail are used. As the patient improves, he/she should practice using only one cane and no handrail. This prepares the patient for situations in which no handrail is available. Patients who have only one functional upper extremity may have to use this method even if a handrail is available. In the illustrations for this section, the patient demonstrates the use of only one cane without using a handrail.

1. Positioned in stride behind the patient, the physical therapist grasps the patient's gait belt and the handrail. To ascend stairs, the patient stands facing up the stairs with their feet and cane parallel to the base of the first stair. The uninvolved lower extremity is moved to the next higher stair and weight is shifted onto this extremity.

2. The patient extends the uninvolved lower extremity, lifting the body. The involved lower extremity and cane are placed on the same stair as the uninvolved lower extremity. The cane and involved lower extremity should be moved simultaneously to avoid having the patient lean backward.
3. The sequence is repeated to ascend the remaining stairs.

Descending Using One Cane

In the illustrations for this section, the patient demonstrates the use of only one cane without using a handrail.

1. Positioned in stride in front of the patient, the physical therapist grasps the patient's gait belt and the handrail. To descend stairs, the patient starts facing down the stairs, with the feet and cane parallel to the stair. The cane and involved lower extremity are lowered to the next lower stair and placed securely on the stair tread.

2. Weight is shifted to the involved lower extremity and cane and the uninvolved lower extremity is lowered to the same stair as the cane and involved lower extremity.
3. The sequence is repeated to descend the remaining stairs.

PROCEDURE 9-18

AMBULATING THROUGH DOORWAYS WITH ONE CANE

Doorways With Automatic Door Closers

In each of the sections concerning ambulating through doorways with a cane, the patient is demonstrating the use of two functional upper extremities. When patients have only one functional upper extremity, the cane must be held by the hand of the functional extremity while it manipulates the door handle and door.

Door Opens Toward Patient—Cane at Hinge Edge

In the illustrations for this section, a cane is used in the patient's left hand, the hand closest to the hinge edge of the door when facing the door.

1. Patients approach the door and stand at the latch edge of the door, out of the arc of the opening door. Patients place their right hand on the door handle.

2. Patients open the door wide enough to permit movement into the doorway before the door closes. Unlike the sequences for a walker or crutches, a door is not opened completely in a single motion. Opening a door in a single motion when using one cane is often not possible when patients must move the upper extremity across the body. Attempting to do so can compromise a patient's safety.

3. The door is opened further, and the tip of the cane is placed on the floor to serve as a door stop.

4. As patients move through a doorway, the tip of the cane is placed progressively closer to the hinge edge of the door to serve as a door stop. Patients may need to use a hand or hip to maintain an open door. Physical therapists and patients must be aware that as the tip of a cane is placed closer to the hinge edge of the door, the door becomes more difficult to block. Once a patient has moved completely through the doorway, the door closes behind the patient.

Door Opens Away From Patient—Cane at Hinge Edge

In the illustrations for this section, a cane is used in the patient's left hand, the hand closest to the hinge edge when facing the door.

1. Patients approach the door and place their right hand on the door handle.

2. The door is opened wide enough to permit a patient to enter the doorway. The tip of the cane is placed on the floor to serve as a door stop. A door is not opened completely in a single motion. As patients move through a doorway, the tip of the cane is placed progressively closer to the latch edge of the door to serve as a door stop. Patients may need to use a hand or hip to maintain an open door. Once patients have moved completely through a doorway, the door closes behind them.

Door Opens Away From Patient—Cane at Latch Edge

In the illustrations for this section, a cane is used in the patient's left hand, the hand closest to the latch edge of the door when facing the door.

1. Patients approach the door and place the right hand on the door handle.

2. The door is pushed open wide enough to permit movement into the doorway. Patients move the right hand from the door handle to the door and use this hand to hold open the door.

3. Patients continue to move through the doorway, using the hand to hold open the door. Once patient have moved completely through the doorway, the door closes behind them.

PROCEDURE 9-19

IN AND OUT OF A WHEELCHAIR WITH TWO CANES

Assuming standing and sitting when using two canes is performed in a manner similar to these maneuvers when using one cane.

 AMBULATING ON LEVEL SURFACES WITH TWO CANES

Three-Point Gait Pattern

1. Positioned in stride, behind and to one side of a patient, the physical therapist grasps the patient's gait belt and shoulder. In the starting position, the patient stands with one cane in each hand in the same position used for measuring cane fit. The patient's feet are side by side.

2. To ambulate, both canes are advanced, and then the involved lower extremity is advanced to the canes. As the patient improves, canes and involved lower extremity can be advanced simultaneously the same amount.

3. The physical therapist advances the outside foot, either at the same time or immediately after the canes are advanced.

4. The patient then advances the uninvolved lower extremity beyond the canes. Initially, the patient may "step to" the involved lower extremity, rather than "step through." Stepping through is the normal gait pattern and should be encouraged. The physical therapist advances the inside foot as the patient moves the uninvolved lower extremity.
5. The sequence is repeated for continued progression.

Four-Point Gait Pattern

1. Positioned in stride, behind and to one side of the patient, the physical therapist grasps the patient's gait belt. In the starting position the patient stands with one cane in each hand in the same position used for measuring cane fit. The patient's feet are side by side.

2. To ambulate, the patient advances one cane. In this example, the right cane is advanced first.

(continued)

3. The patient then advances the opposite lower extremity to a point even with the tip of the right cane. The physical therapist advances the inside foot.

4. The patient shifts weight to the right cane and left lower extremity and advances the left cane beyond the right cane.

5. The patient then advances the right lower extremity to a point even with the tip of the left cane. The physical therapist advances the outside foot.
6. The sequence is repeated for continued progression.

Two-Point Gait Pattern

1. Positioned in stride, behind and to one side of a patient, the physical therapist grasps the patient's gait belt. In the starting position the patient stands with one cane in each hand in the same position used for measuring cane fit. The patient's feet are side by side.

2. The patient advances one cane and the opposite lower extremity simultaneously, placing the toes even with the tip of the cane. The patient then shifts weight onto this cane and lower extremity. In this example, the right cane and left foot have been advanced together. The physical therapist moves the inside foot at this time.

3. The patient then advances the left cane and right lower extremity together. This cane and lower extremity are advanced beyond the other cane and lower extremity in a normal stride length. The physical therapist moves the outside foot at this time.

4. The sequence is repeated for continued progression.

PROCEDURE 9-20

AMBULATING ON STAIRS WITH TWO CANES

Holding the Canes

Ambulation on stairs can be performed using two canes, with or without the use of a handrail. Use of a handrail provides stability and is an added safety factor. When using a handrail, the handrail takes the place of the cane on one side. There are several methods of holding canes when using a handrail. Whatever method of holding canes is used, the sequence of movements for the lower extremities and ambulatory assistive devices is the same.

A practical method of holding two canes while using a handrail is to place both canes in one hand. There are two methods of holding a cane in the hand that is grasping a handrail and cane simultaneously.

One method of grasping a cane and handrail in the same hand is to hold the cane at mid-shaft parallel to the handrail.

A second method of grasping a cane and handrail in the same hand is to hold the cane at mid-shaft in a vertical orientation.

The cane on the side opposite the handrail is used in the usual manner.

Three-Point Gait Pattern

Ascending Stairs

1. To ascend stairs, the patient stands facing up the stairs with feet and canes parallel to the base of the first stair. Positioned in stride behind a patient, the physical therapist grasps the patient's gait belt and the handrail. For the method presented in this section, the patient grasps one cane in each hand.

2. The patient places the uninvolved lower extremity on the next higher stair and weight is shifted onto this extremity.

3. The patient extends the uninvolved lower extremity to raise the body to the same stair. The canes and involved lower extremity are advanced to the same stair simultaneously. The canes must be properly placed on the stair for stability and to provide room for patients to maneuver.

4. The sequence is repeated to ascend the remaining stairs.

Descending Stairs

1. To descend stairs, the patient stands facing down the stairs. Positioned in stride in front of the patient, the physical therapist grasps the patient's gait belt and the handrail. For the method presented in this section, the patient grasps one cane in each hand.

2. The patient lowers the two canes to the next lower stair.

3. The involved lower extremity is lowered to the same stair as the two canes. Weight is shifted to the involved lower extremity and canes and the uninvolved lower extremity is moved to the same stair.

4. The sequence is repeated to descend the remaining stairs.

Four-Point Gait Pattern

Ascending Stairs

1. To ascend stairs, the patient stands facing up the stairs with feet and canes parallel to the base of the stair. Positioned in stride behind the patient, the physical therapist grasps the patient's gait belt and the handrail. For the method presented in this section, the patient grasps one cane in each hand.

2. The patient advances one cane to the next higher stair.

(continued)

3. The patient then advances the opposite lower extremity to the same stair and weight is shifted onto the cane and lower extremity that have been placed on the next higher stair.

4. The patient advances the second cane to the same stair.

5. The patient then extends the lower extremity on the higher stair to lift the body. The second lower extremity is placed on the same stair. Thus, both lower extremities and both canes are on the same stair.
6. The sequence is repeated to ascend the remaining stairs.

Descending Stairs

1. To descend stairs, the patient stands facing down the stairs. Positioned in stride in front of the patient, the physical therapist grasps the patient's gait belt and the handrail. For the method presented in this section, the patient grasps one cane in each hand.

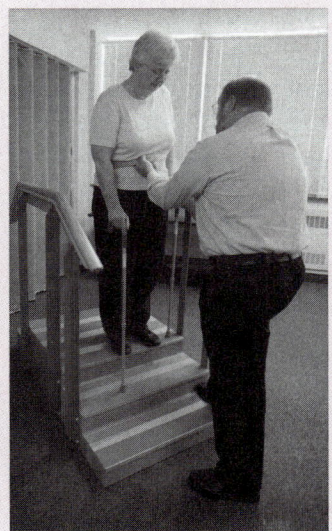

2. The patient moves one cane to the next lower stair.

(continued)

3. The patient flexes the lower extremity on the same side to lower the body, placing the opposite lower extremity on the same stair as the lowered cane.

4. Shifting weight onto the cane and lower extremity on the lower stair, the second cane is moved to the same lower stair.

5. The opposite lower extremity is moved to the same lower stair. Thus, both lower extremities and both canes are on the same stair.
6. The sequence is repeated to descend the remaining stairs.

Two-Point Gait Pattern

Ascending Stairs

Ascending stairs using two canes and a two-point gait pattern is very similar to using a four-point gait pattern. The difference is that in a two-point gait pattern one cane and the opposite lower extremity are moved simultaneously.

1. To ascend stairs, the patient stands facing up the stairs with feet and canes parallel to the base of the stair. Positioned in stride behind the patient, the physical therapist grasps the patient's gait belt and the handrail. For the method presented in this section, the patient grasps one cane in each hand.

2. One cane and the opposite lower extremity are moved to the next higher stair.

3. The second cane and opposite lower extremity are then moved to the same stair.
4. The sequence is repeated to ascend the remaining stairs.

Descending Stairs

Descending stairs using two canes and a two-point gait pattern is very similar to using a four-point gait pattern. The difference is that in a two-point gait pattern one cane and the opposite lower extremity are moved simultaneously.

1. To descend stairs, the patient stands facing down the stairs. Positioned in stride in front of the patient, the physical therapist grasps the patient's gait belt and the handrail. For the method presented in this section, the patient grasps one cane in each hand.

2. One cane and the opposite lower extremity are moved to the next lower stair.

3. The second cane and opposite lower extremity are then lowered to the same stair.
4. The sequence is repeated to descend the remaining stairs.

PROCEDURE 9-21

AMBULATING THROUGH DOORWAYS WITH TWO CANES

Door With Automatic Door Closer

When moving through a doorway, patients can use one cane in each hand, or may place both canes in one hand. The method of moving through doorways with both canes in one hand is the same as when using one cane. In the illustrations for this section the patient is demonstrating the use of two canes.

Door Opens Away From Patient

1. The patient faces the door and shift the weight onto the cane away from the hand that is closest to the door handle. Holding the cane, the unweighted hand grasps the door handle.

2. Using a pushing motion, the door is opened part way, and the door is blocked by the tip of the cane closest to the door.

3. As the patient moves through a doorway, the door is pushed open in increments. Continuing to use the tip of the cane as a door stop, the patient progresses through the doorway. The door closes behind the patient.

Door Opens Toward Patient

1. The patient approaches the latch edge of the door, standing outside the arc through which the opening door will move. The patient shifts weight onto the cane on the side away from the hand that will be placed on the door handle. Holding the cane, the unweighted hand grasps the door handle. Preferably, weight is shifted to the side closest to the door handle, and the hand toward the hinge edge is used to pull open the door.

2. Using a pulling motion, the door is opened wider than the width of the patient. Opening the door wider than the patient is necessary because the door will start to close automatically before the patient can progress through the doorway. To block the automatic closing of the door, the patient moves into the doorway and place the tip of the cane closest to the door on the floor in the path of the door. This serves as a door stop, permitting the patient to move into the doorway without being struck by the closing door.

3. Continuing to use the tip of the cane as a door stop, the patient progresses through the doorway using an appropriate gait pattern. As the patient moves through the doorway, the tip of the cane is used as a door stop by placing it progressively closer to the hinge edge of the door. The physical therapist and patient must be aware that as the tip of a cane gets closer to the hinge edge of the door, it becomes more difficult to hold open the door.
4. Once the patient has moved completely through the doorway, the door closes behind the patient.

Doors Without Automatic Closers

Patients using two canes can negotiate doorways without automatic door closers using the same sequences presented earlier in this chapter in the section *Axillary Crutches.*

REVIEW QUESTIONS

1. What are the general guidelines for instructing a patient in the use of ambulatory assistive devices and gait patterns?

2. Which components of ambulatory assistive devices should be checked for safety?

3. What activities should be taught to a patient learning to use an ambulatory assistive device?

4. List ambulatory assistive devices in the order a) providing the most stability to the least stability, b) requiring the most patient coordination to the least patient coordination.

5. What are the indications for the selection of specific ambulatory assistive devices?

6. Describe the five major gait patterns used with ambulatory assistive devices.

7. Describe which gait patterns can be used with each assistive device.

8. What are the criteria for selection of gait patterns when using ambulatory assistive devices?

9. What is the purpose of using the tilt table in gait training?

10. Describe how to fit each ambulatory assistive device.

11. Describe how a therapist guards a patient ambulating using an assistive device on level surfaces, stairs, and through doorways.

12. How is the wheelchair properly prepared for a patient to move in or out of the wheelchair when using ambulatory assistive devices?

SUGGESTED ACTIVITIES

1. Working in pairs, practice the procedures presented in this chapter. Rotate partners during the practice session.

2. Practice fitting each assistive device to at least three different people.

3. Practice demonstrating gait patterns with each assistive device.

4. Practice guarding partners using each assistive device with various appropriate gait patterns on level surfaces, stairs and curbs, the assumption of sitting from standing and standing from sitting, moving through doorways, falling without injury, and resumption of ambulation after falling.

5. Practice teaching partners how to use ambulatory assistive devices on level surfaces, stairs and curbs, the assumption of sitting from standing and standing from sitting, moving through doorways, falling without injury, and resumption of ambulation after falling, as partners role-play various diagnoses. Students role-playing a patient can add "character" to the role-play by being cooperative, noncooperative, in pain, hard of hearing, or faint to enhance the activity. The patient must role-play the diagnosis and character consistently (see *Case Studies* for suggested patient roles).

6. Monitor vital signs and check for signs of circulatory problems of the lower extremities as appropriate.

7. Document treatment using the SOAP note format.

CASE STUDIES

Use these case studies to complete Activity #5 above.

1. The patient is a 16-year-old male high school soccer player who sustained a left knee injury in a game the previous night. He is to ambulate using axillary crutches with a non-weight-bearing gait pattern until a diagnosis is determined following a MRI in 2 days.
2. The patient is a 63-year-old female with a left CVA, presenting with right hemiplegia. She has sufficient motor control and balance to ambulate with a small-base quad cane.
3. The patient is a 78-year-old male who had a left total hip replacement 1 day ago. He is to ambulate using a walker, with weight bearing as tolerated.
4. The patient is a 49-year-old female with severe rheumatoid arthritis who received a right total knee joint replacement 2 days ago. She is to ambulate using a platform walker, with weight bearing as tolerated.
5. The patient is a 21-year-old male with a complete L3–4 spinal cord injury. He is ready to begin gait training using Lofstrand (forearm) crutches and knee-ankle-foot orthoses (KAFOs). His upper extremity strength is adequate for ambulating with these ambulatory assistive devices.

10

AMERICANS WITH DISABILITIES ACT

LEARNING OBJECTIVES

Upon completion of this chapter, you will be able to:

1. State the purpose of the Americans with Disabilities Act (ADA).
2. List the government agencies responsible for developing rules and regulations, and enforcing the ADA law.
3. List sources of updated information on ADA.
4. Be able to locate specific requirements for an accessible environment: accessible routes, alarms, assembly and auditorium areas, business and mercantile areas, clear space areas, control mechanisms, curb ramps, doors and doorways, drinking fountains, elevators, grab bars, ground and floor surfaces, handrails, hotels, libraries, parking spaces, platform lifts, ramps, reach heights, restaurant and food service areas, restrooms and bathrooms, signage, stairs, telephones, and transportation facilities.

MEDIALINK

A companion CD-ROM, included free with each new copy of this book, supplements the techniques presented in the book. Insert the CD-ROM to watch video clips of patient care skills being demonstrated. This multimedia feature is designed to help you add a new dimension to your learning.

KEY TERMS

Accessible route
Americans with Disabilities Act (1990)
Architectural Barriers Act (1968)
Clear space areas
Control mechanisms
Curb cut
Department of Justice

Equal Employment Opportunity
  Commission
Guidelines
Grab bar
Nosing
Platform lifts
Ramp

Reach range
Regulations
Riser
Rules
Transitions
Tread
United States Access Board

INTRODUCTION

In 1990, Congress passed the **Americans with Disabilities Act (ADA)** (public Law 101–336). The law contains five titles:

Title I—Employment
Title II—Public Services and Transportation
Title III—Public Accommodations
Title IV—Telecommunications
Title V—Other Provisions

The purpose of the ADA is to provide "a clear and comprehensive national mandate for the elimination of discrimination against individuals with disabilities."

Titles II and III address physical accessibility. Title II provides for accessible transportation which permits individuals with disabilities "to gain employment," and which "allows individuals with disabilities to enjoy cultural, recreational, commercial and other benefits that society has to offer." Title III provides individuals with disabilities the "full and equal enjoyment of the goods, services, facilities, privileges, advantages, or accommodations of any place of public accommodation."[1]

The purpose of this chapter is to provide basic information concerning how requirements of the ADA affect accessibility. This chapter will examine the basic requirements of accessibility as they apply to Title II (Public Services and Transportation) and Title III (Public Accommodations) because it is primarily in these areas that accessibility guidelines are addressed. This chapter contains specifics of space and configuration as required by the ADA. The philosophy of interpretation of ADA guidelines is *not* discussed.

The ADA was passed on July 2, 1990. Phased implementation of Titles II and III has been completed and the ADA is now fully implemented. Initial development of guidelines for accessibility was distributed among several public and professional organizations, such as United States Access Board, Building Officials and Code Administrators International, Inc. (BOCA), Council of American Building Officials (CABO), and American National Standards Institute (ANSI). These organizations provided expertise as the requirements known as the Uniform Federal Accessibility Standards (UFAS) and the Americans with Disabilities Accessibility Guidelines (ADAG) were developed.

In July 2004, the **United States Access Board** (USAB) promulgated updated accessibility guidelines for new or renovated facilities. During this review, USAB combined requirements of the ADA and of the **Architectural Barriers Act** (ABA) of 1968. Combining the requirements of the ADA and the ABA represents an effort to ensure consistency of accessibility guidelines for a wide range of facilities in the private and public sectors. The USAB guidelines now appear as *The New ADA–ABA Accessibility Guidelines*.

It is not appropriate, nor is it possible, for the language of the law to contain provisions for every potential situation intended to be covered by the law. Therefore, **rules**, **regulations**, and **guidelines** for implementation of laws are promulgated following passage of a new law. In the case of the ADA, the government agencies primarily responsible for developing rules and regulations and enforcing the law are the **Equal Employment Opportunity Commission (EEOC)** and the **Department of Justice (DOJ)**. More specific interpretation of the law and its rules, regulations, and guidelines occur as the result of administrative rulings and legal opinions in response to complaints and lawsuits filed by those who believe they have been subjected to discrimination as defined by the ADA. Definitive interpretations of specific requirements of the ADA become known as the result of such administrative rulings or legal opinions.

RESOURCES

USAB material, including *A Guide to the New ADA–ABA Accessibility Guidelines* and the full text and diagrams of the *Guidelines* are available from the USAB. The text and diagrams can be downloaded directly from the Internet.

United States Access Board
1331 F Street, N.W., Suite 1000
Washington, DC 20004–1111
(800) 872–2253 (voice)
(800) 993–2822 (TTY)
www.access-board.gov

In addition to access to the USAB, several private reporting services provide monthly updates regarding changes and recent legal opinions. One such service is provided below. This is a proprietary service with which the authors are most familiar. The listing of this service does not imply an endorsement of this service by the authors. The cost of a service such as this is higher than government or quasi-government publications. The benefits of such services are more timely and in-depth research and information.

Thompson Publishing Group, Inc.
Americans with Disabilities Act-ADA Compliance Guide
1725 K Street N. W., Suite 200
Washington, D.C. 20006
(800) 424–2959

GENERAL CONSIDERATIONS FOR ACCESSIBILITY

Requirements for accessibility must take into account a variety of disabilities resulting from a range of impairments. For example, requirements for ground and floor surface guidelines must take into account their effect on wheelchair users and the visually impaired. Curb cuts may be advantageous for wheelchair users but may present a hazard to the visually impaired. Accessibility designs must accommodate a broad spectrum of disabilities, rather than identifying each barrier to accessibility with a single impairment.

SPECIFIC REQUIREMENTS

Within each area of public accommodation, such as an office or a restroom, there are specific components that must be examined and criteria must be met for each component. For example, when a public accommodation encompasses a collection of areas, such as both an office and a restroom, then the criteria for doorways must be applied to both areas, but the criteria for toilets need only be applied to the restroom. In the case of door widths, the clear open width of a door must be no less than 32 inches. This requirement is true of all doors, whether they are for an entry into an office or restroom.

Listed on the following pages are the requirements for the many specific areas of accessibility that may be encountered in public accommodations. Each area is listed as a heading. Specific components and criteria for a given area are listed under the area heading. The list of area headings is alphabetical. Under each area heading, specific components, and criteria for each component, are also listed alphabetically.

In the following list, reference may be made to areas previously listed, or to areas that follow later in the list. These are areas that appear in a number of environments and have common criteria, regardless of the area in which they are required. This method is used to reduce redundancy, but is limited to avoid the need for constant cross-reference searching. While certain components or criteria are applied in a large variety of circumstances, there are some components or criteria that are not applied very often. For this reason, and because of space considerations, the following list does not include every individual requirement for accessibility.

The following guidelines are taken from the USAB *Guide*.[2] For a list of every requirement, and additional details concerning each requirement, referencing the USAB *Guide* is strongly recommended.

ACCESSIBLE ROUTE

A minimum of one route within the path from public access via public transportation, accessible parking spaces, and public streets must be available. Such a route must also be available to connect additional accessible buildings at the same site. Stairs, steps, ramps, or escalators are separate considerations from an accessible route, and have their own specific requirements.

An accessible route may not have a grade (slope) greater than 1:20 (5%) in the direction of travel. Its cross slope shall not be greater than 1:48. The vertical height may not be less than 80 inches. When vertical clearance along an accessible route is less than 80 inches, a warning barrier must be provided. The required floor dimensions of an accessible route are presented in Figure 10–1.

FIGURE 10–1   Clear width of an accessible route.

In all cases, protrusions along an accessible route may not reduce the minimum required clear width as previously presented. Because of the potential for injury, even protrusions that do not limit clear width to less than 36 inches may not be greater than 4 inches in the horizontal dimension, and are limited to specific areas in the vertical dimensions.

When 180-degree turns are encountered on an accessible route, guidelines for clear areas must be followed. These dimensions are presented in Figure 10–2.

FIGURE 10–2   Clear width for turning 180 degrees on an accessible route.

ASSEMBLY AND AUDITORIUM AREAS FOR WHEELCHAIR SEATING

Clear areas that provide seating for patrons using wheelchairs are presented in the following two figures. Figure 10–3 presents the width of seating areas.

(a)
single space

(b)
two spaces

FIGURE 10–3 Width of wheelchair spaces.

Figure 10–4 presents the depth of seating areas, which is dependent upon the direction of wheelchair access to the seating area.

(a)
front or rear
entry

(b)
side
entry

FIGURE 10–4 Depth of wheelchair spaces.

Wheelchair seating locations must be configured in conjunction with assistive listening systems, must be on (but not overlap with) an accessible route with access to accessible emergency exits, and must have access to accessible restrooms. In assembly areas with capacity greater than 300, accessible wheelchair areas must be located in more than one location.

Appropriate lines of sight must be provided for patrons using wheelchairs. In areas where patrons are expected to remain seated, elevations must provide lines of sight either over the heads of patrons (Figure 10–5) or off-set spacing to provide lines of sight over the shoulders but between the heads of patrons in the row immediately in front.

FIGURE 10–5   Sight-line elevation over the heads of seated patrons.

In areas where patrons are expected to rise from their seats, elevations must provide lines of sight either over the heads, or off-set spacing to provide lines of sight over the shoulders but between the heads of patrons (Figure 10–6), in the row immediately in front when patrons are standing.

FIGURE 10–6   Sight-line elevation between the heads of standing patrons.

CHECK-OUT COUNTERS

Check-out counters must be situated on accessible routes within the business or commercial facility. Security barriers used to prevent shopping carts from being removed from stores may not prevent access for users of wheelchairs. Vertical dimensions of check-out counter surfaces and protective edges are presented in Figure 10–7.

FIGURE 10–7   Check-out aisle counters.

CLEAR SPACE AREAS

Clear space areas include the floor dimensions of an accessible route and clearances for use of certain facilities, such as toilet stalls and drinking fountains. For accessible routes, the minimum width for passing is 60 inches. If the width of an accessible route is less than 60 inches, then a passing area must be provided. A passing area shall be not less than 60 inches by 60 inches, and must be provided not less than every 200 feet along the accessible route.

Landings on an accessible route must also have a clear area of not less than 60 inches by 60 inches. Such landings provide a clear space for turning and other maneuvers. Dimensions for a T-shaped turning space are presented in Figure 10–8.

FIGURE 10–8 T-shaped turning spaces.

Clear space areas for positioning of wheelchairs must be not less than 30 inches by 48 inches, as presented in Figure 10–9.

FIGURE 10–9 Clear area requirements for wheelchairs.

The orientation of such clear space is dependent upon position of wheelchair placement with respect to the closest wall, as presented in Figure 10–10.

FIGURE 10–10 Orientation of clear area for wheelchairs.

(a) forward

(b) parallel

Toe clearances shall be between 17 and 25 inches deep under an element, and a minimum width of 30 inches, as presented in Figure 10–11.

FIGURE 10–11 Toe clearance requirements.

(a) elevation

(b) plan

Knee clearance height (vertical dimension) is generally not less than 27 inches from the floor (Figure 10–12). Knee clearance depths must not be less than 11 inches in the horizontal dimension at a point 9 inches above the floor, and not less than 8 inches in the horizontal dimension at a point 27 inches above the floor. This takes into account angulation of wheelchair leg rests, which extend farther from a wheelchair as they extend toward the floor. Maximum knee clearance in the horizontal dimension must be no greater than 25 inches under any element at a point 9 inches from the floor.

FIGURE 10–12 Knee clearance requirements.

(a) elevation

(b) plan

CONTROL MECHANISMS

Control mechanisms must be easy to grasp with one hand and must not require tight grasping, tight pinching, or twisting of a wrist to operate.

CURB CUTS

Curb cuts may not have a grade greater than 1:12 (8.3%) for new construction, with a vertical rise of not greater than 30 inches. For existing sites, a grade may not be greater than 1:10 (10%), with a vertical rise of not greater than 6 inches if space does not permit construction of a grade of 1:12 or less, or not greater than 1:8 (12.5%) for existing sites, with a vertical rise of not greater than 3 inches if space does not permit construction of a grade of 1:12 or less. In all cases, the width of the curb cut, exclusive of the flared sides, must be not less than 36 inches, the same width as an accessible route.

DOORS AND DOORWAYS

Access to all facilities requires that entrances be accessible. Revolving doors and turnstiles shall not be part of an accessible route and may not be the only method of entrance. Gates must meet requirements when on an accessible route. For double-leaf doorways, at least one leaf must meet the requirements, and this leaf must be the active leaf.

Handles must be easy to grasp, must not require tight grasping, tight pinching, or twisting of wrist to operate, and must be mounted not higher than 48 inches above the floor. When automatic door mechanisms are used for opening, the time to open must not be greater than 3 seconds and the force to stop movement must not be greater than 15 pounds. When automatic door mechanisms are used for closing, the time to close must not be greater than 3 seconds for closing from 70 degrees open to a point where the leading edge of the door is 3 inches from the latch.

Fire door opening forces must be the minimum required by the local administrative entity (i.e., Fire Department, Department of Public Safety, etc.), and not greater than 5 pounds force for interior hinged doors, sliding doors, or folding doors. Latches or other hardware do not come under these force requirements.

The depth of an opening in which a door is placed should not be greater than 24 inches. If the depth is greater than 24 inches, this area must be considered part of an accessible route, requiring application of all minimal width and depth requirements.

As presented in the following figures, clear width openings of not less than 32 inches are required for almost all doorways. No projections into the clear opening width may occur within 34 inches of the floor or ground. Between 34 inches from the floor to a height of 80 inches from the floor, projections may not be greater than 4 inches.

There are a large number of doorway configurations. In all cases, clear space for maneuvering a wheelchair when a door opens toward the person and the ability to get close to a door when it opens away from the person must be provided. This is true for swing doors and gates and sliding doors.

Table 10–1 presents the clear space requirements at manual swinging doors.

TABLE 10–1	Clear Space Requirements for Manual Swinging Doors		
Type of Use		**Minimum Maneuvering Clearance**	
Approach Direction	**Door or Gate Side**	**Perpendicular to Doorway**	**Parallel to Doorway (beyond latch side unless noted)**
From front	Pull	60 inches (1525 mm)	18 inches (455 mm)
From front	Push	48 inches (1220 mm)	0 inches (0 mm)[1]
From hinge side	Pull	60 inches (1525 mm)	36 inches (915 mm)
From hinge side	Pull	54 inches (1370 mm)	42 inches (1065 mm)
From hinge side	Push	42 inches (1065 mm)[2]	22 inches (560 mm)[3]
From latch side	Pull	48 inches (1220 mm)[4]	24 inches (610 mm)
From latch side	Push	42 inches (1065 mm)[4]	24 inches (610 mm)

1. Add 12 inches (305 mm) if closer and latch are provided.
2. Add 6 inches (150 mm) if closer and latch are provided.
3. Beyond hinge side.
4. Add 6 inches (150 mm) if closer is provided.

Figure 10–13 presents eleven clear area configurations for maneuvering at swinging doors.

Table 10–2 presents the clear space requirements at sliding and folding doors.

TABLE 10–2	Clear Space Requirements for Sliding and Folding Doors	
	Minimum Maneuvering Clearance	
Approach Direction	**Perpendicular to Doorway**	**Parallel to Doorway (beyond stop/latch side unless noted)**
From front	48 inches (1220 mm)	0 inches (0 mm)
From side[1]	42 inches (1065 mm)	0 inches (0 mm)
From pocket/hinge side	42 inches (1065 mm)	22 inches (560 mm)[2]
From stop/latch side	42 inches (1065 mm)	24 inches (610 mm)

1. Doorway with no door only.
2. Beyond pocket/hinge side.

(a)
front approach, pull side

(b)
front approach, push side

(c)
front approach, push side, door
provided with both closer and latch

(d)
hinge approach, pull side

(e)
hinge approach, pull side

(f)
hinge approach, push side

FIGURE 10–13   Clear space configurations for manual swinging doors.

(g)
hinge approach, push side, door
provided with both closer and latch

(h)
latch approach, pull side

(i)
latch approach, pull side,
door provided with closer

(j)
latch approach, push side

(k)
latch approach, push side,
door provided with closer

FIGURE 10–13 (continued)

FIGURE 10–14 Clear space configurations for sliding and folding doors.

Figure 10–14 presents four clear area configurations for maneuvering at sliding and folding doors. Figure 10–15 presents three clear area configurations for maneuvering at recessed doors.

FIGURE 10–15 Clear space configurations for recessed doors.

FIGURE 10–16 Clear space configurations for doors in series.

When swinging doors are in series, specific dimensions, as presented in Figure 10–16, are required. These dimensions permit the opening of doors in series while maintaining clear space for maneuvering without hindrance from opening/closing doors.

DRINKING FOUNTAINS

Spout outlet height for drinking fountains must not be greater than 36 inches, with not less than 27 inches vertical clear space beneath the unit (Figure 10–17). Spout location not less than 15 inches from the fountains vertical support, and not greater than 5 inches from the front edge of the fountain unit. Water ejection must be no less than 4 inches high. Toe and knee clearances must conform to dimensions provided previously in *Clear Space Areas*. Controls must be mounted on the front of the unit, or on the side of the unit near the front, and must conform to the requirements previously presented for *Control Mechanisms*.

FIGURE 10–17 Positioning requirements for drinking fountains.

ELEVATORS

To be considered accessible, an elevator must be on an accessible route. Unless freight elevators are used for the general public as combination passenger and freight elevators, freight elevators may not be used to meet the requirement of an accessible elevator. All elevators considered accessible must be automatic control elevators.

Car controls must be placed in readily accessible locations, and within the reach dimensions presented later in this chapter under *Reach Ranges*. For cars with the door opening in the center of the front wall, controls must be on a front wall. For

TABLE 10–3	Elevator Car Dimensions			
		Minimum Dimensions		
Door Location	**Door Clear Width**	**Inside Car, Side to Side**	**Inside Car, Back Wall to Front Return**	**Inside Car, Back Wall to Inside Face of Door**
Centered	42 inches (1065 mm)	80 inches (2030 mm)	51 inches (1295 mm)	54 inches (1370 mm)
Side (off-centered)	36 inches (915 mm)[1]	68 inches (1725 mm)	51 inches (1295 mm)	54 inches (1370 mm)
Any	36 inches (915 mm)[1]	54 inches (1370 mm)	80 inches (2030 mm)	80 inches (2030 mm)
Any	36 inches (915 mm)[1]	60 inches (1525 mm)[2]	60 inches (1525 mm)[2]	60 inches (1525 mm)[2]

1. A tolerance of minus 5/8 inch (16 mm) is permitted.
2. Other car configurations that provide a turning *space* complying with 304 with the door closed shall be permitted.

cars with the door opening set to one side of the front wall, controls must be located on the front wall, or on the side wall nearest the door.

Elevator dimensions are presented in Table 10–3, with five possible configurations presented in Figures 10–18.

The center point of hall call buttons must be 42 inches above the floor, and must not be recessed. Projections greater than 4 inches in the horizontal dimension mounted below hall call buttons must be avoided. The up button must be on top. All buttons must have both raised and Braille signage.

Hall signals must contain visual and audible signal at each hoistway, centered not less than 72 inches above the floor level. Audible signal must sound once for up and twice for down, or must have verbal annunciators capable of saying "up" or "down." Signals within the elevator must also be audible, either tone or annunciator, indicating the passage of each floor.

(a)
centered door

(b)
side (off-centered) door

FIGURE 10–18 Elevator car configurations.

GRAB BARS

Circular grab bars must have a diameter not less than 1 1/4 inches and not more than 2 inches. Non-circular grab bar dimensions, both cross section and perimeter, are presented in Figure 10–19. The horizontal distance between grab bars and wall, or vertical distance between grab bars and vertical projections below grab bars must be 1 1/2 inches. The vertical distance between grab bars and horizontal projections above grab bars must be not less than 12 inches.

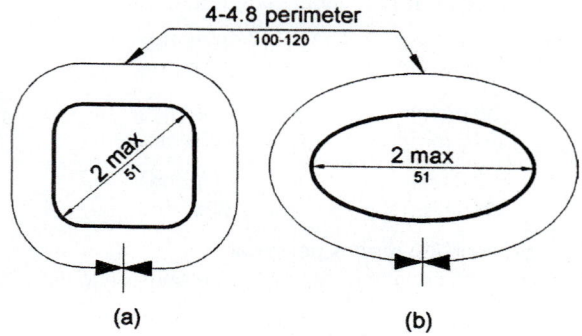

FIGURE 10–19 Noncircular grab bar dimensions.

GROUND AND FLOOR SURFACES

Ground and floor surfaces must be stable, firm, and slip resistant. Carpet must be securely attached, with exposed edges fastened to the floor, and have trim along the full length of exposed edges. Pile thickness must not be greater than 1/2 inch.

Grating spaces must be no greater than 1/2 inch in any dimension. If elongated openings are used, the long dimension of the opening must be oriented perpendicular to the dominant direction of travel.

Transitions between connected surfaces up to 1/4 inch may be left untreated. Transitions between 1/4 inch and 1/2 inch must have a beveled edge with a slope no greater than 1:2 (50%). *Ramp* guidelines, presented later in the chapter, must be used to accommodate transitions greater than 1/2 inch.

HANDRAILS

Circular handrails must have a diameter not less than 1 1/4 inches and not more than 2 inches. Non-circular handrail dimensions, both cross section and perimeter, are presented in Figure 10–20. The horizontal distance between handrails and wall and

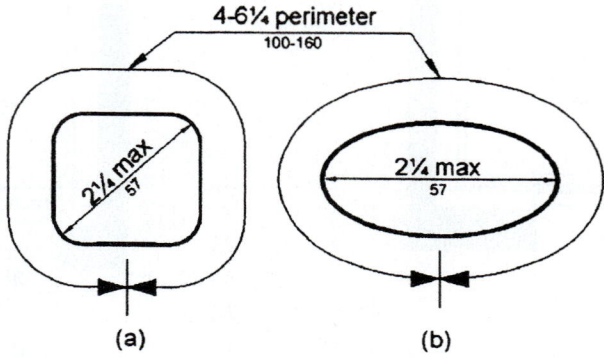

FIGURE 10–20 Noncircular handrail dimensions.

vertical distance between handrails and horizontal projections below handrails must be 1 1/2 inches. The top gripping surface of handrails must not be less than 34 inches or greater than 38 inches in the vertical dimension from the floor or stair tread.

Handrails must have extensions beyond the stairs or ramps they serve. Ramps must have handrail extensions not less than 12 inches from the start and end of the ramp, as presented in Figure 10–21. Handrails along stairs must have an extension not less than 12 inches at the top of stairs and an extension not less than one tread depth at the bottom of the stairs. Handrail extensions must be parallel to the level floor surface at the ends of ramps and at the tops of stairs, but must be parallel to the slope of the stair flight (not parallel to the floor) at the bottom of stairs, as presented in Figures 10–21 through 10–23. The ends of handrails must be rounded,

FIGURE 10–21 Handrail extensions for ramps.

FIGURE 10–22 Handrail extensions at the tops of stair flights.

Note: X = tread depth

FIGURE 10–23 Handrail extensions at the bottom of stair flights.

or returned smoothly to the floor, a wall, or a post. All handrails must be secured, and must not rotate within fittings.

HOTELS (TRANSIENT LODGING)

Hotel accommodations must meet general accessibility guidelines for public areas. Complete specifications for each component area are available in the USAB *Guide*. Accessible areas must include the guest room and bathroom, public restrooms, dining and meeting facilities, entrances, hallways and accessible routes, and elevators, Available guest units must be dispersed among the entire range of units available to the general public in terms of facilities and size, cost, and number of beds provided.

A unique guideline for guest rooms is that there must be not less than 36 inches clear space on each side of a bed. In rooms with two beds, a common clear space between them may be shared, maintaining the 36-inch clear space on the unshared side of each bed.

MEDICAL FACILITIES

In general, each specific area of a medical facility must comply with the appropriate requirements for the designated type of area. There are some specific differences, however. The bathroom in each patient room must comply with the requirements for an accessible toilet and sink. Clear space areas must not be less than 36 inches along each side of a bed, with an accessible path to each side of the bed that allows for a parallel approach to the bed and includes a maneuvering area (preferably between the two beds in a double room) of not less than 60 inches in diameter.

PARKING SPACES

Accessible parking spaces must be designated to be on the shortest possible path from the parking area to an accessible entrance via an accessible route. Access to parking spaces should not be behind other parked cars. Such spaces must be designated with a posted sign not less than 60 inches high, measured from the ground to the bottom of the sign. A sign or symbol painted on the ground alone is not acceptable.

Car parking spaces must not be less than 96 inches wide and van parking spaces must not be less than 132 inches wide. Access aisles between vehicles must not be less than 60 inches wide. An exception is that a van parking space may be only 96 inches wide if the access aisle is not less than 96 inches wide. Access aisles must run the full length of the marked parking space and not less than 240 inches long. Vertical clearance for vehicle access routes to accessible spaces, and the vertical clearance for such parking spaces must not be less than 98 inches. Vertical clearance for vehicle access routes to passenger loading zones must not be less than 114 inches. Accessible curb ramps that are not obstructed by a parking space must also be available when necessary.

PLATFORM LIFTS

Platform lifts are used for building entrances, in building interiors, and with transportation vehicles. In any of these settings, the requirements for platform lifts must be followed. Clear space areas for approaches and landings adjacent to platform lifts must meet the requirements previously presented in *Clear Space Areas*. Controls must be placed within the dimensions presented later in this chapter in *Reach Ranges*. The minimum dimensions and configuration of platform lifts is presented in Figure 10–24.

FIGURE 10–24   Dimensions and configuration of platform lifts.

RAMPS

Any portion of an accessible route with a grade greater than 1:20 (5%) must be considered a ramp. Any transition between two connected surfaces greater than 1/2 inch must be considered a ramp. Ramps must use the least slope possible, must not exceed the guidelines previously presented for curb cuts, must have a cross slope no greater than 1:50 (2%), and must not exceed a rise of 30 inches in any single run. Ramp width must not be less than 36 inches.

Landings must be provided at the top and bottom of each run. They must be not less than 60 inches in length, and at least as wide as the ramp. If a change in ramp direction or doorway occurs at a landing, the landing must meet the required landing clear space of 60 inches by 60 inches.

Handrails are required for a rise of 6 inches or more, or for a horizontal run of 72 inches or more. They must be provided along both sides of the ramp, and must meet the general requirements listed above under *Handrails*.

REACH RANGES

Reach ranges, within which control mechanisms must be placed, are dependent upon the direction of reach, forward or side, and whether a reach is obstructed or unobstructed. Specific requirements for each type of reach are presented in Figures 10–25 through 10–28.

FIGURE 10–25   Reach range—unobstructed forward reach.

FIGURE 10–26   Reach range—obstructed high forward reach.

FIGURE 10–27   Reach range—unobstructed side reach.

FIGURE 10–28   Reach range—obstructed high side reach.

RESTROOMS AND BATHROOMS

Accessible restrooms and bathrooms must be on an accessible route to conform to the definition of accessible restrooms or bathrooms. Restrooms or bathrooms that are designed with dimensions and fixtures that are appropriate for accessible restrooms or bathrooms, but are not on an accessible route, cannot be considered accessible. Guidelines for *Accessible Route, Clear Space Areas,* and *Doorways,* as examples, are general guidelines that must be applied to restrooms and bathrooms in general.

There is a significant number of specific dimensions and configurations for lavatories (sinks), water closets and urinals (toilets), showers and tubs. Other fixtures, such as grab bars, toilet paper dispensers, and mirrors add to the myriad combinations of applicable guidelines. For the sake of brevity and clarity, a number of configurations are presented as Figures 10–29 through 10–46, without text. Additional detail can be found in the USAB *Guide.*

FIGURE 10–29   Clearance for water closets.

FIGURE 10–30   Overlap of water closet clearance in residential bathrooms.

FIGURE 10–31   Sidewall placement of grab bars in water closets.

FIGURE 10–32   Rear wall placement of grab bars in water closets.

FIGURE 10–33   Placement of toilet paper dispenser in water closets.

(a)
adult wall hung
water closet

(b)
adult floor mounted water closet
and children's water closet

FIGURE 10–34   Dimensions of wheelchair accessible water closets.

FIGURE 10–35 Door dimensions of wheelchair accessible water closets.

FIGURE 10–36 Placement dimensions for urinals.

FIGURE 10–37 Clearance dimensions for bathtubs.

FIGURE 10–38 Placement of grab bars for bathtubs with permanent seats.

FIGURE 10–39 Placement of grab bars for bathtubs with removable seats.

FIGURE 10–40
Placement of
water controls in
bathtubs.

Note: inside finished dimensions measured at the center points
of opposing sides

FIGURE 10–41 Dimensions for transfer type
shower compartments.

FIGURE 10–42 Dimensions for standard roll-in type shower compartments.

Note: inside finished dimensions measured at the center points of opposing sides

FIGURE 10–43 Placement of grab bars in transfer type shower compartments.

FIGURE 10–44 Placement of grab bars for standard roll-in type shower compartments.

FIGURE 10–45 Placement of water controls for transfer type shower compartments.

FIGURE 10–46 Placement of water controls for roll-in type shower compartments.

Stairs

Riser (vertical dimension) height must be not less than 4 inches or greater than 7 inches. Angulation of risers (lowest point to highest point for each stair) must not exceed 30 degrees. Open risers are not permitted. **Tread** (horizontal dimension) must be not less than 11 inches. Tread **nosing**, the front edge of a tread, must not project greater than 1 1/2 inches, with a radius of curvature for the nosing of not greater than 1/2 inch. For any given set of stairs, dimensions and configuration must be consistent for all stairs. Outdoor stairs and paths must be designed to avoid accumulation of moisture. Handrails must be provided along both sides of the stairway, except in assembly areas, and must conform to the guidelines previously presented in this chapter under *Handrails*.

Transportation Facilities

Many areas and components within transportation facilities appear elsewhere on this list, such as *Accessible Routes, Reach Ranges,* and *Restrooms,* and must meet all individually listed criteria.

Clear space areas must be on an accessible route. For entry onto buses, a clear space area of not less than 96 inches in length parallel to the path of bus travel is required. The width of such a clear space area must be not less than 60 inches in width from curb, although this may be limited by site constraints.

Fare gates must be on an accessible route and automatic fare gates may not prohibit accessible entry to a transit system. At least one accessible fare gate must be available. Accessible fare gates must be not less than 32 inches in width at fare collection. Controls for such fare gates must conform to *Reach Range* requirements presented earlier in this chapter.

To greatest extent possible, accessible routes should follow paths comparable to paths used by the general public, with distances along accessible route minimized to the greatest extent possible. Platform edges must be protected by screens or guard rails. When not protected by screens or guard rails, detectable warnings must be in place. Shelters must be on an accessible route, with clear space areas of not less than 30 inches by 48 inches available entirely within the shelter.

Review Questions

1. What is the purpose of the Americans with Disabilities Act (ADA)?

2. What are the years in which the ADA, the ABA, and the most recent USAB guidelines were promulgated?

3. List general considerations and specific requirements of the ADA.

4. How does the ADA improve accessibility of facilities for people with physical impairments?

Suggested Activites

1. Access the USAB website and find the *New ADA–ABA Accessibility Guidelines*.

2. Examine specific areas for accessibility. Suggested areas are classrooms, restrooms, library, building entry, cafeteria, dormitory rooms, and access to floors other than the ground floor.

3. Examine assigned areas playing the role of physical therapist or patient. Suggested modes of ambulation when role-playing as patient include using crutches, wheelchair, or a walker.

4. Spend at least 2 hours in a public area while using an assistive device for ambulation. Consistently and appropriately role-play the need for the assistive device. Observe and write a report about the public reaction to your presence, your own reaction to using assistive devices in a public place, and any architectural barriers encountered.

REFERENCE

1. United States Congress (101st), Americans with Disabilities Act (PL 101–336), 1990.
2. United States Access Board, A Guide to the New ADA-ABA Accessibility Guidelines. www.access-board.gov; July 23, 2004.

GLOSSARY OF ABBREVIATIONS

A

A: Assessment
ALS   Amyotrophic lateral sclerosis

B

B or bil   Bilateral
B/C   Because
B/S   Bedside
BE   Below elbow
BID or bid   Twice a day
BK   Below knee
BM   Bowel movement
BOS   Base of support
BP   Blood pressure
bpm   Beats per minute
BR   Bedrest

C

c̄   With
C&S   Culture and sensitivity
c/o   Complains of
CA   Cancer
CABG   Coronary artery bypass graft
CAD   Coronary artery disease
CAT   Computerized axial tomography
CBC   Complete blood cell count
CC, C/C   Chief complaint
CG   Contact guard
CHF   Congestive heart failure
CNS   Central nervous system
Cont. or cont'd   continue, continued
COLD   Chronic obstructive lung disease
COPD   Chronic obstructive pulmonary disease
COTA   Certified occupational therapy assistant
CPM or cpm   Continuous passive motion
CPR   Cardiopulmonary resuscitation
CPT   Chest physical therapy
CS   Close supervision

D

D/C   Discontinue or discharge
DJD   Degenerative joint disease
DM   Diabetes mellitus
DME   Durable medical equipment
DNR   Do not resuscitate
DO   Doctor of osteopathy
DOB   Date of birth
DOE   Dyspnea on exertion
DTR   Deep tendon reflex
DVT   Deep vein thrombosis
Dx or dx   Diagnosis

E

ECF   Extended care facility
ECG or EKG   Electrocardiogram
EEG   Electroencephalogram
EENT   Ear, eyes, nose, throat
EMG   Electromyogram
eval   Evaluation
ex   Exercise
ext.   Extension, external
e-stim   Electrical stimulation
ER   External rotation

F

F   Fair (as a muscle grade)
FBS   Fasting blood sugar
FES   Functional electrical stimulation
FEV   Forced expiratory volume
FH   Family history
fl or flex   Flexion
FRC   Functional residual capacity
FUO   Fever, unknown origin
FVC   Forced vital capacity
F/U   Follow-up
FWB   Full weight bearing
Fx   Fracture, function

G

G   Good (as a muscle grade)
GCS   Glasgow Coma Scale
GI   Gastrointestinal
G-tube   Gastrointestinal tube
GSW   Gun shot wound
GYN   Gynecology

H

H, hr.   Hour
H&P   History and physical
H/A or h/o   History of
HA, H/A   Headache
HEENT   Head, ear, eye, nose, throat
HEP   Home exercise program
HHA   Home health aide
HNP   Herniated nucleus pulposus
HOB   Head of bed
HR   Heart rate
HTN   Hypertension
hs   At bedtime
ht.   Height
Hx or hx   History

I

I or indep   Independent
I&O or IO   Intake and output
ICU   Intensive care unit
Imp.   Impression
inf   Inferior
int rot or IR   Internal rotation
IP   Interphalangeal joint
IV   Intravenous

J

J-tube   Jejunsotomy tube

K

KAFO   Knee ankle foot orthosis

L

L or Ⓛ   Left
Lat   Lateral
LBBB   Left bundle branch block
LBP   Low back pain
LBQC   Large base quad cane
LE   Lower extremity

LLL   Left lower lobe
LLQ   Left lower quadrant
Lig   Ligament
LMN   Lower motor neuron
LOB   Loss of balance
LOC   Loss of consciousness; level of consciousness
LOS   Length of stay
LTG   Long term goal
LTC   Long term care
LUL   Left upper lobe
LUQ   Left upper quadrant
LVH   Left ventricular hypertrophy

M

Max   Maximum, maximal
MCA   Middle cerebral artery
MCP   Metacarpal phalangeal joint
MD   Medical doctor
MED   Minimal erythemal dose
Meds.   Medications
min   Minimum, minimal
MMT   Manual muscle test
mod   Moderate
MRI   Magnetic resonance imaging
MS   Multiple sclerosis
MVA   Motor vehicle accident
mvt   Movement

N

N   Normal (as a muscle grade)
N/A   Not applicable
NBCQ   Narrow base quad cane
NDT   Neurodevelopmental treatment
neg.   Negative
NG   Nasogastric
NICU   Neonatal intensive care unit
nn   Nerve
noc   Night, at night
NPO or npo   Nothing by mouth
NSR   Normal sinus rhythm
N/T   Not tested
NWB   Non-weight bearing

O

O: Objective
OA   Osteoarthritis
OB   Obstetrics

OBS   Organic brain syndrome

od   Once daily

OOB   Out of bed

O.P.   Out patient

O.R. or OR   Operating room

ORIF   Open reduction internal fixation

OT, OTR   Occupational therapy, occupational therapist

P

p̄   After

P   Poor (as a muscle grade)

P: Plan

P.A.   Physician's assistant

PA   Posterior/anterior

para   Paraplegia

pc   after meals

PCA   Posterior cerebral artery

PE   Pulmonary embolus

per   by/through

PERRLA   Pupils equal, round, reactive to light, and accommodation

PET   Positron emission tomography

PF   Plantar flexion

PH   Past history

PIP   Proximal interphalangeal joint

PMH   Past medical history

PNF   Proprioceptive neuromuscular facilitation

PNI   Peripheral nerve injury

PO   Per oral (by mouth)

POMR   Problem-oriented medical record

pos.   Positive

post   Posterior

post op   Postoperative

PRE   Progressive resistive exercise

pre op   before surgery

prn   As often as necessary

PROM   Passive range of motion

prox   Proximal

Pt   Patient

PT   Physical therapy, physical therapist

PTA   Physical therapist assistant, prior to admission

PVD   Peripheral vascular disease

PWB   Partial weight bearing

Q

q   Every

qd   Every day

qh   Every hour

qid   Four times a day

qn   Every night

quads   Quadriceps

R

R or Ⓡ   Right

RA   Rheumatoid arthritis

RBBB   Right bundle branch block

re   concerning, about

RBC   Red blood cell

R.D.   Registered dietician

Rehab   Rehabilitation

reps   Repetitions

resp   Respiratory, respiration

RLL   Right lower lobe

RLQ   Right lower quadrant

RML   Right middle lobe

RN   Registered nurse

R/O or r/o   Rule out

ROM   Range of motion

ROS   Review of systems

RR   Respiratory rate

RROM   Resistive range of motion

R.T.   Respiratory therapy, respiratory therapist

R/T   Related to

RUQ   Right upper quadrant

Rx   Prescription, treatment, orders, intervention, therapy

S

S   Supervision

s̄   Without

S: Subjective

SAQ   Short arc quads

SBA   Stand by assist

SBQC   Small base quad cane

SCI   Spinal cord injury

SED   Suberythemal dose

SLE   Systemic lupus erythematosus

SLP   Speech language pathologist

sig   Significant

SLR   Straight leg raise

SNF   Skilled nursing facility

SOAP   Subjective, objective, assessment, plan

S/O   Standing order

SOB   Short of breath

SOS Step over step
s/p Status post
stat Immediately, at once
STG Short term goal
STNR Symmetrical tonic neck reflex
sup Superior
surg Surgical, surgery
sx Symptoms

T

T Trace (as a muscle grade)
TBA To be assessed
TBI Traumatic brain injury
TDWB Touch down weight bearing
temp Temperature
TENS Transcutaneous electrical nerve stimulator
ther. ex Therapeutic exercise
THR Total hip replacement
TIA Transient ischemic attack
tid Three times a day
TKA Total knee arthroplasty
TKR Total knee replacement
TMJ Temporomandibular joint
TNR Tonic neck reflex
t.o. Telephone order
T/O Throughout
TPR Temperature, pulse, and respiration
TTWB Toe touch weight bearing
Tx Treatment, traction

U

UA Urine analysis
UE Upper extremity
U/L Unilateral

UMN Upper motor neuron
URI Upper respiratory infection
US Ultrasound
UTI Urinary tract infection
UV Ultraviolet

V

VAS Visual analog scale
VC Vital capacity, verbal cues
v.o., VO, V/O Verbal orders
vol. Volume
v.s., VS Vital signs
Vtach Ventricular tachycardia

W

WB Weight bearing
WBAT Weight bearing as tolerated
WBQC Wide base quad cane
w/c Wheelchair
WBC White blood cell
wk. Week
WFL Within functional limits
WNL Within normal limits
wt. Weight

X

x Times

Y

y/o or y.o. Years old
yr. Year

Z

Z Zero (as a muscle grade)

Index

SINGLE PC LICENSE AGREEMENT AND LIMITED WARRANTY

READ THIS LICENSE CAREFULLY BEFORE OPENING THIS PACKAGE. BY OPENING THIS PACKAGE, YOU ARE AGREEING TO THE TERMS AND CONDITIONS OF THIS LICENSE. IF YOU DO NOT AGREE, DO NOT OPEN THE PACKAGE. PROMPTLY RETURN THE UNOPENED PACKAGE AND ALL ACCOMPANYING ITEMS TO THE PLACE YOU OBTAINED THEM. *THESE TERMS APPLY TO ALL LICENSED SOFTWARE ON THE DISK EXCEPT THAT THE TERMS FOR USE OF ANY SHAREWARE OR FREEWARE ON THE DISKETTES ARE AS SET FORTH IN THE ELECTRONIC LICENSE LOCATED ON THE DISK:*

1. GRANT OF LICENSE and OWNERSHIP: The enclosed computer programs and data ("Software") are licensed, not sold, to you by Pearson Education, Inc. ("We" or the "Company") and in consideration of your purchase or adoption of the accompanying Company textbooks and/or other materials, and your agreement to these terms. We reserve any rights not granted to you. You own only the disk(s) but we and/or our licensors own the Software itself. This license allows you to use and display your copy of the Software on a single computer (i.e., with a single CPU) at a single location for academic use only, so long as you comply with the terms of this Agreement. You may make one copy for back up, or transfer your copy to another CPU, provided that the Software is usable on only one computer

2. RESTRICTIONS: You may not transfer or distribute the Software or documentation to anyone else. Except for backup, you may not copy the documentation or the Software. You may not network the Software or otherwise use it on more than one computer or computer terminal at the same time. You may not reverse engineer, disassemble, decompile, modify, adapt, translate, or create derivative works based on the Software or the Documentation. You may be held legally responsible for any copying or copyright infringement which is caused by your failure to abide by the terms of these restrictions.

3. TERMINATION: This license is effective until terminated. This license will terminate automatically without notice from the Company if you fail to comply with any provisions or limitations of this license. Upon termination, you shall destroy the Documentation and all copies of the Software. All provisions of this Agreement as to limitation and disclaimer of warranties, limitation of liability, remedies or damages, and our ownership rights shall survive termination.

4. LIMITED WARRANTY AND DISCLAIMER OF WARRANTY: Company warrants that for a period of 60 days from the date you purchase this SOFTWARE (or purchase or adopt the accompanying textbook), the Software, when properly installed and used in accordance with the Documentation, will operate in substantial conformity with the description of the Software set forth in the Documentation, and that for a period of 30 days the disk(s) on which the Software is delivered shall be free from defects in materials and workmanship under normal use. The Company does not warrant that the Software will meet your requirements or that the operation of the Software will be uninterrupted or error-free. Your only remedy and the Company's only obligation under these limited warranties is, at the Company's

option, return of the disk for a refund of any amounts paid for it by you or replacement of the disk. THIS LIMITED WARRANTY IS THE ONLY WARRANTY PROVIDED BY THE COMPANY AND ITS LICENSORS, AND THE COMPANY AND ITS LICENSORS DISCLAIM ALL OTHER WARRANTIES, EXPRESS OR IMPLIED, INCLUDING WITHOUT LIMITATION, THE IMPLIED WARRANTIES OF MERCHANTABILITY AND FITNESS FOR A PARTICULAR PURPOSE. THE COMPANY DOES NOT WARRANT, GUARANTEE OR MAKE ANY REPRESENTATION REGARDING THE ACCURACY, RELIABILITY, CURRENTNESS, USE, OR RESULTS OF USE, OF THE SOFTWARE.

5. LIMITATION OF REMEDIES AND DAMAGES: IN NO EVENT, SHALL THE COMPANY OR ITS EMPLOYEES, AGENTS, LICENSORS, OR CONTRACTORS BE LIABLE FOR ANY INCIDENTAL, INDIRECT, SPECIAL, OR CONSEQUENTIAL DAMAGES ARISING OUT OF OR IN CONNECTION WITH THIS LICENSE OR THE SOFTWARE, INCLUDING FOR LOSS OF USE, LOSS OF DATA, LOSS OF INCOME OR PROFIT, OR OTHER LOSSES, SUSTAINED AS A RESULT OF INJURY TO ANY PERSON, OR LOSS OF OR DAMAGE TO PROPERTY, OR CLAIMS OF THIRD PARTIES, EVEN IF THE COMPANY OR AN AUTHORIZED REPRESENTATIVE OF THE COMPANY HAS BEEN ADVISED OF THE POSSIBILITY OF SUCH DAMAGES. IN NO EVENT SHALL THE LIABILITY OF THE COMPANY FOR DAMAGES WITH RESPECT TO THE SOFTWARE EXCEED THE AMOUNTS ACTUALLY PAID BY YOU, IF ANY, FOR THE SOFTWARE OR THE ACCOMPANYING TEXTBOOK. BECAUSE SOME JURISDICTIONS DO NOT ALLOW THE LIMITATION OF LIABILITY IN CERTAIN CIRCUMSTANCES, THE ABOVE LIMITATIONS MAY NOT ALWAYS APPLY TO YOU.

6. GENERAL: THIS AGREEMENT SHALL BE CONSTRUED IN ACCORDANCE WITH THE LAWS OF THE UNITED STATES OF AMERICA AND THE STATE OF NEW YORK, APPLICABLE TO CONTRACTS MADE IN NEW YORK, AND SHALL BENEFIT THE COMPANY, ITS AFFILIATES AND ASSIGNEES. HIS AGREEMENT IS THE COMPLETE AND EXCLUSIVE STATEMENT OF THE AGREEMENT BETWEEN YOU AND THE COMPANY AND SUPERSEDES ALL PROPOSALS OR PRIOR AGREEMENTS, ORAL, OR WRITTEN, AND ANY OTHER COMMUNICATIONS BETWEEN YOU AND THE COMPANY OR ANY REPRESENTATIVE OF THE COMPANY RELATING TO THE SUBJECT MATTER OF THIS AGREEMENT. If you are a U.S. Government user, this Software is licensed with "restricted rights" as set forth in subparagraphs (a)-(d) of the Commercial Computer-Restricted Rights clause at FAR 52.227-19 or in subparagraphs (c)(1)(ii) of the Rights in Technical Data and Computer Software clause at DFARS 252.227-7013, and similar clauses, as applicable.

Should you have any questions concerning this agreement or if you wish to contact the Company for any reason, please contact in writing: Prentice-Hall, New Media Department, One Lake Street, Upper Saddle River, NJ 07458.

Preface

ICD-9-CM for Physicians has been designed with the physician office professional in mind. The most recent official government versions of volumes 1 and 2 have been combined to provide physicians and their office staff with an ICD-9-CM book that is easy to use.

In addition, our technical experts have drawn upon their extensive hands-on experience to enhance the government's official version with valuable features essential to correct coding and reimbursement. With these enhancements, physician office health information professionals will increase the efficiency and timeliness of claim submission for both Medicare and other third-party payers.

As you review the content, you'll find the following:

- All the official ICD-9-CM codes, indexes, notes, footnotes and symbols
- Complete official coding guidelines
- Our exclusive color coding, symbols, and footnotes that alert coders to coding and reimbursement issues. Medicare outpatient code edits, such as invalid fourth or fifth digit for diagnosis codes are identified.
- Illustrations and clinically oriented definitions to aid in correct code assignment
- Coding tips based upon the official coding guidelines and advice found in AHA's *Coding Clinic for ICD-9-CM*
- Symbols identifying new codes and text revisions
- Exclusive QuickFlip Color Tabs for quick, easy location of terms and codes in the Alphabetic Index and Tabular List

Use of Official Sources

This *ICD-9-CM for Physicians* contains the official U.S. Department of Health and Human Services, ICD-9-CM codes, effective for the current year.

The color coding, footnotes and symbols, which identify coding and reimbursement issues, are derived from official federal government sources, including the Medicare Outpatient Code Editor as well as the knowledge of our technical experts.

The American Hospital Association's (AHA) *Coding Clinic for ICD-9-CM* references are used with permission of the AHA.

Technical Editors

Anita Schmidt, BS, RHIT, *Clinical Technical Editor*
Ms. Schmidt has expertise in Level I Adult and Pediatric Trauma hospital coding, specializing in ICD-9-CM, DRG, and CPT coding. Her experience includes analysis of medical record documentation and assignment of ICD-9-CM codes and DRGs, and CPT code assignments for same-day surgery cases. She has conducted coding training and auditing inclusive of DRG validation, conducted electronic health record training, and worked with clinical documentation specialists to identify documentation needs and potential areas for physician education. Ms. Schmidt is an active member of the American Health Information Management Association (AHIMA) and the Minnesota Health Information Management Association (MNHIMA).

Karen Schmidt, BSN, *Clinical Technical Director*
Ms. Schmidt has more than 25 years of health care experience beginning with a strong clinical background in critical care nursing and later functioning as director of case management, including the components of quality assurance, utilization management, concurrent coding, case-mix analysis, and discharge planning. Her areas of expertise include ICD-9-CM/DRG coding, outpatient observation, billing compliance, implementation of concurrent coding methodology, and physician documentation education. She is an active member of the American Health Information Management Association (AHIMA).

In addition to the editors, the following people have contributed to this book:

Stacy Perry, *Manager, Desktop Publishing*
Tracy Betzler, *Senior Desktop Publishing Specialist*
Hope M. Dunn, *Senior Desktop Publishing Specialist*
Katie Russell, *Desktop Publishing Specialist*
Kate Holden, *Editor*

What to Do If You Have Questions

If you have any questions call our customer service department toll-free at 800-464-3649, option 1.

If you have comments on the content of this book, please e-mail them to accuracy@optum.com.

Additional Copies

Contact the customer service order department toll-free at 800-464-3649, option 1.

Introduction

History and Future of ICD-9-CM

The International Classification of Diseases, Ninth Revision, Clinical Modification (ICD-9-CM) is based on the official version of the World Health Organization's Ninth Revision, International Classification of Diseases (ICD-9). ICD-9-CM classifies morbidity and mortality information for statistical purposes, indexing of hospital records by disease and operations, data storage, and retrieval.

This modification of ICD-9 supplants the Eighth Revision International Classification of Diseases, Adapted for Use in the United States (ICDA-8) and the Hospital Adaptation of ICDA (H-ICDA).

The concept of extending the International Classification of Diseases for use in hospital indexing was originally developed in response to a need for a more efficient basis for storage and retrieval of diagnostic data. In 1950, the U.S. Public Health Service and the Veterans Administration began independent tests of the International Classification of Diseases for hospital indexing purposes. The following year, the Columbia Presbyterian Medical Center in New York City adopted the International Classification of Diseases, Sixth Revision, with some modifications for use in its medical record department. A few years later, the Commission on Professional and Hospital Activities (CPHA) in Ann Arbor, Mich., adopted the International Classification of Diseases with similar modifications for use in hospitals participating in the Professional Activity Study.

The problem of adapting ICD for indexing hospital records was addressed by the U.S. National Committee on Vital and Health Statistics through its subcommittee on hospital statistics. The subcommittee reviewed the modifications made by the various users of ICD and proposed that uniform changes be made. This was done by a small working party.

In view of the growing interest in the use of the International Classification of Diseases for hospital indexing, a study was undertaken in 1956 by the American Hospital Association and the American Medical Record Association (then the American Association of Medical Record Librarians) of the relative efficiencies of coding systems for diagnostic indexing. This study indicated the International Classification of Diseases provided a suitable and efficient framework for indexing hospital records. The major users of the International Classification of Diseases for hospital indexing purposes then consolidated their experiences, and an adaptation was first published in December 1959. A revision was issued in 1962 and the first "Classification of Operations and Treatments" was included.

In 1966, the international conference for revising the International Classification of Diseases noted the eighth revision of ICD had been constructed with hospital indexing in mind and considered the revised classification suitable, in itself, for hospital use in some countries. However, it was recognized that the basic classification might provide inadequate detail for diagnostic indexing in other countries. A group of consultants was asked to study the eighth revision of ICD (ICD-8) for applicability to various users in the United States. This group recommended that further detail be provided for coding of hospital and morbidity data. The American Hospital Association was requested to develop the needed adaptation proposals. This was done by an advisory committee (the Advisory Committee to the Central Office on ICDA). In 1968 the United States Public Health Service published the product, Eighth Revision International Classification of Diseases, Adapted for Use in the United States. This became commonly known as ICDA-8, and beginning in 1968 it served as the basis for coding diagnostic data for both official morbidity and mortality statistics in the United States.

In 1968, the CPHA published the Hospital Adaptation of ICDA (H-ICDA) based on both the original ICD-8 and ICDA-8. In 1973, CPHA published a revision of H-ICDA, referred to as H-ICDA-2. Hospitals throughout the United States were divided in their use of these classifications until January 1979, when ICD-9-CM was made the single classification intended primarily for use in the United States, replacing these earlier related, but somewhat dissimilar, classifications.

Physicians have been required by law to submit diagnosis codes for Medicare reimbursement since the passage of the Medicare Catastrophic Coverage Act of 1988. This act requires physician offices to include the appropriate diagnosis codes when billing for services provided to Medicare beneficiaries on or after April 1, 1989. The Centers for Medicare and Medicaid Services (CMS) designated ICD-9-CM as the coding system physicians must use.

The ICD-10-CM classification system was developed by the National Center for Health Statistics (NCHS) as a clinical modification to the ICD-10 system developed by the World Health Organization (WHO), primarily as a unique system for use in the United States for morbidity and mortality reporting. Although ICD-10-CM has not yet been implemented for use in the United States, ICD-10 has been adopted for use in the coding and classification or mortality data from death certificates. ICD-10 replaced ICD-9 for this purpose as of January 1, 1999. The Department of Health and Human Services (HHS) published the final rule regarding the adoption of both ICD-10-CM and ICD-10-PCS in the January 16, 2009 *Federal Register* (45 CFR part 162 [CMS—0013—F]). On April 2, 2014, Congress enacted the Protecting Access to Medicare Act of 2014, which contained a provision to delay the implementation of ICD-10-CM/PCS by at least one year. The act prohibits the Department of Health and Human Services (HHS) from adopting the ICD–10-CM/PCS code sets as the mandatory standard until at least October 1, 2015.

ICD-9-CM Background

In February 1977, a steering committee was convened by the National Center for Health Statistics to provide advice and counsel in developing a clinical modification of ICD-9. The organizations represented on the steering committee included the following:

- American Association of Health Data Systems
- American Hospital Association
- American Medical Record Association
- Association for Health Records
- Council on Clinical Classifications
- Centers for Medicare and Medicaid Services, Department of Health and Human Services
- WHO Center for Classification of Diseases for North America, sponsored by the National Center for Health Statistics, Department of Health and Human Services

The Council on Clinical Classifications was sponsored by the following:

- American Academy of Pediatrics
- American College of Obstetricians and Gynecologists
- American College of Physicians
- American College of Surgeons
- American Psychiatric Association
- Commission on Professional and Hospital Activities

The steering committee met periodically in 1977. Clinical guidance and technical input were provided by task forces on classification from the Council on Clinical Classification's sponsoring organizations.

ICD-9-CM is a clinical modification of the World Health Organization's ICD-9. The term "clinical" is used to emphasize the modification's intent: to serve as a useful tool to classify morbidity data for indexing medical records, medical care review, and ambulatory and other medical care programs, as well as for basic health statistics. To describe the clinical picture of the patient, the codes must be more precise than those needed only for statistical groupings and trend analysis.

Characteristics of ICD-9-CM

ICD-9-CM far exceeds its predecessors in the number of codes provided. The disease classification has been expanded to include health-related conditions and to provide greater specificity at the fifth-digit level of detail. These fifth digits are not optional; they are intended for use in recording the information substantiated in the clinical record.

Volume I (Tabular List) of ICD-9-CM contains four appendixes:

Appendix A	Morphology of Neoplasms
Appendix B	Deleted effective October 1, 2004
Appendix C	Classification of Drugs by American Hospital Formulary Service List Number and Their ICD-9-CM Equivalents
Appendix D	Classification of Industrial Accidents According to Agency
Appendix E	List of Three-Digit Categories

These appendixes are included as a reference to provide further information about the patient's clinical picture, to further define a diagnostic statement, to aid in classifying new drugs or to reference three-digit categories.

Volume 2 (Alphabetic Index) of ICD-9-CM contains many diagnostic terms that do not appear in volume I since the index includes most diagnostic terms currently in use.

The Disease Classification

ICD-9-CM is totally compatible with its parent system, ICD-9, thus meeting the need for comparability of morbidity and mortality statistics at the international level. A few fourth-digit codes were created in existing three-digit rubrics only when the necessary detail could not be accommodated by the use of a fifth-digit subclassification. To ensure that each rubric of ICD-9-CM collapses back to its ICD-9 counterpart the following specifications governed the ICD-9-CM disease classification:

Specifications for the Tabular List:

1. Three-digit rubrics and their contents are unchanged from ICD-9.

2. The sequence of three-digit rubrics is unchanged from ICD-9.

3. Three-digit rubrics are not added to the main body of the classification.

4. Unsubdivided three-digit rubrics are subdivided where necessary to

   • add clinical detail

   • isolate terms for clinical accuracy

5. The modification in ICD-9-CM is accomplished by adding a fifth digit to existing ICD-9 rubrics, except as noted under #7 below.

6. The optional dual classification in ICD-9 is modified.

   • Duplicate rubrics are deleted:

     – four-digit manifestation categories duplicating etiology entries

     – manifestation inclusion terms duplicating etiology entries

   • Manifestations of disease are identified, to the extent possible, by creating five-digit codes in the etiology rubrics.

   • When the manifestation of a disease cannot be included in the etiology rubrics, provision for its identification is made by retaining the ICD-9 rubrics used for classifying manifestations of disease.

7. The format of ICD-9-CM is revised from that used in ICD-9.

   • American spelling of medical terms is used.

   • Inclusion terms are indented beneath the titles of codes.

   • Codes not to be used for primary tabulation of disease are printed in italics with the notation, "code first underlying disease."

Specifications for the Alphabetic Index:

1. The format of the Alphabetic Index follows that of ICD-9.

2. When two codes are required to indicate etiology and manifestation, the manifestation code appears in brackets (e.g., diabetic cataract 250.5 [*366.41*]).

The ICD-9-CM Coordination and Maintenance Committee

The ICD-9-CM Coordination and Maintenance Committee, a federal committee, was created as a forum for proposals to update International Classification of Diseases, Ninth Revision, Clinical Modification, Sixth Edition (ICD-9-CM). A representative from the National Center for Health Statistics (NCHS) and one from the Centers for Medicare and Medicaid Services (CMS) co-chair the ICD-9-CM Coordination and Maintenance Committee meetings. Responsibility for maintaining ICD-9-CM is divided between the two agencies, with NCHS classifying diagnoses (volumes 1 and 2) and CMS classifying procedures (volume 3).

Proposals for changes to the ICD-9-CM classification system are submitted and discussed in open forum meetings held in March and September of each year at the headquarters of CMS in Baltimore. Comments received during or after the meetings are then reviewed and evaluated. All final decisions are made by the director of NCHS and the administrator of CMS. The complete official document of changes to the classification system is released as the Addenda for the International Classification of Disease, Ninth Revision, Clinical Modification, Sixth Edition, Volume 1, 2, & 3.

The *ICD-9-CM for Physicians, Volumes 1 & 2,* is based on the official version of the International Classification of Diseases, Ninth Revision, Clinical Modification, Sixth Edition, issued by the U.S. Department of Health and Human Services. Annual code changes are implemented by the government and are effective October 1 and valid through September 30 of the following year. If a convincing case is made that requires a new code to capture new technology or an emerging disease, this new code may be implemented on April 1 of the following year.

Effective March 2014, the ICD-9-CM Coordination and Maintenance Committee was renamed the ICD-10 Coordination and Maintenance Committee.

How to Use the ICD-9-CM for Physicians (Volumes 1 & 2)

ICD-9-CM for Physicians is based on the official version of the International Classification of Diseases, Ninth Revision, Clinical Modification, Sixth Edition, issued by the U.S. Department of Health and Human Services. Annual code changes are implemented by the government and are effective Oct. 1 and valid through Sept. 30 of the following year.

To accommodate the coder's approach to coding, the Alphabetic Index (Volume 2) has been placed before the Tabular List (Volume 1). This allows the user to locate the term in the index, then confirm the accuracy of the code in the Tabular List.

10 Steps to Correct Coding

To code accurately, it is necessary to have a working knowledge of medical terminology and to understand the characteristics, terminology and conventions of ICD-9-CM. Transforming descriptions of diseases, injuries, conditions and procedures into numerical designations (coding) is a complex activity and should not be undertaken without proper training.

Originally, coding allowed retrieval of medical information by diagnoses and operations for medical research, education and administration. Coding today is used to describe the medical necessity of a procedure and facilitate payment of health services, to evaluate utilization patterns and to study the appropriateness of health care costs. Coding provides the basis for epidemiological studies and research into the quality of health care. Incorrect or inaccurate coding can lead to investigations of fraud and abuse. Therefore, coding must be performed correctly and consistently to produce meaningful statistics to aid in planning for the health needs of the nation.

Follow the steps below to code correctly:

Step 1: Identify the reason for the visit (e.g., sign, symptom, diagnosis, condition to be coded).

Physicians describe the patient's condition using terminology that includes specific diagnoses as well as symptoms, problems or reasons for the encounter. If symptoms are present but a definitive diagnosis has not yet been determined, code the symptoms. Do not code conditions that are referred to as "rule out," "suspected," "probable" or "questionable."

Step 2: Always consult the Alphabetic Index, Volume 2, before turning to the Tabular List.

The most critical rule is to begin a code search in the index. Never turn first to the Tabular List (Volume 1), as this will lead to coding errors and less specificity in code assignments. To prevent coding errors, use both the Alphabetic Index and the Tabular List when locating and assigning a code.

Step 3: Locate the main entry term.

The Alphabetic Index is arranged by condition. Conditions may be expressed as nouns, adjectives and eponyms. Some conditions have multiple entries under their synonyms. Main terms are identified using boldface type.

Step 4: Read and interpret any notes listed with the main term.

Notes are identified using italicized type.

Step 5: Review entries for modifiers.

Nonessential modifiers are in parentheses. These parenthetical terms are supplementary words or explanatory information that may either be present or absent in the diagnostic statement and do not affect code assignment.

Step 6: Interpret abbreviations, cross-references, symbols and brackets.

Cross-references used are "*see*," "*see* category," or "*see* also." The abbreviation NEC may follow main terms or subterms. NEC (not elsewhere classified) indicates that there is no specific code for the condition even though the medical documentation may be very specific. The ☑ box indicates the code requires an additional digit. If the appropriate digits are not found in the index, in a box beneath the main term, you MUST refer to the Tabular List. Italicized brackets [ ], are used to enclose a second code number that must be used with the code immediately preceding it and in that sequence.

Step 7: Choose a tentative code and locate it in the Tabular List.

Be guided by any inclusion or exclusion terms, notes or other instructions, such as "*code first*" and "use additional code," that would direct the use of a different or additional code from that selected in the index for a particular diagnosis, condition or disease.

Step 8: Determine whether the code is at the highest level of specificity.

Assign three-digit codes (category codes) if there are no four-digit codes within the code category. Assign four-digit codes (subcategory codes) if there are no five-digit codes for that category. Assign five-digit codes (fifth-digit subclassification codes) for those categories where they are available.

Step 9: Consult the color coding and reimbursement prompts, including the age and sex edits.

Consult the official ICD-9-CM guidelines for coding and reporting, and refer to the AHA's *Coding Clinic for ICD-9-CM* for coding guidelines governing the use of specific codes.

Step 10: Assign the code.

Organization

Introduction

The introductory material in this book includes the history and future of ICD-9-CM as well as an overview of the classification system

Official ICD-9-CM Conventions

This section provides a full explanation of all the official footnotes, symbols, instructional notes, and conventions found in the official government version

Additional Conventions

Exclusive color-coding, symbols, and notations have been included in the *ICD-9-CM for Physicians, Volumes 1 and 2* to alert coders to important coding and reimbursement issues. This section provides a full explanation of the additional conventions used throughout this book.

ICD-10-CM Coding Proficiency and Documentation Self-Assessment

Use this self-assessment to identify the areas that may require additional coding training or documentation improvement before ICD-10-CM is implemented.

Coding Guidelines

Included in this book are the official ICD-9-CM coding guidelines as approved by the four cooperating parties of the ICD-9-CM Coordination and Maintenance Committee. Failure to comply with these official coding guidelines may result in denied or delayed claims.

Disease Classification: Alphabetic Index to Diseases

The Alphabetic Index to Diseases is separated by tabs labeled with the letters of the alphabet, contains diagnostic terms for illnesses, injuries and reasons for encounters with health care professionals. Both the Table of Drugs and Chemicals and the Alphabetic Index to External Causes of Injury and Poisoning are easily located with the tabs in this section.

The warning statement at the bottom of every page of the index, Subterms under main terms may continue to next column or page, is a reminder to always check for additional subterms before making final selection.

Disease Classification: Tabular List of Diseases

The Tabular List of Diseases arranges the ICD-9-CM codes and descriptors numerically. Tabs divide this section into chapters, identified by the code range on the tab.

The Tabular List includes two supplementary classifications:

- V Codes–Supplementary Classification of Factors Influencing Health Status and Contact with Health Services (V01–V91)

- E Codes–Supplementary Classification of External Causes of Injury and Poisoning (E000–E999)

ICD-9-CM includes four official appendixes.

- Appendix A   Morphology of Neoplasms
- Appendix B   Deleted effective October 1, 2004
- Appendix C   Classification of Drugs by AHFS List
- Appendix D   Classification of Industrial Accidents According to Agency
- Appendix E   List of Three-digit Categories

These appendixes are included as a reference to provide further information about the patient's circumstances, help further define a diagnostic statement, maintain a tumor registry and aid in classifying new drugs.

Resources

Listed below are the exclusive resources found **ONLY** in the *ICD-9-CM Expert for Physicians, Volumes 1 & 2.*

10 Steps to Correct Coding

This is a valuable resource that takes the coder step by step through the coding process with detailed explanations accompanied by coding examples that demonstrate the practical application of ICD-9-CM conventions and coding guidelines in 10 steps.

Valid Three-digit Code Table

ICD-9-CM is composed of codes with either 3, 4, or 5 digits. A code is invalid if it has not been coded to the full number of digits required for that code. There are a certain number codes that are valid for reporting as three digit codes. A list of these valid three-digit code is included as a convenient reference when auditing claims.

Code Tables

Exclusive coding tables covering abortion, burns, complications, diabetes, hernia, pregnancy, and others are provided to simplify those complex coding issues.

ICD-9-CM Official Conventions

ICD-9-CM Footnotes, Symbols, Instructional Notes and Conventions

This *ICD-9-CM for Physicians* preserves all the footnotes, symbols, instructional notes and conventions found in the government's official version. Accurate coding depends upon understanding the meaning of these elements.

The following appear in the disease Tabular List, unless otherwise noted.

Official Government Symbols

§   The section mark preceding a code denotes a footnote on the page. This symbol is used in the Tabular List of Diseases.

ICD-9-CM Conventions Used in the Tabular List

In addition to the symbols and footnotes above, the ICD-9-CM disease tabular has certain abbreviations, punctuation, symbols and other conventions. Our *ICD-9-CM for Physicians* preserves these conventions. Proper use of the conventions will lead to efficient and accurate coding.

Abbreviations

NEC   Not elsewhere classifiable
This abbreviation is used when the ICD-9-CM system does not provide a code specific for the patient's condition.

NOS   Not otherwise specified
This abbreviation is the equivalent of "unspecified" and is used only when the coder lacks the information necessary to code to a more specific four-digit subcategory.

[ ]   Brackets enclose synonyms, alternative terminology or explanatory phrases:

482.2   Pneumonia due to Hemophilus influenzae [H. influenzae]

Brackets that appear beneath a code indicate the fifth digits that are considered valid fifth digits for the code. This convention is applied for those instances in ICD-9-CM where not all common fifth digits are considered valid for each subcategory within a category.

715.0   Osteoarthrosis, generalized
[0,4,9]

Generalized arthrosis can only be assigned in cases for which the degenerative joint disease involves multiple joints. Therefore, this code is considered for arthrosis in the sites described as unspecified, hand (which consists of multiple joints), or multiple sites. Therefore, only fifth digits 0, 4, and 9 are valid with subcategory 715.0.

[ ]   Slanted brackets that appear in the Alphabetic Index indicate mandatory multiple coding. Both codes must be assigned to fully describe the condition and are sequenced in the order listed.

Tachycardia
ventricular (paroxysmal)
psychogenic 316 *[427.1]*

Psychogenic paroxysmal tachycardia is reported using both 316, Psychogenic factors associated with diseases classified elsewhere, and 427.1, Paroxysmal ventricular tachycardia.

( )   Parentheses enclose supplementary words, called nonessential modifiers, that may be present in the narrative description of a disease without affecting the code assignment:

198.4   Other parts of nervous system
Meninges (cerebral) (spinal)

:   Colons are used in the Tabular List after an incomplete term that needs one or more of the modifiers that follow in order to make it assignable to a given category:

021.1   Enteric tularemia
Tularemia:
cryptogenic
intestinal
typhoidal

}   Braces enclose a series of terms, each of which is modified by the statement appearing to the right of the brace:

560.2   Volvulus
Knotting
Strangulation   } of intestine, bowel, or
Torsion   colon
Twist

Other Conventions

Boldface   Boldface type is used for all codes and titles in the Tabular List.

Italicized   Italicized type is used for all exclusion notes and to identify codes that should not be used for describing the primary diagnosis.

General Notes Used in the Tabular List

These notes appear only in the Tabular List of Diseases:

Includes   An includes note further defines or clarifies the content of the chapter, subchapter, category, subcategory or subclassification. The includes note in the example below applies only to category 461.

Excludes   Terms following the word "Excludes" are not classified to the chapter, subchapter, category, subcategory or specific subclassification code under which it is found. The note also may provide the location of the excluded diagnosis. Excludes notes are italicized.

461   Acute sinusitis
INCLUDES   abscess
empyema
infection   } acute, of sinus
inflammation   (accessory)
suppuration   (nasal)
EXCLUDES   chronic or unspecified sinusitis (473.0-473.9)

Instructional Notes

The following official instructional notes are critical to correct coding practices. The instructional notes appear in red type in the Tabular List.

Use additional code:
This instruction signals the coder that an additional code should be used if the information is available to provide a more complete picture of that diagnosis.

362.13   Changes in vascular appearance
Vascular sheathing of retina
Use additional code for any associated atherosclerosis (440.8)

For emphasis this instructional note appears in red type in the tabular section.

There are coding circumstances outside of the etiology/ manifestation convention when multiple coding for a single condition is required. The "Use additional code" note will be found under the associated condition code in the tabular. In the index, the multiple coding requirement is indicated by the use of the slanted bracket. The two codes are to be sequenced as listed in the index. For example, retinal arteriosclerosis must be coded using two codes sequenced as listed in the index.

Arteriosclerosis, arteriosclerotic
retinal (vascular) 440.8 *[362.13]*

Code first underlying disease:

The *"Code first underlying"* instructional note found under certain codes is a sequencing rule. Most often this sequencing rule applies to the etiology/manifestation convention and is found under the manifestation code. The manifestation code may never be used alone or as a primary diagnosis (i.e., sequenced first). The instructional note, the code and its descriptor appear in italics in the Tabular List.

> ### 590.81 Pyelitis or pyelonephritis in diseases classified elsewhere
> > *Code first underlying disease as:*
> > tuberculosis (016.0)

Not all codes with a "Code first underlying disease" instructional note are part of the etiology/manifestation convention. The `Code first' note will appear, but the title of the code and the instructional note are not in italics. These codes may be reported alone or as the secondary diagnosis. For example, disseminated chorioretinitis may be reported as a principal or first-listed diagnosis. However, if the underlying condition that caused disseminated chorioretinitis is known, such as tuberculous disseminated chorioretinitis, two codes are required and sequenced as listed in the index.

> ### 363.13 Disseminated choroiditis and chorioretinitis, generalized
> > Code first underlying disease as:
> > tuberculosis (017.3)

For emphasis this instructional note appears in red type in the tabular section.

Code, if applicable, any causal condition first:

A code with this note indicates that this code may be assigned as a principal diagnosis when the causal condition is unknown or not applicable. If a causal condition is known, then the code for that condition should be sequenced as the principal or first-listed diagnosis.

> ### 590.0 Chronic pyelonephritis
> > Chronic pyelitis
> > Chronic pyonephrosis
> > Code, if applicable, any causal condition first

For emphasis this instructional note appears in red type in the tabular section.

Instructional Notes Used in the Index

Omit code:

"Omit code" is used to instruct the coder that no code is to be assigned.

When this instruction is found in the Alphabetic Index to Diseases the medical term should not be coded as a diagnosis.

> **Metaplasia**
> cervix — *omit code*

See Condition:

The "see condition" note found in the Alphabetic Index to Disease instructs the coder to refer to a main term for the condition. This note will follow index terms that are nouns for anatomical sites or adjectival forms of disease term. In the example below, the index terms "Cervix" and "Diffuse" are followed by the — see condition. Coders should search the index using a condition term such as atrophy or prolapse.

> **Cervix** — *see* condition
> **Diffuse** — *see* condition

Morphology Codes:

For each neoplastic disease listed in the index, a morphology code is provided that identifies histological type and behavior.

> *Example:*

> **Myelolipoma** (M8870/0) — *see* Neoplasm, by site, benign

The histology is identified by the first four digits and the behavior is identified by the digit following the slash. Appendix A of Volume 1 contains a listing of morphology codes. This appendix is helpful when the pathology report identifies the neoplasm by using an M code. The coder may refer to Appendix A to determine the nomenclature of the neoplasm that will be the main term to search in the Index. The behavior classification is as follows:

0 Benign

1 Uncertain whether benign or malignant
  Borderline malignancy

2 Carcinoma in situ
  Intraepithelial
  Noninfiltrating
  Noninvasive

3 Malignant, primary site

6 Malignant, metastatic site
  Secondary site

9 Malignant, uncertain whether primary or metastatic site

Additional Conventions

Symbols and Notations

New and Revised Text Symbols

●   A bullet at a code or line of text indicates that the entry is new.

▲   A triangle in the Tabular List indicates that the code title is revised. In the Alphabetic Index the triangle indicates that a code has changed.

►◄   These symbols appear at the beginning and at the end of a section of new or revised text.

Additional Digits Required

✓4ᵗʰ   This symbol indicates that the code requires a fourth digit.

✓5ᵗʰ   This symbol indicates that a code requires a fifth digit.

✓   This symbol found only in the Alphabetic Index sections and the Table of Drugs and Chemicals indicates that an additional digit is required. Referring to the tabular section is essential to locate the appropriate additional digit.

AHA's *Coding Clinic for ICD-9-CM* References

The four cooperating parties have designated the AHA's *Coding Clinic for ICD-9-CM* as the official publication for coding guidelines. The references are identified by the notation **AHA:** followed by the issue, year and page number.

In the example below, AHA's *Coding Clinic for ICD-9-CM*, third quarter 1991, page 15, contains a discussion on code assignment for vitreous hemorrhage:

379.23 Vitreous hemorrhage
AHA: 3Q, '91, 15

The table below explains the abbreviations in the *Coding Clinic* references:

J-F	January/February
M-A	March/April
M-J	May/June
J-A	July/August
S-O	September/October
N-D	November/December
1Q	First quarter
2Q	Second quarter
3Q	Third quarter
4Q	Fourth quarter

AHA's *Coding Clinic for ICD-9-CM* references appear in blue type in the Tabular List.

Age and Sex Edit Symbols

The age edits below address OCE edits and are used to detect inconsistencies between the patient's age and diagnosis. They appear in the Tabular List of Diseases to the right of the code description.

Newborn Age: 0   N

These diagnoses are intended for newborns and neonates and the patient's age must be 0 years.

Pediatric Age: 0-17   P

These diagnoses are intended for children and the patient's age must between 0 and 17 years.

Maternity Age: 12-55   M

These diagnoses are intended for the patients between the age of 12 and 55 years.

Adult Age: 15-124   A

These diagnoses are intended for the patients between the age of 15 and 124 years.

The sex symbols below address OCE edits and are used to detect inconsistencies between the patient's sex and diagnosis. They appear in the Tabular List of Diseases to the right of the code description:

♂   **Male diagnosis only**

This symbol appears to the right of the code description. This reference appears in the disease Tabular List.

♀   **Female diagnosis only**

This symbol appears to the right of the code description. This reference appears in the disease Tabular List.

Color Coding

For a quick reference to the color codes and their meaning, refer to the color/symbol legend located at the bottom of each page.

To alert the coder to Medicare outpatient code edits and other important reimbursement issues, color bars have been added over the code descriptors in the Tabular List. Some codes carry more than one color.

Carriers use the Medicare Outpatient Code Editor (OCE) to examine claims for coding and billing accuracy and completeness. Color codes in this book signify Medicare code edits for manifestation codes not to be reported as a primary diagnosis, and when a more specific diagnosis code should be used.

Manifestation Code

These codes will appear in italic type as well as with a blue color bar over the code title. A manifestation code is not allowed to be reported as a first-listed diagnosis because each describes a manifestation of some other underlying disease, not the disease itself. This is referred to as mandatory multiple coding of etiology and manifestation. Code the underlying disease first. A *Code first underlying disease* instructional note will appear with underlying disease codes identified. In the Alphabetic Index these codes are listed as the secondary code in slanted brackets with the code for the underlying disease listed first.

Other Specified Code

These codes will appear with a gray color bar over the code title. Use these codes when the documentation indicates a specified diagnosis, but the ICD-9-CM system does not have a specific code that describes the diagnosis. These codes may be stated as "Other" or "Not elsewhere classified (NEC)."

Unspecified Code

These codes will have a yellow color bar over the code title. Use these codes when the neither the diagnostic statement nor the documentation provides enough information to assign a more specified diagnosis code. These codes may be stated as "Unspecified" or "Not otherwise specified (NOS)." Note: Do not assign these codes when a more specific diagnosis has been determined.

Other Notations

DEF: This symbol indicates a definition of disease term. The definition will appear in blue type in the Disease Tabular Lists.

TIPS: This symbol precedes official coding advice found in the official coding guidelines and AHA's *Coding Clinic for ICD-9-CM*. Coding tips appear in blue type in the Tabular List.

I-10   In preparation for the transition to coding using the ICD-10-CM classification system, examples of ICD-10-CM codes have been provided for selected ICD-9-CM diagnosis codes. This symbol indicates that the code provided is an ICD-10-CM code to which the selected ICD-9-CM code is mapped.

Note: Coding professionals should keep in mind the following points when referring to the ICD-10-CM codes provided:

- ICD-10-CM codes are not currently valid for reporting purposes.
- The ICD-10-CM code may represent only one possible coding option. Since mappings between ICD-9-CM and ICD-10-CM are not always straightforward one-to-one correspondences due to the differences in

terminology and clinical concepts, the mapping may result in a one-to-many code option. Not all code options for a particular ICD-9-CM code are provided. For cases in which many code alternatives are possible in ICD-10-CM, only one example is provided.

- The ICD-10-CM code examples are provided only for the most frequently reported ICD-9-CM codes in each chapter.
- The ICD-10-CM codes are examples only and are provided to ease the transition to the new classification system.

PDx

This symbol identifies a V code that generally is for use as a first listed diagnosis only (primary) but may be used as an additional diagnosis if the patient has more than one encounter on one day or there is more than one reason for the encounter.

The instructions for V code use contained in the new official coding guidelines identify those V codes that can only be used as a PDx. All other V codes may either be SDx or PDx depending upon circumstances of the encounter, by meeting the definition of first-listed or principal diagnosis, and by following any specific V code guidelines in section I.C.18 a-e. With the elimination of the V Code Table, the responsibility of those assigning the V codes as PDx is to make sure the circumstances of the encounter meet the definition of first-listed or principal diagnosis, follow all coding instructions, and follow the V code specific guidelines. Optum does not include the SDx edit since it is no longer based on an official source and the V code use is determined by circumstances of the encounter.

Note: Please note that the symbols indicating the V code designation and the V codes that may be principal or first listed (primary) diagnoses included in the official coding guidelines [Section I.C.18.e] are consistent with reporting guidelines for health care encounters *excluding acute care inpatient admissions*. These V code edits are often in conflict with the inpatient prospective payment system (IPPS) edits. For example, V22.0 Encounter for supervision of a normal first pregnancy, may be an appropriate primary reason for an outpatient encounter. However, supervision for a normal pregnancy is not an acceptable principal diagnosis for an inpatient admission and will have an unacceptable principal diagnosis edit under IPPS.

V29 Observation Code Category

The V29 observation codes are used to report circumstances when a newborn is being observed for a suspected condition resulting from exposure from the mother or birth process that after examination and observation is found not to exist. These codes are to be used as the first-listed or principal diagnosis with one exception. When the first-listed or principal diagnosis is required to be a code from the V30 category then the V29 observation code is sequenced after the V30. A footnote (1) in the Tabular section is an alert to this coding guideline.

Wrong Surgery Edit (MCE Inpatient Only)

When a particular surgical or other invasive procedure is indicated to treat a medical condition and the wrong procedure is performed, the procedure is not considered reasonable and necessary. Assign E codes to report these wrong surgery incidents. A Wrong Surgery edit associated with the E code will be triggered and the claim will be denied and returned to the provider. The wrong surgery E codes are identified with an asterisk (*) and a footnote.

Alphabetic Indexes

▽ **Subterms under main terms may continue to next column/page.**

This warning statement is a reminder to always check for additional subterms and information that may continue on to the next page or column before making a final selection.

ICD-10-CM Coding and Documentation Proficiency Self-Assessment

Introduction

This self-assessment covers ICD-10-CM coding guidance and the required level of detail for clinical documentation of heart disease, diabetes, and pneumonia. These high-volume diagnoses have numerous coding guidelines and documentation requirements. The assessment also covers ICD-10-CM conventions that are new or problematic. Use this self-assessment to identify the areas that may require additional coding training or documentation improvement.

Instructions

Code assignments are based upon the 2015 ICD-10-CM diagnosis code set for all reportable diagnoses, including external causes of morbidity (V00–Y99), as appropriate, according to the instructions in ICD-10-CM conventions and the 2015 *ICD-10-CM Draft Official Guidelines for Coding and Reporting*. Answer each question based on the information provided. Note that for some questions, the codes in the answer are not based upon the information provided, requiring that the provider be queried for specific information because the documentation is insufficient to assign codes correctly.

The answers to the questions can be found immediately following the assessment on page xviii.

Self-Assessment Questions

1. **There are two classifications of pneumonia by anatomical site rather than cause. What are the anatomical classifications and which site of the lung does each affect?**

   _____ pneumonia affecting _____ (sites) of lung
   _____ pneumonia affecting _____ (sites) of lung

2. **The attending physician's final diagnosis on the progress note on the day of discharge: atypical pneumonia. Sputum results: normal flora. Chest x-ray: bilateral lower lobe consolidation.**

   A   Assign J18.9 Pneumonia, unspecified organism.

   B   Documentation does not follow guidelines and/or the physician must be queried to determine the following:
   - Clinical significance of the sputum results
   - Clinical significance of the chest x-ray

3. **What is the appropriate diagnosis code assignment(s) for ESRD due to type I diabetes on chronic dialysis via right arm AV shunt and hypertension as documented by the provider?**

   Code assignment:_____

4. **Attending admission note: Patient is a 42-year-old female who presents with diabetes with hypoglycemia.**

   A   Assign E11.649 Type II diabetes mellitus with hypoglycemia without coma.

   B   Documentation does not follow guidelines and/or the physician must be queried to determine the following:
   - Type of diabetes mellitus
   - Cause of the hypoglycemia

5. **Assign the appropriate code(s) for a diagnosis by the provider of ischemic heart disease and coronary artery disease without history of coronary bypass and current smoker.**

   Code assignment:_____

6. **Assign the appropriate code(s) for a patient diagnosed by the provider with community-acquired pneumonia who presented with hemoptysis, productive cough, fever, and an increased respiratory rate with sputum culture stain showing gram-negative bacilli.**

   Code assignment:_____

7. **Discharge summary: 1. VAP, with sputum stain identifying *Klebsiella pneumoniae*, sensitivity performed and Keflex administered. 2. Vent-dependent patient.**

   A   Assign J95.851 Ventilator associated pneumonia, B96.1 Klebsiella pneumoniae [K. pneumoniae] as the cause of diseases classified elsewhere, and Z99.11 Dependence on respirator [ventilator] status.

   B   Documentation does not follow guidelines and/or the physician must be queried to determine the following:
   - Clinical significance of the sputum results
   - Pneumonia: present on admission or post admission

8. **Assign the appropriate diagnosis code(s) for diabetes II with Charcôt joint, left hallux with ulcer, with dry gangrene and with chronic osteomyelitis. The patient is admitted for amputation due to osteomyelitis documented in the surgeon's admission note.**

   Code assignment:_____

9. **What is the appropriate code assignment for a diagnosis of ischemic cardiomyopathy and coronary artery disease, as documented by the provider?**

   Code assignment:_____

10. **Discharge summary: Patient was admitted from the ED for work-up of precordial chest pain, elevated troponin; history of CABG, congestive heart failure, hypertension. Final diagnosis: ASCAD with USA, s/p CABG, CHF. Most recent diagnostic left heart catheterization showed clean vein and mammary grafts with 90% atherosclerotic stenosis of the native LAD portion. Plans are for future coronary angioplasty as an outpatient. Continue Lasix, Norvasc, and Nitrolingual.**

    A   Assign I25.110 Atherosclerotic heart disease of native coronary artery with unstable angina, I11.9 Hypertensive heart disease without heart failure, I50.9 Heart failure, unspecified, Z95.1 Presence of aortocoronary bypass graft.

    B   Documentation does not follow guidelines and/or the physician must be queried to determine the following:
    - Description of relationship between the hypertension and congestive heart failure
    - Type of congestive heart failure

11. What is the appropriate diagnosis code assignment for the postobstructive pneumonia, right middle lobe, due to hilar lung cancer right lobe when the treatment is directed only toward the pneumonia as documented in the admission note by the resident?

    Code assignment:_____

12. Discharge summary: RSV pneumonia with acute bronchiolitis in one-month-old, high-risk due to being ex-35-week preemie.

    A   Assign J12.1 Respiratory syncytial virus pneumonia, J21.0 Acute bronchiolitis due to RSV, P07.38 Preterm newborn, gestational age 35 completed weeks.

    B   Documentation does not follow guidelines and/or the physician must be queried to determine the following:

        · Clinical significance of the history of prematurity

        · Identification of the causal organism of the bronchiolitis

13. Assign the appropriate diagnosis code(s) for a subsequent encounter for a patient on prescribed steroids with steroid-induced diabetes mellitus, requiring insulin regimen, determined to be inadequately controlled due to dietary noncompliance as documented by the provider.

    Code assignment:_____

14. What is the appropriate code assignment for a diagnosis of unstable angina in a patient who is a nonsmoker with coronary artery disease due to second-hand smoke, as documented by the provider?

    Code assignment:_____

15. Order for outpatient pre-op labs via telephone by office manager of surgeon's office; registrar sends a fax-back form that confirms the order with physician signature. Both office and lab enter note into medical record of phone order. Reason for the surgery and history are furnished by the patient at registration: angioplasty of AV fistula, right arm due to stenosis, end-stage kidney disease, hypertension, on weekly dialysis.

    A   Assign Z01.812 Encounter for preprocedural laboratory examination, T82.858A Stenosis of vascular prosthetic devices, implants and grafts, initial encounter, I12.0 Hypertensive chronic kidney disease with stage 5 chronic kidney disease or end-stage renal disease, N18.6 End-stage renal disease, and Z99.2 Dependence on renal dialysis.

    B   Documentation does not follow guidelines and/or the physician must be queried to determine the following:

        · Etiology of the end-stage renal failure

        · Hypertension, further qualified

16. What is the appropriate code assignment for the diagnosis of mixed bacterial pneumonia due to *Streptococcus pneumoniae* and *Hemophilus influenzae* identified on sputum culture stain and confirmed by the attending physician in the discharge summary?

    Code assignment:_____

17. Discharge summary: Atypical pneumonia, based on presentation clinical indicators and chest CT showing bronchial wall thickening. Last progress note: Awaiting immunoassay results. Addendum to last progress note by PA: Change antibiotic to Azithromycin. At the time of coding, the immunoassay report is posted to the chart and indicates mycoplasma pneumonia. Upon review of the sensitivity test post discharge, the provider's PA ordered a different antibiotic after consulting the attending by phone.

    A   Assign J18.9 Pneumonia, unspecified organism.

    B   Documentation does not follow guidelines and/or the physician must be queried to determine the following:

        · Clinical significance of the immunoassay results and treatment re-evaluation

        · Provide an addendum if the type of pneumonia can be further specified

18. What is the appropriate diagnosis code assignment for physician documentation of a 15-year-old with diabetes on insulin regimen?

    Code assignment:_____

19. Discharge summary signed by attending: A diagnosis of borderline diabetes is listed and body of summary notes FPG test of 124 mg/dl and indicates a need for follow-up testing in three months with diabetic counseling on next office visit recommended.

    Code assignment:_____

20. What is the appropriate diagnosis code assignment for an admission documented by the resident as due to decompensated congestive heart failure with chronic diastolic heart failure, due to patient not refilling her prescription for Lanoxin because she cannot afford the medication this month?

    Code assignment:_____

21. Order for outpatient echocardiogram. Reason: O90.3, with stamped signature of treating physician. Patient presents to testing facility with order. States order is for monitoring since she is being treated for congestive heart failure and is two months post delivery.

    A   Assign O90.3 Peripartum cardiomyopathy, I50.9 Heart failure.

    B   Documentation does not follow guidelines and/or the physician must be queried to determine the following:

        · Provide signed/dated order

        · Provide a written diagnostic statement

22. Which code is appropriate for the diagnosis of gram-positive pneumonia: J15.8 Pneumonia due to other specified bacteria, or J15.9 Unspecified bacterial pneumonia?

    Code assignment:_____

23. What is the appropriate diagnosis code to reflect physician documentation of an office visit of a 14-year-old female G1P0 for evaluation of diet-controlled gestational diabetes, second trimester at 26 weeks?

    Code assignment:_____

24. **Progress note: Patient with chronic deep ulcer on right heel. Schedule surgery to debride and consult wound care. Monitor glucose levels for patient's diabetes 2.**

   A   Assign E11.621 Type 2 diabetes mellitus with foot ulcer, and L97.419 Non-pressure chronic ulcer of right heel and midfoot with unspecified severity.

   B   Documentation does not follow guidelines and/or the physician must be queried to determine the following:

   • Etiology of the ulcer

   • Stage or severity of the ulcer

25. **What is the appropriate diagnosis code when the PA documents a history of congestive heart failure and combined diastolic and systolic dysfunction under treatment?**

   Code assignment:_____

26. **Office note by provider: Patient presents today for prenatal visit. Patient is 36-year-old G1P2, at 32 weeks, with history of essential hypertension, currently treated and monitored for signs of pre-eclampsia, asymptomatic mitral valve prolapse, history of smoking that ceased prior to pregnancy.**

   A   Assign O09.523 Supervision of elderly multigravida, third trimester, O10.013 Pre-existing essential hypertension complicating pregnancy, third trimester, I34.1 Nonrheumatic mitral (valve) prolapse, Z3A.32 32 weeks gestation of pregnancy.

   B   Documentation does not follow guidelines and/or the physician must be queried to determine the following:

   • Type of hypertension

   • Significance of patient's age affecting the pregnancy

27. **Which of these two coding conventions means the information is insufficient to assign a more specific code; for example, for the diagnosis of bacterial pneumonia?**

   A   NOS

   B   NEC

28. **Discharge summary: CMV pneumonia right lung, s/p right lung transplant in 2010 for end-stage emphysema. History of smoking. Continue outpatient pulmonary rehab.**

   A   Assign T86.812 Lung transplant infection, B25.0 Cytomegaloviral pneumonitis, J43.9 Emphysema, unspecified.

   B   Documentation does not follow guidelines and/or the physician must be queried to determine the following:

   • Whether the CMV infection of the right lung transplant is a complication of the transplant or unrelated to the transplant

   • Whether the emphysema is a current diagnosis or by history only

   • History of smoking: former history of use or dependence

29. **What is the appropriate diagnosis code for an emergency department visit for an 89-year-old patient with bleeding of a left calf ulcer due to diabetes 2 with diabetic peripheral angiopathy, exacerbated by Coumadin use for chronic atrial fibrillation. The bleeding could not be controlled by pressure at nursing home as documented by the ED physician.**

   Code assignment:_____

30. **Physician office visit note by provider: Weekly obstetric visit. 27-year-old G4P2A1, now at 30 weeks with history of miscarriage, current gestational diabetes, being treated with insulin.**

   A   Assign O09.293 Supervision of pregnancy with other poor reproductive or obstetric history, third trimester, O24.414 Gestational diabetes mellitus in pregnancy, insulin controlled, Z3A.30 30 weeks gestation of pregnancy.

   B   Documentation does not follow guidelines and/or the physician must be queried to determine the following:

   • Insulin as a long-term medication

   • Clinical significance of previous miscarriage

31. **What is the appropriate code assignment for a diagnosis of hypertensive heart disease with congestive heart failure, as documented by the emergency department physician?**

   Code assignment:_____

32. **Observation record final diagnosis by nephrologist: Admitted to observation from emergency department due to fluid overload from missing weekly dialysis, acute renal failure, end-stage renal failure, hypertension, history of congestive heart failure on Lasix (compensated). Treated with dialysis.**

   A   Assign E87.70 Fluid overload unspecified, N17.9 Acute kidney failure, I50.9 heart failure, I12.0 Hypertensive chronic kidney disease with stage 5 chronic kidney disease or end-stage renal disease, N18.6 End-stage renal disease, Z91.15 Patient's noncompliance with renal dialysis.

   B   Documentation does not follow guidelines and/or the physician must be queried to determine the following:

   • End-stage renal failure relationship to hypertension

   • Etiology of the fluid overload

33. **Which of these two coding conventions means the information provides detail for which a specific code does not exist. An example of when the convention is used is for the diagnosis *Moraxella catarrhalis* pneumonia.**

   A   NOS

   B   NEC

34. **Admitting note LTCH: 1. Gram-negative pneumonia, resolving: Admit to continue antibiotics three days more to complete regimen ordered during acute inpatient admission, then repeat chest x-ray to evaluate for presence of previously seen consolidation.**

   A   Assign J15.9 Unspecified bacterial pneumonia.

   B   Documentation does not follow guidelines and/or the physician must be queried to determine the following:

   • Whether the diagnosis of pneumonia is current (acute phase) for this encounter or resolved on admission and sequela of illness is under treatment (specify residual)

   • Clinical significance of the repeat chest x-ray (results)

35. **What are the appropriate diagnosis codes for admission to the ASC, as documented by the procedure physician, for pancreatic transplant biopsy to evaluate ongoing rejection. The patient has diabetes type 1 with severe nonproliferative retinopathy and gastroparesis and is on the transplant list awaiting a second pancreas transplant. The patient has a functioning kidney allograft with CKD stage 1, due to diabetic renal disease.**

   Code assignment:_____

36. Wound care note by wound care nurse: 32-year-old male with diabetes 1 (poly)neuropathic ulcer, 2cmx1cm improvement from last week of 2cmx2xm, right lateral 5th toe, Grade 2 subcutaneous tissue involvement, presented with dry, clean dressing, no drainage present, no odor, granular tissue present, no signs of infection, will continue enzymatic debridement. Note: patient is status post kidney/pancreas transplants, which are functioning.

A   Assign E10.621 Type 1 diabetes mellitus with foot ulcer, E10.42 Type 1 diabetes mellitus with diabetic polyneuropathy, L97.512 Non-pressure chronic ulcer of other part of right foot with fat layer exposed, Z94.0 Kidney transplant status, Z94.83 Pancreas transplant status.

B   Documentation does not follow guidelines and/or the physician must be queried to determine the following:

   • Physician must co-sign wound care note

   • Diabetes current diagnosis

37. What is the appropriate diagnosis code for Hospital B for a transfer for therapeutic intervention due to an acute STEMI inferior wall myocardial infarction where the patient suffered an acute subendocardial myocardial infarction prior to discharge, as the physician documented in the discharge summary?

   Code assignment:_____

38. Script written by PCP for outpatient chest x-ray: Productive cough, increased respiratory rate, crackles on inspiration, fever, rule out pneumonia. Script written by PCP for outpatient urinalysis and culture: Fever, tachypnea, history of recurrent urinary tract infections. Radiologist final reading: Pneumonia, COPD. Lab results: Urinalysis was abnormal, culture showed *E. coli*. Sensitivity test results were also performed.

A   Radiology: Assign J18.9 Pneumonia, unspecified organism. Lab: Assign R50.9 Fever, unspecified, R06.82 Tachypnea, not elsewhere classified, Z87.440 Personal history of urinary (tract) infections.

B   Documentation does not follow guidelines and/or the physician must be queried to determine the following:

   • PCP: Etiology for the presenting symptoms identified

   • PCP: Clinical significance of the finding of COPD

39. What is the appropriate diagnosis code for a patient with diabetes 1, inadequately controlled, with an insulin pump who is admitted as an outpatient to evaluate insulin pump function. Insulin pump was found to be functioning. The insulin dosage and titration were changed, as documented by the procedure physician.

   Code assignment:_____

40. What is the appropriate diagnosis code for an encounter the emergency department physician documents as for cardiac arrest due to ventricular fibrillation with cardiogenic shock?

   Code assignment:_____

41. ED record, signed by ED attending: Cardiac arrest, history of coronary artery disease, s/p CABG in 2011, hypertension, history of myocardial infarction in 2011. Patient admitted in cardiac arrest, CPR and defibrillation in the ED, resuscitation was unsuccessful and patient expired. Labs: CK-MB: 12.6, troponin I: 5.0. EKG: ST segment elevation and ventricular fibrillation.

A   Assign I46.9 Cardiac arrest, cause unspecified, I25.10 Atherosclerotic heart disease of native coronary artery without angina pectoris, I10 Essential (primary) hypertension, Z95.1 Presence of aortocoronary bypass graft, I25.2 Old myocardial infarction.

B   Documentation does not follow guidelines and/or the physician must be queried to determine the following:

   • Etiology of cardiac arrest

   • Clinical significance of the lab results and EKG reading

42. What is the appropriate diagnosis code for the second episode in six months of *Pneumocystis jiroveci* pneumonia in a patient who is noted to be HIV positive, as documented by the provider?

   Code assignment:_____

43. Office visit note: Follow-up for recent pneumonia, course of antibiotics completed last week. Patient without complaint. Repeat chest x-ray is negative.

A   Assign Z09 Encounter for follow-up examination after completed treatment for conditions other than malignant neoplasm, Z87.01 Personal history of pneumonia (recurrent).

B   Documentation does not follow guidelines and/or the physician must be queried to determine the following:

   • Type of pneumonia be further specified

   • Pneumonia current or by history only

44. Emergency department record, signed by ED attending: Fractured nose, right black eye of eyelid/ocular area, due to battery assault by boyfriend during domestic abuse incident; apartment residence. Patient is 20-year-old female, G3P2 at 35 weeks with diabetes 1, on insulin, with poor control due to noncompliance and financial difficulties. Admit to labor and delivery observation.

A   Assign O9A.313 Physical abuse complicating pregnancy, third trimester, S02.2XXA Fracture of nasal bones, initial encounter for closed fracture, S00.11XA Contusion of right eyelid and periocular area, initial encounter, O24.013 Pre-existing diabetes mellitus, type 1, in pregnancy, third trimester, E10.65 Type 1 diabetes mellitus with hyperglycemia, T38.3X6A Underdosing of insulin and oral hypoglycemic [antidiabetic] drugs, initial encounter, Z3A.35 35 weeks gestation of pregnancy, Y04.0XXA Assault by unarmed brawl or fight, Y07.03 Male partner, perpetrator of maltreatment and neglect, Z91.14 Patient's other noncompliance with medication regimen, Z91.120 Patient's intentional underdosing of medication regimen due to financial hardship, Z79.4 Long-term (current) use of insulin, Y92.039 Unspecified place in apartment as the place of occurrence of the external cause.

B   Documentation does not follow guidelines and/or the physician must be queried to determine the following:

   • Medical significance of noncompliance

   • Effects of trauma on pregnancy

45. **Progress note by critical care physician: Code blue called after patient arrived on floor after cardiac catheterization with stent placement for coronary artery disease stenosis, history of recent myocardial infarction, no intraop complications noted. Nurse found patient in cardiac arrest; responding team initiated CPR, defibrillation, endotrachial intubation, epinephrine administered. Patient was resuscitated successfully; admit to inpatient status.**

    A   Assign I46.9 Cardiac arrest cause unspecified.

    B   Documentation does not follow guidelines and/or the physician must be queried to determine the following:

    - Cause of cardiac arrest

    - Whether the cardiac arrest was a complication of the procedure

46. **What is the correct code if the resident documents the diagnosis of pneumonia due to mechanical ventilation and the lab record shows vent cultures growing yeast?**

    Code assignment:_____

47. **What is the appropriate diagnosis code when a surgeon documents that a newborn infant was delivered by cesarean on this encounter with macrosomia and the newborn has a diagnosis of syndrome of infant of a diabetic mother?**

    Code assignment:_____

48. **Visit to endocrinologist: Progress note, signed by provider: diabetes 2; 4 months postpartum who had developed gestational diabetes, now with peripartum diabetes 2, under treatment with metaformin.**

    A   Assign E11.9 Type 2 diabetes mellitus without complications, Z86.32 Personal history of gestational diabetes, and O94 Sequela of complication of pregnancy, childbirth, and the puerperium.

    B   Documentation does not follow guidelines and/or the physician must be queried to determine the following:

    - Risk factors for diabetes

    - Diabetic complications

49. **What is the appropriate diagnosis code assignment as documented by the emergency department physician for an encounter with a woman who had acute chest pain on inspiration while surveying the damage in the yard of her former home, with acute emotional stress reaction due to surviving a tornado and losing her home to it today?**

    Code assignment:_____

50. **Admit note by resident: PMH: h/o cardiac arrest due to acute myocardial infarction in 2010, treated by thrombolysis. Admit note: Found to have coronary artery disease, treated medically until now. Admitted today for CABG due to progressive angina. What past history would be appropriate to assign?**

    A   Assign Z86.74 Personal history of sudden cardiac arrest, and I25.2 Old myocardial infarction.

    B   Documentation does not follow guidelines and/or the physician must be queried to determine the following:

    - Type of angina

    - Significance of history of myocardial infarction treatment

Coding and Documentation Review Answers

1. *Answer:* **Lobar pneumonia affects an area of a lobe of the lung; Bronch(o)(ial) pneumonia affects the walls of the bronchioles.**

   Rationale: Under the ICD-10-CM Alphabetic Index entry for pneumonia, the subterms that indicate anatomical areas, such as alveolar, apex, confluent, diffuse, etc., index to *"see"* references. The two *"see"* references are *"see* Pneumonia, lobar" or *"see* Pneumonia, broncho." These two terms are anatomical classifications of pneumonia that indicate the sites in the lung where clinical indicators of consolidation can be seen on radiologic displays. Since these types of pneumonia are identified by radiological findings rather than causal organism, they are classified as pneumonia caused by unspecified organism. Lobar affects an area of the lung lobe. Bronch(o)(ial)pneumonia or lobular pneumonia affects the walls of the bronchioles with multiple foci of isolated consolidation in one or more basal lobes of the lung.

2. *Answer:* **A Assign J18.9 Pneumonia, unspecified organism.**

   Rationale: The type of pneumonia is identified only as "atypical," and no specific organism is attributable; the Alphabetic Index entry for "Pneumonia, atypical" lists J18.9 Pneumonia, unspecified organism. Normal flora identified in a culture indicates a mixture of bacteria normally found at specific body sites and does not represent pathogens and is not clinically significant. The chest x-ray shows bilateral lower lobe consolidation, which can also be seen in congestive heart failure and empyema, among other causes. OCG.I.C.18.b states that signs or symptoms routinely associated with a disease process should not be identified with additional codes unless the physician instructs otherwise.

3. *Answer:* **E10.22 Type 1 diabetes mellitus with diabetic chronic kidney disease, I12.0 Hypertensive chronic kidney disease with stage 5 chronic kidney disease or end-stage renal disease, N18.6 End-stage renal disease, Z99.2 Dependence on renal dialysis**

   Rationale: The type of diabetes is stated as type I, and the chronic kidney disease is due to the diabetes; therefore, assign a code from category E10. ICD-10-CM assumes a cause-and-effect relationship when both hypertension and chronic kidney disease are present (*Official Coding Guidelines* [OCG], section I.C.9.a.2); consequently a code from category I12 is assigned. The tabular "code also" note indicates that the coder should assign an additional code to identify the stage of chronic kidney disease, in this case, end-stage renal disease, N18.6. An instructional note under code N18.6 instructs the coder to use an additional code to identify dialysis status, which is Z99.2 Dependence on renal dialysis.

4. *Answer:* **A E11.649 Type II diabetes mellitus with hypoglycemia without coma**

   Rationale: ICD-10-CM OCG section I.C.4.a.2 states that E11- Type 2 diabetes mellitus, is assigned as the default when the type is not specified. Guideline section I.A.15 indicates that the word "with" means "due to" in the Alphabetic Index; therefore, the documentation links the diabetes and hypoglycemia. Diabetes mellitus codes are combination codes, and the Alphabetic Index entry for diabetes with hypoglycemia, Type 2, refers to E11.649 Type II diabetes mellitus with hypoglycemia without coma.

5. *Answer:* **I25.10 Atherosclerotic heart disease of native coronary artery without angina pectoris, Z72.0 Tobacco use**

   Rationale: The ICD-10-CM Alphabetic Index main term "Disease, coronary (artery)" directs the coder to *"see"* Disease, heart, ischemic, atherosclerotic. Under "Disease/heart/ischemic/atherosclerotic," the code default is I25.10. Both stated conditions are classified to the single code I25.10 Atherosclerotic heart disease of native coronary artery without angina pectoris. When there is no history or documentation of a previous coronary artery bypass graft (CABG) or heart transplant, a code for atherosclerosis of native artery should be assigned. The Alphabetic Index lists code Z72.0 under "Tobacco, use."

6. *Answer:* **J18.9 Pneumonia, unspecified organism, R04.2 Hemoptysis**

   Rationale: The ICD-10-CM Alphabetic Index does not list the nonessential modifier "hemorrhagic" after the term "pneumonia." Therefore, unless documentation links this symptom to the pneumonia, the hemoptysis would be assigned as an additional code. The provider/documentation does not confirm that the sputum culture stain showing gram-negative bacilli is clinically significant. See OCG 1.C.18.b, "Use of a symptom code with a definitive diagnosis," and OCG III, "Reporting Additional Findings, B. Abnormal findings."

7. *Answer:* **A Assign J95.851 Ventilator associated pneumonia, B96.1 Klebsiella pneumoniae [K. pneumoniae] as the cause of diseases classified elsewhere, Z99.11 Dependence on respirator [ventilator] status.**

   Rationale: The ICD-10-CM OCG section I.C.10.d.1 states that the assignment of a complication code is based on the provider's documentation of the relationship between the pneumonia and the mechanical ventilation. In this case, the documentation describes the pneumonia as due to the ventilator. An additional code is assigned if an identified organism is attributed to the VAP, but not a pneumonia code from J12–J18.

8. *Answer:* **E11.610 Type 2 diabetes mellitus with diabetic neuropathic arthropathy, E11.621 Type 2 diabetes mellitus with foot ulcer, E11.52 Type 2 diabetes mellitus with diabetic peripheral angiopathy with gangrene, L97.524 Non-pressure chronic ulcer of other part of left foot with necrosis of bone**

   Rationale: ICD-10-CM OCG section I.A.15 states that the use of the term "with" is to be interpreted to mean "associated with" or "due to" when it appears in a code title, the Alphabetic Index, or an instructional note in the Tabular List. Therefore, the listed conditions are coded as diabetic complications. Guideline section I.C.4.a states that as many codes within a particular category should be assigned as describe all the complications, with sequencing based on the reason for a particular encounter. E11.610 Type 2 diabetes mellitus with diabetic neuropathic arthropathy is sequenced first since this describes the osteomyelitis.

9. *Answer:* **I25.5 Ischemic cardiomyopathy and I25.10 Atherosclerotic heart disease of native coronary artery without angina pectoris**

   Rationale: Ischemic cardiomyopathy is an extrinsic cardiomyopathy due to reduced blood flow to the heart muscle. The ICD-10-CM Alphabetic Index lists I25.5 Ischemic cardiomyopathy under the term "Cardiomyopathy, ischemic to." The "excludes2" note under I25.5 indicates that coronary atherosclerosis (I25.1-, I25.7-) is not included; therefore, these two conditions can be coded together when documented.

10. *Answer:* **B Documentation does not follow guidelines and/or the physician must be queried to determine the following: description of relationship between the hypertension and congestive heart failure, and specify type of the congestive heart failure.**

    Rationale: The relationship between hypertension and congestive heart failure is not assumed in ICD-10-CM and must be documented. Second, if the type of heart failure can be further specified as diastolic, systolic, or both, a more accurate code can be assigned from category I50 Heart failure. Heart disease without a stated causal relationship to hypertension is coded separately.

11. **Answer:** J18.9 Pneumonia, unspecified organism, and C34.01 Malignant neoplasm of right main bronchus or lung

Rationale: There is no specific entry in the Alphabetic Index for postobstructive pneumonia; therefore, only the term "Pneumonia" is listed. When a specified type of pneumonia is not documented, J18.9 Pneumonia, unspecified organism, is the default code and should be assigned. The malignancy is sequenced as an additional code according to OCG section C.2.l.4.

12. **Answer:** <u>A</u> Assign J12.1 Respiratory syncytial virus pneumonia, J21.0 Acute bronchiolitis due to RSV, P07.38 Preterm newborn, gestational age 35 completed weeks.

Rationale: The ICD-10-CM Alphabetic Index entry for "Pneumonia, respiratory syncytial virus" lists J12.1. Respiratory syncytial virus is a common community-acquired infection in children. OCG section I.C.16.a.5 states that if a newborn condition is community-acquired, a code from chapter 16, "Certain Conditions Originating in the Perinatal Period," is not assigned. RSV bronchiolitis is also documented and is also assigned. Both are acute conditions, and when the patient is admitted for both and both are equal in work-up, focus, and treatment, either can be sequenced as the principal diagnosis, following OCG section II.B. The additional information that the patient is a former preemie is coded as its clinical significance is documented and OCG section I.C.16.e states that prematurity is coded when it affects the patient's current health status.

13. **Answer:** E09.65 Drug or chemical induced diabetes mellitus with hyperglycemia, T38.0X5D Adverse effect of glucocorticoids and synthetic analogues subsequent encounter, Z79.4 Long term (current) use of insulin, Z91.11 Patient's noncompliance with dietary regimen

Rationale: Since the steroid use is prescribed and there is no indication of incorrect usage, this is considered an adverse effect and not a poisoning. The diabetes is drug-induced, and according to OCG section I.C.4.a.6.b, sequencing is to "code first" E09 Drug or chemical induced diabetes mellitus, followed by an additional code for the adverse effect to identify the drug T36–T50 with a fifth/sixth character of 5. ICD-10-CM does not use the terms "uncontrolled," "inadequately controlled," or "out of control, poorly controlled." The index instructs the user to "code Diabetes, by type, with hyperglycemia." Therefore, the first-listed code is E09.65 Drug or chemical induced diabetes mellitus with hyperglycemia. This is followed by T38.0X5- Adverse effect of glucocorticoids and synthetic analogues, which is located in the Table of Drugs and Chemicals under the main term "Steroid" with the appropriate additional character requirement, which in this case is a character for a subsequent encounter (D). The patient is maintained on insulin, Z79.4, which OCG section I.C.4.a.6.a, indicates is coded when documented. The diabetes is inadequately controlled due to dietary noncompliance, Z91.11, which is located in the Alphabetic Index under "Noncompliance, with, dietary regimen."

14. **Answer:** I25.110 Atherosclerotic heart disease of native coronary artery with unstable angina pectoris, Z77.22 Contact with and (suspected) exposure to environmental tobacco smoke (acute) (chronic)

Rationale: OCG section I.C.9.b states that ICD-10-CM provides combination codes that link coronary artery disease with angina since the relationship between them is to be assumed unless otherwise documented. No separate code is assigned from category I20 Angina pectoris. Code Z77.22 Contact with and (suspected) exposure to environmental tobacco smoke (acute) (chronic) is assigned as a secondary code when the provider documents that the second-hand smoke is the external cause of the patient's condition. Locate the code in the Alphabetic Index under the term "Exposure, second hand tobacco smoke (acute) (chronic)." When there is no history or documentation of a previous coronary artery bypass graft (CABG) or heart transplant, a code for atherosclerosis of native artery is assigned.

15. **Answer:** <u>A</u> Assign Z01.812 Encounter for preprocedural laboratory examination, T82.858A Stenosis of vascular prosthetic devices, implants and grafts, initial encounter, I12.0 Hypertensive chronic kidney disease with stage 5 chronic kidney disease or end-stage renal disease, N18.6 End-stage renal disease, and Z99.2 Dependence on renal dialysis.

Rationale: A telephone call from the treating physician's office to the testing facility to order a diagnostic outpatient service is acceptable if, as required by the Centers for Medicare and Medicaid Services, payer, state, conditions of participation bylaws, Joint Commission and Office of Inspector General requirements, both the treating physician/office and the testing facility document the phone call in their copies of the patient's medical record. This information may be obtained from the patient or the medical record, but the coder should attempt to confirm this information with the physician, and it is recommended to have a "fax-back" policy in place for the registration sites. In the example, the reason for the order is to have pre-op lab testing performed; "Examination, pre-procedural (pre-operative), laboratory" in the Alphabetic Index lists Z01.812 Encounter for preprocedural laboratory examination. OCG section I.C.21.c.16 indicates that category Z01 is a "first-listed" diagnosis and therefore should be sequenced first followed by the reason for the surgery/procedure.

16. **Answer:** J13 Pneumonia due to Streptococcus pneumoniae, and J14 Pneumonia due to Haemophilus influenzae

Rationale: Since the attending physician confirmed both identified infective organisms, both individual codes are assigned. If the organisms were not identified, then only pneumonia, bacterial (unspecified organism) would be assigned, not the "bacterial, specified" code, since the terms "mixed bacterial" do not identify specified organisms not elsewhere classified.

17. **Answer:** <u>B</u> Documentation does not follow guidelines and/or the physician must be queried to determine the following: the clinical significance of the immunoassay results and treatment re-evaluation and provide an addendum if the type of pneumonia can be further specified.

Rationale: After the documentation is reviewed, a query is warranted to further specify the type of pneumonia. The physician assistant documented a change in treatment based upon the results of the immunoassay test. Although the test results are posted to the chart, the coder should ask about their clinical significance and the reason behind the change in medication. Additionally, the findings on chest x-ray further support a more specific pneumonia as due to the identified organism. Coders are responsible for querying when the clinical documentation as a whole suggests a higher level of specificity.

18. **Answer:** E11.9 Type 2 diabetes mellitus without complications, and Z79.4 Long-term (current) use of insulin

Rationale: According to OCG section I.C.4.a.2.3, the type of diabetes mellitus cannot be determined by patient age or the use of insulin. The guideline further states that when the type of diabetes is not documented, the default is diabetes mellitus type 2 and that insulin documented as a maintenance drug is assigned as an additional code.

19. **Answer:** Assign R73.09 Other abnormal glucose.

Rationale: Without further documentation of a diagnosis of diabetes, the attending's attestation to the discharge summary confirming the lab findings and the indication of clinical significance, only a code from subcategory "abnormal glucose" can be assigned. This can be found in the Alphabetic Index under the main term "Findings, abnormal, inconclusive, without findings, glucose" or by the documentation of borderline diabetes mellitus or diabetes, latent. Code R73.09 Other abnormal glucose, lists "prediabetes" and "latent diabetes" as inclusion terms.

20. *Answer:* I50.33 Acute on chronic diastolic (congestive) heart failure, T46.0X6A Underdosing of cardiac-stimulant glycosides and drugs of similar action initial encounter, and Z91.120 Patient's intentional underdosing of medication regimen due to financial hardship

Rationale: The code for "chronic on acute (i.e., acute on chronic)" is assigned because the acute exacerbation of a chronic condition is coded as acute on chronic, and when a combination code is available, only a single code is assigned. The exacerbation of the congestive heart failure was due to the lack of Lanoxin and is sequenced before the code for the underdosing, according to OCG section I.C.19.e.5.c. The seventh-character assignment of A, indicating the initial encounter, is required to complete code T46.0X6. An additional code to represent noncompliance and the reason and intent is assigned: Z91.120 Patient's intentional underdosing of medication regimen due to financial hardship. The ICD-10-CM Alphabetic Index and Tabular List now provide the nonessential modifier "congestive" in the descriptor of the diastolic and systolic types of heart failure. Therefore an additional code for "congestive heart failure" is not assigned.

21. *Answer:* **B** Documentation does not follow guidelines and/or the physician must be queried to determine the following: provide signed/dated order and provide a written diagnostic statement.

Rationale: A valid order must follow CMS, payer, state, conditions of participation, bylaws and Joint Commission and OIG requirements. Signatures are required for certain diagnostic tests, and CMS Transmittal 327 states that stamped signatures are not acceptable. The introduction to the OCG states that ICD-10-CM is a morbidity classification for classifying diagnoses and reason for health care visits. Codes are not diagnoses—they may not be used as a substitute for a written diagnostic statement within the medical record.

22. *Answer:* J15.9 Unspecified bacterial pneumonia

Rationale: Since the term "gram-positive" is nonspecific and does not identify a specific organism, assign J15.9 Unspecified bacterial pneumonia. When a specific bacterial organism is identified but has no specific entry in the Alphabetic Index or a corresponding ICD-10-CM diagnosis code, the default is J15.8 Pneumonia due to other specified bacteria. The same applies to viral pneumonia coding.

23. *Answer:* O09.612 Supervision of young primigravida, second trimester, O24.410 Gestational diabetes mellitus in pregnancy, diet controlled, Z3A.26, 26 weeks gestation of pregnancy

Rationale: OCG section I.C.15.i covers gestational diabetes. Since the patient is 14 years old and this is her first pregnancy (identified by "G1P0"), the coder would look in the index under "Pregnancy, supervision of, young mother, primigravida." The sixth character "2" specifies second trimester as defined by the note at the introduction to chapter 15. The Alphabetic Index lists the main term "Diabetes" with the subterm "gestational, diet controlled," which references code O24.410. Follow the instructional note for chapter 15 and use an additional code from category Z3A to describe the number of weeks of gestation.

24. *Answer:* **B** Documentation does not follow guidelines and/or the physician must be queried to determine the following: etiology of the ulcer and stage or severity of the ulcer.

Rationale: If the ulcer is of diabetic origin, the link to diabetes must be stated before the ulcer can be coded. The term "deep" does not indicate the tissues involved, and the tissues need to be documented to further classify the stage or level of necrosis for code severity specificity.

25. *Answer:* I50.42 Chronic combined systolic (congestive) and diastolic (congestive) heart failure

Rationale: The ICD-10-CM Alphabetic Index does not have entries for diastolic or systolic under the main term "Dysfunction." Diastolic dysfunction is the decline in performance of one or both ventricles of the heart during the time phase of diastole; left/systemic/body and right/pulmonary/lungs. Dysfunction has a subterm "ventricular/with congestive heart failure," which references I50.9 Heart failure unspecified. However, when there is diastolic or systolic dysfunction in the presence of heart failure, the relationship is assumed. In this example, the heart failure is specified as combined diastolic and systolic. Code I50.42 is the appropriate code. If diastolic or systolic dysfunction is documented without documentation of heart failure, assign I51.9 Heart disease, unspecified. In this case, however, because of the known history of heart failure, the case is coded as chronic.

26. *Answer:* **A** Assign O09.523 Supervision of elderly multigravida, third trimester, O10.013 Pre-existing essential hypertension complicating pregnancy third trimester, I34.1 Nonrheumatic mitral (valve) prolapse, Z3A.32 32 weeks gestation of pregnancy.

Rationale: For this scenario, OCG section I.C.15.b.2 states that the principal diagnosis should be a code from category O09 for supervision of a high-risk (elderly) pregnancy. The patient is 36 years old and has delivered once (G1P2). Assign code O09.523 as the first-listed diagnosis. The sixth character indicates the third trimester, as defined by the note in the introduction to chapter 15. Code Z3A.32 32 weeks gestation of pregnancy, is assigned according to the instructional note for chapter 15. Code O10.013 Pre-existing essential hypertension complicating pregnancy, third trimester, would be assigned as a secondary diagnosis code. Mitral valve prolapse, although asymptomatic, is coded because it is medically significant during pregnancy.

27. *Answer:* **A** NOS

Rationale: The coding convention NOS, or not otherwise specified, is the equivalent of "unspecified" and is assigned when the documentation does not provide more specific information about the condition. In the example, the term bacterial pneumonia means that the specified bacterial organism causing the pneumonia is unknown, or cannot be determined. What is known is that the causal organism is bacterial as opposed to viral. The Alphabetic Index lists the terms "Pneumonia, bacterial"; therefore, the default is J15.9 Unspecified bacterial pneumonia.

28. *Answer:* **A** Assign T86.812 Lung transplant infection, B25.0 Cytomegaloviral pneumonitis, J43.9 Emphysema, unspecified.

Rationale: According to OCG section I.C.19.g.3.a, the code for transplant complications is assigned only if the complication affects the function of the transplanted organ. The complication requires two codes, one from category T86 to identify the type of complication and a second to identify the manifestation. Cytomegaloviral pneumonitis, or CMV, is an opportunistic pneumonia. Since the pneumonitis is in the allograft, it is coded as a lung transplant complication, specifically as an infection. The transplant was performed only on the right, so the emphysema is not "cured" and is still present. Therefore, the emphysema is assigned as an additional diagnosis. Only history of tobacco dependence, not history of smoking or tobacco use, has an index entry. Therefore, the history of smoking is not coded.

29. *Answer:* E11.622 Type 2 diabetes mellitus with other skin ulcer, T45.515A Adverse effect of anticoagulants, E11.51 Type 2 diabetes mellitus with diabetic peripheral angiopathy without gangrene, L97.229 Non-pressure chronic ulcer of left calf with unspecified severity, I48.2 Chronic atrial fibrillation

Rationale: As the bleeding from the ulcer is an adverse effect of the prescribed Coumadin, follow the guidelines in OCG section I.C.19.e.5.a and sequence the nature of the adverse effect first, which in this case is also a diabetic complication, E11.622 Type 2 diabetes mellitus with other skin ulcer. This is followed by the code identifying the drug and adverse effect, T45.515A Adverse effect of anticoagulants, found in the Table of Drugs and Chemicals. Code also all other diabetic complications, E11.51 Type 2 diabetes mellitus with diabetic peripheral angiopathy without gangrene. Also list code L97.229 Non-pressure chronic ulcer of left calf with unspecified severity to identify the site and severity of the ulcer per the "use additional code" instruction note under E11.622. Code I48.2 Chronic atrial fibrillation, indicates the condition for which the Coumadin is taken.

30. *Answer:* **A** Assign O09.293 Supervision of pregnancy with other poor reproductive or obstetric history, third trimester, O24.414 Gestational diabetes mellitus in pregnancy, insulin controlled, Z3A.30, 30 weeks gestation of pregnancy.

Rationale: The provider's documentation indicates this is a routine prenatal visit for a high-risk pregnancy due to a history of miscarriage with current gestational diabetes. OCG section I.C.15.b.2 states that a code from category O09 Supervision of high-risk pregnancy, should be assigned as the first-listed diagnosis, followed by any other applicable chapter 15 codes to describe comorbid conditions affecting the pregnancy. The code for gestational diabetes does not indicate trimester, but the fourth character does represent "in pregnancy." From the instructional note "use additional code from category Z3A" for chapter 15, code Z3A.30 30 weeks gestation of pregnancy, is assigned. OCG section I.C.15.i notes that additional code Z79.4 Long-term (current) use of insulin, should not be assigned with codes from subcategory O24.4.

31. *Answer:* **I11.0 Hypertensive heart disease with heart failure, I50.9 Heart failure, unspecified**

Rationale: According to OCG section I.C.9.1, when a causal relationship between hypertension and heart failure (I50.-) or heart disease (I51.4.-I51.9) is stated (due to) or implied (hypertensive), assign a code from category I11 Hypertensive heart disease. Also the OCG section I.A.15 states that in the Alphabetic Index, the subentry term "with" means "associated with" or "due to." Therefore, a diagnostic statement of "with" provides the link between two conditions. The tabular note instructs the coder to "use additional code to identify type of heart failure I50.-." In the example, the type is not documented; therefore an additional code for heart failure, unspecified is assigned.

32. *Answer:* **A** Assign E87.70 Fluid overload unspecified, N17.9 Acute kidney failure, I50.9 Heart failure, I12.0 Hypertensive chronic kidney disease with stage 5 chronic kidney disease or end-stage renal disease, N18.6 End-stage renal disease, Z91.15 Patient's noncompliance with renal dialysis.

Rationale: The acute conditions necessitating admission were the fluid overload and the acute renal failure. Since the dialysis is treatment for both conditions, according to OCG section II.C either may be sequenced as the principal diagnosis unless one is considered the more significant problem. As long as the admission is clearly documented as to treat the fluid overload and as not related to the history of congestive heart failure, the fluid overload can be coded separately. The congestive heart failure is noted to be "compensated," meaning it is not in acute exacerbation; note that unspecified heart failure I50.9 makes no distinction between acute or decompensated and compensated. If the record indicates that the type of heart failure can be specified further, the coder should query the physician for the type as well as a possible relationship between the heart failure and hypertension. Acute renal failure can be coded in the presence of end-stage kidney disease as there are no excludes or includes notes or instructional notes that indicate otherwise. The cause of the fluid overload was the noncompliance with dialysis, which is in the Alphabetic Index as "Noncompliance, with, dialysis," Z91.15. The dialysis status code is not assigned when the noncompliance is coded, Z91.15, as indicated by the "excludes1" note under Z99.2 Dependence on renal dialysis.

33. *Answer:* **B** NEC

Rationale: The coding convention NEC, or not elsewhere classified, is the equivalent of "specified (other, other specified)" and applies when the

documentation specifies a condition but there is no individual code for that condition. In the example, the type of bacteria causing the pneumonia is identified (specified), but the ICD-10-CM Alphabetic Index does not list an individual code for that particular organism. Therefore, the user would look in the index under "Pneumonia, specified, bacterium NEC," leading to J15.8 Pneumonia due to other specified bacteria.

34. *Answer:* **B** Documentation does not follow guidelines and/or the physician must be queried to determine the following: diagnosis of pneumonia current (acute phase) for this encounter or resolved on admission and sequela of illness is under treatment (specify residual); and clinical significance of the repeat chest x-ray (results).

Rationale: Long-term care hospitals may assign codes for acute unresolved conditions, sequelae, or rehab. The selection of principal diagnosis follows the guidelines in OCG section II. When the patient is admitted for continuation of treatment of an acute condition, OCG section I.B.10 may apply if the acute phase has resolved and it is the sequela that is being treated. This provider must document that the residual condition is being treated and is the reason for admission. If the patient no longer has the clinical indicators of the acute disease, the coder should query the physician for clarification as to whether the acute condition is present or if a sequela is receiving the continuation of care and treatment. As long as an acute condition is the target of treatment, it is coded. For this example, the facility must decide how to address the issue of acute condition versus sequela for "resolving" conditions that may or may not have clinical indicators.

35. *Answer:* **T86.890 Other transplanted tissue rejection, E10.349 Type 1 diabetes mellitus with severe nonproliferative diabetic retinopathy without macular edema, E10.43 Type 1 diabetes mellitus with diabetic autonomic (poly)neuropathy (gastroparesis), E10.22 Type 1 diabetes mellitus with diabetic chronic kidney disease, N18.1 Chronic kidney disease, stage 1, Z94.0 Kidney transplant status, and Z76.82 Awaiting organ transplant status**

Rationale: Rejection affects the transplanted pancreas and is a complication of the pancreas transplant. As the reason for the encounter, the transplant rejection is sequenced first. The patient has ongoing complications of retinopathy and gastroparesis due to diabetes 1, which must also be coded. The patient is also status post kidney transplant due to diabetic renal disease, and the transplanted kidney is functioning with mild CKD stage 1, which is not documented as a complication but is residual renal disease. OCG section I.C.14.a.2 indicates that the CKD stage with kidney transplant status should be assigned. Also indicate that the patient is awaiting transplant by looking in the index under "Transplant, awaiting organ," code Z76.82.

36. *Answer:* **A** Assign E10.621 Type 1 diabetes mellitus with foot ulcer, E10.42 Type 1 diabetes mellitus with diabetic polyneuropathy, L97.512 Non-pressure chronic ulcer of other part of right foot with fat layer exposed, Z94.0 Kidney transplant status, Z94.83 Pancreas transplant status.

Rationale: The term provider is used throughout the *Official Coding Guidelines* to indicate a physician or any qualified health care practitioner who is legally accountable for establishing the patient's diagnosis. State laws define the scope of practice and, for health care entities, regulatory laws establish who may provide documentation; wound care nursing documentation is recognized as valid. Although the patient has a functioning pancreas transplant, diabetes is coded since there are related complications. The diabetes 1 is linked to the ulcer by its description as diabetes 1 neuropathic ulcer. Because the Wagner non-pressure foot ulcer classification grade 2 is penetration through the subcutaneous tissue, the severity chosen is "with fat layer exposed." The ulcer is sequenced first before the neuropathy because it is the reason for the encounter.

37. *Answer:* I21.19 ST elevation (STEMI) myocardial infarction involving other coronary artery of inferior wall, and I22.2 Subsequent non-ST elevation (NSTEMI) myocardial infarction

Rationale: OCG section I.C.9.e.1 states that a code for the site is assigned for an acute STEMI myocardial infarction for encounters occurring when the MI is equal to or less than four weeks old, including transfers during this timeframe. New for ICD-10-CM, OCG section I.C.9.e.4 states that after an initial myocardial infarction, a subsequent or new acute myocardial infarction during the same four-week timeframe is coded to category I22 Subsequent ST elevation (STEMI) and non-ST elevation (NSTEMI) myocardial infarction. When there are both an initial and subsequent acute myocardial infarction, codes from both I21 and I22 are assigned, sequenced based on the circumstances of the encounter.

38. *Answer:* **A** Radiology: Assign J18.9 Pneumonia, unspecified organism. Lab: Assign R50.9 Fever, unspecified, R06.82 Tachypnea, not elsewhere classified, Z87.440 Personal history of urinary (tract) infections.

Rationale: In the outpatient setting, uncertain diagnoses cannot be assigned (OCG section IV.H). The referring provider should document signs, symptoms, and abnormal findings that prompt the outpatient encounter. If a physician has interpreted a diagnostic test and the results are available, the confirmed or definitive diagnosis is coded; the related or integral signs and symptoms are not coded, according to OCG section IV.K.. The second script lists signs and symptoms and history, but the test results are by lab only. Therefore, the signs and symptoms and history codes are assigned. When possible, the coder should ask the PCP to clarify the lab results. Until the PCP confirms the test results for the scripts, only the codes for the symptoms for which the tests were ordered are assigned.

39. *Answer:* E10.65 Type 1 diabetes mellitus with hyperglycemia and Z46.81 Encounter for fitting and adjustment of insulin pump

Rationale: The ICD-10-CM Alphabetic Index lists the terms inadequately controlled, out of control, and poorly controlled to represent diabetes mellitus uncontrolled, with the instruction to assign diabetes, by type, with hyperglycemia. Therefore, assign E10.65 Type 1 diabetes mellitus with hyperglycemia as the first diagnosis as the diabetes was symptomatic and the reason for the encounter, not just an evaluation of the insulin pump or for titration adjustment. Add Z46.81 Encounter for fitting and adjustment of insulin pump, since titration adjustment was performed. The status code Z96.41 Presence of insulin pump (external) (internal) is not assigned since the reason for encounter code indicates the type of status according to OCG section I.C.21.c.3.

40. *Answer:* I49.01 Ventricular fibrillation, I46.2 Cardiac arrest due to underlying cardiac condition, and R57.0 Cardiogenic shock

Rationale: The ICD-10-CM Alphabetic Index now provides separate codes for cardiac arrest due to underlying cardiac condition, due to (other) specified underlying condition (trauma, overdose, etc.) or unspecified cause. Codes for both the cardiac arrest and the underlying condition should be assigned, when the condition is known. In the example for the ED encounter, the ventricular fibrillation is known and should be sequenced first, followed by the code for the cardiac arrest as instructed by the tabular "code first" note under category I46 Cardiac arrest. If further work-up determines the cause of the ventricular fibrillation, such as cardiac ischemia or coronary artery disease, cardiomyopathy, acute myocardial infarction, trauma, overdose, etc., that condition is the principal diagnosis and the appropriate code from category I46 Cardiac arrest, is secondary, along with I49.01 Ventricular fibrillation. Since the cardiogenic shock is not integral to the ventricular fibrillation or the cardiac arrest, the code for shock is assigned even though it is not a chapter 18 code (OCG section I.C.18.b). Review and apply the guidelines in the OCG section II introduction for the UHDDS definition of principal diagnosis for inpatient, and in OCG section IV.G, IV.k and IV.I for the reason of the outpatient encounter. Keep in mind that, according to OCG section IV.A, the coding conventions and the general

and disease-specific guidelines take precedence over the outpatient guidelines.

41. *Answer:* **A** Assign I46.9 Cardiac arrest, cause unspecified, I25.10 Atherosclerotic heart disease of native coronary artery without angina pectoris, I10 Essential (primary) hypertension, Z95.1 Presence of aortocoronary bypass graft, I25.2 Old myocardial infarction.

Rationale: When an emergency department patient dies before the cause of a cardiac arrest is known, the code for the cardiac arrest is the first-listed diagnosis. When the underlying condition is known, the code for the condition is sequenced first, with the code for cardiac arrest as an additional diagnosis. In ICD-10-CM, cardiac arrest now has three subcategories based on whether the underlying condition is known or not and whether it is cardiac or other specified condition. Since there is no documentation of recent cardiac catheterization, the coronary artery disease post CABG is assumed to be of native vessel without angina pectoris.

42. *Answer:* B20 Human immunodeficiency virus [HIV] disease and B59 Pneumocystosis

Rationale: ICD-10-CM OCG section I.C.1.a.1 instructs that confirmation of HIV status can be made by the provider's statement that the patient has an HIV-related illness. Also, section I.C.1.a.2.f states that cases involving patients with any known prior diagnosis of an HIV-related illness are assigned code B20 Human immunodeficiency virus [HIV] disease. The Centers for Disease Control (CDC) classifies *Pneumocystis jiroveci* pneumonia, an opportunistic pneumonia, as an AIDS-defining condition and one of the clinical criteria for HIV stage 3 or AIDS. Another clinical criterion is an HIV-positive patient having bacterial pneumonia twice within one year.

43. *Answer:* **A** Assign Z09 Encounter for follow-up examination after completed treatment for conditions other than malignant neoplasm, Z87.01 Personal history of pneumonia (recurrent).

Rationale: OCG section I.C.21.c.8 states that follow-up codes are assigned when the encounter is for surveillance following completed treatment and the condition no longer exists. Follow-up codes are not used for sequelae or ongoing care of a condition that is healing or resolving. A history code representing the healed/resolved condition is assigned as a secondary code to fully explain the reason for the encounter. The follow-up code is not assigned if the condition is found to have recurred on the follow-up encounter, and instead the code for the condition is listed first.

44. *Answer:* **A** Assign O9A.313 Physical abuse complicating pregnancy, third trimester, S02.2XXA Fracture of nasal bones, initial encounter for closed fracture, S00.11XA Contusion of right eyelid and periocular area, initial encounter, O24.013 Pre-existing diabetes mellitus, type 1, in pregnancy, third trimester, E10.65 Type 1 diabetes mellitus with hyperglycemia, T38.3X6A Underdosing of insulin and oral hypoglycemic [antidiabetic] drugs, initial encounter, Z3A.35 35 weeks gestation of pregnancy, Y04.0XXA Assault by unarmed brawl or fight, Y07.03 Male partner, perpetrator of maltreatment and neglect, Z91.120 Patient's intentional underdosing of medication regimen due to financial hardship, Z79.4 Long term (current) use of insulin, Y92.039 Unspecified place in apartment as the place of occurrence of the external cause

Rationale: The ED provider documentation that is attested by signature confirms the injuries are due to physical abuse. The *Official Coding Guidelines* section I.C.15.r states that abuse in a pregnant patient is sequenced first and coded to category O9A Physical abuse complicating pregnancy, childbirth, and the puerperium, when suspected or confirmed; associated injuries are coded as additional diagnoses. Pre-existing diabetes 1 with poor control is assigned to category O24

Diabetes mellitus in pregnancy, childbirth, and the puerperium, with an additional code from category E10 Type 1 diabetes mellitus, to further identify manifestation of hyperglycemia, indicated in the Alphabetic Index as poor control. Underdosing of medication is covered in OCG section I.C.19.e.5.c and is assigned from category T38 with the sixth character of 6. Sequencing of multiple codes from chapter 20, "External Causes of Morbidity," is explained in OCG section I.C.20.f.

45. *Answer:* <u>B</u> Documentation does not follow guidelines and/or the physician must be queried to determine the following: cause of cardiac arrest and whether the cardiac arrest a complication of the procedure.

Rationale: When a cardiac arrest occurs during an inpatient hospitalization and the patient is resuscitated, a code from category I46 Cardiac arrest, is assigned as an additional diagnosis. It would be appropriate to ask the physician the cause or contributing cause if it is not stated when there is clinical evidence to support the query. When a cardiac arrest is the reason for an inpatient death (the patient is not resuscitated) and the cause or contributing cause is known, the code for cardiac arrest is not assigned.

46. *Answer:* J95.851 Ventilator associated pneumonia

Rationale: ICD-10-CM OCG section I.C.10.d.1 states that the code for a complication is based on the provider's documentation of the relationship between the complication and the cause, in this case, the pneumonia and the mechanical ventilation. Therefore, code J95.851 Ventilator associated pneumonia, is assigned only when the link is expressly stated and not merely when a patient on a mechanical ventilator has pneumonia. An additional code is assigned if an identified organism is attributed to the VAP, but not a code from J12—J18. In the example, since the yeast cultures are identified only as a lab value and are not documented by the provider as related to the VAP, a code for the yeast organism is not assigned. The coder should ask the provider to state the clinical significance of the lab results; if the results are related to the VAP, B37.9 Candidiasis, unspecified, would be assigned.

47. *Answer:* Z38.01 Single liveborn infant, delivered by cesarean, P70.1 Syndrome of infant of a diabetic mother

Rationale: The code for a newborn delivered by cesarean on this admission is found by looking in the Alphabetic Index under "Newborn, born in hospital, by cesarean," code Z38.01. Macrosomia is not listed in the ICD-10-CM Alphabetic Index but is synonymous with "large for gestational age," or LGA, which the index entry for "Large, baby" indicates is coded with P08.1. This is not assigned, however, because subcategory E08.1 has an "excludes1" note indicating that LGA in "syndrome of diabetic mother" is to be included in P70.1.

48. *Answer:* <u>A</u> Assign E11.9 Type 2 diabetes mellitus without complications, Z86.32 Personal history of gestational diabetes, and O94 Sequela of complication of pregnancy, childbirth, and the puerperium.

Rationale: When diagnosed with gestational diabetes mellitus, patients have a high risk of developing diabetes 2 post delivery, which is why clinical guidelines recommend the patients return for postpartum glucose testing. When the postpartum impaired glucose regulation indicates diabetes, the case is coded as diabetes and no other abnormal glucose finding. OCG section I.C.15.o.3 states that if the provider documents a condition as related to pregnancy, codes from chapter 15 may be assigned. OCG section I.C.15.p states that when an initial complication of a pregnancy develops a sequela requiring care or treatment, code O94 is assigned and sequenced after the code identifying the sequela condition. The documented personal history of gestational diabetes is also coded.

49. *Answer:* R07.1 Chest pain on breathing, F43.0 Acute stress reaction, X37.1XXA Tornado, and Y92.017 Garden or yard in a single-family (private) house as the place of occurrence of the external cause

Rationale: The ICD-10-CM Alphabetic Index no longer provides a separate code for other acute pain for use with a specified site of pain. Instead, only the pain of the site is coded when stated as acute of a specified site. The index entry for "Pain, acute" shows R52 Pain, unspecified, which has an "excludes1" note instructing the user to code to pain by site for localized pain of unspecified type. The chest pain is described as "on inspiration"; the Alphabetic Index lists "Pain, chest, on breathing or pleurodynia," R07.1. Always review the entire record for a description of the chest pain and assign a code of the highest level of specificity based on physician documentation; query when appropriate. Since the chest pain is not linked to the stress the patient is experiencing, code F43.9 Acute stress reaction is assigned. To describe the situation related to the diagnoses, assign X37.1XXA Tornado, and Y92.017 Garden or yard in a single-family (private) house, as the place of occurrence of the external cause, for this initial encounter, according to OCG section I.C.20.b.

50. *Answer:* <u>A</u> Assign Z86.74 Personal history of sudden cardiac arrest, and I25.2 Old myocardial infarction.

Rationale: The past medical history documents a past cardiac arrest and myocardial infarction. Since the patient presents for CABG due to progressive angina for which the history of cardiac arrest and myocardial infarction would be relevant, assign the personal history code for both. The Alphabetic Index lists "History, personal, cardiac arrest (death) successfully resuscitated," code Z86.74. The index entry for history of myocardial infarction is "History, personal, myocardial infarction (old)," code I25.2. History codes are appropriate for an encounter when facility policy requires them or when the history is significant to the encounter based on medical significance or in relationship to other diagnoses or conditions. OCG section III.A states that previous conditions may be coded as additional diagnoses when they affect current care or treatment.

Official ICD-9-CM Guidelines for Coding and Reporting

Effective October 1, 2011

Note: Since no official ICD-9-CM addendum to the guidelines has been released since 2011, the guidelines included in this book stand as the official guidelines effective October 1, 2014, through September 30, 2015.

The Centers for Medicare and Medicaid Services (CMS) and the National Center for Health Statistics (NCHS), two departments within the U.S. Federal Government's Department of Health and Human Services (DHHS) provide the following guidelines for coding and reporting using the International Classification of Diseases, 9th Revision, Clinical Modification (ICD-9-CM). These guidelines should be used as a companion document to the official version of the ICD-9-CM as published on CD-ROM by the U.S. Government Printing Office (GPO).

These guidelines have been approved by the four organizations that make up the Cooperating Parties for the ICD-9-CM: the American Hospital Association (AHA), the American Health Information Management Association (AHIMA), CMS, and NCHS. These guidelines are included on the official government version of the ICD-9-CM, and also appear in *"Coding Clinic for ICD-9-CM"* published by the AHA.

These guidelines are a set of rules that have been developed to accompany and complement the official conventions and instructions provided within the ICD-9-CM itself. The instructions and conventions of the classification take precedence over guidelines. These guidelines are based on the coding and sequencing instructions in Volumes I, II and III of ICD-9-CM, but provide additional instruction. Adherence to these guidelines when assigning ICD-9-CM diagnosis and procedure codes is required under the Health Insurance Portability and Accountability Act (HIPAA). The diagnosis codes (Volumes 1-2) have been adopted under HIPAA for all healthcare settings. Volume 3 procedure codes have been adopted for inpatient procedures reported by hospitals. A joint effort between the healthcare provider and the coder is essential to achieve complete and accurate documentation, code assignment, and reporting of diagnoses and procedures. These guidelines have been developed to assist both the healthcare provider and the coder in identifying those diagnoses and procedures that are to be reported. The importance of consistent, complete documentation in the medical record cannot be overemphasized. Without such documentation accurate coding cannot be achieved. The entire record should be reviewed to determine the specific reason for the encounter and the conditions treated.

The term encounter is used for all settings, including hospital admissions. In the context of these guidelines, the term provider is used throughout the guidelines to mean physician or any qualified health care practitioner who is legally accountable for establishing the patient's diagnosis. Only this set of guidelines, approved by the Cooperating Parties, is official.

The guidelines are organized into sections. Section I includes the structure and conventions of the classification and general guidelines that apply to the entire classification, and chapter-specific guidelines that correspond to the chapters as they are arranged in the classification. Section II includes guidelines for selection of principal diagnosis for non-outpatient settings. Section III includes guidelines for reporting additional diagnoses in non-outpatient settings. Section IV is for outpatient coding and reporting.

Section I. Conventions, general coding guidelines and chapter specific guidelines

A. Conventions for the ICD-9-CM
  1. Format:
  2. Abbreviations
    a. Index abbreviations
    b. Tabular abbreviations
  3. Punctuation
  4. Includes and Excludes Notes and Inclusion terms
  5. Other and Unspecified codes
    a. "Other" codes
    b. "Unspecified" codes
  6. Etiology/manifestation convention ("code first", "use additional code" and "in diseases classified elsewhere" notes)
  7. "And"

8. "With"
9. "See" and "See Also"

B. General Coding Guidelines
  1. Use of Both Alphabetic Index and Tabular List
  2. Locate each term in the Alphabetic Index
  3. Level of Detail in Coding
  4. Code or codes from 001.0 through V91.99
  5. Selection of codes 001.0 through 999.9
  6. Signs and symptoms
  7. Conditions that are an integral part of a disease process
  8. Conditions that are not an integral part of a disease process
  9. Multiple coding for a single condition
  10. Acute and Chronic Conditions
  11. Combination Code
  12. Late Effects
  13. Impending or Threatened Condition
  14. Reporting Same Diagnosis Code More than Once
  15. Admissions/Encounters for Rehabilitation
  16. Documentation for BMI and Pressure Ulcer Stages
  17. Syndromes
  18. Documentation of Complications of Care

C. Chapter-Specific Coding Guidelines
  1. Chapter 1: Infectious and Parasitic Diseases (001-139)
    a. Human Immunodeficiency Virus (HIV) Infections
    b. Septicemia, Systemic Inflammatory Response Syndrome (SIRS), Sepsis, Severe Sepsis and Septic Shock
    c. Methicillin Resistant *Staphylococcus aureus* (MRSA) Conditions
  2. Chapter 2: Neoplasms (140-239)
    a. Treatment directed at the malignancy
    b. Treatment of secondary site
    c. Coding and sequencing of complications
    d. Primary malignancy previously excised
    e. Admissions/Encounters involving chemotherapy, immunotherapy and radiation therapy
    f. Admission/encounter to determine extent of malignancy
    g. Symptoms, signs, and ill-defined conditions listed in Chapter 16 associated with neoplasms
    h. Admission/encounter for pain control/management
    i. Malignant neoplasm associated with transplanted organ
  3. Chapter 3: Endocrine, Nutritional, and Metabolic Diseases and Immunity Disorders (240-279)
    a. Diabetes mellitus
  4. Chapter 4: Diseases of Blood and Blood Forming Organs (280-289)
    a. Anemia of chronic disease
  5. Chapter 5: Mental Disorders (290-319)
    Reserved for future guideline expansion
  6. Chapter 6: Diseases of Nervous System and Sense Organs (320-389)
    a. Pain - Category 338
    b. Glaucoma
  7. Chapter 7: Diseases of Circulatory System (390-459)
    a. Hypertension
    b. Cerebral infarction/stroke/ from cerebrovascular accident (CVA)
    c. Postoperative cerebrovascular accident
    d. Late Effects of Cerebrovascular Disease
    e. Acute myocardial infarction (AMI)

Section II. Selection of Principal Diagnosis

A. Codes for symptoms, signs, and ill-defined conditions
B. Two or more interrelated conditions, each potentially meeting the definition for principal diagnosis
C. Two or more diagnoses that equally meet the definition for principal diagnosis
D. Two or more comparative or contrasting conditions
E. A symptom(s) followed by contrasting/comparative diagnoses
F. Original treatment plan not carried out
G. Complications of surgery and other medical care
H. Uncertain Diagnosis
I. Admission from Observation Unit
    1. Admission Following Medical Observation
    2. Admission Following Post-Operative Observation
J. Admission from Outpatient Surgery

Section III. Reporting Additional Diagnoses

A. Previous conditions
B. Abnormal findings
C. Uncertain diagnosis

Section IV. Diagnostic Coding and Reporting Guidelines for Outpatient Services

A. Selection of first-listed condition
    1. Outpatient Surgery
    2. Observation Stay
B. Codes from 001.0 through V91.99
C. Accurate reporting of ICD-9-CM diagnosis codes
D. Selection of codes 001.0 through 999.9
E. Codes that describe symptoms and signs
F. Encounters for circumstances other than a disease or injury
G. Level of Detail in Coding
    1. ICD-9-CM codes with 3, 4, or 5 digits
    2. Use of full number of digits required for a code
H. ICD-9-CM code for the diagnosis, condition, problem, or other reason for encounter/visit
I. Uncertain diagnosis
J. Chronic diseases
K. Code all documented conditions that coexist
L. Patients receiving diagnostic services only
M. Patients receiving therapeutic services only
N. Patients receiving preoperative evaluations only
O. Ambulatory surgery
P. Routine outpatient prenatal visits

Appendix I: Present on Admission Reporting Guidelines

Section I. Conventions, general coding guidelines and chapter specific guidelines

The conventions, general guidelines and chapter-specific guidelines are applicable to all health care settings unless otherwise indicated. The conventions and instructions of the classification take precedence over guidelines.

A. Conventions for the ICD-9-CM

The conventions for the ICD-9-CM are the general rules for use of the classification independent of the guidelines. These conventions are incorporated within the index and tabular of the ICD-9-CM as instructional notes. The conventions are as follows:

1. **Format:**

   The ICD-9-CM uses an indented format for ease in reference

2. **Abbreviations**

   a. **Index abbreviations**

      NEC "Not elsewhere classifiable"

      This abbreviation in the index represents "other specified" when a specific code is not available for a condition the index directs the coder to the "other specified" code in the tabular.

   b. **Tabular abbreviations**

      NEC "Not elsewhere classifiable"

      This abbreviation in the tabular represents "other specified". When a specific code is not available for a condition the tabular includes an NEC entry under a code to identify the code as the "other specified" code.
      (See Section I.A.5.a. "Other" codes).

      NOS "Not otherwise specified"

      This abbreviation is the equivalent of unspecified.
      (See Section I.A.5.b., "Unspecified" codes)

3. **Punctuation**

   [ ] Brackets are used in the tabular list to enclose synonyms, alternative wording or explanatory phrases. Brackets are used in the index to identify manifestation codes.
        (See Section I.A.6. "Etiology/manifestations")

   ( ) Parentheses are used in both the index and tabular to enclose supplementary words that may be present or absent in the statement of a disease or procedure without affecting the code number to which it is assigned. The terms within the parentheses are referred to as nonessential modifiers.

   :   Colons are used in the Tabular list after an incomplete term which needs one or more of the modifiers following the colon to make it assignable to a given category.

4. **Includes and Excludes Notes and Inclusion terms**

   Includes: This note appears immediately under a three-digit code title to further define, or give examples of, the content of the category.

   Excludes: An excludes note under a code indicates that the terms excluded from the code are to be coded elsewhere. In some cases the codes for the excluded terms should not be used in conjunction with the code from which it is excluded. An example of this is a congenital condition excluded from an acquired form of the same condition. The congenital and acquired codes should not be used together. In other cases, the excluded terms may be used together with an excluded code. An example of this is when fractures of different bones are coded to different codes. Both codes may be used together if both types of fractures are present.

   Inclusion terms: List of terms is included under certain four and five digit codes. These terms are the conditions for which that code number is to be used. The terms may be synonyms of the code title, or, in the case of "other specified" codes, the terms are a list of the various conditions assigned to that code. The inclusion terms are not necessarily exhaustive. Additional terms found only in the index may also be assigned to a code.

5. **Other and Unspecified codes**

   a. **"Other" codes**

      Codes titled "other" or "other specified" (usually a code with a 4th digit 8 or fifth-digit 9 for diagnosis codes) are for use when the information in the medical record provides detail for which a specific code does not exist. Index entries with NEC in the line designate "other" codes in the tabular. These index entries represent specific disease entities for which no specific code exists so the term is included within an "other" code.

   b. **"Unspecified" codes**

      Codes (usually a code with a 4th digit 9 or 5th digit 0 for diagnosis codes) titled "unspecified" are for use when the information in the medical record is insufficient to assign a more specific code.

6. **Etiology/manifestation convention ("code first", "use additional code" and "in diseases classified elsewhere" notes)**

   Certain conditions have both an underlying etiology and multiple body system manifestations due to the underlying etiology. For such conditions, the ICD-9-CM has a coding convention that requires the underlying condition be sequenced first followed by the manifestation. Wherever such a combination exists, there is a "use additional code" note at the etiology code, and a "code first" note at the manifestation code. These instructional notes indicate the proper sequencing order of the codes, etiology followed by manifestation.

   In most cases the manifestation codes will have in the code title, "in diseases classified elsewhere." Codes with this title are a component of the etiology/ manifestation convention. The code title indicates that it is a manifestation code. "In diseases classified elsewhere" codes are never permitted to be used as first listed or principal diagnosis codes. They must be used in conjunction with an underlying condition code and they must be listed following the underlying condition.

   There are manifestation codes that do not have "in diseases classified elsewhere" in the title. For such codes a "use additional code" note will still be present and the rules for sequencing apply.

   In addition to the notes in the tabular, these conditions also have a specific index entry structure. In the index both conditions are listed together with the etiology code first followed by the manifestation codes in brackets. The code in brackets is always to be sequenced second.

   The most commonly used etiology/manifestation combinations are the codes for Diabetes mellitus, category 250. For each code under category 250 there is a use additional code note for the manifestation that is specific for that particular diabetic manifestation. Should a patient have more than one manifestation of diabetes, more than one code from category 250 may be used with as many manifestation codes as are needed to fully describe the patient's complete diabetic condition. The category 250 diabetes codes should be sequenced first, followed by the manifestation codes.

   "Code first" and "Use additional code" notes are also used as sequencing rules in the classification for certain codes that are not part of an etiology/ manifestation combination.
   See - Section I.B.9. "Multiple coding for a single condition".

7. **"And"**

   The word "and" should be interpreted to mean either "and" or "or" when it appears in a title.

8. **"With"**

   The word "with" should be interpreted to mean "associated with" or "due to" when it appears in a code title, the Alphabetic Index, or an instructional note in the Tabular List.

   The word "with" in the alphabetic index is sequenced immediately following the main term, not in alphabetical order.

9. **"See" and "See Also"**

   The "see" instruction following a main term in the index indicates that another term should be referenced. It is necessary to go to the main term referenced with the "see" note to locate the correct code.

   A "see also" instruction following a main term in the index instructs that there is another main term that may also be referenced that may provide additional index entries that may be useful. It is not necessary to follow the "see also" note when the original main term provides the necessary code.

B. General Coding Guidelines

1. Use of Both Alphabetic Index and Tabular List

Use both the Alphabetic Index and the Tabular List when locating and assigning a code. Reliance on only the Alphabetic Index or the Tabular List leads to errors in code assignments and less specificity in code selection.

2. Locate each term in the Alphabetic Index

Locate each term in the Alphabetic Index and verify the code selected in the Tabular List. Read and be guided by instructional notations that appear in both the Alphabetic Index and the Tabular List.

3. Level of Detail in Coding

Diagnosis and procedure codes are to be used at their highest number of digits available.

ICD-9-CM diagnosis codes are composed of codes with 3, 4, or 5 digits. Codes with three digits are included in ICD-9-CM as the heading of a category of codes that may be further subdivided by the use of fourth and/or fifth digits, which provide greater detail.

A three-digit code is to be used only if it is not further subdivided. Where fourth-digit subcategories and/or fifth-digit subclassifications are provided, they must be assigned. A code is invalid if it has not been coded to the full number of digits required for that code. For example, Acute myocardial infarction, code 410, has fourth digits that describe the location of the infarction (e.g., 410.2, Of inferolateral wall), and fifth digits that identify the episode of care. It would be incorrect to report a code in category 410 without a fourth and fifth digit.

ICD-9-CM Volume 3 procedure codes are composed of codes with either 3 or 4 digits. Codes with two digits are included in ICD-9-CM as the heading of a category of codes that may be further subdivided by the use of third and/or fourth digits, which provide greater detail.

4. Code or codes from 001.0 through V91.99

The appropriate code or codes from 001.0 through V91.99 must be used to identify diagnoses, symptoms, conditions, problems, complaints or other reason(s) for the encounter/visit.

5. Selection of codes 001.0 through 999.9

The selection of codes 001.0 through 999.9 will frequently be used to describe the reason for the admission/encounter. These codes are from the section of ICD-9-CM for the classification of diseases and injuries (e.g., infectious and parasitic diseases; neoplasms; symptoms, signs, and ill-defined conditions, etc.).

6. Signs and symptoms

Codes that describe symptoms and signs, as opposed to diagnoses, are acceptable for reporting purposes when a related definitive diagnosis has not been established (confirmed) by the provider. Chapter 16 of ICD-9-CM, Symptoms, Signs, and Ill-defined conditions (codes 780.0 - 799.9) contain many, but not all codes for symptoms.

7. Conditions that are an integral part of a disease process

Signs and symptoms that are associated routinely with a disease process should not be assigned as additional codes, unless otherwise instructed by the classification.

8. Conditions that are not an integral part of a disease process

Additional signs and symptoms that may not be associated routinely with a disease process should be coded when present.

9. Multiple coding for a single condition

In addition to the etiology/manifestation convention that requires two codes to fully describe a single condition that affects multiple body systems, there are other single conditions that also require more than one code. "Use additional code" notes are found in the tabular at codes that are not part of an etiology/manifestation pair where a secondary code is useful to fully describe a condition. The sequencing rule is the same as the etiology/manifestation pair - "use additional code" indicates that a secondary code should be added.

For example, for infections that are not included in chapter 1, a secondary code from category 041, Bacterial infection in conditions classified elsewhere and of unspecified site, may be required to

identify the bacterial organism causing the infection. A "use additional code" note will normally be found at the infectious disease code, indicating a need for the organism code to be added as a secondary code.

"Code first" notes are also under certain codes that are not specifically manifestation codes but may be due to an underlying cause. When a "code first" note is present and an underlying condition is present the underlying condition should be sequenced first.

"Code, if applicable, any causal condition first", notes indicate that this code may be assigned as a principal diagnosis when the causal condition is unknown or not applicable. If a causal condition is known, then the code for that condition should be sequenced as the principal or first-listed diagnosis.

Multiple codes may be needed for late effects, complication codes and obstetric codes to more fully describe a condition. See the specific guidelines for these conditions for further instruction.

10. Acute and Chronic Conditions

If the same condition is described as both acute (subacute) and chronic, and separate subentries exist in the Alphabetic Index at the same indentation level, code both and sequence the acute (subacute) code first.

11. Combination Code

A combination code is a single code used to classify:

- Two diagnoses, or
- A diagnosis with an associated secondary process (manifestation)
- A diagnosis with an associated complication

Combination codes are identified by referring to subterm entries in the Alphabetic Index and by reading the inclusion and exclusion notes in the Tabular List.

Assign only the combination code when that code fully identifies the diagnostic conditions involved or when the Alphabetic Index so directs. Multiple coding should not be used when the classification provides a combination code that clearly identifies all of the elements documented in the diagnosis. When the combination code lacks necessary specificity in describing the manifestation or complication, an additional code should be used as a secondary code.

12. Late Effects

A late effect is the residual effect (condition produced) after the acute phase of an illness or injury has terminated. There is no time limit on when a late effect code can be used. The residual may be apparent early, such as in cerebrovascular accident cases, or it may occur months or years later, such as that due to a previous injury. Coding of late effects generally requires two codes sequenced in the following order: The condition or nature of the late effect is sequenced first. The late effect code is sequenced second.

Exceptions to the above guidelines are those instances the late effect code has been expanded (at the fourth and fifth-digit levels) to include the manifestation(s) or the classification instructs otherwise. The code for the acute phase of an illness or injury that led to the late effect is never used with a code for the late effect.

13. Impending or Threatened Condition

Code any condition described at the time of discharge as "impending" or "threatened" as follows:

If it did occur, code as confirmed diagnosis.
If it did not occur, reference the Alphabetic Index to determine if the condition has a subentry term for "impending" or "threatened" and also reference main term entries for "Impending" and for "Threatened."
If the subterms are listed, assign the given code.
If the subterms are not listed, code the existing underlying condition(s) and not the condition described as impending or threatened.

14. Reporting Same Diagnosis Code More than Once

Each unique ICD-9-CM diagnosis code may be reported only once for an encounter. This applies to bilateral conditions or two different conditions classified to the same ICD-9-CM diagnosis code.

15. Admissions/Encounters for Rehabilitation

When the purpose for the admission/encounter is rehabilitation, sequence the appropriate V code from category V57, Care involving use of rehabilitation procedures, as the principal/first-listed diagnosis. The code for the condition for which the service is being performed should be reported as an additional diagnosis.

Only one code from category V57 is required. Code V57.89, Other specified rehabilitation procedures, should be assigned if more than one type of rehabilitation is performed during a single encounter. A procedure code should be reported to identify each type of rehabilitation therapy actually performed.

16. Documentation for BMI and Pressure Ulcer Stages

For the Body Mass Index (BMI) and pressure ulcer stage codes, code assignment may be based on medical record documentation from clinicians who are not the patient's provider (i.e., physician or other qualified healthcare practitioner legally accountable for establishing the patient's diagnosis), since this information is typically documented by other clinicians involved in the care of the patient (e.g., a dietitian often documents the BMI and nurses often documents the pressure ulcer stages). However, the associated diagnosis (such as overweight, obesity, or pressure ulcer) must be documented by the patient's provider. If there is conflicting medical record documentation, either from the same clinician or different clinicians, the patient's attending provider should be queried for clarification.

The BMI and pressure ulcer stage codes should only be reported as secondary diagnoses. As with all other secondary diagnosis codes, the BMI and pressure ulcer stage codes should only be assigned when they meet the definition of a reportable additional diagnosis (see Section III, Reporting Additional Diagnoses).

17. Syndromes

Follow the Alphabetic Index guidance when coding syndromes. In the absence of index guidance, assign codes for the documented manifestations of the syndrome.

18. Documentation of complications of care

Code assignment is based on the provider's documentation of the relationship between the condition and the care or procedure. The guideline extends to any complications of care, regardless of the chapter the code is located in. It is important to note that not all conditions that occur during or following medical care or surgery are classified as complications. There must be a cause-and-effect relationship between the care provided and the condition, and an indication in the documentation that it is a complication. Query the provider for clarification, if the complication is not clearly documented.

C. Chapter-Specific Coding Guidelines

In addition to general coding guidelines, there are guidelines for specific diagnoses and/or conditions in the classification. Unless otherwise indicated, these guidelines apply to all health care settings. Please refer to Section II for guidelines on the selection of principal diagnosis.

1. Chapter 1: Infectious and Parasitic Diseases (001-139)

a. Human Immunodeficiency Virus (HIV) Infections

1) Code only confirmed cases

Code only confirmed cases of HIV infection/illness. This is an exception to the hospital inpatient guideline Section II, H.

In this context, "confirmation" does not require documentation of positive serology or culture for HIV; the provider's diagnostic statement that the patient is HIV positive, or has an HIV-related illness is sufficient.

2) Selection and sequencing of HIV codes

(a) Patient admitted for HIV-related condition

If a patient is admitted for an HIV-related condition, the principal diagnosis should be 042, followed by additional diagnosis codes for all reported HIV-related conditions.

(b) Patient with HIV disease admitted for unrelated condition

If a patient with HIV disease is admitted for an unrelated condition (such as a traumatic injury), the code for the unrelated condition (e.g., the nature of injury code) should be the principal diagnosis. Other diagnoses would be 042 followed by additional diagnosis codes for all reported HIV-related conditions.

(c) Whether the patient is newly diagnosed

Whether the patient is newly diagnosed or has had previous admissions/encounters for HIV conditions is irrelevant to the sequencing decision.

(d) Asymptomatic human immunodeficiency virus

V08 Asymptomatic human immunodeficiency virus [HIV] infection, is to be applied when the patient without any documentation of symptoms is listed as being "HIV positive," "known HIV," "HIV test positive," or similar terminology. Do not use this code if the term "AIDS" is used or if the patient is treated for any HIV-related illness or is described as having any condition(s) resulting from his/her HIV positive status; use 042 in these cases.

(e) Patients with inconclusive HIV serology

Patients with inconclusive HIV serology, but no definitive diagnosis or manifestations of the illness, may be assigned code 795.71, Inconclusive serologic test for Human Immunodeficiency Virus [HIV].

(f) Previously diagnosed HIV-related illness

Patients with any known prior diagnosis of an HIV-related illness should be coded to 042. Once a patient has developed an HIV-related illness, the patient should always be assigned code 042 on every subsequent admission/encounter. Patients previously diagnosed with any HIV illness (042) should never be assigned to 795.71 or V08.

(g) HIV Infection in Pregnancy, Childbirth and the Puerperium

During pregnancy, childbirth or the puerperium, a patient admitted (or presenting for a health care encounter) because of an HIV-related illness should receive a principal diagnosis code of 647.6x, Other specified infectious and parasitic diseases in the mother classifiable elsewhere, but complicating the pregnancy, childbirth or the puerperium, followed by 042 and the code(s) for the HIV-related illness(es). Codes from Chapter 15 always take sequencing priority.

Patients with asymptomatic HIV infection status admitted (or presenting for a health care encounter) during pregnancy, childbirth, or the puerperium should receive codes of 647.6x and V08.

(h) Encounters for testing for HIV

If a patient is being seen to determine his/her HIV status, use code V73.89, Screening for other specified viral disease. Use code V69.8, Other problems related to lifestyle, as a secondary code if an asymptomatic patient is in a known high risk group for HIV. Should a patient with signs or symptoms or illness, or a confirmed HIV related diagnosis be tested for HIV, code the signs and symptoms or the diagnosis. An additional counseling code V65.44 may be used if counseling is provided during the encounter for the test.

When a patient returns to be informed of his/her HIV test results use code V65.44, HIV counseling, if the results of the test are negative.

If the results are positive but the patient is asymptomatic use code V08, Asymptomatic HIV infection. If the results are positive and the patient is symptomatic use code 042, HIV infection, with codes for the HIV related symptoms or diagnosis. The HIV counseling code may also be used if counseling is provided for patients with positive test results.

b. Septicemia, Systemic Inflammatory Response Syndrome (SIRS), Sepsis, Severe Sepsis, and Septic Shock

1) SIRS, Septicemia, and Sepsis

(a) The terms *septicemia* and *sepsis* are often used interchangeably by providers, however they are not considered synonymous terms. The following descriptions are provided for reference but do not preclude querying the provider for clarification about terms used in the documentation:

(i) Septicemia generally refers to a systemic disease associated with the presence of pathological microorganisms or toxins in the blood, which can include bacteria, viruses, fungi or other organisms.

(ii) Systemic inflammatory response syndrome (SIRS) generally refers to the systemic response to infection, trauma/burns, or other insult (such as cancer) with symptoms including fever, tachycardia, tachypnea, and leukocytosis.

(iii) Sepsis generally refers to SIRS due to infection.

(iv) Severe sepsis generally refers to sepsis with associated acute organ dysfunction.

(b) The Coding of SIRS, sepsis and severe sepsis

The coding of SIRS, sepsis and severe sepsis requires a minimum of 2 codes: a code for the underlying cause (such as infection or trauma) and a code from subcategory 995.9 Systemic inflammatory response syndrome (SIRS).

(i) The code for the underlying cause (such as infection or trauma) must be sequenced before the code from subcategory 995.9 Systemic inflammatory response syndrome (SIRS).

(ii) Sepsis and severe sepsis require a code for the systemic infection (038.xx, 112.5, etc.) and either code 995.91, Sepsis, or 995.92, Severe sepsis. If the causal organism is not documented, assign code 038.9, Unspecified septicemia.

(iii) Severe sepsis requires additional code(s) for the associated acute organ dysfunction(s).

(iv) If a patient has sepsis with multiple organ dysfunctions, follow the instructions for coding severe sepsis.

(v) Either the term sepsis or SIRS must be documented to assign a code from subcategory 995.9.

(vi) *See Section I.C.17.g), Injury and poisoning, for information regarding systemic inflammatory response syndrome (SIRS) due to trauma/burns and other non-infectious processes.*

(c) Due to the complex nature of sepsis and severe sepsis, some cases may require querying the provider prior to assignment of the codes.

2) Sequencing sepsis and severe sepsis

(a) Sepsis and severe sepsis as principal diagnosis

If sepsis or severe sepsis is present on admission, and meets the definition of principal diagnosis, the systemic infection code (e.g., 038.xx, 112.5, etc) should be assigned as the principal diagnosis, followed by code 995.91, Sepsis, or 995.92, Severe sepsis, as required by the sequencing rules in the Tabular List. Codes from subcategory 995.9 can never be assigned as a principal diagnosis. A code should also be assigned for any localized infection, if present.

If the sepsis or severe sepsis is due to a postprocedural infection, see Section I.C.1.b.10 for guidelines related to sepsis due to postprocedural infection.

(b) Sepsis and severe sepsis as secondary diagnoses

When sepsis or severe sepsis develops during the encounter (it was not present on admission), the systemic infection code and code 995.91 or 995.92 should be assigned as secondary diagnoses.

(c) Documentation unclear as to whether sepsis or severe sepsis is present on admission

Sepsis or severe sepsis may be present on admission but the diagnosis may not be confirmed until sometime after admission. If the documentation is not clear whether the sepsis or severe sepsis was present on admission, the provider should be queried.

3) Sepsis/SIRS with Localized Infection

If the reason for admission is both sepsis, severe sepsis, or SIRS and a localized infection, such as pneumonia or cellulitis, a code for the systemic infection (038.xx, 112.5, etc) should be assigned first, then code 995.91 or 995.92, followed by the code for the localized infection. If the patient is admitted with a localized infection, such as pneumonia, and sepsis/SIRS doesn't develop until after admission, see guideline I.C.1.b.2.b).

If the localized infection is postprocedural, *see Section I.C.1.b.10 for guidelines related to sepsis due to postprocedural infection.*

Note: The term urosepsis is a nonspecific term. If that is the only term documented then only code 599.0 should be assigned based on the default for the term in the ICD-9-CM index, in addition to the code for the causal organism if known.

4) Bacterial Sepsis and Septicemia

In most cases, it will be a code from category 038, Septicemia, that will be used in conjunction with a code from subcategory 995.9 such as the following:

(a) Streptococcal sepsis

If the documentation in the record states streptococcal sepsis, codes 038.0, Streptococcal septicemia, and code 995.91 should be used, in that sequence.

(b) Streptococcal septicemia

If the documentation states streptococcal septicemia, only code 038.0 should be assigned, however, the provider should be queried whether the patient has sepsis, an infection with SIRS.

5) Acute organ dysfunction that is not clearly associated with the sepsis

If a patient has sepsis and an acute organ dysfunction, but the medical record documentation indicates that the acute organ dysfunction is related to a medical condition other than the sepsis, do not assign code 995.92, Severe sepsis. An acute organ dysfunction must be associated with the sepsis in order to assign the severe sepsis code. If the documentation is not clear as to whether an acute organ dysfunction is related to the sepsis or another medical condition, query the provider.

6) Septic shock

(a) Sequencing of septic shock

Septic shock generally refers to circulatory failure associated with severe sepsis, and, therefore, it represents a type of acute organ dysfunction.

For cases of septic shock, the code for the systemic infection should be sequenced first, followed by codes 995.92, Severe sepsis and 785.52, Septic shock or 998.02, Postoperative septic shock. Any additional codes for other acute organ dysfunctions should also be assigned. As noted in the sequencing instructions in the Tabular List, the code for septic shock cannot be assigned as a principal diagnosis.

(b) Septic Shock without documentation of severe sepsis

Since septic shock indicates the presence of severe sepsis, code 995.92, Severe sepsis, can be assigned with code 785.52, Septic shock, or code 998.02 Postoperative shock, septic, even if the term severe sepsis is not documented in the record.

7) Sepsis and septic shock complicating abortion and pregnancy

Sepsis and septic shock complicating abortion, ectopic pregnancy, and molar pregnancy are classified to category codes in Chapter 11 (630-639).

See section I.C.11.i.7. for information on the coding of puerperal sepsis.

8) Negative or inconclusive blood cultures

Negative or inconclusive blood cultures do not preclude a diagnosis of septicemia or sepsis in patients with clinical evidence of the condition, however, the provider should be queried.

9) Newborn sepsis

See Section I.C.15.j for information on the coding of newborn sepsis.

10) Sepsis due to a Postprocedural Infection

(a) Documentation of causal relationship

As with all postprocedural complications, code assignment is based on the provider's documentation of the relationship between the infection and the procedure.

(b) Sepsis due to postprocedural infection

In cases of postprocedural sepsis, the complication code, such as code 998.59, Other postoperative infection, or 674.3x, Other complications of obstetrical surgical wounds should be coded first followed by the appropriate sepsis codes (systemic infection code and either code 995.91 or 995.92). An additional code(s) for any acute organ dysfunction should also be assigned for cases of severe sepsis.

See Section see Section I.C.1.b.6 if the sepsis or severe sepsis results in postprocedural septic shock.

(c) Postprocedural infection and postprocedural septic shock

In cases where a postprocedural infection has occurred and has resulted in severe sepsis and postprocedural septic shock, the code for the precipitating complication such as code 998.59, Other postoperative infection, or 674.3x, Other complications of obstetrical surgical wounds should be coded first followed by the appropriate sepsis codes (systemic infection code and code 995.92). Code 998.02, Postoperative septic shock, should be assigned as an additional code. In cases of severe sepsis, an additional code(s) for any acute organ dysfunction should also be assigned.

11) External cause of injury codes with SIRS

Refer to Section I.C.19.a.7 for instruction on the use of external cause of injury codes with codes for SIRS resulting from trauma.

12) Sepsis and Severe Sepsis Associated with Non-infectious Process

In some cases, a non-infectious process, such as trauma, may lead to an infection which can result in sepsis or severe sepsis. If sepsis or severe sepsis is documented as associated with a non-infectious condition, such as a burn or serious injury, and this condition meets the definition for principal diagnosis, the code for the non-infectious condition should be sequenced first, followed by the code for the systemic infection and either code 995.91, Sepsis, or 995.92, Severe sepsis. Additional codes for any associated acute organ dysfunction(s) should also be assigned for cases of severe sepsis. If the sepsis or severe sepsis meets the definition of

principal diagnosis, the systemic infection and sepsis codes should be sequenced before the non-infectious condition. When both the associated non-infectious condition and the sepsis or severe sepsis meet the definition of principal diagnosis, either may be assigned as principal diagnosis.

See Section I.C.1.b.2.a. for guidelines pertaining to sepsis or severe sepsis as the principal diagnosis.

Only one code from subcategory 995.9 should be assigned. Therefore, when a non-infectious condition leads to an infection resulting in sepsis or severe sepsis, assign either code 995.91 or 995.92. Do not additionally assign code 995.93, Systemic inflammatory response syndrome due to non-infectious process without acute organ dysfunction, or 995.94, Systemic inflammatory response syndrome with acute organ dysfunction.

See Section I.C.17.g for information on the coding of SIRS due to trauma/burns or other non-infectious disease processes.

c. Methicillin Resistant Staphylococcus aureus (MRSA) Conditions

1) Selection and sequencing of MRSA codes

(a) Combination codes for MRSA infection

When a patient is diagnosed with an infection that is due to methicillin resistant *Staphylococcus aureus* (MRSA), and that infection has a combination code that includes the causal organism (e.g., septicemia, pneumonia) assign the appropriate code for the condition (e.g., code 038.12, Methicillin resistant Staphylococcus aureus septicemia or code 482.42, Methicillin resistant pneumonia due to Staphylococcus aureus). Do not assign code 041.12, Methicillin resistant Staphylococcus aureus, as an additional code because the code includes the type of infection and the MRSA organism. Do not assign a code from subcategory V09.0, Infection with microorganisms resistant to penicillins, as an additional diagnosis.

See Section C.1.b.1 for instructions on coding and sequencing of septicemia.

(b) Other codes for MRSA infection

When there is documentation of a current infection (e.g., wound infection, stitch abscess, urinary tract infection) due to MRSA, and that infection does not have a combination code that includes the causal organism, select the appropriate code to identify the condition along with code 041.12, Methicillin resistant Staphylococcus aureus, for the MRSA infection. Do not assign a code from subcategory V09.0, Infection with microorganisms resistant to penicillins.

(c) Methicillin susceptible Staphylococcus aureus (MSSA) and MRSA colonization

The condition or state of being colonized or carrying MSSA or MRSA is called colonization or carriage, while an individual person is described as being colonized or being a carrier. Colonization means that MSSA or MSRA is present on or in the body without necessarily causing illness. A positive MRSA colonization test might be documented by the provider as "MRSA screen positive" or "MRSA nasal swab positive".

Assign code V02.54, Carrier or suspected carrier, Methicillin resistant Staphylococcus aureus, for patients documented as having MRSA colonization. Assign code V02.53, Carrier or suspected carrier, Methicillin susceptible Staphylococcus aureus, for patient documented as having MSSA colonization. Colonization is not necessarily indicative of a disease process or as the cause of a specific condition the patient may have unless documented as such by the provider.

Code V02.59, Other specified bacterial diseases, should be assigned for other types of staphylococcal colonization (e.g., S. *epidermidis*, S. *saprophyticus*)**.** Code

V02.59 should not be assigned for colonization with any type of *Staphylococcus aureus* (MRSA, MSSA).

(d) MRSA colonization and infection

If a patient is documented as having both MRSA colonization and infection during a hospital admission, code V02.54, Carrier or suspected carrier, Methicillin resistant *Staphylococcus aureus*, and a code for the MRSA infection may both be assigned.

2. Chapter 2: Neoplasms (140-239)

General guidelines

Chapter 2 of the ICD-9-CM contains the codes for most benign and all malignant neoplasms. Certain benign neoplasms, such as prostatic adenomas, may be found in the specific body system chapters. To properly code a neoplasm it is necessary to determine from the record if the neoplasm is benign, in-situ, malignant, or of uncertain histologic behavior. If malignant, any secondary (metastatic) sites should also be determined.

The neoplasm table in the Alphabetic Index should be referenced first. However, if the histological term is documented, that term should be referenced first, rather than going immediately to the Neoplasm Table, in order to determine which column in the Neoplasm Table is appropriate. For example, if the documentation indicates "adenoma," refer to the term in the Alphabetic Index to review the entries under this term and the instructional note to "see also neoplasm, by site, benign." The table provides the proper code based on the type of neoplasm and the site. It is important to select the proper column in the table that corresponds to the type of neoplasm. The tabular should then be referenced to verify that the correct code has been selected from the table and that a more specific site code does not exist.

See Section I. C. 18.d.4. for information regarding V codes for genetic susceptibility to cancer.

a. Treatment directed at the malignancy

If the treatment is directed at the malignancy, designate the malignancy as the principal diagnosis.

The only exception to this guideline is if a patient admission/encounter is solely for the administration of chemotherapy, immunotherapy or radiation therapy, assign the appropriate V58.x code as the first-listed or principal diagnosis, and the diagnosis or problem for which the service is being performed as a secondary diagnosis.

b. Treatment of secondary site

When a patient is admitted because of a primary neoplasm with metastasis and treatment is directed toward the secondary site only, the secondary neoplasm is designated as the principal diagnosis even though the primary malignancy is still present.

c. Coding and sequencing of complications

Coding and sequencing of complications associated with the malignancies or with the therapy thereof are subject to the following guidelines:

1) Anemia associated with malignancy

When admission/encounter is for management of an anemia associated with the malignancy, and the treatment is only for anemia, the appropriate anemia code (such as code 285.22, Anemia in neoplastic disease) is designated as the principal diagnosis and is followed by the appropriate code(s) for the malignancy.

Code 285.22 may also be used as a secondary code if the patient suffers from anemia and is being treated for the malignancy.

If anemia in neoplastic disease and anemia due to antineoplastic chemotherapy are both documented, assign codes for both conditions.

2) Anemia associated with chemotherapy, immunotherapy and radiation therapy

When the admission/encounter is for management of an anemia associated with chemotherapy, immunotherapy or radiotherapy and the only treatment is for the anemia, the

anemia is sequenced first. The appropriate neoplasm code should be assigned as an additional code.

3) Management of dehydration due to the malignancy

When the admission/encounter is for management of dehydration due to the malignancy or the therapy, or a combination of both, and only the dehydration is being treated (intravenous rehydration), the dehydration is sequenced first, followed by the code(s) for the malignancy.

4) Treatment of a complication resulting from a surgical procedure

When the admission/encounter is for treatment of a complication resulting from a surgical procedure, designate the complication as the principal or first-listed diagnosis if treatment is directed at resolving the complication.

d. Primary malignancy previously excised

When a primary malignancy has been previously excised or eradicated from its site and there is no further treatment directed to that site and there is no evidence of any existing primary malignancy, a code from category V10, Personal history of malignant neoplasm, should be used to indicate the former site of the malignancy. Any mention of extension, invasion, or metastasis to another site is coded as a secondary malignant neoplasm to that site. The secondary site may be the principal or first-listed with the V10 code used as a secondary code.

e. Admissions/Encounters involving chemotherapy, immunotherapy and radiation therapy

1) Episode of care involves surgical removal of neoplasm

When an episode of care involves the surgical removal of a neoplasm, primary or secondary site, followed by adjunct chemotherapy or radiation treatment during the same episode of care, the neoplasm code should be assigned as principal or first-listed diagnosis, using codes in the 140-198 series or where appropriate in the 200-203 series.

2) Patient admission/encounter solely for administration of chemotherapy, immunotherapy and radiation therapy

If a patient admission/encounter is solely for the administration of chemotherapy, immunotherapy or radiation therapy assign code V58.0, Encounter for radiation therapy, or V58.11, Encounter for antineoplastic chemotherapy, or V58.12, Encounter for antineoplastic immunotherapy as the first-listed or principal diagnosis. If a patient receives more than one of these therapies during the same admission more than one of these codes may be assigned, in any sequence.

The malignancy for which the therapy is being administered should be assigned as a secondary diagnosis.

3) Patient admitted for radiotherapy/chemotherapy and immunotherapy and develops complications

When a patient is admitted for the purpose of radiotherapy, immunotherapy or chemotherapy and develops complications such as uncontrolled nausea and vomiting or dehydration, the principal or first-listed diagnosis is V58.0, Encounter for radiotherapy, or V58.11, Encounter for antineoplastic chemotherapy, or V58.12, Encounter for antineoplastic immunotherapy followed by any codes for the complications.

f. Admission/encounter to determine extent of malignancy

When the reason for admission/encounter is to determine the extent of the malignancy, or for a procedure such as paracentesis or thoracentesis, the primary malignancy or appropriate metastatic site is designated as the principal or first-listed diagnosis, even though chemotherapy or radiotherapy is administered.

g. Symptoms, signs, and ill-defined conditions listed in Chapter 16 associated with neoplasms

Symptoms, signs, and ill-defined conditions listed in Chapter 16 characteristic of, or associated with, an existing primary or secondary site malignancy cannot be used to replace the malignancy as principal or first-listed diagnosis, regardless of the number of admissions or encounters for treatment and care of the neoplasm.

h. Admission/encounter for pain control/management

See Section I.C.6.a.5 for information on coding admission/encounter for pain control/management.

i. Malignant neoplasm associated with transplanted organ

A malignant neoplasm of a transplanted organ should be coded as a transplant complication. Assign first the appropriate code from subcategory 996.8, Complications of transplanted organ, followed by code 199.2, Malignant neoplasm associated with transplanted organ. Use an additional code for the specific malignancy.

3. Chapter 3: Endocrine, Nutritional, and Metabolic Diseases and Immunity Disorders (240-279)

a. Diabetes mellitus

Codes under category 250, Diabetes mellitus, identify complications/manifestations associated with diabetes mellitus. A fifth-digit is required for all category 250 codes to identify the type of diabetes mellitus and whether the diabetes is controlled or uncontrolled.

See I.C.3.a.7 for secondary diabetes

1) Fifth-digits for category 250:

The following are the fifth-digits for the codes under category 250:

0   type II or unspecified type, not stated as uncontrolled

1   type I, [juvenile type], not stated as uncontrolled

2   type II or unspecified type, uncontrolled

3   type I, [juvenile type], uncontrolled

The age of a patient is not the sole determining factor, though most type I diabetics develop the condition before reaching puberty. For this reason type I diabetes mellitus is also referred to as juvenile diabetes.

2) Type of diabetes mellitus not documented

If the type of diabetes mellitus is not documented in the medical record the default is type II.

3) Diabetes mellitus and the use of insulin

All type I diabetics must use insulin to replace what their bodies do not produce. However, the use of insulin does not mean that a patient is a type I diabetic. Some patients with type II diabetes mellitus are unable to control their blood sugar through diet and oral medication alone and do require insulin. If the documentation in a medical record does not indicate the type of diabetes but does indicate that the patient uses insulin, the appropriate fifth-digit for type II must be used. For type II patients who routinely use insulin, code V58.67, Long-term (current) use of insulin, should also be assigned to indicate that the patient uses insulin. Code V58.67 should not be assigned if insulin is given temporarily to bring a type II patient's blood sugar under control during an encounter.

4) Assigning and sequencing diabetes codes and associated conditions

When assigning codes for diabetes and its associated conditions, the code(s) from category 250 must be sequenced before the codes for the associated conditions. The diabetes codes and the secondary codes that correspond to them are paired codes that follow the etiology/manifestation convention of the classification *(See Section I.A.6., Etiology/manifestation convention).* Assign as many codes from category 250 as needed to identify all of the associated conditions that the patient has. The corresponding secondary codes are listed under each of the diabetes codes.

(a) Diabetic retinopathy/diabetic macular edema

Diabetic macular edema, code 362.07, is only present with diabetic retinopathy. Another code from subcategory 362.0, Diabetic retinopathy, must be used with code 362.07. Codes under subcategory 362.0 are diabetes manifestation codes, so they must be used following the appropriate diabetes code.

5) Diabetes mellitus in pregnancy and gestational diabetes

(a) For diabetes mellitus complicating pregnancy, *see Section I.C.11.f., Diabetes mellitus in pregnancy.*

(b) For gestational diabetes, *see Section I.C.11, g., Gestational diabetes.*

6) Insulin pump malfunction

(a) Underdose of insulin due insulin pump failure

An underdose of insulin due to an insulin pump failure should be assigned 996.57, Mechanical complication due to insulin pump, as the principal or first listed code, followed by the appropriate diabetes mellitus code based on documentation.

(b) Overdose of insulin due to insulin pump failure

The principal or first listed code for an encounter due to an insulin pump malfunction resulting in an overdose of insulin, should also be 996.57, Mechanical complication due to insulin pump, followed by code 962.3, Poisoning by insulins and antidiabetic agents, and the appropriate diabetes mellitus code based on documentation.

7) Secondary Diabetes Mellitus

Codes under category 249, Secondary diabetes mellitus, identify complications/manifestations associated with secondary diabetes mellitus. Secondary diabetes is always caused by another condition or event (e.g., cystic fibrosis, malignant neoplasm of pancreas, pancreatectomy, adverse effect of drug, or poisoning).

(a) Fifth-digits for category 249:

A fifth-digit is required for all category 249 codes to identify whether the diabetes is controlled or uncontrolled.

(b) Secondary diabetes mellitus and the use of insulin

For patients who routinely use insulin, code V58.67, Long-term (current) use of insulin, should also be assigned. Code V58.67 should not be assigned if insulin is given temporarily to bring a patient's blood sugar under control during an encounter.

(c) Assigning and sequencing secondary diabetes codes and associated conditions

When assigning codes for secondary diabetes and its associated conditions (e.g. renal manifestations), the code(s) from category 249 must be sequenced before the codes for the associated conditions. The secondary diabetes codes and the diabetic manifestation codes that correspond to them are paired codes that follow the etiology/manifestation convention of the classification. Assign as many codes from category 249 as needed to identify all of the associated conditions that the patient has. The corresponding codes for the associated conditions are listed under each of the secondary diabetes codes. For example, secondary diabetes with diabetic nephrosis is assigned to code 249.40, followed by 581.81.

(d) Assigning and sequencing secondary diabetes codes and its causes

The sequencing of the secondary diabetes codes in relationship to codes for the cause of the diabetes is based on the reason for the encounter, applicable

ICD-9-CM sequencing conventions, and chapter-specific guidelines.

If a patient is seen for treatment of the secondary diabetes or one of its associated conditions, a code from category 249 is sequenced as the principal or first-listed diagnosis, with the cause of the secondary diabetes (e.g. cystic fibrosis) sequenced as an additional diagnosis.

If, however, the patient is seen for the treatment of the condition causing the secondary diabetes (e.g., malignant neoplasm of pancreas), the code for the cause of the secondary diabetes should be sequenced as the principal or first-listed diagnosis followed by a code from category 249.

(i) Secondary diabetes mellitus due to pancreatectomy

For postpancreatectomy diabetes mellitus (lack of insulin due to the surgical removal of all or part of the pancreas), assign code 251.3, Postsurgical hypoinsulinemia. Assign a code from subcategory 249, Secondary diabetes mellitus and a code from subcategory V88.1, Acquired absence of pancreas as additional codes. Code also any diabetic manifestations (e.g. diabetic nephrosis 581.81).

(ii) Secondary diabetes due to drugs

Secondary diabetes may be caused by an adverse effect of correctly administered medications, poisoning or late effect of poisoning.

See section I.C.17.e for coding of adverse effects and poisoning, and section I.C.19 for E code reporting.

4. Chapter 4: Diseases of Blood and Blood Forming Organs (280-289)

a. Anemia of chronic disease

Subcategory 285.2, Anemia in chronic illness, has codes for anemia in chronic kidney disease, code 285.21; anemia in neoplastic disease, code 285.22; and anemia in other chronic illness, code 285.29. These codes can be used as the principal/first listed code if the reason for the encounter is to treat the anemia. They may also be used as secondary codes if treatment of the anemia is a component of an encounter, but not the primary reason for the encounter. When using a code from subcategory 285 it is also necessary to use the code for the chronic condition causing the anemia.

1) Anemia in chronic kidney disease

When assigning code 285.21, Anemia in chronic kidney disease, it is also necessary to assign a code from category 585, Chronic kidney disease, to indicate the stage of chronic kidney disease.

See I.C.10.a. Chronic kidney disease (CKD).

2) Anemia in neoplastic disease

When assigning code 285.22, Anemia in neoplastic disease, it is also necessary to assign the neoplasm code that is responsible for the anemia. Code 285.22 is for use for anemia that is due to the malignancy, not for anemia due to antineoplastic chemotherapy drugs. Assign the appropriate code for anemia due to antineoplastic chemotherapy.

See I.C.2.c.1 Anemia associated with malignancy.

See I.C.2.c.2 Anemia associated with chemotherapy, immunotherapy and radiation therapy.

5. Chapter 5: Mental Disorders (290-319)

Reserved for future guideline expansion

6. Chapter 6: Diseases of Nervous System and Sense Organs (320-389)

a. Pain - Category 338

1) General coding information

Codes in category 338 may be used in conjunction with codes from other categories and chapters to provide more detail about acute or chronic pain and neoplasm-related pain, unless otherwise indicated below.

If the pain is not specified as acute or chronic, do not assign codes from category 338, except for post-thoracotomy pain, postoperative pain, neoplasm related pain, or central pain syndrome.

A code from subcategories 338.1 and 338.2 should not be assigned if the underlying (definitive) diagnosis is known, unless the reason for the encounter is pain control/management and not management of the underlying condition.

(a) Category 338 Codes as Principal or First-Listed Diagnosis

Category 338 codes are acceptable as principal diagnosis or the first-listed code:

- When pain control or pain management is the reason for the admission/encounter (e.g., a patient with displaced intervertebral disc, nerve impingement and severe back pain presents for injection of steroid into the spinal canal). The underlying cause of the pain should be reported as an additional diagnosis, if known.

- When an admission or encounter is for a procedure aimed at treating the underlying condition (e.g., spinal fusion, kyphoplasty), a code for the underlying condition (e.g., vertebral fracture, spinal stenosis) should be assigned as the principal diagnosis. No code from category 338 should be assigned.

- When a patient is admitted for the insertion of a neurostimulator for pain control, assign the appropriate pain code as the principal or first listed diagnosis. When an admission or encounter is for a procedure aimed at treating the underlying condition and a neurostimulator is inserted for pain control during the same admission/encounter, a code for the underlying condition should be assigned as the principal diagnosis and the appropriate pain code should be assigned as a secondary diagnosis.

(b) Use of Category 338 Codes in Conjunction with Site Specific Pain Codes

(i) Assigning Category 338 Codes and Site-Specific Pain Codes

Codes from category 338 may be used in conjunction with codes that identify the site of pain (including codes from chapter 16) if the category 338 code provides additional information. For example, if the code describes the site of the pain, but does not fully describe whether the pain is acute or chronic, then both codes should be assigned.

(ii) Sequencing of Category 338 Codes with Site-Specific Pain Codes

The sequencing of category 338 codes with site-specific pain codes (including chapter 16 codes), is dependent on the circumstances of the encounter/admission as follows:

- If the encounter is for pain control or pain management, assign the code from category 338 followed by the code identifying the specific site of pain (e.g., encounter for pain management for acute neck pain from trauma is assigned code 338.11, Acute pain due to trauma, followed by code 723.1, Cervicalgia, to identify the site of pain).

- If the encounter is for any other reason except pain control or pain management, and a related definitive diagnosis has not been established (confirmed) by the provider, assign the code for the specific site of pain first, followed by the appropriate code from category 338.

2) Pain due to devices, implants and grafts

Pain associated with devices, implants or grafts left in a surgical site (for example painful hip prosthesis) is assigned to the appropriate code(s) found in Chapter 17, Injury and Poisoning. Use additional code(s) from category 338 to identify acute or chronic pain due to presence of the device, implant or graft (338.18-338.19 or 338.28-338.29).

3) Postoperative Pain

Post-thoracotomy pain and other postoperative pain are classified to subcategories 338.1 and 338.2, depending on whether the pain is acute or chronic. The default for post-thoracotomy and other postoperative pain not specified as acute or chronic is the code for the acute form.

Routine or expected postoperative pain immediately after surgery should not be coded.

(a) Postoperative pain not associated with specific postoperative complication

Postoperative pain not associated with a specific postoperative complication is assigned to the appropriate postoperative pain code in category 338.

(b) Postoperative pain associated with specific postoperative complication

Postoperative pain associated with a specific postoperative complication (such as painful wire sutures) is assigned to the appropriate code(s) found in Chapter 17, Injury and Poisoning. If appropriate, use additional code(s) from category 338 to identify acute or chronic pain (338.18 or 338.28). If pain control/management is the reason for the encounter, a code from category 338 should be assigned as the principal or first-listed diagnosis in accordance with *Section I.C.6.a.1.a above.*

(c) Postoperative pain as principal or first-listed diagnosis

Postoperative pain may be reported as the principal or first-listed diagnosis when the stated reason for the admission/encounter is documented as postoperative pain control/ management.

(d) Postoperative pain as secondary diagnosis

Postoperative pain may be reported as a secondary diagnosis code when a patient presents for outpatient surgery and develops an unusual or inordinate amount of postoperative pain.

The provider's documentation should be used to guide the coding of postoperative pain, as well as *Section III. Reporting Additional Diagnoses and Section IV. Diagnostic Coding and Reporting in the Outpatient Setting.*

See Section II.I.2 for information on sequencing of diagnoses for patients admitted to hospital inpatient care following post-operative observation.

See Section II.J for information on sequencing of diagnoses for patients admitted to hospital inpatient care from outpatient surgery.

See Section IV.A.2 for information on sequencing of diagnoses for patients admitted for observation.

4) Chronic pain

Chronic pain is classified to subcategory 338.2. There is no time frame defining when pain becomes chronic pain. The provider's documentation should be used to guide use of these codes.

5) Neoplasm Related Pain

Code 338.3 is assigned to pain documented as being related, associated or due to cancer, primary or secondary malignancy, or tumor. This code is assigned regardless of whether the pain is acute or chronic.

This code may be assigned as the principal or first-listed code when the stated reason for the admission/encounter is documented as pain control/pain management. The underlying neoplasm should be reported as an additional diagnosis.

When the reason for the admission/encounter is management of the neoplasm and the pain associated with the neoplasm is also documented, code 338.3 may be assigned as an additional diagnosis.

See Section I.C.2 for instructions on the sequencing of neoplasms for all other stated reasons for the admission/encounter (except for pain control/pain management).

6) Chronic pain syndrome

This condition is different than the term "chronic pain," and therefore this code should only be used when the provider has specifically documented this condition.

b. Glaucoma

1) Glaucoma

For types of glaucoma classified to subcategories 365.1-365.6, an additional code should be assigned from subcategory 365.7, Glaucoma stage, to identify the glaucoma stage. Codes from 365.7, Glaucoma stage, may not be assigned as a principal or first-listed diagnosis.

2) Bilateral glaucoma with same stage

When a patient has bilateral glaucoma and both are documented as being the same type and stage, report only the code for the type of glaucoma and one code for the stage.

3) Bilateral glaucoma stage with different stages

When a patient has bilateral glaucoma and each eye is documented as having a different stage, assign one code for the type of glaucoma and one code for the highest glaucoma stage.

4) Bilateral glaucoma with different types and different stages

When a patient has bilateral glaucoma and each eye is documented as having a different type and a different stage, assign one code for each type of glaucoma and one code for the highest glaucoma stage.

5) Patient admitted with glaucoma and stage evolves during the admission

If a patient is admitted with glaucoma and the stage progresses during the admission, assign the code for highest stage documented.

6) Indeterminate stage glaucoma

Assignment of code 365.74, Indeterminate stage glaucoma, should be based on the clinical documentation. Code 365.74 is used for glaucoma whose stage cannot be clinically determined. This code should not be confused with code 365.70, Glaucoma stage, unspecified. Code 365.70 should be assigned when there is no documentation regarding the stage of the glaucoma.

7. Chapter 7: Diseases of Circulatory System (390-459)

a. Hypertension

Hypertension Table

The Hypertension Table, found under the main term, "Hypertension", in the Alphabetic Index, contains a complete listing of all conditions due to or associated with hypertension and classifies them according to malignant, benign, and unspecified.

1) Hypertension, Essential, or NOS

Assign hypertension (arterial) (essential) (primary) (systemic) (NOS) to category code 401 with the appropriate fourth digit to indicate malignant (.0), benign (.1), or unspecified (.9). Do not use either .0 malignant or .1 benign unless medical record documentation supports such a designation.

2) Hypertension with Heart Disease

Heart conditions (425.8, 429.0-429.3, 429.8, 429.9) are assigned to a code from category 402 when a causal relationship is stated (due to hypertension) or implied (hypertensive). Use an additional code from category 428 to identify the type of heart failure in those patients with heart failure. More than one code from category 428 may be assigned if the patient has systolic or diastolic failure and congestive heart failure.

The same heart conditions (425.8, 429.0-429.3, 429.8, 429.9) with hypertension, but without a stated causal relationship, are coded separately. Sequence according to the circumstances of the admission/encounter.

3) Hypertensive Chronic Kidney Disease

Assign codes from category 403, Hypertensive chronic kidney disease, when conditions classified to category 585 or code 587 are present with hypertension. Unlike hypertension with heart disease, ICD-9-CM presumes a cause-and-effect relationship and classifies chronic kidney disease (CKD) with hypertension as hypertensive chronic kidney disease.

Fifth digits for category 403 should be assigned as follows:

- 0 with CKD stage I through stage IV, or unspecified.
- 1 with CKD stage V or end stage renal disease.

The appropriate code from category 585, Chronic kidney disease, should be used as a secondary code with a code from category 403 to identify the stage of chronic kidney disease.

See Section I.C.10.a for information on the coding of chronic kidney disease.

4) Hypertensive Heart and Chronic Kidney Disease

Assign codes from combination category 404, Hypertensive heart and chronic kidney disease, when both hypertensive kidney disease and hypertensive heart disease are stated in the diagnosis. Assume a relationship between the hypertension and the chronic kidney disease, whether or not the condition is so designated. Assign an additional code from category 428, to identify the type of heart failure. More than one code from category 428 may be assigned if the patient has systolic or diastolic failure and congestive heart failure.

Fifth digits for category 404 should be assigned as follows:

- 0 without heart failure and with chronic kidney disease (CKD) stage I through stage IV, or unspecified
- 1 with heart failure and with CKD stage I through stage IV, or unspecified
- 2 without heart failure and with CKD stage V or end stage renal disease
- 3 with heart failure and with CKD stage V or end stage renal disease

The appropriate code from category 585, Chronic kidney disease, should be used as a secondary code with a code from category 404 to identify the stage of kidney disease.

See Section I.C.10.a for information on the coding of chronic kidney disease.

5) Hypertensive Cerebrovascular Disease

First assign codes from 430-438, Cerebrovascular disease, then the appropriate hypertension code from categories 401-405.

6) Hypertensive Retinopathy

Two codes are necessary to identify the condition. First assign the code from subcategory 362.11, Hypertensive retinopathy, then the appropriate code from categories 401-405 to indicate the type of hypertension.

7) Hypertension, Secondary

Two codes are required: one to identify the underlying etiology and one from category 405 to identify the hypertension. Sequencing of codes is determined by the reason for admission/encounter.

8) Hypertension, Transient

Assign code 796.2, Elevated blood pressure reading without diagnosis of hypertension, unless patient has an established diagnosis of hypertension. Assign code 642.3x for transient hypertension of pregnancy.

9) Hypertension, Controlled

Assign appropriate code from categories 401-405. This diagnostic statement usually refers to an existing state of hypertension under control by therapy.

10) Hypertension, Uncontrolled

Uncontrolled hypertension may refer to untreated hypertension or hypertension not responding to current therapeutic regimen. In either case, assign the appropriate code from categories 401-405 to designate the stage and type of hypertension. Code to the type of hypertension.

11) Elevated Blood Pressure

For a statement of elevated blood pressure without further specificity, assign code 796.2, Elevated blood pressure reading without diagnosis of hypertension, rather than a code from category 401.

b. Cerebral infarction/stroke/cerebrovascular accident (CVA)

The terms stroke and CVA are often used interchangeably to refer to a cerebral infarction. The terms stroke, CVA, and cerebral infarction NOS are all indexed to the default code 434.91, Cerebral artery occlusion, unspecified, with infarction.

Additional code(s) should be assigned for any neurologic deficits associated with the acute CVA, regardless of whether or not the neurologic deficit resolves prior to discharge.

See Section I.C.18.d.3 for information on coding status post administration of tPA in a different facility within the last 24 hours.

c. Postoperative cerebrovascular accident

A cerebrovascular hemorrhage or infarction that occurs as a result of medical intervention is coded to 997.02, Iatrogenic cerebrovascular infarction or hemorrhage. Medical record documentation should clearly specify the cause- and-effect relationship between the medical intervention and the cerebrovascular accident in order to assign this code. A secondary code from the code range 430-432 or from a code from subcategories 433 or 434 with a fifth digit of "1" should also be used to identify the type of hemorrhage or infarct.

This guideline conforms to the use additional code note instruction at category 997. Code 436, Acute, but ill-defined, cerebrovascular disease, should not be used as a secondary code with code 997.02.

d. Late Effects of Cerebrovascular Disease

1) Category 438, Late Effects of Cerebrovascular disease

Category 438 is used to indicate conditions classifiable to categories 430-437 as the causes of late effects (neurologic deficits), themselves classified elsewhere. These "late effects" include neurologic deficits that persist after initial onset of conditions classifiable to 430-437. The neurologic deficits caused by cerebrovascular disease may be present from the onset or may arise at any time after the onset of the condition classifiable to 430-437.

Codes in category 438 are only for use for late effects of cerebrovascular disease, not for neurologic deficits associated with an acute CVA.

2) Codes from category 438 with codes from 430-437

Codes from category 438 may be assigned on a health care record with codes from 430-437, if the patient has a current cerebrovascular accident (CVA) and deficits from an old CVA.

3)   Code V12.54

Assign code V12.54, Transient ischemic attack (TIA), and cerebral infarction without residual deficits (and not a code from category 438) as an additional code for history of cerebrovascular disease when no neurologic deficits are present.

e.   Acute myocardial infarction (AMI)

1)   ST elevation myocardial infarction (STEMI) and non ST elevation myocardial infarction (NSTEMI)

The ICD-9-CM codes for acute myocardial infarction (AMI) identify the site, such as anterolateral wall or true posterior wall. Subcategories 410.0-410.6 and 410.8 are used for ST elevation myocardial infarction (STEMI). Subcategory 410.7, Subendocardial infarction, is used for non ST elevation myocardial infarction (NSTEMI) and nontransmural MIs.

2)   Acute myocardial infarction, unspecified

Subcategory 410.9 is the default for the unspecified term acute myocardial infarction. If only STEMI or transmural MI without the site is documented, query the provider as to the site, or assign a code from subcategory 410.9.

3)   AMI documented as nontransmural or subendocardial but site provided

If an AMI is documented as nontransmural or subendocardial, but the site is provided, it is still coded as a subendocardial AMI. If NSTEMI evolves to STEMI, assign the STEMI code. If STEMI converts to NSTEMI due to thrombolytic therapy, it is still coded as STEMI.

See Section I.C.18.d.3 for information on coding status post administration of tPA in a different facility within the last 24 hours.

8.   Chapter 8: Diseases of Respiratory System (460-519)

See I.C.17.f. for ventilator-associated pneumonia.

a.   Chronic Obstructive Pulmonary Disease [COPD] and Asthma

1)   Conditions that comprise COPD and Asthma

The conditions that comprise COPD are obstructive chronic bronchitis, subcategory 491.2, and emphysema, category 492. All asthma codes are under category 493, Asthma. Code 496, Chronic airway obstruction, not elsewhere classified, is a nonspecific code that should only be used when the documentation in a medical record does not specify the type of COPD being treated.

2)   Acute exacerbation of chronic obstructive bronchitis and asthma

The codes for chronic obstructive bronchitis and asthma distinguish between uncomplicated cases and those in acute exacerbation. An acute exacerbation is a worsening or a decompensation of a chronic condition. An acute exacerbation is not equivalent to an infection superimposed on a chronic condition, though an exacerbation may be triggered by an infection.

3)   Overlapping nature of the conditions that comprise COPD and asthma

Due to the overlapping nature of the conditions that make up COPD and asthma, there are many variations in the way these conditions are documented. Code selection must be based on the terms as documented. When selecting the correct code for the documented type of COPD and asthma, it is essential to first review the index, and then verify the code in the tabular list. There are many instructional notes under the different COPD subcategories and codes. It is important that all such notes be reviewed to assure correct code assignment.

4)   Acute exacerbation of asthma and status asthmaticus

An acute exacerbation of asthma is an increased severity of the asthma symptoms, such as wheezing and shortness of breath. Status asthmaticus refers to a patient's failure to respond to therapy administered during an asthmatic episode and is a life threatening complication that requires emergency care. If status asthmaticus is documented by the provider with any type of COPD or with acute bronchitis, the status asthmaticus should be sequenced first. It supersedes any type of COPD including that with acute exacerbation or acute bronchitis. It is inappropriate to assign an asthma code with 5th digit 2, with acute exacerbation, together with an asthma code with 5th digit 1, with status asthmatics. Only the 5th digit 1 should be assigned.

b.   Chronic Obstructive Pulmonary Disease [COPD] and Bronchitis

1)   Acute bronchitis with COPD

Acute bronchitis, code 466.0, is due to an infectious organism. When acute bronchitis is documented with COPD, code 491.22, Obstructive chronic bronchitis with acute bronchitis, should be assigned. It is not necessary to also assign code 466.0. If a medical record documents acute bronchitis with COPD with acute exacerbation, only code 491.22 should be assigned. The acute bronchitis included in code 491.22 supersedes the acute exacerbation. If a medical record documents COPD with acute exacerbation without mention of acute bronchitis, only code 491.21 should be assigned.

c.   Acute Respiratory Failure

1)   Acute respiratory failure as principal diagnosis

Code 518.81, Acute respiratory failure, may be assigned as a principal diagnosis when it is the condition established after study to be chiefly responsible for occasioning the admission to the hospital, and the selection is supported by the Alphabetic Index and Tabular List. However, chapter-specific coding guidelines (such as obstetrics, poisoning, HIV, newborn) that provide sequencing direction take precedence.

2)   Acute respiratory failure as secondary diagnosis

Respiratory failure may be listed as a secondary diagnosis if it occurs after admission, or if it is present on admission, but does not meet the definition of principal diagnosis.

3)   Sequencing of acute respiratory failure and another acute condition

When a patient is admitted with respiratory failure and another acute condition, (e.g., myocardial infarction, cerebrovascular accident, aspiration pneumonia), the principal diagnosis will not be the same in every situation. This applies whether the other acute condition is a respiratory or nonrespiratory condition. Selection of the principal diagnosis will be dependent on the circumstances of admission. If both the respiratory failure and the other acute condition are equally responsible for occasioning the admission to the hospital, and there are no chapter-specific sequencing rules, the guideline regarding two or more diagnoses that equally meet the definition for principal diagnosis *(Section II, C.)* may be applied in these situations.

If the documentation is not clear as to whether acute respiratory failure and another condition are equally responsible for occasioning the admission, query the provider for clarification.

d.   Influenza due to certain identified viruses

Code only confirmed cases of avian influenza (codes 488.01-488.02, 488.09, Influenza due to identified avian influenza virus), 2009 H1N1 influenza virus (codes 488.11-488.12, 488.19), or novel influenza A (codes 488.81-488.82, 488.89, Influenza due to identified novel influenza A virus). This is an exception to the hospital inpatient guideline Section II, H. (Uncertain Diagnosis).

In this context, "confirmation" does not require documentation of positive laboratory testing specific for avian, 2009 H1N1 or novel influenza A virus. However, coding should be based on the provider's diagnostic statement that the patient has avian influenza, 2009 H1N1 influenza, or novel influenza A.

If the provider records "suspected" or "possible" or "probable" avian, 2009 H1N1, or novel influenza A, the appropriate influenza code from category 487, Influenza should be assigned. A code from category 488, Influenza due to certain identified influenza viruses, should not be assigned.

9. **Chapter 9: Diseases of Digestive System (520-579)**

Reserved for future guideline expansion

10. **Chapter 10: Diseases of Genitourinary System (580-629)**

a. **Chronic kidney disease**

1) **Stages of chronic kidney disease (CKD)**

The ICD-9-CM classifies CKD based on severity. The severity of CKD is designated by stages I-V. Stage II, code 585.2, equates to mild CKD; stage III, code 585.3, equates to moderate CKD; and stage IV, code 585.4, equates to severe CKD. Code 585.6, End stage renal disease (ESRD), is assigned when the provider has documented end-stage-renal disease (ESRD).

If both a stage of CKD and ESRD are documented, assign code 585.6 only.

2) **Chronic kidney disease and kidney transplant status**

Patients who have undergone kidney transplant may still have some form of CKD, because the kidney transplant may not fully restore kidney function. Therefore, the presence of CKD alone does not constitute a transplant complication. Assign the appropriate 585 code for the patient's stage of CKD and code V42.0. If a transplant complication such as failure or rejection is documented, see section I.C.17.f.2.b for information on coding complications of a kidney transplant. If the documentation is unclear as to whether the patient has a complication of the transplant, query the provider.

3) **Chronic kidney disease with other conditions**

Patients with CKD may also suffer from other serious conditions, most commonly diabetes mellitus and hypertension. The sequencing of the CKD code in relationship to codes for other contributing conditions is based on the conventions in the tabular list.

See I.C.3.a.4 for sequencing instructions for diabetes.
See I.C.4.a.1 for anemia in CKD.
See I.C.7.a.3 for hypertensive chronic kidney disease.
See I.C.17.f.2.b, Kidney transplant complications, for instructions on coding of documented rejection or failure.

11. **Chapter 11: Complications of Pregnancy, Childbirth, and the Puerperium (630-679)**

a. **General Rules for Obstetric Cases**

1) **Codes from chapter 11 and sequencing priority**

Obstetric cases require codes from chapter 11, codes in the range 630-679, Complications of Pregnancy, Childbirth, and the Puerperium. Chapter 11 codes have sequencing priority over codes from other chapters. Additional codes from other chapters may be used in conjunction with chapter 11 codes to further specify conditions. Should the provider document that the pregnancy is incidental to the encounter, then code V22.2 should be used in place of any chapter 11 codes. It is the provider's responsibility to state that the condition being treated is not affecting the pregnancy.

2) **Chapter 11 codes used only on the maternal record**

Chapter 11 codes are to be used only on the maternal record, never on the record of the newborn.

3) **Chapter 11 fifth-digits**

Categories 640-648, 651-676 have required fifth-digits, which indicate whether the encounter is antepartum, postpartum and whether a delivery has also occurred.

4) **Fifth-digits, appropriate for each code**

The fifth-digits, which are appropriate for each code number, are listed in brackets under each code. The fifth-digits on each code should all be consistent with each other. That is, should a delivery occur all of the fifth-digits should indicate the delivery.

b. **Selection of OB Principal or First-listed Diagnosis**

1) **Routine outpatient prenatal visits**

For routine outpatient prenatal visits when no complications are present codes V22.0, Supervision of normal first pregnancy, and V22.1, Supervision of other normal pregnancy, should be used as the first-listed diagnoses. These codes should not be used in conjunction with chapter 11 codes.

2) **Prenatal outpatient visits for high-risk patients**

For routine prenatal outpatient visits for patients with high-risk pregnancies, a code from category V23, Supervision of high-risk pregnancy, should be used as the first-listed diagnosis. Secondary chapter 11 codes may be used in conjunction with these codes if appropriate.

3) **Episodes when no delivery occurs**

In episodes when no delivery occurs, the principal diagnosis should correspond to the principal complication of the pregnancy, which necessitated the encounter. Should more than one complication exist, all of which are treated or monitored, any of the complications codes may be sequenced first.

4) **When a delivery occurs**

When a delivery occurs, the principal diagnosis should correspond to the main circumstances or complication of the delivery. In cases of cesarean delivery, the selection of the principal diagnosis should be the condition established after study that was responsible for the patient's admission. If the patient was admitted with a condition that resulted in the performance of a cesarean procedure, that condition should be selected as the principal diagnosis. If the reason for the admission/encounter was unrelated to the condition resulting in the cesarean delivery, the condition related to the reason for the admission/encounter should be selected as the principal diagnosis, even if a cesarean was performed.

5) **Outcome of delivery**

An outcome of delivery code, V27.0-V27.9, should be included on every maternal record when a delivery has occurred. These codes are not to be used on subsequent records or on the newborn record.

c. **Fetal Conditions Affecting the Management of the Mother**

1) **Codes from categories 655 and 656**

Codes from categories 655, Known or suspected fetal abnormality affecting management of the mother, and 656, Other known or suspected fetal and placental problems affecting the management of the mother, are assigned only when the fetal condition is actually responsible for modifying the management of the mother, i.e., by requiring diagnostic studies, additional observation, special care, or termination of pregnancy. The fact that the fetal condition exists does not justify assigning a code from this series to the mother's record.

See I.C.18.d. for suspected maternal and fetal conditions not found

2) **In utero surgery**

In cases when surgery is performed on the fetus, a diagnosis code from category 655, Known or suspected fetal abnormalities affecting management of the mother, should be assigned identifying the fetal condition. Procedure code 75.36, Correction of fetal defect, should be assigned on the hospital inpatient record.

No code from Chapter 15, the perinatal codes, should be used on the mother's record to identify fetal conditions. Surgery performed in utero on a fetus is still to be coded as an obstetric encounter.

d. **HIV Infection in Pregnancy, Childbirth and the Puerperium**

During pregnancy, childbirth or the puerperium, a patient admitted because of an HIV-related illness should receive a principal diagnosis of 647.6x, Other specified infectious and parasitic diseases in the mother classifiable elsewhere, but complicating the pregnancy, childbirth or the puerperium, followed by 042 and the code(s) for the HIV-related illness(es).

Patients with asymptomatic HIV infection status admitted during pregnancy, childbirth, or the puerperium should receive codes of 647.6x and V08.

e. Current Conditions Complicating Pregnancy

Assign a code from subcategory 648.x for patients that have current conditions when the condition affects the management of the pregnancy, childbirth, or the puerperium. Use additional secondary codes from other chapters to identify the conditions, as appropriate.

f. Diabetes mellitus in pregnancy

Diabetes mellitus is a significant complicating factor in pregnancy. Pregnant women who are diabetic should be assigned code 648.0x, Diabetes mellitus complicating pregnancy, and a secondary code from category 250, Diabetes mellitus, or category 249, Secondary diabetes to identify the type of diabetes.

Code V58.67, Long-term (current) use of insulin, should also be assigned if the diabetes mellitus is being treated with insulin.

g. Gestational diabetes

Gestational diabetes can occur during the second and third trimester of pregnancy in women who were not diabetic prior to pregnancy. Gestational diabetes can cause complications in the pregnancy similar to those of pre-existing diabetes mellitus. It also puts the woman at greater risk of developing diabetes after the pregnancy. Gestational diabetes is coded to 648.8x, Abnormal glucose tolerance. Codes 648.0x and 648.8x should never be used together on the same record.

Code V58.67, Long-term (current) use of insulin, should also be assigned if the gestational diabetes is being treated with insulin.

h. Normal Delivery, Code 650

1) Normal delivery

Code 650 is for use in cases when a woman is admitted for a full-term normal delivery and delivers a single, healthy infant without any complications antepartum, during the delivery, or postpartum during the delivery episode. Code 650 is always a principal diagnosis. It is not to be used if any other code from chapter 11 is needed to describe a current complication of the antenatal, delivery, or perinatal period. Additional codes from other chapters may be used with code 650 if they are not related to or are in any way complicating the pregnancy.

2) Normal delivery with resolved antepartum complication

Code 650 may be used if the patient had a complication at some point during her pregnancy, but the complication is not present at the time of the admission for delivery.

3) V27.0, Single liveborn, outcome of delivery

V27.0, Single liveborn, is the only outcome of delivery code appropriate for use with 650.

i. The Postpartum and Peripartum Periods

1) Postpartum and peripartum periods

The postpartum period begins immediately after delivery and continues for six weeks following delivery. The peripartum period is defined as the last month of pregnancy to five months postpartum.

2) Postpartum complication

A postpartum complication is any complication occurring within the six-week period.

3) Pregnancy-related complications after 6 week period

Chapter 11 codes may also be used to describe pregnancy-related complications after the six-week period should the provider document that a condition is pregnancy related.

4) Postpartum complications occurring during the same admission as delivery

Postpartum complications that occur during the same admission as the delivery are identified with a fifth digit of "2." Subsequent admissions/encounters for postpartum complications should be identified with a fifth digit of "4."

5) Admission for routine postpartum care following delivery outside hospital

When the mother delivers outside the hospital prior to admission and is admitted for routine postpartum care and no complications are noted, code V24.0, Postpartum care and examination immediately after delivery, should be assigned as the principal diagnosis.

6) Admission following delivery outside hospital with postpartum conditions

A delivery diagnosis code should not be used for a woman who has delivered prior to admission to the hospital. Any postpartum conditions and/or postpartum procedures should be coded.

7) Puerperal sepsis

Code 670.2x, Puerperal sepsis, should be assigned with a secondary code to identify the causal organism (e.g., for a bacterial infection, assign a code from category 041, Bacterial infections in conditions classified elsewhere and of unspecified site). A code from category 038, Septicemia, should not be used for puerperal sepsis. Do not assign code 995.91, Sepsis, as code 670.2x describes the sepsis. If applicable, use additional codes to identify severe sepsis (995.92) and any associated acute organ dysfunction.

j. Code 677, Late effect of complication of pregnancy

1) Code 677

Code 677, Late effect of complication of pregnancy, childbirth, and the puerperium is for use in those cases when an initial complication of a pregnancy develops a sequelae requiring care or treatment at a future date.

2) After the initial postpartum period

This code may be used at any time after the initial postpartum period.

3) Sequencing of Code 677

This code, like all late effect codes, is to be sequenced following the code describing the sequelae of the complication.

k. Abortions

1) Fifth-digits required for abortion categories

Fifth-digits are required for abortion categories 634-637. Fifth digit assignment is based on the status of the patient at the beginning (or start) of the encounter. Fifth-digit 1, incomplete, indicates that all of the products of conception have not been expelled from the uterus. Fifth-digit 2, complete, indicates that all products of conception have been expelled from the uterus.

2) Code from categories 640-648 and 651-659

A code from categories 640-648 and 651-659 may be used as additional codes with an abortion code to indicate the complication leading to the abortion.

Fifth digit 3 is assigned with codes from these categories when used with an abortion code because the other fifth digits will not apply. Codes from the 660-669 series are not to be used for complications of abortion.

3) Code 639 for complications

Code 639 is to be used for all complications following abortion. Code 639 cannot be assigned with codes from categories 634-638.

4) Abortion with Liveborn Fetus

When an attempted termination of pregnancy results in a liveborn fetus assign code 644.21, Early onset of delivery, with an appropriate code from category V27, Outcome of Delivery. The procedure code for the attempted termination of pregnancy should also be assigned.

5) Retained Products of Conception following an abortion

Subsequent admissions for retained products of conception following a spontaneous or legally induced abortion are assigned the appropriate code from category 634, Spontaneous abortion, or 635 Legally induced abortion, with a fifth digit of "1" (incomplete). This advice is appropriate even when the patient was discharged previously with a discharge diagnosis of complete abortion.

12. Chapter 12: Diseases Skin and Subcutaneous Tissue (680-709)

a. Pressure ulcer stage codes

1) Pressure ulcer stages

Two codes are needed to completely describe a pressure ulcer: A code from subcategory 707.0, Pressure ulcer, to identify the site of the pressure ulcer and a code from subcategory 707.2, Pressure ulcer stages.

The codes in subcategory 707.2, Pressure ulcer stages, are to be used as an additional diagnosis with a code(s) from subcategory 707.0, Pressure Ulcer. Codes from 707.2, Pressure ulcer stages, may not be assigned as a principal or first-listed diagnosis. The pressure ulcer stage codes should only be used with pressure ulcers and not with other types of ulcers (e.g., stasis ulcer).

The ICD-9-CM classifies pressure ulcer stages based on severity, which is designated by stages I-IV and unstageable.

2) Unstageable pressure ulcers

Assignment of code 707.25, Pressure ulcer, unstageable, should be based on the clinical documentation. Code 707.25 is used for pressure ulcers whose stage cannot be clinically determined (e.g., the ulcer is covered by eschar or has been treated with a skin or muscle graft) and pressure ulcers that are documented as deep tissue injury but not documented as due to trauma. This code should not be confused with code 707.20, Pressure ulcer, stage unspecified. Code 707.20 should be assigned when there is no documentation regarding the stage of the pressure ulcer.

3) Documented pressure ulcer stage

Assignment of the pressure ulcer stage code should be guided by clinical documentation of the stage or documentation of the terms found in the index. For clinical terms describing the stage that are not found in the index, and there is no documentation of the stage, the provider should be queried.

4) Bilateral pressure ulcers with same stage

When a patient has bilateral pressure ulcers (e.g., both buttocks) and both pressure ulcers are documented as being the same stage, only the code for the site and one code for the stage should be reported.

5) Bilateral pressure ulcers with different stages

When a patient has bilateral pressure ulcers at the same site (e.g., both buttocks) and each pressure ulcer is documented as being at a different stage, assign one code for the site and the appropriate codes for the pressure ulcer stage.

6) Multiple pressure ulcers of different sites and stages

When a patient has multiple pressure ulcers at different sites (e.g., buttock, heel, shoulder) and each pressure ulcer is documented as being at different stages (e.g., stage 3 and stage 4), assign the appropriate codes for each different site and a code for each different pressure ulcer stage.

7) Patients admitted with pressure ulcers documented as healed

No code is assigned if the documentation states that the pressure ulcer is completely healed.

8) Patients admitted with pressure ulcers documented as healing

Pressure ulcers described as healing should be assigned the appropriate pressure ulcer stage code based on the documentation in the medical record. If the documentation does not provide information about the stage of the healing pressure ulcer, assign code 707.20, Pressure ulcer stage, unspecified.

If the documentation is unclear as to whether the patient has a current (new) pressure ulcer or if the patient is being treated for a healing pressure ulcer, query the provider.

9) Patient admitted with pressure ulcer evolving into another stage during the admission

If a patient is admitted with a pressure ulcer at one stage and it progresses to a higher stage, assign the code for highest stage reported for that site.

13. Chapter 13: Diseases of Musculoskeletal and Connective Tissue (710-739)

a. Coding of Pathologic Fractures

1) Acute Fractures vs. Aftercare

Pathologic fractures are reported using subcategory 733.1, when the fracture is newly diagnosed. Subcategory 733.1 may be used while the patient is receiving active treatment for the fracture. Examples of active treatment are: surgical treatment, emergency department encounter, evaluation and treatment by a new physician.

Fractures are coded using the aftercare codes (subcategories V54.0, V54.2, V54.8 or V54.9) for encounters after the patient has completed active treatment of the fracture and is receiving routine care for the fracture during the healing or recovery phase. Examples of fracture aftercare are: cast change or removal, removal of external or internal fixation device, medication adjustment, and follow up visits following fracture treatment.

Care for complications of surgical treatment for fracture repairs during the healing or recovery phase should be coded with the appropriate complication codes.

Care of complications of fractures, such as malunion and nonunion, should be reported with the appropriate codes.

See Section I. C. 17.b for information on the coding of traumatic fractures.

14. Chapter 14: Congenital Anomalies (740-759)

a. Codes in categories 740-759, Congenital Anomalies

Assign an appropriate code(s) from categories 740-759, Congenital Anomalies, when an anomaly is documented. A congenital anomaly may be the principal/first listed diagnosis on a record or a secondary diagnosis.

When a congenital anomaly does not have a unique code assignment, assign additional code(s) for any manifestations that may be present.

When the code assignment specifically identifies the congenital anomaly, manifestations that are an inherent component of the anomaly should not be coded separately. Additional codes should be assigned for manifestations that are not an inherent component.

Codes from Chapter 14 may be used throughout the life of the patient. If a congenital anomaly has been corrected, a personal history code should be used to identify the history of the anomaly. Although present at birth, a congenital anomaly may not be identified until later in life. Whenever the condition is diagnosed by the physician, it is appropriate to assign a code from codes 740-759.

For the birth admission, the appropriate code from category V30, Liveborn infants, according to type of birth should be sequenced as the principal diagnosis, followed by any congenital anomaly codes, 740-759.

15. Chapter 15: Newborn (Perinatal) Guidelines (760-779)

For coding and reporting purposes the perinatal period is defined as before birth through the 28th day following birth. The following guidelines are provided for reporting purposes. Hospitals may record other diagnoses as needed for internal data use.

a. General Perinatal Rules

1) Chapter 15 Codes

They are never for use on the maternal record. Codes from Chapter 11, the obstetric chapter, are never permitted on the newborn record. Chapter 15 code may be used throughout the life of the patient if the condition is still present.

2) Sequencing of perinatal codes

Generally, codes from Chapter 15 should be sequenced as the principal/first-listed diagnosis on the newborn record, with the exception of the appropriate V30 code for the birth episode, followed by codes from any other chapter that provide additional detail. The "use additional code" note at the beginning of the chapter supports this guideline. If the index does not provide a specific code for a perinatal condition, assign code 779.89, Other specified conditions originating in the perinatal period, followed by the code from another chapter that specifies the condition. Codes for signs and symptoms may be assigned when a definitive diagnosis has not been established.

3) Birth process or community acquired conditions

If a newborn has a condition that may be either due to the birth process or community acquired and the documentation does not indicate which it is, the default is due to the birth process and the code from Chapter 15 should be used. If the condition is community-acquired, a code from Chapter 15 should not be assigned.

4) Code all clinically significant conditions

All clinically significant conditions noted on routine newborn examination should be coded. A condition is clinically significant if it requires:

- clinical evaluation; or
- therapeutic treatment; or
- diagnostic procedures; or
- extended length of hospital stay; or
- increased nursing care and/or monitoring; or
- has implications for future health care needs

Note: The perinatal guidelines listed above are the same as the general coding guidelines for "additional diagnoses", except for the final point regarding implications for future health care needs. Codes should be assigned for conditions that have been specified by the provider as having implications for future health care needs. Codes from the perinatal chapter should not be assigned unless the provider has established a definitive diagnosis.

b. Use of codes V30-V39

When coding the birth of an infant, assign a code from categories V30-V39, according to the type of birth. A code from this series is assigned as a principal diagnosis, and assigned only once to a newborn at the time of birth.

c. Newborn transfers

If the newborn is transferred to another institution, the V30 series is not used at the receiving hospital.

d. Use of category V29

1) Assigning a code from category V29

Assign a code from category V29, Observation and evaluation of newborns and infants for suspected conditions not found, to identify those instances when a healthy newborn is evaluated for a suspected condition that is determined after study not to be present. Do not use a code from category V29 when the patient has identified signs or symptoms of a suspected problem; in such cases, code the sign or symptom.

A code from category V29 may also be assigned as a principal code for readmissions or encounters when the V30 code no longer applies. Codes from category V29 are for use only for healthy newborns and infants for which no condition after study is found to be present.

2) V29 code on a birth record

A V29 code is to be used as a secondary code after the V30, Outcome of delivery, code.

e. Use of other V codes on perinatal records

V codes other than V30 and V29 may be assigned on a perinatal or newborn record code. The codes may be used as a principal or first-listed diagnosis for specific types of encounters or for readmissions or encounters when the V30 code no longer applies.

See Section I.C.18 for information regarding the assignment of V codes.

f. Maternal Causes of Perinatal Morbidity

Codes from categories 760-763, Maternal causes of perinatal morbidity and mortality, are assigned only when the maternal condition has actually affected the fetus or newborn. The fact that the mother has an associated medical condition or experiences some complication of pregnancy, labor or delivery does not justify the routine assignment of codes from these categories to the newborn record.

g. Congenital Anomalies in Newborns

For the birth admission, the appropriate code from category V30, Liveborn infants according to type of birth, should be used, followed by any congenital anomaly codes, categories 740-759. Use additional secondary codes from other chapters to specify conditions associated with the anomaly, if applicable.

Also, see Section I.C.14 for information on the coding of congenital anomalies.

h. Coding Additional Perinatal Diagnoses

1) Assigning codes for conditions that require treatment

Assign codes for conditions that require treatment or further investigation, prolong the length of stay, or require resource utilization.

2) Codes for conditions specified as having implications for future health care needs

Assign codes for conditions that have been specified by the provider as having implications for future health care needs.

Note: This guideline should not be used for adult patients.

3) Codes for newborn conditions originating in the perinatal period

Assign a code for newborn conditions originating in the perinatal period (categories 760-779), as well as complications arising during the current episode of care classified in other chapters, only if the diagnoses have been documented by the responsible provider at the time of transfer or discharge as having affected the fetus or newborn.

i. Prematurity and Fetal Growth Retardation

Providers utilize different criteria in determining prematurity. A code for prematurity should not be assigned unless it is documented. The 5th digit assignment for codes from category 764 and subcategories 765.0 and 765.1 should be based on the recorded birth weight and estimated gestational age.

A code from subcategory 765.2, Weeks of gestation, should be assigned as an additional code with category 764 and codes from 765.0 and 765.1 to specify weeks of gestation as documented by the provider in the record.

j. Newborn sepsis

Code 771.81, Septicemia [sepsis] of newborn, should be assigned with a secondary code from category 041, Bacterial infections in conditions classified elsewhere and of unspecified site, to identify the organism. A code from category 038, Septicemia, should not be used on a newborn record. Do not assign code 995.91, Sepsis, as code 771.81 describes the sepsis. If applicable, use additional codes to identify severe sepsis (995.92) and any associated acute organ dysfunction.

16. **Chapter 16: Signs, Symptoms and Ill-Defined Conditions (780-799)**

    Reserved for future guideline expansion

17. **Chapter 17: Injury and Poisoning (800-999)**

    a. **Coding of Injuries**

    When coding injuries, assign separate codes for each injury unless a combination code is provided, in which case the combination code is assigned. Multiple injury codes are provided in ICD-9-CM, but should not be assigned unless information for a more specific code is not available. These traumatic injury codes are not to be used for normal, healing surgical wounds or to identify complications of surgical wounds.

    The code for the most serious injury, as determined by the provider and the focus of treatment, is sequenced first.

    1) **Superficial injuries**

        Superficial injuries such as abrasions or contusions are not coded when associated with more severe injuries of the same site.

    2) **Primary injury with damage to nerves/blood vessels**

        When a primary injury results in minor damage to peripheral nerves or blood vessels, the primary injury is sequenced first with additional code(s) from categories 950-957, Injury to nerves and spinal cord, and/or 900-904, Injury to blood vessels. When the primary injury is to the blood vessels or nerves, that injury should be sequenced first.

    b. **Coding of Traumatic Fractures**

    The principles of multiple coding of injuries should be followed in coding fractures. Fractures of specified sites are coded individually by site in accordance with both the provisions within categories 800-829 and the level of detail furnished by medical record content. Combination categories for multiple fractures are provided for use when there is insufficient detail in the medical record (such as trauma cases transferred to another hospital), when the reporting form limits the number of codes that can be used in reporting pertinent clinical data, or when there is insufficient specificity at the fourth-digit or fifth-digit level. More specific guidelines are as follows:

    1) **Acute Fractures vs. Aftercare**

        Traumatic fractures are coded using the acute fracture codes (800-829) while the patient is receiving active treatment for the fracture. Examples of active treatment are: surgical treatment, emergency department encounter, and evaluation and treatment by a new physician.

        Fractures are coded using the aftercare codes (subcategories V54.0, V54.1, V54.8, or V54.9) for encounters after the patient has completed active treatment of the fracture and is receiving routine care for the fracture during the healing or recovery phase. Examples of fracture aftercare are: cast change or removal, removal of external or internal fixation device, medication adjustment, and follow up visits following fracture treatment.

        Care for complications of surgical treatment for fracture repairs during the healing or recovery phase should be coded with the appropriate complication codes.

        Care of complications of fractures, such as malunion and nonunion, should be reported with the appropriate codes.

        Pathologic fractures are not coded in the 800-829 range, but instead are assigned to subcategory 733.1. *See Section I.C.13.a for additional information.*

    2) **Multiple fractures of same limb**

        Multiple fractures of same limb classifiable to the same three-digit or four-digit category are coded to that category.

    3) **Multiple unilateral or bilateral fractures of same bone**

        Multiple unilateral or bilateral fractures of same bone(s) but classified to different fourth-digit subdivisions (bone part) within the same three-digit category are coded individually by site.

    4) **Multiple fracture categories 819 and 828**

        Multiple fracture categories 819 and 828 classify bilateral fractures of both upper limbs (819) and both lower limbs (828), but without any detail at the fourth-digit level other than open and closed type of fractures.

    5) **Multiple fractures sequencing**

        Multiple fractures are sequenced in accordance with the severity of the fracture. The provider should be asked to list the fracture diagnoses in the order of severity.

    c. **Coding of Burns**

    Current burns (940-948) are classified by depth, extent and by agent (E code). Burns are classified by depth as first degree (erythema), second degree (blistering), and third degree (full-thickness involvement).

    1) **Sequencing of burn and related condition codes**

        Sequence first the code that reflects the highest degree of burn when more than one burn is present.

        a. When the reason for the admission or encounter is for treatment of external multiple burns, sequence first the code that reflects the burn of the highest degree.

        b. When a patient has both internal and external burns, the circumstances of admission govern the selection of the principal diagnosis or first-listed diagnosis.

        c. When a patient is admitted for burn injuries and other related conditions such as smoke inhalation and/or respiratory failure, the circumstances of admission govern the selection of the principal or first-listed diagnosis.

    2) **Burns of the same local site**

        Classify burns of the same local site (three-digit category level, 940-947) but of different degrees to the subcategory identifying the highest degree recorded in the diagnosis.

    3) **Non-healing burns**

        Non-healing burns are coded as acute burns.

        Necrosis of burned skin should be coded as a non-healed burn.

    4) **Code 958.3, Posttraumatic wound infection**

        Assign code 958.3, Posttraumatic wound infection, not elsewhere classified, as an additional code for any documented infected burn site.

    5) **Assign separate codes for each burn site**

        When coding burns, assign separate codes for each burn site. Category 946 Burns of Multiple specified sites, should only be used if the location of the burns are not documented.

        Category 949, Burn, unspecified, is extremely vague and should rarely be used.

    6) **Assign codes from category 948, Burns**

        Burns classified according to extent of body surface involved, when the site of the burn is not specified or when there is a need for additional data. It is advisable to use category 948 as additional coding when needed to provide data for evaluating burn mortality, such as that needed by burn units. It is also advisable to use category 948 as an additional code for reporting purposes when there is mention of a third-degree burn involving 20 percent or more of the body surface.

        In assigning a code from category 948:

        Fourth-digit codes are used to identify the percentage of total body surface involved in a burn (all degree).

Fifth-digits are assigned to identify the percentage of body surface involved in third-degree burn.

Fifth-digit zero (0) is assigned when less than 10 percent or when no body surface is involved in a third-degree burn.

Category 948 is based on the classic "rule of nines" in estimating body surface involved: head and neck are assigned nine percent, each arm nine percent, each leg 18 percent, the anterior trunk 18 percent, posterior trunk 18 percent, and genitalia one percent. Providers may change these percentage assignments where necessary to accommodate infants and children who have proportionately larger heads than adults and patients who have large buttocks, thighs, or abdomen that involve burns.

7) Encounters for treatment of late effects of burns

Encounters for the treatment of the late effects of burns (i.e., scars or joint contractures) should be coded to the residual condition (sequelae) followed by the appropriate late effect code (906.5-906.9). A late effect E code may also be used, if desired.

8) Sequelae with a late effect code and current burn

When appropriate, both a sequelae with a late effect code, and a current burn code may be assigned on the same record (when both a current burn and sequelae of an old burn exist).

d. Coding of Debridement of Wound, Infection, or Burn

Excisional debridement involves surgical removal or cutting away, as opposed to a mechanical (brushing, scrubbing, washing) debridement.

For coding purposes, excisional debridement is assigned to code 86.22.

Nonexcisional debridement is assigned to code 86.28.

e. Adverse Effects, Poisoning and Toxic Effects

The properties of certain drugs, medicinal and biological substances or combinations of such substances, may cause toxic reactions. The occurrence of drug toxicity is classified in ICD-9-CM as follows:

1) Adverse Effect

When the drug was correctly prescribed and properly administered, code the reaction plus the appropriate code from the E930-E949 series. Codes from the E930-E949 series must be used to identify the causative substance for an adverse effect of drug, medicinal and biological substances, correctly prescribed and properly administered. The effect, such as tachycardia, delirium, gastrointestinal hemorrhaging, vomiting, hypokalemia, hepatitis, renal failure, or respiratory failure, is coded and followed by the appropriate code from the E930-E949 series.

Adverse effects of therapeutic substances correctly prescribed and properly administered (toxicity, synergistic reaction, side effect, and idiosyncratic reaction) may be due to (1) differences among patients, such as age, sex, disease, and genetic factors, and (2) drug-related factors, such as type of drug, route of administration, duration of therapy, dosage, and bioavailability.

2) Poisoning

(a) Error was made in drug prescription

Errors made in drug prescription or in the administration of the drug by provider, nurse, patient, or other person, use the appropriate poisoning code from the 960-979 series.

(b) Overdose of a drug intentionally taken

If an overdose of a drug was intentionally taken or administered and resulted in drug toxicity, it would be coded as a poisoning (960-979 series).

(c) Nonprescribed drug taken with correctly prescribed and properly administered drug

If a nonprescribed drug or medicinal agent was taken in combination with a correctly prescribed and properly administered drug, any drug toxicity or other reaction resulting from the interaction of the two drugs would be classified as a poisoning.

(d) Interaction of drug(s) and alcohol

When a reaction results from the interaction of a drug(s) and alcohol, this would be classified as poisoning.

(e) Sequencing of poisoning

When coding a poisoning or reaction to the improper use of a medication (e.g., wrong dose, wrong substance, wrong route of administration) the poisoning code is sequenced first, followed by a code for the manifestation. If there is also a diagnosis of drug abuse or dependence to the substance, the abuse or dependence is coded as an additional code.

See Section I.C.3.a.6.b. if poisoning is the result of insulin pump malfunctions and Section I.C.19 for general use of E-codes.

3) Toxic Effects

(a) Toxic effect codes

When a harmful substance is ingested or comes in contact with a person, this is classified as a toxic effect. The toxic effect codes are in categories 980-989.

(b) Sequencing toxic effect codes

A toxic effect code should be sequenced first, followed by the code(s) that identify the result of the toxic effect.

(c) External cause codes for toxic effects

An external cause code from categories E860-E869 for accidental exposure, codes E950.6 or E950.7 for intentional self-harm, category E962 for assault, or categories E980-E982, for undetermined, should also be assigned to indicate intent.

f. Complications of care

1) Complications of care

(a) Documentation of complications of care

See Section I.B.18. for information on documentation of complications of care.

(b) Use additional code to identify nature of complication

An additional code identifying the complication should be assigned with codes in categories 996-999, Complications of Surgical and Medical Care NEC, when the additional code provides greater specificity as to the nature of the condition. If the complication code fully describes the condition, no additional code is necessary.

2) Transplant complications

(a) Transplant complications other than kidney

Codes under subcategory 996.8, Complications of transplanted organ, are for use for both complications and rejection of transplanted organs. A transplant complication code is only assigned if the complication affects the function of the transplanted organ. Two codes are required to fully describe a transplant complication, the appropriate code from subcategory 996.8 and a secondary code that identifies the complication.

Pre-existing conditions or conditions that develop after the transplant are not coded as complications unless they affect the function of the transplanted organs.

See I.C.18.d.3 for transplant organ removal status

See I.C.2.i for malignant neoplasm associated with transplanted organ.

(b) Chronic kidney disease and kidney transplant complications

Patients who have undergone kidney transplant may still have some form of chronic kidney disease (CKD) because the kidney transplant may not fully restore kidney function. Code 996.81 should be assigned for documented complications of a kidney transplant, such as transplant failure or rejection or other transplant complication. Code 996.81 should not be assigned for post kidney transplant patients who have chronic kidney (CKD) unless a transplant complication such as transplant failure or rejection is documented. If the documentation is unclear as to whether the patient has a complication of the transplant, query the provider.

Conditions that affect the function of the transplanted kidney, other than CKD, should be assigned code 996.81, Complications of transplanted organ, Kidney, and a secondary code that identifies the complication.

For patients with CKD following a kidney transplant, but who do not have a complication such as failure or rejection, *see section I.C.10.a.2, Chronic kidney disease and kidney transplant status.*

3) Ventilator associated pneumonia

(a) Documentation of Ventilator associated Pneumonia

As with all procedural or postprocedural complications, code assignment is based on the provider's documentation of the relationship between the condition and the procedure.

Code 997.31, Ventilator associated pneumonia, should be assigned only when the provider has documented ventilator associated pneumonia (VAP). An additional code to identify the organism (e.g., Pseudomonas aeruginosa, code 041.7) should also be assigned. Do not assign an additional code from categories 480-484 to identify the type of pneumonia.

Code 997.31 should not be assigned for cases where the patient has pneumonia and is on a mechanical ventilator but the provider has not specifically stated that the pneumonia is ventilator-associated pneumonia.

If the documentation is unclear as to whether the patient has a pneumonia that is a complication attributable to the mechanical ventilator, query the provider.

(b) Patient admitted with pneumonia and develops VAP

A patient may be admitted with one type of pneumonia (e.g., code 481, Pneumococcal pneumonia) and subsequently develop VAP. In this instance, the principal diagnosis would be the appropriate code from categories 480-484 for the pneumonia diagnosed at the time of admission. Code 997.31, Ventilator associated pneumonia, would be assigned as an additional diagnosis when the provider has also documented the presence of ventilator associated pneumonia.

g. SIRS due to Non-infectious Process

The systemic inflammatory response syndrome (SIRS) can develop as a result of certain non-infectious disease processes, such as trauma, malignant neoplasm, or pancreatitis. When SIRS is documented with a noninfectious condition, and no subsequent infection is documented, the code for the underlying condition, such as an injury, should be assigned, followed by code 995.93, Systemic inflammatory response syndrome due to noninfectious process without acute organ dysfunction, or 995.94, Systemic inflammatory response syndrome due to non-infectious process with acute organ dysfunction. If an acute organ dysfunction is documented, the appropriate code(s) for the associated acute organ dysfunction(s) should be assigned in addition to code 995.94. If acute organ dysfunction is documented, but it cannot be determined if the acute organ

dysfunction is associated with SIRS or due to another condition (e.g., directly due to the trauma), the provider should be queried.

When the non-infectious condition has led to an infection that results in SIRS, *see Section I.C.1.b.12 for the guideline for sepsis and severe sepsis associated with a non-infectious process.*

18. Classification of Factors Influencing Health Status and Contact with Health Service (Supplemental V01-V91)

Note: The chapter specific guidelines provide additional information about the use of V codes for specified encounters.

a. Introduction

ICD-9-CM provides codes to deal with encounters for circumstances other than a disease or injury. The Supplementary Classification of Factors Influencing Health Status and Contact with Health Services (V01.0 - V91.99) is provided to deal with occasions when circumstances other than a disease or injury (codes 001-999) are recorded as a diagnosis or problem.

There are four primary circumstances for the use of V codes:

1) A person who is not currently sick encounters the health services for some specific reason, such as to act as an organ donor, to receive prophylactic care, such as inoculations or health screenings, or to receive counseling on health related issues.

2) A person with a resolving disease or injury, or a chronic, long-term condition requiring continuous care, encounters the health care system for specific aftercare of that disease or injury (e.g., dialysis for renal disease; chemotherapy for malignancy; cast change). A diagnosis/symptom code should be used whenever a current, acute, diagnosis is being treated or a sign or symptom is being studied.

3) Circumstances or problems influence a person's health status but are not in themselves a current illness or injury.

4) Newborns, to indicate birth status

b. V codes use in any healthcare setting

V codes are for use in any healthcare setting. V codes may be used as either a first listed (principal diagnosis code in the inpatient setting) or secondary code, depending on the circumstances of the encounter. Certain V codes may only be used as first listed, others only as secondary codes.

See Section I.C.18.e, V Codes That May Only be Principal/First-Listed Diagnosis.

c. V Codes indicate a reason for an encounter

They are not procedure codes. A corresponding procedure code must accompany a V code to describe the procedure performed.

d. Categories of V Codes

1) Contact/Exposure

Category V01 indicates contact with or exposure to communicable diseases. These codes are for patients who do not show any sign or symptom of a disease but have been exposed to it by close personal contact with an infected individual or are in an area where a disease is epidemic. These codes may be used as a first listed code to explain an encounter for testing, or, more commonly, as a secondary code to identify a potential risk.

Codes V15.84 – V15.86 describe contact with or (suspected) exposure to asbestos, potentially hazardous body fluids, and lead.

Subcategories V87.0 – V87.3 describe contact with or (suspected) exposure to hazardous metals, aromatic compounds, other potentially hazardous chemicals, and other potentially hazardous substances.

2) Inoculations and vaccinations

Categories V03-V06 are for encounters for inoculations and vaccinations. They indicate that a patient is being seen to receive a prophylactic inoculation against a disease. The injection itself must be represented by the appropriate procedure code. A code from V03-V06 may be used as a secondary code if the inoculation is given as a routine part of preventive health care, such as a well-baby visit.

3) Status

Status codes indicate that a patient is a carrier of a disease, has the sequelae or residual of a past disease or condition, or has another factor influencing a person's health status. This includes such things as the presence of prosthetic or mechanical devices resulting from past treatment. A status code is informative, because the status may affect the course of treatment and its outcome. A status code is distinct from a history code. The history code indicates that the patient no longer has the condition.

A status code should not be used with a diagnosis code from one of the body system chapters, if the diagnosis code includes the information provided by the status code. For example, code V42.1, Heart transplant status, should not be used with code 996.83, Complications of transplanted heart. The status code does not provide additional information. The complication code indicates that the patient is a heart transplant patient.

The status V codes/categories are:

V02   Carrier or suspected carrier of infectious diseases

Carrier status indicates that a person harbors the specific organisms of a disease without manifest symptoms and is capable of transmitting the infection.

V07.5x   Use of agents affecting estrogen receptors and estrogen level

This code indicates when a patient is receiving a drug that affects estrogen receptors and estrogen levels for prevention of cancer.

V08   Asymptomatic HIV infection status

This code indicates that a patient has tested positive for HIV but has manifested no signs or symptoms of the disease.

V09   Infection with drug-resistant microorganisms

This category indicates that a patient has an infection that is resistant to drug treatment. Sequence the infection code first.

V21   Constitutional states in development

V22.2   Pregnant state, incidental

This code is a secondary code only for use when the pregnancy is in no way complicating the reason for visit. Otherwise, a code from the obstetric chapter is required.

V26.5x   Sterilization status

V42   Organ or tissue replaced by transplant

V43   Organ or tissue replaced by other means

V44   Artificial opening status

V45   Other postsurgical states

Assign code V45.87, Transplant organ removal status, to indicate that a transplanted organ has been previously removed. This code should not be assigned for the encounter in which the transplanted organ is removed. The complication necessitating removal of the transplant organ should be assigned for that encounter.

See section I.C17.f.2. for information on the coding of organ transplant complications.

Assign code V45.88, Status post administration of tPA (rtPA) in a different facility within the last 24 hours prior to admission to the current facility, as a secondary diagnosis when a patient is received by transfer into a facility and documentation indicates they were administered tissue plasminogen activator (tPA) within the last 24 hours prior to admission to the current facility.

This guideline applies even if the patient is still receiving the tPA at the time they are received into the current facility.

The appropriate code for the condition for which the tPA was administered (such as cerebrovascular disease or myocardial infarction) should be assigned first.

Code V45.88 is only applicable to the receiving facility record and not to the transferring facility record.

V46   Other dependence on machines

V49.6   Upper limb amputation status

V49.7   Lower limb amputation status

Note: Categories V42-V46, and subcategories V49.6, V49.7 are for use only if there are no complications or malfunctions of the organ or tissue replaced, the amputation site or the equipment on which the patient is dependent.

V49.81   Asymptomatic postmenopausal status (age-related) (natural)

V49.82   Dental sealant status

V49.83   Awaiting organ transplant status

V49.86   Do not resuscitate status

This code may be used when it is documented by the provider that a patient is on do not resuscitate status at any time during the stay.

V49.87   Physical restraint status

This code may be used when it is documented by the provider that a patient has been put in restraints during the current encounter. Please note that this code should not be reported when it is documented by the provider that a patient is temporarily restrained during a procedure.

V58.6x   Long-term (current) drug use

Codes from this subcategory indicate a patient's continuous use of a prescribed drug (including such things as aspirin therapy) for the long-term treatment of a condition or for prophylactic use. It is not for use for patients who have addictions to drugs. This subcategory is not for use of medications for detoxification or maintenance programs to prevent withdrawal symptoms in patients with drug dependence (e.g., methadone maintenance for opiate dependence). Assign the appropriate code for the drug dependence instead.

Assign a code from subcategory V58.6, Long-term (current) drug use, if the patient is receiving a medication for an extended period as a prophylactic measure (such as for the prevention of deep vein thrombosis) or as treatment of a chronic condition (such as arthritis) or a disease requiring a lengthy course of treatment (such as cancer). Do not assign a code from subcategory V58.6 for medication being administered for a brief period of time to treat an acute illness or injury (such as a course of antibiotics to treat acute bronchitis).

V83   Genetic carrier status

Genetic carrier status indicates that a person carries a gene, associated with a particular disease, which may be passed to offspring who may develop that disease. The person does not have the disease and is not at risk of developing the disease.

V84   Genetic susceptibility status

Genetic susceptibility indicates that a person has a gene that increases the risk of that person developing the disease.

Codes from category V84, Genetic susceptibility to disease, should not be used as principal or first-listed codes. If the patient has the condition to which he/she is susceptible, and that condition is the reason for the encounter, the code for the current condition should be sequenced first. If the patient is being seen for follow-up after completed treatment for this condition, and the condition no longer exists, a follow-up code should be sequenced first, followed by the appropriate personal history and genetic susceptibility codes. If the purpose of the encounter is genetic counseling associated with procreative management, a code from subcategory V26.3, Genetic counseling and testing, should be assigned as the first-listed code, followed by a code from category V84. Additional codes should be assigned for any applicable family or personal history.

See Section I.C. 18.d.14 for information on prophylactic organ removal due to a genetic susceptibility.

V85   Body Mass Index (BMI)

V86   Estrogen receptor status

V88   Acquired absence of other organs and tissue

V90   Retained foreign body

4) **History (of)**

There are two types of history V codes, personal and family. Personal history codes explain a patient's past medical condition that no longer exists and is not receiving any treatment, but that has the potential for recurrence, and therefore may require continued monitoring. The exceptions to this general rule are category V14, Personal history of allergy to medicinal agents, and subcategory V15.0, Allergy, other than to medicinal agents. A person who has had an allergic episode to a substance or food in the past should always be considered allergic to the substance.

Family history codes are for use when a patient has a family member(s) who has had a particular disease that causes the patient to be at higher risk of also contracting the disease.

Personal history codes may be used in conjunction with follow-up codes and family history codes may be used in conjunction with screening codes to explain the need for a test or procedure. History codes are also acceptable on any medical record regardless of the reason for visit. A history of an illness, even if no longer present, is important information that may alter the type of treatment ordered.

The history V code categories are:

V10   Personal history of malignant neoplasm

V12   Personal history of certain other diseases

V13   Personal history of other diseases

Except: V13.4, Personal history of arthritis, and subcategory V13.6, Personal history of congenital (corrected) malformations. These conditions are life-long so are not true history codes.

V14   Personal history of allergy to medicinal agents

V15   Other personal history presenting hazards to health

Except: Codes V15.7, Personal history of contraception; V15.84, Contact with and (suspected) exposure to asbestos; V15.85, Contact with and (suspected) exposure to potentially hazardous body fluids; V15.86, Contact with and (suspected) exposure to lead.

V16   Family history of malignant neoplasm

V17   Family history of certain chronic disabling diseases

V18   Family history of certain other specific diseases

V19   Family history of other conditions

V87   Other specified personal exposures and history presenting hazards to health

Except: Subcategories V87.0, Contact with and (suspected) exposure to hazardous metals; V87.1, Contact with and (suspected) exposure to hazardous aromatic compounds; V87.2, Contact with and (suspected) exposure to other potentially

hazardous chemicals; and V87.3, Contact with and (suspected) exposure to other potentially hazardous substances.

5) **Screening**

Screening is the testing for disease or disease precursors in seemingly well individuals so that early detection and treatment can be provided for those who test positive for the disease. Screenings that are recommended for many subgroups in a population include: routine mammograms for women over 40, a fecal occult blood test for everyone over 50, an amniocentesis to rule out a fetal anomaly for pregnant women over 35, because the incidence of breast cancer and colon cancer in these subgroups is higher than in the general population, as is the incidence of Down's syndrome in older mothers.

The testing of a person to rule out or confirm a suspected diagnosis because the patient has some sign or symptom is a diagnostic examination, not a screening. In these cases, the sign or symptom is used to explain the reason for the test.

A screening code may be a first listed code if the reason for the visit is specifically the screening exam. It may also be used as an additional code if the screening is done during an office visit for other health problems. A screening code is not necessary if the screening is inherent to a routine examination, such as a pap smear done during a routine pelvic examination.

Should a condition be discovered during the screening then the code for the condition may be assigned as an additional diagnosis.

The V code indicates that a screening exam is planned. A procedure code is required to confirm that the screening was performed.

The screening V code categories:

V28   Antenatal screening

V73-V82 Special screening examinations

6) **Observation**

There are three observation V code categories. They are for use in very limited circumstances when a person is being observed for a suspected condition that is ruled out. The observation codes are not for use if an injury or illness or any signs or symptoms related to the suspected condition are present. In such cases the diagnosis/symptom code is used with the corresponding E code to identify any external cause. The observation codes are to be used as principal diagnosis only. The only exception to this is when the principal diagnosis is required to be a code from the V30, Live born infant, category. Then the V29 observation code is sequenced after the V30 code. Additional codes may be used in addition to the observation code but only if they are unrelated to the suspected condition being observed.

Codes from subcategory V89.0, Suspected maternal and fetal conditions not found, may either be used as a first listed or as an additional code assignment depending on the case. They are for use in very limited circumstances on a maternal record when an encounter is for a suspected maternal or fetal condition that is ruled out during that encounter (for example, a maternal or fetal condition may be suspected due to an abnormal test result). These codes should not be used when the condition is confirmed. In those cases, the confirmed condition should be coded. In addition, these codes are not for use if an illness or any signs or symptoms related to the suspected condition or problem are present. In such cases the diagnosis/symptom code is used.

Additional codes may be used in addition to the code from subcategory V89.0, but only if they are unrelated to the suspected condition being evaluated.

Codes from subcategory V89.0 may not be used for encounters for antenatal screening of mother. *See Section I.C.18.d., Screening.*

For encounters for suspected fetal condition that are inconclusive following testing and evaluation, assign the appropriate code from category 655, 656, 657 or 658.

The observation V code categories:

V29   Observation and evaluation of newborns for suspected condition not found

      For the birth encounter, a code from category V30 should be sequenced before the V29 code.

V71   Observation and evaluation for suspected condition not found

V89   Suspected maternal and fetal conditions not found

7) Aftercare

Aftercare visit codes cover situations when the initial treatment of a disease or injury has been performed and the patient requires continued care during the healing or recovery phase, or for the long-term consequences of the disease. The aftercare V code should not be used if treatment is directed at a current, acute disease or injury. The diagnosis code is to be used in these cases. Exceptions to this rule are codes V58.0, Radiotherapy, and codes from subcategory V58.1, Encounter for chemotherapy and immunotherapy for neoplastic conditions. These codes are to be first listed, followed by the diagnosis code when a patient's encounter is solely to receive radiation therapy or chemotherapy for the treatment of a neoplasm. Should a patient receive both chemotherapy and radiation therapy during the same encounter code V58.0 and V58.1 may be used together on a record with either one being sequenced first.

The aftercare codes are generally first listed to explain the specific reason for the encounter. An aftercare code may be used as an additional code when some type of aftercare is provided in addition to the reason for admission and no diagnosis code is applicable. An example of this would be the closure of a colostomy during an encounter for treatment of another condition.

Aftercare codes should be used in conjunction with any other aftercare codes or other diagnosis codes to provide better detail on the specifics of an aftercare encounter visit, unless otherwise directed by the classification. The sequencing of multiple aftercare codes is discretionary.

Certain aftercare V code categories need a secondary diagnosis code to describe the resolving condition or sequelae, for others, the condition is inherent in the code title.

Additional V code aftercare category terms include fitting and adjustment, and attention to artificial openings.

Status V codes may be used with aftercare V codes to indicate the nature of the aftercare. For example code V45.81, Aortocoronary bypass status, may be used with code V58.73, Aftercare following surgery of the circulatory system, NEC, to indicate the surgery for which the aftercare is being performed. Also, a transplant status code may be used following code V58.44, Aftercare following organ transplant, to identify the organ transplanted. A status code should not be used when the aftercare code indicates the type of status, such as using V55.0, Attention to tracheostomy with V44.0, Tracheostomy status.

See Section I. B.16 Admissions/Encounter for Rehabilitation

The aftercare V category/codes:

V51.0   Encounter for breast reconstruction following mastectomy

V52   Fitting and adjustment of prosthetic device and implant

V53   Fitting and adjustment of other device

V54   Other orthopedic aftercare

V55   Attention to artificial openings

V56   Encounter for dialysis and dialysis catheter care

V57   Care involving the use of rehabilitation procedures

V58.0   Radiotherapy

V58.11   Encounter for antineoplastic chemotherapy

V58.12   Encounter for antineoplastic immunotherapy

V58.3x   Attention to dressings and sutures

V58.41   Encounter for planned post-operative wound closure

V58.42   Aftercare, surgery, neoplasm

V58.43   Aftercare, surgery, trauma

V58.44   Aftercare involving organ transplant

V58.49   Other specified aftercare following surgery

V58.7x   Aftercare following surgery

V58.81   Fitting and adjustment of vascular catheter

V58.82   Fitting and adjustment of non-vascular catheter

V58.83   Monitoring therapeutic drug

V58.89   Other specified aftercare

8) Follow-up

The follow-up codes are used to explain continuing surveillance following completed treatment of a disease, condition, or injury. They imply that the condition has been fully treated and no longer exists. They should not be confused with aftercare codes that explain current treatment for a healing condition or its sequelae. Follow-up codes may be used in conjunction with history codes to provide the full picture of the healed condition and its treatment. The follow-up code is sequenced first, followed by the history code.

A follow-up code may be used to explain repeated visits. Should a condition be found to have recurred on the follow-up visit, then the diagnosis code should be used in place of the follow-up code.

The follow-up V code categories:

V24   Postpartum care and evaluation

V67   Follow-up examination

9) Donor

Category V59 is the donor codes. They are used for living individuals who are donating blood or other body tissue. These codes are only for individuals donating for others, not for self donations. They are not for use to identify cadaveric donations.

10) Counseling

Counseling V codes are used when a patient or family member receives assistance in the aftermath of an illness or injury, or when support is required in coping with family or social problems. They are not necessary for use in conjunction with a diagnosis code when the counseling component of care is considered integral to standard treatment.

The counseling V categories/codes:

V25.0   General counseling and advice for contraceptive management

V26.3   Genetic counseling

V26.4   General counseling and advice for procreative management

V61.x   Other family circumstances

V65.1   Person consulted on behalf of another person

V65.3   Dietary surveillance and counseling

V65.4   Other counseling, not elsewhere classified

11) Obstetrics and related conditions

See Section I.C.11., the Obstetrics guidelines for further instruction on the use of these codes.

V codes for pregnancy are for use in those circumstances when none of the problems or complications included in the codes from the Obstetrics chapter exist (a routine prenatal visit or postpartum care). Codes V22.0, Supervision of normal first pregnancy, and V22.1, Supervision of other normal pregnancy, are always first listed and are not to be used with any other code from the OB chapter.

The outcome of delivery, category V27, should be included on all maternal delivery records. It is always a secondary code.

V codes for family planning (contraceptive) or procreative management and counseling should be included on an obstetric record either during the pregnancy or the postpartum stage, if applicable.

Obstetrics and related conditions V code categories:

V22	Normal pregnancy
V23	Supervision of high-risk pregnancy
	Except: V23.2, Pregnancy with history of abortion. Code 646.3, Recurrent pregnancy loss, from the OB chapter is required to indicate a history of abortion during a pregnancy.
V24	Postpartum care and evaluation
V25	Encounter for contraceptive management
	Except V25.0x
	(See Section I.C.18.d.11, Counseling)
V26	Procreative management
	Except: V26.5x, Sterilization status, V26.3 and V26.4
	(See Section I.C.18.d.11., Counseling)
V27	Outcome of delivery
V28	Antenatal screening
	(See Section I.C.18.d.6., Screening)
V91	Multiple gestation placenta status

12) Newborn, infant and child

See Section I.C.15, the Newborn guidelines for further instruction on the use of these codes.

Newborn V code categories:

V20	Health supervision of infant or child
V29	Observation and evaluation of newborns for suspected condition not found
	(See Section I.C.18.d.7, Observation)
V30-V39	Liveborn infant according to type of birth

13) Routine and administrative examinations

The V codes allow for the description of encounters for routine examinations, such as, a general check-up, or examinations for administrative purposes, such as a pre-employment physical. The codes are not to be used if the examination is for diagnosis of a suspected condition or for treatment purposes. In such cases the diagnosis code is used. During a routine exam, should a diagnosis or condition be discovered, it should be coded as an additional code. Pre-existing and chronic conditions and history codes may also be included as additional codes as long as the examination is for administrative purposes and not focused on any particular condition.

Pre-operative examination and pre-procedural laboratory examination V codes are for use only in those situations when a patient is being cleared for a procedure or surgery and no treatment is given.

The V codes categories/code for routine and administrative examinations:

V20.2	Routine infant or child health check
	Any injections given should have a corresponding procedure code.
V70	General medical examination
V72	Special investigations and examinations
	Codes V72.5 and V72.62 may be used if the reason for the patient encounter is for routine laboratory/radiology testing in the absence of any signs, symptoms, or associated diagnosis. If routine testing is performed during the same encounter as

a test to evaluate a sign, symptom, or diagnosis, it is appropriate to assign both the V code and the code describing the reason for the non-routine test.

14) Miscellaneous V codes

The miscellaneous V codes capture a number of other health care encounters that do not fall into one of the other categories. Certain of these codes identify the reason for the encounter, others are for use as additional codes that provide useful information on circumstances that may affect a patient's care and treatment.

Prophylactic Organ Removal

For encounters specifically for prophylactic removal of breasts, ovaries, or another organ due to a genetic susceptibility to cancer or a family history of cancer, the principal or first listed code should be a code from subcategory V50.4, Prophylactic organ removal, followed by the appropriate genetic susceptibility code and the appropriate family history code.

If the patient has a malignancy of one site and is having prophylactic removal at another site to prevent either a new primary malignancy or metastatic disease, a code for the malignancy should also be assigned in addition to a code from subcategory V50.4. A V50.4 code should not be assigned if the patient is having organ removal for treatment of a malignancy, such as the removal of the testes for the treatment of prostate cancer.

Miscellaneous V code categories/codes:

V07	Need for isolation and other prophylactic or treatment measures
	Except V07.5X, Use of agents affecting estrogen receptors and estrogen levels
V40.31	Wandering in diseases classified elsewhere
V50	Elective surgery for purposes other than remedying health states
V58.5	Orthodontics
V60	Housing, household, and economic circumstances
V62	Other psychosocial circumstances
V63	Unavailability of other medical facilities for care
V64	Persons encountering health services for specific procedures, not carried out
V66	Convalescence and Palliative Care
V68	Encounters for administrative purposes
V69	Problems related to lifestyle

15) Nonspecific V codes

Certain V codes are so non-specific, or potentially redundant with other codes in the classification, that there can be little justification for their use in the inpatient setting. Their use in the outpatient setting should be limited to those instances when there is no further documentation to permit more precise coding. Otherwise, any sign or symptom or any other reason for visit that is captured in another code should be used.

Nonspecific V code categories/codes:

V11	Personal history of mental disorder
	A code from the mental disorders chapter, with an in remission fifth-digit, should be used.
V13.4	Personal history of arthritis
V13.6	Personal history of congenital malformations
V15.7	Personal history of contraception
V23.2	Pregnancy with history of abortion
V40	Mental and behavioral problems
	Exception: V40.31 Wandering in diseases classified elsewhere
V41	Problems with special senses and other special functions
V47	Other problems with internal organs

V48	Problems with head, neck, and trunk
V49	Problems with limbs and other problems

Exceptions:

V49.6	Upper limb amputation status
V49.7	Lower limb amputation status
V49.81	Asymptomatic postmenopausal status (age-related) (natural)
V49.82	Dental sealant status
V49.83	Awaiting organ transplant status
V49.86	Do not resuscitate status
V49.87	Physical restraints status

V51.8	Other aftercare involving the use of plastic surgery
V58.2	Blood transfusion, without reported diagnosis
V58.9	Unspecified aftercare

See Section IV.K. and Section IV.L. of the Outpatient guidelines.

e. V Codes That May Only be Principal/First-Listed Diagnosis

The list of V codes/categories below may only be reported as the principal/first-listed diagnosis, except when there are multiple encounters on the same day and the medical records for the encounters are combined or when there is more than one V code that meets the definition of principal diagnosis (e.g., a patient is admitted to home healthcare for both aftercare and rehabilitation and they equally meet the definition of principal diagnosis). These codes should not be reported if they do not meet the definition of principal or first-listed diagnosis.

See Section II and Section IV.A for information on selection of principal and first-listed diagnosis.

See Section II.C for information on two or more diagnoses that equally meet the definition for principal diagnosis.

V20.x	Health supervision of infant or child
V22.0	Supervision of normal first pregnancy
V22.1	Supervision of other normal pregnancy
V24.x	Postpartum care and examination
V26.81	Encounter for assisted reproductive fertility procedure cycle
V26.82	Encounter for fertility preservation procedure
V30.x	Single liveborn
V31.x	Twin, mate liveborn
V32.x	Twin, mate stillborn
V33.x	Twin, unspecified
V34.x	Other multiple, mates all liveborn
V35.x	Other multiple, mates all stillborn
V36.x	Other multiple, mates live- and stillborn
V37.x	Other multiple, unspecified
V39.x	Unspecified
V46.12	Encounter for respirator dependence during power failure
V46.13	Encounter for weaning from respirator [ventilator]
V51.0	Encounter for breast reconstruction following mastectomy
V56.0	Extracorporeal dialysis
V57.x	Care involving use of rehabilitation procedures
V58.0	Radiotherapy
V58.11	Encounter for antineoplastic chemotherapy
V58.12	Encounter for antineoplastic immunotherapy
V59.x	Donors
V66.0	Convalescence and palliative care following surgery
V66.1	Convalescence and palliative care following radiotherapy
V66.2	Convalescence and palliative care following chemotherapy
V66.3	Convalescence and palliative care following psychotherapy and other treatment for mental disorder
V66.4	Convalescence and palliative care following treatment of fracture
V66.5	Convalescence and palliative care following other treatment
V66.6	Convalescence and palliative care following combined treatment
V66.9	Unspecified convalescence
V68.x	Encounters for administrative purposes
V70.0	Routine general medical examination at a health care facility
V70.1	General psychiatric examination, requested by the authority
V70.2	General psychiatric examination, other and unspecified
V70.3	Other medical examination for administrative purposes
V70.4	Examination for medicolegal reasons
V70.5	Health examination of defined subpopulations
V70.6	Health examination in population surveys
V70.8	Other specified general medical examinations
V70.9	Unspecified general medical examination
V71.x	Observation and evaluation for suspected conditions not found

19. Supplemental Classification of External Causes of Injury and Poisoning (E-codes, E000-E999)

Introduction: These guidelines are provided for those who are currently collecting E codes in order that there will be standardization in the process. If your institution plans to begin collecting E codes, these guidelines are to be applied. The use of E codes is supplemental to the application of ICD-9-CM diagnosis codes.

External causes of injury and poisoning codes (categories E000 and E800-E999) are intended to provide data for injury research and evaluation of injury prevention strategies. Activity codes (categories E001-E030) are intended to be used to describe the activity of a person seeking care for injuries as well as other health conditions, when the injury or other health condition resulted from an activity or the activity contributed to a condition. E codes capture how the injury, poisoning, or adverse effect happened (cause), the intent (unintentional or accidental; or intentional, such as suicide or assault), the person's status (e.g. civilian, military), the associated activity and the place where the event occurred.

Some major categories of E codes include:

transport accidents

poisoning and adverse effects of drugs, medicinal substances and biologicals

accidental falls

accidents caused by fire and flames

accidents due to natural and environmental factors

late effects of accidents, assaults or self injury

assaults or purposely inflicted injury

suicide or self inflicted injury

These guidelines apply for the coding and collection of E codes from records in hospitals, outpatient clinics, emergency departments, other ambulatory care settings and provider offices, and nonacute care settings, except when other specific guidelines apply.

a. General E Code Coding Guidelines

1) Used with any code in the range of 001-V91

An E code from categories E800-E999 may be used with any code in the range of 001-V91, which indicates an injury, poisoning, or adverse effect due to an external cause.

An activity E code (categories E001-E030) may be used with any code in the range of 001-V91 that indicates an injury, or other health condition that resulted from an activity, or the activity contributed to a condition.

2)   Assign the appropriate E code for all initial treatments

Assign the appropriate E code for the initial encounter of an injury, poisoning, or adverse effect of drugs, not for subsequent treatment.

External cause of injury codes (E-codes) may be assigned while the acute fracture codes are still applicable.

See Section I.C.17.b.1 for coding of acute fractures.

3)   Use the full range of E codes

Use the full range of E codes (E800 – E999) to completely describe the cause, the intent and the place of occurrence, if applicable, for all injuries, poisonings, and adverse effects of drugs.

See a.1.), j.), and k.) in this section for information on the use of status and activity E codes.

4)   Assign as many E codes as necessary

Assign as many E codes as necessary to fully explain each cause.

5)   The selection of the appropriate E code

The selection of the appropriate E code is guided by the Index to External Causes, which is located after the alphabetical index to diseases and by Inclusion and Exclusion notes in the Tabular List.

6)   E code can never be a principal diagnosis

An E code can never be a principal (first listed) diagnosis.

7)   External cause code(s) with systemic inflammatory response syndrome (SIRS)

An external cause code is not appropriate with a code from subcategory 995.9, unless the patient also has another condition for which an E code would be appropriate (such as an injury, poisoning, or adverse effect of drugs).

8)   Multiple Cause E Code Coding Guidelines

More than one E-code is required to fully describe the external cause of an illness, injury or poisoning. The assignment of E-codes should be sequenced in the following priority:

If two or more events cause separate injuries, an E code should be assigned for each cause. The first listed E code will be selected in the following order:

E codes for child and adult abuse take priority over all other E codes.

See Section I.C.19.e., Child and Adult abuse guidelines.

E codes for terrorism events take priority over all other E codes except child and adult abuse.

E codes for cataclysmic events take priority over all other E codes except child and adult abuse and terrorism.

E codes for transport accidents take priority over all other E codes except cataclysmic events, child and adult abuse and terrorism.

Activity and external cause status codes are assigned following all causal (intent) E codes.

The first-listed E code should correspond to the cause of the most serious diagnosis due to an assault, accident, or self-harm, following the order of hierarchy listed above.

9)   If the reporting format limits the number of E codes

If the reporting format limits the number of E codes that can be used in reporting clinical data, report the code for the cause/intent most related to the principal diagnosis. If the format permits capture of additional E codes, the cause/intent, including medical misadventures, of the additional events should be reported rather than the codes for place, activity or external status.

b.   Place of Occurrence Guideline

Use an additional code from category E849 to indicate the Place of Occurrence. The Place of Occurrence describes the place where

the event occurred and not the patient's activity at the time of the event.

Do not use E849.9 if the place of occurrence is not stated.

c.   Adverse Effects of Drugs, Medicinal and Biological Substances Guidelines

1)   Do not code directly from the Table of Drugs

Do not code directly from the Table of Drugs and Chemicals. Always refer back to the Tabular List.

2)   Use as many codes as necessary to describe

Use as many codes as necessary to describe completely all drugs, medicinal or biological substances.

If the reporting format limits the number of E codes, and there are different fourth digit codes in the same three digit category, use the code for "Other specified" of that category of drugs, medicinal or biological substances. If there is no "Other specified" code in that category, use the appropriate "Unspecified" code in that category.

If the reporting format limits the number of E codes, and the codes are in different three digit categories, assign the appropriate E code for other multiple drugs and medicinal substances.

3)   If the same E code would describe the causative agent

If the same E code would describe the causative agent for more than one adverse reaction, assign the code only once.

4)   If two or more drugs, medicinal or biological substances

If two or more drugs, medicinal or biological substances are reported, code each individually unless the combination code is listed in the Table of Drugs and Chemicals. In that case, assign the E code for the combination.

5)   When a reaction results from the interaction of a drug(s)

When a reaction results from the interaction of a drug(s) and alcohol, use poisoning codes and E codes for both.

6)   Codes from the E930-E949 series

Codes from the E930-E949 series must be used to identify the causative substance for an adverse effect of drug, medicinal and biological substances, correctly prescribed and properly administered. The effect, such as tachycardia, delirium, gastrointestinal hemorrhaging, vomiting, hypokalemia, hepatitis, renal failure, or respiratory failure, is coded and followed by the appropriate code from the E930-E949 series.

d.   Child and Adult Abuse Guideline

1)   Intentional injury

When the cause of an injury or neglect is intentional child or adult abuse, the first listed E code should be assigned from categories E960-E968, Homicide and injury purposely inflicted by other persons, (except category E967). An E code from category E967, Child and adult battering and other maltreatment, should be added as an additional code to identify the perpetrator, if known.

2)   Accidental intent

In cases of neglect when the intent is determined to be accidental E code E904.0, Abandonment or neglect of infant and helpless person, should be the first listed E code.

e.   Unknown or Suspected Intent Guideline

1)   If the intent (accident, self-harm, assault) of the cause of an injury or poisoning is unknown

If the intent (accident, self-harm, assault) of the cause of an injury or poisoning is unknown or unspecified, code the intent as undetermined E980-E989.

2)   If the intent (accident, self-harm, assault) of the cause of an injury or poisoning is questionable

If the intent (accident, self-harm, assault) of the cause of an injury or poisoning is questionable, probable or suspected, code the intent as undetermined E980-E989.

f. **Undetermined Cause**

When the intent of an injury or poisoning is known, but the cause is unknown, use codes: E928.9, Unspecified accident, E958.9, Suicide and self-inflicted injury by unspecified means, and E968.9, Assault by unspecified means.

These E codes should rarely be used, as the documentation in the medical record, in both the inpatient outpatient and other settings, should normally provide sufficient detail to determine the cause of the injury.

g. **Late Effects of External Cause Guidelines**

1) **Late effect E codes**

Late effect E codes exist for injuries and poisonings but not for adverse effects of drugs, misadventures and surgical complications.

2) **Late effect E codes (E929, E959, E969, E977, E989, or E999.1)**

A late effect E code (E929, E959, E969, E977, E989, or E999.1) should be used with any report of a late effect or sequela resulting from a previous injury or poisoning (905-909).

3) **Late effect E code with a related current injury**

A late effect E code should never be used with a related current nature of injury code.

4) **Use of late effect E codes for subsequent visits**

Use a late effect E code for subsequent visits when a late effect of the initial injury or poisoning is being treated. There is no late effect E code for adverse effects of drugs.

Do not use a late effect E code for subsequent visits for follow-up care (e.g., to assess healing, to receive rehabilitative therapy) of the injury or poisoning when no late effect of the injury has been documented.

h. **Misadventures and Complications of Care Guidelines**

1) **Code range E870-E876**

Assign a code in the range of E870-E876 if misadventures are stated by the provider. When applying the E code guidelines pertaining to sequencing, these E codes are considered causal codes.

2) **Code range E878-E879**

Assign a code in the range of E878-E879 if the provider attributes an abnormal reaction or later complication to a surgical or medical procedure, but does not mention misadventure at the time of the procedure as the cause of the reaction.

i. **Terrorism Guidelines**

1) **Cause of injury identified by the Federal Government (FBI) as terrorism**

When the cause of an injury is identified by the Federal Government (FBI) as terrorism, the first-listed E-code should be a code from category E979, Terrorism. The definition of terrorism employed by the FBI is found at the inclusion note at E979. The terrorism E-code is the only E-code that should be assigned. Additional E codes from the assault categories should not be assigned.

2) **Cause of an injury is suspected to be the result of terrorism**

When the cause of an injury is suspected to be the result of terrorism a code from category E979 should not be assigned. Assign a code in the range of E codes based circumstances on the documentation of intent and mechanism.

3) **Code E979.9, Terrorism, secondary effects**

Assign code E979.9, Terrorism, secondary effects, for conditions occurring subsequent to the terrorist event. This code should not be assigned for conditions that are due to the initial terrorist act.

4) **Statistical tabulation of terrorism codes**

For statistical purposes these codes will be tabulated within the category for assault, expanding the current category from E960-E969 to include E979 and E999.1.

j. **Activity Code Guidelines**

Assign a code from category E001-E030 to describe the activity that caused or contributed to the injury or other health condition.

Unlike other E codes, activity E codes may be assigned to indicate a health condition (not just injuries) resulted from an activity, or the activity contributed to the condition.

The activity codes are not applicable to poisonings, adverse effects, misadventures or late effects.

Do not assign E030, Unspecified activity, if the activity is not stated.

k. **External cause status**

A code from category E000, External cause status, should be assigned whenever any other E code is assigned for an encounter, including an Activity E code, except for the events noted below. Assign a code from category E000, External cause status, to indicate the work status of the person at the time the event occurred. The status code indicates whether the event occurred during military activity, whether a non-military person was at work, whether an individual including a student or volunteer was involved in a non-work activity at the time of the causal event.

A code from E000, External cause status, should be assigned, when applicable, with other external cause codes, such as transport accidents and falls. The external cause status codes are not applicable to poisonings, adverse effects, misadventures or late effects.

Do not assign a code from category E000 if no other E codes (cause, activity) are applicable for the encounter.

Do not assign code E000.9, Unspecified external cause status, if the status is not stated.

Section II. Selection of Principal Diagnosis

The circumstances of inpatient admission always govern the selection of principal diagnosis. The principal diagnosis is defined in the Uniform Hospital Discharge Data Set (UHDDS) as "that condition established after study to be chiefly responsible for occasioning the admission of the patient to the hospital for care."

The UHDDS definitions are used by hospitals to report inpatient data elements in a standardized manner. These data elements and their definitions can be found in the July 31, 1985, Federal Register (Vol. 50, No, 147), pp. 31038-40.

Since that time the application of the UHDDS definitions has been expanded to include all non-outpatient settings (acute care, short term, long term care and psychiatric hospitals; home health agencies; rehab facilities; nursing homes, etc).

In determining principal diagnosis the coding conventions in the ICD-9-CM, Volumes I and II take precedence over these official coding guidelines.

(See Section I.A., Conventions for the ICD-9-CM)

The importance of consistent, complete documentation in the medical record cannot be overemphasized. Without such documentation the application of all coding guidelines is a difficult, if not impossible, task.

A. **Codes for symptoms, signs, and ill-defined conditions**

Codes for symptoms, signs, and ill-defined conditions from Chapter 16 are not to be used as principal diagnosis when a related definitive diagnosis has been established.

B. **Two or more interrelated conditions, each potentially meeting the definition for principal diagnosis.**

When there are two or more interrelated conditions (such as diseases in the same ICD-9-CM chapter or manifestations characteristically associated with a certain disease) potentially meeting the definition of principal diagnosis, either condition may be sequenced first, unless the circumstances of the admission, the therapy provided, the Tabular List, or the Alphabetic Index indicate otherwise.

C. **Two or more diagnoses that equally meet the definition for principal diagnosis**

In the unusual instance when two or more diagnoses equally meet the criteria for principal diagnosis as determined by the circumstances of admission, diagnostic workup and/or therapy provided, and the Alphabetic Index, Tabular List, or another coding guidelines does not provide sequencing direction, any one of the diagnoses may be sequenced first.

D. **Two or more comparative or contrasting conditions.**

In those rare instances when two or more contrasting or comparative diagnoses are documented as "either/or" (or similar terminology), they are coded as if the diagnoses were confirmed and the diagnoses are sequenced according to the circumstances of the admission. If no further determination can be made as to which diagnosis should be principal, either diagnosis may be sequenced first.

E. **A symptom(s) followed by contrasting/comparative diagnoses**

When a symptom(s) is followed by contrasting/comparative diagnoses, the symptom code is sequenced first. All the contrasting/comparative diagnoses should be coded as additional diagnoses.

F. **Original treatment plan not carried out**

Sequence as the principal diagnosis the condition, which after study occasioned the admission to the hospital, even though treatment may not have been carried out due to unforeseen circumstances.

G. **Complications of surgery and other medical care**

When the admission is for treatment of a complication resulting from surgery or other medical care, the complication code is sequenced as the principal diagnosis. If the complication is classified to the 996-999 series and the code lacks the necessary specificity in describing the complication, an additional code for the specific complication should be assigned.

H. **Uncertain Diagnosis**

If the diagnosis documented at the time of discharge is qualified as "probable", "suspected", "likely", "questionable", "possible", or "still to be ruled out", or other similar terms indicating uncertainty, code the condition as if it existed or was established. The bases for these guidelines are the diagnostic workup, arrangements for further workup or observation, and initial therapeutic approach that correspond most closely with the established diagnosis.

Note: This guideline is applicable only to inpatient admissions to short-term, acute, long-term care and psychiatric hospitals.

I. **Admission from Observation Unit**

1. **Admission Following Medical Observation**

   When a patient is admitted to an observation unit for a medical condition, which either worsens or does not improve, and is subsequently admitted as an inpatient of the same hospital for this same medical condition, the principal diagnosis would be the medical condition which led to the hospital admission.

2. **Admission Following Post-Operative Observation**

   When a patient is admitted to an observation unit to monitor a condition (or complication) that develops following outpatient surgery, and then is subsequently admitted as an inpatient of the same hospital, hospitals should apply the Uniform Hospital Discharge Data Set (UHDDS) definition of principal diagnosis as "that condition established after study to be chiefly responsible for occasioning the admission of the patient to the hospital for care."

J. **Admission from Outpatient Surgery**

When a patient receives surgery in the hospital's outpatient surgery department and is subsequently admitted for continuing inpatient care at the same hospital, the following guidelines should be followed in selecting the principal diagnosis for the inpatient admission:

- If the reason for the inpatient admission is a complication, assign the complication as the principal diagnosis.
- If no complication, or other condition, is documented as the reason for the inpatient admission, assign the reason for the outpatient surgery as the principal diagnosis.
- If the reason for the inpatient admission is another condition unrelated to the surgery, assign the unrelated condition as the principal diagnosis.

Section III. Reporting Additional Diagnoses
GENERAL RULES FOR OTHER (ADDITIONAL) DIAGNOSES

For reporting purposes the definition for "other diagnoses" is interpreted as additional conditions that affect patient care in terms of requiring:

clinical evaluation; or

therapeutic treatment; or

diagnostic procedures; or

extended length of hospital stay; or

increased nursing care and/or monitoring.

The UHDDS item #11-b defines Other Diagnoses as "all conditions that coexist at the time of admission, that develop subsequently, or that affect the treatment received and/or the length of stay. Diagnoses that relate to an earlier episode which have no bearing on the current hospital stay are to be excluded." UHDDS definitions apply to inpatients in acute care, short-term, long term care and psychiatric hospital setting. The UHDDS definitions are used by acute care short-term hospitals to report inpatient data elements in a standardized manner. These data elements and their definitions can be found in the July 31, 1985, Federal Register (Vol. 50, No, 147), pp. 31038-40.

Since that time the application of the UHDDS definitions has been expanded to include all non-outpatient settings (acute care, short term, long term care and psychiatric hospitals; home health agencies; rehab facilities; nursing homes, etc).

The following guidelines are to be applied in designating "other diagnoses" when neither the Alphabetic Index nor the Tabular List in ICD-9-CM provide direction. The listing of the diagnoses in the patient record is the responsibility of the attending provider.

A. **Previous conditions**

If the provider has included a diagnosis in the final diagnostic statement, such as the discharge summary or the face sheet, it should ordinarily be coded. Some providers include in the diagnostic statement resolved conditions or diagnoses and status-post procedures from previous admission that have no bearing on the current stay. Such conditions are not to be reported and are coded only if required by hospital policy.

However, history codes (V10-V19) may be used as secondary codes if the historical condition or family history has an impact on current care or influences treatment.

B. **Abnormal findings**

Abnormal findings (laboratory, x-ray, pathologic, and other diagnostic results) are not coded and reported unless the provider indicates their clinical significance. If the findings are outside the normal range and the attending provider has ordered other tests to evaluate the condition or prescribed treatment, it is appropriate to ask the provider whether the abnormal finding should be added.

Please note: This differs from the coding practices in the outpatient setting for coding encounters for diagnostic tests that have been interpreted by a provider.

C. **Uncertain Diagnosis**

If the diagnosis documented at the time of discharge is qualified as "probable", "suspected", "likely", "questionable", "possible", or "still to be ruled out" or other similar terms indicating uncertainty, code the condition as if it existed or was established. The bases for these guidelines are the diagnostic workup, arrangements for further workup or observation, and initial therapeutic approach that correspond most closely with the established diagnosis.

Note: This guideline is applicable only to inpatient admissions to short-term, acute, long-term care and psychiatric hospitals.

Section IV. Diagnostic Coding and Reporting Guidelines for Outpatient Services

These coding guidelines for outpatient diagnoses have been approved for use by hospitals/ providers in coding and reporting hospital-based outpatient services and provider-based office visits.

Information about the use of certain abbreviations, punctuation, symbols, and other conventions used in the ICD-9-CM Tabular List (code numbers and titles), can be found in Section IA of these guidelines, under "Conventions Used in the Tabular List." Information about the correct sequence to use in finding a code is also described in Section I.

The terms encounter and visit are often used interchangeably in describing outpatient service contacts and, therefore, appear together in these guidelines without distinguishing one from the other.

Though the conventions and general guidelines apply to all settings, coding guidelines for outpatient and provider reporting of diagnoses will vary in a number of instances from those for inpatient diagnoses, recognizing that:

> The Uniform Hospital Discharge Data Set (UHDDS) definition of principal diagnosis applies only to inpatients in acute, short-term, long-term care and psychiatric hospitals.

> Coding guidelines for inconclusive diagnoses (probable, suspected, rule out, etc.) were developed for inpatient reporting and do not apply to outpatients.

A. Selection of first-listed condition

In the outpatient setting, the term first-listed diagnosis is used in lieu of principal diagnosis.

In determining the first-listed diagnosis the coding conventions of ICD-9-CM, as well as the general and disease specific guidelines take precedence over the outpatient guidelines.

Diagnoses often are not established at the time of the initial encounter/visit. It may take two or more visits before the diagnosis is confirmed.

The most critical rule involves beginning the search for the correct code assignment through the Alphabetic Index. Never begin searching initially in the Tabular List as this will lead to coding errors.

1. Outpatient Surgery

When a patient presents for outpatient surgery, code the reason for the surgery as the first-listed diagnosis (reason for the encounter), even if the surgery is not performed due to a contraindication.

2. Observation Stay

When a patient is admitted for observation for a medical condition, assign a code for the medical condition as the first-listed diagnosis.

When a patient presents for outpatient surgery and develops complications requiring admission to observation, code the reason for the surgery as the first reported diagnosis (reason for the encounter), followed by codes for the complications as secondary diagnoses.

B. Codes from 001.0 through V91.99

The appropriate code or codes from 001.0 through V91.99 must be used to identify diagnoses, symptoms, conditions, problems, complaints, or other reason(s) for the encounter/visit.

C. Accurate reporting of ICD-9-CM diagnosis codes

For accurate reporting of ICD-9-CM diagnosis codes, the documentation should describe the patient's condition, using terminology which includes specific diagnoses as well as symptoms, problems, or reasons for the encounter. There are ICD-9-CM codes to describe all of these.

D. Selection of codes 001.0 through 999.9

The selection of codes 001.0 through 999.9 will frequently be used to describe the reason for the encounter. These codes are from the section of ICD-9-CM for the classification of diseases and injuries (e.g. infectious and parasitic diseases; neoplasms; symptoms, signs, and ill-defined conditions, etc.).

E. Codes that describe symptoms and signs

Codes that describe symptoms and signs, as opposed to diagnoses, are acceptable for reporting purposes when a diagnosis has not been established (confirmed) by the provider. Chapter 16 of ICD-9-CM, Symptoms, Signs, and Ill-defined conditions (codes 780.0 - 799.9) contain many, but not all codes for symptoms.

F. Encounters for circumstances other than a disease or injury

ICD-9-CM provides codes to deal with encounters for circumstances other than a disease or injury. The Supplementary Classification of factors Influencing Health Status and Contact with Health Services (V01.0- V91.99) is provided to deal with occasions when circumstances other than a disease or injury are recorded as diagnosis or problems. *See Section I.C. 18 for information on V-codes.*

G. Level of Detail in Coding

1. ICD-9-CM codes with 3, 4, or 5 digits

ICD-9-CM is composed of codes with either 3, 4, or 5 digits. Codes with three digits are included in ICD-9-CM as the heading of a category of codes that may be further subdivided by the use of fourth and/or fifth digits, which provide greater specificity.

2. Use of full number of digits required for a code

A three-digit code is to be used only if it is not further subdivided. Where fourth-digit subcategories and/or fifth-digit subclassifications are provided, they must be assigned. A code is invalid if it has not been coded to the full number of digits required for that code.

See also discussion under Section I.b.3., General Coding Guidelines, Level of Detail in Coding.

H. ICD-9-CM code for the diagnosis, condition, problem, or other reason for encounter/visit

List first the ICD-9-CM code for the diagnosis, condition, problem, or other reason for encounter/visit shown in the medical record to be chiefly responsible for the services provided. List additional codes that describe any coexisting conditions. In some cases the first-listed diagnosis may be a symptom when a diagnosis has not been established (confirmed) by the physician.

I. Uncertain diagnosis

Do not code diagnoses documented as "probable", "suspected," "questionable," "rule out," or "working diagnosis" or other similar terms indicating uncertainty. Rather, code the condition(s) to the highest degree of certainty for that encounter/visit, such as symptoms, signs, abnormal test results, or other reason for the visit.

Please note: This differs from the coding practices used by short-term, acute care, long-term care and psychiatric hospitals.

J. Chronic diseases

Chronic diseases treated on an ongoing basis may be coded and reported as many times as the patient receives treatment and care for the condition(s)

K. Code all documented conditions that coexist

Code all documented conditions that coexist at the time of the encounter/visit, and require or affect patient care treatment or management. Do not code conditions that were previously treated and no longer exist. However, history codes (V10-V19) may be used as secondary codes if the historical condition or family history has an impact on current care or influences treatment.

L. Patients receiving diagnostic services only

For patients receiving diagnostic services only during an encounter/visit, sequence first the diagnosis, condition, problem, or other reason for encounter/visit shown in the medical record to be chiefly responsible for the outpatient services provided during the encounter/visit. Codes for other diagnoses (e.g., chronic conditions) may be sequenced as additional diagnoses.

For encounters for routine laboratory/radiology testing in the absence of any signs, symptoms, or associated diagnosis, assign V72.5 and/or a code from subcategory V72.6. If routine testing is performed during the same encounter as a test to evaluate a sign, symptom, or diagnosis, it is appropriate to assign both the V code and the code describing the reason for the non-routine test.

For outpatient encounters for diagnostic tests that have been interpreted by a physician, and the final report is available at the time of coding, code any confirmed or definitive diagnosis(es) documented in the interpretation. Do not code related signs and symptoms as additional diagnoses.

Please note: This differs from the coding practice in the hospital inpatient setting regarding abnormal findings on test results.

M. Patients receiving therapeutic services only

For patients receiving therapeutic services only during an encounter/visit, sequence first the diagnosis, condition, problem, or other reason for encounter/visit shown in the medical record to be chiefly responsible for the outpatient services provided during the encounter/visit. Codes for other diagnoses (e.g., chronic conditions) may be sequenced as additional diagnoses.

The only exception to this rule is that when the primary reason for the admission/encounter is chemotherapy, radiation therapy, or rehabilitation, the appropriate V code for the service is listed first, and the diagnosis or problem for which the service is being performed listed second.

N. Patients receiving preoperative evaluations only

For patients receiving preoperative evaluations only, sequence first a code from category V72.8, Other specified examinations, to describe the pre-op consultations. Assign a code for the condition to describe the reason for the surgery as an additional diagnosis. Code also any findings related to the pre-op evaluation.

O. Ambulatory surgery

For ambulatory surgery, code the diagnosis for which the surgery was performed. If the postoperative diagnosis is known to be different from the preoperative diagnosis at the time the diagnosis is confirmed, select the postoperative diagnosis for coding, since it is the most definitive.

P. Routine outpatient prenatal visits

For routine outpatient prenatal visits when no complications are present, codes V22.0, Supervision of normal first pregnancy, or V22.1, Supervision of other normal pregnancy, should be used as the principal diagnosis. These codes should not be used in conjunction with chapter 11 codes.

APPENDIX I. PRESENT ON ADMISSION REPORTING GUIDELINES

Introduction

These guidelines are to be used as a supplement to the *ICD-9-CM Official Guidelines for Coding and Reporting* to facilitate the assignment of the Present on Admission (POA) indicator for each diagnosis and external cause of injury code reported on claim forms (UB-04 and 837 Institutional).

These guidelines are not intended to replace any guidelines in the main body of the *ICD-9-CM Official Guidelines for Coding and Reporting*. The POA guidelines are not intended to provide guidance on when a condition should be coded, but rather, how to apply the POA indicator to the final set of diagnosis codes that have been assigned in accordance with Sections I, II, and III of the official coding guidelines. Subsequent to the assignment of the ICD-9-CM codes, the POA indicator should then be assigned to those conditions that have been coded.

As stated in the Introduction to the ICD-9-CM Official Guidelines for Coding and Reporting, a joint effort between the healthcare provider and the coder is essential to achieve complete and accurate documentation, code assignment, and reporting of diagnoses and procedures. The importance of consistent, complete documentation in the medical record cannot be overemphasized. Medical record documentation from any provider involved in the care and treatment of the patient may be used to support the determination of whether a condition was present on admission or not. In the context of the official coding guidelines, the term "provider" means a physician or any qualified healthcare practitioner who is legally accountable for establishing the patient's diagnosis.

These guidelines are not a substitute for the provider's clinical judgment as to the determination of whether a condition was/was not present on admission. The provider should be queried regarding issues related to the linking of signs/symptoms, timing of test results, and the timing of findings.

General Reporting Requirements

All claims involving inpatient admissions to general acute care hospitals or other facilities that are subject to a law or regulation mandating collection of present on admission information.

Present on admission is defined as present at the time the order for inpatient admission occurs -- conditions that develop during an outpatient encounter, including emergency department, observation, or outpatient surgery, are considered as present on admission.

POA indicator is assigned to principal and secondary diagnoses (as defined in Section II of the Official Guidelines for Coding and Reporting) and the external cause of injury codes.

Issues related to inconsistent, missing, conflicting or unclear documentation must still be resolved by the provider.

If a condition would not be coded and reported based on UHDDS definitions and current official coding guidelines, then the POA indicator would not be reported.

Reporting Options

Y - Yes

N - No

U - Unknown

W – Clinically undetermined

Unreported/Not used (or "1" for Medicare usage) – (Exempt from POA reporting)

Reporting Definitions

Y = present at the time of inpatient admission

N = not present at the time of inpatient admission

U = documentation is insufficient to determine if condition is present on admission

W = provider is unable to clinically determine whether condition was present on admission or not

Timeframe for POA Identification and Documentation

There is no required timeframe as to when a provider (per the definition of "provider" used in these guidelines) must identify or document a condition to be present on admission. In some clinical situations, it may not be possible for a provider to make a definitive diagnosis (or a condition may not be recognized or reported by the patient) for a period of time after admission. In some cases it may be several days before the provider arrives at a definitive diagnosis. This does not mean that the condition was not present on admission. Determination of whether the condition was present on admission or not will be based on the applicable POA guideline as identified in this document, or on the provider's best clinical judgment.

If at the time of code assignment the documentation is unclear as to whether a condition was present on admission or not, it is appropriate to query the provider for clarification.

ASSIGNING THE POA INDICATOR

Condition is on the "Exempt from Reporting" list

Leave the "present on admission" field blank if the condition is on the list of ICD-9-CM codes for which this field is not applicable. This is the only circumstance in which the field maybe left blank.

POA explicitly documented

Assign Y for any condition the provider explicitly documents as being present on admission.

Assign N for any condition the provider explicitly documents as not present at the time of admission.

Conditions diagnosed prior to inpatient admission

Assign "Y" for conditions that were diagnosed prior to admission (example: hypertension, diabetes mellitus, asthma)

Conditions diagnosed during the admission but clearly present before admission

Assign "Y" for conditions diagnosed during the admission that were clearly present but not diagnosed until after admission occurred.

Diagnoses subsequently confirmed after admission are considered present on admission if at the time of admission they are documented as suspected, possible, rule out, differential diagnosis, or constitute an underlying cause of a symptom that is present at the time of admission.

Condition develops during outpatient encounter prior to inpatient admission

Assign Y for any condition that develops during an outpatient encounter prior to a written order for inpatient admission.

Documentation does not indicate whether condition was present on admission

Assign "U" when the medical record documentation is unclear as to whether the condition was present on admission. "U" should not be routinely assigned and used only in very limited circumstances. Coders are encouraged to query the providers when the documentation is unclear.

Documentation states that it cannot be determined whether the condition was or was not present on admission

Assign "W" when the medical record documentation indicates that it cannot be clinically determined whether or not the condition was present on admission.

Chronic condition with acute exacerbation during the admission

If the code is a combination code that identifies both the chronic condition and the acute exacerbation, see POA guidelines pertaining to combination codes.

If the combination code only identifies the chronic condition and not the acute exacerbation (e.g., acute exacerbation of chronic leukemia), assign "Y."

Conditions documented as possible, probable, suspected, or rule out at the time of discharge

If the final diagnosis contains a possible, probable, suspected, or rule out diagnosis, and this diagnosis was based on signs, symptoms or clinical findings suspected at the time of inpatient admission, assign "Y."

If the final diagnosis contains a possible, probable, suspected, or rule out diagnosis, and this diagnosis was based on signs, symptoms or clinical findings that were not present on admission, assign "N."

Conditions documented as impending or threatened at the time of discharge

If the final diagnosis contains an impending or threatened diagnosis, and this diagnosis is based on symptoms or clinical findings that were present on admission, assign "Y".

If the final diagnosis contains an impending or threatened diagnosis, and this diagnosis is based on symptoms or clinical findings that were not present on admission, assign "N".

Acute and chronic conditions

Assign "Y" for acute conditions that are present at time of admission and N for acute conditions that are not present at time of admission.

Assign "Y" for chronic conditions, even though the condition may not be diagnosed until after admission.

If a single code identifies both an acute and chronic condition, see the POA guidelines for combination codes.

Combination codes

Assign "N" if any part of the combination code was not present on admission (e.g., obstructive chronic bronchitis with acute exacerbation and the exacerbation was not present on admission; gastric ulcer that does not start bleeding until after admission; asthma patient develops status asthmaticus after admission)

Assign "Y" if all parts of the combination code were present on admission (e.g., patient with diabetic nephropathy is admitted with uncontrolled diabetes).

If the final diagnosis includes comparative or contrasting diagnoses, and both were present, or suspected, at the time of admission, assign "Y."

For infection codes that include the causal organism, assign "Y" if the infection (or signs of the infection) was present on admission, even though the culture results may not be known until after admission (e.g., patient is admitted with pneumonia and the provider documents pseudomonas as the causal organism a few days later).

Same diagnosis code for two or more conditions

When the same ICD-9-CM diagnosis code applies to two or more conditions during the same encounter (e.g. bilateral condition, or two separate conditions classified to the same ICD-9-CM diagnosis code):

Assign "Y" if all conditions represented by the single ICD-9-CM code were present on admission (e.g. bilateral fracture of the same bone, same site, and both fractures were present on admission)

Assign "N" if any of the conditions represented by the single ICD-9-CM code was not present on admission (e.g. dehydration with hyponatremia is assigned to code 276.1, but only one of these conditions was present on admission).

Obstetrical conditions

Whether or not the patient delivers during the current hospitalization does not affect assignment of the POA indicator. The determining factor for POA assignment is whether the pregnancy complication or obstetrical condition described by the code was present at the time of admission or not.

If the pregnancy complication or obstetrical condition was present on admission (e.g., patient admitted in preterm labor), assign "Y".

If the pregnancy complication or obstetrical condition was not present on admission (e.g., 2nd degree laceration during delivery, postpartum hemorrhage that occurred during current hospitalization, fetal distress develops after admission), assign "N".

If the obstetrical code includes more than one diagnosis and any of the diagnoses identified by the code were not present on admission assign "N". (e.g., Code 642.7, Pre-eclampsia or eclampsia superimposed on pre-existing hypertension).

If the obstetrical code includes information that is not a diagnosis, do not consider that information in the POA determination. (e.g. Code 652.1x, Breech or other malpresentation successfully converted to cephalic presentation should be reported as present on admission if the fetus was breech on admission but was converted to cephalic presentation after admission (since the conversion to cephalic presentation does not represent a diagnosis, the fact that the conversion occurred after admission has no bearing on the POA determination).

Perinatal conditions

Newborns are not considered to be admitted until after birth. Therefore, any condition present at birth or that developed in utero is considered present at admission and should be assigned "Y". This includes conditions that occur during delivery (e.g., injury during delivery, meconium aspiration, exposure to streptococcus B in the vaginal canal).

Congenital conditions and anomalies

Assign "Y" for congenital conditions and anomalies, **except for categories 740-759, Congenital anomalies, which are on the exempt list.** Congenital conditions are always considered present on admission.

External cause of injury codes

Assign "Y" for any E code representing an external cause of injury or poisoning that occurred prior to inpatient admission (e.g., patient fell out of bed at home, patient fell out of bed in emergency room prior to admission)

Assign "N" for any E code representing an external cause of injury or poisoning that occurred during inpatient hospitalization (e.g., patient fell out of hospital bed during hospital stay, patient experienced an adverse reaction to a medication administered after inpatient admission)

CATEGORIES AND CODES EXEMPT FROM DIAGNOSIS PRESENT ON ADMISSION REQUIREMENT

Note: *"Diagnosis present on admission" for these code categories are exempt because they represent circumstances regarding the healthcare encounter or factors influencing health status that do not represent a current disease or injury or are always present on admission.*

Categories or subcategories listed are inclusive of all codes within those categories or subcategories, unless otherwise indicated. In order to streamline the POA exempt list and make it easier to read, where all of the codes in a code range are POA exempt, only the code range is shown, rather than listing each of the individual codes in the range.

137-139	Late effects of infectious and parasitic diseases
268.1	Rickets, late effect
326	Late effects of intracranial abscess or pyogenic infection
412	Old myocardial infarction
438	Late effects of cerebrovascular disease
650	Normal delivery
660.7	Failed forceps or vacuum extractor, unspecified
677	Late effect of complication of pregnancy, childbirth, and the puerperium
740-759	Congenital anomalies
905-909	Late effects of injuries, poisonings, toxic effects, and other external causes
V02	Carrier or suspected carrier of infectious diseases
V03	Need for prophylactic vaccination and inoculation against bacterial diseases
V04	Need for prophylactic vaccination and inoculation against certain viral diseases
V05	Need for other prophylactic vaccination and inoculation against single diseases
V06	Need for prophylactic vaccination and inoculation against combinations of diseases
V07	Need for isolation and other prophylactic or treatment measures

V10	Personal history of malignant neoplasm
V11	Personal history of mental disorder
V12	Personal history of certain other diseases
V13	Personal history of other diseases
V14	Personal history of allergy to medicinal agents
V15	Other personal history presenting hazards to health
V16	Family history of malignant neoplasm
V17	Family history of certain chronic disabling diseases
V18	Family history of certain other specific conditions
V19	Family history of other conditions
V20	Health supervision of infant or child
V21	Constitutional states in development
V22	Normal pregnancy
V23	Supervision of high-risk pregnancy
V24	Postpartum care and examination
V25	Encounter for contraceptive management
V26	Procreative management
V27	Outcome of delivery
V28	Antenatal screening
V29	Observation and evaluation of newborns for suspected condition not found
V30-V39	Liveborn infants according to type of birth
V42	Organ or tissue replaced by transplant
V43	Organ or tissue replaced by other means
V44	Artificial opening status
V45	Other postprocedural states
V46	Other dependence on machines and devices
V49.60-V49.77	Upper and lower limb amputation status
V49.81-V49.85	Other specified conditions influencing health status
V50	Elective surgery for purposes other than remedying health states
V51	Aftercare involving the use of plastic surgery
V52	Fitting and adjustment of prosthetic device and implant
V53	Fitting and adjustment of other device
V54	Other orthopedic aftercare
V55	Attention to artificial openings
V56	Encounter for dialysis and dialysis catheter care
V57	Care involving use of rehabilitation procedures
V58	Encounter for other and unspecified procedures and aftercare
V59	Donors
V60	Housing, household, and economic circumstances
V61	Other family circumstances
V62	Other psychosocial circumstances
V64	Persons encountering health services for specific procedures, not carried out
V65	Other persons seeking consultation
V66	Convalescence and palliative care
V67	Follow-up examination
V68	Encounters for administrative purposes
V69	Problems related to lifestyle
V70	General medical examination
V71	Observation and evaluation for suspected condition not found
V72	Special investigations and examinations
V73	Special screening examination for viral and chlamydial diseases
V74	Special screening examination for bacterial and spirochetal diseases
V75	Special screening examination for other infectious diseases
V76	Special screening for malignant neoplasms
V77	Special screening for endocrine, nutritional, metabolic, and immunity disorders
V78	Special screening for disorders of blood and blood-forming organs
V79	Special screening for mental disorders and developmental handicaps
V80	Special screening for neurological, eye, and ear diseases
V81	Special screening for cardiovascular, respiratory, and genitourinary diseases
V82	Special screening for other conditions
V83	Genetic carrier status
V84	Genetic susceptibility to disease
V85	Body Mass Index
V86	Estrogen receptor status
V87.32	Contact with and (suspected) exposure to algae bloom
V87.4	Personal history of drug therapy

V88	Acquired absence of other organs and tissue
V89	Suspected maternal and fetal conditions not found
V90	Retained foreign body
V91	Multiple gestation placenta status
E000	External cause status
E001-E030	Activity
E800-E807	Railway accidents
E810-E819	Motor vehicle traffic accidents
E820-E825	Motor vehicle nontraffic accidents
E826-E829	Other road vehicle accidents
E830-E838	Water transport accidents
E840-E845	Air and space transport accidents
E846-E848	Vehicle accidents not elsewhere classifiable
E849	Place of occurrence (Except E849.7)
E883.1	Accidental fall into well
E883.2	Accidental fall into storm drain or manhole
E884.0	Fall from playground equipment
E884.1	Fall from cliff
E885.0	Fall from (nonmotorized) scooter
E885.1	Fall from roller skates
E885.2	Fall from skateboard
E885.3	Fall from skis
E885.4	Fall from snowboard
E886.0	Fall on same level from collision, pushing, or shoving, by or with other person, In sports
E890.0-E890.9	Conflagration in private dwelling
E893.0	Accident caused by ignition of clothing, from controlled fire in private dwelling
E893.2	Accident caused by ignition of clothing, from controlled fire not in building or structure
E894	Ignition of highly inflammable material
E895	Accident caused by controlled fire in private dwelling
E897	Accident caused by controlled fire not in building or structure
E917.0	Striking against or struck accidentally by objects or persons, in sports without subsequent fall
E917.1	Striking against or struck accidentally by objects or persons, caused by a crowd, by collective fear or panic without subsequent fall
E917.2	Striking against or struck accidentally by objects or persons, in running water without subsequent fall
E917.5	Striking against or struck accidentally by objects or persons, object in sports with subsequent fall
E917.6	Striking against or struck accidentally by objects or persons, caused by a crowd, by collective fear or panic with subsequent fall
E919	Accident caused by machinery (Except E919.2)
E921	Accident caused by explosion of pressure vessel
E922	Accident caused by firearm and air gun missile
E926.2	Visible and ultraviolet light sources
E928.0-E928.8	Other and unspecified environmental and accidental causes
E929.0-E929.9	Late effects of accidental injury
E959	Late effects of self-inflicted injury
E970-E978	Legal intervention
E979	Terrorism
E981	Poisoning by gases in domestic use, undetermined whether accidentally or purposely inflicted
E982	Poisoning by other gases, undetermined whether accidentally or purposely inflicted
E985	Injury by firearms, air guns and explosives, undetermined whether accidentally or purposely inflicted
E987.0	Falling from high place, undetermined whether accidentally or purposely inflicted, residential premises
E987.2	Falling from high place, undetermined whether accidentally or purposely inflicted, natural sites
E989	Late effects of injury, undetermined whether accidentally or purposely inflicted
E990-E999	Injury resulting from operations of war

A

AAT (alpha-1 antitrypsin) deficiency 273.4
AAV (disease) (illness) (infection) — *see* Human immunodeficiency virus (disease) (illness) (infection)
Abactio — *see* Abortion, induced
Abactus venter — *see* Abortion, induced
Abarognosis 781.99
Abasia (-astasia) 307.9
   atactica 781.3
   choreic 781.3
   hysterical 300.11
   paroxysmal trepidant 781.3
   spastic 781.3
   trembling 781.3
   trepidans 781.3
Abderhalden-Kaufmann-Lignac syndrome (cystinosis) 270.0
Abdomen, abdominal — *see also* condition
   accordion 306.4
   acute 789.0
   angina 557.1
   burst 868.00
   convulsive equivalent (*see also* Epilepsy) 345.5 ☑
   heart 746.87
   muscle deficiency syndrome 756.79
   obstipum 756.79
Abdominalgia 789.0 ☑
   periodic 277.31
Abduction contracture, hip or other joint — *see* Contraction, joint
Abercrombie's syndrome (amyloid degeneration) 277.39
Aberrant (congenital) — *see also* Malposition, congenital
   adrenal gland 759.1
   blood vessel NEC 747.60
     arteriovenous NEC 747.60
     cerebrovascular 747.81
     gastrointestinal 747.61
     lower limb 747.64
     renal 747.62
     spinal 747.82
     upper limb 747.63
   breast 757.6
   endocrine gland NEC 759.2
   gastrointestinal vessel (peripheral) 747.61
   hepatic duct 751.69
   lower limb vessel (peripheral) 747.64
   pancreas 751.7
   parathyroid gland 759.2
   peripheral vascular vessel NEC 747.60
   pituitary gland (pharyngeal) 759.2
   renal blood vessel 747.62
   sebaceous glands, mucous membrane, mouth 750.26
   spinal vessel 747.82
   spleen 759.0
   testis (descent) 752.51
   thymus gland 759.2
   thyroid gland 759.2
   upper limb vessel (peripheral) 747.63
Aberratio
   lactis 757.6
   testis 752.51
Aberration — *see also* Anomaly
   chromosome — *see* Anomaly, chromosome(s)
   distantial 368.9
   mental (*see also* Disorder, mental, nonpsychotic) 300.9
Abetalipoproteinemia 272.5
Abionarce 780.79
Abiotrophy 799.89
Ablatio
   placentae — *see* Placenta, ablatio
   retinae (*see also* Detachment, retina) 361.9
Ablation
   pituitary (gland) (with hypofunction) 253.7
   placenta — *see* Placenta, ablatio
   uterus 621.8
Ablepharia, ablepharon, ablephary 743.62
Ablepsia — *see* Blindness
Ablepsy — *see* Blindness

Ablutomania 300.3
Abnormal, abnormality, abnormalities — *see also* Anomaly
   acid-base balance 276.4
     fetus or newborn — *see* Distress, fetal
   adaptation curve, dark 368.63
   alveolar ridge 525.9
   amnion 658.9 ☑
     affecting fetus or newborn 762.9
   anatomical relationship NEC 759.9
   apertures, congenital, diaphragm 756.6
   auditory perception NEC 388.40
   autosomes NEC 758.5
     13 758.1
     18 758.2
     21 or 22 758.0
     D_1 758.1
     E_3 758.2
     G 758.0
   ballistocardiogram 794.39
   basal metabolic rate (BMR) 794.7
   biosynthesis, testicular androgen 257.2
   blood level (of)
     cobalt 790.6
     copper 790.6
     iron 790.6
     lead 790.6
     lithium 790.6
     magnesium 790.6
     mineral 790.6
     zinc 790.6
   blood pressure
     elevated (without diagnosis of hypertension) 796.2
     low (*see also* Hypotension) 458.9
       reading (incidental) (isolated) (nonspecific) 796.3
   blood sugar 790.29
   bowel sounds 787.5
   breathing behavior — *see* Respiration
   caloric test 794.19
   cervix (acquired) NEC 622.9
     congenital 752.40
     in pregnancy or childbirth 654.6 ☑
       causing obstructed labor 660.2 ☑
         affecting fetus or newborn 763.1
   chemistry, blood NEC 790.6
   chest sounds 786.7
   chorion 658.9 ☑
     affecting fetus or newborn 762.9
   chromosomal NEC 758.89
     analysis, nonspecific result 795.2
     autosomes (*see also* Abnormal, autosomes NEC) 758.5
     fetal, (suspected) affecting management of pregnancy 655.1 ☑
     sex 758.81
   clinical findings NEC 796.4
   communication — *see* Fistula
   configuration of pupils 379.49
   coronary
     artery 746.85
     vein 746.9
   cortisol-binding globulin 255.8
   course, Eustachian tube 744.24
   creatinine clearance 794.4
   dentofacial NEC 524.9
     functional 524.50
     specified type NEC 524.89
   development, developmental NEC 759.9
     bone 756.9
     central nervous system 742.9
   direction, teeth 524.30
   Dynia (*see also* Defect, coagulation) 286.9
   Ebstein 746.2
   echocardiogram 793.2
   echoencephalogram 794.01
   echogram NEC — *see* Findings, abnormal, structure
   electrocardiogram (ECG) (EKG) 794.31
   electroencephalogram (EEG) 794.02
   electromyogram (EMG) 794.17
     ocular 794.14
   electro-oculogram (EOG) 794.12
   electroretinogram (ERG) 794.11
   erythrocytes 289.9

Abnormal, abnormality, abnormalities — *see also* Anomaly — *continued*
   erythrocytes — *continued*
     congenital, with perinatal jaundice 282.9 *[774.0]*
   Eustachian valve 746.9
   excitability under minor stress 301.9
   fat distribution 782.9
   feces 787.7
   fetal heart rate — *see* Distress, fetal
   fetus NEC
     affecting management of pregnancy — *see* Pregnancy, management affected by, fetal
     causing disproportion 653.7 ☑
       affecting fetus or newborn 763.1
       causing obstructed labor 660.1 ☑
         affecting fetus or newborn 763.1
   findings without manifest disease — *see* Findings, abnormal
   fluid
     amniotic 792.3
     cerebrospinal 792.0
     peritoneal 792.9
     pleural 792.9
     synovial 792.9
     vaginal 792.9
   forces of labor NEC 661.9 ☑
     affecting fetus or newborn 763.7
   form, teeth 520.2
   function studies
     auditory 794.15
     bladder 794.9
     brain 794.00
     cardiovascular 794.30
     endocrine NEC 794.6
     kidney 794.4
     liver 794.8
     nervous system
       central 794.00
       peripheral 794.19
     oculomotor 794.14
     pancreas 794.9
     placenta 794.9
     pulmonary 794.2
     retina 794.11
     special senses 794.19
     spleen 794.9
     thyroid 794.5
     vestibular 794.16
   gait 781.2
     hysterical 300.11
   gastrin secretion 251.5
   globulin
     cortisol-binding 255.8
     thyroid-binding 246.8
   glucagon secretion 251.4
   glucose 790.29
     in pregnancy, childbirth, or puerperium 648.8 ☑
     fetus or newborn 775.0
     non-fasting 790.29
   gravitational (G) forces or states 994.9
   hair NEC 704.2
   hard tissue formation in pulp 522.3
   head movement 781.0
   heart
     rate
       fetus, affecting liveborn infant
         before the onset of labor 763.81
         during labor 763.82
         unspecified as to time of onset 763.83
       intrauterine
         before the onset of labor 763.81
         during labor 763.82
         unspecified as to time of onset 763.83
       newborn
         before the onset of labor 763.81
         during labor 763.82
         unspecified as to time of onset 763.83
     shadow 793.2
     sounds NEC 785.3

Abnormal, abnormality, abnormalities — *see also* Anomaly — *continued*
   hemoglobin (*see also* Disease, hemoglobin) 282.7
     trait — *see* Trait, hemoglobin, abnormal
   hemorrhage, uterus — *see* Hemorrhage, uterus
   histology NEC 795.4
   increase
     in
       appetite 783.6
       development 783.9
   involuntary movement 781.0
   jaw closure 524.51
   karyotype 795.2
   knee jerk 796.1
   laboratory findings — *see* Findings, abnormal
   labor NEC 661.9 ☑
     affecting fetus or newborn 763.7
   length, organ or site, congenital — *see* Distortion
   liver function test 790.6
   loss of height 781.91
   loss of weight 783.21
   lung shadow 793.19
   mammogram 793.80
     calcification 793.89
     calculus 793.89
     microcalcification 793.81
   Mantoux test 795.51
   membranes (fetal)
     affecting fetus or newborn 762.9
     complicating pregnancy 658.8 ☑
   menstruation — *see* Menstruation
   metabolism (*see also* condition) 783.9
   movement 781.0
     disorder NEC 333.90
       sleep related, unspecified 780.58
       specified NEC 333.99
     head 781.0
     involuntary 781.0
     specified type NEC 333.99
   muscle contraction, localized 728.85
   myoglobin (Aberdeen) (Annapolis) 289.9
   narrowness, eyelid 743.62
   optokinetic response 379.57
   organs or tissues of pelvis NEC
     in pregnancy or childbirth 654.9 ☑
       affecting fetus or newborn 763.89
       causing obstructed labor 660.2 ☑
         affecting fetus or newborn 763.1
   origin — *see* Malposition, congenital
   palmar creases 757.2
   Papanicolaou (smear)
     anus 796.70
       with
         atypical squamous cells
           cannot exclude high grade squamous intraepithelial lesion (ASC-H) 796.72
           of undetermined significance (ASC-US) 796.71
         cytologic evidence of malignancy 796.76
         high grade squamous intraepithelial lesion (HGSIL) 796.74
         low grade squamous intraepithelial lesion (LGSIL) 796.73
       glandular 796.70
       specified finding NEC 796.79
     cervix 795.00
       with
         atypical squamous cells
           cannot exclude high grade squamous intraepithelial lesion (ASC-H) 795.02
           of undetermined significance (ASC-US) 795.01
         cytologic evidence of malignancy 795.06
         high grade squamous intraepithelial lesion (HGSIL) 795.04

Abnormal, abnormality, abnormalities —
see also Anomaly — continued
  Papanicolaou — continued
    cervix — continued
      with — continued
        low grade squamous intraepithelial lesion (LGSIL) 795.03
        nonspecific finding NEC 795.09
      other site 796.9
      vagina 795.10
        with
          atypical squamous cells
            cannot exclude high grade squamous intraepithelial lesion (ASC-H) 795.12
            of undetermined significance (ASC-US) 795.11
          cytologic evidence of malignancy 795.16
          high grade squamous intraepithelial lesion (HGSIL) 795.14
          low grade squamous intraepithelial lesion (LGSIL) 795.13
        glandular 795.10
        specified finding NEC 795.19
  parturition
    affecting fetus or newborn 763.9
    mother — see Delivery, complicated
  pelvis (bony) — see Deformity, pelvis
  percussion, chest 786.7
  periods (grossly) (see also Menstruation) 626.9
  phonocardiogram 794.39
  placenta — see Placenta, abnormal
  plantar reflex 796.1
  plasma protein — see Deficiency, plasma, protein
  pleural folds 748.8
  position (see also Malposition)
    gravid uterus 654.4 ☑
      causing obstructed labor 660.2 ☑
        affecting fetus or newborn 763.1
  posture NEC 781.92
  presentation (fetus) — see Presentation, fetus, abnormal
  product of conception NEC 631.8
  puberty — see Puberty
  pulmonary
    artery 747.39
    function, newborn 770.89
    test results 794.2
    ventilation, newborn 770.89
      hyperventilation 786.01
  pulsations in neck 785.1
  pupil reflexes 379.40
  quality of milk 676.8 ☑
  radiological examination 793.99
    abdomen NEC 793.6
    biliary tract 793.3
    breast 793.89
      mammogram NOS 793.80
      mammographic
        calcification 793.89
        calculus 793.89
        microcalcification 793.81
    gastrointestinal tract 793.4
    genitourinary organs 793.5
    head 793.0
    image test inconclusive due to excess body fat 793.91
    intrathoracic organ NEC 793.2
    lung (field) 793.19
    musculoskeletal system 793.7
    retroperitoneum 793.6
    skin and subcutaneous tissue 793.99
    skull 793.0
  red blood cells 790.09
    morphology 790.09
    volume 790.09
  reflex NEC 796.1
  renal function test 794.4
  respiration signs — see Respiration
  response to nerve stimulation 794.10
  retinal correspondence 368.34
  rhythm, heart (see also Arrhythmia)

Abnormal, abnormality, abnormalities —
see also Anomaly — continued
  rhythm, heart (see also Arrhythmia) — continued
    fetus — see Distress, fetal
  saliva 792.4
  scan
    brain 794.09
    kidney 794.4
    liver 794.8
    lung 794.2
    thyroid 794.5
  secretion
    gastrin 251.5
    glucagon 251.4
  semen 792.2
  serum level (of)
    acid phosphatase 790.5
    alkaline phosphatase 790.5
    amylase 790.5
    enzymes NEC 790.5
    lipase 790.5
  shape
    cornea 743.41
    gallbladder 751.69
    gravid uterus 654.4 ☑
      affecting fetus or newborn 763.89
      causing obstructed labor 660.2 ☑
        affecting fetus or newborn 763.1
    head (see also Anomaly, skull) 756.0
    organ or site, congenital NEC — see Distortion
  sinus venosus 747.40
  size
    fetus, complicating delivery 653.5 ☑
      causing obstructed labor 660.1 ☑
    gallbladder 751.69
    head (see also Anomaly, skull) 756.0
    organ or site, congenital NEC — see Distortion
    teeth 520.2
  skin and appendages, congenital NEC 757.9
  soft parts of pelvis — see Abnormal, organs or tissues of pelvis
  spermatozoa 792.2
  sputum (amount) (color) (excessive) (odor) (purulent) 786.4
  stool NEC 787.7
    bloody 578.1
      occult 792.1
    bulky 787.7
    color (dark) (light) 792.1
    content (fat) (mucus) (pus) 792.1
    occult blood 792.1
  synchondrosis 756.9
  test results without manifest disease — see Findings, abnormal
  thebesian valve 746.9
  thermography — see Findings, abnormal, structure
  threshold, cones or rods (eye) 368.63
  thyroid-binding globulin 246.8
  thyroid product 246.8
  toxicology (findings) NEC 796.0
  tracheal cartilage (congenital) 748.3
  transport protein 273.8
  ultrasound results — see Findings, abnormal, structure
  umbilical cord
    affecting fetus or newborn 762.6
    complicating delivery 663.9 ☑
    specified NEC 663.8 ☑
  union
    cricoid cartilage and thyroid cartilage 748.3
    larynx and trachea 748.3
    thyroid cartilage and hyoid bone 748.3
  urination NEC 788.69
    psychogenic 306.53
    stream
      intermittent 788.61
      slowing 788.62
      splitting 788.61
      weak 788.62
    urgency 788.63
  urine (constituents) NEC 791.9

Abnormal, abnormality, abnormalities —
see also Anomaly — continued
  uterine hemorrhage (see also Hemorrhage, uterus) 626.9
    climacteric 627.0
    postmenopausal 627.1
  vagina (acquired) (congenital)
    in pregnancy or childbirth 654.7 ☑
      affecting fetus or newborn 763.89
      causing obstructed labor 660.2 ☑
        affecting fetus or newborn 763.1
  vascular sounds 785.9
  vectorcardiogram 794.39
  visually evoked potential (VEP) 794.13
  vulva (acquired) (congenital)
    in pregnancy or childbirth 654.8 ☑
      affecting fetus or newborn 763.89
      causing obstructed labor 660.2 ☑
        affecting fetus or newborn 763.1
  weight
    gain 783.1
      of pregnancy 646.1 ☑
        with hypertension — see Toxemia, of pregnancy
    loss 783.21
  x-ray examination — see Abnormal, radiological examination

Abnormally formed uterus — see Anomaly, uterus

Abnormity (any organ or part) — see Anomaly

ABO
  hemolytic disease 773.1
  incompatibility (due to transfusion of blood or blood products)
    with hemolytic transfusion reaction (HTR) (not specified as acute or delayed) 999.61
      24 hours or more after transfusion 999.63
      acute 999.62
      delayed 999.63
      less than 24 hours after transfusion 999.62
      unspecified time after transfusion 999.61
    reaction 999.60
      specified NEC 999.69

Abocclusion 524.20

Abolition, language 784.69

Aborter, habitual or recurrent NEC
  without current pregnancy 629.81
  current abortion (see also Abortion, spontaneous) 634.9 ☑
  affecting fetus or newborn 761.8
  observation in current pregnancy 646.3 ☑

Abortion (complete) (incomplete) (inevitable) (with retained products of conception) 637.9 ☑

> Note — Use the following fifth-digit subclassification with categories 634–637:
>
> 0   unspecified
>
> 1   incomplete
>
> 2   complete

  with
    complication(s) (any) following previous abortion — see category 639 ☑
    damage to pelvic organ (laceration) (rupture) (tear) 637.2 ☑
    embolism (air) (amniotic fluid) (blood clot) (pulmonary) (pyemic) (septic) (soap) 637.6 ☑
    genital tract and pelvic infection 637.0 ☑
    hemorrhage, delayed or excessive 637.1 ☑
    metabolic disorder 637.4 ☑
    renal failure (acute) 637.3 ☑
    sepsis (genital tract) (pelvic organ) 637.0 ☑
      urinary tract 637.7 ☑
    shock (postoperative) (septic) 637.5 ☑
    specified complication NEC 637.7 ☑

Abortion — continued
  with — continued
    toxemia 637.3 ☑
    unspecified complication(s) 637.8 ☑
    urinary tract infection 637.7 ☑
  accidental — see Abortion, spontaneous
  artificial — see Abortion, induced
  attempted (failed) — see Abortion, failed
  criminal — see Abortion, illegal
  early — see Abortion, spontaneous
  elective — see Abortion, legal
  failed (legal) 638.9
    with
      damage to pelvic organ (laceration) (rupture) (tear) 638.2
      embolism (air) (amniotic fluid) (blood clot) (pulmonary) (pyemic) (septic) (soap) 638.6
      genital tract and pelvic infection 638.0
      hemorrhage, delayed or excessive 638.1
      metabolic disorder 638.4
      renal failure (acute) 638.3
      sepsis (genital tract) (pelvic organ) 638.0
        urinary tract 638.7
      shock (postoperative) (septic) 638.5
      specified complication NEC 638.7
      toxemia 638.3
      unspecified complication(s) 638.8
      urinary tract infection 638.7
  fetal indication — see Abortion, legal
  fetus 779.6
  following threatened abortion — see Abortion, by type
  habitual or recurrent (care during pregnancy) 646.3 ☑
    with current abortion (see also Abortion, spontaneous) 634.9 ☑
      affecting fetus or newborn 761.8
    without current pregnancy 629.81
  homicidal — see Abortion, illegal
  illegal 636.9 ☑
    with
      damage to pelvic organ (laceration) (rupture) (tear) 636.2 ☑
      embolism (air) (amniotic fluid) (blood clot) (pulmonary) (pyemic) (septic) (soap) 636.6 ☑
      genital tract and pelvic infection 636.0 ☑
      hemorrhage, delayed or excessive 636.1 ☑
      metabolic disorder 636.4 ☑
      renal failure 636.3 ☑
      sepsis (genital tract) (pelvic organ) 636.0 ☑
        urinary tract 636.7 ☑
      shock (postoperative) (septic) 636.5 ☑
      specified complication NEC 636.7 ☑
      toxemia 636.3 ☑
      unspecified complication(s) 636.8 ☑
      urinary tract infection 636.7 ☑
    fetus 779.6
  induced 637.9 ☑
    illegal — see Abortion, illegal
    legal indications — see Abortion, legal
    medical indications — see Abortion, legal
    therapeutic — see Abortion, legal
  late — see Abortion, spontaneous
  legal (legal indication) (medical indication) (under medical supervision) 635.9 ☑
    with
      damage to pelvic organ (laceration) (rupture) (tear) 635.2 ☑
      embolism (air) (amniotic fluid) (blood clot) (pulmonary) (pyemic) (septic) (soap) 635.6 ☑
      genital tract and pelvic infection 635.0 ☑
      hemorrhage, delayed or excessive 635.1 ☑

☑ Additional Digit Required — Refer to the Tabular List for Digit Selection   ▼ Subterms under main terms may continue to next column or page

Abortion — *continued*
  legal — *continued*
    with — *continued*
      metabolic disorder 635.4 ☑
      renal failure (acute) 635.3 ☑
      sepsis (genital tract) (pelvic organ) 635.0 ☑
        urinary tract 635.7 ☑
      shock (postoperative) (septic) 635.5 ☑
      specified complication NEC 635.7 ☑
      toxemia 635.3 ☑
      unspecified complication(s) 635.8 ☑
      urinary tract infection 635.7 ☑
    fetus 779.6
  medical indication — *see* Abortion, legal
  mental hygiene problem — *see* Abortion, legal
  missed 632
  operative — *see* Abortion, legal
  psychiatric indication — *see* Abortion, legal
  recurrent — *see* Abortion, spontaneous
  self-induced — *see* Abortion, illegal
  septic — *see* Abortion, by type, with sepsis
  spontaneous 634.9 ☑
    with
      damage to pelvic organ (laceration) (rupture) (tear) 634.2 ☑
      embolism (air) (amniotic fluid) (blood clot) (pulmonary) (pyemic) (septic) (soap) 634.6 ☑
      genital tract and pelvic infection 634.0 ☑
      hemorrhage, delayed or excessive 634.1 ☑
      metabolic disorder 634.4 ☑
      renal failure 634.3 ☑
      sepsis (genital tract) (pelvic organ) 634.0 ☑
        urinary tract 634.7 ☑
      shock (postoperative) (septic) 634.5 ☑
      specified complication NEC 634.7 ☑
      toxemia 634.3 ☑
      unspecified complication(s) 634.8 ☑
      urinary tract infection 634.7 ☑
    fetus 761.8
    threatened 640.0 ☑
      affecting fetus or newborn 762.1
  surgical — *see* Abortion, legal
  therapeutic — *see* Abortion, legal
  threatened 640.0 ☑
    affecting fetus or newborn 762.1
  tubal — *see* Pregnancy, tubal
  voluntary — *see* Abortion, legal
Abortus fever 023.9
Aboulomania 301.6
Abrachia 755.20
Abrachiatism 755.20
Abrachiocephalia 759.89
Abrachiocephalus 759.89
Abrami's disease (acquired hemolytic jaundice) 283.9
Abramov-Fiedler myocarditis (acute isolated myocarditis) 422.91
Abrasion — *see also* Injury, superficial, by site
  cornea 918.1
  dental 521.20
    extending into
      dentine 521.22
      pulp 521.23
    generalized 521.25
    limited to enamel 521.21
    localized 521.24
  teeth, tooth (dentifrice) (habitual) (hard tissues) (occupational) (ritual) (traditional) (wedge defect) (*see also* Abrasion, dental) 521.20
Abrikossov's tumor (M9580/0) — *see also* Neoplasm, connective tissue, benign
  malignant (M9580/3) — *see* Neoplasm, connective tissue, malignant
Abrism 988.8
Abruption, placenta — *see* Placenta, abruptio
Abruptio placentae — *see* Placenta, abruptio

Abscess (acute) (chronic) (infectional) (lymphangitic) (metastatic) (multiple) (pyogenic) (septic) (with lymphangitis) — *see also* Cellulitis 682.9
  abdomen, abdominal
    cavity 567.22
    wall 682.2
  abdominopelvic 567.22
  accessory sinus (chronic) (*see also* Sinusitis) 473.9
  adrenal (capsule) (gland) 255.8
  alveolar 522.5
    with sinus 522.7
  ambic 006.3
    bladder 006.8
    brain (with liver or lung abscess) 006.5
    liver (without mention of brain or lung abscess) 006.3
      with
        brain abscess (and lung abscess) 006.5
        lung abscess 006.4
    lung (with liver abscess) 006.4
      with brain abscess 006.5
    seminal vesicle 006.8
    specified site NEC 006.8
    spleen 006.8
  anaerobic 040.0
  ankle 682.6
  anorectal 566
  antecubital space 682.3
  antrum (chronic) (Highmore) (*see also* Sinusitis, maxillary) 473.0
  anus 566
  apical (tooth) 522.5
    with sinus (alveolar) 522.7
  appendix 540.1
  areola (acute) (chronic) (nonpuerperal) 611.0
    puerperal, postpartum 675.1 ☑
  arm (any part, above wrist) 682.3
  artery (wall) 447.2
  atheromatous 447.2
  auditory canal (external) 380.10
  auricle (ear) (staphylococcal) (streptococcal) 380.10
  axilla, axillary (region) 682.3
    lymph gland or node 683
  back (any part) 682.2
  Bartholin's gland 616.3
    with
      abortion — *see* Abortion, by type, with sepsis
      ectopic pregnancy (*see also* categories 633.0–633.9) 639.0
      molar pregnancy (*see also* categories 630–632) 639.0
    complicating pregnancy or puerperium 646.6 ☑
    following
      abortion 639.0
      ectopic or molar pregnancy 639.0
  bartholinian 616.3
  Bezold's 383.01
  bile, biliary, duct or tract (*see also* Cholecystitis) 576.8
  bilharziasis 120.1
  bladder (wall) 595.89
    amebic 006.8
  bone (subperiosteal) (*see also* Osteomyelitis) 730.0 ☑
    accessory sinus (chronic) (*see also* Sinusitis) 473.9
    acute 730.0 ☑
    chronic or old 730.1 ☑
    jaw (lower) (upper) 526.4
    mastoid — *see* Mastoiditis, acute
    petrous (*see also* Petrositis) 383.20
    spinal (tuberculous) (*see also* Tuberculosis) 015.0 ☑ *[730.88]*
      nontuberculous 730.08
  bowel 569.5
  brain (any part) 324.0
    amebic (with liver or lung abscess) 006.5
    cystic 324.0
    late effect — *see* category 326

Abscess — *see also* Cellulitis — *continued*
  brain — *continued*
    otogenic 324.0
    tuberculous (*see also* Tuberculosis) 013.3 ☑
  breast (acute) (chronic) (nonpuerperal) 611.0
    newborn 771.5
    puerperal, postpartum 675.1 ☑
    tuberculous (*see also* Tuberculosis) 017.9 ☑
  broad ligament (chronic) (*see also* Disease, pelvis, inflammatory) 614.4
    acute 614.3
  Brodie's (chronic) (localized) (*see also* Osteomyelitis) 730.1 ☑
  bronchus 519.19
  buccal cavity 528.3
  bulbourethral gland 597.0
  bursa 727.89
    pharyngeal 478.29
  buttock 682.5
  canaliculus, breast 611.0
  canthus 372.20
  cartilage 733.99
  cecum 569.5
    with appendicitis 540.1
  cerebellum, cerebellar 324.0
    late effect — *see* category 326
  cerebral (embolic) 324.0
    late effect — *see* category 326
  cervical (neck region) 682.1
    lymph gland or node 683
    stump (*see also* Cervicitis) 616.0
  cervix (stump) (uteri) (*see also* Cervicitis) 616.0
  cheek, external 682.0
    inner 528.3
  chest 510.9
    with fistula 510.0
    wall 682.2
  chin 682.0
  choroid 363.00
  ciliary body 364.3
  circumtonsillar 475
  cold (tuberculous) (*see also* Tuberculosis, abscess)
    articular — *see* Tuberculosis, joint
  colon (wall) 569.5
  colostomy or enterostomy 569.61
  conjunctiva 372.00
  connective tissue NEC 682.9
  cornea 370.55
    with ulcer 370.00
  corpus
    cavernosum 607.2
    luteum (*see also* Salpingo-oophoritis) 614.2
  Cowper's gland 597.0
  cranium 324.0
  cul-de-sac (Douglas') (posterior) (*see also* Disease, pelvis, inflammatory) 614.4
    acute 614.3
  dental 522.5
    with sinus (alveolar) 522.7
  dentoalveolar 522.5
    with sinus (alveolar) 522.7
  diaphragm, diaphragmatic 567.22
  digit NEC 681.9
  Douglas' cul-de-sac or pouch (*see also* Disease, pelvis, inflammatory) 614.4
    acute 614.3
  Dubois' 090.5
  ductless gland 259.8
  ear
    acute 382.00
    external 380.10
    inner 386.30
    middle — *see* Otitis media
  elbow 682.3
  endamebic — *see* Abscess, amebic
  entamebic — *see* Abscess, amebic
  enterostomy 569.61
  epididymis 604.0
  epidural 324.9
    brain 324.0

Abscess — *see also* Cellulitis — *continued*
  epidural — *continued*
    late effect — *see* category 326
    spinal cord 324.1
  epiglottis 478.79
  epiploon, epiploic 567.22
  erysipelatous (*see also* Erysipelas) 035
  esophagostomy 530.86
  esophagus 530.19
  ethmoid (bone) (chronic) (sinus) (*see also* Sinusitis, ethmoidal) 473.2
  external auditory canal 380.10
  extradural 324.9
    brain 324.0
    late effect — *see* category 326
    spinal cord 324.1
  extraperitoneal — *see* Abscess, peritoneum
  eye 360.00
  eyelid 373.13
  face (any part, except eye) 682.0
  fallopian tube (*see also* Salpingo-oophoritis) 614.2
  fascia 728.89
  fauces 478.29
  fecal 569.5
  femoral (region) 682.6
  filaria, filarial (*see also* Infestation, filarial) 125.9
  finger (any) (intrathecal) (periosteal) (subcutaneous) (subcuticular) 681.00
  fistulous NEC 682.9
  flank 682.2
  foot (except toe) 682.7
  forearm 682.3
  forehead 682.0
  frontal (sinus) (chronic) (*see also* Sinusitis, frontal) 473.1
  gallbladder (*see also* Cholecystitis, acute) 575.0
  gastric 535.0 ☑
  genital organ or tract NEC
    female 616.9
      with
        abortion — *see* Abortion, by type, with sepsis
        ectopic pregnancy (*see also* categories 633.0–633.9) 639.0
        molar pregnancy (*see also* categories 630–632) 639.0
      following
        abortion 639.0
        ectopic or molar pregnancy 639.0
      puerperal, postpartum, childbirth 670.8 ☑
    male 608.4
  genitourinary system, tuberculous (*see also* Tuberculosis) 016.9 ☑
  gingival 523.30
  gland, glandular (lymph) (acute) NEC 683
  glottis 478.79
  gluteal (region) 682.5
  gonorrheal NEC (*see also* Gonococcus) 098.0
  groin 682.2
  gum 523.30
  hand (except finger or thumb) 682.4
  head (except face) 682.8
  heart 429.89
  heel 682.7
  helminthic (*see also* Infestation, by specific parasite) 128.9
  hepatic 572.0
    amebic (*see also* Abscess, liver, amebic) 006.3
    duct 576.8
  hip 682.6
    tuberculous (active) (*see also* Tuberculosis) 015.1 ☑
  ileocecal 540.1
  ileostomy (bud) 569.61
  iliac (region) 682.2
    fossa 540.1
  iliopsoas 567.31
    nontuberculous 728.89
    tuberculous (*see also* Tuberculosis) 015.0 ☑ *[730.88]*
  infraclavicular (fossa) 682.3

☑ Additional Digit Required — Refer to the Tabular List for Digit Selection
    ⬒ Subterms under main terms may continue to next column or page

2015 ICD-9-CM
  ▶◀ Revised Text
  ● New Line
  ▲ Revised Code
  Volume 2 — 3

Abscess — *see also* Cellulitis — *continued*
inguinal (region) 682.2
lymph gland or node 683
intersphincteric (anus) 566
intestine, intestinal 569.5
rectal 566
intra-abdominal (*see also* Abscess, peritoneum) 567.22
postoperative 998.59
intracranial 324.0
late effect — *see* category 326
intramammary — *see* Abscess, breast
intramastoid (*see also* Mastoiditis, acute) 383.00
intraorbital 376.01
intraperitoneal 567.22
intraspinal 324.1
late effect — *see* category 326
intratonsillar 475
iris 364.3
ischiorectal 566
jaw (bone) (lower) (upper) 526.4
skin 682.0
joint (*see also* Arthritis, pyogenic) 711.0 ☑
vertebral (tuberculous) (*see also* Tuberculosis) 015.0 ☑ [730.88]
nontuberculous 724.8
kidney 590.2
with
abortion — *see* Abortion, by type, with urinary tract infection
calculus 592.0
ectopic pregnancy (*see also* categories 633.0–633.9) 639.8
molar pregnancy (*see also* categories 630–632) 639.8
complicating pregnancy or puerperium 646.6 ☑
affecting fetus or newborn 760.1
following
abortion 639.8
ectopic or molar pregnancy 639.8
knee 682.6
joint 711.06
tuberculous (active) (*see also* Tuberculosis) 015.2 ☑
labium (majus) (minus) 616.4
complicating pregnancy, childbirth, or puerperium 646.6 ☑
lacrimal (passages) (sac) (*see also* Dacryocystitis) 375.30
caruncle 375.30
gland (*see also* Dacryoadenitis) 375.00
lacunar 597.0
larynx 478.79
lateral (alveolar) 522.5
with sinus 522.7
leg, except foot 682.6
lens 360.00
lid 373.13
lingual 529.0
tonsil 475
lip 528.5
Littre's gland 597.0
liver 572.0
amebic 006.3
with
brain abscess (and lung abscess) 006.5
lung abscess 006.4
due to Entamoeba histolytica 006.3
dysenteric (*see also* Abscess, liver, amebic) 006.3
pyogenic 572.0
tropical (*see also* Abscess, liver, amebic) 006.3
loin (region) 682.2
lumbar (tuberculous) (*see also* Tuberculosis) 015.0 ☑ [730.88]
nontuberculous 682.2
lung (miliary) (putrid) 513.0
amebic (with liver abscess) 006.4
with brain abscess 006.5
lymphangitic, acute — *see* Cellulitis
lymph, lymphatic, gland or node (acute) 683
any site, except mesenteric 683

Abscess — *see also* Cellulitis — *continued*
lymph, lymphatic, gland or node — *continued*
mesentery 289.2
malar 526.4
mammary gland — *see* Abscess, breast
marginal (anus) 566
mastoid (process) (*see also* Mastoiditis, acute) 383.00
subperiosteal 383.01
maxilla, maxillary 526.4
molar (tooth) 522.5
with sinus 522.7
premolar 522.5
sinus (chronic) (*see also* Sinusitis, maxillary) 473.0
mediastinum 513.1
meibomian gland 373.12
meninges (*see also* Meningitis) 320.9
mesentery, mesenteric 567.22
mesosalpinx (*see also* Salpingo-oophoritis) 614.2
milk 675.1 ☑
Monro's (psoriasis) 696.1
mons pubis 682.2
mouth (floor) 528.3
multiple sites NEC 682.9
mural 682.2
muscle 728.89
psoas 567.31
myocardium 422.92
nabothian (follicle) (*see also* Cervicitis) 616.0
nail (chronic) (with lymphangitis) 681.9
finger 681.02
toe 681.11
nasal (fossa) (septum) 478.19
sinus (chronic) (*see also* Sinusitis) 473.9
nasopharyngeal 478.29
nates 682.5
navel 682.2
newborn NEC 771.4
neck (region) 682.1
lymph gland or node 683
nephritic (*see also* Abscess, kidney) 590.2
nipple 611.0
puerperal, postpartum 675.0 ☑
nose (septum) 478.19
external 682.0
omentum 567.22
operative wound 998.59
orbit, orbital 376.01
ossifluent — *see* Abscess, bone
ovary, ovarian (corpus luteum) (*see also* Salpingo-oophoritis) 614.2
oviduct (*see also* Salpingo-oophoritis) 614.2
palate (soft) 528.3
hard 526.4
palmar (space) 682.4
pancreas (duct) 577.0
paradontal 523.30
parafrenal 607.2
parametric, parametrium (chronic) (*see also* Disease, pelvis, inflammatory) 614.4
acute 614.3
paranephric 590.2
parapancreatic 577.0
parapharyngeal 478.22
pararectal 566
parasinus (*see also* Sinusitis) 473.9
parauterine (*see also* Disease, pelvis, inflammatory) 614.4
acute 614.3
paravaginal (*see also* Vaginitis) 616.10
parietal region 682.8
parodontal 523.30
parotid (duct) (gland) 527.3
region 528.3
parumbilical 682.2
newborn 771.4
pectoral (region) 682.2
pelvirectal 567.22
pelvis, pelvic
female (chronic) (*see also* Disease, pelvis, inflammatory) 614.4
acute 614.3

Abscess — *see also* Cellulitis — *continued*
pelvis, pelvic — *continued*
male, peritoneal (cellular tissue) — *see* Abscess, peritoneum
tuberculous (*see also* Tuberculosis) 016.9 ☑
penis 607.2
gonococcal (acute) 098.0
chronic or duration of 2 months or over 098.2
perianal 566
periapical 522.5
with sinus (alveolar) 522.7
periappendiceal 540.1
pericardial 420.99
pericecal 540.1
pericemental 523.30
pericholecystic (*see also* Cholecystitis, acute) 575.0
pericoronal 523.30
peridental 523.30
perigastric 535.0 ☑
perimetric (*see also* Disease, pelvis, inflammatory) 614.4
acute 614.3
perinephric, perinephritic (*see also* Abscess, kidney) 590.2
perineum, perineal (superficial) 682.2
deep (with urethral involvement) 597.0
urethra 597.0
periodontal (parietal) 523.31
apical 522.5
periosteum, periosteal (*see also* Periostitis) 730.3 ☑
with osteomyelitis (*see also* Osteomyelitis) 730.2 ☑
acute or subacute 730.0 ☑
chronic or old 730.1 ☑
peripleuritic 510.9
with fistula 510.0
periproctic 566
periprostatic 601.2
perirectal (staphylococcal) 566
perirenal (tissue) (*see also* Abscess, kidney) 590.2
perisinuous (nose) (*see also* Sinusitis) 473.9
peritoneum, peritoneal (perforated) (ruptured) 567.22
with
abortion — *see* Abortion, by type, with sepsis
appendicitis 540.1
ectopic pregnancy (*see also* categories 633.0–633.9) 639.0
molar pregnancy (*see also* categories 630–632) 639.0
following
abortion 639.0
ectopic or molar pregnancy 639.0
pelvic, female (*see also* Disease, pelvis, inflammatory) 614.4
acute 614.3
postoperative 998.59
puerperal, postpartum, childbirth 670.8 ☑
tuberculous (*see also* Tuberculosis) 014.0 ☑
peritonsillar 475
perityphlic 540.1
periureteral 593.89
periurethral 597.0
gonococcal (acute) 098.0
chronic or duration of 2 months or over 098.2
periuterine (*see also* Disease, pelvis, inflammatory) 614.4
acute 614.3
perivesical 595.89
pernicious NEC 682.9
petrous bone — *see* Petrositis
phagedenic NEC 682.9
chancroid 099.0
pharynx, pharyngeal (lateral) 478.29
phlegmonous NEC 682.9
pilonidal 685.0
pituitary (gland) 253.8

Abscess — *see also* Cellulitis — *continued*
pleura 510.9
with fistula 510.0
popliteal 682.6
postanal 566
postcecal 540.1
postlaryngeal 478.79
postnasal 478.19
postpharyngeal 478.24
posttonsillar 475
posttyphoid 002.0
Pott's (*see also* Tuberculosis) 015.0 ☑ [730.88]
pouch of Douglas (chronic) (*see also* Disease, pelvis, inflammatory) 614.4
premammary — *see* Abscess, breast
prepatellar 682.6
prostate (*see also* Prostatitis) 601.2
gonococcal (acute) 098.12
chronic or duration of 2 months or over 098.32
psoas 567.31
nontuberculous 728.89
tuberculous (*see also* Tuberculosis) 015.0 ☑ [730.88]
pterygopalatine fossa 682.8
pubis 682.2
puerperal — *see* Puerperal, abscess, by site
pulmonary — *see* Abscess, lung
pulp, pulpal (dental) 522.0
finger 681.01
toe 681.10
pyemic — *see* Septicemia
pyloric valve 535.0 ☑
rectovaginal septum 569.5
rectovesical 595.89
rectum 566
regional NEC 682.9
renal (*see also* Abscess, kidney) 590.2
retina 363.00
retrobulbar 376.01
retrocecal 567.22
retrolaryngeal 478.79
retromammary — *see* Abscess, breast
retroperineal 682.2
retroperitoneal 567.38
postprocedural 998.59
retropharyngeal 478.24
tuberculous (*see also* Tuberculosis) 012.8 ☑
retrorectal 566
retrouterine (*see also* Disease, pelvis, inflammatory) 614.4
acute 614.3
retrovesical 595.89
root, tooth 522.5
with sinus (alveolar) 522.7
round ligament (*see also* Disease, pelvis, inflammatory) 614.4
acute 614.3
rupture (spontaneous) NEC 682.9
sacrum (tuberculous) (*see also* Tuberculosis) 015.0 ☑ [730.88]
nontuberculous 730.08
salivary duct or gland 527.3
scalp (any part) 682.8
scapular 730.01
sclera 379.09
scrofulous (*see also* Tuberculosis) 017.2 ☑
scrotum 608.4
seminal vesicle 608.0
amebic 006.8
septal, dental 522.5
with sinus (alveolar) 522.7
septum (nasal) 478.19
serous (*see also* Periostitis) 730.3 ☑
shoulder 682.3
side 682.2
sigmoid 569.5
sinus (accessory) (chronic) (nasal) (*see also* Sinusitis) 473.9
intracranial venous (any) 324.0
late effect — *see* category 326
Skene's duct or gland 597.0
skin NEC 682.9

Abscess — *see also* Cellulitis — *continued*
skin — *continued*
tuberculous (primary) (*see also* Tuberculosis) 017.0 ☑
sloughing NEC 682.9
specified site NEC 682.8
amebic 006.8
spermatic cord 608.4
sphenoidal (sinus) (*see also* Sinusitis, sphenoidal) 473.3
spinal
cord (any part) (staphylococcal) 324.1
tuberculous (*see also* Tuberculosis) 013.5 ☑
epidural 324.1
spine (column) (tuberculous) (*see also* Tuberculosis) 015.0 ☑ *[730.88]*
nontuberculous 730.08
spleen 289.59
amebic 006.8
staphylococcal NEC 682.9
stitch 998.59
stomach (wall) 535.0 ☑
strumous (tuberculous) (*see also* Tuberculosis) 017.2 ☑
subarachnoid 324.9
brain 324.0
cerebral 324.0
late effect — *see* category 326
spinal cord 324.1
subareolar (*see also* Abscess, breast)
puerperal, postpartum 675.1 ☑
subcecal 540.1
subcutaneous NEC 682.9
subdiaphragmatic 567.22
subdorsal 682.2
subdural 324.9
brain 324.0
late effect — *see* category 326
spinal cord 324.1
subgaleal 682.8
subhepatic 567.22
sublingual 528.3
gland 527.3
submammary — *see* Abscess, breast
submandibular (region) (space) (triangle) 682.0
gland 527.3
submaxillary (region) 682.0
gland 527.3
submental (pyogenic) 682.0
gland 527.3
subpectoral 682.2
subperiosteal — *see* Abscess, bone
subperitoneal 567.22
subphrenic (*see also* Abscess, peritoneum) 567.22
postoperative 998.59
subscapular 682.2
subungual 681.9
suburethral 597.0
sudoriparous 705.89
suppurative NEC 682.9
supraclavicular (fossa) 682.3
suprahepatic 567.22
suprapelvic (*see also* Disease, pelvis, inflammatory) 614.4
acute 614.3
suprapubic 682.2
suprarenal (capsule) (gland) 255.8
sweat gland 705.89
syphilitic 095.8
teeth, tooth (root) 522.5
with sinus (alveolar) 522.7
supporting structures NEC 523.30
temple 682.0
temporal region 682.0
temporosphenoidal 324.0
late effect — *see* category 326
tendon (sheath) 727.89
testicle — *see* Orchitis
thecal 728.89
thigh (acquired) 682.6
thorax 510.9
with fistula 510.0
throat 478.29

Abscess — *see also* Cellulitis — *continued*
thumb (intrathecal) (periosteal) (subcutaneous) (subcuticular) 681.00
thymus (gland) 254.1
thyroid (gland) 245.0
toe (any) (intrathecal) (periosteal) (subcutaneous) (subcuticular) 681.10
tongue (staphylococcal) 529.0
tonsil(s) (lingual) 475
tonsillopharyngeal 475
tooth, teeth (root) 522.5
with sinus (alveolar) 522.7
supporting structure NEC 523.30
trachea 478.9
trunk 682.2
tubal (*see also* Salpingo-oophoritis) 614.2
tuberculous — *see* Tuberculosis, abscess
tubo-ovarian (*see also* Salpingo-oophoritis) 614.2
tunica vaginalis 608.4
umbilicus NEC 682.2
newborn 771.4
upper arm 682.3
upper respiratory 478.9
urachus 682.2
urethra (gland) 597.0
urinary 597.0
uterus, uterine (wall) (*see also* Endometritis) 615.9
ligament (*see also* Disease, pelvis, inflammatory) 614.4
acute 614.3
neck (*see also* Cervicitis) 616.0
uvula 528.3
vagina (wall) (*see also* Vaginitis) 616.10
vaginorectal (*see also* Vaginitis) 616.10
vas deferens 608.4
vermiform appendix 540.1
vertebra (column) (tuberculous) (*see also* Tuberculosis) 015.0 ☑ *[730.88]*
nontuberculous 730.0 ☑
vesical 595.89
vesicouterine pouch (*see also* Disease, pelvis, inflammatory) 614.4
vitreous (humor) (pneumococcal) 360.04
vocal cord 478.5
von Bezold's 383.01
vulva 616.4
complicating pregnancy, childbirth, or puerperium 646.6 ☑
vulvovaginal gland (*see also* Vaginitis) 616.3
web-space 682.4
wrist 682.4
Absence (organ or part) (complete or partial)
acoustic nerve 742.8
adrenal (gland) (congenital) 759.1
acquired V45.79
albumin (blood) 273.8
alimentary tract (complete) (congenital) (partial) 751.8
lower 751.5
upper 750.8
alpha-fucosidase 271.8
alveolar process (acquired) 525.8
congenital 750.26
anus, anal (canal) (congenital) 751.2
aorta (congenital) 747.22
aortic valve (congenital) 746.89
appendix, congenital 751.2
arm (acquired) V49.60
above elbow V49.66
below elbow V49.65
congenital (*see also* Deformity, reduction, upper limb) 755.20
lower — *see* Absence, forearm, congenital
upper (complete) (partial) (with absence of distal elements, incomplete) 755.24
with
complete absence of distal elements 755.21
forearm (incomplete) 755.23
artery (congenital) (peripheral) NEC (*see also* Anomaly, peripheral vascular system) 747.60

Absence — *continued*
artery (*see also* Anomaly, peripheral vascular system) — *continued*
brain 747.81
cerebral 747.81
coronary 746.85
pulmonary 747.31
umbilical 747.5
atrial septum 745.69
auditory canal (congenital) (external) 744.01
auricle (ear) (with stenosis or atresia of auditory canal), congenital 744.01
bile, biliary duct (common) or passage (congenital) 751.61
bladder (acquired) V45.74
congenital 753.8
bone (congenital) NEC 756.9
marrow 284.9
acquired (secondary) 284.89
congenital 284.09
hereditary 284.09
idiopathic 284.9
skull 756.0
bowel sounds 787.5
brain 740.0
specified part 742.2
breast(s) (acquired) V45.71
congenital 757.6
broad ligament (congenital) 752.19
bronchus (congenital) 748.3
calvarium, calvaria (skull) 756.0
canaliculus lacrimalis, congenital 743.65
carpal(s) (congenital) (complete) (partial) (with absence of distal elements, incomplete) (*see also* Deformity, reduction, upper limb) 755.28
with complete absence of distal elements 755.21
cartilage 756.9
caudal spine 756.13
cecum (acquired) (postoperative) (posttraumatic) V45.72
congenital 751.2
cementum 520.4
cerebellum (congenital) (vermis) 742.2
cervix (acquired) (uteri) V88.01
with remaining uterus V88.03
and uterus V88.01
congenital 752.43
chin, congenital 744.89
cilia (congenital) 743.63
acquired 374.89
circulatory system, part NEC 747.89
clavicle 755.51
clitoris (congenital) 752.49
coccyx, congenital 756.13
cold sense (*see also* Disturbance, sensation) 782.0
colon (acquired) (postoperative) V45.72
congenital 751.2
congenital
lumen — *see* Atresia
organ or site NEC — *see* Agenesis
septum — *see* Imperfect, closure
corpus callosum (congenital) 742.2
cricoid cartilage 748.3
diaphragm (congenital) (with hernia) 756.6
with obstruction 756.6
digestive organ(s) or tract, congenital (complete) (partial) 751.8
acquired V45.79
lower 751.5
upper 750.8
ductus arteriosus 747.89
duodenum (acquired) (postoperative) V45.72
congenital 751.1
ear, congenital 744.09
acquired V45.79
auricle 744.01
external 744.01
inner 744.05
lobe, lobule 744.21
middle, except ossicles 744.03
ossicles 744.04
ossicles 744.04

Absence — *continued*
ejaculatory duct (congenital) 752.89
endocrine gland NEC (congenital) 759.2
epididymis (congenital) 752.89
acquired V45.77
epiglottis, congenital 748.3
epileptic (atonic) (typical) (*see also* Epilepsy) 345.0 ☑
erythrocyte 284.9
erythropoiesis 284.9
congenital 284.01
esophagus (congenital) 750.3
Eustachian tube (congenital) 744.24
extremity (acquired)
congenital (*see also* Deformity, reduction) 755.4
lower V49.70
upper V49.60
extrinsic muscle, eye 743.69
eye (acquired) V45.78
adnexa (congenital) 743.69
congenital 743.00
muscle (congenital) 743.69
eyelid (fold), congenital 743.62
acquired 374.89
face
bones NEC 756.0
specified part NEC 744.89
fallopian tube(s) (acquired) V45.77
congenital 752.19
femur, congenital (complete) (partial) (with absence of distal elements, incomplete) (*see also* Deformity, reduction, lower limb) 755.34
with
complete absence of distal elements 755.31
tibia and fibula (incomplete) 755.33
fibrin 790.92
fibrinogen (congenital) 286.3
acquired 286.6
fibula, congenital (complete) (partial) (with absence of distal elements, incomplete) (*see also* Deformity, reduction, lower limb) 755.37
with
complete absence of distal elements 755.31
tibia 755.35
with
complete absence of distal elements 755.31
femur (incomplete) 755.33
with complete absence of distal elements 755.31
finger (acquired) V49.62
congenital (complete) (partial) (*see also* Deformity, reduction, upper limb) 755.29
meaning all fingers (complete) (partial) 755.21
transverse 755.21
fissures of lungs (congenital) 748.5
foot (acquired) V49.73
congenital (complete) 755.31
forearm (acquired) V49.65
congenital (complete) (partial) (with absence of distal elements, incomplete) (*see also* Deformity, reduction, upper limb) 755.25
with
complete absence of distal elements (hand and fingers) 755.21
humerus (incomplete) 755.23
fovea centralis 743.55
fucosidase 271.8
gallbladder (acquired) V45.79
congenital 751.69
gamma globulin (blood) 279.00
genital organs
acquired V45.77
congenital
female 752.89
external 752.49

☑ **Additional Digit Required** — Refer to the Tabular List for Digit Selection ▽ **Subterms under main terms may continue to next column or page**

2015 ICD-9-CM ►◄ Revised Text ● New Line ▲ Revised Code **Volume 2 — 5**

☑ **Additional Digit Required** — Refer to the Tabular List for Digit Selection   ▽ **Subterms under main terms may continue to next column or page**

6 — Volume 2   ▶◀ Revised Text   ● New Line   ▲ Revised Code   2015 ICD-9-CM

Absence — *continued*
  uterus (acquired) V88.01
    with remaining cervical stump V88.02
    and cervix V88.01
    congenital 752.31
  uvula (congenital) 750.26
  vagina, congenital 752.45
    acquired V45.77
  vas deferens (congenital) 752.89
    acquired V45.77
  vein (congenital) (peripheral) NEC (*see also*
    Anomaly, peripheral vascular system)
    747.60
    brain 747.81
    great 747.49
    portal 747.49
    pulmonary 747.49
  vena cava (congenital) (inferior) (superior)
    747.49
  ventral horn cell 742.59
  ventricular septum 745.3
  vermis of cerebellum 742.2
  vertebra, congenital 756.13
  vulva, congenital 752.49
Absentia epileptica — *see also* Epilepsy
  345.0 ☑
Absinthemia — *see also* Dependence 304.6 ☑
Absinthism — *see also* Dependence 304.6 ☑
Absorbent system disease 459.89
Absorption
  alcohol, through placenta or breast milk
    760.71
  antibiotics, through placenta or breast milk
    760.74
  anticonvulsants, through placenta or breast
    milk 760.77
  antifungals, through placenta or breast milk
    760.74
  anti-infective, through placenta or breast
    milk 760.74
  antimetabolics, through placenta or breast
    milk 760.78
  chemical NEC 989.9
    specified chemical or substance — *see*
      Table of Drugs and Chemicals
    through placenta or breast milk (fetus
      or newborn) 760.70
      alcohol 760.71
      anticonvulsants 760.77
      antifungals 760.74
      anti-infective agents 760.74
      antimetabolics 760.78
      cocaine 760.75
      "crack" 760.75
      diethylstilbestrol [DES] 760.76
      hallucinogenic agents 760.73
      medicinal agents NEC 760.79
      narcotics 760.72
      obstetric anesthetic or analgesic drug
        763.5
      specified agent NEC 760.79
      suspected, affecting management of
        pregnancy 655.5 ☑
  cocaine, through placenta or breast milk
    760.75
  drug NEC (*see also* Reaction, drug)
    through placenta or breast milk (fetus
      or newborn) 760.70
      alcohol 760.71
      anticonvulsants 760.77
      antifungals 760.74
      anti-infective agents 760.74
      antimetabolics 760.78
      cocaine 760.75
      "crack" 760.75
      diethylstilbestrol [DES] 760.76
      hallucinogenic agents 760.73
      medicinal agents NEC 760.79
      narcotics 760.72
      obstetric anesthetic or analgesic drug
        763.5
      specified agent NEC 760.79
      suspected, affecting management of
        pregnancy 655.5 ☑
  fat, disturbance 579.8

Absorption — *continued*
  hallucinogenic agents, through placenta or
    breast milk 760.73
  immune sera, through placenta or breast
    milk 760.79
  lactose defect 271.3
  medicinal agents NEC, through placenta or
    breast milk 760.79
  narcotics, through placenta or breast milk
    760.72
  noxious substance — *see* Absorption,
    chemical
  protein, disturbance 579.8
  pus or septic, general — *see* Septicemia
  quinine, through placenta or breast milk
    760.74
  toxic substance — *see* Absorption, chemical
  uremic — *see* Uremia
Abstinence symptoms or syndrome
  alcohol 291.81
  drug 292.0
  neonatal 779.5
Abt-Letterer-Siwe syndrome (acute histiocytosis X) (M9722/3) 202.5 ☑
Abulia 799.89
Abulomania 301.6
Abuse
  adult 995.80
    emotional 995.82
    multiple forms 995.85
    neglect (nutritional) 995.84
    physical 995.81
    psychological 995.82
    sexual 995.83
  alcohol — *see also* Alcoholism 305.0 ☑
    dependent 303.9 ☑
    non-dependent 305.0 ☑
  child 995.50
    counseling
      perpetrator
        non-parent V62.83
        parent V61.22
      victim V61.21
    emotional 995.51
    multiple forms 995.59
    neglect (nutritional) 995.52
    physical 995.54
      shaken infant syndrome 995.55
    psychological 995.51
    sexual 995.53
  drugs, nondependent 305.9 ☑

> *Note* — Use the following fifth-digit
> subclassification with the following
> codes: 305.0, 305.2–305.9:
>
> 0   unspecified
>
> 1   continuous
>
> 2   episodic
>
> 3   in remission

    amphetamine type 305.7 ☑
    antidepressants 305.8 ☑
    anxiolytic 305.4 ☑
    barbiturates 305.4 ☑
    caffeine 305.9 ☑
    cannabis 305.2 ☑
    cocaine type 305.6 ☑
    hallucinogens 305.3 ☑
    hashish 305.2 ☑
    hypnotic 305.4 ☑
    inhalant 305.9 ☑
    LSD 305.3 ☑
    marijuana 305.2 ☑
    mixed 305.9 ☑
    morphine type 305.5 ☑
    opioid type 305.5 ☑
    phencyclidine (PCP) 305.9 ☑
    sedative 305.4 ☑
    specified NEC 305.9 ☑
    tranquilizers 305.4 ☑
  spouse 995.80
  tobacco 305.1
Acalcerosis 275.40
Acalcicosis 275.40
Acalculia 784.69

Acalculia — *continued*
  developmental 315.1
Acanthocheilonemiasis 125.4
Acanthocytosis 272.5
Acanthokeratodermia 701.1
Acantholysis 701.8
  bullosa 757.39
Acanthoma (benign) (M8070/0) — *see also*
  Neoplasm, by site, benign
  malignant (M8070/3) — *see* Neoplasm, by
    site, malignant
Acanthosis (acquired) (nigricans) 701.2
  adult 701.2
  benign (congenital) 757.39
  congenital 757.39
  glycogenic
    esophagus 530.89
  juvenile 701.2
  tongue 529.8
Acanthrocytosis 272.5
Acapnia 276.3
Acarbia 276.2
Acardia 759.89
Acardiacus amorphus 759.89
Acardiotrophia 429.1
Acardius 759.89
Acariasis 133.9
  sarcoptic 133.0
Acaridiasis 133.9
Acarinosis 133.9
Acariosis 133.9
Acarodermatitis 133.9
  urticarioides 133.9
Acarophobia 300.29
Acatalasemia 277.89
Acatalasia 277.89
Acatamathesia 784.69
Acataphasia 784.59
Acathisia 781.0
  due to drugs 333.99
Acceleration, accelerated
  atrioventricular conduction 426.7
  idioventricular rhythm 427.89
Accessory (congenital)
  adrenal gland 759.1
  anus 751.5
  appendix 751.5
  atrioventricular conduction 426.7
  auditory ossicles 744.04
  auricle (ear) 744.1
  autosome(s) NEC 758.5
    21 or 22 758.0
  biliary duct or passage 751.69
  bladder 753.8
  blood vessels (peripheral) (congenital) NEC
    (*see also* Anomaly, peripheral vascu-
    lar system) 747.60
    cerebral 747.81
    coronary 746.85
  bone NEC 756.9
    foot 755.67
  breast tissue, axilla 757.6
  carpal bones 755.56
  cecum 751.5
  cervix 752.44
  chromosome(s) NEC 758.5
    13-15 758.1
    16-18 758.2
    21 or 22 758.0
    autosome(s) NEC 758.5
    D_1 758.1
    E_3 758.2
    G 758.0
    sex 758.81
  coronary artery 746.85
  cusp(s), heart valve NEC 746.89
    pulmonary 746.09
  cystic duct 751.69
  digits 755.00
  ear (auricle) (lobe) 744.1
  endocrine gland NEC 759.2
  external os 752.44
  eyelid 743.62
  eye muscle 743.69
  face bone(s) 756.0
  fallopian tube (fimbria) (ostium) 752.19

Accessory — *continued*
  fingers 755.01
  foreskin 605
  frontonasal process 756.0
  gallbladder 751.69
  genital organ(s)
    female 752.89
      external 752.49
      internal NEC 752.89
    male NEC 752.89
      penis 752.69
  genitourinary organs NEC 752.89
  heart 746.89
    valve NEC 746.89
      pulmonary 746.09
  hepatic ducts 751.69
  hymen 752.49
  intestine (large) (small) 751.5
  kidney 753.3
  lacrimal canal 743.65
  leaflet, heart valve NEC 746.89
    pulmonary 746.09
  ligament, broad 752.19
  liver (duct) 751.69
  lobule (ear) 744.1
  lung (lobe) 748.69
  muscle 756.82
  navicular of carpus 755.56
  nervous system, part NEC 742.8
  nipple 757.6
  nose 748.1
  organ or site NEC — *see* Anomaly, specified
    type NEC
  ovary 752.0
  oviduct 752.19
  pancreas 751.7
  parathyroid gland 759.2
  parotid gland (and duct) 750.22
  pituitary gland 759.2
  placental lobe — *see* Placenta, abnormal
  preauricular appendage 744.1
  prepuce 605
  renal arteries (multiple) 747.62
  rib 756.3
    cervical 756.2
  roots (teeth) 520.2
  salivary gland 750.22
  sesamoids 755.8
  sinus — *see* condition
  skin tags 757.39
  spleen 759.0
  sternum 756.3
  submaxillary gland 750.22
  tarsal bones 755.67
  teeth, tooth 520.1
    causing crowding 524.31
  tendon 756.89
  thumb 755.01
  thymus gland 759.2
  thyroid gland 759.2
  toes 755.02
  tongue 750.13
  tragus 744.1
  ureter 753.4
  urethra 753.8
  urinary organ or tract NEC 753.8
  uterus 752.2
  vagina 752.49
  valve, heart NEC 746.89
    pulmonary 746.09
  vertebra 756.19
  vocal cords 748.3
  vulva 752.49
Accident, accidental — *see also* condition
  birth NEC 767.9
  cardiovascular (*see also* Disease, cardiovas-
    cular) 429.2
  cerebral (*see also* Disease, cerebrovascular,
    acute) 434.91
  cerebrovascular (current) (CVA) (*see also*
    Disease, cerebrovascular, acute)
    434.91
    aborted 434.91
    embolic 434.11
    healed or old V12.54
    hemorrhagic — *see* Hemorrhage, brain

☑ **Additional Digit Required — Refer to the Tabular List for Digit Selection**   ᴺᵁ **Subterms under main terms may continue to next column or page**

2015 ICD-9-CM   ▶◀ Revised Text   ● New Line   ▲ Revised Code   Volume 2 — 7

Accident, accidental — *see also* condition — *continued*
  cerebrovascular (*see also* Disease, cerebrovascular, acute) — *continued*
    impending 435.9
    ischemic 434.91
    late effect — *see* Late effect(s) (of) cerebrovascular disease
    postoperative 997.02
    thrombotic 434.01
  coronary (*see also* Infarct, myocardium) 410.9 ☑
  craniovascular (*see also* Disease, cerebrovascular, acute) 436
  during pregnancy, to mother, affecting fetus or newborn 760.5
  heart, cardiac (*see also* Infarct, myocardium) 410.9 ☑
  intrauterine 779.89
  vascular — *see* Disease, cerebrovascular, acute
Accommodation
  disorder of 367.51
    drug-induced 367.89
    toxic 367.89
  insufficiency of 367.4
  paralysis of 367.51
    hysterical 300.11
  spasm of 367.53
Accouchement — *see* Delivery
Accreta placenta (without hemorrhage) 667.0 ☑
  with hemorrhage 666.0 ☑
Accretio cordis (nonrheumatic) 423.1
Accretions on teeth 523.6
Accumulation secretion, prostate 602.8
Acephalia, acephalism, acephaly 740.0
Acephalic 740.0
Acephalobrachia 759.89
Acephalocardia 759.89
Acephalocardius 759.89
Acephalochiria 759.89
Acephalochirus 759.89
Acephalogaster 759.89
Acephalostomus 759.89
Acephalothorax 759.89
Acephalus 740.0
Acetonemia 790.6
  diabetic 250.1 ☑
    due to secondary diabetes 249.1 ☑
Acetonglycosuria 982.8
Acetonuria 791.6
Achalasia 530.0
  cardia 530.0
  digestive organs congenital NEC 751.8
  esophagus 530.0
  pelvirectal 751.3
  psychogenic 306.4
  pylorus 750.5
  sphincteral NEC 564.89
Achard-Thiers syndrome (adrenogenital) 255.2
Ache(s) — *see* Pain
Acheilia 750.26
Acheiria 755.21
Achillobursitis 726.71
Achillodynia 726.71
Achlorhydria, achlorhydric 536.0
  anemia 280.9
  diarrhea 536.0
  neurogenic 536.0
  postvagotomy 564.2
  psychogenic 306.4
  secondary to vagotomy 564.2
Achloroblepsia 368.52
Achloropsia 368.52
Acholia 575.8
Acholuric jaundice (familial) (splenomegalic) — *see also* Spherocytosis 282.0
  acquired 283.9
Achondroplasia 756.4
Achrestic anemia 281.8
Achroacytosis, lacrimal gland 375.00
  tuberculous (*see also* Tuberculosis) 017.3 ☑
Achroma, cutis 709.00
Achromate (congenital) 368.54

Achromatopia 368.54
Achromatopsia (congenital) 368.54
Achromia
  congenital 270.2
  parasitica 111.0
  unguium 703.8
Achylia
  gastrica 536.8
    neurogenic 536.3
    psychogenic 306.4
  pancreatica 577.1
Achylosis 536.8
Acid
  burn (*see also* Burn, by site)
    from swallowing acid — *see* Burn, internal organs
  deficiency
    amide nicotinic 265.2
    amino 270.9
    ascorbic 267
    folic 266.2
    nicotinic (amide) 265.2
    pantothenic 266.2
  intoxication 276.2
  peptic disease 536.8
  stomach 536.8
    psychogenic 306.4
Acidemia 276.2
  arginosuccinic 270.6
  fetal
    affecting management of pregnancy 656.3 ☑
    before onset of labor, in liveborn infant 768.2
    during labor and delivery in liveborn infant 768.3
    intrauterine 656.3 ☑
    unspecified as to time of onset, in liveborn infant 768.4
  newborn 775.81
  pipecolic 270.7
Acidity, gastric (high) (low) 536.8
  psychogenic 306.4
Acidocytopenia 288.59
Acidocytosis 288.3
Acidopenia 288.59
Acidosis 276.2
  diabetic 250.1 ☑
    due to secondary diabetes 249.1 ☑
  fetal, affecting management of pregnancy 656.8 ☑
  fetal, affecting newborn 775.81
  kidney tubular 588.89
    newborn 775.81
  lactic 276.2
  metabolic NEC 276.2
    with respiratory acidosis 276.4
      of newborn 775.81
    late, of newborn 775.7
  newborn 775.81
  renal
    hyperchloremic 588.89
    tubular (distal) (proximal) 588.89
  respiratory 276.2
    complicated by
      metabolic acidosis 276.4
        of newborn 775.81
      metabolic alkalosis 276.4
Aciduria 791.9
  arginosuccinic 270.6
  beta-aminoisobutyric (BAIB) 277.2
  glutaric
    type I 270.7
    type II (type IIA, IIB, IIC) 277.85
    type III 277.86
  glycolic 271.8
  methylmalonic 270.3
    with glycinemia 270.7
  organic 270.9
  orotic (congenital) (hereditary) (pyrimidine deficiency) 281.4
Acladiosis 111.8
  skin 111.8
Aclasis
  diaphyseal 756.4
  tarsoepiphyseal 756.59

Acleistocardia 745.5
Aclusion 524.4
Acmesthesia 782.0
Acne (pustular) (vulgaris) 706.1
  agminata (*see also* Tuberculosis) 017.0 ☑
  artificialis 706.1
  atrophica 706.0
  cachecticorum (Hebra) 706.1
  conglobata 706.1
  conjunctiva 706.1
  cystic 706.1
  decalvans 704.09
  erythematosa 695.3
  eyelid 706.1
  frontalis 706.0
  indurata 706.1
  keloid 706.1
  lupoid 706.0
  necrotic, necrotica 706.0
    miliaris 704.8
  neonatal 706.1
  nodular 706.1
  occupational 706.1
  papulosa 706.1
  rodens 706.0
  rosacea 695.3
  scorbutica 267
  scrofulosorum (Bazin) (*see also* Tuberculosis) 017.0 ☑
  summer 692.72
  tropical 706.1
  varioliformis 706.0
Acneiform drug eruptions 692.3
Acnitis (primary) — *see also* Tuberculosis 017.0 ☑
Acomia 704.00
Acontractile bladder 344.61
Aconuresis — *see also* Incontinence 788.30
Acosta's disease 993.2
Acousma 780.1
Acoustic — *see* condition
Acousticophobia 300.29
Acquired — *see* condition
Acquired immune deficiency syndrome — *see* Human immunodeficiency virus (disease) (illness) (infection)
Acquired immunodeficiency syndrome — *see* Human immunodeficiency virus (disease) (illness) (infection)
Acragnosis 781.99
Acrania 740.0
Acroagnosis 781.99
Acroangiodermatitis 448.9
Acroasphyxia, chronic 443.89
Acrobrachycephaly 756.0
Acrobystiolith 608.89
Acrobystitis 607.2
Acrocephalopolysyndactyly 755.55
Acrocephalosyndactyly 755.55
Acrocephaly 756.0
Acrochondrohyperplasia 759.82
Acrocyanosis 443.89
  newborn 770.83
    meaning transient blue hands and feet — *omit code*
Acrodermatitis 686.8
  atrophicans (chronica) 701.8
  continua (Hallopeau) 696.1
  enteropathica 686.8
  Hallopeau's 696.1
  perstans 696.1
  pustulosa continua 696.1
  recalcitrant pustular 696.1
Acrodynia 985.0
Acrodysplasia 755.55
Acrohyperhidrosis — *see also* Hyperhidrosis 780.8
Acrokeratosis verruciformis 757.39
Acromastitis 611.0
Acromegaly, acromegalia (skin) 253.0
Acromelalgia 443.82
Acromicria, acromikria 756.59
Acronyx 703.0
Acropachyderma 757.39
Acropachy, thyroid — *see also* Thyrotoxicosis 242.9 ☑

Acroparesthesia 443.89
  simple (Schultz's type) 443.89
  vasomotor (Nothnagel's type) 443.89
Acropathy thyroid — *see also* Thyrotoxicosis 242.9 ☑
Acrophobia 300.29
Acroposthitis 607.2
Acroscleriasis — *see also* Scleroderma 710.1
Acroscleroderma — *see also* Scleroderma 710.1
Acrosclerosis — *see also* Scleroderma 710.1
Acrosphacelus 785.4
Acrosphenosyndactylia 755.55
Acrospiroma, eccrine (M8402/0) — *see* Neoplasm, skin, benign
Acrostealgia 732.9
Acrosyndactyly — *see also* Syndactylism 755.10
Acrotrophodynia 991.4
Actinic — *see also* condition
  cheilitis (due to sun) 692.72
    chronic NEC 692.74
    due to radiation, except from sun 692.82
  conjunctivitis 370.24
  dermatitis (due to sun) (*see also* Dermatitis, actinic) 692.70
    due to
      roentgen rays or radioactive substance 692.82
      ultraviolet radiation, except from sun 692.82
      sun NEC 692.70
  elastosis solare 692.74
  granuloma 692.73
  keratitis 370.24
  ophthalmia 370.24
  reticuloid 692.73
Actinobacillosis, general 027.8
Actinobacillus
  lignieresii 027.8
  mallei 024
  muris 026.1
Actinocutitis NEC — *see also* Dermatitis, actinic 692.70
Actinodermatitis NEC — *see also* Dermatitis, actinic 692.70
Actinomyces
  israelii (infection) — *see* Actinomycosis
  muris-ratti (infection) 026.1
Actinomycosis, actinomycotic 039.9
  with
    pneumonia 039.1
  abdominal 039.2
  cervicofacial 039.3
  cutaneous 039.0
  pulmonary 039.1
  specified site NEC 039.8
  thoracic 039.1
Actinoneuritis 357.89
Action, heart
  disorder 427.9
    postoperative 997.1
  irregular 427.9
    postoperative 997.1
    psychogenic 306.2
Active — *see* condition
Activity decrease, functional 780.99
Acute — *see also* condition
  abdomen NEC 789.0 ☑
  gallbladder (*see also* Cholecystitis, acute) 575.0
Acyanoblepsia 368.53
Acyanopsia 368.53
Acystia 753.8
Acystinervia — *see* Neurogenic, bladder
Acystineuria — *see* Neurogenic, bladder
Adactylia, adactyly (congenital) 755.4
  lower limb (complete) (intercalary) (partial) (terminal) (*see also* Deformity, reduction, lower limb) 755.39
    meaning all digits (complete) (partial) 755.31
    transverse (complete) (partial) 755.31
  upper limb (complete) (intercalary) (partial) (terminal) (*see also* Deformity, reduction, upper limb) 755.29

☑ **Additional Digit Required** — Refer to the Tabular List for Digit Selection   ☂ **Subterms under main terms may continue to next column or page**

Adactylia, adactyly — *continued*
  upper limb (*see also* Deformity, reduction, upper limb) — *continued*
    meaning all digits (complete) (partial) 755.21
    transverse (complete) (partial) 755.21
Adair-Dighton syndrome (brittle bones and blue sclera, deafness) 756.51
Adamantinoblastoma (M9310/0) — *see* Ameloblastoma
Adamantinoma (M9310/0) — *see* Ameloblastoma
Adamantoblastoma (M9310/0) — *see* Ameloblastoma
Adams-Stokes (-Morgagni) disease or syndrome (syncope with heart block) 426.9
Adaptation reaction — *see also* Reaction, adjustment 309.9
Addiction — *see also* Dependence
  absinthe 304.6 ☑
  alcoholic (ethyl) (methyl) (wood) 303.9 ☑
    complicating pregnancy, childbirth, or puerperium 648.4 ☑
      affecting fetus or newborn 760.71
      suspected damage to fetus affecting management of pregnancy 655.4 ☑
  drug (*see also* Dependence) 304.9 ☑
  ethyl alcohol 303.9 ☑
  heroin 304.0 ☑
  hospital 301.51
  methyl alcohol 303.9 ☑
  methylated spirit 303.9 ☑
  morphine (-like substances) 304.0 ☑
  nicotine 305.1
  opium 304.0 ☑
  tobacco 305.1
  wine 303.9 ☑
Addison's
  anemia (pernicious) 281.0
  disease (bronze) (primary adrenal insufficiency) 255.41
    tuberculous (*see also* Tuberculosis) 017.6 ☑
  keloid (morphea) 701.0
  melanoderma (adrenal cortical hypofunction) 255.41
Addison-Biermer anemia (pernicious) 281.0
Addison-Gull disease — *see* Xanthoma
Addisonian crisis or melanosis (acute adrenocortical insufficiency) 255.41
Additional — *see also* Accessory
  chromosome(s) 758.5
    13-15 758.1
    16-18 758.2
    21 758.0
    autosome(s) NEC 758.5
    sex 758.81
Adduction contracture, hip or other joint — *see* Contraction, joint
ADEM (acute disseminated encephalomyelitis) (postinfectious) 136.9 *[323.61]*
  infectious 136.9 *[323.61]*
  noninfectious 323.81
Adenasthenia gastrica 536.0
Aden fever 061
Adenitis — *see also* Lymphadenitis 289.3
  acute, unspecified site 683
    epidemic infectious 075
  axillary 289.3
    acute 683
    chronic or subacute 289.1
  Bartholin's gland 616.89
  bulbourethral gland (*see also* Urethritis) 597.89
  cervical 289.3
    acute 683
    chronic or subacute 289.1
  chancroid (Ducrey's bacillus) 099.0
  chronic (any lymph node, except mesenteric) 289.1
    mesenteric 289.2
  Cowper's gland (*see also* Urethritis) 597.89
  epidemic, acute 075
  gangrenous 683
  gonorrheal NEC 098.89

Adenitis — *see also* Lymphadenitis — *continued*
  groin 289.3
    acute 683
    chronic or subacute 289.1
  infectious 075
  inguinal (region) 289.3
    acute 683
    chronic or subacute 289.1
  lymph gland or node, except mesenteric 289.3
    acute 683
    chronic or subacute 289.1
      mesenteric (acute) (chronic) (nonspecific) (subacute) 289.2
    mesenteric (acute) (chronic) (nonspecific) (subacute) 289.2
      due to Pasteurella multocida (P. septica) 027.2
  parotid gland (suppurative) 527.2
  phlegmonous 683
  salivary duct or gland (any) (recurring) (suppurative) 527.2
  scrofulous (*see also* Tuberculosis) 017.2 ☑
  septic 289.3
  Skene's duct or gland (*see also* Urethritis) 597.89
  strumous, tuberculous (*see also* Tuberculosis) 017.2 ☑
  subacute, unspecified site 289.1
  sublingual gland (suppurative) 527.2
  submandibular gland (suppurative) 527.2
  submaxillary gland (suppurative) 527.2
  suppurative 683
  tuberculous — *see* Tuberculosis, lymph gland
  urethral gland (*see also* Urethritis) 597.89
  venereal NEC 099.8
  Wharton's duct (suppurative) 527.2
Adenoacanthoma (M8570/3) — *see* Neoplasm, by site, malignant
Adenoameloblastoma (M9300/0) 213.1
  upper jaw (bone) 213.0
Adenocarcinoma (M8140/3) — *see also* Neoplasm, by site, malignant

Note — *The list of adjectival modifiers below is not exhaustive. A description of adenocarcinoma that does not appear in this list should be coded in the same manner as carcinoma with that description. Thus, "mixed acidophil-basophil adenocarcinoma," should be coded in the same manner as "mixed acidophil-basophil carcinoma," which appears in the list under "Carcinoma."*

Except where otherwise indicated, the morphological varieties of adenocarcinoma in the list below should be coded by site as for "Neoplasm, malignant."

  with
    apocrine metaplasia (M8573/3)
    cartilaginous (and osseous) metaplasia (M8571/3)
    osseous (and cartilaginous) metaplasia (M8571/3)
    spindle cell metaplasia (M8572/3)
    squamous metaplasia (M8570/3)
  acidophil (M8280/3)
    specified site — *see* Neoplasm, by site, malignant
    unspecified site 194.3
  acinar (M8550/3)
  acinic cell (M8550/3)
  adrenal cortical (M8370/3) 194.0
  alveolar (M8251/3)
    and
      epidermoid carcinoma, mixed (M8560/3)
      squamous cell carcinoma, mixed (M8560/3)
  apocrine (M8401/3)
    breast — *see* Neoplasm, breast, malignant
    specified site NEC — *see* Neoplasm, skin, malignant

Adenocarcinoma — *see also* Neoplasm, by site, malignant — *continued*
  apocrine — *continued*
    unspecified site 173.99
  basophil (M8300/3)
    specified site — *see* Neoplasm, by site, malignant
    unspecified site 194.3
  bile duct type (M8160/3)
    liver 155.1
    specified site NEC — *see* Neoplasm, by site, malignant
    unspecified site 155.1
  bronchiolar (M8250/3) — *see* Neoplasm, lung, malignant
  ceruminous (M8420/3) 173.29
  chromophobe (M8270/3)
    specified site — *see* Neoplasm, by site, malignant
    unspecified site 194.3
  clear cell (mesonephroid type) (M8310/3)
  colloid (M8480/3)
  cylindroid type (M8200/3)
  diffuse type (M8145/3)
    specified site — *see* Neoplasm, by site, malignant
    unspecified site 151.9
  duct (infiltrating) (M8500/3)
    with Paget's disease (M8541/3) — *see* Neoplasm, breast, malignant
    specified site — *see* Neoplasm, by site, malignant
    unspecified site 174.9
  embryonal (M9070/3)
  endometrioid (M8380/3) — *see* Neoplasm, by site, malignant
  eosinophil (M8280/3)
    specified site — *see* Neoplasm, by site, malignant
    unspecified site 194.3
  follicular (M8330/3)
    and papillary (M8340/3) 193
    moderately differentiated type (M8332/3) 193
    pure follicle type (M8331/3) 193
    specified site — *see* Neoplasm, by site, malignant
    trabecular type (M8332/3) 193
    unspecified type 193
    well differentiated type (M8331/3) 193
  gelatinous (M8480/3)
  granular cell (M8320/3)
  Hürthle cell (M8290/3) 193
  in
    adenomatous
      polyp (M8210/3)
      polyposis coli (M8220/3) 153.9
    polypoid adenoma (M8210/3)
    tubular adenoma (M8210/3)
    villous adenoma (M8261/3)
  infiltrating duct (M8500/3)
    with Paget's disease (M8541/3) — *see* Neoplasm, breast, malignant
    specified site — *see* Neoplasm, by site, malignant
    unspecified site 174.9
  inflammatory (M8530/3)
    specified site — *see* Neoplasm, by site, malignant
    unspecified site 174.9
  in situ (M8140/2) — *see* Neoplasm, by site, in situ
  intestinal type (M8144/3)
    specified site — *see* Neoplasm, by site, malignant
    unspecified site 151.9
  intraductal (noninfiltrating) (M8500/2)
    papillary (M8503/2)
      specified site — *see* Neoplasm, by site, in situ
      unspecified site 233.0
    specified site — *see* Neoplasm, by site, in situ
    unspecified site 233.0

Adenocarcinoma — *see also* Neoplasm, by site, malignant — *continued*
  islet cell (M8150/3)
    and exocrine, mixed (M8154/3)
      specified site — *see* Neoplasm, by site, malignant
      unspecified site 157.9
    pancreas 157.4
    specified site NEC — *see* Neoplasm, by site, malignant
    unspecified site 157.4
  lobular (M8520/3)
    specified site — *see* Neoplasm, by site, malignant
    unspecified site 174.9
  medullary (M8510/3)
  mesonephric (M9110/3)
  mixed cell (M8323/3)
  mucinous (M8480/3)
  mucin-producing (M8481/3)
  mucoid (M8480/3) (*see also* Neoplasm, by site, malignant)
    cell (M8300/3)
      specified site — *see* Neoplasm, by site, malignant
      unspecified site 194.3
  nonencapsulated sclerosing (M8350/3) 193
  oncocytic (M8290/3)
  oxyphilic (M8290/3)
  papillary (M8260/3) 193
    and follicular (M8340/3) 193
    intraductal (noninfiltrating) (M8503/2)
      specified site — *see* Neoplasm, by site, in situ
      unspecified site 233.0
    serous (M8460/3)
      specified site — *see* Neoplasm, by site, malignant
      unspecified site 183.0
  papillocystic (M8450/3)
    specified site — *see* Neoplasm, by site, malignant
    unspecified site 183.0
  pseudomucinous (M8470/3)
    specified site — *see* Neoplasm, by site, malignant
    unspecified site 183.0
  renal cell (M8312/3) 189.0
  sebaceous (M8410/3)
  serous (M8441/3) (*see also* Neoplasm, by site, malignant)
    papillary
      specified site — *see* Neoplasm, by site, malignant
      unspecified site 183.0
  signet ring cell (M8490/3)
  superficial spreading (M8143/3)
  sweat gland (M8400/3) — *see* Neoplasm, skin, malignant
  trabecular (M8190/3)
  tubular (M8211/3)
  villous (M8262/3)
  water-clear cell (M8322/3) 194.1
Adenofibroma (M9013/0)
  clear cell (M8313/0) — *see* Neoplasm, by site, benign
  endometrioid (M8381/0) 220
    borderline malignancy (M8381/1) 236.2
    malignant (M8381/3) 183.0
  mucinous (M9015/0)
    specified site — *see* Neoplasm, by site, benign
    unspecified site 220
  prostate
    with
      other lower urinary tract symptoms (LUTS) 600.21
      urinary
        obstruction 600.21
        retention 600.21
  serous (M9014/0)
    specified site — *see* Neoplasm, by site, benign
    unspecified site 220
  specified site — *see* Neoplasm, by site, benign

Subterms under main terms may continue to next column or page

---

☑ **Additional Digit Required** — **Refer to the Tabular List for Digit Selection**

Adenofibroma — *continued*
  unspecified site 220
Adenofibrosis
  breast 610.2
  endometrioid 617.0
Adenoiditis 474.01
  acute 463
  chronic 474.01
    with chronic tonsillitis 474.02
Adenoids (congenital) (of nasal fossa) 474.9
  hypertrophy 474.12
  vegetations 474.2
Adenolipomatosis (symmetrical) 272.8
Adenolymphoma (M8561/0)
  specified site — *see* Neoplasm, by site, benign
  unspecified 210.2
Adenomatosis (M8220/0)
  endocrine (multiple) (M8360/1)
    single specified site — *see* Neoplasm, by site, uncertain behavior
    two or more specified sites 237.4
    unspecified site 237.4
  erosive of nipple (M8506/0) 217
  pluriendocrine — *see* Adenomatosis, endocrine
  pulmonary (M8250/1) 235.7
    malignant (M8250/3) — *see* Neoplasm, lung, malignant
  specified site — *see* Neoplasm, by site, benign
  unspecified site 211.3
Adenomatous
  cyst, thyroid (gland) — *see* Goiter, nodular
  goiter (nontoxic) (*see also* Goiter, nodular) 241.9
    toxic or with hyperthyroidism 242.3 ☑
Adenoma (sessile) (M8140/0) — *see also* Neoplasm, by site, benign

Note — Except where otherwise indicated, the morphological varieties of adenoma in the list below should be coded by site as for "Neoplasm, benign."

  acidophil (M8280/0)
    specified site — *see* Neoplasm, by site, benign
    unspecified site 227.3
  acinar (cell) (M8550/0)
  acinic cell (M8550/0)
  adrenal (cortex) (cortical) (functioning) (M8370/0) 227.0
    clear cell type (M8373/0) 227.0
    compact cell type (M8371/0) 227.0
    glomerulosa cell type (M8374/0) 227.0
    heavily pigmented variant (M8372/0) 227.0
    mixed cell type (M8375/0) 227.0
  alpha cell (M8152/0)
    pancreas 211.7
    specified site NEC — *see* Neoplasm, by site, benign
    unspecified site 211.7
  alveolar (M8251/0)
  apocrine (M8401/0)
    breast 217
    specified site NEC — *see* Neoplasm, skin, benign
    unspecified site 216.9
  basal cell (M8147/0)
  basophil (M8300/0)
    specified site — *see* Neoplasm, by site, benign
    unspecified site 227.3
  beta cell (M8151/0)
    pancreas 211.7
    specified site NEC — *see* Neoplasm, by site, benign
    unspecified site 211.7
  bile duct (M8160/0) 211.5
  black (M8372/0) 227.0
  bronchial (M8140/1) 235.7
    carcinoid type (M8240/3) — *see* Neoplasm, lung, malignant
    cylindroid type (M8200/3) — *see* Neoplasm, lung, malignant
  ceruminous (M8420/0) 216.2

Adenoma — *see also* Neoplasm, by site, benign — *continued*
  chief cell (M8321/0) 227.1
  chromophobe (M8270/0)
    specified site — *see* Neoplasm, by site, benign
    unspecified site 227.3
  clear cell (M8310/0)
  colloid (M8334/0)
    specified site — *see* Neoplasm, by site, benign
    unspecified site 226
  cylindroid type, bronchus (M8200/3) — *see* Neoplasm, lung, malignant
  duct (M8503/0)
  embryonal (M8191/0)
  endocrine, multiple (M8360/1)
    single specified site — *see* Neoplasm, by site, uncertain behavior
    two or more specified sites 237.4
    unspecified site 237.4
  endometrioid (M8380/0) (*see also* Neoplasm, by site, benign)
    borderline malignancy (M8380/1) — *see* Neoplasm, by site, uncertain behavior
  eosinophil (M8280/0)
    specified site — *see* Neoplasm, by site, benign
    unspecified site 227.3
  fetal (M8333/0)
    specified site — *see* Neoplasm, by site, benign
    unspecified site 226
  follicular (M8330/0)
    specified site — *see* Neoplasm, by site, benign
    unspecified site 226
  hepatocellular (M8170/0) 211.5
  Hürthle cell (M8290/0) 226
  intracystic papillary (M8504/0)
  islet cell (functioning) (M8150/0)
    pancreas 211.7
    specified site NEC — *see* Neoplasm, by site, benign
    unspecified site 211.7
  liver cell (M8170/0) 211.5
  macrofollicular (M8334/0)
    specified site NEC — *see* Neoplasm, by site, benign
    unspecified site 226
  malignant, malignum (M8140/3) — *see* Neoplasm, by site, malignant
  mesonephric (M9110/0)
  microfollicular (M8333/0)
    specified site — *see* Neoplasm, by site, benign
    unspecified site 226
  mixed cell (M8323/0)
  monomorphic (M8146/0)
  mucinous (M8480/0)
  mucoid cell (M8300/0)
    specified site — *see* Neoplasm, by site, benign
    unspecified site 227.3
  multiple endocrine (M8360/1)
    single specified site — *see* Neoplasm, by site, uncertain behavior
    two or more specified sites 237.4
    unspecified site 237.4
  nipple (M8506/0) 217
  oncocytic (M8290/0)
  oxyphilic (M8290/0)
  papillary (M8260/0) (*see also* Neoplasm, by site, benign)
    intracystic (M8504/0)
  papillotubular (M8263/0)
  Pick's tubular (M8640/0)
    specified site — *see* Neoplasm, by site, benign
    unspecified site
      female 220
      male 222.0
  pleomorphic (M8940/0)
  polypoid (M8210/0)
  prostate (benign) 600.20

Adenoma — *see also* Neoplasm, by site, benign — *continued*
  prostate — *continued*
    with
      other lower urinary tract symptoms (LUTS) 600.21
      urinary
        obstruction 600.21
        retention 600.21
  rete cell 222.0
  sebaceous, sebaceum (gland) (senile) (M8410/0) (*see also* Neoplasm, skin, benign)
    disseminata 759.5
  Sertoli cell (M8640/0)
    specified site — *see* Neoplasm, by site, benign
    unspecified site
      female 220
      male 222.0
  skin appendage (M8390/0) — *see* Neoplasm, skin, benign
  sudoriferous gland (M8400/0) — *see* Neoplasm, skin, benign
  sweat gland or duct (M8400/0) — *see* Neoplasm, skin, benign
  testicular (M8640/0)
    specified site — *see* Neoplasm, by site, benign
    unspecified site
      female 220
      male 222.0
  thyroid 226
  trabecular (M8190/0)
  tubular (M8211/0) (*see also* Neoplasm, by site, benign)
    papillary (M8460/3)
    Pick's (M8640/0)
      specified site — *see* Neoplasm, by site, benign
      unspecified site
        female 220
        male 222.0
  tubulovillous (M8263/0)
  villoglandular (M8263/0)
  villous (M8261/1) — *see* Neoplasm, by site, uncertain behavior
  water-clear cell (M8322/0) 227.1
  wolffian duct (M9110/0)
Adenomyoma (M8932/0) — *see also* Neoplasm, by site, benign
  prostate 600.20
    with
      other lower urinary tract symptoms (LUTS) 600.21
      urinary
        obstruction 600.21
        retention 600.21
Adenomyometritis 617.0
Adenomyosis (uterus) (internal) 617.0
Adenopathy (lymph gland) 785.6
  inguinal 785.6
  mediastinal 785.6
  mesentery 785.6
  syphilitic (secondary) 091.4
  tracheobronchial 785.6
    tuberculous (*see also* Tuberculosis) 012.1 ☑
      primary, progressive 010.8 ☑
    tuberculous (*see also* Tuberculosis, lymph gland) 017.2 ☑
      tracheobronchial 012.1 ☑
        primary, progressive 010.8 ☑
Adenopharyngitis 462
Adenophlegmon 683
Adenosalpingitis 614.1
Adenosarcoma (M8960/3) 189.0
Adenosclerosis 289.3
Adenosis
  breast (sclerosing) 610.2
  vagina, congenital 752.49
Adentia (complete) (partial) — *see also* Absence, teeth 520.0
Adherent
  labium (minus) 624.4
  pericardium (nonrheumatic) 423.1

Adherent — *continued*
  pericardium — *continued*
    rheumatic 393
  placenta 667.0 ☑
    with hemorrhage 666.0 ☑
  prepuce 605
  scar (skin) NEC 709.2
  tendon in scar 709.2
Adhesion(s), adhesive (postinfectional) (postoperative)
  abdominal (wall) (*see also* Adhesions, peritoneum) 568.0
  amnion to fetus 658.8 ☑
    affecting fetus or newborn 762.8
  appendix 543.9
  arachnoiditis — *see* Meningitis
  auditory tube (Eustachian) 381.89
  bands (*see also* Adhesions, peritoneum)
    cervix 622.3
    uterus 621.5
  bile duct (any) 576.8
  bladder (sphincter) 596.89
  bowel (*see also* Adhesions, peritoneum) 568.0
  cardiac 423.1
    rheumatic 398.99
  cecum (*see also* Adhesions, peritoneum) 568.0
  cervicovaginal 622.3
    congenital 752.49
    postpartal 674.8 ☑
    old 622.3
  cervix 622.3
  clitoris 624.4
  colon (*see also* Adhesions, peritoneum) 568.0
  common duct 576.8
  congenital (*see also* Anomaly, specified type NEC)
    fingers (*see also* Syndactylism, fingers) 755.11
    labium (majus) (minus) 752.49
    omental, anomalous 751.4
    ovary 752.0
    peritoneal 751.4
    toes (*see also* Syndactylism, toes) 755.13
    tongue (to gum or roof of mouth) 750.12
  conjunctiva (acquired) (localized) 372.62
    congenital 743.63
    extensive 372.63
  cornea — *see* Opacity, cornea
  cystic duct 575.8
  diaphragm (*see also* Adhesions, peritoneum) 568.0
  due to foreign body — *see* Foreign body
  duodenum (*see also* Adhesions, peritoneum) 568.0
    with obstruction 537.3
  ear, middle — *see* Adhesions, middle ear
  epididymis 608.89
  epidural — *see* Adhesions, meninges
  epiglottis 478.79
  Eustachian tube 381.89
  eyelid 374.46
    postoperative 997.99
      surgically created V45.69
  gallbladder (*see also* Disease, gallbladder) 575.8
  globe 360.89
  heart 423.1
    rheumatic 398.99
  ileocecal (coil) (*see also* Adhesions, peritoneum) 568.0
  ileum (*see also* Adhesions, peritoneum) 568.0
  intestine (postoperative) (*see also* Adhesions, peritoneum) 568.0
    with obstruction 560.81
      with hernia (*see also* Hernia, by site, with obstruction)
        gangrenous — *see* Hernia, by site, with gangrene
  intra-abdominal (*see also* Adhesions, peritoneum) 568.0
  iris 364.70
    to corneal graft 996.79

☑ **Additional Digit Required** — Refer to the Tabular List for Digit Selection   ▽ **Subterms under main terms may continue to next column or page**

Adhesion(s), adhesive — *continued*
  joint (*see also* Ankylosis) 718.5 ☑
  kidney 593.89
  labium (majus) (minus), congenital 752.49
  liver 572.8
  lung 511.0
  mediastinum 519.3
  meninges 349.2
    cerebral (any) 349.2
      congenital 742.4
    congenital 742.8
    spinal (any) 349.2
      congenital 742.59
    tuberculous (cerebral) (spinal) (*see also* Tuberculosis, meninges) 013.0 ☑
  mesenteric (*see also* Adhesions, peritoneum) 568.0
  middle ear (fibrous) 385.10
    drum head 385.19
      to
        incus 385.11
        promontorium 385.13
        stapes 385.12
    specified NEC 385.19
  nasal (septum) (to turbinates) 478.19
  nerve NEC 355.9
    spinal 355.9
      root 724.9
        cervical NEC 723.4
        lumbar NEC 724.4
        lumbosacral 724.4
        thoracic 724.4
  ocular muscle 378.60
  omentum (*see also* Adhesions, peritoneum) 568.0
  organ or site, congenital NEC — *see* Anomaly, specified type NEC
  ovary 614.6
    congenital (to cecum, kidney, or omentum) 752.0
  parauterine 614.6
  parovarian 614.6
  pelvic (peritoneal)
    female (postoperative) (postinfection) 614.6
    male (postoperative) (postinfection) (*see also* Adhesions, peritoneum) 568.0
    postpartal (old) 614.6
    tuberculous (*see also* Tuberculosis) 016.9 ☑
  penis to scrotum (congenital) 752.69
  periappendiceal (*see also* Adhesions, peritoneum) 568.0
  pericardium (nonrheumatic) 423.1
    rheumatic 393
    tuberculous (*see also* Tuberculosis) 017.9 ☑ *[420.0]*
  pericholecystic 575.8
  perigastric (*see also* Adhesions, peritoneum) 568.0
  periovarian 614.6
  periprostatic 602.8
  perirectal (*see also* Adhesions, peritoneum) 568.0
  perirenal 593.89
  peritoneum, peritoneal (fibrous) (postoperative) 568.0
    with obstruction (intestinal) 560.81
      with hernia (*see also* Hernia, by site, with obstruction)
        gangrenous — *see* Hernia, by site, with gangrene
    duodenum 537.3
    congenital 751.4
    female (postoperative) (postinfective) 614.6
    pelvic, female 614.6
    pelvic, male 568.0
    postpartal, pelvic 614.6
    to uterus 614.6
  peritubal 614.6
  periureteral 593.89
  periuterine 621.5
  perivesical 596.89
  perivesicular (seminal vesicle) 608.89

Adhesion(s), adhesive — *continued*
  pleura, pleuritic 511.0
    tuberculous (*see also* Tuberculosis, pleura) 012.0 ☑
  pleuropericardial 511.0
  postoperative (gastrointestinal tract) (*see also* Adhesions, peritoneum) 568.0
    eyelid 997.99
      surgically created V45.69
    pelvic female 614.9
    pelvic male 568.0
    urethra 598.2
  postpartal, old 624.4
  preputial, prepuce 605
  pulmonary 511.0
  pylorus (*see also* Adhesions, peritoneum) 568.0
  Rosenmüller's fossa 478.29
  sciatic nerve 355.0
  seminal vesicle 608.89
  shoulder (joint) 726.0
  sigmoid flexure (*see also* Adhesions, peritoneum) 568.0
  spermatic cord (acquired) 608.89
    congenital 752.89
  spinal canal 349.2
    nerve 355.9
      root 724.9
        cervical NEC 723.4
        lumbar NEC 724.4
        lumbosacral 724.4
        thoracic 724.4
  stomach (*see also* Adhesions, peritoneum) 568.0
  subscapular 726.2
  tendonitis 726.90
    shoulder 726.0
  testicle 608.89
  tongue (congenital) (to gum or roof of mouth) 750.12
    acquired 529.8
  trachea 519.19
  tubo-ovarian 614.6
  tunica vaginalis 608.89
  ureter 593.89
  uterus 621.5
    to abdominal wall 614.6
      in pregnancy or childbirth 654.4 ☑
        affecting fetus or newborn 763.89
  vagina (chronic) (postoperative) (postradiation) 623.2
  vaginitis (congenital) 752.49
  vesical 596.89
  vitreomacular adhesion 379.27
  vitreous 379.29

Adie (-Holmes) syndrome (tonic pupillary reaction) 379.46
Adiponecrosis neonatorum 778.1
Adiposa dolorosa 272.8
Adiposalgia 272.8
Adiposis
  cerebralis 253.8
  dolorosa 272.8
  tuberosa simplex 272.8
Adiposity 278.02
  heart (*see also* Degeneration, myocardial) 429.1
  localized 278.1
Adiposogenital dystrophy 253.8
Adjustment
  prosthesis or other device — *see* Fitting of
  reaction — *see* Reaction, adjustment
Administration, prophylactic
  antibiotics, long-term V58.62
    short-term use — *omit code*
  antitoxin, any V07.2
  antivenin V07.2
  chemotherapeutic agent NEC V07.39
  chemotherapy NEC V07.39
  diphtheria antitoxin V07.2
  fluoride V07.31
  gamma globulin V07.2
  immune sera (gamma globulin) V07.2
  passive immunization agent V07.2
  RhoGAM V07.2

Admission (encounter)
  as organ donor — *see* Donor
  by mistake V68.9
  for
    adequacy testing (for)
      hemodialysis V56.31
      peritoneal dialysis V56.32
    adjustment (of)
      artificial
        arm (complete) (partial) V52.0
        eye V52.2
        leg (complete) (partial) V52.1
      brain neuropacemaker V53.02
      breast
        implant V52.4
          exchange (different material) (different size) V52.4
        prosthesis V52.4
      cardiac device V53.39
        defibrillator, automatic implantable (with synchronous cardiac pacemaker) V53.32
        pacemaker V53.31
          carotid sinus V53.39
      catheter
        non-vascular V58.82
        vascular V58.81
      cerebral ventricle (communicating) shunt V53.01
      colostomy belt V55.3
      contact lenses V53.1
      cystostomy device V53.6
      dental prosthesis V52.3
      device, unspecified type V53.90
        abdominal V53.59
        cardiac V53.39
          defibrillator, automatic implantable (with synchronous cardiac pacemaker V53.32
          pacemaker V53.31
          carotid sinus V53.39
        cerebral ventricle (communicating) shunt V53.01
        gastrointestinal NEC V53.59
        insulin pump V53.91
        intestinal V53.50
        nervous system V53.09
        orthodontic V53.4
        other device V53.99
        prosthetic V52.9
          breast V52.4
          dental V52.3
          eye V52.2
          specified type NEC V52.8
        special senses V53.09
      substitution
        auditory V53.09
        nervous system V53.09
        visual V53.09
      urinary V53.6
    dialysis catheter
      extracorporeal V56.1
      peritoneal V56.2
    diaphragm (contraceptive) V25.02
    gastric lap band V53.51
    gastrointestinal appliance and device NEC V53.59
    growth rod V54.02
    hearing aid V53.2
    ileostomy device V55.2
    intestinal appliance and device V53.50
    neuropacemaker (brain) (peripheral nerve) (spinal cord) V53.02
    orthodontic device V53.4
    orthopedic (device) V53.7
      brace V53.7
      cast V53.7
      shoes V53.7
    pacemaker
      brain V53.02
      cardiac V53.31
      carotid sinus V53.39
      peripheral nerve V53.02

Admission — *continued*
  for — *continued*
    adjustment — *continued*
      pacemaker — *continued*
        spinal cord V53.02
      prosthesis V52.9
        arm (complete) (partial) V52.0
        breast V52.4
        dental V52.3
        eye V52.2
        leg (complete) (partial) V52.1
        specified type NEC V52.8
      spectacles V53.1
      wheelchair V53.8
    adoption referral or proceedings V68.89
    aftercare (*see also* Aftercare) V58.9
      cardiac pacemaker V53.31
      chemotherapy (oral) (intravenous) V58.11
      dialysis
        extracorporeal (renal) V56.0
        peritoneal V56.8
        renal V56.0
      fracture (*see also* Aftercare, fracture) V54.9
      medical NEC V58.89
      organ transplant V58.44
      orthopedic V54.9
        following explanation of joint prosthesis (for joint prosthesis insertion) (staged procedure) V54.82
        specified care NEC V54.89
      pacemaker device
        brain V53.02
        cardiac V53.31
        carotid sinus V53.39
        nervous system V53.02
        spinal cord V53.02
      postoperative NEC V58.49
        wound closure, planned V58.41
      postpartum
        immediately after delivery V24.0
        routine follow-up V24.2
      postradiation V58.0
      radiation therapy V58.0
      removal of
        non-vascular catheter V58.82
        vascular catheter V58.81
      specified NEC V58.89
      surgical NEC V58.49
        wound closure, planned V58.41
    antineoplastic
      chemotherapy (oral) (intravenous) V58.11
      immunotherapy V58.12
    artificial insemination V26.1
    assisted reproductive fertility procedure cycle V26.81
    attention to artificial opening (of) V55.9
      artificial vagina V55.7
      colostomy V55.3
      cystostomy V55.5
      enterostomy V55.4
      gastrostomy V55.1
      ileostomy V55.2
      jejunostomy V55.4
      nephrostomy V55.6
      specified site NEC V55.8
        intestinal tract V55.4
        urinary tract V55.6
      tracheostomy V55.0
      ureterostomy V55.6
      urethrostomy V55.6
    battery replacement
      cardiac pacemaker V53.31
    blood typing V72.86
      Rh typing V72.86
    boarding V65.0
    breast
      augmentation or reduction V50.1
      implant exchange (different material) (different size) V52.4
      reconstruction following mastectomy V51.0

☑ **Additional Digit Required** — Refer to the Tabular List for Digit Selection   ⁿᵉʷ **Subterms under main terms may continue to next column or page**

Admission — *continued*
  for — *continued*
    breast — *continued*
      removal
        prophylactic V50.41
        tissue expander without synchronous insertion of permanent implant V52.4
    change of
      cardiac pacemaker (battery) V53.31
      carotid sinus pacemaker V53.39
      catheter in artificial opening — *see* Attention to, artificial, opening
      drains V58.49
      dressing
        wound V58.30
          nonsurgical V58.30
          surgical V58.31
      fixation device
        external V54.89
        internal V54.01
      Kirschner wire V54.89
      neuropacemaker device (brain) (peripheral nerve) (spinal cord) V53.02
      nonsurgical wound dressing V58.30
      pacemaker device
        brain V53.02
        cardiac V53.31
        carotid sinus V53.39
        nervous system V53.02
      plaster cast V54.89
      splint, external V54.89
      Steinmann pin V54.89
      surgical wound dressing V58.31
      traction device V54.89
      wound packing V58.30
        nonsurgical V58.30
        surgical V58.31
    checkup only V70.0
    chemotherapy, (oral) (intravenous) antineoplastic V58.11
    circumcision, ritual or routine (in absence of medical indication) V50.2
    clinical research investigation (control) (normal comparison) (participant) V70.7
    closure of artificial opening — *see* Attention to, artificial, opening
    contraceptive
      counseling V25.09
        emergency V25.03
        postcoital V25.03
      management V25.9
        specified type NEC V25.8
    convalescence following V66.9
      chemotherapy V66.2
      psychotherapy V66.3
      radiotherapy V66.1
      surgery V66.0
      treatment (for) V66.5
        combined V66.6
        fracture V66.4
        mental disorder NEC V66.3
        specified condition NEC V66.5
    cosmetic surgery NEC V50.1
      breast reconstruction following mastectomy V51.0
      following healed injury or operation V51.8
    counseling (*see also* Counseling) V65.40
      without complaint or sickness V65.49
      contraceptive management V25.09
        emergency V25.03
        postcoital V25.03
      dietary V65.3
      exercise V65.41
      fertility preservation (prior to cancer therapy) (prior to surgical removal of gonads) V26.42
      for
        nonattending third party V65.19

Admission — *continued*
  for — *continued*
    counseling (*see also* Counseling) — *continued*
      for — *continued*
        pediatric
          pre-adoption visit for adoptive parent(s) V65.11
          pre-birth visit for expectant parent(s) V65.11
          victim of abuse
            child V61.21
            partner or spouse V61.11
        genetic V26.33
        gonorrhea V65.45
        HIV V65.44
        human immunodeficiency virus V65.44
        injury prevention V65.43
        insulin pump training V65.46
        natural family planning
          procreative V26.41
          to avoid pregnancy V25.04
        procreative management V26.49
          using natural family planning V26.41
        sexually transmitted disease NEC V65.45
          HIV V65.44
        specified reason NEC V65.49
        substance use and abuse V65.42
        syphilis V65.45
        victim of abuse
          child V61.21
          partner or spouse V61.11
    desensitization to allergens V07.1
    dialysis V56.0
      catheter
        fitting and adjustment
          extracorporeal V56.1
          peritoneal V56.2
        removal or replacement
          extracorporeal V56.1
          peritoneal V56.2
      extracorporeal (renal) V56.0
      peritoneal V56.8
      renal V56.0
    dietary surveillance and counseling V65.3
    drug monitoring, therapeutic V58.83
    ear piercing V50.3
    elective surgery V50.9
      breast
        augmentation or reduction V50.1
        reconstruction following mastectomy V51.0
        removal, prophylactic V50.41
      circumcision, ritual or routine (in absence of medical indication) V50.2
      cosmetic NEC V50.1
        breast reconstruction following mastectomy V51.0
        following healed injury or operation V51.8
      ear piercing V50.3
      face-lift V50.1
      hair transplant V50.0
      plastic
        breast reconstruction following mastectomy V51.0
        cosmetic NEC V50.1
        following healed injury or operation V51.8
      prophylactic organ removal V50.49
        breast V50.41
        ovary V50.42
      repair of scarred tissue (following healed injury or operation) V51.8
      specified type NEC V50.8
    end-of-life care V66.7
    examination (*see also* Examination) V70.9
      administrative purpose NEC V70.3
      adoption V70.3

Admission — *continued*
  for — *continued*
    examination (*see also* Examination) — *continued*
      allergy V72.7
      antibody response V72.61
      at health care facility V70.0
      athletic team V70.3
      camp V70.3
      cardiovascular, preoperative V72.81
      clinical research investigation (control) (participant) V70.7
      dental V72.2
      developmental testing (child) (infant) V20.2
      donor (potential) V70.8
      driver's license V70.3
      ear V72.19
      employment V70.5
      eye V72.0
      fertility preservation (prior to cancer therapy) (prior to surgical removal of gonads) V26.82
      follow-up (routine) — *see* Examination, follow-up
      for admission to
        old age home V70.3
        school V70.3
      general V70.9
        specified reason NEC V70.8
      gynecological V72.31
      health supervision
        child (over 28 days old) V20.2
        infant (over 28 days old) V20.2
        newborn
          8 to 28 days old V20.32
          under 8 days old V20.31
      hearing V72.19
        following failed hearing screening V72.11
      immigration V70.3
      infant
        8 to 28 days old V20.32
        over 28 days old, routine V20.2
        under 8 days old V20.31
      insurance certification V70.3
      laboratory V72.60
        ordered as part of a routine general medical examination V72.62
        pre-operative V72.63
        pre-procedural V72.63
        specified NEC V72.69
      marriage license V70.3
      medical (general) (*see also* Examination, medical) V70.9
      medicolegal reasons V70.4
      naturalization V70.3
      pelvic (annual) (periodic) V72.31
      postpartum checkup V24.2
      pregnancy (possible) (unconfirmed) V72.40
        negative result V72.41
        positive result V72.42
      preoperative V72.84
        cardiovascular V72.81
        respiratory V72.82
        specified NEC V72.83
      preprocedural V72.84
        cardiovascular V72.81
        general physical V72.83
        respiratory V72.82
        specified NEC V72.83
      prior to chemotherapy V72.83
      prison V70.3
      psychiatric (general) V70.2
        requested by authority V70.1
      radiological NEC V72.5
      respiratory, preoperative V72.82
      school V70.3
      screening — *see* Screening
      skin hypersensitivity V72.7
      specified type NEC V72.85
      sport competition V70.3
      vision V72.0
      well baby and child care V20.2

Admission — *continued*
  for — *continued*
    exercise therapy V57.1
    face-lift, cosmetic reason V50.1
    fertility preservation (prior to cancer therapy) (prior to surgical removal of gonads) V26.82
    fitting (of)
      artificial
        arm (complete) (partial) V52.0
        eye V52.2
        leg (complete) (partial) V52.1
      biliary drainage tube V58.82
      brain neuropacemaker V53.02
      breast V52.4
        implant V52.4
        prosthesis V52.4
      cardiac pacemaker V53.31
      catheter
        non-vascular V58.82
        vascular V58.81
      cerebral ventricle (communicating) shunt V53.01
      chest tube V58.82
      colostomy belt V55.2
      contact lenses V53.1
      cystostomy device V53.6
      dental prosthesis V52.3
      device, unspecified type V53.90
        abdominal V53.59
        cerebral ventricle (communicating) shunt V53.01
        gastrointestinal NEC V53.59
        insulin pump V53.91
        intestinal V53.50
        intrauterine contraceptive
          insertion V25.11
          removal V25.12
            and reinsertion V25.13
          replacement V25.13
        nervous system V53.09
        orthodontic V53.4
        other device V53.99
        prosthetic V52.9
          breast V52.4
          dental V52.3
          eye V52.2
          special senses V53.09
        substitution
          auditory V53.09
          nervous system V53.09
          visual V53.09
      diaphragm (contraceptive) V25.02
      fistula (sinus tract) drainage tube V58.82
      gastric lap band V53.51
      gastrointestinal appliance and device NEC V53.59
      growth rod V54.02
      hearing aid V53.2
      ileostomy device V55.2
      intestinal appliance and device V53.50
      intrauterine contraceptive device
        insertion V25.11
        removal V25.12
          and reinsertion V25.13
        replacement V25.13
      neuropacemaker (brain) (peripheral nerve) (spinal cord) V53.02
      orthodontic device V53.4
      orthopedic (device) V53.7
        brace V53.7
        cast V53.7
        shoes V53.7
      pacemaker
        brain V53.02
        cardiac V53.31
        carotid sinus V53.39
        spinal cord V53.02
      pleural drainage tube V58.82
      portacath V58.81
      prosthesis V52.9
        arm (complete) (partial) V52.0
        breast V52.4
        dental V52.3

☑ **Additional Digit Required — Refer to the Tabular List for Digit Selection**   🔺 **Subterms under main terms may continue to next column or page**

12 — Volume 2   ▶◀ **Revised Text**   ● **New Line**   ▲ **Revised Code**   **2015 ICD-9-CM**

Admission — *continued*
  for — *continued*
    fitting — *continued*
      prosthesis — *continued*
        eye V52.2
        leg (complete) (partial) V52.1
        specified type NEC V52.8
      spectacles V53.1
      wheelchair V53.8
    follow-up examination (routine) (following) V67.9
      cancer chemotherapy V67.2
      chemotherapy V67.2
      high-risk medication NEC V67.51
      injury NEC V67.59
      psychiatric V67.3
      psychotherapy V67.3
      radiotherapy V67.1
      specified surgery NEC V67.09
      surgery V67.00
        vaginal pap smear V67.01
      treatment (for) V67.9
        combined V67.6
        fracture V67.4
        involving high-risk medication NEC V67.51
        mental disorder V67.3
        specified NEC V67.59
    hair transplant, for cosmetic reason V50.0
    health advice, education, or instruction V65.4 ☑
    hearing conservation and treatment V72.12
    hormone replacement therapy (postmenopausal) V07.4
    hospice care V66.7
    immunizations (childhood) appropriate for age V20.2
    immunotherapy, antineoplastic V58.12
    insertion (of)
      intrauterine contraceptive device V25.11
      subdermal implantable contraceptive V25.5
    insulin pump titration V53.91
    insulin pump training V65.46
    intrauterine device
      insertion V25.11
      management V25.42
      removal V25.12
        and reinsertion V25.13
      replacement V25.13
    investigation to determine further disposition V63.8
    in vitro fertilization cycle V26.81
    isolation V07.0
    issue of
      disability examination certificate V68.01
      medical certificate NEC V68.09
      repeat prescription NEC V68.1
        contraceptive device NEC V25.49
    kidney dialysis V56.0
    lengthening of growth rod V54.02
    mental health evaluation V70.2
      requested by authority V70.1
    natural family planning counseling and advice
      procreative V26.41
      to avoid pregnancy V25.04
    nonmedical reason NEC V68.89
    nursing care evaluation V63.8
    observation (without need for further medical care) (*see also* Observation) V71.9
      accident V71.4
      alleged rape or seduction V71.5
      criminal assault V71.6
      following accident V71.4
        at work V71.3
      foreign body ingestion V71.89
      growth and development variations, childhood V21.0
      inflicted injury NEC V71.6

Admission — *continued*
  for — *continued*
    observation (*see also* Observation) — *continued*
      ingestion of deleterious agent or foreign body V71.89
      injury V71.6
      malignant neoplasm V71.1
      mental disorder V71.09
      newborn — *see* Observation, suspected, condition, newborn
      rape V71.5
      specified NEC V71.89
      suspected
        abuse V71.81
        accident V71.4
          at work V71.3
        benign neoplasm V71.89
        cardiovascular V71.7
        disorder V71.9
        exposure
          anthrax V71.82
          biological agent NEC V71.83
          SARS V71.83
        heart V71.7
        inflicted injury NEC V71.6
        malignant neoplasm V71.1
        maternal and fetal problem not found
          amniotic cavity and membrane V89.01
          cervical shortening V89.05
          fetal anomaly V89.03
          fetal growth V89.04
          oligohydramnios V89.01
          other specified NEC V89.09
          placenta V89.02
          polyhydramnios V89.01
        mental NEC V71.09
        neglect V71.81
        specified condition NEC V71.89
        tuberculosis V71.2
      tuberculosis V71.2
    occupational therapy V57.21
    organ transplant, donor — *see* Donor
    ovary, ovarian removal, prophylactic V50.42
    palliative care V66.7
    Papanicolaou smear
      cervix V76.2
        for suspected malignant neoplasm V76.2
        no disease found V71.1
        routine, as part of gynecological examination V72.31
        to confirm findings of recent normal smear following initial abnormal smear V72.32
      vaginal V76.47
        following hysterectomy for malignant condition V67.01
    passage of sounds or bougie in artificial opening — *see* Attention to, artificial, opening
    paternity testing V70.4
    peritoneal dialysis V56.32
    physical therapy NEC V57.1
    plastic surgery
      breast reconstruction following mastectomy V51.0
      cosmetic NEC V50.1
      following healed injury or operation V51.8
    postmenopausal hormone replacement therapy V07.4
    postpartum observation
      immediately after delivery V24.0
      routine follow-up V24.2
    poststerilization (for restoration) V26.0
    procreative management V26.9
      assisted reproductive fertility procedure cycle V26.81
      in vitro fertilization cycle V26.81
      specified type NEC V26.89

Admission — *continued*
  for — *continued*
    prophylactic
      administration of
        antibiotics, long-term V58.62
          short-term use — *omit code*
        antitoxin, any V07.2
        antivenin V07.2
        chemotherapeutic agent NEC V07.39
        chemotherapy NEC V07.39
        diphtheria antitoxin V07.2
        fluoride V07.31
        gamma globulin V07.2
        immune sera (gamma globulin) V07.2
        RhoGAM V07.2
        tetanus antitoxin V07.2
      breathing exercises V57.0
      chemotherapy NEC V07.39
        fluoride V07.31
      measure V07.9
        specified type NEC V07.8
      organ removal V50.49
        breast V50.41
        ovary V50.42
    psychiatric examination (general) V70.2
      requested by authority V70.1
    radiation management V58.0
    radiotherapy V58.0
    reconstruction following mastectomy V51.0
    reforming of artificial opening — *see* Attention to, artificial, opening
    rehabilitation V57.9
      multiple types V57.89
      occupational V57.21
      orthoptic V57.4
      orthotic V57.81
      physical NEC V57.1
      specified type NEC V57.89
      speech (-language) V57.3
      vocational V57.22
    removal of
      breast tissue expander without synchronous insertion of permanent implant V52.4
      cardiac pacemaker V53.31
      cast (plaster) V54.89
      catheter from artificial opening — *see* Attention to, artificial, opening
      cerebral ventricle (communicating) shunt V53.01
      cystostomy catheter V55.5
      device
        cerebral ventricle (communicating) shunt V53.01
        fixation
          external V54.89
          internal V54.01
        intrauterine contraceptive V25.12
        traction, external V54.89
      drains V58.49
      dressing
        wound V58.30
          nonsurgical V58.30
          surgical V58.31
      fixation device
        external V54.89
        internal V54.01
      intrauterine contraceptive device V25.12
      Kirschner wire V54.89
      neuropacemaker (brain) (peripheral nerve) (spinal cord) V53.02
      nonsurgical wound dressing V58.30
      orthopedic fixation device
        external V54.89
        internal V54.01
      pacemaker device
        brain V53.02
        cardiac V53.31
        carotid sinus V53.39
        nervous system V53.02
      plaster cast V54.89

Admission — *continued*
  for — *continued*
    removal of — *continued*
      plate (fracture) V54.01
      rod V54.01
      screw (fracture) V54.01
      splint, traction V54.89
      staples V58.32
      Steinmann pin V54.89
      subdermal implantable contraceptive V25.43
      surgical wound dressing V58.31
      sutures V58.32
      traction device, external V54.89
      ureteral stent V53.6
      wound packing V58.30
        nonsurgical V58.30
        surgical V58.31
    repair of scarred tissue (following healed injury or operation) V51.8
    replacement of intrauterine contraceptive device V25.13
    reprogramming of cardiac pacemaker V53.31
    respirator [ventilator] dependence during
      mechanical failure V46.14
      power failure V46.12
      for weaning V46.13
    restoration of organ continuity (poststerilization) (tuboplasty) (vasoplasty) V26.0
    Rh typing V72.86
    routine infant and child vision and hearing testing V20.2
    sensitivity test (*see also* Test, skin)
      allergy NEC V72.7
      bacterial disease NEC V74.9
      Dick V74.8
      Kveim V82.89
      Mantoux V74.1
      mycotic infection NEC V75.4
      parasitic disease NEC V75.8
      Schick V74.3
      Schultz-Charlton V74.8
    social service (agency) referral or evaluation V63.8
    speech (-language) therapy V57.3
    sterilization V25.2
    suspected disorder (ruled out) (without need for further care) — *see* Observation
    terminal care V66.7
    tests only — *see* Test
    therapeutic drug monitoring V58.83
    therapy
      blood transfusion, without reported diagnosis V58.2
      breathing exercises V57.0
      chemotherapy, antineoplastic V58.11
        prophylactic NEC V07.39
        fluoride V07.31
      dialysis (intermittent) (treatment)
        extracorporeal V56.0
        peritoneal V56.8
        renal V56.0
        specified type NEC V56.8
      exercise (remedial) NEC V57.1
        breathing V57.0
      immunotherapy, antineoplastic V58.12
      long-term (current) (prophylactic) drug use NEC V58.69
        antibiotics V58.62
          short-term use — *omit code*
        anticoagulants V58.61
        anti-inflammatories, non-steroidal (NSAID) V58.64
        antiplatelets V58.63
        antithrombotics V58.63
        aspirin V58.66
        bisphosphonates V58.68
        high-risk medications NEC V58.69
        insulin V58.67
        methadone for pain control V58.69

☑ **Additional Digit Required — Refer to the Tabular List for Digit Selection**
▽ **Subterms under main terms may continue to next column or page**

Admission — *continued*
  for — *continued*
    therapy — *continued*
      long-term drug use — *continued*
        opiate analgesic V58.69
        steroids V58.65
      occupational V57.21
      orthoptic V57.4
      physical NEC V57.1
      radiation V58.0
      speech (-language) V57.3
      vocational V57.22
    toilet or cleaning
      of artificial opening — *see* Attention
        to, artificial, opening
      of non-vascular catheter V58.82
      of vascular catheter V58.81
    treatment
      measure V07.9
        specified type NEC V07.8
    tubal ligation V25.2
    tuboplasty for previous sterilization
      V26.0
    ultrasound, routine fetal V28.3
    vaccination, prophylactic (against)
      arthropod-borne virus, viral NEC
        V05.1
        disease NEC V05.1
        encephalitis V05.0
      Bacille Calmette Guérin (BCG) V03.2
      BCG V03.2
      chickenpox V05.4
      cholera alone V03.0
        with typhoid-paratyphoid
          (cholera + TAB) V06.0
      common cold V04.7
      dengue V05.1
      diphtheria alone V03.5
      diphtheria-tetanus-pertussis (DTP)
        (DTaP) V06.1
        with
          poliomyelitis (DTP + polio)
            V06.3
          typhoid-paratyphoid (DTP +
            TAB) V06.2
      diphtheria-tetanus [Td] [DT] without
        pertussis V06.5
      disease (single) NEC V05.9
        bacterial NEC V03.9
          specified type NEC V03.89
        combinations NEC V06.9
          specified type NEC V06.8
        specified type NEC V05.8
        viral NEC V04.89
      encephalitis, viral, arthropod-borne
        V05.0
      Hemophilus influenzae, type B [Hib]
        V03.81
      hepatitis, viral V05.3
      human papillomavirus (HPV) V04.89
      immune sera (gamma globulin)
        V07.2
      influenza V04.81
        with
          Streptococcus pneumoniae
            [pneumococcus] V06.6
      Leishmaniasis V05.2
      measles alone V04.2
      measles-mumps-rubella (MMR) V06.4
      mumps alone V04.6
        with measles and rubella (MMR)
          V06.4
      not done because of contraindication
        V64.09
      pertussis alone V03.6
      plague V03.3
      pneumonia V03.82
      poliomyelitis V04.0
        with diphtheria-tetanus-pertussis
          (DTP+ polio) V06.3
      rabies V04.5
      respiratory syncytial virus (RSV)
        V04.82
      rubella alone V04.3
        with measles and mumps (MMR)
          V06.4

Admission — *continued*
  for — *continued*
    vaccination, prophylactic — *continued*
      smallpox V04.1
      specified type NEC V05.8
      Streptococcus pneumoniae [pneumo-
        coccus] V03.82
        with
          influenza V06.6
      tetanus toxoid alone V03.7
        with diphtheria [Td] [DT] V06.5
          and pertussis (DTP) (DTaP)
            V06.1
      tuberculosis (BCG) V03.2
      tularemia V03.4
      typhoid alone V03.1
        with diphtheria-tetanus-pertussis
          (TAB + DTP) V06.2
      typhoid-paratyphoid alone (TAB)
        V03.1
      typhus V05.8
      varicella (chicken pox) V05.4
      viral encephalitis, arthropod-borne
        V05.0
      viral hepatitis V05.3
      yellow fever V04.4
    vasectomy V25.2
    vasoplasty for previous sterilization
      V26.0
    vision examination V72.0
    vocational therapy V57.22
    waiting period for admission to other
      facility V63.2
      undergoing social agency investiga-
        tion V63.8
    well baby and child care V20.2
    x-ray of chest
      for suspected tuberculosis V71.2
      routine V72.5
Adnexitis (suppurative) — *see also* Salpingo-
  oophoritis 614.2
Adolescence NEC V21.2
Adoption
  agency referral V68.89
  examination V70.3
  held for V68.89
Adrenal gland — *see* condition
Adrenalism 255.9
  tuberculous (*see also* Tuberculosis) 017.6 ☑
Adrenalitis, adrenitis 255.8
  meningococcal hemorrhagic 036.3
Adrenarche, precocious 259.1
Adrenocortical syndrome 255.2
Adrenogenital syndrome (acquired) (congen-
  ital) 255.2
  iatrogenic, fetus or newborn 760.79
Adrenoleukodystrophy 277.86
  neonatal 277.86
  x-linked 277.86
Adrenomyeloneuropathy 277.86
Adventitious bursa — *see* Bursitis
Adynamia (episodica) (hereditary) (periodic)
  359.3
Adynamic
  ileus or intestine (*see also* Ileus) 560.1
  ureter 753.22
Aeration lung, imperfect, newborn 770.5
Aerobullosis 993.3
Aerocele — *see* Embolism, air
Aerodermectasia
  subcutaneous (traumatic) 958.7
    surgical 998.81
  surgical 998.81
Aerodontalgia 993.2
Aeroembolism 993.3
Aerogenes capsulatus infection — *see also*
  Gangrene, gas 040.0
Aero-otitis media 993.0
Aerophagy, aerophagia 306.4
  psychogenic 306.4
Aerosinusitis 993.1
Aerotitis 993.0
Affection, affections — *see also* Disease
  sacroiliac (joint), old 724.6
  shoulder region NEC 726.2

Afibrinogenemia 286.3
  acquired 286.6
  congenital 286.3
  postpartum 666.3 ☑
African
  sleeping sickness 086.5
  tick fever 087.1
  trypanosomiasis 086.5
    Gambian 086.3
    Rhodesian 086.4
Aftercare V58.9
  amputation stump V54.89
  artificial openings — *see* Attention to, artifi-
    cial, opening
  blood transfusion without reported diagno-
    sis V58.2
  breathing exercise V57.0
  cardiac device V53.39
    defibrillator, automatic implantable
      (with synchronous cardiac pace-
      maker) V53.32
    pacemaker V53.31
      carotid sinus V53.39
  carotid sinus pacemaker V53.39
  cerebral ventricle (communicating) shunt
    V53.01
  chemotherapy (oral) (intravenous) session
    (adjunctive) (maintenance) V58.11
  defibrillator, automatic implantable cardiac
    (with synchronous cardiac pacemak-
    er) V53.32
  exercise (remedial) (therapeutic) V57.1
    breathing V57.0
  extracorporeal dialysis (intermittent)
    (treatment) V56.0
  following surgery NEC V58.49
    for
      injury V58.43
      neoplasm V58.42
      organ transplant V58.44
      trauma V58.43
    joint
      explantation of prosthesis (staged
        procedure) V54.82
      replacement V54.81
    of
      circulatory system V58.73
      digestive system V58.75
      genital organs V58.76
      genitourinary system V58.76
      musculoskeletal system V58.78
      nervous system V58.72
      oral cavity V58.75
      respiratory system V58.74
      sense organs V58.71
      skin V58.77
      subcutaneous tissue V58.77
      teeth V58.75
      urinary system V58.76
    spinal — *see* Aftercare, following
      surgery, of, specified body system
    wound closure, planned V58.41
  fracture V54.9
    healing V54.89
      pathologic
        ankle V54.29
        arm V54.20
          lower V54.22
          upper V54.21
        finger V54.29
        foot V54.29
        hand V54.29
        hip V54.23
        leg V54.24
          lower V54.26
          upper V54.25
        pelvis V54.29
        specified site NEC V54.29
        toe(s) V54.29
        vertebrae V54.27
        wrist V54.29
      traumatic
        ankle V54.19
        arm V54.10
          lower V54.12
          upper V54.11

Aftercare — *continued*
  fracture — *continued*
    healing — *continued*
      traumatic — *continued*
        finger V54.19
        foot V54.19
        hand V54.19
        hip V54.13
        leg V54.14
          lower V54.16
          upper V54.15
        pelvis V54.19
        specified site NEC V54.19
        toe(s) V54.19
        vertebrae V54.17
        wrist V54.19
    removal of
      external fixation device V54.89
      internal fixation device V54.01
    specified care NEC V54.89
  gait training V57.1
    for use of artificial limb(s) V57.81
  internal fixation device V54.09
  involving
    dialysis (intermittent) (treatment)
      extracorporeal V56.0
      peritoneal V56.8
      renal V56.0
    gait training V57.1
      for use of artificial limb(s) V57.81
    growth rod
      adjustment V54.02
      lengthening V54.02
    internal fixation device V54.09
    orthoptic training V57.4
    orthotic training V57.81
    radiotherapy session V58.0
    removal of
      drains V58.49
      dressings
        wound V58.30
          nonsurgical V58.30
          surgical V58.31
      fixation device
        external V54.89
        internal V54.01
      fracture plate V54.01
      nonsurgical wound dressing V58.30
      pins V54.01
      plaster cast V54.89
      rods V54.01
      screws V58.32
      staples V58.32
      surgical wound dressings V58.31
      sutures V58.32
      traction device, external V54.89
      wound packing V58.30
        nonsurgical V58.30
        surgical V58.31
  neuropacemaker (brain) (peripheral nerve)
    (spinal cord) V53.02
  occupational therapy V57.21
  orthodontic V58.5
  orthopedic V54.9
    change of external fixation or traction
      device V54.89
    following joint
      explantation of prosthesis (staged
        procedure) V54.82
      replacement V54.81
    internal fixation device V54.09
    removal of fixation device
      external V54.89
      internal V54.01
    specified care NEC V54.89
  orthoptic training V57.4
  orthotic training V57.81
  pacemaker
    brain V53.02
    cardiac V53.31
    carotid sinus V53.39
    peripheral nerve V53.02
    spinal cord V53.02
  peritoneal dialysis (intermittent) (treatment)
    V56.8
  physical therapy NEC V57.1

☑ **Additional Digit Required** — Refer to the Tabular List for Digit Selection   ▽ **Subterms under main terms may continue to next column or page**

14 — Volume 2   ▶◀ **Revised Text**   ● **New Line**   ▲ **Revised Code**   2015 ICD-9-CM

Aftercare — *continued*
- physical therapy — *continued*
  - breathing exercises V57.0
- radiotherapy session V58.0
- rehabilitation procedure V57.9
  - breathing exercises V57.0
  - multiple types V57.89
  - occupational V57.21
  - orthoptic V57.4
  - orthotic V57.81
  - physical therapy NEC V57.1
  - remedial exercises V57.1
  - specified type NEC V57.89
  - speech (-language) V57.3
  - therapeutic exercises V57.1
  - vocational V57.22
- renal dialysis (intermittent) (treatment) V56.0
- specified type NEC V58.89
  - removal of non-vascular catheter V58.82
  - removal of vascular catheter V58.81
- speech (-language) therapy V57.3
- stump, amputation V54.89
- vocational rehabilitation V57.22

After-cataract 366.50
- obscuring vision 366.53
- specified type, not obscuring vision 366.52

Agalactia 676.4 ☑

Agammaglobulinemia 279.00
- with lymphopenia 279.2
- acquired (primary) (secondary) 279.06
- Bruton's X-linked 279.04
- infantile sex-linked (Bruton's) (congenital) 279.04
- Swiss-type 279.2

Aganglionosis (bowel) (colon) 751.3

Age (old) — *see also* Senile 797

Agenesis — *see also* Absence, by site, congenital
- acoustic nerve 742.8
- adrenal (gland) 759.1
- alimentary tract (complete) (partial) NEC 751.8
  - lower 751.2
  - upper 750.8
- anus, anal (canal) 751.2
- aorta 747.22
- appendix 751.2
- arm (complete) (partial) (*see also* Deformity, reduction, upper limb) 755.20
- artery (peripheral) NEC (*see also* Anomaly, peripheral vascular system) 747.60
  - brain 747.81
  - coronary 746.85
  - pulmonary 747.31
  - umbilical 747.5
- auditory (canal) (external) 744.01
- auricle (ear) 744.01
- bile, biliary duct or passage 751.61
- bone NEC 756.9
- brain 740.0
  - specified part 742.2
- breast 757.6
- bronchus 748.3
- canaliculus lacrimalis 743.65
- carpus NEC (*see also* Deformity, reduction, upper limb) 755.28
- cartilage 756.9
- cecum 751.2
- cerebellum 742.2
- cervix 752.43
- chin 744.89
- cilia 743.63
- circulatory system, part NEC 747.89
- clavicle 755.51
- clitoris 752.49
- coccyx 756.13
- colon 751.2
- corpus callosum 742.2
- cricoid cartilage 748.3
- diaphragm (with hernia) 756.6
- digestive organ(s) or tract (complete) (partial) NEC 751.8
  - lower 751.2
  - upper 750.8
- ductus arteriosus 747.89

Agenesis — *see also* Absence, by site, congenital — *continued*
- duodenum 751.1
- ear NEC 744.09
  - auricle 744.01
  - lobe 744.21
- ejaculatory duct 752.89
- endocrine (gland) NEC 759.2
- epiglottis 748.3
- esophagus 750.3
- Eustachian tube 744.24
- extrinsic muscle, eye 743.69
- eye 743.00
  - adnexa 743.69
- eyelid (fold) 743.62
- face
  - bones NEC 756.0
  - specified part NEC 744.89
- fallopian tube 752.19
- femur NEC (*see also* Absence, femur, congenital) 755.34
- fibula NEC (*see also* Absence, fibula, congenital) 755.37
- finger NEC (*see also* Absence, finger, congenital) 755.29
- foot (complete) (*see also* Deformity, reduction, lower limb) 755.31
- gallbladder 751.69
- gastric 750.8
- genitalia, genital (organ)
  - female 752.89
    - external 752.49
    - internal NEC 752.89
  - male 752.89
    - penis 752.69
- glottis 748.3
- gonadal 758.6
- hair 757.4
- hand (complete) (*see also* Deformity, reduction, upper limb) 755.21
- heart 746.89
  - valve NEC 746.89
    - aortic 746.89
    - mitral 746.89
    - pulmonary 746.01
- hepatic 751.69
- humerus NEC (*see also* Absence, humerus, congenital) 755.24
- hymen 752.49
- ileum 751.1
- incus 744.04
- intestine (small) 751.1
  - large 751.2
- iris (dilator fibers) 743.45
- jaw 524.09
- jejunum 751.1
- kidney(s) (partial) (unilateral) 753.0
- labium (majus) (minus) 752.49
- labyrinth, membranous 744.05
- lacrimal apparatus (congenital) 743.65
- larynx 748.3
- leg NEC (*see also* Deformity, reduction, lower limb) 755.30
- lens 743.35
- limb (complete) (partial) (*see also* Deformity, reduction) 755.4
  - lower NEC 755.30
  - upper 755.20
- lip 750.26
- liver 751.69
- lung (bilateral) (fissures) (lobe) (unilateral) 748.5
- mandible 524.09
- maxilla 524.09
- metacarpus NEC 755.28
- metatarsus NEC 755.38
- muscle (any) 756.81
- musculoskeletal system NEC 756.9
- nail(s) 757.5
- neck, part 744.89
- nerve 742.8
- nipple 757.6
- nose 748.1
- nuclear 742.8

Agenesis — *see also* Absence, by site, congenital — *continued*
- organ
  - of Corti 744.05
  - or site not listed — *see* Anomaly, specified type NEC
- osseous meatus (ear) 744.03
- ovary 752.0
- oviduct 752.19
- pancreas 751.7
- parathyroid (gland) 759.2
- patella 755.64
- pelvic girdle (complete) (partial) 755.69
- penis 752.69
- pericardium 746.89
- perineal body 756.81
- pituitary (gland) 759.2
- prostate 752.89
- pulmonary
  - artery 747.31
  - trunk 747.31
  - vein 747.49
- punctum lacrimale 743.65
- radioulnar NEC (*see also* Absence, forearm, congenital) 755.25
- radius NEC (*see also* Absence, radius, congenital) 755.26
- rectum 751.2
- renal 753.0
- respiratory organ NEC 748.9
- rib 756.3
- roof of orbit 742.0
- round ligament 752.89
- sacrum 756.13
- salivary gland 750.21
- scapula 755.59
- scrotum 752.89
- seminal duct or tract 752.89
- septum
  - atrial 745.69
  - between aorta and pulmonary artery 745.0
  - ventricular 745.3
- shoulder girdle (complete) (partial) 755.59
- skull (bone) 756.0
  - with
    - anencephalus 740.0
    - encephalocele 742.0
    - hydrocephalus 742.3
      - with spina bifida (*see also* Spina bifida) 741.0 ☑
    - microcephalus 742.1
- spermatic cord 752.89
- spinal cord 742.59
- spine 756.13
  - lumbar 756.13
    - isthmus 756.11
    - pars articularis 756.11
- spleen 759.0
- sternum 756.3
- stomach 750.7
- tarsus NEC 755.38
- tendon 756.81
- testicular 752.89
- testis 752.89
- thymus (gland) 759.2
- thyroid (gland) 243
  - cartilage 748.3
- tibia NEC (*see also* Absence, tibia, congenital) 755.36
- tibiofibular NEC 755.35
- toe (complete) (partial) (*see also* Absence, toe, congenital) 755.39
- tongue 750.11
- trachea (cartilage) 748.3
- ulna NEC (*see also* Absence, ulna, congenital) 755.27
- ureter 753.4
- urethra 753.8
- urinary tract NEC 753.8
- uterus 752.31
- uvula 750.26
- vagina (total) (partial) 752.45
- vas deferens 752.89
- vein(s) (peripheral) NEC (*see also* Anomaly, peripheral vascular system) 747.60

Agenesis — *see also* Absence, by site, congenital — *continued*
- vein(s) (*see also* Anomaly, peripheral vascular system) — *continued*
  - brain 747.81
  - great 747.49
  - portal 747.49
  - pulmonary 747.49
  - vena cava (inferior) (superior) 747.49
- vermis of cerebellum 742.2
- vertebra 756.13
  - lumbar 756.13
    - isthmus 756.11
    - pars articularis 756.11
- vulva 752.49

Ageusia — *see also* Disturbance, sensation 781.1

Aggressiveness 301.3

Aggressive outburst — *see also* Disturbance, conduct 312.0 ☑
- in children or adolescents 313.9

Aging skin 701.8

Agitated — *see* condition

Agitation 307.9
- catatonic (*see also* Schizophrenia) 295.2 ☑

Aglossia (congenital) 750.11

Aglycogenosis 271.0

Agnail (finger) (with lymphangitis) 681.02

Agnosia (body image) (tactile) 784.69
- verbal 784.69
  - auditory 784.69
    - secondary to organic lesion 784.69
  - developmental 315.8
  - secondary to organic lesion 784.69
- visual 368.16
  - object 368.16

Agoraphobia 300.22
- with panic disorder 300.21

Agrammatism 784.69

Agranulocytopenia — *see also* Agranulocytosis 288.09

Agranulocytosis — *see also* Neutropenia 288.09
- chronic 288.09
- cyclical 288.02
- due to infection 288.04
- genetic 288.01
- infantile 288.01
- periodic 288.02
- pernicious 288.09

Agraphia (absolute) 784.69
- with alexia 784.61
- developmental 315.39

Agrypnia — *see also* Insomnia 780.52

Ague — *see also* Malaria 084.6
- brass-founders' 985.8
- dumb 084.6
- tertian 084.1

Agyria 742.2

AHTR (acute hemolytic transfusion reaction) — *see* Complications, transfusion

Ahumada-del Castillo syndrome (nonpuerperal galactorrhea and amenorrhea) 253.1

AIDS 042

AIDS-associated retrovirus (disease) (illness) 042
- infection — *see* Human immunodeficiency virus, infection

AIDS-associated virus (disease) (illness) 042
- infection — *see* Human immunodeficiency virus, infection

AIDS-like disease (illness) (syndrome) 042

AIDS-related complex 042

AIDS-related conditions 042

AIDS-related virus (disease) (illness) 042
- infection — *see* Human immunodeficiency virus, infection

AIDS virus (disease) (illness) 042
- infection — *see* Human immunodeficiency virus, infection

Ailment, heart — *see* Disease, heart

Ailurophobia 300.29

Ainhum (disease) 136.0

AIN I (anal intraepithelial neoplasia I) (histologically confirmed) 569.44

☑ **Additional Digit Required** — Refer to the Tabular List for Digit Selection   ▽ **Subterms under main terms may continue to next column or page**

AIN II (anal intraepithelial neoplasia II) (histologically confirmed) 569.44
AIN III (anal intraepithelial neoplasia III) 230.6
  anal canal 230.5
AIPHI (acute idiopathic pulmonary hemorrhage in infants (over 28 days old)) 786.31
Air
  anterior mediastinum 518.1
  compressed, disease 993.3
  embolism (any site) (artery) (cerebral) 958.0
    with
      abortion — see Abortion, by type, with embolism
      ectopic pregnancy (see also categories 633.0–633.9) 639.6
      molar pregnancy (see also categories 630–632) 639.6
    due to implanted device — see Complications, due to (presence of) any device, implant, or graft classified to 996.0–996.5 NEC
    following
      abortion 639.6
      ectopic or molar pregnancy 639.6
    infusion, perfusion, or transfusion 999.1
    in pregnancy, childbirth, or puerperium 673.0 ☑
    traumatic 958.0
  hunger 786.09
    psychogenic 306.1
  leak (lung) (pulmonary) (thorax) 512.84
    iatrogenic 512.1
    persistent 512.84
    postoperative 512.2
  rarefied, effects of — see Effect, adverse, high altitude
  sickness 994.6
Airplane sickness 994.6
Akathisia, acathisia 781.0
  due to drugs 333.99
  neuroleptic-induced acute 333.99
Akinesia algeria 352.6
Akiyami 100.89
Akureyri disease (epidemic neuromyasthenia) 049.8
Alacrima (congenital) 743.65
Alactasia (hereditary) 271.3
Alagille syndrome 759.89
Alalia 784.3
  developmental 315.31
    receptive-expressive 315.32
  secondary to organic lesion 784.3
Alaninemia 270.8
Alastrim 050.1
Albarrán's disease (colibacilluria) 791.9
Albers-Schönberg's disease (marble bones) 756.52
Albert's disease 726.71
Albinism, albino (choroid) (cutaneous) (eye) (generalized) (isolated) (ocular) (oculocutaneous) (partial) 270.2
Albinismus 270.2
Albright (-Martin) (-Bantam) disease (pseudohypoparathyroidism) 275.49
Albright (-McCune) (-Sternberg) syndrome (osteitis fibrosa disseminata) 756.59
Albuminous — see condition
Albuminuria, albuminuric (acute) (chronic) (subacute) 791.0
  Bence-Jones 791.0
  cardiac 785.9
  complicating pregnancy, childbirth, or puerperium 646.2 ☑
    with hypertension — see Toxemia, of pregnancy
    affecting fetus or newborn 760.1
  cyclic 593.6
  gestational 646.2 ☑
  gravidarum 646.2 ☑
    with hypertension — see Toxemia, of pregnancy
    affecting fetus or newborn 760.1
  heart 785.9
  idiopathic 593.6
  orthostatic 593.6

Albuminuria, albuminuric — continued
  postural 593.6
  pre-eclamptic (mild) 642.4 ☑
    affecting fetus or newborn 760.0
    severe 642.5 ☑
      affecting fetus or newborn 760.0
  recurrent physiologic 593.6
  scarlatinal 034.1
Albumosuria 791.0
  Bence-Jones 791.0
  myelopathic (M9730/3) 203.0 ☑
Alcaptonuria 270.2
Alcohol, alcoholic
  abstinence 291.81
  acute intoxication 305.0 ☑
    with dependence 303.0 ☑
  addiction (see also Alcoholism) 303.9 ☑
    maternal
      with suspected fetal damage affecting management of pregnancy 655.4 ☑
      affecting fetus or newborn 760.71
  amnestic disorder, persisting 291.1
  anxiety 291.89
  brain syndrome, chronic 291.2
  cardiopathy 425.5
  chronic (see also Alcoholism) 303.9 ☑
  cirrhosis (liver) 571.2
  delirium 291.0
    acute 291.0
    chronic 291.1
    tremens 291.0
    withdrawal 291.0
  dementia NEC 291.2
  deterioration 291.2
  drunkenness (simple) 305.0 ☑
  hallucinosis (acute) 291.3
  induced
    circadian rhythm sleep disorder 291.82
    hypersomnia 291.82
    insomnia 291.82
    mental disorder 291.9
      anxiety 291.89
      mood 291.89
      sexual 291.89
      sleep 291.82
      specified type 291.89
    parasomnia 291.82
    persisting
      amnestic disorder 291.1
      dementia 291.2
    psychotic disorder
      with
        delusions 291.5
        hallucinations 291.3
    sleep disorder 291.82
  insanity 291.9
  intoxication (acute) 305.0 ☑
    with dependence 303.0 ☑
    pathological 291.4
  jealousy 291.5
  Korsakoff's, Korsakov's, Korsakow's 291.1
  liver NEC 571.3
    acute 571.1
    chronic 571.2
  mania (acute) (chronic) 291.9
  mood 291.89
  paranoia 291.5
  paranoid (type) psychosis 291.5
  pellagra 265.2
  poisoning, accidental (acute) NEC 980.9
    specified type of alcohol — see Table of Drugs and Chemicals
  psychosis (see also Psychosis, alcoholic) 291.9
    Korsakoff's, Korsakov's, Korsakow's 291.1
    polyneuritic 291.1
      with
        delusions 291.5
        hallucinations 291.3
  related disorder 291.9
  withdrawal symptoms, syndrome NEC 291.81
    delirium 291.0
    hallucinosis 291.3

Alcoholism 303.9 ☑

> *Note* — Use the following fifth-digit subclassification with category 303:
>
> 0   unspecified
> 1   continuous
> 2   episodic
> 3   in remission

  with psychosis (see also Psychosis, alcoholic) 291.9
  acute 303.0 ☑
  chronic 303.9 ☑
    with psychosis 291.9
  complicating pregnancy, childbirth, or puerperium 648.4 ☑
    affecting fetus or newborn 760.71
  history V11.3
  Korsakoff's, Korsakov's, Korsakow's 291.1
  suspected damage to fetus affecting management of pregnancy 655.4 ☑
Alder's anomaly or syndrome (leukocyte granulation anomaly) 288.2
Alder-Reilly anomaly (leukocyte granulation) 288.2
Aldosteronism (primary) 255.10
  congenital 255.10
  familial type I 255.11
  glucocorticoid-remediable 255.11
  secondary 255.14
Aldosteronoma (M8370/1) 237.2
Aldrich (-Wiskott) syndrome (eczema-thrombocytopenia) 279.12
Aleppo boil 085.1
Aleukemic — see condition
Aleukia
  congenital 288.09
  hemorrhagica 284.9
    acquired (secondary) 284.89
    congenital 284.09
    idiopathic 284.9
  splenica 289.4
Alexia (congenital) (developmental) 315.01
  secondary to organic lesion 784.61
Algoneurodystrophy 733.7
Algophobia 300.29
Alibert-Bazin disease (M9700/3) 202.1 ☑
Alibert's disease (mycosis fungoides) (M9700/3) 202.1 ☑
Alice in Wonderland syndrome 293.89
Alienation, mental — see also Psychosis 298.9
Alkalemia 276.3
Alkalosis 276.3
  metabolic 276.3
    with respiratory acidosis 276.4
  respiratory 276.3
Alkaptonuria 270.2
Allen-Masters syndrome 620.6
Allergic bronchopulmonary aspergillosis 518.6
Allergy, allergic (reaction) 995.3
  air-borne substance — see also Fever, hay 477.9
    specified allergen NEC 477.8
  alveolitis (extrinsic) 495.9
    due to
      Aspergillus clavatus 495.4
      cryptostroma corticale 495.6
      organisms (fungal, thermophilic actinomycete, other) growing in ventilation (air conditioning systems) 495.7
    specified type NEC 495.8
  anaphylactic reaction or shock 995.0
    due to food — see Anaphylactic reaction or shock, due to, food
  angioderma 995.1
  angioneurotic edema 995.1
  animal (cat) (dog) (epidermal) 477.8
    dander 477.2
    hair 477.2
  arthritis (see also Arthritis, allergic) 716.2 ☑
  asthma — see Asthma
  bee sting (anaphylactic shock) 989.5
  biological — see Allergy, drug

Allergy, allergic — continued
  bronchial asthma — see Asthma
  conjunctivitis (eczematous) 372.14
  dander, animal (cat) (dog) 477.2
  dandruff 477.8
  dermatitis (venenata) — see Dermatitis
  diathesis V15.09
  drug, medicinal substance, and biological (any) (correct medicinal substance properly administered) (external) (internal) 995.27
    wrong substance given or taken NEC 977.9
      specified drug or substance — see Table of Drugs and Chemicals
  dust (house) (stock) 477.8
  eczema — see Eczema
  endophthalmitis 360.19
  epidermal (animal) 477.8
  existing dental restorative material
  feathers 477.8
  food (any) (ingested) 693.1
    atopic 691.8
    in contact with skin 692.5
  gastritis 535.4 ☑
  gastroenteritis 558.3
  gastrointestinal 558.3
  grain 477.0
  grass (pollen) 477.0
    asthma (see also Asthma) 493.0 ☑
    hay fever 477.0
  hair, animal (cat) (dog) 477.2
  hay fever (grass) (pollen) (ragweed) (tree) (see also Fever, hay) 477.9
  history (of) V15.09
    to
      arachnid bite V15.06
      eggs V15.03
      food additives V15.05
      insect bite V15.06
      latex V15.07
      milk products V15.02
      nuts V15.05
        peanuts V15.01
      radiographic dye V15.08
      seafood V15.04
      specified food NEC V15.05
      spider bite V15.06
  horse serum — see Allergy, serum
  inhalant 477.9
    dust 477.8
    pollen 477.0
    specified allergen other than pollen 477.8
  kapok 477.8
  medicine — see Allergy, drug
  migraine 339.00
  milk protein 558.3
  pannus 370.62
  pneumonia 518.3
  pollen (any) (hay fever) 477.0
    asthma (see also Asthma) 493.0 ☑
  primrose 477.0
  primula 477.0
  purpura 287.0
  ragweed (pollen) (Senecio jacobae) 477.0
    asthma (see also Asthma) 493.0 ☑
    hay fever 477.0
  respiratory (see also Allergy, inhalant) 477.9
    due to
      drug — see Allergy, drug
      food — see Allergy, food
  rhinitis (see also Fever, hay) 477.9
    due to food 477.1
  rose 477.0
  Senecio jacobae 477.0
  serum (prophylactic) (therapeutic) 999.59
    anaphylactic reaction or shock 999.49
  shock (anaphylactic) (due to adverse effect of correct medicinal substance properly administered) 995.0
    food — see Anaphylactic reaction or shock, due to, food
    from
      administration of blood and blood products 999.41

☑ Additional Digit Required — Refer to the Tabular List for Digit Selection   ⓦ Subterms under main terms may continue to next column or page

16 — Volume 2   ►◄ Revised Text   ● New Line   ▲ Revised Code   **2015 ICD-9-CM**

Allergy, allergic — *continued*
  shock — *continued*
    from — *continued*
      immunization 999.42
      serum NEC 999.49
  sinusitis (*see also* Fever, hay) 477.9
  skin reaction 692.9
    specified substance — *see* Dermatitis, due to
  tree (any) (hay fever) (pollen) 477.0
    asthma (*see also* Asthma) 493.0 ☑
  upper respiratory (*see also* Fever, hay) 477.9
  urethritis 597.89
  urticaria 708.0
  vaccine — *see* Allergy, serum
Allescheriosis 117.6
Alligator skin disease (ichthyosis congenita) 757.1
  acquired 701.1
Allocheiria, allochiria — *see also* Disturbance, sensation 782.0
Almeida's disease (Brazilian blastomycosis) 116.1
Alopecia (atrophicans) (pregnancy) (premature) (senile) 704.00
  adnata 757.4
  areata 704.01
  celsi 704.01
  cicatrisata 704.09
  circumscripta 704.01
  congenital, congenitalis 757.4
  disseminata 704.01
  effluvium (telogen) 704.02
  febrile 704.09
  generalisata 704.09
  hereditaria 704.09
  marginalis 704.01
  mucinosa 704.09
  postinfectional 704.09
  seborrheica 704.09
  specific 091.82
  syphilitic (secondary) 091.82
  telogen effluvium 704.02
  totalis 704.09
  toxica 704.09
  universalis 704.09
  x-ray 704.09
Alpers' disease 330.8
Alpha-lipoproteinemia 272.4
Alpha thalassemia 282.43
Alphos 696.1
Alpine sickness 993.2
Alport's syndrome (hereditary hematuria-nephropathy-deafness) 759.89
ALPS (autoimmune lymphoproliferative syndrome) 279.41
ALTE (apparent life threatening event) **in newborn and infant** 799.82
Alteration (of), altered
  awareness 780.09
    transient 780.02
  consciousness 780.09
    persistent vegetative state 780.03
    transient 780.02
  mental status 780.97
    amnesia (retrograde) 780.93
    memory loss 780.93
Alternaria (infection) 118
Alternating — *see* condition
Altitude, high (effects) — *see* Effect, adverse, high altitude
Aluminosis (of lung) 503
Alvarez syndrome (transient cerebral ischemia) 435.9
Alveolar capillary block syndrome 516.64
Alveolus, alveolar — *see* condition
Alymphocytosis (pure) 279.2
Alymphoplasia, thymic 279.2
Alzheimer's
  dementia (senile)
    with behavioral disturbance 331.0 [294.11]
    without behavioral disturbance 331.0 [294.10]
  disease or sclerosis 331.0

Alzheimer's — *continued*
  disease or sclerosis — *continued*
    with dementia — *see* Alzheimer's, dementia
Amastia — *see also* Absence, breast 611.89
Amaurosis (acquired) (congenital) — *see also* Blindness 369.00
  fugax 362.34
  hysterical 300.11
  Leber's (congenital) 362.76
  tobacco 377.34
  uremic — *see* Uremia
Amaurotic familial idiocy (infantile) (juvenile) (late) 330.1
Ambisexual 752.7
Amblyopia (acquired) (congenital) (partial) 368.00
  color 368.59
    acquired 368.55
  deprivation 368.02
  ex anopsia 368.00
  hysterical 300.11
  nocturnal 368.60
    vitamin A deficiency 264.5
  refractive 368.03
  strabismic 368.01
  suppression 368.01
  tobacco 377.34
  toxic NEC 377.34
  uremic — *see* Uremia
Ameba, amebic (histolytica) — *see also* Amebiasis
  abscess 006.3
    bladder 006.8
    brain (with liver and lung abscess) 006.5
    liver 006.3
      with
        brain abscess (and lung abscess) 006.5
        lung abscess 006.4
    lung (with liver abscess) 006.4
      with brain abscess 006.5
    seminal vesicle 006.8
    spleen 006.8
  carrier (suspected of) V02.2
  meningoencephalitis
    due to Naegleria (gruberi) 136.29
    primary 136.29
Amebiasis NEC 006.9
  with
    brain abscess (with liver or lung abscess) 006.5
    liver abscess (without mention of brain or lung abscess) 006.3
    lung abscess (with liver abscess) 006.4
      with brain abscess 006.5
  acute 006.0
  bladder 006.8
  chronic 006.1
  cutaneous 006.6
  cutis 006.6
  due to organism other than Entamoeba histolytica 007.8
  hepatic (*see also* Abscess, liver, amebic) 006.3
  nondysenteric 006.2
  seminal vesicle 006.8
  specified
    organism NEC 007.8
    site NEC 006.8
Ameboma 006.8
Amelia 755.4
  lower limb 755.31
  upper limb 755.21
Ameloblastoma (M9310/0) 213.1
  jaw (bone) (lower) 213.1
    upper 213.0
  long bones (M9261/3) — *see* Neoplasm, bone, malignant
  malignant (M9310/3) 170.1
    jaw (bone) (lower) 170.1
      upper 170.0
  mandible 213.1
  tibial (M9261/3) 170.7
Amelogenesis imperfecta 520.5
  nonhereditaria (segmentalis) 520.4

Amenorrhea (primary) (secondary) 626.0
  due to ovarian dysfunction 256.8
  hyperhormonal 256.8
Amentia — *see also* Disability, intellectual 319
  Meynert's (nonalcoholic) 294.0
    alcoholic 291.1
  nevoid 759.6
American
  leishmaniasis 085.5
  mountain tick fever 066.1
  trypanosomiasis — *see* Trypanosomiasis, American
Ametropia — *see also* Disorder, accommodation 367.9
Amianthosis 501
Amimia 784.69
Amino acid
  deficiency 270.9
    anemia 281.4
  metabolic disorder (*see also* Disorder, amino acid) 270.9
Aminoaciduria 270.9
  imidazole 270.5
Amnesia (retrograde) 780.93
  auditory 784.69
    developmental 315.31
    secondary to organic lesion 784.69
  dissociative 300.12
  hysterical or dissociative type 300.12
  psychogenic 300.12
  transient global 437.7
Amnestic (confabulatory) **syndrome** 294.0
  alcohol-induced persisting 291.1
  drug-induced persisting 292.83
  posttraumatic 294.0
Amniocentesis screening (for) V28.2
  alphafetoprotein level, raised V28.1
  chromosomal anomalies V28.0
Amnion, amniotic — *see also* condition
  nodosum 658.8 ☑
Amnionitis (complicating pregnancy) 658.4 ☑
  affecting fetus or newborn 762.7
Amoral trends 301.7
Amotio retinae — *see also* Detachment, retina 361.9
Ampulla
  lower esophagus 530.89
  phrenic 530.89
Amputation
  any part of fetus, to facilitate delivery 763.89
  cervix (supravaginal) (uteri) 622.8
    in pregnancy or childbirth 654.6 ☑
      affecting fetus or newborn 763.89
  clitoris — *see* Wound, open, clitoris
  congenital
    lower limb 755.31
    upper limb 755.21
  neuroma (traumatic) (*see also* Injury, nerve, by site)
    surgical complication (late) 997.61
  penis — *see* Amputation, traumatic, penis
  status (without complication) — *see* Absence, by site, acquired
  stump (surgical) (posttraumatic)
    abnormal, painful, or with complication (late) 997.60
    healed or old NEC (*see also* Absence, by site, acquired)
      lower V49.70
      upper V49.60
  traumatic (complete) (partial)

> *Note* — "Complicated" includes traumatic amputation with delayed healing, delayed treatment, foreign body, or infection.

    arm 887.4
      at or above elbow 887.2
        complicated 887.3
      below elbow 887.0
        complicated 887.1
      both (bilateral) (any level(s)) 887.6
        complicated 887.7
        complicated 887.5
      finger(s) (one or both hands) 886.0
        with thumb(s) 885.0
          complicated 885.1

Amputation — *continued*
  traumatic — *continued*
    finger(s) — *continued*
      complicated 886.1
    foot (except toe(s) only) 896.0
      and other leg 897.6
        complicated 897.7
      both (bilateral) 896.2
        complicated 896.3
      complicated 896.1
      toe(s) only (one or both feet) 895.0
        complicated 895.1
    genital organ(s) (external) NEC 878.8
      complicated 878.9
    hand (except finger(s) only) 887.0
      and other arm 887.6
        complicated 887.7
      both (bilateral) 887.6
        complicated 887.7
      complicated 887.1
    finger(s) (one or both hands) 886.0
      with thumb(s) 885.0
        complicated 885.1
      complicated 886.1
    thumb(s) (with fingers of either hand) 885.0
      complicated 885.1
    head 874.9
    late effect — *see* Late, effects (of), amputation
    leg 897.4
      and other foot 897.6
        complicated 897.7
      at or above knee 897.2
        complicated 897.3
      below knee 897.0
        complicated 897.1
      both (bilateral) 897.6
        complicated 897.7
      complicated 897.5
    lower limb(s) except toe(s) — *see* Amputation, traumatic, leg
    nose — *see* Wound, open, nose
    penis 878.0
      complicated 878.1
    sites other than limbs — *see* Wound, open, by site
    thumb(s) (with finger(s) of either hand) 885.0
      complicated 885.1
    toe(s) (one or both feet) 895.0
      complicated 895.1
    upper limb(s) — *see* Amputation, traumatic, arm
Amputee (bilateral) (old) — *see also* Absence, by site, acquired V49.70
Amusia 784.69
  developmental 315.39
  secondary to organic lesion 784.69
Amyelencephalus 740.0
Amyelia 742.59
Amygdalitis — *see* Tonsillitis
Amygdalolith 474.8
Amyloid disease or degeneration 277.30
  heart 277.39 [425.7]
Amyloidosis (familial) (general) (generalized) (genetic) (primary) 277.30
  with lung involvement 277.39 [517.8]
  cardiac, hereditary 277.39
  heart 277.39 [425.7]
  nephropathic 277.39 [583.81]
  neuropathic (Portuguese) (Swiss) 277.39 [357.4]
  pulmonary 277.39 [517.8]
  secondary 277.39
  systemic, inherited 277.39
Amylopectinosis (brancher enzyme deficiency) 271.0
Amylophagia 307.52
Amyoplasia, congenita 756.89
Amyotonia 728.2
  congenita 358.8
Amyotrophia, amyotrophy, amyotrophic 728.2
  congenita 756.89
  diabetic 250.6 ☑ [353.5]

☑ Additional Digit Required — Refer to the Tabular List for Digit Selection   ▽ Subterms under main terms may continue to next column or page

2015 ICD-9-CM   ▶◀ Revised Text   ● New Line   ▲ Revised Code   Volume 2 — 17

Allergy, allergic — Amyotrophia, amyotrophy, amyotrophic

Amyotrophia, amyotrophy, amyotrophic —
continued
  diabetic — *continued*
    due to secondary diabetes
      249.6 ☑ *[353.5]*
  lateral sclerosis (syndrome) 335.20
  neuralgic 353.5
  sclerosis (lateral) 335.20
  spinal progressive 335.21
Anacidity, gastric 536.0
  psychogenic 306.4
Anaerosis of newborn 770.88
Analbuminemia 273.8
Analgesia — *see also* Anesthesia 782.0
Analphalipoproteinemia 272.5
Anaphylactic reaction or shock (correct
  substance properly administered) 995.0
  due to
    administration of blood and blood
      products 999.41
    chemical — *see* Table of Drugs and
      Chemicals
    correct medicinal substance properly
      administered 995.0
    drug or medicinal substance
      correct substance properly adminis-
        tered 995.0
      overdose or wrong substance given
        or taken 977.9
      specified drug — *see* Table of
        Drugs and Chemicals
  following sting(s) 989.5
  food 995.60
    additives 995.66
    crustaceans 995.62
    eggs 995.68
    fish 995.65
    fruits 995.63
    milk products 995.67
    nuts (tree) 995.64
    peanuts 995.61
    seeds 995.64
    specified NEC 995.69
    tree nuts 995.64
    vegetables 995.63
  immunization 999.42
  overdose or wrong substance given or
    taken 977.9
    specified drug — *see* Table of Drugs
      and Chemicals
  serum NEC 999.49
  following sting(s) 989.5
  purpura 287.0
  serum NEC 999.49
Anaphylactoid reaction or shock — *see*
  Anaphylactic reaction or shock
Anaphylaxis — *see* Anaphylactic reaction or
  shock
Anaplasia, cervix 622.10
Anaplasmosis, human 082.49
Anarthria 784.51
Anarthritic rheumatoid disease 446.5
Anasarca 782.3
  cardiac (*see also* Failure, heart) 428.0
  fetus or newborn 778.0
  lung 514
  nutritional 262
  pulmonary 514
  renal (*see also* Nephrosis) 581.9
Anaspadias 752.62
Anastomosis
  aneurysmal — *see* Aneurysm
  arteriovenous, congenital NEC (*see also*
    Anomaly, arteriovenous) 747.60
    ruptured, of brain (*see also* Hemorrhage,
      subarachnoid) 430
  intestinal 569.89
    complicated NEC 997.49
      involving urinary tract 997.5
  retinal and choroidal vessels 743.58
    acquired 362.17
Anatomical narrow angle (glaucoma) 365.02
Ancylostoma (infection) (infestation) 126.9
  americanus 126.1
  braziliense 126.2
  caninum 126.8

Ancylostoma — *continued*
  ceylanicum 126.3
  duodenale 126.0
  Necator americanus 126.1
Ancylostomiasis (intestinal) 126.9
  ancylostoma
    americanus 126.1
    caninum 126.8
    ceylanicum 126.3
    duodenale 126.0
  braziliense 126.2
  Necator americanus 126.1
Anders' disease or syndrome (adiposis
  tuberosa simplex) 272.8
Andersen's glycogen storage disease 271.0
Anderson's disease 272.7
Andes disease 993.2
Andrews' disease (bacterid) 686.8
Androblastoma (M8630/1)
  benign (M8630/0)
    specified site — *see* Neoplasm, by site,
      benign
    unspecified site
      female 220
      male 222.0
  malignant (M8630/3)
    specified site — *see* Neoplasm, by site,
      malignant
    unspecified site
      female 183.0
      male 186.9
  specified site — *see* Neoplasm, by site, un-
    certain behavior
  tubular (M8640/0)
    with lipid storage (M8641/0)
      specified site — *see* Neoplasm, by
        site, benign
      unspecified site
        female 220
        male 222.0
    specified site — *see* Neoplasm, by site,
      benign
    unspecified site
      female 220
      male 222.0
  unspecified site
    female 236.2
    male 236.4
Android pelvis 755.69
  with disproportion (fetopelvic) 653.3 ☑
    affecting fetus or newborn 763.1
    causing obstructed labor 660.1 ☑
      affecting fetus or newborn 763.1
Anectasis, pulmonary (newborn or fetus)
  770.5
Anemia 285.9
  with
    disorder of
      anaerobic glycolysis 282.3
      pentose phosphate pathway 282.2
    koilonychia 280.9
  6-phosphogluconic dehydrogenase deficien-
    cy 282.2
  achlorhydric 280.9
  achrestic 281.8
  Addison's (pernicious) 281.0
  Addison-Biermer (pernicious) 281.0
  agranulocytic 288.09
  amino acid deficiency 281.4
  antineoplastic chemotherapy induced 285.3
  aplastic 284.9
    acquired (secondary) 284.89
    congenital 284.01
    constitutional 284.01
    due to
      antineoplastic chemotherapy 284.89
      chronic systemic disease 284.89
      drugs 284.89
      infection 284.89
      radiation 284.89
    idiopathic 284.9
    myxedema 244.9
    of or complicating pregnancy 648.2 ☑
    red cell (acquired) (adult) (with thymo-
      ma) 284.81
      congenital 284.01

Anemia — *continued*
  aplastic — *continued*
    red cell — *continued*
      pure 284.01
      specified type NEC 284.89
      toxic (paralytic) 284.89
  aregenerative 284.9
    congenital 284.01
  asiderotic 280.9
  atypical (primary) 285.9
  autohemolysis of Selwyn and Dacie (type I)
    282.2
  autoimmune hemolytic 283.0
  Baghdad Spring 282.2
  Balantidium coli 007.0
  Biermer's (pernicious) 281.0
  blood loss (chronic) 280.0
    acute 285.1
  bothriocephalus 123.4
  brickmakers' (*see also* Ancylostomiasis)
    126.9
  cerebral 437.8
  childhood 282.9
  chlorotic 280.9
  chronic 285.9
    blood loss 280.0
    hemolytic 282.9
      idiopathic 283.9
    simple 281.9
  chronica congenita aregenerativa 284.01
  combined system disease NEC 281.0 *[336.2]*
    due to dietary deficiency 281.1 *[336.2]*
  complicating pregnancy or childbirth
    648.2 ☑
  congenital (following fetal blood loss) 776.5
    aplastic 284.01
    due to isoimmunization NEC 773.2
    Heinz-body 282.7
    hereditary hemolytic NEC 282.9
    nonspherocytic
      Type I 282.2
      Type II 282.3
    pernicious 281.0
    spherocytic (*see also* Spherocytosis)
      282.0
  Cooley's (erythroblastic) 282.44
  crescent — *see* Disease, sickle-cell
  cytogenic 281.0
  Dacie's (nonspherocytic)
    type I 282.2
    type II 282.3
  Davidson's (refractory) 284.9
  deficiency 281.9
    2, 3 diphosphoglycurate mutase 282.3
    2, 3 PG 282.3
    6-PGD 282.2
    6-phosphogluronic dehydrogenase
      282.2
    amino acid 281.4
    combined B_{12} and folate 281.3
    enzyme, drug-induced (hemolytic) 282.2
    erythrocytic glutathione 282.2
    folate 281.2
      dietary 281.2
      drug-induced 281.2
    folic acid 281.2
      dietary 281.2
      drug-induced 281.2
    G-6-PD 282.2
    GGS-R 282.2
    glucose-6-phosphate dehydrogenase
      (G-6-PD) 282.2
    glucose-phosphate isomerase 282.3
    glutathione peroxidase 282.2
    glutathione reductase 282.2
    glyceraldehyde phosphate dehydroge-
      nase 282.3
    GPI 282.3
    G SH 282.2
    hexokinase 282.3
    iron (Fe) 280.9
      specified NEC 280.8
    nutritional 281.9
      with
        poor iron absorption 280.9
        specified deficiency NEC 281.8

Anemia — *continued*
  deficiency — *continued*
    nutritional — *continued*
      due to inadequate dietary iron intake
        280.1
      specified type NEC 281.8
    of or complicating pregnancy 648.2 ☑
    pentose phosphate pathway 282.2
    PFK 282.3
    phosphofructo-aldolase 282.3
    phosphofructokinase 282.3
    phosphoglycerate kinase 282.3
    PK 282.3
    protein 281.4
    pyruvate kinase (PK) 282.3
    TPI 282.3
    triosephosphate isomerase 282.3
    vitamin B_{12} NEC 281.1
      dietary 281.1
      pernicious 281.0
  Diamond-Blackfan (congenital hypoplastic)
    284.01
  dibothriocephalus 123.4
  dimorphic 281.9
  diphasic 281.8
  diphtheritic 032.89
  Diphyllobothrium 123.4
  drepanocytic (*see also* Disease, sickle-cell)
    282.60
  due to
    antineoplastic chemotherapy 285.3
    blood loss (chronic) 280.0
      acute 285.1
    chemotherapy, antineoplastic 285.3
    defect of Embden-Meyerhof pathway
      glycolysis 282.3
    disorder of glutathione metabolism
      282.2
    drug — *see* Anemia, by type (*see also*
      Table of Drugs and Chemicals)
      chemotherapy, antineoplastic 285.3
    fetal blood loss 776.5
    fish tapeworm (D. latum) infestation
      123.4
    glutathione metabolism disorder 282.2
    hemorrhage (chronic) 280.0
      acute 285.1
    hexose monophosphate (HMP) shunt
      deficiency 282.2
    impaired absorption 280.9
    loss of blood (chronic) 280.0
      acute 285.1
    myxedema 244.9
    Necator americanus 126.1
    prematurity 776.6
    selective vitamin B_{12} malabsorption with
      proteinuria 281.1
  Dyke-Young type (secondary)
    (symptomatic) 283.9
  dyserythropoietic (congenital) (types I, II,
    III) 285.8
  dyshemopoietic (congenital) 285.8
  Egypt (*see also* Ancylostomiasis) 126.9
  elliptocytosis (*see also* Elliptocytosis) 282.1
  enzyme deficiency, drug-induced 282.2
  epidemic (*see also* Ancylostomiasis) 126.9
  EPO resistant 285.21
  erythroblastic
    familial 282.44
    fetus or newborn (*see also* Disease,
      hemolytic) 773.2
    late 773.5
  erythrocytic glutathione deficiency 282.2
  erythropoietin-resistant (EPO resistant ane-
    mia) 285.21
  essential 285.9
  Faber's (achlorhydric anemia) 280.9
  factitious (self-induced blood letting) 280.0
  familial erythroblastic (microcytic) 282.44
  Fanconi's (congenital pancytopenia) 284.09
  favism 282.2
  fetal 678.0 ☑
    following blood loss, affecting newborn
      776.5

☑ **Additional Digit Required** — Refer to the Tabular List for Digit Selection   **Subterms under main terms may continue to next column or page**

18 — Volume 2   ▶◀ **Revised Text**   ● **New Line**   ▲ **Revised Code**   **2015 ICD-9-CM**

Anemia — *continued*
fetus or newborn
due to
ABO
antibodies 773.1
incompatibility, maternal/fetal 773.1
isoimmunization 773.1
Rh
antibodies 773.0
incompatibility, maternal/fetal 773.0
isoimmunization 773.0
following fetal blood loss 776.5
fish tapeworm (D. latum) infestation 123.4
folate (folic acid) deficiency 281.2
dietary 281.2
drug-induced 281.2
folate malabsorption, congenital 281.2
folic acid deficiency 281.2
dietary 281.2
drug-induced 281.2
G-6-PD 282.2
general 285.9
glucose-6-phosphate dehydrogenase deficiency 282.2
glutathione-reductase deficiency 282.2
goat's milk 281.2
granulocytic 288.09
Heinz-body, congenital 282.7
hemoglobin deficiency 285.9
hemolytic 283.9
acquired 283.9
with hemoglobinuria NEC 283.2
autoimmune (cold type) (idiopathic) (primary) (secondary) (symptomatic) (warm type) 283.0
due to
cold reactive antibodies 283.0
drug exposure 283.0
warm reactive antibodies 283.0
fragmentation 283.19
idiopathic (chronic) 283.9
infectious 283.19
autoimmune 283.0
non-autoimmune 283.10
toxic 283.19
traumatic cardiac 283.19
acute 283.9
due to enzyme deficiency NEC 282.3
fetus or newborn (*see also* Disease, hemolytic) 773.2
late 773.5
Lederer's (acquired infectious hemolytic anemia) 283.19
autoimmune (acquired) 283.0
chronic 282.9
idiopathic 283.9
cold type (secondary) (symptomatic) 283.0
congenital (spherocytic) (*see also* Spherocytosis) 282.0
nonspherocytic — *see* Anemia, hemolytic, nonspherocytic, congenital
drug-induced 283.0
enzyme deficiency 282.2
due to
cardiac conditions 283.19
drugs 283.0
enzyme deficiency NEC 282.3
drug-induced 282.2
presence of shunt or other internal prosthetic device 283.19
thrombotic thrombocytopenic purpura 446.6
elliptocytotic (*see also* Elliptocytosis) 282.1
familial 282.9
hereditary 282.9
due to enzyme deficiency NEC 282.3
specified NEC 282.8
idiopathic (chronic) 283.9
infectious (acquired) 283.19
mechanical 283.19
microangiopathic 283.19

Anemia — *continued*
hemolytic — *continued*
non-autoimmune NEC 283.10
nonspherocytic
congenital or hereditary NEC 282.3
glucose-6-phosphate dehydrogenase deficiency 282.2
pyruvate kinase (PK) deficiency 282.3
type I 282.2
type II 282.3
type I 282.2
type II 282.3
of or complicating pregnancy 648.2 ☑
resulting from presence of shunt or other internal prosthetic device 283.19
secondary 283.19
autoimmune 283.0
sickle-cell — *see* Disease, sickle-cell
Stransky-Regala type (Hb-E) (*see also* Disease, hemoglobin) 282.7
symptomatic 283.19
autoimmune 283.0
toxic (acquired) 283.19
uremic (adult) (child) 283.11
warm type (secondary) (symptomatic) 283.0
hemorrhagic (chronic) 280.0
acute 285.1
HEMPAS 285.8
hereditary erythroblast multinuclearity-positive acidified serum test 285.8
Herrick's (hemoglobin S disease) 282.61
hexokinase deficiency 282.3
high A$_2$ 282.46
hookworm (*see also* Ancylostomiasis) 126.9
hypochromic (idiopathic) (microcytic) (normoblastic) 280.9
with iron loading 285.0
due to blood loss (chronic) 280.0
acute 285.1
familial sex linked 285.0
pyridoxine-responsive 285.0
hypoplasia, red blood cells 284.81
congenital or familial 284.01
hypoplastic (idiopathic) 284.9
congenital 284.01
familial 284.01
of childhood 284.09
idiopathic 285.9
hemolytic, chronic 283.9
in (due to) (with)
chronic illness NEC 285.29
chronic kidney disease 285.21
end-stage renal disease 285.21
neoplastic disease 285.22
infantile 285.9
infective, infectional 285.9
intertropical (*see also* Ancylostomiasis) 126.9
iron (Fe) deficiency 280.9
due to blood loss (chronic) 280.0
acute 285.1
of or complicating pregnancy 648.2 ☑
specified NEC 280.8
Jaksch's (pseudoleukemia infantum) 285.8
Joseph-Diamond-Blackfan (congenital hypoplastic) 284.01
labyrinth 386.50
Lederer's (acquired infectious hemolytic anemia) 283.19
leptocytosis (hereditary) 282.40
leukoerythroblastic 284.2
macrocytic 281.9
nutritional 281.2
of or complicating pregnancy 648.2 ☑
tropical 281.2
malabsorption (familial), selective B$_{12}$ with proteinuria 281.1
malarial (*see also* Malaria) 084.6
malignant (progressive) 281.0
malnutrition 281.9
marsh (*see also* Malaria) 084.6
Mediterranean 282.40
with hemoglobinopathy 282.49
megaloblastic 281.9

Anemia — *continued*
megaloblastic — *continued*
combined B$_{12}$ and folate deficiency 281.3
nutritional (of infancy) 281.2
of infancy 281.2
of or complicating pregnancy 648.2 ☑
refractory 281.3
specified NEC 281.3
megalocytic 281.9
microangiopathic hemolytic 283.19
microcytic (hypochromic) 280.9
due to blood loss (chronic) 280.0
acute 285.1
familial 282.49
hypochromic 280.9
microdrepanocytosis 282.41
miners' (*see also* Ancylostomiasis) 126.9
myelopathic 285.8
myelophthisic (normocytic) 284.2
newborn (*see also* Disease, hemolytic) 773.2
due to isoimmunization (*see also* Disease, hemolytic) 773.2
late, due to isoimmunization 773.5
posthemorrhagic 776.5
nonregenerative 284.9
nonspherocytic hemolytic — *see* Anemia, hemolytic, nonspherocytic
normocytic (infectional) (not due to blood loss) 285.9
due to blood loss (chronic) 280.0
acute 285.1
myelophthisic 284.2
nutritional (deficiency) 281.9
with
poor iron absorption 280.9
specified deficiency NEC 281.8
due to inadequate dietary iron intake 280.1
megaloblastic (of infancy) 281.2
of childhood 282.9
of chronic
disease NEC 285.29
illness NEC 285.29
of or complicating pregnancy 648.2 ☑
affecting fetus or newborn 760.8
of prematurity 776.6
orotic aciduric (congenital) (hereditary) 281.4
osteosclerotic 289.89
ovalocytosis (hereditary) (*see also* Elliptocytosis) 282.1
paludal (*see also* Malaria) 084.6
pentose phosphate pathway deficiency 282.2
pernicious (combined system disease) (congenital) (dorsolateral spinal degeneration) (juvenile) (myelopathy) (neuropathy) (posterior sclerosis) (primary) (progressive) (spleen) 281.0
of or complicating pregnancy 648.2 ☑
pleochromic 285.9
of sprue 281.8
portal 285.8
posthemorrhagic (chronic) 280.0
acute 285.1
newborn 776.5
postoperative
due to (acute) blood loss 285.1
chronic blood loss 280.0
other 285.9
postpartum 648.2 ☑
pressure 285.9
primary 285.9
profound 285.9
progressive 285.9
malignant 281.0
pernicious 281.0
protein-deficiency 281.4
pseudoleukemica infantum 285.8
puerperal 648.2 ☑
pure red cell 284.81
congenital 284.01
pyridoxine-responsive (hypochromic) 285.0
pyruvate kinase (PK) deficiency 282.3
refractoria sideroblastica 238.72

Anemia — *continued*
refractory (primary) 238.72
with
excess
blasts-1 (RAEB-1) 238.72
blasts-2 (RAEB-2) 238.73
hemochromatosis 238.72
ringed sideroblasts (RARS) 238.72
due to
drug 285.0
myelodysplastic syndrome 238.72
toxin 285.0
hereditary 285.0
idiopathic 238.72
megaloblastic 281.3
sideroblastic 238.72
hereditary 285.0
sideropenic 280.9
Rietti-Greppi-Micheli (thalassemia minor) 282.46
scorbutic 281.8
secondary (to) 285.9
blood loss (chronic) 280.0
acute 285.1
hemorrhage 280.0
acute 285.1
inadequate dietary iron intake 280.1
semiplastic 284.9
septic 285.9
sickle-cell (*see also* Disease, sickle-cell) 282.60
sideroachrestic 285.0
sideroblastic (acquired) (any type) (congenital) (drug-induced) (due to disease) (hereditary) (primary) (secondary) (sex-linked hypochromic) (vitamin B$_6$ responsive) 285.0
refractory 238.72
congenital 285.0
drug-induced 285.0
hereditary 285.0
sex-linked hypochromic 285.0
vitamin B$_6$-responsive 285.0
sideropenic (refractory) 280.9
due to blood loss (chronic) 280.0
acute 285.1
simple chronic 281.9
specified type NEC 285.8
spherocytic (hereditary) (*see also* Spherocytosis) 282.0
splenic 285.8
familial (Gaucher's) 272.7
splenomegalic 285.8
stomatocytosis 282.8
syphilitic 095.8
target cell (oval) 285.8
with thalassemia — *see* Thalassemia
thalassemia 282.40
thrombocytopenic (*see also* Thrombocytopenia) 287.5
toxic 284.89
triosephosphate isomerase deficiency 282.3
tropical, macrocytic 281.2
tuberculous (*see also* Tuberculosis) 017.9 ☑
vegan's 281.1
vitamin
B$_6$-responsive 285.0
B$_{12}$ deficiency (dietary) 281.1
pernicious 281.0
von Jaksch's (pseudoleukemia infantum) 285.8
Witts' (achlorhydric anemia) 280.9
Zuelzer (-Ogden) (nutritional megaloblastic anemia) 281.2
Anencephalus, anencephaly 740.0
fetal, affecting management of pregnancy 655.0 ☑
Anergasia — *see also* Psychosis, organic 294.9
senile 290.0
Anesthesia, anesthetic 782.0
complication or reaction NEC 995.22
due to
correct substance properly administered 995.22

Anesthesia, anesthetic — *continued*
  complication or reaction — *continued*
    due to — *continued*
      overdose or wrong substance given 968.4
      specified anesthetic — *see* Table of Drugs and Chemicals
  cornea 371.81
  death from
    correct substance properly administered 995.4
    during delivery 668.9 ☑
    overdose or wrong substance given 968.4
    specified anesthetic — *see* Table of Drugs and Chemicals
  eye 371.81
  functional 300.11
  hyperesthetic, thalamic 338.0
  hysterical 300.11
  local skin lesion 782.0
  olfactory 781.1
  sexual (psychogenic) 302.72
  shock
    due to
      correct substance properly administered 995.4
      overdose or wrong substance given 968.4
      specified anesthetic — *see* Table of Drugs and Chemicals
  skin 782.0
  tactile 782.0
  testicular 608.9
  thermal 782.0
Anetoderma (maculosum) 701.3
Aneuploidy NEC 758.5
Aneurin deficiency 265.1
Aneurysm (anastomotic) (artery) (cirsoid) (diffuse) (false) (fusiform) (multiple) (ruptured) (saccular) (varicose) 442.9
  abdominal (aorta) 441.4
    ruptured 441.3
    syphilitic 093.0
  aorta, aortic (nonsyphilitic) 441.9
    abdominal 441.4
      dissecting 441.02
      ruptured 441.3
      syphilitic 093.0
    arch 441.2
      ruptured 441.1
    arteriosclerotic NEC 441.9
      ruptured 441.5
    ascending 441.2
      ruptured 441.1
    congenital 747.29
    descending 441.9
      abdominal 441.4
        ruptured 441.3
      ruptured 441.5
      thoracic 441.2
        ruptured 441.1
    dissecting 441.00
      abdominal 441.02
      thoracic 441.01
      thoracoabdominal 441.03
    due to coarctation (aorta) 747.10
    ruptured 441.5
    sinus, right 747.29
    syphilitic 093.0
    thoracoabdominal 441.7
      ruptured 441.6
    thorax, thoracic (arch) (nonsyphilitic) 441.2
      dissecting 441.01
      ruptured 441.1
      syphilitic 093.0
    transverse 441.2
      ruptured 441.1
    valve (heart) (*see also* Endocarditis, aortic) 424.1
  arteriosclerotic NEC 442.9
    cerebral 437.3
      ruptured (*see also* Hemorrhage, subarachnoid) 430

Aneurysm — *continued*
  arteriovenous (congenital) (peripheral) NEC (*see also* Anomaly, arteriovenous) 747.60
    acquired NEC 447.0
      brain 437.3
        ruptured (*see also* Hemorrhage, subarachnoid) 430
      coronary 414.11
      pulmonary 417.0
    brain (cerebral) 747.81
      ruptured (*see also* Hemorrhage, subarachnoid) 430
    coronary 746.85
    pulmonary 747.32
    retina 743.58
    specified site NEC 747.89
      acquired 447.0
    traumatic (*see also* Injury, blood vessel, by site) 904.9
  basal — *see* Aneurysm, brain
  berry (congenital) (ruptured) (*see also* Hemorrhage, subarachnoid) 430
    nonruptured 437.3
  brain 437.3
    arteriosclerotic 437.3
      ruptured (*see also* Hemorrhage, subarachnoid) 430
    arteriovenous 747.81
      acquired 437.3
        ruptured (*see also* Hemorrhage, subarachnoid) 430
      ruptured (*see also* Hemorrhage, subarachnoid) 430
    berry (congenital) (ruptured) (*see also* Hemorrhage, subarachnoid) 430
      nonruptured 437.3
    congenital 747.81
      ruptured (*see also* Hemorrhage, subarachnoid) 430
    meninges 437.3
      ruptured (*see also* Hemorrhage, subarachnoid) 430
    miliary (congenital) (ruptured) (*see also* Hemorrhage, subarachnoid) 430
    mycotic 421.0
      ruptured (*see also* Hemorrhage, subarachnoid) 430
    nonruptured 437.3
    ruptured (*see also* Hemorrhage, subarachnoid) 430
    syphilitic 094.87
    syphilitic (hemorrhage) 094.87
    traumatic — *see* Injury, intracranial
  cardiac (false) (*see also* Aneurysm, heart) 414.10
  carotid artery (common) (external) 442.81
    internal (intracranial portion) 437.3
      extracranial portion 442.81
      ruptured into brain (*see also* Hemorrhage, subarachnoid) 430
    syphilitic 093.89
      intracranial 094.87
  cavernous sinus (*see also* Aneurysm, brain) 437.3
    arteriovenous 747.81
      ruptured (*see also* Hemorrhage, subarachnoid) 430
    congenital 747.81
      ruptured (*see also* Hemorrhage, subarachnoid) 430
  celiac 442.84
  central nervous system, syphilitic 094.89
  cerebral — *see* Aneurysm, brain
  chest — *see* Aneurysm, thorax
  circle of Willis (*see also* Aneurysm, brain) 437.3
    congenital 747.81
      ruptured (*see also* Hemorrhage, subarachnoid) 430
    ruptured (*see also* Hemorrhage, subarachnoid) 430
  common iliac artery 442.2
  congenital (peripheral) NEC 747.60
    brain 747.81

Aneurysm — *continued*
  congenital — *continued*
    brain — *continued*
      ruptured (*see also* Hemorrhage, subarachnoid) 430
    cerebral — *see* Aneurysm, brain, congenital
    coronary 746.85
    gastrointestinal 747.61
    lower limb 747.64
    pulmonary 747.32
    renal 747.62
    retina 743.58
    specified site NEC 747.89
    spinal 747.82
    upper limb 747.63
  conjunctiva 372.74
  conus arteriosus (*see also* Aneurysm, heart) 414.10
  coronary (arteriosclerotic) (artery) (vein) (*see also* Aneurysm, heart) 414.11
    arteriovenous 746.85
    congenital 746.85
    syphilitic 093.89
  cylindrical 441.9
    ruptured 441.5
    syphilitic 093.9
  dissecting 442.9
    aorta 441.00
      abdominal 441.02
      thoracic 441.01
      thoracoabdominal 441.03
    syphilitic 093.9
  ductus arteriosus 747.0
  embolic — *see* Embolism, artery
  endocardial, infective (any valve) 421.0
  femoral 442.3
  gastroduodenal 442.84
  gastroepiploic 442.84
  heart (chronic or with a stated duration of over 8 weeks) (infectional) (wall) 414.10
    acute or with a stated duration of 8 weeks or less (*see also* Infarct, myocardium) 410.9 ☑
    congenital 746.89
    valve — *see* Endocarditis
  hepatic 442.84
  iliac (common) 442.2
  infective (any valve) 421.0
  innominate (nonsyphilitic) 442.89
    syphilitic 093.89
  interauricular septum (*see also* Aneurysm, heart) 414.10
  interventricular septum (*see also* Aneurysm, heart) 414.10
  intracranial — *see* Aneurysm, brain
  intrathoracic (nonsyphilitic) 441.2
    ruptured 441.1
    syphilitic 093.0
  jugular vein (acute) 453.89
    chronic 453.76
  lower extremity 442.3
  lung (pulmonary artery) 417.1
  malignant 093.9
  mediastinal (nonsyphilitic) 442.89
    syphilitic 093.89
  miliary (congenital) (ruptured) (*see also* Hemorrhage, subarachnoid) 430
  mitral (heart) (valve) 424.0
  mural (arteriovenous) (heart) (*see also* Aneurysm, heart) 414.10
  mycotic, any site 421.0
    without endocarditis — *see* Aneurysm by site
    ruptured, brain (*see also* Hemorrhage, subarachnoid) 430
  myocardium (*see also* Aneurysm, heart) 414.10
  neck 442.81
  pancreaticoduodenal 442.84
  patent ductus arteriosus 747.0
  peripheral NEC 442.89
    congenital NEC (*see also* Aneurysm, congenital) 747.60
  popliteal 442.3

Aneurysm — *continued*
  pulmonary 417.1
    arteriovenous 747.32
      acquired 417.0
    syphilitic 093.89
    valve (heart) (*see also* Endocarditis, pulmonary) 424.3
  racemose 442.9
    congenital (peripheral) NEC 747.60
  radial 442.0
  Rasmussen's (*see also* Tuberculosis) 011.2 ☑
  renal 442.1
  retinal (acquired) 362.17
    congenital 743.58
    diabetic 250.5 ☑ *[362.01]*
      due to secondary diabetes 249.5 ☑ *[362.01]*
  sinus, aortic (of Valsalva) 747.29
  specified site NEC 442.89
  spinal (cord) 442.89
    congenital 747.82
    syphilitic (hemorrhage) 094.89
  spleen, splenic 442.83
  subclavian 442.82
    syphilitic 093.89
  superior mesenteric 442.84
  syphilitic 093.9
    aorta 093.0
    central nervous system 094.89
    congenital 090.5
    spine, spinal 094.89
  thoracoabdominal 441.7
    ruptured 441.6
  thorax, thoracic (arch) (nonsyphilitic) 441.2
    dissecting 441.01
    ruptured 441.1
    syphilitic 093.0
  traumatic (complication) (early) — *see* Injury, blood vessel, by site
  tricuspid (heart) (valve) — *see* Endocarditis, tricuspid
  ulnar 442.0
  upper extremity 442.0
  valve, valvular — *see* Endocarditis
  venous 456.8
    congenital NEC (*see also* Aneurysm, congenital) 747.60
  ventricle (arteriovenous) (*see also* Aneurysm, heart) 414.10
  visceral artery NEC 442.84
Angiectasis 459.89
Angiectopia 459.9
Angiitis 447.6
  allergic granulomatous 446.4
  hypersensitivity 446.20
    Goodpasture's syndrome 446.21
    specified NEC 446.29
  necrotizing 446.0
  Wegener's (necrotizing respiratory granulomatosis) 446.4
Angina (attack) (cardiac) (chest) (effort) (heart) (pectoris) (syndrome) (vasomotor) 413.9
  abdominal 557.1
  accelerated 411.1
  agranulocytic 288.03
  aphthous 074.0
  catarrhal 462
  crescendo 411.1
  croupous 464.4
  cruris 443.9
    due to atherosclerosis NEC (*see also* Arteriosclerosis, extremities) 440.20
  decubitus 413.0
  diphtheritic (membranous) 032.0
  equivalent 413.9
  erysipelatous 034.0
  erythematous 462
  exudative, chronic 476.0
  faucium 478.29
  gangrenous 462
    diphtheritic 032.0
  infectious 462
  initial 411.1
  intestinal 557.1
  ludovici 528.3
  Ludwig's 528.3

☑ Additional Digit Required — Refer to the Tabular List for Digit Selection   ▽ Subterms under main terms may continue to next column or page

20 — Volume 2   ▶◀ Revised Text   ● New Line   ▲ Revised Code   2015 ICD-9-CM

Angina — *continued*
  malignant 462
    diphtheritic 032.0
  membranous 464.4
    diphtheritic 032.0
  mesenteric 557.1
  monocytic 075
  nocturnal 413.0
  phlegmonous 475
    diphtheritic 032.0
  preinfarctional 411.1
  Prinzmetal's 413.1
  progressive 411.1
  pseudomembranous 101
  psychogenic 306.2
  pultaceous, diphtheritic 032.0
  scarlatinal 034.1
  septic 034.0
  simple 462
  stable NEC 413.9
  staphylococcal 462
  streptococcal 034.0
  stridulous, diphtheritic 032.3
  syphilitic 093.9
    congenital 090.5
  tonsil 475
  trachealis 464.4
  unstable 411.1
  variant 413.1
  Vincent's 101
Angioblastoma (M9161/1) — *see* Neoplasm, connective tissue, uncertain behavior
Angiocholecystitis — *see also* Cholecystitis, acute 575.0
Angiocholitis — *see also* Cholecystitis, acute 576.1
Angiodysgensis spinalis 336.1
Angiodysplasia (intestinalis) (intestine) 569.84
  with hemorrhage 569.85
  duodenum 537.82
    with hemorrhage 537.83
  stomach 537.82
    with hemorrhage 537.83
Angioedema (allergic) (any site) (with urticaria) 995.1
  hereditary 277.6
Angioendothelioma (M9130/1) — *see also* Neoplasm, by site, uncertain behavior
  benign (M9130/0) (*see also* Hemangioma, by site) 228.00
  bone (M9260/3) — *see* Neoplasm, bone, malignant
  Ewing's (M9260/3) — *see* Neoplasm, bone, malignant
  nervous system (M9130/0) 228.09
Angiofibroma (M9160/0) — *see also* Neoplasm, by site, benign
  juvenile (M9160/0) 210.7
    specified site — *see* Neoplasm, by site, benign
    unspecified site 210.7
Angiohemophilia (A) (B) 286.4
Angioid streaks (choroid) (retina) 363.43
Angiokeratoma (M9141/0) — *see also* Neoplasm, skin, benign
  corporis diffusum 272.7
Angiokeratosis
  diffuse 272.7
Angioleiomyoma (M8894/0) — *see* Neoplasm, connective tissue, benign
Angioleucitis 683
Angiolipoma (M8861/0) — *see also* Lipoma, by site 214.9
  infiltrating (M8861/1) — *see* Neoplasm, connective tissue, uncertain behavior
Angioma (M9120/0) — *see also* Hemangioma, by site 228.00
  capillary 448.1
  hemorrhagicum hereditaria 448.0
  malignant (M9120/3) — *see* Neoplasm, connective tissue, malignant
  pigmentosum et atrophicum 757.33
  placenta — *see* Placenta, abnormal
  plexiform (M9131/0) — *see* Hemangioma, by site
  senile 448.1

Angioma — *see also* Hemangioma, by site — *continued*
  serpiginosum 709.1
  spider 448.1
  stellate 448.1
Angiomatosis 757.32
  bacillary 083.8
  corporis diffusum universale 272.7
  cutaneocerebral 759.6
  encephalocutaneous 759.6
  encephalofacial 759.6
  encephalotrigeminal 759.6
  hemorrhagic familial 448.0
  hereditary familial 448.0
  heredofamilial 448.0
  meningo-oculofacial 759.6
  multiple sites 228.09
  neuro-oculocutaneous 759.6
  retina (Hippel's disease) 759.6
  retinocerebellosa 759.6
  retinocerebral 759.6
  systemic 228.09
Angiomyolipoma (M8860/0)
  specified site — *see* Neoplasm, connective tissue, benign
  unspecified site 223.0
Angiomyoliposarcoma (M8860/3) — *see* Neoplasm, connective tissue, malignant
Angiomyoma (M8894/0) — *see* Neoplasm, connective tissue, benign
Angiomyosarcoma (M8894/3) — *see* Neoplasm, connective tissue, malignant
Angioneurosis 306.2
Angioneurotic edema (allergic) (any site) (with urticaria) 995.1
  hereditary 277.6
Angiopathia, angiopathy 459.9
  diabetic (peripheral) 250.7 ☑ [443.81]
    due to secondary diabetes 249.7 ☑ [443.81]
  peripheral 443.9
    diabetic 250.7 ☑ [443.81]
      due to secondary diabetes 249.7 ☑ [443.81]
    specified type NEC 443.89
  retinae syphilitica 093.89
  retinalis (juvenilis) 362.18
    background 362.10
    diabetic 250.5 ☑ [362.01]
      due to secondary diabetes 249.5 ☑ [362.01]
    proliferative 362.29
    tuberculous (*see also* Tuberculosis) 017.3 ☑ [362.18]
Angiosarcoma (M9120/3) — *see* Neoplasm, connective tissue, malignant
Angiosclerosis — *see* Arteriosclerosis
Angioscotoma, enlarged 368.42
Angiospasm 443.9
  brachial plexus 353.0
  cerebral 435.9
  cervical plexus 353.2
  nerve
    arm 354.9
      axillary 353.0
      median 354.1
      ulnar 354.2
    autonomic (*see also* Neuropathy, peripheral, autonomic) 337.9
    axillary 353.0
    leg 355.8
      plantar 355.6
    lower extremity — *see* Angiospasm, nerve, leg
    median 354.1
    peripheral NEC 355.9
    spinal NEC 355.9
    sympathetic (*see also* Neuropathy, peripheral, autonomic) 337.9
    ulnar 354.2
    upper extremity — *see* Angiospasm, nerve, arm
  peripheral NEC 443.9
  traumatic 443.9
    foot 443.9
    leg 443.9

Angiospasm — *continued*
  vessel 443.9
Angiospastic disease or edema 443.9
Angle's
  class I 524.21
  class II 524.22
  class III 524.23
Anguillulosis 127.2
Angulation
  cecum (*see also* Obstruction, intestine) 560.9
  coccyx (acquired) 738.6
    congenital 756.19
  femur (acquired) 736.39
    congenital 755.69
  intestine (large) (small) (*see also* Obstruction, intestine) 560.9
  sacrum (acquired) 738.5
    congenital 756.19
  sigmoid (flexure) (*see also* Obstruction, intestine) 560.9
  spine (*see also* Curvature, spine) 737.9
  tibia (acquired) 736.89
    congenital 755.69
  ureter 593.3
  wrist (acquired) 736.09
    congenital 755.59
Angulus infectiosus 686.8
Anhedonia 780.99
Anhidrosis (lid) (neurogenic) (thermogenic) 705.0
Anhydration 276.51
  with
    hypernatremia 276.0
    hyponatremia 276.1
Anhydremia 276.52
  with
    hypernatremia 276.0
    hyponatremia 276.1
Anidrosis 705.0
Aniridia (congenital) 743.45
Anisakiasis (infection) (infestation) 127.1
Anisakis larva infestation 127.1
Aniseikonia 367.32
Anisocoria (pupil) 379.41
  congenital 743.46
Anisocytosis 790.09
Anisometropia (congenital) 367.31
Ankle — *see* condition
Ankyloblepharon (acquired) (eyelid) 374.46
  filiforme (adnatum) (congenital) 743.62
  total 743.62
Ankylodactly — *see also* Syndactylism 755.10
Ankyloglossia 750.0
Ankylosis (fibrous) (osseous) 718.50
  ankle 718.57
  any joint, produced by surgical fusion V45.4
  cricoarytenoid (cartilage) (joint) (larynx) 478.79
  dental 521.6
  ear ossicle NEC 385.22
    malleus 385.21
  elbow 718.52
  finger 718.54
  hip 718.55
  incostapedial joint (infectional) 385.22
  joint, produced by surgical fusion NEC V45.4
  knee 718.56
  lumbosacral (joint) 724.6
  malleus 385.21
  multiple sites 718.59
  postoperative (status) V45.4
  sacroiliac (joint) 724.6
  shoulder 718.51
  specified site NEC 718.58
  spine NEC 724.9
  surgical V45.4
  teeth, tooth (hard tissues) 521.6
  temporomandibular joint 524.61
  wrist 718.53
Ankylostoma — *see* Ancylostoma
Ankylostomiasis (intestinal) — *see* Ancylostomiasis
Ankylurethria — *see also* Stricture, urethra 598.9
Annular — *see also* condition
  detachment, cervix 622.8

Annular — *see also* condition — *continued*
  organ or site, congenital NEC — *see* Distortion
  pancreas (congenital) 751.7
Anodontia (complete) (partial) (vera) 520.0
  with abnormal spacing 524.30
  acquired 525.10
    causing malocclusion 524.30
    due to
      caries 525.13
      extraction 525.10
      periodontal disease 525.12
      trauma 525.11
Anomaly, anomalous (congenital) (unspecified type) 759.9
  abdomen 759.9
  abdominal wall 756.70
  acoustic nerve 742.9
  adrenal (gland) 759.1
  Alder (-Reilly) (leukocyte granulation) 288.2
  alimentary tract 751.9
    lower 751.5
      specified type NEC 751.8
    upper (any part, except tongue) 750.9
      tongue 750.10
        specified type NEC 750.19
  alveolar 524.70
    ridge (process) 525.8
    specified NEC 524.79
  ankle (joint) 755.69
  anus, anal (canal) 751.5
  aorta, aortic 747.20
    arch 747.21
    coarctation (postductal) (preductal) 747.10
    cusp or valve NEC 746.9
    septum 745.0
    specified type NEC 747.29
  aorticopulmonary septum 745.0
  apertures, diaphragm 756.6
  appendix 751.5
  aqueduct of Sylvius 742.3
    with spina bifida (*see also* Spina bifida) 741.0 ☑
  arm 755.50
    reduction (*see also* Deformity, reduction, upper limb) 755.20
  arteriovenous (congenital) (peripheral) NEC 747.60
    brain 747.81
    cerebral 747.81
    coronary 746.85
    gastrointestinal 747.61
      acquired — *see* Angiodysplasia
    lower limb 747.64
    renal 747.62
    specified site NEC 747.69
    spinal 747.82
    upper limb 747.63
  artery (*see also* Anomaly, peripheral vascular system) NEC 747.60
    brain 747.81
    cerebral 747.81
    coronary 746.85
    eye 743.9
    pulmonary 747.39
    renal 747.62
    retina 743.9
    umbilical 747.5
  arytenoepiglottic folds 748.3
  atrial
    bands 746.9
    folds 746.9
    septa 745.5
  atrioventricular
    canal 745.69
    common 745.69
    conduction 426.7
    excitation 426.7
    septum 745.4
  atrium — *see* Anomaly, atrial
  auditory canal 744.3
    specified type NEC 744.29
      with hearing impairment 744.02
  auricle
    ear 744.3

☑ Additional Digit Required — Refer to the Tabular List for Digit Selection   ▼ Subterms under main terms may continue to next column or page

2015 ICD-9-CM   ►◄ Revised Text   ● New Line   ▲ Revised Code   Volume 2 — 21

☑ **Additional Digit Required** — Refer to the Tabular List for Digit Selection   ⬩ Subterms under main terms may continue to next column or page

22 — Volume 2   ▶◀ Revised Text   ● New Line   ▲ Revised Code   **2015 ICD-9-CM**

Anomaly, anomalous — *continued*
 heart — *continued*
  malposition 746.87
  maternal, affecting fetus or newborn 760.3
  obstructive NEC 746.84
  patent ductus arteriosus (Botalli) 747.0
  septum 745.9
   acquired 429.71
   aortic 745.0
   aorticopulmonary 745.0
   atrial 745.5
   auricular 745.5
   between aorta and pulmonary artery 745.0
   endocardial cushion type 745.60
    specified type NEC 745.69
   interatrial 745.5
   interventricular 745.4
    with pulmonary stenosis or atresia, dextraposition of aorta, and hypertrophy of right ventricle 745.2
    acquired 429.71
   specified type NEC 745.8
   ventricular 745.4
    with pulmonary stenosis or atresia, dextraposition of aorta, and hypertrophy of right ventricle 745.2
    acquired 429.71
  specified type NEC 746.89
  tetralogy of Fallot 745.2
  valve NEC 746.9
   aortic 746.9
    atresia 746.89
    bicuspid valve 746.4
    insufficiency 746.4
    specified type NEC 746.89
    stenosis 746.3
     subaortic 746.81
     supravalvular 747.22
   mitral 746.9
    atresia 746.89
    insufficiency 746.6
    specified type NEC 746.89
    stenosis 746.5
   pulmonary 746.00
    atresia 746.01
    insufficiency 746.09
    stenosis 746.02
     infundibular 746.83
     subvalvular 746.83
   tricuspid 746.9
    atresia 746.1
    stenosis 746.1
  ventricle 746.9
 heel 755.67
 Hegglin's 288.2
 hemianencephaly 740.0
 hemicephaly 740.0
 hemicrania 740.0
 hepatic duct 751.60
 hip (joint) 755.63
 hourglass
  bladder 753.8
  gallbladder 751.69
  stomach 750.7
 humerus 755.50
 hymen 752.40
 hypersegmentation of neutrophils, hereditary 288.2
 hypophyseal 759.2
 ileocecal (coil) (valve) 751.5
 ileum (intestine) 751.5
 ilium 755.60
 integument 757.9
  specified type NEC 757.8
 interarch distance (excessive) (inadequate) 524.28
 intervertebral cartilage or disc 756.10
 intestine (large) (small) 751.5
  fixational type 751.4
 iris 743.9
  specified type NEC 743.46
 ischium 755.60

Anomaly, anomalous — *continued*
 jaw-cranial base relationship 524.10
  specified NEC 524.19
 jaw NEC 524.9
  closure 524.51
  size (major) NEC 524.00
  specified type NEC 524.89
 jejunum 751.5
 joint 755.9
  hip
   dislocation (*see also* Dislocation, hip, congenital) 754.30
   predislocation (*see also* Subluxation, congenital, hip) 754.32
   preluxation (*see also* Subluxation, congenital, hip) 754.32
   subluxation (*see also* Subluxation, congenital, hip) 754.32
  lumbosacral 756.10
   spondylolisthesis 756.12
   spondylosis 756.11
  multiple arthrogryposis 754.89
  sacroiliac 755.69
 Jordan's 288.2
 kidney(s) (calyx) (pelvis) 753.9
  vessel 747.62
 Klippel-Feil (brevicollis) 756.16
 knee (joint) 755.64
 labium (majus) (minus) 752.40
 labyrinth, membranous (causing impairment of hearing) 744.05
 lacrimal
  apparatus, duct or passage 743.9
   specified type NEC 743.65
  gland 743.9
   specified type NEC 743.64
 Langdon Down (mongolism) 758.0
 larynx, laryngeal (muscle) 748.3
  web, webbed 748.2
 leg (lower) (upper) 755.60
  reduction NEC (*see also* Deformity, reduction, lower limb) 755.30
 lens 743.9
  shape 743.36
  specified type NEC 743.39
 leukocytes, genetic 288.2
  granulation (constitutional) 288.2
 lid (fold) 743.9
 ligament 756.9
  broad 752.10
  round 752.9
 limb, except reduction deformity 755.9
  lower 755.60
   reduction deformity (*see also* Deformity, reduction, lower limb) 755.30
   specified type NEC 755.69
  upper 755.50
   reduction deformity (*see also* Deformity, reduction, upper limb) 755.20
   specified type NEC 755.59
 lip 750.9
  harelip (*see also* Cleft, lip) 749.10
  specified type NEC 750.26
 liver (duct) 751.60
  atresia 751.69
 lower extremity 755.60
  vessel 747.64
 lumbosacral (joint) (region) 756.10
 lung (fissure) (lobe) NEC 748.60
  agenesis 748.5
  specified type NEC 748.69
 lymphatic system 759.9
 Madelung's (radius) 755.54
 mandible 524.9
  size NEC 524.00
 maxilla 524.9
  size NEC 524.00
 May (-Hegglin) 288.2
 meatus urinarius 753.9
  specified type NEC 753.8
 meningeal bands or folds, constriction of 742.8
 meninges 742.9
  brain 742.4

Anomaly, anomalous — *continued*
 meninges — *continued*
  spinal 742.59
 meningocele (*see also* Spina bifida) 741.9 ☑
  acquired 349.2
 mesentery 751.9
 metacarpus 755.50
 metatarsus 755.67
 middle ear, except ossicles (causing impairment of hearing) 744.03
  ossicles 744.04
 mitral (leaflets) (valve) 746.9
  atresia 746.89
  insufficiency 746.6
  specified type NEC 746.89
  stenosis 746.5
 mouth 750.9
  specified type NEC 750.26
 multiple NEC 759.7
  specified type NEC 759.89
 muscle 756.9
  eye 743.9
   specified type NEC 743.69
  specified type NEC 756.89
 musculoskeletal system, except limbs 756.9
  specified type NEC 756.9
 nail 757.9
  specified type NEC 757.5
 narrowness, eyelid 743.62
 nasal sinus or septum 748.1
 neck (any part) 744.9
  specified type NEC 744.89
 nerve 742.9
  acoustic 742.9
   specified type NEC 742.8
  optic 742.9
   specified type NEC 742.8
 nervous system NEC 742.9
  brain 742.9
   specified type NEC 742.4
  specified type NEC 742.8
 neurological 742.9
 nipple 757.6
 nonteratogenic NEC 754.89
 nose, nasal (bone) (cartilage) (septum) (sinus) 748.1
 ocular muscle 743.9
 omphalomesenteric duct 751.0
 opening, pulmonary veins 747.49
 optic
  disc 743.9
   specified type NEC 743.57
  nerve 742.9
 opticociliary vessels 743.9
 orbit (eye) 743.9
  specified type NEC 743.66
 organ
  of Corti (causing impairment of hearing) 744.05
  or site 759.9
   specified type NEC 759.89
 origin
  both great arteries from same ventricle 745.11
  coronary artery 746.85
  innominate artery 747.69
  left coronary artery from pulmonary artery 746.85
  pulmonary artery 747.39
  renal vessels 747.62
  subclavian artery (left) (right) 747.21
 osseous meatus (ear) 744.03
 ovary 752.0
 oviduct 752.10
 palate (hard) (soft) 750.9
  cleft (*see also* Cleft, palate) 749.00
 pancreas (duct) 751.7
 papillary muscles 746.9
 parathyroid gland 759.2
 paraurethral ducts 753.9
 parotid (gland) 750.9
 patella 755.64
 Pelger-Huët (hereditary hyposegmentation) 288.2
 pelvic girdle 755.60

Anomaly, anomalous — *continued*
 pelvic girdle — *continued*
  specified type NEC 755.69
 pelvis (bony) 755.60
  complicating delivery 653.0 ☑
   rachitic 268.1
    fetal 756.4
 penis (glans) 752.69
 pericardium 746.89
 peripheral vascular system NEC 747.60
  gastrointestinal 747.61
  lower limb 747.64
  renal 747.62
  specified site NEC 747.69
  spinal 747.82
  upper limb 747.63
 Peter's 743.44
 pharynx 750.9
  branchial cleft 744.41
  specified type NEC 750.29
 Pierre Robin 756.0
 pigmentation 709.00
  congenital 757.33
  specified NEC 709.09
 pituitary (gland) 759.2
 pleural folds 748.8
 portal vein 747.40
 position tooth, teeth 524.30
  crowding 524.31
  displacement 524.30
   horizontal 524.33
   vertical 524.34
  distance
   interocclusal
    excessive 524.37
    insufficient 524.36
  excessive spacing 524.32
  rotation 524.35
  specified NEC 524.39
 preauricular sinus 744.46
 prepuce 752.9
 prostate 752.9
 pulmonary 748.60
  artery 747.39
  circulation 747.39
  specified type NEC 748.69
  valve 746.00
   atresia 746.01
   insufficiency 746.09
   specified type NEC 746.09
   stenosis 746.02
    infundibular 746.83
    subvalvular 746.83
  vein 747.40
  venous
   connection 747.49
    partial 747.42
    total 747.41
   return 747.49
    partial 747.42
    total (TAPVR) (complete) (subdiaphragmatic) (supradiaphragmatic) 747.41
 pupil 743.9
 pylorus 750.9
  hypertrophy 750.5
  stenosis 750.5
 rachitic, fetal 756.4
 radius 755.50
 rectovaginal (septum) 752.40
 rectum 751.5
 refraction 367.9
 renal 753.9
  vessel 747.62
 respiratory system 748.9
  specified type NEC 748.8
 rib 756.3
  cervical 756.2
 Rieger's 743.44
 rings, trachea 748.3
 rotation (*see also* Malrotation)
  hip or thigh (*see also* Subluxation, congenital, hip) 754.32
 round ligament 752.9
 sacroiliac (joint) 755.69
 sacrum 756.10

☑ **Additional Digit Required — Refer to the Tabular List for Digit Selection**   Subterms under main terms may continue to next column or page

Anomaly, anomalous — *continued*
saddle
  back 754.2
  nose 754.0
    syphilitic 090.5
salivary gland or duct 750.9
  specified type NEC 750.26
scapula 755.50
sclera 743.9
  specified type NEC 743.47
scrotum 752.9
sebaceous gland 757.9
seminal duct or tract 752.9
sense organs 742.9
  specified type NEC 742.8
septum
  heart — *see* Anomaly, heart, septum
  nasal 748.1
sex chromosomes NEC (*see also* Anomaly, chromosomes) 758.81
shoulder (girdle) (joint) 755.50
  specified type NEC 755.59
sigmoid (flexure) 751.5
sinus of Valsalva 747.29
site NEC 759.9
skeleton generalized NEC 756.50
skin (appendage) 757.9
  specified type NEC 757.39
skull (bone) 756.0
  with
    anencephalus 740.0
    encephalocele 742.0
    hydrocephalus 742.3
      with spina bifida (*see also* Spina bifida) 741.0 ☑
    microcephalus 742.1
specified type NEC
  adrenal (gland) 759.1
  alimentary tract (complete) (partial) 751.8
    lower 751.5
    upper 750.8
  ankle 755.69
  anus, anal (canal) 751.5
  aorta, aortic 747.29
    arch 747.21
  appendix 751.5
  arm 755.59
  artery (peripheral) NEC (*see also* Anomaly, peripheral vascular system) 747.60
    brain 747.81
    coronary 746.85
    eye 743.58
    pulmonary 747.39
    retinal 743.58
    umbilical 747.5
  auditory canal 744.29
    causing impairment of hearing 744.02
  bile duct or passage 751.69
  bladder 753.8
    neck 753.8
  bone(s) 756.9
    arm 755.59
    face 756.0
    leg 755.69
    pelvic girdle 755.69
    shoulder girdle 755.59
    skull 756.0
      with
        anencephalus 740.0
        encephalocele 742.0
        hydrocephalus 742.3
          with spina bifida (*see also* Spina bifida) 741.0 ☑
        microcephalus 742.1
  brain 742.4
  breast 757.6
  broad ligament 752.19
  bronchus 748.3
  canal of Nuck 752.89
  cardiac septal closure 745.8
  carpus 755.59
  cartilaginous 756.9

Anomaly, anomalous — *continued*
specified type — *continued*
  cecum 751.5
  cervix 752.49
  chest (wall) 756.3
  chin 744.89
  ciliary body 743.46
  circulatory system 747.89
  clavicle 755.51
  clitoris 752.49
  coccyx 756.19
  colon 751.5
  common duct 751.69
  connective tissue 756.89
  cricoid cartilage 748.3
  cystic duct 751.69
  diaphragm 756.6
  digestive organ(s) or tract 751.8
    lower 751.5
    upper 750.8
  duodenum 751.5
  ear 744.29
    auricle 744.29
      causing impairment of hearing 744.02
    causing impairment of hearing 744.09
    inner (causing impairment of hearing) 744.05
    middle, except ossicles 744.03
      ossicles 744.04
  ejaculatory duct 752.89
  endocrine 759.2
  epiglottis 748.3
  esophagus 750.4
  Eustachian tube 744.24
  eye 743.8
    lid 743.63
    muscle 743.69
  face 744.89
    bone(s) 756.0
  fallopian tube 752.19
  fascia 756.89
  femur 755.69
  fibula 755.69
  finger 755.59
  foot 755.67
  fovea centralis 743.55
  gallbladder 751.69
  Gartner's duct 752.89
  gastrointestinal tract 751.8
  genitalia, genital organ(s)
    female 752.89
      external 752.49
      internal NEC 752.89
    male 752.89
      penis 752.69
      scrotal transposition 752.81
  genitourinary tract NEC 752.89
  glottis 748.3
  hair 757.4
  hand 755.59
  heart 746.89
    valve NEC 746.89
      pulmonary 746.09
  hepatic duct 751.69
  hydatid of Morgagni 752.89
  hymen 752.49
  integument 757.8
  intestine (large) (small) 751.5
    fixational type 751.4
  iris 743.46
  jejunum 751.5
  joint 755.8
  kidney 753.3
  knee 755.64
  labium (majus) (minus) 752.49
  labyrinth, membranous 744.05
  larynx 748.3
  leg 755.69
  lens 743.39
  limb, except reduction deformity 755.8
    lower 755.69
      reduction deformity (*see also* Deformity, reduction, lower limb) 755.30

Anomaly, anomalous — *continued*
specified type — *continued*
  limb, except reduction deformity — *continued*
    upper 755.59
      reduction deformity (*see also* Deformity, reduction, upper limb) 755.20
  lip 750.26
  liver 751.69
  lung (fissure) (lobe) 748.69
  meatus urinarius 753.8
  metacarpus 755.59
  mouth 750.26
  Müllerian
    cervix 752.49
    uterus 752.39
    vagina 752.49
  muscle 756.89
    eye 743.69
  musculoskeletal system, except limbs 756.9
  nail 757.5
  neck 744.89
  nerve 742.8
    acoustic 742.8
    optic 742.8
  nervous system 742.8
  nipple 757.6
  nose 748.1
  organ NEC 759.89
    of Corti 744.05
  osseous meatus (ear) 744.03
  ovary 752.0
  oviduct 752.19
  pancreas 751.7
  parathyroid 759.2
  patella 755.64
  pelvic girdle 755.69
  penis 752.69
  pericardium 746.89
  peripheral vascular system NEC (*see also* Anomaly, peripheral vascular system) 747.60
  pharynx 750.29
  pituitary 759.2
  prostate 752.89
  radius 755.59
  rectum 751.5
  respiratory system 748.8
  rib 756.3
  round ligament 752.89
  sacrum 756.19
  salivary duct or gland 750.26
  scapula 755.59
  sclera 743.47
  scrotum 752.89
    transposition 752.81
  seminal duct or tract 752.89
  shoulder girdle 755.59
  site NEC 759.89
  skin 757.39
  skull (bone(s)) 756.0
    with
      anencephalus 740.0
      encephalocele 742.0
      hydrocephalus 742.3
        with spina bifida (*see also* Spina bifida) 741.0 ☑
      microcephalus 742.1
  specified organ or site NEC 759.89
  spermatic cord 752.89
  spinal cord 742.59
  spine 756.19
  spleen 759.0
  sternum 756.3
  stomach 750.7
  tarsus 755.67
  tendon 756.89
  testis 752.89
  thorax (wall) 756.3
  thymus 759.2
  thyroid (gland) 759.2
    cartilage 748.3
  tibia 755.69
  toe 755.66

Anomaly, anomalous — *continued*
specified type — *continued*
  tongue 750.19
  trachea (cartilage) 748.3
  ulna 755.59
  urachus 753.7
  ureter 753.4
    obstructive 753.29
  urethra 753.8
    obstructive 753.6
  urinary tract 753.8
  uterus (Müllerian) 752.39
  uvula 750.26
  vagina 752.49
  vascular NEC (*see also* Anomaly, peripheral vascular system) 747.60
    brain 747.81
  vas deferens 752.89
  vein(s) (peripheral) NEC (*see also* Anomaly, peripheral vascular system) 747.60
    brain 747.81
    great 747.49
    portal 747.49
    pulmonary 747.49
  vena cava (inferior) (superior) 747.49
  vertebra 756.19
  vulva 752.49
spermatic cord 752.9
spine, spinal 756.10
  column 756.10
  cord 742.9
    meningocele (*see also* Spina bifida) 741.9 ☑
    specified type NEC 742.59
    spina bifida (*see also* Spina bifida) 741.9 ☑
    vessel 747.82
  meninges 742.59
  nerve root 742.9
spleen 759.0
Sprengel's 755.52
sternum 756.3
stomach 750.9
  specified type NEC 750.7
submaxillary gland 750.9
superior vena cava 747.40
talipes — *see* Talipes
tarsus 755.67
  with complete absence of distal elements 755.31
teeth, tooth NEC 520.9
  position 524.30
    crowding 524.31
    displacement 524.30
      horizontal 524.33
      vertical 524.34
    distance
      interocclusal
        excessive 524.37
        insufficient 524.36
    excessive spacing 524.32
    rotation 524.35
    specified NEC 524.39
  spacing 524.30
tendon 756.9
  specified type NEC 756.89
termination
  coronary artery 746.85
testis 752.9
thebesian valve 746.9
thigh 755.60
  flexion (*see also* Subluxation, congenital, hip) 754.32
thorax (wall) 756.3
throat 750.9
thumb 755.50
  supernumerary 755.01
thymus gland 759.2
thyroid (gland) 759.2
  cartilage 748.3
tibia 755.60
  saber 090.5
toe 755.66
  supernumerary 755.02

☑ **Additional Digit Required — Refer to the Tabular List for Digit Selection**   ⟱ **Subterms under main terms may continue to next column or page**

24 — Volume 2   ▶◀ Revised Text   ● New Line   ▲ Revised Code   **2015 ICD-9-CM**

Anomaly, anomalous — *continued*
toe — *continued*
  webbed (*see also* Syndactylism, toes)
    755.13
tongue 750.10
  specified type NEC 750.19
trachea, tracheal 748.3
  cartilage 748.3
  rings 748.3
tragus 744.3
transverse aortic arch 747.21
trichromata 368.59
trichromatopsia 368.59
tricuspid (leaflet) (valve) 746.9
  atresia 746.1
  Ebstein's 746.2
  specified type NEC 746.89
  stenosis 746.1
trunk 759.9
Uhl's (hypoplasia of myocardium, right
  ventricle) 746.84
ulna 755.50
umbilicus 759.9
  artery 747.5
union, trachea with larynx 748.3
unspecified site 759.9
upper extremity 755.50
  vessel 747.63
urachus 753.7
  specified type NEC 753.7
ureter 753.9
  obstructive 753.20
  specified type NEC 753.4
    obstructive 753.29
urethra (valve) 753.9
  obstructive 753.6
  specified type NEC 753.8
urinary tract or system (any part, except
  urachus) 753.9
  specified type NEC 753.8
  urachus 753.7
uterus 752.39
  with only one functioning horn 752.33
  in pregnancy or childbirth 654.0 ☑
    affecting fetus or newborn 763.89
    causing obstructed labor 660.2 ☑
      affecting fetus or newborn 763.1
uvula 750.9
vagina 752.40
valleculae 748.3
valve (heart) NEC 746.9
  formation, ureter 753.29
  pulmonary 746.00
  specified type NEC 746.89
vascular NEC (*see also* Anomaly, peripheral
  vascular system) 747.60
  ring 747.21
vas deferens 752.9
vein(s) (peripheral) NEC (*see also* Anomaly,
  peripheral vascular system) 747.60
  brain 747.81
  cerebral 747.81
  coronary 746.89
  great 747.40
    specified type NEC 747.49
  portal 747.40
  pulmonary 747.40
  retina 743.9
vena cava (inferior) (superior) 747.40
venous — *see* Anomaly, vein
venous return (pulmonary) 747.49
  partial 747.42
  total 747.41
ventricle, ventricular (heart) 746.9
  bands 746.9
  folds 746.9
  septa 745.4
vertebra 756.10
vesicourethral orifice 753.9
vessels NEC (*see also* Anomaly, peripheral
  vascular system) 747.60
  optic papilla 743.9
vitelline duct 751.0
vitreous humor 743.9
  specified type NEC 743.51
vulva 752.40

Anomaly, anomalous — *continued*
wrist (joint) 755.50
Anomia 784.69
Anonychia 757.5
  acquired 703.8
Anophthalmos, anophthalmus (clinical)
  (congenital) (globe) 743.00
  acquired V45.78
Anopsia (altitudinal) (quadrant) 368.46
Anorchia 752.89
Anorchism, anorchidism 752.89
Anorexia 783.0
  hysterical 300.11
  nervosa 307.1
Anosmia — *see also* Disturbance, sensation
  781.1
  hysterical 300.11
  postinfectional 478.9
  psychogenic 306.7
  traumatic 951.8
Anosognosia 780.99
Anosphrasia 781.1
Anosteoplasia 756.50
Anotia 744.09
Anovulatory cycle 628.0
Anoxemia 799.02
  newborn 770.88
Anoxia 799.02
  altitude 993.2
  cerebral 348.1
    with
      abortion — *see* Abortion, by type,
        with specified complication
        NEC
      ectopic pregnancy (*see also* cate-
        gories 633.0–633.9) 639.8
      molar pregnancy (*see also* categories
        630–632) 639.8
    complicating
      delivery (cesarean) (instrumental)
        669.4 ☑
    ectopic or molar pregnancy 639.8
    obstetric anesthesia or sedation
      668.2 ☑
    during or resulting from a procedure
      997.01
    following
      abortion 639.8
      ectopic or molar pregnancy 639.8
    newborn (*see also* Distress, fetal, liveborn
      infant) 770.88
  due to drowning 994.1
  fetal, affecting newborn 770.88
  heart — *see* Insufficiency, coronary
  high altitude 993.2
  intrauterine
    fetal death (before onset of labor) 768.0
      during labor 768.1
    liveborn infant — *see* Distress, fetal,
      liveborn infant
  myocardial — *see* Insufficiency, coronary
  newborn 768.9
    mild or moderate 768.6
    severe 768.5
  pathological 799.02
Anteflexion — *see* Anteversion
Antenatal
  care, normal pregnancy V22.1
    first V22.0
  sampling
    chorionic villus V28.89
  screening of mother (for) V28.9
    based on amniocentesis NEC V28.2
      chromosomal anomalies V28.0
      raised alphafetoprotein levels V28.1
    chromosomal anomalies V28.0
    fetal growth retardation using ulatrason-
      ics V28.4
    genomic V28.89
    isoimmunization V28.5
    malformations using ultrasonics V28.3
    proteomic V28.89
    raised alphafetoprotein levels in amniot-
      ic fluid V28.1
    risk
      pre-term labor V28.82

Antenatal — *continued*
  screening of mother — *continued*
    specified condition NEC V28.89
    Streptococcus B V28.6
  survey
    fetal anatomic V28.81
  testing
    nuchal translucency V28.89
Antepartum — *see* condition
Anterior — *see also* condition
  spinal artery compression syndrome 721.1
Antero-occlusion 524.24
Anteversion
  cervix — *see* Anteversion, uterus
  femur (neck), congenital 755.63
  uterus, uterine (cervix) (postinfectional)
    (postpartal, old) 621.6
    congenital 752.39
    in pregnancy or childbirth 654.4 ☑
      affecting fetus or newborn 763.89
      causing obstructed labor 660.2 ☑
        affecting fetus or newborn 763.1
Anthracosilicosis (occupational) 500
Anthracosis (lung) (occupational) 500
  lingua 529.3
Anthrax 022.9
  with pneumonia 022.1 *[484.5]*
  colitis 022.2
  cutaneous 022.0
  gastrointestinal 022.2
  intestinal 022.2
  pulmonary 022.1
  respiratory 022.1
  septicemia 022.3
  specified manifestation NEC 022.8
Anthropoid pelvis 755.69
  with disproportion (fetopelvic) 653.2 ☑
    affecting fetus or newborn 763.1
    causing obstructed labor 660.1 ☑
      affecting fetus or newborn 763.1
Anthropophobia 300.29
Antibioma, breast 611.0
Antibodies
  maternal (blood group) (*see also* Incompat-
    ibility) 656.2 ☑
  anti-D, cord blood 656.1 ☑
    fetus or newborn 773.0
Antibody
  anticardiolipin 795.79
    with
      hemorrhagic disorder 286.53
      hypercoagulable state 289.81
  antiphosphatidylglycerol 795.79
    with
      hemorrhagic disorder 286.53
      hypercoagulable state 289.81
  antiphosphatidylinositol 795.79
    with
      hemorrhagic disorder 286.53
      hypercoagulable state 289.81
  antiphosphatidylserine 795.79
    with
      hemorrhagic disorder 286.53
      hypercoagulable state 289.81
  antiphospholipid 795.79
    with
      hemorrhagic disorder 286.53
      hypercoagulable state 289.81
  deficiency syndrome
    agammaglobulinemic 279.00
    congenital 279.04
    hypogammaglobulinemic 279.00
Anticoagulant
  intrinsic, circulating, causing hemorrhagic
    disorder (*see also* Circulating, antico-
    agulants) 286.59
  lupus (LAC) 795.79
    with
      hemorrhagic disorder 286.53
      hypercoagulable state 289.81
Antimongolism syndrome 758.39
Antimonial cholera 985.4
Antisocial personality 301.7
Antithrombinemia — *see also* Circulating an-
  ticoagulants 286.59

Antithromboplastinemia — *see also* Circulat-
  ing anticoagulants 286.59
Antithromboplastinogenemia — *see also*
  Circulating anticoagulants 286.59
Antitoxin complication or reaction — *see*
  Complications, vaccination
Anton (-Babinski) syndrome (hemiasomatognosia) 307.9
Antritis (chronic) 473.0
  maxilla 473.0
  acute 461.0
  stomach 535.4 ☑
Antrum, antral — *see* condition
Anuria 788.5
  with
    abortion — *see* Abortion, by type, with
      renal failure
    ectopic pregnancy (*see also* categories
      633.0–633.9) 639.3
    molar pregnancy (*see also* categories
      630–632) 639.3
  calculus (impacted) (recurrent) 592.9
    kidney 592.0
    ureter 592.1
  congenital 753.3
  due to a procedure 997.5
  following
    abortion 639.3
    ectopic or molar pregnancy 639.3
  newborn 753.3
  postrenal 593.4
  puerperal, postpartum, childbirth 669.3 ☑
  specified as due to a procedure 997.5
  sulfonamide
    correct substance properly administered
      788.5
    overdose or wrong substance given or
      taken 961.0
  traumatic (following crushing) 958.5
Anus, anal — *see also* condition
  high risk human papillomavirus (HPV) DNA
    test positive 796.75
  low risk human papillomavirus (HPV) DNA
    test positive 796.79
Anusitis 569.49
Anxiety (neurosis) (reaction) (state) 300.00
  alcohol-induced 291.89
  depression 300.4
  drug-induced 292.89
  due to or associated with physical condition
    293.84
  generalized 300.02
  hysteria 300.20
  in
    acute stress reaction 308.0
    transient adjustment reaction 309.24
  panic type 300.01
  separation, abnormal 309.21
  syndrome (organic) (transient) 293.84
Aorta, aortic — *see* condition
Aortectasia — *see also* Ectasia, aortic 447.70
  with aneurysm 441.9
Aortitis (nonsyphilitic) 447.6
  arteriosclerotic 440.0
  calcific 447.6
  Döhle-Heller 093.1
  luetic 093.1
  rheumatic (*see also* Endocarditis, acute,
    rheumatic) 391.1
  rheumatoid — *see* Arthritis, rheumatoid
  specific 093.1
  syphilitic 093.1
    congenital 090.5
Apathetic 799.25
  thyroid storm (*see also* Thyrotoxicosis)
    242.9 ☑
Apathy 799.25
Apepsia 536.8
  achlorhydric 536.0
  psychogenic 306.4
Aperistalsis, esophagus 530.0
Apert-Gallais syndrome (adrenogenital) 255.2
Apertognathia 524.20
Apert's syndrome (acrocephalosyndactyly)
  755.55
Aphagia 787.20

Aphagia — *continued*
psychogenic 307.1
Aphakia (acquired) (bilateral) (postoperative)
(unilateral) 379.31
congenital 743.35
Aphalangia (congenital) 755.4
lower limb (complete) (intercalary) (partial)
(terminal) 755.39
meaning all digits (complete) (partial)
755.31
transverse 755.31
upper limb (complete) (intercalary) (partial)
(terminal) 755.29
meaning all digits (complete) (partial)
755.21
transverse 755.21
Aphasia (amnestic) (ataxic) (auditory) (Broca's)
(choreatic) (classic) (expressive) (global)
(ideational) (ideokinetic) (ideomotor)
(jargon) (motor) (nominal) (receptive)
(semantic) (sensory) (syntactic) (verbal)
(visual) (Wernicke's) 784.3
developmental 315.31
syphilis, tertiary 094.89
uremic — *see* Uremia
Aphemia 784.3
uremic — *see* Uremia
Aphonia 784.41
clericorum 784.49
hysterical 300.11
organic 784.41
psychogenic 306.1
Aphthae, aphthous — *see also* condition
Bednar's 528.2
cachectic 529.0
epizootic 078.4
fever 078.4
oral 528.2
stomatitis 528.2
thrush 112.0
ulcer (oral) (recurrent) 528.2
genital organ(s) NEC
female 616.50
male 608.89
larynx 478.79
Apical — *see* condition
Apical ballooning syndrome 429.83
Aplasia — *see also* Agenesis
alveolar process (acquired) 525.8
congenital 750.26
aorta (congenital) 747.22
aortic valve (congenital) 746.89
axialis extracorticalis (congenital) 330.0
bone marrow (myeloid) 284.9
acquired (secondary) 284.89
congenital 284.01
idiopathic 284.9
brain 740.0
specified part 742.2
breast 757.6
bronchus 748.3
cementum 520.4
cerebellar 742.2
congenital (pure) red cell 284.01
corpus callosum 742.2
erythrocyte 284.81
congenital 284.01
extracortical axial 330.0
eye (congenital) 743.00
fovea centralis (congenital) 743.55
germinal (cell) 606.0
iris 743.45
labyrinth, membranous 744.05
limb (congenital) 755.4
lower NEC 755.30
upper NEC 755.20
lung (bilateral) (congenital) (unilateral)
748.5
nervous system NEC 742.8
nuclear 742.8
ovary 752.0
Pelizaeus-Merzbacher 330.0
prostate (congenital) 752.89
red cell (with thymoma) 284.81
acquired (secondary) 284.81
due to drugs 284.81

Aplasia — *see also* Agenesis — *continued*
red cell — *continued*
adult 284.81
congenital 284.01
hereditary 284.01
of infants 284.01
primary 284.01
pure 284.01
due to drugs 284.81
round ligament (congenital) 752.89
salivary gland 750.21
skin (congenital) 757.39
spinal cord 742.59
spleen 759.0
testis (congenital) 752.89
thymic, with immunodeficiency 279.2
thyroid 243
uterus 752.39
ventral horn cell 742.59
Apleuria 756.3
Apnea, apneic (spells) 786.03
newborn, neonatorum 770.81
essential 770.81
obstructive 770.82
primary 770.81
sleep 770.81
specified NEC 770.82
psychogenic 306.1
sleep, unspecified 780.57
with
hypersomnia, unspecified 780.53
hyposomnia, unspecified 780.51
insomnia, unspecified 780.51
sleep disturbance 780.57
central, in conditions classified elsewhere 327.27
obstructive (adult) (pediatric) 327.23
organic 327.20
other 327.29
primary central 327.21
Apneumatosis newborn 770.4
Apodia 755.31
Aponeurosis 726.90
Apophysitis (bone) — *see also* Osteochondrosis 732.9
calcaneus 732.5
juvenile 732.6
Apoplectiform convulsions — *see also* Disease, cerebrovascular, acute 436
Apoplexia, apoplexy, apoplectic — *see also*
Disease, cerebrovascular, acute 436
abdominal 569.89
adrenal 036.3
attack 436
basilar (*see also* Disease, cerebrovascular,
acute) 436
brain (*see also* Disease, cerebrovascular,
acute) 436
bulbar (*see also* Disease, cerebrovascular,
acute) 436
capillary (*see also* Disease, cerebrovascular,
acute) 436
cardiac (*see also* Infarct, myocardium)
410.9 ☑
cerebral (*see also* Disease, cerebrovascular,
acute) 436
chorea (*see also* Disease, cerebrovascular,
acute) 436
congestive (*see also* Disease, cerebrovascular, acute) 436
newborn 767.4
embolic (*see also* Embolism, brain) 434.1 ☑
fetus 767.0
fit (*see also* Disease, cerebrovascular, acute)
436
healed or old V12.54
heart (auricle) (ventricle) (*see also* Infarct,
myocardium) 410.9 ☑
heat 992.0
hemiplegia (*see also* Disease, cerebrovascular, acute) 436
hemorrhagic (stroke) (*see also* Hemorrhage,
brain) 432.9
ingravescent (*see also* Disease, cerebrovascular, acute) 436

Apoplexia, apoplexy, apoplectic — *see also*
Disease, cerebrovascular, acute —
continued
late effect — *see* Late effect(s) (of) cerebrovascular disease
lung — *see* Embolism, pulmonary
meninges, hemorrhagic (*see also* Hemorrhage, subarachnoid) 430
neonatorum 767.0
newborn 767.0
pancreatitis 577.0
placenta 641.2 ☑
progressive (*see also* Disease, cerebrovascular, acute) 436
pulmonary (artery) (vein) — *see* Embolism,
pulmonary
sanguineous (*see also* Disease, cerebrovascular, acute) 436
seizure (*see also* Disease, cerebrovascular,
acute) 436
serous (*see also* Disease, cerebrovascular,
acute) 436
spleen 289.59
stroke (*see also* Disease, cerebrovascular,
acute) 436
thrombotic (*see also* Thrombosis, brain)
434.0 ☑
uremic — *see* Uremia
uteroplacental 641.2 ☑
Appendage
fallopian tube (cyst of Morgagni) 752.11
intestine (epiploic) 751.5
preauricular 744.1
testicular (organ of Morgagni) 752.89
Appendicitis 541
with
perforation, peritonitis (generalized), or
rupture 540.0
with peritoneal abscess 540.1
peritoneal abscess 540.1
acute (catarrhal) (fulminating) (gangrenous)
(inflammatory) (obstructive) (retrocecal) (suppurative) 540.9
with
perforation, peritonitis, or rupture
540.0
with peritoneal abscess 540.1
peritoneal abscess 540.1
amebic 006.8
chronic (recurrent) 542
exacerbation — *see* Appendicitis, acute
fulminating — *see* Appendicitis, acute
gangrenous — *see* Appendicitis, acute
healed (obliterative) 542
interval 542
neurogenic 542
obstructive 542
pneumococcal 541
recurrent 542
relapsing 542
retrocecal 541
subacute (adhesive) 542
subsiding 542
suppurative — *see* Appendicitis, acute
tuberculous (*see also* Tuberculosis 014.8 ☑
Appendiclausis 543.9
Appendicolithiasis 543.9
Appendicopathia oxyurica 127.4
Appendix, appendicular — *see also* condition
Morgagni (male) 752.89
fallopian tube 752.11
Appetite
depraved 307.52
excessive 783.6
psychogenic 307.51
lack or loss (*see also* Anorexia) 783.0
nonorganic origin 307.59
perverted 307.52
hysterical 300.11
Apprehension, apprehensiveness (abnormal)
(state) 300.00
specified type NEC 300.09
Approximal wear 521.10
Apraxia (classic) (ideational) (ideokinetic)
(ideomotor) (motor) 784.69
oculomotor, congenital 379.51

Apraxia — *continued*
verbal 784.69
Aptyalism 527.7
Aqueous misdirection 365.83
Arabicum elephantiasis — *see also* Infesta-
tion, filarial 125.9
Arachnidism 989.5
Arachnitis — *see* Meningitis
Arachnodactyly 759.82
Arachnoidism 989.5
Arachnoiditis (acute) (adhesive) (basic) (brain)
(cerebrospinal) (chiasmal) (chronic)
(spinal) — *see also* Meningitis 322.9
meningococcal (chronic) 036.0
syphilitic 094.2
tuberculous (*see also* Tuberculosis,
meninges) 013.0 ☑
Araneism 989.5
Arboencephalitis, Australian 062.4
Arborization block (heart) 426.6
Arbor virus, arbovirus (infection) NEC 066.9
ARC 042
Arches — *see* condition
Arcuate uterus 752.36
Arcuatus uterus 752.36
Arcus (cornea)
juvenilis 743.43
interfering with vision 743.42
senilis 371.41
Arc-welders' lung 503
Arc-welders' syndrome (photokeratitis) 370.24
Areflexia 796.1
Areola — *see* condition
Argentaffinoma (M8241/1) — *see also* Neo-
plasm, by site, uncertain behavior
benign (M8241/0) — *see* Neoplasm, by site,
benign
malignant (M8241/3) — *see* Neoplasm, by
site, malignant
syndrome 259.2
Argentinian hemorrhagic fever 078.7
Arginosuccinicaciduria 270.6
Argonz-Del Castillo syndrome (nonpuerperal
galactorrhea and amenorrhea) 253.1
Argyll-Robertson phenomenon, pupil, or
syndrome (syphilitic) 094.89
atypical 379.45
nonluetic 379.45
nonsyphilitic 379.45
reversed 379.45
Argyria, argyriasis NEC 985.8
conjunctiva 372.55
cornea 371.16
from drug or medicinal agent
correct substance properly administered
709.09
overdose or wrong substance given or
taken 961.2
Arhinencephaly 742.2
Arias-Stella phenomenon 621.30
Ariboflavinosis 266.0
Arizona enteritis 008.1
Arm — *see* condition
Armenian disease 277.31
Arnold-Chiari obstruction or syndrome —
see also Spina bifida 741.0 ☑
type I 348.4
type II (*see also* Spina bifida) 741.0 ☑
type III 742.0
type IV 742.2
Arousals
confusional 327.41
Arrest, arrested
active phase of labor 661.1 ☑
affecting fetus or newborn 763.7
any plane in pelvis
complicating delivery 660.1 ☑
affecting fetus or newborn 763.1
bone marrow (*see also* Anemia, aplastic)
284.9
cardiac 427.5
with
abortion — *see* Abortion, by type,
with specified complication
NEC

☑ **Additional Digit Required** — Refer to the Tabular List for Digit Selection

▽ **Subterms under main terms may continue to next column or page**

Arrest, arrested — *continued*
- cardiac — *continued*
  - with — *continued*
    - ectopic pregnancy (*see also* categories 633.0–633.9) 639.8
    - molar pregnancy (*see also* categories 630–632) 639.8
  - complicating
    - anesthesia
      - correct substance properly administered 427.5
      - obstetric 668.1 ☑
      - overdose or wrong substance given 968.4
      - specified anesthetic — *see* Table of Drugs and Chemicals
    - delivery (cesarean) (instrumental) 669.4 ☑
    - ectopic or molar pregnancy 639.8
    - surgery (nontherapeutic) (therapeutic) 997.1
  - fetus or newborn 779.85
  - following
    - abortion 639.8
    - ectopic or molar pregnancy 639.8
  - personal history, successfully resuscitated V12.53
  - postoperative (immediate) 997.1
    - long-term effect of cardiac surgery 429.4
- cardiorespiratory (*see also* Arrest, cardiac) 427.5
- deep transverse 660.3 ☑
  - affecting fetus or newborn 763.1
- development or growth
  - bone 733.91
  - child 783.40
  - fetus 764.9 ☑
    - affecting management of pregnancy 656.5 ☑
  - tracheal rings 748.3
- epiphyseal 733.91
- granulopoiesis 288.09
- heart — *see* Arrest, cardiac
- respiratory 799.1
  - newborn 770.87
- sinus 426.6
- transverse (deep) 660.3 ☑
  - affecting fetus or newborn 763.1
Arrhenoblastoma (M8630/1)
- benign (M8630/0)
  - specified site — *see* Neoplasm, by site, benign
  - unspecified site
    - female 220
    - male 222.0
- malignant (M8630/3)
  - specified site — *see* Neoplasm, by site, malignant
  - unspecified site
    - female 183.0
    - male 186.9
- specified site — *see* Neoplasm, by site, uncertain behavior
- unspecified site
  - female 236.2
  - male 236.4
Arrhinencephaly 742.2
- due to
  - trisomy 13 (13-15) 758.1
  - trisomy 18 (16-18) 758.2
Arrhythmia (auricle) (cardiac) (cordis) (gallop rhythm) (juvenile) (nodal) (reflex) (sinus) (supraventricular) (transitory) (ventricle) 427.9
- bigeminal rhythm 427.89
- block 426.9
- bradycardia 427.89
- contractions, premature 427.60
- coronary sinus 427.89
- ectopic 427.89
- extrasystolic 427.60
- postoperative 997.1
- psychogenic 306.2
- vagal 780.2

Arrillaga-Ayerza syndrome (pulmonary artery sclerosis with pulmonary hypertension) 416.0
Arsenical
- dermatitis 692.4
- keratosis 692.4
- pigmentation 985.1
  - from drug or medicinal agent
    - correct substance properly administered 709.09
    - overdose or wrong substance given or taken 961.1
Arsenism 985.1
- from drug or medicinal agent
  - correct substance properly administered 692.4
  - overdose or wrong substance given or taken 961.1
Arterial — *see* condition
Arteriectasis 447.8
Arteriofibrosis — *see* Arteriosclerosis
Arteriolar sclerosis — *see* Arteriosclerosis
Arteriolith — *see* Arteriosclerosis
Arteriolitis 447.6
- necrotizing, kidney 447.5
- renal — *see* Hypertension, kidney
Arteriolosclerosis — *see* Arteriosclerosis
Arterionephrosclerosis — *see also* Hypertension, kidney 403.90
Arteriopathy 447.9
Arteriosclerosis, arteriosclerotic (artery) (deformans) (diffuse) (disease) (endarteritis) (general) (obliterans) (obliterative) (occlusive) (senile) (with calcification) 440.9
- with
  - gangrene 440.24
  - psychosis (*see also* Psychosis, arteriosclerotic) 290.40
  - ulceration 440.23
- aorta 440.0
- arteries of extremities — *see* Arteriosclerosis, extremities
- basilar (artery) (*see also* Occlusion, artery, basilar) 433.0 ☑
- brain 437.0
- bypass graft
  - coronary artery 414.05
    - autologous artery (gastroepiploic) (internal mammary) 414.04
    - autologous vein 414.02
    - nonautologous biological 414.03
    - of transplanted heart 414.07
  - extremity 440.30
    - autologous vein 440.31
    - nonautologous biological 440.32
- cardiac — *see* Arteriosclerosis, coronary
- cardiopathy — *see* Arteriosclerosis, coronary
- cardiorenal (*see also* Hypertension, cardiorenal) 404.90
- cardiovascular (*see also* Disease, cardiovascular) 429.2
- carotid (artery) (common) (internal) (*see also* Occlusion, artery, carotid) 433.1 ☑
- central nervous system 437.0
- cerebral 437.0
  - late effect — *see* Late effect(s) (of) cerebrovascular disease
- cerebrospinal 437.0
- cerebrovascular 437.0
- coronary (artery) 414.00
  - due to
    - calcified coronary lesion (severely) 414.4
    - lipid rich plaque 414.3
  - graft — *see* Arteriosclerosis, bypass graft
  - native artery 414.01
    - of transplanted heart 414.06
- extremities (native artery) NEC 440.20
  - bypass graft 440.30
    - autologous vein 440.31
    - nonautologous biological 440.32
  - claudication (intermittent) 440.21
    - and
      - gangrene 440.24
      - rest pain 440.22

Arteriosclerosis, arteriosclerotic — *continued*
- extremities — *continued*
  - claudication — *continued*
    - and — *continued*
      - rest pain — *continued*
        - and
          - gangrene 440.24
          - ulceration 440.23
            - and gangrene 440.24
  - ulceration 440.23
    - and gangrene 440.24
  - gangrene 440.24
  - rest pain 440.22
    - and
      - gangrene 440.24
      - ulceration 440.23
        - and gangrene 440.24
  - specified site NEC 440.29
  - ulceration 440.23
    - and gangrene 440.24
- heart (disease) (*see also* Arteriosclerosis, coronary)
  - valve 424.99
    - aortic 424.1
    - mitral 424.0
    - pulmonary 424.3
    - tricuspid 424.2
- iliac 440.8
- kidney (*see also* Hypertension, kidney) 403.90
- labyrinth, labyrinthine 388.00
- medial NEC (*see also* Arteriosclerosis, extremities) 440.20
- mesentery (artery) 557.1
- Mönckeberg's (*see also* Arteriosclerosis, extremities) 440.20
- myocarditis 429.0
- nephrosclerosis (*see also* Hypertension, kidney) 403.90
- peripheral (of extremities) — *see* Arteriosclerosis, extremities
- precerebral 433.9 ☑
  - specified artery NEC 433.8 ☑
- pulmonary (idiopathic) 416.0
- renal (artery) (*see also* Hypertension, kidney) 403.90
  - arterioles (*see also* Hypertension, kidney) 403.90
  - artery 440.1
- retinal (vascular) 440.8 [362.13]
- specified artery NEC 440.8
  - with gangrene 440.8 [785.4]
- spinal (cord) 437.0
- vertebral (artery) (*see also* Occlusion, artery, vertebral) 433.2 ☑
Arteriospasm 443.9
Arteriovenous — *see* condition
Arteritis 447.6
- allergic (*see also* Angiitis, hypersensitivity) 446.20
- aorta (nonsyphilitic) 447.6
  - syphilitic 093.1
- aortic arch 446.7
- brachiocephalica 446.7
- brain 437.4
  - syphilitic 094.89
- branchial 446.7
- cerebral 437.4
  - late effect — *see* Late effect(s) (of) cerebrovascular disease
  - syphilitic 094.89
- coronary (artery) (*see also* Arteriosclerosis, coronary)
  - rheumatic 391.9
    - chronic 398.99
  - syphilitic 093.89
- cranial (left) (right) 446.5
- deformans — *see* Arteriosclerosis
- giant cell 446.5
- necrosing or necrotizing 446.0
- nodosa 446.0
- obliterans (*see also* Arteriosclerosis)
  - subclaviocarotica 446.7
- pulmonary 417.8
- retina 362.18
- rheumatic — *see* Fever, rheumatic

Arteritis — *continued*
- senile — *see* Arteriosclerosis
- suppurative 447.2
- syphilitic (general) 093.89
  - brain 094.89
  - coronary 093.89
  - spinal 094.89
- temporal 446.5
- young female, syndrome 446.7
Artery, arterial — *see* condition
Arthralgia — *see also* Pain, joint 719.4 ☑
- allergic (*see also* Pain, joint) 719.4 ☑
- in caisson disease 993.3
- psychogenic 307.89
- rubella 056.71
- Salmonella 003.23
- temporomandibular joint 524.62
Arthritis, arthritic (acute) (chronic) (subacute) 716.9 ☑
- meaning Osteoarthritis — *see* Osteoarthrosis

Note — Use the following fifth-digit subclassification with categories 711–712, 715–716:

0	site unspecified
1	shoulder region
2	upper arm
3	forearm
4	hand
5	pelvic region and thigh
6	lower leg
7	ankle and foot
8	other specified sites
9	multiple sites

- allergic 716.2 ☑
- ankylosing (crippling) (spine) 720.0
  - sites other than spine 716.9 ☑
- atrophic 714.0
  - spine 720.9
- back (*see also* Arthritis, spine) 721.90
- Bechterew's (ankylosing spondylitis) 720.0
- blennorrhagic 098.50
- cervical, cervicodorsal (*see also* Spondylosis, cervical) 721.0
- Charcôt's 094.0 [713.5]
  - diabetic 250.6 ☑ [713.5]
    - due to secondary diabetes 249.6 ☑ [713.5]
  - syringomyelic 336.0 [713.5]
  - tabetic 094.0 [713.5]
- chylous (*see also* Filariasis) 125.9 [711.7] ☑
- climacteric NEC 716.3 ☑
- coccyx 721.8
- cricoarytenoid 478.79
- crystal (-induced) — *see* Arthritis, due to crystals
- deformans (*see also* Osteoarthrosis) 715.9 ☑
  - spine 721.90
    - with myelopathy 721.91
- degenerative (*see also* Osteoarthrosis) 715.9 ☑
  - idiopathic 715.09
  - polyarticular 715.09
  - spine 721.90
    - with myelopathy 721.91
- dermatoarthritis, lipoid 272.8 [713.0]
- due to or associated with
  - acromegaly 253.0 [713.0]
  - actinomycosis 039.8 [711.4] ☑
  - amyloidosis 277.39 [713.7]
  - bacterial disease NEC 040.89 [711.4] ☑
  - Behçet's syndrome 136.1 [711.2] ☑
  - blastomycosis 116.0 [711.6] ☑
  - brucellosis (*see also* Brucellosis) 023.9 [711.4] ☑
  - caisson disease 993.3
  - coccidioidomycosis 114.3 [711.6] ☑
  - coliform (Escherichia coli) 711.0 ☑
  - colitis, ulcerative (*see also* Colitis, ulcerative) 556.9 [713.1]

☑ **Additional Digit Required** — Refer to the Tabular List for Digit Selection   ᵂ **Subterms under main terms may continue to next column or page**

Index

Arthritis, arthritic — Arthus phenomenon

Arthritis, arthritic — *continued*
  due to or associated with — *continued*
    cowpox 051.01 *[711.5]* ☑
    crystals (*see also* Gout)
      dicalcium phosphate 275.49 *[712.1]* ☑
      pyrophosphate 275.49 *[712.2]* ☑
      specified NEC 275.49 *[712.8]* ☑
    dermatoarthritis, lipoid 272.8 *[713.0]*
    dermatological disorder NEC 709.9 *[713.3]*
    diabetes 250.6 ☑ *[713.5]*
      due to secondary diabetes 249.6 ☑ *[713.5]*
    diphtheria 032.89 *[711.4]* ☑
    dracontiasis 125.7 *[711.7]* ☑
    dysentery 009.0 *[711.3]* ☑
    endocrine disorder NEC 259.9 *[713.0]*
    enteritis NEC 009.1 *[711.3]* ☑
      infectious (*see also* Enteritis, infectious) 009.0 *[711.3]* ☑
        specified organism NEC 008.8 *[711.3]* ☑
      regional (*see also* Enteritis, regional) 555.9 *[713.1]*
        specified organism NEC 008.8 *[711.3]* ☑
    epiphyseal slip, nontraumatic (old) 716.8 ☑
    erysipelas 035 *[711.4]* ☑
    erythema
      epidemic 026.1
      multiforme 695.10 *[713.3]*
      nodosum 695.2 *[713.3]*
    Escherichia coli 711.0 ☑
    filariasis NEC 125.9 *[711.7]* ☑
    gastrointestinal condition NEC 569.9 *[713.1]*
    glanders 024 *[711.4]* ☑
    Gonococcus 098.50
    gout 274.00
    helminthiasis NEC 128.9 *[711.7]* ☑
    hematological disorder NEC 289.9 *[713.2]*
    hemochromatosis 275.03 *[713.0]*
    hemoglobinopathy NEC (*see also* Disease, hemoglobin) 282.7 *[713.2]*
    hemophilia (*see also* Hemophilia) 286.0 *[713.2]*
    Hemophilus influenzae (H. influenzae) 711.0 ☑
    Henoch (-Schönlein) purpura 287.0 *[713.6]*
    H. influenzae 711.0 ☑
    histoplasmosis NEC (*see also* Histoplasmosis) 115.99 *[711.6]* ☑
    human parvovirus 079.83 *[711.5]* ☑
    hyperparathyroidism 252.00 *[713.0]*
    hypersensitivity reaction NEC 995.3 *[713.6]*
    hypogammaglobulinemia (*see also* Hypogamma-globulinemia) 279.00 *[713.0]*
    hypothyroidism NEC 244.9 *[713.0]*
    infection (*see also* Arthritis, infectious) 711.9 ☑
    infectious disease NEC 136.9 *[711.8]* ☑
    leprosy (*see also* Leprosy) 030.9 *[711.4]* ☑
    leukemia NEC (M9800/3) 208.9 *[713.2]*
    lipoid dermatoarthritis 272.8 *[713.0]*
    Lyme disease 088.81 *[711.8]* ☑
    Mediterranean fever, familial 277.31 *[713.7]*
    meningococcal infection 036.82
    metabolic disorder NEC 277.9 *[713.0]*
    multiple myelomatosis (M9730/3) 203.0 *[713.2]*
    mumps 072.79 *[711.5]* ☑
    mycobacteria 031.8 *[711.4]* ☑
    mycosis NEC 117.9 *[711.6]* ☑
    neurological disorder NEC 349.9 *[713.5]*
    ochronosis 270.2 *[713.0]*
    O'Nyong Nyong 066.3 *[711.5]* ☑
    parasitic disease NEC 136.9 *[711.8]* ☑

Arthritis, arthritic — *continued*
  due to or associated with — *continued*
    paratyphoid fever (*see also* Fever, paratyphoid) 002.9 *[711.3]* ☑
    parvovirus B19 079.83 *[711.5]* ☑
    Pneumococcus 711.0 ☑
    poliomyelitis (*see also* Poliomyelitis) 045.9 *[711.5]* ☑
    Pseudomonas 711.0 ☑
    psoriasis 696.0
    pyogenic organism (E. coli) (H. influenzae) (Pseudomonas) (Streptococcus) 711.0 ☑
    rat-bite fever 026.1 *[711.4]* ☑
    regional enteritis (*see also* Enteritis, regional) 555.9 *[713.1]*
    Reiter's disease 099.3 *[711.1]* ☑
    respiratory disorder NEC 519.9 *[713.4]*
    reticulosis, malignant (M9720/3) 202.3 *[713.2]*
    rubella 056.71
    salmonellosis 003.23
    sarcoidosis 135 *[713.7]*
    serum sickness 999.59 *[713.6]*
    Staphylococcus 711.0 ☑
    Streptococcus 711.0 ☑
    syphilis (*see also* Syphilis) 094.0 *[711.4]* ☑
    syringomyelia 336.0 *[713.5]*
    thalassemia (*see also* Thalassemia) 282.40 *[713.2]*
    tuberculosis (*see also* Tuberculosis, arthritis) 015.9 ☑ *[711.4]* ☑
    typhoid fever 002.0 *[711.3]* ☑
    ulcerative colitis (*see also* Colitis, ulcerative) 556.9 *[713.1]*
    urethritis
      nongonococcal (*see also* Urethritis, nongonococcal) 099.40 *[711.1]* ☑
      nonspecific (*see also* Urethritis, nongonococcal) 099.40 *[711.1]* ☑
      Reiter's 099.3
    viral disease NEC 079.99 *[711.5]* ☑
  erythema epidemic 026.1
  gonococcal 098.50
  gouty 274.00
    acute 274.01
  hypertrophic (*see also* Osteoarthrosis) 715.9 ☑
    spine 721.90
      with myelopathy 721.91
  idiopathic, blennorrheal 099.3
  in caisson disease 993.3 *[713.8]*
  infectious or infective (acute) (chronic) (subacute) NEC 711.9 ☑
    nonpyogenic 711.9 ☑
    spine 720.9
  inflammatory NEC 714.9
  juvenile rheumatoid (chronic) (polyarticular) 714.30
    acute 714.31
    monoarticular 714.33
    pauciarticular 714.32
  lumbar (*see also* Spondylosis, lumbar) 721.3
  meningococcal 036.82
  menopausal NEC 716.3 ☑
  migratory — *see* Fever, rheumatic
  neuropathic (Charcôt's) 094.0 *[713.5]*
    diabetic 250.6 ☑ *[713.5]*
      due to secondary diabetes 249.6 ☑ *[713.5]*
    nonsyphilitic NEC 349.9 *[713.5]*
    syringomyelic 336.0 *[713.5]*
    tabetic 094.0 *[713.5]*
  nodosa (*see also* Osteoarthrosis) 715.9 ☑
    spine 721.90
      with myelopathy 721.91
  nonpyogenic NEC 716.9 ☑
    spine 721.90
      with myelopathy 721.91
  ochronotic 270.2 *[713.0]*
  palindromic (*see also* Rheumatism, palindromic) 719.3 ☑
  pneumococcal 711.0 ☑

Arthritis, arthritic — *continued*
  postdysenteric 009.0 *[711.3]* ☑
  postrheumatic, chronic (Jaccoud's) 714.4
  primary progressive 714.0
    spine 720.9
  proliferative 714.0
    spine 720.0
  psoriatic 696.0
  purulent 711.0 ☑
  pyogenic or pyemic 711.0 ☑
  reactive 099.3
  rheumatic 714.0
    acute or subacute — *see* Fever, rheumatic
    chronic 714.0
    spine 720.9
  rheumatoid (nodular) 714.0
    with
      splenoadenomegaly and leukopenia 714.1
      visceral or systemic involvement 714.2
    aortitis 714.89
    carditis 714.2
    heart disease 714.2
    juvenile (chronic) (polyarticular) 714.30
      acute 714.31
      monoarticular 714.33
      pauciarticular 714.32
    spine 720.0
  rubella 056.71
  sacral, sacroiliac, sacrococcygeal (*see also* Spondylosis, sacral) 721.3
  scorbutic 267
  senile or senescent (*see also* Osteoarthrosis) 715.9 ☑
    spine 721.90
      with myelopathy 721.91
  septic 711.0 ☑
  serum (nontherapeutic) (therapeutic) 999.59 *[713.6]*
  specified form NEC 716.8 ☑
  spine 721.90
    with myelopathy 721.91
    atrophic 720.9
    degenerative 721.90
      with myelopathy 721.91
    hypertrophic (with deformity) 721.90
      with myelopathy 721.91
    infectious or infective NEC 720.9
    Marie-Strümpell 720.0
    nonpyogenic 721.90
      with myelopathy 721.91
    pyogenic 720.9
    rheumatoid 720.0
    traumatic (old) 721.7
    tuberculous (*see also* Tuberculosis) 015.0 ☑ *[720.81]*
  staphylococcal 711.0 ☑
  streptococcal 711.0 ☑
  suppurative 711.0 ☑
  syphilitic 094.0 *[713.5]*
    congenital 090.49 *[713.5]*
  syphilitica deformans (Charcôt) 094.0 *[713.5]*
  temporomandibular joint 524.69
  thoracic (*see also* Spondylosis, thoracic) 721.2
  toxic of menopause 716.3 ☑
  transient 716.4 ☑
  traumatic (chronic) (old) (post) 716.1 ☑
    current injury — *see* nature of injury
  tuberculous (*see also* Tuberculosis, arthritis) 015.9 ☑ *[711.4]* ☑
  urethritica 099.3 *[711.1]* ☑
  urica, uratic 274.00
  venereal 099.3 *[711.1]* ☑
  vertebral (*see also* Arthritis, spine) 721.90
  villous 716.8 ☑
  von Bechterew's 720.0

Arthrocele — *see also* Effusion, joint 719.0 ☑
Arthrochondritis — *see* Arthritis
Arthrodesis status V45.4
Arthrodynia — *see also* Pain, joint 719.4 ☑
  psychogenic 307.89
Arthrodysplasia 755.9

Arthrofibrosis joint — *see also* Ankylosis 718.5
Arthrogryposis 728.3
  multiplex, congenita 754.89
Arthrokatadysis 715.35
Arthrolithiasis 274.00
Arthro-onychodysplasia 756.89
Arthro-osteo-onychodysplasia 756.89
Arthropathy — *see also* Arthritis 716.9 ☑

Note — Use the following fifth-digit
subclassification with categories
711–712, 716:

  0   site unspecified
  1   shoulder region
  2   upper arm
  3   forearm
  4   hand
  5   pelvic region and thigh
  6   lower leg
  7   ankle and foot
  8   other specified sites
  9   multiple sites

  Behçet's 136.1 *[711.2]* ☑
  Charcôt's 094.0 *[713.5]*
    diabetic 250.6 ☑ *[713.5]*
      due to secondary diabetes 249.6 ☑ *[713.5]*
    syringomyelic 336.0 *[713.5]*
    tabetic 094.0 *[713.5]*
  crystal (-induced) — *see* Arthritis, due to crystals
  gouty 274.00
    acute 274.01
    chronic (without mention of tophus (tophi)) 274.02
      with tophus (tophi) 274.03
  neurogenic, neuropathic (Charcôt's) (tabetic) 094.0 *[713.5]*
    diabetic 250.6 ☑ *[713.5]*
      due to secondary diabetes 249.6 ☑ *[713.5]*
    nonsyphilitic NEC 349.9 *[713.5]*
    syringomyelic 336.0 *[713.5]*
  postdysenteric NEC 009.0 *[711.3]* ☑
  postrheumatic, chronic (Jaccoud's) 714.4
  psoriatic 696.0
  pulmonary 731.2
  specified NEC 716.8 ☑
  syringomyelia 336.0 *[713.5]*
  tabes dorsalis 094.0 *[713.5]*
  tabetic 094.0 *[713.5]*
  transient 716.4 ☑
  traumatic 716.1 ☑
  uric acid 274.00
Arthrophyte — *see also* Loose, body, joint 718.1 ☑
Arthrophytis 719.80
  ankle 719.87
  elbow 719.82
  foot 719.87
  hand 719.84
  hip 719.85
  knee 719.86
  multiple sites 719.89
  pelvic region 719.85
  shoulder (region) 719.81
  specified site NEC 719.88
  wrist 719.83
Arthropyosis — *see also* Arthritis, pyogenic 711.0 ☑
Arthroscopic surgical procedure converted to open procedure V64.43
Arthrosis (deformans) (degenerative) — *see also* Osteoarthrosis 715.9 ☑
  Charcôt's 094.0 *[713.5]*
  polyarticular 715.09
  spine (*see also* Spondylosis) 721.90
Arthus phenomenon 995.21

☑ Additional Digit Required — Refer to the Tabular List for Digit Selection ⬛ Subterms under main terms may continue to next column or page

28 — Volume 2 ▶◀ Revised Text ● New Line ▲ Revised Code 2015 ICD-9-CM

Arthus phenomenon — continued
  due to
    correct substance properly administered 995.21
    overdose or wrong substance given or taken 977.9
      specified drug — see Table of Drugs and Chemicals
  serum 999.59
Articular — see also condition
  disc disorder (reducing or non-reducing) 524.63
  spondylolisthesis 756.12
Articulation
  anterior 524.27
  posterior 524.27
  reverse 524.27
Artificial
  device (prosthetic) — see Fitting, device
  insemination V26.1
  menopause (states) (symptoms) (syndrome) 627.4
  opening status (functioning) (without complication) V44.9
    anus (colostomy) V44.3
    colostomy V44.3
    cystostomy V44.50
      appendico-vesicostomy V44.52
      cutaneous-vesicostomy V44.51
      specified type NEC V44.59
    enterostomy V44.4
    gastrostomy V44.1
    ileostomy V44.2
    intestinal tract NEC V44.4
    jejunostomy V44.4
    nephrostomy V44.6
    specified site NEC V44.8
    tracheostomy V44.0
    ureterostomy V44.6
    urethrostomy V44.6
    urinary tract NEC V44.6
    vagina V44.7
    vagina status V44.7
ARV (disease) (illness) (infection) — see Human immunodeficiency virus (disease) (illness) (infection)
Arytenoid — see condition
Asbestosis (occupational) 501
Asboe-Hansen's disease (incontinentia pigmenti) 757.33
Ascariasis (intestinal) (lung) 127.0
Ascaridiasis 127.0
Ascaridosis 127.0
Ascaris 127.0
  lumbricoides (infestation) 127.0
  pneumonia 127.0
Ascending — see condition
ASC-H (atypical squamous cells cannot exclude high grade squamous intraepithelial lesion)
  anus 796.72
  cervix 795.02
  vagina 795.12
Aschoff's bodies — see also Myocarditis, rheumatic 398.0
Ascites 789.59
  abdominal NEC 789.59
  cancerous (M8000/6) 789.51
  cardiac 428.0
  chylous (nonfilarial) 457.8
    filarial (see also Infestation, filarial) 125.9
  congenital 778.0
  due to S. japonicum 120.2
  fetal, causing fetopelvic disproportion 653.7 ☑
  heart 428.0
  joint (see also Effusion, joint) 719.0 ☑
  malignant (M8000/6) 789.51
  pseudochylous 789.59
  syphilitic 095.2
  tuberculous (see also Tuberculosis) 014.0 ☑
Ascorbic acid (vitamin C) **deficiency** (scurvy) 267
ASC-US (atypical squamous cells of undetermined significance)
  anus 796.71

ASC-US — continued
  cervix 795.01
  vagina 795.11
ASCVD (arteriosclerotic cardiovascular disease) 429.2
Aseptic — see condition
Asherman's syndrome 621.5
Asialia 527.7
Asiatic cholera — see also Cholera 001.9
Asocial personality or trends 301.7
Asomatognosia 781.8
Aspergillosis 117.3
  with pneumonia 117.3 [484.6]
  allergic bronchopulmonary 518.6
  nonsyphilitic NEC 117.3
Aspergillus (flavus) (fumigatus) (infection) (terreus) 117.3
Aspermatogenesis 606.0
Aspermia (testis) 606.0
Asphyxia, asphyxiation (by) 799.01
  antenatal — see Distress, fetal
  bedclothes 994.7
  birth (see also Asphyxia, newborn) 768.9
  bunny bag 994.7
  carbon monoxide 986
  caul (see also Asphyxia, newborn) 768.9
  cave-in 994.7
    crushing — see Injury, internal, intrathoracic organs
  constriction 994.7
  crushing — see Injury, internal, intrathoracic organs
  drowning 994.1
  fetal, affecting newborn 768.9
  food or foreign body (in larynx) 933.1
    bronchioles 934.8
    bronchus (main) 934.1
    lung 934.8
    nasopharynx 933.0
    nose, nasal passages 932
    pharynx 933.0
    respiratory tract 934.9
      specified part NEC 934.8
    throat 933.0
    trachea 934.0
  gas, fumes, or vapor NEC 987.9
    specified — see Table of Drugs and Chemicals
  gravitational changes 994.7
  hanging 994.7
  inhalation — see Inhalation
  intrauterine
    fetal death (before onset of labor) 768.0
      during labor 768.1
    liveborn infant — see Distress, fetal, liveborn infant
  local 443.0
  mechanical 994.7
    during birth (see also Distress, fetal) 768.9
  mucus 933.1
    bronchus (main) 934.1
    larynx 933.1
    lung 934.8
    nasal passages 932
    newborn 770.18
    pharynx 933.0
    respiratory tract 934.9
      specified part NEC 934.8
    throat 933.0
    trachea 934.0
    vaginal (fetus or newborn) 770.18
  newborn 768.9
    with neurologic involvement 768.5
    blue 768.6
    livida 768.6
    mild or moderate 768.6
    pallida 768.5
    severe 768.5
    white 768.5
  pathological 799.01
  plastic bag 994.7
  postnatal (see also Asphyxia, newborn) 768.9
    mechanical 994.7
  pressure 994.7
  reticularis 782.61

Asphyxia, asphyxiation — continued
  strangulation 994.7
  submersion 994.1
  traumatic NEC — see Injury, internal, intrathoracic organs
  vomiting, vomitus — see Asphyxia, food or foreign body
Aspiration
  acid pulmonary (syndrome) 997.39
    obstetric 668.0 ☑
  amniotic fluid 770.13
    with respiratory symptoms 770.14
  bronchitis 507.0
  clear amniotic fluid 770.13
    with
      pneumonia 770.14
      pneumonitis 770.14
      respiratory symptoms 770.14
  contents of birth canal 770.17
    with respiratory symptoms 770.18
  fetal 770.10
    blood 770.15
      with
        pneumonia 770.16
        pneumonitis 770.16
    pneumonitis 770.18
  food, foreign body, or gasoline (with asphyxiation) — see Asphyxia, food or foreign body
  meconium 770.11
    with
      pneumonia 770.12
      pneumonitis 770.12
      respiratory symptoms 770.12
    below vocal cords 770.11
      with respiratory symptoms 770.12
  mucus 933.1
    into
      bronchus (main) 934.1
      lung 934.8
      respiratory tract 934.9
        specified part NEC 934.8
      trachea 934.0
    newborn 770.17
    vaginal (fetus or newborn) 770.17
  newborn 770.10
    with respiratory symptoms 770.18
    blood 770.15
      with
        pneumonia 770.16
        pneumonitis 770.16
        respiratory symptoms 770.16
  pneumonia 507.0
    fetus or newborn 770.18
    meconium 770.12
  pneumonitis 507.0
    fetus or newborn 770.18
    meconium 770.12
    obstetric 668.0 ☑
  postnatal stomach contents 770.85
    with
      pneumonia 770.86
      pneumonitis 770.86
      respiratory symptoms 770.86
  syndrome of newborn (massive) 770.18
    meconium 770.12
  vernix caseosa 770.12
Asplenia 759.0
  with mesocardia 746.87
Assam fever 085.0
Assimilation, pelvis
  with disproportion 653.2 ☑
    affecting fetus or newborn 763.1
    causing obstructed labor 660.1 ☑
      affecting fetus or newborn 763.1
Assmann's focus — see also Tuberculosis 011.0 ☑
Astasia (-abasia) 307.9
  hysterical 300.11
Asteatosis 706.8
  cutis 706.8
Astereognosis 780.99
Asterixis 781.3
  in liver disease 572.8
Asteroid hyalitis 379.22
Asthenia, asthenic 780.79

Asthenia, asthenic — continued
  cardiac (see also Failure, heart) 428.9
    psychogenic 306.2
  cardiovascular (see also Failure, heart) 428.9
    psychogenic 306.2
  heart (see also Failure, heart) 428.9
    psychogenic 306.2
  hysterical 300.11
  myocardial (see also Failure, heart) 428.9
    psychogenic 306.2
  nervous 300.5
  neurocirculatory 306.2
  neurotic 300.5
  psychogenic 300.5
  psychoneurotic 300.5
  psychophysiologic 300.5
  reaction, psychoneurotic 300.5
  senile 797
  Stiller's 780.79
  tropical anhidrotic 705.1
Asthenopia 368.13
  accommodative 367.4
  hysterical (muscular) 300.11
  psychogenic 306.7
Asthenospermia 792.2
Asthma, asthmatic (bronchial) (catarrh) (spasmodic) 493.9 ☑

Note — Use the following fifth-digit subclassification with codes 493.0–493.2, 493.9:

0 without mention of status asthmaticus or acute exacerbation or unspecified

1 with status asthmaticus

2 with acute exacerbation

  with
    chronic obstructive pulmonary disease (COPD) 493.2 ☑
      hay fever 493.0 ☑
      rhinitis, allergic 493.0 ☑
  allergic 493.9 ☑
    stated cause (external allergen) 493.0 ☑
  atopic 493.0 ☑
  cardiac (see also Failure, ventricular, left) 428.1
  cardiobronchial (see also Failure, ventricular, left) 428.1
  cardiorenal (see also Hypertension, cardiorenal) 404.90
  childhood 493.0 ☑
  Colliers' 500
  cough variant 493.82
  croup 493.9 ☑
  detergent 507.8
  due to
    detergent 507.8
    inhalation of fumes 506.3
    internal immunological process 493.0 ☑
  endogenous (intrinsic) 493.1 ☑
  eosinophilic 518.3
  exercise induced bronchospasm 493.81
  exogenous (cosmetics) (dander or dust) (drugs) (dust) (feathers) (food) (hay) (platinum) (pollen) 493.0 ☑
  extrinsic 493.0 ☑
  grinders' 502
  hay 493.0 ☑
  heart (see also Failure, ventricular, left) 428.1
  IgE 493.0 ☑
  infective 493.1 ☑
  intrinsic 493.1 ☑
  Kopp's 254.8
  late-onset 493.1 ☑
  meat-wrappers' 506.9
  Millar's (laryngismus stridulus) 478.75
  millstone makers' 502
  miners' 500
  Monday morning 504
  New Orleans (epidemic) 493.0 ☑
  platinum 493.0 ☑
  pneumoconiotic (occupational) NEC 505
  potters' 502
  psychogenic 316 [493.9] ☑

☑ Additional Digit Required — Refer to the Tabular List for Digit Selection   ▽ Subterms under main terms may continue to next column or page

2015 ICD-9-CM   ▶◀ Revised Text   ● New Line   ▲ Revised Code   Volume 2 — 29

Arthus phenomenon — Asthma, asthmatic

Asthma, asthmatic — *continued*
 pulmonary eosinophilic 518.3
 red cedar 495.8
 Rostan's (*see also* Failure, ventricular, left)
  428.1
 sandblasters' 502
 sequoiosis 495.8
 stonemasons' 502
 thymic 254.8
 tuberculous (*see also* Tuberculosis, pulmonary) 011.9 ☑
 Wichmann's (laryngismus stridulus) 478.75
 wood 495.8
Astigmatism (compound) (congenital) 367.20
 irregular 367.22
 regular 367.21
Astroblastoma (M9430/3)
 nose 748.1
 specified site — *see* Neoplasm, by site, malignant
 unspecified site 191.9
Astrocytoma (cystic) (M9400/3)
 anaplastic type (M9401/3)
  specified site — *see* Neoplasm, by site,
   malignant
  unspecified site 191.9
 fibrillary (M9420/3)
  specified site — *see* Neoplasm, by site,
   malignant
  unspecified site 191.9
 fibrous (M9420/3)
  specified site — *see* Neoplasm, by site,
   malignant
  unspecified site 191.9
 gemistocytic (M9411/3)
  specified site — *see* Neoplasm, by site,
   malignant
  unspecified site 191.9
 juvenile (M9421/3)
  specified site — *see* Neoplasm, by site,
   malignant
  unspecified site 191.9
 nose 748.1
 pilocytic (M9421/3)
  specified site — *see* Neoplasm, by site,
   malignant
  unspecified site 191.9
 piloid (M9421/3)
  specified site — *see* Neoplasm, by site,
   malignant
  unspecified site 191.9
 protoplasmic (M9410/3)
  specified site — *see* Neoplasm, by site,
   malignant
  unspecified site 191.9
 specified site — *see* Neoplasm, by site, malignant
 subependymal (M9383/1) 237.5
  giant cell (M9384/1) 237.5
 unspecified site 191.9
Astroglioma (M9400/3)
 nose 748.1
 specified site — *see* Neoplasm, by site, malignant
 unspecified site 191.9
Asymbolia 784.60
Asymmetrical breathing 786.09
Asymmetry — *see also* Distortion
 breast, between native and reconstructed
  612.1
 chest 786.9
 face 754.0
 jaw NEC 524.12
  maxillary 524.11
 pelvis with disproportion 653.0 ☑
  affecting fetus or newborn 763.1 ☑
  causing obstructed labor 660.1 ☑
   affecting fetus or newborn 763.1
Asynergia 781.3
Asynergy 781.3
 ventricular 429.89
Asystole (heart) — *see also* Arrest, cardiac
 427.5
Ataxia, ataxy, ataxic 781.3
 acute 781.3
 brain 331.89

Ataxia, ataxy, ataxic — *continued*
 cerebellar 334.3
  hereditary (Marie's) 334.2
  in
   alcoholism 303.9 ☑ *[334.4]*
   myxedema (*see also* Myxedema)
    244.9 *[334.4]*
   neoplastic disease NEC 239.9 *[334.4]*
 cerebral 331.89
 family, familial 334.2
  cerebral (Marie's) 334.2
  spinal (Friedreich's) 334.0
 Friedreich's (heredofamilial) (spinal) 334.0
 frontal lobe 781.3
 gait 781.2
  hysterical 300.11
 general 781.3
 hereditary NEC 334.2
  cerebellar 334.2
  spastic 334.1
  spinal 334.0
 heredofamilial (Marie's) 334.2
 hysterical 300.11
 locomotor (progressive) 094.0
  diabetic 250.6 ☑ *[337.1]*
   due to secondary diabetes
    249.6 ☑ *[337.1]*
 Marie's (cerebellar) (heredofamilial) 334.2
 nonorganic origin 307.9
 partial 094.0
 postchickenpox 052.7
 progressive locomotor 094.0
 psychogenic 307.9
 Sanger-Brown's 334.2
 spastic 094.0
  hereditary 334.1
  syphilitic 094.0
 spinal
  hereditary 334.0
  progressive locomotor 094.0
 telangiectasia 334.8
Ataxia-telangiectasia 334.8
Atelectasis (absorption collapse) (complete)
 (compression) (massive) (partial)
 (postinfective) (pressure collapse) (pulmonary) (relaxation) 518.0
 newborn (congenital) (partial) 770.5
  primary 770.4
 primary 770.4
 tuberculous (*see also* Tuberculosis, pulmonary) 011.9 ☑
Ateleiosis, ateliosis 253.3
Atelia — *see* Distortion
Ateliosis 253.3
Atelocardia 746.9
Atelomyelia 742.59
Athelia 757.6
Atheroembolism
 extremity
  lower 445.02
  upper 445.01
 kidney 445.81
 specified site NEC 445.89
Atheroma, atheromatous — *see also* Arteriosclerosis 440.9
 aorta, aortic 440.0
  valve (*see also* Endocarditis, aortic) 424.1
 artery — *see* Arteriosclerosis
 basilar (artery) (*see also* Occlusion, artery,
  basilar) 433.0 ☑
 carotid (artery) (common) (internal) (*see also*
  Occlusion, artery, carotid) 433.1 ☑
 cerebral (arteries) 437.0
 coronary (artery) — *see* Arteriosclerosis,
  coronary
 degeneration — *see* Arteriosclerosis
 heart, cardiac — *see* Arteriosclerosis, coronary
 mitral (valve) 424.0
 myocardium, myocardial — *see* Arteriosle-
  rosis, coronary
 pulmonary valve (heart) (*see also* Endocarditis, pulmonary) 424.3
 skin 706.2
 tricuspid (heart) (valve) 424.2
 valve, valvular — *see* Endocarditis

Atheroma, atheromatous — *see also*
 Arteriosclerosis — *continued*
  vertebral (artery) (*see also* Occlusion, artery,
   vertebral) 433.2 ☑
Atheromatosis — *see also* Arteriosclerosis
 arterial, congenital 272.8
Atherosclerosis — *see* Arteriosclerosis
Athetosis (acquired) 781.0
 bilateral 333.79
 congenital (bilateral) 333.6
 double 333.71
 unilateral 781.0
Athlete's
 foot 110.4
 heart 429.3
Athletic team examination V70.3
Athrepsia 261
Athrea (acquired) — *see also* Hypothyroidism
 244.9
 congenital 243
Athyreosis (congenital) 243
 acquired — *see* Hypothyroidism
Athyroidism (acquired) — *see also* Hypothyroidism 244.9
 congenital 243
Atmospheric pyrexia 992.0
Atonia, atony, atonic
 abdominal wall 728.2
 bladder (sphincter) 596.4
  neurogenic NEC 596.54
   with cauda equina syndrome 344.61
 capillary 448.9
 cecum 564.89
  psychogenic 306.4
 colon 564.89
  psychogenic 306.4
 congenital 779.89
 dyspepsia 536.3
  psychogenic 306.4
 intestine 564.89
  psychogenic 306.4
 stomach 536.3
  neurotic or psychogenic 306.4
  psychogenic 306.4
 uterus 661.2 ☑
  with hemorrhage (postpartum) 666.1 ☑
  without hemorrhage
   intrapartum 661.2 ☑
   postpartum 669.8 ☑
 vesical 596.4
Atopy NEC V15.09
Atransferrinemia, congenital 273.8
Atresia, atretic (congenital) 759.89
 alimentary organ or tract NEC 751.8
  lower 751.2
  upper 750.8
 ani, anus, anal (canal) 751.2
 aorta 747.22
  with hypoplasia of ascending aorta and
   defective development of left
   ventricle (with mitral valve atresia) 746.7
  arch 747.11
  ring 747.21
 aortic (orifice) (valve) 746.89
  arch 747.11
 aqueduct of Sylvius 742.3
  with spina bifida (*see also* Spina bifida)
   741.0 ☑
 artery NEC (*see also* Atresia, blood vessel)
  747.60
  cerebral 747.81
  coronary 746.85
  eye 743.58
  pulmonary 747.31
  umbilical 747.5
 auditory canal (external) 744.02
 bile, biliary duct (common) or passage
  751.61
  acquired (*see also* Obstruction, biliary)
   576.2
 bladder (neck) 753.6
 blood vessel (peripheral) NEC 747.60
  cerebral 747.81
  gastrointestinal 747.61
  lower limb 747.64

Atresia, atretic — *continued*
 blood vessel — *continued*
  pulmonary artery 747.31
  renal 747.62
  spinal 747.82
  upper limb 747.63
 bronchus 748.3
 canal, ear 744.02
 cardiac
  valve 746.89
   aortic 746.89
   mitral 746.89
   pulmonary 746.01
   tricuspid 746.1
 cecum 751.2
 cervix (acquired) 622.4
  congenital 752.43
  in pregnancy or childbirth 654.6 ☑
   affecting fetus or newborn 763.89
   causing obstructed labor 660.2 ☑
    affecting fetus or newborn 763.1
 choana 748.0
 colon 751.2
 cystic duct 751.61
  acquired 575.8
   with obstruction (*see also* Obstruc-
    tion, gallbladder) 575.2
 digestive organs NEC 751.8
 duodenum 751.1
 ear canal 744.02
 ejaculatory duct 752.89
 epiglottis 748.3
 esophagus 750.3
 Eustachian tube 744.24
 fallopian tube (acquired) 628.2
  congenital 752.19
 follicular cyst 620.0
 foramen of
  Luschka 742.3
   with spina bifida (*see also* Spina bifi-
    da) 741.0 ☑
  Magendie 742.3
   with spina bifida (*see also* Spina bifi-
    da) 741.0 ☑
 gallbladder 751.69
 genital organ
  external
   female 752.49
   male NEC 752.89
    penis 752.69
  internal
   female 752.89
   male 752.89
 glottis 748.3
 gullet 750.3
 heart
  valve NEC 746.89
   aortic 746.89
   mitral 746.89
   pulmonary 746.01
   tricuspid 746.1
 hymen 752.42
  acquired 623.3
  postinfective 623.3
 ileum 751.1
 intestine (small) 751.1
  large 751.2
 iris, filtration angle (*see also* Buphthalmia)
  743.20
 jejunum 751.1
 kidney 753.3
 lacrimal, apparatus 743.65
  acquired — *see* Stenosis, lacrimal
 larynx 748.3
 ligament, broad 752.19
 lung 748.5
 meatus urinarius 753.6
 mitral valve 746.89
  with atresia or hypoplasia of aortic orifice or valve, with hypoplasia of
   ascending aorta and defective
   development of left ventricle
   746.7
 nares (anterior) (posterior) 748.0
 nasolacrimal duct 743.65
 nasopharynx 748.8

☑ **Additional Digit Required** — Refer to the Tabular List for Digit Selection ▽ **Subterms under main terms may continue to next column or page**

30 — Volume 2   ▶◀ Revised Text   ● New Line   ▲ Revised Code   **2015 ICD-9-CM**

Atresia, atretic — *continued*
  nose, nostril 748.0
    acquired 738.0
  organ or site NEC — *see* Anomaly, specified type NEC
  osseous meatus (ear) 744.03
  oviduct (acquired) 628.2
    congenital 752.19
  parotid duct 750.23
    acquired 527.8
  pulmonary (artery) 747.31
    valve 746.01
    vein 747.49
  pulmonic 746.01
  pupil 743.46
  rectum 751.2
  salivary duct or gland 750.23
    acquired 527.8
  sublingual duct 750.23
    acquired 527.8
  submaxillary duct or gland 750.23
    acquired 527.8
  trachea 748.3
  tricuspid valve 746.1
  ureter 753.29
  ureteropelvic junction 753.21
  ureterovesical orifice 753.22
  urethra (valvular) 753.6
  urinary tract NEC 753.29
  uterus 752.31
    acquired 621.8
  vagina (acquired) 623.2
    congenital (total) (partial) 752.45
    postgonococcal (old) 098.2
    postinfectional 623.2
    senile 623.2
  vascular NEC (*see also* Atresia, blood vessel) 747.60
    cerebral 747.81
  vas deferens 752.89
  vein NEC (*see also* Atresia, blood vessel) 747.60
    cardiac 746.89
    great 747.49
    portal 747.49
    pulmonary 747.49
    vena cava (inferior) (superior) 747.49
  vesicourethral orifice 753.6
  vulva 752.49
    acquired 624.8

Atrichia, atrichosis 704.00
  congenital (universal) 757.4

Atrioventricularis commune 745.69

At risk for falling V15.88

Atrophia — *see also* Atrophy
  alba 709.09
  cutis 701.8
    idiopathica progressiva 701.8
    senilis 701.8
  dermatological, diffuse (idiopathic) 701.8
  flava hepatis (acuta) (subacuta) (*see also* Necrosis, liver) 570
  gyrata of choroid and retina (central) 363.54
    generalized 363.57
  senilis 797
    dermatological 701.8
  unguium 703.8
    congenita 757.5

Atrophoderma, atrophodermia 701.9
  diffusum (idiopathic) 701.8
  maculatum 701.3
    et striatum 701.3
      due to syphilis 095.8
    syphilitic 091.3
  neuriticum 701.8
  pigmentosum 757.33
  reticulatum symmetricum faciei 701.8
  senile 701.8
  symmetrical 701.8
  vermiculata 701.8

Atrophy, atrophic
  adrenal (autoimmune) (capsule) (cortex) (gland) 255.41
    with hypofunction 255.41
  alveolar process or ridge (edentulous) 525.20

Atrophy, atrophic — *continued*
  alveolar process or ridge — *continued*
    mandible 525.20
      minimal 525.21
      moderate 525.22
      severe 525.23
    maxilla 525.20
      minimal 525.24
      moderate 525.25
      severe 525.26
  appendix 543.9
  Aran-Duchenne muscular 335.21
  arm 728.2
  arteriosclerotic — *see* Arteriosclerosis
  arthritis 714.0
    spine 720.9
  bile duct (any) 576.8
  bladder 596.89
  blanche (of Milian) 701.3
  bone (senile) 733.99
    due to
      disuse 733.7
      infection 733.99
      tabes dorsalis (neurogenic) 094.0
    posttraumatic 733.99
  brain (cortex) (progressive) 331.9
    with dementia 290.10
    Alzheimer's 331.0
      with dementia — *see* Alzheimer's, dementia
    circumscribed (Pick's) 331.11
      with dementia
        with behavioral disturbance 331.11 *[294.11]*
        without behavioral disturbance 331.11 *[294.10]*
    congenital 742.4
    hereditary 331.9
    senile 331.2
  breast 611.4
    puerperal, postpartum 676.3 ☑
  buccal cavity 528.9
  cardiac (brown) (senile) (*see also* Degeneration, myocardial) 429.1
  cartilage (infectional) (joint) 733.99
  cast, plaster of Paris 728.2
  cerebellar — *see* Atrophy, brain
  cerebral — *see* Atrophy, brain
  cervix (endometrium) (mucosa) (myometrium) (senile) (uteri) 622.8
    menopausal 627.8
  Charcôt-Marie-Tooth 356.1
  choroid 363.40
    diffuse secondary 363.42
    hereditary (*see also* Dystrophy, choroid) 363.50
      gyrate
        central 363.54
        diffuse 363.57
        generalized 363.57
    senile 363.41
  ciliary body 364.57
  colloid, degenerative 701.3
  conjunctiva (senile) 372.89
  corpus cavernosum 607.89
  cortical (*see also* Atrophy, brain) 331.9
  Cruveilhier's 335.21
  cystic duct 576.8
  dacryosialadenopathy 710.2
  degenerative
    colloid 701.3
    senile 701.3
  Déjérine-Thomas 333.0
  diffuse idiopathic, dermatological 701.8
  disuse
    bone 733.7
    muscle 728.2
    pelvic muscles and anal sphincter 618.83
  Duchenne-Aran 335.21
  ear 388.9
  edentulous alveolar ridge 525.20
    mandible 525.20
      minimal 525.21
      moderate 525.22
      severe 525.23
    maxilla 525.20

Atrophy, atrophic — *continued*
  edentulous alveolar ridge — *continued*
    maxilla — *continued*
      minimal 525.24
      moderate 525.25
      severe 525.26
  emphysema, lung 492.8
  endometrium (senile) 621.8
    cervix 622.8
  enteric 569.89
  epididymis 608.3
  eyeball, cause unknown 360.41
  eyelid (senile) 374.50
  facial (skin) 701.9
  facioscapulohumeral (Landouzy-Déjérine) 359.1
  fallopian tube (senile), acquired 620.3
  fatty, thymus (gland) 254.8
  gallbladder 575.8
  gastric 537.89
    gastritis (chronic) 535.1 ☑
  gastrointestinal 569.89
  genital organ, male 608.89
  glandular 289.3
  globe (phthisis bulbi) 360.41
  gum (*see also* Recession, gingival) 523.20
  hair 704.2
  heart (brown) (senile) (*see also* Degeneration, myocardial) 429.1
  hemifacial 754.0
    Romberg 349.89
  hydronephrosis 591
  infantile 261
    paralysis, acute (*see also* Poliomyelitis, with paralysis) 045.1 ☑
  intestine 569.89
  iris (generalized) (postinfectional) (sector shaped) 364.59
    essential 364.51
    progressive 364.51
    sphincter 364.54
  kidney (senile) (*see also* Sclerosis, renal) 587
    with hypertension (*see also* Hypertension, kidney) 403.90
    congenital 753.0
    hydronephrotic 591
    infantile 753.0
  lacrimal apparatus (primary) 375.13
    secondary 375.14
  Landouzy-Déjérine 359.1
  laryngitis, infection 476.0
  larynx 478.79
  Leber's optic 377.16
  lip 528.5
  liver (acute) (subacute) (*see also* Necrosis, liver) 570
    chronic (yellow) 571.8
    yellow (congenital) 570
      with
        abortion — *see* Abortion, by type, with specified complication NEC
        ectopic pregnancy (*see also* categories 633.0–633.9) 639.8
        molar pregnancy (*see also* categories 630–632) 639.8
    chronic 571.8
    complicating pregnancy 646.7 ☑
    following
      abortion 639.8
      ectopic or molar pregnancy 639.8
    from injection, inoculation or transfusion (onset within 8 months after administration) — *see* Hepatitis, viral
    healed 571.5
    obstetric 646.7 ☑
    postabortal 639.8
    postimmunization — *see* Hepatitis, viral
    posttransfusion — *see* Hepatitis, viral
    puerperal, postpartum 674.8 ☑
  lung (senile) 518.89
    congenital 748.69
  macular (dermatological) 701.3
    syphilitic, skin 091.3

Atrophy, atrophic — *continued*
  macular — *continued*
    syphilitic, skin — *continued*
      striated 095.8
  muscle, muscular 728.2
    disuse 728.2
    Duchenne-Aran 335.21
    extremity (lower) (upper) 728.2
    familial spinal 335.11
    general 728.2
    idiopathic 728.2
    infantile spinal 335.0
    myelopathic (progressive) 335.10
    myotonic 359.21
    neuritic 356.1
    neuropathic (peroneal) (progressive) 356.1
    peroneal 356.1
    primary (idiopathic) 728.2
    progressive (familial) (hereditary) (pure) 335.21
      adult (spinal) 335.19
      infantile (spinal) 335.0
      juvenile (spinal) 335.11
      spinal 335.10
        adult 335.19
        hereditary or familial 335.11
        infantile 335.0
    pseudohypertrophic 359.1
    spinal (progressive) 335.10
      adult 335.19
      Aran-Duchenne 335.21
      familial 335.11
      hereditary 335.11
      infantile 335.0
      juvenile 335.11
    syphilitic 095.6
  myocardium (*see also* Degeneration, myocardial) 429.1
  myometrium (senile) 621.8
    cervix 622.8
  myotatic 728.2
  myotonia 359.21
  nail 703.8
    congenital 757.5
  nasopharynx 472.2
  nerve (*see also* Disorder, nerve)
    abducens 378.54
    accessory 352.4
    acoustic or auditory 388.5
    cranial 352.9
      first (olfactory) 352.0
      second (optic) (*see also* Atrophy, optic nerve) 377.10
      third (oculomotor) (partial) 378.51
        total 378.52
      fourth (trochlear) 378.53
      fifth (trigeminal) 350.8
      sixth (abducens) 378.54
      seventh (facial) 351.8
      eighth (auditory) 388.5
      ninth (glossopharyngeal) 352.2
      tenth (pneumogastric) (vagus) 352.3
      eleventh (accessory) 352.4
      twelfth (hypoglossal) 352.5
    facial 351.8
    glossopharyngeal 352.2
    hypoglossal 352.5
    oculomotor (partial) 378.51
      total 378.52
    olfactory 352.0
    peripheral 355.9
    pneumogastric 352.3
    trigeminal 350.8
    trochlear 378.53
    vagus (pneumogastric) 352.3
  nervous system, congenital 742.8
  neuritic (*see also* Disorder, nerve) 355.9
  neurogenic NEC 355.9
    bone
      tabetic 094.0
  nutritional 261
  old age 797
  olivopontocerebellar 333.0

☑ **Additional Digit Required** — Refer to the Tabular List for Digit Selection   ▽ **Subterms under main terms may continue to next column or page**

Atrophy, atrophic — *continued*
　optic nerve (ascending) (descending) (infectional) (nonfamilial) (papillomacular bundle) (postretinal) (secondary NEC) (simple) 377.10
　　associated with retinal dystrophy 377.13
　　dominant hereditary 377.16
　　glaucomatous 377.14
　　hereditary (dominant) (Leber's) 377.16
　　Leber's (hereditary) 377.16
　　partial 377.15
　　postinflammatory 377.12
　　primary 377.11
　　syphilitic 094.84
　　　congenital 090.49
　　　tabes dorsalis 094.0
　orbit 376.45
　ovary (senile), acquired 620.3
　oviduct (senile), acquired 620.3
　palsy, diffuse 335.20
　pancreas (duct) (senile) 577.8
　papillary muscle 429.81
　paralysis 355.9
　parotid gland 527.0
　patches skin 701.3
　　senile 701.8
　penis 607.89
　pharyngitis 472.1
　pharynx 478.29
　pluriglandular 258.8
　polyarthritis 714.0
　prostate 602.2
　pseudohypertrophic 359.1
　renal (*see also* Sclerosis, renal) 587
　reticulata 701.8
　retina (*see also* Degeneration, retina) 362.60
　　hereditary (*see also* Dystrophy, retina) 362.70
　rhinitis 472.0
　salivary duct or gland 527.0
　scar NEC 709.2
　sclerosis, lobar (of brain) 331.0
　　with dementia
　　　with behavioral disturbance 331.0 *[294.11]*
　　　without behavioral disturbance 331.0 *[294.10]*
　scrotum 608.89
　seminal vesicle 608.89
　senile 797
　　degenerative, of skin 701.3
　skin (patches) (senile) 701.8
　spermatic cord 608.89
　spinal (cord) 336.8
　　acute 336.8
　　muscular (chronic) 335.10
　　　adult 335.19
　　　familial 335.11
　　　juvenile 335.10
　　paralysis 335.10
　　　acute (*see also* Poliomyelitis, with paralysis) 045.1 ☑
　spine (column) 733.99
　spleen (senile) 289.59
　spots (skin) 701.3
　　senile 701.8
　stomach 537.89
　striate and macular 701.3
　　syphilitic 095.8
　subcutaneous 701.9
　　due to injection 999.9
　sublingual gland 527.0
　submaxillary gland 527.0
　Sudeck's 733.7
　suprarenal (autoimmune) (capsule) (gland) 255.41
　　with hypofunction 255.41
　tarso-orbital fascia, congenital 743.66
　testis 608.3
　thenar, partial 354.0
　throat 478.29
　thymus (fat) 254.8
　thyroid (gland) 246.8
　　with
　　　cretinism 243
　　　myxedema 244.9

Atrophy, atrophic — *continued*
　thyroid — *continued*
　　congenital 243
　tongue (senile) 529.8
　　papillae 529.4
　　smooth 529.4
　trachea 519.19
　tunica vaginalis 608.89
　turbinate 733.99
　tympanic membrane (nonflaccid) 384.82
　　flaccid 384.81
　ulcer (*see also* Ulcer, skin) 707.9
　upper respiratory tract 478.9
　uterus, uterine (acquired) (senile) 621.8
　　cervix 622.8
　　due to radiation (intended effect) 621.8
　vagina (senile) 627.3
　vascular 459.89
　vas deferens 608.89
　vertebra (senile) 733.99
　vulva (primary) (senile) 624.1
　Werdnig-Hoffmann 335.0
　yellow (acute) (congenital) (liver) (subacute) (*see also* Necrosis, liver) 570
　　chronic 571.8
　　resulting from administration of blood, plasma, serum, or other biological substance (within 8 months of administration) — *see* Hepatitis, viral

Attack
　akinetic (*see also* Epilepsy) 345.0 ☑
　angina — *see* Angina
　apoplectic (*see also* Disease, cerebrovascular, acute) 436
　benign shuddering 333.93
　bilious — *see* Vomiting
　cataleptic 300.11
　cerebral (*see also* Disease, cerebrovascular, acute) 436
　coronary (*see also* Infarct, myocardium) 410.9 ☑
　cyanotic, newborn 770.83
　epileptic (*see also* Epilepsy) 345.9 ☑
　epileptiform 780.39
　heart (*see also* Infarct, myocardium) 410.9 ☑
　hemiplegia (*see also* Disease, cerebrovascular, acute) 436
　hysterical 300.11
　jacksonian (*see also* Epilepsy) 345.5 ☑
　myocardium, myocardial (*see also* Infarct, myocardium) 410.9 ☑
　myoclonic (*see also* Epilepsy) 345.1 ☑
　panic 300.01
　paralysis (*see also* Disease, cerebrovascular, acute) 436
　paroxysmal 780.39
　psychomotor (*see also* Epilepsy) 345.4 ☑
　salaam (*see also* Epilepsy) 345.6 ☑
　schizophreniform (*see also* Schizophrenia) 295.4 ☑
　sensory and motor 780.39
　syncope 780.2
　toxic, cerebral 780.39
　transient ischemic (TIA) 435.9
　unconsciousness 780.2
　　hysterical 300.11
　vasomotor 780.2
　vasovagal (idiopathic) (paroxysmal) 780.2

Attention to
　artificial opening (of) V55.9
　　digestive tract NEC V55.4
　　specified site NEC V55.8
　　urinary tract NEC V55.6
　　vagina V55.7
　colostomy V55.3
　cystostomy V55.5
　dressing
　　wound V58.30
　　　nonsurgical V58.30
　　　surgical V58.31
　gastrostomy V55.1
　ileostomy V55.2
　jejunostomy V55.4
　nephrostomy V55.6

Attention to — *continued*
　surgical dressings V58.31
　sutures V58.32
　tracheostomy V55.0
　ureterostomy V55.6
　urethrostomy V55.6

Attrition
　gum (*see also* Recession, gingival) 523.20
　teeth (hard tissues) 521.10
　　excessive 521.10
　　　extending into
　　　　dentine 521.12
　　　　pulp 521.13
　　　generalized 521.15
　　　limited to enamel 521.11
　　　localized 521.14

Atypical — *see also* condition
　cells
　　endocervical 795.00
　　endometrial 795.00
　　glandular
　　　anus 796.70
　　　cervical 795.00
　　　vaginal 795.10
　　distribution, vessel (congenital) (peripheral) NEC 747.60
　endometrium 621.9
　kidney 593.89

Atypism, cervix 622.10
Audible tinnitus — *see also* Tinnitus 388.30
Auditory — *see* condition
Audry's syndrome (acropachyderma) 757.39
Aujeszky's disease 078.89
Aura
　jacksonian (*see also* Epilepsy) 345.5 ☑
　persistent migraine 346.5 ☑
　　with cerebral infarction 346.6 ☑
　　without cerebral infarction 346.5 ☑

Aurantiasis, cutis 278.3
Auricle, auricular — *see* condition
Auriculotemporal syndrome 350.8
Australian
　Q fever 083.0
　X disease 062.4
Autism, autistic (child) (infantile) 299.0 ☑
Autodigestion 799.89
Autoerythrocyte sensitization 287.2
Autographism 708.3
Autoimmune
　cold sensitivity 283.0
　disease NEC 279.49
　hemolytic anemia 283.0
　inhibitors to clotting factors 286.52
　lymphoproliferative syndrome (ALPS) 279.41
　thyroiditis 245.2
Autoinfection, septic — *see* Septicemia
Autointoxication 799.89
Automatism 348.89
　with temporal sclerosis 348.81
　epileptic (*see also* Epilepsy) 345.4 ☑
　paroxysmal, idiopathic (*see also* Epilepsy) 345.4 ☑
Autonomic, autonomous
　bladder 596.54
　　neurogenic 596.54
　　　with cauda equina 344.61
　dysreflexia 337.3
　faciocephalalgia (*see also* Neuropathy, peripheral, autonomic) 337.9
　hysterical seizure 300.11
　imbalance (*see also* Neuropathy, peripheral, autonomic) 337.9
Autophony 388.40
Autosensitivity, erythrocyte 287.2
Autotopagnosia 780.99
Autotoxemia 799.89
Autumn — *see* condition
Avellis' syndrome 344.89
Aversion
　oral 783.3
　　newborn 779.31
　　nonorganic origin 307.59
Aviators
　disease or sickness (*see also* Effect, adverse, high altitude) 993.2

Aviators — *continued*
　ear 993.0
　effort syndrome 306.2
Avitaminosis (multiple NEC) — *see also* Deficiency, vitamin 269.2
　A 264.9
　B 266.9
　　with
　　　beriberi 265.0
　　　pellagra 265.2
　B₁ 265.1
　B₂ 266.0
　B₆ 266.1
　B₁₂ 266.2
　C (with scurvy) 267
　D 268.9
　　with
　　　osteomalacia 268.2
　　　rickets 268.0
　E 269.1
　G 266.0
　H 269.1
　K 269.0
　multiple 269.2
　nicotinic acid 265.2
　P 269.1
Avulsion (traumatic) 879.8
　blood vessel — *see* Injury, blood vessel, by site
　cartilage (*see also* Dislocation, by site)
　　knee, current (*see also* Tear, meniscus) 836.2
　　symphyseal (inner), complicating delivery 665.6 ☑
　complicated 879.9
　diaphragm — *see* Injury, internal, diaphragm
　ear — *see* Wound, open, ear
　epiphysis of bone — *see* Fracture, by site
　external site other than limb — *see* Wound, open, by site
　eye 871.3
　fingernail — *see* Wound, open, finger
　fracture — *see* Fracture, by site
　genital organs, external — *see* Wound, open, genital organs
　head (intracranial) NEC (*see also* Injury, intracranial, with open intracranial wound)
　　complete 874.9
　　external site NEC 873.8
　　　complicated 873.9
　internal organ or site — *see* Injury, internal, by site
　joint (*see also* Dislocation, by site)
　　capsule — *see* Sprain, by site
　ligament — *see* Sprain, by site
　limb (*see also* Amputation, traumatic, by site)
　　skin and subcutaneous tissue — *see* Wound, open, by site
　muscle — *see* Sprain, by site
　nerve (root) — *see* Injury, nerve, by site
　scalp — *see* Wound, open, scalp
　skin and subcutaneous tissue — *see* Wound, open, by site
　symphyseal cartilage (inner), complicating delivery 665.6 ☑
　tendon (*see also* Sprain, by site)
　　with open wound — *see* Wound, open, by site
　toenail — *see* Wound, open, toe(s)
　tooth 873.63
　　complicated 873.73
Awaiting organ transplant status V49.83
Awareness of heart beat 785.1
Axe grinders' disease 502
Axenfeld's anomaly or syndrome 743.44
Axilla, axillary — *see also* condition
　breast 757.6
Axonotmesis — *see* Injury, nerve, by site
Ayala's disease 756.89
Ayerza's disease or syndrome (pulmonary artery sclerosis with pulmonary hypertension) 416.0

☑ **Additional Digit Required** — Refer to the Tabular List for Digit Selection　　　　　　▽ **Subterms under main terms may continue to next column or page**

Azoospermia 606.0
Azorean disease (of the nervous system) 334.8
Azotemia 790.6
  meaning uremia (see also Uremia) 586
Aztec ear 744.29
Azygos lobe, lung (fissure) 748.69

B

Baader's syndrome (erythema multiforme exudativum) 695.19
Baastrup's syndrome 721.5
Babesiasis 088.82
Babesiosis 088.82
Babington's disease (familial hemorrhagic telangiectasia) 448.0
Babinski-Fröhlich syndrome (adiposogenital dystrophy) 253.8
Babinski-Nageotte syndrome 344.89
Babinski's syndrome (cardiovascular syphilis) 093.89
Bacillary — see condition
Bacilluria 791.9
  asymptomatic, in pregnancy or puerperium 646.5 ☑
  tuberculous (see also Tuberculosis) 016.9 ☑
Bacillus — see also Infection, bacillus
  abortus infection 023.1
  anthracis infection 022.9
  coli
    infection 041.49
      generalized 038.42
      intestinal 008.00
    pyemia 038.42
    septicemia 038.42
  Flexner's 004.1
  fusiformis infestation 101
  mallei infection 024
  Shiga's 004.0
  suipestifer infection (see also Infection, Salmonella) 003.9
Back — see condition
Backache (postural) 724.5
  psychogenic 307.89
  sacroiliac 724.6
Backflow (pyelovenous) — see Disease, renal 593.9
Backknee — see also Genu, recurvatum 736.5
Bacteremia 790.7
  newborn 771.83
Bacteria
  in blood (see also Bacteremia) 790.7
  in urine (see also Bacteriuria) 599.0
Bacterial — see condition
Bactericholia — see also Cholecystitis, acute 575.0
Bacterid, bacteride (Andrews' pustular) 686.8
Bacteriuria, bacteruria 791.9
  with
    urinary tract infection 599.0
  asymptomatic 791.9
    in pregnancy or puerperium 646.5 ☑
      affecting fetus or newborn 760.1
Bad
  breath 784.99
  heart — see Disease, heart
  trip (see also Abuse, drugs, nondependent) 305.3 ☑
Baehr-Schiffrin disease (thrombotic thrombocytopenic purpura) 446.6
Baelz's disease (cheilitis glandularis apostematosa) 528.5
Baerensprung's disease (eczema marginatum) 110.3
Bagassosis (occupational) 495.1
Baghdad boil 085.1
Bagratuni's syndrome (temporal arteritis) 446.5
Baker's
  cyst (knee) 727.51
    tuberculous (see also Tuberculosis) 015.2 ☑
  itch 692.89
Bakwin-Krida syndrome (craniometaphyseal dysplasia) 756.89
Balanitis (circinata) (gangraenosa) (infectious) (vulgaris) 607.1

Balanitis — continued
  amebic 006.8
  candidal 112.2
  chlamydial 099.53
  due to Ducrey's bacillus 099.0
  erosiva circinata et gangraenosa 607.1
  gangrenous 607.1
  gonococcal (acute) 098.0
    chronic or duration of 2 months or over 098.2
  nongonococcal 607.1
  phagedenic 607.1
  venereal NEC 099.8
  xerotica obliterans 607.81
Balanoposthitis 607.1
  chlamydial 099.53
  gonococcal (acute) 098.0
    chronic or duration of 2 months or over 098.2
  ulcerative NEC 099.8
Balanorrhagia — see Balanitis
Balantidiasis 007.0
Balantidiosis 007.0
Balbuties, balbutio — see also Disorder, fluency 315.35
Bald
  patches on scalp 704.00
  tongue 529.4
Baldness — see also Alopecia 704.00
Balfour's disease (chloroma) 205.3 ☑
Balint's syndrome (psychic paralysis of visual fixation) 368.16
Balkan grippe 083.0
Ball
  food 938
  hair 938
Ballantyne (-Runge) syndrome (postmaturity) 766.22
Balloon disease — see also Effect, adverse, high altitude 993.2
Ballooning posterior leaflet syndrome 424.0
Baló's disease or concentric sclerosis 341.1
Bamberger's disease (hypertrophic pulmonary osteoarthropathy) 731.2
Bamberger-Marie disease (hypertrophic pulmonary osteoarthropathy) 731.2
Bamboo spine 720.0
Bancroft's filariasis 125.0
Band(s)
  adhesive (see also Adhesions, peritoneum) 568.0
  amniotic 658.8 ☑
    affecting fetus or newborn 762.8
  anomalous or congenital (see also Anomaly, specified type NEC)
    atrial 746.9
    heart 746.9
    intestine 751.4
    omentum 751.4
    ventricular 746.9
  cervix 622.3
  gallbladder (congenital) 751.69
  intestinal (adhesive) (see also Adhesions, peritoneum) 568.0
    congenital 751.4
  obstructive (see also Obstruction, intestine) 560.81
  periappendiceal (congenital) 751.4
  peritoneal (adhesive) (see also Adhesions, peritoneum) 568.0
    with intestinal obstruction 560.81
    congenital 751.4
  uterus 621.5
  vagina 623.2
Bandemia (without diagnosis of specific infection) 288.66
Bandl's ring (contraction)
  complicating delivery 661.4 ☑
    affecting fetus or newborn 763.7
Bang's disease (Brucella abortus) 023.1
Bangkok hemorrhagic fever 065.4
Bannister's disease 995.1
Bantam-Albright-Martin disease (pseudohypoparathyroidism) 275.49

Banti's disease or syndrome (with cirrhosis) (with portal hypertension) — see Cirrhosis, liver
Bar
  calcaneocuboid 755.67
  calcaneonavicular 755.67
  cubonavicular 755.67
  prostate 600.90
    with
      other lower urinary tract symptoms (LUTS) 600.91
      urinary
        obstruction 600.91
        retention 600.91
  talocalcaneal 755.67
Baragnosis 780.99
Barasheh, barashek 266.2
Barcoo disease or rot — see also Ulcer, skin 707.9
Bard-Pic syndrome (carcinoma, head of pancreas) 157.0
Bärensprung's disease (eczema marginatum) 110.3
Baritosis 503
Barium lung disease 503
Barlow (-Möller) disease or syndrome (meaning infantile scurvy) 267
Barlow's syndrome (meaning mitral valve prolapse) 424.0
Barodontalgia 993.2
Baron Münchausen syndrome 301.51
Barosinusitis 993.1
Barotitis 993.0
Barotrauma 993.2
  odontalgia 993.2
  otitic 993.0
  sinus 993.1
Barraquer's disease or syndrome (progressive lipodystrophy) 272.6
Barré-Guillain syndrome 357.0
Barrel chest 738.3
Barré-Liéou syndrome (posterior cervical sympathetic) 723.2
Barrett's esophagus 530.85
Barrett's syndrome or ulcer (chronic peptic ulcer of esophagus) 530.85
Bársony-Polgár syndrome (corkscrew esophagus) 530.5
Bársony-Teschendorf syndrome (corkscrew esophagus) 530.5
Bartholin's
  adenitis (see also Bartholinitis) 616.89
  gland — see condition
Bartholinitis (suppurating) 616.89
  gonococcal (acute) 098.0
    chronic or duration of 2 months or over 098.2
Barth syndrome 759.89
Bartonellosis 088.0
Bartter's syndrome (secondary hyperaldosteronism with juxtaglomerular hyperplasia) 255.13
Basal — see condition
Basan's (hidrotic) **ectodermal dysplasia** 757.31
Baseball finger 842.13
Basedow's disease or syndrome (exophthalmic goiter) 242.0 ☑
Basic — see condition
Basilar — see condition
Bason's (hidrotic) **ectodermal dysplasia** 757.31
Basopenia 288.59
Basophilia 288.65
Basophilism (corticoadrenal) (Cushing's) (pituitary) (thymic) 255.0
Bassen-Kornzweig syndrome (abetalipoproteinemia) 272.5
Bat ear 744.29
Bateman's
  disease 078.0
  purpura (senile) 287.2
Bathing cramp 994.1
Bathophobia 300.23
Batten's disease, retina 330.1 [362.71]
Batten-Mayou disease 330.1 [362.71]

Batten-Steinert syndrome 359.21
Battered
  adult (syndrome) 995.81
  baby or child (syndrome) 995.54
  spouse (syndrome) 995.81
Battey mycobacterium infection 031.0
Battledore placenta — see Placenta, abnormal
Battle exhaustion — see also Reaction, stress, acute 308.9
Baumgarten-Cruveilhier (cirrhosis) **disease, or syndrome** 571.5
Bauxite
  fibrosis (of lung) 503
  workers' disease 503
Bayle's disease (dementia paralytica) 094.1
Bazin's disease (primary) — see also Tuberculosis 017.1 ☑
Beach ear 380.12
Beaded hair (congenital) 757.4
Beals syndrome 759.82
Beard's disease (neurasthenia) 300.5
Bearn-Kunkel (-Slater) syndrome (lupoid hepatitis) 571.49
Beat
  elbow 727.2
  hand 727.2
  knee 727.2
Beats
  ectopic 427.60
  escaped, heart 427.60
    postoperative 997.1
  premature (nodal) 427.60
    atrial 427.61
    auricular 427.61
    postoperative 997.1
    specified type NEC 427.69
    supraventricular 427.61
    ventricular 427.69
Beau's
  disease or syndrome (see also Degeneration, myocardial) 429.1
  lines (transverse furrows on fingernails) 703.8
Bechterew's disease (ankylosing spondylitis) 720.0
Bechterew-Strümpell-Marie syndrome (ankylosing spondylitis) 720.0
Becker's
  disease
    idiopathic mural endomyocardial disease 425.2
    myotonia congenita, recessive form 359.22
  dystrophy 359.22
Beck's syndrome (anterior spinal artery occlusion) 433.8 ☑
Beckwith (-Wiedemann) syndrome 759.89
Bedbugs bite(s) — see Injury, superficial, by site
Bedclothes, asphyxiation or suffocation by 994.7
Bed confinement status V49.84
Bednar's aphthae 528.2
Bedsore (see also Ulcer, pressure) 707.00
  with gangrene 707.00 [785.4]
Bedwetting — see also Enuresis 788.36
Beer-drinkers' heart (disease) 425.5
Bee sting (with allergic or anaphylactic shock) 989.5
Begbie's disease (exophthalmic goiter) 242.0 ☑
Behavior disorder, disturbance — see also Disturbance, conduct
  antisocial, without manifest psychiatric disorder
    adolescent V71.02
    adult V71.01
    child V71.02
  dyssocial, without manifest psychiatric disorder
    adolescent V71.02
    adult V71.01
    child V71.02
  high risk — see Problem
Behçet's syndrome 136.1
Behr's disease 362.50

☑ **Additional Digit Required** — Refer to the Tabular List for Digit Selection   ▽ **Subterms under main terms may continue to next column or page**

2015 ICD-9-CM   ▶◀ **Revised Text**   ● **New Line**   ▲ **Revised Code**   **Volume 2 — 33**

Beigel's disease or morbus (white piedra)
111.2
Bejel 104.0
Bekhterev's disease (ankylosing spondylitis)
720.0
Bekhterev-Strümpell-Marie syndrome
(ankylosing spondylitis) 720.0
Belching — *see also* Eructation 787.3
Bell's
disease (*see also* Psychosis, affective)
296.0 ☑
mania (*see also* Psychosis, affective) 296.0 ☑
palsy, paralysis 351.0
infant 767.5
newborn 767.5
syphilitic 094.89
spasm 351.0
**Bence-Jones albuminuria, albuminosuria,
or proteinuria** 791.0
Bends 993.3
Benedikt's syndrome (paralysis) 344.89
Benign — *see also* condition
cellular changes, cervix 795.09
prostate
with
other lower urinary tract symptoms
(LUTS) 600.21
urinary
obstruction 600.21
retention 600.21
hyperplasia 600.20
neoplasm 222.2
Bennett's
disease (leukemia) 208.9 ☑
fracture (closed) 815.01
open 815.11
Benson's disease 379.22
Bent
back (hysterical) 300.11
nose 738.0
congenital 754.0
Bereavement V62.82
as adjustment reaction 309.0
Bergeron's disease (hysteroepilepsy) 300.11
Berger's paresthesia (lower limb) 782.0
Beriberi (acute) (atrophic) (chronic) (dry)
(subacute) (wet) 265.0
with polyneuropathy 265.0 [357.4]
heart (disease) 265.0 [425.7]
leprosy 030.1
neuritis 265.0 [357.4]
Berlin's disease or edema (traumatic) 921.3
Berloque dermatitis 692.72
Bernard-Horner syndrome — *see also* Neuropathy, peripheral, autonomic 337.9
Bernard-Sergent syndrome (acute adrenocor-
tical insufficiency) 255.41
Bernard-Soulier disease or thrombopathy
287.1
Bernhardt's disease or paresthesia 355.1
Bernhardt-Roth disease or syndrome
(paresthesia) 355.1
Bernheim's syndrome — *see also* Failure,
heart 428.0
Bertielliasis 123.8
Bertolotti's syndrome (sacralization of fifth
lumbar vertebra) 756.15
Berylliosis (acute) (chronic) (lung) (occupation-
al) 503
Besnier's
lupus pernio 135
prurigo (atopic dermatitis) (infantile
eczema) 691.8
Besnier-Boeck disease or sarcoid 135
Besnier-Boeck-Schaumann disease (sarcoido-
sis) 135
Best's disease 362.76
Bestiality 302.1
**Beta-adrenergic hyperdynamic circulatory
state** 429.82
Beta-aminoisobutyric aciduria 277.2
Beta-mercaptolactate-cysteine disulfiduria
270.0
Beta thalassemia (mixed) 282.44
major 282.44
minor 282.46

Beurmann's disease (sporotrichosis) 117.1
Bezoar 938
intestine 936
stomach 935.2
Bezold's abscess — *see also* Mastoiditis 383.01
Bianchi's syndrome (aphasia-apraxia-alexia)
784.69
Bicornuate or bicornis uterus (complete)
(partial) 752.34
in pregnancy or childbirth 654.0 ☑
with obstructed labor 660.2 ☑
affecting fetus or newborn 763.1
affecting fetus or newborn 763.89
Bicuspid aortic valve 746.4
Biedl-Bardet syndrome 759.89
Bielschowsky's disease 330.1
Bielschowsky-Jansky
amaurotic familial idiocy 330.1
disease 330.1
Biemond's syndrome (obesity, polydactyly,
and intellectual disabilities) 759.89
Biermer's anemia or disease (pernicious
anemia) 281.0
Biett's disease 695.4
Bifid (congenital) — *see also* Imperfect, closure
apex, heart 746.89
clitoris 752.49
epiglottis 748.3
kidney 753.3
nose 748.1
patella 755.64
scrotum 752.89
toe 755.66
tongue 750.13
ureter 753.4
uterus 752.34
uvula 749.02
with cleft lip (*see also* Cleft, palate, with
cleft lip) 749.20
Biforis uterus (suprasimplex) 752.34
Bifurcation (congenital) — *see also* Imperfect,
closure
gallbladder 751.69
kidney pelvis 753.3
renal pelvis 753.3
rib 756.3
tongue 750.13
trachea 748.3
ureter 753.4
urethra 753.8
uvula 749.02
with cleft lip (*see also* Cleft, palate, with
cleft lip) 749.20
vertebra 756.19
Bigeminal pulse 427.89
Bigeminy 427.89
Big spleen syndrome 289.4
Bilateral — *see* condition
Bile duct — *see* condition
Bile pigments in urine 791.4
Bilharziasis — *see also* Schistosomiasis 120.9
chyluria 120.0
cutaneous 120.3
galacturia 120.0
hematochyluria 120.0
intestinal 120.1
lipemia 120.9
lipuria 120.0
Oriental 120.2
piarhemia 120.9
pulmonary 120.2
tropical hematuria 120.0
vesical 120.0
Biliary — *see* condition
Bilious (attack) — *see also* Vomiting
fever, hemoglobinuric 084.8
Bilirubinuria 791.4
Biliuria 791.4
Billroth's disease
meningocele (*see also* Spina bifida) 741.9 ☑
Bilobate placenta — *see* Placenta, abnormal
Bilocular
heart 745.7
stomach 536.8
Bing-Horton syndrome (histamine cephalgia)
339.00

Binswanger's disease or dementia 290.12
Biörck (-Thorson) syndrome (malignant carcinoid) 259.2
Biparta, bipartite — *see also* Imperfect, closure
carpal scaphoid 755.59
patella 755.64
placenta — *see* Placenta, abnormal
vagina 752.49
Bird
face 756.0
fanciers' lung or disease 495.2
flu — *see also* Influenza, avian 488.02
Bird's disease (oxaluria) 271.8
Birth
abnormal fetus or newborn 763.9
accident, fetus or newborn — *see* Birth, injury
complications in mother — *see* Delivery,
complicated
compression during NEC 767.9
defect — *see* Anomaly
delayed, fetus 763.9
difficult NEC, affecting fetus or newborn
763.9
dry, affecting fetus or newborn 761.1
forced, NEC, affecting fetus or newborn
763.89
forceps, affecting fetus or newborn 763.2
hematoma of sternomastoid 767.8
immature 765.1 ☑
extremely 765.0 ☑
inattention, after or at 995.52
induced, affecting fetus or newborn 763.89
infant — *see* Newborn
injury NEC 767.9
adrenal gland 767.8
basal ganglia 767.0
brachial plexus (paralysis) 767.6
brain (compression) (pressure) 767.0
cerebellum 767.0
cerebral hemorrhage 767.0
conjunctiva 767.8
eye 767.8
fracture
bone, any except clavicle or spine
767.3
clavicle 767.2
femur 767.3
humerus 767.3
long bone 767.3
radius and ulna 767.3
skeleton NEC 767.3
skull 767.3
spine 767.4
tibia and fibula 767.3
hematoma 767.8
liver (subcapsular) 767.8
mastoid 767.8
skull 767.19
sternomastoid 767.8
testes 767.8
vulva 767.8
intracranial (edema) 767.0
laceration
brain 767.0
by scalpel 767.8
peripheral nerve 767.7
liver 767.8
meninges
brain 767.0
spinal cord 767.4
nerves (cranial, peripheral) 767.7
brachial plexus 767.6
facial 767.5
paralysis 767.7
brachial plexus 767.6
Erb (-Duchenne) 767.6
facial nerve 767.5
Klumpke (-Déjérine) 767.6
radial nerve 767.6
spinal (cord) (hemorrhage) (laceration) (rupture) 767.4
rupture
intracranial 767.0
liver 767.8

Birth — *continued*
injury — *continued*
rupture — *continued*
spinal cord 767.4
spleen 767.8
viscera 767.8
scalp 767.19
scalpel wound 767.8
skeleton NEC 767.3
specified NEC 767.8
spinal cord 767.4
spleen 767.8
subdural hemorrhage 767.0
tentorial, tear 767.0
testes 767.8
vulva 767.8
instrumental, NEC, affecting fetus or newborn 763.2
lack of care, after or at 995.52
multiple
affected by maternal complications of
pregnancy 761.5
healthy liveborn — *see* Newborn, multiple
neglect, after or at 995.52
newborn — *see* Newborn
palsy or paralysis NEC 767.7
precipitate, fetus or newborn 763.6
premature (infant) 765.1 ☑
prolonged, affecting fetus or newborn 763.9
retarded, fetus or newborn 763.9
shock, newborn 779.89
strangulation or suffocation
due to aspiration of clear amniotic fluid
770.13
with respiratory symptoms 770.14
mechanical 767.8
trauma NEC 767.9
triplet
affected by maternal complications of
pregnancy 761.5
healthy liveborn — *see* Newborn, multiple
twin
affected by maternal complications of
pregnancy 761.5
healthy liveborn — *see* Newborn, twin
ventouse, affecting fetus or newborn 763.3
Birthmark 757.32
Birt-Hogg-Dube syndrome 759.89
Bisalbuminemia 273.8
Biskra button 085.1
Bite(s)
with intact skin surface — *see* Contusion
animal — *see* Wound, open, by site
intact skin surface — *see* Contusion
bedbug — *see* Injury, superficial, by site
centipede 989.5
chigger 133.8
fire ant 989.5
flea — *see* Injury, superficial, by site
human (open wound) (*see also* Wound,
open, by site)
intact skin surface — *see* Contusion
insect
nonvenomous — *see* Injury, superficial,
by site
venomous 989.5
mad dog (death from) 071
open
anterior 524.24
posterior 524.25
poisonous 989.5
red bug 133.8
reptile 989.5
nonvenomous — *see* Wound, open, by
site
snake 989.5
nonvenomous — *see* Wound, open, by
site
spider (venomous) 989.5
nonvenomous — *see* Injury, superficial,
by site
venomous 989.5
Biting
cheek or lip 528.9

☑ Additional Digit Required — Refer to the Tabular List for Digit Selection
▽ Subterms under main terms may continue to next column or page

34 — Volume 2   ▶◀ Revised Text   ● New Line   ▲ Revised Code   2015 ICD-9-CM

Biting — continued
nail 307.9
Black
death 020.9
eye NEC 921.0
hairy tongue 529.3
heel 924.20
lung disease 500
palm 923.20
Blackfan-Diamond anemia or syndrome
(congenital hypoplastic anemia) 284.01
Blackhead 706.1
Blackout 780.2
Blackwater fever 084.8
Bladder — see condition
Blast
blindness 921.3
concussion — see Blast, injury
injury 869.0
with open wound into cavity 869.1
abdomen or thorax — see Injury, internal, by site
brain (see also Concussion, brain) 850.9
with skull fracture — see Fracture, skull
ear (acoustic nerve trauma) 951.5
with perforation, tympanic membrane — see Wound, open, ear, drum
lung (see also Injury, internal, lung) 861.20
otitic (explosive) 388.11
Blastomycosis, blastomycotic (chronic) (cutaneous) (disseminated) (lung) (pulmonary) (systemic) 116.0
Brazilian 116.1
European 117.5
keloidal 116.2
North American 116.0
primary pulmonary 116.0
South American 116.1
Bleb(s) 709.8
emphysematous (bullous) (diffuse) (lung) (ruptured) (solitary) 492.0
filtering, eye (postglaucoma) (status) V45.69
with complication 997.99
postcataract extraction (complication) 997.99
lung (ruptured) 492.0
congenital 770.5
subpleural (emphysematous) 492.0
Bleeder (familial) (hereditary) — see also Defect, coagulation 286.9
nonfamilial 286.9
Bleeding — see also Hemorrhage 459.0
anal 569.3
anovulatory 628.0
atonic, following delivery 666.1 ☑
capillary 448.9
due to subinvolution 621.1
puerperal 666.2 ☑
ear 388.69
excessive, associated with menopausal onset 627.0
familial (see also Defect, coagulation) 286.9
following intercourse 626.7
gastrointestinal 578.9
gums 523.8
hemorrhoids — see Hemorrhoids, bleeding
intermenstrual
irregular 626.6
regular 626.5
intraoperative 998.11
irregular NEC 626.4
menopausal 627.0
mouth 528.9
nipple 611.79
nose 784.7
ovulation 626.5
postclimacteric 627.1
postcoital 626.7
postmenopausal 627.1
following induced menopause 627.4
postoperative 998.11
preclimacteric 627.0
puberty 626.3

Bleeding — see also Hemorrhage — continued
puberty — continued
excessive, with onset of menstrual periods 626.3
rectum, rectal 569.3
tendencies (see also Defect, coagulation) 286.9
throat 784.8
umbilical stump 772.3
umbilicus 789.9
unrelated to menstrual cycle 626.6
uterus, uterine 626.9
climacteric 627.0
dysfunctional 626.8
functional 626.8
unrelated to menstrual cycle 626.6
vagina, vaginal 623.8
functional 626.8
vicarious 625.8
Blennorrhagia, blennorrhagic — see Blennorrhea
Blennorrhea (acute) 098.0
adultorum 098.40
alveolaris 523.40
chronic or duration of 2 months or over 098.2
gonococcal (neonatorum) 098.40
inclusion (neonatal) (newborn) 771.6
neonatorum 098.40
Blepharelosis — see also Entropion 374.00
Blepharitis (eyelid) 373.00
angularis 373.01
ciliaris 373.00
with ulcer 373.01
marginal 373.00
with ulcer 373.01
scrofulous (see also Tuberculosis) 017.3 ☑ [373.00]
squamous 373.02
ulcerative 373.01
Blepharochalasis 374.34
congenital 743.62
Blepharoclonus 333.81
Blepharoconjunctivitis — see also Conjunctivitis 372.20
angular 372.21
contact 372.22
Blepharophimosis (eyelid) 374.46
congenital 743.62
Blepharoplegia 374.89
Blepharoptosis 374.30
congenital 743.61
Blepharopyorrhea 098.49
Blepharospasm 333.81
due to drugs 333.85
Blessig's cyst 362.62
Blighted ovum 631.8
Blind
bronchus (congenital) 748.3
eye (see also Blindness)
hypertensive 360.42
hypotensive 360.41
loop syndrome (postoperative) 579.2
sac, fallopian tube (congenital) 752.19
spot, enlarged 368.42
tract or tube (congenital) NEC — see Atresia
Blindness (acquired) (congenital) (both eyes) 369.
with deafness V49.85
blast 921.3
with nerve injury — see Injury, nerve, optic
Bright's — see Uremia
color (congenital) 368.59
acquired 368.55
blue 368.53
green 368.52
red 368.51
total 368.54
concussion 950.9
cortical 377.75
day 368.10
acquired 368.10
congenital 368.10
hereditary 368.10

Blindness — continued
day — continued
specified type NEC 368.10
due to
injury NEC 950.9
refractive error — see Error, refractive
eclipse (total) 363.31
emotional 300.11
face 368.16
hysterical 300.11
legal (both eyes) (USA definition) 369.4
with impairment of better (less impaired) eye
near-total 369.02
with
lesser eye impairment 369.02
near-total 369.04
total 369.03
profound 369.05
with
lesser eye impairment 369.05
near-total 369.07
profound 369.08
total 369.06
severe 369.21
with
lesser eye impairment 369.21
blind 369.11
near-total 369.13
profound 369.14
severe 369.22
total 369.12
total
with lesser eye impairment
total 369.01
mind 784.69
moderate
both eyes 369.25
with impairment of lesser eye (specified as)
blind, not further specified 369.15
low vision, not further specified 369.23
near-total 369.17
profound 369.18
severe 369.24
total 369.16
one eye 369.74
with vision of other eye (specified as)
near-normal 369.75
normal 369.76
near-total
both eyes 369.04
with impairment of lesser eye (specified as)
blind, not further specified 369.02
total 369.03
one eye 369.64
with vision of other eye (specified as)
near-normal 369.65
normal 369.66
night 368.60
acquired 368.62
congenital (Japanese) 368.61
hereditary 368.61
specified type NEC 368.69
vitamin A deficiency 264.5
nocturnal — see Blindness, night
one eye 369.60
with low vision of other eye 369.10
profound
both eyes 369.08
with impairment of lesser eye (specified as)
blind, not further specified 369.05
near-total 369.07
total 369.06
one eye 369.67
with vision of other eye (specified as)
near-normal 369.68
normal 369.69
psychic 784.69
severe
both eyes 369.22

Blindness — continued
severe — continued
both eyes — continued
with impairment of lesser eye (specified as)
blind, not further specified 369.11
low vision, not further specified 369.21
near-total 369.13
profound 369.14
total 369.12
one eye 369.71
with vision of other eye (specified as)
near-normal 369.72
normal 369.73
snow 370.24
sun 363.31
temporary 368.12
total
both eyes 369.01
one eye 369.61
with vision of other eye (specified as)
near-normal 369.62
normal 369.63
transient 368.12
traumatic NEC 950.9
word (developmental) 315.01
acquired 784.61
secondary to organic lesion 784.61
Blister — see also Injury, superficial, by site
beetle dermatitis 692.89
due to burn — see Burn, by site, second degree
fever 054.9
fracture — omit code
multiple, skin, nontraumatic 709.8
Bloating 787.3
Bloch-Siemens syndrome (incontinentia pigmenti) 757.33
Bloch-Stauffer dyshormonal dermatosis 757.33
Bloch-Sulzberger disease or syndrome (incontinentia pigmenti) (melanoblastosis) 757.33
Block
alveolar capillary 516.8
arborization (heart) 426.6
arrhythmic 426.9
atrioventricular (AV) (incomplete) (partial) 426.10
with
2:1 atrioventricular response block 426.13
atrioventricular dissociation 426.0
first degree (incomplete) 426.11
second degree (Mobitz type I) 426.13
Mobitz (type) II 426.12
third degree 426.0
complete 426.0
congenital 746.86
Mobitz (incomplete)
type I (Wenckebach's) 426.13
type II 426.12
partial 426.13
auriculoventricular (see also Block, atrioventricular) 426.10
complete 426.0
congenital 746.86
congenital 746.86
bifascicular (cardiac) 426.53
bundle branch (complete) (false) (incomplete) 426.50
bilateral 426.53
left (complete) (main stem) 426.3
with right bundle branch block 426.53
anterior fascicular 426.2
with
posterior fascicular block 426.3
right bundle branch block 426.52
hemiblock 426.2
incomplete 426.2

Block — *continued*
  bundle branch — *continued*
    left — *continued*
      incomplete — *continued*
        with right bundle branch block 426.53
        posterior fascicular 426.2
          with
            anterior fascicular block 426.3
            right bundle branch block 426.51
    right 426.4
      with
        left bundle branch block (incomplete) (main stem) 426.53
        left fascicular block 426.53
          anterior 426.52
          posterior 426.51
      Wilson's type 426.4
  cardiac 426.9
  conduction 426.9
    complete 426.0
  Eustachian tube (*see also* Obstruction, Eustachian tube) 381.60
  fascicular (left anterior) (left posterior) 426.2
  foramen Magendie (acquired) 331.3
    congenital 742.3
      with spina bifida (*see also* Spina bifida) 741.0 ☑
  heart 426.9
    first degree (atrioventricular) 426.11
    second degree (atrioventricular) 426.13
    third degree (atrioventricular) 426.0
    bundle branch (complete) (false) (incomplete) 426.50
      bilateral 426.53
      left (*see also* Block, bundle branch, left) 426.3
      right (*see also* Block, bundle branch, right) 426.4
    complete (atrioventricular) 426.0
    congenital 746.86
    incomplete 426.13
    intra-atrial 426.6
    intraventricular NEC 426.6
    sinoatrial 426.6
    specified type NEC 426.6
  hepatic vein 453.0
  intraventricular (diffuse) (myofibrillar) 426.6
    bundle branch (complete) (false) (incomplete) 426.50
      bilateral 426.53
      left (*see also* Block, bundle branch, left) 426.3
      right (*see also* Block, bundle branch, right) 426.4
  kidney (*see also* Disease, renal) 593.9
    postcystoscopic 997.5
  myocardial (*see also* Block, heart) 426.9
  nodal 426.10
  optic nerve 377.49
  organ or site (congenital) NEC — *see* Atresia
  parietal 426.6
  peri-infarction 426.6
  portal (vein) 452
  sinoatrial 426.6
  sinoauricular 426.6
  spinal cord 336.9
  trifascicular 426.54
  tubal 628.2
  vein NEC 453.9
Blocq's disease or syndrome (astasia-abasia) 307.9
Blood
  constituents, abnormal NEC 790.6
  disease 289.9
    specified NEC 289.89
  donor V59.01
    other blood components V59.09
    stem cells V59.02
    whole blood V59.01
  dyscrasia 289.9
    with
      abortion — *see* Abortion, by type, with hemorrhage, delayed or excessive

Blood — *continued*
  dyscrasia — *continued*
    with — *continued*
      ectopic pregnancy (*see also* categories 633.0–633.9) 639.1
      molar pregnancy (*see also* categories 630–632) 639.1
    following
      abortion 639.1
      ectopic or molar pregnancy 639.1
    newborn NEC 776.9
    puerperal, postpartum 666.3 ☑
  flukes NEC (*see also* Infestation, Schistosoma) 120.9
  in
    feces (*see also* Melena) 578.1
      occult 792.1
    urine (*see also* Hematuria) 599.70
  mole 631.8
  occult 792.1
  poisoning (*see also* Septicemia) 038.9
  pressure
    decreased, due to shock following injury 958.4
    fluctuating 796.4
    high (*see also* Hypertension) 401.9
      borderline 796.2
      incidental reading (isolated) (nonspecific), without diagnosis of hypertension 796.2
    low (*see also* Hypotension) 458.9
      incidental reading (isolated) (nonspecific), without diagnosis of hypotension 796.3
  spitting (*see also* Hemoptysis) 786.30
  staining cornea 371.12
  transfusion
    without reported diagnosis V58.2
    donor V59.01
      stem cells V59.02
    reaction or complication — *see* Complications, transfusion
  tumor — *see* Hematoma
  vessel rupture — *see* Hemorrhage
  vomiting (*see also* Hematemesis) 578.0
Blood-forming organ disease 289.9
Bloodgood's disease 610.1
Bloodshot eye 379.93
Bloom (-Machacek) (-Torre) syndrome 757.39
Blotch, palpebral 372.55
Blount-Barber syndrome (tibia vara) 732.4
Blount's disease (tibia vara) 732.4
Blue
  baby 746.9
  bloater 491.20
    with
      acute bronchitis 491.22
      exacerbation (acute) 491.21
  diaper syndrome 270.0
  disease 746.9
  dome cyst 610.0
  drum syndrome 381.02
  sclera 743.47
    with fragility of bone and deafness 756.51
  toe syndrome 445.02
Blueness — *see also* Cyanosis 782.5
Blurring, visual 368.8
Blushing (abnormal) (excessive) 782.62
BMI (body mass index)
  adult
    25.0-25.9 V85.21
    26.0-26.9 V85.22
    27.0-27.9 V85.23
    28.0-28.9 V85.24
    29.0-29.9 V85.25
    30.0-30.9 V85.30
    31.0-31.9 V85.31
    32.0-32.9 V85.32
    33.0-33.9 V85.33
    34.0-34.9 V85.34
    35.0-35.9 V85.35
    36.0-36.9 V85.36
    37.0-37.9 V85.37
    38.0-38.9 V85.38
    39.0-39.9 V85.39

BMI — *continued*
  adult — *continued*
    40.0-44.9 V85.41
    45.0-49.9 V85.42
    50.0-59.9 V85.43
    60.0-69.9 V85.44
    70 and over V85.45
    between 19-24 V85.1
    less than 19 V85.0
  pediatric
    5th percentile to less than 85th percentile for age V85.52
    85th percentile to less than 95th percentile for age V85.53
    greater than or equal to 95th percentile for age V85.54
    less than 5th percentile for age V85.51
Boarder, hospital V65.0
  infant V65.0
Bockhart's impetigo (superficial folliculitis) 704.8
Bodechtel-Guttmann disease (subacute sclerosing panencephalitis) 046.2
Boder-Sedgwick syndrome (ataxia-telangiectasia) 334.8
Body, bodies
  Aschoff (*see also* Myocarditis, rheumatic) 398.0
  asteroid, vitreous 379.22
  choroid, colloid (degenerative) 362.57
    hereditary 362.77
  cytoid (retina) 362.82
  drusen (retina) (*see also* Drusen) 362.57
    optic disc 377.21
  fibrin, pleura 511.0
  foreign — *see* Foreign body
  Hassall-Henle 371.41
  loose
    joint (*see also* Loose, body, joint) 718.1 ☑
      knee 717.6
    knee 717.6
    sheath, tendon 727.82
  Mallory's 034.1
  mass index (BMI)
    adult
      25.0-25.9 V85.21
      26.0-26.9 V85.22
      27.0-27.9 V85.23
      28.0-28.9 V85.24
      29.0-29.9 V85.25
      30.0-30.9 V85.30
      31.0-31.9 V85.31
      32.0-32.9 V85.32
      33.0-33.9 V85.33
      34.0-34.9 V85.34
      35.0-35.9 V85.35
      36.0-36.9 V85.36
      37.0-37.9 V85.37
      38.0-38.9 V85.38
      39.0-39.9 V85.39
      40.0-44.9 V85.41
      45.0-49.9 V85.42
      50.0-59.9 V85.43
      60.0-69.9 V85.44
      70 and over V85.45
      between 19-24 V85.1
      less than 19 V85.0
    pediatric
      5th percentile to less than 85th percentile for age V85.52
      85th percentile to less than 95th percentile for age V85.53
      greater than or equal to 95th percentile for age V85.54
      less than 5th percentile for age V85.51
  Mooser 081.0
  Negri 071
  rice (joint) (*see also* Loose, body, joint) 718.1 ☑
    knee 717.6
  rocking 307.3
Boeck's
  disease (sarcoidosis) 135
  lupoid (miliary) 135

Boeck's — *continued*
  sarcoid 135
Boerhaave's syndrome (spontaneous esophageal rupture) 530.4
Boggy
  cervix 622.8
  uterus 621.8
Boil — *see also* Carbuncle 680.9
  abdominal wall 680.2
  Aleppo 085.1
  ankle 680.6
  anus 680.5
  arm (any part, above wrist) 680.3
  auditory canal, external 680.0
  axilla 680.3
  back (any part) 680.2
  Baghdad 085.1
  breast 680.2
  buttock 680.5
  chest wall 680.2
  corpus cavernosum 607.2
  Delhi 085.1
  ear (any part) 680.0
  eyelid 373.13
  face (any part, except eye) 680.0
  finger (any) 680.4
  flank 680.2
  foot (any part) 680.7
  forearm 680.3
  Gafsa 085.1
  genital organ, male 608.4
  gluteal (region) 680.5
  groin 680.2
  hand (any part) 680.4
  head (any part, except face) 680.8
  heel 680.7
  hip 680.6
  knee 680.6
  labia 616.4
  lacrimal (*see also* Dacryocystitis) 375.30
    gland (*see also* Dacryoadenitis) 375.00
    passages (duct) (sac) (*see also* Dacryocystitis) 375.30
  leg, any part, except foot 680.6
  multiple sites 680.9
  natal 085.1
  neck 680.1
  nose (external) (septum) 680.0
  orbit, orbital 376.01
  partes posteriores 680.5
  pectoral region 680.2
  penis 607.2
  perineum 680.2
  pinna 680.0
  scalp (any part) 680.8
  scrotum 608.4
  seminal vesicle 608.0
  shoulder 680.3
  skin NEC 680.9
  specified site NEC 680.8
  spermatic cord 608.4
  temple (region) 680.0
  testis 608.4
  thigh 680.6
  thumb 680.4
  toe (any) 680.7
  tropical 085.1
  trunk 680.2
  tunica vaginalis 608.4
  umbilicus 680.2
  upper arm 680.3
  vas deferens 608.4
  vulva 616.4
  wrist 680.4
Bold hives — *see also* Urticaria 708.9
Bolivian hemorrhagic fever 078.7
Bombé, iris 364.74
Bomford-Rhoads anemia (refractory) 238.72
Bone — *see* condition
Bonnevie-Ullrich syndrome 758.6
Bonnier's syndrome 386.19
Bonvale Dam fever 780.79
Bony block of joint 718.80
  ankle 718.87
  elbow 718.82
  foot 718.87

Bony block of joint — *continued*
  hand 718.84
  hip 718.85
  knee 718.86
  multiple sites 718.89
  pelvic region 718.85
  shoulder (region) 718.81
  specified site NEC 718.88
  wrist 718.83
BOOP (bronchiolitis obliterans organized pneumonia) 516.8
Borderline
  diabetes mellitus 790.29
  hypertension 796.2
  intellectual functioning V62.89
  osteopenia 733.90
  pelvis 653.1 ☑
    with obstruction during labor 660.1 ☑
      affecting fetus or newborn 763.1
  psychosis (*see also* Schizophrenia) 295.5 ☑
    of childhood (*see also* Psychosis, childhood) 299.8 ☑
  schizophrenia (*see also* Schizophrenia) 295.5 ☑
Borna disease 062.9
Bornholm disease (epidemic pleurodynia) 074.1
Borrelia vincentii (mouth) (pharynx) (tonsils) 101
Bostock's catarrh — *see also* Fever, hay 477.9
Boston exanthem 048
Botalli, ductus (patent) (persistent) 747.0
Bothriocephalus latus infestation 123.4
Botulism 005.1
  food poisoning 005.1
  infant 040.41
  non-foodborne 040.42
  wound 040.42
Bouba — *see also* Yaws 102.9
Bouffée délirante 298.3
Bouillaud's disease or syndrome (rheumatic heart disease) 391.9
Bourneville's disease (tuberous sclerosis) 759.5
Boutonneuse fever 082.1
Boutonniere
  deformity (finger) 736.21
  hand (intrinsic) 736.21
Bouveret (-Hoffmann) disease or syndrome (paroxysmal tachycardia) 427.2
Bovine heart — *see* Hypertrophy, cardiac
Bowel — *see* condition
Bowen's
  dermatosis (precancerous) (M8081/2) — *see* Neoplasm, skin, in situ
  disease (M8081/2) — *see* Neoplasm, skin, in situ
  epithelioma (M8081/2) — *see* Neoplasm, skin, in situ
  type
    epidermoid carcinoma in situ (M8081/2) — *see* Neoplasm, skin, in situ
    intraepidermal squamous cell carcinoma (M8081/2) — *see* Neoplasm, skin, in situ
Bowing
  femur 736.89
    congenital 754.42
  fibula 736.89
    congenital 754.43
  forearm 736.09
    away from midline (cubitus valgus) 736.01
    toward midline (cubitus varus) 736.02
  leg(s), long bones, congenital 754.44
  radius 736.09
    away from midline (cubitus valgus) 736.01
    toward midline (cubitus varus) 736.02
  tibia 736.89
    congenital 754.43
Bowleg(s) 736.42
  congenital 754.44
  rachitic 268.1
Boyd's dysentery 004.2
Brachial — *see* condition

Brachman-de Lange syndrome (Amsterdam dwarf, intellectual disabilities, and brachycephaly) 759.89
Brachycardia 427.89
Brachycephaly 756.0
Brachymorphism and ectopia lentis 759.89
Bradley's disease (epidemic vomiting) 078.82
Bradycardia 427.89
  chronic (sinus) 427.81
  newborn 779.81
  nodal 427.89
  postoperative 997.1
  reflex 337.09
  sinoatrial 427.89
    with paroxysmal tachyarrhythmia or tachycardia 427.81
    chronic 427.81
  sinus 427.89
    with paroxysmal tachyarrhythmia or tachycardia 427.81
    chronic 427.81
    persistent 427.81
    severe 427.81
  tachycardia syndrome 427.81
  vagal 427.89
Bradykinesia 781.0
Bradypnea 786.09
Brailsford's disease 732.3
  radial head 732.3
  tarsal scaphoid 732.5
Brailsford-Morquio disease or syndrome (mucopolysaccharidosis IV) 277.5
Brain — *see also* condition
  death 348.82
  syndrome (acute) (chronic) (nonpsychotic) (organic) (with neurotic reaction) (with behavioral reaction) (*see also* Syndrome, brain) 310.9
    with
      presenile brain disease 290.10
      psychosis, psychotic reaction (*see also* Psychosis, organic) 294.9
    congenital (*see also* Disability, intellectual) 319
Branched-chain amino-acid disease 270.3
Branchial — *see* condition
Brandt's syndrome (acrodermatitis enteropathica) 686.8
Brash (water) 787.1
Brass-founders' ague 985.8
Bravais-Jacksonian epilepsy — *see also* Epilepsy 345.5 ☑
Braziers' disease 985.8
Brazilian
  blastomycosis 116.1
  leishmaniasis 085.5
BRBPR (bright red blood per rectum) 569.3
Break
  cardiorenal — *see* Hypertension, cardiorenal
  retina (*see also* Defect, retina) 361.30
Breakbone fever 061
Breakdown
  device, implant, or graft — *see* Complications, mechanical
  nervous (*see also* Disorder, mental, nonpsychotic) 300.9
  perineum 674.2 ☑
Breast — *see also* condition
  buds 259.1
    in newborn 779.89
  dense 793.82
  nodule 793.89
Breast feeding difficulties 676.8 ☑
Breath
  foul 784.99
  holder, child 312.81
  holding spells 786.9
  shortness 786.05
Breathing
  asymmetrical 786.09
  bronchial 786.09
  exercises V57.0
  labored 786.09
  mouth 784.99
    causing malocclusion 524.59

Breathing — *continued*
  periodic 786.09
    high altitude 327.22
  tic 307.20
Breathlessness 786.09
Breda's disease — *see also* Yaws 102.9
Breech
  delivery, affecting fetus or newborn 763.0
  extraction, affecting fetus or newborn 763.0
  presentation (buttocks) (complete) (frank) 652.2 ☑
    with successful version 652.1 ☑
    before labor, affecting fetus or newborn 761.7
    during labor, affecting fetus or newborn 763.0
Breisky's disease (kraurosis vulvae) 624.09
Brennemann's syndrome (acute mesenteric lymphadenitis) 289.2
Brenner's
  tumor (benign) (M9000/0) 220
    borderline malignancy (M9000/1) 236.2
    malignant (M9000/3) 183.0
    proliferating (M9000/1) 236.2
Bretonneau's disease (diphtheritic malignant angina) 032.0
Breus' mole 631.8
Brevicollis 756.16
Bricklayers' itch 692.89
Brickmakers' anemia 126.9
Bridge
  myocardial 746.85
Bright's
  blindness — *see* Uremia
  disease (*see also* Nephritis) 583.9
    arteriosclerotic (*see also* Hypertension, kidney) 403.90
Bright red blood per rectum (BRBPR) 569.3
Brill's disease (recrudescent typhus) 081.1
  flea-borne 081.0
  louse-borne 081.1
Brill-Symmers disease (follicular lymphoma) (M9690/3) 202.0 ☑
Brill-Zinsser disease (recrudescent typhus) 081.1
Brinton's disease (linitis plastica) (M8142/3) 151.9
Brion-Kayser disease — *see also* Fever, paratyphoid 002.9
Briquet's disorder or syndrome 300.81
Brissaud's
  infantilism (infantile myxedema) 244.9
  motor-verbal tic 307.23
Brissaud-Meige syndrome (infantile myxedema) 244.9
Brittle
  bones (congenital) 756.51
  nails 703.8
    congenital 757.5
Broad — *see also* condition
  beta disease 272.2
  ligament laceration syndrome 620.6
Brock's syndrome (atelectasis due to enlarged lymph nodes) 518.0
Brocq's disease 691.8
  atopic (diffuse) neurodermatitis 691.8
  lichen simplex chronicus 698.3
  parakeratosis psoriasiformis 696.2
  parapsoriasis 696.2
Brocq-Duhring disease (dermatitis herpetiformis) 694.0
Brodie's
  abscess (localized) (chronic) (*see also* Osteomyelitis) 730.1 ☑
  disease (joint) (*see also* Osteomyelitis) 730.1 ☑
Broken
  arches 734
    congenital 755.67
  back — *see* Fracture, vertebra, by site
  bone — *see* Fracture, by site
  compensation — *see* Disease, heart
  heart syndrome 429.83
  implant or internal device — *see* listing under Complications, mechanical
  neck — *see* Fracture, vertebra, cervical

Broken — *continued*
  nose 802.0
    open 802.1
  tooth, teeth 873.63
    complicated 873.73
Bromhidrosis 705.89
Bromidism, bromism
  acute 967.3
    correct substance properly administered 349.82
    overdose or wrong substance given or taken 967.3
  chronic (*see also* Dependence) 304.1 ☑
Bromidrosiphobia 300.23
Bromidrosis 705.89
Bronchi, bronchial — *see* condition
Bronchiectasis (cylindrical) (diffuse) (fusiform) (localized) (moniliform) (postinfectious) (recurrent) (saccular) 494.0
  with acute exacerbation 494.1
  congenital 748.61
  tuberculosis (*see also* Tuberculosis) 011.5 ☑
Bronchiolectasis — *see* Bronchiectasis
Bronchiolitis (acute) (infectious) (subacute) 466.19
  with
    bronchospasm or obstruction 466.19
    influenza, flu, or grippe (*see also* Influenza) 487.1
  catarrhal (acute) (subacute) 466.19
  chemical 506.0
    chronic 506.4
  chronic (obliterative) 491.8
  due to external agent — *see* Bronchitis, acute, due to
  fibrosa obliterans 491.8
  influenzal (*see also* Influenza) 487.1
  obliterans 491.8
    with organizing pneumonia (BOOP) 516.8
    status post lung transplant 996.84
  obliterative (chronic) (diffuse) (subacute) 491.8
    due to fumes or vapors 506.4
  respiratory syncytial virus 466.11
  vesicular — *see* Pneumonia, broncho-
Bronchitis (diffuse) (hypostatic) (infectious) (inflammatory) (simple) 490
  with
    emphysema — *see* Emphysema
    influenza, flu, or grippe (*see also* Influenza) 487.1
    obstruction airway, chronic 491.20
      with
        acute bronchitis 491.22
        exacerbation (acute) 491.21
    tracheitis 490
      acute or subacute 466.0
        with bronchospasm or obstruction 466.0
      chronic 491.8
  acute or subacute 466.0
    with
      bronchiectasis 494.1
      bronchospasm 466.0
      obstruction 466.0
      tracheitis 466.0
    chemical (due to fumes or vapors) 506.0
    due to
      fumes or vapors 506.0
      radiation 508.8
  allergic (acute) (*see also* Asthma) 493.9 ☑
  arachidic 934.1
  aspiration 507.0
    due to fumes or vapors 506.0
  asthmatic (acute) 493.90
    with
      acute exacerbation 493.92
      status asthmaticus 493.91
    chronic 493.2 ☑
  capillary 466.11
    with bronchospasm or obstruction 466.19
    chronic 491.8
  caseous (*see also* Tuberculosis) 011.3 ☑
  Castellani's 104.8

☑ Additional Digit Required — Refer to the Tabular List for Digit Selection   ▽ Subterms under main terms may continue to next column or page

2015 ICD-9-CM   ▶◀ Revised Text   ● New Line   ▲ Revised Code   Volume 2 — 37

Bronchitis — continued
catarrhal 490
    acute — see Bronchitis, acute
    chronic 491.0
chemical (acute) (subacute) 506.0
    chronic 506.4
    due to fumes or vapors (acute) (subacute) 506.0
        chronic 506.4
chronic 491.9
    with
        tracheitis (chronic) 491.8
    asthmatic 493.2 ☑
    catarrhal 491.0
    chemical (due to fumes and vapors) 506.4
    due to
        fumes or vapors (chemical) (inhalation) 506.4
        radiation 508.8
        tobacco smoking 491.0
    mucopurulent 491.1
    obstructive 491.20
        with
            acute bronchitis 491.22
            exacerbation (acute) 491.21
        purulent 491.1
        simple 491.0
        specified type NEC 491.8
croupous 466.0
    with bronchospasm or obstruction 466.0
    due to fumes or vapors 506.0
emphysematous 491.20
    with
        acute bronchitis 491.22
        exacerbation (acute) 491.21
exudative 466.0
fetid (chronic) (recurrent) 491.1
fibrinous, acute or subacute 466.0
    with bronchospasm or obstruction 466.0
grippal (see also Influenza) 487.1
influenzal (see also Influenza) 487.1
membranous, acute or subacute 466.0
    with bronchospasm or obstruction 466.0
moulders' 502
mucopurulent (chronic) (recurrent) 491.1
    acute or subacute 466.0
obliterans 491.8
obstructive (chronic) 491.20
    with
        acute bronchitis 491.22
        exacerbation (acute) 491.21
pituitous 491.1
plastic (inflammatory) 466.0
pneumococcal, acute or subacute 466.0
    with bronchospasm or obstruction 466.0
pseudomembranous 466.0
purulent (chronic) (recurrent) 491.1
    acute or subacute 466.0
        with bronchospasm or obstruction 466.0
putrid 491.1
scrofulous (see also Tuberculosis) 011.3 ☑
senile 491.9
septic, acute or subacute 466.0
    with bronchospasm or obstruction 466.0
smokers' 491.0
spirochetal 104.8
suffocative, acute or subacute 466.0
summer (see also Asthma) 493.9 ☑
suppurative (chronic) 491.1
    acute or subacute 466.0
tuberculous (see also Tuberculosis) 011.3 ☑
ulcerative 491.8
    Vincent's 101
Vincent's 101
viral, acute or subacute 466.0
Bronchoalveolitis 485
Bronchoaspergillosis 117.3
Bronchocele
    meaning
        dilatation of bronchus 519.19
        goiter 240.9
Bronchogenic carcinoma 162.9
Bronchohemisporosis 117.9
Broncholithiasis 518.89

Broncholithiasis — continued
    tuberculous (see also Tuberculosis) 011.3 ☑
Bronchomalacia 748.3
Bronchomoniliasis 112.89
Bronchomycosis 112.89
Bronchonocardiosis 039.1
Bronchopleuropneumonia — see Pneumonia, broncho-
Bronchopneumonia — see Pneumonia, broncho-
Bronchopneumonitis — see Pneumonia, broncho-
Bronchopulmonary — see condition
Bronchopulmonitis — see Pneumonia, broncho-
Bronchorrhagia 786.30
    newborn 770.3
    tuberculous (see also Tuberculosis) 011.3 ☑
Bronchorrhea (chronic) (purulent) 491.0
    acute 466.0
Bronchospasm 519.11
    with
        asthma — see Asthma
        bronchiolitis, acute 466.19
            due to respiratory syncytial virus 466.11
        bronchitis — see Bronchitis
        chronic obstructive pulmonary disease (COPD) 496
        emphysema — see Emphysema
            due to external agent — see Condition, respiratory, acute, due to
    acute 519.11
    exercise induced 493.81
Bronchospirochetosis 104.8
Bronchostenosis 519.19
Bronchus — see condition
Bronze, bronzed
    diabetes 275.01
    disease (Addison's) (skin) 255.41
        tuberculous (see also Tuberculosis) 017.6 ☑
Brooke's disease or tumor (M8100/0) — see Neoplasm, skin, benign
Brown enamel of teeth (hereditary) 520.5
Brown-Séquard's paralysis (syndrome) 344.89
Brown's tendon sheath syndrome 378.61
Brow presentation complicating delivery 652.4 ☑
Brucella, brucellosis (infection) 023.9
    abortus 023.1
    canis 023.3
    dermatitis, skin 023.9
    melitensis 023.0
    mixed 023.8
    suis 023.2
Bruck-de Lange disease or syndrome (Amsterdam dwarf, intellectual disabilities, and brachycephaly) 759.89
Bruck's disease 733.99
Brugada syndrome 746.89
Brug's filariasis 125.1
Brugsch's syndrome (acropachyderma) 757.39
Bruhl's disease (splenic anemia with fever) 285.8
Bruise (skin surface intact) — see also Contusion
    with
        fracture — see Fracture, by site
        open wound — see Wound, open, by site
    internal organ (abdomen, chest, or pelvis) — see Injury, internal, by site
    umbilical cord 663.6 ☑
        affecting fetus or newborn 762.6
Bruit 785.9
    arterial (abdominal) (carotid) 785.9
    supraclavicular 785.9
Brushburn — see Injury, superficial, by site
Bruton's X-linked agammaglobulinemia 279.04
Bruxism 306.8
    sleep related 327.53
Bubbly lung syndrome 770.7
Bubo 289.3
    blennorrhagic 098.89

Bubo — continued
    chancroidal 099.0
    climatic 099.1
    due to Hemophilus ducreyi 099.0
    gonococcal 098.89
    indolent NEC 099.8
    inguinal NEC 099.8
        chancroidal 099.0
        climatic 099.1
        due to H. ducreyi 099.0
    scrofulous (see also Tuberculosis) 017.2 ☑
    soft chancre 099.0
    suppurating 683
    syphilitic 091.0
        congenital 090.0
    tropical 099.1
    venereal NEC 099.8
    virulent 099.0
Bubonic plague 020.0
Bubonocele — see Hernia, inguinal
Buccal — see condition
Buchanan's disease (juvenile osteochondrosis of iliac crest) 732.1
Buchem's syndrome (hyperostosis corticalis) 733.3
Buchman's disease (osteochondrosis, juvenile) 732.1
Bucket handle fracture (semilunar cartilage) — see also Tear, meniscus 836.2
Budd-Chiari syndrome (hepatic vein thrombosis) 453.0
Budgerigar-fanciers' disease or lung 495.2
Büdinger-Ludloff-Läwen disease 717.89
Buds
    breast 259.1
    in newborn 779.89
Buerger's disease (thromboangiitis obliterans) 443.1
Bulbar — see condition
Bulbus cordis 745.9
    persistent (in left ventricle) 745.8
Bulging fontanels (congenital) 756.0
Bulimia 783.6
    nervosa 307.51
    nonorganic origin 307.51
Bulky uterus 621.2
Bulla(e) 709.8
    lung (emphysematous) (solitary) 492.0
Bullet wound — see also Wound, open, by site
    fracture — see Fracture, by site, open
    internal organ (abdomen, chest, or pelvis) — see Injury, internal, by site, with open wound
    intracranial — see Laceration, brain, with open wound
Bullis fever 082.8
Bullying — see also Disturbance, conduct 312.0 ☑
Bundle
    branch block (complete) (false) (incomplete) 426.50
        bilateral 426.53
        left (see also Block, bundle branch, left) 426.3
            hemiblock 426.2
        right (see also Block, bundle branch, right) 426.4
    of His — see condition
    of Kent syndrome (anomalous atrioventricular excitation) 426.7
Bungpagga 040.81
Bunion 727.1
Bunionette 727.1
Bunyamwera fever 066.3
Buphthalmia, buphthalmos (congenital) 743.20
    associated with
        keratoglobus, congenital 743.22
        megalocornea 743.22
        ocular anomalies NEC 743.22
    isolated 743.21
    simple 743.21
Bürger-Grütz disease or syndrome (essential familial hyperlipemia) 272.3
Buried roots 525.3

Burke's syndrome 577.8
Burkitt's
    tumor (M9750/3) 200.2 ☑
    type malignant, lymphoma, lymphoblastic, or undifferentiated (M9750/3) 200.2 ☑
Burn (acid) (cathode ray) (caustic) (chemical) (electric heating appliance) (electricity) (fire) (flame) (hot liquid or object) (irradiation) (lime) (radiation) (steam) (thermal) (x-ray) 949.0

> Note — Use the following fifth-digit subclassification with category 948 to indicate the percent of body surface with third degree burn:
>
> 0   Less than 10% or unspecified
> 1   10–19%
> 2   20–29%
> 3   30–39%
> 4   40–49%
> 5   50–59%
> 6   60–69%
> 7   70–79%
> 8   80–89%
> 9   90% or more of body surface

with
    blisters — see Burn, by site, second degree
    erythema — see Burn, by site, first degree
    skin loss (epidermal) (see also Burn, by site, second degree)
    full thickness (see also Burn, by site, third degree)
        with necrosis of underlying tissues — see Burn, by site, third degree, deep
first degree — see Burn, by site, first degree
second degree — see Burn, by site, second degree
third degree — see Burn, by site, third degree
    deep — see Burn, by site, third degree, deep
abdomen, abdominal (muscle) (wall) 942.03
    with
        trunk — see Burn, trunk, multiple sites
    first degree 942.13
    second degree 942.23
    third degree 942.33
        deep 942.43
            with loss of body part 942.53
ankle 945.03
    with
        lower limb(s) — see Burn, leg, multiple sites
    first degree 945.13
    second degree 945.23
    third degree 945.33
        deep 945.43
            with loss of body part 945.53
anus — see Burn, trunk, specified site NEC
arm(s) 943.00
    first degree 943.10
    second degree 943.20
    third degree 943.30
        deep 943.40
            with loss of body part 943.50
    lower — see Burn, forearm(s)
    multiple sites, except hand(s) or wrist(s) 943.09
        first degree 943.19
        second degree 943.29
        third degree 943.39
            deep 943.49
                with loss of body part 943.59
    upper 943.03
        first degree 943.13
        second degree 943.23
        third degree 943.33

☑ **Additional Digit Required** — Refer to the Tabular List for Digit Selection

ⓥ **Subterms under main terms may continue to next column or page**

Burn — *continued*
  arm(s) — *continued*
    upper — *continued*
      third degree — *continued*
        deep 943.43
          with loss of body part 943.53
  auditory canal (external) — *see* Burn, ear
  auricle (ear) — *see* Burn, ear
  axilla 943.04
    with
      upper limb(s), except hand(s) or
        wrist(s) — *see* Burn, arm(s),
        multiple sites
    first degree 943.14
    second degree 943.24
    third degree 943.34
      deep 943.44
        with loss of body part 943.54
  back 942.04
    with
      trunk — *see* Burn, trunk, multiple
        sites
    first degree 942.14
    second degree 942.24
    third degree 942.34
      deep 942.44
        with loss of body part 942.54
  biceps
    brachii — *see* Burn, arm(s), upper
    femoris — *see* Burn, thigh
  breast(s) 942.01
    with
      trunk — *see* Burn, trunk, multiple
        sites
    first degree 942.11
    second degree 942.21
    third degree 942.31
      deep 942.41
        with loss of body part 942.51
  brow — *see* Burn, forehead
  buttock(s) — *see* Burn, back
  canthus (eye) 940.1
    chemical 940.0
  cervix (uteri) 947.4
  cheek (cutaneous) 941.07
    with
      face or head — *see* Burn, head, mul-
        tiple sites
    first degree 941.17
    second degree 941.27
    third degree 941.37
      deep 941.47
        with loss of body part 941.57
  chest wall (anterior) 942.02
    with
      trunk — *see* Burn, trunk, multiple
        sites
    first degree 942.12
    second degree 942.22
    third degree 942.32
      deep 942.42
        with loss of body part 942.52
  chin 941.04
    with
      face or head — *see* Burn, head, mul-
        tiple sites
    first degree 941.14
    second degree 941.24
    third degree 941.34
      deep 941.44
        with loss of body part 941.54
  clitoris — *see* Burn, genitourinary organs,
    external
  colon 947.3
  conjunctiva (and cornea) 940.4
    chemical
      acid 940.3
      alkaline 940.2
  cornea (and conjunctiva) 940.4
    chemical
      acid 940.3
      alkaline 940.2
  costal region — *see* Burn, chest wall
  due to ingested chemical agent — *see* Burn,
    internal organs
  ear (auricle) (canal) (drum) (external) 941.01

Burn — *continued*
  ear — *continued*
    with
      face or head — *see* Burn, head, mul-
        tiple sites
    first degree 941.11
    second degree 941.21
    third degree 941.31
      deep 941.41
        with loss of a body part 941.51
  elbow 943.02
    with
      hand(s) and wrist(s) — *see* Burn,
        multiple specified sites
      upper limb(s), except hand(s) or
        wrist(s) (*see also* Burn, arm(s),
        multiple sites)
    first degree 943.12
    second degree 943.22
    third degree 943.32
      deep 943.42
        with loss of body part 943.52
  electricity, electric current — *see* Burn, by
    site
  entire body — *see* Burn, multiple, specified
    sites
  epididymis — *see* Burn, genitourinary or-
    gans, external
  epigastric region — *see* Burn, abdomen
  epiglottis 947.1
  esophagus 947.2
  extent (percent of body surface)
    less than 10 percent 948.0 ☑
    10-19 percent 948.1 ☑
    20-29 percent 948.2 ☑
    30-39 percent 948.3 ☑
    40-49 percent 948.4 ☑
    50-59 percent 948.5 ☑
    60-69 percent 948.6 ☑
    70-79 percent 948.7 ☑
    80-89 percent 948.8 ☑
    90 percent or more 948.9 ☑
  extremity
    lower — *see* Burn, leg
    upper — *see* Burn, arm(s)
  eye(s) (and adnexa) (only) 940.9
    with
      face, head, or neck 941.02
        first degree 941.12
        second degree 941.22
        third degree 941.32
          deep 941.42
            with loss of body part
              941.52
      other sites (classifiable to more than
        one category in 940–945) —
        see Burn, multiple, specified
        sites
      resulting rupture and destruction of
        eyeball 940.5
    specified part — *see* Burn, by site
  eyeball (*see also* Burn, eye)
    with resulting rupture and destruction
      of eyeball 940.5
  eyelid(s) 940.1
    chemical 940.0
  face — *see* Burn, head
  finger (nail) (subungual) 944.01
    with
      hand(s) — *see* Burn, hand(s), multi-
        ple sites
      other sites — *see* Burn, multiple,
        specified sites
      thumb 944.04
        first degree 944.14
        second degree 944.24
        third degree 944.34
          deep 944.44
            with loss of body part
              944.54
    first degree 944.11
    second degree 944.21
    third degree 944.31
      deep 944.41
        with loss of body part 944.51
    multiple (digits) 944.03

Burn — *continued*
  finger — *continued*
    multiple — *continued*
      with thumb — *see* Burn, finger, with
        thumb
      first degree 944.13
      second degree 944.23
      third degree 944.33
        deep 944.43
          with loss of body part 944.53
  flank — *see* Burn, abdomen
  foot 945.02
    with
      lower limb(s) — *see* Burn, leg, multi-
        ple sites
    first degree 945.12
    second degree 945.22
    third degree 945.32
      deep 945.42
        with loss of body part 945.52
  forearm(s) 943.01
    with
      upper limb(s), except hand(s) or
        wrist(s) — *see* Burn, arm(s),
        multiple sites
    first degree 943.11
    second degree 943.21
    third degree 943.31
      deep 943.41
        with loss of body part 943.51
  forehead 941.07
    with
      face or head — *see* Burn, head, mul-
        tiple sites
    first degree 941.17
    second degree 941.27
    third degree 941.37
      deep 941.47
        with loss of body part 941.57
  fourth degree — *see* Burn, by site, third de-
    gree, deep
  friction — *see* Injury, superficial, by site
  from swallowing caustic or corrosive sub-
    stance NEC — *see* Burn, internal or-
    gans
  full thickness — *see* Burn, by site, third de-
    gree
  gastrointestinal tract 947.3
  genitourinary organs
    external 942.05
      with
        trunk — *see* Burn, trunk, multiple
          sites
      first degree 942.15
      second degree 942.25
      third degree 942.35
        deep 942.45
          with loss of body part 942.55
    internal 947.8
  globe (eye) — *see* Burn, eyeball
  groin — *see* Burn, abdomen
  gum 947.0
  hand(s) (phalanges) (and wrist) 944.00
    first degree 944.10
    second degree 944.20
    third degree 944.30
      deep 944.40
        with loss of body part 944.50
    back (dorsal surface) 944.06
      first degree 944.16
      second degree 944.26
      third degree 944.36
        deep 944.46
          with loss of body part 944.56
    multiple sites 944.08
      first degree 944.18
      second degree 944.28
      third degree 944.38
        deep 944.48
          with loss of body part 944.58
  head (and face) 941.00
    first degree 941.10
    second degree 941.20
    third degree 941.30
      deep 941.40
        with loss of body part 941.50

Burn — *continued*
  head — *continued*
    eye(s) only 940.9
      specified part — *see* Burn, by site
    multiple sites 941.09
      with eyes — *see* Burn, eyes, with
        face, head, or neck
      first degree 941.19
      second degree 941.29
      third degree 941.39
        deep 941.49
          with loss of body part 941.59
  heel — *see* Burn, foot
  hip — *see* Burn, trunk, specified site NEC
  iliac region — *see* Burn, trunk, specified site
    NEC
  infected 958.3
  inhalation (*see also* Burn, internal organs)
    947.9
  internal organs 947.9
    from caustic or corrosive substance
      (swallowing) NEC 947.9
    specified NEC (*see also* Burn, by site)
      947.8
  interscapular region — *see* Burn, back
  intestine (large) (small) 947.3
  iris — *see* Burn, eyeball
  knee 945.05
    with
      lower limb(s) — *see* Burn, leg, multi-
        ple sites
    first degree 945.15
    second degree 945.25
    third degree 945.35
      deep 945.45
        with loss of body part 945.55
  labium (majus) (minus) — *see* Burn, geni-
    tourinary organs, external
  lacrimal apparatus, duct, gland, or sac 940.1
    chemical 940.0
  larynx 947.1
  late effect — *see* Late, effects (of), burn
  leg 945.00
    first degree 945.10
    second degree 945.20
    third degree 945.30
      deep 945.40
        with loss of body part 945.50
    lower 945.04
      with other part(s) of lower limb(s) —
        see Burn, leg, multiple sites
      first degree 945.14
      second degree 945.24
      third degree 945.34
        deep 945.44
          with loss of body part 945.54
    multiple sites 945.09
      first degree 945.19
      second degree 945.29
      third degree 945.39
        deep 945.49
          with loss of body part 945.59
    upper — *see* Burn, thigh
  lightning — *see* Burn, by site
  limb(s)
    lower (including foot or toe(s)) — *see*
      Burn, leg
    upper (except wrist and hand) — *see*
      Burn, arm(s)
  lip(s) 941.03
    with
      face or head — *see* Burn, head, mul-
        tiple sites
    first degree 941.13
    second degree 941.23
    third degree 941.33
      deep 941.43
        with loss of body part 941.53
  lumbar region — *see* Burn, back
  lung 947.1
  malar region — *see* Burn, cheek
  mastoid region — *see* Burn, scalp
  membrane, tympanic — *see* Burn, ear
  midthoracic region — *see* Burn, chest wall
  mouth 947.0
  multiple (*see also* Burn, unspecified) 949.0

☑ **Additional Digit Required** — Refer to the Tabular List for Digit Selection   ▽ **Subterms under main terms may continue to next column or page**

Burn — continued

multiple (see also Burn, unspecified) — continued

  specified sites classifiable to more than one category in

    940-945 ☑, 946.0

     first degree 946.1

     second degree 946.2

     third degree 946.3

      deep 946.4

       with loss of body part 946.5

muscle, abdominal — see Burn, abdomen

nasal (septum) — see Burn, nose

neck 941.08

  with

    face or head — see Burn, head, multiple sites

  first degree 941.18

  second degree 941.28

  third degree 941.38

    deep 941.48

     with loss of body part 941.58

nose (septum) 941.05

  with

    face or head — see Burn, head, multiple sites

  first degree 941.15

  second degree 941.25

  third degree 941.35

    deep 941.45

     with loss of body part 941.55

occipital region — see Burn, scalp

orbit region 940.1

  chemical 940.0

oronasopharynx 947.0

palate 947.0

palm(s) 944.05

  with

    hand(s) and wrist(s) — see Burn, hand(s), multiple sites

  first degree 944.15

  second degree 944.25

  third degree 944.35

    deep 944.45

     with loss of a body part 944.55

parietal region — see Burn, scalp

penis — see Burn, genitourinary organs, external

perineum — see Burn, genitourinary organs, external

periocular area 940.1

  chemical 940.0

pharynx 947.0

pleura 947.1

popliteal space — see Burn, knee

prepuce — see Burn, genitourinary organs, external

pubic region — see Burn, genitourinary organs, external

pudenda — see Burn, genitourinary organs, external

rectum 947.3

sac, lacrimal 940.1

  chemical 940.0

sacral region — see Burn, back

salivary (ducts) (glands) 947.0

scalp 941.06

  with

    face or neck — see Burn, head, multiple sites

  first degree 941.16

  second degree 941.26

  third degree 941.36

    deep 941.46

     with loss of body part 941.56

scapular region 943.06

  with

    upper limb(s), except hand(s) or wrist(s) — see Burn, arm(s), multiple sites

  first degree 943.16

  second degree 943.26

  third degree 943.36

    deep 943.46

     with loss of body part 943.56

sclera — see Burn, eyeball

Burn — continued

scrotum — see Burn, genitourinary organs, external

septum, nasal — see Burn, nose

shoulder(s) 943.05

  with

    hand(s) and wrist(s) — see Burn, multiple, specified sites

    upper limb(s), except hand(s) or wrist(s) — see Burn, arm(s), multiple sites

  first degree 943.15

  second degree 943.25

  third degree 943.35

    deep 943.45

     with loss of body part 943.55

skin NEC (see also Burn, unspecified) 949.0

skull — see Burn, head

small intestine 947.3

sternal region — see Burn, chest wall

stomach 947.3

subconjunctival — see Burn, conjunctiva

subcutaneous — see Burn, by site, third degree

submaxillary region — see Burn, head

submental region — see Burn, chin

sun — see Sunburn

supraclavicular fossa — see Burn, neck

supraorbital — see Burn, forehead

temple — see Burn, scalp

temporal region — see Burn, scalp

testicle — see Burn, genitourinary organs, external

testis — see Burn, genitourinary organs, external

thigh 945.06

  with

    lower limb(s) — see Burn, leg, multiple sites

  first degree 945.16

  second degree 945.26

  third degree 945.36

    deep 945.46

     with loss of body part 945.56

thorax (external) — see Burn, chest wall

throat 947.0

thumb(s) (nail) (subungual) 944.02

  with

    finger(s) — see Burn, finger, with other sites, thumb

    hand(s) and wrist(s) — see Burn, hand(s), multiple sites

  first degree 944.12

  second degree 944.22

  third degree 944.32

    deep 944.42

     with loss of body part 944.52

toe (nail) (subungual) 945.01

  with

    lower limb(s) — see Burn, leg, multiple sites

  first degree 945.11

  second degree 945.21

  third degree 945.31

    deep 945.41

     with loss of body part 945.51

tongue 947.0

tonsil 947.0

trachea 947.1

trunk 942.00

  first degree 942.10

  second degree 942.20

  third degree 942.30

    deep 942.40

     with loss of body part 942.50

  multiple sites 942.09

    first degree 942.19

    second degree 942.29

    third degree 942.39

     deep 942.49

      with loss of body part 942.59

  specified site NEC 942.09

    first degree 942.19

    second degree 942.29

    third degree 942.39

     deep 942.49

Burn — continued

trunk — continued

  specified site — continued

    third degree — continued

     deep — continued

      with loss of body part 942.59

tunica vaginalis — see Burn, genitourinary organs, external

tympanic membrane — see Burn, ear

tympanum — see Burn, ear

ultraviolet 692.82

unspecified site (multiple) 949.0

  with extent of body surface involved specified

    less than 10 percent 948.0 ☑

    10-19 percent 948.1 ☑

    20-29 percent 948.2 ☑

    30-39 percent 948.3 ☑

    40-49 percent 948.4 ☑

    50-59 percent 948.5 ☑

    60-69 percent 948.6 ☑

    70-79 percent 948.7 ☑

    80-89 percent 948.8 ☑

    90 percent or more 948.9 ☑

  first degree 949.1

  second degree 949.2

  third degree 949.3

    deep 949.4

     with loss of body part 949.5

uterus 947.4

uvula 947.0

vagina 947.4

vulva — see Burn, genitourinary organs, external

wrist(s) 944.07

  with

    hand(s) — see Burn, hand(s), multiple sites

  first degree 944.17

  second degree 944.27

  third degree 944.37

    deep 944.47

     with loss of body part 944.57

Burnett's syndrome (milk-alkali) 275.42

Burnier's syndrome (hypophyseal dwarfism) 253.3

Burning

  feet syndrome 266.2

  sensation (see also Disturbance, sensation) 782.0

  tongue 529.6

Burns' disease (osteochondrosis, lower ulna) 732.3

Bursa — see also condition

  pharynx 478.29

Bursitis NEC 727.3

  Achilles tendon 726.71

  adhesive 726.90

    shoulder 726.0

  ankle 726.79

  buttock 726.5

  calcaneal 726.79

  collateral ligament

    fibular 726.63

    tibial 726.62

  Duplay's 726.2

  elbow 726.33

  finger 726.8

  foot 726.79

  gonococcal 098.52

  hand 726.4

  hip 726.5

  infrapatellar 726.69

  ischiogluteal 726.5

  knee 726.60

  occupational NEC 727.2

  olecranon 726.33

  pes anserinus 726.61

  pharyngeal 478.29

  popliteal 727.51

  prepatellar 726.65

  radiohumeral 727.3

  scapulohumeral 726.19

    adhesive 726.0

  shoulder 726.10

    adhesive 726.0

Bursitis — continued

  subacromial 726.19

    adhesive 726.0

  subcoracoid 726.19

  subdeltoid 726.19

    adhesive 726.0

  subpatellar 726.69

  syphilitic 095.7

  Thornwaldt's, Tornwaldt's (pharyngeal) 478.29

  toe 726.79

  trochanteric area 726.5

  wrist 726.4

Burst stitches or sutures (complication of surgery) (external) (see also Dehiscence) 998.32

  internal 998.31

Buruli ulcer 031.1

Bury's disease (erythema elevatum diutinum) 695.89

Buschke's disease or scleredema (adultorum) 710.1

Busquet's disease (osteoperiostitis) — see also Osteomyelitis 730.1 ☑

Busse-Buschke disease (cryptococcosis) 117.5

Buttock — see condition

Button

  Biskra 085.1

  Delhi 085.1

  oriental 085.1

Buttonhole hand (intrinsic) 736.21

Bwamba fever (encephalitis) 066.3

Byssinosis (occupational) 504

Bywaters' syndrome 958.5

C

Cacergasia 300.9

Cachexia 799.4

  cancerous (see also Neoplasm, by site, malignant) 799.4

  cardiac — see Disease, heart

  dehydration 276.51

    with

     hypernatremia 276.0

     hyponatremia 276.1

  due to malnutrition 799.4

  exophthalmic 242.0 ☑

  heart — see Disease, heart

  hypophyseal 253.2

  hypopituitary 253.2

  lead 984.9

    specified type of lead — see Table of Drugs and Chemicals

  malaria 084.9

  malignant (see also Neoplasm, by site, malignant) 799.4

  marsh 084.9

  nervous 300.5

  old age 797

  pachydermic — see Hypothyroidism

  paludal 084.9

  pituitary (postpartum) 253.2

  renal (see also Disease, renal) 593.9

  saturnine 984.9

    specified type of lead — see Table of Drugs and Chemicals

  senile 797

  Simmonds' (pituitary cachexia) 253.2

  splenica 289.59

  strumipriva (see also Hypothyroidism) 244.9

  tuberculous NEC (see also Tuberculosis) 011.9 ☑

Café au lait spots 709.09

Caffey's disease or syndrome (infantile cortical hyperostosis) 756.59

Caisson disease 993.3

Caked breast (puerperal, postpartum) 676.2 ☑

Cake kidney 753.3

Calabar swelling 125.2

Calcaneal spur 726.73

Calcaneoapophysitis 732.5

Calcaneonavicular bar 755.67

Calcareous — see condition

Calcicosis (occupational) 502

Calciferol (vitamin D) **deficiency** 268.9

☑ Additional Digit Required — Refer to the Tabular List for Digit Selection

▽ Subterms under main terms may continue to next column or page

40 — Volume 2

▶◀ Revised Text

● New Line

▲ Revised Code

2015 ICD-9-CM

Calciferol (vitamin D) **deficiency** — *continued*
  with
    osteomalacia 268.2
    rickets (*see also* Rickets) 268.0

Calcification
  adrenal (capsule) (gland) 255.41
    tuberculous (*see also* Tuberculosis)
      017.6 ☑
  aorta 440.0
  artery (annular) — *see* Arteriosclerosis
  auricle (ear) 380.89
  bladder 596.89
    due to S. hematobium 120.0
  brain (cortex) — *see* Calcification, cerebral
  bronchus 519.19
  bursa 727.82
  cardiac (*see also* Degeneration, myocardial) 429.1
  cartilage (postinfectional) 733.99
  cerebral (cortex) 348.89
    artery 437.0
  cervix (uteri) 622.8
  choroid plexus 349.2
  conjunctiva 372.54
  corpora cavernosa (penis) 607.89
  cortex (brain) — *see* Calcification, cerebral
  dental pulp (nodular) 522.2
  dentinal papilla 520.4
  disc, intervertebral 722.90
    cervical, cervicothoracic 722.91
    lumbar, lumbosacral 722.93
    thoracic, thoracolumbar 722.92
  fallopian tube 620.8
  falx cerebri — *see* Calcification, cerebral
  fascia 728.89
  gallbladder 575.8
  general 275.40
  heart (*see also* Degeneration, myocardial) 429.1
    valve — *see* Endocarditis
  intervertebral cartilage or disc (postinfectional) 722.90
    cervical, cervicothoracic 722.91
    lumbar, lumbosacral 722.93
    thoracic, thoracolumbar 722.92
  intracranial — *see* Calcification, cerebral
  intraspinal ligament 728.89
  joint 719.80
    ankle 719.87
    elbow 719.82
    foot 719.87
    hand 719.84
    hip 719.85
    knee 719.86
    multiple sites 719.89
    pelvic region 719.85
    shoulder (region) 719.81
    specified site NEC 719.88
    wrist 719.83
  kidney 593.89
    tuberculous (*see also* Tuberculosis) 016.0 ☑
  larynx (senile) 478.79
  lens 366.8
  ligament 728.89
    intraspinal 728.89
    knee (medial collateral) 717.89
  lung 518.89
    active 518.89
    postinfectional 518.89
    tuberculous (*see also* Tuberculosis, pulmonary) 011.9 ☑
  lymph gland or node (postinfectional) 289.3
    tuberculous (*see also* Tuberculosis, lymph gland) 017.2 ☑
  mammographic 793.89
  massive (paraplegic) 728.10
  medial NEC (*see also* Arteriosclerosis, extremities) 440.20
  meninges (cerebral) 349.2
  metastatic 275.40
  Mönckeberg's — *see* Arteriosclerosis
  muscle 728.10
    heterotopic, postoperative 728.13

Calcification — *continued*
  myocardium, myocardial (*see also* Degeneration, myocardial) 429.1
  ovary 620.8
  pancreas 577.8
  penis 607.89
  periarticular 728.89
  pericardium (*see also* Pericarditis) 423.8
  pineal gland 259.8
  pleura 511.0
    postinfectional 518.89
    tuberculous (*see also* Tuberculosis, pleura) 012.0 ☑
  pulp (dental) (nodular) 522.2
  renal 593.89
  Rider's bone 733.99
  sclera 379.16
  semilunar cartilage 717.89
  spleen 289.59
  subcutaneous 709.3
  suprarenal (capsule) (gland) 255.41
  tendon (sheath) 727.82
    with bursitis, synovitis or tenosynovitis 727.82
  trachea 519.19
  ureter 593.89
  uterus 621.8
  vitreous 379.29

Calcified — *see also* Calcification
  hematoma NEC 959.9

Calcinosis (generalized) (interstitial) (tumoral) (universalis) 275.49
  circumscripta 709.3
  cutis 709.3
  intervertebralis 275.49 *[722.90]*
  Raynaud's phenomenonsclerodactylytelangiectasis (CRST) 710.1

Calciphylaxis — *see also* Calcification, by site 275.49

Calcium
  blood
    high (*see also* Hypercalcemia) 275.42
    low (*see also* Hypocalcemia) 275.41
  deposits (*see also* Calcification, by site)
    in bursa 727.82
    in tendon (sheath) 727.82
      with bursitis, synovitis or tenosynovitis 727.82
  salts or soaps in vitreous 379.22

Calciuria 791.9

Calculi — *see* Calculus

Calculosis, intrahepatic — *see* Choledocholithiasis

Calculus, calculi, calculous 592.9
  ampulla of Vater — *see* Choledocholithiasis
  anuria (impacted) (recurrent) 592.0
  appendix 543.9
  bile duct (any) — *see* Choledocholithiasis
  biliary — *see* Cholelithiasis
  bilirubin, multiple — *see* Cholelithiasis
  bladder (encysted) (impacted) (urinary) 594.1
    diverticulum 594.0
  bronchus 518.89
  calyx (kidney) (renal) 592.0
    congenital 753.3
  cholesterol (pure) (solitary) — *see* Cholelithiasis
  common duct (bile) — *see* Choledocholithiasis
  conjunctiva 372.54
  cystic 594.1
    duct — *see* Cholelithiasis
  dental 523.6
    subgingival 523.6
    supragingival 523.6
  epididymis 608.89
  gallbladder (*see also* Cholelithiasis)
    congenital 751.69
  hepatic (duct) — *see* Choledocholithiasis
  intestine (impaction) (obstruction) 560.39
  kidney (impacted) (multiple) (pelvis) (recurrent) (staghorn) 592.0
    congenital 753.3
  lacrimal (passages) 375.57
  liver (impacted) — *see* Choledocholithiasis

Calculus, calculi, calculous — *continued*
  lung 518.89
  mammographic 793.89
  nephritic (impacted) (recurrent) 592.0
  nose 478.19
  pancreas (duct) 577.8
  parotid gland 527.5
  pelvis, encysted 592.0
  prostate 602.0
  pulmonary 518.89
  renal (impacted) (recurrent) 592.0
    congenital 753.3
  salivary (duct) (gland) 527.5
  seminal vesicle 608.89
  staghorn 592.0
  Stensen's duct 527.5
  sublingual duct or gland 527.5
    congenital 750.26
  submaxillary duct, gland, or region 527.5
  suburethral 594.8
  tonsil 474.8
  tooth, teeth 523.6
  tunica vaginalis 608.89
  ureter (impacted) (recurrent) 592.1
  urethra (impacted) 594.2
  urinary (duct) (impacted) (passage) (tract) 592.9
    lower tract NEC 594.9
      specified site 594.8
  vagina 623.8
  vesical (impacted) 594.1
  Wharton's duct 527.5

Caliectasis 593.89

California
  disease 114.0
  encephalitis 062.5

Caligo cornea 371.03

Callositas, callosity (infected) 700

Callus (infected) 700
  bone 726.91
  excessive, following fracture (*see also* Late, effect (of), fracture)

Calvé (-Perthes) disease (osteochondrosis, femoral capital) 732.1

Calvities — *see also* Alopecia 704.00

Cameroon fever — *see also* Malaria 084.6

Camptocormia 300.11

Camptodactyly (congenital) 755.59

Camurati-Engelmann disease (diaphyseal sclerosis) 756.59

Canal — *see* condition

Canaliculitis (lacrimal) (acute) 375.31
  Actinomyces 039.8
  chronic 375.41

Canavan's disease 330.0

Cancer (M8000/3) — *see also* Neoplasm, by site, malignant

> *Note* — The term "cancer" when modified by an adjective or adjectival phrase indicating a morphological type should be coded in the same manner as "carcinoma" with that adjective or phrase. Thus, "squamous-cell cancer" should be coded in the same manner as "squamous-cell carcinoma," which appears in the list under "Carcinoma."

  bile duct type (M8160/3), liver 155.1
  hepatocellular (M8170/3) 155.0

Cancerous (M8000/3) — *see* Neoplasm, by site, malignant

Cancerphobia 300.29

Cancrum oris 528.1

Candidiasis, candidal 112.9
  with pneumonia 112.4
  balanitis 112.2
  congenital 771.7
  disseminated 112.5
  endocarditis 112.81
  esophagus 112.84
  intertrigo 112.3
  intestine 112.85
  lung 112.4
  meningitis 112.83
  mouth 112.0
  nails 112.3
  neonatal 771.7

Candidiasis, candidal — *continued*
  onychia 112.3
  otitis externa 112.82
  otomycosis 112.82
  paronychia 112.3
  perionyxis 112.3
  pneumonia 112.4
  pneumonitis 112.4
  skin 112.3
  specified site NEC 112.89
  systemic 112.5
  urogenital site NEC 112.2
  vagina 112.1
  vulva 112.1
  vulvovaginitis 112.1

Candidosis — *see* Candidiasis

Candiru infection or infestation 136.8

Canities (premature) 704.3
  congenital 757.4

Canker (mouth) (sore) 528.2
  rash 034.1

Cannabinosis 504

Canton fever 081.9

Cap
  cradle 690.11

Capillariasis 127.5

Capillary — *see* condition

Caplan-Colinet syndrome 714.81

Caplan's syndrome 714.81

Capsule — *see* condition

Capsulitis (joint) 726.90
  adhesive (shoulder) 726.0
  hip 726.5
  knee 726.60
  labyrinthine 387.8
  thyroid 245.9
  wrist 726.4

Caput
  crepitus 756.0
  medusae 456.8
  succedaneum 767.19

Carapata disease 087.1

Carate — *see* Pinta

Carbohydrate-deficient glycoprotein syndrome (CGDS) 271.8

Carboxyhemoglobinemia 986

Carbuncle 680.9
  abdominal wall 680.2
  ankle 680.6
  anus 680.5
  arm (any part, above wrist) 680.3
  auditory canal, external 680.0
  axilla 680.3
  back (any part) 680.2
  breast 680.2
  buttock 680.5
  chest wall 680.2
  corpus cavernosum 607.2
  ear (any part) (external) 680.0
  eyelid 373.13
  face (any part, except eye) 680.0
  finger (any) 680.4
  flank 680.2
  foot (any part) 680.7
  forearm 680.3
  genital organ (male) 608.4
  gluteal (region) 680.5
  groin 680.2
  hand (any part) 680.4
  head (any part, except face) 680.8
  heel 680.7
  hip 680.6
  kidney (*see also* Abscess, kidney) 590.2
  knee 680.6
  labia 616.4
  lacrimal
    gland (*see also* Dacryoadenitis) 375.00
    passages (duct) (sac) (*see also* Dacryocystitis) 375.30
  leg, any part except foot 680.6
  lower extremity, any part except foot 680.6
  malignant 022.0
  multiple sites 680.9
  neck 680.1
  nose (external) (septum) 680.0
  orbit, orbital 376.01

☑ **Additional Digit Required** — Refer to the Tabular List for Digit Selection   ᵛ⁴ **Subterms under main terms may continue to next column or page**

2015 ICD-9-CM   ▶◀ Revised Text   ● New Line   ▲ Revised Code   **Volume 2 — 41**

Carbuncle — *continued*
partes posteriores 680.5
pectoral region 680.2
penis 607.2
perineum 680.2
pinna 680.0
scalp (any part) 680.8
scrotum 608.4
seminal vesicle 608.0
shoulder 680.3
skin NEC 680.9
specified site NEC 680.8
spermatic cord 608.4
temple (region) 680.0
testis 608.4
thigh 680.6
thumb 680.4
toe (any) 680.7
trunk 680.2
tunica vaginalis 608.4
umbilicus 680.2
upper arm 680.3
urethra 597.0
vas deferens 608.4
vulva 616.4
wrist 680.4
Carbunculus — *see also* Carbuncle 680.9
Carcinoid (tumor) (M8240/1) — *see* Tumor, carcinoid
Carcinoidosis 259.2
Carcinomaphobia 300.29
Carcinomatosis
peritonei (M8010/6) 197.6
specified site NEC (M8010/3) — *see* Neoplasm, by site, malignant
unspecified site (M8010/6) 199.0
Carcinoma (M8010/3) — *see also* Neoplasm, by site, malignant

---

Note — *Except where otherwise indicated, the morphological varieties of carcinoma in the list below should be coded by site as for "Neoplasm, malignant."*

---

with
apocrine metaplasia (M8573/3)
cartilaginous (and osseous) metaplasia (M8571/3)
osseous (and cartilaginous) metaplasia (M8571/3)
productive fibrosis (M8141/3)
spindle cell metaplasia (M8572/3)
squamous metaplasia (M8570/3)
acidophil (M8280/3)
specified site — *see* Neoplasm, by site, malignant
unspecified site 194.3
acidophil-basophil, mixed (M8281/3)
specified site — *see* Neoplasm, by site, malignant
unspecified site 194.3
acinar (cell) (M8550/3)
acinic cell (M8550/3)
adenocystic (M8200/3)
adenoid
cystic (M8200/3)
squamous cell (M8075/3)
adenosquamous (M8560/3)
adnexal (skin) (M8390/3) — *see* Neoplasm, skin, malignant
adrenal cortical (M8370/3) 194.0
alveolar (M8251/3)
cell (M8250/3) — *see* Neoplasm, lung, malignant
anaplastic type (M8021/3)
apocrine (M8401/3)
breast — *see* Neoplasm, breast, malignant
specified site NEC — *see* Neoplasm, skin, malignant
unspecified site 173.99
basal cell (pigmented) (M8090/3) (*see also* Neoplasm, skin, malignant) 173.91
fibro-epithelial type (M8093/3) — *see* Neoplasm, skin, malignant
morphea type (M8092/3) — *see* Neoplasm, skin, malignant

Carcinoma — *see also* Neoplasm, by site, malignant — *continued*
basal cell (*see also* Neoplasm, skin, malignant) — *continued*
multicentric (M8091/3) — *see* Neoplasm, skin, malignant
basaloid (M8123/3)
basal-squamous cell, mixed (M8094/3) — *see* Neoplasm, skin, malignant
basophil (M8300/3)
specified site — *see* Neoplasm, by site, malignant
unspecified site 194.3
basophil-acidophil, mixed (M8281/3)
specified site — *see* Neoplasm, by site, malignant
unspecified site 194.3
basosquamous (M8094/3) — *see* Neoplasm, skin, malignant
bile duct type (M8160/3)
and hepatocellular, mixed (M8180/3) 155.0
liver 155.1
specified site NEC — *see* Neoplasm, by site, malignant
unspecified site 155.1
branchial or branchiogenic 146.8
bronchial or bronchogenic — *see* Neoplasm, lung, malignant
bronchiolar (terminal) (M8250/3) — *see* Neoplasm, lung, malignant
bronchiolo-alveolar (M8250/3) — *see* Neoplasm, lung, malignant
bronchogenic (epidermoid) 162.9
C cell (M8510/3)
specified site — *see* Neoplasm, by site, malignant
unspecified site 193
ceruminous (M8420/3) 173.29
chorionic (M9100/3)
specified site — *see* Neoplasm, by site, malignant
unspecified site
female 181
male 186.9
chromophobe (M8270/3)
specified site — *see* Neoplasm, by site, malignant
unspecified site 194.3
clear cell (mesonephroid type) (M8310/3)
cloacogenic (M8124/3)
specified site — *see* Neoplasm, by site, malignant
unspecified site 154.8
colloid (M8480/3)
cribriform (M8201/3)
cylindroid type (M8200/3)
diffuse type (M8145/3)
specified site — *see* Neoplasm, by site, malignant
unspecified site 151.9
duct (cell) (M8500/3)
with Paget's disease (M8541/3) — *see* Neoplasm, breast, malignant
infiltrating (M8500/3)
specified site — *see* Neoplasm, by site, malignant
unspecified site 174.9
ductal (M8500/3)
ductular, infiltrating (M8521/3)
embryonal (M9070/3)
and teratoma, mixed (M9081/3)
combined with choriocarcinoma (M9101/3) — *see* Neoplasm, by site, malignant
infantile type (M9071/3)
liver 155.0
polyembryonal type (M9072/3)
endometrioid (M8380/3)
eosinophil (M8280/3)
specified site — *see* Neoplasm, by site, malignant
unspecified site 194.3
epidermoid (M8070/3) (*see also* Carcinoma, squamous cell)

Carcinoma — *see also* Neoplasm, by site, malignant — *continued*
epidermoid (*see also* Carcinoma, squamous cell) — *continued*
and adenocarcinoma, mixed (M8560/3)
in situ, Bowen's type (M8081/2) — *see* Neoplasm, skin, in situ
intradermal — *see* Neoplasm, skin, in situ
fibroepithelial type basal cell (M8093/3) — *see* Neoplasm, skin, malignant
follicular (M8330/3)
and papillary (mixed) (M8340/3) 193
moderately differentiated type (M8332/3) 193
pure follicle type (M8331/3) 193
specified site — *see* Neoplasm, by site, malignant
trabecular type (M8332/3) 193
unspecified site 193
well differentiated type (M8331/3) 193
gelatinous (M8480/3)
giant cell (M8031/3)
and spindle cell (M8030/3)
granular cell (M8320/3)
granulosa cell (M8620/3) 183.0
hepatic cell (M8170/3) 155.0
hepatocellular (M8170/3) 155.0
and bile duct, mixed (M8180/3) 155.0
hepatocholangiolitic (M8180/3) 155.0
Hürthle cell (thyroid) 193
hypernephroid (M8311/3)
in
adenomatous
polyp (M8210/3)
polyposis coli (M8220/3) 153.9
pleomorphic adenoma (M8940/3)
polypoid adenoma (M8210/3)
situ (M8010/2) — *see* Carcinoma, in situ
tubular adenoma (M8210/3)
villous adenoma (M8261/3)
infiltrating duct (M8500/3)
with Paget's disease (M8541/3) — *see* Neoplasm, breast, malignant
specified site — *see* Neoplasm, by site, malignant
unspecified site 174.9
inflammatory (M8530/3)
specified site — *see* Neoplasm, by site, malignant
unspecified site 174.9
in situ (M8010/2) (*see also* Neoplasm, by site, in situ)
epidermoid (M8070/2) (*see also* Neoplasm, by site, in situ)
with questionable stromal invasion (M8076/2)
specified site — *see* Neoplasm, by site, in situ
unspecified site 233.1
Bowen's type (M8081/2) — *see* Neoplasm, skin, in situ
intraductal (M8500/2)
specified site — *see* Neoplasm, by site, in situ
unspecified site 233.0
lobular (M8520/2)
specified site — *see* Neoplasm, by site, in situ
unspecified site 233.0
papillary (M8050/2) — *see* Neoplasm, by site, in situ
squamous cell (M8070/2) (*see also* Neoplasm, by site, in situ)
with questionable stromal invasion (M8076/2)
specified site — *see* Neoplasm, by site, in situ
unspecified site 233.1
transitional cell (M8120/2) — *see* Neoplasm, by site, in situ
intestinal type (M8144/3)
specified site — *see* Neoplasm, by site, malignant
unspecified site 151.9

Carcinoma — *see also* Neoplasm, by site, malignant — *continued*
intraductal (noninfiltrating) (M8500/2)
papillary (M8503/2)
specified site — *see* Neoplasm, by site, in situ
unspecified site 233.0
specified site — *see* Neoplasm, by site, in situ
unspecified site 233.0
intraepidermal (M8070/2) (*see also* Neoplasm, skin, in situ)
squamous cell, Bowen's type (M8081/2) — *see* Neoplasm, skin, in situ
intraepithelial (M8010/2) (*see also* Neoplasm, by site, in situ)
squamous cell (M8072/2) — *see* Neoplasm, by site, in situ
intraosseous (M9270/3) 170.1
upper jaw (bone) 170.0
islet cell (M8150/3)
and exocrine, mixed (M8154/3)
specified site — *see* Neoplasm, by site, malignant
unspecified site 157.9
pancreas 157.4
specified site NEC — *see* Neoplasm, by site, malignant
unspecified site 157.4
juvenile, breast (M8502/3) — *see* Neoplasm, breast, malignant
Kulchitsky's cell (carcinoid tumor of intestine) 259.2
large cell (M8012/3)
squamous cell, non-keratinizing type (M8072/3)
Leydig cell (testis) (M8650/3)
specified site — *see* Neoplasm, by site, malignant
unspecified site 186.9
female 183.0
male 186.9
liver cell (M8170/3) 155.0
lobular (infiltrating) (M8520/3)
non-infiltrating (M8520/3)
specified site — *see* Neoplasm, by site, in situ
unspecified site 233.0
specified site — *see* Neoplasm, by site, malignant
unspecified site 174.9
lymphoepithelial (M8082/3)
medullary (M8510/3)
with
amyloid stroma (M8511/3)
specified site — *see* Neoplasm, by site, malignant
unspecified site 193
lymphoid stroma (M8512/3)
specified site — *see* Neoplasm, by site, malignant
unspecified site 174.9
Merkel cell 209.36
buttock 209.36
ear 209.31
eyelid, including canthus 209.31
face 209.31
genitals 209.36
lip 209.31
lower limb 209.34
neck 209.32
nodal presentation 209.75
scalp 209.32
secondary (any site) 209.75
specified site NEC 209.36
trunk 209.35
unknown primary site 209.75
upper limb 209.33
visceral metastatic presentation 209.75
mesometanephric (M9110/3)
mesonephric (M9110/3)
metastatic (M8010/6) — *see* Metastasis, cancer
metatypical (M8095/3) — *see* Neoplasm, skin, malignant

Carcinoma — *see also* Neoplasm, by site, malignant — *continued*
  morphea type basal cell (M8092/3) — *see* Neoplasm, skin, malignant
  mucinous (M8480/3)
  mucin-producing (M8481/3)
  mucin-secreting (M8481/3)
  mucoepidermoid (M8430/3)
  mucoid (M8480/3)
    cell (M8300/3)
      specified site — *see* Neoplasm, by site, malignant
      unspecified site 194.3
  mucous (M8480/3)
  neuroendocrine
    high grade (M8240/3) 209.30
    malignant poorly differentiated (M8240/3) 209.30
  nonencapsulated sclerosing (M8350/3) 193
  noninfiltrating
    intracystic (M8504/2) — *see* Neoplasm, by site, in situ
    intraductal (M8500/2)
      papillary (M8503/2)
        specified site — *see* Neoplasm, by site, in situ
        unspecified site 233.0
      specified site — *see* Neoplasm, by site, in situ
      unspecified site 233.0
    lobular (M8520/2)
      specified site — *see* Neoplasm, by site, in situ
      unspecified site 233.0
  oat cell (M8042/3)
    specified site — *see* Neoplasm, by site, malignant
    unspecified site 162.9
  odontogenic (M9270/3) 170.1
    upper jaw (bone) 170.0
  onocytic (M8290/3)
  oxyphilic (M8290/3)
  papillary (M8050/3)
    and follicular (mixed) (M8340/3) 193
    epidermoid (M8052/3)
    intraductal (noninfiltrating) (M8503/2)
      specified site — *see* Neoplasm, by site, in situ
      unspecified site 233.0
    serous (M8460/3)
      specified site — *see* Neoplasm, by site, malignant
      surface (M8461/3)
        specified site — *see* Neoplasm, by site, malignant
        unspecified site 183.0
      unspecified site 183.0
    squamous cell (M8052/3)
    transitional cell (M8130/3)
  papillocystic (M8450/3)
    specified site — *see* Neoplasm, by site, malignant
    unspecified site 183.0
  parafollicular cell (M8510/3)
    specified site — *see* Neoplasm, by site, malignant
    unspecified site 193
  pleomorphic (M8022/3)
  polygonal cell (M8034/3)
  prickle cell (M8070/3)
  pseudoglandular, squamous cell (M8075/3)
  pseudomucinous (M8470/3)
    specified site — *see* Neoplasm, by site, malignant
    unspecified site 183.0
  pseudosarcomatous (M8033/3)
  regaud type (M8082/3) — *see* Neoplasm, nasopharynx, malignant
  renal cell (M8312/3) 189.0
  reserve cell (M8041/3)
  round cell (M8041/3)
  Schmincke (M8082/3) — *see* Neoplasm, nasopharynx, malignant
  Schneiderian (M8121/3)
    specified site — *see* Neoplasm, by site, malignant

Carcinoma — *see also* Neoplasm, by site, malignant — *continued*
  Schneiderian –– *continued*
    unspecified site 160.0
  scirrhous (M8141/3)
  sebaceous (M8410/3) — *see* Neoplasm, skin, malignant
  secondary (M8010/6) — *see* Neoplasm, by site, malignant, secondary
  secretory, breast (M8502/3) — *see* Neoplasm, breast, malignant
  serous (M8441/3)
    papillary (M8460/3)
      specified site — *see* Neoplasm, by site, malignant
      unspecified site 183.0
    surface, papillary (M8461/3)
      specified site — *see* Neoplasm, by site, malignant
      unspecified site 183.0
  Sertoli cell (M8640/3)
    specified site — *see* Neoplasm, by site, malignant
    unspecified site 186.9
  signet ring cell (M8490/3)
    metastatic (M8490/6) — *see* Neoplasm, by site, secondary
  simplex (M8231/3)
  skin appendage (M8390/3) — *see* Neoplasm, skin, malignant
  small cell (M8041/3)
    fusiform cell type (M8043/3)
    squamous cell, non-keratinizing type (M8073/3)
  solid (M8230/3)
    with amyloid stroma (M8511/3)
      specified site — *see* Neoplasm, by site, malignant
      unspecified site 193
  spheroidal cell (M8035/3)
  spindle cell (M8032/3)
    and giant cell (M8030/3)
  spinous cell (M8070/3)
  squamous (cell) (M8070/3)
    adenoid type (M8075/3)
    and adenocarcinoma, mixed (M8560/3)
    intraepidermal, Bowen's type — *see* Neoplasm, skin, in situ
    keratinizing type (large cell) (M8071/3)
    large cell, non-keratinizing type (M8072/3)
    microinvasive (M8076/3)
      specified site — *see* Neoplasm, by site, malignant
      unspecified site 180.9
    non-keratinizing type (M8072/3)
    papillary (M8052/3)
    pseudoglandular (M8075/3)
    skin (*see also* Neoplasm, skin, malignant) 173.92
    small cell, non-keratinizing type (M8073/3)
    spindle cell type (M8074/3)
    verrucous (M8051/3)
  superficial spreading (M8143/3)
  sweat gland (M8400/3) — *see* Neoplasm, skin, malignant
  theca cell (M8600/3) 183.0
  thymic (M8580/3) 164.0
  trabecular (M8190/3)
  transitional (cell) (M8120/3)
    papillary (M8130/3)
    spindle cell type (M8122/3)
  tubular (M8211/3)
  undifferentiated type (M8020/3)
  urothelial (M8120/3)
  ventriculi (M8211/3)
  verrucous (epidermoid) (squamous cell) (M8051/3)
  villous (M8262/3)
  water-clear cell (M8322/3) 194.1
  wolffian duct (M9110/3)

Carcinosarcoma (M8980/3) — *see also* Neoplasm, by site, malignant
  embryonal type (M8981/3) — *see* Neoplasm, by site, malignant

Cardiac — *see also* condition
  death — *see* Disease, heart
  device
    defibrillator, automatic implantable (with synchronous cardiac pacemaker) V45.02
      in situ NEC V45.00
    pacemaker
      cardiac
        fitting or adjustment V53.31
        in situ V45.01
      carotid sinus
        fitting or adjustment V53.39
        in situ V45.09
    pacemaker — *see* Cardiac, device, pacemaker
    tamponade 423.3
Cardia, cardial — *see* condition
Cardialgia — *see also* Pain, precordial 786.51
Cardiectasis — *see* Hypertrophy, cardiac
Cardiochalasia 530.81
Cardiomalacia — *see also* Degeneration, myocardial 429.1
Cardiomegalia glycogenica diffusa 271.0
Cardiomegaly — *see also* Hypertrophy, cardiac 429.3
  congenital 746.89
  glycogen 271.0
  hypertensive (*see also* Hypertension, heart) 402.90
  idiopathic 429.3
Cardiomyoliposis — *see also* Degeneration, myocardial 429.1
Cardiomyopathy (congestive) (constrictive) (familial) (infiltrative) (obstructive) (restrictive) (sporadic) 425.4
  alcoholic 425.5
  amyloid 277.39 *[425.7]*
  beriberi 265.0 *[425.7]*
  cobalt-beer 425.5
  congenital 425.3
  due to
    amyloidosis 277.39 *[425.7]*
    beriberi 265.0 *[425.7]*
    cardiac glycogenosis 271.0 *[425.7]*
    Chagas' disease 086.0
    Friedreich's ataxia 334.0 *[425.8]*
    hypertension — *see* Hypertension, with, heart involvement
    mucopolysaccharidosis 277.5 *[425.7]*
    myotonia atrophica 359.21 *[425.8]*
    progressive muscular dystrophy 359.1 *[425.8]*
    sarcoidosis 135 *[425.8]*
  glycogen storage 271.0 *[425.7]*
  hypertensive — *see* Hypertension, with, heart involvement
  hypertrophic 425.18
    nonobstructive 425.18
    obstructive 425.11
      congenital 746.84
  idiopathic (concentric) 425.4
  in
    Chagas' disease 086.0
    sarcoidosis 135 *[425.8]*
  ischemic 414.8
  metabolic NEC 277.9 *[425.7]*
    amyloid 277.39 *[425.7]*
    thyrotoxic (*see also* Thyrotoxicosis) 242.9 ☑ *[425.7]*
    thyrotoxicosis (*see also* Thyrotoxicosis) 242.9 ☑ *[425.7]*
  newborn 425.4
    congenital 425.3
  nutritional 269.9 *[425.7]*
    beriberi 265.0 *[425.7]*
  obscure of Africa 425.2
  peripartum 674.5 ☑
  postpartum 674.5 ☑
  primary 425.4
  secondary 425.9
  stress inuced 429.83
  takotsubo 429.83
  thyrotoxic (*see also* Thyrotoxicosis) 242.9 ☑ *[425.7]*
  toxic NEC 425.9

Cardiomyopathy — *continued*
  tuberculous (*see also* Tuberculosis) 017.9 ☑ *[425.8]*
Cardionephritis — *see* Hypertension, cardiorenal
Cardionephropathy — *see* Hypertension, cardiorenal
Cardionephrosis — *see* Hypertension, cardiorenal
Cardioneurosis 306.2
Cardiopathia nigra 416.0
Cardiopathy — *see also* Disease, heart 429.9
  hypertensive (*see also* Hypertension, heart) 402.90
  idiopathic 425.4
  mucopolysaccharidosis 277.5 *[425.7]*
Cardiopericarditis — *see also* Pericarditis 423.9
Cardiophobia 300.29
Cardioptosis 746.87
Cardiorenal — *see* condition
Cardiorrhexis — *see also* Infarct, myocardium 410.9 ☑
Cardiosclerosis — *see* Arteriosclerosis, coronary
Cardiosis — *see* Disease, heart
Cardiospasm (esophagus) (reflex) (stomach) 530.0
  congenital 750.7
Cardiostenosis — *see* Disease, heart
Cardiosymphysis 423.1
Cardiothyrotoxicosis — *see* Hyperthyroidism
Cardiovascular — *see* condition
Carditis (acute) (bacterial) (chronic) (subacute) 429.89
  Coxsackie 074.20
  hypertensive (*see also* Hypertension, heart) 402.90
  meningococcal 036.40
  rheumatic — *see* Disease, heart, rheumatic
  rheumatoid 714.2
Care (of)
  child (routine) V20.1
  convalescent following V66.9
    chemotherapy V66.2
    medical NEC V66.5
    psychotherapy V66.3
    radiotherapy V66.1
    surgery V66.0
    surgical NEC V66.0
    treatment (for) V66.5
      combined V66.6
      fracture V66.4
      mental disorder NEC V66.3
      specified type NEC V66.5
  end-of-life V66.7
  family member (handicapped) (sick)
    creating problem for family V61.49
    provided away from home for holiday relief V60.5
    unavailable, due to
      absence (person rendering care) (sufferer) V60.4
      inability (any reason) of person rendering care V60.4
  holiday relief V60.5
  hospice V66.7
  lack of (at or after birth) (infant) (child) 995.52
    adult 995.84
  lactation of mother V24.1
  palliative V66.7
  postpartum
    immediately after delivery V24.0
    routine follow-up V24.2
  prenatal V22.1
    first pregnancy V22.0
    high-risk pregnancy V23.9
      inconclusive fetal viability V23.87
      specified problem NEC V23.89
  terminal V66.7
  unavailable, due to
    absence of person rendering care V60.4
    inability (any reason) of person rendering care V60.4
  well baby V20.1

☑ Additional Digit Required — Refer to the Tabular List for Digit Selection   ▽ Subterms under main terms may continue to next column or page

2015 ICD-9-CM   ►◄ Revised Text   ● New Line   ▲ Revised Code   **Volume 2 — 43**

Caries (bone) — *see also* Tuberculosis, bone
  015.9 ☑ *[730.8]* ☑
  arrested 521.04
  cementum 521.03
  cerebrospinal (tuberculous)
    015.0 *[730.88]*
  dental (acute) (chronic) (incipient) (infected)
    521.00
    with pulp exposure 521.03
    extending to
      dentine 521.02
      pulp 521.03
    other specified NEC 521.09
    pit and fissure 521.06
    primary
      pit and fissure origin 521.06
      root surface 521.08
      smooth surface origin 521.07
    root surface 521.08
    smooth surface 521.07
  dentin (acute) (chronic) 521.02
  enamel (acute) (chronic) (incipient) 521.01
  external meatus 380.89
  hip (*see also* Tuberculosis) 015.1 *[730.85]*
  initial 521.01
  knee 015.2 ☑ *[730.86]*
  labyrinth 386.8
  limb NEC 015.7 ☑ *[730.88]*
  mastoid (chronic) (process) 383.1
  middle ear 385.89
  nose 015.7 ☑ *[730.88]*
  orbit 015.7 ☑ *[730.88]*
  ossicle 385.24
  petrous bone 383.20
  sacrum (tuberculous) 015.0 ☑ *[730.88]*
  spine, spinal (column) (tuberculous)
    015.0 ☑ *[730.88]*
  syphilitic 095.5
    congenital 090.0 *[730.8]* ☑
  teeth (internal) 521.00
    initial 521.01
  vertebra (column) (tuberculous)
    015.0 ☑ *[730.88]*
Carini's syndrome (ichthyosis congenita) 757.1
Carious teeth 521.00
Carneous mole 631.8
Carnosinemia 270.5
Carotid body or sinus syndrome 337.01
Carotidynia 337.01
Carotinemia (dietary) 278.3
Carotinosis (cutis) (skin) 278.3
Carpal tunnel syndrome 354.0
Carpenter's syndrome 759.89
Carpopedal spasm — *see also* Tetany 781.7
Carpoptosis 736.05
Carrier (suspected) **of**
  amebiasis V02.2
  bacterial disease (meningococcal, staphylo-
    coccal) NEC V02.59
  cholera V02.0
  cystic fibrosis gene V83.81
  defective gene V83.89
  diphtheria V02.4
  dysentery (bacillary) V02.3
    amebic V02.2
  Endamoeba histolytica V02.2
  gastrointestinal pathogens NEC V02.3
  genetic defect V83.89
  gonorrhea V02.7
  group B streptococcus V02.51
  HAA (hepatitis Australian-antigen) V02.61
  hemophilia A (asymptomatic) V83.01
    symptomatic V83.02
  hepatitis V02.60
    Australian-antigen (HAA) V02.61
    B V02.61
    C V02.62
    serum V02.61
    specified type NEC V02.69
    viral V02.60
  infective organism NEC V02.9
  malaria V02.9
  paratyphoid V02.3
  Salmonella V02.3
    typhosa V02.1
  serum hepatitis V02.61

Carrier (suspected) **of** — *continued*
  Shigella V02.3
  Staphylococcus NEC V02.59
    methicillin
      resistant Staphylococcus aureus
        V02.54
      susceptible Staphylococcus aureus
        V02.53
  Streptococcus NEC V02.52
    group B V02.51
  typhoid V02.1
  venereal disease NEC V02.8
Carrión's disease (Bartonellosis) 088.0
Car sickness 994.6
Carter's
  relapsing fever (Asiatic) 087.0
Cartilage — *see* condition
Caruncle (inflamed)
  abscess, lacrimal (*see also* Dacryocystitis)
    375.30
  conjunctiva 372.00
    acute 372.00
  eyelid 373.00
  labium (majus) (minus) 616.89
  lacrimal 375.30
  urethra (benign) 599.3
  vagina (wall) 616.89
Cascade stomach 537.6
Caseation lymphatic gland — *see also* Tuberculosis 017.2 ☑
Caseous
  bronchitis — *see* Tuberculosis, pulmonary
  meningitis 013.0 ☑
  pneumonia — *see* Tuberculosis, pulmonary
Cassidy (-Scholte) syndrome (malignant carcinoid) 259.2
Castellani's bronchitis 104.8
Castleman's tumor or lymphoma (mediastinal lymph node hyperplasia) 785.6
Castration, traumatic 878.2
  complicated 878.3
Casts in urine 791.7
Catalepsy 300.11
  catatonic (acute) (*see also* Schizophrenia)
    295.2 ☑
  hysterical 300.11
  schizophrenic (*see also* Schizophrenia)
    295.2 ☑
Cataphasia — *see also* Disorder, fluency 315.35
Cataplexy (idiopathic) — *see* Narcolepsy
Cataract (anterior cortical) (anterior polar)
  (black) (capsular) (central) (cortical) (hypermature) (immature) (incipient) (mature) 366.9
  anterior
    and posterior axial embryonal 743.33
    pyramidal 743.31
    subcapsular polar
      infantile, juvenile, or presenile 366.01
      senile 366.13
  associated with
    calcinosis 275.40 *[366.42]*
    craniofacial dysostosis 756.0 *[366.44]*
    galactosemia 271.1 *[366.44]*
    hypoparathyroidism 252.1 *[366.42]*
    myotonic disorders 359.21 *[366.43]*
    neovascularization 366.33
  blue dot 743.39
  cerulean 743.39
  complicated NEC 366.30
  congenital 743.30
    capsular or subcapsular 743.31
    cortical 743.32
    nuclear 743.33
    specified type NEC 743.39
    total or subtotal 743.34
    zonular 743.32
  coronary (congenital) 743.39
    acquired 366.12
  cupuliform 366.14
  diabetic 250.5 ☑ *[366.41]*
    due to secondary diabetes
      249.5 ☑ *[366.41]*
  drug-induced 366.45
  due to
    chalcosis 360.24 *[366.34]*

Cataract — *continued*
  due to — *continued*
    chronic choroiditis (*see also* Choroiditis)
      363.20 *[366.32]*
    degenerative myopia 360.21 *[366.34]*
    glaucoma (*see also* Glaucoma)
      365.9 *[366.31]*
    infection, intraocular NEC 366.32
    inflammatory ocular disorder NEC 366.32
    iridocyclitis, chronic 364.10 *[366.33]*
    pigmentary retinal dystrophy
      362.74 *[366.34]*
    radiation 366.46
  electric 366.46
  glassblowers' 366.46
  heat ray 366.46
  heterochromic 366.33
  in eye disease NEC 366.30
  infantile (*see also* Cataract, juvenile) 366.00
  intumescent 366.12
  irradiational 366.46
  juvenile 366.00
    anterior subcapsular polar 366.01
    combined forms 366.09
    cortical 366.03
    lamellar 366.03
    nuclear 366.04
    posterior subcapsular polar 366.02
    specified NEC 366.09
    zonular 366.03
  lamellar 743.32
    infantile, juvenile, or presenile 366.03
  morgagnian 366.18
  myotonic 359.21 *[366.43]*
  myxedema 244.9 *[366.44]*
  nuclear 366.16
  posterior, polar (capsular) 743.31
    infantile, juvenile, or presenile 366.02
    senile 366.14
  presenile (*see also* Cataract, juvenile) 366.00
  punctate
    acquired 366.12
    congenital 743.39
  secondary (membrane) 366.50
    obscuring vision 366.53
    specified type, not obscuring vision
      366.52
  senile 366.10
    anterior subcapsular polar 366.13
    combined forms 366.19
    cortical 366.15
    hypermature 366.18
    immature 366.12
    incipient 366.12
    mature 366.17
    nuclear 366.16
    posterior subcapsular polar 366.14
    specified NEC 366.19
    total or subtotal 366.17
  snowflake 250.5 ☑ *[366.41]*
    due to secondary diabetes
      249.5 ☑ *[366.41]*
  specified NEC 366.8
  subtotal (senile) 366.17
    congenital 743.34
  sunflower 360.24 *[366.34]*
  tetanic NEC 252.1 *[366.42]*
  total (mature) (senile) 366.17
    congenital 743.34
    localized 366.21
    traumatic 366.22
  toxic 366.45
  traumatic 366.20
    partially resolved 366.23
    total 366.22
  zonular (perinuclear) 743.32
    infantile, juvenile, or presenile 366.03
Cataracta 366.10
  brunescens 366.16
  cerulea 743.39
  complicata 366.30
  congenita 743.30
  coralliformis 743.39
  coronaria (congenital) 743.39
    acquired 366.12
  diabetic 250.5 ☑ *[366.41]*

Cataracta — *continued*
  diabetic — *continued*
    due to secondary diabetes
      249.5 ☑ *[366.41]*
  floriformis 360.24 *[366.34]*
  membranacea
    accreta 366.50
    congenita 743.39
  nigra 366.16
Catarrh, catarrhal (inflammation) — *see also*
  condition 460
  acute 460
  asthma, asthmatic (*see also* Asthma)
    493.9 ☑
  Bostock's (*see also* Fever, hay) 477.9
  bowel — *see* Enteritis
  bronchial 490
    acute 466.0
    chronic 491.0
    subacute 466.0
  cervix, cervical (canal) (uteri) — *see* Cervicitis
  chest (*see also* Bronchitis) 490
  chronic 472.0
  congestion 472.0
  conjunctivitis 372.03
  due to syphilis 095.9
    congenital 090.0
  enteric — *see* Enteritis
  epidemic (*see also* Influenza) 487.1
  Eustachian 381.50
  eye (acute) (vernal) 372.03
  fauces (*see also* Pharyngitis) 462
  febrile 460
  fibrinous acute 466.0
  gastroenteric — *see* Enteritis
  gastrointestinal — *see* Enteritis
  gingivitis 523.00
  hay (*see also* Fever, hay) 477.9
  infectious 460
  intestinal — *see* Enteritis
  larynx (*see also* Laryngitis, chronic) 476.0
  liver 070.1
    with hepatic coma 070.0
  lung (*see also* Bronchitis) 490
    acute 466.0
    chronic 491.0
  middle ear (chronic) — *see* Otitis media,
    chronic
  mouth 528.00
  nasal (chronic) (*see also* Rhinitis) 472.0
    acute 460
  nasobronchial 472.2
  nasopharyngeal (chronic) 472.2
    acute 460
  nose — *see* Catarrh, nasal
  ophthalmia 372.03
  pneumococcal, acute 466.0
  pulmonary (*see also* Bronchitis) 490
    acute 466.0
    chronic 491.0
  spring (eye) 372.13
  suffocating (*see also* Asthma) 493.9 ☑
  summer (hay) (*see also* Fever, hay) 477.9
  throat 472.1
  tracheitis 464.10
    with obstruction 464.11
  tubotympanal 381.4
    acute (*see also* Otitis media, acute, non-
      suppurative) 381.00
    chronic 381.10
  vasomotor (*see also* Fever, hay) 477.9
  vesical (bladder) — *see* Cystitis
Catarrhus aestivus — *see also* Fever, hay 477.9
Catastrophe, cerebral — *see also* Disease,
  cerebrovascular, acute 436
Catatonia, catatonic (acute) 781.99
  with
    affective psychosis — *see* Psychosis, af-
      fective
  agitation 295.2 ☑
  dementia (praecox) 295.2 ☑
  due to or associated with physical condition
    293.89
  excitation 295.2 ☑
  excited type 295.2 ☑
  in conditions classified elsewhere 293.89

☑ Additional Digit Required — Refer to the Tabular List for Digit Selection   ▽ Subterms under main terms may continue to next column or page

44 — Volume 2   ▶◀ Revised Text   ● New Line   ▲ Revised Code   2015 ICD-9-CM

Catatonia, catatonic — *continued*
  schizophrenia 295.2 ☑
  stupor 295.2 ☑
Cat's ear 744.29
Cat-scratch — *see also* Injury, superficial
  disease or fever 078.3
Cauda equina — *see also* condition
  syndrome 344.60
Cauliflower ear 738.7
Caul over face 768.9
Causalgia 355.9
  lower limb 355.71
  upper limb 354.4
Cause
  external, general effects NEC 994.9
  not stated 799.9
  unknown 799.9
Caustic burn — *see also* Burn, by site
  from swallowing caustic or corrosive sub-
    stance — *see* Burn, internal organs
Cavare's disease (familial periodic paralysis)
  359.3
Cave-in, injury
  crushing (severe) (*see also* Crush, by site)
    869.1
  suffocation 994.7
Cavernitis (penis) 607.2
  lymph vessel — *see* Lymphangioma
Cavernositis 607.2
Cavernous — *see* condition
Cavitation of lung — *see also* Tuberculosis
  011.2 ☑
  nontuberculous 518.89
  primary, progressive 010.8 ☑
Cavity
  lung — *see* Cavitation of lung
  optic papilla 743.57
  pulmonary — *see* Cavitation of lung
  teeth 521.00
  vitreous (humor) 379.21
Cavovarus foot, congenital 754.59
Cavus foot (congenital) 754.71
  acquired 736.73
Cazenave's
  disease (pemphigus) NEC 694.4
  lupus (erythematosus) 695.4
CDGS (carbohydrate-deficient glycoprotein
  syndrome) 271.8
Cecitis — *see* Appendicitis
Cecocele — *see* Hernia
Cecum — *see* condition
Celiac
  artery compression syndrome 447.4
  disease 579.0
  infantilism 579.0
Cell, cellular — *see also* condition
  anterior chamber (eye) (positive aqueous
    ray) 364.04
Cellulitis (diffuse) (with lymphangitis) — *see*
  also Abscess 682.9
  abdominal wall 682.2
  anaerobic (*see also* Gas gangrene) 040.0
  ankle 682.6
  anus 566
  areola 611.0
  arm (any part, above wrist) 682.3
  auditory canal (external) 380.10
  axilla 682.3
  back (any part) 682.2
  breast 611.0
    postpartum 675.1 ☑
  broad ligament (*see also* Disease, pelvis, in-
    flammatory) 614.4
    acute 614.3
  buttock 682.5
  cervical (neck region) 682.1
  cervix (uteri) (*see also* Cervicitis) 616.0
  cheek, external 682.0
    internal 528.3
  chest wall 682.2
  chronic NEC 682.9
  colostomy 569.61
  corpus cavernosum 607.2
  digit 681.9

Cellulitis — *see also* Abscess — *continued*
  Douglas' cul-de-sac or pouch (chronic) (*see*
    also Disease, pelvis, inflammatory)
    614.4
    acute 614.3
  drainage site (following operation) 998.59
  ear, external 380.10
  enterostomy 569.61
  erysipelar (*see also* Erysipelas) 035
  esophagostomy 530.86
  eyelid 373.13
  face (any part, except eye) 682.0
  finger (intrathecal) (periosteal) (subcuta-
    neous) (subcuticular) 681.00
  flank 682.2
  foot (except toe) 682.7
  forearm 682.3
  gangrenous (*see also* Gangrene) 785.4
  genital organ NEC
    female — *see* Abscess, genital organ,
      female
    male 608.4
  glottis 478.71
  gluteal (region) 682.5
  gonococcal NEC 098.0
  groin 682.2
  hand (except finger or thumb) 682.4
  head (except face) NEC 682.8
  heel 682.7
  hip 682.6
  jaw (region) 682.0
  knee 682.6
  labium (majus) (minus) (*see also* Vulvitis)
    616.10
  larynx 478.71
  leg, except foot 682.6
  lip 528.5
  mammary gland 611.0
  mouth (floor) 528.3
  multiple sites NEC 682.9
  nasopharynx 478.21
  navel 682.2
    newborn NEC 771.4
  neck (region) 682.1
  nipple 611.0
  nose 478.19
    external 682.0
  orbit, orbital 376.01
  palate (soft) 528.3
  pectoral (region) 682.2
  pelvis, pelvic
    with
      abortion — *see* Abortion, by type,
        with sepsis
      ectopic pregnancy (*see also* cate-
        gories 633.0–633.9) 639.0
      molar pregnancy (*see also* categories
        630–632) 639.0
    female (*see also* Disease, pelvis, inflam-
      matory) 614.4
      acute 614.3
    following
      abortion 639.0
      ectopic or molar pregnancy 639.0
    male 567.21
    puerperal, postpartum, childbirth
      670.8 ☑
  penis 607.2
  perineal, perineum 682.2
  perirectal 566
  peritonsillar 475
  periurethral 597.0
  periuterine (*see also* Disease, pelvis, inflam-
    matory) 614.4
    acute 614.3
  pharynx 478.21
  phlegmonous NEC 682.9
  rectum 566
  retromammary 611.0
  retroperitoneal (*see also* Peritonitis)
    567.2 ☑, 567.38
  round ligament (*see also* Disease, pelvis, in-
    flammatory) 614.4
    acute 614.3
  scalp (any part) 682.8
    dissecting 704.8

Cellulitis — *see also* Abscess — *continued*
  scrotum 608.4
  seminal vesicle 608.0
  septic NEC 682.9
  shoulder 682.3
  specified sites NEC 682.8
  spermatic cord 608.4
  submandibular (region) (space) (triangle)
    682.0
    gland 527.3
  submaxillary 528.3
    gland 527.3
  submental (pyogenic) 682.0
    gland 527.3
  suppurative NEC 682.9
  testis 608.4
  thigh 682.6
  thumb (intrathecal) (periosteal) (subcuta-
    neous) (subcuticular) 681.00
  toe (intrathecal) (periosteal) (subcutaneous)
    (subcuticular) 681.10
  tonsil 475
  trunk 682.2
  tuberculous (primary) (*see also* Tuberculosis)
    017.0 ☑
  tunica vaginalis 608.4
  umbilical 682.2
    newborn NEC 771.4
  vaccinal 999.39
  vagina — *see* Vaginitis
  vas deferens 608.4
  vocal cords 478.5
  vulva (*see also* Vulvitis) 616.10
  wrist 682.4
Cementoblastoma, benign (M9273/0) 213.1
  upper jaw (bone) 213.0
Cementoma (M9273/0) 213.1
  gigantiform (M9275/0) 213.1
    upper jaw (bone) 213.0
  upper jaw (bone) 213.0
Cementoperiostitis 523.40
  acute 523.33
  apical 523.40
Cephalgia, cephalagia — *see also* Headache
  784.0
  histamine 339.00
  nonorganic origin 307.81
  other trigeminal autonomic (TACS) 339.09
  psychogenic 307.81
  tension 307.81
Cephalhematocele, cephalematocele
  due to birth injury 767.19
  fetus or newborn 767.19
  traumatic (*see also* Contusion, head) 920
Cephalhematoma, cephalematoma (calcified)
  due to birth injury 767.19
  fetus or newborn 767.19
  traumatic (*see also* Contusion, head) 920
Cephalic — *see* condition
Cephalitis — *see* Encephalitis
Cephalocele 742.0
Cephaloma — *see* Neoplasm, by site, malig-
  nant
Cephalomenia 625.8
Cephalopelvic — *see* condition
Cercomoniasis 007.3
Cerebellitis — *see* Encephalitis
Cerebellum (cerebellar) — *see* condition
Cerebral — *see* condition
Cerebritis — *see* Encephalitis
Cerebrohepatorenal syndrome 759.89
Cerebromacular degeneration 330.1
Cerebromalacia — *see also* Softening, brain
  348.89
  due to cerebrovascular accident 438.89
Cerebrosidosis 272.7
Cerebrospasticity — *see* Palsy, cerebral
Cerebrospinal — *see* condition
Cerebrum — *see* condition
Ceroid storage disease 272.7
Cerumen (accumulation) (impacted) 380.4
Cervical — *see also* condition
  auricle 744.43
  high risk human papillomavirus (HPV) DNA
    test positive 795.05

Cervical — *see also* condition — *continued*
  intraepithelial glandular neoplasia 233.1
  low risk human papillomavirus (HPV) DNA
    test positive 795.09
  rib 756.2
  shortening — *see* Short, cervical
Cervicalgia 723.1
Cervicitis (acute) (chronic) (nonvenereal)
  (subacute) (with erosion or ectropion)
  616.0
  with
    abortion — *see* Abortion, by type, with
      sepsis
    ectopic pregnancy (*see also* categories
      633.0–633.9) 639.0
    molar pregnancy (*see also* categories
      630–632) 639.0
    ulceration 616.0
  chlamydial 099.53
  complicating pregnancy or puerperium
    646.6 ☑
    affecting fetus or newborn 760.8
  following
    abortion 639.0
    ectopic or molar pregnancy 639.0
  gonococcal (acute) 098.15
    chronic or duration of 2 months or more
      098.35
  senile (atrophic) 616.0
  syphilitic 095.8
  trichomonal 131.09
  tuberculous (*see also* Tuberculosis) 016.7 ☑
Cervicoaural fistula 744.49
Cervicocolpitis (emphysematosa) — *see also*
  Cervicitis 616.0
Cervix — *see* condition
Cesarean delivery, operation or section NEC
  669.7 ☑
  affecting fetus or newborn 763.4
  (planned) occurring after 37 completed
    weeks of gestation but before 39
    completed weeks gestation due to
    (spontaneous) onset of labor
    649.8 ☑
  post mortem, affecting fetus or newborn
    761.6
  previous, affecting management of pregnan-
    cy 654.2 ☑
Céstan-Chenais paralysis 344.89
Céstan-Raymond syndrome 433.8 ☑
Céstan's syndrome 344.89
Cestode infestation NEC 123.9
  specified type NEC 123.8
Cestodiasis 123.9
CGF (congenital generalized fibromatosis)
  759.89
Chabert's disease 022.9
Chacaleh 266.2
Chafing 709.8
Chagas' disease — *see also* Trypanosomiasis,
  American 086.2
  with heart involvement 086.0
Chagres fever 084.0
Chalasia (cardiac sphincter) 530.81
Chalazion 373.2
Chalazoderma 757.39
Chalcosis 360.24
  cornea 371.15
  crystalline lens 360.24 *[366.34]*
  retina 360.24
Chalicosis (occupational) (pulmonum) 502
Chancre (any genital site) (hard) (indurated)
  (infecting) (primary) (recurrent) 091.0
  congenital 090.0
  conjunctiva 091.2
  Ducrey's 099.0
  extragenital 091.2
  eyelid 091.2
  Hunterian 091.0
  lip (syphilis) 091.2
  mixed 099.8
  nipple 091.2
  Nisbet's 099.0
  of
    carate 103.0
    pinta 103.0

☑ **Additional Digit Required — Refer to the Tabular List for Digit Selection**   ▽ **Subterms under main terms may continue to next column or page**

Chancre — *continued*
  of — *continued*
    yaws 102.0
  palate, soft 091.2
  phagedenic 099.0
  Ricord's 091.0
  Rollet's (syphilitic) 091.0
  seronegative 091.0
  seropositive 091.0
  simple 099.0
  soft 099.0
    bubo 099.0
  urethra 091.0
  yaws 102.0
Chancriform syndrome 114.1
Chancroid 099.0
  anus 099.0
  penis (Ducrey's bacillus) 099.0
  perineum 099.0
  rectum 099.0
  scrotum 099.0
  urethra 099.0
  vulva 099.0
Chandipura fever 066.8
Chandler's disease (osteochondritis dissecans, hip) 732.7
Change(s) (of) — *see also* Removal of —
  arteriosclerotic — *see* Arteriosclerosis
  battery
    cardiac pacemaker V53.31
  bone 733.90
    diabetic 250.8 ☑ [731.8]
      due to secondary diabetes
        249.8 ☑ [731.8]
    in disease, unknown cause 733.90
  bowel habits 787.99
  cardiorenal (vascular) (*see also* Hypertension, cardiorenal) 404.90
  cardiovascular — *see* Disease, cardiovascular
  circulatory 459.9
  cognitive or personality change of other type, nonpsychotic 310.1
  color, teeth, tooth
    during formation 520.8
    extrinsic 523.6
    intrinsic posteruptive 521.7
  contraceptive device V25.42
  cornea, corneal
    degenerative NEC 371.40
    membrane NEC 371.30
    senile 371.41
  coronary (*see also* Ischemia, heart) 414.9
  degenerative
    chamber angle (anterior) (iris) 364.56
    ciliary body 364.57
    spine or vertebra (*see also* Spondylosis) 721.90
  dental pulp, regressive 522.2
  drains V58.49
  dressing
    wound V58.30
      nonsurgical V58.30
      surgical V58.31
  fixation device V54.89
    external V54.89
    internal V54.01
  heart (*see also* Disease, heart)
  hip joint 718.95
  hyperplastic larynx 478.79
  hypertrophic
    nasal sinus (*see also* Sinusitis) 473.9
    turbinate, nasal 478.0
    upper respiratory tract 478.9
  inflammatory — *see* Inflammation
  joint (*see also* Derangement, joint) 718.90
    sacroiliac 724.6
  Kirschner wire V54.89
  knee 717.9
  macular, congenital 743.55

Change(s) — *see also* Removal of —
  continued
  malignant (M — — /3) (*see also* Neoplasm, by site, malignant)

> *Note* — for malignant change occurring in a neoplasm, use the appropriate M code with behavior digit /3 e.g., malignant change in uterine fibroid — M8890/3. For malignant change occurring in a nonneoplastic condition (e.g., gastric ulcer) use the M code M8000/3.

  mental (status) NEC 780.97
    due to or associated with physical condition — *see* Syndrome, brain
  myocardium, myocardial — *see* Degeneration, myocardial
  of life (*see also* Menopause) 627.2
  pacemaker battery (cardiac) V53.31
  peripheral nerve 355.9
  personality (nonpsychotic) NEC 310.1
  plaster cast V54.89
  refractive, transient 367.81
  regressive, dental pulp 522.2
  retina 362.9
    myopic (degenerative) (malignant) 360.21
    vascular appearance 362.13
  sacroiliac joint 724.6
  scleral 379.19
    degenerative 379.16
  senile (*see also* Senility) 797
  sensory (*see also* Disturbance, sensation) 782.0
  skin texture 782.8
  spinal cord 336.9
  splint, external V54.89
  subdermal implantable contraceptive V25.5
  suture V58.32
  traction device V54.89
  trophic 355.9
    arm NEC 354.9
    leg NEC 355.8
    lower extremity NEC 355.8
    upper extremity NEC 354.9
  vascular 459.9
  vasomotor 443.9
  voice 784.49
    psychogenic 306.1
  wound packing V58.30
    nonsurgical V58.30
    surgical V58.31
Changing sleep-work schedule, affecting sleep 327.36
Changuinola fever 066.0
Chapping skin 709.8
Character
  depressive 301.12
Charcôt's
  arthropathy 094.0 [713.5]
  cirrhosis — *see* Cirrhosis, biliary
  disease 094.0
    spinal cord 094.0
  fever (biliary) (hepatic) (intermittent) — *see* Choledocholithiasis
  joint (disease) 094.0 [713.5]
    diabetic 250.6 ☑ [713.5]
      due to secondary diabetes
        249.6 ☑ [713.5]
    syringomyelic 336.0 [713.5]
  syndrome (intermittent claudication) 443.9
    due to atherosclerosis 440.21
Charcôt-Marie-Tooth disease, paralysis, or syndrome 356.1
CHARGE association (syndrome) 759.89
Charleyhorse (quadriceps) 843.8
  muscle, except quadriceps — *see* Sprain, by site
Charlouis' disease — *see also* Yaws 102.9
Chauffeur's fracture — *see* Fracture, ulna, lower end
Cheadle (-Möller) (-Barlow) disease or syndrome (infantile scurvy) 267
Checking (of)
  contraceptive device (intrauterine) V25.42
  device
    fixation V54.89

Checking — *continued*
  device — *continued*
    fixation — *continued*
      external V54.89
      internal V54.09
      traction V54.89
    Kirschner wire V54.89
    plaster cast V54.89
    splint, external V54.89
Checkup
  following treatment — *see* Examination
  health V70.0
  infant (over 28 days old) (not sick) V20.2
  newborn, routine
    8 to 28 days old V20.32
    over 28 days old, routine V20.2
    under 8 days old V20.31
    weight V20.32
  pregnancy (normal) V22.1
    first V22.0
    high-risk pregnancy V23.9
      inconclusive fetal viability V23.87
      specified problem NEC V23.89
Chédiak-Higashi (-Steinbrinck) anomaly, disease, or syndrome (congenital gigantism of peroxidase granules) 288.2
Cheek — *see also* condition
  biting 528.9
Cheese itch 133.8
Cheese washers' lung 495.8
Cheilitis 528.5
  actinic (due to sun) 692.72
    chronic NEC 692.74
      due to radiation, except from sun 692.82
    due to radiation, except from sun 692.82
  acute 528.5
  angular 528.5
  catarrhal 528.5
  chronic 528.5
  exfoliative 528.5
  gangrenous 528.5
  glandularis apostematosa 528.5
  granulomatosa 351.8
  infectional 528.5
  membranous 528.5
  Miescher's 351.8
  suppurative 528.5
  ulcerative 528.5
  vesicular 528.5
Cheilodynia 528.5
Cheilopalatoschisis — *see also* Cleft, palate, with cleft lip 749.20
Cheilophagia 528.9
Cheiloschisis — *see also* Cleft, lip 749.10
Cheilosis 528.5
  with pellagra 265.2
  angular 528.5
  due to
    dietary deficiency 266.0
    vitamin deficiency 266.0
Cheiromegaly 729.89
Cheiropompholyx 705.81
Cheloid — *see also* Keloid 701.4
Chemical burn — *see also* Burn, by site
  from swallowing chemical — *see* Burn, internal organs
Chemodectoma (M8693/1) — *see* Paraganglioma, nonchromaffin
Chemoprophylaxis NEC V07.39
Chemosis, conjunctiva 372.73
Chemotherapy
  convalescence V66.2
  encounter (for) (oral) (intravenous) V58.11
  maintenance (oral) (intravenous) V58.11
  prophylactic NEC V07.39
    fluoride V07.31
Cherubism 526.89
Chest — *see* condition
Cheyne-Stokes respiration (periodic) 786.04
Chiari's
  disease or syndrome (hepatic vein thrombosis) 453.0
  malformation
    type I 348.4
    type II (*see also* Spina bifida) 741.0 ☑

Chiari's — *continued*
  malformation — *continued*
    type III 742.0
    type IV 742.2
    network 746.89
Chiari-Frommel syndrome 676.6 ☑
Chicago disease (North American blastomycosis) 116.0
Chickenpox — *see also* Varicella 052.9
  exposure to V01.71
  vaccination and inoculation (prophylactic) V05.4
Chiclero ulcer 085.4
Chiggers 133.8
Chignon 111.2
  fetus or newborn (from vacuum extraction) 767.19
Chigoe disease 134.1
Chikungunya fever 066.3
Chilaiditi's syndrome (subphrenic displacement, colon) 751.4
Chilblains 991.5
  lupus 991.5
Child
  behavior causing concern V61.20
    adopted child V61.24
    biological child V61.23
    foster child V61.25
Childbed fever 670.8 ☑
Childbirth — *see also* Delivery
  puerperal complications — *see* Puerperal
Childhood, period of rapid growth V21.0
Chill(s) 780.64
  with fever 780.60
  without fever 780.64
  congestive 780.99
    in malarial regions 084.6
  septic — *see* Septicemia
  urethral 599.84
Chilomastigiasis 007.8
Chin — *see* condition
Chinese dysentery 004.9
Chiropractic dislocation — *see also* Lesion, nonallopathic, by site 739.9
Chitral fever 066.0
Chlamydia, chlamydial — *see* condition
Chloasma 709.09
  cachecticorum 709.09
  eyelid 374.52
    congenital 757.33
    hyperthyroid 242.0 ☑
  gravidarum 646.8 ☑
  idiopathic 709.09
  skin 709.09
  symptomatic 709.09
Chloroma (M9930/3) 205.3 ☑
Chlorosis 280.9
  Egyptian (*see also* Ancylostomiasis) 126.9
  miners' (*see also* Ancylostomiasis) 126.9
Chlorotic anemia 280.9
Chocolate cyst (ovary) 617.1
Choked
  disk or disc — *see* Papilledema
  on food, phlegm, or vomitus NEC (*see also* Asphyxia, food) 933.1
  phlegm 933.1
  while vomiting NEC (*see also* Asphyxia, food) 933.1
Chokes (resulting from bends) 993.3
Choking sensation 784.99
Cholangiectasis — *see also* Disease, gallbladder 575.8
Cholangiocarcinoma (M8160/3)
  and hepatocellular carcinoma, combined (M8180/3) 155.0
  liver 155.1
  specified site NEC — *see* Neoplasm, by site, malignant
  unspecified site 155.1
Cholangiohepatitis 575.8
  due to fluke infestation 121.1
Cholangiohepatoma (M8180/3) 155.0
Cholangiolitis (acute) (chronic) (extrahepatic) (gangrenous) 576.1
  intrahepatic 575.8

☑ **Additional Digit Required** — Refer to the Tabular List for Digit Selection   ⛛ **Subterms under main terms may continue to next column or page**

Cholangiolitis — *continued*
  paratyphoidal (*see also* Fever, paratyphoid)
    002.9
  typhoidal 002.0
Cholangioma (M8160/0) 211.5
  malignant — *see* Cholangiocarcinoma
Cholangitis (acute) (ascending) (catarrhal)
  (chronic) (infective) (malignant) (primary) (recurrent) (sclerosing) (secondary)
  (stenosing) (suppurative) 576.1
  chronic nonsuppurative destructive 571.6
  nonsuppurative destructive (chronic) 571.6
Cholecystdocholithiasis — *see* Choledocholithiasis
Cholecystitis 575.10
  with
    calculus, stones in
      bile duct (common) (hepatic) — *see*
        Choledocholithiasis
      gallbladder — *see* Cholelithiasis
  acute 575.0
  acute and chronic 575.12
  chronic 575.11
  emphysematous (acute) (*see also* Cholecys-
    titis, acute) 575.0
  gangrenous (*see also* Cholecystitis, acute)
    575.0
  paratyphoidal, current (*see also* Fever,
    paratyphoid) 002.9
  suppurative (*see also* Cholecystitis, acute)
    575.0
  typhoidal 002.0
Choledochitis (suppurative) 576.1
Choledocholith — *see* Choledocholithiasis
Choledocholithiasis 574.5 ☑

Note — Use the following fifth-digit
subclassification with category 574:

0   *without mention of obstruction*

1   *with obstruction*

  with
    cholecystitis 574.4 ☑
      acute 574.3 ☑
      chronic 574.4 ☑
    cholelithiasis 574.9 ☑
      with
        cholecystitis 574.7 ☑
          acute 574.6 ☑
          and chronic 574.8 ☑
        chronic 574.7 ☑
Cholelithiasis (impacted) (multiple) 574.2 ☑

Note — Use the following fifth-digit
subclassification with category 574:

0   *without mention of obstruction*

1   *with obstruction*

  with
    cholecystitis 574.1 ☑
      acute 574.0 ☑
      chronic 574.1 ☑
    choledocholithiasis 574.9 ☑
      with
        cholecystitis 574.7 ☑
          acute 574.6 ☑
          and chronic 574.8 ☑
        chronic cholecystitis 574.7 ☑
Cholemia — *see also* Jaundice 782.4
  familial 277.4
  Gilbert's (familial nonhemolytic) 277.4
Cholemic gallstone — *see* Cholelithiasis
Choleperitoneum, choleperitonitis — *see
  also* Disease, gallbladder 567.81
Cholera (algid) (Asiatic) (asphyctic) (epidemic)
  (gravis) (Indian) (malignant) (morbus)
  (pestilential) (spasmodic) 001.9
  antimonial 985.4
  carrier (suspected) of V02.0
  classical 001.0
  contact V01.0
  due to
    Vibrio
      cholerae (Inaba, Ogawa, Hikojima
        serotypes) 001.0
      El Tor 001.1

Cholera — *continued*
  El Tor 001.1
  exposure to V01.0
  vaccination, prophylactic (against) V03.0
Cholerine — *see also* Cholera 001.9
Cholestasis 576.8
  due to total parenteral nutrition (TPN) 573.8
Cholesteatoma (ear) 385.30
  attic (primary) 385.31
  diffuse 385.35
  external ear (canal) 380.21
  marginal (middle ear) 385.32
    with involvement of mastoid cavity
      385.33
    secondary (with middle ear involvement)
      385.33
  mastoid cavity 385.30
  middle ear (secondary) 385.32
    with involvement of mastoid cavity
      385.33
  postmastoidectomy cavity (recurrent)
    383.32
  primary 385.31
  recurrent, postmastoidectomy cavity 383.32
  secondary (middle ear) 385.32
    with involvement of mastoid cavity
      385.33
Cholesteatosis (middle ear) — *see also*
  Cholesteatoma 385.30
  diffuse 385.35
Cholesteremia 272.0
Cholesterin
  granuloma, middle ear 385.82
  in vitreous 379.22
Cholesterol
  deposit
    retina 362.82
    vitreous 379.22
  elevated (high) 272.0
    with elevated (high) triglycerides 272.2
  imbibition of gallbladder (*see also* Disease,
    gallbladder) 575.6
Cholesterolemia 272.0
  essential 272.0
  familial 272.0
  hereditary 272.0
Cholesterosis, cholesterolosis (gallbladder)
  575.6
  with
    cholecystitis — *see* Cholecystitis
    cholelithiasis — *see* Cholelithiasis
  middle ear (*see also* Cholesteatoma) 385.30
Cholocolic fistula — *see also* Fistula, gallbladder 575.5
Choluria 791.4
Chondritis (purulent) 733.99
  auricle 380.03
  costal 733.6
    Tietze's 733.6
  patella, posttraumatic 717.7
  pinna 380.03
  posttraumatica patellae 717.7
  tuberculous (active) (*see also* Tuberculosis)
    015.9 ☑
    intervertebral 015.0 ☑ *[730.88]*
Chondroangiopathia calcarea seu punctate
  756.59
Chondroblastoma (M9230/0) — *see also*
  Neoplasm, bone, benign
  malignant (M9230/3) — *see* Neoplasm,
    bone, malignant
Chondrocalcinosis (articular) (crystal deposition) (dihydrate) — *see also* Arthritis, due
  to, crystals 275.49 *[712.3]* ☑
  due to
    calcium pyrophosphate
      275.49 *[712.2]* ☑
    dicalcium phosphate crystals
      275.49 *[712.1]* ☑
    pyrophosphate crystals 275.49 *[712.2]* ☑
Chondrodermatitis nodularis helicis 380.00
Chondrodysplasia 756.4
  angiomatose 756.4
  calcificans congenita 756.59
  epiphysialis punctata 756.59
  hereditary deforming 756.4

Chondrodysplasia — *continued*
  rhizomelic punctata 277.86
Chondrodystrophia (fetalis) 756.4
  calcarea 756.4
  calcificans congenita 756.59
  fetalis hypoplastica 756.59
  hypoplastica calcinosa 756.59
  punctata 756.59
  tarda 277.5
Chondrodystrophy (familial) (hypoplastic)
  756.4
  myotonic (congenital) 359.23
Chondroectodermal dysplasia 756.55
Chondrolysis 733.99
Chondroma (M9220/0) — *see also* Neoplasm,
  cartilage, benign
  juxtacortical (M9221/0) — *see* Neoplasm,
    bone, benign
  periosteal (M9221/0) — *see* Neoplasm,
    bone, benign
Chondromalacia 733.92
  epiglottis (congenital) 748.3
  generalized 733.92
  knee 717.7
  larynx (congenital) 748.3
  localized, except patella 733.92
  patella, patellae 717.7
  systemic 733.92
  tibial plateau 733.92
  trachea (congenital) 748.3
Chondromatosis (M9220/1) — *see* Neoplasm,
  cartilage, uncertain behavior
Chondromyxosarcoma (M9220/3) — *see*
  Neoplasm, cartilage, malignant
Chondro-osteodysplasia (Morquio-Brailsford
  type) 277.5
Chondro-osteodystrophy 277.5
Chondro-osteoma (M9210/0) — *see* Neoplasm, bone, benign
Chondropathia tuberosa 733.6
Chondrosarcoma (M9220/3) — *see also* Neoplasm, cartilage, malignant
  juxtacortical (M9221/3) — *see* Neoplasm,
    bone, malignant
  mesenchymal (M9240/3) — *see* Neoplasm,
    connective tissue, malignant
Chordae tendineae rupture (chronic) 429.5
Chordee (nonvenereal) 607.89
  congenital 752.63
  gonococcal 098.2
Chorditis (fibrinous) (nodosa) (tuberosa) 478.5
Chordoma (M9370/3) — *see* Neoplasm, by site,
  malignant
Chorea (gravis) (minor) (spasmodic) 333.5
  with
    heart involvement — *see* Chorea with
      rheumatic heart disease
    rheumatic heart disease (chronic, inac-
      tive, or quiescent) (conditions
      classifiable to 393–398) (*see*
      rheumatic heart condition in-
      volved)
      active or acute (conditions classifi-
        able to 391) 392.0
  acute — *see* Chorea, Sydenham's
  apoplectic (*see also* Disease, cerebrovascu-
    lar, acute) 436
  chronic 333.4
  electric 049.8
  gravidarum — *see* Eclampsia, pregnancy
  habit 307.22
  hereditary 333.4
  Huntington's 333.4
  posthemiplegic 344.89
  pregnancy — *see* Eclampsia, pregnancy
  progressive 333.4
    chronic 333.4
    hereditary 333.4
  rheumatic (chronic) 392.9
    with heart disease or involvement — *see*
      Chorea, with rheumatic heart
      disease
  senile 333.5
  Sydenham's 392.9
    with heart involvement — *see* Chorea,
      with rheumatic heart disease

Chorea — *continued*
  Sydenham's — *continued*
    nonrheumatic 333.5
    variabilis 307.23
Choreoathetosis (paroxysmal) 333.5
Chorioadenoma (destruens) (M9100/1) 236.1
Chorioamnionitis 658.4 ☑
  affecting fetus or newborn 762.7
Chorioangioma (M9120/0) 219.8
Choriocarcinoma (M9100/3)
  combined with
    embryonal carcinoma (M9101/3) — *see*
      Neoplasm, by site, malignant
    teratoma (M9101/3) — *see* Neoplasm,
      by site, malignant
  specified site — *see* Neoplasm, by site, ma-
    lignant
  unspecified site
    female 181
    male 186.9
Chorioencephalitis, lymphocytic (acute)
  (serous) 049.0
Chorioepithelioma (M9100/3) — *see* Choriocarcinoma
Choriomeningitis (acute) (benign) (lymphocytic) (serous) 049.0
Chorionepithelioma (M9100/3) — *see* Choriocarcinoma
Chorionitis — *see also* Scleroderma 710.1
Chorioretinitis 363.20
  disseminated 363.10
    generalized 363.13
    in
      neurosyphilis 094.83
      secondary syphilis 091.51
    peripheral 363.12
    posterior pole 363.11
    tuberculous (*see also* Tuberculosis)
      017.3 ☑ *[363.13]*
  due to
    histoplasmosis (*see also* Histoplasmosis)
      115.92
    toxoplasmosis (acquired) 130.2
      congenital (active) 771.2
  focal 363.00
    juxtapapillary 363.01
    peripheral 363.04
    posterior pole NEC 363.03
  juxtapapillaris, juxtapapillary 363.01
  progressive myopia (degeneration) 360.21
  syphilitic (secondary) 091.51
    congenital (early) 090.0 *[363.13]*
      late 090.5 *[363.13]*
    late 095.8 *[363.13]*
  tuberculous (*see also* Tuberculosis)
    017.3 ☑ *[363.13]*
Choristoma — *see* Neoplasm, by site, benign
Choroid — *see* condition
Choroideremia, choroidermia (initial stage)
  (late stage) (partial or total atrophy)
  363.55
Choroiditis — *see also* Chorioretinitis 363.20
  leprous 030.9 *[363.13]*
  senile guttate 363.41
  sympathetic 360.11
  syphilitic (secondary) 091.51
    congenital (early) 090.0 *[363.13]*
      late 090.5 *[363.13]*
    late 095.8 *[363.13]*
  Tay's 363.41
  tuberculous (*see also* Tuberculosis)
    017.3 ☑ *[363.13]*
Choroidopathy NEC 363.9
  degenerative (*see also* Degeneration,
    choroid) 363.40
  hereditary (*see also* Dystrophy, choroid)
    363.50
  specified type NEC 363.8
Choroidoretinitis — *see* Chorioretinitis
Choroidosis, central serous 362.41
Choroidretinopathy, serous 362.41
Christian's syndrome (chronic histiocytosis X)
  277.89
Christian-Weber disease (nodular nonsuppu-
  rative panniculitis) 729.30
Christmas disease 286.1

☑ **Additional Digit Required — Refer to the Tabular List for Digit Selection**   ▽ **Subterms under main terms may continue to next column or page**

Chromaffinoma (M8700/0) — *see also* Neoplasm, by site, benign
  malignant (M8700/3) — *see* Neoplasm, by site, malignant
Chromatopsia 368.59
Chromhidrosis, chromidrosis 705.89
Chromoblastomycosis 117.2
Chromomycosis 117.2
Chromophytosis 111.0
Chromotrichomycosis 111.8
Chronic — *see* condition
Churg-Strauss syndrome 446.4
Chyle cyst, mesentery 457.8
Chylocele (nonfilarial) 457.8
  filarial (*see also* Infestation, filarial) 125.9
  tunica vaginalis (nonfilarial) 608.84
    filarial (*see also* Infestation, filarial) 125.9
Chylomicronemia (fasting) (with hyperprebetalipoproteinemia) 272.3
Chylopericardium (acute) 420.90
Chylothorax (nonfilarial) 457.8
  filarial (*see also* Infestation, filarial) 125.9
Chylous
  ascites 457.8
  cyst of peritoneum 457.8
  hydrocele 603.9
  hydrothorax (nonfilarial) 457.8
    filarial (*see also* Infestation, filarial) 125.9
Chyluria 791.1
  bilharziasis 120.0
  due to
    Brugia (malayi) 125.1
    Wuchereria (bancrofti) 125.0
      malayi 125.1
  filarial (*see also* Infestation, filarial) 125.9
  filariasis (*see also* Infestation, filarial) 125.9
  nonfilarial 791.1
Cicatricial (deformity) — *see* Cicatrix
Cicatrix (adherent) (contracted) (painful) (vicious) 709.2
  adenoid 474.8
  alveolar process 525.8
  anus 569.49
  auricle 380.89
  bile duct (*see also* Disease, biliary) 576.8
  bladder 596.89
  bone 733.99
  brain 348.89
  cervix (postoperative) (postpartal) 622.3
    in pregnancy or childbirth 654.6 ☑
      causing obstructed labor 660.2 ☑
  chorioretinal 363.30
    disseminated 363.35
    macular 363.32
    peripheral 363.34
    posterior pole NEC 363.33
  choroid — *see* Cicatrix, chorioretinal
  common duct (*see also* Disease, biliary) 576.8
  congenital 757.39
  conjunctiva 372.64
  cornea 371.00
    tuberculous (*see also* Tuberculosis) 017.3 ☑ [371.05]
  duodenum (bulb) 537.3
  esophagus 530.3
  eyelid 374.46
    with
      ectropion — *see* Ectropion
      entropion — *see* Entropion
  hypopharynx 478.29
  knee, semilunar cartilage 717.5
  lacrimal
    canaliculi 375.53
    duct
      acquired 375.56
      neonatal 375.55
    punctum 375.52
    sac 375.54
  larynx 478.79
  limbus (cystoid) 372.64
  lung 518.89
  macular 363.32
    disseminated 363.35
    peripheral 363.34
  middle ear 385.89

Cicatrix — *continued*
  mouth 528.9
  muscle 728.89
  nasolacrimal duct
    acquired 375.56
    neonatal 375.55
  nasopharynx 478.29
  palate (soft) 528.9
  penis 607.89
  prostate 602.8
  rectum 569.49
  retina 363.30
    disseminated 363.35
    macular 363.32
    peripheral 363.34
    posterior pole NEC 363.33
  semilunar cartilage — *see* Derangement, meniscus
  seminal vesicle 608.89
  skin 709.2
    infected 686.8
    postinfectional 709.2
    tuberculous (*see also* Tuberculosis) 017.0 ☑
  specified site NEC 709.2
  throat 478.29
  tongue 529.8
  tonsil (and adenoid) 474.8
  trachea 478.9
  tuberculous NEC (*see also* Tuberculosis) 011.9 ☑
  ureter 593.89
  urethra 599.84
  uterus 621.8
  vagina 623.4
    in pregnancy or childbirth 654.7 ☑
      causing obstructed labor 660.2 ☑
  vocal cord 478.5
  wrist, constricting (annular) 709.2
CIDP (chronic inflammatory demyelinating polyneuropathy) 357.81
CIN I (cervical intraepithelial neoplasia I) 622.11
CIN II (cervical intraepithelial neoplasia II) 622.12
CIN III (cervical intraepithelial neoplasia III) 233.1
Cinchonism
  correct substance properly administered 386.9
  overdose or wrong substance given or taken 961.4
Circine herpes 110.5
Circle of Willis — *see* condition
Circular — *see also* condition
  hymen 752.49
Circulating anticoagulants, antibodies, or inhibitors — *see also* Anticoagulants 286.59
  extrinsic 287.8
  following childbirth 666.3 ☑
  intrinsic, causing hemorrhagic disorder 286.59
    with
      acquired hemophilia 286.52
      antiphospholipid antibody 286.53
  postpartum 666.3 ☑
Circulation
  collateral (venous), any site 459.89
  defective 459.9
    congenital 747.9
    lower extremity 459.89
  embryonic 747.9
  failure 799.89
    fetus or newborn 779.89
    peripheral 785.59
  fetal, persistent 747.83
  heart, incomplete 747.9
Circulatory system — *see* condition
Circulus senilis 371.41
Circumcision
  in absence of medical indication V50.2
  ritual V50.2
  routine V50.2
  status (post), female 629.20
Circumscribed — *see* condition

Circumvallata placenta — *see* Placenta, abnormal
Cirrhosis, cirrhotic 571.5
  with alcoholism 571.2
  alcoholic (liver) 571.2
  atrophic (of liver) — *see* Cirrhosis, portal
  Baumgarten-Cruveilhier 571.5
  biliary (cholangiolitic) (cholangitic) (cholestatic) (extrahepatic) (hypertrophic) (intrahepatic) (nonobstructive) (obstructive) (pericholangiolitic) (posthepatic) (primary) (secondary) (xanthomatous) 571.6
    due to
      clonorchiasis 121.1
      flukes 121.3
  brain 331.9
  capsular — *see* Cirrhosis, portal
  cardiac 571.5
    alcoholic 571.2
  central (liver) — *see* Cirrhosis, liver
  Charcôt's 571.6
  cholangiolitic — *see* Cirrhosis, biliary
  cholangitic — *see* Cirrhosis, biliary
  cholestatic — *see* Cirrhosis, biliary
  clitoris (hypertrophic) 624.2
  coarsely nodular 571.5
  congestive (liver) — *see* Cirrhosis, cardiac
  Cruveilhier-Baumgarten 571.5
  cryptogenic (of liver) 571.5
    alcoholic 571.2
  dietary (*see also* Cirrhosis, portal) 571.5
  due to
    bronzed diabetes 275.01
    congestive hepatomegaly — *see* Cirrhosis, cardiac
    cystic fibrosis 277.00
    hemochromatosis (*see also* Hemochromatosis) 275.03
    hepatolenticular degeneration 275.1
    passive congestion (chronic) — *see* Cirrhosis, cardiac
    Wilson's disease 275.1
    xanthomatosis 272.2
  extrahepatic (obstructive) — *see* Cirrhosis, biliary
  fatty 571.8
    alcoholic 571.0
  florid 571.2
  Glisson's — *see* Cirrhosis, portal
  Hanot's (hypertrophic) — *see* Cirrhosis, biliary
  hepatic — *see* Cirrhosis, liver
  hepatolienal — *see* Cirrhosis, liver
  hobnail — *see* Cirrhosis, portal
  hypertrophic (*see also* Cirrhosis, liver)
    biliary — *see* Cirrhosis, biliary
    Hanot's — *see* Cirrhosis, biliary
  infectious NEC — *see* Cirrhosis, portal
  insular — *see* Cirrhosis, portal
  intrahepatic (obstructive) (primary) (secondary) — *see* Cirrhosis, biliary
  juvenile (*see also* Cirrhosis, portal) 571.5
  kidney (*see also* Sclerosis, renal) 587
  Laennec's (of liver) 571.2
    nonalcoholic 571.5
  liver (chronic) (hepatolienal) (hypertrophic) (nodular) (splenomegalic) (unilobar) 571.5
    with alcoholism 571.2
    alcoholic 571.2
    congenital (due to failure of obliteration of umbilical vein) 777.8
    cryptogenic 571.5
      alcoholic 571.2
    fatty 571.8
      alcoholic 571.0
    macronodular 571.5
      alcoholic 571.2
    micronodular 571.5
      alcoholic 571.2
    nodular, diffuse 571.5
      alcoholic 571.2
    pigmentary 275.01
    portal 571.5
      alcoholic 571.2

Cirrhosis, cirrhotic — *continued*
  liver — *continued*
    postnecrotic 571.5
      alcoholic 571.2
    syphilitic 095.3
  lung (chronic) (*see also* Fibrosis, lung) 515
  macronodular (of liver) 571.5
    alcoholic 571.2
  malarial 084.9
  metabolic NEC 571.5
  micronodular (of liver) 571.5
    alcoholic 571.2
  monolobular — *see* Cirrhosis, portal
  multilobular — *see* Cirrhosis, portal
  nephritis (*see also* Sclerosis, renal) 587
  nodular — *see* Cirrhosis, liver
  nutritional (fatty) 571.5
  obstructive (biliary) (extrahepatic) (intrahepatic) — *see* Cirrhosis, biliary
  ovarian 620.8
  paludal 084.9
  pancreas (duct) 577.8
  pericholangiolitic — *see* Cirrhosis, biliary
  periportal — *see* Cirrhosis, portal
  pigment, pigmentary (of liver) 275.01
  portal (of liver) 571.5
    alcoholic 571.2
  posthepatitic (*see also* Cirrhosis, postnecrotic) 571.5
  postnecrotic (of liver) 571.5
    alcoholic 571.2
  primary (intrahepatic) — *see* Cirrhosis, biliary
  pulmonary (*see also* Fibrosis, lung) 515
  renal (*see also* Sclerosis, renal) 587
  septal (*see also* Cirrhosis, postnecrotic) 571.5
  spleen 289.51
  splenomegalic (of liver) — *see* Cirrhosis, liver
  stasis (liver) — *see* Cirrhosis, liver
  stomach 535.4 ☑
  Todd's (*see also* Cirrhosis, biliary) 571.6
  toxic (nodular) — *see* Cirrhosis, postnecrotic
  trabecular — *see* Cirrhosis, postnecrotic
  unilobar — *see* Cirrhosis, liver
  vascular (of liver) — *see* Cirrhosis, liver
  xanthomatous (biliary) (*see also* Cirrhosis, biliary) 571.6
    due to xanthomatosis (familial) (metabolic) (primary) 272.2
Cistern, subarachnoid 793.0
Citrullinemia 270.6
Citrullinuria 270.6
Ciuffini-Pancoast tumor (M8010/3) (carcinoma, pulmonary apex) 162.3
Civatte's disease or poikiloderma 709.09
CJD (Creutzfeldt-Jakob disease) 046.19
  variant (vCJD) 046.11
CLABSI (central line-associated bloodstream infection) 999.32
Clam diggers' itch 120.3
Clap — *see* Gonorrhea
Clarke-Hadfield syndrome (pancreatic infantilism) 577.8
Clark's paralysis 343.9
Clastothrix 704.2
Claude Bernard-Horner syndrome — *see also* Neuropathy, peripheral, autonomic 337.9
Claude's syndrome 352.6
Claudication, intermittent 443.9
  cerebral (artery) (*see also* Ischemia, cerebral, transient) 435.9
  due to atherosclerosis 440.21
  spinal cord (arteriosclerotic) 435.1
    syphilitic 094.89
  spinalis 435.1
  venous (axillary) 453.89
Claudicatio venosa intermittens 453.89
Claustrophobia 300.29
Clavus (infected) 700
Clawfoot (congenital) 754.71
  acquired 736.74
Clawhand (acquired) 736.06
  congenital 755.59
Clawtoe (congenital) 754.71

☑ **Additional Digit Required — Refer to the Tabular List for Digit Selection**   ▽ **Subterms under main terms may continue to next column or page**

48 — Volume 2   ▶◀ Revised Text   ● New Line   ▲ Revised Code   **2015 ICD-9-CM**

Clawtoe — *continued*
acquired 735.5
Clay eating 307.52
Clay shovelers' fracture — *see* Fracture, vertebra, cervical
Cleansing of artificial opening — *see also* Attention to artificial opening V55.9
Cleft (congenital) — *see also* Imperfect, closure
alveolar process 525.8
branchial (persistent) 744.41
cyst 744.42
clitoris 752.49
cricoid cartilage, posterior 748.3
facial (*see also* Cleft, lip) 749.10
lip 749.10
with cleft palate 749.20
bilateral (lip and palate) 749.24
with unilateral lip or palate 749.25
complete 749.23
incomplete 749.24
unilateral (lip and palate) 749.22
with bilateral lip or palate 749.25
complete 749.21
incomplete 749.22
bilateral 749.14
with cleft palate, unilateral 749.25
complete 749.13
incomplete 749.14
unilateral 749.12
with cleft palate, bilateral 749.25
complete 749.11
incomplete 749.12
nose 748.1
palate 749.00
with cleft lip 749.20
bilateral (lip and palate) 749.24
with unilateral lip or palate 749.25
complete 749.23
incomplete 749.24
unilateral (lip and palate) 749.22
with bilateral lip or palate 749.25
complete 749.21
incomplete 749.22
bilateral 749.04
with cleft lip, unilateral 749.25
complete 749.03
incomplete 749.04
unilateral 749.02
with cleft lip, bilateral 749.25
complete 749.01
incomplete 749.02
penis 752.69
posterior, cricoid cartilage 748.3
scrotum 752.89
sternum (congenital) 756.3
thyroid cartilage (congenital) 748.3
tongue 750.13
uvula 749.02
with cleft lip (*see also* Cleft, lip, with cleft palate) 749.20
water 366.12
Cleft hand (congenital) 755.58
Cleidocranial dysostosis 755.59
Cleidotomy, fetal 763.89
Cleptomania 312.32
Clérambault's syndrome 297.8
erotomania 302.89
Clergyman's sore throat 784.49
Click, clicking
systolic syndrome 785.2
Clifford's syndrome (postmaturity) 766.22
Climacteric — *see also* Menopause 627.2
arthritis NEC (*see also* Arthritis, climacteric) 716.3 ☑
depression (*see also* Psychosis, affective) 296.2 ☑
disease 627.2
recurrent episode 296.3 ☑
single episode 296.2 ☑
female (symptoms) 627.2
male (symptoms) (syndrome) 608.89
melancholia (*see also* Psychosis, affective) 296.2 ☑
recurrent episode 296.3 ☑

Climacteric — *see also* Menopause — *continued*
melancholia (*see also* Psychosis, affective) — *continued*
single episode 296.2 ☑
paranoid state 297.2
paraphrenia 297.2
polyarthritis NEC 716.39
male 608.89
symptoms (female) 627.2
Clinical research investigation (control) (participant) V70.7
Clinodactyly 755.59
Clitoris — *see* condition
Cloaca, persistent 751.5
Clonorchiasis 121.1
Clonorchiosis 121.1
Clonorchis infection, liver 121.1
Clonus 781.0
Closed bite 524.20
Closed surgical procedure converted to open procedure
arthroscopic V64.43
laparoscopic V64.41
thoracoscopic V64.42
Closure
artificial opening (*see also* Attention to artificial opening) V55.9
congenital, nose 748.0
cranial sutures, premature 756.0
defective or imperfect NEC — *see* Imperfect, closure
fistula, delayed — *see* Fistula
fontanelle, delayed 756.0
foramen ovale, imperfect 745.5
hymen 623.3
interauricular septum, defective 745.5
interventricular septum, defective 745.4
lacrimal duct 375.56
congenital 743.65
neonatal 375.55
nose (congenital) 748.0
acquired 738.0
primary angle without glaucoma damage 365.06
vagina 623.2
valve — *see* Endocarditis
vulva 624.8
Clot (blood)
artery (obstruction) (occlusion) (*see also* Embolism) 444.9
atrial appendage 429.89
bladder 596.7
brain (extradural or intradural) (*see also* Thrombosis, brain) 434.0 ☑
late effect — *see* Late effect(s) (of) cerebrovascular disease
circulation 444.9
heart (*see also* Infarct, myocardium) 410.9 ☑
without myocardial infarction 429.89
vein (*see also* Thrombosis) 453.9
Clotting defect NEC — *see also* Defect, coagulation 286.9
Clouded state 780.09
epileptic (*see also* Epilepsy) 345.9 ☑
paroxysmal (idiopathic) (*see also* Epilepsy) 345.9 ☑
Clouding
corneal graft 996.51
Cloudy
antrum, antra 473.0
dialysis effluent 792.5
Clouston's (hidrotic) ectodermal dysplasia 757.31
Clubbing of fingers 781.5
Clubfinger 736.29
acquired 736.29
congenital 754.89
Clubfoot (congenital) 754.70
acquired 736.71
equinovarus 754.51
paralytic 736.71
Club hand (congenital) 754.89
acquired 736.07
Clubnail (acquired) 703.8

Clubnail — *continued*
congenital 757.5
Clump kidney 753.3
Clumsiness 781.3
syndrome 315.4
Cluttering — *see also* Disorder, fluency 315.35
Clutton's joints 090.5
Coagulation, intravascular (diffuse) (disseminated) — *see also* Fibrinolysis 286.6
newborn 776.2
Coagulopathy — *see also* Defect, coagulation 286.9
consumption 286.6
intravascular (disseminated) NEC 286.6
newborn 776.2
Coalition
calcaneoscaphoid 755.67
calcaneus 755.67
tarsal 755.67
Coal miners'
elbow 727.2
lung 500
Coal workers' lung or pneumoconiosis 500
Coarctation
aorta (postductal) (preductal) 747.10
pulmonary artery 747.31
Coated tongue 529.3
Coats' disease 362.12
Cocainism — *see also* Dependence 304.2 ☑
Coccidioidal granuloma 114.3
Coccidioidomycosis 114.9
with pneumonia 114.0
cutaneous (primary) 114.1
disseminated 114.3
extrapulmonary (primary) 114.1
lung 114.5
acute 114.0
chronic 114.4
primary 114.0
meninges 114.2
primary (pulmonary) 114.0
acute 114.0
prostate 114.3
pulmonary 114.5
acute 114.0
chronic 114.4
primary 114.0
specified site NEC 114.3
Coccidioidosis 114.9
lung 114.5
acute 114.0
chronic 114.4
primary 114.0
meninges 114.2
Coccidiosis (colitis) (diarrhea) (dysentery) 007.2
Cocciuria 791.9
Coccus in urine 791.9
Coccydynia 724.79
Coccygodynia 724.79
Coccyx — *see* condition
Cochin-China
diarrhea 579.1
anguilluliasis 127.2
ulcer 085.1
Cockayne's disease or syndrome (microcephaly and dwarfism) 759.89
Cockayne-Weber syndrome (epidermolysis bullosa) 757.39
Cocked-up toe 735.2
Cock's peculiar tumor 706.2
Codman's tumor (benign chondroblastoma) (M9230/0) — *see* Neoplasm, bone, benign
Coenurosis 123.8
Coffee workers' lung 495.8
Cogan's syndrome 370.52
congenital oculomotor apraxia 379.51
nonsyphilitic interstitial keratitis 370.52
Coiling, umbilical cord — *see* Complications, umbilical cord
Coitus, painful (female) 625.0
male 608.89
psychogenic 302.76
Cold 460
with influenza, flu, or grippe (*see also* Influenza) 487.1

Cold — *continued*
abscess (*see also* Tuberculosis, abscess)
articular — *see* Tuberculosis, joint
agglutinin
disease (chronic) or syndrome 283.0
hemoglobinuria 283.0
paroxysmal (cold) (nocturnal) 283.2
allergic (*see also* Fever, hay) 477.9
bronchus or chest — *see* Bronchitis
with grippe or influenza (*see also* Influenza) 487.1
common (head) 460
vaccination, prophylactic (against) V04.7
deep 464.10
effects of 991.9
specified effect NEC 991.8
excessive 991.9
specified effect NEC 991.8
exhaustion from 991.8
exposure to 991.9
specified effect NEC 991.8
grippy (*see also* Influenza) 487.1
head 460
injury syndrome (newborn) 778.2
intolerance 780.99
on lung — *see* Bronchitis
rose 477.0
sensitivity, autoimmune 283.0
virus 460
Coldsore — *see also* Herpes, simplex 054.9
Colibacillosis 041.49
generalized 038.42
Colibacilluria 791.9
Colic (recurrent) 789.7
abdomen 789.7
psychogenic 307.89
appendicular 543.9
appendix 543.9
bile duct — *see* Choledocholithiasis
biliary — *see* Cholelithiasis
bilious — *see* Cholelithiasis
common duct — *see* Choledocholithiasis
Devonshire NEC 984.9
specified type of lead — *see* Table of Drugs and Chemicals
flatulent 787.3
gallbladder or gallstone — *see* Cholelithiasis
gastric 536.8
hepatic (duct) — *see* Choledocholithiasis
hysterical 300.11
in
adult 789.0 ☑
child over 12 months old 789.0 ☑
infant 789.7
infantile 789.7
intestinal 789.7
kidney 788.0
lead NEC 984.9
specified type of lead — *see* Table of Drugs and Chemicals
liver (duct) — *see* Choledocholithiasis
mucous 564.9
psychogenic 316 [564.9]
nephritic 788.0
painter's NEC 984.9
pancreas 577.8
psychogenic 306.4
renal 788.0
saturnine NEC 984.9
specified type of lead — *see* Table of Drugs and Chemicals
spasmodic 789.7
ureter 788.0
urethral 599.84
due to calculus 594.2
uterus 625.8
menstrual 625.3
vermicular 543.9
virus 460
worm NEC 128.9
Colicystitis — *see also* Cystitis 595.9
Colitis (acute) (catarrhal) (croupous) (cystica superficialis) (exudative) (hemorrhagic) (noninfectious) (phlegmonous) (presumed noninfectious) 558.9
adaptive 564.9

☑ Additional Digit Required — Refer to the Tabular List for Digit Selection

⟶ Subterms under main terms may continue to next column or page

2015 ICD-9-CM

▶◀ Revised Text

● New Line

▲ Revised Code

Volume 2 — 49

Clawtoe — Colitis

Index

Colitis — Complications

Colitis — *continued*
allergic 558.3
amebic (*see also* Amebiasis) 006.9
  nondysenteric 006.2
anthrax 022.2
bacillary (*see also* Infection, Shigella) 004.9
balantidial 007.0
chronic 558.9
  ulcerative (*see also* Colitis, ulcerative)
  556.9
coccidial 007.2
dietetic 558.9
due to radiation 558.1
eosinophilic 558.42
functional 558.9
gangrenous 009.0
giardial 007.1
granulomatous 555.1
gravis (*see also* Colitis, ulcerative) 556.9
infectious (*see also* Enteritis, due to, specific
  organism) 009.0
  presumed 009.1
ischemic 557.9
  acute 557.0
  chronic 557.1
  due to mesenteric artery insufficiency
  557.1
membranous 564.9
  psychogenic 316 [564.9]
mucous 564.9
  psychogenic 316 [564.9]
necrotic 009.0
polyposa (*see also* Colitis, ulcerative) 556.9
protozoal NEC 007.9
pseudomembranous 008.45
pseudomucinous 564.9
regional 555.1
segmental 555.1
septic (*see also* Enteritis, due to, specific organism) 009.0
spastic 564.9
  psychogenic 316 [564.9]
Staphylococcus 008.41
  food 005.0
thromboulcerative 557.0
toxic 558.2
transmural 555.1
trichomonal 007.3
tuberculous (ulcerative) 014.8 ☑
ulcerative (chronic) (idiopathic) (nonspecific)
  556.9
  entero- 556.0
  fulminant 557.0
  ileo- 556.1
  left-sided 556.5
  procto- 556.2
  proctosigmoid 556.3
  psychogenic 316 [556] ☑
  specified NEC 556.8
  universal 556.6
Collagen disease NEC 710.9
  nonvascular 710.9
  vascular (allergic) (*see also* Angiitis, hypersensitivity) 446.20
Collagenosis — *see also* Collagen disease 710.9
  cardiovascular 425.4
  mediastinal 519.3
Collapse 780.2
  adrenal 255.8
  cardiorenal (*see also* Hypertension, cardiorenal) 404.90
  cardiorespiratory 785.51
  fetus or newborn 779.85
  cardiovascular (*see also* Disease, heart)
  785.51
  fetus or newborn 779.85
  circulatory (peripheral) 785.59
    with
      abortion — *see* Abortion, by type,
      with shock
      ectopic pregnancy (*see also* cate-
      gories 633.0–633.9) 639.5
      molar pregnancy (*see also* categories
      630–632) 639.5
    during or after labor and delivery
    669.1 ☑

Collapse — *continued*
  circulatory — *continued*
    fetus or newborn 779.85
    following
      abortion 639.5
      ectopic or molar pregnancy 639.5
    during or after labor and delivery 669.1 ☑
      fetus or newborn 779.89
    during or resulting from a surgical proce-
    dure 998.00
    external ear canal 380.50
      secondary to
        inflammation 380.53
        surgery 380.52
        trauma 380.51
    general 780.2
    heart — *see* Disease, heart
    heat 992.1
    hysterical 300.11
    labyrinth, membranous (congenital) 744.05
    lung (massive) (*see also* Atelectasis) 518.0
      pressure, during labor 668.0 ☑
    myocardial — *see* Disease, heart
    nervous (*see also* Disorder, mental, nonpsy-
    chotic) 300.9
    neurocirculatory 306.2
    nose 738.0
    postoperative (cardiovascular) 998.09
    pulmonary (*see also* Atelectasis) 518.0
      fetus or newborn 770.5
        partial 770.5
        primary 770.4
    thorax 512.89
      iatrogenic 512.1
      postoperative 512.1
    trachea 519.19
    valvular — *see* Endocarditis
    vascular (peripheral) 785.59
      with
        abortion — *see* Abortion, by type,
        with shock
        ectopic pregnancy (*see also* cate-
        gories 633.0–633.9) 639.5
        molar pregnancy (*see also* categories
        630–632) 639.5
      cerebral (*see also* Disease, cerebrovascu-
      lar, acute) 436
      during or after labor and delivery
      669.1 ☑
      fetus or newborn 779.89
      following
        abortion 639.5
        ectopic or molar pregnancy 639.5
    vasomotor 785.59
    vertebra 733.13
Collateral — *see also* condition
  circulation (venous) 459.89
  dilation, veins 459.89
Colles' fracture (closed) (reversed) (separation)
  813.41
  open 813.51
Collet-Sicard syndrome 352.6
Collet's syndrome 352.6
Colliculitis urethralis — *see also* Urethritis
  597.89
Colliers'
  asthma 500
  lung 500
  phthisis (*see also* Tuberculosis) 011.4 ☑
Collodion baby (ichthyosis congenita) 757.1
Colloid milium 709.3
Coloboma NEC 743.49
  choroid 743.59
  fundus 743.52
  iris 743.46
  lens 743.36
  lids 743.62
  optic disc (congenital) 743.57
    acquired 377.23
  retina 743.56
  sclera 743.47
Coloenteritis — *see* Enteritis
Colon — *see* condition
Colonization
  MRSA (methicillin resistant Staphylococcus
    aureus) V02.54

Colonization — *continued*
  MSSA (methicillin susceptible Staphylococ-
    cus aureus) V02.53
Coloptosis 569.89
Color
  amblyopia NEC 368.59
    acquired 368.55
  blindness NEC (congenital) 368.59
    acquired 368.55
Colostomy
  attention to V55.3
  fitting or adjustment V55.3
  malfunctioning 569.62
  status V44.3
Colpitis — *see also* Vaginitis 616.10
Colpocele 618.6
Colpocystitis — *see also* Vaginitis 616.10
Colporrhexis 665.4 ☑
Colpospasm 625.1
Column, spinal, vertebral — *see* condition
Coma 780.01
  apoplectic (*see also* Disease, cerebrovascular, acute) 436
  diabetic (with ketoacidosis) 250.3 ☑
    due to secondary diabetes 249.3 ☑
    hyperosmolar 250.2 ☑
      due to secondary diabetes 249.2 ☑
  eclamptic (*see also* Eclampsia) 780.39
  epileptic 345.3
  hepatic 572.2
  hyperglycemic 250.3 ☑
    due to secondary diabetes 249.3 ☑
  hyperosmolar (diabetic) (nonketotic)
    250.2 ☑
    due to secondary diabetes 249.2 ☑
  hypoglycemic 251.0
    diabetic 250.3 ☑
      due to secondary diabetes 249.3 ☑
  insulin 250.3 ☑
    due to secondary diabetes 249.3 ☑
    hyperosmolar 250.2 ☑
      due to secondary diabetes 249.2 ☑
    non-diabetic 251.0
    organic hyperinsulinism 251.0
  Kussmaul's (diabetic) 250.3 ☑
    due to secondary diabetes 249.3 ☑
  liver 572.2
  newborn 779.2
  prediabetic 250.2 ☑
    due to secondary diabetes 249.2 ☑
  uremic — *see* Uremia
Combat fatigue — *see also* Reaction, stress,
  acute 308.9
Combined — *see* condition
Comedo 706.1
Comedocarcinoma (M8501/3) — *see also*
  Neoplasm, breast, malignant
  noninfiltrating (M8501/2)
    specified site — *see* Neoplasm, by site,
    in situ
    unspecified site 233.0
Comedomastitis 610.4
Comedones 706.1
  lanugo 757.4
Comma bacillus, carrier (suspected) of V02.3
Comminuted fracture — *see* Fracture, by site
Common
  aortopulmonary trunk 745.0
  atrioventricular canal (defect) 745.69
  atrium 745.69
  cold (head) 460
    vaccination, prophylactic (against) V04.7
  truncus (arteriosus) 745.0
  ventricle 745.3
Commotio (current)
  cerebri (*see also* Concussion, brain) 850.9
    with skull fracture — *see* Fracture, skull,
    by site
  retinae 921.3
  spinalis — *see* Injury, spinal, by site
Commotion (current)
  brain (without skull fracture) (*see also* Concussion, brain) 850.9
    with skull fracture — *see* Fracture, skull,
    by site
  spinal cord — *see* Injury, spinal, by site

Communication
  abnormal (*see also* Fistula)
    between
      base of aorta and pulmonary artery
      745.0
      left ventricle and right atrium 745.4
      pericardial sac and pleural sac 748.8
      pulmonary artery and pulmonary
      vein 747.39
    congenital, between uterus and anterior
    abdominal wall 752.39
      bladder 752.39
      intestine 752.39
      rectum 752.39
  left ventricular — right atrial 745.4
  pulmonary artery-pulmonary vein 747.39
Compartment syndrome — *see* Syndrome,
  compartment
Compensation
  broken — *see* Failure, heart
  failure — *see* Failure, heart
  neurosis, psychoneurosis 300.11
Complaint — *see also* Disease
  bowel, functional 564.9
    psychogenic 306.4
  intestine, functional 564.9
    psychogenic 306.4
  kidney (*see also* Disease, renal) 593.9
  liver 573.9
  miners' 500
Complete — *see* condition
Complex
  cardiorenal (*see also* Hypertension, cardiorenal) 404.90
  castration 300.9
  Costen's 524.60
  ego-dystonic homosexuality 302.0
  Eisenmenger's (ventricular septal defect)
  745.4
  homosexual, ego-dystonic 302.0
  hypersexual 302.89
  inferiority 301.9
  jumped process
    spine — *see* Dislocation, vertebra
  primary, tuberculosis (*see also* Tuberculosis)
    010.0 ☑
  regional pain syndrome 355.9
    type I 337.20
      lower limb 337.22
      specified site NEC 337.29
      upper limb 337.21
    type II
      lower limb 355.71
      upper limb 354.4
  Taussig-Bing (transposition, aorta and
    overriding pulmonary artery) 745.11
Complications
  abortion NEC — *see* categories 634–639 ☑
  accidental puncture or laceration during a
  procedure 998.2
  amniocentesis, fetal 679.1 ☑
  amputation stump (late) (surgical) 997.60
    traumatic — *see* Amputation, traumatic
  anastomosis (and bypass) (*see also* Complications, due to (presence of) any device, implant, or graft classified to
  996.0–996.5 NEC)
    hemorrhage NEC 998.11
    intestinal (internal) NEC 997.49
      involving urinary tract 997.5
    mechanical — *see* Complications, me-
    chanical, graft
    urinary tract (involving intestinal tract)
    997.5
  anesthesia, anesthetic NEC (*see also* Anesthesia, complication) 995.22
    in labor and delivery 668.9 ☑
      affecting fetus or newborn 763.5
      cardiac 668.1 ☑
      central nervous system 668.2 ☑
      pulmonary 668.0 ☑
      specified type NEC 668.8 ☑
  aortocoronary (bypass) graft 996.03
    atherosclerosis — *see* Arteriosclerosis,
    coronary
    embolism 996.72

☑ **Additional Digit Required** — Refer to the Tabular List for Digit Selection   ꙮ **Subterms under main terms may continue to next column or page**

Complications — *continued*
  aortocoronary graft — *continued*
    occlusion NEC 996.72
    thrombus 996.72
  arthroplasty (*see also* Complications, prosthetic joint) 996.49
  artificial opening
    cecostomy 569.60
    colostomy 569.60
    cystostomy 596.83
      infection 596.81
      mechanical 596.82
      specified complication NEC 596.83
    enterostomy 569.60
    esophagostomy 530.87
      infection 530.86
      mechanical 530.87
    gastrostomy 536.40
    ileostomy 569.60
    jejunostomy 569.60
    nephrostomy 997.5
    tracheostomy 519.00
    ureterostomy 997.5
    urethrostomy 997.5
  bariatric surgery
    gastric band procedure 539.09
      infection 539.01
    specified procedure NEC 539.89
      infection 539.81
  bile duct implant (prosthetic) NEC 996.79
    infection or inflammation 996.69
    mechanical 996.59
  bleeding (intraoperative) (postoperative) 998.11
  blood vessel graft 996.1
    aortocoronary 996.03
      atherosclerosis — *see* Arteriosclerosis, coronary
      embolism 996.72
      occlusion NEC 996.72
      thrombus 996.72
    atherosclerosis — *see* Arteriosclerosis, extremities
    embolism 996.74
    occlusion NEC 996.74
    thrombus 996.74
  bone growth stimulator NEC 996.78
    infection or inflammation 996.67
  bone marrow transplant 996.85
  breast implant (prosthetic) NEC 996.79
    infection or inflammation 996.69
    mechanical 996.54
  bypass (*see also* Complications, anastomosis)
    aortocoronary 996.03
      atherosclerosis — *see* Arteriosclerosis, coronary
      embolism 996.72
      occlusion NEC 996.72
      thrombus 996.72
    carotid artery 996.1
      atherosclerosis — *see* Arteriosclerosis, extremities
      embolism 996.74
      occlusion NEC 996.74
      thrombus 996.74
  cardiac (*see also* Disease, heart) 429.9
    device, implant, or graft NEC 996.72
      infection or inflammation 996.61
      long-term effect 429.4
      mechanical (*see also* Complications, mechanical, by type) 996.00
        valve prosthesis 996.71
          infection or inflammation 996.61
    postoperative NEC 997.1
      long-term effect 429.4
  cardiorenal (*see also* Hypertension, cardiorenal) 404.90
  carotid artery bypass graft 996.1
    atherosclerosis — *see* Arteriosclerosis, extremities
    embolism 996.74
    occlusion NEC 996.74
    thrombus 996.74
  cataract fragments in eye 998.82

Complications — *continued*
  catheter device NEC (*see also* Complications, due to (presence of) any device, implant, or graft classified to 996.0–996.5 NEC)
    mechanical — *see* Complications, mechanical, catheter
  cecostomy 569.60
  cesarean section wound 674.3 ☑
  chemotherapy (antineoplastic) 995.29
  chin implant (prosthetic) NEC 996.79
    infection or inflammation 996.69
    mechanical 996.59
  colostomy (enterostomy) 569.60
    specified type NEC 569.69
  contraceptive device, intrauterine NEC 996.76
    infection 996.65
    inflammation 996.65
    mechanical 996.32
  cord (umbilical) — *see* Complications, umbilical cord
  cornea
    due to
      contact lens 371.82
  coronary (artery) bypass (graft) NEC 996.03
    atherosclerosis — *see* Arteriosclerosis, coronary
    embolism 996.72
    infection or inflammation 996.61
    mechanical 996.03
    occlusion NEC 996.72
    specified type NEC 996.72
    thrombus 996.72
  cystostomy 596.83
    infection 596.81
    mechanical 596.82
    specified complication NEC 596.83
  delivery 669.9 ☑
    procedure (instrumental) (manual) (surgical) 669.4 ☑
    specified type NEC 669.8 ☑
  dialysis (hemodialysis) (peritoneal) (renal) NEC 999.9
    catheter NEC (*see also* Complications, due to (presence of) any device, implant, or graft classified to 996.0–996.5 NEC)
      infection or inflammation 996.62
        peritoneal 996.68
      mechanical 996.1
        peritoneal 996.56
  drug NEC 995.29
  due to (presence of) any device, implant, or graft classified to 996.0–996.5 NEC 996.70
    with infection or inflammation — *see* Complications, infection or inflammation, due to (presence of) any device, implant, or graft classified to 996.0–996.5 NEC
    arterial NEC 996.74
      coronary NEC 996.03
        atherosclerosis — *see* Arteriosclerosis, coronary
        embolism 996.72
        occlusion NEC 996.72
        specified type NEC 996.72
        thrombus 996.72
      renal dialysis 996.73
    arteriovenous fistula or shunt NEC 996.74
    bone growth stimulator 996.78
    breast NEC 996.79
    cardiac NEC 996.72
      defibrillator 996.72
      pacemaker 996.72
      valve prosthesis 996.71
    catheter NEC 996.79
      spinal 996.75
      urinary, indwelling 996.76
      vascular NEC 996.74
        renal dialysis 996.73
      ventricular shunt 996.75
    coronary (artery) bypass (graft) NEC 996.03

Complications — *continued*
  due to any device, implant, or graft classified to 996.0–996.5 — *continued*
    coronary bypass — *continued*
      atherosclerosis — *see* Arteriosclerosis, coronary
      embolism 996.72
      occlusion NEC 996.72
      thrombus 996.72
    electrodes
      brain 996.75
      heart 996.72
    esophagostomy 530.87
    gastrointestinal NEC 996.79
    genitourinary NEC 996.76
    heart valve prosthesis NEC 996.71
    infusion pump 996.74
    insulin pump 996.57
    internal
      joint prosthesis 996.77
      orthopedic NEC 996.78
      specified type NEC 996.79
    intrauterine contraceptive device NEC 996.76
    joint prosthesis, internal NEC 996.77
    mechanical — *see* Complications, mechanical
    nervous system NEC 996.75
    ocular lens NEC 996.79
    orbital NEC 996.79
    orthopedic NEC 996.78
      joint, internal 996.77
    renal dialysis 996.73
    specified type NEC 996.79
    urinary catheter, indwelling 996.76
    vascular NEC 996.74
    ventricular shunt 996.75
  during dialysis NEC 999.9
  ectopic or molar pregnancy NEC 639.9
  electroshock therapy NEC 999.9
  enterostomy 569.60
    specified type NEC 569.69
  esophagostomy 530.87
    infection 530.86
    mechanical 530.87
  external (fixation) device with internal component(s) NEC 996.78
    infection or inflammation 996.67
    mechanical 996.49
  extracorporeal circulation NEC 999.9
  eye implant (prosthetic) NEC 996.79
    infection or inflammation 996.69
    mechanical
      ocular lens 996.53
      orbital globe 996.59
  fetal, from amniocentesis 679.1 ☑
  gastrointestinal, postoperative NEC (*see also* Complications, surgical procedures) 997.49
  gastrostomy 536.40
    specified type NEC 536.49
  genitourinary device, implant or graft NEC 996.76
    erosion of implanted vaginal mesh 629.31
    exposure of implanted vaginal mesh 629.32
    infection or inflammation 996.65
      urinary catheter, indwelling 996.64
    mechanical (*see also* Complications, mechanical, by type) 996.30
      specified NEC 996.39
  graft (bypass) (patch) (*see also* Complications, due to (presence of) any device, implant, or graft classified to 996.0–996.5 NEC)
    bone marrow 996.85
    corneal NEC 996.79
      infection or inflammation 996.69
      rejection or reaction 996.51
      retroprosthetic membrane 996.51
    mechanical — *see* Complications, mechanical, graft
    organ (immune or nonimmune cause) (partial) (total) 996.80
      bone marrow 996.85

Complications — *continued*
  graft (*see also* Complications, due to any device, implant, or graft classified to 996.0–996.5) — *continued*
    organ — *continued*
      heart 996.83
      intestines 996.87
      kidney 996.81
      liver 996.82
      lung 996.84
      pancreas 996.86
      specified NEC 996.89
    skin NEC 996.79
      infection or inflammation 996.69
      rejection 996.52
        artificial 996.55
        decellularized allodermis 996.55
  heart (*see also* Disease, heart transplant (immune or nonimmune cause)) 996.83
  hematoma (intraoperative) (postoperative) 998.12
  hemorrhage (intraoperative) (postoperative) 998.11
  hyperalimentation therapy NEC 999.9
  immunization (procedure) — *see* Complications, vaccination
  implant (*see also* Complications, due to (presence of) any device, implant, or graft classified to 996.0–996.5 NEC)
    dental placement, hemorrhagic 525.71
    mechanical — *see* Complications, mechanical, implant
  infection and inflammation
    due to (presence of) any device, implant or graft classified to 996.0–996.5 NEC 996.60
      arterial NEC 996.62
        coronary 996.61
        renal dialysis 996.62
      arteriovenous fistula or shunt 996.62
      artificial heart 996.61
      bone growth stimulator 996.67
      breast 996.69
      cardiac 996.61
      catheter NEC 996.69
        central venous 999.31
          bloodstream 999.32
          localized 999.33
        Hickman 999.31
          bloodstream 999.32
          localized 999.33
        peripherally inserted central (PICC) 999.31
          bloodstream 999.32
          localized 999.33
        peritoneal 996.68
        portacath (port-a-cath) 999.31
          bloodstream 999.32
          localized 999.33
        spinal 996.63
        triple lumen 999.31
          bloodstream 999.32
          localized 999.33
        umbilical venous 999.31
          bloodstream 999.32
          localized 999.33
        urinary, indwelling 996.64
        vascular (arterial) (dialysis) (peripheral venous) NEC 996.62
        ventricular shunt 996.63
      central venous catheter 999.31
        bloodstream 999.32
        localized 999.33
      coronary artery bypass 996.61
      electrodes
        brain 996.63
        heart 996.61
      gastrointestinal NEC 996.69
      genitourinary NEC 996.65
        indwelling urinary catheter 996.64
      heart assist device 996.61
      heart valve 996.61
      Hickman catheter 999.31

☑ **Additional Digit Required** — Refer to the Tabular List for Digit Selection   ▽ **Subterms under main terms may continue to next column or page**

2015 ICD-9-CM   ▶◀ Revised Text   ● New Line   ▲ Revised Code   **Volume 2 — 51**

Complications — *continued*
  infection and inflammation — *continued*
    due to any device, implant or graft classified to 996.0–996.5 — *continued*
      Hickman catheter — *continued*
        bloodstream 999.32
        localized 999.33
      infusion pump 996.62
      insulin pump 996.69
      intrauterine contraceptive device 996.65
      joint prosthesis, internal 996.66
      ocular lens 996.69
      orbital (implant) 996.69
      orthopedic NEC 996.67
        joint, internal 996.66
      peripherally inserted central catheter (PICC) 999.31
        bloodstream 999.32
        localized 999.33
      portacath (port-a-cath) 999.31
        bloodstream 999.32
        localized 999.33
      specified type NEC 996.69
      triple lumen catheter 999.31
        bloodstream 999.32
        localized 999.33
      umbilical venous catheter 999.31
        bloodstream 999.32
        localized 999.33
      urinary catheter, indwelling 996.64
      ventricular shunt 996.63
  infusion (procedure) 999.88
    blood — *see* Complications, transfusion
    infection NEC 999.39
    sepsis NEC 999.39
  inhalation therapy NEC 999.9
  injection (procedure) 999.9
    drug reaction (*see also* Reaction, drug) 995.27
    infection NEC 999.39
    sepsis NEC 999.39
    serum (prophylactic) (therapeutic) — *see* Complications, vaccination
    vaccine (any) — *see* Complications, vaccination
  inoculation (any) — *see* Complications, vaccination
  insulin pump 996.57
  internal device (catheter) (electronic) (fixation) (prosthetic) (*see also* Complications, due to (presence of) any device, implant, or graft classified to 996.0–996.5 NEC)
    mechanical — *see* Complications, mechanical
  intestinal pouch, specified NEC 569.79
  intestinal transplant (immune or nonimmune cause) 996.87
  intraoperative bleeding or hemorrhage 998.11
  intrauterine contraceptive device (*see also* Complications, contraceptive device) 996.76
    with fetal damage affecting management of pregnancy 655.8 ☑
    infection or inflammation 996.65
  in utero procedure
    fetal 679.1 ☑
    maternal 679.0 ☑
  jejunostomy 569.60
  kidney transplant (immune or nonimmune cause) 996.81
  labor 669.9 ☑
    specified condition NEC 669.8 ☑
  liver transplant (immune or nonimmune cause) 996.82
  lumbar puncture 349.0
  mechanical
    anastomosis — *see* Complications, mechanical, graft
    artificial heart 996.09
    bypass — *see* Complications, mechanical, graft

Complications — *continued*
  mechanical — *continued*
    catheter NEC 996.59
      cardiac 996.09
      cystostomy 596.82
      dialysis (hemodialysis) 996.1
        peritoneal 996.56
      during a procedure 998.2
      urethral, indwelling 996.31
    colostomy 569.62
    device NEC 996.59
      balloon (counterpulsation), intra-aortic 996.1
      cardiac 996.00
        automatic implantable defibrillator 996.04
        long-term effect 429.4
        specified NEC 996.09
      contraceptive, intrauterine 996.32
      counterpulsation, intra-aortic 996.1
      fixation, external, with internal components 996.49
      fixation, internal (nail, rod, plate) 996.40
      genitourinary 996.30
        specified NEC 996.39
      insulin pump 996.57
      nervous system 996.2
      orthopedic, internal 996.40
        prosthetic joint (*see also* Complications, mechanical, device, orthopedic, prosthetic, joint) 996.47
      prosthetic NEC 996.59
        joint 996.47
          articular bearing surface wear 996.46
          aseptic loosening 996.41
          breakage 996.43
          dislocation 996.42
          failure 996.47
          fracture 996.43
            around prosthetic 996.44
            peri-prosthetic 996.44
          instability 996.42
          loosening 996.41
          peri-prosthetic osteolysis 996.45
          subluxation 996.42
          wear 996.46
      umbrella, vena cava 996.1
      vascular 996.1
    dorsal column stimulator 996.2
    electrode NEC 996.59
      brain 996.2
      cardiac 996.01
      spinal column 996.2
    enterostomy 569.62
    esophagostomy 530.87
    fistula, arteriovenous, surgically created 996.1
    gastrostomy 536.42
    graft NEC 996.52
      aortic (bifurcation) 996.1
      aortocoronary bypass 996.03
      blood vessel NEC 996.1
      bone 996.49
      cardiac 996.00
      carotid artery bypass 996.1
      cartilage 996.49
      corneal 996.51
      coronary bypass 996.03
      decellularized allodermis 996.55
      genitourinary 996.30
        specified NEC 996.39
      muscle 996.49
      nervous system 996.2
      organ (immune or nonimmune cause) 996.80
        heart 996.83
        intestines 996.87
        kidney 996.81
        liver 996.82
        lung 996.84
        pancreas 996.86
        specified NEC 996.89

Complications — *continued*
  mechanical — *continued*
    graft — *continued*
      orthopedic, internal 996.49
      peripheral nerve 996.2
      prosthetic NEC 996.59
      skin 996.52
        artificial 996.55
      specified NEC 996.59
      tendon 996.49
      tissue NEC 996.52
      tooth 996.59
      ureter, without mention of resection 996.39
      vascular 996.1
    heart valve prosthesis 996.02
      long-term effect 429.4
    implant NEC 996.59
      cardiac 996.00
        automatic implantable defibrillator 996.04
        long-term effect 429.4
        specified NEC 996.09
      electrode NEC 996.59
        brain 996.2
        cardiac 996.01
        spinal column 996.2
      genitourinary 996.30
      nervous system 996.2
      orthopedic, internal 996.49
      prosthetic NEC 996.59
        in
          bile duct 996.59
          breast 996.54
          chin 996.59
          eye
            ocular lens 996.53
            orbital globe 996.59
      vascular 996.1
    insulin pump 996.57
    nonabsorbable surgical material 996.59
    pacemaker NEC 996.59
      brain 996.2
      cardiac 996.01
      nerve (phrenic) 996.2
    patch — *see* Complications, mechanical, graft
    prosthesis NEC 996.59
      bile duct 996.59
      breast 996.54
      chin 996.59
      ocular lens 996.53
      reconstruction, vas deferens 996.39
    reimplant NEC 996.59
      extremity (*see also* Complications, reattached, extremity) 996.90
      organ (*see also* Complications, transplant, organ, by site) 996.80
    repair — *see* Complications, mechanical, graft
    respirator [ventilator] V46.14
    shunt NEC 996.59
      arteriovenous, surgically created 996.1
      ventricular (communicating) 996.2
    stent NEC 996.59
    tracheostomy 519.02
    vas deferens reconstruction 996.39
    ventilator [respirator] V46.14
  medical care NEC 999.9
    cardiac NEC 997.1
    gastrointestinal NEC 997.49
    nervous system NEC 997.00
    peripheral vascular NEC 997.2
    respiratory NEC 997.39
    urinary NEC 997.5
    vascular
      mesenteric artery 997.71
      other vessels 997.79
      peripheral vessels 997.2
      renal artery 997.72
  nephrostomy 997.5
  nervous system
    device, implant, or graft NEC 349.1
      mechanical 996.2
    postoperative NEC 997.00

Complications — *continued*
  obstetric 669.9 ☑
    procedure (instrumental) (manual) (surgical) 669.4 ☑
    specified NEC 669.8 ☑
    surgical wound 674.3 ☑
  ocular lens implant NEC 996.79
    infection or inflammation 996.69
    mechanical 996.53
  organ transplant — *see* Complications, transplant, organ, by site
  orthopedic device, implant, or graft
    internal (fixation) (nail) (plate) (rod) NEC 996.78
      infection or inflammation 996.67
      joint prosthesis 996.77
        infection or inflammation 996.66
      mechanical 996.40
  pacemaker (cardiac) 996.72
    infection or inflammation 996.61
    mechanical 996.01
  pancreas transplant (immune or nonimmune cause) 996.86
  perfusion NEC 999.9
  perineal repair (obstetrical) 674.3 ☑
    disruption 674.2 ☑
  pessary (uterus) (vagina) — *see* Complications, contraceptive device
  phototherapy 990
  postcystoscopic 997.5
  postmastoidectomy NEC 383.30
  postoperative — *see* Complications, surgical procedures
  pregnancy NEC 646.9 ☑
    affecting fetus or newborn 761.9
  prosthetic device, internal (*see also* Complications, due to (presence of) any device, implant or graft classified to 996.0–996.5 NEC)
    mechanical NEC (*see also* Complications, mechanical) 996.59
  puerperium NEC (*see also* Puerperal) 674.9 ☑
  puncture, spinal 349.0
  pyelogram 997.5
  radiation 990
  radiotherapy 990
  reattached
    body part, except extremity 996.99
    extremity (infection) (rejection) 996.90
      arm(s) 996.94
      digit(s) (hand) 996.93
        foot 996.95
      finger(s) 996.93
      foot 996.95
      forearm 996.91
      hand 996.92
      leg 996.96
      lower NEC 996.96
      toe(s) 996.95
      upper NEC 996.94
  reimplant NEC (*see also* Complications, due to (presence of) any device, implant, or graft classified to 996.0–996.5 NEC)
    bone marrow 996.85
    extremity (*see also* Complications, reattached, extremity) 996.90
      due to infection 996.90
    mechanical — *see* Complications, mechanical, reimplant
    organ (immune or nonimmune cause) (partial) (total) (*see also* Complications, transplant, organ, by site) 996.80
  renal allograft 996.81
  renal dialysis — *see* Complications, dialysis
  respirator [ventilator], mechanical V46.14
  respiratory 519.9
    device, implant or graft NEC 996.79
      infection or inflammation 996.69
      mechanical 996.59
    distress syndrome, adult, following trauma and surgery 518.52
    insufficiency, acute, postoperative 518.52

☑ **Additional Digit Required — Refer to the Tabular List for Digit Selection**   ▽ **Subterms under main terms may continue to next column or page**

52 — Volume 2   ▶◀ Revised Text   ● New Line   ▲ Revised Code   2015 ICD-9-CM

Complications — *continued*
  respiratory — *continued*
    postoperative NEC 997.39
    therapy NEC 999.9
  sedation during labor and delivery 668.9 ☑
    affecting fetus or newborn 763.5
    cardiac 668.1 ☑
    central nervous system 668.2 ☑
    pulmonary 668.0 ☑
    specified type NEC 668.8 ☑
  seroma (intraoperative) (postoperative) (noninfected) 998.13
    infected 998.51
  shunt (*see also* Complications, due to (presence of) any device, implant, or graft classified to 996.0–996.5 NEC)
    mechanical — *see* Complications, mechanical, shunt
  specified body system NEC
    device, implant, or graft — *see* Complications, due to (presence of) any device, implant, or graft classified to 996.0–996.5 NEC
    postoperative NEC 997.99
  spinal puncture or tap 349.0
  stoma, external
    gastrointestinal tract
      colostomy 569.60
      enterostomy 569.60
      esophagostomy 530.87
        infection 530.86
        mechanical 530.87
      gastrostomy 536.40
    urinary tract 997.5
  stomach banding 539.09
  stomach stapling 539.89
  surgical procedures 998.9
    accidental puncture or laceration 998.2
    amputation stump (late) 997.60
    anastomosis — *see* Complications, anastomosis
    burst stitches or sutures (external) (*see also* Dehiscence) 998.32
      internal 998.31
    cardiac 997.1
      long-term effect following cardiac surgery 429.4
    cataract fragments in eye 998.82
    catheter device — *see* Complications, catheter device
    cecostomy malfunction 569.62
    colostomy malfunction 569.62
    cystostomy malfunction 596.82
      infection 596.81
      mechanical 596.82
      specified complication NEC 596.83
    dehiscence (of incision) (external) (*see also* Dehiscence) 998.32
      internal 998.31
    dialysis NEC (*see also* Complications, dialysis) 999.9
    disruption (*see also* Dehiscence)
      anastomosis (internal) — *see* Complications, mechanical, graft
      internal suture (line) 998.31
      wound (external) 998.32
        internal 998.31
    dumping syndrome (postgastrectomy) 564.2
    elephantiasis or lymphedema 997.99
      postmastectomy 457.0
    emphysema (surgical) 998.81
    enterostomy malfunction 569.62
    esophagostomy malfunction 530.87
    evisceration 998.32
    fistula (persistent postoperative) 998.6
    foreign body inadvertently left in wound (sponge) (suture) (swab) 998.4
    from nonabsorbable surgical material (Dacron) (mesh) (permanent suture) (reinforcing) (Teflon) — *see* Complications, due to (presence of) any device, implant, or graft classified to 996.0–996.5 NEC
    gastrointestinal NEC 997.49
    gastrostomy malfunction 536.42

Complications — *continued*
  surgical procedures — *continued*
    hematoma 998.12
    hemorrhage 998.11
    ileostomy malfunction 569.62
    internal prosthetic device NEC (*see also* Complications, internal device) 996.70
      hemolytic anemia 283.19
      infection or inflammation 996.60
      malfunction — *see* Complications, mechanical
      mechanical complication — *see* Complications, mechanical
      thrombus 996.70
    jejunostomy malfunction 569.62
    nervous system NEC 997.00
    obstruction, internal anastomosis — *see* Complications, mechanical, graft
    other body system NEC 997.99
    peripheral vascular NEC 997.2
    postcardiotomy syndrome 429.4
    postcholecystectomy syndrome 576.0
    postcommissurotomy syndrome 429.4
    postgastrectomy dumping syndrome 564.2
    postmastectomy lymphedema syndrome 457.0
    postmastoidectomy 383.30
      cholesteatoma, recurrent 383.32
      cyst, mucosal 383.31
      granulation 383.33
      inflammation, chronic 383.33
    postvagotomy syndrome 564.2
    postvalvulotomy syndrome 429.4
    reattached extremity (infection) (rejection) (*see also* Complications, reattached, extremity) 996.90
    respiratory NEC 997.39
    seroma 998.13
    shock (endotoxic) (septic) 998.02
      hypovolemic 998.09
    shunt, prosthetic (thrombus) (*see also* Complications, due to (presence of) any device, implant, or graft classified to 996.0–996.5 NEC)
      hemolytic anemia 283.19
    specified complication NEC 596.83
    specified complication NEC 998.89
    stitch abscess 998.59
    transplant — *see* Complications, graft
    ureterostomy malfunction 997.5
    urethrostomy malfunction 997.5
    urinary NEC 997.5
    vascular
      mesenteric artery 997.71
      other vessels 997.79
      peripheral vessels 997.2
      renal artery 997.72
    wound infection 998.59
  therapeutic misadventure NEC 999.9
    surgical treatment 998.9
  tracheostomy 519.00
  transfusion (blood) (lymphocytes) (plasma) 999.80
    acute lung injury (TRALI) 518.7
    atrophy, liver, yellow, subacute (within 8 months of administration) — *see* Hepatitis, viral
    bone marrow 996.85
    embolism
      air 999.1
      thrombus 999.2
    febrile nonhemolytic reaction (FNHTR) 780.66
    hemolysis NEC 999.89
      bone marrow 996.85
    hemolytic reaction, incompatibility unspecified 999.83
      acute 999.84
      delayed 999.85
    hepatitis (serum) (type B) (within 8 months after administration) — *see* Hepatitis, viral
    incompatibility reaction
      ABO 999.60

Complications — *continued*
  transfusion — *continued*
    incompatibility reaction — *continued*
      ABO — *continued*
        with hemolytic transfusion reaction (HTR) (not specified as acute or delayed) 999.61
          acute 999.62
          delayed 999.63
        specified type NEC 999.69
      minor blood group 999.89
      non-ABO (minor antigens) (Duffy) (Kell) (Kidd) (Lewis) (M) (N) (P) (S) 999.75
        with hemolytic transfusion reaction (HTR) (not specified as acute or delayed) 999.76
          acute 999.77
          delayed 999.78
        specified type NEC 999.79
      Rh antigen (C) (c) (D) (E) (e) (factor) 999.70
        with hemolytic transfusion reaction (HTR) (not specified as acute or delayed) 999.71
          acute 999.72
          delayed 999.73
        specified type NEC 999.74
    infection 999.39
      acute 999.34
    jaundice (serum) (within 8 months after administration) — *see* Hepatitis, viral
    sepsis 999.39
    shock or reaction NEC 999.89
      bone marrow 996.85
    specified reaction NEC 999.89
    subacute yellow atrophy of liver (within 8 months after administration) — *see* Hepatitis, viral
    thromboembolism 999.2
  transplant NEC (*see also* Complications, due to (presence of) any device, implant, or graft classified to 996.0–996.5 NEC)
    bone marrow 996.85
    organ (immune or nonimmune cause) (partial) (total) 996.80
      bone marrow 996.85
      heart 996.83
      intestines 996.87
      kidney 996.81
      liver 996.82
      lung 996.84
      pancreas 996.86
      specified NEC 996.89
    stem cell(s) 996.88
      from
        peripheral blood 996.88
        umbilical cord 996.88
  trauma NEC (early) 958.8
  ultrasound therapy NEC 999.9
  umbilical cord
    affecting fetus or newborn 762.6
    complicating delivery 663.9 ☑
      affecting fetus or newborn 762.6
      specified type NEC 663.8 ☑
  urethral catheter NEC 996.76
    infection or inflammation 996.64
    mechanical 996.31
  urinary, postoperative NEC 997.5
  vaccination 999.9
    anaphylaxis NEC 999.42
    cellulitis 999.39
    encephalitis or encephalomyelitis 323.51
    hepatitis (serum) (type B) (within 8 months after administration) — *see* Hepatitis, viral
    infection (general) (local) NEC 999.39
    jaundice (serum) (within 8 months after administration) — *see* Hepatitis, viral
    meningitis 997.09 *[321.8]*
    myelitis 323.52
    protein sickness 999.52

Complications — *continued*
  vaccination — *continued*
    reaction (allergic) 999.52
      serum 999.52
    sepsis 999.39
    serum intoxication, sickness, rash, or other serum reaction NEC 999.52
    shock (allergic) (anaphylactic) 999.49
    subacute yellow atrophy of liver (within 8 months after administration) — *see* Hepatitis, viral
    vaccinia (generalized) 999.0
      localized 999.39
  vascular
    device, implant, or graft NEC 996.74
      infection or inflammation 996.62
      mechanical NEC 996.1
        cardiac (*see also* Complications, mechanical, by type) 996.00
    following infusion, perfusion, or transfusion 999.2
    postoperative NEC 997.2
      mesenteric artery 997.71
      other vessels 997.79
      peripheral vessels 997.2
      renal artery 997.72
  ventilation therapy NEC 999.9
  ventilator [respirator], mechanical V46.14
Compound presentation, complicating delivery 652.8 ☑
  causing obstructed labor 660.0 ☑
Compressed air disease 993.3
Compression
  with injury — *see* specific injury
  arm NEC 354.9
  artery 447.1
    celiac, syndrome 447.4
  brachial plexus 353.0
  brain (stem) 348.4
    due to
      contusion, brain — *see* Contusion, brain
      injury NEC (*see also* Hemorrhage, brain, traumatic)
        birth — *see* Birth, injury, brain
      laceration, brain — *see* Laceration, brain
    osteopathic 739.0
  bronchus 519.19
  by cicatrix — *see* Cicatrix
  cardiac 423.9
  cauda equina 344.60
    with neurogenic bladder 344.61
  celiac (artery) (axis) 447.4
  cerebral — *see* Compression, brain
  cervical plexus 353.2
  cord (umbilical) — *see* Compression, umbilical cord
  cranial nerve 352.9
    second 377.49
    third (partial) 378.51
      total 378.52
    fourth 378.53
    fifth 350.8
    sixth 378.54
    seventh 351.8
  divers' squeeze 993.3
  duodenum (external) (*see also* Obstruction, duodenum) 537.3
  during birth 767.9
  esophagus 530.3
    congenital, external 750.3
  Eustachian tube 381.63
  facies (congenital) 754.0
  fracture — *see* Fracture, by site
  heart — *see* Disease, heart
  intestine (*see also* Obstruction, intestine) 560.9
    with hernia — *see* Hernia, by site, with obstruction
  laryngeal nerve, recurrent 478.79
  leg NEC 355.8
  lower extremity NEC 355.8
  lumbosacral plexus 353.1
  lung 518.89

☑ **Additional Digit Required** — Refer to the Tabular List for Digit Selection   ▽ **Subterms under main terms may continue to next column or page**

Compression — *continued*
  lymphatic vessel 457.1
  medulla — *see* Compression, brain
  nerve NEC (*see also* Disorder, nerve)
    arm NEC 354.9
    autonomic nervous system (*see also*
      Neuropathy, peripheral, autonom-
      ic) 337.9
    axillary 353.0
    cranial NEC 352.9
    due to displacement of intervertebral
      disc 722.2
      with myelopathy 722.70
      cervical 722.0
        with myelopathy 722.71
      lumbar, lumbosacral 722.10
        with myelopathy 722.73
      thoracic, thoracolumbar 722.11
        with myelopathy 722.72
    iliohypogastric 355.79
    ilioinguinal 355.79
    leg NEC 355.8
    lower extremity NEC 355.8
    median (in carpal tunnel) 354.0
    obturator 355.79
    optic 377.49
    plantar 355.6
    posterior tibial (in tarsal tunnel) 355.5
    root (by scar tissue) NEC 724.9
      cervical NEC 723.4
      lumbar NEC 724.4
      lumbosacral 724.4
      thoracic 724.4
    saphenous 355.79
    sciatic (acute) 355.0
    sympathetic 337.9
    traumatic — *see* Injury, nerve
    ulnar 354.2
    upper extremity NEC 354.9
  peripheral — *see* Compression, nerve
  spinal (cord) (old or nontraumatic) 336.9
    by displacement of intervertebral disc
      — *see* Displacement, interverte-
      bral disc
    nerve
      root NEC 724.9
        postoperative 722.80
          cervical region 722.81
          lumbar region 722.83
          thoracic region 722.82
        traumatic — *see* Injury, nerve,
          spinal
    traumatic — *see* Injury, nerve, spinal
    spondylogenic 721.91
      cervical 721.1
      lumbar, lumbosacral 721.42
      thoracic 721.41
    traumatic (*see also* Injury, spinal, by site)
      with fracture, vertebra — *see* Frac-
        ture, vertebra, by site, with
        spinal cord injury
  spondylogenic — *see* Compression, spinal
    cord, spondylogenic
  subcostal nerve (syndrome) 354.8
  sympathetic nerve NEC 337.9
  syndrome 958.5
  thorax 512.89
    iatrogenic 512.1
    postoperative 512.1
  trachea 519.19
    congenital 748.3
  ulnar nerve (by scar tissue) 354.2
  umbilical cord
    affecting fetus or newborn 762.5
      cord prolapsed 762.4
    complicating delivery 663.2 ☑
      cord around neck 663.1 ☑
      cord prolapsed 663.0 ☑
  upper extremity NEC 354.9
  ureter 593.3
  urethra — *see* Stricture, urethra
  vein 459.2
  vena cava (inferior) (superior) 459.2
  vertebral NEC — *see* Compression, spinal
    (cord)

Compulsion, compulsive
  eating 307.51
  neurosis (obsessive) 300.3
  personality 301.4
  states (mixed) 300.3
  swearing 300.3
    in Gilles de la Tourette's syndrome
      307.23
  tics and spasms 307.22
  water drinking NEC (syndrome) 307.9
Concato's disease (pericardial polyserositis)
  423.2
  peritoneal 568.82
  pleural — *see* Pleurisy
Concavity, chest wall 738.3
Concealed
  hemorrhage NEC 459.0
  penis 752.65
Concentric fading 368.12
Concern (normal) **about sick person in family**
  V61.49
Concrescence (teeth) 520.2
Concretio cordis 423.1
  rheumatic 393
Concretion — *see also* Calculus
  appendicular 543.9
  canaliculus 375.57
  clitoris 624.8
  conjunctiva 372.54
  eyelid 374.56
  intestine (impaction) (obstruction) 560.39
  lacrimal (passages) 375.57
  prepuce (male) 605
    female (clitoris) 624.8
  salivary gland (any) 527.5
  seminal vesicle 608.89
  stomach 537.89
  tonsil 474.8
Concussion (current) 850.9
  with
    loss of consciousness 850.5
      brief (less than one hour)
        30 minutes or less 850.11
        31-59 minutes 850.12
      moderate (1-24 hours) 850.2
      prolonged (more than 24 hours)
        (with complete recovery)
        (with return to pre-existing
        conscious level) 850.3
        without return to pre-existing
        conscious level 850.4
    mental confusion or disorientation
      (without loss of consciousness)
      850.0
    with loss of consciousness — *see*
      Concussion, with, loss of con-
      sciousness
  without loss of consciousness 850.0
  blast (air) (hydraulic) (immersion) (underwa-
    ter) 869.0
    with open wound into cavity 869.1
    abdomen or thorax — *see* Injury, inter-
      nal, by site
    brain — *see* Concussion, brain
    ear (acoustic nerve trauma) 951.5
      with perforation, tympanic mem-
        brane — *see* Wound, open,
        ear drum
    thorax — *see* Injury, internal, intratho-
      racic organs NEC
  brain or cerebral (without skull fracture)
    850.9
    with
      loss of consciousness 850.5
        brief (less than one hour)
          30 minutes or less 850.11
          31-59 minutes 850.12
        moderate (1-24 hours) 850.2
        prolonged (more than 24 hours)
          (with complete recovery)
          (with return to pre-exist-
          ing conscious level) 850.3
          without return to pre-existing
          conscious level 850.4

Concussion — *continued*
  brain or cerebral — *continued*
    with — *continued*
      mental confusion or disorientation
        (without loss of conscious-
        ness) 850.0
        with loss of consciousness — *see*
          Concussion, brain, with,
          loss of consciousness
      skull fracture — *see* Fracture, skull,
        by site
    without loss of consciousness 850.0
  cauda equina 952.4
  cerebral — *see* Concussion, brain
  conus medullaris (spine) 952.4
  hydraulic — *see* Concussion, blast
  internal organs — *see* Injury, internal, by
    site
  labyrinth — *see* Injury, intracranial
  ocular 921.3
  osseous labyrinth — *see* Injury, intracranial
  spinal (cord) (*see also* Injury, spinal, by site)
    due to
      broken
        back — *see* Fracture, vertebra, by
          site, with spinal cord injury
        neck — *see* Fracture, vertebra,
          cervical, with spinal cord
          injury
      fracture, fracture dislocation, or
        compression fracture of spine
        or vertebra — *see* Fracture,
        vertebra, by site, with spinal
        cord injury
  syndrome 310.2
  underwater blast — *see* Concussion, blast
Condition — *see also* Disease
  fetal hematologic 678.0 ☑
  psychiatric 298.9
  respiratory NEC 519.9
    acute or subacute NEC 519.9
      due to
        external agent 508.9
          specified type NEC 508.8
        fumes or vapors (chemical) (in-
          halation) 506.3
        radiation 508.0
    chronic NEC 519.9
      due to
        external agent 508.9
          specified type NEC 508.8
        fumes or vapors (chemical) (in-
          halation) 506.4
        radiation 508.1
    due to
      external agent 508.9
        specified type NEC 508.8
      fumes or vapors (chemical) (inhala-
        tion) 506.9
      smoke inhalation 508.2
Conduct disturbance — *see also* Disturbance,
  conduct 312.9
  adjustment reaction 309.3
  hyperkinetic 314.2
Condyloma NEC 078.11
  acuminatum 078.11
  gonorrheal 098.0
  latum 091.3
  syphilitic 091.3
    congenital 090.0
  venereal, syphilitic 091.3
Confinement — *see* Delivery
Conflagration — *see also* Burn, by site
  asphyxia (by inhalation of gases, fumes, or
    vapors) 987.9
  specified agent — *see* Table of Drugs
    and Chemicals
Conflict
  family V61.9
    specified circumstance NEC V61.8
  interpersonal NEC V62.81
  marital V61.10
    involving
      divorce V61.03
      estrangement V61.09
  parent (guardian)-child V61.20

Conflict — *continued*
  parent-child — *continued*
    adopted child V61.24
    biological child V61.23
    foster child V61.25
  partner V61.10
Confluent — *see* condition
Confusional arousals 327.41
Confusion, confused (mental) (state) — *see*
  also State, confusional 298.9
  acute 293.0
  epileptic 293.0
  postoperative 293.9
  psychogenic 298.2
  reactive (from emotional stress, psycholog-
    ical trauma) 298.2
  subacute 293.1
Congelation 991.9
Congenital — *see also* condition
  aortic septum 747.29
  generalized fibromatosis (CGF) 759.89
  intrinsic factor deficiency 281.0
  malformation — *see* Anomaly
Congestion, congestive
  asphyxia, newborn 768.9
  bladder 596.89
  bowel 569.89
  brain (*see also* Disease, cerebrovascular NEC)
    437.8
    malarial 084.9
  breast 611.79
  bronchi 519.19
  bronchial tube 519.19
  catarrhal 472.0
  cerebral — *see* Congestion, brain
  cerebrospinal — *see* Congestion, brain
  chest 786.9
  chill 780.99
    malarial (*see also* Malaria) 084.6
  circulatory NEC 459.9
  conjunctiva 372.71
  due to disturbance of circulation 459.9
  duodenum 537.3
  enteritis — *see* Enteritis
  eye 372.71
  fibrosis syndrome (pelvic) 625.5
  gastroenteritis — *see* Enteritis
  general 799.89
  glottis 476.0
  heart (*see also* Failure, heart) 428.0
  hepatic 573.0
  hypostatic (lung) 514
  intestine 569.89
  intracranial — *see* Congestion, brain
  kidney 593.89
  labyrinth 386.50
  larynx 476.0
  liver 573.0
  lung 786.9
    active or acute (*see also* Pneumonia) 486
      congenital 770.0
    chronic 514
    hypostatic 514
    idiopathic, acute 518.52
    passive 514
  malaria, malarial (brain) (fever) (*see also*
    Malaria) 084.6
  medulla — *see* Congestion, brain
  nasal 478.19
  nose 478.19
  orbit, orbital 376.33
    inflammatory (chronic) 376.10
      acute 376.00
  ovary 620.8
  pancreas 577.8
  pelvic, female 625.5
  pleural 511.0
  prostate (active) 602.1
  pulmonary — *see* Congestion, lung
  renal 593.89
  retina 362.89
  seminal vesicle 608.89
  spinal cord 336.1
  spleen 289.51
    chronic 289.51
  stomach 537.89

☑ **Additional Digit Required — Refer to the Tabular List for Digit Selection**   ▽ **Subterms under main terms may continue to next column or page**

54 — Volume 2   ▶◀ Revised Text   ● New Line   ▲ Revised Code   **2015 ICD-9-CM**

Congestion, congestive — *continued*
trachea 464.11
urethra 599.84
uterus 625.5
with subinvolution 621.1
viscera 799.89
Congestive — *see* Congestion
Conical
cervix 622.6
cornea 371.60
teeth 520.2
Conjoined twins 759.4
causing disproportion (fetopelvic) 678.1 ☑
fetal 678.1 ☑
Conjugal maladjustment V61.10
involving
divorce V61.03
estrangement V61.09
Conjunctiva — *see* condition
Conjunctivitis (exposure) (infectious)
(nondiphtheritic) (pneumococcal) (pustular) (staphylococcal) (streptococcal)
NEC 372.30
actinic 370.24
acute 372.00
atopic 372.05
chemical 372.06
contagious 372.03
follicular 372.02
hemorrhagic (viral) 077.4
toxic 372.06
adenoviral (acute) 077.3
allergic (chronic) 372.14
with hay fever 372.05
anaphylactic 372.05
angular 372.03
Apollo (viral) 077.4
atopic 372.05
blennorrhagic (neonatorum) 098.40
catarrhal 372.03
chemical 372.06
allergic 372.05
meaning corrosion — *see* Burn, conjunctiva
chlamydial 077.98
due to
Chlamydia trachomatis — *see* Trachoma
paratrachoma 077.0
chronic 372.10
allergic 372.14
follicular 372.12
simple 372.11
specified type NEC 372.14
vernal 372.13
diphtheritic 032.81
due to
dust 372.05
enterovirus type 70 077.4
erythema multiforme 695.10 *[372.33]*
filariasis (*see also* Filariasis) 125.9 *[372.15]*
mucocutaneous
disease NEC 372.33
leishmaniasis 085.5 *[372.15]*
Reiter's disease 099.3 *[372.33]*
syphilis 095.8 *[372.10]*
toxoplasmosis (acquired) 130.1
congenital (active) 771.2
trachoma — *see* Trachoma
dust 372.05
eczematous 370.31
epidemic 077.1
hemorrhagic 077.4
follicular (acute) 372.02
adenoviral (acute) 077.3
chronic 372.12
glare 370.24
gonococcal (neonatorum) 098.40
granular (trachomatous) 076.1
late effect 139.1
hemorrhagic (acute) (epidemic) 077.4
herpetic (simplex) 054.43
zoster 053.21
inclusion 077.0
infantile 771.6
influenzal 372.03

Conjunctivitis — *continued*
Koch-Weeks 372.03
light 372.05
medicamentosa 372.05
membranous 372.04
meningococcic 036.89
Morax-Axenfeld 372.02
mucopurulent NEC 372.03
neonatal 771.6
gonococcal 098.40
Newcastle's 077.8
nodosa 360.14
of Beal 077.3
parasitic 372.15
filariasis (*see also* Filariasis) 125.9 *[372.15]*
mucocutaneous leishmaniasis
085.5 *[372.15]*
Parinaud's 372.02
petrificans 372.39
phlyctenular 370.31
pseudomembranous 372.04
diphtheritic 032.81
purulent 372.03
Reiter's 099.3 *[372.33]*
rosacea 695.3 *[372.31]*
serous 372.01
viral 077.99
simple chronic 372.11
specified NEC 372.39
sunlamp 372.04
swimming pool 077.0
toxic 372.06
trachomatous (follicular) 076.1
acute 076.0
late effect 139.1
traumatic NEC 372.39
tuberculous (*see also* Tuberculosis)
017.3 ☑ *[370.31]*
tularemic 021.3
tularensis 021.3
vernal 372.13
limbar 372.13 *[370.32]*
viral 077.99
acute hemorrhagic 077.4
specified NEC 077.8
Conjunctivochalasis 372.81
Conjunctoblepharitis — *see* Conjunctivitis
Connective tissue — *see* condition
Conn (-Louis) syndrome (primary aldosteronism) 255.12
Conradi (-Hünermann) syndrome or disease (chondrodysplasia calcificans congenita) 756.59
Consanguinity V19.7
Consecutive — *see* condition
Consolidated lung (base) — *see* Pneumonia, lobar
Constipation 564.00
atonic 564.09
drug induced
correct substance properly administered 564.09
overdose or wrong substance given or taken 977.9
specified drug — *see* Table of Drugs and Chemicals
neurogenic 564.09
other specified NEC 564.09
outlet dysfunction 564.02
psychogenic 306.4
simple 564.00
slow transit 564.01
spastic 564.09
Constitutional — *see also* condition
arterial hypotension (*see also* Hypotension) 458.9
obesity 278.00
morbid 278.01
psychopathic state 301.9
short stature in childhood 783.43
state, developmental V21.9
specified development NEC V21.8
substandard 301.6
Constitutionally substandard 301.6
Constriction
anomalous, meningeal bands or folds 742.8

Constriction — *continued*
aortic arch (congenital) 747.10
asphyxiation or suffocation by 994.7
bronchus 519.19
canal, ear (*see also* Stricture, ear canal, acquired) 380.50
duodenum 537.3
gallbladder (*see also* Obstruction, gallbladder) 575.2
congenital 751.69
intestine (*see also* Obstruction, intestine) 560.9
larynx 478.74
congenital 748.3
meningeal bands or folds, anomalous 742.8
organ or site, congenital NEC — *see* Atresia
prepuce (congenital) 605
pylorus 537.0
adult hypertrophic 537.0
congenital or infantile 750.5
newborn 750.5
ring (uterus) 661.4 ☑
affecting fetus or newborn 763.7
spastic (*see also* Spasm)
ureter 593.3
urethra — *see* Stricture, urethra
stomach 537.89
ureter 593.3
urethra — *see* Stricture, urethra
visual field (functional) (peripheral) 368.45
Constrictive — *see* condition
Consultation
without complaint or sickness V65.9
feared complaint unfounded V65.5
specified reason NEC V65.8
medical (*see also* Counseling, medical)
specified reason NEC V65.8
Consumption — *see* Tuberculosis
Contact — *see also* Exposure (suspected)
with
AIDS virus V01.79
anthrax V01.81
asbestos V15.84
cholera V01.0
communicable disease V01.9
specified type NEC V01.89
viral NEC V01.79
Escherichia coli (E. coli) V01.83
German measles V01.4
gonorrhea V01.6
HIV V01.79
human immunodeficiency virus V01.79
lead V15.86
meningococcus V01.84
parasitic disease NEC V01.89
poliomyelitis V01.2
potentially hazardous body fluids V15.85
rabies V01.5
rubella V01.4
SARS-associated coronavirus V01.82
smallpox V01.3
syphilis V01.6
tuberculosis V01.1
varicella V01.71
venereal disease V01.6
viral disease NEC V01.79
dermatitis — *see* Dermatitis
Contamination, food — *see also* Poisoning, food 005.9
Contraception, contraceptive
advice NEC V25.09
family planning V25.09
fitting of diaphragm V25.02
prescribing or use of
oral contraceptive agent V25.01
specified agent NEC V25.02
counseling NEC V25.09
emergency V25.03
family planning V25.09
fitting of diaphragm V25.02
prescribing or use of
oral contraceptive agent V25.01
emergency V25.03
postcoital V25.03
specified agent NEC V25.02
device (in situ) V45.59

Contraception, contraceptive —
continued
device — *continued*
causing menorrhagia 996.76
checking V25.42
complications 996.32
insertion V25.11
intrauterine V45.51
reinsertion V25.13
removal V25.12
and reinsertion V25.13
replacement V25.13
subdermal V45.52
fitting of diaphragm V25.02
insertion
intrauterine contraceptive device V25.11
subdermal implantable V25.5
maintenance V25.40
examination V25.40
oral contraceptive V25.41
specified method NEC V25.49
subdermal implantable V25.43
intrauterine device V25.42
intrauterine device V25.42
oral contraceptive V25.41
specified method NEC V25.49
subdermal implantable V25.43
management NEC V25.49
prescription
oral contraceptive agent V25.01
emergency V25.03
postcoital V25.03
repeat V25.41
specified agent NEC V25.02
repeat V25.49
sterilization V25.2
surveillance V25.40
intrauterine device V25.42
oral contraceptive agent V25.41
subdermal implantable V25.43
specified method NEC V25.49
Contraction, contracture, contracted
Achilles tendon (*see also* Short, tendon, Achilles) 727.81
anus 564.89
axilla 729.90
bile duct (*see also* Disease, biliary) 576.8
bladder 596.89
neck or sphincter 596.0
bowel (*see also* Obstruction, intestine) 560.9
Braxton Hicks 644.1 ☑
breast implant, capsular 611.83
bronchus 519.19
burn (old) — *see* Cicatrix
capsular, of breast implant 611.83
cecum (*see also* Obstruction, intestine) 560.9
cervix (*see also* Stricture, cervix) 622.4
congenital 752.49
cicatricial — *see* Cicatrix
colon (*see also* Obstruction, intestine) 560.9
conjunctiva trachomatous, active 076.1
late effect 139.1
Dupuytren's 728.6
eyelid 374.41
eye socket (after enucleation) 372.64
face 729.90
fascia (lata) (postural) 728.89
Dupuytren's 728.6
palmar 728.6
plantar 728.71
finger NEC 736.29
congenital 755.59
joint (*see also* Contraction, joint) 718.44
flaccid, paralytic
joint (*see also* Contraction, joint)
718.4 ☑
muscle 728.85
ocular 378.50
gallbladder (*see also* Obstruction, gallbladder) 575.2
hamstring 728.89
tendon 727.81
heart valve — *see* Endocarditis
Hicks' 644.1 ☑
hip (*see also* Contraction, joint) 718.4 ☑

☑ **Additional Digit Required — Refer to the Tabular List for Digit Selection**   ▽ **Subterms under main terms may continue to next column or page**

Contraction, contracture, contracted — *continued*
hourglass
  bladder 596.89
    congenital 753.8
  gallbladder (*see also* Obstruction, gall-
    bladder) 575.2
    congenital 751.69
  stomach 536.8
    congenital 750.7
    psychogenic 306.4
  uterus 661.4 ☑
    affecting fetus or newborn 763.7
hysterical 300.11
infantile (*see also* Epilepsy) 345.6 ☑
internal os (*see also* Stricture, cervix) 622.4
intestine (*see also* Obstruction, intestine)
    560.9
joint (abduction) (acquired) (adduction)
    (flexion) (rotation) 718.40
  ankle 718.47
  congenital NEC 755.8
    generalized or multiple 754.89
      lower limb joints 754.89
    hip (*see also* Subluxation, congenital,
      hip) 754.32
    lower limb (including pelvic girdle)
      not involving hip 754.89
    upper limb (including shoulder gir-
      dle) 755.59
  elbow 718.42
  foot 718.47
  hand 718.44
  hip 718.45
  hysterical 300.11
  knee 718.46
  multiple sites 718.49
  pelvic region 718.45
  shoulder (region) 718.41
  specified site NEC 718.48
  wrist 718.43
kidney (granular) (secondary) (*see also*
    Sclerosis, renal) 587
  congenital 753.3
  hydronephritic 591
  pyelonephritic (*see also* Pyelitis, chronic)
    590.00
  tuberculous (*see also* Tuberculosis)
    016.0 ☑
ligament 728.89
  congenital 756.89
liver — *see* Cirrhosis, liver
muscle (postinfectional) (postural) NEC
    728.85
  congenital 756.89
    sternocleidomastoid 754.1
  extraocular 378.60
  eye (extrinsic) (*see also* Strabismus) 378.9
    paralytic (*see also* Strabismus, paralyt-
      ic) 378.50
  flaccid 728.85
  hysterical 300.11
  ischemic (Volkmann's) 958.6
  paralytic 728.85
  posttraumatic 958.6
  psychogenic 306.0
    specified as conversion reaction
      300.11
myotonic 728.85
neck (*see also* Torticollis) 723.5
  congenital 754.1
  psychogenic 306.0
ocular muscle (*see also* Strabismus) 378.9
  paralytic (*see also* Strabismus, paralytic)
    378.50
organ or site, congenital NEC — *see* Atresia
outlet (pelvis) — *see* Contraction, pelvis
palmar fascia 728.6
paralytic
  joint (*see also* Contraction, joint)
    718.4 ☑
  muscle 728.85
    ocular (*see also* Strabismus, paralytic)
      378.50
pelvis (acquired) (general) 738.6
  affecting fetus or newborn 763.1

Contraction, contracture, contracted — *continued*
pelvis — *continued*
  complicating delivery 653.1 ☑
    causing obstructed labor 660.1 ☑
    generally contracted 653.1 ☑
      causing obstructed labor
        660.1 ☑
    inlet 653.2 ☑
      causing obstructed labor
        660.1 ☑
    midpelvic 653.8 ☑
      causing obstructed labor
        660.1 ☑
    midplane 653.8 ☑
      causing obstructed labor
        660.1 ☑
    outlet 653.3 ☑
      causing obstructed labor
        660.1 ☑
plantar fascia 728.71
premature
  atrial 427.61
  auricular 427.61
  auriculoventricular 427.61
  heart (junctional) (nodal) 427.60
  supraventricular 427.61
  ventricular 427.69
prostate 602.8
pylorus (*see also* Pylorospasm) 537.81
rectosigmoid (*see also* Obstruction, intes-
    tine) 560.9
rectum, rectal (sphincter) 564.89
  psychogenic 306.4
ring (Bandl's) 661.4 ☑
  affecting fetus or newborn 763.7
scar — *see* Cicatrix
sigmoid (*see also* Obstruction, intestine)
    560.9
socket, eye 372.64
spine (*see also* Curvature, spine) 737.9
stomach 536.8
  hourglass 536.8
    congenital 750.7
  psychogenic 306.4
tendon (sheath) (*see also* Short, tendon)
    727.81
toe 735.8
ureterovesical orifice (postinfectional) 593.3
urethra 599.84
uterus 621.8
  abnormal 661.9 ☑
    affecting fetus or newborn 763.7
  clonic, hourglass or tetanic 661.4 ☑
    affecting fetus or newborn 763.7
  dyscoordinate 661.4 ☑
    affecting fetus or newborn 763.7
  hourglass 661.4 ☑
    affecting fetus or newborn 763.7
  hypotonic NEC 661.2 ☑
    affecting fetus or newborn 763.7
  incoordinate 661.4 ☑
    affecting fetus or newborn 763.7
  inefficient or poor 661.2 ☑
    affecting fetus or newborn 763.7
  irregular 661.2 ☑
    affecting fetus or newborn 763.7
  tetanic 661.4 ☑
    affecting fetus or newborn 763.7
vagina (outlet) 623.2
vesical 596.89
  neck or urethral orifice 596.0
visual field, generalized 368.45
Volkmann's (ischemic) 958.6
Contusion (skin surface intact) 924.9
with
  crush injury — *see* Crush
  dislocation — *see* Dislocation, by site
  fracture — *see* Fracture, by site
  internal injury (*see also* Injury, internal,
    by site)
    heart — *see* Contusion, cardiac
    kidney — *see* Contusion, kidney
    liver — *see* Contusion, liver
    lung — *see* Contusion, lung
    spleen — *see* Contusion, spleen

Contusion — *continued*
with — *continued*
  intracranial injury — *see* Injury, intracra-
    nial
  nerve injury — *see* Injury, nerve
  open wound — *see* Wound, open, by
    site
abdomen, abdominal (muscle) (wall) 922.2
  organ(s) NEC 868.00
adnexa, eye NEC 921.9
ankle 924.21
  with other parts of foot 924.20
arm 923.9
  lower (with elbow) 923.10
  upper 923.03
    with shoulder or axillary region
      923.09
auditory canal (external) (meatus) (and
    other part(s) of neck, scalp, or face,
    except eye) 920
auricle, ear (and other part(s) of neck, scalp,
    or face except eye) 920
axilla 923.02
  with shoulder or upper arm 923.09
back 922.31
bone NEC 924.9
brain (cerebral) (membrane) (with hemor-
    rhage) 851.8 ☑

> Note — Use the following fifth-digit
> subclassification with categories
> 851–854:
>
> 0   unspecified state of consciousness
>
> 1   with no loss of consciousness
>
> 2   with brief [less than one hour]
>   loss of consciousness
>
> 3   with moderate [1–24 hours] loss
>   of consciousness
>
> 4   with prolonged [more than 24
>   hours] loss of consciousness and
>   return to pre-existing conscious
>   level
>
> 5   with prolonged [more than 24
>   hours] loss of consciousness,
>   without return to pre-existing
>   conscious level
>
> Use fifth-digit 5 to designate when a
> patient is unconscious and dies before
> regaining consciousness, regardless of
> the duration of the loss of consciousness
>
> 6   with loss of consciousness of un-
>   specified duration
>
> 9   with concussion, unspecified

  with
    open intracranial wound 851.9 ☑
    skull fracture — *see* Fracture, skull,
      by site
  cerebellum 851.4 ☑
    with open intracranial wound
      851.5 ☑
  cortex 851.0 ☑
    with open intracranial wound
      851.1 ☑
  occipital lobe 851.4 ☑
    with open intracranial wound
      851.5 ☑
  stem 851.4 ☑
    with open intracranial wound
      851.5 ☑
breast 922.0
brow (and other part(s) of neck, scalp, or
    face, except eye) 920
buttock 922.32
canthus 921.1
cardiac 861.01
  with open wound into thorax 861.11
cauda equina (spine) 952.4
cerebellum — *see* Contusion, brain, cerebel-
    lum
cerebral — *see* Contusion, brain
cheek(s) (and other part(s) of neck, scalp, or
    face, except eye) 920

Contusion — *continued*
chest (wall) 922.1
chin (and other part(s) of neck, scalp, or face,
    except eye) 920
clitoris 922.4
conjunctiva 921.1
conus medullaris (spine) 952.4
cornea 921.3
corpus cavernosum 922.4
cortex (brain) (cerebral) — *see* Contusion,
    brain, cortex
costal region 922.1
ear (and other part(s) of neck, scalp, or face
    except eye) 920
elbow 923.11
  with forearm 923.10
epididymis 922.4
epigastric region 922.2
eyeball 921.3
eyelid(s) (and periocular area) 921.1
eye NEC 921.9
face (and neck, or scalp, any part, except
    eye) 920
femoral triangle 922.2
fetus or newborn 772.6
finger(s) (nail) (subungual) 923.3
flank 922.2
foot (with ankle) (excluding toe(s)) 924.20
forearm (and elbow) 923.10
forehead (and other part(s) of neck, scalp,
    or face, except eye) 920
genital organs, external 922.4
globe (eye) 921.3
groin 922.2
gum(s) (and other part(s) of neck, scalp, or
    face, except eye) 920
hand(s) (except fingers alone) 923.20
head (any part, except eye) (and face) (and
    neck) 920
heart — *see* Contusion, cardiac
heel 924.20
hip 924.01
  with thigh 924.00
iliac region 922.2
inguinal region 922.2
internal organs (abdomen, chest, or pelvis)
    NEC — *see* Injury, internal, by site
interscapular region 922.33
iris (eye) 921.3
kidney 866.01
  with open wound into cavity 866.11
knee 924.11
  with lower leg 924.10
labium (majus) (minus) 922.4
lacrimal apparatus, gland, or sac 921.1
larynx (and other part(s) of neck, scalp, or
    face, except eye) 920
late effect — *see* Late, effects (of), contusion
leg 924.5
  lower (with knee) 924.10
lens 921.3
lingual (and other part(s) of neck, scalp, or
    face, except eye) 920
lip(s) (and other part(s) of neck, scalp, or
    face, except eye) 920
liver 864.01
  with
    laceration — *see* Laceration, liver
    open wound into cavity 864.11
lower extremity 924.5
  multiple sites 924.4
lumbar region 922.31
lung 861.21
  with open wound into thorax 861.31
malar region (and other part(s) of neck,
    scalp, or face, except eye) 920
mandibular joint (and other part(s) of neck,
    scalp, or face, except eye) 920
mastoid region (and other part(s) of neck,
    scalp, or face, except eye) 920
membrane, brain — *see* Contusion, brain
midthoracic region 922.1
mouth (and other part(s) of neck, scalp, or
    face, except eye) 920
multiple sites (not classifiable to same three-
    digit category) 924.8

☑ Additional Digit Required — Refer to the Tabular List for Digit Selection   ▽ Subterms under main terms may continue to next column or page

56 — Volume 2   ▶◀ Revised Text   ● New Line   ▲ Revised Code   2015 ICD-9-CM

Contusion — *continued*
    multiple sites — *continued*
        lower limb 924.4
        trunk 922.8
        upper limb 923.8
    muscle NEC 924.9
    myocardium — *see* Contusion, cardiac
    nasal (septum) (and other part(s) of neck, scalp, or face, except eye) 920
    neck (and scalp or face, any part, except eye) 920
    nerve — *see* Injury, nerve, by site
    nose (and other part(s) of neck, scalp, or face, except eye) 920
    occipital region (scalp) (and neck or face, except eye) 920
        lobe — *see* Contusion, brain, occipital lobe
    orbit (region) (tissues) 921.2
    palate (soft) (and other part(s) of neck, scalp, or face, except eye) 920
    parietal region (scalp) (and neck, or face, except eye) 920
        lobe — *see* Contusion, brain
    penis 922.4
    pericardium — *see* Contusion, cardiac
    perineum 922.4
    periocular area 921.1
    pharynx (and other part(s) of neck, scalp, or face, except eye) 920
    popliteal space (*see also* Contusion, knee) 924.11
    prepuce 922.4
    pubic region 922.4
    pudenda 922.4
    pulmonary — *see* Contusion, lung
    quadriceps femoralis 924.00
    rib cage 922.1
    sacral region 922.32
    salivary ducts or glands (and other part(s) of neck, scalp, or face, except eye) 920
    scalp (and neck, or face any part, except eye) 920
    scapular region 923.01
        with shoulder or upper arm 923.09
    sclera (eye) 921.3
    scrotum 922.4
    shoulder 923.00
        with upper arm or axillar regions 923.09
    skin NEC 924.9
    skull 920
    spermatic cord 922.4
    spinal cord (*see also* Injury, spinal, by site)
        cauda equina 952.4
        conus medullaris 952.4
    spleen 865.01
        with open wound into cavity 865.11
    sternal region 922.1
    stomach — *see* Injury, internal, stomach
    subconjunctival 921.1
    subcutaneous NEC 924.9
    submaxillary region (and other part(s) of neck, scalp, or face, except eye) 920
    submental region (and other part(s) of neck, scalp, or face, except eye) 920
    subperiosteal NEC 924.9
    supraclavicular fossa (and other part(s) of neck, scalp, or face, except eye) 920
    supraorbital (and other part(s) of neck, scalp, or face, except eye) 920
    temple (region) (and other part(s) of neck, scalp, or face, except eye) 920
    testis 922.4
    thigh (and hip) 924.00
    thorax 922.1
        organ — *see* Injury, internal, intrathoracic
    throat (and other part(s) of neck, scalp, or face, except eye) 920
    thumb(s) (nail) (subungual) 923.3
    toe(s) (nail) (subungual) 924.3
    tongue (and other part(s) of neck, scalp, or face, except eye) 920
    trunk 922.9
        multiple sites 922.8

Contusion — *continued*
    trunk — *continued*
        specified site — *see* Contusion, by site
    tunica vaginalis 922.4
    tympanum (membrane) (and other part(s) of neck, scalp, or face, except eye) 920
    upper extremity 923.9
        multiple sites 923.8
    uvula (and other part(s) of neck, scalp, or face, except eye) 920
    vagina 922.4
    vocal cord(s) (and other part(s) of neck, scalp, or face, except eye) 920
    vulva 922.4
    wrist 923.21
        with hand(s), except finger(s) alone 923.20
Conus (any type) (congenital) 743.57
    acquired 371.60
    medullaris syndrome 336.8
Convalescence (following) V66.9
    chemotherapy V66.2
    medical NEC V66.5
    psychotherapy V66.3
    radiotherapy V66.1
    surgery NEC V66.0
    treatment (for) NEC V66.5
        combined V66.6
        fracture V66.4
        mental disorder NEC V66.3
        specified disorder NEC V66.5
Conversion
    closed surgical procedure to open procedure
        arthroscopic V64.43
        laparoscopic V64.41
        thoracoscopic V64.42
    hysteria, hysterical, any type 300.11
    neurosis, any 300.11
    reaction, any 300.11
Converter, tuberculosis (test reaction) 795.51
Convulsions (idiopathic) 780.39
    apoplectiform (*see also* Disease, cerebrovascular, acute) 436
    brain 780.39
    cerebral 780.39
    cerebrospinal 780.39
    due to trauma NEC — *see* Injury, intracranial
    eclamptic (*see also* Eclampsia) 780.39
    epileptic (*see also* Epilepsy) 345.9 ☑
    epileptiform (*see also* Seizure, epileptiform) 780.39
    epileptoid (*see also* Seizure, epileptiform) 780.39
    ether
        anesthetic
            correct substance properly administered 780.39
            overdose or wrong substance given 968.2
        other specified type — *see* Table of Drugs and Chemicals
    febrile (simple) 780.31
        complex 780.32
    generalized 780.39
    hysterical 300.11
    infantile 780.39
        epilepsy — *see* Epilepsy
    internal 780.39
    jacksonian (*see also* Epilepsy) 345.5 ☑
    myoclonic 333.2
    newborn 779.0
    paretic 094.1
    pregnancy (nephritic) (uremic) — *see* Eclampsia, pregnancy
    psychomotor (*see also* Epilepsy) 345.4 ☑
    puerperal, postpartum — *see* Eclampsia, pregnancy
    recurrent 780.39
        epileptic — *see* Epilepsy
    reflex 781.0
    repetitive 780.39
        epileptic — *see* Epilepsy
    salaam (*see also* Epilepsy) 345.6 ☑
    scarlatinal 034.1

Convulsions — *continued*
    spasmodic 780.39
    tetanus, tetanic (*see also* Tetanus) 037
    thymic 254.8
    uncinate 780.39
    uremic 586
Convulsive — *see also* Convulsions
    disorder or state 780.39
        epileptic — *see* Epilepsy
    equivalent, abdominal (*see also* Epilepsy) 345.5 ☑
Cooke-Apert-Gallais syndrome (adrenogenital) 255.2
Cooley's anemia (erythroblastic) 282.44
Coolie itch 126.9
Cooper's
    disease 610.1
    hernia — *see* Hernia, Cooper's
Coordination disturbance 781.3
Copper wire arteries, retina 362.13
Copra itch 133.8
Coprolith 560.39
Coprophilia 302.89
Coproporphyria, hereditary 277.1
Coprostasis 560.32
    with hernia (*see also* Hernia, by site, with obstruction)
        gangrenous — *see* Hernia, by site, with gangrene
Cor
    biloculare 745.7
    bovinum — *see* Hypertrophy, cardiac
    bovis (*see also* Hypertrophy, cardiac)
    pulmonale (chronic) 416.9
        acute 415.0
    triatriatum, triatrium 746.82
    triloculare 745.8
        biatriatum 745.3
        biventriculare 745.69
Corbus' disease 607.1
Cord — *see also* condition
    around neck (tightly) (with compression)
        affecting fetus or newborn 762.5
        complicating delivery 663.1 ☑
            without compression 663.3 ☑
            affecting fetus or newborn 762.6
    bladder NEC 344.61
        tabetic 094.0
    prolapse
        affecting fetus or newborn 762.4
        complicating delivery 663.0 ☑
Cord's angiopathy — *see also* Tuberculosis 017.3 ☑ *[362.18]*
Cordis ectopia 746.87
Corditis (spermatic) 608.4
Corectopia 743.46
Cori type glycogen storage disease — *see* Disease, glycogen storage
Cork-handlers' disease or lung 495.3
Corkscrew esophagus 530.5
Corlett's pyosis (impetigo) 684
Corn (infected) 700
Cornea — *see also* condition
    donor V59.5
    guttata (dystrophy) 371.57
    plana 743.41
Cornelia de Lange's syndrome (Amsterdam dwarf, intellectual disabilities, and brachycephaly) 759.89
Cornual gestation or pregnancy — *see* Pregnancy, cornual
Cornu cutaneum 702.8
Coronary (artery) — *see also* condition
    arising from aorta or pulmonary trunk 746.85
Corpora — *see also* condition
    amylacea (prostate) 602.8
    cavernosa — *see* condition
Corpulence — *see* Obesity
Corpus — *see* condition
Corrigan's disease — *see* Insufficiency, aortic
Corrosive burn — *see* Burn, by site
Corsican fever — *see also* Malaria 084.6
Cortical — *see also* condition
    blindness 377.75
    necrosis, kidney (bilateral) 583.6

Corticoadrenal — *see* condition
Corticosexual syndrome 255.2
Coryza (acute) 460
    with grippe or influenza (*see also* Influenza) 487.1
    syphilitic 095.8
        congenital (chronic) 090.0
Costen's syndrome or complex 524.60
Costiveness — *see* Constipation 564.00
Costochondritis 733.6
Cotard's syndrome (paranoia) 297.1
Cot death 798.0
Cotia virus 059.8
Cotun90's disease 724.3
Cough 786.2
    with hemorrhage (*see also* Hemoptysis) 786.39
    affected 786.2
    bronchial 786.2
        with grippe or influenza (*see also* Influenza) 487.1
    chronic 786.2
    epidemic 786.2
    functional 306.1
    hemorrhagic 786.39
    hysterical 300.11
    laryngeal, spasmodic 786.2
    nervous 786.2
    psychogenic 306.1
    smokers' 491.0
    tea tasters' 112.89
Counseling NEC V65.40
    without complaint or sickness V65.49
    abuse victim NEC V62.89
        child V61.21
        partner V61.11
        spouse V61.11
    child abuse, maltreatment, or neglect V61.21
    contraceptive NEC V25.09
        device (intrauterine) V25.02
        maintenance V25.40
            intrauterine contraceptive device V25.42
            oral contraceptive (pill) V25.41
            specified type NEC V25.49
            subdermal implantable V25.43
        management NEC V25.9
        oral contraceptive (pill) V25.01
            emergency V25.03
            postcoital V25.03
        prescription NEC V25.02
            oral contraceptive (pill) V25.01
                emergency V25.03
                postcoital V25.03
                repeat prescription V25.41
            repeat prescription V25.40
        subdermal implantable V25.43
        surveillance NEC V25.40
    dietary V65.3
    exercise V65.41
    expectant parent(s)
        pediatric pre-adoption visit V65.11
        pediatric pre-birth visit V65.11
    explanation of
        investigation finding NEC V65.49
        medication NEC V65.49
    family planning V25.09
        natural
            procreative V26.41
            to avoid pregnancy V25.04
    for nonattending third party V65.19
    genetic V26.33
    gonorrhea V65.45
    health (advice) (education) (instruction) NEC V65.49
    HIV V65.44
    human immunodeficiency virus V65.44
    injury prevention V65.43
    insulin pump training V65.46
    marital V61.10
    medical (for) V65.9
        boarding school resident V60.6
        condition not demonstrated V65.5
        feared complaint and no disease found V65.5

☑ **Additional Digit Required** — Refer to the Tabular List for Digit Selection   ⬇ **Subterms under main terms may continue to next column or page**

Counseling — *continued*
  medical — *continued*
    institutional resident V60.6
    on behalf of another V65.19
    person living alone V60.3
  natural family planning
    procreative V26.41
    to avoid pregnancy V25.04
  parent (guardian)-child conflict V61.20
    adopted child V61.24
    biological child V61.23
    foster child V61.25
    specified problem NEC V61.29
  partner abuse
    perpetrator V61.12
    victim V61.11
  pediatric
    pre-adoption visit for adoptive parent(s)
      V65.11
    pre-birth visit for expectant parents
      V65.11
  perpetrator of
    child abuse V62.83
      parental V61.22
    partner abuse V61.12
    spouse abuse V61.12
  procreative V65.49
  sex NEC V65.49
    transmitted disease NEC V65.45
      HIV V65.44
  specified reason NEC V65.49
  spousal abuse
    perpetrator V61.12
    victim V61.11
  substance use and abuse V65.42
  syphilis V65.45
  victim (of)
    abuse NEC V62.89
    child abuse V61.21
    partner abuse V61.11
    spousal abuse V61.11
Coupled rhythm 427.89
Couvelaire uterus (complicating delivery) —
  see Placenta, separation
Cowper's gland — *see* condition
Cowperitis — *see also* Urethritis 597.89
  gonorrheal (acute) 098.0
    chronic or duration of 2 months or over
      098.2
Cowpox (abortive) 051.01
  due to vaccination 999.0
    eyelid 051.01 *[373.5]*
      postvaccination 999.0 *[373.5]*
Coxa
  plana 732.1
  valga (acquired) 736.31
    congenital 755.61
    late effect of rickets 268.1
  vara (acquired) 736.32
    congenital 755.62
    late effect of rickets 268.1
Coxae malum senilis 715.25
Coxalgia (nontuberculous) 719.45
  tuberculous (*see also* Tuberculosis)
    015.1 ☑ *[730.85]*
Coxalgic pelvis 736.30
Coxitis 716.65
Coxsackie (infection) (virus) 079.2
  central nervous system NEC 048
  endocarditis 074.22
  enteritis 008.67
  meningitis (aseptic) 047.0
  myocarditis 074.23
  pericarditis 074.21
  pharyngitis 074.0
  pleurodynia 074.1
  specific disease NEC 074.8
Crabs, meaning pubic lice 132.2
Crack baby 760.75
Cracked
  nipple 611.2
    puerperal, postpartum 676.1 ☑
  tooth 521.81
Cradle cap 690.11
Craft neurosis 300.89
Craigiasis 007.8

Cramp(s) 729.82
  abdominal 789.0 ☑
  bathing 994.1
  colic 789.7
    infantile 789.7
    psychogenic 306.4
  due to immersion 994.1
  extremity (lower) (upper) NEC 729.82
  fireman 992.2
  heat 992.2
  hysterical 300.11
  immersion 994.1
  intestinal 789.0 ☑
    psychogenic 306.4
  linotypist's 300.89
    organic 333.84
  muscle (extremity) (general) 729.82
    due to immersion 994.1
    hysterical 300.11
  occupational (hand) 300.89
    organic 333.84
  psychogenic 307.89
  salt depletion 276.1
  sleep related leg 327.52
  stoker 992.2
  stomach 789.0 ☑
  telegraphers' 300.89
    organic 333.84
  typists' 300.89
    organic 333.84
  uterus 625.8
    menstrual 625.3
  writers' 333.84
    organic 333.84
    psychogenic 300.89
Cranial — *see* condition
Cranioclasis, fetal 763.89
Craniocleidodysostosis 755.59
Craniofenestria (skull) 756.0
Craniolacunia (skull) 756.0
Craniopagus 759.4
Craniopathy, metabolic 733.3
Craniopharyngeal — *see* condition
Craniopharyngioma (M9350/1) 237.0
Craniorachischisis (totalis) 740.1
Cranioschisis 756.0
Craniostenosis 756.0
Craniosynostosis 756.0
Craniotabes (cause unknown) 733.3
  rachitic 268.1
  syphilitic 090.5
Craniotomy, fetal 763.89
Cranium — *see* condition
Craw-craw 125.3
CRBSI (catheter-related bloodstream infection)
  999.31
Creaking joint 719.60
  ankle 719.67
  elbow 719.62
  foot 719.67
  hand 719.64
  hip 719.65
  knee 719.66
  multiple sites 719.69
  pelvic region 719.65
  shoulder (region) 719.61
  specified site NEC 719.68
  wrist 719.63
Creeping
  eruption 126.9
  palsy 335.21
  paralysis 335.21
Crenated tongue 529.8
Creotoxism 005.9
Crepitus
  caput 756.0
  joint 719.60
    ankle 719.67
    elbow 719.62
    foot 719.67
    hand 719.64
    hip 719.65
    knee 719.66
    multiple sites 719.69
    pelvic region 719.65
    shoulder (region) 719.61

Crepitus — *continued*
  joint — *continued*
    specified site NEC 719.68
    wrist 719.63
Crescent or conus choroid, congenital 743.57
Cretin, cretinism (athyrotic) (congenital) (endemic) (metabolic) (nongoitrous) (sporadic) 243
  goitrous (sporadic) 246.1
  pelvis (dwarf type) (male type) 243
    with disproportion (fetopelvic) 653.1 ☑
      affecting fetus or newborn 763.1
      causing obstructed labor 660.1 ☑
        affecting fetus or newborn 763.1
  pituitary 253.3
Cretinoid degeneration 243
Creutzfeldt-Jakob disease (CJD) (syndrome)
  046.19
  with dementia
    with behavioral disturbance
      046.19 *[294.11]*
    without behavioral disturbance
      046.19 *[294.10]*
  familial 046.19
  iatrogenic 046.19
  specified NEC 046.19
  sporadic 046.19
  variant (vCJD) 046.11
    with dementia
      with behavioral disturbance
        046.11 *[294.11]*
      without behavioral disturbance
        046.11 *[294.10]*
Crib death 798.0
Cribriform hymen 752.49
Cri-du-chat syndrome 758.31
Crigler-Najjar disease or syndrome (congenital hyperbilirubinemia) 277.4
Crimean hemorrhagic fever 065.0
Criminalism 301.7
Crisis
  abdomen 789.0 ☑
  addisonian (acute adrenocortical insufficien-
    cy) 255.41
  adrenal (cortical) 255.41
  asthmatic — *see* Asthma
  brain, cerebral (*see also* Disease, cerebrovas-
    cular, acute) 436
  celiac 579.0
  Dietl's 593.4
  emotional NEC 309.29
    acute reaction to stress 308.0
    adjustment reaction 309.9
    specific to childhood or adolescence
      313.9
  gastric (tabetic) 094.0
  glaucomatocyclitic 364.22
  heart (*see also* Failure, heart) 428.9
  hypertensive — *see* Hypertension
  nitritoid
    correct substance properly administered
      458.29
    overdose or wrong substance given or
      taken 961.1
  oculogyric 378.87
    psychogenic 306.7
  Pel's 094.0
  psychosexual identity 302.6
  rectum 094.0
  renal 593.81
  sickle cell 282.62
  stomach (tabetic) 094.0
  tabetic 094.0
  thyroid (*see also* Thyrotoxicosis) 242.9 ☑
  thyrotoxic (*see also* Thyrotoxicosis) 242.9 ☑
  vascular — *see* Disease, cerebrovascular,
    acute
Crocq's disease (acrocyanosis) 443.89
Crohn's disease — *see also* Enteritis, regional
  555.9
Cronkhite-Canada syndrome 211.3
Crooked septum, nasal 470
Cross
  birth (of fetus) complicating delivery
    652.3 ☑
    with successful version 652.1 ☑

Cross — *continued*
  birth complicating delivery — *continued*
    causing obstructed labor 660.0 ☑
  bite, anterior or posterior 524.27
  eye (*see also* Esotropia) 378.00
Crossed ectopia of kidney 753.3
Crossfoot 754.50
Croup, croupous (acute) (angina) (catarrhal)
  (infective) (inflammatory) (laryngeal)
  (membranous) (nondiphtheritic) (pseudomembranous) 464.4
  asthmatic (*see also* Asthma) 493.9 ☑
  bronchial 466.0
  diphtheritic (membranous) 032.3
  false 478.75
  spasmodic 478.75
    diphtheritic 032.3
  stridulous 478.75
    diphtheritic 032.3
Crouzon's disease (craniofacial dysostosis)
  756.0
Crowding, teeth 524.31
CRST syndrome (cutaneous systemic sclerosis)
  710.1
Cruchet's disease (encephalitis lethargica)
  049.8
Cruelty in children — *see also* Disturbance,
  conduct 312.9
Crural ulcer — *see also* Ulcer, lower extremity
  707.10
Crush, crushed, crushing (injury) 929.9
  abdomen 926.19
    internal — *see* Injury, internal, abdomen
  ankle 928.21
    with other parts of foot 928.20
  arm 927.9
    lower (and elbow) 927.10
    upper 927.03
      with shoulder or axillary region
        927.09
  axilla 927.02
    with shoulder or upper arm 927.09
  back 926.11
  breast 926.19
  buttock 926.12
  cheek 925.1
  chest — *see* Injury, internal, chest
  ear 925.1
  elbow 927.11
    with forearm 927.10
  face 925.1
  finger(s) 927.3
    with hand(s) 927.20
      and wrist(s) 927.21
  flank 926.19
  foot, excluding toe(s) alone (with ankle)
    928.20
  forearm (and elbow) 927.10
  genitalia, external (female) (male) 926.0
    internal — *see* Injury, internal, genital
      organ NEC
  hand, except finger(s) alone (and wrist)
    927.20
  head — *see* Fracture, skull, by site
  heel 928.20
  hip 928.01
    with thigh 928.00
  internal organ (abdomen, chest, or pelvis)
    — *see* Injury, internal, by site
  knee 928.11
    with leg, lower 928.10
  labium (majus) (minus) 926.0
  larynx 925.2
  late effect — *see* Late, effects (of), crushing
  leg 928.9
    lower 928.10
      and knee 928.11
    upper 928.00
  limb
    lower 928.9
      multiple sites 928.8
    upper 927.9
      multiple sites 927.8
  multiple sites NEC 929.0
  neck 925.2
  nerve — *see* Injury, nerve, by site

☑ **Additional Digit Required** — Refer to the Tabular List for Digit Selection   ▽ **Subterms under main terms may continue to next column or page**

58 — Volume 2   ▶◀ Revised Text   ● New Line   ▲ Revised Code   2015 ICD-9-CM

Crush, crushed, crushing — *continued*
  nose 802.0
    open 802.1
  penis 926.0
  pharynx 925.2
  scalp 925.1
  scapular region 927.01
    with shoulder or upper arm 927.09
  scrotum 926.0
  shoulder 927.00
    with upper arm or axillary region 927.09
  skull or cranium — *see* Fracture, skull, by site
  spinal cord — *see* Injury, spinal, by site
  syndrome (complication of trauma) 958.5
  testis 926.0
  thigh (with hip) 928.00
  throat 925.2
  thumb(s) (and fingers) 927.3
  toe(s) 928.3
    with foot 928.20
      and ankle 928.21
  tonsil 925.2
  trunk 926.9
    chest — *see* Injury, internal, intrathoracic organs NEC
    internal organ — *see* Injury, internal, by site
    multiple sites 926.8
    specified site NEC 926.19
  vulva 926.0
  wrist 927.21
    with hand(s), except fingers alone 927.20
Crusta lactea 690.11
Crusts 782.8
Crutch paralysis 953.4
Cruveilhier-Baumgarten cirrhosis, disease, or syndrome 571.5
Cruveilhier's disease 335.21
Cruz-Chagas disease — *see also* Trypanosomiasis 086.2
Crying
  constant, continuous
    adolescent 780.95
    adult 780.95
    baby 780.92
    child 780.95
    infant 780.92
    newborn 780.92
  excessive
    adolescent 780.95
    adult 780.95
    baby 780.92
    child 780.95
    infant 780.92
    newborn 780.92
Cryofibrinogenemia 273.2
Cryoglobulinemia (mixed) 273.2
Crypt (anal) (rectal) 569.49
Cryptitis (anal) (rectal) 569.49
Cryptococcosis (European) (pulmonary) (systemic) 117.5
Cryptococcus 117.5
  epidermicus 117.5
  neoformans, infection by 117.5
Cryptopapillitis (anus) 569.49
Cryptophthalmos (eyelid) 743.06
Cryptorchid, cryptorchism, cryptorchidism 752.51
Cryptosporidiosis 007.4
  hepatobiliary 136.8
  respiratory 136.8
Cryptotia 744.29
Crystallopathy
  calcium pyrophosphate (*see also* Arthritis) 275.49 [712.2] ☑
  dicalcium phosphate (*see also* Arthritis) 275.49 [712.1] ☑
  gouty 274.00
  pyrophosphate NEC (*see also* Arthritis) 275.49 [712.2] ☑
  uric acid 274.00
Crystalluria 791.9
Csillag's disease (lichen sclerosis et atrophicus) 701.0
Cuban itch 050.1

Cubitus
  valgus (acquired) 736.01
    congenital 755.59
    late effect of rickets 268.1
  varus (acquired) 736.02
    congenital 755.59
    late effect of rickets 268.1
Cultural deprivation V62.4
Cupping of optic disc 377.14
Curling esophagus 530.5
Curling's ulcer — *see* Ulcer, duodenum
Curschmann (-Batten) (-Steinert) disease or syndrome 359.21
Curvature
  organ or site, congenital NEC — *see* Distortion
  penis (lateral) 752.69
  Pott's (spinal) (*see also* Tuberculosis) 015.0 ☑ [737.43]
  radius, idiopathic, progressive (congenital) 755.54
  spine (acquired) (angular) (idiopathic) (incorrect) (postural) 737.9
    congenital 754.2
    due to or associated with
      Charcôt-Marie-Tooth disease 356.1 [737.40]
      mucopolysaccharidosis 277.5 [737.40]
      neurofibromatosis 237.71 [737.40]
      osteitis
        deformans 731.0 [737.40]
        fibrosa cystica 252.01 [737.40]
      osteoporosis (*see also* Osteoporosis) 733.00 [737.40]
      poliomyelitis (*see also* Poliomyelitis) 138 [737.40]
      tuberculosis (Pott's curvature) (*see also* Tuberculosis) 015.0 ☑ [737.43]
    kyphoscoliotic (*see also* Kyphoscoliosis) 737.30
    kyphotic (*see also* Kyphosis) 737.10
    late effect of rickets 268.1 [737.40]
    Pott's 015.0 ☑ [737.40]
    scoliotic (*see also* Scoliosis) 737.30
    specified NEC 737.8
    tuberculous 015.0 ☑ [737.40]
Cushing's
  basophilism, disease, or syndrome (iatrogenic) (idiopathic) (pituitary basophilism) (pituitary dependent) 255.0
  ulcer — *see* Ulcer, peptic
Cushingoid due to steroid therapy
  correct substance properly administered 255.0
  overdose or wrong substance given or taken 962.0
Cut (external) — *see* Wound, open, by site
Cutaneous — *see also* condition
  hemorrhage 782.7
  horn (cheek) (eyelid) (mouth) 702.8
  larva migrans 126.9
Cutis — *see also* condition
  hyperelastic 756.83
    acquired 701.8
  laxa 756.83
    senilis 701.8
  marmorata 782.61
  osteosis 709.3
  pendula 756.83
    acquired 701.8
  rhomboidalis nuchae 701.8
  verticis gyrata 757.39
    acquired 701.8
Cyanopathy, newborn 770.83
Cyanosis 782.5
  autotoxic 289.7
  common atrioventricular canal 745.69
  congenital 770.83
  conjunctiva 372.71
  due to
    endocardial cushion defect 745.60
    nonclosure, foramen botalli 745.5
    patent foramen botalli 745.5

Cyanosis — *continued*
  due to — *continued*
    persistent foramen ovale 745.5
    enterogenous 289.7
    fetus or newborn 770.83
    ostium primum defect 745.61
    paroxysmal digital 443.0
    retina, retinal 362.10
Cycle
  anovulatory 628.0
  menstrual, irregular 626.4
Cyclencephaly 759.89
Cyclical vomiting 536.2
  associated with migraine 346.2 ☑
  psychogenic 306.4
Cyclitic membrane 364.74
Cyclitis — *see also* Iridocyclitis 364.3
  acute 364.00
    primary 364.01
    recurrent 364.02
  chronic 364.10
    in
      sarcoidosis 135 [364.11]
      tuberculosis (*see also* Tuberculosis) 017.3 ☑ [364.11]
  Fuchs' heterochromic 364.21
  granulomatous 364.10
  lens induced 364.23
  nongranulomatous 364.00
  posterior 363.21
  primary 364.01
  recurrent 364.02
  secondary (noninfectious) 364.04
    infectious 364.03
  subacute 364.00
    primary 364.01
    recurrent 364.02
Cyclokeratitis — *see* Keratitis
Cyclophoria 378.44
Cyclopia, cyclops 759.89
Cycloplegia 367.51
Cyclospasm 367.53
Cyclosporiasis 007.5
Cyclothymia 301.13
Cyclothymic personality 301.13
Cyclotropia 378.33
Cyesis — *see* Pregnancy
Cylindroma (M8200/3) — *see also* Neoplasm, by site, malignant
  eccrine dermal (M8200/0) — *see* Neoplasm, skin, benign
  skin (M8200/0) — *see* Neoplasm, skin, benign
Cylindruria 791.7
Cyllosoma 759.89
Cynanche
  diphtheritic 032.3
  tonsillaris 475
Cynorexia 783.6
Cyphosis — *see* Kyphosis
Cyprus fever — *see also* Brucellosis 023.9
Cyriax's syndrome (slipping rib) 733.99
Cyst (mucus) (retention) (serous) (simple)

> *Note* — *In general, cysts are not neoplastic and are classified to the appropriate category for disease of the specified anatomical site. This generalization does not apply to certain types of cysts which are neoplastic in nature, for example, dermoid, nor does it apply to cysts of certain structures, for example, branchial cleft, which are classified as developmental anomalies.*
>
> *The following listing includes some of the most frequently reported sites of cysts as well as qualifiers which indicate the type of cyst. The latter qualifiers usually are not repeated under the anatomical sites. Since the code assignment for a given site may vary depending upon the type of cyst, the coder should refer to the listings under the specified type of cyst before consideration is given to the site.*

  accessory, fallopian tube 752.11

Cyst — *continued*
  adenoid (infected) 474.8
  adrenal gland 255.8
    congenital 759.1
  air, lung 518.89
  allantoic 753.7
  alveolar process (jaw bone) 526.2
  amnion, amniotic 658.8 ☑
  anterior chamber (eye) 364.60
    exudative 364.62
    implantation (surgical) (traumatic) 364.61
    parasitic 360.13
  anterior nasopalatine 526.1
  antrum 478.19
  anus 569.49
  apical (periodontal) (tooth) 522.8
  appendix 543.9
  arachnoid, brain 348.0
  arytenoid 478.79
  auricle 706.2
  Baker's (knee) 727.51
    tuberculous (*see also* Tuberculosis) 015.2 ☑
  Bartholin's gland or duct 616.2
  bile duct (*see also* Disease, biliary) 576.8
  bladder (multiple) (trigone) 596.89
  Blessig's 362.62
  blood, endocardial (*see also* Endocarditis) 424.90
  blue dome 610.0
  bone (local) 733.20
    aneurysmal 733.22
    jaw 526.2
      developmental (odontogenic) 526.0
      fissural 526.1
      latent 526.89
    solitary 733.21
    unicameral 733.21
  brain 348.0
    congenital 742.4
    hydatid (*see also* Echinococcus) 122.9
    third ventricle (colloid) 742.4
  branchial (cleft) 744.42
  branchiogenic 744.42
  breast (benign) (blue dome) (pedunculated) (solitary) (traumatic) 610.0
    involution 610.4
    sebaceous 610.8
  broad ligament (benign) 620.8
    embryonic 752.11
  bronchogenic (mediastinal) (sequestration) 518.89
    congenital 748.4
  buccal 528.4
  bulbourethral gland (Cowper's) 599.89
  bursa, bursal 727.49
    pharyngeal 478.26
  calcifying odontogenic (M9301/0) 213.1
    upper jaw (bone) 213.0
  canal of Nuck (acquired) (serous) 629.1
    congenital 752.41
  canthus 372.75
  carcinomatous (M8010/3) — *see* Neoplasm, by site, malignant
  cartilage (joint) — *see* Derangement, joint
  cauda equina 336.8
  cavum septi pellucidi NEC 348.0
  celomic (pericardium) 746.89
  cerebellopontine (angle) — *see* Cyst, brain
  cerebellum — *see* Cyst, brain
  cerebral — *see* Cyst, brain
  cervical lateral 744.42
  cervix 622.8
    embryonal 752.41
    nabothian (gland) 616.0
  chamber, anterior (eye) 364.60
    exudative 364.62
    implantation (surgical) (traumatic) 364.61
    parasitic 360.13
  chiasmal, optic NEC (*see also* Lesion, chiasmal) 377.54
  chocolate (ovary) 617.1
  choledochal (congenital) 751.69
    acquired 576.8

☑ **Additional Digit Required** — **Refer to the Tabular List for Digit Selection**   ▽ **Subterms under main terms may continue to next column or page**

2015 ICD-9-CM   ▶◀ Revised Text   ● New Line   ▲ Revised Code   **Volume 2 — 59**

Cyst — continued
- choledochus 751.69
- chorion 658.8 ☑
- choroid plexus 348.0
- chyle, mesentery 457.8
- ciliary body 364.60
  - exudative 364.64
  - implantation 364.61
  - primary 364.63
- clitoris 624.8
- coccyx (see also Cyst, bone) 733.20
- colloid
  - third ventricle (brain) 742.4
  - thyroid gland — see Goiter
- colon 569.89
- common (bile) duct (see also Disease, biliary) 576.8
- congenital NEC 759.89
  - adrenal glands 759.1
  - epiglottis 748.3
  - esophagus 750.4
  - fallopian tube 752.11
  - kidney 753.10
    - multiple 753.19
    - single 753.11
  - larynx 748.3
  - liver 751.62
  - lung 748.4
  - mediastinum 748.8
  - ovary 752.0
  - oviduct 752.11
  - pancreas 751.7
  - periurethral (tissue) 753.8
  - prepuce NEC 752.69
    - penis 752.69
  - sublingual 750.26
  - submaxillary gland 750.26
  - thymus (gland) 759.2
  - tongue 750.19
  - ureterovesical orifice 753.4
  - vulva 752.41
- conjunctiva 372.75
- cornea 371.23
- corpora quadrigemina 348.0
- corpus
  - albicans (ovary) 620.2
  - luteum (ruptured) 620.1
- Cowper's gland (benign) (infected) 599.89
- cranial meninges 348.0
- craniobuccal pouch 253.8
- craniopharyngeal pouch 253.8
- cystic duct (see also Disease, gallbladder) 575.8
- Cysticercus (any site) 123.1
- Dandy-Walker 742.3
  - with spina bifida (see also Spina bifida) 741.0 ☑
- dental 522.8
  - developmental 526.0
  - eruption 526.0
  - lateral periodontal 526.0
  - primordial (keratocyst) 526.0
  - root 522.8
- dentigerous 526.0
  - mandible 526.0
  - maxilla 526.0
- dermoid (M9084/0) (see also Neoplasm, by site, benign)
  - with malignant transformation (M9084/3) 183.0
  - implantation
    - external area or site (skin) NEC 709.8
    - iris 364.61
    - skin 709.8
    - vagina 623.8
    - vulva 624.8
  - mouth 528.4
  - oral soft tissue 528.4
  - sacrococcygeal 685.1
    - with abscess 685.0
- developmental of ovary, ovarian 752.0
- dura (cerebral) 348.0
  - spinal 349.2
- ear (external) 706.2
- echinococcal (see also Echinococcus) 122.9

Cyst — continued
- embryonal
  - cervix uteri 752.41
  - genitalia, female external 752.41
  - uterus 752.39
  - vagina 752.41
- endometrial 621.8
  - ectopic 617.9
- endometrium (uterus) 621.8
  - ectopic — see Endometriosis
- enteric 751.5
- enterogenous 751.5
- epidermal (inclusion) (see also Cyst, skin) 706.2
- epidermoid (inclusion) (see also Cyst, skin) 706.2
  - mouth 528.4
  - not of skin — see Cyst, by site
  - oral soft tissue 528.4
- epididymis 608.89
- epiglottis 478.79
- epiphysis cerebri 259.8
- epithelial (inclusion) (see also Cyst, skin) 706.2
- epoophoron 752.11
- eruption 526.0
- esophagus 530.89
- ethmoid sinus 478.19
- eye (retention) 379.8
  - congenital 743.03
  - posterior segment, congenital 743.54
- eyebrow 706.2
- eyelid (sebaceous) 374.84
  - infected 373.13
  - sweat glands or ducts 374.84
- falciform ligament (inflammatory) 573.8
- fallopian tube 620.8
  - congenital 752.11
- female genital organs NEC 629.89
- fimbrial (congenital) 752.11
- fissural (oral region) 526.1
- follicle (atretic) (graafian) (ovarian) 620.0
  - nabothian (gland) 616.0
- follicular (atretic) (ovarian) 620.0
  - dentigerous 526.0
- frontal sinus 478.19
- gallbladder or duct 575.8
- ganglion 727.43
- Gartner's duct 752.41
- gas, of mesentery 568.89
- gingiva 523.8
- gland of moll 374.84
- globulomaxillary 526.1
- graafian follicle 620.0
- granulosal lutein 620.2
- hemangiomatous (M9121/0) (see also Hemangioma) 228.00
- hydatid (see also Echinococcus) 122.9
  - fallopian tube (Morgagni) 752.11
  - liver NEC 122.8
  - lung NEC 122.9
  - Morgagni 752.89
    - fallopian tube 752.11
  - specified site NEC 122.9
- hymen 623.8
  - embryonal 752.41
- hypopharynx 478.26
- hypophysis, hypophyseal (duct) (recurrent) 253.8
  - cerebri 253.8
- implantation (dermoid)
  - anterior chamber (eye) 364.61
  - external area or site (skin) NEC 709.8
  - iris 364.61
  - vagina 623.8
  - vulva 624.8
- incisor, incisive canal 526.1
- inclusion (epidermal) (epithelial) (epidermoid) (mucous) (squamous) (see also Cyst, skin) 706.2
  - not of skin — see Neoplasm, by site, benign
- intestine (large) (small) 569.89
- intracranial — see Cyst, brain
- intraligamentous 728.89
  - knee 717.89

Cyst — continued
- intrasellar 253.8
- iris (idiopathic) 364.60
  - exudative 364.62
  - implantation (surgical) (traumatic) 364.61
  - miotic pupillary 364.55
  - parasitic 360.13
- Iwanoff's 362.62
- jaw (bone) (aneurysmal) (extravasation) (hemorrhagic) (traumatic) 526.2
  - developmental (odontogenic) 526.0
  - fissural 526.1
- keratin 706.2
- kidney (congenital) 753.10
  - acquired 593.2
  - calyceal (see also Hydronephrosis) 591
  - multiple 753.19
  - pyelogenic (see also Hydronephrosis) 591
  - simple 593.2
  - single 753.11
  - solitary (not congenital) 593.2
- labium (majus) (minus) 624.8
  - sebaceous 624.8
- lacrimal
  - apparatus 375.43
  - gland or sac 375.12
- larynx 478.79
- lens 379.39
  - congenital 743.39
- lip (gland) 528.5
- liver 573.8
  - congenital 751.62
  - hydatid (see also Echinococcus) 122.8
    - granulosis 122.0
    - multilocularis 122.5
- lung 518.89
  - congenital 748.4
  - giant bullous 492.0
- lutein 620.1
- lymphangiomatous (M9173/0) 228.1
- lymphoepithelial
  - mouth 528.4
  - oral soft tissue 528.4
- macula 362.54
- malignant (M8000/3) — see Neoplasm, by site, malignant
- mammary gland (sweat gland) (see also Cyst, breast) 610.0
- mandible 526.2
  - dentigerous 526.0
  - radicular 522.8
- maxilla 526.2
  - dentigerous 526.0
  - radicular 522.8
- median
  - anterior maxillary 526.1
  - palatal 526.1
- mediastinum (congenital) 748.8
- meibomian (gland) (retention) 373.2
  - infected 373.12
- membrane, brain 348.0
- meninges (cerebral) 348.0
  - spinal 349.2
- meniscus knee 717.5
- mesentery, mesenteric (gas) 568.89
  - chyle 457.8
  - gas 568.89
- mesonephric duct 752.89
- mesothelial
  - peritoneum 568.89
  - pleura (peritoneal) 568.89
- milk 611.5
- miotic pupillary (iris) 364.55
- Morgagni (hydatid) 752.89
  - fallopian tube 752.11
- mouth 528.4
- Müllerian duct 752.89
  - appendix testis 608.89
  - cervix (embryonal) 752.41
  - fallopian tube 752.11
  - prostatic utricle 599.89
  - vagina (embryonal) 752.41
- multilocular (ovary) (M8000/1) 239.5
- myometrium 621.8

Cyst — continued
- nabothian (follicle) (ruptured) 616.0
- nasal sinus 478.19
- nasoalveolar 528.4
- nasolabial 528.4
- nasopalatine (duct) 526.1
  - anterior 526.1
- nasopharynx 478.26
- neoplastic (M8000/1) (see also Neoplasm, by site, unspecified nature)
  - benign (M8000/0) — see Neoplasm, by site, benign
  - uterus 621.8
- nervous system — see Cyst, brain
- neuroenteric 742.59
- neuroepithelial ventricle 348.0
- nipple 610.0
- nose 478.19
  - skin of 706.2
- odontogenic, developmental 526.0
- omentum (lesser) 568.89
  - congenital 751.8
- oral soft tissue (dermoid) (epidermoid) (lymphoepithelial) 528.4
- ora serrata 361.19
- orbit 376.81
- ovary, ovarian (twisted) 620.2
  - adherent 620.2
  - chocolate 617.1
  - corpus
    - albicans 620.2
    - luteum 620.1
  - dermoid (M9084/0) 220
  - developmental 752.0
  - due to failure of involution NEC 620.2
  - endometrial 617.1
  - follicular (atretic) (graafian) (hemorrhagic) 620.0
  - hemorrhagic 620.2
  - in pregnancy or childbirth 654.4 ☑
    - affecting fetus or newborn 763.89
    - causing obstructed labor 660.2 ☑
      - affecting fetus or newborn 763.1
  - multilocular (M8000/1) 239.5
  - pseudomucinous (M8470/0) 220
  - retention 620.2
  - serous 620.2
  - theca lutein 620.2
  - tuberculous (see also Tuberculosis) 016.6 ☑
  - unspecified 620.2
- oviduct 620.8
- palatal papilla (jaw) 526.1
- palate 526.1
  - fissural 526.1
  - median (fissural) 526.1
- palatine, of papilla 526.1
- pancreas, pancreatic 577.2
  - congenital 751.7
  - false 577.2
  - hemorrhagic 577.2
  - true 577.2
- paralabral
  - hip 718.85
  - shoulder 840.7
- paramesonephric duct — see Cyst, Müllerian duct
- paranephric 593.2
- para ovarian 752.11
- paraphysis, cerebri 742.4
- parasitic NEC 136.9
- parathyroid (gland) 252.8
- paratubal (fallopian) 620.8
- paraurethral duct 599.89
- paroophoron 752.11
- parotid gland 527.6
  - mucous extravasation or retention 527.6
- parovarian 752.11
- pars planus 364.60
  - exudative 364.64
  - primary 364.63
- pelvis, female
  - in pregnancy or childbirth 654.4 ☑
    - affecting fetus or newborn 763.89
    - causing obstructed labor 660.2 ☑
      - affecting fetus or newborn 763.1

☑ **Additional Digit Required** — Refer to the Tabular List for Digit Selection   ▽ **Subterms under main terms may continue to next column or page**

Cyst — *continued*
penis (sebaceous) 607.89
periapical 522.8
pericardial (congenital) 746.89
acquired (secondary) 423.8
pericoronal 526.0
perineural (Tarlov's) 355.9
periodontal 522.8
lateral 526.0
peripancreatic 577.2
peripelvic (lymphatic) 593.2
peritoneum 568.89
chylous 457.8
pharynx (wall) 478.26
pilar 704.41
pilonidal (infected) (rectum) 685.1
with abscess 685.0
malignant (M9084/3) 173.59
pituitary (duct) (gland) 253.8
placenta (amniotic) — *see* Placenta, abnormal
pleura 519.8
popliteal 727.51
porencephalic 742.4
acquired 348.0
postanal (infected) 685.1
with abscess 685.0
posterior segment of eye, congenital 743.54
postmastoidectomy cavity 383.31
preauricular 744.47
prepuce 607.89
congenital 752.69
primordial (jaw) 526.0
prostate 600.3
pseudomucinous (ovary) (M8470/0) 220
pudenda (sweat glands) 624.8
pupillary, miotic 364.55
sebaceous 624.8
radicular (residual) 522.8
radiculodental 522.8
ranular 527.6
Rathke's pouch 253.8
rectum (epithelium) (mucous) 569.49
renal — *see* Cyst, kidney
residual (radicular) 522.8
retention (ovary) 620.2
retina 361.19
macular 362.54
parasitic 360.13
primary 361.13
secondary 361.14
retroperitoneal 568.89
sacrococcygeal (dermoid) 685.1
with abscess 685.0
salivary gland or duct 527.6
mucous extravasation or retention 527.6
Sampson's 617.1
sclera 379.19
scrotum (sebaceous) 706.2
sweat glands 706.2
sebaceous (duct) (gland) 706.2
breast 610.8
eyelid 374.84
genital organ NEC
female 629.89
male 608.89
scrotum 706.2
semilunar cartilage (knee) (multiple) 717.5
seminal vesicle 608.89
serous (ovary) 620.2
sinus (antral) (ethmoidal) (frontal) (maxillary) (nasal) (sphenoidal) 478.19
Skene's gland 599.89
skin (epidermal) (epidermoid, inclusion) (epithelial) (inclusion) (retention) (sebaceous) 706.2
breast 610.8
eyelid 374.84
genital organ NEC
female 629.89
male 608.89
neoplastic 216.3
scrotum 706.2
sweat gland or duct 705.89
solitary
bone 733.21

Cyst — *continued*
solitary — *continued*
kidney 593.2
spermatic cord 608.89
sphenoid sinus 478.19
spinal meninges 349.2
spine (*see also* Cyst, bone) 733.20
spleen NEC 289.59
congenital 759.0
hydatid (*see also* Echinococcus) 122.9
spring water (pericardium) 746.89
subarachnoid 348.0
intrasellar 793.0
subdural (cerebral) 348.0
spinal cord 349.2
sublingual gland 527.6
mucous extravasation or retention 527.6
submaxillary gland 527.6
mucous extravasation or retention 527.6
suburethral 599.89
suprarenal gland 255.8
suprasellar — *see* Cyst, brain
sweat gland or duct 705.89
sympathetic nervous system 337.9
synovial 727.40
popliteal space 727.51
Tarlov's 355.9
tarsal 373.2
tendon (sheath) 727.42
testis 608.89
theca-lutein (ovary) 620.2
Thornwaldt's, Tornwaldt's 478.26
thymus (gland) 254.8
thyroglossal (duct) (infected) (persistent) 759.2
thyroid 246.2
adenomatous — *see* Goiter, nodular
colloid (*see also* Goiter) 240.9
thyrolingual duct (infected) (persistent) 759.2
tongue (mucous) 529.8
tonsil 474.8
tooth (dental root) 522.8
trichilemmal (proliferating) 704.42
tubo-ovarian 620.8
inflammatory 614.1
tunica vaginalis 608.89
turbinate (nose) (*see also* Cyst, bone) 733.20
Tyson's gland (benign) (infected) 607.89
umbilicus 759.89
urachus 753.7
ureter 593.89
ureterovesical orifice 593.89
congenital 753.4
urethra 599.84
urethral gland (Cowper's) 599.89
uterine
ligament 620.8
embryonic 752.11
tube 620.8
uterus (body) (corpus) (recurrent) 621.8
embryonal 752.39
utricle (ear) 386.8
prostatic 599.89
utriculus masculinus 599.89
vagina, vaginal (squamous cell) (wall) 623.8
embryonal 752.41
implantation 623.8
inclusion 623.8
vallecula, vallecular 478.79
ventricle, neuroepithelial 348.0
verumontanum 599.89
vesical (orifice) 596.89
vitreous humor 379.29
vulva (sweat glands) 624.8
congenital 752.41
implantation 624.8
inclusion 624.8
sebaceous gland 624.8
vulvovaginal gland 624.8
wolffian 752.89
Cystadenocarcinoma (M8440/3) — *see also* Neoplasm, by site, malignant
bile duct type (M8161/3) 155.1
endometrioid (M8380/3) — *see* Neoplasm, by site, malignant

Cystadenocarcinoma — *see also* Neoplasm, by site, malignant — *continued*
mucinous (M8470/3)
papillary (M8471/3)
specified site — *see* Neoplasm, by site, malignant
unspecified site 183.0
specified site — *see* Neoplasm, by site, malignant
unspecified site 183.0
papillary (M8450/3)
mucinous (M8471/3)
specified site — *see* Neoplasm, by site, malignant
unspecified site 183.0
pseudomucinous (M8471/3)
specified site — *see* Neoplasm, by site, malignant
unspecified site 183.0
serous (M8460/3)
specified site — *see* Neoplasm, by site, malignant
unspecified site 183.0
specified site — *see* Neoplasm, by site, malignant
unspecified 183.0
pseudomucinous (M8470/3)
papillary (M8471/3)
specified site — *see* Neoplasm, by site, malignant
unspecified site 183.0
specified site — *see* Neoplasm, by site, malignant
unspecified site 183.0
serous (M8441/3)
papillary (M8460/3)
specified site — *see* Neoplasm, by site, malignant
unspecified site 183.0
specified site — *see* Neoplasm, by site, malignant
unspecified site 183.0
Cystadenofibroma (M9013/0)
clear cell (M8313/0) — *see* Neoplasm, by site, benign
endometrioid (M8381/0) 220
borderline malignancy (M8381/1) 236.2
malignant (M8381/3) 183.0
mucinous (M9015/0)
specified site — *see* Neoplasm, by site, benign
unspecified site 220
serous (M9014/0)
specified site — *see* Neoplasm, by site, benign
unspecified site 220
specified site — *see* Neoplasm, by site, benign
unspecified site 220
Cystadenoma (M8440/0) — *see also* Neoplasm, by site, benign
bile duct (M8161/0) 211.5
endometrioid (M8380/0) (*see also* Neoplasm, by site, benign)
borderline malignancy (M8380/1) — *see* Neoplasm, by site, uncertain behavior
malignant (M8440/3) — *see* Neoplasm, by site, malignant
mucinous (M8470/0)
borderline malignancy (M8470/1)
specified site — *see* Neoplasm, uncertain behavior
unspecified site 236.2
papillary (M8471/0)
borderline malignancy (M8471/1)
specified site — *see* Neoplasm, by site, uncertain behavior
unspecified site 236.2
specified site — *see* Neoplasm, by site, benign
unspecified site 220
specified site — *see* Neoplasm, by site, benign
unspecified site 220

Cystadenoma — *see also* Neoplasm, by site, benign — *continued*
papillary (M8450/0)
borderline malignancy (M8450/1)
specified site — *see* Neoplasm, by site, uncertain behavior
unspecified site 236.2
lymphomatosum (M8561/0) 210.2
mucinous (M8471/0)
borderline malignancy (M8471/1)
specified site — *see* Neoplasm, by site, uncertain behavior
unspecified site 236.2
specified site — *see* Neoplasm, by site, benign
unspecified site 220
pseudomucinous (M8471/0)
borderline malignancy (M8471/1)
specified site — *see* Neoplasm, by site, uncertain behavior
unspecified site 236.2
specified site — *see* Neoplasm, by site, benign
unspecified site 220
serous (M8460/0)
borderline malignancy (M8460/1)
specified site — *see* Neoplasm, by site, uncertain behavior
unspecified site 236.2
specified site — *see* Neoplasm, by site, benign
unspecified site 220
specified site — *see* Neoplasm, by site, benign
unspecified site 220
pseudomucinous (M8470/0)
borderline malignancy (M8470/1)
specified site — *see* Neoplasm, by site, uncertain behavior
unspecified site 236.2
papillary (M8471/0)
borderline malignancy (M8471/1)
specified site — *see* Neoplasm, by site, uncertain behavior
unspecified site 236.2
specified site — *see* Neoplasm, by site, benign
unspecified site 220
specified site — *see* Neoplasm, by site, benign
unspecified site 220
serous (M8441/0)
borderline malignancy (M8441/1)
specified site — *see* Neoplasm, by site, uncertain behavior
unspecified site 236.2
papillary (M8460/0)
borderline malignancy (M8460/1)
specified site — *see* Neoplasm, by site, uncertain behavior
unspecified site 236.2
specified site — *see* Neoplasm, by site, benign
unspecified site 220
specified site — *see* Neoplasm, by site, benign
unspecified site 220
thyroid 226
Cystathioninemia 270.4
Cystathioninuria 270.4
Cystic — *see also* condition
breast, chronic 610.1
corpora lutea 620.1
degeneration, congenital
brain 742.4
kidney (*see also* Cystic, disease, kidney) 753.10
disease
breast, chronic 610.1
kidney, congenital 753.10
medullary 753.16
multiple 753.19
polycystic — *see* Polycystic, kidney
single 753.11
specified NEC 753.19
liver, congenital 751.62

☑ Additional Digit Required — Refer to the Tabular List for Digit Selection
▽ Subterms under main terms may continue to next column or page
2015 ICD-9-CM   ▶◀ Revised Text   ● New Line   ▲ Revised Code   Volume 2 — 61

Cyst — Cystic

Cystic — *see also* condition — *continued*
  disease — *continued*
    lung 518.89
      congenital 748.4
    pancreas, congenital 751.7
    semilunar cartilage 717.5
  duct — *see* condition
  eyeball, congenital 743.03
  fibrosis (pancreas) 277.00
    with
      manifestations
        gastrointestinal 277.03
        pulmonary 277.02
        specified NEC 277.09
      meconium ileus 277.01
      pulmonary exacerbation 277.02
  hygroma (M9173/0) 228.1
  kidney, congenital 753.10
    medullary 753.16
    multiple 753.19
    polycystic — *see* Polycystic, kidney
    single 753.11
    specified NEC 753.19
  liver, congenital 751.62
  lung 518.89
    congenital 748.4
  mass — *see* Cyst
  mastitis, chronic 610.1
  ovary 620.2
  pancreas, congenital 751.7
Cysticerciasis 123.1
Cysticercosis (mammary) (subretinal) 123.1
Cysticercus 123.1
  cellulosae infestation 123.1
Cystinosis (malignant) 270.0
Cystinuria 270.0
Cystitis (bacillary) (colli) (diffuse) (exudative)
  (hemorrhagic) (purulent) (recurrent)
  (septic) (suppurative) (ulcerative) 595.9
  with
    abortion — *see* Abortion, by type, with
      urinary tract infection
    ectopic pregnancy (*see also* categories
      633.0–633.9) 639.8

Cystitis — *continued*
  with — *continued*
    fibrosis 595.1
    leukoplakia 595.1
    malakoplakia 595.1
    metaplasia 595.1
    molar pregnancy (*see also* categories
      630–632) 639.8
  actinomycotic 039.8 *[595.4]*
  acute 595.0
    of trigone 595.3
  allergic 595.89
  amebic 006.8 *[595.4]*
  bilharzial 120.9 *[595.4]*
  blennorrhagic (acute) 098.11
    chronic or duration of 2 months or more
      098.31
  bullous 595.89
  calculous 594.1
  chlamydial 099.53
  chronic 595.2
    interstitial 595.1
    of trigone 595.3
  complicating pregnancy, childbirth, or
    puerperium 646.6 ☑
    affecting fetus or newborn 760.1
  cystic(a) 595.81
  diphtheritic 032.84
  echinococcal
    granulosus 122.3 *[595.4]*
    multilocularis 122.6 *[595.4]*
  emphysematous 595.89
  encysted 595.81
  follicular 595.3
  following
    abortion 639.8
    ectopic or molar pregnancy 639.8
  gangrenous 595.89
  glandularis 595.89
  gonococcal (acute) 098.11
    chronic or duration of 2 months or more
      098.31
  incrusted 595.89
  interstitial 595.1

Cystitis — *continued*
  irradiation 595.82
  irritation 595.89
  malignant 595.89
  monilial 112.2
  of trigone 595.3
  panmural 595.1
  polyposa 595.89
  prostatic 601.3
  radiation 595.82
  Reiter's (abacterial) 099.3
  specified NEC 595.89
  subacute 595.2
  submucous 595.1
  syphilitic 095.8
  trichomoniasis 131.09
  tuberculous (*see also* Tuberculosis) 016.1 ☑
  ulcerative 595.1
Cystocele
  female (without uterine prolapse) 618.01
    with uterine prolapse 618.4
      complete 618.3
      incomplete 618.2
    lateral 618.02
    midline 618.01
    paravaginal 618.02
  in pregnancy or childbirth 654.4 ☑
    affecting fetus or newborn 763.89
    causing obstructed labor 660.2 ☑
      affecting fetus or newborn 763.1
  male 596.89
Cystoid
  cicatrix limbus 372.64
  degeneration macula 362.53
Cystolithiasis 594.1
Cystoma (M8440/0) — *see also* Neoplasm, by
  site, benign
  endometrial, ovary 617.1
  mucinous (M8470/0)
    specified site — *see* Neoplasm, by site,
      benign
    unspecified site 220

Cystoma — *see also* Neoplasm, by site, benign
  — *continued*
  serous (M8441/0)
    specified site — *see* Neoplasm, by site,
      benign
    unspecified site 220
  simple (ovary) 620.2
Cystoplegia 596.53
Cystoptosis 596.89
Cystopyelitis — *see also* Pyelitis 590.80
Cystorrhagia 596.89
Cystosarcoma phyllodes (M9020/1) 238.3
  benign (M9020/0) 217
  malignant (M9020/3) — *see* Neoplasm,
    breast, malignant
Cystostomy status V44.50
  with complication 596.83
    infection 596.81
    mechanical 596.82
    specified complication NEC 596.83
  appendico-vesicostomy V44.52
  cutaneous-vesicostomy V44.51
  specified type NEC V44.59
Cystourethritis — *see also* Urethritis 597.89
Cystourethrocele — *see also* Cystocele
  female (without uterine prolapse) 618.09
    with uterine prolapse 618.4
      complete 618.3
      incomplete 618.2
  male 596.89
Cytomegalic inclusion disease 078.5
  congenital 771.1
Cytomycosis, reticuloendothelial — *see also*
  Histoplasmosis, American 115.00
Cytopenia 289.9
  refractory
    with
      multilineage dysplasia (RCMD)
        238.72
      and ringed sideroblasts (RCMD-
        RS) 238.72

☑ **Additional Digit Required — Refer to the Tabular List for Digit Selection**
▽ **Subterms under main terms may continue to next column or page**

62 — Volume 2   ▶◀ **Revised Text**   ● **New Line**   ▲ **Revised Code**   2015 ICD-9-CM

D

Daae (-Finsen) disease (epidemic pleurodynia) 074.1
Dabney's grip 074.1
Da Costa's syndrome (neurocirculatory asthenia) 306.2
Dacryoadenitis, dacryadenitis 375.00
  acute 375.01
  chronic 375.02
Dacryocystitis 375.30
  acute 375.32
  chronic 375.42
  neonatal 771.6
  phlegmonous 375.33
  syphilitic 095.8
    congenital 090.0
  trachomatous, active 076.1
    late effect 139.1
  tuberculous (see also Tuberculosis) 017.3 ☑
Dacryocystoblenorrhea 375.42
Dacryocystocele 375.43
Dacryolith, dacryolithiasis 375.57
Dacryoma 375.43
Dacryopericystitis (acute) (subacute) 375.32
  chronic 375.42
Dacryops 375.11
Dacryosialadenopathy, atrophic 710.2
Dacryostenosis 375.56
  congenital 743.65
Dactylitis
  bone (see also Osteomyelitis) 730.2 ☑
  sickle-cell 282.62
    Hb-C 282.64
    Hb-SS 282.62
    specified NEC 282.69
  syphilitic 095.5
  tuberculous (see also Tuberculosis) 015.5 ☑
Dactylolysis spontanea 136.0
Dactylosymphysis — see also Syndactylism 755.10
Damage
  arteriosclerotic — see Arteriosclerosis
  brain 348.9
    anoxic, hypoxic 348.1
      during or resulting from a procedure 997.01
    ischemic, in newborn 768.70
      mild 768.71
      moderate 768.72
      severe 768.73
    child NEC 343.9
    due to birth injury 767.0
    minimal (child) (see also Hyperkinesia) 314.9
    newborn 767.0
  cardiac (see also Disease, heart)
  cardiorenal (vascular) (see also Hypertension, cardiorenal) 404.90
  central nervous system — see Damage, brain
  cerebral NEC — see Damage, brain
  coccyx, complicating delivery 665.6 ☑
  coronary (see also Ischemia, heart) 414.9
  eye, birth injury 767.8
  heart (see also Disease, heart)
    valve — see Endocarditis
  hypothalamus NEC 348.9
  liver 571.9
    alcoholic 571.3
  medication 995.20
  myocardium (see also Degeneration, myocardial) 429.1
  pelvic
    joint or ligament, during delivery 665.6 ☑
    organ NEC
      with
        abortion — see Abortion, by type, with damage to pelvic organs
        ectopic pregnancy (see also categories 633.0–633.9) 639.2
        molar pregnancy (see also categories 630–632) 639.2
      during delivery 665.5 ☑

Damage — continued
  pelvic — continued
    organ — continued
      following
        abortion 639.2
        ectopic or molar pregnancy 639.2
  renal (see also Disease, renal) 593.9
  skin, solar 692.79
    acute 692.72
    chronic 692.74
  subendocardium, subendocardial (see also Degeneration, myocardial) 429.1
  vascular 459.9
Dameshek's syndrome (erythroblastic anemia) 282.49
Dana-Putnam syndrome (subacute combined sclerosis with pernicious anemia) 281.0 [336.2]
Danbolt (-Closs) syndrome (acrodermatitis enteropathica) 686.8
Dandruff 690.18
Dandy fever 061
Dandy-Walker deformity or syndrome (atresia, foramen of Magendie) 742.3
  with spina bifida (see also Spina bifida) 741.0 ☑
Dangle foot 736.79
Danielssen's disease (anesthetic leprosy) 030.1
Danlos' syndrome 756.83
Darier's disease (congenital) (keratosis follicularis) 757.39
  due to vitamin A deficiency 264.8
  meaning erythema annulare centrifugum 695.0
Darier-Roussy sarcoid 135
Dark area on retina 239.81
Darling's
  disease (see also Histoplasmosis, American) 115.00
  histoplasmosis (see also Histoplasmosis, American) 115.00
Dartre 054.9
Darwin's tubercle 744.29
Davidson's anemia (refractory) 284.9
Davies-Colley syndrome (slipping rib) 733.99
Davies' disease 425.0
Dawson's encephalitis 046.2
Day blindness — see also Blindness, day 368.60
Dead
  fetus
    retained (in utero) 656.4 ☑
      early pregnancy (death before 22 completed weeks gestation) 632
      late (death after 22 completed weeks gestation) 656.4 ☑
    syndrome 641.3 ☑
  labyrinth 386.50
  ovum, retained 631.8
Deaf and dumb NEC 389.7
Deaf mutism (acquired) (congenital) NEC 389.7
  endemic 243
  hysterical 300.11
  syphilitic, congenital 090.0
Deafness (acquired) (complete) (congenital) (hereditary) (middle ear) (partial) 389.9
  with
    blindness V49.85
    blue sclera and fragility of bone 756.51
  auditory fatigue 389.9
  aviation 993.0
    nerve injury 951.5
  boilermakers' 951.5
  central 389.14
    with conductive hearing loss 389.20
      bilateral 389.22
      unilateral 389.21
  conductive (air) 389.00
    with sensorineural hearing loss 389.20
      bilateral 389.22
      unilateral 389.21
    bilateral 389.06
    combined types 389.08
    external ear 389.01

Deafness — continued
  conductive — continued
    inner ear 389.04
    middle ear 389.03
    multiple types 389.08
    tympanic membrane 389.02
    unilateral 389.05
  emotional (complete) 300.11
  functional (complete) 300.11
  high frequency 389.8
  hysterical (complete) 300.11
  injury 951.5
  low frequency 389.8
  mental 784.69
  mixed conductive and sensorineural 389.20
    bilateral 389.22
    unilateral 389.21
  nerve
    with conductive hearing loss 389.20
      bilateral 389.22
      unilateral 389.21
    bilateral 389.12
    unilateral 389.13
  neural
    with conductive hearing loss 389.20
      bilateral 389.22
      unilateral 389.21
    bilateral 389.12
    unilateral 389.13
  noise-induced 388.12
    nerve injury 951.5
  nonspeaking 389.7
  perceptive 389.10
    with conductive hearing loss 389.20
      bilateral 389.22
      unilateral 389.21
    central 389.14
    neural
      bilateral 389.12
      unilateral 389.13
    sensorineural 389.10
      asymmetrical 389.16
      bilateral 389.18
      unilateral 389.15
    sensory
      bilateral 389.11
      unilateral 389.17
  psychogenic (complete) 306.7
  sensorineural (see also Deafness, perceptive) 389.10
    asymmetrical 389.16
    bilateral 389.18
    unilateral 389.15
  sensory
    with conductive hearing loss 389.20
      bilateral 389.22
      unilateral 389.21
    bilateral 389.11
    unilateral 389.17
  specified type NEC 389.8
  sudden NEC 388.2
  syphilitic 094.89
  transient ischemic 388.02
  transmission — see Deafness, conductive
  traumatic 951.5
  word (secondary to organic lesion) 784.69
    developmental 315.31
Death
  after delivery (cause not stated) (sudden) 674.9 ☑
  anesthetic
    due to
      correct substance properly administered 995.4
      overdose or wrong substance given 968.4
      specified anesthetic — see Table of Drugs and Chemicals
    during delivery 668.9 ☑
  brain 348.82
  cardiac (sudden) (SCD) — code to underlying condition
    family history of V17.41
    personal history of, successfully resuscitated V12.53
  cause unknown 798.2

Death — continued
  cot (infant) 798.0
  crib (infant) 798.0
  fetus, fetal (cause not stated) (intrauterine) 779.9
    early, with retention (before 22 completed weeks gestation) 632
    from asphyxia or anoxia (before labor) 768.0
      during labor 768.1
    late, affecting management of pregnancy (after 22 completed weeks gestation) 656.4 ☑
  from pregnancy NEC 646.9 ☑
  instantaneous 798.1
  intrauterine (see also Death, fetus) 779.9
    complicating pregnancy 656.4 ☑
  maternal, affecting fetus or newborn 761.6
  neonatal NEC 779.9
  sudden (cause unknown) 798.1
    cardiac (SCD)
      family history of V17.41
      personal history of, successfully resuscitated V12.53
    during delivery 669.9 ☑
      under anesthesia NEC 668.9 ☑
    infant, syndrome (SIDS) 798.0
    puerperal, during puerperium 674.9 ☑
  unattended (cause unknown) 798.9
  under anesthesia NEC
    due to
      correct substance properly administered 995.4
      overdose or wrong substance given 968.4
      specified anesthetic — see Table of Drugs and Chemicals
    during delivery 668.9 ☑
  violent 798.1
de Beurmann-Gougerot disease (sporotrichosis) 117.1
Debility (general) (infantile) (postinfectional) 799.3
  with nutritional difficulty 269.9
  congenital or neonatal NEC 779.9
  nervous 300.5
  old age 797
  senile 797
Débove's disease (splenomegaly) 789.2
Decalcification
  bone (see also Osteoporosis) 733.00
  teeth 521.89
Decapitation 874.9
  fetal (to facilitate delivery) 763.89
Decapsulation, kidney 593.89
Decay
  dental 521.00
  senile 797
  tooth, teeth 521.00
Decensus, uterus — see Prolapse, uterus
Deciduitis (acute)
  with
    abortion — see Abortion, by type, with sepsis
    ectopic pregnancy (see also categories 633.0–633.9) 639.0
    molar pregnancy (see also categories 630–632) 639.0
  affecting fetus or newborn 760.8
  following
    abortion 639.0
    ectopic or molar pregnancy 639.0
  in pregnancy 646.6 ☑
  puerperal, postpartum 670.1 ☑
Deciduoma malignum (M9100/3) 181
Deciduous tooth (retained) 520.6
Decline (general) — see also Debility 799.3
Decompensation
  cardiac (acute) (chronic) (see also Disease, heart) 429.9
    failure — see Failure, heart
  cardiorenal (see also Hypertension, cardiorenal) 404.90
  cardiovascular (see also Disease, cardiovascular) 429.2
  heart (see also Disease, heart) 429.9

☑ Additional Digit Required — Refer to the Tabular List for Digit Selection   ▽ Subterms under main terms may continue to next column or page

2015 ICD-9-CM   ▶◀ Revised Text   ● New Line   ▲ Revised Code   Volume 2 — 63

Decompensation — *continued*
　heart (*see also* Disease, heart) — *contin-ued*
　　failure — *see* Failure, heart
　hepatic 572.2
　myocardial (acute) (chronic) (*see also* Disease, heart) 429.9
　　failure — *see* Failure, heart
　respiratory 519.9
Decompression sickness 993.3
Decrease, decreased
　blood
　　platelets (*see also* Thrombocytopenia) 287.5
　　pressure 796.3
　　　due to shock following
　　　　injury 958.4
　　　　operation 998.00
　　white cell count 288.50
　　specified NEC 288.59
　cardiac reserve — *see* Disease, heart
　estrogen 256.39
　　postablative 256.2
　fetal movements 655.7 ☑
　fragility of erythrocytes 289.89
　function
　　adrenal (cortex) 255.41
　　　medulla 255.5
　　ovary in hypopituitarism 253.4
　　parenchyma of pancreas 577.8
　　pituitary (gland) (lobe) (anterior) 253.2
　　　posterior (lobe) 253.8
　functional activity 780.99
　glucose 790.29
　haptoglobin (serum) NEC 273.8
　leukocytes 288.50
　libido 799.81
　lymphocytes 288.51
　platelets (*see also* Thrombocytopenia) 287.5
　pulse pressure 785.9
　respiration due to shock following injury 958.4
　sexual desire 799.81
　tear secretion NEC 375.15
　tolerance
　　fat 579.8
　　salt and water 276.9
　vision NEC 369.9
　white blood cell count 288.50
Decubital gangrene — *see also* Ulcer, pressure 707.00 [785.4]
Decubiti — *see also* Ulcer, pressure 707.00
Decubitus (ulcer) — *see also* Ulcer, pressure 707.00
　with gangrene 707.00 [785.4]
　ankle 707.06
　back
　　lower 707.03
　　upper 707.02
　buttock 707.05
　coccyx 707.03
　elbow 707.01
　head 707.09
　heel 707.07
　hip 707.04
　other site 707.09
　sacrum 707.03
　shoulder blades 707.02
Deepening acetabulum 718.85
Defect, defective 759.9
　3-beta-hydroxysteroid dehydrogenase 255.2
　11-hydroxylase 255.2
　21-hydroxylase 255.2
　abdominal wall, congenital 756.70
　aorticopulmonary septum 745.0
　aortic septal 745.0
　atrial septal (ostium secundum type) 745.5
　　acquired 429.71
　　ostium primum type 745.61
　　sinus venosus 745.8
　atrioventricular
　　canal 745.69
　　septum 745.4
　　　acquired 429.71
　atrium secundum 745.5
　　acquired 429.71

Defect, defective — *continued*
　auricular septal 745.5
　　acquired 429.71
　bilirubin excretion 277.4
　biosynthesis, testicular androgen 257.2
　bridge 525.60
　bulbar septum 745.0
　butanol-insoluble iodide 246.1
　chromosome — *see* Anomaly, chromosome
　circulation (acquired) 459.9
　　congenital 747.9
　　newborn 747.9
　clotting NEC (*see also* Defect, coagulation) 286.9
　coagulation (factor) (*see also* Deficiency, coagulation factor) 286.9
　　with
　　　abortion — *see* Abortion, by type, with hemorrhage
　　　ectopic pregnancy (*see also* categories 634–638) 639.1
　　　molar pregnancy (*see also* categories 630–632) 639.1
　　acquired (any) 286.7
　　antepartum or intrapartum 641.3 ☑
　　　affecting fetus or newborn 762.1
　　causing hemorrhage of pregnancy or delivery 641.3 ☑
　　complicating pregnancy, childbirth, or puerperium 649.3 ☑
　　due to
　　　liver disease 286.7
　　　vitamin K deficiency 286.7
　　newborn, transient 776.3
　　postpartum 666.3 ☑
　　specified type NEC 286.9
　conduction (heart) 426.9
　　bone (*see also* Deafness, conductive) 389.00
　congenital, organ or site NEC (*see also* Anomaly)
　　circulation 747.9
　　Descemet's membrane 743.9
　　　specified type NEC 743.49
　　diaphragm 756.6
　　ectodermal 757.9
　　esophagus 750.9
　　pulmonic cusps — *see* Anomaly, heart valve
　　respiratory system 748.9
　　　specified type NEC 748.8
　crown 525.60
　cushion endocardial 745.60
　dental restoration 525.60
　dentin (hereditary) 520.5
　Descemet's membrane (congenital) 743.9
　　acquired 371.30
　　specific type NEC 743.49
　deutan 368.52
　developmental (*see also* Anomaly, by site)
　　cauda equina 742.59
　　left ventricle 746.9
　　　with atresia or hypoplasia of aortic orifice or valve, with hypoplasia of ascending aorta 746.7
　　　in hypoplastic left heart syndrome 746.7
　　testis 752.9
　　vessel 747.9
　diaphragm
　　with elevation, eventration, or hernia — *see* Hernia, diaphragm
　　congenital 756.6
　　　with elevation, eventration, or hernia 756.6
　　　gross (with elevation, eventration, or hernia) 756.6
　ectodermal, congenital 757.9
　Eisenmenger's (ventricular septal defect) 745.4
　endocardial cushion 745.60
　　specified type NEC 745.69
　esophagus, congenital 750.9
　extensor retinaculum 728.9
　fibrin polymerization (*see also* Defect, coagulation) 286.3

Defect, defective — *continued*
　filling
　　biliary tract 793.3
　　bladder 793.5
　　dental 525.60
　　gallbladder 793.3
　　kidney 793.5
　　stomach 793.4
　　ureter 793.5
　fossa ovalis 745.5
　gene, carrier (suspected) of V83.89
　Gerbode 745.4
　glaucomatous, without elevated tension 365.89
　Hageman (factor) (*see also* Defect, coagulation) 286.3
　hearing (*see also* Deafness) 389.9
　high grade 317
　homogentisic acid 270.2
　interatrial septal 745.5
　　acquired 429.71
　interauricular septal 745.5
　　acquired 429.71
　interventricular septal 745.4
　　with pulmonary stenosis or atresia, dextraposition of aorta, and hypertrophy of right ventricle 745.2
　　acquired 429.71
　　in tetralogy of Fallot 745.2
　iodide trapping 246.1
　iodotyrosine dehalogenase 246.1
　kynureninase 270.2
　learning, specific 315.2
　major osseous 731.3
　mental (*see also* Disability, intellectual) 319
　osseous, major 731.3
　osteochondral NEC 738.8
　ostium
　　primum 745.61
　　secundum 745.5
　pericardium 746.89
　peroxidase-binding 246.1
　placental blood supply — *see* Placenta, insufficiency
　platelet (qualitative) 287.1
　　constitutional 286.4
　postural, spine 737.9
　protan 368.51
　pulmonic cusps, congenital 746.00
　renal pelvis 753.9
　　obstructive 753.29
　　specified type NEC 753.3
　respiratory system, congenital 748.9
　　specified type NEC 748.8
　retina, retinal 361.30
　　with detachment (*see also* Detachment, retina, with retinal defect) 361.00
　　multiple 361.33
　　　with detachment 361.02
　　nerve fiber bundle 362.85
　　single 361.30
　　　with detachment 361.01
　septal (closure) (heart) NEC 745.9
　　acquired 429.71
　　atrial 745.5
　　specified type NEC 745.8
　speech NEC 784.59
　　developmental 315.39
　　late effect of cerebrovascular disease — *see* Late effect(s) (of) cerebrovascular disease, speech and language deficit
　　secondary to organic lesion 784.59
　Taussig-Bing (transposition, aorta and overriding pulmonary artery) 745.11
　teeth, wedge 521.20
　thyroid hormone synthesis 246.1
　tritan 368.53
　ureter 753.9
　　obstructive 753.29
　vascular (acquired) (local) 459.9
　　congenital (peripheral) NEC 747.60
　　　gastrointestinal 747.61
　　　lower limb 747.64
　　　renal 747.62
　　　specified NEC 747.69

Defect, defective — *continued*
　vascular — *continued*
　　congenital — *continued*
　　　spinal 747.82
　　　upper limb 747.63
　　ventricular septal 745.4
　　　with pulmonary stenosis or atresia, dextraposition of aorta, and hypertrophy of right ventricle 745.2
　　　acquired 429.71
　　　atrioventricular canal type 745.69
　　　between infundibulum and anterior portion 745.4
　　　in tetralogy of Fallot 745.2
　　　isolated anterior 745.4
　vision NEC 369.9
　visual field 368.40
　　arcuate 368.43
　　heteronymous, bilateral 368.47
　　homonymous, bilateral 368.46
　　localized NEC 368.44
　　nasal step 368.44
　　peripheral 368.44
　　sector 368.43
　voice and resonance 784.40
　wedge, teeth (abrasion) 521.20
Defeminization syndrome 255.2
Deferentitis 608.4
　gonorrheal (acute) 098.14
　　chronic or duration of 2 months or over 098.34
Defibrination syndrome — *see also* Fibrinolysis 286.6
Deficiency, deficient
　3-beta-hydroxysteroid dehydrogenase 255.2
　6-phosphogluconic dehydrogenase (anemia) 282.2
　11-beta-hydroxylase 255.2
　17-alpha-hydroxylase 255.2
　18-hydroxysteroid dehydrogenase 255.2
　20-alpha-hydroxylase 255.2
　21-hydroxylase 255.2
　AAT (alpha-1 antitrypsin) 273.4
　abdominal muscle syndrome 756.79
　accelerator globulin (Ac G) (blood) (*see also* Defect, coagulation) 286.3
　AC globulin (congenital) (*see also* Defect, coagulation) 286.3
　　acquired 286.7
　activating factor (blood) (*see also* Defect, coagulation) 286.3
　adenohypophyseal 253.2
　adenosine deaminase 277.2
　aldolase (hereditary) 271.2
　alpha-1-antitrypsin 273.4
　alpha-1-trypsin inhibitor 273.4
　alpha-fucosidase 271.8
　alpha-lipoprotein 272.5
　alpha-mannosidase 271.8
　amino acid 270.9
　anemia — *see* Anemia, deficiency
　aneurin 265.1
　　with beriberi 265.0
　antibody NEC 279.00
　antidiuretic hormone 253.5
　antihemophilic
　　factor (A) 286.0
　　　B 286.1
　　　C 286.2
　　globulin (AHG) NEC 286.0
　antithrombin III 289.81
　antitrypsin 273.4
　argininosuccinate synthetase or lyase 270.6
　ascorbic acid (with scurvy) 267
　autoprothrombin
　　I (*see also* Defect, coagulation) 286.3
　　II 286.1
　　C (*see also* Defect, coagulation) 286.3
　bile salt 579.8
　biotin 266.2
　biotinidase 277.6
　bradykinase-1 277.6
　brancher enzyme (amylopectinosis) 271.0
　calciferol 268.9
　　with
　　　osteomalacia 268.2

☑ **Additional Digit Required** — Refer to the Tabular List for Digit Selection
▽ **Subterms under main terms may continue to next column or page**

64 — Volume 2　　　　▶◀ Revised Text　　　　● New Line　　　▲ Revised Code　　　　2015 ICD-9-CM

Deficiency, deficient — *continued*
 calciferol — *continued*
  with — *continued*
   rickets (*see also* Rickets) 268.0
 calcium 275.40
  dietary 269.3
 calorie, severe 261
 carbamyl phosphate synthetase 270.6
 cardiac (*see also* Insufficiency, myocardial) 428.0
 carnitine 277.81
  due to
   hemodialysis 277.83
   inborn errors of metabolism 277.82
   valproic acid therapy 277.83
  iatrogenic 277.83
  palmitoyltransferase (CPT1, CPT2) 277.85
  palmityl transferase (CPT1, CPT2) 277.85
  primary 277.81
  secondary 277.84
 carotene 264.9
 Carr factor (*see also* Defect, coagulation) 286.9
 central nervous system 349.9
 ceruloplasmin 275.1
 cevitamic acid (with scurvy) 267
 choline 266.2
 Christmas factor 286.1
 chromium 269.3
 citrin 269.1
 clotting (blood) (*see also* Defect, coagulation) 286.9
 coagulation factor NEC 286.9
  with
   abortion — *see* Abortion, by type, with hemorrhage
   ectopic pregnancy (*see also* categories 634–638) 639.1
   molar pregnancy (*see also* categories 630–632) 639.1
  acquired (any) 286.7
  antepartum or intrapartum 641.3 ☑
   affecting fetus or newborn 762.1
  complicating pregnancy, childbirth, or puerperium 649.3 ☑
  due to
   liver disease 286.7
   vitamin K deficiency 286.7
  newborn, transient 776.3
  postpartum 666.3 ☑
  specified type NEC 286.3
 color vision (congenital) 368.59
  acquired 368.55
 combined glucocorticoid and mineralocorticoid 255.41
 combined, two or more coagulation factors (*see also* Defect, coagulation) 286.9
 complement factor NEC 279.8
 contact factor (*see also* Defect, coagulation) 286.3
 copper NEC 275.1
 corticoadrenal 255.41
 craniofacial axis 756.0
 cyanocobalamin (vitamin B_{12}) 266.2
 debrancher enzyme (limit dextrinosis) 271.0
 desmolase 255.2
 diet 269.9
 dihydrofolate reductase 281.2
 dihydropteridine reductase 270.1
 dihydropyrimidine dehydrogenase (DPD) 277.6
 disaccharidase (intestinal) 271.3
 disease NEC 269.9
 ear(s) V48.8
 edema 262
 endocrine 259.9
 enzymes, circulating NEC (*see also* Deficiency, by specific enzyme) 277.6
 ergosterol 268.9
  with
   osteomalacia 268.2
   rickets (*see also* Rickets) 268.0
 erythrocytic glutathione (anemia) 282.2
 eyelid(s) V48.8
 factor (*see also* Defect, coagulation) 286.9
  I (congenital) (fibrinogen) 286.3

Deficiency, deficient — *continued*
 factor (*see also* Defect, coagulation) — *continued*
  I — *continued*
   antepartum or intrapartum 641.3 ☑
    affecting fetus or newborn 762.1
   newborn, transient 776.3
   postpartum 666.3 ☑
  II (congenital) (prothrombin) 286.3
  V (congenital) (labile) 286.3
  VII (congenital) (stable) 286.3
  VIII (congenital) (functional) 286.0
   with
    functional defect 286.0
    vascular defect 286.4
  IX (Christmas) (congenital) (functional) 286.1
  X (congenital) (Stuart-Prower) 286.3
  XI (congenital) (plasma thromboplastin antecedent) 286.2
  XII (congenital) (Hageman) 286.3
  XIII (congenital) (fibrin stabilizing) 286.3
  Hageman 286.3
  multiple (congenital) 286.9
   acquired 286.7
 fibrinase (*see also* Defect, coagulation) 286.3
 fibrinogen (congenital) (*see also* Defect, coagulation) 286.3
  acquired 286.6
 fibrin-stabilizing factor (congenital) (*see also* Defect, coagulation) 286.3
 finger — *see* Absence, finger
 fletcher factor (*see also* Defect, coagulation) 286.9
 fluorine 269.3
 folate, anemia 281.2
 folic acid (vitamin B_c) 266.2
  anemia 281.2
 follicle-stimulating hormone (FSH) 253.4
 fructokinase 271.2
 fructose-1, 6-diphosphate 271.2
 fructose-1-phosphate aldolase 271.2
 FSH (follicle-stimulating hormone) 253.4
 fucosidase 271.8
 galactokinase 271.1
 galactose-1-phosphate uridyl transferase 271.1
 gamma globulin in blood 279.00
 glass factor (*see also* Defect, coagulation) 286.3
 glucocorticoid 255.41
 glucose-6-phosphatase 271.0
 glucose-6-phosphate dehydrogenase anemia 282.2
 glucuronyl transferase 277.4
 glutathione-reductase (anemia) 282.2
 glycogen synthetase 271.0
 growth hormone 253.3
 Hageman factor (congenital) (*see also* Defect, coagulation) 286.3
 head V48.0
 hemoglobin (*see also* Anemia) 285.9
 hepatophosphorylase 271.0
 hexose monophosphate (HMP) shunt 282.2
 HGH (human growth hormone) 253.3
 HG-PRT 277.2
 homogentisic acid oxidase 270.2
 hormone (*see also* Deficiency, by specific hormone)
  anterior pituitary (isolated) (partial) NEC 253.4
   growth (human) 253.3
  follicle-stimulating 253.4
  growth (human) (isolated) 253.3
  human growth 253.3
  interstitial cell-stimulating 253.4
  luteinizing 253.4
  melanocyte-stimulating 253.4
  testicular 257.2
 human growth hormone 253.3
 humoral 279.00
  with
   hyper-IgM 279.05
    autosomal recessive 279.05
    X-linked 279.05
   increased IgM 279.05

Deficiency, deficient — *continued*
 humoral — *continued*
  congenital hypogammaglobulinemia 279.04
  non-sex-linked 279.06
  selective immunoglobulin NEC 279.03
   IgA 279.01
   IgG 279.03
   IgM 279.02
    increased 279.05
  specified NEC 279.09
 hydroxylase 255.2
 hypoxanthine-guanine phosphoribosyltransferase (HG-PRT) 277.2
 ICSH (interstitial cell-stimulating hormone) 253.4
 immunity NEC 279.3
  cell-mediated 279.10
   with
    hyperimmunoglobulinemia 279.2
    thrombocytopenia and eczema 279.12
   specified NEC 279.19
  combined (severe) 279.2
   syndrome 279.2
  common variable 279.06
  humoral NEC 279.00
   IgA (secretory) 279.01
   IgG 279.03
   IgM 279.02
 immunoglobulin, selective NEC 279.03
  IgA 279.01
  IgG 279.03
  IgM 279.02
 inositol (B complex) 266.2
 interferon 279.49
 internal organ V47.0
 interstitial cell-stimulating hormone (ICSH) 253.4
 intrinsic factor (Castle's) (congenital) 281.0
 intrinsic (urethral) sphincter (ISD) 599.82
 invertase 271.3
 iodine 269.3
 iron, anemia 280.9
 labile factor (congenital) (*see also* Defect, coagulation) 286.3
  acquired 286.7
 lacrimal fluid (acquired) 375.15
  congenital 743.64
 lactase 271.3
 Laki-Lorand factor (*see also* Defect, coagulation) 286.3
 lecithin-cholesterol acyltranferase 272.5
 LH (luteinizing hormone) 253.4
 limb V49.0
  lower V49.0
   congenital (*see also* Deficiency, lower limb, congenital) 755.30
  upper V49.0
   congenital (*see also* Deficiency, upper limb, congenital) 755.20
 lipocaic 577.8
 lipoid (high-density) 272.5
 lipoprotein (familial) (high density) 272.5
 liver phosphorylase 271.0
 long chain 3-hydroxyacyl CoA dehydrogenase (LCHAD) 277.85
 long chain/very long chain acyl CoA dehydrogenase (LCAD, VLCAD) 277.85
 lower limb V49.0
  congenital 755.30
   with complete absence of distal elements 755.31
   longitudinal (complete) (partial) (with distal deficiencies, incomplete) 755.32
    with complete absence of distal elements 755.31
    combined femoral, tibial, fibular (incomplete) 755.33
    femoral 755.34
    fibular 755.37
    metatarsal(s) 755.38
    phalange(s) 755.39
     meaning all digits 755.31
    tarsal(s) 755.38

Deficiency, deficient — *continued*
 lower limb — *continued*
  congenital — *continued*
   longitudinal — *continued*
    tibia 755.36
    tibiofibular 755.35
    transverse 755.31
 luteinizing hormone (LH) 253.4
 lysosomal alpha-1, 4 glucosidase 271.0
 magnesium 275.2
 mannosidase 271.8
 medium chain acyl CoA dehydrogenase (MCAD) 277.85
 melanocyte-stimulating hormone (MSH) 253.4
 menadione (vitamin K) 269.0
  newborn 776.0
 mental (familial) (hereditary) (*see also* Disability, intellectual) 319
 methylenetetrahydrofolate reductase (MTHFR) 270.4
 mineralocorticoid 255.42
 mineral NEC 269.3
 molybdenum 269.3
 moral 301.7
 multiple, syndrome 260
 myocardial (*see also* Insufficiency, myocardial) 428.0
 myophosphorylase 271.0
 NADH-diaphorase or reductase (congenital) 289.7
 NADH (DPNH)-methemoglobin-reductase (congenital) 289.7
 neck V48.1
 niacin (amide) (-tryptophan) 265.2
 nicotinamide 265.2
 nicotinic acid (amide) 265.2
 nose V48.8
 number of teeth (*see also* Anodontia) 520.0
 nutrition, nutritional 269.9
  specified NEC 269.8
 ornithine transcarbamylase 270.6
 ovarian 256.39
 oxygen (*see also* Anoxia) 799.02
 pantothenic acid 266.2
 parathyroid (gland) 252.1
 phenylalanine hydroxylase 270.1
 phosphoenolpyruvate carboxykinase 271.8
 phosphofructokinase 271.2
 phosphoglucomutase 271.0
 phosphohexosisomerase 271.0
 phosphomannomutase 271.8
 phosphomannose isomerase 271.8
 phosphomannosyl mutase 271.8
 phosphorylase kinase, liver 271.0
 pituitary (anterior) 253.2
  posterior 253.5
 placenta — *see* Placenta, insufficiency
 plasma
  cell 279.00
  protein (paraproteinemia) (pyroglobulinemia) 273.8
   gamma globulin 279.00
  thromboplastin
   antecedent (PTA) 286.2
   component (PTC) 286.1
 platelet NEC 287.1
  constitutional 286.4
 polyglandular 258.9
 potassium (K) 276.8
 proaccelerin (congenital) (*see also* Defect, congenital) 286.3
  acquired 286.7
 proconvertin factor (congenital) (*see also* Defect, coagulation) 286.3
  acquired 286.7
 prolactin 253.4
 protein 260
  anemia 281.4
  C 289.81
   plasma — *see* Deficiency, plasma, protein
  S 289.81
 prothrombin (congenital) (*see also* Defect, coagulation) 286.3
  acquired 286.7

☑ **Additional Digit Required — Refer to the Tabular List for Digit Selection**   ▽ **Subterms under main terms may continue to next column or page**

2015 ICD-9-CM   ▶◀ **Revised Text**   ● **New Line**   ▲ **Revised Code**   Volume 2 — 65

Deficiency, deficient — *continued*

Prower factor (*see also* Defect, coagulation) 286.3
PRT 277.2
pseudocholinesterase 289.89
psychobiological 301.6
PTA 286.2
PTC 286.1
purine nucleoside phosphorylase 277.2
pyracin (alpha) (beta) 266.1
pyridoxal 266.1
pyridoxamine 266.1
pyridoxine (derivatives) 266.1
pyruvate carboxylase 271.8
pyruvate dehydrogenase 271.8
pyruvate kinase (PK) 282.3
riboflavin (vitamin B_2) 266.0
saccadic eye movements 379.57
salivation 527.7
salt 276.1
secretion
  ovary 256.39
  salivary gland (any) 527.7
  urine 788.5
selenium 269.3
serum
  antitrypsin, familial 273.4
  protein (congenital) 273.8
short chain acyl CoA dehydrogenase (SCAD) 277.85
short stature homeobox gene (SHOX)
  with
    dyschondrosteosis 756.89
    short stature (idiopathic) 783.43
    Turner's syndrome 758.6
smooth pursuit movements (eye) 379.58
sodium (Na) 276.1
SPCA (*see also* Defect, coagulation) 286.3
specified NEC 269.8
stable factor (congenital) (*see also* Defect, coagulation) 286.3
  acquired 286.7
Stuart (-Prower) factor (*see also* Defect, coagulation) 286.3
sucrase 271.3
sucrase-isomaltase 271.3
sulfite oxidase 270.0
syndrome, multiple 260
thiamine, thiaminic (chloride) 265.1
thrombokinase (*see also* Defect, coagulation) 286.3
  newborn 776.0
thrombopoieten 287.39
thymolymphatic 279.2
thyroid (gland) 244.9
tocopherol 269.1
toe — *see* Absence, toe
tooth bud (*see also* Anodontia) 520.0
trunk V48.1
UDPG-glycogen transferase 271.0
upper limb V49.0
  congenital 755.20
    with complete absence of distal elements 755.21
    longitudinal (complete) (partial) (with distal deficiencies, incomplete) 755.22
      carpal(s) 755.28
      combined humeral, radial, ulnar (incomplete) 755.23
      humeral 755.24
      metacarpal(s) 755.28
      phalange(s) 755.29
        meaning all digits 755.21
      radial 755.26
      radioulnar 755.25
      ulnar 755.27
    transverse (complete) (partial) 755.21
vascular 459.9
vasopressin 253.5
viosterol (*see also* Deficiency, calciferol) 268.9
vitamin (multiple) NEC 269.2
  A 264.9
    with
      Bitôt's spot 264.1

Deficiency, deficient — *continued*

vitamin — *continued*
  A — *continued*
    with — *continued*
      Bitôt's spot — *continued*
        corneal 264.2
        with corneal ulceration 264.3
      keratomalacia 264.4
      keratosis, follicular 264.8
      night blindness 264.5
      scar of cornea, xerophthalmic 264.6
      specified manifestation NEC 264.8
        ocular 264.7
      xeroderma 264.8
      xerophthalmia 264.7
      xerosis
        conjunctival 264.0
          with Bitôt's spot 264.1
        corneal 264.2
          with corneal ulceration 264.3
  B_1 NEC 265.1
    beriberi 265.0
  B_2 266.0
  B_6 266.1
  B_{12} 266.2
  B_c (folic acid) 266.2
  B (complex) NEC 266.9
    with
      beriberi 265.0
      pellagra 265.2
    specified type NEC 266.2
  C (ascorbic acid) (with scurvy) 267
  D (calciferol) (ergosterol) 268.9
    with
      osteomalacia 268.2
      rickets (*see also* Rickets) 268.0
  E 269.1
  folic acid 266.2
  G 266.0
  H 266.2
  K 269.0
    of newborn 776.0
  nicotinic acid 265.2
  P 269.1
  PP 265.2
  specified NEC 269.1
  zinc 269.3

Deficient — *see also* Deficiency
  blink reflex 374.45
  craniofacial axis 756.0
  number of teeth (*see also* Anodontia) 520.0
  secretion of urine 788.5

Deficit
  attention 799.51
  cognitive communication 799.52
  concentration 799.51
  executive function 799.55
  frontal lobe 799.55
  neurologic NEC 781.99
    due to
      cerebrovascular lesion (*see also* Disease, cerebrovascular, acute) 436
      late effect — *see* Late effect(s) (of) cerebrovascular disease
      transient ischemic attack 435.9
    ischemic
      reversible (RIND) 434.91
        history of (personal) V12.54
      prolonged (PRIND) 434.91
        history of (personal) V12.54
  oxygen 799.02
  psychomotor 799.54
  visuospatial 799.53

Deflection
  radius 736.09
  septum (acquired) (nasal) (nose) 470
  spine — *see* Curvature, spine
  turbinate (nose) 470

Defluvium
  capillorum (*see also* Alopecia) 704.00
  ciliorum 374.55

Defluvium — *continued*
  unguium 703.8

Deformity 738.9
abdomen, congenital 759.9
abdominal wall
  acquired 738.8
  congenital 756.70
  muscle deficiency syndrome 756.79
acquired (unspecified site) 738.9
  specified site NEC 738.8
adrenal gland (congenital) 759.1
alimentary tract, congenital 751.9
  lower 751.5
    specified type NEC 751.8
  upper (any part, except tongue) 750.9
    specified type NEC 750.8
    tongue 750.10
      specified type NEC 750.19
ankle (joint) (acquired) 736.70
  abduction 718.47
  congenital 755.69
  contraction 718.47
  specified NEC 736.79
anus (congenital) 751.5
  acquired 569.49
aorta (congenital) 747.20
  acquired 447.8
  arch 747.21
    acquired 447.8
  coarctation 747.10
aortic
  arch 747.21
    acquired 447.8
  cusp or valve (congenital) 746.9
    acquired (*see also* Endocarditis, aortic) 424.1
  ring 747.21
appendix 751.5
arm (acquired) 736.89
  congenital 755.50
arteriovenous (congenital) (peripheral) NEC 747.60
  gastrointestinal 747.61
  lower limb 747.64
  renal 747.62
  specified NEC 747.69
  spinal 747.82
  upper limb 747.63
artery (congenital) (peripheral) NEC (*see also* Deformity, vascular) 747.60
  acquired 447.8
  cerebral 747.81
  coronary (congenital) 746.85
    acquired (*see also* Ischemia, heart) 414.9
  retinal 743.9
  umbilical 747.5
atrial septal (congenital) (heart) 745.5
auditory canal (congenital) (external) (*see also* Deformity, ear) 744.3
  acquired 380.50
auricle
  ear (congenital) (*see also* Deformity, ear) 744.3
    acquired 380.32
  heart (congenital) 746.9
back (acquired) — *see* Deformity, spine
Bartholin's duct (congenital) 750.9
bile duct (congenital) 751.60
  acquired 576.8
    with calculus, choledocholithiasis, or stones — *see* Choledocholithiasis
biliary duct or passage (congenital) 751.60
  acquired 576.8
    with calculus, choledocholithiasis, or stones — *see* Choledocholithiasis
bladder (neck) (sphincter) (trigone) (acquired) 596.89
  congenital 753.9
bone (acquired) NEC 738.9
  congenital 756.9
  turbinate 738.0
boutonniere (finger) 736.21
brain (congenital) 742.9

Deformity — *continued*
brain — *continued*
  acquired 348.89
  multiple 742.4
  reduction 742.2
  vessel (congenital) 747.81
breast (acquired) 611.89
  congenital 757.6
  reconstructed 612.0
bronchus (congenital) 748.3
  acquired 519.19
bursa, congenital 756.9
canal of Nuck 752.9
canthus (congenital) 743.9
  acquired 374.89
capillary (acquired) 448.9
  congenital NEC (*see also* Deformity, vascular) 747.60
cardiac — *see* Deformity, heart
cardiovascular system (congenital) 746.9
caruncle, lacrimal (congenital) 743.9
  acquired 375.69
cascade, stomach 537.6
cecum (congenital) 751.5
  acquired 569.89
cerebral (congenital) 742.9
  acquired 348.89
cervix (acquired) (uterus) 622.8
  congenital 752.40
cheek (acquired) 738.19
  congenital 744.9
chest (wall) (acquired) 738.3
  congenital 754.89
  late effect of rickets 268.1
chin (acquired) 738.19
  congenital 744.9
choroid (congenital) 743.9
  acquired 363.8
  plexus (congenital) 742.9
    acquired 349.2
cicatricial — *see* Cicatrix
cilia (congenital) 743.9
  acquired 374.89
circulatory system (congenital) 747.9
clavicle (acquired) 738.8
  congenital 755.51
clitoris (congenital) 752.40
  acquired 624.8
clubfoot — *see* Clubfoot
coccyx (acquired) 738.6
  congenital 756.10
colon (congenital) 751.5
  acquired 569.89
concha (ear) (congenital) (*see also* Deformity, ear) 744.3
  acquired 380.32
congenital, organ or site not listed (*see also* Anomaly) 759.9
cornea (congenital) 743.9
  acquired 371.70
coronary artery (congenital) 746.85
  acquired (*see also* Ischemia, heart) 414.9
cranium (acquired) 738.19
  congenital (*see also* Deformity, skull, congenital) 756.0
cricoid cartilage (congenital) 748.3
  acquired 478.79
cystic duct (congenital) 751.60
  acquired 575.8
Dandy-Walker 742.3
  with spina bifida (*see also* Spina bifida) 741.0 ☑
diaphragm (congenital) 756.6
  acquired 738.8
digestive organ(s) or system (congenital) NEC 751.9
  specified type NEC 751.8
ductus arteriosus 747.0
duodenal bulb 537.89
duodenum (congenital) 751.5
  acquired 537.89
dura (congenital) 742.9
  brain 742.4
    acquired 349.2
  spinal 742.59
    acquired 349.2

☑ **Additional Digit Required** — Refer to the Tabular List for Digit Selection   ▽ **Subterms under main terms may continue to next column or page**

Deformity — *continued*
 ear (congenital) 744.3
  acquired 380.32
  auricle 744.3
   causing impairment of hearing
    744.02
  causing impairment of hearing 744.00
  external 744.3
   causing impairment of hearing
    744.02
  internal 744.05
  lobule 744.3
  middle 744.03
   ossicles 744.04
  ossicles 744.04
 ectodermal (congenital) NEC 757.9
  specified type NEC 757.8
 ejaculatory duct (congenital) 752.9
  acquired 608.89
 elbow (joint) (acquired) 736.00
  congenital 755.50
  contraction 718.42
 endocrine gland NEC 759.2
 epididymis (congenital) 752.9
  acquired 608.89
  torsion 608.24
 epiglottis (congenital) 748.3
  acquired 478.79
 esophagus (congenital) 750.9
  acquired 530.89
 Eustachian tube (congenital) NEC 744.3
  specified type NEC 744.24
 extremity (acquired) 736.9
  congenital, except reduction deformity
   755.9
   lower 755.60
   upper 755.50
  reduction — *see* Deformity, reduction
 eye (congenital) 743.9
  acquired 379.8
  muscle 743.9
 eyebrow (congenital) 744.89
 eyelid (congenital) 743.9
  acquired 374.89
  specified type NEC 743.62
 face 738.19
  congenital (any part) 744.9
   due to intrauterine malposition and
    pressure 754.0
 fallopian tube (congenital) 752.10
  acquired 620.8
 femur (acquired) 736.89
  congenital 755.60
 fetal
  with fetopelvic disproportion 653.7 ☑
   affecting fetus or newborn 763.1
  causing obstructed labor 660.1 ☑
   affecting fetus or newborn 763.1
  known or suspected, affecting management of pregnancy 655.9 ☑
 finger (acquired) 736.20
  boutonniere type 736.21
  congenital 755.50
  flexion contracture 718.44
  swan neck 736.22
 flexion (joint) (acquired) 736.9
  congenital NEC 755.9
  hip or thigh (acquired) 736.39
   congenital (*see also* Subluxation,
    congenital, hip) 754.32
 foot (acquired) 736.70
  cavovarus 736.75
   congenital 754.59
  congenital NEC 754.70
   specified type NEC 754.79
  valgus (acquired) 736.79
   congenital 754.60
    specified type NEC 754.69
  varus (acquired) 736.79
   congenital 754.50
    specified type NEC 754.59
 forearm (acquired) 736.00
  congenital 755.50
 forehead (acquired) 738.19
  congenital (*see also* Deformity, skull,
   congenital) 756.0

Deformity — *continued*
 frontal bone (acquired) 738.19
  congenital (*see also* Deformity, skull,
   congenital) 756.0
 gallbladder (congenital) 751.60
  acquired 575.8
 gastrointestinal tract (congenital) NEC 751.9
  acquired 569.89
  specified type NEC 751.8
 genitalia, genital organ(s) or system NEC
  congenital 752.9
  female (congenital) 752.9
   acquired 629.89
   external 752.40
   internal 752.9
  male (congenital) 752.9
   acquired 608.89
 globe (eye) (congenital) 743.9
  acquired 360.89
 gum (congenital) 750.9
  acquired 523.9
 gunstock 736.02
 hand (acquired) 736.00
  claw 736.06
  congenital 755.50
  minus (and plus) (intrinsic) 736.09
  pill roller (intrinsic) 736.09
  plus (and minus) (intrinsic) 736.09
  swan neck (intrinsic) 736.09
 head (acquired) 738.10
  congenital (*see also* Deformity, skull
   congenital) 756.0
  specified NEC 738.19
 heart (congenital) 746.9
  auricle (congenital) 746.9
  septum 745.9
   auricular 745.5
   specified type NEC 745.8
   ventricular 745.4
  valve (congenital) NEC 746.9
   acquired — *see* Endocarditis
   pulmonary (congenital) 746.00
   specified type NEC 746.89
  ventricle (congenital) 746.9
 heel (acquired) 736.76
  congenital 755.67
 hepatic duct (congenital) 751.60
  acquired 576.8
   with calculus, choledocholithiasis, or
    stones — *see* Choledocholithi-
    asis
 hip (joint) (acquired) 736.30
  congenital NEC 755.63
  flexion 718.45
   congenital (*see also* Subluxation,
    congenital, hip) 754.32
 hourglass — *see* Contraction, hourglass
 humerus (acquired) 736.89
  congenital 755.50
 hymen (congenital) 752.40
 hypophyseal (congenital) 759.2
 ileocecal (coil) (valve) (congenital) 751.5
  acquired 569.89
 ileum (intestine) (congenital) 751.5
  acquired 569.89
 ilium (acquired) 738.6
  congenital 755.60
 integument (congenital) 757.9
 intervertebral cartilage or disc (acquired)
  (*see also* Displacement, intervertebral
  disc)
  congenital 756.10
 intestine (large) (small) (congenital) 751.5
  acquired 569.89
 iris (acquired) 364.75
  congenital 743.9
  prolapse 364.89
 ischium (acquired) 738.6
  congenital 755.60
 jaw (acquired) (congenital) NEC 524.9
  due to intrauterine malposition and
   pressure 754.0
 joint (acquired) NEC 738.8
  congenital 755.9

Deformity — *continued*
 joint — *continued*
  contraction (abduction) (adduction)
   (extension) (flexion) — *see* Contraction, joint
 kidney(s) (calyx) (pelvis) (congenital) 753.9
  acquired 593.89
  vessel 747.62
  acquired 459.9
 Klippel-Feil (brevicollis) 756.16
 knee (acquired) NEC 736.6
  congenital 755.64
 labium (majus) (minus) (congenital) 752.40
  acquired 624.8
 lacrimal apparatus or duct (congenital)
  743.9
  acquired 375.69
 larynx (muscle) (congenital) 748.3
  acquired 478.79
  web (glottic) (subglottic) 748.2
 leg (lower) (upper) (acquired) NEC 736.89
  congenital 755.60
   reduction — *see* Deformity, reduc-
    tion, lower limb
 lens (congenital) 743.9
  acquired 379.39
 lid (fold) (congenital) 743.9
  acquired 374.89
 ligament (acquired) 728.9
  congenital 756.9
 limb (acquired) 736.9
  congenital, except reduction deformity
   755.9
  lower 755.60
   reduction (*see also* Deformity,
    reduction, lower limb)
    755.30
  upper 755.50
   reduction (*see also* Deformity, re-
    duction, upper limb)
    755.20
  specified NEC 736.89
 lip (congenital) NEC 750.9
  acquired 528.5
  specified type NEC 750.26
 liver (congenital) 751.60
  acquired 573.8
  duct (congenital) 751.60
   acquired 576.8
    with calculus, choledocholithiasis,
     or stones — *see* Choledo-
     cholithi-asis
 lower extremity — *see* Deformity, leg
 lumbosacral (joint) (region) (congenital)
  756.10
  acquired 738.5
 lung (congenital) 748.60
  acquired 518.89
  specified type NEC 748.69
 lymphatic system, congenital 759.9
 Madelung's (radius) 755.54
 maxilla (acquired) (congenital) 524.9
 meninges or membrane (congenital) 742.9
  brain 742.4
   acquired 349.2
  spinal (cord) 742.59
   acquired 349.2
 mesentery (congenital) 751.9
  acquired 568.89
 metacarpus (acquired) 736.00
  congenital 755.50
 metatarsus (acquired) 736.70
  congenital 754.70
 middle ear, except ossicles (congenital)
  744.03
  ossicles 744.04
 mitral (leaflets) (valve) (congenital) 746.9
  acquired — *see* Endocarditis, mitral
  Ebstein's 746.89
  parachute 746.5
  specified type NEC 746.89
  stenosis, congenital 746.5
 mouth (acquired) 528.9
  congenital NEC 750.9
   specified type NEC 750.26
 multiple, congenital NEC 759.7

Deformity — *continued*
 multiple, congenital — *continued*
  specified type NEC 759.89
 muscle (acquired) 728.9
  congenital 756.9
   specified type NEC 756.89
   sternocleidomastoid (due to intrauter-
    ine malposition and pressure)
    754.1
 musculoskeletal system, congenital NEC
  756.9
  specified type NEC 756.9
 nail (acquired) 703.9
  congenital 757.9
 nasal — *see* Deformity, nose
 neck (acquired) NEC 738.2
  congenital (any part) 744.9
   sternocleidomastoid 754.1
 nervous system (congenital) 742.9
 nipple (congenital) 757.6
  acquired 611.89
 nose, nasal (cartilage) (acquired) 738.0
  bone (turbinate) 738.0
  congenital 748.1
   bent 754.0
   squashed 754.0
  saddle 738.0
   syphilitic 090.5
  septum 470
   congenital 748.1
  sinus (wall) (congenital) 748.1
   acquired 738.0
  syphilitic (congenital) 090.5
   late 095.8
 ocular muscle (congenital) 743.9
  acquired 378.60
 opticociliary vessels (congenital) 743.9
 orbit (congenital) (eye) 743.9
  acquired NEC 376.40
   associated with craniofacial deformi-
    ties 376.44
   due to
    bone disease 376.43
    surgery 376.47
    trauma 376.47
 organ of Corti (congenital) 744.05
 ovary (congenital) 752.0
  acquired 620.8
 oviduct (congenital) 752.10
  acquired 620.8
 palate (congenital) 750.9
  acquired 526.89
  cleft (congenital) (*see also* Cleft, palate)
   749.00
  hard, acquired 526.89
  soft, acquired 528.9
 pancreas (congenital) 751.7
  acquired 577.8
 parachute, mitral valve 746.5
 parathyroid (gland) 759.2
 parotid (gland) (congenital) 750.9
  acquired 527.8
 patella (acquired) 736.6
  congenital 755.64
 pelvis, pelvic (acquired) (bony) 738.6
  with disproportion (fetopelvic) 653.0 ☑
   affecting fetus or newborn 763.1
   causing obstructed labor 660.1 ☑
    affecting fetus or newborn 763.1
  congenital 755.60
  rachitic (late effect) 268.1
 penis (glans) (congenital) 752.9
  acquired 607.89
 pericardium (congenital) 746.9
  acquired — *see* Pericarditis
 pharynx (congenital) 750.9
  acquired 478.29
 Pierre Robin (congenital) 756.0
 pinna (acquired) 380.32
  congenital 744.3
 pituitary (congenital) 759.2
 pleural folds (congenital) 748.8
 portal vein (congenital) 747.40
 posture — *see* Curvature, spine
 prepuce (congenital) 752.9
  acquired 607.89

☑ **Additional Digit Required** — **Refer to the Tabular List for Digit Selection**

🅦 **Subterms under main terms may continue to next column or page**

2015 ICD-9-CM ▶◀ **Revised Text** ● **New Line** ▲ **Revised Code** **Volume 2 — 67**

Deformity — Degeneration, degenerative

Deformity — continued
prostate (congenital) 752.9
acquired 602.8
pulmonary valve — see Endocarditis, pulmonary
pupil (congenital) 743.9
acquired 364.75
pylorus (congenital) 750.9
acquired 537.89
rachitic (acquired), healed or old 268.1
radius (acquired) 736.00
congenital 755.50
reduction — see Deformity, reduction, upper limb
rectovaginal septum (congenital) 752.40
acquired 623.8
rectum (congenital) 751.5
acquired 569.49
reduction (extremity) (limb) 755.4
brain 742.2
lower limb 755.30
with complete absence of distal elements 755.31
longitudinal (complete) (partial) (with distal deficiencies, incomplete) 755.32
with complete absence of distal elements 755.31
combined femoral, tibial, fibular (incomplete) 755.33
femoral 755.34
fibular 755.37
metatarsal(s) 755.38
phalangal(s) 755.39
meaning all digits 755.31
tarsal(s) 755.38
tibia 755.36
tibiofibular 755.35
transverse 755.31
upper limb 755.20
with complete absence of distal elements 755.21
longitudinal (complete) (partial) (with distal deficiencies, incomplete) 755.22
with complete absence of distal elements 755.21
carpal(s) 755.28
combined humeral, radial, ulnar (incomplete) 755.23
humeral 755.24
metacarpal(s) 755.28
phalange(s) 755.29
meaning all digits 755.21
radial 755.26
radioulnar 755.25
ulnar 755.27
transverse (complete) (partial) 755.21
renal — see Deformity, kidney
respiratory system (congenital) 748.9
specified type NEC 748.8
rib (acquired) 738.3
congenital 756.3
cervical 756.2
rotation (joint) (acquired) 736.9
congenital 755.9
hip or thigh 736.39
congenital (see also Subluxation, congenital, hip) 754.32
sacroiliac joint (congenital) 755.69
acquired 738.5
sacrum (acquired) 738.5
congenital 756.10
saddle
back 737.8
nose 738.0
syphilitic 090.5
salivary gland or duct (congenital) 750.9
acquired 527.8
scapula (acquired) 736.89
congenital 755.50
scrotum (congenital) 752.9
acquired 608.89
sebaceous gland, acquired 706.8
seminal tract or duct (congenital) 752.9
acquired 608.89

Deformity — continued
septum (nasal) (acquired) 470
congenital 748.1
shoulder (joint) (acquired) 736.89
congenital 755.50
specified type NEC 755.59
contraction 718.41
sigmoid (flexure) (congenital) 751.5
acquired 569.89
sinus of Valsalva 747.29
skin (congenital) 757.9
acquired NEC 709.8
skull (acquired) 738.19
congenital 756.0
with
anencephalus 740.0
encephalocele 742.0
hydrocephalus 742.3
with spina bifida (see also Spina bifida) 741.0 ☑
microcephalus 742.1
due to intrauterine malposition and pressure 754.0
soft parts, organs or tissues (of pelvis)
in pregnancy or childbirth NEC 654.9 ☑
affecting fetus or newborn 763.89
causing obstructed labor 660.2 ☑
affecting fetus or newborn 763.1
spermatic cord (congenital) 752.9
acquired 608.89
torsion 608.22
extravaginal 608.21
intravaginal 608.22
spinal
column — see Deformity, spine
cord (congenital) 742.9
acquired 336.8
vessel (congenital) 747.82
nerve root (congenital) 742.9
acquired 724.9
spine (acquired) NEC 738.5
congenital 756.10
due to intrauterine malposition and pressure 754.2
kyphoscoliotic (see also Kyphoscoliosis) 737.30
kyphotic (see also Kyphosis) 737.10
lordotic (see also Lordosis) 737.20
rachitic 268.1
scoliotic (see also Scoliosis) 737.30
spleen
acquired 289.59
congenital 759.0
Sprengel's (congenital) 755.52
sternum (acquired) 738.3
congenital 756.3
stomach (congenital) 750.9
acquired 537.89
submaxillary gland (congenital) 750.9
acquired 527.8
swan neck (acquired)
finger 736.22
hand 736.09
talipes — see Talipes
teeth, tooth NEC 520.9
testis (congenital) 752.9
acquired 608.89
torsion 608.20
thigh (acquired) 736.89
congenital 755.60
thorax (acquired) (wall) 738.3
congenital 754.89
late effect of rickets 268.1
thumb (acquired) 736.20
congenital 755.50
thymus (tissue) (congenital) 759.2
thyroid (gland) (congenital) 759.2
cartilage 748.3
acquired 478.79
tibia (acquired) 736.89
congenital 755.60
saber 090.5
toe (acquired) 735.9
congenital 755.66
specified NEC 735.8
tongue (congenital) 750.10

Deformity — continued
tongue — continued
acquired 529.8
tooth, teeth NEC 520.9
trachea (rings) (congenital) 748.3
acquired 519.19
transverse aortic arch (congenital) 747.21
tricuspid (leaflets) (valve) (congenital) 746.9
acquired — see Endocarditis, tricuspid
atresia or stenosis 746.1
specified type NEC 746.89
trunk (acquired) 738.3
congenital 759.9
ulna (acquired) 736.00
congenital 755.50
upper extremity — see Deformity, arm
urachus (congenital) 753.7
ureter (opening) (congenital) 753.9
acquired 593.89
urethra (valve) (congenital) 753.9
acquired 599.84
urinary tract or system (congenital) 753.9
urachus 753.7
uterus (congenital) 752.39
acquired 621.8
uvula (congenital) 750.9
acquired 528.9
vagina (congenital) 752.40
acquired 623.8
valve, valvular (heart) (congenital) 746.9
acquired — see Endocarditis
pulmonary 746.00
specified type NEC 746.89
vascular (congenital) (peripheral) NEC 747.60
acquired 459.9
gastrointestinal 747.61
lower limb 747.64
renal 747.62
specified site NEC 747.69
spinal 747.82
upper limb 747.63
vas deferens (congenital) 752.9
acquired 608.89
vein (congenital) NEC (see also Deformity, vascular) 747.60
brain 747.81
coronary 746.9
great 747.40
vena cava (inferior) (superior) (congenital) 747.40
vertebra — see Deformity, spine
vesicourethral orifice (acquired) 596.89
congenital NEC 753.9
specified type NEC 753.8
vessels of optic papilla (congenital) 743.9
visual field (contraction) 368.45
vitreous humor (congenital) 743.9
acquired 379.29
vulva (congenital) 752.40
acquired 624.8
wrist (joint) (acquired) 736.00
congenital 755.50
contraction 718.43
valgus 736.03
congenital 755.59
varus 736.04
congenital 755.59

Degeneration, degenerative
adrenal (capsule) (gland) 255.8
with hypofunction 255.41
fatty 255.8
hyaline 255.8
infectional 255.8
lardaceous 277.39
amyloid (any site) (general) 277.39
anterior cornua, spinal cord 336.8
anterior labral 840.8
aorta, aortic 440.0
fatty 447.8
valve (heart) (see also Endocarditis, aortic) 424.1
arteriovascular — see Arteriosclerosis
artery, arterial (atheromatous) (calcareous) (see also Arteriosclerosis)
amyloid 277.39

Degeneration, degenerative — continued
artery, arterial (see also Arteriosclerosis) — continued
lardaceous 277.39
medial NEC (see also Arteriosclerosis, extremities) 440.20
articular cartilage NEC (see also Disorder, cartilage, articular) 718.0 ☑
elbow 718.02
knee 717.5
patella 717.7
shoulder 718.01
spine (see also Spondylosis) 721.90
atheromatous — see Arteriosclerosis
bacony (any site) 277.39
basal nuclei or ganglia NEC 333.0
bone 733.90
brachial plexus 353.0
brain (cortical) (progressive) 331.9
arteriosclerotic 437.0
childhood 330.9
specified type NEC 330.8
congenital 742.4
cystic 348.0
congenital 742.4
familial NEC 331.89
grey matter 330.8
heredofamilial NEC 331.89
in
alcoholism 303.9 ☑ [331.7]
beriberi 265.0 [331.7]
cerebrovascular disease 437.9 [331.7]
congenital hydrocephalus 742.3 [331.7]
with spina bifida (see also Spina bifida) 741.0 ☑ [331.7]
Fabry's disease 272.7 [330.2]
Gaucher's disease 272.7 [330.2]
Hunter's disease or syndrome 277.5 [330.3]
lipidosis
cerebral 330.1
generalized 272.7 [330.2]
mucopolysaccharidosis 277.5 [330.3]
myxedema (see also Myxedema) 244.9 [331.7]
neoplastic disease NEC (M8000/1) 239.9 [331.7]
Niemann-Pick disease 272.7 [330.2]
sphingolipidosis 272.7 [330.2]
vitamin B_{12} deficiency 266.2 [331.7]
motor centers 331.89
senile 331.2
specified type NEC 331.89
breast — see Disease, breast
Bruch's membrane 363.40
bundle of His 426.50
left 426.3
right 426.4
calcareous NEC 275.49
capillaries 448.9
amyloid 277.39
fatty 448.9
lardaceous 277.39
cardiac (brown) (calcareous) (fatty) (fibrous) (hyaline) (mural) (muscular) (pigmentary) (senile) (with arteriosclerosis) (see also Degeneration, myocardial) 429.1
valve, valvular — see Endocarditis
cardiorenal (see also Hypertension, cardiorenal) 404.90
cardiovascular (see also Disease, cardiovascular) 429.2
renal (see also Hypertension, cardiorenal) 404.90
cartilage (joint) — see Derangement, joint
cerebellar NEC 334.9
primary (hereditary) (sporadic) 334.2
cerebral — see Degeneration, brain
cerebromacular 330.1
cerebrovascular 437.1
due to hypertension 437.2
late effect — see Late effect(s) (of) cerebrovascular disease
cervical plexus 353.2

☑ Additional Digit Required — Refer to the Tabular List for Digit Selection   ▽ Subterms under main terms may continue to next column or page

68 — Volume 2   ▶◀ Revised Text   ● New Line   ▲ Revised Code   2015 ICD-9-CM

Degeneration, degenerative — continued
- cervix 622.8
  - due to radiation (intended effect) 622.8
    - adverse effect or misadventure 622.8
- changes, spine or vertebra (see also Spondylosis) 721.90
- chitinous 277.39
- chorioretinal 363.40
  - congenital 743.53
  - hereditary 363.50
- choroid (colloid) (drusen) 363.40
  - hereditary 363.50
  - senile 363.41
    - diffuse secondary 363.42
- cochlear 386.8
- collateral ligament (knee) (medial) 717.82
  - lateral 717.81
- combined (spinal cord) (subacute) 266.2 [336.2]
  - with anemia (pernicious) 281.0 [336.2]
    - due to dietary deficiency 281.1 [336.2]
    - due to vitamin B₁₂ deficiency anemia (dietary) 281.1 [336.2]
- conjunctiva 372.50
  - amyloid 277.39 [372.50]
- cornea 371.40
  - calcerous 371.44
  - familial (hereditary) (see also Dystrophy, cornea) 371.50
    - macular 371.55
    - reticular 371.54
  - hyaline (of old scars) 371.41
  - marginal (Terrien's) 371.48
  - mosaic (shagreen) 371.41
  - nodular 371.46
  - peripheral 371.48
  - senile 371.41
- cortical (cerebellar) (parenchymatous) 334.2
  - alcoholic 303.9 ☑ [334.4]
  - diffuse, due to arteriopathy 437.0
- corticobasal 331.6
- corticostriatal-spinal 334.8
- cretinoid 243
- cruciate ligament (knee) (posterior) 717.84
  - anterior 717.83
- cutis 709.3
  - amyloid 277.39
- dental pulp 522.2
- disc disease — see Degeneration, intervertebral disc
- dorsolateral (spinal cord) — see Degeneration, combined
- endocardial 424.90
- extrapyramidal NEC 333.90
- eye NEC 360.40
  - macular (see also Degeneration, macula) 362.50
    - congenital 362.75
    - hereditary 362.76
- fatty (diffuse) (general) 272.8
  - liver 571.8
    - alcoholic 571.0
  - localized site — see Degeneration, by site, fatty
  - placenta — see Placenta, abnormal
- globe (eye) NEC 360.40
  - macular — see Degeneration, macula
- grey matter 330.8
- heart (brown) (calcareous) (fatty) (fibrous) (hyaline) (mural) (muscular) (pigmentary) (senile) (with arteriosclerosis) (see also Degeneration, myocardial) 429.1
  - amyloid 277.39 [425.7]
  - atheromatous — see Arteriosclerosis, coronary
  - gouty 274.82
  - hypertensive (see also Hypertension, heart) 402.90
  - ischemic 414.9
  - valve, valvular — see Endocarditis
- hepatolenticular (Wilson's) 275.1
- hepatorenal 572.4
- heredofamilial
  - brain NEC 331.89

Degeneration, degenerative — continued
- heredofamilial — continued
  - spinal cord NEC 336.8
- hyaline (diffuse) (generalized) 728.9
  - localized (see also Degeneration, by site)
    - cornea 371.41
      - keratitis 371.41
- hypertensive vascular — see Hypertension
- infrapatellar fat pad 729.31
- internal semilunar cartilage 717.3
- intervertebral disc 722.6
  - with myelopathy 722.70
  - cervical, cervicothoracic 722.4
    - with myelopathy 722.71
  - lumbar, lumbosacral 722.52
    - with myelopathy 722.73
  - thoracic, thoracolumbar 722.51
    - with myelopathy 722.72
- intestine 569.89
  - amyloid 277.39
  - lardaceous 277.39
- iris (generalized) (see also Atrophy, iris) 364.59
  - pigmentary 364.53
  - pupillary margin 364.54
- ischemic — see Ischemia
- joint disease (see also Osteoarthrosis) 715.9 ☑
  - multiple sites 715.09
  - spine (see also Spondylosis) 721.90
- kidney (see also Sclerosis, renal) 587
  - amyloid 277.39 [583.81]
  - cyst, cystic (multiple) (solitary) 593.2
    - congenital (see also Cystic, disease, kidney) 753.10
  - fatty 593.89
  - fibrocystic (congenital) 753.19
  - lardaceous 277.39 [583.81]
  - polycystic (congenital) 753.12
    - adult type (APKD) 753.13
    - autosomal dominant 753.13
    - autosomal recessive 753.14
    - childhood type (CPKD) 753.14
    - infantile type 753.14
  - waxy 277.39 [583.81]
- Kuhnt-Junius (retina) 362.52
- labyrinth, osseous 386.8
- lacrimal passages, cystic 375.12
- lardaceous (any site) 277.39
- lateral column (posterior), spinal cord (see also Degeneration, combined) 266.2 [336.2]
- lattice 362.63
- lens 366.9
  - infantile, juvenile, or presenile 366.00
  - senile 366.10
- lenticular (familial) (progressive) (Wilson's) (with cirrhosis of liver) 275.1
  - striate artery 437.0
- lethal ball, prosthetic heart valve 996.02
- ligament
  - collateral (knee) (medial) 717.82
    - lateral 717.81
  - cruciate (knee) (posterior) 717.84
    - anterior 717.83
- liver (diffuse) 572.8
  - amyloid 277.39
  - congenital (cystic) 751.62
  - cystic 572.8
    - congenital 751.62
  - fatty 571.8
    - alcoholic 571.0
  - hypertrophic 572.8
  - lardaceous 277.39
  - parenchymatous, acute or subacute (see also Necrosis, liver) 570
  - pigmentary 572.8
  - toxic (acute) 573.8
  - waxy 277.39
- lung 518.89
- lymph gland 289.3
  - hyaline 289.3
  - lardaceous 277.39
- macula (acquired) (senile) 362.50
  - atrophic 362.51
  - Best's 362.76

Degeneration, degenerative — continued
- macula — continued
  - congenital 362.75
  - cystic 362.54
  - cystoid 362.53
  - disciform 362.52
  - dry 362.51
  - exudative 362.52
  - familial pseudoinflammatory 362.77
  - hereditary 362.76
  - hole 362.54
  - juvenile (Stargardt's) 362.75
  - nonexudative 362.51
  - pseudohole 362.54
  - wet 362.52
- medullary — see Degeneration, brain
- membranous labyrinth, congenital (causing impairment of hearing) 744.05
- meniscus — see Derangement, joint
- microcystoid 362.62
- mitral — see Insufficiency, mitral
- Mönckeberg's (see also Arteriosclerosis, extremities) 440.20
- moral 301.7
- motor centers, senile 331.2
- mural (see also Degeneration, myocardial) 429.1
  - heart, cardiac (see also Degeneration, myocardial) 429.1
  - myocardium, myocardial (see also Degeneration, myocardial) 429.1
- muscle 728.9
  - fatty 728.9
  - fibrous 728.9
  - heart (see also Degeneration, myocardial) 429.1
  - hyaline 728.9
- muscular progressive 728.2
- myelin, central nervous system NEC 341.9
- myocardium, myocardial (brown) (calcareous) (fatty) (fibrous) (hyaline) (mural) (muscular) (pigmentary) (senile) (with arteriosclerosis) 429.1
  - with rheumatic fever (conditions classifiable to 390) 398.0
    - active, acute, or subacute 391.2
      - with chorea 392.0
    - inactive or quiescent (with chorea) 398.0
  - amyloid 277.39 [425.7]
  - congenital 746.89
  - fetus or newborn 779.89
  - gouty 274.82
  - hypertensive (see also Hypertension, heart) 402.90
  - ischemic 414.8
  - rheumatic (see also Degeneration, myocardium, with rheumatic fever) 398.0
  - syphilitic 093.82
- nasal sinus (mucosa) (see also Sinusitis) 473.9
  - frontal 473.1
  - maxillary 473.0
- nerve — see Disorder, nerve
- nervous system 349.89
  - amyloid 277.39 [357.4]
  - autonomic (see also Neuropathy, peripheral, autonomic) 337.9
  - fatty 349.89
  - peripheral autonomic NEC (see also Neuropathy, peripheral, autonomic) 337.9
- nipple 611.9
- nose 478.19
- oculoacusticocerebral, congenital (progressive) 743.8
- olivopontocerebellar (familial) (hereditary) 333.0
- osseous labyrinth 386.8
- ovary 620.8
  - cystic 620.2
  - microcystic 620.2
- pallidal, pigmentary (progressive) 333.0
- pancreas 577.8

Degeneration, degenerative — continued
- pancreas — continued
  - tuberculous (see also Tuberculosis) 017.9 ☑
- papillary muscle 429.81
- paving stone 362.61
- penis 607.89
- peritoneum 568.89
- pigmentary (diffuse) (general)
  - localized — see Degeneration, by site
  - pallidal (progressive) 333.0
  - secondary 362.65
- pineal gland 259.8
- pituitary (gland) 253.8
- placenta (fatty) (fibrinoid) (fibroid) — see Placenta, abnormal
- popliteal fat pad 729.31
- posterolateral (spinal cord) (see also Degeneration, combined) 266.2 [336.2]
- pulmonary valve (heart) (see also Endocarditis, pulmonary) 424.3
- pulp (tooth) 522.2
- pupillary margin 364.54
- renal (see also Sclerosis, renal) 587
  - fibrocystic 753.19
  - polycystic 753.12
    - adult type (APKD) 753.13
    - autosomal dominant 753.13
    - autosomal recessive 753.14
    - childhood type (CPKD) 753.14
    - infantile type 753.14
- reticuloendothelial system 289.89
- retina (peripheral) 362.60
  - with retinal defect (see also Detachment, retina, with retinal defect) 361.00
  - cystic (senile) 362.50
  - cystoid 362.53
  - hereditary (see also Dystrophy, retina) 362.70
    - cerebroretinal 362.71
    - congenital 362.75
    - juvenile (Stargardt's) 362.75
    - macula 362.76
  - Kuhnt-Junius 362.52
  - lattice 362.63
  - macular (see also Degeneration, macula) 362.50
  - microcystoid 362.62
  - palisade 362.63
  - paving stone 362.61
  - pigmentary (primary) 362.74
    - secondary 362.65
  - posterior pole (see also Degeneration, macula) 362.50
  - secondary 362.66
  - senile 362.60
    - cystic 362.53
    - reticular 362.64
- saccule, congenital (causing impairment of hearing) 744.05
- sacculocochlear 386.8
- senile 797
  - brain 331.2
  - cardiac, heart, or myocardium (see also Degeneration, myocardial) 429.1
  - motor centers 331.2
  - reticule 362.64
  - retina, cystic 362.50
  - vascular — see Arteriosclerosis
- silicone rubber poppet (prosthetic valve) 996.02
- sinus (cystic) (see also Sinusitis) 473.9
  - polypoid 471.1
- skin 709.3
  - amyloid 277.39
  - colloid 709.3
- spinal (cord) 336.8
  - amyloid 277.39
  - column 733.90
  - combined (subacute) (see also Degeneration, combined) 266.2 [336.2]
    - with anemia (pernicious) 281.0 [336.2]
  - dorsolateral (see also Degeneration, combined) 266.2 [336.2]
  - familial NEC 336.8

☑ Additional Digit Required — Refer to the Tabular List for Digit Selection   ▽ Subterms under main terms may continue to next column or page

2015 ICD-9-CM   ▶◀ Revised Text   ● New Line   ▲ Revised Code   Volume 2 — 69

Degeneration, degenerative — *continued*
spinal — *continued*
fatty 336.8
funicular (*see also* Degeneration, combined) 266.2 *[336.2]*
heredofamilial NEC 336.8
posterolateral (*see also* Degeneration, combined) 266.2 *[336.2]*
subacute combined — *see* Degeneration, combined
tuberculous (*see also* Tuberculosis) 013.8 ☑
spine 733.90
spleen 289.59
amyloid 277.39
lardaceous 277.39
stomach 537.89
lardaceous 277.39
strionigral 333.0
sudoriparous (cystic) 705.89
suprarenal (capsule) (gland) 255.8
with hypofunction 255.41
sweat gland 705.89
synovial membrane (pulpy) 727.9
tapetoretinal 362.74
adult or presenile form 362.50
testis (postinfectional) 608.89
thymus (gland) 254.8
fatty 254.8
lardaceous 277.39
thyroid (gland) 246.8
tricuspid (heart) (valve) — *see* Endocarditis, tricuspid
tuberculous NEC (*see also* Tuberculosis) 011.9 ☑
turbinate 733.90
uterus 621.8
cystic 621.8
vascular (senile) (*see also* Arteriosclerosis)
hypertensive — *see* Hypertension
vitreoretinal (primary) 362.73
secondary 362.66
vitreous humor (with infiltration) 379.21
wallerian NEC — *see* Disorder, nerve
waxy (any site) 277.39
Wilson's hepatolenticular 275.1
Deglutition
paralysis 784.99
hysterical 300.11
pneumonia 507.0
Degos' disease or syndrome 447.8
Degradation disorder, branched-chain amino acid 270.3
Dehiscence
anastomosis — *see* Complications, anastomosis
cesarean wound 674.1 ☑
closure of
cornea 998.32
fascia, superficial or muscular 998.31
internal organ 998.31
mucosa 998.32
muscle or muscle flap 998.31
ribs or rib cage 998.31
skin 998.32
skull or craniotomy 998.31
sternum or sternotomy 998.31
subcutaneous tissue 998.32
tendon or ligament 998.31
traumatic laceration (external) (internal) 998.33
episiotomy 674.2 ☑
operation wound 998.32
deep 998.31
external 998.32
internal 998.31
superficial 998.32
perineal wound (postpartum) 674.2 ☑
postoperative 998.32
abdomen 998.32
internal 998.31
internal 998.31
traumatic injury wound repair 998.33
uterine wound 674.1 ☑
Dehydration (cachexia) 276.51

Dehydration — *continued*
with
hypernatremia 276.0
hyponatremia 276.1
newborn 775.5
Deiters' nucleus syndrome 386.19
Déjérine's disease 356.0
Déjérine-Klumpke paralysis 767.6
Déjérine-Roussy syndrome 338.0
Déjérine-Sottas disease or neuropathy (hypertrophic) 356.0
Déjérine-Thomas atrophy or syndrome 333.0
de Lange's syndrome (Amsterdam dwarf, intellectual disabilities, and brachycephaly) 759.89
Delay, delayed
adaptation, cones or rods 368.63
any plane in pelvis
affecting fetus or newborn 763.1
complicating delivery 660.1 ☑
birth or delivery NEC 662.1 ☑
affecting fetus or newborn 763.89
second twin, triplet, or multiple mate 662.3 ☑
closure (*see also* Fistula)
cranial suture 756.0
fontanel 756.0
coagulation NEC 790.92
conduction (cardiac) (ventricular) 426.9
delivery NEC 662.1 ☑
second twin, triplet, etc. 662.3 ☑
affecting fetus or newborn 763.89
development
in childhood 783.40
physiological 783.40
intellectual NEC 315.9
learning NEC 315.2
reading 315.00
sexual 259.0
speech 315.39
and language due to hearing loss 315.34
associated with hyperkinesis 314.1
spelling 315.09
gastric emptying 536.8
menarche 256.39
due to pituitary hypofunction 253.4
menstruation (cause unknown) 626.8
milestone in childhood 783.42
motility — *see* Hypomotility
passage of meconium (newborn) 777.1
primary respiration 768.9
puberty 259.0
separation of umbilical cord 779.83
sexual maturation, female 259.0
vaccination V64.00
Del Castillo's syndrome (germinal aplasia) 606.0
Déleage's disease 359.89
Deletion syndrome
5p 758.31
22q11.2 758.32
autosomal NEC 758.39
constitutional 5q deletion 758.39
Delhi (boil) (button) (sore) 085.1
Delinquency (juvenile) 312.9
group (*see also* Disturbance, conduct) 312.2 ☑
neurotic 312.4
Delirium, delirious 780.09
acute 780.09
due to conditions classified elsewhere 293.0
alcoholic 291.0
acute 291.0
chronic 291.1
alcoholicum 291.0
chronic (*see also* Psychosis) 293.89
due to or associated with physical condition — *see* Psychosis, organic
drug-induced 292.81
due to conditions classified elsewhere 293.0
eclamptic (*see also* Eclampsia) 780.39
exhaustion (*see also* Reaction, stress, acute) 308.9
hysterical 300.11

Delirium, delirious — *continued*
in
presenile dementia 290.11
senile dementia 290.3
induced by drug 292.81
manic, maniacal (acute) (*see also* Psychosis, affective) 296.0 ☑
recurrent episode 296.1 ☑
single episode 296.0 ☑
puerperal 293.9
senile 290.3
subacute (psychotic) 293.1
thyroid (*see also* Thyrotoxicosis) 242.9 ☑
traumatic (*see also* Injury, intracranial)
with
lesion, spinal cord — *see* Injury, spinal, by site
shock, spinal — *see* Injury, spinal, by site
tremens (impending) 291.0
uremic — *see* Uremia
withdrawal
alcoholic (acute) 291.0
chronic 291.1
drug 292.0

Delivery

Note — Use the following fifth-digit subclassification with categories 640–649, 651–676:

0   unspecified as to episode of care

1   delivered, with or without mention of antepartum condition

2   delivered, with mention of postpartum complication

3   antepartum condition or complication

4   postpartum condition or complication

breech (assisted) (buttocks) (complete) (frank) (spontaneous) 652.2 ☑
affecting fetus or newborn 763.0
extraction NEC 669.6 ☑
cesarean (for) 669.7 ☑
abnormal
cervix 654.6 ☑
pelvic organs or tissues 654.9 ☑
pelvis (bony) (major) NEC 653.0 ☑
presentation or position 652.9 ☑
in multiple gestation 652.6 ☑
size, fetus 653.5 ☑
soft parts (of pelvis) 654.9 ☑
uterus, congenital 654.0 ☑
vagina 654.7 ☑
vulva 654.8 ☑
abruptio placentae 641.2 ☑
acromion presentation 652.8 ☑
affecting fetus or newborn 763.4
anteversion, cervix or uterus 654.4 ☑
atony, uterus 661.2 ☑
with hemorrhage 666.1 ☑
bicornis or bicornuate uterus 654.0 ☑
breech presentation (buttocks) (complete) (frank) 652.2 ☑
brow presentation 652.4 ☑
cephalopelvic disproportion (normally formed fetus) 653.4 ☑
chin presentation 652.4 ☑
cicatrix of cervix 654.6 ☑
contracted pelvis (general) 653.1 ☑
inlet 653.2 ☑
outlet 653.3 ☑
cord presentation or prolapse 663.0 ☑
cystocele 654.4 ☑
deformity (acquired) (congenital)
pelvic organs or tissues NEC 654.9 ☑
pelvis (bony) NEC 653.0 ☑
displacement, uterus NEC 654.4 ☑
disproportion NEC 653.9 ☑
distress
fetal 656.8 ☑
maternal 669.0 ☑
eclampsia 642.6 ☑

Delivery — *continued*
cesarean — *continued*
face presentation 652.4 ☑
failed
forceps 660.7 ☑
trial of labor NEC 660.6 ☑
vacuum extraction 660.7 ☑
ventouse 660.7 ☑
fetal deformity 653.7 ☑
fetal-maternal hemorrhage 656.0 ☑
fetus, fetal
distress 656.8 ☑
prematurity 656.8 ☑
fibroid (tumor) (uterus) 654.1 ☑
footling 652.8 ☑
with successful version 652.1 ☑
hemorrhage (antepartum) (intrapartum) NEC 641.9 ☑
hydrocephalic fetus 653.6 ☑
incarceration of uterus 654.3 ☑
incoordinate uterine action 661.4 ☑
inertia, uterus 661.2 ☑
primary 661.0 ☑
secondary 661.1 ☑
lateroversion, uterus or cervix 654.4 ☑
mal lie 652.9 ☑
malposition
fetus 652.9 ☑
in multiple gestation 652.6 ☑
pelvic organs or tissues NEC 654.9 ☑
uterus NEC or cervix 654.4 ☑
malpresentation NEC 652.9 ☑
in multiple gestation 652.6 ☑
maternal
diabetes mellitus (conditions classifiable to 249 and 250) 648.0 ☑
heart disease NEC 648.6 ☑
meconium in liquor 656.8 ☑
staining only 792.3
oblique presentation 652.3 ☑
oversize fetus 653.5 ☑
pelvic tumor NEC 654.9 ☑
placental insufficiency 656.5 ☑
placenta previa 641.0 ☑
with hemorrhage 641.1 ☑
(planned) occurring after 37 completed weeks of gestation but before 39 completed weeks gestation due to (spontaneous) onset of labor 649.8 ☑
poor dilation, cervix 661.0 ☑
pre-eclampsia 642.4 ☑
severe 642.5 ☑
previous
cesarean delivery, section 654.2 ☑
surgery (to)
cervix 654.6 ☑
gynecological NEC 654.9 ☑
rectum 654.8 ☑
uterus NEC 654.9 ☑
previous cesarean delivery, section 654.2 ☑
vagina 654.7 ☑
prolapse
arm or hand 652.7 ☑
uterus 654.4 ☑
prolonged labor 662.1 ☑
rectocele 654.4 ☑
retroversion, uterus or cervix 654.3 ☑
rigid
cervix 654.6 ☑
pelvic floor 654.4 ☑
perineum 654.8 ☑
vagina 654.7 ☑
vulva 654.8 ☑
sacculation, pregnant uterus 654.4 ☑
scar(s)
cervix 654.6 ☑
cesarean delivery, section 654.2 ☑
uterus NEC 654.9 ☑
due to previous cesarean delivery, section 654.2 ☑
Shirodkar suture in situ 654.5 ☑
shoulder presentation 652.8 ☑

Delivery — *continued*
  cesarean — *continued*
    stenosis or stricture, cervix 654.6 ☑
    transverse presentation or lie 652.3 ☑
    tumor, pelvic organs or tissues NEC 654.4 ☑
    umbilical cord presentation or prolapse 663.0 ☑
  completely normal case — *see* category 650
  complicated (by) NEC 669.9 ☑
    abdominal tumor, fetal 653.7 ☑
      causing obstructed labor 660.1 ☑
    abnormal, abnormality of
      cervix 654.6 ☑
        causing obstructed labor 660.2 ☑
      forces of labor 661.9 ☑
      formation of uterus 654.0 ☑
      pelvic organs or tissues 654.9 ☑
        causing obstructed labor 660.2 ☑
      pelvis (bony) (major) NEC 653.0 ☑
        causing obstructed labor 660.1 ☑
      presentation or position NEC 652.9 ☑
        causing obstructed labor 660.0 ☑
      size, fetus 653.5 ☑
        causing obstructed labor 660.1 ☑
      soft parts (of pelvis) 654.9 ☑
        causing obstructed labor 660.2 ☑
      uterine contractions NEC 661.9 ☑
      uterus (formation) 654.0 ☑
        causing obstructed labor 660.2 ☑
      vagina 654.7 ☑
        causing obstructed labor 660.2 ☑
    abnormally formed uterus (any type) (congenital) 654.0 ☑
      causing obstructed labor 660.2 ☑
    acromion presentation 652.8 ☑
      causing obstructed labor 660.0 ☑
    adherent placenta 667.0 ☑
      with hemorrhage 666.0 ☑
    adhesions, uterus (to abdominal wall) 654.4 ☑
    advanced maternal age NEC 659.6 ☑
      multigravida 659.6 ☑
      primigravida 659.5 ☑
    air embolism 673.0 ☑
    amnionitis 658.4 ☑
    amniotic fluid embolism 673.1 ☑
    anesthetic death 668.9 ☑
    annular detachment, cervix 665.3 ☑
    antepartum hemorrhage — *see* Delivery, complicated, hemorrhage
    anteversion, cervix or uterus 654.4 ☑
      causing obstructed labor 660.2 ☑
    apoplexy 674.0 ☑
      placenta 641.2 ☑
    arrested active phase 661.1 ☑
    asymmetrical pelvis bone 653.0 ☑
      causing obstructed labor 660.1 ☑
    atony, uterus with hemorrhage (hypotonic) (inertia) 666.1 ☑
      hypertonic 661.4 ☑
    Bandl's ring 661.4 ☑
    battledore placenta — *see* Placenta, abnormal
    bicornis or bicornuate uterus 654.0 ☑
      causing obstructed labor 660.2 ☑
    birth injury to mother NEC 665.9 ☑
    bleeding (*see also* Delivery, complicated, hemorrhage) 641.9 ☑
    breech presentation (assisted) (buttocks) (complete) (frank) (spontaneous) 652.2 ☑
      with successful version 652.1 ☑
    brow presentation 652.4 ☑

Delivery — *continued*
  complicated — *continued*
    cephalopelvic disproportion (normally formed fetus) 653.4 ☑
      causing obstructed labor 660.1 ☑
    cerebral hemorrhage 674.0 ☑
    cervical dystocia 661.2 ☑
    chin presentation 652.4 ☑
      causing obstructed labor 660.0 ☑
    cicatrix
      cervix 654.6 ☑
        causing obstructed labor 660.2 ☑
      vagina 654.7 ☑
        causing obstructed labor 660.2 ☑
    coagulation defect 649.3 ☑
    colporrhexis 665.4 ☑
      with perineal laceration 664.0 ☑
    compound presentation 652.8 ☑
      causing obstructed labor 660.0 ☑
    compression of cord (umbilical) 663.2 ☑
      around neck 663.1 ☑
      cord prolapsed 663.0 ☑
    contraction, contracted pelvis 653.1 ☑
      causing obstructed labor 660.1 ☑
      general 653.1 ☑
        causing obstructed labor 660.1 ☑
      inlet 653.2 ☑
        causing obstructed labor 660.1 ☑
      midpelvic 653.8 ☑
        causing obstructed labor 660.1 ☑
      midplane 653.8 ☑
        causing obstructed labor 660.1 ☑
      outlet 653.3 ☑
        causing obstructed labor 660.1 ☑
    contraction ring 661.4 ☑
    cord (umbilical) 663.9 ☑
      around neck, tightly or with compression 663.1 ☑
        without compression 663.3 ☑
      bruising 663.6 ☑
      complication NEC 663.9 ☑
        specified type NEC 663.8 ☑
      compression NEC 663.2 ☑
      entanglement NEC 663.3 ☑
        with compression 663.2 ☑
      forelying 663.0 ☑
      hematoma 663.6 ☑
      marginal attachment 663.8 ☑
      presentation 663.0 ☑
      prolapse (complete) (occult) (partial) 663.0 ☑
      short 663.4 ☑
      specified complication NEC 663.8 ☑
      thrombosis (vessels) 663.6 ☑
      vascular lesion 663.6 ☑
      velamentous insertion 663.8 ☑
    Couvelaire uterus 641.2 ☑
    cretin pelvis (dwarf type) (male type) 653.1 ☑
      causing obstructed labor 660.1 ☑
    crossbirth 652.3 ☑
      with successful version 652.1 ☑
      causing obstructed labor 660.0 ☑
    cyst (Gartner's duct) 654.7 ☑
    cystocele 654.4 ☑
      causing obstructed labor 660.2 ☑
    death of fetus (near term) 656.4 ☑
      early (before 22 completed weeks gestation) 632
    deformity (acquired) (congenital)
      fetus 653.7 ☑
        causing obstructed labor 660.1 ☑
      pelvic organs or tissues NEC 654.9 ☑
        causing obstructed labor 660.2 ☑
      pelvis (bony) NEC 653.0 ☑

Delivery — *continued*
  complicated — *continued*
    deformity — *continued*
      pelvis — *continued*
        causing obstructed labor 660.1 ☑
    delay, delayed
      delivery in multiple pregnancy 662.3 ☑
      due to locked mates 660.5 ☑
      following rupture of membranes (spontaneous) 658.2 ☑
        artificial 658.3 ☑
    depressed fetal heart tones 659.7 ☑
    diastasis recti 665.8 ☑
    dilatation
      bladder 654.4 ☑
        causing obstructed labor 660.2 ☑
      cervix, incomplete, poor or slow 661.0 ☑
    diseased placenta 656.7 ☑
    displacement uterus NEC 654.4 ☑
      causing obstructed labor 660.2 ☑
    disproportion NEC 653.9 ☑
      causing obstructed labor 660.1 ☑
    disruptio uteri — *see* Delivery, complicated, rupture, uterus
    distress
      fetal 656.8 ☑
      maternal 669.0 ☑
    double uterus (congenital) 654.0 ☑
      causing obstructed labor 660.2 ☑
    dropsy amnion 657.0 ☑
    dysfunction, uterus 661.9 ☑
      hypertonic 661.4 ☑
      hypotonic 661.2 ☑
        primary 661.0 ☑
        secondary 661.1 ☑
      incoordinate 661.4 ☑
    dystocia
      cervical 661.2 ☑
      fetal — *see* Delivery, complicated, abnormal, presentation
      maternal — *see* Delivery, complicated, prolonged labor
      pelvic — *see* Delivery, complicated, contraction pelvis
      positional 652.8 ☑
      shoulder girdle 660.4 ☑
    eclampsia 642.6 ☑
    ectopic kidney 654.4 ☑
      causing obstructed labor 660.2 ☑
    edema, cervix 654.6 ☑
      causing obstructed labor 660.2 ☑
    effusion, amniotic fluid 658.1 ☑
    elderly multigravida 659.6 ☑
    elderly primigravida 659.5 ☑
    embolism (pulmonary) 673.2 ☑
      air 673.0 ☑
      amniotic fluid 673.1 ☑
      blood clot 673.2 ☑
      cerebral 674.0 ☑
      fat 673.8 ☑
      pyemic 673.3 ☑
      septic 673.3 ☑
    entanglement, umbilical cord 663.3 ☑
      with compression 663.2 ☑
      around neck (with compression) 663.1 ☑
    eversion, cervix or uterus 665.2 ☑
    excessive
      fetal growth 653.5 ☑
        causing obstructed labor 660.1 ☑
      size of fetus 653.5 ☑
        causing obstructed labor 660.1 ☑
    face presentation 652.4 ☑
      causing obstructed labor 660.0 ☑
      to pubes 660.3 ☑
    failure, fetal head to enter pelvic brim 652.5 ☑
      causing obstructed labor 660.0 ☑

Delivery — *continued*
  complicated — *continued*
    female genital mutilation 660.8 ☑
    fetal
      acid-base balance 656.8 ☑
      death (near term) NEC 656.4 ☑
        early (before 22 completed weeks gestation) 632
      deformity 653.7 ☑
        causing obstructed labor 660.1 ☑
      distress 656.8 ☑
      heart rate or rhythm 659.7 ☑
      reduction of multiple fetuses reduced to single fetus 651.7 ☑
    fetopelvic disproportion 653.4 ☑
      causing obstructed labor 660.1 ☑
    fever during labor 659.2 ☑
    fibroid (tumor) (uterus) 654.1 ☑
      causing obstructed labor 660.2 ☑
    fibromyomata 654.1 ☑
      causing obstructed labor 660.2 ☑
    forelying umbilical cord 663.0 ☑
    fracture of coccyx 665.6 ☑
    hematoma 664.5 ☑
      broad ligament 665.7 ☑
      ischial spine 665.7 ☑
      pelvic 665.7 ☑
      perineum 664.5 ☑
      soft tissues 665.7 ☑
      subdural 674.0 ☑
      umbilical cord 663.6 ☑
      vagina 665.7 ☑
      vulva or perineum 664.5 ☑
    hemorrhage (uterine) (antepartum) (intrapartum) (pregnancy) 641.9 ☑
      accidental 641.2 ☑
      associated with
        afibrinogenemia 641.3 ☑
        coagulation defect 641.3 ☑
          hyperfibrinolysis 641.3 ☑
          hypofibrinogenemia 641.3 ☑
      cerebral 674.0 ☑
      due to
        low-lying placenta 641.1 ☑
        placenta previa 641.1 ☑
        premature separation of placenta (normally implanted) 641.2 ☑
        retained placenta 666.0 ☑
        trauma 641.8 ☑
        uterine leiomyoma 641.8 ☑
      marginal sinus rupture 641.2 ☑
      placenta NEC 641.9 ☑
      postpartum (atonic) (immediate) (within 24 hours) 666.1 ☑
        with retained or trapped placenta 666.0 ☑
        delayed 666.2 ☑
        secondary 666.2 ☑
        third stage 666.0 ☑
    hourglass contraction, uterus 661.4 ☑
    hydramnios 657.0 ☑
    hydrocephalic fetus 653.6 ☑
      causing obstructed labor 660.1 ☑
    hydrops fetalis 653.7 ☑
      causing obstructed labor 660.1 ☑
    hypertension — *see* Hypertension, complicating pregnancy
    hypertonic uterine dysfunction 661.4 ☑
    hypotonic uterine dysfunction 661.2 ☑
    impacted shoulders 660.4 ☑
    incarceration, uterus 654.3 ☑
      causing obstructed labor 660.2 ☑
    incomplete dilation (cervix) 661.0 ☑
    incoordinate uterus 661.4 ☑
    indication NEC 659.9 ☑
      specified type NEC 659.8 ☑
    inertia, uterus 661.2 ☑
      hypertonic 661.4 ☑
      hypotonic 661.2 ☑
        primary 661.0 ☑
        secondary 661.1 ☑

☑ Additional Digit Required — Refer to the Tabular List for Digit Selection

Ⓦ Subterms under main terms may continue to next column or page

Delivery — *continued*
  complicated — *continued*
    infantile
      genitalia 654.4 ☑
        causing obstructed labor
          660.2 ☑
      uterus (os) 654.4 ☑
        causing obstructed labor
          660.2 ☑
    injury (to mother) NEC 665.9 ☑
    intrauterine fetal death (near term) NEC
      656.4 ☑
      early (before 22 completed weeks
        gestation) 632
    inversion, uterus 665.2 ☑
    kidney, ectopic 654.4 ☑
      causing obstructed labor 660.2 ☑
    knot (true), umbilical cord 663.2 ☑
    labor
      onset (spontaneous) after 37 complet-
        ed weeks of gestation but be-
        fore 39 completed weeks
        gestation with delivery by
        (planned) cesarean section
        649.8 ☑
      premature (before 37 completed
        weeks gestation) 644.2 ☑
    laceration 664.9 ☑
      anus (sphincter) (healed) (old)
        654.8 ☑
        with mucosa 664.3 ☑
        not associated with third-degree
          perineal laceration
          664.6 ☑
      bladder (urinary) 665.5 ☑
      bowel 665.5 ☑
      central 664.4 ☑
      cervix (uteri) 665.3 ☑
      fourchette 664.0 ☑
      hymen 664.0 ☑
      labia (majora) (minora) 664.0 ☑
      pelvic
        floor 664.1 ☑
        organ NEC 665.5 ☑
      perineum, perineal 664.4 ☑
        first degree 664.0 ☑
        second degree 664.1 ☑
        third degree 664.2 ☑
        fourth degree 664.3 ☑
        central 664.4 ☑
        extensive NEC 664.4 ☑
        muscles 664.1 ☑
        skin 664.0 ☑
        slight 664.0 ☑
      peritoneum (pelvic) 665.5 ☑
      periurethral tissue 664.8 ☑
      rectovaginal (septum) (without per-
        ineal laceration) 665.4 ☑
        with perineum 664.2 ☑
          with anal or rectal mucosa
          664.3 ☑
      skin (perineum) 664.0 ☑
      specified site or type NEC 664.8 ☑
      sphincter ani (healed) (old) 654.8 ☑
        with mucosa 664.3 ☑
        not associated with third-degree
          perineal laceration
          664.6 ☑
      urethra 665.5 ☑
      uterus 665.1 ☑
        before labor 665.0 ☑
      vagina, vaginal (deep) (high) (sulcus)
        (wall) (without perineal lacer-
        ation) 665.4 ☑
        with perineum 664.0 ☑
        muscles, with perineum 664.1 ☑
      vulva 664.0 ☑
    lateroversion, uterus or cervix 654.4 ☑
      causing obstructed labor 660.2 ☑
    locked mates 660.5 ☑
    low implantation of placenta — *see* De-
      livery, complicated, placenta,
      previa
    mal lie 652.9 ☑

Delivery — *continued*
  complicated — *continued*
    malposition
      fetus NEC 652.9 ☑
        causing obstructed labor
          660.0 ☑
      pelvic organs or tissues NEC 654.9 ☑
        causing obstructed labor
          660.2 ☑
      placenta 641.1 ☑
        without hemorrhage 641.0 ☑
      uterus NEC or cervix 654.4 ☑
        causing obstructed labor
          660.2 ☑
    malpresentation 652.9 ☑
      causing obstructed labor 660.0 ☑
    marginal sinus (bleeding) (rupture)
      641.2 ☑
    maternal hypotension syndrome
      669.2 ☑
    meconium in liquor 656.8 ☑
    membranes, retained — *see* Delivery,
      complicated, placenta, retained
    mentum presentation 652.4 ☑
      causing obstructed labor 660.0 ☑
    metrorrhagia (myopathia) — *see* Deliv-
      ery, complicated, hemorrhage
    metrorrhexis — *see* Delivery, complicat-
      ed, rupture, uterus
    multiparity (grand) 659.4 ☑
    myelomeningocele, fetus 653.7 ☑
      causing obstructed labor 660.1 ☑
    Nägele's pelvis 653.0 ☑
      causing obstructed labor 660.1 ☑
    nonengagement, fetal head 652.5 ☑
      causing obstructed labor 660.0 ☑
    oblique presentation 652.3 ☑
      causing obstructed labor 660.0 ☑
    obstetric
      shock 669.1 ☑
      trauma NEC 665.9 ☑
    obstructed labor 660.9 ☑
      due to
        abnormality of pelvic organs or
          tissues (conditions classifi-
          able to 654.0–654.9)
          660.2 ☑
        deep transverse arrest 660.3 ☑
        impacted shoulders 660.4 ☑
        locked twins 660.5 ☑
        malposition and malpresentation
          of fetus (conditions classi-
          fiable to 652.0–652.9)
          660.0 ☑
        persistent occipitoposterior
          660.3 ☑
        shoulder dystocia 660.4 ☑
    occult prolapse of umbilical cord
      663.0 ☑
    oversize fetus 653.5 ☑
      causing obstructed labor 660.1 ☑
    pathological retraction ring, uterus
      661.4 ☑
    pelvic
      arrest (deep) (high) (of fetal head)
        (transverse) 660.3 ☑
      deformity (bone) (*see also* Deformity,
        pelvis, with disproportion)
      soft tissue 654.9 ☑
        causing obstructed labor
          660.2 ☑
      tumor NEC 654.9 ☑
        causing obstructed labor
          660.2 ☑
    penetration, pregnant uterus by instru-
      ment 665.1 ☑
    perforation — *see* Delivery, complicated,
      laceration
    persistent
      hymen 654.8 ☑
        causing obstructed labor
          660.2 ☑
      occipitoposterior 660.3 ☑

Delivery — *continued*
  complicated — *continued*
    placenta, placental
      ablatio 641.2 ☑
      abnormality 656.7 ☑
        with hemorrhage 641.2 ☑
      abruptio 641.2 ☑
      accreta 667.0 ☑
        with hemorrhage 666.0 ☑
      adherent (without hemorrhage)
        667.0 ☑
        with hemorrhage 666.0 ☑
      apoplexy 641.2 ☑
      battledore placenta — *see* Placenta,
        abnormal
      detachment (premature) 641.2 ☑
      disease 656.7 ☑
      hemorrhage NEC 641.9 ☑
      increta (without hemorrhage)
        667.0 ☑
        with hemorrhage 666.0 ☑
      low (implantation) 641.1 ☑
        without hemorrhage 641.0 ☑
      malformation 656.7 ☑
        with hemorrhage 641.2 ☑
      malposition 641.1 ☑
        without hemorrhage 641.0 ☑
      marginal sinus rupture 641.2 ☑
      percreta 667.0 ☑
        with hemorrhage 666.0 ☑
      premature separation 641.2 ☑
      previa (central) (lateral) (marginal)
        (partial) 641.1 ☑
        without hemorrhage 641.0 ☑
      retained (with hemorrhage) 666.0 ☑
        without hemorrhage 667.0 ☑
      rupture of marginal sinus 641.2 ☑
      separation (premature) 641.2 ☑
      trapped 666.0 ☑
        without hemorrhage 667.0 ☑
      vicious insertion 641.1 ☑
    polyhydramnios 657.0 ☑
    polyp, cervix 654.6 ☑
      causing obstructed labor 660.2 ☑
    precipitate labor 661.3 ☑
    premature
      labor (before 37 completed weeks
        gestation) 644.2 ☑
      rupture, membranes 658.1 ☑
        delayed delivery following
          658.2 ☑
    presenting umbilical cord 663.0 ☑
    previous
      cesarean delivery, section 654.2 ☑
      surgery
        cervix 654.6 ☑
          causing obstructed labor
            660.2 ☑
        gynecological NEC 654.9 ☑
          causing obstructed labor
            660.2 ☑
        perineum 654.8 ☑
        rectum 654.8 ☑
        uterus NEC 654.9 ☑
          due to previous cesarean de-
            livery, section 654.2 ☑
        vagina 654.7 ☑
          causing obstructed labor
            660.2 ☑
        vulva 654.8 ☑
    primary uterine inertia 661.0 ☑
    primipara, elderly or old 659.5 ☑
    prolapse
      arm or hand 652.7 ☑
        causing obstructed labor
          660.0 ☑
      cord (umbilical) 663.0 ☑
      fetal extremity 652.8 ☑
      foot or leg 652.8 ☑
        causing obstructed labor
          660.0 ☑
      umbilical cord (complete) (occult)
        (partial) 663.0 ☑
      uterus 654.4 ☑

Delivery — *continued*
  complicated — *continued*
    prolapse — *continued*
      uterus — *continued*
        causing obstructed labor
          660.2 ☑
    prolonged labor 662.1 ☑
      first stage 662.0 ☑
      second stage 662.2 ☑
      active phase 661.2 ☑
      due to
        cervical dystocia 661.2 ☑
        contraction ring 661.4 ☑
        tetanic uterus 661.4 ☑
        uterine inertia 661.2 ☑
          primary 661.0 ☑
          secondary 661.1 ☑
      latent phase 661.0 ☑
    pyrexia during labor 659.2 ☑
    rachitic pelvis 653.2 ☑
      causing obstructed labor 660.1 ☑
    rectocele 654.4 ☑
      causing obstructed labor 660.2 ☑
    retained membranes or portions of pla-
      centa 666.2 ☑
      without hemorrhage 667.1 ☑
    retarded (prolonged) birth 662.1 ☑
    retention secundines (with hemorrhage)
      666.2 ☑
      without hemorrhage 667.1 ☑
    retroversion, uterus or cervix 654.3 ☑
      causing obstructed labor 660.2 ☑
    rigid
      cervix 654.6 ☑
        causing obstructed labor
          660.2 ☑
      pelvic floor 654.4 ☑
        causing obstructed labor
          660.2 ☑
      perineum or vulva 654.8 ☑
        causing obstructed labor
          660.2 ☑
      vagina 654.7 ☑
        causing obstructed labor
          660.2 ☑
    Robert's pelvis 653.0 ☑
      causing obstructed labor 660.1 ☑
    rupture (*see also* Delivery, complicated,
      laceration)
      bladder (urinary) 665.5 ☑
      cervix 665.3 ☑
      marginal sinus 641.2 ☑
      membranes, premature 658.1 ☑
      pelvic organ NEC 665.5 ☑
      perineum (without mention of other
        laceration) — *see* Delivery,
        complicated, laceration, per-
        ineum
      peritoneum (pelvic) 665.5 ☑
      urethra 665.5 ☑
      uterus (during labor) 665.1 ☑
        before labor 665.0 ☑
    sacculation, pregnant uterus 654.4 ☑
    sacral teratomas, fetal 653.7 ☑
      causing obstructed labor 660.1 ☑
    scar(s)
      cervix 654.6 ☑
        causing obstructed labor
          660.2 ☑
      cesarean delivery, section 654.2 ☑
        causing obstructed labor
          660.2 ☑
      perineum 654.8 ☑
        causing obstructed labor
          660.2 ☑
      uterus NEC 654.9 ☑
        causing obstructed labor
          660.2 ☑
        due to previous cesarean delivery,
          section 654.2 ☑
      vagina 654.7 ☑
        causing obstructed labor
          660.2 ☑
      vulva 654.8 ☑

☑ **Additional Digit Required** — Refer to the Tabular List for Digit Selection   ▽ **Subterms under main terms may continue to next column or page**

72 — Volume 2   ►◄ Revised Text   ● New Line   ▲ Revised Code   **2015 ICD-9-CM**

Delivery — *continued*
  complicated — *continued*
    scar(s) — *continued*
      vulva — *continued*
        causing obstructed labor 660.2 ☑
    scoliotic pelvis 653.0 ☑
      causing obstructed labor 660.1 ☑
    secondary uterine inertia 661.1 ☑
    secundines, retained — *see* Delivery, complicated, placenta, retained
    separation
      placenta (premature) 641.2 ☑
      pubic bone 665.6 ☑
      symphysis pubis 665.6 ☑
    septate vagina 654.7 ☑
      causing obstructed labor 660.2 ☑
    shock (birth) (obstetric) (puerperal) 669.1 ☑
    short cord syndrome 663.4 ☑
    shoulder
      girdle dystocia 660.4 ☑
      presentation 652.8 ☑
        causing obstructed labor 660.0 ☑
    Siamese twins 678.1 ☑
    slow slope active phase 661.2 ☑
    spasm
      cervix 661.4 ☑
      uterus 661.4 ☑
    spondylolisthesis, pelvis 653.3 ☑
      causing obstructed labor 660.1 ☑
    spondylolysis (lumbosacral) 653.3 ☑
      causing obstructed labor 660.1 ☑
    spondylosis 653.0 ☑
      causing obstructed labor 660.1 ☑
    stenosis or stricture
      cervix 654.6 ☑
        causing obstructed labor 660.2 ☑
      vagina 654.7 ☑
        causing obstructed labor 660.2 ☑
    sudden death, unknown cause 669.9 ☑
    tear (pelvic organ) (*see also* Delivery, complicated, laceration) 664.9 ☑
      anal sphincter (healed) (old) 654.8 ☑
        not associated with third-degree perineal laceration 664.6 ☑
    teratomas, sacral, fetal 653.7 ☑
      causing obstructed labor 660.1 ☑
    tetanic uterus 661.4 ☑
    tipping pelvis 653.0 ☑
      causing obstructed labor 660.1 ☑
    transverse
      arrest (deep) 660.3 ☑
      presentation or lie 652.3 ☑
        with successful version 652.1 ☑
        causing obstructed labor 660.0 ☑
    trauma (obstetrical) NEC 665.9 ☑
      periurethral 664.8 ☑
    tumor
      abdominal, fetal 653.7 ☑
        causing obstructed labor 660.1 ☑
      pelvic organs or tissues NEC 654.9 ☑
        causing obstructed labor 660.2 ☑
    umbilical cord (*see also* Delivery, complicated, cord) 663.9 ☑
      around neck tightly, or with compression 663.1 ☑
      entanglement NEC 663.3 ☑
        with compression 663.2 ☑
      prolapse (complete) (occult) (partial) 663.0 ☑
    unstable lie 652.0 ☑
      causing obstructed labor 660.0 ☑
    uterine
      inertia (*see also* Delivery, complicated, inertia, uterus) 661.2 ☑
      spasm 661.4 ☑

Delivery — *continued*
  complicated — *continued*
    vasa previa 663.5 ☑
    velamentous insertion of cord 663.8 ☑
    young maternal age 659.8 ☑
  delayed NEC 662.1 ☑
    following rupture of membranes (spontaneous) 658.2 ☑
      artificial 658.3 ☑
    second twin, triplet, etc. 662.3 ☑
  difficult NEC 669.9 ☑
    previous, affecting management of pregnancy or childbirth V23.49
    specified type NEC 669.8 ☑
  early onset (spontaneous) 644.2 ☑
  footling 652.8 ☑
    with successful version 652.1 ☑
  forceps NEC 669.5 ☑
    affecting fetus or newborn 763.2
  missed (at or near term) 656.4 ☑
  multiple gestation NEC 651.9 ☑
    with fetal loss and retention of one or more fetus(es) 651.6 ☑
    following (elective) fetal reduction 651.7 ☑
    specified type NEC 651.8 ☑
      with fetal loss and retention of one or more fetus(es) 651.6 ☑
      following (elective) fetal reduction 651.7 ☑
  nonviable infant 656.4 ☑
  normal — *see* category 650
  precipitate 661.3 ☑
    affecting fetus or newborn 763.6
  premature NEC (before 37 completed weeks gestation) 644.2 ☑
    previous, affecting management of pregnancy V23.41
  quadruplet NEC 651.2 ☑
    with fetal loss and retention of one or more fetus(es) 651.5 ☑
    following (elective) fetal reduction 651.7 ☑
  quintuplet NEC 651.8 ☑
    with fetal loss and retention of one or more fetus(es) 651.6 ☑
    following (elective) fetal reduction 651.7 ☑
  sextuplet NEC 651.8 ☑
    with fetal loss and retention of one or more fetus(es) 651.6 ☑
    following (elective) fetal reduction 651.7 ☑
  specified complication NEC 669.8 ☑
  stillbirth (near term) NEC 656.4 ☑
    early (before 22 completed weeks gestation) 632
  term pregnancy (live birth) NEC — *see* category 650
  stillbirth NEC 656.4 ☑
  threatened premature 644.2 ☑
  triplets NEC 651.1 ☑
    with fetal loss and retention of one or more fetus(es) 651.4 ☑
    delayed delivery (one or more mates) 662.3 ☑
    following (elective) fetal reduction 651.7 ☑
    locked mates 660.5 ☑
  twins NEC 651.0 ☑
    with fetal loss and retention of one fetus 651.3 ☑
    delayed delivery (one or more mates) 662.3 ☑
    following (elective) fetal reduction 651.7 ☑
    locked mates 660.5 ☑
  uncomplicated — *see* category 650
  vacuum extractor NEC 669.5 ☑
    affecting fetus or newborn 763.3
  ventouse NEC 669.5 ☑
    affecting fetus or newborn 763.3
Dellen, cornea 371.41
Delusions (paranoid) 297.9

Delusions — *continued*
  grandiose 297.1
  parasitosis 300.29
  systematized 297.1
Dementia 294.20
  with behavioral disturbance (aggressive) (combative) (violent) 294.21
  alcohol-induced persisting (*see also* Psychosis, alcoholic) 291.2
  Alzheimer's — *see* Alzheimer's, dementia
  arteriosclerotic (simple type) (uncomplicated) 290.40
    with
      acute confusional state 290.41
      delirium 290.41
      delusions 290.42
      depressed mood 290.43
    depressed type 290.43
    paranoid type 290.42
  Binswanger's 290.12
  catatonic (acute) (*see also* Schizophrenia) 295.2
  congenital (*see also* Disability, intellectual) 319
  degenerative 290.9
    presenile-onset — *see* Dementia, presenile
    senile-onset — *see* Dementia, senile
  developmental (*see also* Schizophrenia) 295.9 ☑
  dialysis 294.8
    transient 293.9
  drug-induced persisting (*see also* Psychosis, drug) 292.82
  due to or associated with condition(s) classified elsewhere
    Alzheimer's
      with behavioral disturbance 331.0 [294.11]
      without behavioral disturbance 331.0 [294.10]
    cerebral lipidoses
      with behavioral disturbance 330.1 [294.11]
      without behavioral disturbance 330.1 [294.10]
    epilepsy
      with behavioral disturbance 345.9 ☑ [294.11]
      without behavioral disturbance 345.9 ☑ [294.10]
    hepatolenticular degeneration
      with behavioral disturbance 275.1 [294.11]
      without behavioral disturbance 275.1 [294.10]
    HIV
      with behavioral disturbance 042 [294.11]
      without behavioral disturbance 042 [294.10]
    Huntington's chorea
      with behavioral disturbance 333.4 [294.11]
      without behavioral disturbance 333.4 [294.10]
    Jakob-Creutzfeldt disease (CJD)
      with behavioral disturbance 046.19 [294.11]
      without behavioral disturbance 046.19 [294.10]
      variant (vCJD) 046.11
        with dementia
          with behavioral disturbance 046.11 [294.11]
          without behavioral disturbance 046.11 [294.10]
    Lewy bodies
      with behavioral disturbance 331.82 [294.11]
      without behavioral disturbance 331.82 [294.10]
    multiple sclerosis
      with behavioral disturbance 340 [294.11]

Dementia — *continued*
  due to or associated with condition(s) classified elsewhere — *continued*
    multiple sclerosis — *continued*
      without behavioral disturbance 340 [294.10]
    neurosyphilis
      with behavioral disturbance 094.9 [294.11]
      without behavioral disturbance 094.9 [294.10]
    Parkinsonism
      with behavioral disturbance 331.82 [294.11]
      without behavioral disturbance 331.82 [294.10]
    Parkinson's disease
      with behavioral disturbance 332.0 [294.11]
      without behavioral disturbance 332.0 [294.10]
    Pelizaeus-Merzbacher disease
      with behavioral disturbance 333.0 [294.11]
      without behavioral disturbance 333.0 [294.10]
    Pick's disease
      with behavioral disturbance 331.11 [294.11]
      without behavioral disturbance 331.11 [294.10]
    polyarteritis nodosa
      with behavioral disturbance 446.0 [294.11]
      without behavioral disturbance 446.0 [294.10]
    syphilis
      with behavioral disturbance 094.1 [294.11]
      without behavioral disturbance 094.1 [294.10]
    Wilson's disease
      with behavioral disturbance 275.1 [294.11]
      without behavioral disturbance 275.1 [294.10]
  frontal 331.19
    with behavioral disturbance 331.19 [294.11]
    without behavioral disturbance 331.19 [294.10]
  frontotemporal 331.19
    with behavioral disturbance 331.19 [294.11]
    without behavioral disturbance 331.19 [294.10]
  hebephrenic (acute) 295.1 ☑
  Heller's (infantile psychosis) (*see also* Psychosis, childhood) 299.1 ☑
  idiopathic 290.9
    presenile-onset — *see* Dementia, presenile
    senile-onset — *see* Dementia, senile
  in
    arteriosclerotic brain disease 290.40
    senility 290.0
  induced by drug 292.82
  infantile, infantilia (*see also* Psychosis, childhood) 299.0 ☑
  Lewy body 331.82
    with behavioral disturbance 331.82 [294.11]
    without behavioral disturbance 331.82 [294.10]
  multi-infarct (cerebrovascular) (*see also* Dementia, arteriosclerotic) 290.40
  old age 290.0
  paralytica, paralytic 094.1
    juvenilis 090.40
    syphilitic 094.1
      congenital 090.40
    tabetic form 094.1
  paranoid (*see also* Schizophrenia) 295.3 ☑
  paraphrenic (*see also* Schizophrenia) 295.3 ☑
  paretic 094.1

☑ **Additional Digit Required — Refer to the Tabular List for Digit Selection**   ▽ **Subterms under main terms may continue to next column or page**

Dementia — Dependence

Dementia — *continued*
praecox (*see also* Schizophrenia) 295.9 ☑
presenile 290.10
   with
      acute confusional state 290.11
      delirium 290.11
      delusional features 290.12
      depressive features 290.13
   depressed type 290.13
   paranoid type 290.12
   simple type 290.10
   uncomplicated 290.10
primary (acute) (*see also* Schizophrenia) 295.0 ☑
progressive, syphilitic 094.1
puerperal — *see* Psychosis, puerperal
schizophrenic (*see also* Schizophrenia) 295.9 ☑
senile 290.0
   with
      acute confusional state 290.3
      delirium 290.3
      delusional features 290.20
      depressive features 290.21
   depressed type 290.21
   exhaustion 290.0
   paranoid type 290.20
simple type (acute) (*see also* Schizophrenia) 295.0 ☑
simplex (acute) (*see also* Schizophrenia) 295.0 ☑
syphilitic 094.1
uremic — *see* Uremia
vascular 290.40
   with
      delirium 290.41
      delusions 290.42
      depressed mood 290.43
Demerol dependence — *see also* Dependence 304.0 ☑
Demineralization, ankle — *see also* Osteoporosis 733.00
Demodex folliculorum (infestation) 133.8
Demoralization 799.25
de Morgan's spots (senile angiomas) 448.1
Demyelinating
polyneuritis, chronic inflammatory 357.81
Demyelination, demyelinization
central nervous system 341.9
   specified NEC 341.8
corpus callosum (central) 341.8
global 340
Dengue (fever) 061
sandfly 061
vaccination, prophylactic (against) V05.1
virus hemorrhagic fever 065.4
Dens
evaginatus 520.2
in dente 520.2
invaginatus 520.2
Dense
breast(s) 793.82
Density
increased, bone (disseminated) (generalized) (spotted) 733.99
lung (nodular) 518.89
Dental — *see also* condition
examination only V72.2
Dentia praecox 520.6
Denticles (in pulp) 522.2
Dentigerous cyst 526.0
Dentin
irregular (in pulp) 522.3
opalescent 520.5
secondary (in pulp) 522.3
sensitive 521.89
Dentinogenesis imperfecta 520.5
Dentinoma (M9271/0) 213.1
upper jaw (bone) 213.0
Dentition 520.7
abnormal 520.6
anomaly 520.6
delayed 520.6
difficult 520.7
disorder of 520.6
precocious 520.6

Dentition — *continued*
retarded 520.6
Denture sore (mouth) 528.9
Dependence

Note — Use the following fifth-digit subclassification with category 304:

0   unspecified

1   continuous

2   episodic

3   in remission

with
   withdrawal symptoms
      alcohol 291.81
      drug 292.0
14-hydroxy-dihydromorphinone 304.0 ☑
absinthe 304.6 ☑
acemorphan 304.0 ☑
acetanilid(e) 304.6 ☑
acetophenetidin 304.6 ☑
acetorphine 304.0 ☑
acetyldihydrocodeine 304.0 ☑
acetyldihydrocodeinone 304.0 ☑
Adalin 304.1 ☑
Afghanistan black 304.3 ☑
agrypnal 304.1 ☑
alcohol, alcoholic (ethyl) (methyl) (wood) 303.9 ☑
   maternal, with suspected fetal damage affecting management of pregnancy 655.4 ☑
allobarbitone 304.1 ☑
allonal 304.1 ☑
allylisopropylacetylurea 304.1 ☑
alphaprodine (hydrochloride) 304.0 ☑
Alurate 304.1 ☑
Alvodine 304.0 ☑
amethocaine 304.6 ☑
amidone 304.0 ☑
amidopyrine 304.6 ☑
aminopyrine 304.6 ☑
amobarbital 304.1 ☑
amphetamine(s) (type) (drugs classifiable to 969.7) 304.4 ☑
amylene hydrate 304.6 ☑
amylobarbitone 304.1 ☑
amylocaine 304.6 ☑
Amytal (sodium) 304.1 ☑
analgesic (drug) NEC 304.6 ☑
   synthetic with morphine-like effect 304.0 ☑
anesthetic (agent) (drug) (gas) (general) (local) NEC 304.6 ☑
Angel dust 304.6 ☑
anileridine 304.0 ☑
antipyrine 304.6 ☑
anxiolytic 304.1 ☑
aprobarbital 304.1 ☑
aprobarbitone 304.1 ☑
atropine 304.6 ☑
Avertin (bromide) 304.6 ☑
barbenyl 304.1 ☑
barbital(s) 304.1 ☑
barbitone 304.1 ☑
barbiturate(s) (compounds) (drugs classifiable to 967.0) 304.1 ☑
barbituric acid (and compounds) 304.1 ☑
benzedrine 304.4 ☑
benzylmorphine 304.0 ☑
Beta-chlor 304.1 ☑
bhang 304.3 ☑
blue velvet 304.0 ☑
Brevital 304.1 ☑
bromal (hydrate) 304.1 ☑
bromide(s) NEC 304.1 ☑
bromine compounds NEC 304.1 ☑
bromisovalum 304.1 ☑
bromoform 304.1 ☑
Bromo-seltzer 304.1 ☑
bromural 304.1 ☑
butabarbital (sodium) 304.1 ☑
butabarpal 304.1 ☑

Dependence — *continued*
butallylonal 304.1 ☑
butethal 304.1 ☑
buthalitone (sodium) 304.1 ☑
Butisol 304.1 ☑
butobarbitone 304.1 ☑
butyl chloral (hydrate) 304.1 ☑
caffeine 304.4 ☑
cannabis (indica) (sativa) (resin) (derivatives) (type) 304.3 ☑
carbamazepine 304.6 ☑
Carbrital 304.1 ☑
carbromal 304.1 ☑
carisoprodol 304.6 ☑
Catha (edulis) 304.4 ☑
chloral (betaine) (hydrate) 304.1 ☑
chloralamide 304.1 ☑
chloralformamide 304.1 ☑
chloralose 304.1 ☑
chlordiazepoxide 304.1 ☑
Chloretone 304.1 ☑
chlorobutanol 304.1 ☑
chlorodyne 304.1 ☑
chloroform 304.6 ☑
Cliradon 304.0 ☑
coca (leaf) and derivatives 304.2 ☑
cocaine 304.2 ☑
   hydrochloride 304.2 ☑
   salt (any) 304.2 ☑
codeine 304.0 ☑
combination of drugs (excluding morphine or opioid type drug) NEC 304.8 ☑
   morphine or opioid type drug with any other drug 304.7 ☑
croton-chloral 304.1 ☑
cyclobarbital 304.1 ☑
cyclobarbitone 304.1 ☑
dagga 304.3 ☑
Delvinal 304.1 ☑
Demerol 304.0 ☑
desocodeine 304.0 ☑
desomorphine 304.0 ☑
desoxyephedrine 304.4 ☑
DET 304.5 ☑
dexamphetamine 304.4 ☑
dexedrine 304.4 ☑
dextromethorphan 304.0 ☑
dextromoramide 304.0 ☑
dextronorpseudoephedrine 304.4 ☑
dextrorphan 304.0 ☑
diacetylmorphine 304.0 ☑
Dial 304.1 ☑
diallylbarbituric acid 304.1 ☑
diamorphine 304.0 ☑
diazepam 304.1 ☑
dibucaine 304.6 ☑
dichloroethane 304.6 ☑
diethyl barbituric acid 304.1 ☑
diethylsulfone-diethylmethane 304.1 ☑
difencloxazine 304.0 ☑
dihydrocodeine 304.0 ☑
dihydrocodeinone 304.0 ☑
dihydrohydroxycodeinone 304.0 ☑
dihydroisocodeine 304.0 ☑
dihydromorphine 304.0 ☑
dihydromorphinone 304.0 ☑
dihydroxcodeinone 304.0 ☑
Dilaudid 304.0 ☑
dimenhydrinate 304.6 ☑
dimethylmeperidine 304.0 ☑
dimethyltriptamine 304.5 ☑
Dionin 304.0 ☑
diphenoxylate 304.6 ☑
dipipanone 304.0 ☑
d-lysergic acid diethylamide 304.5 ☑
DMT 304.5 ☑
Dolophine 304.0 ☑
DOM 304.2 ☑
Doriden 304.1 ☑
dormiral 304.1 ☑
Dormison 304.1 ☑
Dromoran 304.0 ☑
drug NEC 304.9 ☑

Dependence — *continued*
drug — *continued*
   analgesic NEC 304.6 ☑
   combination (excluding morphine or opioid type drug) NEC 304.8 ☑
      morphine or opioid type drug with any other drug 304.7 ☑
   complicating pregnancy, childbirth, or puerperium 648.3 ☑
      affecting fetus or newborn 779.5
   hallucinogenic 304.5 ☑
   hypnotic NEC 304.1 ☑
   narcotic NEC 304.9 ☑
   psychostimulant NEC 304.4 ☑
   sedative 304.1 ☑
   soporific NEC 304.1 ☑
   specified type NEC 304.6 ☑
   suspected damage to fetus affecting management of pregnancy 655.5 ☑
   synthetic, with morphine-like effect 304.0 ☑
   tranquilizing 304.1 ☑
duboisine 304.6 ☑
ectylurea 304.1 ☑
Endocaine 304.6 ☑
Equanil 304.1 ☑
Eskabarb 304.1 ☑
etchlorvynol 304.1 ☑
ether (ethyl) (liquid) (vapor) (vinyl) 304.6 ☑
ethidene 304.6 ☑
ethinamate 304.1 ☑
ethoheptazine 304.6 ☑
ethyl
   alcohol 303.9 ☑
   bromide 304.6 ☑
   carbamate 304.6 ☑
   chloride 304.6 ☑
   morphine 304.0 ☑
ethylene (gas) 304.6 ☑
   dichloride 304.6 ☑
ethylidene chloride 304.6 ☑
etilfen 304.1 ☑
etorphine 304.0 ☑
etoval 304.1 ☑
eucodal 304.0 ☑
euneryl 304.1 ☑
Evipal 304.1 ☑
Evipan 304.1 ☑
fentanyl 304.0 ☑
ganja 304.3 ☑
gardenal 304.1 ☑
gardenpanyl 304.1 ☑
gelsemine 304.6 ☑
Gelsemium 304.6 ☑
Gemonil 304.1 ☑
glucochloral 304.1 ☑
glue (airplane) (sniffing) 304.6 ☑
glutethimide 304.1 ☑
hallucinogenics 304.5 ☑
hashish 304.3 ☑
headache powder NEC 304.6 ☑
Heavenly Blue 304.5 ☑
hedonal 304.1 ☑
hemp 304.3 ☑
heptabarbital 304.1 ☑
Heptalgin 304.0 ☑
heptobarbitone 304.1 ☑
heroin 304.0 ☑
   salt (any) 304.0 ☑
hexethal (sodium) 304.1 ☑
hexobarbital 304.1 ☑
Hycodan 304.0 ☑
hydrocodone 304.0 ☑
hydromorphinol 304.0 ☑
hydromorphinone 304.0 ☑
hydromorphone 304.0 ☑
hydroxycodeine 304.0 ☑
hypnotic NEC 304.1 ☑
Indian hemp 304.3 ☑
inhalant 304.6 ☑
intranarcon 304.1 ☑
Kemithal 304.1 ☑

☑ **Additional Digit Required** — Refer to the Tabular List for Digit Selection

▽ **Subterms under main terms may continue to next column or page**

Dependence — *continued*
ketobemidone 304.0 ☑
khat 304.4 ☑
kif 304.3 ☑
Lactuca (virosa) extract 304.1 ☑
lactucarium 304.1 ☑
laudanum 304.0 ☑
Lebanese red 304.3 ☑
Leritine 304.0 ☑
lettuce opium 304.1 ☑
Levanil 304.1 ☑
Levo-Dromoran 304.0 ☑
levo-iso-methadone 304.0 ☑
levorphanol 304.0 ☑
Librium 304.1 ☑
Lomotil 304.6 ☑
Lotusate 304.1 ☑
LSD (-25) (and derivatives) 304.5 ☑
Luminal 304.1 ☑
lysergic acid 304.5 ☑
    amide 304.5 ☑
maconha 304.3 ☑
magic mushroom 304.5 ☑
marihuana 304.3 ☑
MDA (methylene dioxyamphetamine) 304.4 ☑
Mebaral 304.1 ☑
Medinal 304.1 ☑
Medomin 304.1 ☑
megahallucinogenics 304.5 ☑
meperidine 304.0 ☑
mephobarbital 304.1 ☑
meprobamate 304.1 ☑
mescaline 304.5 ☑
methadone 304.0 ☑
methamphetamine(s) 304.4 ☑
methaqualone 304.1 ☑
metharbital 304.1 ☑
methitural 304.1 ☑
methobarbitone 304.1 ☑
methohexital 304.1 ☑
methopholine 304.6 ☑
methyl
    alcohol 303.9 ☑
    bromide 304.6 ☑
    morphine 304.0 ☑
    sulfonal 304.1 ☑
methylaparafynol 304.1 ☑
methylated spirit 303.9 ☑
methylbutinol 304.6 ☑
methyldihydromorphinone 304.0 ☑
methylene
    chloride 304.6 ☑
    dichloride 304.6 ☑
    dioxyamphetamine (MDA) 304.4 ☑
methylphenidate 304.4 ☑
methyprylone 304.1 ☑
metopon 304.0 ☑
Miltown 304.1 ☑
morning glory seeds 304.5 ☑
morphinan(s) 304.0 ☑
morphine (sulfate) (sulfite) (type) (drugs classifiable to 965.00–965.09) 304.0 ☑
morphine or opioid type drug (drugs classifiable to 965.00–965.09) with any other drug 304.7 ☑
morphinol(s) 304.0 ☑
morphinon 304.0 ☑
morpholinylethylmorphine 304.0 ☑
mylomide 304.1 ☑
myristicin 304.5 ☑
narcotic (drug) NEC 304.9 ☑
nealbarbital 304.1 ☑
nealbarbitone 304.1 ☑
Nembutal 304.1 ☑
Neonal 304.1 ☑
Neraval 304.1 ☑
Neravan 304.1 ☑
neurobarb 304.1 ☑
nicotine 305.1
Nisentil 304.0 ☑
nitrous oxide 304.6 ☑

Dependence — *continued*
Noctec 304.1 ☑
Noludar 304.1 ☑
nonbarbiturate sedatives and tranquilizers with similar effect 304.1 ☑
noptil 304.1 ☑
normorphine 304.0 ☑
noscapine 304.0 ☑
Novocaine 304.6 ☑
Numorphan 304.0 ☑
nunol 304.1 ☑
Nupercaine 304.6 ☑
Oblivon 304.1 ☑
on
    aspirator V46.0
    hemodialysis V45.11
    hyperbaric chamber V46.8
    iron lung V46.11
    machine (enabling) V46.9
        specified type NEC V46.8
    peritoneal dialysis V45.11
    Possum (Patient-Operated-Selector-Mechanism) V46.8
    renal dialysis machine V45.11
    respirator [ventilator] V46.11
        encounter
            during
                mechanical failure V46.14
                power failure V46.12
            for weaning V46.13
    supplemental oxygen V46.2
    wheelchair V46.3
opiate 304.0 ☑
opioids 304.0 ☑
opioid type drug 304.0 ☑
    with any other drug 304.7 ☑
opium (alkaloids) (derivatives) (tincture) 304.0 ☑
ortal 304.1 ☑
Oxazepam 304.1 ☑
oxycodone 304.0 ☑
oxymorphone 304.0 ☑
Palfium 304.0 ☑
Panadol 304.6 ☑
pantopium 304.0 ☑
pantopon 304.0 ☑
papaverine 304.0 ☑
paracetamol 304.6 ☑
paracodin 304.0 ☑
paraldehyde 304.1 ☑
paregoric 304.0 ☑
Parzone 304.0 ☑
PCP (phencyclidine) 304.6 ☑
Pearly Gates 304.5 ☑
pentazocine 304.0 ☑
pentobarbital 304.1 ☑
pentobarbitone (sodium) 304.1 ☑
Pentothal 304.1 ☑
Percaine 304.6 ☑
Percodan 304.0 ☑
Perichlor 304.1 ☑
Pernocton 304.1 ☑
Pernoston 304.1 ☑
peronine 304.0 ☑
pethidine (hydrochloride) 304.0 ☑
petrichloral 304.1 ☑
peyote 304.5 ☑
Phanodron 304.1 ☑
phenacetin 304.6 ☑
phenadoxone 304.0 ☑
phenaglycodol 304.1 ☑
phenazocine 304.0 ☑
phencyclidine 304.6 ☑
phenmetrazine 304.4 ☑
phenobal 304.1 ☑
phenobarbital 304.1 ☑
phenobarbitone 304.1 ☑
phenomorphan 304.0 ☑
phenonyl 304.1 ☑
phenoperidine 304.0 ☑
pholcodine 304.0 ☑
piminodine 304.0 ☑
Pipadone 304.0 ☑
Pitkin's solution 304.6 ☑

Dependence — *continued*
Placidyl 304.1 ☑
polysubstance 304.8 ☑
Pontocaine 304.6 ☑
pot 304.3 ☑
potassium bromide 304.1 ☑
Preludin 304.4 ☑
Prinadol 304.0 ☑
probarbital 304.1 ☑
procaine 304.6 ☑
propanal 304.1 ☑
propoxyphene 304.6 ☑
psilocibin 304.5 ☑
psilocin 304.5 ☑
psilocybin 304.5 ☑
psilocyline 304.5 ☑
psilocyn 304.5 ☑
psychedelic agents 304.5 ☑
psychostimulant NEC 304.4 ☑
psychotomimetic agents 304.5 ☑
pyrahexyl 304.3 ☑
Pyramidon 304.6 ☑
quinalbarbitone 304.1 ☑
racemoramide 304.0 ☑
racemorphan 304.0 ☑
Rela 304.6 ☑
scopolamine 304.6 ☑
secobarbital 304.1 ☑
Seconal 304.1 ☑
sedative NEC 304.1 ☑
    nonbarbiturate with barbiturate effect 304.1 ☑
Sedormid 304.1 ☑
sernyl 304.1 ☑
sodium bromide 304.1 ☑
Soma 304.6 ☑
Somnal 304.1 ☑
Somnos 304.1 ☑
Soneryl 304.1 ☑
soporific (drug) NEC 304.1 ☑
specified drug NEC 304.6 ☑
speed 304.4 ☑
spinocaine 304.6 ☑
Stovaine 304.6 ☑
STP 304.5 ☑
stramonium 304.6 ☑
Sulfonal 304.1 ☑
sulfonethylmethane 304.1 ☑
sulfonmethane 304.1 ☑
Surital 304.1 ☑
synthetic drug with morphine-like effect 304.0 ☑
talbutal 304.1 ☑
tetracaine 304.6 ☑
tetrahydrocannabinol 304.3 ☑
tetronal 304.1 ☑
THC 304.3 ☑
thebacon 304.0 ☑
thebaine 304.0 ☑
thiamil 304.1 ☑
thiamylal 304.1 ☑
thiopental 304.1 ☑
tobacco 305.1
toluene, toluol 304.6 ☑
tranquilizer NEC 304.1 ☑
    nonbarbiturate with barbiturate effect 304.1 ☑
tribromacetaldehyde 304.6 ☑
tribromethanol 304.6 ☑
tribromomethane 304.6 ☑
trichloroethanol 304.6 ☑
trichoroethyl phosphate 304.1 ☑
triclofos 304.1 ☑
Trional 304.1 ☑
Tuinal 304.1 ☑
Turkish Green 304.3 ☑
urethan(e) 304.6 ☑
Valium 304.1 ☑
Valmid 304.1 ☑
veganin 304.0 ☑
veramon 304.1 ☑
Veronal 304.1 ☑
versidyne 304.6 ☑

Dependence — *continued*
vinbarbital 304.1 ☑
vinbarbitone 304.1 ☑
vinyl bitone 304.1 ☑
vitamin B_6 266.1
wine 303.9 ☑
Zactane 304.6 ☑
Dependency
passive 301.6
reactions 301.6
Depersonalization (episode, in neurotic state) (neurotic) (syndrome) 300.6
Depletion
carbohydrates 271.9
complement factor 279.8
extracellular fluid 276.52
plasma 276.52
potassium 276.8
    nephropathy 588.89
salt or sodium 276.1
    causing heat exhaustion or prostration 992.4
    nephropathy 593.9
volume 276.50
    extracellular fluid 276.52
    plasma 276.52
Deployment (military)
personal history of V62.22
returned from V62.22
status V62.21
Deposit
argentous, cornea 371.16
bone, in Boeck's sarcoid 135
calcareous, calcium — *see* Calcification
cholesterol
    retina 362.82
    skin 709.3
    vitreous (humor) 379.22
conjunctival 372.56
cornea, corneal NEC 371.10
    argentous 371.16
    in
        cystinosis 270.0 *[371.15]*
        mucopolysaccharidosis 277.5 *[371.15]*
crystalline, vitreous (humor) 379.22
hemosiderin, in old scars of cornea 371.11
metallic, in lens 366.45
skin 709.3
teeth, tooth (betel) (black) (green) (materia alba) (orange) (soft) (tobacco) 523.6
urate, in kidney (*see also* Disease, renal) 593.9
Depraved appetite 307.52
Depression 311
acute (*see also* Psychosis, affective) 296.2 ☑
    recurrent episode 296.3 ☑
    single episode 296.2 ☑
agitated (*see also* Psychosis, affective) 296.2 ☑
    recurrent episode 296.3 ☑
    single episode 296.2 ☑
anaclitic 309.21
anxiety 300.4
arches 734
    congenital 754.61
autogenous (*see also* Psychosis, affective) 296.2 ☑
    recurrent episode 296.3 ☑
    single episode 296.2 ☑
basal metabolic rate (BMR) 794.7
bone marrow 289.9
central nervous system 799.1
    newborn 779.2
cerebral 331.9
    newborn 779.2
cerebrovascular 437.8
    newborn 779.2
chest wall 738.3
endogenous (*see also* Psychosis, affective) 296.2 ☑
    recurrent episode 296.3 ☑
    single episode 296.2 ☑
functional activity 780.99
hysterical 300.11

☑ **Additional Digit Required** — **Refer to the Tabular List for Digit Selection**

▽ᵇ **Subterms under main terms may continue to next column or page**

Depression — continued
  involutional, climacteric, or menopausal (see
      also Psychosis, affective) 296.2 ☑
    recurrent episode 296.3 ☑
    single episode 296.2 ☑
  major 296.2 ☑
    recurrent episode 296.3 ☑
    single episode 296.2 ☑
  manic (see also Psychosis, affective) 296.80
  medullary 348.89
    newborn 779.2
  mental 300.4
  metatarsal heads — see Depression, arches
  metatarsus — see Depression, arches
  monopolar (see also Psychosis, affective)
      296.2 ☑
    recurrent episode 296.3 ☑
    single episode 296.2 ☑
  nervous 300.4
  neurotic 300.4
  nose 738.0
  postpartum 648.4 ☑
  psychogenic 300.4
    reactive 298.0
  psychoneurotic 300.4
  psychotic (see also Psychosis, affective)
      296.2 ☑
    reactive 298.0
    recurrent episode 296.3 ☑
    single episode 296.2 ☑
  reactive 300.4
    neurotic 300.4
    psychogenic 298.0
    psychoneurotic 300.4
    psychotic 298.0
  recurrent 296.3 ☑
  respiratory center 348.89
    newborn 770.89
  scapula 736.89
  senile 290.21
  situational (acute) (brief) 309.0
    prolonged 309.1
  skull 754.0
  sternum 738.3
  visual field 368.40
Depressive reaction — see also Reaction, de-
    pressive
  acute (transient) 309.0
    with anxiety 309.28
  prolonged 309.1
  situational (acute) 309.0
    prolonged 309.1
Deprivation
  cultural V62.4
  emotional V62.89
    affecting
      adult 995.82
      infant or child 995.51
  food 994.2
    specific substance NEC 269.8
  protein (familial) (kwashiorkor) 260
  sleep V69.4
  social V62.4
    affecting
      adult 995.82
      infant or child 995.51
  symptoms, syndrome
    alcohol 291.81
    drug 292.0
  vitamins (see also Deficiency, vitamin) 269.2
  water 994.3
de Quervain's
  disease (tendon sheath) 727.04
  syndrome 259.51
  thyroiditis (subacute granulomatous thy-
      roiditis) 245.1
Derangement
  ankle (internal) 718.97
    current injury (see also Dislocation, an-
        kle) 837.0
    recurrent 718.37
  cartilage (articular) NEC (see also Disorder,
      cartilage, articular) 718.0 ☑
    knee 717.9
      recurrent 718.36
    recurrent 718.3 ☑

Derangement — continued
  collateral ligament (knee) (medial) (tibial)
      717.82
    current injury 844.1
      lateral (fibular) 844.0
    lateral (fibular) 717.81
      current injury 844.0
  cruciate ligament (knee) (posterior) 717.84
    anterior 717.83
      current injury 844.2
    current injury 844.2
  elbow (internal) 718.92
    current injury (see also Dislocation, el-
        bow) 832.00
    recurrent 718.32
  gastrointestinal 536.9
  heart — see Disease, heart
  hip (joint) (internal) (old) 718.95
    current injury (see also Dislocation, hip)
        835.00
    recurrent 718.35
  intervertebral disc — see Displacement, in-
      tervertebral disc
  joint (internal) 718.90
    ankle 718.97
    current injury (see also Dislocation, by
        site)
      knee, meniscus or cartilage (see also
          Tear, meniscus) 836.2
    elbow 718.92
    foot 718.97
    hand 718.94
    hip 718.95
    knee 717.9
    multiple sites 718.99
    pelvic region 718.95
    recurrent 718.30
      ankle 718.37
      elbow 718.32
      foot 718.37
      hand 718.34
      hip 718.35
      knee 718.36
      multiple sites 718.39
      pelvic region 718.35
      shoulder (region) 718.31
      specified site NEC 718.38
      temporomandibular (old) 524.69
      wrist 718.33
    shoulder (region) 718.91
    specified site NEC 718.98
    spine NEC 724.9
    temporomandibular 524.69
    wrist 718.93
  knee (cartilage) (internal) 717.9
    current injury (see also Tear, meniscus)
        836.2
    ligament 717.89
      capsular 717.85
      collateral — see Derangement, collat-
          eral ligament
      cruciate — see Derangement, cruci-
          ate ligament
      specified NEC 717.85
    recurrent 718.36
  low back NEC 724.9
  meniscus NEC (knee) 717.5
    current injury (see also Tear, meniscus)
        836.2
    lateral 717.40
      anterior horn 717.42
      posterior horn 717.43
      specified NEC 717.49
    medial 717.3
      anterior horn 717.1
      posterior horn 717.2
    recurrent 718.3 ☑
    site other than knee — see Disorder,
        cartilage, articular
  mental (see also Psychosis) 298.9
  rotator cuff (recurrent) (tear) 726.10
    current 840.4
  sacroiliac (old) 724.6
    current — see Dislocation, sacroiliac
  semilunar cartilage (knee) 717.5
    current injury 836.2

Derangement — continued
  semilunar cartilage — continued
    current injury — continued
      lateral 836.1
      medial 836.0
    recurrent 718.3 ☑
  shoulder (internal) 718.91
    current injury (see also Dislocation,
        shoulder) 831.00
    recurrent 718.31
  spine (recurrent) NEC 724.9
    current — see Dislocation, spine
  temporomandibular (internal) (joint) (old)
      524.69
    current — see Dislocation, jaw
Dercum's disease or syndrome (adiposis do-
    lorosa) 272.8
Derealization (neurotic) 300.6
Dermal — see condition
Dermaphytid — see Dermatophytosis
Dermatergosis — see Dermatitis
Dermatitis (allergic) (contact) (occupational)
    (venenata) 692.9
  ab igne 692.82
  acneiform 692.9
  actinic (due to sun) 692.70
    acute 692.72
    chronic NEC 692.74
    other than from sun NEC 692.82
  ambustionis
    due to
      burn or scald — see Burn, by site
      sunburn (see also Sunburn) 692.71
  amebic 006.6
  ammonia 691.0
  anaphylactoid NEC 692.9
  arsenical 692.4
  artefacta 698.4
    psychogenic 316 [698.4]
  asthmatic 691.8
  atopic (allergic) (intrinsic) 691.8
    psychogenic 316 [691.8]
  atrophicans 701.8
    diffusa 701.8
    maculosa 701.3
  autoimmune progesterone 279.49
  berlock, berloque 692.72
  blastomycetic 116.0
  blister beetle 692.89
  Brucella NEC 023.9
  bullosa 694.9
    striata pratensis 692.6
  bullous 694.9
    mucosynechial, atrophic 694.60
      with ocular involvement 694.61
    seasonal 694.8
  calorica
    due to
      burn or scald — see Burn, by site
      cold 692.89
      sunburn (see also Sunburn) 692.71
  caterpillar 692.89
  cercarial 120.3
  combustionis
    due to
      burn or scald — see Burn, by site
      sunburn (see also Sunburn) 692.71
  congelationis 991.5
  contusiformis 695.2
  diabetic 250.8 ☑
  diaper 691.0
  diphtheritica 032.85
  due to
    acetone 692.2
    acids 692.4
    adhesive plaster 692.4
    alcohol (skin contact) (substances classi-
        fiable to 980.0–980.9) 692.4
      taken internally 693.8
    alkalis 692.4
    allergy NEC 692.9
    ammonia (household) (liquid) 692.4
    animal
      dander (cat) (dog) 692.84
      hair (cat) (dog) 692.84
    arnica 692.3

Dermatitis — continued
  due to — continued
    arsenic 692.4
      taken internally 693.8
    blister beetle 692.89
    cantharides 692.3
    carbon disulphide 692.2
    caterpillar 692.89
    caustics 692.4
    cereal (ingested) 693.1
      contact with skin 692.5
    chemical(s) NEC 692.4
      internal 693.8
      irritant NEC 692.4
      taken internally 693.8
    chlorocompounds 692.2
    coffee (ingested) 693.1
      contact with skin 692.5
    cold weather 692.89
    cosmetics 692.81
    cyclohexanes 692.2
    dander, animal (cat) (dog) 692.84
    deodorant 692.81
    detergents 692.0
    dichromate 692.4
    drugs and medicinals (correct substance
        properly administered) (internal
        use) 693.0
      external (in contact with skin) 692.3
        wrong substance given or taken
            976.9
      specified substance — see
          Table of Drugs and
          Chemicals
      wrong substance given or taken
          977.9
        specified substance — see Table
            of Drugs and Chemicals
    dyes 692.89
      hair 692.89
    epidermophytosis — see Dermatophyto-
        sis
    esters 692.2
    external irritant NEC 692.9
      specified agent NEC 692.89
    eye shadow 692.81
    fish (ingested) 693.1
      contact with skin 692.5
    flour (ingested) 693.1
      contact with skin 692.5
    food (ingested) 693.1
      in contact with skin 692.5
    fruit (ingested) 693.1
      contact with skin 692.5
    fungicides 692.3
    furs 692.84
    glycols 692.2
    greases NEC 692.1
    hair, animal (cat) (dog) 692.84
    hair dyes 692.89
    hot
      objects and materials — see Burn, by
          site
      weather or places 692.89
    hydrocarbons 692.2
    infrared rays, except from sun 692.82
      solar NEC (see also Dermatitis, due to,
          sun) 692.70
    ingested substance 693.9
      drugs and medicinals (see also Der-
          matitis, due to, drugs and
          medicinals) 693.0
      food 693.1
      specified substance NEC 693.8
    ingestion or injection of chemical 693.8
      drug (correct substance properly ad-
          ministered) 693.0
      wrong substance given or taken
          977.9
        specified substance — see Table
            of Drugs and Chemicals
    insecticides 692.4
    internal agent 693.9
      drugs and medicinals (see also Der-
          matitis, due to, drugs and
          medicinals) 693.0

☑ **Additional Digit Required** — Refer to the Tabular List for Digit Selection   ⑩ **Subterms under main terms may continue to next column or page**

76 — Volume 2   ▶◀ **Revised Text**   ● **New Line**   ▲ **Revised Code**   **2015 ICD-9-CM**

Dermatitis — continued
  due to — continued
    internal agent — continued
      food (ingested) 693.1
        in contact with skin 692.5
        specified agent NEC 693.8
    iodine 692.3
    iodoform 692.3
    irradiation 692.82
    jewelry 692.83
    keratolytics 692.3
    ketones 692.2
    lacquer tree (Rhus verniciflua) 692.6
    light (sun) NEC (see also Dermatitis, due to, sun) 692.70
      other 692.82
    low temperature 692.89
    mascara 692.81
    meat (ingested) 693.1
      contact with skin 692.5
    mercury, mercurials 692.3
    metals 692.83
    milk (ingested) 693.1
      contact with skin 692.5
    Neomycin 692.3
    nylon 692.4
    oils NEC 692.1
    paint solvent 692.2
    pediculocides 692.3
    petroleum products (substances classifiable to 981) 692.4
    phenol 692.3
    photosensitiveness, photosensitivity (sun) 692.72
      other light 692.82
    plants NEC 692.6
    plasters, medicated (any) 692.3
    plastic 692.4
    poison
      ivy (Rhus toxicodendron) 692.6
      oak (Rhus diversiloba) 692.6
      plant or vine 692.6
      sumac (Rhus venenata) 692.6
      vine (Rhus radicans) 692.6
    preservatives 692.89
    primrose (primula) 692.6
    primula 692.6
    radiation 692.82
      sun NEC (see also Dermatitis, due to, sun) 692.70
      tanning bed 692.82
    radioactive substance 692.82
    radium 692.82
    ragweed (Senecio jacobae) 692.6
    Rhus (diversiloba) (radicans) (toxicodendron) (venenata) (verniciflua) 692.6
    rubber 692.4
    scabicides 692.3
    Senecio jacobae 692.6
    solar radiation — see Dermatitis, due to, sun
    solvents (any) (substances classifiable to 982.0–982.8) 692.2
      chlorocompound group 692.2
      cyclohexane group 692.2
      ester group 692.2
      glycol group 692.2
      hydrocarbon group 692.2
      ketone group 692.2
      paint 692.2
    specified agent NEC 692.89
    sun 692.70
      acute 692.72
      chronic NEC 692.74
      specified NEC 692.79
    sunburn (see also Sunburn) 692.71
    sunshine NEC (see also Dermatitis, due to, sun) 692.70
    tanning bed 692.82
    tetrachlorethylene 692.2
    toluene 692.2
    topical medications 692.3
    turpentine 692.2
    ultraviolet rays, except from sun 692.82

Dermatitis — continued
  due to — continued
    ultraviolet rays, except from sun — continued
      sun NEC (see also Dermatitis, due to, sun) 692.70
    vaccine or vaccination (correct substance properly administered) 693.0
      wrong substance given or taken
        bacterial vaccine 978.8
          specified — see Table of Drugs and Chemicals
        other vaccines NEC 979.9
          specified — see Table of Drugs and Chemicals
    varicose veins (see also Varicose, vein, inflamed or infected) 454.1
    x-rays 692.82
  dyshydrotic 705.81
  dysmenorrheica 625.8
  eczematoid NEC 692.9
    infectious 690.8
  eczematous NEC 692.9
  epidemica 695.89
  erysipelatosa 695.81
  escharotica — see Burn, by site
  exfoliativa, exfoliative 695.89
    generalized 695.89
    infantum 695.81
    neonatorum 695.81
  eyelid 373.31
    allergic 373.32
    contact 373.32
    eczematous 373.31
    herpes (zoster) 053.20
      simplex 054.41
    infective 373.5
      due to
        actinomycosis 039.3 [373.5]
        herpes
          simplex 054.41
          zoster 053.20
        impetigo 684 [373.5]
        leprosy (see also Leprosy) 030.0 [373.4]
        lupus vulgaris (tuberculous) (see also Tuberculosis) 017.0 ☑ [373.4]
        mycotic dermatitis (see also Dermatomycosis) 111.9 [373.5]
        vaccinia 051.02 [373.5]
          postvaccination 999.0 [373.5]
        yaws (see also Yaws) 102.9 [373.4]
  facta, factitia 698.4
    psychogenic 316 [698.4]
  ficta 698.4
    psychogenic 316 [698.4]
  flexural 691.8
  follicularis 704.8
  friction 709.8
  fungus 111.9
    specified type NEC 111.8
  gangrenosa, gangrenous (infantum) (see also Gangrene) 785.4
  gestationis 646.8 ☑
  gonococcal 098.89
  gouty 274.89
  harvest mite 133.8
  heat 692.89
  herpetiformis (bullous) (erythematous) (pustular) (vesicular) 694.0
    juvenile 694.2
    senile 694.5
  hiemalis 692.89
  hypostatic, hypostatica 454.1
    with ulcer 454.2
  impetiginosa 684
  infantile (acute) (chronic) (intertriginous) (intrinsic) (seborrheic) 690.12
  infectiosa eczematoides 690.8
  infectious (staphylococcal) (streptococcal) 686.9
    eczematoid 690.8
  infective eczematoid 690.8
  Jacquet's (diaper dermatitis) 691.0

Dermatitis — continued
  leptus 133.8
  lichenified NEC 692.9
  lichenoid, chronic 701.0
  lichenoides purpurica pigmentosa 709.1
  meadow 692.6
  medicamentosa (correct substance properly administered) (internal use) (see also Dermatitis, due to, drugs or medicinals) 693.0
    due to contact with skin 692.3
  mite 133.8
  multiformis 694.0
    juvenile 694.2
    senile 694.5
  napkin 691.0
  neuro 698.3
  neurotica 694.0
  nummular NEC 692.9
  osteatosis, osteatotic 706.8
  papillaris capillitii 706.1
  pellagrous 265.2
  perioral 695.3
  perstans 696.1
  photosensitivity (sun) 692.72
    other light 692.82
  pigmented purpuric lichenoid 709.1
  polymorpha dolorosa 694.0
  primary irritant 692.9
  pruriginosa 694.0
  pruritic NEC 692.9
  psoriasiform nodularis 696.2
  psychogenic 316
  purulent 686.00
  pustular contagious 051.2
  pyococcal 686.00
  pyocyaneus 686.09
  pyogenica 686.00
  radiation 692.82
  repens 696.1
  Ritter's (exfoliativa) 695.81
  Schamberg's (progressive pigmentary dermatosis) 709.09
  schistosome 120.3
  seasonal bullous 694.8
  seborrheic 690.10
    infantile 690.12
  sensitization NEC 692.9
  septic (see also Septicemia) 686.00
    gonococcal 098.89
  solar, solare NEC (see also Dermatitis, due to, sun) 692.70
  stasis 454.1
    due to
      postphlebitic syndrome 459.12
        with ulcer 459.13
      varicose veins — see Varicose
    ulcerated or with ulcer (varicose) 454.2
  sunburn (see also Sunburn) 692.71
  suppurative 686.00
  traumatic NEC 709.8
  trophoneurotica 694.0
  ultraviolet, except from sun 692.82
    due to sun NEC (see also Dermatitis, due to, sun) 692.82
  varicose 454.1
    with ulcer 454.2
  vegetans 686.8
  verrucosa 117.2
  xerotic 706.8
Dermatoarthritis, lipoid 272.8 [713.0]
Dermatochalasia, dermatochalasis 374.87
Dermatofibroma (lenticulare) (M8832/0) — see also Neoplasm, skin, benign
  protuberans (M8832/1) — see Neoplasm, skin, uncertain behavior
Dermatofibrosarcoma (protuberans) (M8832/3) — see Neoplasm, skin, malignant
Dermatographia 708.3
Dermatolysis (congenital) (exfoliativa) 757.39
  acquired 701.8
  eyelids 374.34
  palpebrarum 374.34
  senile 701.8
Dermatomegaly NEC 701.8

Dermatomucomyositis 710.3
Dermatomycosis 111.9
  furfuracea 111.0
  specified type NEC 111.8
Dermatomyositis (acute) (chronic) 710.3
Dermatoneuritis of children 985.0
Dermatophiliasis 134.1
Dermatophytide — see Dermatophytosis
Dermatophytosis (Epidermophyton) (infection) (microsporum) (tinea) (Trichophyton) 110.9
  beard 110.0
  body 110.5
  deep seated 110.6
  fingernails 110.1
  foot 110.4
  groin 110.3
  hand 110.2
  nail 110.1
  perianal (area) 110.3
  scalp 110.0
  scrotal 110.8
  specified site NEC 110.8
  toenails 110.1
  vulva 110.8
Dermatopolyneuritis 985.0
Dermatorrhexis 756.83
  acquired 701.8
Dermatosclerosis — see also Scleroderma 710.1
  localized 701.0
Dermatosis 709.9
  Andrews' 686.8
  atopic 691.8
  Bowen's (M8081/2) — see Neoplasm, skin, in situ
  bullous 694.9
    specified type NEC 694.8
  erythematosquamous 690.8
  exfoliativa 695.89
  factitial 698.4
  gonococcal 098.89
  herpetiformis 694.0
    juvenile 694.2
    senile 694.5
  hysterical 300.11
  linear IgA 694.8
  menstrual NEC 709.8
  neutrophilic, acute febrile 695.89
  occupational (see also Dermatitis) 692.9
  papulosa nigra 709.8
  pigmentary NEC 709.00
    progressive 709.09
      Schamberg's 709.09
    Siemens-Bloch 757.33
  progressive pigmentary 709.09
  psychogenic 316
  pustular subcorneal 694.1
  Schamberg's (progressive pigmentary) 709.09
  senile NEC 709.3
  specified NEC 702.8
  Unna's (seborrheic dermatitis) 690.10
Dermographia 708.3
Dermographism 708.3
Dermoid (cyst) (M9084/0) — see also Neoplasm, by site, benign
  with malignant transformation (M9084/3) 183.0
Dermopathy
  infiltrative, with thyrotoxicosis 242.0 ☑
  nephrogenic fibrosing 701.8
  senile NEC 709.3
Dermophytosis — see Dermatophytosis
Descemet's membrane — see condition
Descemetocele 371.72
Descending — see condition
Descensus uteri (complete) (incomplete) (partial) (without vaginal wall prolapse) 618.1
  with mention of vaginal wall prolapse — see Prolapse, uterovaginal
Desensitization to allergens V07.1
Desert
  rheumatism 114.0
  sore (see also Ulcer, skin) 707.9

☑ Additional Digit Required — Refer to the Tabular List for Digit Selection ▽ Subterms under main terms may continue to next column or page

2015 ICD-9-CM   ▶◀ Revised Text   ● New Line   ▲ Revised Code   Volume 2 — 77

Desertion (child) (newborn) 995.52
  adult 995.84
Desmoid (extra-abdominal) (tumor) (M8821/1)
  — see also Neoplasm, connective tissue,
    uncertain behavior
  abdominal (M8822/1) — see Neoplasm,
    connective tissue, uncertain behavior
Despondency 300.4
Desquamative dermatitis NEC 695.89
Destruction
  articular facet (see also Derangement, joint)
    718.9 ☑
    vertebra 724.9
  bone 733.90
    syphilitic 095.5
  joint (see also Derangement, joint) 718.9 ☑
    sacroiliac 724.6
  kidney 593.89
  live fetus to facilitate birth NEC 763.89
  ossicles (ear) 385.24
  rectal sphincter 569.49
  septum (nasal) 478.19
  tuberculous NEC (see also Tuberculosis)
    011.9 ☑
  tympanic membrane 384.82
  tympanum 385.89
  vertebral disc — see Degeneration, interver-
    tebral disc
Destructiveness — see also Disturbance, conduct 312.9
  adjustment reaction 309.3
Detachment
  cartilage (see also Sprain, by site)
    knee — see Tear, meniscus
  cervix, annular 622.8
    complicating delivery 665.3 ☑
  choroid (old) (postinfectional) (simple)
    (spontaneous) 363.70
    hemorrhagic 363.72
    serous 363.71
  knee, medial meniscus (old) 717.3
    current injury 836.0
  ligament — see Sprain, by site
  placenta (premature) — see Placenta, sepa-
    ration
  retina (recent) 361.9
    with retinal defect (rhegmatogenous)
      361.00
      giant tear 361.03
      multiple 361.02
      partial
        with
          giant tear 361.03
          multiple defects 361.02
          retinal dialysis (juvenile)
            361.04
          single defect 361.01
      retinal dialysis (juvenile) 361.04
      single 361.01
      subtotal 361.05
      total 361.05
    delimited (old) (partial) 361.06
    old
      delimited 361.06
      partial 361.06
      total or subtotal 361.07
    pigment epithelium (RPE) (serous)
      362.42
      exudative 362.42
      hemorrhagic 362.43
    rhegmatogenous (see also Detachment,
      retina, with retinal defect) 361.00
    serous (without retinal defect) 361.2
    specified type NEC 361.89
    traction (with vitreoretinal organization)
      361.81
  vitreous humor 379.21
Detergent asthma 507.8
Deterioration
  epileptic
    with behavioral disturbance
      345.9 ☑ [294.11]
    without behavioral disturbance
      345.9 ☑ [294.10]
  heart, cardiac (see also Degeneration, my-
    ocardial) 429.1

Deterioration — continued
  mental (see also Psychosis) 298.9
  myocardium, myocardial (see also Degener-
    ation, myocardial) 429.1
  senile (simple) 797
  transplanted organ — see Complications,
    transplant, organ, by site
de Toni-Fanconi syndrome (cystinosis) 270.0
Deuteranomaly 368.52
Deuteranopia (anomalous trichromat) (complete) (incomplete) 368.52
Deutschländer's disease — see Fracture, foot
Development
  abnormal, bone 756.9
  arrested 783.40
    bone 733.91
    child 783.40
    due to malnutrition (protein-calorie)
      263.2
    fetus or newborn 764.9 ☑
    tracheal rings (congenital) 748.3
  defective, congenital (see also Anomaly)
    cauda equina 742.59
    left ventricle 746.9
      with atresia or hypoplasia of aortic
        orifice or valve with hypopla-
        sia of ascending aorta 746.7
      in hypoplastic left heart syndrome
        746.7
  delayed (see also Delay, development)
    783.40
    arithmetical skills 315.1
    language (skills) 315.31
      and speech due to hearing loss
        315.34
      expressive 315.31
      mixed receptive-expressive 315.32
    learning skill, specified NEC 315.2
    mixed skills 315.5
    motor coordination 315.4
    reading 315.00
    specified
      learning skill NEC 315.2
      type NEC, except learning 315.8
    speech 315.39
      and language due to hearing loss
        315.34
      associated with hyperkinesia 314.1
      phonological 315.39
    spelling 315.09
    written expression 315.2
  imperfect, congenital (see also Anomaly)
    heart 746.9
    lungs 748.60
  improper (fetus or newborn) 764.9 ☑
  incomplete (fetus or newborn) 764.9 ☑
    affecting management of pregnancy
      656.5 ☑
    bronchial tree 748.3
    organ or site not listed — see Hypoplasia
    respiratory system 748.9
  sexual, precocious NEC 259.1
  tardy, mental (see also Disability, intellectu-
    al) 319
Developmental — see condition
Devergie's disease (pityriasis rubra pilaris)
  696.4
Deviation
  conjugate (eye) 378.87
    palsy 378.81
    spasm, spastic 378.82
  esophagus 530.89
  eye, skew 378.87
  mandible, opening and closing 524.53
  midline (jaw) (teeth) 524.29
    specified site NEC — see Malposition
  occlusal plane 524.76
  organ or site, congenital NEC — see Malpo-
    sition, congenital
  septum (acquired) (nasal) 470
    congenital 754.0
  sexual 302.9
    bestiality 302.1
    coprophilia 302.89
    ego-dystonic
      homosexuality 302.0

Deviation — continued
  sexual — continued
    ego-dystonic — continued
      lesbianism 302.0
    erotomania 302.89
      Clérambault's 297.8
    exhibitionism (sexual) 302.4
    fetishism 302.81
      transvestic 302.3
    frotteurism 302.89
    homosexuality, ego-dystonic 302.0
      pedophilic 302.2
    lesbianism, ego-dystonic 302.0
    masochism 302.83
    narcissism 302.89
    necrophilia 302.89
    nymphomania 302.89
    pederosis 302.2
    pedophilia 302.2
    sadism 302.84
    sadomasochism 302.84
    satyriasis 302.89
    specified type NEC 302.89
    transvestic fetishism 302.3
    transvestism 302.3
    voyeurism 302.82
    zoophilia (erotica) 302.1
  teeth, midline 524.29
  trachea 519.19
  ureter (congenital) 753.4
Devic's disease 341.0
Device
  cerebral ventricle (communicating) in situ
    V45.2
  contraceptive — see Contraceptive, device
  drainage, cerebrospinal fluid V45.2
Devil's
  grip 074.1
  pinches (purpura simplex) 287.2
Devitalized tooth 522.9
Devonshire colic 984.9
  specified type of lead — see Table of Drugs
    and Chemicals
Dextraposition, aorta 747.21
  with ventricular septal defect, pulmonary
    stenosis or atresia, and hypertrophy
    of right ventricle 745.2
  in tetralogy of Fallot 745.2
Dextratransposition, aorta 745.11
Dextrinosis, limit (debrancher enzyme deficiency) 271.0
Dextrocardia (corrected) (false) (isolated)
  (secondary) (true) 746.87
  with
    complete transposition of viscera 759.3
    situs inversus 759.3
Dextroversion, kidney (left) 753.3
Dhobie itch 110.3
DHTR (delayed hemolytic transfusion reaction)
  — see Complications, transfusion
Diabetes, diabetic (brittle) (congenital) (familial) (mellitus) (severe) (slight) (without
  complication) 250.0 ☑

   Note — Use the following fifth-digit
   subclassification with category 250:

   0   *type II or unspecified type, not*
       stated as uncontrolled

   Fifth-digit 0 is for use for type II pa-
   tients, even if the patient requires insulin

   1   *type I [juvenile type], not stated*
       as uncontrolled

   2   *type II or unspecified type, uncon-*
       trolled

   Fifth-digit 2 is for use for type II pa-
   tients, even if the patient requires insulin

   3   *type I [juvenile type], uncontrolled*

  with
    coma (with ketoacidosis) 250.3 ☑
      due to secondary diabetes 249.3 ☑
      hyperosmolar (nonketotic) 250.2 ☑
        due to secondary diabetes
          249.2 ☑

Diabetes, diabetic — continued
  with — continued
    complication NEC 250.9 ☑
      due to secondary diabetes 249.9 ☑
      specified NEC 250.8 ☑
        due to secondary diabetes
          249.8 ☑
    gangrene 250.7 ☑ [785.4]
      due to secondary diabetes
        249.7 ☑ [785.4]
    hyperglycemia — code to Diabetes, by
      type, with 5th digit for not stated
      as uncontrolled
    hyperosmolarity 250.2 ☑
      due to secondary diabetes 249.2 ☑
    ketosis, ketoacidosis 250.1 ☑
      due to secondary diabetes 249.1 ☑
    loss of protective sensation (LOPS) —
      see Diabetes, neuropathy
    osteomyelitis 250.8 ☑ [731.8]
      due to secondary diabetes
        249.8 ☑ [731.8]
    specified manisfestations NEC 250.8 ☑
      due to secondary diabetes 249.8 ☑
  acetonemia 250.1 ☑
    due to secondary diabetes 249.1 ☑
  acidosis 250.1 ☑
    due to secondary diabetes 249.1 ☑
  amyotrophy 250.6 ☑ [353.5]
    due to secondary diabetes
      249.6 ☑ [353.5]
  angiopathy, peripheral 250.7 ☑ [443.81]
    due to secondary diabetes
      249.7 ☑ [443.81]
  asymptomatic 790.29
  autonomic neuropathy (peripheral)
    250.6 ☑ [337.1]
    due to secondary diabetes
      249.6 ☑ [337.1]
  bone change 250.8 ☑ [731.8]
    due to secondary diabetes
      249.8 ☑ [731.8]
  borderline 790.29
  bronze, bronzed 275.01
  cataract 250.5 ☑ [366.41]
    due to secondary diabetes
      249.5 ☑ [366.41]
  chemical induced — see Diabetes, sec-
    ondary
  complicating pregnancy, childbirth, or
    puerperium 648.0 ☑
  coma (with ketoacidosis) 250.3 ☑
    due to secondary diabetes 249.3 ☑
    hyperglycemic 250.3 ☑
      due to secondary diabetes 249.3 ☑
    hyperosmolar (nonketotic) 250.2 ☑
      due to secondary diabetes 249.2 ☑
    hypoglycemic 250.3 ☑
      due to secondary diabetes 249.3 ☑
    insulin 250.3 ☑
      due to secondary diabetes 249.3 ☑
  complicating pregnancy, childbirth, or
    puerperium (maternal) (conditions
    classifiable to 249 and 250) 648.0 ☑
    affecting fetus or newborn 775.0
  complication NEC 250.9 ☑
    due to secondary diabetes 249.9 ☑
    specified NEC 250.8 ☑
      due to secondary diabetes 249.8 ☑
  dorsal sclerosis 250.6 ☑ [340]
    due to secondary diabetes
      249.6 ☑ [340]
  drug-induced — see also Diabetes, sec-
    ondary
    overdose or wrong substance given or
      taken — see Table of Drugs and
      Chemicals
  due to
    cystic fibrosis — see Diabetes, secondary
    infection — see Diabetes, secondary
  dwarfism-obesity syndrome 258.1
  gangrene 250.7 ☑ [785.4]
    due to secondary diabetes
      249.7 ☑ [785.4]

☑ **Additional Digit Required** — Refer to the Tabular List for Digit Selection   ▽ **Subterms under main terms may continue to next column or page**

Diabetes, diabetic — *continued*
gastroparesis 250.6 ☑ *[536.3]*
  due to secondary diabetes
    249.6 *[536.3]*
gestational 648.8 ☑
  complicating pregnancy, childbirth, or
    puerperium 648.8 ☑
glaucoma 250.5 *[365.44]*
  due to secondary diabetes
    249.5 *[365.44]*
glomerulosclerosis (intercapillary)
    250.4 ☑ *[581.81]*
  due to secondary diabetes
    249.4 ☑ *[581.81]*
glycogenosis, secondary 250.8 ☑ *[259.8]*
  due to secondary diabetes
    249.8 ☑ *[259.8]*
hemochromatosis (*see also* Hemochromatosis) 275.03
hyperosmolar coma 250.2 ☑
  due to secondary diabetes 249.2 ☑
hyperosmolarity 250.2 ☑
  due to secondary diabetes 249.2 ☑
hypertension-nephrosis syndrome
    250.4 ☑ *[581.81]*
  due to secondary diabetes
    249.4 ☑ *[581.81]*
hypoglycemia 250.8 ☑
  due to secondary diabetes 249.8 ☑
hypoglycemic shock 250.8 ☑
  due to secondary diabetes 249.8 ☑
inadequately controlled — code to Diabetes, by type, with 5th digit for not stated as uncontrolled
insipidus 253.5
  nephrogenic 588.1
  pituitary 253.5
  vasopressin-resistant 588.1
intercapillary glomerulosclerosis
    250.4 ☑ *[581.81]*
  due to secondary diabetes
    249.4 ☑ *[581.81]*
iritis 250.5 *[364.42]*
  due to secondary diabetes
    249.5 *[364.42]*
ketosis, ketoacidosis 250.1 ☑
  due to secondary diabetes 249.1 ☑
Kimmelstiel (-Wilson) disease or syndrome (intercapillary glomerulosclerosis) 250.4 ☑ *[581.81]*
  due to secondary diabetes
    249.4 ☑ *[581.81]*
Lancereaux's (diabetes mellitus with marked emaciation) 250.8 ☑ *[261]*
  due to secondary diabetes
    249.8 ☑ *[261]*
latent (chemical) — *see* Diabetes, secondary
complicating pregnancy, childbirth, or puerperium 648.8 ☑
lipoidosis 250.8 ☑ *[272.7]*
  due to secondary diabetes
    249.8 ☑ *[272.7]*
macular edema 250.5 ☑ *[362.07]*
  due to secondary diabetes
    249.5 *[362.07]*
maternal
  with manifest disease in the infant 775.1
  affecting fetus or newborn 775.0
microaneurysms, retinal 250.5 ☑ *[362.01]*
  due to secondary diabetes
    249.5 ☑ *[362.01]*
mononeuropathy 250.6 ☑ *[355.9]*
  due to secondary diabetes
    249.6 ☑ *[355.9]*
neonatal, transient 775.1
nephropathy 250.4 ☑ *[583.81]*
  due to secondary diabetes
    249.4 ☑ *[583.81]*
nephrosis (syndrome) 250.4 ☑ *[581.81]*
  due to secondary diabetes
    249.4 ☑ *[581.81]*
neuralgia 250.6 ☑ *[357.2]*
  due to secondary diabetes
    249.6 ☑ *[357.2]*

Diabetes, diabetic — *continued*
neuritis 250.6 ☑ *[357.2]*
  due to secondary diabetes
    249.6 ☑ *[357.2]*
neurogenic arthropathy 250.6 ☑ *[713.5]*
  due to secondary diabetes
    249.6 ☑ *[713.5]*
neuropathy 250.6 ☑ *[357.2]*
  autonomic (peripheral) 250.6 ☑ *[337.1]*
    due to secondary diabetes
     249.6 ☑ *[337.1]*
  due to secondary diabetes
    249.6 ☑ *[357.2]*
nonclinical 790.29
osteomyelitis 250.8 ☑ *[731.8]*
  due to secondary diabetes
    249.8 ☑ *[731.8]*
out of control — code to Diabetes, by type, with 5th digit for uncontrolled
peripheral autonomic neuropathy
    250.6 ☑ *[337.1]*
  due to secondary diabetes
    249.6 ☑ *[337.1]*
phosphate 275.3
polyneuropathy 250.6 ☑ *[357.2]*
  due to secondary diabetes
    249.6 ☑ *[357.2]*
poorly controlled — code to Diabetes, by type, with 5th digit for not stated as uncontrolled
renal (true) 271.4
retinal
  edema 250.5 ☑ *[362.07]*
    due to secondary diabetes
     249.5 ☑ *[362.07]*
  hemorrhage 250.5 ☑ *[362.01]*
    due to secondary diabetes
     249.5 ☑ *[362.01]*
  microaneurysms 250.5 ☑ *[362.01]*
    due to secondary diabetes
     249.5 ☑ *[362.01]*
  retinitis 250.5 ☑ *[362.01]*
    due to secondary diabetes
     249.5 ☑ *[362.01]*
  retinopathy 250.5 ☑ *[362.01]*
    background 250.5 ☑ *[362.01]*
     due to secondary diabetes
      249.5 ☑ *[362.01]*
    due to secondary diabetes
     249.5 ☑ *[362.01]*
    nonproliferative 250.5 ☑ *[362.03]*
     due to secondary diabetes
      249.5 ☑ *[362.03]*
     mild 250.5 ☑ *[362.04]*
      due to secondary diabetes
       249.5 ☑ *[362.04]*
     moderate 250.5 ☑ *[362.05]*
      due to secondary diabetes
       249.5 ☑ *[362.05]*
     severe 250.5 ☑ *[362.06]*
      due to secondary diabetes
       249.5 ☑ *[362.06]*
    proliferative 250.5 ☑ *[362.02]*
     due to secondary diabetes
      249.5 ☑ *[362.02]*
secondary (chemical-induced) (due to chronic condition) (due to infection) (drug-induced) 249.0 ☑
  with
    coma (with ketoacidosis) 249.3 ☑
     hyperosmolar (nonketotic)
      249.2 ☑
    complication NEC 249.9 ☑
     specified NEC 249.8 ☑
    gangrene 249.7 ☑ *[785.4]*
    hyperosmolarity 249.2 ☑
    ketosis, ketoacidosis 249.1 ☑
    osteomyelitis 249.8 ☑ *[731.8]*
    specified manifestations NEC
     249.8 ☑
  acetonemia 249.1 ☑
  acidosis 249.1 ☑
  amyotrophy 249.6 ☑ *[353.5]*
  angiopathy, peripheral 249.7 ☑ *[443.81]*

Diabetes, diabetic — *continued*
secondary — *continued*
  autonomic neuropathy (peripheral)
    249.6 ☑ *[337.1]*
  bone change 249.8 ☑ *[731.8]*
  cataract 249.5 ☑ *[366.41]*
  coma (with ketoacidosis) 249.3 ☑
    hyperglycemic 249.3 ☑
    hyperosmolar (nonketotic) 249.2 ☑
    hypoglycemic 249.3 ☑
    insulin 249.3 ☑
  complicating pregnancy, childbirth, or puerperium (maternal) 648.0 ☑
    affecting fetus or newborn 775.0
  complication NEC 249.9 ☑
    specified NEC 249.8 ☑
  dorsal sclerosis 249.6 ☑ *[340]*
  due to overdose or wrong substance given or taken — *see* Table of Drugs and Chemicals
  gangrene 249.7 ☑ *[785.4]*
  gastroparesis 249.6 ☑ *[536.3]*
  glaucoma 249.5 ☑ *[365.44]*
  glomerulosclerosis (intercapillary)
    249.4 ☑ *[581.81]*
  glycogenosis, secondary 249.8 ☑ *[259.8]*
  hyperosmolar coma 249.2 ☑
  hyperosmolarity 249.2 ☑
  hypertension-nephrosis syndrome
    249.4 ☑ *[581.81]*
  hypoglycemia 249.8 ☑
  hypoglycemic shock 249.8 ☑
  intercapillary glomerulosclerosis
    249.4 ☑ *[581.81]*
  iritis 249.5 ☑ *[364.42]*
  ketosis, ketoacidosis 249.1 ☑
  Kimmelstiel (-Wilson) disease or syndrome (intercapillary glomerulosclerosis) 249.4 ☑ *[581.81]*
  Lancereaux's (diabetes mellitus with marked emaciation)
    249.8 ☑ *[261]*
  lipoidosis 249.8 ☑ *[272.7]*
  macular edema 249.5 ☑ *[362.07]*
  maternal
    with manifest disease in the infant 775.1
    affecting fetus or newborn 775.0
  microaneurysms, retinal
    249.5 ☑ *[362.01]*
  mononeuropathy 249.6 ☑ *[355.9]*
  nephropathy 249.4 ☑ *[583.81]*
  nephrosis (syndrome) 249.4 ☑ *[581.81]*
  neuralgia 249.6 ☑ *[357.2]*
  neuritis 249.6 ☑ *[357.2]*
  neurogenic arthropathy 249.6 ☑ *[713.5]*
  neuropathy 249.6 ☑ *[357.2]*
    autonomic (peripheral)
     249.6 ☑ *[337.1]*
  osteomyelitis 249.8 ☑ *[731.8]*
  peripheral autonomic neuropathy
    249.6 ☑ *[337.1]*
  polyneuropathy 249.6 ☑ *[357.2]*
  retinal
    edema 249.5 ☑ *[362.07]*
    hemorrhage 249.5 ☑ *[362.01]*
    microaneurysms 249.5 ☑ *[362.01]*
    retinitis 249.5 ☑ *[362.01]*
    retinopathy 249.5 ☑ *[362.01]*
     background 249.5 ☑ *[362.01]*
     nonproliferative 249.5 ☑ *[362.03]*
      mild 249.5 ☑ *[362.04]*
      moderate 249.5 ☑ *[362.05]*
      severe 249.5 ☑ *[362.06]*
     proliferative 249.5 ☑ *[362.02]*
  ulcer (skin) 249.8 ☑ *[707.9]*
    lower extremity 249.8 ☑ *[707.10]*
     ankle 249.8 ☑ *[707.13]*
     calf 249.8 ☑ *[707.12]*
     foot 249.8 ☑ *[707.15]*
     heel 249.8 ☑ *[707.14]*
     knee 249.8 ☑ *[707.19]*
     specified site NEC
      249.8 ☑ *[707.19]*

Diabetes, diabetic — *continued*
secondary — *continued*
  ulcer — *continued*
    lower extemity — *continued*
     thigh 249.8 ☑ *[707.11]*
     toes 249.8 ☑ *[707.15]*
     specified site NEC 249.8 ☑ *[707.8]*
    xanthoma 249.8 ☑ *[272.2]*
  steroid induced — *see also* Diabetes, secondary
  overdose or wrong substance given or taken 962.0
  stress 790.29
  subclinical 790.29
  subliminal 790.29
  sugar 250.0 ☑
  ulcer (skin) 250.8 ☑ *[707.9]*
    due to secondary diabetes
     249.8 ☑ *[707.9]*
    lower extremity 250.8 ☑ *[707.10]*
     ankle 250.8 ☑ *[707.13]*
      due to secondary diabetes
       249.8 ☑ *[707.13]*
     calf 250.8 ☑ *[707.12]*
      due to secondary diabetes
       249.8 ☑ *[707.12]*
      due to secondary diabetes
       249.8 ☑ *[707.10]*
     foot 250.8 ☑ *[707.15]*
      due to secondary diabetes
       249.8 ☑ *[707.15]*
     heel 250.8 ☑ *[707.14]*
      due to secondary diabetes
       249.8 ☑ *[707.14]*
     knee 250.8 ☑ *[707.19]*
      due to secondary diabetes
       249.8 ☑ *[707.19]*
     specified site NEC 250.8 ☑ *[707.19]*
      due to secondary diabetes
       249.8 ☑ *[707.19]*
     thigh 250.8 ☑ *[707.11]*
      due to secondary diabetes
       249.8 ☑ *[707.11]*
     toes 250.8 ☑ *[707.15]*
      due to secondary diabetes
       249.8 ☑ *[707.15]*
    specified site NEC 250.8 ☑ *[707.8]*
     due to secondary diabetes
      249.8 ☑ *[707.8]*
  xanthoma 250.8 ☑ *[272.2]*
    due to secondary diabetes
     249.8 ☑ *[272.2]*
Diacyclothrombopathia 287.1
Diagnosis deferred 799.9
Dialysis (intermittent) (treatment)
  anterior retinal (juvenile) (with detachment) 361.04
  extracorporeal V56.0
  hemodialysis V56.0
    status only V45.11
  peritoneal V56.8
    status only V45.11
  renal V56.0
    status only V45.11
  specified type NEC V56.8
Diamond-Blackfan anemia or syndrome (congenital hypoplastic anemia) 284.01
Diamond-Gardener syndrome (autoerythrocyte sensitization) 287.2
Diaper rash 691.0
Diaphoresis (excessive) NEC — *see also* Hyperhidrosis 780.8
Diaphragm — *see* condition
Diaphragmalgia 786.52
Diaphragmitis 519.4
Diaphyseal aclasis 756.4
Diaphysitis 733.99
Diarrhea, diarrheal (acute) (autumn) (bilious) (bloody) (catarrhal) (choleraic) (chronic) (gravis) (green) (infantile) (lienteric) (noninfectious) (presumed noninfectious) (putrefactive) (secondary) (sporadic) (summer) (symptomatic) (thermic) 787.91
achlorhydric 536.0

☑ Additional Digit Required — Refer to the Tabular List for Digit Selection   ▼ Subterms under main terms may continue to next column or page

2015 ICD-9-CM   ▶◀ Revised Text   ● New Line   ▲ Revised Code   Volume 2 — 79

Diabetes, diabetic — Diarrhea, diarrheal

Diarrhea, diarrheal — *continued*
allergic 558.3
amebic (*see also* Amebiasis) 006.9
　with abscess — *see* Abscess, amebic
　acute 006.0
　chronic 006.1
　nondysenteric 006.2
bacillary — *see* Dysentery, bacillary
bacterial NEC 008.5
balantidial 007.0
bile salt-induced 579.8
cachectic NEC 787.91
chilomastix 007.8
choleriformis 001.1
coccidial 007.2
Cochin-China 579.1
　anguilluliasis 127.2
　psilosis 579.1
Dientamoeba 007.8
dietetic 787.91
due to
　achylia gastrica 536.8
　Aerobacter aerogenes 008.2
　Bacillus coli — *see* Enteritis, E. coli
　bacteria NEC 008.5
　bile salts 579.8
　Capillaria
　　hepatica 128.8
　　philippinensis 127.5
　Clostridium perfringens (C) (F) 008.46
　Enterobacter aerogenes 008.2
　enterococci 008.49
　Escherichia coli — *see* Enteritis, E. coli
　Giardia lamblia 007.1
　Heterophyes heterophyes 121.6
　irritating foods 787.91
　Metagonimus yokogawai 121.5
　Necator americanus 126.1
　Paracolobactrum arizonae 008.1
　Paracolon bacillus NEC 008.47
　　Arizona 008.1
　Proteus (bacillus) (mirabilis) (Morganii) 008.3
　Pseudomonas aeruginosa 008.42
　S. japonicum 120.2
　specified organism NEC 008.8
　　bacterial 008.49
　　viral NEC 008.69
　Staphylococcus 008.41
　Streptococcus 008.49
　　anaerobic 008.46
　Strongyloides stercoralis 127.2
　Trichuris trichiuria 127.3
　virus NEC (*see also* Enteritis, viral) 008.69
dysenteric 009.2
　due to specified organism NEC 008.8
dyspeptic 787.91
endemic 009.3
　due to specified organism NEC 008.8
epidemic 009.2
　due to specified organism NEC 008.8
fermentative 787.91
flagellate 007.9
Flexner's (ulcerative) 004.1
functional 564.5
　following gastrointestinal surgery 564.4
　psychogenic 306.4
giardial 007.1
Giardia lamblia 007.1
hill 579.1
hyperperistalsis (nervous) 306.4
infectious 009.2
　due to specified organism NEC 008.8
　presumed 009.3
inflammatory 787.91
　due to specified organism NEC 008.8
malarial (*see also* Malaria) 084.6
mite 133.8
mycotic 117.9
nervous 306.4
neurogenic 564.5
parenteral NEC 009.2
postgastrectomy 564.4
postvagotomy 564.4
prostaglandin induced 579.8
protozoal NEC 007.9

Diarrhea, diarrheal — *continued*
psychogenic 306.4
septic 009.2
　due to specified organism NEC 008.8
specified organism NEC 008.8
　bacterial 008.49
　viral NEC 008.69
Staphylococcus 008.41
Streptococcus 008.49
　anaerobic 008.46
toxic 558.2
travelers' 009.2
　due to specified organism NEC 008.8
trichomonal 007.3
tropical 579.1
tuberculous 014.8 ☑
ulcerative (chronic) (*see also* Colitis, ulcerative) 556.9
viral (*see also* Enteritis, viral) 008.8
zymotic NEC 009.2
Diastasis
cranial bones 733.99
　congenital 756.0
joint (traumatic) — *see* Dislocation, by site
muscle 728.84
　congenital 756.89
recti (abdomen) 728.84
　complicating delivery 665.8 ☑
　congenital 756.79
Diastema, teeth, tooth 524.30
Diastematomyelia 742.51
Diataxia, cerebral, infantile 343.0
Diathesis
allergic V15.09
bleeding (familial) 287.9
cystine (familial) 270.0
gouty 274.9
hemorrhagic (familial) 287.9
　newborn NEC 776.0
oxalic 271.8
scrofulous (*see also* Tuberculosis) 017.2 ☑
spasmophilic (*see also* Tetany) 781.7
ulcer 536.9
uric acid 274.9
Diaz's disease or osteochondrosis 732.5
Dibothriocephaliasis 123.4
larval 123.5
Dibothriocephalus (infection) (infestation) (latus) 123.4
larval 123.5
Dicephalus 759.4
Dichotomy, teeth 520.2
Dichromat, dichromata (congenital) 368.59
Dichromatopsia (congenital) 368.59
Dichuchwa 104.0
Dicroceliasis 121.8
Didelphys, didelphic — *see also* Double uterus 752.2
Didymitis — *see also* Epididymitis 604.90
Died — *see also* Death
without
　medical attention (cause unknown) 798.9
　sign of disease 798.2
Dientamoeba diarrhea 007.8
Dietary
inadequacy or deficiency 269.9
surveillance and counseling V65.3
Dietl's crisis 593.4
Dieulafoy lesion (hemorrhagic)
of
　duodenum 537.84
　esophagus 530.82
　intestine 569.86
　stomach 537.84
Difficult
birth, affecting fetus or newborn 763.9
delivery NEC 669.9 ☑
Difficulty
feeding 783.3
　adult 783.3
　breast 676.8 ☑
　child 783.3
　elderly 783.3
　infant 783.3
　newborn 779.31

Difficulty — *continued*
feeding — *continued*
　nonorganic (infant) NEC 307.59
mechanical, gastroduodenal stoma 537.89
reading 315.00
specific, spelling 315.09
swallowing (*see also* Dysphagia) 787.20
walking 719.7
Diffuse — *see* condition
Diffused ganglion 727.42
Di George's syndrome (thymic hypoplasia) 279.11
Digestive — *see* condition
Di Guglielmo's disease or syndrome (M9841/3) 207.0 ☑
Dihydropyrimidine dehydrogenase disease (DPD) 277.6
Diktyoma (M9051/3) — *see* Neoplasm, by site, malignant
Dilaceration, tooth 520.4
Dilatation
anus 564.89
　venule — *see* Hemorrhoids
aorta (focal) (general) (*see also* Ectasia, aortic) 447.70
　with aneurysm 441.9
　congenital 747.29
　infectional 093.0
　ruptured 441.5
　syphilitic 093.0
appendix (cystic) 543.9
artery 447.8
bile duct (common) (congenital) 751.69
　acquired 576.8
bladder (sphincter) 596.89
　congenital 753.8
　in pregnancy or childbirth 654.4 ☑
　　causing obstructed labor 660.2 ☑
　　　affecting fetus or newborn 763.1
blood vessel 459.89
bronchus, bronchi 494.0
　with acute exacerbation 494.1
calyx (due to obstruction) 593.89
capillaries 448.9
cardiac (acute) (chronic) (*see also* Hypertrophy, cardiac) 429.3
　congenital 746.89
　　valve NEC 746.89
　　　pulmonary 746.09
　hypertensive (*see also* Hypertension, heart) 402.90
cavum septi pellucidi 742.4
cecum 564.89
　psychogenic 306.4
cervix (uteri) (*see also* Incompetency, cervix)
　incomplete, poor, slow
　　affecting fetus or newborn 763.7
　　complicating delivery 661.0 ☑
　　　affecting fetus or newborn 763.7
colon 564.7
　congenital 751.3
　due to mechanical obstruction 560.89
　psychogenic 306.4
common bile duct (congenital) 751.69
　acquired 576.8
　　with calculus, choledocholithiasis, or stones — *see* Choledocholithiasis
cystic duct 751.69
　acquired (any bile duct) 575.8
duct, mammary 610.4
duodenum 564.89
esophagus 530.89
　congenital 750.4
　due to
　　achalasia 530.0
　　cardiospasm 530.0
Eustachian tube, congenital 744.24
fontanel 756.0
gallbladder 575.8
　congenital 751.69
gastric 536.8
　acute 536.1
　psychogenic 306.4
heart (acute) (chronic) (*see also* Hypertrophy, cardiac) 429.3

Dilatation — *continued*
heart (*see also* Hypertrophy, cardiac) — *continued*
　congenital 746.89
　hypertensive (*see also* Hypertension, heart) 402.90
　valve (*see also* Endocarditis)
　　congenital 746.89
ileum 564.89
　psychogenic 306.4
inguinal rings — *see* Hernia, inguinal
jejunum 564.89
　psychogenic 306.4
kidney (calyx) (collecting structures) (cystic) (parenchyma) (pelvis) 593.89
lacrimal passages 375.69
lymphatic vessel 457.1
mammary duct 610.4
Meckel's diverticulum (congenital) 751.0
meningeal vessels, congenital 742.8
myocardium (acute) (chronic) (*see also* Hypertrophy, cardiac) 429.3
organ or site, congenital NEC — *see* Distortion
pancreatic duct 577.8
pelvis, kidney 593.89
pericardium — *see* Pericarditis
pharynx 478.29
prostate 602.8
pulmonary
　artery (idiopathic) 417.8
　　congenital 747.39
　valve, congenital 746.09
pupil 379.43
rectum 564.89
renal 593.89
saccule vestibularis, congenital 744.05
salivary gland (duct) 527.8
sphincter ani 564.89
stomach 536.8
　acute 536.1
　psychogenic 306.4
submaxillary duct 527.8
trachea, congenital 748.3
ureter (idiopathic) 593.89
　congenital 753.20
　due to obstruction 593.5
urethra (acquired) 599.84
vasomotor 443.9
vein 459.89
ventricular, ventricle (acute) (chronic) (*see also* Hypertrophy, cardiac) 429.3
　cerebral, congenital 742.4
　hypertensive (*see also* Hypertension, heart) 402.90
venule 459.89
　anus — *see* Hemorrhoids
vesical orifice 596.89
Dilated, dilation — *see* Dilatation
Diminished
hearing (acuity) (*see also* Deafness) 389.9
pulse pressure 785.9
vision NEC 369.9
vital capacity 794.2
Diminuta taenia 123.6
Diminution, sense or sensation (cold) (heat) (tactile) (vibratory) — *see also* Disturbance, sensation 782.0
Dimitri-Sturge-Weber disease (encephalocutaneous angiomatosis) 759.6
Dimple
parasacral 685.1
　with abscess 685.0
pilonidal 685.1
　with abscess 685.0
postanal 685.1
　with abscess 685.0
Dioctophyma renale (infection) (infestation) 128.8
Dipetalonemiasis 125.4
Diphallus 752.69
Diphtheria, diphtheritic (gangrenous) (hemorrhagic) 032.9
carrier (suspected) of V02.4
cutaneous 032.85
cystitis 032.84

☑ **Additional Digit Required — Refer to the Tabular List for Digit Selection**　　　　　　　　　　　Ⓝ **Subterms under main terms may continue to next column or page**

Diphtheria, diphtheritic — *continued*
  faucial 032.0
  infection of wound 032.85
  inoculation (anti) (not sick) V03.5
  laryngeal 032.3
  myocarditis 032.82
  nasal anterior 032.2
  nasopharyngeal 032.1
  neurological complication 032.89
  peritonitis 032.83
  specified site NEC 032.89
Diphyllobothriasis (intestine) 123.4
  larval 123.5
Diplacusis 388.41
Diplegia (upper limbs) 344.2
  brain or cerebral 437.8
  congenital 343.0
  facial 351.0
    congenital 352.6
  infantile or congenital (cerebral) (spastic) (spinal) 343.0
  lower limbs 344.1
  syphilitic, congenital 090.49
Diplococcus, diplococcal — *see* condition
Diplomyelia 742.59
Diplopia 368.2
  refractive 368.15
Dipsomania — *see also* Alcoholism 303.9 ☑
  with psychosis (*see also* Psychosis, alcoholic) 291.9
Dipylidiasis 123.8
  intestine 123.8
Direction, teeth, abnormal 524.30
Dirt-eating child 307.52
Disability, disabilities
  heart — *see* Disease, heart
  intellectual 319
    borderline V62.89
    mild, IQ 50-70 317
    moderate, IQ 35-49 318.0
    profound, IQ under 20 318.2
    severe, IQ 20-34 318.1
  learning NEC 315.2
  special spelling 315.09
Disarticulation — *see also* Derangement, joint 718.9 ☑
  meaning
    amputation
      status — *see* Absence, by site
      traumatic — *see* Amputation, traumatic
    dislocation, traumatic or congenital — *see* Dislocation
Disaster, cerebrovascular — *see also* Disease, cerebrovascular, acute 436
Discharge
  anal NEC 787.99
  breast (female) (male) 611.79
  conjunctiva 372.89
  continued locomotor idiopathic (*see also* Epilepsy) 345.5 ☑
  diencephalic autonomic idiopathic (*see also* Epilepsy) 345.5 ☑
  ear 388.60
    blood 388.69
    cerebrospinal fluid 388.61
  excessive urine 788.42
  eye 379.93
  nasal 478.19
  nipple 611.79
  patterned motor idiopathic (*see also* Epilepsy) 345.5 ☑
  penile 788.7
  postnasal — *see* Sinusitis
  sinus, from mediastinum 510.0
  umbilicus 789.9
  urethral 788.7
    bloody 599.84
  vaginal 623.5
Discitis 722.90
  cervical, cervicothoracic 722.91
  lumbar, lumbosacral 722.93
  thoracic, thoracolumbar 722.92
Discogenic syndrome — *see* Displacement, intervertebral disc

Discoid
  kidney 753.3
  meniscus, congenital 717.5
  semilunar cartilage 717.5
Discoloration
  mouth 528.9
  nails 703.8
  teeth 521.7
    due to
      drugs 521.7
      metals (copper) (silver) 521.7
      pulpal bleeding 521.7
    during formation 520.8
    extrinsic 523.6
    intrinsic posteruptive 521.7
Discomfort
  chest 786.59
  visual 368.13
Discomycosis — *see* Actinomycosis
Discontinuity, ossicles, ossicular chain 385.23
Discrepancy
  centric occlusion
    maximum intercuspation 524.55
    of teeth 524.55
  leg length (acquired) 736.81
    congenital 755.30
  uterine size-date 649.6 ☑
Discrimination
  political V62.4
  racial V62.4
  religious V62.4
  sex V62.4
Disease, diseased — *see also* Syndrome
  Abrami's (acquired hemolytic jaundice) 283.9
  absorbent system 459.89
  accumulation — *see* Thesaurismosis
  acid-peptic 536.8
  Acosta's 993.2
  Adams-Stokes (-Morgagni) (syncope with heart block) 426.9
  Addison's (bronze) (primary adrenal insufficiency) 255.41
    anemia (pernicious) 281.0
    tuberculous (*see also* Tuberculosis) 017.6 ☑
  Addison-Gull — *see* Xanthoma
  adenoids (and tonsils) (chronic) 474.9
  adrenal (gland) (capsule) (cortex) 255.9
    hyperfunction 255.3
    hypofunction 255.41
    specified type NEC 255.8
  ainhum (dactylolysis spontanea) 136.0
  akamushi (scrub typhus) 081.2
  Akureyri (epidemic neuromyasthenia) 049.8
  Albarrán's (colibacilluria) 791.9
  Albers-Schönberg's (marble bones) 756.52
  Albert's 726.71
  Albright (-Martin) (-Bantam) 275.49
  Alibert's (mycosis fungoides) (M9700/3) 202.1 ☑
  Alibert-Bazin (M9700/3) 202.1 ☑
  alimentary canal 569.9
  alligator skin (ichthyosis congenita) 757.1
    acquired 701.1
  Almeida's (Brazilian blastomycosis) 116.1
  Alpers' 330.8
  alpine 993.2
  altitude 993.2
  alveoli, teeth 525.9
  Alzheimer's — *see* Alzheimer's
  amyloid (any site) 277.30
  anarthritic rheumatoid 446.5
  Anders' (adiposis tuberosa simplex) 272.8
  Andersen's (glycogenosis IV) 271.0
  Anderson's (angiokeratoma corporis diffusum) 272.7
  Andes 993.2
  Andrews' (bacterid) 686.8
  angiospastic, angiospasmodic 443.9
    cerebral 435.9
      with transient neurologic deficit 435.9
    vein 459.89

Disease, diseased — *see also* Syndrome — *continued*
  anterior
    chamber 364.9
    horn cell 335.9
      specified type NEC 335.8
  antral (chronic) 473.0
    acute 461.0
  anus NEC 569.49
  aorta (nonsyphilitic) 447.9
    syphilitic NEC 093.89
  aortic (heart) (valve) (*see also* Endocarditis, aortic) 424.1
  apollo 077.4
  aponeurosis 726.90
  appendix 543.9
  aqueous (chamber) 364.9
  arc-welders' lung 503
  Armenian 277.31
  Arnold-Chiari (*see also* Spina bifida) 741.0 ☑
  arterial 447.9
    occlusive (*see also* Occlusion, by site) 444.22
      with embolus or thrombus — *see* Occlusion, by site
    due to stricture or stenosis 447.1
    specified type NEC 447.8
  arteriocardiorenal — *see* Hypertension, cardiorenal
  arteriolar (generalized) (obliterative) 447.9
    specified type NEC 447.8
  arteriorenal — *see* Hypertension, kidney
  arteriosclerotic (*see also* Arteriosclerosis)
    cardiovascular 429.2
    coronary — *see* Arteriosclerosis, coronary
    heart — *see* Arteriosclerosis, coronary
    vascular — *see* Arteriosclerosis
  artery 447.9
    cerebral 437.9
    coronary — *see* Arteriosclerosis, coronary
    specified type NEC 447.8
  arthropod-borne NEC 088.9
    specified type NEC 088.89
  Asboe-Hansen's (incontinentia pigmenti) 757.33
  atticoantral, chronic (with posterior or superior marginal perforation of ear drum) 382.2
  auditory canal, ear 380.9
  Aujeszky's 078.89
  auricle, ear NEC 380.30
  autoimmune NEC 279.49
    hemolytic (cold type) (warm type) 283.0
    parathyroid 252.1
    thyroid 245.2
  aviators' (*see also* Effect, adverse, high altitude) 993.2
  ax(e)-grinders' 502
  Ayala's 756.89
  Ayerza's (pulmonary artery sclerosis with pulmonary hypertension) 416.0
  Azorean (of the nervous system) 334.8
  Babington's (familial hemorrhagic telangiectasia) 448.0
  back bone NEC 733.90
  bacterial NEC 040.89
    zoonotic NEC 027.9
      specified type NEC 027.8
  Baehr-Schiffrin (thrombotic thrombocytopenic purpura) 446.6
  Baelz's (cheilitis glandularis apostematosa) 528.5
  Baerensprung's (eczema marginatum) 110.3
  Balfour's (chloroma) 205.3 ☑
  balloon (*see also* Effect, adverse, high altitude) 993.2
  Baló's 341.1
  Bamberger (-Marie) (hypertrophic pulmonary osteoarthropathy) 731.2
  Bang's (Brucella abortus) 023.1
  Bannister's 995.1
  Banti's (with cirrhosis) (with portal hypertension) — *see* Cirrhosis, liver

Disease, diseased — *see also* Syndrome — *continued*
  Barcoo (*see also* Ulcer, skin) 707.9
  barium lung 503
  Barlow (-Möller) (infantile scurvy) 267
  barometer makers' 985.0
  Barraquer (-Simons) (progressive lipodystrophy) 272.6
  basal ganglia 333.90
    degenerative NEC 333.0
    specified NEC 333.89
  Basedow's (exophthalmic goiter) 242.0 ☑
  basement membrane NEC 583.89
    with
      pulmonary hemorrhage (Goodpasture's syndrome) 446.21 [583.81]
  Bateman's 078.0
    purpura (senile) 287.2
  Batten's 330.1 [362.71]
  Batten-Mayou (retina) 330.1 [362.71]
  Batten-Steinert 359.21
  Battey 031.0
  Baumgarten-Cruveilhier (cirrhosis of liver) 571.5
  bauxite-workers' 503
  Bayle's (dementia paralytica) 094.1
  Bazin's (primary) (*see also* Tuberculosis) 017.1 ☑
  Beard's (neurasthenia) 300.5
  Beau's (*see also* Degeneration, myocardial) 429.1
  Bechterew's (ankylosing spondylitis) 720.0
  Becker's
    idiopathic mural endomyocardial disease 425.2
    myotonia congenita, recessive form 359.22
  Begbie's (exophthalmic goiter) 242.0 ☑
  Behr's 362.50
  Beigel's (white piedra) 111.2
  Bekhterev's (ankylosing spondylitis) 720.0
  Bell's (*see also* Psychosis, affective) 296.0 ☑
  Bennett's (leukemia) 208.9 ☑
  Benson's 379.22
  Bergeron's (hysteroepilepsy) 300.11
  Berlin's 921.3
  Bernard-Soulier (thrombopathy) 287.1
  Bernhardt (-Roth) 355.1
  beryllium 503
  Besnier-Boeck (-Schaumann) (sarcoidosis) 135
  Best's 362.76
  Beurmann's (sporotrichosis) 117.1
  Bielschowsky (-Jansky) 330.1
  Biermer's (pernicious anemia) 281.0
  Biett's (discoid lupus erythematosus) 695.4
  bile duct (*see also* Disease, biliary) 576.9
  biliary (duct) (tract) 576.9
    with calculus, choledocholithiasis, or stones — *see* Choledocholithiasis
  Billroth's (meningocele) (*see also* Spina bifida) 741.9 ☑
  Binswanger's 290.12
  Bird's (oxaluria) 271.8
  bird fanciers' 495.2
  black lung 500
  bladder 596.9
    specified NEC 596.89
  bleeder's 286.0
  Bloch-Sulzberger (incontinentia pigmenti) 757.33
  Blocq's (astasia-abasia) 307.9
  blood (-forming organs) 289.9
    specified NEC 289.89
    vessel 459.9
  Bloodgood's 610.1
  Blount's (tibia vara) 732.4
  blue 746.9
  Bodechtel-Guttmann (subacute sclerosing panencephalitis) 046.2
  Boeck's (sarcoidosis) 135
  bone 733.90
    fibrocystic NEC 733.29
      jaw 526.2
    marrow 289.9

☑ **Additional Digit Required** — Refer to the Tabular List for Digit Selection

◪ **Subterms under main terms may continue to next column or page**

Disease, diseased — *see also* Syndrome — *continued*

bone — *continued*
  Paget's (osteitis deformans) 731.0
    specified type NEC 733.99
  von Recklinghausen's (osteitis fibrosa cystica) 252.01
Bonfils' — *see* Disease, Hodgkin's
Borna 062.9
Bornholm (epidemic pleurodynia) 074.1
Bostock's (*see also* Fever, hay) 477.9
Bouchard's (myopathic dilatation of the stomach) 536.1
Bouillaud's (rheumatic heart disease) 391.9
Bourneville (-Brissaud) (tuberous sclerosis) 759.5
Bouveret (-Hoffmann) (paroxysmal tachycardia) 427.2
bowel 569.9
  functional 564.9
    psychogenic 306.4
Bowen's (M8081/2) — *see* Neoplasm, skin, in situ
Bozzolo's (multiple myeloma) (M9730/3) 203.0 ☑
Bradley's (epidemic vomiting) 078.82
Brailsford's 732.3
  radius, head 732.3
  tarsal, scaphoid 732.5
Brailsford-Morquio (mucopolysaccharidosis IV) 277.5
brain 348.9
  Alzheimer's 331.0
    with dementia — *see* Alzheimer's, dementia
  arterial, artery 437.9
  arteriosclerotic 437.0
  congenital 742.9
  degenerative — *see* Degeneration, brain
  inflammatory (*see also* Encephalitis)
    late effect — *see* category 326
  organic 348.9
    arteriosclerotic 437.0
  parasitic NEC 123.9
  Pick's 331.11
    with dementia
      with behavioral disturbance 331.11 [294.11]
      without behavioral disturbance 331.11 [294.10]
  senile 331.2
braziers' 985.8
breast 611.9
  cystic (chronic) 610.1
  fibrocystic 610.1
  inflammatory 611.0
  Paget's (M8540/3) 174.0
  puerperal, postpartum NEC 676.3 ☑
  specified NEC 611.89
Breda's (*see also* Yaws) 102.9
Breisky's (kraurosis vulvae) 624.09
Bretonneau's (diphtheritic malignant angina) 032.0
Bright's (*see also* Nephritis) 583.9
  arteriosclerotic (*see also* Hypertension, kidney) 403.90
Brill's (recrudescent typhus) 081.1
  flea-borne 081.0
  louse-borne 081.1
Brill-Symmers (follicular lymphoma) (M9690/3) 202.0 ☑
Brill-Zinsser (recrudescent typhus) 081.1
Brinton's (leather bottle stomach) (M8142/3) 151.9
Brion-Kayser (*see also* Fever, paratyphoid) 002.9
broad
  beta 272.2
  ligament, noninflammatory 620.9
    specified NEC 620.8
Brocq's 691.8
  meaning
    atopic (diffuse) neurodermatitis 691.8
    dermatitis herpetiformis 694.0
    lichen simplex chronicus 698.3

Disease, diseased — *see also* Syndrome — *continued*

Brocq's — *continued*
  meaning — *continued*
    parapsoriasis 696.2
    prurigo 698.2
Brocq-Duhring (dermatitis herpetiformis) 694.0
Brodie's (joint) (*see also* Osteomyelitis) 730.1 ☑
bronchi 519.19
bronchopulmonary 519.19
bronze (Addison's) 255.41
  tuberculous (*see also* Tuberculosis) 017.6 ☑
Brown-Séquard 344.89
Bruck's 733.99
Bruck-de Lange (Amsterdam dwarf, intellectual disabilities, and brachycephaly) 759.89
Bruhl's (splenic anemia with fever) 285.8
Bruton's (X-linked agammaglobulinemia) 279.04
buccal cavity 528.9
Buchanan's (juvenile osteochondrosis, iliac crest) 732.1
Buchman's (osteochondrosis juvenile) 732.1
Budgerigar-Fanciers' 495.2
Büdinger-Ludloff-Läwen 717.89
Buerger's (thromboangiitis obliterans) 443.1
Bürger-Grütz (essential familial hyperlipemia) 272.3
Burns' (lower ulna) 732.3
bursa 727.9
Bury's (erythema elevatum diutinum) 695.89
Buschke's 710.1
Busquet's (*see also* Osteomyelitis) 730.1 ☑
Busse-Buschke (cryptococcosis) 117.5
C₂ (*see also* Alcoholism) 303.9 ☑
Caffey's (infantile cortical hyperostosis) 756.59
caisson 993.3
calculous 592.9
California 114.0
Calvé (-Perthes) (osteochondrosis, femoral capital) 732.1
Camurati-Engelmann (diaphyseal sclerosis) 756.59
Canavan's 330.0
capillaries 448.9
Carapata 087.1
cardiac — *see* Disease, heart
cardiopulmonary, chronic 416.9
cardiorenal (arteriosclerotic) (hepatic) (hypertensive) (vascular) (*see also* Hypertension, cardiorenal) 404.90
cardiovascular (arteriosclerotic) 429.2
  congenital 746.9
  hypertensive (*see also* Hypertension, heart) 402.90
    benign 402.10
    malignant 402.00
  renal (*see also* Hypertension, cardiorenal) 404.90
  syphilitic (asymptomatic) 093.9
carotid gland 259.8
Carrión's (Bartonellosis) 088.0
cartilage NEC 733.90
  specified NEC 733.99
Castellani's 104.8
cat-scratch 078.3
Cavare's (familial periodic paralysis) 359.3
Cazenave's (pemphigus) 694.4
cecum 569.9
celiac (adult) 579.0
  infantile 579.0
cellular tissue NEC 709.9
central core 359.0
cerebellar, cerebellum — *see* Disease, brain
cerebral (*see also* Disease, brain) 348.9
  arterial, artery 437.9
  degenerative — *see* Degeneration, brain
cerebrospinal 349.9
cerebrovascular NEC 437.9
  acute 436
    embolic — *see* Embolism, brain

Disease, diseased — *see also* Syndrome — *continued*

cerebrovascular — *continued*
  acute — *continued*
    late effect — *see* Late effect(s) (of) cerebrovascular disease
    puerperal, postpartum, childbirth 674.0 ☑
    thrombotic — *see* Thrombosis, brain
  arteriosclerotic 437.0
  embolic — *see* Embolism, brain
  ischemic, generalized NEC 437.1
  late effect — *see* Late effect(s) (of) cerebrovascular disease
  occlusive 437.1
  puerperal, postpartum, childbirth 674.0 ☑
  specified type NEC 437.8
  thrombotic — *see* Thrombosis, brain
ceroid storage 272.7
cervix (uteri)
  inflammatory 616.0
  noninflammatory 622.9
    specified NEC 622.8
Chabert's 022.9
Chagas' (*see also* Trypanosomiasis, American) 086.2
Chandler's (osteochondritis dissecans, hip) 732.7
Charcôt-Marie-Tooth 356.1
Charcôt's (joint) 094.0 [713.5]
  spinal cord 094.0
Charlouis' (*see also* Yaws) 102.9
Cheadle (-Möller) (-Barlow) (infantile scurvy) 267
Chédiak-Steinbrinck (-Higashi) (congenital gigantism of peroxidase granules) 288.2
cheek, inner 528.9
chest 519.9
Chiari's (hepatic vein thrombosis) 453.0
Chicago (North American blastomycosis) 116.0
chignon (white piedra) 111.2
chigoe, chigo (jigger) 134.1
childhood granulomatous 288.1
Chinese liver fluke 121.1
chlamydial NEC 078.88
cholecystic (*see also* Disease, gallbladder) 575.9
choroid 363.9
  degenerative (*see also* Degeneration, choroid) 363.40
  hereditary (*see also* Dystrophy, choroid) 363.50
  specified type NEC 363.8
Christian's (chronic histiocytosis X) 277.89
Christian-Weber (nodular nonsuppurative panniculitis) 729.30
Christmas 286.1
ciliary body 364.9
  specified NEC 364.89
circulatory (system) NEC 459.9
  chronic, maternal, affecting fetus or newborn 760.3
  specified NEC 459.89
  syphilitic 093.9
    congenital 090.5
Civatte's (poikiloderma) 709.09
climacteric 627.2
  male 608.89
coagulation factor deficiency (congenital) (*see also* Defect, coagulation) 286.9
Coats' 362.12
coccidioidal pulmonary 114.5
  acute 114.0
  chronic 114.4
  primary 114.0
  residual 114.4
Cockayne's (microcephaly and dwarfism) 759.89
Cogan's 370.52
cold
  agglutinin 283.0
    or hemoglobinuria 283.0

Disease, diseased — *see also* Syndrome — *continued*

cold — *continued*
  agglutinin — *continued*
    or hemoglobinuria — *continued*
      paroxysmal (cold) (nocturnal) 283.2
  hemagglutinin (chronic) 283.0
collagen NEC 710.9
  nonvascular 710.9
  specified NEC 710.8
  vascular (allergic) (*see also* Angiitis, hypersensitivity) 446.20
colon 569.9
  functional 564.9
    congenital 751.3
  ischemic 557.0
combined system (of spinal cord) 266.2 [336.2]
  with anemia (pernicious) 281.0 [336.2]
compressed air 993.3
Concato's (pericardial polyserositis) 423.2
  peritoneal 568.82
  pleural — *see* Pleurisy
congenital NEC 799.89
conjunctiva 372.9
  chlamydial 077.98
    specified NEC 077.8
  specified type NEC 372.89
  viral 077.99
    specified NEC 077.8
connective tissue, diffuse (*see also* Disease, collagen) 710.9
Conor and Bruch's (boutonneuse fever) 082.1
Conradi (-Hünermann) 756.59
Cooley's (erythroblastic anemia) 282.44
Cooper's 610.1
Corbus' 607.1
cork-handlers' 495.3
cornea (*see also* Keratopathy) 371.9
coronary (*see also* Ischemia, heart) 414.9
  congenital 746.85
  ostial, syphilitic 093.20
    aortic 093.22
    mitral 093.21
    pulmonary 093.24
    tricuspid 093.23
Corrigan's — *see* Insufficiency, aortic
Cotugno's 724.3
Coxsackie (virus) NEC 074.8
cranial nerve NEC 352.9
Creutzfeldt-Jakob (CJD) 046.19
  with dementia
    with behavioral disturbance 046.19 [294.11]
    without behavioral disturbance 046.19 [294.10]
  familial 046.19
  iatrogenic 046.19
  specified NEC 046.19
  sporadic 046.19
  variant (vCJD) 046.11
    with dementia
      with behavioral disturbance 046.11 [294.11]
      without behavioral disturbance 046.11 [294.10]
Crigler-Najjar (congenital hyperbilirubinemia) 277.4
Crocq's (acrocyanosis) 443.89
Crohn's (intestine) (*see also* Enteritis, regional) 555.9
Crouzon's (craniofacial dysostosis) 756.0
Cruchet's (encephalitis lethargica) 049.8
Cruveilhier's 335.21
Cruz-Chagas (*see also* Trypanosomiasis, American) 086.2
crystal deposition (*see also* Arthritis, due to, crystals) 712.9 ☑
Csillag's (lichen sclerosus et atrophicus) 701.0
Curschmann's 359.21
Cushing's (pituitary basophilism) 255.0
cystic
  breast (chronic) 610.1

☑ **Additional Digit Required** — Refer to the Tabular List for Digit Selection   ▽ **Subterms under main terms may continue to next column or page**

82 — Volume 2   ▶◀ **Revised Text**   ● **New Line**   ▲ **Revised Code**   **2015 ICD-9-CM**

Disease, diseased — *see also* Syndrome — *continued*
cystic — *continued*
kidney, congenital (*see also* Cystic, disease, kidney) 753.10
liver, congenital 751.62
lung 518.89
congenital 748.4
pancreas 577.2
congenital 751.7
renal, congenital (*see also* Cystic, disease, kidney) 753.10
semilunar cartilage 717.5
cysticercus 123.1
cystine storage (with renal sclerosis) 270.0
cytomegalic inclusion (generalized) 078.5
with
pneumonia 078.5 [484.1]
congenital 771.1
Daae (-Finsen) (epidemic pleurodynia) 074.1
dancing 297.8
Danielssen's (anesthetic leprosy) 030.1
Darier's (congenital) (keratosis follicularis) 757.39
erythema annulare centrifugum 695.0
vitamin A deficiency 264.8
Darling's (histoplasmosis) (*see also* Histoplasmosis, American) 115.00
Davies' 425.0
de Beurmann-Gougerot (sporotrichosis) 117.1
Débove's (splenomegaly) 789.2
deer fly (*see also* Tularemia) 021.9
deficiency 269.9
degenerative (*see also* Degeneration)
disc — *see* Degeneration, intervertebral disc
Degos' 447.8
Déjérine (-Sottas) 356.0
Déleage's 359.89
demyelinating, demyelinizing (brain stem) (central nervous system) 341.9
multiple sclerosis 340
specified NEC 341.8
de Quervain's (tendon sheath) 727.04
thyroid (subacute granulomatous thyroiditis) 245.1
Dercum's (adiposis dolorosa) 272.8
Deutschländer's — *see* Fracture, foot
Devergie's (pityriasis rubra pilaris) 696.4
Devic's 341.0
diaphorase deficiency 289.7
diaphragm 519.4
diarrheal, infectious 009.2
diatomaceous earth 502
Diaz's (osteochondrosis astragalus) 732.5
digestive system 569.9
Di Guglielmo's (erythemic myelosis) (M9841/3) 207.0 ☑
Dimitri-Sturge-Weber (encephalocutaneous angiomatosis) 759.6
disc, degenerative — *see* Degeneration, intervertebral disc
discogenic (*see also* Disease, intervertebral disc) 722.90
diverticular — *see* Diverticula
Down's (mongolism) 758.0
Dubini's (electric chorea) 049.8
Dubois' (thymus gland) 090.5
Duchenne's 094.0
locomotor ataxia 094.0
muscular dystrophy 359.1
paralysis 335.22
pseudohypertrophy, muscles 359.1
Duchenne-Griesinger 359.1
ductless glands 259.9
Duhring's (dermatitis herpetiformis) 694.0
Dukes (-Filatov) 057.8
duodenum NEC 537.9
specified NEC 537.89
Duplay's 726.2
Dupré's (meningism) 781.6
Dupuytren's (muscle contracture) 728.6
Durand-Nicolas-Favre (climatic bubo) 099.1
Duroziez's (congenital mitral stenosis) 746.5
Dutton's (trypanosomiasis) 086.9

Disease, diseased — *see also* Syndrome — *continued*
Eales' 362.18
ear (chronic) (inner) NEC 388.9
middle 385.9
adhesive (*see also* Adhesions, middle ear) 385.10
specified NEC 385.89
Eberth's (typhoid fever) 002.0
Ebstein's
heart 746.2
meaning diabetes 250.4 ☑ [581.81]
due to secondary diabetes 249.4 ☑ [581.81]
Echinococcus (*see also* Echinococcus) 122.9
ECHO virus NEC 078.89
Economo's (encephalitis lethargica) 049.8
Eddowes' (brittle bones and blue sclera) 756.51
Edsall's 992.2
Eichstedt's (pityriasis versicolor) 111.0
Ellis-van Creveld (chondroectodermal dysplasia) 756.55
endocardium — *see* Endocarditis
endocrine glands or system NEC 259.9
specified NEC 259.8
endomyocardial, idiopathic mural 425.2
Engelmann's (diaphyseal sclerosis) 756.59
Engel-von Recklinghausen (osteitis fibrosa cystica) 252.01
English (rickets) 268.0
Engman's (infectious eczematoid dermatitis) 690.8
enteroviral, enterovirus NEC 078.89
central nervous system NEC 048
epidemic NEC 136.9
epididymis 608.9
epigastric, functional 536.9
psychogenic 306.4
Erb (-Landouzy) 359.1
Erb-Goldflam 358.00
Erdheim-Chester (ECD) 277.89
Erichsen's (railway spine) 300.16
esophagus 530.9
functional 530.5
psychogenic 306.4
Eulenburg's (congenital paramyotonia) 359.29
Eustachian tube 381.9
Evans' (thrombocytopenic purpura) 287.32
external auditory canal 380.9
extrapyramidal NEC 333.90
eye 379.90
anterior chamber 364.9
inflammatory NEC 364.3
muscle 378.9
eyeball 360.9
eyelid 374.9
eyeworm of Africa 125.2
Fabry's (angiokeratoma corporis diffusum) 272.7
facial nerve (seventh) 351.9
newborn 767.5
Fahr-Volhard (malignant nephrosclerosis) 403.00
fallopian tube, noninflammatory 620.9
specified NEC 620.8
familial periodic 277.31
paralysis 359.3
Fanconi's (congenital pancytopenia) 284.09
Farber's (disseminated lipogranulomatosis) 272.8
fascia 728.9
inflammatory 728.9
Fauchard's (periodontitis) 523.40
Favre-Durand-Nicolas (climatic bubo) 099.1
Favre-Racouchot (elastoidosis cutanea nodularis) 701.8
Fede's 529.0
Feer's 985.0
Felix's (juvenile osteochondrosis, hip) 732.1
Fenwick's (gastric atrophy) 537.89
Fernels' (aortic aneurysm) 441.9
fibrocaseous, of lung (*see also* Tuberculosis, pulmonary) 011.9 ☑
fibrocystic (*see also* Fibrocystic, disease)

Disease, diseased — *see also* Syndrome — *continued*
fibrocystic (*see also* Fibrocystic, disease) — *continued*
newborn 277.01
Fiedler's (leptospiral jaundice) 100.0
fifth 057.0
Filatoff's (infectious mononucleosis) 075
Filatov's (infectious mononucleosis) 075
file-cutters' 984.9
specified type of lead — *see* Table of Drugs and Chemicals
filterable virus NEC 078.89
fish skin 757.1
acquired 701.1
Flajani (-Basedow) (exophthalmic goiter) 242.0 ☑
Flatau-Schilder 341.1
flax-dressers' 504
Fleischner's 732.3
flint 502
fluke — *see* Infestation, fluke
Følling's (phenylketonuria) 270.1
foot and mouth 078.4
foot process 581.3
Forbes' (glycogenosis III) 271.0
Fordyce's (ectopic sebaceous glands) (mouth) 750.26
Fordyce-Fox (apocrine miliaria) 705.82
Fothergill's
meaning scarlatina anginosa 034.1
neuralgia (*see also* Neuralgia, trigeminal) 350.1
Fournier's 608.83
female 616.89
fourth 057.8
Fox (-Fordyce) (apocrine miliaria) 705.82
Francis' (*see also* Tularemia) 021.9
Franklin's (heavy chain) 273.2
Frei's (climatic bubo) 099.1
Freiberg's (flattening metatarsal) 732.5
Friedländer's (endarteritis obliterans) — *see* Arteriosclerosis
Friedreich's
combined systemic or ataxia 334.0
facial hemihypertrophy 756.0
myoclonia 333.2
Fröhlich's (adiposogenital dystrophy) 253.8
Frommel's 676.6 ☑
frontal sinus (chronic) 473.1
acute 461.1
Fuller's earth 502
fungus, fungous NEC 117.9
Gaisböck's (polycythemia hypertonica) 289.0
gallbladder 575.9
congenital 751.60
Gamna's (sideretic splenomegaly) 289.51
Gamstorp's (adynamia episodica hereditaria) 359.3
Gandy-Nanta (siderotic splenomegaly) 289.51
Gannister (occupational) 502
Garré's (*see also* Osteomyelitis) 730.1 ☑
gastric (*see also* Disease, stomach) 537.9
gastroesophageal reflux (GERD) 530.81
gastrointestinal (tract) 569.9
amyloid 277.39
functional 536.9
psychogenic 306.4
Gaucher's (adult) (cerebroside lipidosis) (infantile) 272.7
Gayet's (superior hemorrhagic polioencephalitis) 265.1
Gee (-Herter) (-Heubner) (-Thaysen) (nontropical sprue) 579.0
generalized neoplastic (M8000/6) 199.0
genital organs NEC
female 629.9
specified NEC 629.89
male 608.9
Gerhardt's (erythromelalgia) 443.82
Gerlier's (epidemic vertigo) 078.81
Gibert's (pityriasis rosea) 696.3
Gibney's (perispondylitis) 720.9
Gierke's (glycogenosis I) 271.0

Disease, diseased — *see also* Syndrome — *continued*
Gilbert's (familial nonhemolytic jaundice) 277.4
Gilchrist's (North American blastomycosis) 116.0
Gilford (-Hutchinson) (progeria) 259.8
Gilles de la Tourette's (motor-verbal tic) 307.23
Giovannini's 117.9
gland (lymph) 289.9
Glanzmann's (hereditary hemorrhagic thrombasthenia) 287.1
glassblowers' 527.1
Glénard's (enteroptosis) 569.89
Glisson's (*see also* Rickets) 268.0
glomerular
membranous, idiopathic 581.1
minimal change 581.3
glycogen storage (Andersen's) (Cori types 1-7) (Forbes') (McArdle-Schmid-Pearson) (Pompe's) (types I-VII) 271.0
cardiac 271.0 [425.7]
generalized 271.0
glucose–6–phosphatase deficiency 271.0
heart 271.0 [425.7]
hepatorenal 271.0
liver and kidneys 271.0
myocardium 271.0 [425.7]
von Gierke's (glycogenosis I) 271.0
Goldflam-Erb 358.00
Goldscheider's (epidermolysis bullosa) 757.39
Goldstein's (familial hemorrhagic telangiectasia) 448.0
gonococcal NEC 098.0
Goodall's (epidemic vomiting) 078.82
Gordon's (exudative enteropathy) 579.8
Gougerot's (trisymptomatic) 709.1
Gougerot-Carteaud (confluent reticulate papillomatosis) 701.8
Gougerot-Hailey-Hailey (benign familial chronic pemphigus) 757.39
graft-versus-host 279.50
acute 279.51
on chronic 279.53
chronic 279.52
grain-handlers' 495.8
Grancher's (splenopneumonia) — *see* Pneumonia
granulomatous (childhood) (chronic) 288.1
graphite lung 503
Graves' (exophthalmic goiter) 242.0 ☑
Greenfield's 330.0
green monkey 078.89
Griesinger's (*see also* Ancylostomiasis) 126.9
grinders' 502
Grisel's 723.5
Gruby's (tinea tonsurans) 110.0
Guertin's (electric chorea) 049.8
Guillain-Barré 357.0
Guinon's (motor-verbal tic) 307.23
Gull's (thyroid atrophy with myxedema) 244.8
Gull and Sutton's — *see* Hypertension, kidney
gum NEC 523.9
Günther's (congenital erythropoietic porphyria) 277.1
gynecological 629.9
specified NEC 629.89
H 270.0
Haas' 732.3
Habermann's (acute parapsoriasis varioliformis) 696.2
Haff 985.1
Hageman (congenital factor XII deficiency) (*see also* Defect, congenital) 286.3
Haglund's (osteochondrosis os tibiale externum) 732.5
Hagner's (hypertrophic pulmonary osteoarthropathy) 731.2
Hailey-Hailey (benign familial chronic pemphigus) 757.39
hair (follicles) NEC 704.9

Disease, diseased — *see also* Syndrome — *continued*
   hair — *continued*
      specified type NEC 704.8
   Hallervorden-Spatz 333.0
   Hallopeau's (lichen sclerosus et atrophicus) 701.0
   Hamman's (spontaneous mediastinal emphysema) 518.1
   hand, foot, and mouth 074.3
   Hand-Schüller-Christian (chronic histiocytosis X) 277.89
   Hanot's — *see* Cirrhosis, biliary
   Hansen's (leprosy) 030.9
      benign form 030.1
      malignant form 030.0
   Harada's 363.22
   Harley's (intermittent hemoglobinuria) 283.2
   Hartnup (pellagra-cerebellar ataxia-renal aminoaciduria) 270.0
   Hart's (pellagra-cerebellar ataxia-renal aminoaciduria) 270.0
   Hashimoto's (struma lymphomatosa) 245.2
   Hb — *see* Disease, hemoglobin
   heart (organic) 429.9
      with
         acute pulmonary edema (*see also* Failure, ventricular, left) 428.1
         hypertensive 402.91
            with renal failure 404.93
            benign 402.11
               with renal failure 404.13
            malignant 402.01
               with renal failure 404.03
         kidney disease — *see* Hypertension, cardiorenal
         rheumatic fever (conditions classifiable to 390)
            active 391.9
               with chorea 392.0
            inactive or quiescent (with chorea) 398.90
      amyloid 277.39 *[425.7]*
      aortic (valve) (*see also* Endocarditis, aortic) 424.1
      arteriosclerotic or sclerotic (minimal) (senile) — *see* Arteriosclerosis, coronary
      artery, arterial — *see* Arteriosclerosis, coronary
      atherosclerotic — *see* Arteriosclerosis, coronary
      beer drinkers' 425.5
      beriberi 265.0 *[425.7]*
      black 416.0
      congenital NEC 746.9
         cyanotic 746.9
         maternal, affecting fetus or newborn 760.3
         specified type NEC 746.89
      congestive (*see also* Failure, heart) 428.0
      coronary 414.9
      cryptogenic 429.9
      due to
         amyloidosis 277.39 *[425.7]*
         beriberi 265.0 *[425.7]*
         cardiac glycogenosis 271.0 *[425.7]*
         Friedreich's ataxia 334.0 *[425.8]*
         gout 274.82
         mucopolysaccharidosis 277.5 *[425.7]*
         myotonia atrophica 359.21 *[425.8]*
         progressive muscular dystrophy 359.1 *[425.8]*
         sarcoidosis 135 *[425.8]*
      fetal 746.9
         inflammatory 746.89
      fibroid (*see also* Myocarditis) 429.0
      functional 427.9
         postoperative 997.1
         psychogenic 306.2
      glycogen storage 271.0 *[425.7]*
      gonococcal NEC 098.85
      gouty 274.82
      hypertensive (*see also* Hypertension, heart) 402.90

Disease, diseased — *see also* Syndrome — *continued*
   heart — *continued*
      hypertensive (*see also* Hypertension, heart) — *continued*
         benign 402.10
         malignant 402.00
      hyperthyroid (*see also* Hyperthyroidism) 242.9 ☑ *[425.7]*
      incompletely diagnosed — *see* Disease, heart
      ischemic (chronic) (*see also* Ischemia, heart) 414.9
         acute (*see also* Infarct, myocardium) 410.9 ☑
            without myocardial infarction 411.89
               with coronary (artery) occlusion 411.81
         asymptomatic 412
         diagnosed on ECG or other special investigation but currently presenting no symptoms 412
      kyphoscoliotic 416.1
      mitral (*see also* Endocarditis, mitral) 394.9
      muscular (*see also* Degeneration, myocardial) 429.1
      postpartum 674.8 ☑
      psychogenic (functional) 306.2
      pulmonary (chronic) 416.9
         acute 415.0
         specified NEC 416.8
      rheumatic (chronic) (inactive) (old) (quiescent) (with chorea) 398.90
         active or acute 391.9
            with chorea (active) (rheumatic) (Sydenham's) 392.0
            specified type NEC 391.8
         maternal, affecting fetus or newborn 760.3
      rheumatoid — *see* Arthritis, rheumatoid
      sclerotic — *see* Arteriosclerosis, coronary
      senile (*see also* Myocarditis) 429.0
      specified type NEC 429.89
      syphilitic 093.89
         aortic 093.1
            aneurysm 093.0
         asymptomatic 093.89
         congenital 090.5
      thyroid (gland) (*see also* Hyperthyroidism) 242.9 ☑ *[425.7]*
      thyrotoxic (*see also* Thyrotoxicosis) 242.9 ☑ *[425.7]*
      tuberculous (*see also* Tuberculosis) 017.9 ☑ *[425.8]*
      valve, valvular (obstructive) (regurgitant) (*see also* Endocarditis)
         congenital NEC (*see also* Anomaly, heart, valve) 746.9
            pulmonary 746.00
            specified type NEC 746.89
      vascular — *see* Disease, cardiovascular
   heavy-chain (gamma G) 273.2
   Heberden's 715.04
   Hebra's
      dermatitis exfoliativa 695.89
      erythema multiforme exudativum 695.19
      pityriasis
         maculata et circinata 696.3
         rubra 695.89
         pilaris 696.4
      prurigo 698.2
   Heerfordt's (uveoparotitis) 135
   Heidenhain's 290.10
      with dementia 290.10
   Heilmeyer-Schöner (M9842/3) 207.1 ☑
   Heine-Medin (*see also* Poliomyelitis) 045.9 ☑
   Heller's (*see also* Psychosis, childhood) 299.1 ☑
   Heller-Döhle (syphilitic aortitis) 093.1
   hematopoietic organs 289.9
   hemoglobin (Hb) 282.7
      with thalassemia 282.49

Disease, diseased — *see also* Syndrome — *continued*
   hemoglobin — *continued*
      abnormal (mixed) NEC 282.7
         with thalassemia 282.49
      AS genotype 282.5
      Bart's 282.43
      C (Hb-C) 282.7
         with other abnormal hemoglobin NEC 282.7
         elliptocytosis 282.7
         Hb-S (without crisis) 282.63
            with
               crisis 282.64
               vaso-occlusive pain 282.64
         sickle-cell (without crisis) 282.63
            with
               crisis 282.64
               vaso-occlusive pain 282.64
         thalassemia 282.49
      constant spring 282.7
      D (Hb-D) 282.7
         with other abnormal hemoglobin NEC 282.7
         Hb-S (without crisis) 282.68
            with crisis 282.69
         sickle-cell (without crisis) 282.68
            with crisis 282.69
         thalassemia 282.49
      E (Hb-E) 282.7
         with other abnormal hemoglobin NEC 282.7
         Hb-S (without crisis) 282.68
            with crisis 282.69
         sickle-cell (without crisis) 282.68
            with crisis 282.69
         thalassemia 282.47
      elliptocytosis 282.7
      F (Hb-F) 282.7
      G (Hb-G) 282.7
      H (Hb-H) 282.43
      hereditary persistence, fetal (HPFH) ("Swiss variety") 282.7
      high fetal gene 282.7
      I thalassemia 282.49
      M 289.7
      S (*see also* Disease, sickle-cell, Hb-S)
         thalassemia (without crisis) 282.41
            with
               crisis 282.42
               vaso-occlusive pain 282.42
      spherocytosis 282.7
      unstable, hemolytic 282.7
      Zurich (Hb-Zurich) 282.7
   hemolytic (fetus) (newborn) 773.2
      autoimmune (cold type) (warm type) 283.0
      due to or with
         incompatibility
            ABO (blood group) 773.1
            blood (group) (Duffy) (Kell) (Kidd) (Lewis) (M) (S) NEC 773.2
            Rh (blood group) (factor) 773.0
         Rh negative mother 773.0
      unstable hemoglobin 282.7
   hemorrhagic 287.9
      newborn 776.0
   Henoch (-Schönlein) (purpura nervosa) 287.0
   hepatic — *see* Disease, liver
   hepatolenticular 275.1
   heredodegenerative NEC
      brain 331.89
      spinal cord 336.8
   Hers' (glycogenosis VI) 271.0
   Herter (-Gee) (-Heubner) (nontropical sprue) 579.0
   Herxheimer's (diffuse idiopathic cutaneous atrophy) 701.8
   Heubner's 094.89
   Heubner-Herter (nontropical sprue) 579.0
   high fetal gene or hemoglobin thalassemia (*see also* Thalassemia) 282.40
   Hildenbrand's (typhus) 081.9
   Hippel's (retinocerebral angiomatosis) 759.6
   hip (joint) NEC 719.95

Disease, diseased — *see also* Syndrome — *continued*
   hip — *continued*
      congenital 755.63
      suppurative 711.05
      tuberculous (*see also* Tuberculosis) 015.1 ☑ *[730.85]*
   Hirschfeld's (acute diabetes mellitus) (*see also* Diabetes) 250.0 ☑
      due to secondary diabetes 249.0 ☑
   Hirschsprung's (congenital megacolon) 751.3
   His (-Werner) (trench fever) 083.1
   HIV 042
   Hodgkin's (M9650/3) 201.9 ☑

   Note — *Use the following fifth-digit subclassification with category 201:*
0	*unspecified site*
1	*lymph nodes of head, face, and neck*
2	*intrathoracic lymph nodes*
3	*intra-abdominal lymph nodes*
4	*lymph nodes of axilla and upper limb*
5	*lymph nodes of inguinal region and lower limb*
6	*intrapelvic lymph nodes*
7	*spleen*
8	*lymph nodes of multiple sites*

      lymphocytic
         depletion (M9653/3) 201.7 ☑
            diffuse fibrosis (M9654/3) 201.7 ☑
            reticular type (M9655/3) 201.7 ☑
         predominance (M9651/3) 201.4 ☑
      lymphocytic-histiocytic predominance (M9651/3) 201.4 ☑
      mixed cellularity (M9652/3) 201.6 ☑
      nodular sclerosis (M9656/3) 201.5 ☑
         cellular phase (M9657/3) 201.5 ☑
   Hodgson's 441.9
      ruptured 441.5
   Hoffa (-Kastert) (liposynovitis prepatellaris) 272.8
   Holla (*see also* Spherocytosis) 282.0
   homozygous-Hb-S 282.61
   hoof and mouth 078.4
   hookworm (*see also* Ancylostomiasis) 126.9
   Horton's (temporal arteritis) 446.5
   host-versus-graft (immune or nonimmune cause) 279.50
   HPFH (hereditary persistence of fetal hemoglobin) ("Swiss variety") 282.7
   Huchard's disease (continued arterial hypertension) 401.9
   Huguier's (uterine fibroma) 218.9
   human immunodeficiency (virus) 042
   hunger 251.1
   Hunt's
      dyssynergia cerebellaris myoclonica 334.2
      herpetic geniculate ganglionitis 053.11
   Huntington's 333.4
   Huppert's (multiple myeloma) (M9730/3) 203.0 ☑
   Hurler's (mucopolysaccharidosis I) 277.5
   Hutchinson-Boeck (sarcoidosis) 135
   Hutchinson-Gilford (progeria) 259.8
   Hutchinson's, meaning
      angioma serpiginosum 709.1
      cheiropompholyx 705.81
      prurigo estivalis 692.72
   hyaline (diffuse) (generalized) 728.9
      membrane (lung) (newborn) 769
   hydatid (*see also* Echinococcus) 122.9
   Hyde's (prurigo nodularis) 698.3
   hyperkinetic (*see also* Hyperkinesia) 314.9
      heart 429.82
   hypertensive (*see also* Hypertension) 401.9
   hypophysis 253.9
      hyperfunction 253.1

Disease, diseased — *see also* Syndrome — *continued*
  hypophysis — *continued*
    hypofunction 253.2
  Iceland (epidemic neuromyasthenia) 049.8
  I cell 272.7
  ill-defined 799.89
  immunologic NEC 279.9
  immunoproliferative 203.8 ☑
  inclusion 078.5
    salivary gland 078.5
  infancy, early NEC 779.9
  infective NEC 136.9
  inguinal gland 289.9
  internal semilunar cartilage, cystic 717.5
  intervertebral disc 722.90
    with myelopathy 722.70
    cervical, cervicothoracic 722.91
      with myelopathy 722.71
    lumbar, lumbosacral 722.93
      with myelopathy 722.73
    thoracic, thoracolumbar 722.92
      with myelopathy 722.72
  intestine 569.9
    functional 564.9
      congenital 751.3
      psychogenic 306.4
    lardaceous 277.39
    organic 569.9
    protozoal NEC 007.9
  iris 364.9
    specified NEC 364.89
  iron
    metabolism (*see also* Hemochromatosis) 275.09
    storage (*see also* Hemochromatosis) 275.03
  Isambert's (*see also* Tuberculosis, larynx) 012.3 ☑
  Iselin's (osteochondrosis, fifth metatarsal) 732.5
  island (scrub typhus) 081.2
  itai-itai 985.5
  Jadassohn's (maculopapular erythroderma) 696.2
  Jadassohn-Pellizari's (anetoderma) 701.3
  Jakob-Creutzfeldt (CJD) 046.19
    with dementia
      with behavioral disturbance 046.19 *[294.11]*
      without behavioral disturbance 046.19 *[294.10]*
    familial 046.19
    iatrogenic 046.19
    specified NEC 046.19
    sporadic 046.19
    variant (vCJD) 046.11
      with dementia
        with behavioral disturbance 046.11 *[294.11]*
        without behavioral disturbance 046.11 *[294.10]*
  Jaksch (-Luzet) (pseudoleukemia infantum) 285.8
  Janet's 300.89
  Jansky-Bielschowsky 330.1
  jaw NEC 526.9
    fibrocystic 526.2
  Jensen's 363.05
  Jeune's (asphyxiating thoracic dystrophy) 756.4
  jigger 134.1
  Johnson-Stevens (erythema multiforme exudativum) 695.13
  joint NEC 719.9 ☑
    ankle 719.97
    Charcôt 094.0 *[713.5]*
    degenerative (*see also* Osteoarthrosis) 715.9 ☑
      multiple 715.09
      spine (*see also* Spondylosis) 721.90
    elbow 719.92
    foot 719.97
    hand 719.94
    hip 719.95

Disease, diseased — *see also* Syndrome — *continued*
  joint — *continued*
    hypertrophic (chronic) (degenerative) (*see also* Osteoarthrosis) 715.9 ☑
      spine (*see also* Spondylosis) 721.90
    knee 719.96
    Luschka 721.90
    multiple sites 719.99
    pelvic region 719.95
    sacroiliac 724.6
    shoulder (region) 719.91
    specified site NEC 719.98
    spine NEC 724.9
      pseudarthrosis following fusion 733.82
      sacroiliac 724.6
    wrist 719.93
  Jourdain's (acute gingivitis) 523.00
  Jüngling's (sarcoidosis) 135
  Kahler (-Bozzolo) (multiple myeloma) (M9730/3) 203.0 ☑
  Kalischer's 759.6
  Kaposi's 757.33
    lichen ruber 697.8
      acuminatus 696.4
      moniliformis 697.8
    xeroderma pigmentosum 757.33
  Kaschin-Beck (endemic polyarthritis) 716.00
    ankle 716.07
    arm 716.02
      lower (and wrist) 716.03
      upper (and elbow) 716.02
    foot (and ankle) 716.07
    forearm (and wrist) 716.03
    hand 716.04
    leg 716.06
      lower 716.06
      upper 716.05
    multiple sites 716.09
    pelvic region (hip) (thigh) 716.05
    shoulder region 716.01
    specified site NEC 716.08
  Katayama 120.2
  Kawasaki 446.1
  Kedani (scrub typhus) 081.2
  kidney (functional) (pelvis) (*see also* Disease, renal) 593.9
    chronic 585.9
      requiring chronic dialysis 585.6
      stage
        I 585.1
        II (mild) 585.2
        III (moderate) 585.3
        IV (severe) 585.4
        V 585.5
    cystic (congenital) 753.10
      multiple 753.19
      single 753.11
      specified NEC 753.19
    fibrocystic (congenital) 753.19
    in gout 274.10
    polycystic (congenital) 753.12
      adult type (APKD) 753.13
      autosomal dominant 753.13
      autosomal recessive 753.14
      childhood type (CPKD) 753.14
      infantile type 753.14
  Kienböck's (carpal lunate) (wrist) 732.3
  Kimmelstiel (-Wilson) (intercapillary glomerulosclerosis) 250.4 ☑ *[581.81]*
    due to secondary diabetes 249.4 ☑ *[581.81]*
  Kinnier Wilson's (hepatolenticular degeneration) 275.1
  kissing 075
  Kleb's (*see also* Nephritis) 583.9
  Klinger's 446.4
  Klippel's 723.8
  Klippel-Feil (brevicollis) 756.16
  knight's 911.1
  Köbner's (epidermolysis bullosa) 757.39
  Koenig-Wichmann (pemphigus) 694.4
  Köhler's
    first (osteoarthrosis juvenilis) 732.5

Disease, diseased — *see also* Syndrome — *continued*
  Köhler's — *continued*
    second (Freiberg's infraction, metatarsal head) 732.5
    patellar 732.4
    tarsal navicular (bone) (osteoarthrosis juvenilis) 732.5
  Köhler-Freiberg (infraction, metatarsal head) 732.5
  Köhler-Mouchet (osteoarthrosis juvenilis) 732.5
  Köhler-Pellegrini-Stieda (calcification, knee joint) 726.62
  Kok 759.89
  König's (osteochondritis dissecans) 732.7
  Korsakoff's (nonalcoholic) 294.0
    alcoholic 291.1
  Kostmann's (infantile genetic agranulocytosis) 288.01
  Krabbe's 330.0
  Kraepelin-Morel (*see also* Schizophrenia) 295.9 ☑
  Kraft-Weber-Dimitri 759.6
  Kufs' 330.1
  Kugelberg-Welander 335.11
  Kuhnt-Junius 362.52
  Kümmell's (-Verneuil) (spondylitis) 721.7
  Kundrat's (lymphosarcoma) 200.1 ☑
  kuru 046.0
  Kussmaul (-Meier) (polyarteritis nodosa) 446.0
  Kyasanur Forest 065.2
  Kyrle's (hyperkeratosis follicularis in cutem penetrans) 701.1
  labia
    inflammatory 616.10
    noninflammatory 624.9
      specified NEC 624.8
  labyrinth, ear 386.8
  lacrimal system (apparatus) (passages) 375.9
    gland 375.00
      specified NEC 375.89
  Lafora's 333.2
  Lagleyze-von Hippel (retinocerebral angiomatosis) 759.6
  Lancereaux-Mathieu (leptospiral jaundice) 100.0
  Landry's 357.0
  Lane's 569.89
  lardaceous (any site) 277.39
  Larrey-Weil (leptospiral jaundice) 100.0
  Larsen (-Johansson) (juvenile osteopathia patellae) 732.4
  larynx 478.70
  Lasègue's (persecution mania) 297.9
  Leber's 377.16
  Lederer's (acquired infectious hemolytic anemia) 283.19
  Legg's (capital femoral osteochondrosis) 732.1
  Legg-Calvé-Perthes (capital femoral osteochondrosis) 732.1
  Legg-Calvé-Waldenström (femoral capital osteochondrosis) 732.1
  Legg-Perthes (femoral capital osteochondrosis) 732.1
  Legionnaires' 482.84
  Leigh's 330.8
  Leiner's (exfoliative dermatitis) 695.89
  Leloir's (lupus erythematosus) 695.4
  Lenegre's 426.0
  lens (eye) 379.39
  Leriche's (osteoporosis, posttraumatic) 733.7
  Letterer-Siwe (acute histiocytosis X) (M9722/3) 202.5 ☑
  Lev's (acquired complete heart block) 426.0
  Lewandowski's (*see also* Tuberculosis) 017.0 ☑
  Lewandowski-Lutz (epidermodysplasia verruciformis) 078.19
  Lewy body 331.82
    with dementia
      with behavioral disturbance 331.82 *[294.11]*

Disease, diseased — *see also* Syndrome — *continued*
  Lewy body — *continued*
    with dementia — *continued*
      without behavioral disturbance 331.82 *[294.10]*
  Leyden's (periodic vomiting) 536.2
  Libman-Sacks (verrucous endocarditis) 710.0 *[424.91]*
  Lichtheim's (subacute combined sclerosis with pernicious anemia) 281.0 *[336.2]*
  ligament 728.9
  light chain 203.0 ☑
  Lightwood's (renal tubular acidosis) 588.89
  Lignac's (cystinosis) 270.0
  Lindau's (retinocerebral angiomatosis) 759.6
  Lindau-von Hippel (angiomatosis retinocerebellosa) 759.6
  lipidosis 272.7
  lipoid storage NEC 272.7
  Lipschütz's 616.50
  lip NEC 528.5
  Little's — *see* Palsy, cerebral
  liver 573.9
    alcoholic 571.3
      acute 571.1
      chronic 571.3
    chronic 571.9
      alcoholic 571.3
    cystic, congenital 751.62
    drug-induced 573.3
    due to
      chemicals 573.3
      fluorinated agents 573.3
      hypersensitivity drugs 573.3
      isoniazids 573.3
    end stage NEC 572.8
      due to hepatitis — *see* Hepatitis
    fibrocystic (congenital) 751.62
    glycogen storage 271.0
    organic 573.9
    polycystic (congenital) 751.62
  Lobo's (keloid blastomycosis) 116.2
  Lobstein's (brittle bones and blue sclera) 756.51
  locomotor system 334.9
  Lorain's (pituitary dwarfism) 253.3
  Lou Gehrig's 335.20
  Lucas-Championnière (fibrinous bronchitis) 466.0
  Ludwig's (submaxillary cellulitis) 528.3
  luetic — *see* Syphilis
  lumbosacral region 724.6
  lung NEC 518.89
    black 500
    congenital 748.60
    cystic 518.89
      congenital 748.4
    fibroid (chronic) (*see also* Fibrosis, lung) 515
    fluke 121.2
      oriental 121.2
    in
      amyloidosis 277.39 *[517.8]*
      polymyositis 710.4 *[517.8]*
      sarcoidosis 135 *[517.8]*
      Sjögren's syndrome 710.2 *[517.8]*
      syphilis 095.1
      systemic lupus erythematosus 710.0 *[517.8]*
      systemic sclerosis 710.1 *[517.2]*
    interstitial (chronic) 515
      acute 136.3
      respiratory bronchiolitis 516.34
    nonspecific, chronic 496
    obstructive (chronic) (COPD) 496
      with
        acute
          bronchitis 491.22
          exacerbation NEC 491.21
        alveolitis, allergic (*see also* Alveolitis, allergic) 495.9
        asthma (chronic) (obstructive) 493.2 ☑
        bronchiectasis 494.0
          with acute exacerbation 494.1

☑ Additional Digit Required — Refer to the Tabular List for Digit Selection   ⃤ Subterms under main terms may continue to next column or page

Disease, diseased — *see also* Syndrome — *continued*
lung — *continued*
    obstructive — *continued*
        with — *continued*
            bronchitis (chronic) 491.20
                with
                    acute bronchitis 491.22
                    exacerbation (acute) 491.21
                decompensated 491.21
                    with exacerbation 491.21
            emphysema NEC 492.8
        diffuse (with fibrosis) 496
        of childhood, specific NEC 516.69
        polycystic 518.89
            asthma (chronic) (obstructive) 493.2 ☑
            congenital 748.4
        purulent (cavitary) 513.0
        restrictive 518.89
        rheumatoid 714.81
            diffuse interstitial 714.81
        specified NEC 518.89
    Lutembacher's (atrial septal defect with mitral stenosis) 745.5
    Lutz-Miescher (elastosis perforans serpiginosa) 701.1
    Lutz-Splendore-de Almeida (Brazilian blastomycosis) 116.1
    Lyell's (toxic epidermal necrolysis) 695.15
        due to drug
            correct substance properly administered 695.15
            overdose or wrong substance given or taken 977.9
            specific drug — *see* Table of Drugs and Chemicals
    Lyme 088.81
    lymphatic (gland) (system) 289.9
        channel (noninfective) 457.9
        vessel (noninfective) 457.9
            specified NEC 457.8
    lymphoproliferative (chronic) (M9970/1) 238.79
        X linked 759.89
    Machado-Joseph 334.8
    Madelung's (lipomatosis) 272.8
    Madura (actinomycotic) 039.9
        mycotic 117.4
    Magitot's 526.4
    Majocchi's (purpura annularis telangiectodes) 709.1
    malarial (*see also* Malaria) 084.6
    Malassez's (cystic) 608.89
    Malibu 919.8
        infected 919.9
    malignant (M8000/3) (*see also* Neoplasm, by site, malignant)
        previous, affecting management of pregnancy V23.89
    Manson's 120.1
    maple bark 495.6
    maple syrup (urine) 270.3
    Marburg (virus) 078.89
    Marchiafava (-Bignami) 341.8
    Marfan's 090.49
        congenital syphilis 090.49
        meaning Marfan's syndrome 759.82
    Marie-Bamberger (hypertrophic pulmonary osteoarthropathy) (secondary) 731.2
        primary or idiopathic (acropachyderma) 757.39
        pulmonary (hypertrophic osteoarthropathy) 731.2
    Marie-Strümpell (ankylosing spondylitis) 720.0
    Marion's (bladder neck obstruction) 596.0
    Marsh's (exophthalmic goiter) 242.0 ☑
    Martin's 715.27
    mast cell 757.33
        systemic (M9741/3) 202.6 ☑
    mastoid (*see also* Mastoiditis) 383.9
        process 385.9
    maternal, unrelated to pregnancy NEC, affecting fetus or newborn 760.9

Disease, diseased — *see also* Syndrome — *continued*
    Mathieu's (leptospiral jaundice) 100.0
    Mauclaire's 732.3
    Mauriac's (erythema nodosum syphiliticum) 091.3
    Maxcy's 081.0
    McArdle (-Schmid-Pearson) (glycogenosis V) 271.0
    mediastinum NEC 519.3
    Medin's (*see also* Poliomyelitis) 045.9 ☑
    Mediterranean 282.40
        with hemoglobinopathy 282.49
    medullary center (idiopathic) (respiratory) 348.89
    Meige's (chronic hereditary edema) 757.0
    Meleda 757.39
    Ménétrier's (hypertrophic gastritis) 535.2 ☑
    Ménière's (active) 386.00
        cochlear 386.02
        cochleovestibular 386.01
        inactive 386.04
        in remission 386.04
        vestibular 386.03
    meningeal — *see* Meningitis
    mental (*see also* Psychosis) 298.9
    Merzbacher-Pelizaeus 330.0
    mesenchymal 710.9
    mesenteric embolic 557.0
    metabolic NEC 277.9
    metal polishers' 502
    metastatic — *see* Metastasis
    Mibelli's 757.39
    microdrepanocytic 282.41
    microvascular — code to condition
    microvillus
        atrophy 751.5
        inclusion (MVD) 751.5
    Miescher's 709.3
    Mikulicz's (dryness of mouth, absent or decreased lacrimation) 527.1
    Milkman (-Looser) (osteomalacia with pseudofractures) 268.2
    Miller's (osteomalacia) 268.2
    Mills' 335.29
    Milroy's (chronic hereditary edema) 757.0
    Minamata 985.0
    Minor's 336.1
    Minot's (hemorrhagic disease, newborn) 776.0
    Minot-von Willebrand-Jürgens (angiohemophilia) 286.4
    Mitchell's (erythromelalgia) 443.82
    mitral — *see* Endocarditis, mitral
    Mljet (mal de Meleda) 757.39
    Möbius', Moebius' 346.2 ☑
    Moeller's 267
    Möller (-Barlow) (infantile scurvy) 267
    Mönckeberg's (*see also* Arteriosclerosis, extremities) 440.20
    Mondor's (thrombophlebitis of breast) 451.89
    Monge's 993.2
    Morel-Kraepelin (*see also* Schizophrenia) 295.9 ☑
    Morgagni's (syndrome) (hyperostosis frontalis interna) 733.3
    Morgagni-Adams-Stokes (syncope with heart block) 426.9
    Morquio (-Brailsford) (-Ullrich) (mucopolysaccharidosis IV) 277.5
    Morton's (with metatarsalgia) 355.6
    Morvan's 336.0
    rnotor neuron (bulbar) (mixed type) 335.20
    Mouchet's (juvenile osteochondrosis, foot) 732.5
    mouth 528.9
    Moyamoya 437.5
    Mucha's (acute parapsoriasis varioliformis) 696.2
    mu-chain 273.2
    mucolipidosis (I) (II) (III) 272.7
    Münchmeyer's (exostosis luxurians) 728.11
    Murri's (intermittent hemoglobinuria) 283.2
    muscle 359.9
        inflammatory 728.9

Disease, diseased — *see also* Syndrome — *continued*
    muscle — *continued*
        ocular 378.9
    musculoskeletal system 729.90
    mushroom workers' 495.5
    Myà's (congenital dilation, colon) 751.3
    mycotic 117.9
    myeloproliferative (chronic) (M9960/1) 238.79
    myocardium, myocardial (*see also* Degeneration, myocardial) 429.1
        hypertensive (*see also* Hypertension, heart 402.90
        primary (idiopathic) 425.4
    myoneural 358.9
    Naegeli's 287.1
    nail 703.9
        specified type NEC 703.8
    Nairobi sheep 066.1
    nasal 478.19
        cavity NEC 478.19
        sinus (chronic) — *see* Sinusitis
    navel (newborn) NEC 779.89
        delayed separation of umbilical cord 779.83
    nemaline body 359.0
    neoplastic, generalized (M8000/6) 199.0
    nerve — *see* Disorder, nerve
    nervous system (central) 349.9
        autonomic, peripheral (*see also* Neuropathy, peripheral, autonomic) 337.9
        congenital 742.9
        inflammatory — *see* Encephalitis
        parasympathetic (*see also* Neuropathy, peripheral, autonomic) 337.9
        peripheral NEC 355.9
        prion NEC 046.79
        specified NEC 349.89
        sympathetic (*see also* Neuropathy, peripheral, autonomic) 337.9
        vegetative (*see also* Neuropathy, peripheral, autonomic) 337.9
    Nettleship's (urticaria pigmentosa) 757.33
    Neumann's (pemphigus vegetans) 694.4
    neurologic (central) NEC (*see also* Disease, nervous system) 349.9
        peripheral NEC 355.9
    neuromuscular system NEC 358.9
    Newcastle 077.8
    Nicolas (-Durand) — Favre (climatic bubo) 099.1
    Niemann-Pick (lipid histiocytosis) 272.7
    nipple 611.9
        Paget's (M8540/3) 174.0
    Nishimoto (-Takeuchi) 437.5
    nonarthropod-borne NEC 078.89
        central nervous system NEC 049.9
        enterovirus NEC 078.89
    nonautoimmune hemolytic NEC 283.10
    Nonne-Milroy-Meige (chronic hereditary edema) 757.0
    Norrie's (congenital progressive oculoacousticocerebral degeneration) 743.8
    nose 478.19
    nucleus pulposus — *see* Disease, intervertebral disc
    nutritional 269.9
        maternal, affecting fetus or newborn 760.4
    oasthouse, urine 270.2
    obliterative vascular 447.1
    Odelberg's (juvenile osteochondrosis) 732.1
    Oguchi's (retina) 368.61
    Ohara's (*see also* Tularemia) 021.9
    Ollier's (chondrodysplasia) 756.4
    Opitz's (congestive splenomegaly) 289.51
    Oppenheim's 358.8
    Oppenheim-Urbach (necrobiosis lipoidica diabeticorum) 250.8 ☑ *[709.3]*
        due to secondary diabetes 249.8 ☑ *[709.3]*
    optic nerve NEC 377.49
    orbit 376.9
        specified NEC 376.89
    Oriental liver fluke 121.1

Disease, diseased — *see also* Syndrome — *continued*
    Oriental lung fluke 121.2
    Ormond's 593.4
    Osgood-Schlatter 732.4
    Osgood's tibia (tubercle) 732.4
    Osler (-Vaquez) (polycythemia vera) (M9950/1) 238.4
    Osler-Rendu (familial hemorrhagic telangiectasia) 448.0
    osteofibrocystic 252.01
    Otto's 715.35
    outer ear 380.9
    ovary (noninflammatory) NEC 620.9
        cystic 620.2
        polycystic 256.4
        specified NEC 620.8
    Owren's (congenital) (*see also* Defect, coagulation) 286.3
    Paas' 756.59
    Paget's (osteitis deformans) 731.0
        with infiltrating duct carcinoma of the breast (M8541/3) — *see* Neoplasm, breast, malignant
        bone 731.0
            osteosarcoma in (M9184/3) — *see* Neoplasm, bone, malignant
        breast (M8540/3) 174.0
            extramammary (M8542/3) (*see also* Neoplasm, skin, malignant)
                anus 154.3
                skin 173.59
            malignant (M8540/3)
                breast 174.0
                specified site NEC (M8542/3) — *see* Neoplasm, skin, malignant
                unspecified site 174.0
            mammary (M8540/3) 174.0
            nipple (M8540/3) 174.0
        palate (soft) 528.9
    Paltauf-Sternberg 201.9 ☑
    pancreas 577.9
        cystic 577.2
            congenital 751.7
        fibrocystic 277.00
    Panner's 732.3
        capitellum humeri 732.3
        head of humerus 732.3
        tarsal navicular (bone) (osteochondrosis) 732.5
    panvalvular — *see* Endocarditis, mitral
    parametrium 629.9
    parasitic NEC 136.9
        cerebral NEC 123.9
        intestinal NEC 129
        mouth 112.0
        skin NEC 134.9
        specified type — *see* Infestation
        tongue 112.0
    parathyroid (gland) 252.9
        specified NEC 252.8
    Parkinson's 332.0
    parodontal 523.9
    Parrot's (syphilitic osteochondritis) 090.0
    Parry's (exophthalmic goiter) 242.0 ☑
    Parson's (exophthalmic goiter) 242.0 ☑
    Pavy's 593.6
    Paxton's (white piedra) 111.2
    Payr's (splenic flexure syndrome) 569.89
    pearl-workers' (chronic osteomyelitis) (*see also* Osteomyelitis) 730.1 ☑
    Pel-Ebstein — *see* Disease, Hodgkin's
    Pelizaeus-Merzbacher 330.0
        with dementia
            with behavioral disturbance 330.0 *[294.11]*
            without behavioral disturbance 330.0 *[294.10]*
    Pellegrini-Stieda (calcification, knee joint) 726.62
    pelvis, pelvic
        female NEC 629.9
            specified NEC 629.89
        gonococcal (acute) 098.19
            chronic or duration of 2 months or over 098.39

☑ Additional Digit Required — Refer to the Tabular List for Digit Selection   ▽ Subterms under main terms may continue to next column or page

86 — Volume 2   ▶◀ Revised Text   ● New Line   ▲ Revised Code   2015 ICD-9-CM

Disease, diseased — *see also* Syndrome — *continued*
  pelvis, pelvic — *continued*
    infection (*see also* Disease, pelvis, inflammatory) 614.9
    inflammatory (female) (PID) 614.9
      with
        abortion — *see* Abortion, by type, with sepsis
        ectopic pregnancy (*see also* categories 633.0–633.9) 639.0
        molar pregnancy (*see also* categories 630–632) 639.0
      acute 614.3
      chronic 614.4
      complicating pregnancy 646.6 ☑
        affecting fetus or newborn 760.8
      following
        abortion 639.0
        ectopic or molar pregnancy 639.0
      peritonitis (acute) 614.5
        chronic NEC 614.7
      puerperal, postpartum, childbirth 670.8 ☑
      specified NEC 614.8
    organ, female NEC 629.9
      specified NEC 629.89
    peritoneum, female NEC 629.9
      specified NEC 629.89
  penis 607.9
    inflammatory 607.2
  peptic NEC 536.9
    acid 536.8
  periapical tissues NEC 522.9
  pericardium 423.9
    specified type NEC 423.8
  perineum
    female
      inflammatory 616.9
        specified NEC 616.89
      noninflammatory 624.9
        specified NEC 624.8
    male (inflammatory) 682.2
  periodic (familial) (Reimann's) NEC 277.31
    paralysis 359.3
  periodontal NEC 523.9
    specified NEC 523.8
  periosteum 733.90
  peripheral
    arterial 443.9
    autonomic nervous system (*see also* Neuropathy, autonomic) 337.9
    nerve NEC (*see also* Neuropathy) 356.9
      multiple — *see* Polyneuropathy
    vascular 443.9
      specified type NEC 443.89
  peritoneum 568.9
    pelvic, female 629.9
      specified NEC 629.89
  Perrin-Ferraton (snapping hip) 719.65
  persistent mucosal (middle ear) (with posterior or superior marginal perforation of ear drum) 382.2
  Perthes' (capital femoral osteochondrosis) 732.1
  Petit's (*see also* Hernia, lumbar) 553.8
  Peutz-Jeghers 759.6
  Peyronie's 607.85
  Pfeiffer's (infectious mononucleosis) 075
  pharynx 478.20
  Phocas' 610.1
  photochromogenic (acid-fast bacilli) (pulmonary) 031.0
    nonpulmonary 031.9
  Pick's
    brain 331.11
      with dementia
        with behavioral disturbance 331.11 *[294.11]*
        without behavioral disturbance 331.11 *[294.10]*
    cerebral atrophy 331.11
      with dementia
        with behavioral disturbance 331.11 *[294.11]*

Disease, diseased — *see also* Syndrome — *continued*
  Pick's — *continued*
    cerebral atrophy — *continued*
      with dementia — *continued*
        without behavioral disturbance 331.11 *[294.10]*
    lipid histiocytosis 272.7
    liver (pericardial pseudocirrhosis of liver) 423.2
    pericardium (pericardial pseudocirrhosis of liver) 423.2
    polyserositis (pericardial pseudocirrhosis of liver) 423.2
  Pierson's (osteochondrosis) 732.1
  pigeon fanciers' or breeders' 495.2
  pineal gland 259.8
  pink 985.0
  Pinkus' (lichen nitidus) 697.1
  pinworm 127.4
  pituitary (gland) 253.9
    hyperfunction 253.1
    hypofunction 253.2
  pituitary snuff-takers' 495.8
  placenta
    affecting fetus or newborn 762.2
    complicating pregnancy or childbirth 656.7 ☑
  pleura (cavity) (*see also* Pleurisy) 511.0
  Plummer's (toxic nodular goiter) 242.3 ☑
  pneumatic
    drill 994.9
    hammer 994.9
  policeman's 729.2
  Pollitzer's (hidradenitis suppurativa) 705.83
  polycystic (congenital) 759.89
    congenital 748.4
    kidney or renal 753.12
      adult type (APKD) 753.13
      autosomal dominant 753.13
      autosomal recessive 753.14
      childhood type (CPKD) 753.14
      infantile type 753.14
    liver or hepatic 751.62
    lung or pulmonary 518.89
    ovary, ovaries 256.4
    spleen 759.0
  polyethylene 996.45
  Pompe's (glycogenosis II) 271.0
  Poncet's (tuberculous rheumatism) (*see also* Tuberculosis) 015.9 ☑
  Posada-Wernicke 114.9
  Potain's (pulmonary edema) 514
  Pott's (*see also* Tuberculosis) 015.0 ☑ *[730.88]*
    osteomyelitis 015.0 ☑ *[730.88]*
    paraplegia 015.0 ☑ *[730.88]*
    spinal curvature 015.0 ☑ *[737.43]*
    spondylitis 015.0 ☑ *[720.81]*
  Potter's 753.0
  Poulet's 714.2
  pregnancy NEC (*see also* Pregnancy) 646.9 ☑
  Preiser's (osteoporosis) 733.09
  Pringle's (tuberous sclerosis) 759.5
  Profichet's 729.90
  prostate 602.9
    specified type NEC 602.8
  protozoal NEC 136.8
    intestine, intestinal NEC 007.9
  pseudo-Hurler's (mucolipidosis III) 272.7
  psychiatric (*see also* Psychosis) 298.9
  psychotic (*see also* Psychosis) 298.9
  Puente's (simple glandular cheilitis) 528.5
  puerperal NEC (*see also* Puerperal) 674.9 ☑
  pulmonary (*see also* Disease, lung)
    amyloid 277.39 *[517.8]*
    artery 417.9
    circulation, circulatory 417.9
      specified NEC 417.8
    diffuse obstructive (chronic) 496
      with
        acute bronchitis 491.22
        asthma (chronic) (obstructive) 493.2 ☑
        exacerbation NEC (acute) 491.21

Disease, diseased — *see also* Syndrome — *continued*
  pulmonary (*see also* Disease, lung) — *continued*
    heart (chronic) 416.9
      specified NEC 416.8
    hypertensive (vascular) 416.0
      cardiovascular 416.0
    obstructive diffuse (chronic) 496
      with
        acute bronchitis 491.22
        asthma (chronic) (obstructive) 493.2 ☑
        bronchitis (chronic) 491.20
        with
          exacerbation (acute) 491.21
          acute 491.22
          exacerbation NEC (acute) 491.21
        decompensated 491.21
          with exacerbation 491.21
    valve (*see also* Endocarditis, pulmonary) 424.3
  pulp (dental) NEC 522.9
  pulseless 446.7
  Putnam's (subacute combined sclerosis with pernicious anemia) 281.0 *[336.2]*
  Pyle (-Cohn) (craniometaphyseal dysplasia) 756.89
  pyramidal tract 333.90
  Quervain's
    tendon sheath 727.04
    thyroid (subacute granulomatous thyroiditis) 245.1
  Quincke's — *see* Edema, angioneurotic
  Quinquaud (acne decalvans) 704.09
  rag sorters' 022.1
  Raynaud's (paroxysmal digital cyanosis) 443.0
  reactive airway — *see* Asthma
  Recklinghausen's (M9540/1) 237.71
    bone (osteitis fibrosa cystica) 252.01
  Recklinghausen-Applebaum (hemochromatosis) (*see also* Hemochromatosis) 275.03
  Reclus' (cystic) 610.1
  rectum NEC 569.49
  Refsum's (heredopathia atactica polyneuritiformis) 356.3
  Reichmann's (gastrosuccorrhea) 536.8
  Reimann's (periodic) 277.31
  Reiter's 099.3
  renal (functional) (pelvis) (*see also* Disease, kidney) 593.9
    with
      edema (*see also* Nephrosis) 581.9
      exudative nephritis 583.89
      lesion of interstitial nephritis 583.89
      stated generalized cause — *see* Nephritis
    acute 593.9
    basement membrane NEC 583.89
      with
        pulmonary hemorrhage (Goodpasture's syndrome) 446.21 *[583.81]*
    chronic (*see also* Disease, kidney, chronic) 585.9
    complicating pregnancy or puerperium NEC 646.2 ☑
      with hypertension — *see* Toxemia, of pregnancy
      affecting fetus or newborn 760.1
    cystic, congenital (*see also* Cystic, disease, kidney) 753.10
    diabetic 250.4 ☑ *[583.81]*
      due to secondary diabetes 249.4 ☑ *[581.81]*
    due to
      amyloidosis 277.39 *[583.81]*
      diabetes mellitus 250.4 ☑ *[583.81]*
        due to secondary diabetes 249.4 ☑ *[581.81]*
      systemic lupus erythematosis 710.0 *[583.81]*

Disease, diseased — *see also* Syndrome — *continued*
  renal (*see also* Disease, kidney) — *continued*
    end-stage 585.6
    exudative 583.89
    fibrocystic (congenital) 753.19
    gonococcal 098.19 *[583.81]*
    gouty 274.10
    hypertensive (*see also* Hypertension, kidney) 403.90
    immune complex NEC 583.89
    interstitial (diffuse) (focal) 583.89
    lupus 710.0 *[583.81]*
    maternal, affecting fetus or newborn 760.1
      hypertensive 760.0
    phosphate-losing (tubular) 588.0
    polycystic (congenital) 753.12
      adult type (APKD) 753.13
      autosomal dominant 753.13
      autosomal recessive 753.14
      childhood type (CPKD) 753.14
      infantile type 753.14
    specified lesion or cause NEC (*see also* Glomerulonephritis) 583.89
    subacute 581.9
    syphilitic 095.4
    tuberculous (*see also* Tuberculosis) 016.0 ☑ *[583.81]*
    tubular (*see also* Nephrosis, tubular) 584.5
  Rendu-Osler-Weber (familial hemorrhagic telangiectasia) 448.0
  renovascular (arteriosclerotic) (*see also* Hypertension, kidney) 403.90
  respiratory (tract) 519.9
    acute or subacute (upper) NEC 465.9
      due to fumes or vapors 506.3
      multiple sites NEC 465.8
      noninfectious 478.9
      streptococcal 034.0
    chronic 519.9
      arising in the perinatal period 770.7
      due to fumes or vapors 506.4
    due to
      aspiration of liquids or solids 508.9
      external agents NEC 508.9
        specified NEC 508.8
      fumes or vapors 506.9
        acute or subacute NEC 506.3
        chronic 506.4
    fetus or newborn NEC 770.9
    obstructive 496
    smoke inhalation 508.2
    specified type NEC 519.8
    upper (acute) (infectious) NEC 465.9
      multiple sites NEC 465.8
      noninfectious NEC 478.9
      streptococcal 034.0
  retina, retinal NEC 362.9
    Batten's or Batten-Mayou 330.1 *[362.71]*
    degeneration 362.89
    vascular lesion 362.17
  rheumatic (*see also* Arthritis) 716.8 ☑
    heart — *see* Disease, heart, rheumatic
  rheumatoid (heart) — *see* Arthritis, rheumatoid
  rickettsial NEC 083.9
    specified type NEC 083.8
  Riedel's (ligneous thyroiditis) 245.3
  Riga (-Fede) (cachectic aphthae) 529.0
  Riggs' (compound periodontitis) 523.40
  Ritter's 695.81
  Rivalta's (cervicofacial actinomycosis) 039.3
  Robles' (onchocerciasis) 125.3 *[360.13]*
  Roger's (congenital interventricular septal defect) 745.4
  Rokitansky's (*see also* Necrosis, liver) 570
  Romberg's 349.89
  Rosenthal's (factor XI deficiency) 286.2
  Rossbach's (hyperchlorhydria) 536.8
    psychogenic 306.4
  Roth (-Bernhardt) 355.1
  Runeberg's (progressive pernicious anemia) 281.0

☑ **Additional Digit Required** — Refer to the Tabular List for Digit Selection   ▵ **Subterms under main terms may continue to next column or page**

2015 ICD-9-CM   ►◄ **Revised Text**   ● **New Line**   ▲ **Revised Code**   Volume 2 — 87

Disease, diseased — Disease, diseased

Disease, diseased — *see also* Syndrome — *continued*

Rust's (tuberculous spondylitis) (*see also* Tuberculosis) 015.0 ☑ *[720.81]*
Rustitskii's (multiple myeloma) (M9730/3) 203.0 ☑
Ruysch's (Hirschsprung's disease) 751.3
Sachs (-Tay) 330.1
sacroiliac NEC 724.6
salivary gland or duct NEC 527.9
   inclusion 078.5
      streptococcal 034.0
   virus 078.5
Sander's (paranoia) 297.1
Sandhoff's 330.1
sandworm 126.9
Savill's (epidemic exfoliative dermatitis) 695.89
Schamberg's (progressive pigmentary dermatosis) 709.09
Schaumann's (sarcoidosis) 135
Schenck's (sporotrichosis) 117.1
Scheuermann's (osteochondrosis) 732.0
Schilder (-Flatau) 341.1
Schimmelbusch's 610.1
Schlatter-Osgood 732.4
Schlatter's tibia (tubercle) 732.4
Schmorl's 722.30
   cervical 722.39
   lumbar, lumbosacral 722.32
   specified region NEC 722.39
   thoracic, thoracolumbar 722.31
Scholz's 330.0
Schönlein (-Henoch) (purpura rheumatica) 287.0
Schottmüller's (*see also* Fever, paratyphoid) 002.9
Schüller-Christian (chronic histiocytosis X) 277.89
Schultz's (agranulocytosis) 288.09
Schwalbe-Ziehen-Oppenheimer 333.6
Schwartz-Jampel 359.23
Schweninger-Buzzi (macular atrophy) 701.3
sclera 379.19
scrofulous (*see also* Tuberculosis) 017.2 ☑
scrotum 608.9
sebaceous glands NEC 706.9
Secretan's (posttraumatic edema) 782.3
semilunar cartilage, cystic 717.5
seminal vesicle 608.9
Senear-Usher (pemphigus erythematosus) 694.4
serum NEC 999.59
Sever's (osteochondrosis calcaneum) 732.5
sexually transmitted — *see* Disease, venereal
Sézary's (reticulosis) (M9701/3) 202.2 ☑
Shaver's (bauxite pneumoconiosis) 503
Sheehan's (postpartum pituitary necrosis) 253.2
shimamushi (scrub typhus) 081.2
shipyard 077.1
sickle cell 282.60
   with
      crisis 282.62
      Hb-S disease 282.61
      other abnormal hemoglobin (Hb-D) (Hb-E) (Hb-G) (Hb-J) (Hb-K) (Hb-O) (Hb-P) (high fetal gene) (without crisis) 282.68
         with crisis 282.69
   elliptocytosis 282.60
   Hb-C (without crisis) 282.63
      with
         crisis 282.64
         vaso-occlusive pain 282.64
   Hb-S 282.61
      with
         crisis 282.62
         Hb-C (without crisis) 282.63
            with
               crisis 282.64
               vaso-occlusive pain 282.64

Disease, diseased — *see also* Syndrome — *continued*

sickle cell — *continued*
   Hb-S — *continued*
      with — *continued*
         other abnormal hemoglobin (Hb-D) (Hb-E) (Hb-G) (Hb-J) (Hb-K) (Hb-O) (Hb-P) (high fetal gene) (without crisis) 282.68
            with crisis 282.69
   spherocytosis 282.60
   thalassemia (without crisis) 282.41
      with
         crisis 282.42
         vaso-occlusive pain 282.42
Siegal-Cattan-Mamou (periodic) 277.31
silo fillers' 506.9
Simian B 054.3
Simmonds' (pituitary cachexia) 253.2
Simons' (progressive lipodystrophy) 272.6
Sinding-Larsen (juvenile osteopathia patellae) 732.4
sinus (*see also* Sinusitis)
   brain 437.9
   specified NEC 478.19
Sirkari's 085.0
sixth (*see also* Exanthem subitum) 058.10
Sjögren (-Gougerot) 710.2
   with lung involvement 710.2 *[517.8]*
Skevas-Zerfus 989.5
skin NEC 709.9
   due to metabolic disorder 277.9
   specified type NEC 709.8
sleeping (*see also* Narcolepsy) 347.00
   meaning sleeping sickness (*see also* Trypanosomiasis) 086.5
small vessel 443.9
Smith-Strang (oasthouse urine) 270.2
Sneddon-Wilkinson (subcorneal pustular dermatosis) 694.1
South African creeping 133.8
Spencer's (epidemic vomiting) 078.82
Spielmeyer-Stock 330.1
Spielmeyer-Vogt 330.1
spine, spinal 733.90
   combined system (*see also* Degeneration, combined) 266.2 *[336.2]*
      with pernicious anemia 281.0 *[336.2]*
   cord NEC 336.9
      congenital 742.9
   demyelinating NEC 341.8
   joint (*see also* Disease, joint, spine) 724.9
   tuberculous 015.0 ☑ *[730.8]* ☑
spinocerebellar 334.9
   specified NEC 334.8
spleen (organic) (postinfectional) 289.50
   amyloid 277.39
   lardaceous 277.39
   polycystic 759.0
   specified NEC 289.59
sponge divers' 989.5
Stanton's (melioidosis) 025
Stargardt's 362.75
Startle 759.89
Steinert's 359.21
Sternberg's — *see* Disease, Hodgkin's
Stevens-Johnson (erythema multiforme exudativum) 695.13
Sticker's (erythema infectiosum) 057.0
Stieda's (calcification, knee joint) 726.62
Still's (juvenile rheumatoid arthritis) 714.30
   adult onset 714.2
Stiller's (asthenia) 780.79
Stokes' (exophthalmic goiter) 242.0 ☑
Stokes-Adams (syncope with heart block) 426.9
Stokvis (-Talma) (enterogenous cyanosis) 289.7
stomach NEC (organic) 537.9
   functional 536.9
      psychogenic 306.4
   lardaceous 277.39
stonemasons' 502

Disease, diseased — *see also* Syndrome — *continued*

storage
   glycogen (*see also* Disease, glycogen storage) 271.0
   lipid 272.7
   mucopolysaccharide 277.5
striatopallidal system 333.90
   specified NEC 333.89
Strümpell-Marie (ankylosing spondylitis) 720.0
Stuart's (congenital factor X deficiency) (*see also* Defect, coagulation) 286.3
Stuart-Prower (congenital factor X deficiency) (*see also* Defect, coagulation) 286.3
Sturge (-Weber) (-Dimitri) (encephalocutaneous angiomatosis) 759.6
Stuttgart 100.89
Sudeck's 733.7
supporting structures of teeth NEC 525.9
suprarenal (gland) (capsule) 255.9
   hyperfunction 255.3
   hypofunction 255.41
Sutton's 709.09
Sutton and Gull's — *see* Hypertension, kidney
sweat glands NEC 705.9
   specified type NEC 705.89
sweating 078.2
Sweeley-Klionsky 272.7
Swift (-Feer) 985.0
swimming pool (bacillus) 031.1
swineherd's 100.89
Sylvest's (epidemic pleurodynia) 074.1
Symmers (follicular lymphoma) (M9690/3) 202.0 ☑
sympathetic nervous system (*see also* Neuropathy, peripheral, autonomic) 337.9
synovium 727.9
syphilitic — *see* Syphilis
systemic tissue mast cell (M9741/3) 202.6 ☑
Taenzer's 757.4
Takayasu's (pulseless) 446.7
Talma's 728.85
Tangier (familial high-density lipoprotein deficiency) 272.5
Tarral-Besnier (pityriasis rubra pilaris) 696.4
Taylor's 701.8
Tay-Sachs 330.1
tear duct 375.69
teeth, tooth 525.9
   hard tissues 521.9
      specified NEC 521.89
   pulp NEC 522.9
tendon 727.9
   inflammatory NEC 727.9
terminal vessel 443.9
testis 608.9
Thaysen-Gee (nontropical sprue) 579.0
Thomsen's 359.22
Thomson's (congenital poikiloderma) 757.33
Thornwaldt's, Tornwaldt's (pharyngeal bursitis) 478.29
throat 478.20
   septic 034.0
thromboembolic (*see also* Embolism) 444.9
thymus (gland) 254.9
   specified NEC 254.8
thyroid (gland) NEC 246.9
   heart (*see also* Hyperthyroidism) 242.9 ☑ *[425.7]*
   lardaceous 277.39
   specified NEC 246.8
Tietze's 733.6
Tommaselli's
   correct substance properly administered 599.70
   overdose or wrong substance given or taken 961.4
tongue 529.9
tonsils, tonsillar (and adenoids) (chronic) 474.9
   specified NEC 474.8
tooth, teeth 525.9

Disease, diseased — *see also* Syndrome — *continued*

tooth, teeth — *continued*
   hard tissues 521.9
      specified NEC 521.89
   pulp NEC 522.9
Tornwaldt's (pharyngeal bursitis) 478.29
Tourette's 307.23
trachea 519.19
tricuspid — *see* Endocarditis, tricuspid
triglyceride-storage, type I, II, III 272.7
triple vessel (coronary arteries) — *see* Arteriosclerosis, coronary
trisymptomatic, Gourgerot's 709.1
trophoblastic (*see also* Hydatidiform mole) 630
   previous, affecting management of pregnancy V23.1
tsutsugamushi (scrub typhus) 081.2
tube (fallopian), noninflammatory 620.9
   specified NEC 620.8
tuberculous NEC (*see also* Tuberculosis) 011.9 ☑
tubo-ovarian
   inflammatory (*see also* Salpingo-oophoritis) 614.2
   noninflammatory 620.9
      specified NEC 620.8
tubotympanic, chronic (with anterior perforation of ear drum) 382.1
tympanum 385.9
Uhl's 746.84
umbilicus (newborn) NEC 779.89
   delayed separation 779.83
Underwood's (sclerema neonatorum) 778.1
undiagnosed 799.9
Unna's (seborrheic dermatitis) 690.18
unstable hemoglobin hemolytic 282.7
Unverricht (-Lundborg) 345.1 ☑
Urbach-Oppenheim (necrobiosis lipoidica diabeticorum) 250.8 ☑ *[709.3]*
   due to secondary diabetes 249.8 ☑ *[709.3]*
Urbach-Wiethe (lipoid proteinosis) 272.8
ureter 593.9
urethra 599.9
   specified type NEC 599.84
urinary (tract) 599.9
   bladder 596.9
      specified NEC 596.89
   maternal, affecting fetus or newborn 760.1
Usher-Senear (pemphigus erythematosus) 694.4
uterus (organic) 621.9
   infective (*see also* Endometritis) 615.9
   inflammatory (*see also* Endometritis) 615.9
   noninflammatory 621.9
      specified type NEC 621.8
uveal tract
   anterior 364.9
   posterior 363.9
vagabonds' 132.1
vagina, vaginal
   inflammatory 616.10
   noninflammatory 623.9
      specified NEC 623.8
Valsuani's (progressive pernicious anemia, puerperal) 648.2 ☑
   complicating pregnancy or puerperium 648.2 ☑
valve, valvular — *see also* Endocarditis
   congenital NEC (*see also* Anomaly, heart, valve) 746.9
   pulmonary 746.00
      specified type NEC 746.89
van Bogaert-Nijssen (-Peiffer) 330.0
van Creveld-von Gierke (glycogenosis I) 271.0
van den Bergh's (enterogenous cyanosis) 289.7
van Neck's (juvenile osteochondrosis) 732.1
Vaquez (-Osler) (polycythemia vera) (M9950/1) 238.4
vascular 459.9

☑ **Additional Digit Required** — Refer to the Tabular List for Digit Selection   ▽ **Subterms under main terms may continue to next column or page**

88 — Volume 2   ▶◀ Revised Text   ● New Line   ▲ Revised Code   2015 ICD-9-CM

Disease, diseased — *see also* Syndrome — *continued*
vascular — *continued*
  arteriosclerotic — *see* Arteriosclerosis
  hypertensive — *see* Hypertension
  obliterative 447.1
    peripheral 443.9
  occlusive 459.9
  peripheral (occlusive) 443.9
    in (due to) (with) diabetes mellitus 250.7 ☑ [443.81]
      in (due to) (with) secondary diabetes 249.7 ☑ [443.81]
    specified type NEC 443.89
vas deferens 608.9
vasomotor 443.9
vasospastic 443.9
vein 459.9
venereal 099.9
  chlamydial NEC 099.50
    anus 099.52
    bladder 099.53
    cervix 099.53
    epididymis 099.54
    genitourinary NEC 099.55
      lower 099.53
      specified NEC 099.54
    pelvic inflammatory disease 099.54
    perihepatic 099.56
    peritoneum 099.56
    pharynx 099.51
    rectum 099.52
    specified site NEC 099.59
    testis 099.54
    vagina 099.53
    vulva 099.53
  complicating pregnancy, childbirth, or puerperium 647.2 ☑
  fifth 099.1
  sixth 099.1
  specified nature or type NEC 099.8
    chlamydial — *see* Disease, venereal, chlamydial
Verneuil's (syphilitic bursitis) 095.7
Verse's (calcinosis intervertebralis) 275.49 [722.90]
vertebra, vertebral NEC 733.90
  disc — *see* Disease, Intervertebral disc
vibration NEC 994.9
Vidal's (lichen simplex chronicus) 698.3
Vincent's (trench mouth) 101
Virchow's 733.99
virus (filterable) NEC 078.89
  arbovirus NEC 066.9
  arthropod-borne NEC 066.9
  central nervous system NEC 049.9
    specified type NEC 049.8
  complicating pregnancy, childbirth, or puerperium 647.6 ☑
  contact (with) V01.79
    varicella V01.71
  exposure to V01.79
    varicella V01.71
  Marburg 078.89
  maternal
    with fetal damage affecting management of pregnancy 655.3 ☑
  nonarthropod-borne NEC 078.89
    central nervous system NEC 049.9
      specified NEC 049.8
  vaccination, prophylactic (against) V04.89
vitreous 379.29
vocal cords NEC 478.5
Vogt's (Cecile) 333.71
Vogt-Spielmeyer 330.1
Volhard-Fahr (malignant nephrosclerosis) 403.90
Volkmann's
  acquired 958.6
von Bechterew's (ankylosing spondylitis) 720.0
von Economo's (encephalitis lethargica) 049.8
von Eulenburg's (congenital paramyotonia) 359.29

Disease, diseased — *see also* Syndrome — *continued*
von Gierke's (glycogenosis I) 271.0
von Graefe's 378.72
von Hippel's (retinocerebral angiomatosis) 759.6
von Hippel-Lindau (angiomatosis retinocerebellosa) 759.6
von Jaksch's (pseudoleukemia infantum) 285.8
von Recklinghausen's (M9540/1) 237.71
  bone (osteitis fibrosa cystica) 252.01
von Recklinghausen-Applebaum (hemochromatosis) (*see also* Hemochromatosis) 275.03
von Willebrand (-Jürgens) (angiohemophilia) 286.4
von Zambusch's (lichen sclerosus et atrophicus) 701.0
Voorhoeve's (dyschondroplasia) 756.4
Vrolik's (osteogenesis imperfecta) 756.51
vulva
  inflammatory 616.10
  noninflammatory 624.9
    specified NEC 624.8
Wagner's (colloid milium) 709.3
Waldenström's (osteochondrosis capital femoral) 732.1
Wallgren's (obstruction of splenic vein with collateral circulation) 459.89
Wardrop's (with lymphangitis) 681.9
  finger 681.02
  toe 681.11
Wassilieff's (leptospiral jaundice) 100.0
wasting NEC 799.4
  due to malnutrition 261
  paralysis 335.21
Waterhouse-Friderichsen 036.3
waxy (any site) 277.39
Weber-Christian (nodular nonsuppurative panniculitis) 729.30
Wegner's (syphilitic osteochondritis) 090.0
Weil's (leptospiral jaundice) 100.0
  of lung 100.0
Weir Mitchell's (erythromelalgia) 443.82
Werdnig-Hoffmann 335.0
Werlhof's (*see also* Purpura, thrombocytopenic) 287.39
Wermer's 258.01
Werner's (progeria adultorum) 259.8
Werner-His (trench fever) 083.1
Werner-Schultz (agranulocytosis) 288.09
Wernicke's (superior hemorrhagic polioencephalitis) 265.1
Wernicke-Posadas 114.9
Whipple's (intestinal lipodystrophy) 040.2
whipworm 127.3
white
White's (congenital) (keratosis follicularis) 757.39
  blood cell 288.9
    specified NEC 288.8
  spot 701.0
Whitmore's (melioidosis) 025
Widal-Abrami (acquired hemolytic jaundice) 283.9
Wilkie's 557.1
Wilkinson-Sneddon (subcorneal pustular dermatosis) 694.1
Willis' (diabetes mellitus) (*see also* Diabetes) 250.0 ☑
  due to secondary diabetes 249.0 ☑
Wilson's (hepatolenticular degeneration) 275.1
Wilson-Brocq (dermatitis exfoliativa) 695.89
winter vomiting 078.82
Wise's 696.2
Wohlfart-Kugelberg-Welander 335.11
Woillez's (acute idiopathic pulmonary congestion) 518.52
Wolman's (primary familial xanthomatosis) 272.7
wool-sorters' 022.1
Zagari's (xerostomia) 527.7
Zahorsky's (exanthem subitum) 058.10
Ziehen-Oppenheim 333.6

Disease, diseased — *see also* Syndrome — *continued*
zoonotic, bacterial NEC 027.9
  specified type NEC 027.8
Disfigurement (due to scar) 709.2
  head V48.6
  limb V49.4
  neck V48.7
  trunk V48.7
Disgerminoma — *see* Dysgerminoma
Disinsertion, retina 361.04
Disintegration, complete, of the body 799.89
  traumatic 869.1
Disk kidney 753.3
Dislocatable hip, congenital — *see also* Dislocation, hip, congenital 754.30
Dislocation (articulation) (closed) (displacement) (simple) (subluxation) 839.8

> *Note* — *"Closed" includes simple, complete, partial, uncomplicated, and unspecified dislocation.*
>
> *"Open" includes dislocation specified as infected or compound and dislocation with foreign body.*
>
> *"Chronic," "habitual," "old," or "recurrent" dislocations should be coded as indicated under the entry "Dislocation, recurrent," and "pathological" as indicated under the entry "Dislocation, pathological."*
>
> *For late effect of dislocation see Late, effect, dislocation.*

  with fracture — *see* Fracture, by site
  acromioclavicular (joint) (closed) 831.04
    open 831.14
  anatomical site (closed)
    specified NEC 839.69
      open 839.79
    unspecified or ill-defined 839.8
      open 839.9
  ankle (scaphoid bone) (closed) 837.0
    open 837.1
  arm (closed) 839.8
    open 839.9
  astragalus (closed) 837.0
    open 837.1
  atlanto-axial (closed) 839.01
    open 839.11
  atlas (closed) 839.01
    open 839.11
  axis (closed) 839.02
    open 839.12
  back (closed) 839.8
    open 839.9
  Bell-Daly 723.8
  breast bone (closed) 839.61
    open 839.71
  capsule, joint — *see* Dislocation, by site
  carpal (bone) — *see* Dislocation, wrist
  carpometacarpal (joint) (closed) 833.04
    open 833.14
  cartilage (joint) (*see also* Dislocation, by site)
    knee — *see* Tear, meniscus
  cervical, cervicodorsal, or cervicothoracic (spine) (vertebra) — *see* Dislocation, vertebra, cervical
  chiropractic (*see also* Lesion, nonallopathic) 739.9
  chondrocostal — *see* Dislocation, costochondral
  chronic — *see* Dislocation, recurrent
  clavicle (closed) 831.04
    open 831.14
  coccyx (closed) 839.41
    open 839.51
  collar bone (closed) 831.04
    open 831.14
  compound (open) NEC 839.9
  congenital NEC 755.8
    hip (*see also* Dislocation, hip, congenital) 754.30
    lens 743.37
    rib 756.3
    sacroiliac 755.69

Dislocation — *continued*
congenital — *continued*
    spine NEC 756.19
    vertebra 756.19
  coracoid (closed) 831.09
    open 831.19
  costal cartilage (closed) 839.69
    open 839.79
  costochondral (closed) 839.69
    open 839.79
  cricoarytenoid articulation (closed) 839.69
    open 839.79
  cricothyroid (cartilage) articulation (closed) 839.69
    open 839.79
  dorsal vertebrae (closed) 839.21
    open 839.31
  ear ossicle 385.23
  elbow (closed) 832.00
    anterior (closed) 832.01
      open 832.11
    congenital 754.89
    divergent (closed) 832.09
      open 832.19
    lateral (closed) 832.04
      open 832.14
    medial (closed) 832.03
      open 832.13
    open 832.10
    posterior (closed) 832.02
      open 832.12
    recurrent 718.32
    specified type NEC 832.09
      open 832.19
  eye 360.81
    lateral 376.36
  eyeball 360.81
    lateral 376.36
  femur
    distal end (closed) 836.50
      anterior 836.52
        open 836.62
      lateral 836.54
        open 836.64
      medial 836.53
        open 836.63
      open 836.60
      posterior 836.51
        open 836.61
    proximal end (closed) 835.00
      anterior (pubic) 835.03
        open 835.13
      obturator 835.02
        open 835.12
      open 835.10
      posterior 835.01
        open 835.11
  fibula
    distal end (closed) 837.0
      open 837.1
    proximal end (closed) 836.59
      open 836.69
  finger(s) (phalanx) (thumb) (closed) 834.00
    interphalangeal (joint) 834.02
      open 834.12
    metacarpal (bone), distal end 834.01
      open 834.11
    metacarpophalangeal (joint) 834.01
      open 834.11
    open 834.10
    recurrent 718.34
  foot (closed) 838.00
    open 838.10
    recurrent 718.37
  forearm (closed) 839.8
    open 839.9
  fracture — *see* Fracture, by site
  glenoid (closed) 831.09
    open 831.19
  habitual — *see* Dislocation, recurrent
  hand (closed) 839.8
    open 839.9
  hip (closed) 835.00
    anterior 835.03
      obturator 835.02
      open 835.12

☑ **Additional Digit Required** — Refer to the Tabular List for Digit Selection   ▽ **Subterms under main terms may continue to next column or page**

2015 ICD-9-CM   ▶◀ Revised Text   ● New Line   ▲ Revised Code   Volume 2 — 89

Dislocation — *continued*
  hip — *continued*
    anterior — *continued*
      open 835.13
    congenital (unilateral) 754.30
      with subluxation of other hip 754.35
      bilateral 754.31
    developmental 718.75
    open 835.10
    posterior 835.01
      open 835.11
    recurrent 718.35
  humerus 831.00
    distal end (*see also* Dislocation, elbow) 832.00
      open 831.10
    proximal end (closed) 831.00
      anterior (subclavicular) (subcoracoid) (subglenoid) (closed) 831.01
        open 831.11
      inferior (closed) 831.03
        open 831.13
      open 831.10
      posterior (closed) 831.02
        open 831.12
  implant — *see* Complications, mechanical
  incus 385.23
  infracoracoid (closed) 831.01
    open 831.11
  innominate (pubic junction) (sacral junction) (closed) 839.69
    acetabulum (*see also* Dislocation, hip) 835.00
    open 839.79
  interphalangeal (joint)
    finger or hand (closed) 834.02
      open 834.12
    foot or toe (closed) 838.06
      open 838.16
  jaw (cartilage) (meniscus) (closed) 830.0
    open 830.1
    recurrent 524.69
  joint NEC (closed) 839.8
    developmental 718.7 ☑
    open 839.9
    pathological — *see* Dislocation, pathological
    recurrent — *see* Dislocation, recurrent
  knee (closed) 836.50
    anterior 836.51
      open 836.61
    congenital (with genu recurvatum) 754.41
    habitual 718.36
    lateral 836.54
      open 836.64
    medial 836.53
      open 836.63
    old 718.36
    open 836.60
    posterior 836.52
      open 836.62
    recurrent 718.36
    rotatory 836.59
      open 836.69
  lacrimal gland 375.16
  leg (closed) 839.8
    open 839.9
  lens (crystalline) (complete) (partial) 379.32
    anterior 379.33
    congenital 743.37
    ocular implant 996.53
    posterior 379.34
    traumatic 921.3
  ligament — *see* Dislocation, by site
  lumbar (vertebrae) (closed) 839.20
    open 839.30
  lumbosacral (vertebrae) (closed) 839.20
    congenital 756.19
    open 839.30
  mandible (closed) 830.0
    open 830.1
  maxilla (inferior) (closed) 830.0
    open 830.1
  meniscus (knee) (*see also* Tear, meniscus)
    other sites — *see* Dislocation, by site

Dislocation — *continued*
  metacarpal (bone)
    distal end (closed) 834.01
      open 834.11
    proximal end (closed) 833.05
      open 833.15
  metacarpophalangeal (joint) (closed) 834.01
    open 834.11
  metatarsal (bone) (closed) 838.04
    open 838.14
  metatarsophalangeal (joint) (closed) 838.05
    open 838.15
  midcarpal (joint) (closed) 833.03
    open 833.13
  midtarsal (joint) (closed) 838.02
    open 838.12
  Monteggia's — *see* Dislocation, hip
  multiple locations (except fingers only or toes only) (closed) 839.8
    open 839.9
  navicular (bone) foot (closed) 837.0
    open 837.1
  neck (*see also* Dislocation, vertebra, cervical) 839.00
  Nélaton's — *see* Dislocation, ankle
  nontraumatic (joint) — *see* Dislocation, pathological
  nose (closed) 839.69
    open 839.79
  not recurrent, not current injury — *see* Dislocation, pathological
  occiput from atlas (closed) 839.01
    open 839.11
  old — *see* Dislocation, recurrent
  open (compound) NEC 839.9
  ossicle, ear 385.23
  paralytic (flaccid) (spastic) — *see* Dislocation, pathological
  patella (closed) 836.3
    congenital 755.64
    open 836.4
  pathological NEC 718.20
    ankle 718.27
    elbow 718.22
    foot 718.27
    hand 718.24
    hip 718.25
    knee 718.26
    lumbosacral joint 724.6
    multiple sites 718.29
    pelvic region 718.25
    sacroiliac 724.6
    shoulder (region) 718.21
    specified site NEC 718.28
    spine 724.8
      sacroiliac 724.6
    wrist 718.23
  pelvis (closed) 839.69
    acetabulum (*see also* Dislocation, hip) 835.00
    open 839.79
  phalanx
    foot or toe (closed) 838.09
      open 838.19
    hand or finger (*see also* Dislocation, finger) 834.00
  postpoliomyelitic — *see* Dislocation, pathological
  prosthesis, internal — *see* Complications, mechanical
  radiocarpal (joint) (closed) 833.02
    open 833.12
  radioulnar (joint)
    distal end (closed) 833.01
      open 833.11
    proximal end (*see also* Dislocation, elbow) 832.00
  radius
    distal end (closed) 833.00
      open 833.10
    proximal end (closed) 832.01
      open 832.11
  recurrent (*see also* Derangement, joint, recurrent) 718.3 ☑
    elbow 718.32
    hip 718.35

Dislocation — *continued*
  recurrent (*see also* Derangement, joint, recurrent) — *continued*
    joint NEC 718.38
    knee 718.36
    lumbosacral (joint) 724.6
    patella 718.36
    sacroiliac 724.6
    shoulder 718.31
    temporomandibular 524.69
  rib (cartilage) (closed) 839.69
    congenital 756.3
    open 839.79
  sacrococcygeal (closed) 839.42
    open 839.52
  sacroiliac (joint) (ligament) (closed) 839.42
    congenital 755.69
    open 839.52
    recurrent 724.6
  sacrum (closed) 839.42
    open 839.52
  scaphoid (bone)
    ankle or foot (closed) 837.0
      open 837.1
    wrist (closed) (*see also* Dislocation, wrist) 833.00
      open 833.10
  scapula (closed) 831.09
    open 831.19
  semilunar cartilage, knee — *see* Tear, meniscus
  septal cartilage (nose) (closed) 839.69
    open 839.79
  septum (nasal) (old) 470
  sesamoid bone — *see* Dislocation, by site
  shoulder (blade) (ligament) (closed) 831.00
    anterior (subclavicular) (subcoracoid) (subglenoid) (closed) 831.01
      open 831.11
    chronic 718.31
    inferior 831.03
      open 831.13
    open 831.10
    posterior (closed) 831.02
      open 831.12
    recurrent 718.31
  skull — *see* Injury, intracranial
  Smith's — *see* Dislocation, foot
  spine (articular process) (*see also* Dislocation, vertebra) (closed) 839.40
    atlanto-axial (closed) 839.01
      open 839.11
      recurrent 723.8
    cervical, cervicodorsal, cervicothoracic (closed) (*see also* Dislocation, vertebrae, cervical) 839.00
      open 839.10
      recurrent 723.8
    coccyx 839.41
      open 839.51
    congenital 756.19
    due to birth trauma 767.4
    open 839.50
    recurrent 724.9
    sacroiliac 839.42
      recurrent 724.6
    sacrum (sacrococcygeal) (sacroiliac) 839.42
      open 839.52
  spontaneous — *see* Dislocation, pathological
  sternoclavicular (joint) (closed) 839.61
    open 839.71
  sternum (closed) 839.61
    open 839.71
  subastragalar — *see* Dislocation, foot
  subglenoid (closed) 831.01
    open 831.11
  symphysis
    jaw (closed) 830.0
      open 830.1
    mandibular (closed) 830.0
      open 830.1
    pubis (closed) 839.69
      open 839.79
  tarsal (bone) (joint) 838.01

Dislocation — *continued*
  tarsal — *continued*
    open 838.11
  tarsometatarsal (joint) 838.03
    open 838.13
  temporomandibular (joint) (closed) 830.0
    open 830.1
    recurrent 524.69
  thigh
    distal end (*see also* Dislocation, femur, distal end) 836.50
    proximal end (*see also* Dislocation, hip) 835.00
  thoracic (vertebrae) (closed) 839.21
    open 839.31
  thumb(s) (*see also* Dislocation, finger) 834.00
  thyroid cartilage (closed) 839.69
    open 839.79
  tibia
    distal end (closed) 837.0
      open 837.1
    proximal end (closed) 836.50
      anterior 836.51
        open 836.61
      lateral 836.54
        open 836.64
      medial 836.53
        open 836.63
      open 836.60
      posterior 836.52
        open 836.62
      rotatory 836.59
        open 836.69
  tibiofibular
    distal (closed) 837.0
      open 837.1
    superior (closed) 836.59
      open 836.69
  toe(s) (closed) 838.09
    open 838.19
  trachea (closed) 839.69
    open 839.79
  ulna
    distal end (closed) 833.09
      open 833.19
    proximal end — *see* Dislocation, elbow
  vertebra (articular process) (body) (closed) (traumatic) 839.40
    cervical, cervicodorsal or cervicothoracic (closed) 839.00
      first (atlas) 839.01
        open 839.11
      second (axis) 839.02
        open 839.12
      third 839.03
        open 839.13
      fourth 839.04
        open 839.14
      fifth 839.05
        open 839.15
      sixth 839.06
        open 839.16
      seventh 839.07
        open 839.17
      congenital 756.19
      multiple sites 839.08
        open 839.18
      open 839.10
    congenital 756.19
    dorsal 839.21
      open 839.31
      recurrent 724.9
    lumbar, lumbosacral 839.20
      open 839.30
    non-traumatic — *see* Displacement, intervertebral disc
    open NEC 839.50
    recurrent 724.9
    specified region NEC 839.49
      open 839.59
    thoracic 839.21
      open 839.31
  wrist (carpal bone) (scaphoid) (semilunar) (closed) 833.00
    carpometacarpal (joint) 833.04
      open 833.14

☑ **Additional Digit Required** — Refer to the Tabular List for Digit Selection   ▽ **Subterms under main terms may continue to next column or page**

90 — Volume 2   ►◄ Revised Text   ● New Line   ▲ Revised Code   2015 ICD-9-CM

Dislocation — *continued*
  wrist — *continued*
    metacarpal bone, proximal end 833.05
      open 833.15
    midcarpal (joint) 833.03
      open 833.13
    open 833.10
    radiocarpal (joint) 833.02
      open 833.12
    radioulnar (joint) 833.01
      open 833.11
    recurrent 718.33
    specified site NEC 833.09
      open 833.19
  xiphoid cartilage (closed) 839.61
    open 839.71
Dislodgement
  artificial skin graft 996.55
  decellularized allodermis graft 996.55
Disobedience, hostile (covert) (overt) — *see also* Disturbance, conduct 312.0 ☑
Disorder — *see also* Disease
  academic underachievement, childhood and adolescence 313.83
  accommodation 367.51
    drug-induced 367.89
    toxic 367.89
  adjustment (*see also* Reaction, adjustment) 309.9
    with
      anxiety 309.24
      anxiety and depressed mood 309.28
      depressed mood 309.0
      disturbance of conduct 309.3
      disturbance of emotions and conduct 309.4
  adrenal (capsule) (cortex) (gland) 255.9
    specified type NEC 255.8
  adrenogenital 255.2
  affective (*see also* Psychosis, affective) 296.90
    atypical 296.81
  aggressive, unsocialized (*see also* Disturbance, conduct) 312.0 ☑
  alcohol, alcoholic (*see also* Alcohol) 291.9
    induced mood 291.89
  allergic — *see* Allergy
  amino acid (metabolic) (*see also* Disturbance, metabolism, amino acid) 270.9
    albinism 270.2
    alkaptonuria 270.2
    argininosuccinicaciduria 270.6
    beta-amino-isobutyricaciduria 277.2
    cystathioninuria 270.4
    cystinosis 270.0
    cystinuria 270.0
    glycinuria 270.0
    homocystinuria 270.4
    imidazole 270.5
    maple syrup (urine) disease 270.3
    neonatal, transitory 775.89
    oasthouse urine disease 270.2
    ochronosis 270.2
    phenylketonuria 270.1
    phenylpyruvic oligophrenia 270.1
    purine NEC 277.2
    pyrimidine NEC 277.2
    renal transport NEC 270.0
    specified type NEC 270.8
    transport NEC 270.0
      renal 270.0
    xanthinuria 277.2
  amnestic (*see also* Amnestic syndrome) 294.8
    alcohol-induced persisting 291.1
    drug-induced persisting 292.83
    in conditions classified elsewhere 294.0
  anaerobic glycolysis with anemia 282.3
  anxiety (*see also* Anxiety) 300.00
    due to or associated with physical condition 293.84
  arteriole 447.9
    specified type NEC 447.8
  artery 447.9
    specified type NEC 447.8

Disorder — *see also* Disease — *continued*
  articulation — *see* Disorder, joint
  Asperger's 299.8 ☑
  attachment of infancy or early childhood 313.89
  attention deficit 314.00
    with hyperactivity 314.01
    predominantly
      combined hyperactive/inattentive 314.01
      hyperactive/impulsive 314.01
      inattentive 314.00
    residual type 314.8
  auditory processing disorder 388.45
    acquired 388.45
    developmental 315.32
  autistic 299.0 ☑
  autoimmune NEC 279.49
    hemolytic (cold type) (warm type) 283.0
    parathyroid 252.1
    thyroid 245.2
  avoidant, childhood or adolescence 313.21
  balance
    acid-base 276.9
      mixed (with hypercapnia) 276.4
    electrolyte 276.9
    fluid 276.9
  behavior NEC (*see also* Disturbance, conduct) 312.9
    disruptive 312.9
  bilirubin excretion 277.4
  bipolar (affective) (alternating) 296.80

> *Note* — *Use the following fifth-digit subclassification with categories 296.0–296.6:*
>
> 0   *unspecifed*
>
> 1   *mild*
>
> 2   *moderate*
>
> 3   *severe, without mention of psychotic behavior*
>
> 4   *severe, specified as with psychotic behavior*
>
> 5   *in partial or unspecified remission*
>
> 6   *in full remission*

    atypical 296.7
    currently
      depressed 296.5 ☑
      hypomanic 296.4 ☑
      manic 296.4 ☑
    mixed 296.6 ☑
    specified type NEC 296.89
    type I 296.7
      most recent episode (or current)
        depressed 296.5 ☑
        hypomanic 296.4 ☑
        manic 296.4 ☑
        mixed 296.6 ☑
        unspecified 296.7
      single manic episode 296.0 ☑
    type II (recurrent major depressive episodes with hypomania) 296.89
  bladder 596.9
    functional NEC 596.59
    specified NEC 596.89
  bleeding 286.9
  bone NEC 733.90
    specified NEC 733.99
  brachial plexus 353.0
  branched-chain amino-acid degradation 270.3
  breast 611.9
    puerperal, postpartum 676.3 ☑
    specified NEC 611.89
  Briquet's 300.81
  bursa 727.9
    shoulder region 726.10
  carbohydrate metabolism, congenital 271.9
  cardiac, functional 427.9
    postoperative 997.1
    psychogenic 306.2
  cardiovascular, psychogenic 306.2
  cartilage NEC 733.90

Disorder — *see also* Disease — *continued*
  cartilage — *continued*
    articular 718.00
      ankle 718.07
      elbow 718.02
      foot 718.07
      hand 718.04
      hip 718.05
      knee 717.9
      multiple sites 718.09
      pelvic region 718.05
      shoulder region 718.01
      specified
        site NEC 718.08
        type NEC 733.99
      wrist 718.03
  catatonic — *see* Catatonia
  central auditory processing 315.32
    acquired 388.45
    developmental 315.32
  cervical region NEC 723.9
  cervical root (nerve) NEC 353.2
  character NEC (*see also* Disorder, personality) 301.9
  ciliary body 364.9
    specified NEC 364.89
  coagulation (factor) (*see also* Defect, coagulation) 286.9
    factor VIII (congenital) (functional) 286.0
    factor IX (congenital) (functional) 286.1
    neonatal, transitory 776.3
  coccyx 724.70
    specified NEC 724.79
  cognitive 294.9
  colon 569.9
    functional 564.9
      congenital 751.3
  communication 307.9
  conduct (*see also* Disturbance, conduct) 312.9
    adjustment reaction 309.3
    adolescent onset type 312.82
    childhood onset type 312.81
    compulsive 312.30
      specified type NEC 312.39
    hyperkinetic 314.2
    onset unspecified 312.89
    socialized (type) 312.20
      aggressive 312.23
      unaggressive 312.21
    specified NEC 312.89
  conduction, heart 426.9
    specified NEC 426.89
  conflict
    sexual orientation 302.0
  congenital
    glycosylation (CDG) 271.8
  convulsive (secondary) (*see also* Convulsions) 780.39
    due to injury at birth 767.0
    idiopathic 780.39
  coordination 781.3
  cornea NEC 371.89
    due to contact lens 371.82
  corticosteroid metabolism NEC 255.2
  cranial nerve — *see* Disorder, nerve, cranial
  cyclothymic 301.13
  degradation, branched-chain amino acid 270.3
  delusional 297.1
  dentition 520.6
  depersonalization 300.6
  depressive NEC 311
    atypical 296.82
    major (*see also* Psychosis, affective) 296.2 ☑
      recurrent episode 296.3 ☑
      single episode 296.2 ☑
  development, specific 315.9
    associated with hyperkinesia 314.1
    coordination 315.4
    language 315.31
      and speech due to hearing loss 315.34
    learning 315.2
      arithmetical 315.1

Disorder — *see also* Disease — *continued*
  development, specific — *continued*
    learning — *continued*
      reading 315.00
    mixed 315.5
    motor coordination 315.4
    specified type NEC 315.8
    speech 315.39
      and language due to hearing loss 315.34
  diaphragm 519.4
  digestive 536.9
    fetus or newborn 777.9
      specified NEC 777.8
    psychogenic 306.4
  disintegrative, childhood 299.1 ☑
  dissociative 300.15
    identity 300.14
    nocturnal 307.47
  drug-related 292.9
  dysmorphic body 300.7
  dysthymic 300.4
  ear 388.9
    degenerative NEC 388.00
    external 380.9
      specified 380.89
    pinna 380.30
    specified type NEC 388.8
    vascular NEC 388.00
  eating NEC 307.50
  electrolyte NEC 276.9
    with
      abortion — *see* Abortion, by type, with metabolic disorder
      ectopic pregnancy (*see also* categories 633.0–633.9) 639.4
      molar pregnancy (*see also* categories 630–632) 639.4
    acidosis 276.2
      metabolic 276.2
      respiratory 276.2
    alkalosis 276.3
      metabolic 276.3
      respiratory 276.3
    following
      abortion 639.4
      ectopic or molar pregnancy 639.4
    neonatal, transitory NEC 775.5
  emancipation as adjustment reaction 309.22
  emotional (*see also* Disorder, mental, nonpsychotic) V40.9
  endocrine 259.9
    specified type NEC 259.8
  esophagus 530.9
    functional 530.5
    psychogenic 306.4
  explosive
    intermittent 312.34
    isolated 312.35
  expressive language 315.31
  eye 379.90
    globe — *see* Disorder, globe
    ill-defined NEC 379.99
    limited duction NEC 378.63
    specified NEC 379.8
  eyelid 374.9
    degenerative 374.50
    sensory 374.44
    specified type NEC 374.89
    vascular 374.85
  factitious (with combined psychological and physical signs and symptoms) (with predominantly physical signs and symptoms) 300.19
    with predominantly psychological signs and symptoms 300.16
  factor, coagulation (*see also* Defect, coagulation) 286.9
    IX (congenital) (functional) 286.1
    VIII (congenital) (functional) 286.0
  fascia 728.9
  fatty acid oxidation 277.85
  feeding — *see* Feeding
  female sexual arousal 302.72
  fluency 315.35
    adult onset 307.0

☑ **Additional Digit Required** — Refer to the Tabular List for Digit Selection   ᴺᴱᶜ **Subterms under main terms may continue to next column or page**

2015 ICD-9-CM   ▶◀ Revised Text   ● New Line   ▲ Revised Code   Volume 2 — 91

Disorder — *see also* Disease — *continued*
fluency — *continued*
   childhood onset 315.35
   due to late effect of cerebrovascular accident 438.14
   in conditions classified elsewhere 784.52
fluid NEC 276.9
gastric (functional) 536.9
   motility 536.8
   psychogenic 306.4
   secretion 536.8
gastrointestinal (functional) NEC 536.9
   newborn (neonatal) 777.9
      specified NEC 777.8
   psychogenic 306.4
gender (child) 302.6
   adult 302.85
gender identity (childhood) 302.6
   adolescents 302.85
   adults (-life) 302.85
genitourinary system, psychogenic 306.50
globe 360.9
   degenerative 360.20
      specified NEC 360.29
   specified type NEC 360.89
hearing (*see also* Deafness)
   conductive type (air) (*see also* Deafness, conductive) 389.00
   mixed conductive and sensorineural 389.20
      bilateral 389.22
      unilateral 389.21
   nerve
      bilateral 389.12
      unilateral 389.13
   perceptive (*see also* Deafness, perceptive) 389.10
   sensorineural type NEC (*see also* Deafness, sensorineural 389.10
heart action 427.9
   postoperative 997.1
hematological, transient neonatal 776.9
   specified type NEC 776.8
hematopoietic organs 289.9
hemorrhagic NEC 287.9
   due to intrinsic circulating anticoagulants, antibodies, or inhibitors 286.59
   with
      acquired hemophilia 286.52
      antiphospholipid antibody 286.53
   specified type NEC 287.8
hemostasis (*see also* Defect, coagulation) 286.9
homosexual conflict 302.0
hypomanic (chronic) 301.11
identity
   childhood and adolescence 313.82
      gender 302.6
immune mechanism (immunity) 279.9
   single complement (C1-C9) 279.8
   specified type NEC 279.8
impulse control (*see also* Disturbance, conduct, compulsive) 312.30
infant sialic acid storage 271.8
integument, fetus or newborn 778.9
   specified type NEC 778.8
interactional psychotic (childhood) (*see also* Psychosis, childhood) 299.1 ☑
intermittent explosive 312.34
intervertebral disc 722.90
   cervical, cervicothoracic 722.91
   lumbar, lumbosacral 722.93
   thoracic, thoracolumbar 722.92
intestinal 569.9
   functional NEC 564.9
      congenital 751.3
      postoperative 564.4
   psychogenic 306.4
introverted, of childhood and adolescence 313.22
involuntary emotional expression (IEED) 310.81
iris 364.9
   specified NEC 364.89
iron, metabolism 275.09

Disorder — *see also* Disease — *continued*
iron, metabolism — *continued*
   specified type NEC 275.09
isolated explosive 312.35
joint NEC 719.90
   ankle 719.97
   elbow 719.92
   foot 719.97
   hand 719.94
   hip 719.95
   knee 719.96
   multiple sites 719.99
   pelvic region 719.95
   psychogenic 306.0
   shoulder (region) 719.91
   specified site NEC 719.98
   temporomandibular 524.60
      sounds on opening or closing 524.64
      specified NEC 524.69
   wrist 719.93
kidney 593.9
   functional 588.9
      specified NEC 588.89
labyrinth, labyrinthine 386.9
   specified type NEC 386.8
lactation 676.9 ☑
language (developmental) (expressive) 315.31
   mixed receptive-expressive 315.32
learning 315.9
ligament 728.9
ligamentous attachments, peripheral (*see also* Enthesopathy)
   spine 720.1
limb NEC 729.90
   psychogenic 306.0
lipid
   metabolism, congenital 272.9
   storage 272.7
lipoprotein deficiency (familial) 272.5
low back NEC 724.9
   psychogenic 306.0
lumbosacral
   plexus 353.1
   root (nerve) NEC 353.4
lymphoproliferative (chronic) NEC (M9970/1) 238.79
   post-transplant (PTLD) 238.77
major depressive (*see also* Psychosis, affective) 296.2 ☑
   recurrent episode 296.3 ☑
   single episode 296.2 ☑
male erectile 607.84
   nonorganic origin 302.72
manic (*see also* Psychosis, affective) 296.0 ☑
   atypical 296.81
mathematics 315.1
meniscus NEC (*see also* Disorder, cartilage, articular) 718.0 ☑
menopausal 627.9
   specified NEC 627.8
menstrual 626.9
   psychogenic 306.52
   specified NEC 626.8
mental (nonpsychotic) 300.9
   affecting management of pregnancy, childbirth, or puerperium 648.4 ☑
   drug-induced 292.9
      hallucinogen persisting perception 292.89
      specified type NEC 292.89
   due to or associated with
      alcoholism 291.9
      drug consumption NEC 292.9
         specified type NEC 292.89
      physical condition NEC 293.9
   induced by drug 292.9
      specified type NEC 292.89
   neurotic (*see also* Neurosis) 300.9
   of infancy, childhood or adolescence 313.9
   persistent
      other
         due to conditions classified elsewhere 294.8

Disorder — *see also* Disease — *continued*
mental — *continued*
   persistent — *continued*
      unspecified
         due to conditions classified elsewhere 294.9
   presenile 310.1
      psychotic NEC 290.10
   previous, affecting management of pregnancy V23.89
   psychoneurotic (*see also* Neurosis) 300.9
   psychotic (*see also* Psychosis) 298.9
      brief 298.8
      senile 290.20
   specific, following organic brain damage 310.9
      cognitive or personality change of other type 310.1
      frontal lobe syndrome 310.0
      postconcussional syndrome 310.2
      specified type NEC 310.89
   transient
      in conditions classified elsewhere 293.9
metabolism NEC 277.9
   with
      abortion — *see* Abortion, by type, with metabolic disorder
      ectopic pregnancy (*see also* categories 633.0–633.9) 639.4
      molar pregnancy (*see also* categories 630–632) 639.4
   alkaptonuria 270.2
   amino acid (*see also* Disorder, amino acid) 270.9
      specified type NEC 270.8
   ammonia 270.6
   arginine 270.6
   argininosuccinic acid 270.6
   basal 794.7
   bilirubin 277.4
   calcium 275.40
   carbohydrate 271.9
      specified type NEC 271.8
   cholesterol 272.9
   citrulline 270.6
   copper 275.1
   corticosteroid 255.2
   cystine storage 270.0
   cystinuria 270.0
   fat 272.9
   fatty acid oxidation 277.85
   following
      abortion 639.4
      ectopic or molar pregnancy 639.4
   fructosemia 271.2
   fructosuria 271.2
   fucosidosis 271.8
   galactose-1-phosphate uridyl transferase 271.1
   glutamine 270.7
   glycine 270.7
   glycogen storage NEC 271.0
      hepatorenal 271.0
   hemochromatosis (*see also* Hemochromatosis) 275.03
   in labor and delivery 669.0 ☑
   iron 275.09
   lactose 271.3
   lipid 272.9
      specified type NEC 272.8
      storage 272.7
   lipoprotein (*see also* Hyperlipemia deficiency (familial)) 272.5
   lysine 270.7
   magnesium 275.2
   mannosidosis 271.8
   mineral 275.9
      specified type NEC 275.8
   mitochondrial 277.87
   mucopolysaccharide 277.5
   nitrogen 270.9
   ornithine 270.6
   oxalosis 271.8
   pentosuria 271.8
   phenylketonuria 270.1

Disorder — *see also* Disease — *continued*
metabolism — *continued*
   phosphate 275.3
   phosphorous 275.3
   plasma protein 273.9
      specified type NEC 273.8
   porphyrin 277.1
   purine 277.2
   pyrimidine 277.2
   serine 270.7
   sodium 276.9
   specified type NEC 277.89
   steroid 255.2
   threonine 270.7
   urea cycle 270.6
   xylose 271.8
micturition NEC 788.69
   psychogenic 306.53
misery and unhappiness, of childhood and adolescence 313.1
mitochondrial metabolism 277.87
mitral valve 424.0
mood (*see also* Disorder, bipolar) 296.90
   alcohol-induced 291.89
   episodic 296.90
      specified NEC 296.99
   in conditions classified elsewhere 293.83
motor tic 307.20
   chronic 307.22
   transient (childhood) 307.21
movement NEC 333.90
   hysterical 300.11
   medication-induced 333.90
   periodic limb 327.51
   sleep related, unspecified 780.58
      other organic 327.59
   specified type NEC 333.99
   stereotypic 307.3
mucopolysaccharide 277.5
muscle 728.9
   psychogenic 306.0
   specified type NEC 728.3
muscular attachments, peripheral (*see also* Enthesopathy)
   spine 720.1
musculoskeletal system NEC 729.90
   psychogenic 306.0
myeloproliferative (chronic) NEC (M9960/1) 238.79
myoneural 358.9
   due to lead 358.2
   specified type NEC 358.8
   toxic 358.2
myotonic 359.29
neck region NEC 723.9
nerve 349.9
   abducens NEC 378.54
   accessory 352.4
   acoustic 388.5
   auditory 388.5
   auriculotemporal 350.8
   axillary 353.0
   cerebral — *see* Disorder, nerve, cranial
   cranial 352.9
      first 352.0
      second 377.49
      third
         partial 378.51
         total 378.52
      fourth 378.53
      fifth 350.9
      sixth 378.54
      seventh NEC 351.9
      eighth 388.5
      ninth 352.2
      tenth 352.3
      eleventh 352.4
      twelfth 352.5
      multiple 352.6
   entrapment — *see* Neuropathy, entrapment
   facial 351.9
      specified NEC 351.8
   femoral 355.2
   glossopharyngeal NEC 352.2
   hypoglossal 352.5

Disorder — *see also* Disease — *continued*
  nerve — *continued*
    iliohypogastric 355.79
    ilioinguinal 355.79
    intercostal 353.8
    lateral
      cutaneous of thigh 355.1
      popliteal 355.3
    lower limb NEC 355.8
    medial, popliteal 355.4
    median NEC 354.1
    obturator 355.79
    oculomotor
      partial 378.51
      total 378.52
    olfactory 352.0
    optic 377.49
      hypoplasia 377.43
      ischemic 377.41
      nutritional 377.33
      toxic 377.34
    peroneal 355.3
    phrenic 354.8
    plantar 355.6
    pneumogastric 352.3
    posterior tibial 355.5
    radial 354.3
    recurrent laryngeal 352.3
    root 353.9
      specified NEC 353.8
    saphenous 355.79
    sciatic NEC 355.0
    specified NEC 355.9
      lower limb 355.79
      upper limb 354.8
    spinal 355.9
    sympathetic NEC 337.9
    trigeminal 350.9
      specified NEC 350.8
    trochlear 378.53
    ulnar 354.2
    upper limb NEC 354.9
    vagus 352.3
  nervous system NEC 349.9
    autonomic (peripheral) (*see also* Neuropathy, peripheral, autonomic) 337.9
    cranial 352.9
    parasympathetic (*see also* Neuropathy, peripheral, autonomic) 337.9
    specified type NEC 349.89
    sympathetic (*see also* Neuropathy, peripheral, autonomic) 337.9
    vegetative (*see also* Neuropathy, peripheral, autonomic) 337.9
  neurohypophysis NEC 253.6
  neurological NEC 781.99
    peripheral NEC 355.9
  neuromuscular NEC 358.9
    hereditary NEC 359.1
    specified NEC 358.8
    toxic 358.2
  neurotic 300.9
    specified type NEC 300.89
  neutrophil, polymorphonuclear (functional) 288.1
  nightmare 307.47
  night terror 307.46
  obsessive-compulsive 300.3
  oppositional defiant, childhood and adolescence 313.81
  optic
    chiasm 377.54
      associated with
        inflammatory disorders 377.54
        neoplasm NEC 377.52
          pituitary 377.51
        pituitary disorders 377.51
        vascular disorders 377.53
    nerve 377.49
    radiations 377.63
    tracts 377.63
  orbit 376.9
    specified NEC 376.89
  orgasmic
    female 302.73
    male 302.74

Disorder — *see also* Disease — *continued*
  overanxious, of childhood and adolescence 313.0
  oxidation, fatty acid 277.85
  pancreas, internal secretion (other than diabetes mellitus) 251.9
    specified type NEC 251.8
  panic 300.01
    with agoraphobia 300.21
  papillary muscle NEC 429.81
  paranoid 297.9
    induced 297.3
    shared 297.3
  parathyroid 252.9
    specified type NEC 252.8
  paroxysmal, mixed 780.39
  pentose phosphate pathway with anemia 282.2
  periodic limb movement 327.51
  peroxisomal 277.86
  personality 301.9
    affective 301.10
    aggressive 301.3
    amoral 301.7
    anancastic, anankastic 301.4
    antisocial 301.7
    asocial 301.7
    asthenic 301.6
    avoidant 301.82
    borderline 301.83
    compulsive 301.4
    cyclothymic 301.13
    dependent-passive 301.6
    dyssocial 301.7
    emotional instability 301.59
    epileptoid 301.3
    explosive 301.3
    following organic brain damage 310.1
    histrionic 301.50
    hyperthymic 301.11
    hypomanic (chronic) 301.11
    hypothymic 301.12
    hysterical 301.50
    immature 301.89
    inadequate 301.6
    introverted 301.21
    labile 301.59
    moral deficiency 301.7
    narcissistic 301.81
    obsessional 301.4
    obsessive-compulsive 301.4
    overconscientious 301.4
    paranoid 301.0
    passive (-dependent) 301.6
    passive-aggressive 301.84
    pathological NEC 301.9
    pseudosocial 301.7
    psychopathic 301.9
    schizoid 301.20
      introverted 301.21
      schizotypal 301.22
    schizotypal 301.22
    seductive 301.59
    type A 301.4
    unstable 301.59
  pervasive developmental 299.9 ☑
    childhood-onset 299.8 ☑
    specified NEC 299.8 ☑
  phonological 315.39
  pigmentation, choroid (congenital) 743.53
  pinna 380.30
    specified type NEC 380.39
  pituitary, thalamic 253.9
    anterior NEC 253.4
    iatrogenic 253.7
    postablative 253.7
    specified NEC 253.8
  pityriasis-like NEC 696.8
  platelets (blood) 287.1
  polymorphonuclear neutrophils (functional) 288.1
  porphyrin metabolism 277.1
  postmenopausal 627.9
    specified type NEC 627.8
  post-transplant lymphoproliferative (PTLD) 238.77

Disorder — *see also* Disease — *continued*
  post-traumatic stress (PTSD) 309.81
  posttraumatic stress 309.81
    acute 309.81
    brief 309.81
    chronic 309.81
  premenstrual dysphoric (PMDD) 625.4
  psoriatic-like NEC 696.8
  psychic, with diseases classified elsewhere 316
  psychogenic NEC (*see also* condition) 300.9
    allergic NEC
      respiratory 306.1
    anxiety 300.00
      atypical 300.00
      generalized 300.02
    appetite 307.59
    articulation, joint 306.0
    asthenic 300.5
    blood 306.8
    cardiovascular (system) 306.2
    compulsive 300.3
    cutaneous 306.3
    depressive 300.4
    digestive (system) 306.4
    dysmenorrheic 306.52
    dyspneic 306.1
    eczematous 306.3
    endocrine (system) 306.6
    eye 306.7
    feeding 307.59
    functional NEC 306.9
    gastric 306.4
    gastrointestinal (system) 306.4
    genitourinary (system) 306.50
    heart (function) (rhythm) 306.2
    hemic 306.8
    hyperventilatory 306.1
    hypochondriacal 300.7
    hysterical 300.10
    intestinal 306.4
    joint 306.0
    learning 315.2
    limb 306.0
    lymphatic (system) 306.8
    menstrual 306.52
    micturition 306.53
    monoplegic NEC 306.0
    motor 307.9
    muscle 306.0
    musculoskeletal 306.0
    neurocirculatory 306.2
    obsessive 300.3
    occupational 300.89
    organ or part of body NEC 306.9
    organs of special sense 306.7
    paralytic NEC 306.0
    phobic 300.20
    physical NEC 306.9
    pruritic 306.3
    rectal 306.4
    respiratory (system) 306.1
    rheumatic 306.0
    sexual (function) 302.70
      specified type NEC 302.79
    sexual orientation conflict 302.0
    skin (allergic) (eczematous) (pruritic) 306.3
    sleep 307.40
      initiation or maintenance 307.41
        persistent 307.42
        transient 307.41
      movement 780.58
      sleep terror 307.46
      specified type NEC 307.49
    specified part of body NEC 306.8
    stomach 306.4
  psychomotor NEC 307.9
    hysterical 300.11
  psychoneurotic (*see also* Neurosis) 300.9
    mixed NEC 300.89
  psychophysiologic (*see also* Disorder, psychosomatic) 306.9
  psychosexual identity (childhood) 302.6
    adult-life 302.85
  psychosomatic NEC 306.9

Disorder — *see also* Disease — *continued*
  psychosomatic — *continued*
    allergic NEC
      respiratory 306.1
    articulation, joint 306.0
    cardiovascular (system) 306.2
    cutaneous 306.3
    digestive (system) 306.4
    dysmenorrheic 306.52
    dyspneic 306.1
    endocrine (system) 306.6
    eye 306.7
    gastric 306.4
    gastrointestinal (system) 306.4
    genitourinary (system) 306.50
    heart (functional) (rhythm) 306.2
    hyperventilatory 306.1
    intestinal 306.4
    joint 306.0
    limb 306.0
    lymphatic (system) 306.8
    menstrual 306.52
    micturition 306.53
    monoplegic NEC 306.0
    muscle 306.0
    musculoskeletal 306.0
    neurocirculatory 306.2
    organs of special sense 306.7
    paralytic NEC 306.0
    pruritic 306.3
    rectal 306.4
    respiratory (system) 306.1
    rheumatic 306.0
    sexual (function) 302.70
    skin 306.3
    specified part of body NEC 306.8
    specified type NEC 302.79
    stomach 306.4
  psychotic (*see also* Psychosis) 298.9
    brief 298.8
  purine metabolism NEC 277.2
  pyrimidine metabolism NEC 277.2
  reactive attachment of infancy or early childhood 313.89
  reading, developmental 315.00
  reflex 796.1
  REM sleep behavior 327.42
  renal function, impaired 588.9
    specified type NEC 588.89
  renal transport NEC 588.89
  respiration, respiratory NEC 519.9
    due to
      aspiration of liquids or solids 508.9
      inhalation of fumes or vapors 506.9
      smoke inhalation 508.2
    psychogenic 306.1
  retina 362.9
    specified type NEC 362.89
  rumination 307.53
  sacroiliac joint NEC 724.6
  sacrum 724.6
  schizo-affective (*see also* Schizophrenia) 295.7 ☑
  schizoid, childhood or adolescence 313.22
  schizophreniform 295.4 ☑
  schizotypal personality 301.22
  secretion, thyrocalcitonin 246.0
  seizure 345.9 ☑
    recurrent 345.9 ☑
    epileptic — *see* Epilepsy
  semantic pragmatic 315.39
    with autism 299.0 ☑
  sense of smell 781.1
    psychogenic 306.7
  separation anxiety 309.21
  sexual (*see also* Deviation, sexual) 302.9
    aversion 302.79
    desire, hypoactive 302.71
    function, psychogenic 302.70
  shyness, of childhood and adolescence 313.21
  single complement (C1-C9) 279.8
  skin NEC 709.9
    fetus or newborn 778.9
      specified type 778.8

☑ Additional Digit Required — Refer to the Tabular List for Digit Selection   ▽ Subterms under main terms may continue to next column or page

2015 ICD-9-CM   ▶◀ Revised Text   ● New Line   ▲ Revised Code   Volume 2 — 93

Disorder — see also Disease — continued
skin — continued
  psychogenic (allergic) (eczematous) (pruritic) 306.3
  specified type NEC 709.8
  vascular 709.1
sleep 780.50
  with apnea — see Apnea, sleep
  alcohol induced 291.82
  arousal 307.46
    confusional 327.41
  circadian rhythm 327.30
    advanced sleep phase type 327.32
    alcohol induced 291.82
    delayed sleep phase type 327.31
    drug induced 292.85
    free running type 327.34
    in conditions classified elsewhere 327.37
    irregular sleep-wake type 327.33
    jet lag type 327.35
    other 327.39
    shift work type 327.36
  drug induced 292.85
  initiation or maintenance (see also Insomnia) 780.52
    nonorganic origin (transient) 307.41
      persistent 307.42
  nonorganic origin 307.40
    specified type NEC 307.49
  organic specified type NEC 327.8
  periodic limb movement 327.51
  specified NEC 780.59
  wake
    cycle — see Disorder, sleep, circadian rhythm
    schedule — see Disorer, sleep, circadian rhythm
social, of childhood and adolescence 313.22
soft tissue 729.90
  specified type NEC 729.99
somatization 300.81
somatoform (atypical) (undifferentiated) 300.82
  severe 300.81
  specified type NEC 300.89
speech NEC 784.59
  nonorganic origin 307.9
spine NEC 724.9
  ligamentous or muscular attachments, peripheral 720.1
steroid metabolism NEC 255.2
stomach (functional) (see also Disorder, gastric) 536.9
  psychogenic 306.4
storage, iron 275.09
stress (see also Reaction, stress, acute) 308.3
  posttraumatic
    acute 309.81
    brief 309.81
    chronic 309.81
substitution 300.11
suspected — see Observation
synovium 727.9
temperature regulation, fetus or newborn 778.4
temporomandibular joint NEC 524.60
  sounds on opening or closing 524.64
  specified NEC 524.69
tendon 727.9
  shoulder region 726.10
thoracic root (nerve) NEC 353.3
thyrocalcitonin secretion 246.0
thyroid (gland) NEC 246.9
  specified type NEC 246.8
tic 307.20
  chronic (motor or vocal) 307.22
  motor-verbal 307.23
  organic origin 333.1
  transient (of childhood) 307.21
tooth NEC 525.9
  development NEC 520.9
    specified type NEC 520.8
  eruption 520.6
  specified type NEC 525.8
Tourette's 307.23

Disorder — see also Disease — continued
transport, carbohydrate 271.9
  specified type NEC 271.8
tubular, phosphate-losing 588.0
tympanic membrane 384.9
unaggressive, unsocialized (see also Disturbance, conduct) 312.1 ☑
undersocialized, unsocialized (see also Disturbance, conduct)
  aggressive (type) 312.0 ☑
  unaggressive (type) 312.1 ☑
vision, visual NEC 368.9
  binocular NEC 368.30
  cortex 377.73
    associated with
      inflammatory disorders 377.73
      neoplasms 377.71
      vascular disorders 377.72
  pathway NEC 377.63
    associated with
      inflammatory disorders 377.63
      neoplasms 377.61
      vascular disorders 377.62
vocal tic
  chronic 307.22
wakefulness (see also Hypersomnia) 780.54
  nonorganic origin (transient) 307.43
    persistent 307.44
written expression 315.2
Disorganized globe 360.29
Displacement, displaced

Note — For acquired displacement of bones, cartilage, joints, tendons, due to injury, see also Dislocation.

Displacements at ages under one year should be considered congenital, provided there is no indication the condition was acquired after birth.

  acquired traumatic of bone, cartilage, joint, tendon NEC (without fracture) (see also Dislocation) 839.8
    with fracture — see Fracture, by site
  adrenal gland (congenital) 759.1
  alveolus and teeth, vertical 524.75
  appendix, retrocecal (congenital) 751.5
  auricle (congenital) 744.29
  bladder (acquired) 596.89
    congenital 753.8
  brachial plexus (congenital) 742.8
  brain stem, caudal 742.4
  canaliculus lacrimalis 743.65
  cardia, through esophageal hiatus 750.6
  cerebellum, caudal 742.4
  cervix — see Displacement, uterus
  colon (congenital) 751.4
  device, implant, or graft — see Complications, mechanical
  epithelium
    columnar of cervix 622.10
    cuboidal, beyond limits of external os (uterus) 752.49
  esophageal mucosa into cardia of stomach, congenital 750.4
  esophagus (acquired) 530.89
    congenital 750.4
  eyeball (acquired) (old) 376.36
    congenital 743.8
    current injury 871.3
    lateral 376.36
  fallopian tube (acquired) 620.4
    congenital 752.19
    opening (congenital) 752.19
  gallbladder (congenital) 751.69
  gastric mucosa 750.7
    into
      duodenum 750.7
      esophagus 750.7
      Meckel's diverticulum, congenital 750.7
  globe (acquired) (lateral) (old) 376.36
    current injury 871.3
  graft
    artificial skin graft 996.55
    decellularized allodermis graft 996.55
  heart (congenital) 746.87

Displacement, displaced — continued
heart — continued
  acquired 429.89
hymen (congenital) (upward) 752.49
internal prosthesis NEC — see Complications, mechanical
intervertebral disc (with neuritis, radiculitis, sciatica, or other pain) 722.2
  with myelopathy 722.70
  cervical, cervicodorsal, cervicothoracic 722.0
    with myelopathy 722.71
    due to major trauma — see Dislocation, vertebra, cervical
  due to trauma — see Dislocation, vertebra
  lumbar, lumbosacral 722.10
    with myelopathy 722.73
    due to major trauma — see Dislocation, vertebra, lumbar
  thoracic, thoracolumbar 722.11
    with myelopathy 722.72
    due to major trauma — see Dislocation, vertebra, thoracic
intrauterine device 996.32
kidney (acquired) 593.0
  congenital 753.3
lacrimal apparatus or duct (congenital) 743.65
macula (congenital) 743.55
Meckel's diverticulum (congenital) 751.0
nail (congenital) 757.5
  acquired 703.8
opening of Wharton's duct in mouth 750.26
organ or site, congenital NEC — see Malposition, congenital
ovary (acquired) 620.4
  congenital 752.0
  free in peritoneal cavity (congenital) 752.0
  into hernial sac 620.4
oviduct (acquired) 620.4
  congenital 752.19
parathyroid (gland) 252.8
parotid gland (congenital) 750.26
punctum lacrimale (congenital) 743.65
sacroiliac (congenital) (joint) 755.69
  current injury — see Dislocation, sacroiliac
  old 724.6
spine (congenital) 756.19
spleen, congenital 759.0
stomach (congenital) 750.7
  acquired 537.89
subglenoid (closed) 831.01
sublingual duct (congenital) 750.26
teeth, tooth 524.30
  horizontal 524.33
  vertical 524.34
tongue (congenital) (downward) 750.19
trachea (congenital) 748.3
ureter or ureteric opening or orifice (congenital) 753.4
uterine opening of oviducts or fallopian tubes 752.19
uterus, uterine (see also Malposition, uterus) 621.6
  congenital 752.39
ventricular septum 746.89
  with rudimentary ventricle 746.89
xyphoid bone (process) 738.3
Disproportion 653.9 ☑
affecting fetus or newborn 763.1
breast, reconstructed 612.1
  between native and reconstructed 612.1
caused by
  conjoined twins 678.1 ☑
  contraction, pelvis (general) 653.1 ☑
    inlet 653.2 ☑
    midpelvic 653.8 ☑
    midplane 653.8 ☑
    outlet 653.3 ☑
  fetal
    ascites 653.7 ☑
    hydrocephalus 653.6 ☑
    hydrops 653.7 ☑

Disproportion — continued
caused by — continued
  fetal — continued
    meningomyelocele 653.7 ☑
    sacral teratoma 653.7 ☑
    tumor 653.7 ☑
  hydrocephalic fetus 653.6 ☑
  pelvis, pelvic, abnormality (bony) NEC 653.0 ☑
  unusually large fetus 653.5 ☑
causing obstructed labor 660.1 ☑
cephalopelvic, normally formed fetus 653.4 ☑
  causing obstructed labor 660.1 ☑
fetal NEC 653.5 ☑
  causing obstructed labor 660.1 ☑
fetopelvic, normally formed fetus 653.4 ☑
  causing obstructed labor 660.1 ☑
mixed maternal and fetal origin, normally formed fetus 653.4 ☑
pelvis, pelvic (bony) NEC 653.1 ☑
  causing obstructed labor 660.1 ☑
specified type NEC 653.8 ☑
Disruption
cesarean wound 674.1 ☑
family V61.09
  due to
    child in
      care of non-parental family member V61.06
      foster care V61.06
      welfare custody V61.05
    death of family member V61.07
    divorce V61.03
    estrangement V61.09
      parent-child V61.04
    extended absence of family member NEC V61.08
    family member
      on military deployment V61.01
      return from military deployment V61.02
    legal separation V61.03
gastrointestinal anastomosis 997.49
ligament(s) (see also Sprain)
  knee
    current injury — see Dislocation, knee
    old 717.89
      capsular 717.85
      collateral (medial) 717.82
        lateral 717.81
      cruciate (posterior) 717.84
        anterior 717.83
      specified site NEC 717.85
marital V61.10
  involving
    divorce V61.03
    estrangement V61.09
operation wound (external) (see also Dehiscence) 998.32
  internal 998.31
organ transplant, anastomosis site — see Complications, transplant, organ, by site
ossicles, ossicular chain 385.23
  traumatic — see Fracture, skull, base
parenchyma
  liver (hepatic) — see Laceration, liver, major
  spleen — see Laceration, spleen, parenchyma, massive
phase-shift, of 24-hour sleep-wake cycle, unspecified 780.55
  nonorganic origin 307.45
sleep-wake cycle (24-hour), unspecified 780.55
  circadian rhythm 327.33
  nonorganic origin 307.45
suture line (external) (see also Dehiscence) 998.32
  internal 998.31
wound 998.30
  cesarean operation 674.1 ☑
  episiotomy 674.2 ☑
  operation (surgical) 998.32

☑ Additional Digit Required — Refer to the Tabular List for Digit Selection

▽ Subterms under main terms may continue to next column or page

Disruption — *continued*
  wound — *continued*
    operation — *continued*
      cesarean 674.1 ☑
      internal 998.31
     perineal (obstetric) 674.2 ☑
     uterine 674.1 ☑
Disruptio uteri — *see also* Rupture, uterus
  complicating delivery — *see* Delivery, complicated, rupture, uterus
Dissatisfaction with
  employment V62.29
  school environment V62.3
Dissecting — *see* condition
Dissection
  aorta 441.00
    abdominal 441.02
    thoracic 441.01
    thoracoabdominal 441.03
  artery, arterial
    carotid 443.21
    coronary 414.12
    iliac 443.22
    renal 443.23
    specified NEC 443.29
    vertebral 443.24
  vascular 459.9
  wound — *see* Wound, open, by site
Disseminated — *see* condition
Dissociated personality NEC 300.15
Dissociation
  auriculoventricular or atrioventricular (any degree) (AV) 426.89
    with heart block 426.0
  interference 426.89
  isorhythmic 426.89
  rhythm
    atrioventricular (AV) 426.89
    interference 426.89
Dissociative
  identity disorder 300.14
  reaction NEC 300.15
Dissolution, vertebra — *see also* Osteoporosis 733.00
Distention
  abdomen (gaseous) 787.3
  bladder 596.89
  cecum 569.89
  colon 569.89
  gallbladder 575.8
  gaseous (abdomen) 787.3
  intestine 569.89
  kidney 593.89
  liver 573.9
  seminal vesicle 608.89
  stomach 536.8
    acute 536.1
    psychogenic 306.4
  ureter 593.5
  uterus 621.8
Distichia, distichiasis (eyelid) 743.63
Distoma hepaticum infestation 121.3
Distomiasis 121.9
  bile passages 121.3
    due to Clonorchis sinensis 121.1
  hemic 120.9
  hepatic (liver) 121.3
    due to Clonorchis sinensis (clonorchiasis) 121.1
  intestinal 121.4
  liver 121.3
    due to Clonorchis sinensis 121.1
  lung 121.2
  pulmonary 121.2
Distomolar (fourth molar) 520.1
  causing crowding 524.31
Disto-occlusion (division I) (division II) 524.22
Distortion (congenital)
  adrenal (gland) 759.1
  ankle (joint) 755.69
  anus 751.5
  aorta 747.29
  appendix 751.5
  arm 755.59
  artery (peripheral) NEC (*see also* Distortion, peripheral vascular system) 747.60

Distortion — *continued*
  artery (*see also* Distortion, peripheral vascular system) — *continued*
    cerebral 747.81
    coronary 746.85
    pulmonary 747.39
    retinal 743.58
    umbilical 747.5
  auditory canal 744.29
    causing impairment of hearing 744.02
  bile duct or passage 751.69
  bladder 753.8
  brain 742.4
  bronchus 748.3
  cecum 751.5
  cervix (uteri) 752.49
  chest (wall) 756.3
  clavicle 755.51
  clitoris 752.49
  coccyx 756.19
  colon 751.5
  common duct 751.69
  cornea 743.41
  cricoid cartilage 748.3
  cystic duct 751.69
  duodenum 751.5
  ear 744.29
    auricle 744.29
      causing impairment of hearing 744.02
    causing impairment of hearing 744.09
    external 744.29
      causing impairment of hearing 744.02
    inner 744.05
    middle, except ossicles 744.03
      ossicles 744.04
    ossicles 744.04
  endocrine (gland) NEC 759.2
  epiglottis 748.3
  Eustachian tube 744.24
  eye 743.8
    adnexa 743.69
  face bone(s) 756.0
  fallopian tube 752.19
  femur 755.69
  fibula 755.69
  finger(s) 755.59
  foot 755.67
  gallbladder 751.69
  genitalia, genital organ(s)
    female 752.89
      external 752.49
      internal NEC 752.89
    male 752.89
      penis 752.69
  glottis 748.3
  gyri 742.4
  hand bone(s) 755.59
  heart (auricle) (ventricle) 746.89
    valve (cusp) 746.89
  hepatic duct 751.69
  humerus 755.59
  hymen 752.49
  ileum 751.5
  intestine (large) (small) 751.5
    with anomalous adhesions, fixation or malrotation 751.4
  jaw NEC 524.89
  jejunum 751.5
  kidney 753.3
  knee (joint) 755.64
  labium (majus) (minus) 752.49
  larynx 748.3
  leg 755.69
  lens 743.36
  liver 751.69
  lumbar spine 756.19
    with disproportion (fetopelvic) 653.0 ☑
      affecting fetus or newborn 763.1
      causing obstructed labor 660.1 ☑
  lumbosacral (joint) (region) 756.19
  lung (fissures) (lobe) 748.69
  nerve 742.8
  nose 748.1

Distortion — *continued*
  organ
    of Corti 744.05
    of site not listed — *see* Anomaly, specified type NEC
  ossicles, ear 744.04
  ovary 752.0
  oviduct 752.19
  pancreas 751.7
  parathyroid (gland) 759.2
  patella 755.64
  peripheral vascular system NEC 747.60
    gastrointestinal 747.61
    lower limb 747.64
    renal 747.62
    spinal 747.82
    upper limb 747.63
  pituitary (gland) 759.2
  radius 755.59
  rectum 751.5
  rib 756.3
  sacroiliac joint 755.69
  sacrum 756.19
  scapula 755.59
  shoulder girdle 755.59
  site not listed — *see* Anomaly, specified type NEC
  skull bone(s) 756.0
    with
      anencephalus 740.0
      encephalocele 742.0
      hydrocephalus 742.3
        with spina bifida (*see also* Spina bifida) 741.0 ☑
      microcephalus 742.1
  spinal cord 742.59
  spine 756.19
  spleen 759.0
  sternum 756.3
  thorax (wall) 756.3
  thymus (gland) 759.2
  thyroid (gland) 759.2
    cartilage 748.3
  tibia 755.69
  toe(s) 755.66
  tongue 750.19
  trachea (cartilage) 748.3
  ulna 755.59
  ureter 753.4
    causing obstruction 753.20
  urethra 753.8
    causing obstruction 753.6
  uterus 752.39
  vagina 752.49
  vein (peripheral) NEC (*see also* Distortion, peripheral vascular system) 747.60
    great 747.49
    portal 747.49
    pulmonary 747.49
  vena cava (inferior) (superior) 747.49
  vertebra 756.19
  visual NEC 368.15
    shape or size 368.14
  vulva 752.49
  wrist (bones) (joint) 755.59
Distress
  abdomen 789.0 ☑
  colon 564.9
  emotional V40.9
  epigastric 789.0 ☑
  fetal (syndrome) 768.4
    affecting management of pregnancy or childbirth 656.8 ☑
    liveborn infant 768.4
      first noted
        before onset of labor 768.2
        during labor and delivery 768.3
    stillborn infant (death before onset of labor) 768.0
      death during labor 768.1
  gastrointestinal (functional) 536.9
    psychogenic 306.4
  intestinal (functional) NEC 564.9
    psychogenic 306.4
  intrauterine — *see* Distress, fetal
  leg 729.5

Distress — *continued*
  maternal 669.0 ☑
  mental V40.9
  respiratory 786.09
    acute (adult) 518.82
    adult syndrome (following trauma and surgery) 518.52
      specified NEC 518.82
    fetus or newborn 770.89
    syndrome (idiopathic) (newborn) 769
  stomach 536.9
    psychogenic 306.4
Distribution vessel, atypical NEC 747.60
  coronary artery 746.85
  spinal 747.82
Districhiasis 704.2
Disturbance — *see also* Disease
  absorption NEC 579.9
    calcium 269.3
    carbohydrate 579.8
    fat 579.8
    protein 579.8
    specified type NEC 579.8
    vitamin (*see also* Deficiency, vitamin) 269.2
  acid-base equilibrium 276.9
  activity and attention, simple, with hyperkinesis 314.01
  amino acid (metabolic) (*see also* Disorder, amino acid) 270.9
    imidazole 270.5
    maple syrup (urine) disease 270.3
    transport 270.0
  assimilation, food 579.9
  attention, simple 314.00
    with hyperactivity 314.01
  auditory, nerve, except deafness 388.5
  behavior (*see also* Disturbance, conduct) 312.9
  blood clotting (hypoproteinemia) (mechanism) (*see also* Defect, coagulation) 286.9
  central nervous system NEC 349.9
  cerebral nerve NEC 352.9
  circulatory 459.9
  conduct 312.9

> *Note* — Use the following fifth-digit subclassification with categories 312.0–312.2:
>
> 0   unspecified
>
> 1   mild
>
> 2   moderate
>
> 3   severe

    adjustment reaction 309.3
    adolescent onset type 312.82
    childhood onset type 312.81
    compulsive 312.30
      intermittent explosive disorder 312.34
      isolated explosive disorder 312.35
      kleptomania 312.32
      pathological gambling 312.31
      pyromania 312.33
    hyperkinetic 314.2
    intermittent explosive 312.34
    isolated explosive 312.35
    mixed with emotions 312.4
    socialized (type) 312.20
      aggressive 312.23
      unaggressive 312.21
    specified type NEC 312.89
    undersocialized, unsocialized
      aggressive (type) 312.0 ☑
      unaggressive (type) 312.1 ☑
  coordination 781.3
  cranial nerve NEC 352.9
  deep sensibility — *see* Disturbance, sensation
  digestive 536.9
    psychogenic 306.4
  electrolyte — *see* Imbalance, electrolyte
  emotions specific to childhood or adolescence 313.9

☑ Additional Digit Required — Refer to the Tabular List for Digit Selection   ⬚ Subterms under main terms may continue to next column or page

2015 ICD-9-CM   ▶◀ Revised Text   ● New Line   ▲ Revised Code   Volume 2 — 95

Disturbance — *see also* Disease —
   continued
  emotions specific to childhood or adoles-
    cence — *continued*
    with
      academic underachievement 313.83
      anxiety and fearfulness 313.0
      elective mutism 313.23
      identity disorder 313.82
      jealousy 313.3
      misery and unhappiness 313.1
      oppositional defiant disorder 313.81
      overanxiousness 313.0
      sensitivity 313.21
      shyness 313.21
      social withdrawal 313.22
      withdrawal reaction 313.22
    involving relationship problems 313.3
    mixed 313.89
    specified type NEC 313.89
  endocrine (gland) 259.9
    neonatal, transitory 775.9
      specified NEC 775.89
  equilibrium 780.4
  feeding (elderly) (infant) 783.3
    newborn 779.31
    nonorganic origin NEC 307.59
    psychogenic NEC 307.59
  fructose metabolism 271.2
  gait 781.2
    hysterical 300.11
  gastric (functional) 536.9
    motility 536.8
    psychogenic 306.4
    secretion 536.8
  gastrointestinal (functional) 536.9
    psychogenic 306.4
  habit, child 307.9
  hearing, except deafness 388.40
  heart, functional (conditions classifiable to
    426, 427, 428)
    due to presence of (cardiac) prosthesis
      429.4
    postoperative (immediate) 997.1
      long-term effect of cardiac surgery
        429.4
    psychogenic 306.2
  hormone 259.9
  innervation uterus, sympathetic, parasym-
    pathetic 621.8
  keratinization NEC
    gingiva 523.10
    lip 528.5
    oral (mucosa) (soft tissue) 528.79
      residual ridge mucosa
        excessive 528.72
        minimal 528.71
    tongue 528.79
  labyrinth, labyrinthine (vestibule) 386.9
  learning, specific NEC 315.2
  memory (*see also* Amnesia) 780.93
    mild, following organic brain damage
      310.89
  mental (*see also* Disorder, mental) 300.9
    associated with diseases classified else-
      where 316
  metabolism (acquired) (congenital) (*see also*
    Disorder, metabolism) 277.9
    with
      abortion — *see* Abortion, by type,
        with metabolic disorder
      ectopic pregnancy (*see also* cate-
        gories 633.0–633.9) 639.4
      molar pregnancy (*see also* categories
        630–632) 639.4
    amino acid (*see also* Disorder, amino
      acid) 270.9
      aromatic NEC 270.2
      branched-chain 270.3
      specified type NEC 270.8
      straight-chain NEC 270.7
      sulfur-bearing 270.4
      transport 270.0
    ammonia 270.6
    arginine 270.6
    argininosuccinic acid 270.6

Disturbance — *see also* Disease —
   continued
  metabolism (*see also* Disorder, metabolism)
    — *continued*
    carbohydrate NEC 271.9
    cholesterol 272.9
    citrulline 270.6
    cystathionine 270.4
    fat 272.9
    following
      abortion 639.4
      ectopic or molar pregnancy 639.4
    general 277.9
      carbohydrate 271.9
      iron 275.09
      phosphate 275.3
      sodium 276.9
    glutamine 270.7
    glycine 270.7
    histidine 270.5
    homocystine 270.4
    in labor or delivery 669.0 ☑
    iron 275.09
    isoleucine 270.3
    leucine 270.3
    lipoid 272.9
      specified type NEC 272.8
    lysine 270.7
    methionine 270.4
    neonatal, transitory 775.9
      specified type NEC 775.89
    nitrogen 788.99
    ornithine 270.6
    phosphate 275.3
    phosphatides 272.7
    serine 270.7
    sodium NEC 276.9
    threonine 270.7
    tryptophan 270.2
    tyrosine 270.2
    urea cycle 270.6
    valine 270.3
  motor 796.1
  nervous functional 799.21
  neuromuscular mechanism (eye) due to
    syphilis 094.84
  nutritional 269.9
    nail 703.8
  ocular motion 378.87
    psychogenic 306.7
  oculogyric 378.87
    psychogenic 306.7
  oculomotor NEC 378.87
    psychogenic 306.7
  olfactory nerve 781.1
  optic nerve NEC 377.49
  oral epithelium, including tongue 528.79
    residual ridge mucosa
      excessive 528.72
      minimal 528.71
  personality (pattern) (trait) (*see also* Disor-
    der, personality) 301.9
    following organic brain damage 310.1
  polyglandular 258.9
  psychomotor 307.9
  pupillary 379.49
  reflex 796.1
  rhythm, heart 427.9
    postoperative (immediate) 997.1
      long-term effect of cardiac surgery
        429.4
    psychogenic 306.2
  salivary secretion 527.7
  sensation (cold) (heat) (localization) (tactile
    discrimination localization) (texture)
    (vibratory) NEC 782.0
    hysterical 300.11
    skin 782.0
    smell 781.1
    taste 781.1
  sensory (*see also* Disturbance, sensation)
    782.0
    innervation 782.0
  situational (transient) (*see also* Reaction,
    adjustment) 309.9
    acute 308.3

Disturbance — *see also* Disease —
   continued
  sleep 780.50
    with apnea — *see* Apnea, sleep
    initiation or maintenance (*see also* Insom-
      nia) 780.52
      nonorganic origin 307.41
    nonorganic origin 307.40
      specified type NEC 307.49
    specified NEC 780.59
      nonorganic origin 307.49
    wakefulness (*see also* Hypersomnia)
      780.54
      nonorganic origin 307.43
  sociopathic 301.7
  speech NEC 784.59
    developmental 315.39
      associated with hyperkinesis 314.1
    secondary to organic lesion 784.59
  stomach (functional) (*see also* Disturbance,
    gastric) 536.9
  sympathetic (nerve) (*see also* Neuropathy,
    peripheral, autonomic) 337.9
  temperature sense 782.0
    hysterical 300.11
  tooth
    eruption 520.6
    formation 520.4
    structure, hereditary NEC 520.5
  touch (*see also* Disturbance, sensation) 782.0
  vascular 459.9
    arteriosclerotic — *see* Arteriosclerosis
  vasomotor 443.9
  vasospastic 443.9
  vestibular labyrinth 386.9
  vision, visual NEC 368.9
    psychophysical 368.16
    specified NEC 368.8
    subjective 368.10
  voice and resonance 784.40
  wakefulness (initiation or maintenance) (*see
    also* Hypersomnia) 780.54
    nonorganic origin 307.43
Disulfiduria, beta-mercaptolactate-cysteine
  270.0
Disuse atrophy, bone 733.7
Ditthomska syndrome 307.81
Diuresis 788.42
Divers'
  palsy or paralysis 993.3
  squeeze 993.3
Diverticula, diverticulosis, diverticulum
  (acute) (multiple) (perforated) (ruptured)
    562.10
  with diverticulitis 562.11
  aorta (Kommerell's) 747.21
  appendix (noninflammatory) 543.9
  bladder (acquired) (sphincter) 596.3
    congenital 753.8
  broad ligament 620.8
  bronchus (congenital) 748.3
    acquired 494.0
      with acute exacerbation 494.1
  calyx, calyceal (kidney) 593.89
  cardia (stomach) 537.1
  cecum 562.10
    with
      diverticulitis 562.11
        with hemorrhage 562.13
      hemorrhage 562.12
    congenital 751.5
  colon (acquired) 562.10
    with
      diverticulitis 562.11
        with hemorrhage 562.13
      hemorrhage 562.12
    congenital 751.5
  duodenum 562.00
    with
      diverticulitis 562.01
        with hemorrhage 562.03
      hemorrhage 562.02
    congenital 751.5
  ephrenic (esophagus) 530.6
  esophagus (congenital) 750.4
    acquired 530.6

Diverticula, diverticulosis, diverticulum —
   continued
  esophagus — *continued*
    epiphrenic 530.6
    pulsion 530.6
    traction 530.6
    Zenker's 530.6
  Eustachian tube 381.89
  fallopian tube 620.8
  gallbladder (congenital) 751.69
  gastric 537.1
  heart (congenital) 746.89
  ileum 562.00
    with
      diverticulitis 562.01
        with hemorrhage 562.03
      hemorrhage 562.02
  intestine (large) 562.10
    with
      diverticulitis 562.11
        with hemorrhage 562.13
      hemorrhage 562.12
    congenital 751.5
    small 562.00
      with
        diverticulitis 562.01
          with hemorrhage 562.03
        hemorrhage 562.02
      congenital 751.5
  jejunum 562.00
    with
      diverticulitis 562.01
        with hemorrhage 562.03
      hemorrhage 562.02
  kidney (calyx) (pelvis) 593.89
    with calculus 592.0
  Kommerell's 747.21
  laryngeal ventricle (congenital) 748.3
  Meckel's (displaced) (hypertrophic) 751.0
  midthoracic 530.6
  organ or site, congenital NEC — *see* Distor-
    tion
  pericardium (conginital) (cyst) 746.89
    acquired (true) 423.8
  pharyngoesophageal (pulsion) 530.6
  pharynx (congenital) 750.27
  pulsion (esophagus) 530.6
  rectosigmoid 562.10
    with
      diverticulitis 562.11
        with hemorrhage 562.13
      hemorrhage 562.12
    congenital 751.5
  rectum 562.10
    with
      diverticulitis 562.11
        with hemorrhage 562.13
      hemorrhage 562.12
  renal (calyces) (pelvis) 593.89
    with calculus 592.0
  Rokitansky's 530.6
  seminal vesicle 608.0
  sigmoid 562.10
    with
      diverticulitis 562.11
        with hemorrhage 562.13
      hemorrhage 562.12
    congenital 751.5
  small intestine 562.00
    with
      diverticulitis 562.01
        with hemorrhage 562.03
      hemorrhage 562.02
  stomach (cardia) (juxtacardia) (juxtapyloric)
    (acquired) 537.1
    congenital 750.7
  subdiaphragmatic 530.6
  trachea (congenital) 748.3
    acquired 519.19
  traction (esophagus) 530.6
  ureter (acquired) 593.89
    congenital 753.4
  ureterovesical orifice 593.89
  urethra (acquired) 599.2
    congenital 753.8
  ventricle, left (congenital) 746.89

☑ **Additional Digit Required** — Refer to the Tabular List for Digit Selection   ▽ **Subterms under main terms may continue to next column or page**

Index (side tab)
Disturbance — Diverticula, diverticulosis (side tab)

Diverticula, diverticulosis, diverticulum — *continued*
  vesical (urinary) 596.3
    congenital 753.8
  Zenker's (esophagus) 530.6
Diverticulitis (acute) — *see also* Diverticula 562.11
  with hemorrhage 562.13
  bladder (urinary) 596.3
  cecum (perforated) 562.11
    with hemorrhage 562.13
  colon (perforated) 562.11
    with hemorrhage 562.13
  duodenum 562.01
    with hemorrhage 562.03
  esophagus 530.6
  ileum (perforated) 562.01
    with hemorrhage 562.03
  intestine (large) (perforated) 562.11
    with hemorrhage 562.13
    small 562.01
      with hemorrhage 562.03
  jejunum (perforated) 562.01
    with hemorrhage 562.03
  Meckel's (perforated) 751.0
  pharyngoesophageal 530.6
  rectosigmoid (perforated) 562.11
    with hemorrhage 562.13
  rectum 562.11
    with hemorrhage 562.13
  sigmoid (old) (perforated) 562.11
    with hemorrhage 562.13
  small intestine (perforated) 562.01
    with hemorrhage 562.03
  vesical (urinary) 596.3
Diverticulosis — *see* Diverticula
Division
  cervix uteri 622.8
    external os into two openings by frenum 752.44
  external (cervical) into two openings by frenum 752.44
  glans penis 752.69
  hymen 752.49
  labia minora (congenital) 752.49
  ligament (partial or complete) (current) (*see also* Sprain, by site)
    with open wound — *see* Wound, open, by site
  muscle (partial or complete) (current) (*see also* Sprain, by site)
    with open wound — *see* Wound, open, by site
  nerve — *see* Injury, nerve, by site
  penis glans 752.69
  spinal cord — *see* Injury, spinal, by site
  vein 459.9
    traumatic — *see* Injury, vascular, by site
Divorce V61.03
Dix-Hallpike neurolabyrinthitis 386.12
Dizziness 780.4
  hysterical 300.11
  psychogenic 306.9
Doan-Wiseman syndrome (primary splenic neutropenia) 289.53
Dog bite — *see* Wound, open, by site
Döhle body-panmyelopathic syndrome 288.2
Döhle-Heller aortitis 093.1
Dolichocephaly, dolichocephalus 754.0
Dolichocolon 751.5
Dolichostenomelia 759.82
Donohue's syndrome (leprechaunism) 259.8
Donor
  blood V59.01
    other blood components V59.09
    stem cells V59.02
    whole blood V59.01
  bone V59.2
    marrow V59.3
  cornea V59.5
  egg (oocyte) (ovum) V59.70
    over age 35 V59.73
      anonymous recipient V59.73
      designated recipient V59.74
    under age 35 V59.71

Donor — *continued*
  egg — *continued*
    under age 35 — *continued*
      anonymous recipient V59.71
      designated recipient V59.72
  heart V59.8
  kidney V59.4
  liver V59.6
  lung V59.8
  lymphocyte V59.8
  organ V59.9
    specified NEC V59.8
  potential, examination of V70.8
  skin V59.1
  specified organ or tissue NEC V59.8
  sperm V59.8
  stem cells V59.02
  tissue V59.9
    specified type NEC V59.8
Donovanosis (granuloma venereum) 099.2
DOPS (diffuse obstructive pulmonary syndrome) 496
Double
  albumin 273.8
  aortic arch 747.21
  auditory canal 744.29
  auricle (heart) 746.82
  bladder 753.8
  external (cervical) os 752.44
  kidney with double pelvis (renal) 753.3
  larynx 748.3
  meatus urinarius 753.8
  organ or site NEC — *see* Accessory
  orifice
    heart valve NEC 746.89
      pulmonary 746.09
  outlet, right ventricle 745.11
  pelvis (renal) with double ureter 753.4
  penis 752.69
  tongue 750.13
  ureter (one or both sides) 753.4
    with double pelvis (renal) 753.4
  urethra 753.8
  urinary meatus 753.8
  uterus (any degree) 752.2
    with doubling of cervix and vagina 752.2
    in pregnancy or childbirth 654.0 ☑
      affecting fetus or newborn 763.89
  vagina 752.47
    with doubling of cervix and uterus 752.2
  vision 368.2
  vocal cords 748.3
  vulva 752.49
  whammy (syndrome) 360.81
Douglas' pouch, cul-de-sac — *see* condition
Down's disease or syndrome (mongolism) 758.0
Down-growth, epithelial (anterior chamber) 364.61
DPD (dihydropyrimidine dehydrogenase deficiency) 277.6
Dracontiasis 125.7
Dracunculiasis 125.7
Dracunculosis 125.7
Drainage
  abscess (spontaneous) — *see* Abscess
  anomalous pulmonary veins to hepatic veins or right atrium 747.41
  stump (amputation) (surgical) 997.62
  suprapubic, bladder 596.89
Dream state, hysterical 300.13
Drepanocytic anemia — *see also* Disease, sickle cell 282.60
Dresbach's syndrome (elliptocytosis) 282.1
Dreschlera (infection) 118
  hawaiiensis 117.8
Dressler's syndrome (postmyocardial infarction) 411.0
Dribbling (post-void) 788.35
Drift, ulnar 736.09
Drinking (alcohol) — *see also* Alcoholism
  excessive, to excess NEC (*see also* Abuse, drugs, nondependent) 305.0 ☑
    bouts, periodic 305.0 ☑
    continual 303.9 ☑
    episodic 305.0 ☑

Drinking (alcohol) — *see also* Alcoholism — *continued*
  excessive, to excess (*see also* Abuse, drugs, nondependent) — *continued*
    habitual 303.9 ☑
    periodic 305.0 ☑
Drip, postnasal (chronic) 784.91
  due to
    allergic rhinitis — *see* Rhinitis, allergic
    common cold 460
    gastroesophageal reflux — *see* Reflux, gastroesophageal
    nasopharyngitis — *see* Nasopharyngitis
    other known condition — code to condition
    sinusitis — *see* Sinusitis
Drivers' license examination V70.3
Droop
  Cooper's 611.81
  facial 781.94
Drop
  finger 736.29
  foot 736.79
  hematocrit (precipitous) 790.01
  hemoglobin 790.01
  toe 735.8
  wrist 736.05
Dropped
  dead 798.1
  heart beats 426.6
Dropsy, dropsical — *see also* Edema 782.3
  abdomen 789.59
  amnion (*see also* Hydramnios) 657.0 ☑
  brain — *see* Hydrocephalus
  cardiac (*see also* Failure, heart) 428.0
  cardiorenal (*see also* Hypertension, cardiorenal) 404.90
  chest 511.9
  fetus or newborn 778.0
    due to isoimmunization 773.3
  gangrenous (*see also* Gangrene) 785.4
  heart (*see also* Failure, heart) 428.0
  hepatic — *see* Cirrhosis, liver
  infantile — *see* Hydrops, fetalis
  kidney (*see also* Nephrosis) 581.9
  liver — *see* Cirrhosis, liver
  lung 514
  malarial (*see also* Malaria) 084.9
  neonatorum — *see* Hydrops, fetalis
  nephritic 581.9
  newborn — *see* Hydrops, fetalis
  nutritional 269.9
  ovary 620.8
  pericardium (*see also* Pericarditis) 423.9
  renal (*see also* Nephrosis) 581.9
  uremic — *see* Uremia
Drowned, drowning (near) 994.1
  lung 518.52
Drowsiness 780.09
Drug — *see also* condition
  addiction (*see also* listing under Dependence) 304.9 ☑
  adverse effect, correct substance properly administered 995.20
  allergy 995.27
  dependence (*see also* listing under Dependence) 304.9 ☑
  habit (*see also* listing under Dependence) 304.9 ☑
  hypersensitivity 995.27
  induced
    circadian rhythm sleep disorder 292.85
    hypersomnia 292.85
    insomnia 292.85
    mental disorder 292.9
      anxiety 292.89
      mood 292.84
      sexual 292.89
      sleep 292.85
      specified type 292.89
    parasomnia 292.85
    persisting
      amnestic disorder 292.83
      dementia 292.82

Drug — *see also* condition — *continued*
  induced — *continued*
    psychotic disorder
      with
        delusions 292.11
        hallucinations 292.12
    sleep disorder 292.85
  intoxication 292.89
  overdose — *see* Table of Drugs and Chemicals
  poisoning — *see* Table of Drugs and Chemicals
  therapy (maintenance) status NEC
    chemotherapy, antineoplastic V58.11
    immunotherapy, antineoplastic V58.12
    long-term (current) (prophylactic) use V58.69
      antibiotics V58.62
      anticoagulants V58.61
      anti-inflammatories, non-steroidal (NSAID) V58.64
      antiplatelets V58.63
      antithrombotics V58.63
      aspirin V58.66
      bisphosphonates V58.68
      high-risk medications NEC V58.69
      insulin V58.67
      methadone for pain control V58.69
      opiate analgesic V58.69
      steroids V58.65
    methadone 304.00
  wrong substance given or taken in error — *see* Table of Drugs and Chemicals
Drunkenness — *see also* Abuse, drugs, nondependent 305.0 ☑
  acute in alcoholism (*see also* Alcoholism) 303.0 ☑
  chronic (*see also* Alcoholism) 303.9 ☑
  pathologic 291.4
  simple (acute) 305.0 ☑
    in alcoholism 303.0 ☑
  sleep 307.47
Drusen
  optic disc or papilla 377.21
  retina (colloid) (hyaloid degeneration) 362.57
    hereditary 362.77
Drusenfieber 075
Dry, dryness — *see also* condition
  eye 375.15
    syndrome 375.15
  larynx 478.79
  mouth 527.7
  nose 478.19
  skin syndrome 701.1
  socket (teeth) 526.5
  throat 478.29
DSAP (disseminated superficial actinic porokeratosis) 692.75
DSTR (delayed serologic transfusion reaction)
  due to or resulting from
    incompatibility
      ABO 999.69
      non-ABO antigen (minor) (Duffy) (Kell) (Kidd) (Lewis) (M) (N) (P) (S) 999.79
      Rh antigen (C) (c) (D) (E) (e) 999.74
Duane's retraction syndrome 378.71
Duane-Stilling-Türk syndrome (ocular retraction syndrome) 378.71
Dubini's disease (electric chorea) 049.8
Dubin-Johnson disease or syndrome 277.4
Dubois' abscess or disease 090.5
Duchenne's
  disease 094.0
    locomotor ataxia 094.0
    muscular dystrophy 359.1
    pseudohypertrophy, muscles 359.1
  paralysis 335.22
  syndrome 335.22
Duchenne-Aran myelopathic, muscular atrophy (nonprogressive) (progressive) 335.21
Duchenne-Griesinger disease 359.1
Ducrey's
  bacillus 099.0

☑ **Additional Digit Required** — Refer to the Tabular List for Digit Selection   Ⓝ **Subterms under main terms may continue to next column or page**

Index

Ducrey's — Dysfunction

☑ **Additional Digit Required** — Refer to the Tabular List for Digit Selection   ▽ **Subterms under main terms may continue to next column or page**

98 — Volume 2   ▶◀ **Revised Text**   ● **New Line**   ▲ **Revised Code**   **2015 ICD-9-CM**

Dysfunction — continued
  senile 797
  sexual 302.70
  sinoatrial node 427.81
  somatic 739.9
    abdomen 739.9
    acromioclavicular 739.7
    cervical 739.1
    cervicothoracic 739.1
    costochondral 739.8
    costovertebral 739.8
    extremities
      lower 739.6
      upper 739.7
    head 739.0
    hip 739.5
    lumbar, lumbosacral 739.3
    occipitocervical 739.0
    pelvic 739.5
    pubic 739.5
    rib cage 739.8
    sacral 739.4
    sacrococcygeal 739.4
    sacroiliac 739.4
    specified site NEC 739.9
    sternochondral 739.8
    sternoclavicular 739.7
    temporomandibular 739.0
    thoracic, thoracolumbar 739.2
  stomach 536.9
    psychogenic 306.4
  suprarenal 255.9
    hyperfunction 255.3
    hypofunction 255.41
  symbolic NEC 784.60
    specified type NEC 784.69
  systolic 429.9
    with heart failure — see Failure, heart
  temporomandibular (joint) (joint-pain-syn-
      drome) NEC 524.60
    sounds on opening or closing 524.64
    specified NEC 524.69
  testicular 257.9
    hyperfunction 257.0
    hypofunction 257.2
    specified type NEC 257.8
  thymus 254.9
  thyroid 246.9
    complicating pregnancy, childbirth, or
        puerperium 648.1 ☑
    hyperfunction — see Hyperthyroidism
    hypofunction — see Hypothyroidism
  uterus, complicating delivery 661.9 ☑
    affecting fetus or newborn 763.7
    hypertonic 661.4 ☑
    hypotonic 661.2 ☑
      primary 661.0 ☑
      secondary 661.1 ☑
  velopharyngeal (acquired) 528.9
    congenital 750.29
  ventricular 429.9
    with congestive heart failure (see also
        Failure, heart) 428.0
    due to
      cardiomyopathy — see Cardiomyopa-
          thy
      hypertension — see Hypertension,
          heart
    left, reversible following sudden emo-
        tional stress 429.83
  vesicourethral NEC 596.59
  vestibular 386.50
    specified type NEC 386.58
Dysgammaglobulinemia 279.06
Dysgenesis
  gonadal (due to chromosomal anomaly)
      758.6
    pure 752.7
  kidney(s) 753.0
  ovarian 758.6
  renal 753.0
  reticular 279.2
  seminiferous tubules 758.6
  tidal platelet 287.31

Dysgerminoma (M9060/3)
  specified site — see Neoplasm, by site, ma-
      lignant
  unspecified site
    female 183.0
    male 186.9
Dysgeusia 781.1
Dysgraphia 781.3
Dyshidrosis 705.81
Dysidrosis 705.81
Dysinsulinism 251.8
Dyskaryotic cervical smear 795.09
Dyskeratosis — see also Keratosis 701.1
  bullosa hereditaria 757.39
  cervix 622.10
  congenital 757.39
  follicularis 757.39
    vitamin A deficiency 264.8
  gingiva 523.8
  oral soft tissue NEC 528.79
  tongue 528.79
  uterus NEC 621.8
Dyskinesia 781.3
  biliary 575.8
  esophagus 530.5
  hysterical 300.11
  intestinal 564.89
  neuroleptic-induced tardive 333.85
  nonorganic origin 307.9
  orofacial 333.82
    due to drugs 333.85
  psychogenic 307.9
  subacute, due to drugs 333.85
  tardive (oral) 333.85
Dyslalia 784.59
  developmental 315.39
Dyslexia 784.61
  developmental 315.02
  secondary to organic lesion 784.61
Dyslipidemia 272.4
Dysmaturity — see also Immaturity 765.1 ☑
  lung 770.4
  pulmonary 770.4
Dysmenorrhea (essential) (exfoliative) (func-
      tional) (intrinsic) (membranous) (prima-
      ry) (secondary) 625.3
  psychogenic 306.52
Dysmetabolic syndrome X 277.7
Dysmetria 781.3
**Dysmorodystrophia mesodermalis congeni-
    ta** 759.82
Dysnomia 784.3
Dysorexia 783.0
  hysterical 300.11
Dysostosis
  cleidocranial, cleidocranialis 755.59
  craniofacial 756.0
  Fairbank's (idiopathic familial generalized
      osteophytosis) 756.50
  mandibularis 756.0
  mandibulofacial, incomplete 756.0
  multiplex 277.5
  orodigitofacial 759.89
Dyspareunia (female) 625.0
  male 608.89
  psychogenic 302.76
Dyspepsia (allergic) (congenital) (fermentative)
      (flatulent) (functional) (gastric) (gastroin-
      testinal) (neurogenic) (occupational)
      (reflex) 536.8
  acid 536.8
  atonic 536.3
    psychogenic 306.4
  diarrhea 787.91
    psychogenic 306.4
  intestinal 564.89
    psychogenic 306.4
  nervous 306.4
  neurotic 306.4
    psychogenic 306.4
Dysphagia 787.20
  cervical 787.29
  functional 300.11
  hysterical 300.11
  nervous 300.11
  neurogenic 787.29

Dysphagia — continued
  oral phase 787.21
  oropharyngeal phase 787.22
  pharyngeal phase 787.23
  pharyngoesophageal phase 787.24
  psychogenic 306.4
  sideropenic 280.8
  spastica 530.5
  specified NEC 787.29
Dysphagocytosis, congenital 288.1
Dysphasia 784.59
Dysphonia 784.42
  clericorum 784.49
  functional 300.11
  hysterical 300.11
  psychogenic 306.1
  spastica 478.79
Dyspigmentation — see also Pigmentation
  eyelid (acquired) 374.52
Dyspituitarism 253.9
  hyperfunction 253.1
  hypofunction 253.2
  posterior lobe 253.6
Dysplasia — see also Anomaly
  alveolar capillary, with vein misalignment
      516.64
  anus 569.44
    intraepithelial neoplasia I (AIN I) (histo-
        logically confirmed) 569.44
    intraepithelial neoplasia II (AIN II) (histo-
        logically confirmed) 569.44
    intraepithelial neoplasia III (AIN III) 230.6
      anal canal 230.5
    mild (histologically confirmed) 569.44
    moderate (histologically confirmed)
        569.44
    severe 230.6
      anal canal 230.5
  artery
    fibromuscular NEC 447.8
      carotid 447.8
      renal 447.3
  bladder 596.89
  bone (fibrous) NEC 733.29
    diaphyseal, progressive 756.59
    jaw 526.89
    monostotic 733.29
    polyostotic 756.54
    solitary 733.29
  brain 742.9
  bronchopulmonary, fetus or newborn 770.7
  cervix (uteri) 622.10
    cervical intraepithelial neoplasia I (CIN
        I) 622.11
    cervical intraepithelial neoplasia II (CIN
        II) 622.12
    cervical intraepithelial neoplasia III (CIN
        III) 233.1
    CIN I 622.11
    CIN II 622.12
    CIN III 233.1
    mild 622.11
    moderate 622.12
    severe 233.1
  chondroectodermal 756.55
  chondromatose 756.4
  colon 211.3
  craniocarpotarsal 759.89
  craniometaphyseal 756.89
  dentinal 520.5
  diaphyseal, progressive 756.59
  ectodermal (anhidrotic) (Bason) (Clouston's)
      (congenital) (Feinmesser) (heredi-
      tary) (hidrotic) (Marshall) (Robin-
      son's) 757.31
  epiphysealis 756.9
    multiplex 756.56
    punctata 756.59
  epiphysis 756.9
    multiple 756.56
  epithelial
    epiglottis 478.79
    uterine cervix 622.10
  erythroid NEC 289.89
  eye (see also Microphthalmos) 743.10
  familial metaphyseal 756.89

Dysplasia — see also Anomaly —
    continued
  fibromuscular, artery NEC 447.8
    carotid 447.8
    renal 447.3
  fibrous
    bone NEC 733.29
    diaphyseal, progressive 756.59
    jaw 526.89
    monostotic 733.29
    polyostotic 756.54
    solitary 733.29
  high-grade, focal — see Neoplasm, by site,
      benign
  hip (congenital) 755.63
    with dislocation (see also Dislocation,
        hip, congenital) 754.30
  hypohidrotic ectodermal 757.31
  joint 755.8
  kidney 753.15
  leg 755.69
  linguofacialis 759.89
  lung 748.5
  macular 743.55
  mammary (benign) (gland) 610.9
    cystic 610.1
    specified type NEC 610.8
  metaphyseal 756.9
    familial 756.89
  monostotic fibrous 733.29
  muscle 756.89
  myeloid NEC 289.89
  nervous system (general) 742.9
  neuroectodermal 759.6
  oculoauriculovertebral 756.0
  oculodentodigital 759.89
  olfactogenital 253.4
  osteo-onycho-arthro (hereditary) 756.89
  periosteum 733.99
  polyostotic fibrous 756.54
  progressive diaphyseal 756.59
  prostate 602.3
    intraepithelial neoplasia I [PIN I] 602.3
    intraepithelial neoplasia II [PIN II] 602.3
    intraepithelial neoplasia III [PIN III] 233.4
  renal 753.15
  renofacialis 753.0
  retinal NEC 743.56
  retrolental (see also Retinopathy of prema-
      turity) 362.21
  skin 709.8
  spinal cord 742.9
  thymic, with immunodeficiency 279.2
  vagina 623.0
    mild 623.0
    moderate 623.0
    severe 233.31
  vocal cord 478.5
  vulva 624.8
    intraepithelial neoplasia I (VIN I) 624.01
    intraepithelial neoplasia II (VIN II) 624.02
    intraepithelial neoplasia III (VIN III)
        233.32
    mild 624.01
    moderate 624.02
    severe 233.32
    VIN I 624.01
    VIN II 624.02
    VIN III 233.32
Dyspnea (nocturnal) (paroxysmal) 786.09
  asthmatic (bronchial) (see also Asthma)
      493.9 ☑
    with bronchitis (see also Asthma)
        493.9 ☑
      chronic 493.2 ☑
  cardiac (see also Failure, ventricular, left)
      428.1
  cardiac (see also Failure, ventricular, left)
      428.1
  functional 300.11
  hyperventilation 786.01
  hysterical 300.11
  Monday morning 504
  newborn 770.89
  psychogenic 306.1
  uremic — see Uremia

☑ Additional Digit Required — Refer to the Tabular List for Digit Selection   ▽ Subterms under main terms may continue to next column or page

Dyspraxia 781.3
   syndrome 315.4
Dysproteinemia 273.8
   transient with copper deficiency 281.4
Dysprothrombinemia (constitutional) — *see also* Defect, coagulation 286.3
Dysreflexia, autonomic 337.3
Dysrhythmia
   cardiac 427.9
      postoperative (immediate) 997.1
         long-term effect of cardiac surgery 429.4
      specified type NEC 427.89
   cerebral or cortical 348.30
Dyssecretosis, mucoserous 710.2
Dyssocial reaction, without manifest psychiatric disorder
   adolescent V71.02
   adult V71.01
   child V71.02
Dyssomnia NEC 780.56
   nonorganic origin 307.47
Dyssplenism 289.4
Dyssynergia
   biliary (*see also* Disease, biliary) 576.8
   cerebellaris myoclonica 334.2
   detrusor sphincter (bladder) 596.55
   ventricular 429.89
Dystasia, hereditary areflexic 334.3
Dysthymia 300.4
Dysthymic disorder 300.4
Dysthyroidism 246.9
Dystocia 660.9 ☑
   affecting fetus or newborn 763.1
   cervical 661.2 ☑
      affecting fetus or newborn 763.7
   contraction ring 661.4 ☑
      affecting fetus or newborn 763.7
   fetal 660.9 ☑
      abnormal size 653.5 ☑
      affecting fetus or newborn 763.1
      deformity 653.7 ☑
   maternal 660.9 ☑
      affecting fetus or newborn 763.1
   positional 660.0 ☑
      affecting fetus or newborn 763.1
   shoulder (girdle) 660.4 ☑
      affecting fetus or newborn 763.1
   uterine NEC 661.4 ☑
      affecting fetus or newborn 763.7
Dystonia
   acute
      due to drugs 333.72
         neuroleptic-induced acute 333.72
   deformans progressiva 333.6
   lenticularis 333.6
   musculorum deformans 333.6
   torsion (idiopathic) 333.6
      acquired 333.79
      fragments (of) 333.89
      genetic 333.6
      symptomatic 333.79
Dystonic
   movements 781.0
Dystopia kidney 753.3
Dystrophia myotonica 359.2 ☑
Dystrophy, dystrophia 783.9
   adiposogenital 253.8
   asphyxiating thoracic 756.4
   Becker's type 359.22
   brevicollis 756.16
   Bruch's membrane 362.77
   cervical (sympathetic) NEC 337.09
   chondro-osseus with punctate epiphyseal dysplasia 756.59
   choroid (hereditary) 363.50
      central (areolar) (partial) 363.53
         total (gyrate) 363.54
      circinate 363.53
      circumpapillary (partial) 363.51
         total 363.52
      diffuse
         partial 363.56
         total 363.57
      generalized
         partial 363.56

Dystrophy, dystrophia — *continued*
   choroid — *continued*
      generalized — *continued*
         total 363.57
      gyrate
         central 363.54
         generalized 363.57
      helicoid 363.52
      peripapillary — *see* Dystrophy, choroid, circumpapillary
      serpiginous 363.54
   cornea (hereditary) 371.50
      anterior NEC 371.52
      Cogan's 371.52
      combined 371.57
      crystalline 371.56
      endothelial (Fuchs') 371.57
      epithelial 371.50
         juvenile 371.51
         microscopic cystic 371.52
      granular 371.53
      lattice 371.54
      macular 371.55
      marginal (Terrien's) 371.48
      Meesman's 371.51
      microscopic cystic (epithelial) 371.52
      nodular, Salzmann's 371.46
      polymorphous 371.58
      posterior NEC 371.58
      ring-like 371.52
      Salzmann's nodular 371.46
      stromal NEC 371.56
   dermatochondrocorneal 371.50
   Duchenne's 359.1
   due to malnutrition 263.9
   Erb's 359.1
   familial
      hyperplastic periosteal 756.59
      osseous 277.5
   foveal 362.77
   Fuchs', cornea 371.57
   Gowers' muscular 359.1
   hair 704.2
   hereditary, progressive muscular 359.1
   hypogenital, with diabetic tendency 759.81
   Landouzy-Déjérine 359.1
   Leyden-Möbius 359.1
   mesodermalis congenita 759.82
   muscular 359.1
      congenital (hereditary) 359.0
         myotonic 359.22
      distal 359.1
      Duchenne's 359.1
      Erb's 359.1
      fascioscapulohumeral 359.1
      Gowers' 359.1
      hereditary (progressive) 359.1
      Landouzy-Déjérine 359.1
      limb-girdle 359.1
      myotonic 359.21
      progressive (hereditary) 359.1
         Charcôt-Marie-Tooth 356.1
      pseudohypertrophic (infantile) 359.1
   myocardium, myocardial (*see also* Degeneration, myocardial) 429.1
   myotonic 359.21
   myotonica 359.21
   nail 703.8
      congenital 757.5
   neurovascular (traumatic) (*see also* Neuropathy, peripheral, autonomic) 337.9
   nutritional 263.9
   ocular 359.1
   oculocerebrorenal 270.8
   oculopharyngeal 359.1
   ovarian 620.8
   papillary (and pigmentary) 701.1
   pelvicrural atrophic 359.1
   pigmentary (*see also* Acanthosis) 701.2
   pituitary (gland) 253.8
   polyglandular 258.8
   posttraumatic sympathetic — *see* Dystrophy, sympathetic
   progressive ophthalmoplegic 359.1
   reflex neuromuscular — *see* Dystrophy, sympathetic

Dystrophy, dystrophia — *continued*
   retina, retinal (hereditary) 362.70
      albipunctate 362.74
      Bruch's membrane 362.77
      cone, progressive 362.75
      hyaline 362.77
      in
         Bassen-Kornzweig syndrome 272.5 *[362.72]*
         cerebroretinal lipidosis 330.1 *[362.71]*
         Refsum's disease 356.3 *[362.72]*
         systemic lipidosis 272.7 *[362.71]*
      juvenile (Stargardt's) 362.75
      pigmentary 362.74
      pigment epithelium 362.76
      progressive cone (-rod) 362.75
      pseudoinflammatory foveal 362.77
      rod, progressive 362.75
      sensory 362.75
      vitelliform 362.76
   Salzmann's nodular 371.46
   scapuloperoneal 359.1
   skin NEC 709.9
   sympathetic (posttraumatic) (reflex) 337.20
      lower limb 337.22
      specified site NEC 337.29
      upper limb 337.21
   tapetoretinal NEC 362.74
   thoracic asphyxiating 756.4
   unguium 703.8
      congenital 757.5
   vitreoretinal (primary) 362.73
      secondary 362.66
   vulva 624.09
Dysuria 788.1
   psychogenic 306.53

E

Eagle-Barrett syndrome 756.71
Eales' disease (syndrome) 362.18
Ear — *see also* condition
   ache 388.70
      otogenic 388.71
      referred 388.72
   lop 744.29
   piercing V50.3
   swimmers' acute 380.12
      tank 380.12
   tropical 111.8 *[380.15]*
   wax 380.4
Earache 388.70
   otogenic 388.71
   referred 388.72
Early satiety 780.94
Eaton-Lambert syndrome — *see also* Syndrome, Lambert-Eaton) 358.30
Eberth's disease (typhoid fever) 002.0
Ebstein's
   anomaly or syndrome (downward displacement, tricuspid valve into right ventricle) 746.2
   disease (diabetes) 250.4 ☑ *[581.81]*
      due to secondary diabetes 249.4 ☑ *[581.81]*
Eccentro-osteochondrodysplasia 277.5
Ecchondroma (M9210/0) — *see* Neoplasm, bone, benign
Ecchondrosis (M9210/1) 238.0
Ecchordosis physaliphora 756.0
Ecchymosis (multiple) 459.89
   conjunctiva 372.72
   eye (traumatic) 921.0
   eyelids (traumatic) 921.1
   newborn 772.6
   spontaneous 782.7
   traumatic — *see* Contusion
ECD (Erdheim-Chester disease) 277.89
Echinococciasis — *see* Echinococcus
Echinococcosis — *see* Echinococcus
Echinococcus (infection) 122.9
   granulosus 122.4
      liver 122.0
      lung 122.1
      orbit 122.3 *[376.13]*
      specified site NEC 122.3
      thyroid 122.2

Echinococcus — *continued*
   liver NEC 122.8
      granulosus 122.0
      multilocularis 122.5
   lung NEC 122.9
      granulosus 122.1
      multilocularis 122.6
   multilocularis 122.7
      liver 122.5
      specified site NEC 122.6
   orbit 122.9 *[376.13]*
      granulosus 122.3 *[376.13]*
      multilocularis 122.6 *[376.13]*
   specified site NEC 122.9
      granulosus 122.3
      multilocularis 122.6 *[376.13]*
   thyroid NEC 122.9
      granulosus 122.2
      multilocularis 122.6
Echinorhynchiasis 127.7
Echinostomiasis 121.8
Echolalia 784.69
ECHO virus infection NEC 079.1
Eclampsia, eclamptic (coma) (convulsions) (delirium) 780.39
   female, child-bearing age NEC — *see* Eclampsia, pregnancy
   gravidarum — *see* Eclampsia, pregnancy
   male 780.39
   not associated with pregnancy or childbirth 780.39
   pregnancy, childbirth, or puerperium 642.6 ☑
      with pre-existing hypertension 642.7 ☑
      affecting fetus or newborn 760.0
   uremic 586
Eclipse blindness (total) 363.31
Economic circumstance affecting care V60.9
   specified type NEC V60.89
Economo's disease (encephalitis lethargica) 049.8
Ectasia, ectasis
   annuloaortic 424.1
   aorta (*see also* Ectasia, aortic) 447.70
      with aneurysm 441.9
      ruptured 441.5
   aortic 447.70
      with aneurysm 441.9
      abdominal 447.72
      thoracic 447.71
      thoracoabdominal 447.73
   breast 610.4
   capillary 448.9
   cornea (marginal) (postinfectional) 371.71
   duct (mammary) 610.4
   gastric antral vascular (GAVE) 537.82
      with hemorrhage 537.83
      without hemorrhage 537.82
   kidney 593.89
   mammary duct (gland) 610.4
   papillary 448.9
   renal 593.89
   salivary gland (duct) 527.8
   scar, cornea 371.71
   sclera 379.11
Ecthyma 686.8
   contagiosum 051.2
   gangrenosum 686.09
   infectiosum 051.2
Ectocardia 746.87
Ectodermal dysplasia, congenital 757.31
Ectodermosis erosiva pluriorificialis 695.19
Ectopic, ectopia (congenital) 759.89
   abdominal viscera 751.8
      due to defect in anterior abdominal wall 756.79
   ACTH syndrome 255.0
   adrenal gland 759.1
   anus 751.5
   auricular beats 427.61
   beats 427.60
   bladder 753.5
   bone and cartilage in lung 748.69
   brain 742.4
   breast tissue 757.6
   cardiac 746.87

☑ Additional Digit Required — Refer to the Tabular List for Digit Selection   ▼ **Subterms under main terms may continue to next column or page**

100 — Volume 2   ▶◀ Revised Text   ● New Line   ▲ Revised Code   **2015 ICD-9-CM**

Ectopic, ectopia — *continued*
  cerebral 742.4
  cordis 746.87
  endometrium 617.9
  gallbladder 751.69
  gastric mucosa 750.7
  gestation — *see* Pregnancy, ectopic
  heart 746.87
  hormone secretion NEC 259.3
  hyperparathyroidism 259.3
  kidney (crossed) (intrathoracic) (pelvis) 753.3
    in pregnancy or childbirth 654.4 ☑
      causing obstructed labor 660.2 ☑
  lens 743.37
  lentis 743.37
  mole — *see* Pregnancy, ectopic
  organ or site NEC — *see* Malposition, congenital
  ovary 752.0
  pancreas, pancreatic tissue 751.7
  pregnancy — *see* Pregnancy, ectopic
  pupil 364.75
  renal 753.3
  sebaceous glands of mouth 750.26
  secretion
    ACTH 255.0
    adrenal hormone 259.3
    adrenalin 259.3
    adrenocorticotropin 255.0
    antidiuretic hormone (ADH) 259.3
    epinephrine 259.3
    hormone NEC 259.3
    norepinephrine 259.3
    pituitary (posterior) 259.3
  spleen 759.0
  testis 752.51
  thyroid 759.2
  ureter 753.4
  ventricular beats 427.69
  vesicae 753.5
Ectrodactyly 755.4
  finger (*see also* Absence, finger, congenital) 755.29
  toe (*see also* Absence, toe, congenital) 755.39
Ectromelia 755.4
  lower limb 755.30
  upper limb 755.20
Ectropion 374.10
  anus 569.49
  cervix 622.0
    with mention of cervicitis 616.0
  cicatricial 374.14
  congenital 743.62
  eyelid 374.10
    cicatricial 374.14
    congenital 743.62
    mechanical 374.12
    paralytic 374.12
    senile 374.11
    spastic 374.13
  iris (pigment epithelium) 364.54
  lip (congenital) 750.26
    acquired 528.5
  mechanical 374.12
  paralytic 374.12
  rectum 569.49
  senile 374.11
  spastic 374.13
  urethra 599.84
  uvea 364.54
Eczema (acute) (allergic) (chronic) (erythematous) (fissum) (occupational) (rubrum) (squamous) 692.9
  asteatotic 706.8
  atopic 691.8
  contact NEC 692.9
  dermatitis NEC 692.9
  due to specified cause — *see* Dermatitis, due to
  dyshidrotic 705.81
  external ear 380.22
  flexural 691.8
  gouty 274.89
  herpeticum 054.0

Eczema — *continued*
  hypertrophicum 701.8
  hypostatic — *see* Varicose, vein
  impetiginous 684
  infantile (acute) (chronic) (due to any substance) (intertriginous) (seborrheic) 690.12
  intertriginous NEC 692.9
    infantile 690.12
  intrinsic 691.8
  lichenified NEC 692.9
  marginatum 110.3
  nummular 692.9
  pustular 686.8
  seborrheic 690.18
    infantile 690.12
  solare 692.72
  stasis (lower extremity) 454.1
    ulcerated 454.2
  vaccination, vaccinatum 999.0
  varicose (lower extremity) — *see* Varicose, vein
  verrucosum callosum 698.3
Eczematoid, exudative 691.8
Eddowes' syndrome (brittle bones and blue sclera) 756.51
Edema, edematous 782.3
  with nephritis (*see also* Nephrosis) 581.9
  allergic 995.1
  angioneurotic (allergic) (any site) (with urticaria) 995.1
    hereditary 277.6
  angiospastic 443.9
  Berlin's (traumatic) 921.3
  brain (cytotoxic) (vasogenic) 348.5
    due to birth injury 767.8
    fetus or newborn 767.8
  cardiac (*see also* Failure, heart) 428.0
  cardiovascular (*see also* Failure, heart) 428.0
  cerebral — *see* Edema, brain
  cerebrospinal vessel — *see* Edema, brain
  cervix (acute) (uteri) 622.8
    puerperal, postpartum 674.8 ☑
  chronic hereditary 757.0
  circumscribed, acute 995.1
    hereditary 277.6
  complicating pregnancy (gestational) 646.1 ☑
    with hypertension — *see* Toxemia, of pregnancy
  conjunctiva 372.73
  connective tissue 782.3
  cornea 371.20
    due to contact lenses 371.24
    idiopathic 371.21
    secondary 371.22
  cystoid macular 362.53
  due to
    lymphatic obstruction — *see* Edema, lymphatic
    salt retention 276.0
  epiglottis — *see* Edema, glottis
  essential, acute 995.1
    hereditary 277.6
  extremities, lower — *see* Edema, legs
  eyelid NEC 374.82
  familial, hereditary (legs) 757.0
  famine 262
  fetus or newborn 778.5
  genital organs
    female 629.89
    male 608.86
  gestational 646.1 ☑
    with hypertension — *see* Toxemia, of pregnancy
  glottis, glottic, glottides (obstructive) (passive) 478.6
    allergic 995.1
      hereditary 277.6
    due to external agent — *see* Condition, respiratory, acute, due to specified agent
  heart (*see also* Failure, heart) 428.0
    newborn 779.89
  heat 992.7
  hereditary (legs) 757.0

Edema, edematous — *continued*
  inanition 262
  infectious 782.3
  intracranial 348.5
    due to injury at birth 767.8
  iris 364.89
  joint (*see also* Effusion, joint) 719.0 ☑
  larynx (*see also* Edema, glottis) 478.6
  legs 782.3
    due to venous obstruction 459.2
    hereditary 757.0
  localized 782.3
    due to venous obstruction 459.2
      lower extremity 459.2
  lower extremities — *see* Edema, legs
  lung 514
    acute 518.4
      with heart disease or failure (*see also* Failure, ventricular, left) 428.1
        congestive 428.0
      chemical (due to fumes or vapors) 506.1
      due to
        external agent(s) NEC 508.9
          specified NEC 508.8
        fumes and vapors (chemical) (inhalation) 506.1
        radiation 508.0
    chemical (acute) 506.1
      chronic 506.4
    chronic 514
      chemical (due to fumes or vapors) 506.4
      due to
        external agent(s) NEC 508.9
          specified NEC 508.8
        fumes or vapors (chemical) (inhalation) 506.4
        radiation 508.1
    due to
      external agent 508.9
        specified NEC 508.8
      high altitude 993.2
      near drowning 994.1
    postoperative 518.4
    terminal 514
  lymphatic 457.1
    due to mastectomy operation 457.0
  macula 362.83
    cystoid 362.53
    diabetic 250.5 ☑ *[362.07]*
      due to secondary diabetes 249.5 ☑ *[362.07]*
  malignant (*see also* Gangrene, gas) 040.0
  Milroy's 757.0
  nasopharynx 478.25
  neonatorum 778.5
  nutritional (newborn) 262
    with dyspigmentation, skin and hair 260
  optic disc or nerve — *see* Papilledema
  orbit 376.33
    circulatory 459.89
  palate (soft) (hard) 528.9
  pancreas 577.8
  penis 607.83
  periodic 995.1
    hereditary 277.6
  pharynx 478.25
  pitting 782.3
  pulmonary — *see* Edema, lung
  Quincke's 995.1
    hereditary 277.6
  renal (*see also* Nephrosis) 581.9
  retina (localized) (macular) (peripheral) 362.83
    cystoid 362.53
    diabetic 250.5 ☑ *[362.07]*
      due to secondary diabetes 249.5 ☑ *[362.07]*
  salt 276.0
  scrotum 608.86
  seminal vesicle 608.86
  spermatic cord 608.86
  spinal cord 336.1
  starvation 262
  stasis (*see also* Hypertension, venous) 459.30

Edema, edematous — *continued*
  subconjunctival 372.73
  subglottic (*see also* Edema, glottis) 478.6
  supraglottic (*see also* Edema, glottis) 478.6
  testis 608.86
  toxic NEC 782.3
  traumatic NEC 782.3
  tunica vaginalis 608.86
  vas deferens 608.86
  vocal cord — *see* Edema, glottis
  vulva (acute) 624.8
Edentia (complete) (partial) — *see also* Absence, tooth 520.0
  acquired (*see also* Edentulism) 525.40
    due to
      caries 525.13
      extraction 525.10
      periodontal disease 525.12
      specified NEC 525.19
      trauma 525.11
  causing malocclusion 524.30
  congenital (deficiency of tooth buds) 520.0
Edentulism 525.40
  complete 525.40
    class I 525.41
    class II 525.42
    class III 525.43
    class IV 525.44
  partial 525.50
    class I 525.51
    class II 525.52
    class III 525.53
    class IV 525.54
Edsall's disease 992.2
Educational handicap V62.3
Edwards' syndrome 758.2
Effect, adverse NEC
  abnormal gravitational (G) forces or states 994.9
  air pressure — *see* Effect, adverse, atmospheric pressure
  altitude (high) — *see* Effect, adverse, high altitude
  anesthetic
    in labor and delivery NEC 668.9 ☑
      affecting fetus or newborn 763.5
  antitoxin — *see* Complications, vaccination
  atmospheric pressure 993.9
    due to explosion 993.4
    high 993.3
    low — *see* Effect, adverse, high altitude
    specified effect NEC 993.8
  biological, correct substance properly administered (*see also* Effect, adverse, drug) 995.20
  blood (derivatives) (serum) (transfusion) — *see* Complications, transfusion
  chemical substance NEC 989.9
    specified — *see* Table of Drugs and Chemicals
  cobalt, radioactive (*see also* Effect, adverse, radioactive substance) 990
  cold (temperature) (weather) 991.9
    chilblains 991.5
    frostbite — *see* Frostbite
    specified effect NEC 991.8
  drugs and medicinals 995.20
    correct substance properly administered 995.20
    overdose or wrong substance given or taken 977.9
      specified drug — *see* Table of Drugs and Chemicals
  electric current (shock) 994.8
    burn — *see* Burn, by site
  electricity (electrocution) (shock) 994.8
    burn — *see* Burn, by site
  exertion (excessive) 994.5
  exposure 994.9
    exhaustion 994.4
  external cause NEC 994.9
  fallout (radioactive) NEC 990
  fluoroscopy NEC 990

☑ **Additional Digit Required** — Refer to the Tabular List for Digit Selection   ⬚ **Subterms under main terms may continue to next column or page**

Effect, adverse — *continued*
- foodstuffs
  - anaphylactic reaction or shock due to food NEC — *see* Anaphylactic reaction or shock, due to food
  - noxious 988.9
    - specified type NEC (*see also* Poisoning, by name of noxious foodstuff) 988.8
  - gases, fumes, or vapors — *see* Table of Drugs and Chemicals
- glue (airplane) sniffing 304.6 ☑
- heat — *see* Heat
- high altitude NEC 993.2
  - anoxia 993.2
  - on
    - ears 993.0
    - sinuses 993.1
  - polycythemia 289.0
- hot weather — *see* Heat
- hunger 994.2
- immersion, foot 991.4
- immunization — *see* Complications, vaccination
- immunological agents — *see* Complications, vaccination
- implantation (removable) of isotope or radium NEC 990
- infrared (radiation) (rays) NEC 990
  - burn — *see* Burn, by site
  - dermatitis or eczema 692.82
- infusion — *see* Complications, infusion
- ingestion or injection of isotope (therapeutic) NEC 990
- irradiation NEC (*see also* Effect, adverse, radiation) 990
- isotope (radioactive) NEC 990
- lack of care (child) (infant) (newborn) 995.52
  - adult 995.84
- lightning 994.0
  - burn — *see* Burn, by site
- Lirugin — *see* Complications, vaccination
- medicinal substance, correct, properly administered (*see also* Effect, adverse, drugs) 995.20
- mesothorium NEC 990
- motion 994.6
- noise, inner ear 388.10
- other drug, medicinal and biological substance 995.29
- overheated places — *see* Heat
- polonium NEC 990
- psychosocial, of work environment V62.1
- radiation (diagnostic) (fallout) (infrared) (natural source) (therapeutic) (tracer) (ultraviolet) (x-ray) NEC 990
  - with pulmonary manifestations
    - acute 508.0
    - chronic 508.1
  - dermatitis or eczema 692.82
    - due to sun NEC (*see also* Dermatitis, due to, sun) 692.70
  - fibrosis of lungs 508.1
  - maternal with suspected damage to fetus affecting management of pregnancy 655.6 ☑
  - pneumonitis 508.0
- radioactive substance NEC 990
  - dermatitis or eczema 692.82
- radioactivity NEC 990
- radiotherapy NEC 990
  - dermatitis or eczema 692.82
- radium NEC 990
- reduced temperature 991.9
  - frostbite — *see* Frostbite
  - immersion, foot (hand) 991.4
  - specified effect NEC 991.8
- roentgenography NEC 990
- roentgenoscopy NEC 990
- roentgen rays NEC 990
- serum (prophylactic) (therapeutic) NEC 999.59
- specified NEC 995.89
  - external cause NEC 994.9
- strangulation 994.7
- submersion 994.1

Effect, adverse — *continued*
- teletherapy NEC 990
- thirst 994.3
- transfusion — *see* Complications, transfusion
- ultraviolet (radiation) (rays) NEC 990
  - burn (*see also* Burn, by site)
    - from sun (*see also* Sunburn) 692.71
  - dermatitis or eczema 692.82
    - due to sun NEC (*see also* Dermatitis, due to, sun) 692.70
- uranium NEC 990
- vaccine (any) — *see* Complications, vaccination
- weightlessness 994.9
- whole blood (*see also* Complications, transfusion)
  - overdose or wrong substance given (*see also* Table of Drugs and Chemicals) 964.7
- working environment V62.1
- x-rays NEC 990
  - dermatitis or eczema 692.82

Effect, remote
- of cancer — *see* condition

Effects, late — *see* Late, effect (of)

Effluvium, telogen 704.02

Effort
- intolerance 306.2
- syndrome (aviators) (psychogenic) 306.2

Effusion
- amniotic fluid (*see also* Rupture, membranes, premature) 658.1 ☑
- brain (serous) 348.5
- bronchial (*see also* Bronchitis) 490
- cerebral 348.5
- cerebrospinal (*see also* Meningitis) 322.9
  - vessel 348.5
- chest — *see* Effusion, pleura
- intracranial 348.5
- joint 719.00
  - ankle 719.07
  - elbow 719.02
  - foot 719.07
  - hand 719.04
  - hip 719.05
  - knee 719.06
  - multiple sites 719.09
  - pelvic region 719.05
  - shoulder (region) 719.01
  - specified site NEC 719.08
  - wrist 719.03
- meninges (*see also* Meningitis) 322.9
- pericardium, pericardial (*see also* Pericarditis) 423.9
  - acute 420.90
- peritoneal (chronic) 568.82
- pleura, pleurisy, pleuritic, pleuropericardial 511.9
  - bacterial, nontuberculous 511.1
  - fetus or newborn 511.9
  - malignant 511.81
  - nontuberculous 511.9
    - bacterial 511.1
  - pneumococcal 511.1
  - staphylococcal 511.1
  - streptococcal 511.1
  - traumatic 862.29
    - with open wound 862.39
  - tuberculous (*see also* Tuberculosis, pleura) 012.0 ☑
    - primary progressive 010.1 ☑
- pulmonary — *see* Effusion, pleura
- spinal (*see also* Meningitis) 322.9
- thorax, thoracic — *see* Effusion, pleura

Egg (oocyte) (ovum)
- donor V59.70
  - over age 35 V59.73
    - anonymous recipient V59.73
    - designated recipient V59.74
  - under age 35 V59.71
    - anonymous recipient V59.71
    - designated recipient V59.72

Eggshell nails 703.8
- congenital 757.5

Ego-dystonic
- homosexuality 302.0
- lesbianism 302.0
- sexual orientation 302.0

Egyptian splenomegaly 120.1

Ehlers-Danlos syndrome 756.83

Ehrlichiosis 082.40
- chaffeensis 082.41
- specified type NEC 082.49

Eichstedt's disease (pityriasis versicolor) 111.0

EIN (endometrial intraepithelial neoplasia) 621.35

Eisenmenger's complex or syndrome (ventricular septal defect) 745.4

Ejaculation, semen
- painful 608.89
  - psychogenic 306.59
- premature 302.75
- retrograde 608.87

Ekbom syndrome (restless legs) 333.94

Ekman's syndrome (brittle bones and blue sclera) 756.51

Elastic skin 756.83
- acquired 701.8

Elastofibroma (M8820/0) — *see* Neoplasm, connective tissue, benign

Elastoidosis
- cutanea nodularis 701.8
- cutis cystica et comedonica 701.8

Elastoma 757.39
- juvenile 757.39
- Miescher's (elastosis perforans serpiginosa) 701.1

Elastomyofibrosis 425.3

Elastosis 701.8
- atrophicans 701.8
- perforans serpiginosa 701.1
- reactive perforating 701.1
- senilis 701.8
- solar (actinic) 692.74

Elbow — *see* condition

Electric
- current, electricity, effects (concussion) (fatal) (nonfatal) (shock) 994.8
  - burn — *see* Burn, by site
- feet (foot) syndrome 266.2
- shock from electroshock gun (taser) 994.8

Electrocution 994.8

Electrolyte imbalance 276.9
- with
  - abortion — *see* Abortion, by type, with metabolic disorder
  - ectopic pregnancy (*see also* categories 633.0–633.9) 639.4
  - hyperemesis gravidarum (before 22 completed weeks gestation) 643.1 ☑
  - molar pregnancy (*see also* categories 630–632) 639.4
- following
  - abortion 639.4
  - ectopic or molar pregnancy 639.4

Elephantiasis (nonfilarial) 457.1
- arabicum (*see also* Infestation, filarial) 125.9
- congenita hereditaria 757.0
- congenital (any site) 757.0
- due to
  - Brugia (malayi) 125.1
  - mastectomy operation 457.0
  - Wuchereria (bancrofti) 125.0
    - malayi 125.1
- eyelid 374.83
- filarial (*see also* Infestation, filarial) 125.9
- filariensis (*see also* Infestation, filarial) 125.9
- gingival 523.8
- glandular 457.1
- graecorum 030.9
- lymphangiectatic 457.1
- lymphatic vessel 457.1
  - due to mastectomy operation 457.0
- neuromatosa 237.71
- postmastectomy 457.0
- scrotum 457.1
- streptococcal 457.1
- surgical 997.99
  - postmastectomy 457.0

Elephantiasis — *continued*
- telangiectodes 457.1
- vulva (nonfilarial) 624.8

Elephant man syndrome 237.71

Elevated — *see* Elevation
- findings on laboratory examination — *see* Findings, abnormal, without diagnosis (examination) (laboratory test)
- GFR (glomerular filtration rate) — *see* Findings, abnormal, without diagnosis (examination) (laboratory test)

Elevation
- 17-ketosteroids 791.9
- acid phosphatase 790.5
- alkaline phosphatase 790.5
- amylase 790.5
- antibody titers 795.79
- basal metabolic rate (BMR) 794.7
- blood pressure (*see also* Hypertension) 401.9
  - reading (incidental) (isolated) (nonspecific), no diagnosis of hypertension 796.2
- blood sugar 790.29
- body temperature (of unknown origin) (*see also* Pyrexia) 780.60
- cancer antigen 125 [CA 125] 795.82
- carcinoembryonic antigen [CEA] 795.81
- cholesterol 272.0
  - with high triglycerides 272.2
- conjugate, eye 378.81
- C-reactive protein (CRP) 790.95
- CRP (C-reactive protein) 790.95
- diaphragm, congenital 756.6
- GFR (glomerular filtration rate) — *see* Findings, abnormal, without diagnosis (examination) (laboratory test)
- glucose
  - fasting 790.21
  - tolerance test 790.22
- immunoglobulin level 795.79
- indolacetic acid 791.9
- lactic acid dehydrogenase (LDH) level 790.4
- leukocytes 288.60
- lipase 790.5
- lipoprotein a level 272.8
- liver function test (LFT) 790.6
  - alkaline phosphatase 790.5
  - aminotransferase 790.4
  - bilirubin 782.4
  - hepatic enzyme NEC 790.5
  - lactate dehydrogenase 790.4
- lymphocytes 288.61
- prostate specific antigen (PSA) 790.93
- renin 790.99
  - in hypertension (*see also* Hypertension, renovascular) 405.91
- Rh titer (*see also* Complications, transfusion) 999.70
- scapula, congenital 755.52
- sedimentation rate 790.1
- SGOT 790.4
- SGPT 790.4
- transaminase 790.4
- triglycerides 272.1
  - with high cholesterol 272.2
- vanillylmandelic acid 791.9
- venous pressure 459.89
- VMA 791.9
- white blood cell count 288.60
  - specified NEC 288.69

Elliptocytosis (congenital) (hereditary) 282.1
- Hb-C (disease) 282.7
- hemoglobin disease 282.7
- sickle-cell (disease) 282.60
  - trait 282.5

Ellison-Zollinger syndrome (gastric hypersecretion with pancreatic islet cell tumor) 251.5

Ellis-van Creveld disease or syndrome (chondroectodermal dysplasia) 756.55

Elongation, elongated (congenital) — *see also* Distortion
- bone 756.9
- cervix (uteri) 752.49
  - acquired 622.6
  - hypertrophic 622.6

Elongation, elongated — *see also* Distortion
  — *continued*
  colon 751.5
  common bile duct 751.69
  cystic duct 751.69
  frenulum, penis 752.69
  labia minora, acquired 624.8
  ligamentum patellae 756.89
  petiolus (epiglottidis) 748.3
  styloid bone (process) 733.99
  tooth, teeth 520.2
  uvula 750.26
    acquired 528.9
Elschnig bodies or pearls 366.51
El Tor cholera 001.1
Emaciation (due to malnutrition) 261
Emancipation disorder 309.22
Embadomoniasis 007.8
Embarrassment heart, cardiac — *see* Disease, heart
Embedded
  fragment (status) — *see* Foreign body, retained
  splinter (status) — *see* Foreign body, retained
  tooth, teeth 520.6
    root only 525.3
Embolic — *see* condition
Embolism 444.9
  with
    abortion — *see* Abortion, by type, with embolism
    ectopic pregnancy (*see also* categories 633.0–633.9) 639.6
    molar pregnancy (*see also* categories 630–632) 639.6
  air (any site) 958.0
    with
      abortion — *see* Abortion, by type, with embolism
      ectopic pregnancy (*see also* categories 633.0–633.9) 639.6
      molar pregnancy (*see also* categories 630–632) 639.6
    due to implanted device — *see* Complications, due to (presence of) any device, implant, or graft classified to 996.0–996.5 NEC
    following
      abortion 639.6
      ectopic or molar pregnancy 639.6
      infusion, perfusion, or transfusion 999.1
    in pregnancy, childbirth, or puerperium 673.0 ☑
    traumatic 958.0
  amniotic fluid (pulmonary) 673.1 ☑
    with
      abortion — *see* Abortion, by type, with embolism
      ectopic pregnancy (*see also* categories 633.0–633.9) 639.6
      molar pregnancy (*see also* categories 630–632) 639.6
    following
      abortion 639.6
      ectopic or molar pregnancy 639.6
  aorta, aortic 444.1
    abdominal 444.09
      saddle 444.01
    bifurcation 444.09
    saddle 444.01
    thoracic 444.1
  artery 444.9
    auditory, internal 433.8 ☑
    basilar (*see also* Occlusion, artery, basilar) 433.0 ☑
    bladder 444.89
    carotid (common) (internal) (*see also* Occlusion, artery, carotid) 433.1 ☑
    cerebellar (anterior inferior) (posterior inferior) (superior) 433.8 ☑
    cerebral (*see also* Embolism, brain) 434.1 ☑
    choroidal (anterior) 433.8 ☑

Embolism — *continued*
  artery — *continued*
    communicating posterior 433.8 ☑
    coronary (*see also* Infarct, myocardium) 410.9 ☑
      without myocardial infarction 411.81
    extremity 444.22
      lower 444.22
      upper 444.21
    hypophyseal 433.8 ☑
    mesenteric (with gangrene) 557.0
    ophthalmic (*see also* Occlusion, retina) 362.30
    peripheral 444.22
    pontine 433.8 ☑
    precerebral NEC — *see* Occlusion, artery, precerebral
    pulmonary — *see* Embolism, pulmonary
    pyemic 449
      pulmonary 415.12
    renal 593.81
    retinal (*see also* Occlusion, retina) 362.30
    septic 449
      pulmonary 415.12
    specified site NEC 444.89
    vertebral (*see also* Occlusion, artery, vertebral) 433.2 ☑
  auditory, internal 433.8 ☑
  basilar (artery) (*see also* Occlusion, artery, basilar) 433.0 ☑
  birth, mother — *see* Embolism, obstetrical
  blood-clot
    with
      abortion — *see* Abortion, by type, with embolism
      ectopic pregnancy (*see also* categories 633.0–633.9) 639.6
      molar pregnancy (*see also* categories 630–632) 639.6
    following
      abortion 639.6
      ectopic or molar pregnancy 639.6
    in pregnancy, childbirth, or puerperium 673.2 ☑
  brain 434.1 ☑
    with
      abortion — *see* Abortion, by type, with embolism
      ectopic pregnancy (*see also* categories 633.0–633.9) 639.6
      molar pregnancy (*see also* categories 630–632) 639.6
    following
      abortion 639.6
      ectopic or molar pregnancy 639.6
    late effect — *see* Late effect(s) (of) cerebrovascular disease
    puerperal, postpartum, childbirth 674.0 ☑
  capillary 448.9
  cardiac (*see also* Infarct, myocardium) 410.9 ☑
  carotid (artery) (common) (internal) (*see also* Occlusion, artery, carotid) 433.1 ☑
  cavernous sinus (venous) — *see* Embolism, intracranial venous sinus
  cerebral (*see also* Embolism, brain) 434.1 ☑
  cholesterol — *see* Atheroembolism
  choroidal (anterior) (artery) 433.8 ☑
  coronary (artery or vein) (systemic) (*see also* Infarct, myocardium) 410.9 ☑
    without myocardial infarction 411.81
  due to (presence of) any device, implant, or graft classifiable to 996.0–996.5 — *see* Complications, due to (presence of) any device, implant, or graft classified to 996.0–996.5 NEC
  encephalomalacia (*see also* Embolism, brain) 434.1 ☑
  extremities 444.22
    lower 444.22
    upper 444.21
  eye 362.30
  fat (cerebral) (pulmonary) (systemic) 958.1

Embolism — *continued*
  fat — *continued*
    with
      abortion — *see* Abortion, by type, with embolism
      ectopic pregnancy (*see also* categories 633.0–633.9) 639.6
      molar pregnancy (*see also* categories 630–632) 639.6
    complicating delivery or puerperium 673.8 ☑
    following
      abortion 639.6
      ectopic or molar pregnancy 639.6
    in pregnancy, childbirth, or the puerperium 673.8 ☑
  femoral (artery) 444.22
    vein 453.6
      deep 453.41
  following
    abortion 639.6
    ectopic or molar pregnancy 639.6
    infusion, perfusion, or transfusion
      air 999.1
      thrombus 999.2
  heart (fatty) (*see also* Infarct, myocardium) 410.9 ☑
  hepatic (vein) 453.0
  iliac (artery) 444.81
  iliofemoral 444.81
  in pregnancy, childbirth, or puerperium (pulmonary) — *see* Embolism, obstetrical
  intestine (artery) (vein) (with gangrene) 557.0
  intracranial (*see also* Embolism, brain) 434.1 ☑
    venous sinus (any) 325
      late effect — *see* category 326
      nonpyogenic 437.6
        in pregnancy or puerperium 671.5 ☑
  kidney (artery) 593.81
  lateral sinus (venous) — *see* Embolism, intracranial venous sinus
  longitudinal sinus (venous) — *see* Embolism, intracranial venous sinus
  lower extremity 444.22
  lung (massive) — *see* Embolism, pulmonary
  meninges (*see also* Embolism, brain) 434.1 ☑
  mesenteric (artery) (with gangrene) 557.0
  multiple NEC 444.9
  obstetrical (pulmonary) 673.2 ☑
    air 673.0 ☑
    amniotic fluid (pulmonary) 673.1 ☑
    blood-clot 673.2 ☑
    cardiac 674.8 ☑
    fat 673.8 ☑
    heart 674.8 ☑
    pyemic 673.3 ☑
    septic 673.3 ☑
    specified NEC 674.8 ☑
  ophthalmic (*see also* Occlusion, retina) 362.30
  paradoxical NEC 444.9
  penis 607.82
  peripheral arteries NEC 444.22
    lower 444.22
    upper 444.21
  pituitary 253.8
  popliteal (artery) 444.22
  portal (vein) 452
  postoperative NEC 997.2
    cerebral 997.02
    mesenteric artery 997.71
    other vessels 997.79
    peripheral vascular 997.2
    pulmonary 415.11
      septic 415.11
    renal artery 997.72
  precerebral artery (*see also* Occlusion, artery, precerebral) 433.9 ☑
  puerperal — *see* Embolism, obstetrical
  pulmonary (acute) (artery) (vein) 415.19

Embolism — *continued*
  pulmonary — *continued*
    with
      abortion — *see* Abortion, by type, with embolism
      ectopic pregnancy (*see also* categories 633.0–633.9) 639.6
      molar pregnancy (*see also* categories 630–632) 639.6
    chronic 416.2
    following
      abortion 639.6
      ectopic or molar pregnancy 639.6
    healed or old V12.55
    iatrogenic 415.11
    in pregnancy, childbirth, or puerperium — *see* Embolism, obstetrical
    personal history of V12.55
    postoperative 415.11
    septic 415.12
  pyemic (multiple) (*see also* Septicemia) 415.12
    with
      abortion — *see* Abortion, by type, with embolism
      ectopic pregnancy (*see also* categories 633.0–633.9) 639.6
      molar pregnancy (*see also* categories 630–632) 639.6
    Aerobacter aerogenes 415.12
    enteric gram-negative bacilli 415.12
    Enterobacter aerogenes 415.12
    Escherichia coli 415.12
    following
      abortion 639.6
      ectopic or molar pregnancy 639.6
    Hemophilus influenzae 415.12
    pneumococcal 415.12
    Proteus vulgaris 415.12
    Pseudomonas (aeruginosa) 415.12
    puerperal, postpartum, childbirth (any organism) 673.3 ☑
    Serratia 415.12
    specified organism NEC 415.12
    staphylococcal 415.12
      aureus 415.12
      specified organism NEC 415.12
    streptococcal 415.12
  renal (artery) 593.81
    vein 453.3
  retina, retinal (*see also* Occlusion, retina) 362.30
  saddle
    abdominal aorta 444.01
    pulmonary artery 415.13
  septic 415.12
    arterial 449
  septicemic — *see* Embolism, pyemic
  sinus — *see* Embolism, intracranial venous sinus
  soap
    with
      abortion — *see* Abortion, by type, with embolism
      ectopic pregnancy (*see also* categories 633.0–633.9) 639.6
      molar pregnancy (*see also* categories 630–632) 639.6
    following
      abortion 639.6
      ectopic or molar pregnancy 639.6
  spinal cord (nonpyogenic) 336.1
    in pregnancy or puerperium 671.5 ☑
    pyogenic origin 324.1
    late effect — *see* category 326
  spleen, splenic (artery) 444.89
  thrombus (thromboembolism) following infusion, perfusion, or transfusion 999.2
  upper extremity 444.21
  vein 453.9
    with inflammation or phlebitis — *see* Thrombophlebitis
    antecubital (acute) 453.81
      chronic 453.71
    axillary (acute) 453.84

☑ Additional Digit Required — Refer to the Tabular List for Digit Selection   ▽ Subterms under main terms may continue to next column or page

Embolism — *continued*
vein — *continued*
axillary — *continued*
chronic 453.74
basilic (acute) 453.81
chronic 453.71
brachial (acute) 453.82
chronic 453.72
brachiocephalic (acute) (innominate)
453.87
chronic 453.77
cephalic (acute) 453.81
chronic 453.71
cerebral (*see also* Embolism, brain)
434.1 ☑
coronary (*see also* Infarct, myocardium)
410.9 ☑
without myocardial infarction 411.81
hepatic 453.0
internal jugular (acute) 453.86
chronic 453.76
lower extremity (superficial) 453.6
deep 453.40
acute 453.40
calf 453.42
distal (lower leg) 453.42
femoral 453.41
iliac 453.41
lower leg 453.42
peroneal 453.42
popliteal 453.41
proximal (upper leg) 453.41
thigh 453.41
tibial 453.42
chronic 453.50
calf 453.52
disal (lower leg) 453.52
femoral 453.51
iliac 453.51
lower leg 453.52
peroneal 453.52
popliteal 453.51
proximal (upper leg) 453.51
thigh 453.51
tibial 453.52
saphenous (greater) (lesser) 453.6
superficial 453.6
mesenteric (with gangrene) 557.0
portal 452
pulmonary — *see* Embolism, pulmonary
radial (acute) 453.82
chronic 453.72
renal 453.3
saphenous (greater) (lesser) 453.6
specified NEC (acute) 453.89
with inflammation or phlebitis — *see*
Thrombophlebitis
chronic 453.79
subclavian (acute) 453.85
chronic 453.75
superior vena cava (acute) 453.87
chronic 453.77
thoracic (acute) 453.87
chronic 453.77
ulnar (acute) 453.82
chronic 453.72
upper extremity (acute) 453.83
chronic 453.73
deep 453.72
superficial 453.71
deep 453.82
superficial 453.81
vena cava
inferior 453.2
superior (acute) 453.87
chronic 453.77
vessels of brain (*see also* Embolism, brain)
434.1 ☑
Embolization — *see* Embolism
Embolus — *see* Embolism
Embryoma (M9080/1) — *see also* Neoplasm,
by site, uncertain behavior
benign (M9080/0) — *see* Neoplasm, by site,
benign
kidney (M8960/3) 189.0
liver (M8970/3) 155.0

Embryoma (M9080/1) — *see also* Neoplasm,
by site, uncertain behavior —
continued
malignant (M9080/3) (*see also* Neoplasm,
by site, malignant)
kidney (M8960/3) 189.0
liver (M8970/3) 155.0
testis (M9070/3) 186.9
undescended 186.0
testis (M9070/3) 186.9
undescended 186.0
Embryonic
circulation 747.9
heart 747.9
vas deferens 752.89
Embryopathia NEC 759.9
Embryotomy, fetal 763.89
Embryotoxon 743.43
interfering with vision 743.42
Emesis — *see also* Vomiting
bilious 787.04
gravidarum — *see* Hyperemesis, gravidarum
Emissions, nocturnal (semen) 608.89
Emotional
crisis — *see* Crisis, emotional
disorder (*see also* Disorder, mental) 300.9
instability (excessive) 301.3
lability 799.24
overlay — *see* Reaction, adjustment
upset 300.9
Emotionality, pathological 301.3
Emotogenic disease — *see also* Disorder,
psychogenic 306.9
Emphysema (atrophic) (centriacinar) (centrilobular) (chronic) (diffuse) (essential) (hypertrophic) (interlobular) (lung) (obstructive) (panlobular) (paracicatricial)
(paracinar) (postural) (pulmonary) (senile) (subpleural) (traction) (unilateral)
(unilobular) (vesicular) 492.8
with bronchitis
chronic 491.20
with
acute bronchitis 491.22
exacerbation (acute) 491.21
bullous (giant) 492.0
cellular tissue 958.7
surgical 998.81
compensatory 518.2
congenital 770.2
conjunctiva 372.89
connective tissue 958.7
surgical 998.81
due to fumes or vapors 506.4
eye 376.89
eyelid 374.85
surgical 998.81
traumatic 958.7
fetus or newborn (interstitial) (mediastinal)
(unilobular) 770.2
heart 416.9
interstitial 518.1
congenital 770.2
fetus or newborn 770.2
laminated tissue 958.7
surgical 998.81
mediastinal 518.1
fetus or newborn 770.2
newborn (interstitial) (mediastinal) (unilobular) 770.2
obstructive diffuse with fibrosis 492.8
orbit 376.89
subcutaneous 958.7
due to trauma 958.7
nontraumatic 518.1
surgical 998.81
surgical 998.81
thymus (gland) (congenital) 254.8
traumatic 958.7
tuberculous (*see also* Tuberculosis, pulmonary) 011.9 ☑
Employment examination (certification) V70.5
Empty sella (turcica) syndrome 253.8

Empyema (chest) (diaphragmatic) (double)
(encapsulated) (general) (interlobar)
(lung) (medial) (necessitatis) (perforating
chest wall) (pleura) (pneumococcal)
(residual) (sacculated) (streptococcal)
(supradiaphragmatic) 510.9
with fistula 510.0
accessory sinus (chronic) (*see also* Sinusitis)
473.9
acute 510.9
with fistula 510.0
antrum (chronic) (*see also* Sinusitis, maxillary) 473.0
brain (any part) (*see also* Abscess, brain)
324.0
ethmoidal (sinus) (chronic) (*see also* Sinusitis, ethmoidal) 473.2
extradural (*see also* Abscess, extradural)
324.9
frontal (sinus) (chronic) (*see also* Sinusitis,
frontal) 473.1
gallbladder (*see also* Cholecystitis, acute)
575.0
mastoid (process) (acute) (*see also* Mastoiditis, acute) 383.00
maxilla, maxillary 526.4
sinus (chronic) (*see also* Sinusitis, maxillary) 473.0
nasal sinus (chronic) (*see also* Sinusitis) 473.9
sinus (accessory) (nasal) (*see also* Sinusitis)
473.9
sphenoidal (chronic) (sinus) (*see also* Sinusitis, sphenoidal) 473.3
subarachnoid (*see also* Abscess, extradural)
324.9
subdural (*see also* Abscess, extradural) 324.9
tuberculous (*see also* Tuberculosis, pleura)
012.0 ☑
ureter (*see also* Ureteritis) 593.89
ventricular (*see also* Abscess, brain) 324.0
Enameloma 520.2
Encephalitis (bacterial) (chronic) (hemorrhagic)
(idiopathic) (nonepidemic) (spurious)
(subacute) 323.9
acute (*see also* Encephalitis, viral)
disseminated (postinfectious) NEC
136.9 [323.61]
postimmunization or postvaccination
323.51
inclusional 049.8
inclusion body 049.8
necrotizing 049.8
arboviral, arbovirus NEC 064
arthropod-borne (*see also* Encephalitis, viral,
arthropod-borne) 064
Australian X 062.4
Bwamba fever 066.3
California (virus) 062.5
Central European 063.2
Czechoslovakian 063.2
Dawson's (inclusion body) 046.2
diffuse sclerosing 046.2
due to
actinomycosis 039.8 [323.41]
cat-scratch disease 078.3 [323.01]
human herpesvirus 6 058.21
human herpesvirus 7 058.29
human herpesvirus NEC 058.29
human immunodeficiency virus (HIV)
disease 042 [323.01]
infectious mononucleosis 075 [323.01]
malaria (*see also* Malaria) 084.6 [323.2]
Negishi virus 064
ornithosis 073.7 [323.01]
other infection classified elsewhere
136.9 [323.41]
prophylactic inoculation against smallpox 323.51
rickettsiosis (*see also* Rickettsiosis)
083.9 [323.1]
rubella 056.01
toxoplasmosis (acquired) 130.0
congenital (active) 771.2 [323.41]
typhus (fever) (*see also* Typhus)
081.9 [323.1]
vaccination (smallpox) 323.51

Encephalitis — *continued*
Eastern equine 062.2
endemic 049.8
epidemic 049.8
equine (acute) (infectious) (viral) 062.9
Eastern 062.2
Venezuelan 066.2
Western 062.1
Far Eastern 063.0
following vaccination or other immunization
procedure 323.51
herpes 054.3
human herpesvirus 6 058.21
human herpesvirus 7 058.29
human herpesvirus NEC 058.29
Ilheus (virus) 062.8
inclusion body 046.2
infectious (acute) (virus) NEC 049.8
influenzal (*see also* Influenza) 487.8 [323.41]
lethargic 049.8
Japanese (B type) 062.0
La Crosse 062.5
Langat 063.8
late effect — *see* Late, effect, encephalitis
lead 984.9 [323.71]
lethargic (acute) (infectious) (influenzal)
049.8
lethargica 049.8
louping ill 063.1
lupus 710.0 [323.81]
lymphatica 049.0
Mengo 049.8
meningococcal 036.1
mumps 072.2
Murray Valley 062.4
myoclonic 049.8
Negishi virus 064
otitic NEC 382.4 [323.41]
parasitic NEC 123.9 [323.41]
periaxialis (concentrica) (diffusa) 341.1
postchickenpox 052.0
postexanthematous NEC 057.9 [323.62]
postimmunization 323.51
postinfectious NEC 136.9 [323.62]
postmeasles 055.0
posttraumatic 323.81
postvaccinal (smallpox) 323.51
postvaricella 052.0
postviral NEC 079.99 [323.62]
postexanthematous 057.9 [323.62]
specified NEC 057.8 [323.62]
Powassan 063.8
progressive subcortical (Binswanger's)
290.12
Rasmussen 323.81
Rio Bravo 049.8
rubella 056.01
Russian
autumnal 062.0
spring-summer type (taiga) 063.0
saturnine 984.9 [323.71]
Semliki Forest 062.8
serous 048
slow-acting virus NEC 046.8
specified cause NEC 323.81
St. Louis type 062.3
subacute sclerosing 046.2
subcorticalis chronica 290.12
summer 062.0
suppurative 324.0
syphilitic 094.81
congenital 090.41
tick-borne 063.9
torula, torular 117.5 [323.41]
toxic NEC 989.9 [323.71]
toxoplasmic (acquired) 130.0
congenital (active) 771.2 [323.41]
trichinosis 124 [323.41]
Trypanosomiasis (*see also* Trypanosomiasis)
086.9 [323.2]
tuberculous (*see also* Tuberculosis) 013.6 ☑
type B (Japanese) 062.0
type C 062.3
van Bogaert's 046.2
Venezuelan 066.2
Vienna type 049.8

☑ **Additional Digit Required** — Refer to the Tabular List for Digit Selection   ▽ **Subterms under main terms may continue to next column or page**

104 — Volume 2   ▶◀ **Revised Text**   ● **New Line**   ▲ **Revised Code**   **2015 ICD-9-CM**

Encephalitis — *continued*
viral, virus 049.9
arthropod-borne NEC 064
mosquito-borne 062.9
Australian X disease 062.4
California virus 062.5
Eastern equine 062.2
Ilheus virus 062.8
Japanese (B type) 062.0
Murray Valley 062.4
specified type NEC 062.8
St. Louis 062.3
type B 062.0
type C 062.3
Western equine 062.1
tick-borne 063.9
biundulant 063.2
Central European 063.2
Czechoslovakian 063.2
diphasic meningoencephalitis 063.2
Far Eastern 063.0
Langat 063.8
louping ill 063.1
Powassan 063.8
Russian spring-summer (taiga) 063.0
specified type NEC 063.8
vector unknown 064
Western equine 062.1
slow acting NEC 046.8
specified type NEC 049.8
vaccination, prophylactic (against) V05.0
von Economo's 049.8
Western equine 062.1
West Nile type 066.41
Encephalocele 742.0
orbit 376.81
Encephalocystocele 742.0
Encephaloduroarteriomyosynangiosis (EDAMS) 437.5
Encephalomalacia (brain) (cerebellar) (cerebral) (cerebrospinal) — *see also* Softening, brain 348.89
due to
hemorrhage (*see also* Hemorrhage, brain) 431
recurrent spasm of artery 435.9
embolic (cerebral) (*see also* Embolism, brain) 434.1 ☑
subcorticalis chronica arteriosclerotica 290.12
thrombotic (*see also* Thrombosis, brain) 434.0 ☑
Encephalomeningitis — *see* Meningoencephalitis
Encephalomeningocele 742.0
Encephalomeningomyelitis — *see* Meningoencephalitis
Encephalomeningopathy — *see also* Meningoencephalitis 349.9
Encephalomyelitis (chronic) (granulomatous) (myalgic, benign) — *see also* Encephalitis 323.9
abortive disseminated 049.8
acute disseminated (ADEM) (postinfectious) 136.9 [323.61]
infectious 136.9 [323.61]
noninfectious 323.81
postimmunization 323.51
due to
cat-scratch disease 078.3 [323.01]
infectious mononucleosis 075 [323.01]
ornithosis 073.7 [323.01]
vaccination (any) 323.51
equine (acute) (infectious) 062.9
Eastern 062.2
Venezuelan 066.2
Western 062.1
funicularis infectiosa 049.8
late effect — *see* Late, effect, encephalitis
Munch-Peterson's 049.8
postchickenpox 052.0
postimmunization 323.51
postmeasles 055.0
postvaccinal (smallpox) 323.51

Encephalomyelitis — *see also* Encephalitis — *continued*
rubella 056.01
specified cause NEC 323.81
syphilitic 094.81
West Nile 066.41
Encephalomyelocele 742.0
Encephalomyelomeningitis — *see* Meningoencephalitis
Encephalomyeloneuropathy 349.9
Encephalomyelopathy 349.9
subacute necrotizing (infantile) 330.8
Encephalomyeloradiculitis (acute) 357.0
Encephalomyeloradiculoneuritis (acute) 357.0
Encephalomyeloradiculopathy 349.9
Encephalomyocarditis 074.23
Encephalopathia hyperbilirubinemica, newborn 774.7
due to isoimmunization (conditions classifiable to 773.0–773.2) 773.4
Encephalopathy (acute) 348.30
alcoholic 291.2
anoxic — *see* Damage, brain, anoxic
arteriosclerotic 437.0
late effect — *see* Late effect(s) (of) cerebrovascular disease
bilirubin, newborn 774.7
due to isoimmunization 773.4
congenital 742.9
demyelinating (callosal) 341.8
due to
birth injury (intracranial) 767.8
dialysis 294.8
transient 293.9
drugs — (*see also* Table of Drugs and Chemicals) 349.82
hyperinsulinism — *see* Hyperinsulinism
influenza (virus) (*see also* Influenza) 487.8
identified
avian 488.09
(novel) 2009 H1N1 488.19
lack of vitamin (*see also* Deficiency, vitamin) 269.2
nicotinic acid deficiency 291.2
serum (nontherapeutic) (therapeutic) 999.59
syphilis 094.81
trauma (postconcussional) 310.2
current (*see also* Concussion, brain) 850.9
with skull fracture — *see* Fracture, skull, by site, with intracranial injury
vaccination 323.51
hepatic 572.2
hyperbilirubinemic, newborn 774.7
due to isoimmunization (conditions classifiable to 773.0–773.2) 773.4
hypertensive 437.2
hypoglycemic 251.2
hypoxic (*see also* Damage, brain, anoxic)
ischemic (HIE) 768.70
mild 768.71
moderate 768.72
severe 768.73
infantile cystic necrotizing (congenital) 341.8
lead 984.9 [323.71]
leukopolio 330.0
metabolic (*see also* Delirium) 348.31
drug induced 349.82
toxic 349.82
necrotizing
hemorrhagic (acute) 323.61
subacute 330.8
other specified type NEC 348.39
pellagrous 265.2
portal-systemic 572.2
postcontusional 310.2
posttraumatic 310.2
saturnine 984.9 [323.71]
septic 348.31
spongiform, subacute (viral) 046.19

Encephalopathy — *continued*
subacute
necrotizing 330.8
spongiform 046.19
viral, spongioform 046.19
subcortical progressive (Schilder) 341.1
chronic (Binswanger's) 290.12
toxic 349.82
metabolic 349.82
traumatic (postconcussional) 310.2
current (*see also* Concussion, brain) 850.9
with skull fracture — *see* Fracture, skull, by site, with intracranial injury
vitamin B deficiency NEC 266.9
Wernicke's (superior hemorrhagic polioencephalitis) 265.1
Encephalorrhagia — *see also* Hemorrhage, brain 432.9
healed or old V12.54
late effect — *see* Late effect(s) (of) cerebrovascular disease
Encephalosis, posttraumatic 310.2
Enchondroma (M9220/0) — *see also* Neoplasm, bone, benign
multiple, congenital 756.4
Enchondromatosis (cartilaginous) (congenital) (multiple) 756.4
Enchondroses, multiple (cartilaginous) (congenital) 756.4
Encopresis — *see also* Incontinence, feces 787.60
nonorganic origin 307.7
Encounter for — *see also* Admission for
administrative purpose only V68.9
referral of patient without examination or treatment V68.81
specified purpose NEC V68.89
chemotherapy, (oral) (intravenous), antineoplastic V58.11
determination of fetal viability of pregnancy V23.87
dialysis
extracorporeal (renal) V56.0
peritoneal V56.8
disability examination V68.01
end-of-life care V66.7
hospice care V66.7
immunizations (childhood) appropriate for age V20.2
immunotherapy, antineoplastic V58.12
joint prosthesis insertion following prior explantation of joint prosthesis V54.82
palliative care V66.7
paternity testing V70.4
radiotherapy V58.0
respirator [ventilator] dependence
during
mechanical failure V46.14
power failure V46.12
for weaning V46.13
routine infant and child vision and hearing testing V20.2
school examination V70.3
following surgery V67.09
screening mammogram NEC V76.12
for high-risk patient V76.11
terminal care V66.7
weaning from respirator [ventilator] V46.13
Encystment — *see* Cyst
Endamebiasis — *see* Amebiasis
Endamoeba — *see* Amebiasis
Endarteritis (bacterial, subacute) (infective) (septic) 447.6
brain, cerebral or cerebrospinal 437.4
late effect — *see* Late effect(s) (of) cerebrovascular disease
coronary (artery) — *see* Arteriosclerosis, coronary
deformans — *see* Arteriosclerosis
embolic (*see also* Embolism) 444.9
obliterans (*see also* Arteriosclerosis)
pulmonary 417.8
pulmonary 417.8
retina 362.18

Endarteritis — *continued*
senile — *see* Arteriosclerosis
syphilitic 093.89
brain or cerebral 094.89
congenital 090.5
spinal 094.89
tuberculous (*see also* Tuberculosis) 017.9 ☑
Endemic — *see* condition
Endocarditis (chronic) (indeterminate) (interstitial) (marantic) (nonbacterial thrombotic) (residual) (sclerotic) (sclerous) (senile) (valvular) 424.90
with
rheumatic fever (conditions classifiable to 390)
active — *see* Endocarditis, acute, rheumatic
inactive or quiescent (with chorea) 397.9
acute or subacute 421.9
rheumatic (aortic) (mitral) (pulmonary) (tricuspid) 391.1
with chorea (acute) (rheumatic) (Sydenham's) 392.0
aortic (heart) (nonrheumatic) (valve) 424.1
with
mitral (valve) disease 396.9
active or acute 391.1
with chorea (acute) (rheumatic) (Sydenham's) 392.0
bacterial 421.0
rheumatic fever (conditions classifiable to 390)
active — *see* Endocarditis, acute, rheumatic
inactive or quiescent (with chorea) 395.9
with mitral disease 396.9
acute or subacute 421.9
arteriosclerotic 424.1
congenital 746.89
hypertensive 424.1
rheumatic (chronic) (inactive) 395.9
with mitral (valve) disease 396.9
active or acute 391.1
with chorea (acute) (rheumatic) (Sydenham's) 392.0
active or acute 391.1
with chorea (acute) (rheumatic) (Sydenham's) 392.0
specified cause, except rheumatic 424.1
syphilitic 093.22
arteriosclerotic or due to arteriosclerosis 424.99
atypical verrucous (Libman-Sacks) 710.0 [424.91]
bacterial (acute) (any valve) (chronic) (subacute) 421.0
blastomycotic 116.0 [421.1]
candidal 112.81
congenital 425.3
constrictive 421.0
Coxsackie 074.22
due to
blastomycosis 116.0 [421.1]
candidiasis 112.81
Coxsackie (virus) 074.22
disseminated lupus erythematosus 710.0 [424.91]
histoplasmosis (*see also* Histoplasmosis) 115.94
hypertension (benign) 424.99
moniliasis 112.81
prosthetic cardiac valve 996.61
Q fever 083.0 [421.1]
serratia marcescens 421.0
typhoid (fever) 002.0 [421.1]
fetal 425.3
gonococcal 098.84
hypertensive 424.99
infectious or infective (acute) (any valve) (chronic) (subacute) 421.0
lenta (acute) (any valve) (chronic) (subacute) 421.0

Endocarditis — continued
Libman-Sacks 710.0 [424.91]
Loeffler's (parietal fibroplastic) 421.0
malignant (acute) (any valve) (chronic)
    (subacute) 421.0
meningococcal 036.42
mitral (chronic) (double) (fibroid) (heart)
    (inactive) (valve) (with chorea) 394.9
    with
      aortic (valve) disease 396.9
        active or acute 391.1
          with chorea (acute) (Syden-
            ham's) 392.0
        rheumatic fever (conditions classifi-
        able to 390)
          active — see Endocarditis, acute,
           rheumatic
          inactive or quiescent (with
           chorea) 394.9
        with aortic valve disease 396.9
      active or acute 391.1
        with chorea (acute) (rheumatic)
          (Sydenham's) 392.0
        bacterial 421.0
    arteriosclerotic 424.0
    congenital 746.89
    hypertensive 424.0
    nonrheumatic 424.0
      acute or subacute 421.9
    syphilitic 093.21
monilial 112.81
mycotic (acute) (any valve) (chronic) (suba-
    cute) 421.0
pneumococcic (acute) (any valve) (chronic)
    (subacute) 421.0
pulmonary (chronic) (heart) (valve) 424.3
    with
      rheumatic fever (conditions classifi-
        able to 390)
        active — see Endocarditis, acute,
          rheumatic
        inactive or quiescent (with
          chorea) 397.1
    acute or subacute 421.9
      rheumatic 391.1
        with chorea (acute) (rheumatic)
          (Sydenham's) 392.0
    arteriosclerotic or due to arteriosclerosis
      424.3
    congenital 746.09
    hypertensive or due to hypertension
      (benign) 424.3
    rheumatic (chronic) (inactive) (with
      chorea) 397.1
      active or acute 391.1
        with chorea (acute) (rheumatic)
          (Sydenham's) 392.0
    syphilitic 093.24
purulent (acute) (any valve) (chronic) (suba-
    cute) 421.0
rheumatic (chronic) (inactive) (with chorea)
    397.9
    active or acute (aortic) (mitral) (pul-
      monary) (tricuspid) 391.1
      with chorea (acute) (rheumatic)
        (Sydenham's) 392.0
septic (acute) (any valve) (chronic) (suba-
    cute) 421.0
specified cause, except rheumatic 424.99
streptococcal (acute) (any valve) (chronic)
    (subacute) 421.0
subacute — see Endocarditis, acute
suppurative (any valve) (acute) (chronic)
    (subacute) 421.0
syphilitic NEC 093.20
toxic (see also Endocarditis, acute) 421.9
tricuspid (chronic) (heart) (inactive)
    (rheumatic) (valve) (with chorea)
    397.0
    with
      rheumatic fever (conditions classifi-
        able to 390)
        active — see Endocarditis, acute,
          rheumatic

Endocarditis — continued
tricuspid — continued
    with — continued
      rheumatic fever — continued
        inactive or quiescent (with
          chorea) 397.0
    active or acute 391.1
      with chorea (acute) (rheumatic)
        (Sydenham's) 392.0
    arteriosclerotic 424.2
    congenital 746.89
    hypertensive 424.2
    nonrheumatic 424.2
      acute or subacute 421.9
    specified cause, except rheumatic 424.2
    syphilitic 093.23
    tuberculous (see also Tuberculosis)
      017.9 ☑ [424.91]
typhoid 002.0 [421.1]
ulcerative (acute) (any valve) (chronic)
    (subacute) 421.0
vegetative (acute) (any valve) (chronic)
    (subacute) 421.0
verrucous (acute) (any valve) (chronic)
    (subacute) NEC 710.0 [424.91]
    nonbacterial 710.0 [424.91]
    nonrheumatic 710.0 [424.91]
Endocardium, endocardial — see also condi-
    tion
cushion defect 745.60
specified type NEC 745.69
Endocervicitis — see also Cervicitis 616.0
    due to
      intrauterine (contraceptive) device
        996.65
    gonorrheal (acute) 098.15
      chronic or duration of 2 months or over
        098.35
    hyperplastic 616.0
    syphilitic 095.8
    trichomonal 131.09
    tuberculous (see also Tuberculosis) 016.7 ☑
Endocrine — see condition
Endocrinopathy, pluriglandular 258.9
Endodontitis 522.0
End-of-life care V66.7
Endomastoiditis — see also Mastoiditis 383.9
Endometrioma 617.9
Endometriosis 617.9
    appendix 617.5
    bladder 617.8
    bowel 617.5
    broad ligament 617.3
    cervix 617.0
    colon 617.5
    cul-de-sac (Douglas') 617.3
    exocervix 617.0
    fallopian tube 617.2
    female genital organ NEC 617.8
    gallbladder 617.8
    in scar of skin 617.6
    internal 617.0
    intestine 617.5
    lung 617.8
    myometrium 617.0
    ovary 617.1
    parametrium 617.3
    pelvic peritoneum 617.3
    peritoneal (pelvic) 617.3
    rectovaginal septum 617.4
    rectum 617.5
    round ligament 617.3
    skin 617.6
    specified site NEC 617.8
    stromal (M8931/1) 236.0
    umbilicus 617.8
    uterus 617.0
      internal 617.0
    vagina 617.4
    vulva 617.8
Endometritis (nonspecific) (purulent) (septic)
    (suppurative) 615.9
    with
      abortion — see Abortion, by type, with
        sepsis

Endometritis — continued
    with — continued
      ectopic pregnancy (see also categories
        633.0–633.9) 639.0
      molar pregnancy (see also categories
        630–632) 639.0
    acute 615.0
    blennorrhagic 098.16
      acute 098.16
      chronic or duration of 2 months or over
        098.36
    cervix, cervical (see also Cervicitis) 616.0
      hyperplastic 616.0
    chronic 615.1
    complicating pregnancy 670.1 ☑
      affecting fetus or newborn 760.8
      septic 670.2 ☑
    decidual 615.9
    following
      abortion 639.0
      ectopic or molar pregnancy 639.0
    gonorrheal (acute) 098.16
      chronic or duration of 2 months or over
        098.36
    hyperplastic (see also Hyperplasia, en-
      dometrium) 621.30
      cervix 616.0
    polypoid — see Endometritis, hyperplastic
    puerperal, postpartum, childbirth 670.1 ☑
      septic 670.2 ☑
    senile (atrophic) 615.9
    subacute 615.0
    tuberculous (see also Tuberculosis) 016.7 ☑
Endometrium — see condition
Endomyocardiopathy, South African 425.2
Endomyocarditis — see Endocarditis
Endomyofibrosis 425.0
Endomyometritis — see also Endometritis
    615.9
Endopericarditis — see Endocarditis
Endoperineuritis — see Disorder, nerve
Endophlebitis — see also Phlebitis 451.9
    leg 451.2
      deep (vessels) 451.19
      superficial (vessels) 451.0
    portal (vein) 572.1
    retina 362.18
    specified site NEC 451.89
    syphilitic 093.89
Endophthalmia — see also Endophthalmitis
    360.00
    gonorrheal 098.42
Endophthalmitis (globe) (infective)
    (metastatic) (purulent) (subacute) 360.00
    acute 360.01
    bleb associated 379.63
    chronic 360.03
    parasitic 360.13
    phacoanaphylactic 360.19
    specified type NEC 360.19
    sympathetic 360.11
Endosalpingioma (M9111/1) 236.2
Endosalpingiosis 629.89
Endosteitis — see Osteomyelitis
Endothelioma, bone (M9260/3) — See Neo-
    plasm, bone, malignant
Endotheliosis 287.8
    hemorrhagic infectional 287.8
Endotoxemia — code to condition
Endotoxic shock 785.52
    postoperative 998.02
Endotrachelitis — see also Cervicitis 616.0
Enema rash 692.89
Engelmann's disease (diaphyseal sclerosis)
    756.9
**Engel-von Recklinghausen disease or syn-
    drome** (osteitis fibrosa cystica) 252.01
English disease — see also Rickets 268.0
Engman's disease (infectious eczematoid
    dermatitis) 690.8
Engorgement
    breast 611.79
      newborn 778.7
      puerperal, postpartum 676.2 ☑
    liver 573.9
    lung 514

Engorgement — continued
    pulmonary 514
    retina, venous 362.37
    stomach 536.8
    venous, retina 362.37
Enlargement, enlarged — see also Hypertro-
    phy
    abdomen 789.3 ☑
    adenoids 474.12
      and tonsils 474.10
    alveolar process or ridge 525.8
    apertures of diaphragm (congenital) 756.6
    blind spot, visual field 368.42
    gingival 523.8
    heart, cardiac (see also Hypertrophy, cardiac)
      429.3
    lacrimal gland, chronic 375.03
    liver (see also Hypertrophy, liver) 789.1
    lymph gland or node 785.6
    orbit 376.46
    organ or site, congenital NEC — see
      Anomaly, specified type NEC
    parathyroid (gland) 252.01
    pituitary fossa 793.0
    prostate (simple) (soft) 600.00
      with
        other lower urinary tract symptoms
          (LUTS) 600.01
        urinary
          obstruction 600.01
          retention 600.01
    sella turcica 793.0
    spleen (see also Splenomegaly) 789.2
      congenital 759.0
    thymus (congenital) (gland) 254.0
    thyroid (gland) (see also Goiter) 240.9
    tongue 529.8
    tonsils 474.11
      and adenoids 474.10
    uterus 621.2
Enophthalmos 376.50
    due to
      atrophy of orbital tissue 376.51
      surgery 376.52
      trauma 376.52
Enostosis 526.89
Entamebiasis — see Amebiasis
Entamebic — see Amebiasis
Entanglement, umbilical cord(s) 663.3 ☑
    with compression 663.2 ☑
    affecting fetus or newborn 762.5
    around neck with compression 663.1 ☑
    twins in monoamniotic sac 663.2 ☑
Enteralgia 789.0 ☑
Enteric — see condition
Enteritis (acute) (catarrhal) (choleraic) (chronic)
    (congestive) (diarrheal) (exudative) (fol-
    licular) (hemorrhagic) (infantile) (lienter-
    ic) (noninfectious) (perforative) (phleg-
    monous) (presumed noninfectious)
    (pseudomembranous) 558.9
    adaptive 564.9
    aertrycke infection 003.0
    allergic 558.3
    amebic (see also Amebiasis) 006.9
      with abscess — see Abscess, amebic
      acute 006.0
        with abscess — see Abscess, amebic
        nondysenteric 006.2
      chronic 006.1
        with abscess — see Abscess, amebic
        nondysenteric 006.2
      nondysenteric 006.2
    anaerobic (cocci) (gram-negative) (gram-
      positive) (mixed) NEC 008.46
    bacillary NEC 004.9
    bacterial NEC 008.5
      specified NEC 008.49
    Bacteroides (fragilis) (melaninogeniscus)
      (oralis) 008.46
    Butyrivibrio (fibriosolvens) 008.46
    Campylobacter 008.43
    Candida 112.85
    Chilomastix 007.8
    choleriformis 001.1
    chronic 558.9

☑ **Additional Digit Required — Refer to the Tabular List for Digit Selection**   ▽ **Subterms under main terms may continue to next column or page**

Enteritis — *continued*
chronic — *continued*
   ulcerative (*see also* Colitis, ulcerative) 556.9
cicatrizing (chronic) 555.0
Clostridium
   botulinum 005.1
   difficile 008.45
   haemolyticum 008.46
   novyi 008.46
   perfringens (C) (F) 008.46
   specified type NEC 008.46
coccidial 007.2
dietetic 558.9
due to
   achylia gastrica 536.8
   adenovirus 008.62
   Aerobacter aerogenes 008.2
   anaerobes (*see also* Enteritis, anaerobic) 008.46
   Arizona (bacillus) 008.1
   astrovirus 008.66
   Bacillus coli — *see* Enteritis, E. coli
   bacteria NEC 008.5
      specified NEC 008.49
   Bacteroides (*see also* Enteritis, Bacteroides) 008.46
   Butyrivibrio (fibriosolvens) 008.46
   calicivirus 008.65
   Camplyobacter 008.43
   Clostridium — *see* Enteritis, Clostridium
   Cockle agent 008.64
   Coxsackie (virus) 008.67
   Ditchling agent 008.64
   ECHO virus 008.67
   Enterobacter aerogenes 008.2
   enterococci 008.49
   enterovirus NEC 008.67
   Escherichia coli — *see* Enteritis, E. coli
   Eubacterium 008.46
   Fusobacterium (nucleatum) 008.46
   gram-negative bacteria NEC 008.47
      anaerobic NEC 008.46
   Hawaii agent 008.63
   irritating foods 558.9
   Klebsiella aerogenes 008.47
   Marin County agent 008.66
   Montgomery County agent 008.63
   norovirus 008.63
   Norwalk-like agent 008.63
   Norwalk virus 008.63
   Otofuke agent 008.63
   Paracolobactrum arizonae 008.1
   paracolon bacillus NEC 008.47
      Arizona 008.1
   Paramatta agent 008.64
   Peptococcus 008.46
   Peptostreptococcus 008.46
   Proprionibacterium 008.46
   Proteus (bacillus) (mirabilis) (morganii) 008.3
   Pseudomonas aeruginosa 008.42
   Rotavirus 008.61
   Sapporo agent 008.63
   small round virus (SRV) NEC 008.64
      featureless NEC 008.63
      structured NEC 008.63
   Snow Mountain (SM) agent 008.63
   specified
      bacteria NEC 008.49
      organism, nonbacterial NEC 008.8
      virus NEC 008.69
   Staphylococcus 008.41
   Streptococcus 008.49
      anaerobic 008.46
   Taunton agent 008.63
   Torovirus 008.69
   Treponema 008.46
   Veillonella 008.46
   virus 008.8
      specified type NEC 008.69
   Wollan (W) agent 008.64
   Yersinia enterocolitica 008.44
dysentery — *see* Dysentery
E. coli 008.00
   enterohemorrhagic 008.04

Enteritis — *continued*
E. coli — *continued*
   enteroinvasive 008.03
   enteropathogenic 008.01
   enterotoxigenic 008.02
   specified type NEC 008.09
el tor 001.1
embadomonial 007.8
eosinophilic 558.41
epidemic 009.0
Eubacterium 008.46
fermentative 558.9
fulminant 557.0
Fusobacterium (nucleatum) 008.46
gangrenous (*see also* Enteritis, due to, by organism) 009.0
giardial 007.1
gram-negative bacteria NEC 008.47
   anaerobic NEC 008.46
infectious NEC (*see also* Enteritis, due to, by organism) 009.0
   presumed 009.1
influenzal (*see also* Influenza) 487.8
ischemic 557.9
   acute 557.0
   chronic 557.1
   due to mesenteric artery insufficiency 557.1
membranous 564.9
mucous 564.9
myxomembranous 564.9
necrotic (*see also* Enteritis, due to, by organism) 009.0
necroticans 005.2
necrotizing of fetus or newborn (*see also* Enterocolitis, necrotizing, newborn) 777.50
neurogenic 564.9
newborn 777.8
   necrotizing (*see also* Enterocolitis, necrotizing, newborn) 777.50
parasitic NEC 129
paratyphoid (fever) (*see also* Fever, paratyphoid) 002.9
Peptococcus 008.46
Peptostreptococcus 008.46
Proprionibacterium 008.46
protozoal NEC 007.9
radiation 558.1
regional (of) 555.9
   intestine
      large (bowel, colon, or rectum) 555.1
         with small intestine 555.2
      small (duodenum, ileum, or jejunum) 555.0
         with large intestine 555.2
Salmonella infection 003.0
salmonellosis 003.0
segmental (*see also* Enteritis, regional) 555.9
septic (*see also* Enteritis, due to, by organism) 009.0
Shigella 004.9
simple 558.9
spasmodic 564.9
spastic 564.9
staphylococcal 008.41
   due to food 005.0
streptococcal 008.49
   anaerobic 008.46
toxic 558.2
Treponema (denticola) (macrodentium) 008.46
trichomonal 007.3
tuberculous (*see also* Tuberculosis) 014.8 ☑
typhosa 002.0
ulcerative (chronic) (*see also* Colitis, ulcerative) 556.9
Veillonella 008.46
viral 008.8
   adenovirus 008.62
   enterovirus 008.67
   specified virus NEC 008.69
Yersinia enterocolitica 008.44
zymotic 009.0
Enteroarticular syndrome 099.3
Enterobiasis 127.4

Enterobius vermicularis 127.4
Enterocele — *see also* Hernia 553.9
   pelvis, pelvic (acquired) (congenital) 618.6
   vagina, vaginal (acquired) (congenital) 618.6
Enterocolitis — *see also* Enteritis
   fetus or newborn (*see also* Enterocolitis, necrotizing, newborn) 777.8
      necrotizing 777.50
   fulminant 557.0
   granulomatous 555.2
   hemorrhagic (acute) 557.0
      chronic 557.1
   necrotizing (acute) (membranous) 557.0
      newborn 777.50
         with
            perforation 777.53
            pneumatosis and perforation 777.53
            pneumatosis without perforation 777.52
         without pneumatosis, without perforation 777.51
         stage I 777.51
         stage II 777.52
         stage III 777.53
   primary necrotizing (*see also* Enterocolitis, necrotizing, newborn) 777.50
   pseudomembranous 008.45
      newborn 008.45
   radiation 558.1
      newborn (*see also* Enterocolitis, necrotizing, newborn) 777.50
   ulcerative 556.0
Enterocystoma 751.5
Enterogastritis — *see* Enteritis
Enterogenous cyanosis 289.7
Enterolith, enterolithiasis (impaction) 560.39
   with hernia (*see also* Hernia, by site, with obstruction)
      gangrenous — *see* Hernia, by site, with gangrene
Enteropathy 569.9
   exudative (of Gordon) 579.8
   gluten 579.0
   hemorrhagic, terminal 557.0
   protein-losing 579.8
Enteroperitonitis — *see also* Peritonitis 567.9
Enteroptosis 569.89
Enterorrhagia 578.9
Enterospasm 564.9
   psychogenic 306.4
Enterostenosis — *see also* Obstruction, intestine 560.9
Enterostomy status V44.4
   with complication 569.60
Enthesopathy 726.90
   ankle and tarsus 726.70
   elbow region 726.30
      specified NEC 726.39
   hip 726.5
   knee 726.60
   peripheral NEC 726.8
   shoulder region 726.10
      adhesive 726.0
   spinal 720.1
   wrist and carpus 726.4
Entrance, air into vein — *see* Embolism, air
Entrapment, nerve — *see* Neuropathy, entrapment
Entropion (eyelid) 374.00
   cicatricial 374.04
   congenital 743.62
   late effect of trachoma (healed) 139.1
   mechanical 374.02
   paralytic 374.02
   senile 374.01
   spastic 374.03
Enucleation of eye (current) (traumatic) 871.3
Enuresis 788.30
   habit disturbance 307.6
   nocturnal 788.36
      psychogenic 307.6
   nonorganic origin 307.6
   psychogenic 307.6
Enzymopathy 277.9
Eosinopenia 288.59

Eosinophilia 288.3
   with
      angiolymphoid hyperplasia (ALHE) 228.01
   allergic 288.3
   hereditary 288.3
   idiopathic 288.3
   infiltrative 518.3
   Loeffler's 518.3
   myalgia syndrome 710.5
   pulmonary (tropical) 518.3
   secondary 288.3
   tropical 518.3
Eosinophilic — *see also* condition
   fasciitis 728.89
   granuloma (bone) 277.89
   infiltration lung 518.3
Ependymitis (acute) (cerebral) (chronic) (granular) — *see also* Meningitis 322.9
Ependymoblastoma (M9392/3)
   specified site — *see* Neoplasm, by site, malignant
   unspecified site 191.9
Ependymoma (epithelial) (malignant) (M9391/3)
   anaplastic type (M9392/3)
      specified site — *see* Neoplasm, by site, malignant
      unspecified site 191.9
   benign (M9391/0)
      specified site — *see* Neoplasm, by site, benign
      unspecified site 225.0
   myxopapillary (M9394/1) 237.5
   papillary (M9393/1) 237.5
   specified site — *see* Neoplasm, by site, malignant
   unspecified site 191.9
Ependymopathy 349.2
   spinal cord 349.2
Ephelides, ephelis 709.09
Ephemeral fever — *see also* Pyrexia 780.60
Epiblepharon (congenital) 743.62
Epicanthus, epicanthic fold (congenital) (eyelid) 743.63
Epicondylitis (elbow) (lateral) 726.32
   medial 726.31
Epicystitis — *see also* Cystitis 595.9
Epidemic — *see* condition
Epidermidalization, cervix — *see* condition
Epidermidization, cervix — *see* condition
Epidermis, epidermal — *see* condition
Epidermization, cervix — *see* condition
Epidermodysplasia verruciformis 078.19
Epidermoid
   cholesteatoma — *see* Cholesteatoma
   inclusion (*see also* Cyst, skin) 706.2
Epidermolysis
   acuta (combustiformis) (toxica) 695.15
   bullosa 757.39
   necroticans combustiformis 695.15
      due to drug
         correct substance properly administered 695.15
         overdose or wrong substance given or taken 977.9
         specified drug — *see* Table of Drugs and Chemicals
Epidermophytid — *see* Dermatophytosis
Epidermophytosis (infected) — *see* Dermatophytosis
Epidermosis, ear (middle) — *see also* Cholesteatoma 385.30
Epididymis — *see* condition
Epididymitis (nonvenereal) 604.90
   with abscess 604.0
   acute 604.99
   blennorrhagic (acute) 098.0
      chronic or duration of 2 months or over 098.2
   caseous (*see also* Tuberculosis) 016.4 ☑
   chlamydial 099.54
   diphtheritic 032.89 [604.91]
   filarial 125.9 [604.91]
   gonococcal (acute) 098.0

☑ **Additional Digit Required** — Refer to the Tabular List for Digit Selection   ▽ **Subterms under main terms may continue to next column or page**

2015 ICD-9-CM   ▶◀ **Revised Text**   ● **New Line**   ▲ **Revised Code**   **Volume 2 — 107**

Epididymitis — *continued*
  gonococcal — *continued*
    chronic or duration of 2 months or over
      098.2
    recurrent 604.99
    residual 604.99
    syphilitic 095.8 *[604.91]*
    tuberculous (*see also* Tuberculosis) 016.4 ☑
Epididymo-orchitis — *see also* Epididymitis
  604.90
  with abscess 604.0
  chlamydial 099.54
  gonococcal (acute) 098.13
    chronic or duration of 2 months or over
      098.33
Epidural — *see* condition
Epigastritis — *see also* Gastritis 535.5 ☑
Epigastrium, epigastric — *see* condition
Epigastrocele — *see also* Hernia, epigastric
  553.29
Epiglottiditis (acute) 464.30
  with obstruction 464.31
  chronic 476.1
  viral 464.30
    with obstruction 464.31
Epiglottis — *see* condition
Epiglottitis (acute) 464.30
  with obstruction 464.31
  chronic 476.1
  viral 464.30
    with obstruction 464.31
Epignathus 759.4
Epilepsia
  partialis continua (*see also* Epilepsy)
    345.7 ☑
  procursiva (*see also* Epilepsy) 345.8 ☑
Epilepsy, epileptic (idiopathic) 345.9 ☑

Note — use the following fifth-digit subclassification with categories 345.0, 345.1, 345.4–345.9:

0   without mention of intractable epilepsy

1   with intractable epilepsy

    pharmacoresistant (pharmacologically resistant)

    poorly controlled

    refractory (medically)

    treatment resistant

  abdominal 345.5 ☑
  absence (attack) 345.0 ☑
  akinetic 345.0 ☑
    psychomotor 345.4 ☑
  automatism 345.4 ☑
  autonomic diencephalic 345.5 ☑
  brain 345.9 ☑
  Bravais-Jacksonian 345.5 ☑
  cerebral 345.9 ☑
  climacteric 345.9 ☑
  clonic 345.1 ☑
  clouded state 345.9 ☑
  coma 345.3
  communicating 345.4 ☑
  complicating pregnancy, childbirth, or the
    puerperium 649.4 ☑
  congenital 345.9 ☑
  convulsions 345.9 ☑
  cortical (focal) (motor) 345.5 ☑
  cursive (running) 345.8 ☑
  cysticercosis 123.1
  deterioration
    with behavioral disturbance
      345.9 ☑ *[294.11]*
    without behavioral disturbance
      345.9 ☑ *[294.10]*
  due to syphilis 094.89
  equivalent 345.5 ☑
  fit 345.9 ☑
  focal (motor) 345.5 ☑
  gelastic 345.8 ☑
  generalized 345.9 ☑
    convulsive 345.1 ☑

Epilepsy, epileptic — *continued*
  generalized — *continued*
    flexion 345.1 ☑
    nonconvulsive 345.0 ☑
  grand mal (idiopathic) 345.1 ☑
  Jacksonian (motor) (sensory) 345.5 ☑
  Kojevnikoff's, Kojevnikov's, Kojewnikoff's
    345.7 ☑
  laryngeal 786.2
  limbic system 345.4 ☑
  localization related (focal) (partial) and
    epileptic syndromes
    with
      complex partial seizures 345.4 ☑
      simple partial seizures 345.5 ☑
  major (motor) 345.1 ☑
  minor 345.0 ☑
  mixed (type) 345.9 ☑
  motor partial 345.5 ☑
  musicogenic 345.1 ☑
  myoclonus, myoclonic 345.1 ☑
    progressive (familial) 345.1 ☑
  nonconvulsive, generalized 345.0 ☑
  parasitic NEC 123.9
  partial (focalized) 345.5 ☑
    with
      impairment of consciousness
        345.4 ☑
      memory and ideational disturbances
        345.4 ☑
    without impairment of consciousness
      345.5 ☑
    abdominal type 345.5 ☑
    motor type 345.5 ☑
    psychomotor type 345.4 ☑
    psychosensory type 345.4 ☑
    secondarily generalized 345.4 ☑
    sensory type 345.5 ☑
    somatomotor type 345.5 ☑
    somatosensory type 345.5 ☑
    temporal lobe type 345.4 ☑
    visceral type 345.5 ☑
    visual type 345.5 ☑
  peripheral 345.9 ☑
  petit mal 345.0 ☑
  photokinetic 345.8 ☑
  progressive myoclonic (familial) 345.1 ☑
  psychic equivalent 345.5 ☑
  psychomotor 345.4 ☑
  psychosensory 345.4 ☑
  reflex 345.1 ☑
  seizure 345.9 ☑
  senile 345.9 ☑
  sensory-induced 345.5 ☑
  sleep (*see also* Narcolepsy) 347.00
  somatomotor type 345.5 ☑
  somatosensory 345.5 ☑
  specified type NEC 345.8 ☑
  status (grand mal) 345.3
    focal motor 345.7 ☑
    petit mal 345.2
    psychomotor 345.7 ☑
    temporal lobe 345.7 ☑
  symptomatic 345.9 ☑
  temporal lobe 345.4 ☑
  tonic (-clonic) 345.1 ☑
  traumatic (injury unspecified) 907.0
    injury specified — *see* Late, effect (of)
      specified injury
  twilight 293.0
  uncinate (gyrus) 345.4 ☑
  Unverricht (-Lundborg) (familial myoclonic)
    345.1 ☑
  visceral 345.5 ☑
  visual 345.5 ☑
Epileptiform
  convulsions 780.39
  seizure 780.39
Epiloia 759.5
Epimenorrhea 626.2
Epipharyngitis — *see also* Nasopharyngitis
  460
Epiphora 375.20

Epiphora — *continued*
  due to
    excess lacrimation 375.21
    insufficient drainage 375.22
Epiphyseal arrest 733.91
  femoral head 732.2
Epiphyseolysis, epiphysiolysis — *see also*
  Osteochondrosis 732.9
Epiphysitis — *see also* Osteochondrosis 732.9
  juvenile 732.6
  marginal (Scheuermann's) 732.0
  os calcis 732.5
  syphilitic (congenital) 090.0
  vertebral (Scheuermann's) 732.0
Epiplocele — *see also* Hernia 553.9
Epiploitis — *see also* Peritonitis 567.9
Epiplosarcomphalocele — *see also* Hernia,
  umbilicus 553.1
Episcleritis 379.00
  gouty 274.89 *[379.09]*
  nodular 379.02
  periodica fugax 379.01
    angioneurotic — *see* Edema, angioneurotic
  specified NEC 379.09
  staphylococcal 379.00
  suppurative 379.00
  syphilitic 095.0
  tuberculous (*see also* Tuberculosis)
    017.3 ☑ *[379.09]*
Episode
  brain (*see also* Disease, cerebrovascular,
    acute) 436
  cerebral (*see also* Disease, cerebrovascular,
    acute) 436
  depersonalization (in neurotic state) 300.6
  hyporesponsive 780.09
  psychotic (*see also* Psychosis) 298.9
    organic, transient 293.9
  schizophrenic (acute) NEC (*see also*
    Schizophrenia) 295.4 ☑
Epispadias
  female 753.8
  male 752.62
Episplenitis 289.59
Epistaxis (multiple) 784.7
  hereditary 448.0
  vicarious menstruation 625.8
Epithelioma (malignant) (M8011/3) — *see also*
  Neoplasm, by site, malignant
  adenoides cysticum (M8100/0) — *see* Neoplasm, skin, benign
  basal cell (M8090/3) — *see* Neoplasm, skin,
    malignant
  benign (M8011/0) — *see* Neoplasm, by site,
    benign
  Bowen's (M8081/2) — *see* Neoplasm, skin,
    in situ
  calcifying (benign) (Malherbe's) (M8110/0)
    — *see* Neoplasm, skin, benign
  external site — *see* Neoplasm, skin, malignant
  intraepidermal, Jadassohn (M8096/0) — *see*
    Neoplasm, skin, benign
  squamous cell (M8070/3) — *see* Neoplasm,
    by site, malignant
Epitheliopathy
  pigment, retina 363.15
  posterior multifocal placoid (acute) 363.15
Epithelium, epithelial — *see* condition
Epituberculosis (allergic) (with atelectasis) —
  see also Tuberculosis 010.8 ☑
Eponychia 757.5
Epstein's
  nephrosis or syndrome (*see also* Nephrosis)
    581.9
  pearl (mouth) 528.4
Epstein-Barr infection (viral) 075
  chronic 780.79 *[139.8]*
Epulis (giant cell) (gingiva) 523.8
Equinia 024
Equinovarus (congenital) 754.51
  acquired 736.71
Equivalent
  angina 413.9

Equivalent — *continued*
  convulsive (abdominal) (*see also* Epilepsy)
    345.5 ☑
  epileptic (psychic) (*see also* Epilepsy)
    345.5 ☑
Erb's
  disease 359.1
  palsy, paralysis (birth) (brachial) (newborn)
    767.6
    spinal (spastic) syphilitic 094.89
  pseudohypertrophic muscular dystrophy
    359.1
Erb-Goldflam disease or syndrome 358.00
Erb (-Duchenne) paralysis (birth injury)
  (newborn) 767.6
Erdheim-Chester disease (ECD) 277.89
Erdheim's syndrome (acromegalic
  macrospondylitis) 253.0
Erection, painful (persistent) 607.3
Ergosterol deficiency (vitamin D) 268.9
  with
    osteomalacia 268.2
    rickets (*see also* Rickets) 268.0
Ergotism (ergotized grain) 988.2
  from ergot used as drug (migraine therapy)
    correct substance properly administered
      349.82
    overdose or wrong substance given or
      taken 975.0
Erichsen's disease (railway spine) 300.16
Erlacher-Blount syndrome (tibia vara) 732.4
Erosio interdigitalis blastomycetica 112.3
Erosion
  arteriosclerotic plaque — *see* Arteriosclerosis, by site
  artery NEC 447.2
    without rupture 447.8
  bone 733.99
  bronchus 519.19
  cartilage (joint) 733.99
  cervix (uteri) (acquired) (chronic) (congenital) 622.0
    with mention of cervicitis 616.0
  cornea (recurrent) (*see also* Keratitis) 371.42
    traumatic 918.1
  dental (idiopathic) (occupational) 521.30
    extending into
      dentine 521.32
      pulp 521.33
    generalized 521.35
    limited to enamel 521.31
    localized 521.34
  duodenum, postpyloric — *see* Ulcer, duodenum
  esophagus 530.89
  gastric 535.4 ☑
  implanted vaginal mesh
    in, into
      pelvic floor muscles 629.31
      surrounding organ(s) or tissue 629.31
  intestine 569.89
  lymphatic vessel 457.8
  pylorus, pyloric (ulcer) 535.4 ☑
  sclera 379.16
  spine, aneurysmal 094.89
  spleen 289.59
  stomach 535.4 ☑
  teeth (idiopathic) (occupational) (*see also*
    Erosion, dental) 521.30
    due to
      medicine 521.30
      persistent vomiting 521.30
  urethra 599.84
  uterus 621.8
  vaginal prosthetic materials NEC
    in, into
      pelvic floor muscles 629.31
      surrounding organ(s) or tissue 629.31
  vertebra 733.99
Erotomania 302.89
  Clérambault's 297.8
Error
  in diet 269.9
  refractive 367.9
    astigmatism (*see also* Astigmatism)
      367.20

☑ **Additional Digit Required — Refer to the Tabular List for Digit Selection**   ▽ **Subterms under main terms may continue to next column or page**

108 — Volume 2   ▶◀ Revised Text   ● New Line   ▲ Revised Code   **2015 ICD-9-CM**

Error — *continued*
  refractive — *continued*
    drug-induced 367.89
    hypermetropia 367.0
    hyperopia 367.0
    myopia 367.1
    presbyopia 367.4
    toxic 367.89
Eructation 787.3
  nervous 306.4
  psychogenic 306.4
Eruption
  creeping 126.9
  drug — *see* Dermatitis, due to, drug
  Hutchinson, summer 692.72
  Kaposi's varicelliform 054.0
  napkin (psoriasiform) 691.0
  polymorphous
    light (sun) 692.72
    other source 692.82
  psoriasiform, napkin 691.0
  recalcitrant pustular 694.8
  ringed 695.89
  skin (*see also* Dermatitis) 782.1
    creeping (meaning hookworm) 126.9
    due to
      chemical(s) NEC 692.4
        internal use 693.8
      drug — *see* Dermatitis, due to, drug
      prophylactic inoculation or vaccination against disease — *see* Dermatitis, due to, vaccine
      smallpox vaccination NEC — *see* Dermatitis, due to, vaccine
    erysipeloid 027.1
    feigned 698.4
    Hutchinson, summer 692.72
    Kaposi's, varicelliform 054.0
      vaccinia 999.0
    lichenoid, axilla 698.3
    polymorphous, due to light 692.72
    toxic NEC 695.0
    vesicular 709.8
  teeth, tooth
    accelerated 520.6
    delayed 520.6
    difficult 520.6
    disturbance of 520.6
    in abnormal sequence 520.6
    incomplete 520.6
    late 520.6
    natal 520.6
    neonatal 520.6
    obstructed 520.6
    partial 520.6
    persistent primary 520.6
    premature 520.6
    prenatal 520.6
  vesicular 709.8
Erysipelas (gangrenous) (infantile) (newborn) (phlegmonous) (suppurative) 035
  external ear 035 *[380.13]*
  puerperal, postpartum, childbirth 670.8 ☑
Erysipelatoid (Rosenbach's) 027.1
Erysipeloid (Rosenbach's) 027.1
Erythema, erythematous (generalized) 695.9
  ab igne — *see* Burn, by site, first degree
  annulare (centrifugum) (rheumaticum) 695.0
  arthriticum epidemicum 026.1
  brucellum (*see also* Brucellosis) 023.9
  bullosum 695.19
  caloricum — *see* Burn, by site, first degree
  chronicum migrans 088.81
  circinatum 695.19
  diaper 691.0
  due to
    chemical (contact) NEC 692.4
      internal 693.8
    drug (internal use) 693.0
      contact 692.3
  elevatum diutinum 695.89
  endemic 265.2
  epidemic, arthritic 026.1
  figuratum perstans 695.0
  gluteal 691.0

Erythema, erythematous — *continued*
  gyratum (perstans) (repens) 695.19
  heat — *see* Burn, by site, first degree
  ichthyosiforme congenitum 757.1
  induratum (primary) (scrofulosorum) (*see also* Tuberculosis) 017.1 ☑
    nontuberculous 695.2
  infantum febrile 057.8
  infectional NEC 695.9
  infectiosum 057.0
  inflammation NEC 695.9
  intertrigo 695.89
  iris 695.10
  lupus (discoid) (localized) (*see also* Lupus, erythematosus) 695.4
  marginatum 695.0
    rheumaticum — *see* Fever, rheumatic
  medicamentosum — *see* Dermatitis, due to, drug
  migrans 529.1
    chronicum 088.81
  multiforme 695.10
    bullosum 695.19
    conjunctiva 695.19
    exudativum (Hebra) 695.19
    major 695.12
    minor 695.11
    pemphigoides 694.5
  napkin 691.0
  neonatorum 778.8
  nodosum 695.2
    tuberculous (*see also* Tuberculosis) 017.1 ☑
  nummular, nummulare 695.19
  palmar 695.0
  palmaris hereditarium 695.0
  pernio 991.5
  perstans solare 692.72
  rash, newborn 778.8
  scarlatiniform (exfoliative) (recurrent) 695.0
  simplex marginatum 057.8
  solare (*see also* Sunburn) 692.71
  streptogenes 696.5
  toxic, toxicum NEC 695.0
    newborn 778.8
  tuberculous (primary) (*see also* Tuberculosis) 017.0 ☑
  venenatum 695.0
Erythematosus — *see* condition
Erythematous — *see* condition
Erythermalgia (primary) 443.82
Erythralgia 443.82
Erythrasma 039.0
Erythredema 985.0
  polyneuritica 985.0
  polyneuropathy 985.0
Erythremia (acute) (M9841/3) 207.0 ☑
  chronic (M9842/3) 207.1 ☑
  secondary 289.0
Erythroblastopenia (acquired) 284.89
  congenital 284.01
Erythroblastophthisis 284.01
Erythroblastosis (fetalis) (newborn) 773.2
  due to
    ABO
      antibodies 773.1
      incompatibility, maternal/fetal 773.1
      isoimmunization 773.1
    Rh
      antibodies 773.0
      incompatibility, maternal/fetal 773.0
      isoimmunization 773.0
Erythrocyanosis (crurum) 443.89
Erythrocythemia — *see* Erythremia
Erythrocytopenia 285.9
Erythrocytosis (megalosplenic)
  familial 289.6
  oval, hereditary (*see also* Elliptocytosis) 282.1
  secondary 289.0
  stress 289.0
Erythroderma — *see also* Erythema 695.9
  desquamativa (in infants) 695.89
  exfoliative 695.89
  ichthyosiform, congenital 757.1
  infantum 695.89

Erythroderma — *see also* Erythema — *continued*
  maculopapular 696.2
  neonatorum 778.8
  psoriaticum 696.1
  secondary 695.9
Erythrodysesthesia, palmar plantar (PPE) 693.0
Erythrogenesis imperfecta 284.09
Erythroleukemia (M9840/3) 207.0 ☑
Erythromelalgia 443.82
Erythromelia 701.8
Erythropenia 285.9
Erythrophagocytosis 289.9
Erythrophobia 300.23
Erythroplakia
  oral mucosa 528.79
  tongue 528.79
Erythroplasia (Queyrat) (M8080/2)
  specified site — *see* Neoplasm, skin, in situ
  unspecified site 233.5
Erythropoiesis, idiopathic ineffective 285.0
Escaped beats, heart 427.60
  postoperative 997.1
Escherichia coli (E. coli) — *see* Infection, Escherichia coli
Esoenteritis — *see* Enteritis
Esophagalgia 530.89
Esophagectasis 530.89
  due to cardiospasm 530.0
Esophagismus 530.5
Esophagitis (alkaline) (chemical) (chronic) (infectional) (necrotic) (peptic) (postoperative) (regurgitant) 530.10
  acute 530.12
  candidal 112.84
  eosinophilic 530.13
  reflux 530.11
  specified NEC 530.19
  tuberculous (*see also* Tuberculosis) 017.8 ☑
  ulcerative 530.19
Esophagocele 530.6
Esophagodynia 530.89
Esophagomalacia 530.89
Esophagoptosis 530.89
Esophagospasm 530.5
Esophagostenosis 530.3
Esophagostomiasis 127.7
Esophagostomy
  complication 530.87
    infection 530.86
    malfunctioning 530.87
    mechanical 530.87
Esophagotracheal — *see* condition
Esophagus — *see* condition
Esophoria 378.41
  convergence, excess 378.84
  divergence, insufficiency 378.85
Esotropia (nonaccommodative) 378.00
  accommodative 378.35
  alternating 378.05
    with
      A pattern 378.06
      specified noncomitancy NEC 378.08
      V pattern 378.07
      X pattern 378.08
      Y pattern 378.08
    intermittent 378.22
  intermittent 378.20
    alternating 378.22
    monocular 378.21
  monocular 378.01
    with
      A pattern 378.02
      specified noncomitancy NEC 378.04
      V pattern 378.03
      X pattern 378.04
      Y pattern 378.04
    intermittent 378.21
Espundia 085.5
Essential — *see* condition
Esterapenia 289.89
Esthesioneuroblastoma (M9522/3) 160.0
Esthesioneurocytoma (M9521/3) 160.0
Esthesioneuroepithelioma (M9523/3) 160.0
Esthiomene 099.1

Estivo-autumnal
  fever 084.0
  malaria 084.0
Estrangement V61.09
Estriasis 134.0
Ethanolaminuria 270.8
Ethanolism — *see also* Alcoholism 303.9 ☑
Ether dependence, dependency — *see also* Dependence 304.6 ☑
Etherism — *see also* Dependence 304.6 ☑
Ethmoid, ethmoidal — *see* condition
Ethmoiditis (chronic) (nonpurulent) (purulent) — *see also* Sinusitis, ethmoidal 473.2
  influenzal (*see also* Influenza) 487.1
  Woakes' 471.1
Ethylism — *see also* Alcoholism 303.9 ☑
Eulenburg's disease (congenital paramyotonia) 359.29
Eunuchism 257.2
Eunuchoidism 257.2
  hypogonadotropic 257.2
European blastomycosis 117.5
Eustachian — *see* condition
Euthyroidism 244.9
Euthyroid sick syndrome 790.94
Evaluation
  fetal lung maturity 659.8 ☑
  for suspected condition (*see also* Observation) V71.9
    abuse V71.81
    exposure
      anthrax V71.82
      biologic agent NEC V71.83
      SARS V71.83
    neglect V71.81
    newborn — *see* Observation, suspected, condition, newborn
    specified condition NEC V71.89
  mental health V70.2
    requested by authority V70.1
  nursing care V63.8
  social service V63.8
Evans' syndrome (thrombocytopenic purpura) 287.32
Event, apparent life threatening in newborn and infant (ALTE) 799.82
Eventration
  colon into chest — *see* Hernia, diaphragm
  diaphragm (congenital) 756.6
Eversion
  bladder 596.89
  cervix (uteri) 622.0
    with mention of cervicitis 616.0
  foot NEC 736.79
    congenital 755.67
  lacrimal punctum 375.51
  punctum lacrimale (postinfectional) (senile) 375.51
  ureter (meatus) 593.89
  urethra (meatus) 599.84
  uterus 618.1
    complicating delivery 665.2 ☑
      affecting fetus or newborn 763.89
    puerperal, postpartum 674.8 ☑
Evidence
  of malignancy
    cytologic
      without histologic confirmation
        anus 796.76
        cervix 795.06
        vagina 795.16
Evisceration
  birth injury 767.8
  bowel (congenital) — *see* Hernia, ventral
  congenital (*see also* Hernia, ventral) 553.29
  operative wound 998.32
  traumatic NEC 869.1
    eye 871.3
Evulsion — *see* Avulsion
Ewing's
  angioendothelioma (M9260/3) — *see* Neoplasm, bone, malignant
  sarcoma (M9260/3) — *see* Neoplasm, bone, malignant
  tumor (M9260/3) — *see* Neoplasm, bone, malignant

☑ **Additional Digit Required — Refer to the Tabular List for Digit Selection**

▼ **Subterms under main terms may continue to next column or page**

Exaggerated lumbosacral angle (with imping-
ing spine) 756.12
Examination (general) (routine) (of) (for) V70.9
allergy V72.7
annual V70.0
cardiovascular preoperative V72.81
cervical Papanicolaou smear V76.2
as a part of routine gynecological examination V72.31
to confirm findings of recent normal
smear following initial abnormal
smear V72.32
child care (routine) V20.2
clinical research investigation (normal control patient) (participant) V70.7
dental V72.2
developmental testing (child) (infant) V20.2
donor (potential) V70.8
ear V72.19
eye V72.0
following
accident (motor vehicle) V71.4
alleged rape or seduction (victim or culprit) V71.5
inflicted injury (victim or culprit) NEC
V71.6
rape or seduction, alleged (victim or
culprit) V71.5
treatment (for) V67.9
combined V67.6
fracture V67.4
involving high-risk medication NEC
V67.51
mental disorder V67.3
specified condition NEC V67.59
follow-up (routine) (following) V67.9
cancer chemotherapy V67.2
chemotherapy V67.2
disease NEC V67.59
high-risk medication NEC V67.51
injury NEC V67.59
population survey V70.6
postpartum V24.2
psychiatric V67.3
psychotherapy V67.3
radiotherapy V67.1
specified surgery NEC V67.09
surgery V67.00
vaginal pap smear V67.01
gynecological V72.31
for contraceptive maintenance V25.40
intrauterine device V25.42
pill V25.41
specified method NEC V25.49
health (of)
armed forces personnel V70.5
checkup V70.0
child, routine V20.2
defined subpopulation NEC V70.5
inhabitants of institutions V70.5
occupational V70.5
pre-employment screening V70.5
preschool children V70.5
for admission to school V70.3
prisoners V70.5
for entrance into prison V70.3
prostitutes V70.5
refugees V70.5
school children V70.5
students V70.5
hearing V72.19
following failed hearing screening
V72.11
infant
8 to 28 days old V20.32
over 28 days old, routine V20.2
under 8 days old V20.31
laboratory V72.60
ordered as part of a routine general
medical examination V72.62
pre-operative V72.63
pre-procedural V72.63
specified NEC V72.69
lactating mother V24.1
medical (for) (of) V70.9
administrative purpose NEC V70.3

Examination — continued
medical — continued
admission to
old age home V70.3
prison V70.3
school V70.3
adoption V70.3
armed forces personnel V70.5
at health care facility V70.0
camp V70.3
child, routine V20.2
clinical research (control) (normal comparison) (participant) V70.7
defined subpopulation NEC V70.5
donor (potential) V70.8
driving license V70.3
general V70.9
routine V70.0
specified reason NEC V70.8
immigration V70.3
inhabitants of institutions V70.5
insurance certification V70.3
marriage V70.3
medicolegal reasons V70.4
naturalization V70.3
occupational V70.5
population survey V70.6
pre-employment V70.5
preschool children V70.5
for admission to school V70.3
prison V70.3
prisoners V70.5
for entrance into prison V70.3
prostitutes V70.5
refugees V70.5
school children V70.5
specified reason NEC V70.8
sport competition V70.3
students V70.5
medicolegal reason V70.4
pelvic (annual) (periodic) V72.31
periodic (annual) (routine) V70.0
postpartum
immediately after delivery V24.0
routine follow-up V24.2
pregnancy (unconfirmed) (possible) V72.40
negative result V72.41
positive result V72.42
prenatal V22.1
first pregnancy V22.0
high-risk pregnancy V23.9
specified problem NEC V23.89
to determine fetal viability V23.87
preoperative V72.84
cardiovascular V72.81
respiratory V72.82
specified NEC V72.83
preprocedural V72.84
cardiovascular V72.81
general physical V72.83
respiratory V72.82
specified NEC V72.83
prior to chemotherapy V72.83
psychiatric V70.2
follow-up not needing further care V67.3
requested by authority V70.1
radiological NEC V72.5
respiratory preoperative V72.82
screening — see Screening
sensitization V72.7
skin V72.7
hypersensitivity V72.7
special V72.9
specified type or reason NEC V72.85
preoperative V72.83
specified NEC V72.83
teeth V72.2
vaginal Papanicolaou smear V76.47
following hysterectomy for malignant
condition V67.01
victim or culprit following
alleged rape or seduction V71.5
inflicted injury NEC V71.6
vision V72.0
well baby V20.2
Exanthem, exanthema — see also Rash 782.1

Exanthem, exanthema — see also Rash —
continued
Boston 048
epidemic, with meningitis 048
lichenoid psoriasiform 696.2
subitum 058.10
due to
human herpesvirus 6 058.11
human herpesvirus 7 058.12
viral, virus NEC 057.9
specified type NEC 057.8
Excess, excessive, excessively
alcohol level in blood 790.3
carbohydrate tissue, localized 278.1
carotene (dietary) 278.3
cold 991.9
specified effect NEC 991.8
convergence 378.84
crying 780.95
of
adolescent 780.95
adult 780.95
baby 780.92
child 780.95
infant (baby) 780.92
newborn 780.92
development, breast 611.1
diaphoresis (see also Hyperhidrosis) 780.8
distance, interarch 524.28
divergence 378.85
drinking (alcohol) NEC (see also Abuse,
drugs, nondependent) 305.0
continual (see also Alcoholism) 303.9
habitual (see also Alcoholism) 303.9
eating 783.6
eyelid fold (congenital) 743.62
fat 278.02
in heart (see also Degeneration, myocardial) 429.1
tissue, localized 278.1
foreskin 605
gas 787.3
gastrin 251.5
glucagon 251.4
heat (see also Heat) 992.9
horizontal
overjet 524.26
overlap 524.26
interarch distance 524.28
intermaxillary vertical dimension 524.37
interocclusal distance of teeth 524.37
large
colon 564.7
congenital 751.3
fetus or infant 766.0
with obstructed labor 660.1
affecting management of pregnancy
656.6
causing disproportion 653.5
newborn (weight of 4500 grams or
more) 766.0
organ or site, congenital NEC — see
Anomaly, specified type NEC
lid fold (congenital) 743.62
long
colon 751.5
organ or site, congenital NEC — see
Anomaly, specified type NEC
umbilical cord (entangled)
affecting fetus or newborn 762.5
in pregnancy or childbirth 663.3
with compression 663.2
menstruation 626.2
number of teeth 520.1
causing crowding 524.31
nutrients (dietary) NEC 783.6
potassium (K) 276.7
salivation (see also Ptyalism) 527.7
secretion (see also Hypersecretion)
milk 676.6
sputum 786.4
sweat (see also Hyperhidrosis) 780.8
short
organ or site, congenital NEC — see
Anomaly, specified type NEC

Excess, excessive, excessively —
continued
short — continued
umbilical cord
affecting fetus or newborn 762.6
in pregnancy or childbirth 663.4
skin NEC 701.9
eyelid 743.62
acquired 374.30
sodium (Na) 276.0
spacing of teeth 524.32
sputum 786.4
sweating (see also Hyperhidrosis) 780.8
tearing (ducts) (eye) (see also Epiphora)
375.20
thirst 783.5
due to deprivation of water 994.3
tissue in reconstructed breast 612.0
tuberosity 524.07
vitamin
A (dietary) 278.2
administered as drug (chronic) (prolonged excessive intake) 278.2
reaction to sudden overdose
963.5
D (dietary) 278.4
administered as drug (chronic) (prolonged excessive intake) 278.4
reaction to sudden overdose
963.5
weight 278.02
gain 783.1
of pregnancy 646.1
loss 783.21
Excitability, abnormal, under minor stress
309.29
Excitation
catatonic (see also Schizophrenia) 295.2
psychogenic 298.1
reactive (from emotional stress, psychological trauma) 298.1
Excitement
manic (see also Psychosis, affective) 296.0
recurrent episode 296.1
single episode 296.0
mental, reactive (from emotional stress,
psychological trauma) 298.1
state, reactive (from emotional stress, psychological trauma) 298.1
Excluded pupils 364.76
Excoriation (traumatic) — see also Injury, superficial, by site 919.8
neurotic 698.4
Excyclophoria 378.44
Excyclotropia 378.33
Exencephalus, exencephaly 742.0
Exercise
breathing V57.0
remedial NEC V57.1
therapeutic NEC V57.1
Exfoliation
skin
due to erythematous condition 695.50
involving (percent of body surface)
less than 10 percent 695.50
10-19 percent 695.51
20-29 percent 695.52
30-39 percent 695.53
40-49 percent 695.54
50-59 percent 695.55
60-69 percent 695.56
70-79 percent 695.57
80-89 percent 695.58
90 percent or more 695.59
teeth
due to systemic causes 525.0
Exfoliative — see also condition
dermatitis 695.89
Exhaustion, exhaustive (physical NEC) 780.79
battle (see also Reaction, stress, acute) 308.9
cardiac (see also Failure, heart) 428.9
delirium (see also Reaction, stress, acute)
308.9
due to
cold 991.8
excessive exertion 994.5

☑ Additional Digit Required — Refer to the Tabular List for Digit Selection   ▽ Subterms under main terms may continue to next column or page

110 — Volume 2   ▶◀ Revised Text   ● New Line   ▲ Revised Code   2015 ICD-9-CM

Exhaustion, exhaustive — *continued*
due to — *continued*
exposure 994.4
overexertion 994.5
fetus or newborn 779.89
heart (*see also* Failure, heart) 428.9
heat 992.5
due to
salt depletion 992.4
water depletion 992.3
manic (*see also* Psychosis, affective) 296.0 ☑
recurrent episode 296.1 ☑
single episode 296.0 ☑
maternal, complicating delivery 669.8 ☑
affecting fetus or newborn 763.89
mental 300.5
myocardium, myocardial (*see also* Failure, heart) 428.9
nervous 300.5
old age 797
postinfectional NEC 780.79
psychogenic 300.5
psychosis (*see also* Reaction, stress, acute) 308.9
senile 797
dementia 290.0
Exhibitionism (sexual) 302.4
Exomphalos 756.72
Exophoria 378.42
convergence, insufficiency 378.83
divergence, excess 378.85
Exophthalmic
cachexia 242.0 ☑
goiter 242.0 ☑
ophthalmoplegia 242.0 ☑ *[376.22]*
Exophthalmos 376.30
congenital 743.66
constant 376.31
endocrine NEC 259.9 *[376.22]*
hyperthyroidism 242.0 ☑ *[376.21]*
intermittent NEC 376.34
malignant 242.0 ☑ *[376.21]*
pulsating 376.35
endocrine NEC 259.9 *[376.22]*
thyrotoxic 242.0 ☑ *[376.21]*
Exostosis 726.91
cartilaginous (M9210/0) — *see* Neoplasm, bone, benign
congenital 756.4
ear canal, external 380.81
gonococcal 098.89
hip 726.5
intracranial 733.3
jaw (bone) 526.81
luxurians 728.11
multiple (cancellous) (congenital) (hereditary) 756.4
nasal bones 726.91
orbit, orbital 376.42
osteocartilaginous (M9210/0) — *see* Neoplasm, bone, benign
spine 721.8
with spondylosis — *see* Spondylosis
syphilitic 095.5
wrist 726.4
Exotropia 378.10
alternating 378.15
with
A pattern 378.16
specified noncomitancy NEC 378.18
V pattern 378.17
X pattern 378.18
Y pattern 378.18
intermittent 378.24
intermittent 378.20
alternating 378.24
monocular 378.23
monocular 378.11
with
A pattern 378.12
specified noncomitancy NEC 378.14
V pattern 378.13
X pattern 378.14
Y pattern 378.14
intermittent 378.23

Explanation of
investigation finding V65.4 ☑
medication V65.4 ☑
Exposure (suspected) 994.9
algae bloom V87.32
cold 991.9
specified effect NEC 991.8
effects of 994.9
exhaustion due to 994.4
implanted vaginal mesh
into vagina 629.32
through vaginal wall 629.32
to
AIDS virus V01.79
anthrax V01.81
aromatic
amines V87.11
dyes V87.19
arsenic V87.01
asbestos V15.84
benzene V87.12
body fluids (hazardous) V15.85
cholera V01.0
chromium compounds V87.09
communicable disease V01.9
specified type NEC V01.89
dyes V87.2
aromatic V87.19
Escherichia coli (E. coli) V01.83
German measles V01.4
gonorrhea V01.6
hazardous
aromatic compounds NEC V87.19
body fluids V15.85
chemicals V87.2
metals V87.09
substances V87.39
HIV V01.79
human immunodeficiency virus V01.79
lead V15.86
meningococcus V01.84
mold V87.31
nickel dust V87.09
parasitic disease V01.89
poliomyelitis V01.2
polycyclic aromatic hydrocarbons V87.19
potentially hazardous body fluids V15.85
rabies V01.5
rubella V01.4
SARS-associated coronavirus V01.82
smallpox V01.3
syphilis V01.6
tuberculosis V01.1
uranium V87.02
varicella V01.71
venereal disease V01.6
viral disease NEC V01.79
varicella V01.71
vaginal prosthetic materials NEC
into vagina 629.32
through vaginal wall 629.32
Exsanguination, fetal 772.0
Exstrophy
abdominal content 751.8
bladder (urinary) 753.5
Extensive — *see* condition
Extra — *see also* Accessory
rib 756.3
cervical 756.2
Extraction
with hook 763.89
breech NEC 669.6 ☑
affecting fetus or newborn 763.0
cataract postsurgical V45.61
manual NEC 669.8 ☑
affecting fetus or newborn 763.89
Extrasystole 427.60
atrial 427.61
postoperative 997.1
ventricular 427.69
Extrauterine gestation or pregnancy — *see* Pregnancy, ectopic
Extravasation
blood 459.0
lower extremity 459.0
chemotherapy, vesicant 999.81

Extravasation — *continued*
chyle into mesentery 457.8
pelvicalyceal 593.4
pyelosinus 593.4
urine 788.8
from ureter 788.8
vesicant
agent NEC 999.82
chemotherapy 999.81
Extremity — *see* condition
Extrophy — *see* Exstrophy
Extroversion
bladder 753.5
uterus 618.1
complicating delivery 665.2 ☑
affecting fetus or newborn 763.89
postpartal (old) 618.1
Extruded tooth 524.34
Extrusion
alveolus and teeth 524.75
breast implant (prosthetic) 996.54
device, implant, or graft — *see* Complications, mechanical
eye implant (ball) (globe) 996.59
intervertebral disc — *see* Displacement, intervertebral disc
lacrimal gland 375.43
mesh (reinforcing) 996.59
ocular lens implant 996.53
prosthetic device NEC — *see* Complications, mechanical
vitreous 379.26
Exudate, pleura — *see* Effusion, pleura
Exudates, retina 362.82
Exudative — *see* condition
Eye, eyeball, eyelid — *see* condition
Eyestrain 368.13
Eyeworm disease of Africa 125.2

F

Faber's anemia or syndrome (achlorhydric anemia) 280.9
Fabry's disease (angiokeratoma corporis diffusum) 272.7
Face, facial — *see* condition
Facet of cornea 371.44
Faciocephalalgia, autonomic — *see also* Neuropathy, peripheral, autonomic 337.9
Facioscapulohumeral myopathy 359.1
Factitious disorder, illness — *see* Illness, factitious
Factor
deficiency — *see* Deficiency, factor
psychic, associated with diseases classified elsewhere 316
risk — *see* Problem
V Leiden mutation 289.81
Fahr-Volhard disease (malignant nephrosclerosis) 403.00
Failure, failed
adenohypophyseal 253.2
attempted abortion (legal) (*see also* Abortion, failed) 638.9
bone marrow (anemia) 284.9
acquired (secondary) 284.89
congenital 284.09
idiopathic 284.9
cardiac (*see also* Failure, heart) 428.9
newborn 779.89
cardiorenal (chronic) 428.9
hypertensive (*see also* Hypertension, cardiorenal) 404.93
cardiorespiratory 799.1
specified during or due to a procedure 997.1
long-term effect of cardiac surgery 429.4
cardiovascular (chronic) 428.9
cerebrovascular 437.8
cervical dilatation in labor 661.0 ☑
affecting fetus or newborn 763.7
circulation, circulatory 799.89
fetus or newborn 779.89
peripheral 785.50
postoperative 998.00

Failure, failed — *continued*
compensation — *see* Disease, heart
congestive (*see also* Failure, heart) 428.0
conscious sedation, during procedure 995.24
coronary (*see also* Insufficiency, coronary) 411.89
dental implant 525.79
due to
infection 525.71
lack of attached gingiva 525.72
occlusal trauma (caused by poor prosthetic design) 525.72
parafunctional habits 525.72
periodontal infection (peri-implantitis) 525.72
poor oral hygiene 525.72
unintentional loading 525.71
endosseous NEC 525.79
mechanical 525.73
osseointegration 525.71
due to
complications of systemic disease 525.71
poor bone quality 525.71
premature loading 525.71
iatrogenic 525.71
prior to intentional prosthetic loading 525.71
post-osseointegration
biological 525.72
iatrogenic 525.72
due to complications of systemic disease 525.72
mechanical 525.73
pre-integration 525.71
pre-osseointegration 525.71
dental prosthesis causing loss of dental implant 525.73
dental restoration
marginal integrity 525.61
periodontal anatomical integrity 525.65
descent of head (at term) 652.5 ☑
affecting fetus or newborn 763.1
in labor 660.0 ☑
affecting fetus or newborn 763.1
device, implant, or graft — *see* Complications, mechanical
engagement of head NEC 652.5 ☑
in labor 660.0 ☑
affecting fetus or newborn 763.1
extrarenal 788.99
fetal head to enter pelvic brim 652.5 ☑
affecting fetus or newborn 763.1
in labor 660.0 ☑
affecting fetus or newborn 763.1
forceps NEC 660.7 ☑
affecting fetus or newborn 763.1
fusion (joint) 996.49
growth in childhood 783.43
heart (acute) (sudden) 428.9
with
abortion — *see* Abortion, by type, with specified complication NEC
acute pulmonary edema (*see also* Failure, ventricular, left) 428.1
with congestion (*see also* Failure, heart) 428.0
decompensation (*see also* Failure, heart) 428.0
dilation — *see* Disease, heart
ectopic pregnancy (*see also* categories 633.0–633.9) 639.8
molar pregnancy (*see also* categories 630–632) 639.8
arteriosclerotic 440.9
combined left-right sided 428.0
combined systolic and diastolic 428.40
acute 428.41
acute on chronic 428.43
chronic 428.42
compensated (*see also* Failure, heart) 428.0

☑ Additional Digit Required — Refer to the Tabular List for Digit Selection   ▽ Subterms under main terms may continue to next column or page

2015 ICD-9-CM   ▶◀ Revised Text   ● New Line   ▲ Revised Code   Volume 2 — 111

Exhaustion, exhaustive — Failure, failed

Failure, failed — *continued*
  heart — *continued*
    complicating
      abortion — *see* Abortion, by type, with specified complication NEC
      delivery (cesarean) (instrumental) 669.4 ☑
      ectopic pregnancy (*see also* categories 633.0–633.9) 639.8
      molar pregnancy (*see also* categories 630–632) 639.8
      obstetric anesthesia or sedation 668.1 ☑
      surgery 997.1
    congestive (compensated) (decompensated) (*see also* Failure, heart) 428.0
      with rheumatic fever (conditions classifiable to 390)
        active 391.8
        inactive or quiescent (with chorea) 398.91
      fetus or newborn 779.89
      hypertensive (*see also* Hypertension, heart) 402.91
        with renal disease (*see also* Hypertension, cardiorenal) 404.91
          with renal failure 404.93
        benign 402.11
        malignant 402.01
      rheumatic (chronic) (inactive) (with chorea) 398.91
        active or acute 391.8
          with chorea (Sydenham's) 392.0
    decompensated (*see also* Failure, heart) 428.0
    degenerative (*see also* Degeneration, myocardial) 429.1
    diastolic 428.30
      acute 428.31
      acute on chronic 428.33
      chronic 428.32
    due to presence of (cardiac) prosthesis 429.4
    fetus or newborn 779.89
    following
      abortion 639.8
      cardiac surgery 429.4
      ectopic or molar pregnancy 639.8
    high output NEC 428.9
    hypertensive (*see also* Hypertension, heart) 402.91
      with renal disease (*see also* Hypertension, cardiorenal) 404.91
        with renal failure 404.93
      benign 402.11
      malignant 402.01
    left (ventricular) (*see also* Failure, ventricular, left) 428.1
      with right-sided failure (see also Failure, heart) 428.0
    low output (syndrome) NEC 428.9
    organic — *see* Disease, heart
    postoperative (immediate) 997.1
      long term effect of cardiac surgery 429.4
    rheumatic (chronic) (congestive) (inactive) 398.91
    right (secondary to left heart failure, conditions classifiable to 428.1) (ventricular) (*see also* Failure, heart) 428.0
    senile 797
    specified during or due to a procedure 997.1
      long-term effect of cardiac surgery 429.4
    systolic 428.20
      acute 428.21
      acute on chronic 428.23
      chronic 428.22
    thyrotoxic (*see also* Thyrotoxicosis) 242.9 ☑ *[425.7]*

Failure, failed — *continued*
  heart — *continued*
    valvular — *see* Endocarditis
  hepatic 572.8
    acute 570
    due to a procedure 997.49
  hepatorenal 572.4
  hypertensive heart (*see also* Hypertension, heart) 402.91
    benign 402.11
    malignant 402.01
  induction (of labor) 659.1 ☑
    abortion (legal) (*see also* Abortion, failed) 638.9
    affecting fetus or newborn 763.89
    by oxytocic drugs 659.1 ☑
    instrumental 659.0 ☑
    mechanical 659.0 ☑
    medical 659.1 ☑
    surgical 659.0 ☑
  initial alveolar expansion, newborn 770.4
  involution, thymus (gland) 254.8
  kidney — *see* Failure, renal
  lactation 676.4 ☑
  Leydig's cell, adult 257.2
  liver 572.8
    acute 570
  medullary 799.89
  mitral — *see* Endocarditis, mitral
  moderate sedation, during procedure 995.24
  myocardium, myocardial (*see also* Failure, heart) 428.9
    chronic (*see also* Failure, heart) 428.0
    congestive (*see also* Failure, heart) 428.0
  ovarian (primary) 256.39
    iatrogenic 256.2
    postablative 256.2
    postirradiation 256.2
    postsurgical 256.2
  ovulation 628.0
  prerenal 788.99
  renal (kidney) 586
    with
      abortion — *see* Abortion, by type, with renal failure
      ectopic pregnancy (*see also* categories 633.0–633.9) 639.3
      edema (*see also* Nephrosis) 581.9
      hypertension (*see also* Hypertension, kidney) 403.91
      hypertensive heart disease (conditions classifiable to 402) 404.92
        with heart failure 404.93
        benign 404.12
          with heart failure 404.13
        malignant 404.02
          with heart failure 404.03
      molar pregnancy (*see also* categories 630–632) 639.3
      tubular necrosis (acute) 584.5
    acute 584.9
      with lesion of
        necrosis
          cortical (renal) 584.6
          medullary (renal) (papillary) 584.7
          tubular 584.5
        specified pathology NEC 584.8
    chronic 585.9
      hypertensive or with hypertension (*see also* Hypertension, kidney) 403.91
    due to a procedure 997.5
    following
      abortion 639.3
      crushing 958.5
      ectopic or molar pregnancy 639.3
      labor and delivery (acute) 669.3 ☑
    hypertensive (*see also* Hypertension, kidney) 403.91
    puerperal, postpartum 669.3 ☑
  respiration, respiratory 518.81
    acute 518.81
      following trauma and surgery 518.51

Failure, failed — *continued*
  respiration, respiratory — *continued*
    acute and chronic 518.84
      following trauma and surgery 518.53
    center 348.89
      newborn 770.84
    chronic 518.83
      following trauma and surgery or shock 518.51
      newborn 770.84
  rotation
    cecum 751.4
    colon 751.4
    intestine 751.4
    kidney 753.3
  sedation, during procedure
    conscious 995.24
    moderate 995.24
  segmentation (*see also* Fusion)
    fingers (*see also* Syndactylism, fingers) 755.11
    toes (*see also* Syndactylism, toes) 755.13
  seminiferous tubule, adult 257.2
  senile (general) 797
    with psychosis 290.20
  testis, primary (seminal) 257.2
  to progress 661.2 ☑
  to thrive
    adult 783.7
    child 783.41
    newborn 779.34
  transplant 996.80
    bone marrow 996.85
    organ (immune or nonimmune cause) 996.80
      bone marrow 996.85
      heart 996.83
      intestines 996.87
      kidney 996.81
      liver 996.82
      lung 996.84
      pancreas 996.86
      specified NEC 996.89
    skin 996.52
      artificial 996.55
      decellularized allodermis 996.55
      temporary allograft or pigskin graft — omit code
    stem cell(s) 996.88
      from
        peripheral blood 996.88
        umbilical cord 996.88
  trial of labor NEC 660.6 ☑
    affecting fetus or newborn 763.1
  tubal ligation 998.89
  urinary 586
  vacuum extraction
    abortion — *see* Abortion, failed
    delivery NEC 660.7 ☑
      affecting fetus or newborn 763.1
  vasectomy 998.89
  ventouse NEC 660.7 ☑
    affecting fetus or newborn 763.1
  ventricular (*see also* Failure, heart) 428.9
    left 428.1
      with rheumatic fever (conditions classifiable to 390)
        active 391.8
          with chorea 392.0
        inactive or quiescent (with chorea) 398.91
      hypertensive (*see also* Hypertension, heart) 402.91
        benign 402.11
        malignant 402.01
      rheumatic (chronic) (inactive) (with chorea) 398.91
        active or acute 391.8
          with chorea 392.0
    right (*see also* Failure, heart) 428.0
  vital centers, fetus or newborn 779.89
  weight gain in childhood 783.41
Fainting (fit) (spell) 780.2
Falciform hymen 752.49
Fallen arches 734
Falling, any organ or part — *see* Prolapse

Fall, maternal, affecting fetus or newborn 760.5
Fallopian
  insufflation
    fertility testing V26.21
    following sterilization reversal V26.22
  tube — *see* condition
Fallot's
  pentalogy 745.2
  tetrad or tetralogy 745.2
  triad or trilogy 746.09
Fallout, radioactive (adverse effect) NEC 990
False — *see also* condition
  bundle branch block 426.50
  bursa 727.89
  croup 478.75
  joint 733.82
  labor (pains) 644.1 ☑
  opening, urinary, male 752.69
  passage, urethra (prostatic) 599.4
  positive
    serological test for syphilis 795.6
    Wassermann reaction 795.6
  pregnancy 300.11
Family, familial — *see also* condition
  affected by
    family member
      currently on deployment (military) V61.01
      returned from deployment (military) (current or past conflict) V61.02
  disruption (*see also* Disruption, family) V61.09
  estrangement V61.09
  hemophagocytic
    lymphohistiocytosis 288.4
    reticulosis 288.4
  Li-Fraumeni (syndrome) V84.01
  planning advice V25.09
    natural
      procreative V26.41
      to avoid pregnancy V25.04
  problem V61.9
    specified circumstance NEC V61.8
  retinoblastoma (syndrome) 190.5
Famine 994.2
  edema 262
Fanconi's anemia (congenital pancytopenia) 284.09
Fanconi (-de Toni) (-Debré) syndrome (cystinosis) 270.0
Farber (-Uzman) syndrome or disease (disseminated lipogranulomatosis) 272.8
Farcin 024
Farcy 024
Farmers'
  lung 495.0
  skin 692.74
Farsightedness 367.0
Fascia — *see* condition
Fasciculation 781.0
Fasciculitis optica 377.32
Fasciitis 729.4
  eosinophilic 728.89
  necrotizing 728.86
  nodular 728.79
  perirenal 593.4
  plantar 728.71
  pseudosarcomatous 728.79
  traumatic (old) NEC 728.79
    current — *see* Sprain, by site
Fasciola hepatica infestation 121.3
Fascioliasis 121.3
Fasciolopsiasis (small intestine) 121.4
Fasciolopsis (small intestine) 121.4
Fast pulse 785.0
Fat
  embolism (cerebral) (pulmonary) (systemic) 958.1
    with
      abortion — *see* Abortion, by type, with embolism
      ectopic pregnancy (*see also* categories 633.0–633.9) 639.6

☑ **Additional Digit Required** — Refer to the Tabular List for Digit Selection

▽ **Subterms under main terms may continue to next column or page**

Fat — *continued*
  embolism — *continued*
    with — *continued*
      molar pregnancy (*see also* categories 630–632) 639.6
      complicating delivery or puerperium 673.8 ☑
      following
        abortion 639.6
        ectopic or molar pregnancy 639.6
      in pregnancy, childbirth, or the puerperium 673.8 ☑
  excessive 278.02
    in heart (*see also* Degeneration, myocardial) 429.1
  general 278.02
  hernia, herniation 729.30
    eyelid 374.34
    knee 729.31
    orbit 374.34
    retro-orbital 374.34
    retropatellar 729.31
    specified site NEC 729.39
  indigestion 579.8
  in stool 792.1
  localized (pad) 278.1
    heart (*see also* Degeneration, myocardial) 429.1
    knee 729.31
    retropatellar 729.31
  necrosis (*see also* Fatty, degeneration)
    breast (aseptic) (segmental) 611.3
    mesentery 567.82
    omentum 567.82
    peritoneum 567.82
  pad 278.1
Fatal familial insomnia (FFI) 046.72
Fatal syncope 798.1
Fatigue 780.79
  auditory deafness (*see also* Deafness) 389.9
  chronic, syndrome 780.71
  combat (*see also* Reaction, stress, acute) 308.9
  during pregnancy 646.8 ☑
  general 780.79
    psychogenic 300.5
  heat (transient) 992.6
  muscle 729.89
  myocardium (*see also* Failure, heart) 428.9
  nervous 300.5
  neurosis 300.5
  operational 300.89
  postural 729.89
  posture 729.89
  psychogenic (general) 300.5
  senile 797
  syndrome NEC 300.5
    chronic 780.71
  undue 780.79
  voice 784.49
Fatness 278.02
Fatty — *see also* condition
  apron 278.1
  degeneration (diffuse) (general) NEC 272.8
    localized — *see* Degeneration, by site, fatty
    placenta — *see* Placenta, abnormal
  heart (enlarged) (*see also* Degeneration, myocardial) 429.1
  infiltration (diffuse) (general) (*see also* Degeneration, by site, fatty) 272.8
    heart (enlarged) (*see also* Degeneration, myocardial) 429.1
  liver 571.8
    alcoholic 571.0
  necrosis — *see* Degeneration, fatty
  phanerosis 272.8
Fauces — *see* condition
Fauchard's disease (periodontitis) 523.40
Faucitis 478.29
Faulty — *see also* condition
  position of teeth 524.30
Favism (anemia) 282.2
Favre-Racouchot disease (elastoidosis cutanea nodularis) 701.8
Favus 110.9

Favus — *continued*
  beard 110.0
  capitis 110.0
  corporis 110.5
  eyelid 110.8
  foot 110.4
  hand 110.2
  scalp 110.0
  specified site NEC 110.8
Feared complaint unfounded V65.5
Fear, fearfulness (complex) (reaction) 300.20
  child 313.0
  of
    animals 300.29
    closed spaces 300.29
    crowds 300.29
    eating in public 300.23
    heights 300.29
    open spaces 300.22
      with panic attacks 300.21
    public speaking 300.23
    streets 300.22
      with panic attacks 300.21
    travel 300.22
      with panic attacks 300.21
    washing in public 300.23
  transient 308.0
Febricula (continued) (simple) — *see also* Pyrexia 780.60
Febrile — *see also* Pyrexia 780.60
  convulsion (simple) 780.31
    complex 780.32
  nonhemolytic transfusion reaction (FNHTR) 780.66
  seizure (simple) 780.31
    atypical 780.32
    complex 780.32
    complicated 780.32
Febris — *see also* Fever 780.60
  aestiva (*see also* Fever, hay) 477.9
  flava (*see also* Fever, yellow) 060.9
  melitensis 023.0
  pestis (*see also* Plague) 020.9
  puerperalis 672.0 ☑
  recurrens (*see also* Fever, relapsing) 087.9
    pediculo vestimenti 087.0
  rubra 034.1
  typhoidea 002.0
  typhosa 002.0
Fecal — *see* condition
Fecalith (impaction) 560.32
  with hernia (*see also* Hernia, by site, with obstruction)
    gangrenous — *see* Hernia, by site, with gangrene
  appendix 543.9
  congenital 777.1
Fede's disease 529.0
Feeble-minded 317
Feeble rapid pulse due to shock following injury 958.4
Feeding
  faulty (elderly) (infant) 783.3
    newborn 779.31
  formula check V20.2
  improper (elderly) (infant) 783.3
    newborn 779.31
  problem (elderly) (infant) 783.3
    newborn 779.31
    nonorganic origin 307.59
Feeling of foreign body in throat 784.99
Feer's disease 985.0
Feet — *see* condition
Feigned illness V65.2
Feil-Klippel syndrome (brevicollis) 756.16
Feinmesser's (hidrotic) **ectodermal dysplasia** 757.31
Felix's disease (juvenile osteochondrosis, hip) 732.1
Felon (any digit) (with lymphangitis) 681.01
  herpetic 054.6
Felty's syndrome (rheumatoid arthritis with splenomegaly and leukopenia) 714.1
Feminism in boys 302.6
Feminization, testicular 259.51
  with pseudohermaphroditism, male 259.51

Femoral hernia — *see* Hernia, femoral
Femora vara 736.32
Femur, femoral — *see* condition
Fenestrata placenta — *see* Placenta, abnormal
Fenestration, fenestrated — *see also* Imperfect, closure
  aorta-pulmonary 745.0
  aorticopulmonary 745.0
  aortopulmonary 745.0
  cusps, heart valve NEC 746.89
    pulmonary 746.09
  hymen 752.49
  pulmonic cusps 746.09
Fenwick's disease 537.89
Fermentation (gastric) (gastrointestinal) (stomach) 536.8
  intestine 564.89
    psychogenic 306.4
  psychogenic 306.4
Fernell's disease (aortic aneurysm) 441.9
Fertile eunuch syndrome 257.2
Fertility, meaning multiparity — *see* Multiparity
Fetal
  alcohol syndrome 760.71
  anemia 678.0 ☑
  thrombocytopenia 678.0 ☑
  twin to twin transfusion 678.0 ☑
Fetalis uterus 752.39
Fetid
  breath 784.99
  sweat 705.89
Fetishism 302.81
  transvestic 302.3
Fetomaternal hemorrhage
  affecting management of pregnancy 656.0 ☑
  fetus or newborn 772.0
Fetus, fetal — *see also* condition
  papyraceous 779.89
  type lung tissue 770.4
Fever 780.60
  with chills 780.60
    in malarial regions (*see also* Malaria) 084.6
  abortus NEC 023.9
  aden 061
  African tick-borne 087.1
  American
    mountain tick 066.1
    spotted 082.0
  and ague (*see also* Malaria) 084.6
  aphthous 078.4
  arbovirus hemorrhagic 065.9
  Assam 085.0
  Australian A or Q 083.0
  Bangkok hemorrhagic 065.4
  biliary, Charcôt's intermittent — *see* Choledocholithiasis
  bilious, hemoglobinuric 084.8
  blackwater 084.8
  blister 054.9
  Bonvale Dam 780.79
  boutonneuse 082.1
  brain 323.9
    late effect — *see* category 326
  breakbone 061
  Bullis 082.8
  Bunyamwera 066.3
  Burdwan 085.0
  Bwamba (encephalitis) 066.3
  Cameroon (*see also* Malaria) 084.6
  Canton 081.9
  catarrhal (acute) 460
    chronic 472.0
  cat-scratch 078.3
  cerebral 323.9
    late effect — *see* category 326
  cerebrospinal (meningococcal) (*see also* Meningitis, cerebrospinal) 036.0
  Chagres 084.0
  Chandipura 066.8
  changuinola 066.0
  Charcôt's (biliary) (hepatic) (intermittent) — *see* Choledocholithiasis
  Chikungunya (viral) 066.3

Fever — *continued*
  Chikungunya — *continued*
    hemorrhagic 065.4
  childbed 670.8 ☑
  Chitral 066.0
  Colombo (*see also* Fever, paratyphoid) 002.9
  Colorado tick (virus) 066.1
  congestive
    malarial (*see also* Malaria) 084.6
    remittent (*see also* Malaria) 084.6
  Congo virus 065.0
  continued 780.60
    malarial 084.0
  Corsican (*see also* Malaria) 084.6
  Crimean hemorrhagic 065.0
  Cyprus (*see also* Brucellosis) 023.9
  dandy 061
  deer fly (*see also* Tularemia) 021.9
  dehydration, newborn 778.4
  dengue (virus) 061
    hemorrhagic 065.4
  desert 114.0
  due to heat 992.0
  Dumdum 085.0
  enteric 002.0
  ephemeral (of unknown origin) (*see also* Pyrexia) 780.60
  epidemic, hemorrhagic of the Far East 065.0
  erysipelatous (*see also* Erysipelas) 035
  estivo-autumnal (malarial) 084.0
  etiocholanolone 277.31
  famine (*see also* Fever, relapsing)
    meaning typhus — *see* Typhus
  Far Eastern hemorrhagic 065.0
  five day 083.1
  Fort Bragg 100.89
  gastroenteric 002.0
  gastromalarial (*see also* Malaria) 084.6
  Gibraltar (*see also* Brucellosis) 023.9
  glandular 075
  Guama (viral) 066.3
  Haverhill 026.1
  hay (allergic) (with rhinitis) 477.9
    with
      asthma (bronchial) (*see also* Asthma) 493.0 ☑
    due to
      dander, animal (cat) (dog) 477.2
      dust 477.8
      fowl 477.8
      hair, animal (cat) (dog) 477.2
      pollen, any plant or tree 477.0
      specified allergen other than pollen 477.8
  heat (effects) 992.0
  hematuric, bilious 084.8
  hemoglobinuric (malarial) 084.8
    bilious 084.8
  hemorrhagic (arthropod-borne) NEC 065.9
    with renal syndrome 078.6
    arenaviral 078.7
    Argentine 078.7
    Bangkok 065.4
    Bolivian 078.7
    Central Asian 065.0
    chikungunya 065.4
    Crimean 065.0
    dengue (virus) 065.4
    Ebola 065.8
    epidemic 078.6
      of Far East 065.0
    Far Eastern 065.0
    Junin virus 078.7
    Korean 078.6
    Kyasanur forest 065.2
    Machupo virus 078.7
    mite-borne NEC 065.8
    mosquito-borne 065.4
    Omsk 065.1
    Philippine 065.4
    Russian (Yaroslav) 078.6
    Singapore 065.4
    Southeast Asia 065.4
    Thailand 065.4
    tick-borne NEC 065.3
  hepatic (*see also* Cholecystitis) 575.8

☑ **Additional Digit Required** — Refer to the Tabular List for Digit Selection   ▽ **Subterms under main terms may continue to next column or page**

2015 ICD-9-CM   ►◄ **Revised Text**   ● **New Line**   ▲ **Revised Code**   **Volume 2 — 113**

Fat — Fever

Fever — continued
  hepatic (see also Cholecystitis) — continued
    intermittent (Charcôt's) — see Choledocholithiasis
  herpetic (see also Herpes) 054.9
  Hyalomma tick 065.0
  icterohemorrhagic 100.0
  inanition 780.60
    newborn 778.4
  in conditions classified elsewhere 780.61
  infective NEC 136.9
  intermittent (bilious) (see also Malaria) 084.6
    hepatic (Charcôt) — see Choledocholithiasis
    of unknown origin (see also Pyrexia) 780.60
    pernicious 084.0
  iodide
    correct substance properly administered 780.60
    overdose or wrong substance given or taken 975.5
  Japanese river 081.2
  jungle yellow 060.0
  Junin virus, hemorrhagic 078.7
  Katayama 120.2
  Kedani 081.2
  Kenya 082.1
  Korean hemorrhagic 078.6
  Lassa 078.89
  Lone Star 082.8
  lung — see Pneumonia
  Machupo virus, hemorrhagic 078.7
  malaria, malarial (see also Malaria) 084.6
  Malta (see also Brucellosis) 023.9
  Marseilles 082.1
  marsh (see also Malaria) 084.6
  Mayaro (viral) 066.3
  Mediterranean (see also Brucellosis) 023.9
    familial 277.31
    tick 082.1
  meningeal — see Meningitis
  metal fumes NEC 985.8
  Meuse 083.1
  Mexican — see Typhus, Mexican
  Mianeh 087.1
  miasmatic (see also Malaria) 084.6
  miliary 078.2
  milk, female 672.0 ☑
  mill 504
  mite-borne hemorrhagic 065.8
  Monday 504
  mosquito-borne NEC 066.3
    hemorrhagic NEC 065.4
  mountain 066.1
    meaning
      Rocky Mountain spotted 082.0
      undulant fever (see also Brucellosis) 023.9
    tick (American) 066.1
  Mucambo (viral) 066.3
  mud 100.89
  Neapolitan (see also Brucellosis) 023.9
  neutropenic 288.00
  newborn (environmentally-induced) 778.4
  nine-mile 083.0
  nonexanthematous tick 066.1
  North Asian tick-borne typhus 082.2
  Omsk hemorrhagic 065.1
  O'nyong-nyong (viral) 066.3
  Oropouche (viral) 066.3
  Oroya 088.0
  paludal (see also Malaria) 084.6
  Panama 084.0
  pappataci 066.0
  paratyphoid 002.9
    A 002.1
    B (Schottmüller's) 002.2
    C (Hirschfeld) 002.3
  parrot 073.9
  periodic 277.31
  pernicious, acute 084.0
  persistent (of unknown origin) (see also Pyrexia) 780.60
  petechial 036.0

Fever — continued
  pharyngoconjunctival 077.2
    adenoviral type 3 077.2
  Philippine hemorrhagic 065.4
  phlebotomus 066.0
  Piry 066.8
  Pixuna (viral) 066.3
  Plasmodium ovale 084.3
  pleural (see also Pleurisy) 511.0
  pneumonic — see Pneumonia
  polymer fume 987.8
  postimmunization 780.63
  postoperative 780.62
    due to infection 998.59
  posttransfusion 780.66
  postvaccination 780.63
  pretibial 100.89
  puerperal, postpartum 672.0 ☑
  putrid — see Septicemia
  pyemic — see Septicemia
  Q 083.0
    with pneumonia 083.0 [484.8]
  quadrilateral 083.0
  quartan (malaria) 084.2
  Queensland (coastal) 083.0
    seven-day 100.89
  Quintan (A) 083.1
  quotidian 084.0
  rabbit (see also Tularemia) 021.9
  rat-bite 026.9
    due to
      Spirillum minor or minus 026.0
      Spirochaeta morsus muris 026.0
      Streptobacillus moniliformis 026.1
  recurrent — see Fever, relapsing
  relapsing 087.9
    Carter's (Asiatic) 087.0
    Dutton's (West African) 087.1
    Koch's 087.9
    louse-borne (epidemic) 087.0
    Novy's (American) 087.1
    Obermeyer's (European) 087.0
    spirillum NEC 087.9
    tick-borne (endemic) 087.1
  remittent (bilious) (congestive) (gastric) (see also Malaria) 084.6
  rheumatic (active) (acute) (chronic) (subacute) 390
    with heart involvement 391.9
      carditis 391.9
      endocarditis (aortic) (mitral) (pulmonary) (tricuspid) 391.1
      multiple sites 391.8
      myocarditis 391.2
      pancarditis, acute 391.8
      pericarditis 391.0
      specified type NEC 391.8
      valvulitis 391.1
    cardiac hypertrophy 398.99
    inactive or quiescent
      with cardiac hypertrophy 398.99
        carditis 398.90
      endocarditis 397.9
        aortic (valve) 395.9
          with mitral (valve) disease 396.9
        mitral (valve) 394.9
          with aortic (valve) disease 396.9
        pulmonary (valve) 397.1
        tricuspid (valve) 397.0
      heart conditions (classifiable to 429.3, 429.6, 429.9) 398.99
      failure (congestive) (conditions classifiable to 428.0, 428.9) 398.91
      left ventricular failure (conditions classifiable to 428.1) 398.91
      myocardial degeneration (conditions classifiable to 429.1) 398.0
      myocarditis (conditions classifiable to 429.0) 398.0
      pancarditis 398.99
      pericarditis 393
  Rift Valley (viral) 066.3
  Rocky Mountain spotted 082.0

Fever — continued
  rose 477.0
  Ross river (viral) 066.3
  Russian hemorrhagic 078.6
  sandfly 066.0
  San Joaquin (valley) 114.0
  São Paulo 082.0
  scarlet 034.1
  septic — see Septicemia
  seven-day 061
    Japan 100.89
    Queensland 100.89
  shin bone 083.1
  Singapore hemorrhagic 065.4
  solar 061
  sore 054.9
  South African tick-bite 087.1
  Southeast Asia hemorrhagic 065.4
  spinal — see Meningitis
  spirillary 026.0
  splenic (see also Anthrax) 022.9
  spotted (Rocky Mountain) 082.0
    American 082.0
    Brazilian 082.0
    Colombian 082.0
    meaning
      cerebrospinal meningitis 036.0
      typhus 082.9
  spring 309.23
  steroid
    correct substance properly administered 780.60
    overdose or wrong substance given or taken 962.0
  streptobacillary 026.1
  subtertian 084.0
  Sumatran mite 081.2
  sun 061
  swamp 100.89
  sweating 078.2
  swine 003.8
  sylvatic yellow 060.0
  Tahyna 062.5
  tertian — see Malaria, tertian
  Thailand hemorrhagic 065.4
  thermic 992.0
  three day 066.0
    with Coxsackie exanthem 074.8
  tick
    American mountain 066.1
    Colorado 066.1
    Kemerovo 066.1
    Mediterranean 082.1
    mountain 066.1
    nonexanthematous 066.1
    Quaranfil 066.1
  tick-bite NEC 066.1
  tick-borne NEC 066.1
    hemorrhagic NEC 065.3
  transitory of newborn 778.4
  trench 083.1
  tsutsugamushi 081.2
  typhogastric 002.0
  typhoid (abortive) (ambulant) (any site) (hemorrhagic) (infection) (intermittent) (malignant) (rheumatic) 002.0
  typhomalarial (see also Malaria) 084.6
  typhus — see Typhus
  undulant (see also Brucellosis) 023.9
  unknown origin (see also Pyrexia) 780.60
  uremic — see Uremia
  uveoparotid 135
  valley (Coccidioidomycosis) 114.0
  Venezuelan equine 066.2
  Volhynian 083.1
  Wesselsbron (viral) 066.3
  West
    African 084.8
    Nile (viral) 066.40
      with
        cranial nerve disorders 066.42
        encephalitis 066.41
        optic neuritis 066.42
        other complications 066.49
        other neurologic manifestations 066.42

Fever — continued
  West — continued
    Nile — continued
      with — continued
        polyradiculitis 066.42
  Whitmore's 025
  Wolhynian 083.1
  worm 128.9
  Yaroslav hemorrhagic 078.6
  yellow 060.9
    jungle 060.0
    sylvatic 060.0
    urban 060.1
    vaccination, prophylactic (against) V04.4
  Zika (viral) 066.3

Fibrillation
  atrial (established) (paroxysmal) 427.31
  auricular (atrial) (established) 427.31
  cardiac (ventricular) 427.41
  coronary (see also Infarct, myocardium) 410.9 ☑
  heart (ventricular) 427.41
  muscular 728.9
  postoperative 997.1
  ventricular 427.41

Fibrin
  ball or bodies, pleural (sac) 511.0
  chamber, anterior (eye) (gelatinous exudate) 364.04

Fibrinogenolysis (hemorrhagic) — see Fibrinolysis

Fibrinogenopenia (congenital) (hereditary) — see also Defect, coagulation 286.3
  acquired 286.6

Fibrinolysis (acquired) (hemorrhagic) (pathologic) 286.6
  with
    abortion — see Abortion, by type, with hemorrhage, delayed or excessive
    ectopic pregnancy (see also categories 633.0–633.9) 639.1
    molar pregnancy (see also categories 630–632) 639.1
  antepartum or intrapartum 641.3 ☑
    affecting fetus or newborn 762.1
  following
    abortion 639.1
    ectopic or molar pregnancy 639.1
  newborn, transient 776.2
  postpartum 666.3 ☑

Fibrinopenia (hereditary) — see also Defect, coagulation 286.3
  acquired 286.6

Fibrinopurulent — see condition

Fibrinous — see condition

Fibroadenoma (M9010/0)
  cellular intracanalicular (M9020/0) 217
  giant (intracanalicular) (M9020/0) 217
  intracanalicular (M9011/0)
    cellular (M9020/0) 217
    giant (M9020/0) 217
    specified site — see Neoplasm, by site, benign
    unspecified site 217
  juvenile (M9030/0) 217
  pericanicular (M9012/0)
    specified site — see Neoplasm, by site, benign
    unspecified site 217
  phyllodes (M9020/0) 217
  prostate 600.20
    with
      other lower urinary tract symptoms (LUTS) 600.21
      urinary
        obstruction 600.21
        retention 600.21
  specified site — see Neoplasm, by site, benign
  unspecified site 217

Fibroadenosis, breast (chronic) (cystic) (diffuse) (periodic) (segmental) 610.2

Fibroangioma (M9160/0) — see also Neoplasm, by site, benign

☑ Additional Digit Required — Refer to the Tabular List for Digit Selection   ▽ **Subterms under main terms may continue to next column or page**

114 — Volume 2   ▶◀ Revised Text   ● New Line   ▲ Revised Code   2015 ICD-9-CM

Fibroangioma — *see also* Neoplasm, by site, benign — *continued*
> juvenile (M9160/0)
>> specified site — *see* Neoplasm, by site, benign
>> unspecified site 210.7

Fibrocellulitis progressiva ossificans 728.11

Fibrochondrosarcoma (M9220/3) — *see* Neoplasm, cartilage, malignant

Fibrocystic
> disease 277.00
>> bone NEC 733.29
>> breast 610.1
>> jaw 526.2
>> kidney (congenital) 753.19
>> liver 751.62
>> lung 518.89
>>> congenital 748.4
>> pancreas 277.00
> kidney (congenital) 753.19

Fibrodysplasia ossificans multiplex (progressiva) 728.11

Fibroelastosis (cordis) (endocardial) (endomyocardial) 425.3

Fibroid (tumor) (M8890/0) — *see also* Neoplasm, connective tissue, benign
> disease, lung (chronic) (*see also* Fibrosis, lung) 515
> heart (disease) (*see also* Myocarditis) 429.0
> induration, lung (chronic) (*see also* Fibrosis, lung) 515
> in pregnancy or childbirth 654.1 ☑
>> affecting fetus or newborn 763.89
>> causing obstructed labor 660.2 ☑
>>> affecting fetus or newborn 763.1
> liver — *see* Cirrhosis, liver
> lung (*see also* Fibrosis, lung) 515
> pneumonia (chronic) (*see also* Fibrosis, lung) 515
> uterus (M8890/0) (*see also* Leiomyoma, uterus) 218.9

Fibrolipoma (M8851/0) — *see also* Lipoma, by site 214.9

Fibroliposarcoma (M8850/3) — *see* Neoplasm, connective tissue, malignant

Fibroma (M8810/0) — *see also* Neoplasm, connective tissue, benign
> ameloblastic (M9330/0) 213.1
>> upper jaw (bone) 213.0
> bone (nonossifying) 733.99
>> ossifying (M9262/0) — *see* Neoplasm, bone, benign
> cementifying (M9274/0) — *see* Neoplasm, bone, benign
> chondromyxoid (M9241/0) — *see* Neoplasm, bone, benign
> desmoplastic (M8823/1) — *see* Neoplasm, connective tissue, uncertain behavior
> facial (M8813/0) — *see* Neoplasm, connective tissue, benign
> invasive (M8821/1) — *see* Neoplasm, connective tissue, uncertain behavior
> molle (M8851/0) (*see also* Lipoma, by site) 214.9
> myxoid (M8811/0) — *see* Neoplasm, connective tissue, benign
> nasopharynx, nasopharyngeal (juvenile) (M9160/0) 210.7
> nonosteogenic (nonossifying) — *see* Dysplasia, fibrous
> odontogenic (M9321/0) 213.1
>> upper jaw (bone) 213.0
> ossifying (M9262/0) — *see* Neoplasm, bone, benign
> periosteal (M8812/0) — *see* Neoplasm, bone, benign
> prostate 600.20
>> with
>>> other lower urinary tract symptoms (LUTS) 600.21
>>> urinary
>>>> obstruction 600.21
>>>> retention 600.21
> soft (M8851/0) (*see also* Lipoma, by site) 214.9

Fibromatosis 728.79

Fibromatosis — *continued*
> abdominal (M8822/1) — *see* Neoplasm, connective tissue, uncertain behavior
> aggressive (M8821/1) — *see* Neoplasm, connective tissue, uncertain behavior
> congenital generalized (CGF) 759.89
> Dupuytren's 728.6
> gingival 523.8
> plantar fascia 728.71
> proliferative 728.79
> pseudosarcomatous (proliferative) (subcutaneous) 728.79
> subcutaneous pseudosarcomatous (proliferative) 728.79

Fibromyalgia 729.1

Fibromyoma (M8890/0) — *see also* Neoplasm, connective tissue, benign
> uterus (corpus) (*see also* Leiomyoma, uterus) 218.9
>> in pregnancy or childbirth 654.1 ☑
>>> affecting fetus or newborn 763.89
>>> causing obstructed labor 660.2 ☑
>>>> affecting fetus or newborn 763.1

Fibromyositis — *see also* Myositis 729.1
> scapulohumeral 726.2

Fibromyxolipoma (M8852/0) — *see also* Lipoma, by site 214.9

Fibromyxoma (M8811/0) — *see* Neoplasm, connective tissue, benign

Fibromyxosarcoma (M8811/3) — *see* Neoplasm, connective tissue, malignant

Fibro-odontoma, ameloblastic (M9290/0) 213.1
> upper jaw (bone) 213.0

Fibro-osteoma (M9262/0) — *see* Neoplasm, bone, benign

Fibroplasia, retrolental (*see also* Retinopathy of prematurity) 362.21

Fibropurulent — *see* condition

Fibrosarcoma (M8810/3) — *see also* Neoplasm, connective tissue, malignant
> ameloblastic (M9330/3) 170.1
>> upper jaw (bone) 170.0
> congenital (M8814/3) — *see* Neoplasm, connective tissue, malignant
> fascial (M8813/3) — *see* Neoplasm, connective tissue, malignant
> infantile (M8814/3) — *see* Neoplasm, connective tissue, malignant
> odontogenic (M9330/3) 170.1
>> upper jaw (bone) 170.0
> periosteal (M8812/3) — *see* Neoplasm, bone, malignant

Fibrosclerosis
> breast 610.3
> corpora cavernosa (penis) 607.89
> familial multifocal NEC 710.8
> multifocal (idiopathic) NEC 710.8
> penis (corpora cavernosa) 607.89

Fibrosis, fibrotic
> adrenal (gland) 255.8
> alveolar (diffuse) 516.31
> amnion 658.8 ☑
> anal papillae 569.49
> anus 569.49
> appendix, appendiceal, noninflammatory 543.9
> arteriocapillary — *see* Arteriosclerosis
> bauxite (of lung) 503
> biliary 576.8
>> due to Clonorchis sinensis 121.1
> bladder 596.89
>> interstitial 595.1
>> localized submucosal 595.1
>> panmural 595.1
> bone, diffuse 756.59
> breast 610.3
> capillary (*see also* Arteriosclerosis)
>> lung (chronic) (*see also* Fibrosis, lung) 515
> cardiac (*see also* Myocarditis) 429.0
> cervix 622.8
> chorion 658.8 ☑
> corpus cavernosum 607.89
> cystic (of pancreas) 277.00

Fibrosis, fibrotic — *continued*
> cystic — *continued*
>> with
>>> manifestations
>>>> gastrointestinal 277.03
>>>> pulmonary 277.02
>>>> specified NEC 277.09
>>> meconium ileus 277.01
>>> pulmonary exacerbation 277.02
> due to (presence of) any device, implant, or graft — *see* Complications, due to (presence of) any device, implant, or graft classified to 996.0–996.5 NEC
> ejaculatory duct 608.89
> endocardium (*see also* Endocarditis) 424.90
> endomyocardial (African) 425.0
> epididymis 608.89
> eye muscle 378.62
> graphite (of lung) 503
> heart (*see also* Myocarditis) 429.0
> hepatic (*see also* Cirrhosis, liver)
>> due to Clonorchis sinensis 121.1
> hepatolienal — *see* Cirrhosis, liver
> hepatosplenic — *see* Cirrhosis, liver
> infrapatellar fat pad 729.31
> interstitial pulmonary, newborn 770.7
> intrascrotal 608.89
> kidney (*see also* Sclerosis, renal) 587
> liver — *see* Cirrhosis, liver
> lung (atrophic) (capillary) (chronic) (confluent) (massive) (perialveolar) (peribronchial) 515
>> with
>>> anthracosilicosis (occupational) 500
>>> anthracosis (occupational) 500
>>> asbestosis (occupational) 501
>>> bagassosis (occupational) 495.1
>>> bauxite 503
>>> berylliosis (occupational) 503
>>> byssinosis (occupational) 504
>>> calcicosis (occupational) 502
>>> chalicosis (occupational) 502
>>> dust reticulation (occupational) 504
>>> farmers' lung 495.0
>>> gannister disease (occupational) 502
>>> graphite 503
>>> pneumonoconiosis (occupational) 505
>>> pneumosiderosis (occupational) 503
>>> siderosis (occupational) 503
>>> silicosis (occupational) 502
>>> tuberculosis (*see also* Tuberculosis) 011.4 ☑
>> diffuse (idiopathic) (interstitial) 516.31
>> due to
>>> bauxite 503
>>> fumes or vapors (chemical) (inhalation) 506.4
>>> graphite 503
>> following radiation 508.1
>> postinflammatory 515
>> silicotic (massive) (occupational) 502
>> tuberculous (*see also* Tuberculosis) 011.4 ☑
> lymphatic gland 289.3
> median bar 600.90
>> with
>>> other lower urinary tract symptoms (LUTS) 600.91
>>> urinary
>>>> obstruction 600.91
>>>> retention 600.91
> mediastinum (idiopathic) 519.3
> meninges 349.2
> muscle NEC 728.2
>> iatrogenic (from injection) 999.9
> myocardium, myocardial (*see also* Myocarditis) 429.0
> oral submucous 528.8
> ovary 620.8
> oviduct 620.8
> pancreas 577.8
>> cystic 277.00
>>> with
>>>> manifestations
>>>>> gastrointestinal 277.03

Fibrosis, fibrotic — *continued*
> pancreas — *continued*
>> cystic — *continued*
>>> with — *continued*
>>>> manifestations — *continued*
>>>>> pulmonary 277.02
>>>>> specified NEC 277.09
>>>> meconium ileus 277.01
>>>> pulmonary exacerbation 277.02
> penis 607.89
> periappendiceal 543.9
> periarticular (*see also* Ankylosis) 718.5 ☑
> pericardium 423.1
> perineum, in pregnancy or childbirth 654.8 ☑
>> affecting fetus or newborn 763.89
>> causing obstructed labor 660.2 ☑
>>> affecting fetus or newborn 763.1
> perineural NEC 355.9
>> foot 355.6
> periureteral 593.89
> placenta — *see* Placenta, abnormal
> pleura 511.0
> popliteal fat pad 729.31
> preretinal 362.56
> prostate (chronic) 600.90
>> with
>>> other lower urinary tract symptoms (LUTS) 600.91
>>> urinary
>>>> obstruction 600.91
>>>> retention 600.91
> pulmonary (chronic) (*see also* Fibrosis, lung) 515
>> alveolar capillary block 516.8
>> idiopathic 516.31
>> interstitial
>>> diffuse (idiopathic) 516.31
>>> newborn 770.7
> radiation — *see* Effect, adverse, radiation
> rectal sphincter 569.49
> retroperitoneal, idiopathic 593.4
> sclerosing mesenteric (idiopathic) 567.82
> scrotum 608.89
> seminal vesicle 608.89
> senile 797
> skin NEC 709.2
> spermatic cord 608.89
> spleen 289.59
>> bilharzial (*see also* Schistosomiasis) 120.9
> subepidermal nodular (M8832/0) — *see* Neoplasm, skin, benign
> submucous NEC 709.2
>> oral 528.8
>> tongue 528.8
> syncytium — *see* Placenta, abnormal
> testis 608.89
>> chronic, due to syphilis 095.8
> thymus (gland) 254.8
> tunica vaginalis 608.89
> ureter 593.89
> urethra 599.84
> uterus (nonneoplastic) 621.8
>> bilharzial (*see also* Schistosomiasis) 120.9
>> neoplastic (*see also* Leiomyoma, uterus) 218.9
> vagina 623.8
> valve, heart (*see also* Endocarditis) 424.90
> vas deferens 608.89
> vein 459.89
>> lower extremities 459.89
> vesical 595.1

Fibrositis (periarticular) (rheumatoid) 729.0
> humeroscapular region 726.2
> nodular, chronic
>> Jaccoud's 714.4
>> rheumatoid 714.4
> ossificans 728.11
> scapulohumeral 726.2

Fibrothorax 511.0

Fibrotic — *see* Fibrosis

Fibrous — *see* condition

Fibroxanthoma (M8831/0) — *see also* Neoplasm, connective tissue, benign
> atypical (M8831/1) — *see* Neoplasm, connective tissue, uncertain behavior

☑ Additional Digit Required — Refer to the Tabular List for Digit Selection ▽ Subterms under main terms may continue to next column or page

2015 ICD-9-CM ▶◀ Revised Text ● New Line ▲ Revised Code Volume 2 — 115

Findings, (abnormal), without diagnosis — *continued*

scan — *continued*
  brain 794.09
  kidney 794.4
  liver 794.8
  lung 794.2
  pancreas 794.9
  placental 794.9
  spleen 794.9
  thyroid 794.5
sedimentation rate, elevated 790.1
semen 792.2
serological (for)
  human immunodeficiency virus (HIV)
    inconclusive 795.71
    positive V08
  syphilis — *see* Findings, serology for syphilis
serology for syphilis
  false positive 795.6
  positive 097.1
    false 795.6
    follow-up of latent syphilis — *see* Syphilis, latent
    only finding — *see* Syphilis, latent
serum 790.99
  blood NEC 790.99
  enzymes NEC 790.5
  proteins 790.99
SGOT 790.4
SGPT 790.4
sickling of red blood cells 790.09
skin test, positive 795.79
  tuberculin (without active tuberculosis) 795.51
sodium 790.6
  deficiency 276.1
  excess 276.0
specified NEC 796.9
spermatozoa 792.2
spinal fluid 792.0
  culture, positive 792.0
sputum culture, positive 795.39
  for acid-fast bacilli 795.39
stool NEC 792.1
  bloody 578.1
    occult 792.1
  color 792.1
  culture, positive 792.1
  occult blood 792.1
stress test 794.39
structure, body (echogram) (thermogram) (ultrasound) (x-ray) NEC 793.99
  abdomen 793.6
  breast 793.89
    abnormal mammogram 793.80
    mammographic
      calcification 793.89
      calculus 793.89
      microcalcification 793.81
  gastrointestinal tract 793.4
  genitourinary organs 793.5
  head 793.0
    echogram (ultrasound) 794.01
  intrathoracic organs NEC 793.2
  lung 793.19
  musculoskeletal 793.7
  placenta 793.99
  retroperitoneum 793.6
  skin 793.99
  subcutaneous tissue NEC 793.99
synovial fluid 792.9
thermogram — *see* Findings, abnormal, structure
throat culture, positive 795.39
thyroid (function) 794.5
  metabolism (rate) 794.5
  scan 794.5
  uptake 794.5
total proteins 790.99
toxicology (drugs) (heavy metals) 796.0
transarninase (level) 790.4
triglycerides 272.9
  high 272.1
    with high cholesterol 272.2

Findings, (abnormal), without diagnosis — *continued*

tuberculin skin test (without active tuberculosis) 795.51
tumor markers NEC 795.89
ultrasound (*see also* Findings, abnormal, structure)
  cardiogram 793.2
uric acid, blood 790.6
urine, urinary constituents 791.9
  acetone 791.6
  albumin 791.0
  bacteria 791.9
  bile 791.4
  blood 599.70
  casts or cells 791.7
  chyle 791.1
  culture, positive 791.9
  glucose 791.5
  hemoglobin 791.2
  ketone 791.6
  protein 791.0
  pus 791.9
  sugar 791.5
  vaginal
    fluid 792.9
    high risk human papillomavirus (HPV) DNA test positive 795.15
    low risk human papillomavirus (HPV) DNA test positive 795.19
vanillylmandelic acid, elevated 791.9
vectorcardiogram (VCG) 794.39
ventriculogram (cerebral) 793.0
VMA, elevated 791.9
Wassermann reaction
  false positive 795.6
  positive 097.1
    follow-up of latent syphilis — *see* Syphilis, latent
    only finding — *see* Syphilis, latent
white blood cell 288.9
  count 288.9
    elevated 288.60
    low 288.50
  differential 288.9
  morphology 288.9
wound culture 795.39
xerography 793.89
zinc, blood 790.6
Finger — *see* condition
Finnish type nephrosis (congenital) 759.89
Fire, St. Anthony's — *see also* Erysipelas 035
Fish
  hook stomach 537.89
  meal workers' lung 495.8
Fisher's syndrome 357.0
Fissure, fissured
  abdominal wall (congenital) 756.79
  anus, anal 565.0
    congenital 751.5
  buccal cavity 528.9
  clitoris (congenital) 752.49
  ear, lobule (congenital) 744.29
  epiglottis (congenital) 748.3
  larynx 478.79
    congenital 748.3
  lip 528.5
    congenital (*see also* Cleft, lip) 749.10
  nipple 611.2
    puerperal, postpartum 676.1 ☑
  palate (congenital) (*see also* Cleft, palate) 749.00
  postanal 565.0
  rectum 565.0
  skin 709.8
    streptococcal 686.9
  spine (congenital) (*see also* Spina bifida) 741.9 ☑
  sternum (congenital) 756.3
  tongue (acquired) 529.5
    congenital 750.13
Fistula (sinus) 686.9
  abdomen (wall) 569.81
    bladder 596.2
    intestine 569.81
    ureter 593.82

Fistula — *continued*

abdomen — *continued*
  uterus 619.2
abdominorectal 569.81
abdominosigmoidal 569.81
abdominothoracic 510.0
abdominouterine 619.2
  congenital 752.39
abdominovesical 596.2
accessory sinuses (*see also* Sinusitis) 473.9
actinomycotic — *see* Actinomycosis
alveolar
  antrum (*see also* Sinusitis, maxillary) 473.0
  process 522.7
anorectal 565.1
antrobuccal (*see also* Sinusitis, maxillary) 473.0
antrum (*see also* Sinusitis, maxillary) 473.0
anus, anal (infectional) (recurrent) 565.1
  congenital 751.5
  tuberculous (*see also* Tuberculosis) 014.8 ☑
aortic sinus 747.29
aortoduodenal 447.2
appendix, appendicular 543.9
arteriovenous (acquired) 447.0
  brain 437.3
    congenital 747.81
      ruptured (*see also* Hemorrhage, subarachnoid) 430
    ruptured (*see also* Hemorrhage, subarachnoid) 430
  cerebral 437.3
    congenital 747.81
  congenital (peripheral) 747.60
    brain — *see* Fistula, arteriovenous, brain, congenital
    coronary 746.85
    gastrointestinal 747.61
    lower limb 747.64
    pulmonary 747.39
    renal 747.62
    specified site NEC 747.69
    upper limb 747.63
  coronary 414.19
    congenital 746.85
  heart 414.19
  pulmonary (vessels) 417.0
    congenital 747.39
  surgically created (for dialysis) V45.11
    complication NEC 996.73
      atherosclerosis — *see* Arteriosclerosis, extremities
      embolism 996.74
      infection or inflammation 996.62
      mechanical 996.1
      occlusion NEC 996.74
      thrombus 996.74
    traumatic — *see* Injury, blood vessel, by site
artery 447.2
aural 383.81
  congenital 744.49
auricle 383.81
  congenital 744.49
Bartholin's gland 619.8
bile duct (*see also* Fistula, biliary) 576.4
biliary (duct) (tract) 576.4
  congenital 751.69
bladder (neck) (sphincter) 596.2
  into seminal vesicle 596.2
bone 733.99
brain 348.89
  arteriovenous — *see* Fistula, arteriovenous, brain
branchial (cleft) 744.41
branchiogenous 744.41
breast 611.0
  puerperal, postpartum 675.1 ☑
bronchial 510.0
bronchocutaneous, bronchomediastinal, bronchopleural, bronchopleuromediastinal (infective) 510.0
  tuberculous (*see also* Tuberculosis) 011.3 ☑

Fistula — *continued*

bronchoesophageal 530.89
  congenital 750.3
buccal cavity (infective) 528.3
canal, ear 380.89
carotid-cavernous
  congenital 747.81
    with hemorrhage 430
  traumatic 900.82
    with hemorrhage (*see also* Hemorrhage, brain, traumatic) 853.0 ☑
    late effect 908.3
cecosigmoidal 569.81
cecum 569.81
cerebrospinal (fluid) 349.81
cervical, lateral (congenital) 744.41
cervicoaural (congenital) 744.49
cervicosigmoidal 619.1
cervicovesical 619.0
cervix 619.8
chest (wall) 510.0
cholecystocolic (*see also* Fistula, gallbladder) 575.5
cholecystocolonic (*see also* Fistula, gallbladder) 575.5
cholecystoduodenal (*see also* Fistula, gallbladder) 575.5
cholecystoenteric (*see also* Fistula, gallbladder) 575.5
cholecystogastric (*see also* Fistula, gallbladder) 575.5
cholecystointestinal (*see also* Fistula, gallbladder) 575.5
choledochoduodenal 576.4
cholocolic (*see also* Fistula, gallbladder) 575.5
coccyx 685.1
  with abscess 685.0
colon 569.81
colostomy 569.69
colovaginal (acquired) 619.1
common duct (bile duct) 576.4
congenital, NEC — *see* Anomaly, specified type NEC
cornea, causing hypotony 360.32
coronary, arteriovenous 414.19
  congenital 746.85
costal region 510.0
cul-de-sac, Douglas' 619.8
cutaneous 686.9
cystic duct (*see also* Fistula, gallbladder) 575.5
  congenital 751.69
cystostomy 596.83
dental 522.7
diaphragm 510.0
  bronchovisceral 510.0
  pleuroperitoneal 510.0
  pulmonoperitoneal 510.0
duodenum 537.4
ear (canal) (external) 380.89
enterocolic 569.81
enterocutaneous 569.81
enteroenteric 569.81
entero-uterine 619.1
  congenital 752.39
enterovaginal 619.1
  congenital 752.49
enterovesical 596.1
epididymis 608.89
  tuberculous (*see also* Tuberculosis) 016.4 ☑
esophagobronchial 530.89
  congenital 750.3
esophagocutaneous 530.89
esophagopleurocutaneous 530.89
esophagotracheal 530.84
  congenital 750.3
esophagus 530.89
  congenital 750.4
ethmoid (*see also* Sinusitis, ethmoidal) 473.2
eyeball (cornea) (sclera) 360.32
eyelid 373.11
fallopian tube (external) 619.2
fecal 569.81

☑ **Additional Digit Required** — Refer to the Tabular List for Digit Selection

▽ **Subterms under main terms may continue to next column or page**

Fistula — continued
  fecal — continued
    congenital 751.5
  from periapical lesion 522.7
  frontal sinus (see also Sinusitis, frontal) 473.1
  gallbladder 575.5
    with calculus, cholelithiasis, stones (see
      also Cholelithiasis) 574.2 ☑
    congenital 751.69
  gastric 537.4
  gastrocolic 537.4
    congenital 750.7
    tuberculous (see also Tuberculosis)
      014.8 ☑
  gastroenterocolic 537.4
  gastroesophageal 537.4
  gastrojejunal 537.4
  gastrojejunocolic 537.4
  genital
    organs
      female 619.9
        specified site NEC 619.8
      male 608.89
    tract-skin (female) 619.2
  hepatopleural 510.0
  hepatopulmonary 510.0
  horseshoe 565.1
  ileorectal 569.81
  ileosigmoidal 569.81
  ileostomy 569.69
  ileovesical 596.1
  ileum 569.81
  in ano 565.1
    tuberculous (see also Tuberculosis)
      014.8 ☑
  inner ear (see also Fistula, labyrinth) 386.40
  intestine 569.81
  intestinocolonic (abdominal) 569.81
  intestinoureteral 593.82
  intestinouterine 619.1
  intestinovaginal 619.1
    congenital 752.49
  intestinovesical 596.1
  involving female genital tract 619.9
    digestive-genital 619.1
    genital tract-skin 619.2
    specified site NEC 619.8
    urinary-genital 619.0
  ischiorectal (fossa) 566
  jejunostomy 569.69
  jejunum 569.81
  joint 719.80
    ankle 719.87
    elbow 719.82
    foot 719.87
    hand 719.84
    hip 719.85
    knee 719.86
    multiple sites 719.89
    pelvic region 719.85
    shoulder (region) 719.81
    specified site NEC 719.88
    tuberculous — see Tuberculosis, joint
    wrist 719.83
  kidney 593.89
  labium (majus) (minus) 619.8
  labyrinth, labyrinthine NEC 386.40
    combined sites 386.48
    multiple sites 386.48
    oval window 386.42
    round window 386.41
    semicircular canal 386.43
  lacrimal, lachrymal (duct) (gland) (sac)
    375.61
  lacrimonasal duct 375.61
  laryngotracheal 748.3
  larynx 478.79
  lip 528.5
    congenital 750.25
  lumbar, tuberculous (see also Tuberculosis)
    015.0 ☑ [730.8] ☑
  lung 510.0
  lymphatic (node) (vessel) 457.8
  mamillary 611.0
  mammary (gland) 611.0
    puerperal, postpartum 675.1 ☑

Fistula — continued
  mastoid (process) (region) 383.1
  maxillary (see also Sinusitis, maxillary) 473.0
  mediastinal 510.0
  mediastinobronchial 510.0
  mediastinocutaneous 510.0
  middle ear 385.89
  mouth 528.3
  nasal 478.19
    sinus (see also Sinusitis) 473.9
  nasopharynx 478.29
  nipple — see Fistula, breast
  nose 478.19
  oral (cutaneous) 528.3
    maxillary (see also Sinusitis, maxillary)
      473.0
    nasal (with cleft palate) (see also Cleft,
      palate) 749.00
  orbit, orbital 376.10
  oro-antral (see also Sinusitis, maxillary) 473.0
  oval window (internal ear) 386.42
  oviduct (external) 619.2
  palate (hard) 526.89
    soft 528.9
  pancreatic 577.8
  pancreaticoduodenal 577.8
  parotid (gland) 527.4
    region 528.3
  pelvoabdominointestinal 569.81
  penis 607.89
  perianal 565.1
  pericardium (pleura) (sac) (see also Pericardi-
    tis) 423.8
  pericecal 569.81
  perineal — see Fistula, perineum
  perineorectal 569.81
  perineosigmoidal 569.81
  perineo-urethroscrotal 608.89
  perineum, perineal (with urethral involve-
    ment) NEC 599.1
    tuberculous (see also Tuberculosis)
      017.9 ☑
    ureter 593.82
  perirectal 565.1
    tuberculous (see also Tuberculosis)
      014.8 ☑
  peritoneum (see also Peritonitis) 567.22
  periurethral 599.1
  pharyngo-esophageal 478.29
  pharynx 478.29
    branchial cleft (congenital) 744.41
  pilonidal (infected) (rectum) 685.1
    with abscess 685.0
  pleura, pleural, pleurocutaneous, pleuroperi-
    toneal 510.0
    stomach 510.0
    tuberculous (see also Tuberculosis)
      012.0 ☑
  pleuropericardial 423.8
  postauricular 383.81
  postoperative, persistent 998.6
  preauricular (congenital) 744.46
  prostate 602.8
  pulmonary 510.0
    arteriovenous 417.0
      congenital 747.39
    tuberculous (see also Tuberculosis, pul-
      monary) 011.9 ☑
  pulmonoperitoneal 510.0
  rectolabial 619.1
  rectosigmoid (intercommunicating) 569.81
  rectoureteral 593.82
  rectourethral 599.1
    congenital 753.8
  rectouterine 619.1
    congenital 752.39
  rectovaginal 619.1
    congenital 752.49
    old, postpartal 619.1
    tuberculous (see also Tuberculosis)
      014.8 ☑
  rectovesical 596.1
    congenital 753.8
  rectovesicovaginal 619.1
  rectovulvar 619.1
    congenital 752.49

Fistula — continued
  rectum (to skin) 565.1
    tuberculous (see also Tuberculosis)
      014.8 ☑
  renal 593.89
  retroauricular 383.81
  round window (internal ear) 386.41
  salivary duct or gland 527.4
    congenital 750.24
  sclera 360.32
  scrotum (urinary) 608.89
    tuberculous (see also Tuberculosis)
      016.5 ☑
  semicircular canals (internal ear) 386.43
  sigmoid 569.81
    vesicoabdominal 596.1
  sigmoidovaginal 619.1
    congenital 752.49
  skin 686.9
    ureter 593.82
    vagina 619.2
  sphenoidal sinus (see also Sinusitis, sphe-
    noidal) 473.3
  splenocolic 289.59
  stercoral 569.81
  stomach 537.4
  sublingual gland 527.4
    congenital 750.24
  submaxillary
    gland 527.4
      congenital 750.24
    region 528.3
  thoracic 510.0
    duct 457.8
  thoracicoabdominal 510.0
  thoracicogastric 510.0
  thoracicointestinal 510.0
  thoracoabdominal 510.0
  thoracogastric 510.0
  thorax 510.0
  thyroglossal duct 759.2
  thyroid 246.8
  trachea (congenital) (external) (internal)
    748.3
  tracheoesophageal 530.84
    congenital 750.3
    following tracheostomy 519.09
  traumatic
    arteriovenous (see also Injury, blood
      vessel, by site) 904.9
      brain — see Injury, intracranial
  tuberculous — see Tuberculosis, by site
  typhoid 002.0
  umbilical 759.89
  umbilico-urinary 753.8
  urachal, urachus 753.7
  ureter (persistent) 593.82
  ureteroabdominal 593.82
  ureterocervical 593.82
  ureterorectal 593.82
  ureterosigmoido-abdominal 593.82
  ureterovaginal 619.0
  ureterovesical 596.2
  urethra 599.1
    congenital 753.8
    tuberculous (see also Tuberculosis)
      016.3 ☑
  urethroperineal 599.1
  urethroperineovesical 596.2
  urethrorectal 599.1
    congenital 753.8
  urethroscrotal 608.89
  urethrovaginal 619.0
  urethrovesical 596.2
  urethrovesicovaginal 619.0
  urinary (persistent) (recurrent) 599.1
  uteroabdominal (anterior wall) 619.2
    congenital 752.39
  uteroenteric 619.1
  uterofecal 619.1
  uterointestinal 619.1
    congenital 752.39
  uterorectal 619.1
    congenital 752.39
  uteroureteric 619.0
  uterovaginal 619.8

Fistula — continued
  uterovesical 619.0
    congenital 752.39
  uterus 619.8
  vagina (wall) 619.8
    postpartal, old 619.8
  vaginocutaneous (postpartal) 619.2
  vaginoileal (acquired) 619.1
  vaginoperineal 619.2
  vesical NEC 596.2
  vesicoabdominal 596.2
  vesicocervicovaginal 619.0
  vesicocolic 596.1
  vesicocutaneous 596.2
  vesicoenteric 596.1
  vesicointestinal 596.1
  vesicometrorectal 619.1
  vesicoperineal 596.2
  vesicorectal 596.1
    congenital 753.8
  vesicosigmoidal 596.1
  vesicosigmoidovaginal 619.1
  vesicoureteral 596.2
  vesicoureterovaginal 619.0
  vesicourethral 596.2
  vesicourethrorectal 596.1
  vesicouterine 619.0
    congenital 752.39
  vesicovaginal 619.0
  vulvorectal 619.1
    congenital 752.49
Fit 780.39
  apoplectic (see also Disease, cerebrovascu-
    lar, acute) 436
    late effect — see Late effect(s) (of) cere-
      brovascular disease
  epileptic (see also Epilepsy) 345.9 ☑
  fainting 780.2
  hysterical 300.11
  newborn 779.0
Fitting (of)
  artificial
    arm (complete) (partial) V52.0
    breast V52.4
      implant exchange (different material)
        (different size) V52.4
    eye(s) V52.2
    leg(s) (complete) (partial) V52.1
  brain neuropacemaker V53.02
  cardiac pacemaker V53.31
  carotid sinus pacemaker V53.39
  cerebral ventricle (communicating) shunt
    V53.01
  colostomy belt V53.5 ☑
  contact lenses V53.1
  cystostomy device V53.6
  defibrillator, automatic implantable cardiac
    (with synchronous cardiac pacemak-
    er) V53.32
  dentures V52.3
  device, unspecified type V53.90
    abdominal V53.59
    cardiac
      defibrillator, automatic implantable
        (with synchronous cardiac
        pacemaker) V53.32
      pacemaker V53.31
      specified NEC V53.39
    cerebral ventricle (communicating)
      shunt V53.01
    gastrointestinal NEC V53.59
    insulin pump V53.91
    intestinal V53.50
    intrauterine contraceptive
      insertion V25.11
      removal V25.12
        and reinsertion V25.13
      replacement V25.13
    nervous system V53.09
    orthodontic V53.4
    orthoptic V53.1
    other device V53.99
    prosthetic V52.9
      breast V52.4
      dental V52.3
      eye V52.2

☑ **Additional Digit Required** — Refer to the Tabular List for Digit Selection   ▽ **Subterms under main terms may continue to next column or page**

☑ **Additional Digit Required** — Refer to the Tabular List for Digit Selection   ⑩ **Subterms under main terms may continue to next column or page**

2015 ICD-9-CM   ▶◀ **Revised Text**   ● **New Line**   ▲ **Revised Code**   **Volume 2 — 119**

Foreign body — *continued*
  entering through orifice — *continued*
    eye — *continued*
      intraocular — *see* Foreign body, by site
      specified site NEC 930.8
    eyeball 930.8
      intraocular — *see* Foreign body, in-traocular
    eyelid 930.1
      retained or old 374.86
    frontal sinus 932
    gastrointestinal tract 938
    genitourinary tract 939.9
    globe 930.8
      penetrating 871.6
        magnetic 871.5
          retained or old 360.50
        retained or old 360.60
    gum 935.0
    Highmore's antrum 932
    hypopharynx 933.0
    ileocecal coil 936
    ileum 936
    inspiration (of) 933.1
    intestine (large) (small) 936
    lacrimal apparatus, duct, gland, or sac 930.2
    larynx 933.1
    lung 934.8
    maxillary sinus 932
    mouth 935.0
    nasal sinus 932
    nasopharynx 933.0
    nose (passage) 932
    nostril 932
    oral cavity 935.0
    palate 935.0
    penis 939.3
    pharynx 933.0
    pyriform sinus 933.0
    rectosigmoid 937
      junction 937
    rectum 937
    respiratory tract 934.9
      specified part NEC 934.8
    sclera 930.1
    sinus 932
      accessory 932
      frontal 932
      maxillary 932
      nasal 932
      pyriform 933.0
    small intestine 936
    stomach (hairball) 935.2
    suffocation by (*see also* Asphyxia, food) 933.1
    swallowed 938
      tongue 933.0
    tear ducts or glands 930.2
    throat 933.0
    tongue 935.0
      swallowed 933.0
    tonsil, tonsillar 933.0
      fossa 933.0
    trachea 934.0
    ureter 939.0
    urethra 939.0
    uterus (any part) 939.1
    vagina 939.2
    vulva 939.2
    wind pipe 934.0
  feeling of, in throat 784.99
  granuloma (old) 728.82
    bone 733.99
    in operative wound (inadvertently left) 998.4
      due to surgical material intentionally left — *see* Complications, due to (presence of) any device, implant, or graft classified to 996.0–996.5 NEC
    muscle 728.82
    skin 709.4
    soft tissue 709.4
    subcutaneous tissue 709.4

Foreign body — *continued*
  in
    bone (residual) 733.99
    open wound — *see* Wound, open, by site complicated
    soft tissue (residual) 729.6
  inadvertently left in operation wound (causing adhesions, obstruction, or perforation) 998.4
  ingestion, ingested NEC 938
  inhalation or inspiration (*see also* Asphyxia, food) 933.1
  internal organ, not entering through an orifice — *see* Injury, internal, by site, with open wound
  intraocular (nonmagnetic) 871.6
    combined sites 871.6
      magnetic 871.5
        retained or old 360.59
      retained or old 360.69
    magnetic 871.5
      retained or old 360.50
    retained or old 360.60
    specified site NEC 871.6
      magnetic 871.5
        retained or old 360.59
      retained or old 360.69
    iris (nonmagnetic) 871.6
      magnetic 871.5
        retained or old 360.52
      retained or old 360.62
    lens (nonmagnetic) 871.6
      magnetic 871.5
        retained or old 360.53
      retained or old 360.63
  lid, eye 930.1
  ocular muscle 870.4
    retained or old 376.6
  old or residual
    bone 733.99
    eyelid 374.86
    middle ear 385.83
    muscle 729.6
      ocular 376.6
    retrobulbar 376.6
    skin 729.6
      with granuloma 709.4
    soft tissue 729.6
      with granuloma 709.4
    subcutaneous tissue 729.6
      with granuloma 709.4
  operation wound, left accidentally 998.4
  orbit 870.4
    retained or old 376.6
  posterior wall, eye 871.6
    magnetic 871.5
      retained or old 360.55
    retained or old 360.65
  respiratory tree 934.9
    specified site NEC 934.8
  retained (old) (nonmagnetic) (in) V90.9
    anterior chamber (eye) 360.61
      magnetic 360.51
    ciliary body 360.62
      magnetic 360.52
    eyelid 374.86
    fragment(s)
      acrylics V90.2
      animal quills V90.31
      animal spines V90.31
      cement V90.83
      concrete V90.83
      crystalline V90.83
      depleted
        isotope V90.09
        uranium V90.01
      diethylhexylphthalates V90.2
      glass V90.81
      isocyanate V90.2
      metal V90.10
        magnetic V90.11
        nonmagnetic V90.12
      organic NEC V90.39
      plastic V90.2
      radioactive
        nontherapeutic V90.09

Foreign body — *continued*
  retained — *continued*
    fragment(s) — *continued*
      radioactive — *continued*
        specified NEC V90.09
      stone V90.83
      tooth V90.32
      wood V90.33
    globe 360.60
      magnetic 360.50
    intraocular 360.60
      magnetic 360.50
      specified site NEC 360.69
        magnetic 360.59
    iris 360.62
      magnetic 360.52
    lens 360.63
      magnetic 360.53
    muscle 729.6
    orbit 376.6
    posterior wall of globe 360.65
      magnetic 360.55
    retina 360.65
      magnetic 360.55
    retrobulbar 376.6
    skin 729.6
      with granuloma 709.4
    soft tissue 729.6
      with granuloma 709.4
    specified NEC V90.89
    subcutaneous tissue 729.6
      with granuloma 709.4
    vitreous 360.64
      magnetic 360.54
  retina 871.6
    magnetic 871.5
      retained or old 360.55
    retained or old 360.65
  superficial, without major open wound (*see also* Injury, superficial, by site) 919.6
  swallowed NEC 938
  throat, feeling of 784.99
  vitreous (humor) 871.6
    magnetic 871.5
      retained or old 360.54
    retained or old 360.64
Forking, aqueduct of Sylvius 742.3
  with spina bifida (*see also* Spina bifida) 741.0 ☑
Formation
  bone in scar tissue (skin) 709.3
  connective tissue in vitreous 379.25
  Elschnig pearls (postcataract extraction) 366.51
  hyaline in cornea 371.49
  sequestrum in bone (due to infection) (*see also* Osteomyelitis) 730.1 ☑
  valve
    colon, congenital 751.5
    ureter (congenital) 753.29
Formication 782.0
Fort Bragg fever 100.89
Fossa — *see also* condition
  pyriform — *see* condition
Foster care (status) V60.81
Foster-Kennedy syndrome 377.04
Fothergill's
  disease, meaning scarlatina anginosa 034.1
  neuralgia (*see also* Neuralgia, trigeminal) 350.1
Foul breath 784.99
Found dead (cause unknown) 798.9
Foundling V20.0
Fournier's disease (idiopathic gangrene) 608.83
  female 616.89
Fourth
  cranial nerve — *see* condition
  disease 057.8
  molar 520.1
Foville's syndrome 344.89
Fox's
  disease (apocrine miliaria) 705.82
  impetigo (contagiosa) 684
Fox-Fordyce disease (apocrine miliaria) 705.82

Fracture (abduction) (adduction) (avulsion) (compression) (crush) (dislocation) (oblique) (separation) (closed) 829.0

Note — For fracture of any of the following sites with fracture of other bones — *see* Fracture, multiple.

"Closed" includes the following descriptions of fractures, with or without delayed healing, unless they are specified as open or compound:

comminuted	linear
depressed	simple
elevated	slipped epiphysis
fissured	spiral
greenstick	unspecified
impacted	

"Open" includes the following descriptions of fractures, with or without delayed healing:

compound	puncture
infected	with foreign body
missile	

For late effect of fracture, see Late, effect, fracture, by site.

  with
    internal injuries in same region (conditions classifiable to 860–869) (*see also* Injury, internal, by site)
    pelvic region — *see* Fracture, pelvis
  acetabulum (with visceral injury) (closed) 808.0
    open 808.1
  acromion (process) (closed) 811.01
    open 811.11
  alveolus (closed) 802.8
    open 802.9
  ankle (malleolus) (closed) 824.8
    bimalleolar (Dupuytren's) (Pott's) 824.4
      open 824.5
    bone 825.21
      open 825.31
    lateral malleolus only (fibular) 824.2
      open 824.3
    medial malleolus only (tibial) 824.0
      open 824.1
    open 824.9
    pathologic 733.16
    talus 825.21
      open 825.31
    trimalleolar 824.6
      open 824.7
  antrum — *see* Fracture, skull, base
  arm (closed) 818.0
    and leg(s) (any bones) 828.0
      open 828.1
    both (any bones) (with rib(s)) (with sternum) 819.0
      open 819.1
    lower 813.80
      open 813.90
    open 818.1
    upper — *see* Fracture, humerus
  astragalus (closed) 825.21
    open 825.31
  atlas — *see* Fracture, vertebra, cervical, first
  axis — *see* Fracture, vertebra, cervical, second
  back — *see* Fracture, vertebra, by site
  Barton's — *see* Fracture, radius, lower end
  basal (skull) — *see* Fracture, skull, base
  Bennett's (closed) 815.01
    open 815.11
  bimalleolar (closed) 824.4
    open 824.5
  bone (closed) NEC 829.0
    birth injury NEC 767.3
    open 829.1
    pathologic NEC (*see also* Fracture, pathologic) 733.10

Fracture — *continued*
bone — *continued*
 stress NEC (*see also* Fracture, stress)
  733.95
boot top — *see* Fracture, fibula
boxers' — *see* Fracture, metacarpal bone(s)
breast bone — *see* Fracture, sternum
bucket handle (semilunar cartilage) — *see*
 Tear, meniscus
buckle — *see* Fracture, torus
burst — *see* Fracture, traumatic, by site
bursting — *see* Fracture, phalanx, hand,
 distal
calcaneus (closed) 825.0
 open 825.1
capitate (bone) (closed) 814.07
 open 814.17
capitellum (humerus) (closed) 812.49
 open 812.59
carpal bone(s) (wrist NEC) (closed) 814.00
 open 814.10
 specified site NEC 814.09
  open 814.19
cartilage, knee (semilunar) — *see* Tear,
 meniscus
cervical — *see* Fracture, vertebra, cervical
chauffeur's — *see* Fracture, ulna, lower end
chisel — *see* Fracture, radius, upper end
chronic — *see* Fracture, pathologic
clavicle (interligamentous part) (closed)
 810.00
 acromial end 810.03
  open 810.13
 due to birth trauma 767.2
 open 810.10
 shaft (middle third) 810.02
  open 810.12
 sternal end 810.01
  open 810.11
clayshovelers' — *see* Fracture, vertebra,
 cervical
coccyx (*see also* Fracture, vertebra, coccyx)
 complicating delivery 665.6 ☑
collar bone — *see* Fracture, clavicle
Colles' (reversed) (closed) 813.41
 open 813.51
comminuted — *see* Fracture, by site
compression (*see also* Fracture, by site)
 nontraumatic — *see* Fracture, pathologic
congenital 756.9
coracoid process (closed) 811.02
 open 811.12
coronoid process (ulna) (closed) 813.02
 mandible (closed) 802.23
  open 802.33
 open 813.12
corpus cavernosum penis 959.13
costochondral junction — *see* Fracture, rib
costosternal junction — *see* Fracture, rib
cranium — *see* Fracture, skull, by site
cricoid cartilage (closed) 807.5
 open 807.6
cuboid (ankle) (closed) 825.23
 open 825.33
cuneiform
 foot (closed) 825.24
  open 825.34
 wrist (closed) 814.03
  open 814.13
dental implant 525.73
dental restorative material
 with loss of material 525.64
 without loss of material 525.63
due to
 birth injury — *see* Birth injury, fracture
 gunshot — *see* Fracture, by site, open
 neoplasm — *see* Fracture, pathologic
 osteoporosis — *see* Fracture, pathologic
Dupuytren's (ankle) (fibula) (closed) 824.4
 open 824.5
 radius 813.42
  open 813.52
Duverney's — *see* Fracture, ilium
elbow (*see also* Fracture, humerus, lower
 end)
 olecranon (process) (closed) 813.01

Fracture — *continued*
elbow (*see also* Fracture, humerus, lower
 end) — *continued*
 olecranon — *continued*
  open 813.11
 supracondylar (closed) 812.41
  open 812.51
ethmoid (bone) (sinus) — *see* Fracture, skull,
 base
face bone(s) (closed) NEC 802.8
 with
  other bone(s) — *see* Fracture, multiple, skull
  skull (*see also* Fracture, skull)
   involving other bones — *see*
    Fracture, multiple, skull
 open 802.9
fatigue — *see* Fracture, march
femur, femoral (closed) 821.00
 cervicotrochanteric 820.03
  open 820.13
 condyles, epicondyles 821.21
  open 821.31
 distal end — *see* Fracture, femur, lower
  end
 epiphysis (separation)
  capital 820.01
   open 820.11
  head 820.01
   open 820.11
  lower 821.22
   open 821.32
  trochanteric 820.01
   open 820.11
  upper 820.01
   open 820.11
 head 820.09
  open 820.19
 lower end or extremity (distal end)
  (closed) 821.20
  condyles, epicondyles 821.21
   open 821.31
  epiphysis (separation) 821.22
   open 821.32
  multiple sites 821.29
   open 821.39
  open 821.30
  specified site NEC 821.29
   open 821.39
  supracondylar 821.23
   open 821.33
  T-shaped 821.21
   open 821.31
 neck (closed) 820.8
  base (cervicotrochanteric) 820.03
   open 820.13
  extracapsular 820.20
   open 820.30
  intertrochanteric (section) 820.21
   open 820.31
  intracapsular 820.00
   open 820.10
  intratrochanteric 820.21
   open 820.31
  midcervical 820.02
   open 820.12
  open 820.9
  pathologic 733.14
   specified part NEC 733.15
  specified site NEC 820.09
   open 820.19
  stress 733.96
  transcervical 820.02
   open 820.12
  transtrochanteric 820.20
   open 820.30
 open 821.10
 pathologic 733.14
  specified part NEC 733.15
 peritrochanteric (section) 820.20
  open 820.30
 shaft (lower third) (middle third) (upper
  third) 821.01
  open 821.11
  stress 733.97
 subcapital 820.09

Fracture — *continued*
femur, femoral — *continued*
 subcapital — *continued*
  open 820.19
 subtrochanteric (region) (section) 820.22
  open 820.32
 supracondylar 821.23
  open 821.33
 transepiphyseal 820.01
  open 820.11
 trochanter (greater) (lesser) (*see also*
  Fracture, femur, neck, by site)
  820.20
  open 820.30
 T-shaped, into knee joint 821.21
  open 821.31
 upper end 820.8
  open 820.9
fibula (closed) 823.81
 with tibia 823.82
  open 823.92
 distal end 824.8
  open 824.9
 epiphysis
  lower 824.8
   open 824.9
  upper — *see* Fracture, fibula, upper
   end
 head — *see* Fracture, fibula, upper end
 involving ankle 824.2
  open 824.3
 lower end or extremity 824.8
  open 824.9
 malleolus (external) (lateral) 824.2
  open 824.3
 open NEC 823.91
 pathologic 733.16
 proximal end — *see* Fracture, fibula,
  upper end
 shaft 823.21
  with tibia 823.22
   open 823.32
  open 823.31
  stress 733.93
 torus 823.41
  with tibia 823.42
 upper end or extremity (epiphysis)
  (head) (proximal end) (styloid)
  823.01
  with tibia 823.02
   open 823.12
  open 823.11
finger(s), of one hand (closed) (*see also*
 Fracture, phalanx, hand) 816.00
 with
  metacarpal bone(s), of same hand
   817.0
   open 817.1
  thumb of same hand 816.03
   open 816.13
 open 816.10
foot, except toe(s) alone (closed) 825.20
 open 825.30
forearm (closed) NEC 813.80
 lower end (distal end) (lower epiphysis)
  813.40
  open 813.50
 open 813.90
 shaft 813.20
  open 813.30
 upper end (proximal end) (upper epiphysis) 813.00
  open 813.10
fossa, anterior, middle, or posterior — *see*
 Fracture, skull, base
Fracture (abduction) (adduction) (avulsion)
 (compression) (crush) (dislocation)
 (oblique) (separation) 829.0
frontal (bone) (*see also* Fracture, skull, vault)
 sinus — *see* Fracture, skull, base
Galeazzi's — *see* Fracture, radius, lower end
glenoid (cavity) (fossa) (scapula) (closed)
 811.03
 open 811.13
Gosselin's — *see* Fracture, ankle
greenstick — *see* Fracture, by site

Fracture — *continued*
grenade-throwers' — *see* Fracture, humerus,
 shaft
gutter — *see* Fracture, skull, vault
hamate (closed) 814.08
 open 814.18
hand, one (closed) 815.00
 carpals 814.00
  open 814.10
  specified site NEC 814.09
   open 814.19
 metacarpals 815.00
  open 815.10
 multiple, bones of one hand 817.0
  open 817.1
 open 815.10
 phalanges (*see also* Fracture, phalanx,
  hand) 816.00
  open 816.10
healing
 aftercare (*see also* Aftercare, fracture)
  V54.89
 change of cast V54.89
 complications — *see* condition
 convalescence V66.4
 removal of
  cast V54.89
  fixation device
   external V54.89
   internal V54.01
heel bone (closed) 825.0
 open 825.1
Hill-Sachs 812.09
hip (closed) (*see also* Fracture, femur, neck)
 820.8
 open 820.9
 pathologic 733.14
humerus (closed) 812.20
 anatomical neck 812.02
  open 812.12
 articular process (*see also* Fracture
  humerus, condyle(s)) 812.44
  open 812.54
 capitellum 812.49
  open 812.59
 condyle(s) 812.44
  lateral (external) 812.42
   open 812.52
  medial (internal epicondyle) 812.43
   open 812.53
  open 812.54
 distal end — *see* Fracture, humerus,
  lower end
 epiphysis
  lower (*see also* Fracture, humerus,
   condyle(s)) 812.44
   open 812.54
  upper 812.09
   open 812.19
 external condyle 812.42
  open 812.52
 great tuberosity 812.03
  open 812.13
 head 812.09
  open 812.19
 internal epicondyle 812.43
  open 812.53
 lesser tuberosity 812.09
  open 812.19
 lower end or extremity (distal end) (*see
  also* Fracture, humerus, by site)
  812.40
  multiple sites NEC 812.49
   open 812.59
  open 812.50
  specified site NEC 812.49
   open 812.59
 neck 812.01
  open 812.11
 open 812.30
 pathologic 733.11
 proximal end — *see* Fracture, humerus,
  upper end
 shaft 812.21
  open 812.31
 supracondylar 812.41

☑ **Additional Digit Required** — Refer to the Tabular List for Digit Selection ▽ **Subterms under main terms may continue to next column or page**

2015 ICD-9-CM ▶◀ Revised Text ● New Line ▲ Revised Code Volume 2 — 121

Fracture — continued
humerus — continued
   supracondylar — continued
      open 812.51
   surgical neck 812.01
      open 812.11
   trochlea 812.49
      open 812.59
   T-shaped 812.44
      open 812.54
   tuberosity — see Fracture, humerus, upper end
   upper end or extremity (proximal end) (see also Fracture, humerus, by site) 812.00
      open 812.10
      specified site NEC 812.09
         open 812.19
hyoid bone (closed) 807.5
   open 807.6
hyperextension — see Fracture, radius, lower end
ilium (with visceral injury) (closed) 808.41
   open 808.51
impaction, impacted — see Fracture, by site
incus — see Fracture, skull, base
innominate bone (with visceral injury) (closed) 808.49
   open 808.59
instep, of one foot (closed) 825.20
   with toe(s) of same foot 827.0
      open 827.1
   open 825.30
insufficiency — see Fracture, pathologic, by site
internal
   ear — see Fracture, skull, base
   semilunar cartilage, knee — see Tear, meniscus, medial
intertrochanteric — see Fracture, femur, neck, intertrochanteric
ischium (with visceral injury) (closed) 808.42
   open 808.52
jaw (bone) (lower) (closed) (see also Fracture, mandible) 802.20
   angle 802.25
      open 802.35
   open 802.30
   upper — see Fracture, maxilla
knee
   cap (closed) 822.0
      open 822.1
   cartilage (semilunar) — see Tear, meniscus
labyrinth (osseous) — see Fracture, skull, base
larynx (closed) 807.5
   open 807.6
late effect — see Late, effects (of), fracture
Le Fort's — see Fracture, maxilla
leg (closed) 827.0
   with rib(s) or sternum 828.0
      open 828.1
   both (any bones) 828.0
      open 828.1
   lower — see Fracture, tibia
   open 827.1
   upper — see Fracture, femur
limb
   lower (multiple) (closed) NEC 827.0
      open 827.1
   upper (multiple) (closed) NEC 818.0
      open 818.1
long bones, due to birth trauma — see Birth injury, fracture
lower end or extremity (anterior lip) (posterior) 824.8
   open 824.9
lumbar — see Fracture, vertebra, lumbar
lunate bone (closed) 814.02
   open 814.12
malar bone (closed) 802.4
   open 802.5
Malgaigne's (closed) 808.43
   open 808.53
malleolus (closed) 824.8

Fracture — continued
malleolus — continued
   bimalleolar 824.4
      open 824.5
   lateral 824.2
      and medial (see also Fracture, malleolus, bimalleolar)
         with lip of tibia — see Fracture, malleolus, trimalleolar
      open 824.3
   medial (closed) 824.0
      and lateral (see also Fracture, malleolus, bimalleolar)
         with lip of tibia — see Fracture, malleolus, trimalleolar
      open 824.1
   open 824.9
   trimalleolar (closed) 824.6
      open 824.7
malleus — see Fracture, skull, base
malunion 733.81
mandible (closed) 802.20
   angle 802.25
      open 802.35
   body 802.28
      alveolar border 802.27
         open 802.37
      open 802.38
      symphysis 802.26
         open 802.36
   condylar process 802.21
      open 802.31
   coronoid process 802.23
      open 802.33
   multiple sites 802.29
      open 802.39
   open 802.30
   ramus NEC 802.24
      open 802.34
   subcondylar 802.22
      open 802.32
manubrium — see Fracture, sternum
march 733.95
   femoral neck 733.96
   fibula 733.93
   metatarsals 733.94
   pelvis 733.98
   shaft of femur 733.97
   tibia 733.93
maxilla, maxillary (superior) (upper jaw) (closed) 802.4
   inferior — see Fracture, mandible
   open 802.5
meniscus, knee — see Tear, meniscus
metacarpus, metacarpal (bone(s)), of one hand (closed) 815.00
   with phalanx, phalanges, hand (finger(s)) (thumb) of same hand 817.0
      open 817.1
   base 815.02
      first metacarpal 815.01
         open 815.11
      open 815.12
      thumb 815.01
         open 815.11
   multiple sites 815.09
      open 815.19
   neck 815.04
      open 815.14
   open 815.10
   shaft 815.03
      open 815.13
metatarsus, metatarsal (bone(s)), of one foot (closed) 825.25
   with tarsal bone(s) 825.29
      open 825.39
   open 825.35
Monteggia's (closed) 813.03
   open 813.13
Moore's — see Fracture, radius, lower end
multangular bone (closed)
   larger 814.05
      open 814.15
   smaller 814.06
      open 814.16

Fracture — continued
multiple (closed) 829.0

Note — Multiple fractures of sites classifiable to the same three- or four-digit category are coded to that category, except for sites classifiable to 810–818 or 820–827 in different limbs.

Multiple fractures of sites classifiable to different fourth-digit subdivisions within the same three–digit category should be dealt with according to coding rules.

Multiple fractures of sites classifiable to different three–digit categories (identifiable from the listing under "Fracture"), and of sites classifiable to 810–818 or 820–827 in different limbs should be coded according to the following list, which should be referred to in the following priority order: skull or face bones, pelvis or vertebral column, legs, arms.

   arm (multiple bones in same arm except in hand alone) (sites classifiable to 810–817 with sites classifiable to a different three–digit category in 810–817 in same arm) (closed) 818.0
      open 818.1
   arms, both or arm(s) with rib(s) or sternum (sites classifiable to 810–818 with sites classifiable to same range of categories in other limb or to 807) (closed) 819.0
      open 819.1
   bones of trunk NEC (closed) 809.0
      open 809.1
   hand, metacarpal bone(s) with phalanx or phalanges of same hand (sites classifiable to 815 with sites classifiable to 816 in same hand) (closed) 817.0
      open 817.1
   leg (multiple bones in same leg) (sites classifiable to 820–826 with sites classifiable to a different three–digit category in that range in same leg) (closed) 827.0
      open 827.1
   legs, both or leg(s) with arm(s), rib(s), or sternum (sites classifiable to 820–827 with sites classifiable to same range of categories in other leg or to 807 or 810–819) (closed) 828.0
      open 828.1
   open 829.1
   pelvis with other bones except skull or face bones (sites classifiable to 808 with sites classifiable to 805–807 or 810–829) (closed) 809.0
      open 809.1

Fracture — continued
multiple — continued
   skull, specified or unspecified bones, or face bone(s) with any other bone(s) (sites classifiable to 800–803 with sites classifiable to 805–829) (closed) 804.0 ☑

Note — Use the following fifth-digit subclassification with categories 800, 801, 803, and 804:

0   unspecified state of consciousness

1   with no loss of consciousness

2   with brief [less than one hour] loss of consciousness

3   with moderate [1–24 hours] loss of consciousness

4   with prolonged [more than 24 hours] loss of consciousness and return to pre–existing conscious level

5   with prolonged [more than 24 hours] loss of consciousness, without return to pre–existing conscious level

Use fifth-digit 5 to designate when a patient is unconscious and dies before regaining consciousness, regardless of the duration of the loss of consciousness

6   with loss of consciousness of un-specified duration

9   with concussion, unspecified

   with
      contusion, cerebral 804.1 ☑
      epidural hemorrhage 804.2 ☑
      extradural hemorrhage 804.2 ☑
      hemorrhage (intracranial) NEC 804.3 ☑
      intracranial injury NEC 804.4 ☑
      laceration, cerebral 804.1 ☑
      subarachnoid hemorrhage 804.2 ☑
      subdural hemorrhage 804.2 ☑
   open 804.5 ☑
      with
         contusion, cerebral 804.6 ☑
         epidural hemorrhage 804.7 ☑
         extradural hemorrhage 804.7 ☑
         hemorrhage (intracranial) NEC 804.8 ☑
         intracranial injury NEC 804.9 ☑
         laceration, cerebral 804.6 ☑
         subarachnoid hemorrhage 804.7 ☑
         subdural hemorrhage 804.7 ☑
   vertebral column with other bones, except skull or face bones (sites classifiable to 805 or 806 with sites classifiable to 807–808 or 810–829) (closed) 809.0
      open 809.1
nasal (bone(s)) (closed) 802.0
   open 802.1
   sinus — see Fracture, skull, base
navicular
   carpal (wrist) (closed) 814.01
      open 814.11
   tarsal (ankle) (closed) 825.22
      open 825.32
neck — see Fracture, vertebra, cervical
neural arch — see Fracture, vertebra, by site
nonunion 733.82
nose, nasal, (bone) (septum) (closed) 802.0
   open 802.1
occiput — see Fracture, skull, base
odontoid process — see Fracture, vertebra, cervical
olecranon (process) (ulna) (closed) 813.01

☑ Additional Digit Required — Refer to the Tabular List for Digit Selection   ✔ Subterms under main terms may continue to next column or page

122 — Volume 2   ▶◀ Revised Text   ● New Line   ▲ Revised Code   2015 ICD-9-CM

Fracture — *continued*
  olecranon — *continued*
    open 813.11
  open 829.1
  orbit, orbital (bone) (region) (closed) 802.8
    floor (blow-out) 802.6
      open 802.7
    open 802.9
    roof — *see* Fracture, skull, base
    specified part NEC 802.8
      open 802.9
  os
    calcis (closed) 825.0
      open 825.1
    magnum (closed) 814.07
      open 814.17
    pubis (with visceral injury) (closed) 808.2
      open 808.3
    triquetrum (closed) 814.03
      open 814.13
  osseous
    auditory meatus — *see* Fracture, skull, base
    labyrinth — *see* Fracture, skull, base
    ossicles, auditory (incus) (malleus) (stapes) — *see* Fracture, skull, base
  osteoporotic — *see* Fracture, pathologic
  palate (closed) 802.8
    open 802.9
  paratrooper — *see* Fracture, tibia, lower end
  parietal bone — *see* Fracture, skull, vault
  parry — *see* Fracture, Monteggia's
  patella (closed) 822.0
    open 822.1
  pathologic (cause unknown) 733.10
    ankle 733.16
    femur (neck) 733.14
      specified NEC 733.15
    fibula 733.16
    hip 733.14
    humerus 733.11
    radius (distal) 733.12
    specified site NEC 733.19
    tibia 733.16
    ulna 733.12
    vertebrae (collapse) 733.13
    wrist 733.12
  pedicle (of vertebral arch) — *see* Fracture, vertebra, by site
  pelvis, pelvic (bone(s)) (with visceral injury) (closed) 808.8
    multiple
      with
        disruption of pelvic circle 808.43
          open 808.53
        disruption of pelvic ring 808.43
          open 808.53
      without
        disruption of pelvic circle 808.44
          open 808.54
        disruption of pelvic ring 808.44
          open 808.54
    open 808.9
    rim (closed) 808.49
      open 808.59
    stress 733.98
  peritrochanteric (closed) 820.20
    open 820.30
  phalanx, phalanges, of one
    foot (closed) 826.0
      with bone(s) of same lower limb 827.0
        open 827.1
      open 826.1
    hand (closed) 816.00
      with metacarpal bone(s) of same hand 817.0
        open 817.1
      distal 816.02
        open 816.12
      middle 816.01
        open 816.11
      multiple sites NEC 816.03
        open 816.13
      open 816.10
      proximal 816.01

Fracture — *continued*
  phalanx, phalanges, of one — *continued*
    hand — *continued*
      proximal — *continued*
        open 816.11
  pisiform (closed) 814.04
    open 814.14
  pond — *see* Fracture, skull, vault
  Pott's (closed) 824.4
    open 824.5
  prosthetic device, internal — *see* Complications, mechanical
  pubis (with visceral injury) (closed) 808.2
    open 808.3
  Quervain's (closed) 814.01
    open 814.11
  radius (alone) (closed) 813.81
    with ulna NEC 813.83
      open 813.93
    distal end — *see* Fracture, radius, lower end
    epiphysis
      lower — *see* Fracture, radius, lower end
      upper — *see* Fracture, radius, upper end
    head — *see* Fracture, radius, upper end
    lower end or extremity (distal end) (lower epiphysis) 813.42
      with ulna (lower end) 813.44
        open 813.54
      open 813.52
      torus 813.45
        with ulna 813.47
    neck — *see* Fracture, radius, upper end
    open NEC 813.91
    pathologic 733.12
    proximal end — *see* Fracture, radius, upper end
    shaft (closed) 813.21
      with ulna (shaft) 813.23
        open 813.33
      open 813.31
    upper end 813.07
      with ulna (upper end) 813.08
        open 813.18
      epiphysis 813.05
        open 813.15
      head 813.05
        open 813.15
      multiple sites 813.07
        open 813.17
      neck 813.06
        open 813.16
      open 813.17
      specified site NEC 813.07
        open 813.17
  ramus
    inferior or superior (with visceral injury) (closed) 808.2
      open 808.3
    ischium — *see* Fracture, ischium
    mandible 802.24
      open 802.34
  rib(s) (closed) 807.0 ☑

Note — *Use the following fifth-digit subclassification with categories 807.0–807.1:*

0   rib(s), unspecified

1   one rib

2   two ribs

3   three ribs

4   four ribs

5   five ribs

6   six ribs

7   seven ribs

8   eight or more ribs

9   multiple ribs, unspecified

    with flail chest (open) 807.4
    open 807.1 ☑
  root, tooth 873.63

Fracture — *continued*
  root, tooth — *continued*
    complicated 873.73
  sacrum — *see* Fracture, vertebra, sacrum
  scaphoid
    ankle (closed) 825.22
      open 825.32
    wrist (closed) 814.01
      open 814.11
  scapula (closed) 811.00
    acromial, acromion (process) 811.01
      open 811.11
    body 811.09
      open 811.19
    coracoid process 811.02
      open 811.12
    glenoid (cavity) (fossa) 811.03
      open 811.13
    neck 811.03
      open 811.13
    open 811.10
  semilunar
    bone, wrist (closed) 814.02
      open 814.12
    cartilage (interior) (knee) — *see* Tear, meniscus
  sesamoid bone — *see* Fracture, by site
  Shepherd's (closed) 825.21
    open 825.31
  shoulder (*see also* Fracture, humerus, upper end)
    blade — *see* Fracture, scapula
  silverfork — *see* Fracture, radius, lower end
  sinus (ethmoid) (frontal) (maxillary) (nasal) (sphenoidal) — *see* Fracture, skull, base
  Skillern's — *see* Fracture, radius, shaft
  skull (multiple NEC) (with face bones) (closed) 803.0 ☑

Note — *Use the following fifth-digit subclassification with categories 800, 801, 803, and 804:*

0   *unspecified state of consciousness*

1   *with no loss of consciousness*

2   *with brief [less than one hour] loss of consciousness*

3   *with moderate [1-24 hours] loss of consciousness*

4   *with prolonged [more than 24 hours] loss of consciousness and return to pre-existing conscious level*

5   *with prolonged [more than 24 hours] loss of consciousness, without return to pre-existing conscious level*

Use fifth-digit 5 to designate when a patient is unconscious and dies before regaining consciousness, regardless of the duration of the loss of consciousness

6   *with loss of consciousness of unspecified duration*

9   *with concussion, unspecified*

    with
      contusion, cerebral 803.1 ☑
      epidural hemorrhage 803.2 ☑
      extradural hemorrhage 803.2 ☑
      hemorrhage (intracranial) NEC 803.3 ☑
      intracranial injury NEC 803.4 ☑
      laceration, cerebral 803.1 ☑
      other bones — *see* Fracture, multiple, skull
      subarachnoid hemorrhage 803.2 ☑
      subdural hemorrhage 803.2 ☑
    base (antrum) (ethmoid bone) (fossa) (internal ear) (nasal sinus) (occiput) (sphenoid) (temporal bone) (closed) 801.0 ☑

Fracture — *continued*
  skull — *continued*
    base — *continued*
      with
        contusion, cerebral 801.1 ☑
        epidural hemorrhage 801.2 ☑
        extradural hemorrhage 801.2 ☑
        hemorrhage (intracranial) NEC 801.3 ☑
        intracranial injury NEC 801.4 ☑
        laceration, cerebral 801.1 ☑
        subarachnoid hemorrhage 801.2 ☑
        subdural hemorrhage 801.2 ☑
      open 801.5 ☑
        with
          contusion, cerebral 801.6 ☑
          epidural hemorrhage 801.7 ☑
          extradural hemorrhage 801.7 ☑
          hemorrhage (intracranial) NEC 801.8 ☑
          intracranial injury NEC 801.9 ☑
          laceration, cerebral 801.6 ☑
          subarachnoid hemorrhage 801.7 ☑
          subdural hemorrhage 801.7 ☑
    birth injury 767.3
    face bones — *see* Fracture, face bones
    open 803.5 ☑
      with
        contusion, cerebral 803.6 ☑
        epidural hemorrhage 803.7 ☑
        extradural hemorrhage 803.7 ☑
        hemorrhage (intracranial) NEC 803.8 ☑
        intracranial injury NEC 803.9 ☑
        laceration, cerebral 803.6 ☑
        subarachnoid hemorrhage 803.7 ☑
        subdural hemorrhage 803.7 ☑
    vault (frontal bone) (parietal bone) (vertex) (closed) 800.0 ☑
      with
        contusion, cerebral 800.1 ☑
        epidural hemorrhage 800.2 ☑
        extradural hemorrhage 800.2 ☑
        hemorrhage (intracranial) NEC 800.3 ☑
        intracranial injury NEC 800.4 ☑
        laceration, cerebral 800.1 ☑
        subarachnoid hemorrhage 800.2 ☑
        subdural hemorrhage 800.2 ☑
      open 800.5 ☑
        with
          contusion, cerebral 800.6 ☑
          epidural hemorrhage 800.7 ☑
          extradural hemorrhage 800.7 ☑
          hemorrhage (intracranial) NEC 800.8 ☑
          intracranial injury NEC 800.9 ☑
          laceration, cerebral 800.6 ☑
          subarachnoid hemorrhage 800.7 ☑
          subdural hemorrhage 800.7 ☑
  Smith's 813.41
    open 813.51
  sphenoid (bone) (sinus) — *see* Fracture, skull, base
  spine (*see also* Fracture, vertebra, by site due to birth trauma) 767.4
  spinous process — *see* Fracture, vertebra, by site
  spontaneous — *see* Fracture, pathologic
  sprinters' — *see* Fracture, ilium
  stapes — *see* Fracture, skull, base

☑ **Additional Digit Required** — Refer to the Tabular List for Digit Selection   ▽ **Subterms under main terms may continue to next column or page**

Fracture — Fracture

Fracture — *continued*

stave (*see also* Fracture, metacarpus, metacarpal bone(s))
   spine — *see* Fracture, tibia, upper end
sternum (closed) 807.2
   with flail chest (open) 807.4
   open 807.3
Stieda's — *see* Fracture, femur, lower end
stress 733.95
   femoral neck 733.96
   fibula 733.93
   metatarsals 733.94
   pelvis 733.98
   shaft of femur 733.97
   specified site NEC 733.95
   tibia 733.93
styloid process
   metacarpal (closed) 815.02
      open 815.12
   radius — *see* Fracture, radius, lower end
   temporal bone — *see* Fracture, skull, base
   ulna — *see* Fracture, ulna, lower end
supracondylar, elbow 812.41
   open 812.51
symphysis pubis (with visceral injury) (closed) 808.2
   open 808.3
talus (ankle bone) (closed) 825.21
   open 825.31
tarsus, tarsal bone(s) (with metatarsus) of one foot (closed) NEC 825.29
   open 825.39
temporal bone (styloid) — *see* Fracture, skull, base
tendon — *see* Sprain, by site
thigh — *see* Fracture, femur, shaft
thumb (and finger(s)) of one hand (closed) (*see also* Fracture, phalanx, hand) 816.00
   with metacarpal bone(s) of same hand 817.0
      open 817.1
   metacarpal(s) — *see* Fracture, metacarpus
   open 816.10
thyroid cartilage (closed) 807.5
   open 807.6
tibia (closed) 823.80
   with fibula 823.82
      open 823.92
   condyles — *see* Fracture, tibia, upper end
   distal end 824.8
      open 824.9
   epiphysis
      lower 824.8
         open 824.9
      upper — *see* Fracture, tibia, upper end
   head (involving knee joint) — *see* Fracture, tibia, upper end
   intercondyloid eminence — *see* Fracture, tibia, upper end
   involving ankle 824.0
      open 824.9
   lower end or extremity (anterior lip) (posterior lip) 824.8
      open 824.9
   malleolus (internal) (medial) 824.0
      open 824.1
   open NEC 823.90
   pathologic 733.16
   proximal end — *see* Fracture, tibia, upper end
   shaft 823.20
      with fibula 823.22
         open 823.32
      open 823.30
   spine — *see* Fracture, tibia, upper end
   stress 733.93
   torus 823.40
      with fibula 823.42
   tuberosity — *see* Fracture, tibia, upper end

Fracture — *continued*

tibia — *continued*
   upper end or extremity (condyle) (epiphysis) (head) (spine) (proximal end) (tuberosity) 823.00
      with fibula 823.02
         open 823.12
      open 823.10
toe(s), of one foot (closed) 826.0
   with bone(s) of same lower limb 827.0
      open 827.1
   open 826.1
tooth (root) 873.63
   complicated 873.73
torus
   fibula 823.41
      with tibia 823.42
   humerus 812.49
   radius (alone) 813.45
      with ulna 813.47
   tibia 823.40
      with fibula 823.42
   ulna (alone) 813.46
      with radius 813.47
trachea (closed) 807.5
   open 807.6
transverse process — *see* Fracture, vertebra, by site
trapezium (closed) 814.05
   open 814.15
trapezoid bone (closed) 814.06
   open 814.16
trimalleolar (closed) 824.6
   open 824.7
triquetral (bone) (closed) 814.03
   open 814.13
trochanter (greater) (lesser) (closed) (*see also* Fracture, femur, neck, by site) 820.20
   open 820.30
trunk (bones) (closed) 809.0
   open 809.1
tuberosity (external) — *see* Fracture, by site
ulna (alone) (closed) 813.82
   with radius NEC 813.83
      open 813.93
   coronoid process (closed) 813.02
      open 813.12
   distal end — *see* Fracture, ulna, lower end
   epiphysis
      lower — *see* Fracture, ulna, lower end
      upper — *see* Fracture, ulna, upper end
   head — *see* Fracture, ulna, lower end
   lower end (distal end) (head) (lower epiphysis) (styloid process) 813.43
      with radius (lower end) 813.44
         open 813.54
      open 813.53
   olecranon process (closed) 813.01
      open 813.11
   open NEC 813.92
   pathologic 733.12
   proximal end — *see* Fracture, ulna, upper end
   shaft 813.22
      with radius (shaft) 813.23
         open 813.33
      open 813.32
   styloid process — *see* Fracture, ulna, lower end
   torus 813.46
      with radius 813.47
   transverse — *see* Fracture, ulna, by site
   upper end (epiphysis) 813.04
      with radius (upper end) 813.08
         open 813.18
      multiple sites 813.04
         open 813.14
      specified site NEC 813.04
         open 813.14
unciform (closed) 814.08
   open 814.18

Fracture — *continued*

vertebra, vertebral (back) (body) (column) (neural arch) (pedicle) (spine) (spinous process) (transverse process) (closed) 805.8
   with
      hematomyelia — *see* Fracture, vertebra, by site, with spinal cord injury
      injury to
         cauda equina — *see* Fracture, vertebra, sacrum, with spinal cord injury
         nerve — *see* Fracture, vertebra, by site, with spinal cord injury
      paralysis — *see* Fracture, vertebra, by site, with spinal cord injury
      paraplegia — *see* Fracture, vertebra, by site, with spinal cord injury
      quadriplegia — *see* Fracture, vertebra, by site, with spinal cord injury
      spinal concussion — *see* Fracture, vertebra, by site, with spinal cord injury
      spinal cord injury (closed) NEC 806.8

> *Note* — *Use the following fifth-digit subclassification with categories 806.0–806.3:*
>
> C_1–C_4 *or unspecified level and* D_1–D_6 (T_1–T_6) *or unspecified level with*
>
> 0   *unspecified spinal cord injury*
> 1   *complete lesion of cord*
> 2   *anterior cord syndrome*
> 3   *central cord syndrome*
> 4   *specified injury NEC*
>
> C_5–C_7 *level and* D_7–D_{12} *level with:*
>
> 5   *unspecified spinal cord injury*
> 6   *complete lesion of cord*
> 7   *anterior cord syndrome*
> 8   *central cord syndrome*
> 9   *specified injury NEC*

      cervical 806.0 ☑
         open 806.1 ☑
      dorsal, dorsolumbar 806.2 ☑
         open 806.3 ☑
      open 806.9
      thoracic, thoracolumbar 806.2 ☑
         open 806.3 ☑
   atlanto-axial — *see* Fracture, vertebra, cervical
   cervical (hangman) (teardrop) (closed) 805.00
      with spinal cord injury — *see* Fracture, vertebra, with spinal cord injury, cervical
      first (atlas) 805.01
         open 805.11
      second (axis) 805.02
         open 805.12
      third 805.03
         open 805.13
      fourth 805.04
         open 805.14
      fifth 805.05
         open 805.15
      sixth 805.06
         open 805.16
      seventh 805.07
         open 805.17
      multiple sites 805.08
         open 805.18
      open 805.10
   chronic 733.13
   coccyx (closed) 805.6
      with spinal cord injury (closed) 806.60
         cauda equina injury 806.62

Fracture — *continued*

vertebra, vertebral — *continued*
   coccyx — *continued*
      with spinal cord injury — *continued*
         cauda equina injury — *continued*
            complete lesion 806.61
               open 806.71
            open 806.72
         open 806.70
         specified type NEC 806.69
            open 806.79
      open 805.7
   collapsed 733.13
   compression, not due to trauma 733.13
   dorsal (closed) 805.2
      with spinal cord injury — *see* Fracture, vertebra, with spinal cord injury, dorsal
      open 805.3
   dorsolumbar (closed) 805.2
      with spinal cord injury — *see* Fracture, vertebra, with spinal cord injury, dorsal
      open 805.3
   due to osteoporosis 733.13
   fetus or newborn 767.4
   lumbar (closed) 805.4
      with spinal cord injury (closed) 806.4
         open 806.5
      open 805.5
   nontraumatic 733.13
   open NEC 805.9
   pathologic (any site) 733.13
   sacrum (closed) 805.6
      with spinal cord injury 806.60
         cauda equina injury 806.62
            complete lesion 806.61
               open 806.71
            open 806.72
         open 806.70
         specified type NEC 806.69
            open 806.79
      open 805.7
   site unspecified (closed) 805.8
      with spinal cord injury (closed) 806.8
         open 806.9
      open 805.9
   stress (any site) 733.95
   thoracic (closed) 805.2
      with spinal cord injury — *see* Fracture, vertebra, with spinal cord injury, thoracic
      open 805.3
   vertex — *see* Fracture, skull, vault
   vomer (bone) 802.0
      open 802.1
   Wagstaffe's — *see* Fracture, ankle
   wrist (closed) 814.00
      open 814.10
      pathologic 733.12
   xiphoid (process) — *see* Fracture, sternum
   zygoma (zygomatic arch) (closed) 802.4
      open 802.5

Fragile X syndrome 759.83

Fragilitas
   crinium 704.2
   hair 704.2
   ossium 756.51
      with blue sclera 756.51
   unguium 703.8
      congenital 757.5

Fragility
   bone 756.51
      with deafness and blue sclera 756.51
   capillary (hereditary) 287.8
   hair 704.2
   nails 703.8

Fragmentation — *see* Fracture, by site

Frailty 797

Frambesia, frambesial (tropica) — *see also* Yaws 102.9
   initial lesion or ulcer 102.0
   primary 102.0

☑ **Additional Digit Required** — Refer to the Tabular List for Digit Selection   ▽ **Subterms under main terms may continue to next column or page**

124 — Volume 2   ▶◀ Revised Text   ● New Line   ▲ Revised Code   2015 ICD-9-CM

Frambeside
  gummatous 102.4
  of early yaws 102.2
Frambesioma 102.1
Franceschetti's syndrome (mandibulofacial dysostosis) 756.0
Francis' disease — *see also* Tularemia 021.9
Franklin's disease (heavy chain) 273.2
Frank's essential thrombocytopenia — *see also* Purpura, thrombocytopenic 287.39
Fraser's syndrome 759.89
Freckle 709.09
  malignant melanoma in (M8742/3) — *see* Melanoma
  melanotic (of Hutchinson) (M8742/2) — *see* Neoplasm, skin, in situ
  retinal 239.81
Freeman-Sheldon syndrome 759.89
Freezing 991.9
  specified effect NEC 991.8
Freiberg's
  disease (osteochondrosis, second metatarsal) 732.5
  infraction of metatarsal head 732.5
  osteochondrosis 732.5
Frei's disease (climatic bubo) 099.1
Fremitus, friction, cardiac 785.3
Frenulum linguae 750.0
Frenum
  external os 752.44
  tongue 750.0
Frequency (urinary) NEC 788.41
  micturition 788.41
  nocturnal 788.43
  polyuria 788.42
  psychogenic 306.53
Frey's syndrome (auriculotemporal syndrome) 705.22
Friction
  burn (*see also* Injury, superficial, by site) 919.0
  fremitus, cardiac 785.3
  precordial 785.3
  sounds, chest 786.7
Friderichsen-Waterhouse syndrome or disease 036.3
Friedländer's
  B (bacillus) NEC (*see also* condition) 041.3
    sepsis or septicemia 038.49
  disease (endarteritis obliterans) — *see* Arteriosclerosis
Friedreich's
  ataxia 334.0
  combined systemic disease 334.0
  disease 333.2
    combined systemic 334.0
  myoclonia 333.2
  sclerosis (spinal cord) 334.0
Friedrich-Erb-Arnold syndrome (acropachyderma) 757.39
Frigidity 302.72
  psychic or psychogenic 302.72
Fröhlich's disease or syndrome (adiposogenital dystrophy) 253.8
Froin's syndrome 336.8
Frommel-Chiari syndrome 676.6 ☑
Frommel's disease 676.6 ☑
Frontal — *see also* condition
  lobe syndrome 310.0

Frostbite 991.3
  face 991.0
  foot 991.2
  hand 991.1
  specified site NEC 991.3
Frotteurism 302.89
Frozen 991.9
  pelvis 620.8
  shoulder 726.0
Fructosemia 271.2
Fructosuria (benign) (essential) 271.2
Fuchs'
  black spot (myopic) 360.21
  corneal dystrophy (endothelial) 371.57
  heterochromic cyclitis 364.21
Fucosidosis 271.8
Fugue 780.99
  dissociative 300.13
  hysterical (dissociative) 300.13
  reaction to exceptional stress (transient) 308.1
Fukuhara syndrome 277.87
Fuller Albright's syndrome (osteitis fibrosa disseminata) 756.59
Fuller's earth disease 502
Fulminant, fulminating — *see* condition
Functional — *see* condition
Functioning
  borderline intellectual V62.89
Fundus — *see also* condition
  flavimaculatus 362.76
Fungemia 117.9
Fungus, fungous
  cerebral 348.89
  disease NEC 117.9
  infection — *see* Infection, fungus
  testis (*see also* Tuberculosis) 016.5 ☑ *[608.81]*
Funiculitis (acute) 608.4
  chronic 608.4
  endemic 608.4
  gonococcal (acute) 098.14
    chronic or duration of 2 months or over 098.34
  tuberculous (*see also* Tuberculosis) 016.5 ☑
Funnel
  breast (acquired) 738.3
    congenital 754.81
    late effect of rickets 268.1
  chest (acquired) 738.3
    congenital 754.81
    late effect of rickets 268.1
  pelvis (acquired) 738.6
    with disproportion (fetopelvic) 653.3 ☑
      affecting fetus or newborn 763.1
    causing obstructed labor 660.1 ☑
      affecting fetus or newborn 763.1
    congenital 755.69
    tuberculous (*see also* Tuberculosis) 016.9 ☑
FUO — *see also* Pyrexia 780.60
Furfur 690.18
  microsporon 111.0
Furor, paroxysmal (idiopathic) — *see also* Epilepsy 345.8 ☑
Furriers' lung 495.8
Furrowed tongue 529.5
  congenital 750.13
Furrowing nail(s) (transverse) 703.8

Furrowing nail(s) — *continued*
  congenital 757.5
Furuncle 680.9
  abdominal wall 680.2
  ankle 680.6
  anus 680.5
  arm (any part, above wrist) 680.3
  auditory canal, external 680.0
  axilla 680.3
  back (any part) 680.2
  breast 680.2
  buttock 680.5
  chest wall 680.2
  corpus cavernosum 607.2
  ear (any part) 680.0
  eyelid 373.13
  face (any part, except eye) 680.0
  finger (any) 680.4
  flank 680.2
  foot (any part) 680.7
  forearm 680.3
  gluteal (region) 680.5
  groin 680.2
  hand (any part) 680.4
  head (any part, except face) 680.8
  heel 680.7
  hip 680.6
  kidney (*see also* Abscess, kidney) 590.2
  knee 680.6
  labium (majus) (minus) 616.4
  lacrimal
    gland (*see also* Dacryoadenitis) 375.00
    passages (duct) (sac) (*see also* Dacryocystitis) 375.30
  leg, any part except foot 680.6
  malignant 022.0
  multiple sites 680.9
  neck 680.1
  nose (external) (septum) 680.0
  orbit 376.01
  partes posteriores 680.5
  pectoral region 680.2
  penis 607.2
  perineum 680.2
  pinna 680.0
  scalp (any part) 680.8
  scrotum 608.4
  seminal vesicle 608.0
  shoulder 680.3
  skin NEC 680.9
  specified site NEC 680.8
  spermatic cord 608.4
  temple (region) 680.0
  testis 604.90
  thigh 680.6
  thumb 680.4
  toe (any) 680.7
  trunk 680.2
  tunica vaginalis 608.4
  umbilicus 680.2
  upper arm 680.3
  vas deferens 608.4
  vulva 616.4
  wrist 680.4
Furunculosis — *see also* Furuncle 680.9
  external auditory meatus 680.0 *[380.13]*
Fusarium (infection) 118
Fusion, fused (congenital)
  anal (with urogenital canal) 751.5

Fusion, fused — *continued*
  aorta and pulmonary artery 745.0
  astragaloscaphoid 755.67
  atria 745.5
  atrium and ventricle 745.69
  auditory canal 744.02
  auricles, heart 745.5
  binocular, with defective stereopsis 368.33
  bone 756.9
  cervical spine — *see* Fusion, spine
  choanal 748.0
  commissure, mitral valve 746.5
  cranial sutures, premature 756.0
  cusps, heart valve NEC 746.89
    mitral 746.5
    tricuspid 746.89
  ear ossicles 744.04
  fingers (*see also* Syndactylism, fingers) 755.11
  hymen 752.42
  hymeno-urethral 599.89
    causing obstructed labor 660.1 ☑
      affecting fetus or newborn 763.1
  joint (acquired) (*see also* Ankylosis)
    congenital 755.8
  kidneys (incomplete) 753.3
  labium (majus) (minus) 752.49
  larynx and trachea 748.3
  limb 755.8
    lower 755.69
    upper 755.59
  lobe, lung 748.5
  lumbosacral (acquired) 724.6
    congenital 756.15
    surgical V45.4
  nares (anterior) (posterior) 748.0
  nose, nasal 748.0
  nostril(s) 748.0
  organ or site NEC — *see* Anomaly, specified type NEC
  ossicles 756.9
    auditory 744.04
  pulmonary valve segment 746.02
  pulmonic cusps 746.02
  ribs 756.3
  sacroiliac (acquired) (joint) 724.6
    congenital 755.69
    surgical V45.4
  skull, imperfect 756.0
  spine (acquired) 724.9
    arthrodesis status V45.4
    congenital (vertebra) 756.15
    postoperative status V45.4
  sublingual duct with submaxillary duct at opening in mouth 750.26
  talonavicular (bar) 755.67
  teeth, tooth 520.2
  testes 752.89
  toes (*see also* Syndactylism, toes) 755.13
  trachea and esophagus 750.3
  twins 759.4
  urethral-hymenal 599.89
  vagina 752.49
  valve cusps — *see* Fusion, cusps, heart valve
  ventricles, heart 745.4
  vertebra (arch) — *see* Fusion, spine
  vulva 752.49
Fusospirillosis (mouth) (tongue) (tonsil) 101
Fussy infant (baby) 780.91

☑ **Additional Digit Required** — Refer to the Tabular List for Digit Selection   ▽ **Subterms under main terms may continue to next column or page**

G

Gafsa boil 085.1
Gain, weight (abnormal) (excessive) — *see also* Weight, gain 783.1
Gaisböck's disease or syndrome (polycythemia hypertonica) 289.0
Gait
  abnormality 781.2
    hysterical 300.11
  ataxic 781.2
    hysterical 300.11
  disturbance 781.2
    hysterical 300.11
  paralytic 781.2
  scissor 781.2
  spastic 781.2
  staggering 781.2
    hysterical 300.11
Galactocele (breast) (infected) 611.5
  puerperal, postpartum 676.8 ☑
Galactophoritis 611.0
  puerperal, postpartum 675.2 ☑
Galactorrhea 676.6 ☑
  not associated with childbirth 611.6
Galactosemia (classic) (congenital) 271.1
Galactosuria 271.1
Galacturia 791.1
  bilharziasis 120.0
Galen's vein — *see* condition
Gallbladder — *see also* condition
  acute (*see also* Disease, gallbladder) 575.0
Gall duct — *see* condition
Gallop rhythm 427.89
Gallstone (cholemic) (colic) (impacted) — *see also* Cholelithiasis
  causing intestinal obstruction 560.31
Gambling, pathological 312.31
Gammaloidosis 277.39
Gammopathy 273.9
  macroglobulinemia 273.3
  monoclonal (benign) (essential) (idiopathic) (with lymphoplasmacytic dyscrasia) 273.1
Gamna's disease (siderotic splenomegaly) 289.51
Gampsodactylia (congenital) 754.71
Gamstorp's disease (adynamia episodica hereditaria) 359.3
Gandy-Nanta disease (siderotic splenomegaly) 289.51
Gang activity, without manifest psychiatric disorder V71.09
  adolescent V71.02
  adult V71.01
  child V71.02
Gangliocytoma (M9490/0) — *see* Neoplasm, connective tissue, benign
Ganglioglioma (M9505/1) — *see* Neoplasm, by site, uncertain behavior
Ganglion 727.43
  joint 727.41
  of yaws (early) (late) 102.6
  periosteal (*see also* Periostitis) 730.3 ☑
  tendon sheath (compound) (diffuse) 727.42
  tuberculous (*see also* Tuberculosis) 015.9 ☑
Ganglioneuroblastoma (M9490/3) — *see* Neoplasm, connective tissue, malignant
Ganglioneuroma (M9490/0) — *see also* Neoplasm, connective tissue, benign
  malignant (M9490/3) — *see* Neoplasm, connective tissue, malignant
Ganglioneuromatosis (M9491/0) — *see* Neoplasm, connective tissue, benign
Ganglionitis
  fifth nerve (*see also* Neuralgia, trigeminal) 350.1
  gasserian 350.1
  geniculate 351.1
    herpetic 053.11
    newborn 767.5
  herpes zoster 053.11
  herpetic geniculate (Hunt's syndrome) 053.11
Gangliosidosis 330.1
Gangosa 102.5

Gangrene, gangrenous (anemia) (artery) (cellulitis) (dermatitis) (dry) (infective) (moist) (pemphigus) (septic) (skin) (stasis) (ulcer) 785.4
  with
    arteriosclerosis (native artery) 440.24
      bypass graft 440.30
        autologous vein 440.31
        nonautologous biological 440.32
    diabetes (mellitus) 250.7 ☑ *[785.4]*
      due to secondary diabetes 249.7 ☑ *[785.4]*
  abdomen (wall) 785.4
  adenitis 683
  alveolar 526.5
  angina 462
    diphtheritic 032.0
  anus 569.49
  appendices epiploicae — *see* Gangrene, mesentery
  appendix — *see* Appendicitis, acute
  arteriosclerotic — *see* Arteriosclerosis, with, gangrene
  auricle 785.4
  Bacillus welchii (*see also* Gangrene, gas) 040.0
  bile duct (*see also* Cholangitis) 576.8
  bladder 595.89
  bowel — *see* Gangrene, intestine
  cecum — *see* Gangrene, intestine
  Clostridium perfringens or welchii (*see also* Gangrene, gas) 040.0
  colon — *see* Gangrene, intestine
  connective tissue 785.4
  cornea 371.40
  corpora cavernosa (infective) 607.2
    noninfective 607.89
  cutaneous, spreading 785.4
  decubital (*see also* Ulcer, pressure) 707.00 *[785.4]*
  diabetic (any site) 250.7 ☑ *[785.4]*
    due to secondary diabetes 249.7 ☑ *[785.4]*
  dropsical 785.4
  emphysematous (*see also* Gangrene, gas) 040.0
  epidemic (ergotized grain) 988.2
  epididymis (infectional) (*see also* Epididymitis) 604.99
  erysipelas (*see also* Erysipelas) 035
  extremity (lower) (upper) 785.4
  gallbladder or duct (*see also* Cholecystitis, acute) 575.0
  gas (bacillus) 040.0
    with
      abortion — *see* Abortion, by type, with sepsis
      ectopic pregnancy (*see also* categories 633.0–633.9) 639.0
      molar pregnancy (*see also* categories 630–632) 639.0
    following
      abortion 639.0
      ectopic or molar pregnancy 639.0
    puerperal, postpartum, childbirth 670.8 ☑
  glossitis 529.0
  gum 523.8
  hernia — *see* Hernia, by site, with gangrene
  hospital noma 528.1
  intestine, intestinal (acute) (hemorrhagic) (massive) 557.0
    with
      hernia — *see* Hernia, by site, with gangrene
      mesenteric embolism or infarction 557.0
      obstruction (*see also* Obstruction, intestine) 560.9
  laryngitis 464.00
    with obstruction 464.01
  liver 573.8
  lung 513.0
    spirochetal 104.8
  lymphangitis 457.2
  Meleney's (cutaneous) 686.09

Gangrene, gangrenous — *continued*
  mesentery 557.0
    with
      embolism or infarction 557.0
      intestinal obstruction (*see also* Obstruction, intestine) 560.9
  mouth 528.1
  noma 528.1
  orchitis 604.90
  ovary (*see also* Salpingo-oophoritis) 614.2
  pancreas 577.0
  penis (infectional) 607.2
    noninfective 607.89
  perineum 785.4
  pharynx 462
  pneumonia 513.0
  Pott's 440.24
  presenile 443.1
  pulmonary 513.0
  pulp, tooth 522.1
  quinsy 475
  Raynaud's (symmetric gangrene) 443.0 *[785.4]*
  rectum 569.49
  retropharyngeal 478.24
  rupture — *see* Hernia, by site, with gangrene
  scrotum 608.4
    noninfective 608.83
  senile 440.24
  septic 034.0
  septic 034.0
  sore throat 462
  spermatic cord 608.4
    noninfective 608.89
  spine 785.4
  spirochetal NEC 104.8
  spreading cutaneous 785.4
  stomach 537.89
  stomatitis 528.1
  symmetrical 443.0 *[785.4]*
  testis (infectional) (*see also* Orchitis) 604.99
    noninfective 608.89
  throat 462
    diphtheritic 032.0
  thyroid (gland) 246.8
  tonsillitis (acute) 463
  tooth (pulp) 522.1
  tuberculous NEC (*see also* Tuberculosis) 011.9 ☑
  tunica vaginalis 608.4
    noninfective 608.89
  umbilicus 785.4
  uterus (*see also* Endometritis) 615.9
  uvulitis 528.3
  vas deferens 608.4
    noninfective 608.89
  vulva (*see also* Vulvitis) 616.10
Gannister disease (occupational) 502
  with tuberculosis — *see* Tuberculosis, pulmonary
Ganser's syndrome, hysterical 300.16
Gardner-Diamond syndrome (autoerythrocyte sensitization) 287.2
Gargoylism 277.5
Garré's
  disease (*see also* Osteomyelitis) 730.1 ☑
  osteitis (sclerosing) (*see also* Osteomyelitis) 730.1 ☑
  osteomyelitis (*see also* Osteomyelitis) 730.1 ☑
Garrod's pads, knuckle 728.79
Gartner's duct
  cyst 752.41
  persistent 752.41
Gas 787.3
  asphyxia, asphyxiation, inhalation, poisoning, suffocation NEC 987.9
    specified gas — *see* Table of Drugs and Chemicals
  bacillus gangrene or infection — *see* Gas, gangrene
  cyst, mesentery 568.89
  excessive 787.3
  gangrene 040.0

Gas — *continued*
  gangrene — *continued*
    with
      abortion — *see* Abortion, by type, with sepsis
      ectopic pregnancy (*see also* categories 633.0–633.9) 639.0
      molar pregnancy (*see also* categories 630–632) 639.0
    following
      abortion 639.0
      ectopic or molar pregnancy 639.0
    puerperal, postpartum, childbirth 670.8 ☑
  on stomach 787.3
  pains 787.3
Gastradenitis 535.0 ☑
Gastralgia 536.8
  psychogenic 307.89
Gastrectasis, gastrectasia 536.1
  psychogenic 306.4
Gastric — *see* condition
Gastrinoma (M8153/1)
  malignant (M8153/3)
    pancreas 157.4
    specified site NEC — *see* Neoplasm, by site, malignant
    unspecified site 157.4
  specified site — *see* Neoplasm, by site, uncertain behavior
  unspecified site 235.5
Gastritis 535.5 ☑

> *Note* — Use the following fifth-digit subclassification for category 535:
> 0   without mention of hemorrhage
> 1   with hemorrhage

  acute 535.0 ☑
  alcoholic 535.3 ☑
  allergic 535.4 ☑
  antral 535.4 ☑
  atrophic 535.1 ☑
  atrophic-hyperplastic 535.1 ☑
  bile-induced 535.4 ☑
  catarrhal 535.0 ☑
  chronic (atrophic) 535.1 ☑
  cirrhotic 535.4 ☑
  corrosive (acute) 535.4 ☑
  dietetic 535.4 ☑
  due to diet deficiency 269.9 *[535.4]* ☑
  eosinophilic 535.7 ☑
  erosive 535.4 ☑
  follicular 535.4 ☑
    chronic 535.1 ☑
  giant hypertrophic 535.2 ☑
  glandular 535.4 ☑
    chronic 535.1 ☑
  hypertrophic (mucosa) 535.2 ☑
    chronic giant 211.1
  irritant 535.4 ☑
  nervous 306.4
  phlegmonous 535.0 ☑
  psychogenic 306.4
  sclerotic 535.4 ☑
  spastic 536.8
  subacute 535.0 ☑
  superficial 535.4 ☑
  suppurative 535.0 ☑
  toxic 535.4 ☑
  tuberculous (*see also* Tuberculosis) 017.9 ☑
Gastrocarcinoma (M8010/3) 151.9
Gastrocolic — *see* condition
Gastrocolitis — *see* Enteritis
Gastrodisciasis 121.8
Gastroduodenitis — *see also* Gastritis 535.5 ☑
  catarrhal 535.0 ☑
  infectional 535.0 ☑
  virus, viral 008.8
    specified type NEC 008.69
Gastrodynia 536.8
Gastroenteritis (acute) (catarrhal) (congestive) (hemorrhagic) (noninfectious) — *see also* Enteritis 558.9
  aertrycke infection 003.0

☑ Additional Digit Required — Refer to the Tabular List for Digit Selection   ᴺᴱᶜ Subterms under main terms may continue to next column or page

2015 ICD-9-CM   ▶◀ Revised Text   ● New Line   ▲ Revised Code   Volume 2 — 127

Gastroenteritis — *see also* Enteritis —
  continued
  allergic 558.3
  chronic 558.9
    ulcerative (*see also* Colitis, ulcerative)
      556.9
  dietetic 558.9
  due to
    antineoplastic chemotherapy 558.9
    food poisoning (*see also* Poisoning, food)
      005.9
    radiation 558.1
  eosinophilic 558.41
  epidemic 009.0
  functional 558.9
  infectious (*see also* Enteritis, due to, by or-
    ganism) 009.0
    presumed 009.1
  salmonella 003.0
  septic (*see also* Enteritis, due to, by organ-
    ism) 009.0
  toxic 558.2
  tuberculous (*see also* Tuberculosis) 014.8 ☑
  ulcerative (*see also* Colitis, ulcerative) 556.9
  viral NEC 008.8
    specified type NEC 008.69
  zymotic 009.0
Gastroenterocolitis — *see* Enteritis
Gastroenteropathy, protein-losing 579.8
Gastroenteroptosis 569.89
Gastroesophageal laceration-hemorrhage
  syndrome 530.7
Gastroesophagitis 530.19
Gastrohepatitis — *see also* Gastritis 535.5 ☑
Gastrointestinal — *see* condition
Gastrojejunal — *see* condition
Gastrojejunitis — *see also* Gastritis 535.5 ☑
Gastrojejunocolic — *see* condition
Gastroliths 537.89
Gastromalacia 537.89
Gastroparalysis 536.3
  diabetic 250.6 ☑ [536.3]
    due to secondary diabetes
      249.6 ☑ [536.3]
Gastroparesis 536.3
  diabetic 250.6 ☑ [536.3]
    due to secondary diabetes
      249.6 ☑ [536.3]
Gastropathy 537.9
  congestive portal 537.89
  erythematous 535.5 ☑
  exudative 579.8
  portal hypertensive 537.89
Gastroptosis 537.5
Gastrorrhagia 578.0
Gastrorrhea 536.8
  psychogenic 306.4
Gastroschisis (congenital) 756.73
  acquired 569.89
Gastrospasm (neurogenic) (reflex) 536.8
  neurotic 306.4
  psychogenic 306.4
Gastrostaxis 578.0
Gastrostenosis 537.89
Gastrostomy
  attention to V55.1
  complication 536.40
    specified type 536.49
  infection 536.41
  malfunctioning 536.42
  status V44.1
Gastrosuccorrhea (continuous) (intermittent)
  536.8
  neurotic 306.4
  psychogenic 306.4
Gaucher's
  disease (adult) (cerebroside lipidosis) (infan-
    tile) 272.7
  hepatomegaly 272.7
  splenomegaly (cerebroside lipidosis) 272.7
GAVE (gastric antral vascular ectasia) 537.82
  with hemorrhage 537.83
  without hemorrhage 537.82
Gayet's disease (superior hemorrhagic polioencephalitis) 265.1

Gayet-Wernicke's syndrome (superior hemorrhagic polioencephalitis) 265.1
Gee (-Herter) (-Heubner) (-Thaysen) disease
  or syndrome (nontropical sprue) 579.0
Gélineau's syndrome — *see also* Narcolepsy
  347.00
Gemination, teeth 520.2
Gemistocytoma (M9411/3)
  specified site — *see* Neoplasm, by site, ma-
    lignant
  unspecified site 191.9
General, generalized — *see* condtion
Genetic
  susceptibility to
    MEN (multiple endocrine neoplasia)
      V84.81
    neoplasia
      multiple endocrine (MEN) V84.81
    neoplasm
      malignant, of
        breast V84.01
        endometrium V84.04
        other V84.09
        ovary V84.02
        prostate V84.03
    specified disease NEC V84.89
Genital — *see* condition
  warts 078.11
Genito-anorectal syndrome 099.1
Genitourinary system — *see* condition
Genu
  congenital 755.64
  extrorsum (acquired) 736.42
    congenital 755.64
    late effects of rickets 268.1
  introrsum (acquired) 736.41
    congenital 755.64
    late effects of rickets 268.1
  rachitic (old) 268.1
  recurvatum (acquired) 736.5
    congenital 754.40
      with dislocation of knee 754.41
    late effects of rickets 268.1
  valgum (acquired) (knock-knee) 736.41
    congenital 755.64
    late effects of rickets 268.1
  varum (acquired) (bowleg) 736.42
    congenital 755.64
    late effect of rickets 268.1
Geographic tongue 529.1
Geophagia 307.52
Geotrichosis 117.9
  intestine 117.9
  lung 117.9
  mouth 117.9
Gephyrophobia 300.29
Gerbode defect 745.4
GERD (gastroesophageal reflux disease) 530.81
Gerhardt's
  disease (erythromelalgia) 443.82
  syndrome (vocal cord paralysis) 478.30
Gerlier's disease (epidemic vertigo) 078.81
German measles 056.9
  exposure to V01.4
Germinoblastoma (diffuse) (M9614/3)
  202.8 ☑
  follicular (M9692/3) 202.0 ☑
Germinoma (M9064/3) — *see* Neoplasm, by
  site, malignant
Gerontoxon 371.41
Gerstmann-Sträussler-Scheinker syndrome
  (GSS) 046.71
Gerstmann's syndrome (finger agnosia)
  784.69
Gestation (period) — *see also* Pregnancy
  ectopic NEC (*see also* Pregnancy, ectopic)
    633.90
    with intrauterine pregnancy 633.91
  multiple
    placenta status
      quadruplet
        two or more monoamniotic fetus-
          es V91.22
        two or more monochorionic fetus-
          es V91.21

Gestation — *see also* Pregnancy —
  continued
  multiple — *continued*
    placenta status — *continued*
      quadruplet — *continued*
        unable to determine number of
          placenta and number of
          amniotic sacs V91.29
        unspecified number of placenta
          and unspecified number
          of amniotic sacs V91.20
      specified (greater than quadruplets)
        NEC
      two or more monoamniotic fetus-
        es V91.92
      two or more monochorionic fetus-
        es V91.91
      unable to determine number of
        placenta and number of
        amniotic sacs V91.99
      unspecified number of placenta
        and unspecified number
        of amniotic sacs V91.90
    triplet
      two or more monoamniotic fetus-
        es V91.12
      two or more monochorionic fetus-
        es V91.11
      unable to determine number of
        placenta and number of
        amniotic sacs V91.19
      unspecified number of placenta,
        unspecified number of
        amniotic sacs V91.10
    twin
      dichorionic/diamniotic (two pla-
        centae, two amniotic sacs)
        V91.03
      monochorionic/diamniotic (one
        placenta, two amniotic
        sacs) V91.02
      monochorionic/monoamniotic
        (one placenta, one amniot-
        ic sac) V91.01
      unable to determine number of
        placenta and number of
        amniotic sacs V91.09
      unspecified number of placenta,
        unspecified number of
        amniotic sacs V91.00
Gestational proteinuria 646.2 ☑
  with hypertension — *see* Toxemia, of preg-
    nancy
Ghon tubercle primary infection — *see also*
  Tuberculosis 010.0 ☑
Ghost
  teeth 520.4
  vessels, cornea 370.64
Ghoul hand 102.3
Gianotti Crosti syndrome 057.8
  due to known virus — *see* Infection, virus
  due to unknown virus 057.8
Giant
  cell
    epulis 523.8
    peripheral (gingiva) 523.8
    tumor, tendon sheath 727.02
  colon (congenital) 751.3
  esophagus (congenital) 750.4
  kidney 753.3
  urticaria 995.1
    hereditary 277.6
Giardia lamblia infestation 007.1
Giardiasis 007.1
Gibert's disease (pityriasis rosea) 696.3
Gibraltar fever — *see* Brucellosis
Giddiness 780.4
  hysterical 300.11
  psychogenic 306.9
Gierke's disease (glycogenosis I) 271.0
Gigantism (cerebral) (hypophyseal) (pituitary)
  253.0
Gilbert's disease or cholemia (familial nonhemolytic jaundice) 277.4
Gilchrist's disease (North American blastomy-
  cosis) 116.0

Gilford (-Hutchinson) disease or syndrome
  (progeria) 259.8
Gilles de la Tourette's disease (motor-verbal
  tic) 307.23
Gillespie's syndrome (dysplasia oculodentodigitalis) 759.89
Gingivitis 523.10
  acute 523.00
    necrotizing 101
    non-plaque induced 523.01
    plaque induced 523.00
  catarrhal 523.00
  chronic 523.10
    non-plaque induced 523.11
  desquamative 523.10
  expulsiva 523.40
  hyperplastic 523.10
  marginal, simple 523.10
  necrotizing, acute 101
  non-plaque induced 523.11
  pellagrous 265.2
  plaque induced 523.10
  ulcerative 523.10
    acute necrotizing 101
  Vincent's 101
Gingivoglossitis 529.0
Gingivopericementitis 523.40
Gingivosis 523.10
Gingivostomatitis 523.10
  herpetic 054.2
Giovannini's disease 117.9
GISA (glycopeptide intermediate staphylococcus aureus) V09.8 ☑
Glanders 024
Gland, glandular — *see* condition
Glanzmann (-Naegeli) disease or thrombas-
  thenia 287.1
Glassblowers' disease 527.1
Glaucoma (capsular) (inflammatory) (noninflammatory) (primary) 365.9
  with increased episcleral venous pressure
    365.82
  absolute 360.42
  acute 365.22
    narrow angle 365.22
    secondary 365.60
  angle closure 365.20
    acute 365.22
    attack 365.22
    chronic 365.23
    crisis 365.22
    intermittent 365.21
    interval 365.21
    primary 365.20
      chronic 365.23
    residual stage 365.24
    subacute 365.21
  angle recession 365.65
  borderline 365.00
  chronic 365.11
    noncongestive 365.11
    open angle 365.11
    simple 365.11
  closed angle — *see* Glaucoma, angle closure
  congenital 743.20
    associated with other eye anomalies
      743.22
    simple 743.21
  congestive — *see* Glaucoma, narrow angle
  corticosteroid-induced (glaucomatous
    stage) 365.31
    residual stage 365.32
  exfoliation 365.52
  hemorrhagic 365.60
  hypersecretion 365.81
  infantile 365.14
    congenital 743.20
      associated with other eye anomalies
        743.22
      simple 743.21
  inflammatory 365.62
  in or with
    aniridia 365.42
    Axenfeld's anomaly 365.41
    congenital syndromes NEC
      759.89 [365.44]

☑ **Additional Digit Required** — Refer to the Tabular List for Digit Selection   ▽ **Subterms under main terms may continue to next column or page**

128 — Volume 2   ▶◀ **Revised Text**   ● **New Line**   ▲ **Revised Code**   **2015 ICD-9-CM**

Glaucoma — *continued*
- in or with — *continued*
  - disorder of lens NEC 365.59
  - inflammation, ocular 365.62
  - iris
    - anomalies NEC 365.42
    - atrophy, essential 365.42
    - bombé 365.61
  - microcornea 365.43
  - neurofibromatosis 237.71 [365.44]
  - ocular
    - cysts NEC 365.64
    - disorders NEC 365.60
    - trauma 365.65
    - tumors NEC 365.64
  - pupillary block or seclusion 365.61
  - Rieger's anomaly or syndrome 365.41
  - seclusion of pupil 365.61
  - Sturge-Weber (-Dimitri) syndrome 759.6 [365.44]
  - systemic syndrome NEC 365.44
  - tumor of globe 365.64
  - vascular disorders NEC 365.63
- juvenile 365.14
- low tension 365.12
- malignant 365.83
- narrow angle (primary) 365.20
  - acute 365.22
  - chronic 365.23
  - intermittent 365.21
  - interval 365.21
  - residual stage 365.24
  - subacute 365.21
- neovascular 365.63
- newborn 743.20
  - associated with other eye anomalies 743.22
  - simple 743.21
- noncongestive (chronic) 365.11
- nonobstructive (chronic) 365.11
- normal tension 365.12
- obstructive 365.60
  - due to lens changes 365.59
- open angle 365.10
  - with
    - abnormal optic disc appearance or asymmetry 365.01
    - borderline findings
      - high risk 365.05
      - intraocular pressure 365.01
      - low risk 365.01
    - cupping of optic discs 365.01
    - thin central corneal thickness (pachymetry) 365.01
  - high risk 365.05
  - low risk 365.01
  - primary 365.11
  - residual stage 365.15
- phacoanaphylactic 365.59
- phacolytic 365.51
- phacomorphic
  - acute 365.22
  - borderline 365.06
- pigmentary 365.13
- pigment dispersion 365.13
- postinfectious 365.60
- pseudoexfoliation 365.52
- secondary NEC 365.60
  - due to
    - steroids 365.31
    - surgery 365.60
- simple (chronic) 365.11
- simplex 365.11
- stage
  - advanced 365.73
  - early 365.71
  - end-stage 365.73
  - indeterminate 365.74
  - mild 365.71
  - moderate 365.72
  - severe 365.73
  - unspecified 365.70
- steroid
  - induced 365.31
  - responders 365.03
- suspect 365.00

Glaucoma — *continued*
- suspect — *continued*
  - primary angle closure 365.02
  - syphilitic 095.8
  - traumatic NEC 365.65
    - newborn 767.8
  - uveitic 365.62
  - wide angle (*see also* Glaucoma, open angle) 365.10
Glaucomatous flecks (subcapsular) 366.31
Glazed tongue 529.4
Gleet 098.2
Glénard's disease or syndrome (enteroptosis) 569.89
Glinski-Simmonds syndrome (pituitary cachexia) 253.2
Glioblastoma (multiforme) (M9440/3)
- with sarcomatous component (M9442/3)
  - specified site — *see* Neoplasm, by site, malignant
  - unspecified site 191.9
- giant cell (M9441/3)
  - specified site — *see* Neoplasm, by site, malignant
  - unspecified site 191.9
- specified site — *see* Neoplasm, by site, malignant
- unspecified site 191.9
Glioma (malignant) (M9380/3)
- astrocytic (M9400/3)
  - specified site — *see* Neoplasm, by site, malignant
  - unspecified site 191.9
- mixed (M9382/3)
  - specified site — *see* Neoplasm, by site, malignant
  - unspecified site 191.9
- nose 748.1
- specified site NEC — *see* Neoplasm, by site, malignant
- subependymal (M9383/1) 237.5
- unspecified site 191.9
Gliomatosis cerebri (M9381/3) 191.0
Glioneuroma (M9505/1) — *see* Neoplasm, by site, uncertain behavior
Gliosarcoma (M9380/3)
- specified site — *see* Neoplasm, by site, malignant
- unspecified site 191.9
Gliosis (cerebral) 349.89
- spinal 336.0
Glisson's
- cirrhosis — *see* Cirrhosis, portal
- disease (*see also* Rickets) 268.0
Glissonitis 573.3
Globinuria 791.2
Globus 306.4
- hystericus 300.11
Glomangioma (M8712/0) — *see also* Hemangioma 228.00
Glomangiosarcoma (M8710/3) — *see* Neoplasm, connective tissue, malignant
Glomerular nephritis — *see also* Nephritis 583.9
Glomerulitis — *see also* Nephritis 583.9
Glomerulonephritis — *see also* Nephritis 583.9
- with
  - edema (*see also* Nephrosis) 581.9
  - lesion of
    - exudative nephritis 583.89
    - interstitial nephritis (diffuse) (focal) 583.89
    - necrotizing glomerulitis 583.4
      - acute 580.4
      - chronic 582.4
    - renal necrosis 583.9
      - cortical 583.6
      - medullary 583.7
    - specified pathology NEC 583.89
      - acute 580.89
      - chronic 582.89
  - necrosis, renal 583.9
    - cortical 583.6
    - medullary (papillary) 583.7
  - specified pathology or lesion NEC 583.89
- acute 580.9

Glomerulonephritis — *see also* Nephritis — *continued*
- acute — *continued*
  - with
    - exudative nephritis 580.89
    - interstitial nephritis (diffuse) (focal) 580.89
    - necrotizing glomerulitis 580.4
    - extracapillary with epithelial crescents 580.4
    - poststreptococcal 580.0
    - proliferative (diffuse) 580.0
    - rapidly progressive 580.4
    - specified pathology NEC 580.89
- arteriolar (*see also* Hypertension, kidney) 403.90
- arteriosclerotic (*see also* Hypertension, kidney) 403.90
- ascending (*see also* Pyelitis) 590.80
- basement membrane NEC 583.89
  - with
    - pulmonary hemorrhage (Goodpasture's syndrome) 446.21 [583.81]
- chronic 582.9
  - with
    - exudative nephritis 582.89
    - interstitial nephritis (diffuse) (focal) 582.89
    - necrotizing glomerulitis 582.4
    - specified pathology or lesion NEC 582.89
  - endothelial 582.2
  - extracapillary with epithelial crescents 582.4
  - hypocomplementemic persistent 582.2
  - lobular 582.2
  - membranoproliferative 582.2
  - membranous 582.1
    - and proliferative (mixed) 582.2
    - sclerosing 582.1
  - mesangiocapillary 582.2
  - mixed membranous and proliferative 582.2
  - proliferative (diffuse) 582.0
  - rapidly progressive 582.4
  - sclerosing 582.1
- cirrhotic — *see* Sclerosis, renal
- desquamative — *see* Nephrosis
- due to or associated with
  - amyloidosis 277.39 [583.81]
    - with nephrotic syndrome 277.39 [581.81]
    - chronic 277.39 [582.81]
  - diabetes mellitus 250.4 ☑ [583.81]
    - with nephrotic syndrome 250.4 ☑ [581.81]
    - due to secondary diabetes 249.4 ☑ [581.81]
    - due to secondary diabetes 249.4 ☑ [581.81]
  - diphtheria 032.89 [580.81]
  - gonococcal infection (acute) 098.19 [583.81]
    - chronic or duration of 2 months or over 098.39 [583.81]
  - infectious hepatitis 070.9 [580.81]
  - malaria (with nephrotic syndrome) 084.9 [581.81]
  - mumps 072.79 [580.81]
  - polyarteritis (nodosa) (with nephrotic syndrome) 446.0 [581.81]
  - specified pathology NEC 583.89
    - acute 580.89
    - chronic 582.89
  - streptotrichosis 039.8 [583.81]
  - subacute bacterial endocarditis 421.0 [580.81]
  - syphilis (late) 095.4
    - congenital 090.5 [583.81]
    - early 091.69 [583.81]
  - systemic lupus erythematosus 710.0 [583.81]
    - with nephrotic syndrome 710.0 [581.81]
    - chronic 710.0 [582.81]

Glomerulonephritis — *see also* Nephritis — *continued*
- due to or associated with — *continued*
  - tuberculosis (*see also* Tuberculosis) 016.0 [583.81]
  - typhoid fever 002.0 [580.81]
- extracapillary with epithelial crescents 583.4
  - acute 580.4
  - chronic 582.4
- exudative 583.89
  - acute 580.89
  - chronic 582.89
- focal (*see also* Nephritis) 583.9
  - embolic 580.4
- granular 582.89
- granulomatous 582.89
- hydremic (*see also* Nephrosis) 581.9
- hypocomplementemic persistent 583.2
  - with nephrotic syndrome 581.2
  - chronic 582.2
- immune complex NEC 583.89
- infective (*see also* Pyelitis) 590.80
- interstitial (diffuse) (focal) 583.89
  - with nephrotic syndrome 581.89
  - acute 580.89
  - chronic 582.89
- latent or quiescent 582.9
- lobular 583.2
  - with nephrotic syndrome 581.2
  - chronic 582.2
- membranoproliferative 583.2
  - with nephrotic syndrome 581.2
  - chronic 582.2
- membranous 583.1
  - with nephrotic syndrome 581.1
  - and proliferative (mixed) 583.2
    - with nephrotic syndrome 581.2
    - chronic 582.2
  - chronic 582.1
  - sclerosing 582.1
    - with nephrotic syndrome 581.1
- mesangiocapillary 583.2
  - with nephrotic syndrome 581.2
  - chronic 582.2
- minimal change 581.3
- mixed membranous and proliferative 583.2
  - with nephrotic syndrome 581.2
  - chronic 582.2
- necrotizing 583.4
  - acute 580.4
  - chronic 582.4
- nephrotic (*see also* Nephrosis) 581.9
- old — *see* Glomerulonephritis, chronic
- parenchymatous 581.89
- poststreptococcal 580.0
- proliferative (diffuse) 583.0
  - with nephrotic syndrome 581.0
  - acute 580.0
  - chronic 582.0
- purulent (*see also* Pyelitis) 590.80
- quiescent — *see* Nephritis, chronic
- rapidly progressive 583.4
  - acute 580.4
  - chronic 582.4
- sclerosing membranous (chronic) 582.1
  - with nephrotic syndrome 581.1
- septic (*see also* Pyelitis) 590.80
- specified pathology or lesion NEC 583.89
  - with nephrotic syndrome 581.89
  - acute 580.89
  - chronic 582.89
- suppurative (acute) (disseminated) (*see also* Pyelitis) 590.80
- toxic — *see* Nephritis, acute
- tubal, tubular — *see* Nephrosis, tubular
- type II (Ellis) — *see* Nephrosis
- vascular — *see* Hypertension, kidney
Glomerulosclerosis — *see also* Sclerosis, renal 587
- focal 582.1
  - with nephrotic syndrome 581.1
- intercapillary (nodular) (with diabetes) 250.4 ☑ [581.81]
  - due to secondary diabetes 249.4 ☑ [581.81]
Glossagra 529.6

☑ **Additional Digit Required** — Refer to the Tabular List for Digit Selection   ▽ **Subterms under main terms may continue to next column or page**

Glossalgia 529.6
Glossitis 529.0
  areata exfoliativa 529.1
  atrophic 529.4
  benign migratory 529.1
  gangrenous 529.0
  Hunter's 529.4
  median rhomboid 529.2
  Moeller's 529.4
  pellagrous 265.2
Glossocele 529.8
Glossodynia 529.6
  exfoliativa 529.4
Glossoncus 529.8
Glossophytia 529.3
Glossoplegia 529.8
Glossoptosis 529.8
Glossopyrosis 529.6
Glossotrichia 529.3
Glossy skin 701.9
Glottis — *see* condition
Glottitis — *see* Glossitis
Glucagonoma (M8152/0)
  malignant (M8152/3)
    pancreas 157.4
    specified site NEC — *see* Neoplasm, by
      site, malignant
    unspecified site 157.4
  pancreas 211.7
  specified site NEC — *see* Neoplasm, by site,
    benign
  unspecified site 211.7
Glucoglycinuria 270.7
Glue ear syndrome 381.20
Glue sniffing (airplane glue) — *see also* Dependence 304.6 ☑
Glycinemia (with methylmalonic acidemia)
  270.7
Glycinuria (renal) (with ketosis) 270.0
Glycogen
  infiltration (*see also* Disease, glycogen storage) 271.0
  storage disease (*see also* Disease, glycogen
    storage) 271.0
Glycogenosis — *see also* Disease, glycogen
  storage 271.0
  cardiac 271.0 *[425.7]*
  Cori, types I-VII 271.0
  diabetic, secondary 250.8 ☑ *[259.8]*
    due to secondary diabetes
      249.8 ☑ *[259.8]*
  diffuse (with hepatic cirrhosis) 271.0
  generalized 271.0
  glucose-6-phosphatase deficiency 271.0
  hepatophosphorylase deficiency 271.0
  hepatorenal 271.0
  myophosphorylase deficiency 271.0
  pulmonary interstitial 516.62
Glycopenia 251.2
Glycopeptide
  intermediate staphylococcus aureus (GISA)
    V09.8 ☑
  resistant
    enterococcus V09.8 ☑
    staphylococcus aureus (GRSA) V09.8 ☑
Glycoprolinuria 270.8
Glycosuria 791.5
  renal 271.4
Gnathostoma (spinigerum) (infection) (infestation) 128.1
  wandering swellings from 128.1
Gnathostomiasis 128.1
Goiter (adolescent) (colloid) (diffuse) (dipping)
  (due to iodine deficiency) (endemic)
  (euthyroid) (heart) (hyperplastic) (internal) (intrathoracic) (juvenile) (mixed
  type) (nonendemic) (parenchymatous)
  (plunging) (sporadic) (subclavicular)
  (substernal) 240.9
  with
    hyperthyroidism (recurrent) (*see also*
      Goiter, toxic) 242.0 ☑
    thyrotoxicosis (*see also* Goiter, toxic)
      242.0 ☑
  adenomatous (*see also* Goiter, nodular)
    241.9

Goiter — *continued*
  cancerous (M8000/3) 193
  complicating pregnancy, childbirth, or
    puerperium 648.1 ☑
  congenital 246.1
  cystic (*see also* Goiter, nodular) 241.9
  due to enzyme defect in synthesis of thyroid
    hormone (butane-insoluble iodine)
    (coupling) (deiodinase) (iodide trapping or organification) (iodotyrosine
    dehalogenase) (peroxidase) 246.1
  dyshormonogenic 246.1
  exophthalmic (*see also* Goiter, toxic)
    242.0 ☑
  familial (with deaf-mutism) 243
  fibrous 245.3
  lingual 759.2
  lymphadenoid 245.2
  malignant (M8000/3) 193
  multinodular (nontoxic) 241.1
    toxic or with hyperthyroidism (*see also*
      Goiter, toxic) 242.2 ☑
  nodular (nontoxic) 241.9
    with
      hyperthyroidism (*see also* Goiter,
        toxic) 242.3 ☑
      thyrotoxicosis (*see also* Goiter, toxic)
        242.3 ☑
    endemic 241.9
    exophthalmic (diffuse) (*see also* Goiter,
      toxic) 242.0 ☑
    multinodular (nontoxic) 241.1
    sporadic 241.9
    toxic (*see also* Goiter, toxic) 242.3 ☑
    uninodular (nontoxic) 241.0
  nontoxic (nodular) 241.9
    multinodular 241.1
    uninodular 241.0
  pulsating (*see also* Goiter, toxic) 242.0 ☑
  simple 240.0
  toxic 242.0 ☑

> *Note* — *Use the following fifth-digit*
> *subclassification with category 242:*
>
> 0   *without mention of thyrotoxic*
>   *crisis or storm*
>
> 1   *with mention of thyrotoxic crisis*
>   *or storm*

    adenomatous 242.3 ☑
      multinodular 242.2 ☑
      uninodular 242.1 ☑
    multinodular 242.2 ☑
    nodular 242.3 ☑
      multinodular 242.2 ☑
      uninodular 242.1 ☑
    uninodular 242.1 ☑
  uninodular (nontoxic) 241.0
    toxic or with hyperthyroidism (*see also*
      Goiter, toxic) 242.1 ☑
Goldberg (-Maxwell) (-Morris) syndrome
  (testicular feminization) 259.51
Goldblatt's
  hypertension 440.1
  kidney 440.1
Goldenhar's syndrome (oculoauriculovertebral dysplasia) 756.0
Goldflam-Erb disease or syndrome 358.00
Goldscheider's disease (epidermolysis bullosa)
  757.39
Goldstein's disease (familial hemorrhagic
  telangiectasia) 448.0
Golfer's elbow 726.32
Goltz-Gorlin syndrome (dermal hypoplasia)
  757.39
Gonadoblastoma (M9073/1)
  specified site — *see* Neoplasm, by site uncertain behavior
  unspecified site
    female 236.2
    male 236.4
Gonecystitis — *see also* Vesiculitis 608.4
Gongylonemiasis 125.6
  mouth 125.6
Goniosynechiae 364.73
Gonococcemia 098.89

Gonococcus, gonococcal (disease) (infection)
  — *see also* condition 098.0
  anus 098.7
  bursa 098.52
  chronic NEC 098.2
  complicating pregnancy, childbirth, or
    puerperium 647.1 ☑
    affecting fetus or newborn 760.2
  conjunctiva, conjunctivitis (neonatorum)
    098.40
  dermatosis 098.89
  endocardium 098.84
  epididymo-orchitis 098.13
    chronic or duration of 2 months or over
      098.33
  eye (newborn) 098.40
  fallopian tube (chronic) 098.37
    acute 098.17
  genitourinary (acute) (organ) (system) (tract)
    (*see also* Gonorrhea) 098.0
    lower 098.0
      chronic 098.2
    upper 098.10
      chronic 098.30
  heart NEC 098.85
  joint 098.50
  keratoderma 098.81
  keratosis (blennorrhagica) 098.81
  lymphatic (gland) (node) 098.89
  meninges 098.82
  orchitis (acute) 098.13
    chronic or duration of 2 months or over
      098.33
  pelvis (acute) 098.19
    chronic or duration of 2 months or over
      098.39
  pericarditis 098.83
  peritonitis 098.86
  pharyngitis 098.6
  pharynx 098.6
  proctitis 098.7
  pyosalpinx (chronic) 098.37
    acute 098.17
  rectum 098.7
  septicemia 098.89
  skin 098.89
  specified site NEC 098.89
  synovitis 098.51
  tendon sheath 098.51
  throat 098.6
  urethra (acute) 098.0
    chronic or duration of 2 months or over
      098.2
  vulva (acute) 098.0
    chronic or duration of 2 months or over
      098.2
Gonocytoma (M9073/1)
  specified site — *see* Neoplasm, by site, uncertain behavior
  unspecified site
    female 236.2
    male 236.4
Gonorrhea 098.0
  acute 098.0
  Bartholin's gland (acute) 098.0
    chronic or duration of 2 months or over
      098.2
  bladder (acute) 098.11
    chronic or duration of 2 months or over
      098.31
  carrier (suspected of) V02.7
  cervix (acute) 098.15
    chronic or duration of 2 months or over
      098.35
  chronic 098.2
  complicating pregnancy, childbirth, or
    puerperium 647.1 ☑
    affecting fetus or newborn 760.2
  conjunctiva, conjunctivitis (neonatorum)
    098.40
  contact V01.6
  Cowper's gland (acute) 098.0
    chronic or duration of 2 months or over
      098.2
  duration of two months or over 098.2
  exposure to V01.6

Gonorrhea — *continued*
  fallopian tube (chronic) 098.37
    acute 098.17
  genitourinary (acute) (organ) (system) (tract)
    098.0
    chronic 098.2
    duration of two months or over 098.2
  kidney (acute) 098.19
    chronic or duration of 2 months or over
      098.39
  ovary (acute) 098.19
    chronic or duration of 2 months or over
      098.39
  pelvis (acute) 098.19
    chronic or duration of 2 months or over
      098.39
  penis (acute) 098.0
    chronic or duration of 2 months or over
      098.2
  prostate (acute) 098.12
    chronic or duration of 2 months or over
      098.32
  seminal vesicle (acute) 098.14
    chronic or duration of 2 months or over
      098.34
  specified site NEC — *see* Gonococcus
  spermatic cord (acute) 098.14
    chronic or duration of 2 months or over
      098.34
  urethra (acute) 098.0
    chronic or duration of 2 months or over
      098.2
  vagina (acute) 098.0
    chronic or duration of 2 months or over
      098.2
  vas deferens (acute) 098.14
    chronic or duration of 2 months or over
      098.34
  vulva (acute) 098.0
    chronic or duration of 2 months or over
      098.2
Goodpasture's syndrome (pneumorenal)
  446.21
Good's syndrome 279.06
Gopalan's syndrome (burning feet) 266.2
Gordon's disease (exudative enteropathy)
  579.8
Gorlin-Chaudhry-Moss syndrome 759.89
Gougerot-Blum syndrome (pigmented purpuric lichenoid dermatitis) 709.1
Gougerot-Carteaud disease or syndrome
  (confluent reticulate papillomatosis)
  701.8
Gougerot-Hailey-Hailey disease (benign familial chronic pemphigus) 757.39
Gougerot (-Houwer) -Sjögren syndrome
  (keratoconjunctivitis sicca) 710.2
Gougerot's syndrome (trisymptomatic) 709.1
Gouley's syndrome (constrictive pericarditis)
  423.2
Goundou 102.6
Gout, gouty 274.9
  with
    specified manifestations NEC 274.89
    tophi (tophus) 274.03
  acute 274.01
  arthritis 274.00
    acute 274.01
  arthropathy 274.00
    acute 274.01
    chronic (without mention of tophus
      (tophi)) 274.02
      with tophus (tophi) 274.03
  attack 274.01
  chronic 274.02
    tophaceous 274.03
  degeneration, heart 274.82
  diathesis 274.9
  eczema 274.89
  episcleritis 274.89 *[379.09]*
  external ear (tophus) 274.81
  flare 274.01
  glomerulonephritis 274.10
  iritis 274.89 *[364.11]*
  joint 274.00
  kidney 274.10

☑ **Additional Digit Required** — Refer to the Tabular List for Digit Selection   ⍩ **Subterms under main terms may continue to next column or page**

130 — Volume 2   ▶◀ **Revised Text**   ● **New Line**   ▲ **Revised Code**   **2015 ICD-9-CM**

Gout, gouty — *continued*
  lead 984.9
    specified type of lead — *see* Table of
      Drugs and Chemicals
  nephritis 274.10
  neuritis 274.89 [357.4]
  phlebitis 274.89 [451.9]
  rheumatic 714.0
  saturnine 984.9
    specified type of lead — *see* Table of
      Drugs and Chemicals
  spondylitis 274.00
  synovitis 274.00
  syphilitic 095.8
  tophi 274.03
    ear 274.81
    heart 274.82
    specified site NEC 274.82
Gowers'
  muscular dystrophy 359.1
  syndrome (vasovagal attack) 780.2
Gowers-Paton-Kennedy syndrome 377.04
Gradenigo's syndrome 383.02
Graft-versus-host disease 279.50
  due to organ transplant NEC — *see* Complications, transplant, organ
Graham Steell's murmur (pulmonic regurgitation) — *see also* Endocarditis, pulmonary 424.3
Grain-handlers' disease or lung 495.8
Grain mite (itch) 133.8
Grand
  mal (idiopathic) (*see also* Epilepsy) 345.1 ☑
    hysteria of Charcôt 300.11
    nonrecurrent or isolated 780.39
  multipara
    affecting management of labor and delivery 659.4 ☑
    status only (not pregnant) V61.5
Granite workers' lung 502
Granular — *see also* condition
  inflammation, pharynx 472.1
  kidney (contracting) (*see also* Sclerosis, renal) 587
  liver — *see* Cirrhosis, liver
  nephritis — *see* Nephritis
Granulation tissue, abnormal — *see also* Granuloma
  abnormal or excessive 701.5
  postmastoidectomy cavity 383.33
  postoperative 701.5
  skin 701.5
Granulocytopenia, granulocytopenic (primary) 288.00
  malignant 288.09
Granulomatosis NEC 686.1
  disciformis chronica et progressiva 709.3
  infantiseptica 771.2
  lipoid 277.89
  lipophagic, intestinal 040.2
  miliary 027.0
  necrotizing, respiratory 446.4
  progressive, septic 288.1
  Wegener's (necrotizing respiratory) 446.4
Granulomatous tissue — *see* Granuloma
Granuloma NEC 686.1
  abdomen (wall) 568.89
    skin (pyogenicum) 686.1
      from residual foreign body 709.4
  annulare 695.89
  anus 569.49
  apical 522.6
  appendix 543.9
  aural 380.23
  beryllium (skin) 709.4
    lung 503
  bone (*see also* Osteomyelitis) 730.1 ☑
    eosinophilic 277.89
    from residual foreign body 733.99
  canaliculus lacrimalis 375.81
  cerebral 348.89
  cholesterin, middle ear 385.82
  coccidioidal (progressive) 114.3
    lung 114.4
    meninges 114.2
    primary (lung) 114.0

Granuloma — *continued*
  colon 569.89
  conjunctiva 372.61
  dental 522.6
  ear, middle (cholesterin) 385.82
    with otitis media — *see* Otitis media
  eosinophilic 277.89
    bone 277.89
    lung 277.89
    oral mucosa 528.9
  exuberant 701.5
  eyelid 374.89
  facial
    lethal midline 446.3
    malignant 446.3
  faciale 701.8
  fissuratum (gum) 523.8
  foot NEC 686.1
  foreign body (in soft tissue) NEC 728.82
    bone 733.99
    in operative wound 998.4
    muscle 728.82
    skin 709.4
    subcutaneous tissue 709.4
  fungoides 202.1 ☑
  gangraenescens 446.3
  giant cell (central) (jaw) (reparative) 526.3
    gingiva 523.8
    peripheral (gingiva) 523.8
  gland (lymph) 289.3
  Hodgkin's (M9661/3) 201.1 ☑
  ileum 569.89
  infectious NEC 136.9
  inguinale (Donovan) 099.2
    venereal 099.2
  intestine 569.89
  iridocyclitis 364.10
  jaw (bone) 526.3
    reparative giant cell 526.3
  kidney (*see also* Infection, kidney) 590.9
  lacrimal sac 375.81
  larynx 478.79
  lethal midline 446.3
  lipid 277.89
  lipoid 277.89
  liver 572.8
  lung (infectious) (*see also* Fibrosis, lung) 515
    coccidioidal 114.4
    eosinophilic 277.89
  lymph gland 289.3
  Majocchi's 110.6
  malignant, face 446.3
  mandible 526.3
  mediastinum 519.3
  midline 446.3
  monilial 112.3
  muscle 728.82
    from residual foreign body 728.82
  nasal sinus (*see also* Sinusitis) 473.9
  operation wound 998.59
    foreign body 998.4
    stitch (external) 998.89
      internal wound 998.89
    talc 998.7
  oral mucosa, eosinophilic or pyogenic 528.9
  orbit, orbital 376.11
  paracoccidioidal 116.1
  penis, venereal 099.2
  periapical 522.6
  peritoneum 568.89
    due to ova of helminths NEC (*see also* Helminthiasis) 128.9
  postmastoidectomy cavity 383.33
  postoperative — *see* Granuloma, operation wound
  prostate 601.8
  pudendi (ulcerating) 099.2
  pudendorum (ulcerative) 099.2
  pulp, internal (tooth) 521.49
  pyogenic, pyogenicum (skin) 686.1
    maxillary alveolar ridge 522.6
    oral mucosa 528.9
  rectum 569.49
  reticulohistiocytic 277.89
  rubrum nasi 705.89
  sarcoid 135

Granuloma — *continued*
  Schistosoma 120.9
  septic (skin) 686.1
  silica (skin) 709.4
  sinus (accessory) (infectional) (nasal) (*see also* Sinusitis) 473.9
  skin (pyogenicum) 686.1
    from foreign body or material 709.4
  sperm 608.89
  spine
    syphilitic (epidural) 094.89
    tuberculous (*see also* Tuberculosis) 015.0 ☑ [730.88]
  stitch (postoperative) 998.89
    internal wound 998.89
  suppurative (skin) 686.1
  suture (postoperative) 998.89
    internal wound 998.89
  swimming pool 031.1
  talc 728.82
    in operation wound 998.7
  telangiectaticum (skin) 686.1
  tracheostomy 519.09
  trichophyticum 110.6
  tropicum 102.4
  umbilicus 686.1
    newborn 771.4
  urethra 599.84
  uveitis 364.10
  vagina 099.2
  venereum 099.2
  vocal cords 478.5
  Wegener's (necrotizing respiratory granulomatosis) 446.4
Granulosis rubra nasi 705.89
Graphite fibrosis (of lung) 503
Graphospasm 300.89
  organic 333.84
Grating scapula 733.99
Gravel (urinary) — *see also* Calculus 592.9
Graves' disease (exophthalmic goiter) — *see also* Goiter, toxic 242.0 ☑
Gravis — *see* condition
Grawitz's tumor (hypernephroma) (M8312/3) 189.0
Grayness, hair (premature) 704.3
  congenital 757.4
Gray or grey syndrome (chloramphenicol) (newborn) 779.4
Greenfield's disease 330.0
Green sickness 280.9
Greenstick fracture — *see* Fracture, by site
Greig's syndrome (hypertelorism) 756.0
Grief 309.0
Griesinger's disease — *see also* Ancylostomiasis 126.9
Grinders'
  asthma 502
  lung 502
  phthisis (*see also* Tuberculosis) 011.4 ☑
Grinding, teeth 306.8
Grip
  Dabney's 074.1
  devil's 074.1
Grippe, grippal — *see also* Influenza
  Balkan 083.0
  intestinal (*see also* Influenza) 487.8
  summer 074.8
Grippy cold — *see also* Influenza 487.1
Grisel's disease 723.5
Groin — *see* condition
Grooved
  nails (transverse) 703.8
  tongue 529.5
    congenital 750.13
Ground itch 126.9
Growing pains, children 781.99
Growth (fungoid) (neoplastic) (new) (M8000/1) — *see also* Neoplasm, by site, unspecified nature
  adenoid (vegetative) 474.12
  benign (M8000/0) — *see* Neoplasm, by site, benign
  fetal, poor 764.9 ☑
    affecting management of pregnancy 656.5 ☑

Growth — *see also* Neoplasm, by site, unspecified nature — *continued*
  malignant (M8000/3) — *see* Neoplasm, site, malignant
  rapid, childhood V21.0
  secondary (M8000/6) — *see* Neoplasm, by site, malignant, secondary
GRSA (glycopeptide resistant staphylococcus aureus) V09.8 ☑
Gruber's hernia — *see* Hernia, Gruber's
Gruby's disease (tinea tonsurans) 110.0
GSS (Gerstmann-Sträussler-Scheinker syndrome) 046.71
G-trisomy 758.0
Guama fever 066.3
Gubler (-Millard) paralysis or syndrome 344.89
Guérin-Stern syndrome (arthrogryposis multiplex congenita) 754.89
Guertin's disease (electric chorea) 049.8
Guillain-Barré disease or syndrome 357.0
Guinea worms (infection) (infestation) 125.7
Guinon's disease (motor-verbal tic) 307.23
Gull and Sutton's disease — *see* Hypertension, kidney
Gull's disease (thyroid atrophy with myxedema) 244.8
Gum — *see* condition
Gumboil 522.7
Gumma (syphilitic) 095.9
  artery 093.89
    cerebral or spinal 094.89
  bone 095.5
    of yaws (late) 102.6
  brain 094.89
  cauda equina 094.89
  central nervous system NEC 094.9
  ciliary body 095.8 [364.11]
  congenital 090.5
    testis 090.5
  eyelid 095.8 [373.5]
  heart 093.89
  intracranial 094.89
  iris 095.8 [364.11]
  kidney 095.4
  larynx 095.8
  leptomeninges 094.2
  liver 095.3
  meninges 094.2
  myocardium 093.82
  nasopharynx 095.8
  neurosyphilitic 094.9
  nose 095.8
  orbit 095.8
  palate (soft) 095.8
  penis 095.8
  pericardium 093.81
  pharynx 095.8
  pituitary 095.8
  scrofulous (see also Tuberculosis) 017.0 ☑
  skin 095.8
  specified site NEC 095.8
  spinal cord 094.89
  tongue 095.8
  tonsil 095.8
  trachea 095.8
  tuberculous (see also Tuberculosis) 017.0 ☑
  ulcerative due to yaws 102.4
  ureter 095.8
  yaws 102.4
    bone 102.6
Gunn's syndrome (jaw-winking syndrome) 742.8
Gunshot wound — *see also* Wound, open, by site
  fracture — *see* Fracture, by site, open
  internal organs (abdomen, chest, or pelvis) — *see* Injury, internal, by site, with open wound
  intracranial — *see* Laceration, brain, with open intracranial wound
Günther's disease or syndrome (congenital erythropoietic porphyria) 277.1
Gustatory hallucination 780.1
Gynandrism 752.7

☑ **Additional Digit Required** — Refer to the Tabular List for Digit Selection   ▽ **Subterms under main terms may continue to next column or page**

2015 ICD-9-CM   ▶◀ **Revised Text**   ● **New Line**   ▲ **Revised Code**   **Volume 2 — 131**

Gynandroblastoma (M8632/1)
　specified site — see Neoplasm, by site, uncertain behavior
　unspecified site
　　female 236.2
　　male 236.4
Gynandromorphism 752.7
Gynatresia (congenital) 752.49
Gynecoid pelvis, male 738.6
Gynecological examination V72.31
　for contraceptive maintenance V25.40
Gynecomastia 611.1
Gynephobia 300.29
Gyrate scalp 757.39

H

Haas' disease (osteochondrosis head of humerus) 732.3
Habermann's disease (acute parapsoriasis varioliformis) 696.2
Habit, habituation
　chorea 307.22
　disturbance, child 307.9
　drug (see also Dependence) 304.9 ☑
　laxative (see also Abuse, drugs, nondependent) 305.9 ☑
　spasm 307.20
　　chronic 307.22
　　transient (of childhood) 307.21
　tic 307.20
　　chronic 307.22
　　transient (of childhood) 307.21
　use of
　　nonprescribed drugs (see also Abuse, drugs, nondependent) 305.9 ☑
　　patent medicines (see also Abuse, drugs, nondependent) 305.9 ☑
　vomiting 536.2
Hadfield-Clarke syndrome (pancreatic infantilism) 577.8
Haff disease 985.1
Hageman factor defect, deficiency, or disease — see also Defect, coagulation 286.3
Haglund's disease (osteochondrosis os tibiale externum) 732.5
Haglund-Läwen-Fründ syndrome 717.89
Hagner's disease (hypertrophic pulmonary osteoarthropathy) 731.2
Hag teeth, tooth 524.39
Hailey-Hailey disease (benign familial chronic pemphigus) 757.39
Hair — see also condition
　plucking 307.9
Hairball in stomach 935.2
Hairy black tongue 529.3
Half vertebra 756.14
Halitosis 784.99
Hallermann-Streiff syndrome 756.0
Hallervorden-Spatz disease or syndrome 333.0
Hallopeau's
　acrodermatitis (continua) 696.1
　disease (lichen sclerosis et atrophicus) 701.0
Hallucination (auditory) (gustatory) (olfactory) (tactile) 780.1
　alcohol-induced 291.3
　drug-induced 292.12
　visual 368.16
Hallucinosis 298.9
　alcohol-induced (acute) 291.3
　drug-induced 292.12
Hallus — see Hallux
Hallux 735.9
　limitus 735.8
　malleus (acquired) 735.3
　rigidus (acquired) 735.2
　　congenital 755.66
　　late effects of rickets 268.1
　valgus (acquired) 735.0
　　congenital 755.66
　varus (acquired) 735.1
　　congenital 755.66
Halo, visual 368.15
Hamartoblastoma 759.6
Hamartoma 759.6

Hamartoma — continued
　epithelial (gingival), odontogenic, central, or peripheral (M9321/0) 213.1
　　upper jaw (bone) 213.0
　vascular 757.32
Hamartosis, hamartoses NEC 759.6
Hamman's disease or syndrome (spontaneous mediastinal emphysema) 518.1
Hamman-Rich syndrome (diffuse interstitial pulmonary fibrosis) 516.33
Hammer toe (acquired) 735.4
　congenital 755.66
　late effects of rickets 268.1
Hand — see condition
Hand-foot syndrome 693.0
Hand-Schüller-Christian disease or syndrome (chronic histiocytosis x) 277.89
Hanging (asphyxia) (strangulation) (suffocation) 994.7
Hangnail (finger) (with lymphangitis) 681.02
Hangover (alcohol) — see also Abuse, drugs, nondependent 305.0 ☑
Hanot-Chauffard (-Troisier) syndrome (bronze diabetes) 275.01
Hanot's cirrhosis or disease — see Cirrhosis, biliary
Hansen's disease (leprosy) 030.9
　benign form 030.1
　malignant form 030.0
Harada's disease or syndrome 363.22
Hard chancre 091.0
Hardening
　artery — see Arteriosclerosis
　brain 348.89
　liver 571.8
Hard firm prostate 600.10
　with
　　urinary
　　　obstruction 600.11
　　　retention 600.11
Harelip — see also Cleft, lip 749.10
Hare's syndrome (M8010/3) (carcinoma, pulmonary apex) 162.3
Harkavy's syndrome 446.0
Harlequin (fetus) 757.1
　color change syndrome 779.89
Harley's disease (intermittent hemoglobinuria) 283.2
Harris'
　lines 733.91
　syndrome (organic hyperinsulinism) 251.1
Hart's disease or syndrome (pellagra-cerebellar ataxia-renal aminoaciduria) 270.0
Hartmann's pouch (abnormal sacculation of gallbladder neck) 575.8
　of intestine V44.3
　　attention to V55.3
Hartnup disease (pellagra-cerebellar ataxia-renal aminoaciduria) 270.0
Harvester lung 495.0
Hashimoto's disease or struma (struma lymphomatosa) 245.2
Hassall-Henle bodies (corneal warts) 371.41
Haut mal — see also Epilepsy 345.1 ☑
Haverhill fever 026.1
Hawaiian wood rose dependence 304.5 ☑
Hawkins' keloid 701.4
Hay
　asthma (see also Asthma) 493.0 ☑
　fever (allergic) (with rhinitis) 477.9
　　with asthma (bronchial) (see also Asthma) 493.0 ☑
　　allergic, due to grass, pollen, ragweed, or tree 477.0
　　conjunctivitis 372.05
　　due to
　　　dander, animal (cat) (dog) 477.2
　　　dust 477.8
　　　fowl 477.8
　　　hair, animal (cat) (dog) 477.2
　　　pollen 477.0
　　　specified allergen other than pollen 477.8
Hayem-Faber syndrome (achlorhydric anemia) 280.9

Hayem-Widal syndrome (acquired hemolytic jaundice) 283.9
Haygarth's nodosities 715.04
Hazard-Crile tumor (M8350/3) 193
Hb (abnormal)
　disease — see Disease, hemoglobin
　trait — see Trait
H disease 270.0
Head — see also condition
　banging 307.3
Headache 784.0
　allergic 339.00
　associated with sexual activity 339.82
　cluster 339.00
　　chronic 339.02
　　episodic 339.01
　daily
　　chronic 784.0
　　new persistent (NPDH) 339.42
　drug induced 339.3
　due to
　　loss, spinal fluid 349.0
　　lumbar puncture 349.0
　　saddle block 349.0
　emotional 307.81
　histamine 339.00
　hypnic 339.81
　lumbar puncture 349.0
　medication overuse 339.3
　menopausal 627.2
　menstrual 346.4 ☑
　migraine 346.9 ☑
　nasal septum 784.0
　nonorganic origin 307.81
　orgasmic 339.82
　postspinal 349.0
　post-traumatic 339.20
　　acute 339.21
　　chronic 339.22
　premenstrual 346.4 ☑
　preorgasmic 339.82
　primary
　　cough 339.83
　　exertional 339.84
　　stabbing 339.85
　　thunderclap 339.43
　psychogenic 307.81
　psychophysiologic 307.81
　rebound 339.3
　short lasting unilateral neuralgiform with conjunctival injection and tearing (SUNCT) 339.05
　sick 346.9 ☑
　spinal 349.0
　　complicating labor and delivery 668.8 ☑
　　postpartum 668.8 ☑
　spinal fluid loss 349.0
　syndrome
　　cluster 339.00
　　complicated NEC 339.44
　　periodic in child or adolescent 346.2 ☑
　　specified NEC 339.89
　tension 307.81
　　type 339.10
　　　chronic 339.12
　　　episodic 339.11
　vascular 784.0
　　migraine type 346.9 ☑
　vasomotor 346.9 ☑
Health
　advice V65.4 ☑
　audit V70.0
　checkup V70.0
　education V65.4 ☑
　hazard (see also History of) V15.9
　　falling V15.88
　　specified cause NEC V15.89
　instruction V65.4 ☑
　services provided because (of)
　　boarding school residence V60.6
　　holiday relief for person providing home care V60.5
　　inadequate
　　　housing V60.1
　　　resources V60.2
　　lack of housing V60.0

Health — continued
　services provided because — continued
　　no care available in home V60.4
　　person living alone V60.3
　　poverty V60.3
　　residence in institution V60.6
　　specified cause NEC V60.89
　　vacation relief for person providing home care V60.5
Healthy
　donor (see also Donor) V59.9
　infant or child
　　accompanying sick mother V65.0
　　receiving care V20.1
　person
　　accompanying sick relative V65.0
　　admitted for sterilization V25.2
　　receiving prophylactic inoculation or vaccination (see also Vaccination, prophylactic) V05.9
Hearing
　conservation and treatment V72.12
　examination V72.19
　　following failed hearing screening V72.11
Heart — see condition
Heartburn 787.1
　psychogenic 306.4
Heat (effects) 992.9
　apoplexy 992.0
　burn (see also Burn, by site)
　　from sun (see also Sunburn) 692.71
　collapse 992.1
　cramps 992.2
　dermatitis or eczema 692.89
　edema 992.7
　erythema — see Burn, by site
　excessive 992.9
　　specified effect NEC 992.8
　exhaustion 992.5
　　anhydrotic 992.3
　　due to
　　　salt (and water) depletion 992.4
　　　water depletion 992.3
　fatigue (transient) 992.6
　fever 992.0
　hyperpyrexia 992.0
　prickly 705.1
　prostration — see Heat, exhaustion
　pyrexia 992.0
　rash 705.1
　specified effect NEC 992.8
　stroke 992.0
　sunburn (see also Sunburn) 692.71
　syncope 992.1
Heavy-chain disease 273.2
Heavy-for-dates (fetus or infant) 766.1
　4500 grams or more 766.0
　exceptionally 766.0
Hebephrenia, hebephrenic (acute) — see also Schizophrenia 295.1 ☑
　dementia (praecox) (see also Schizophrenia) 295.1 ☑
　schizophrenia (see also Schizophrenia) 295.1 ☑
Heberden's
　disease or nodes 715.04
　syndrome (angina pectoris) 413.9
Hebra's disease
　dermatitis exfoliativa 695.89
　erythema multiforme exudativum 695.19
　pityriasis 695.89
　　maculata et circinata 696.3
　　rubra 695.89
　　　pilaris 696.4
　prurigo 698.2
Hebra, nose 040.1
Hedinger's syndrome (malignant carcinoid) 259.2
Heel — see condition
Heerfordt's disease or syndrome (uveoparotitis) 135
Hegglin's anomaly or syndrome 288.2
Heidenhain's disease 290.10
　with dementia 290.10

☑ **Additional Digit Required** — Refer to the Tabular List for Digit Selection　　　　　　　　　▽ **Subterms under main terms may continue to next column or page**

Heilmeyer-Schöner disease (M9842/3) 207.1 ☑
Heine-Medin disease — *see also* Poliomyelitis 045.9 ☑
Heinz-body anemia, congenital 282.7
Heller's disease or syndrome (infantile psychosis) — *see also* Psychosis, childhood 299.1 ☑
H.E.L.L.P 642.5 ☑
Helminthiasis — *see also* Infestation, by specific parasite 128.9
  Ancylostoma (*see also* Ancylostoma) 126.9
  intestinal 127.9
    mixed types (types classifiable to more than one of the categories 120.0–127.7) 127.8
    specified type 127.7
  mixed types (intestinal) (types classifiable to more than one of the categories 120.0–127.7) 127.8
  Necator americanus 126.1
  specified type NEC 128.8
  Trichinella 124
Heloma 700
Hemangioblastoma (M9161/1) — *see also* Neoplasm, connective tissue, uncertain behavior
  malignant (M9161/3) — *see* Neoplasm, connective tissue, malignant
Hemangioblastomatosis, cerebelloretinal 759.6
Hemangioendothelioma (M9130/1) — *see also* Neoplasm, by site, uncertain behavior
  benign (M9130/0) 228.00
  bone (diffuse) (M9130/3) — *see* Neoplasm, bone, malignant
  malignant (M9130/3) — *see* Neoplasm, connective tissue, malignant
  nervous system (M9130/0) 228.09
Hemangioendotheliosarcoma (M9130/3) — *see* Neoplasm, connective tissue, malignant
Hemangiofibroma (M9160/0) — *see* Neoplasm, by site, benign
Hemangiolipoma (M8861/0) — *see* Lipoma
Hemangioma (M9120/0) 228.00
  arteriovenous (M9123/0) — *see* Hemangioma, by site
  brain 228.02
  capillary (M9131/0) — *see* Hemangioma, by site
  cavernous (M9121/0) — *see* Hemangioma, by site
  central nervous system NEC 228.09
  choroid 228.09
  heart 228.09
  infantile (M9131/0) — *see* Hemangioma, by site
  intra-abdominal structures 228.04
  intracranial structures 228.02
  intramuscular (M9132/0) — *see* Hemangioma, by site
  iris 228.09
  juvenile (M9131/0) — *see* Hemangioma, by site
  malignant (M9120/3) — *see* Neoplasm, connective tissue, malignant
  meninges 228.09
    brain 228.02
    spinal cord 228.09
  peritoneum 228.04
  placenta — *see* Placenta, abnormal
  plexiform (M9131/0) — *see* Hemangioma, by site
  racemose (M9123/0) — *see* Hemangioma, by site
  retina 228.03
  retroperitoneal tissue 228.04
  sclerosing (M8832/0) — *see* Neoplasm, skin, benign
  simplex (M9131/0) — *see* Hemangioma, by site
  skin and subcutaneous tissue 228.01
  specified site NEC 228.09
  spinal cord 228.09

Hemangioma — *continued*
  venous (M9122/0) — *see* Hemangioma, by site
  verrucous keratotic (M9142/0) — *see* Hemangioma, by site
Hemangiomatosis (systemic) 757.32
  involving single site — *see* Hemangioma
Hemangiopericytoma (M9150/1) — *see also* Neoplasm, connective tissue, uncertain behavior
  benign (M9150/0) — *see* Neoplasm, connective tissue, benign
  malignant (M9150/3) — *see* Neoplasm, connective tissue, malignant
Hemangiosarcoma (M9120/3) — *see* Neoplasm, connective tissue, malignant
Hemarthrosis (nontraumatic) 719.10
  ankle 719.17
  elbow 719.12
  foot 719.17
  hand 719.14
  hip 719.15
  knee 719.16
  multiple sites 719.19
  pelvic region 719.15
  shoulder (region) 719.11
  specified site NEC 719.18
  traumatic — *see* Sprain, by site
  wrist 719.13
Hematemesis 578.0
  with ulcer — *see* Ulcer, by site, with hemorrhage
  due to S. japonicum 120.2
  Goldstein's (familial hemorrhagic telangiectasia) 448.0
  newborn 772.4
    due to swallowed maternal blood 777.3
Hematidrosis 705.89
Hematinuria — *see also* Hemoglobinuria 791.2
  malarial 084.8
  paroxysmal 283.2
Hematite miners' lung 503
Hematobilia 576.8
Hematocele (congenital) (diffuse) (idiopathic) 608.83
  broad ligament 620.7
  canal of Nuck 629.0
  cord, male 608.83
  fallopian tube 620.8
  female NEC 629.0
  ischiorectal 569.89
  male NEC 608.83
  ovary 629.0
  pelvis, pelvic
    female 629.0
      with ectopic pregnancy (*see also* Pregnancy, ectopic) 633.90
      with intrauterine pregnancy 633.91
    male 608.83
  periuterine 629.0
  retrouterine 629.0
  scrotum 608.83
  spermatic cord (diffuse) 608.83
  testis 608.84
  traumatic — *see* Injury, internal, pelvis
  tunica vaginalis 608.83
  uterine ligament 629.0
  uterus 621.4
  vagina 623.6
  vulva 624.5
Hematocephalus 742.4
Hematochezia — *see also* Melena 578.1
Hematochyluria — *see also* Infestation, filarial 125.9
Hematocolpos 626.8
Hematocornea 371.12
Hematogenous — *see* condition

Hematoma (skin surface intact) (traumatic) — *see also* Contusion

Note — Hematomas are coded according to origin and the nature and site of the hematoma or the accompanying injury. Hematomas of unspecified origin are coded as injuries of the sites involved, except:

(a) hematomas of genital organs which are coded as diseases of the organ involved unless they complicate pregnancy or delivery

(b) hematomas of the eye which are coded as diseases of the eye.

For late effect of hematoma classifiable to 920–924 see Late, effect, contusion

  with
    crush injury — *see* Crush
    fracture — *see* Fracture, by site
    injury of internal organs (*see also* Injury, internal, by site)
      kidney — *see* Hematoma, kidney, traumatic
      liver — *see* Hematoma, liver, traumatic
      spleen — *see* Hematoma, spleen
    nerve injury — *see* Injury, nerve
    open wound — *see* Wound, open, by site
    skin surface intact — *see* Contusion
  abdomen (wall) — *see* Contusion, abdomen
  amnion 658.8 ☑
  aorta, dissecting 441.00
    abdominal 441.02
    thoracic 441.01
    thoracoabdominal 441.03
  aortic intramural — *see* Dissection, aorta
  arterial (complicating trauma) 904.9
    specified site — *see* Injury, blood vessel, by site
  auricle (ear) 380.31
  birth injury 767.8
    skull 767.19
  brain (traumatic) 853.0 ☑

Note — Use the following fifth-digit subclassification with categories 851–854:

0   unspecified state of consciousness

1   with no loss of consciousness

2   with brief [less than one hour] loss of consciousness

3   with moderate [1–24 hours] loss of consciousness

4   with prolonged [more than 24 hours] loss of consciousness and return to pre–existing conscious level

5   with prolonged [more than 24 hours] loss of consciousness, without return to pre–existing conscious level

Use fifth-digit 5 to designate when a patient is unconscious and dies before regaining consciousness, regardless of the duration of the loss of consciousness

6   with loss of consciousness of unspecified duration

9   with concussion, unspecified

    with
      cerebral
        contusion — *see* Contusion, brain
        laceration — *see* Laceration, brain
      open intracranial wound 853.1 ☑
      skull fracture — *see* Fracture, skull, by site
    extradural or epidural 852.4 ☑
      with open intracranial wound 852.5 ☑
      fetus or newborn 767.0

Hematoma — *see also* Contusion — *continued*
  brain — *continued*
    extradural or epidural — *continued*
      nontraumatic 432.0
    fetus or newborn NEC 767.0
    nontraumatic (*see also* Hemorrhage, brain) 431
      epidural or extradural 432.0
      newborn NEC 772.8
      subarachnoid, arachnoid, or meningeal (*see also* Hemorrhage, subarachnoid) 430
      subdural (*see also* Hemorrhage, subdural) 432.1
    subarachnoid, arachnoid, or meningeal 852.0 ☑
      with open intracranial wound 852.1 ☑
      fetus or newborn 772.2
      nontraumatic (*see also* Hemorrhage, subarachnoid) 430
    subdural 852.2 ☑
      with open intracranial wound 852.3 ☑
      fetus or newborn (localized) 767.0
      nontraumatic (*see also* Hemorrhage, subdural) 432.1
  breast (nontraumatic) 611.89
  broad ligament (nontraumatic) 620.7
    complicating delivery 665.7 ☑
    traumatic — *see* Injury, internal, broad ligament
  calcified NEC 959.9
  capitis 920
    due to birth injury 767.19
    newborn 767.19
  cerebral — *see* Hematoma, brain
  cesarean section wound 674.3 ☑
  chorion — *see* Placenta, abnormal
  complicating delivery (perineum) (vulva) 664.5 ☑
    pelvic 665.7 ☑
    vagina 665.7 ☑
  corpus
    cavernosum (nontraumatic) 607.82
    luteum (nontraumatic) (ruptured) 620.1
  dura (mater) — *see* Hematoma, brain, subdural
  epididymis (nontraumatic) 608.83
  epidural (traumatic) (*see also* Hematoma, brain, extradural)
    spinal — *see* Injury, spinal, by site
  episiotomy 674.3 ☑
  external ear 380.31
  extradural (*see also* Hematoma, brain, extradural)
    fetus or newborn 767.0
    nontraumatic 432.0
      fetus or newborn 767.0
  fallopian tube 620.8
  genital organ (nontraumatic)
    female NEC 629.89
    male NEC 608.83
    traumatic (external site) 922.4
      internal — *see* Injury, internal, genital organ
  graafian follicle (ruptured) 620.0
  internal organs (abdomen, chest, or pelvis) (*see also* Injury, internal, by site)
    kidney — *see* Hematoma, kidney, traumatic
    liver — *see* Hematoma, liver, traumatic
    spleen — *see* Hematoma, spleen
  intracranial — *see* Hematoma, brain
  kidney, cystic 593.81
    traumatic 866.01
      with open wound into cavity 866.11
  labia (nontraumatic) 624.5
  lingual (and other parts of neck, scalp, or face, except eye) 920
  liver (subcapsular) 573.8
    birth injury 767.8
    fetus or newborn 767.8
    traumatic NEC 864.01

☑ **Additional Digit Required** — Refer to the Tabular List for Digit Selection
▽ **Subterms under main terms may continue to next column or page**

2015 ICD-9-CM   ►◄ **Revised Text**   ● **New Line**   ▲ **Revised Code**   **Volume 2 — 133**

Hematoma — *see also* Contusion — *continued*
liver — *continued*
traumatic — *continued*
with
laceration — *see* Laceration, liver
open wound into cavity 864.11
mediastinum — *see* Injury, internal, mediastinum
meninges, meningeal (brain) (*see also* Hematoma, brain, subarachnoid)
spinal — *see* Injury, spinal, by site
mesosalpinx (nontraumatic) 620.8
traumatic — *see* Injury, internal, pelvis
muscle (traumatic) — *see* Contusion, by site
nontraumatic 729.92
nasal (septum) (and other part(s) of neck, scalp, or face, except eye) 920
obstetrical surgical wound 674.3 ☑
orbit, orbital (nontraumatic) 376.32
traumatic 921.2
ovary (corpus luteum) (nontraumatic) 620.1
traumatic — *see* Injury, internal, ovary
pelvis (female) (nontraumatic) 629.89
complicating delivery 665.7 ☑
male 608.83
traumatic (*see also* Injury, internal, pelvis)
specified organ NEC (*see also* Injury, internal, pelvis) 867.6
penis (nontraumatic) 607.82
pericranial (and neck, or face any part, except eye) 920
due to injury at birth 767.19
perineal wound (obstetrical) 674.3 ☑
complicating delivery 664.5 ☑
perirenal, cystic 593.81
pinna 380.31
placenta — *see* Placenta, abnormal
postoperative 998.12
retroperitoneal (nontraumatic) 568.81
traumatic — *see* Injury, internal, retroperitoneum
retropubic, male 568.81
scalp (and neck, or face any part, except eye) 920
fetus or newborn 767.19
scrotum (nontraumatic) 608.83
traumatic 922.4
seminal vesicle (nontraumatic) 608.83
traumatic — *see* Injury, internal, seminal, vesicle
soft tissue 729.92
spermatic cord (*see also* Injury, internal, spermatic cord)
nontraumatic 608.83
spinal (cord) (meninges) (*see also* Injury, spinal, by site)
fetus or newborn 767.4
nontraumatic 336.1
spleen 865.01
with
laceration — *see* Laceration, spleen
open wound into cavity 865.11
sternocleidomastoid, birth injury 767.8
sternomastoid, birth injury 767.8
subarachnoid (*see also* Hematoma, brain, subarachnoid)
fetus or newborn 772.2
nontraumatic (*see also* Hemorrhage, subarachnoid) 430
newborn 772.2
subdural (*see also* Hematoma, brain, subdural)
fetus or newborn (localized) 767.0
nontraumatic (*see also* Hemorrhage, subdural) 432.1
subperiosteal (syndrome) 267
traumatic — *see* Hematoma, by site
superficial, fetus or newborn 772.6
syncytium — *see* Placenta, abnormal
testis (nontraumatic) 608.83
birth injury 767.8
traumatic 922.4
tunica vaginalis (nontraumatic) 608.83
umbilical cord 663.6 ☑
affecting fetus or newborn 762.6

Hematoma — *see also* Contusion — *continued*
uterine ligament (nontraumatic) 620.7
traumatic — *see* Injury, internal, pelvis
uterus 621.4
traumatic — *see* Injury, internal, pelvis
vagina (nontraumatic) (ruptured) 623.6
complicating delivery 665.7 ☑
traumatic 922.4
vas deferens (nontraumatic) 608.83
traumatic — *see* Injury, internal, vas deferens
vitreous 379.23
vocal cord 920
vulva (nontraumatic) 624.5
complicating delivery 664.5 ☑
fetus or newborn 767.8
traumatic 922.4
Hematometra 621.4
Hematomyelia 336.1
with fracture of vertebra (*see also* Fracture, vertebra, by site, with spinal cord injury) 806.8
fetus or newborn 767.4
Hematomyelitis 323.9
late effect — *see* category 326
Hematoperitoneum — *see also* Hemoperitoneum 568.81
Hematopneumothorax — *see also* Hemothorax 511.89
Hematopoiesis, cyclic 288.02
Hematoporphyria (acquired) (congenital) 277.1
Hematoporphyrinuria (acquired) (congenital) 277.1
Hematorachis, hematorrhachis 336.1
fetus or newborn 767.4
Hematosalpinx 620.8
with
ectopic pregnancy (*see also* categories 633.0–633.9) 639.2
infectional (*see also* Salpingo-oophoritis) 614.2
molar pregnancy (*see also* categories 630–632) 639.2
Hematospermia 608.82
Hematothorax — *see also* Hemothorax 511.89
Hematotympanum 381.03
Hematuria (benign) (essential) (idiopathic) 599.70
due to S. hematobium 120.0
endemic 120.0
gross 599.71
intermittent 599.70
malarial 084.8
microscopic 599.72
paroxysmal 599.70
sulfonamide
correct substance properly administered 599.70
overdose or wrong substance given or taken 961.0
tropical (bilharziasis) 120.0
tuberculous (*see also* Tuberculosis) 016.9 ☑
Hematuric bilious fever 084.8
Hemeralopia 368.10
Hemiabiotrophy 799.89
Hemi-akinesia 781.8
Hemianalgesia — *see also* Disturbance, sensation 782.0
Hemianencephaly 740.0
Hemianesthesia — *see also* Disturbance, sensation 782.0
Hemianopia, hemianopsia (altitudinal) (homonymous) 368.46
binasal 368.47
bitemporal 368.47
heteronymous 368.47
syphilitic 095.8
Hemiasomatognosia 307.9
Hemiathetosis 781.0
Hemiatrophy 799.89
cerebellar 334.8
face 349.89
progressive 349.89
fascia 728.9

Hemiatrophy — *continued*
leg 728.2
tongue 529.8
Hemiballism (us) 333.5
Hemiblock (cardiac) (heart) (left) 426.2
Hemicardia 746.89
Hemicephalus, hemicephaly 740.0
Hemichorea 333.5
Hemicrania 346.9 ☑
congenital malformation 740.0
continua 339.41
paroxysmal 339.03
chronic 339.04
episodic 339.03
Hemidystrophy — *see* Hemiatrophy
Hemiectromelia 755.4
Hemihypalgesia — *see also* Disturbance, sensation 782.0
Hemihypertrophy (congenital) 759.89
cranial 756.0
Hemihypesthesia — *see also* Disturbance, sensation 782.0
Hemi-inattention 781.8
Hemimelia 755.4
lower limb 755.30
paraxial (complete) (incomplete) (intercalary) (terminal) 755.32
fibula 755.37
tibia 755.36
transverse (complete) (partial) 755.31
upper limb 755.20
paraxial (complete) (incomplete) (intercalary) (terminal) 755.22
radial 755.26
ulnar 755.27
transverse (complete) (partial) 755.21
Hemiparalysis — *see also* Hemiplegia 342.9 ☑
Hemiparesis — *see also* Hemiplegia 342.9 ☑
Hemiparesthesia — *see also* Disturbance, sensation 782.0
Hemiplegia 342.9 ☑
acute (*see also* Disease, cerebrovascular, acute) 436
alternans facialis 344.89
apoplectic (*see also* Disease, cerebrovascular, acute) 436
late effect or residual
affecting
dominant side 438.21
nondominant side 438.22
unspecified side 438.20
arteriosclerotic 437.0
late effect or residual
affecting
dominant side 438.21
nondominant side 438.22
unspecified side 438.20
ascending (spinal) NEC 344.89
attack (*see also* Disease, cerebrovascular, acute) 436
brain, cerebral (current episode) 437.8
congenital 343.1
cerebral — *see* Hemiplegia, brain
congenital (cerebral) (spastic) (spinal) 343.1
conversion neurosis (hysterical) 300.11
cortical — *see* Hemiplegia, brain
due to
arteriosclerosis 437.0
late effect or residual
affecting
dominant side 438.21
nondominant side 438.22
unspecified side 438.20
cerebrovascular lesion (*see also* Disease, cerebrovascular, acute) 436
late effect
affecting
dominant side 438.21
nondominant side 438.22
unspecified side 438.20
embolic (current) (*see also* Embolism, brain) 434.1 ☑
late effect
affecting
dominant side 438.21
nondominant side 438.22

Hemiplegia — *continued*
embolic (*see also* Embolism, brain) — *continued*
late effect — *continued*
affecting — *continued*
unspecified side 438.20
flaccid 342.0 ☑
hypertensive (current episode) 437.8
infantile (postnatal) 343.4
late effect
birth injury, intracranial or spinal 343.4
cerebrovascular lesion — *see* Late effect(s) (of) cerebrovascular disease
viral encephalitis 139.0
middle alternating NEC 344.89
newborn NEC 767.0
seizure (current episode) (*see also* Disease, cerebrovascular, acute) 436
spastic 342.1 ☑
congenital or infantile 343.1
specified NEC 342.8 ☑
thrombotic (current) (*see also* Thrombosis, brain) 434.0 ☑
late effect — *see* Late effect(s) (of) cerebrovascular disease
Hemisection, spinal cord — *see* Fracture, vertebra, by site, with spinal cord injury
Hemispasm 781.0
facial 781.0
Hemispatial neglect 781.8
Hemisporosis 117.9
Hemitremor 781.0
Hemivertebra 756.14
Hemobilia 576.8
Hemocholecyst 575.8
Hemochromatosis (acquired) (liver) (myocardium) (secondary) 275.03
with refractory anemia 238.72
diabetic 275.03
due to repeated red blood cell transfusions 275.02
hereditary 275.01
primary idiopathic 275.01
specified NEC 275.03
transfusion associated (red blood cell) 275.02
Hemodialysis V56.0
Hemoglobin — *see also* condition
abnormal (disease) — *see* Disease, hemoglobin
AS genotype 282.5
fetal, hereditary persistence 282.7
H Constant Spring 282.43
H disease 282.43
high-oxygen-affinity 289.0
low NEC 285.9
S (Hb-S), heterozygous 282.5
Hemoglobinemia 283.2
due to blood transfusion NEC 999.89
bone marrow 996.85
paroxysmal 283.2
Hemoglobinopathy (mixed) — *see also* Disease, hemoglobin 282.7
with thalassemia 282.49
sickle-cell 282.60
with thalassemia (without crisis) 282.41
with
crisis 282.42
vaso-occlusive pain 282.42
Hemoglobinuria, hemoglobinuric 791.2
with anemia, hemolytic, acquired (chronic) NEC 283.2
cold (agglutinin) (paroxysmal) (with Raynaud's syndrome) 283.2
due to
exertion 283.2
hemolysis (from external causes) NEC 283.2
exercise 283.2
fever (malaria) 084.8
infantile 791.2
intermittent 283.2
malarial 084.8
march 283.2
nocturnal (paroxysmal) 283.2

Hemoglobinuria, hemoglobinuric —
    continued
    paroxysmal (cold) (nocturnal) 283.2
Hemolymphangioma (M9175/0) 228.1
Hemolysis
    fetal — *see* Jaundice, fetus or newborn
    intravascular (disseminated) NEC 286.6
        with
            abortion — *see* Abortion, by type,
                with hemorrhage, delayed or
                excessive
            ectopic pregnancy (*see also* cate-
                gories 633.0–633.9) 639.1
            hemorrhage of pregnancy 641.3 ☑
                affecting fetus or newborn 762.1
            molar pregnancy (*see also* categories
                630–632) 639.1
        acute 283.2
        following
            abortion 639.1
            ectopic or molar pregnancy 639.1
    neonatal — *see* Jaundice, fetus or newborn
    transfusion NEC 999.89
        bone marrow 996.85
Hemolytic — *see also* condition
    anemia — *see* Anemia, hemolytic
    uremic syndrome 283.11
Hemometra 621.4
Hemopericardium (with effusion) 423.0
    newborn 772.8
    traumatic (*see also* Hemothorax, traumatic)
        860.2
        with open wound into thorax 860.3
Hemoperitoneum 568.81
    infectional (*see also* Peritonitis) 567.29
    traumatic — *see* Injury, internal, peritoneum
Hemophagocytic syndrome 288.4
    infection-associated 288.4
Hemophilia (familial) (hereditary) 286.0
    A 286.0
        carrier (asymptomatic) V83.01
            symptomatic V83.02
    acquired 286.52
    autoimmune 286.52
    B (Leyden) 286.1
    C 286.2
    calcipriva (*see also* Fibrinolysis) 286.7
    classical 286.0
    nonfamilial 286.7
    secondary 286.52
    vascular 286.4
Hemophilus influenzae NEC 041.5
    arachnoiditis (basic) (brain) (spinal) 320.0
        late effect — *see* category 326
    bronchopneumonia 482.2
    cerebral ventriculitis 320.0
        late effect — *see* category 326
    cerebrospinal inflammation 320.0
        late effect — *see* category 326
    infection NEC 041.5
    leptomeningitis 320.0
        late effect — *see* category 326
    meningitis (cerebral) (cerebrospinal) (spinal)
        320.0
        late effect — *see* category 326
    meningomyelitis 320.0
        late effect — *see* category 326
    pachymeningitis (adhesive) (fibrous) (hem-
        orrhagic) (hypertrophic) (spinal)
        320.0
        late effect — *see* category 326
    pneumonia (broncho-) 482.2
Hemophthalmos 360.43
Hemopneumothorax — *see also* Hemothorax
    511.89
    traumatic 860.4
        with open wound into thorax 860.5
Hemoptysis 786.30
    due to Paragonimus (westermani) 121.2
    newborn 770.3
    specified NEC 786.39
    tuberculous (*see also* Tuberculosis, pul-
        monary) 011.9 ☑
Hemorrhage, hemorrhagic (nontraumatic)
    459.0
    abdomen 459.0

Hemorrhage, hemorrhagic — *continued*
    accidental (antepartum) 641.2 ☑
        affecting fetus or newborn 762.1
    adenoid 474.8
    adrenal (capsule) (gland) (medulla) 255.41
        newborn 772.5
    after labor — *see* Hemorrhage, postpartum
    alveolar
        lung, newborn 770.3
        process 525.8
    alveolus 525.8
    amputation stump (surgical) 998.11
        secondary 997.69
    anemia (chronic) 280.0
        acute 285.1
    antepartum — *see* Hemorrhage, pregnancy
    anus (sphincter) 569.3
    apoplexy (stroke) 432.9
    arachnoid — *see* Hemorrhage, subarach-
        noid
    artery NEC 459.0
        brain (*see also* Hemorrhage, brain) 431
        middle meningeal — *see* Hemorrhage,
            subarachnoid
    basilar (ganglion) (*see also* Hemorrhage,
        brain) 431
    bladder 596.89
    blood dyscrasia 289.9
    bowel 578.9
        newborn 772.4
    brain (miliary) (nontraumatic) 431
        with
            birth injury 767.0
            arachnoid — *see* Hemorrhage, subarach-
                noid
            due to
                birth injury 767.0
                rupture of aneurysm (congenital) (*see*
                    also Hemorrhage, subarach-
                    noid) 430
                mycotic 431
                syphilis 094.89
        epidural or extradural — *see* Hemor-
            rhage, extradural
        fetus or newborn (anoxic) (hypoxic) (due
            to birth trauma) (nontraumatic)
            767.0
            intraventricular 772.10
                grade I 772.11
                grade II 772.12
                grade III 772.13
                grade IV 772.14
        iatrogenic 997.02
        postoperative 997.02
        puerperal, postpartum, childbirth
            674.0 ☑
        stem 431
        subarachnoid, arachnoid, or meningeal
            — *see* Hemorrhage, subarach-
            noid
        subdural — *see* Hemorrhage, subdural

Hemorrhage, hemorrhagic — *continued*
    brain — *continued*
        traumatic NEC 853.0 ☑

> *Note* — Use the following fifth-digit
> subclassification with categories
> 851–854:
>
> 0   unspecified state of consciousness
>
> 1   with no loss of consciousness
>
> 2   with brief [less than one hour]
>   loss of consciousness
>
> 3   with moderate [1–24 hours] loss
>   of consciousness
>
> 4   with prolonged [more than 24
>   hours] loss of consciousness and
>   return to pre-existing conscious
>   level
>
> 5   with prolonged [more than 24
>   hours] loss of consciousness,
>   without return to pre-existing
>   conscious level
>
> Use fifth-digit 5 to designate when a
> patient is unconscious and dies before
> regaining consciousness, regardless of
> the duration of the loss of consciousness
>
> 6   with loss of consciousness of un-
>   specified duration
>
> 9   with concussion, unspecified

        with
            cerebral
                contusion — *see* Contusion,
                    brain
                laceration — *see* Laceration,
                    brain
            open intracranial wound 853.1 ☑
            skull fracture — *see* Fracture,
                skull, by site
        extradural or epidural 852.4 ☑
            with open intracranial wound
                852.5 ☑
        subarachnoid 852.0 ☑
            with open intracranial wound
                852.1 ☑
        subdural 852.2 ☑
            with open intracranial wound
                852.3 ☑
    breast 611.79
    bronchial tube — *see* Hemorrhage, lung
    bronchopulmonary — *see* Hemorrhage,
        lung
    bronchus (cause unknown) (*see also* Hemor-
        rhage, lung) 786.30
    bulbar (*see also* Hemorrhage, brain) 431
    bursa 727.89
    capillary 448.9
        primary 287.8
    capsular — *see* Hemorrhage, brain
    cardiovascular 429.89
    cecum 578.9
    cephalic (*see also* Hemorrhage, brain) 431
    cerebellar (*see also* Hemorrhage, brain) 431
    cerebellum (*see also* Hemorrhage, brain) 431
    cerebral (*see also* Hemorrhage, brain) 431
        fetus or newborn (anoxic) (traumatic)
        767.0
    cerebromeningeal (*see also* Hemorrhage,
        brain) 431
    cerebrospinal (*see also* Hemorrhage, brain)
        431
    cerebrovascular accident — *see* Hemor-
        rhage, brain
    cerebrum (*see also* Hemorrhage, brain) 431
    cervix (stump) (uteri) 622.8
    cesarean section wound 674.3 ☑
    chamber, anterior (eye) 364.41
    childbirth — *see* Hemorrhage, complicating,
        delivery
    choroid 363.61
        expulsive 363.62
    ciliary body 364.41
    cochlea 386.8
    colon — *see* Hemorrhage, intestine

Hemorrhage, hemorrhagic — *continued*
    complicating
        delivery 641.9 ☑
            affecting fetus or newborn 762.1
            associated with
                afibrinogenemia 641.3 ☑
                    affecting fetus or newborn
                      763.89
                coagulation defect 641.3 ☑
                    affecting fetus or newborn
                      763.89
                hyperfibrinolysis 641.3 ☑
                    affecting fetus or newborn
                      763.89
                hypofibrinogenemia 641.3 ☑
                    affecting fetus or newborn
                      763.89
            due to
                low-lying placenta 641.1 ☑
                  affecting fetus or newborn
                    762.0
                placenta previa 641.1 ☑
                  affecting fetus or newborn
                    762.0
                premature separation of placenta
                  641.2 ☑
                  affecting fetus or newborn
                    762.1
                retained
                  placenta 666.0 ☑
                  secundines 666.2 ☑
                trauma 641.8 ☑
                  affecting fetus or newborn
                    763.89
                uterine leiomyoma 641.8 ☑
                  affecting fetus or newborn
                    763.89
        surgical procedure 998.11
    complication(s)
        of dental implant placement 525.71
    concealed NEC 459.0
    congenital 772.9
    conjunctiva 372.72
        newborn 772.8
    cord, newborn 772.0
        slipped ligature 772.3
        stump 772.3
    corpus luteum (ruptured) 620.1
    cortical (*see also* Hemorrhage, brain) 431
    cranial 432.9
    cutaneous 782.7
        newborn 772.6
    cystitis — *see* Cystitis
    cyst, pancreas 577.2
    delayed
        with
            abortion — *see* Abortion, by type,
                with hemorrhage, delayed or
                excessive
            ectopic pregnancy (*see also* cate-
                gories 633.0–633.9) 639.1
            molar pregnancy (*see also* categories
                630–632) 639.1
        following
            abortion 639.1
            ectopic or molar pregnancy 639.1
        postpartum 666.2 ☑
    diathesis (familial) 287.9
        newborn 776.0
    disease 287.9
        newborn 776.0
        specified type NEC 287.8
    disorder 287.9
        due to intrinsic circulating anticoagu-
            lants, antibodies, or inhibitors
            286.59
            with
                acquired hemophilia 286.52
                antiphospholipid antibody 286.53
        specified type NEC 287.8
    due to
        any device, implant or graft (presence
            of) classifiable to 996.0–996.5 —
            see Complications, due to (pres-
            ence of) any device, implant, or
            graft classified to 996.0–996.5NEC

☑ **Additional Digit Required** — Refer to the Tabular List for Digit Selection   ▽ **Subterms under main terms may continue to next column or page**

Index

Hemorrhage, hemorrhagic — Hemorrhage, hemorrhagic

Hemorrhage, hemorrhagic — *continued*
due to — *continued*
  intrinsic circulating anticoagulant, anti-
    bodies, or inhibitors 286.59
    with
      acquired hemophilia 286.52
      antiphospholipid antibody 286.53
  duodenum, duodenal 537.89
    ulcer — *see* Ulcer, duodenum, with
      hemorrhage
  dura mater — *see* Hemorrhage, subdural
  endotracheal — *see* Hemorrhage, lung
  epicranial subaponeurotic (massive) 767.11
  epidural — *see* Hemorrhage, extradural
  episiotomy 674.3 ☑
  esophagus 530.82
    varix (*see also* Varix, esophagus, bleed-
      ing) 456.0
  excessive
    with
      abortion — *see* Abortion, by type,
        with hemorrhage, delayed or
        excessive
      ectopic pregnancy (*see also* cate-
        gories 633.0–633.9) 639.1
      molar pregnancy (*see also* categories
        630–632) 639.1
    following
      abortion 639.1
      ectopic or molar pregnancy 639.1
  external 459.0
  extradural (traumatic) (*see also* Hemorrhage,
    brain, traumatic, extradural)
    birth injury 767.0
    fetus or newborn (anoxic) (traumatic)
      767.0
    nontraumatic 432.0
  eye 360.43
    chamber (anterior) (aqueous) 364.41
    fundus 362.81
  eyelid 374.81
  fallopian tube 620.8
  fetomaternal 772.0
    affecting management of pregnancy or
      puerperium 656.0 ☑
  fetus, fetal, affecting newborn 772.0
    from
      cut end of co-twin's cord 772.0
      placenta 772.0
      ruptured cord 772.0
      vasa previa 772.0
    into
      co-twin 772.0
      mother's circulation 772.0
        affecting management of preg-
          nancy or puerperium
          656.0 ☑
  fever (*see also* Fever, hemorrhagic) 065.9
    with renal syndrome 078.6
    arthropod-borne NEC 065.9
    Bangkok 065.4
    Crimean 065.0
    dengue virus 065.4
    epidemic 078.6
    Junin virus 078.7
    Korean 078.6
    Machupo virus 078.7
    mite-borne 065.8
    mosquito-borne 065.4
    Philippine 065.4
    Russian (Yaroslav) 078.6
    Singapore 065.4
    southeast Asia 065.4
    Thailand 065.4
    tick-borne NEC 065.3
  fibrinogenolysis (*see also* Fibrinolysis) 286.6
  fibrinolytic (acquired) (*see also* Fibrinolysis)
    286.6
  fontanel 767.19
  from tracheostomy stoma 519.09
  fundus, eye 362.81
  funis
    affecting fetus or newborn 772.0
    complicating delivery 663.8 ☑
  gastric (*see also* Hemorrhage, stomach)
    578.9

Hemorrhage, hemorrhagic — *continued*
gastroenteric 578.9
  newborn 772.4
gastrointestinal (tract) 578.9
  newborn 772.4
genitourinary (tract) NEC 599.89
gingiva 523.8
globe 360.43
gravidarum — *see* Hemorrhage, pregnancy
gum 523.8
heart 429.89
hypopharyngeal (throat) 784.8
intermenstrual 626.6
  irregular 626.6
  regular 626.5
internal (organs) 459.0
  capsule (*see also* Hemorrhage, brain) 431
  ear 386.8
  newborn 772.8
intestine 578.9
  congenital 772.4
  newborn 772.4
into
  bladder wall 596.7
  bursa 727.89
  corpus luysii (*see also* Hemorrhage,
    brain) 431
intra-abdominal 459.0
  during or following surgery 998.11
intra-alveolar, newborn (lung) 770.3
intracerebral (*see also* Hemorrhage, brain)
  431
intracranial NEC 432.9
  puerperal, postpartum, childbirth
    674.0 ☑
  traumatic — *see* Hemorrhage, brain,
    traumatic
intramedullary NEC 336.1
intraocular 360.43
intraoperative 998.11
intrapartum — *see* Hemorrhage, complicating, delivery
intrapelvic
  female 629.89
  male 459.0
intraperitoneal 459.0
intrapontine (*see also* Hemorrhage, brain)
  431
intrauterine 621.4
  complicating delivery — *see* Hemor-
    rhage, complicating, delivery
  in pregnancy or childbirth — *see* Hemor-
    rhage, pregnancy
  postpartum (*see also* Hemorrhage,
    postpartum) 666.1 ☑
intraventricular (*see also* Hemorrhage, brain)
  431
  fetus or newborn (anoxic) (traumatic)
    772.10
    grade I 772.11
    grade II 772.12
    grade III 772.13
    grade IV 772.14
intravesical 596.7
iris (postinfectional) (postinflammatory)
  (toxic) 364.41
joint (nontraumatic) 719.10
  ankle 719.17
  elbow 719.12
  foot 719.17
  forearm 719.13
  hand 719.14
  hip 719.15
  knee 719.16
  lower leg 719.16
  multiple sites 719.19
  pelvic region 719.15
  shoulder (region) 719.11
  specified site NEC 719.18
  thigh 719.15
  upper arm 719.12
  wrist 719.13
kidney 593.81
knee (joint) 719.16
labyrinth 386.8
leg NEC 459.0

Hemorrhage, hemorrhagic — *continued*
lenticular striate artery (*see also* Hemorrhage, brain) 431
ligature, vessel 998.11
liver 573.8
lower extremity NEC 459.0
lung 786.30
  newborn 770.3
  tuberculous (*see also* Tuberculosis, pul-
    monary) 011.9 ☑
malaria 084.8
marginal sinus 641.2 ☑
massive subaponeurotic, birth injury 767.11
maternal, affecting fetus or newborn 762.1
mediastinum 786.30
medulla (*see also* Hemorrhage, brain) 431
membrane (brain) (*see also* Hemorrhage,
  subarachnoid) 430
  spinal cord — *see* Hemorrhage, spinal
    cord
meninges, meningeal (brain) (middle) (*see
  also* Hemorrhage, subarachnoid) 430
  spinal cord — *see* Hemorrhage, spinal
    cord
mesentery 568.81
metritis 626.8
midbrain (*see also* Hemorrhage, brain) 431
mole 631.8
mouth 528.9
mucous membrane NEC 459.0
  newborn 772.8
muscle 728.89
nail (subungual) 703.8
nasal turbinate 784.7
  newborn 772.8
nasopharynx 478.29
navel, newborn 772.3
newborn 772.9
  adrenal 772.5
  alveolar (lung) 770.3
  brain (anoxic) (hypoxic) (due to birth
    trauma) 767.0
  cerebral (anoxic) (hypoxic) (due to birth
    trauma) 767.0
  conjunctiva 772.8
  cutaneous 772.6
  diathesis 776.0
    due to vitamin K deficiency 776.0
  epicranial subaponeurotic (massive)
    767.11
  gastrointestinal 772.4
  internal (organs) 772.8
  intestines 772.4
  intra-alveolar (lung) 770.3
  intracranial (from any perinatal cause)
    767.0
  intraventricular (from any perinatal
    cause) 772.10
    grade I 772.11
    grade II 772.12
    grade III 772.13
    grade IV 772.14
  lung 770.3
  pulmonary (massive) 770.3
  spinal cord, traumatic 767.4
  stomach 772.4
  subaponeurotic (massive) 767.11
  subarachnoid (from any perinatal cause)
    772.2
  subconjunctival 772.8
  subgaleal 767.11
  umbilicus 772.0
    slipped ligature 772.3
    vasa previa 772.0
nipple 611.79
nose 784.7
  newborn 772.8
obstetrical surgical wound 674.3 ☑
omentum 568.89
  newborn 772.4
optic nerve (sheath) 377.42
orbit 376.32
ovary 620.1
oviduct 620.8
pancreas 577.8
parathyroid (gland) (spontaneous) 252.8

Hemorrhage, hemorrhagic — *continued*
parturition — *see* Hemorrhage, complicating, delivery
penis 607.82
pericardium, pericarditis 423.0
perineal wound (obstetrical) 674.3 ☑
peritoneum, peritoneal 459.0
peritonsillar tissue 474.8
  after operation on tonsils 998.11
  due to infection 475
petechial 782.7
pituitary (gland) 253.8
placenta NEC 641.9 ☑
  affecting fetus or newborn 762.1
  from surgical or instrumental damage
    641.8 ☑
    affecting fetus or newborn 762.1
  previa 641.1 ☑
    affecting fetus or newborn 762.0
pleura — *see* Hemorrhage, lung
polioencephalitis, superior 265.1
polymyositis — *see* Polymyositis
pons (*see also* Hemorrhage, brain) 431
pontine (*see also* Hemorrhage, brain) 431
popliteal 459.0
postcoital 626.7
postextraction (dental) 998.11
postmenopausal 627.1
postnasal 784.7
postoperative 998.11
postpartum (atonic) (following delivery of
  placenta) 666.1 ☑
  delayed or secondary (after 24 hours)
    666.2 ☑
  retained placenta 666.0 ☑
  third stage 666.0 ☑
pregnancy (concealed) 641.9 ☑
  accidental 641.2 ☑
    affecting fetus or newborn 762.1
  affecting fetus or newborn 762.1
  before 22 completed weeks gestation
    640.9 ☑
    affecting fetus or newborn 762.1
  due to
    abruptio placenta 641.2 ☑
      affecting fetus or newborn 762.1
    afibrinogenemia or other coagula-
      tion defect (conditions classifi-
      able to 286.0–286.9) 641.3 ☑
      affecting fetus or newborn 762.1
    coagulation defect 641.3 ☑
      affecting fetus or newborn 762.1
    hyperfibrinolysis 641.3 ☑
      affecting fetus or newborn 762.1
    hypofibrinogenemia 641.3 ☑
      affecting fetus or newborn 762.1
    leiomyoma, uterus 641.8 ☑
      affecting fetus or newborn 762.1
    low-lying placenta 641.1 ☑
      affecting fetus or newborn 762.1
    marginal sinus (rupture) 641.2 ☑
      affecting fetus or newborn 762.1
    placenta previa 641.1 ☑
      affecting fetus or newborn 762.0
    premature separation of placenta
      (normally implanted) 641.2 ☑
      affecting fetus or newborn 762.1
    threatened abortion 640.0 ☑
      affecting fetus or newborn 762.1
    trauma 641.8 ☑
      affecting fetus or newborn 762.1
  early (before 22 completed weeks gesta-
    tion) 640.9 ☑
    affecting fetus or newborn 762.1
  previous, affecting management of
    pregnancy or childbirth V23.49
  unavoidable — *see* Hemorrhage, preg-
    nancy, due to placenta previa
prepartum (mother) — *see* Hemorrhage,
  pregnancy
preretinal, cause unspecified 362.81
prostate 602.1
puerperal (*see also* Hemorrhage, postpartum) 666.1 ☑

☑ **Additional Digit Required** — Refer to the Tabular List for Digit Selection   ▽ **Subterms under main terms may continue to next column or page**

136 — Volume 2   ▶◀ **Revised Text**   ● **New Line**   ▲ **Revised Code**   **2015 ICD-9-CM**

Hemorrhage, hemorrhagic — *continued*
pulmonary (*see also* Hemorrhage, lung) 786.30
  acute idiopathic in infants (AIPHI) (over 28 days old) 786.31
  newborn (massive) 770.3
  renal syndrome 446.21
purpura (primary) (*see also* Purpura, thrombocytopenic) 287.39
rectum (sphincter) 569.3
recurring, following initial hemorrhage at time of injury 958.2
renal 593.81
  pulmonary syndrome 446.21
respiratory tract (*see also* Hemorrhage, lung) 786.30
retina, retinal (deep) (superficial) (vessels) 362.81
  diabetic 250.5 ☑ [362.01]
    due to secondary diabetes 249.5 ☑ [362.01]
  due to birth injury 772.8
retrobulbar 376.89
retroperitoneal 459.0
retroplacental (*see also* Placenta, separation) 641.2 ☑
scalp 459.0
  due to injury at birth 767.19
scrotum 608.83
secondary (nontraumatic) 459.0
  following initial hemorrhage at time of injury 958.2
seminal vesicle 608.83
skin 782.7
  newborn 772.6
spermatic cord 608.83
spinal (cord) 336.1
  aneurysm (ruptured) 336.1
    syphilitic 094.89
  due to birth injury 767.4
  fetus or newborn 767.4
spleen 289.59
spontaneous NEC 459.0
  petechial 782.7
stomach 578.9
  newborn 772.4
  ulcer — *see* Ulcer, stomach, with hemorrhage
subaponeurotic, newborn 767.11
  massive (birth injury) 767.11
subarachnoid (nontraumatic) 430
  fetus or newborn (anoxic) (traumatic) 772.2
  puerperal, postpartum, childbirth 674.0 ☑
  traumatic — *see* Hemorrhage, brain, traumatic, subarachnoid
subconjunctival 372.72
  due to birth injury 772.8
  newborn 772.8
subcortical (*see also* Hemorrhage, brain) 431
subcutaneous 782.7
subdiaphragmatic 459.0
subdural (nontraumatic) 432.1
  due to birth injury 767.0
  fetus or newborn (anoxic) (hypoxic) (due to birth trauma) 767.0
  puerperal, postpartum, childbirth 674.0 ☑
  spinal 336.1
  traumatic — *see* Hemorrhage, brain, traumatic, subdural
subgaleal 767.11
subhyaloid 362.81
subperiosteal 733.99
subretinal 362.81
subtentorial (*see also* Hemorrhage, subdural) 432.1
subungual 703.8
  due to blood dyscrasia 287.8
suprarenal (capsule) (gland) 255.41
  fetus or newborn 772.5
tentorium (traumatic) (*see also* Hemorrhage, brain, traumatic)
  fetus or newborn 767.0

Hemorrhage, hemorrhagic — *continued*
tentorium (*see also* Hemorrhage, brain, traumatic) — *continued*
  nontraumatic — *see* Hemorrhage, subdural
testis 608.83
thigh 459.0
third stage 666.0 ☑
thorax — *see* Hemorrhage, lung
throat 784.8
thrombocythemia 238.71
thymus (gland) 254.8
thyroid (gland) 246.3
  cyst 246.3
tongue 529.8
tonsil 474.8
  postoperative 998.11
tooth socket (postextraction) 998.11
trachea — *see* Hemorrhage, lung
traumatic (*see also* nature of injury)
  brain — *see* Hemorrhage, brain, traumatic
  recurring or secondary (following initial hemorrhage at time of injury) 958.2
tuberculous NEC (*see also* Tuberculosis, pulmonary) 011.9 ☑
tunica vaginalis 608.83
ulcer — *see* Ulcer, by site, with hemorrhage
umbilicus, umbilical cord 772.0
  after birth, newborn 772.3
  complicating delivery 663.8 ☑
    affecting fetus or newborn 772.0
  slipped ligature 772.3
  stump 772.3
unavoidable (due to placenta previa) 641.1 ☑
  affecting fetus or newborn 762.0
upper extremity 459.0
urethra (idiopathic) 599.84
uterus, uterine (abnormal) 626.9
  climacteric 627.0
  complicating delivery — *see* Hemorrhage, complicating, delivery
  due to
    intrauterine contraceptive device 996.76
    perforating uterus 996.32
  functional or dysfunctional 626.8
  in pregnancy — *see* Hemorrhage, pregnancy
  intermenstrual 626.6
    irregular 626.6
    regular 626.5
  postmenopausal 627.1
  postpartum (*see also* Hemorrhage, postpartum) 666.1 ☑
  prepubertal 626.8
  pubertal 626.3
  puerperal (immediate) 666.1 ☑
vagina 623.8
vasa previa 663.5 ☑
  affecting fetus or newborn 772.0
vas deferens 608.83
ventricular (*see also* Hemorrhage, brain) 431
vesical 596.89
viscera 459.0
  newborn 772.8
vitreous (humor) (intraocular) 379.23
vocal cord 478.5
vulva 624.8

Hemorrhoids (anus) (rectum) (without complication) 455.6
bleeding, prolapsed, strangulated, or ulcerated NEC 455.8
  external 455.5
  internal 455.2
complicated NEC 455.8
complicating pregnancy and puerperium 671.8 ☑
external 455.3
  with complication NEC 455.5
  bleeding, prolapsed, strangulated, or ulcerated 455.5
  thrombosed 455.4
internal 455.0

Hemorrhoids — *continued*
internal — *continued*
  with complication NEC 455.2
  bleeding, prolapsed, strangulated, or ulcerated 455.2
  thrombosed 455.1
residual skin tag 455.9
sentinel pile 455.9
thrombosed NEC 455.7
  external 455.4
  internal 455.1

Hemosalpinx 620.8
Hemosiderosis 275.09
dietary 275.09
pulmonary (idiopathic) 275.09 [516.1]
transfusion NEC 275.02
  bone marrow 996.85
Hemospermia 608.82
Hemothorax 511.89
bacterial, nontuberculous 511.1
newborn 772.8
nontuberculous 511.89
  bacterial 511.1
pneumococcal 511.1
postoperative 998.11
staphylococcal 511.1
streptococcal 511.1
traumatic 860.2
  with
    open wound into thorax 860.3
    pneumothorax 860.4
      with open wound into thorax 860.5
tuberculous (*see also* Tuberculosis, pleura) 012.0 ☑
Hemotympanum 385.89
Hench-Rosenberg syndrome (palindromic arthritis) — *see also* Rheumatism, palindromic 719.3 ☑
Henle's warts 371.41
Henoch (-Schönlein)
disease or syndrome (allergic purpura) 287.0
purpura (allergic) 287.0
Henpue, henpuye 102.6
Heparin-induced thrombocytopenia (HIT) 289.84
Heparitinuria 277.5
Hepar lobatum 095.3
Hepatalgia 573.8
Hepatic — *see also* condition
flexure syndrome 569.89
Hepatitis 573.3
acute (*see also* Necrosis, liver) 570
  alcoholic 571.1
  infective 070.1
    with hepatic coma 070.0
alcoholic 571.1
amebic — *see* Abscess, liver, amebic
anicteric (acute) — *see* Hepatitis, viral
antigen-associated (HAA) — *see* Hepatitis, viral, type B
Australian antigen (positive) — *see* Hepatitis, viral, type B
autoimmune 571.42
catarrhal (acute) 070.1
  with hepatic coma 070.0
  chronic 571.40
  newborn 070.1
    with hepatic coma 070.0
chemical 573.3
cholangiolitic 573.8
cholestatic 573.8
chronic 571.40
  active 571.49
    viral — *see* Hepatitis, viral
  aggressive 571.49
  persistent 571.41
  viral — *see* Hepatitis, viral
cytomegalic inclusion virus 078.5 [573.1]
diffuse 573.3
"dirty needle" — *see* Hepatitis, viral
drug-induced 573.3
due to
  Coxsackie 074.8 [573.1]
  cytomegalic inclusion virus 078.5 [573.1]
  infectious mononucleosis 075 [573.1]

Hepatitis — *continued*
due to — *continued*
  malaria 084.9 [573.2]
  mumps 072.71
  secondary syphilis 091.62
  toxoplasmosis (acquired) 130.5
    congenital (active) 771.2
epidemic — *see* Hepatitis, viral, type A
fetus or newborn 774.4
fibrous (chronic) 571.49
  acute 570
from injection, inoculation, or transfusion (blood) (other substance) (plasma) (serum) (onset within 8 months after administration) — *see* Hepatitis, viral
fulminant (viral) (*see also* Hepatitis, viral) 070.9
  with hepatic coma 070.6
  type A 070.1
    with hepatic coma 070.0
  type B — *see* Hepatitis, viral, type B
giant cell (neonatal) 774.4
hemorrhagic 573.8
history of
  B V12.09
  C V12.09
homologous serum — *see* Hepatitis, viral
hypertrophic (chronic) 571.49
  acute 570
infectious, infective (acute) (chronic) (subacute) 070.1
  with hepatic coma 070.0
inoculation — *see* Hepatitis, viral
interstitial (chronic) 571.49
  acute 570
lupoid 571.49
malarial 084.9 [573.2]
malignant (*see also* Necrosis, liver) 570
neonatal (toxic) 774.4
newborn 774.4
parenchymatous (acute) (*see also* Necrosis, liver) 570
peliosis 573.3
persistent, chronic 571.41
plasma cell 571.49
postimmunization — *see* Hepatitis, viral
postnecrotic 571.49
posttransfusion — *see* Hepatitis, viral
recurrent 571.49
septic 573.3
serum — *see* Hepatitis, viral
  carrier (suspected of) V02.61
subacute (*see also* Necrosis, liver) 570
suppurative (diffuse) 572.0
syphilitic (late) 095.3
  congenital (early) 090.0 [573.2]
    late 090.5 [573.2]
  secondary 091.62
toxic (noninfectious) 573.3
  fetus or newborn 774.4
tuberculous (*see also* Tuberculosis) 017.9 ☑
viral (acute) (anicteric) (cholangiolitic) (cholestatic) (chronic) (subacute) 070.9
  with hepatic coma 070.6
  AU-SH type virus — *see* Hepatitis, viral, type B
  Australian antigen — *see* Hepatitis, viral, type B
  B-antigen — *see* Hepatitis, viral, type B
  Coxsackie 074.8 [573.1]
  cytomegalic inclusion 078.5 [573.1]
  IH (virus) — *see* Hepatitis, viral, type A
  infectious hepatitis virus — *see* Hepatitis, viral, type A
  serum hepatitis virus — *see* Hepatitis, viral, type B
  SH — *see* Hepatitis, viral, type B
  specified type NEC 070.59
    with hepatic coma 070.49
  type A 070.1
    with hepatic coma 070.0
  type B (acute) 070.30
    with
      hepatic coma 070.20
        with hepatitis delta 070.21

☑ **Additional Digit Required — Refer to the Tabular List for Digit Selection**

▽ **Subterms under main terms may continue to next column or page**

Hepatitis — continued
  viral — continued
    type B — continued
      with — continued
        hepatitis delta 070.31
          with hepatic coma 070.21
      carrier status V02.61
      chronic 070.32
        with
          hepatic coma 070.22
            with hepatitis delta 070.23
          hepatitis delta 070.33
            with hepatic coma 070.23
    type C
      acute 070.51
        with hepatic coma 070.41
      carrier status V02.62
      chronic 070.54
        with hepatic coma 070.44
      in remission 070.54
      unspecified 070.70
        with hepatic coma 070.71
    type delta (with hepatitis B carrier state)
      070.52
      with
        active hepatitis B disease — see
          Hepatitis, viral, type B
        hepatic coma 070.42
    type E 070.53
      with hepatic coma 070.43
  vaccination and inoculation (prophylactic) V05.3
  Waldenström's (lupoid hepatitis) 571.49
Hepatization, lung (acute) — see also Pneumonia, lobar
  chronic (see also Fibrosis, lung) 515
Hepatoblastoma (M8970/3) 155.0
Hepatocarcinoma (M8170/3) 155.0
Hepatocholangiocarcinoma (M8180/3) 155.0
Hepatocholangioma, benign (M8180/0) 211.5
Hepatocholangitis 573.8
Hepatocystitis — see also Cholecystitis 575.10
Hepatodystrophy 570
Hepatolenticular degeneration 275.1
Hepatolithiasis — see Choledocholithiasis
Hepatoma (malignant) (M8170/3) 155.0
  benign (M8170/0) 211.5
  congenital (M8970/3) 155.0
  embryonal (M8970/3) 155.0
Hepatomegalia glycogenica diffusa 271.0
Hepatomegaly — see also Hypertrophy, liver
  789.1
  congenital 751.69
    syphilitic 090.0
  due to Clonorchis sinensis 121.1
  Gaucher's 272.7
  syphilitic (congenital) 090.0
Hepatoptosis 573.8
Hepatorrhexis 573.8
Hepatosis, toxic 573.8
Hepatosplenomegaly 571.8
  due to S. japonicum 120.2
  hyperlipemic (Bürger-Grutz type) 272.3
Herald patch 696.3
Hereditary — see condition
Heredodegeneration 330.9
  macular 362.70
Heredopathia atactica polyneuritiformis 356.3
Heredosyphilis — see also Syphilis, congenital
  090.9
Hermaphroditism (true) 752.7
  with specified chromosomal anomaly —
    see Anomaly, chromosomes, sex
Hernia, hernial (acquired) (recurrent) 553.9
  with
    gangrene (obstructed) NEC 551.9
    obstruction NEC 552.9
      and gangrene 551.9
  abdomen (wall) — see Hernia, ventral
  abdominal, specified site NEC 553.8
    with
      gangrene (obstructed) 551.8
      obstruction 552.8
        and gangrene 551.8
  appendix 553.8

Hernia, hernial — continued
  appendix — continued
    with
      gangrene (obstructed) 551.8
      obstruction 552.8
        and gangrene 551.8
  bilateral (inguinal) — see Hernia, inguinal
  bladder (sphincter)
    congenital (female) (male) 756.71
    female (see also Cystocele, female)
      618.01
    male 596.89
  brain 348.4
    congenital 742.0
  broad ligament 553.8
  cartilage, vertebral — see Displacement,
    intervertebral disc
  cerebral 348.4
    congenital 742.0
    endaural 742.0
  ciliary body 364.89
    traumatic 871.1
  colic 553.9
    with
      gangrene (obstructed) 551.9
      obstruction 552.9
        and gangrene 551.9
  colon 553.9
    with
      gangrene (obstructed) 551.9
      obstruction 552.9
        and gangrene 551.9
  colostomy (stoma) 569.69
  Cooper's (retroperitoneal) 553.8
    with
      gangrene (obstructed) 551.8
      obstruction 552.8
        and gangrene 551.8
  crural — see Hernia, femoral
  cystostomy 596.83
  diaphragm, diaphragmatic 553.3
    with
      gangrene (obstructed) 551.3
      obstruction 552.3
        and gangrene 551.3
    congenital 756.6
    due to gross defect of diaphragm 756.6
    traumatic 862.0
      with open wound into cavity 862.1
  direct (inguinal) — see Hernia, inguinal
  disc, intervertebral — see Displacement,
    intervertebral disc
  diverticulum, intestine 553.9
    with
      gangrene (obstructed) 551.9
      obstruction 552.9
        and gangrene 551.9
  double (inguinal) — see Hernia, inguinal
  due to adhesion with obstruction 552.9
  duodenojejunal 553.8
    with
      gangrene (obstructed) 551.8
      obstruction 552.8
        and gangrene 551.8
  en glissade — see Hernia, inguinal
  enterostomy (stoma) 569.69
  epigastric 553.29
    with
      gangrene (obstruction) 551.29
      obstruction 552.29
        and gangrene 551.29
    recurrent 553.21
      with
        gangrene (obstructed) 551.21
        obstruction 552.21
          and gangrene 551.21
  esophageal hiatus (sliding) 553.3
    with
      gangrene (obstructed) 551.3
      obstruction 552.3
        and gangrene 551.3
    congenital 750.6
  external (inguinal) — see Hernia, inguinal
  fallopian tube 620.4
  fascia 728.89
  fat 729.30

Hernia, hernial — continued
  fat — continued
    eyelid 374.34
    orbital 374.34
    pad 729.30
      eye, eyelid 374.34
      knee 729.31
      orbit 374.34
      popliteal (space) 729.31
      specified site NEC 729.39
  femoral (unilateral) 553.00
    with
      gangrene (obstructed) 551.00
      obstruction 552.00
        with gangrene 551.00
    bilateral 553.02
      gangrenous (obstructed) 551.02
      obstructed 552.02
        with gangrene 551.02
      recurrent 553.03
        gangrenous (obstructed) 551.03
        obstructed 552.03
          with gangrene 551.03
    recurrent (unilateral) 553.01
      bilateral 553.03
        gangrenous (obstructed) 551.03
        obstructed 552.03
          with gangrene 551.01
      gangrenous (obstructed) 551.01
      obstructed 552.01
        with gangrene 551.01
  foramen
    Bochdalek 553.3
      with
        gangrene (obstructed) 551.3
        obstruction 552.3
          and gangrene 551.3
      congenital 756.6
    magnum 348.4
    Morgagni, Morgagnian 553.3
      with
        gangrene 551.3
        obstruction 552.3
          and gangrene 551.3
      congenital 756.6
  funicular (umbilical) 553.1
    with
      gangrene (obstructed) 551.1
      obstruction 552.1
        and gangrene 551.1
    spermatic cord — see Hernia, inguinal
  gangrenous — see Hernia, by site, with
    gangrene
  gastrointestinal tract 553.9
    with
      gangrene (obstructed) 551.9
      obstruction 552.9
        and gangrene 551.9
  gluteal — see Hernia, femoral
  Gruber's (internal mesogastric) 553.8
    with
      gangrene (obstructed) 551.8
      obstruction 552.8
        and gangrene 551.8
  Hesselbach's 553.8
    with
      gangrene (obstructed) 551.8
      obstruction 552.8
        and gangrene 551.8
  hiatal (esophageal) (sliding) 553.3
    with
      gangrene (obstructed) 551.3
      obstruction 552.3
        and gangrene 551.3
    congenital 750.6
  incarcerated (see also Hernia, by site, with
    obstruction) 552.9
    gangrenous (see also Hernia, by site, with
      gangrene) 551.9
  incisional 553.21
    with
      gangrene (obstructed) 551.21
      obstruction 552.21
        and gangrene 551.21
    lumbar — see Hernia, lumbar
    recurrent 553.21

Hernia, hernial — continued
  incisional — continued
    recurrent — continued
      with
        gangrene (obstructed) 551.21
        obstruction 552.21
          and gangrene 551.21
  indirect (inguinal) — see Hernia, inguinal
  infantile — see Hernia, inguinal
  infrapatellar fat pad 729.31
  inguinal (direct) (double) (encysted) (external) (funicular) (indirect) (infantile) (internal) (interstitial) (oblique) (scrotal) (sliding) 550.9 ☑

> Note — Use the following fifth-digit
> subclassification with category 550:
>
> 0   unilateral or unspecified (not
>   specified as recurrent)
>
> 1   unilateral or unspecified, recurrent
>
> 2   bilateral (not specified as recurrent)
>
> 3   bilateral, recurrent

    with
      gangrene (obstructed) 550.0 ☑
      obstruction 550.1 ☑
        and gangrene 550.0 ☑
  internal 553.8
    with
      gangrene (obstructed) 551.8
      obstruction 552.8
        and gangrene 551.8
    inguinal — see Hernia, inguinal
  interstitial 553.9
    with
      gangrene (obstructed) 551.9
      obstruction 552.9
        and gangrene 551.9
    inguinal — see Hernia, inguinal
  intervertebral cartilage or disc — see Displacement, intervertebral disc
  intestine, intestinal 553.9
    with
      gangrene (obstructed) 551.9
      obstruction 552.9
        and gangrene 551.9
  intra-abdominal 553.9
    with
      gangrene (obstructed) 551.9
      obstruction 552.9
        and gangrene 551.9
  intraparietal 553.9
    with
      gangrene (obstructed) 551.9
      obstruction 552.9
        and gangrene 551.9
  iris 364.89
    traumatic 871.1
  irreducible (see also Hernia, by site, with
    obstruction) 552.9
    gangrenous (with obstruction) (see also
      Hernia, by site, with gangrene)
      551.9
  ischiatic 553.8
    with
      gangrene (obstructed) 551.8
      obstruction 552.8
        and gangrene 551.8
  ischiorectal 553.8
    with
      gangrene (obstructed) 551.8
      obstruction 552.8
        and gangrene 551.8
  lens 379.32
    traumatic 871.1
  linea
    alba — see Hernia, epigastric
    semilunaris — see Hernia, spigelian
  Littre's (diverticular) 553.9
    with
      gangrene (obstructed) 551.9
      obstruction 552.9
        and gangrene 551.9
  lumbar 553.8

☑ Additional Digit Required — Refer to the Tabular List for Digit Selection   ⍜ Subterms under main terms may continue to next column or page

138 — Volume 2   ▶◀ Revised Text   ● New Line   ▲ Revised Code   2015 ICD-9-CM

Hernia, hernial — *continued*
  lumbar — *continued*
    with
      gangrene (obstructed) 551.8
        obstruction 552.8
          and gangrene 551.8
      intervertebral disc 722.10
  lung (subcutaneous) 518.89
    congenital 748.69
  mediastinum 519.3
  mesenteric (internal) 553.8
    with
      gangrene (obstructed) 551.8
        obstruction 552.8
          and gangrene 551.8
  mesocolon 553.8
    with
      gangrene (obstructed) 551.8
        obstruction 552.8
          and gangrene 551.8
  muscle (sheath) 728.89
  nucleus pulposus — *see* Displacement, intervertebral disc
  oblique (inguinal) — *see* Hernia, inguinal
  obstructive (*see also* Hernia, by site, with obstruction) 552.9
    gangrenous (with obstruction) (*see also* Hernia, by site, with gangrene) 551.9
  obturator 553.8
    with
      gangrene (obstructed) 551.8
        obstruction 552.8
          and gangrene 551.8
  omental 553.8
    with
      gangrene (obstructed) 551.8
        obstruction 552.8
          and gangrene 551.8
  orbital fat (pad) 374.34
  ovary 620.4
  oviduct 620.4
  paracolostomy (stoma) 569.69
  paraduodenal 553.8
    with
      gangrene (obstructed) 551.8
        obstruction 552.8
          and gangrene 551.8
  paraesophageal 553.3
    with
      gangrene (obstructed) 551.3
        obstruction 552.3
          and gangrene 551.3
    congenital 750.6
  parahiatal 553.3
    with
      gangrene (obstructed) 551.3
        obstruction 552.3
          and gangrene 551.3
  paraumbilical 553.1
    with
      gangrene (obstructed) 551.1
        obstruction 552.1
          and gangrene 551.1
  parietal 553.9
    with
      gangrene (obstructed) 551.9
        obstruction 552.9
          and gangrene 551.9
  perineal 553.8
    with
      gangrene (obstructed) 551.8
        obstruction 552.8
          and gangrene 551.8
  peritoneal sac, lesser 553.8
    with
      gangrene (obstructed) 551.8
        obstruction 552.8
          and gangrene 551.8
  popliteal fat pad 729.31
  postoperative 553.21
    with
      gangrene (obstructed) 551.21
        obstruction 552.21
          and gangrene 551.21
  pregnant uterus 654.4 ☑

Hernia, hernial — *continued*
  prevesical 596.89
  properitoneal 553.8
    with
      gangrene (obstructed) 551.8
        obstruction 552.8
          and gangrene 551.8
  pudendal 553.8
    with
      gangrene (obstructed) 551.8
        obstruction 552.8
          and gangrene 551.8
  rectovaginal 618.6
  retroperitoneal 553.8
    with
      gangrene (obstructed) 551.8
        obstruction 552.8
          and gangrene 551.8
  Richter's (parietal) 553.9
    with
      gangrene (obstructed) 551.9
        obstruction 552.9
          and gangrene 551.9
  Rieux's, Riex's (retrocecal) 553.8
    with
      gangrene (obstructed) 551.8
        obstruction 552.8
          and gangrene 551.8
  sciatic 553.8
    with
      gangrene (obstructed) 551.8
        obstruction 552.8
          and gangrene 551.8
  scrotum, scrotal — *see* Hernia, inguinal
  sliding (inguinal) (*see also* Hernia, inguinal)
    hiatus — *see* Hernia, hiatal
  spigelian 553.29
    with
      gangrene (obstructed) 551.29
        obstruction 552.29
          and gangrene 551.29
  spinal (*see also* Spina bifida) 741.9 ☑
    with hydrocephalus 741.0 ☑
  strangulated (*see also* Hernia, by site, with obstruction) 552.9
    gangrenous (with obstruction) (*see also* Hernia, by site, with gangrene) 551.9
  supraumbilicus (linea alba) — *see* Hernia, epigastric
  tendon 727.9
  testis (nontraumatic) 550.9 ☑
    meaning
      scrotal hernia 550.9 ☑
      symptomatic late syphilis 095.8
  Treitz's (fossa) 553.8
    with
      gangrene (obstructed) 551.8
        obstruction 552.8
          and gangrene 551.8
  tunica
    albuginea 608.89
    vaginalis 752.89
  umbilicus, umbilical 553.1
    with
      gangrene (obstructed) 551.1
        obstruction 552.1
          and gangrene 551.1
  ureter 593.89
    with obstruction 593.4
  uterus 621.8
    pregnant 654.4 ☑
  vaginal (posterior) 618.6
  Velpeau's (femoral) (*see also* Hernia, femoral) 553.00
  ventral 553.20
    with
      gangrene (obstructed) 551.20
        obstruction 552.20
          and gangrene 551.20
    incisional 553.21
    recurrent 553.21
      with
        gangrene (obstructed) 551.21
          obstruction 552.21
            and gangrene 551.21

Hernia, hernial — *continued*
  vesical
    congenital (female) (male) 756.71
    female (*see also* Cystocele, female) 618.01
    male 596.89
  vitreous (into anterior chamber) 379.21
    traumatic 871.1
Herniation — *see also* Hernia
  brain (stem) 348.4
  cerebral 348.4
  gastric mucosa (into duodenal bulb) 537.89
  mediastinum 519.3
  nucleus pulposus — *see* Displacement, intervertebral disc
Herpangina 074.0
Herpes, herpetic 054.9
  auricularis (zoster) 053.71
    simplex 054.73
  blepharitis (zoster) 053.20
    simplex 054.41
  circinate 110.5
  circinatus 110.5
    bullous 694.5
  conjunctiva (simplex) 054.43
    zoster 053.21
  cornea (simplex) 054.43
    disciform (simplex) 054.43
    zoster 053.21
  encephalitis 054.3
  eye (zoster) 053.29
    simplex 054.40
  eyelid (zoster) 053.20
    simplex 054.41
  febrilis 054.9
  fever 054.9
  geniculate ganglionitis 053.11
  genital, genitalis 054.10
    specified site NEC 054.19
  gestationis 646.8 ☑
  gingivostomatitis 054.2
  iridocyclitis (simplex) 054.44
    zoster 053.22
  iris (any site) 695.10
  iritis (simplex) 054.44
  keratitis (simplex) 054.43
    dendritic 054.42
    disciform 054.43
    interstitial 054.43
    zoster 053.21
  keratoconjunctivitis (simplex) 054.43
    zoster 053.21
  labialis 054.9
    meningococcal 036.89
  lip 054.9
  meningitis (simplex) 054.72
    zoster 053.0
  ophthalmicus (zoster) 053.20
    simplex 054.40
  otitis externa (zoster) 053.71
    simplex 054.73
  penis 054.13
  perianal 054.10
  pharyngitis 054.79
  progenitalis 054.10
  scrotum 054.19
  septicemia 054.5
  simplex 054.9
    complicated 054.8
      ophthalmic 054.40
        specified NEC 054.49
      specified NEC 054.79
    congenital 771.2
    external ear 054.73
    keratitis 054.43
      dendritic 054.42
    meningitis 054.72
    myelitis 054.74
    neuritis 054.79
    specified complication NEC 054.79
      ophthalmic 054.49
    visceral 054.71
  stomatitis 054.2
  tonsurans 110.0
    maculosus (of Hebra) 696.3
  visceral 054.71

Herpes, herpetic — *continued*
  vulva 054.12
  vulvovaginitis 054.11
  whitlow 054.6
  zoster 053.9
    auricularis 053.71
    complicated 053.8
      specified NEC 053.79
    conjunctiva 053.21
    cornea 053.21
    ear 053.71
    eye 053.29
    geniculate 053.11
    keratitis 053.21
      interstitial 053.21
    myelitis 053.14
    neuritis 053.10
    ophthalmicus(a) 053.20
    oticus 053.71
    otitis externa 053.71
    specified complication NEC 053.79
    specified site NEC 053.9
    zosteriform, intermediate type 053.9
Herrick's
  anemia (hemoglobin S disease) 282.61
  syndrome (hemoglobin S disease) 282.61
Hers' disease (glycogenosis VI) 271.0
Herter (-Gee) disease or syndrome (nontropical sprue) 579.0
Herter's infantilism (nontropical sprue) 579.0
Herxheimer's disease (diffuse idiopathic cutaneous atrophy) 701.8
Herxheimer's reaction 995.91
Hesitancy, urinary 788.64
Hesselbach's hernia — *see* Hernia, Hesselbach's
Heterochromia (congenital) 743.46
  acquired 364.53
  cataract 366.33
  cyclitis 364.21
  hair 704.3
  iritis 364.21
  retained metallic foreign body 360.62
    magnetic 360.52
  uveitis 364.21
Heterophoria 378.40
  alternating 378.45
  vertical 378.43
Heterophyes, small intestine 121.6
Heterophyiasis 121.6
Heteropsia 368.8
Heterotopia, heterotopic — *see also* Malposition, congenital
  cerebralis 742.4
  pancreas, pancreatic 751.7
  spinalis 742.59
Heterotropia 378.30
  intermittent 378.20
    vertical 378.31
  vertical (constant) (intermittent) 378.31
Heubner's disease 094.89
Heubner-Herter disease or syndrome (nontropical sprue) 579.0
Hexadactylism 755.0 ☑
Heyd's syndrome (hepatorenal) 572.4
HGSIL (high grade squamous intraepithelial lesion) (cytologic finding) (Pap smear finding)
  anus 796.74
  cervix 795.04
    biopsy finding — code to CIN II or CIN III
  vagina 795.14
Hibernoma (M8880/0) — *see* Lipoma
Hiccough 786.8
  epidemic 078.89
  psychogenic 306.1
Hiccup — *see also* Hiccough 786.8
Hicks (-Braxton) contractures 644.1 ☑
Hidden penis 752.65
Hidradenitis (axillaris) (suppurative) 705.83
Hidradenoma (nodular) (M8400/0) — *see also* Neoplasm, skin, benign
  clear cell (M8402/0) — *see* Neoplasm, skin, benign

☑ Additional Digit Required — Refer to the Tabular List for Digit Selection   ▽ Subterms under main terms may continue to next column or page

2015 ICD-9-CM   ▶◀ Revised Text   ● New Line   ▲ Revised Code   **Volume 2 — 139**

Hidradenoma — *see also* Neoplasm, skin, benign — *continued*
  papillary (M8405/0) — *see* Neoplasm, skin, benign
Hidrocystoma (M8404/0) — *see* Neoplasm, skin, benign
HIE (hypoxic-ischemic encephalopathy) 768.70
  mild 768.71
  moderate 768.72
  severe 768.73
High
  A₂ anemia 282.46
  altitude effects 993.2
    anoxia 993.2
    on
      ears 993.0
      sinuses 993.1
    polycythemia 289.0
  arch
    foot 755.67
    palate 750.26
  artery (arterial) tension (*see also* Hypertension) 401.9
    without diagnosis of hypertension 796.2
  basal metabolic rate (BMR) 794.7
  blood pressure (*see also* Hypertension) 401.9
    borderline 796.2
    incidental reading (isolated) (nonspecific), no diagnosis of hypertension 796.2
  cholesterol 272.0
    with high triglycerides 272.2
  compliance bladder 596.4
  diaphragm (congenital) 756.6
  frequency deafness (congenital) (regional) 389.8
  head at term 652.5 ☑
    affecting fetus or newborn 763.1
  output failure (cardiac) (*see also* Failure, heart) 428.9
  oxygen-affinity hemoglobin 289.0
  palate 750.26
  risk
    behavior — *see* Problem
    family situation V61.9
      specified circumstance NEC V61.8
    human papillomavirus (HPV) DNA test positive
      anal 796.75
      cervical 795.05
      vaginal 795.15
    individual NEC V62.89
    infant NEC V20.1
    patient taking drugs (prescribed) V67.51
      nonprescribed (*see also* Abuse, drugs, nondependent) 305.9 ☑
    pregnancy V23.9
      inadequate prenatal care V23.7
      inconclusive fetal viability V23.87
      specified problem NEC V23.89
  temperature (of unknown origin) (*see also* Pyrexia) 780.60
  thoracic rib 756.3
  triglycerides 272.1
    with high cholesterol 272.2
Hildenbrand's disease (typhus) 081.9
Hilger's syndrome 337.09
Hill diarrhea 579.1
Hilliard's lupus — *see also* Tuberculosis 017.0 ☑
Hilum — *see* condition
Hip — *see* condition
Hippel's disease (retinocerebral angiomatosis) 759.6
Hippus 379.49
Hirschfeld's disease (acute diabetes mellitus) — *see also* Diabetes 250.0 ☑
  due to secondary diabetes 249.0 ☑
Hirschsprung's disease or megacolon (congenital) 751.3
Hirsuties — *see also* Hypertrichosis 704.1
Hirsutism — *see also* Hypertrichosis 704.1
Hirudiniasis (external) (internal) 134.2
Hiss-Russell dysentery 004.1
Histamine cephalgia 339.00
Histidinemia 270.5

Histidinuria 270.5
Histicytic syndromes 288.4
Histiocytoma (M8832/0) — *see also* Neoplasm, skin, benign
  fibrous (M8830/0) (*see also* Neoplasm, skin, benign)
    atypical (M8830/1) — *see* Neoplasm, connective tissue, uncertain behavior
    malignant (M8830/3) — *see* Neoplasm, connective tissue, malignant
Histiocytosis (acute) (chronic) (subacute) 277.89
  acute differentiated progressive (M9722/3) 202.5 ☑
  adult pulmonary Langerhans cell (PLCH) 516.5
  cholesterol 277.89
  essential 277.89
  lipid, lipoid (essential) 272.7
  lipochrome (familial) 288.1
  malignant (M9720/3) 202.3 ☑
  non-Langerhans cell 277.89
  polyostotic sclerosing 277.89
  X (chronic) 277.89
    acute (progressive) (M9722/3) 202.5 ☑
Histoplasmosis 115.90
  with
    endocarditis 115.94
    meningitis 115.91
    pericarditis 115.93
    pneumonia 115.95
    retinitis 115.92
    specified manifestation NEC 115.99
  African (due to Histoplasma duboisii) 115.10
    with
      endocarditis 115.14
      meningitis 115.11
      pericarditis 115.13
      pneumonia 115.15
      retinitis 115.12
      specified manifestation NEC 115.19
  American (due to Histoplasma capsulatum) 115.00
    with
      endocarditis 115.04
      meningitis 115.01
      pericarditis 115.03
      pneumonia 115.05
      retinitis 115.02
      specified manifestation NEC 115.09
  Darling's — *see* Histoplasmosis, American
  large form (*see also* Histoplasmosis, African) 115.10
  lung 115.05
  small form (*see also* Histoplasmosis, American) 115.00
History (personal) of
  abuse
    emotional V15.42
    neglect V15.42
    physical V15.41
    sexual V15.41
  affective psychosis V11.1
  alcoholism V11.3
    specified as drinking problem (*see also* Abuse, drugs, nondependent) 305.0 ☑
  allergy to V15.09
    analgesic agent NEC V14.6
    anesthetic NEC V14.4
    antibiotic agent NEC V14.1
      penicillin V14.0
    anti-infective agent NEC V14.3
    arachnid bite V15.06
    diathesis V15.09
    drug V14.9
      specified type NEC V14.8
    eggs V15.03
    food additives V15.05
    insect bite V15.06
    latex V15.07
    medicinal agents V14.9
      specified type NEC V14.8
    milk products V15.02
    narcotic agent NEC V14.5

History of — *continued*
  allergy to — *continued*
    nuts V15.05
      peanuts V15.01
    penicillin V14.0
    radiographic dye V15.08
    seafood V15.04
    serum V14.7
    specified food NEC V15.05
    specified nonmedicinal agents NEC V15.09
    spider bite V15.06
    sulfa V14.2
    sulfonamides V14.2
    therapeutic agent NEC V15.09
    vaccine V14.7
  anaphylactic reaction or shock V13.81
  anaphylaxis V13.81
  anemia V12.3
  arrest, sudden cardiac V12.53
  arthritis V13.4
  attack, transient ischemic (TIA) V12.54
  benign neoplasm of brain V12.41
  blood disease V12.3
  calculi, urinary V13.01
  cardiovascular disease V12.50
    myocardial infarction 412
  chemotherapy, antineoplastic V87.41
  child abuse V15.41
  cigarette smoking V15.82
  circulatory system disease V12.50
    myocardial infarction 412
  cleft lip and palate, corrected V13.64
  combat and operational stress reaction V11.4
  congenital malformation (corrected)
    circulatory system V13.65
    digestive system V13.67
    ear V13.64
    eye V13.64
    face V13.64
    genitourinary system V13.62
    heart V13.65
    integument V13.68
    limbs V13.68
    musculoskeletal V13.68
    neck V13.64
    nervous system V13.63
    respiratory system V13.66
    specified type NEC V13.69
  contraception V15.7
  death, sudden, successfully resuscitated V12.53
  deficit
    prolonged reversible ischemic neurologic (PRIND) V12.54
    reversible ischemic neurologic (RIND) V12.54
  diathesis, allergic V15.09
  digestive system disease V12.70
    peptic ulcer V12.71
    polyps, colonic V12.72
    specified NEC V12.79
  disease (of) V13.9
    blood V12.3
    blood-forming organs V12.3
    cardiovascular system V12.50
    circulatory system V12.50
      specified NEC V12.59
    digestive system V12.70
      peptic ulcer V12.71
      polyps, colonic V12.72
      specified NEC V12.79
    infectious V12.00
      malaria V12.03
      methicillin resistant Staphylococcus aureus (MRSA) V12.04
      MRSA (methicillin resistant Staphylococcus aureus) V12.04
      poliomyelitis V12.02
      specified NEC V12.09
      tuberculosis V12.01
    parasitic V12.00
      specified NEC V12.09
    respiratory system V12.60
      pneumonia V12.61

History of — *continued*
  disease — *continued*
    respiratory system — *continued*
      specified NEC V12.69
    skin V13.3
    specified site NEC V13.89
    subcutaneous tissue V13.3
    trophoblastic V13.1
      affecting management of pregnancy V23.1
  disorder (of) V13.9
    endocrine V12.29
      gestational diabetes V12.21
    genital system V13.29
    hematological V12.3
    immunity V12.29
    mental V11.9
      affective type V11.1
      manic-depressive V11.1
      neurosis V11.2
      schizophrenia V11.0
      specified type NEC V11.8
    metabolic V12.29
    musculoskeletal NEC V13.59
    nervous system V12.40
      specified type NEC V12.49
    obstetric V13.29
      affecting management of current pregnancy V23.49
      ectopic pregnancy V23.42
      pre-term labor V23.41
    pre-term labor V13.21
    sense organs V12.40
      specified type NEC V12.49
    specified site NEC V13.89
    urinary system V13.00
      calculi V13.01
      infection V13.02
      nephrotic syndrome V13.03
      specified NEC V13.09
  drug use
    nonprescribed (*see also* Abuse, drugs, nondependent) 305.9 ☑
    patent (*see also* Abuse, drugs, non-dependent) 305.9 ☑
  dysplasia
    cervical (conditions classifiable to 622.10-622.12) V13.22
    vaginal (conditions classifiable to 623.0) V13.23
    vulvar (conditions classifiable to 624.01-624.02) V13.24
  effect NEC of external cause V15.89
  embolism V12.51
    pulmonary V12.55
  emotional abuse V15.42
  encephalitis V12.42
  endocrine disorder V12.29
    gestational diabetes V12.21
  estrogen therapy V87.43
  extracorporeal membrane oxygenation (ECMO) V15.87
  failed
    conscious sedation V15.80
    moderate sedation V15.80
  falling V15.88
  family
    allergy V19.6
    anemia V18.2
    arteriosclerosis V17.49
    arthritis V17.7
    asthma V17.5
    blindness V19.0
    blood disorder NEC V18.3
    cardiovascular disease V17.49
    carrier, genetic disease V18.9
    cerebrovascular disease V17.1
    chronic respiratory condition NEC V17.6
    colonic polyps V18.51
    congenital anomalies V19.5
    consanguinity V19.7
    coronary artery disease V17.3
    cystic fibrosis V18.19
    deafness V19.2
    diabetes mellitus V18.0
    digestive disorders V18.59

☑ **Additional Digit Required** — Refer to the Tabular List for Digit Selection   ▽ **Subterms under main terms may continue to next column or page**

140 — Volume 2   ▶◀ **Revised Text**   ● **New Line**   ▲ **Revised Code**   **2015 ICD-9-CM**

History of — *continued*
  family — *continued*
    disabilities, intellectual V18.4
    disease or disorder (of)
      allergic V19.6
      blood NEC V18.3
      cardiovascular NEC V17.49
      cerebrovascular V17.1
      colonic polyps V18.51
      coronary artery V17.3
      death, sudden cardiac (SCD) V17.41
      digestive V18.59
      ear NEC V19.3
      endocrine V18.19
        multiple neoplasia (MEN) syndrome V18.11
      eye NEC V19.19
        glaucoma V19.11
      genitourinary NEC V18.7
      glaucoma V19.11
      hypertensive V17.49
      infectious V18.8
      ischemic heart V17.3
      kidney V18.69
        polycystic V18.61
      mental V17.0
      metabolic V18.19
      musculoskeletal NEC V17.89
        osteoporosis V17.81
      neurological NEC V17.2
      parasitic V18.8
      psychiatric condition V17.0
      skin condition V19.4
    ear disorder NEC V19.3
    endocrine disease V18.19
      multiple neoplasia (MEN) syndrome V18.11
    epilepsy V17.2
    eye disorder NEC V19.19
      glaucoma V19.11
    genetic disease carrier V18.9
    genitourinary disease NEC V18.7
    glaucoma V19.11
    glomerulonephritis V18.69
    gout V18.19
    hay fever V17.6
    hearing loss V19.2
    hematopoietic neoplasia V16.7
    Hodgkin's disease V16.7
    Huntington's chorea V17.2
    hydrocephalus V19.5
    hypertension V17.49
    infarction, myocardial V17.3
    infectious disease V18.8
    intellectual disabilities V18.4
    ischemic heart disease V17.3
    kidney disease V18.69
      polycystic V18.61
    leukemia V16.6
    lymphatic malignant neoplasia NEC V16.7
    malignant neoplasm (of) NEC V16.9
      anorectal V16.0
      anus V16.0
      appendix V16.0
      bladder V16.52
      bone V16.8
      brain V16.8
      breast V16.3
        male V16.8
      bronchus V16.1
      cecum V16.0
      cervix V16.49
      colon V16.0
      duodenum V16.0
      esophagus V16.0
      eye V16.8
      gallbladder V16.0
      gastrointestinal tract V16.0
      genital organs V16.40
      hemopoietic NEC V16.7
      ileum V16.0
      ilium V16.8
      intestine V16.0
      intrathoracic organs NEC V16.2
      kidney V16.51

History of — *continued*
  family — *continued*
    malignant neoplasm — *continued*
      larynx V16.2
      liver V16.0
      lung V16.1
      lymphatic NEC V16.7
      ovary V16.41
      oviduct V16.41
      pancreas V16.0
      penis V16.49
      prostate V16.42
      rectum V16.0
      respiratory organs NEC V16.2
      skin V16.8
      specified site NEC V16.8
      stomach V16.0
      testis V16.43
      trachea V16.1
      ureter V16.59
      urethra V16.59
      urinary organs V16.59
      uterus V16.49
      vagina V16.49
      vulva V16.49
    MEN (multiple endocrine neoplasia syndrome) V18.11
    mental retardation — *see* History, family, intellectual disabilities
    metabolic disease NEC V18.19
    mongolism V19.5
    multiple
      endocrine neoplasia (MEN) syndrome V18.11
      myeloma V16.7
    musculoskeletal disease NEC V17.89
      osteoporosis V17.81
    myocardial infarction V17.3
    nephritis V18.69
    nephrosis V18.69
    osteoporosis V17.81
    parasitic disease V18.8
    polycystic kidney disease V18.61
    psychiatric disorder V17.0
    psychosis V17.0
    retinitis pigmentosa V19.19
    schizophrenia V17.0
    skin conditions V19.4
    specified condition NEC V19.8
    stroke (cerebrovascular) V17.1
    sudden cardiac death (SCD) V17.41
    visual loss V19.0
  foreign body fully removed V15.53
  fracture, healed
    pathologic V13.51
    stress V13.52
    traumatic V15.51
  genital system disorder V13.29
    pre-term labor V13.21
  gestational diabetes V12.21
  health hazard V15.9
    falling V15.88
    specified cause NEC V15.89
  hepatitis
    B V12.09
    C V12.09
  Hodgkin's disease V10.72
  hypospadias (corrected) V13.61
  immunity disorder V12.29
  immunosuppression therapy V87.46
  infarction, cerebral, without residual deficits V12.54
  infection
    central nervous system V12.42
    urinary (tract) V13.02
  infectious disease V12.00
    malaria V12.03
    methicillin resistant Staphylococcus aureus (MRSA) V12.04
    MRSA (methicillin resistant Staphylococcus aureus) V12.04
    poliomyelitis V12.02
    specified NEC V12.09
    tuberculosis V12.01
  injury NEC V15.59
    traumatic brain V15.52

History of — *continued*
  insufficient prenatal care V23.7
  in utero procedure
    during pregnancy V15.21
    while a fetus V15.22
  irradiation V15.3
  leukemia V10.60
    lymphoid V10.61
    monocytic V10.63
    myeloid V10.62
    specified type NEC V10.69
  little or no prenatal care V23.7
  low birth weight (*see also* Status, low birth weight) V21.30
  lymphosarcoma V10.71
  malaria V12.03
  malignant carcinoid tumor V10.91
  malignant neoplasm (of) V10.90
    accessory sinus V10.22
    adrenal V10.88
    anus V10.06
    bile duct V10.09
    bladder V10.51
    bone V10.81
    brain V10.85
    breast V10.3
    bronchus V10.11
    cervix uteri V10.41
    colon V10.05
    connective tissue NEC V10.89
    corpus uteri V10.42
    digestive system V10.00
      specified part NEC V10.09
    duodenum V10.09
    endocrine gland NEC V10.88
    epididymis V10.48
    esophagus V10.03
    eye V10.84
    fallopian tube V10.44
    female genital organ V10.40
      specified site NEC V10.44
    gallbladder V10.09
    gastrointestinal tract V10.00
    gum V10.02
    hematopoietic NEC V10.79
    hypopharynx V10.02
    ileum V10.09
    intrathoracic organs NEC V10.20
    jejunum V10.09
    kidney V10.52
    large intestine V10.05
    larynx V10.21
    lip V10.02
    liver V10.07
    lung V10.11
    lymphatic NEC V10.79
    lymph glands or nodes NEC V10.79
    male genital organ V10.45
      specified site NEC V10.49
    mediastinum V10.29
    melanoma (of skin) V10.82
    middle ear V10.22
    mouth V10.02
      specified part NEC V10.02
    nasal cavities V10.22
    nasopharynx V10.02
    nervous system NEC V10.86
    nose V10.22
    oropharynx V10.02
    ovary V10.43
    pancreas V10.09
    parathyroid V10.88
    penis V10.49
    pharynx V10.02
    pineal V10.88
    pituitary V10.88
    placenta V10.44
    pleura V10.29
    prostate V10.46
    rectosigmoid junction V10.06
    rectum V10.06
    renal pelvis V10.53
    respiratory organs NEC V10.20
    salivary gland V10.02
    skin V10.83
      melanoma V10.82

History of — *continued*
  malignant neoplasm — *continued*
    small intestine NEC V10.09
    soft tissue NEC V10.89
    specified site NEC V10.89
    stomach V10.04
    testis V10.47
    thymus V10.29
    thyroid V10.87
    tongue V10.01
    trachea V10.12
    ureter V10.59
    urethra V10.59
    urinary organ V10.50
    uterine adnexa V10.44
    uterus V10.42
    vagina V10.44
    vulva V10.44
  malignant neuroendocrine tumor V10.91
  manic-depressive psychosis V11.1
  meningitis V12.42
  mental disorder V11.9
    affective type V11.1
    manic-depressive V11.1
    neurosis V11.2
    schizophrenia V11.0
    specified type NEC V11.8
  Merkel cell carcinoma V10.91
  metabolic disorder V12.29
  methicillin resistant Staphylococcus aureus (MRSA) V12.04
  MRSA (methicillin resistant Staphylococcus aureus) V12.04
  musculoskeletal disorder NEC V13.59
  myocardial infarction 412
  neglect (emotional) V15.42
  nephrotic syndrome V13.03
  nervous system disorder V12.40
    specified type NEC V12.49
  neurosis V11.2
  noncompliance with medical treatment V15.81
  nutritional deficiency V12.1
  obstetric disorder V13.29
    affecting management of current pregnancy V23.49
      ectopic pregnancy V23.42
      pre-term labor V23.41
    pre-term labor V13.21
  parasitic disease V12.00
    specified NEC V12.09
  perinatal problems V13.7
    low birth weight (*see also* Status, low birth weight) V21.30
  physical abuse V15.41
  poisoning V15.6
  poliomyelitis V12.02
  polyps, colonic V12.72
  poor obstetric V13.29
    affecting management of current pregnancy V23.49
      ectopic pregnancy V23.42
      pre-term labor V23.41
    pre-term labor V13.21
  prolonged reversible ischemic neurologic deficit (PRIND) V12.54
  psychiatric disorder V11.9
    affective type V11.1
    manic-depressive V11.1
    neurosis V11.2
    schizophrenia V11.0
    specified type NEC V11.8
  psychological trauma V15.49
    emotional abuse V15.42
    neglect V15.42
    physical abuse V15.41
    rape V15.41
  psychoneurosis V11.2
  radiation therapy V15.3
  rape V15.41
  respiratory system disease V12.60
    pneumonia V12.61
    specified NEC V12.69
  reticulosarcoma V10.71
  return from military deployment V62.22

☑ **Additional Digit Required — Refer to the Tabular List for Digit Selection**   ▽ **Subterms under main terms may continue to next column or page**

2015 ICD-9-CM   ▶◀ **Revised Text**   ● **New Line**   ▲ **Revised Code**   **Volume 2 — 141**

History of — continued
reversible ischemic neurologic deficit (RIND)
V12.54
schizophrenia V11.0
skin disease V13.3
smoking (tobacco) V15.82
steroid therapy V87.45
inhaled V87.44
systemic V87.45
stroke without residual deficits V12.54
subcutaneous tissue disease V13.3
sudden
cardiac
arrest V12.53
death (successfully resuscitated)
V12.53
surgery to
great vessels V15.1
heart V15.1
in utero
during pregnancy V15.21
while a fetus V15.22
organs NEC V15.29
syndrome, nephrotic V13.03
therapy
antineoplastic drug V87.41
drug NEC V87.49
estrogen V87.43
immunosuppression V87.46
monoclonal drug V87.42
steroid V87.45
inhaled V87.44
systemic V87.45
thrombophlebitis V12.52
thrombosis V12.51
pulmonary V12.55
tobacco use V15.82
trophoblastic disease V13.1
affecting management of pregnancy
V23.1
tuberculosis V12.01
ulcer, peptic V12.71
urinary system disorder V13.00
calculi V13.01
infection V13.02
nephrotic syndrome V13.03
specified NEC V13.09
His-Werner disease (trench fever) 083.1
HIT (heparin-induced thrombocytopenia)
289.84
Hives (bold) — see also Urticaria 708.9
HIV infection (disease) (illness) — see Human
immunodeficiency virus (disease) (illness) (infection)
Hoarseness 784.42
Hobnail liver — see Cirrhosis, portal
Hobo, hoboism V60.0
Hodgkin's
disease (M9650/3) 201.9 ☑
lymphocytic
depletion (M9653/3) 201.7 ☑
diffuse fibrosis (M9654/3)
201.7 ☑
reticular type (M9655/3) 201.7 ☑
predominance (M9651/3) 201.4 ☑
lymphocytic-histiocytic predominance
(M9651/3) 201.4 ☑
mixed cellularity (M9652/3) 201.6 ☑
nodular sclerosis (M9656/3) 201.5 ☑
cellular phase (M9657/3) 201.5 ☑
granuloma (M9661/3) 201.1 ☑
lymphogranulomatosis (M9650/3) 201.9 ☑
lymphoma (M9650/3) 201.9 ☑
lymphosarcoma (M9650/3) 201.9 ☑
paragranuloma (M9660/3) 201.0 ☑
sarcoma (M9662/3) 201.2 ☑
Hodgson's disease (aneurysmal dilatation of
aorta) 441.9
ruptured 441.5
Hodi-potsy 111.0
Hoffa (-Kastert) disease or syndrome (liposynovitis prepatellaris) 272.8
Hoffmann-Bouveret syndrome (paroxysmal
tachycardia) 427.2
Hoffman's syndrome 244.9 [359.5]

Hole
macula 362.54
optic disc, crater-like 377.22
retina (macula) 362.54
round 361.31
with detachment 361.01
Holla disease — see also Spherocytosis 282.0
Holländer-Simons syndrome (progressive
lipodystrophy) 272.6
Hollow foot (congenital) 754.71
acquired 736.73
Holmes' syndrome (visual disorientation)
368.16
Holoprosencephaly 742.2
due to
trisomy 13 758.1
trisomy 18 758.2
Holthouse's hernia — see Hernia, inguinal
Homesickness 309.89
Homicidal ideation V62.85
Homocystinemia 270.4
Homocystinuria 270.4
Homologous serum jaundice (prophylactic)
(therapeutic) — see Hepatitis, viral
Homosexuality — omit code
ego-dystonic 302.0
pedophilic 302.2
problems with 302.0
Homozygous Hb-S disease 282.61
Honeycomb lung 518.89
congenital 748.4
Hong Kong ear 117.3
HOOD (hereditary osteo-onychodysplasia)
756.89
Hooded
clitoris 752.49
penis 752.69
Hookworm (anemia) (disease) (infestation) —
see Ancylostomiasis
Hoppe-Goldflam syndrome 358.00
Hordeolum (external) (eyelid) 373.11
internal 373.12
Horn
cutaneous 702.8
cheek 702.8
eyelid 702.8
penis 702.8
iliac 756.89
nail 703.8
congenital 757.5
papillary 700
Horner's
syndrome (see also Neuropathy, peripheral,
autonomic) 337.9
traumatic 954.0
teeth 520.4
Horseshoe kidney (congenital) 753.3
Horton's
disease (temporal arteritis) 446.5
headache or neuralgia 339.00
Hospice care V66.7
Hospitalism (in children) NEC 309.83
Hourglass contraction, contracture
bladder 596.89
gallbladder 575.2
congenital 751.69
stomach 536.8
congenital 750.7
psychogenic 306.4
uterus 661.4 ☑
affecting fetus or newborn 763.7
Household circumstance affecting care V60.9
specified type NEC V60.89
Housemaid's knee 727.2
Housing circumstance affecting care V60.9
specified type NEC V60.89
HTLV-I infection 079.51
HTLV-II infection 079.52
HTLV-III/LAV (disease) (illness) (infection) —
see Human immunodeficiency virus
(disease) (illness) (infection)
HTLV-III (disease) (illness) (infection) — see
Human immunodeficiency virus (disease) (illness) (infection)

HTR (hemolytic transfusion reaction)
due to or resulting from
incompatibility
ABO 999.61
acute 999.62
delayed 999.63
non-ABO antigen (minor) (Duffy)
(Kell) (Kidd) (Lewis) (M) (N) (P)
(S) 999.76
acute 999.77
delayed 999.78
Rh antigen (C) (c) (D) (E) (e) 999.71
acute 999.72
delayed 999.73
Huchard's disease (continued arterial hypertension) 401.9
Hudson-Ståhli lines 371.11
Huguier's disease (uterine fibroma) 218.9
Human bite (open wound) — see also Wound,
open, by site
intact skin surface — see Contusion
Human immunodeficiency virus (disease)
(illness) 042
infection V08
with symptoms, symptomatic 042
Human immunodeficiency virus-2 infection
079.53
Human immunovirus (disease) (illness) (infection) — see Human immunodeficiency
virus (disease) (illness) (infection)
Human papillomavirus 079.4
high risk, DNA test positive
anal 796.75
cervical 795.05
vaginal 795.15
low risk, DNA test positive
anal 796.79
cervical 795.09
vaginal 795.19
Human parvovirus 079.83
Human T-cell lymphotrophic virus-I infection 079.51
Human T-cell lymphotrophic virus-II infection 079.52
Human T-cell lymphotrophic virus-III (disease) (illness) (infection) — see Human
immunodeficiency virus (disease) (illness) (infection)
Humpback (acquired) 737.9
congenital 756.19
Hum, venous — omit code
Hunchback (acquired) 737.9
congenital 756.19
Hunger 994.2
air, psychogenic 306.1
disease 251.1
Hungry bone syndrome 275.5
Hunner's ulcer — see also Cystitis 595.1
Hunt's
neuralgia 053.11
syndrome (herpetic geniculate ganglionitis)
053.11
dyssynergia cerebellaris myoclonica
334.2
Hunter's glossitis 529.4
Hunterian chancre 091.0
Hunter (-Hurler) syndrome (mucopolysaccharidosis II) 277.5
Huntington's
chorea 333.4
disease 333.4
Huppert's disease (multiple myeloma)
(M9730/3) 203.0 ☑
Hurler (-Hunter) disease or syndrome (mucopolysaccharidosis II) 277.5
Hürthle cell
adenocarcinoma (M8290/3) 193
adenoma (M8290/0) 226
carcinoma (M8290/3) 193
tumor (M8290/0) 226
Hutchinson's
disease meaning
angioma serpiginosum 709.1
cheiropompholyx 705.81
prurigo estivalis 692.72

Hutchinson's — continued
disease meaning — continued
summer eruption, or summer prurigo
692.72
incisors 090.5
melanotic freckle (M8742/2) (see also Neoplasm, skin, in situ)
malignant melanoma in (M8742/3) —
see Melanoma
teeth or incisors (congenital syphilis) 090.5
Hutchinson-Boeck disease or syndrome
(sarcoidosis) 135
Hutchinson-Gilford disease or syndrome
(progeria) 259.8
Hyaline
degeneration (diffuse) (generalized) 728.9
localized — see Degeneration, by site
membrane (disease) (lung) (newborn) 769
Hyalinosis cutis et mucosae 272.8
Hyalin plaque, sclera, senile 379.16
Hyalitis (asteroid) 379.22
syphilitic 095.8
Hydatid
cyst or tumor (see also Echinococcus)
fallopian tube 752.11
mole — see Hydatidiform mole
Morgagni (congenital) 752.89
fallopian tube 752.11
Hydatidiform mole (benign) (complicating
pregnancy) (delivered) (undelivered) 630
invasive (M9100/1) 236.1
malignant (M9100/1) 236.1
previous, affecting management of pregnancy V23.1
Hydatidosis — see Echinococcus
Hyde's disease (prurigo nodularis) 698.3
Hydradenitis 705.83
Hydradenoma (M8400/0) — see Hidradenoma
Hydralazine lupus or syndrome
correct substance properly administered
695.4
overdose or wrong substance given or taken
972.6
Hydramnios 657.0 ☑
affecting fetus or newborn 761.3
Hydrancephaly 742.3
with spina bifida (see also Spina bifida)
741.0 ☑
Hydranencephaly 742.3
with spina bifida (see also Spina bifida)
741.0 ☑
Hydrargyrism NEC 985.0
Hydrarthrosis — see also Effusion, joint
719.0 ☑
gonococcal 098.50
intermittent (see also Rheumatism, palindromic) 719.3 ☑
of yaws (early) (late) 102.6
syphilitic 095.8
congenital 090.5
Hydremia 285.9
Hydrencephalocele (congenital) 742.0
Hydrencephalomeningocele (congenital)
742.0
Hydroa 694.0
aestivale 692.72
gestationis 646.8 ☑
herpetiformis 694.0
pruriginosa 694.0
vacciniforme 692.72
Hydroadenitis 705.83
Hydrocalycosis — see also Hydronephrosis 591
congenital 753.29
Hydrocalyx — see also Hydronephrosis 591
Hydrocele (calcified) (chylous) (idiopathic)
(infantile) (inguinal canal) (recurrent)
(senile) (spermatic cord) (testis) (tunica
vaginalis) 603.9
canal of Nuck (female) 629.1
male 603.9
congenital 778.6
encysted 603.0
congenital 778.6
female NEC 629.89
infected 603.1
round ligament 629.89

Hydrocele — *continued*
  specified type NEC 603.8
    congenital 778.6
  spinalis (*see also* Spina bifida) 741.9 ☑
  vulva 624.8
Hydrocephalic fetus
  affecting management or pregnancy
    655.0 ☑
  causing disproportion 653.6 ☑
    with obstructed labor 660.1 ☑
      affecting fetus or newborn 763.1
Hydrocephalus (acquired) (external) (internal)
  (malignant) (noncommunicating) (obstructive) (recurrent) 331.4
  aqueduct of Sylvius stricture 742.3
    with spina bifida (*see also* Spina bifida)
      741.0 ☑
  chronic 742.3
    with spina bifida (*see also* Spina bifida)
      741.0 ☑
  communicating 331.3
  congenital (external) (internal) 742.3
    with spina bifida (*see also* Spina bifida)
      741.0 ☑
  due to
    stricture of aqueduct of Sylvius 742.3
      with spina bifida (*see also* Spina bifi-
        da) 741.0 ☑
    toxoplasmosis (congenital) 771.2
  fetal affecting management of pregnancy
    655.0 ☑
  foramen Magendie block (acquired) 331.3
    congenital 742.3
      with spina bifida (*see also* Spina bifi-
        da) 741.0 ☑
  newborn 742.3
    with spina bifida (*see also* Spina bifida)
      741.0 ☑
  normal pressure 331.5
    idiopathic (INPH) 331.5
    secondary 331.3
  otitic 348.2
  syphilitic, congenital 090.49
  tuberculous (*see also* Tuberculosis) 013.8 ☑
Hydrocolpos (congenital) 623.8
Hydrocystoma (M8404/0) — *see* Neoplasm,
  skin, benign
Hydroencephalocele (congenital) 742.0
Hydroencephalomeningocele (congenital)
  742.0
Hydrohematopneumothorax — *see also*
  Hemothorax 511.89
Hydromeningitis — *see* Meningitis
Hydromeningocele (spinal) — *see also* Spina
  bifida 741.9 ☑
  cranial 742.0
Hydrometra 621.8
Hydrometrocolpos 623.8
Hydromicrocephaly 742.1
Hydromphalus (congenital) (since birth)
  757.39
Hydromyelia 742.53
Hydromyelocele — *see also* Spina bifida
  741.9 ☑
Hydronephrosis 591
  atrophic 591
  congenital 753.29
  due to S. hematobium 120.0
  early 591
  functionless (infected) 591
  infected 591
  intermittent 591
  primary 591
  secondary 591
  tuberculous (*see also* Tuberculosis) 016.0 ☑
Hydropericarditis — *see also* Pericarditis 423.9
Hydropericardium — *see also* Pericarditis
  423.9
Hydroperitoneum 789.59
Hydrophobia 071
Hydrophthalmos — *see also* Buphthalmia
  743.20
Hydropneumohemothorax — *see also*
  Hemothorax 511.89
Hydropneumopericarditis — *see also* Pericarditis 423.9

Hydropneumopericardium — *see also* Pericarditis 423.9
Hydropneumothorax 511.89
  nontuberculous 511.89
    bacterial 511.1
  pneumococcal 511.1
  staphylococcal 511.1
  streptococcal 511.1
  traumatic 860.0
    with open wound into thorax 860.1
  tuberculous (*see also* Tuberculosis, pleura)
    012.0 ☑
Hydrops 782.3
  abdominis 789.59
  amnii (complicating pregnancy) (*see also*
    Hydramnios) 657.0 ☑
  articulorum intermittens (*see also* Rheuma-
    tism, palindromic) 719.3 ☑
  cardiac (*see also* Failure, heart) 428.0
  congenital — *see* Hydrops, fetalis
  endolymphatic (*see also* Disease, Ménière's)
    386.00
  fetal, fetalis or newborn 778.0
    due to
      alpha thalassemia 282.43
      isoimmunization 773.3
    not due to isoimmunization 778.0
  gallbladder 575.3
  idiopathic (fetus or newborn) 778.0
  joint (*see also* Effusion, joint) 719.0 ☑
  labyrinth (*see also* Disease, Ménière's) 386.00
  meningeal NEC 331.4
  nutritional 262
  pericardium — *see* Pericarditis
  pleura (*see also* Hydrothorax) 511.89
  renal (*see also* Nephrosis) 581.9
  spermatic cord (*see also* Hydrocele) 603.9
Hydropyonephrosis — *see also* Pyelitis 590.80
  chronic 590.00
Hydrorachis 742.53
Hydrorrhea (nasal) 478.19
  gravidarum 658.1 ☑
  pregnancy 658.1 ☑
Hydrosadenitis 705.83
Hydrosalpinx (fallopian tube) (follicularis)
  614.1
Hydrothorax (double) (pleural) 511.89
  chylous (nonfilarial) 457.8
    filaria (*see also* Infestation, filarial) 125.9
  nontuberculous 511.89
    bacterial 511.1
  pneumococcal 511.1
  staphylococcal 511.1
  streptococcal 511.1
  traumatic 862.29
    with open wound into thorax 862.39
  tuberculous (*see also* Tuberculosis, pleura)
    012.0 ☑
Hydroureter 593.5
  congenital 753.22
Hydroureteronephrosis — *see also* Hydronephrosis 591
Hydrourethra 599.84
Hydroxykynureninuria 270.2
Hydroxyprolinemia 270.8
Hydroxyprolinuria 270.8
Hygroma (congenital) (cystic) (M9173/0) 228.1
  prepatellar 727.3
  subdural — *see* Hematoma, subdural
Hymen — *see* condition
Hymenolepiasis (diminuta) (infection) (infestation) (nana) 123.6
Hymenolepsis (diminuta) (infection) (infesta-
  tion) (nana) 123.6
Hypalgesia — *see also* Disturbance, sensation
  782.0
Hyperabduction syndrome 447.8
Hyperacidity, gastric 536.8
  psychogenic 306.4
Hyperactive, hyperactivity 314.01
  basal cell, uterine cervix 622.10
  bladder 596.51
  bowel (syndrome) 564.9
    sounds 787.5
  cervix epithelial (basal) 622.10
  child 314.01

Hyperactive, hyperactivity — *continued*
  colon 564.9
  gastrointestinal 536.8
    psychogenic 306.4
  intestine 564.9
  labyrinth (unilateral) 386.51
    with loss of labyrinthine reactivity 386.58
    bilateral 386.52
  nasal mucous membrane 478.19
  stomach 536.8
  thyroid (gland) (*see also* Thyrotoxicosis)
    242.9 ☑
Hyperacusis 388.42
Hyperadrenalism (cortical) 255.3
  medullary 255.6
Hyperadrenocorticism 255.3
  congenital 255.2
  iatrogenic
    correct substance properly administered
      255.3
    overdose or wrong substance given or
      taken 962.0
Hyperaffectivity 301.11
Hyperaldosteronism (atypical) (hyperplastic)
  (normoaldosteronal) (normotensive)
  (primary) 255.10
  secondary 255.14
Hyperalgesia — *see also* Disturbance, sensation 782.0
Hyperalimentation 783.6
  carotene 278.3
  specified NEC 278.8
  vitamin A 278.2
  vitamin D 278.4
Hyperaminoaciduria 270.9
  arginine 270.6
  citrulline 270.6
  cystine 270.0
  glycine 270.0
  lysine 270.7
  ornithine 270.6
  renal (types I, II, III) 270.0
Hyperammonemia (congenital) 270.6
Hyperamnesia 780.99
Hyperamylasemia 790.5
Hyperaphia 782.0
Hyperazotemia 791.9
Hyperbetalipoproteinemia (acquired) (essential) (familial) (hereditary) (primary)
  (secondary) 272.0
  with prebetalipoproteinemia 272.2
Hyperbilirubinemia 782.4
  congenital 277.4
  constitutional 277.4
  neonatal (transient) (*see also* Jaundice, fetus
    or newborn) 774.6
    of prematurity 774.2
Hyperbilirubinemica encephalopathia,
  newborn 774.7
  due to isoimmunization 773.4
Hypercalcemia, hypercalcemic (idiopathic)
  275.42
  nephropathy 588.89
Hypercalcinuria 275.40
Hypercapnia 786.09
  with mixed acid-based disorder 276.4
  fetal, affecting newborn 770.89
Hypercarotinemia 278.3
Hypercementosis 521.5
Hyperchloremia 276.9
Hyperchlorhydria 536.8
  neurotic 306.4
  psychogenic 306.4
Hypercholesterinemia — *see* Hypercholesterolemia
Hypercholesterolemia 272.0
  with hyperglyceridemia, endogenous 272.2
  essential 272.0
  familial 272.0
  hereditary 272.0
  primary 272.0
  pure 272.0
Hypercholesterolosis 272.0
Hyperchylia gastrica 536.8
  psychogenic 306.4

Hyperchylomicronemia (familial) (with hyperbetalipoproteinemia) 272.3
Hypercoagulation syndrome (primary) 289.81
  secondary 289.82
Hypercorticosteronism
  correct substance properly administered
    255.3
  overdose or wrong substance given or taken
    962.0
Hypercortisonism
  correct substance properly administered
    255.3
  overdose or wrong substance given or taken
    962.0
Hyperdynamic beta-adrenergic state or
  syndrome (circulatory) 429.82
Hyperekplexia 759.89
Hyperelectrolytemia 276.9
Hyperemesis 536.2
  arising during pregnancy — *see* Hypereme-
    sis, gravidarum
  gravidarum (mild) (before 22 completed
    weeks gestation) 643.0 ☑
    with
      carbohydrate depletion 643.1 ☑
      dehydration 643.1 ☑
      electrolyte imbalance 643.1 ☑
      metabolic disturbance 643.1 ☑
    affecting fetus or newborn 761.8
    severe (with metabolic disturbance)
      643.1 ☑
  psychogenic 306.4
Hyperemia (acute) 780.99
  anal mucosa 569.49
  bladder 596.7
  cerebral 437.8
  conjunctiva 372.71
  ear, internal, acute 386.30
  enteric 564.89
  eye 372.71
  eyelid (active) (passive) 374.82
  intestine 564.89
  iris 364.41
  kidney 593.81
  labyrinth 386.30
  liver (active) (passive) 573.8
  lung 514
  ovary 620.8
  passive 780.99
  pulmonary 514
  renal 593.81
  retina 362.89
  spleen 289.59
  stomach 537.89
Hyperesthesia (body surface) — *see also* Disturbance, sensation 782.0
  larynx (reflex) 478.79
    hysterical 300.11
  pharynx (reflex) 478.29
Hyperestrinism 256.0
Hyperestrogenism 256.0
Hyperestrogenosis 256.0
Hyperexplexia 759.89
Hyperextension, joint 718.80
  ankle 718.87
  elbow 718.82
  foot 718.87
  hand 718.84
  hip 718.85
  knee 718.86
  multiple sites 718.89
  pelvic region 718.85
  shoulder (region) 718.81
  specified site NEC 718.88
  wrist 718.83
Hyperfibrinolysis — *see* Fibrinolysis
Hyperfolliculinism 256.0
Hyperfructosemia 271.2
Hyperfunction
  adrenal (cortex) 255.3
    androgenic, acquired benign 255.3
    medulla 255.6
    virilism 255.2
  corticoadrenal NEC 255.3
  labyrinth — *see* Hyperactive, labyrinth
  medulloadrenal 255.6

☑ **Additional Digit Required — Refer to the Tabular List for Digit Selection** ▽ **Subterms under main terms may continue to next column or page**

2015 ICD-9-CM   ▶◀ Revised Text   ● New Line   ▲ Revised Code   Volume 2 — 143

Hyperfunction — *continued*
  ovary 256.1
    estrogen 256.0
  pancreas 577.8
  parathyroid (gland) 252.00
  pituitary (anterior) (gland) (lobe) 253.1
  testicular 257.0
Hypergammaglobulinemia 289.89
  monoclonal, benign (BMH) 273.1
  polyclonal 273.0
  Waldenström's 273.0
Hyperglobulinemia 273.8
Hyperglycemia 790.29
  maternal
    affecting fetus or newborn 775.0
    manifest diabetes in infant 775.1
  postpancreatectomy (complete) (partial)
    251.3
Hyperglyceridemia 272.1
  endogenous 272.1
  essential 272.1
  familial 272.1
  hereditary 272.1
  mixed 272.3
  pure 272.1
Hyperglycinemia 270.7
Hypergonadism
  ovarian 256.1
  testicular (infantile) (primary) 257.0
Hyperheparinemia — *see also* Circulating, in-
    trinsic anticoagulants 287.5
Hyperhidrosis, hyperidrosis 705.21
  axilla 705.21
  face 705.21
  focal (localized) 705.21
    primary 705.21
      axilla 705.21
      face 705.21
      palms 705.21
      soles 705.21
    secondary 705.22
      axilla 705.22
      face 705.22
      palms 705.22
      soles 705.22
  generalized 780.8
  palms 705.21
  psychogenic 306.3
  secondary 780.8
  soles 705.21
Hyperhistidinemia 270.5
Hyperinsulinism (ectopic) (functional) (organ-
    ic) NEC 251.1
  iatrogenic 251.0
  reactive 251.2
  spontaneous 251.2
  therapeutic misadventure (from administra-
    tion of insulin) 962.3
Hyperiodemia 276.9
Hyperirritability (cerebral), in newborn 779.1
Hyperkalemia 276.7
Hyperkeratosis — *see also* Keratosis 701.1
  cervix 622.2
  congenital 757.39
  cornea 371.89
  due to yaws (early) (late) (palmar or plantar)
    102.3
  eccentrica 757.39
  figurata centrifuga atrophica 757.39
  follicularis 757.39
    in cutem penetrans 701.1
  limbic (cornea) 371.89
  palmoplantaris climacterica 701.1
  pinta (carate) 103.1
  senile (with pruritus) 702.0
  tongue 528.79
  universalis congenita 757.1
  vagina 623.1
  vocal cord 478.5
  vulva 624.09
Hyperkinesia, hyperkinetic (disease) (reac-
    tion) (syndrome) 314.9
  with
    attention deficit — *see* Disorder, atten-
      tion deficit
    conduct disorder 314.2

Hyperkinesia, hyperkinetic — *continued*
  with
    continued
      developmental delay 314.1
      simple disturbance of activity and atten-
        tion 314.01
      specified manifestation NEC 314.8
  heart (disease) 429.82
  of childhood or adolescence NEC 314.9
Hyperlacrimation — *see also* Epiphora 375.20
Hyperlipemia — *see also* Hyperlipidemia 272.4
Hyperlipidemia 272.4
  carbohydrate-induced 272.1
  combined 272.2
  endogenous 272.1
  exogenous 272.3
  fat-induced 272.3
  group
    A 272.0
    B 272.1
    C 272.2
    D 272.3
    mixed 272.2
  specified type NEC 272.4
Hyperlipidosis 272.7
  hereditary 272.7
Hyperlipoproteinemia (acquired) (essential)
    (familial) (hereditary) (primary) (sec-
    ondary) 272.4
  Fredrickson type
    I 272.3
    IIa 272.0
    IIb 272.2
    III 272.2
    IV 272.1
    V 272.3
  low-density-lipoid-type (LDL) 272.0
  very-low-density-lipoid-type (VLDL) 272.1
Hyperlucent lung, unilateral 492.8
Hyperluteinization 256.1
Hyperlysinemia 270.7
Hypermagnesemia 275.2
  neonatal 775.5
Hypermaturity (fetus or newborn)
  post-term infant 766.21
  prolonged gestation infant 766.22
Hypermenorrhea 626.2
Hypermetabolism 794.7
Hypermethioninemia 270.4
Hypermetropia (congenital) 367.0
Hypermobility
  cecum 564.9
  coccyx 724.71
  colon 564.9
    psychogenic 306.4
  ileum 564.89
  joint (acquired) 718.80
    ankle 718.87
    elbow 718.82
    foot 718.87
    hand 718.84
    hip 718.85
    knee 718.86
    multiple sites 718.89
    pelvic region 718.85
    shoulder (region) 718.81
    specified site NEC 718.88
    wrist 718.83
  kidney, congenital 753.3
  meniscus (knee) 717.5
  scapula 718.81
  stomach 536.8
    psychogenic 306.4
  syndrome 728.5
  testis, congenital 752.52
  urethral 599.81
Hypermotility
  gastrointestinal 536.8
  intestine 564.9
    psychogenic 306.4
  stomach 536.8
Hypernasality 784.43
Hypernatremia 276.0
  with water depletion 276.0
Hypernephroma (M8312/3) 189.0
Hyperopia 367.0
Hyperorexia 783.6

Hyperornithinemia 270.6
Hyperosmia — *see also* Disturbance, sensation
    781.1
Hyperosmolality 276.0
Hyperosteogenesis 733.99
Hyperostosis 733.99
  calvarial 733.3
  cortical 733.3
    infantile 756.59
  frontal, internal of skull 733.3
  interna frontalis 733.3
  monomelic 733.99
  skull 733.3
    congenital 756.0
  vertebral 721.8
    with spondylosis — *see* Spondylosis
    ankylosing 721.6
Hyperovarianism 256.1
Hyperovarism, hyperovaria 256.1
Hyperoxaluria (primary) 271.8
Hyperoxia 987.8
Hyperparathyroidism 252.00
  ectopic 259.3
  other 252.08
  primary 252.01
  secondary (of renal origin) 588.81
    non-renal 252.02
  tertiary 252.08
Hyperpathia — *see also* Disturbance, sensation
    782.0
  psychogenic 307.80
Hyperperistalsis 787.4
  psychogenic 306.4
Hyperpermeability, capillary 448.9
Hyperphagia 783.6
Hyperphenylalaninemia 270.1
Hyperphoria 378.40
  alternating 378.45
Hyperphosphatemia 275.3
Hyperpiesia — *see also* Hypertension 401.9
Hyperpiesis — *see also* Hypertension 401.9
Hyperpigmentation — *see* Pigmentation
Hyperpinealism 259.8
Hyperpipecolatemia 270.7
Hyperpituitarism 253.1
Hyperplasia, hyperplastic
  adenoids (lymphoid tissue) 474.12
    and tonsils 474.10
  adrenal (capsule) (cortex) (gland) 255.8
    with
      sexual precocity (male) 255.2
      virilism, adrenal 255.2
      virilization (female) 255.2
    congenital 255.2
    due to excess ACTH (ectopic) (pituitary)
      255.0
    medulla 255.8
  alpha cells (pancreatic)
    with
      gastrin excess 251.5
      glucagon excess 251.4
  angiolymphoid, with eosinophilia (ALHE)
    228.01
  appendix (lymphoid) 543.0
  artery, fibromuscular NEC 447.8
    carotid 447.8
    renal 447.3
  bone 733.99
    marrow 289.9
  breast (*see also* Hypertrophy, breast) 611.1
    ductal 610.8
      atypical 610.8
  carotid artery 447.8
  cementation, cementum (teeth) (tooth)
    521.5
  cervical gland 785.6
  cervix (uteri) 622.10
    basal cell 622.10
    congenital 752.49
    endometrium 622.10
    polypoid 622.10
  chin 524.05
  clitoris, congenital 752.49
  dentin 521.5
  endocervicitis 616.0

Hyperplasia, hyperplastic — *continued*
  endometrium, endometrial (adenomatous)
    (atypical) (cystic) (glandular) (poly-
    poid) (uterus) 621.30
    with atypia 621.33
    without atypia
      complex 621.32
      simple 621.31
    benign 621.34
  cervix 622.10
  epithelial 709.8
    focal, oral, including tongue 528.79
    mouth (focal) 528.79
    nipple 611.89
    skin 709.8
    tongue (focal) 528.79
    vaginal wall 623.0
  erythroid 289.9
  faswith ossificans (progressiva) 728.11
  fibromuscular, artery NEC 447.8
    carotid 447.8
    renal 447.3
  genital
    female 629.89
    male 608.89
  gingiva 523.8
  glandularis
    cystica uteri 621.30
    endometrium (uterus) 621.30
    interstitialis uteri 621.30
  granulocytic 288.69
  gum 523.8
  hymen, congenital 752.49
  islands of Langerhans 251.1
  islet cell (pancreatic) 251.9
    alpha cells
      with excess
        gastrin 251.5
        glucagon 251.4
      beta cells 251.1
  juxtaglomerular (complex) (kidney) 593.89
  kidney (congenital) 753.3
  liver (congenital) 751.69
  lymph node (gland) 785.6
  lymphoid (diffuse) (nodular) 785.6
    appendix 543.0
    intestine 569.89
  mandibular 524.02
    alveolar 524.72
    unilateral condylar 526.89
  Marchand multiple nodular (liver) — *see*
    Cirrhosis, postnecrotic
  maxillary 524.01
    alveolar 524.71
  medulla, adrenal 255.8
  myometrium, myometrial 621.2
  neuroendocrine cell, of infancy 516.61
  nose (lymphoid) (polypoid) 478.19
  oral soft tissue (inflammatory) (irritative)
    (mucosa) NEC 528.9
    gingiva 523.8
    tongue 529.8
  organ or site, congenital NEC — *see*
    Anomaly, specified type NEC
  ovary 620.8
  palate, papillary 528.9
  pancreatic islet cells 251.9
    alpha
      with excess
        gastrin 251.5
        glucagon 251.4
      beta 251.1
  parathyroid (gland) 252.01
  persistent, vitreous (primary) 743.51
  pharynx (lymphoid) 478.29
  prostate 600.90
    with
      other lower urinary tract symptoms
        (LUTS) 600.91
      urinary
        obstruction 600.91
        retention 600.91
    adenofibromatous 600.20
      with
        other lower urinary tract symp-
          toms (LUTS) 600.21

☑ **Additional Digit Required** — Refer to the Tabular List for Digit Selection   ▽ **Subterms under main terms may continue to next column or page**

144 — Volume 2   ▶◀ Revised Text   ● New Line   ▲ Revised Code   2015 ICD-9-CM

Hyperplasia, hyperplastic — *continued*
  prostate — *continued*
    adenofibromatous — *continued*
      with — *continued*
        urinary
          obstruction 600.21
          retention 600.21
      nodular 600.10
        with
          urinary
            obstruction 600.11
            retention 600.11
  renal artery (fibromuscular) 447.3
  reticuloendothelial (cell) 289.9
  salivary gland (any) 527.1
  Schimmelbusch's 610.1
  suprarenal (capsule) (gland) 255.8
  thymus (gland) (persistent) 254.0
  thyroid (*see also* Goiter) 240.9
    primary 242.0 ☑
    secondary 242.2 ☑
  tonsil (lymphoid tissue) 474.11
    and adenoids 474.10
  urethrovaginal 599.89
  uterus, uterine (myometrium) 621.2
    endometrium (*see also* Hyperplasia, en-
      dometrium) 621.30
  vitreous (humor), primary persistent 743.51
  vulva 624.3
  zygoma 738.11
Hyperpnea — *see also* Hyperventilation 786.01
Hyperpotassemia 276.7
Hyperprebetalipoproteinemia 272.1
  with chylomicronemia 272.3
  familial 272.1

Hyperprolactinemia 253.1
Hyperprolinemia 270.8
Hyperproteinemia 273.8
Hyperprothrombinemia 289.89
Hyperpselaphesia 782.0
Hyperpyrexia 780.60
  heat (effects of) 992.0
  malarial (*see also* Malaria) 084.6
  malignant, due to anesthetic 995.86
  rheumatic — *see* Fever, rheumatic
  unknown origin (*see also* Pyrexia) 780.60
Hyperreactor, vascular 780.2
Hyperreflexia 796.1
  bladder, autonomic 596.54
    with cauda equina 344.61
  detrusor 344.61
Hypersalivation — *see also* Ptyalism 527.7
Hypersarcosinemia 270.8
Hypersecretion
  ACTH 255.3
  androgens (ovarian) 256.1
  calcitonin 246.0
  corticoadrenal 255.3
  cortisol 255.0
  estrogen 256.0
  gastric 536.8
    psychogenic 306.4
  gastrin 251.5
  glucagon 251.4
  hormone
    ACTH 255.3
    anterior pituitary 253.1
    growth NEC 253.0
    ovarian androgen 256.1
    testicular 257.0

Hypersecretion — *continued*
  hormone — *continued*
    thyroid stimulating 242.8 ☑
  insulin — *see* Hyperinsulinism
  lacrimal glands (*see also* Epiphora) 375.20
  medulloadrenal 255.6
  milk 676.6 ☑
  ovarian androgens 256.1
  pituitary (anterior) 253.1
  salivary gland (any) 527.7
  testicular hormones 257.0
  thyrocalcitonin 246.0
  upper respiratory 478.9
Hypersegmentation, hereditary 288.2
  eosinophils 288.2
  neutrophil nuclei 288.2
**Hypersensitive, hypersensitiveness, hyper-
  sensitivity** — *see also* Allergy
  angiitis 446.20
    specified NEC 446.29
  carotid sinus 337.01
  colon 564.9
    psychogenic 306.4
  DNA (deoxyribonucleic acid) NEC 287.2
  drug (*see also* Allergy, drug) 995.27
  due to correct medical substance properly
    administered 995.27
  esophagus 530.89
  insect bites — *see* Injury, superficial, by site
  labyrinth 386.58
  pain (*see also* Disturbance, sensation) 782.0
  pneumonitis NEC 495.9
  reaction (*see also* Allergy) 995.3
    upper respiratory tract NEC 478.8
  stomach (allergic) (nonallergic) 536.8

**Hypersensitive, hypersensitiveness,
  hypersensitivity** — *see also* Allergy —
  continued
  stomach — *continued*
    psychogenic 306.4
Hypersomatotropism (classic) 253.0
Hypersomnia, unspecified 780.54
  with sleep apnea, unspecified 780.53
  alcohol induced 291.82
  drug induced 292.85
  due to
    medical condition classified elsewhere
      327.14
    mental disorder 327.15
  idiopathic
    with long sleep time 327.11
    without long sleep time 327.12
  menstrual related 327.13
  nonorganic origin 307.43
    persistent (primary) 307.44
    transient 307.43
  organic 327.10
    other 327.19
  primary 307.44
  recurrent 327.13
Hypersplenia 289.4
Hypersplenism 289.4
Hypersteatosis 706.3
Hyperstimulation, ovarian 256.1
Hypersuprarenalism 255.3
Hypersusceptibility — *see* Allergy
Hyper-TBG-nemia 246.8
Hypertelorism 756.0
  orbit, orbital 376.41

☑ **Additional Digit Required** — Refer to the Tabular List for Digit Selection   ▽ **Subterms under main terms may continue to next column or page**

2015 ICD-9-CM   ►◄ Revised Text   ● New Line   ▲ Revised Code   Volume 2 — 145

Hypertension, hypertensive	Malignant	Benign	Unspecified
Hypertension, hypertensive (arterial) (arteriolar) (crisis) (degeneration) (disease) (essential) (fluctuating) (idiopathic) (intermittent) (labile) (low renin) (orthostatic) (paroxysmal) (primary) (systemic) (uncontrolled) (vascular)	401.0	401.1	401.9
with			
chronic kidney disease			
stage I through stage IV, or unspecified	403.00	403.10	403.90
stage V or end stage renal disese	403.01	403.11	403.91
heart involvement (conditions classifiable to 429.0–429.3, 429.8, 429.9 due to hypertension) (see also Hypertension, heart)	402.00	402.10	402.90
with kidney involvement — see Hypertension, cardiorenal			
renal (kidney) involvement (only conditions classifiable to 585, 587) (excludes conditions classifiable to 584) (see also Hypertension, kidney)	403.00	403.10	403.90
with heart involvement — see Hypertension, cardiorenal			
failure (and sclerosis) (see also Hypertension, kidney)	403.01	403.11	403.91
sclerosis without failure (see also Hypertension, kidney)	403.00	403.10	403.90
accelerated (see also Hypertension, by type, malignant))	401.0	—	—
antepartum — see Hypertension, complicating pregnancy, childbirth, or the puerperium			
borderline	—	—	796.2
cardiorenal (disease)	404.00	404.10	404.90
with			
chronic kidney disease			
stage I through stage IV, or unspecified	404.00	404.10	404.90
and heart failure	404.01	404.11	404.91
stage V or end stage renal disease	404.02	404.12	404.92
and heart failure	404.03	404.13	404.93
heart failure	404.01	404.11	404.91
and chronic kidney disease	404.01	404.11	404.91
stage I through stage IV or unspecified	404.01	404.11	404.91
stave V or end stage renal disease	404.03	404.13	404.93
cardiovascular disease (arteriosclerotic) (sclerotic)	402.00	402.10	402.90
with			
heart failure	402.01	402.11	402.91
renal involvement (conditions classifiable to 403) (see also Hypertension, cardiorenal)	404.00	404.10	404.90
cardiovascular renal (disease) (sclerosis) (see also Hypertension, cardiorenal)	404.00	404.10	404.90
cerebrovascular disease NEC	437.2	—	—
complicating pregnancy, childbirth, or the puerperium	642.2	642.0	642.9
with			
albuminuria (and edema) (mild)	—	—	642.4
severe	—	—	642.5
chronic kidney disesae	642.2	—	—
and heart disease	642.2	—	—
edema (mild)	—	—	642.4
severe	—	—	642.5
heart disease	642.2	—	—
and chronic kidney disease	642.2	—	—
renal disease	642.2	—	—
and heart disease	642.2	—	—
chronic	642.2	642.0	—
with pre-eclampsia or eclampsia	642.7	—	—
fetus or newborn	760.0	—	—
essential	—	642.0	—
with pre-eclampsia or eclampsia	—	642.7	—
fetus or newborn	760.0	—	—
fetus or newborn	760.0	—	—
gestational	—	—	642.3
pre-existing	642.2	642.0	—
with pre-eclampsia or eclampsia	642.7	—	—
fetus or newborn	760.0	—	—
secondary to renal disease	642.1	—	—
with pre-eclampsia or eclampsia	642.7	—	—
fetus or newborn	760.0	—	—
transient	—	—	642.3
due to			
aldosteronism, primary	405.09	405.19	405.99
brain tumor	405.09	405.19	405.99
bulbar poliomyelitis	405.09	405.19	405.99
calculus			
kidney	405.09	405.19	405.99

Hypertension, hypertensive — continued	Malignant	Benign	Unspecified
due to — continued			
calculus — continued			
ureter	405.09	405.19	405.99
coarctation, aorta	405.09	405.19	405.99
Cushing's disease	405.09	405.19	405.99
glomerulosclerosis (see also Hypertension, kidney)	403.00	403.10	403.90
periarteritis nodosa	405.09	405.19	405.99
pheochromocytoma	405.09	405.19	405.99
polycystic kidney(s)	405.09	405.19	405.99
polycythemia	405.09	405.19	405.99
porphyria	405.09	405.19	405.99
pyelonephritis	405.09	405.19	405.99
renal (artery)			
aneurysm	405.01	405.11	405.91
anomaly	405.01	405.11	405.91
embolism	405.01	405.11	405.91
fibromuscular hyperplasia	405.01	405.11	405.91
occlusion	405.01	405.11	405.91
stenosis	405.01	405.11	405.91
thrombosis	405.01	405.11	405.91
encephalopathy	437.2	—	—
gestational (transient) NEC	—	—	642.3
Goldblatt's	440.1	—	—
heart (disease) (conditions classifiable to 429.0–429.3, 429.8, 429.9 due to hypertension)	402.00	402.10	402.90
with heart failure	402.01	402.11	402.91
hypertensive kidney disease (conditions classifiable to 403) (see also Hypertension, cardiorenal)	404.00	404.10	404.90
renal sclerosis (see also Hypertension, cardiorenal)	404.00	404.10	404.90
intracranial, benign	—	348.2	—
intraocular	—	—	365.04
kidney	403.00	403.10	403.90
with			
chronic kidney disease			
stage I through stage IV, or unspecified	403.00	403.10	403.90
stage V or end stage renal disese	403.01	403.11	403.91
heart involvement (conditions classifiable to 429.0–429.3, 429.8, 429.9 due to hypertension) (see also Hypertension, cardiorenal)	404.00	404.10	404.90
hypertensive heart (disease) (conditions classifiable to 402) (see also Hypertension, cardiorenal)	404.00	404.10	404.90
lesser circulation	—	—	416.0
necrotizing	401.0	—	—
ocular	—	—	365.04
pancreatic duct — code to underlying condition			
with			
chronic pancreatitis	—	—	577.1
portal (due to chronic liver disease)	—	—	572.3
postoperative	—	—	997.91
psychogenic	—	—	306.2
puerperal, postpartum — see Hypertension, complicating pregnancy, childbirth, or the puerperium			
pulmonary (artery) (secondary)	—	—	416.8
with			
cor pulmonale (chronic)	—	—	416.8
acute	—	—	415.0
right heart ventricular strain/failure	—	—	416.8
acute	—	—	415.0
idiopathic	—	—	416.0
primary	—	—	416.0
of newborn	—	—	747.83
secondary	—	—	416.8
renal (disease) (see also Hypertension, kidney)	403.00	403.10	403.90
renovascular NEC	405.01	405.11	405.91
secondary NEC	405.09	405.19	405.99
due to			
aldosteronism, primary	405.09	405.19	405.99
brain tumor	405.09	405.19	405.99
bulbar poliomyelitis	405.09	405.19	405.99
calculus			
kidney	405.09	405.19	405.99
ureter	405.09	405.19	405.99
coarctation, aorta	405.09	405.19	405.99
Cushing's disease	405.09	405.19	405.99
glomerulosclerosis (see also Hypertension, kidney)	403.00	403.10	403.90

☑ **Additional Digit Required — Refer to the Tabular List for Digit Selection**   ▽ **Subterms under main terms may continue to next column or page**

	Malignant	Benign	Unspecified
Hypertension, hypertensive — *continued*			
secondary — *continued*			
due to — *continued*			
periarteritis nodosa	405.09	405.19	405.99
pheochromocytoma	405.09	405.19	405.99
polycystic kidney(s)	405.09	405.19	405.99
polycythemia	405.09	405.19	405.99
porphyria	405.09	405.19	405.99
pyelonephritis	405.09	405.19	405.99
renal (artery)			
aneurysm	405.01	405.11	405.91
anomaly	405.01	405.11	405.91
embolism	405.01	405.11	405.91
fibromuscular hyperplasia	405.01	405.11	405.91
occlusion	405.01	405.11	405.91
stenosis	405.01	405.11	405.91
thrombosis	405.01	405.11	405.91
transient	—	—	796.2
of pregnancy	—	—	642.3
vascular degeneration	401.0	401.1	401.9
venous, chronic (asymptomatic) (idiopathic)	—	—	459.30
with			
complication, NEC	—	—	459.39
inflammation	—	—	459.32
with ulcer	—	—	459.33
ulcer	—	—	459.31
with inflammation	—	—	459.33
due to			
deep vein thrombosis (*see also* Syndrome, postphlebetic)	—	—	459.10

Hypertensive urgency — see Hypertension
Hyperthecosis, ovary 256.8
Hyperthermia (of unknown origin) — see also
    Pyrexia 780.60
    malignant (due to anesthesia) 995.86
    newborn 778.4
Hyperthymergasia — see also Psychosis, affec-
    tive 296.0 ☑
    reactive (from emotional stress, psycholog-
      ical trauma) 298.1
    recurrent episode 296.1 ☑
    single episode 296.0 ☑
Hyperthymism 254.8
Hyperthyroid (recurrent) — see Hyperthy-
    roidism
Hyperthyroidism (latent) (preadult) (recurrent)
    (without goiter) 242.9 ☑

> Note — Use the following fifth-digit
> subclassification with category 242:
> 0   without mention of thyrotoxic
>   crisis or storm
> 1   with mention of thyrotoxic crisis
>   or storm

    with
      goiter (diffuse) 242.0 ☑
        adenomatous 242.3 ☑
          multinodular 242.2 ☑
          uninodular 242.1 ☑
        nodular 242.3 ☑
          multinodular 242.2 ☑
          uninodular 242.1 ☑
        thyroid nodule 242.1 ☑
    complicating pregnancy, childbirth, or
      puerperium 648.1 ☑
    neonatal (transient) 775.3
Hypertonia — see Hypertonicity
Hypertonicity
    bladder 596.51
    fetus or newborn 779.89
    gastrointestinal (tract) 536.8
    infancy 779.89
      due to electrolyte imbalance 779.89
    muscle 728.85
    stomach 536.8
      psychogenic 306.4
    uterus, uterine (contractions) 661.4 ☑
      affecting fetus or newborn 763.7
Hypertony — see Hypertonicity
Hypertransaminemia 790.4
Hypertrichosis 704.1
    congenital 757.4
    eyelid 374.54
    lanuginosa 757.4
      acquired 704.1
Hypertriglyceridemia, essential 272.1
Hypertrophy, hypertrophic
    adenoids (infectional) 474.12
      and tonsils (faucial) (infective) (lingual)
        (lymphoid) 474.10
    adrenal 255.8
    alveolar process or ridge 525.8
    anal papillae 569.49
    apocrine gland 705.82
    artery NEC 447.8
      carotid 447.8
      congenital (peripheral) NEC 747.60
        gastrointestinal 747.61
        lower limb 747.64
        renal 747.62
        specified NEC 747.69
        spinal 747.82
        upper limb 747.63
      renal 447.3
    arthritis (chronic) (see also Osteoarthrosis)
      715.9 ☑
      spine (see also Spondylosis) 721.90
    arytenoid 478.79
    asymmetrical (heart) 429.9
    auricular — see Hypertrophy, cardiac
    Bartholin's gland 624.8
    bile duct 576.8
    bladder (sphincter) (trigone) 596.89
    blind spot, visual field 368.42
    bone 733.99

Hypertrophy, hypertrophic — continued
    brain 348.89
    breast 611.1
      cystic 610.1
      fetus or newborn 778.7
      fibrocystic 610.1
      massive pubertal 611.1
      puerperal, postpartum 676.3 ☑
      senile (parenchymatous) 611.1
    cardiac (chronic) (idiopathic) 429.3
      with
        rheumatic fever (conditions classifi-
          able to 390)
          active 391.8
            with chorea 392.0
          inactive or quiescent (with
            chorea) 398.99
      congenital NEC 746.89
      fatty (see also Degeneration, myocardial)
        429.1
      hypertensive (see also Hypertension,
        heart) 402.90
      rheumatic (with chorea) 398.99
        active or acute 391.8
          with chorea 392.0
      valve (see also Endocarditis) 424.90
        congenital NEC 746.89
    cartilage 733.99
    cecum 569.89
    cervix (uteri) 622.6
      congenital 752.49
      elongation 622.6
    clitoris (cirrhotic) 624.2
      congenital 752.49
    colon 569.89
      congenital 751.3
    conjunctiva, lymphoid 372.73
    cornea 371.89
    corpora cavernosa 607.89
    duodenum 537.89
    endometrium (uterus) (see also Hyperplasia,
      endometrium) 621.30
      cervix 622.6
    epididymis 608.89
    esophageal hiatus (congenital) 756.6
      with hernia — see Hernia, diaphragm
    eyelid 374.30
    falx, skull 733.99
    fat pad 729.30
      infrapatellar 729.31
      knee 729.31
      orbital 374.34
      popliteal 729.31
      prepatellar 729.31
      retropatellar 729.31
      specified site NEC 729.39
    foot (congenital) 755.67
    frenum, frenulum (tongue) 529.8
      linguae 529.8
      lip 528.5
    gallbladder or cystic duct 575.8
    gastric mucosa 535.2 ☑
    gingiva 523.8
    gland, glandular (general) NEC 785.6
    gum (mucous membrane) 523.8
    heart (idiopathic) (see also Hypertrophy,
      cardiac)
      valve (see also Endocarditis)
        congenital NEC 746.89
    hemifacial 754.0
    hepatic — see Hypertrophy, liver
    hiatus (esophageal) 756.6
    hilus gland 785.6
    hymen, congenital 752.49
    ileum 569.89
    infrapatellar fat pad 729.31
    intestine 569.89
    jejunum 569.89
    kidney (compensatory) 593.1
      congenital 753.3
    labial frenulum 528.5
    labium (majus) (minus) 624.3
    lacrimal gland, chronic 375.03
    ligament 728.9
      spinal 724.8
    linguae frenulum 529.8

Hypertrophy, hypertrophic — continued
    lingual tonsil (infectional) 474.11
    lip (frenum) 528.5
      congenital 744.81
    liver 789.1
      acute 573.8
      cirrhotic — see Cirrhosis, liver
      congenital 751.69
      fatty — see Fatty, liver
    lymph gland 785.6
      tuberculous — see Tuberculosis, lymph
        gland
    mammary gland — see Hypertrophy, breast
    maxillary frenulum 528.5
    Meckel's diverticulum (congenital) 751.0
    medial meniscus, acquired 717.3
    median bar 600.90
      with
        other lower urinary tract symptoms
          (LUTS) 600.91
        urinary
          obstruction 600.91
          retention 600.91
    mediastinum 519.3
    meibomian gland 373.2
    meniscus, knee, congenital 755.64
    metatarsal head 733.99
    metatarsus 733.99
    mouth 528.9
    mucous membrane
      alveolar process 523.8
      nose 478.19
      turbinate (nasal) 478.0
    muscle 728.9
    muscular coat, artery NEC 447.8
      carotid 447.8
      renal 447.3
    myocardium (see also Hypertrophy, cardiac)
      429.3
      idiopathic 425.18
    myometrium 621.2
    nail 703.8
      congenital 757.5
    nasal 478.19
      alae 478.19
      bone 738.0
      cartilage 478.19
      mucous membrane (septum) 478.19
      sinus (see also Sinusitis) 473.9
      turbinate 478.0
    nasopharynx, lymphoid (infectional) (tissue)
      (wall) 478.29
    neck, uterus 622.6
    nipple 611.1
    normal aperture diaphragm (congenital)
      756.6
    nose (see also Hypertrophy, nasal) 478.19
    orbit 376.46
    organ or site, congenital NEC — see
      Anomaly, specified type NEC
    osteoarthropathy (pulmonary) 731.2
    ovary 620.8
    palate (hard) 526.89
      soft 528.9
    pancreas (congenital) 751.7
    papillae
      anal 569.49
      tongue 529.3
    parathyroid (gland) 252.01
    parotid gland 527.1
    penis 607.89
    phallus 607.89
      female (clitoris) 624.2
    pharyngeal tonsil 474.12
    pharyngitis 472.1
    pharynx 478.29
      lymphoid (infectional) (tissue) (wall)
        478.29
    pituitary (fossa) (gland) 253.8
    popliteal fat pad 729.31
    preauricular (lymph) gland (Hampstead)
      785.6
    prepuce (congenital) 605
      female 624.2
    prostate (asymptomatic) (early) (recurrent)
      600.90

Hypertrophy, hypertrophic — continued
    prostate — continued
      with
        other lower urinary tract symptoms
          (LUTS) 600.91
        urinary
          obstruction 600.91
          retention 600.91
      adenofibromatous 600.20
        with
          other lower urinary tract symp-
            toms (LUTS) 600.21
          urinary
            obstruction 600.21
            retention 600.21
      benign 600.00
        with
          other lower urinary tract symp-
            toms (LUTS) 600.01
          urinary
            obstruction 600.01
            retention 600.01
      congenital 752.89
    pseudoedematous hypodermal 757.0
    pseudomuscular 359.1
    pylorus (muscle) (sphincter) 537.0
      congenital 750.5
      infantile 750.5
    rectal sphincter 569.49
    rectum 569.49
    renal 593.1
    rhinitis (turbinate) 472.0
    salivary duct or gland 527.1
      congenital 750.26
    scaphoid (tarsal) 733.99
    scar 701.4
    scrotum 608.89
    sella turcica 253.8
    seminal vesicle 608.89
    sigmoid 569.89
    skin condition NEC 701.9
    spermatic cord 608.89
    spinal ligament 724.8
    spleen — see Splenomegaly
    spondylitis (spine) (see also Spondylosis)
      721.90
    stomach 537.89
    subaortic stenosis (idiopathic) 425.11
    sublingual gland 527.1
      congenital 750.26
    submaxillary gland 527.1
    suprarenal (gland) 255.8
    tendon 727.9
    testis 608.89
      congenital 752.89
    thymic, thymus (congenital) (gland) 254.0
    thyroid (gland) (see also Goiter) 240.9
      primary 242.0 ☑
      secondary 242.2 ☑
    toe (congenital) 755.65
      acquired 735.8
    tongue 529.8
      congenital 750.15
      frenum 529.8
      papillae (foliate) 529.3
    tonsil (faucial) (infective) (lingual) (lym-
      phoid) 474.11
      with
        adenoiditis 474.01
        tonsillitis 474.00
          and adenoiditis 474.02
      and adenoids 474.10
    tunica vaginalis 608.89
    turbinate (mucous membrane) 478.0
    ureter 593.89
    urethra 599.84
    uterus 621.2
      puerperal, postpartum 674.8 ☑
    uvula 528.9
    vagina 623.8
    vas deferens 608.89
    vein 459.89
    ventricle, ventricular (heart) (left) (right) (see
      also Hypertrophy, cardiac)
      congenital 746.89

☑ Additional Digit Required — Refer to the Tabular List for Digit Selection   ▧ Subterms under main terms may continue to next column or page

148 — Volume 2   ▶◀ Revised Text   ● New Line   ▲ Revised Code   2015 ICD-9-CM

Hypertrophy, hypertrophic — *continued*
  ventricle, ventricular (*see also* Hypertrophy, cardiac) — *continued*
    due to hypertension (left) (right) (*see also* Hypertension, heart) 402.90
      benign 402.10
      malignant 402.00
    right with ventricular septal defect, pulmonary stenosis or atresia, and dextraposition of aorta 745.2
  verumontanum 599.89
  vesical 596.89
  vocal cord 478.5
  vulva 624.3
    stasis (nonfilarial) 624.3
Hypertropia (intermittent) (periodic) 378.31
Hypertyrosinemia 270.2
Hyperuricemia 790.6
Hypervalinemia 270.3
Hyperventilation (tetany) 786.01
  hysterical 300.11
  psychogenic 306.1
  syndrome 306.1
Hyperviscidosis 277.00
Hyperviscosity (of serum) (syndrome) NEC 273.3
  polycythemic 289.0
  sclerocythemic 282.8
Hypervitaminosis (dietary) NEC 278.8
  A (dietary) 278.2
  D (dietary) 278.4
  from excessive administration or use of vitamin preparations (chronic) 278.8
    reaction to sudden overdose 963.5
    vitamin A 278.2
      reaction to sudden overdose 963.5
    vitamin D 278.4
      reaction to sudden overdose 963.5
    vitamin K
      correct substance properly administered 278.8
      overdose or wrong substance given or taken 964.3
Hypervolemia 276.69
Hypesthesia — *see also* Disturbance, sensation 782.0
  cornea 371.81
Hyphema (anterior chamber) (ciliary body) (iris) 364.41
  traumatic 921.3
Hyphemia — *see* Hyphema
Hypoacidity, gastric 536.8
  psychogenic 306.4
Hypoactive labyrinth (function) — *see* Hypofunction, labyrinth
Hypoadrenalism 255.41
  tuberculous (*see also* Tuberculosis) 017.6 ☑
Hypoadrenocorticism 255.41
  pituitary 253.4
Hypoalbuminemia 273.8
Hypoaldosteronism 255.42
Hypoalphalipoproteinemia 272.5
Hypobarism 993.2
Hypobaropathy 993.2
Hypobetalipoproteinemia (familial) 272.5
Hypocalcemia 275.41
  cow's milk 775.4
  dietary 269.3
  neonatal 775.4
  phosphate-loading 775.4
Hypocalcification, teeth 520.4
Hypochloremia 276.9
Hypochlorhydria 536.8
  neurotic 306.4
  psychogenic 306.4
Hypocholesteremia 272.5
Hypochondria (reaction) 300.7
Hypochondriac 300.7
Hypochondriasis 300.7
Hypochromasia blood cells 280.9
Hypochromic anemia 280.9
  due to blood loss (chronic) 280.0
    acute 285.1
  microcytic 280.9
Hypocoagulability — *see also* Defect, coagulation 286.9

Hypocomplementemia 279.8
Hypocythemia (progressive) 284.9
Hypodontia — *see also* Anodontia 520.0
Hypoeosinophilia 288.59
Hypoesthesia — *see also* Disturbance, sensation 782.0
  cornea 371.81
  tactile 782.0
Hypoestrinism 256.39
Hypoestrogenism 256.39
Hypoferremia 280.9
  due to blood loss (chronic) 280.0
Hypofertility
  female 628.9
  male 606.1
Hypofibrinogenemia 286.3
  acquired 286.6
  congenital 286.3
Hypofunction
  adrenal (gland) 255.41
    cortex 255.41
    medulla 255.5
    specified NEC 255.5
  cerebral 331.9
  corticoadrenal NEC 255.41
  intestinal 564.89
  labyrinth (unilateral) 386.53
    with loss of labyrinthine reactivity 386.55
    bilateral 386.54
      with loss of labyrinthine reactivity 386.56
  Leydig cell 257.2
  ovary 256.39
    postablative 256.2
  pituitary (anterior) (gland) (lobe) 253.2
    posterior 253.5
  testicular 257.2
    iatrogenic 257.1
    postablative 257.1
    postirradiation 257.1
    postsurgical 257.1
Hypogammaglobulinemia 279.00
  acquired primary 279.06
  non-sex-linked, congenital 279.06
  sporadic 279.06
  transient of infancy 279.09
Hypogenitalism (congenital) (female) (male) 752.89
  penis 752.69
Hypoglycemia (spontaneous) 251.2
  coma 251.0
    diabetic 250.3 ☑
      due to secondary diabetes 249.3 ☑
  diabetic 250.8 ☑
    due to secondary diabetes 249.8 ☑
  due to insulin 251.0
    therapeutic misadventure 962.3
  familial (idiopathic) 251.2
  following gastrointestinal surgery 579.3
  infantile (idiopathic) 251.2
  in infant of diabetic mother 775.0
  leucine-induced 270.3
  neonatal 775.6
  reactive 251.2
  specified NEC 251.1
Hypoglycemic shock 251.0
  diabetic 250.8 ☑
    due to secondary diabetes 249.8 ☑
  due to insulin 251.0
  functional (syndrome) 251.1
Hypogonadism
  female 256.39
  gonadotrophic (isolated) 253.4
  hypogonadotropic (isolated) (with anosmia) 253.4
  isolated 253.4
  male 257.2
    hereditary familial (Reifenstein's syndrome) 259.52
  ovarian (primary) 256.39
  pituitary (secondary) 253.4
  testicular (primary) (secondary) 257.2
Hypohidrosis 705.0
Hypohidrotic ectodermal dysplasia 757.31
Hypoidrosis 705.0
Hypoinsulinemia, postsurgical 251.3

Hypoinsulinemia, postsurgical — *continued*
  postpancreatectomy (complete) (partial) 251.3
Hypokalemia 276.8
Hypokinesia 780.99
Hypoleukia splenica 289.4
Hypoleukocytosis 288.50
Hypolipidemia 272.5
Hypolipoproteinemia 272.5
Hypomagnesemia 275.2
  neonatal 775.4
Hypomania, hypomanic reaction — *see also* Psychosis, affective 296.0 ☑
  recurrent episode 296.1 ☑
  single episode 296.0 ☑
Hypomastia (congenital) 611.82
Hypomenorrhea 626.1
Hypometabolism 783.9
Hypomotility
  gastrointestinal tract 536.8
    psychogenic 306.4
  intestine 564.89
    psychogenic 306.4
  stomach 536.8
    psychogenic 306.4
Hyponasality 784.44
Hyponatremia 276.1
Hypo-ovarianism 256.39
Hypo-ovarism 256.39
Hypoparathyroidism (idiopathic) (surgically induced) 252.1
  neonatal 775.4
Hypoperfusion (in)
  newborn 779.89
Hypopharyngitis 462
Hypophoria 378.40
Hypophosphatasia 275.3
Hypophosphatemia (acquired) (congenital) (familial) 275.3
  renal 275.3
Hypophyseal, hypophysis — *see also* condition
  dwarfism 253.3
  gigantism 253.0
  syndrome 253.8
Hypophyseothalamic syndrome 253.8
Hypopiesis — *see* Hypotension
Hypopigmentation 709.00
  eyelid 374.53
Hypopinealism 259.8
Hypopituitarism (juvenile) (syndrome) 253.2
  due to
    hormone therapy 253.7
    hypophysectomy 253.7
    radiotherapy 253.7
  postablative 253.7
  postpartum hemorrhage 253.2
Hypoplasia, hypoplasis 759.89
  adrenal (gland) 759.1
  alimentary tract 751.8
    lower 751.2
    upper 750.8
  angiolymphoid, with eosinophilia (ALHE) 228.01
  anus, anal (canal) 751.2
  aorta 747.22
  aortic
    arch (tubular) 747.10
    orifice or valve with hypoplasia of ascending aorta and defective development of left ventricle (with mitral valve atresia) 746.7
  appendix 751.2
  areola 757.6
  arm (*see also* Absence, arm, congenital) 755.20
  artery (congenital) (peripheral) 747.60
    brain 747.81
    cerebral 747.81
    coronary 746.85
    gastrointestinal 747.61
    lower limb 747.64
    pulmonary 747.31
    renal 747.62
    retinal 743.58

Hypoplasia, hypoplasis — *continued*
  artery — *continued*
    specified NEC 747.69
    spinal 747.82
    umbilical 747.5
    upper limb 747.63
  auditory canal 744.29
    causing impairment of hearing 744.02
  biliary duct (common) or passage 751.61
  bladder 753.8
  bone NEC 756.9
    face 756.0
    malar 756.0
    mandible 524.04
      alveolar 524.74
    marrow 284.9
      acquired (secondary) 284.89
      congenital 284.09
      idiopathic 284.9
    maxilla 524.03
      alveolar 524.73
    skull (*see also* Hypoplasia, skull) 756.0
  brain 742.1
    gyri 742.2
    specified part 742.2
  breast (areola) 611.82
  bronchus (tree) 748.3
  cardiac 746.89
    valve — *see* Hypoplasia, heart, valve
    vein 746.89
  carpus (*see also* Absence, carpal, congenital) 755.28
  cartilaginous 756.9
  cecum 751.2
  cementum 520.4
    hereditary 520.5
  cephalic 742.1
  cerebellum 742.2
  cervix (uteri) 752.43
  chin 524.06
  clavicle 755.51
  coccyx 756.19
  colon 751.2
  corpus callosum 742.2
  cricoid cartilage 748.3
  dermal, focal (Goltz) 757.39
  digestive organ(s) or tract NEC 751.8
    lower 751.2
    upper 750.8
  ear 744.29
    auricle 744.23
    lobe 744.29
    middle, except ossicles 744.03
      ossicles 744.04
    ossicles 744.04
  enamel of teeth (neonatal) (postnatal) (prenatal) 520.4
    hereditary 520.5
  endocrine (gland) NEC 759.2
  endometrium 621.8
  epididymis 752.89
  epiglottis 748.3
  erythroid, congenital 284.01
  erythropoietic, chronic acquired 284.81
  esophagus 750.3
  Eustachian tube 744.24
  eye (*see also* Microphthalmos) 743.10
    lid 743.62
  face 744.89
    bone(s) 756.0
  fallopian tube 752.19
  femur (*see also* Absence, femur, congenital) 755.34
  fibula (*see also* Absence, fibula, congenital) 755.37
  finger (*see also* Absence, finger, congenital) 755.29
  focal dermal 757.39
  foot 755.31
  gallbladder 751.69
  genitalia, genital organ(s)
    female 752.89
      external 752.49
      internal NEC 752.89
    in adiposogenital dystrophy 253.8
    male 752.89

☑ Additional Digit Required — Refer to the Tabular List for Digit Selection   ⬝ Subterms under main terms may continue to next column or page

2015 ICD-9-CM   ▶◀ Revised Text   ● New Line   ▲ Revised Code   Volume 2 — 149

Hypoplasia, hypoplasis — continued
  genitalia, genital organ(s) — continued
    male — continued
      penis 752.69
  glottis 748.3
  hair 757.4
  hand 755.21
  heart 746.89
    left (complex) (syndrome) 746.7
    valve NEC 746.89
      pulmonary 746.01
  humerus (see also Absence, humerus, congenital) 755.24
  hymen 752.49
  intestine (small) 751.1
    large 751.2
  iris 743.46
  jaw 524.09
  kidney(s) 753.0
  labium (majus) (minus) 752.49
  labyrinth, membranous 744.05
  lacrimal duct (apparatus) 743.65
  larynx 748.3
  leg (see also Absence, limb, congenital, lower) 755.30
  limb 755.4
    lower (see also Absence, limb, congenital, lower) 755.30
    upper (see also Absence, limb, congenital, upper) 755.20
  liver 751.69
  lung (lobe) 748.5
  mammary (areolar) 611.82
  mandibular 524.04
    alveolar 524.74
    unilateral condylar 526.89
  maxillary 524.03
    alveolar 524.73
  medullary 284.9
  megakaryocytic 287.30
  metacarpus (see also Absence, metacarpal, congenital) 755.28
  metatarsus (see also Absence, metatarsal, congenital) 755.38
  muscle 756.89
    eye 743.69
  myocardium (congenital) (Uhl's anomaly) 746.84
  nail(s) 757.5
  nasolacrimal duct 743.65
  nervous system NEC 742.8
  neural 742.8
  nose, nasal 748.1
  ophthalmic (see also Microphthalmos) 743.10
  optic nerve 377.43
  organ
    of Corti 744.05
    or site NEC — see Anomaly, by site
  osseous meatus (ear) 744.03
  ovary 752.0
  oviduct 752.19
  pancreas 751.7
  parathyroid (gland) 759.2
  parotid gland 750.26
  patella 755.64
  pelvis, pelvic girdle 755.69
  penis 752.69
  peripheral vascular system (congenital) NEC 747.60
    gastrointestinal 747.61
    lower limb 747.64
    renal 747.62
    specified NEC 747.69
    spinal 747.82
    upper limb 747.63
  pituitary (gland) 759.2
  pulmonary 748.5

Hypoplasia, hypoplasis — continued
  pulmonary — continued
    arteriovenous 747.32
    artery 747.31
    valve 746.01
  punctum lacrimale 743.65
  radioulnar (see also Absence, radius, congenital, with ulna) 755.25
  radius (see also Absence, radius, congenital) 755.26
  rectum 751.2
  respiratory system NEC 748.9
  rib 756.3
  sacrum 756.19
  scapula 755.59
  shoulder girdle 755.59
  skin 757.39
  skull (bone) 756.0
    with
      anencephalus 740.0
      encephalocele 742.0
      hydrocephalus 742.3
        with spina bifida (see also Spina bifida) 741.0 ☑
      microcephalus 742.1
  spinal (cord) (ventral horn cell) 742.59
    vessel 747.82
  spine 756.19
  spleen 759.0
  sternum 756.3
  tarsus (see also Absence, tarsal, congenital) 755.38
  testis, testicle 752.89
  thymus (gland) 279.11
  thyroid (gland) 243
    cartilage 748.3
  tibiofibular (see also Absence, tibia, congenital, with fibula) 755.35
  toe (see also Absence, toe, congenital) 755.39
  tongue 750.16
  trachea (cartilage) (rings) 748.3
  Turner's (tooth) 520.4
  ulna (see also Absence, ulna, congenital) 755.27
  umbilical artery 747.5
  ureter 753.29
  uterus 752.32
  vagina 752.45
  vascular (peripheral) NEC (see also Hypoplasia, peripheral vascular system) 747.60
    brain 747.81
  vein(s) (peripheral) NEC (see also Hypoplasia, peripheral vascular system) 747.60
    brain 747.81
    cardiac 746.89
    great 747.49
    portal 747.49
    pulmonary 747.49
  vena cava (inferior) (superior) 747.49
  vertebra 756.19
  vulva 752.49
  zonule (ciliary) 743.39
  zygoma 738.12
Hypopotassemia 276.8
Hypoproaccelerinemia — see also Defect, coagulation 286.3
Hypoproconvertinemia (congenital) — see also Defect, coagulation 286.3
Hypoproteinemia (essential) (hypermetabolic) (idiopathic) 273.8
Hypoproteinosis 260
Hypoprothrombinemia (congenital) (hereditary) (idiopathic) — see also Defect, coagulation 286.3
  acquired 286.7
  newborn 776.3

Hypopselaphesia 782.0
Hypopyon (anterior chamber) (eye) 364.05
  iritis 364.05
  ulcer (cornea) 370.04
Hypopyrexia 780.99
Hyporeflex 796.1
Hyporeninemia, extreme 790.99
  in primary aldosteronism 255.10
Hyporesponsive episode 780.09
Hyposecretion
  ACTH 253.4
  ovary 256.39
    postablative 256.2
  salivary gland (any) 527.7
Hyposegmentation of neutrophils, hereditary 288.2
Hyposiderinemia 280.9
Hyposmolality 276.1
  syndrome 276.1
Hyposomatotropism 253.3
Hyposomnia, unspecified — see also Insomnia 780.52
  with sleep apnea, unspecified 780.51
Hypospadias (male) 752.61
  female 753.8
Hypospermatogenesis 606.1
Hyposphagma 372.72
Hyposplenism 289.59
Hypostasis, pulmonary 514
Hypostatic — see condition
Hyposthenuria 593.89
Hyposuprarenalism 255.41
Hypo-TBG-nemia 246.8
Hypotension (arterial) (constitutional) 458.9
  chronic 458.1
  iatrogenic 458.29
  maternal, syndrome (following labor and delivery) 669.2 ☑
  of hemodialysis 458.21
  orthostatic (chronic) 458.0
    dysautonomic-dyskinetic syndrome 333.0
  permanent idiopathic 458.1
  postoperative 458.29
  postural 458.0
  specified type NEC 458.8
  transient 796.3
Hypothermia (accidental) 991.6
  anesthetic 995.89
  associated with low environmental temperature 991.6
  newborn NEC 778.3
  not associated with low environmental temperature 780.65
Hypothymergasia — see also Psychosis, affective 296.2 ☑
  recurrent episode 296.3 ☑
  single episode 296.2 ☑
Hypothyroidism (acquired) 244.9
  complicating pregnancy, childbirth, or puerperium 648.1 ☑
  congenital 243
  due to
    ablation 244.1
      radioactive iodine 244.1
      surgical 244.0
    iodine (administration) (ingestion) 244.2
      radioactive 244.1
    irradiation therapy 244.1
    p-aminosalicylic acid (PAS) 244.3
    phenylbutazone 244.3
    resorcinol 244.3
    specified cause NEC 244.8
    surgery 244.0
  goitrous (sporadic) 246.1
  iatrogenic NEC 244.3
  iodine 244.2

Hypothyroidism — continued
  pituitary 244.8
  postablative NEC 244.1
  postsurgical 244.0
  primary 244.9
  secondary NEC 244.8
  specified cause NEC 244.8
  sporadic goitrous 246.1
Hypotonia, hypotonicity, hypotony 781.3
  benign congenital 358.8
  bladder 596.4
  congenital 779.89
    benign 358.8
  eye 360.30
    due to
      fistula 360.32
      ocular disorder NEC 360.33
    following loss of aqueous or vitreous 360.33
    primary 360.31
  infantile muscular (benign) 359.0
  muscle 728.9
  uterus, uterine (contractions) — see Inertia, uterus
Hypotrichosis 704.09
  congenital 757.4
  lid (congenital) 757.4
    acquired 374.55
  postinfectional NEC 704.09
Hypotropia 378.32
Hypoventilation 786.09
  congenital central alveolar syndrome 327.25
  idiopathic sleep related nonobstructive alveolar 327.24
  obesity 278.03
  sleep related, in conditions classifiable elsewhere 327.26
Hypovitaminosis — see also Deficiency, vitamin 269.2
Hypovolemia 276.52
  surgical shock 998.09
  traumatic (shock) 958.4
Hypoxemia — see also Anoxia 799.02
  sleep related, in conditions classifiable elsewhere 327.26
Hypoxia — see also Anoxia 799.02
  cerebral 348.1
    during or resulting from a procedure 997.01
    newborn 770.88
      mild or moderate 768.6
      severe 768.5
  fetal, affecting newborn 770.88
  intrauterine — see Distress, fetal
  myocardial (see also Insufficiency, coronary) 411.89
    arteriosclerotic — see Arteriosclerosis, coronary
  newborn 770.88
  sleep related 327.24
Hypoxic-ischemic encephalopathy (HIE) 768.70
  mild 768.71
  moderate 768.72
  severe 768.73
Hypsarrhythmia — see also Epilepsy 345.6 ☑
Hysteralgia, pregnant uterus 646.8 ☑
Hysteria, hysterical 300.10
  anxiety 300.20
  Charcôt's gland 300.11
  conversion (any manifestation) 300.11
  dissociative type NEC 300.15
  psychosis, acute 298.1
Hysteroepilepsy 300.11
Hysterotomy, affecting fetus or newborn 763.89

☑ Additional Digit Required — Refer to the Tabular List for Digit Selection   ▽ᵀᴱ Subterms under main terms may continue to next column or page

I

Iatrogenic syndrome of excess cortisol 255.0
IBM (inclusion body myositis) 359.71
Iceland disease (epidemic neuromyasthenia) 049.8
Ichthyosis (congenita) 757.1
  acquired 701.1
  fetalis gravior 757.1
  follicularis 757.1
  hystrix 757.39
  lamellar 757.1
  lingual 528.6
  palmaris and plantaris 757.39
  simplex 757.1
  vera 757.1
  vulgaris 757.1
Ichthyotoxism 988.0
  bacterial (see also Poisoning, food) 005.9
Icteroanemia, hemolytic (acquired) 283.9
  congenital (see also Spherocytosis) 282.0
Icterus — see also Jaundice 782.4
  catarrhal — see Icterus, infectious
  conjunctiva 782.4
    newborn 774.6
  epidemic — see Icterus, infectious
  febrilis — see Icterus, infectious
  fetus or newborn — see Jaundice, fetus or newborn
  gravis (see also Necrosis, liver) 570
    complicating pregnancy 646.7 ☑
      affecting fetus or newborn 760.8
    fetus or newborn NEC 773.0
    obstetrical 646.7 ☑
      affecting fetus or newborn 760.8
  hematogenous (acquired) 283.9
  hemolytic (acquired) 283.9
    congenital (see also Spherocytosis) 282.0
  hemorrhagic (acute) 100.0
    leptospiral 100.0
    newborn 776.0
    spirochetal 100.0
  infectious 070.1
    with hepatic coma 070.0
    leptospiral 100.0
    spirochetal 100.0
  intermittens juvenilis 277.4
  malignant (see also Necrosis, liver) 570
  neonatorum (see also Jaundice, fetus or newborn) 774.6
  pernicious (see also Necrosis, liver) 570
  spirochetal 100.0
Ictus solaris, solis 992.0
Ideation
  homicidal V62.85
  suicidal V62.84
Identity disorder 313.82
  dissociative 300.14
  gender role (child) 302.6
    adult 302.85
  psychosexual (child) 302.6
    adult 302.85
Idioglossia 307.9
Idiopathic — see condition
Idiosyncrasy — see also Allergy 995.3
  drug, medicinal substance, and biological — see Allergy, drug
Idiot, idiocy (congenital) 318.2
  amaurotic (Bielschowsky) (-Jansky) (family) (infantile) (late) (juvenile) (late) (Vogt-Spielmeyer) 330.1
  microcephalic 742.1
  Mongolian 758.0
  oxycephalic 756.0
Id reaction (due to bacteria) 692.89
IEED (involuntary emotional expression disorder) 310.81
IFIS (intraoperative floppy iris syndrome) 364.81
IgE asthma 493.0 ☑
Ileitis (chronic) — see also Enteritis 558.9
  infectious 009.0
  noninfectious 558.9
  regional (ulcerative) 555.0
    with large intestine 555.2
  segmental 555.0

Ileitis — see also Enteritis — continued
  segmental — continued
    with large intestine 555.2
  terminal (ulcerative) 555.0
    with large intestine 555.2
Ileocolitis — see also Enteritis 558.9
  infectious 009.0
  regional 555.2
  ulcerative 556.1
Ileostomy status V44.2
  with complication 569.60
Ileotyphus 002.0
Ileum — see condition
Ileus (adynamic) (bowel) (colon) (inhibitory) (intestine) (neurogenic) (paralytic) 560.1
  arteriomesenteric duodenal 537.2
  due to gallstone (in intestine) 560.31
  duodenal, chronic 537.2
  following gastrointestinal surgery 997.49
  gallstone 560.31
  mechanical (see also Obstruction, intestine) 560.9
  meconium 777.1
    due to cystic fibrosis 277.01
  myxedema 564.89
  postoperative 997.49
  transitory, newborn 777.4
Iliac — see condition
Iliotibial band friction syndrome 728.89
Illegitimacy V61.6
Ill, louping 063.1
Illness — see also Disease
  factitious 300.19
    with
      combined psychological and physical signs and symptoms 300.19
      predominantly
        physical signs and symptoms 300.19
        psychological symptoms 300.16
  chronic (with physical signs) 301.51
  heart — see Disease, heart
  manic-depressive (see also Psychosis, affective) 296.80
  mental (see also Disorder, mental) 300.9
Imbalance 781.2
  autonomic (see also Neuropathy, peripheral, autonomic) 337.9
  electrolyte 276.9
    with
      abortion — see Abortion, by type, with metabolic disorder
      ectopic pregnancy (see also categories 633.0–633.9) 639.4
      hyperemesis gravidarum (before 22 completed weeks gestation) 643.1 ☑
      molar pregnancy (see also categories 630–632) 639.4
    following
      abortion 639.4
      ectopic or molar pregnancy 639.4
    neonatal, transitory NEC 775.5
  endocrine 259.9
  eye muscle NEC 378.9
    heterophoria — see Heterophoria
  glomerulotubular NEC 593.89
  hormone 259.9
  hysterical (see also Hysteria) 300.10
  labyrinth NEC 386.50
  posture 729.90
  sympathetic (see also Neuropathy, peripheral, autonomic) 337.9
Imbecile, imbecility 318.0
  moral 301.7
  old age 290.9
  senile 290.9
  specified IQ — see IQ
  unspecified IQ 318.0
Imbedding, intrauterine device 996.32
Imbibition, cholesterol (gallbladder) 575.6
Imerslund (-Gräsbeck) syndrome (anemia due to familial selective vitamin B_{12} malabsorption) 281.1
Iminoacidopathy 270.8
Iminoglycinuria, familial 270.8

Immature — see also Immaturity
  personality 301.89
Immaturity 765.1 ☑
  extreme 765.0 ☑
  fetus or infant light-for-dates — see Light-for-dates
  lung, fetus or newborn 770.4
  organ or site NEC — see Hypoplasia
  pulmonary, fetus or newborn 770.4
  reaction 301.89
  sexual (female) (male) 259.0
Immersion 994.1
  foot 991.4
  hand 991.4
Immobile, immobility
  complete
    due to severe physical disability or frailty 780.72
  intestine 564.89
  joint — see Ankylosis
  syndrome (paraplegic) 728.3
Immunization
  ABO
    affecting management of pregnancy 656.2 ☑
      fetus or newborn 773.1
  complication — see Complications, vaccination
  Rh factor
    affecting management of pregnancy 656.1 ☑
      fetus or newborn 773.0
    from transfusion (see also Complications, transfusion) 999.70
Immunodeficiency 279.3
  with
    adenosine-deaminase deficiency 279.2
    defect, predominant
      B-cell 279.00
      T-cell 279.10
    hyperimmunoglobulinemia 279.2
    lymphopenia, hereditary 279.2
    thrombocytopenia and eczema 279.12
    thymic
      aplasia 279.2
      dysplasia 279.2
  autosomal recessive, Swiss-type 279.2
  common variable 279.06
  severe combined (SCID) 279.2
  to Rh factor
    affecting management of pregnancy 656.1 ☑
      fetus or newborn 773.0
  X-linked, with increased IgM 279.05
Immunotherapy, prophylactic V07.2
  antineoplastic V58.12
Impaction, impacted
  bowel, colon, rectum 560.30
    with hernia (see also Hernia, by site, with obstruction)
      gangrenous — see Hernia, by site, with gangrene
    by
      calculus 560.32
      gallstone 560.31
    fecal 560.32
    specified type NEC 560.32
  calculus — see Calculus
  cerumen (ear) (external) 380.4
  cuspid 520.6
  dental 520.6
  fecal, feces 560.32
    with hernia (see also Hernia, by site, with obstruction)
      gangrenous — see Hernia, by site, with gangrene
  fracture — see Fracture, by site
  gallbladder — see Cholelithiasis
  gallstone(s) — see Cholelithiasis
    in intestine (any part) 560.31
  intestine(s) 560.30
    with hernia (see also Hernia, by site, with obstruction)
      gangrenous — see Hernia, by site, with gangrene

Impaction, impacted — continued
  intestine(s) — continued
    by
      calculus 560.32
      gallstone 560.31
    fecal 560.32
    specified type NEC 560.32
  intrauterine device (IUD) 996.32
  molar 520.6
  shoulder 660.4 ☑
    affecting fetus or newborn 763.1
  tooth, teeth 520.6
  turbinate 733.99
Impaired, impairment (function)
  arm V49.1
    movement, involving
      musculoskeletal system V49.1
      nervous system V49.2
  auditory discrimination 388.43
  back V48.3
  body (entire) V49.89
  cognitive, mild, so stated 331.83
  combined visual hearing V49.85
  dual sensory V49.85
  glucose
    fasting 790.21
    tolerance test (oral) 790.22
  hearing (see also Deafness) 389.9
    combined with visual impairment V49.85
  heart — see Disease, heart
  kidney (see also Disease, renal) 593.9
    disorder resulting from 588.9
      specified NEC 588.89
  leg V49.1
    movement, involving
      musculoskeletal system V49.1
      nervous system V49.2
  limb V49.1
    movement, involving
      musculoskeletal system V49.1
      nervous system V49.2
  liver 573.8
  mastication 524.9
  mild cognitive, so stated 331.83
  mobility
    ear ossicles NEC 385.22
    incostapedial joint 385.22
    malleus 385.21
  myocardium, myocardial (see also Insufficiency, myocardial) 428.0
  neuromusculoskeletal NEC V49.89
    back V48.3
    head V48.2
    limb V49.2
    neck V48.3
    spine V48.3
    trunk V48.3
  rectal sphincter 787.99
  renal (see also Disease, renal) 593.9
    disorder resulting from 588.9
      specified NEC 588.89
  spine V48.3
  vision NEC 369.9
    both eyes NEC 369.3
    combined with hearing impairment V49.85
    moderate 369.74
      both eyes 369.25
        with impairment of lesser eye (specified as)
          blind, not further specified 369.15
          low vision, not further specified 369.23
          near-total 369.17
          profound 369.18
          severe 369.24
          total 369.16
      one eye 369.74
        with vision of other eye (specified as)
          near-normal 369.75
          normal 369.76
    near-total 369.64
      both eyes 369.04

☑ Additional Digit Required — Refer to the Tabular List for Digit Selection   ▽ Subterms under main terms may continue to next column or page

2015 ICD-9-CM   ▶◀ Revised Text   ● New Line   ▲ Revised Code   Volume 2 — 151

Impaired, impairment — *continued*
vision — *continued*
near-total — *continued*
both eyes — *continued*
with impairment of lesser eye
(specified as)
blind, not further specified
369.02
total 369.03
one eye 369.64
with vision of other eye (specified
as)
near normal 369.65
normal 369.66
one eye 369.60
with low vision of other eye 369.10
profound 369.67
both eyes 369.08
with impairment of lesser eye
(specified as)
blind, not further specified
369.05
near-total 369.07
total 369.06
one eye 369.67
with vision of other eye (specified
as)
near-normal 369.68
normal 369.69
severe 369.71
both eyes 369.22
with impairment of lesser eye
(specified as)
blind, not further specified
369.11
low vision, not further specified 369.21
near-total 369.13
profound 369.14
total 369.12
one eye 369.71
with vision of other eye (specified
as)
near-normal 369.72
normal 369.73
total
both eyes 369.01
one eye 369.61
with vision of other eye (specified
as)
near-normal 369.62
normal 369.63
Impaludism — *see* Malaria
Impediment, speech NEC 784.59
psychogenic 307.9
secondary to organic lesion 784.59
Impending
cerebrovascular accident or attack 435.9
coronary syndrome 411.1
delirium tremens 291.0
myocardial infarction 411.1
Imperception, auditory (acquired) (congenital) 389.9
Imperfect
aeration, lung (newborn) 770.5
closure (congenital)
alimentary tract NEC 751.8
lower 751.5
upper 750.8
atrioventricular ostium 745.69
atrium (secundum) 745.5
primum 745.61
branchial cleft or sinus 744.41
choroid 743.59
cricoid cartilage 748.3
cusps, heart valve NEC 746.89
pulmonary 746.09
ductus
arteriosus 747.0
Botalli 747.0
ear drum 744.29
causing impairment of hearing
744.03
endocardial cushion 745.60
epiglottis 748.3

Imperfect — *continued*
closure — *continued*
esophagus with communication to
bronchus or trachea 750.3
Eustachian valve 746.89
eyelid 743.62
face, facial (*see also* Cleft, lip) 749.10
foramen
Botalli 745.5
ovale 745.5
genitalia, genital organ(s) or system
female 752.89
external 752.49
internal NEC 752.89
uterus 752.39
male 752.89
penis 752.69
glottis 748.3
heart valve (cusps) NEC 746.89
interatrial ostium or septum 745.5
interauricular ostium or septum 745.5
interventricular ostium or septum 745.4
iris 743.46
kidney 753.3
larynx 748.3
lens 743.36
lip (*see also* Cleft, lip) 749.10
nasal septum or sinus 748.1
nose 748.1
omphalomesenteric duct 751.0
optic nerve entry 743.57
organ or site NEC — *see* Anomaly, specified type, by site
ostium
interatrial 745.5
interauricular 745.5
interventricular 745.4
palate (*see also* Cleft, palate) 749.00
preauricular sinus 744.46
retina 743.56
roof of orbit 742.0
sclera 743.47
septum
aortic 745.0
aorticopulmonary 745.0
atrial (secundum) 745.5
primum 745.61
between aorta and pulmonary artery
745.0
heart 745.9
interatrial (secundum) 745.5
primum 745.61
interauricular (secundum) 745.5
primum 745.61
interventricular 745.4
with pulmonary stenosis or atresia, dextraposition of aorta, and hypertrophy of
right ventricle 745.2
in tetralogy of Fallot 745.2
nasal 748.1
ventricular 745.4
with pulmonary stenosis or atresia, dextraposition of aorta, and hypertrophy of
right ventricle 745.2
in tetralogy of Fallot 745.2
skull 756.0
with
anencephalus 740.0
encephalocele 742.0
hydrocephalus 742.3
with spina bifida (*see also*
Spina bifida) 741.0 ☑
microcephalus 742.1
spine (with meningocele) (*see also* Spina
bifida) 741.90
thyroid cartilage 748.3
trachea 748.3
tympanic membrane 744.29
causing impairment of hearing
744.03
uterus (with communication to bladder,
intestine, or rectum) 752.39
uvula 749.02

Imperfect — *continued*
closure — *continued*
uvula — *continued*
with cleft lip (*see also* Cleft, palate,
with cleft lip) 749.20
vitelline duct 751.0
development — *see* Anomaly, by site
erection 607.84
fusion — *see* Imperfect, closure
inflation lung (newborn) 770.5
intestinal canal 751.5
poise 729.90
rotation — *see* Malrotation
septum, ventricular 745.4
Imperfectly descended testis 752.51
Imperforate (congenital) — *see also* Atresia
anus 751.2
bile duct 751.61
cervix (uteri) 752.49
esophagus 750.3
hymen 752.42
intestine (small) 751.1
large 751.2
jejunum 751.1
pharynx 750.29
rectum 751.2
salivary duct 750.23
urethra 753.6
urinary meatus 753.6
vagina 752.49
Impervious (congenital) — *see also* Atresia
anus 751.2
bile duct 751.61
esophagus 750.3
intestine (small) 751.1
large 751.5
rectum 751.2
urethra 753.6
Impetiginization of other dermatoses 684
Impetigo (any organism) (any site) (bullous)
(circinate) (contagiosa) (neonatorum)
(simplex) 684
Bockhart's (superficial folliculitis) 704.8
external ear 684 [380.13]
eyelid 684 [373.5]
Fox's (contagiosa) 684
furfuracea 696.5
herpetiformis 694.3
nonobstetrical 694.3
staphylococcal infection 684
ulcerative 686.8
vulgaris 684
Impingement, soft tissue between teeth
524.89
anterior 524.81
posterior 524.82
Implantation
anomalous (*see also* Anomaly, specified
type, by site)
ureter 753.4
cyst
external area or site (skin) NEC 709.8
iris 364.61
vagina 623.8
vulva 624.8
dermoid (cyst)
external area or site (skin) NEC 709.8
iris 364.61
vagina 623.8
vulva 624.8
placenta, low or marginal — *see* Placenta
previa
Implant, endometrial 617.9
Impotence (sexual) 607.84
organic origin NEC 607.84
psychogenic 302.72
Impoverished blood 285.9
Impression, basilar 756.0
Imprisonment V62.5
Improper
development, infant 764.9 ☑
Improperly tied umbilical cord (causing
hemorrhage) 772.3
Impulses, obsessional 300.3
Impulsive 799.23
neurosis 300.3

Impulsiveness 799.23
Inaction, kidney — *see also* Disease, renal
593.9
Inactive — *see* condition
Inadequate, inadequacy
aesthetics of dental restoration 525.67
biologic 301.6
cardiac and renal — *see* Hypertension, cardiorenal
constitutional 301.6
development
child 783.40
fetus 764.9 ☑
affecting management of pregnancy
656.5 ☑
genitalia
after puberty NEC 259.0
congenital — *see* Hypoplasia, genitalia
lungs 748.5
organ or site NEC — *see* Hypoplasia, by
site
dietary 269.9
distance, interarch 524.28
education V62.3
environment
economic problem V60.2
household condition NEC V60.1
poverty V60.2
unemployment V62.0
functional 301.6
household care, due to
family member
handicapped or ill V60.4
temporarily away from home V60.4
on vacation V60.5
technical defects in home V60.1
temporary absence from home of person
rendering care V60.4
housing (heating) (space) V60.1
interarch distance 524.28
material resources V60.2
mental (*see also* Disability, intellectual) 319
nervous system 799.29
personality 301.6
prenatal care in current pregnancy V23.7
pulmonary
function 786.09
newborn 770.89
ventilation, newborn 770.89
respiration 786.09
newborn 770.89
sample
cytology
anal 796.78
cervical 795.08
vaginal 795.18
social 301.6
Inanition 263.9
with edema 262
due to
deprivation of food 994.2
malnutrition 263.9
fever 780.60
Inappropriate
change in quantitative human chorionic
gonadotropin (hCG) in early pregnancy 631.0
level of quantitative human chorionic gonadotropin (hCG) for gestational age
in early pregnancy 631.0
secretion
ACTH 255.0
antidiuretic hormone (ADH) (excessive)
253.6
deficiency 253.5
ectopic hormone NEC 259.3
pituitary (posterior) 253.6
Inattention after or at birth 995.52
Inborn errors of metabolism — *see* Disorder,
metabolism
Incarceration, incarcerated
bubonocele (*see also* Hernia, inguinal, with
obstruction)
gangrenous — *see* Hernia, inguinal, with
gangrene

☑ **Additional Digit Required** — Refer to the Tabular List for Digit Selection   ▽ **Subterms under main terms may continue to next column or page**

152 — Volume 2   ▶◀ Revised Text   ● New Line   ▲ Revised Code   **2015 ICD-9-CM**

Incarceration, incarcerated — *continued*
  colon (by hernia) (*see also* Hernia, by site, with obstruction)
    gangrenous — *see* Hernia, by site, with gangrene
  enterocele 552.9
    gangrenous 551.9
  epigastrocele 552.29
    gangrenous 551.29
  epiplocele 552.9
    gangrenous 551.9
  exomphalos 552.1
    gangrenous 551.1
  fallopian tube 620.8
  hernia (*see also* Hernia, by site, with obstruction)
    gangrenous — *see* Hernia, by site, with gangrene
  iris, in wound 871.1
  lens, in wound 871.1
  merocele (*see also* Hernia, femoral, with obstruction) 552.00
  omentum (by hernia) (*see also* Hernia, by site, with obstruction)
    gangrenous — *see* Hernia, by site, with gangrene
  omphalocele 756.72
  rupture (meaning hernia) (*see also* Hernia, by site, with obstruction) 552.9
    gangrenous (*see also* Hernia, by site, with gangrene) 551.9
  sarcoepiplocele 552.9
    gangrenous 551.9
  sarcoepiplomphalocele 552.1
    with gangrene 551.1
  uterus 621.8
    gravid 654.3 ☑
      causing obstructed labor 660.2 ☑
        affecting fetus or newborn 763.1
Incident, cerebrovascular — *see also* Disease, cerebrovascular, acute 436
Incineration (entire body) (from fire, conflagration, electricity, or lightning) — *see* Burn, multiple, specified sites
Incised wound
  external — *see* Wound, open, by site
  internal organs (abdomen, chest, or pelvis) — *see* Injury, internal, by site, with open wound
Incision, incisional
  hernia — *see* Hernia, incisional
  surgical, complication — *see* Complications, surgical procedures
  traumatic
    external — *see* Wound, open, by site
    internal organs (abdomen, chest, or pelvis) — *see* Injury, internal, by site, with open wound
Inclusion
  azurophilic leukocytic 288.2
  blennorrhea (neonatal) (newborn) 771.6
  cyst — *see* Cyst, skin
  gallbladder in liver (congenital) 751.69
Incompatibility
  ABO
    affecting management of pregnancy 656.2 ☑
    fetus or newborn 773.1
    infusion or transfusion reaction (*see also* Complications, transfusion) 999.60
  blood (group) (Duffy) (E) (K(ell)) (Kidd) (Lewis) (M) (N) (P) (S) NEC
    affecting management of pregnancy 656.2 ☑
    fetus or newborn 773.2
    infusion or transfusion reaction (*see also* Complications, transfusion) 999.75
  contour of existing restoration of tooth with oral health 525.65
  marital V61.10
    involving
      divorce V61.03
      estrangement V61.09

Incompatibility — *continued*
  non-ABO (*see also* Complications, transfusion) 999.75
  Rh (antigen) (C) (c) (D) (E) (e) (blood group) (factor)
    affecting management of pregnancy 656.1 ☑
    fetus or newborn 773.0
    infusion or transfusion reaction (*see also* Complications, transfusion) 999.70
  Rhesus — *see* Incompatibility, Rh
Incompetency, incompetence, incompetent
  annular
    aortic (valve) (*see also* Insufficiency, aortic) 424.1
    mitral (valve) (*see also* Insufficiency, mitral) 424.0
    pulmonary valve (heart) (*see also* Endocarditis, pulmonary) 424.3
  aortic (valve) (*see also* Insufficiency, aortic) 424.1
    syphilitic 093.22
  cardiac (orifice) 530.0
    valve — *see* Endocarditis
  cervix, cervical (os) 622.5
    in pregnancy 654.5 ☑
      affecting fetus or newborn 761.0
  chronotropic 426.89
    with
      autonomic dysfunction 337.9
      ischemic heart disease 414.9
      left ventricular dysfunction 429.89
      sinus node dysfunction 427.81
  esophagogastric (junction) (sphincter) 530.0
  heart valve, congenital 746.89
  mitral (valve) — *see* Insufficiency, mitral
  papillary muscle (heart) 429.81
  pelvic fundus
    pubocervical tissue 618.81
    rectovaginal tissue 618.82
  pulmonary valve (heart) (*see also* Endocarditis, pulmonary) 424.3
    congenital 746.09
  tricuspid (annular) (rheumatic) (valve) (*see also* Endocarditis, tricuspid) 397.0
  valvular — *see* Endocarditis
  vein, venous (saphenous) (varicose) (*see also* Varicose, vein) 454.9
  velopharyngeal (closure)
    acquired 528.9
    congenital 750.29
Incomplete — *see also* condition
  bladder emptying 788.21
  defecation 787.61
  expansion lungs (newborn) 770.5
  gestation (liveborn) — *see* Immaturity
  rotation — *see* Malrotation
Inconclusive
  image test due to excess body fat 793.91
  mammogram, mammography 793.82
    due to dense breasts 793.82
Incontinence 788.30
  without sensory awareness 788.34
  anal sphincter 787.60
  continuous leakage 788.37
  feces, fecal 787.60
    due to hysteria 300.11
    nonorganic origin 307.7
  hysterical 300.11
  mixed (male) (female) (urge and stress) 788.33
  overflow 788.38
  paradoxical 788.39
  rectal 787.60
  specified NEC 788.39
  stress (female) 625.6
    male NEC 788.32
  urethral sphincter 599.84
  urge 788.31
    and stress (male) (female) 788.33
  urine 788.30
    active 788.30
    due to
      cognitive impairment 788.91
      immobility 788.91

Incontinence — *continued*
  urine — *continued*
    due to — *continued*
      severe physical disability 788.91
    functional 788.91
    male 788.30
      stress 788.32
        and urge 788.33
    neurogenic 788.39
    nonorganic origin 307.6
    stress (female) 625.6
      male NEC 788.32
    urge 788.31
      and stress 788.33
Incontinentia pigmenti 757.33
Incoordinate
  uterus (action) (contractions) 661.4 ☑
    affecting fetus or newborn 763.7
Incoordination
  esophageal-pharyngeal (newborn) 787.24
  muscular 781.3
  papillary muscle 429.81
Increase, increased
  abnormal, in development 783.9
  androgens (ovarian) 256.1
  anticoagulants (antithrombin) (anti-II) (anti-VIIIa) (anti-IXa) (anti-XIa) (prothrombin) (*see also* Anticoagulants 286.59
    anti-IIa 287.8
    anti-Xa 287.8
    extrinsic 287.8
    postpartum 666.3 ☑
  cold sense (*see also* Disturbance, sensation) 782.0
  estrogen 256.0
  function
    adrenal (cortex) 255.3
      medulla 255.6
    pituitary (anterior) (gland) (lobe) 253.1
      posterior 253.6
  heat sense (*see also* Disturbance, sensation) 782.0
  intracranial pressure 781.99
    injury at birth 767.8
  light reflex of retina 362.13
  permeability, capillary 448.9
  pressure
    intracranial 781.99
      injury at birth 767.8
    intraocular 365.00
  pulsations 785.9
  pulse pressure 785.9
  sphericity, lens 743.36
  splenic activity 289.4
  venous pressure 459.89
    portal 572.3
Incrustation, cornea, lead or zinc 930.0
Incyclophoria 378.44
Incyclotropia 378.33
Indeterminate sex 752.7
India rubber skin 756.83
Indicanuria 270.2
Indigestion (bilious) (functional) 536.8
  acid 536.8
  catarrhal 536.8
  due to decomposed food NEC 005.9
  fat 579.8
  nervous 306.4
  psychogenic 306.4
Indirect — *see* condition
Indolent bubo NEC 099.8
Induced
  abortion — *see* Abortion, induced
  birth, affecting fetus or newborn 763.89
  delivery — *see* Delivery
  labor — *see* Delivery
Induration, indurated
  brain 348.89
  breast (fibrous) 611.79
    puerperal, postpartum 676.3 ☑
  broad ligament 620.8
  chancre 091.0
    anus 091.1
    congenital 090.0
    extragenital NEC 091.2
  corpora cavernosa (penis) (plastic) 607.89

Induration, indurated — *continued*
  liver (chronic) 573.8
    acute 573.8
  lung (black) (brown) (chronic) (fibroid) (*see also* Fibrosis, lung) 515
    essential brown 275.09 *[516.1]*
  penile 607.89
  phlebitic — *see* Phlebitis
  skin 782.8
  stomach 537.89
Induratio penis plastica 607.89
Industrial — *see* condition
Inebriety — *see also* Abuse, drugs, nondependent 305.0 ☑
Inefficiency
  kidney (*see also* Disease, renal) 593.9
  thyroid (acquired) (gland) 244.9
Inelasticity, skin 782.8
Inequality, leg (acquired) (length) 736.81
  congenital 755.30
Inertia
  bladder 596.4
    neurogenic 596.54
      with cauda equina syndrome 344.61
  stomach 536.8
    psychogenic 306.4
  uterus, uterine 661.2 ☑
    affecting fetus or newborn 763.7
    primary 661.0 ☑
    secondary 661.1 ☑
  vesical 596.4
    neurogenic 596.54
      with cauda equina 344.61
Infant — *see also* condition
  excessive crying of 780.92
  fussy (baby) 780.91
  held for adoption V68.89
  newborn — *see* Newborn
  post-term (gestation period over 40 completed weeks to 42 completed weeks) 766.21
  prolonged gestation of (period over 42 completed weeks) 766.22
  syndrome of diabetic mother 775.0
"Infant Hercules" syndrome 255.2
Infantile — *see also* condition
  genitalia, genitals 259.0
    in pregnancy or childbirth NEC 654.4 ☑
      affecting fetus or newborn 763.89
      causing obstructed labor 660.2 ☑
        affecting fetus or newborn 763.1
  heart 746.9
  kidney 753.3
  lack of care 995.52
  macula degeneration 362.75
  melanodontia 521.05
  os, uterus (*see also* Infantile, genitalia) 259.0
  pelvis 738.6
    with disproportion (fetopelvic) 653.1 ☑
      affecting fetus or newborn 763.1
      causing obstructed labor 660.1 ☑
        affecting fetus or newborn 763.1
  penis 259.0
  testis 257.2
  uterus (*see also* Infantile, genitalia) 259.0
  vulva 752.49
Infantilism 259.9
  with dwarfism (hypophyseal) 253.3
  Brissaud's (infantile myxedema) 244.9
  celiac 579.0
  Herter's (nontropical sprue) 579.0
  hypophyseal 253.3
  hypothalamic (with obesity) 253.8
  idiopathic 259.9
  intestinal 579.0
  pancreatic 577.8
  pituitary 253.3
  renal 588.0
  sexual (with obesity) 259.0
Infants, healthy liveborn — *see* Newborn
Infarct, infarction
  adrenal (capsule) (gland) 255.41
  amnion 658.8 ☑
  anterior (with contiguous portion of intraventricular septum) NEC (*see also* Infarct, myocardium) 410.1 ☑

☑ Additional Digit Required — Refer to the Tabular List for Digit Selection   ⟱ Subterms under main terms may continue to next column or page

2015 ICD-9-CM   ▶◀ Revised Text   ● New Line   ▲ Revised Code   Volume 2 — 153

Infarct, infarction — continued

appendices epiploicae 557.0
bowel 557.0
brain (stem) 434.91
  embolic (see also Embolism, brain) 434.11
  healed or old without residuals V12.54
  iatrogenic 997.02
  lacunar 434.91
  late effect — see Late effect(s) (of) cerebrovascular disease
  postoperative 997.02
  puerperal, postpartum, childbirth 674.0 ☑
  thrombotic (see also Thrombosis, brain) 434.01
breast 611.89
Brewer's (kidney) 593.81
cardiac (see also Infarct, myocardium) 410.9 ☑
cerebellar (see also Infarct, brain) 434.91
  embolic (see also Embolism, brain) 434.11
cerebral (see also Infarct, brain) 434.91
  aborted 434.91
  embolic (see also Embolism, brain) 434.11
  thrombotic (see also Infarct, brain) 434.01
chorion 658.8 ☑
colon (acute) (agnogenic) (embolic) (hemorrhagic) (nonocclusive) (nonthrombotic) (occlusive) (segmental) (thrombotic) (with gangrene) 557.0
coronary artery (see also Infarct, myocardium) 410.9 ☑
cortical 434.91
embolic (see also Embolism) 444.9
fallopian tube 620.8
gallbladder 575.8
heart (see also Infarct, myocardium) 410.9 ☑
hepatic 573.4
hypophysis (anterior lobe) 253.8
impending (myocardium) 411.1
intestine (acute) (agnogenic) (embolic) (hemorrhagic) (nonocclusive) (nonthrombotic) (occlusive) (thrombotic) (with gangrene) 557.0
kidney 593.81
lacunar 434.91
liver 573.4
lung (embolic) (thrombotic) 415.19
  with
    abortion — see Abortion, by type, with, embolism
    ectopic pregnancy (see also categories 633.0–633.9) 639.6
    molar pregnancy (see also categories 630–632) 639.6
  following
    abortion 639.6
    ectopic or molar pregnancy 639.6
  iatrogenic 415.11
  in pregnancy, childbirth, or puerperium — see Embolism, obstetrical
  postoperative 415.11
  septic 415.12
lymph node or vessel 457.8
medullary (brain) — see Infarct, brain
meibomian gland (eyelid) 374.85
mesentery, mesenteric (embolic) (thrombotic) (with gangrene) 557.0
midbrain — see Infarct, brain
myocardium, myocardial (acute or with a stated duration of 8 weeks or less) (with hypertension) 410.9 ☑

> Note — Use the following fifth-digit subclassification with category 410:
> 0   episode unspecified
> 1   initial episode
> 2   subsequent episode without recurrence

Infarct, infarction — continued

myocardium, myocardial — continued
  with symptoms after 8 weeks from date of infarction 414.8
  anterior (wall) (with contiguous portion of intraventricular septum) NEC 410.1 ☑
  anteroapical (with contiguous portion of intraventricular septum) 410.1 ☑
  anterolateral (wall) 410.0 ☑
  anteroseptal (with contiguous portion of intraventricular septum) 410.1 ☑
  apical-lateral 410.5 ☑
  atrial 410.8 ☑
  basal-lateral 410.5 ☑
  chronic (with symptoms after 8 weeks from date of infarction) 414.8
  diagnosed on ECG, but presenting no symptoms 412
  diaphragmatic wall (with contiguous portion of intraventricular septum) 410.4 ☑
  healed or old, currently presenting no symptoms 412
  high lateral 410.5 ☑
  impending 411.1
  inferior (wall) (with contiguous portion of intraventricular septum) 410.4 ☑
  inferolateral (wall) 410.2 ☑
  inferoposterior wall 410.3 ☑
  intraoperative 997.1
  lateral wall 410.5 ☑
  non-Q wave 410.7 ☑
  non-ST elevation (NSTEMI) 410.7 ☑
  nontransmural 410.7 ☑
  papillary muscle 410.8 ☑
  past (diagnosed on ECG or other special investigation, but currently presenting no symptoms) 412
    with symptoms NEC 414.8
  posterior (strictly) (true) (wall) 410.6 ☑
  posterobasal 410.6 ☑
  posteroinferior 410.3 ☑
  posterolateral 410.5 ☑
  postprocedural 997.1
  previous, currently presenting no symptoms 412
  Q wave (see also Infarct, myo-cardium, by site) 410.9 ☑
  septal 410.8 ☑
  specified site NEC 410.8 ☑
  ST elevation (STEMI) 410.9 ☑
    anterior (wall) 410.1 ☑
    anterolateral (wall) 410.0 ☑
    inferior (wall) 410.4 ☑
    inferolateral (wall) 410.2 ☑
    inferoposterior wall 410.3 ☑
    lateral wall 410.5 ☑
    posterior (strictly) (true) (wall) 410.6 ☑
    specified site NEC 410.8 ☑
  subendocardial 410.7 ☑
  syphilitic 093.82
  non-ST elevation myocardial infarction (NSTEMI) 410.7 ☑
nontransmural 410.7 ☑
omentum 557.0
ovary 620.8
pancreas 577.8
papillary muscle (see also Infarct, myocardium) 410.8 ☑
parathyroid gland 252.8
pituitary (gland) 253.8
placenta (complicating pregnancy) 656.7 ☑
  affecting fetus or newborn 762.2
pontine — see Infarct, brain
posterior NEC (see also Infarct, myocardium) 410.6 ☑
prostate 602.8
pulmonary (artery) (hemorrhagic) (vein) 415.19

Infarct, infarction — continued

pulmonary — continued
  with
    abortion — see Abortion, by type, with embolism
    ectopic pregnancy (see also categories 633.0–633.9) 639.6
    molar pregnancy (see also categories 630–632) 639.6
  following
    abortion 639.6
    ectopic or molar pregnancy 639.6
  iatrogenic 415.11
  in pregnancy, childbirth, or puerperium — see Embolism, obstetrical
  postoperative 415.11
  septic 415.12
renal 593.81
  embolic or thrombotic 593.81
retina, retinal 362.84
  with occlusion — see Occlusion, retina
spinal (acute) (cord) (embolic) (nonembolic) 336.1
spleen 289.59
  embolic or thrombotic 444.89
subchorionic — see Infarct, placenta
subendocardial (see also Infarct, myocardium) 410.7 ☑
suprarenal (capsule) (gland) 255.41
syncytium — see Infarct, placenta
testis 608.83
thrombotic (see also Thrombosis) 453.9
  artery, arterial — see Embolism
thyroid (gland) 246.3
ventricle (heart) (see also Infarct, myocardium) 410.9 ☑

Infecting — see condition

Infection, infected, infective (opportunistic) 136.9

with
  influenza viruses occurring in pigs or other animals — see Influenza, due to identified, novel influenza A virus
  lymphangitis — see Lymphangitis
abortion — see Abortion, by type, with, sepsis
abscess (skin) — see Abscess, by site
Absidia 117.7
acanthamoeba 136.21
Acanthocheilonema (perstans) 125.4
  streptocerca 125.6
accessory sinus (chronic) (see also Sinusitis) 473.9
Achorion — see Dermatophytosis
Acremonium falciforme 117.4
acromioclavicular (joint) 711.91
actinobacillus
  lignieresii 027.8
  mallei 024
  muris 026.1
actinomadura — see Actinomycosis
Actinomyces (israelii) (see also Actinomycosis)
  muris-ratti 026.1
Actinomycetales (actinomadura) (Actinomyces) (Nocardia) (Streptomyces) — see Actinomycosis
actinomycotic NEC (see also Actinomycosis) 039.9
adenoid (chronic) 474.01
  acute 463
  and tonsil (chronic) 474.02
    acute or subacute 463
adenovirus NEC 079.0
  in diseases classified elsewhere — see category 079 ☑
  unspecified nature or site 079.0
Aerobacter aerogenes NEC 041.85
  enteritis 008.2
aerogenes capsulatus (see also Gangrene, gas) 040.0
aertrycke (see also Infection, Salmonella) 003.9
ajellomyces dermatitidis 116.0

Infection, infected, infective — continued

alimentary canal NEC (see also Enteritis, due to, by organism) 009.0
Allescheria boydii 117.6
Alternaria 118
alveolus, alveolar (process) (pulpal origin) 522.4
ameba, amebic (histolytica) (see also Amebiasis) 006.9
  acute 006.0
  chronic 006.1
  free-living 136.29
  hartmanni 007.8
  specified
    site NEC 006.8
    type NEC 007.8
amniotic fluid or cavity 658.4 ☑
  affecting fetus or newborn 762.7
anaerobes (cocci) (gram-negative) (gram-positive) (mixed) NEC 041.84
anal canal 569.49
Ancylostoma braziliense 126.2
Angiostrongylus cantonensis 128.8
anisakiasis 127.1
Anisakis larva 127.1
anthrax (see also Anthrax) 022.9
antrum (chronic) (see also Sinusitis, maxillary) 473.0
anus (papillae) (sphincter) 569.49
arbor virus NEC 066.9
arbovirus NEC 066.9
argentophil-rod 027.0
Ascaris lumbricoides 127.0
ascomycetes 117.4
Aspergillus (flavus) (fumigatus) (terreus) 117.3
atypical
  acid-fast (bacilli) (see also Mycobacterium, atypical) 031.9
  mycobacteria (see also Mycobacterium, atypical) 031.9
auditory meatus (circumscribed) (diffuse) (external) (see also Otitis, externa) 380.10
auricle (ear) (see also Otitis, externa) 380.10
axillary gland 683
Babesiasis 088.82
Babesiosis 088.82
Bacillus NEC 041.89
  abortus 023.1
  anthracis (see also Anthrax) 022.9
  cereus (food poisoning) 005.89
  coli — see Infection, Escherichia coli
  coliform NEC 041.85
  Ducrey's (any location) 099.0
  Flexner's 004.1
  Friedländer's NEC 041.3
  fusiformis 101
  gas (gangrene) (see also Gangrene, gas) 040.0
  mallei 024
  melitensis 023.0
  paratyphoid, paratyphosus 002.9
    A 002.1
    B 002.2
    C 002.3
  Schmorl's 040.3
  Shiga 004.0
  suipestifer (see also Infection, Salmonella) 003.9
  swimming pool 031.1
  typhosa 002.0
  welchii (see also Gangrene, gas) 040.0
  Whitmore's 025
bacterial NEC 041.9
  specified NEC 041.89
    anaerobic NEC 041.84
    gram-negative NEC 041.85
      anaerobic NEC 041.84
Bacterium
  paratyphosum 002.9
    A 002.1
    B 002.2
    C 002.3
  typhosum 002.0

☑ **Additional Digit Required** — Refer to the Tabular List for Digit Selection

Ⓣ **Subterms under main terms may continue to next column or page**

Infection, infected, infective — *continued*

Bacteroides (fragilis) (melaninogenicus) (oralis) NEC 041.82

balantidium coli 007.0

Bartholin's gland 616.89

Basidiobolus 117.7

Bedsonia 079.98

    specified NEC 079.88

bile duct 576.1

bladder (*see also* Cystitis) 595.9

Blastomyces, blastomycotic 116.0

    brasiliensis 116.1

    dermatitidis 116.0

    European 117.5

    loboi 116.2

    North American 116.0

    South American 116.1

bleb

    postprocedural 379.60

        stage 1 379.61

        stage 2 379.62

        stage 3 379.63

blood stream (*see also* Septicemia)

    catheter-related (CRBSI) 999.31

    central line-associated (CLABSI) 999.32

    due to central venous catheter 999.32

bone 730.9 ☑

    specified — *see* Osteomyelitis

Bordetella 033.9

    bronchiseptica 033.8

    parapertussis 033.1

    pertussis 033.0

Borrelia

    bergdorfi 088.81

    vincentii (mouth) (pharynx) (tonsil) 101

bovine stomatitis 059.11

brain (*see also* Encephalitis) 323.9

    late effect — *see* category 326

    membranes (*see also* Meningitis) 322.9

    septic 324.0

        late effect — *see* category 326

        meninges (*see also* Meningitis) 320.9

branchial cyst 744.42

breast 611.0

    puerperal, postpartum 675.2 ☑

        with nipple 675.9 ☑

            specified type NEC 675.8 ☑

        nonpurulent 675.2 ☑

        purulent 675.1 ☑

bronchus (*see also* Bronchitis) 490

    fungus NEC 117.9

Brucella 023.9

    abortus 023.1

    canis 023.3

    melitensis 023.0

    mixed 023.8

    suis 023.2

Brugia (Wuchereria) malayi 125.1

bursa — *see* Bursitis

buttocks (skin) 686.9

Candida (albicans) (tropicalis) (*see also* Candidiasis) 112.9

    congenital 771.7

Candiru 136.8

Capillaria

    hepatica 128.8

    philippinensis 127.5

cartilage 733.99

catheter-related bloodstream (CRBSI) 999.31

cat liver fluke 121.0

cellulitis — *see* Cellulitis, by site

central line-associated 999.31

    bloodstream 999.32

Cephalosporum falciforme 117.4

Cercomonas hominis (intestinal) 007.3

cerebrospinal (*see also* Meningitis) 322.9

    late effect — *see* category 326

cervical gland 683

cervix (*see also* Cervicitis) 616.0

cesarean section wound 674.3 ☑

Chilomastix (intestinal) 007.8

Chlamydia 079.98

    specified NEC 079.88

cholera (*see also* Cholera) 001.9

chorionic plate 658.8 ☑

Infection, infected, infective — *continued*

Cladosporium

    bantianum 117.8

    carrionii 117.2

    mansoni 111.1

    trichoides 117.8

    wernecki 111.1

Clonorchis (sinensis) (liver) 121.1

Clostridium (haemolyticum) (novyi) NEC 041.84

    botulinum 005.1

    histolyticum (*see also* Gangrene, gas) 040.0

    oedematiens (*see also* Gangrene, gas) 040.0

    perfringens 041.83

        due to food 005.2

    septicum (*see also* Gangrene, gas) 040.0

    sordellii (*see also* Gangrene, gas) 040.0

    welchii (*see also* Gangrene, gas) 040.0

        due to food 005.2

Coccidioides (immitis) (*see also* Coccidioidomycosis) 114.9

coccus NEC 041.89

colon (*see also* Enteritis, due to, by organism) 009.0

    bacillus — *see* Infection, Escherichia coli

colostomy or enterostomy 569.61

common duct 576.1

complicating pregnancy, childbirth, or puerperium NEC 647.9 ☑

    affecting fetus or newborn 760.2

Condiobolus 117.7

congenital NEC 771.89

    Candida albicans 771.7

    chronic 771.2

    cytomegalovirus 771.1

    hepatitis, viral 771.2

    herpes simplex 771.2

    listeriosis 771.2

    malaria 771.2

    poliomyelitis 771.2

    rubella 771.0

    toxoplasmosis 771.2

    tuberculosis 771.2

    urinary (tract) 771.82

    vaccinia 771.2

coronavirus 079.89

    SARS-associated 079.82

corpus luteum (*see also* Salpingo-oophoritis) 614.2

Corynebacterium diphtheriae — *see* Diphtheria

cotia virus 059.8

Coxsackie (*see also* Coxsackie) 079.2

    endocardium 074.22

    heart NEC 074.20

    in diseases classified elsewhere — *see* category 079 ☑

    meninges 047.0

    myocardium 074.23

    pericardium 074.21

    pharynx 074.0

    specified disease NEC 074.8

    unspecified nature or site 079.2

Cryptococcus neoformans 117.5

Cryptosporidia 007.4

Cunninghamella 117.7

cyst — *see* Cyst

Cysticercus cellulosae 123.1

cystostomy 596.83

cytomegalovirus 078.5

    congenital 771.1

dental (pulpal origin) 522.4

deuteromycetes 117.4

Dicrocoelium dendriticum 121.8

Dipetalonema (perstans) 125.4

    streptocerca 125.6

diphtherial — *see* Diphtheria

Diphyllobothrium (adult) (latum) (pacificum) 123.4

    larval 123.5

Diplogonoporus (grandis) 123.8

Dipylidium (caninum) 123.8

Dirofilaria 125.6

dog tapeworm 123.8

Infection, infected, infective — *continued*

Dracunculus medinensis 125.7

Dreschlera 118

    hawaiiensis 117.8

Ducrey's bacillus (any site) 099.0

due to or resulting from

    central venous catheter (*see also* Complications, due to, catheter, central venous) 999.31

        bloodstream 999.32

        localized 999.33

    device, implant, or graft (any) (presence of) — *see* Complications, infection and inflammation, due to (presence of) any device, implant, or graft classified to 996.0–996.5 NEC

    injection, inoculation, infusion, transfusion, or vaccination (prophylactic) (therapeutic) 999.39

    blood and blood products

        acute 999.34

    injury NEC — *see* Wound, open, by site, complicated

    surgery 998.59

duodenum 535.6 ☑

ear (*see also* Otitis)

    external (*see also* Otitis, externa) 380.10

    inner (*see also* Labyrinthitis) 386.30

    middle — *see* Otitis, media

Eaton's agent NEC 041.81

Eberthella typhosa 002.0

Ebola 078.89

echinococcosis 122.9

Echinococcus (*see also* Echinococcus) 122.9

Echinostoma 121.8

ECHO virus 079.1

    in diseases classified elsewhere — *see* category 079 ☑

    unspecified nature or site 079.1

Ehrlichiosis 082.40

    chaffeensis 082.41

    specified type NEC 082.49

Endamoeba — *see* Infection, ameba

endocardium (*see also* Endocarditis) 421.0

endocervix (*see also* Cervicitis) 616.0

Entamoeba — *see* Infection, ameba

enteric (*see also* Enteritis, due to, by organism) 009.0

Enterobacter aerogenes NEC 041.85

Enterobacter sakazakii 041.85

Enterobius vermicularis 127.4

enterococcus NEC 041.04

enterovirus NEC 079.89

    central nervous system NEC 048

    enteritis 008.67

    meningitis 047.9

Entomophthora 117.7

Epidermophyton — *see* Dermatophytosis

epidermophytosis — *see* Dermatophytosis

episiotomy 674.3 ☑

Epstein-Barr virus 075

    chronic 780.79 [139.8]

erysipeloid 027.1

Erysipelothrix (insidiosa) (rhusiopathiae) 027.1

erythema infectiosum 057.0

Escherichia coli (E. coli) 041.49

    enteritis — *see* Enteritis, E. coli

    generalized 041.49

    intestinal — *see* Enteritis, E. coli

    non-Shiga toxin-producing 041.49

    Shiga toxin-producing (STEC) 041.43

        with

            unspecified O group 041.43

            non-O157 (with known O group) 041.43

            O157 (with confirmation of Shiga toxin when H antigen is unknown, or is not H7) 041.41

            O157:H7 with or without confirmation of Shiga toxin-production 041.41

            O157H:- (nonmotile) with confirmation of Shiga toxin 041.41

        specified NEC 041.42

Infection, infected, infective — *continued*

esophagostomy 530.86

ethmoidal (chronic) (sinus) (*see also* Sinusitis, ethmoidal) 473.2

Eubacterium 041.84

Eustachian tube (ear) 381.50

    acute 381.51

    chronic 381.52

exanthema subitum (*see also* Exanthem subitum) 058.10

exit site 999.33

external auditory canal (meatus) (*see also* Otitis, externa) 380.10

eyelid 373.9

    specified NEC 373.8

eye NEC 360.00

fallopian tube (*see also* Salpingo-oophoritis) 614.2

fascia 728.89

Fasciola

    gigantica 121.3

    hepatica 121.3

Fasciolopsis (buski) 121.4

fetus (intra-amniotic) — *see* Infection, congenital

filarial — *see* Infestation, filarial

finger (skin) 686.9

    abscess (with lymphangitis) 681.00

        pulp 681.01

    cellulitis (with lymphangitis) 681.00

    distal closed space (with lymphangitis) 681.00

    nail 681.02

        fungus 110.1

fish tapeworm 123.4

    larval 123.5

flagellate, intestinal 007.9

fluke — *see* Infestation, fluke

focal

    teeth (pulpal origin) 522.4

    tonsils 474.00

        and adenoids 474.02

Fonsecaea

    compactum 117.2

    pedrosoi 117.2

food (*see also* Poisoning, food) 005.9

foot (skin) 686.9

    fungus 110.4

Francisella tularensis (*see also* Tularemia) 021.9

frontal sinus (chronic) (*see also* Sinusitis, frontal) 473.1

fungus NEC 117.9

    beard 110.0

    body 110.5

    dermatiacious NEC 117.8

    foot 110.4

    groin 110.3

    hand 110.2

    nail 110.1

    pathogenic to compromised host only 118

    perianal (area) 110.3

    scalp 110.0

    scrotum 110.8

    skin 111.9

        foot 110.4

        hand 110.2

    toenails 110.1

    trachea 117.9

Fusarium 118

Fusobacterium 041.84

gallbladder (*see also* Cholecystitis, acute) 575.0

Gardnerella vaginalis 041.89

gas bacillus (*see also* Gas, gangrene) 040.0

gastric (*see also* Gastritis) 535.5 ☑

Gastrodiscoides hominis 121.8

gastroenteric (*see also* Enteritis, due to, by organism) 009.0

gastrointestinal (*see also* Enteritis, due to, by organism) 009.0

gastrostomy 536.41

generalized NEC (*see also* Septicemia) 038.9

genital organ or tract NEC

    female 614.9

☑ Additional Digit Required — Refer to the Tabular List for Digit Selection   ▽ Subterms under main terms may continue to next column or page

2015 ICD-9-CM   ▶◀ Revised Text   ● New Line   ▲ Revised Code   Volume 2 — 155

Infection, infected, infective — *continued*

genital organ or tract — *continued*
  female — *continued*
    with
      abortion — *see* Abortion, by type, with sepsis
      ectopic pregnancy (*see also* categories 633.0–633.9) 639.0
      molar pregnancy (*see also* categories 630–632) 639.0
    complicating pregnancy 646.6 ☑
      affecting fetus or newborn 760.8
    following
      abortion 639.0
      ectopic or molar pregnancy 639.0
      puerperal, postpartum, childbirth 670.8 ☑
    minor or localized 646.6 ☑
      affecting fetus or newborn 760.8
  male 608.4
genitourinary tract NEC 599.0
Ghon tubercle, primary (*see also* Tuberculosis) 010.0 ☑
Giardia lamblia 007.1
gingival (chronic) 523.10
  acute 523.00
  Vincent's 101
glanders 024
Glenosporopsis amazonica 116.2
Gnathostoma spinigerum 128.1
Gongylonema 125.6
gonococcal NEC (*see also* Gonococcus) 098.0
gram-negative bacilli NEC 041.85
  anaerobic 041.84
guinea worm 125.7
gum (*see also* Infection, gingival) 523.10
Hantavirus 079.81
heart 429.89
Helicobacter pylori [H. pylori] 041.86
helminths NEC 128.9
  intestinal 127.9
    mixed (types classifiable to more than one category in 120.0–127.7) 127.8
    specified type NEC 127.7
  specified type NEC 128.8
Hemophilus influenzae NEC 041.5
  generalized 038.41
herpes (simplex) (*see also* Herpes, simplex) 054.9
  congenital 771.2
  zoster (*see also* Herpes, zoster) 053.9
    eye NEC 053.29
Heterophyes heterophyes 121.6
Histoplasma (*see also* Histoplasmosis) 115.90
  capsulatum (*see also* Histoplasmosis, American) 115.00
  duboisii (*see also* Histoplasmosis, African) 115.10
HIV V08
  with symptoms, symptomatic 042
hookworm (*see also* Ancylostomiasis) 126.9
human herpesvirus 6 058.81
human herpesvirus 7 058.82
human herpesvirus 8 058.89
human herpesvirus NEC 058.89
human immunodeficiency virus V08
  with symptoms, symptomatic 042
human papillomavirus 079.4
hydrocele 603.1
hydronephrosis 591
Hymenolepis 123.6
hypopharynx 478.29
inguinal glands 683
  due to soft chancre 099.0
insertion site 999.33
intestine, intestinal (*see also* Enteritis, due to, by organism) 009.0
intrauterine (*see also* Endometritis) 615.9
  complicating delivery 646.6 ☑
isospora belli or hominis 007.2
Japanese B encephalitis 062.0
jaw (bone) (acute) (chronic) (lower) (subacute) (upper) 526.4
joint — *see* Arthritis, infectious or infective

Kaposi's sarcoma-associated herpesvirus 058.89
kidney (cortex) (hematogenous) 590.9
  with
    abortion — *see* Abortion, by type, with urinary tract infection
    calculus 592.0
    ectopic pregnancy (*see also* categories 633.0–633.9) 639.8
    molar pregnancy (*see also* categories 630–632) 639.8
  complicating pregnancy or puerperium 646.6 ☑
    affecting fetus or newborn 760.1
  following
    abortion 639.8
    ectopic or molar pregnancy 639.8
  pelvis and ureter 590.3
Klebsiella pneumoniae NEC 041.3
knee (skin) NEC 686.9
  joint — *see* Arthritis, infectious
Koch's (*see also* Tuberculosis, pulmonary) 011.9 ☑
labia (majora) (minora) (*see also* Vulvitis) 616.10
lacrimal
  gland (*see also* Dacryoadenitis) 375.00
  passages (duct) (sac) (*see also* Dacryocystitis) 375.30
larynx NEC 478.79
leg (skin) NEC 686.9
Leishmania (*see also* Leishmaniasis) 085.9
  braziliensis 085.5
  donovani 085.0
  ethiopica 085.3
  furunculosa 085.1
  infantum 085.0
  mexicana 085.4
  tropica (minor) 085.1
    major 085.2
Leptosphaeria senegalensis 117.4
leptospira (*see also* Leptospirosis) 100.9
  Australis 100.89
  Bataviae 100.89
  pyrogenes 100.89
  specified type NEC 100.89
leptospirochetal NEC (*see also* Leptospirosis) 100.9
Leptothrix — *see* Actinomycosis
Listeria monocytogenes (listeriosis) 027.0
  congenital 771.2
liver fluke — *see* Infestation, fluke, liver
Loa loa 125.2
  eyelid 125.2 *[373.6]*
Loboa loboi 116.2
local, skin (staphylococcal) (streptococcal) NEC 686.9
  abscess — *see* Abscess, by site
  cellulitis — *see* Cellulitis, by site
  ulcer (*see also* Ulcer, skin) 707.9
Loefflerella
  mallei 024
  whitmori 025
lung 518.89
  atypical Mycobacterium 031.0
    tuberculous (*see also* Tuberculosis, pulmonary) 011.9 ☑
  basilar 518.89
  chronic 518.89
  fungus NEC 117.9
  spirochetal 104.8
  virus — *see* Pneumonia, virus
lymph gland (axillary) (cervical) (inguinal) 683
  mesenteric 289.2
lymphoid tissue, base of tongue or posterior pharynx, NEC 474.00
madurella
  grisea 117.4
  mycetomii 117.4
major
  with
    abortion — *see* Abortion, by type, with sepsis

major — *continued*
  with — *continued*
    ectopic pregnancy (*see also* categories 633.0–633.9) 639.0
    molar pregnancy (*see also* categories 630–632) 639.0
  following
    abortion 639.0
    ectopic or molar pregnancy 639.0
  puerperal, postpartum, childbirth 670.0 ☑
Malassezia furfur 111.0
Malleomyces
  mallei 024
  pseudomallei 025
mammary gland 611.0
  puerperal, postpartum 675.2 ☑
Mansonella (ozzardi) 125.5
mastoid (suppurative) — *see* Mastoiditis
maxilla, maxillary 526.4
  sinus (chronic) (*see also* Sinusitis, maxillary) 473.0
mediastinum 519.2
medina 125.7
meibomian
  cyst 373.12
  gland 373.12
melioidosis 025
meninges (*see also* Meningitis) 320.9
meningococcal (*see also* condition) 036.9
  brain 036.1
  cerebrospinal 036.0
  endocardium 036.42
  generalized 036.2
  meninges 036.0
  meningococcemia 036.2
  specified site NEC 036.89
mesenteric lymph nodes or glands NEC 289.2
Metagonimus 121.5
metatarsophalangeal 711.97
methicillin
  resistant Staphylococcus aureus (MRSA) 041.12
  susceptible Staphylococcus aureus (MSSA) 041.11
microorganism resistant to drugs — *see* Resistance (to), drugs by microorganisms
Microsporidia 136.8
microsporum, microsporic — *see* Dermatophytosis
Mima polymorpha NEC 041.85
mixed flora NEC 041.89
Monilia (*see also* Candidiasis) 112.9
  neonatal 771.7
monkeypox 059.01
Monosporium apiospermum 117.6
mouth (focus) NEC 528.9
  parasitic 136.9
MRSA (methicillin resistant Staphylococcus aureus) 041.12
MSSA (methicillin susceptible Staphylococcus aureus) 041.11
Mucor 117.7
muscle NEC 728.89
mycelium NEC 117.9
mycetoma
  actinomycotic NEC (*see also* Actinomycosis) 039.9
  mycotic NEC 117.4
Mycobacterium, mycobacterial (*see also* Mycobacterium) 031.9
Mycoplasma NEC 041.81
mycotic NEC 117.9
  pathogenic to compromised host only 118
  skin NEC 111.9
  systemic 117.9
myocardium NEC 422.90
nail (chronic) (with lymphangitis) 681.9
  finger 681.02
    fungus 110.1
    ingrowing 703.0
  toe 681.11

nail — *continued*
  toe — *continued*
    fungus 110.1
nasal sinus (chronic) (*see also* Sinusitis) 473.9
nasopharynx (chronic) 478.29
  acute 460
navel 686.9
  newborn 771.4
Neisserian — *see* Gonococcus
Neotestudina rosatii 117.4
newborn, generalized 771.89
nipple 611.0
  puerperal, postpartum 675.0 ☑
    with breast 675.9 ☑
      specified type NEC 675.8 ☑
Nocardia — *see* Actinomycosis
nose 478.19
nostril 478.19
obstetrical surgical wound 674.3 ☑
Oesophagostomum (apiostomum) 127.7
Oestrus ovis 134.0
Oidium albicans (*see also* Candidiasis) 112.9
Onchocerca (volvulus) 125.3
  eye 125.3 *[360.13]*
  eyelid 125.3 *[373.6]*
operation wound 998.59
Opisthorchis (felineus) (tenuicollis) (viverrini) 121.0
orbit 376.00
  chronic 376.10
orthopoxvirus 059.00
  specified NEC 059.09
ovary (*see also* Salpingo-oophoritis) 614.2
Oxyuris vermicularis 127.4
pancreas 577.0
Paracoccidioides brasiliensis 116.1
Paragonimus (westermani) 121.2
parainfluenza virus 079.89
parameningococcus NEC 036.9
  with meningitis 036.0
parapoxvirus 059.10
  specified NEC 059.19
parasitic NEC 136.9
paratyphoid 002.9
  type A 002.1
  type B 002.2
  type C 002.3
paraurethral ducts 597.89
parotid gland 527.2
Pasteurella NEC 027.2
  multocida (cat-bite) (dog-bite) 027.2
  pestis (*see also* Plague) 020.9
  pseudotuberculosis 027.2
  septica (cat-bite) (dog-bite) 027.2
  tularensis (*see also* Tularemia) 021.9
pelvic, female (*see also* Disease, pelvis, inflammatory) 614.9
penis (glans) (retention) NEC 607.2
  herpetic 054.13
Peptococcus 041.84
Peptostreptococcus 041.84
periapical (pulpal origin) 522.4
peridental 523.30
perineal wound (obstetrical) 674.3 ☑
periodontal 523.31
periorbital 376.00
  chronic 376.10
perirectal 569.49
perirenal (*see also* Infection, kidney) 590.9
peritoneal (*see also* Peritonitis) 567.9
periureteral 593.89
periurethral 597.89
Petriellidium boydii 117.6
pharynx 478.29
  Coxsackie virus 074.0
  phlegmonous 462
  posterior, lymphoid 474.00
Phialophora
  gougerotii 117.8
  jeanselmei 117.8
  verrucosa 117.2
Piedraia hortai 111.3
pinna, acute 380.11
pinta 103.9
  intermediate 103.1

☑ **Additional Digit Required** — Refer to the Tabular List for Digit Selection   ▽ **Subterms under main terms may continue to next column or page**

156 — Volume 2   ▶◀ Revised Text   ● New Line   ▲ Revised Code   2015 ICD-9-CM

Infection, infected, infective — *continued*

pinta — *continued*
  late 103.2
  mixed 103.3
  primary 103.0
pinworm 127.4
pityrosporum furfur 111.0
pleuropneumonia-like organisms NEC (PP-LO) 041.81
pneumococcal NEC 041.2
  generalized (purulent) 038.2
Pneumococcus NEC 041.2
port 999.33
postoperative wound 998.59
posttraumatic NEC 958.3
postvaccinal 999.39
poxvirus 059.9
  specified NEC 059.8
prepuce NEC 607.1
Proprionibacterium 041.84
prostate (capsule) (*see also* Prostatitis) 601.9
Proteus (mirabilis) (morganii) (vulgaris) NEC 041.6
  enteritis 008.3
protozoal NEC 136.8
  intestinal NEC 007.9
Pseudomonas NEC 041.7
  mallei 024
  pneumonia 482.1
  pseudomallei 025
psittacosis 073.9
puerperal, postpartum (major) 670.0 ☑
  minor 646.6 ☑
pulmonary — *see* Infection, lung
purulent — *see* Abscess
putrid, generalized — *see* Septicemia
pyemic — *see* Septicemia
Pyrenochaeta romeroi 117.4
Q fever 083.0
rabies 071
rectum (sphincter) 569.49
renal (*see also* Infection, kidney) 590.9
  pelvis and ureter 590.3
reservoir 999.33
resistant (to) drugs — *see* Resistance (to), drugs by microorganisms
respiratory 519.8
  chronic 519.8
  influenzal (acute) (upper) (*see also* Influenza) 487.1
  lung 518.89
  rhinovirus 460
  syncytial virus 079.6
  upper (acute) (infectious) NEC 465.9
    with flu, grippe, or influenza (*see also* Influenza) 487.1
    influenzal (*see also* Influenza) 487.1
    multiple sites NEC 465.8
    streptococcal 034.0
    viral NEC 465.9
respiratory syncytial virus (RSV) 079.6
resulting from presence of shunt or other internal prosthetic device — *see* Complications, infection and inflammation, due to (presence of) any device, implant, or graft classified to 996.0–996.5 NEC
retroperitoneal 567.39
retrovirus 079.50
  human immunodeficiency virus type 2 (HIV2) 079.53
  human T-cell lymphotrophic virus type I (HTLV-I) 079.51
  human T-cell lymphotrophic virus type II (HTLV-II) 079.52
  specified NEC 079.59
Rhinocladium 117.1
Rhinosporidium — *see beri* 117.0
rhinovirus
  in diseases classified elsewhere — *see* category 079 ☑
  unspecified nature or site 079.3
Rhizopus 117.7
rickettsial 083.9
rickettsialpox 083.2
rubella (*see also* Rubella) 056.9

Infection, infected, infective — *continued*

rubella (*see also* Rubella) — *continued*
  congenital 771.0
Saccharomyces (*see also* Candidiasis) 112.9
Saksenaea 117.7
salivary duct or gland (any) 527.2
Salmonella (aertrycke) (callinarum) (choleraesuis) (enteritidis) (suipestifer) (typhimurium) 003.9
  with
    arthritis 003.23
    gastroenteritis 003.0
    localized infection 003.20
      specified type NEC 003.29
    meningitis 003.21
    osteomyelitis 003.24
    pneumonia 003.22
    septicemia 003.1
    specified manifestation NEC 003.8
  due to food (poisoning) (any serotype) (*see also* Poisoning, food, due to, Salmonella)
  hirschfeldii 002.3
  localized 003.20
    specified type NEC 003.29
  paratyphi 002.9
    A 002.1
    B 002.2
    C 002.3
  schottmuelleri 002.2
  specified type NEC 003.8
  typhi 002.0
  typhosa 002.0
saprophytic 136.8
Sarcocystis, lindemanni 136.5
SARS-associated coronavirus 079.82
scabies 133.0
Schistosoma — *see* Infestation, Schistosoma
Schmorl's bacillus 040.3
scratch or other superficial injury — *see* Injury, superficial, by site
scrotum (acute) NEC 608.4
sealpox 059.12
secondary, burn or open wound (dislocation) (fracture) 958.3
seminal vesicle (*see also* Vesiculitis) 608.0
septic
  generalized — *see* Septicemia
  localized, skin — *see* Abscess
septicemic — *see* Septicemia
seroma 998.51
Serratia (marcescens) 041.85
  generalized 038.44
sheep liver fluke 121.3
Shigella 004.9
  boydii 004.2
  dysenteriae 004.0
  flexneri 004.1
  group
    A 004.0
    B 004.1
    C 004.2
    D 004.3
  Schmitz (-Stutzer) 004.0
  schmitzii 004.0
  Shiga 004.0
  sonnei 004.3
  specified type NEC 004.8
Sin Nombre virus 079.81
sinus (*see also* Sinusitis) 473.9
  pilonidal 685.1
    with abscess 685.0
  skin NEC 686.9
Skene's duct or gland (*see also* Urethritis) 597.89
skin (local) (staphylococcal) (streptococcal) NEC 686.9
  abscess — *see* Abscess, by site
  cellulitis — *see* Cellulitis, by site
  due to fungus 111.9
    specified type NEC 111.8
  mycotic 111.9
    specified type NEC 111.8
  ulcer (*see also* Ulcer, skin) 707.9
slow virus 046.9
  specified condition NEC 046.8

Infection, infected, infective — *continued*

Sparganum (mansoni) (proliferum) 123.5
spermatic cord NEC 608.4
sphenoidal (chronic) (sinus) (*see also* Sinusitis, sphenoidal) 473.3
Spherophorus necrophorus 040.3
spinal cord NEC (*see also* Encephalitis) 323.9
  abscess 324.1
    late effect — *see* category 326
  late effect — *see* category 326
  meninges — *see* Meningitis
  streptococcal 320.2
Spirillum
  minus or minor 026.0
  morsus muris 026.0
  obermeieri 087.0
spirochetal NEC 104.9
  lung 104.8
  specified nature or site NEC 104.8
spleen 289.59
Sporothrix schenckii 117.1
Sporotrichum (schenckii) 117.1
Sporozoa 136.8
staphylococcal NEC 041.10
  aureus 041.11
    methicillin
      resistant (MRSA) 041.12
      susceptible (MSSA) 041.11
  food poisoning 005.0
  generalized (purulent) 038.10
    aureus 038.11
      methicillin
        resistant 038.12
        susceptible 038.11
    specified organism NEC 038.19
  pneumonia 482.40
    aureus 482.41
      methicillin
        resistant (MRSA) 482.42
        susceptible (MSSA) 482.41
    MRSA (methicillin resistant Staphylococcus aureus) 482.42
    MSSA (methicillin susceptible Staphylococcus aureus) 482.41
    specified type NEC 482.49
  septicemia 038.10
    aureus 038.11
      methicillin
        resistant (MRSA) 038.12
        susceptible (MSSA) 038.11
    MRSA (methicillin resistant Staphylococcus aureus) 038.12
    MSSA (methicillin susceptible Staphylococcus aureus) 038.11
    specified organism NEC 038.19
  specified NEC 041.19
steatoma 706.2
Stellantchasmus falcatus 121.6
Streptobacillus moniliformis 026.1
streptococcal NEC 041.00
  generalized (purulent) 038.0
  Group
    A 041.01
    B 041.02
    C 041.03
    D [enterococcus] 041.04
    G 041.05
  pneumonia — *see* Pneumonia, streptococcal
  septicemia 038.0
  sore throat 034.0
  specified NEC 041.09
Streptomyces — *see* Actinomycosis
streptotrichosis — *see* Actinomycosis
Strongyloides (stercoralis) 127.2
stump (amputation) (posttraumatic) (surgical) 997.62
  traumatic — *see* Amputation, traumatic, by site, complicated
subcutaneous tissue, local NEC 686.9
submaxillary region 528.3
suipestifer (*see also* Infection, Salmonella) 003.9
swimming pool bacillus 031.1

Infection, infected, infective — *continued*

syphilitic — *see* Syphilis
systemic — *see* Septicemia
Taenia — *see* Infestation, Taenia
Taeniarhynchus saginatus 123.2
tanapox 059.21
tapeworm — *see* Infestation, tapeworm
tendon (sheath) 727.89
Ternidens diminutus 127.7
testis (*see also* Orchitis) 604.90
thigh (skin) 686.9
threadworm 127.4
throat 478.29
  pneumococcal 462
  staphylococcal 462
  streptococcal 034.0
  viral NEC (*see also* Pharyngitis) 462
thumb (skin) 686.9
  abscess (with lymphangitis) 681.00
    pulp 681.01
  cellulitis (with lymphangitis) 681.00
  nail 681.02
thyroglossal duct 529.8
toe (skin) 686.9
  abscess (with lymphangitis) 681.10
  cellulitis (with lymphangitis) 681.10
  nail 681.11
    fungus 110.1
tongue NEC 529.0
  parasitic 112.0
tonsil (faucial) (lingual) (pharyngeal) 474.00
  acute or subacute 463
  and adenoid 474.02
  tag 474.00
tooth, teeth 522.4
  periapical (pulpal origin) 522.4
  peridental 523.30
  periodontal 523.31
  pulp 522.0
  socket 526.5
TORCH — *see* Infection, congenital NEC
  without active infection 760.2
Torula histolytica 117.5
Toxocara (cani) (cati) (felis) 128.0
Toxoplasma gondii (*see also* Toxoplasmosis) 130.9
trachea, chronic 491.8
  fungus 117.9
traumatic NEC 958.3
trematode NEC 121.9
trench fever 083.1
Treponema
  denticola 041.84
  macrodenticum 041.84
  pallidum (*see also* Syphilis) 097.9
Trichinella (spiralis) 124
Trichomonas 131.9
  bladder 131.09
  cervix 131.09
  hominis 007.3
  intestine 007.3
  prostate 131.03
  specified site NEC 131.8
  urethra 131.02
  urogenitalis 131.00
  vagina 131.01
  vulva 131.01
Trichophyton, trichophytid — *see* Dermatophytosis
Trichosporon (beigelii) cutaneum 111.2
Trichostrongylus 127.6
Trichuris (trichiuria) 127.3
Trombicula (irritans) 133.8
Trypanosoma (*see also* Trypanosomiasis) 086.9
  cruzi 086.2
tubal (*see also* Salpingo-oophoritis) 614.2
tuberculous NEC (*see also* Tuberculosis) 011.9 ☑
tubo-ovarian (*see also* Salpingo-oophoritis) 614.2
tunica vaginalis 608.4
tunnel 999.33
tympanic membrane — *see* Myringitis
typhoid (abortive) (ambulant) (bacillus) 002.0

Infection, infected, infective — *continued*
  typhus 081.9
    flea-borne (endemic) 081.0
    louse-borne (epidemic) 080
    mite-borne 081.2
    recrudescent 081.1
    tick-borne 082.9
      African 082.1
      North Asian 082.2
  umbilicus (septic) 686.9
    newborn NEC 771.4
  ureter 593.89
  urethra (*see also* Urethritis) 597.80
  urinary (tract) NEC 599.0
    with
      abortion — *see* Abortion, by type,
          with urinary tract infection
      ectopic pregnancy (*see also* cate-
          gories 633.0–633.9) 639.8
      molar pregnancy (*see also* categories
          630–632) 639.8
    candidal 112.2
    complicating pregnancy, childbirth, or
        puerperium 646.6 ☑
      affecting fetus or newborn 760.1
      asymptomatic 646.5 ☑
        affecting fetus or newborn 760.1
    diplococcal (acute) 098.0
      chronic 098.2
    due to Trichomonas (vaginalis) 131.00
      following
        abortion 639.8
        ectopic or molar pregnancy 639.8
    gonococcal (acute) 098.0
      chronic or duration of 2 months
          or over 098.2
    newborn 771.82
    trichomonal 131.00
    tuberculous (*see also* Tuberculosis)
        016.3 ☑
  uterus, uterine (*see also* Endometritis)
      615.9
  utriculus masculinus NEC 597.89
  vaccination 999.39
  vagina (granulation tissue) (wall) (*see
      also* Vaginitis) 616.10
  varicella 052.9
  varicose veins — *see* Varicose, veins
  variola 050.9
    major 050.0
    minor 050.1
  vas deferens NEC 608.4
  Veillonella 041.84
  verumontanum 597.89
  vesical (*see also* Cystitis) 595.9
  Vibrio
    cholerae 001.0
      El Tor 001.1
    parahaemolyticus (food poisoning)
        005.4
    vulnificus 041.85
  Vincent's (gums) (mouth) (tonsil) 101
  vaccination 999.39
  virus, viral 079.99
    adenovirus
      in diseases classified elsewhere —
          see category 079 ☑
      unspecified nature or site 079.0
    central nervous system NEC 049.9
      enterovirus 048
        meningitis 047.9
          specified type NEC 047.8
      slow virus 046.9
      specified condition NEC 046.8
    chest 519.8
    conjunctivitis 077.99
      specified type NEC 077.8
    coronavirus 079.89
      SARS-associated 079.82
    Coxsackie (*see also* Infection, Coxsackie)
        079.2
    Ebola 065.8
    ECHO
      in diseases classified elsewhere —
          see category 079 ☑
      unspecified nature or site 079.1

Infection, infected, infective — *continued*
  virus, viral — *continued*
    encephalitis 049.9
      arthropod-borne NEC 064
      tick-borne 063.9
        specified type NEC 063.8
    enteritis NEC (*see also* Enteritis, viral)
        008.8
    exanthem NEC 057.9
    Hantavirus 079.81
    human papilloma 079.4
    in diseases classified elsewhere — *see*
        category 079 ☑
    intestine (*see also* Enteritis, viral) 008.8
    lung — *see* Pneumonia, viral
    respiratory syncytial (RSV) 079.6
    retrovirus 079.50
    rhinovirus
      in diseases classified elsewhere —
          see category 079 ☑
      unspecified nature or site 079.3
    salivary gland disease 078.5
    slow 046.9
      specified condition NEC 046.8
    specified type NEC 079.89
      in diseases classified elsewhere —
          see category 079 ☑
    unspecified nature or site 079.99
    warts 078.10
      specified type NEC 078.19
    yaba monkey tumor 059.22
  vulva (*see also* Vulvitis) 616.10
  whipworm 127.3
  Whitmore's bacillus 025
  wound (local) (posttraumatic) NEC 958.3
    with
      dislocation — *see* Dislocation, by site,
          open
      fracture — *see* Fracture, by site, open
      open wound — *see* Wound, open,
          by site, complicated
    postoperative 998.59
    surgical 998.59
  Wuchereria 125.0
    bancrofti 125.0
    malayi 125.1
  yaba monkey tumor virus 059.22
  yatapoxvirus 059.20
  yaws — *see* Yaws
  yeast (*see also* Candidiasis) 112.9
  yellow fever (*see also* Fever, yellow) 060.9
  Yersinia pestis (*see also* Plague) 020.9
  Zeis' gland 373.12
  zoonotic bacterial NEC 027.9
  Zopfia senegalensis 117.4
Infective, infectious — *see* condition
Inferiority complex 301.9
  constitutional psychopathic 301.9
Infertility
  female 628.9
    age related 628.8
    associated with
      adhesions, peritubal 614.6 [628.2]
      anomaly
        cervical mucus 628.4
        congenital
          cervix 628.4
          fallopian tube 628.2
          uterus 628.3
          vagina 628.4
      anovulation 628.0
      dysmucorrhea 628.4
      endometritis, tuberculous (*see also*
          Tuberculosis) 016.7 ☑ [628.3]
      Stein-Leventhal syndrome
          256.4 [628.0]
    due to
      adiposogenital dystrophy
          253.8 [628.1]
      anterior pituitary disorder NEC
          253.4 [628.1]
        hyperfunction 253.1 [628.1]
      cervical anomaly 628.4
      fallopian tube anomaly 628.2
      ovarian failure 256.39 [628.0]

Infertility — *continued*
  female — *continued*
    due to — *continued*
      Stein-Leventhal syndrome
          256.4 [628.0]
      uterine anomaly 628.3
      vaginal anomaly 628.4
    nonimplantation 628.3
    origin
      cervical 628.4
      pituitary-hypothalamus NEC
          253.8 [628.1]
        anterior pituitary NEC
            253.4 [628.1]
          hyperfunction NEC
              253.1 [628.1]
          dwarfism 253.3 [628.1]
          panhypopituitarism 253.2 [628.1]
      specified NEC 628.8
      tubal (block) (occlusion) (stenosis)
          628.2
        adhesions 614.6 [628.2]
      uterine 628.3
      vaginal 628.4
    previous, requiring supervision of preg-
        nancy V23.0
  male 606.9
    absolute 606.0
    due to
      azoospermia 606.0
      drug therapy 606.8
      extratesticular cause NEC 606.8
      germinal cell
        aplasia 606.0
        desquamation 606.1
      hypospermatogenesis 606.1
      infection 606.8
      obstruction, afferent ducts 606.8
      oligospermia 606.1
      radiation 606.8
      spermatogenic arrest (complete)
          606.0
        incomplete 606.1
      systemic disease 606.8
Infestation 134.9
  Acanthocheilonema (perstans) 125.4
    streptocerca 125.6
  Acariasis 133.9
    demodex folliculorum 133.8
    Sarcoptes scabiei 133.0
    trombiculae 133.8
  Agamofilaria streptocerca 125.6
  Ancylostoma, Ankylostoma 126.9
    americanum 126.1
    braziliense 126.2
    canium 126.8
    ceylanicum 126.3
    duodenale 126.0
    new world 126.1
    old world 126.0
  Angiostrongylus cantonensis 128.8
  anisakiasis 127.1
  Anisakis larva 127.1
  arthropod NEC 134.1
  Ascaris lumbricoides 127.0
  Bacillus fusiformis 101
  Balantidium coli 007.0
  beef tapeworm 123.2
  Bothriocephalus (latus) 123.4
    larval 123.5
  broad tapeworm 123.4
    larval 123.5
  Brugia malayi 125.1
  Candiru 136.8
  Capillaria
    hepatica 128.8
    philippinensis 127.5
  cat liver fluke 121.0
  Cercomonas hominis (intestinal) 007.3
  cestodes 123.9
    specified type NEC 123.8
  chigger 133.8
  chigoe 134.1
  Chilomastix 007.8
  Clonorchis (sinensis) (liver) 121.1
  coccidia 007.2

Infestation — *continued*
  complicating pregnancy, childbirth, or
      puerperium 647.9 ☑
    affecting fetus or newborn 760.8
  Cysticercus cellulosae 123.1
  Demodex folliculorum 133.8
  Dermatobia (hominis) 134.0
  Dibothriocephalus (latus) 123.4
    larval 123.5
  Dicrocoelium dendriticum 121.8
  Diphyllobothrium (adult) (intestinal) (latum)
      (pacificum) 123.4
    larval 123.5
  Diplogonoporus (grandis) 123.8
  Dipylidium (caninum) 123.8
  Distoma hepaticum 121.3
  dog tapeworm 123.8
  Dracunculus medinensis 125.7
  dragon worm 125.7
  dwarf tapeworm 123.6
  Echinococcus (*see also* Echinococcus) 122.9
  Echinostoma ilocanum 121.8
  Embadomonas 007.8
  Endamoeba (histolytica) — *see* Infection,
      ameba
  Entamoeba (histolytica) — *see* Infection,
      ameba
  Enterobius vermicularis 127.4
  Epidermophyton — *see* Dermatophytosis
  eyeworm 125.2
  Fasciola
    gigantica 121.3
    hepatica 121.3
  Fasciolopsis (buski) (small intestine) 121.4
    blood NEC (*see also* Schistosomiasis)
        120.9
    cat liver 121.0
    filarial 125.9
      due to
        Acanthocheilonema (perstans)
            125.4
          streptocerca 125.6
        Brugia (Wuchereria) malayi 125.1
        Dracunculus medinensis 125.7
        guinea worms 125.7
        Mansonella (ozzardi) 125.5
        Onchocerca volvulus 125.3
          eye 125.3 [360.13]
          eyelid 125.3 [373.6]
        Wuchereria (bancrofti) 125.0
          malayi 125.1
      specified type NEC 125.6
  fish tapeworm 123.4
    larval 123.5
  fluke 121.9
  intestinal (giant) 121.4
  liver (sheep) 121.3
    cat 121.0
    Chinese 121.1
    clonorchiasis 121.1
    fascioliasis 121.3
    Oriental 121.1
  lung (oriental) 121.2
  sheep liver 121.3
  fly larva 134.0
  Gasterophilus (intestinalis) 134.0
  Gastrodiscoides hominis 121.8
  Giardia lamblia 007.1
  Gnathostoma (spinigerum) 128.1
  Gongylonema 125.6
  guinea worm 125.7
  helminth NEC 128.9
    intestinal 127.9
      mixed (types classifiable to more
          than one category in
          120.0–127.7) 127.8
      specified type NEC 127.7
    specified type NEC 128.8
  Heterophyes heterophyes (small intestine)
      121.6
  hookworm (*see also* Infestation, ancy-
      lostoma) 126.9
  Hymenolepis (diminuta) (nana) 123.6
  intestinal NEC 129
  leeches (aquatic) (land) 134.2
  Leishmania — *see* Leishmaniasis

☑ Additional Digit Required — Refer to the Tabular List for Digit Selection   ᵀᴮˢ Subterms under main terms may continue to next column or page

Infestation — *continued*
  lice (*see also* Infestation, pediculus) 132.9
  Linguatulidae, linguatula (pentastoma)
    (serrata) 134.1
  Loa loa 125.2
    eyelid 125.2 *[373.6]*
  louse (*see also* Infestation, pediculus) 132.9
    body 132.1
    head 132.0
    pubic 132.2
  maggots 134.0
  Mansonella (ozzardi) 125.5
  medina 125.7
  Metagonimus yokogawai (small intestine)
    121.5
  Microfilaria streptocerca 125.3
    eye 125.3 *[360.13]*
    eyelid 125.3 *[373.6]*
  Microsporon furfur 111.0
  microsporum — *see* Dermatophytosis
  mites 133.9
    scabic 133.0
    specified type NEC 133.8
  monilia (albicans) (*see also* Candidiasis)
    112.9
    vagina 112.1
    vulva 112.1
  mouth 112.0
  Necator americanus 126.1
  nematode (intestinal) 127.9
    Ancylostoma (*see also* Ancylostoma)
      126.9
    Ascaris lumbricoides 127.0
    conjunctiva NEC 128.9
    Dioctophyma 128.8
    Enterobius vermicularis 127.4
    Gnathostoma spinigerum 128.1
    Oesophagostomum (apiostomum) 127.7
    Physaloptera 127.4
    specified type NEC 127.7
    Strongyloides stercoralis 127.2
    Ternidens diminutus 127.7
    Trichinella spiralis 124
    Trichostrongylus 127.6
    Trichuris (trichiuria) 127.3
  Oesophagostomum (apiostomum) 127.7
  Oestrus ovis 134.0
  Onchocerca (volvulus) 125.3
    eye 125.3 *[360.13]*
    eyelid 125.3 *[373.6]*
  Opisthorchis (felineus) (tenuicollis) (viverri-
    ni) 121.0
  Oxyuris vermicularis 127.4
  Paragonimus (westermani) 121.2
  parasite, parasitic NEC 136.9
    eyelid 134.9 *[373.6]*
    intestinal 129
    mouth 112.0
    orbit 376.13
    skin 134.9
    tongue 112.0
  pediculus 132.9
    capitis (humanus) (any site) 132.0
    corporis (humanus) (any site) 132.1
    eyelid 132.0 *[373.6]*
    mixed (classifiable to more than one
      category in 132.0–132.2) 132.3
    pubis (any site) 132.2
  phthirus (pubis) (any site) 132.2
    with any infestation classifiable to 132.0,
      132.1 and 132.3
  pinworm 127.4
  pork tapeworm (adult) 123.0
  protozoal NEC 136.8
  pubic louse 132.2
  rat tapeworm 123.6
  red bug 133.8
  roundworm (large) NEC 127.0
  sand flea 134.1
  saprophytic NEC 136.8
  Sarcoptes scabiei 133.0
  scabies 133.0
  Schistosoma 120.9
    bovis 120.8
    cercariae 120.3
    hematobium 120.0

Infestation — *continued*
  Schistosoma — *continued*
    intercalatum 120.8
    japonicum 120.2
    mansoni 120.1
    mattheii 120.8
    specified
      site — *see* Schistosomiasis
      type NEC 120.8
    spindale 120.8
  screw worms 134.0
  skin NEC 134.9
  Sparganum (mansoni) (proliferum) 123.5
    larval 123.5
  specified type NEC 134.8
  Spirometra larvae 123.5
  Sporozoa NEC 136.8
  Stellantchasmus falcatus 121.6
  Strongyloides 127.2
  Strongylus (gibsoni) 127.7
  Taenia 123.3
    diminuta 123.6
    Echinococcus (*see also* Echinococcus)
      122.9
    mediocanellata 123.2
    nana 123.6
    saginata (mediocanellata) 123.2
    solium (intestinal form) 123.0
      larval form 123.1
  Taeniarhynchus saginatus 123.2
  tapeworm 123.9
    beef 123.2
    broad 123.4
      larval 123.5
    dog 123.8
    dwarf 123.6
    fish 123.4
      larval 123.5
    pork 123.0
    rat 123.6
  Ternidens diminutus 127.7
  Tetranychus molestissimus 133.8
  threadworm 127.4
  tongue 112.0
  Toxocara (cani) (cati) (felis) 128.0
  trematode(s) NEC 121.9
  Trichina spiralis 124
  Trichinella spiralis 124
  Trichocephalus 127.3
  Trichomonas 131.9
    bladder 131.09
    cervix 131.09
    intestine 007.3
    prostate 131.03
    specified site NEC 131.8
    urethra (female) (male) 131.02
    urogenital 131.00
    vagina 131.01
    vulva 131.01
  Trichophyton — *see* Dermatophytosis
  Trichostrongylus instabilis 127.6
  Trichuris (trichiuria) 127.3
  Trombicula (irritans) 133.8
  Trypanosoma — *see* Trypanosomiasis
  Tunga penetrans 134.1
  Uncinaria americana 126.1
  whipworm 127.3
  worms NEC 128.9
    intestinal 127.9
  Wuchereria 125.9
    bancrofti 125.0
    malayi 125.1

Infiltrate, infiltration
  with an iron compound 275.09
  amyloid (any site) (generalized) 277.39
  calcareous (muscle) NEC 275.49
    localized — *see* Degeneration, by site
  calcium salt (muscle) 275.49
  chemotherapy, vesicant 999.81
  corneal (*see also* Edema, cornea) 371.20
  eyelid 373.9
  fatty (diffuse) (generalized) 272.8
    localized — *see* Degeneration, by site,
      fatty
  glycogen, glycogenic (*see also* Disease,
    glycogen storage) 271.0

Infiltrate, infiltration — *continued*
  heart, cardiac
    fatty (*see also* Degeneration, myocardial)
      429.1
    glycogenic 271.0 *[425.7]*
  inflammatory in vitreous 379.29
  kidney (*see also* Disease, renal) 593.9
  leukemic (M9800/3) — *see* Leukemia
  liver 573.8
    fatty — *see* Fatty, liver
    glycogen (*see also* Disease, glycogen
      storage) 271.0
  lung (*see also* Infiltrate, pulmonary) 793.19
    eosinophilic 518.3
    x-ray finding only 793.19
  lymphatic (*see also* Leukemia, lymphatic)
    204.9 ☑
    gland, pigmentary 289.3
  muscle, fatty 728.9
  myelogenous (*see also* Leukemia, myeloid)
    205.9 ☑
  myocardium, myocardial
    fatty (*see also* Degeneration, myocardial)
      429.1
    glycogenic 271.0 *[425.7]*
  pulmonary 793.19
    with
      eosinophilia 518.3
      pneumonia — *see* Pneumonia, by
        type
    x-ray finding only 793.19
    Ranke's primary (*see also* Tuberculosis)
      010.0 ☑
  skin, lymphocytic (benign) 709.8
  thymus (gland) (fatty) 254.8
  urine 788.8
  vesicant
    agent NEC 999.82
    chemotherapy 999.81
  vitreous humor 379.29
Infirmity 799.89
  senile 797
Inflammation, inflamed, inflammatory (with
  exudation)
  abducens (nerve) 378.54
  accessory sinus (chronic) (*see also* Sinusitis)
    473.9
  adrenal (gland) 255.8
  alimentary canal — *see* Enteritis
  alveoli (teeth) 526.5
    scorbutic 267
  amnion — *see* Amnionitis
  anal canal 569.49
  antrum (chronic) (*see also* Sinusitis, maxil-
    lary) 473.0
  anus 569.49
  appendix (*see also* Appendicitis) 541
  arachnoid — *see* Meningitis
  areola 611.0
    puerperal, postpartum 675.0 ☑
  areolar tissue NEC 686.9
  artery — *see* Arteritis
  auditory meatus (external) (*see also* Otitis,
    externa) 380.10
  Bartholin's gland 616.89
  bile duct or passage 576.1
  bladder (*see also* Cystitis) 595.9
  bleb
    postprocedural 379.60
      stage 1 379.61
      stage 2 379.62
      stage 3 379.63
  bone — *see* Osteomyelitis
  bowel (*see also* Enteritis) 558.9
  brain (*see also* Encephalitis) 323.9
    late effect — *see* category 326
    membrane — *see* Meningitis
  breast 611.0
    puerperal, postpartum 675.2 ☑
  broad ligament (*see also* Disease, pelvis, in-
    flammatory) 614.4
    acute 614.3
  bronchus — *see* Bronchitis
  bursa — *see* Bursitis
  capsule
    liver 573.3

Inflammation, inflamed, inflammatory —
  continued
  capsule — *continued*
    spleen 289.59
  catarrhal (*see also* Catarrh) 460
    vagina 616.10
  cecum (*see also* Appendicitis) 541
  cerebral (*see also* Encephalitis) 323.9
    late effect — *see* category 326
    membrane — *see* Meningitis
  cerebrospinal (*see also* Meningitis) 322.9
    late effect — *see* category 326
    meningococcal 036.0
    tuberculous (*see also* Tuberculosis)
      013.6 ☑
  cervix (uteri) (*see also* Cervicitis) 616.0
  chest 519.9
  choroid NEC (*see also* Choroiditis) 363.20
  cicatrix (tissue) — *see* Cicatrix
  colon (*see also* Enteritis) 558.9
    granulomatous 555.1
    newborn 558.9
  connective tissue (diffuse) NEC 728.9
  cornea (*see also* Keratitis) 370.9
    with ulcer (*see also* Ulcer, cornea) 370.00
  corpora cavernosa (penis) 607.2
  cranial nerve — *see* Disorder, nerve, cranial
  diarrhea — *see* Diarrhea
  disc (intervertebral) (space) 722.90
    cervical, cervicothoracic 722.91
    lumbar, lumbosacral 722.93
    thoracic, thoracolumbar 722.92
  Douglas' cul-de-sac or pouch (chronic) (*see
    also* Disease, pelvis, inflammatory)
    614.4
    acute 614.3
  due to (presence of) any device, implant, or
    graft classifiable to 996.0–996.5 —
    see Complications, infection and in-
    flammation, due to (presence of) any
    device, implant, or graft classified to
    996.0–996.5 NEC
  duodenum 535.6 ☑
  dura mater — *see* Meningitis
  ear (*see also* Otitis)
    external (*see also* Otitis, externa) 380.10
    inner (*see also* Labyrinthitis) 386.30
    middle — *see* Otitis media
  esophagus 530.10
  ethmoidal (chronic) (sinus) (*see also* Sinusi-
    tis, ethmoidal) 473.2
  Eustachian tube (catarrhal) 381.50
    acute 381.51
    chronic 381.52
  extrarectal 569.49
  eye 379.99
  eyelid 373.9
    specified NEC 373.8
  fallopian tube (*see also* Salpingo-oophoritis)
    614.2
  fascia 728.9
  fetal membranes (acute) 658.4 ☑
    affecting fetus or newborn 762.7
  follicular, pharynx 472.1
  frontal (chronic) (sinus) (*see also* Sinusitis,
    frontal) 473.1
  gallbladder (*see also* Cholecystitis, acute)
    575.0
  gall duct (*see also* Cholecystitis) 575.10
  gastrointestinal (*see also* Enteritis) 558.9
  genital organ (diffuse) (internal)
    female 614.9
      with
        abortion — *see* Abortion, by type,
          with sepsis
        ectopic pregnancy (*see also* cate-
          gories 633.0–633.9) 639.0
        molar pregnancy (*see also* cate-
          gories 630–632) 639.0
      complicating pregnancy, childbirth,
        or puerperium 646.6 ☑
        affecting fetus or newborn 760.8
      following
        abortion 639.0
        ectopic or molar pregnancy 639.0
    male 608.4

☑ Additional Digit Required — Refer to the Tabular List for Digit Selection   ▽ Subterms under main terms may continue to next column or page

2015 ICD-9-CM   ▶◀ Revised Text   ● New Line   ▲ Revised Code   Volume 2 — 159

Inflammation, inflamed, inflammatory — continued

gland (lymph) (see also Lymphadenitis) 289.3
glottis (see also Laryngitis) 464.00
  with obstruction 464.01
granular, pharynx 472.1
gum 523.10
heart (see also Carditis) 429.89
hepatic duct 576.8
hernial sac — see Hernia, by site
ileum (see also Enteritis) 558.9
  terminal or regional 555.0
    with large intestine 555.2
intervertebral disc 722.90
  cervical, cervicothoracic 722.91
  lumbar, lumbosacral 722.93
  thoracic, thoracolumbar 722.92
intestine (see also Enteritis) 558.9
jaw (acute) (bone) (chronic) (lower) (suppurative) (upper) 526.4
jejunum — see Enteritis
joint NEC (see also Arthritis) 716.9 ☑
  sacroiliac 720.2
kidney (see also Nephritis) 583.9
knee (joint) 716.66
  tuberculous (active) (see also Tuberculosis) 015.2 ☑
labium (majus) (minus) (see also Vulvitis) 616.10
lacrimal
  gland (see also Dacryoadenitis) 375.00
  passages (duct) (sac) (see also Dacryocystitis) 375.30
larynx (see also Laryngitis) 464.00
  with obstruction 464.01
  diphtheritic 032.3
leg NEC 686.9
lip 528.5
liver (capsule) (see also Hepatitis) 573.3
  acute 570
  chronic 571.40
  suppurative 572.0
lung (acute) (see also Pneumonia) 486
  chronic (interstitial) 518.89
lymphatic vessel (see also Lymphangitis) 457.2
lymph node or gland (see also Lymphadenitis) 289.3
mammary gland 611.0
  puerperal, postpartum 675.2 ☑
maxilla, maxillary 526.4
  sinus (chronic) (see also Sinusitis, maxillary) 473.0
membranes of brain or spinal cord — see Meningitis
meninges — see Meningitis
mouth 528.00
muscle 728.9
myocardium (see also Myocarditis) 429.0
nasal sinus (chronic) (see also Sinusitis) 473.9
nasopharynx — see Nasopharyngitis
navel 686.9
  newborn NEC 771.4
nerve NEC 729.2
nipple 611.0
  puerperal, postpartum 675.0 ☑
nose 478.19
  suppurative 472.0
oculomotor nerve 378.51
optic nerve 377.30
orbit (chronic) 376.10
  acute 376.00
  chronic 376.10
ovary (see also Salpingo-oophoritis) 614.2
oviduct (see also Salpingo-oophoritis) 614.2
pancreas — see Pancreatitis
parametrium (chronic) (see also Disease, pelvis, inflammatory) 614.4
  acute 614.3
parotid region 686.9
  gland 527.2
pelvis, female (see also Disease, pelvis, inflammatory) 614.9
penis (corpora cavernosa) 607.2
perianal 569.49

Inflammation, inflamed, inflammatory — continued

pericardium (see also Pericarditis) 423.9
perineum (female) (male) 686.9
perirectal 569.49
peritoneum (see also Peritonitis) 567.9
periuterine (see also Disease, pelvis, inflammatory) 614.9
perivesical (see also Cystitis) 595.9
petrous bone (see also Petrositis) 383.20
pharynx (see also Pharyngitis) 462
  follicular 472.1
  granular 472.1
pia mater — see Meningitis
pleura — see Pleurisy
postmastoidectomy cavity 383.30
  chronic 383.33
pouch, internal ileoanal 569.71
prostate (see also Prostatitis) 601.9
rectosigmoid — see Rectosigmoiditis
rectum (see also Proctitis) 569.49
respiratory, upper (see also Infection, respiratory, upper) 465.9
  chronic, due to external agent — see Condition, respiratory, chronic, due to, external agent
  due to
    fumes or vapors (chemical) (inhalation) 506.2
    radiation 508.1
retina (see also Retinitis) 363.20
retrocecal (see also Appendicitis) 541
retroperitoneal (see also Peritonitis) 567.9
salivary duct or gland (any) (suppurative) 527.2
scorbutic, alveoli, teeth 267
scrotum 608.4
sigmoid — see Enteritis
sinus (see also Sinusitis) 473.9
Skene's duct or gland (see also Urethritis) 597.89
skin 686.9
spermatic cord 608.4
sphenoidal (sinus) (see also Sinusitis, sphenoidal) 473.3
spinal
  cord (see also Encephalitis) 323.9
    late effect — see category 326
  membrane — see Meningitis
  nerve — see Disorder, nerve
spine (see also Spondylitis) 720.9
spleen (capsule) 289.59
stomach — see Gastritis
stricture, rectum 569.49
subcutaneous tissue NEC 686.9
suprarenal (gland) 255.8
synovial (fringe) (membrane) — see Bursitis
tendon (sheath) NEC 726.90
testis (see also Orchitis) 604.90
thigh 686.9
throat (see also Sore throat) 462
thymus (gland) 254.8
thyroid (gland) (see also Thyroiditis) 245.9
tongue 529.0
tonsil — see Tonsillitis
trachea — see Tracheitis
trochlear nerve 378.53
tubal (see also Salpingo-oophoritis) 614.2
tuberculous NEC (see also Tuberculosis) 011.9 ☑
tubo-ovarian (see also Salpingo-oophoritis) 614.2
tunica vaginalis 608.4
tympanic membrane — see Myringitis
umbilicus, umbilical 686.9
  newborn NEC 771.4
uterine ligament (see also Disease, pelvis, inflammatory) 614.4
  acute 614.3
uterus (catarrhal) (see also Endometritis) 615.9
uveal tract (anterior) (see also Iridocyclitis) 364.3
  posterior — see Chorioretinitis
  sympathetic 360.11
vagina (see also Vaginitis) 616.10

Inflammation, inflamed, inflammatory — continued

vas deferens 608.4
vein (see also Phlebitis) 451.9
  thrombotic 451.9
    cerebral (see also Thrombosis, brain) 434.0 ☑
    leg 451.2
      deep (vessels) NEC 451.19
      superficial (vessels) 451.0
    lower extremity 451.2
      deep (vessels) NEC 451.19
      superficial (vessels) 451.0
vocal cord 478.5
vulva (see also Vulvitis) 616.10
Inflation, lung imperfect (newborn) 770.5
Influenza, influenzal 487.1
  with
    bronchitis 487.1
    bronchopneumonia 487.0
    cold (any type) 487.1
    digestive manifestations 487.8
    hemoptysis 487.1
    involvement of
      gastrointestinal tract 487.8
      nervous system 487.8
    laryngitis 487.1
    manifestations NEC 487.8
      respiratory 487.1
        pneumonia 487.0
    pharyngitis 487.1
    pneumonia (any form classifiable to 480–483, 485–486) 487.0
    respiratory manifestations NEC 487.1
    sinusitis 487.1
    sore throat 487.1
    tonsillitis 487.1
    tracheitis 487.1
    upper respiratory infection (acute) 487.1
  abdominal 487.8
  A/H5N1 (see also Influenza, avian) 488.02
  Asian 487.1
  avian 488.02
    with involvement of gastrointestinal tract 488.09
    bronchopneumonia 488.01
    laryngitis 488.02
    manifestations NEC 488.09
      respiratory 488.02
    pharyngitis 488.02
    pneumonia (any form classifiable to 480–483, 485–486) 488.01
    respiratory infection (acute) (upper) 488.02
  bronchial 487.1
  bronchopneumonia 487.0
  catarrhal 487.1
  due to identified
    animal origin influenza virus — see Influenza, due to identified, novel influenza A virus
    avian influenza virus 488.02
      with
        manifestations NEC 488.09
          respiratory 488.02
        pneumonia (any form classifiable to 480–483, 485–486) 488.01
    (novel 2009) H1N1 influenza virus 488.12
      with
        manifestations NEC 488.19
          respiratory 488.12
        pneumonia 488.11
    novel influenza A virus 488.82
      with
        encephalopathy 488.89
        involvement of gastrointestinal tract 488.89
        laryngitis 488.82
        manifestations NEC 488.89
          respiratory (acute) (upper) 488.82
        pharyngitis 488.82
        pneumonia 488.81
  epidemic 487.1
  gastric 487.8

Influenza, influenzal — continued

  intestinal 487.8
  laryngitis 487.1
  maternal affecting fetus or newborn 760.2
    manifest influenza in infant 771.2
  (novel) 2009 H1N1 488.12
    with involvement of gastrointestinal tract 488.19
    bronchopneumonia 488.11
    laryngitis 488.12
    manifestations NEC 488.19
      respiratory 488.12
    pharyngitis 488.12
    pneumonia (any form classifiable to 480–483, 485–486) 488.11
    respiratory infection (acute) (upper) 488.12
  novel A/H1N1 (see also Influenza, (novel) 2009 H1N1) 488.12
  novel influenza A viruses not previously found in humans — see Influenza, due to identified, novel influenza A virus
  pharyngitis 487.1
  pneumonia (any form) 487.0
  respiratory (upper) 487.1
  specified NEC 487.1
  stomach 487.8
  vaccination, prophylactic (against) V04.81
Influenza-like disease — see also Influenza 487.1
Infraction, Freiberg's (metatarsal head) 732.5
Infraeruption, teeth 524.34
Infusion complication, misadventure, or reaction — see Complication, infusion
Ingestion
  chemical — see Table of Drugs and Chemicals
  drug or medicinal substance
    overdose or wrong substance given or taken 977.9
      specified drug — see Table of Drugs and Chemicals
  foreign body NEC (see also Foreign body) 938
Ingrowing
  hair 704.8
  nail (finger) (toe) (infected) 703.0
Inguinal — see also condition
  testis 752.51
Inhalation
  carbon monoxide 986
  flame
    lung 947.1
    mouth 947.0
  food or foreign body (see also Asphyxia, food or foreign body) 933.1
  gas, fumes, or vapor (noxious) 987.9
    specified agent — see Table of Drugs and Chemicals
  liquid or vomitus (see also Asphyxia, food or foreign body) 933.1
    lower respiratory tract NEC 934.9
  meconium (fetus or newborn) 770.11
    with respiratory symptoms 770.12
  mucus (see also Asphyxia, mucus) 933.1
  oil (causing suffocation) (see also Asphyxia, food or foreign body) 933.1
  pneumonia — see Pneumonia, aspiration
  smoke 508.2
  steam 987.9
  stomach contents or secretions (see also Asphyxia, food or foreign body) 933.1
    in labor and delivery 668.0 ☑
Inhibition, inhibited
  academic as adjustment reaction 309.23
  orgasm
    female 302.73
    male 302.74
  sexual
    desire 302.71
    excitement 302.72
  work as adjustment reaction 309.23
Inhibitor
  autoimmune, to clotting factors 286.52

☑ **Additional Digit Required** — Refer to the Tabular List for Digit Selection   ▽ **Subterms under main terms may continue to next column or page**

160 — Volume 2   ▶◀ **Revised Text**   ● **New Line**   ▲ **Revised Code**   **2015 ICD-9-CM**

Inhibitor — continued
  systemic lupus erythematosus (presence of) 795.79
    with
      hemorrhagic disorder 286.53
      hypercoagulable state 289.81
Iniencephalus, iniencephaly 740.2
Injected eye 372.74
Injury 959.9

> Note — For abrasion, insect bite (non-venomous), blister, or scratch, see Injury, superficial.
>
> For laceration, traumatic rupture, tear, or penetrating wound of internal organs, such as heart, lung, liver, kidney, pelvic organs, whether or not accompanied by open wound in the same region, see Injury, internal.
>
> For nerve injury, see Injury, nerve.
>
> For late effect of injuries classifiable to 850–854, 860–869, 900–919, 950–959, see Late, effect, injury, by type.

  abdomen, abdominal (viscera) (see also Injury, internal, abdomen)
    muscle or wall 959.12
  acoustic, resulting in deafness 951.5
  adenoid 959.09
  adrenal (gland) — see Injury, internal, adrenal
  alveolar (process) 959.09
  ankle (and foot) (and knee) (and leg, except thigh) 959.7
  anterior chamber, eye 921.3
  anus 959.19
  aorta (thoracic) 901.0
    abdominal 902.0
  appendix — see Injury, internal, appendix
  arm, upper (and shoulder) 959.2
  artery (complicating trauma) (see also Injury, blood vessel, by site) 904.9
    cerebral or meningeal (see also Hemorrhage, brain, traumatic, subarachnoid) 852.0 ☑
  auditory canal (external) (meatus) 959.09
  auricle, auris, ear 959.09
  axilla 959.2
  back 959.19
  bile duct — see Injury, internal, bile duct
  birth (see also Birth, injury)
    canal NEC, complicating delivery 665.9 ☑
  bladder (sphincter) — see Injury, internal, bladder
  blast (air) (hydraulic) (immersion) (underwater) NEC 869.0
    with open wound into cavity NEC 869.1
    abdomen or thorax — see Injury, internal, by site
    brain — see Concussion, brain
    ear (acoustic nerve trauma) 951.5
      with perforation of tympanic membrane — see Wound, open, ear, drum
  blood vessel NEC 904.9
    abdomen 902.9
      multiple 902.87
      specified NEC 902.89
    aorta (thoracic) 901.0
      abdominal 902.0
    arm NEC 903.9
    axillary 903.00
      artery 903.01
      vein 903.02
    azygos vein 901.89
    basilic vein 903.1
    brachial (artery) (vein) 903.1
    bronchial 901.89
    carotid artery 900.00
      common 900.01
      external 900.02
      internal 900.03
    celiac artery 902.20
      specified branch NEC 902.24
    cephalic vein (arm) 903.1

Injury — continued
  blood vessel — continued
    colica dextra 902.26
    cystic
      artery 902.24
      vein 902.39
    deep plantar 904.6
    digital (artery) (vein) 903.5
    due to accidental puncture or laceration during procedure 998.2
    extremity
      lower 904.8
        multiple 904.7
        specified NEC 904.7
      upper 903.9
        multiple 903.8
        specified NEC 903.8
    femoral
      artery (superficial) 904.1
        above profunda origin 904.0
        common 904.0
      vein 904.2
    gastric
      artery 902.21
      vein 902.39
    head 900.9
      intracranial — see Injury, intracranial
      multiple 900.82
      specified NEC 900.89
    hemiazygos vein 901.89
    hepatic
      artery 902.22
      vein 902.11
    hypogastric 902.59
      artery 902.51
      vein 902.52
    ileocolic
      artery 902.26
      vein 902.31
    iliac 902.50
      artery 902.53
      specified branch NEC 902.59
      vein 902.54
    innominate
      artery 901.1
      vein 901.3
    intercostal (artery) (vein) 901.81
    jugular vein (external) 900.81
      internal 900.1
    leg NEC 904.8
    mammary (artery) (vein) 901.82
    mesenteric
      artery 902.20
        inferior 902.27
        specified branch NEC 902.29
        superior (trunk) 902.25
          branches, primary 902.26
      vein 902.39
        inferior 902.32
        superior (and primary subdivisions) 902.31
    neck 900.9
      multiple 900.82
      specified NEC 900.89
    ovarian 902.89
      artery 902.81
      vein 902.82
    palmar artery 903.4
    pelvis 902.9
      multiple 902.87
      specified NEC 902.89
    plantar (deep) (artery) (vein) 904.6
    popliteal 904.40
      artery 904.41
      vein 904.42
    portal 902.33
    pulmonary 901.40
      artery 901.41
      vein 901.42
    radial (artery) (vein) 903.2
    renal 902.40
      artery 902.41
      specified NEC 902.49
      vein 902.42
    saphenous
      artery 904.7

Injury — continued
  blood vessel — continued
    saphenous — continued
      vein (greater) (lesser) 904.3
    splenic
      artery 902.23
      vein 902.34
    subclavian
      artery 901.1
      vein 901.3
    suprarenal 902.49
    thoracic 901.9
      multiple 901.83
      specified NEC 901.89
    tibial 904.50
      artery 904.50
        anterior 904.51
        posterior 904.53
      vein 904.50
        anterior 904.52
        posterior 904.54
    ulnar (artery) (vein) 903.3
    uterine 902.59
      artery 902.55
      vein 902.56
    vena cava
      inferior 902.10
        specified branches NEC 902.19
      superior 901.2
  brachial plexus 953.4
    newborn 767.6
  brain (traumatic) NEC (see also Injury, intracranial) 854.0 ☑
    due to fracture of skull — see Fracture, skull, by site
  breast 959.19
  broad ligament — see Injury, internal, broad ligament
  bronchus, bronchi — see Injury, internal, bronchus
  brow 959.09
  buttock 959.19
  canthus, eye 921.1
  cathode ray 990
  cauda equina 952.4
    with fracture, vertebra — see Fracture, vertebra, sacrum
  cavernous sinus (see also Injury, intracranial) 854.0 ☑
  cecum — see Injury, internal, cecum
  celiac ganglion or plexus 954.1
  cerebellum (see also Injury, intracranial) 854.0 ☑
  cervix (uteri) — see Injury, internal, cervix
  cheek 959.09
  chest (see also Injury, internal, chest)
    wall 959.11
  childbirth (see also Birth, injury)
    maternal NEC 665.9 ☑
  chin 959.09
  choroid (eye) 921.3
  clitoris 959.14
  coccyx 959.19
    complicating delivery 665.6 ☑
  colon — see Injury, internal, colon
  common duct — see Injury, internal, common duct
  conjunctiva 921.1
    superficial 918.2
  cord
    spermatic — see Injury, internal, spermatic cord
    spinal — see Injury, spinal, by site
  cornea 921.3
    abrasion 918.1
    due to contact lens 371.82
    penetrating — see Injury, eyeball, penetrating
    superficial 918.1
      due to contact lens 371.82
  cortex (cerebral) (see also Injury, intracranial) 854.0 ☑
    visual 950.3
  costal region 959.11
  costochondral 959.11

Injury — continued
  cranial
    bones — see Fracture, skull, by site
    cavity (see also Injury, intracranial) 854.0 ☑
    nerve — see Injury, nerve, cranial
  crushing — see Crush
  cutaneous sensory nerve
    lower limb 956.4
    upper limb 955.5
  deep tissue — see Contusion, by site
    meaning pressure ulcer 707.25
  delivery (see also Birth, injury)
    maternal NEC 665.9 ☑
  Descemet's membrane — see Injury, eyeball, penetrating
  diaphragm — see Injury, internal, diaphragm
  diffuse axonal — see Injury, intracranial
  duodenum — see Injury, internal, duodenum
  ear (auricle) (canal) (drum) (external) 959.09
  elbow (and forearm) (and wrist) 959.3
  epididymis 959.14
  epigastric region 959.12
  epiglottis 959.09
  epiphyseal, current — see Fracture, by site
  esophagus — see Injury, internal, esophagus
  Eustachian tube 959.09
  extremity (lower) (upper) NEC 959.8
  eye 921.9
    penetrating eyeball — see Injury, eyeball, penetrating
    superficial 918.9
  eyeball 921.3
    penetrating 871.7
      with
        partial loss (of intraocular tissue) 871.2
        prolapse or exposure (of intraocular tissue) 871.1
      without prolapse 871.0
      foreign body (nonmagnetic) 871.6
        magnetic 871.5
    superficial 918.9
  eyebrow 959.09
  eyelid(s) 921.1
    laceration — see Laceration, eyelid
    superficial 918.0
  face (and neck) 959.09
  fallopian tube — see Injury, internal, fallopian tube
  finger(s) (nail) 959.5
  flank 959.19
  foot (and ankle) (and knee) (and leg, except thigh) 959.7
  forceps NEC 767.9
    scalp 767.19
  forearm (and elbow) (and wrist) 959.3
  forehead 959.09
  gallbladder — see Injury, internal, gallbladder
  gasserian ganglion 951.2
  gastrointestinal tract — see Injury, internal, gastrointestinal tract
  genital organ(s)
    with
      abortion — see Abortion, by type, with, damage to pelvic organs
      ectopic pregnancy (see also categories 633.0–633.9) 639.2
      molar pregnancy (see also categories 630–632) 639.2
    external 959.14
      fracture of corpus cavernosum penis 959.13
    following
      abortion 639.2
      ectopic or molar pregnancy 639.2
    internal — see Injury, internal, genital organs
    obstetrical trauma NEC 665.9 ☑
      affecting fetus or newborn 763.89
  gland
    lacrimal 921.1

☑ Additional Digit Required — Refer to the Tabular List for Digit Selection   ▽ Subterms under main terms may continue to next column or page

2015 ICD-9-CM   ▶◀ Revised Text   ● New Line   ▲ Revised Code   Volume 2 — 161

Injury — *continued*
  gland — *continued*
    lacrimal — *continued*
      laceration 870.8
    parathyroid 959.09
    salivary 959.09
    thyroid 959.09
  globe (eye) (*see also* Injury, eyeball) 921.3
  grease gun — *see* Wound, open, by site, complicated
  groin 959.19
  gum 959.09
  hand(s) (except fingers) 959.4
  head NEC 959.01
    with
      loss of consciousness 850.5
      skull fracture — *see* Fracture, skull, by site
  heart — *see* Injury, internal, heart
  heel 959.7
  hip (and thigh) 959.6
  hymen 959.14
  hyperextension (cervical) (vertebra) 847.0
  ileum — *see* Injury, internal, ileum
  iliac region 959.19
  infrared rays NEC 990
  instrumental (during surgery) 998.2
    birth injury — *see* Birth, injury
    nonsurgical (*see also* Injury, by site) 959.9
    obstetrical 665.9 ☑
      affecting fetus or newborn 763.89
      bladder 665.5 ☑
      cervix 665.3 ☑
      high vaginal 665.4 ☑
      perineal NEC 664.9 ☑
      urethra 665.5 ☑
      uterus 665.5 ☑
    internal 869.0

> *Note* — For injury of internal organ(s) by foreign body entering body through a natural orifice (e.g., inhaled, ingested, or swallowed) — *see* Foreign body, entering through orifice.
>
> For internal injury of any of the following sites with internal injury of any other of the sites — *see* Injury, internal, multiple.

    with
      fracture
        pelvis — *see* Fracture, pelvis
        specified site, except pelvis — *see* Injury, internal, by site
      open wound into cavity 869.1
    abdomen, abdominal (viscera) NEC 868.00
      with
        fracture, pelvis — *see* Fracture, pelvis
        open wound into cavity 868.10
      specified site NEC 868.09
        with open wound into cavity 868.19
    adrenal (gland) 868.01
      with open wound into cavity 868.11
    aorta (thoracic) 901.0
      abdominal 902.0
    appendix 863.85
      with open wound into cavity 863.95
    bile duct 868.02
      with open wound into cavity 868.12
    bladder (sphincter) 867.0
      with
        abortion — *see* Abortion, by type, with damage to pelvic organs
        ectopic pregnancy (*see also* categories 633.0–633.9) 639.2
        molar pregnancy (*see also* categories 630–632) 639.2
        open wound into cavity 867.1
      following
        abortion 639.2
        ectopic or molar pregnancy 639.2
      obstetrical trauma 665.5 ☑

Injury — *continued*
  internal — *continued*
    bladder — *continued*
      obstetrical trauma — *continued*
        affecting fetus or newborn 763.89
    blood vessel — *see* Injury, blood vessel, by site
    broad ligament 867.6
      with open wound into cavity 867.7
    bronchus, bronchi 862.21
      with open wound into cavity 862.31
    cecum 863.89
      with open wound into cavity 863.99
    cervix (uteri) 867.4
      with
        abortion — *see* Abortion, by type, with damage to pelvic organs
        ectopic pregnancy (*see also* categories 633.0–633.9) 639.2
        molar pregnancy (*see also* categories 630–632) 639.2
        open wound into cavity 867.5
      following
        abortion 639.2
        ectopic or molar pregnancy 639.2
      obstetrical trauma 665.3 ☑
        affecting fetus or newborn 763.89
    chest (*see also* Injury, internal, intrathoracic organs) 862.8
      with open wound into cavity 862.9
    colon 863.40
      with
        open wound into cavity 863.50
        rectum 863.46
          with open wound into cavity 863.56
      ascending (right) 863.41
        with open wound into cavity 863.51
      descending (left) 863.43
        with open wound into cavity 863.53
      multiple sites 863.46
        with open wound into cavity 863.56
      sigmoid 863.44
        with open wound into cavity 863.54
      specified site NEC 863.49
        with open wound into cavity 863.59
      transverse 863.42
        with open wound into cavity 863.52
    common duct 868.02
      with open wound into cavity 868.12
    complicating delivery 665.9 ☑
      affecting fetus or newborn 763.89
    diaphragm 862.0
      with open wound into cavity 862.1
    duodenum 863.21
      with open wound into cavity 863.31
    esophagus (intrathoracic) 862.22
      with open wound into cavity 862.32
      cervical region 874.4
        complicated 874.5
    fallopian tube 867.6
      with open wound into cavity 867.7
    gallbladder 868.02
      with open wound into cavity 868.12
    gastrointestinal tract NEC 863.80
      with open wound into cavity 863.90
    genital organ NEC 867.6
      with open wound into cavity 867.7
    heart 861.00
      with open wound into thorax 861.10
    ileum 863.29
      with open wound into cavity 863.39
    intestine NEC 863.89
      with open wound into cavity 863.99
      large NEC 863.40
        with open wound into cavity 863.50
      small NEC 863.20

Injury — *continued*
  internal — *continued*
    intestine — *continued*
      small — *continued*
        with open wound into cavity 863.30
    intra-abdominal (organ) 868.00
      with open wound into cavity 868.10
      multiple sites 868.09
        with open wound into cavity 868.19
      specified site NEC 868.09
        with open wound into cavity 868.19
    intrathoracic organs (multiple) 862.8
      with open wound into cavity 862.9
      diaphragm (only) — *see* Injury, internal, diaphragm
      heart (only) — *see* Injury, internal, heart
      lung (only) — *see* Injury, internal, lung
      specified site NEC 862.29
        with open wound into cavity 862.39
    intrauterine (*see also* Injury, internal, uterus) 867.4
      with open wound into cavity 867.5
    jejunum 863.29
      with open wound into cavity 863.39
    kidney (subcapsular) 866.00
      with
        disruption of parenchyma (complete) 866.03
          with open wound into cavity 866.13
        hematoma (without rupture of capsule) 866.01
          with open wound into cavity 866.11
        laceration 866.02
          with open wound into cavity 866.12
        open wound into cavity 866.10
    liver 864.00
      with
        contusion 864.01
          with open wound into cavity 864.11
        hematoma 864.01
          with open wound into cavity 864.11
        laceration 864.05
          with open wound into cavity 864.15
          major (disruption of hepatic parenchyma) 864.04
            with open wound into cavity 864.14
          minor (capsule only) 864.02
            with open wound into cavity 864.12
          moderate (involving parenchyma) 864.03
            with open wound into cavity 864.13
          multiple 864.04
          stellate 864.04
            with open wound into cavity 864.14
        open wound into cavity 864.10
    lung 861.20
      with open wound into thorax 861.30
      aspiration 507.0
      hemopneumothorax — *see* Hemopneumothorax, traumatic
      hemothorax — *see* Hemothorax, traumatic
      pneumohemothorax — *see* Pneumohemothorax, traumatic
      pneumothorax — *see* Pneumothorax, traumatic
      transfusion related, acute (TRALI) 518.7
    mediastinum 862.29
      with open wound into cavity 862.39

Injury — *continued*
  internal — *continued*
    mesentery 863.89
      with open wound into cavity 863.99
    mesosalpinx 867.6
      with open wound into cavity 867.7
    multiple 869.0

> *Note* — Multiple internal injuries of sites classifiable to the same three- or four-digit category should be classified to that category.
>
> Multiple injuries classifiable to different fourth-digit subdivisions of 861 (heart and lung injuries) should be dealt with according to coding rules.

      internal
        with open wound into cavity 869.1
      intra-abdominal organ (sites classifiable to 863–868)
        with
          intrathoracic organ(s) (sites classifiable to 861–862) 869.0
            with open wound into cavity 869.1
          other intra–abdominal organ(s) (sites classifiable to 863–868, except where classifiable to the same three–digit category) 868.09
            with open wound into cavity 868.19
      intrathoracic organ (sites classifiable to 861–862)
        with
          intra–abdominal organ(s) (sites classifiable to 863–868) 869.0
            with open wound into cavity 869.1
          other intrathoracic organ(s) (sites classifiable to 861–862, except where classifiable to the same three–digit category) 862.8
            with open wound into cavity 862.9
    myocardium — *see* Injury, internal, heart
    ovary 867.6
      with open wound into cavity 867.7
    pancreas (multiple sites) 863.84
      with open wound into cavity 863.94
      body 863.82
        with open wound into cavity 863.92
      head 863.81
        with open wound into cavity 863.91
      tail 863.83
        with open wound into cavity 863.93
    pelvis, pelvic (organs) (viscera) 867.8
      with
        fracture, pelvis — *see* Fracture, pelvis
        open wound into cavity 867.9
      specified site NEC 867.6
        with open wound into cavity 867.7
    peritoneum 868.03
      with open wound into cavity 868.13
    pleura 862.29
      with open wound into cavity 862.39
    prostate 867.6
      with open wound into cavity 867.7
    rectum 863.45
      with
        colon 863.46
          with open wound into cavity 863.56
        open wound into cavity 863.55
    retroperitoneum 868.04

☑ **Additional Digit Required** — Refer to the Tabular List for Digit Selection   ▿ **Subterms under main terms may continue to next column or page**

162 — Volume 2   ▶◀ Revised Text   ● New Line   ▲ Revised Code   **2015 ICD-9-CM**

Injury — *continued*
  internal — *continued*
    retroperitoneum — *continued*
      with open wound into cavity 868.14
    round ligament 867.6
      with open wound into cavity 867.7
    seminal vesicle 867.6
      with open wound into cavity 867.7
    spermatic cord 867.6
      with open wound into cavity 867.7
      scrotal — *see* Wound, open, spermatic cord
    spleen 865.00
      with
        disruption of parenchyma (massive) 865.04
          with open wound into cavity 865.14
        hematoma (without rupture of capsule) 865.01
          with open wound into cavity 865.11
        open wound into cavity 865.10
        tear, capsular 865.02
          with open wound into cavity 865.12
          extending into parenchyma 865.03
            with open wound into cavity 865.13
    stomach 863.0
      with open wound into cavity 863.1
    suprarenal gland (multiple) 868.01
      with open wound into cavity 868.11
    thorax, thoracic (cavity) (organs) (multiple) (*see also* Injury, internal, intrathoracic organs) 862.8
      with open wound into cavity 862.9
    thymus (gland) 862.29
      with open wound into cavity 862.39
    trachea (intrathoracic) 862.29
      with open wound into cavity 862.39
      cervical region (*see also* Wound, open, trachea) 874.02
    ureter 867.2
      with open wound into cavity 867.3
    urethra (sphincter) 867.0
      with
        abortion — *see* Abortion, by type, with damage to pelvic organs
        ectopic pregnancy (*see also* categories 633.0–633.9) 639.2
        molar pregnancy (*see also* categories 630–632) 639.2
        open wound into cavity 867.1
      following
        abortion 639.2
        ectopic or molar pregnancy 639.2
      obstetrical trauma 665.5 ☑
        affecting fetus or newborn 763.89
    uterus 867.4
      with
        abortion — *see* Abortion, by type, with damage to pelvic organs
        ectopic pregnancy (*see also* categories 633.0–633.9) 639.2
        molar pregnancy (*see also* categories 630–632) 639.2
        open wound into cavity 867.5
      following
        abortion 639.2
        ectopic or molar pregnancy 639.2
      obstetrical trauma NEC 665.5 ☑
        affecting fetus or newborn 763.89
    vas deferens 867.6
      with open wound into cavity 867.7
    vesical (sphincter) 867.0
      with open wound into cavity 867.1
    viscera (abdominal) (*see also* Injury, internal, multiple) 868.00
      with
        fracture, pelvis — *see* Fracture, pelvis
        open wound into cavity 868.10

Injury — *continued*
  internal — *continued*
    viscera (*see also* Injury, internal, multiple) — *continued*
      thoracic NEC (*see also* Injury, internal, intrathoracic organs) 862.8
        with open wound into cavity 862.9
    interscapular region 959.19
    intervertebral disc 959.19
    intestine — *see* Injury, internal, intestine
    intra-abdominal (organs) NEC — *see* Injury, internal, intra-abdominal
    intracranial (traumatic) 854.0 ☑

> *Note* — Use the following fifth-digit subclassification with categories 851–854:
>
> 0   *unspecified state of consciousness*
>
> 1   *with no loss of consciousness*
>
> 2   *with brief [less than one hour] loss of consciousness*
>
> 3   *with moderate [1–24 hours] loss of consciousness*
>
> 4   *with prolonged [more than 24 hours] loss of consciousness and return to pre–existing conscious level*
>
> 5   *with prolonged [more than 24 hours] loss of consciousness, without return to pre–existing conscious level*
>
> *Use fifth-digit 5 to designate when a patient is unconscious and dies before regaining consciousness, regardless of the duration of the loss of consciousness*
>
> 6   *with loss of consciousness of unspecified duration*
>
> 9   *with concussion, unspecified*

      with
        open intracranial wound 854.1 ☑
        skull fracture — *see* Fracture, skull, by site
      contusion 851.8 ☑
        with open intracranial wound 851.9 ☑
        brain stem 851.4 ☑
          with open intracranial wound 851.5 ☑
        cerebellum 851.4 ☑
          with open intracranial wound 851.5 ☑
        cortex (cerebral) 851.0 ☑
          with open intracranial wound 851.2 ☑
      hematoma — *see* Injury, intracranial, hemorrhage
      hemorrhage 853.0 ☑
        with
          laceration — *see* Injury, intracranial, laceration
          open intracranial wound 853.1 ☑
        extradural 852.4 ☑
          with open intracranial wound 852.5 ☑
        subarachnoid 852.0 ☑
          with open intracranial wound 852.1 ☑
        subdural 852.2 ☑
          with open intracranial wound 852.3 ☑
      laceration 851.8 ☑
        with open intracranial wound 851.9 ☑
        brain stem 851.6 ☑
          with open intracranial wound 851.7 ☑
        cerebellum 851.6 ☑
          with open intracranial wound 851.7 ☑
        cortex (cerebral) 851.2 ☑

Injury — *continued*
  intracranial — *continued*
    laceration — *continued*
      cortex — *continued*
        with open intracranial wound 851.3 ☑
    intraocular — *see* Injury, eyeball, penetrating
    intraocular — *see* Injury, eyeball, penetrating
    intrathoracic organs (multiple) — *see* Injury, internal, intrathoracic organs
    intrauterine — *see* Injury, internal, intrauterine
    iris 921.3
      penetrating — *see* Injury, eyeball, penetrating
    jaw 959.09
    jejunum — *see* Injury, internal, jejunum
    joint NEC 959.9
      old or residual 718.80
        ankle 718.87
        elbow 718.82
        foot 718.87
        hand 718.84
        hip 718.85
        knee 718.86
        multiple sites 718.89
        pelvic region 718.85
        shoulder (region) 718.81
        specified site NEC 718.88
        wrist 718.83
    kidney — *see* Injury, internal, kidney
      acute (nontraumatic) 584.9
    knee (and ankle) (and foot) (and leg, except thigh) 959.7
    labium (majus) (minus) 959.14
    labyrinth, ear 959.09
    lacrimal apparatus, gland, or sac 921.1
      laceration 870.8
    larynx 959.09
    late effect — *see* Late, effects (of), injury
    leg, except thigh (and ankle) (and foot) (and knee) 959.7
      upper or thigh 959.6
    lens, eye 921.3
      penetrating — *see* Injury, eyeball, penetrating
    lid, eye — *see* Injury, eyelid
    lip 959.09
    liver — *see* Injury, internal, liver
    lobe, parietal — *see* Injury, intracranial
    lumbar (region) 959.19
      plexus 953.5
    lumbosacral (region) 959.19
      plexus 953.5
    lung — *see* Injury, internal, lung
    malar region 959.09
    mastoid region 959.09
    maternal, during pregnancy, affecting fetus or newborn 760.5
    maxilla 959.09
    mediastinum — *see* Injury, internal, mediastinum
    membrane
      brain (*see also* Injury, intracranial) 854.0 ☑
      tympanic 959.09
    meningeal artery — *see* Hemorrhage, brain, traumatic, subarachnoid
    meninges (cerebral) — *see* Injury, intracranial
    mesenteric
      artery — *see* Injury, blood vessel, mesenteric, artery
      plexus, inferior 954.1
      vein — *see* Injury, blood vessel, mesenteric, vein
    mesentery — *see* Injury, internal, mesentery
    mesosalpinx — *see* Injury, internal, mesosalpinx
    middle ear 959.09
    midthoracic region 959.11
    mouth 959.09
    multiple (sites not classifiable to the same four–digit category in 959.0–959.7) 959.8
      internal 869.0

Injury — *continued*
  multiple — *continued*
    internal — *continued*
      with open wound into cavity 869.1
    musculocutaneous nerve 955.4
    nail
      finger 959.5
      toe 959.7
    nasal (septum) (sinus) 959.09
    nasopharynx 959.09
    neck (and face) 959.09
    nerve 957.9
      abducens 951.3
      abducent 951.3
      accessory 951.6
      acoustic 951.5
      ankle and foot 956.9
      anterior crural, femoral 956.1
      arm (*see also* Injury, nerve, upper limb) 955.9
      auditory 951.5
      axillary 955.0
      brachial plexus 953.4
      cervical sympathetic 954.0
      cranial 951.9
        first or olfactory 951.8
        second or optic 950.0
        third or oculomotor 951.0
        fourth or trochlear 951.1
        fifth or trigeminal 951.2
        sixth or abducens 951.3
        seventh or facial 951.4
        eighth, acoustic, or auditory 951.5
        ninth or glossopharyngeal 951.8
        tenth, pneumogastric, or vagus 951.8
        eleventh or accessory 951.6
        twelfth or hypoglossal 951.7
        newborn 767.7
      cutaneous sensory
        lower limb 956.4
        upper limb 955.5
      digital (finger) 955.6
        toe 956.5
      facial 951.4
        newborn 767.5
      femoral 956.1
      finger 955.9
      foot and ankle 956.9
      forearm 955.9
      glossopharyngeal 951.8
      hand and wrist 955.9
      head and neck, superficial 957.0
      hypoglossal 951.7
      involving several parts of body 957.8
      leg (*see also* Injury, nerve, lower limb) 956.9
      lower limb 956.9
        multiple 956.8
        specified site NEC 956.5
      lumbar plexus 953.5
      lumbosacral plexus 953.5
      median 955.1
        forearm 955.1
        wrist and hand 955.1
      multiple (in several parts of body) (sites not classifiable to the same three-digit category) 957.8
      musculocutaneous 955.4
      musculospiral 955.3
        upper arm 955.3
      oculomotor 951.0
      olfactory 951.8
      optic 950.0
      pelvic girdle 956.9
        multiple sites 956.8
        specified site NEC 956.5
      peripheral 957.9
        multiple (in several regions) (sites not classifiable to the same three-digit category) 957.8
        specified site NEC 957.1
      peroneal 956.3
        ankle and foot 956.3
        lower leg 956.3
      plantar 956.5
      plexus 957.9

☑ **Additional Digit Required** — Refer to the Tabular List for Digit Selection
2015 ICD-9-CM   ▶◀ Revised Text   ● New Line   ▲ Revised Code

Subterms under main terms may continue to next column or page
Volume 2 — 163

Injury — *continued*
  nerve — *continued*
    plexus — *continued*
      celiac 954.1
      mesenteric, inferior 954.1
      spinal 953.9
        brachial 953.4
        lumbosacral 953.5
        multiple sites 953.8
      sympathetic NEC 954.1
    pneumogastric 951.8
    radial 955.3
      wrist and hand 955.3
    sacral plexus 953.5
    sciatic 956.0
      thigh 956.0
    shoulder girdle 955.9
      multiple 955.8
      specified site NEC 955.7
    specified site NEC 957.1
    spinal 953.9
      plexus — *see* injury, nerve, plexus, spinal
      root 953.9
        cervical 953.0
        dorsal 953.1
        lumbar 953.2
        muitiple sites 953.8
        sacral 953.3
    splanchnic 954.1
    sympathetic NEC 954.1
      cervical 954.0
    thigh 956.9
    tibial 956.5
      ankle and foot 956.2
      lower leg 956.5
      posterior 956.2
    toe 956.9
    trigeminal 951.2
    trochlear 951.1
    trunk, excluding shoulder and pelvic girdles 954.9
      specified site NEC 954.8
      sympathetic NEC 954.1
    ulnar 955.2
      forearm 955.2
      wrist (and hand) 955.2
    upper limb 955.9
      multiple 955.8
      specified site NEC 955.7
    vagus 951.8
    wrist and hand 955.9
  nervous system, diffuse 957.8
  nose (septum) 959.09
  obstetrical NEC 665.9 ☑
    affecting fetus or newborn 763.89
  occipital (region) (scalp) 959.09
    lobe (*see also* Injury, intracranial) 854.0 ☑
  optic 950.9
    chiasm 950.1
    cortex 950.3
    nerve 950.0
    pathways 950.2
  orbit, orbital (region) 921.2
    penetrating 870.3
      with foreign body 870.4
  ovary — *see* Injury, internal, ovary
  paint-gun — *see* Wound, open, by site, complicated
  palate (soft) 959.09
  pancreas — *see* Injury, internal, pancreas
  parathyroid (gland) 959.09
  parietal (region) (scalp) 959.09
    lobe — *see* Injury, intracranial
  pelvic
    floor 959.19
      complicating delivery 664.1 ☑
        affecting fetus or newborn 763.89
    joint or ligament, complicating delivery 665.6 ☑
      affecting fetus or newborn 763.89
    organs (*see also* Injury, internal, pelvis)

Injury — *continued*
  pelvic — *continued*
    organs (*see also* Injury, internal, pelvis) — *continued*
      with
        abortion — *see* Abortion, by type, with damage to pelvic organs
        ectopic pregnancy (*see also* categories 633.0–633.9) 639.2
        molar pregnancy (*see also* categories 633.0–633.9) 639.2
      following
        abortion 639.2
        ectopic or molar pregnancy 639.2
      obstetrical trauma 665.5 ☑
        affecting fetus or newborn 763.89
  pelvis 959.19
  penis 959.14
    fracture of corpus cavernosum 959.13
  perineum 959.14
  peritoneum — *see* Injury, internal, peritoneum
  periurethral tissue
    with
      abortion — *see* Abortion, by type, with damage to pelvic organs
      ectopic pregnancy (*see also* categories 633.0–633.9) 639.2
      molar pregnancy (*see also* categories 630–632) 639.2
    complicating delivery 664.8 ☑
      affecting fetus or newborn 763.89
    following
      abortion 639.2
      ectopic or molar pregnancy 639.2
  phalanges
    foot 959.7
    hand 959.5
  pharynx 959.09
  pleura — *see* Injury, internal, pleura
  popliteal space 959.7
  post-cardiac surgery (syndrome) 429.4
  prepuce 959.14
  prostate — *see* Injury, internal, prostate
  pubic region 959.19
  pudenda 959.14
  radiation NEC 990
  radioactive substance or radium NEC 990
  rectovaginal septum 959.14
  rectum — *see* Injury, internal, rectum
  retina 921.3
    penetrating — *see* Injury, eyeball, penetrating
  retroperitoneal — *see* Injury, internal, retroperitoneum
  roentgen rays NEC 990
  round ligament — *see* Injury, internal, round ligament
  sacral (region) 959.19
    plexus 953.5
  sacroiliac ligament NEC 959.19
  sacrum 959.19
  salivary ducts or glands 959.09
  scalp 959.09
    due to birth trauma 767.19
    fetus or newborn 767.19
  scapular region 959.2
  sclera 921.3
    penetrating — *see* Injury, eyeball, penetrating
    superficial 918.2
  scrotum 959.14
  seminal vesicle — *see* Injury, internal, seminal vesicle
  shoulder (and upper arm) 959.2
  sinus
    cavernous (*see also* Injury, intracranial) 854.0 ☑
    nasal 959.09
  skeleton NEC, birth injury 767.3
  skin NEC 959.9
  skull — *see* Fracture, skull, by site
  soft tissue (of external sites) (severe) — *see* Wound, open, by site
  specified site NEC 959.8

Injury — *continued*
  spermatic cord — *see* Injury, internal, spermatic cord
  spinal (cord) 952.9
    with fracture, vertebra — *see* Fracture, vertebra, by site, with spinal cord injury
    cervical (C_1-C_4) 952.00
      with
        anterior cord syndrome 952.02
        central cord syndrome 952.03
        complete lesion of cord 952.01
        incomplete lesion NEC 952.04
        posterior cord syndrome 952.04
    C_5-C_7 level 952.05
      with
        anterior cord syndrome 952.07
        central cord syndrome 952.08
        complete lesion of cord 952.06
        incomplete lesion NEC 952.09
        posterior cord syndrome 952.09
      specified type NEC 952.09
    specified type NEC 952.04
    dorsal (D_1-D_6) (T_1-T_6) (thoracic) 952.10
      with
        anterior cord syndrome 952.12
        central cord syndrome 952.13
        complete lesion of cord 952.11
        incomplete lesion NEC 952.14
        posterior cord syndrome 952.14
    D_7-D_{12} level (T_7-T_{12}) 952.15
      with
        anterior cord syndrome 952.17
        central cord syndrome 952.18
        complete lesion of cord 952.16
        incomplete lesion NEC 952.19
        posterior cord syndrome 952.19
      specified type NEC 952.19
      specified type NEC 952.14
    lumbar 952.2
    multiple sites 952.8
    nerve (root) NEC — *see* Injury, nerve, spinal, root
    plexus 953.9
      brachial 953.4
      lumbosacral 953.5
      multiple sites 953.8
    sacral 952.3
    thoracic (*see also* Injury, spinal, dorsal) 952.10
  spleen — *see* Injury, internal, spleen
  stellate ganglion 954.1
  sternal region 959.11
  stomach — *see* Injury, internal, stomach
  subconjunctival 921.1
  subcutaneous 959.9
  subdural — *see* Injury, intracranial
  submaxillary region 959.09
  submental region 959.09
  subungual
    fingers 959.5
    toes 959.7

Injury — *continued*
  superficial 919 ☑

> **Note** — Use the following fourth-digit subdivisions with categories 910–919:
>
> 0   Abrasion or friction burn without mention of infection
> 1   Abrasion or friction burn, infected
> 2   Blister without mention of infection
> 3   Blister, infected
> 4   Insect bite, nonvenomous, without mention of infection
> 5   Insect bite, nonvenomous, infected
> 6   Superficial foreign body (splinter) without major open wound and without mention of infection
> 7   Superficial foreign body (splinter) without major open wound, infected
> 8   Other and unspecified superficial injury without mention of infection
> 9   Other and unspecified superficial injury, infected
>
> For late effects of superficial injury, see category 906.2.

    abdomen, abdominal (muscle) (wall) (and other part(s) of trunk) 911 ☑
    ankle (and hip, knee, leg, or thigh) 916 ☑
    anus (and other part(s) of trunk) 911 ☑
    arm 913 ☑
      upper (and shoulder) 912 ☑
    auditory canal (external) (meatus) (and other part(s) of face, neck, or scalp, except eye) 910 ☑
    axilla (and upper arm) 912 ☑
    back (and other part(s) of trunk) 911 ☑
    breast (and other part(s) of trunk) 911 ☑
    brow (and other part(s) of face, neck, or scalp, except eye) 910 ☑
    buttock (and other part(s) of trunk) 911 ☑
    canthus, eye 918.0
    cheek(s) (and other part(s) of face, neck, or scalp, except eye) 910 ☑
    chest wall (and other part(s) of trunk) 911 ☑
    chin (and other part(s) of face, neck, or scalp, except eye) 910 ☑
    clitoris (and other part(s) of trunk) 911 ☑
    conjunctiva 918.2
    cornea 918.1
      due to contact lens 371.82
    costal region (and other part(s) of trunk) 911 ☑
    ear(s) (auricle) (canal) (drum) (external) (and other part(s) of face, neck, or scalp, except eye) 910 ☑
    elbow (and forearm) (and wrist) 913 ☑
    epididymis (and other part(s) of trunk) 911 ☑
    epigastric region (and other part(s) of trunk) 911 ☑
    epiglottis (and other part(s) of face, neck, or scalp, except eye) 910 ☑
    eyelid(s) (and periocular area) 918.0
    eye(s) (and adnexa) NEC 918.9
    face (any part(s), except eye) (and neck or scalp) 910 ☑
    finger(s) (nail) (any) 915 ☑
    flank (and other part(s) of trunk) 911 ☑
    foot (phalanges) (and toe(s)) 917 ☑
    forearm (and elbow) (and wrist) 913 ☑
    forehead (and other part(s) of face, neck, or scalp, except eye) 910 ☑
    globe (eye) 918.9

☑ **Additional Digit Required — Refer to the Tabular List for Digit Selection**   ▽ **Subterms under main terms may continue to next column or page**

Injury — *continued*
  superficial — *continued*
    groin (and other part(s) of trunk) 911 ☑
    gum(s) (and other part(s) of face, neck, or scalp, except eye) 910 ☑
    hand(s) (except fingers alone) 914 ☑
    head (and other part(s) of face, neck, or scalp, except eye) 910 ☑
    heel (and foot or toe) 917 ☑
    hip (and ankle, knee, leg, or thigh) 916 ☑
    iliac region (and other part(s) of trunk) 911 ☑
    interscapular region (and other part(s) of trunk) 911 ☑
    iris 918.9
    knee (and ankle, hip, leg, or thigh) 916 ☑
    labium (majus) (minus) (and other part(s) of trunk) 911 ☑
    lacrimal (apparatus) (gland) (sac) 918.0
    leg (lower) (upper) (and ankle, hip, knee, or thigh) 916 ☑
    lip(s) (and other part(s) of face, neck, or scalp, except eye) 910 ☑
    lower extremity (except foot) 916 ☑
    lumbar region (and other part(s) of trunk) 911 ☑
    malar region (and other part(s) of face, neck, or scalp, except eye) 910 ☑
    mastoid region (and other part(s) of face, neck, or scalp, except eye) 910 ☑
    midthoracic region (and other part(s) of trunk) 911 ☑
    mouth (and other part(s) of face, neck, or scalp, except eye) 910 ☑
    multiple sites (not classifiable to the same three-digit category) 919 ☑
    nasal (septum) (and other part(s) of face, neck, or scalp, except eye) 910 ☑
    neck (and face or scalp, any part(s), except eye) 910 ☑
    nose (septum) (and other part(s) of face, neck, or scalp, except eye) 910 ☑
    occipital region (and other part(s) of face, neck, or scalp, except eye) 910 ☑
    orbital region 918.0
    palate (soft) (and other part(s) of face, neck, or scalp, except eye) 910 ☑
    parietal region (and other part(s) of face, neck, or scalp, except eye) 910 ☑
    penis (and other part(s) of trunk) 911 ☑
    perineum (and other part(s) of trunk) 911 ☑
    periocular area 918.0
    pharynx (and other part(s) of face, neck, or scalp, except eye) 910 ☑
    popliteal space (and ankle, hip, leg, or thigh) 916 ☑
    prepuce (and other part(s) of trunk) 911 ☑
    pubic region (and other part(s) of trunk) 911 ☑
    pudenda (and other part(s) of trunk) 911 ☑
    sacral region (and other part(s) of trunk) 911 ☑
    salivary (ducts) (glands) (and other part(s) of face, neck, or scalp, except eye) 910 ☑
    scalp (and other part(s) of face or neck, except eye) 910 ☑
    scapular region (and upper arm) 912 ☑
    sclera 918.2
    scrotum (and other part(s) of trunk) 911 ☑
    shoulder (and upper arm) 912 ☑
    skin NEC 919 ☑
    specified site(s) NEC 919 ☑
    sternal region (and other part(s) of trunk) 911 ☑
    subconjunctival 918.2
    subcutaneous NEC 919 ☑

Injury — *continued*
  superficial — *continued*
    submaxillary region (and other part(s) of face, neck, or scalp, except eye) 910 ☑
    submental region (and other part(s) of face, neck, or scalp, except eye) 910 ☑
    supraclavicular fossa (and other part(s) of face, neck, or scalp, except eye) 910 ☑
    supraorbital 918.0
    temple (and other part(s) of face, neck, or scalp, except eye) 910 ☑
    temporal region (and other part(s) of face, neck, or scalp, except eye) 910 ☑
    testis (and other part(s) of trunk) 911 ☑
    thigh (and ankle, hip, knee, or leg) 916 ☑
    thorax, thoracic (external) (and other part(s) of trunk) 911 ☑
    throat (and other part(s) of face, neck, or scalp, except eye) 910 ☑
    thumb(s) (nail) 915 ☑
    toe(s) (nail) (subungual) (and foot) 917 ☑
    tongue (and other part(s) of face, neck, or scalp, except eye) 910 ☑
    tooth, teeth (*see also* Abrasion, dental) 521.20
    trunk (any part(s)) 911 ☑
    tunica vaginalis 959.14
    tympanum, tympanic membrane (and other part(s) of face, neck, or scalp, except eye) 910 ☑
    upper extremity NEC 913 ☑
    uvula (and other part(s) of face, neck, or scalp, except eye) 910 ☑
    vagina (and other part(s) of trunk) 911 ☑
    vulva (and other part(s) of trunk) 911 ☑
    wrist (and elbow) (and forearm) 913 ☑
  supraclavicular fossa 959.19
  supraorbital 959.09
  surgical complication (external or internal site) 998.2
  symphysis pubis 959.19
    complicating delivery 665.6 ☑
      affecting fetus or newborn 763.89
  temple 959.09
  temporal region 959.09
  testis 959.14
  thigh (and hip) 959.6
  thorax, thoracic (external) 959.11
    cavity — *see* Injury, internal, thorax
    internal — *see* Injury, internal, intrathoracic organs
  throat 959.09
  thumb(s) (nail) 959.5
  thymus — *see* Injury, internal, thymus
  thyroid (gland) 959.09
  toe (nail) (any) 959.7
  tongue 959.09
  tonsil 959.09
  tooth NEC 873.63
    complicated 873.73
  trachea — *see* Injury, internal, trachea
  trunk 959.19
  tunica vaginalis 959.14
  tympanum, tympanic membrane 959.09
  ultraviolet rays NEC 990
  ureter — *see* Injury, internal, ureter
  urethra (sphincter) — *see* Injury, internal, urethra
  uterus — *see* Injury, internal, uterus
  uvula 959.09
  vagina 959.14
  vascular — *see* Injury, blood vessel
  vas deferens — *see* Injury, internal, vas deferens
  vein (*see also* Injury, blood vessel, by site) 904.9
  vena cava
    inferior 902.10
    superior 901.2

Injury — *continued*
  vesical (sphincter) — *see* Injury, internal, vesical
  viscera (abdominal) — *see* Injury, internal, viscera
    with fracture, pelvis — *see* Fracture, pelvis
  visual 950.9
    cortex 950.3
  vitreous (humor) 871.2
  vulva 959.14
  whiplash (cervical spine) 847.0
  wringer — *see* Crush, by site
  wrist (and elbow) (and forearm) 959.3
  x-ray NEC 990
Inoculation — *see also* Vaccination
  complication or reaction — *see* Complication, vaccination
INPH (idiopathic normal pressure hydrocephalus) 331.5
Insanity, insane — *see also* Psychosis 298.9
  adolescent (*see also* Schizophrenia) 295.9 ☑
  alternating (*see also* Psychosis, affective, circular) 296.7
  confusional 298.9
    acute 293.0
    subacute 293.1
  delusional 298.9
  paralysis, general 094.1
    progressive 094.1
  paresis, general 094.1
  senile 290.20
Insect
  bite — *see* Injury, superficial, by site
  venomous, poisoning by 989.5
Insemination, artificial V26.1
Insensitivity
  adrenocorticotropin hormone (ACTH) 255.41
  androgen 259.50
    complete 259.51
    partial 259.52
Insertion
  cord (umbilical) lateral or velamentous 663.8 ☑
    affecting fetus or newborn 762.6
  intrauterine contraceptive device V25.11
  placenta, vicious — *see* Placenta, previa
  subdermal implantable contraceptive V25.5
  velamentous, umbilical cord 663.8 ☑
    affecting fetus or newborn 762.6
Insolation 992.0
  meaning sunstroke 992.0
Insomnia, unspecified 780.52
  with sleep apnea, unspecified 780.51
  adjustment 307.41
  alcohol induced 291.82
  behavioral, of childhood V69.5
  drug induced 292.85
  due to
    medical condition classified elsewhere 327.01
    mental disorder 327.02
  fatal familial (FFI) 046.72
  idiopathic 307.42
  nonorganic origin 307.41
    persistent (primary) 307.42
    transient 307.41
  organic 327.00
    other 327.09
  paradoxical 307.42
  primary 307.42
  psychophysiological 307.42
  subjective complaint 307.49
Inspiration
  food or foreign body (*see also* Asphyxia, food or foreign body) 933.1
  mucus (*see also* Asphyxia, mucus) 933.1
Inspissated bile syndrome, newborn 774.4
Instability
  detrusor 596.59
  emotional (excessive) 301.3
  joint (posttraumatic) 718.80
    ankle 718.87
    elbow 718.82
    foot 718.87

Instability — *continued*
  joint — *continued*
    hand 718.84
    hip 718.85
    knee 718.86
    lumbosacral 724.6
    multiple sites 718.89
    pelvic region 718.85
    sacroiliac 724.6
    shoulder (region) 718.81
    specified site NEC 718.88
    wrist 718.83
  lumbosacral 724.6
  nervous 301.89
  personality (emotional) 301.59
  thyroid, paroxysmal 242.9 ☑
  urethral 599.83
  vasomotor 780.2
Insufficiency, insufficient
  accommodation 367.4
  adrenal (gland) (acute) (chronic) 255.41
    medulla 255.5
    primary 255.41
    specified site NEC 255.5
  adrenocortical 255.41
  anterior (occlusal) guidance 524.54
  anus 569.49
  aortic (valve) 424.1
    with
      mitral (valve) disease 396.1
        insufficiency, incompetence, or regurgitation 396.3
        stenosis or obstruction 396.1
      stenosis or obstruction 424.1
        with mitral (valve) disease 396.8
    congenital 746.4
    rheumatic 395.1
      with
        mitral (valve) disease 396.1
          insufficiency, incompetence, or regurgitation 396.3
          stenosis or obstruction 396.1
        stenosis or obstruction 395.2
          with mitral (valve) disease 396.8
    specified cause NEC 424.1
    syphilitic 093.22
  arterial 447.1
    basilar artery 435.0
    carotid artery 435.8
    cerebral 437.1
    coronary (acute or subacute) 411.89
    mesenteric 557.1
    peripheral 443.9
    precerebral 435.9
    vertebral artery 435.1
    vertebrobasilar 435.3
  arteriovenous 459.9
  basilar artery 435.0
  biliary 575.8
  cardiac (*see also* Insufficiency, myocardial) 428.0
    complicating surgery 997.1
    due to presence of (cardiac) prosthesis 429.4
    postoperative 997.1
      long-term effect of cardiac surgery 429.4
    specified during or due to a procedure 997.1
      long-term effect of cardiac surgery 429.4
  cardiorenal (*see also* Hypertension, cardiorenal) 404.90
  cardiovascular (*see also* Disease, cardiovascular) 429.2
    renal (*see also* Hypertension, cardiorenal) 404.90
  carotid artery 435.8
  cerebral (vascular) 437.9
  cerebrovascular 437.9
    with transient focal neurological signs and symptoms 435.9
    acute 437.1
      with transient focal neurological signs and symptoms 435.9

☑ Additional Digit Required — Refer to the Tabular List for Digit Selection   ⓦ Subterms under main terms may continue to next column or page

2015 ICD-9-CM   ▶◀ Revised Text   ● New Line   ▲ Revised Code   Volume 2 — 165

Insufficiency, insufficient — *continued*
  circulatory NEC 459.9
    fetus or newborn 779.89
  convergence 378.83
  coronary (acute or subacute) 411.89
    chronic or with a stated duration of over
      8 weeks 414.8
  corticoadrenal 255.41
  dietary 269.9
  divergence 378.85
  food 994.2
  gastroesophageal 530.89
  gonadal
    ovary 256.39
    testis 257.2
  gonadotropic hormone secretion 253.4
  heart (*see also* Insufficiency, myocardial)
    fetus or newborn 779.89
    valve (*see also* Endocarditis) 424.90
      congenital NEC 746.89
  hepatic 573.8
  idiopathic autonomic 333.0
  interocclusal distance of teeth (ridge) 524.36
  kidney
    acute 593.9
    chronic 585.9
  labyrinth, labyrinthine (function) 386.53
    bilateral 386.54
    unilateral 386.53
  lacrimal 375.15
  liver 573.8
  lung (acute) (*see also* Insufficiency, pul-
    monary) 518.82
    following trauma and surgery 518.52
    newborn 770.89
  mental (congenital) (*see also* Disability, intel-
    lectual) 319
  mesenteric 557.1
  mitral (valve) 424.0
    with
      aortic (valve) disease 396.3
        insufficiency, incompetence, or
          regurgitation 396.3
        stenosis or obstruction 396.2
      obstruction or stenosis 394.2
        with aortic valve disease 396.8
    congenital 746.6
    rheumatic 394.1
      with
        aortic (valve) disease 396.3
          insufficiency, incompetence,
            or regurgitation 396.3
          stenosis or obstruction 396.2
        obstruction or stenosis 394.2
          with aortic valve disease 396.8
      active or acute 391.1
        with chorea, rheumatic (Syden-
          ham's) 392.0
    specified cause, except rheumatic 424.0
  muscle
    heart — *see* Insufficiency, myocardial
    ocular (*see also* Strabismus) 378.9
  myocardial, myocardium (with arterioscle-
    rosis) 428.0
    with rheumatic fever (conditions classifi-
      able to 390)
      active, acute, or subacute 391.2
        with chorea 392.0
      inactive or quiescent (with chorea)
        398.0
    congenital 746.89
    due to presence of (cardiac) prosthesis
      429.4
    fetus or newborn 779.89
    following cardiac surgery 429.4
    hypertensive (*see also* Hypertension,
      heart) 402.91
      benign 402.11
      malignant 402.01
    postoperative 997.1
      long-term effect of cardiac surgery
        429.4
    rheumatic 398.0
      active, acute, or subacute 391.2
        with chorea (Sydenham's) 392.0
  syphilitic 093.82

Insufficiency, insufficient — *continued*
  nourishment 994.2
  organic 799.89
  ovary 256.39
    postablative 256.2
  pancreatic 577.8
  parathyroid (gland) 252.1
  peripheral vascular (arterial) 443.9
  pituitary (anterior) 253.2
    posterior 253.5
  placental — *see* Placenta, insufficiency
  platelets 287.5
  prenatal care in current pregnancy V23.7
  progressive pluriglandular 258.9
  pseudocholinesterase 289.89
  pulmonary (acute) 518.82
    following
      shock 518.52
      surgery 518.52
      trauma 518.52
    newborn 770.89
    valve (*see also* Endocarditis, pulmonary)
      424.3
      congenital 746.09
  pyloric 537.0
  renal 593.9
    acute 593.9
    chronic 585.9
    due to a procedure 997.5
  respiratory 786.09
    acute 518.82
      following trauma and surgery 518.52
    newborn 770.89
  rotation — *see* Malrotation
  suprarenal 255.41
    medulla 255.5
  tarso-orbital fascia, congenital 743.66
  tear film 375.15
  testis 257.2
  thyroid (gland) (acquired) (*see also* Hypothy-
    roidism)
    congenital 243
  tricuspid (*see also* Endocarditis, tricuspid)
    397.0
    congenital 746.89
    syphilitic 093.23
  urethral sphincter 599.84
  valve, valvular (heart) (*see also* Endocarditis)
    424.90
  vascular 459.9
    intestine NEC 557.9
    mesenteric 557.1
    peripheral 443.9
    renal (*see also* Hypertension, kidney)
      403.90
  velopharyngeal
    acquired 528.9
    congenital 750.29
  venous (peripheral) 459.81
  ventricular — *see* Insufficiency, myocardial
  vertebral artery 435.1
  vertebrobasilar artery 435.3
  weight gain during pregnancy 646.8 ☑
  zinc 269.3
Insufflation
  fallopian
    fertility testing V26.21
    following sterilization reversal V26.22
  meconium 770.11
    with respiratory symptoms 770.12
Insular — *see* condition
Insulinoma (M8151/0)
  malignant (M8151/3)
    pancreas 157.4
    specified site — *see* Neoplasm, by site,
      malignant
    unspecified site 157.4
  pancreas 211.7
  specified site — *see* Neoplasm, by site, be-
    nign
  unspecified site 211.7
Insuloma — *see* Insulinoma
Insult
  brain 437.9
    acute 436
  cerebral 437.9

Insult — *continued*
  cerebral — *continued*
    acute 436
  cerebrovascular 437.9
    acute 436
  vascular NEC 437.9
    acute 436
Insurance examination (certification) V70.3
Intemperance — *see also* Alcoholism 303.9 ☑
Interception of pregnancy (menstrual extraction) V25.3
Interference
  balancing side 524.56
  non-working side 524.56
Intermenstrual
  bleeding 626.6
    irregular 626.6
    regular 626.5
  hemorrhage 626.6
    irregular 626.6
    regular 626.5
  pain(s) 625.2
Intermittent — *see* condition
Internal — *see* condition
Interproximal wear 521.10
Interrogation
  cardiac defibrillator (automatic) (im-
    plantable) V53.32
  cardiac pacemaker V53.31
  cardiac (event) (loop) recorder V53.39
  infusion pump (implanted) (intrathecal)
    V53.09
  neurostimulator V53.02
Interruption
  aortic arch 747.11
  bundle of His 426.50
  fallopian tube (for sterilization) V25.2
  phase-shift, sleep cycle 307.45
  repeated REM-sleep 307.48
  sleep
    due to perceived environmental distur-
      bances 307.48
    phase-shift, of 24-hour sleep-wake cycle
      307.45
    repeated REM-sleep type 307.48
  vas deferens (for sterilization) V25.2
Intersexuality 752.7
Interstitial — *see* condition
Intertrigo 695.89
  labialis 528.5
Intervertebral disc — *see* condition
Intestine, intestinal — *see also* condition
  flu 487.8
Intolerance
  carbohydrate NEC 579.8
  cardiovascular exercise, with pain (at rest)
    (with less than ordinary activity)
    (with ordinary activity) V47.2
  cold 780.99
  dissacharide (hereditary) 271.3
  drug
    correct substance properly administered
      995.27
    wrong substance given or taken in error
      977.9
    specified drug — *see* Table of Drugs
      and Chemicals
  effort 306.2
  fat NEC 579.8
  foods NEC 579.8
  fructose (hereditary) 271.2
  glucose (-galactose) (congenital) 271.3
  gluten 579.0
  lactose (hereditary) (infantile) 271.3
  lysine (congenital) 270.7
  milk NEC 579.8
  protein (familial) 270.7
  starch NEC 579.8
  sucrose (-isomaltose) (congenital) 271.3
Intoxicated NEC — *see also* Alcoholism
  305.0 ☑
Intoxication
  acid 276.2
  acute
    alcoholic 305.0 ☑
      with alcoholism 303.0 ☑

Intoxication — *continued*
  acute — *continued*
    alcoholic — *continued*
      hangover effects 305.0 ☑
    caffeine 305.9 ☑
    hallucinogenic (*see also* Abuse, drugs,
      nondependent) 305.3 ☑
  alcohol (acute) 305.0 ☑
    with alcoholism 303.0 ☑
    hangover effects 305.0 ☑
    idiosyncratic 291.4
    pathological 291.4
  alimentary canal 558.2
  ammonia (hepatic) 572.2
  caffeine 305.9 ☑
  chemical (*see also* Table of Drugs and
    Chemicals)
    via placenta or breast milk 760.70
      alcohol 760.71
      anticonvulsants
      antifungals
      anti-infective agents 760.74
      antimetabolics
      cocaine 760.75
      "crack" 760.75
      hallucinogenic agents NEC 760.73
      medicinal agents NEC 760.79
      narcotics 760.72
      obstetric anesthetic or analgesic drug
        763.5
      specified agent NEC 760.79
      suspected, affecting management of
        pregnancy 655.5 ☑
  cocaine, through placenta or breast milk
    760.75
  delirium
    alcohol 291.0
    drug 292.81
  drug 292.89
    with delirium 292.81
    correct substance properly administered
      (*see also* Allergy, drug) 995.27
    newborn 779.4
    obstetric anesthetic or sedation 668.9 ☑
      affecting fetus or newborn 763.5
    overdose or wrong substance given or
      taken — *see* Table of Drugs and
      Chemicals
    pathologic 292.2
    specific to newborn 779.4
    via placenta or breast milk 760.70
      alcohol 760.71
      anticonvulsants 760.77
      antifungals 760.74
      anti-infective agents 760.74
      antimetabolics 760.78
      cocaine 760.75
      "crack" 760.75
      hallucinogenic agents 760.73
      medicinal agents NEC 760.79
      narcotics 760.72
      obstetric anesthetic or analgesic drug
        763.5
      specified agent NEC 760.79
      suspected, affecting management of
        pregnancy 655.5 ☑
  enteric — *see* Intoxication, intestinal
  fetus or newborn, via placenta or breast milk
    760.70
    alcohol 760.71
    anticonvulsants 760.77
    antifungals 760.74
    anti-infective agents 760.74
    antimetabolics 760.78
    cocaine 760.75
    "crack" 760.75
    hallucinogenic agents 760.73
    medicinal agents NEC 760.79
    narcotics 760.72
    obstetric anesthetic or analgesic drug
      763.5
    specified agent NEC 760.79
    suspected, affecting management of
      pregnancy 655.5 ☑
  food — *see* Poisoning, food
  gastrointestinal 558.2

☑ **Additional Digit Required** — Refer to the Tabular List for Digit Selection   ▽ **Subterms under main terms may continue to next column or page**

Intoxication — *continued*
- hallucinogenic (acute) 305.3 ☑
- hepatocerebral 572.2
- idiosyncratic alcohol 291.4
- intestinal 569.89
  - due to putrefaction of food 005.9
- methyl alcohol (*see also* Alcoholism) 305.0 ☑
  - with alcoholism 303.0 ☑
- non-foodborne due to toxins of Clostridium botulinum [C. botulinum] — *see* Botulism
- pathologic 291.4
  - drug 292.2
- potassium (K) 276.7
- septic
  - with
    - abortion — *see* Abortion, by type, with sepsis
    - ectopic pregnancy (*see also* categories 633.0–633.9) 639.0
    - molar pregnancy (*see also* categories 630–632) 639.0
  - during labor 659.3 ☑
  - following
    - abortion 639.0
    - ectopic or molar pregnancy 639.0
  - generalized — *see* Septicemia
  - puerperal, postpartum, childbirth 670.2 ☑
- serum (prophylactic) (therapeutic) 999.59
- uremic — *see* Uremia
- water 276.69

Intracranial — *see* condition
Intrahepatic gallbladder 751.69
Intraligamentous — *see also* condition
- pregnancy — *see* Pregnancy, cornual

Intraocular — *see also* condition
- sepsis 360.00

Intrathoracic — *see also* condition
- kidney 753.3
- stomach — *see* Hernia, diaphragm

Intrauterine contraceptive device
- checking V25.42
- insertion V25.11
- in situ V45.51
- management V25.42
- prescription V25.02
  - repeat V25.42
- reinsertion V25.13
- removal V25.12
  - and reinsertion V25.13
- replacement V25.13

Intraventricular — *see* condition
Intrinsic deformity — *see* Deformity
Intruded tooth 524.34
Intrusion, repetitive, of sleep (due to environmental disturbances) (with atypical polysomnographic features) 307.48
Intumescent, lens (eye) NEC 366.9
- senile 366.12
Intussusception (colon) (enteric) (intestine) (rectum) 560.0
- appendix 543.9
- congenital 751.5
- fallopian tube 620.8
- ileocecal 560.0
- ileocolic 560.0
- ureter (with obstruction) 593.4
Invagination
- basilar 756.0
- colon or intestine 560.0
Invalid (since birth) 799.89
Invalidism (chronic) 799.89
Inversion
- albumin-globulin (A-G) ratio 273.8
- bladder 596.89
- cecum (*see also* Intussusception) 560.0
- cervix 622.8
- nipple 611.79
  - congenital 757.6
  - puerperal, postpartum 676.3 ☑
- optic papilla 743.57
- organ or site, congenital NEC — *see* Anomaly, specified type NEC
- sleep rhythm 327.39

Inversion — *continued*
- sleep rhythm — *continued*
  - nonorganic origin 307.45
- testis (congenital) 752.51
- uterus (postinfectional) (postpartal, old) 621.7
  - chronic 621.7
  - complicating delivery 665.2 ☑
    - affecting fetus or newborn 763.89
- vagina — *see* Prolapse, vagina
Investigation
- allergens V72.7
- clinical research (control) (normal comparison) (participant) V70.7
Inviability — *see* Immaturity
Involuntary movement, abnormal 781.0
Involution, involutional — *see also* condition
- breast, cystic or fibrocystic 610.1
- depression (*see also* Psychosis, affective) 296.2 ☑
  - recurrent episode 296.3 ☑
  - single episode 296.2 ☑
- melancholia (*see also* Psychosis, affective) 296.2 ☑
  - recurrent episode 296.3 ☑
  - single episode 296.2 ☑
- ovary, senile 620.3
- paranoid state (reaction) 297.2
- paraphrenia (climacteric) (menopause) 297.2
- psychosis 298.8
- thymus failure 254.8
IQ
- under 20 318.2
- 20-34 318.1
- 35-49 318.0
- 50-70 317
IRDS 769
Irideremia 743.45
Iridis rubeosis 364.42
- diabetic 250.5 ☑ *[364.42]*
  - due to secondary diabetes 249.5 ☑ *[364.42]*
Iridochoroiditis (panuveitis) 360.12
Iridocyclitis NEC 364.3
- acute 364.00
  - primary 364.01
  - recurrent 364.02
- chronic 364.10
  - in
    - lepromatous leprosy 030.0 *[364.11]*
    - sarcoidosis 135 *[364.11]*
    - tuberculosis (*see also* Tuberculosis) 017.3 ☑ *[364.11]*
- due to allergy 364.04
- endogenous 364.01
- gonococcal 098.41
- granulomatous 364.10
- herpetic (simplex) 054.44
  - zoster 053.22
- hypopyon 364.05
- lens induced 364.23
- nongranulomatous 364.00
- primary 364.01
- recurrent 364.02
- rheumatic 364.10
- secondary 364.04
  - infectious 364.03
  - noninfectious 364.04
- subacute 364.00
  - primary 364.01
  - recurrent 364.02
- sympathetic 360.11
- syphilitic (secondary) 091.52
- tuberculous (chronic) (*see also* Tuberculosis) 017.3 ☑ *[364.11]*
Iridocyclochoroiditis (panuveitis) 360.12
Iridodialysis 364.76
Iridodonesis 364.89
Iridoplegia (complete) (partial) (reflex) 379.49
Iridoschisis 364.52
IRIS (Immune Reconstitution Inflammatory Syndrome) 995.90
Iris — *see* condition
Iritis 364.3
- acute 364.00

Iritis — *continued*
- acute — *continued*
  - primary 364.01
  - recurrent 364.02
- chronic 364.10
  - in
    - sarcoidosis 135 *[364.11]*
    - tuberculosis (*see also* Tuberculosis) 017.3 ☑ *[364.11]*
- diabetic 250.5 ☑ *[364.42]*
  - due to secondary diabetes 249.5 ☑ *[364.42]*
- due to
  - allergy 364.04
  - herpes simplex 054.44
  - leprosy 030.0 *[364.11]*
- endogenous 364.01
- gonococcal 098.41
- gouty 274.89 *[364.11]*
- granulomatous 364.10
- hypopyon 364.05
- lens induced 364.23
- nongranulomatous 364.00
- papulosa 095.8 *[364.11]*
- primary 364.01
- recurrent 364.02
- rheumatic 364.10
- secondary 364.04
  - infectious 364.03
  - noninfectious 364.04
- subacute 364.00
  - primary 364.01
  - recurrent 364.02
- sympathetic 360.11
- syphilitic (secondary) 091.52
  - congenital 090.0 *[364.11]*
  - late 095.8 *[364.11]*
- tuberculous (*see also* Tuberculosis) 017.3 ☑ *[364.11]*
- uratic 274.89 *[364.11]*
Iron
- deficiency anemia 280.9
- metabolism disease 275.09
- storage disease 275.09
Iron-miners' lung 503
Irradiated enamel (tooth, teeth) 521.89
Irradiation
- burn — *see* Burn, by site
- effects, adverse 990
Irreducible, irreducibility — *see* condition
Irregular, irregularity
- action, heart 427.9
- alveolar process 525.8
- bleeding NEC 626.4
- breathing 786.09
- colon 569.89
- contour
  - acquired 371.70
  - of cornea 743.41
    - acquired 371.70
  - reconstructed breast 612.0
- dentin in pulp 522.3
- eye movements NEC 379.59
- menstruation (cause unknown) 626.4
- periods 626.4
- prostate 602.9
- pupil 364.75
- respiratory 786.09
- septum (nasal) 470
- shape, organ or site, congenital NEC — *see* Distortion
- sleep-wake rhythm (non-24-hour) 327.39
  - nonorganic origin 307.45
- vertebra 733.99
Irritability 799.22
- bladder 596.89
  - neurogenic 596.54
    - with cauda equina syndrome 344.61
- bowel (syndrome) 564.1
- bronchial (*see also* Bronchitis) 490
- cerebral, newborn 779.1
- colon 564.1
  - psychogenic 306.4
- duodenum 564.89
- heart (psychogenic) 306.2
- ileum 564.89

Irritability — *continued*
- jejunum 564.89
- myocardium 306.2
- nervousness 799.21
- rectum 564.89
- stomach 536.9
  - psychogenic 306.4
- sympathetic (nervous system) (*see also* Neuropathy, peripheral, autonomic) 337.9
- urethra 599.84
- ventricular (heart) (psychogenic) 306.2
Irritable — *see also* Irritability 799.22
Irritation
- anus 569.49
- axillary nerve 353.0
- bladder 596.89
- brachial plexus 353.0
- brain (traumatic) (*see also* Injury, intracranial) 854.0 ☑
  - nontraumatic — *see* Encephalitis
- bronchial (*see also* Bronchitis) 490
- cerebral (traumatic) (*see also* Injury, intracranial) 854.0 ☑
  - nontraumatic — *see* Encephalitis
- cervical plexus 353.2
- cervix (*see also* Cervicitis) 616.0
- choroid, sympathetic 360.11
- cranial nerve — *see* Disorder, nerve, cranial
- digestive tract 536.9
  - psychogenic 306.4
- gastric 536.9
  - psychogenic 306.4
- gastrointestinal (tract) 536.9
  - functional 536.9
  - psychogenic 306.4
- globe, sympathetic 360.11
- intestinal (bowel) 564.9
- labyrinth 386.50
- lumbosacral plexus 353.1
- meninges (traumatic) (*see also* Injury, intracranial) 854.0 ☑
  - nontraumatic — *see* Meningitis
- myocardium 306.2
- nerve — *see* Disorder, nerve
- nervous 799.21
- nose 478.19
- penis 607.89
- perineum 709.9
- peripheral
  - autonomic nervous system (*see also* Neuropathy, peripheral, autonomic) 337.9
  - nerve — *see* Disorder, nerve
- peritoneum (*see also* Peritonitis) 567.9
- pharynx 478.29
- plantar nerve 355.6
- spinal (cord) (traumatic) (*see also* Injury, spinal, by site)
  - nerve (*see also* Disorder, nerve)
    - root NEC 724.9
    - traumatic — *see* Injury, nerve, spinal
  - nontraumatic — *see* Myelitis
- stomach 536.9
  - psychogenic 306.4
- sympathetic nerve NEC (*see also* Neuropathy, peripheral, autonomic) 337.9
- ulnar nerve 354.2
- vagina 623.9
Isambert's disease 012.3 ☑
Ischemia, ischemic 459.9
- basilar artery (with transient neurologic deficit) 435.0
- bone NEC 733.40
- bowel (transient) 557.9
  - acute 557.0
  - chronic 557.1
  - due to mesenteric artery insufficiency 557.1
- brain (*see also* Ischemia, cerebral)
  - recurrent focal 435.9
- cardiac (*see also* Ischemia, heart) 414.9
- cardiomyopathy 414.8
- carotid artery (with transient neurologic deficit) 435.8
- cerebral (chronic) (generalized) 437.1

Ischemia, ischemic — *continued*
cerebral — *continued*
arteriosclerotic 437.0
intermittent (with transient neurologic deficit) 435.9
newborn 779.2
puerperal, postpartum, childbirth 674.0 ☑
recurrent focal (with transient neurologic deficit) 435.9
transient (with transient neurologic deficit) 435.9
colon 557.9
acute 557.0
chronic 557.1
due to mesenteric artery insufficiency 557.1
coronary (chronic) (*see also* Ischemia, heart) 414.9
demand 411.89
heart (chronic or with a stated duration of over 8 weeks) 414.9
acute or with a stated duration of 8 weeks or less (*see also* Infarct, myocardium) 410.9 ☑
without myocardial infarction 411.89
with coronary (artery) occlusion 411.81
subacute 411.89
intestine (transient) 557.9
acute 557.0
chronic 557.1
due to mesenteric artery insufficiency 557.1
kidney 593.81
labyrinth 386.50

Ischemia, ischemic — *continued*
muscles, leg 728.89
myocardium, myocardial (chronic or with a stated duration of over 8 weeks) 414.8
acute (*see also* Infarct, myocardium) 410.9 ☑
without myocardial infarction 411.89
with coronary (artery) occlusion 411.81
renal 593.81
retina, retinal 362.84
small bowel 557.9
acute 557.0
chronic 557.1
due to mesenteric artery insufficiency 557.1
spinal cord 336.1
subendocardial (*see also* Insufficiency, coronary) 411.89
supply (*see also* Angina) 414.9
vertebral artery (with transient neurologic deficit) 435.1
Ischialgia — *see also* Sciatica 724.3
Ischiopagus 759.4
Ischium, ischial — *see* condition
Ischomenia 626.8
Ischuria 788.5
Iselin's disease or osteochondrosis 732.5
Islands of
parotid tissue in
lymph nodes 750.26
neck structures 750.26
submaxillary glands in
fascia 750.26
lymph nodes 750.26

Islands of — *continued*
submaxillary glands in — *continued*
neck muscles 750.26
Islet cell tumor, pancreas (M8150/0) 211.7
Isoimmunization NEC — *see also* Incompatibility 656.2 ☑
anti-E 656.2 ☑
fetus or newborn 773.2
ABO blood groups 773.1
Rhesus (Rh) factor 773.0
Isolation V07.0
social V62.4
Isosporosis 007.2
Issue
medical certificate NEC V68.09
cause of death V68.09
disability examination V68.01
fitness V68.09
incapacity V68.09
repeat prescription NEC V68.1
appliance V68.1
contraceptive V25.40
device NEC V25.49
intrauterine V25.42
specified type NEC V25.49
pill V25.41
glasses V68.1
medicinal substance V68.1
Itch — *see also* Pruritus 698.9
bakers' 692.89
barbers' 110.0
bricklayers' 692.89
cheese 133.8
clam diggers' 120.3
coolie 126.9
copra 133.8

Itch — *see also* Pruritus — *continued*
Cuban 050.1
dew 126.9
dhobie 110.3
eye 379.99
filarial (*see also* Infestation, filarial) 125.9
grain 133.8
grocers' 133.8
ground 126.9
harvest 133.8
jock 110.3
Malabar 110.9
beard 110.0
foot 110.4
scalp 110.0
meaning scabies 133.0
Norwegian 133.0
perianal 698.0
poultrymen's 133.8
sarcoptic 133.0
scrub 134.1
seven year V61.10
meaning scabies 133.0
straw 133.8
swimmers' 120.3
washerwoman's 692.4
water 120.3
winter 698.8
Itsenko-Cushing syndrome (pituitary basophilism) 255.0
Ivemark's syndrome (asplenia with congenital heart disease) 759.0
Ivory bones 756.52
Ixodes 134.8
Ixodiasis 134.8

J

Jaccoud's nodular fibrositis, chronic (Jaccoud's syndrome) 714.4
Jackson's
  membrane 751.4
  paralysis or syndrome 344.89
  veil 751.4
Jacksonian
  epilepsy (see also Epilepsy) 345.5 ☑
  seizures (focal) (see also Epilepsy) 345.5 ☑
Jacob's ulcer (M8090/3) — see Neoplasm, skin, malignant, by site
Jacquet's dermatitis (diaper dermatitis) 691.0
Jadassohn's
  blue nevus (M8780/0) — see Neoplasm, skin, benign
  disease (maculopapular erythroderma) 696.2
  intraepidermal epithelioma (M8096/0) — see Neoplasm, skin, benign
Jadassohn-Lewandowski syndrome (pachyonychia congenita) 757.5
Jadassohn-Pellizari's disease (anetoderma) 701.3
Jadassohn-Tièche nevus (M8780/0) — see Neoplasm, skin, benign
Jaffe-Lichtenstein (-Uehlinger) syndrome 252.01
Jahnke's syndrome (encephalocutaneous angiomatosis) 759.6
Jakob-Creutzfeldt disease (CJD) (syndrome) 046.19
  with dementia
    with behavioral disturbance 046.19 [294.11]
    without behavioral disturbance 046.19 [294.10]
  familial 046.19
  iatrogenic 046.19
  specified NEC 046.19
  sporadic 046.19
  variant (vCJD) 046.11
    with dementia
      with behavioral disturbance 046.11 [294.11]
      without behavioral disturbance 046.11 [294.10]
Jaksch (-Luzet) disease or syndrome (pseudoleukemia infantum) 285.8
Jamaican
  neuropathy 349.82
  paraplegic tropical ataxic-spastic syndrome 349.82
Janet's disease (psychasthenia) 300.89
Janiceps 759.4
Jansky-Bielschowsky amaurotic familial idiocy 330.1
Japanese
  B type encephalitis 062.0
  river fever 081.2
  seven-day fever 100.89
Jaundice (yellow) 782.4
  acholuric (familial) (splenomegalic) (see also Spherocytosis) 282.0
    acquired 283.9
  breast milk 774.39
  catarrhal (acute) 070.1
    with hepatic coma 070.0
    chronic 571.9
    epidemic — see Jaundice, epidemic
  cholestatic (benign) 782.4
  chronic idiopathic 277.4
  epidemic (catarrhal) 070.1
    with hepatic coma 070.0
    leptospiral 100.0
    spirochetal 100.0
  febrile (acute) 070.1
    with hepatic coma 070.0
    leptospiral 100.0
    spirochetal 100.0
  fetus or newborn 774.6
    due to or associated with
      ABO
        absence or deficiency of enzyme system for bilirubin conjugation (congenital) 774.39

Jaundice — continued
  fetus or newborn — continued
    due to or associated with — continued
      antibodies 773.1
      blood group incompatibility NEC 773.2
      breast milk inhibitors to conjugation 774.39
        associated with preterm delivery 774.2
      bruising 774.1
      Crigler-Najjar syndrome 277.4 [774.31]
      delayed conjugation 774.30
        associated with preterm delivery 774.2
        development 774.39
      drugs or toxins transmitted from mother 774.1
      G-6-PD deficiency 282.2 [774.0]
      galactosemia 271.1 [774.5]
      Gilbert's syndrome 277.4 [774.31]
      hepatocellular damage 774.4
      hereditary hemolytic anemia (see also Anemia, hemolytic) 282.9 [774.0]
      hypothyroidism, congenital 243 [774.31]
      incompatibility, maternal/fetal 773.1
      incompatibility, maternal/fetal NEC 773.2
      infection 774.1
      inspissated bile syndrome 774.4
      isoimmunization 773.1
      isoimmunization NEC 773.2
      mucoviscidosis 277.01 [774.5]
      obliteration of bile duct, congenital 751.61 [774.5]
      polycythemia 774.1
      preterm delivery 774.2
      red cell defect 282.9 [774.0]
      Rh
        antibodies 773.0
        incompatibility, maternal/fetal 773.0
        isoimmunization 773.0
      spherocytosis (congenital) 282.0 [774.0]
      swallowed maternal blood 774.1
    physiological NEC 774.6
  from injection, inoculation, infusion, or transfusion (blood) (plasma) (serum) (other substance) (onset within 8 months after administration) — see Hepatitis, viral
  Gilbert's (familial nonhemolytic) 277.4
  hematogenous 283.9
  hemolytic (acquired) 283.9
    congenital (see also Spherocytosis) 282.0
  hemorrhagic (acute) 100.0
    leptospiral 100.0
    newborn 776.0
    spirochetal 100.0
  hepatocellular 573.8
  homologous (serum) — see Hepatitis, viral
  idiopathic, chronic 277.4
  infectious (acute) (subacute) 070.1
    with hepatic coma 070.0
    leptospiral 100.0
    spirochetal 100.0
  leptospiral 100.0
  malignant (see also Necrosis, liver) 570
  newborn (physiological) (see also Jaundice, fetus or newborn) 774.6
  nonhemolytic, congenital familial (Gilbert's) 277.4
  nuclear, newborn (see also Kernicterus of newborn) 774.7
  obstructive NEC (see also Obstruction, biliary) 576.8
  postimmunization — see Hepatitis, viral
  posttransfusion — see Hepatitis, viral
  regurgitation (see also Obstruction, biliary) 576.8

Jaundice — continued
  serum (homologous) (prophylactic) (therapeutic) — see Hepatitis, viral
  spirochetal (hemorrhagic) 100.0
  symptomatic 782.4
    newborn 774.6
Jaw — see condition
Jaw-blinking 374.43
  congenital 742.8
Jaw-winking phenomenon or syndrome 742.8
Jealousy
  alcoholic 291.5
  childhood 313.3
  sibling 313.3
Jejunitis — see also Enteritis 558.9
Jejunostomy status V44.4
Jejunum, jejunal — see condition
Jensen's disease 363.05
Jericho boil 085.1
Jerks, myoclonic 333.2
Jervell-Lange-Nielsen syndrome 426.82
Jeune's disease or syndrome (asphyxiating thoracic dystrophy) 756.4
Jigger disease 134.1
Job's syndrome (chronic granulomatous disease) 288.1
Jod-Basedow phenomenon 242.8 ☑
Johnson-Stevens disease (erythema multiforme exudativum) 695.13
Joint — see also condition
  Charcôt's 094.0 [713.5]
  false 733.82
  flail — see Flail, joint
  mice — see Loose, body, joint, by site
  sinus to bone 730.9 ☑
  von Gies' 095.8
Jordan's anomaly or syndrome 288.2
Josephs-Diamond-Blackfan anemia (congenital hypoplastic) 284.01
Joubert syndrome 759.89
Jumpers' knee 727.2
Jungle yellow fever 060.0
Jüngling's disease (sarcoidosis) 135
Junin virus hemorrhagic fever 078.7
Juvenile — see also condition
  delinquent 312.9
    group (see also Disturbance, conduct) 312.2 ☑
  neurotic 312.4

K

Kabuki syndrome 759.89
Kahler (-Bozzolo) disease (multiple myeloma) (M9730/3) 203.0 ☑
Kakergasia 300.9
Kakke 265.0
Kala-azar (Indian) (infantile) (Mediterranean) (Sudanese) 085.0
Kalischer's syndrome (encephalocutaneous angiomatosis) 759.6
Kallmann's syndrome (hypogonadotropic hypogonadism with anosmia) 253.4
Kanner's syndrome (autism) — see also Psychosis, childhood 299.0 ☑
Kaolinosis 502
Kaposi's
  disease 757.33
    lichen ruber 696.4
      acuminatus 696.4
      moniliformis 697.8
    xeroderma pigmentosum 757.33
  sarcoma (M9140/3) 176.9
    adipose tissue 176.1
    aponeurosis 176.1
    artery 176.1
    associated herpesvirus infection 058.89
    blood vessel 176.1
    bursa 176.1
    connective tissue 176.1
    external genitalia 176.8
    fascia 176.1
    fatty tissue 176.1
    fibrous tissue 176.1
    gastrointestinal tract NEC 176.3
    ligament 176.1

Kaposi's — continued
  sarcoma — continued
    lung 176.4
    lymph
      gland(s) 176.5
      node(s) 176.5
    lymphatic(s) NEC 176.1
    muscle (skeletal) 176.1
    oral cavity NEC 176.8
    palate 176.2
    scrotum 176.8
    skin 176.0
    soft tissue 176.1
    specified site NEC 176.8
    subcutaneous tissue 176.1
    synovia 176.1
    tendon (sheath) 176.1
    vein 176.1
    vessel 176.1
    viscera NEC 176.9
    vulva 176.8
  varicelliform eruption 054.0
    vaccinia 999.0
Kartagener's syndrome or triad (sinusitis, bronchiectasis, situs inversus) 759.3
Kasabach-Merritt syndrome (capillary hemangioma associated with thrombocytopenic purpura) 287.39
Kaschin-Beck disease (endemic polyarthritis) — see Disease, Kaschin-Beck
Kast's syndrome (dyschondroplasia with hemangiomas) 756.4
Katatonia — see Catatonia
Katayama disease or fever 120.2
Kathisophobia 781.0
Kawasaki disease 446.1
Kayser-Fleischer ring (cornea) (pseudosclerosis) 275.1 [371.14]
Kaznelson's syndrome (congenital hypoplastic anemia) 284.01
Kearns-Sayre syndrome 277.87
Kedani fever 081.2
Kelis 701.4
Kelly (-Patterson) syndrome (sideropenic dysphagia) 280.8
Keloid, cheloid 701.4
  Addison's (morphea) 701.0
  cornea 371.00
  Hawkins' 701.4
  scar 701.4
Keloma 701.4
Kenya fever 082.1
Keratectasia 371.71
  congenital 743.41
Keratinization NEC
  alveolar ridge mucosa
    excessive 528.72
    minimal 528.71
Keratitis (nodular) (nonulcerative) (simple) (zonular) NEC 370.9
  with ulceration (see also Ulcer, cornea) 370.00
  actinic 370.24
  arborescens 054.42
  areolar 370.22
  bullosa 370.8
  deep — see Keratitis, interstitial
  dendritic(a) 054.42
  desiccation 370.34
  diffuse interstitial 370.52
  disciform(is) 054.43
    varicella 052.7 [370.44]
  epithelialis vernalis 372.13 [370.32]
  exposure 370.34
  filamentary 370.23
  gonococcal (congenital) (prenatal) 098.43
  herpes, herpetic (simplex) NEC 054.43
    zoster 053.21
  hypopyon 370.04
  in
    chickenpox 052.7 [370.44]
    exanthema (see also Exanthem) 057.9 [370.44]
    paravaccinia (see also Paravaccinia) 051.9 [370.44]

☑ Additional Digit Required — Refer to the Tabular List for Digit Selection   ᵂ Subterms under main terms may continue to next column or page

2015 ICD-9-CM   ▶◀ Revised Text   ● New Line   ▲ Revised Code   Volume 2 — 169

☑ **Additional Digit Required — Refer to the Tabular List for Digit Selection**   ▽ **Subterms under main terms may continue to next column or page**

Kyphosis, kyphotic — *continued*
due to or associated with — *continued*
osteitis
deformans 731.0 *[737.41]*
fibrosa cystica 252.01 *[737.41]*
osteoporosis (*see also* Osteoporosis)
733.0 ✔ *[737.41]*
poliomyelitis (*see also* Poliomyelitis)
138 *[737.41]*
radiation 737.11
tuberculosis (*see also* Tuberculosis)
015.0 ✔ *[737.41]*
Kümmell's 721.7
late effect of rickets 268.1 *[737.41]*
Morquio-Brailsford type (spinal)
277.5 *[737.41]*
pelvis 738.6
postlaminectomy 737.12
specified cause NEC 737.19
syphilitic, congenital 090.5 *[737.41]*
tuberculous (*see also* Tuberculosis)
015.0 ✔ *[737.41]*
Kyrle's disease (hyperkeratosis follicularis in
cutem penetrans) 701.1

L

Labia, labium — *see* condition
Labiated hymen 752.49
Labile
blood pressure 796.2
emotions, emotionality 301.3
vasomotor system 443.9
Lability, emotional 799.24
Labioglossal paralysis 335.22
Labium leporinum — *see also* Cleft, lip 749.10
Labor — *see also* Delivery
with complications — *see* Delivery, complicated
abnormal NEC 661.9 ✔
affecting fetus or newborn 763.7
arrested active phase 661.1 ✔
affecting fetus or newborn 763.7
desultory 661.2 ✔
affecting fetus or newborn 763.7
dyscoordinate 661.4 ✔
affecting fetus or newborn 763.7
early onset (22-36 weeks gestation)
644.2 ✔
failed
induction 659.1 ✔
mechanical 659.0 ✔
medical 659.1 ✔
surgical 659.0 ✔
trial (vaginal delivery) 660.6 ✔
false 644.1 ✔
forced or induced, affecting fetus or newborn 763.89
hypertonic 661.4 ✔
affecting fetus or newborn 763.7
hypotonic 661.2 ✔
affecting fetus or newborn 763.7
primary 661.0 ✔
affecting fetus or newborn 763.7
secondary 661.1 ✔
affecting fetus or newborn 763.7
incoordinate 661.4 ✔
affecting fetus or newborn 763.7
irregular 661.2 ✔
affecting fetus or newborn 763.7
long — *see* Labor, prolonged
missed (at or near term) 656.4 ✔
obstructed NEC 660.9 ✔
affecting fetus or newborn 763.1
due to female genital mutilation
660.8 ✔
specified cause NEC 660.8 ✔
affecting fetus or newborn 763.1
pains, spurious 644.1 ✔
precipitate 661.3 ✔
affecting fetus or newborn 763.6
premature 644.2 ✔
threatened 644.0 ✔
prolonged or protracted 662.1 ✔
first stage 662.0 ✔
affecting fetus or newborn 763.89

Labor — *see also* Delivery — *continued*
prolonged or protracted — *continued*
second stage 662.2 ✔
affecting fetus or newborn 763.89
affecting fetus or newborn 763.89
threatened NEC 644.1 ✔
undelivered 644.1 ✔
Labored breathing — *see also* Hyperventilation 786.09
Labyrinthitis (inner ear) (destructive) (latent)
386.30
circumscribed 386.32
diffuse 386.31
focal 386.32
purulent 386.33
serous 386.31
suppurative 386.33
syphilitic 095.8
toxic 386.34
viral 386.35
Laceration — *see also* Wound, open, by site
accidental, complicating surgery 998.2
Achilles tendon 845.09
with open wound 892.2
anus (sphincter) 879.6
with
abortion — *see* Abortion, by type,
with damage to pelvic organs
ectopic pregnancy (*see also* categories 633.0–633.9) 639.2
molar pregnancy (*see also* categories
630–632) 639.2
complicated 879.7
complicating delivery (healed) (old)
654.8 ✔
with laceration of anal or rectal mucosa 664.3 ✔
not associated with third-degree
perineal laceration 664.6 ✔
following
abortion 639.2
ectopic or molar pregnancy 639.2
nontraumatic, nonpuerperal (healed)
(old) 569.43
bladder (urinary)
with
abortion — *see* Abortion, by type,
with damage to pelvic organs
ectopic pregnancy (*see also* categories 633.0–633.9) 639.2
molar pregnancy (*see also* categories
630–632) 639.2
following
abortion 639.2
ectopic or molar pregnancy 639.2
obstetrical trauma 665.5 ✔
blood vessel — *see* Injury, blood vessel, by
site
bowel
with
abortion — *see* Abortion, by type,
with damage to pelvic organs
ectopic pregnancy (*see also* categories 633.0–633.9) 639.2
molar pregnancy (*see also* categories
630–632) 639.2
following
abortion 639.2
ectopic or molar pregnancy 639.2
obstetrical trauma 665.5 ✔

Laceration — *see also* Wound, open, by site —
continued
brain (cerebral) (membrane) (with hemorrhage) 851.8 ✔

> *Note* — Use the following fifth-digit
> subclassification with categories
> 851–854:
>
> 0   unspecified state of consciousness
>
> 1   with no loss of consciousness
>
> 2   with brief [less than one hour]
>   loss of consciousness
>
> 3   with moderate [1–24 hours] loss
>   of consciousness
>
> 4   with prolonged [more than 24
>   hours] loss of consciousness and
>   return to pre–existing conscious
>   level
>
> 5   with prolonged [more than 24
>   hours] loss of consciousness,
>   without return to pre–existing
>   conscious level
>
> *Use fifth-digit 5 to designate when a
> patient is unconscious and dies before
> regaining consciousness, regardless of
> the duration of the loss of consciousness*
>
> 6   with loss of consciousness of un-
>   specified duration
>
> 9   with concussion, unspecified

with
open intracranial wound 851.9 ✔
skull fracture — *see* Fracture, skull,
by site
cerebellum 851.6 ✔
with open intracranial wound
851.7 ✔
cortex 851.2 ✔
with open intracranial wound
851.3 ✔
during birth 767.0
stem 851.6 ✔
with open intracranial wound
851.7 ✔
broad ligament
with
abortion — *see* Abortion, by type,
with damage to pelvic organs
ectopic pregnancy (*see also* categories 633.0–633.9) 639.2
molar pregnancy (*see also* categories
630–632) 639.2
following
abortion 639.2
ectopic or molar pregnancy 639.2
nontraumatic 620.6
obstetrical trauma 665.6 ✔
syndrome (nontraumatic) 620.6
capsule, joint — *see* Sprain, by site
cardiac — *see* Laceration, heart
causing eversion of cervix uteri (old) 622.0
central, complicating delivery 664.4 ✔
cerebellum — *see* Laceration, brain, cerebellum
cerebral (*see also* Laceration, brain)
during birth 767.0
cervix (uteri)
with
abortion — *see* Abortion, by type,
with damage to pelvic organs
ectopic pregnancy (*see also* categories 633.0–633.9) 639.2
molar pregnancy (*see also* categories
630–632) 639.2
following
abortion 639.2
ectopic or molar pregnancy 639.2
nonpuerperal, nontraumatic 622.3
obstetrical trauma (current) 665.3 ✔
old (postpartal) 622.3
traumatic — *see* Injury, internal, cervix
chordae heart 429.5
complicated 879.9

Laceration — *see also* Wound, open, by site —
continued
cornea — *see* Laceration, eyeball
superficial 918.1
cortex (cerebral) — *see* Laceration, brain,
cortex
esophagus 530.89
eye(s) — *see* Laceration, ocular
eyeball NEC 871.4
with prolapse or exposure of intraocular
tissue 871.1
penetrating — *see* Penetrating wound,
eyeball
specified as without prolapse of intraocular tissue 871.0
eyelid NEC 870.8
full thickness 870.1
involving lacrimal passages 870.2
skin (and periocular area) 870.0
penetrating — *see* Penetrating
wound, orbit
fourchette
with
abortion — *see* Abortion, by type,
with damage to pelvic organs
ectopic pregnancy (*see also* categories 633.0–633.9) 639.2
molar pregnancy (*see also* categories
630–632) 639.2
complicating delivery 664.0 ✔
following
abortion 639.2
ectopic or molar pregnancy 639.2
heart (without penetration of heart chambers) 861.02
with
open wound into thorax 861.12
penetration of heart chambers
861.03
with open wound into thorax
861.13
hernial sac — *see* Hernia, by site
internal organ (abdomen) (chest) (pelvis)
NEC — *see* Injury, internal, by site
NEC — *see* Injury, internal, by site
kidney (parenchyma) 866.02
with
complete disruption of parenchyma
(rupture) 866.03
with open wound into cavity
866.13
open wound into cavity 866.12
labia
complicating delivery 664.0 ✔
ligament (*see also* Sprain, by site)
with open wound — *see* Wound, open,
by site
liver 864.05
with open wound into cavity 864.15
major (disruption of hepatic parenchyma) 864.04
with open wound into cavity 864.14
minor (capsule only) 864.02
with open wound into cavity 864.12
moderate (involving parenchyma without major disruption) 864.03
with open wound into cavity 864.13
multiple 864.04
with open wound into cavity
864.14
stellate 864.04
with open wound into cavity 864.14
lung 861.22
with open wound into thorax 861.32
meninges — *see* Laceration, brain
meniscus (knee) (*see also* Tear, meniscus)
836.2
old 717.5
site other than knee (*see also* Sprain, by
site)
old NEC (*see also* Disorder, cartilage,
articular) 718.0 ✔
muscle (*see also* Sprain, by site)
with open wound — *see* Wound, open,
by site
myocardium — *see* Laceration, heart

✔ **Additional Digit Required** — Refer to the Tabular List for Digit Selection   ⵣ **Subterms under main terms may continue to next column or page**

Laceration — *see also* Wound, open, by site — *continued*

nerve — *see* Injury, nerve, by site
ocular NEC (*see also* Laceration, eyeball) 871.4
  adnexa NEC 870.8
    penetrating 870.3
      with foreign body 870.4
  orbit (eye) 870.8
    penetrating 870.3
      with foreign body 870.4
pelvic
  floor (muscles)
    with
      abortion — *see* Abortion, by type, with damage to pelvic organs
      ectopic pregnancy (*see also* categories 633.0–633.9) 639.2
      molar pregnancy (*see also* categories 630–632) 639.2
    complicating delivery 664.1 ☑
    following
      abortion 639.2
      ectopic or molar pregnancy 639.2
    nonpuerperal 618.7
    old (postpartal) 618.7
  organ NEC
    with
      abortion — *see* Abortion, by type, with damage to pelvic organs
      ectopic pregnancy (*see also* categories 633.0–633.9) 639.2
      molar pregnancy (*see also* categories 630–632) 639.2
    complicating delivery 665.5 ☑
      affecting fetus or newborn 763.89
    following
      abortion 639.2
      ectopic or molar pregnancy 639.2
    obstetrical trauma 665.5 ☑
perineum, perineal (old) (postpartal) 618.7
  with
    abortion — *see* Abortion, by type, with damage to pelvic floor
    ectopic pregnancy (*see also* categories 633.0–633.9) 639.2
    molar pregnancy (*see also* categories 630–632) 639.2
  complicating delivery 664.4 ☑
    first degree 664.0 ☑
    second degree 664.1 ☑
    third degree 664.2 ☑
    fourth degree 664.3 ☑
    anal sphincter (healed) (old) 654.8 ☑
      not associated with third-degree perineal laceration 664.6 ☑
    sphincter (anal) (healed) (old) 654.8 ☑
      not associated with third-degree perineal laceration 664.6 ☑
    central 664.4 ☑
    involving
      anal sphincter 664.2 ☑
      fourchette 664.0 ☑
      hymen 664.0 ☑
      labia 664.0 ☑
      pelvic floor 664.1 ☑
      perineal muscles 664.1 ☑
      rectovaginal septum 664.2 ☑
        with anal mucosa 664.3 ☑
      skin 664.0 ☑
      sphincter (anal) 664.2 ☑
        with anal mucosa 664.3 ☑
      vagina 664.0 ☑
      vaginal muscles 664.1 ☑
      vulva 664.0 ☑
    secondary 674.2 ☑
  following
    abortion 639.2
    ectopic or molar pregnancy 639.2
  male 879.6

Laceration — *see also* Wound, open, by site — *continued*

perineum, perineal — *continued*
  male — *continued*
    complicated 879.7
  muscles, complicating delivery 664.1 ☑
  nonpuerperal, current injury 879.6
    complicated 879.7
  secondary (postpartal) 674.2 ☑
peritoneum
  with
    abortion — *see* Abortion, by type, with damage to pelvic organs
    ectopic pregnancy (*see also* categories 633.0–633.9) 639.2
    molar pregnancy (*see also* categories 630–632) 639.2
  following
    abortion 639.2
    ectopic or molar pregnancy 639.2
  obstetrical trauma 665.5 ☑
periurethral tissue
  with
    abortion — *see* Abortion, by type, with damage to pelvic organs
    ectopic pregnancy (*see also* categories 633.0–633.9) 639.2
    molar pregnancy (*see also* categories 630–632) 639.2
  following
    abortion 639.2
    ectopic or molar pregnancy 639.2
  obstetrical trauma 664.8 ☑
rectovaginal (septum)
  with
    abortion — *see* Abortion, by type, with damage to pelvic organs
    ectopic pregnancy (*see also* categories 633.0–633.9) 639.2
    molar pregnancy (*see also* categories 630–632) 639.2
  complicating delivery 665.4 ☑
    with perineum 664.2 ☑
      involving anal or rectal mucosa 664.3 ☑
  following
    abortion 639.2
    ectopic or molar pregnancy 639.2
  nonpuerperal 623.4
  old (postpartal) 623.4
spinal cord (meninges) (*see also* Injury, spinal, by site)
  due to injury at birth 767.4
  fetus or newborn 767.4
spleen 865.09
  with
    disruption of parenchyma (massive) 865.04
      with open wound into cavity 865.14
    open wound into cavity 865.19
  capsule (without disruption of parenchyma) 865.02
    with open wound into cavity 865.12
  parenchyma 865.03
    with open wound into cavity 865.13
    massive disruption (rupture) 865.04
      with open wound into cavity 865.14
tendon 848.9
  with open wound — *see* Wound, open, by site
  Achilles 845.09
    with open wound 892.2
  lower limb NEC 844.9
    with open wound NEC 894.2
  upper limb NEC 840.9
    with open wound NEC 884.2
tentorium cerebelli — *see* Laceration, brain, cerebellum
tongue 873.64
  complicated 873.74
urethra
  with
    abortion — *see* Abortion, by type, with damage to pelvic organs

Laceration — *see also* Wound, open, by site — *continued*

urethra — *continued*
  with — *continued*
    ectopic pregnancy (*see also* categories 633.0–633.9) 639.2
    molar pregnancy (*see also* categories 630–632) 639.2
  following
    abortion 639.2
    ectopic or molar pregnancy 639.2
  nonpuerperal, nontraumatic 599.84
  obstetrical trauma 665.5 ☑
uterus
  with
    abortion — *see* Abortion, by type, with damage to pelvic organs
    ectopic pregnancy (*see also* categories 633.0–633.9) 639.2
    molar pregnancy (*see also* categories 630–632) 639.2
  following
    abortion 639.2
    ectopic or molar pregnancy 639.2
  nonpuerperal, nontraumatic 621.8
  obstetrical trauma NEC 665.5 ☑
  old (postpartal) 621.8
vagina
  with
    abortion — *see* Abortion, by type, with damage to pelvic organs
    ectopic pregnancy (*see also* categories 633.0–633.9) 639.2
    molar pregnancy (*see also* categories 630–632) 639.2
    perineal involvement, complicating delivery 664.0 ☑
  complicating delivery 665.4 ☑
    first degree 664.0 ☑
    second degree 664.1 ☑
    third degree 664.2 ☑
    fourth degree 664.3 ☑
    high 665.4 ☑
    muscles 664.1 ☑
    sulcus 665.4 ☑
    wall 665.4 ☑
  following
    abortion 639.2
    ectopic or molar pregnancy 639.2
  nonpuerperal, nontraumatic 623.4
  old (postpartal) 623.4
valve, heart — *see* Endocarditis
vulva
  with
    abortion — *see* Abortion, by type, with damage to pelvic organs
    ectopic pregnancy (*see also* categories 633.0–633.9) 639.2
    molar pregnancy (*see also* categories 630–632) 639.2
  complicating delivery 664.0 ☑
  following
    abortion 639.2
    ectopic or molar pregnancy 639.2
  nonpuerperal, nontraumatic 624.4
  old (postpartal) 624.4
Lachrymal — *see* condition
Lachrymonasal duct — *see* condition
Lack of
  adequate intermaxillary vertical dimension 524.36
  appetite (*see also* Anorexia) 783.0
  care
    in home V60.4
    of adult 995.84
    of infant (at or after birth) 995.52
  coordination 781.3
  development (*see also* Hypoplasia)
    physiological in childhood 783.40
  education V62.3
  energy 780.79
  financial resources V60.2
  food 994.2
    in environment V60.89
  growth in childhood 783.43
  heating V60.1

Lack of — *continued*
  housing (permanent) (temporary) V60.0
    adequate V60.1
  material resources V60.2
  medical attention 799.89
  memory (*see also* Amnesia) 780.93
    mild, following organic brain damage 310.89
  ovulation 628.0
  person able to render necessary care V60.4
  physical exercise V69.0
  physiologic development in childhood 783.40
  posterior occlusal support 524.57
  prenatal care in current pregnancy V23.7
  shelter V60.0
  sleep V69.4
  water 994.3
Lacrimal — *see* condition
Lacrimation, abnormal — *see also* Epiphora 375.20
Lacrimonasal duct — *see* condition
Lactation, lactating (breast) (puerperal) (postpartum)
  defective 676.4 ☑
  disorder 676.9 ☑
    specified type NEC 676.8 ☑
  excessive 676.6 ☑
  failed 676.4 ☑
  mastitis NEC 675.2 ☑
  mother (care and/or examination) V24.1
  nonpuerperal 611.6
  suppressed 676.5 ☑
Lacticemia 271.3
  excessive 276.2
Lactosuria 271.3
Lacunar skull 756.0
Laennec's cirrhosis (alcoholic) 571.2
  nonalcoholic 571.5
Lafora's disease 333.2
Lagleyze-von Hippel disease (retinocerebral angiomatosis) 759.6
Lag, lid (nervous) 374.41
Lagophthalmos (eyelid) (nervous) 374.20
  cicatricial 374.23
  keratitis (*see also* Keratitis) 370.34
  mechanical 374.22
  paralytic 374.21
La grippe — *see* Influenza
Lahore sore 085.1
Lakes, venous (cerebral) 437.8
Laki-Lorand factor deficiency — *see also* Defect, coagulation 286.3
Lalling 307.9
Lambliasis 007.1
Lame back 724.5
Lancereaux's diabetes (diabetes mellitus with marked emaciation) 250.8 ☑ *[261]*
  due to secondary diabetes 249.8 ☑ *[261]*
Landau-Kleffner syndrome 345.8 ☑
Landouzy-Déjérine dystrophy (fascioscapulohumeral atrophy) 359.1
Landry's disease or paralysis 357.0
Landry-Guillain-Barré syndrome 357.0
Lane's
  band 751.4
  disease 569.89
  kink (*see also* Obstruction, intestine) 560.9
Langdon Down's syndrome (mongolism) 758.0
Language abolition 784.69
Lanugo (persistent) 757.4
Laparoscopic surgical procedure converted to open procedure V64.41
Lardaceous
  degeneration (any site) 277.39
  disease 277.39
  kidney 277.39 *[583.81]*
  liver 277.39
Large
  baby (regardless of gestational age) 766.1
    exceptionally (weight of 4500 grams or more) 766.0
    of diabetic mother 775.0
  ear 744.22
  fetus (*see also* Oversize, fetus)

☑ **Additional Digit Required** — Refer to the Tabular List for Digit Selection   ▽ **Subterms under main terms may continue to next column or page**

Large — *continued*
  fetus (*see also* Oversize, fetus) — *continued*
    causing disproportion 653.5 ☑
      with obstructed labor 660.1 ☑
    for dates
      fetus or newborn (regardless of gestational age) 766.1
      affecting management of pregnancy 656.6 ☑
      exceptionally (weight of 4500 grams or more) 766.0
  physiological cup 743.57
  stature 783.9
  waxy liver 277.39
  white kidney — *see* Nephrosis
Larsen-Johansson disease (juvenile osteopathia patellae) 732.4
Larsen's syndrome (flattened facies and multiple congenital dislocations) 755.8
Larva migrans
  cutaneous NEC 126.9
    ancylostoma 126.9
  of Diptera in vitreous 128.0
  visceral NEC 128.0
Laryngeal — *see also* condition 786.2
  syncope 786.2
Laryngismus (acute) (infectious) (stridulous) 478.75
  congenital 748.3
  diphtheritic 032.3
Laryngitis (acute) (edematous) (fibrinous) (gangrenous) (infective) (infiltrative) (malignant) (membranous) (phlegmonous) (pneumococcal) (pseudomembranous) (septic) (subglottic) (suppurative) (ulcerative) (viral) 464.00
  with
    influenza, flu, or grippe (*see also* Influenza) 487.1
    obstruction 464.01
    tracheitis (*see also* Laryngotracheitis) 464.20
      with obstruction 464.21
      acute 464.20
        with obstruction 464.21
      chronic 476.1
  atrophic 476.0
  Borrelia vincentii 101
  catarrhal 476.0
  chronic 476.0
    with tracheitis (chronic) 476.1
    due to external agent — *see* Condition, respiratory, chronic, due to
  diphtheritic (membranous) 032.3
  due to external agent — *see* Inflammation, respiratory, upper, due to
  Hemophilus influenzae 464.00
    with obstruction 464.01
  H. influenzae 464.00
    with obstruction 464.01
  hypertrophic 476.0
  influenzal (*see also* Influenza) 487.1
  pachydermic 478.79
  sicca 476.0
  spasmodic 478.75
    acute 464.00
      with obstruction 464.01
  streptococcal 034.0
  stridulous 478.75
  syphilitic 095.8
    congenital 090.5
  tuberculous (*see also* Tuberculosis, larynx) 012.3 ☑
  Vincent's 101
Laryngocele (congenital) (ventricular) 748.3
Laryngofissure 478.79
  congenital 748.3
Laryngomalacia (congenital) 748.3
Laryngopharyngitis (acute) 465.0
  chronic 478.9
    due to external agent — *see* Condition, respiratory, chronic, due to
    due to external agent — *see* Inflammation, respiratory, upper, due to
  septic 034.0

Laryngoplegia — *see also* Paralysis, vocal cord 478.30
Laryngoptosis 478.79
Laryngospasm 478.75
  due to external agent — *see* Condition, respiratory, acute, due to
Laryngostenosis 478.74
  congenital 748.3
Laryngotracheitis (acute) (infectional) (viral) — *see also* Laryngitis 464.20
  with obstruction 464.21
  atrophic 476.1
  Borrelia vincenti 101
  catarrhal 476.1
  chronic 476.1
    due to external agent — *see* Condition, respiratory, chronic, due to
  diphtheritic (membranous) 032.3
  due to external agent — *see* Inflammation, respiratory, upper, due to
  H. influenzae 464.20
    with obstruction 464.21
  hypertrophic 476.1
  influenzal (*see also* Influenza) 487.1
  pachydermic 478.75
  sicca 476.1
  spasmodic 478.75
    acute 464.20
      with obstruction 464.21
  streptococcal 034.0
  stridulous 478.75
  syphilitic 095.8
    congenital 090.5
  tuberculous (*see also* Tuberculosis, larynx) 012.3 ☑
  Vincent's 101
Laryngotracheobronchitis — *see also* Bronchitis 490
  acute 466.0
  chronic 491.8
  viral 466.0
Laryngotracheobronchopneumonitis — *see* Pneumonia, broncho-
Larynx, laryngeal — *see* condition
Lasègue's disease (persecution mania) 297.9
Lassa fever 078.89
Lassitude — *see also* Weakness 780.79
Late — *see also* condition
  effect(s) (of) (*see also* condition)
    abscess
      intracranial or intraspinal (conditions classifiable to 324) — *see* category 326
    adverse effect of drug, medicinal or biological substance 909.5
    allergic reaction 909.9
    amputation
      postoperative (late) 997.60
      traumatic (injury classifiable to 885–887 and 895–897) 905.9
    burn (injury classifiable to 948–949) 906.9
      extremities NEC (injury classifiable to 943 or 945) 906.7
      hand or wrist (injury classifiable to 944) 906.6
      eye (injury classifiable to 940) 906.5
      face, head, and neck (injury classifiable to 941) 906.5
      specified site NEC (injury classifiable to 942 and 946–947) 906.8
    cerebrovascular disease (conditions classifiable to 430–437) 438.9
      with
        alterations of sensations 438.6
        aphasia 438.11
        apraxia 438.81
        ataxia 438.84
        cognitive deficits 438.0
        disturbances of vision 438.7
        dysarthria 438.13
        dysphagia 438.82
        dysphasia 438.12
        facial droop 438.83
        facial weakness 438.83
        fluency disorder 438.14

Late — *see also* condition — *continued*
  effect(s) (*see also* condition) — *continued*
    cerebrovascular disease — *continued*
      with — *continued*
        hemiplegia/hemiparesis
          affecting
            dominant side 438.21
            nondominant side 438.22
            unspecified side 438.20
        monoplegia of lower limb
          affecting
            dominant side 438.41
            nondominant side 438.42
            unspecified side 438.40
        monoplegia of upper limb
          affecting
            dominant side 438.31
            nondominant side 438.32
            unspecified side 438.30
        paralytic syndrome NEC
          affecting
            bilateral 438.53
            dominant side 438.51
            nondominant side 438.52
            unspecified side 438.50
        speech and language deficit 438.10
          specified type NEC 438.19
          stuttering 438.14
        vertigo 438.85
      specified type NEC 438.89
    childbirth complication(s) 677
    complication(s) of
      childbirth 677
      delivery 677
      pregnancy 677
      puerperium 677
      surgical and medical care (conditions classifiable to 996–999) 909.3
      trauma (conditions classifiable to 958) 908.6
    contusion (injury classifiable to 920–924) 906.3
    crushing (injury classifiable to 925–929) 906.4
    delivery complication(s) 677
    dislocation (injury classifiable to 830–839) 905.6
    encephalitis or encephalomyelitis (conditions classifiable to 323) — *see* category 326
      in infectious diseases 139.8
        viral (conditions classifiable to 049.8, 049.9, 062–064) 139.0
    external cause NEC (conditions classifiable to 995) 909.9
      certain conditions classifiable to categories 991–994 909.4
    foreign body in orifice (injury classifiable to 930–939) 908.5
    fracture (multiple) (injury classifiable to 828–829) 905.5
      extremity
        lower (injury classifiable to 821–827) 905.4
          neck of femur (injury classifiable to 820) 905.3
        upper (injury classifiable to 810–819) 905.2
      face and skull (injury classifiable to 800–804) 905.0
      skull and face (injury classifiable to 800–804) 905.0
      spine and trunk (injury classifiable to 805 and 807–809) 905.1
        with spinal cord lesion (injury classifiable to 806) 907.2
    infection
      pyogenic, intracranial — *see* category 326
    infectious diseases (conditions classifiable to 001–136) NEC 139.8
    injury (injury classifiable to 959) 908.9

Late — *see also* condition — *continued*
  effect(s) (*see also* condition) — *continued*
    injury — *continued*
      blood vessel 908.3
        abdomen and pelvis (injury classifiable to 902) 908.4
        extremity (injury classifiable to 903–904) 908.3
        head and neck (injury classifiable to 900) 908.3
        intracranial (injury classifiable to 850–854) 907.0
          with skull fracture 905.0
        thorax (injury classifiable to 901) 908.4
      internal organ NEC (injury classifiable to 867 and 869) 908.2
        abdomen (injury classifiable to 863–866 and 868) 908.1
        thorax (injury classifiable to 860–862) 908.0
      intracranial (injury classifiable to 850–854) 907.0
        with skull fracture (injury classifiable to 800–801 and 803–804) 905.0
      nerve NEC (injury classifiable to 957) 907.9
        cranial (injury classifiable to 950–951) 907.1
        peripheral NEC (injury classifiable to 957) 907.9
          lower limb and pelvic girdle (injury classifiable to 956) 907.5
          upper limb and shoulder girdle (injury classifiable to 955) 907.4
        roots and plexus(es), spinal (injury classifiable to 953) 907.3
        trunk (injury classifiable to 954) 907.3
      spinal
        cord (injury classifiable to 806 and 952) 907.2
        nerve root(s) and plexus(es) (injury classifiable to 953) 907.3
      superficial (injury classifiable to 910–919) 906.2
      tendon (tendon injury classifiable to 840–848, 880–884 with .2, and 890–894 with .2) 905.8
    meningitis
      bacterial (conditions classifiable to 320) — *see* category 326
      unspecified cause (conditions classifiable to 322) — *see* category 326
    myelitis (*see also* Late, effect(s) (of), encephalitis) — *see* category 326
    parasitic diseases (conditions classifiable to 001–136 NEC) 139.8
    phlebitis or thrombophlebitis of intracranial venous sinuses (conditions classifiable to 325) — *see* category 326
    poisoning due to drug, medicinal or biological substance (conditions classifiable to 960–979) 909.0
    poliomyelitis, acute (conditions classifiable to 045) 138
    pregnancy complication(s) 677
    puerperal complication(s) 677
    radiation (conditions classifiable to 990) 909.2
    rickets 268.1
    sprain and strain without mention of tendon injury (injury classifiable to 840–848, except tendon injury) 905.7
      tendon involvement 905.8

☑ **Additional Digit Required — Refer to the Tabular List for Digit Selection**   ▽ **Subterms under main terms may continue to next column or page**

2015 ICD-9-CM   ▶◀ **Revised Text**   ● **New Line**   ▲ **Revised Code**   **Volume 2 — 173**

Late — see also condition — continued
  effect(s) (see also condition) — continued
    toxic effect of
      drug, medicinal or biological substance (conditions classifiable to 960–979) 909.0
      nonmedical substance (conditions classifiable to 980–989) 909.1
      trachoma (conditions classifiable to 076) 139.1
      tuberculosis 137.0
        bones and joints (conditions classifiable to 015) 137.3
        central nervous system (conditions classifiable to 013) 137.1
        genitourinary (conditions classifiable to 016) 137.2
        pulmonary (conditions classifiable to 010–012) 137.0
        specified organs NEC (conditions classifiable to 014, 017–018) 137.4
        viral encephalitis (conditions classifiable to 049.8, 049.9, 062–064) 139.0
      wound, open
        extremity (injury classifiable to 880–884 and 890–894, except .2) 906.1
          tendon (injury classifiable to 880–884 with .2 and 890–894 with .2) 905.8
        head, neck, and trunk (injury classifiable to 870–879) 906.0
  infant
    post-term (gestation period over 40 completed weeks to 42 completed weeks) 766.21
    prolonged gestation (period over 42 completed weeks) 766.22
Latent — see condition
Lateral — see condition
Laterocession — see Lateroversion
Lateroflexion — see Lateroversion
Lateroversion
  cervix — see Lateroversion, uterus
  uterus, uterine (cervix) (postinfectional) (postpartal, old) 621.6
    congenital 752.39
    in pregnancy or childbirth 654.4 ☑
      affecting fetus or newborn 763.89
Lathyrism 988.2
Launois-Bensaude's lipomatosis 272.8
Launois-Cléret syndrome (adiposogenital dystrophy) 253.8
Launois' syndrome (pituitary gigantism) 253.0
Laurence-Moon-Biedl syndrome (obesity, polydactyly, and intellectual disabilities) 759.89
LAV (disease) (illness) (infection) — see Human immunodeficiency virus (disease) (illness) (infection)
LAV/HTLV-III (disease) (illness) (infection) — see Human immunodeficiency virus (disease) (illness) (infection)
Lawford's syndrome (encephalocutaneous angiomatosis) 759.6
Laxative habit — see also Abuse, drugs, nondependent 305.9 ☑
Lax, laxity — see also Relaxation
  ligament 728.4
  skin (acquired) 701.8
    congenital 756.83
Lazy leukocyte syndrome 288.09
LCAD (long chain/very long chain acyl CoA dehydrogenase deficiency, VLCAD) 277.85
LCHAD (long chain 3-hydroxyacyl CoA dehydrogenase deficiency) 277.85
Lead — see also condition
  exposure (suspected) to V15.86
  incrustation of cornea 371.15
  poisoning 984.9
    specified type of lead — see Table of Drugs and Chemicals
Lead miners' lung 503

Leakage
  amniotic fluid 658.1 ☑
    with delayed delivery 658.2 ☑
      affecting fetus or newborn 761.1
  bile from drainage tube (T tube) 997.49
  blood (microscopic), fetal, into maternal circulation 656.0 ☑
    affecting management of pregnancy or puerperium 656.0 ☑
  device, implant, or graft — see Complications, mechanical
  spinal fluid at lumbar puncture site 997.09
  urine, continuous 788.37
Leaky heart — see Endocarditis
Learning defect, specific NEC (strephosymbolia) 315.2
Leather bottle stomach (M8142/3) 151.9
Leber's
  congenital amaurosis 362.76
  optic atrophy (hereditary) 377.16
Lederer's anemia or disease (acquired infectious hemolytic anemia) 283.19
Lederer-Brill syndrome (acquired infectious hemolytic anemia) 283.19
Leeches (aquatic) (land) 134.2
Left-sided neglect 781.8
Leg — see condition
Legal investigation V62.5
Legg (-Calvé) -Perthes disease or syndrome (osteochondrosis, femoral capital) 732.1
Legionnaires' disease 482.84
Leigh's disease 330.8
Leiner's disease (exfoliative dermatitis) 695.89
Leiofibromyoma (M8890/0) — see also Leiomyoma
  uterus (cervix) (corpus) (see also Leiomyoma, uterus) 218.9
Leiomyoblastoma (M8891/1) — see Neoplasm, connective tissue, uncertain behavior
Leiomyofibroma (M8890/0) — see also Neoplasm, connective tissue, benign
  uterus (cervix) (corpus) (see also Leiomyoma, uterus) 218.9
Leiomyoma (M8890/0) — see also Neoplasm, connective tissue, benign
  bizarre (M8893/0) — see Neoplasm, connective tissue, benign
  cellular (M8892/1) — see Neoplasm, connective tissue, uncertain behavior
  epithelioid (M8891/1) — see Neoplasm, connective tissue, uncertain behavior
  prostate (polypoid) 600.20
    with
      other lower urinary tract symptoms (LUTS) 600.21
      urinary
        obstruction 600.21
        retention 600.21
  uterus (cervix) (corpus) 218.9
    interstitial 218.1
    intramural 218.1
    submucous 218.0
    subperitoneal 218.2
    subserous 218.2
    vascular (M8894/0) — see Neoplasm, connective tissue, benign
Leiomyomatosis (intravascular) (M8890/1) — see Neoplasm, connective tissue, uncertain behavior
Leiomyosarcoma (M8890/3) — see also Neoplasm, connective tissue, malignant
  epithelioid (M8891/3) — see Neoplasm, connective tissue, malignant
Leishmaniasis 085.9
  American 085.5
    cutaneous 085.4
    mucocutaneous 085.5
  Asian desert 085.2
  Brazilian 085.5
  cutaneous 085.9
    acute necrotizing 085.2
    American 085.4
    Asian desert 085.2
    diffuse 085.3
    dry form 085.1

Leishmaniasis — continued
  cutaneous — continued
    Ethiopian 085.3
    eyelid 085.5 [373.6]
    late 085.1
    lepromatous 085.3
    recurrent 085.1
    rural 085.2
    ulcerating 085.1
    urban 085.1
    wet form 085.2
    zoonotic form 085.2
  dermal (see also Leishmaniasis, cutaneous) post kala-azar 085.0
  eyelid 085.5 [373.6]
  infantile 085.0
  Mediterranean 085.0
  mucocutaneous (American) 085.5
  naso-oral 085.5
  nasopharyngeal 085.5
  Old World 085.1
  tegumentaria diffusa 085.4
  vaccination, prophylactic (against) V05.2
  visceral (Indian) 085.0
Leishmanoid, dermal — see also Leishmaniasis, cutaneous
  post kala-azar 085.0
Leloir's disease 695.4
Lemiere syndrome 451.89
Lenegre's disease 426.0
Lengthening, leg 736.81
Lennox-Gastaut syndrome 345.0 ☑
  with tonic seizures 345.1 ☑
Lennox's syndrome — see also Epilepsy 345.0 ☑
Lens — see condition
Lenticonus (anterior) (posterior) (congenital) 743.36
Lenticular degeneration, progressive 275.1
Lentiglobus (posterior) (congenital) 743.36
Lentigo (congenital) 709.09
  juvenile 709.09
  Maligna (M8742/2) (see also Neoplasm, skin, in situ)
    melanoma (M8742/3) — see Melanoma
  senile 709.09
Leonine leprosy 030.0
Leontiasis
  ossium 733.3
  syphilitic 095.8
    congenital 090.5
Léopold-Lévi's syndrome (paroxysmal thyroid instability) 242.9 ☑
Lepore hemoglobin syndrome 282.45
Lepothrix 039.0
Lepra 030.9
  Willan's 696.1
Leprechaunism 259.8
Lepromatous leprosy 030.0
Leprosy 030.9
  anesthetic 030.1
  beriberi 030.1
  borderline (group B) (infiltrated) (neuritic) 030.3
  cornea (see also Leprosy, by type) 030.9 [371.89]
  dimorphous (group B) (infiltrated) (lepromatous) (neuritic) (tuberculoid) 030.3
  eyelid 030.0 [373.4]
  indeterminate (group I) (macular) (neuritic) (uncharacteristic) 030.2
  leonine 030.0
  lepromatous (diffuse) (infiltrated) (macular) (neuritic) (nodular) (type L) 030.0
  macular (early) (neuritic) (simple) 030.2
  maculoanesthetic 030.1
  mixed 030.0
  neuro 030.1
  nodular 030.0
  primary neuritic 030.3
  specified type or group NEC 030.8
  tubercular 030.1
  tuberculoid (macular) (maculoanesthetic) (major) (minor) (neuritic) (type T) 030.1
Leptocytosis, hereditary 282.40

Leptomeningitis (chronic) (circumscribed) (hemorrhagic) (nonsuppurative) — see also Meningitis 322.9
  aseptic 047.9
    adenovirus 049.1
    Coxsackie virus 047.0
    ECHO virus 047.1
    enterovirus 047.9
    lymphocytic choriomeningitis 049.0
  epidemic 036.0
  late effect — see category 326
  meningococcal 036.0
  pneumococcal 320.1
  syphilitic 094.2
  tuberculous (see also Tuberculosis, meninges) 013.0 ☑
Leptomeningopathy — see also Meningitis 322.9
Leptospiral — see condition
Leptospirochetal — see condition
Leptospirosis 100.9
  autumnalis 100.89
  canicula 100.89
  grippotyphosa 100.89
  hebdomidis 100.89
  icterohemorrhagica 100.0
  nanukayami 100.89
  pomona 100.89
  Weil's disease 100.0
Leptothricosis — see Actinomycosis
Leptothrix infestation — see Actinomycosis
Leptotricosis — see Actinomycosis
Leptus dermatitis 133.8
Leriche's syndrome (aortic bifurcation occlusion) 444.09
Léris pleonosteosis 756.89
Léri-Weill syndrome 756.59
Lermoyez's syndrome — see also Disease, Ménière's 386.00
Lesbianism — omit code
  ego-dystonic 302.0
  problems with 302.0
Lesch-Nyhan syndrome (hypoxanthineguanine-phosphoribosyltransferase deficiency) 277.2
Lesion(s)
  abducens nerve 378.54
  alveolar process 525.8
  anorectal 569.49
  aortic (valve) — see Endocarditis, aortic
  auditory nerve 388.5
  basal ganglion 333.90
  bile duct (see also Disease, biliary) 576.8
  bladder 596.9
  bone 733.90
  brachial plexus 353.0
  brain 348.89
    congenital 742.9
    vascular (see also Lesion, cerebrovascular) 437.9
      degenerative 437.1
      healed or old without residuals V12.54
      hypertensive 437.2
      late effect — see Late effect(s) (of) cerebrovascular disease
  buccal 528.9
  calcified — see Calcification
  canthus 373.9
  carate — see Pinta, lesions
  cardia 537.89
  cardiac — see also Disease, heart
    congenital 746.9
    valvular — see Endocarditis
  cauda equina 344.60
    with neurogenic bladder 344.61
  cecum 569.89
  cerebral — see Lesion, brain
  cerebrovascular (see also Disease, cerebrovascular NEC) 437.9
    degenerative 437.1
    healed or old without residuals V12.54
    hypertensive 437.2
    specified type NEC 437.8
  cervical root (nerve) NEC 353.2

Note – Use the following fifth-digit
subclassification for categories 203–208:

0 without mention of having
   achieved remission

   failed remission

1 with remission

2 in relapse

☑ **Additional Digit Required** — Refer to the Tabular List for Digit Selection ⑳ **Subterms under main terms may continue to next column or page**

Leukemia, leukemic — continued
Schilling-type monocytic (M9890/3) — see Leukemia, monocytic
stem cell (M9801/3) 208.0 ☑
subacute NEC (M9802/3) 208.2 ☑
subleukemic NEC (M9804/3) 208.8 ☑
thrombocytic (M9910/3) 207.2 ☑
undifferentiated (M9801/3) 208.0 ☑
Leukemoid reaction (basophilic) (lymphocytic) (monocytic) (myelocytic) (neutrophilic) 288.62
Leukoaraiosis (hypertensive) 437.1
Leukoariosis — see Leukoaraiosis
Leukoclastic vasculitis 446.29
Leukocoria 360.44
Leukocythemia — see Leukemia
Leukocytopenia 288.50
Leukocytosis 288.60
basophilic 288.8
eosinophilic 288.3
lymphocytic 288.8
monocytic 288.8
neutrophilic 288.8
Leukoderma 709.09
syphilitic 091.3
late 095.8
Leukodermia — see also Leukoderma 709.09
Leukodystrophy (cerebral) (globoid cell) (metachromatic) (progressive) (sudanophilic) 330.0
Leukoedema, mouth or tongue 528.79
Leukoencephalitis
acute hemorrhagic (postinfectious) NEC 136.9 [323.61]
postimmunization or postvaccinal 323.51
subacute sclerosing 046.2
van Bogaert's 046.2
van Bogaert's (sclerosing) 046.2
Leukoencephalopathy — see also Encephalitis 323.9
acute necrotizing hemorrhagic (postinfectious) 136.9 [323.61]
postimmunization or postvaccinal 323.51
arteriosclerotic 437.0
Binswanger's 290.12
metachromatic 330.0
multifocal (progressive) 046.3
progressive multifocal 046.3
reversible, posterior 348.5
Leukoerythroblastosis 289.9
Leukoerythrosis 289.0
Leukokeratosis — see also Leukoplakia 702.8
mouth 528.6
nicotina palati 528.79
tongue 528.6
Leukokoria 360.44
Leukokraurosis vulva, vulvae 624.09
Leukolymphosarcoma (M9850/3) 207.8 ☑
Leukoma (cornea) (interfering with central vision) 371.03
adherent 371.04
Leukomalacia, periventricular 779.7
Leukomelanopathy, hereditary 288.2
Leukonychia (punctata) (striata) 703.8
congenital 757.5
Leukopathia
unguium 703.8
congenital 757.5
Leukopenia 288.50
basophilic 288.59
cyclic 288.02
eosinophilic 288.59
familial 288.59
malignant (see also Agranulocytosis) 288.09
periodic 288.02
transitory neonatal 776.7
Leukopenic — see condition
Leukoplakia 702.8
anus 569.49
bladder (postinfectional) 596.89
buccal 528.6
cervix (uteri) 622.2
esophagus 530.83
gingiva 528.6

Leukoplakia — continued
kidney (pelvis) 593.89
larynx 478.79
lip 528.6
mouth 528.6
oral soft tissue (including tongue) (mucosa) 528.6
palate 528.6
pelvis (kidney) 593.89
penis (infectional) 607.0
rectum 569.49
syphilitic 095.8
tongue 528.6
tonsil 478.29
ureter (postinfectional) 593.89
urethra (postinfectional) 599.84
uterus 621.8
vagina 623.1
vesical 596.89
vocal cords 478.5
vulva 624.09
Leukopolioencephalopathy 330.0
Leukorrhea (vagina) 623.5
due to trichomonas (vaginalis) 131.00
trichomonal (Trichomonas vaginalis) 131.00
Leukosarcoma (M9850/3) 207.8 ☑
Leukosis (M9800/3) — see Leukemia
Lev's disease or syndrome (acquired complete heart block) 426.0
Levi's syndrome (pituitary dwarfism) 253.3
Levocardia (isolated) 746.87
with situs inversus 759.3
Levulosuria 271.2
Lewandowski's disease (primary) — see also Tuberculosis 017.0 ☑
Lewandowski-Lutz disease (epidermodysplasia verruciformis) 078.19
Lewy body dementia 331.82
Lewy body disease 331.82
Leyden's disease (periodic vomiting) 536.2
Leyden-Möbius dystrophy 359.1
Leydig cell
carcinoma (M8650/3)
specified site — see Neoplasm, by site, malignant
unspecified site
female 183.0
male 186.9
tumor (M8650/1)
benign (M8650/0)
specified site — see Neoplasm, by site, benign
unspecified site
female 220
male 186.9
malignant (M8650/3)
specified site — see Neoplasm, by site, malignant
unspecified site
female 183.0
male 186.9
specified site — see Neoplasm, by site, uncertain behavior
unspecified site
female 236.2
male 236.4
Leydig-Sertoli cell tumor (M8631/0)
specified site — see Neoplasm, by site, benign
unspecified site
female 220
male 222.0
LGSIL (low grade squamous intraepithelial lesion)
anus 796.73
cervix 795.03
vagina 795.13
Liar, pathologic 301.7
Libman-Sacks disease or syndrome 710.0 [424.91]
Lice (infestation) 132.9
body (pediculus corporis) 132.1
crab 132.2
head (pediculus capitis) 132.0
mixed (classifiable to more than one of the categories 132.0–132.2) 132.3

Lice — continued
pubic (pediculus pubis) 132.2
Lichen 697.9
albus 701.0
annularis 695.89
atrophicus 701.0
corneus obtusus 698.3
myxedematous 701.8
nitidus 697.1
pilaris 757.39
acquired 701.1
planopilaris 697.0
planus (acute) (chronicus) (hypertrophic) (verrucous) 697.0
morphoeicus 701.0
sclerosus (et atrophicus) 701.0
ruber 696.4
acuminatus 696.4
moniliformis 697.8
obtusus corneus 698.3
of Wilson 697.0
planus 697.0
sclerosus (et atrophicus) 701.0
scrofulosus (primary) (see also Tuberculosis) 017.0 ☑
simplex (Vidal's) 698.3
chronicus 698.3
circumscriptus 698.3
spinulosus 757.39
mycotic 117.9
striata 697.8
urticatus 698.2
Lichenification 698.3
nodular 698.3
Lichenoides tuberculosis (primary) — see also Tuberculosis 017.0 ☑
Lichtheim's disease or syndrome (subacute combined sclerosis with pernicious anemia) 281.0 [336.2]
Lien migrans 289.59
Lientery — see also Diarrhea 787.91
infectious 009.2
Life circumstance problem NEC V62.89
Li-Fraumeni cancer syndrome V84.01
Ligament — see condition
Light-for-dates (infant) 764.0 ☑
with signs of fetal malnutrition 764.1 ☑
affecting management of pregnancy 656.5 ☑
Light-headedness 780.4
Lightning (effects) (shock) (stroke) (struck by) 994.0
burn — see Burn, by site
foot 266.2
Lightwood's disease or syndrome (renal tubular acidosis) 588.89
Lignac's disease (cystinosis) 270.0
Lignac (-de Toni) (-Fanconi) (-Debré) syndrome (cystinosis) 270.0
Lignac (-Fanconi) syndrome (cystinosis) 270.0
Ligneous thyroiditis 245.3
Likoff's syndrome (angina in menopausal women) 413.9
Limb — see condition
Limitation of joint motion — see also Stiffness, joint 719.5 ☑
sacroiliac 724.6
Limit dextrinosis 271.0
Limited
cardiac reserve — see Disease, heart
duction, eye NEC 378.63
mandibular range of motion 524.52
Lindau's disease (retinocerebral angiomatosis) 759.6
Lindau (-von Hippel) disease (angiomatosis retinocerebellosa) 759.6
Linea corneae senilis 371.41
Lines
Beau's (transverse furrows on fingernails) 703.8
Harris' 733.91
Hudson-Stähli 371.11
Stähli's 371.11
Lingua
geographical 529.1
nigra (villosa) 529.3

Lingua — continued
plicata 529.5
congenital 750.13
tylosis 528.6
Lingual (tongue) — see also condition
thyroid 759.2
Linitis (gastric) 535.4 ☑
plastica (M8142/3) 151.9
Lioderma essentialis (cum melanosis et telangiectasia) 757.33
Lip — see also condition
biting 528.9
Lipalgia 272.8
Lipedema — see Edema
Lipemia — see also Hyperlipidemia 272.4
retina, retinalis 272.3
Lipidosis 272.7
cephalin 272.7
cerebral (infantile) (juvenile) (late) 330.1
cerebroretinal 330.1 [362.71]
cerebroside 272.7
cerebrospinal 272.7
chemically-induced 272.7
cholesterol 272.7
diabetic 250.8 ☑ [272.7]
due to secondary diabetes 249.8 ☑ [272.7]
dystopic (hereditary) 272.7
glycolipid 272.7
hepatosplenomegalic 272.3
hereditary, dystopic 272.7
sulfatide 330.0
Lipoadenoma (M8324/0) — see Neoplasm, by site, benign
Lipoblastoma (M8881/0) — see Lipoma, by site
Lipoblastomatosis (M8881/0) — see Lipoma, by site
Lipochondrodystrophy 277.5
Lipochrome histiocytosis (familial) 288.1
Lipodermatosclerosis 729.39
Lipodystrophia progressiva 272.6
Lipodystrophy (progressive) 272.6
insulin 272.6
intestinal 040.2
mesenteric 567.82
Lipofibroma (M8851/0) — see Lipoma, by site
Lipoglycoproteinosis 272.8
Lipogranuloma, sclerosing 709.8
Lipogranulomatosis (disseminated) 272.8
kidney 272.8
Lipoid — see also condition
histiocytosis 272.7
essential 272.7
nephrosis (see also Nephrosis) 581.3
proteinosis of Urbach 272.8
Lipoidemia — see also Hyperlipidemia 272.4
Lipoidosis — see also Lipidosis 272.7
Lipoma (M8850/0) 214.9
breast (skin) 214.1
face 214.0
fetal (M8881/0) (see also Lipoma, by site)
fat cell (M8880/0) — see Lipoma, by site
infiltrating (M8856/0) — see Lipoma, by site
intra-abdominal 214.3
intramuscular (M8856/0) — see Lipoma, by site
intrathoracic 214.2
kidney 214.3
mediastinum 214.2
muscle 214.8
peritoneum 214.3
retroperitoneum 214.3
skin 214.1
face 214.0
spermatic cord 214.4
spindle cell (M8857/0) — see Lipoma, by site
stomach 214.3
subcutaneous tissue 214.1
face 214.0
thymus 214.2
thyroid gland 214.2
Lipomatosis (dolorosa) 272.8
epidural 214.8
fetal (M8881/0) — see Lipoma, by site

☑ Additional Digit Required — Refer to the Tabular List for Digit Selection   ▽ Subterms under main terms may continue to next column or page

176 — Volume 2   ►◄ Revised Text   ● New Line   ▲ Revised Code   2015 ICD-9-CM

Lipomatosis — *continued*
  Launois-Bensaude's 272.8
Lipomyohemangioma (M8860/0)
  specified site — *see* Neoplasm, connective tissue, benign
  unspecified site 223.0
Lipomyoma (M8860/0)
  specified site — *see* Neoplasm, connective tissue, benign
  unspecified site 223.0
Lipomyxoma (M8852/0) — *see* Lipoma, by site
Lipomyxosarcoma (M8852/3) — *see* Neoplasm, connective tissue, malignant
Lipophagocytosis 289.89
Lipoproteinemia (alpha) 272.4
  broad-beta 272.2
  floating-beta 272.2
  hyper-pre-beta 272.1
Lipoproteinosis (Rössle-Urbach-Wiethe) 272.8
Liposarcoma (M8850/3) — *see also* Neoplasm, connective tissue, malignant
  differentiated type (M8851/3) — *see* Neoplasm, connective tissue, malignant
  embryonal (M8852/3) — *see* Neoplasm, connective tissue, malignant
  mixed type (M8855/3) — *see* Neoplasm, connective tissue, malignant
  myxoid (M8852/3) — *see* Neoplasm, connective tissue, malignant
  pleomorphic (M8854/3) — *see* Neoplasm, connective tissue, malignant
  round cell (M8853/3) — *see* Neoplasm, connective tissue, malignant
  well differentiated type (M8851/3) — *see* Neoplasm, connective tissue, malignant
Liposynovitis prepatellaris 272.8
Lipping
  cervix 622.0
  spine (*see also* Spondylosis) 721.90
  vertebra (*see also* Spondylosis) 721.90
Lip pits (mucus), congenital 750.25
Lipschütz disease or ulcer 616.50
Lipuria 791.1
  bilharziasis 120.0
Liquefaction, vitreous humor 379.21
Lisping 307.9
Lissauer's paralysis 094.1
Lissencephalia, lissencephaly 742.2
Listerellose 027.0
Listeriose 027.0
Listeriosis 027.0
  congenital 771.2
  fetal 771.2
  suspected fetal damage affecting management of pregnancy 655.4 ☑
Listlessness 780.79
Lithemia 790.6
Lithiasis — *see also* Calculus
  hepatic (duct) — *see* Choledocholithiasis
  urinary 592.9
Lithopedion 779.9
  affecting management of pregnancy 656.8 ☑
Lithosis (occupational) 502
  with tuberculosis — *see* Tuberculosis, pulmonary
Lithuria 791.9
Litigation V62.5
Little
  league elbow 718.82
  stroke syndrome 435.9
Little's disease — *see* Palsy, cerebral
Littre's
  gland — *see* condition
  hernia — *see* Hernia, Littre's
Littritis — *see also* Urethritis 597.89
Livedo 782.61
  annularis 782.61
  racemose 782.61
  reticularis 782.61
Live flesh 781.0
Liver — *see also* condition
  donor V59.6
Livida, asphyxia
  newborn 768.6

Living
  alone V60.3
    with handicapped person V60.4
Lloyd's syndrome 258.1
Loa loa 125.2
Loasis 125.2
Lobe, lobar — *see* condition
Lobo's disease or blastomycosis 116.2
Lobomycosis 116.2
Lobotomy syndrome 310.0
Lobstein's disease (brittle bones and blue sclera) 756.51
Lobster-claw hand 755.58
Lobulation (congenital) — *see also* Anomaly, specified type NEC, by site
  kidney, fetal 753.3
  liver, abnormal 751.69
  spleen 759.0
Lobule, lobular — *see* condition
Local, localized — *see* condition
Locked bowel or intestine — *see also* Obstruction, intestine 560.9
Locked-in state 344.81
Locked twins 660.5 ☑
  affecting fetus or newborn 763.1
Locking
  joint (*see also* Derangement, joint) 718.90
  knee 717.9
Lockjaw — *see also* Tetanus 037
Locomotor ataxia (progressive) 094.0
Löffler's
  endocarditis 421.0
  eosinophilia or syndrome 518.3
  pneumonia 518.3
  syndrome (eosinophilic pneumonitis) 518.3
Löfgren's syndrome (sarcoidosis) 135
Loiasis 125.2
  eyelid 125.2 [373.6]
Loneliness V62.89
Lone star fever 082.8
Longitudinal stripes or grooves, nails 703.8
  congenital 757.5
Long labor 662.1 ☑
  affecting fetus or newborn 763.89
  first stage 662.0 ☑
  second stage 662.2 ☑
Long-term (current) (prophylactic) **drug use** V58.69
  antibiotics V58.62
  anticoagulants V58.61
  anti-inflammatories, non-steroidal (NSAID) V58.64
  antiplatelets/antithrombotics V58.63
  aspirin V58.66
  bisphosphonates V58.68
  high-risk medications NEC V58.69
  insulin V58.67
  methadone for pain control V58.69
  opiate analgesic V58.69
  pain killers V58.69
    anti-inflammatories, non-steroidal (NSAID) V58.64
    aspirin V58.66
  steroids V58.65
  tamoxifen V07.51
Loop
  intestine (*see also* Volvulus) 560.2
  intrascleral nerve 379.29
  vascular on papilla (optic) 743.57
Loose — *see also* condition
  body
    in tendon sheath 727.82
    joint 718.10
      ankle 718.17
      elbow 718.12
      foot 718.17
      hand 718.14
      hip 718.15
      knee 717.6
      multiple sites 718.19
      pelvic region 718.15
      prosthetic implant — *see* Complications, mechanical
      shoulder (region) 718.11
      specified site NEC 718.18
      wrist 718.13

Loose — *see also* condition — *continued*
  cartilage (joint) (*see also* Loose, body, joint) 718.1 ☑
    knee 717.6
  facet (vertebral) 724.9
  prosthetic implant — *see* Complications, mechanical
  sesamoid, joint (*see also* Loose, body, joint) 718.1 ☑
  tooth, teeth 525.8
Loosening epiphysis 732.9
Looser (-Debray)-Milkman syndrome (osteomalacia with pseudofractures) 268.2
Lop ear (deformity) 744.29
Lorain's disease or syndrome (pituitary dwarfism) 253.3
Lorain-Levi syndrome (pituitary dwarfism) 253.3
Lordosis (acquired) (postural) 737.20
  congenital 754.2
  due to or associated with
    Charcôt-Marie-Tooth disease 356.1 [737.42]
    mucopolysaccharidosis 277.5 [737.42]
    neurofibromatosis 237.71 [737.42]
    osteitis
      deformans 731.0 [737.42]
      fibrosa cystica 252.01 [737.42]
    osteoporosis (*see also* Osteoporosis) 733.00 [737.42]
    poliomyelitis (*see also* Poliomyelitis) 138 [737.42]
    tuberculosis (*see also* Tuberculosis) 015.0 ☑ [737.42]
  late effect of rickets 268.1 [737.42]
  postlaminectomy 737.21
  postsurgical NEC 737.22
  rachitic 268.1 [737.42]
  specified NEC 737.29
  tuberculous (*see also* Tuberculosis) 015.0 ☑ [737.42]
Loss
  appetite 783.0
    hysterical 300.11
    nonorganic origin 307.59
    psychogenic 307.59
  blood — *see* Hemorrhage
  central vision 368.41
  consciousness 780.09
    transient 780.2
  control, sphincter, rectum 787.60
    nonorganic origin 307.7
  ear ossicle, partial 385.24
  elasticity, skin 782.8
  extremity or member, traumatic, current — *see* Amputation, traumatic
  fluid (acute) 276.50
    with
      hypernatremia 276.0
      hyponatremia 276.1
    fetus or newborn 775.5
  hair 704.00
  hearing (*see also* Deafness)
    central 389.14
    conductive (air) 389.00
      with sensorineural hearing loss 389.20
        bilateral 389.22
        unilateral 389.21
      bilateral 389.06
      combined types 389.08
      external ear 389.01
      inner ear 389.04
      middle ear 389.03
      multiple types 389.08
      tympanic membrane 389.02
      unilateral 389.05
    mixed conductive and sensorineural 389.20
      bilateral 389.22
      unilateral 389.21
    mixed type 389.20
      bilateral 389.22
      unilateral 389.21
    nerve
      bilateral 389.12

Loss — *continued*
  hearing (*see also* Deafness) — *continued*
    nerve — *continued*
      unilateral 389.13
    neural
      bilateral 389.12
      unilateral 389.13
    noise-induced 388.12
    perceptive NEC (*see also* Loss, hearing, sensorineural) 389.10
    sensorineural 389.10
      with conductive hearing loss 389.20
        bilateral 389.22
        unilateral 389.21
      asymmetrical 389.16
      bilateral 389.18
      central 389.14
      neural 389.12
        bilateral 389.12
        unilateral 389.13
      sensory
        bilateral 389.11
        unilateral 389.17
      unilateral 389.15
    sensory
      bilateral 389.11
      unilateral 389.17
    specified type NEC 389.8
    sudden NEC 388.2
  height 781.91
  labyrinthine reactivity (unilateral) 386.55
    bilateral 386.56
  memory (*see also* Amnesia) 780.93
    mild, following organic brain damage 310.89
  mind (*see also* Psychosis) 298.9
  occlusal vertical dimension 524.37
  organ or part — *see* Absence, by site, acquired
  recurrent pregnancy — *see* Pregnancy, management affected by, abortion, habitual
  sensation 782.0
  sense of
    smell (*see also* Disturbance, sensation) 781.1
    taste (*see also* Disturbance, sensation) 781.1
    touch (*see also* Disturbance, sensation) 781.1
  sight (acquired) (complete) (congenital) — *see* Blindness
  spinal fluid
    headache 349.0
  substance of
    bone (*see also* Osteoporosis) 733.00
    cartilage 733.99
    ear 380.32
    vitreous (humor) 379.26
  tooth, teeth
    acquired 525.10
      due to
        caries 525.13
        extraction 525.10
        periodontal disease 525.12
        specified NEC 525.19
        trauma 525.11
  vision, visual (*see also* Blindness) 369.9
    both eyes (*see also* Blindness, both eyes) 369.3
    complete (*see also* Blindness, both eyes) 369.00
    one eye 369.8
    sudden 368.11
    transient 368.12
  vitreous 379.26
  voice (*see also* Aphonia) 784.41
  weight (cause unknown) 783.21
Lou Gehrig's disease 335.20
Louis-Bar syndrome (ataxia-telangiectasia) 334.8
Louping ill 063.1
Lousiness — *see* Lice
Low
  back syndrome 724.2
  basal metabolic rate (BMR) 794.7

☑ **Additional Digit Required** — Refer to the Tabular List for Digit Selection

▽ **Subterms under main terms may continue to next column or page**

Low — *continued*
  birthweight 765.1 ✓
    extreme (less than 1000 grams) 765.0 ✓
    for gestational age 764.0 ✓
    status (*see also* Status, low birth weight)
      V21.30
  bladder compliance 596.52
  blood pressure (*see also* Hypotension) 458.9
    reading (incidental) (isolated) (nonspecific) 796.3
  cardiac reserve — *see* Disease, heart
  compliance bladder 596.52
  frequency deafness — *see* Disorder, hearing
  function (*see also* Hypofunction)
    kidney (*see also* Disease, renal) 593.9
    liver 573.9
  hemoglobin 285.9
  implantation, placenta — *see* Placenta, previa
  insertion, placenta — *see* Placenta, previa
  lying
    kidney 593.0
    organ or site, congenital — *see* Malposition, congenital
    placenta — *see* Placenta, previa
  output syndrome (cardiac) (*see also* Failure, heart) 428.9
  platelets (blood) (*see also* Thrombocytopenia) 287.5
  reserve, kidney (*see also* Disease, renal) 593.9
  risk
    human papillomavirus (HPA) DNA test positive
      anal 796.79
      cervical 795.09
      vaginal 795.19
  salt syndrome 593.9
  tension glaucoma 365.12
  vision 369.9
    both eyes 369.20
    one eye 369.70
Lower extremity — *see* condition
Lowe (-Terrey-MacLachlan) syndrome (oculocerebrorenal dystrophy) 270.8
Lown (-Ganong) -Levine syndrome (short P-R interval, normal QRS complex, and paroxysmal supraventricular tachycardia) 426.81
LSD reaction — *see also* Abuse, drugs, nondependent 305.3 ✓
L-shaped kidney 753.3
Lucas-Championnière disease (fibrinous bronchitis) 466.0
Lucey-Driscoll syndrome (jaundice due to delayed conjugation) 774.30
Ludwig's
  angina 528.3
  disease (submaxillary cellulitis) 528.3
Lues (venerea), **luetic** — *see* Syphilis
Luetscher's syndrome (dehydration) 276.51
Lumbago 724.2
  due to displacement, intervertebral disc 722.10
Lumbalgia 724.2
  due to displacement, intervertebral disc 722.10
Lumbar — *see* condition
Lumbarization, vertebra 756.15
Lumbermen's itch 133.8
Lump — *see also* Mass
  abdominal 789.3 ✓
  breast 611.72
  chest 786.6
  epigastric 789.3 ✓
  head 784.2
  kidney 753.3
  liver 789.1
  lung 786.6
  mediastinal 786.6
  neck 784.2
  nose or sinus 784.2
  pelvic 789.3 ✓
  skin 782.2
  substernal 786.6
  throat 784.2

Lump — *see also* Mass — *continued*
  umbilicus 789.3 ✓
Lunacy — *see also* Psychosis 298.9
Lunatomalacia 732.3
Lung — *see also* condition
  donor V59.8
  drug addict's 417.8
  mainliners' 417.8
  vanishing 492.0
Lupoid (miliary) **of Boeck** 135
Lupus 710.0
  anticoagulant 795.79
    with
      hemorrhagic disorder 286.53
      hypercoagulable state 289.81
  Cazenave's (erythematosus) 695.4
  discoid (local) 695.4
  disseminated 710.0
  erythematodes (discoid) (local) 695.4
  erythematosus (discoid) (local) 695.4
    disseminated 710.0
    eyelid 373.34
    systemic 710.0
      with
        encephalitis 710.0 [323.81]
        lung involvement 710.0 [517.8]
      inhibitor (presence of) 795.79
        with hypercoagulable state 289.81
  exedens 017.0 ✓
  eyelid (*see also* Tuberculosis)
    017.0 ✓ [373.4]
  Hilliard's 017.0 ✓
  hydralazine
    correct substance properly administered 695.4
    overdose or wrong substance given or taken 972.6
  miliaris disseminatus faciei 017.0 ✓
  nephritis 710.0 [583.81]
    acute 710.0 [580.81]
    chronic 710.0 [582.81]
  nontuberculous, not disseminated 695.4
  pernio (Besnier) 135
  tuberculous (*see also* Tuberculosis) 017.0 ✓
    eyelid (*see also* Tuberculosis)
      017.0 ✓ [373.4]
  vulgaris 017.0 ✓
Luschka's joint disease 721.90
Luteinoma (M8610/0) 220
Lutembacher's disease or syndrome (atrial septal defect with mitral stenosis) 745.5
Luteoma (M8610/0) 220
Lutz-Miescher disease (elastosis perforans serpiginosa) 701.1
Lutz-Splendore-de Almeida disease (Brazilian blastomycosis) 116.1
Luxatio
  bulbi due to birth injury 767.8
  coxae congenita (*see also* Dislocation, hip, congenital) 754.30
  erecta — *see* Dislocation, shoulder
  imperfecta — *see* Sprain, by site
  perinealis — *see* Dislocation, hip
Luxation — *see also* Dislocation, by site
  eyeball 360.81
    due to birth injury 767.8
    lateral 376.36
  genital organs (external) NEC — *see* Wound, open, genital organs
  globe (eye) 360.81
    lateral 376.36
  lacrimal gland (postinfectional) 375.16
  lens (old) (partial) 379.32
    congenital 743.37
      syphilitic 090.49 [379.32]
    Marfan's disease 090.49
    spontaneous 379.32
  penis — *see* Wound, open, penis
  scrotum — *see* Wound, open, scrotum
  testis — *see* Wound, open, testis
L-xyloketosuria 271.8
Lycanthropy — *see also* Psychosis 298.9
Lyell's disease or syndrome (toxic epidermal necrolysis) 695.15

Lyell's disease or syndrome — *continued*
  due to drug
    correct substance properly administered 695.15
    overdose or wrong substance given or taken 977.9
    specified drug — *see* Table of Drugs and Chemicals
Lyme disease 088.81
Lymph
  gland or node — *see* condition
  scrotum (*see also* Infestation, filarial) 125.9
Lymphadenitis 289.3
  with
    abortion — *see* Abortion, by type, with sepsis
    ectopic pregnancy (*see also* categories 633.0–633.9) 639.0
    molar pregnancy (*see also* categories 630–632) 639.0
  acute 683
    mesenteric 289.2
  any site, except mesenteric 289.3
    acute 683
    chronic 289.1
    mesenteric (acute) (chronic) (nonspecific) (subacute) 289.2
    subacute 289.1
      mesenteric 289.2
  breast, puerperal, postpartum 675.2 ✓
  chancroidal (congenital) 099.0
  chronic 289.1
    mesenteric 289.2
  dermatopathic 695.89
  due to
    anthracosis (occupational) 500
    Brugia (Wuchereria) malayi 125.1
    diphtheria (toxin) 032.89
    lymphogranuloma venereum 099.1
    Wuchereria bancrofti 125.0
  following
    abortion 639.0
    ectopic or molar pregnancy 639.0
  generalized 289.3
  gonorrheal 098.89
  granulomatous 289.1
  infectional 683
  mesenteric (acute) (chronic) (nonspecific) (subacute) 289.2
    due to Bacillus typhi 002.0
    tuberculous (*see also* Tuberculosis) 014.8 ✓
  mycobacterial 031.8
  purulent 683
  pyogenic 683
  regional 078.3
  septic 683
  streptococcal 683
  subacute, unspecified site 289.1
  suppurative 683
  syphilitic (early) (secondary) 091.4
    late 095.8
  tuberculous — *see* Tuberculosis, lymph gland
  venereal 099.1
Lymphadenoid goiter 245.2
Lymphadenopathy (general) 785.6
  due to toxoplasmosis (acquired) 130.7
  congenital (active) 771.2
Lymphadenopathy-associated virus (disease) (illness) (infection) — *see* Human immunodeficiency virus (disease) (illness) (infection)
Lymphadenosis 785.6
  acute 075
Lymphangiectasis 457.1
  conjunctiva 372.89
  postinfectional 457.1
  scrotum 457.1
Lymphangiectatic elephantiasis, nonfilarial 457.1
Lymphangioendothelioma (M9170/0) 228.1
  malignant (M9170/3) — *see* Neoplasm, connective tissue, malignant
Lymphangioleiomyomatosis 516.4
Lymphangioma (M9170/0) 228.1

Lymphangioma — *continued*
  capillary (M9171/0) 228.1
  cavernous (M9172/0) 228.1
  cystic (M9173/0) 228.1
  malignant (M9170/3) — *see* Neoplasm, connective tissue, malignant
Lymphangiomyoma (M9174/0) 228.1
Lymphangiomyomatosis 516.4
Lymphangiosarcoma (M9170/3) — *see* Neoplasm, connective tissue, malignant
Lymphangitis 457.2
  with
    abortion — *see* Abortion, by type, with sepsis
    abscess — *see* Abscess, by site
    cellulitis — *see* Abscess, by site
    ectopic pregnancy (*see also* categories 633.0–633.9) 639.0
    molar pregnancy (*see also* categories 630–632) 639.0
  acute (with abscess or cellulitis) 682.9
    specified site — *see* Abscess, by site
  breast, puerperal, postpartum 675.2 ✓
  chancroidal 099.0
  chronic (any site) 457.2
  due to
    Brugia (Wuchereria) malayi 125.1
    Wuchereria bancrofti 125.0
  following
    abortion 639.0
    ectopic or molar pregnancy 639.0
  gangrenous 457.2
  penis
    acute 607.2
    gonococcal (acute) 098.0
      chronic or duration of 2 months or more 098.2
  puerperal, postpartum, childbirth 670.8 ✓
  strumous, tuberculous (*see also* Tuberculosis) 017.2 ✓
  subacute (any site) 457.2
  tuberculous — *see* Tuberculosis, lymph gland
Lymphatic (vessel) — *see* condition
Lymphatism 254.8
  scrofulous (*see also* Tuberculosis) 017.2 ✓
Lymphectasia 457.1
Lymphedema — *see also* Elephantiasis 457.1
  acquired (chronic) 457.1
  chronic hereditary 757.0
  congenital 757.0
  idiopathic hereditary 757.0
  praecox 457.1
  secondary 457.1
  surgical NEC 997.99
    postmastectomy (syndrome) 457.0
Lymph-hemangioma (M9120/0) — *see* Hemangioma, by site
Lymphoblastic — *see* condition
Lymphoblastoma (diffuse) (M9630/3) 200.1 ✓
  giant follicular (M9690/3) 202.0 ✓
  macrofollicular (M9690/3) 202.0 ✓
Lymphoblastosis, acute benign 075
Lymphocele 457.8
Lymphocythemia 288.51
Lymphocytic — *see also* condition
  chorioencephalitis (acute) (serous) 049.0
  choriomeningitis (acute) (serous) 049.0
Lymphocytoma (diffuse) (malignant) (M9620/3) 200.1 ✓
Lymphocytomatosis (M9620/3) 200.1 ✓
Lymphocytopenia 288.51
Lymphocytosis (symptomatic) 288.61
  infectious (acute) 078.89
Lymphoepithelioma (M8082/3) — *see* Neoplasm, by site, malignant
Lymphogranuloma (malignant) (M9650/3) 201.9 ✓
  inguinale 099.1
  venereal (any site) 099.1
    with stricture of rectum 099.1
  venereum 099.1
Lymphogranulomatosis (malignant) (M9650/3) 201.9 ✓
  benign (Boeck's sarcoid) (Schaumann's) 135
  Hodgkin's (M9650/3) 201.9 ✓

Lymphohistiocytosis, familial hemophagocytic 288.4

Lymphoid — *see* condition

Lympholeukoblastoma (M9850/3) 207.8 ☑

Lympholeukosarcoma (M9850/3) 207.8 ☑

Lymphoma (malignant) (M9590/3) 202.8 ☑

Note — *Use the following fifth-digit subclassification with categories 200–202:*

0   *unspecified site, extranodal and solid organ sites*

1   *lymph nodes of head, face, and neck*

2   *intrathoracic lymph nodes*

3   *intra–abdominal lymph nodes*

4   *lymph nodes of axilla and upper limb*

5   *lymph nodes of inguinal region and lower limb*

6   *intrapelvic lymph nodes*

7   *spleen*

8   *lymph nodes of multiple sites*

benign (M9590/0) — *see* Neoplasm, by site, benign
Burkitt's type (lymphoblastic) (undifferentiated) (M9750/3) 200.2 ☑
Castleman's (mediastinal lymph node hyperplasia) 785.6
centroblastic-centrocytic
  diffuse (M9614/3) 202.8 ☑
  follicular (M9692/3) 202.0 ☑
centroblastic type (diffuse) (M9632/3) 202.8 ☑
  follicular (M9697/3) 202.0 ☑
centrocytic (M9622/3) 202.8 ☑
compound (M9613/3) 200.8 ☑
convoluted cell type (lymphoblastic) (M9602/3) 202.8 ☑
diffuse NEC (M9590/3) 202.8 ☑
  large B cell 202.8 ☑
follicular (giant) (M9690/3) 202.0 ☑
  center cell (diffuse) (M9615/3) 202.8 ☑
    cleaved (diffuse) (M9623/3) 202.8 ☑
      follicular (M9695/3) 202.0 ☑
    non-cleaved (diffuse) (M9633/3) 202.8 ☑
      follicular (M9698/3) 202.0 ☑
  centroblastic-centrocytic (M9692/3) 202.0 ☑
  centroblastic type (M9697/3) 202.0 ☑
  large cell 202.0 ☑
  lymphocytic
    intermediate differentiation (M9694/3) 202.0 ☑
    poorly differentiated (M9696/3) 202.0 ☑
  mixed (cell type) (lymphocytic-histiocytic) (small cell and large cell) (M9691/3) 202.0 ☑
germinocytic (M9622/3) 202.8 ☑
giant, follicular or follicle (M9690/3) 202.0 ☑
histiocytic (diffuse) (M9640/3) 200.0 ☑
  nodular (M9642/3) 200.0 ☑
  pleomorphic cell type (M9641/3) 200.0 ☑
Hodgkin's (M9650/3) (*see also* Disease, Hodgkin's) 201.9 ☑
immunoblastic (type) (M9612/3) 200.8 ☑
large cell (M9640/3) 200.7 ☑
  anaplastic 200.6 ☑
  nodular (M9642/3) 202.0 ☑
  pleomorphic cell type (M9641/3) 200.0 ☑
lymphoblastic (diffuse) (M9630/3) 200.1 ☑
  Burkitt's type (M9750/3) 200.2 ☑
  convoluted cell type (M9602/3) 202.8 ☑
lymphocytic (cell type) (diffuse) (M9620/3) 200.1 ☑

Lymphoma — *continued*
lymphocytic — *continued*
  with plasmacytoid differentiation, diffuse (M9611/3) 200.8 ☑
  intermediate differentiation (diffuse) (M9621/3) 200.1 ☑
    follicular (M9694/3) 202.0 ☑
    nodular (M9694/3) 202.0 ☑
  nodular (M9690/3) 202.0 ☑
  poorly differentiated (diffuse) (M9630/3) 200.1 ☑
    follicular (M9696/3) 202.0 ☑
    nodular (M9696/3) 202.0 ☑
  well differentiated (diffuse) (M9620/3) 200.1 ☑
    follicular (M9693/3) 202.0 ☑
    nodular (M9693/3) 202.0 ☑
lymphocytic-histiocytic, mixed (diffuse) (M9613/3) 200.8 ☑
  follicular (M9691/3) 202.0 ☑
  nodular (M9691/3) 202.0 ☑
lymphoplasmacytoid type (M9611/3) 200.8 ☑
lymphosarcoma type (M9610/3) 200.1 ☑
macrofollicular (M9690/3) 202.0 ☑
mantle cell 200.4 ☑
marginal zone 200.3 ☑
  extranodal B-cell 200.3 ☑
  nodal B-cell 200.3 ☑
  splenic B-cell 200.3 ☑
mixed cell type (diffuse) (M9613/3) 200.8 ☑
  follicular (M9691/3) 202.0 ☑
  nodular (M9691/3) 202.0 ☑
nodular (M9690/3) 202.0 ☑
  histiocytic (M9642/3) 200.0 ☑
  lymphocytic (M9690/3) 202.0 ☑
    intermediate differentiation (M9694/3) 202.0 ☑
    poorly differentiated (M9696/3) 202.0 ☑
  mixed (cell type) (lymphocytic-histiocytic) (small cell and large cell) (M9691/3) 202.0 ☑
non-Hodgkin's type NEC (M9591/3) 202.8 ☑
peripheral T-cell 202.7 ☑
primary central nervous system 200.5 ☑
reticulum cell (type) (M9640/3) 200.0 ☑
small cell and large cell, mixed (diffuse) (M9613/3) 200.8 ☑
  follicular (M9691/3) 202.0 ☑
  nodular (M9691/3) 202.0 ☑
stem cell (type) (M9601/3) 202.8 ☑
T-cell 202.1 ☑
  peripheral 202.7 ☑
undifferentiated (cell type) (non-Burkitt's) (M9600/3) 202.8 ☑
  Burkitt's type (M9750/3) 200.2 ☑

Lymphomatosis (M9590/3) — *see also* Lymphoma
granulomatous 099.1

Lymphopathia
venereum 099.1
veneris 099.1

Lymphopenia 288.51
familial 279.2

Lymphoreticulosis, benign (of inoculation) 078.3

Lymphorrhea 457.8

Lymphosarcoma (M9610/3) 200.1 ☑
diffuse (M9610/3) 200.1 ☑
  with plasmacytoid differentiation (M9611/3) 200.8 ☑
  lymphoplasmacytic (M9611/3) 200.8 ☑
follicular (giant) (M9690/3) 202.0 ☑
  lymphoblastic (M9696/3) 202.0 ☑
  lymphocytic, intermediate differentiation (M9694/3) 202.0 ☑
  mixed cell type (M9691/3) 202.0 ☑
giant follicular (M9690/3) 202.0 ☑
Hodgkin's (M9650/3) 201.9 ☑
immunoblastic (M9612/3) 200.8 ☑
lymphoblastic (diffuse) (M9630/3) 200.1 ☑
  follicular (M9696/3) 202.0 ☑
  nodular (M9696/3) 202.0 ☑

Lymphosarcoma — *continued*
lymphocytic (diffuse) (M9620/3) 200.1 ☑
  intermediate differentiation (diffuse) (M9621/3) 200.1 ☑
    follicular (M9694/3) 202.0 ☑
    nodular (M9694/3) 202.0 ☑
mixed cell type (diffuse) (M9613/3) 200.8 ☑
  follicular (M9691/3) 202.0 ☑
  nodular (M9691/3) 202.0 ☑
nodular (M9690/3) 202.0 ☑
  lymphoblastic (M9696/3) 202.0 ☑
  lymphocytic, intermediate differentiation (M9694/3) 202.0 ☑
  mixed cell type (M9691/3) 202.0 ☑
prolymphocytic (M9631/3) 200.1 ☑
reticulum cell (M9640/3) 200.0 ☑

Lymphostasis 457.8

Lypemania — *see also* Melancholia 296.2 ☑

Lyssa 071

M

Macacus ear 744.29

Maceration
fetus (cause not stated) 779.9
wet feet, tropical (syndrome) 991.4

Machado-Joseph disease 334.8

Machupo virus hemorrhagic fever 078.7

Macleod's syndrome (abnormal transradiancy, one lung) 492.8

Macrocephalia, macrocephaly 756.0

Macrocheilia (congenital) 744.81

Macrochilia (congenital) 744.81

Macrocolon (congenital) 751.3

Macrocornea 743.41
associated with buphthalmos 743.22

Macrocytic — *see* condition

Macrocytosis 289.89

Macrodactylia, macrodactylism (fingers) (thumbs) 755.57
toes 755.65

Macrodontia 520.2

Macroencephaly 742.4

Macrogenia 524.05

Macrogenitosomia (female) (male) (praecox) 255.2

Macrogingivae 523.8

Macroglobulinemia (essential) (idiopathic) (monoclonal) (primary) (syndrome) (Waldenström's) 273.3

Macroglossia (congenital) 750.15
acquired 529.8

Macrognathia, macrognathism (congenital) 524.00
mandibular 524.02
  alveolar 524.72
maxillary 524.01
  alveolar 524.71

Macrogyria (congenital) 742.4

Macrohydrocephalus — *see also* Hydrocephalus 331.4

Macromastia — *see also* Hypertrophy, breast 611.1

Macrophage activation syndrome 288.4

Macropsia 368.14

Macrosigmoid 564.7
congenital 751.3

Macrospondylitis, acromegalic 253.0

Macrostomia (congenital) 744.83

Macrotia (external ear) (congenital) 744.22

Macula
cornea, corneal
  congenital 743.43
    interfering with vision 743.42
  interfering with central vision 371.03
  not interfering with central vision 371.02
degeneration (*see also* Degeneration, macula) 362.50
hereditary (*see also* Dystrophy, retina) 362.70
edema, cystoid 362.53

Maculae ceruleae 132.1

Macules and papules 709.8

Maculopathy, toxic 362.55

Madarosis 374.55

Madelung's
deformity (radius) 755.54
disease (lipomatosis) 272.8
lipomatosis 272.8

Madness — *see also* Psychosis 298.9
myxedema (acute) 293.0
  subacute 293.1

Madura
disease (actinomycotic) 039.9
  mycotic 117.4
foot (actinomycotic) 039.4
  mycotic 117.4

Maduromycosis (actinomycotic) 039.9
mycotic 117.4

Maffucci's syndrome (dyschondroplasia with hemangiomas) 756.4

Magenblase syndrome 306.4

Main en griffe (acquired) 736.06
congenital 755.59

Maintenance
chemotherapy regimen or treatment V58.11
dialysis regimen or treatment
  extracorporeal (renal) V56.0
  peritoneal V56.8
  renal V56.0
drug therapy or regimen
  chemotherapy, antineoplastic V58.11
  immunotherapy, antineoplastic V58.12
external fixation NEC V54.89
methadone 304.00
radiotherapy V58.0
traction NEC V54.89

Majocchi's
disease (purpura annularis telangiectodes) 709.1
granuloma 110.6

Major — *see* condition

Mal
cerebral (idiopathic) (*see also* Epilepsy) 345.9 ☑
comital (*see also* Epilepsy) 345.9 ☑
de los pintos (*see also* Pinta) 103.9
de Meleda 757.39
de mer 994.6
lie — *see* Presentation, fetal
perforant (*see also* Ulcer, lower extremity) 707.15

Malabar itch 110.9
beard 110.0
foot 110.4
scalp 110.0

Malabsorption 579.9
calcium 579.8
carbohydrate 579.8
disaccharide 271.3
drug-induced 579.8
due to bacterial overgrowth 579.8
fat 579.8
folate, congenital 281.2
galactose 271.1
glucose-galactose (congenital) 271.3
intestinal 579.9
isomaltose 271.3
lactose (hereditary) 271.3
methionine 270.4
monosaccharide 271.8
postgastrectomy 579.3
postsurgical 579.3
protein 579.8
sucrose (-isomaltose) (congenital) 271.3
syndrome 579.9
  postgastrectomy 579.3
  postsurgical 579.3

Malacia, bone 268.2
juvenile (*see also* Rickets) 268.0
Kienböck's (juvenile) (lunate) (wrist) 732.3
  adult 732.8

Malacoplakia
bladder 596.89
colon 569.89
pelvis (kidney) 593.89
ureter 593.89
urethra 599.84

Malacosteon 268.2
juvenile (*see also* Rickets) 268.0

Maladaptation — *see* Maladjustment

☑ **Additional Digit Required — Refer to the Tabular List for Digit Selection**   ⬚ **Subterms under main terms may continue to next column or page**

2015 ICD-9-CM   ▶◀ **Revised Text**   ● **New Line**   ▲ **Revised Code**   **Volume 2 — 179**

Maladie de Roger 745.4
Maladjustment
  conjugal V61.10
    involving
        divorce V61.03
        estrangement V61.09
  educational V62.3
  family V61.9
    specified circumstance NEC V61.8
  marital V61.10
    involving
        divorce V61.03
        estrangement V61.09
  occupational V62.29
    current military deployment status
        V62.21
  simple, adult (see also Reaction, adjustment)
        309.9
  situational acute (see also Reaction, adjust-
        ment) 309.9
  social V62.4
Malaise 780.79
Malakoplakia — see Malacoplakia
Malaria, malarial (fever) 084.6
  algid 084.9
  any type, with
    algid malaria 084.9
    blackwater fever 084.8
    fever
        blackwater 084.8
        hemoglobinuric (bilious) 084.8
    hemoglobinuria, malarial 084.8
    hepatitis 084.9 [573.2]
    nephrosis 084.9 [581.81]
    pernicious complication NEC 084.9
        cardiac 084.9
        cerebral 084.9
  cardiac 084.9
  carrier (suspected) of V02.9
  cerebral 084.9
  complicating pregnancy, childbirth, or
        puerperium 647.4 ☑
  congenital 771.2
  congestion, congestive 084.6
    brain 084.9
  continued 084.0
  estivo-autumnal 084.0
  falciparum (malignant tertian) 084.0
  hematinuria 084.8
  hematuria 084.8
  hemoglobinuria 084.8
  hemorrhagic 084.6
  induced (therapeutically) 084.7
    accidental — see Malaria, by type
  liver 084.9 [573.2]
  malariae (quartan) 084.2
  malignant (tertian) 084.0
  mixed infections 084.5
  monkey 084.4
  ovale 084.3
  pernicious, acute 084.0
  Plasmodium, P.
    falciparum 084.0
    malariae 084.2
    ovale 084.3
    vivax 084.1
  quartan 084.2
  quotidian 084.0
  recurrent 084.6
    induced (therapeutically) 084.7
        accidental — see Malaria, by type
  remittent 084.6
  specified types NEC 084.4
  spleen 084.6
  subtertian 084.0
  tertian (benign) 084.1
    malignant 084.0
  tropical 084.0
  typhoid 084.6
  vivax (benign tertian) 084.1
Malassez's disease (testicular cyst) 608.89
Malassimilation 579.9
Maldescent, testis 752.51
Maldevelopment — see also Anomaly, by site
  brain 742.9
  colon 751.5

Maldevelopment — see also Anomaly, by site
  — continued
  hip (joint) 755.63
    congenital dislocation (see also Disloca-
        tion, hip, congenital) 754.30
  mastoid process 756.0
  middle ear, except ossicles 744.03
    ossicles 744.04
  newborn (not malformation) 764.9 ☑
  ossicles, ear 744.04
  spine 756.10
  toe 755.66
Male type pelvis 755.69
  with disproportion (fetopelvic) 653.2 ☑
    affecting fetus or newborn 763.1
    causing obstructed labor 660.1 ☑
        affecting fetus or newborn 763.1
Malformation (congenital) — see also
  Anomaly
  arteriovenous
    pulmonary 747.32
  bone 756.9
  bursa 756.9
  Chiari
    type I 348.4
    type II (see also Spina bifida) 741.0 ☑
    type III 742.0
    type IV 742.2
  circulatory system NEC 747.9
    specified type NEC 747.89
  cochlea 744.05
  digestive system NEC 751.9
    lower 751.5
    specified type NEC 751.8
    upper 750.9
  eye 743.9
  gum 750.9
  heart NEC 746.9
    specified type NEC 746.89
    valve 746.9
  internal ear 744.05
  joint NEC 755.9
    specified type NEC 755.8
  Mondini's (congenital) (malformation,
        cochlea) 744.05
  muscle 756.9
  nervous system (central) 742.9
  pelvic organs or tissues
    in pregnancy or childbirth 654.9 ☑
        affecting fetus or newborn 763.89
        causing obstructed labor 660.2 ☑
            affecting fetus or newborn 763.1
  placenta (see also Placenta, abnormal)
        656.7 ☑
  respiratory organs 748.9
    specified type NEC 748.8
  Rieger's 743.44
  sense organs NEC 742.9
    specified type NEC 742.8
  skin 757.9
    specified type NEC 757.8
  spinal cord 742.9
  teeth, tooth NEC 520.9
  tendon 756.9
  throat 750.9
  umbilical cord (complicating delivery)
        663.9 ☑
    affecting fetus or newborn 762.6
  umbilicus 759.9
  urinary system NEC 753.9
    specified type NEC 753.8
  venous — see Anomaly, vein
Malfunction — see also Dysfunction
  arterial graft 996.1
  cardiac pacemaker 996.01
  catheter device — see Complications, me-
        chanical, catheter
  colostomy 569.62
    valve 569.62
  cystostomy 596.82
    infection 596.81
    mechanical 596.82
    specified complication NEC 596.83
  device, implant, or graft NEC — see Compli-
        cations, mechanical
  enteric stoma 569.62

Malfunction — see also Dysfunction —
  continued
  enterostomy 569.62
  esophagostomy 530.87
  gastroenteric 536.8
  gastrostomy 536.42
  ileostomy
    valve 569.62
  nephrostomy 997.5
  pacemaker — see Complications, mechani-
        cal, pacemaker
  prosthetic device, internal — see Complica-
        tions, mechanical
  tracheostomy 519.02
  valve
    colostomy 569.62
    ileostomy 569.62
  vascular graft or shunt 996.1
Malgaigne's fracture (closed) 808.43
  open 808.53
Malherbe's
  calcifying epithelioma (M8110/0) — see
        Neoplasm, skin, benign
  tumor (M8110/0) — see Neoplasm, skin,
        benign
Malibu disease 919.8
  infected 919.9
Malignancy (M8000/3) — see Neoplasm, by
  site, malignant
Malignant — see condition
Malingerer, malingering V65.2
Mallet, finger (acquired) 736.1
  congenital 755.59
  late effect of rickets 268.1
Malleus 024
Mallory's bodies 034.1
Mallory-Weiss syndrome 530.7
Malnutrition (calorie) 263.9
  complicating pregnancy 648.9 ☑
  degree
    first 263.1
    second 263.0
    third 262
    mild (protein) 263.1
    moderate (protein) 263.0
    severe 261
        protein-calorie 262
  fetus 764.2 ☑
    "light-for-dates" 764.1 ☑
  following gastrointestinal surgery 579.3
  intrauterine or fetal 764.2 ☑
    fetus or infant "light-for-dates" 764.1 ☑
  lack of care, or neglect (child) (infant) 995.52
    adult 995.84
  malignant 260
  mild (protein) 263.1
  moderate (protein) 263.0
  protein 260
  protein-calorie 263.9
    mild 263.1
    moderate 263.0
    severe 262
    specified type NEC 263.8
  severe 261
    protein-calorie NEC 262
Malocclusion (teeth) 524.4
  angle's class I 524.21
  angle's class II 524.22
  angle's class III 524.23
  due to
    abnormal swallowing 524.59
    accessory teeth (causing crowding)
        524.31
    dentofacial abnormality NEC 524.89
    impacted teeth (causing crowding) 520.6
    missing teeth 524.30
    mouth breathing 524.59
    sleep postures 524.59
    supernumerary teeth (causing crowding)
        524.31
    thumb sucking 524.59
    tongue, lip, or finger habits 524.59
  temporomandibular (joint) 524.69
Malposition
  cardiac apex (congenital) 746.87
  cervix — see Malposition, uterus

Malposition — continued
  congenital
    adrenal (gland) 759.1
    alimentary tract 751.8
        lower 751.5
        upper 750.8
    aorta 747.21
    appendix 751.5
    arterial trunk 747.29
    artery (peripheral) NEC (see also Malposi-
        tion, congenital, peripheral vascu-
        lar system) 747.60
        coronary 746.85
        pulmonary 747.39
    auditory canal 744.29
        causing impairment of hearing
            744.02
    auricle (ear) 744.29
        causing impairment of hearing
            744.02
    cervical 744.43
    biliary duct or passage 751.69
    bladder (mucosa) 753.8
        exteriorized or extroverted 753.5
    brachial plexus 742.8
    brain tissue 742.4
    breast 757.6
    bronchus 748.3
    cardiac apex 746.87
    cecum 751.5
    clavicle 755.51
    colon 751.5
    digestive organ or tract NEC 751.8
        lower 751.5
        upper 750.8
    ear (auricle) (external) 744.29
        ossicles 744.04
    endocrine (gland) NEC 759.2
    epiglottis 748.3
    Eustachian tube 744.24
    eye 743.8
    facial features 744.89
    fallopian tube 752.19
    finger(s) 755.59
        supernumerary 755.01
    foot 755.67
    gallbladder 751.69
    gastrointestinal tract 751.8
    genitalia, genital organ(s) or tract
        female 752.89
            external 752.49
            internal NEC 752.89
        male 752.89
            penis 752.69
            scrotal transposition 752.81
    glottis 748.3
    hand 755.59
    heart 746.87
        dextrocardia 746.87
            with complete transposition of
                viscera 759.3
    hepatic duct 751.69
    hip (joint) (see also Dislocation, hip,
        congenital) 754.30
    intestine (large) (small) 751.5
        with anomalous adhesions, fixation,
            or malrotation 751.4
    joint NEC 755.8
    kidney 753.3
    larynx 748.3
    limb 755.8
        lower 755.69
        upper 755.59
    liver 751.69
    lung (lobe) 748.69
    nail(s) 757.5
    nerve 742.8
    nervous system NEC 742.8
    nose, nasal (septum) 748.1
    organ or site NEC — see Anomaly, spec-
        ified type NEC, by site
    ovary 752.0
    pancreas 751.7
    parathyroid (gland) 759.2
    patella 755.64
    peripheral vascular system 747.60

☑ **Additional Digit Required** — Refer to the Tabular List for Digit Selection   ▽ **Subterms under main terms may continue to next column or page**

180 — Volume 2   ►◄ Revised Text   ● New Line   ▲ Revised Code   2015 ICD-9-CM

Malposition — *continued*
  congenital — *continued*
    peripheral vascular system — *continued*
      gastrointestinal 747.61
      lower limb 747.64
      renal 747.62
      specified NEC 747.69
      spinal 747.82
      upper limb 747.63
    pituitary (gland) 759.2
    respiratory organ or system NEC 748.9
    rib (cage) 756.3
      supernumerary in cervical region 756.2
    scapula 755.59
    shoulder 755.59
    spinal cord 742.59
    spine 756.19
    spleen 759.0
    sternum 756.3
    stomach 750.7
    symphysis pubis 755.69
    testis (undescended) 752.51
    thymus (gland) 759.2
    thyroid (gland) (tissue) 759.2
      cartilage 748.3
    toe(s) 755.66
      supernumerary 755.02
    tongue 750.19
    trachea 748.3
    uterus 752.39
    vein(s) (peripheral) NEC (*see also* Malposition, congenital, peripheral vascular system) 747.60
      great 747.49
      portal 747.49
      pulmonary 747.49
    vena cava (inferior) (superior) 747.49
  device, implant, or graft — *see* Complications, mechanical
  fetus NEC (*see also* Presentation, fetal) 652.9 ☑
    with successful version 652.1 ☑
    affecting fetus or newborn 763.1
    before labor, affecting fetus or newborn 761.7
    causing obstructed labor 660.0 ☑
    in multiple gestation (one fetus or more) 652.6 ☑
      with locking 660.5 ☑
      causing obstructed labor 660.0 ☑
  gallbladder (*see also* Disease, gallbladder) 575.8
  gastrointestinal tract 569.89
    congenital 751.8
  heart (*see also* Malposition, congenital, heart) 746.87
  intestine 569.89
    congenital 751.5
  pelvic organs or tissues
    in pregnancy or childbirth 654.4 ☑
      affecting fetus or newborn 763.89
      causing obstructed labor 660.2 ☑
        affecting fetus or newborn 763.1
  placenta — *see* Placenta, previa
  stomach 537.89
    congenital 750.7
  tooth, teeth 524.30
    with impaction 520.6
  uterus (acquired) (acute) (adherent) (any degree) (asymptomatic) (postinfectional) (postpartal, old) 621.6
    anteflexion or anteversion (*see also* Anteversion, uterus) 621.6
    congenital 752.39
    flexion 621.6
      lateral (*see also* Lateroversion, uterus) 621.6
    in pregnancy or childbirth 654.4 ☑
      affecting fetus or newborn 763.89
      causing obstructed labor 660.2 ☑
        affecting fetus or newborn 763.1
    inversion 621.6
    lateral (flexion) (version) (*see also* Lateroversion, uterus) 621.6

Malposition — *continued*
  uterus — *continued*
    lateroflexion (*see also* Lateroversion, uterus) 621.6
    lateroversion (*see also* Lateroversion, uterus) 621.6
    retroflexion or retroversion (*see also* Retroversion, uterus) 621.6
Malposture 729.90
Malpresentation, fetus — *see also* Presentation, fetal 652.9 ☑
Malrotation
  cecum 751.4
  colon 751.4
  intestine 751.4
  kidney 753.3
MALT (mucosa associated lymphoid tissue) 200.3 ☑
Malta fever — *see also* Brucellosis 023.9
Maltosuria 271.3
Maltreatment (of)
  adult 995.80
    emotional 995.82
    multiple forms 995.85
    neglect (nutritional) 995.84
    physical 995.81
    psychological 995.82
    sexual 995.83
  child 995.50
    emotional 995.51
    multiple forms 995.59
    neglect (nutritional) 995.52
    physical 995.54
      shaken infant syndrome 995.55
    psychological 995.51
    sexual 995.53
  spouse (*see also* Maltreatment, adult) 995.80
Malt workers' lung 495.4
Malum coxae senilis 715.25
Malunion, fracture 733.81
Mammillitis — *see also* Mastitis 611.0
  puerperal, postpartum 675.2 ☑
Mammitis — *see also* Mastitis 611.0
  puerperal, postpartum 675.2 ☑
Mammographic
  calcification 793.89
  calculus 793.89
  microcalcification 793.81
Mammoplasia 611.1
Management
  contraceptive V25.9
    specified type NEC V25.8
  procreative V26.9
    specified type NEC V26.89
Mangled NEC — *see also* nature and site of injury 959.9
Mania (monopolar) — *see also* Psychosis, affective 296.0 ☑
  alcoholic (acute) (chronic) 291.9
  Bell's — *see* Mania, chronic
  chronic 296.0 ☑
    recurrent episode 296.1 ☑
    single episode 296.0 ☑
  compulsive 300.3
  delirious (acute) 296.0 ☑
    recurrent episode 296.1 ☑
    single episode 296.0 ☑
  epileptic (*see also* Epilepsy) 345.4 ☑
  hysterical 300.10
  inhibited 296.89
  puerperal (after delivery) 296.0 ☑
    recurrent episode 296.1 ☑
    single episode 296.0 ☑
  recurrent episode 296.1 ☑
  senile 290.8
  single episode 296.0 ☑
  stupor 296.89
  stuporous 296.89
  unproductive 296.89
Manic-depressive insanity, psychosis, reaction, or syndrome — *see also* Psychosis, affective 296.80
  circular (alternating) 296.7
    currently
      depressed 296.5 ☑
      episode unspecified 296.7

Manic-depressive insanity, psychosis, reaction, or syndrome — *see also* Psychosis, affective — *continued*
  circular — *continued*
    currently — *continued*
      hypomanic, previously depressed 296.4 ☑
      manic 296.4 ☑
      mixed 296.6 ☑
  depressed (type), depressive 296.2 ☑
    atypical 296.82
    recurrent episode 296.3 ☑
    single episode 296.2 ☑
  hypomanic 296.0 ☑
    recurrent episode 296.1 ☑
    single episode 296.0 ☑
  manic 296.0 ☑
    atypical 296.81
    recurrent episode 296.1 ☑
    single episode 296.0 ☑
  mixed NEC 296.89
  perplexed 296.89
  stuporous 296.89
Manifestations, rheumatoid
  lungs 714.81
  pannus — *see* Arthritis, rheumatoid
  subcutaneous nodules — *see* Arthritis, rheumatoid
Mankowsky's syndrome (familial dysplastic osteopathy) 731.2
Mannoheptulosuria 271.8
Mannosidosis 271.8
Manson's
  disease (schistosomiasis) 120.1
  pyosis (pemphigus contagiosus) 684
  schistosomiasis 120.1
Mansonellosis 125.5
Manual — *see* condition
Maple bark disease 495.6
Maple bark-strippers' lung 495.6
Maple syrup (urine) disease or syndrome 270.3
Marable's syndrome (celiac artery compression) 447.4
Marasmus 261
  brain 331.9
  due to malnutrition 261
  intestinal 569.89
  nutritional 261
  senile 797
  tuberculous NEC (*see also* Tuberculosis) 011.9 ☑
Marble
  bones 756.52
  skin 782.61
Marburg disease (virus) 078.89
March
  foot 733.94
  hemoglobinuria 283.2
Marchand multiple nodular hyperplasia (liver) 571.5
Marchesani (-Weill) syndrome (brachymorphism and ectopia lentis) 759.89
Marchiafava (-Bignami) disease or syndrome 341.8
Marchiafava-Micheli syndrome (paroxysmal nocturnal hemoglobinuria) 283.2
Marcus Gunn's syndrome (jaw-winking syndrome) 742.8
Marfan's
  congenital syphilis 090.49
  disease 090.49
  syndrome (arachnodactyly) 759.82
    meaning congenital syphilis 090.49
      with luxation of lens 090.49 [379.32]
Marginal
  implantation, placenta — *see* Placenta, previa
  placenta — *see* Placenta, previa
  sinus (hemorrhage) (rupture) 641.2 ☑
    affecting fetus or newborn 762.1
Marie's
  cerebellar ataxia 334.2
  syndrome (acromegaly) 253.0

Marie-Bamberger disease or syndrome (hypertrophic) (pulmonary) (secondary) 731.2
  idiopathic (acropachyderma) 757.39
  primary (acropachyderma) 757.39
Marie-Charcôt-Tooth neuropathic atrophy, muscle 356.1
Marie-Strümpell arthritis or disease (ankylosing spondylitis) 720.0
Marihuana, marijuana
  abuse (*see also* Abuse, drugs, nondependent) 305.2 ☑
  dependence (*see also* Dependence) 304.3 ☑
Marion's disease (bladder neck obstruction) 596.0
Marital conflict V61.10
Mark
  port wine 757.32
  raspberry 757.32
  strawberry 757.32
  stretch 701.3
  tattoo 709.09
Maroteaux-Lamy syndrome (mucopolysaccharidosis VI) 277.5
Marriage license examination V70.3
Marrow (bone)
  arrest 284.9
  megakaryocytic 287.30
  poor function 289.9
Marseilles fever 082.1
Marshall's (hidrotic) **ectodermal dysplasia** 757.31
Marsh's disease (exophthalmic goiter) 242.0 ☑
Marsh fever — *see also* Malaria 084.6
Martin-Albright syndrome (pseudohypoparathyroidism) 275.49
Martin's disease 715.27
Martorell-Fabre syndrome (pulseless disease) 446.7
Masculinization, female, with adrenal hyperplasia 255.2
Masculinovoblastoma (M8670/0) 220
Masochism 302.83
Masons' lung 502
Mass
  abdominal 789.3 ☑
  anus 787.99
  bone 733.90
  breast 611.72
  cheek 784.2
  chest 786.6
  cystic — *see* Cyst
  ear 388.8
  epigastric 789.3 ☑
  eye 379.92
  female genital organ 625.8
  gum 784.2
  head 784.2
  intracranial 784.2
  joint 719.60
    ankle 719.67
    elbow 719.62
    foot 719.67
    hand 719.64
    hip 719.65
    knee 719.66
    multiple sites 719.69
    pelvic region 719.65
    shoulder (region) 719.61
    specified site NEC 719.68
    wrist 719.63
  kidney (*see also* Disease, kidney) 593.9
  lung 786.6
  lymph node 785.6
  malignant (M8000/3) — *see* Neoplasm, by site, malignant
  mediastinal 786.6
  mouth 784.2
  muscle (limb) 729.89
  neck 784.2
  nose or sinus 784.2
  palate 784.2
  pelvis, pelvic 789.3 ☑
  penis 607.89
  perineum 625.8

☑ **Additional Digit Required** — Refer to the Tabular List for Digit Selection   ⚐ **Subterms under main terms may continue to next column or page**

2015 ICD-9-CM   ►◄ **Revised Text**   ● **New Line**   ▲ **Revised Code**   **Volume 2 — 181**

Mass — *continued*
  rectum 787.99
  scrotum 608.89
  skin 782.2
  specified organ NEC — *see* Disease of specified organ or site
  splenic 789.2
  substernal 786.6
    thyroid (*see also* Goiter) 240.9
  superficial (localized) 782.2
  testes 608.89
  throat 784.2
  tongue 784.2
  umbilicus 789.3 ☑
  uterus 625.8
  vagina 625.8
  vulva 625.8
Massive — *see* condition
Mastalgia 611.71
  psychogenic 307.89
Mast cell
  disease 757.33
    systemic (M9741/3) 202.6 ☑
  leukemia (M9900/3) 207.8 ☑
  sarcoma (M9740/3) 202.6 ☑
  tumor (M9740/1) 238.5
    malignant (M9740/3) 202.6 ☑
Masters-Allen syndrome 620.6
Mastitis (acute) (adolescent) (diffuse) (interstitial) (lobular) (nonpuerperal) (nonsuppurative) (parenchymatous) (phlegmonous) (simple) (subacute) (suppurative) 611.0
  chronic (cystic) (fibrocystic) 610.1
  cystic 610.1
    Schimmelbusch's type 610.1
  fibrocystic 610.1
  infective 611.0
  lactational 675.2 ☑
  lymphangitis 611.0
  neonatal (noninfective) 778.7
    infective 771.5
  periductal 610.4
  plasma cell 610.4
  puerperalis 675.2 ☑
  puerperal, postpartum, (interstitial) (nonpurulent) (parenchymatous) 675.2 ☑
    purulent 675.1 ☑
    stagnation 676.2 ☑
  retromammary 611.0
    puerperal, postpartum 675.1 ☑
  submammary 611.0
    puerperal, postpartum 675.1 ☑
Mastocytoma (M9740/1) 238.5
  malignant (M9740/3) 202.6 ☑
Mastocytosis 757.33
  malignant (M9741/3) 202.6 ☑
  systemic (M9741/3) 202.6 ☑
Mastodynia 611.71
  psychogenic 307.89
Mastoid — *see* condition
Mastoidalgia — *see also* Otalgia 388.70
Mastoiditis (coalescent) (hemorrhagic) (pneumococcal) (streptococcal) (suppurative) 383.9
  acute or subacute 383.00
    with
      Gradenigo's syndrome 383.02
      petrositis 383.02
      specified complication NEC 383.02
      subperiosteal abscess 383.01
  chronic (necrotic) (recurrent) 383.1
  tuberculous (*see also* Tuberculosis) 015.6 ☑
Mastopathy, mastopathia 611.9
  chronica cystica 610.1
  diffuse cystic 610.1
  estrogenic 611.89
  ovarian origin 611.89
Mastoplasia 611.1
Masturbation 307.9
Maternal condition, affecting fetus or newborn
  acute yellow atrophy of liver 760.8
  albuminuria 760.1
  anesthesia or analgesia 763.5
  blood loss 762.1

Maternal condition, affecting fetus or newborn — *continued*
  chorioamnionitis 762.7
  circulatory disease, chronic (conditions classifiable to 390–459, 745–747) 760.3
  congenital heart disease (conditions classifiable to 745–746) 760.3
  cortical necrosis of kidney 760.1
  death 761.6
  diabetes mellitus 775.0
    manifest diabetes in the infant 775.1
  disease NEC 760.9
    circulatory system, chronic (conditions classifiable to 390–459, 745–747) 760.3
    genitourinary system (conditions classifiable to 580–599) 760.1
    respiratory (conditions classifiable to 490–519, 748) 760.3
  eclampsia 760.0
  hemorrhage NEC 762.1
  hepatitis acute, malignant, or subacute 760.8
  hyperemesis (gravidarum) 761.8
  hypertension (arising during pregnancy) (conditions classifiable to 642) 760.0
  infection
    disease classifiable to 001-136 ☑, 760.2
    genital tract NEC 760.8
    urinary tract 760.1
  influenza 760.2
    manifest influenza in the infant 771.2
  injury (conditions classifiable to 800–996) 760.5
  malaria 760.2
    manifest malaria in infant or fetus 771.2
  malnutrition 760.4
  necrosis of liver 760.8
  nephritis (conditions classifiable to 580–583) 760.1
  nephrosis (conditions classifiable to 581) 760.1
  noxious substance transmitted via breast milk or placenta 760.70
    alcohol 760.71
    anticonvulsants 760.77
    antifungals 760.74
    anti-infective agents 760.74
    antimetabolics 760.78
    cocaine 760.75
    "crack" 760.75
    diethylstilbestrol [DES] 760.76
    hallucinogenic agents 760.73
    medicinal agents NEC 760.79
    narcotics 760.72
    obstetric anesthetic or analgesic drug 760.72
    specified agent NEC 760.79
  nutritional disorder (conditions classifiable to 260–269) 760.4
  operation unrelated to current delivery (*see also* Newborn, affected by) 760.64
  pre-eclampsia 760.0
  pyelitis or pyelonephritis, arising during pregnancy (conditions classifiable to 590) 760.1
  renal disease or failure 760.1
  respiratory disease, chronic (conditions classifiable to 490–519, 748) 760.3
  rheumatic heart disease (chronic) (conditions classifiable to 393–398) 760.3
  rubella (conditions classifiable to 056) 760.2
    manifest rubella in the infant or fetus 771.0
  surgery unrelated to current delivery (*see also* Newborn, affected by) 760.64
    to uterus or pelvic organs 760.64
  syphilis (conditions classifiable to 090–097) 760.2
    manifest syphilis in the infant or fetus 090.0
  thrombophlebitis 760.3
  toxemia (of pregnancy) 760.0
    pre-eclamptic 760.0

Maternal condition, affecting fetus or newborn — *continued*
  toxoplasmosis (conditions classifiable to 130) 760.2
    manifest toxoplasmosis in the infant or fetus 771.2
  transmission of chemical substance through the placenta 760.70
    alcohol 760.71
    anticonvulsants 760.77
    antifungals 760.74
    anti-infective 760.74
    antimetabolics 760.78
    cocaine 760.75
    "crack" 760.75
    diethylstilbestrol [DES] 760.76
    hallucinogenic agents 760.73
    narcotics 760.72
    specified substance NEC 760.79
  uremia 760.1
  urinary tract conditions (conditions classifiable to 580–599) 760.1
  vomiting (pernicious) (persistent) (vicious) 761.8
Maternity — *see* Delivery
Matheiu's disease (leptospiral jaundice) 100.0
Mauclaire's disease or osteochondrosis 732.3
Maxcy's disease 081.0
Maxilla, maxillary — *see* condition
May (-Hegglin) anomaly or syndrome 288.2
Mayaro fever 066.3
Mazoplasia 610.8
MBD (minimal brain dysfunction), child — *see also* Hyperkinesia 314.9
MCAD (medium chain acyl CoA dehydrogenase deficiency) 277.85
McArdle (-Schmid-Pearson) disease or syndrome (glycogenosis V) 271.0
McCune-Albright syndrome (osteitis fibrosa disseminata) 756.59
MCLS (mucocutaneous lymph node syndrome) 446.1
McQuarrie's syndrome (idiopathic familial hypoglycemia) 251.2
Measles (black) (hemorrhagic) (suppressed) 055.9
  with
    encephalitis 055.0
    keratitis 055.71
    keratoconjunctivitis 055.71
    otitis media 055.2
    pneumonia 055.1
  complication 055.8
    specified type NEC 055.79
  encephalitis 055.0
  French 056.9
  German 056.9
  keratitis 055.71
  keratoconjunctivitis 055.71
  liberty 056.9
  otitis media 055.2
  pneumonia 055.1
  specified complications NEC 055.79
  vaccination, prophylactic (against) V04.2
Meatitis, urethral — *see also* Urethritis 597.89
Meat poisoning — *see* Poisoning, food
Meatus, meatal — *see* condition
Meat-wrappers' asthma 506.9
Meckel's
  diverticulitis 751.0
  diverticulum (displaced) (hypertrophic) 751.0
Meconium
  aspiration 770.11
    with
      pneumonia 770.12
      pneumonitis 770.12
      respiratory symptoms 770.12
    below vocal cords 770.11
      with respiratory symptoms 770.12
    syndrome 770.12
  delayed passage in newborn 777.1
  ileus 777.1
    due to cystic fibrosis 277.01
  in liquor 792.3
    noted during delivery 656.8 ☑

Meconium — *continued*
  insufflation 770.11
    with respiratory symptoms 770.12
  obstruction
    fetus or newborn 777.1
      in mucoviscidosis 277.01
  passage of 792.3
    noted during delivery 763.84
  peritonitis 777.6
  plug syndrome (newborn) NEC 777.1
  staining 779.84
Median — *see also* condition
  arcuate ligament syndrome 447.4
  bar (prostate) 600.90
    with
      other lower urinary tract symptoms (LUTS) 600.91
      urinary
        obstruction 600.91
        retention 600.91
  rhomboid glossitis 529.2
  vesical orifice 600.90
    with
      other lower urinary tract symptoms (LUTS) 600.91
      urinary
        obstruction 600.91
        retention 600.91
Mediastinal shift 793.2
Mediastinitis (acute) (chronic) 519.2
  actinomycotic 039.8
  syphilitic 095.8
  tuberculous (*see also* Tuberculosis) 012.8 ☑
Mediastinopericarditis — *see also* Pericarditis 423.9
  acute 420.90
  chronic 423.8
    rheumatic 393
  rheumatic, chronic 393
Mediastinum, mediastinal — *see* condition
Medical services provided for — *see* Health, services provided because (of)
Medicine poisoning (by overdose) (wrong substance given or taken in error) 977.9
  specified drug or substance — *see* Table of Drugs and Chemicals
Medin's disease (poliomyelitis) 045.9 ☑
Mediterranean
  anemia 282.40
    with other hemoglobinopathy 282.49
  disease or syndrome (hemopathic) 282.40
    with other hemoglobinopathy 282.49
  fever (*see also* Brucellosis) 023.9
    familial 277.31
  kala-azar 085.0
  leishmaniasis 085.0
  tick fever 082.1
Medulla — *see* condition
Medullary
  cystic kidney 753.16
  sponge kidney 753.17
Medullated fibers
  optic (nerve) 743.57
  retina 362.85
Medulloblastoma (M9470/3)
  desmoplastic (M9471/3) 191.6
  specified site — *see* Neoplasm, by site, malignant
  unspecified site 191.6
Medulloepithelioma (M9501/3) — *see also* Neoplasm, by site, malignant
  teratoid (M9502/3) — *see* Neoplasm, by site, malignant
Medullomyoblastoma (M9472/3)
  specified site — *see* Neoplasm, by site, malignant
  unspecified site 191.6
Meekeren-Ehlers-Danlos syndrome 756.83
Megacaryocytic — *see* condition
Megacolon (acquired) (functional) (not Hirschsprung's disease) 564.7
  aganglionic 751.3
  congenital, congenitum 751.3
  Hirschsprung's (disease) 751.3
  psychogenic 306.4
  toxic (*see also* Colitis, ulcerative) 556.9

☑ **Additional Digit Required — Refer to the Tabular List for Digit Selection**   ⚑ **Subterms under main terms may continue to next column or page**

Megaduodenum 537.3
Megaesophagus (functional) 530.0
  congenital 750.4
Megakaryocytic — *see* condition
Megalencephaly 742.4
Megalerythema (epidermicum) (infectiosum)
  057.0
Megalia, cutis et ossium 757.39
Megaloappendix 751.5
Megalocephalus, megalocephaly NEC 756.0
Megalocornea 743.41
  associated with buphthalmos 743.22
Megalocytic anemia 281.9
Megalodactylia (fingers) (thumbs) 755.57
  toes 755.65
Megaloduodenum 751.5
Megaloesophagus (functional) 530.0
  congenital 750.4
Megalogastria (congenital) 750.7
Megalomania 307.9
Megalophthalmos 743.8
Megalopsia 368.14
Megalosplenia — *see also* Splenomegaly 789.2
Megaloureter 593.89
  congenital 753.22
Megarectum 569.49
Megasigmoid 564.7
  congenital 751.3
Megaureter 593.89
  congenital 753.22
Megrim 346.9 ☑
Meibomian
  cyst 373.2
    infected 373.12
  gland — *see* condition
  infarct (eyelid) 374.85
  stye 373.11
Meibomitis 373.12
Meige
  -Milroy disease (chronic hereditary edema)
    757.0
  syndrome (blepharospasm-oromandibular
    dystonia) 333.82
Melalgia, nutritional 266.2
Melancholia — *see also* Psychosis, affective
  296.90
  climacteric 296.2 ☑
    recurrent episode 296.3 ☑
    single episode 296.2 ☑
  hypochondriac 300.7
  intermittent 296.2 ☑
    recurrent episode 296.3 ☑
    single episode 296.2 ☑
  involutional 296.2 ☑
    recurrent episode 296.3 ☑
    single episode 296.2 ☑
  menopausal 296.2 ☑
    recurrent episode 296.3 ☑
    single episode 296.2 ☑
  puerperal 296.2 ☑
  reactive (from emotional stress, psycholog-
    ical trauma) 298.0
  recurrent 296.3 ☑
  senile 290.21
  stuporous 296.2 ☑
    recurrent episode 296.3 ☑
    single episode 296.2 ☑
Melanemia 275.09
Melanoameloblastoma (M9363/0) — *see*
  Neoplasm, bone, benign
Melanoblastoma (M8720/3) — *see* Melanoma
Melanoblastosis
  Block-Sulzberger 757.33
  cutis linearis sive systematisata 757.33
Melanocarcinoma (M8720/3) — *see*
  Melanoma
Melanocytoma, eyeball (M8726/0) 224.0
Melanocytosis, neurocutaneous 757.33
Melanoderma, melanodermia 709.09
  Addison's (primary adrenal insufficiency)
    255.41
Melanodontia, infantile 521.05
Melanodontoclasia 521.05
Melanoepithelioma (M8720/3) — *see*
  Melanoma

Melanoma (malignant) (M8720/3) 172.9

Note — Except where otherwise indicated, the morphological varieties of
melanoma in the list below should be
coded by site as for "Melanoma (malignant)". Internal sites should be coded
to malignant neoplasm of those sites.

  abdominal wall 172.5
  ala nasi 172.3
  amelanotic (M8730/3) — *see* Melanoma, by
    site
  ankle 172.7
  anus, anal 154.3
    canal 154.2
  arm 172.6
  auditory canal (external) 172.2
  auricle (ear) 172.2
  auricular canal (external) 172.2
  axilla 172.5
  axillary fold 172.5
  back 172.5
  balloon cell (M8722/3) — *see* Melanoma,
    by site
  benign (M8720/0) — *see* Neoplasm, skin,
    benign
  breast (female) (male) 172.5
  brow 172.3
  buttock 172.5
  canthus (eye) 172.1
  cheek (external) 172.3
  chest wall 172.5
  chin 172.3
  choroid 190.6
  conjunctiva 190.3
  ear (external) 172.2
  epithelioid cell (M8771/3) (*see also*
    Melanoma, by site)
    and spindle cell, mixed (M8775/3) — *see*
      Melanoma, by site
  external meatus (ear) 172.2
  eye 190.9
  eyebrow 172.3
  eyelid (lower) (upper) 172.1
  face NEC 172.3
  female genital organ (external) NEC 184.4
  finger 172.6
  flank 172.5
  foot 172.7
  forearm 172.6
  forehead 172.3
  foreskin 187.1
  gluteal region 172.5
  groin 172.5
  hand 172.6
  heel 172.7
  helix 172.2
  hip 172.7
  in
    giant pigmented nevus (M8761/3) —
      see Melanoma, by site
    Hutchinson's melanotic freckle
      (M8742/3) — *see* Melanoma, by
      site
    junctional nevus (M8740/3) — *see*
      Melanoma, by site
    precancerous melanosis (M8741/3) —
      see Melanoma, by site
  in situ — *see* Melanoma, by site
    skin 172.9
  interscapular region 172.5
  iris 190.0
  jaw 172.3
  juvenile (M8770/0) — *see* Neoplasm, skin,
    benign
  knee 172.7
  labium
    majus 184.1
    minus 184.2
  lacrimal gland 190.2
  leg 172.7
  lip (lower) (upper) 172.0
  liver 197.7
  lower limb NEC 172.7
  male genital organ (external) NEC 187.9
  meatus, acoustic (external) 172.2
  meibomian gland 172.1

Melanoma — *continued*
  metastatic
    of or from specified site — *see*
      Melanoma, by site
    site not of skin — *see* Neoplasm, by site,
      malignant, secondary
    to specified site — *see* Neoplasm, by site,
      malignant, secondary
    unspecified site 172.9
  nail 172.9
    finger 172.6
    toe 172.7
  neck 187.4
  nodular (M8721/3) — *see* Melanoma, by site
  nose, external 172.3
  orbit 190.1
  penis 187.4
  perianal skin 172.5
  perineum 172.5
  pinna 172.2
  popliteal (fossa) (space) 172.7
  prepuce 187.1
  pubes 172.5
  pudendum 184.4
  retina 190.5
  scalp 172.4
  scrotum 187.7
  septum nasal (skin) 172.3
  shoulder 172.6
  skin NEC 172.8
    in situ 172.9
  spindle cell (M8772/3) (*see also* Melanoma,
    by site)
    type A (M8773/3) 190.0
    type B (M8774/3) 190.0
  submammary fold 172.5
  superficial spreading (M8743/3) — *see*
    Melanoma, by site
  temple 172.3
  thigh 172.7
  toe 172.7
  trunk NEC 172.5
  umbilicus 172.5
  upper limb NEC 172.6
  vagina vault 184.0
  vulva 184.4
Melanoplakia 528.9
Melanosarcoma (M8720/3) — *see also*
  Melanoma
  epithelioid cell (M8771/3) — *see* Melanoma
Melanosis 709.09
  addisonian (primary adrenal insufficiency)
    255.41
    tuberculous (*see also* Tuberculosis)
      017.6 ☑
  adrenal 255.41
  colon 569.89
  conjunctiva 372.55
    congenital 743.49
  corii degenerativa 757.33
  cornea (presenile) (senile) 371.12
    congenital 743.43
      interfering with vision 743.42
  eye 372.55
    congenital 743.49
  jute spinners' 709.09
  lenticularis progressiva 757.33
  liver 573.8
  precancerous (M8741/2) (*see also* Neoplasm,
    skin, in situ)
    malignant melanoma in (M8741/3) —
      see Melanoma
  prenatal 743.43
    interfering with vision 743.42
  Riehl's 709.09
  sclera 379.19
    congenital 743.47
  suprarenal 255.41
  tar 709.09
  toxic 709.09
Melanuria 791.9
Melasma 709.09
  adrenal (gland) 255.41
  suprarenal (gland) 255.41

MELAS syndrome (mitochondrial encephalopa-
  thy, lactic acidosis and stroke-like
  episodes) 277.87
Melena 578.1
  due to
    swallowed maternal blood 777.3
    ulcer — *see* Ulcer, by site, with hemor-
      rhage
  newborn 772.4
    due to swallowed maternal blood 777.3
Meleney's
  gangrene (cutaneous) 686.09
  ulcer (chronic undermining) 686.09
Melioidosis 025
Melitensis, febris 023.0
Melitococcosis 023.0
Melkersson (-Rosenthal) syndrome 351.8
Mellitus, diabetes — *see* Diabetes
Melorheostosis (bone) (leri) 733.99
Meloschisis 744.83
Melotia 744.29
Membrana
  capsularis lentis posterior 743.39
  epipapillaris 743.57
Membranacea placenta — *see* Placenta, abnormal
Membranaceous uterus 621.8
Membrane, membranous — *see also* condi-
  tion
  folds, congenital — *see* Web
  Jackson's 751.4
  over face (causing asphyxia), fetus or new-
    born 768.9
  premature rupture — *see* Rupture, mem-
    branes, premature
  pupillary 364.74
    persistent 743.46
  retained (complicating delivery) (with
    hemorrhage) 666.2 ☑
    without hemorrhage 667.1 ☑
  secondary (eye) 366.50
  unruptured (causing asphyxia) 768.9
  vitreous humor 379.25
Membranitis, fetal 658.4 ☑
  affecting fetus or newborn 762.7
Memory disturbance, loss or lack — *see also*
  Amnesia 780.93
  mild, following organic brain damage
    310.89
MEN (multiple endocrine neoplasia) (syndromes)
  type I 258.01
  type IIA 258.02
  type IIB 258.03
Menadione (vitamin K) **deficiency** 269.0
Menarche, precocious 259.1
Mendacity, pathologic 301.7
Mendelson's syndrome (resulting from a
  procedure) 997.32
  obstetric 668.0 ☑
Mende's syndrome (ptosis-epicanthus) 270.2
Ménétrier's disease or syndrome (hypertrophic gastritis) 535.2 ☑
Ménière's disease, syndrome, or vertigo
  386.00
  cochlear 386.02
  cochleovestibular 386.01
  inactive 386.04
  in remission 386.04
  vestibular 386.03
Meninges, meningeal — *see* condition
Meningioma (M9530/0) — *see also* Neoplasm,
  meninges, benign
  angioblastic (M9535/0) — *see* Neoplasm,
    meninges, benign
  angiomatous (M9534/0) — *see* Neoplasm,
    meninges, benign
  endotheliomatous (M9531/0) — *see* Neo-
    plasm, meninges, benign
  fibroblastic (M9532/0) — *see* Neoplasm,
    meninges, benign
  fibrous (M9532/0) — *see* Neoplasm,
    meninges, benign
  hemangioblastic (M9535/0) — *see* Neo-
    plasm, meninges, benign

☑ **Additional Digit Required** — Refer to the Tabular List for Digit Selection

▽ **Subterms under main terms may continue to next column or page**

Meningioma — see also Neoplasm, meninges, benign — continued
  hemangiopericytic (M9536/0) — see Neoplasm, meninges, benign
  malignant (M9530/3) — see Neoplasm, meninges, malignant
  meningiothelial (M9531/0) — see Neoplasm, meninges, benign
  meningotheliomatous (M9531/0) — see Neoplasm, meninges, benign
  mixed (M9537/0) — see Neoplasm, meninges, benign
  multiple (M9530/1) 237.6
  papillary (M9538/1) 237.6
  psammomatous (M9533/0) — see Neoplasm, meninges, benign
  syncytial (M9531/0) — see Neoplasm, meninges, benign
  transitional (M9537/0) — see Neoplasm, meninges, benign
Meningiomatosis (diffuse) (M9530/1) 237.6
Meningism — see also Meningismus 781.6
Meningismus (infectional) (pneumococcal) 781.6
  due to serum or vaccine 997.09 [321.8]
  influenzal NEC (see also Influenza) 487.8
Meningitis (basal) (basic) (basilar) (brain) (cerebral) (cervical) (congestive) (diffuse) (hemorrhagic) (infantile) (membranous) (metastatic) (nonspecific) (pontine) (progressive) (simple) (spinal) (subacute) (sympathetica) (toxic) 322.9
  abacterial NEC (see also Meningitis, aseptic) 047.9
  actinomycotic 039.8 [320.7]
  adenoviral 049.1
  Aerobacter aerogenes 320.82
    anaerobes (cocci) (gram-negative) (gram-positive) (mixed) (NEC) 320.81
  arbovirus NEC 066.9 [321.2]
    specified type NEC 066.8 [321.2]
  aseptic (acute) NEC 047.9
    adenovirus 049.1
    Coxsackie virus 047.0
    due to
      adenovirus 049.1
      Coxsackie virus 047.0
      ECHO virus 047.1
      enterovirus 047.9
      mumps 072.1
      poliovirus (see also Poliomyelitis) 045.2 ☑ [321.2]
    ECHO virus 047.1
    herpes (simplex) virus 054.72
      zoster 053.0
    leptospiral 100.81
    lymphocytic choriomeningitis 049.0
    noninfective 322.0
  Bacillus pyocyaneus 320.89
  bacterial NEC 320.9
    anaerobic 320.81
    gram-negative 320.82
      anaerobic 320.81
  Bacteroides (fragilis) (oralis) (melaninogenicus) 320.81
  cancerous (M8000/6) 198.4
  candidal 112.83
  carcinomatous (M8010/6) 198.4
  caseous (see also Tuberculosis, meninges) 013.0 ☑
  cerebrospinal (acute) (chronic) (diplococcal) (endemic) (epidemic) (fulminant) (infectious) (malignant) (meningococcal) (sporadic) 036.0
    carrier (suspected) of V02.59
  chronic NEC 322.2
  clear cerebrospinal fluid NEC 322.0
  Clostridium (haemolyticum) (novyi) NEC 320.81
  coccidioidomycosis 114.2
  Coxsackie virus 047.0
  cryptococcal 117.5 [321.0]
  diplococcal 036.0
    gram-negative 036.0
    gram-positive 320.1

Meningitis — continued
  Diplococcus pneumoniae 320.1
  due to
    actinomycosis 039.8 [320.7]
    adenovirus 049.1
    coccidiomycosis 114.2
    enterovirus 047.9
      specified NEC 047.8
    histoplasmosis (see also Histoplasmosis) 115.91
    Listerosis 027.0 [320.7]
    Lyme disease 088.81 [320.7]
    moniliasis 112.83
    mumps 072.1
    neurosyphilis 094.2
    nonbacterial organisms NEC 321.8
    oidiomycosis 112.83
    poliovirus (see also Poliomyelitis) 045.2 ☑ [321.2]
    preventive immunization, inoculation, or vaccination 997.09 [321.8]
    sarcoidosis 135 [321.4]
    sporotrichosis 117.1 [321.1]
    syphilis 094.2
      acute 091.81
      congenital 090.42
      secondary 091.81
    trypanosomiasis (see also Trypanosomiasis) 086.9 [321.3]
    whooping cough 033.9 [320.7]
  ECHO virus 047.1
  E. coli 320.82
  endothelial-leukocytic, benign, recurrent 047.9
  Enterobacter aerogenes 320.82
  enteroviral 047.9
    specified type NEC 047.8
  enterovirus 047.9
    specified NEC 047.8
  eosinophilic 322.1
  epidemic NEC 036.0
  Escherichia coli (E. coli) 320.82
  Eubacterium 320.81
  fibrinopurulent NEC 320.9
    specified type NEC 320.89
  Friedländer (bacillus) 320.82
  fungal NEC 117.9 [321.1]
  Fusobacterium 320.81
  gonococcal 098.82
  gram-negative bacteria NEC 320.82
    anaerobic 320.81
    cocci 036.0
      specified NEC 320.82
  gram-negative cocci NEC 036.0
    specified NEC 320.82
  gram-positive cocci NEC 320.9
  herpes (simplex) virus 054.72
    zoster 053.0
  H. influenzae 320.0
  infectious NEC 320.9
  influenzal 320.0
  Klebsiella pneumoniae 320.82
  late effect — see Late, effect, meningitis
  leptospiral (aseptic) 100.81
  Listerella (monocytogenes) 027.0 [320.7]
  Listeria monocytogenes 027.0 [320.7]
  lymphocytic (acute) (benign) (serous) 049.0
    choriomeningitis virus 049.0
  meningococcal (chronic) 036.0
  Mima polymorpha 320.82
  Mollaret's 047.9
  monilial 112.83
  mumps (virus) 072.1
  mycotic NEC 117.9 [321.1]
  Neisseria 036.0
  neurosyphilis 094.2
  nonbacterial NEC (see also Meningitis, aseptic) 047.9
  nonpyogenic NEC 322.0
  oidiomycosis 112.83
  ossificans 349.2
  Peptococcus 320.81
  Peptostreptococcus 320.81
  pneumococcal 320.1
  poliovirus (see also Poliomyelitis) 045.2 ☑ [321.2]

Meningitis — continued
  Proprionibacterium 320.81
  Proteus morganii 320.82
  Pseudomonas (aeruginosa) (pyocyaneus) 320.82
  purulent NEC 320.9
    specified organism NEC 320.89
  pyogenic NEC 320.9
    specified organism NEC 320.89
  Salmonella 003.21
  septic NEC 320.9
    specified organism NEC 320.89
  serosa circumscripta NEC 322.0
  serous NEC (see also Meningitis, aseptic) 047.9
    lymphocytic 049.0
    syndrome 348.2
  Serratia (marcescens) 320.82
  specified organism NEC 320.89
  sporadic cerebrospinal 036.0
  sporotrichosis 117.1 [321.1]
  staphylococcal 320.3
  sterile 997.09
  streptococcal (acute) 320.2
  suppurative 320.9
    specified organism NEC 320.89
  syphilitic 094.2
    acute 091.81
    congenital 090.42
    secondary 091.81
  torula 117.5 [321.0]
  traumatic (complication of injury) 958.8
  Treponema (denticola) (macrodenticum) 320.81
  trypanosomiasis 086.1 [321.3]
  tuberculous (see also Tuberculosis, meninges) 013.0 ☑
  typhoid 002.0 [320.7]
  Veillonella 320.81
  Vibrio vulnificus 320.82
  viral, virus NEC (see also Meningitis, aseptic) 047.9
  Wallgren's (see also Meningitis, aseptic) 047.9
Meningocele (congenital) (spinal) — see also Spina bifida 741.9 ☑
  acquired (traumatic) 349.2
  cerebral 742.0
  cranial 742.0
Meningocerebritis — see Meningoencephalitis
Meningococcemia (acute) (chronic) 036.2
Meningococcus, meningococcal — see also condition 036.9
  adrenalitis, hemorrhagic 036.3
  carditis 036.40
  carrier (suspected) of V02.59
  cerebrospinal fever 036.0
  encephalitis 036.1
  endocarditis 036.42
  exposure to V01.84
  infection NEC 036.9
  meningitis (cerebrospinal) 036.0
  myocarditis 036.43
  optic neuritis 036.81
  pericarditis 036.41
  septicemia (chronic) 036.2
Meningoencephalitis — see also Encephalitis 323.9
  acute NEC 048
  bacterial, purulent, pyogenic, or septic — see Meningitis
  chronic NEC 094.1
  diffuse NEC 094.1
  diphasic 063.2
  due to
    actinomycosis 039.8 [320.7]
    blastomycosis NEC (see also Blastomycosis) 116.0 [323.41]
    free-living amebae 136.29
    Listeria monocytogenes 027.0 [320.7]
    Lyme disease 088.81 [320.7]
    mumps 072.2
    Naegleria (amebae) (gruberi) (organisms) 136.29
    rubella 056.01

Meningoencephalitis — see also Encephalitis — continued
  due to — continued
    sporotrichosis 117.1 [321.1]
    toxoplasmosis (acquired) 130.0
      congenital (active) 771.2 [323.41]
    Trypanosoma 086.1 [323.2]
  epidemic 036.0
  herpes 054.3
  herpetic 054.3
  H. influenzae 320.0
  infectious (acute) 048
  influenzal 320.0
  late effect — see category 326
  Listeria monocytogenes 027.0 [320.7]
  lymphocytic (serous) 049.0
  mumps 072.2
  parasitic NEC 123.9 [323.41]
  pneumococcal 320.1
  primary amebic 136.29
  rubella 056.01
  serous 048
    lymphocytic 049.0
  specific 094.2
  staphylococcal 320.3
  streptococcal 320.2
  syphilitic 094.2
  toxic NEC 989.9 [323.71]
    due to
      carbon tetrachloride (vapor) 987.8 [323.71]
      hydroxyquinoline derivatives poisoning 961.3 [323.71]
      lead 984.9 [323.71]
      mercury 985.0 [323.71]
      thallium 985.8 [323.71]
  toxoplasmosis (acquired) 130.0
  trypanosomic 086.1 [323.2]
  tuberculous (see also Tuberculosis, meninges) 013.0 ☑
  virus NEC 048
Meningoencephalocele 742.0
  syphilitic 094.89
  congenital 090.49
Meningoencephalomyelitis — see also Meningoencephalitis 323.9
  acute NEC 048
    disseminated (postinfectious) 136.9 [323.61]
      postimmunization or postvaccination 323.51
  due to
    actinomycosis 039.8 [320.7]
    torula 117.5 [323.41]
    toxoplasma or toxoplasmosis (acquired) 130.0
      congenital (active) 771.2 [323.41]
  late effect — see category 326
Meningoencephalomyelopathy — see also Meningoencephalomyelitis 349.9
Meningoencephalopathy — see also Meningoencephalitis 348.39
Meningoencephalopoliomyelitis — see also Poliomyelitis, bulbar 045.0 ☑
  late effect 138
Meningomyelitis — see also Meningoencephalitis 323.9
  blastomycotic NEC (see also Blastomycosis) 116.0 [323.41]
  due to
    actinomycosis 039.8 [320.7]
    blastomycosis (see also Blastomycosis) 116.0 [323.41]
    Meningococcus 036.0
    sporotrichosis 117.1 [323.41]
    torula 117.5 [323.41]
  late effect — see category 326
  lethargic 049.8
  meningococcal 036.0
  syphilitic 094.2
  tuberculous (see also Tuberculosis, meninges) 013.0 ☑
Meningomyelocele — see also Spina bifida 741.9 ☑
  syphilitic 094.89

Meningomyeloneuritis — *see* Meningoencephalitis

Meningoradiculitis — *see* Meningitis

Meningovascular — *see* condition

Meniscocytosis 282.60

Menkes' syndrome — *see* Syndrome, Menkes'

Menolipsis 626.0

Menometrorrhagia 626.2

Menopause, menopausal (symptoms) (syndrome) 627.2

  arthritis (any site) NEC 716.3 ☑

  artificial 627.4

  bleeding 627.0

  crisis 627.2

  depression (*see also* Psychosis, affective) 296.2 ☑

    agitated 296.2 ☑

      recurrent episode 296.3 ☑

      single episode 296.2 ☑

    psychotic 296.2 ☑

      recurrent episode 296.3 ☑

      single episode 296.2 ☑

    recurrent episode 296.3 ☑

    single episode 296.2 ☑

  melancholia (*see also* Psychosis, affective) 296.2 ☑

    recurrent episode 296.3 ☑

    single episode 296.2 ☑

  paranoid state 297.2

  paraphrenia 297.2

  postsurgical 627.4

  premature 256.31

    postirradiation 256.2

    postsurgical 256.2

  psychoneurosis 627.2

  psychosis NEC 298.8

  surgical 627.4

  toxic polyarthritis NEC 716.39

Menorrhagia (primary) 626.2

  climacteric 627.0

  menopausal 627.0

  postclimacteric 627.1

  postmenopausal 627.1

  preclimacteric 627.0

  premenopausal 627.0

  puberty (menses retained) 626.3

Menorrhalgia 625.3

Menoschesis 626.8

Menostaxis 626.2

Menses, retention 626.8

Menstrual — *see also* Menstruation

  cycle, irregular 626.4

  disorders NEC 626.9

  extraction V25.3

  fluid, retained 626.8

  molimen 625.4

  period, normal V65.5

  regulation V25.3

Menstruation

  absent 626.0

  anovulatory 628.0

  delayed 626.8

  difficult 625.3

  disorder 626.9

    psychogenic 306.52

    specified NEC 626.8

  during pregnancy 640.8 ☑

  excessive 626.2

  frequent 626.2

  infrequent 626.1

  irregular 626.4

  latent 626.8

  membranous 626.8

  painful (primary) (secondary) 625.3

    psychogenic 306.52

  passage of clots 626.2

  precocious 259.1

  protracted 626.8

  retained 626.8

  retrograde 626.8

  scanty 626.1

  suppression 626.8

  vicarious (nasal) 625.8

Mentagra — *see also* Sycosis 704.8

Mental — *see also* condition

Mental — *see also* condition — *continued*

  deficiency (*see also* Disability, intellectual) 319

  deterioration (*see also* Psychosis) 298.9

  disorder (*see also* Disorder, mental) 300.9

  exhaustion 300.5

  insufficiency (congenital) (*see also* Disability, intellectual) 319

  observation without need for further medical care NEC V71.09

  retardation — *see* Disability, intellectual

  subnormality (*see also* Disability, intellectual) 319

    mild 317

    moderate 318.0

    profound 318.2

    severe 318.1

  upset (*see also* Disorder, mental) 300.9

Meralgia paresthetica 355.1

Mercurial — *see* condition

Mercurialism NEC 985.0

Merergasia 300.9

Merkel cell tumor — *see* Carcinoma, Merkel cell

Merocele — *see also* Hernia, femoral 553.00

Meromelia 755.4

  lower limb 755.30

    intercalary 755.32

      femur 755.34

        tibiofibular (complete) (incomplete) 755.33

      fibula 755.37

      metatarsal(s) 755.38

      tarsal(s) 755.38

      tibia 755.36

      tibiofibular 755.35

    terminal (complete) (partial) (transverse) 755.31

    longitudinal 755.32

      metatarsal(s) 755.38

      phalange(s) 755.39

      tarsal(s) 755.38

    transverse 755.31

  upper limb 755.20

    intercalary 755.22

      carpal(s) 755.28

      humeral 755.24

        radioulnar (complete) (incomplete) 755.23

      metacarpal(s) 755.28

      phalange(s) 755.29

      radial 755.26

      radioulnar 755.25

      ulnar 755.27

    terminal (complete) (partial) (transverse) 755.21

    longitudinal 755.22

      carpal(s) 755.28

      metacarpal(s) 755.28

      phalange(s) 755.29

    transverse 755.21

Merosmia 781.1

MERRF syndrome (myoclonus with epilepsy and with ragged red fibers) 277.87

Merycism — *see also* Vomiting

  psychogenic 307.53

Merzbacher-Pelizaeus disease 330.0

Mesaortitis — *see* Aortitis

Mesarteritis — *see* Arteritis

Mesencephalitis — *see also* Encephalitis 323.9

  late effect — *see* category 326

Mesenchymoma (M8990/1) — *see also* Neoplasm, connective tissue, uncertain behavior

  benign (M8990/0) — *see* Neoplasm, connective tissue, benign

  malignant (M8990/3) — *see* Neoplasm, connective tissue, malignant

Mesenteritis

  retractile 567.82

  sclerosing 567.82

Mesentery, mesenteric — *see* condition

Mesiodens, mesiodentes 520.1

  causing crowding 524.31

Mesio-occlusion 524.23

Mesocardia (with asplenia) 746.87

Mesocolon — *see* condition

Mesonephroma (malignant) (M9110/3) — *see also* Neoplasm, by site, malignant

  benign (M9110/0) — *see* Neoplasm, by site, benign

Mesophlebitis — *see* Phlebitis

Mesostromal dysgenesis 743.51

Mesothelioma (malignant) (M9050/3) — *see also* Neoplasm, by site, malignant

  benign (M9050/0) — *see* Neoplasm, by site, benign

  biphasic type (M9053/3) (*see also* Neoplasm, by site, malignant)

    benign (M9053/0) — *see* Neoplasm, by site, benign

  epithelioid (M9052/3) (*see also* Neoplasm, by site, malignant)

    benign (M9052/0) — *see* Neoplasm, by site, benign

  fibrous (M9051/3) (*see also* Neoplasm, by site, malignant)

    benign (M9051/0) — *see* Neoplasm, by site, benign

Metabolic syndrome 277.7

Metabolism disorder 277.9

  specified type NEC 277.89

Metagonimiasis 121.5

Metagonimus infestation (small intestine) 121.5

Metal

  pigmentation (skin) 709.00

  polishers' disease 502

Metalliferous miners' lung 503

Metamorphopsia 368.14

Metaplasia

  bone, in skin 709.3

  breast 611.89

  cervix — *omit code*

  endometrium (squamous) 621.8

  esophagus 530.85

  intestinal, of gastric mucosa 537.89

  kidney (pelvis) (squamous) (*see also* Disease, renal) 593.89

  myelogenous 289.89

  myeloid 289.89

    agnogenic 238.76

    megakaryocytic 238.76

  spleen 289.59

  squamous cell

    amnion 658.8 ☑

    bladder 596.89

    cervix — *see* condition

    trachea 519.19

    tracheobronchial tree 519.19

    uterus 621.8

    cervix — *see* condition

Metastasis, metastatic

  abscess — *see* Abscess

  calcification 275.40

  cancer, neoplasm, or disease

    from specified site (M8000/3) — *see* Neoplasm, by site, malignant

    to specified site (M8000/6) — *see* Neoplasm, by site, secondary

  deposits (in) (M8000/6) — *see* Neoplasm, by site, secondary

  mesentery, of neuroendocrine tumor 209.74

  pneumonia 038.8 [484.8]

  spread (to) (M8000/6) — *see* Neoplasm, by site, secondary

Metatarsalgia 726.70

  anterior 355.6

  due to Freiberg's disease 732.5

  Morton's 355.6

Metatarsus, metatarsal — *see also* condition

  abductus valgus (congenital) 754.60

  adductus varus (congenital) 754.53

  primus varus 754.52

  valgus (adductus) (congenital) 754.60

  varus (abductus) (congenital) 754.53

    primus 754.52

Methadone use 304.00

Methemoglobinemia 289.7

  acquired (with sulfhemoglobinemia) 289.7

  congenital 289.7

  enzymatic 289.7

Methemoglobinemia — *continued*

  Hb-M disease 289.7

  hereditary 289.7

  toxic 289.7

Methemoglobinuria — *see also* Hemoglobinuria 791.2

Methicillin

  resistant staphyloccocus aureus (MRSA) 041.12

    colonization V02.54

    personal history of V12.04

  susceptible staphylococcus aureus (MSSA) 041.11

    colonization V02.53

Methioninemia 270.4

Metritis (catarrhal) (septic) (suppurative) — *see also* Endometritis 615.9

  blennorrhagic 098.16

    chronic or duration of 2 months or over 098.36

  cervical (*see also* Cervicitis) 616.0

  gonococcal 098.16

    chronic or duration of 2 months or over 098.36

  hemorrhagic 626.8

  puerperal, postpartum, childbirth 670.1 ☑

    septic 670.2 ☑

  tuberculous (*see also* Tuberculosis) 016.7 ☑

Metropathia hemorrhagica 626.8

Metroperitonitis — *see also* Peritonitis, pelvic, female 614.5

Metrorrhagia 626.6

  arising during pregnancy — *see* Hemorrhage, pregnancy

  postpartum NEC 666.2 ☑

  primary 626.6

  psychogenic 306.59

  puerperal 666.2 ☑

Metrorrhexis — *see* Rupture, uterus

Metrosalpingitis — *see also* Salpingo-oophoritis 614.2

Metrostaxis 626.6

Metrovaginitis — *see also* Endometritis 615.9

  gonococcal (acute) 098.16

    chronic or duration of 2 months or over 098.36

Mexican fever — *see* Typhus, Mexican

Meyenburg-Altherr-Uehlinger syndrome 733.99

Meyer-Schwickerath and Weyers syndrome (dysplasia oculodentodigitalis) 759.89

Meynert's amentia (nonalcoholic) 294.0

  alcoholic 291.1

Mibelli's disease 757.39

Mice, joint — *see also* Loose, body, joint 718.1 ☑

  knee 717.6

Micheli-Rietti syndrome (thalassemia minor) 282.46

Michotte's syndrome 721.5

Micrencephalon, micrencephaly 742.1

Microalbuminuria 791.0

Microaneurysm, retina 362.14

  diabetic 250.5 ☑ [362.01]

    due to secondary diabetes 249.5 ☑ [362.01]

Microangiopathy 443.9

  diabetic (peripheral) 250.7 ☑ [443.81]

    due to secondary diabetes 249.7 ☑ [443.81]

    retinal 250.5 ☑ [362.01]

      due to secondary diabetes 249.5 ☑ [362.01]

  peripheral 443.9

    diabetic 250.7 ☑ [443.81]

      due to secondary diabetes 249.7 ☑ [443.81]

  retinal 362.18

    diabetic 250.5 ☑ [362.01]

      due to secondary diabetes 249.5 ☑ [362.01]

  thrombotic 446.6

    Moschcowitz's (thrombotic thrombocytopenic purpura) 446.6

Microcalcification, mammographic 793.81

☑ Additional Digit Required — Refer to the Tabular List for Digit Selection   ᵂ Subterms under main terms may continue to next column or page

2015 ICD-9-CM   ▶◀ Revised Text   ● New Line   ▲ Revised Code   Volume 2 — 185

Meningomyeloneuritis — Microcalcification, mammographic

Microcephalus, microcephalic, microcephaly 742.1
  due to toxoplasmosis (congenital) 771.2
Microcheilia 744.82
Microcolon (congenital) 751.5
Microcornea (congenital) 743.41
Microcytic — see condition
Microdeletions NEC 758.33
Microdontia 520.2
Microdrepanocytosis (thalassemia-Hb-S disease) 282.41
  with sickle cell crisis 282.42
Microembolism
  atherothrombotic — see Atheroembolism
  retina 362.33
Microencephalon 742.1
Microfilaria streptocerca infestation 125.3
Microgastria (congenital) 750.7
Microgenia 524.06
Microgenitalia (congenital) 752.89
  penis 752.64
Microglioma (M9710/3)
  specified site — see Neoplasm, by site, malignant
  unspecified site 191.9
Microglossia (congenital) 750.16
Micrognathia, micrognathism (congenital) 524.00
  mandibular 524.04
    alveolar 524.74
  maxillary 524.03
    alveolar 524.73
Microgyria (congenital) 742.2
Microinfarct, heart — see also Insufficiency, coronary 411.89
Microlithiasis, alveolar, pulmonary 516.2
Micromastia 611.82
Micromyelia (congenital) 742.59
Micropenis 752.64
Microphakia (congenital) 743.36
Microphthalmia (congenital) — see also Microphthalmos 743.10
Microphthalmos (congenital) 743.10
  associated with eye and adnexal anomalies NEC 743.12
  due to toxoplasmosis (congenital) 771.2
  isolated 743.11
  simple 743.11
  syndrome 759.89
Micropsia 368.14
Microsporidiosis 136.8
Microsporon furfur infestation 111.0
Microsporosis — see also Dermatophytosis 110.9
  nigra 111.1
Microstomia (congenital) 744.84
Microthelia 757.6
Microthromboembolism — see Embolism
Microtia (congenital) (external ear) 744.23
Microtropia 378.34
Microvillus inclusion disease (MVD) 751.5
Micturition
  disorder NEC 788.69
    psychogenic 306.53
  frequency 788.41
    psychogenic 306.53
  nocturnal 788.43
  painful 788.1
    psychogenic 306.53
Middle
  ear — see condition
  lobe (right) syndrome 518.0
Midplane — see condition
Miescher's disease 709.3
  cheilitis 351.8
  granulomatosis disciformis 709.3
Miescher-Leder syndrome or granulomatosis 709.3
Mieten's syndrome 759.89

Migraine (idiopathic) 346.9 ☑

Note — The following fifth digit subclassification is for use with category 346:

0 *without mention of intractable migraine without mention of status migrainosus*

    without mention of refractory migraine without mention of status migrainosus

1 *with intractable migraine, so stated, without mention of status migrainosus*

    with refractory migraine, so stated, without mention of status migrainosus

2 *without mention of intractable migraine with status migrainosus*

    without mention of refractory migraine with status migrainosus

3 *with intractable migraine, so stated, with status migrainosus*

    with refractory migraine, so stated, with status migrainosus

  with aura (acute-onset) (without headache) (prolonged) (typical) 346.0 ☑
  without aura 346.1 ☑
    chronic 346.7 ☑
    transformed 346.7 ☑
  abdominal (syndrome) 346.2 ☑
  allergic (histamine) 346.2 ☑
  atypical 346.8 ☑
  basilar 346.0 ☑
  chronic without aura 346.7 ☑
  classic(al) 346.0 ☑
  common 346.1 ☑
  complicated 346.0 ☑
  hemiplegic 346.3 ☑
    familial 346.3 ☑
    sporadic 346.3 ☑
  lower-half 339.00
  menstrual 346.4 ☑
  menstrually related 346.4 ☑
  ophthalmic 346.8 ☑
  ophthalmoplegic 346.2 ☑
  premenstrual 346.4 ☑
  pure menstrual 346.4 ☑
  retinal 346.0 ☑
  specified form NEC 346.8 ☑
  transformed without aura 346.7 ☑
  variant 346.2 ☑
Migrant, social V60.0
Migratory, migrating — see also condition
  person V60.0
  testis, congenital 752.52
Mikulicz's disease or syndrome (dryness of mouth, absent or decreased lacrimation) 527.1
Milian atrophia blanche 701.3
Miliaria (crystallina) (rubra) (tropicalis) 705.1
  apocrine 705.82
Miliary — see condition
Milium — see also Cyst, sebaceous 706.2
  colloid 709.3
  eyelid 374.84
Milk
  crust 690.11
  excess secretion 676.6 ☑
  fever, female 672.0 ☑
  poisoning 988.8
  retention 676.2 ☑
  sickness 988.8
  spots 423.1
Milkers' nodes 051.1
Milk-leg (deep vessels) 671.4 ☑
  complicating pregnancy 671.3 ☑
  nonpuerperal 451.19
  puerperal, postpartum, childbirth 671.4 ☑
Milkman (-Looser) disease or syndrome (osteomalacia with pseudofractures) 268.2

Milky urine — see also Chyluria 791.1
Millar's asthma (laryngismus stridulus) 478.75
Millard-Gubler-Foville paralysis 344.89
Millard-Gubler paralysis or syndrome 344.89
Miller-Dieker syndrome 758.33
Miller's disease (osteomalacia) 268.2
Miller Fisher's syndrome 357.0
Milles' syndrome (encephalocutaneous angiomatosis) 759.6
Mills' disease 335.29
Millstone makers' asthma or lung 502
Milroy's disease (chronic hereditary edema) 757.0
Miners' — see also condition
  asthma 500
  elbow 727.2
  knee 727.2
  lung 500
  nystagmus 300.89
  phthisis (see also Tuberculosis) 011.4 ☑
  tuberculosis (see also Tuberculosis) 011.4 ☑
Minkowski-Chauffard syndrome — see also Spherocytosis 282.0
Minor — see condition
Minor's disease 336.1
Minot's disease (hemorrhagic disease, newborn) 776.0
Minot-von Willebrand (-Jürgens) disease or syndrome (angiohemophilia) 286.4
Minus (and plus) hand (intrinsic) 736.09
Miosis (persistent) (pupil) 379.42
Mirizzi's syndrome (hepatic duct stenosis) — see also Obstruction, biliary 576.2
  with calculus, cholelithiasis, or stones — see Choledocholithiasis
Mirror writing 315.09
  secondary to organic lesion 784.69
Misadventure (prophylactic) (therapeutic) — see also Complications 999.9
  administration of insulin 962.3
  infusion — see Complications, infusion
  local applications (of fomentations, plasters, etc.) 999.9
    burn or scald — see Burn, by site
  medical care (early) (late) NEC 999.9
    adverse effect of drugs or chemicals — see Table of Drugs and Chemicals
    burn or scald — see Burn, by site
  radiation NEC 990
  radiotherapy NEC 990
  surgical procedure (early) (late) — see Complications, surgical procedure
  transfusion — see Complications, transfusion
  vaccination or other immunological procedure — see Complications, vaccination
Misanthropy 301.7
Miscarriage — see Abortion, spontaneous
Mischief, malicious, child — see also Disturbance, conduct 312.0 ☑
Misdirection
  aqueous 365.83
Mismanagement, feeding 783.3
Misplaced, misplacement
  kidney (see also Disease, renal) 593.0
    congenital 753.3
  organ or site, congenital NEC — see Malposition, congenital
Missed
  abortion 632
  delivery (at or near term) 656.4 ☑
  labor (at or near term) 656.4 ☑
Misshapen reconstructed breast 612.0
Missing — see also Absence
  teeth (acquired) 525.10
    congenital (see also Anodontia) 520.0
    due to
      caries 525.13
      extraction 525.10
      periodontal disease 525.12
      specified NEC 525.19
      trauma 525.11
  vertebrae (congenital) 756.13
Misuse of drugs NEC — see also Abuse, drug, nondependent 305.9 ☑

Mitchell's disease (erythromelalgia) 443.82
Mite(s)
  diarrhea 133.8
  grain (itch) 133.8
  hair follicle (itch) 133.8
  in sputum 133.8
Mitochondrial encephalopathy, lactic acidosis and stroke-like episodes (MELAS syndrome) 277.87
Mitochondrial neurogastrointestinal encephalopathy syndrome (MNGIE) 277.87
Mitral — see condition
Mittelschmerz 625.2
Mixed — see condition
Mljet disease (mal de Meleda) 757.39
Mobile, mobility
  cecum 751.4
  coccyx 733.99
  excessive — see Hypermobility
  gallbladder 751.69
  kidney 593.0
    congenital 753.3
  organ or site, congenital NEC — see Malposition, congenital
  spleen 289.59
Mobitz heart block (atrioventricular) 426.10
  type I (Wenckebach's) 426.13
  type II 426.12
Möbius'
  disease 346.2 ☑
  syndrome
    congenital oculofacial paralysis 352.6
    ophthalmoplegic migraine 346.2 ☑
Moeller(-Barlow) disease (infantile scurvy) 267
  glossitis 529.4
Mohr's syndrome (types I and II) 759.89
Mola destruens (M9100/1) 236.1
Molarization, premolars 520.2
Molar pregnancy 631.8
  hydatidiform (delivered) (undelivered) 630
Molding, head (during birth) — omit code
Mold(s) in vitreous 117.9
Mole (pigmented) (M8720/0) — see also Neoplasm, skin, benign
  blood 631.8
  Breus' 631.8
  cancerous (M8720/3) — see Melanoma
  carneous 631.8
  destructive (M9100/1) 236.1
  ectopic — see Pregnancy, ectopic
  fleshy 631.8
  hemorrhagic 631.8
  hydatid, hydatidiform (benign) (complicating pregnancy) (delivered) (undelivered) (see also Hydatidiform mole) 630
    invasive (M9100/1) 236.1
    malignant (M9100/1) 236.1
    previous, affecting management of pregnancy V23.1
  invasive (hydatidiform) (M9100/1) 236.1
  malignant
    meaning
      malignant hydatidiform mole (M9100/1) 236.1
      melanoma (M8720/3) — see Melanoma
  nonpigmented (M8730/0) — see Neoplasm, skin, benign
  pregnancy NEC 631.8
  skin (M8720/0) — see Neoplasm, skin, benign
  stone 631.8
  tubal — see Pregnancy, tubal
  vesicular (see also Hydatidiform mole) 630
Molimen, molimina (menstrual) 625.4
Mollaret's meningitis 047.9
Mollities (cerebellar) (cerebral) 437.8
  ossium 268.2
Molluscum
  contagiosum 078.0
  epitheliale 078.0
  fibrosum (M8851/0) — see Lipoma, by site
  pendulum (M8851/0) — see Lipoma, by site

☑ **Additional Digit Required** — Refer to the Tabular List for Digit Selection
▽ **Subterms under main terms may continue to next column or page**

186 — Volume 2   ▶◀ Revised Text   ● New Line   ▲ Revised Code   2015 ICD-9-CM

Mönckeberg's arteriosclerosis, degeneration, disease, or sclerosis — see also Arteriosclerosis, extremities 440.20
Monday fever 504
Monday morning dyspnea or asthma 504
Mondini's malformation (cochlea) 744.05
Mondor's disease (thrombophlebitis of breast) 451.89
Mongolian, mongolianism, mongolism, mongoloid 758.0
   spot 757.33
Monilethrix (congenital) 757.4
Monilia infestation — see Candidiasis
Moniliasis — see also Candidiasis
   neonatal 771.7
   vulvovaginitis 112.1
Monkeypox 059.01
Monoarthritis 716.60
   ankle 716.67
   arm 716.62
      lower (and wrist) 716.63
      upper (and elbow) 716.62
   foot (and ankle) 716.67
   forearm (and wrist) 716.63
   hand 716.64
   leg 716.66
      lower 716.66
      upper 716.65
   pelvic region (hip) (thigh) 716.65
   shoulder (region) 716.61
   specified site NEC 716.68
Monoblastic — see condition
Monochromatism (cone) (rod) 368.54
Monocytic — see condition
Monocytopenia 288.59
Monocytosis (symptomatic) 288.63
Monofixation syndrome 378.34
Monomania — see also Psychosis 298.9
Mononeuritis 355.9
   cranial nerve — see Disorder, nerve, cranial
   femoral nerve 355.2
   lateral
      cutaneous nerve of thigh 355.1
      popliteal nerve 355.3
   lower limb 355.8
      specified nerve NEC 355.79
   medial popliteal nerve 355.4
   median nerve 354.1
   multiplex 354.5
   plantar nerve 355.6
   posterior tibial nerve 355.5
   radial nerve 354.3
   sciatic nerve 355.0
   ulnar nerve 354.2
   upper limb 354.9
      specified nerve NEC 354.8
   vestibular 388.5
Mononeuropathy — see also Mononeuritis 355.9
   diabetic NEC 250.6 ☑ [355.9]
      due to secondary diabetes 249.6 ☑ [355.9]
      lower limb 250.6 ☑ [355.8]
         due to secondary diabetes 249.6 ☑ [355.8]
      upper limb 250.6 ☑ [354.9]
         due to secondary diabetes 249.6 ☑ [354.9]
   iliohypogastric nerve 355.79
   ilioinguinal nerve 355.79
   obturator nerve 355.79
   saphenous nerve 355.79
Mononucleosis, infectious 075
   with hepatitis 075 [573.1]
Monoplegia 344.5
   brain (current episode) (see also Paralysis, brain) 437.8
      fetus or newborn 767.8
   cerebral (current episode) (see also Paralysis, brain) 437.8
   congenital or infantile (cerebral) (spastic) (spinal) 343.3
   embolic (current) (see also Embolism, brain) 434.1 ☑
      late effect — see Late effect(s) (of) cerebrovascular disease

Monoplegia — continued
   infantile (cerebral) (spastic) (spinal) 343.3
   lower limb 344.30
      affecting
         dominant side 344.31
         nondominant side 344.32
      due to late effect of cerebrovascular accident — see Late effect(s) (of) cerebrovascular accident
   newborn 767.8
   psychogenic 306.0
      specified as conversion reaction 300.11
   thrombotic (current) (see also Thrombosis, brain) 434.0 ☑
      late effect — see Late effect(s) (of) cerebrovascular disease
   transient 781.4
   upper limb 344.40
      affecting
         dominant side 344.41
         nondominant side 344.42
      due to late effect of cerebrovascular accident — see Late effect(s) (of) cerebrovascular accident
Monorchism, monorchidism 752.89
Monteggia's fracture (closed) 813.03
   open 813.13
Mood swings
   brief compensatory 296.99
   rebound 296.99
Mooren's ulcer (cornea) 370.07
Moore's syndrome — see also Epilepsy 345.9 ☑
Mooser bodies 081.0
Mooser-Neill reaction 081.0
Moral
   deficiency 301.7
   imbecility 301.7
Morax-Axenfeld conjunctivitis 372.03
Morbilli — see also Measles 055.9
Morbus
   anglicus, anglorum 268.0
   Beigel 111.2
   caducus (see also Epilepsy) 345.9 ☑
   caeruleus 746.89
   celiacus 579.0
   comitialis (see also Epilepsy) 345.9 ☑
   cordis (see also Disease, heart)
      valvulorum — see Endocarditis
   coxae 719.95
      tuberculous (see also Tuberculosis) 015.1 ☑
   hemorrhagicus neonatorum 776.0
   maculosus neonatorum 772.6
   renum 593.0
   senilis (see also Osteoarthrosis) 715.9 ☑
Morel-Kraepelin disease — see also Schizophrenia 295.9 ☑
Morel-Moore syndrome (hyperostosis frontalis interna) 733.3
Morel-Morgagni syndrome (hyperostosis frontalis interna) 733.3
Morgagni
   cyst, organ, hydatid, or appendage 752.89
      fallopian tube 752.11
   disease or syndrome (hyperostosis frontalis interna) 733.3
Morgagni-Adams-Stokes syndrome (syncope with heart block) 426.9
Morgagni-Stewart-Morel syndrome (hyperostosis frontalis interna) 733.3
Moria — see also Psychosis 298.9
Morning sickness 643.0 ☑
Moron 317
Morphea (guttate) (linear) 701.0
Morphine dependence — see also Dependence 304.0 ☑
Morphinism — see also Dependence 304.0 ☑
Morphinomania — see also Dependence 304.0 ☑
Morphoea 701.0
Morquio (-Brailsford) (-Ullrich) disease or syndrome (mucopolysaccharidosis IV) 277.5
   kyphosis 277.5

Morris syndrome (testicular feminization) 259.51
Morsus humanus (open wound) — see also Wound, open, by site
   skin surface intact — see Contusion
Mortification (dry) (moist) — see also Gangrene 785.4
Morton's
   disease 355.6
   foot 355.6
   metatarsalgia (syndrome) 355.6
   neuralgia 355.6
   neuroma 355.6
   syndrome (metatarsalgia) (neuralgia) 355.6
   toe 355.6
Morvan's disease 336.0
Mosaicism, mosaic (chromosomal) 758.9
   autosomal 758.5
   sex 758.81
Moschcowitz's syndrome (thrombotic thrombocytopenic purpura) 446.6
Mother yaw 102.0
Motion sickness (from travel, any vehicle) (from roundabouts or swings) 994.6
Mottled teeth (enamel) (endemic) (nonendemic) 520.3
Mottling enamel (endemic) (nonendemic) (teeth) 520.3
Mouchet's disease 732.5
Mould(s) (in vitreous) 117.9
Moulders'
   bronchitis 502
   tuberculosis (see also Tuberculosis) 011.4 ☑
Mounier-Kuhn syndrome 748.3
   with
      acute exacerbation 494.1
      bronchiectasis 494.0
         with (acute) exacerbation 494.1
   acquired 519.19
      with bronchiectasis 494.0
         with (acute) exacerbation 494.1
Mountain
   fever — see Fever, mountain
   sickness 993.2
      with polycythemia, acquired 289.0
      acute 289.0
   tick fever 066.1
Mouse, joint — see also Loose, body, joint 718.1 ☑
   knee 717.6
Mouth — see condition
Movable
   coccyx 724.71
   kidney (see also Disease, renal) 593.0
      congenital 753.3
   organ or site, congenital NEC — see Malposition, congenital
   spleen 289.59
Movement
   abnormal (dystonic) (involuntary) 781.0
   decreased fetal 655.7 ☑
   paradoxical facial 374.43
Moya Moya disease 437.5
Mozart's ear 744.29
MRSA (methicillin-resistant staphylococcus aureus) 041.12
   colonization V02.54
   personal history of V12.04
MSSA (methicillin susceptible staphylococcus aureus) 041.11
   colonization V02.53
Mucha's disease (acute parapsoriasis varioliformis) 696.2
Mucha-Haberman syndrome (acute parapsoriasis varioliformis) 696.2
Mu-chain disease 273.2
Mucinosis (cutaneous) (papular) 701.8
Mucocele
   appendix 543.9
   buccal cavity 528.9
   gallbladder (see also Disease, gallbladder) 575.3
   lacrimal sac 375.43
   orbit (eye) 376.81
   salivary gland (any) 527.6
   sinus (accessory) (nasal) 478.19

Mucocele — continued
   turbinate (bone) (middle) (nasal) 478.19
   uterus 621.8
Mucocutaneous lymph node syndrome (acute) (febrile) (infantile) 446.1
Mucoenteritis 564.9
Mucolipidosis I, II, III 272.7
Mucopolysaccharidosis (types 1-6) 277.5
   cardiopathy 277.5 [425.7]
Mucormycosis (lung) 117.7
Mucosa associated lymphoid tissue (MALT) 200.3 ☑
Mucositis — see also Inflammation, by site 528.00
   cervix (ulcerative) 616.81
   due to
      antineoplastic therapy (ulcerative) 528.01
      other drugs (ulcerative) 528.02
      specified NEC 528.09
   gastrointestinal (ulcerative) 538
   nasal (ulcerative) 478.11
   necroticans agranulocytica (see also Agranulocytosis) 288.09
   ulcerative 528.00
   vagina (ulcerative) 616.81
   vulva (ulcerative) 616.81
Mucous — see also condition
   patches (syphilitic) 091.3
      congenital 090.0
Mucoviscidosis 277.00
   with meconium obstruction 277.01
Mucus
   asphyxia or suffocation (see also Asphyxia, mucus) 933.1
      newborn 770.18
   in stool 792.1
   plug (see also Asphyxia, mucus) 933.1
      aspiration, of newborn 770.17
      tracheobronchial 519.19
      newborn 770.18
Muguet 112.0
Mulberry molars 090.5
Müllerian mixed tumor (M8950/3) — see Neoplasm, by site, malignant
Multicystic kidney 753.19
Multilobed placenta — see Placenta, abnormal
Multinodular prostate 600.10
   with
      urinary
         obstruction 600.11
         retention 600.11
Multiparity V61.5
   affecting
      fetus or newborn 763.89
      management of
         labor and delivery 659.4 ☑
         pregnancy V23.3
   requiring contraceptive management (see also Contraception) V25.9
Multipartita placenta — see Placenta, abnormal
Multiple, multiplex — see also condition
   birth
      affecting fetus or newborn 761.5
      healthy liveborn — see Newborn, multiple
   digits (congenital) 755.00
      fingers 755.01
      toes 755.02
   organ or site NEC — see Accessory
   personality 300.14
   renal arteries 747.62
Mumps 072.9
   with complication 072.8
      specified type NEC 072.79
   encephalitis 072.2
   hepatitis 072.71
   meningitis (aseptic) 072.1
   meningoencephalitis 072.2
   oophoritis 072.79
   orchitis 072.0
   pancreatitis 072.3
   polyneuropathy 072.72
   vaccination, prophylactic (against) V04.6

☑ **Additional Digit Required** — Refer to the Tabular List for Digit Selection
▽ **Subterms under main terms may continue to next column or page**

Mumu — see also Infestation, filarial 125.9
Münchausen syndrome 301.51
Münchmeyer's disease or syndrome (exostosis luxurians) 728.11
Mural — see condition
Murmur (cardiac) (heart) (nonorganic) (organic) 785.2
  abdominal 787.5
  aortic (valve) (see also Endocarditis, aortic) 424.1
  benign — omit code
  cardiorespiratory 785.2
  diastolic — see condition
  Flint (see also Endocarditis, aortic) 424.1
  functional — omit code
  Graham Steell (pulmonic regurgitation) (see also Endocarditis, pulmonary) 424.3
  innocent — omit code
  insignificant — omit code
  midsystolic 785.2
  mitral (valve) — see Stenosis, mitral
  physiologic — see condition
  presystolic, mitral — see Insufficiency, mitral
  pulmonic (valve) (see also Endocarditis, pulmonary) 424.3
  Still's (vibratory) — omit code
  systolic (valvular) — see condition
  tricuspid (valve) — see Endocarditis, tricuspid
  undiagnosed 785.2
  valvular — see condition
  vibratory — omit code
Murri's disease (intermittent hemoglobinuria) 283.2
Muscae volitantes 379.24
Muscle, muscular — see condition
Musculoneuralgia 729.1
Mushrooming hip 718.95
Mushroom workers' (pickers') lung 495.5
Mutation(s)
  factor V Leiden 289.81
  prothrombin gene 289.81
  surfactant, of lung 516.63
Mutism — see also Aphasia 784.3
  akinetic 784.3
  deaf (acquired) (congenital) 389.7
  hysterical 300.11
  selective (elective) 313.23
    adjustment reaction 309.83
MVD (microvillus inclusion disease) 751.5
MVID (microvillus inclusion disease) 751.5
Myà's disease (congenital dilation, colon) 751.3
Myalgia (intercostal) 729.1
  eosinophilia syndrome 710.5
  epidemic 074.1
    cervical 078.89
  psychogenic 307.89
  traumatic NEC 959.9
Myasthenia 358.00
  cordis — see Failure, heart
  gravis 358.00
    with exacerbation (acute) 358.01
    in crisis 358.01
    neonatal 775.2
    pseudoparalytica 358.00
  stomach 536.8
    psychogenic 306.4
  syndrome
    in
      botulism 005.1 [358.1]
      diabetes mellitus 250.6 ☑ [358.1]
        due to secondary diabetes 249.6 ☑ [358.1]
      hypothyroidism (see also Hypothyroidism) 244.9 [358.1]
      malignant neoplasm NEC 199.1 [358.1]
      pernicious anemia 281.0 [358.1]
      thyrotoxicosis (see also Thyrotoxicosis) 242.9 ☑ [358.1]
Myasthenic 728.87
Mycelium infection NEC 117.9
Mycetismus 988.1
Mycetoma (actinomycotic) 039.9
  bone 039.8

Mycetoma — continued
  bone — continued
    mycotic 117.4
  foot 039.4
    mycotic 117.4
  madurae 039.9
    mycotic 117.4
  maduromycotic 039.9
    mycotic 117.4
  mycotic 117.4
  nocardial 039.9
Mycobacteriosis — see Mycobacterium
Mycobacterium, mycobacterial (infection) 031.9
  acid-fast (bacilli) 031.9
  anonymous (see also Mycobacterium, atypical) 031.9
  atypical (acid-fast bacilli) 031.9
    cutaneous 031.1
    pulmonary 031.0
      tuberculous (see also Tuberculosis, pulmonary) 011.9 ☑
    specified site NEC 031.8
  avium 031.0
    intracellulare complex bacteremia (MAC) 031.2
  balnei 031.1
  Battey 031.0
  cutaneous 031.1
  disseminated 031.2
    avium-intracellulare complex (DMAC) 031.2
  fortuitum 031.0
  intracellulare (battey bacillus) 031.0
  kakerifu 031.8
  kansasii 031.0
  kasongo 031.8
  leprae — see Leprosy
  luciflavum 031.0
  marinum 031.1
  pulmonary 031.0
    tuberculous (see also Tuberculosis, pulmonary) 011.9 ☑
  scrofulaceum 031.1
  tuberculosis (human, bovine) (see also Tuberculosis)
    avian type 031.0
  ulcerans 031.1
  xenopi 031.0
Mycosis, mycotic 117.9
  cutaneous NEC 111.9
  ear 111.8 [380.15]
  fungoides (M9700/3) 202.1 ☑
  mouth 112.0
  pharynx 117.9
  skin NEC 111.9
  stomatitis 112.0
  systemic NEC 117.9
  tonsil 117.9
  vagina, vaginitis 112.1
Mydriasis (persistent) (pupil) 379.43
Myelatelia 742.59
Myelinoclasis, perivascular, acute (postinfectious) NEC 136.9 [323.61]
  postimmunization or postvaccinal 323.51
Myelinosis, central pontine 341.8
Myelitis (ascending) (cerebellar) (childhood) (chronic) (descending) (diffuse) (disseminated) (pressure) (progressive) (spinal cord) (subacute) — see also Encephalitis 323.9
  acute (transverse) 341.20
    idiopathic 341.22
    in conditions classified elsewhere 341.21
  due to
    other infection classified elsewhere 136.9 [323.42]
    specified cause NEC 323.82
    vaccination (any) 323.52
    viral diseases classified elsewhere 323.02
  herpes simplex 054.74
  herpes zoster 053.14
  late effect — see category 326
  optic neuritis in 341.0
  postchickenpox 052.2
  postimmunization 323.52

Myelitis — see also Encephalitis — continued
  postinfectious 136.9 [323.63]
  postvaccinal 323.52
  postvaricella 052.2
  syphilitic (transverse) 094.89
  toxic 989.9 [323.72]
  transverse 323.82
    acute 341.20
      idiopathic 341.22
      in conditions classified elsewhere 341.21
    idiopathic 341.22
  tuberculous (see also Tuberculosis) 013.6 ☑
  virus 049.9
Myeloblastic — see condition
Myelocele — see also Spina bifida 741.9 ☑
  with hydrocephalus 741.0 ☑
Myelocystocele — see also Spina bifida 741.9 ☑
Myelocytic — see condition
Myelocytoma 205.1 ☑
Myelodysplasia (spinal cord) 742.59
  meaning myelodysplastic syndrome — see Syndrome, myelodysplastic
Myeloencephalitis — see Encephalitis
Myelofibrosis 289.83
  with myeloid metaplasia 238.76
  idiopathic (chronic) 238.76
  megakaryocytic 238.79
  primary 238.76
  secondary 289.83
Myelogenous — see condition
Myeloid — see condition
Myelokathexis 288.09
Myeloleukodystrophy 330.0
Myelolipoma (M8870/0) — see Neoplasm, by site, benign
Myeloma (multiple) (plasma cell) (plasmacytic) (M9730/3) 203.0 ☑
  monostotic (M9731/1) 238.6
  solitary (M9731/1) 238.6
Myelomalacia 336.8
Myelomata, multiple (M9730/3) 203.0 ☑
Myelomatosis (M9730/3) 203.0 ☑
Myelomeningitis — see Meningoencephalitis
Myelomeningocele (spinal cord) — see also Spina bifida 741.9 ☑
  fetal, causing fetopelvic disproportion 653.7 ☑
Myelo-osteo-musculodysplasia hereditaria 756.89
Myelopathic — see condition
Myelopathy (spinal cord) 336.9
  cervical 721.1
  diabetic 250.6 ☑ [336.3]
    due to secondary diabetes 249.6 ☑ [336.3]
  drug-induced 336.8
  due to or with
    carbon tetrachloride 987.8 [323.72]
    degeneration or displacement, intervertebral disc 722.70
      cervical, cervicothoracic 722.71
      lumbar, lumbosacral 722.73
      thoracic, thoracolumbar 722.72
    hydroxyquinoline derivatives 961.3 [323.72]
    infection — see Encephalitis
    intervertebral disc disorder 722.70
      cervical, cervicothoracic 722.71
      lumbar, lumbosacral 722.73
      thoracic, thoracolumbar 722.72
    lead 984.9 [323.72]
    mercury 985.0 [323.72]
    neoplastic disease (see also Neoplasm, by site) 239.9 [336.3]
    pernicious anemia 281.0 [336.3]
    spondylosis 721.91
      cervical 721.1
      lumbar, lumbosacral 721.42
      thoracic 721.41
    thallium 985.8 [323.72]
  lumbar, lumbosacral 721.42
  necrotic (subacute) 336.1
  radiation-induced 336.8

Myelopathy — continued
  spondylogenic NEC 721.91
    cervical 721.1
    lumbar, lumbosacral 721.42
    thoracic 721.41
  thoracic 721.41
  toxic NEC 989.9 [323.72]
  transverse (see also Myelitis) 323.82
  vascular 336.1
Myelophthisis 284.2
Myeloproliferative disease (M9960/1) 238.79
Myeloradiculitis — see also Polyneuropathy 357.0
Myeloradiculodysplasia (spinal) 742.59
Myelosarcoma (M9930/3) 205.3 ☑
Myelosclerosis 289.89
  with myeloid metaplasia (M9961/1) 238.76
  disseminated, of nervous system 340
  megakaryocytic (M9961/1) 238.79
Myelosis (M9860/3) — see also Leukemia, myeloid 205.9 ☑
  acute (M9861/3) 205.0 ☑
  aleukemic (M9864/3) 205.8 ☑
  chronic (M9863/3) 205.1 ☑
  erythremic (M9840/3) 207.0 ☑
    acute (M9841/3) 207.0 ☑
  megakaryocytic (M9920/3) 207.2 ☑
  nonleukemic (chronic) 288.8
  subacute (M9862/3) 205.2 ☑
Myesthenia — see Myasthenia
Myiasis (cavernous) 134.0
  orbit 134.0 [376.13]
Myoadenoma, prostate 600.20
  with
    other lower urinary tract symptoms (LUTS) 600.21
    urinary
      obstruction 600.21
      retention 600.21
Myoblastoma
  granular cell (M9580/0) (see also Neoplasm, connective tissue, benign)
    malignant (M9580/3) — see Neoplasm, connective tissue, malignant
  tongue (M9580/0) 210.1
Myocardial — see condition
Myocardiopathy (congestive) (constrictive) (familial) (idiopathic) (infiltrative) (obstructive) (primary) (restrictive) (sporadic) 425.4
  alcoholic 425.5
  amyloid 277.39 [425.7]
  beriberi 265.0 [425.7]
  cobalt-beer 425.5
  due to
    amyloidosis 277.39 [425.7]
    beriberi 265.0 [425.7]
    cardiac glycogenosis 271.0 [425.7]
    Chagas' disease 086.0
    Friedreich's ataxia 334.0 [425.8]
    influenza (see also Influenza) 487.8 [425.8]
    mucopolysaccharidosis 277.5 [425.7]
    myotonia atrophica 359.21 [425.8]
    progressive muscular dystrophy 359.1 [425.8]
    sarcoidosis 135 [425.8]
  glycogen storage 271.0 [425.7]
  hypertrophic 425.18
    nonobstructive 425.18
    obstructive 425.11
  metabolic NEC 277.9 [425.7]
  nutritional 269.9 [425.7]
  obscure (African) 425.2
  peripartum 674.5 ☑
  postpartum 674.5 ☑
  secondary 425.9
  thyrotoxic (see also Thyrotoxicosis) 242.9 ☑ [425.7]
  toxic NEC 425.9
Myocarditis (fibroid) (interstitial) (old) (progressive) (senile) (with arteriosclerosis) 429.0
  with
    rheumatic fever (conditions classifiable to 390) 398.0

☑ **Additional Digit Required** — Refer to the Tabular List for Digit Selection   ▽ **Subterms under main terms may continue to next column or page**

188 — Volume 2   ▶◀ **Revised Text**   ● **New Line**   ▲ **Revised Code**   **2015 ICD-9-CM**

Myocarditis — *continued*
　with — *continued*
　　rheumatic fever — *continued*
　　　active (*see also* Myocarditis, acute, rheumatic) 391.2
　　　inactive or quiescent (with chorea) 398.0
　active (nonrheumatic) 422.90
　　rheumatic 391.2
　　　with chorea (acute) (rheumatic) (Sydenham's) 392.0
　acute or subacute (interstitial) 422.90
　　due to Streptococcus (beta-hemolytic) 391.2
　　idiopathic 422.91
　　rheumatic 391.2
　　　with chorea (acute) (rheumatic) (Sydenham's) 392.0
　　specified type NEC 422.99
　aseptic of newborn 074.23
　bacterial (acute) 422.92
　chagasic 086.0
　chronic (interstitial) 429.0
　congenital 746.89
　constrictive 425.4
　Coxsackie (virus) 074.23
　diphtheritic 032.82
　due to or in
　　Coxsackie (virus) 074.23
　　diphtheria 032.82
　　epidemic louse-borne typhus 080 [422.0]
　　influenza (*see also* Influenza) 487.8 [422.0]
　　Lyme disease 088.81 [422.0]
　　scarlet fever 034.1 [422.0]
　　toxoplasmosis (acquired) 130.3
　　tuberculosis (*see also* Tuberculosis) 017.9 ☑ [422.0]
　　typhoid 002.0 [422.0]
　　typhus NEC 081.9 [422.0]
　eosinophilic 422.91
　epidemic of newborn 074.23
　Fiedler's (acute) (isolated) (subacute) 422.91
　giant cell (acute) (subacute) 422.91
　gonococcal 098.85
　granulomatous (idiopathic) (isolated) (nonspecific) 422.91
　hypertensive (*see also* Hypertension, heart) 402.90
　idiopathic 422.91
　　granulomatous 422.91
　infective 422.92
　influenzal (*see also* Influenza) 487.8 [422.0]
　isolated (diffuse) (granulomatous) 422.91
　malignant 422.99
　meningococcal 036.43
　nonrheumatic, active 422.90
　parenchymatous 422.90
　pneumococcal (acute) (subacute) 422.92
　rheumatic (chronic) (inactive) (with chorea) 398.0
　　active or acute 391.2
　　　with chorea (acute) (rheumatic) (Sydenham's) 392.0
　septic 422.92
　specific (giant cell) (productive) 422.91
　staphylococcal (acute) (subacute) 422.92
　suppurative 422.92
　syphilitic (chronic) 093.82
　toxic 422.93
　　rheumatic (*see also* Myocarditis, acute, rheumatic) 391.2
　tuberculous (*see also* Tuberculosis) 017.9 ☑ [422.0]
　typhoid 002.0 [422.0]
　valvular — *see* Endocarditis
　viral, except Coxsackie 422.91
　　Coxsackie 074.23
　　of newborn (Coxsackie) 074.23
Myocardium, myocardial — *see* condition
Myocardosis — *see also* Cardiomyopathy 425.4
Myoclonia (essential) 333.2
　epileptica 345.1 ☑
　Friedrich's 333.2
　massive 333.2

Myoclonic
　epilepsy, familial (progressive) 345.1 ☑
　jerks 333.2
Myoclonus (familial essential) (multifocal) (simplex) 333.2
　with epilepsy and with ragged red fibers (MERRF syndrome) 277.87
　facial 351.8
　massive (infantile) 333.2
　palatal 333.2
　pharyngeal 333.2
Myocytolysis 429.1
Myodiastasis 728.84
Myoendocarditis — *see also* Endocarditis
　acute or subacute 421.9
Myoepithelioma (M8982/0) — *see* Neoplasm, by site, benign
Myofascitis (acute) 729.1
　low back 724.2
Myofibroma (M8890/0) — *see also* Neoplasm, connective tissue, benign
　uterus (cervix) (corpus) (*see also* Leiomyoma) 218.9
Myofibromatosis
　infantile 759.89
Myofibrosis 728.2
　heart (*see also* Myocarditis) 429.0
　humeroscapular region 726.2
　scapulohumeral 726.2
Myofibrositis — *see also* Myositis 729.1
　scapulohumeral 726.2
Myogelosis (occupational) 728.89
Myoglobinuria 791.3
Myoglobulinuria, primary 791.3
Myokymia — *see also* Myoclonus
　facial 351.8
Myolipoma (M8860/0)
　specified site — *see* Neoplasm, connective tissue, benign
　unspecified site 223.0
Myoma (M8895/0) — *see also* Neoplasm, connective tissue, benign
　cervix (stump) (uterus) (*see also* Leiomyoma) 218.9
　malignant (M8895/3) — *see* Neoplasm, connective tissue, malignant
　prostate 600.20
　　with
　　　other lower urinary tract symptoms (LUTS) 600.21
　　　urinary
　　　　obstruction 600.21
　　　　retention 600.21
　uterus (cervix) (corpus) (*see also* Leiomyoma) 218.9
　　in pregnancy or childbirth 654.1 ☑
　　　affecting fetus or newborn 763.89
　　　causing obstructed labor 660.2 ☑
　　　　affecting fetus or newborn 763.1
Myomalacia 728.9
　cordis, heart (*see also* Degeneration, myocardial) 429.1
Myometritis — *see also* Endometritis 615.9
Myometrium — *see* condition
Myonecrosis, clostridial 040.0
Myopathy 359.9
　alcoholic 359.4
　amyloid 277.39 [359.6]
　benign, congenital 359.0
　central core 359.0
　centronuclear 359.0
　congenital (benign) 359.0
　critical illness 359.81
　distal 359.1
　due to drugs 359.4
　endocrine 259.9 [359.5]
　　specified type NEC 259.8 [359.5]
　extraocular muscles 376.82
　facioscapulohumeral 359.1
　in
　　Addison's disease 255.41 [359.5]
　　amyloidosis 277.39 [359.6]
　　cretinism 243 [359.5]
　　Cushing's syndrome 255.0 [359.5]
　　disseminated lupus erythematosus 710.0 [359.6]

Myopathy — *continued*
　in — *continued*
　　giant cell arteritis 446.5 [359.6]
　　hyperadrenocorticism NEC 255.3 [359.5]
　　hyperparathyroidism 252.01 [359.5]
　　hypopituitarism 253.2 [359.5]
　　hypothyroidism (*see also* Hypothyroidism) 244.9 [359.5]
　　malignant neoplasm NEC (M8000/3) 199.1 [359.6]
　　myxedema (*see also* Myxedema) 244.9 [359.5]
　　polyarteritis nodosa 446.0 [359.6]
　　rheumatoid arthritis 714.0 [359.6]
　　sarcoidosis 135 [359.6]
　　scleroderma 710.1 [359.6]
　　Sjögren's disease 710.2 [359.6]
　　thyrotoxicosis (*see also* Thyrotoxicosis) 242.9 ☑ [359.5]
　inflammatory 359.79
　　immune NEC 359.79
　　specified NEC 359.79
　intensive care (ICU) 359.81
　limb-girdle 359.1
　myotubular 359.0
　necrotizing, acute 359.81
　nemaline 359.0
　ocular 359.1
　oculopharyngeal 359.1
　of critical illness 359.81
　primary 359.89
　progressive NEC 359.89
　proximal myotonic (PROMM) 359.21
　quadriplegic, acute 359.81
　rod body 359.0
　scapulohumeral 359.1
　specified type NEC 359.89
　toxic 359.4
Myopericarditis — *see also* Pericarditis 423.9
Myopia (axial) (congenital) (increased curvature or refraction, nucleus of lens) 367.1
　degenerative, malignant 360.21
　malignant 360.21
　progressive high (degenerative) 360.21
Myosarcoma (M8895/3) — *see* Neoplasm, connective tissue, malignant
Myosis (persistent) 379.42
　stromal (endolymphatic) (M8931/1) 236.0
Myositis 729.1
　clostridial 040.0
　due to posture 729.1
　epidemic 074.1
　fibrosa or fibrous (chronic) 728.2
　　Volkmann's (complicating trauma) 958.6
　inclusion body (IBM) 359.71
　infective 728.0
　interstitial 728.81
　multiple — *see* Polymyositis
　occupational 729.1
　orbital, chronic 376.12
　ossificans 728.12
　　circumscribed 728.12
　　progressive 728.11
　　traumatic 728.12
　progressive fibrosing 728.11
　purulent 728.0
　rheumatic 729.1
　rheumatoid 729.1
　suppurative 728.0
　syphilitic 095.6
　traumatic (old) 729.1
Myospasia impulsiva 307.23
Myotonia (acquisita) (intermittens) 728.85
　atrophica 359.21
　congenita 359.22
　　acetazolamide responsive 359.22
　　dominant form 359.22
　　recessive form 359.22
　drug-induced 359.24
　dystrophica 359.21
　fluctuans 359.29
　levior 359.22
　permanens 359.29
Myotonic pupil 379.46
Myriapodiasis 134.1

Myringitis
　with otitis media — *see* Otitis media
　acute 384.00
　　specified type NEC 384.09
　bullosa hemorrhagica 384.01
　bullous 384.01
　chronic 384.1
Mysophobia 300.29
Mytilotoxism 988.0
Myxadenitis labialis 528.5
Myxedema (adult) (idiocy) (infantile) (juvenile) (thyroid gland) — *see also* Hypothyroidism 244.9
　circumscribed 242.9 ☑
　congenital 243
　cutis 701.8
　localized (pretibial) 242.9 ☑
　madness (acute) 293.0
　　subacute 293.1
　papular 701.8
　pituitary 244.8
　postpartum 674.8 ☑
　pretibial 242.9 ☑
　primary 244.9
Myxochondrosarcoma (M9220/3) — *see* Neoplasm, cartilage, malignant
Myxofibroma (M8811/0) — *see also* Neoplasm, connective tissue, benign
　odontogenic (M9320/0) 213.1
　　upper jaw (bone) 213.0
Myxofibrosarcoma (M8811/3) — *see* Neoplasm, connective tissue, malignant
Myxolipoma (M8852/0) — *see also* Lipoma, by site 214.9
Myxoliposarcoma (M8852/3) — *see* Neoplasm, connective tissue, malignant
Myxoma (M8840/0) — *see also* Neoplasm, connective tissue, benign
　odontogenic (M9320/0) 213.1
　　upper jaw (bone) 213.0
Myxosarcoma (M8840/3) — *see* Neoplasm, connective tissue, malignant

N

Naegeli's
　disease (hereditary hemorrhagic thrombasthenia) 287.1
　leukemia, monocytic (M9863/3) 205.1 ☑
　syndrome (incontinentia pigmenti) 757.33
Naffziger's syndrome 353.0
Naga sore — *see also* Ulcer, skin 707.9
Nägele's pelvis 738.6
　with disproportion (fetopelvic) 653.0 ☑
　　affecting fetus or newborn 763.1
　　causing obstructed labor 660.1 ☑
　　　affecting fetus or newborn 763.1
Nager-de Reynier syndrome (dysostosis mandibularis) 756.0
Nail — *see also* condition
　biting 307.9
　patella syndrome (hereditary osteoonychodysplasia) 756.89
Nanism, nanosomia — *see also* Dwarfism 259.4
　hypophyseal 253.3
　pituitary 253.3
　renis, renalis 588.0
Nanukayami 100.89
Napkin rash 691.0
Narcissism 301.81
Narcolepsy 347.00
　with cataplexy 347.01
　in conditions classified elsewhere 347.10
　　with cataplexy 347.11
Narcosis
　carbon dioxide (respiratory) 786.09
　due to drug
　　correct substance properly administered 780.09
　　overdose or wrong substance given or taken 977.9
　　　specified drug — *see* Table of Drugs and Chemicals
Narcotism (chronic) — *see also* Dependence 304.9 ☑

Narcotism (chronic) — *see also* Dependence
— *continued*
  acute
    correct substance properly administered 349.82
    overdose or wrong substance given or taken 967.8
      specified drug — *see* Table of Drugs and Chemicals
NARP (ataxia and retinitis pigmentosa) 277.87
Narrow
  anterior chamber angle 365.02
  pelvis (inlet) (outlet) — *see* Contraction, pelvis
Narrowing
  artery NEC 447.1
    auditory, internal 433.8 ☑
    basilar 433.0 ☑
      with other precerebral artery 433.3 ☑
        bilateral 433.3 ☑
    carotid 433.1 ☑
      with other precerebral artery 433.3 ☑
        bilateral 433.3 ☑
    cerebellar 433.8 ☑
    choroidal 433.8 ☑
    communicating posterior 433.8 ☑
    coronary (*see also* Arteriosclerosis, coronary)
      congenital 746.85
        due to syphilis 090.5
    hypophyseal 433.8 ☑
    pontine 433.8 ☑
    precerebral NEC 433.9 ☑
      multiple or bilateral 433.3 ☑
      specified NEC 433.8 ☑
    vertebral 433.2 ☑
      with other precerebral artery 433.3 ☑
        bilateral 433.3 ☑
  auditory canal (external) (*see also* Stricture, ear canal, acquired) 380.50
  cerebral arteries 437.0
  cicatricial — *see* Cicatrix
  congenital — *see* Anomaly, congenital
  coronary artery — *see* Narrowing, artery, coronary
  ear, middle 385.22
  Eustachian tube (*see also* Obstruction, Eustachian tube) 381.60
  eyelid 374.46
    congenital 743.62
  intervertebral disc or space NEC — *see* Degeneration, intervertebral disc
  joint space, hip 719.85
  larynx 478.74
  lids 374.46
    congenital 743.62
  mesenteric artery (with gangrene) 557.0
  palate 524.89
  palpebral fissure 374.46
  retinal artery 362.13
  ureter 593.3
  urethra (*see also* Stricture, urethra) 598.9
Narrowness, abnormal, eyelid 743.62
Nasal — *see* condition
Nasolacrimal — *see* condition
Nasopharyngeal — *see also* condition
  bursa 478.29
  pituitary gland 759.2
  torticollis 723.5
Nasopharyngitis (acute) (infective) (subacute) 460
  chronic 472.2
    due to external agent — *see* Condition, respiratory, chronic, due to
  due to external agent — *see* Condition, respiratory, due to
  septic 034.0
  streptococcal 034.0
  suppurative (chronic) 472.2
  ulcerative (chronic) 472.2
Nasopharynx, nasopharyngeal — *see* condition
Natal tooth, teeth 520.6

Nausea — *see also* Vomiting 787.02
  with vomiting 787.01
  epidemic 078.82
  gravidarum — *see* Hyperemesis, gravidarum
  marina 994.6
Navel — *see* condition
Neapolitan fever — *see also* Brucellosis 023.9
Near drowning 994.1
Nearsightedness 367.1
Near-syncope 780.2
Nebécourt's syndrome 253.3
Nebula, cornea (eye) 371.01
  congenital 743.43
    interfering with vision 743.42
Necator americanus infestation 126.1
Necatoriasis 126.1
Neck — *see* condition
Necrencephalus — *see also* Softening, brain 437.8
Necrobacillosis 040.3
Necrobiosis 799.89
  brain or cerebral (*see also* Softening, brain) 437.8
  lipoidica 709.3
    diabeticorum 250.8 ☑ [709.3]
      due to secondary diabetes 249.8 ☑ [709.3]
Necrodermolysis 695.15
Necrolysis, toxic epidermal 695.15
  due to drug
    correct substance properly administered 695.15
    overdose or wrong substance given or taken 977.9
      specified drug — *see* Table of Drugs and Chemicals
  Stevens-Johnson syndrome overlap (SJS-TEN overlap syndrome) 695.14
Necrophilia 302.89
Necrosis, necrotic
  adrenal (capsule) (gland) 255.8
  antrum, nasal sinus 478.19
  aorta (hyaline) (*see also* Aneurysm, aorta) 441.9
    cystic medial 441.00
      abdominal 441.02
      thoracic 441.01
      thoracoabdominal 441.03
    ruptured 441.5
  arteritis 446.0
  artery 447.5
  aseptic, bone 733.40
    femur (head) (neck) 733.42
      medial condyle 733.43
    humoral head 733.41
    jaw 733.45
    medial femoral condyle 733.43
    specific site NEC 733.49
    talus 733.44
  avascular, bone NEC (*see also* Necrosis, aseptic, bone) 733.40
  bladder (aseptic) (sphincter) 596.89
  bone (*see also* Osteomyelitis) 730.1 ☑
    acute 730.0 ☑
    aseptic or avascular 733.40
      femur (head) (neck) 733.42
        medial condyle 733.43
      humoral head 733.41
      jaw 733.45
      medial femoral condyle 733.43
      specified site NEC 733.49
      talus 733.44
    ethmoid 478.19
    ischemic 733.40
    jaw 526.4
      asceptic 733.45
    marrow 289.89
    Paget's (osteitis deformans) 731.0
    tuberculous — *see* Tuberculosis, bone
  brain (softening) (*see also* Softening, brain) 437.8
  breast (aseptic) (fat) (segmental) 611.3
  bronchus, bronchi 519.19
  central nervous system NEC (*see also* Softening, brain) 437.8
  cerebellar (*see also* Softening, brain) 437.8

Necrosis, necrotic — *continued*
  cerebral (softening) (*see also* Softening, brain) 437.8
  cerebrospinal (softening) (*see also* Softening, brain) 437.8
  colon 557.0
  cornea (*see also* Keratitis) 371.40
  cortical, kidney 583.6
  cystic medial (aorta) 441.00
    abdominal 441.02
    thoracic 441.01
    thoracoabdominal 441.03
  dental 521.09
    pulp 522.1
  due to swallowing corrosive substance — *see* Burn, by site
  ear (ossicle) 385.24
  esophagus 530.89
  ethmoid (bone) 478.19
  eyelid 374.50
  fat, fatty (generalized) (*see also* Degeneration, fatty) 272.8
    abdominal wall 567.82
    breast (aseptic) (segmental) 611.3
    intestine 569.89
    localized — *see* Degeneration, by site, fatty
    mesentery 567.82
    omentum 567.82
    pancreas 577.8
    peritoneum 567.82
    skin (subcutaneous) 709.3
      newborn 778.1
  femur (aseptic) (avascuiar) 733.42
    head 733.42
    medial condyle 733.43
    neck 733.42
  gallbladder (*see also* Cholecystitis, acute) 575.0
  gangrenous 785.4
  gastric 537.89
  glottis 478.79
  heart (myocardium) — *see* Infarct, myocardium
  hepatic (*see also* Necrosis, liver) 570
  hip (aseptic) (avascular) 733.42
  intestine (acute) (hemorrhagic) (massive) 557.0
  ischemic 785.4
  jaw 526.4
    asceptic 733.45
  kidney (bilateral) 583.9
    acute 584.9
    cortical 583.6
      acute 584.6
        with
          abortion — *see* Abortion, by type, with renal failure
          ectopic pregnancy (*see also* categories 633.0–633.9) 639.3
          molar pregnancy (*see also* categories 630–632) 639.3
        complicating pregnancy 646.2 ☑
          affecting fetus or newborn 760.1
        following labor and delivery 669.3 ☑
    medullary (papillary) (*see also* Pyelitis) 590.80
      in
        acute renal failure 584.7
        nephritis, nephropathy 583.7
    papillary (*see also* Pyelitis) 590.80
      in
        acute renal failure 584.7
        nephritis, nephropathy 583.7
    tubular 584.5
      with
        abortion — *see* Abortion, by type, with renal failure
        ectopic pregnancy (*see also* categories 633.0–633.9) 639.3
        molar pregnancy (*see also* categories 630–632) 639.3

Necrosis, necrotic — *continued*
  kidney — *continued*
    tubular — *continued*
      complicating
        abortion 639.3
        ectopic or molar pregnancy 639.3
        pregnancy 646.2 ☑
          affecting fetus or newborn 760.1
      following labor and delivery 669.3 ☑
      traumatic 958.5
  larynx 478.79
  liver (acute) (congenital) (diffuse) (massive) (subacute) 570
    with
      abortion — *see* Abortion, by type, with specified complication NEC
      ectopic pregnancy (*see also* categories 633.0–633.9) 639.8
      molar pregnancy (*see also* categories 630–632) 639.8
    complicating pregnancy 646.7 ☑
      affecting fetus or newborn 760.8
    following
      abortion 639.8
      ectopic or molar pregnancy 639.8
    obstetrical 646.7 ☑
    postabortal 639.8
    puerperal, postpartum 674.8 ☑
    toxic 573.3
  lung 513.0
  lymphatic gland 683
  mammary gland 611.3
  mastoid (chronic) 383.1
  mesentery 557.0
    fat 567.82
  mitral valve — *see* Insufficiency, mitral
  myocardium, myocardial — *see* Infarct, myocardium
  nose (septum) 478.19
  omentum 557.0
    with mesenteric infarction 557.0
    fat 567.82
  orbit, orbital 376.10
  ossicles, ear (aseptic) 385.24
  ovary (*see also* Salpingo-oophoritis) 614.2
  pancreas (aseptic) (duct) (fat) 577.8
    acute 577.0
    infective 577.0
  papillary, kidney (*see also* Pyelitis) 590.80
  perineum 624.8
  peritoneum 557.0
    with mesenteric infarction 557.0
    fat 567.82
  pharynx 462
    in granulocytopenia 288.09
  phosphorus 983.9
  pituitary (gland) (postpartum) (Sheehan) 253.2
  placenta (*see also* Placenta, abnormal) 656.7 ☑
  pneumonia 513.0
  pulmonary 513.0
  pulp (dental) 522.1
  pylorus 537.89
  radiation — *see* Necrosis, by site
  radium — *see* Necrosis, by site
  renal — *see* Necrosis, kidney
  sclera 379.19
  scrotum 608.89
  skin or subcutaneous tissue 709.8
    due to burn — *see* Burn, by site
    gangrenous 785.4
  spine, spinal (column) 730.18
    acute 730.18
    cord 336.1
  spleen 289.59
  stomach 537.89
  stomatitis 528.1
  subcutaneous fat 709.3
    fetus or newborn 778.1
  subendocardial — *see* Infarct, myocardium
  suprarenal (capsule) (gland) 255.8
  teeth, tooth 521.09
  testis 608.89

☑ Additional Digit Required — Refer to the Tabular List for Digit Selection   ▽ Subterms under main terms may continue to next column or page

190 — Volume 2   ▶◀ Revised Text   ● New Line   ▲ Revised Code   2015 ICD-9-CM

Necrosis, necrotic — *continued*
thymus (gland) 254.8
tonsil 474.8
trachea 519.19
tuberculous NEC — *see* Tuberculosis
tubular (acute) (anoxic) (toxic) 584.5
    due to a procedure 997.5
umbilical cord, affecting fetus or newborn
    762.6
vagina 623.8
vertebra (lumbar) 730.18
    acute 730.18
    tuberculous (*see also* Tuberculosis)
      015.0 ☑ [730.8] ☑
vesical (aseptic) (bladder) 596.89
vulva 624.8

Necrosis, necrotic — *continued*
  x-ray — *see* Necrosis, by site
Necrospermia 606.0
Necrotizing angiitis 446.0
Negativism 301.7
Neglect (child) (newborn) NEC 995.52
  adult 995.84
  after or at birth 995.52
  hemispatial 781.8
  left-sided 781.8
  sensory 781.8
  visuospatial 781.8
Negri bodies 071
Neill-Dingwall syndrome (microcephaly and
  dwarfism) 759.89
Neisserian infection NEC — *see* Gonococcus

Nematodiasis NEC — *see also* Infestation, Nematode 127.9
  ancylostoma (*see also* Ancylostomiasis)
    126.9
Neoformans cryptococcus infection 117.5
Neonatal — *see also* condition
  abstinence syndrome 779.5
  adrenoleukodystrophy 277.86
  teeth, tooth 520.6
Neonatorum — *see* condition
Neoplasia
  anal intraepithelial I (AIN I) (histologically
    confirmed) 569.44
  anal intraepithelial II (AIN II) (histologically
    confirmed) 569.44
  anal intraepithelial III (AIN III) 230.6

Neoplasia — *continued*
  anal intraepithelial III — *continued*
    anal canal 230.5
  endometrial intraepithelial (EIN) 621.35
  multiple endocrine (MEN)
    type I 258.01
    type IIA 258.02
    type IIB 258.03
  vaginal intraepithelial I (VAIN I) 623.0
  vaginal intraepithelial II (VAIN II) 623.0
  vaginal intraepithelial III (VAIN III) 233.31
  vulvular intraepithelial I (VIN I) 624.01
  vulvular intraepithelial II (VIN II) 624.02
  vulvular intraepithelial III (VIN III) 233.32

☑ **Additional Digit Required** — Refer to the Tabular List for Digit Selection ⓥ **Subterms under main terms may continue to next column or page**

2015 ICD-9-CM ▶◀ Revised Text ● New Line ▲ Revised Code Volume 2 — 191

Necrosis, necrotic — Neoplasia

	Malignant			Benign	Uncertain Behavior	Unspecified
	Primary	Secondary	Ca in situ			
Neoplasm, neoplastic	199.1	—	234.9	229.9	238.9	239.9

Notes — 1. The list below gives the code numbers for neoplasms by anatomical site. For each site there are six possible code numbers according to whether the neoplasm in question is malignant, benign, in situ, of uncertain behavior, or of unspecified nature. The description of the neoplasm will often indicate which of the six columns is appropriate; e.g., malignant melanoma of skin, benign fibroadenoma of breast, carcinoma in situ of cervix uteri.

Where such descriptors are not present, the remainder of the Index should be consulted where guidance is given to the appropriate column for each morphological (histological) variety listed; e.g., Mesonephroma — see Neoplasm, malignant; Embryoma — see also Neoplasm, uncertain behavior; Disease, Bowen's — see Neoplasm, skin, in situ. However, the guidance in the Index can be overridden if one of the descriptors mentioned above is present; e.g., malignant adenoma of colon is coded to 153.9 and not to 211.3 as the adjective "malignant" overrides the Index entry "Adenoma — see also Neoplasm, benign."

2. Sites marked with the sign * (e.g., face NEC*) should be classified to malignant neoplasm of skin of these sites if the variety of neoplasm is a squamous cell carcinoma or an epidermoid carcinoma, and to benign neoplasm of skin of these sites if the variety of neoplasm is a papilloma (any type).

	Primary	Secondary	Ca in situ	Benign	Uncertain Behavior	Unspecified
abdomen, abdominal	195.2	198.89	234.8	229.8	238.8	239.89
cavity	195.2	198.89	234.8	229.8	238.8	239.89
organ	195.2	198.89	234.8	229.8	238.8	239.89
viscera	195.2	198.89	234.8	229.8	238.8	239.89
wall	173.50	198.2	232.5	216.5	238.2	239.2
basal cell carcinoma	173.51	—	—	—	—	—
connective tissue	171.5	198.89	—	215.5	238.1	239.2
specified type NEC	173.59	—	—	—	—	—
squamous cell carcinoma	173.52	—	—	—	—	—
abdominopelvic	195.8	198.89	234.8	229.8	238.8	239.89
accessory sinus — see Neoplasm, sinus						
acoustic nerve	192.0	198.4	—	225.1	237.9	239.7
acromion (process)	170.4	198.5	—	213.4	238.0	239.2
adenoid (pharynx) (tissue)	147.1	198.89	230.0	210.7	235.1	239.0
adipose tissue (see also Neoplasm, connective tissue)	171.9	198.89	—	215.9	238.1	239.2
adnexa (uterine)	183.9	198.82	233.39	221.8	236.3	239.5
adrenal (cortex) (gland) (medulla)	194.0	198.7	234.8	227.0	237.2	239.7
ala nasi (external)	173.30	198.2	232.3	216.3	238.2	239.2
alimentary canal or tract NEC	159.9	197.8	230.9	211.9	235.5	239.0
alveolar	143.9	198.89	230.0	210.4	235.1	239.0
mucosa	143.9	198.89	230.0	210.4	235.1	239.0
lower	143.1	198.89	230.0	210.4	235.1	239.0
upper	143.0	198.89	230.0	210.4	235.1	239.0
ridge or process	170.1	198.5	—	213.1	238.0	239.2
carcinoma	143.9	—	—	—	—	—
lower	143.1	—	—	—	—	—
upper	143.0	—	—	—	—	—
lower	170.1	198.5	—	213.1	238.0	239.2
mucosa	143.9	198.89	230.0	210.4	235.1	239.0
lower	143.1	198.89	230.0	210.4	235.1	239.0
upper	143.0	198.89	230.0	210.4	235.1	239.0
upper	170.0	198.5	—	213.0	238.0	239.2
sulcus	145.1	198.89	230.0	210.4	235.1	239.0
alveolus	143.9	198.89	230.0	210.4	235.1	239.0
lower	143.1	198.89	230.0	210.4	235.1	239.0
upper	143.0	198.89	230.0	210.4	235.1	239.0
ampulla of Vater	156.2	197.8	230.8	211.5	235.3	239.0
ankle NEC*	195.5	198.89	232.7	229.8	238.8	239.89
anorectum, anorectal (junction)	154.8	197.5	230.7	211.4	235.2	239.0
antecubital fossa or space*	195.4	198.89	232.6	229.8	238.8	239.89

	Malignant			Benign	Uncertain Behavior	Unspecified
	Primary	Secondary	Ca in situ			
Neoplasm, neoplastic — continued						
antrum (Highmore) (maxillary)	160.2	197.3	231.8	212.0	235.9	239.1
pyloric	151.2	197.8	230.2	211.1	235.2	239.0
tympanicum	160.1	197.3	231.8	212.0	235.9	239.1
anus, anal	154.3	197.5	230.6	211.4	235.5	239.0
canal	154.2	197.5	230.5	211.4	235.5	239.0
contiguous sites with rectosigmoid junction or rectum	154.8	—	—	—	—	—
margin (see also Neoplasm, anus, skin)	173.50	198.2	232.5	216.6	238.2	239.2
skin	173.50	198.2	232.5	216.5	238.2	239.2
basal cell carcinoma	173.51	—	—	—	—	—
specified type NEC	173.59	—	—	—	—	—
squamous cell carcinoma	173.52	—	—	—	—	—
sphincter	154.2	197.5	230.5	211.4	235.5	239.0
aorta (thoracic)	171.4	198.89	—	215.4	238.1	239.2
abdominal	171.5	198.89	—	215.5	238.1	239.2
aortic body	194.6	198.89	—	227.6	237.3	239.7
aponeurosis	171.9	198.89	—	215.9	238.1	239.2
palmar	171.2	198.89	—	215.2	238.1	239.2
plantar	171.3	198.89	—	215.3	238.1	239.2
appendix	153.5	197.5	230.3	211.3	235.2	239.0
arachnoid (cerebral)	192.1	198.4	—	225.2	237.6	239.7
spinal	192.3	198.4	—	225.4	237.6	239.7
areola (female)	174.0	198.81	233.0	217	238.3	239.3
male	175.0	198.81	233.0	217	238.3	239.3
arm NEC*	195.4	198.89	232.6	229.8	238.8	239.89
artery — see Neoplasm, connective tissue						
aryepiglottic fold	148.2	198.89	230.0	210.8	235.1	239.0
hypopharyngeal aspect	148.2	198.89	230.0	210.8	235.1	239.0
laryngeal aspect	161.1	197.3	231.0	212.1	235.6	239.1
marginal zone	148.2	198.89	230.0	210.8	235.1	239.0
arytenoid (cartilage)	161.3	197.3	231.0	212.1	235.6	239.1
fold — see Neoplasm, aryepiglottic						
associated with transplanted organ	199.2	—		—	—	—
atlas	170.2	198.5	—	213.2	238.0	239.2
atrium, cardiac	164.1	198.89	—	212.7	238.8	239.89
auditory canal (external) (skin) (see also Neoplasm, skin, ear)	173.20	198.2	232.2	216.2	238.2	239.2
internal	160.1	197.3	231.8	212.0	235.9	239.1
nerve	192.0	198.4	—	225.1	237.9	239.7
tube	160.1	197.3	231.8	212.0	235.9	239.1
Eustachian	160.1	197.3	231.8	212.0	235.9	239.1
opening	147.2	198.89	230.0	210.7	235.1	239.0
auricle, ear see also Neoplasm, skin, ear)	173.20	198.2	232.2	216.2	238.2	239.2
cartilage	171.0	198.89	—	215.0	238.1	239.2
auricular canal (external) (see also Neoplasm, skin, ear)	173.20	198.2	232.2	216.2	238.2	239.2
internal	160.1	197.3	231.8	212.0	235.9	239.1
autonomic nerve or nervous system NEC	171.9	198.89	—	215.9	238.1	239.2
axilla, axillary	195.1	198.89	234.8	229.8	238.8	239.89
fold (see also Neoplasm, skin, trunk)	173.50	198.2	232.5	216.5	238.2	239.2

☑ **Additional Digit Required — Refer to the Tabular List for Digit Selection**   ▽ **Subterms under main terms may continue to next column or page**

	Malignant					
	Primary	Secondary	Ca in situ	Benign	Uncertain Behavior	Unspecified
Neoplasm, neoplastic— *continued*						
back NEC*	195.8	198.89	232.5	229.8	238.8	239.89
Bartholin's gland	184.1	198.82	233.32	221.2	236.3	239.5
basal ganglia	191.0	198.3	—	225.0	237.5	239.6
basis pedunculi	191.7	198.3	—	225.0	237.5	239.6
bile or biliary (tract)	156.9	197.8	230.8	211.5	235.3	239.0
canaliculi (biliferi) (intrahepatic)	155.1	197.8	230.8	211.5	235.3	239.0
canals, interlobular	155.1	197.8	230.8	211.5	235.3	239.0
contiguous sites	156.8	—	—	—	—	—
duct or passage (common) (cystic) (extrahepatic)	156.1	197.8	230.8	211.5	235.3	239.0
contiguous sites with gallbladder	156.8	—	—	—	—	—
interlobular	155.1	197.8	230.8	211.5	235.3	239.0
intrahepatic	155.1	197.8	230.8	211.5	235.3	239.0
and extrahepatic	156.9	197.8	230.8	211.5	235.3	239.0
bladder (urinary)	188.9	198.1	233.7	223.3	236.7	239.4
contiguous sites	188.8	—	—	—	—	—
dome	188.1	198.1	233.7	223.3	236.7	239.4
neck	188.5	198.1	233.7	223.3	236.7	239.4
orifice	188.9	198.1	233.7	223.3	236.7	239.4
ureteric	188.6	198.1	233.7	223.3	236.7	239.4
urethral	188.5	198.1	233.7	223.3	236.7	239.4
sphincter	188.8	198.1	233.7	223.3	236.7	239.4
trigone	188.0	198.1	233.7	223.3	236.7	239.4
urachus	188.7	—	233.7	223.3	236.7	239.4
wall	188.9	198.1	233.7	223.3	236.7	239.4
anterior	188.3	198.1	233.7	223.3	236.7	239.4
lateral	188.2	198.1	233.7	223.3	236.7	239.4
posterior	188.4	198.1	233.7	223.3	236.7	239.4
blood vessel — see Neoplasm, connective tissue						
bone (periosteum)	170.9	198.5	—	213.9	238.0	239.2

> *Note* — Carcinomas and adenocarcinomas, of any type other than intraosseous or odontogenic, of the sites listed under "Neoplasm, bone" should be considered as constituting metastatic spread from an unspecified primary site and coded to 198.5 for morbidity coding.

	Primary	Secondary	Ca in situ	Benign	Uncertain Behavior	Unspecified
acetabulum	170.6	198.5	—	213.6	238.0	239.2
acromion (process)	170.4	198.5	—	213.4	238.0	239.2
ankle	170.8	198.5	—	213.8	238.0	239.2
arm NEC	170.4	198.5	—	213.4	238.0	239.2
astragalus	170.8	198.5	—	213.8	238.0	239.2
atlas	170.2	198.5	—	213.2	238.0	239.2
axis	170.2	198.5	—	213.2	238.0	239.2
back NEC	170.2	198.5	—	213.2	238.0	239.2
calcaneus	170.8	198.5	—	213.8	238.0	239.2
calvarium	170.0	198.5	—	213.0	238.0	239.2
carpus (any)	170.5	198.5	—	213.5	238.0	239.2
cartilage NEC	170.9	198.5	—	213.9	238.0	239.2
clavicle	170.3	198.5	—	213.3	238.0	239.2
clivus	170.0	198.5	—	213.0	238.0	239.2
coccygeal vertebra	170.6	198.5	—	213.6	238.0	239.2
coccyx	170.6	198.5	—	213.6	238.0	239.2
costal cartilage	170.3	198.5	—	213.3	238.0	239.2
costovertebral joint	170.3	198.5	—	213.3	238.0	239.2
cranial	170.0	198.5	—	213.0	238.0	239.2
cuboid	170.8	198.5	—	213.8	238.0	239.2
cuneiform	170.9	198.5	—	213.9	238.0	239.2
ankle	170.8	198.5	—	213.8	238.0	239.2
wrist	170.5	198.5	—	213.5	238.0	239.2
digital	170.9	198.5	—	213.9	238.0	239.2
finger	170.5	198.5	—	213.5	238.0	239.2
toe	170.8	198.5	—	213.8	238.0	239.2

	Malignant					
	Primary	Secondary	Ca in situ	Benign	Uncertain Behavior	Unspecified
Neoplasm, neoplastic— *continued*						
bone — *continued*						
elbow	170.4	198.5	—	213.4	238.0	239.2
ethmoid (labyrinth)	170.0	198.5	—	213.0	238.0	239.2
face	170.0	198.5	—	213.0	238.0	239.2
lower jaw	170.1	198.5	—	213.1	238.0	239.2
femur (any part)	170.7	198.5	—	213.7	238.0	239.2
fibula (any part)	170.7	198.5	—	213.7	238.0	239.2
finger (any)	170.5	198.5	—	213.5	238.0	239.2
foot	170.8	198.5	—	213.8	238.0	239.2
forearm	170.4	198.5	—	213.4	238.0	239.2
frontal	170.0	198.5	—	213.0	238.0	239.2
hand	170.5	198.5	—	213.5	238.0	239.2
heel	170.8	198.5	—	213.8	238.0	239.2
hip	170.6	198.5	—	213.6	238.0	239.2
humerus (any part)	170.4	198.5	—	213.4	238.0	239.2
hyoid	170.0	198.5	—	213.0	238.0	239.2
ilium	170.6	198.5	—	213.6	238.0	239.2
innominate	170.6	198.5	—	213.6	238.0	239.2
intervertebral cartilage or disc	170.2	198.5	—	213.2	238.0	239.2
ischium	170.6	198.5	—	213.6	238.0	239.2
jaw (lower)	170.1	198.5	—	213.1	238.0	239.2
upper	170.0	198.5	—	213.0	238.0	239.2
knee	170.7	198.5	—	213.7	238.0	239.2
leg NEC	170.7	198.5	—	213.7	238.0	239.2
limb NEC	170.9	198.5	—	213.9	238.0	239.2
lower (long bones)	170.7	198.5	—	213.7	238.0	239.2
short bones	170.8	198.5	—	213.8	238.0	239.2
upper (long bones)	170.4	198.5	—	213.4	238.0	239.2
short bones	170.5	198.5	—	213.5	238.0	239.2
long	170.9	198.5	—	213.9	238.0	239.2
lower limbs NEC	170.7	198.5	—	213.7	238.0	239.2
upper limbs NEC	170.4	198.5	—	213.4	238.0	239.2
malar	170.0	198.5	—	213.0	238.0	239.2
mandible	170.1	198.5	—	213.1	238.0	239.2
marrow NEC	202.9	198.5	—	—	—	238.79
mastoid	170.0	198.5	—	213.0	238.0	239.2
maxilla, maxillary (superior)	170.0	198.5	—	213.0	238.0	239.2
inferior	170.1	198.5	—	213.1	238.0	239.2
metacarpus (any)	170.5	198.5	—	213.5	238.0	239.2
metatarsus (any)	170.8	198.5	—	213.8	238.0	239.2
navicular (ankle)	170.8	198.5	—	213.8	238.0	239.2
hand	170.5	198.5	—	213.5	238.0	239.2
nose, nasal	170.0	198.5	—	213.0	238.0	239.2
occipital	170.0	198.5	—	213.0	238.0	239.2
orbit	170.0	198.5	—	213.0	238.0	239.2
parietal	170.0	198.5	—	213.0	238.0	239.2
patella	170.8	198.5	—	213.8	238.0	239.2
pelvic	170.6	198.5	—	213.6	238.0	239.2
phalanges	170.9	198.5	—	213.9	238.0	239.2
foot	170.8	198.5	—	213.8	238.0	239.2
hand	170.5	198.5	—	213.5	238.0	239.2
pubic	170.6	198.5	—	213.6	238.0	239.2
radius (any part)	170.4	198.5	—	213.4	238.0	239.2
rib	170.3	198.5	—	213.3	238.0	239.2
sacral vertebra	170.6	198.5	—	213.6	238.0	239.2
sacrum	170.6	198.5	—	213.6	238.0	239.2
scaphoid (of hand)	170.5	198.5	—	213.5	238.0	239.2
of ankle	170.8	198.5	—	213.8	238.0	239.2
scapula (any part)	170.4	198.5	—	213.4	238.0	239.2
sella turcica	170.0	198.5	—	213.0	238.0	239.2
short	170.9	198.5	—	213.9	238.0	239.2
lower limb	170.8	198.5	—	213.8	238.0	239.2

☑ Additional Digit Required — Refer to the Tabular List for Digit Selection   ▽ Subterms under main terms may continue to next column or page

194— Volume 2   ▶◀ Revised Text   ● New Line   ▲ Revised Code   2015 ICD-9-CM

	Malignant					
	Primary	Secondary	Ca in situ	Benign	Uncertain Behavior	Unspecified
Neoplasm, neoplastic — *continued*						
bone — *continued*						
short — *continued*						
upper limb	170.5	198.5	—	213.5	238.0	239.2
shoulder	170.4	198.5	—	213.4	238.0	239.2
skeleton, skeletal NEC	170.9	198.5	—	213.9	238.0	239.2
skull	170.0	198.5	—	213.0	238.0	239.2
sphenoid	170.0	198.5	—	213.0	238.0	239.2
spine, spinal (column)	170.2	198.5	—	213.2	238.0	239.2
coccyx	170.6	198.5	—	213.6	238.0	239.2
sacrum	170.6	198.5	—	213.6	238.0	239.2
sternum	170.3	198.5	—	213.3	238.0	239.2
tarsus (any)	170.8	198.5	—	213.8	238.0	239.2
temporal	170.0	198.5	—	213.0	238.0	239.2
thumb	170.5	198.5	—	213.5	238.0	239.2
tibia (any part)	170.7	198.5	—	213.7	238.0	239.2
toe (any)	170.8	198.5	—	213.8	238.0	239.2
trapezium	170.5	198.5	—	213.5	238.0	239.2
trapezoid	170.5	198.5	—	213.5	238.0	239.2
turbinate	170.0	198.5	—	213.0	238.0	239.2
ulna (any part)	170.4	198.5	—	213.4	238.0	239.2
unciform	170.5	198.5	—	213.5	238.0	239.2
vertebra (column)	170.2	198.5	—	213.2	238.0	239.2
coccyx	170.6	198.5	—	213.6	238.0	239.2
sacrum	170.6	198.5	—	213.6	238.0	239.2
vomer	170.0	198.5	—	213.0	238.0	239.2
wrist	170.5	198.5	—	213.5	238.0	239.2
xiphoid process	170.3	198.5	—	213.3	238.0	239.2
zygomatic	170.0	198.5	—	213.0	238.0	239.2
book-leaf (mouth)	145.8	198.89	230.0	210.4	235.1	239.0
bowel — *see* Neoplasm, intestine						
brachial plexus	171.2	198.89	—	215.2	238.1	239.2
brain NEC	191.9	198.3	—	225.0	237.5	239.6
basal ganglia	191.0	198.3	—	225.0	237.5	239.6
cerebellopontine angle	191.6	198.3	—	225.0	237.5	239.6
cerebellum NOS	191.6	198.3	—	225.0	237.5	239.6
cerebrum	191.0	198.3	—	225.0	237.5	239.6
choroid plexus	191.5	198.3	—	225.0	237.5	239.6
contiguous sites	191.8	—	—	—	—	—
corpus callosum	191.8	198.3	—	225.0	237.5	239.6
corpus striatum	191.0	198.3	—	225.0	237.5	239.6
cortex (cerebral)	191.0	198.3	—	225.0	237.5	239.6
frontal lobe	191.1	198.3	—	225.0	237.5	239.6
globus pallidus	191.0	198.3	—	225.0	237.5	239.6
hippocampus	191.2	198.3	—	225.0	237.5	239.6
hypothalamus	191.0	198.3	—	225.0	237.5	239.6
internal capsule	191.0	198.3	—	225.0	237.5	239.6
medulla oblongata	191.7	198.3	—	225.0	237.5	239.6
meninges	192.1	198.4	—	225.2	237.6	239.7
midbrain	191.7	198.3	—	225.0	237.5	239.6
occipital lobe	191.4	198.3	—	225.0	237.5	239.6
parietal lobe	191.3	198.3	—	225.0	237.5	239.6
peduncle	191.7	198.3	—	225.0	237.5	239.6
pons	191.7	198.3	—	225.0	237.5	239.6
stem	191.7	198.3	—	225.0	237.5	239.6
tapetum	191.8	198.3	—	225.0	237.5	239.6
temporal lobe	191.2	198.3	—	225.0	237.5	239.6
thalamus	191.0	198.3	—	225.0	237.5	239.6
uncus	191.2	198.3	—	225.0	237.5	239.6
ventricle (floor)	191.5	198.3	—	225.0	237.5	239.6
branchial (cleft) (vestiges)	146.8	198.89	230.0	210.6	235.1	239.0
breast (connective tissue) (female) (glandular tissue) (soft parts)	174.9	198.81	233.0	217	238.3	239.3
areola	174.0	198.81	233.0	217	238.3	239.3
male	175.0	198.81	233.0	217	238.3	239.3
axillary tail	174.6	198.81	233.0	217	238.3	239.3

	Malignant					
	Primary	Secondary	Ca in situ	Benign	Uncertain Behavior	Unspecified
Neoplasm, neoplastic — *continued*						
breast — *continued*						
central portion	174.1	198.81	233.0	217	238.3	239.3
contiguous sites	174.8	—	—	—	—	—
ectopic sites	174.8	198.81	233.0	217	238.3	239.3
inner	174.8	198.81	233.0	217	238.3	239.3
lower	174.8	198.81	233.0	217	238.3	239.3
lower-inner quadrant	174.3	198.81	233.0	217	238.3	239.3
lower-outer quadrant	174.5	198.81	233.0	217	238.3	239.3
male	175.9	198.81	233.0	217	238.3	239.3
areola	175.0	198.81	233.0	217	238.3	239.3
ectopic tissue	175.9	198.81	233.0	217	238.3	239.3
nipple	175.0	198.81	233.0	217	238.3	239.3
mastectomy site (skin) (*see also* Neoplasm, mastectomy site)	173.50	198.2	—	—	—	—
specified as breast tissue	174.8	198.81	—	—	—	—
midline	174.8	198.81	233.0	217	238.3	239.3
nipple	174.0	198.81	233.0	217	238.3	239.3
male	175.0	198.81	233.0	217	238.3	239.3
outer	174.8	198.81	233.0	217	238.3	239.3
skin (*see also* Neoplasm, mastectomy site)	173.50	198.2	232.5	216.5	238.2	239.2
tail (axillary)	174.6	198.81	233.0	217	238.3	239.3
upper	174.8	198.81	233.0	217	238.3	239.3
upper-inner quadrant	174.2	198.81	233.0	217	238.3	239.3
upper-outer quadrant	174.4	198.81	233.0	217	238.3	239.3
broad ligament	183.3	198.82	233.39	221.0	236.3	239.5
bronchiogenic, bronchogenic (lung)	162.9	197.0	231.2	212.3	235.7	239.1
bronchiole	162.9	197.0	231.2	212.3	235.7	239.1
bronchus	162.9	197.0	231.2	212.3	235.7	239.1
carina	162.2	197.0	231.2	212.3	235.7	239.1
contiguous sites with lung or trachea	162.8	—	—	—	—	—
lower lobe of lung	162.5	197.0	231.2	212.3	235.7	239.1
main	162.2	197.0	231.2	212.3	235.7	239.1
middle lobe of lung	162.4	197.0	231.2	212.3	235.7	239.1
upper lobe of lung	162.3	197.0	231.2	212.3	235.7	239.1
brow	173.30	198.2	232.3	216.3	238.2	239.2
basal cell carcinoma	173.31	—	—	—	—	—
specified type NEC	173.39	—	—	—	—	—
squamous cell carcinoma	173.32	—	—	—	—	—
buccal (cavity)	145.9	198.89	230.0	210.4	235.1	239.0
commissure	145.0	198.89	230.0	210.4	235.1	239.0
groove (lower) (upper)	145.1	198.89	230.0	210.4	235.1	239.0
mucosa	145.0	198.89	230.0	210.4	235.1	239.0
sulcus (lower) (upper)	145.1	198.89	230.0	210.4	235.1	239.0
bulbourethral gland	189.3	198.1	233.9	223.81	236.99	239.5
bursa — *see* Neoplasm, connective tissue						
buttock NEC*	195.3	198.89	232.5	229.8	238.8	239.89
calf*	195.5	198.89	232.7	229.8	238.8	239.89
calvarium	170.0	198.5	—	213.0	238.0	239.2
calyx, renal	189.1	198.0	233.9	223.1	236.91	239.5
canal						
anal	154.2	197.5	230.5	211.4	235.5	239.0

☑ **Additional Digit Required — Refer to the Tabular List for Digit Selection**

▽ **Subterms under main terms may continue to next column or page**

Neoplasm, neoplastic —	Malignant Primary	Secondary	Ca in situ	Benign	Uncertain Behavior	Unspecified
continued						
canal — continued						
auditory (external) (see also Neoplasm, skin, ear)	173.20	198.2	232.2	216.2	238.2	239.2
auricular (external) (see also Neoplasm, skin, ear)	173.20	198.2	232.2	216.2	238.2	239.2
canaliculi, biliary (biliferi) (intrahepatic)	155.1	197.8	230.8	211.5	235.3	239.0
canthus (eye) (inner) (outer)	173.10	198.2	232.1	216.1	238.2	239.2
basal cell carcinoma	173.11	—	—	—	—	—
specified type NEC	173.19	—	—	—	—	—
squamous cell carcinoma	173.12	—	—	—	—	—
capillary — see Neoplasm, connective tissue						
caput coli	153.4	197.5	230.3	211.3	235.2	239.0
cardia (gastric)	151.0	197.8	230.2	211.1	235.2	239.0
cardiac orifice (stomach)	151.0	197.8	230.2	211.1	235.2	239.0
cardio-esophageal junction	151.0	197.8	230.2	211.1	235.2	239.0
cardio-esophagus	151.0	197.8	230.2	211.1	235.2	239.0
carina (bronchus)	162.2	197.0	231.2	212.3	235.7	239.1
carotid (artery)	171.0	198.89	—	215.0	238.1	239.2
body	194.5	198.89	—	227.5	237.3	239.7
carpus (any bone)	170.5	198.5	—	213.5	238.0	239.2
cartilage (articular) (joint) NEC (see also Neoplasm, bone)	170.9	198.5	—	213.9	238.0	239.2
arytenoid	161.3	197.3	231.0	212.1	235.6	239.1
auricular	171.0	198.89	—	215.0	238.1	239.2
bronchi	162.2	197.3	—	212.3	235.7	239.1
connective tissue — see Neoplasm, connective tissue						
costal	170.3	198.5	—	213.3	238.0	239.2
cricoid	161.3	197.3	231.0	212.1	235.6	239.1
cuneiform	161.3	197.3	231.0	212.1	235.6	239.1
ear (external)	171.0	198.89	—	215.0	238.1	239.2
ensiform	170.3	198.5	—	213.3	238.0	239.2
epiglottis	161.1	197.3	231.0	212.1	235.6	239.1
anterior surface	146.4	198.89	230.0	210.6	235.1	239.0
eyelid	171.0	198.89	—	215.0	238.1	239.2
intervertebral	170.2	198.5	—	213.2	238.0	239.2
larynx, laryngeal	161.3	197.3	231.0	212.1	235.6	239.1
nose, nasal	160.0	197.3	231.8	212.0	235.9	239.1
pinna	171.0	198.89	—	215.0	238.1	239.2
rib	170.3	198.5	—	213.3	238.0	239.2
semilunar (knee)	170.7	198.5	—	213.7	238.0	239.2
thyroid	161.3	197.3	231.0	212.1	235.6	239.1
trachea	162.0	197.3	231.1	212.2	235.7	239.1
cauda equina	192.2	198.3	—	225.3	237.5	239.7
cavity						
buccal	145.9	198.89	230.0	210.4	235.1	239.0
nasal	160.0	197.3	231.8	212.0	235.9	239.1
oral	145.9	198.89	230.0	210.4	235.1	239.0
peritoneal	158.9	197.6	—	211.8	235.4	239.0
tympanic	160.1	197.3	231.8	212.0	235.9	239.1
cecum	153.4	197.5	230.3	211.3	235.2	239.0
central nervous system — see Neoplasm, nervous system						
white matter	191.0	198.3	—	225.0	237.5	239.6
cerebellopontine (angle)	191.6	198.3	—	225.0	237.5	239.6
cerebellum, cerebellar	191.6	198.3	—	225.0	237.5	239.6
cerebrum, cerebral (cortex) (hemisphere) (white matter)	191.0	198.3	—	225.0	237.5	239.6
meninges	192.1	198.4	—	225.2	237.6	239.7
peduncle	191.7	198.3	—	225.0	237.5	239.6
ventricle (any)	191.5	198.3	—	225.0	237.5	239.6
cervical region	195.0	198.89	234.8	229.8	238.8	239.89
cervix (cervical) (uteri) (uterus)	180.9	198.82	233.1	219.0	236.0	239.5
canal	180.0	198.82	233.1	219.0	236.0	239.5
contiguous sites	180.8	—	—	—	—	—
endocervix (canal) (gland)	180.0	198.82	233.1	219.0	236.0	239.5
exocervix	180.1	198.82	233.1	219.0	236.0	239.5
external os	180.1	198.82	233.1	219.0	236.0	239.5
internal os	180.0	198.82	233.1	219.0	236.0	239.5
nabothian gland	180.0	198.82	233.1	219.0	236.0	239.5
squamocolumnar junction	180.8	198.82	233.1	219.0	236.0	239.5
stump	180.8	198.82	233.1	219.0	236.0	239.5
cheek	195.0	198.89	234.8	229.8	238.8	239.89
external	173.30	198.2	232.3	216.3	238.2	239.2
basal cell carcinoma	173.31	—	—	—	—	—
specified type NEC	173.39	—	—	—	—	—
squamous cell carcinoma	173.32	—	—	—	—	—
inner aspect	145.0	198.89	230.0	210.4	235.1	239.0
internal	145.0	198.89	230.0	210.4	235.1	239.0
mucosa	145.0	198.89	230.0	210.4	235.1	239.0
chest (wall) NEC	195.1	198.89	234.8	229.8	238.8	239.89
chiasma opticum	192.0	198.4	—	225.1	237.9	239.7
chin	173.30	198.2	232.3	216.3	238.2	239.2
basal cell carcinoma	173.31	—	—	—	—	—
specified type NEC	173.39	—	—	—	—	—
squamous cell carcinoma	173.32	—	—	—	—	—
choana	147.3	198.89	230.0	210.7	235.1	239.0
cholangiole	155.1	197.8	230.8	211.5	235.3	239.0
choledochal duct	156.1	197.8	230.8	211.5	235.3	239.0
choroid	190.6	198.4	234.0	224.6	238.8	239.81
plexus	191.5	198.3	—	225.0	237.5	239.6
ciliary body	190.0	198.4	234.0	224.0	238.8	239.89
clavicle	170.3	198.5	—	213.3	238.0	239.2
clitoris	184.3	198.82	233.32	221.2	236.3	239.5
clivus	170.0	198.5	—	213.0	238.0	239.2
cloacogenic zone	154.8	197.5	230.7	211.4	235.5	239.0
coccygeal body or glomus	194.6	198.89	—	227.6	237.3	239.7
vertebra	170.6	198.5	—	213.6	238.0	239.2
coccyx	170.6	198.5	—	213.6	238.0	239.2
colon — see also Neoplasm, intestine, large	153.9	197.5	230.3	211.3	235.2	239.0
with rectum	154.0	197.5	230.4	211.4	235.2	239.0
columnella (see also Neoplasm, skin, face)	173.30	198.2	232.3	216.3	238.2	239.2
column, spinal — see Neoplasm, spine						
commissure						
labial, lip	140.6	198.89	230.0	210.4	235.1	239.0
laryngeal	161.0	197.3	231.0	212.1	235.6	239.1
common (bile) duct	156.1	197.8	230.8	211.5	235.3	239.0

☑ Additional Digit Required — Refer to the Tabular List for Digit Selection · Subterms under main terms may continue to next column or page

	Malignant			Benign	Uncertain Behavior	Unspecified
	Primary	Secondary	Ca in situ			
Neoplasm, neoplastic — *continued*						
concha (*see also* Neoplasm, skin, ear)	173.20	198.2	232.2	216.2	238.2	239.2
nose	160.0	197.3	231.8	212.0	235.9	239.1
conjunctiva	190.3	198.4	234.0	224.3	238.8	239.89
connective tissue NEC	171.9	198.89	—	215.9	238.1	239.2

Note — For neoplasms of connective tissue (blood vessel, bursa, fascia, ligament, muscle, peripheral nerves, sympathetic and parasympathetic nerves and ganglia, synovia, tendon, etc.) or of morphological types that indicate connective tissue, code according to the list under "Neoplasm, connective tissue"; for sites that do not appear in this list, code to neoplasm of that site; e.g.,

liposarcoma, shoulder 171.2

leiomyosarcoma, stomach 151.9

neurofibroma, chest wall 215.4

Morphological types that indicate connective tissue appear in the proper place in the alphabetic index with the instruction "see Neoplasm, connective tissue..."

	Malignant			Benign	Uncertain Behavior	Unspecified
	Primary	Secondary	Ca in situ			
abdomen	171.5	198.89	—	215.5	238.1	239.2
abdominal wall	171.5	198.89	—	215.5	238.1	239.2
ankle	171.3	198.89	—	215.3	238.1	239.2
antecubital fossa or space	171.2	198.89	—	215.2	238.1	239.2
arm	171.2	198.89	—	215.2	238.1	239.2
auricle (ear)	171.0	198.89	—	215.0	238.1	239.2
axilla	171.4	198.89	—	215.4	238.1	239.2
back	171.7	198.89	—	215.7	238.1	239.2
breast (female) (*see also* Neoplasm, breast)	174.9	198.81	233.0	217	238.3	239.3
male	175.9	198.81	233.0	217	238.3	239.3
buttock	171.6	198.89	—	215.6	238.1	239.2
calf	171.3	198.89	—	215.3	238.1	239.2
cervical region	171.0	198.89	—	215.0	238.1	239.2
cheek	171.0	198.89	—	215.0	238.1	239.2
chest (wall)	171.4	198.89	—	215.4	238.1	239.2
chin	171.0	198.89	—	215.0	238.1	239.2
contiguous sites	171.8	—	—	—	—	—
diaphragm	171.4	198.89	—	215.4	238.1	239.2
ear (external)	171.0	198.89	—	215.0	238.1	239.2
elbow	171.2	198.89	—	215.2	238.1	239.2
extrarectal	171.6	198.89	—	215.6	238.1	239.2
extremity	171.8	198.89	—	215.8	238.1	239.2
lower	171.3	198.89	—	215.3	238.1	239.2
upper	171.2	198.89	—	215.2	238.1	239.2
eyelid	171.0	198.89	—	215.0	238.1	239.2
face	171.0	198.89	—	215.0	238.1	239.2
finger	171.2	198.89	—	215.2	238.1	239.2
flank	171.7	198.89	—	215.7	238.1	239.2
foot	171.3	198.89	—	215.3	238.1	239.2
forearm	171.2	198.89	—	215.2	238.1	239.2
forehead	171.0	198.89	—	215.0	238.1	239.2
gastric	171.5	198.89	—	215.5	238.1	—
gastrointestinal	171.5	198.89	—	215.5	238.1	—
gluteal region	171.6	198.89	—	215.6	238.1	239.2
great vessels NEC	171.4	198.89	—	215.4	238.1	239.2
groin	171.6	198.89	—	215.6	238.1	239.2
hand	171.2	198.89	—	215.2	238.1	239.2
head	171.0	198.89	—	215.0	238.1	239.2
heel	171.3	198.89	—	215.3	238.1	239.2
hip	171.3	198.89	—	215.3	238.1	239.2
hypochondrium	171.5	198.89	—	215.5	238.1	239.2
iliopsoas muscle	171.6	198.89	—	215.5	238.1	239.2
infraclavicular region	171.4	198.89	—	215.4	238.1	239.2
inguinal (canal) (region)	171.6	198.89	—	215.6	238.1	239.2
intestine	171.5	198.89	—	215.5	238.1	—
intrathoracic	171.4	198.89	—	215.4	238.1	239.2
ischorectal fossa	171.6	198.89	—	215.6	238.1	239.2
jaw	143.9	198.89	230.0	210.4	235.1	239.0

	Malignant			Benign	Uncertain Behavior	Unspecified
	Primary	Secondary	Ca in situ			
Neoplasm, neoplastic — *continued* connective tissue — *continued*						
knee	171.3	198.89	—	215.3	238.1	239.2
leg	171.3	198.89	—	215.3	238.1	239.2
limb NEC	171.9	198.89	—	215.8	238.1	239.2
lower	171.3	198.89	—	215.3	238.1	239.2
upper	171.2	198.89	—	215.2	238.1	239.2
nates	171.6	198.89	—	215.6	238.1	239.2
neck	171.0	198.89	—	215.0	238.1	239.2
orbit	190.1	198.4	234.0	224.1	238.8	239.89
pararectal	171.6	198.89	—	215.6	238.1	239.2
para-urethral	171.6	198.89	—	215.6	238.1	239.2
paravaginal	171.6	198.89	—	215.6	238.1	239.2
pelvis (floor)	171.6	198.89	—	215.6	238.1	239.2
pelvo-abdominal	171.8	198.89	—	215.8	238.1	239.2
perineum	171.6	198.89	—	215.6	238.1	239.2
perirectal (tissue)	171.6	198.89	—	215.6	238.1	239.2
periurethral (tissue)	171.6	198.89	—	215.6	238.1	239.2
popliteal fossa or space	171.3	198.89	—	215.3	238.1	239.2
presacral	171.6	198.89	—	215.6	238.1	239.2
psoas muscle	171.5	198.89	—	215.5	238.1	239.2
pterygoid fossa	171.0	198.89	—	215.0	238.1	239.2
rectovaginal septum or wall	171.6	198.89	—	215.6	238.1	239.2
rectovesical	171.6	198.89	—	215.6	238.1	239.2
retroperitoneum	158.0	197.6	—	211.8	235.4	239.0
sacrococcygeal region	171.6	198.89	—	215.6	238.1	239.2
scalp	171.0	198.89	—	215.0	238.1	239.2
scapular region	171.4	198.89	—	215.4	238.1	239.2
shoulder	171.2	198.89	—	215.2	238.1	239.2
skin (dermis) NEC	173.90	198.2	232.9	216.9	238.2	239.2
stomach	171.5	198.89	—	215.5	238.1	—
submental	171.0	198.89	—	215.0	238.1	239.2
supraclavicular region	171.0	198.89	—	215.0	238.1	239.2
temple	171.0	198.89	—	215.0	238.1	239.2
temporal region	171.0	198.89	—	215.0	238.1	239.2
thigh	171.3	198.89	—	215.3	238.1	239.2
thoracic (duct) (wall)	171.4	198.89	—	215.4	238.1	239.2
thorax	171.4	198.89	—	215.4	238.1	239.2
thumb	171.2	198.89	—	215.2	238.1	239.2
toe	171.3	198.89	—	215.3	238.1	239.2
trunk	171.7	198.89	—	215.7	238.1	239.2
umbilicus	171.5	198.89	—	215.5	238.1	239.2
vesicorectal	171.6	198.89	—	215.6	238.1	239.2
wrist	171.2	198.89	—	215.2	238.1	239.2
conus medullaris	192.2	198.3	—	225.3	237.5	239.7
cord (true) (vocal)	161.0	197.3	231.0	212.1	235.6	239.1
false	161.1	197.3	231.0	212.1	235.6	239.1
spermatic	187.6	198.82	233.6	222.8	236.6	239.5
spinal (cervical) (lumbar) (thoracic)	192.2	198.3	—	225.3	237.5	239.7
cornea (limbus)	190.4	198.4	234.0	224.4	238.8	239.89
corpus						
albicans	183.0	198.6	233.39	220	236.2	239.5
callosum, brain	191.8	198.3	—	225.0	237.5	239.6
cavernosum	187.3	198.82	233.5	222.1	236.6	239.5
gastric	151.4	197.8	230.2	211.1	235.2	239.0
penis	187.3	198.82	233.5	222.1	236.6	239.5
striatum, cerebrum	191.0	198.3	—	225.0	237.5	239.6
uteri	182.0	198.82	233.2	219.1	236.0	239.5
isthmus	182.1	198.82	233.2	219.1	236.0	239.5
cortex						
adrenal	194.0	198.7	234.8	227.0	237.2	239.7
cerebral	191.0	198.3	—	225.0	237.5	239.6
costal cartilage	170.3	198.5	—	213.3	238.0	239.2

☑ **Additional Digit Required** — Refer to the Tabular List for Digit Selection   ▽ **Subterms under main terms may continue to next column or page**

2015 ICD-9-CM   ▶◀ **Revised Text**   ● **New Line**   ▲ **Revised Code**   **Volume 2 — 197**

	Malignant			Benign	Uncertain Behavior	Unspecified
	Primary	Secondary	Ca in situ			
Neoplasm, neoplastic — *continued*						
costovertebral joint	170.3	198.5	—	213.3	238.0	239.2
Cowper's gland	189.3	198.1	233.9	223.81	236.99	239.5
cranial (fossa, any)	191.9	198.3	—	225.0	237.5	239.6
meninges	192.1	198.4	—	225.2	237.6	239.7
nerve (any)	192.0	198.4	—	225.1	237.9	239.7
craniobuccal pouch	194.3	198.89	234.8	227.3	237.0	239.7
craniopharyngeal (duct) (pouch)	194.3	198.89	234.8	227.3	237.0	239.7
cricoid	148.0	198.89	230.0	210.8	235.1	239.0
cartilage	161.3	197.3	231.0	212.1	235.6	239.1
cricopharynx	148.0	198.89	230.0	210.8	235.1	239.0
crypt of Morgagni	154.8	197.5	230.7	211.4	235.2	239.0
crystalline lens	190.0	198.4	234.0	224.0	238.8	239.89
cul-de-sac (Douglas')	158.8	197.6	—	211.8	235.4	239.0
cuneiform cartilage	161.3	197.3	231.0	212.1	235.6	239.1
cutaneous — *see* Neoplasm, skin						
cutis — *see* Neoplasm, skin						
cystic (bile) duct (common)	156.1	197.8	230.8	211.5	235.3	239.0
dermis — *see* Neoplasm, skin						
diaphragm	171.4	198.89	—	215.4	238.1	239.2
digestive organs, system, tube, or tract NEC	159.9	197.8	230.9	211.9	235.5	239.0
contiguous sites with peritoneum	159.8	—	—	—	—	—
disc, intervertebral	170.2	198.5	—	213.2	238.0	239.2
disease, generalized	199.0	—	234.9	229.9	238.9	—
disseminated	199.0	—	234.9	229.9	238.9	—
Douglas' cul-de-sac or pouch	158.8	197.6	—	211.8	235.4	239.0
duodenojejunal junction	152.8	197.4	230.7	211.2	235.2	239.0
duodenum	152.0	197.4	230.7	211.2	235.2	239.0
dura (cranial) (mater)	192.1	198.4	—	225.2	237.6	239.7
cerebral	192.1	198.4	—	225.2	237.6	239.7
spinal	192.3	198.4	—	225.4	237.6	239.7
ear (external) (*see also* Neoplasm, ear, skin)	173.20	198.2	232.2	216.2	238.2	239.2
auricle or auris (*see also* Neoplasm, ear, skin)	173.20	198.2	232.2	216.2	238.2	239.2
canal, external (*see also* Neoplasm, ear, skin)	173.20	198.2	232.2	216.2	238.2	239.2
cartilage	171.0	198.89	—	215.0	238.1	239.2
external meatus (*see also* Neoplasm, ear, skin)	173.20	198.2	232.2	216.2	238.2	239.2
inner	160.1	197.3	231.8	212.0	235.9	239.89
lobule (*see also* Neoplasm, ear, skin)	173.20	198.2	232.2	216.2	238.2	239.2
middle	160.1	197.3	231.8	212.0	235.9	239.89
contiguous sites with accessory sinuses or nasal cavities	160.8	—	—	—	—	—
skin	173.20	198.2	232.2	216.2	238.2	239.2
basal cell carcinoma	173.21	—	—	—	—	—
specified type NEC	173.29	—	—	—	—	—
squamous cell carcinoma	173.22	—	—	—	—	—
earlobe	173.20	198.2	232.2	216.2	238.2	239.2

	Malignant			Benign	Uncertain Behavior	Unspecified
	Primary	Secondary	Ca in situ			
Neoplasm, neoplastic — *continued*						
earlobe — *continued*						
basal cell carcinoma	173.21	—	—	—	—	—
specified type NEC	173.29	—	—	—	—	—
squamous cell carcinoma	173.22	—	—	—	—	—
ejaculatory duct	187.8	198.82	233.6	222.8	236.6	239.5
elbow NEC*	195.4	198.89	232.6	229.8	238.8	239.89
endocardium	164.1	198.89	—	212.7	238.8	239.89
endocervix (canal) (gland)	180.0	198.82	233.1	219.0	236.0	239.5
endocrine gland NEC	194.9	198.89	—	227.9	237.4	239.7
pluriglandular NEC	194.8	198.89	234.8	227.8	237.4	239.7
endometrium (gland) (stroma)	182.0	198.82	233.2	219.1	236.0	239.5
ensiform cartilage	170.3	198.5	—	213.3	238.0	239.2
enteric — *see* Neoplasm, intestine						
ependyma (brain)	191.5	198.3	—	225.0	237.5	239.6
epicardium	164.1	198.89	—	212.7	238.8	239.89
epididymis	187.5	198.82	233.6	222.3	236.6	239.5
epidural	192.9	198.4	—	225.9	237.9	239.7
epiglottis	161.1	197.3	231.0	212.1	235.6	239.1
anterior aspect or surface	146.4	198.89	230.0	210.6	235.1	239.0
cartilage	161.3	197.3	231.0	212.1	235.6	239.1
free border (margin)	146.4	198.89	230.0	210.6	235.1	239.0
junctional region	146.5	198.89	230.0	210.6	235.1	239.0
posterior (laryngeal) surface	161.1	197.3	231.0	212.1	235.6	239.1
suprahyoid portion	161.1	197.3	231.0	212.1	235.6	239.1
esophagogastric junction	151.0	197.8	230.2	211.1	235.2	239.0
esophagus	150.9	197.8	230.1	211.0	235.5	239.0
abdominal	150.2	197.8	230.1	211.0	235.5	239.0
cervical	150.0	197.8	230.1	211.0	235.5	239.0
contiguous sites	150.8	—	—	—	—	—
distal (third)	150.5	197.8	230.1	211.0	235.5	239.0
lower (third)	150.5	197.8	230.1	211.0	235.5	239.0
middle (third)	150.4	197.8	230.1	211.0	235.5	239.0
proximal (third)	150.3	197.8	230.1	211.0	235.5	239.0
specified part NEC	150.8	197.8	230.1	211.0	235.5	239.0
thoracic	150.1	197.8	230.1	211.0	235.5	239.0
upper (third)	150.3	197.8	230.1	211.0	235.5	239.0
ethmoid (sinus)	160.3	197.3	231.8	212.0	235.9	239.1
bone or labyrinth	170.0	198.5	—	213.0	238.0	239.2
Eustachian tube	160.1	197.3	231.8	212.0	235.9	239.1
exocervix	180.1	198.82	233.1	219.0	236.0	239.5
external meatus (ear) (*see also* Neoplasm, skin, ear)	173.20	198.2	232.2	216.2	238.2	239.2
os, cervix uteri	180.1	198.82	233.1	219.0	236.0	239.5
extradural	192.9	198.4	—	225.9	237.9	239.7
extrahepatic (bile) duct	156.1	197.8	230.8	211.5	235.3	239.0
contiguous sites with gallbladder	156.8	—	—	—	—	—
extraocular muscle	190.1	198.4	234.0	224.1	238.8	239.89
extrarectal	195.3	198.89	234.8	229.8	238.8	239.89
extremity*	195.8	198.89	232.8	229.8	238.8	239.89
lower*	195.5	198.89	232.7	229.8	238.8	239.89
upper*	195.4	198.89	232.6	229.8	238.8	239.89
eye NEC	190.9	198.4	234.0	224.9	238.8	239.89
contiguous sites	190.8	—	—	—	—	—

☑ **Additional Digit Required — Refer to the Tabular List for Digit Selection**   ▽ **Subterms under main terms may continue to next column or page**

198— Volume 2   ▶◀ Revised Text   ● New Line   ▲ Revised Code   2015 ICD-9-CM

Neoplasm, neoplastic — continued

	Malignant					
	Primary	Secondary	Ca in situ	Benign	Uncertain Behavior	Unspecified
eye — continued						
specified sites						
NEC	190.8	198.4	234.0	224.8	238.8	239.89
eyeball	190.0	198.4	234.0	224.0	238.8	239.89
eyebrow	173.30	198.2	232.3	216.3	238.2	239.2
basal cell						
carcinoma	173.31	—	—	—	—	—
specified type						
NEC	173.39	—	—	—	—	—
squamous cell						
carcinoma	173.32	—	—	—	—	—
eyelid (lower) (skin) (upper)	173.10	198.2	232.1	216.1	238.2	239.2
basal cell						
carcinoma	173.11	—	—	—	—	—
cartilage	171.0	198.89	—	215.0	238.1	239.2
specified type						
NEC	173.19	—	—	—	—	—
squamous cell						
carcinoma	173.12	—	—	—	—	—
face NEC*	195.0	198.89	232.3	229.8	238.8	239.89
fallopian tube (accessory)	183.2	198.82	233.39	221.0	236.3	239.5
falx (cerebelli) (cerebri)	192.1	198.4	—	225.2	237.6	239.7
fascia (see also Neoplasm, connective tissue)						
palmar	171.2	198.89	—	215.2	238.1	239.2
plantar	171.3	198.89	—	215.3	238.1	239.2
fatty tissue — see Neoplasm, connective tissue						
fauces, faucial NEC	146.9	198.89	230.0	210.6	235.1	239.0
pillars	146.2	198.89	230.0	210.6	235.1	239.0
tonsil	146.0	198.89	230.0	210.5	235.1	239.0
femur (any part)	170.7	198.5	—	213.7	238.0	239.2
fetal membrane	181	198.82	233.2	219.8	236.1	239.5
fibrous tissue — see Neoplasm, connective tissue						
fibula (any part)	170.7	198.5	—	213.7	238.0	239.2
filum terminale	192.2	198.3	—	225.3	237.5	239.7
finger NEC*	195.4	198.89	232.6	229.8	238.8	239.89
flank NEC*	195.8	198.89	232.5	229.8	238.8	239.89
follicle, nabothian	180.0	198.82	233.1	219.0	236.0	239.5
foot NEC*	195.5	198.89	232.7	229.8	238.8	239.89
forearm NEC*	195.4	198.89	232.6	229.8	238.8	239.89
forehead (skin)	173.30	198.2	232.3	216.3	238.2	239.2
basal cell						
carcinoma	173.31	—	—	—	—	—
specified type						
NEC	173.39	—	—	—	—	—
squamous cell						
carcinoma	173.32	—	—	—	—	—
foreskin	187.1	198.82	233.5	222.1	236.6	239.5
fornix						
pharyngeal	147.3	198.89	230.0	210.7	235.1	239.0
vagina	184.0	198.82	233.31	221.1	236.3	239.5
fossa (of)						
anterior (cranial)	191.9	198.3	—	225.0	237.5	239.6
cranial	191.9	198.3	—	225.0	237.5	239.6
ischiorectal	195.3	198.89	234.8	229.8	238.8	239.89
middle (cranial)	191.9	198.3	—	225.0	237.5	239.6
pituitary	194.3	198.89	234.8	227.3	237.0	239.7
posterior (cranial)	191.9	198.3	—	225.0	237.5	239.6
pterygoid	171.0	198.89	—	215.0	238.1	239.2
pyriform	148.1	198.89	230.0	210.8	235.1	239.0
Rosenmüller	147.2	198.89	230.0	210.7	235.1	239.0
tonsillar	146.1	198.89	230.0	210.6	235.1	239.0
fourchette	184.4	198.82	233.32	221.2	236.3	239.5
frenulum						
labii — see Neoplasm, lip, internal						

Neoplasm, neoplastic — continued

	Malignant					
	Primary	Secondary	Ca in situ	Benign	Uncertain Behavior	Unspecified
frenulum — continued						
linguae	141.3	198.89	230.0	210.1	235.1	239.0
frontal						
bone	170.0	198.5	—	213.0	238.0	239.2
lobe, brain	191.1	198.3	—	225.0	237.5	239.6
meninges	192.1	198.4	—	225.2	237.6	239.7
pole	191.1	198.3	—	225.0	237.5	239.6
sinus	160.4	197.3	231.8	212.0	235.9	239.1
fundus						
stomach	151.3	197.8	230.2	211.1	235.2	239.0
uterus	182.0	198.82	233.2	219.1	236.0	239.5
gallbladder	156.0	197.8	230.8	211.5	235.3	239.0
contiguous sites with extrahepatic bile ducts	156.8	—	—	—	—	—
gall duct (extrahepatic)	156.1	197.8	230.8	211.5	235.3	239.0
intrahepatic	155.1	197.8	230.8	211.5	235.3	239.0
ganglia (see also Neoplasm, connective tissue)	171.9	198.89	—	215.9	238.1	239.2
basal	191.0	198.3	—	225.0	237.5	239.6
ganglion (see also Neoplasm, connective tissue)	171.9	198.89	—	215.9	238.1	239.2
cranial nerve	192.0	198.4	—	225.1	237.9	239.7
Gartner's duct	184.0	198.82	233.31	221.1	236.3	239.5
gastric — see Neoplasm, stomach						
gastrocolic	159.8	197.8	230.9	211.9	235.5	239.0
gastroesophageal junction	151.0	197.8	230.2	211.1	235.2	239.0
gastrointestinal (tract) NEC	159.9	197.8	230.9	211.9	235.5	239.0
generalized	199.0	—	234.9	229.9	238.9	—
genital organ or tract						
female NEC	184.9	198.82	233.39	221.9	236.3	239.5
contiguous sites	184.8	—	—	—	—	—
specified site NEC	184.8	198.82	233.39	221.8	236.3	239.5
male NEC	187.9	198.82	233.6	222.9	236.6	239.5
contiguous sites	187.8	—	—	—	—	—
specified site NEC	187.8	198.82	233.6	222.8	236.6	239.5
genitourinary tract						
female	184.9	198.82	233.39	221.9	236.3	239.5
male	187.9	198.82	233.6	222.9	236.6	239.5
gingiva (alveolar) (marginal)	143.9	198.89	230.0	210.4	235.1	239.0
lower	143.1	198.89	230.0	210.4	235.1	239.0
mandibular	143.1	198.89	230.0	210.4	235.1	239.0
maxillary	143.0	198.89	230.0	210.4	235.1	239.0
upper	143.0	198.89	230.0	210.4	235.1	239.0
gland, glandular (lymphatic) (system) (see also Neoplasm, lymph gland)						
endocrine NEC	194.9	198.89	—	227.9	237.4	239.7
salivary — see Neoplasm, salivary, gland						
glans penis	187.2	198.82	233.5	222.1	236.6	239.5
globus pallidus	191.0	198.3	—	225.0	237.5	239.6
glomus						
coccygeal	194.6	198.89	—	227.6	237.3	239.7
jugularis	194.6	198.89	—	227.6	237.3	239.7
glosso-epiglottic fold(s)	146.4	198.89	230.0	210.6	235.1	239.0
glossopalatine fold	146.2	198.89	230.0	210.6	235.1	239.0
glossopharyngeal sulcus	146.1	198.89	230.0	210.6	235.1	239.0

☑ **Additional Digit Required — Refer to the Tabular List for Digit Selection**   ▽ **Subterms under main terms may continue to next column or page**

Neoplasm, neoplastic — continued	Malignant			Benign	Uncertain Behavior	Unspecified
	Primary	Secondary	Ca in situ			
glottis	161.0	197.3	231.0	212.1	235.6	239.1
gluteal region*	195.3	198.89	232.5	229.8	238.8	239.89
great vessels NEC	171.4	198.89	—	215.4	238.1	239.2
groin NEC	195.3	198.89	232.5	229.8	238.8	239.89
gum	143.9	198.89	230.0	210.4	235.1	239.0
contiguous sites	143.8	—	—	—	—	—
lower	143.1	198.89	230.0	210.4	235.1	239.0
upper	143.0	198.89	230.0	210.4	235.1	239.0
hand NEC*	195.4	198.89	232.6	229.8	238.8	239.89
head NEC*	195.0	198.89	232.4	229.8	238.8	239.89
heart	164.1	198.89	—	212.7	238.8	239.89
contiguous sites with mediastinum or thymus	164.8	—	—	—	—	—
heel NEC*	195.5	198.89	232.7	229.8	238.8	239.89
helix (see also Neoplasm, skin, ear)	173.20	198.2	232.2	216.2	238.2	239.2
hematopoietic, hemopoietic tissue NEC	202.8	198.89	—	—	—	238.79
hemisphere, cerebral	191.0	198.3	—	225.0	237.5	239.6
hemorrhoidal zone	154.2	197.5	230.5	211.4	235.5	239.0
hepatic	155.2	197.7	230.8	211.5	235.3	239.0
duct (bile)	156.1	197.8	230.8	211.5	235.3	239.0
flexure (colon)	153.0	197.5	230.3	211.3	235.2	239.0
primary	155.0	—	—	—	—	—
hilus of lung	162.2	197.0	231.2	212.3	235.7	239.1
hip NEC*	195.5	198.89	232.7	229.8	238.8	239.89
hippocampus, brain	191.2	198.3	—	225.0	237.5	239.6
humerus (any part)	170.4	198.5	—	213.4	238.0	239.2
hymen	184.0	198.82	233.31	221.1	236.3	239.5
hypopharynx, hypopharyngeal NEC	148.9	198.89	230.0	210.8	235.1	239.0
contiguous sites	148.8	—	—	—	—	—
postcricoid region	148.0	198.89	230.0	210.8	235.1	239.0
posterior wall	148.3	198.89	230.0	210.8	235.1	239.0
pyriform fossa (sinus)	148.1	198.89	230.0	210.8	235.1	239.0
specified site NEC	148.8	198.89	230.0	210.8	235.1	239.0
wall	148.9	198.89	230.0	210.8	235.1	239.0
posterior	148.3	198.89	230.0	210.8	235.1	239.0
hypophysis	194.3	198.89	234.8	227.3	237.0	239.7
hypothalamus	191.0	198.3	—	225.0	237.5	239.6
ileocecum, ileocecal (coil) (junction) (valve)	153.4	197.5	230.3	211.3	235.2	239.0
ileum	152.2	197.4	230.7	211.2	235.2	239.0
ilium	170.6	198.5	—	213.6	238.0	239.2
immunoproliferative NEC	203.8	—	—	—	—	—
infraclavicular (region)*	195.1	198.89	232.5	229.8	238.8	239.89
inguinal (region)*	195.3	198.89	232.5	229.8	238.8	239.89
insula	191.0	198.3	—	225.0	237.5	239.6
insular tissue (pancreas)	157.4	197.8	230.9	211.7	235.5	239.0
brain	191.0	198.3	—	225.0	237.5	239.6
interarytenoid fold	148.2	198.89	230.0	210.8	235.1	239.0
hypopharyngeal aspect	148.2	198.89	230.0	210.8	235.1	239.0
laryngeal aspect	161.1	197.3	231.0	212.1	235.6	239.1
marginal zone	148.2	198.89	230.0	210.8	235.1	239.0
interdental papillae	143.9	198.89	230.0	210.4	235.1	239.0
lower	143.1	198.89	230.0	210.4	235.1	239.0
upper	143.0	198.89	230.0	210.4	235.1	239.0
internal capsule	191.0	198.3	—	225.0	237.5	239.6
os (cervix)	180.0	198.82	233.1	219.0	236.0	239.5

Neoplasm, neoplastic — continued	Malignant			Benign	Uncertain Behavior	Unspecified
	Primary	Secondary	Ca in situ			
intervertebral cartilage or disc	170.2	198.5	—	213.2	238.0	239.2
intestine, intestinal	159.0	197.8	230.7	211.9	235.2	239.0
large	153.9	197.5	230.3	211.3	235.2	239.0
appendix	153.5	197.5	230.3	211.3	235.2	239.0
caput coli	153.4	197.5	230.3	211.3	235.2	239.0
cecum	153.4	197.5	230.3	211.3	235.2	239.0
colon	153.9	197.5	230.3	211.3	235.2	239.0
and rectum	154.0	197.5	230.4	211.4	235.2	239.0
ascending	153.6	197.5	230.3	211.3	235.2	239.0
caput	153.4	197.5	230.3	211.3	235.2	239.0
contiguous sites	153.8	—	—	—	—	—
descending	153.2	197.5	230.3	211.3	235.2	239.0
distal	153.2	197.5	230.3	211.3	235.2	239.0
left	153.2	197.5	230.3	211.3	235.2	239.0
pelvic	153.3	197.5	230.3	211.3	235.2	239.0
right	153.6	197.5	230.3	211.3	235.2	239.0
sigmoid (flexure)	153.3	197.5	230.3	211.3	235.2	239.0
transverse	153.1	197.5	230.3	211.3	235.2	239.0
contiguous sites	153.8	—	—	—	—	—
hepatic flexure	153.0	197.5	230.3	211.3	235.2	239.0
ileocecum, ileocecal (coil) (valve)	153.4	197.5	230.3	211.3	235.2	239.0
sigmoid flexure (lower) (upper)	153.3	197.5	230.3	211.3	235.2	239.0
splenic flexure	153.7	197.5	230.3	211.3	235.2	239.0
small	152.9	197.4	230.7	211.2	235.2	239.0
contiguous sites	152.8	—	—	—	—	—
duodenum	152.0	197.4	230.7	211.2	235.2	239.0
ileum	152.2	197.4	230.7	211.2	235.2	239.0
jejunum	152.1	197.4	230.7	211.2	235.2	239.0
tract NEC	159.0	197.8	230.7	211.9	235.2	239.0
intra-abdominal	195.2	198.89	234.8	229.8	238.8	239.89
intracranial NEC	191.9	198.3	—	225.0	237.5	239.6
intrahepatic (bile) duct	155.1	197.8	230.8	211.5	235.3	239.0
intraocular	190.0	198.4	234.0	224.0	238.8	239.89
intraorbital	190.1	198.4	234.0	224.1	238.8	239.89
intrasellar	194.3	198.89	234.8	227.3	237.0	239.7
intrathoracic (cavity) (organs NEC)	195.1	198.89	234.8	229.8	238.8	239.89
contiguous sites with respiratory organs	165.8	—	—	—	—	—
iris	190.0	198.4	234.0	224.0	238.8	239.89
ischiorectal (fossa)	195.3	198.89	234.8	229.8	238.8	239.89
ischium	170.6	198.5	—	213.6	238.0	239.2
island of Reil	191.0	198.3	—	225.0	237.5	239.6
islands or islets of Langerhans	157.4	197.8	230.9	211.7	235.5	239.0
isthmus uteri	182.1	198.82	233.2	219.1	236.0	239.5
jaw	195.0	198.89	234.8	229.8	238.8	239.89
bone	170.1	198.5	—	213.1	238.0	239.2
carcinoma	143.9	—	—	—	—	—
lower	143.1	—	—	—	—	—
upper	143.0	—	—	—	—	—
lower	170.1	198.5	—	213.1	238.0	239.2
upper	170.0	198.5	—	213.0	238.0	239.2
carcinoma (any type) (lower) (upper)	195.0	—	—	—	—	—
skin (see also Neoplasm, skin, face)	173.30	198.2	232.3	216.3	238.2	239.2
soft tissues	143.9	198.89	230.0	210.4	235.1	239.0
lower	143.1	198.89	230.0	210.4	235.1	239.0
upper	143.0	198.89	230.0	210.4	235.1	239.0
jejunum	152.1	197.4	230.7	211.2	235.2	239.0

☑ Additional Digit Required — Refer to the Tabular List for Digit Selection   ⓦ Subterms under main terms may continue to next column or page

200 — Volume 2   ►◄ Revised Text   ● New Line   ▲ Revised Code   2015 ICD-9-CM

	Malignant					
	Primary	Secondary	Ca in situ	Benign	Uncertain Behavior	Unspecified
Neoplasm, neoplastic — *continued*						
joint NEC (*see also* Neoplasm, bone)	170.9	198.5	—	213.9	238.0	239.2
acromioclavicular	170.4	198.5	—	213.4	238.0	239.2
bursa or synovial membrane — *see* Neoplasm, connective tissue						
costovertebral	170.3	198.5	—	213.3	238.0	239.2
sternocostal	170.3	198.5	—	213.3	238.0	239.2
temporomandibular	170.1	198.5	—	213.1	238.0	239.2
junction						
anorectal	154.8	197.5	230.7	211.4	235.5	239.0
cardioesophageal	151.0	197.8	230.2	211.1	235.2	239.0
esophagogastric	151.0	197.8	230.2	211.1	235.2	239.0
gastroesophageal	151.0	197.8	230.2	211.1	235.2	239.0
hard and soft palate	145.5	198.89	230.0	210.4	235.1	239.0
ileocecal	153.4	197.5	230.3	211.3	235.2	239.0
pelvirectal	154.0	197.5	230.4	211.4	235.2	239.0
pelviureteric	189.1	198.0	233.9	223.1	236.91	239.5
rectosigmoid	154.0	197.5	230.4	211.4	235.2	239.0
squamocolumnar, of cervix	180.8	198.82	233.1	219.0	236.0	239.5
kidney (parenchyma)	189.0	198.0	233.9	223.0	236.91	239.5
calyx	189.1	198.0	233.9	223.1	236.91	239.5
hilus	189.1	198.0	233.9	223.1	236.91	239.5
pelvis	189.1	198.0	233.9	223.1	236.91	239.5
knee NEC*	195.5	198.89	232.7	229.8	238.8	239.89
labia (skin)	184.4	198.82	233.32	221.2	236.3	239.5
majora	184.1	198.82	233.32	221.2	236.3	239.5
minora	184.2	198.82	233.32	221.2	236.3	239.5
labial (*see also* Neoplasm, lip)						
sulcus (lower) (upper)	145.1	198.89	230.0	210.4	235.1	239.0
labium (skin)	184.4	198.82	233.32	221.2	236.3	239.5
majus	184.1	198.82	233.32	221.2	236.3	239.5
minus	184.2	198.82	233.32	221.2	236.3	239.5
lacrimal						
canaliculi	190.7	198.4	234.0	224.7	238.8	239.89
duct (nasal)	190.7	198.4	234.0	224.7	238.8	239.89
gland	190.2	198.4	234.0	224.2	238.8	239.89
punctum	190.7	198.4	234.0	224.7	238.8	239.89
sac	190.7	198.4	234.0	224.7	238.8	239.89
Langerhans, islands or islets	157.4	197.8	230.9	211.7	235.5	239.0
laryngopharynx	148.9	198.89	230.0	210.8	235.1	239.0
larynx, laryngeal NEC	161.9	197.3	231.0	212.1	235.6	239.1
aryepiglottic fold	161.1	197.3	231.0	212.1	235.6	239.1
cartilage (arytenoid) (cricoid) (cuneiform) (thyroid)	161.3	197.3	231.0	212.1	235.6	239.1
commissure (anterior) (posterior)	161.0	197.3	231.0	212.1	235.6	239.1
contiguous sites	161.8	—	—	—	—	—
extrinsic NEC	161.1	197.3	231.0	212.1	235.6	239.1
meaning hypopharynx	148.9	198.89	230.0	210.8	235.1	239.0
interarytenoid fold	161.1	197.3	231.0	212.1	235.6	239.1
intrinsic	161.0	197.3	231.0	212.1	235.6	239.1
ventricular band	161.1	197.3	231.0	212.1	235.6	239.1
leg NEC*	195.5	198.89	232.7	229.8	238.8	239.89
lens, crystalline	190.0	198.4	234.0	224.0	238.8	239.89
lid (lower) (upper)	173.10	198.2	232.1	216.1	238.2	239.2
basal cell carcinoma	173.11	—	—	—	—	—
specified type NEC	173.19	—	—	—	—	—
squamous cell carcinoma	173.12	—	—	—	—	—
Neoplasm, neoplastic — *continued*						
ligament (*see also* Neoplasm, connective tissue)						
broad	183.3	198.82	233.39	221.0	236.3	239.5
Mackenrodt's	183.8	198.82	233.39	221.8	236.3	239.5
non-uterine — *see* Neoplasm, connective tissue						
round	183.5	198.82	—	221.0	236.3	239.5
sacro-uterine	183.4	198.82	—	221.0	236.3	239.5
uterine	183.4	198.82	—	221.0	236.3	239.5
utero-ovarian	183.8	198.82	233.39	221.8	236.3	239.5
uterosacral	183.4	198.82	—	221.0	236.3	239.5
limb*	195.8	198.89	232.8	229.8	238.8	239.89
lower*	195.5	198.89	232.7	229.8	238.8	239.89
upper*	195.4	198.89	232.6	229.8	238.8	239.89
limbus of cornea	190.4	198.4	234.0	224.4	238.8	239.89
lingual NEC (*see also* Neoplasm, tongue)	141.9	198.89	230.0	210.1	235.1	239.0
lingula, lung	162.3	197.0	231.2	212.3	235.7	239.1
lip (external) (lipstick area) (vermillion border)	140.9	198.89	230.0	210.0	235.1	239.0
buccal aspect — *see* Neoplasm, lip, internal						
commissure	140.6	198.89	230.0	210.4	235.1	239.0
contiguous sites	140.8	—	—	—	—	—
with oral cavity or pharynx	149.8	—	—	—	—	—
frenulum — *see* Neoplasm, lip, internal						
inner aspect — *see* Neoplasm, lip, internal						
internal (buccal) (frenulum) (mucosa) (oral)	140.5	198.89	230.0	210.0	235.1	239.0
lower	140.4	198.89	230.0	210.0	235.1	239.0
upper	140.3	198.89	230.0	210.0	235.1	239.0
lower	140.1	198.89	230.0	210.0	235.1	239.0
internal (buccal) (frenulum) (mucosa) (oral)	140.4	198.89	230.0	210.0	235.1	239.0
mucosa — *see* Neoplasm, lip, internal						
oral aspect — *see* Neoplasm, lip, internal						
skin (commissure) (lower) (upper)	173.00	198.2	232.0	216.0	238.2	239.2
basal cell carcinoma	173.01	—	—	—	—	—
specified type NEC	173.09	—	—	—	—	—
squamous cell carcinoma	173.02	—	—	—	—	—
upper	140.0	198.89	230.0	210.0	235.1	239.0
internal (buccal) (frenulum) (mucosa) (oral)	140.3	198.89	230.0	210.0	235.1	239.0
liver	155.2	197.7	230.8	211.5	235.3	239.0
primary	155.0	—	—	—	—	—
lobe						
azygos	162.3	197.0	231.2	212.3	235.7	239.1
frontal	191.1	198.3	—	225.0	237.5	239.6
lower	162.5	197.0	231.2	212.3	235.7	239.1
middle	162.4	197.0	231.2	212.3	235.7	239.1
occipital	191.4	198.3	—	225.0	237.5	239.6

	Malignant					
	Primary	Secondary	Ca in situ	Benign	Uncertain Behavior	Unspecified
Neoplasm, neoplastic — *continued*						
lobe — *continued*						
parietal	191.3	198.3	—	225.0	237.5	239.6
temporal	191.2	198.3	—	225.0	237.5	239.6
upper	162.3	197.0	231.2	212.3	235.7	239.1
lumbosacral plexus	171.6	198.4	—	215.6	238.1	239.2
lung	162.9	197.0	231.2	212.3	235.7	239.1
azygos lobe	162.3	197.0	231.2	212.3	235.7	239.1
carina	162.2	197.0	231.2	212.3	235.7	239.1
contiguous sites with bronchus or trachea	162.8	—	—	—	—	—
hilus	162.2	197.0	231.2	212.3	235.7	239.1
lingula	162.3	197.0	231.2	212.3	235.7	239.1
lobe NEC	162.9	197.0	231.2	212.3	235.7	239.1
lower lobe	162.5	197.0	231.2	212.3	235.7	239.1
main bronchus	162.2	197.0	231.2	212.3	235.7	239.1
middle lobe	162.4	197.0	231.2	212.3	235.7	239.1
upper lobe	162.3	197.0	231.2	212.3	235.7	239.1
lymph, lymphatic						
channel NEC (*see also* Neoplasm, connective tissue)	171.9	198.89	—	215.9	238.1	239.2
gland						
(secondary)	—	196.9	—	229.0	238.8	239.89
abdominal	—	196.2	—	229.0	238.8	239.89
aortic	—	196.2	—	229.0	238.8	239.89
arm	—	196.3	—	229.0	238.8	239.89
auricular (anterior) (posterior)	—	196.0	—	229.0	238.8	239.89
axilla, axillary	—	196.3	—	229.0	238.8	239.89
brachial	—	196.3	—	229.0	238.8	239.89
bronchial	—	196.1	—	229.0	238.8	239.89
bronchopulmonary	—	196.1	—	229.0	238.8	239.89
celiac	—	196.2	—	229.0	238.8	239.89
cervical	—	196.0	—	229.0	238.8	239.89
cervicofacial	—	196.0	—	229.0	238.8	239.89
Cloquet	—	196.5	—	229.0	238.8	239.89
colic	—	196.2	—	229.0	238.8	239.89
common duct	—	196.2	—	229.0	238.8	239.89
cubital	—	196.3	—	229.0	238.8	239.89
diaphragmatic	—	196.1	—	229.0	238.8	239.89
epigastric, inferior	—	196.6	—	229.0	238.8	239.89
epitrochlear	—	196.3	—	229.0	238.8	239.89
esophageal	—	196.1	—	229.0	238.8	239.89
face	—	196.0	—	229.0	238.8	239.89
femoral	—	196.5	—	229.0	238.8	239.89
gastric	—	196.2	—	229.0	238.8	239.89
groin	—	196.5	—	229.0	238.8	239.89
head	—	196.0	—	229.0	238.8	239.89
hepatic	—	196.2	—	229.0	238.8	239.89
hilar (pulmonary)	—	196.1	—	229.0	238.8	239.89
splenic	—	196.2	—	229.0	238.8	239.89
hypogastric	—	196.6	—	229.0	238.8	239.89
ileocolic	—	196.2	—	229.0	238.8	239.89
iliac	—	196.6	—	229.0	238.8	239.89
infraclavicular	—	196.3	—	229.0	238.8	239.89
inguina, inguinal	—	196.5	—	229.0	238.8	239.89
innominate	—	196.1	—	229.0	238.8	239.89
intercostal	—	196.1	—	229.0	238.8	239.89
intestinal	—	196.2	—	229.0	238.8	239.89
intra-abdominal	—	196.2	—	229.0	238.8	239.89
intrapelvic	—	196.6	—	229.0	238.8	239.89
intrathoracic	—	196.1	—	229.0	238.8	239.9
jugular	—	196.0	—	229.0	238.8	239.89
leg	—	196.5	—	229.0	238.8	239.89
limb, lower	—	196.5	—	229.0	238.8	239.9
upper	—	196.3	—	229.0	238.8	239.89
lower limb	—	196.5	—	229.0	238.8	239.9
lumbar	—	196.2	—	229.0	238.8	239.89

	Malignant					
	Primary	Secondary	Ca in situ	Benign	Uncertain Behavior	Unspecified
Neoplasm, neoplastic — *continued*						
lymph, lymphatic — *continued*						
gland — *continued*						
mandibular	—	196.0	—	229.0	238.8	239.89
mediastinal	—	196.1	—	229.0	238.8	239.89
mesenteric (inferior) (superior)	—	196.2	—	229.0	238.8	239.89
midcolic	—	196.2	—	229.0	238.8	239.89
multiple sites in categories 196.0–196.6	—	196.8	—	229.0	238.8	239.89
neck	—	196.0	—	229.0	238.8	239.89
obturator	—	196.6	—	229.0	238.8	239.89
occipital	—	196.0	—	229.0	238.8	239.89
pancreatic	—	196.2	—	229.0	238.8	239.89
para-aortic	—	196.2	—	229.0	238.8	239.89
paracervical	—	196.6	—	229.0	238.8	239.89
parametrial	—	196.6	—	229.0	238.8	239.89
parasternal	—	196.1	—	229.0	238.8	239.89
parotid	—	196.0	—	229.0	238.8	239.89
pectoral	—	196.3	—	229.0	238.8	239.89
pelvic	—	196.6	—	229.0	238.8	239.89
peri-aortic	—	196.2	—	229.0	238.8	239.89
peripancreatic	—	196.2	—	229.0	238.8	239.89
popliteal	—	196.5	—	229.0	238.8	239.89
porta hepatis	—	196.2	—	229.0	238.8	239.89
portal	—	196.2	—	229.0	238.8	239.89
preauricular	—	196.0	—	229.0	238.8	239.89
prelaryngeal	—	196.0	—	229.0	238.8	239.89
presymphysial	—	196.6	—	229.0	238.8	239.89
pretracheal	—	196.0	—	229.0	238.8	239.89
primary (any site) NEC	202.9	—		—	—	—
pulmonary (hiler)	—	196.1	—	229.0	238.8	239.89
pyloric	—	196.2	—	229.0	238.8	239.89
retroperitoneal	—	196.2	—	229.0	238.8	239.89
retropharyngeal	—	196.0	—	229.0	238.8	239.89
Rosenmüller's	—	196.5	—	229.0	238.8	239.89
sacral	—	196.6	—	229.0	238.8	239.89
scalene	—	196.0	—	229.0	238.8	239.89
site NEC	—	196.9	—	229.0	238.8	239.89
splenic (hilar)	—	196.2	—	229.0	238.8	239.89
subclavicular	—	196.3	—	229.0	238.8	239.89
subinguinal	—	196.5	—	229.0	238.8	239.89
sublingual	—	196.0	—	229.0	238.8	239.89
submandibular	—	196.0	—	229.0	238.8	239.89
submaxillary	—	196.0	—	229.0	238.8	239.89
submental	—	196.0	—	229.0	238.8	239.89
subscapular	—	196.3	—	229.0	238.8	239.89
supraclavicular	—	196.0	—	229.0	238.8	239.89
thoracic	—	196.1	—	229.0	238.8	239.89
tibial	—	196.5	—	229.0	238.8	239.89
tracheal	—	196.1	—	229.0	238.8	239.89
tracheobronchial	—	196.1	—	229.0	238.8	239.89
upper limb	—	196.3	—	229.0	238.8	239.89
Virchow's	—	196.0	—	229.0	238.8	239.89
node (*see also* Neoplasm, lymph gland)						
primary NEC	202.9	—	—	—	—	—
vessel (*see also* Neoplasm, connective tissue)	171.9	198.89	—	215.9	238.1	239.2
Mackenrodt's ligament	183.8	198.82	233.39	221.8	236.3	239.5
malar	170.0	198.5	—	213.0	238.0	239.2
region — *see* Neoplasm, cheek						
mammary gland — *see* Neoplasm, breast						
mandible	170.1	198.5	—	213.1	238.0	239.2
alveolar						

☑ Additional Digit Required — Refer to the Tabular List for Digit Selection　　　　　　▽ Subterms under main terms may continue to next column or page

202 — Volume 2　　　　▶◀ Revised Text　　　● New Line　　　▲ Revised Code　　　2015 ICD-9-CM

	Malignant					
	Primary	**Secondary**	**Ca in situ**	**Benign**	**Uncertain Behavior**	**Unspecified**
Neoplasm, neoplastic — *continued*						
mandible — *continued*						
alveolar — *continued*						
mucosa	143.1	198.89	230.0	210.4	235.1	239.0
mucose	143.1	198.89	230.0	210.4	235.1	239.0
ridge or process	170.1	198.5	—	213.1	238.0	239.2
carcinoma	143.1	—	—	—	—	—
carcinoma	143.1	—	—	—	—	—
marrow (bone) NEC	202.9	198.5	—	—	—	238.79
mastectomy site (skin)	173.50	198.2				
basal cell carcinoma	173.51	—	—	—	—	—
specified as breast tissue	174.8	198.81				
specified type NEC	173.59	—	—	—	—	—
squamous cell carcinoma	173.52	—	—	—	—	—
mastoid (air cells) (antrum) (cavity)	160.1	197.3	231.8	212.0	235.9	239.1
bone or process	170.0	198.5	—	213.0	238.0	239.2
maxilla, maxillary (superior)	170.0	198.5	—	213.0	238.0	239.2
alveolar						
mucosa	143.0	198.89	230.0	210.4	235.1	239.0
ridge or process	170.0	198.5	—	213.0	238.0	239.2
carcinoma	143.0	—	—	—	—	—
antrum	160.2	197.3	231.8	212.0	235.9	239.1
carcinoma	143.0	—	—	—	—	—
inferior — *see* Neoplasm, mandible						
sinus	160.2	197.3	231.8	212.0	235.9	239.1
meatus						
external (ear) (*see also* Neoplasm, skin, ear)	173.20	198.2	232.2	216.2	238.2	239.2
Meckel's diverticulum	152.3	197.4	230.7	211.2	235.2	239.0
mediastinum, mediastinal	164.9	197.1	—	212.5	235.8	239.89
anterior	164.2	197.1	—	212.5	235.8	239.89
contiguous sites with heart and thymus	164.8	—	—	—	—	—
posterior	164.3	197.1	—	212.5	235.8	239.89
medulla						
adrenal	194.0	198.7	234.8	227.0	237.2	239.7
oblongata	191.7	198.3	—	225.0	237.5	239.6
meibomian gland	173.10	198.2	232.1	216.1	238.2	239.2
basal cell carcinoma	173.11	—	—	—	—	—
specified type NEC	173.19	—	—	—	—	—
squamous cell carcinoma	173.12	—	—	—	—	—
meninges (brain) (cerebral) (cranial) (intracranial)	192.1	198.4		225.2	237.6	239.7
spinal (cord)	192.3	198.4		225.4	237.6	239.7
meniscus, knee joint (lateral) (medial)	170.7	198.5		213.7	238.0	239.2
mesentery, mesenteric	158.8	197.6	—	211.8	235.4	239.0
mesoappendix	158.8	197.6	—	211.8	235.4	239.0
mesocolon	158.8	197.6	—	211.8	235.4	239.0
mesopharynx — *see* Neoplasm, oropharynx						
mesosalpinx	183.3	198.82	233.39	221.0	236.3	239.5
mesovarium	183.3	198.82	233.39	221.0	236.3	239.5

	Malignant					
	Primary	**Secondary**	**Ca in situ**	**Benign**	**Uncertain Behavior**	**Unspecified**
Neoplasm, neoplastic — *continued*						
metacarpus (any bone)	170.5	198.5	—	213.5	238.0	239.2
metastatic NEC (*see also* Neoplasm, by site, secondary)	—	199.1	—	—	—	—
metatarsus (any bone)	170.8	198.5	—	213.8	238.0	239.2
midbrain	191.7	198.3	—	225.0	237.5	239.6
milk duct — *see* Neoplasm, breast						
mons						
pubis	184.4	198.82	233.32	221.2	236.3	239.5
veneris	184.4	198.82	233.32	221.2	236.3	239.5
motor tract	192.9	198.4	—	225.9	237.9	239.7
brain	191.9	198.3	—	225.0	237.5	239.6
spinal	192.2	198.3	—	225.3	237.5	239.7
mouth	145.9	198.89	230.0	210.4	235.1	239.0
contiguous sites	145.8	—	—	—	—	—
floor	144.9	198.89	230.0	210.3	235.1	239.0
anterior portion	144.0	198.89	230.0	210.3	235.1	239.0
contiguous sites	144.8	—	—	—	—	—
lateral portion	144.1	198.89	230.0	210.3	235.1	239.0
roof	145.5	198.89	230.0	210.4	235.1	239.0
specified part NEC	145.8	198.89	230.0	210.4	235.1	239.0
vestibule	145.1	198.89	230.0	210.4	235.1	239.0
mucosa						
alveolar (ridge or process)	143.9	198.89	230.0	210.4	235.1	239.0
lower	143.1	198.89	230.0	210.4	235.1	239.0
upper	143.0	198.89	230.0	210.4	235.1	239.0
buccal	145.0	198.89	230.0	210.4	235.1	239.0
cheek	145.0	198.89	230.0	210.4	235.1	239.0
lip — *see* Neoplasm, lip, internal						
nasal	160.0	197.3	231.8	212.0	235.9	239.1
oral	145.0	198.89	230.0	210.4	235.1	239.0
Müllerian duct						
female	184.8	198.82	233.39	221.8	236.3	239.5
male	187.8	198.82	233.6	222.8	236.6	239.5
multiple sites NEC	199.0	—	234.9	229.9	238.9	—
muscle (*see also* Neoplasm, connective tissue)						
extraocular	190.1	198.4	234.0	224.1	238.8	239.89
myocardium	164.1	198.89	—	212.7	238.8	239.89
myometrium	182.0	198.82	233.2	219.1	236.0	239.5
myopericardium	164.1	198.89	—	212.7	238.8	239.89
nabothian gland (follicle)	180.0	198.82	233.1	219.0	236.0	239.5
nail	173.90	198.2	232.9	216.9	238.2	239.2
finger (*see also* Neoplasm, skin, limb, upper)	173.60	198.2	232.6	216.6	238.2	239.2
toe (*see also* Neoplasm, skin, limb, lower)	173.70	198.2	232.7	216.7	238.2	239.2
nares, naris (anterior) (posterior)	160.0	197.3	231.8	212.0	235.9	239.1
nasal — *see* Neoplasm, nose						
nasolabial groove (*see also* Neoplasm, skin, face)	173.30	198.2	232.3	216.3	238.2	239.2
nasolacrimal duct	190.7	198.4	234.0	224.7	238.8	239.89
nasopharynx, nasopharyngeal	147.9	198.89	230.0	210.7	235.1	239.0
contiguous sites	147.8	—	—	—	—	—
floor	147.3	198.89	230.0	210.7	235.1	239.0
roof	147.0	198.89	230.0	210.7	235.1	239.0
specified site NEC	147.8	198.89	230.0	210.7	235.1	239.0
wall	147.9	198.89	230.0	210.7	235.1	239.0

☑ **Additional Digit Required** — **Refer to the Tabular List for Digit Selection**   ⓦ **Subterms under main terms may continue to next column or page**

2015 ICD-9-CM   ▶◀ **Revised Text**   ● **New Line**   ▲ **Revised Code**   **Volume 2 — 203**

	Malignant			Benign	Uncertain Behavior	Unspecified
	Primary	Secondary	Ca in situ			

Neoplasm, neoplastic — *continued*
nasopharynx, nasopharyngeal — *continued*
wall — *continued*

	Primary	Secondary	Ca in situ	Benign	Uncertain Behavior	Unspecified
anterior	147.3	198.89	230.0	210.7	235.1	239.0
lateral	147.2	198.89	230.0	210.7	235.1	239.0
posterior	147.1	198.89	230.0	210.7	235.1	239.0
superior	147.0	198.89	230.0	210.7	235.1	239.0
nates (*see also* Neoplasm, skin, trunk)	173.50	198.2	232.5	216.5	238.2	239.2
neck NEC*	195.0	198.89	234.8	229.8	238.8	239.89
skin	173.40	198.2	232.4	216.4	238.2	239.2
basal cell carcinoma	173.41	—	—	—	—	—
specified type NEC	173.49	—	—	—	—	—
squamous cell carcinoma	173.42	—	—	—	—	—
nerve (autonomic) (ganglion) (parasympathetic) (peripheral) (sympathetic) (*see also* Neoplasm, connective tissue)						
abducens	192.0	198.4	—	225.1	237.9	239.7
accessory (spinal)	192.0	198.4	—	225.1	237.9	239.7
acoustic	192.0	198.4	—	225.1	237.9	239.7
auditory	192.0	198.4	—	225.1	237.9	239.7
brachial	171.1	198.89	—	215.2	238.1	239.2
cranial (any)	192.0	198.4	—	225.1	237.9	239.7
facial	192.0	198.4	—	225.1	237.9	239.7
femoral	171.3	198.89	—	215.3	238.1	239.2
glossopharyngeal	192.0	198.4	—	225.1	237.9	239.7
hypoglossal	192.0	198.4	—	225.1	237.9	239.7
intercostal	171.4	198.89	—	215.4	238.1	239.2
lumbar	171.7	198.89	—	215.7	238.1	239.2
median	171.2	198.89	—	215.2	238.1	239.2
obturator	171.3	198.89	—	215.3	238.1	239.2
oculomotor	192.0	198.4	—	225.1	237.9	239.7
olfactory	192.0	198.4	—	225.1	237.9	239.7
optic	192.0	198.4	—	225.1	237.9	239.7
peripheral NEC	171.9	198.89	—	215.9	238.1	239.2
radial	171.2	198.89	—	215.2	238.1	239.2
sacral	171.6	198.89	—	215.6	238.1	239.2
sciatic	171.3	198.89	—	215.3	238.1	239.2
spinal NEC	171.9	198.89	—	215.9	238.1	239.2
trigeminal	192.0	198.4	—	225.1	237.9	239.7
trochlear	192.0	198.4	—	225.1	237.9	239.7
ulnar	171.2	198.89	—	215.2	238.1	239.2
vagus	192.0	198.4	—	225.1	237.9	239.7
nervous system (central) NEC	192.9	198.4	—	225.9	237.9	239.7
autonomic NEC	171.9	198.89	—	215.9	238.1	239.2
brain (*see also* Neoplasm, brain)						
membrane or meninges	192.1	198.4	—	225.2	237.6	239.7
contiguous sites	192.8	—	—	—	—	—
parasympathetic NEC	171.9	198.89	—	215.9	238.1	239.2
sympathetic NEC	171.9	198.89	—	215.9	238.1	239.2
nipple (female)	174.0	198.81	233.0	217	238.3	239.3
male	175.0	198.81	233.0	217	238.3	239.3
nose, nasal	195.0	198.89	234.8	229.8	238.8	239.89
ala (external) (*see also* Neoplasm, nose, skin)	173.30	198.2	232.3	216.3	238.2	239.2
bone	170.0	198.5	—	213.0	238.0	239.2
cartilage	160.0	197.3	231.8	212.0	235.9	239.1

Neoplasm, neoplastic — *continued*
nose, nasal — *continued*

	Primary	Secondary	Ca in situ	Benign	Uncertain Behavior	Unspecified
cavity	160.0	197.3	231.8	212.0	235.9	239.1
contiguous sites with accessory sinuses or middle ear	160.8	—	—	—	—	—
choana	147.3	198.89	230.0	210.7	235.1	239.0
external (skin) (*see also* Neoplasm, nose, skin)	173.30	198.2	232.3	216.3	238.2	239.2
fossa	160.0	197.3	231.8	212.0	235.9	239.1
internal	160.0	197.3	231.8	212.0	235.9	239.1
mucosa	160.0	197.3	231.8	212.0	235.9	239.1
septum	160.0	197.3	231.8	212.0	235.9	239.1
posterior margin	147.3	198.89	230.0	210.7	235.1	239.0
sinus — *see* Neoplasm, sinus						
skin	173.30	198.2	232.3	216.3	238.2	239.2
basal cell carcinoma	173.31	—	—	—	—	—
specified type NEC	173.39	—	—	—	—	—
squamous cell carcinoma	173.32	—	—	—	—	—
turbinate (mucosa)	160.0	197.3	231.8	212.0	235.9	239.1
bone	170.0	198.5	—	213.0	238.0	239.2
vestibule	160.0	197.3	231.8	212.0	235.9	239.1
nostril	160.0	197.3	231.8	212.0	235.9	239.1
nucleus pulposus	170.2	198.5	—	213.2	238.0	239.2
occipital						
bone	170.0	198.5	—	213.0	238.0	239.2
lobe or pole, brain	191.4	198.3	—	225.0	237.5	239.6
odontogenic — *see* Neoplasm, jaw bone						
oesophagus — *see* Neoplasm, esophagus						
olfactory nerve or bulb	192.0	198.4	—	225.1	237.9	239.7
olive (brain)	191.7	198.3	—	225.0	237.5	239.6
omentum	158.8	197.6	—	211.8	235.4	239.0
operculum (brain)	191.0	198.3	—	225.0	237.5	239.6
optic nerve, chiasm, or tract	192.0	198.4	—	225.1	237.9	239.7
oral (cavity)	145.9	198.89	230.0	210.4	235.1	239.0
contiguous sites with lip or pharynx	149.8	—	—	—	—	—
ill-defined	149.9	198.89	230.0	210.4	235.1	239.0
mucosa	145.9	198.89	230.0	210.4	235.1	239.0
orbit	190.1	198.4	234.0	224.1	238.8	239.89
bone	170.0	198.5	—	213.0	238.0	239.2
eye	190.1	198.4	234.0	224.1	238.8	239.89
soft parts	190.1	198.4	234.0	224.1	238.8	239.89
organ of Zuckerkandl	194.6	198.89	—	227.6	237.3	239.7
oropharynx	146.9	198.89	230.0	210.6	235.1	239.0
branchial cleft (vestige)	146.8	198.89	230.0	210.6	235.1	239.0
contiguous sites	146.8	—	—	—	—	—
junctional region	146.5	198.89	230.0	210.6	235.1	239.0
lateral wall	146.6	198.89	230.0	210.6	235.1	239.0
pillars of fauces	146.2	198.89	230.0	210.6	235.1	239.0
posterior wall	146.7	198.89	230.0	210.6	235.1	239.0
specified part NEC	146.8	198.89	230.0	210.6	235.1	239.0
vallecula	146.3	198.89	230.0	210.6	235.1	239.0
os						
external	180.1	198.82	233.1	219.0	236.0	239.5

☑ **Additional Digit Required — Refer to the Tabular List for Digit Selection**   ▽ **Subterms under main terms may continue to next column or page**

204— Volume 2   ►◄ **Revised Text**   ● **New Line**   ▲ **Revised Code**   **2015 ICD-9-CM**

	Malignant					
	Primary	Secondary	Ca in situ	Benign	Uncertain Behavior	Unspecified
Neoplasm, neoplastic — *continued*						
os — *continued*						
internal	180.0	198.82	233.1	219.0	236.0	239.5
ovary	183.0	198.6	233.39	220	236.2	239.5
oviduct	183.2	198.82	233.39	221.0	236.3	239.5
palate	145.5	198.89	230.0	210.4	235.1	239.0
hard	145.2	198.89	230.0	210.4	235.1	239.0
junction of hard and soft palate	145.5	198.89	230.0	210.4	235.1	239.0
soft	145.3	198.89	230.0	210.4	235.1	239.0
nasopharyngeal surface	147.3	198.89	230.0	210.7	235.1	239.0
posterior surface	147.3	198.89	230.0	210.7	235.1	239.0
superior surface	147.3	198.89	230.0	210.7	235.1	239.0
palatoglossal arch	146.2	198.89	230.0	210.6	235.1	239.0
palatopharyngeal arch	146.2	198.89	230.0	210.6	235.1	239.0
pallium	191.0	198.3	—	225.0	237.5	239.6
palpebra	173.10	198.2	232.1	216.1	238.2	239.2
basal cell carcinoma	173.11	—	—	—	—	—
specified type NEC	173.19	—	—	—	—	—
squamous cell carcinoma	173.12	—	—	—	—	—
pancreas	157.9	197.8	230.9	211.6	235.5	239.0
body	157.1	197.8	230.9	211.6	235.5	239.0
contiguous sites	157.8	—	—	—	—	—
duct (of Santorini) (of Wirsung)	157.3	197.8	230.9	211.6	235.5	239.0
ectopic tissue	157.8	197.8	230.9	211.6	235.5	239.0
head	157.0	197.8	230.9	211.6	235.5	239.0
islet cells	157.4	197.8	230.9	211.7	235.5	239.0
neck	157.8	197.8	230.9	211.6	235.5	239.0
tail	157.2	197.8	230.9	211.6	235.5	239.0
para-aortic body	194.6	198.89	—	227.6	237.3	239.7
paraganglion NEC	194.6	198.89	—	227.6	237.3	239.7
parametrium	183.4	198.82	—	221.0	236.3	239.5
paranephric	158.0	197.6	—	211.8	235.4	239.0
pararectal	195.3	198.89	—	229.8	238.8	239.89
parasagittal (region)	195.0	198.89	234.8	229.8	238.8	239.89
parasellar	192.9	198.4	—	225.9	237.9	239.7
parathyroid (gland)	194.1	198.89	234.8	227.1	237.4	239.7
paraurethral	195.3	198.89	—	229.8	238.8	239.89
gland	189.4	198.1	233.9	223.89	236.99	239.5
paravaginal	195.3	198.89	—	229.8	238.8	239.89
parenchyma, kidney	189.0	198.0	233.9	223.0	236.91	239.5
parietal						
bone	170.0	198.5	—	213.0	238.0	239.2
lobe, brain	191.3	198.3	—	225.0	237.5	239.6
paroophoron	183.3	198.82	233.39	221.0	236.3	239.5
parotid (duct) (gland)	142.0	198.89	230.0	210.2	235.0	239.0
parovarium	183.3	198.82	233.39	221.0	236.3	239.5
patella	170.8	198.5	—	213.8	238.0	239.2
peduncle, cerebral	191.7	198.3	—	225.0	237.5	239.6
pelvirectal junction	154.0	197.5	230.4	211.4	235.2	239.0
pelvis, pelvic	195.3	198.89	234.8	229.8	238.8	239.89
bone	170.6	198.5	—	213.6	238.0	239.2
floor	195.3	198.89	234.8	229.8	238.8	239.89
renal	189.1	198.0	233.9	223.1	236.91	239.5
viscera	195.3	198.89	234.8	229.8	238.8	239.89
wall	195.3	198.89	234.8	229.8	238.8	239.89
pelvo-abdominal	195.8	198.89	234.8	229.8	238.8	239.89
penis	187.4	198.82	233.5	222.1	236.6	239.5
body	187.3	198.82	233.5	222.1	236.6	239.5
corpus (cavernosum)	187.3	198.82	233.5	222.1	236.6	239.5
glans	187.2	198.82	233.5	222.1	236.6	239.5
skin NEC	187.4	198.82	233.5	222.1	236.6	239.5
periadrenal (tissue)	158.0	197.6	—	211.8	235.4	239.0

	Malignant					
	Primary	Secondary	Ca in situ	Benign	Uncertain Behavior	Unspecified
Neoplasm, neoplastic — *continued*						
perianal (skin) (*see also* Neoplasm, skin, anus)	173.50	198.2	232.5	216.5	238.2	239.2
pericardium	164.1	198.89	—	212.7	238.8	239.89
perinephric	158.0	197.6	—	211.8	235.4	239.0
perineum	195.3	198.89	234.8	229.8	238.8	239.89
periodontal tissue NEC	143.9	198.89	230.0	210.4	235.1	239.0
periosteum — *see* Neoplasm, bone						
peripancreatic	158.0	197.6	—	211.8	235.4	239.0
peripheral nerve NEC	171.9	198.89	—	215.9	238.1	239.2
perirectal (tissue)	195.3	198.89	—	229.8	238.8	239.89
perirenal (tissue)	158.0	197.6	—	211.8	235.4	239.0
peritoneum, peritoneal (cavity)	158.9	197.6	—	211.8	235.4	239.0
contiguous sites	158.8	—	—	—	—	—
with digestive organs	159.8	—	—	—	—	—
parietal	158.8	197.6	—	211.8	235.4	239.0
pelvic	158.8	197.6	—	211.8	235.4	239.0
specified part NEC	158.8	197.6	—	211.8	235.4	239.0
peritonsillar (tissue)	195.0	198.89	234.8	229.8	238.8	239.89
periurethral tissue	195.3	198.89	—	229.8	238.8	239.89
phalanges	170.9	198.5	—	213.9	238.0	239.2
foot	170.8	198.5	—	213.8	238.0	239.2
hand	170.5	198.5	—	213.5	238.0	239.2
pharynx, pharyngeal	149.0	198.89	230.0	210.9	235.1	239.0
bursa	147.1	198.89	230.0	210.7	235.1	239.0
fornix	147.3	198.89	230.0	210.7	235.1	239.0
recess	147.2	198.89	230.0	210.7	235.1	239.0
region	149.0	198.89	230.0	210.9	235.1	239.0
tonsil	147.1	198.89	230.0	210.7	235.1	239.0
wall (lateral) (posterior)	149.0	198.89	230.0	210.9	235.1	239.0
pia mater (cerebral) (cranial)	192.1	198.4	—	225.2	237.6	239.7
spinal	192.3	198.4	—	225.4	237.6	239.7
pillars of fauces	146.2	198.89	230.0	210.6	235.1	239.0
pineal (body) (gland)	194.4	198.89	234.8	227.4	237.1	239.7
pinna (ear) NEC (*see also* Neoplasm, skin, ear)	173.20	198.2	232.2	216.2	238.2	239.2
cartilage	171.0	198.89	—	215.0	238.1	239.2
piriform fossa or sinus	148.1	198.89	230.0	210.8	235.1	239.0
pituitary (body) (fossa) (gland) (lobe)	194.3	198.89	234.8	227.3	237.0	239.7
placenta	181	198.82	233.2	219.8	236.1	239.5
pleura, pleural (cavity)	163.9	197.2	—	212.4	235.8	239.1
contiguous sites	163.8	—	—	—	—	—
parietal	163.0	197.2	—	212.4	235.8	239.1
visceral	163.1	197.2	—	212.4	235.8	239.1
plexus						
brachial	171.2	198.89	—	215.2	238.1	239.2
cervical	171.0	198.89	—	215.0	238.1	239.2
choroid	191.5	198.3	—	225.0	237.5	239.6
lumbosacral	171.6	198.89	—	215.6	238.1	239.2
sacral	171.6	198.89	—	215.6	238.1	239.2
pluri-endocrine	194.8	198.89	234.8	227.8	237.4	239.7
pole						
frontal	191.1	198.3	—	225.0	237.5	239.6
occipital	191.4	198.3	—	225.0	237.5	239.6
pons (varolii)	191.7	198.3	—	225.0	237.5	239.6
popliteal fossa or space*	195.5	198.89	234.8	229.8	238.8	239.89
postcricoid (region)	148.0	198.89	230.0	210.8	235.1	239.0

☑ Additional Digit Required — Refer to the Tabular List for Digit Selection   ▽ Subterms under main terms may continue to next column or page

2015 ICD-9-CM   ►◄ Revised Text   ● New Line   ▲ Revised Code   Volume 2 — 205

Neoplasm, neoplastic — continued	Malignant			Benign	Uncertain Behavior	Unspecified
	Primary	Secondary	Ca in situ	Benign	Uncertain Behavior	Unspecified
posterior fossa (cranial)	191.9	198.3	—	225.0	237.5	239.6
postnasal space	147.9	198.89	230.0	210.7	235.1	239.0
prepuce	187.1	198.82	233.5	222.1	236.6	239.5
prepylorus	151.1	197.8	230.2	211.1	235.2	239.0
presacral (region)	195.3	198.89	—	229.8	238.8	239.89
prostate (gland)	185	198.82	233.4	222.2	236.5	239.5
utricle	189.3	198.1	233.9	223.81	236.99	239.5
pterygoid fossa	171.0	198.89	—	215.0	238.1	239.2
pubic bone	170.6	198.5	—	213.6	238.0	239.2
pudenda, pudendum (female)	184.4	198.82	233.32	221.2	236.3	239.5
pulmonary	162.9	197.0	231.2	212.3	235.7	239.1
putamen	191.0	198.3	—	225.0	237.5	239.6
pyloric antrum	151.2	197.8	230.2	211.1	235.2	239.0
canal	151.1	197.8	230.2	211.1	235.2	239.0
pylorus	151.1	197.8	230.2	211.1	235.2	239.0
pyramid (brain)	191.7	198.3	—	225.0	237.5	239.6
pyriform fossa or sinus	148.1	198.89	230.0	210.8	235.1	239.0
radius (any part)	170.4	198.5	—	213.4	238.0	239.2
Rathke's pouch	194.3	198.89	234.8	227.3	237.0	239.7
rectosigmoid (colon) (junction)	154.0	197.5	230.4	211.4	235.2	239.0
contiguous sites with anus or rectum	154.8	—	—	—	—	—
rectouterine pouch	158.8	197.6	—	211.8	235.4	239.0
rectovaginal septum or wall	195.3	198.89	234.8	229.8	238.8	239.89
rectovesical septum	195.3	198.89	234.8	229.8	238.8	239.89
rectum (ampulla)	154.1	197.5	230.4	211.4	235.2	239.0
and colon	154.0	197.5	230.4	211.4	235.2	239.0
contiguous sites with anus or rectosigmoid junction	154.8	—	—	—	—	—
renal	189.0	198.0	233.9	223.0	236.91	239.5
calyx	189.1	198.0	233.9	223.1	236.91	239.5
hilus	189.1	198.0	233.9	223.1	236.91	239.5
parenchyma	189.0	198.0	233.9	223.0	236.91	239.5
pelvis	189.1	198.0	233.9	223.1	236.91	239.5
respiratory organs or system NEC	165.9	197.3	231.9	212.9	235.9	239.1
contiguous sites with intrathoracic organs	165.8	—	—	—	—	—
specified sites NEC	165.8	197.3	231.8	212.8	235.9	239.1
tract NEC	165.9	197.3	231.9	212.9	235.9	239.1
upper	165.0	197.3	231.9	212.9	235.9	239.1
retina	190.5	198.4	234.0	224.5	238.8	239.81
retrobulbar	190.1	198.4	234.0	224.1	238.8	239.89
retrocecal	158.0	197.6	—	211.8	235.4	239.0
retromolar (area) (triangle) (trigone)	145.6	198.89	230.0	210.4	235.1	239.0
retro-orbital	195.0	198.89	234.8	229.8	238.8	239.89
retroperitoneal (space) (tissue)	158.0	197.6	—	211.8	235.4	239.0
contiguous sites	158.8	—	—	—	—	—
retroperitoneum	158.0	197.6	—	211.8	235.4	239.0
contiguous sites	158.8	—	—	—	—	—
retropharyngeal	149.0	198.89	230.0	210.9	235.1	239.0
retrovesical (septum)	195.3	198.89	234.8	229.8	238.8	239.89
rhinencephalon	191.0	198.3	—	225.0	237.5	239.6
rib	170.3	198.5	—	213.3	238.0	239.2
Rosenmüller's fossa	147.2	198.89	230.0	210.7	235.1	239.0
round ligament	183.5	198.82	—	221.0	236.3	239.5
Neoplasm, neoplastic — continued						
sacrococcyx, sacrococcygeal	170.6	198.5	—	213.6	238.0	239.2
region	195.3	198.89	234.8	229.8	238.8	239.89
sacrouterine ligament	183.4	198.82	—	221.0	236.3	239.5
sacrum, sacral (vertebra)	170.6	198.5	—	213.6	238.0	239.2
salivary gland or duct (major)	142.9	198.89	230.0	210.2	235.0	239.0
contiguous sites	142.8	—	—	—	—	—
minor NEC	145.9	198.89	230.0	210.4	235.1	239.0
parotid	142.0	198.89	230.0	210.2	235.0	239.0
pluriglandular	142.8	198.89	—	210.2	235.0	239.0
sublingual	142.2	198.89	230.0	210.2	235.0	239.0
submandibular	142.1	198.89	230.0	210.2	235.0	239.0
submaxillary	142.1	198.89	230.0	210.2	235.0	239.0
salpinx (uterine)	183.2	198.82	233.39	221.0	236.3	239.5
Santorini's duct	157.3	197.8	230.9	211.6	235.5	239.0
scalp	173.40	198.2	232.4	216.4	238.2	239.2
basal cell carcinoma	173.41	—	—	—	—	—
specified type NEC	173.49	—	—	—	—	—
squamous cell carcinoma	173.42	—	—	—	—	—
scapula (any part)	170.4	198.5	—	213.4	238.0	239.2
scapular region	195.1	198.89	234.8	229.8	238.8	239.89
scar NEC (see also Neoplasm, skin)	173.90	198.2	232.9	216.9	238.2	239.2
sciatic nerve	171.3	198.89	—	215.3	238.1	239.2
sclera	190.0	198.4	234.0	224.0	238.8	239.89
scrotum (skin)	187.7	198.82	—	222.4	236.6	239.5
sebaceous gland — see Neoplasm, skin						
sella turcica	194.3	198.89	234.8	227.3	237.0	239.7
bone	170.0	198.5	—	213.0	238.0	239.2
semilunar cartilage (knee)	170.7	198.5	—	213.7	238.0	239.2
seminal vesicle	187.8	198.82	233.6	222.8	236.6	239.5
septum nasal	160.0	197.3	231.8	212.0	235.9	239.1
posterior margin	147.3	198.89	230.0	210.7	235.1	239.0
rectovaginal	195.3	198.89	234.8	229.8	238.8	239.89
rectovesical	195.3	198.89	234.8	229.8	238.8	239.89
urethrovaginal	184.9	198.82	233.39	221.9	236.3	239.5
vesicovaginal	184.9	198.82	233.39	221.9	236.3	239.5
shoulder NEC*	195.4	198.89	232.6	229.8	238.8	239.89
sigmoid flexure (lower) (upper)	153.3	197.5	230.3	211.3	235.2	239.0
sinus (accessory)	160.9	197.3	231.8	212.0	235.9	239.1
bone (any)	170.0	198.5	—	213.0	238.0	239.2
contiguous sites with middle ear or nasal cavities	160.8	—	—	—	—	—
ethmoidal	160.3	197.3	231.8	212.0	235.9	239.1
frontal	160.4	197.3	231.8	212.0	235.9	239.1
maxillary	160.2	197.3	231.8	212.0	235.9	239.1
nasal, paranasal NEC	160.9	197.3	231.8	212.0	235.9	239.1
pyriform	148.1	198.89	230.0	210.8	235.1	239.0
sphenoidal	160.5	197.3	231.8	212.0	235.9	239.1
skeleton, skeletal NEC	170.9	198.5	—	213.9	238.0	239.2
Skene's gland	189.4	198.1	233.9	223.89	236.99	239.5
skin NOS	173.90	198.2	232.9	216.9	238.2	239.2
abdominal wall	173.50	198.2	232.5	216.5	238.2	239.2
basal cell carcinoma	173.51	—	—	—	—	—
specified type NEC	173.59	—	—	—	—	—
squamous cell carcinoma	173.52	—	—	—	—	—

☑ Additional Digit Required — Refer to the Tabular List for Digit Selection   ▽ Subterms under main terms may continue to next column or page

Neoplasm, neoplastic— *continued*	Malignant Primary	Malignant Secondary	Malignant Ca in situ	Benign	Uncertain Behavior	Unspecified
skin — *continued*						
ala nasi (*see also* Neoplasm, skin, face)	173.30	198.2	232.3	216.3	238.2	239.2
ankle (*see also* Neoplasm, skin, limb, lower)	173.70	198.2	232.7	216.7	238.2	239.2
antecubital space (*see also* Neoplasm, skin, limb, upper)	173.60	198.2	232.6	216.6	238.2	239.2
anus	173.50	198.2	232.5	216.5	238.2	239.2
basal cell carcinoma	173.51	—	—	—	—	—
specified type NEC	173.59	—	—	—	—	—
squamous cell carcinoma	173.52	—	—	—	—	—
arm (*see also* Neoplasm, skin, limb, upper)	173.60	198.2	232.6	216.6	238.2	239.2
auditory canal (external) (*see also* Neoplasm, skin, ear)	173.20	198.2	232.2	216.2	238.2	239.2
auricle (ear) (*see also* Neoplasm, skin, ear)	173.20	198.2	232.2	216.2	238.2	239.2
auricular canal (external) (*see also* Neoplasm, skin, ear)	173.20	198.2	232.2	216.2	238.2	239.2
axilla, axillary fold (*see also* Neoplasm, skin, trunk)	173.50	198.2	232.5	216.5	238.2	239.2
back	173.50	198.2	232.5	216.5	238.2	239.2
basal cell carcinoma	173.51	—	—	—	—	—
specified type NEC	173.59	—	—	—	—	—
squamous cell carcinoma	173.52	—	—	—	—	—
basal cell carcinoma, unspecified site	173.91	—	—	—	—	—
breast (*see also* Neoplasm, skin, trunk)	173.50	198.2	232.5	216.5	238.2	239.2
brow (*see also* Neoplasm, skin, face)	173.30	198.2	232.3	216.3	238.2	239.2
buttock (*see also* Neoplasm, skin, trunk)	173.50	198.2	232.5	216.5	238.2	239.2
calf (*see also* Neoplasm, skin, limb, lower)	173.70	198.2	232.7	216.7	238.2	239.2
canthus (eye) (inner) (outer)	173.10	198.2	232.1	216.1	238.2	239.2
basal cell carcinoma	173.11	—	—	—	—	—
specified type NEC	173.19	—	—	—	—	—
squamous cell carcinoma	173.12	—	—	—	—	—
cervical region (*see also* Neoplasm, skin, neck)	173.40	198.2	232.4	216.4	238.2	239.2
cheek (external) (*see also* Neoplasm, skin, face)	173.30	198.2	232.3	216.3	238.2	239.2
chest (wall) (*see also* Neoplasm, skin, trunk)	173.50	198.2	232.5	216.5	238.2	239.2
chin (*see also* Neoplasm, skin, face)	173.30	198.2	232.3	216.3	238.2	239.2

Neoplasm, neoplastic— *continued*	Malignant Primary	Malignant Secondary	Malignant Ca in situ	Benign	Uncertain Behavior	Unspecified
skin — *continued*						
clavicular area (*see also* Neoplasm, skin, trunk)	173.50	198.2	232.5	216.5	238.2	239.2
clitoris	—	198.82	233.32	221.2	236.3	239.5
columnella (*see also* Neoplasm, skin, face)	173.30	198.2	232.3	216.3	238.2	239.2
concha (*see also* Neoplasm, skin, ear)	173.20	198.2	232.2	216.2	238.2	239.2
contiguous sites	173.80	—	—	—	—	—
basal cell carcinoma	173.81	—	—	—	—	—
specified type NEC	173.89	—	—	—	—	—
squamous cell carcinoma	173.82	—	—	—	—	—
ear (external)	173.20	198.2	232.2	216.2	238.2	239.2
basal cell carcinoma	173.21	—	—	—	—	—
specified type NEC	173.29	—	—	—	—	—
squamous cell carcinoma	173.22	—	—	—	—	—
elbow (*see also* Neoplasm, skin, limb, upper)	173.60	198.2	232.6	216.6	238.2	239.2
eyebrow (*see also* Neoplasm, skin, face)	173.30	198.2	232.3	216.3	238.2	239.2
eyelid	173.10	198.2	232.1	—	238.2	239.2
basal cell carcinoma	173.11	—	—	—	—	—
specified type NEC	173.19	—	—	—	—	—
squamous cell carcinoma	173.12	—	—	—	—	—
face NEC	173.30	198.2	232.3	216.3	238.2	239.2
basal cell carcinoma	173.31	—	—	—	—	—
specified type NEC	173.39	—	—	—	—	—
squamous cell carcinoma	173.32	—	—	—	—	—
female genital organs (external)	184.4	198.82	233.30	221.2	236.3	239.5
clitoris	184.3	198.82	233.32	221.2	236.3	239.5
labium NEC	184.4	198.82	233.32	221.2	236.3	239.5
majus	184.1	198.82	233.32	221.2	236.3	239.5
minus	184.2	198.82	233.32	221.2	236.3	239.5
pudendum	184.4	198.82	233.32	221.2	236.3	239.5
vulva	184.4	198.82	233.32	221.2	236.3	239.5
finger (*see also* Neoplasm, skin, limb, upper)	173.60	198.2	232.6	216.6	238.2	239.2
flank (*see also* Neoplasm, skin, trunk)	173.50	198.2	232.5	216.5	238.2	239.2
foot (*see also* Neoplasm, skin, limb, lower)	173.70	198.2	232.7	216.7	238.2	239.2
forearm (*see also* Neoplasm, skin, limb, upper)	173.60	198.2	232.6	216.6	238.2	239.2
forehead (*see also* Neoplasm, skin, face)	173.30	198.2	232.3	216.3	238.2	239.2
glabella (*see also* Neoplasm, skin, face)	173.30	198.2	232.3	216.3	238.2	239.2
gluteal region (*see also* Neoplasm, skin, trunk)	173.50	198.2	232.5	216.5	238.2	239.2
groin (*see also* Neoplasm, skin, trunk)	173.50	198.2	232.5	216.5	238.2	239.2

☑ Additional Digit Required — Refer to the Tabular List for Digit Selection   ▽ Subterms under main terms may continue to next column or page

2015 ICD-9-CM   ▶◀ Revised Text   ● New Line   ▲ Revised Code   Volume 2 — 207

Neoplasm, neoplastic— continued
skin — continued

	Malignant			Benign	Uncertain Behavior	Unspecified
	Primary	Secondary	Ca in situ			
hand (see also Neoplasm, skin, limb, upper)	173.60	198.2	232.6	216.6	238.2	239.2
head NEC (see also Neoplasm, skin, scalp)	173.40	198.2	232.4	216.4	238.2	239.2
heel (see also Neoplasm, skin, limb, lower)	173.70	198.2	232.7	216.7	238.2	239.2
helix (see also Neoplasm, skin, ear)	173.20	198.2	—	216.2	238.2	239.2
hip	173.70	198.2	232.7	216.7	238.2	239.2
basal cell carcinoma	173.71	—	—	—	—	—
specified type NEC	173.79	—	—	—	—	—
squamous cell carcinoma	173.72	—	—	—	—	—
infraclavicular region (see also Neoplasm, skin, trunk)	173.50	198.2	232.5	216.5	238.2	239.2
inguinal region (see also Neoplasm, skin, trunk)	173.50	198.2	232.5	216.5	238.2	239.2
jaw (see also Neoplasm, skin, face)	173.30	198.2	232.3	216.3	238.2	239.2
knee (see also Neoplasm, skin, limb, lower)	173.70	198.2	232.7	216.7	238.2	239.2
labia						
majora	184.1	198.82	233.32	221.2	236.3	239.5
minora	184.2	198.82	233.32	221.2	236.3	239.5
leg (see also Neoplasm, skin, limb, lower)	173.70	198.2	232.7	216.7	238.2	239.2
lid (lower) (upper)	173.10	198.2	232.1	216.1	238.2	239.2
basal cell carcinoma	173.11	—	—	—	—	—
specified type NEC	173.19	—	—	—	—	—
squamous cell carcinoma	173.12	—	—	—	—	—
limb NEC	173.90	198.2	232.9	216.9	238.2	239.5
lower	173.70	198.2	232.7	216.7	238.2	239.2
basal cell carcinoma	173.71	—	—	—	—	—
specified type NEC	173.79	—	—	—	—	—
squamous cell carcinoma	173.72	—	—	—	—	—
upper	173.60	198.2	232.6	216.6	238.2	239.2
basal cell carcinoma	173.61	—	—	—	—	—
specified type NEC	173.69	—	—	—	—	—
squamous cell carcinoma	173.62	—	—	—	—	—
lip (lower) (upper)	173.00	198.2	232.0	216.0	238.2	239.2
basal cell carcinoma	173.01	—	—	—	—	—
specified type NEC	173.09	—	—	—	—	—
squamous cell carcinoma	173.02	—	—	—	—	—
male genital organs	187.9	198.82	233.6	222.9	236.6	239.5
penis	187.4	198.82	233.5	222.1	236.6	239.5
prepuce	187.1	198.82	233.5	222.1	236.6	239.5
scrotum	187.7	198.82	233.6	222.4	236.6	239.5

Neoplasm, neoplastic— continued
skin — continued

	Malignant			Benign	Uncertain Behavior	Unspecified
	Primary	Secondary	Ca in situ			
mastectomy site (see also Neoplasm, skin, trunk)	173.50	198.2	—	—	—	—
specified as breast tissue	174.8	198.81	—	—	—	—
meatus, acoustic (external) (see also Neoplasm, skin, ear)	173.20	198.2	232.2	216.2	238.2	239.2
nates (see also Neoplasm, skin, trunk)	173.50	198.2	232.5	216.5	238.2	239.0
neck	173.40	198.2	232.4	216.4	238.2	239.2
basal cell carcinoma	173.41	—	—	—	—	—
specified type NEC	173.49	—	—	—	—	—
squamous cell carcinoma	173.42	—	—	—	—	—
nose (external) (see also Neoplasm, skin, face)	173.30	198.2	232.3	216.3	238.2	239.2
palm (see also Neoplasm, skin, limb, upper)	173.60	198.2	232.6	216.6	238.2	239.2
palpebra	173.10	198.2	232.1	216.1	238.2	239.2
basal cell carcinoma	173.11	—	—	—	—	—
specified type NEC	173.19	—	—	—	—	—
squamous cell carcinoma	173.12	—	—	—	—	—
penis NEC	187.4	198.82	233.5	222.1	236.6	239.5
perianal (see also Neoplasm, skin, anus)	173.50	198.2	232.5	216.5	238.2	239.2
perineum (see also Neoplasm, skin, anus)	173.50	198.2	232.5	216.5	238.2	239.2
pinna (see also Neoplasm, skin, ear)	173.20	198.2	232.2	216.2	238.2	239.2
plantar (see also Neoplasm, skin, iimb, lower)	173.70	198.2	232.7	216.7	238.2	239.2
popliteal fossa or space (see also Neoplasm, skin, limb, lower)	173.70	198.2	232.7	216.7	238.2	239.2
prepuce	187.1	198.82	233.5	222.1	236.6	239.5
pubes (see also Neoplasm, skin, trunk)	173.50	198.2	232.5	216.5	238.2	239.2
sacrococcygeal region (see also Neoplasm, skin, trunk)	173.50	198.2	232.5	216.5	238.2	239.2
scalp	173.40	198.2	232.4	216.4	238.2	239.2
basal cell carcinoma	173.41	—	—	—	—	—
specified type NEC	173.49	—	—	—	—	—
squamous cell carcinoma	173.42	—	—	—	—	—
scapular region (see also Neoplasm, skin, trunk)	173.50	198.2	232.5	216.5	238.2	239.2
scrotum	187.7	198.82	233.6	222.4	236.6	239.5
shoulder	173.60	198.2	232.6	216.6	238.2	239.2
basal cell carcinoma	173.61	—	—	—	—	—
specified type NEC	173.69	—	—	—	—	—
squamous cell carcinoma	173.62	—	—	—	—	—

☑ **Additional Digit Required** — Refer to the Tabular List for Digit Selection   ▽ **Subterms under main terms may continue to next column or page**

	Malignant					
	Primary	Secondary	Ca in situ	Benign	Uncertain Behavior	Unspecified
Neoplasm, neoplastic— *continued*						
skin — *continued*						
sole (foot) (see also Neoplasm, skin, limb, lower)	173.70	198.2	232.7	216.7	238.2	239.2
specified sites NEC	173.80	198.2	232.8	216.8	—	239.2
basal cell carcinoma	173.81	—	—	—	—	—
specified type NEC	173.89	—	—	—	—	—
squamous cell carcinoma	173.82	—	—	—	—	—
specified type NEC, unspecified site	173.99	—	—	—	—	—
squamous cell carcinoma, unspecified site	173.92	—	—	—	—	—
submammary fold (see also Neoplasm, skin, trunk)	173.50	198.2	232.5	216.5	238.2	239.2
supraclavicular region (see also Neoplasm, skin, neck)	173.40	198.2	232.4	216.4	238.2	239.2
temple (see also Neoplasm, skin, face)	173.30	198.2	232.3	216.3	238.2	239.2
thigh (see also Neoplasm, skin, limb, lower)	173.70	198.2	232.7	216.7	238.2	239.2
thoracic wall (see also Neoplasm, skin, trunk)	173.50	198.2	232.5	216.5	238.2	239.2
thumb (see also Neoplasm, skin, limb, upper)	173.60	198.2	232.6	216.6	238.2	239.2
toe (see also Neoplasm, skin, limb, lower)	173.70	198.2	232.7	216.7	238.2	239.2
tragus (see also Neoplasm, skin, ear)	173.20	198.2	232.2	216.2	238.2	239.2
trunk	173.50	198.2	232.5	216.5	238.2	239.2
basal cell carcinoma	173.51	—	—	—	—	—
specified type NEC	173.59	—	—	—	—	—
squamous cell carcinoma	173.52	—	—	—	—	—
umbilicus (see also Neoplasm, skin, trunk)	173.50	198.2	232.5	216.5	238.2	239.2
vulva	184.4	198.82	233.32	221.2	236.3	239.5
wrist (see also Neoplasm, skin, limb, upper)	173.60	198.2	232.6	216.6	238.2	239.2
skull	170.0	198.5	—	213.0	238.0	239.2
soft parts or tissues — see Neoplasm, connective tissue						
specified site NEC	195.8	198.89	234.8	229.8	238.8	239.89
specified site — see Neoplasm, skin						
spermatic cord	187.6	198.82	233.6	222.8	236.6	239.5
sphenoid	160.5	197.3	231.8	212.0	235.9	239.1
bone	170.0	198.5	—	213.0	238.0	239.2
sinus	160.5	197.3	231.8	212.0	235.9	239.1
sphincter						
anal	154.2	197.5	230.5	211.4	235.5	239.0
of Oddi	156.1	197.8	230.8	211.5	235.3	239.0
spine, spinal (column)	170.2	198.5	—	213.2	238.0	239.2
bulb	191.7	198.3	—	225.0	237.5	239.6
coccyx	170.6	198.5	—	213.6	238.0	239.2
Neoplasm, neoplastic— *continued*						
spine, spinal — *continued*						
cord (cervical) (lumbar) (sacral) (thoracic)	192.2	198.3	—	225.3	237.5	239.7
dura mater	192.3	198.4	—	225.4	237.6	239.7
lumbosacral	170.2	198.5	—	213.2	238.0	239.2
membrane	192.3	198.4	—	225.4	237.6	239.7
meninges	192.3	198.4	—	225.4	237.6	239.7
nerve (root)	171.9	198.89	—	215.9	238.1	239.2
pia mater	192.3	198.4	—	225.4	237.6	239.7
root	171.9	198.89	—	215.9	238.1	239.2
sacrum	170.6	198.5	—	213.6	238.0	239.2
spleen, splenic NEC	159.1	197.8	230.9	211.9	235.5	239.0
flexure (colon)	153.7	197.5	230.3	211.3	235.2	239.0
stem, brain	191.7	198.3	—	225.0	237.5	239.6
Stensen's duct	142.0	198.89	230.0	210.2	235.0	239.0
sternum	170.3	198.5	—	213.3	238.0	239.2
stomach	151.9	197.8	230.2	211.1	235.2	239.0
antrum (pyloric)	151.2	197.8	230.2	211.1	235.2	239.0
body	151.4	197.8	230.2	211.1	235.2	239.0
cardia	151.0	197.8	230.2	211.1	235.2	239.0
cardiac orifice	151.0	197.8	230.2	211.1	235.2	239.0
contiguous sites	151.8	—	—	—	—	—
corpus	151.4	197.8	230.2	211.1	235.2	239.0
fundus	151.3	197.8	230.2	211.1	235.2	239.0
greater curvature NEC	151.6	197.8	230.2	211.1	235.2	239.0
lesser curvature NEC	151.5	197.8	230.2	211.1	235.2	239.0
prepylorus	151.1	197.8	230.2	211.1	235.2	239.0
pylorus	151.1	197.8	230.2	211.1	235.2	239.0
wall NEC	151.9	197.8	230.2	211.1	235.2	239.0
anterior NEC	151.8	197.8	230.2	211.1	235.2	239.0
posterior NEC	151.8	197.8	230.2	211.1	235.2	239.0
stroma, endometrial	182.0	198.82	233.2	219.1	236.0	239.5
stump, cervical	180.8	198.82	233.1	219.0	236.0	239.5
subcutaneous (nodule) (tissue) NEC — see Neoplasm, connective tissue						
subdural	192.1	198.4	—	225.2	237.6	239.7
subglottis, subglottic	161.2	197.3	231.0	212.1	235.6	239.1
sublingual	144.9	198.89	230.0	210.3	235.1	239.0
gland or duct	142.2	198.89	230.0	210.2	235.0	239.0
submandibular gland	142.1	198.89	230.0	210.2	235.0	239.0
submaxillary gland or duct	142.1	198.89	230.0	210.2	235.0	239.0
submental	195.0	198.89	234.8	229.8	238.8	239.89
subpleural	162.9	197.0	—	212.3	235.7	239.1
substernal	164.2	197.1	—	212.5	235.8	239.89
sudoriferous, sudoriparous gland, site unspecified	173.90	198.2	232.9	216.9	238.2	239.2
specified site — see Neoplasm, skin						
supraclavicular region	195.0	198.89	234.8	229.8	238.8	239.89
supraglottis	161.1	197.3	231.0	212.1	235.6	239.1
suprarenal (capsule) (cortex) (gland) (medulla)	194.0	198.7	234.8	227.0	237.2	239.7
suprasellar (region)	191.9	198.3	—	225.0	237.5	239.6
sweat gland (apocrine) (eccrine), site unspecified	173.90	198.2	232.9	216.9	238.2	239.2
sympathetic nerve or nervous system NEC	171.9	198.89	—	215.9	238.1	239.2

Neoplasm, neoplastic —	Malignant			Benign	Uncertain Behavior	Unspecified
	Primary	Secondary	Ca in situ			
continued						
symphysis pubis	170.6	198.5	—	213.6	238.0	239.2
synovial membrane — *see* Neoplasm, connective tissue						
tapetum, brain	191.8	198.3	—	225.0	237.5	239.6
tarsus (any bone)	170.8	198.5	—	213.8	238.0	239.2
temple (skin) (*see also* Neoplasm, skin, face)	173.30	198.2	232.3	216.3	238.2	239.2
temporal						
bone	170.0	198.5	—	213.0	238.0	239.2
lobe or pole	191.2	198.3	—	225.0	237.5	239.6
region	195.0	198.89	234.8	229.8	238.8	239.89
skin (*see also* Neoplasm, skin, face)	173.30	198.2	232.3	216.3	238.2	239.2
tendon (sheath) — *see* Neoplasm, connective tissue						
tentorium (cerebelli)	192.1	198.4	—	225.2	237.6	239.7
testis, testes (descended) (scrotal)	186.9	198.82	233.6	222.0	236.4	239.5
ectopic	186.0	198.82	233.6	222.0	236.4	239.5
retained	186.0	198.82	233.6	222.0	236.4	239.5
undescended	186.0	198.82	233.6	222.0	236.4	239.5
thalamus	191.0	198.3	—	225.0	237.5	239.6
thigh NEC*	195.5	198.89	234.8	229.8	238.8	239.89
thorax, thoracic (cavity) (organs NEC)	195.1	198.89	234.8	229.8	238.8	239.89
duct	171.4	198.89	—	215.4	238.1	239.2
wall NEC	195.1	198.89	234.8	229.8	238.8	239.89
throat	149.0	198.89	230.0	210.9	235.1	239.0
thumb NEC*	195.4	198.89	232.6	229.8	238.8	239.89
thymus (gland)	164.0	198.89	—	212.6	235.8	239.89
contiguous sites with heart and mediastinum	164.8	—	—	—	—	—
thyroglossal duct	193	198.89	234.8	226	237.4	239.7
thyroid (gland)	193	198.89	234.8	226	237.4	239.7
cartilage	161.3	197.3	231.0	212.1	235.6	239.1
tibia (any part)	170.7	198.5	—	213.7	238.0	239.2
toe NEC*	195.5	198.89	232.7	229.8	238.8	239.89
tongue	141.9	198.89	230.0	210.1	235.1	239.0
anterior (two-thirds) NEC	141.4	198.89	230.0	210.1	235.1	239.0
dorsal surface	141.1	198.89	230.0	210.1	235.1	239.0
ventral surface	141.3	198.89	230.0	210.1	235.1	239.0
base (dorsal surface)	141.0	198.89	230.0	210.1	235.1	239.0
border (lateral)	141.2	198.89	230.0	210.1	235.1	239.0
contiguous sites	141.8	—	—	—	—	—
dorsal surface NEC	141.1	198.89	230.0	210.1	235.1	239.0
fixed part NEC	141.0	198.89	230.0	210.1	235.1	239.0
foreamen cecum	141.1	198.89	230.0	210.1	235.1	239.0
frenulum linguae	141.3	198.89	230.0	210.1	235.1	239.0
junctional zone	141.5	198.89	230.0	210.1	235.1	239.0
margin (lateral)	141.2	198.89	230.0	210.1	235.1	239.0
midline NEC	141.1	198.89	230.0	210.1	235.1	239.0
mobile part NEC	141.4	198.89	230.0	210.1	235.1	239.0
posterior (third)	141.0	198.89	230.0	210.1	235.1	239.0
root	141.0	198.89	230.0	210.1	235.1	239.0
surface (dorsal)	141.1	198.89	230.0	210.1	235.1	239.0
base	141.0	198.89	230.0	210.1	235.1	239.0
ventral	141.3	198.89	230.0	210.1	235.1	239.0
tip	141.2	198.89	230.0	210.1	235.1	239.0
tonsil	141.6	198.89	230.0	210.1	235.1	239.0
tonsil	146.0	198.89	230.0	210.5	235.1	239.0
fauces, faucial	146.0	198.89	230.0	210.5	235.1	239.0
lingual	141.6	198.89	230.0	210.1	235.1	239.0
palatine	146.0	198.89	230.0	210.5	235.1	239.0
pharyngeal	147.1	198.89	230.0	210.7	235.1	239.0

Neoplasm, neoplastic —	Malignant			Benign	Uncertain Behavior	Unspecified
	Primary	Secondary	Ca in situ			
continued						
tonsil — *continued*						
pillar (anterior) (posterior)	146.2	198.89	230.0	210.6	235.1	239.0
tonsillar fossa	146.1	198.89	230.0	210.6	235.1	239.0
tooth socket NEC	143.9	198.89	230.0	210.4	235.1	239.0
trachea (cartilage) (mucosa)	162.0	197.3	231.1	212.2	235.7	239.1
contiguous sites with bronchus or lung	162.8	—	—	—	—	—
tracheobronchial	162.8	197.3	231.1	212.2	235.7	239.1
contiguous sites with lung	162.8	—	—	—	—	—
tragus (*see also* Neoplasm, skin, ear)	173.20	198.2	232.2	216.2	238.2	239.2
trunk NEC*	195.8	198.89	232.5	229.8	238.8	239.89
tubo-ovarian	183.8	198.82	233.39	221.8	236.3	239.5
tunica vaginalis	187.8	198.82	233.6	222.8	236.6	239.5
turbinate (bone)	170.0	198.5	—	213.0	238.0	239.2
nasal	160.0	197.3	231.8	212.0	235.9	239.1
tympanic cavity	160.1	197.3	231.8	212.0	235.9	239.1
ulna (any part)	170.4	198.5	—	213.4	238.0	239.2
umbilicus, umbilical (*see also* Neoplasm, skin, trunk)	173.50	198.2	232.5	216.5	238.2	239.2
uncus, brain	191.2	198.3	—	225.0	237.5	239.6
unknown site or unspecified	199.1	199.1	234.9	229.9	238.9	239.9
urachus	188.7	198.1	233.7	223.3	236.7	239.4
ureter-bladder (junction)	188.6	198.1	233.7	223.3	236.7	239.4
ureter, ureteral	189.2	198.1	233.9	223.2	236.91	239.5
orifice (bladder)	188.6	198.1	233.7	223.3	236.7	239.4
urethra, urethral (gland)	189.3	198.1	233.9	223.81	236.99	239.5
orifice, internal	188.5	198.1	233.7	223.3	236.7	239.4
urethrovaginal (septum)	184.9	198.82	233.39	221.9	236.3	239.5
urinary organ or system NEC	189.9	198.1	233.9	223.9	236.99	239.5
bladder — *see* Neoplasm, bladder						
contiguous sites	189.8	—	—	—	—	—
specified sites NEC	189.8	198.1	233.9	223.89	236.99	239.5
utero-ovarian	183.8	198.82	233.39	221.8	236.3	239.5
ligament	183.3	198.82	—	221.0	236.3	239.5
uterosacral ligament	183.4	198.82	—	221.0	236.3	239.5
uterus, uteri, uterine	179	198.82	233.2	219.9	236.0	239.5
adnexa NEC	183.9	198.82	233.39	221.8	236.3	239.5
contiguous sites	183.8	—	—	—	—	—
body	182.0	198.82	233.2	219.1	236.0	239.5
contiguous sites	182.8	—	—	—	—	—
cervix	180.9	198.82	233.1	219.0	236.0	239.5
cornu	182.0	198.82	233.2	219.1	236.0	239.5
corpus	182.0	198.82	233.2	219.1	236.0	239.5
endocervix (canal) (gland)	180.0	198.82	233.1	219.0	236.0	239.5
endometrium	182.0	198.82	233.2	219.1	236.0	239.5
exocervix	180.1	198.82	233.1	219.0	236.0	239.5
external os	180.1	198.82	233.1	219.0	236.0	239.5
fundus	182.0	198.82	233.2	219.1	236.0	239.5
internal os	180.0	198.82	233.1	219.0	236.0	239.5
isthmus	182.1	198.82	233.2	219.1	236.0	239.5
ligament	183.4	198.82	—	221.0	236.3	239.5
broad	183.3	198.82	233.39	221.0	236.3	239.5
round	183.5	198.82	—	221.0	236.3	239.5
lower segment	182.1	198.82	233.2	219.1	236.0	239.5
myometrium	182.0	198.82	233.2	219.1	236.0	239.5

☑ **Additional Digit Required** — Refer to the Tabular List for Digit Selection　　　　▼ **Subterms under main terms may continue to next column or page**

210— Volume 2　　　　　▶◀ **Revised Text**　　　　● **New Line**　　　▲ **Revised Code**　　　　**2015 ICD-9-CM**

Neoplasm, neoplastic — continued	Malignant			Benign	Uncertain Behavior	Unspecified
	Primary	Secondary	Ca in situ			
uterus, uteri, uterine — continued						
squamocolumnar junction	180.8	198.82	233.1	219.0	236.0	239.5
tube	183.2	198.82	233.39	221.0	236.3	239.5
utricle, prostatic	189.3	198.1	233.9	223.81	236.99	239.5
uveal tract	190.0	198.4	234.0	224.0	238.8	239.89
uvula	145.4	198.89	230.0	210.4	235.1	239.0
vagina, vaginal (fornix) (vault) (wall)	184.0	198.82	233.31	221.1	236.3	239.5
vaginovesical	184.9	198.82	233.39	221.9	236.3	239.5
septum	184.9	198.82	233.39	221.9	236.3	239.5
vallecula (epiglottis)	146.3	198.89	230.0	210.6	235.1	239.0
vascular — see Neoplasm, connective tissue						
vas deferens	187.6	198.82	233.6	222.8	236.6	239.5
Vater's ampulla	156.2	197.8	230.8	211.5	235.3	239.0
vein, venous — see Neoplasm, connective tissue						
vena cava (abdominal) (inferior)	171.5	198.89	—	215.5	238.1	239.2
superior	171.4	198.89	—	215.4	238.1	239.2
ventricle (cerebral) (floor) (fourth) (lateral) (third)	191.5	198.3	—	225.0	237.5	239.6
cardiac (left) (right)	164.1	198.89	—	212.7	238.8	239.89
ventricular band of larynx	161.1	197.3	231.0	212.1	235.6	239.1
ventriculus — see Neoplasm, stomach						
vermillion border — see Neoplasm, lip						
vermis, cerebellum	191.6	198.3	—	225.0	237.5	239.6
vertebra (column)	170.2	198.5	—	213.2	238.0	239.2
coccyx	170.6	198.5	—	213.6	238.0	239.2
sacrum	170.6	198.5	—	213.6	238.0	239.2
vesical — see Neoplasm, bladder						
vesicle, seminal	187.8	198.82	233.6	222.8	236.6	239.5
vesicocervical tissue	184.9	198.82	233.39	221.9	236.3	239.5
vesicorectal	195.3	198.89	234.8	229.8	238.8	239.89
vesicovaginal	184.9	198.82	233.39	221.9	236.3	239.5
septum	184.9	198.82	233.39	221.9	236.3	239.5
vessel (blood) — see Neoplasm, connective tissue						
vestibular gland, greater	184.1	198.82	233.32	221.2	236.3	239.5
vestibule						
mouth	145.1	198.89	230.0	210.4	235.1	239.0
nose	160.0	197.3	231.8	212.0	235.9	239.1
Virchow's gland	—	196.0		229.0	238.8	239.89
viscera NEC	195.8	198.89	234.8	229.8	238.8	239.89
vocal cords (true)	161.0	197.3	231.0	212.1	235.6	239.1
false	161.1	197.3	231.0	212.1	235.6	239.1
vomer	170.0	198.5	—	213.0	238.0	239.2
vulva	184.4	198.82	233.32	221.2	236.3	239.5
vulvovaginal gland	184.4	198.82	233.32	221.2	236.3	239.5
Waldeyer's ring	149.1	198.89	230.0	210.9	235.1	239.0
Wharton's duct	142.1	198.89	230.0	210.2	235.0	239.0
white matter (central) (cerebral)	191.0	198.3	—	225.0	237.5	239.6
windpipe	162.0	197.3	231.1	212.2	235.7	239.1
Wirsung's duct	157.3	197.8	230.9	211.6	235.5	239.0
wolffian (body) (duct) female	184.8	198.82	233.39	221.8	236.3	239.5
male	187.8	198.82	233.6	222.8	236.6	239.5
womb — see Neoplasm, uterus						

Neoplasm, neoplastic — continued	Malignant			Benign	Uncertain Behavior	Unspecified
	Primary	Secondary	Ca in situ			
wrist NEC*	195.4	198.89	232.6	229.8	238.8	239.89
xiphoid process	170.3	198.5	—	213.3	238.0	239.2
Zuckerkandl's organ	194.6	198.89	—	227.6	237.3	239.7

Neovascularization — Nephrosis, nephrotic

Neovascularization
choroid 362.16
ciliary body 364.42
cornea 370.60
deep 370.63
localized 370.61
iris 364.42
retina 362.16
subretinal 362.16
Nephralgia 788.0
Nephritis, nephritic (albuminuric) (azotemic)
(congenital) (degenerative) (diffuse)
(disseminated) (epithelial) (familial) (focal) (granulomatous) (hemorrhagic) (infantile) (nonsuppurative, excretory)
(uremic) 583.9
with
edema — see Nephrosis
lesion of
glomerulonephritis
hypocomplementemic persistent
583.2
with nephrotic syndrome
581.2
chronic 582.2
lobular 583.2
with nephrotic syndrome
581.2
chronic 582.2
membranoproliferative 583.2
with nephrotic syndrome
581.2
chronic 582.2
membranous 583.1
with nephrotic syndrome
581.1
chronic 582.1
mesangiocapillary 583.2
with nephrotic syndrome
581.2
chronic 582.2
mixed membranous and proliferative 583.2
with nephrotic syndrome
581.2
chronic 582.2
proliferative (diffuse) 583.0
with nephrotic syndrome
581.0
acute 580.0
chronic 582.0
rapidly progressive 583.4
acute 580.4
chronic 582.4
interstitial nephritis (diffuse) (focal)
583.89
with nephrotic syndrome 581.89
acute 580.89
chronic 582.89
necrotizing glomerulitis 583.4
acute 580.4
chronic 582.4
renal necrosis 583.9
cortical 583.6
medullary 583.7
specified pathology NEC 583.89
with nephrotic syndrome 581.89
acute 580.89
chronic 582.89
necrosis, renal 583.9
cortical 583.6
medullary (papillary) 583.7
nephrotic syndrome (see also Nephrosis)
581.9
papillary necrosis 583.7
specified pathology NEC 583.89
acute 580.9
extracapillary with epithelial crescents
580.4
hypertensive (see also Hypertension,
kidney) 403.90
necrotizing 580.4
poststreptococcal 580.0
proliferative (diffuse) 580.0
rapidly progressive 580.4
specified pathology NEC 580.89

Nephritis, nephritic — continued
amyloid 277.39 [583.81]
chronic 277.39 [582.81]
arteriolar (see also Hypertension, kidney)
403.90
arteriosclerotic (see also Hypertension, kidney) 403.90
ascending (see also Pyelitis) 590.80
atrophic 582.9
basement membrane NEC 583.89
with
pulmonary hemorrhage (Goodpasture's syndrome)
446.21 [583.81]
calculous, calculus 592.0
cardiac (see also Hypertension, kidney)
403.90
cardiovascular (see also Hypertension, kidney) 403.90
chronic 582.9
arteriosclerotic (see also Hypertension,
kidney) 403.90
hypertensive (see also Hypertension,
kidney) 403.90
cirrhotic (see also Sclerosis, renal) 587
complicating pregnancy, childbirth, or
puerperium 646.2 ☑
with hypertension 642.1 ☑
affecting fetus or newborn 760.0
affecting fetus or newborn 760.1
croupous 580.9
desquamative — see Nephrosis
due to
amyloidosis 277.39 [583.81]
chronic 277.39 [582.81]
arteriosclerosis (see also Hypertension,
kidney) 403.90
diabetes mellitus 250.4 ☑ [583.81]
with nephrotic syndrome
250.4 ☑ [581.81]
due to secondary diabetes
249.4 ☑ [583.81]
due to secondary diabetes
249.4 ☑ [583.81]
diphtheria 032.89 [580.81]
gonococcal infection (acute)
098.19 [583.81]
chronic or duration of 2 months or
over 098.39 [583.81]
gout 274.10
infectious hepatitis 070.9 [580.81]
mumps 072.79 [580.81]
specified kidney pathology NEC 583.89
acute 580.89
chronic 582.89
streptotrichosis 039.8 [583.81]
subacute bacterial endocarditis
421.0 [580.81]
systemic lupus erythematosus
710.0 [583.81]
chronic 710.0 [582.81]
typhoid fever 002.0 [580.81]
endothelial 582.2
end stage (chronic) (terminal) NEC 585.6
epimembranous 581.1
exudative 583.89
with nephrotic syndrome 581.89
acute 580.89
chronic 582.89
gonococcal (acute) 098.19 [583.81]
chronic or duration of 2 months or over
098.39 [583.81]
gouty 274.10
hereditary (Alport's syndrome) 759.89
hydremic — see Nephrosis
hypertensive (see also Hypertension, kidney)
403.90
hypocomplementemic persistent 583.2
with nephrotic syndrome 581.2
chronic 582.2
immune complex NEC 583.89
infective (see also Pyelitis) 590.80
interstitial (diffuse) (focal) 583.89
with nephrotic syndrome 581.89
acute 580.89
chronic 582.89

Nephritis, nephritic — continued
latent or quiescent — see Nephritis, chronic
lead 984.9
specified type of lead — see Table of
Drugs and Chemicals
lobular 583.2
with nephrotic syndrome 581.2
chronic 582.2
lupus 710.0 [583.81]
acute 710.0 [580.81]
chronic 710.0 [582.81]
membranoproliferative 583.2
with nephrotic syndrome 581.2
chronic 582.2
membranous 583.1
with nephrotic syndrome 581.1
chronic 582.1
mesangiocapillary 583.2
with nephrotic syndrome 581.2
chronic 582.2
minimal change 581.3
mixed membranous and proliferative 583.2
with nephrotic syndrome 581.2
chronic 582.2
necrotic, necrotizing 583.4
acute 580.4
chronic 582.4
nephrotic — see Nephrosis
old — see Nephritis, chronic
parenchymatous 581.89
polycystic 753.12
adult type (APKD) 753.13
autosomal dominant 753.13
autosomal recessive 753.14
childhood type (CPKD) 753.14
infantile type 753.14
poststreptococcal 580.0
pregnancy — see Nephritis, complicating
pregnancy
proliferative 583.0
with nephrotic syndrome 581.0
acute 580.0
chronic 582.0
purulent (see also Pyelitis) 590.80
rapidly progressive 583.4
acute 580.4
chronic 582.4
salt-losing or salt-wasting (see also Disease,
renal) 593.9
saturnine 584.9
specified type of lead — see Table of
Drugs and Chemicals
septic (see also Pyelitis) 590.80
specified pathology 583.89
acute 580.89
chronic 582.89
staphylococcal (see also Pyelitis) 590.80
streptotrichosis 039.8 [583.81]
subacute (see also Nephrosis) 581.9
suppurative (see also Pyelitis) 590.80
syphilitic (late) 095.4
congenital 090.5 [583.81]
early 091.69 [583.81]
terminal (chronic) (end-stage) NEC 585.6
toxic — see Nephritis, acute
tubal, tubular — see Nephrosis, tubular
tuberculous (see also Tuberculosis)
016.0 ☑ [583.81]
type II (Ellis) — see Nephrosis
vascular — see Hypertension, kidney
war 580.9
Nephroblastoma (M8960/3) 189.0
epithelial (M8961/3) 189.0
mesenchymal (M8962/3) 189.0
Nephrocalcinosis 275.49
Nephrocystitis, pustular — see also Pyelitis
590.80
Nephrolithiasis (congenital) (pelvis) (recurrent)
592.0
uric acid 274.11
Nephroma (M8960/3) 189.0
mesoblastic (M8960/1) 236.9 ☑
Nephronephritis — see also Nephrosis 581.9
Nephronopthisis 753.16
Nephropathy — see also Nephritis 583.9

Nephropathy — see also Nephritis —
continued
with
exudative nephritis 583.89
interstitial nephritis (diffuse) (focal)
583.89
medullary necrosis 583.7
necrosis 583.9
cortical 583.6
medullary or papillary 583.7
papillary necrosis 583.7
specified lesion or cause NEC 583.89
analgesic 583.89
with medullary necrosis, acute 584.7
arteriolar (see also Hypertension, kidney)
403.90
arteriosclerotic (see also Hypertension, kidney) 403.90
complicating pregnancy 646.2 ☑
diabetic 250.4 ☑ [583.81]
due to secondary diabetes
249.4 ☑ [583.81]
gouty 274.10
specified type NEC 274.19
hereditary amyloid 277.31
hypercalcemic 588.89
hypertensive (see also Hypertension, kidney)
403.90
hypokalemic (vacuolar) 588.89
IgA 583.9
obstructive 593.89
congenital 753.20
phenacetin 584.7
phosphate-losing 588.0
potassium depletion 588.89
proliferative (see also Nephritis, proliferative)
583.0
protein-losing 588.89
salt-losing or salt-wasting (see also Disease,
renal) 593.9
sickle-cell (see also Disease, sickle-cell)
282.60 [583.81]
toxic 584.5
vasomotor 584.5
water-losing 588.89
Nephroptosis — see also Disease, renal 593.0
congenital (displaced) 753.3
Nephropyosis — see also Abscess, kidney
590.2
Nephrorrhagia 593.81
Nephrosclerosis (arteriolar) (arteriosclerotic)
(chronic) (hyaline) — see also Hypertension, kidney 403.90
gouty 274.10
hyperplastic (arteriolar) (see also Hypertension, kidney) 403.90
senile (see also Sclerosis, renal) 587
Nephrosis, nephrotic (Epstein's) (syndrome)
581.9
with
lesion of
focal glomerulosclerosis 581.1
glomerulonephritis
endothelial 581.2
hypocomplementemic persistent
581.2
lobular 581.2
membranoproliferative 581.2
membranous 581.1
mesangiocapillary 581.2
minimal change 581.3
mixed membranous and proliferative 581.2
proliferative 581.0
segmental hyalinosis 581.1
specified pathology NEC 581.89
acute — see Nephrosis, tubular
anoxic — see Nephrosis, tubular
arteriosclerotic (see also Hypertension, kidney) 403.90
chemical — see Nephrosis, tubular
cholemic 572.4
complicating pregnancy, childbirth, or
puerperium — see Nephritis, complicating pregnancy
diabetic 250.4 ☑ [581.81]

☑ **Additional Digit Required** — Refer to the Tabular List for Digit Selection   ▽ **Subterms under main terms may continue to next column or page**

212 — **Volume 2**   ▶◀ **Revised Text**   ● **New Line**   ▲ **Revised Code**   **2015 ICD-9-CM**

Nephrosis, nephrotic — *continued*
  diabetic — *continued*
    due to secondary diabetes
      249.4 ☑ *[581.81]*
  Finnish type (congenital) 759.89
  hemoglobinuric — *see* Nephrosis, tubular
  in
    amyloidosis 277.39 *[581.81]*
    diabetes mellitus 250.4 ☑ *[581.81]*
      due to secondary diabetes
        249.4 ☑ *[581.81]*
    epidemic hemorrhagic fever 078.6
    malaria 084.9 *[581.81]*
    polyarteritis 446.0 *[581.81]*
    systemic lupus erythematosus
      710.0 *[581.81]*
  ischemic — *see* Nephrosis, tubular
  lipoid 581.3
  lower nephron — *see* Nephrosis, tubular
  lupoid 710.0 *[581.81]*
  lupus 710.0 *[581.81]*
  malarial 084.9 *[581.81]*
  minimal change 581.3
  necrotizing — *see* Nephrosis, tubular
  osmotic (sucrose) 588.89
  polyarteritic 446.0 *[581.81]*
  radiation 581.9
  specified lesion or cause NEC 581.89
  syphilitic 095.4
  toxic — *see* Nephrosis, tubular
  tubular (acute) 584.5
    due to a procedure 997.5
    radiation 581.9
Nephrosonephritis hemorrhagic (endemic) 078.6
Nephrostomy status V44.6
  with complication 997.5
Nerve — *see* condition
Nerves 799.21
Nervous — *see also* condition 799.21
  breakdown 300.9
  heart 306.2
  stomach 306.4
  tension 799.21
Nervousness 799.21
Nesidioblastoma (M8150/0)
  pancreas 211.7
  specified site NEC — *see* Neoplasm, by site, benign
  unspecified site 211.7
Netherton's syndrome (ichthyosiform erythroderma) 757.1
Nettle rash 708.8
Nettleship's disease (urticaria pigmentosa) 757.33
Neumann's disease (pemphigus vegetans) 694.4
Neuralgia, neuralgic (acute) — *see also* Neuritis 729.2
  accessory (nerve) 352.4
  acoustic (nerve) 388.5
  ankle 355.8
  anterior crural 355.8
  anus 787.99
  arm 723.4
  auditory (nerve) 388.5
  axilla 353.0
  bladder 788.1
  brachial 723.4
  brain — *see* Disorder, nerve, cranial
  broad ligament 625.9
  cerebral — *see* Disorder, nerve, cranial
  ciliary 339.00
  cranial nerve (*see also* Disorder, nerve, cranial)
    fifth or trigeminal (*see also* Neuralgia, trigeminal) 350.1
  ear 388.71
    middle 352.1
  facial 351.8
  finger 354.9
  flank 355.8
  foot 355.8
  forearm 354.9
  Fothergill's (*see also* Neuralgia, trigeminal) 350.1

Neuralgia, neuralgic — *see also* Neuritis — *continued*
  Fothergill's (*see also* Neuralgia, trigeminal) — *continued*
    postherpetic 053.12
  glossopharyngeal (nerve) 352.1
  groin 355.8
  hand 354.9
  heel 355.8
  Horton's 339.00
  Hunt's 053.11
  hypoglossal 352.5
  iliac region 355.8
  infraorbital (*see also* Neuralgia, trigeminal) 350.1
  inguinal 355.8
  intercostal (nerve) 353.8
    postherpetic 053.19
  jaw 352.1
  kidney 788.0
  knee 355.8
  loin 355.8
  malarial (*see also* Malaria) 084.6
  mastoid 385.89
  maxilla 352.1
  median thenar 354.1
  metatarsal 355.6
  middle ear 352.1
  migrainous 339.00
  Morton's 355.6
  nerve, cranial — *see* Disorder, nerve, cranial
  nose 352.0
  occipital 723.8
  olfactory (nerve) 352.0
  ophthalmic 377.30
    postherpetic 053.19
  optic (nerve) 377.30
  penis 607.9
  perineum 355.8
  pleura 511.0
  postherpetic NEC 053.19
    geniculate ganglion 053.11
    ophthalmic 053.19
    trifacial 053.12
    trigeminal 053.12
  pubic region 355.8
  radial (nerve) 723.4
  rectum 787.99
  sacroiliac joint 724.3
  sciatic (nerve) 724.3
  scrotum 608.9
  seminal vesicle 608.9
  shoulder 354.9
  Sluder's 337.09
  specified nerve NEC — *see* Disorder, nerve
  spermatic cord 608.9
  sphenopalatine (ganglion) 337.09
  subscapular (nerve) 723.4
  suprascapular (nerve) 723.4
  testis 608.89
  thenar (median) 354.1
  thigh 355.8
  tongue 352.5
  trifacial (nerve) (*see also* Neuralgia, trigeminal) 350.1
  trigeminal (nerve) 350.1
    postherpetic 053.12
  tympanic plexus 388.71
  ulnar (nerve) 723.4
  vagus (nerve) 352.3
  wrist 354.9
  writers' 300.89
    organic 333.84
Neurapraxia — *see* Injury, nerve, by site
Neurasthenia 300.5
  cardiac 306.2
  gastric 306.4
  heart 306.2
  postfebrile 780.79
  postviral 780.79
Neurilemmoma (M9560/0) — *see also* Neoplasm, connective tissue, benign
  acoustic (nerve) 225.1
  malignant (M9560/3) (*see also* Neoplasm, connective tissue, malignant)
    acoustic (nerve) 192.0

Neurilemmosarcoma (M9560/3) — *see* Neoplasm, connective tissue, malignant
Neurilemoma — *see* Neurilemmoma
Neurinoma (M9560/0) — *see* Neurilemmoma
Neurinomatosis (M9560/1) — *see also* Neoplasm, connective tissue, uncertain behavior
  centralis 759.5
Neuritis — *see also* Neuralgia 729.2
  abducens (nerve) 378.54
  accessory (nerve) 352.4
  acoustic (nerve) 388.5
    syphilitic 094.86
  alcoholic 357.5
    with psychosis 291.1
  amyloid, any site 277.39 *[357.4]*
  anterior crural 355.8
  arising during pregnancy 646.4 ☑
  arm 723.4
  ascending 355.2
  auditory (nerve) 388.5
  brachial (nerve) NEC 723.4
    due to displacement, intervertebral disc 722.0
  cervical 723.4
  chest (wall) 353.8
  costal region 353.8
  cranial nerve (*see also* Disorder, nerve, cranial)
    first or olfactory 352.0
    second or optic 377.30
    third or oculomotor 378.52
    fourth or trochlear 378.53
    fifth or trigeminal (*see also* Neuralgia, trigeminal) 350.1
    sixth or abducens 378.54
    seventh or facial 351.8
      newborn 767.5
    eighth or acoustic 388.5
    ninth or glossopharyngeal 352.1
    tenth or vagus 352.3
    eleventh or accessory 352.4
    twelfth or hypoglossal 352.5
  Déjérine-Sottas 356.0
  diabetic 250.6 ☑ *[357.2]*
    due to secondary diabetes
      249.6 ☑ *[357.2]*
  diphtheritic 032.89 *[357.4]*
  due to
    beriberi 265.0 *[357.4]*
    displacement, prolapse, protrusion, or rupture of intervertebral disc 722.2
      cervical 722.0
      lumbar, lumbosacral 722.10
      thoracic, thoracolumbar 722.11
    herniation, nucleus pulposus 722.2
      cervical 722.0
      lumbar, lumbosacral 722.10
      thoracic, thoracolumbar 722.11
  endemic 265.0 *[357.4]*
  facial (nerve) 351.8
    newborn 767.5
  general — *see* Polyneuropathy
  geniculate ganglion 351.1
    due to herpes 053.11
  glossopharyngeal (nerve) 352.1
  gouty 274.89 *[357.4]*
  hypoglossal (nerve) 352.5
  ilioinguinal (nerve) 355.8
  in diseases classified elsewhere — *see* Polyneuropathy, in
  infectious (multiple) 357.0
  intercostal (nerve) 353.8
  interstitial hypertrophic progressive NEC 356.9
  leg 355.8
  lumbosacral NEC 724.4
  median (nerve) 354.1
    thenar 354.1
  multiple (acute) (infective) 356.9
    endemic 265.0 *[357.4]*
  multiplex endemica 265.0 *[357.4]*
  nerve root (*see also* Radiculitis) 729.2
  oculomotor (nerve) 378.52
  olfactory (nerve) 352.0

Neuritis — *see also* Neuralgia — *continued*
  optic (nerve) 377.30
    in myelitis 341.0
    meningococcal 036.81
  pelvic 355.8
  peripheral (nerve) (*see also* Neuropathy, peripheral)
    complicating pregnancy or puerperium 646.4 ☑
    specified nerve NEC — *see* Mononeuritis
  pneumogastric (nerve) 352.3
  postchickenpox 052.7
  postherpetic 053.19
  progressive hypertrophic interstitial NEC 356.9
  puerperal, postpartum 646.4 ☑
  radial (nerve) 723.4
  retrobulbar 377.32
    syphilitic 094.85
  rheumatic (chronic) 729.2
  sacral region 355.8
  sciatic (nerve) 724.3
    due to displacement of intervertebral disc 722.10
  serum 999.59
  specified nerve NEC — *see* Disorder, nerve
  spinal (nerve) 355.9
    root (*see also* Radiculitis) 729.2
  subscapular (nerve) 723.4
  suprascapular (nerve) 723.4
  syphilitic 095.8
  thenar (median) 354.1
  thoracic NEC 724.4
  toxic NEC 357.7
  trochlear (nerve) 378.53
  ulnar (nerve) 723.4
  vagus (nerve) 352.3
Neuroangiomatosis, encephalofacial 759.6
Neuroastrocytoma (M9505/1) — *see* Neoplasm, by site, uncertain behavior
Neuro-avitaminosis 269.2
Neuroblastoma (M9500/3) 160.0
  olfactory (M9522/3) 160.0
  specified site — *see* Neoplasm, by site, malignant
  unspecified site 194.0
Neurochorioretinitis — *see also* Chorioretinitis 363.20
Neurocirculatory asthenia 306.2
Neurocytoma (M9506/0) — *see* Neoplasm, by site, benign
Neurodermatitis (circumscribed) (circumscripta) (local) 698.3
  atopic 691.8
  diffuse (Brocq) 691.8
  disseminated 691.8
  nodulosa 698.3
Neuroencephalomyelopathy, optic 341.0
Neuroendocrine tumor — *see* Tumor, neuroendocrine
Neuroepithelioma (M9503/3) — *see also* Neoplasm, by site, malignant
  olfactory (M9521/3) 160.0
Neurofibroma (M9540/0) — *see also* Neoplasm, connective tissue, benign
  melanotic (M9541/0) — *see* Neoplasm, connective tissue, benign
  multiple (M9540/1) 237.70
    type 1 237.71
    type 2 237.72
  plexiform (M9550/0) — *see* Neoplasm, connective tissue, benign
Neurofibromatosis (multiple) (M9540/1) 237.70
  acoustic 237.72
  malignant (M9540/3) — *see* Neoplasm, connective tissue, malignant
  Schwannomatosis 237.73
  specified type NEC 237.79
  type 1 237.71
  type 2 237.72
  von Recklinghausen's 237.71
Neurofibrosarcoma (M9540/3) — *see* Neoplasm, connective tissue, malignant
Neurogenic — *see also* condition

☑ **Additional Digit Required** — Refer to the Tabular List for Digit Selection   ▽ **Subterms under main terms may continue to next column or page**

2015 ICD-9-CM   ▶◀ **Revised Text**   ● **New Line**   ▲ **Revised Code**   **Volume 2 — 213**

Index

Neurogenic — *see also* condition —
  continued
  bladder (atonic) (automatic) (autonomic)
    (flaccid) (hypertonic) (hypotonic)
    (inertia) (infranuclear) (irritable)
    (motor) (nonreflex) (nuclear) (paraly-
    sis) (reflex) (sensory) (spastic)
    (supranuclear) (uninhibited) 596.54
    with cauda equina syndrome 344.61
  bowel 564.81
  heart 306.2
Neuroglioma (M9505/1) — *see* Neoplasm,
  by site, uncertain behavior
Neurolabyrinthitis (of Dix and Hallpike) 386.12
Neurolathyrism 988.2
Neuroleprosy 030.1
Neuroleptic malignant syndrome 333.92
Neurolipomatosis 272.8
Neuroma (M9570/0) — *see also* Neoplasm,
  connective tissue, benign
  acoustic (nerve) (M9560/0) 225.1
  amputation (traumatic) (*see also* Injury,
    nerve, by site)
    surgical complication (late) 997.61
  appendix 211.3
  auditory nerve 225.1
  digital 355.6
    toe 355.6
  interdigital (toe) 355.6
  intermetatarsal 355.6
  Morton's 355.6
  multiple 237.70
    type 1 237.71
    type 2 237.72
  nonneoplastic 355.9
    arm NEC 354.9
    leg NEC 355.8
    lower extremity NEC 355.8
    specified site NEC — *see* Mononeuritis,
      by site
    upper extremity NEC 354.9
  optic (nerve) 225.1
  plantar 355.6
  plexiform (M9550/0) — *see* Neoplasm,
    connective tissue, benign
  surgical (nonneoplastic) 355.9
    arm NEC 354.9
    leg NEC 355.8
    lower extremity NEC 355.8
    upper extremity NEC 354.9
  traumatic (*see also* Injury, nerve, by site)
    old — *see* Neuroma, nonneoplastic
Neuromyalgia 729.1
Neuromyasthenia (epidemic) 049.8
Neuromyelitis 341.8
  ascending 357.0
  optica 341.0
Neuromyopathy NEC 358.9
Neuromyositis 729.1
Neuronevus (M8725/0) — *see* Neoplasm, skin,
  benign
Neuronitis 357.0
  ascending (acute) 355.2
  vestibular 386.12
Neuroparalytic — *see* condition
Neuropathy, neuropathic — *see also* Disorder,
  nerve 355.9
  acute motor 357.82
  alcoholic 357.5
    with psychosis 291.1
  arm NEC 354.9
  ataxia and retinitis pigmentosa (NARP syn-
    drome) 277.87
  autonomic (peripheral) — *see* Neuropathy,
    peripheral, autonomic
  axillary nerve 353.0
  brachial plexus 353.0
  cervical plexus 353.2
  chronic
    progressive segmentally demyelinating
      357.89
    relapsing demyelinating 357.89
  congenital sensory 356.2
  Déjérine-Sottas 356.0
  diabetic 250.6 ☑ *[357.2]*
    autonomic (peripheral) 250.6 ☑ *[337.1]*

Neuropathy, neuropathic — *see also* Disorder,
  nerve — *continued*
  diabetic — *continued*
    due to secondary diabetes
      249.6 ☑ *[357.2]*
      autonomic (peripheral)
        249.6 ☑ *[337.1]*
  entrapment 355.9
    iliohypogastric nerve 355.79
    ilioinguinal nerve 355.79
    lateral cutaneous nerve of thigh 355.1
    median nerve 354.0
    obturator nerve 355.79
    peroneal nerve 355.3
    posterior tibial nerve 355.5
    saphenous nerve 355.79
    ulnar nerve 354.2
  facial nerve 351.9
  hereditary 356.9
    peripheral 356.0
    sensory (radicular) 356.2
  hypertrophic
    Charcôt-Marie-Tooth 356.1
    Déjérine-Sottas 356.0
    interstitial 356.9
    Refsum 356.3
  intercostal nerve 354.8
  ischemic — *see* Disorder, nerve
  Jamaican (ginger) 357.7
  leg NEC 355.8
  lower extremity NEC 355.8
  lumbar plexus 353.1
  median nerve 354.1
  motor
    acute 357.82
  multiple (acute) (chronic) (*see also*
    Polyneuropathy) 356.9
  optic 377.39
    ischemic 377.41
    nutritional 377.33
    toxic 377.34
  peripheral (nerve) (*see also* Polyneuropathy)
    356.9
    arm NEC 354.9
    autonomic 337.9
      amyloid 277.39 *[337.1]*
      idiopathic 337.00
      in
        amyloidosis 277.39 *[337.1]*
        diabetes (mellitus)
          250.6 ☑ *[337.1]*
          due to secondary diabetes
            249.6 ☑ *[337.1]*
        diseases classified elsewhere
          337.1
        gout 274.89 *[337.1]*
        hyperthyroidism 242.9 ☑ *[337.1]*
    due to
      antitetanus serum 357.6
      arsenic 357.7
      drugs 357.6
      lead 357.7
      organophosphate compounds 357.7
      toxic agent NEC 357.7
    hereditary 356.0
    idiopathic 356.9
      progressive 356.4
      specified type NEC 356.8
    in diseases classified elsewhere — *see*
      Polyneuropathy, in
    leg NEC 355.8
    lower extremity NEC 355.8
    upper extremity NEC 354.9
  plantar nerves 355.6
  progressive
    hypertrophic interstitial 356.9
    inflammatory 357.89
  radicular NEC 729.2
    brachial 723.4
    cervical NEC 723.4
    hereditary sensory 356.2
    lumbar 724.4
    lumbosacral 724.4
    thoracic NEC 724.4
  sacral plexus 353.1
  sciatic 355.0

Neuropathy, neuropathic — *see also* Disorder,
  nerve — *continued*
  spinal nerve NEC 355.9
    root (*see also* Radiculitis) 729.2
  toxic 357.7
  trigeminal sensory 350.8
  ulnar nerve 354.2
  upper extremity NEC 354.9
  uremic 585.9 *[357.4]*
  vitamin B$_{12}$ 266.2 *[357.4]*
    with anemia (pernicious) 281.0 *[357.4]*
      due to dietary deficiency
        281.1 *[357.4]*
Neurophthisis — *see also* Disorder, nerve
  diabetic 250.6 ☑ *[357.2]*
    due to secondary diabetes
      249.6 ☑ *[357.2]*
  peripheral 356.9
Neuropraxia — *see* Injury, nerve
Neuroretinitis 363.05
  syphilitic 094.85
Neurosarcoma (M9540/3) — *see* Neoplasm,
  connective tissue, malignant
Neurosclerosis — *see* Disorder, nerve
Neurosis, neurotic 300.9
  accident 300.16
  anancastic, anankastic 300.3
  anxiety (state) 300.00
    generalized 300.02
    panic type 300.01
  asthenic 300.5
  bladder 306.53
  cardiac (reflex) 306.2
  cardiovascular 306.2
  climacteric, unspecified type 627.2
  colon 306.4
  compensation 300.16
  compulsive, compulsion 300.3
  conversion 300.11
  craft 300.89
  cutaneous 306.3
  depersonalization 300.6
  depressive (reaction) (type) 300.4
  endocrine 306.6
  environmental 300.89
  fatigue 300.5
  functional (*see also* Disorder, psychosomat-
    ic) 306.9
  gastric 306.4
  gastrointestinal 306.4
  genitourinary 306.50
  heart 306.2
  hypochondriacal 300.7
  hysterical 300.10
    conversion type 300.11
    dissociative type 300.15
  impulsive 300.3
  incoordination 306.0
    larynx 306.1
    vocal cord 306.1
  intestine 306.4
  larynx 306.1
    hysterical 300.11
    sensory 306.1
  menopause, unspecified type 627.2
  mixed NEC 300.89
  musculoskeletal 306.0
  obsessional 300.3
    phobia 300.3
  obsessive-compulsive 300.3
  occupational 300.89
  ocular 306.7
  oral (*see also* Disorder, fluency) 315.35
  organ (*see also* Disorder, psychosomatic)
    306.9
  pharynx 306.1
  phobic 300.20
  posttraumatic (acute) (situational) 309.81
    chronic 309.81
  psychasthenic (type) 300.89
  railroad 300.16
  rectum 306.4
  respiratory 306.1
  rumination 306.4
  senile 300.89
  sexual 302.70

Neurosis, neurotic — *continued*
  situational 300.89
  specified type NEC 300.89
  state 300.9
    with depersonalization episode 300.6
  stomach 306.4
  vasomotor 306.2
  visceral 306.4
  war 300.16
Neurospongioblastosis diffusa 759.5
Neurosyphilis (arrested) (early) (inactive) (late)
  (latent) (recurrent) 094.9
  with ataxia (cerebellar) (locomotor) (spastic)
    (spinal) 094.0
  acute meningitis 094.2
  aneurysm 094.89
  arachnoid (adhesive) 094.2
  arteritis (any artery) 094.89
  asymptomatic 094.3
  congenital 090.40
  dura (mater) 094.89
  general paresis 094.1
  gumma 094.9
  hemorrhagic 094.9
  juvenile (asymptomatic) (meningeal) 090.40
  leptomeninges (aseptic) 094.2
  meningeal 094.2
  meninges (adhesive) 094.2
  meningovascular (diffuse) 094.2
  optic atrophy 094.84
  parenchymatous (degenerative) 094.1
  paresis (*see also* Paresis, general) 094.1
  paretic (*see also* Paresis, general) 094.1
  relapse 094.9
  remission in (sustained) 094.9
  serological 094.3
  specified nature or site NEC 094.89
  tabes (dorsalis) 094.0
    juvenile 090.40
  tabetic 094.0
    juvenile 090.40
  taboparesis 094.1
    juvenile 090.40
  thrombosis 094.89
  vascular 094.89
Neurotic — *see also* Neurosis 300.9
  excoriation 698.4
    psychogenic 306.3
Neurotmesis — *see* Injury, nerve, by site
Neurotoxemia — *see* Toxemia
Neutro-occlusion 524.21
Neutropenia, neutropenic (idiopathic) (pernicious) (primary) 288.00
  chronic 288.09
    hypoplastic 288.09
  congenital (nontransient) 288.01
  cyclic 288.02
  drug induced 288.03
  due to infection 288.04
  fever 288.00
  genetic 288.01
  immune 288.09
  infantile 288.01
  malignant 288.09
  neonatal, transitory (isoimmune) (maternal
    transfer) 776.7
  periodic 288.02
  splenic 289.53
  splenomegaly 289.53
  toxic 288.09
Neutrophilia, hereditary giant 288.2
Nevocarcinoma (M8720/3) — *see* Melanoma
Nevus (M8720/0) — *see also* Neoplasm, skin,
  benign

Note — Except where otherwise indicated, varieties of nevus in the list below
that are followed by a morphology code
number (M----/0) should be coded by
site as for "Neoplasm, skin, benign."

  acanthotic 702.8
  achromic (M8730/0)
  amelanotic (M8730/0)
  anemic, anemicus 709.09
  angiomatous (M9120/0) (*see also* Heman-
    gioma) 228.00
  araneus 448.1

☑ **Additional Digit Required** — Refer to the Tabular List for Digit Selection   ⬇ **Subterms under main terms may continue to next column or page**

214 — Volume 2   ▶◀ Revised Text   ● New Line   ▲ Revised Code   2015 ICD-9-CM

Index   Neurogenic — Nevus

☑ Additional Digit Required — Refer to the Tabular List for Digit Selection   ◔ Subterms under main terms may continue to next column or page

2015 ICD-9-CM   ▶◀ Revised Text   ● New Line   ▲ Revised Code   Volume 2 — 215

Nonexanthematous tick fever 066.1
Nonexpansion, lung (newborn) NEC 770.4
Nonfunctioning
    cystic duct (see also Disease, gallbladder)
        575.8
    gallbladder (see also Disease, gallbladder)
        575.8
    kidney (see also Disease, renal) 593.9
    labyrinth 386.58
Nonhealing
    stump (surgical) 997.69
    wound, surgical 998.83
Nonimplantation of ovum, causing infertility 628.3
Noninsufflation, fallopian tube 628.2
Nonne-Milroy-Meige syndrome (chronic
    hereditary edema) 757.0
Nonovulation 628.0
Nonpatent fallopian tube 628.2
Nonpneumatization, lung NEC 770.4
Nonreflex bladder 596.54
    with cauda equina 344.61
Nonretention of food — see Vomiting
Nonrotation — see Malrotation
Nonsecretion, urine — see also Anuria 788.5
    newborn 753.3
Nonunion
    fracture 733.82
    organ or site, congenital NEC — see Imperfect, closure
    symphysis pubis, congenital 755.69
    top sacrum, congenital 756.19
Nonviability 765.0 ☑
Nonvisualization, gallbladder 793.3
Nonvitalized tooth 522.9
Non-working side interference 524.56
Normal
    delivery — see category 650
    menses V65.5
    state (feared complaint unfounded) V65.5
Normoblastosis 289.89

Normocytic anemia (infectional) 285.9
    due to blood loss (chronic) 280.0
    acute 285.1
Norrie's disease (congenital) (progressive
    oculoacousticocerebral degeneration)
    743.8
North American blastomycosis 116.0
Norwegian itch 133.0
Nosebleed 784.7
Nose, nasal — see condition
Nosomania 298.9
Nosophobia 300.29
Nostalgia 309.89
Notched lip, congenital — see also Cleft, lip
    749.10
Notching nose, congenital (tip) 748.1
Notch of iris 743.46
Nothnagel's
    syndrome 378.52
    vasomotor acroparesthesia 443.89
Novy's relapsing fever (American) 087.1
Noxious
    foodstuffs, poisoning by
        fish 988.0
        fungi 988.1
        mushrooms 988.1
        plants (food) 988.2
        shellfish 988.0
        specified type NEC 988.8
        toadstool 988.1
    substances transmitted through placenta
        or breast milk (affecting fetus or
        newborn) 760.70
        acetretin 760.78
        alcohol 760.71
        aminopterin 760.78
        antiandrogens 760.79
        anticonvulsant 760.77
        antifungal 760.74
        anti-infective agents 760.74
        antimetabolic 760.78

Noxious — continued
    substances transmitted through placenta or
        breast milk — continued
        atorvastatin 760.78
        carbamazepine 760.77
        cocaine 760.75
        "crack" 760.75
        diethylstilbestrol (DES) 760.76
        divalproex sodium 760.77
        endocrine disrupting chemicals 760.79
        estrogens 760.79
        etretinate 760.78
        fluconazole 760.74
        fluvastatin 760.78
        hallucinogenic agents NEC 760.73
        hormones 760.79
        lithium 760.79
        lovastatin 760.78
        medicinal agents NEC 760.79
        methotrexate 760.78
        misoprostil 760.79
        narcotics 760.72
        obstetric anesthetic or analgesic 763.5
        phenobarbital 760.77
        phenytoin 760.77
        pravastatin 760.78
        progestins 760.79
        retinoic acid 760.78
        simvastatin 760.78
        solvents 760.79
        specified agent NEC 760.79
        statins 760.78
        suspected, affecting management of
            pregnancy 655.5 ☑
        tetracycline 760.74
        thalidomide 760.79
        trimethadione 760.77
        valproate 760.77
        valproic acid 760.77
        vitamin A 760.78
NPDH (new persistent daily headache) 339.42

Nuchal hitch (arm) 652.8 ☑
Nucleus pulposus — see condition
Numbness 782.0
Nuns' knee 727.2
Nursemaid's
    elbow 832.2
    shoulder 831.0 ☑
Nutmeg liver 573.8
Nutrition, deficient or insufficient (particular
    kind of food) 269.9
    due to
        insufficient food 994.2
        lack of
            care (child) (infant) 995.52
            adult 995.84
        food 994.2
Nyctalopia — see also Blindness, night 368.60
    vitamin A deficiency 264.5
Nycturia 788.43
    psychogenic 306.53
Nymphomania 302.89
Nystagmus 379.50
    associated with vestibular system disorders
        379.54
    benign paroxysmal positional 386.11
    central positional 386.2
    congenital 379.51
    deprivation 379.53
    dissociated 379.55
    latent 379.52
    miners' 300.89
    positional
        benign paroxysmal 386.11
        central 386.2
    specified NEC 379.56
    vestibular 379.54
    visual deprivation 379.53

☑ **Additional Digit Required — Refer to the Tabular List for Digit Selection**   ▽ **Subterms under main terms may continue to next column or page**

216 — Volume 2   ▶◀ Revised Text   ● New Line   ▲ Revised Code   **2015 ICD-9-CM**

O

Oasthouse urine disease 270.2
Obermeyer's relapsing fever (European) 087.0
Obesity (constitutional) (exogenous) (familial) (nutritional) (simple) 278.00
  adrenal 255.8
  complicating pregnancy, childbirth, or puerperium 649.1 ☑
  due to hyperalimentation 278.00
  endocrine NEC 259.9
  endogenous 259.9
  Fröhlich's (adiposogenital dystrophy) 253.8
  glandular NEC 259.9
  hypothyroid (see also Hypothyroidism) 244.9
  hypoventilation syndrome 278.03
  morbid 278.01
  of pregnancy 649.1 ☑
  pituitary 253.8
  severe 278.01
  thyroid (see also Hypothyroidism) 244.9
Oblique — see also condition
  lie before labor, affecting fetus or newborn 761.7
Obliquity, pelvis 738.6
Obliteration
  abdominal aorta 446.7
  appendix (lumen) 543.9
  artery 447.1
  ascending aorta 446.7
  bile ducts 576.8
    with calculus, choledocholithiasis, or stones — see Choledocholithiasis
    congenital 751.61
      jaundice from 751.61 [774.5]
  common duct 576.8
    with calculus, choledocholithiasis, or stones — see Choledocholithiasis
    congenital 751.61
  cystic duct 575.8
    with calculus, choledocholithiasis, or stones — see Choledocholithiasis
  disease, arteriolar 447.1
  endometrium 621.8
  eye, anterior chamber 360.34
  fallopian tube 628.2
  lymphatic vessel 457.1
    postmastectomy 457.0
  organ or site, congenital NEC — see Atresia
  placental blood vessels — see Placenta, abnormal
  supra-aortic branches 446.7
  ureter 593.89
  urethra 599.84
  vein 459.9
  vestibule (oral) 525.8
Observation (for) V71.9
  without need for further medical care V71.9
  accident NEC V71.4
    at work V71.3
  criminal assault V71.6
  deleterious agent ingestion V71.89
  disease V71.9
    cardiovascular V71.7
    heart V71.7
    mental V71.09
    specified condition NEC V71.89
  foreign body ingestion V71.89
  growth and development variations V21.8
  injuries (accidental) V71.4
    inflicted NEC V71.6
      during alleged rape or seduction V71.5
  malignant neoplasm, suspected V71.1
  postpartum
    immediately after delivery V24.0
    routine follow-up V24.2
  pregnancy
    high-risk V23.9
      inconclusive fetal viability V23.87
      specified problem NEC V23.89
    normal (without complication) V22.1
      with nonobstetric complication V22.2
      first V22.0
  rape or seduction, alleged V71.5
    injury during V71.5

Observation — continued
  suicide attempt, alleged V71.89
  suspected (undiagnosed) (unproven)
    abuse V71.81
    cardiovascular disease V71.7
    child or wife battering victim V71.6
    concussion (cerebral) V71.6
    condition NEC V71.89
      infant — see Observation, suspected, condition, newborn
      maternal and fetal
        amniotic cavity and membrane problem V89.01
        cervical shortening V89.05
        fetal anomaly V89.03
        fetal growth problem V89.04
        oligohydramnios V89.01
        other specified problem NEC V89.09
        placental problem V89.02
        polyhydramnios V89.01
      newborn V29.9
        cardiovascular disease V29.8
        congenital anomaly V29.8
        genetic V29.3
        infectious V29.0
        ingestion foreign object V29.8
        injury V29.8
        metabolic V29.3
        neoplasm V29.8
        neurological V29.1
        poison, poisoning V29.8
        respiratory V29.2
        specified NEC V29.8
    exposure
      anthrax V71.82
      biologic agent NEC V71.83
      SARS V71.83
    infectious disease not requiring isolation V71.89
    malignant neoplasm V71.1
    mental disorder V71.09
    neglect V71.81
    neoplasm
      benign V71.89
      malignant V71.1
    specified condition NEC V71.89
    tuberculosis V71.2
  tuberculosis, suspected V71.2
Obsession, obsessional 300.3
  ideas and mental images 300.3
  impulses 300.3
  neurosis 300.3
  phobia 300.3
  psychasthenia 300.3
  ruminations 300.3
  state 300.3
  syndrome 300.3
Obsessive-compulsive 300.3
  neurosis 300.3
  personality 301.4
  reaction 300.3
Obstetrical trauma NEC (complicating delivery) 665.9 ☑
  with
    abortion — see Abortion, by type, with damage to pelvic organs
    ectopic pregnancy (see also categories 633.0–633.9) 639.2
    molar pregnancy (see also categories 630–632) 639.2
  affecting fetus or newborn 763.89
  following
    abortion 639.2
    ectopic or molar pregnancy 639.2
Obstipation — see also Constipation 564.00
  psychogenic 306.4
Obstruction, obstructed, obstructive
  airway NEC 519.8
    with
      allergic alveolitis NEC 495.9
      asthma NEC (see also Asthma) 493.9 ☑
      bronchiectasis 494.0
        with acute exacerbation 494.1

Obstruction, obstructed, obstructive — continued
  airway — continued
    with — continued
      bronchitis (chronic) (see also Bronchitis, with, obstruction) 491.20
      emphysema NEC 492.8
      chronic 496
        with
          allergic alveolitis NEC 495.5
          asthma NEC (see also Asthma) 493.2 ☑
          bronchiectasis 494.0
            with acute exacerbation 494.1
          bronchitis (chronic) (see also Bronchitis, with, obstruction) 491.20
          emphysema NEC 492.8
    due to
      bronchospasm 519.11
      foreign body 934.9
      inhalation of fumes or vapors 506.9
      laryngospasm 478.75
  alimentary canal (see also Obstruction, intestine) 560.9
  ampulla of Vater 576.2
    with calculus, cholelithiasis, or stones — see Choledocholithiasis
  aortic (heart) (valve) (see also Stenosis, aortic) 424.1
    rheumatic (see also Stenosis, aortic, rheumatic) 395.0
  aortoiliac 444.09
  aqueduct of Sylvius 331.4
    congenital 742.3
      with spina bifida (see also Spina bifida) 741.0 ☑
  Arnold-Chiari (see also Spina bifida) 741.0 ☑
  artery (see also Embolism, artery) 444.9
    basilar (complete) (partial) (see also Occlusion, artery, basilar) 433.0 ☑
    carotid (complete) (partial) (see also Occlusion, artery, carotid) 433.1 ☑
    precerebral — see Occlusion, artery, precerebral NEC
    retinal (central) (see also Occlusion, retina) 362.30
    vertebral (complete) (partial) (see also Occlusion, artery, vertebral) 433.2 ☑
  asthma (chronic) (with obstructive pulmonary disease) 493.2 ☑
  band (intestinal) 560.81
  bile duct or passage (see also Obstruction, biliary) 576.2
    congenital 751.61
      jaundice from 751.61 [774.5]
  biliary (duct) (tract) 576.2
    with calculus 574.51
      with cholecystitis (chronic) 574.41
        acute 574.31
    congenital 751.61
      jaundice from 751.61 [774.5]
    gallbladder 575.2
      with calculus 574.21
        with cholecystitis (chronic) 574.11
          acute 574.01
  bladder neck (acquired) 596.0
    congenital 753.6
  bowel (see also Obstruction, intestine) 560.9
  bronchus 519.19
  canal, ear (see also Stricture, ear canal, acquired) 380.50
  cardia 537.89
  caval veins (inferior) (superior) 459.2
  cecum (see also Obstruction, intestine) 560.9
  circulatory 459.9
  colon (see also Obstruction, intestine) 560.9
    sympathicotonic 560.89
  common duct (see also Obstruction, biliary) 576.2
    congenital 751.61
  coronary (artery) (heart) (see also Arteriosclerosis, coronary)
    acute (see also Infarct, myocardium) 410.9 ☑

Obstruction, obstructed, obstructive — continued
  coronary (see also Arteriosclerosis, coronary) — continued
    acute (see also Infarct, myocardium) — continued
      without myocardial infarction 411.81
  cystic duct (see also Obstruction, gallbladder) 575.2
    congenital 751.61
  device, implant, or graft — see Complications, due to (presence of) any device, implant, or graft classified to 996.0–996.5 NEC
  due to foreign body accidentally left in operation wound 998.4
  duodenum 537.3
    congenital 751.1
    due to
      compression NEC 537.3
      cyst 537.3
      intrinsic lesion or disease NEC 537.3
      scarring 537.3
      torsion 537.3
      ulcer 532.91
      volvulus 537.3
  ejaculatory duct 608.89
  endocardium 424.90
    arteriosclerotic 424.99
    specified cause, except rheumatic 424.99
  esophagus 530.3
  eustachian tube (complete) (partial) 381.60
    cartilaginous
      extrinsic 381.63
      intrinsic 381.62
    due to
      cholesteatoma 381.61
      osseous lesion NEC 381.61
      polyp 381.61
    osseous 381.61
  fallopian tube (bilateral) 628.2
  fecal 560.32
    with hernia (see also Hernia, by site, with obstruction)
      gangrenous — see Hernia, by site, with gangrene
  foramen of Monro (congenital) 742.3
    with spina bifida (see also Spina bifida) 741.0 ☑
  foreign body — see Foreign body
  gallbladder 575.2
    with calculus, cholelithiasis, or stones 574.21
      with cholecystitis (chronic) 574.11
        acute 574.01
    congenital 751.69
      jaundice from 751.69 [774.5]
  gastric outlet 537.0
  gastrointestinal (see also Obstruction, intestine) 560.9
  glottis 478.79
  hepatic 573.8
    duct (see also Obstruction, biliary) 576.2
      congenital 751.61
  icterus (see also Obstruction, biliary) 576.8
    congenital 751.61
  ileocecal coil (see also Obstruction, intestine) 560.9
  ileum (see also Obstruction, intestine) 560.9
  iliofemoral (artery) 444.81
  internal anastomosis — see Complications, mechanical, graft
  intestine (mechanical) (neurogenic) (paroxysmal) (postinfectional) (reflex) 560.9
    with
      adhesions (intestinal) (peritoneal) 560.81
      hernia (see also Hernia, by site, with obstruction)
        gangrenous — see Hernia, by site, with gangrene
    adynamic (see also Ileus) 560.1
    by gallstone 560.31
    congenital or infantile (small) 751.1
      large 751.2

Obstruction, obstructed, obstructive —
  continued
  intestine — *continued*
    due to
      Ascaris lumbricoides 127.0
      mural thickening 560.89
      procedure 997.49
        involving urinary tract 997.5
    impaction 560.32
    infantile — *see* Obstruction, intestine, congenital
    newborn
      due to
        fecaliths 777.1
        inspissated milk 777.2
        meconium (plug) 777.1
          in mucoviscidosis 277.01
        transitory 777.4
      specified cause NEC 560.89
      transitory, newborn 777.4
    volvulus 560.2
  intracardiac ball valve prosthesis 996.02
  jaundice (*see also* Obstruction, biliary) 576.8
    congenital 751.61
  jejunum (*see also* Obstruction, intestine) 560.9
  kidney 593.89
  labor 660.9 ☑
    affecting fetus or newborn 763.1
    by
      bony pelvis (conditions classifiable to 653.0–653.9) 660.1 ☑
      deep transverse arrest 660.3 ☑
      impacted shoulder 660.4 ☑
      locked twins 660.5 ☑
      malposition (fetus) (conditions classifiable to 652.0–652.9) 660.0 ☑
        head during labor 660.3 ☑
      persistent occipitoposterior position 660.3 ☑
      soft tissue, pelvic (conditions classifiable to 654.0–654.9) 660.2 ☑
  lacrimal
    canaliculi 375.53
      congenital 743.65
      punctum 375.52
      sac 375.54
  lacrimonasal duct 375.56
    congenital 743.65
    neonatal 375.55
  lacteal, with steatorrhea 579.2
  laryngitis (*see also* Laryngitis) 464.01
  larynx 478.79
    congenital 748.3
  liver 573.8
    cirrhotic (*see also* Cirrhosis, liver) 571.5
  lung 518.89
    with
      asthma — *see* Asthma
      bronchitis (chronic) 491.20
      emphysema NEC 492.8
    airway, chronic 496
    chronic NEC 496
      with
        asthma (chronic) (obstructive) 493.2 ☑
    disease, chronic 496
      with
        asthma (chronic) (obstructive) 493.2 ☑
    emphysematous 492.8
  lymphatic 457.1
  meconium
    fetus or newborn 777.1
      in mucoviscidosis 277.01
    newborn due to fecaliths 777.1
  mediastinum 519.3
  mitral (rheumatic) — *see* Stenosis, mitral
  nasal 478.19
    duct 375.56
      neonatal 375.55
    sinus — *see* Sinusitis
  nasolacrimal duct 375.56
    congenital 743.65
    neonatal 375.55

Obstruction, obstructed, obstructive —
  continued
  nasopharynx 478.29
  nose 478.19
  organ or site, congenital NEC — *see* Atresia
  pancreatic duct 577.8
  parotid gland 527.8
  pelviureteral junction (*see also* Obstruction, ureter) 593.4
  pharynx 478.29
  portal (circulation) (vein) 452
  prostate 600.90
    with
      other lower urinary tract symptoms (LUTS) 600.91
      urinary
        obstruction 600.91
        retention 600.91
    valve (urinary) 596.0
  pulmonary
    valve (heart) (*see also* Endocarditis, pulmonary) 424.3
    vein, isolated 747.49
  pyemic — *see* Septicemia
  pylorus (acquired) 537.0
    congenital 750.5
    infantile 750.5
  rectosigmoid (*see also* Obstruction, intestine) 560.9
  rectum 569.49
  renal 593.89
  respiratory 519.8
    chronic 496
  retinal (artery) (vein) (central) (*see also* Occlusion, retina) 362.30
  salivary duct (any) 527.8
    with calculus 527.5
  sigmoid (*see also* Obstruction, intestine) 560.9
  sinus (accessory) (nasal) (*see also* Sinusitis) 473.9
  Stensen's duct 527.8
  stomach 537.89
    acute 536.1
    congenital 750.7
  submaxillary gland 527.8
    with calculus 527.5
  thoracic duct 457.1
  thrombotic — *see* Thrombosis
  tooth eruption 520.6
  trachea 519.19
  tracheostomy airway 519.09
  tricuspid — *see* Endocarditis, tricuspid
  upper respiratory, congenital 748.8
  ureter (functional) 593.4
    congenital 753.20
    due to calculus 592.1
  ureteropelvic junction, congenital 753.21
  ureterovesical junction, congenital 753.22
  urethra 599.60
    congenital 753.6
  urinary (moderate) 599.60
    organ or tract (lower) 599.60
      due to
        benign prostatic hypertrophy (BPH) - see category 600
      specified NEC 599.69
        due to
          benign prostatic hypertrophy (BPH) — see category 600
    prostatic valve 596.0
  uropathy 599.60
  uterus 621.8
  vagina 623.2
  valvular — *see* Endocarditis
  vascular graft or shunt 996.1
    atherosclerosis — *see* Arteriosclerosis, coronary
    embolism 996.74
    occlusion NEC 996.74
    thrombus 996.74
  vein, venous 459.2
    caval (inferior) (superior) 459.2
    thrombotic — *see* Thrombosis
  vena cava (inferior) (superior) 459.2

Obstruction, obstructed, obstructive —
  continued
  ventricular shunt 996.2
  vesical 596.0
  vesicourethral orifice 596.0
  vessel NEC 459.9
Obturator — *see* condition
Occlusal
  plane deviation 524.76
  wear, teeth 521.10
Occlusion
  anus 569.49
    congenital 751.2
    infantile 751.2
  aortoiliac (chronic) 444.09
  aqueduct of Sylvius 331.4
    congenital 742.3
      with spina bifida (*see also* Spina bifida) 741.0
  arteries of extremities, lower 444.22
    without thrombus or embolus (*see also* Arteriosclerosis, extremities) 440.20
    due to stricture or stenosis 447.1
    upper 444.21
      without thrombus or embolus (*see also* Arteriosclerosis, extremities) 440.20
      due to stricture or stenosis 447.1
  artery NEC (*see also* Embolism, artery) 444.9
    auditory, internal 433.8 ☑
    basilar 433.0 ☑
      with other precerebral artery 433.3 ☑
      bilateral 433.3 ☑
    brain or cerebral (*see also* Infarct, brain) 434.9 ☑
    carotid 433.1 ☑
      with other precerebral artery 433.3 ☑
      bilateral 433.3 ☑
    cerebellar (anterior inferior) (posterior inferior) (superior) 433.8 ☑
    cerebral (*see also* Infarct, brain) 434.9 ☑
    choroidal (anterior) 433.8 ☑
    chronic total
      coronary 414.2
      extremity(ies) 440.4
    communicating posterior 433.8 ☑
    complete
      coronary 414.2
      extremity(ies) 440.4
    coronary (thrombotic) (*see also* Infarct, myocardium) 410.9 ☑
      acute 410.9 ☑
        without myocardial infarction 411.81
      chronic total 414.2
      complete 414.2
      healed or old 412
      total 414.2
    extremity(ies)
      chronic total 440.4
      complete 440.4
      total 440.4
    hypophyseal 433.8 ☑
    iliac (artery) 444.81
    mesenteric (embolic) (thrombotic) (with gangrene) 557.0
    pontine 433.8 ☑
    precerebral NEC 433.9 ☑
      late effect — *see* Late effect(s) (of) cerebrovascular disease
      multiple or bilateral 433.3 ☑
      puerperal, postpartum, childbirth 674.0 ☑
      specified NEC 433.8 ☑
    renal 593.81
    retinal — *see* Occlusion, retina, artery
    spinal 433.8 ☑
    vertebral 433.2 ☑
      with other precerebral artery 433.3 ☑
      bilateral 433.3 ☑

Occlusion — *continued*
  basilar (artery) — *see* Occlusion, artery, basilar
  bile duct (any) (*see also* Obstruction, biliary) 576.2
  bowel (*see also* Obstruction, intestine) 560.9
  brain (artery) (vascular) (*see also* Infarct, brain) 434.9 ☑
  breast (duct) 611.89
  carotid (artery) (common) (internal) — *see* Occlusion, artery, carotid
  cerebellar (anterior inferior) (artery) (posterior inferior) (superior) 433.8 ☑
  cerebral (artery) (*see also* Infarct, brain) 434.9 ☑
  cerebrovascular (*see also* Infarct, brain) 434.9 ☑
    diffuse 437.0
  cervical canal (*see also* Stricture, cervix) 622.4
    by falciparum malaria 084.0
  cervix (uteri) (*see also* Stricture, cervix) 622.4
  choanal 748.0
  choroidal (artery) 433.8 ☑
  colon (*see also* Obstruction, intestine) 560.9
  communicating posterior artery 433.8 ☑
  coronary (artery) (thrombotic) (*see also* Infarct, myocardium) 410.9 ☑
    without myocardial infarction 411.81
    acute 410.9 ☑
      without myocardial infarction 411.81
    healed or old 412
  cystic duct (*see also* Obstruction, gallbladder) 575.2
    congenital 751.69
  disto
    division I 524.22
    division II 524.22
  embolic — *see* Embolism
  fallopian tube 628.2
    congenital 752.19
  gallbladder (*see also* Obstruction, gallbladder) 575.2
    congenital 751.69
      jaundice from 751.69 [774.5]
  gingiva, traumatic 523.8
  hymen 623.3
    congenital 752.42
  hypophyseal (artery) 433.8 ☑
  iliac artery 444.81
  intestine (*see also* Obstruction, intestine) 560.9
  kidney 593.89
  lacrimal apparatus — *see* Stenosis, lacrimal
  lung 518.89
  lymph or lymphatic channel 457.1
  mammary duct 611.89
  mesenteric artery (embolic) (thrombotic) (with gangrene) 557.0
  nose 478.1 ☑
    congenital 748.0
  organ or site, congenital NEC — *see* Atresia
  oviduct 628.2
    congenital 752.19
  periodontal, traumatic 523.8
  peripheral arteries (lower extremity) 444.22
    without thrombus or embolus (*see also* Arteriosclerosis, extremities) 440.20
    due to stricture or stenosis 447.1
    upper extremity 444.21
      without thrombus or embolus (*see also* Arteriosclerosis, extremities) 440.20
      due to stricture or stenosis 447.1
  pontine (artery) 433.8 ☑
  posterior lingual, of mandibular teeth 524.29
  precerebral artery — *see* Occlusion, artery, precerebral NEC
  puncta lacrimalia 375.52
  pupil 364.74
  pylorus (*see also* Stricture, pylorus) 537.0
  renal artery 593.81
  retina, retinal (vascular) 362.30
    artery, arterial 362.30

☑ **Additional Digit Required** — Refer to the Tabular List for Digit Selection ▽ **Subterms under main terms may continue to next column or page**

218 — Volume 2 ▶◀ Revised Text ● New Line ▲ Revised Code 2015 ICD-9-CM

Occlusion — *continued*
  retina, retinal — *continued*
    artery, arterial — *continued*
      branch 362.32
      central (total) 362.31
      partial 362.33
      transient 362.34
      tributary 362.32
    vein 362.30
      branch 362.36
      central (total) 362.35
      incipient 362.37
      partial 362.37
      tributary 362.36
  spinal artery 433.8 ✓
  stent
    coronary 996.72
  teeth (mandibular) (posterior lingual) 524.29
  thoracic duct 457.1
  tubal 628.2
  ureter (complete) (partial) 593.4
    congenital 753.29
  urethra (*see also* Stricture, urethra) 598.9
    congenital 753.6
  uterus 621.8
  vagina 623.2
  vascular NEC 459.9
  vein — *see* Thrombosis
  vena cava
    inferior 453.2
    superior (acute) 453.87
      chronic 453.77
  ventricle (brain) NEC 331.4
  vertebral (artery) — *see* Occlusion, artery, vertebral
  vessel (blood) NEC 459.9
  vulva 624.8
Occlusio pupillae 364.74
Occupational
  problems NEC V62.29
  therapy V57.21
Ochlophobia 300.29
Ochronosis (alkaptonuric) (congenital) (endogenous) 270.2
  with chloasma of eyelid 270.2
Ocular muscle — *see also* condition
  myopathy 359.1
  torticollis 781.93
Oculoauriculovertebral dysplasia 756.0
Oculogyric
  crisis or disturbance 378.87
    psychogenic 306.7
Oculomotor syndrome 378.81
Oddi's sphincter spasm 576.5
Odelberg's disease (juvenile osteochondrosis) 732.1
Odontalgia 525.9
Odontoameloblastoma (M9311/0) 213.1
  upper jaw (bone) 213.0
Odontoclasia 521.05
Odontoclasis 873.63
  complicated 873.73
Odontodysplasia, regional 520.4
Odontogenesis imperfecta 520.5
Odontoma (M9280/0) 213.1
  ameloblastic (M9311/0) 213.1
    upper jaw (bone) 213.0
  calcified (M9280/0) 213.1
    upper jaw (bone) 213.0
  complex (M9282/0) 213.1
    upper jaw (bone) 213.0
  compound (M9281/0) 213.1
    upper jaw (bone) 213.0
  fibroameloblastic (M9290/0) 213.1
    upper jaw (bone) 213.0
  follicular 526.0
    upper jaw (bone) 213.0
Odontomyelitis (closed) (open) 522.0
Odontonecrosis 521.09
Odontorrhagia 525.8
Odontosarcoma, ameloblastic (M9290/3) 170.1
  upper jaw (bone) 170.0
Odynophagia 787.20
Oesophagostomiasis 127.7
Oesophagostomum infestation 127.7

Oestriasis 134.0
Ogilvie's syndrome (sympathicotonic colon obstruction) 560.89
Oguchi's disease (retina) 368.61
Ohara's disease — *see also* Tularemia 021.9
Oidiomycosis — *see also* Candidiasis 112.9
Oidiomycotic meningitis 112.83
Oidium albicans infection — *see also* Candidiasis 112.9
Old age 797
  dementia (of) 290.0
Olfactory — *see* condition
Oligemia 285.9
Oligergasia — *see also* Disability, intellectual 319
Oligoamnios 658.0 ✓
  affecting fetus or newborn 761.2
Oligoastrocytoma, mixed (M9382/3)
  specified site — *see* Neoplasm, by site, malignant
  unspecified site 191.9
Oligocythemia 285.9
Oligodendroblastoma (M9460/3)
  specified site — *see* Neoplasm, by site, malignant
  unspecified site 191.9
Oligodendroglioma (M9450/3)
  anaplastic type (M9451/3)
    specified site — *see* Neoplasm, by site, malignant
    unspecified site 191.9
  specified site — *see* Neoplasm, by site, malignant
  unspecified site 191.9
Oligodendroma — *see* Oligodendroglioma
Oligodontia — *see also* Anodontia 520.0
Oligoencephalon 742.1
Oligohydramnios 658.0 ✓
  affecting fetus or newborn 761.2
  due to premature rupture of membranes 658.1 ✓
    affecting fetus or newborn 761.2
Oligohydrosis 705.0
Oligomenorrhea 626.1
Oligophrenia — *see also* Disability, intellectual 319
  phenylpyruvic 270.1
Oligospermia 606.1
Oligotrichia 704.09
  congenita 757.4
Oliguria 788.5
  with
    abortion — *see* Abortion, by type, with renal failure
    ectopic pregnancy (*see also* categories 633.0–633.9) 639.3
    molar pregnancy (*see also* categories 630–632) 639.3
  complicating
    abortion 639.3
    ectopic or molar pregnancy 639.3
    pregnancy 646.2 ✓
      with hypertension — *see* Toxemia, of pregnancy
  due to a procedure 997.5
  following labor and delivery 669.3 ✓
  heart or cardiac — *see* Failure, heart
  puerperal, postpartum 669.3 ✓
  specified due to a procedure 997.5
Ollier's disease (chondrodysplasia) 756.4
Omentitis — *see also* Peritonitis 567.9
Omentocele — *see also* Hernia, omental 553.8
Omentum, omental — *see* condition
Omphalitis (congenital) (newborn) 771.4
  not of newborn 686.9
  tetanus 771.3
Omphalocele 756.72
Omphalomesenteric duct, persistent 751.0
Omphalorrhagia, newborn 772.3
Omsk hemorrhagic fever 065.1
Onanism 307.9
Onchocerciasis 125.3
  eye 125.3 *[360.13]*
Onchocercosis 125.3
Oncocytoma (M8290/0) — *see* Neoplasm, by site, benign

Ondine's curse 348.89
Oneirophrenia — *see also* Schizophrenia 295.4 ✓
Onychauxis 703.8
  congenital 757.5
Onychia (with lymphangitis) 681.9
  dermatophytic 110.1
  finger 681.02
  toe 681.11
Onychitis (with lymphangitis) 681.9
  finger 681.02
  toe 681.11
Onychocryptosis 703.0
Onychodystrophy 703.8
  congenital 757.5
Onychogryphosis 703.8
Onychogryposis 703.8
Onycholysis 703.8
Onychomadesis 703.8
Onychomalacia 703.8
Onychomycosis 110.1
  finger 110.1
  toe 110.1
Onycho-osteodysplasia 756.89
Onychophagy 307.9
Onychoptosis 703.8
Onychorrhexis 703.8
  congenital 757.5
Onychoschizia 703.8
Onychotrophia — *see also* Atrophy, nail 703.8
O'nyong-nyong fever 066.3
Onyxis (finger) (toe) 703.0
Onyxitis (with lymphangitis) 681.9
  finger 681.02
  toe 681.11
Oocyte (egg) (ovum)
  donor V59.70
    over age 35 V59.73
      anonymous recipient V59.73
      designated recipient V59.74
    under age 35 V59.71
      anonymous recipient V59.71
      designated recipient V59.72
Oophoritis (cystic) (infectional) (interstitial) — *see also* Salpingo-oophoritis 614.2
  complicating pregnancy 646.6 ✓
  fetal (acute) 752.0
  gonococcal (acute) 098.19
    chronic or duration of 2 months or over 098.39
  tuberculous (*see also* Tuberculosis) 016.6 ✓
Opacity, opacities
  cornea 371.00
    central 371.03
    congenital 743.43
      interfering with vision 743.42
    degenerative (*see also* Degeneration, cornea) 371.40
    hereditary (*see also* Dystrophy, cornea) 371.50
    inflammatory (*see also* Keratitis) 370.9
    late effect of trachoma (healed) 139.1
    minor 371.01
    peripheral 371.02
  enamel (fluoride) (nonfluoride) (teeth) 520.3
  lens (*see also* Cataract) 366.9
  snowball 379.22
  vitreous (humor) 379.24
    congenital 743.51
Opalescent dentin (hereditary) 520.5
Open, opening
  abnormal, organ or site, congenital — *see* Imperfect, closure
  angle
    with
      borderline findings
        high risk 365.05
        intraocular pressure 365.01
        low risk 365.01
      cupping of discs 365.01
    high risk 365.05
    low risk 365.01
  bite
    anterior 524.24
    posterior 524.25
  false — *see* Imperfect, closure

Open, opening — *continued*
  margin on tooth restoration 525.61
    restoration margins 525.61
  wound — *see* Wound, open, by site
Operation
  causing mutilation of fetus 763.89
  destructive, on live fetus, to facilitate birth 763.89
  for delivery, fetus or newborn 763.89
  maternal, unrelated to current delivery, affecting fetus or newborn (*see also* Newborn, affected by) 760.64
Operational fatigue 300.89
Operative — *see* condition
Operculitis (chronic) 523.40
  acute 523.30
Operculum, retina 361.32
  with detachment 361.01
Ophiasis 704.01
Ophthalmia — *see also* Conjunctivitis 372.30
  actinic rays 370.24
  allergic (acute) 372.05
    chronic 372.14
  blennorrhagic (neonatorum) 098.40
  catarrhal 372.03
  diphtheritic 032.81
  Egyptian 076.1
  electric, electrica 370.24
  gonococcal (neonatorum) 098.40
  metastatic 360.11
  migraine 346.8 ✓
  neonatorum, newborn 771.6
    gonococcal 098.40
  nodosa 360.14
  phlyctenular 370.31
    with ulcer (*see also* Ulcer, cornea) 370.00
  sympathetic 360.11
Ophthalmitis — *see* Ophthalmia
Ophthalmocele (congenital) 743.66
Ophthalmoneuromyelitis 341.0
Ophthalmopathy, infiltrative with thyrotoxicosis 242.0 ✓
Ophthalmoplegia — *see also* Strabismus 378.9
  anterior internuclear 378.86
  ataxia-areflexia syndrome 357.0
  bilateral 378.9
  diabetic 250.5 ✓ *[378.86]*
    due to secondary diabetes 249.5 ✓ *[378.86]*
  exophthalmic 242.0 ✓ *[376.22]*
  external 378.55
    progressive 378.72
    total 378.56
  internal (complete) (total) 367.52
  internuclear 378.86
  migraine 346.2 ✓
  painful 378.55
  Parinaud's 378.81
  progressive external 378.72
  supranuclear, progressive 333.0
  total (external) 378.56
    internal 367.52
  unilateral 378.9
Opisthognathism 524.00
Opisthorchiasis (felineus) (tenuicollis) (viverrini) 121.0
Opisthotonos, opisthotonus 781.0
Opitz's disease (congestive splenomegaly) 289.51
Opiumism — *see also* Dependence 304.0 ✓
Oppenheim's disease 358.8
Oppenheim-Urbach disease or syndrome (necrobiosis lipoidica diabeticorum) 250.8 ✓ *[709.3]*
  due to secondary diabetes 249.8 ✓ *[709.3]*
Opsoclonia 379.59
Optic nerve — *see* condition
Orbit — *see* condition
Orchioblastoma (M9071/3) 186.9
Orchitis (nonspecific) (septic) 604.90
  with abscess 604.0
  blennorrhagic (acute) 098.13
    chronic or duration of 2 months or over 098.33
  diphtheritic 032.89 *[604.91]*
  filarial 125.9 *[604.91]*

✓ **Additional Digit Required** — Refer to the Tabular List for Digit Selection   ᵂ **Subterms under main terms may continue to next column or page**

Orchitis — continued
  gangrenous 604.99
  gonococcal (acute) 098.13
    chronic or duration of 2 months or over 098.33
  mumps 072.0
  parotidea 072.0
  suppurative 604.99
  syphilitic 095.8 [604.91]
  tuberculous (see also Tuberculosis)
    016.5 ☑ [608.81]
Orf 051.2
Organic — see also condition
  heart — see Disease, heart
  insufficiency 799.89
Oriental
  bilharziasis 120.2
  schistosomiasis 120.2
  sore 085.1
Orientation
  ego-dystonic sexual 302.0
Orifice — see condition
Origin, both great vessels from right ventricle 745.11
Ormond's disease or syndrome 593.4
Ornithosis 073.9
  with
    complication 073.8
      specified NEC 073.7
    pneumonia 073.0
    pneumonitis (lobular) 073.0
Orodigitofacial dysostosis 759.89
Oropouche fever 066.3
Orotaciduria, oroticaciduria (congenital) (hereditary) (pyrimidine deficiency) 281.4
Oroya fever 088.0
Orthodontics V58.5
  adjustment V53.4
  aftercare V58.5
  fitting V53.4
Orthopnea 786.02
Orthoptic training V57.4
Osgood-Schlatter
  disease 732.4
  osteochondrosis 732.4
Osler's
  disease (M9950/1) (polycythemia vera) 238.4
  nodes 421.0
Osler-Rendu disease (familial hemorrhagic telangiectasia) 448.0
Osler-Vaquez disease (M9950/1) (polycythemia vera) 238.4
Osler-Weber-Rendu syndrome (familial hemorrhagic telangiectasia) 448.0
Osmidrosis 705.89
Osseous — see condition
Ossification
  artery — see Arteriosclerosis
  auricle (ear) 380.39
  bronchus 519.19
  cardiac (see also Degeneration, myocardial) 429.1
  cartilage (senile) 733.99
  coronary (artery) — see Arteriosclerosis, coronary
  diaphragm 728.10
  ear 380.39
    middle (see also Otosclerosis) 387.9
  falx cerebri 349.2
  fascia 728.10
  fontanel
    defective or delayed 756.0
    premature 756.0
  heart (see also Degeneration, myocardial) 429.1
    valve — see Endocarditis
  larynx 478.79
  ligament
    posterior longitudinal 724.8
      cervical 723.7
  meninges (cerebral) 349.2
    spinal 336.8
  multiple, eccentric centers 733.99
  muscle 728.10

Ossification — continued
  muscle — continued
    heterotopic, postoperative 728.13
  myocardium, myocardial (see also Degeneration, myocardial) 429.1
  penis 607.81
  periarticular 728.89
  sclera 379.16
  tendon 727.82
  trachea 519.19
  tympanic membrane (see also Tympanosclerosis) 385.00
  vitreous (humor) 360.44
Osteitis — see also Osteomyelitis 730.2 ☑
  acute 730.0 ☑
  alveolar 526.5
  chronic 730.1 ☑
  condensans (ilii) 733.5
  deformans (Paget's) 731.0
    due to or associated with malignant neoplasm (see also Neoplasm, bone, malignant) 170.9 [731.1]
  due to yaws 102.6
  fibrosa NEC 733.29
    cystica (generalisata) 252.01
    disseminata 756.59
    osteoplastica 252.01
  fragilitans 756.51
  Garré's (sclerosing) 730.1 ☑
  infectious (acute) (subacute) 730.0 ☑
    chronic or old 730.1 ☑
  jaw (acute) (chronic) (lower) (neonatal) (suppurative) (upper) 526.4
  parathyroid 252.01
  petrous bone (see also Petrositis) 383.20
  pubis 733.5
  sclerotic, nonsuppurative 730.1 ☑
  syphilitic 095.5
  tuberculosa
    cystica (of Jüngling) 135
    multiplex cystoides 135
Osteoarthritica spondylitis (spine) — see also Spondylosis 721.90
Osteoarthritis — see also Osteoarthrosis 715.9 ☑
  distal interphalangeal 715.9 ☑
  hyperplastic 731.2
  interspinalis 715.9 ☑
    spine (see also Spondylosis) 721.90
  spine, spinal NEC (see also Spondylosis) 721.90
Osteoarthropathy — see also Osteoarthrosis 715.9 ☑
  chronic idiopathic hypertrophic 757.39
  familial idiopathic 757.39
  hypertrophic pulmonary 731.2
    secondary 731.2
  idiopathic hypertrophic 757.39
  primary hypertrophic 731.2
  pulmonary hypertrophic 731.2
  secondary hypertrophic 731.2
Osteoarthrosis (degenerative) (hypertrophic) (rheumatoid) 715.9 ☑

> *Note* — Use the following fifth-digit subclassification with category 715:
>
> 0   *site unspecified*
>
> 1   *shoulder region*
>
> 2   *upper arm*
>
> 3   *forearm*
>
> 4   *hand*
>
> 5   *pelvic region and thigh*
>
> 6   *lower leg*
>
> 7   *ankle and foot*
>
> 8   *other specified sites except spine*
>
> 9   *multiple sites*

  Deformans alkaptonurica 270.2
  generalized 715.09
  juvenilis (Köhler's) 732.5
  localized 715.3 ☑
    idiopathic 715.1 ☑
    primary 715.1 ☑

Osteoarthrosis — continued
  localized — continued
    secondary 715.2 ☑
  multiple sites, not specified as generalized 715.89
  polyarticular 715.09
  spine (see also Spondylosis) 721.90
  temporomandibular joint 524.69
Osteoblastoma (M9200/0) — see Neoplasm, bone, benign
Osteochondritis — see also Osteochondrosis 732.9
  dissecans 732.7
    hip 732.7
  ischiopubica 732.1
  multiple 756.59
  syphilitic (congenital) 090.0
Osteochondrodermodysplasia 756.59
Osteochondrodystrophy 277.5
  deformans 277.5
  familial 277.5
  fetalis 756.4
Osteochondrolysis 732.7
Osteochondroma (M9210/0) — see also Neoplasm, bone, benign
  multiple, congenital 756.4
Osteochondromatosis (M9210/1) 238.0
  synovial 727.82
Osteochondromyxosarcoma (M9180/3) — see Neoplasm, bone, malignant
Osteochondropathy NEC 732.9
Osteochondrosarcoma (M9180/3) — see Neoplasm, bone, malignant
Osteochondrosis 732.9
  acetabulum 732.1
  adult spine 732.8
  astragalus 732.5
  Blount's 732.4
  Buchanan's (juvenile osteochondrosis of iliac crest) 732.1
  Buchman's (juvenile osteochondrosis) 732.1
  Burns' 732.3
  calcaneus 732.5
  capitular epiphysis (femur) 732.1
  carpal
    lunate (wrist) 732.3
    scaphoid 732.3
  coxae juvenilis 732.1
  deformans juvenilis (coxae) (hip) 732.1
    Scheuermann's 732.0
    spine 732.0
    tibia 732.4
    vertebra 732.0
  Diaz's (astragalus) 732.5
  dissecans (knee) (shoulder) 732.7
  femoral capital epiphysis 732.1
  femur (head) (juvenile) 732.1
  foot (juvenile) 732.5
  Freiberg's (disease) (second metatarsal) 732.5
  Haas' 732.3
  Haglund's (os tibiale externum) 732.5
  hand (juvenile) 732.3
  head of
    femur 732.1
    humerus (juvenile) 732.3
  hip (juvenile) 732.1
  humerus (juvenile) 732.3
  iliac crest (juvenile) 732.1
  ilium (juvenile) 732.1
  ischiopubic synchondrosis 732.1
  Iselin's (osteochondrosis fifth metatarsal) 732.5
  juvenile, juvenilis 732.6
    arm 732.3
    capital femoral epiphysis 732.1
    capitellum humeri 732.3
    capitular epiphysis 732.1
    carpal scaphoid 732.3
    clavicle, sternal epiphysis 732.6
    coxae 732.1
    deformans 732.1
    foot 732.5
    hand 732.3
    hip and pelvis 732.1
    lower extremity, except foot 732.4

Osteochondrosis — continued
  juvenile, juvenilis — continued
    lunate, wrist 732.3
    medial cuneiform bone 732.5
    metatarsal (head) 732.5
    metatarsophalangeal 732.5
    navicular, ankle 732.5
    patella 732.4
    primary patellar center (of Köhler) 732.4
    specified site NEC 732.6
    spine 732.0
    tarsal scaphoid 732.5
    tibia (epiphysis) (tuberosity) 732.4
    upper extremity 732.3
    vertebra (body) (Calvé) 732.0
      epiphyseal plates (of Scheuermann) 732.0
  Kienböck's (disease) 732.3
  Köhler's (disease) (navicular, ankle) 732.5
    patellar 732.4
    tarsal navicular 732.5
  Legg-Calvé-Perthes (disease) 732.1
  lower extremity (juvenile) 732.4
  lunate bone 732.3
  Mauclaire's 732.3
  metacarpal heads (of Mauclaire) 732.3
  metatarsal (fifth) (head) (second) 732.5
  navicular, ankle 732.5
  os calcis 732.5
  Osgood-Schlatter 732.4
  os tibiale externum 732.5
  Panner's 732.3
  patella (juvenile) 732.4
  patellar center
    primary (of Köhler) 732.4
    secondary (of Sinding-Larsen) 732.4
  pelvis (juvenile) 732.1
  Pierson's 732.1
  radial head (juvenile) 732.3
  Scheuermann's 732.0
  Sever's (calcaneum) 732.5
  Sinding-Larsen (secondary patellar center) 732.4
  spine (juvenile) 732.0
    adult 732.8
  symphysis pubis (of Pierson) (juvenile) 732.1
  syphilitic (congenital) 090.0
  tarsal (navicular) (scaphoid) 732.5
  tibia (proximal) (tubercle) 732.4
  tuberculous — see Tuberculosis, bone
  ulna 732.3
  upper extremity (juvenile) 732.3
  van Neck's (juvenile osteochondrosis) 732.1
  vertebral (juvenile) 732.0
    adult 732.8
Osteoclastoma (M9250/1) 238.0
  malignant (M9250/3) — see Neoplasm, bone, malignant
Osteocopic pain 733.90
Osteodynia 733.90
Osteodystrophy
  azotemic 588.0
  chronica deformans hypertrophica 731.0
  congenital 756.50
    specified type NEC 756.59
  deformans 731.0
  fibrosa localisata 731.0
  parathyroid 252.01
  renal 588.0
Osteofibroma (M9262/0) — see Neoplasm, bone, benign
Osteofibrosarcoma (M9182/3) — see Neoplasm, bone, malignant
Osteogenesis imperfecta 756.51
Osteogenic — see condition
Osteoma (M9180/0) — see also Neoplasm, bone, benign
  osteoid (M9191/0) (see also Neoplasm, bone, benign)
    giant (M9200/0) — see Neoplasm, bone, benign
Osteomalacia 268.2
  chronica deformans hypertrophica 731.0
  due to vitamin D deficiency 268.2
  infantile (see also Rickets) 268.0
  juvenile (see also Rickets) 268.0

☑ **Additional Digit Required** — Refer to the Tabular List for Digit Selection   🖝 **Subterms under main terms may continue to next column or page**

220 — Volume 2   ▶◀ Revised Text   ● New Line   ▲ Revised Code   2015 ICD-9-CM

Osteomalacia — continued
  oncogenic 275.8
  pelvis 268.2
  vitamin D-resistant 275.3
Osteomalacic bone 268.2
Osteomalacosis 268.2
Osteomyelitis (general) (infective) (localized) (neonatal) (purulent) (pyogenic) (septic) (staphylococcal) (streptococcal) (suppurative) (with periostitis) 730.2 ☑

> Note — Use the following fifth-digit subclassification with category 730:
>
> 0   site unspecified
> 1   shoulder region
> 2   upper arm
> 3   forearm
> 4   hand
> 5   pelvic region and thigh
> 6   lower leg
> 7   ankle and foot
> 8   other specified sites
> 9   multiple sites

  acute or subacute 730.0 ☑
  chronic or old 730.1 ☑
  due to or associated with
    diabetes mellitus 250.8 *[731.8]*
      due to secondary diabetes 249.8 ☑ *[731.8]*
    tuberculosis (see also Tuberculosis, bone) 015.9 ☑ *[730.8]* ☑
      limb bones 015.5 ☑ *[730.8]* ☑
      specified bones NEC 015.7 ☑ *[730.8]* ☑
      spine 015.0 ☑ *[730.8]* ☑
    typhoid 002.0 *[730.8]* ☑
  Garré's 730.1 ☑
  jaw (acute) (chronic) (lower) (neonatal) (suppurative) (upper) 526.4
  nonsuppurating 730.1 ☑
  orbital 376.03
  petrous bone (see also Petrositis) 383.20
  Salmonella 003.24
  sclerosing, nonsuppurative 730.1 ☑
  sicca 730.1 ☑
  syphilitic 095.5
    congenital 090.0 *[730.8]* ☑
  tuberculous — see Tuberculosis, bone
  typhoid 002.0 *[730.8]* ☑
Osteomyelofibrosis 289.89
Osteomyelosclerosis 289.89
Osteonecrosis 733.40
  meaning osteomyelitis 730.1 ☑
Osteo-onycho-arthro dysplasia 756.89
Osteo-onychodysplasia, hereditary 756.89
Osteopathia
  condensans disseminata 756.53
  hyperostotica multiplex infantilis 756.59
  hypertrophica toxica 731.2
  striata 756.4
Osteopathy resulting from poliomyelitis — see also Poliomyelitis 045.9 ☑ *[730.7]* ☑
  familial dysplastic 731.2
Osteopecilia 756.53
Osteopenia 733.90
  borderline 733.90
Osteoperiostitis — see also Osteomyelitis 730.2 ☑
  ossificans toxica 731.2
  toxica ossificans 731.2
Osteopetrosis (familial) 756.52
Osteophyte — see Exostosis
Osteophytosis — see Exostosis
Osteopoikilosis 756.53
Osteoporosis (generalized) 733.00
  circumscripta 731.0
  disuse 733.03
  drug-induced 733.09
  idiopathic 733.02
  postmenopausal 733.01
  posttraumatic 733.7

Osteoporosis — continued
  screening V82.81
  senile 733.01
  specified type NEC 733.09
Osteoporosis-osteomalacia syndrome 268.2
Osteopsathyrosis 756.51
Osteoradionecrosis, jaw 526.89
Osteosarcoma (M9180/3) — see also Neoplasm, bone, malignant
  chondroblastic (M9181/3) — see Neoplasm, bone, malignant
  fibroblastic (M9182/3) — see Neoplasm, bone, malignant
  in Paget's disease of bone (M9184/3) — see Neoplasm, bone, malignant
  juxtacortical (M9190/3) — see Neoplasm, bone, malignant
  parosteal (M9190/3) — see Neoplasm, bone, malignant
  telangiectatic (M9183/3) — see Neoplasm, bone, malignant
Osteosclerosis 756.52
  fragilis (generalisata) 756.52
Osteosclerotic anemia 289.89
Osteosis
  acromegaloid 757.39
  cutis 709.3
  parathyroid 252.01
  renal fibrocystic 588.0
Österreicher-Turner syndrome 756.89
Ostium
  atrioventriculare commune 745.69
  primum (arteriosum) (defect) (persistent) 745.61
  secundum (arteriosum) (defect) (patent) (persistent) 745.5
Ostrum-Furst syndrome 756.59
Os, uterus — see condition
Otalgia 388.70
  otogenic 388.71
  referred 388.72
Othematoma 380.31
Otitic hydrocephalus 348.2
Otitis 382.9
  with effusion 381.4
    purulent 382.4
    secretory 381.4
    serous 381.4
    suppurative 382.4
  acute 382.9
  adhesive (see also Adhesions, middle ear) 385.10
  chronic 382.9
    with effusion 381.3
    mucoid, mucous (simple) 381.20
    purulent 382.3
    secretory 381.3
    serous 381.10
    suppurative 382.3
  diffuse parasitic 136.8
  externa (acute) (diffuse) (hemorrhagica) 380.10
    actinic 380.22
    candidal 112.82
    chemical 380.22
    chronic 380.23
      mycotic — see Otitis, externa, mycotic
      specified type NEC 380.23
    circumscribed 380.10
    contact 380.22
    due to
      erysipelas 035 *[380.13]*
      impetigo 684 *[380.13]*
      seborrheic dermatitis 690.10 *[380.13]*
    eczematoid 380.22
    furuncular 680.0 *[380.13]*
    infective 380.10
      chronic 380.16
    malignant 380.14
    mycotic (chronic) 380.15
      due to
        aspergillosis 117.3 *[380.15]*
        moniliasis 112.82
        otomycosis 111.8 *[380.15]*
    reactive 380.22

Otitis — continued
  externa — continued
    specified type NEC 380.22
    tropical 111.8 *[380.15]*
  insidiosa (see also Otosclerosis) 387.9
  interna (see also Labyrinthitis) 386.30
  media (hemorrhagic) (staphylococcal) (streptococcal) 382.9
    acute 382.9
      with effusion 381.00
      allergic 381.04
        mucoid 381.05
        sanguineous 381.06
        serous 381.04
      catarrhal 381.00
      exudative 381.00
      mucoid 381.02
        allergic 381.05
      necrotizing 382.00
        with spontaneous rupture of ear drum 382.01
        in
          influenza (see also Influenza) 487.8 *[382.02]*
          measles 055.2
          scarlet fever 034.1 *[382.02]*
      nonsuppurative 381.00
      purulent 382.00
        with spontaneous rupture of ear drum 382.01
      sanguineous 381.03
        allergic 381.06
      secretory 381.01
      seromucinous 381.02
      serous 381.01
        allergic 381.04
      suppurative 382.00
        with spontaneous rupture of ear drum 382.01
        due to
          influenza (see also Influenza) 487.8 *[382.02]*
          scarlet fever 034.1 *[382.02]*
      transudative 381.00
    adhesive (see also Adhesions, middle ear) 385.10
    allergic 381.4
      acute 381.04
        mucoid 381.05
        sanguineous 381.06
        serous 381.04
      chronic 381.3
    catarrhal 381.4
      acute 381.00
      chronic (simple) 381.10
    chronic 382.9
      with effusion 381.3
      adhesive (see also Adhesions, middle ear) 385.10
      allergic 381.3
      atticoantral, suppurative (with posterior or superior marginal perforation of ear drum) 382.2
      benign suppurative (with anterior perforation of ear drum) 382.1
      catarrhal 381.10
      exudative 381.3
      mucinous 381.3
      mucoid, mucous (simple) 381.20
      mucosanguineous 381.29
      nonsuppurative 381.3
      purulent 382.3
      secretory 381.3
      seromucinous 381.3
      serosanguineous 381.19
      serous (simple) 381.10
      suppurative 382.3
        atticoantral (with posterior or superior marginal perforation of ear drum) 382.2
        benign (with anterior perforation of ear drum) 382.1
        tuberculous (see also Tuberculosis) 017.4 ☑
      tubotympanic 382.1
      transudative 381.3

Otitis — continued
  media — continued
    exudative 381.4
      acute 381.00
      chronic 381.3
    fibrotic (see also Adhesions, middle ear) 385.10
    mucoid, mucous 381.4
      acute 381.02
      chronic (simple) 381.20
    mucosanguineous, chronic 381.29
    nonsuppurative 381.4
      acute 381.00
      chronic 381.3
    postmeasles 055.2
    purulent 382.4
      acute 382.00
        with spontaneous rupture of ear drum 382.01
      chronic 382.3
    sanguineous, acute 381.03
      allergic 381.06
    secretory 381.4
      acute or subacute 381.01
      chronic 381.3
    seromucinous 381.4
      acute or subacute 381.02
      chronic 381.3
    serosanguineous, chronic 381.19
    serous 381.4
      acute or subacute 381.01
      chronic (simple) 381.10
    subacute — see Otitis, media, acute
    suppurative 382.4
      acute 382.00
        with spontaneous rupture of ear drum 382.01
      chronic 382.3
        atticoantral 382.2
        benign 382.1
        tuberculous (see also Tuberculosis) 017.4 ☑
        tubotympanic 382.1
    transudative 381.4
      acute 381.00
      chronic 381.3
    tuberculous (see also Tuberculosis) 017.4 ☑
  postmeasles 055.2
Otoconia 386.8
Otolith syndrome 386.19
Otomycosis 111.8 *[380.15]*
  in
    aspergillosis 117.3 *[380.15]*
    moniliasis 112.82
Otopathy 388.9
Otoporosis — see also Otosclerosis 387.9
Otorrhagia 388.69
  traumatic — see nature of injury
Otorrhea 388.60
  blood 388.69
  cerebrospinal (fluid) 388.61
Otosclerosis (general) 387.9
  cochlear (endosteal) 387.2
  involving
    otic capsule 387.2
    oval window
      nonobliterative 387.0
      obliterative 387.1
    round window 387.2
  nonobliterative 387.0
  obliterative 387.1
  specified type NEC 387.8
Otospongiosis — see also Otosclerosis 387.9
Otto's disease or pelvis 715.35
Outburst, aggressive — see also Disturbance, conduct 312.0 ☑
  in children or adolescents 313.9
Outcome of delivery
  multiple birth NEC V27.9
    all liveborn V27.5
    all stillborn V27.7
    some liveborn V27.6
    unspecified V27.9
  single V27.9
    liveborn V27.0

☑ **Additional Digit Required** — Refer to the Tabular List for Digit Selection   ▽ **Subterms under main terms may continue to next column or page**

Outcome of delivery — *continued*
  single — *continued*
    stillborn V27.1
    twins V27.9
      both liveborn V27.2
      both stillborn V27.4
      one liveborn, one stillborn V27.3
Outlet — *see* condition
  syndrome (thoracic) 353.0
Outstanding ears (bilateral) 744.29
Ovalocytosis (congenital) (hereditary) — *see also* Elliptocytosis 282.1
Ovarian — *see also* condition
  pregnancy — *see* Pregnancy, ovarian
  remnant syndrome 620.8
  vein syndrome 593.4
Ovaritis (cystic) — *see also* Salpingo-oophoritis 614.2
Ovary, ovarian — *see* condition
Overactive — *see also* Hyperfunction
  bladder 596.51
  eye muscle (*see also* Strabismus) 378.9
  hypothalamus 253.8
  thyroid (*see also* Thyrotoxicosis) 242.9 ☑
Overactivity, child 314.01
Overbite (deep) (excessive) (horizontal) (vertical) 524.29
Overbreathing — *see also* Hyperventilation 786.01
Overconscientious personality 301.4
Overdevelopment — *see also* Hypertrophy
  breast (female) (male) 611.1
  nasal bones 738.0
  prostate, congenital 752.89
Overdistention — *see* Distention
Overdose overdosage (drug) 977.9
  specified drug or substance — *see* Table of Drugs and Chemicals
Overeating 783.6
  nonorganic origin 307.51
Overexertion (effects) (exhaustion) 994.5
Overexposure (effects) 994.9
  exhaustion 994.4
Overfeeding — *see also* Overeating 783.6
Overfill, endodontic 526.62
Overgrowth, bone NEC 733.99
Overhanging
  tooth restoration 525.62
  unrepairable, dental restorative materials 525.62
Overheated (effects) (places) — *see* Heat
Overinhibited child 313.0
Overjet 524.29
  excessive horizontal 524.26
Overlaid, overlying (suffocation) 994.7
Overlap
  excessive horizontal 524.26
Overlapping toe (acquired) 735.8
  congenital (fifth toe) 755.66
Overload
  fluid 276.69
    due to transfusion (blood) (blood components) 276.61
  iron, due to repeated red blood cell transfusions 275.02
  potassium (K) 276.7
  sodium (Na) 276.0
  transfusion associated circulatory (TACO) 276.61
Overnutrition — *see also* Hyperalimentation 783.6
Overproduction — *see also* Hypersecretion
  ACTH 255.3
  cortisol 255.0
  growth hormone 253.0
  thyroid-stimulating hormone (TSH) 242.8 ☑
Overriding
  aorta 747.21
  finger (acquired) 736.29
    congenital 755.59
  toe (acquired) 735.8
    congenital 755.66
Oversize
  fetus (weight of 4500 grams or more) 766.0
    affecting management of pregnancy 656.6 ☑

Oversize — *continued*
  fetus — *continued*
    causing disproportion 653.5 ☑
      with obstructed labor 660.1 ☑
    affecting fetus or newborn 763.1
Overstimulation, ovarian 256.1
Overstrained 780.79
  heart — *see* Hypertrophy, cardiac
Overweight — *see also* Obesity 278.02
Overwork 780.79
Oviduct — *see* condition
Ovotestis 752.7
Ovulation (cycle)
  failure or lack of 628.0
  pain 625.2
Ovum
  blighted 631.8
  donor V59.70
    over age 35 V59.73
      anonymous recipient V59.73
      designated recipient V59.74
    under age 35 V59.71
      anonymous recipient V59.71
      designated recipient V59.72
  dropsical 631.8
  pathologic 631.8
Owren's disease or syndrome (parahemophilia) — *see also* Defect, coagulation 286.3
Oxalosis 271.8
Oxaluria 271.8
Ox heart — *see* Hypertrophy, cardiac
OX syndrome 758.6
Oxycephaly, oxycephalic 756.0
  syphilitic, congenital 090.0
Oxyuriasis 127.4
Oxyuris vermicularis (infestation) 127.4
Ozena 472.0

P

Pacemaker syndrome 429.4
Pachyderma, pachydermia 701.8
  laryngis 478.5
  laryngitis 478.79
  larynx (verrucosa) 478.79
Pachydermatitis 701.8
Pachydermatocele (congenital) 757.39
  acquired 701.8
Pachydermatosis 701.8
Pachydermoperiostitis
  secondary 731.2
Pachydermoperiostosis
  primary idiopathic 757.39
  secondary 731.2
Pachymeningitis (adhesive) (basal) (brain) (cerebral) (cervical) (chronic) (circumscribed) (external) (fibrous) (hemorrhagic) (hypertrophic) (internal) (purulent) (spinal) (suppurative) — *see also* Meningitis 322.9
  gonococcal 098.82
Pachyonychia (congenital) 757.5
  acquired 703.8
Pachyperiosteodermia
  primary or idiopathic 757.39
  secondary 731.2
Pachyperiostosis
  primary or idiopathic 757.39
  secondary 731.2
Pacinian tumor (M9507/0) — *see* Neoplasm, skin, benign
Pads, knuckle or Garrod's 728.79
Paget's disease (osteitis deformans) 731.0
  with infiltrating duct carcinoma of the breast (M8541/3) — *see* Neoplasm, breast, malignant
  bone 731.0
    osteosarcoma in (M9184/3) — *see* Neoplasm, bone, malignant
  breast (M8540/3) 174.0
  extramammary (M8542/3) (*see also* Neoplasm, skin, malignant)
    anus 154.3
    skin 173.59
  malignant (M8540/3)
    breast 174.0

Paget's disease — *continued*
  malignant — *continued*
    specified site NEC (M8542/3) — *see* Neoplasm, skin, malignant
    unspecified site 174.0
  mammary (M8540/3) 174.0
  necrosis of bone 731.0
  nipple (M8540/3) 174.0
  osteitis deformans 731.0
Paget-Schroetter syndrome (intermittent venous claudication) 453.89
Pain(s) — *see also* Painful 780.96
  abdominal 789.0 ☑
  acute 338.19
    due to trauma 338.11
    postoperative 338.18
      post-thoracotomy 338.12
  adnexa (uteri) 625.9
  alimentary, due to vascular insufficiency 557.9
  anginoid (*see also* Pain, precordial) 786.51
  anus 569.42
  arch 729.5
  arm 729.5
  axillary 729.5
  back (postural) 724.5
    low 724.2
    psychogenic 307.89
  bile duct 576.9
  bladder 788.99
  bone 733.90
  breast 611.71
    psychogenic 307.89
  broad ligament 625.9
  cancer associated 338.3
  cartilage NEC 733.90
  cecum 789.0 ☑
  cervicobrachial 723.3
  chest (central) 786.50
    atypical 786.59
    midsternal 786.51
    musculoskeletal 786.59
    noncardiac 786.59
    substernal 786.51
    wall (anterior) 786.52
  chronic 338.29
    associated with significant psychosocial dysfunction 338.4
    due to trauma 338.21
    postoperative 338.28
      post-thoracotomy 338.22
    syndrome 338.4
  coccyx 724.79
  colon 789.0 ☑
  common duct 576.9
  coronary — *see* Angina
  costochondral 786.52
  diaphragm 786.52
  due to (presence of) any device, implant, or graft classifiable to 996.0–996.5 — *see* Complications, due to (presence of) any device, implant, or graft classified to 996.0–996.5 NEC
  malignancy (primary) (secondary) 338.3
  ear (*see also* Otalgia) 388.70
  epigastric, epigastrium 789.06
  extremity (lower) (upper) 729.5
  eye 379.91
  face, facial 784.0
    atypical 350.2
    nerve 351.8
  false (labor) 644.1 ☑
  female genital organ NEC 625.9
    psychogenic 307.89
  finger 729.5
  flank 789.0 ☑
  foot 729.5
  gallbladder 575.9
  gas (intestinal) 787.3
  gastric 536.8
  generalized 780.96
  genital organ
    female 625.9
    male 608.9
    psychogenic 307.89
  groin 789.0 ☑

Pain(s) — *see also* Painful — *continued*
  growing 781.99
  hand 729.5
  head (*see also* Headache) 784.0
  heart (see also Pain, precordial) 786.51
  infraorbital (*see also* Neuralgia, trigeminal) 350.1
  intermenstrual 625.2
  jaw 784.92
  joint 719.40
    ankle 719.47
    elbow 719.42
    foot 719.47
    hand 719.44
    hip 719.45
    knee 719.46
    multiple sites 719.49
    pelvic region 719.45
    psychogenic 307.89
    shoulder (region) 719.41
    specified site NEC 719.48
    wrist 719.43
  kidney 788.0
  labor, false or spurious 644.1 ☑
  laryngeal 784.1
  leg 729.5
  limb 729.5
  low back 724.2
  lumbar region 724.2
  mandible, mandibular 784.92
  mastoid (*see also* Otalgia) 388.70
  maxilla 784.92
  menstrual 625.3
  metacarpophalangeal (joint) 719.44
  metatarsophalangeal (joint) 719.47
  mouth 528.9
  muscle 729.1
    intercostal 786.59
  musculoskeletal (see also Pain, by site) 729.1
  nasal 478.19
  nasopharynx 478.29
  neck NEC 723.1
    psychogenic 307.89
  neoplasm related (acute) (chronic) 338.3
  nerve NEC 729.2
  neuromuscular 729.1
  nose 478.19
  ocular 379.91
  ophthalmic 379.91
  orbital region 379.91
  osteocopic 733.90
  ovary 625.9
    psychogenic 307.89
  over heart (*see also* Pain, precordial) 786.51
  ovulation 625.2
  pelvic (female) 625.9
    male NEC 789.0 ☑
      psychogenic 307.89
    psychogenic 307.89
  penis 607.9
    psychogenic 307.89
  pericardial (*see also* Pain, precordial) 786.51
  perineum
    female 625.9
    male 608.9
  pharynx 478.29
  pleura, pleural, pleuritic 786.52
  postoperative 338.18
    acute 338.18
    chronic 338.28
  post-thoracotomy 338.12
    acute 338.12
    chronic 338.22
  preauricular 388.70
  precordial (region) 786.51
    psychogenic 307.89
  premenstrual 625.4
  psychogenic 307.80
    cardiovascular system 307.89
    gastrointestinal system 307.89
    genitourinary system 307.89
    heart 307.89
    musculoskeletal system 307.89
    respiratory system 307.89
    skin 306.3
  radicular (spinal) (*see also* Radiculitis) 729.2

☑ **Additional Digit Required — Refer to the Tabular List for Digit Selection**   ⬚ **Subterms under main terms may continue to next column or page**

Pain(s) — *see also* Painful — *continued*
rectum 569.42
respiration 786.52
retrosternal 786.51
rheumatic NEC 729.0
muscular 729.1
rib 786.50
root (spinal) (*see also* Radiculitis) 729.2
round ligament (stretch) 625.9
sacroiliac 724.6
sciatic 724.3
scrotum 608.9
psychogenic 307.89
seminal vesicle 608.9
sinus 478.19
skin 782.0
spermatic cord 608.9
spinal root (*see also* Radiculitis) 729.2
stomach 536.8
psychogenic 307.89
substernal 786.51
testis 608.9
psychogenic 307.89
thoracic spine 724.1
with radicular and visceral pain 724.4
throat 784.1
tibia 733.90
toe 729.5
tongue 529.6
tooth 525.9
total hip replacement 996.77
total knee replacement 996.77
trigeminal (*see also* Neuralgia, trigeminal) 350.1
tumor associated 338.3
umbilicus 789.05
ureter 788.0
urinary (organ) (system) 788.0
uterus 625.9
psychogenic 307.89
vagina 625.9
vertebrogenic (syndrome) 724.5
vesical 788.99
vulva 625.9
xiphoid 733.90
Painful — *see also* Pain
arc syndrome 726.19
coitus
female 625.0
male 608.89
psychogenic 302.76
ejaculation (semen) 608.89
psychogenic 302.79
erection 607.3
feet syndrome 266.2
menstruation 625.3
psychogenic 306.52
micturition 788.1
ophthalmoplegia 378.55
respiration 786.52
scar NEC 709.2
urination 788.1
wire sutures 998.89
Painters' colic 984.9
specified type of lead — *see* Table of Drugs and Chemicals
Palate — *see* condition
Palatoplegia 528.9
Palatoschisis — *see also* Cleft, palate 749.00
Palilalia 784.69
Palindromic arthritis — *see also* Rheumatism, palindromic 719.3 ☑
Palliative care V66.7
Pallor 782.61
temporal, optic disc 377.15
Palmar — *see also* condition
fascia — *see* condition
Palpable
cecum 569.89
kidney 593.89
liver 573.9
lymph nodes 785.6
ovary 620.8
prostate 602.9
spleen (*see also* Splenomegaly) 789.2
uterus 625.8

Palpitation (heart) 785.1
psychogenic 306.2
Palsy — *see also* Paralysis 344.9
atrophic diffuse 335.20
Bell's 351.0
newborn 767.5
birth 767.7
brachial plexus 353.0
fetus or newborn 767.6
brain (*see also* Palsy, cerebral)
noncongenital or noninfantile 344.89
late effect — *see* Late effect(s) (of) cerebrovascular disease
syphilitic 094.89
congenital 090.49
bulbar (chronic) (progressive) 335.22
pseudo NEC 335.23
supranuclear NEC 344.8 ☑
cerebral (congenital) (infantile) (spastic) 343.9
athetoid 333.71
diplegic 343.0
late effect — *see* Late effect(s) (of) cerebrovascular disease
hemiplegic 343.1
monoplegic 343.3
noncongenital or noninfantile 437.8
late effect — *see* Late effect(s) (of) cerebrovascular disease
paraplegic 343.0
quadriplegic 343.2
spastic, not congenital or infantile 344.89
syphilitic 094.89
congenital 090.49
tetraplegic 343.2
cranial nerve (*see also* Disorder, nerve, cranial)
multiple 352.6
creeping 335.21
divers' 993.3
Erb's (birth injury) 767.6
facial 351.0
newborn 767.5
glossopharyngeal 352.2
Klumpke (-Déjérine) 767.6
lead 984.9
specified type of lead — *see* Table of Drugs and Chemicals
median nerve (tardy) 354.0
peroneal nerve (acute) (tardy) 355.3
progressive supranuclear 333.0
pseudobulbar NEC 335.23
radial nerve (acute) 354.3
seventh nerve 351.0
newborn 767.5
shaking (*see also* Parkinsonism) 332.0
spastic (cerebral) (spinal) 343.9
hemiplegic 343.1
specified nerve NEC — *see* Disorder, nerve
supranuclear NEC 356.8
progressive 333.0
ulnar nerve (tardy) 354.2
wasting 335.21
Paltauf-Sternberg disease 201.9 ☑
Paludism — *see* Malaria
Panama fever 084.0
Panaris (with lymphangitis) 681.9
finger 681.02
toe 681.11
Panaritium (with lymphangitis) 681.9
finger 681.02
toe 681.11
Panarteritis (nodosa) 446.0
brain or cerebral 437.4
Pancake heart 793.2
with cor pulmonale (chronic) 416.9
Pancarditis (acute) (chronic) 429.89
with
rheumatic
fever (active) (acute) (chronic) (subacute) 391.8
inactive or quiescent 398.99
rheumatic, acute 391.8
chronic or inactive 398.99

Pancoast's syndrome or tumor (carcinoma, pulmonary apex) (M8010/3) 162.3
Pancoast-Tobias syndrome (M8010/3) (carcinoma, pulmonary apex) 162.3
Pancolitis 556.6
Pancreas, pancreatic — *see* condition
Pancreatitis 577.0
acute (edematous) (hemorrhagic) (recurrent) 577.0
annular 577.0
apoplectic 577.0
calcerceous 577.0
chronic (infectious) 577.1
recurrent 577.1
cystic 577.2
fibrous 577.8
gangrenous 577.0
hemorrhagic (acute) 577.0
interstitial (chronic) 577.1
acute 577.0
malignant 577.0
mumps 072.3
painless 577.1
recurrent 577.1
relapsing 577.1
subacute 577.0
suppurative 577.0
syphilitic 095.8
Pancreatolithiasis 577.8
Pancytolysis 289.9
Pancytopenia (acquired) 284.19
with
malformations 284.09
myelodysplastic syndrome — *see* Syndrome, myelodysplastic
congenital 284.09
due to
antineoplastic chemotherapy 284.11
drug, specified NEC 284.12
specified NEC 284.19
Panencephalitis — *see also* Encephalitis
subacute, sclerosing 046.2
Panhematopenia 284.81
congenital 284.09
constitutional 284.09
splenic, primary 289.4
Panhemocytopenia 284.81
congenital 284.09
constitutional 284.09
Panhypogonadism 257.2
Panhypopituitarism 253.2
prepubertal 253.3
Panic (attack) (state) 300.01
reaction to exceptional stress (transient) 308.0
Panmyelopathy, familial constitutional 284.09
Panmyelophthisis 284.2
acquired (secondary) 284.81
congenital 284.2
idiopathic 284.9
Panmyelosis (acute) (M9951/1) 238.79
Panner's disease 732.3
capitellum humeri 732.3
head of humerus 732.3
tarsal navicular (bone) (osteochondrosis) 732.5
Panneuritis endemica 265.0 [357.4]
Panniculitis 729.30
back 724.8
knee 729.31
mesenteric 567.82
neck 723.6
nodular, nonsuppurative 729.30
sacral 724.8
specified site NEC 729.39
Panniculus adiposus (abdominal) 278.1
Pannus (corneal) 370.62
abdominal (symptomatic) 278.1
allergic eczematous 370.62
degenerativus 370.62
keratic 370.62
rheumatoid — *see* Arthritis, rheumatoid
trachomatosus, trachomatous (active) 076.1 [370.62]
late effect 139.1

Panophthalmitis 360.02
Panotitis — *see* Otitis media
Pansinusitis (chronic) (hyperplastic) (nonpurulent) (purulent) 473.8
acute 461.8
due to fungus NEC 117.9
tuberculous (*see also* Tuberculosis) 012.8 ☑
Panuveitis 360.12
sympathetic 360.11
Panvalvular disease — *see* Endocarditis, mitral
Papageienkrankheit 073.9
Papanicolaou smear
anus 796.70
with
atypical squamous cells
cannot exclude high grade squamous intraepithelial lesion (ASC-H) 796.72
of undetermined significance (ASC-US) 796.71
cytologic evidence of malignancy 796.76
high grade squamous intraepithelial lesion (HGSIL) 796.74
low grade squamous intraepithelial lesion (LGSIL) 796.73
glandular 796.70
specified finding NEC 796.79
unsatisfactory cytology 796.78
cervix (screening test) V76.2
as part of gynecological examination V72.31
for suspected malignant neoplasm V76.2
no disease found V71.1
inadequate cytology sample 795.08
nonspecific abnormal finding 795.00
with
atypical squamous cells
cannot exclude high grade squamous intraepithelial lesion (ASC-H) 795.02
of undetermined significance (ASC-US) 795.01
cytologic evidence of malignancy 795.06
high grade squamous intraepithelial lesion (HGSIL) 795.04
low grade squamous intraepithelial lesion (LGSIL) 795.03
nonspecific finding NEC 795.09
to confirm findings of recent normal smear following initial abnormal smear V72.32
satisfactory smear but lacking transformation zone 795.07
unsatisfactory cervical cytology 795.08
other specified site (*see also* Screening, malignant neoplasm)
for suspected malignant neoplasm (*see also* Screening, malignant neoplasm)
no disease found V71.1
nonspecific abnormal finding 796.9
vagina V76.47
with
atypical squamous cells
cannot exclude high grade squamous intraepithelial lesion (ASC-H) 795.12
of undetermined significance (ASC-US) 795.11
cytologic evidence of malignancy 795.16
high grade squamous intraepithelial lesion (HGSIL) 795.14
low grade squamous intraepithelial lesion (LGSIL) 795.13
abnormal NEC 795.19
following hysterectomy for malignant condition V67.01
inadequate cytology sample 795.18
unsatisfactory cytology 795.18
Papilledema 377.00
associated with
decreased ocular pressure 377.02

Papilledema — continued
  associated with — continued
    increased intracranial pressure 377.01
    retinal disorder 377.03
  choked disc 377.00
  infectional 377.00
Papillitis 377.31
  anus 569.49
  chronic lingual 529.4
  necrotizing, kidney 584.7
  optic 377.31
  rectum 569.49
  renal, necrotizing 584.7
  tongue 529.0
Papilloma (M8050/0) — see also Neoplasm, by site, benign

> Note — Except where otherwise indicated, the morphological varieties of papilloma in the list below should be coded by site as for "Neoplasm, benign."

  acuminatum (female) (male) 078.11
  bladder (urinary) (transitional cell) (M8120/1) 236.7
    benign (M8120/0) 223.3
  choroid plexus (M9390/0) 225.0
    anaplastic type (M9390/3) 191.5
    malignant (M9390/3) 191.5
  ductal (M8503/0)
  dyskeratotic (M8052/0)
  epidermoid (M8052/0)
  hyperkeratotic (M8052/0)
  intracystic (M8504/0)
  intraductal (M8503/0)
  inverted (M8053/0)
  keratotic (M8052/0)
  parakeratotic (M8052/0)
  pinta (primary) 103.0
  renal pelvis (transitional cell) (M8120/1) 236.99
    benign (M8120/0) 223.1
  Schneiderian (M8121/0)
    specified site — see Neoplasm, by site, benign
    unspecified site 212.0
  serous surface (M8461/0)
    borderline malignancy (M8461/1)
      specified site — see Neoplasm, by site, uncertain behavior
      unspecified site 236.2
    specified site — see Neoplasm, by site, benign
    unspecified site 220
  squamous (cell) (M8052/0)
  transitional (cell) (M8120/0)
    bladder (urinary) (M8120/1) 236.7
    inverted type (M8121/1) — see Neoplasm, by site, uncertain behavior
    renal pelvis (M8120/1) 236.91
    ureter (M8120/1) 236.91
  ureter (transitional cell) (M8120/1) 236.91
    benign (M8120/0) 223.2
  urothelial (M8120/1) — see Neoplasm, by site, uncertain behavior
  verrucous (M8051/0)
  villous (M8261/1) — see Neoplasm, by site, uncertain behavior
  yaws, plantar or palmar 102.1
Papillomata, multiple, of yaws 102.1
Papillomatosis (M8060/0) — see also Neoplasm, by site, benign
  confluent and reticulate 701.8
  cutaneous 701.8
  ductal, breast 610.1
  Gougerot-Carteaud (confluent reticulate) 701.8
  intraductal (diffuse) (M8505/0) — see Neoplasm, by site, benign
  subareolar duct (M8506/0) 217
Papillon-Léage and Psaume syndrome (orodigitofacial dysostosis) 759.89
Papule 709.8
  carate (primary) 103.0
  fibrous, of nose (M8724/0) 216.3
  pinta (primary) 103.0
Papulosis
  lymphomatoid 709.8

Papulosis — continued
  malignant 447.8
Papyraceous fetus 779.89
  complicating pregnancy 646.0 ☑
Paracephalus 759.7
Parachute mitral valve 746.5
Paracoccidioidomycosis 116.1
  mucocutaneous-lymphangitic 116.1
  pulmonary 116.1
  visceral 116.1
Paracoccidiomycosis — see Paracoccidioidomycosis
Paracusis 388.40
Paradentosis 523.5
Paradoxical facial movements 374.43
Paraffinoma 999.9
Paraganglioma (M8680/1)
  adrenal (M8700/0) 227.0
    malignant (M8700/3) 194.0
  aortic body (M8691/1) 237.3
    malignant (M8691/3) 194.6
  carotid body (M8692/1) 237.3
    malignant (M8692/3) 194.5
  chromaffin (M8700/0) (see also Neoplasm, by site, benign)
    malignant (M8700/3) — see Neoplasm, by site, malignant
  extra-adrenal (M8693/1)
    malignant (M8693/3)
      specified site — see Neoplasm, by site, malignant
      unspecified site 194.6
    specified site — see Neoplasm, by site, uncertain behavior
    unspecified site 237.3
  glomus jugulare (M8690/1) 237.3
    malignant (M8690/3) 194.6
  jugular (M8690/1) 237.3
    malignant (M8680/3)
      specified site — see Neoplasm, by site, malignant
      unspecified site 194.6
  nonchromaffin (M8693/1)
    malignant (M8693/3)
      specified site — see Neoplasm, by site, malignant
      unspecified site 194.6
    specified site — see Neoplasm, by site, uncertain behavior
    unspecified site 237.3
  parasympathetic (M8682/1)
    specified site — see Neoplasm, by site, uncertain behavior
    unspecified site 237.3
  specified site — see Neoplasm, by site, uncertain behavior
  sympathetic (M8681/1)
    specified site — see Neoplasm, by site, uncertain behavior
    unspecified site 237.3
  unspecified site 237.3
Parageusia 781.1
  psychogenic 306.7
Paragonimiasis 121.2
Paragranuloma, Hodgkin's (M9660/3) 201.0 ☑
Parahemophilia — see also Defect, coagulation 286.3
Parakeratosis 690.8
  psoriasiformis 696.2
  variegata 696.2
Paralysis, paralytic (complete) (incomplete) 344.9
  with
    broken
      back — see Fracture, vertebra, by site, with spinal cord injury
      neck — see Fracture, vertebra, cervical, with spinal cord injury
    fracture, vertebra — see Fracture, vertebra, by site, with spinal cord injury
    syphilis 094.89
  abdomen and back muscles 355.9
  abdominal muscles 355.9
  abducens (nerve) 378.54

Paralysis, paralytic — continued
  abductor 355.9
    lower extremity 355.8
    upper extremity 354.9
  accessory nerve 352.4
  accommodation 367.51
    hysterical 300.11
  acoustic nerve 388.5
  agitans 332.0
    arteriosclerotic 332.0
  alternating 344.89
    oculomotor 344.89
  amyotrophic 335.20
  ankle 355.8
  anterior serratus 355.9
  anus (sphincter) 569.49
  apoplectic (current episode) (see also Disease, cerebrovascular, acute) 436
    late effect — see Late effect(s) (of) cerebrovascular disease
  arm 344.40
    affecting
      dominant side 344.41
      nondominant side 344.42
    both 344.2
    hysterical 300.11
    late effect — see Late effect(s) (of) cerebrovascular disease
    psychogenic 306.0
      transient 781.4
      traumatic NEC (see also Injury, nerve, upper limb) 955.9
  arteriosclerotic (current episode) 437.0
    late effect — see Late effect(s) (of) cerebrovascular disease
  ascending (spinal), acute 357.0
  associated, nuclear 344.89
  asthenic bulbar 358.00
  ataxic NEC 334.9
    general 094.1
  athetoid 333.71
  atrophic 356.9
    infantile, acute (see also Poliomyelitis, with paralysis) 045.1 ☑
    muscle NEC 355.9
    progressive 335.21
    spinal (acute) (see also Poliomyelitis, with paralysis) 045.1 ☑
  attack (see also Disease, cerebrovascular, acute) 436
  axillary 353.0
  Babinski-Nageotte's 344.89
  Bell's 351.0
    newborn 767.5
  Benedikt's 344.89
  birth (injury) 767.7
    brain 767.0
    intracranial 767.0
    spinal cord 767.4
  bladder (sphincter) 596.53
    neurogenic 596.54
      with cauda equina syndrome 344.61
    puerperal, postpartum, childbirth 665.5 ☑
    sensory 596.54
      with cauda equina 344.61
    spastic 596.54
      with cauda equina 344.61
  bowel, colon, or intestine (see also Ileus) 560.1
  brachial plexus 353.0
    due to birth injury 767.6
    newborn 767.6
  brain
    congenital — see Palsy, cerebral
    current episode 437.8
    diplegia 344.2
    hemiplegia 342.9 ☑
      late effect — see Late effect(s) (of) cerebrovascular disease
    infantile — see Palsy, cerebral
    late effect — see Late effect(s) (of) cerebrovascular disease
    monoplegia (see also Monoplegia)
      late effect — see Late effect(s) (of) cerebrovascular disease

Paralysis, paralytic — continued
  brain — continued
    paraplegia 344.1
    quadriplegia — see Quadriplegia
    syphilitic, congenital 090.49
    triplegia 344.89
  bronchi 519.19
  Brown-Séquard's 344.89
  bulbar (chronic) (progressive) 335.22
    infantile (see also Poliomyelitis, bulbar) 045.0 ☑
    poliomyelitic (see also Poliomyelitis, bulbar) 045.0 ☑
    pseudo 335.23
    supranuclear 344.89
  bulbospinal 358.00
  cardiac (see also Failure, heart) 428.9
  cerebral
    current episode 437.8
    spastic, infantile — see Palsy, cerebral
  cerebrocerebellar 437.8
    diplegic infantile 343.0
  cervical
    plexus 353.2
    sympathetic NEC 337.09
  Céstan-Chenais 344.89
  Charcôt-Marie-Tooth type 356.1
  childhood — see Palsy, cerebral
  Clark's 343.9
  colon (see also Ileus) 560.1
  compressed air 993.3
  compression
    arm NEC 354.9
    cerebral — see Paralysis, brain
    leg NEC 355.8
    lower extremity NEC 355.8
    upper extremity NEC 354.9
  congenital (cerebral) (spastic) (spinal) — see Palsy, cerebral
  conjugate movement (of eye) 378.81
    cortical (nuclear) (supranuclear) 378.81
  convergence 378.83
  cordis (see also Failure, heart) 428.9
  cortical (see also Paralysis, brain) 437.8
  cranial or cerebral nerve (see also Disorder, nerve, cranial) 352.9
  creeping 335.21
  crossed leg 344.89
  crutch 953.4
  deglutition 784.99
    hysterical 300.11
  dementia 094.1
  descending (spinal) NEC 335.9
  diaphragm (flaccid) 519.4
    due to accidental section of phrenic nerve during procedure 998.2
  digestive organs NEC 564.89
  diplegic — see Diplegia
  divergence (nuclear) 378.85
  divers' 993.3
  Duchenne's 335.22
  due to intracranial or spinal birth injury — see Palsy, cerebral
  embolic (current episode) (see also Embolism, brain) 434.1 ☑
    late effect — see Late effect(s) (of) cerebrovascular disease
  enteric (see also Ileus) 560.1
    with hernia — see Hernia, by site, with obstruction
  Erb (-Duchenne) (birth) (newborn) 767.6
  Erb's syphilitic spastic spinal 094.89
  esophagus 530.89
  essential, infancy (see also Poliomyelitis) 045.9 ☑
  extremity
    lower — see Paralysis, leg
    spastic (hereditary) 343.3
      noncongenital or noninfantile 344.1
    transient (cause unknown) 781.4
    upper — see Paralysis, arm
  eye muscle (extrinsic) 378.55
    intrinsic 367.51
  facial (nerve) 351.0
    birth injury 767.5
    congenital 767.5

☑ **Additional Digit Required** — Refer to the Tabular List for Digit Selection   ▽ **Subterms under main terms may continue to next column or page**

224 — Volume 2   ▶◀ **Revised Text**   ● **New Line**   ▲ **Revised Code**   **2015 ICD-9-CM**

Paralysis, paralytic — *continued*
- facial — *continued*
  - following operation NEC 998.2
  - newborn 767.5
- familial 359.3
  - periodic 359.3
  - spastic 334.1
- fauces 478.29
- finger NEC 354.9
- foot NEC 355.8
- gait 781.2
- gastric nerve 352.3
- gaze 378.81
- general 094.1
  - ataxic 094.1
  - insane 094.1
  - juvenile 090.40
  - progressive 094.1
  - tabetic 094.1
- glossopharyngeal (nerve) 352.2
- glottis (*see also* Paralysis, vocal cord) 478.30
- gluteal 353.4
- Gubler (-Millard) 344.89
- hand 354.9
  - hysterical 300.11
  - psychogenic 306.0
- heart (*see also* Failure, heart) 428.9
- hemifacial, progressive 349.89
- hemiplegic — *see* Hemiplegia
- hyperkalemic periodic (familial) 359.3
- hypertensive (current episode) 437.8
- hypoglossal (nerve) 352.5
- hypokalemic periodic 359.3
- Hyrtl's sphincter (rectum) 569.49
- hysterical 300.11
- ileus (*see also* Ileus) 560.1
- infantile (*see also* Poliomyelitis) 045.9 ☑
  - atrophic acute 045.1 ☑
  - bulbar 045.0 ☑
  - cerebral — *see* Palsy, cerebral
  - paralytic 045.1 ☑
  - progressive acute 045.9 ☑
  - spastic — *see* Palsy, cerebral
  - spinal 045.9 ☑
- infective (*see also* Poliomyelitis) 045.9 ☑
- inferior nuclear 344.9
- insane, general or progressive 094.1
- internuclear 378.86
- interosseous 355.9
- intestine (*see also* Ileus) 560.1
- intracranial (current episode) (*see also* Paralysis, brain) 437.8
  - due to birth injury 767.0
- iris 379.49
  - due to diphtheria (toxin) 032.81 [379.49]
- ischemic, Volkmann's (complicating trauma) 958.6
- isolated sleep, recurrent
- Jackson's 344.89
- jake 357.7
- Jamaica ginger (jake) 357.7
- juvenile general 090.40
- Klumpke (-Déjérine) (birth) (newborn) 767.6
- labioglossal (laryngeal) (pharyngeal) 335.22
- Landry's 357.0
- laryngeal nerve (recurrent) (superior) (*see also* Paralysis, vocal cord) 478.30
- larynx (*see also* Paralysis, vocal cord) 478.30
  - due to diphtheria (toxin) 032.3
- late effect
  - due to
    - birth injury, brain or spinal (cord) — *see* Palsy, cerebral
    - edema, brain or cerebral — *see* Paralysis, brain
    - lesion
      - late effect — *see* Late effect(s) (of) cerebrovascular disease
      - spinal (cord) — *see* Paralysis, spinal
- lateral 335.24
- lead 984.1
  - specified type of lead — *see* Table of Drugs and Chemicals
- left side — *see* Hemiplegia
- leg 344.30

Paralysis, paralytic — *continued*
- leg — *continued*
  - affecting
    - dominant side 344.31
    - nondominant side 344.32
  - both (*see also* Paraplegia) 344.1
  - crossed 344.89
  - hysterical 300.11
  - psychogenic 306.0
  - transient or transitory 781.4
    - traumatic NEC (*see also* Injury, nerve, lower limb) 956.9
- levator palpebrae superioris 374.31
- limb NEC 344.5
  - all four — *see* Quadriplegia
  - quadriplegia — *see* Quadriplegia
- lip 528.5
- Lissauer's 094.1
- local 355.9
- lower limb (*see also* Paralysis, leg)
  - both (*see also* Paraplegia) 344.1
- lung 518.89
  - newborn 770.89
- median nerve 354.1
- medullary (tegmental) 344.89
  - tegmental 344.89
- mesencephalic NEC 344.89
  - tegmental 344.89
- middle alternating 344.89
- Millard-Gubler-Foville 344.89
- monoplegic — *see* Monoplegia
- motor NEC 344.9
  - cerebral — *see* Paralysis, brain
  - spinal — *see* Paralysis, spinal
- multiple
  - cerebral — *see* Paralysis, brain
  - spinal — *see* Paralysis, spinal
- muscle (flaccid) 359.9
  - due to nerve lesion NEC 355.9
  - eye (extrinsic) 378.55
    - intrinsic 367.51
    - oblique 378.51
  - iris sphincter 364.89
  - ischemic (complicating trauma) (Volkmann's) 958.6
  - pseudohypertrophic 359.1
- muscular (atrophic) 359.9
  - progressive 335.21
- musculocutaneous nerve 354.9
- musculospiral 354.9
- nerve (*see also* Disorder, nerve)
  - third or oculomotor (partial) 378.51
    - total 378.52
  - fourth or trochlear 378.53
  - sixth or abducens 378.54
  - seventh or facial 351.0
    - birth injury 767.5
    - due to
      - injection NEC 999.9
      - operation NEC 997.09
    - newborn 767.5
  - accessory 352.4
  - auditory 388.5
  - birth injury 767.7
  - cranial or cerebral (*see also* Disorder, nerve, cranial) 352.9
  - facial 351.0
    - birth injury 767.5
    - newborn 767.5
  - laryngeal (*see also* Paralysis, vocal cord) 478.30
  - newborn 767.7
  - phrenic 354.8
    - newborn 767.7
  - radial 354.3
    - birth injury 767.6
    - newborn 767.6
  - syphilitic 094.89
  - traumatic NEC (*see also* Injury, nerve, by site) 957.9
  - trigeminal 350.9
  - ulnar 354.2
- newborn NEC 767.0
- normokalemic periodic 359.3
- obstetrical, newborn 767.7
- ocular 378.9
- oculofacial, congenital 352.6

Paralysis, paralytic — *continued*
- oculomotor (nerve) (partial) 378.51
  - alternating 344.89
  - external bilateral 378.55
  - total 378.52
- olfactory nerve 352.0
- palate 528.9
- palatopharyngolaryngeal 352.6
- paratrigeminal 350.9
- periodic (familial) (hyperkalemic) (hypokalemic) (normokalemic) (potassium sensitive) (secondary) 359.3
- peripheral
  - autonomic nervous system — *see* Neuropathy, peripheral, autonomic
  - nerve NEC 355.9
- peroneal (nerve) 355.3
- pharynx 478.29
- phrenic nerve 354.8
- plantar nerves 355.6
- pneumogastric nerve 352.3
- poliomyelitis (current) (*see also* Poliomyelitis, with paralysis) 045.1 ☑
  - bulbar 045.0 ☑
- popliteal nerve 355.3
- pressure (*see also* Neuropathy, entrapment) 355.9
- progressive 335.21
  - atrophic 335.21
  - bulbar 335.22
  - general 094.1
  - hemifacial 349.89
  - infantile, acute (*see also* Poliomyelitis) 045.9 ☑
  - multiple 335.20
- pseudobulbar 335.23
- pseudohypertrophic 359.1
  - muscle 359.1
- psychogenic 306.0
- pupil, pupillary 379.49
- quadriceps 355.8
- quadriplegic (*see also* Quadriplegia) 344.0 ☑
- radial nerve 354.3
  - birth injury 767.6
- rectum (sphincter) 569.49
- rectus muscle (eye) 378.55
- recurrent
  - isolated sleep 327.43
  - laryngeal nerve (*see also* Paralysis, vocal cord) 478.30
- respiratory (muscle) (system) (tract) 786.09
  - center NEC 344.89
    - fetus or newborn 770.87
  - congenital 768.9
  - newborn 768.9
- right side — *see* Hemiplegia
- Saturday night 354.3
- saturnine 984.9
  - specified type of lead — *see* Table of Drugs and Chemicals
- sciatic nerve 355.0
- secondary — *see* Paralysis, late effect
- seizure (cerebral) (current episode) (*see also* Disease, cerebrovascular, acute) 436
  - late effect — *see* Late effect(s) (of) cerebrovascular disease
- senile NEC 344.9
- serratus magnus 355.9
- shaking (*see also* Parkinsonism) 332.0
- shock (*see also* Disease, cerebrovascular, acute) 436
  - late effect — *see* Late effect(s) (of) cerebrovascular disease
- shoulder 354.9
- soft palate 528.9
- spasmodic — *see* Paralysis, spastic
- spastic 344.9
  - cerebral infantile — *see* Palsy, cerebral
  - congenital (cerebral) — *see* Palsy, cerebral
  - familial 334.1
  - hereditary 334.1
  - infantile 343.9
  - noncongenital or noninfantile, cerebral 344.9

Paralysis, paralytic — *continued*
- spastic — *continued*
  - syphilitic 094.0
    - spinal 094.89
- sphincter, bladder (*see also* Paralysis, bladder) 596.53
- spinal (cord) NEC 344.1
  - accessory nerve 352.4
  - acute (*see also* Poliomyelitis) 045.9 ☑
  - ascending acute 357.0
  - atrophic (acute) (*see also* Poliomyelitis, with paralysis) 045.1 ☑
    - spastic, syphilitic 094.89
  - congenital NEC 343.9
  - hemiplegic — *see* Hemiplegia
  - hereditary 336.8
  - infantile (*see also* Poliomyelitis) 045.9 ☑
  - late effect 344.89
  - monoplegic — *see* Monoplegia
  - nerve 355.9
  - progressive 335.10
  - quadriplegic — *see* Quadriplegia
  - spastic NEC 343.9
  - traumatic — *see* Injury, spinal, by site
- sternomastoid 352.4
- stomach 536.3
  - diabetic 250.6 ☑ [536.3]
    - due to secondary diabetes 249.6 ☑ [536.3]
  - nerve (nondiabetic) 352.3
- stroke (current episode) — *see* Infarct, brain
  - late effect — *see* Late effect(s) (of) cerebrovascular disease
- subscapularis 354.8
- superior nuclear NEC 334.9
- supranuclear 356.8
- sympathetic
  - cervical NEC 337.09
  - nerve NEC (*see also* Neuropathy, peripheral, autonomic) 337.9
  - nervous system — *see* Neuropathy, peripheral, autonomic
- syndrome 344.9
  - specified NEC 344.89
- syphilitic spastic spinal (Erb's) 094.89
- tabetic general 094.1
- thigh 355.8
- throat 478.29
  - diphtheritic 032.0
  - muscle 478.29
- thrombotic (current episode) (*see also* Thrombosis, brain) 434.0 ☑
  - late effect — *see* Late effect(s) (of) cerebrovascular disease
- thumb NEC 354.9
- tick (-bite) 989.5
- Todd's (postepileptic transitory paralysis) 344.89
- toe 355.6
- tongue 529.8
- transient
  - arm or leg NEC 781.4
  - traumatic NEC (*see also* Injury, nerve, by site) 957.9
- trapezius 352.4
- traumatic, transient NEC (*see also* Injury, nerve, by site) 957.9
- trembling (*see also* Parkinsonism) 332.0
- triceps brachii 354.9
- trigeminal nerve 350.9
- trochlear nerve 378.53
- ulnar nerve 354.2
- upper limb (*see also* Paralysis, arm)
  - both (*see also* Diplegia) 344.2
- uremic — *see* Uremia
- uveoparotitic 135
- uvula 528.9
  - hysterical 300.11
  - postdiphtheritic 032.0
- vagus nerve 352.3
- vasomotor NEC 337.9
- velum palati 528.9
- vesical (*see also* Paralysis, bladder) 596.53
- vestibular nerve 388.5
- visual field, psychic 368.16
- vocal cord 478.30

☑ **Additional Digit Required** — Refer to the Tabular List for Digit Selection   ▽ **Subterms under main terms may continue to next column or page**

Paralysis, paralytic — *continued*
  vocal cord — *continued*
    bilateral (partial) 478.33
      complete 478.34
    complete (bilateral) 478.34
    unilateral (partial) 478.31
      complete 478.32
    Volkmann's (complicating trauma) 958.6
  wasting 335.21
  Weber's 344.89
  wrist NEC 354.9
Paramedial orifice, urethrovesical 753.8
Paramenia 626.9
Parametritis (chronic) — *see also* Disease, pelvis, inflammatory 614.4
  acute 614.3
  puerperal, postpartum, childbirth 670.8 ☑
Parametrium, parametric — *see* condition
Paramnesia — *see also* Amnesia 780.93
Paramolar 520.1
  causing crowding 524.31
Paramyloidosis 277.30
Paramyoclonus multiplex 333.2
Paramyotonia 359.29
  congenita (of von Eulenburg) 359.29
Paraneoplastic syndrome — *see* condition
Parangi — *see also* Yaws 102.9
Paranoia 297.1
  alcoholic 291.5
  querulans 297.8
  senile 290.20
Paranoid
  dementia (*see also* Schizophrenia) 295.3 ☑
    praecox (acute) 295.3 ☑
    senile 290.20
  personality 301.0
  psychosis 297.9
    alcoholic 291.5
    climacteric 297.2
    drug-induced 292.11
    involutional 297.2
    menopausal 297.2
    protracted reactive 298.4
    psychogenic 298.4
      acute 298.3
    senile 290.20
  reaction (chronic) 297.9
    acute 298.3
  schizophrenia (acute) (*see also* Schizophrenia) 295.3 ☑
  state 297.9
    alcohol-induced 291.5
    climacteric 297.2
    drug-induced 292.11
    due to or associated with
      arteriosclerosis (cerebrovascular) 290.42
      presenile brain disease 290.12
      senile brain disease 290.20
    involutional 297.2
    menopausal 297.2
    senile 290.20
    simple 297.0
    specified type NEC 297.8
  tendencies 301.0
  traits 301.0
  trends 301.0
  type, psychopathic personality 301.0
Paraparesis — *see also* Paraplegia 344.1
Paraphasia 784.3
Paraphilia — *see also* Deviation, sexual 302.9
Paraphimosis (congenital) 605
  chancroidal 099.0
Paraphrenia, paraphrenic (late) 297.2
  climacteric 297.2
  dementia (*see also* Schizophrenia) 295.3 ☑
  involutional 297.2
  menopausal 297.2
  schizophrenia (acute) (*see also* Schizophrenia) 295.3 ☑
Paraplegia 344.1
  with
    broken back — *see* Fracture, vertebra, by site, with spinal cord injury

Paraplegia — *continued*
  with — *continued*
    fracture, vertebra — *see* Fracture, vertebra, by site, with spinal cord injury
  ataxic — *see* Degeneration, combined, spinal cord
  brain (current episode) (*see also* Paralysis, brain) 437.8
  cerebral (current episode) (*see also* Paralysis, brain) 437.8
  congenital or infantile (cerebral) (spastic) (spinal) 343.0
  cortical — *see* Paralysis, brain
  familial spastic 334.1
  functional (hysterical) 300.11
  hysterical 300.11
  infantile 343.0
  late effect 344.1
  Pott's (*see also* Tuberculosis) 015.0 ☑ *[730.88]*
  psychogenic 306.0
  spastic
    Erb's spinal 094.89
    hereditary 334.1
    not infantile or congenital 344.1
  spinal (cord)
    traumatic NEC — *see* Injury, spinal, by site
  syphilitic (spastic) 094.89
  traumatic NEC — *see* Injury, spinal, by site
Paraproteinemia 273.2
  benign (familial) 273.1
  monoclonal 273.1
  secondary to malignant or inflammatory disease 273.1
Parapsoriasis 696.2
  en plaques 696.2
  guttata 696.2
  lichenoides chronica 696.2
  retiformis 696.2
  varioliformis (acuta) 696.2
Parascarlatina 057.8
Parasitic — *see also* condition
  disease NEC (*see also* Infestation, parasitic) 136.9
    contact V01.89
    exposure to V01.89
    intestinal NEC 129
    skin NEC 134.9
  stomatitis 112.0
  sycosis 110.0
    beard 110.0
    scalp 110.0
  twin 759.4
Parasitism NEC 136.9
  intestinal NEC 129
  skin NEC 134.9
  specified — *see* Infestation
Parasitophobia 300.29
Parasomnia 307.47
  alcohol induced 291.82
  drug induced 292.85
  nonorganic origin 307.47
  organic 327.40
    in conditions classified elsewhere 327.44
    other 327.49
Paraspadias 752.69
Paraspasm facialis 351.8
Parathyroid gland — *see* condition
Parathyroiditis (autoimmune) 252.1
Parathyroprival tetany 252.1
Paratrachoma 077.0
Paratyphilitis — *see also* Appendicitis 541
Paratyphoid (fever) — *see* Fever, paratyphoid
Paratyphus — *see* Fever, paratyphoid
Paraurethral duct 753.8
Para-urethritis 597.89
  gonococcal (acute) 098.0
    chronic or duration of 2 months or over 098.2
Paravaccinia NEC 051.9
  milkers' node 051.1
Paravaginitis — *see also* Vaginitis 616.10
Parencephalitis — *see also* Encephalitis 323.9
  late effect — *see* category 326

Parergasia 298.9
Paresis — *see also* Paralysis 344.9
  accommodation 367.51
  bladder (spastic) (sphincter) (*see also* Paralysis, bladder) 596.53
    tabetic 094.0
  bowel, colon, or intestine (*see also* Ileus) 560.1
  brain or cerebral — *see* Paralysis, brain
  extrinsic muscle, eye 378.55
  general 094.1
    arrested 094.1
    brain 094.1
    cerebral 094.1
    insane 094.1
    juvenile 090.40
      remission 090.49
    progressive 094.1
    remission (sustained) 094.1
    tabetic 094.1
  heart (*see also* Failure, heart) 428.9
  infantile (*see also* Poliomyelitis) 045.9 ☑
  insane 094.1
  juvenile 090.40
  late effect — *see* Paralysis, late effect
  luetic (general) 094.1
  peripheral progressive 356.9
  pseudohypertrophic 359.1
  senile NEC 344.9
  stomach 536.3
    diabetic 250.6 ☑ *[536.3]*
      due to secondary diabetes 249.6 ☑ *[536.3]*
  syphilitic (general) 094.1
    congenital 090.40
  transient, limb 781.4
  vesical (sphincter) NEC 596.53
Paresthesia — *see also* Disturbance, sensation 782.0
  Berger's (paresthesia of lower limb) 782.0
  Bernhardt 355.1
  Magnan's 782.0
Paretic — *see* condition
Parinaud's
  conjunctivitis 372.02
  oculoglandular syndrome 372.02
  ophthalmoplegia 378.81
  syndrome (paralysis of conjugate upward gaze) 378.81
Parkes Weber and Dimitri syndrome (encephalocutaneous angiomatosis) 759.6
Parkinson's disease, syndrome, or tremor — *see* Parkinsonism
Parkinsonism (arteriosclerotic) (idiopathic) (primary) 332.0
  associated with orthostatic hypotension (idiopathic) (symptomatic) 333.0
  due to drugs 332.1
  neuroleptic-induced 332.1
  secondary 332.1
  syphilitic 094.82
Parodontitis 523.40
Parodontosis 523.5
Paronychia (with lymphangitis) 681.9
  candidal (chronic) 112.3
  chronic 681.9
    candidal 112.3
    finger 681.02
    toe 681.11
  finger 681.02
  toe 681.11
  tuberculous (primary) (*see also* Tuberculosis) 017.0 ☑
Parorexia NEC 307.52
  hysterical 300.11
Parosmia 781.1
  psychogenic 306.7
Parotid gland — *see* condition
Parotiditis — *see also* Parotitis 527.2
  epidemic 072.9
  infectious 072.9
Parotitis 527.2
  allergic 527.2
  chronic 527.2
  epidemic (*see also* Mumps) 072.9
  infectious (*see also* Mumps) 072.9

Parotitis — *continued*
  noninfectious 527.2
  nonspecific toxic 527.2
  not mumps 527.2
  postoperative 527.2
  purulent 527.2
  septic 527.2
  suppurative (acute) 527.2
  surgical 527.2
  toxic 527.2
Paroxysmal — *see also* condition
  dyspnea (nocturnal) 786.09
Parrot's disease (syphilitic osteochondritis) 090.0
Parrot fever 073.9
Parry's disease or syndrome (exophthalmic goiter) 242.0 ☑
Parry-Romberg syndrome 349.89
Parsonage-Aldren-Turner syndrome 353.5
Parsonage-Turner syndrome 353.5
Parson's disease (exophthalmic goiter) 242.0 ☑
Pars planitis 363.21
Particolored infant 757.39
Parturition — *see* Delivery
Parvovirus 079.83
  B19 079.83
  human 079.83
Passage
  false, urethra 599.4
  meconium noted during delivery 763.84
  of sounds or bougies (*see also* Attention to artificial opening) V55.9
Passive — *see* condition
Pasteurella septica 027.2
Pasteurellosis — *see also* Infection, Pasteurella 027.2
PAT (paroxysmal atrial tachycardia) 427.0
Patau's syndrome (trisomy D1) 758.1
Patch
  herald 696.3
Patches
  mucous (syphilitic) 091.3
    congenital 090.0
  smokers' (mouth) 528.6
Patellar — *see* condition
Patellofemoral syndrome 719.46
Patent — *see also* Imperfect closure
  atrioventricular ostium 745.69
  canal of Nuck 752.41
  cervix 622.5
    complicating pregnancy 654.5 ☑
      affecting fetus or newborn 761.0
  ductus arteriosus or Botalli 747.0
  Eustachian
    tube 381.7
    valve 746.89
  foramen
    Botalli 745.5
    ovale 745.5
  interauricular septum 745.5
  interventricular septum 745.4
  omphalomesenteric duct 751.0
  os (uteri) — *see* Patent, cervix
  ostium secundum 745.5
  urachus 753.7
  vitelline duct 751.0
Paternity testing V70.4
Paterson-Kelly syndrome or web (sideropenic dysphagia) 280.8
Paterson (-Brown) (-Kelly) syndrome (sideropenic dysphagia) 280.8
Paterson's syndrome (sideropenic dysphagia) 280.8
Pathologic, pathological — *see also* condition
  asphyxia 799.01
  drunkenness 291.4
  emotionality 301.3
  fracture — *see* Fracture, pathologic
  liar 301.7
  personality 301.9
  resorption, tooth 521.40
    external 521.42
    internal 521.41
    specified NEC 521.49
  sexuality (*see also* Deviation, sexual) 302.9

☑ Additional Digit Required — Refer to the Tabular List for Digit Selection   ⁽ᵂ⁾ Subterms under main terms may continue to next column or page

226 — Volume 2   ▶◀ Revised Text   ● New Line   ▲ Revised Code   2015 ICD-9-CM

Pathology (of) — *see also* Disease
   periradicular, associated with previous endodontic treatment 526.69
Patterned motor discharge, idiopathic — *see also* Epilepsy 345.5 ☑
Patulous — *see also* Patent
   anus 569.49
   Eustachian tube 381.7
Pause, sinoatrial 427.81
Pavor nocturnus 307.46
Pavy's disease 593.6
Paxton's disease (white piedra) 111.2
Payr's disease or syndrome (splenic flexure syndrome) 569.89
PBA (pseudobulbar affect) 310.81
Pearls
   Elschnig 366.51
   enamel 520.2
Pearl-workers' disease (chronic osteomyelitis) — *see also* Osteomyelitis 730.1 ☑
Pectenitis 569.49
Pectenosis 569.49
Pectoral — *see* condition
Pectus
   carinatum (congenital) 754.82
     acquired 738.3
     rachitic (*see also* Rickets) 268.0
   excavatum (congenital) 754.81
     acquired 738.3
     rachitic (*see also* Rickets) 268.0
   recurvatum (congenital) 754.81
     acquired 738.3
Pedatrophia 261
Pederosis 302.2
Pediculosis (infestation) 132.9
   capitis (head louse) (any site) 132.0
   corporis (body louse) (any site) 132.1
   eyelid 132.0 [373.6]
   mixed (classifiable to more than one category in 132.0–132.2) 132.3
   pubis (pubic louse) (any site) 132.2
   vestimenti 132.1
   vulvae 132.2
Pediculus (infestation) — *see* Pediculosis
Pedophilia 302.2
Peg-shaped teeth 520.2
Pelade 704.01
Pel's crisis 094.0
Pel-Ebstein disease — *see* Disease, Hodgkin's
Pelger-Huët anomaly or syndrome (hereditary hyposegmentation) 288.2
Peliosis (rheumatica) 287.0
Pelizaeus-Merzbacher
   disease 330.0
   sclerosis, diffuse cerebral 330.0
Pellagra (alcoholic or with alcoholism) 265.2
   with polyneuropathy 265.2 [357.4]
Pellagra-cerebellar-ataxia-renal aminoaciduria syndrome 270.0
Pellegrini's disease (calcification, knee joint) 726.62
Pellegrini (-Stieda) disease or syndrome (calcification, knee joint) 726.62
Pellizzi's syndrome (pineal) 259.8
Pelvic — *see also* condition
   congestion-fibrosis syndrome 625.5
   kidney 753.3
Pelvioectasis 591
Pelviolithiasis 592.0
Pelviperitonitis
   female (*see also* Peritonitis, pelvic, female) 614.5
   male (*see also* Peritonitis) 567.21
Pelvis, pelvic — *see also* condition or type
   infantile 738.6
   Nägele's 738.6
   obliquity 738.6
   Robert's 755.69
Pemphigoid 694.5
   benign, mucous membrane 694.60
     with ocular involvement 694.61
   bullous 694.5
   cicatricial 694.60
     with ocular involvement 694.61
   juvenile 694.2
Pemphigus 694.4

Pemphigus — *continued*
   benign 694.5
     chronic familial 757.39
   Brazilian 694.4
   circinatus 694.0
   congenital, traumatic 757.39
   conjunctiva 694.61
   contagiosus 684
   erythematodes 694.4
   erythematosus 694.4
   foliaceus 694.4
   frambesioides 694.4
   gangrenous (*see also* Gangrene) 785.4
   malignant 694.4
   neonatorum, newborn 684
   ocular 694.61
   papillaris 694.4
   seborrheic 694.4
   South American 694.4
   syphilitic (congenital) 090.0
   vegetans 694.4
   vulgaris 694.4
   wildfire 694.4
Pendred's syndrome (familial goiter with deaf-mutism) 243
Pendulous
   abdomen 701.9
     in pregnancy or childbirth 654.4 ☑
       affecting fetus or newborn 763.89
   breast 611.89
Penetrating wound — *see also* Wound, open, by site
   with internal injury — *see* Injury, internal, by site, with open wound
   eyeball 871.7
     with foreign body (nonmagnetic) 871.6
       magnetic 871.5
   ocular (*see also* Penetrating wound, eyeball) 871.7
     adnexa 870.3
       with foreign body 870.4
   orbit 870.3
     with foreign body 870.4
Penetration, pregnant uterus by instrument
   with
     abortion — *see* Abortion, by type, with damage to pelvic organs
     ectopic pregnancy (*see also* categories 633.0–633.9) 639.2
     molar pregnancy (*see also* categories 630–632) 639.2
   complication of delivery 665.1 ☑
     affecting fetus or newborn 763.89
   following
     abortion 639.2
     ectopic or molar pregnancy 639.2
Penfield's syndrome — *see also* Epilepsy 345.5 ☑
Penicilliosis of lung 117.3
Penis — *see* condition
Penitis 607.2
Pentalogy (of Fallot) 745.2
Penta X syndrome 758.81
Pentosuria (benign) (essential) 271.8
Peptic acid disease 536.8
Peregrinating patient V65.2
Perforated — *see* Perforation
Perforation, perforative (nontraumatic)
   antrum (*see also* Sinusitis, maxillary) 473.0
   appendix 540.0
     with peritoneal abscess 540.1
   atrial septum, multiple 745.5
   attic, ear 384.22
     healed 384.81
   bile duct, except cystic (*see also* Disease, biliary) 576.3
     cystic 575.4
   bladder (urinary) 596.6
     with
       abortion — *see* Abortion, by type, with damage to pelvic organs
       ectopic pregnancy (*see also* categories 633.0–633.9) 639.2
       molar pregnancy (*see also* categories 630–632) 639.2

Perforation, perforative — *continued*
   bladder — *continued*
     following
       abortion 639.2
       ectopic or molar pregnancy 639.2
     obstetrical trauma 665.5 ☑
   bowel 569.83
     with
       abortion — *see* Abortion, by type, with damage to pelvic organs
       ectopic pregnancy (*see also* categories 633.0–633.9) 639.2
       molar pregnancy (*see also* categories 630–632) 639.2
     fetus or newborn 777.6
     following
       abortion 639.2
       ectopic or molar pregnancy 639.2
     obstetrical trauma 665.5 ☑
   broad ligament
     with
       abortion — *see* Abortion, by type, with damage to pelvic organs
       ectopic pregnancy (*see also* categories 633.0–633.9) 639.2
       molar pregnancy (*see also* categories 630–632) 639.2
     following
       abortion 639.2
       ectopic or molar pregnancy 639.2
     obstetrical trauma 665.6 ☑
   by
     device, implant, or graft — *see* Complications, mechanical
     foreign body left accidentally in operation wound 998.4
     instrument (any) during a procedure, accidental 998.2
   cecum 540.0
     with peritoneal abscess 540.1
   cervix (uteri) (*see also* Injury, internal, cervix)
     with
       abortion — *see* Abortion, by type, with damage to pelvic organs
       ectopic pregnancy (*see also* categories 633.0–633.9) 639.2
       molar pregnancy (*see also* categories 630–632) 639.2
     following
       abortion 639.2
       ectopic or molar pregnancy 639.2
     obstetrical trauma 665.3 ☑
   colon 569.83
   common duct (bile) 576.3
   cornea (*see also* Ulcer, cornea) 370.00
     due to ulceration 370.06
   cystic duct 575.4
   diverticulum (*see also* Diverticula) 562.10
     small intestine 562.00
   duodenum, duodenal (ulcer) — *see* Ulcer, duodenum, with perforation
   ear drum — *see* Perforation, tympanum
   enteritis — *see* Enteritis
   esophagus 530.4
   ethmoidal sinus (*see also* Sinusitis, ethmoidal) 473.2
   foreign body (external site) (*see also* Wound, open, by site, complicated)
     internal site, by ingested object — *see* Foreign body
   frontal sinus (*see also* Sinusitis, frontal) 473.1
   gallbladder or duct (*see also* Disease, gallbladder) 575.4
   gastric (ulcer) — *see* Ulcer, stomach, with perforation
   heart valve — *see* Endocarditis
   ileum (*see also* Perforation, intestine) 569.83
   instrumental
     external — *see* Wound, open, by site
     pregnant uterus, complicating delivery 665.9 ☑
     surgical (accidental) (blood vessel) (nerve) (organ) 998.2
   intestine 569.83

Perforation, perforative — *continued*
   intestine — *continued*
     with
       abortion — *see* Abortion, by type, with damage to pelvic organs
       ectopic pregnancy (*see also* categories 633.0–633.9) 639.2
       molar pregnancy (*see also* categories 630–632) 639.2
     fetus or newborn 777.6
     obstetrical trauma 665.5 ☑
     ulcerative NEC 569.83
   jejunum, jejunal 569.83
     ulcer — *see* Ulcer, gastrojejunal, with perforation
   mastoid (antrum) (cell) 383.89
   maxillary sinus (*see also* Sinusitis, maxillary) 473.0
   membrana tympani — *see* Perforation, tympanum
   nasal
     septum 478.19
       congenital 748.1
       syphilitic 095.8
     sinus (*see also* Sinusitis) 473.9
       congenital 748.1
   palate (hard) 526.89
     soft 528.9
       syphilitic 095.8
         syphilitic 095.8
   palatine vault 526.89
     syphilitic 095.8
       congenital 090.5
   pelvic
     floor
       with
         abortion — *see* Abortion, by type, with damage to pelvic organs
         ectopic pregnancy (*see also* categories 633.0–633.9) 639.2
         molar pregnancy (*see also* categories 630–632) 639.2
       obstetrical trauma 664.1 ☑
     organ
       with
         abortion — *see* Abortion, by type, with damage to pelvic organs
         ectopic pregnancy (*see also* categories 633.0–633.9) 639.2
         molar pregnancy (*see also* categories 630–632) 639.2
       following
         abortion 639.2
         ectopic or molar pregnancy 639.2
       obstetrical trauma 665.5 ☑
   perineum — *see* Laceration, perineum
   periurethral tissue
     with
       abortion — *see* Abortion, by type, with damage to pelvic organs
       ectopic pregnancy (*see also* categories 630–632) 639.2
       molar pregnancy (*see also* categories 630–632) 639.2
   pharynx 478.29
   pylorus, pyloric (ulcer) — *see* Ulcer, stomach, with perforation
   rectum 569.49
   root canal space 526.61
   sigmoid 569.83
   sinus (accessory) (chronic) (nasal) (*see also* Sinusitis) 473.9
   sphenoidal sinus (*see also* Sinusitis, sphenoidal) 473.3
   stomach (due to ulcer) — *see* Ulcer, stomach, with perforation
   surgical (accidental) (by instrument) (blood vessel) (nerve) (organ) 998.2
   traumatic
     external — *see* Wound, open, by site
     eye (*see also* Penetrating wound, ocular) 871.7
     internal organ — *see* Injury, internal, by site

☑ **Additional Digit Required** — Refer to the Tabular List for Digit Selection   ▽ **Subterms under main terms may continue to next column or page**

Perforation, perforative — *continued*
　tympanum (membrane) (persistent posttrau-
　　matic) (postinflammatory) 384.20
　　with
　　　otitis media — *see* Otitis media
　　attic 384.22
　　central 384.21
　　healed 384.81
　　marginal NEC 384.23
　　multiple 384.24
　　pars flaccida 384.22
　　total 384.25
　　traumatic — *see* Wound, open, ear,
　　　drum
　typhoid, gastrointestinal 002.0
　ulcer — *see* Ulcer, by site, with perforation
　ureter 593.89
　urethra
　　with
　　　abortion — *see* Abortion, by type,
　　　　with damage to pelvic organs
　　　ectopic pregnancy (*see also* cate-
　　　　gories 633.0–633.9) 639.2
　　　molar pregnancy (*see also* categories
　　　　630–632) 639.2
　　following
　　　abortion 639.2
　　　ectopic or molar pregnancy 639.2
　　obstetrical trauma 665.5 ☑
　uterus (*see also* Injury, internal, uterus)
　　with
　　　abortion — *see* Abortion, by type,
　　　　with damage to pelvic organs
　　　ectopic pregnancy (*see also* cate-
　　　　gories 633.0–633.9) 639.2
　　　molar pregnancy (*see also* categories
　　　　630–632) 639.2
　　by intrauterine contraceptive device
　　　996.32
　　following
　　　abortion 639.2
　　　ectopic or molar pregnancy 639.2
　　obstetrical trauma — *see* Injury, internal,
　　　uterus, obstetrical trauma
　uvula 528.9
　　syphilitic 095.8
　vagina — *see* Laceration, vagina
　viscus NEC 799.89
　　traumatic 868.00
　　　with open wound into cavity 868.10
Periadenitis mucosa necrotica recurrens
　528.2
Periangiitis 446.0
Periantritis 535.4 ☑
Periappendicitis (acute) — *see also* Appendici-
　tis 541
Periarteritis (disseminated) (infectious)
　(necrotizing) (nodosa) 446.0
Periarthritis (joint) 726.90
　Duplay's 726.2
　gonococcal 098.50
　humeroscapularis 726.2
　scapulohumeral 726.2
　shoulder 726.2
　wrist 726.4
Periarthrosis (angioneural) — *see* Periarthritis
Peribronchitis 491.9
　tuberculous (*see also* Tuberculosis) 011.3 ☑
Pericapsulitis, adhesive (shoulder) 726.0
Pericarditis (granular) (with decompensation)
　(with effusion) 423.9
　with
　　rheumatic fever (conditions classifiable
　　　to 390)
　　　active (*see also* Pericarditis,
　　　　rheumatic) 391.0
　　　inactive or quiescent 393
　actinomycotic 039.8 *[420.0]*
　acute (nonrheumatic) 420.90
　　with chorea (acute) (rheumatic) (Syden-
　　　ham's) 392.0
　　bacterial 420.99
　　benign 420.91
　　hemorrhagic 420.90
　　idiopathic 420.91
　　infective 420.90

Pericarditis — *continued*
　acute — *continued*
　　nonspecific 420.91
　　rheumatic 391.0
　　　with chorea (acute) (rheumatic)
　　　　(Sydenham's) 392.0
　　sicca 420.90
　　viral 420.91
　adhesive or adherent (external) (internal)
　　423.1
　　acute — *see* Pericarditis, acute
　　rheumatic (internal) 393
　ambemic 006.8 *[420.0]*
　bacterial (acute) (subacute) (with serous or
　　seropurulent effusion) 420.99
　calcareous 423.2
　cholesterol (chronic) 423.8
　　acute 420.90
　chronic (nonrheumatic) 423.8
　　rheumatic 393
　constrictive 423.2
　Coxsackie 074.21
　due to
　　actinomycosis 039.8 *[420.0]*
　　amebiasis 006.8 *[420.0]*
　　Coxsackie (virus) 074.21
　　histoplasmosis (*see also* Histoplasmosis)
　　　115.93
　　nocardiosis 039.8 *[420.0]*
　　tuberculosis (*see also* Tuberculosis)
　　　017.9 ☑ *[420.0]*
　fibrinocaseous (*see also* Tuberculosis)
　　017.9 ☑ *[420.0]*
　fibrinopurulent 420.99
　fibrinous — *see* Pericarditis, rheumatic
　fibropurulent 420.99
　fibrous 423.1
　gonococcal 098.83
　hemorrhagic 423.0
　idiopathic (acute) 420.91
　infective (acute) 420.90
　meningococcal 036.41
　neoplastic (chronic) 423.8
　　acute 420.90
　nonspecific 420.91
　obliterans, obliterating 423.1
　plastic 423.1
　pneumococcal (acute) 420.99
　postinfarction 411.0
　purulent (acute) 420.99
　rheumatic (active) (acute) (with effusion)
　　(with pneumonia) 391.0
　　with chorea (acute) (rheumatic) (Syden-
　　　ham's) 392.0
　　chronic or inactive (with chorea) 393
　septic (acute) 420.99
　serofibrinous — *see* Pericarditis, rheumatic
　staphylococcal (acute) 420.99
　streptococcal (acute) 420.99
　suppurative (acute) 420.99
　syphilitic 093.81
　tuberculous (acute) (chronic) (*see also* Tuber-
　　culosis) 017.9 ☑ *[420.0]*
　uremic 585.9 *[420.0]*
　viral (acute) 420.91
Pericardium, pericardial — *see* condition
Pericellulitis — *see also* Cellulitis 682.9
Pericementitis 523.40
　acute 523.30
　chronic (suppurative) 523.40
Pericholecystitis — *see also* Cholecystitis
　575.10
Perichondritis
　auricle 380.00
　　acute 380.01
　　chronic 380.02
　bronchus 491.9
　ear (external) 380.00
　　acute 380.01
　　chronic 380.02
　larynx 478.71
　　syphilitic 095.8
　　typhoid 002.0 *[478.71]*
　nose 478.19
　pinna 380.00
　　acute 380.01

Perichondritis — *continued*
　pinna — *continued*
　　chronic 380.02
　　trachea 478.9
Periclasia 523.5
Pericolitis 569.89
Pericoronitis (chronic) 523.40
　acute 523.33
Pericystitis — *see also* Cystitis 595.9
Pericytoma (M9150/1) — *see also* Neoplasm,
　connective tissue, uncertain behavior
　benign (M9150/0) — *see* Neoplasm, connec-
　　tive tissue, benign
　malignant (M9150/3) — *see* Neoplasm,
　　connective tissue, malignant
Peridacryocystitis, acute 375.32
Peridiverticulitis — *see also* Diverticulitis
　562.11
Periduodenitis 535.6 ☑
Periendocarditis — *see also* Endocarditis
　424.90
　acute or subacute 421.9
Periepididymitis — *see also* Epididymitis
　604.90
Perifolliculitis (abscedens) 704.8
　capitis, abscedens et suffodiens 704.8
　dissecting, scalp 704.8
　scalp 704.8
　superficial pustular 704.8
Perigastritis (acute) 535.0 ☑
Perigastrojejunitis (acute) 535.0 ☑
Perihepatitis (acute) 573.3
　chlamydial 099.56
　gonococcal 098.86
Peri-ileitis (subacute) 569.89
Perilabyrinthitis (acute) — *see* Labyrinthitis
Perimeningitis — *see* Meningitis
Perimetritis — *see also* Endometritis 615.9
Perimetrosalpingitis — *see also* Salpingo-
　oophoritis 614.2
Perineocele 618.05
Perinephric — *see* condition
Perinephritic — *see* condition
Perinephritis — *see also* Infection, kidney
　590.9
　purulent (*see also* Abscess, kidney) 590.2
Perineum, perineal — *see* condition
Perineuritis NEC 729.2
Periodic — *see also* condition
　disease (familial) 277.31
　edema 995.1
　　hereditary 277.6
　fever 277.31
　headache syndromes in child or adolescent
　　346.2 ☑
　limb movement disorder 327.51
　paralysis (familial) 359.3
　peritonitis 277.31
　polyserositis 277.31
　somnolence (*see also* Narcolepsy) 347.00
Periodontal
　cyst 522.8
　pocket 523.8
Periodontitis (chronic) (complex) (compound)
　(simplex) 523.40
　acute 523.33
　aggressive 523.30
　　generalized 523.32
　　localized 523.31
　apical 522.6
　　acute (pulpal origin) 522.4
　generalized 523.42
　localized 523.41
Periodontoclasia 523.5
Periodontosis 523.5
Periods — *see also* Menstruation
　heavy 626.2
　irregular 626.4
Perionychia (with lymphangitis) 681.9
　finger 681.02
　toe 681.11
Perioophoritis — *see also* Salpingo-oophoritis
　614.2
Periorchitis — *see also* Orchitis 604.90
Periosteum, periosteal — *see* condition

Periostitis (circumscribed) (diffuse) (infective)
　730.3 ☑

> *Note* — Use the following fifth-digit
> subclassification with category 730:
>
> 0　site unspecified
> 1　shoulder region
> 2　upper arm
> 3　forearm
> 4　hand
> 5　pelvic region and thigh
> 6　lower leg
> 7　ankle and foot
> 8　other specified sites
> 9　multiple sites

　with osteomyelitis (*see also* Osteomyelitis)
　　730.2 ☑
　　acute or subacute 730.0 ☑
　　chronic or old 730.1 ☑
　albuminosa, albuminosus 730.3 ☑
　alveolar 526.5
　alveolodental 526.5
　dental 526.5
　gonorrheal 098.89
　hyperplastica, generalized 731.2
　jaw (lower) (upper) 526.4
　monomelic 733.99
　orbital 376.02
　syphilitic 095.5
　　congenital 090.0 *[730.8]* ☑
　　secondary 091.61
　tuberculous (*see also* Tuberculosis, bone)
　　015.9 ☑ *[730.8]* ☑
　yaws (early) (hypertrophic) (late) 102.6
Periostosis — *see also* Periostitis 730.3 ☑
　with osteomyelitis (*see also* Osteomyelitis)
　　730.2 ☑
　　acute or subacute 730.0 ☑
　　chronic or old 730.1 ☑
　hyperplastic 756.59
Peripartum cardiomyopathy 674.5 ☑
Periphlebitis — *see also* Phlebitis 451.9
　lower extremity 451.2
　　deep (vessels) 451.19
　　superficial (vessels) 451.0
　portal 572.1
　retina 362.18
　superficial (vessels) 451.0
　tuberculous (*see also* Tuberculosis) 017.9 ☑
　　retina 017.3 ☑ *[362.18]*
Peripneumonia — *see* Pneumonia
Periproctitis 569.49
Periprostatitis — *see also* Prostatitis 601.9
Perirectal — *see* condition
Perirenal — *see* condition
Perisalpingitis — *see also* Salpingo-oophoritis
　614.2
Perisigmoiditis 569.89
Perisplenitis (infectional) 289.59
Perispondylitis — *see* Spondylitis
Peristalsis reversed or visible 787.4
Peritendinitis — *see also* Tenosynovitis 726.90
　adhesive (shoulder) 726.0
Perithelioma (M9150/1) — *see* Pericytoma
Peritoneum, peritoneal — *see also* condition
　equilibration test V56.32
Peritonitis (acute) (adhesive) (fibrinous)
　(hemorrhagic) (idiopathic) (localized)
　(perforative) (primary) (with adhesions)
　(with effusion) 567.9
　with or following
　　abortion — *see* Abortion, by type, with
　　　sepsis
　　abscess 567.21
　　appendicitis 540.0
　　　with peritoneal abscess 540.1
　　ectopic pregnancy (*see also* categories
　　　633.0–633.9) 639.0
　　molar pregnancy (*see also* categories
　　　630–632) 639.0
　aseptic 998.7

☑ **Additional Digit Required** — Refer to the Tabular List for Digit Selection　　　　　　　　　⑪ **Subterms under main terms may continue to next column or page**

Petit's
disease (see also Hernia, lumbar) 553.8
Petit mal (idiopathic) — see also Epilepsy
345.0 ☑
status 345.2
Petrellidosis 117.6
Petrositis 383.20
acute 383.21
chronic 383.22
Peutz-Jeghers disease or syndrome 759.6
Peyronie's disease 607.85
Pfeiffer's disease 075
Phacentocele 379.32
traumatic 921.3
Phacoanaphylaxis 360.19
Phacocele (old) 379.32
traumatic 921.3
Phaehyphomycosis 117.8
Phagedena (dry) (moist) — see also Gangrene
785.4
arteriosclerotic 440.24
geometric 686.09
penis 607.89
senile 440.2 ☑ [785.4]
sloughing 785.4
tropical (see also Ulcer, skin) 707.9
vulva 616.50
Phagedenic — see also condition
abscess (see also Abscess)
chancroid 099.0
bubo NEC 099.8
chancre 099.0
ulcer (tropical) (see also Ulcer, skin) 707.9
Phagomania 307.52
Phakoma 362.89
Phantom limb (syndrome) 353.6
Pharyngeal — see also condition
arch remnant 744.41
pouch syndrome 279.11
Pharyngitis (acute) (catarrhal) (gangrenous)
(infective) (malignant) (membranous)
(phlegmonous) (pneumococcal) (pseudomembranous) (simple) (staphylococcal) (subacute) (suppurative) (ulcerative)
(viral) 462
with influenza, flu, or grippe (see also Influenza) 487.1
aphthous 074.0
atrophic 472.1
chlamydial 099.51
chronic 472.1
Coxsackie virus 074.0
diphtheritic (membranous) 032.0
follicular 472.1
fusospirochetal 101
gonococcal 098.6
granular (chronic) 472.1
herpetic 054.79
hypertrophic 472.1
infectional, chronic 472.1
influenzal (see also Influenza) 487.1
lymphonodular, acute 074.8
septic 034.0
streptococcal 034.0
tuberculous (see also Tuberculosis) 012.8 ☑
vesicular 074.0
Pharyngoconjunctival fever 077.2
Pharyngoconjunctivitis, viral 077.2
Pharyngolaryngitis (acute) 465.0
chronic 478.9
septic 034.0
Pharyngoplegia 478.29
Pharyngotonsillitis 465.8
tuberculous 012.8 ☑
Pharyngotracheitis (acute) 465.8
chronic 478.9
Pharynx, pharyngeal — see condition
Phase of life problem NEC V62.89
Phenomenon
Arthus' 995.21
flashback (drug) 292.89
jaw-winking 742.8
Jod-Basedow 242.8 ☑
L. E. cell 710.0
lupus erythematosus cell 710.0

Phenomenon — continued
Pelger-Huët (hereditary hyposegmentation)
288.2
Raynaud's (paroxysmal digital cyanosis)
(secondary) 443.0
Reilly's (see also Neuropathy, peripheral,
autonomic) 337.9
vasomotor 780.2
vasospastic 443.9
vasovagal 780.2
Wenckebach's, heart block (second degree)
426.13
Phenylketonuria (PKU) 270.1
Phenylpyruvicaciduria 270.1
Pheochromoblastoma (M8700/3)
specified site — see Neoplasm, by site, malignant
unspecified site 194.0
Pheochromocytoma (M8700/0)
malignant (M8700/3)
specified site — see Neoplasm, by site,
malignant
unspecified site 194.0
specified site — see Neoplasm, by site, benign
unspecified site 227.0
Phimosis (congenital) 605
chancroidal 099.0
due to infection 605
Phlebectasia — see also Varicose, vein 454.9
congenital NEC 747.60
esophagus (see also Varix, esophagus) 456.1
with hemorrhage (see also Varix, esophagus, bleeding) 456.0
Phlebitis (infective) (pyemic) (septic) (suppurative) 451.9
antecubital vein 451.82
arm NEC 451.84
axillary vein 451.89
basilic vein 451.82
deep 451.83
superficial 451.82
axillary vein 451.89
basilic vein 451.82
blue 451.9
brachial vein 451.83
breast, superficial 451.89
cavernous (venous) sinus — see Phlebitis,
intracranial sinus
cephalic vein 451.82
cerebral (venous) sinus — see Phlebitis, intracranial sinus
chest wall, superficial 451.89
complicating pregnancy or puerperium
671.2 ☑
affecting fetus or newborn 760.3
cranial (venous) sinus — see Phlebitis, intracranial sinus
deep (vessels) 451.19
femoral vein 451.11
specified vessel NEC 451.19
due to implanted device — see Complications, due to (presence of) any device, implant, or graft classified to
996.0–996.5 NEC
during or resulting from a procedure 997.2
femoral vein (deep) (superficial) 451.11
femoropopliteal 451.19
following infusion, perfusion, or transfusion
999.2
gouty 274.89 [451.9]
hepatic veins 451.89
iliac vein 451.81
iliofemoral 451.11
intracranial sinus (any) (venous) 325
late effect — see category 326
nonpyogenic 437.6
in pregnancy or puerperium 671.5 ☑
jugular vein 451.89
lateral (venous) sinus — see Phlebitis, intracranial sinus
leg 451.2
deep (vessels) 451.19
femoral vein 451.11
specified vessel NEC 451.19
superficial (vessels) 451.0

Phlebitis — continued
leg — continued
superficial — continued
femoral vein 451.11
longitudinal sinus — see Phlebitis, intracranial sinus
lower extremity 451.2
deep (vessels) 451.19
femoral vein 451.11
specified vessel NEC 451.19
migrans, migrating (superficial) 453.1
superficial (vessels) 451.0
femoral vein 451.11
pelvic
with
abortion — see Abortion, by type,
with sepsis
ectopic pregnancy (see also categories 633.0–633.9) 639.0
molar pregnancy (see also categories
630–632) 639.0
following
abortion 639.0
ectopic or molar pregnancy 639.0
puerperal, postpartum 671.4 ☑
popliteal vein 451.19
portal (vein) 572.1
postoperative 997.2
pregnancy 671.2 ☑
deep 671.3 ☑
specified type NEC 671.5 ☑
superficial 671.2 ☑
puerperal, postpartum, childbirth 671.2 ☑
deep 671.4 ☑
lower extremities 671.2 ☑
pelvis 671.4 ☑
specified site NEC 671.5 ☑
superficial 671.2 ☑
radial vein 451.83
retina 362.18
saphenous (great) (long) 451.0
accessory or small 451.0
sinus (meninges) — see Phlebitis, intracranial sinus
specified site NEC 451.89
subclavian vein 451.89
syphilitic 093.89
tibial vein 451.19
ulcer, ulcerative 451.9
leg 451.2
deep (vessels) 451.19
femoral vein 451.11
specified vessel NEC 451.19
superficial (vessels) 451.0
femoral vein 451.11
lower extremity 451.2
deep (vessels) 451.19
femoral vein 451.11
specified vessel NEC 451.19
superficial (vessels) 451.0
ulnar vein 451.83
umbilicus 451.89
upper extremity (see also Phlebitis, arm)
deep (veins) 451.83
brachial vein 451.83
radial vein 451.83
ulnar vein 451.83
superficial (veins) 451.82
antecubital vein 451.82
basilica vein 451.82
cephalic vein 451.82
uterus (septic) (see also Endometritis) 615.9
varicose (leg) (lower extremity) (see also
Varicose, vein) 454.1
Phlebofibrosis 459.89
Phleboliths 459.89
Phlebosclerosis 459.89
Phlebothrombosis — see Thrombosis
Phlebotomus fever 066.0
Phlegmasia
alba dolens (deep vessels) 451.19
complicating pregnancy 671.3 ☑
nonpuerperal 451.19
puerperal, postpartum, childbirth
671.4 ☑
cerulea dolens 451.19

Phlegm, choked on 933.1
Phlegmon — see also Abscess 682.9
erysipelatous (see also Erysipelas) 035
iliac 682.2
fossa 540.1
throat 478.29
Phlegmonous — see condition
Phlyctenulosis (allergic) (keratoconjunctivitis)
(nontuberculous) 370.31
cornea 370.31
with ulcer (see also Ulcer, cornea) 370.00
tuberculous (see also Tuberculosis)
017.3 ☑ [370.31]
Phobia, phobic (reaction) 300.20
animal 300.29
isolated NEC 300.29
obsessional 300.3
simple NEC 300.29
social 300.23
specified NEC 300.29
state 300.20
Phocas' disease 610.1
Phocomelia 755.4
lower limb 755.32
complete 755.33
distal 755.35
proximal 755.34
upper limb 755.22
complete 755.23
distal 755.25
proximal 755.24
Phoria — see also Heterophoria 378.40
Phosphate-losing tubular disorder 588.0
Phosphatemia 275.3
Phosphaturia 275.3
Photoallergic response 692.72
Photocoproporphyria 277.1
Photodermatitis (sun) 692.72
light other than sun 692.82
Photokeratitis 370.24
Photo-ophthalmia 370.24
Photophobia 368.13
Photopsia 368.15
Photoretinitis 363.31
Photoretinopathy 363.31
Photosensitiveness (sun) 692.72
light other than sun 692.82
Photosensitization (skin) (sun) 692.72
light other than sun 692.82
Phototoxic response 692.72
Phrenitis 323.9
Phrynoderma 264.8
Phthiriasis (pubis) (any site) 132.2
with any infestation classifiable to
132.0, 132.1, 132.3
Phthirus infestation — see Phthiriasis
Phthisis — see also Tuberculosis 011.9 ☑
bulbi (infectional) 360.41
colliers' 011.4 ☑
cornea 371.05
eyeball (due to infection) 360.41
millstone makers' 011.4 ☑
miners' 011.4 ☑
potters' 011.4 ☑
sandblasters' 011.4 ☑
stonemasons' 011.4 ☑
Phycomycosis 117.7
Physalopteriasis 127.7
Physical therapy NEC V57.1
breathing exercises V57.0
Physiological cup, optic papilla
borderline, glaucoma suspect 365.00
enlarged 377.14
glaucomatous 377.14
Phytobezoar 938
intestine 936
stomach 935.2
Pian — see also Yaws 102.9
Pianoma 102.1
Piarhemia, piarrhemia — see also Hyperlipemia 272.4
bilharziasis 120.9
Pica 307.52
hysterical 300.11
Pick's
cerebral atrophy 331.11

☑ **Additional Digit Required** — Refer to the Tabular List for Digit Selection   ▽ **Subterms under main terms may continue to next column or page**

230 — Volume 2   ▶◀ Revised Text   ● New Line   ▲ Revised Code   2015 ICD-9-CM

Pick's — *continued*
  cerebral atrophy — *continued*
    with dementia
      with behavioral disturbance
        331.11 [294.11]
      without behavioral disturbance
        331.11 [294.10]
  disease
    brain 331.11
      dementia in
        with behavioral disturbance
          331.11 [294.11]
        without behavioral disturbance
          331.11 [294.10]
    lipid histiocytosis 272.7
    liver (pericardial pseudocirrhosis of liver)
      423.2
    pericardium (pericardial pseudocirrhosis
      of liver) 423.2
    polyserositis (pericardial pseudocirrhosis of
      liver) 423.2
  syndrome
    heart (pericardial pseudocirrhosis of liv-
      er) 423.2
    liver (pericardial pseudocirrhosis of liver)
      423.2
  tubular adenoma (M8640/0)
    specified site — *see* Neoplasm, by site,
      benign
    unspecified site
      female 220
      male 222.0
Pick-Herxheimer syndrome (diffuse idiopathic
  cutaneous atrophy) 701.8
Pick-Niemann disease (lipid histiocytosis)
  272.7
Pickwickian syndrome (cardiopulmonary
  obesity) 278.03
Piebaldism, classic 709.09
Piedra 111.2
  beard 111.2
    black 111.3
    white 111.2
  black 111.3
  scalp 111.3
    black 111.3
    white 111.2
  white 111.2
Pierre Marie-Bamberger syndrome (hypertrophic pulmonary osteoarthropathy)
  731.2
Pierre Marie's syndrome (pulmonary hypertrophic osteoarthropathy) 731.2
Pierre Mauriac's syndrome (diabetes-
  dwarfism-obesity) 258.1
Pierre Robin deformity or syndrome (congenital) 756.0
Pierson's disease or osteochondrosis 732.1
Pigeon
  breast or chest (acquired) 738.3
    congenital 754.82
    rachitic (*see also* Rickets) 268.0
  breeders' disease or lung 495.2
  fanciers' disease or lung 495.2
  toe 735.8
Pigmentation (abnormal) 709.00
  anomaly 709.00
    congenital 757.33
    specified NEC 709.09
  conjunctiva 372.55
  cornea 371.10
    anterior 371.11
    posterior 371.13
    stromal 371.12
  lids (congenital) 757.33
    acquired 374.52
  limbus corneae 371.10
  metals 709.00
  optic papilla, congenital 743.57
  retina (congenital) (grouped) (nevoid)
    743.53
    acquired 362.74
  scrotum, congenital 757.33
Piles — *see* Hemorrhoids
Pili
  annulati or torti (congenital) 757.4

Pili — *continued*
  incarnati 704.8
Pill roller hand (intrinsic) 736.09
Pilomatrixoma (M8110/0) — *see* Neoplasm,
  skin, benign
Pilonidal — *see* condition
Pimple 709.8
PIN I (prostatic intraepithelial neoplasia I) 602.3
PIN II (prostatic intraepithelial neoplasia II)
  602.3
PIN III (prostatic intraepithelial neoplasia III)
  233.4
Pinched nerve — *see* Neuropathy, entrapment
Pineal body or gland — *see* condition
Pinealoblastoma (M9362/3) 194.4
Pinealoma (M9360/1) 237.1
  malignant (M9360/3) 194.4
Pineoblastoma (M9362/3) 194.4
Pineocytoma (M9361/1) 237.1
Pinguecula 372.51
Pingueculitis 372.34
Pinhole meatus — *see also* Stricture, urethra
  598.9
Pink
  disease 985.0
  eye 372.03
  puffer 492.8
Pinkus' disease (lichen nitidus) 697.1
Pinpoint
  meatus (*see also* Stricture, urethra) 598.9
  os uteri (*see also* Stricture, cervix) 622.4
Pinselhaare (congenital) 757.4
Pinta 103.9
  cardiovascular lesions 103.2
  chancre (primary) 103.0
  erythematous plaques 103.1
  hyperchromic lesions 103.1
  hyperkeratosis 103.1
  lesions 103.9
    cardiovascular 103.2
    hyperchromic 103.1
    intermediate 103.1
    late 103.2
    mixed 103.3
    primary 103.0
    skin (achromic) (cicatricial) (dyschromic)
      103.2
      hyperchromic 103.1
      mixed (achromic and hyperchromic)
        103.3
  papule (primary) 103.0
  skin lesions (achromic) (cicatricial)
    (dyschromic) 103.2
    hyperchromic 103.1
    mixed (achromic and hyperchromic)
      103.3
  vitiligo 103.2
Pintid 103.0
Pinworms (disease) (infection) (infestation)
  127.4
Piry fever 066.8
Pistol wound — *see* Gunshot wound
Pitchers' elbow 718.82
Pithecoid pelvis 755.69
  with disproportion (fetopelvic) 653.2 ☑
    affecting fetus or newborn 763.1
    causing obstructed labor 660.1 ☑
Pithiatism 300.11
Pit, lip (mucus), **congenital** 750.25
Pitted — *see also* Pitting
  teeth 520.4
Pitting (edema) — *see also* Edema 782.3
  lip 782.3
  nail 703.8
    congenital 757.5
Pituitary gland — *see* condition
Pituitary snuff-takers' disease 495.8
Pityriasis 696.5
  alba 696.5
  capitis 690.11
  circinata (et maculata) 696.3
  Hebra's (exfoliative dermatitis) 695.89
  lichenoides et varioliformis 696.2
  maculata (et circinata) 696.3
  nigra 111.1
  pilaris 757.39

Pityriasis — *continued*
  pilaris — *continued*
    acquired 701.1
    Hebra's 696.4
  rosea 696.3
  rotunda 696.3
  rubra (Hebra) 695.89
    pilaris 696.4
  sicca 690.18
  simplex 690.18
  specified type NEC 696.5
  streptogenes 696.5
  versicolor 111.0
  scrotal 111.0
Placenta, placental
  ablatio 641.2 ☑
    affecting fetus or newborn 762.1
  abnormal, abnormality 656.7 ☑
    with hemorrhage 641.8 ☑
      affecting fetus or newborn 762.1
    affecting fetus or newborn 762.2
  abruptio 641.2 ☑
    affecting fetus or newborn 762.1
  accessory lobe — *see* Placenta, abnormal
  accreta (without hemorrhage) 667.0 ☑
    with hemorrhage 666.0 ☑
  adherent (without hemorrhage) 667.0 ☑
    with hemorrhage 666.0 ☑
  apoplexy — *see* Placenta, separation
  battledore — *see* Placenta, abnormal
  bilobate — *see* Placenta, abnormal
  bipartita –– *see* Placenta, abnormal
  carneous mole 631.8
  centralis — *see* Placenta, previa
  circumvallata — *see* Placenta, abnormal
  cyst (amniotic) — *see* Placenta, abnormal
  deficiency — *see* Placenta, insufficiency
  degeneration — *see* Placenta, insufficiency
  detachment (partial) (premature) (with
    hemorrhage) 641.2 ☑
    affecting fetus or newborn 762.1
  dimidiata — *see* Placenta, abnormal
  disease 656.7 ☑
    affecting fetus or newborn 762.2
  duplex — *see* Placenta, abnormal
  dysfunction — *see* Placenta, insufficiency
  fenestrata — *see* Placenta, abnormal
  fibrosis — *see* Placenta, abnormal
  fleshy mole 631.8
  hematoma — *see* Placenta, abnormal
  hemorrhage NEC — *see* Placenta, separation
  hormone disturbance or malfunction — *see*
    Placenta, abnormal
  hyperplasia — *see* Placenta, abnormal
  increta (without hemorrhage) 667.0 ☑
    with hemorrhage 666.0 ☑
  infarction 656.7 ☑
    affecting fetus or newborn 762.2
  insertion, vicious — *see* Placenta, previa
  insufficiency
    affecting
      fetus or newborn 762.2
      management of pregnancy 656.5 ☑
  lateral — *see* Placenta, previa
  low implantation or insertion — *see* Placen-
    ta, previa
  low-lying — *see* Placenta, previa
  malformation — *see* Placenta, abnormal
  malposition — *see* Placenta, previa
  marginalis, marginata — *see* Placenta, pre-
    via
  marginal sinus (hemorrhage) (rupture)
    641.2 ☑
    affecting fetus or newborn 762.1
  membranacea — *see* Placenta, abnormal
  multilobed — *see* Placenta, abnormal
  multipartita — *see* Placenta, abnormal
  necrosis — *see* Placenta, abnormal
  percreta (without hemorrhage) 667.0 ☑
    with hemorrhage 666.0 ☑
  polyp 674.4 ☑
  previa (central) (centralis) (complete) (later-
    al) (marginal) (marginalis) (partial)
    (partialis) (total) (with hemorrhage)
    641.1 ☑

Placenta, placental — *continued*
  previa — *continued*
    without hemorrhage (before labor and
      delivery) (during pregnancy)
      641.0 ☑
      affecting fetus or newborn 762.0
      noted
        before labor, without hemorrhage
          (with cesarean delivery)
          641.0 ☑
        during pregnancy (without hemor-
          rhage) 641.0 ☑
  retention (with hemorrhage) 666.0 ☑
    without hemorrhage 667.0 ☑
    fragments, complicating puerperium
      (delayed hemorrhage) 666.2 ☑
      without hemorrhage 667.1 ☑
    postpartum, puerperal 666.2 ☑
  separation (normally implanted) (partial)
    (premature) (with hemorrhage)
    641.2 ☑
    affecting fetus or newborn 762.1
  septuplex — *see* Placenta, abnormal
  small — *see* Placenta, insufficiency
  softening (premature) — *see* Placenta, ab-
    normal
  spuria — *see* Placenta, abnormal
  succenturiata — *see* Placenta, abnormal
  syphilitic 095.8
  transfusion syndromes 762.3
  transmission of chemical substance — *see*
    Absorption, chemical, through pla-
    centa
  trapped (with hemorrhage) 666.0 ☑
    without hemorrhage 667.0 ☑
  trilobate — *see* Placenta, abnormal
  tripartita — *see* Placenta, abnormal
  triplex — *see* Placenta, abnormal
  varicose vessel — *see* Placenta, abnormal
  vicious insertion — *see* Placenta, previa
Placentitis
  affecting fetus or newborn 762.7
  complicating pregnancy 658.4 ☑
Plagiocephaly (skull) 754.0
Plague 020.9
  abortive 020.8
  ambulatory 020.8
  bubonic 020.0
  cellulocutaneous 020.1
  lymphatic gland 020.0
  pneumonic 020.5
    primary 020.3
    secondary 020.4
  pulmonary — *see* Plague, pneumonic
  pulmonic — *see* Plague, pneumonic
  septicemic 020.2
  tonsillar 020.9
    septicemic 020.2
  vaccination, prophylactic (against) V03.3
Planning, family V25.09
  contraception V25.9
  natural
    procreative V26.41
    to avoid pregnancy V25.04
  procreation V26.49
    natural V26.41
Plaque
  artery, arterial — *see* Arteriosclerosis
  calcareous — *see* Calcification
  Hollenhorst's (retinal) 362.33
  tongue 528.6
Plasma cell myeloma 203.0 ☑
Plasmacytoma, plasmocytoma (solitary)
  (M9731/1) 238.6
  benign (M9731/0) — *see* Neoplasm, by site,
    benign
  malignant (M9731/3) 203.8 ☑
Plasmacytopenia 288.59
Plasmacytosis 288.64
Plaster ulcer — *see also* Ulcer, pressure 707.00
Plateau iris syndrome (without glaucoma)
  364.82
  with glaucoma 365.23
Platybasia 756.0
Platyonychia (congenital) 757.5
  acquired 703.8

☑ **Additional Digit Required** — Refer to the Tabular List for Digit Selection   ⓦ **Subterms under main terms may continue to next column or page**

232 — Volume 2   ▶◀ Revised Text   ● New Line   ▲ Revised Code   **2015 ICD-9-CM**

Pneumonia — *continued*
due to — *continued*
Eaton's agent 483.0
Escherichia coli (E. coli) 482.82
Friedländer's bacillus 482.0
fumes or vapors (chemical) (inhalation) 506.0
fungus NEC 117.9 *[484.7]*
coccidioidomycosis 114.0
Hemophilus influenzae (H. influenzae) 482.2
Herellea 482.83
influenza (*see also* Influenza) 487.0
Klebsiella pneumoniae 482.0
Mycoplasma (pneumoniae) 483.0
parainfluenza virus 480.2
pleuropneumonia-like organism (PPLO) 483.0
Pneumococcus 481
Pneumocystis carinii 136.3
Pneumocystis jiroveci 136.3
Proteus 482.83
Pseudomonas 482.1
respiratory syncytial virus 480.1
rickettsia 083.9 *[484.8]*
SARS-associated coronavirus 480.3
specified
bacteria NEC 482.89
organism NEC 483.8
virus NEC 480.8
Staphylococcus 482.40
aureus 482.41
methicillin
resistant (MRSA) 482.42
susceptible (MSSA) 482.41
specified type NEC 482.49
Streptococcus (*see also* Pneumonia, streptococcal)
pneumoniae 481
virus (*see also* Pneumonia, viral) 480.9
SARS-associated coronavirus 480.3
Eaton's agent 483.0
embolic, embolism — (*see* Embolism, pulmonary)
eosinophilic 518.3
Escherichia coli (E. coli) 482.82
Eubacterium 482.81
fibrinous — *see* Pneumonia, lobar
fibroid (chronic) (*see also* Fibrosis, lung) 515
fibrous (*see also* Fibrosis, lung) 515
Friedländer's bacillus 482.0
Fusobacterium (nucleatum) 482.81
gangrenous 513.0
giant cell (*see also* Pneumonia, viral) 480.9
gram-negative bacteria NEC 482.83
anaerobic 482.81
grippal (*see also* Influenza) 487.0
Hemophilus influenzae (bronchial) (lobar) 482.2
hypostatic (broncho-) (lobar) 514
in
actinomycosis 039.1
anthrax 022.1 *[484.5]*
aspergillosis 117.3 *[484.6]*
candidiasis 112.4
coccidioidomycosis 114.0
cytomegalic inclusion disease 078.5 *[484.1]*
histoplasmosis (*see also* Histoplasmosis) 115.95
infectious disease NEC 136.9 *[484.8]*
measles 055.1
mycosis, systemic NEC 117.9 *[484.7]*
nocardiasis, nocardiosis 039.1
ornithosis 073.0
pneumocystosis 136.3
psittacosis 073.0
Q fever 083.0 *[484.8]*
salmonellosis 003.22
toxoplasmosis 130.4
tularemia 021.2
typhoid (fever) 002.0 *[484.8]*
varicella 052.1
whooping cough (*see also* Whooping cough) 033.9 *[484.3]*
infective, acquired prenatally 770.0

Pneumonia — *continued*
influenzal (broncho) (lobar) (virus) (*see also* Influenza) 487.0
inhalation (*see also* Pneumonia, aspiration) 507.0
fumes or vapors (chemical) 506.0
interstitial 516.8
with influenzal (*see also* Influenza) 487.0
acute
due to Pneumocystis (carinii) (jiroveci) 136.3
meaning:
acute interstitial pneumonitis 516.33
atypical pneumonia — *see* Pneumonia, atypical
bacterial pneumonia — *see* Pneumonia, bacterial
chronic (*see also* Fibrosis, lung) 515
desquamative 516.37
hypostatic 514
idiopathic 516.30
lymphoid 516.35
lipoid 507.1
lymphoid (due to known underlying cause) 516.8
non-specific (due to known underlying cause) 516.8
organizing (due to known underlying cause) 516.8
plasma cell 136.3
Pseudomonas 482.1
intrauterine (infective) 770.0
aspiration 770.18
blood 770.16
clear amniotic fluid 770.14
meconium 770.12
postnatal stomach contents 770.86
Klebsiella pneumoniae 482.0
Legionnaires' 482.84
lipid, lipoid (exogenous) (interstitial) 507.1
endogenous 516.8
lobar (diplococcal) (disseminated) (double) (interstitial) (pneumococcal, any type) 481
with influenza (*see also* Influenza) 487.0
bacterial 482.9
specified type NEC 482.89
chronic (*see also* Fibrosis, lung) 515
Escherichia coli (E. coli) 482.82
Friedländer's bacillus 482.0
Hemophilus influenzae (H. influenzae) 482.2
hypostatic 514
influenzal (*see also* Influenza) 487.0
Klebsiella 482.0
ornithosis 073.0
Proteus 482.83
Pseudomonas 482.1
psittacosis 073.0
specified organism NEC 483.8
bacterial NEC 482.89
staphylococcal 482.40
aureus 482.41
methicillin
resistant (MRSA) 482.42
susceptible (MSSA) 482.41
specified type NEC 482.49
streptococcal — *see* Pneumonia, streptococcal
viral, virus (*see also* Pneumonia, viral) 480.9
lobular (confluent) — *see* Pneumonia, broncho-
Löffler's 518.3
massive — *see* Pneumonia, lobar
meconium aspiration 770.12
metastatic NEC 038.8 *[484.8]*
methicillin resistant Staphylococcus aureus (MRSA) 482.42
methicillin susceptible Staphylococcus aureus (MSSA) 482.41
MRSA (methicillin resistant Staphylococcus aureus) 482.42
MSSA (methicillin susceptible Staphylococcus aureus) 482.41

Pneumonia — *continued*
multilobar — *see* Pneumonia, by type
Mycoplasma (pneumoniae) 483.0
necrotic 513.0
nitrogen dioxide 506.9
orthostatic 514
parainfluenza virus 480.2
parenchymatous (*see also* Fibrosis, lung) 515
passive 514
patchy — *see* Pneumonia, broncho-
Peptococcus 482.81
Peptostreptococcus 482.81
plasma cell 136.3
pleurolobar — *see* Pneumonia, lobar
pleuropneumonia-like organism (PPLO) 483.0
pneumococcal (broncho) (lobar) 481
Pneumocystis (carinii) (jiroveci) 136.3
postinfectional NEC 136.9 *[484.8]*
postmeasles 055.1
postoperative 997.39
aspiration 997.32
primary atypical 486
Proprionibacterium 482.81
Proteus 482.83
Pseudomonas 482.1
psittacosis 073.0
radiation 508.0
respiratory syncytial virus 480.1
resulting from a procedure 997.39
aspiration 997.32
rheumatic 390 *[517.1]*
Salmonella 003.22
SARS-associated coronavirus 480.3
segmented, segmental — *see* Pneumonia, broncho-
Serratia (marcescens) 482.83
specified
bacteria NEC 482.89
organism NEC 483.8
virus NEC 480.8
spirochetal 104.8 *[484.8]*
staphylococcal (broncho) (lobar) 482.40
aureus 482.41
methicillin
resistant 482.42
susceptible (MSSA) 482.41
specified type NEC 482.49
static, stasis 514
streptococcal (broncho) (lobar) NEC 482.30
Group
A 482.31
B 482.32
specified NEC 482.39
pneumoniae 481
specified type NEC 482.39
Streptococcus pneumoniae 481
traumatic (complication) (early) (secondary) 958.8
tuberculous (any) (*see also* Tuberculosis) 011.6 ☑
tularemic 021.2
TWAR agent 483.1
varicella 052.1
Veillonella 482.81
ventilator associated 997.31
viral, virus (broncho) (interstitial) (lobar) 480.9
with influenza, flu, or grippe (*see also* Influenza) 487.0
adenoviral 480.0
parainfluenza 480.2
respiratory syncytial 480.1
SARS-associated coronavirus 480.3
specified type NEC 480.8
white (congenital) 090.0
Pneumonic — *see* condition
Pneumonitis (acute) (primary) — *see also* Pneumonia 486
allergic 495.9
specified type NEC 495.8
aspiration 507.0
due to fumes or gases 506.0
fetal 770.18
due to
blood 770.16

Pneumonitis — *see also* Pneumonia — *continued*
aspiration — *continued*
fetal — *continued*
due to — *continued*
clear amniotic fluid 770.14
meconium 770.12
postnatal stomach contents 770.86
newborn 770.18
due to
blood 770.16
clear amniotic fluid 770.14
meconium 770.12
postnatal stomach contents 770.86
obstetric 668.0 ☑
chemical 506.0
due to fumes or gases 506.0
resulting from a procedure 997.32
cholesterol 516.8
chronic (*see also* Fibrosis, lung) 515
congenital rubella 771.0
crack 506.0
due to
crack (cocaine) 506.0
fumes or vapors 506.0
inhalation
food (regurgitated), milk, vomitus 507.0
oils, essences 507.1
saliva 507.0
solids, liquids NEC 507.8
toxoplasmosis (acquired) 130.4
congenital (active) 771.2 *[484.8]*
eosinophilic 518.3
fetal aspiration 770.18
due to
blood 770.16
clear amniotic fluid 770.14
meconium 770.12
postnatal stomach contents 770.86
hypersensitivity 495.9
interstitial (chronic) (*see also* Fibrosis, lung) 515
acute 516.33
idiopathic
lymphocytic 516.35
non-specific 516.32
lymphoid 516.8
lymphoid, interstitial 516.8
meconium aspiration 770.12
postanesthetic
correct substance properly administered 507.0
obstetric 668.0 ☑
overdose or wrong substance given 968.4
specified anesthetic — *see* Table of Drugs and Chemicals
postoperative 997.3 ☑
aspiration 997.32
obstetric 668.0 ☑
radiation 508.0
rubella, congenital 771.0
"ventilation" 495.7
ventilator associated 997.31
wood-dust 495.8
Pneumoconiosis — *see* Pneumoconiosis
Pneumoparotid 527.8
Pneumopathy NEC 518.89
alveolar 516.9
specified NEC 516.8
due to dust NEC 504
parietoalveolar 516.9
specified condition NEC 516.8
Pneumopericarditis — *see also* Pericarditis 423.9
acute 420.90
Pneumopericardium — *see also* Pericarditis
congenital 770.2
fetus or newborn 770.2
traumatic (post) (*see also* Pneumothorax, traumatic) 860.0
with open wound into thorax 860.1
Pneumoperitoneum 568.89

Pneumoperitoneum — continued
  fetus or newborn 770.2
Pneumophagia (psychogenic) 306.4
Pneumopleurisy, pneumopleuritis — see
  also Pneumonia 486
Pneumopyopericardium 420.99
Pneumopyothorax — see also Pyopneumothorax 510.9
  with fistula 510.0
Pneumorrhagia 786.30
  newborn 770.3
  tuberculous (see also Tuberculosis, pul-
    monary) 011.9 ☑
Pneumosiderosis (occupational) 503
Pneumothorax 512.89
  acute 512.89
  chronic 512.83
  congenital 770.2
  due to operative injury of chest wall or lung
    512.1
    accidental puncture or laceration 512.1
  fetus or newborn 770.2
  iatrogenic 512.1
  postoperative 512.1
  specified type NEC 512.89
  spontaneous 512.89
    fetus or newborn 770.2
    primary 512.81
    secondary 512.82
    tension 512.0
  sucking 512.89
    iatrogenic 512.1
    postoperative 512.1
  tense valvular, infectional 512.0
  tension 512.0
    iatrogenic 512.1
    postoperative 512.1
    spontaneous 512.0
  traumatic 860.0
    with
      hemothorax 860.4
        with open wound into thorax
          860.5
      open wound into thorax 860.1
  tuberculous (see also Tuberculosis) 011.7 ☑
Pocket(s)
  endocardial (see also Endocarditis) 424.90
  periodontal 523.8
Podagra 274.01
Podencephalus 759.89
Poikilocytosis 790.09
Poikiloderma 709.09
  Civatte's 709.09
  congenital 757.33
  vasculare atrophicans 696.2
Poikilodermatomyositis 710.3
Pointed ear 744.29
Poise imperfect 729.90
Poisoned — see Poisoning
Poisoning (acute) — see also Table of Drugs
  and Chemicals
  Bacillus, B.
    aertrycke (see also Infection, Salmonella)
      003.9
    botulinus 005.1
    cholerae (suis) (see also Infection,
      Salmonella) 003.9
    paratyphosus (see also Infection,
      Salmonella) 003.9
    suipestifer (see also Infection, Salmonel-
      la) 003.9
  bacterial toxins NEC 005.9
  berries, noxious 988.2
  blood (general) — see Septicemia
  botulism 005.1
  bread, moldy, mouldy — see Poisoning,
    food
  Ciguatera 988.0
  damaged meat — see Poisoning, food
  death-cap (Amanita phalloides) (Amanita
    verna) 988.1
  decomposed food — see Poisoning, food
  diseased food — see Poisoning, food
  drug — see Table of Drugs and Chemicals
  epidemic, fish, meat, or other food — see
    Poisoning, food

Poisoning — see also Table of Drugs and
  Chemicals — continued
  fava bean 282.2
  fish (bacterial) (see also Poisoning, food)
    noxious 988.0
  food (acute) (bacterial) (diseased) (infected)
    NEC 005.9
    due to
      bacillus
        aertrycke (see also Poisoning,
          food, due to Salmonella)
          003.9
        botulinus 005.1
        cereus 005.89
        choleraesuis (see also Poisoning,
          food, due to Salmonella)
          003.9
        paratyphosus (see also Poisoning,
          food, due to Salmonella)
          003.9
        suipestifer (see also Poisoning,
          food, due to Salmonella)
          003.9
      Clostridium 005.3
        botulinum 005.1
        perfringens 005.2
        welchii 005.2
      Salmonella (aertrycke) (callinarum)
        (choleraesuis) (enteritidis)
        (paratyphi) (suipestifer) 003.9
        with
          gastroenteritis 003.0
          localized infection(s) (see also
            Infection, Salmonella)
            003.20
          septicemia 003.1
          specified manifestation NEC
            003.8
      specified bacterium NEC 005.89
      Staphylococcus 005.0
      Streptococcus 005.89
      Vibrio parahaemolyticus 005.4
      Vibrio vulnificus 005.81
    noxious or naturally toxic 988.0
      berries 988.2
      fish 988.0
      mushroom 988.1
      plants NEC 988.2
  ice cream — see Poisoning, food
  ichthyotoxism (bacterial) 005.9
  kreotoxism, food 005.9
  malarial — see Malaria
  meat — see Poisoning, food
  mushroom (noxious) 988.1
  mussel (see also Poisoning, food)
    noxious 988.0
  noxious foodstuffs (see also Poisoning, food,
    noxious) 988.9
  specified type NEC 988.8
  plants, noxious 988.2
  pork (see also Poisoning, food)
    specified NEC 988.8
    Trichinosis 124
  ptomaine — see Poisoning, food
  putrefaction, food — see Poisoning, food
  radiation 508.0
  Salmonella (see also Infection, Salmonella)
    003.9
  sausage (see also Poisoning, food)
    Trichinosis 124
  saxitoxin 988.0
  shellfish (see also Poisoning, food)
    noxious (amnesic) (azaspiracid) (diarrhe-
      ic) (neurotoxic) (paralytic) 988.0
  Staphylococcus, food 005.0
  toxic, from disease NEC 799.89
  truffles — see Poisoning, food
  uremic — see Uremia
  uric acid 274.9
  water 276.69
**Poison ivy, oak, sumac or other plant der-
  matitis** 692.6
Poker spine 720.0
Policeman's disease 729.2
Polioencephalitis (acute) (bulbar) — see also
  Poliomyelitis, bulbar 045.0 ☑

Polioencephalitis — see also Poliomyelitis,
  bulbar — continued
  inferior 335.22
  influenzal (see also Influenza) 487.8
  superior hemorrhagic (acute) (Wernicke's)
    265.1
  Wernicke's (superior hemorrhagic) 265.1
Polioencephalomyelitis (acute) (anterior)
  (bulbar) — see also Polioencephalitis
  045.0 ☑
Polioencephalopathy, superior hemorrhagic
  265.1
  with
    beriberi 265.0
    pellagra 265.2
Poliomeningoencephalitis — see Meningoencephalitis
Poliomyelitis (acute) (anterior) (epidemic)
  045.9 ☑

Note — Use the following fifth-digit
subclassification with category 045:

0   poliovirus, unspecified type
1   poliovirus, type I
2   poliovirus, type II
3   poliovirus, type III

  with
    paralysis 045.1 ☑
      bulbar 045.0 ☑
  abortive 045.2 ☑
  ascending 045.9 ☑
    progressive 045.9 ☑
  bulbar 045.0 ☑
  cerebral 045.0 ☑
  chronic 335.21
  congenital 771.2
  contact V01.2
  deformities 138
  exposure to V01.2
  late effect 138
  nonepidemic 045.9 ☑
  nonparalytic 045.2 ☑
  old with deformity 138
  posterior, acute 053.19
  residual 138
  sequelae 138
  spinal, acute 045.9 ☑
  syphilitic (chronic) 094.89
  vaccination, prophylactic (against) V04.0
Poliosis (eyebrow) (eyelashes) 704.3
  circumscripta (congenital) 757.4
    acquired 704.3
  congenital 757.4
Pollakiuria 788.41
  psychogenic 306.53
Pollinosis 477.0
Pollitzer's disease (hidradenitis suppurativa)
  705.83
Polyadenitis — see also Adenitis 289.3
  malignant 020.0
Polyalgia 729.99
Polyangiitis (essential) 446.0
Poiyarteritis (nodosa) (renal) 446.0
Polyarthralgia 719.49
  psychogenic 306.0
Polyarthritis, polyarthropathy NEC 716.59
  due to or associated with other specified
    conditions — see Arthritis, due to or
    associated with
  endemic (see also Disease, Kaschin-Beck)
    716.0 ☑
  inflammatory 714.9
    specified type NEC 714.89
  juvenile (chronic) 714.30
    acute 714.31
  migratory — see Fever, rheumatic
  rheumatic 714.0
    fever (acute) — see Fever, rheumatic
Polycarential syndrome of infancy 260
Polychondritis (atrophic) (chronic) (relapsing)
  733.99
Polycoria 743.46
Polycystic (congenital) (disease) 759.89

Polycystic — continued
  degeneration, kidney — see Polycystic, kid-
    ney
  kidney (congenital) 753.12
    adult type (APKD) 753.13
    autosomal dominant 753.13
    autosomal recessive 753.14
    childhood type (CPKD) 753.14
    infantile type 753.14
  liver 751.62
  lung 518.89
    congenital 748.4
  ovary, ovaries 256.4
  spleen 759.0
Polycythemia (primary) (rubra) (vera)
  (M9950/1) 238.4
  acquired 289.0
  benign 289.0
    familial 289.6
  due to
    donor twin 776.4
    fall in plasma volume 289.0
    high altitude 289.0
    maternal-fetal transfusion 776.4
    stress 289.0
  emotional 289.0
  erythropoietin 289.0
  familial (benign) 289.6
  Gaisböck's (hypertonica) 289.0
  high altitude 289.0
  hypertonica 289.0
  hypoxemic 289.0
  neonatorum 776.4
  nephrogenous 289.0
  relative 289.0
  secondary 289.0
  spurious 289.0
  stress 289.0
Polycytosis cryptogenica 289.0
Polydactylism, polydactyly 755.00
  fingers 755.01
  toes 755.02
Polydipsia 783.5
Polydystrophic oligophrenia 277.5
Polyembryoma (M9072/3) — see Neoplasm,
  by site, malignant
Polygalactia 676.6 ☑
Polyglandular
  deficiency 258.9
  dyscrasia 258.9
  dysfunction 258.9
  syndrome 258.8
Polyhydramnios — see also Hydramnios
  657.0 ☑
Polymastia 757.6
Polymenorrhea 626.2
Polymicrogyria 742.2
Polymyalgia 725
  arteritica 446.5
  rheumatica 725
Polymyositis (acute) (chronic) (hemorrhagic)
  710.4
  with involvement of
    lung 710.4 [517.8]
    skin 710.3
  ossificans (generalisata) (progressiva) 728.19
  Wagner's (dermatomyositis) 710.3
Polyneuritis, polyneuritic — see also
  Polyneuropathy 356.9
  alcoholic 357.5
    with psychosis 291.1
  cranialis 352.6
  demyelinating, chronic inflammatory (CIDP)
    357.81
  diabetic 250.6 ☑ [357.2]
    due to secondary diabetes
      249.6 ☑ [357.2]
  due to lack of vitamin NEC 269.2 [357.4]
  endemic 265.0 [357.4]
  erythredema 985.0
  febrile 357.0
  hereditary ataxic 356.3
  idiopathic, acute 357.0
  infective (acute) 357.0
  nutritional 269.9 [357.4]
  postinfectious 357.0

☑ **Additional Digit Required** — Refer to the Tabular List for Digit Selection   ▽ **Subterms under main terms may continue to next column or page**

Polyneuropathy (peripheral) 356.9
  alcoholic 357.5
  amyloid 277.39 *[357.4]*
  arsenical 357.7
  critical illness 357.82
  demyelinating, chronic inflammatory (CIDP) 357.81
  diabetic 250.6 ☑ *[357.2]*
    due to secondary diabetes 249.6 ☑ *[357.2]*
  due to
    antitetanus serum 357.6
    arsenic 357.7
    drug or medicinal substance 357.6
      correct substance properly administered 357.6
      overdose or wrong substance given or taken 977.9
      specified drug — see Table of Drugs and Chemicals
    lack of vitamin NEC 269.2 *[357.4]*
    lead 357.7
    organophosphate compounds 357.7
    pellagra 265.2 *[357.4]*
    porphyria 277.1 *[357.4]*
    serum 357.6
    toxic agent NEC 357.7
  hereditary 356.0
  idiopathic 356.9
    progressive 356.4
  in
    amyloidosis 277.39 *[357.4]*
    avitaminosis 269.2 *[357.4]*
      specified NEC 269.1 *[357.4]*
    beriberi 265.0 *[357.4]*
    collagen vascular disease NEC 710.9 *[357.1]*
    deficiency
      B-complex NEC 266.2 *[357.4]*
      vitamin B 266.1 *[357.4]*
      vitamin B6 266.9 *[357.4]*
    diabetes 250.6 ☑ *[357.2]*
      due to secondary diabetes 249.6 ☑ *[357.2]*
    diphtheria (see also Diphtheria) 032.89 *[357.4]*
    disseminated lupus erythematosus 710.0 *[357.1]*
    herpes zoster 053.13
    hypoglycemia 251.2 *[357.4]*
    malignant neoplasm (M8000/3) NEC 199.1 *[357.3]*
    mumps 072.72
    pellagra 265.2 *[357.4]*
    polyarteritis nodosa 446.0 *[357.1]*
    porphyria 277.1 *[357.4]*
    rheumatoid arthritis 714.0 *[357.1]*
    sarcoidosis 135 *[357.4]*
    uremia 585.9 *[357.4]*
  lead 357.7
  nutritional 269.9 *[357.4]*
    specified NEC 269.8 *[357.4]*
  postherpetic 053.13
  progressive 356.4
  sensory (hereditary) 356.2
  specified NEC 356.8
Polyonychia 757.5
Polyopia 368.2
  refractive 368.15
Polyorchism, polyorchidism (three testes) 752.89
Polyorrhymenitis (peritoneal) — see also Polyserositis 568.82
  pericardial 423.2
Polyostotic fibrous dysplasia 756.54
Polyotia 744.1
Polyphagia 783.6
Polypoid — see condition
Polyposis — see also Polyp
  coli (adenomatous) (M8220/0) 211.3
    adenocarcinoma in (M8220/3) 153.9
    carcinoma in (M8220/3) 153.9
  familial (M8220/0) 211.3
  intestinal (adenomatous) (M8220/0) 211.3
  multiple (M8221/0) — see Neoplasm, by site, benign

Polyp, polypus

Note — Polyps of organs or sites that do not appear in the list below should be coded to the residual category for diseases of the organ or site concerned.

  accessory sinus 471.8
  adenoid tissue 471.0
  adenomatous (M8210/0) (see also Neoplasm, by site, benign)
    adenocarcinoma in (M8210/3) — see Neoplasm, by site, malignant
    carcinoma in (M8210/3) — see Neoplasm, by site, malignant
    multiple (M8221/0) — see Neoplasm, by site, benign
  antrum 471.8
  anus, anal (canal) (nonadenomatous) 569.0
    adenomatous 211.4
  Bartholin's gland 624.6
  bladder (M8120/1) 236.7
  broad ligament 620.8
  cervix (uteri) 622.7
    adenomatous 219.0
    in pregnancy or childbirth 654.6 ☑
      affecting fetus or newborn 763.89
      causing obstructed labor 660.2 ☑
    mucous 622.7
    nonneoplastic 622.7
  choanal 471.0
  cholesterol 575.6
  clitoris 624.6
  colon (M8210/0) (see also Polyp, adenomatous) 211.3
  corpus uteri 621.0
  dental 522.0
  ear (middle) 385.30
  endometrium 621.0
  ethmoidal (sinus) 471.8
  fallopian tube 620.8
  female genital organs NEC 624.8
  frontal (sinus) 471.8
  gallbladder 575.6
  gingiva 523.8
  gum 523.8
  labia 624.6
  larynx (mucous) 478.4
  malignant (M8000/3) — see Neoplasm, by site, malignant
  maxillary (sinus) 471.8
  middle ear 385.30
  myometrium 621.0
  nares
    anterior 471.9
    posterior 471.0
  nasal (mucous) 471.9
    cavity 471.0
    septum 471.9
  nasopharyngeal 471.0
  neoplastic (M8210/0) — see Neoplasm, by site, benign
  nose (mucous) 471.9
  oviduct 620.8
  paratubal 620.8
  pharynx 478.29
    congenital 750.29
  placenta, placental 674.4 ☑
  prostate 600.20
    with
      other lower urinary tract symptoms (LUTS) 600.21
      urinary
        obstruction 600.21
        retention 600.21
  pudenda 624.6
  pulp (dental) 522.0
  rectosigmoid 211.4
  rectum (nonadenomatous) 569.0
    adenomatous 211.4
  septum (nasal) 471.9
  sinus (accessory) (ethmoidal) (frontal) (maxillary) (sphenoidal) 471.8
  sphenoidal (sinus) 471.8
  stomach (M8210/0) 211.1
  tube, fallopian 620.8
  turbinate, mucous membrane 471.8
  ureter 593.89

Polyp, polypus — continued
  urethra 599.3
  uterine
    ligament 620.8
    tube 620.8
  uterus (body) (corpus) (mucous) 621.0
    in pregnancy or childbirth 654.1 ☑
      affecting fetus or newborn 763.89
      causing obstructed labor 660.2 ☑
  vagina 623.7
  vocal cord (mucous) 478.4
  vulva 624.6
Polyradiculitis (acute) 357.0
Polyradiculoneuropathy (acute) (segmentally demyelinating) 357.0
Polysarcia 278.00
Polyserositis (peritoneal) 568.82
  due to pericarditis 423.2
  paroxysmal (familial) 277.31
  pericardial 423.2
  periodic (familial) 277.31
  pleural — see Pleurisy
  recurrent 277.31
  tuberculous (see also Tuberculosis, polyserositis) 018.9 ☑
Polysialia 527.7
Polysplenia syndrome 759.0
Polythelia 757.6
Polytrichia — see also Hypertrichosis 704.1
Polyunguia (congenital) 757.5
  acquired 703.8
Polyuria 788.42
Pompe's disease (glycogenosis II) 271.0
Pompholyx 705.81
Poncet's disease (tuberculous rheumatism) — see also Tuberculosis 015.9 ☑
Pond fracture — see Fracture, skull, vault
Ponos 085.0
Pons, pontine — see condition
Poor
  aesthetics of existing restoration of tooth 525.67
  contractions, labor 661.2 ☑
    affecting fetus or newborn 763.7
  fetal growth NEC 764.9 ☑
    affecting management of pregnancy 656.5 ☑
  incorporation
    artificial skin graft 996.55
    decellularized allodermis graft 996.55
  obstetrical history V13.29
    affecting management of current pregnancy V23.49
      ectopic pregnancy V23.42
      pre-term labor V23.41
    pre-term labor V13.21
  sucking reflex (newborn) 796.1
  vision NEC 369.9
Poradenitis, nostras 099.1
Porencephaly (congenital) (developmental) (true) 742.4
  acquired 348.0
  nondevelopmental 348.0
  traumatic (post) 310.2
Porocephaliasis 134.1
Porokeratosis 757.39
  disseminated superficial actinic (DSAP) 692.75
Poroma, eccrine (M8402/0) — see Neoplasm, skin, benign
Porphyria (acute) (congenital) (constitutional) (erythropoietic) (familial) (hepatica) (idiopathic) (idiosyncratic) (intermittent) (latent) (mixed hepatic) (photosensitive) (South African genetic) (Swedish) 277.1
  acquired 277.1
  cutaneatarda
    hereditaria 277.1
    symptomatica 277.1
  due to drugs
    correct substance properly administered 277.1
    overdose or wrong substance given or taken 977.9
    specified drug — see Table of Drugs and Chemicals

Porphyria — continued
  secondary 277.1
  toxic NEC 277.1
  variegata 277.1
Porphyrinuria (acquired) (congenital) (secondary) 277.1
Porphyruria (acquired) (congenital) 277.1
Portal — see condition
Port wine nevus or mark 757.32
Posadas-Wernicke disease 114.9
Position
  fetus, abnormal (see also Presentation, fetal) 652.9 ☑
  teeth, faulty (see also Anomaly, position tooth) 524.30
Positive
  culture (nonspecific) 795.39
    AIDS virus V08
    blood 790.7
    HIV V08
    human immunodeficiency virus V08
    nose 795.39
      Staphylococcus — see Carrier (suspected) of, Staphylococcus
    skin lesion NEC 795.39
    spinal fluid 792.0
    sputum 795.39
    stool 792.1
    throat 795.39
    urine 791.9
    wound 795.39
  findings, anthrax 795.31
  HIV V08
  human immunodeficiency virus (HIV) V08
  PPD 795.51
  serology
    AIDS virus V08
      inconclusive 795.71
    HIV V08
      inconclusive 795.71
    human immunodeficiency virus (HIV) V08
      inconclusive 795.71
    syphilis 097.1
      with signs or symptoms — see Syphilis, by site and stage
      false 795.6
  skin test 795.7 ☑
    tuberculin (without active tuberculosis) 795.51
  VDRL 097.1
    with signs or symptoms — see Syphilis, by site and stage
    false 795.6
  Wassermann reaction 097.1
    false 795.6
Postcardiotomy syndrome 429.4
Postcaval ureter 753.4
Postcholecystectomy syndrome 576.0
Postclimacteric bleeding 627.1
Postcommissurotomy syndrome 429.4
Postconcussional syndrome 310.2
Postcontusional syndrome 310.2
Postcricoid region — see condition
Post-dates (pregnancy) — see Pregnancy
Postencephalitic — see also condition
  syndrome 310.89
Posterior — see condition
Posterolateral sclerosis (spinal cord) — see Degeneration, combined
Postexanthematous — see condition
Postfebrile — see condition
Postgastrectomy dumping syndrome 564.2
Posthemiplegic chorea 344.89
Posthemorrhagic anemia (chronic) 280.0
  acute 285.1
  newborn 776.5
Posthepatitis syndrome 780.79
Postherpetic neuralgia (intercostal) (syndrome) (zoster) 053.19
  geniculate ganglion 053.11
  ophthalmica 053.19
  trigeminal 053.12
Posthitis 607.1
Postimmunization complication or reaction — see Complications, vaccination

---

☑ Additional Digit Required — Refer to the Tabular List for Digit Selection   ▼ Subterms under main terms may continue to next column or page

Postinfectious — see condition
Postinfluenzal syndrome 780.79
Postlaminectomy syndrome 722.80
  cervical, cervicothoracic 722.81
  kyphosis 737.12
  lumbar, lumbosacral 722.83
  thoracic, thoracolumbar 722.82
Postleukotomy syndrome 310.0
Postlobectomy syndrome 310.0
Postmastectomy lymphedema (syndrome) 457.0
Postmaturity, postmature (fetus or newborn) (gestation period over 42 completed weeks) 766.22
  affecting management of pregnancy
    post-term pregnancy 645.1 ☑
    prolonged pregnancy 645.2 ☑
  syndrome 766.22
Postmeasles — see also condition
  complication 055.8
  specified NEC 055.79
Postmenopausal
  endometrium (atrophic) 627.8
    suppurative (see also Endometritis) 615.9
  hormone replacement therapy V07.4
  status (age related) (natural) V49.81
Postnasal drip 784.91
Postnatal — see condition
Postoperative — see also condition
  confusion state 293.9
  psychosis 293.9
  status NEC (see also Status (post)) V45.89
Postpancreatectomy hyperglycemia 251.3
Postpartum — see also condition
  anemia 648.2 ☑
  cardiomyopathy 674.5 ☑
  observation
    immediately after delivery V24.0
    routine follow-up V24.2
Postperfusion syndrome NEC 999.89
  bone marrow 996.85
Postpoliomyelitic — see condition
Postsurgery status NEC — see also Status (post V45.89
Post-term (pregnancy) 645.1 ☑
  infant (gestation period over 40 completed weeks to 42 completed weeks) 766.21
Post-transplant lymphoproliferative disorder (PTLD) 238.77
Posttraumatic — see condition
Posttraumatic brain syndrome, nonpsychotic 310.2
Post-traumatic stress disorder (PTSD) 309.81
Post-typhoid abscess 002.0
Postures, hysterical 300.11
Postvaccinal reaction or complication — see Complications, vaccination
Postvagotomy syndrome 564.2
Postvalvulotomy syndrome 429.4
Postvasectomy sperm count V25.8
Potain's disease (pulmonary edema) 514
Potain's syndrome (gastrectasis with dyspepsia) 536.1
Pott's
  curvature (spinal) (see also Tuberculosis) 015.0 ☑ [737.43]
  disease or paraplegia (see also Tuberculosis) 015.0 ☑ [730.88]
  fracture (closed) 824.4
    open 824.5
  gangrene 440.24
  osteomyelitis (see also Tuberculosis) 015.0 ☑ [730.88]
  spinal curvature (see also Tuberculosis) 015.0 ☑ [737.43]
  tumor, puffy (see also Osteomyelitis) 730.2 ☑
Potter's
  asthma 502
  disease 753.0
  facies 754.0
  lung 502
  syndrome (with renal agenesis) 753.0

Pouch
  bronchus 748.3
  Douglas' — see condition
  esophagus, esophageal (congenital) 750.4
    acquired 530.6
  gastric 537.1
  Hartmann's (abnormal sacculation of gallbladder neck) 575.8
    of intestine V44.3
      attention to V55.3
  pharynx, pharyngeal (congenital) 750.27
Pouchitis 569.71
Poulet's disease 714.2
Poultrymen's itch 133.8
Poverty V60.2
PPE (palmar plantar erythrodysesthesia) 693.0
Prader-Labhart-Willi-Fanconi syndrome (hypogenital dystrophy with diabetic tendency) 759.81
Prader-Willi syndrome (hypogenital dystrophy with diabetic tendency) 759.81
Preachers' voice 784.49
Pre-AIDS — see Human immunodeficiency virus (disease) (illness) (infection)
Preauricular appendage 744.1
Prebetalipoproteinemia (acquired) (essential) (familial) (hereditary) (primary) (secondary) 272.1
  with chylomicronemia 272.3
Precipitate labor 661.3 ☑
  affecting fetus or newborn 763.6
Preclimacteric bleeding 627.0
  menorrhagia 627.0
Precocious
  adrenarche 259.1
  menarche 259.1
  menstruation 259.1
  pubarche 259.1
  puberty NEC 259.1
  sexual development NEC 259.1
  thelarche 259.1
Precocity, sexual (constitutional) (cryptogenic) (female) (idiopathic) (male) NEC 259.1
  with adrenal hyperplasia 255.2
Precordial pain 786.51
  psychogenic 307.89
Predeciduous teeth 520.2
Prediabetes, prediabetic 790.29
  complicating pregnancy, childbirth, or puerperium 648.8 ☑
    fetus or newborn 775.89
Predislocation status of hip, at birth — see also Subluxation, congenital, hip 754.32
Preeclampsia (mild) 642.4 ☑
  with pre-existing hypertension 642.7 ☑
  affecting fetus or newborn 760.0
  severe 642.5 ☑
  superimposed on pre-existing hypertensive disease 642.7 ☑
Preeruptive color change, teeth, tooth 520.8
Preexcitation 426.7
  atrioventricular conduction 426.7
  ventricular 426.7
Preglaucoma 365.00
Pregnancy (single) (uterine) (without sickness) V22.2

Note — Use the following fifth-digit subclassification with categories 640–649, 651–679:

0   unspecified as to episode of care

1   delivered, with or without mention of antepartum condition

2   delivered, with mention of postpartum complication

3   antepartum condition or complication

4   postpartum condition or complication

  abdominal (ectopic) 633.00
    with intrauterine pregnancy 633.01
    affecting fetus or newborn 761.4
  abnormal NEC 646.9 ☑
  ampullar — see Pregnancy, tubal

Pregnancy — continued
  biochemical 631.0
  broad ligament — see Pregnancy, cornual
  cervical — see Pregnancy, cornual
  chemical 631.0
  combined (extrauterine and intrauterine) — see Pregnancy, cornual
  complicated (by) 646.9 ☑
    abnormal, abnormality NEC 646.9 ☑
      cervix 654.6 ☑
      cord (umbilical) 663.9 ☑
      glucose tolerance (conditions classifiable to 790.21–790.29) 648.8 ☑
      pelvic organs or tissues NEC 654.9 ☑
      pelvis (bony) 653.0 ☑
      perineum or vulva 654.8 ☑
      placenta, placental (vessel) 656.7 ☑
      position
        cervix 654.4 ☑
        placenta 641.1 ☑
          without hemorrhage 641.0 ☑
        uterus 654.4 ☑
      size, fetus 653.5 ☑
      uterus (congenital) 654.0 ☑
    abscess or cellulitis
      bladder 646.6 ☑
      genitourinary tract (conditions classifiable to 590, 595, 597, 599.0, 614.0–614.5, 614.7–614.9, 615) 646.6 ☑
      kidney 646.6 ☑
      urinary tract NEC 646.6 ☑
    adhesion, pelvic peritoneal 648.9 ☑
    air embolism 673.0 ☑
    albuminuria 646.2 ☑
      with hypertension — see Toxemia, of pregnancy
    amnionitis 658.4 ☑
    amniotic fluid embolism 673.1 ☑
    anemia (conditions classifiable to 280–285) 648.2 ☑
    appendicitis 648.9 ☑
    atrophy, yellow (acute) (liver) (subacute) 646.7 ☑
    bacilluria, asymptomatic 646.5 ☑
    bacteriuria, asymptomatic 646.5 ☑
    bariatric surgery status 649.2 ☑
    bicornis or bicornuate uterus 654.0 ☑
    biliary problems 646.8 ☑
    bone and joint disorders (conditions classifiable to 720–724 or conditions affecting lower limbs classifiable to 711–719, 725–738) 648.7 ☑
    breech presentation (buttocks) (complete) (frank) 652.2 ☑
      with successful version 652.1 ☑
    cardiovascular disease (conditions classifiable to 390–398, 410–429) 648.6 ☑
      congenital (conditions classifiable to 745–747) 648.5 ☑
    cerebrovascular disorders (conditions classifiable to 430–434, 436–437) 674.0 ☑
    cervicitis (conditions classifiable to 616.0) 646.6 ☑
    chloasma (gravidarum) 646.8 ☑
    cholelithiasis 646.8 ☑
    cholestasis 646.7 ☑
    chorea (gravidarum) — see Eclampsia, pregnancy
    coagulation defect 649.3 ☑
    conjoined twins 678.1 ☑
    contraction, pelvis (general) 653.1 ☑
      inlet 653.2 ☑
      outlet 653.3 ☑
    convulsions (eclamptic) (uremic) 642.6 ☑
      with pre-existing hypertension 642.7 ☑

Pregnancy — continued
  complicated — continued
    current disease or condition (nonobstetric)
      abnormal glucose tolerance 648.8 ☑
      anemia 648.2 ☑
      biliary tract 646.7 ☑
      bone and joint (lower limb) 648.7 ☑
      cardiovascular 648.6 ☑
        congenital 648.5 ☑
      cerebrovascular 674.0 ☑
      diabetes (conditions classifiable to 249 and 250) 648.0 ☑
      drug dependence 648.3 ☑
      female genital mutilation 648.9 ☑
      genital organ or tract 646.6 ☑
      gonorrheal 647.1 ☑
      hypertensive 642.2 ☑
        chronic kidney 642.2 ☑
        renal 642.1 ☑
      infectious 647.9 ☑
        specified type NEC 647.8 ☑
      liver 646.7 ☑
      malarial 647.4 ☑
      nutritional deficiency 648.9 ☑
      parasitic NEC 647.8 ☑
      periodontal disease 648.9 ☑
      renal 646.2 ☑
        hypertensive 642.1 ☑
      rubella 647.5 ☑
      specified condition NEC 648.9 ☑
      syphilitic 647.0 ☑
      thyroid 648.1 ☑
      tuberculous 647.3 ☑
      urinary 646.6 ☑
      venereal 647.2 ☑
      viral NEC 647.6 ☑
    cystitis 646.6 ☑
    cystocele 654.4 ☑
    death of fetus (near term) 656.4 ☑
      early pregnancy (before 22 completed weeks gestation) 632
    deciduitis 646.6 ☑
    decreased fetal movements 655.7 ☑
    diabetes (mellitus) (conditions classifiable to 249 and 250) 648.0 ☑
    disorders of liver and biliary tract 646.7 ☑
    displacement, uterus NEC 654.4 ☑
    disproportion — see Disproportion
    double uterus 654.0 ☑
    drug dependence (conditions classifiable to 304) 648.3 ☑
    dysplasia, cervix 654.6 ☑
    early onset of delivery (spontaneous) 644.2 ☑
    eclampsia, eclamptic (coma) (convulsions) (delirium) (nephritis) (uremia) 642.6 ☑
      with pre-existing hypertension 642.7 ☑
    edema 646.1 ☑
      with hypertension — see Toxemia, of pregnancy
    effusion, amniotic fluid 658.1 ☑
      delayed delivery following 658.2 ☑
    embolism
      air 673.0 ☑
      amniotic fluid 673.1 ☑
      blood-clot 673.2 ☑
      cerebral 674.0 ☑
      pulmonary NEC 673.2 ☑
      pyemic 673.3 ☑
      septic 673.3 ☑
    emesis (gravidarum) — see Pregnancy, complicated, vomiting
    endometritis (conditions classifiable to 615.0–615.9) 670.1 ☑
      decidual 646.6 ☑
    epilepsy 649.4 ☑
    excessive weight gain NEC 646.1 ☑
    face presentation 652.4 ☑
    failure, fetal head to enter pelvic brim 652.5 ☑

☑ **Additional Digit Required** — Refer to the Tabular List for Digit Selection   ▽ Subterms under main terms may continue to next column or page

Pregnancy — *continued*
  complicated — *continued*
    false labor (pains) 644.1 ☑
    fatigue 646.8 ☑
    fatty metamorphosis of liver 646.7 ☑
    female genital mutilation 648.9 ☑
    fetal
      anemia 678.0 ☑
      complications from in utero procedure 679.1 ☑
      conjoined twins 678.1 ☑
      death (near term) 656.4 ☑
        early (before 22 completed weeks gestation) 632
      deformity 653.7 ☑
      distress 656.8 ☑
      hematologic conditions 678.0 ☑
      reduction of multiple fetuses reduced to single fetus 651.7 ☑
      thrombocytopenia 678.0 ☑
      twin to twin transfusion 678.0 ☑
    fibroid (tumor) (uterus) 654.1 ☑
    footling presentation 652.8 ☑
      with successful version 652.1 ☑
    gallbladder disease 646.8 ☑
    gastric banding status 649.2 ☑
    gastric bypass status for obesity
    genital herpes (asymptomatic) (history of) (inactive) 647.6 ☑
    goiter 648.1 ☑
    gonococcal infection (conditions classifiable to 098) 647.1 ☑
    gonorrhea (conditions classifiable to 098) 647.1 ☑
    hemorrhage 641.9 ☑
      accidental 641.2 ☑
      before 22 completed weeks gestation NEC 640.9 ☑
      cerebrovascular 674.0 ☑
      due to
        afibrinogenemia or other coagulation defect (conditions classifiable to 286.0–286.9) 641.3 ☑
        leiomyoma, uterine 641.8 ☑
        marginal sinus (rupture) 641.2 ☑
        premature separation, placenta 641.2 ☑
        trauma 641.8 ☑
      early (before 22 completed weeks gestation) 640.9 ☑
      threatened abortion 640.0 ☑
      unavoidable 641.1 ☑
    hepatitis (acute) (malignant) (subacute) 646.7 ☑
      viral 647.6 ☑
    herniation of uterus 654.4 ☑
    high head at term 652.5 ☑
    hydatidiform mole (delivered) (undelivered) 630
    hydramnios 657.0 ☑
    hydrocephalic fetus 653.6 ☑
    hydrops amnii 657.0 ☑
    hydrorrhea 658.1 ☑
    hyperemesis (gravidarum) — *see* Hyperemesis, gravidarum
    hypertension — *see* Hypertension, complicating pregnancy
    hypertensive
      chronic kidney disease 642.2 ☑
      heart and chronic kidney disease 642.2 ☑
      heart and renal disease 642.2 ☑
      heart disease 642.2 ☑
      renal disease 642.2 ☑
      hypertensive heart and chronic kidney disease 642.2 ☑
    hyperthyroidism 648.1 ☑
    hypothyroidism 648.1 ☑
    hysteralgia 646.8 ☑
    icterus gravis 646.7 ☑
    incarceration, uterus 654.3 ☑
    incompetent cervix (os) 654.5 ☑
    infection 647.9 ☑

Pregnancy — *continued*
  complicated — *continued*
    infection — *continued*
      amniotic fluid 658.4 ☑
      bladder 646.6 ☑
      genital organ (conditions classifiable to 614.0–614.5, 614.7–614.9, 615) 646.6 ☑
      kidney (conditions classifiable to 590.0–590.9) 646.6 ☑
      urinary (tract) 646.6 ☑
        asymptomatic 646.5 ☑
    infective and parasitic diseases NEC 647.8 ☑
    inflammation
      bladder 646.6 ☑
      genital organ (conditions classifiable to 614.0–614.5, 614.7–614.9, 615) 646.6 ☑
      urinary tract NEC 646.6 ☑
    insufficient weight gain 646.8 ☑
    insulin resistance 648.8 ☑
    intrauterine fetal death (near term) NEC 656.4 ☑
      early (before 22 completed weeks' gestation) 632
    malaria (conditions classifiable to 084) 647.4 ☑
    malformation, uterus (congenital) 654.0 ☑
    malnutrition (conditions classifiable to 260–269) 648.9 ☑
    malposition
      fetus — *see* Pregnancy, complicated, malpresentation
      uterus or cervix 654.4 ☑
    malpresentation 652.9 ☑
      with successful version 652.1 ☑
      in multiple gestation 652.6 ☑
      specified type NEC 652.8 ☑
    marginal sinus hemorrhage or rupture 641.2 ☑
    maternal complications from in utero procedure 679.0 ☑
    maternal drug abuse 648.4 ☑
    maternal obesity syndrome 646.1 ☑
    menstruation 640.8 ☑
    mental disorders (conditions classifiable to 290–303, 305.0, 305.2-305.9, 306–316, 317–319) 648.4 ☑
    mentum presentation 652.4 ☑
    missed
      abortion 632
      delivery (at or near term) 656.4 ☑
      labor (at or near term) 656.4 ☑
    necrosis
      genital organ or tract (conditions classifiable to 614.0–614.5, 614.7–614.9, 615) 646.6 ☑
      liver (conditions classifiable to 570) 646.7 ☑
      renal, cortical 646.2 ☑
    nephritis or nephrosis (conditions classifiable to 580–589) 646.2 ☑
      with hypertension 642.1 ☑
    nephropathy NEC 646.2 ☑
    neuritis (peripheral) 646.4 ☑
    nutritional deficiency (conditions classifiable to 260–269) 648.9 ☑
    obesity 649.1 ☑
      surgery status 649.2 ☑
    oblique lie or presentation 652.3 ☑
      with successful version 652.1 ☑
    obstetrical trauma 665.9 ☑
    oligohydramnios NEC 658.0 ☑
    onset of contractions before 37 weeks 644.0 ☑
    oversize fetus 653.5 ☑
    papyraceous fetus 646.0 ☑
    patent cervix 654.5 ☑
    pelvic inflammatory disease (conditions classifiable to 614.0–614.5, 614.7–614.9, 615) 646.6 ☑
    pelvic peritoneal adhesion 648.9 ☑

Pregnancy — *continued*
  complicated — *continued*
    placenta, placental
      abnormality 656.7 ☑
      abruptio or ablatio 641.2 ☑
      detachment 641.2 ☑
      disease 656.7 ☑
      infarct 656.7 ☑
      low implantation 641.1 ☑
        without hemorrhage 641.0 ☑
      malformation 656.7 ☑
      malposition 641.1 ☑
        without hemorrhage 641.0 ☑
      marginal sinus hemorrhage 641.2 ☑
      previa 641.1 ☑
        without hemorrhage 641.0 ☑
      separation (premature) (undelivered) 641.2 ☑
    placentitis 658.4 ☑
    pneumonia 648.9 ☑
    polyhydramnios 657.0 ☑
    postmaturity
      post-term 645.1 ☑
      prolonged 645.2 ☑
    prediabetes 648.8 ☑
    pre-eclampsia (mild) 642.4 ☑
      severe 642.5 ☑
      superimposed on pre-existing hypertensive disease 642.7 ☑
    premature rupture of membranes 658.1 ☑
      with delayed delivery 658.2 ☑
    previous
      ectopic pregnancy V23.42
      infertility V23.0
      in utero procedure during previous pregnancy V23.86
      nonobstetric condition V23.89
      poor obstetrical history V23.49
      premature delivery V23.41
      trophoblastic disease (conditions classifiable to 630) V23.1
    prolapse, uterus 654.4 ☑
    proteinuria (gestational) 646.2 ☑
      with hypertension — *see* Toxemia, of pregnancy
    pruritus (neurogenic) 646.8 ☑
    psychosis or psychoneurosis 648.4 ☑
    ptyalism 646.8 ☑
    pyelitis (conditions classifiable to 590.0–590.9) 646.6 ☑
    renal disease or failure NEC 646.2 ☑
      with secondary hypertension 642.1 ☑
      hypertensive 642.2 ☑
    retention, retained dead ovum 631.8
    retroversion, uterus 654.3 ☑
    Rh immunization, incompatibility, or sensitization 656.1 ☑
    rubella (conditions classifiable to 056) 647.5 ☑
    rupture
      amnion (premature) 658.1 ☑
        with delayed delivery 658.2 ☑
      marginal sinus (hemorrhage) 641.2 ☑
      membranes (premature) 658.1 ☑
        with delayed delivery 658.2 ☑
      uterus (before onset of labor) 665.0 ☑
    salivation (excessive) 646.8 ☑
    salpingo–oophoritis (conditions classifiable to 614.0–614.2) 646.6 ☑
    septicemia (conditions classifiable to 038.0–038.9) 647.8 ☑
      postpartum 670.2 ☑
      puerperal 670.2 ☑
    smoking 649.0 ☑
    spasms, uterus (abnormal) 646.8 ☑
    specified condition NEC 646.8 ☑
    spotting 649.5 ☑
    spurious labor pains 644.1 ☑
    status post
      bariatric surgery 649.2 ☑

Pregnancy — *continued*
  complicated — *continued*
    status post — *continued*
      gastric banding 649.2 ☑
      gastric bypass for obesity 649.2 ☑
      obesity surgery 649.2 ☑
    superfecundation 651.9 ☑
    superfetation 651.9 ☑
    syphilis (conditions classifiable to 090–097) 647.0 ☑
    threatened
      abortion 640.0 ☑
      premature delivery 644.2 ☑
      premature labor 644.0 ☑
    thrombophlebitis (superficial) 671.2 ☑
      deep 671.3 ☑
      septic 670.3 ☑
    thrombosis 671.2 ☑
      venous (superficial) 671.2 ☑
        deep 671.3 ☑
    thyroid dysfunction (conditions classifiable to 240–246) 648.1 ☑
    thyroiditis 648.1 ☑
    thyrotoxicosis 648.1 ☑
    tobacco use disorder 649.0 ☑
    torsion of uterus 654.4 ☑
    toxemia — *see* Toxemia, of pregnancy
    transverse lie or presentation 652.3 ☑
      with successful version 652.1 ☑
    trauma 648.9 ☑
      obstetrical 665.9 ☑
    tuberculosis (conditions classifiable to 010–018) 647.3 ☑
    tumor
      cervix 654.6 ☑
      ovary 654.4 ☑
      pelvic organs or tissue NEC 654.4 ☑
      uterus (body) 654.1 ☑
        cervix 654.6 ☑
      vagina 654.7 ☑
      vulva 654.8 ☑
    unstable lie 652.0 ☑
    uremia — *see* Pregnancy, complicated, renal disease
    urethritis 646.6 ☑
    vaginitis or vulvitis (conditions classifiable to 616.1) 646.6 ☑
    varicose
      placental vessels 656.7 ☑
      veins (legs) 671.0 ☑
        perineum 671.1 ☑
        vulva 671.1 ☑
    varicosity, labia or vulva 671.1 ☑
    venereal disease NEC (conditions classifiable to 099) 647.2 ☑
    venous complication 671.9 ☑
    viral disease NEC (conditions classifiable to 042, 050–055, 057–079, 795.05, 795.15, 796.75) 647.6 ☑
    vomiting (incoercible) (pernicious) (persistent) (uncontrollable) (vicious) 643.9 ☑
      due to organic disease or other cause 643.8 ☑
      early — *see* Hyperemesis, gravidarum
      late (after 22 completed weeks gestation) 643.2 ☑
    young maternal age 659.8 ☑
  complications NEC 646.9 ☑
  cornual 633.80
    with intrauterine pregnancy 633.81
    affecting fetus or newborn 761.4
  death, maternal NEC 646.9 ☑
  delivered — *see* Delivery
  ectopic (ruptured) NEC 633.90
    with intrauterine pregnancy 633.91
    abdominal — *see* Pregnancy, abdominal
    affecting fetus or newborn 761.4
    combined (extrauterine and intrauterine) — *see* Pregnancy, cornual
    ovarian — *see* Pregnancy, ovarian
    specified type NEC 633.80
      with intrauterine pregnancy 633.81

☑ Additional Digit Required — Refer to the Tabular List for Digit Selection   Ⓝ Subterms under main terms may continue to next column or page

Pregnancy — *continued*
  ectopic — *continued*
    specified type — *continued*
      affecting fetus or newborn 761.4
    tubal — *see* Pregnancy, tubal
  examination, pregnancy
    negative result V72.41
    not confirmed V72.40
    positive result V72.42
  extrauterine — *see* Pregnancy, ectopic
  fallopian — *see* Pregnancy, tubal
  false 300.11
    labor (pains) 644.1 ☑
  fatigue 646.8 ☑
  illegitimate V61.6
  incidental finding V22.2
  in double uterus 654.0 ☑
  interstitial — *see* Pregnancy, cornual
  intraligamentous — *see* Pregnancy, cornual
  intramural — *see* Pregnancy, cornual
  intraperitoneal — *see* Pregnancy, abdominal
  isthmian — *see* Pregnancy, tubal
  management affected by
    abnormal, abnormality
      fetus (suspected) 655.9 ☑
        specified NEC 655.8 ☑
      placenta 656.7 ☑
    advanced maternal age NEC 659.6 ☑
      multigravida 659.6 ☑
      primigravida 659.5 ☑
    antibodies (maternal)
      anti-c 656.1 ☑
      anti-d 656.1 ☑
      anti-e 656.1 ☑
      blood group (ABO) 656.2 ☑
        Rh(esus) 656.1 ☑
    appendicitis 648.9 ☑
    bariatric surgery status 649.2 ☑
    coagulation defect 649.3 ☑
    elderly multigravida 659.6 ☑
    elderly primigravida 659.5 ☑
    epilepsy 649.4 ☑
    fetal (suspected)
      abnormality 655.9 ☑
        abdominal 655.8 ☑
        acid-base balance 656.8 ☑
        cardiovascular 655.8 ☑
        facial 655.8 ☑
        gastrointestinal 655.8 ☑
        gentourinary 655.8 ☑
        heart rate or rhythm 659.7 ☑
        limb 655.8 ☑
        specified NEC 655.8 ☑
      acidemia 656.3 ☑
      anencephaly 655.0 ☑
      aneuploidy 655.1 ☑
      bradycardia 659.7 ☑
      central nervous system malformation 655.0 ☑
      chromosomal abnormalities (conditions classifiable to 758.0–758.9) 655.1 ☑
      damage from
        drugs 655.5 ☑
          obstetric, anesthetic, or sedative 655.5 ☑
        environmental toxins 655.8 ☑
        intrauterine contraceptive device 655.8 ☑
        maternal
          alcohol addiction 655.4 ☑
          disease NEC 655.4 ☑
          drug use 655.5 ☑
          listeriosis 655.4 ☑
          rubella 655.3 ☑
          toxoplasmosis 655.4 ☑
          viral infection 655.3 ☑
        radiation 655.6 ☑
      death (near term) 656.4 ☑
        early (before 22 completed weeks' gestation) 632
      distress 656.8 ☑
      excessive growth 656.6 ☑

Pregnancy — *continued*
  management affected by — *continued*
    fetal — *continued*
      fetal-maternal hemorrhage 656.0 ☑
      growth retardation 656.5 ☑
      hereditary disease 655.2 ☑
      hereditary disease in family (possibly) affecting fetus 655.2 ☑
      hydrocephalus 655.0 ☑
      incompatibility, blood groups (ABO) 656.2 ☑
      intrauterine death 656.4 ☑
      poor growth 656.5 ☑
      Rh(esus) 656.1 ☑
      spina bifida (with myelomeningocele) 655.0 ☑
    gastric banding status 649.2 ☑
    gastric bypass status for obesity 649.2 ☑
    insufficient prenatal care V23.7
    insulin resistance 648.8 ☑
    intrauterine death 656.4 ☑
    isoimmunization (ABO) 656.2 ☑
      Rh(esus) 656.1 ☑
    large-for-dates fetus 656.6 ☑
    light-for-dates fetus 656.5 ☑
    meconium in liquor 656.8 ☑
    mental disorder (conditions classifiable to 290–303, 305.0, 305.2–305.9, 306–316, 317–319) 648.4 ☑
    multiparity (grand) 659.4 ☑
    obesity 649.1 ☑
      surgery status 649.2 ☑
    poor obstetric history V23.49
      pre-term labor V23.41
    postmaturity
      post-term 645.1 ☑
      prolonged 645.2 ☑
    post-term pregnancy 645.1 ☑
    previous
      abortion V23.2
        habitual 646.3 ☑
      cesarean delivery 654.2 ☑
      difficult delivery V23.49
      ectopic pregnancy V23.42
      forceps delivery V23.49
      habitual abortions 646.3 ☑
      hemorrhage, antepartum or postpartum V23.49
      hydatidiform mole V23.1
      infertility V23.0
      in utero procedure during previous pregnancy V23.86
      malignancy NEC V23.89
      nonobstetrical conditions V23.8 ☑
      premature delivery V23.41
      recurrent pregnancy loss 646.3 ☑
      trophoblastic disease (conditions in 630) V23.1
      vesicular mole V23.1
    prolonged pregnancy 645.2 ☑
    recurrent pregnancy loss 646.3 ☑
    small-for-dates fetus 656.5 ☑
    smoking 649.0 ☑
    spotting 649.5 ☑
    suspected conditions not found
      amniotic cavity and membrane problem V89.01
      cervical shortening V89.05
      fetal anomaly V89.03
      fetal growth problem V89.04
      oligohydramnios V89.01
      other specified problem NEC V89.09
      placental problem V89.02
      polyhydramnios V89.01
    tobacco use disorder 649.0 ☑
    venous complication 671.9 ☑
    young maternal age 659.8 ☑
  maternal death NEC 646.9 ☑
  mesometric (mural) -— *see* Pregnancy, cornual
  molar 631.8
    hydatidiform (*see also* Hydatidiform mole) 630
      previous, affecting management of pregnancy V23.1

Pregnancy — *continued*
  molar — *continued*
    previous, affecting management of pregnancy V23.49
  multiple NEC 651.9 ☑
    with fetal loss and retention of one or more fetus(es) 651.6 ☑
    affecting fetus or newborn 761.5
    following (elective) fetal reduction 651.7 ☑
    specified type NEC 651.8 ☑
      with fetal loss and retention of one or more fetus(es) 651.6 ☑
      following (elective) fetal reduction 651.7 ☑
  mural — *see* Pregnancy, cornual
  observation NEC V22.1
    first pregnancy V22.0
    high-risk V23.9
      inconclusive fetal viability V23.87
      specified problem NEC V23.89
  ovarian 633.20
    with intrauterine pregnancy 633.21
    affecting fetus or newborn 761.4
  possible, not (yet) confirmed V72.40
  postmature
    post-term 645.1 ☑
    prolonged 645.2 ☑
  post-term 645.1 ☑
  prenatal care only V22.1
    first pregnancy V22.0
    high-risk V23.9
      inconclusive fetal viability V23.87
      specified problem NEC V23.89
  prolonged 645.2 ☑
  quadruplet NEC 651.2 ☑
    with fetal loss and retention of one or more fetus(es) 651.5 ☑
    affecting fetus or newborn 761.5
    following (elective) fetal reduction 651.7 ☑
  quintuplet NEC 651.8 ☑
    with fetal loss and retention of one or more fetus(es) 651.6 ☑
    affecting fetus or newborn 761.5
    following (elective) fetal reduction 651.7 ☑
  resulting from
    assisted reproductive technology V23.85
    in vitro fertilization V23.85
  sextuplet NEC 651.8 ☑
    with fetal loss and retention of one or more fetus(es) 651.6 ☑
    affecting fetus or newborn 761.5
    following (elective) fetal reduction 651.7 ☑
  spurious 300.11
  superfecundation NEC 651.9 ☑
    with fetal loss and retention of one or more fetus(es) 651.6 ☑
    following (elective) fetal reduction 651.7 ☑
  superfetation NEC 651.9 ☑
    with fetal loss and retention of one or more fetus(es) 651.6 ☑
    following (elective) fetal reduction 651.7 ☑
  supervision (of) (for) (*see also* Pregnancy, management affected by)
    elderly
      multigravida V23.82
      primigravida V23.81
    high-risk V23.9
      inconclusive fetal viability V23.87
      insufficient prenatal care V23.7
      specified problem NEC V23.89
    inconclusive fetal viability V23.87
    multiparity V23.3
    normal NEC V22.1
      first V22.0
    poor
      obstetric history V23.49
        ectopic pregnancy V23.42
        pre-term labor V23.41
      reproductive history V23.5

Pregnancy — *continued*
  supervision (*see also* Pregnancy, management affected by) — *continued*
    previous
      abortion V23.2
      hydatidiform mole V23.1
      infertility V23.0
      neonatal death V23.5
      stillbirth V23.5
      trophoblastic disease V23.1
      vesicular mole V23.1
    specified problem NEC V23.89
    young
      multigravida V23.84
      primigravida V23.83
  triplet NEC 651.1 ☑
    with fetal loss and retention of one or more fetus(es) 651.4 ☑
    affecting fetus or newborn 761.5
    following (elective) fetal reduction 651.7 ☑
  tubal (with rupture) 633.10
    with intrauterine pregnancy 633.11
    affecting fetus or newborn 761.4
  twin NEC 651.0 ☑
    with fetal loss and retention of one fetus 651.3 ☑
    affecting fetus or newborn 761.5
    conjoined 678.1 ☑
    following (elective) fetal reduction 651.7 ☑
  unconfirmed V72.40
  undelivered (no other diagnosis) V22.2
    with false labor 644.1 ☑
    high-risk V23.9
      specified problem NEC V23.89
  unwanted NEC V61.7

Pregnant uterus — *see* condition
Preiser's disease (osteoporosis) 733.09
Prekwashiorkor 260
Preleukemia 238.75
Preluxation of hip, congenital — *see also* Subluxation, congenital, hip 754.32
Premature — *see also* condition
  beats (nodal) 427.60
    atrial 427.61
    auricular 427.61
    postoperative 997.1
    specified type NEC 427.69
    supraventricular 427.61
    ventricular 427.69
  birth NEC 765.1 ☑
  closure
    cranial suture 756.0
    fontanel 756.0
    foramen ovale 745.8
  contractions 427.60
    atrial 427.61
    auricular 427.61
    auriculoventricular 427.61
    heart (extrasystole) 427.60
    junctional 427.60
    nodal 427.60
    postoperative 997.1
    ventricular 427.69
  ejaculation 302.75
  infant NEC 765.1 ☑
    excessive 765.0 ☑
    light-for-dates — *see* Light-for-dates
  labor 644.2 ☑
    threatened 644.0 ☑
  lungs 770.4
  menopause 256.31
  puberty 259.1
  rupture of membranes or amnion 658.1 ☑
    affecting fetus or newborn 761.1
    delayed delivery following 658.2 ☑
  senility (syndrome) 259.8
  separation, placenta (partial) — *see* Placenta, separation
  ventricular systole 427.69
Prematurity NEC 765.1 ☑
  extreme 765.0 ☑
Premenstrual syndrome 625.4
Premenstrual tension 625.4
Premolarization, cuspids 520.2

☑ **Additional Digit Required** — Refer to the Tabular List for Digit Selection

Ⓦ **Subterms under main terms may continue to next column or page**

Premyeloma 273.1

Prenatal
care, normal pregnancy V22.1
first V22.0
death, cause unknown — *see* Death, fetus
screening — *see* Antenatal, screening
teeth 520.6

Prepartum — *see* condition

Preponderance, left or right ventricular 429.3

Prepuce — *see* condition

PRES (posterior reversible encephalopathy syndrome) 348.39

Presbycardia 797
hypertensive (*see also* Hypertension, heart) 402.90

Presbycusis 388.01

Presbyesophagus 530.89

Presbyophrenia 310.1

Presbyopia 367.4

Prescription of contraceptives NEC V25.02
diaphragm V25.02
oral (pill) V25.01
emergency V25.03
postcoital V25.03
repeat V25.41
repeat V25.40
oral (pill) V25.41

Presenile — *see also* condition
aging 259.8
dementia (*see also* Dementia, presenile) 290.10

Presenility 259.8

Presentation, fetal
abnormal 652.9 ☑
with successful version 652.1 ☑
before labor, affecting fetus or newborn 761.7
causing obstructed labor 660.0 ☑
affecting fetus or newborn, any, except breech 763.1
in multiple gestation (one or more) 652.6 ☑
specified NEC 652.8 ☑
arm 652.7 ☑
causing obstructed labor 660.0 ☑
breech (buttocks) (complete) (frank) 652.2 ☑
with successful version 652.1 ☑
before labor, affecting fetus or newborn 761.7
before labor, affecting fetus or newborn 761.7
brow 652.4 ☑
causing obstructed labor 660.0 ☑
buttocks 652.2 ☑
chin 652.4 ☑
complete 652.2 ☑
compound 652.8 ☑
cord 663.0 ☑
extended head 652.4 ☑
face 652.4 ☑
to pubes 652.8 ☑
footling 652.8 ☑
frank 652.2 ☑
hand, leg, or foot NEC 652.8 ☑
incomplete 652.8 ☑
mentum 652.4 ☑
multiple gestation (one fetus or more) 652.6 ☑
oblique 652.3 ☑
with successful version 652.1 ☑
shoulder 652.8 ☑
affecting fetus or newborn 763.1
transverse 652.3 ☑
with successful version 652.1 ☑
umbilical cord 663.0 ☑
unstable 652.0 ☑

Prespondylolisthesis (congenital) (lumbosacral) 756.11

Pressure
area, skin ulcer (*see also* Ulcer, pressure) 707.00
atrophy, spine 733.99
birth, fetus or newborn NEC 767.9

Pressure — *continued*
brachial plexus 353.0
brain 348.4
injury at birth 767.0
cerebral — *see* Pressure, brain
chest 786.59
cone, tentorial 348.4
injury at birth 767.0
funis — *see* Compression, umbilical cord
hyposystolic (*see also* Hypotension) 458.9
increased
intracranial 781.99
due to
benign intracranial hypertension 348.2
hydrocephalus — *see* hydrocephalus
injury at birth 767.8
intraocular 365.00
lumbosacral plexus 353.1
mediastinum 519.3
necrosis (chronic) (skin) (*see also* Decubitus) 707.00
nerve — *see* Compression, nerve
paralysis (*see also* Neuropathy, entrapment) 355.9
pre-ulcer skin changes limited to persistent focal erythema (*see also* Ulcer, pressure) 707.21
sore (chronic) (*see also* Ulcer, pressure) 707.00
spinal cord 336.9
ulcer (chronic) (*see also* Ulcer, pressure) 707.00
umbilical cord — *see* Compression, umbilical cord
venous, increased 459.89

Pre-syncope 780.2

Preterm infant NEC 765.1 ☑
extreme 765.0 ☑

Priapism (penis) 607.3

Prickling sensation — *see also* Disturbance, sensation 782.0

Prickly heat 705.1

Primary — *see also* condition
angle closure suspect 365.02

Primigravida, elderly
affecting
fetus or newborn 763.89
management of pregnancy, labor, and delivery 659.5 ☑

Primipara, old
affecting
fetus or newborn 763.89
management of pregnancy, labor, and delivery 659.5 ☑

Primula dermatitis 692.6

Primus varus (bilateral) (metatarsus) 754.52

PRIND (prolonged reversible ischemic neurologic deficit) 434.91
history of (personal) V12.54

Pringle's disease (tuberous sclerosis) 759.5

Prinzmetal's angina 413.1

Prinzmetal-Massumi syndrome (anterior chest wall) 786.52

Prizefighter ear 738.7

Problem (with) V49.9
academic V62.3
acculturation V62.4
adopted child V61.24
aged
in-law V61.3
parent V61.3
person NEC V61.8
alcoholism in family V61.41
anger reaction (*see also* Disturbance, conduct) 312.0 ☑
behavioral V40.9
specified NEC V40.39
behavior, child 312.9
betting V69.3
biological child V61.23
cardiorespiratory NEC V47.2
career choice V62.29
care of sick or handicapped person in family or household V61.49

Problem — *continued*
communication V40.1
conscience regarding medical care V62.6
delinquency (juvenile) 312.9
diet, inappropriate V69.1
digestive NEC V47.3
ear NEC V41.3
eating habits, inappropriate V69.1
economic V60.2
affecting care V60.9
specified type NEC V60.89
educational V62.3
enuresis, child 307.6
exercise, lack of V69.0
eye NEC V41.1
family V61.9
specified circumstance NEC V61.8
fear reaction, child 313.0
feeding (elderly) (infant) 783.3
newborn 779.31
nonorganic 307.59
fetal, affecting management of pregnancy 656.9 ☑
specified type NEC 656.8 ☑
financial V60.2
foster child V61.25
functional V41.9
specified type NEC V41.8
gambling V69.3
genital NEC V47.5
head V48.9
deficiency V48.0
disfigurement V48.6
mechanical V48.2
motor V48.2
movement of V48.2
sensory V48.4
specified condition NEC V48.8
hearing V41.2
high-risk sexual behavior V69.2
identity 313.82
influencing health status NEC V49.89
internal organ NEC V47.9
deficiency V47.0
mechanical or motor V47.1
interpersonal NEC V62.81
jealousy, child 313.3
learning V40.0
legal V62.5
life circumstance NEC V62.89
lifestyle V69.9
specified NEC V69.8
limb V49.9
deficiency V49.0
disfigurement V49.4
mechanical V49.1
motor V49.2
movement, involving
musculoskeletal system V49.1
nervous system V49.2
sensory V49.3
specified condition NEC V49.5
litigation V62.5
living alone V60.3
loneliness NEC V62.89
marital V61.10
involving
divorce V61.03
estrangement V61.09
psychosexual disorder 302.9
sexual function V41.7
relationship V61.10
mastication V41.6
medical care, within family V61.49
mental V40.9
specified NEC V40.2
mental hygiene, adult V40.9
multiparity V61.5
nail biting, child 307.9
neck V48.9
deficiency V48.1
disfigurement V48.7
mechanical V48.3
motor V48.3
movement V48.3
sensory V48.5

Problem — *continued*
neck — *continued*
specified condition NEC V48.8
neurological NEC 781.99
none (feared complaint unfounded) V65.5
occupational V62.29
parent-child V61.20
adopted child V61.24
biological child V61.23
foster child V61.25
relationship V61.20
partner V61.10
relationship V61.10
personality (*see also* Disorder, personality) 301.9
personal NEC V62.89
interpersonal conflict NEC V62.81
phase of life V62.89
placenta, affecting management of pregnancy 656.9 ☑
specified type NEC 656.8 ☑
poverty V60.2
presence of sick or handicapped person in family or household V61.49
psychiatric 300.9
psychosocial V62.9
specified type NEC V62.89
relational NEC V62.81
relationship, childhood 313.3
religious or spiritual belief
other than medical care V62.89
regarding medical care V62.6
self-damaging behavior V69.8
sexual
behavior, high-risk V69.2
function NEC V41.7
sibling
relational V61.8
relationship V61.8
sight V41.0
sleep disorder, child 307.40
sleep, lack of V69.4
smell V41.5
speech V40.1
spite reaction, child (*see also* Disturbance, conduct) 312.0 ☑
spoiled child reaction (*see also* Disturbance, conduct) 312.1 ☑
substance abuse in family V61.42
swallowing V41.6
tantrum, child (*see also* Disturbance, conduct) 312.1 ☑
taste V41.5
thumb sucking, child 307.9
tic (child) 307.21
trunk V48.9
deficiency V48.1
disfigurement V48.7
mechanical V48.3
motor V48.3
movement V48.3
sensory V48.5
specified condition NEC V48.8
unemployment V62.0
urinary NEC V47.4
voice production V41.4

Procedure (surgical) **not done** NEC V64.3
because of
contraindication V64.1
patient's decision V64.2
for reasons of conscience or religion V62.6
specified reason NEC V64.3

Procidentia
anus (sphincter) 569.1
rectum (sphincter) 569.1
stomach 537.89
uteri 618.1

Proctalgia 569.42
fugax 564.6
spasmodic 564.6
psychogenic 307.89

Proctitis 569.49
amebic 006.8
chlamydial 099.52
gonococcal 098.7

☑ **Additional Digit Required** — Refer to the Tabular List for Digit Selection

▼ **Subterms under main terms may continue to next column or page**

2015 ICD-9-CM

▶◀ **Revised Text**

● **New Line**

▲ **Revised Code**

Volume 2 — 239

Premyeloma — Proctitis

Index

Proctitis — Pseudobursa

Proctitis — continued
granulomatous 555.1
idiopathic 556.2
  with ulcerative sigmoiditis 556.3
tuberculous (see also Tuberculosis) 014.8 ☑
ulcerative (chronic) (nonspecific) 556.2
  with ulcerative sigmoiditis 556.3
Proctocele
female (without uterine prolapse) 618.04
  with uterine prolapse 618.4
    complete 618.3
    incomplete 618.2
male 569.49
Proctocolitis, idiopathic 556.2
with ulcerative sigmoiditis 556.3
Proctoptosis 569.1
Proctosigmoiditis 569.89
ulcerative (chronic) 556.3
Proctospasm 564.6
psychogenic 306.4
Prodromal-AIDS — see Human immunodeficiency virus (disease) (illness) (infection)
Profichet's disease or syndrome 729.90
Progeria (adultorum) (syndrome) 259.8
Prognathism (mandibular) (maxillary) 524.10
Progonoma (melanotic) (M9363/0) — see Neoplasm, by site, benign
Progressive — see condition
Prolapse, prolapsed
anus, anal (canal) (sphincter) 569.1
arm or hand, complicating delivery 652.7 ☑
  causing obstructed labor 660.0 ☑
    affecting fetus or newborn 763.1
  fetus or newborn 763.1
bladder (acquired) (mucosa) (sphincter)
  congenital (female) (male) 756.71
  female (see also Cystocele, female) 618.01
  male 596.89
breast implant (prosthetic) 996.54
cecostomy 569.69
cecum 569.89
cervix, cervical (hypertrophied) 618.1
  anterior lip, obstructing labor 660.2 ☑
    affecting fetus or newborn 763.1
  congenital 752.49
  postpartal (old) 618.1
  stump 618.84
ciliary body 871.1
colon (pedunculated) 569.89
colostomy 569.69
conjunctiva 372.73
cord — see Prolapse, umbilical cord
cystostomy 596.83
disc (intervertebral) — see Displacement, intervertebral disc
duodenum 537.89
eye implant (orbital) 996.59
  lens (ocular) 996.53
fallopian tube 620.4
fetal extremity, complicating delivery 652.8 ☑
  causing obstructed labor 660.0 ☑
  fetus or newborn 763.1
funis — see Prolapse, umbilical cord
gastric (mucosa) 537.89
genital, female 618.9
  specified NEC 618.89
globe 360.81
ileostomy bud 569.69
intervertebral disc — see Displacement, intervertebral disc
intestine (small) 569.89
iris 364.89
  traumatic 871.1
kidney (see also Disease, renal) 593.0
  congenital 753.3
laryngeal muscles or ventricle 478.79
leg, complicating delivery 652.8 ☑
  causing obstructed labor 660.0 ☑
  fetus or newborn 763.1
liver 573.8
meatus urinarius 599.5
mitral valve 424.0
ocular lens implant 996.53

Prolapse, prolapsed — continued
organ or site, congenital NEC — see Malposition, congenital
ovary 620.4
pelvic (floor), female 618.89
perineum, female 618.89
pregnant uterus 654.4 ☑
rectum (mucosa) (sphincter) 569.1
  due to Trichuris trichiuria 127.3
spleen 289.59
stomach 537.89
umbilical cord
  affecting fetus or newborn 762.4
  complicating delivery 663.0 ☑
ureter 593.89
  with obstruction 593.4
ureterovesical orifice 593.89
urethra (acquired) (infected) (mucosa) 599.5
  congenital 753.8
uterovaginal 618.4
  complete 618.3
  incomplete 618.2
  specified NEC 618.89
uterus (first degree) (second degree) (third degree) (complete) (without vaginal wall prolapse) 618.1
  with mention of vaginal wall prolapse — see Prolapse, uterovaginal
  congenital 752.39
  in pregnancy or childbirth 654.4 ☑
    affecting fetus or newborn 763.1
    causing obstructed labor 660.2 ☑
      affecting fetus or newborn 763.1
  postpartal (old) 618.1
uveal 871.1
vagina (anterior) (posterior) (vault) (wall) (without uterine prolapse) 618.00
  with uterine prolapse 618.4
    complete 618.3
    incomplete 618.2
  paravaginal 618.02
  posthysterectomy 618.5
  specified NEC 618.09
vitreous (humor) 379.26
  traumatic 871.1
womb — see Prolapse, uterus
Prolapsus, female 618.9
Proliferative — see condition
Prolinemia 270.8
Prolinuria 270.8
Prolonged, prolongation
bleeding time (see also Defect, coagulation) 790.92
  "idiopathic" (in von Willebrand's disease) 286.4
coagulation time (see also Defect, coagulation) 790.92
gestation syndrome 766.22
labor 662.1 ☑
  affecting fetus or newborn 763.89
  first stage 662.0 ☑
  second stage 662.2 ☑
pregnancy 645.2 ☑
PR interval 426.11
prothrombin time (see also Defect, coagulation) 790.92
QT interval 794.31
  syndrome 426.82
rupture of membranes (24 hours or more prior to onset of labor) 658.2 ☑
uterine contractions in labor 661.4 ☑
  affecting fetus or newborn 763.7
Prominauris 744.29
Prominence
auricle (ear) (congenital) 744.29
  acquired 380.32
ischial spine or sacral promontory
  with disproportion (fetopelvic) 653.3 ☑
    affecting fetus or newborn 763.1
    causing obstructed labor 660.1 ☑
      affecting fetus or newborn 763.1
nose (congenital) 748.1
  acquired 738.0
PROMM (proximal myotonic myotonia) 359.21
Pronation
ankle 736.79

Pronation — continued
foot 736.79
  congenital 755.67
Prophylactic
administration of
  antibiotics, long-term V58.62
    short-term — omit code
  antitoxin, any V07.2
  antivenin V07.2
  chemotherapeutic agent NEC V07.39
    fluoride V07.31
  diphtheria antitoxin V07.2
  drug V07.39
  exemestar (Aromasin) V07.52
  gamma globulin V07.2
  immune sera (gamma globulin) V07.2
    RhoGAM V07.2
  tetanus antitoxin V07.2
chemotherapy NEC V07.39
  fluoride V07.31
hormone replacement (postmenopausal) V07.4
immunotherapy V07.2
measure V07.9
  specified type NEC V07.8
medication V07.39
postmenopausal hormone replacement V07.4
sterilization V25.2
Proptosis (ocular) — see also Exophthalmos 376.30
thyroid 242.0 ☑
Propulsion
eyeball 360.81
Prosecution, anxiety concerning V62.5
Prosopagnosia 368.16
Prostate, prostatic — see condition
Prostatism 600.90
with
  other lower urinary tract symptoms (LUTS) 600.91
  urinary
    obstruction 600.91
    retention 600.91
Prostatitis (congestive) (suppurative) 601.9
acute 601.0
cavitary 601.8
chlamydial 099.54
chronic 601.1
diverticular 601.8
due to Trichomonas (vaginalis) 131.03
fibrous 600.90
  with
    other lower urinary tract symptoms (LUTS) 600.91
    urinary
      obstruction 600.91
      retention 600.91
gonococcal (acute) 098.12
  chronic or duration of 2 months or over 098.32
granulomatous 601.8
hypertrophic 600.00
  with
    other lower urinary tract symptoms (LUTS) 600.01
    urinary
      obstruction 600.01
      retention 600.01
specified type NEC 601.8
subacute 601.1
trichomonal 131.03
tuberculous (see also Tuberculosis) 016.5 ☑ [601.4]
Prostatocystitis 601.3
Prostatorrhea 602.8
Prostatoseminovesiculitis, trichomonal 131.03
Prostration 780.79
heat 992.5
  anhydrotic 992.3
  due to
    salt (and water) depletion 992.4
    water depletion 992.3
nervous 300.5
newborn 779.89

Prostration — continued
senile 797
Protanomaly 368.51
Protanopia (anomalous trichromat) (complete) (incomplete) 368.51
Protection (against) (from) — see Prophylactic
Protein
deficiency 260
malnutrition 260
sickness (prophylactic) (therapeutic) 999.59
Proteinemia 790.99
Proteinosis
alveolar, lung or pulmonary 516.0
lipid 272.8
lipoid (of Urbach) 272.8
Proteinuria — see also Albuminuria 791.0
Bence-Jones NEC 791.0
gestational 646.2 ☑
  with hypertension — see Toxemia, of pregnancy
orthostatic 593.6
postural 593.6
Proteolysis, pathologic 286.6
Protocoproporphyria 277.1
Protoporphyria (erythrohepatic) (erythropoietic) 277.1
Protrusio acetabuli 718.65
Protrusion
acetabulum (into pelvis) 718.65
device, implant, or graft — see Complications, mechanical
ear, congenital 744.29
intervertebral disc — see Displacement, intervertebral disc
nucleus pulposus — see Displacement, intervertebral disc
Proud flesh 701.5
Prune belly (syndrome) 756.71
Prurigo (ferox) (gravis) (Hebra's) (hebrae) (mitis) (simplex) 698.2
agria 698.3
asthma syndrome 691.8
Besnier's (atopic dermatitis) (infantile eczema) 691.8
eczematodes allergicum 691.8
estivalis (Hutchinson's) 692.72
Hutchinson's 692.72
nodularis 698.3
psychogenic 306.3
Pruritus, pruritic 698.9
ani 698.0
  psychogenic 306.3
conditions NEC 698.9
  psychogenic 306.3
due to Onchocerca volvulus 125.3
ear 698.9
essential 698.9
genital organ(s) 698.1
  psychogenic 306.3
gravidarum 646.8 ☑
hiemalis 698.8
neurogenic (any site) 306.3
perianal 698.0
psychogenic (any site) 306.3
scrotum 698.1
  psychogenic 306.3
senile, senilis 698.8
Trichomonas 131.9
vulva, vulvae 698.1
  psychogenic 306.3
Psammocarcinoma (M8140/3) — see Neoplasm, by site, malignant
Pseudarthrosis, pseudoarthrosis (bone) 733.82
joint following fusion V45.4
Pseudoacanthosis
nigricans 701.8
Pseudoaneurysm — see Aneurysm
Pseudoangina (pectoris) — see Angina
Pseudoangioma 452
Pseudo-Argyll-Robertson pupil 379.45
Pseudoarteriosus 747.89
Pseudoarthrosis — see Pseudarthrosis
Pseudoataxia 799.89
Pseudobulbar affect (PBA) 310.81
Pseudobursa 727.89

☑ **Additional Digit Required** — Refer to the Tabular List for Digit Selection   ꙍ **Subterms under main terms may continue to next column or page**

240 — Volume 2   ▶◀ Revised Text   ● New Line   ▲ Revised Code   2015 ICD-9-CM

Pseudocholera 025
Pseudochromidrosis 705.89
Pseudocirrhosis, liver, pericardial 423.2
Pseudocoarctation 747.21
Pseudocowpox 051.1
Pseudocoxalgia 732.1
Pseudocroup 478.75
Pseudocyesis 300.11
Pseudocyst
　lung 518.89
　pancreas 577.2
　retina 361.19
Pseudodementia 300.16
Pseudoelephantiasis neuroarthritica 757.0
Pseudoemphysema 518.89
Pseudoencephalitis
　superior (acute) hemorrhagic 265.1
Pseudoerosion cervix, congenital 752.49
Pseudoexfoliation, lens capsule 366.11
Pseudofracture (idiopathic) (multiple) (spontaneous) (symmetrical) 268.2
Pseudoglanders 025
Pseudoglioma 360.44
Pseudogout — *see* Chondrocalcinosis
Pseudohallucination 780.1
Pseudohemianesthesia 782.0
Pseudohemophilia (Bernuth's) (hereditary) (typeB) 286.4
　type A 287.8
　vascular 287.8
Pseudohermaphroditism 752.7
　with chromosomal anomaly — *see* Anomaly, chromosomal
　adrenal 255.2
　female (without adrenocortical disorder) 752.7
　　with adrenocortical disorder 255.2
　　　adrenal 255.2
　male (without gonadal disorder) 752.7
　　with
　　　adrenocortical disorder 255.2
　　　cleft scrotum 752.7
　　　feminizing testis 259.51
　　　gonadal disorder 257.9
　　　adrenal 255.2
Pseudohole, macula 362.54
Pseudo-Hurler's disease (mucolipidosis III) 272.7
Pseudohydrocephalus 348.2
Pseudohypertrophic muscular dystrophy (Erb's) 359.1
Pseudohypertrophy, muscle 359.1
Pseudohypoparathyroidism 275.49
Pseudoinfluenza — *see also* Influenza 487.1
Pseudoinsomnia 307.49
Pseudoleukemia 288.8
　infantile 285.8
Pseudomembranous — *see* condition
Pseudomeningocele (cerebral) (infective) 349.2
　postprocedural 997.01
　spinal 349.2
Pseudomenstruation 626.8
Pseudomucinous
　cyst (ovary) (M8470/0) 220
　peritoneum 568.89
Pseudomyeloma 273.1
Pseudomyxoma peritonei (M8480/6) 197.6
Pseudoneuritis optic (nerve) 377.24
　papilla 377.24
　congenital 743.57
Pseudoneuroma — *see* Injury, nerve, by site
Pseudo-obstruction
　intestine (chronic) (idiopathic) (intermittent secondary) (primary) 564.89
　acute 560.89
Pseudopapilledema 377.24
Pseudoparalysis
　arm or leg 781.4
　atonic, congenital 358.8
Pseudopelade 704.09
Pseudophakia V43.1
Pseudopolycythemia 289.0
Pseudopolyposis, colon 556.4
Pseudoporencephaly 348.0
Pseudopseudohypoparathyroidism 275.49

Pseudopsychosis 300.16
Pseudopterygium 372.52
Pseudoptosis (eyelid) 374.34
Pseudorabies 078.89
Pseudoretinitis, pigmentosa 362.65
Pseudorickets 588.0
　senile (Pozzi's) 731.0
Pseudorubella 057.8
Pseudoscarlatina 057.8
Pseudosclerema 778.1
Pseudosclerosis (brain)
　Jakob's 046.19
　of Westphal (-Strümpell) (hepatolenticular degeneration) 275.1
　spastic 046.19
　　with dementia
　　　with behavioral disturbance 046.19 [294.11]
　　　without behavioral disturbance 046.19 [294.10]
Pseudoseizure 780.39
　non-psychiatric 780.39
　psychiatric 300.11
Pseudotabes 799.89
　diabetic 250.6 ☑ [337.1]
　　due to secondary diabetes 249.6 ☑ [337.1]
Pseudotetanus — *see also* Convulsions 780.39
Pseudotetany 781.7
　hysterical 300.11
Pseudothalassemia 285.0
Pseudotrichinosis 710.3
Pseudotruncus arteriosus 747.29
Pseudotuberculosis, pasteurella (infection) 027.2
Pseudotumor
　cerebri 348.2
　orbit (inflammatory) 376.11
Pseudo-Turner's syndrome 759.89
Pseudoxanthoma elasticum 757.39
Psilosis (sprue) (tropical) 579.1
　Monilia 112.89
　nontropical 579.0
　not sprue 704.00
Psittacosis 073.9
Psoitis 728.89
Psora NEC 696.1
Psoriasis 696.1
　any type, except arthropathic 696.1
　arthritic, arthropathic 696.0
　buccal 528.6
　flexural 696.1
　follicularis 696.1
　guttate 696.1
　inverse 696.1
　mouth 528.6
　nummularis 696.1
　psychogenic 316 [696.1]
　punctata 696.1
　pustular 696.1
　rupioides 696.1
　vulgaris 696.1
Psorospermiasis 136.4
Psorospermosis 136.4
　follicularis (vegetans) 757.39
Psychalgia 307.80
Psychasthenia 300.89
　compulsive 300.3
　mixed compulsive states 300.3
　obsession 300.3
Psychiatric disorder or problem NEC 300.9
Psychogenic — *see also* condition
　factors associated with physical conditions 316
Psychoneurosis, psychoneurotic — *see also* Neurosis 300.9
　anxiety (state) 300.00
　climacteric 627.2
　compensation 300.16
　compulsion 300.3
　conversion hysteria 300.11
　depersonalization 300.6
　depressive type 300.4
　dissociative hysteria 300.15
　hypochondriacal 300.7
　hysteria 300.10

Psychoneurosis, psychoneurotic — *see also* Neurosis — *continued*
　hysteria — *continued*
　　conversion type 300.11
　　dissociative type 300.15
　mixed NEC 300.89
　neurasthenic 300.5
　obsessional 300.3
　obsessive-compulsive 300.3
　occupational 300.89
　personality NEC 301.89
　phobia 300.20
　senile NEC 300.89
Psychopathic — *see also* condition
　constitution, posttraumatic 310.2
　　with psychosis 293.9
　personality 301.9
　　amoral trends 301.7
　　antisocial trends 301.7
　　asocial trends 301.7
　　mixed types 301.7
　state 301.9
Psychopathy, sexual — *see also* Deviation, sexual 302.9
Psychophysiologic, psychophysiological condition — *see* Reaction, psychophysiologic
Psychose passionelle 297.8
Psychosexual identity disorder 302.6
　adult-life 302.85
　childhood 302.6
Psychosis 298.9
　acute hysterical 298.1
　affecting management of pregnancy, childbirth, or puerperium 648.4 ☑
　affective (*see also* Disorder, mood) 296.90

> Note — Use the following fifth-digit subclassification with categories 296.0–296.6:
>
> 0　unspecified
>
> 1　mild
>
> 2　moderate
>
> 3　severe, without mention of psychotic behavior
>
> 4　severe, specified as with psychotic behavior
>
> 5　in partial or unspecified remission
>
> 6　in full remission

　　drug-induced 292.84
　　due to or associated with physical condition 293.83
　　involutional 293.83
　　　recurrent episode 296.3 ☑
　　　single episode 296.2 ☑
　　manic-depressive 296.80
　　　circular (alternating) 296.7
　　　　currently depressed 296.5 ☑
　　　　currently manic 296.4 ☑
　　　depressed type 296.2 ☑
　　　　atypical 296.82
　　　　recurrent episode 296.3 ☑
　　　　single episode 296.2 ☑
　　　manic 296.0 ☑
　　　　atypical 296.81
　　　　recurrent episode 296.1 ☑
　　　　single episode 296.0 ☑
　　　mixed type NEC 296.89
　　　specified type NEC 296.89
　　senile 290.21
　　specified type NEC 296.99
　alcoholic 291.9
　　with
　　　anxiety 291.89
　　　delirium tremens 291.0
　　　delusions 291.5
　　　dementia 291.2
　　　hallucinosis 291.3
　　　jealousy 291.5
　　　mood disturbance 291.89
　　　paranoia 291.5
　　　persisting amnesia 291.1
　　　sexual dysfunction 291.89

Psychosis — *continued*
　alcoholic — *continued*
　　with — *continued*
　　　sleep disturbance 291.89
　　amnestic confabulatory 291.1
　　delirium tremens 291.0
　　hallucinosis 291.3
　　Korsakoff's, Korsakov's, Korsakow's 291.1
　　paranoid type 291.5
　　pathological intoxication 291.4
　　polyneuritic 291.1
　　specified type NEC 291.89
　alternating (*see also* Psychosis, manic-depressive, circular) 296.7
　anergastic (*see also* Psychosis, organic) 294.9
　arteriosclerotic 290.40
　　with
　　　acute confusional state 290.41
　　　delirium 290.41
　　　delusions 290.42
　　　depressed mood 290.43
　　depressed type 290.43
　　paranoid type 290.42
　　simple type 290.40
　　uncomplicated 290.40
　atypical 298.9
　　depressive 296.82
　　manic 296.81
　borderline (schizophrenia) (*see also* Schizophrenia) 295.5 ☑
　　of childhood (*see also* Psychosis, childhood) 299.8 ☑
　　prepubertal 299.8 ☑
　brief reactive 298.8
　childhood, with origin specific to 299.9 ☑

> Note — Use the following fifth-digit subclassification with category 299:
>
> 0　current or active state
>
> 1　residual state

　　atypical 299.8 ☑
　　specified type NEC 299.8 ☑
　circular (*see also* Psychosis, manic-depressive, circular) 296.7
　climacteric (*see also* Psychosis, involutional) 298.8
　confusional 298.9
　　acute 293.0
　　reactive 298.2
　　subacute 293.1
　depressive (*see also* Psychosis, affective) 296.2 ☑
　　atypical 296.82
　　involutional 296.2 ☑
　　　with hypomania (bipolar II) 296.89
　　　recurrent episode 296.3 ☑
　　　single episode 296.2 ☑
　　psychogenic 298.0
　　reactive (emotional stress) (psychological trauma) 298.0
　　recurrent episode 296.3 ☑
　　　with hypomania (bipolar II) 296.89
　　single episode 296.2 ☑
　disintegrative, childhood (*see also* Psychosis, childhood) 299.1 ☑
　drug 292.9
　　with
　　　affective syndrome 292.84
　　　amnestic syndrome 292.83
　　　anxiety 292.89
　　　delirium 292.81
　　　　withdrawal 292.0
　　　delusions 292.11
　　　dementia 292.82
　　　depressive state 292.84
　　　hallucinations 292.12
　　　hallucinosis 292.12
　　　mood disorder 292.84
　　　mood disturbance 292.84
　　　organic personality syndrome NEC 292.89
　　　sexual dysfunction 292.89
　　　sleep disturbance 292.89
　　　withdrawal syndrome (and delirium) 292.0

☑ Additional Digit Required — Refer to the Tabular List for Digit Selection　　　　　　　　　　▽ Subterms under main terms may continue to next column or page

Psychosis — *continued*
  drug — *continued*
    affective syndrome 292.84
    delusions 292.11
    hallucinatory state 292.12
    hallucinosis 292.12
    paranoid state 292.11
    specified type NEC 292.89
    withdrawal syndrome (and delirium) 292.0
  due to or associated with physical condition (*see also* Psychosis, organic) 293.9
  epileptic NEC 293.9
  excitation (psychogenic) (reactive) 298.1
  exhaustive (*see also* Reaction, stress, acute) 308.9
  hypomanic (*see also* Psychosis, affective) 296.0 ☑
    recurrent episode 296.1 ☑
    single episode 296.0 ☑
  hysterical 298.8
    acute 298.1
  in
    conditions classified elsewhere
      with
        delusions 293.81
        hallucinations 293.82
    pregnancy, childbirth, or puerperium 648.4 ☑
  incipient 298.8
    schizophrenic (*see also* Schizophrenia) 295.5 ☑
  induced 297.3
  infantile (*see also* Psychosis, childhood) 299.0 ☑
  infective 293.9
    acute 293.0
    subacute 293.1
  interactional (childhood) (*see also* Psychosis, childhood) 299.1 ☑
  involutional 298.8
    depressive (*see also* Psychosis, affective) 296.2 ☑
      recurrent episode 296.3 ☑
      single episode 296.2 ☑
    melancholic 296.2 ☑
      recurrent episode 296.3 ☑
      single episode 296.2 ☑
    paranoid state 297.2
    paraphrenia 297.2
  Korsakoff's, Korakov's, Korsakow's (nonalcoholic) 294.0
    alcoholic 291.1
  mania (phase) (*see also* Psychosis, affective) 296.0 ☑
    recurrent episode 296.1 ☑
    single episode 296.0 ☑
  manic (*see also* Psychosis, affective) 296.0 ☑
    atypical 296.81
    recurrent episode 296.1 ☑
    single episode 296.0 ☑
  manic-depressive 296.80
    circular 296.7
      currently
        depressed 296.5 ☑
        manic 296.4 ☑
      mixed 296.6 ☑
    depressive 296.2 ☑
      recurrent episode 296.3 ☑
        with hypomania (bipolar II) 296.89
      single episode 296.2 ☑
    hypomanic 296.0 ☑
      recurrent episode 296.1 ☑
      single episode 296.0 ☑
    manic 296.0 ☑
      atypical 296.81
      recurrent episode 296.1 ☑
      single episode 296.0 ☑
    mixed NEC 296.89
    perplexed 296.89
    stuporous 296.89
  menopausal (*see also* Psychosis, involutional) 298.8

Psychosis — *continued*
  mixed schizophrenic and affective (*see also* Schizophrenia) 295.7 ☑
  multi-infarct (cerebrovascular) (*see also* Psychosis, arteriosclerotic) 290.40
  organic NEC 294.9
    due to or associated with
      addiction
        alcohol (*see also* Psychosis, alcoholic) 291.9
        drug (*see also* Psychosis, drug) 292.9
      alcohol intoxication, acute (*see also* Psychosis, alcoholic) 291.9
      alcoholism (*see also* Psychosis, alcoholic) 291.9
      arteriosclerosis (cerebral) (*see also* Psychosis, arteriosclerotic) 290.40
      cerebrovascular disease
        acute (psychosis) 293.0
        arteriosclerotic (*see also* Psychosis, arteriosclerotic) 290.40
      childbirth — *see* Psychosis, puerperal
      dependence
        alcohol (*see also* Psychosis, alcoholic) 291.9
        drug 292.9
      disease
        alcoholic liver (*see also* Psychosis, alcoholic) 291.9
        brain
          arteriosclerotic (*see also* Psychosis, arteriosclerotic) 290.40
          cerebrovascular
            acute (psychosis) 293.0
            arteriosclerotic (*see also* Psychosis, arteriosclerotic) 290.40
        endocrine or metabolic 293.9
          acute (psychosis) 293.0
          subacute (psychosis) 293.1
        Jakob-Creutzfeldt 046.19
          with behavioral disturbance 046.19 *[294.11]*
          without behavioral disturbance 046.19 *[294.10]*
          familial 046.19
          iatrogenic 046.19
          specified NEC 046.19
          sporadic 046.19
          variant 046.11
            with dementia
              with behavioral disturbance 046.11 *[294.11]*
              without behavioral disturbance 046.11 *[294.10]*
        liver, alcoholic (*see also* Psychosis, alcoholic) 291.9
      disorder
        cerebrovascular
          acute (psychosis) 293.0
        endocrine or metabolic 293.9
          acute (psychosis) 293.0
          subacute (psychosis) 293.1
      epilepsy
        with behavioral disturbance 345.9 ☑ *[294.11]*
        without behavioral disturbance 345.9 ☑ *[294.10]*
        transient (acute) 293.0
      Huntington's chorea
        with behavioral disturbance 333.4 *[294.11]*
        without behavioral disturbance 333.4 *[294.10]*
      infection
        brain 293.9
          acute (psychosis) 293.0
          chronic 294.8
          subacute (psychosis) 293.1
        intracranial NEC 293.9

Psychosis — *continued*
  organic — *continued*
    due to or associated with — *continued*
      infection — *continued*
        intracranial — *continued*
          acute (psychosis) 293.0
          chronic 294.8
          subacute (psychosis) 293.1
      intoxication
        alcoholic (acute) (*see also* Psychosis, alcoholic) 291.9
        pathological 291.4
        drug (*see also* Psychosis, drug) 292.9
      ischemia
        cerebrovascular (generalized) (*see also* Psychosis, arteriosclerotic) 290.40
      Jakob-Creutzfeldt disease (syndrome) 046.19
        with behavioral disturbance 046.19 *[294.11]*
        without behavioral disturbance 046.19 *[294.10]*
        variant 046.11
          with dementia
            with behavioral disturbance 046.11 *[294.11]*
            without behavioral disturbance 046.11 *[294.10]*
      multiple sclerosis
        with behavioral disturbance 340 *[294.11]*
        without behavioral disturbance 340 *[294.10]*
      physical condition NEC 293.9
        with
          delusions 293.81
          hallucinations 293.82
      presenility 290.10
      puerperium — *see* Psychosis, puerperal
      sclerosis, multiple
        with behavioral disturbance 340 *[294.11]*
        without behavioral disturbance 340 *[294.10]*
      senility 290.20
      status epilepticus
        with behavioral disturbance 345.3 *[294.11]*
        without behavioral disturbance 345.3 *[294.10]*
      trauma
        brain (birth) (from electrical current) (surgical) 293.9
          acute (psychosis) 293.0
          chronic 294.8
          subacute (psychosis) 293.1
        unspecified physical condition 293.9
          with
            delusion 293.81
            hallucinations 293.82
  infective 293.9
    acute (psychosis) 293.0
    subacute 293.1
  posttraumatic 293.9
    acute 293.0
    subacute 293.1
  specified type NEC 294.8
  transient 293.9
    with
      anxiety 293.84
      delusions 293.81
      depression 293.83
      hallucinations 293.82
    depressive type 293.83
    hallucinatory type 293.82
    paranoid type 293.81
    specified type NEC 293.89
  paranoic 297.1
  paranoid (chronic) 297.9

Psychosis — *continued*
  paranoid — *continued*
    alcoholic 291.5
    chronic 297.1
    climacteric 297.2
    involutional 297.2
    menopausal 297.2
    protracted reactive 298.4
    psychogenic 298.4
      acute 298.3
    schizophrenic (*see also* Schizophrenia) 295.3 ☑
    senile 290.20
  paroxysmal 298.9
    senile 290.20
  polyneuritic, alcoholic 291.1
  postoperative 293.9
  postpartum — *see* Psychosis, puerperal
  postpsychotic (*see also* Schizophrenia) 295.5 ☑
  prepsychotic (*see also* Schizophrenia) 295.5 ☑
  presbyophrenic (type) 290.8
  presenile (*see also* Dementia, presenile) 290.10
  prison 300.16
  psychogenic 298.8
    depressive 298.0
    paranoid 298.4
      acute 298.3
  puerperal
    specified type — *see* categories 295-298 ☑
    unspecified type 293.89
      acute 293.0
      chronic 293.89
      subacute 293.1
  reactive (emotional stress) (psychological trauma) 298.8
    brief 298.8
    confusion 298.2
    depressive 298.0
    excitation 298.1
  schizo-affective (depressed) (excited) (*see also* Schizophrenia) 295.7 ☑
  schizophrenia, schizophrenic (*see also* Schizophrenia) 295.9 ☑
    borderline type 295.5 ☑
      of childhood (*see also* Psychosis, childhood) 299.8 ☑
    catatonic (excited) (withdrawn) 295.2 ☑
    childhood type (*see also* Psychosis, childhood) 299.9 ☑
    hebephrenic 295.1 ☑
    incipient 295.5 ☑
    latent 295.5 ☑
    paranoid 295.3 ☑
    prepsychotic 295.5 ☑
    prodromal 295.5 ☑
    pseudoneurotic 295.5 ☑
    pseudopsychopathic 295.5 ☑
    schizophreniform 295.4 ☑
    simple 295.0 ☑
    undifferentiated type 295.9 ☑
  schizophreniform 295.4 ☑
  senile NEC 290.20
    with
      delusional features 290.20
      depressive features 290.21
    depressed type 290.21
    paranoid type 290.20
    simple deterioration 290.20
    specified type — *see* categories 295-298 ☑
  shared 297.3
  situational (reactive) 298.8
  symbiotic (childhood) (*see also* Psychosis, childhood) 299.1 ☑
  toxic (acute) 293.9

Psychotic — *see also* condition 298.9
  episode 298.9
    due to or associated with physical conditions (*see also* Psychosis, organic) 293.9

Pterygium (eye) 372.40
  central 372.43
  colli 744.5

☑ **Additional Digit Required** — Refer to the Tabular List for Digit Selection   🔻 **Subterms under main terms may continue to next column or page**

242 — Volume 2   ▶◀ Revised Text   ● New Line   ▲ Revised Code   2015 ICD-9-CM

Pterygium — continued
   double 372.44
   peripheral (stationary) 372.41
      progressive 372.42
   recurrent 372.45
Ptilosis 374.55
PTLD (post-transplant lymphoproliferative disorder) 238.77
Ptomaine (poisoning) — see also Poisoning, food 005.9
Ptosis (adiposa) 374.30
   breast 611.81
   cecum 569.89
   colon 569.89
   congenital (eyelid) 743.61
      specified site NEC — see Anomaly, specified type NEC
   epicanthus syndrome 270.2
   eyelid 374.30
      congenital 743.61
      mechanical 374.33
      myogenic 374.32
      paralytic 374.31
   gastric 537.5
   intestine 569.89
   kidney (see also Disease, renal) 593.0
      congenital 753.3
   liver 573.8
   renal (see also Disease, renal) 593.0
      congenital 753.3
   splanchnic 569.89
   spleen 289.59
   stomach 537.5
   viscera 569.89
PTP (posttransfusion purpura) 287.41
PTSD (Post-traumatic stress disorder) 309.81
Ptyalism 527.7
   hysterical 300.11
   periodic 527.2
   pregnancy 646.8 ☑
   psychogenic 306.4
Ptyalolithiasis 527.5
Pubalgia 848.8
Pubarche, precocious 259.1
Pubertas praecox 259.1
Puberty V21.1
   abnormal 259.9
   bleeding 626.3
   delayed 259.0
   precocious (constitutional) (cryptogenic) (idiopathic) NEC 259.1
      due to
         adrenal
            cortical hyperfunction 255.2
            hyperplasia 255.2
         cortical hyperfunction 255.2
         ovarian hyperfunction 256.1
            estrogen 256.0
         pineal tumor 259.8
         testicular hyperfunction 257.0
   premature 259.1
      due to
         adrenal cortical hyperfunction 255.2
         pineal tumor 259.8
         pituitary (anterior) hyperfunction 253.1
Puckering, macula 362.56
Pudenda, pudendum — see condition
Puente's disease (simple glandular cheilitis) 528.5
Puerperal
   abscess
      areola 675.1 ☑
      Bartholin's gland 646.6 ☑
      breast 675.1 ☑
      cervix (uteri) 670.8 ☑
      fallopian tube 670.8 ☑
      genital organ 670.8 ☑
      kidney 646.6 ☑
      mammary 675.1 ☑
      mesosalpinx 670.8 ☑
      nabothian 646.6 ☑
      nipple 675.0 ☑
      ovary, ovarian 670.8 ☑
      oviduct 670.8 ☑
      parametric 670.8 ☑

Puerperal — continued
   abscess — continued
      para-uterine 670.8 ☑
      pelvic 670.8 ☑
      perimetric 670.8 ☑
      periuterine 670.8 ☑
      retro-uterine 670.8 ☑
      subareolar 675.1 ☑
      suprapelvic 670.8 ☑
      tubal (ruptured) 670.8 ☑
      tubo-ovarian 670.8 ☑
      urinary tract NEC 646.6 ☑
      uterine, uterus 670.8 ☑
      vagina (wall) 646.6 ☑
      vaginorectal 646.6 ☑
      vulvovaginal gland 646.6 ☑
   accident 674.9 ☑
   adnexitis 670.8 ☑
   afibrinogenemia, or other coagulation defect 666.3 ☑
   albuminuria (acute) (subacute) 646.2 ☑
      pre-eclamptic 642.4 ☑
   anemia (conditions classifiable to 280–285) 648.2 ☑
   anuria 669.3 ☑
   apoplexy 674.0 ☑
   asymptomatic bacteriuria 646.5 ☑
   atrophy, breast 676.3 ☑
   blood dyscrasia 666.3 ☑
   caked breast 676.2 ☑
   cardiomyopathy 674.5 ☑
   cellulitis — see Puerperal, abscess
   cerebrovascular disorder (conditions classifiable to 430–434, 436–437) 674.0 ☑
   cervicitis (conditions classifiable to 616.0) 646.6 ☑
   coagulopathy (any) 666.3 ☑
   complications 674.9 ☑
      specified type NEC 674.8 ☑
   convulsions (eclamptic) (uremic) 642.6 ☑
      with pre-existing hypertension 642.7 ☑
   cracked nipple 676.1 ☑
   cystitis 646.6 ☑
   cystopyelitis 646.6 ☑
   deciduitis (acute) 670.8 ☑
   delirium NEC 293.9
   diabetes (mellitus) (conditions classifiable to 249 and 250) 648.0 ☑
   disease 674.9 ☑
      breast NEC 676.3 ☑
      cerebrovascular (acute) 674.0 ☑
      nonobstetric NEC (see also Pregnancy, complicated, current disease or condition) 648.9 ☑
      pelvis inflammatory 670.8 ☑
      renal NEC 646.2 ☑
      tubo-ovarian 670.8 ☑
      Valsuani's (progressive pernicious anemia) 648.2 ☑
   disorder
      lactation 676.9 ☑
      specified type NEC 676.8 ☑
      nonobstetric NEC (see also Pregnancy, complicated, current disease or condition) 648.9 ☑
   disruption
      cesarean wound 674.1 ☑
      episiotomy wound 674.2 ☑
      perineal laceration wound 674.2 ☑
   drug dependence (conditions classifiable to 304) 648.3 ☑
   eclampsia 642.6 ☑
      with pre-existing hypertension 642.7 ☑
   embolism (pulmonary) 673.2 ☑
      air 673.0 ☑
      amniotic fluid 673.1 ☑
      blood-clot 673.2 ☑
      brain or cerebral 674.0 ☑
      cardiac 674.8 ☑
      fat 673.8 ☑
      intracranial sinus (venous) 671.5 ☑
      pyemic 673.3 ☑
      septic 673.3 ☑
      spinal cord 671.5 ☑

Puerperal — continued
   endometritis (conditions classifiable to 615.0–615.9) 670.1 ☑
   endophlebitis — see Puerperal, phlebitis
   endotrachelitis 646.6 ☑
   engorgement, breasts 676.2 ☑
   erysipelas 670.8 ☑
   failure
      lactation 676.4 ☑
      renal, acute 669.3 ☑
   fever 672 ☑
      meaning pyrexia (of unknown origin) 672.0 ☑
      meaning sepsis 670.2 ☑
   fissure, nipple 676.1 ☑
   fistula
      breast 675.1 ☑
      mammary gland 675.1 ☑
      nipple 675.0 ☑
   galactophoritis 675.2 ☑
   galactorrhea 676.6 ☑
   gangrene
      gas 670.8 ☑
         with sepsis 670.2 ☑
      uterus 670.8 ☑
   gonorrhea (conditions classifiable to 098) 647.1 ☑
   hematoma, subdural 674.0 ☑
   hematosalpinx, infectional 670.8 ☑
   hemiplegia, cerebral 674.0 ☑
   hemorrhage 666.1 ☑
      brain 674.0 ☑
      bulbar 674.0 ☑
      cerebellar 674.0 ☑
      cerebral 674.0 ☑
      cortical 674.0 ☑
      delayed (after 24 hours) (uterine) 666.2 ☑
      extradural 674.0 ☑
      internal capsule 674.0 ☑
      intracranial 674.0 ☑
      intrapontine 674.0 ☑
      meningeal 674.0 ☑
      pontine 674.0 ☑
      subarachnoid 674.0 ☑
      subcortical 674.0 ☑
      subdural 674.0 ☑
      uterine, delayed 666.2 ☑
      ventricular 674.0 ☑
   hemorrhoids 671.8 ☑
   hepatorenal syndrome 674.8 ☑
   hypertrophy
      breast 676.3 ☑
      mammary gland 676.3 ☑
   induration breast (fibrous) 676.3 ☑
   infarction
      lung — see Puerperal, embolism
      pulmonary — see Puerperal, embolism
   infection
      Bartholin's gland 646.6 ☑
      breast 675.2 ☑
         with nipple 675.9 ☑
            specified type NEC 675.8 ☑
      cervix 646.6 ☑
      endocervix 646.6 ☑
      fallopian tube 670.8 ☑
      generalized 670.0 ☑
      genital tract (major) 670.0 ☑
         minor or localized 646.6 ☑
      kidney (bacillus coli) 646.6 ☑
      mammary gland 675.2 ☑
         with nipple 675.9 ☑
            specified type NEC 675.8 ☑
      nipple 675.0 ☑
         with breast 675.9 ☑
            specified type NEC 675.8 ☑
      ovary 670.8 ☑
      pelvic 670.8 ☑
      peritoneum 670.8 ☑
      renal 646.6 ☑
      tubo-ovarian 670.8 ☑
      urinary (tract) NEC 646.6 ☑
         asymptomatic 646.5 ☑

Puerperal — continued
   infection — continued
      uterus, uterine 670.8 ☑
      vagina 646.6 ☑
   inflammation (see also Puerperal, infection)
      areola 675.1 ☑
      Bartholin's gland 646.6 ☑
      breast 675.2 ☑
      broad ligament 670.8 ☑
      cervix (uteri) 646.6 ☑
      fallopian tube 670.8 ☑
      genital organs 670.8 ☑
         localized 646.6 ☑
      mammary gland 675.2 ☑
      nipple 675.0 ☑
      ovary 670.8 ☑
      oviduct 670.8 ☑
      pelvis 670.8 ☑
      periuterine 670.8 ☑
      tubal 670.8 ☑
      vagina 646.6 ☑
      vein — see Puerperal, phlebitis
   inversion, nipple 676.3 ☑
   ischemia, cerebral 674.0 ☑
   lymphangitis 670.8 ☑
      breast 675.2 ☑
   malaria (conditions classifiable to 084) 647.4 ☑
   malnutrition 648.9 ☑
   mammillitis 675.0 ☑
   mammitis 675.2 ☑
   mania 296.0 ☑
      recurrent episode 296.1 ☑
      single episode 296.0 ☑
   mastitis 675.2 ☑
      purulent 675.1 ☑
      retromammary 675.1 ☑
      submammary 675.1 ☑
   melancholia 296.2 ☑
      recurrent episode 296.3 ☑
      single episode 296.2 ☑
   mental disorder (conditions classifiable to 290–303, 305.0, 305.2–305.9, 306–316, 317–319) 648.4 ☑
   metritis (suppurative) 670.1 ☑
      septic 670.2 ☑
   metroperitonitis 670.8 ☑
   metrorrhagia 666.2 ☑
   metrosalpingitis 670.8 ☑
   metrovaginitis 670.8 ☑
   milk leg 671.4 ☑
   monoplegia, cerebral 674.0 ☑
   necrosis
      kidney, tubular 669.3 ☑
      liver (acute) (subacute) (conditions classifiable to 570) 674.8 ☑
      ovary 670.8 ☑
      renal cortex 669.3 ☑
   nephritis or nephrosis (conditions classifiable to 580–589) 646.2 ☑
      with hypertension 642.1 ☑
   nutritional deficiency (conditions classifiable to 260–269) 648.9 ☑
   occlusion, precerebral artery 674.0 ☑
   oliguria 669.3 ☑
   oophoritis 670.8 ☑
   ovaritis 670.8 ☑
   paralysis
      bladder (sphincter) 665.5 ☑
      cerebral 674.0 ☑
   paralytic stroke 674.0 ☑
   parametritis 670.8 ☑
   paravaginitis 646.6 ☑
   pelviperitonitis 670.8 ☑
   perimetritis 670.8 ☑
   perimetrosalpingitis 670.8 ☑
   perinephritis 646.6 ☑
   perioophoritis 670.8 ☑
   periphlebitis — see Puerperal, phlebitis
   perisalpingitis 670.8 ☑
   peritoneal infection 670.8 ☑
   peritonitis (pelvic) 670.8 ☑
   perivaginitis 646.6 ☑

☑ **Additional Digit Required — Refer to the Tabular List for Digit Selection**   ▨ **Subterms under main terms may continue to next column or page**

Puerperal — continued
phlebitis 671.2 ☑
  deep 671.4 ☑
  intracranial sinus (venous) 671.5 ☑
  pelvic 671.4 ☑
  specified site NEC 671.5 ☑
  superficial 671.2 ☑
phlegmasia alba dolens 671.4 ☑
placental polyp 674.4 ☑
pneumonia, embolic — see Puerperal, embolism
prediabetes 648.8 ☑
pre-eclampsia (mild) 642.4 ☑
  with pre-existing hypertension 642.7 ☑
  severe 642.5 ☑
psychosis, unspecified (see also Psychosis, puerperal) 293.89
pyelitis 646.6 ☑
pyelocystitis 646.6 ☑
pyelohydronephrosis 646.6 ☑
pyelonephritis 646.6 ☑
pyelonephrosis 646.6 ☑
pyemia 670.2 ☑
pyocystitis 646.6 ☑
pyohemia 670.2 ☑
pyometra 670.8 ☑
pyonephritis 646.6 ☑
pyonephrosis 646.6 ☑
pyo-oophoritis 670.8 ☑
pyosalpingitis 670.8 ☑
pyosalpinx 670.8 ☑
pyrexia (of unknown origin) 672.0 ☑
renal
  disease NEC 646.2 ☑
  failure, acute 669.3 ☑
retention
  decidua (fragments) (with delayed hemorrhage) 666.2 ☑
    without hemorrhage 667.1 ☑
  placenta (fragments) (with delayed hemorrhage) 666.2 ☑
    without hemorrhage 667.1 ☑
  secundines (fragments) (with delayed hemorrhage) 666.2 ☑
    without hemorrhage 667.1 ☑
retracted nipple 676.0 ☑
rubella (conditions classifiable to 056) 647.5 ☑
salpingitis 670.8 ☑
salpingo-oophoritis 670.8 ☑
salpingo-ovaritis 670.8 ☑
salpingoperitonitis 670.8 ☑
sapremia 670.2 ☑
secondary perineal tear 674.2 ☑
sepsis (pelvic) 670.2 ☑
septicemia 670.2 ☑
subinvolution (uterus) 674.8 ☑
sudden death (cause unknown) 674.9 ☑
suppuration — see Puerperal, abscess
syphilis (conditions classifiable to 090–097) 647.0 ☑
tetanus 670.8 ☑
thelitis 675.0 ☑
thrombocytopenia 666.3 ☑
thrombophlebitis (superficial) 671.2 ☑
  deep 671.4 ☑
  pelvic 671.4 ☑
  septic 670.3 ☑
  specified site NEC 671.5 ☑
thrombosis (venous) — see Thrombosis, puerperal
thyroid dysfunction (conditions classifiable to 240–246) 648.1 ☑
toxemia (see also Toxemia, of pregnancy) 642.4 ☑
  eclamptic 642.6 ☑
    with pre-existing hypertension 642.7 ☑
  pre-eclamptic (mild) 642.4 ☑
    with
      convulsions 642.6 ☑
      pre-existing hypertension 642.7 ☑
      severe 642.5 ☑

Puerperal — continued
tuberculosis (conditions classifiable to 010–018) 647.3 ☑
uremia 669.3 ☑
vaginitis (conditions classifiable to 616.1) 646.6 ☑
varicose veins (legs) 671.0 ☑
  vulva or perineum 671.1 ☑
venous complication 671.9 ☑
vulvitis (conditions classifiable to 616.1) 646.6 ☑
vulvovaginitis (conditions classifiable to 616.1) 646.6 ☑
white leg 671.4 ☑
Pulled muscle — see Sprain, by site
Pulmolithiasis 518.89
Pulmonary — see condition
Pulmonitis (unknown etiology) 486
Pulpitis (acute) (anachoretic) (chronic) (hyperplastic) (putrescent) (suppurative) (ulcerative) 522.0
Pulpless tooth 522.9
Pulse
alternating 427.89
  psychogenic 306.2
bigeminal 427.89
fast 785.0
feeble, rapid, due to shock following injury 958.4
rapid 785.0
slow 427.89
strong 785.9
trigeminal 427.89
water-hammer (see also Insufficiency, aortic) 424.1
weak 785.9
Pulseless disease 446.7
Pulsus
alternans or trigeminy 427.89
  psychogenic 306.2
Punch drunk 310.2
Puncta lacrimalia occlusion 375.52
Punctiform hymen 752.49
Puncture (traumatic) — see also Wound, open, by site
accidental, complicating surgery 998.2
bladder, nontraumatic 596.6
by
  device, implant, or graft — see Complications, mechanical
  foreign body
    internal organs (see also Injury, internal, by site)
      by ingested object — see Foreign body
    left accidentally in operation wound 998.4
  instrument (any) during a procedure, accidental 998.2
internal organs, abdomen, chest, or pelvis — see Injury, internal, by site
kidney, nontraumatic 593.89
Pupil — see condition
Pupillary membrane 364.74
  persistent 743.46
Pupillotonia 379.46
  pseudotabetic 379.46
Purpura 287.2
abdominal 287.0
allergic 287.0
anaphylactoid 287.0
annularis telangiectodes 709.1
arthritic 287.0
autoerythrocyte sensitization 287.2
autoimmune 287.0
bacterial 287.0
Bateman's (senile) 287.2
capillary fragility (hereditary) (idiopathic) 287.8
cryoglobulinemic 273.2
devil's pinches 287.2
fibrinolytic (see also Fibrinolysis) 286.6
fulminans, fulminous 286.6
gangrenous 287.0
hemorrhagic (see also Purpura, thrombocytopenic) 287.39

Purpura — continued
hemorrhagic (see also Purpura, thrombocytopenic) — continued
  nodular 272.7
  nonthrombocytopenic 287.0
  thrombocytopenic 287.39
Henoch's (purpura nervosa) 287.0
Henoch-Schönlein (allergic) 287.0
hypergammaglobulinemic (benign primary) (Waldenström's) 273.0
idiopathic 287.31
  nonthrombocytopenic 287.0
  thrombocytopenic 287.31
immune thrombocytopenic 287.31
infectious 287.0
malignant 287.0
neonatorum 772.6
nervosa 287.0
newborn NEC 772.6
nonthrombocytopenic 287.2
  hemorrhagic 287.0
  idiopathic 287.0
nonthrombopenic 287.2
peliosis rheumatica 287.0
pigmentaria, progressiva 709.09
posttransfusion (PTP) 287.41
  from whole blood (fresh) or blood products 287.41
primary 287.0
primitive 287.0
red cell membrane sensitivity 287.2
rheumatica 287.0
Schönlein (-Henoch) (allergic) 287.0
scorbutic 267
senile 287.2
simplex 287.2
symptomatica 287.0
telangiectasia annularis 709.1
thrombocytopenic (see also Thrombocytopenia) 287.30
  congenital 287.33
  essential 287.30
  hereditary 287.31
  idiopathic 287.31
  immune 287.31
  neonatal, transitory (see also Thrombocytopenia, neonatal transitory) 776.1
  primary 287.30
  puerperal, postpartum 666.3 ☑
  thrombotic 446.6
thrombohemolytic (see also Fibrinolysis) 286.6
thrombopenic (see also Thrombocytopenia) 287.30
  congenital 287.33
  essential 287.30
  thrombotic 446.6
    thrombocytic 446.6
    thrombocytopenic 446.6
toxic 287.0
variolosa 050.0
vascular 287.0
visceral symptoms 287.0
Werlhof's (see also Purpura, thrombocytopenic) 287.39
Purpuric spots 782.7
Purulent — see condition
Pus
absorption, general — see Septicemia
in
  stool 792.1
  urine 791.9
tube (rupture) (see also Salpingo-oophoritis) 614.2
Pustular rash 782.1
Pustule 686.9
malignant 022.0
nonmalignant 686.9
Putnam-Dana syndrome (subacute combined sclerosis with pernicious anemia) 281.0 [336.2]
Putnam's disease (subacute combined sclerosis with pernicious anemia) 281.0 [336.2]
Putrefaction, intestinal 569.89
Putrescent pulp (dental) 522.1

Pyarthritis — see Pyarthrosis
Pyarthrosis — see also Arthritis, pyogenic 711.0 ☑
  tuberculous — see Tuberculosis, joint
Pycnoepilepsy, pycnolepsy (idiopathic) — see also Epilepsy 345.0 ☑
Pyelectasia 593.89
Pyelectasis 593.89
Pyelitis (congenital) (uremic) 590.80
  with
    abortion — see Abortion, by type, with specified complication NEC
  contracted kidney 590.00
  ectopic pregnancy (see also categories 633.0–633.9) 639.8
  molar pregnancy (see also categories 630–632) 639.8
acute 590.10
  with renal medullary necrosis 590.11
chronic 590.00
  with
    renal medullary necrosis 590.01
complicating pregnancy, childbirth, or puerperium 646.6 ☑
  affecting fetus or newborn 760.1
cystica 590.3
  following
    abortion 639.8
    ectopic or molar pregnancy 639.8
gonococcal 098.19
  chronic or duration of 2 months or over 098.39
tuberculous (see also Tuberculosis) 016.0 ☑ [590.81]
Pyelocaliectasis 593.89
Pyelocystitis — see also Pyelitis 590.80
Pyelohydronephrosis 591
Pyelonephritis — see also Pyelitis 590.80
acute 590.10
  with renal medullary necrosis 590.11
chronic 590.00
syphilitic (late) 095.4
tuberculous (see also Tuberculosis) 016.0 ☑ [590.81]
Pyelonephrosis — see also Pyelitis 590.80
chronic 590.00
Pyelophlebitis 451.89
Pyelo-ureteritis cystica 590.3
Pyemia, pyemic (purulent) — see also Septicemia 038.9
abscess — see Abscess
arthritis (see also Arthritis, pyogenic) 711.0 ☑
Bacillus coli 038.42
embolism (see also Septicemia) 415.12
fever 038.9
infection 038.9
joint (see also Arthritis, pyogenic) 711.0 ☑
liver 572.1
meningococcal 036.2
newborn 771.81
phlebitis — see Phlebitis
pneumococcal 038.2
portal 572.1
postvaccinal 999.39
puerperal 670.2 ☑
specified organism NEC 038.8
staphylococcal 038.10
  aureus 038.11
    methicillin
      resistant 038.12
      susceptible 038.11
  specified organism NEC 038.19
streptococcal 038.0
tuberculous — see Tuberculosis, miliary
Pygopagus 759.4
Pykno-epilepsy, pyknolepsy (idiopathic) — see also Epilepsy 345.0 ☑
Pyle (-Cohn) disease (craniometaphyseal dysplasia) 756.89
Pylephlebitis (suppurative) 572.1
Pylethrombophlebitis 572.1
Pylethrombosis 572.1
Pyloritis — see also Gastritis 535.5 ☑
Pylorospasm (reflex) 537.81
  congenital or infantile 750.5

☑ Additional Digit Required — Refer to the Tabular List for Digit Selection

▽ Subterms under main terms may continue to next column or page

244 — Volume 2

▶◀ Revised Text

● New Line

▲ Revised Code

2015 ICD-9-CM

Pylorospasm — *continued*
  neurotic 306.4
  newborn 750.5
  psychogenic 306.4
Pylorus, pyloric — *see* condition
Pyoarthrosis — *see* Pyarthrosis
Pyocele
  mastoid 383.00
  sinus (accessory) (nasal) (*see also* Sinusitis)
    473.9
  turbinate (bone) 473.9
  urethra (*see also* Urethritis) 597.0
Pyococcal dermatitis 686.00
Pyococcide, skin 686.00
Pyocolpos — *see also* Vaginitis 616.10
Pyocyaneus dermatitis 686.09
Pyocystitis — *see also* Cystitis 595.9
Pyoderma, pyodermia 686.00
  gangrenosum 686.01
  specified type NEC 686.09
  vegetans 686.8
Pyodermatitis 686.00
  vegetans 686.8
Pyogenic — *see* condition
Pyohemia — *see* Septicemia
Pyohydronephrosis — *see also* Pyelitis 590.80
Pyometra 615.9
Pyometritis — *see also* Endometritis 615.9
Pyometrium — *see also* Endometritis 615.9
Pyomyositis 728.0
  ossificans 728.19
  tropical (bungpagga) 040.81
Pyonephritis — *see also* Pyelitis 590.80
  chronic 590.00
Pyonephrosis (congenital) — *see also* Pyelitis
  590.80
  acute 590.10
Pyo-oophoritis — *see also* Salpingo-oophoritis
  614.2
Pyo-ovarium — *see also* Salpingo-oophoritis
  614.2
Pyopericarditis 420.99
Pyopericardium 420.99
Pyophlebitis — *see* Phlebitis
Pyopneumopericardium 420.99
Pyopneumothorax (infectional) 510.9
  with fistula 510.0
  subdiaphragmatic (*see also* Peritonitis)
    567.29
  subphrenic (*see also* Peritonitis) 567.29
  tuberculous (*see also* Tuberculosis, pleura)
    012.0 ☑
Pyorrhea (alveolar) (alveolaris) 523.40
  degenerative 523.5
Pyosalpingitis — *see also* Salpingo-oophoritis
  614.2
Pyosalpinx — *see also* Salpingo-oophoritis
  614.2
Pyosepticemia — *see* Septicemia
Pyosis
  Corlett's (impetigo) 684
  Manson's (pemphigus contagiosus) 684
Pyothorax 510.9
  with fistula 510.0
  tuberculous (*see also* Tuberculosis, pleura)
    012.0 ☑
Pyoureter 593.89
  tuberculous (*see also* Tuberculosis) 016.2 ☑
Pyramidopallidonigral syndrome 332.0
Pyrexia (of unknown origin) (P.U.O.) 780.60
  atmospheric 992.0
  during labor 659.2 ☑
  environmentally-induced newborn 778.4
  heat 992.0
  newborn, environmentally-induced 778.4
  puerperal 672.0 ☑
Pyroglobulinemia 273.8
Pyromania 312.33
Pyrosis 787.1
Pyrroloporphyria 277.1
Pyuria (bacterial) 791.9

Q

Q fever 083.0
  with pneumonia 083.0 *[484.8]*
Quadricuspid aortic valve 746.89

Quadrilateral fever 083.0
Quadriparesis — *see* Quadriplegia
  meaning muscle weakness 728.87
Quadriplegia 344.00
  with fracture, vertebra (process) — *see*
    Fracture, vertebra, cervical, with
    spinal cord injury
  brain (current episode) 437.8
  C1-C4
    complete 344.01
    incomplete 344.02
  C5-C7
    complete 344.03
    incomplete 344.04
  cerebral (current episode) 437.8
  congenital or infantile (cerebral) (spastic)
    (spinal) 343.2
  cortical 437.8
  embolic (current episode) (*see also* Em-
    bolism, brain) 434.1 ☑
  functional 780.72
  infantile (cerebral) (spastic) (spinal) 343.2
  newborn NEC 767.0
  specified NEC 344.09
  thrombotic (current episode) (*see also*
    Thrombosis, brain) 434.0 ☑
  traumatic — *see* Injury, spinal, cervical
Quadruplet
  affected by maternal complications of
    pregnancy 761.5
  healthy liveborn — *see* Newborn, multiple
  pregnancy (complicating delivery) NEC
    651.8 ☑
    with fetal loss and retention of one or
      more fetus(es) 651.5 ☑
    following (elective) fetal reduction
      651.7 ☑
Quarrelsomeness 301.3
Quartan
  fever 084.2
  malaria (fever) 084.2
Queensland fever 083.0
  coastal 083.0
  seven-day 100.89
Quervain's disease 727.04
  thyroid (subacute granulomatous thyroidi-
    tis) 245.1
Queyrat's erythroplasia (M8080/2)
  specified site — *see* Neoplasm, skin, in situ
  unspecified site 233.5
Quincke's disease or edema — *see* Edema,
  angioneurotic
Quinquaud's disease (acne decalvans) 704.09
Quinsy (gangrenous) 475
Quintan fever 083.1
Raised — *see* Elevation
Quintuplet
  affected by maternal complications of
    pregnancy 761.5
  healthy liveborn — *see* Newborn, multiple
  pregnancy (complicating delivery) NEC
    651.2 ☑
    with fetal loss and retention of one or
      more fetus(es) 651.6 ☑
    following (elective) fetal reduction
      651.7 ☑
Quotidian
  fever 084.0
  malaria (fever) 084.0

R

Rabbia 071
Rabbit fever — *see also* Tularemia 021.9
Rabies 071
  contact V01.5
  exposure to V01.5
  inoculation V04.5
    reaction — *see* Complications, vaccina-
      tion
  vaccination, prophylactic (against) V04.5
Rachischisis — *see also* Spina bifida 741.9 ☑
Rachitic — *see also* condition
  deformities of spine 268.1
  pelvis 268.1
    with disproportion (fetopelvic) 653.2 ☑
      affecting fetus or newborn 763.1

Rachitic — *see also* condition — *continued*
  pelvis — *continued*
    with disproportion — *continued*
      causing obstructed labor 660.1 ☑
      affecting fetus or newborn 763.1
Rachitis, rachitism — *see also* Rickets
  acute 268.0
  fetalis 756.4
  renalis 588.0
  tarda 268.0
Racket nail 757.5
Radial nerve — *see* condition
Radiation effects or sickness — *see also* Effect, adverse, radiation
  cataract 366.46
  dermatitis 692.82
  sunburn (*see also* Sunburn) 692.71
Radiculitis (pressure) (vertebrogenic) 729.2
  accessory nerve 723.4
  anterior crural 724.4
  arm 723.4
  brachial 723.4
  cervical NEC 723.4
  due to displacement of intervertebral disc
    — *see* Neuritis, due to, displacement
    intervertebral disc
  leg 724.4
  lumbar NEC 724.4
  lumbosacral 724.4
  rheumatic 729.2
  syphilitic 094.89
  thoracic (with visceral pain) 724.4
Radiculomyelitis 357.0
  toxic, due to
    Clostridium tetani 037
    Corynebacterium diphtheriae 032.89
Radiculopathy — *see also* Radiculitis 729.2
Radioactive substances, adverse effect —
  see Effect, adverse, radioactive substance
Radiodermal burns (acute) (chronic) (occupa-
  tional) — *see* Burn, by site
Radiodermatitis 692.82
Radionecrosis — *see* Effect, adverse, radiation
Radiotherapy session V58.0
Radium, adverse effect — *see* Effect, adverse,
  radioactive substance
Raeder-Harbitz syndrome (pulseless disease)
  446.7
Rage — *see also* Disturbance, conduct 312.0 ☑
  meaning rabies 071
Rag sorters' disease 022.1
Raillietiniasis 123.8
Railroad neurosis 300.16
Railway spine 300.16
Raiva 071
Rake teeth, tooth 524.39
Rales 786.7
Ramifying renal pelvis 753.3
Ramsay Hunt syndrome (herpetic geniculate
  ganglionitis) 053.11
  meaning dyssynergia cerebellaris myocloni-
    ca 334.2
Ranke's primary infiltration — *see also* Tuberculosis 010.0 ☑
Ranula 527.6
  congenital 750.26
Rape
  adult 995.83
  alleged, observation or examination V71.5
  child 995.53
Rapid
  feeble pulse, due to shock, following injury
    958.4
  heart (beat) 785.0
    psychogenic 306.2
  respiration 786.06
    psychogenic 306.1
  second stage (delivery) 661.3 ☑
    affecting fetus or newborn 763.6
  time-zone change syndrome 327.35
Rarefaction, bone 733.99
Rash 782.1
  canker 034.1
  diaper 691.0
  drug (internal use) 693.0

Rash — *continued*
  drug — *continued*
    contact 692.3
  ECHO 9 virus 078.89
  enema 692.89
  food (*see also* Allergy, food) 693.1
  heat 705.1
  napkin 691.0
  nettle 708.8
  pustular 782.1
  rose 782.1
    epidemic 056.9
    of infants 057.8
  scarlet 034.1
  serum (prophylactic) (therapeutic) 999.59
  toxic 782.1
  wandering tongue 529.1
Rasmussen's aneurysm — *see also* Tuberculosis 011.2 ☑
Rat-bite fever 026.9
  due to Streptobacillus moniliformis 026.1
  spirochetal (morsus muris) 026.0
Rathke's pouch tumor (M9350/1) 237.0
Raymond (-Céstan) syndrome 433.8 ☑
Raynaud's
  disease or syndrome (paroxysmal digital
    cyanosis) 443.0
  gangrene (symmetric) 443.0 *[785.4]*
  phenomenon (paroxysmal digital cyanosis)
    (secondary) 443.0
RDS 769
Reaction
  acute situational maladjustment (*see also*
    Reaction, adjustment) 309.9
  adaptation (*see also* Reaction, adjustment)
    309.9
  adjustment 309.9
    with
      anxious mood 309.24
        with depressed mood 309.28
      conduct disturbance 309.3
        combined with disturbance of
          emotions 309.4
      depressed mood 309.0
        brief 309.0
          with anxious mood 309.28
        prolonged 309.1
      elective mutism 309.83
      mixed emotions and conduct 309.4
      mutism, elective 309.83
      physical symptoms 309.82
      predominant disturbance (of)
        conduct 309.3
        emotions NEC 309.29
          mixed 309.28
          mixed, emotions and conduct
            309.4
      specified type NEC 309.89
      specific academic or work inhibition
        309.23
      withdrawal 309.83
    depressive 309.0
      with conduct disturbance 309.4
      brief 309.0
      prolonged 309.1
    specified type NEC 309.89
  adverse food NEC 995.7
  affective (*see also* Psychosis, affective)
    296.90
    specified type NEC 296.99
  aggressive 301.3
    unsocialized (*see also* Disturbance, con-
      duct) 312.0 ☑
  allergic (*see also* Allergy) 995.3
    drug, medicinal substance, and biologi-
      cal — *see* Allergy, drug
    due to correct medical substance prop-
      erly administered 995.27
    food — *see* Allergy, food
    serum 999.59
  anaphylactic — *see* Anaphylactic reaction
  anesthesia — *see* Anesthesia, complication
  anger 312.0 ☑
  antisocial 301.7
  antitoxin (prophylactic) (therapeutic) — *see*
    Complications, vaccination

☑ **Additional Digit Required** — Refer to the Tabular List for Digit Selection   ᵂ **Subterms under main terms may continue to next column or page**

2015 ICD-9-CM   ▶◀ Revised Text   ● New Line   ▲ Revised Code   Volume 2 — 245

Reaction — *continued*
anxiety 300.00
Arthus 995.21
asthenic 300.5
compulsive 300.3
conversion (anesthetic) (autonomic) (hyperkinetic) (mixed paralytic) (paresthet-
  ic) 300.11
deoxyribonuclease (DNA) (DNase) hypersensitivity NEC 287.2
depressive 300.4
  acute 309.0
  affective (*see also* Psychosis, affective)
    296.2 ☑
    recurrent episode 296.3 ☑
    single episode 296.2 ☑
  brief 309.0
  manic (*see also* Psychosis, affective)
    296.80
  neurotic 300.4
  psychoneurotic 300.4
  psychotic 298.0
dissociative 300.15
drug NEC (*see also* Table of Drugs and
  Chemicals) 995.20
  allergic (*see also* Allergy, drug) 995.27
  correct substance properly administered
    995.20
  obstetric anesthetic or analgesic NEC
    668.9 ☑
    affecting fetus or newborn 763.5
    specified drug — *see* Table of Drugs
      and Chemicals
  overdose or poisoning 977.9
    specified drug — *see* Table of Drugs
      and Chemicals
  specific to newborn 779.4
  transmitted via placenta or breast milk
    — *see* Absorption, drug, through
      placenta
  withdrawal NEC 292.0
    infant of dependent mother 779.5
  wrong substance given or taken in error
    977.9
    specified drug — *see* Table of Drugs
      and Chemicals
dyssocial 301.7
dystonic, acute, due to drugs 333.72
erysipeloid 027.1
fear 300.20
  child 313.0
fluid loss, cerebrospinal 349.0
food (*see also* Allergy, food)
  adverse NEC 995.7
  anaphylactic shock — *see* Anaphylactic
    reaction or shock, due to, food
foreign
  body NEC 728.82
    in operative wound (inadvertently
      left) 998.4
      due to surgical material intention-
        ally left — *see* Complica-
        tions, due to (presence of)
        any device, implant, or
        graft classified to
        996.0–996.5 NEC
    substance accidentally left during a
      procedure (chemical) (powder)
      (talc) 998.7
    body or object (instrument) (sponge)
      (swab) 998.4
graft-versus-host (GVH) 279.50
grief (acute) (brief) 309.0
  prolonged 309.1
gross stress (*see also* Reaction, stress, acute)
  308.9
group delinquent (*see also* Disturbance,
  conduct) 312.2 ☑
Herxheimer's 995.91
hyperkinetic (*see also* Hyperkinesia) 314.9
hypochondriacal 300.7
hypoglycemic, due to insulin 251.0
  therapeutic misadventure 962.3
hypomanic (*see also* Psychosis, affective)
  296.0 ☑
  recurrent episode 296.1 ☑

Reaction — *continued*
hypomanic (*see also* Psychosis, affective) —
  continued
  single episode 296.0 ☑
hysterical 300.10
  conversion type 300.11
  dissociative 300.15
id (bacterial cause) 692.89
immaturity NEC 301.89
  aggressive 301.3
  emotional instability 301.59
immunization — *see* Complications, vaccination
incompatibility
  blood group (*see also* Complications,
    transfusion) 999.80
    ABO (due to transfusion of blood or
      blood products) (*see also*
      Complications, transfusion)
      999.60
    minor blood group 999.89
    non-ABO — *see also* Complications,
      transfusion 999.75
    Rh antigen (C) (c) (D) (E) (e) (factor) (infu-
      sion) (transfusion) (*see also* Com-
      plications, transfusion) 999.70
inflammatory — *see* Infection
infusion — *see* Complications, infusion
inoculation (immune serum) — *see* Complications, vaccination
insulin 995.23
involutional
  paranoid 297.2
  psychotic (*see also* Psychosis, affective,
    depressive) 296.2 ☑
leukemoid (basophilic) (lymphocytic)
  (monocytic) (myelocytic) (neutrophilic) 288.62
LSD (*see also* Abuse, drugs, nondependent)
  305.3 ☑
lumbar puncture 349.0
manic-depressive (*see also* Psychosis, affective) 296.80
  depressed 296.2 ☑
    recurrent episode 296.3 ☑
    single episode 296.2 ☑
  hypomanic 296.0 ☑
neurasthenic 300.5
neurogenic (*see also* Neurosis) 300.9
neurotic-depressive 300.4
neurotic NEC 300.9
nitritoid — *see* Crisis, nitritoid
nonspecific
  to
    cell mediated immunity measure-
      ment of gamma interferon
      antigen response without ac-
      tive tuberculosis 795.52
    QuantiFERON-TB test (QFT) without
      active tuberculosis 795.52
    tuberculin test (*see also* Reaction, tu-
      berculin skin test) 795.51
obsessive compulsive 300.3
organic 293.9
  acute 293.0
  subacute 293.1
overanxious, child or adolescent 313.0
paranoid (chronic) 297.9
  acute 298.3
  climacteric 297.2
  involutional 297.2
  menopausal 297.2
  senile 290.20
  simple 297.0
passive
  aggressive 301.84
  dependency 301.6
personality (*see also* Disorder, personality)
  301.9
phobic 300.20
postradiation — *see* Effect, adverse, radiation
psychogenic NEC 300.9
psychoneurotic (*see also* Neurosis) 300.9
  anxiety 300.00
  compulsive 300.3

Reaction — *continued*
psychoneurotic (*see also* Neurosis) — continued
  conversion 300.11
  depersonalization 300.6
  depressive 300.4
  dissociative 300.15
  hypochondriacal 300.7
  hysterical 300.10
    conversion type 300.11
    dissociative type 300.15
  neurasthenic 300.5
  obsessive 300.3
  obsessive-compulsive 300.3
  phobic 300.20
  tension state 300.9
psychophysiologic NEC (*see also* Disorder,
  psychosomatic) 306.9
  cardiovascular 306.2
  digestive 306.4
  endocrine 306.6
  gastrointestinal 306.4
  genitourinary 306.50
  heart 306.2
  hemic 306.8
  intestinal (large) (small) 306.4
  laryngeal 306.1
  lymphatic 306.8
  musculoskeletal 306.0
  pharyngeal 306.1
  respiratory 306.1
  skin 306.3
  special sense organs 306.7
psychosomatic (*see also* Disorder, psychosomatic) 306.9
psychotic (*see also* Psychosis) 298.9
  depressive 298.0
  due to or associated with physical condi-
    tion (*see also* Psychosis, organic)
    293.9
  involutional (*see also* Psychosis, affective)
    296.2 ☑
    recurrent episode 296.3 ☑
    single episode 296.2 ☑
pupillary (myotonic) (tonic) 379.46
radiation — *see* Effect, adverse, radiation
runaway (*see also* Disturbance, conduct)
  socialized 312.2 ☑
  undersocialized, unsocialized 312.1 ☑
scarlet fever toxin — *see* Complications,
  vaccination
schizophrenic (*see also* Schizophrenia)
  295.9 ☑
  latent 295.5 ☑
serological for syphilis — *see* Serology for
  syphilis
serum (prophylactic) (therapeutic) 999.59
  anaphylactic 999.49
  due to
    administration of blood and blood
      products 999.51
      anaphylactic 999.41
    vaccination 999.52
      anaphylactic 999.41
  immediate 999.49
situational (*see also* Reaction, adjustment)
  309.9
  acute, to stress 308.3
  adjustment (*see also* Reaction, adjust-
    ment) 309.9
somatization (*see also* Disorder, psychosomatic) 306.9
spinal puncture 349.0
spite, child (*see also* Disturbance, conduct)
  312.0 ☑
stress, acute 308.9
  with predominant disturbance (of)
    consciousness 308.1
    emotions 308.0
    mixed 308.4
    psychomotor 308.2
    specified type NEC 308.3
  bone or cartilage — *see* Fracture, stress
surgical procedure — *see* Complications,
  surgical procedure

Reaction — *continued*
  tetanus antitoxin — *see* Complications,
    vaccination
  toxin-antitoxin — *see* Complications, vacci-
    nation
  transfusion (blood) (bone marrow) (lympho-
    cytes) (allergic) (*see also* Complica-
    tions, transfusion) 999.80
  tuberculin skin test, nonspecific (without
    active tuberculosis) 795.51
    positive (without active tuberculosis)
      795.51
  ultraviolet — *see* Effect, adverse, ultraviolet
  undersocialized, unsocialized (*see also* Dis-
    turbance, conduct)
    aggressive (type) 312.0 ☑
    unaggressive (type) 312.1 ☑
  vaccination (any) — *see* Complications,
    vaccination
  white graft (skin) 996.52
  withdrawing, child or adolescent 313.22
  x-ray — *see* Effect, adverse, x-rays
Reactive depression — *see also* Reaction, depressive 300.4
  neurotic 300.4
  psychoneurotic 300.4
  psychotic 298.0
Rebound tenderness 789.6 ☑
Recalcitrant patient V15.81
Recanalization, thrombus — *see* Thrombosis
Recession, receding
  chamber angle (eye) 364.77
  chin 524.06
  gingival (postinfective) (postoperative)
    523.20
    generalized 523.25
    localized 523.24
    minimal 523.21
    moderate 523.22
    severe 523.23
Recklinghausen-Applebaum disease
  (hemochromatosis) 275.03
Recklinghausen's disease (M9540/1) 237.71
  bones (osteitis fibrosa cystica) 252.01
Reclus' disease (cystic) 610.1
Recrudescent typhus (fever) 081.1
Recruitment, auditory 388.44
Rectalgia 569.42
Rectitis 569.49
Rectocele
  female (without uterine prolapse) 618.04
    with uterine prolapse 618.4
      complete 618.3
      incomplete 618.2
    in pregnancy or childbirth 654.4 ☑
      causing obstructed labor 660.2 ☑
        affecting fetus or newborn 763.1
  male 569.49
  vagina, vaginal (outlet) 618.04
Rectosigmoiditis 569.89
  ulcerative (chronic) 556.3
Rectosigmoid junction — *see* condition
Rectourethral — *see* condition
Rectovaginal — *see* condition
Rectovesical — *see* condition
Rectum, rectal — *see* condition
Recurrent — *see* condition
  pregnancy loss — *see* Pregnancy, manage-
    ment affected by, abortion, habitual
Red bugs 133.8
Red cedar asthma 495.8
Redness
  conjunctiva 379.93
  eye 379.93
  nose 478.19
Reduced ventilatory or vital capacity 794.2
Reduction
  function
    kidney (*see also* Disease, renal) 593.9
    liver 573.8
  ventilatory capacity 794.2
  vital capacity 794.2
Redundant, redundancy
  abdomen 701.9
  anus 751.5
  cardia 537.89

☑ **Additional Digit Required — Refer to the Tabular List for Digit Selection**

▽ **Subterms under main terms may continue to next column or page**

Redundant, redundancy — *continued*
- clitoris 624.2
- colon (congenital) 751.5
- foreskin (congenital) 605
- intestine 751.5
- labia 624.3
- organ or site, congenital NEC — *see* Accessory
- panniculus (abdominal) 278.1
- prepuce (congenital) 605
- pylorus 537.89
- rectum 751.5
- scrotum 608.89
- sigmoid 751.5
- skin (of face) 701.9
  - eyelids 374.30
- stomach 537.89
- uvula 528.9
- vagina 623.8

Reduplication — *see* Duplication

Referral
- adoption (agency) V68.89
- nursing care V63.8
- patient without examination or treatment V68.81
- social services V63.8

Reflex — *see also* condition
- blink, deficient 374.45
- hyperactive gag 478.29
- neurogenic bladder NEC 596.54
  - atonic 596.54
    - with cauda equina syndrome 344.61
- vasoconstriction 443.9
- vasovagal 780.2

Reflux 530.81
- acid 530.81
- esophageal 530.81
  - with esophagitis 530.11
- esophagitis 530.11
- gastroesophageal 530.81
- mitral — *see* Insufficiency, mitral
- ureteral — *see* Reflux, vesicoureteral
- vesicoureteral 593.70
  - with
    - reflux nephropathy 593.73
      - bilateral 593.72
      - unilateral 593.71

Reformed gallbladder 576.0

Reforming, artificial openings — *see also* Attention to, artificial, opening V55.9

Refractive error — *see also* Error, refractive 367.9

Refsum's disease or syndrome (heredopathia atactica polyneuritiformis) 356.3

Refusal of
- food 307.59
  - hysterical 300.11
- treatment because of, due to
  - patient's decision NEC V64.2
  - reason of conscience or religion V62.6

Regaud
- tumor (M8082/3) — *see* Neoplasm, nasopharynx, malignant
- type carcinoma (M8082/3) — *see* Neoplasm, nasopharynx, malignant

Regional — *see* condition

Regulation feeding (elderly) (infant) 783.3
- newborn 779.31

Regurgitated
- food, choked on 933.1
- stomach contents, choked on 933.1

Regurgitation 787.03
- aortic (valve) (*see also* Insufficiency, aortic) 424.1
  - congenital 746.4
  - syphilitic 093.22
- food (*see also* Vomiting)
  - with reswallowing — *see* Rumination
  - newborn 779.33
- gastric contents — *see* Vomiting
- heart — *see* Endocarditis
- mitral (valve) (*see also* Insufficiency, mitral)
  - congenital 746.6
- myocardial — *see* Endocarditis
- pulmonary (heart) (valve) (*see also* Endocarditis, pulmonary) 424.3

Regurgitation — *continued*
- stomach — *see* Vomiting
- tricuspid — *see* Endocarditis, tricuspid
- valve, valvular — *see* Endocarditis
- vesicoureteral — *see* Reflux, vesicoureteral

Rehabilitation V57.9
- multiple types V57.89
- occupational V57.21
- specified type NEC V57.89
- speech (-language) V57.3
- vocational V57.22

Reichmann's disease or syndrome (gastrosuccorrhea) 536.8

Reifenstein's syndrome (hereditary familial hypogonadism, male) 259.52

Reilly's syndrome or phenomenon — *see also* Neuropathy, peripheral, autonomic 337.9

Reimann's periodic disease 277.31

Reinsertion, contraceptive device V25.42
- intrauterine V25.13

Reiter's disease, syndrome, or urethritis 099.3 *[711.1]* ☑

Rejection
- food, hysterical 300.11
- transplant 996.80
  - bone marrow 996.85
  - corneal 996.51
  - organ (immune or nonimmune cause) 996.80
    - bone marrow 996.85
    - heart 996.83
    - intestines 996.87
    - kidney 996.81
    - liver 996.82
    - lung 996.84
    - pancreas 996.86
    - specified NEC 996.89
  - skin 996.52
    - artificial 996.55
    - decellularized allodermis 996.55
  - stem cells(s) 996.88
    - from
      - peripheral blood 996.88
      - umbilical cord 996.88

Relapsing fever 087.9
- Carter's (Asiatic) 087.0
- Dutton's (West African) 087.1
- Koch's 087.9
- louse-borne (epidemic) 087.0
- Novy's (American) 087.1
- Obermeyer's (European) 087.0
- Spirillum 087.9
- tick-borne (endemic) 087.1

Relaxation
- anus (sphincter) 569.49
  - due to hysteria 300.11
- arch (foot) 734
  - congenital 754.61
- back ligaments 728.4
- bladder (sphincter) 596.59
- cardio-esophageal 530.89
- cervix (*see also* Incompetency, cervix) 622.5
- diaphragm 519.4
- inguinal rings — *see* Hernia, inguinal
- joint (capsule) (ligament) (paralytic) (*see also* Derangement, joint) 718.90
  - congenital 755.8
- lumbosacral joint 724.6
- pelvic floor 618.89
- pelvis 618.89
- perineum 618.89
- posture 729.90
- rectum (sphincter) 569.49
- sacroiliac (joint) 724.6
- scrotum 608.89
- urethra (sphincter) 599.84
- uterus (outlet) 618.89
- vagina (outlet) 618.89
- vesical 596.59

Remains
- canal of Cloquet 743.51
- capsule (opaque) 743.51

Remittent fever (malarial) 084.6

Remnant
- canal of Cloquet 743.51

Remnant — *continued*
- capsule (opaque) 743.51
- cervix, cervical stump (acquired) (postoperative) 622.8
- cystic duct, postcholecystectomy 576.0
- fingernail 703.8
  - congenital 757.5
- meniscus, knee 717.5
- thyroglossal duct 759.2
- tonsil 474.8
  - infected 474.00
- urachus 753.7

Remote effect of cancer — *see* condition

Removal (of)
- catheter (urinary) (indwelling) V53.6
  - from artificial opening — *see* Attention to, artificial, opening
  - non-vascular V58.82
  - vascular V58.81
- cerebral ventricle (communicating) shunt V53.01
- device (*see also* Fitting (of))
  - contraceptive V25.12
    - with reinsertion V25.13
  - fixation
    - external V54.89
    - internal V54.01
  - traction V54.89
- drains V58.49
- dressing
  - wound V58.30
    - nonsurgical V58.30
    - surgical V58.31
- ileostomy V55.2
- Kirschner wire V54.89
- nonvascular catheter V58.82
- pin V54.01
- plaster cast V54.89
- plate (fracture) V54.01
- rod V54.01
- screw V54.01
- splint, external V54.89
- staples V58.32
- subdermal implantable contraceptive V25.43
- sutures V58.32
- traction device, external V54.89
- vascular catheter V58.81
- wound packing V58.30
  - nonsurgical V58.30
  - surgical V58.31

Ren
- arcuatus 753.3
- mobile, mobilis (*see also* Disease, renal) 593.0
  - congenital 753.3
- unguliformis 753.3

Renal — *see also* condition
- glomerulohyalinosis-diabetic syndrome 250.4 ☑ *[581.81]*
  - due to secondary diabetes 249.4 ☑ *[581.81]*

Rendu-Osler-Weber disease or syndrome (familial hemorrhagic telangiectasia) 448.0

Reninoma (M8361/1) 236.91

Rénon-Delille syndrome 253.8

Repair
- pelvic floor, previous, in pregnancy or childbirth 654.4 ☑
  - affecting fetus or newborn 763.89
- scarred tissue V51.8

Replacement by artificial or mechanical device or prosthesis of — *see also* Fitting (of)
- artificial skin V43.83
- bladder V43.5
- blood vessel V43.4
- breast V43.82
- eye globe V43.0
- heart
  - with
    - assist device V43.21
    - fully implantable artificial heart V43.22
  - valve V43.3

Replacement by artificial or mechanical device or prosthesis of — *see also* Fitting (of) — *continued*
- intestine V43.89
- joint V43.60
  - ankle V43.66
  - elbow V43.62
  - finger V43.69
  - hip (partial) (total) V43.64
  - knee V43.65
  - shoulder V43.61
  - specified NEC V43.69
  - wrist V43.63
- kidney V43.89
- larynx V43.81
- lens V43.1
- limb(s) V43.7
- liver V43.89
- lung V43.89
- organ NEC V43.89
- pancreas V43.89
- skin (artificial) V43.83
- tissue NEC V43.89

Reprogramming
- cardiac pacemaker V53.31

Request for expert evidence V68.2

Reserve, decreased or low
- cardiac — *see* Disease, heart
- kidney (*see also* Disease, renal) 593.9

Residual — *see also* condition
- bladder 596.89
- foreign body — *see* Retention, foreign body
- state, schizophrenic (*see also* Schizophrenia) 295.6 ☑
- urine 788.69

Resistance, resistant (to)
- activated protein C 289.81

Note — use the following subclassification for categories V09.5, V09.7, V09.8, V09.9:

0   without mention of resistance to multiple drugs

1   with resistance to multiple drugs

    V09.5 quinolones and fluoroquinolones

    V09.7 antimycobacterial agents

    V09.8 specified drugs NEC

    V09.9 unspecified drugs

- drugs by microorganisms V09.9 ☑
  - Amikacin V09.4
  - aminoglycosides V09.4
  - Amodiaquine V09.5 ☑
  - Amoxicillin V09.0
  - Ampicillin V09.0
  - antimycobacterial agents V09.7 ☑
  - Azithromycin V09.2
  - Azlocillin V09.0
  - Aztreonam V09.1
  - Bacampicillin V09.0
  - Bacitracin V09.8 ☑
  - Benznidazole V09.8 ☑
  - B-lactam antibiotics V09.1
  - Capreomycin V09.7 ☑
  - Carbenicillin V09.0
  - Cefaclor V09.1
  - Cefadroxil V09.1
  - Cefamandole V09.1
  - Cefatetan V09.1
  - Cefazolin V09.1
  - Cefixime V09.1
  - Cefonicid V09.1
  - Cefoperazone V09.1
  - Ceforanide V09.1
  - Cefotaxime V09.1
  - Cefoxitin V09.1
  - Ceftazidime V09.1
  - Ceftizoxime V09.1
  - Ceftriaxone V09.1
  - Cefuroxime V09.1
  - Cephalexin V09.1
  - Cephaloglycin V09.1
  - Cephaloridine V09.1

☑ **Additional Digit Required** — Refer to the Tabular List for Digit Selection   ᵂ **Subterms under main terms may continue to next column or page**

2015 ICD-9-CM   ▶◀ **Revised Text**   ● **New Line**   ▲ **Revised Code**   **Volume 2 — 247**

Retinitis — see also Chorioretinitis —
  continued
  focal — *continued*
    peripheral 363.08
    posterior pole NEC 363.07
  gravidarum 646.8 ☑
  hemorrhagica externa 362.12
  juxtapapillary (Jensen's) 363.05
  luetic — see Retinitis, syphilitic
  metastatic 363.14
  pigmentosa 362.74
  proliferans 362.29
  proliferating 362.29
  punctata albescens 362.76
  renal 585.9 [363.13]
  syphilitic (secondary) 091.51
    congenital 090.0 [363.13]
    early 091.51
    late 095.8 [363.13]
  syphilitica, central, recurrent 095.8 [363.13]
  tuberculous (see also Tuberculous)
    017.3 ☑ [363.13]
Retinoblastoma (M9510/3) 190.5
  differentiated type (M9511/3) 190.5
  undifferentiated type (M9512/3) 190.5
Retinochoroiditis — see also Chorioretinitis
  363.20
  central angiospastic 362.41
  disseminated 363.10
    metastatic 363.14
    neurosyphilitic 094.83
    pigment epitheliopathy 363.15
    syphilitic 094.83
  due to toxoplasmosis (acquired) (focal)
    130.2
  focal 363.00
    in histoplasmosis 115.92
      capsulatum 115.02
      duboisii 115.12
    juxtapapillary (Jensen's) 363.05
    macular 363.06
    paramacular 363.06
    peripheral 363.08
    posterior pole NEC 363.07
  juxtapapillaris 363.05
  syphilitic (disseminated) 094.83
Retinopathy (background) 362.10
  arteriosclerotic 440.8 [362.13]
  atherosclerotic 440.8 [362.13]
  central serous 362.41
  circinate 362.10
  Coat's 362.12
  diabetic 250.5 ☑ [362.01]
    due to secondary diabetes
      249.5 ☑ [362.01]
    nonproliferative 250.5 ☑ [362.03]
      due to secondary diabetes
        249.5 ☑ [362.03]
      mild 250.5 ☑ [362.04]
        due to secondary diabetes
          249.5 ☑ [362.04]
      moderate 250.5 ☑ [362.05]
        due to secondary diabetes
          249.5 ☑ [362.05]
      severe 250.5 ☑ [362.06]
        due to secondary diabetes
          249.5 ☑ [362.06]
    proliferative 250.5 ☑ [362.02]
      due to secondary diabetes
        249.5 ☑ [362.02]
  exudative 362.12
  hypertensive 362.11
  nonproliferative
    diabetic 250.5 ☑ [362.03]
      due to secondary diabetes
        249.5 ☑ [362.03]
      mild 250.5 ☑ [362.04]
        due to secondary diabetes
          249.5 ☑ [362.04]
      moderate 250.5 ☑ [362.05]
        due to secondary diabetes
          249.5 ☑ [362.05]
      severe 250.5 ☑ [362.06]
        due to secondary diabetes
          249.5 ☑ [362.06]
  of prematurity 362.20

Retinopathy — *continued*
  of prematurity — *continued*
    cicatricial 362.21
    stage
      0 362.22
      1 362.23
      2 362.24
      3 362.25
      4 362.26
      5 362.27
  pigmentary, congenital 362.74
  proliferative 362.29
    diabetic 250.5 ☑ [362.02]
      due to secondary diabetes
        249.5 ☑ [362.02]
    sickle-cell 282.60 [362.29]
  solar 363.31
Retinoschisis 361.10
  bullous 361.12
  congenital 743.56
  flat 361.11
  juvenile 362.73
Retractile testis 752.52
Retraction
  cervix — see Retraction, uterus
  drum (membrane) 384.82
  eyelid 374.41
  finger 736.29
  head 781.0
  lid 374.41
  lung 518.89
  mediastinum 519.3
  nipple 611.79
    congenital 757.6
    puerperal, postpartum 676.0 ☑
  palmar fascia 728.6
  pleura (see also Pleurisy) 511.0
  ring, uterus (Bandl's) (pathological) 661.4 ☑
    affecting fetus or newborn 763.7
  sternum (congenital) 756.3
    acquired 738.3
    during respiration 786.9
  substernal 738.3
  supraclavicular 738.8
  syndrome (Duane's) 378.71
  uterus 621.6
  valve (heart) — see Endocarditis
Retrobulbar — see condition
Retrocaval ureter 753.4
Retrocecal — see also condition
  appendix (congenital) 751.5
Retrocession — see Retroversion
Retrodisplacement — see Retroversion
Retroflection, retroflexion — see Retrover-
  sion
Retrognathia, retrognathism (mandibular)
  (maxillary) 524.10
Retrograde
  ejaculation 608.87
  menstruation 626.8
Retroiliac ureter 753.4
Retroperineal — see condition
Retroperitoneal — see condition
Retroperitonitis 567.39
Retropharyngeal — see condition
Retroplacental — see condition
Retroposition — see Retroversion
Retroprosthetic membrane 996.51
Retrosternal thyroid (congenital) 759.2
Retroversion, retroverted
  cervix — see Retroversion, uterus
  female NEC (see also Retroversion, uterus)
    621.6
  iris 364.70
  testis (congenital) 752.51
  uterus, uterine (acquired) (acute) (adherent)
    (any degree) (asymptomatic) (cervix)
    (postinfectional) (postpartal) (old)
    621.6
    congenital 752.39
    in pregnancy or childbirth 654.3 ☑
      affecting fetus or newborn 763.89
      causing obstructed labor 660.2 ☑
        affecting fetus or newborn 763.1
Retrusion, premaxilla (developmental) 524.04
Rett's syndrome 330.8

Reverse, reversed
  peristalsis 787.4
Reye-Sheehan syndrome (postpartum pituitary necrosis) 253.2
Reye's syndrome 331.81
Rhabdomyolysis (idiopathic) 728.88
Rhabdomyoma (M8900/0) — see also Neoplasm, connective tissue, benign
  adult (M8904/0) — see Neoplasm, connec-
    tive tissue, benign
  fetal (M8903/0) — see Neoplasm, connec-
    tive tissue, benign
  glycogenic (M8904/0) — see Neoplasm,
    connective tissue, benign
Rhabdomyosarcoma (M8900/3) — see also
  Neoplasm, connective tissue, malignant
  alveolar (M8920/3) — see Neoplasm, con-
    nective tissue, malignant
  embryonal (M8910/3) — see Neoplasm,
    connective tissue, malignant
  mixed type (M8902/3) — see Neoplasm,
    connective tissue, malignant
  pleomorphic (M8901/3) — see Neoplasm,
    connective tissue, malignant
Rhabdosarcoma (M8900/3) — see Rhabdomyosarcoma
Rh antigen (C) (c) (D) (E) (e) (factor)
  hemolytic disease 773.0
  incompatibility, immunization, or sensitiza-
    tion
    affecting management of pregnancy
      656.1 ☑
    fetus or newborn 773.0
    transfusion reaction (see also Complica-
      tions, transfusion) 999.70
  negative mother, affecting fetus or newborn
    773.0
  titer elevated (see also Complications,
    transfusion) 999.70
  transfusion reaction (see also Complications,
    transfusion) 999.70
Rhesus (factor) (Rh) incompatibility — see Rh,
  incompatibility
Rheumaticosis — see Rheumatism
Rheumatism, rheumatic (acute NEC) 729.0
  adherent pericardium 393
  arthritis
    acute or subacute — see Fever,
      rheumatic
    chronic 714.0
      spine 720.0
  articular (chronic) NEC (see also Arthritis)
    716.9 ☑
    acute or subacute — see Fever,
      rheumatic
  back 724.9
  blennorrhagic 098.59
  carditis — see Disease, heart, rheumatic
  cerebral — see Fever, rheumatic
  chorea (acute) — see Chorea, rheumatic
  chronic NEC 729.0
  coronary arteritis 391.9
    chronic 398.99
  degeneration, myocardium (see also Degen-
    eration, myocardium, with rheumatic
    fever) 398.0
  desert 114.0
  febrile — see Fever, rheumatic
  fever — see Fever, rheumatic
  gonococcal 098.59
  gout 714.0
  heart
    disease (see also Disease, heart,
      rheumatic) 398.90
    failure (chronic) (congestive) (inactive)
      398.91
  hemopericardium — see Rheumatic, peri-
    carditis
  hydropericardium — see Rheumatic, peri-
    carditis
  inflammatory (acute) (chronic) (subacute)
    — see Fever, rheumatic
  intercostal 729.0
    meaning Tietze's disease 733.6
  joint (chronic) NEC (see also Arthritis)
    716.9 ☑

Rheumatism, rheumatic — *continued*
  joint (see also Arthritis) — *continued*
    acute — see Fever, rheumatic
  mediastinopericarditis — see Rheumatic,
    pericarditis
  muscular 729.0
  myocardial degeneration (see also Degener-
    ation, myocardium, with rheumatic
    fever) 398.0
  myocarditis (chronic) (inactive) (with
    chorea) 398.0
    active or acute 391.2
      with chorea (acute) (rheumatic)
        (Sydenham's) 392.0
  myositis 729.1
  neck 724.9
  neuralgic 729.0
  neuritis (acute) (chronic) 729.2
  neuromuscular 729.0
  nodose — see Arthritis, nodosa
  nonarticular 729.0
  palindromic 719.30
    ankle 719.37
    elbow 719.32
    foot 719.37
    hand 719.34
    hip 719.35
    knee 719.36
    multiple sites 719.39
    pelvic region 719.35
    shoulder (region) 719.31
    specified site NEC 719.38
    wrist 719.33
  pancarditis, acute 391.8
    with chorea (acute) (rheumatic) (Syden-
      ham's) 392.0
    chronic or inactive 398.99
  pericarditis (active) (acute) (with effusion)
    (with pneumonia) 391.0
    with chorea (acute) (rheumatic) (Syden-
      ham's) 392.0
    chronic or inactive 393
  pericardium — see Rheumatic, pericarditis
  pleuropericarditis — see Rheumatic, peri-
    carditis
  pneumonia 390 [517.1]
  pneumonitis 390 [517.1]
  pneumopericarditis — see Rheumatic,
    pericarditis
  polyarthritis
    acute or subacute — see Fever,
      rheumatic
    chronic 714.0
  polyarticular NEC (see also Arthritis) 716.9 ☑
  psychogenic 306.0
  radiculitis 729.2
  sciatic 724.3
  septic — see Fever, rheumatic
  spine 724.9
  subacute NEC 729.0
  torticollis 723.5
  tuberculous NEC (see also Tuberculosis)
    015.9 ☑
  typhoid fever 002.0
Rheumatoid — see also condition
  lungs 714.81
Rhinitis (atrophic) (catarrhal) (chronic)
  (croupous) (fibrinous) (hyperplastic)
  (hypertrophic) (membranous) (purulent)
  (suppurative) (ulcerative) 472.0
  with
    hay fever (see also Fever, hay) 477.9
      with asthma (bronchial) 493.0 ☑
    sore throat — see Nasopharyngitis
  acute 460
  allergic (nonseasonal) (seasonal) (see also
    Fever, hay) 477.9
    with asthma (see also Asthma) 493.0 ☑
    due to food 477.1
  granulomatous 472.0
  infective 460
  obstructive 472.0
  pneumococcal 460
  syphilitic 095.8
    congenital 090.0
  tuberculous (see also Tuberculosis) 012.8 ☑

Retinitis — Rhinitis

☑ Additional Digit Required — Refer to the Tabular List for Digit Selection   ᴺᴱᶜ Subterms under main terms may continue to next column or page

2015 ICD-9-CM   ▶◀ Revised Text   ● New Line   ▲ Revised Code   Volume 2 — 249

Rhinitis — continued
  vasomotor (see also Fever, hay) 477.9
Rhinoantritis (chronic) 473.0
  acute 461.0
Rhinodacryolith 375.57
Rhinolalia (aperta) (clausa) (open) 784.43
Rhinolith 478.19
  nasal sinus (see also Sinusitis) 473.9
Rhinomegaly 478.19
Rhinopharyngitis (acute) (subacute) — see
    also Nasopharyngitis 460
  chronic 472.2
  destructive ulcerating 102.5
  mutilans 102.5
Rhinophyma 695.3
Rhinorrhea 478.19
  cerebrospinal (fluid) 349.81
  paroxysmal (see also Fever, hay) 477.9
  spasmodic (see also Fever, hay) 477.9
Rhinosalpingitis 381.50
  acute 381.51
  chronic 381.52
Rhinoscleroma 040.1
Rhinosporidiosis 117.0
Rhinovirus infection 079.3
Rhizomelic chrondrodysplasia punctata
    277.86
Rhizomelique, pseudopolyarthritic 446.5
Rhoads and Bomford anemia (refractory)
    238.72
Rhus
  diversiloba dermatitis 692.6
  radicans dermatitis 692.6
  toxicodendron dermatitis 692.6
  venenata dermatitis 692.6
  verniciflua dermatitis 692.6
Rhythm
  atrioventricular nodal 427.89
  disorder 427.9
    coronary sinus 427.89
    ectopic 427.89
    nodal 427.89
  escape 427.89
  heart, abnormal 427.9
    fetus or newborn — see Abnormal, heart
      rate
  idioventricular 426.89
    accelerated 427.89
  nodal 427.89
  sleep, inversion 327.39
    nonorganic origin 307.45
Rhytidosis facialis 701.8
Rib — see also condition
  cervical 756.2
Riboflavin deficiency 266.0
Rice bodies — see also Loose, body, joint
    718.1 ☑
  knee 717.6
Richter's hernia — see Hernia, Richter's
Ricinism 988.2
Rickets (active) (acute) (adolescent) (adult)
    (chest wall) (congenital) (current) (infan-
    tile) (intestinal) 268.0
  celiac 579.0
  fetal 756.4
  hemorrhagic 267
  hypophosphatemic with nephrotic-glyco-
    suric dwarfism 270.0
  kidney 588.0
  late effect 268.1
  renal 588.0
  scurvy 267
  vitamin D-resistant 275.3
Rickettsial disease 083.9
  specified type NEC 083.8
Rickettsialpox 083.2
Rickettsiosis NEC 083.9
  specified type NEC 083.8
  tick-borne 082.9
    specified type NEC 082.8
  vesicular 083.2
Ricord's chancre 091.0
Riddoch's syndrome (visual disorientation)
    368.16
Rider's
  bone 733.99

Rider's — continued
  chancre 091.0
Ridge, alveolus — see also condition
  edentulous
    atrophy 525.20
      mandible 525.20
        minimal 525.21
        moderate 525.22
        severe 525.23
      maxilla 525.20
        minimal 525.24
        moderate 525.25
        severe 525.26
    flabby 525.20
Ridged ear 744.29
Riedel's
  disease (ligneous thyroiditis) 245.3
  lobe, liver 751.69
  struma (ligneous thyroiditis) 245.3
  thyroiditis (ligneous) 245.3
Rieger's anomaly or syndrome (mesodermal
    dysgenesis, anterior ocular segment)
    743.44
Riehl's melanosis 709.09
Rietti-Greppi-Micheli anemia or syndrome
    282.46
Rieux's hernia — see Hernia, Rieux's
Rift Valley fever 066.3
Riga's disease (cachectic aphthae) 529.0
Riga-Fede disease (cachectic aphthae) 529.0
Riggs' disease (compound periodontitis)
    523.40
Right middle lobe syndrome 518.0
Rigid, rigidity — see also condition
  abdominal 789.4 ☑
  articular, multiple congenital 754.89
  back 724.8
  cervix uteri
    in pregnancy or childbirth 654.6 ☑
      affecting fetus or newborn 763.89
      causing obstructed labor 660.2 ☑
        affecting fetus or newborn 763.1
  hymen (acquired) (congenital) 623.3
  nuchal 781.6
  pelvic floor
    in pregnancy or childbirth 654.4 ☑
      affecting fetus or newborn 763.89
      causing obstructed labor 660.2 ☑
        affecting fetus or newborn 763.1
  perineum or vulva
    in pregnancy or childbirth 654.8 ☑
      affecting fetus or newborn 763.89
      causing obstructed labor 660.2 ☑
        affecting fetus or newborn 763.1
  spine 724.8
  vagina
    in pregnancy or childbirth 654.7 ☑
      affecting fetus or newborn 763.89
      causing obstructed labor 660.2 ☑
        affecting fetus or newborn 763.1
Rigors 780.99
Riley-Day syndrome (familial dysautonomia)
    742.8
RIND (reversible ischemic neurological deficit)
    434.91
  history of (personal) V12.54
Ring(s)
  aorta 747.21
  Bandl's, complicating delivery 661.4 ☑
    affecting fetus or newborn 763.7
  contraction, complicating delivery 661.4 ☑
    affecting fetus or newborn 763.7
  esophageal (congenital) 750.3
  Fleischer (-Kayser) (cornea) 275.1 [371.14]
  hymenal, tight (acquired) (congenital) 623.3
  Kayser-Fleischer (cornea) 275.1 [371.14]
  retraction, uterus, pathological 661.4 ☑
    affecting fetus or newborn 763.7
  Schatzki's (esophagus) (congenital) (lower)
    750.3
    acquired 530.3
  Soemmering's 366.51
  trachea, abnormal 748.3
  vascular (congenital) 747.21
  Vossius' 921.3
    late effect 366.21

Ringed hair (congenital) 757.4
Ringing in the ear — see also Tinnitus 388.30
Ringworm 110.9
  beard 110.0
  body 110.5
  Burmese 110.9
  corporeal 110.5
  foot 110.4
  groin 110.3
  hand 110.2
  honeycomb 110.0
  nails 110.1
  perianal (area) 110.3
  scalp 110.0
  specified site NEC 110.8
  Tokelau 110.5
Rise, venous pressure 459.89
Risk
  factor — see Problem
  falling V15.88
  suicidal 300.9
Ritter's disease (dermatitis exfoliativa neona-
    torum) 695.81
Rivalry, sibling 313.3
Rivalta's disease (cervicofacial actinomycosis)
    039.3
River blindness 125.3 [360.13]
Robert's pelvis 755.69
  with disproportion (fetopelvic) 653.0 ☑
    affecting fetus or newborn 763.1
    causing obstructed labor 660.1 ☑
      affecting fetus or newborn 763.1
Robinson's (hidrotic) **ectodermal dysplasia**
    757.31
Robin's syndrome 756.0
Robles' disease (onchocerciasis) 125.3 [360.13]
Rochalimea — see Rickettsial disease
Rocky Mountain fever (spotted) 082.0
Rodent ulcer (M8090/3) — see also Neoplasm,
    skin, malignant
  cornea 370.07
Roentgen ray, adverse effect — see Effect,
    adverse, x-ray
Roetheln 056.9
Roger's disease (congenital interventricular
    septal defect) 745.4
Rokitansky's
  disease (see also Necrosis, liver) 570
  tumor 620.2
Rokitansky-Aschoff sinuses (mucosal out-
    pouching of gallbladder) — see also
    Disease, gallbladder 575.8
Rokitansky-Kuster-Hauser syndrome (con-
    genital absence vagina) 752.45
Rollet's chancre (syphilitic) 091.0
Rolling of head 781.0
Romano-Ward syndrome (prolonged QT inter-
    val syndrome) 426.82
Romanus lesion 720.1
Romberg's disease or syndrome 349.89
Roof, mouth — see condition
Rosacea 695.3
  acne 695.3
  keratitis 695.3 [370.49]
Rosary, rachitic 268.0
Rose
  cold 477.0
  fever 477.0
  rash 782.1
    epidemic 056.9
    of infants 057.8
Rosenbach's erysipelatoid or erysipeloid
    027.1
Rosen-Castleman-Liebow syndrome (pul-
    monary proteinosis) 516.0
Rosenthal's disease (factor XI deficiency) 286.2
Roseola 057.8
  infantum, infantilis (see also Exanthem
    subitum) 058.10
Rossbach's disease (hyperchlorhydria) 536.8
  psychogenic 306.4
Rössle-Urbach-Wiethe lipoproteinosis 272.8
Ross river fever 066.3
Rostan's asthma (cardiac) — see also Failure,
    ventricular, left 428.1

Rot
  Barcoo (see also Ulcer, skin) 707.9
  knife-grinders' (see also Tuberculosis)
    011.4 ☑
Rotation
  anomalous, incomplete or insufficient —
    see Malrotation
  cecum (congenital) 751.4
  colon (congenital) 751.4
  manual, affecting fetus or newborn 763.89
  spine, incomplete or insufficient 737.8
  tooth, teeth 524.35
  vertebra, incomplete or insufficient 737.8
Rot-Bernhardt disease 355.1
Röteln 056.9
Roth-Bernhardt disease or syndrome 355.1
Roth's disease or meralgia 355.1
Rothmund (-Thomson) syndrome 757.33
Rotor's disease or syndrome (idiopathic hy-
    perbilirubinemia) 277.4
Rotundum ulcer — see Ulcer, stomach
Round
  back (with wedging of vertebrae) 737.10
    late effect of rickets 268.1
  hole, retina 361.31
    with detachment 361.01
  ulcer (stomach) — see Ulcer, stomach
  worms (infestation) (large) NEC 127.0
Roussy-Lévy syndrome 334.3
Routine postpartum follow-up V24.2
Roy (-Jutras) syndrome (acropachyderma)
    757.39
Rubella (German measles) 056.9
  complicating pregnancy, childbirth, or
    puerperium 647.5 ☑
  complication 056.8
    neurological 056.00
      encephalomyelitis 056.01
      specified type NEC 056.09
    specified type NEC 056.79
  congenital 771.0
  contact V01.4
  exposure to V01.4
  maternal
    with suspected fetal damage affecting
      management of pregnancy
      655.3 ☑
    affecting fetus or newborn 760.2
      manifest rubella in infant 771.0
  specified complications NEC 056.79
  vaccination, prophylactic (against) V04.3
Rubeola (measles) — see also Measles 055.9
  complicated 055.8
  meaning rubella (see also Rubella) 056.9
  scarlatinosis 057.8
Rubeosis iridis 364.42
  diabetica 250.5 ☑ [364.42]
    due to secondary diabetes
      249.5 ☑ [364.42]
Rubinstein-Taybi's syndrome (brachydactylia,
    short stature and intellectual disabilities
    759.89
Rudimentary (congenital) — see also Agenesis
  arm 755.22
  bone 756.9
  cervix uteri 752.43
  eye (see also Microphthalmos) 743.10
  fallopian tube 752.19
  leg 755.32
  lobule of ear 744.21
  patella 755.64
  respiratory organs in thoracopagus 759.4
  tracheal bronchus 748.3
  uterine horn 752.39
  uterus 752.39
    in male 752.7
    solid or with cavity 752.39
  vagina 752.45
Rud's syndrome (mental deficiency, epilepsy,
    and infantilism) 759.89
Ruiter-Pompen (-Wyers) syndrome (angiok-
    eratoma corporis diffusum) 272.7
Ruled out condition — see also Observation,
    suspected V71.9
Rumination — see also Vomiting
  disorder 307.53

☑ Additional Digit Required — Refer to the Tabular List for Digit Selection   Subterms under main terms may continue to next column or page

250 — Volume 2   ▶◀ Revised Text   ● New Line   ▲ Revised Code   2015 ICD-9-CM

Rumination — *see also* Vomiting — *continued*
  neurotic 300.3
  obsessional 300.3
  psychogenic 307.53
Runaway reaction — *see also* Disturbance, conduct
  socialized 312.2 ☑
  undersocialized, unsocialized 312.1 ☑
Runeberg's disease (progressive pernicious anemia) 281.0
Runge's syndrome (postmaturity) 766.22
Runny nose 784.99
Rupia 091.3
  congenital 090.0
  tertiary 095.9
Rupture, ruptured 553.9
  abdominal viscera NEC 799.89
    obstetrical trauma 665.5 ☑
  abscess (spontaneous) — *see* Abscess, by site
  amnion — *see* Rupture, membranes
  aneurysm — *see* Aneurysm
  anus (sphincter) — *see* Laceration, anus
  aorta, aortic 441.5
    abdominal 441.3
    arch 441.1
    ascending 441.1
    descending 441.5
      abdominal 441.3
      thoracic 441.1
    syphilitic 093.0
    thoracoabdominal 441.6
    thorax, thoracic 441.1
    transverse 441.1
    traumatic (thoracic) 901.0
      abdominal 902.0
    valve or cusp (*see also* Endocarditis, aortic) 424.1
  appendix (with peritonitis) 540.0
    with peritoneal abscess 540.1
    traumatic — *see* Injury, internal, gastrointestinal tract
  arteriovenous fistula, brain (congenital) 430
  artery 447.2
    brain (*see also* Hemorrhage, brain) 431
    coronary (*see also* Infarct, myocardium) 410.9 ☑
    heart (*see also* Infarct, myocardium) 410.9 ☑
    pulmonary 417.8
    traumatic (complication) (*see also* Injury, blood vessel, by site) 904.9
  bile duct, except cystic (*see also* Disease, biliary) 576.3
    cystic 575.4
    traumatic — *see* Injury, internal, intra-abdominal
  bladder (sphincter) 596.6
    with
      abortion — *see* Abortion, by type, with damage to pelvic organs
      ectopic pregnancy (*see also* categories 633.0–633.9) 639.2
      molar pregnancy (*see also* categories 630–632) 639.2
    following
      abortion 639.2
      ectopic or molar pregnancy 639.2
    nontraumatic 596.6
    obstetrical trauma 665.5 ☑
    spontaneous 596.6
    traumatic — *see* Injury, internal, bladder
  blood vessel (*see also* Hemorrhage) 459.0
    brain (*see also* Hemorrhage, brain) 431
    heart (*see also* Infarct, myocardium) 410.9 ☑
    traumatic (complication) (*see also* Injury, blood vessel, by site) 904.9
  bone — *see* Fracture, by site
  bowel 569.89
    traumatic — *see* Injury, internal, intestine
  Bowman's membrane 371.31

Rupture, ruptured — *continued*
  brain
    aneurysm (congenital) (*see also* Hemorrhage, subarachnoid) 430
      late effect — *see* Late effect(s) (of) cerebrovascular disease
    syphilitic 094.87
    hemorrhagic (*see also* Hemorrhage, brain) 431
    injury at birth 767.0
    syphilitic 094.89
  capillaries 448.9
  cardiac (*see also* Infarct, myocardium) 410.9 ☑
  cartilage (articular) (current) (*see also* Sprain, by site)
    knee — *see* Tear, meniscus
    semilunar — *see* Tear, meniscus
  cecum (with peritonitis) 540.0
    with peritoneal abscess 540.1
    traumatic 863.89
      with open wound into cavity 863.99
  cerebral aneurysm (congenital) (*see also* Hemorrhage, subarachnoid) 430
    late effect — *see* Late effect(s) (of) cerebrovascular disease
  cervix (uteri)
    with
      abortion — *see* Abortion, by type, with damage to pelvic organs
      ectopic pregnancy (*see also* categories 633.0–633.9) 639.2
      molar pregnancy (*see also* categories 630–632) 639.2
    following
      abortion 639.2
      ectopic or molar pregnancy 639.2
    obstetrical trauma 665.3 ☑
    traumatic — *see* Injury, internal, cervix
  chordae tendineae 429.5
  choroid (direct) (indirect) (traumatic) 363.63
  circle of Willis (*see also* Hemorrhage, subarachnoid) 430
    late effect — *see* Late effect(s) (of) cerebrovascular disease
  colon 569.89
    traumatic — *see* Injury, internal, colon
  cornea (traumatic) (*see also* Rupture, eye)
    due to ulcer 370.00
  coronary (artery) (thrombotic) (*see also* Infarct, myocardium) 410.9 ☑
  corpus luteum (infected) (ovary) 620.1
  cyst — *see* Cyst
  cystic duct (*see also* Disease, gallbladder) 575.4
  Descemet's membrane 371.33
    traumatic — *see* Rupture, eye
  diaphragm (*see also* Hernia, diaphragm)
    traumatic — *see* Injury, internal, diaphragm
  diverticulum
    bladder 596.3
    intestine (large) (*see also* Diverticula) 562.10
      small 562.00
  duodenal stump 537.89
  duodenum (ulcer) — *see* Ulcer, duodenum, with perforation
  ear drum (*see also* Perforation, tympanum) 384.20
    with otitis media — *see* Otitis media
    traumatic — *see* Wound, open, ear
  esophagus 530.4
    traumatic 862.22
      with open wound into cavity 862.32
      cervical region — *see* Wound, open, esophagus
  eye (without prolapse of intraocular tissue) 871.0
    with
      exposure of intraocular tissue 871.1
      partial loss of intraocular tissue 871.2
      prolapse of intraocular tissue 871.1
    due to burn 940.5
  fallopian tube 620.8

Rupture, ruptured — *continued*
  fallopian tube — *continued*
    due to pregnancy — *see* Pregnancy, tubal
    traumatic — *see* Injury, internal, fallopian tube
  fontanel 767.3
  free wall (ventricle) (*see also* Infarct, myocardium) 410.9 ☑
  gallbladder or duct (*see also* Disease, gallbladder) 575.4
    traumatic — *see* Injury, internal, gallbladder
  gastric (*see also* Rupture, stomach) 537.89
    vessel 459.0
  globe (eye) (traumatic) — *see* Rupture, eye
  graafian follicle (hematoma) 620.0
  heart (auricle) (ventricle) (*see also* Infarct, myocardium) 410.9 ☑
    infectional 422.90
    traumatic — *see* Rupture, myocardium, traumatic
  hymen 623.8
  internal
    organ, traumatic (*see also* Injury, internal, by site)
      heart — *see* Rupture, myocardium, traumatic
      kidney — *see* Rupture, kidney
      liver — *see* Rupture, liver
      spleen — *see* Rupture, spleen, traumatic
      semilunar cartilage — *see* Tear, meniscus
  intervertebral disc — *see* Displacement, intervertebral disc
    traumatic (current) — *see* Dislocation, vertebra
  intestine 569.89
    traumatic — *see* Injury, internal, intestine
  intracranial, birth injury 767.0
  iris 364.76
    traumatic — *see* Rupture, eye
  joint capsule — *see* Sprain, by site
  kidney (traumatic) 866.03
    with open wound into cavity 866.13
    due to birth injury 767.8
    nontraumatic 593.89
  lacrimal apparatus (traumatic) 870.2
  lens (traumatic) 366.20
  ligament (*see also* Sprain, by site)
    with open wound — *see* Wound, open, by site
    old (*see also* Disorder, cartilage, articular) 718.0 ☑
  liver (traumatic) 864.04
    with open wound into cavity 864.14
    due to birth injury 767.8
    nontraumatic 573.8
  lymphatic (node) (vessel) 457.8
  marginal sinus (placental) (with hemorrhage) 641.2 ☑
    affecting fetus or newborn 762.1
  meaning hernia — *see* Hernia
  membrana tympani (*see also* Perforation, tympanum) 384.20
    with otitis media — *see* Otitis media
    traumatic — *see* Wound, open, ear
  membranes (spontaneous)
    artificial
      delayed delivery following 658.3 ☑
        affecting fetus or newborn 761.1
      fetus or newborn 761.1
    delayed delivery following 658.2 ☑
      affecting fetus or newborn 761.1
    premature (less than 24 hours prior to onset of labor) 658.1 ☑
      affecting fetus or newborn 761.1
      delayed delivery following 658.2 ☑
        affecting fetus or newborn 761.1
  meningeal artery (*see also* Hemorrhage, subarachnoid) 430
    late effect — *see* Late effect(s) (of) cerebrovascular disease
  meniscus (knee) (*see also* Tear, meniscus)

Rupture, ruptured — *continued*
  meniscus (*see also* Tear, meniscus) — *continued*
    old (*see also* Derangement, meniscus) 717.5
    site other than knee — *see* Disorder, cartilage, articular
    site other than knee — *see* Sprain, by site
  mesentery 568.89
    traumatic — *see* Injury, internal, mesentery
  mitral — *see* Insufficiency, mitral
  muscle (traumatic) NEC (*see also* Sprain, by site)
    with open wound — *see* Wound, open, by site
    nontraumatic 728.83
  musculotendinous cuff (nontraumatic) (shoulder) 840.4
  mycotic aneurysm, causing cerebral hemorrhage (*see also* Hemorrhage, subarachnoid) 430
    late effect — *see* Late effect(s) (of) cerebrovascular disease
  myocardium, myocardial (*see also* Infarct, myocardium) 410.9 ☑
    traumatic 861.03
      with open wound into thorax 861.13
  nontraumatic (meaning hernia) (*see also* Hernia, by site) 553.9
  obstructed (*see also* Hernia, by site, with obstruction) 552.9
    gangrenous (*see also* Hernia, by site, with gangrene) 551.9
  operation wound (*see also* Dehiscence) 998.32
    internal 998.31
  ovary, ovarian 620.8
    corpus luteum 620.1
    follicle (graafian) 620.0
  oviduct 620.8
    due to pregnancy — *see* Pregnancy, tubal
  pancreas 577.8
    traumatic — *see* Injury, internal, pancreas
  papillary muscle (ventricular) 429.6
  pelvic
    floor, complicating delivery 664.1 ☑
    organ NEC — *see* Injury, pelvic, organs
  penis (traumatic) — *see* Wound, open, penis
  perineum 624.8
    during delivery (*see also* Laceration, perineum, complicating delivery) 664.4 ☑
  pharynx (nontraumatic) (spontaneous) 478.29
  pregnant uterus (before onset of labor) 665.0 ☑
  prostate (traumatic) — *see* Injury, internal, prostate
  pulmonary
    artery 417.8
    valve (heart) (*see also* Endocarditis, pulmonary) 424.3
    vein 417.8
    vessel 417.8
  pupil, sphincter 364.75
  pus tube (*see also* Salpingo-oophoritis) 614.2
  pyosalpinx (*see also* Salpingo-oophoritis) 614.2
  rectum 569.49
    traumatic — *see* Injury, internal, rectum
  retina, retinal (traumatic) (without detachment) 361.30
    with detachment (*see also* Detachment, retina, with retinal defect) 361.00
  rotator cuff (capsule) (traumatic) 840.4
    nontraumatic (complete) 727.61
      partial 726.13
  sclera 871.0
  semilunar cartilage, knee (*see also* Tear, meniscus) 836.2

Rupture, ruptured — *continued*
  semilunar cartilage, knee (*see also* Tear, meniscus) — *continued*
    old (*see also* Derangement, meniscus) 717.5
  septum (cardiac) 410.8 ☑
  sigmoid 569.89
    traumatic — *see* Injury, internal, colon, sigmoid
  sinus of Valsalva 747.29
  spinal cord (*see also* Injury, spinal, by site)
    due to injury at birth 767.4
    fetus or newborn 767.4
    syphilitic 094.89
    traumatic (*see also* Injury, spinal, by site)
      with fracture — *see* Fracture, vertebra, by site, with spinal cord injury
  spleen 289.59
    congenital 767.8
    due to injury at birth 767.8
    malarial 084.9
    nontraumatic 289.59
    spontaneous 289.59
    traumatic 865.04
      with open wound into cavity 865.14
  splenic vein 459.0
  stomach 537.89
    due to injury at birth 767.8
    traumatic — *see* Injury, internal, stomach
    ulcer — *see* Ulcer, stomach, with perforation
  synovium 727.50
    specified site NEC 727.59
  tendon (traumatic) (*see also* Sprain, by site)
    with open wound — *see* Wound, open, by site
    Achilles 845.09
      nontraumatic 727.67
    ankle 845.09
      nontraumatic 727.68
    biceps (long bead) 840.8
      nontraumatic 727.62
    foot 845.10
      interphalangeal (joint) 845.13

Rupture, ruptured — *continued*
  tendon (*see also* Sprain, by site) — *continued*
    foot — *continued*
      metatarsophalangeal (joint) 845.12
      nontraumatic 727.68
      specified site NEC 845.19
      tarsometatarsal (joint) 845.11
    hand 842.10
      carpometacarpal (joint) 842.11
      interphalangeal (joint) 842.13
      metacarpophalangeal (joint) 842.12
      nontraumatic 727.63
        extensors 727.63
        flexors 727.64
      specified site NEC 842.19
    nontraumatic 727.60
      specified site NEC 727.69
    patellar 844.8
      nontraumatic 727.66
    quadriceps 844.8
      nontraumatic 727.65
    rotator cuff (capsule) 840.4
      nontraumatic (complete) 727.61
        partial 726.13
    wrist 842.00
      carpal (joint) 842.01
      nontraumatic 727.63
        extensors 727.63
        flexors 727.64
      radiocarpal (joint) (ligament) 842.02
      radioulnar (joint), distal 842.09
      specified site NEC 842.09
  testis (traumatic) 878.2
    complicated 878.3
    due to syphilis 095.8
  thoracic duct 457.8
  tonsil 474.8
  traumatic
    with open wound — *see* Wound, open, by site
    aorta — *see* Rupture, aorta, traumatic
    ear drum — *see* Wound, open, ear, drum
    external site — *see* Wound, open, by site
    eye 871.2
    globe (eye) — *see* Wound, open, eyeball

Rupture, ruptured — *continued*
  traumatic — *continued*
    internal organ (abdomen, chest, or pelvis) (*see also* Injury, internal, by site)
      heart — *see* Rupture, myocardium, traumatic
      kidney — *see* Rupture, kidney
      liver — *see* Rupture, liver
      spleen — *see* Rupture, spleen, traumatic
    ligament, muscle, or tendon (*see also* Sprain, by site)
      with open wound — *see* Wound, open, by site
    meaning hernia — *see* Hernia
  tricuspid (heart) (valve) — *see* Endocarditis, tricuspid
  tube, tubal 620.8
    abscess (*see also* Salpingo-oophoritis) 614.2
    due to pregnancy — *see* Pregnancy, tubal
  tympanum, tympanic (membrane) (*see also* Perforation, tympanum) 384.20
    with otitis media — *see* Otitis media
    traumatic — *see* Wound, open, ear, drum
  umbilical cord 663.8 ☑
    fetus or newborn 772.0
  ureter (traumatic) (*see also* Injury, internal, ureter) 867.2
    nontraumatic 593.89
  urethra 599.84
    with
      abortion — *see* Abortion, by type, with damage to pelvic organs
      ectopic pregnancy (*see also* categories 633.0–633.9) 639.2
      molar pregnancy (*see also* categories 630–632) 639.2
    following
      abortion 639.2
      ectopic or molar pregnancy 639.2
    obstetrical trauma 665.5 ☑
    traumatic — *see* Injury, internal urethra

Rupture, ruptured — *continued*
  uterosacral ligament 620.8
  uterus (traumatic) (*see also* Injury, internal, uterus)
    affecting fetus or newborn 763.89
    during labor 665.1 ☑
    nonpuerperal, nontraumatic 621.8
    nontraumatic 621.8
    pregnant (during labor) 665.1 ☑
      before labor 665.0 ☑
  vagina 878.6
    complicated 878.7
    complicating delivery — *see* Laceration, vagina, complicating delivery
  valve, valvular (heart) — *see* Endocarditis
  varicose vein — *see* Varicose, vein
  varix — *see* Varix
  vena cava 459.0
  ventricle (free wall) (left) (*see also* Infarct, myocardium) 410.9 ☑
  vesical (urinary) 596.6
    traumatic — *see* Injury, internal, bladder
  vessel (blood) 459.0
    pulmonary 417.8
  viscus 799.89
  vulva 878.4
    complicated 878.5
    complicating delivery 664.0 ☑

Russell's dwarf (uterine dwarfism and craniofacial dysostosis) 759.89

Russell's dysentery 004.8

Russell (-Silver) syndrome (congenital hemihypertrophy and short stature) 759.89

Russian spring-summer type encephalitis 063.0

Rust's disease (tuberculous spondylitis) 015.0 ☑ *[720.81]*

Rustitskii's disease (multiple myeloma) (M9730/3) 203.0 ☑

Ruysch's disease (Hirschsprung's disease) 751.3

Rytand-Lipsitch syndrome (complete atrioventricular block) 426.0

☑ Additional Digit Required — Refer to the Tabular List for Digit Selection   ▽ Subterms under main terms may continue to next column or page

S

Saber
shin 090.5
tibia 090.5
Saccharomyces infection — see also Candidiasis 112.9
Saccharopinuria 270.7
Saccular — see condition
Sacculation
aorta (nonsyphilitic) (see also Aneurysm, aorta) 441.9
ruptured 441.5
syphilitic 093.0
bladder 596.3
colon 569.89
intralaryngeal (congenital) (ventricular) 748.3
larynx (congenital) (ventricular) 748.3
organ or site, congenital — see Distortion
pregnant uterus, complicating delivery 654.4 ☑
affecting fetus or newborn 763.1
causing obstructed labor 660.2 ☑
affecting fetus or newborn 763.1
rectosigmoid 569.89
sigmoid 569.89
ureter 593.89
urethra 599.2
vesical 596.3
Sachs (-Tay) disease (amaurotic familial idiocy) 330.1
Sacks-Libman disease 710.0 [424.91]
Sac, lacrimal — see condition
Sacralgia 724.6
Sacralization
fifth lumbar vertebra 756.15
incomplete (vertebra) 756.15
Sacrodynia 724.6
Sacroiliac joint — see condition
Sacroiliitis NEC 720.2
Sacrum — see condition
Saddle
back 737.8
embolus
abdominal aorta 444.01
pulmonary artery 415.13
injury — code to condition
nose 738.0
congenital 754.0
due to syphilis 090.5
Sadism (sexual) 302.84
Saemisch's ulcer 370.04
Saenger's syndrome 379.46
Sago spleen 277.39
Sailors' skin 692.74
Saint
Anthony's fire (see also Erysipelas) 035
Guy's dance — see Chorea
Louis-type encephalitis 062.3
triad (see also Hernia, diaphragm) 553.3
Vitus' dance — see Chorea
Salicylism
correct substance properly administered 535.4 ☑
overdose or wrong substance given or taken 965.1
Salivary duct or gland — see also condition
virus disease 078.5
Salivation (excessive) — see also Ptyalism 527.7
Salmonella (aertrycke) (choleraesuis) (enteritidis) (gallinarum) (suipestifer) (typhimurium) — see also Infection, Salmonella 003.9
arthritis 003.23
carrier (suspected) of V02.3
meningitis 003.21
osteomyelitis 003.24
pneumonia 003.22
septicemia 003.1
typhosa 002.0
carrier (suspected) of V02.1
Salmonellosis 003.0
with pneumonia 003.22

Salpingitis (catarrhal) (fallopian tube) (nodular) (pseudofollicular) (purulent) (septic) — see also Salpingo-oophoritis 614.2
ear 381.50
acute 381.51
chronic 381.52
Eustachian (tube) 381.50
acute 381.51
chronic 381.52
follicularis 614.1
gonococcal (chronic) 098.37
acute 098.17
interstitial, chronic 614.1
isthmica nodosa 614.1
old — see Salpingo-oophoritis, chronic
puerperal, postpartum, childbirth 670.8 ☑
specific (chronic) 098.37
acute 098.17
tuberculous (acute) (chronic) (see also Tuberculosis) 016.6 ☑
venereal (chronic) 098.37
acute 098.17
Salpingocele 620.4
Salpingo-oophoritis (catarrhal) (purulent) (ruptured) (septic) (suppurative) 614.2
acute 614.0
with
abortion — see Abortion, by type, with sepsis
ectopic pregnancy (see also categories 633.0–633.9) 639.0
molar pregnancy (see also categories 630–632) 639.0
following
abortion 639.0
ectopic or molar pregnancy 639.0
gonococcal 098.17
puerperal, postpartum, childbirth 670.8 ☑
tuberculous (see also Tuberculosis) 016.6 ☑
chronic 614.1
gonococcal 098.37
tuberculous (see also Tuberculosis) 016.6 ☑
complicating pregnancy 646.6 ☑
affecting fetus or newborn 760.8
gonococcal (chronic) 098.37
acute 098.17
old — see Salpingo-oophoritis, chronic
puerperal 670.8 ☑
specific — see Salpingo-oophoritis, gonococcal
subacute (see also Salpingo-oophoritis, acute) 614.0
tuberculous (acute) (chronic) (see also Tuberculosis) 016.6 ☑
venereal — see Salpingo-oophoritis, gonococcal
Salpingo-ovaritis — see also Salpingo-oophoritis 614.2
Salpingoperitonitis — see also Salpingo-oophoritis 614.2
Salt-losing
nephritis (see also Disease, renal) 593.9
syndrome (see also Disease, renal) 593.9
Salt-rheum — see also Eczema 692.9
Salzmann's nodular dystrophy 371.46
Sampling
chorionic villus V28.89
Sampson's cyst or tumor 617.1
Sandblasters'
asthma 502
lung 502
Sander's disease (paranoia) 297.1
Sandfly fever 066.0
Sandhoff's disease 330.1
Sanfilippo's syndrome (mucopolysaccharidosis III) 277.5
Sanger-Brown's ataxia 334.2
San Joaquin Valley fever 114.0
Sao Paulo fever or typhus 082.0
Saponification, mesenteric 567.89
Sapremia — see Septicemia
Sarcocele (benign)
syphilitic 095.8

Sarcocele — continued
syphilitic — continued
congenital 090.5
Sarcoepiplocele — see also Hernia 553.9
Sarcoepiplomphalocele — see also Hernia, umbilicus 553.1
Sarcoid (any site) 135
with lung involvement 135 [517.8]
Boeck's 135
Darier-Roussy 135
Spiegler-Fendt 686.8
Sarcoidosis 135
cardiac 135 [425.8]
lung 135 [517.8]
Sarcoma (M8800/3) — see also Neoplasm, connective tissue, malignant
alveolar soft part (M9581/3) — see Neoplasm, connective tissue, malignant
ameloblastic (M9330/3) 170.1
upper jaw (bone) 170.0
botryoid (M8910/3) — see Neoplasm, connective tissue, malignant
botryoides (M8910/3) — see Neoplasm, connective tissue, malignant
cerebellar (M9480/3) 191.6
circumscribed (arachnoidal) (M9471/3) 191.6
circumscribed (arachnoidal) cerebellar (M9471/3) 191.6
clear cell, of tendons and aponeuroses (M9044/3) — see Neoplasm, connective tissue, malignant
embryonal (M8991/3) — see Neoplasm, connective tissue, malignant
endometrial (stromal) (M8930/3) 182.0
isthmus 182.1
endothelial (M9130/3) (see also Neoplasm, connective tissue, malignant)
bone (M9260/3) — see Neoplasm, bone, malignant
epithelioid cell (M8804/3) — see Neoplasm, connective tissue, malignant
Ewing's (M9260/3) — see Neoplasm, bone, malignant
follicular dendritic cell 202.9 ☑
germinoblastic (diffuse) (M9632/3) 202.8 ☑
follicular (M9697/3) 202.0 ☑
giant cell (M8802/3) (see also Neoplasm, connective tissue, malignant)
bone (M9250/3) — see Neoplasm, bone, malignant
glomoid (M8710/3) — see Neoplasm, connective tissue, malignant
granulocytic (M9930/3) 205.3 ☑
hemangioendothelial (M9130/3) — see Neoplasm, connective tissue, malignant
hemorrhagic, multiple (M9140/3) — see Kaposi's, sarcoma
Hodgkin's (M9662/3) 201.2 ☑
immunoblastic (M9612/3) 200.8 ☑
interdigitating dendritic cell 202.9 ☑
Kaposi's (M9140/3) — see Kaposi's, sarcoma
Kupffer cell (M9124/3) 155.0
Langerhans cell 202.9 ☑
leptomeningeal (M9530/3) — see Neoplasm, meninges, malignant
lymphangioendothelial (M9170/3) — see Neoplasm, connective tissue, malignant
lymphoblastic (M9630/3) 200.1 ☑
lymphocytic (M9620/3) 200.1 ☑
mast cell (M9740/3) 202.6 ☑
melanotic (M8720/3) — see Melanoma
meningeal (M9530/3) — see Neoplasm, meninges, malignant
meningothelial (M9530/3) — see Neoplasm, meninges, malignant
mesenchymal (M8800/3) (see also Neoplasm, connective tissue, malignant)
mixed (M8990/3) — see Neoplasm, connective tissue, malignant
mesothelial (M9050/3) — see Neoplasm, by site, malignant

Sarcoma — see also Neoplasm, connective tissue, malignant — continued
monstrocellular (M9481/3)
specified site — see Neoplasm, by site, malignant
unspecified site 191.9
myeloid (M9930/3) 205.3 ☑
neurogenic (M9540/3) — see Neoplasm, connective tissue, malignant
odontogenic (M9270/3) 170.1
upper jaw (bone) 170.0
osteoblastic (M9180/3) — see Neoplasm, bone, malignant
osteogenic (M9180/3) (see also Neoplasm, bone, malignant)
juxtacortical (M9190/3) — see Neoplasm, bone, malignant
periosteal (M9190/3) — see Neoplasm, bone, malignant
periosteal (M8812/3) (see also Neoplasm, bone, malignant)
osteogenic (M9190/3) — see Neoplasm, bone, malignant
plasma cell (M9731/3) 203.8 ☑
pleomorphic cell (M8802/3) — see Neoplasm, connective tissue, malignant
reticuloendothelial (M9720/3) 202.3 ☑
reticulum cell (M9640/3) 200.0 ☑
nodular (M9642/3) 200.0 ☑
pleomorphic cell type (M9641/3) 200.0 ☑
round cell (M8803/3) — see Neoplasm, connective tissue, malignant
small cell (M8803/3) — see Neoplasm, connective tissue, malignant
spindle cell (M8801/3) — see Neoplasm, connective tissue, malignant
stromal (endometrial) (M8930/3) 182.0
isthmus 182.1
synovial (M9040/3) (see also Neoplasm, connective tissue, malignant)
biphasic type (M9043/3) — see Neoplasm, connective tissue, malignant
epithelioid cell type (M9042/3) — see Neoplasm, connective tissue, malignant
spindle cell type (M9041/3) — see Neoplasm, connective tissue, malignant
Sarcomatosis
meningeal (M9539/3) — see Neoplasm, meninges, malignant
specified site NEC (M8800/3) — see Neoplasm, connective tissue, malignant
unspecified site (M8800/6) 171.9
Sarcosinemia 270.8
Sarcosporidiosis 136.5
Satiety, early 780.94
Satisfactory smear but lacking transformation zone
anal 796.77
cervical 795.07
Saturnine — see condition
Saturnism 984.9
specified type of lead — see Table of Drugs and Chemicals
Satyriasis 302.89
Sauriasis — see Ichthyosis
Sauriderma 757.39
Sauriosis — see Ichthyosis
Savill's disease (epidemic exfoliative dermatitis) 695.89
SBE (subacute bacterial endocarditis) 421.0
Scabies (any site) 133.0
Scabs 782.8
Scaglietti-Dagnini syndrome (acromegalic macrospondylitis) 253.0
Scald, scalded — see also Burn, by site
skin syndrome 695.81
Scalenus anticus (anterior) syndrome 353.0
Scales 782.8
Scalp — see condition
Scaphocephaly 756.0
Scaphoiditis, tarsal 732.5
Scapulalgia 733.90

☑ Additional Digit Required — Refer to the Tabular List for Digit Selection   ▽ Subterms under main terms may continue to next column or page

Scapulohumeral myopathy 359.1
Scarabiasis 134.1
Scarlatina 034.1
  anginosa 034.1
  maligna 034.1
  myocarditis, acute 034.1 [422.0]
    old (see also Myocarditis) 429.0
  otitis media 034.1 [382.02]
  ulcerosa 034.1
Scarlatinella 057.8
Scarlet fever (albuminuria) (angina) (convulsions) (lesions of lid) (rash) 034.1
Scar, scarring — see also Cicatrix 709.2
  adherent 709.2
  atrophic 709.2
  cervix
    in pregnancy or childbirth 654.6 ☑
      affecting fetus or newborn 763.89
      causing obstructed labor 660.2 ☑
        affecting fetus or newborn 763.1
  cheloid 701.4
  chorioretinal 363.30
    disseminated 363.35
    macular 363.32
    peripheral 363.34
    posterior pole NEC 363.33
  choroid (see also Scar, chorioretinal) 363.30
  compression, pericardial 423.9
  congenital 757.39
  conjunctiva 372.64
  cornea 371.00
    xerophthalmic 264.6
  due to previous cesarean delivery, complicating pregnancy or childbirth 654.2 ☑
    affecting fetus or newborn 763.89
  duodenal (bulb) (cap) 537.3
  hypertrophic 701.4
  keloid 701.4
  labia 624.4
  lung (base) 518.89
  macula 363.32
    disseminated 363.35
    peripheral 363.34
  muscle 728.89
  myocardium, myocardial 412
  painful 709.2
  papillary muscle 429.81
  posterior pole NEC 363.33
    macular — see Scar, macula
  postnecrotic (hepatic) (liver) 571.9
  psychic V15.49
  retina (see also Scar, chorioretinal) 363.30
  trachea 478.9
  uterus 621.8
    in pregnancy or childbirth NEC 654.9 ☑
      affecting fetus or newborn 763.89
      due to previous cesarean delivery 654.2 ☑
  vulva 624.4
Schamberg's disease, dermatitis, or dermatosis (progressive pigmentary dermatosis) 709.09
Schatzki's ring (esophagus) (lower) (congenital) 750.3
  acquired 530.3
Schaufenster krankheit 413.9
Schaumann's
  benign lymphogranulomatosis 135
  disease (sarcoidosis) 135
  syndrome (sarcoidosis) 135
Scheie's syndrome (mucopolysaccharidosis IS) 277.5
Schenck's disease (sporotrichosis) 117.1
Scheuermann's disease or osteochondrosis 732.0
Scheuthauer-Marie-Sainton syndrome (cleidocranialis dysostosis) 755.59
Schilder (-Flatau) disease 341.1
Schilling-type monocytic leukemia (M9890/3) 206.9 ☑
Schimmelbusch's disease, cystic mastitis, or hyperplasia 610.1
Schirmer's syndrome (encephalocutaneous angiomatosis) 759.6
Schistocelia 756.79

Schistoglossia 750.13
Schistosoma infestation — see Infestation, Schistosoma
Schistosomiasis 120.9
  Asiatic 120.2
  bladder 120.0
  chestermani 120.8
  colon 120.1
  cutaneous 120.3
  due to
    S. hematobium 120.0
    S. japonicum 120.2
    S. mansoni 120.1
    S. mattheii 120.8
  eastern 120.2
  genitourinary tract 120.0
  intestinal 120.1
  lung 120.2
  Manson's (intestinal) 120.1
  Oriental 120.2
  pulmonary 120.2
  specified type NEC 120.8
  vesical 120.0
Schizencephaly 742.4
Schizo-affective psychosis — see also Schizophrenia 295.7 ☑
Schizodontia 520.2
Schizoid personality 301.20
  introverted 301.21
  schizotypal 301.22
Schizophrenia, schizophrenic (reaction) 295.9 ☑

> Note — Use the following fifth-digit subclassification with category 295:
>
> 0   unspecified
>
> 1   subchronic
>
> 2   chronic
>
> 3   subchronic with acute exacerbation
>
> 4   chronic with acute exacerbation
>
> 5   in remission

  acute (attack) NEC 295.8 ☑
    episode 295.4 ☑
  atypical form 295.8 ☑
  borderline 295.5 ☑
  catalepsy 295.2 ☑
  catatonic (type) (acute) (excited) (withdrawn) 295.2 ☑
  childhood (type) (see also Psychosis, childhood) 299.9 ☑
  chronic NEC 295.6 ☑
  coenesthesiopathic 295.8 ☑
  cyclic (type) 295.7 ☑
  disorganized (type) 295.1 ☑
  flexibilitas cerea 295.2 ☑
  hebephrenic (type) (acute) 295.1 ☑
  incipient 295.5 ☑
  latent 295.5 ☑
  paranoid (type) (acute) 295.3 ☑
  paraphrenic (acute) 295.3 ☑
  prepsychotic 295.5 ☑
  primary (acute) 295.0 ☑
  prodromal 295.5 ☑
  pseudoneurotic 295.5 ☑
  pseudopsychopathic 295.5 ☑
  reaction 295.9 ☑
  residual type (state) 295.6 ☑
  restzustand 295.6 ☑
  schizo-affective (type) (depressed) (excited) 295.7 ☑
  schizophreniform type 295.4 ☑
  simple (type) (acute) 295.0 ☑
  simplex (acute) 295.0 ☑
  specified type NEC 295.8 ☑
  syndrome of childhood NEC (see also Psychosis, childhood) 299.9 ☑
  undifferentiated type 295.9 ☑
    acute 295.8 ☑
    chronic 295.6 ☑
Schizothymia 301.20
  introverted 301.21

Schizothymia — continued
  schizotypal 301.22
Schlafkrankheit 086.5
Schlatter-Osgood disease (osteochondrosis, tibial tubercle) 732.4
Schlatter's tibia (osteochondrosis) 732.4
Schloffer's tumor — see also Peritonitis 567.29
Schmidt's syndrome
  sphallo-pharyngo-laryngeal hemiplegia 352.6
  thyroid-adrenocortical insufficiency 258.1
  vagoaccessory 352.6
Schmincke
  carcinoma (M8082/3) — see Neoplasm, nasopharynx, malignant
  tumor (M8082/3) — see Neoplasm, nasopharynx, malignant
Schmitz (-Stutzer) dysentery 004.0
Schmorl's disease or nodes 722.30
  lumbar, lumbosacral 722.32
  specified region NEC 722.39
  thoracic, thoracolumbar 722.31
Schneiderian
  carcinoma (M8121/3)
    specified site — see Neoplasm, by site, malignant
    unspecified site 160.0
  papilloma (M8121/0)
    specified site — see Neoplasm, by site, benign
    unspecified site 212.0
Schneider's syndrome 047.9
Schnitzler syndrome 273.1
Schoffer's tumor — see also Peritonitis 567.29
Scholte's syndrome (malignant carcinoid) 259.2
Scholz's disease 330.0
Scholz (-Bielschowsky-Henneberg) syndrome 330.0
Schönlein (-Henoch) disease (primary) (purpura) (rheumatic) 287.0
School examination V70.3
  following surgery V67.09
Schottmüller's disease — see also Fever, paratyphoid 002.9
Schroeder's syndrome (endocrine-hypertensive) 255.3
Schüller-Christian disease or syndrome (chronic histiocytosis X) 277.89
Schultz's disease or syndrome (agranulocytosis) 288.09
Schultze's acroparesthesia, simple 443.89
Schwalbe-Ziehen-Oppenheimer disease 333.6
Schwannoma (M9560/0) — see also Neoplasm, connective tissue, benign
  malignant (M9560/3) — see Neoplasm, connective tissue, malignant
Schwannomatosis 237.73
Schwartz-Bartter syndrome (inappropriate secretion of antidiuretic hormone) 253.6
Schwartz (-Jampel) syndrome 359.23
Schweninger-Buzzi disease (macular atrophy) 701.3
Sciatic — see condition
Sciatica (infectional) 724.3
  due to
    displacement of intervertebral disc 722.10
    herniation, nucleus pulposus 722.10
  wallet 724.3
Scimitar syndrome (anomalous venous drainage, right lung to inferior vena cava) 747.49
Sclera — see condition
Sclerectasia 379.11
Scleredema
  adultorum 710.1
  Buschke's 710.1
  newborn 778.1
Sclerema
  adiposum (newborn) 778.1
  adultorum 710.1
  edematosum (newborn) 778.1
  neonatorum 778.1
  newborn 778.1

Scleriasis — see Scleroderma
Scleritis 379.00
  with corneal involvement 379.05
  anterior (annular) (localized) 379.03
  brawny 379.06
  granulomatous 379.09
  posterior 379.07
  specified NEC 379.09
  suppurative 379.09
  syphilitic 095.0
  tuberculous (nodular) (see also Tuberculosis) 017.3 ☑ [379.09]
Sclerochoroiditis — see also Scleritis 379.00
Scleroconjunctivitis — see also Scleritis 379.00
Sclerocystic ovary (syndrome) 256.4
Sclerodactylia 701.0
Scleroderma, sclerodermia (acrosclerotic) (diffuse) (generalized) (progressive) (pulmonary) 710.1
  circumscribed 701.0
  linear 701.0
  localized (linear) 701.0
  newborn 778.1
Sclerokeratitis 379.05
  meaning sclerosing keratitis 370.54
  tuberculous (see also Tuberculosis) 017.3 ☑ [379.09]
Scleromalacia
  multiple 731.0
  perforans 379.04
Scleroma, trachea 040.1
Scleromyxedema 701.8
Scleroperikeratitis 379.05
Sclerose en plaques 340
Sclerosis, sclerotic
  adrenal (gland) 255.8
  Alzheimer's 331.0
    with dementia — see Alzheimer's, dementia
  amyotrophic (lateral) 335.20
  annularis fibrosi
    aortic 424.1
    mitral 424.0
  aorta, aortic 440.0
    valve (see also Endocarditis, aortic) 424.1
  artery, arterial, arteriolar, arteriovascular — see Arteriosclerosis
  ascending multiple 340
  Balo's (concentric) 341.1
  basilar — see Sclerosis, brain
  bone (localized) NEC 733.99
  brain (general) (lobular) 348.89
    Alzheimer's — see Alzheimer's, dementia
    artery, arterial 437.0
    atrophic lobar 331.0
      with dementia
        with behavioral disturbance 331.0 [294.11]
        without behavioral disturbance 331.0 [294.10]
    diffuse 341.1
      familial (chronic) (infantile) 330.0
      infantile (chronic) (familial) 330.0
      Pelizaeus-Merzbacher type 330.0
    disseminated 340
    hereditary 334.2
    hippocampal 348.81
    infantile (degenerative) (diffuse) 330.0
    insular 340
    Krabbe's 330.0
    mesial temporal 348.81
    miliary 340
    multiple 340
    Pelizaeus-Merzbacher 330.0
    progressive familial 330.0
    senile 437.0
    temporal 348.81
      mesial 348.81
    tuberous 759.5
  bulbar, progressive 340
  bundle of His 426.50
    left 426.3
    right 426.4
  cardiac — see Arteriosclerosis, coronary

Sclerosis, sclerotic — continued
cardiorenal (see also Hypertension, cardiorenal) 404.90
cardiovascular (see also Disease, cardiovascular) 429.2
    renal (see also Hypertension, cardiorenal) 404.90
centrolobar, familial 330.0
cerebellar — see Sclerosis, brain
cerebral — see Sclerosis, brain
cerebrospinal 340
    disseminated 340
    multiple 340
cerebrovascular 437.0
choroid 363.40
    diffuse 363.56
combined (spinal cord) (see also Degeneration, combined)
    multiple 340
concentric, Baló's 341.1
cornea 370.54
coronary (artery) — see Arteriosclerosis, coronary
corpus cavernosum
    female 624.8
    male 607.89
Dewitzky's
    aortic 424.1
    mitral 424.0
diffuse NEC 341.1
disease, heart — see Arteriosclerosis, coronary
disseminated 340
dorsal 340
dorsolateral (spinal cord) — see Degeneration, combined
endometrium 621.8
extrapyramidal 333.90
eye, nuclear (senile) 366.16
Friedreich's (spinal cord) 334.0
funicular (spermatic cord) 608.89
gastritis 535.4 ☑
general (vascular) — see Arteriosclerosis
gland (lymphatic) 457.8
hepatic 571.9
hereditary
    cerebellar 334.2
    spinal 334.0
hippocampal 348.81
idiopathic cortical (Garré's) (see also Osteomyelitis) 730.1 ☑
ilium, piriform 733.5
insular 340
    pancreas 251.8
Islands of Langerhans 251.8
kidney — see Sclerosis, renal
larynx 478.79
lateral 335.24
    amyotrophic 335.20
    descending 335.24
    primary 335.24
    spinal 335.24
liver 571.9
lobar, atrophic (of brain) 331.0
    with dementia
        with behavioral disturbance 331.0 [294.11]
        without behavioral disturbance 331.0 [294.10]
lung (see also Fibrosis, lung) 515
mastoid 383.1
mesial temporal 348.81
mitral — see Endocarditis, mitral
Mönckeberg's (medial) (see also Arteriosclerosis, extremities) 440.20
multiple (brain stem) (cerebral) (generalized) (spinal cord) 340
myocardium, myocardial — see Arteriosclerosis, coronary
nuclear (senile), eye 366.16
ovary 620.8
pancreas 577.8
penis 607.89
peripheral arteries (see also Arteriosclerosis, extremities) 440.20
plaques 340

Sclerosis, sclerotic — continued
pluriglandular 258.8
polyglandular 258.8
posterior (spinal cord) (syphilitic) 094.0
posterolateral (spinal cord) — see Degeneration, combined
prepuce 607.89
primary lateral 335.24
progressive systemic 710.1
pulmonary (see also Fibrosis, lung) 515
    artery 416.0
    valve (heart) (see also Endocarditis, pulmonary) 424.3
renal 587
    with
        cystine storage disease 270.0
        hypertension (see also Hypertension, kidney) 403.90
        hypertensive heart disease (conditions classifiable to 402) (see also Hypertension, cardiorenal) 404.90
        arteriolar (hyaline) (see also Hypertension, kidney) 403.90
        hyperplastic (see also Hypertension, kidney) 403.90
retina (senile) (vascular) 362.17
rheumatic
    aortic valve 395.9
    mitral valve 394.9
Schilder's 341.1
senile — see Arteriosclerosis
spinal (cord) (general) (progressive) (transverse) 336.8
    ascending 357.0
    combined (see also Degeneration, combined)
        multiple 340
        syphilitic 094.89
    disseminated 340
    dorsolateral — see Degeneration, combined
    hereditary (Friedreich's) (mixed form) 334.0
    lateral (amyotrophic) 335.24
    multiple 340
    posterior (syphilitic) 094.0
stomach 537.89
subendocardial, congenital 425.3
systemic (progressive) 710.1
    with lung involvement 710.1 [517.2]
temporal 348.81
    mesial 348.81
tricuspid (heart) (valve) — see Endocarditis, tricuspid
tuberous (brain) 759.5
tympanic membrane (see also Tympanosclerosis) 385.00
valve, valvular (heart) — see Endocarditis
vascular — see Arteriosclerosis
vein 459.89
Sclerotenonitis 379.07
Sclerotitis — see also Scleritis 379.00
    syphilitic 095.0
    tuberculous (see also Tuberculosis) 017.3 ☑ [379.09]
Scoliosis (acquired) (postural) 737.30
    congenital 754.2
    due to or associated with
        Charcôt-Marie-Tooth disease 356.1 [737.43]
        mucopolysaccharidosis 277.5 [737.43]
        neurofibromatosis 237.71 [737.43]
        osteitis
            deformans 731.0 [737.43]
            fibrosa cystica 252.01 [737.43]
        osteoporosis (see also Osteoporosis) 733.00 [737.43]
        poliomyelitis 138 [737.43]
        radiation 737.33
        tuberculosis (see also Tuberculosis) 015.0 ☑ [737.43]
    idiopathic 737.30
        infantile
            progressive 737.32
            resolving 737.31

Scoliosis — continued
    paralytic 737.39
    rachitic 268.1
    sciatic 724.3
    specified NEC 737.39
    thoracogenic 737.34
    tuberculous (see also Tuberculosis) 015.0 ☑ [737.43]
Scoliotic pelvis 738.6
    with disproportion (fetopelvic) 653.0 ☑
        affecting fetus or newborn 763.1
        causing obstructed labor 660.1 ☑
            affecting fetus or newborn 763.1
Scorbutus, scorbutic 267
    anemia 281.8
Scotoma (ring) 368.44
    arcuate 368.43
    Bjerrum 368.43
    blind spot area 368.42
    central 368.41
    centrocecal 368.41
    paracecal 368.42
    paracentral 368.41
    scintillating 368.12
    Seidel 368.43
Scratch — see Injury, superficial, by site
Scratchy throat 784.99
Screening (for) V82.9
    alcoholism V79.1
    anemia, deficiency NEC V78.1
        iron V78.0
    anomaly, congenital V82.89
    antenatal, of mother V28.9
        alphafetoprotein levels, raised V28.1
        based on amniocentesis V28.2
            chromosomal anomalies V28.0
            raised alphafetoprotein levels V28.1
        fetal growth retardation using ultrasonics V28.4
        ultrasonics V28.4
        genomic V28.89
        isoimmunization V28.5
        malformations using ultrasonics V28.3
        proteomic V28.89
        raised alphafetoprotein levels V28.1
        risk
            pre-term labor V28.82
        specified condition NEC V28.89
        Streptococcus B V28.6
    arterial hypertension V81.1
    arthropod-borne viral disease NEC V73.5
    asymptomatic bacteriuria V81.5
    bacterial
        and spirochetal sexually transmitted diseases V74.5
        conjunctivitis V74.4
        disease V74.9
            sexually transmitted V74.5
            specified condition NEC V74.8
    bacteriuria, asymptomatic V81.5
    blood disorder NEC V78.9
        specified type NEC V78.8
    bronchitis, chronic V81.3
    brucellosis V74.8
    cancer — see Screening, malignant neoplasm
    cardiovascular disease NEC V81.2
    cataract V80.2
    Chagas' disease V75.3
    chemical poisoning V82.5
    cholera V74.0
    cholesterol level V77.91
    chromosomal
        anomalies
            by amniocentesis, antenatal V28.0
            maternal postnatal V82.4
        athletes V70.3
    colonoscopy V76.51
    condition
        cardiovascular NEC V81.2
        eye NEC V80.2
        genitourinary NEC V81.6
        neurological NEC V80.09
        respiratory NEC V81.4
        skin V82.0
        specified NEC V82.89

Screening — continued
    congenital
        anomaly V82.89
            eye V80.2
        dislocation of hip V82.3
        eye condition or disease V80.2
    conjunctivitis, bacterial V74.4
    contamination NEC (see also Poisoning) V82.5
    coronary artery disease V81.0
    cystic fibrosis V77.6
    deficiency anemia NEC V78.1
        iron V78.0
    dengue fever V73.5
    depression V79.0
    developmental handicap V79.9
        in early childhood V79.3
        specified type NEC V79.8
    diabetes mellitus V77.1
    diphtheria V74.3
    disease or disorder V82.9
        bacterial V74.9
            specified NEC V74.8
        blood V78.9
            specified type NEC V78.8
        blood-forming organ V78.9
            specified type NEC V78.8
        cardiovascular NEC V81.2
            hypertensive V81.1
            ischemic V81.0
        Chagas' V75.3
        chlamydial V73.98
            specified NEC V73.88
        ear NEC V80.3
        endocrine NEC V77.99
        eye NEC V80.2
        genitourinary NEC V81.6
        heart NEC V81.2
            hypertensive V81.1
            ischemic V81.0
        HPV (human papillomavirus) V73.81
        human papillomavirus V73.81
        immunity NEC V77.99
        infectious NEC V75.9
        lipoid NEC V77.91
        mental V79.9
            specified type NEC V79.8
        metabolic NEC V77.99
            inborn NEC V77.7
        neurological NEC V80.09
        nutritional NEC V77.99
        rheumatic NEC V82.2
        rickettsial V75.0
        sexually transmitted V74.5
            bacterial V74.5
            spirochetal V74.5
        sickle-cell V78.2
            trait V78.2
        specified type NEC V82.89
        thyroid V77.0
        vascular NEC V81.2
            ischemic V81.0
        venereal V74.5
        viral V73.99
            arthropod-borne NEC V73.5
            specified type NEC V73.89
    dislocation of hip, congenital V82.3
    drugs in athletes V70.3
    elevated titer V82.9
    emphysema (chronic) V81.3
    encephalitis, viral (mosquito or tick borne) V73.5
    endocrine disorder NEC V77.99
    eye disorder NEC V80.2
        congenital V80.2
    fever
        dengue V73.5
        hemorrhagic V73.5
        yellow V73.4
    filariasis V75.6
    galactosemia V77.4
    genetic V82.79
        disease carrier status V82.71
    genitourinary condition NEC V81.6
    glaucoma V80.1
    gonorrhea V74.5

☑ Additional Digit Required — Refer to the Tabular List for Digit Selection

◹ Subterms under main terms may continue to next column or page

2015 ICD-9-CM

▶◀ Revised Text

● New Line

▲ Revised Code

Volume 2 — 255

Screening — continued

gout V77.5
Hansen's disease V74.2
heart disease NEC V81.2
   hypertensive V81.1
   ischemic V81.0
heavy metal poisoning V82.5
helminthiasis, intestinal V75.7
hematopoietic malignancy V76.89
hemoglobinopathies NEC V78.3
hemorrhagic fever V73.5
Hodgkin's disease V76.89
hormones in athletes V70.3
HPV (human papillomavirus) V73.81
human papillomavirus (HPV) V73.81
hypercholesterolemia V77.91
hyperlipdemia V77.91
hypertension V81.1
immunity disorder NEC V77.99
inborn errors of metabolism NEC V77.7
infection
   bacterial V74.9
      specified type NEC V74.8
   mycotic V75.4
   parasitic NEC V75.8
infectious disease V75.9
   specified type NEC V75.8
ingestion of radioactive substance V82.5
intellectual disabilities V79.2
intestinal helminthiasis V75.7
iron deficiency anemia V78.0
ischemic heart disease V81.0
lead poisoning V82.5
leishmaniasis V75.2
leprosy V74.2
leptospirosis V74.8
leukemia V76.89
lipoid disorder NEC V77.91
lymphoma V76.89
malaria V75.1
malignant neoplasm (of) V76.9
   bladder V76.3
   blood V76.89
   breast V76.10
      mammogram NEC V76.12
         for high-risk patient V76.11
      specified type NEC V76.19
   cervix V76.2
   colon V76.51
   colorectal V76.51
   hematopoietic system V76.89
   intestine V76.50
      colon V76.51
      small V76.52
   lung V76.0
   lymph (glands) V76.89
   nervous system V76.81
   oral cavity V76.42
   other specified neoplasm NEC V76.89
   ovary V76.46
   prostate V76.44
   rectum V76.41
   respiratory organs V76.0
   skin V76.43
   specified sites NEC V76.49
   testis V76.45
   vagina V76.47
      following hysterectomy for malignant condition V67.01
malnutrition V77.2
mammogram NEC V76.12
   for high-risk patient V76.11
maternal postnatal chromosomal anomalies V82.4
measles V73.2
mental
   disorder V79.9
      specified type NEC V79.8
   retardation — see Screening, intellectual disabilities
metabolic disorder NEC V77.99
metabolic errors, inborn V77.7
mucoviscidosis V77.6
multiphasic V82.6
mycosis V75.4
mycotic infection V75.4

Screening — continued

nephropathy V81.5
neurological condition NEC V80.09
nutritional disorder V77.99
obesity V77.8
osteoporosis V82.81
parasitic infection NEC V75.8
phenylketonuria V77.3
plague V74.8
poisoning
   chemical NEC V82.5
   contaminated water supply V82.5
      heavy metal V82.5
poliomyelitis V73.0
postnatal chromosomal anomalies, maternal V82.4
prenatal — see Screening, antenatal
pulmonary tuberculosis V74.1
radiation exposure V82.5
renal disease V81.5
respiratory condition NEC V81.4
rheumatic disorder NEC V82.2
rheumatoid arthritis V82.1
rickettsial disease V75.0
rubella V73.3
schistosomiasis V75.5
senile macular lesions of eye V80.2
sexually transmitted diseases V74.5
   bacterial V74.5
   spirochetal V74.5
sickle-cell anemia, disease, or trait V78.2
skin condition V82.0
sleeping sickness V75.3
smallpox V73.1
special V82.9
   specified condition NEC V82.89
specified type NEC V82.89
spirochetal disease V74.5
   sexually transmitted V74.5
   specified type NEC V74.8
stimulants in athletes V70.3
syphilis V74.5
tetanus V74.8
thyroid disorder V77.0
trachoma V73.6
traumatic brain injury V80.01
trypanosomiasis V75.3
tuberculosis, pulmonary V74.1
venereal disease V74.5
viral encephalitis
   mosquito-borne V73.5
   tick-borne V73.5
whooping cough V74.8
worms, intestinal V75.7
yaws V74.6
yellow fever V73.4
Scrofula — see also Tuberculosis 017.2 ☑
Scrofulide (primary) — see also Tuberculosis 017.0 ☑
Scrofuloderma, scrofulodermia (any site) (primary) — see also Tuberculosis 017.0 ☑
Scrofulosis (universal) — see also Tuberculosis 017.2 ☑
Scrofulosis lichen (primary) — see also Tuberculosis 017.0 ☑
Scrofulous — see condition
Scrotal tongue 529.5
   congenital 750.13
Scrotum — see condition
Scurvy (gum) (infantile) (rickets) (scorbutic) 267
Sea-blue histiocyte syndrome 272.7
Seabright-Bantam syndrome (pseudohypoparathyroidism) 275.49
Sealpox 059.12
Seasickness 994.6
Seatworm 127.4
Sebaceous
   cyst (see also Cyst, sebaceous) 706.2
   gland disease NEC 706.9
Sebocystomatosis 706.2
Seborrhea, seborrheic 706.3
   adiposa 706.3
   capitis 690.11
   congestiva 695.4
   corporis 706.3

Seborrhea, seborrheic — continued

dermatitis 690.10
   infantile 690.12
diathesis in infants 695.89
eczema 690.18
   infantile 690.12
keratosis 702.19
   inflamed 702.11
nigricans 705.89
sicca 690.18
wart 702.19
   inflamed 702.11
Seckel's syndrome 759.89
Seclusion pupil 364.74
Seclusiveness, child 313.22
Secondary — see also condition
   neoplasm — see Neoplasm, by site, malignant, secondary
Secretan's disease or syndrome (posttraumatic edema) 782.3
Secretion
   antidiuretic hormone, inappropriate (syndrome) 253.6
   catecholamine, by pheochromocytoma 255.6
   hormone
      antidiuretic, inappropriate (syndrome) 253.6
      by
         carcinoid tumor 259.2
         pheochromocytoma 255.6
      ectopic NEC 259.3
   urinary
      excessive 788.42
      suppression 788.5
Section
   cesarean
      affecting fetus or newborn 763.4
      post mortem, affecting fetus or newborn 761.6
      previous, in pregnancy or childbirth 654.2 ☑
         affecting fetus or newborn 763.89
   nerve, traumatic — see Injury, nerve, by site
Seeligmann's syndrome (ichthyosis congenita) 757.1
Segmentation, incomplete (congenital) — see also Fusion
   bone NEC 756.9
   lumbosacral (joint) 756.15
   vertebra 756.15
      lumbosacral 756.15
Seizure(s) 780.39
   akinetic (idiopathic) (see also Epilepsy) 345.0 ☑
      psychomotor 345.4 ☑
   apoplexy, apoplectic (see also Disease, cerebrovascular, acute) 436
   atonic (see also Epilepsy) 345.0 ☑
   autonomic 300.11
   brain or cerebral (see also Disease, cerebrovascular, acute) 436
   convulsive (see also Convulsions) 780.39
   cortical (focal) (motor) (see also Epilepsy) 345.5 ☑
   disorder (see also Epilepsy) 345.9 ☑
   due to stroke 438.89
   epilepsy, epileptic (cryptogenic) (see also Epilepsy) 345.9 ☑
   epileptiform, epileptoid 780.39
      focal (see also Epilepsy) 345.5 ☑
   febrile (simple) 780.31
      with status epilepticus 345.3
      atypical 780.32
      complex 780.32
      complicated 780.32
   heart — see Disease, heart
   hysterical 300.11
   Jacksonian (focal) (see also Epilepsy) 345.5 ☑
      motor type 345.5 ☑
      sensory type 345.5 ☑
   migraine triggered 346.0 ☑
   newborn 779.0
   paralysis (see also Disease, cerebrovascular, acute) 436

Seizure(s) — continued

posttraumatic 780.33
recurrent 345.8 ☑
   epileptic — see Epilepsy
repetitive 780.39
   epileptic — see Epilepsy
salaam (see also Epilepsy) 345.6 ☑
uncinate (see also Epilepsy) 345.4 ☑
Self-mutilation 300.9
Semicoma 780.09
Semiconsciousness 780.09
Seminal
   vesicle — see condition
   vesiculitis (see also Vesiculitis) 608.0
Seminoma (M9061/3)
   anaplastic type (M9062/3)
      specified site — see Neoplasm, by site, malignant
      unspecified site 186.9
   specified site — see Neoplasm, by site, malignant
   spermatocytic (M9063/3)
      specified site — see Neoplasm, by site, malignant
      unspecified site 186.9
   unspecified site 186.9
Semliki Forest encephalitis 062.8
Senear-Usher disease or syndrome (pemphigus erythematosus) 694.4
Senecio jacobae dermatitis 692.6
Senectus 797
Senescence 797
Senile — see also condition 797
   cervix (atrophic) 622.8
   degenerative atrophy, skin 701.3
   endometrium (atrophic) 621.8
   fallopian tube (atrophic) 620.3
   heart (failure) 797
   lung 492.8
   ovary (atrophic) 620.3
   syndrome 259.8
   vagina, vaginitis (atrophic) 627.3
   wart 702.0
Senility 797
   with
      acute confusional state 290.3
      delirium 290.3
      mental changes 290.9
      psychosis NEC (see also Psychosis, senile) 290.20
   premature (syndrome) 259.8
Sensation
   burning (see also Disturbance, sensation) 782.0
      tongue 529.6
   choking 784.99
   loss of (see also Disturbance, sensation) 782.0
   prickling (see also Disturbance, sensation) 782.0
   tingling (see also Disturbance, sensation) 782.0
Sense loss (touch) — see also Disturbance, sensation 782.0
   smell 781.1
   taste 781.1
Sensibility disturbance NEC (cortical) (deep) (vibratory) — see also Disturbance, sensation 782.0
Sensitive dentine 521.89
Sensitiver Beziehungswahn 297.8
Sensitivity, sensitization — see also Allergy
   autoerythrocyte 287.2
   carotid sinus 337.01
   child (excessive) 313.21
   cold, autoimmune 283.0
   methemoglobin 289.7
   suxamethonium 289.89
   tuberculin, without clinical or radiological symptoms 795.51
Sensory
   extinction 781.8
   neglect 781.8
Separation
   acromioclavicular — see Dislocation, acromioclavicular

☑ Additional Digit Required — Refer to the Tabular List for Digit Selection   ⬇ Subterms under main terms may continue to next column or page

☑ **Additional Digit Required** — Refer to the Tabular List for Digit Selection

〽 **Subterms under main terms may continue to next column or page**

Shedding
  nail 703.8
  teeth, premature, primary (deciduous) 520.6
Sheehan's disease or syndrome (postpartum pituitary necrosis) 253.2
Shelf, rectal 569.49
Shell
  shock (current) (*see also* Reaction, stress, acute) 308.9
    lasting state 300.16
  teeth 520.5
Shield kidney 753.3
Shifting
  pacemaker 427.89
  sleep-work schedule (affecting sleep) 327.36
Shift, mediastinal 793.2
Shiga's
  bacillus 004.0
  dysentery 004.0
Shigella (dysentery) — *see also* Dysentery, bacillary 004.9
  carrier (suspected) of V02.3
Shigellosis — *see also* Dysentery, bacillary 004.9
Shingles — *see also* Herpes, zoster 053.9
  eye NEC 053.29
Shin splints 844.9
Shipyard eye or disease 077.1
Shirodkar suture, in pregnancy 654.5 ☑
Shock 785.50
  with
    abortion — *see* Abortion, by type, with shock
    ectopic pregnancy (*see also* categories 633.0–633.9) 639.5
    molar pregnancy (*see also* categories 630–632) 639.5
  allergic — *see* Anaphylactic reaction or shock
  anaclitic 309.21
  anaphylactic — *see also* Anaphylactic reaction or shock
    due to administration of blood and blood products 999.41
  anaphylactoid — *see* Anaphylactic reaction or shock
  anesthetic
    correct substance properly administered 995.4
    overdose or wrong substance given 968.4
      specified anesthetic — *see* Table of Drugs and Chemicals
  birth, fetus or newborn NEC 779.89
  cardiogenic 785.51
  chemical substance — *see* Table of Drugs and Chemicals
  circulatory 785.59
  complicating
    abortion — *see* Abortion, by type, with shock
    ectopic pregnancy (*see also* categories 633.0–633.9) 639.5
    labor and delivery 669.1 ☑
    molar pregnancy (*see also* categories 630–632) 639.5
  culture 309.29
  due to
    drug 995.0
      correct substance properly administered 995.0
      overdose or wrong substance given or taken 977.9
      specified drug — *see* Table of Drugs and Chemicals
    food — *see* Anaphylactic shock, due to, food
  during labor and delivery 669.1 ☑
  electric 994.8
    from electroshock gun (taser) 994.8
  endotoxic 785.52
    due to surgical procedure 998.02
    postoperative 998.02
  following
    abortion 639.5
    ectopic or molar pregnancy 639.5

Shock — *continued*
  following — *continued*
    injury (immediate) (delayed) 958.4
    labor and delivery 669.1 ☑
  gram-negative 785.52
    postoperative 998.02
  hematogenic 785.59
  hemorrhagic
    due to
      disease 785.59
      surgery (intraoperative) (postoperative) 998.09
      trauma 958.4
  hypovolemic NEC 785.59
    surgical 998.09
    traumatic 958.4
  insulin 251.0
    therapeutic misadventure 962.3
  kidney 584.5
    traumatic (following crushing) 958.5
  lightning 994.0
  lung 518.82
    related to trauma and surgery 518.52
  nervous (*see also* Reaction, stress, acute) 308.9
  obstetric 669.1 ☑
    with
      abortion — *see* Abortion, by type, with shock
      ectopic pregnancy (*see also* categories 633.0–633.9) 639.5
      molar pregnancy (*see also* categories 630–632) 639.5
    following
      abortion 639.5
      ectopic or molar pregnancy 639.5
  paralysis, paralytic (*see also* Disease, cerebrovascular, acute) 436
    late effect — *see* Late effect(s) (of) cerebrovascular disease
  pleural (surgical) 998.09
    due to trauma 958.4
  postoperative 998.00
    with
      abortion — *see* Abortion, by type, with shock
      ectopic pregnancy (*see also* categories 633.0–633.9) 639.5
      molar pregnancy (*see also* categories 630–632) 639.5
    cardiogenic 998.01
    following
      abortion 639.5
      ectopic or molar pregnancy 639.5
    hypovolemic 998.09
    septic (endotoxic) (gram-negative) 998.02
    specified NEC 998.09
  psychic (*see also* Reaction, stress, acute) 308.9
    past history (of) V15.49
  psychogenic (*see also* Reaction, stress, acute) 308.9
  septic 785.52
    with
      abortion — *see* Abortion, by type, with shock
      ectopic pregnancy (*see also* categories 633.0–633.9) 639.5
      molar pregnancy (*see also* categories 630–632) 639.5
    due to
      surgical procedure 998.02
      transfusion NEC 999.89
        bone marrow 996.85
    following
      abortion 639.5
      ectopic or molar pregnancy 639.5
      surgical procedure 998.02
      transfusion NEC 999.89
        bone marrow 996.85
    postoperative 998.02
  spinal (*see also* Injury, spinal, by site)
    with spinal bone injury — *see* Fracture, vertebra, by site, with spinal cord injury

Shock — *continued*
  surgical 998.00
  therapeutic misadventure NEC (*see also* Complications) 998.89
  thyroxin 962.7
  toxic 040.82
  transfusion — *see* Complications, transfusion
  traumatic (immediate) (delayed) 958.4
Shoemakers' chest 738.3
Short, shortening, shortness
  Achilles tendon (acquired) 727.81
  arm 736.89
    congenital 755.20
  back 737.9
  bowel syndrome 579.3
  breath 786.05
  cervical, cervix 649.7 ☑
    gravid uterus 649.7 ☑
    non-gravid uterus 622.5
      acquired 622.5
      congenital 752.49
  chain acyl CoA dehydrogenase deficiency (SCAD) 277.85
  common bile duct, congenital 751.69
  cord (umbilical) 663.4 ☑
    affecting fetus or newborn 762.6
  cystic duct, congenital 751.69
  esophagus (congenital) 750.4
  femur (acquired) 736.81
    congenital 755.34
  frenulum linguae 750.0
  frenum, lingual 750.0
  hamstrings 727.81
  hip (acquired) 736.39
    congenital 755.63
  leg (acquired) 736.81
    congenital 755.30
  metatarsus (congenital) 754.79
    acquired 736.79
  organ or site, congenital NEC — *see* Distortion
  palate (congenital) 750.26
  P-R interval syndrome 426.81
  radius (acquired) 736.09
    congenital 755.26
  round ligament 629.89
  sleeper 307.49
  stature, constitutional (hereditary) (idiopathic) 783.43
  tendon 727.81
    Achilles (acquired) 727.81
      congenital 754.79
    congenital 756.89
  thigh (acquired) 736.81
    congenital 755.34
  tibialis anticus 727.81
  umbilical cord 663.4 ☑
    affecting fetus or newborn 762.6
  urethra 599.84
  uvula (congenital) 750.26
  vagina 623.8
Shortsightedness 367.1
Shoshin (acute fulminating beriberi) 265.0
Shoulder — *see* condition
Shovel-shaped incisors 520.2
Shower, thromboembolic — *see* Embolism
Shunt (status)
  aortocoronary bypass V45.81
  arterial-venous (dialysis) V45.11
  arteriovenous, pulmonary (acquired) 417.0
    congenital 747.39
    traumatic (complication) 901.40
  cerebral ventricle (communicating) in situ V45.2
  coronary artery bypass V45.81
  surgical, prosthetic, with complications — *see* Complications, shunt
  vascular NEC V45.89
Shutdown
  renal 586
    with
      abortion — *see* Abortion, by type, with renal failure
      ectopic pregnancy (*see also* categories 633.0–633.9) 639.3

Shutdown — *continued*
  renal — *continued*
    with — *continued*
      molar pregnancy (*see also* categories 630–632) 639.3
    complicating
      abortion 639.3
      ectopic or molar pregnancy 639.3
    following labor and delivery 669.3 ☑
Shwachman's syndrome 288.02
Shy-Drager syndrome (orthostatic hypotension with multisystem degeneration) 333.0
Sialadenitis (any gland) (chronic) (suppurative) 527.2
  epidemic — *see* Mumps
Sialadenosis, periodic 527.2
Sialaporia 527.7
Sialectasia 527.8
Sialitis 527.2
Sialoadenitis — *see also* Sialadenitis 527.2
Sialoangitis 527.2
Sialodochitis (fibrinosa) 527.2
Sialodocholithiasis 527.5
Sialolithiasis 527.5
Sialorrhea — *see also* Ptyalism 527.7
  periodic 527.2
Sialosis 527.8
  rheumatic 710.2
Siamese twin 759.4
  complicating pregnancy 678.1 ☑
Sicard's syndrome 352.6
Sicca syndrome (keratoconjunctivitis) 710.2
Sick 799.9
  cilia syndrome 759.89
  or handicapped person in family V61.49
Sickle-cell
  anemia (see also Disease, sickle-cell) 282.60
  disease (see also Disease, sickle-cell) 282.60
  hemoglobin
    C disease (without crisis) 282.63
      with
        crisis 282.64
          vaso-occlusive pain 282.64
    D disease (without crisis) 282.68
      with crisis 282.69
    E disease (without crisis) 282.68
      with crisis 282.69
    thalassemia (without crisis) 282.41
      with
        crisis 282.42
          vaso-occlusive pain 282.42
  trait 282.5
Sicklemia — *see also* Disease, sickle-cell 282.60
  trait 282.5
Sickness
  air (travel) 994.6
  airplane 994.6
  alpine 993.2
  altitude 993.2
  Andes 993.2
  aviators' 993.2
  balloon 993.2
  car 994.6
  compressed air 993.3
  decompression 993.3
  green 280.9
  harvest 100.89
  milk 988.8
  morning 643.0 ☑
  motion 994.6
  mountain 993.2
    acute 289.0
  protein (*see also* Complications, vaccination) 999.59
  radiation NEC 990
  roundabout (motion) 994.6
  sea 994.6
  serum NEC 999.59
  sleeping (African) 086.5
    by Trypanosoma 086.5
      gambiense 086.3
      rhodesiense 086.4
    Gambian 086.3
    late effect 139.8
    Rhodesian 086.4

☑ **Additional Digit Required** — Refer to the Tabular List for Digit Selection   🖝 **Subterms under main terms may continue to next column or page**

Sickness — *continued*
sweating 078.2
swing (motion) 994.6
train (railway) (travel) 994.6
travel (any vehicle) 994.6
Sick sinus syndrome 427.81
Sideropenia — *see also* Anemia, iron deficiency 280.9
Siderosis (lung) (occupational) 503
central nervous system (CNS) 437.8
cornea 371.15
eye (bulbi) (vitreous) 360.23
lens 360.23
Siegal-Cattan-Mamou disease (periodic) 277.31
Siemens' syndrome
ectodermal dysplasia 757.31
keratosis follicularis spinulosa (decalvans) 757.39
Sighing respiration 786.7
Sigmoid
flexure — *see* condition
kidney 753.3
Sigmoiditis — *see* Enteritis
Silfverskiöld's syndrome 756.50
Silicosis, silicotic (complicated) (occupational) (simple) 502
fibrosis, lung (confluent) (massive) (occupational) 502
non-nodular 503
pulmonum 502
Silicotuberculosis — *see also* Tuberculosis 011.4 ☑
Silo fillers' disease 506.9
Silver's syndrome (congenital hemihypertrophy and short stature) 759.89
Silver wire arteries, retina 362.13
Silvestroni-Bianco syndrome (thalassemia minima) 282.49
Simian crease 757.2
Simmonds' cachexia or disease (pituitary cachexia) 253.2
Simons' disease or syndrome (progressive lipodystrophy) 272.6
Simple, simplex — *see* condition
Sinding-Larsen disease (juvenile osteopathia patellae) 732.4
Singapore hemorrhagic fever 065.4
Singers' node or nodule 478.5
Single
atrium 745.69
coronary artery 746.85
umbilical artery 747.5
ventricle 745.3
Singultus 786.8
epidemicus 078.89
Sinus — *see also* Fistula
abdominal 569.81
arrest 426.6
arrhythmia 427.89
bradycardia 427.89
chronic 427.81
branchial cleft (external) (internal) 744.41
coccygeal (infected) 685.1
with abscess 685.0
dental 522.7
dermal (congenital) 685.1
with abscess 685.0
draining — *see* Fistula
infected, skin NEC 686.9
marginal, ruptured or bleeding 641.2 ☑
affecting fetus or newborn 762.1
pause 426.6
pericranii 742.0
pilonidal (infected) (rectum) 685.1
with abscess 685.0
preauricular 744.46
rectovaginal 619.1
sacrococcygeal (dermoid) (infected) 685.1
with abscess 685.0
skin
infected NEC 686.9
noninfected — *see* Ulcer, skin
tachycardia 427.89
tarsi syndrome 726.79
testis 608.89

Sinus — *see also* Fistula — *continued*
tract (postinfectional) — *see* Fistula
urachus 753.7
Sinuses, Rokitansky-Aschoff — *see also* Disease, gallbladder 575.8
Sinusitis (accessory) (nasal) (hyperplastic) (nonpurulent) (purulent) (chronic) 473.9
with influenza, flu, or grippe (*see also* Influenza) 487.1
acute 461.9
ethmoidal 461.2
frontal 461.1
maxillary 461.0
specified type NEC 461.8
sphenoidal 461.3
allergic (*see also* Fever, hay) 477.9
antrum — *see* Sinusitis, maxillary
due to
fungus, any sinus 117.9
high altitude 993.1
ethmoidal 473.2
acute 461.2
frontal 473.1
acute 461.1
influenzal (*see also* Influenza) 487.1
maxillary 473.0
acute 461.0
specified site NEC 473.8
sphenoidal 473.3
acute 461.3
syphilitic, any sinus 095.8
tuberculous, any sinus (*see also* Tuberculosis) 012.8 ☑
Sinusitis-bronchiectasis-situs inversus (syndrome) (triad) 759.3
Sioloangitis 527.2
Sipple's syndrome (medullary thyroid carcinoma-pheochromocytoma) 258.02
Sirenomelia 759.89
Siriasis 992.0
Sirkari's disease 085.0
SIRS (systemic inflammatory response syndrome) 995.90
due to
infectious process 995.91
with acute organ dysfunction 995.92
non-infectious process 995.93
with acute organ dysfunction 995.94
Siti 104.0
Sitophobia 300.29
Situational
disturbance (transient) (*see also* Reaction, adjustment) 309.9
acute 308.3
maladjustment, acute (*see also* Reaction, adjustment) 309.9
reaction (*see also* Reaction, adjustment) 309.9
acute 308.3
Situation, psychiatric 300.9
Situs inversus or transversus 759.3
abdominalis 759.3
thoracis 759.3
Sixth disease
due to
human herpesvirus 6 058.11
human herpesvirus 7 058.12
Sjögren-Larsson syndrome (ichthyosis congenita) 757.1
Sjögren (-Gougerot) syndrome or disease (keratoconjunctivitis sicca) 710.2
with lung involvement 710.2 [517.8]
SJS-TEN (Stevens-Johnson syndrome - toxic epidermal necrolysis overlap syndrome) 695.14
Skeletal — *see* condition
Skene's gland — *see* condition
Skenitis — *see also* Urethritis 597.89
gonorrheal (acute) 098.0
chronic or duration of 2 months or over 098.2
Skerljevo 104.0
Skevas-Zerfus disease 989.5
Skin — *see also* condition
donor V59.1
hidebound 710.9

SLAP lesion (superior glenoid labrum) 840.7
Slate-dressers' lung 502
Slate-miners' lung 502
Sleep
deprivation V69.4
disorder 780.50
with apnea — *see* Apnea, sleep
child 307.40
movement, unspecified 780.58
nonorganic origin 307.40
specified type NEC 307.49
disturbance 780.50
with apnea — *see* Apnea, sleep
nonorganic origin 307.40
specified type NEC 307.49
drunkenness 307.47
movement disorder, unspecified 780.58
paroxysmal (*see also* Narcolepsy) 347.00
related movement disorder, unspecified 780.58
rhythm inversion 327.39
nonorganic origin 307.45
walking 307.46
hysterical 300.13
Sleeping sickness 086.5
late effect 139.8
Sleeplessness — *see also* Insomnia 780.52
menopausal 627.2
nonorganic origin 307.41
Slipped, slipping
epiphysis (postinfectional) 732.9
traumatic (old) 732.9
current — *see* Fracture, by site
upper femoral (nontraumatic) 732.2
intervertebral disc — *see* Displacement, intervertebral disc
ligature, umbilical 772.3
patella 717.89
rib 733.99
sacroiliac joint 724.6
tendon 727.9
ulnar nerve, nontraumatic 354.2
vertebra NEC (*see also* Spondylolisthesis) 756.12
Slocumb's syndrome 255.3
Sloughing (multiple) (skin) 686.9
abscess — *see* Abscess, by site
appendix 543.9
bladder 596.89
fascia 728.9
graft — *see* Complications, graft
phagedena (*see also* Gangrene) 785.4
reattached extremity (*see also* Complications, reattached extremity) 996.90
rectum 569.49
scrotum 608.89
tendon 727.9
transplanted organ (*see also* Rejection, transplant, organ, by site) 996.80
ulcer (*see also* Ulcer, skin) 707.9
Slow
feeding newborn 779.31
fetal, growth NEC 764.9 ☑
affecting management of pregnancy 656.5 ☑
Slowing
heart 427.89
urinary stream 788.62
Sluder's neuralgia or syndrome 337.09
Slurred, slurring, speech 784.59
Small-for-dates — *see also* Light-for-dates 764.0 ☑
affecting management of pregnancy 656.5 ☑
Smallpox 050.9
contact V01.3
exposure to V01.3
hemorrhagic (pustular) 050.0
malignant 050.0
modified 050.2
vaccination
complications — *see* Complications, vaccination
prophylactic (against) V04.1
Small, smallness
cardiac reserve — *see* Disease, heart

Small, smallness — *continued*
for dates
fetus or newborn 764.0 ☑
with malnutrition 764.1 ☑
affecting management of pregnancy 656.5 ☑
infant, term 764.0 ☑
with malnutrition 764.1 ☑
affecting management of pregnancy 656.5 ☑
introitus, vagina 623.3
kidney, unknown cause 589.9
bilateral 589.1
unilateral 589.0
ovary 620.8
pelvis
with disproportion (fetopelvic) 653.1 ☑
affecting fetus or newborn 763.1
causing obstructed labor 660.1 ☑
affecting fetus or newborn 763.1
placenta — *see* Placenta, insufficiency
uterus 621.8
white kidney 582.9
Smearing, fecal 787.62
Smith's fracture (separation) (closed) 813.41
open 813.51
Smith-Lemli Opitz syndrome (cerebrohepatorenal syndrome) 759.89
Smith-Magenis syndrome 758.33
Smith-Strang disease (oasthouse urine) 270.2
Smokers'
bronchitis 491.0
cough 491.0
syndrome (*see also* Abuse, drugs, nondependent) 305.1
throat 472.1
tongue 528.6
Smoking complicating pregnancy, childbirth, or the puerperium 649.0 ☑
Smothering spells 786.09
Snaggle teeth, tooth 524.39
Snapping
finger 727.05
hip 719.65
jaw 524.69
temporomandibular joint sounds on opening or closing 524.64
knee 717.9
thumb 727.05
Sneddon-Wilkinson disease or syndrome (subcorneal pustular dermatosis) 694.1
Sneezing 784.99
intractable 478.19
Sniffing
cocaine (*see also* Dependence) 304.2 ☑
ether (*see also* Dependence) 304.6 ☑
glue (airplane) (*see also* Dependence) 304.6 ☑
Snoring 786.09
Snow blindness 370.24
Snuffles (nonsyphilitic) 460
syphilitic (infant) 090.0
Social migrant V60.0
Sodoku 026.0
Soemmering's ring 366.51
Soft — *see also* condition
enlarged prostate 600.00
with
other lower urinary tract symptoms (LUTS) 600.01
urinary
obstruction 600.01
retention 600.01
nails 703.8
Softening
bone 268.2
brain (necrotic) (progressive) 348.89
arteriosclerotic 437.0
congenital 742.4
due to cerebrovascular accident 438.89
embolic (*see also* Embolism, brain) 434.1 ☑
hemorrhagic (*see also* Hemorrhage, brain) 431
occlusive 434.9 ☑

☑ Additional Digit Required — Refer to the Tabular List for Digit Selection   ▽ Subterms under main terms may continue to next column or page

Softening — *continued*
  brain — *continued*
    thrombotic (*see also* Thrombosis, brain)
      434.0 ☑
  cartilage 733.92
  cerebellar — *see* Softening, brain
  cerebral — *see* Softening, brain
  cerebrospinal — *see* Softening, brain
  myocardial, heart (*see also* Degeneration, myocardial) 429.1
  nails 703.8
  spinal cord 336.8
  stomach 537.89
Soiling, fecal 787.62
Solar fever 061
Soldier's
  heart 306.2
  patches 423.1
Solitary
  cyst
    bone 733.21
    kidney 593.2
  kidney (congenital) 753.0
  tubercle, brain (*see also* Tuberculosis, brain) 013.2 ☑
  ulcer, bladder 596.89
Somatization reaction, somatic reaction — *see also* Disorder, psychosomatic 306.9
  disorder 300.81
Somatoform disorder 300.82
  atypical 300.82
  severe 300.81
  undifferentiated 300.82
Somnambulism 307.46
  hysterical 300.13
Somnolence 780.09
  nonorganic origin 307.43
  periodic 349.89
Sonne dysentery 004.3
Soor 112.0
Sore
  Delhi 085.1
  desert (*see also* Ulcer, skin) 707.9
  eye 379.99
  Lahore 085.1
  mouth 528.9
    canker 528.2
    due to dentures 528.9
  muscle 729.1
  Naga (*see also* Ulcer, skin) 707.9
  oriental 085.1
  pressure (*see also* Ulcer, pressure) 707.00
    with gangrene (*see also* Ulcer, pressure) 707.00 [785.4]
  skin NEC 709.9
  soft 099.0
  throat 462
    with influenza, flu, or grippe (*see also* Influenza) 487.1
    acute 462
    chronic 472.1
    clergyman's 784.49
    coxsackie (virus) 074.0
    diphtheritic 032.0
    epidemic 034.0
    gangrenous 462
    herpetic 054.79
    influenzal (*see also* Influenza) 487.1
    malignant 462
    purulent 462
    putrid 462
    septic 034.0
    streptococcal (ulcerative) 034.0
    ulcerated 462
    viral NEC 462
      Coxsackie 074.0
  tropical (*see also* Ulcer, skin) 707.9
  veldt (*see also* Ulcer, skin) 707.9
Sotos' syndrome (cerebral gigantism) 253.0
Sounds
  friction, pleural 786.7
  succussion, chest 786.7
  temporomandibular joint
    on opening or closing 524.64
South African cardiomyopathy syndrome 425.2

South American
  blastomycosis 116.1
  trypanosomiasis — *see* Trypanosomiasis
Southeast Asian hemorrhagic fever 065.4
Spacing, teeth, abnormal 524.30
  excessive 524.32
Spade-like hand (congenital) 754.89
Spading nail 703.8
  congenital 757.5
Spanemia 285.9
Spanish collar 605
Sparganosis 123.5
Spasmodic — *see* condition
Spasmophilia — *see also* Tetany 781.7
Spasm, spastic, spasticity — *see also* condition 781.0
  accommodation 367.53
  ampulla of Vater (*see also* Disease, gallbladder) 576.8
  anus, ani (sphincter) (reflex) 564.6
    psychogenic 306.4
  artery NEC 443.9
    basilar 435.0
    carotid 435.8
    cerebral 435.9
      specified artery NEC 435.8
    retinal (*see also* Occlusion, retinal, artery) 362.30
    vertebral 435.1
    vertebrobasilar 435.3
  Bell's 351.0
  bladder (sphincter, external or internal) 596.89
  bowel 564.9
    psychogenic 306.4
  bronchus, bronchiole 519.11
  cardia 530.0
  cardiac — *see* Angina
  carpopedal (*see also* Tetany) 781.7
  cecum 564.9
    psychogenic 306.4
  cerebral (arteries) (vascular) 435.9
    specified artery NEC 435.8
  cerebrovascular 435.9
  cervix, complicating delivery 661.4 ☑
    affecting fetus or newborn 763.7
  ciliary body (of accommodation) 367.53
  colon 564.1
    psychogenic 306.4
  common duct (*see also* Disease, biliary) 576.8
  compulsive 307.22
  conjugate 378.82
  convergence 378.84
  coronary (artery) — *see* Angina
  diaphragm (reflex) 786.8
    psychogenic 306.1
  duodenum, duodenal (bulb) 564.89
  esophagus (diffuse) 530.5
    psychogenic 306.4
  facial 351.8
  fallopian tube 620.8
  gait 781.2
  gastrointestinal (tract) 536.8
    psychogenic 306.4
  glottis 478.75
    hysterical 300.11
    psychogenic 306.1
      specified as conversion reaction 300.11
    reflex through recurrent laryngeal nerve 478.75
  habit 307.20
    chronic 307.22
    transient (of childhood) 307.21
  heart — *see* Angina
  hourglass — *see* Contraction, hourglass
  hysterical 300.11
  infantile (*see also* Epilepsy) 345.6 ☑
  internal oblique, eye 378.51
  intestinal 564.9
    psychogenic 306.4
  larynx, laryngeal 478.75
    hysterical 300.11
    psychogenic 306.1

Spasm, spastic, spasticity — *see also* condition — *continued*
  larynx, laryngeal — *continued*
    psychogenic — *continued*
      specified as conversion reaction 300.11
  levator palpebrae superioris 333.81
  lightning (*see also* Epilepsy) 345.6 ☑
  mobile 781.0
  muscle 728.85
    back 724.8
    psychogenic 306.0
  nerve, trigeminal 350.1
  nervous 306.0
  nodding 307.3
    infantile (*see also* Epilepsy) 345.6 ☑
  occupational 300.89
  oculogyric 378.87
  ophthalmic artery 362.30
  orbicularis 781.0
  perineal 625.8
  peroneo-extensor (*see also* Flat, foot) 734
  pharynx (reflex) 478.29
    hysterical 300.11
    psychogenic 306.1
      specified as conversion reaction 300.11
  pregnant uterus, complicating delivery 661.4 ☑
  psychogenic 306.0
  pylorus 537.81
    adult hypertrophic 537.0
    congenital or infantile 750.5
    psychogenic 306.4
  rectum (sphincter) 564.6
    psychogenic 306.4
  retinal artery NEC (*see also* Occlusion, retina, artery) 362.30
  sacroiliac 724.6
  salaam (infantile) (*see also* Epilepsy) 345.6 ☑
  saltatory 781.0
  sigmoid 564.9
    psychogenic 306.4
  sphincter of Oddi (*see also* Disease, gallbladder) 576.5
  stomach 536.8
    neurotic 306.4
  throat 478.29
    hysterical 300.11
    psychogenic 306.1
      specified as conversion reaction 300.11
  tic 307.20
    chronic 307.22
    transient (of childhood) 307.21
  tongue 529.8
  torsion 333.6
  trigeminal nerve 350.1
    postherpetic 053.12
  ureter 593.89
  urethra (sphincter) 599.84
  uterus 625.8
    complicating labor 661.4 ☑
    affecting fetus or newborn 763.7
  vagina 625.1
    psychogenic 306.51
  vascular NEC 443.9
  vasomotor NEC 443.9
  vein NEC 459.89
  vesical (sphincter, external or internal) 596.89
  viscera 789.0 ☑
Spasmus nutans 307.3
Spastic — *see also* Spasm
  child 343.9
Spasticity — *see also* Spasm
  cerebral, child 343.9
Speakers' throat 784.49
Specific, specified — *see* condition
Speech
  defect, disorder, disturbance, impediment NEC 784.59
    psychogenic 307.9
  (language) therapy V57.3
Spells 780.39

Spells — *continued*
  breath-holding 786.9
Spencer's disease (epidemic vomiting) 078.82
Spens' syndrome (syncope with heart block) 426.9
Spermatic cord — *see* condition
Spermatocele 608.1
  congenital 752.89
Spermatocystitis 608.4
Spermatocytoma (M9063/3)
  specified site — *see* Neoplasm, by site, malignant
  unspecified site 186.9
Spermatorrhea 608.89
Sperm counts
  fertility testing V26.21
  following sterilization reversal V26.22
  postvasectomy V25.8
Sphacelus — *see also* Gangrene 785.4
Sphenoidal — *see* condition
Sphenoiditis (chronic) — *see also* Sinusitis, sphenoidal 473.3
Sphenopalatine ganglion neuralgia 337.09
Sphericity, increased, lens 743.36
Spherocytosis (congenital) (familial) (hereditary) 282.0
  hemoglobin disease 282.7
  sickle-cell (disease) 282.60
Spherophakia 743.36
Sphincter — *see* condition
Sphincteritis, sphincter of Oddi — *see also* Cholecystitis 576.8
Sphingolipidosis 272.7
Sphingolipodystrophy 272.7
Sphingomyelinosis 272.7
Spicule tooth 520.2
Spider
  finger 755.59
  nevus 448.1
  vascular 448.1
Spiegler-Fendt sarcoid 686.8
Spielmeyer-Stock disease 330.1
Spielmeyer-Vogt disease 330.1
Spina bifida (aperta) 741.9 ☑

> *Note* — Use the following fifth-digit subclassification with category 741:
>
> 0   unspecified region
>
> 1   cervical region
>
> 2   dorsal [thoracic] region
>
> 3   lumbar region

  with hydrocephalus 741.0 ☑
    fetal (suspected), affecting management of pregnancy 655.0 ☑
  occulta 756.17
Spindle, Krukenberg's 371.13
Spine, spinal — *see* condition
Spiradenoma (eccrine) (M8403/0) — *see* Neoplasm, skin, benign
Spirillosis NEC — *see also* Fever, relapsing 087.9
Spirillum minus 026.0
Spirillum obermeieri infection 087.0
Spirochetal — *see* condition
Spirochetosis 104.9
  arthritic, arthritica 104.9 [711.8] ☑
  bronchopulmonary 104.8
  icterohemorrhagica 100.0
  lung 104.8
Spitting blood — *see also* Hemoptysis 786.30
Splanchnomegaly 569.89
Splanchnoptosis 569.89
Spleen, splenic — *see also* condition
  agenesis 759.0
  flexure syndrome 569.89
  neutropenia syndrome 289.53
  sequestration syndrome 289.52
Splenectasis — *see also* Splenomegaly 789.2
Splenitis (interstitial) (malignant) (nonspecific) 289.59
  malarial (*see also* Malaria) 084.6
  tuberculous (*see also* Tuberculosis) 017.7 ☑
Splenocele 289.59
Splenomegalia — *see* Splenomegaly
Splenomegalic — *see* condition

☑ Additional Digit Required — Refer to the Tabular List for Digit Selection   ▽ Subterms under main terms may continue to next column or page

Splenomegaly 789.2
  Bengal 789.2
  cirrhotic 289.51
  congenital 759.0
  congestive, chronic 289.51
  cryptogenic 789.2
  Egyptian 120.1
  Gaucher's (cerebroside lipidosis) 272.7
  idiopathic 789.2
  malarial (see also Malaria) 084.6
  neutropenic 289.53
  Niemann-Pick (lipid histiocytosis) 272.7
  siderotic 289.51
  syphilitic 095.8
    congenital 090.0
  tropical (Bengal) (idiopathic) 789.2
Splenopathy 289.50
Splenopneumonia — see Pneumonia
Splenoptosis 289.59
Splinter — see Injury, superficial, by site
Split, splitting
  heart sounds 427.89
  lip, congenital (see also Cleft, lip) 749.10
  nails 703.8
  urinary stream 788.61
Spoiled child reaction — see also Disturbance,
    conduct 312.1 ☑
Spondylarthritis — see also Spondylosis
    721.90
Spondylarthrosis — see also Spondylosis
    721.90
Spondylitis 720.9
  ankylopoietica 720.0
  ankylosing (chronic) 720.0
  atrophic 720.9
    ligamentous 720.9
  chronic (traumatic) (see also Spondylosis)
    721.90
  deformans (chronic) (see also Spondylosis)
    721.90
  gonococcal 098.53
  gouty 274.00
  hypertrophic (see also Spondylosis) 721.90
  infectious NEC 720.9
  juvenile (adolescent) 720.0
  Kümmell's 721.7
  Marie-Strümpell (ankylosing) 720.0
  muscularis 720.9
  ossificans ligamentosa 721.6
  osteoarthritica (see also Spondylosis) 721.90
  posttraumatic 721.7
  proliferative 720.0
  rheumatoid 720.0
  rhizomelica 720.0
  sacroiliac NEC 720.2
  senescent (see also Spondylosis) 721.90
  senile (see also Spondylosis) 721.90
  static (see also Spondylosis) 721.90
  traumatic (chronic) (see also Spondylosis)
    721.90
  tuberculous (see also Tuberculosis)
    015.0 ☑ [720.81]
  typhosa 002.0 [720.81]
Spondyloarthrosis — see also Spondylosis
    721.90
Spondylolisthesis (congenital) (lumbosacral)
    756.12
  with disproportion (fetopelvic) 653.3 ☑
    affecting fetus or newborn 763.1
    causing obstructed labor 660.1 ☑
      affecting fetus or newborn 763.1
  acquired 738.4
  degenerative 738.4
  traumatic 738.4
    acute (lumbar) — see Fracture, vertebra,
      lumbar
    site other than lumbosacral — see
      Fracture, vertebra, by site
Spondylolysis (congenital) 756.11
  acquired 738.4
  cervical 756.19
  lumbosacral region 756.11
    with disproportion (fetopelvic) 653.3 ☑
      affecting fetus or newborn 763.1
      causing obstructed labor 660.1 ☑
        affecting fetus or newborn 763.1

Spondylopathy
  inflammatory 720.9
    specified type NEC 720.89
  traumatic 721.7
Spondylose rhizomelique 720.0
Spondylosis 721.90
  with
    disproportion 653.3 ☑
      affecting fetus or newborn 763.1
      causing obstructed labor 660.1 ☑
        affecting fetus or newborn 763.1
    myelopathy NEC 721.91
  cervical, cervicodorsal 721.0
    with myelopathy 721.1
  inflammatory 720.9
  lumbar, lumbosacral 721.3
    with myelopathy 721.42
  sacral 721.3
    with myelopathy 721.42
  thoracic 721.2
    with myelopathy 721.41
  traumatic 721.7
Sponge
  divers' disease 989.5
  inadvertently left in operation wound 998.4
  kidney (medullary) 753.17
Spongioblastoma (M9422/3)
  multiforme (M9440/3)
    specified site — see Neoplasm, by site,
      malignant
    unspecified site 191.9
  polare (M9423/3)
    specified site — see Neoplasm, by site,
      malignant
    unspecified site 191.9
  primitive polar (M9443/3)
    specified site — see Neoplasm, by site,
      malignant
    unspecified site 191.9
  specified site — see Neoplasm, by site, ma-
    lignant
  unspecified site 191.9
Spongiocytoma (M9400/3)
  specified site — see Neoplasm, by site, ma-
    lignant
  unspecified site 191.9
Spongioneuroblastoma (M9504/3) — see
    Neoplasm, by site, malignant
Spontaneous — see also condition
  fracture — see Fracture, pathologic
Spoon nail 703.8
  congenital 757.5
Sporadic — see condition
Sporotrichosis (bones) (cutaneous) (dissemi-
    nated) (epidermal) (lymphatic) (lympho-
    cutaneous) (mucous membranes) (pul-
    monary) (skeletal) (visceral) 117.1
Sporotrichum schenckii infection 117.1
Spots, spotting
  atrophic (skin) 701.3
  Bitôt's (in the young child) 264.1
  café au lait 709.09
  cayenne pepper 448.1
  complicating pregnancy 649.5 ☑
  cotton wool (retina) 362.83
  de Morgan's (senile angiomas) 448.1
  Fúchs' black (myopic) 360.21
  intermenstrual
    irregular 626.6
    regular 626.5
  interpalpebral 372.53
  Koplik's 055.9
  liver 709.09
  Mongolian (pigmented) 757.33
  of pregnancy 649.5 ☑
  purpuric 782.7
  ruby 448.1
Spotted fever — see Fever, spotted
Sprain, strain (joint) (ligament) (muscle) (ten-
    don) 848.9
  abdominal wall (muscle) 848.8
  Achilles tendon 845.09
  acromioclavicular 840.0
  ankle 845.00
    and foot 845.00
  anterior longitudinal, cervical 847.0

Sprain, strain — continued
  arm 840.9
    upper 840.9
      and shoulder 840.9
  astragalus 845.00
  atlanto-axial 847.0
  atlanto-occipital 847.0
  atlas 847.0
  axis 847.0
  back (see also Sprain, spine) 847.9
  breast bone 848.40
  broad ligament — see Injury, internal, broad
    ligament
  calcaneofibular 845.02
  carpal 842.01
  carpometacarpal 842.11
  cartilage
    costal, without mention of injury to
      sternum 848.3
      involving sternum 848.42
    ear 848.8
    knee 844.9
      with current tear (see also Tear,
        meniscus) 836.2
      semilunar (knee) 844.8
      with current tear (see also Tear,
        meniscus) 836.2
    septal, nose 848.0
    thyroid region 848.2
    xiphoid 848.49
  cervical, cervicodorsal, cervicothoracic 847.0
  chondrocostal, without mention of injury
    to sternum 848.3
    involving sternum 848.42
  chondrosternal 848.42
  chronic (joint) — see Derangement, joint
  clavicle 840.9
  coccyx 847.4
  collar bone 840.9
  collateral, knee (medial) (tibial) 844.1
    lateral (fibular) 844.0
      recurrent or old 717.89
      lateral 717.81
      medial 717.82
  coracoacromial 840.8
  coracoclavicular 840.1
  coracohumeral 840.2
  coracoid (process) 840.9
  coronary, knee 844.8
  costal cartilage, without mention of injury
    to sternum 848.3
    involving sternum 848.42
  cricoarytenoid articulation 848.2
  cricothyroid articulation 848.2
  cruciate
    knee 844.2
    old 717.89
      anterior 717.83
      posterior 717.84
  deltoid
    ankle 845.01
    shoulder 840.8
  dorsal (spine) 847.1
  ear cartilage 848.8
  elbow 841.9
    and forearm 841.9
    specified site NEC 841.8
  femur (proximal end) 843.9
    distal end 844.9
  fibula (proximal end) 844.9
    distal end 845.00
  fibulocalcaneal 845.02
  finger(s) 842.10
  foot 845.10
    and ankle 845.00
  forearm 841.9
    and elbow 841.9
    specified site NEC 841.8
  glenoid (shoulder) (see also SLAP lesion)
    840.8
  hand 842.10
  hip 843.9
    and thigh 843.9
  humerus (proximal end) 840.9
    distal end 841.9
  iliofemoral 843.0

Sprain, strain — continued
  infraspinatus 840.3
  innominate
    acetabulum 843.9
    pubic junction 848.5
    sacral junction 846.1
  internal
    collateral, ankle 845.01
    semilunar cartilage 844.8
      with current tear (see also Tear,
        meniscus) 836.2
      old 717.5
  interphalangeal
    finger 842.13
    toe 845.13
  ischiocapsular 843.1
  jaw (cartilage) (meniscus) 848.1
    old 524.69
  knee 844.9
    and leg 844.9
    old 717.5
    collateral
      lateral 717.81
      medial 717.82
    cruciate
      anterior 717.83
      posterior 717.84
  late effect — see Late, effects (of), sprain
  lateral collateral, knee 844.0
    old 717.81
  leg 844.9
    and knee 844.9
  ligamentum teres femoris 843.8
  low back 846.9
  lumbar (spine) 847.2
  lumbosacral 846.0
    chronic or old 724.6
  mandible 848.1
    old 524.69
  maxilla 848.1
  medial collateral, knee 844.1
    old 717.82
  meniscus
    jaw 848.1
      old 524.69
    knee 844.8
      with current tear (see also Tear,
        meniscus) 836.2
      old 717.5
    mandible 848.1
      old 524.69
    specified site NEC 848.8
  metacarpal 842.10
    distal 842.12
    proximal 842.11
  metacarpophalangeal 842.12
  metatarsal 845.10
  metatarsophalangeal 845.12
  midcarpal 842.19
  midtarsal 845.19
  multiple sites, except fingers alone or toes
    alone 848.8
  neck 847.0
  nose (septal cartilage) 848.0
  occiput from atlas 847.0
  old — see Derangement, joint
  orbicular, hip 843.8
  patella(r) 844.8
    old 717.89
  pelvis 848.5
  phalanx
    finger 842.10
    toe 845.10
  radiocarpal 842.02
  radiohumeral 841.2
  radioulnar 841.9
    distal 842.09
  radius, radial (proximal end) 841.9
    and ulna 841.9
      distal 842.09
    collateral 841.0
    distal end 842.00
  recurrent — see Sprain, by site
  rib (cage), without mention of injury to
    sternum 848.3
    involving sternum 848.42

☑ Additional Digit Required — Refer to the Tabular List for Digit Selection
▽ Subterms under main terms may continue to next column or page

Sprain, strain — *continued*
  rotator cuff (capsule) 840.4
  round ligament (*see also* Injury, internal,
      round ligament)
    femur 843.8
  sacral (spine) 847.3
  sacrococcygeal 847.3
  sacroiliac (region) 846.9
    chronic or old 724.6
    ligament 846.1
    specified site NEC 846.8
  sacrospinatus 846.2
  sacrospinous 846.2
  sacrotuberous 846.3
  scaphoid bone, ankle 845.00
  scapula(r) 840.9
  semilunar cartilage (knee) 844.8
    with current tear (*see also* Tear, menis-
        cus) 836.2
    old 717.5
  septal cartilage (nose) 848.0
  shoulder 840.9
    and arm, upper 840.9
    blade 840.9
  specified site NEC 848.8
  spine 847.9
    cervical 847.0
    coccyx 847.4
    dorsal 847.1
    lumbar 847.2
    lumbosacral 846.0
      chronic or old 724.6
    sacral 847.3
    sacroiliac (*see also* Sprain, sacroiliac)
        846.9
      chronic or old 724.6
    thoracic 847.1
  sternoclavicular 848.41
  sternum 848.40
  subglenoid (*see also* SLAP lesion) 840.8
  subscapularis 840.5
  supraspinatus 840.6
  symphysis
    jaw 848.1
      old 524.69
    mandibular 848.1
      old 524.69
    pubis 848.5
  talofibular 845.09
  tarsal 845.10
  tarsometatarsal 845.11
  temporomandibular 848.1
    old 524.69
  teres
    ligamentum femoris 843.8
    major or minor 840.8
  thigh (proximal end) 843.9
    and hip 843.9
    distal end 844.9
  thoracic (spine) 847.1
  thorax 848.8
  thumb 842.10
  thyroid cartilage or region 848.2
  tibia (proximal end) 844.9
    distal end 845.00
  tibiofibular
    distal 845.03
    superior 844.3
  toe(s) 845.10
  trachea 848.8
  trapezoid 840.8
  ulna, ulnar (proximal end) 841.9
    collateral 841.1
    distal end 842.00
  ulnohumeral 841.3
  vertebrae (*see also* Sprain, spine) 847.9
    cervical, cervicodorsal, cervicothoracic
        847.0
  wrist (cuneiform) (scaphoid) (semilunar)
      842.00
  xiphoid cartilage 848.49
Sprengel's deformity (congenital) 755.52
Spring fever 309.23
Sprue 579.1
  celiac 579.0
  idiopathic 579.0

Sprue — *continued*
  meaning thrush 112.0
  nontropical 579.0
  tropical 579.1
Spur — *see also* Exostosis
  bone 726.91
    calcaneal 726.73
  calcaneal 726.73
  iliac crest 726.5
  nose (septum) 478.19
    bone 726.91
  septal 478.19
Spuria placenta — *see* Placenta, abnormal
Spurway's syndrome (brittle bones and blue
    sclera) 756.51
Sputum, abnormal (amount) (color) (exces-
    sive) (odor) (purulent) 786.4
  bloody 786.30
Squamous — *see also* condition
  cell metaplasia
    bladder 596.89
    cervix — *see* condition
  epithelium in
    cervical canal (congenital) 752.49
    uterine mucosa (congenital) 752.39
  metaplasia
    bladder 596.89
    cervix — *see* condition
Squashed nose 738.0
  congenital 754.0
Squeeze, divers' 993.3
Squint — *see also* Strabismus 378.9
  accommodative (*see also* Esotropia) 378.00
  concomitant (*see also* Heterotropia) 378.30
Stab — *see also* Wound, open, by site
  internal organs — *see* Injury, internal, by
      site, with open wound
Staggering gait 781.2
  hysterical 300.11
Staghorn calculus 592.0
Stain, staining
  meconium 779.84
  port wine 757.32
  tooth, teeth (hard tissues) 521.7
    due to
      accretions 523.6
      deposits (betel) (black) (green) (ma-
          teria alba) (orange) (tobacco)
          523.6
      metals (copper) (silver) 521.7
      nicotine 523.6
      pulpal bleeding 521.7
      tobacco 523.6
Stälh's
  ear 744.29
  pigment line (cornea) 371.11
Stälhi's pigment lines (cornea) 371.11
Stammering — *see also* Disorder, fluency
    315.35
Standstill
  atrial 426.6
  auricular 426.6
  cardiac (*see also* Arrest, cardiac) 427.5
  sinoatrial 426.6
  sinus 426.6
  ventricular (*see also* Arrest, cardiac) 427.5
Stannosis 503
Stanton's disease (melioidosis) 025
Staphylitis (acute) (catarrhal) (chronic) (gan-
    grenous) (membranous) (suppurative)
    (ulcerative) 528.3
Staphylococcemia 038.10
  aureus 038.11
  specified organism NEC 038.19
Staphylococcus, staphylococcal — *see* condi-
    tion
Staphyloderma (skin) 686.00
Staphyloma 379.11
  anterior, localized 379.14
  ciliary 379.11
  cornea 371.73
  equatorial 379.13
  posterior 379.12
  posticum 379.12
  ring 379.15
  sclera NEC 379.11

Starch eating 307.52
Stargardt's disease 362.75
Starvation (inanition) (due to lack of food)
    994.2
  edema 262
  voluntary NEC 307.1
Stasis
  bile (duct) (*see also* Disease, biliary) 576.8
  bronchus (*see also* Bronchitis) 490
  cardiac (*see also* Failure, heart) 428.0
  cecum 564.89
  colon 564.89
  dermatitis (*see also* Varix, with stasis dermati-
      tis) 454.1
  duodenal 536.8
  eczema (*see also* Varix, with stasis dermati-
      tis) 454.1
  edema (*see also* Hypertension, venous)
      459.30
  foot 991.4
  gastric 536.3
  ileocecal coil 564.89
  ileum 564.89
  intestinal 564.89
  jejunum 564.89
  kidney 586
  liver 571.9
    cirrhotic — *see* Cirrhosis, liver
  lymphatic 457.8
  pneumonia 514
  portal 571.9
  pulmonary 514
  rectal 564.89
  renal 586
    tubular 584.5
  stomach 536.3
  ulcer
    with varicose veins 454.0
    without varicose veins 459.81
  urine NEC (*see also* Retention, urine) 788.20
  venous 459.81
State
  affective and paranoid, mixed, organic psy-
      chotic 294.8
  agitated 307.9
    acute reaction to stress 308.2
  anxiety (neurotic) (*see also* Anxiety) 300.00
    specified type NEC 300.09
  apprehension (*see also* Anxiety) 300.00
    specified type NEC 300.09
  climacteric, female 627.2
    following induced menopause 627.4
  clouded
    epileptic (*see also* Epilepsy) 345.9 ✓
    paroxysmal (idiopathic) (*see also* Epilep-
        sy) 345.9 ✓
  compulsive (mixed) (with obsession) 300.3
  confusional 298.9
    acute 293.0
      with
        arteriosclerotic dementia 290.41
        presenile brain disease 290.11
        senility 290.3
    alcoholic 291.0
    drug-induced 292.81
  epileptic 293.0
  postoperative 293.9
  reactive (emotional stress) (psychologi-
      cal trauma) 298.2
  subacute 293.1
  constitutional psychopathic 301.9
  convulsive (*see also* Convulsions) 780.39
  depressive NEC 311
    induced by drug 292.84
    neurotic 300.4
  dissociative 300.15
  hallucinatory 780.1
    induced by drug 292.12
  hypercoagulable (primary) 289.81
    secondary 289.82
  hyperdynamic beta-adrenergic circulatory
      429.82
  locked-in 344.81
  menopausal 627.2
    artificial 627.4
    following induced menopause 627.4

State — *continued*
  neurotic NEC 300.9
    with depersonalization episode 300.6
  obsessional 300.3
  oneiroid (*see also* Schizophrenia) 295.4 ✓
  panic 300.01
  paranoid 297.9
    alcohol-induced 291.5
    arteriosclerotic 290.42
    climacteric 297.2
    drug-induced 292.11
    in
      presenile brain disease 290.12
      senile brain disease 290.20
    involutional 297.2
    menopausal 297.2
    senile 290.20
    simple 297.0
  postleukotomy 310.0
  pregnant (*see also* Pregnancy) V22.2
  psychogenic, twilight 298.2
  psychotic, organic (*see also* Psychosis, organ-
      ic) 294.9
    mixed paranoid and affective 294.8
    senile or presenile NEC 290.9
    transient NEC 293.9
      with
        anxiety 293.84
        delusions 293.81
        depression 293.83
        hallucinations 293.82
  residual schizophrenic (*see also*
      Schizophrenia) 295.6 ✓
  tension (*see also* Anxiety) 300.9
  transient organic psychotic 293.9
    anxiety type 293.84
    depressive type 293.83
    hallucinatory type 293.83
    paranoid type 293.81
    specified type NEC 293.89
  twilight
    epileptic 293.0
    psychogenic 298.2
  vegetative (persistent) 780.03
Status (post)
  absence
    epileptic (*see also* Epilepsy) 345.2
    of organ, acquired (postsurgical) — *see*
        Absence, by site, acquired
  administration of tPA(rtPA) in a different
      institution within the last 24 hours
      prior to admission to facility V45.88
  anastomosis of intestine (for bypass) V45.3
  anginosus 413.9
  angioplasty, percutaneous transluminal
      coronary V45.82
  ankle prosthesis V43.66
  aortocoronary bypass or shunt V45.81
  arthrodesis V45.4
  artificially induced condition NEC V45.89
  artificial opening (of) V44.9
    gastrointestinal tract NEC V44.4
    specified site NEC V44.8
    urinary tract NEC V44.6
    vagina V44.7
  aspirator V46.0
  asthmaticus (*see also* Asthma) 493.9 ✓
  awaiting organ transplant V49.83
  bariatric surgery V45.86
    complicating pregnancy, childbirth, or
        the puerperium 649.2 ✓
  bed confinement V49.84
  breast
    correction V43.82
    implant removal V45.83
    reconstruction V43.82
  cardiac
    device (in situ) V45.00
      carotid sinus V45.09
        fitting or adjustment V53.39
      defibrillator, automatic implantable
          (with synchronous cardiac
          pacemaker) V45.02
      pacemaker V45.01
        fitting or adjustment V53.31
  carotid sinus stimulator V45.09

✓ **Additional Digit Required** — Refer to the Tabular List for Digit Selection   ☞ **Subterms under main terms may continue to next column or page**

262 — Volume 2   ▶◀ Revised Text   ● New Line   ▲ Revised Code   2015 ICD-9-CM

Status — *continued*
- cataract extraction V45.61
- chemotherapy V66.2
  - current V58.69
- circumcision, female 629.20
- clitorectomy (female genital mutilation type I) 629.21
  - with excision of labia minora (female genital mutilation type II) 629.22
- colonization — *see* Carrier (suspected) of
- colostomy V44.3
- contraceptive device V45.59
  - intrauterine V45.51
  - subdermal V45.52
- convulsivus idiopathicus (*see also* Epilepsy) 345.3
- coronary artery bypass or shunt V45.81
- cutting
  - female genital 629.20
    - specified NEC 629.29
    - type I 629.21
    - type II 629.22
    - type III 629.23
    - type IV 629.29
- cystostomy V44.50
  - appendico-vesicostomy V44.52
  - cutaneous-vesicostomy V44.51
  - specified type NEC V44.59
- defibrillator, automatic implantable cardiac (with synchronous cardiac pacemaker) V45.02
- delinquent immunization V15.83
- dental crowns V45.84
- dental fillings V45.84
- dental restoration V45.84
- dental sealant V49.82
- dialysis (hemo) (peritoneal) V45.11
- donor V59.9
- do not resuscitate V49.86
- drug therapy or regimen V67.59
  - high-risk medication NEC V67.51
- elbow prosthesis V43.62
- embedded
  - fragment — *see* Foreign body, retained
  - splinter — *see* Foreign body, retained
- enterostomy V44.4
- epileptic, epilepticus (absence) (grand mal) (*see also* Epilepsy) 345.3
  - focal motor 345.7 ☑
  - partial 345.7 ☑
  - petit mal 345.2
  - psychomotor 345.7 ☑
  - temporal lobe 345.7 ☑
- estrogen receptor
  - negative [ER-] V86.1
  - positive [ER+] V86.0
- explantation of joint prosthesis NEC V88.29
  - hip V88.21
  - knee V88.22
- eye (adnexa) surgery V45.69
- female genital
  - cutting 629.20
    - specified NEC 629.29
    - type I 629.21
    - type II 629.22
    - type III 629.23
    - type IV 629.29
  - mutilation 629.20
    - type I 629.21
    - type II 629.22
    - type III 629.23
    - type IV 629.29
- filtering bleb (eye) (postglaucoma) V45.69
  - with rupture or complication 997.99
  - postcataract extraction (complication) 997.99
- finger joint prosthesis V43.69
- foster care V60.81
- gastric
  - banding V45.86
    - complicating pregnancy, childbirth, or the puerperium 649.2 ☑
  - bypass for obesity V45.86
    - complicating pregnancy, childbirth, or the puerperium 649.2 ☑
- gastrostomy V44.1

Status — *continued*
- grand mal 345.3
- heart valve prosthesis V43.3
- hemodialysis V45.11
- hip prosthesis (joint) (partial) (total) V43.64
  - explantation V88.21
- hysterectomy V88.01
  - partial with remaining cervical stump V88.02
  - total V88.01
- ileostomy V44.2
- infibulation (female genital mutilation type III) 629.23
- insulin pump V45.85
- intestinal bypass V45.3
- intrauterine contraceptive device V45.51
- jejunostomy V44.4
- joint prosthesis NEC V43.69
  - explantation V88.29
- knee joint prosthesis V43.65
  - explantation V88.22
- lacunaris 437.8
- lacunosis 437.8
- lapsed immunization schedule V15.83
- low birth weight V21.30
  - less than 500 grams V21.31
  - 1000–1499 grams V21.33
  - 1500–1999 grams V21.34
  - 2000–2500 grams V21.35
  - 500–999 grams V21.32
- lymphaticus 254.8
- malignant neoplasm, ablated or excised — *see* History, malignant neoplasm
- marmoratus 333.79
- military deployment V62.22
- mutilation, female 629.20
  - type I 629.21
  - type II 629.22
  - type III 629.23
  - type IV 629.29
- nephrostomy V44.6
- neuropacemaker NEC V45.89
  - brain V45.89
  - carotid sinus V45.09
  - neurologic NEC V45.89
- obesity surgery V45.86
  - complicating pregnancy, childbirth, or the puerperium 649.2 ☑
- organ replacement
  - by artificial or mechanical device or prosthesis of
    - artery V43.4
    - artificial skin V43.83
    - bladder V43.5
    - blood vessel V43.4
    - breast V43.82
    - eye globe V43.0
    - heart
      - assist device V43.21
      - fully implantable artificial heart V43.22
      - valve V43.3
    - intestine V43.89
    - joint V43.60
      - ankle V43.66
      - elbow V43.62
      - finger V43.69
      - hip (partial) (total) V43.64
      - knee V43.65
      - shoulder V43.61
      - specified NEC V43.69
      - wrist V43.63
    - kidney V43.89
    - larynx V43.81
    - lens V43.1
    - limb(s) V43.7
    - liver V43.89
    - lung V43.89
    - organ NEC V43.89
    - pancreas V43.89
    - skin (artificial) V43.83
    - tissue NEC V43.89
    - vein V43.4
  - by organ transplant (heterologous) (homologous) — *see* Status, transplant

Status — *continued*
- pacemaker
  - brain V45.89
  - cardiac V45.01
  - carotid sinus V45.09
  - neurologic NEC V45.89
  - specified site NEC V45.89
- percutaneous transluminal coronary angioplasty V45.82
- peritoneal dialysis V45.11
- petit mal 345.2
- physical restraints V49.87
- postcommotio cerebri 310.2
- postmenopausal (age related) (natural) V49.81
- postoperative NEC V45.89
- postpartum NEC V24.2
  - care immediately following delivery V24.0
  - routine follow-up V24.2
- postsurgical NEC V45.89
- renal dialysis V45.11
  - noncompliance V45.12
- respirator [ventilator] V46.11
  - encounter
    - during
      - mechanical failure V46.14
      - power failure V46.12
    - for weaning V46.13
- retained foreign body — *see* Foreign body, retained
- reversed jejunal transposition (for bypass) V45.3
- sex reassignment surgery (*see also* Transsexualism) 302.50
- shoulder prosthesis V43.61
- shunt
  - aortocoronary bypass V45.81
  - arteriovenous (for dialysis) V45.11
  - cerebrospinal fluid V45.2
  - vascular NEC V45.89
    - aortocoronary (bypass) V45.81
  - ventricular (communicating) (for drainage) V45.2
- sterilization
  - tubal ligation V26.51
  - vasectomy V26.52
- subdermal contraceptive device V45.52
- thymicolymphaticus 254.8
- thymicus 254.8
- thymolymphaticus 254.8
- tooth extraction 525.10
- tracheostomy V44.0
- transplant
  - blood vessel V42.89
  - bone V42.4
    - marrow V42.81
  - cornea V42.5
  - heart V42.1
    - valve V42.2
  - intestine V42.84
  - kidney V42.0
  - liver V42.7
  - lung V42.6
  - organ V42.9
    - removal (due to complication, failure, rejection or infection) V45.87
    - specified site NEC V42.89
  - pancreas V42.83
  - peripheral stem cells V42.82
  - skin V42.3
  - stem cells, peripheral V42.82
  - tissue V42.9
    - specified type NEC V42.89
  - vessel, blood V42.89
- tubal ligation V26.51
- underimmunization V15.83
- ureterostomy V44.6
- urethrostomy V44.6
- vagina, artificial V44.7
- vascular shunt NEC V45.89
  - aortocoronary (bypass) V45.81
- vasectomy V26.52
- ventilator [respirator] V46.11

Status — *continued*
- ventilator [respirator] — *continued*
  - encounter
    - during
      - mechanical failure V46.14
      - power failure V46.12
    - for weaning V46.13
  - wheelchair confinement V46.3
  - wrist prosthesis V43.63
- **Stave fracture** — *see* Fracture, metacarpus, metacarpal bone(s)
- **Steal**
  - subclavian artery 435.2
  - vertebral artery 435.1
- **Stealing, solitary, child problem** — *see also* Disturbance, conduct 312.1 ☑
- **Steam burn** — *see* Burn, by site
- **Steatocystoma multiplex** 706.2
- **Steatoma** (infected) 706.2
  - eyelid (cystic) 374.84
    - infected 373.13
- **Steatorrhea** (chronic) 579.8
  - with lacteal obstruction 579.2
  - idiopathic 579.0
    - adult 579.0
    - infantile 579.0
  - pancreatic 579.4
  - primary 579.0
  - secondary 579.8
  - specified cause NEC 579.8
  - tropical 579.1
- **Steatosis** 272.8
  - heart (*see also* Degeneration, myocardial) 429.1
  - kidney 593.89
  - liver 571.8
- **Steele-Richardson (-Olszewski) Syndrome** 333.0
- **Steinbrocker's syndrome** — *see also* Neuropathy, peripheral, autonomic 337.9
- **Steinert's disease** 359.21
- **Stein-Leventhal syndrome** (polycystic ovary) 256.4
- **Stein's syndrome** (polycystic ovary) 256.4
- **STEMI** (ST elevation myocardial infarction — *see also* — Infarct, myocardium, ST elevation 410.9 ☑
- **Stenocardia** — *see also* Angina 413.9
- **Stenocephaly** 756.0
- **Stenosis** (cicatricial) — *see also* Stricture
  - ampulla of Vater 576.2
    - with calculus, cholelithiasis, or stones — *see* Choledocholithiasis
  - anus, anal (canal) (sphincter) 569.2
    - congenital 751.2
  - aorta (ascending) 747.22
    - arch 747.10
    - arteriosclerotic 440.0
    - calcified 440.0
  - aortic (valve) 424.1
    - with
      - mitral (valve)
        - insufficiency or incompetence 396.2
        - stenosis or obstruction 396.0
    - atypical 396.0
    - congenital 746.3
    - rheumatic 395.0
      - with
        - insufficiency, incompetency or regurgitation 395.2
          - with mitral (valve) disease 396.8
        - mitral (valve)
          - disease (stenosis) 396.0
          - insufficiency or incompetence 396.2
          - stenosis or obstruction 396.0
    - specified cause, except rheumatic 424.1
    - syphilitic 093.22
  - aqueduct of Sylvius (congenital) 742.3
    - with spina bifida (*see also* Spina bifida) 741.0 ☑
    - acquired 331.4
  - artery NEC (*see also* Arteriosclerosis) 447.1
    - basilar — *see* Narrowing, artery, basilar

☑ Additional Digit Required — Refer to the Tabular List for Digit Selection   ▽ Subterms under main terms may continue to next column or page

2015 ICD-9-CM   ►◄ Revised Text   ● New Line   ▲ Revised Code   Volume 2 — 263

Stenosis — see also Stricture — continued
  artery (see also Arteriosclerosis) — continued
    carotid (common) (internal) — see Narrowing, artery, carotid
    celiac 447.4
    cerebral 437.0
      due to
        embolism (see also Embolism, brain) 434.1 ☑
        thrombus (see also Thrombosis, brain) 434.0 ☑
    extremities 440.20
    precerebral — see Narrowing, artery, precerebral
    pulmonary (congenital) 747.31
      acquired 417.8
    renal 440.1
    vertebral — see Narrowing, artery, vertebral
  bile duct or biliary passage (see also Obstruction, biliary) 576.2
    congenital 751.61
  bladder neck (acquired) 596.0
    congenital 753.6
  brain 348.89
  bronchus 519.19
    syphilitic 095.8
  cardia (stomach) 537.89
    congenital 750.7
  cardiovascular (see also Disease, cardiovascular) 429.2
  carotid artery — see Narrowing, artery, carotid
  cervix, cervical (canal) 622.4
    congenital 752.49
    in pregnancy or childbirth 654.6 ☑
      affecting fetus or newborn 763.89
      causing obstructed labor 660.2 ☑
        affecting fetus or newborn 763.1
  colon (see also Obstruction, intestine) 560.9
    congenital 751.2
  colostomy 569.62
  common bile duct (see also Obstruction, biliary) 576.2
    congenital 751.61
  coronary (artery) — see Arteriosclerosis, coronary
  cystic duct (see also Obstruction, gallbladder) 575.2
    congenital 751.61
  due to (presence of) any device, implant, or graft classifiable to 996.0–996.5 — see Complications, due to (presence of) any device, implant, or graft classified to 996.0–996.5 NEC
  duodenum 537.3
    congenital 751.1
  ejaculatory duct NEC 608.89
  endocervical os — see Stenosis, cervix
  enterostomy 569.62
  esophagostomy 530.87
  esophagus 530.3
    congenital 750.3
    syphilitic 095.8
      congenital 090.5
  external ear canal 380.50
    secondary to
      inflammation 380.53
      surgery 380.52
      trauma 380.51
  gallbladder (see also Obstruction, gallbladder) 575.2
  glottis 478.74
  heart valve (acquired) (see also Endocarditis)
    congenital NEC 746.89
      aortic 746.3
      mitral 746.5
      pulmonary 746.02
      tricuspid 746.1
  hepatic duct (see also Obstruction, biliary) 576.2
  hymen 623.3
  hypertrophic subaortic (idiopathic) 425.11
  infundibulum cardiac 746.83

Stenosis — see also Stricture — continued
  intestine (see also Obstruction, intestine) 560.9
    congenital (small) 751.1
      large 751.2
  lacrimal
    canaliculi 375.53
    duct 375.56
      congenital 743.65
    punctum 375.52
      congenital 743.65
    sac 375.54
      congenital 743.65
  lacrimonasal duct 375.56
    congenital 743.65
    neonatal 375.55
  larynx 478.74
    congenital 748.3
    syphilitic 095.8
      congenital 090.5
  mitral (valve) (chronic) (inactive) 394.0
    with
      aortic (valve)
        disease (insufficiency) 396.1
        insufficiency or incompetence 396.1
        stenosis or obstruction 396.0
      incompetency, insufficiency or regurgitation 394.2
        with aortic valve disease 396.8
    active or acute 391.1
      with chorea (acute) (rheumatic) (Sydenham's) 392.0
    congenital 746.5
    specified cause, except rheumatic 424.0
    syphilitic 093.21
  myocardium, myocardial (see also Degeneration, myocardial) 429.1
    hypertrophic subaortic (idiopathic) 425.11
  nares (anterior) (posterior) 478.19
    congenital 748.0
  nasal duct 375.56
    congenital 743.65
  nasolacrimal duct 375.56
    congenital 743.65
    neonatal 375.55
  organ or site, congenital NEC — see Atresia
  papilla of Vater 576.2
    with calculus, cholelithiasis, or stones — see Choledocholithiasis
  pulmonary (artery) (congenital) 747.31
    with ventricular septal defect, dextraposition of aorta and hypertrophy of right ventricle 745.2
    acquired 417.8
    infundibular 746.83
    in tetralogy of Fallot 745.2
    subvalvular 746.83
    valve (see also Endocarditis, pulmonary) 424.3
      congenital 746.02
    vein 747.49
      acquired 417.8
    vessel NEC 417.8
  pulmonic (congenital) 746.02
    infundibular 746.83
    subvalvular 746.83
  pylorus (hypertrophic) 537.0
    adult 537.0
    congenital 750.5
    infantile 750.5
  rectum (sphincter) (see also Stricture, rectum) 569.2
  renal artery 440.1
  salivary duct (any) 527.8
  sphincter of Oddi (see also Obstruction, biliary) 576.2
  spinal 724.00
    cervical 723.0
    lumbar, lumbosacral (without neurogenic claudication) 724.02
      with neurogenic claudication 724.03
    nerve (root) NEC 724.9
    specified region NEC 724.09
    thoracic, thoracolumbar 724.01

Stenosis — see also Stricture — continued
  stomach, hourglass 537.6
  subaortic 746.81
    hypertrophic (idiopathic) 425.11
  supra (valvular)-aortic 747.22
  trachea 519.19
    congenital 748.3
    syphilitic 095.8
    tuberculous (see also Tuberculosis) 012.8 ☑
  tracheostomy 519.02
  tricuspid (valve) (see also Endocarditis, tricuspid) 397.0
    congenital 746.1
    nonrheumatic 424.2
  tubal 628.2
  ureter (see also Stricture, ureter) 593.3
    congenital 753.29
  urethra (see also Stricture, urethra) 598.9
  vagina 623.2
    congenital 752.49
    in pregnancy or childbirth 654.7 ☑
      affecting fetus or newborn 763.89
      causing obstructed labor 660.2 ☑
        affecting fetus or newborn 763.1
  valve (cardiac) (heart) (see also Endocarditis) 424.90
    congenital NEC 746.89
      aortic 746.3
      mitral 746.5
      pulmonary 746.02
      tricuspid 746.1
      urethra 753.6
  valvular (see also Endocarditis) 424.90
    congenital NEC 746.89
    urethra 753.6
  vascular graft or shunt 996.1
    atherosclerosis — see Arteriosclerosis, extremities
    embolism 996.74
    occlusion NEC 996.74
    thrombus 996.74
  vena cava (inferior) (superior) 459.2
    congenital 747.49
  ventricular shunt 996.2
  vulva 624.8
Stent jail 996.72
Stercolith — see also Fecalith 560.32
  appendix 543.9
Stercoraceous, stercoral ulcer 569.82
  anus or rectum 569.41
Stereopsis, defective
  with fusion 368.33
  without fusion 368.32
Stereotypes NEC 307.3
Sterility
  female — see Infertility, female
  male (see also Infertility, male) 606.9
Sterilization, admission for V25.2
  status
    tubal ligation V26.51
    vasectomy V26.52
Sternalgia — see also Angina 413.9
Sternopagus 759.4
Sternum bifidum 756.3
Sternutation 784.99
Steroid
  effects (adverse) (iatrogenic)
    cushingoid
      correct substance properly administered 255.0
      overdose or wrong substance given or taken 962.0
    diabetes — see Diabetes, secondary
      correct substance properly administered 251.8
      overdose or wrong substance given or taken 962.0
    due to
      correct substance properly administered 255.8
      overdose or wrong substance given or taken 962.0
    fever
      correct substance properly administered 780.60

Steroid — continued
  effects — continued
    fever — continued
      overdose or wrong substance given or taken 962.0
    withdrawal
      correct substance properly administered 255.41
      overdose or wrong substance given or taken 962.0
  responder 365.03
Stevens-Johnson disease or syndrome (erythema multiforme exudativum) 695.13
  toxic epidermal necrolysis overlap (SJS-TEN overlap syndrome) 695.14
Stewart-Morel syndrome (hyperostosis frontalis interna) 733.3
Sticker's disease (erythema infectiosum) 057.0
Stickler syndrome 759.89
Sticky eye 372.03
Stieda's disease (calcification, knee joint) 726.62
Stiff
  back 724.8
  neck (see also Torticollis) 723.5
Stiff-baby 759.89
Stiff-man syndrome 333.91
Stiffness, joint NEC 719.50
  ankle 719.57
  back 724.8
  elbow 719.52
  finger 719.54
  hip 719.55
  knee 719.56
  multiple sites 719.59
  sacroiliac 724.6
  shoulder 719.51
  specified site NEC 719.58
  spine 724.9
  surgical fusion V45.4
  wrist 719.53
Stigmata, congenital syphilis 090.5
Stillbirth, stillborn NEC 779.9
Still's disease or syndrome 714.30
  adult onset 714.2
Stiller's disease (asthenia) 780.79
Still-Felty syndrome (rheumatoid arthritis with splenomegaly and leukopenia) 714.1
Stilling-Türk-Duane syndrome (ocular retraction syndrome) 378.71
Stimulation, ovary 256.1
Sting (animal) (bee) (fish) (insect) (jellyfish) (Portuguese man-o-war) (wasp) (venomous) 989.5
  anaphylactic shock or reaction 989.5
  plant 692.6
Stippled epiphyses 756.59
Stitch
  abscess 998.59
  burst (in external operation wound) (see also Dehiscence) 998.32
    internal 998.31
  in back 724.5
Stojano's (subcostal) **syndrome** 098.86
Stokes-Adams syndrome (syncope with heart block) 426.9
Stokes' disease (exophthalmic goiter) 242.0 ☑
Stokvis' (-Talma) disease (enterogenous cyanosis) 289.7
Stomach — see condition
Stoma malfunction
  colostomy 569.62
  cystostomy 596.82
    infection 596.81
    mechanical 596.82
    specified complication NEC 596.83
  enterostomy 569.62
  esophagostomy 530.87
  gastrostomy 536.42
  ileostomy 569.62
  nephrostomy 997.5
  tracheostomy 519.02
  ureterostomy 997.5
Stomatitis 528.00
  angular 528.5

Stomatitis — *continued*
angular — *continued*
due to dietary or vitamin deficiency 266.0
aphthous 528.2
bovine 059.11
candidal 112.0
catarrhal 528.00
denture 528.9
diphtheritic (membranous) 032.0
due to
dietary deficiency 266.0
thrush 112.0
vitamin deficiency 266.0
epidemic 078.4
epizootic 078.4
follicular 528.00
gangrenous 528.1
herpetic 054.2
herpetiformis 528.2
malignant 528.00
membranous acute 528.00
monilial 112.0
mycotic 112.0
necrotic 528.1
ulcerative 101
necrotizing ulcerative 101
parasitic 112.0
septic 528.00
specified NEC 528.09
spirochetal 101
suppurative (acute) 528.00
ulcerative 528.00
necrotizing 101
ulceromembranous 101
vesicular 528.00
with exanthem 074.3
Vincent's 101
Stomatocytosis 282.8
Stomatomycosis 112.0
Stomatorrhagia 528.9
Stone(s) — *see also* Calculus
bladder 594.1
diverticulum 594.0
cystine 270.0
heart syndrome (*see also* Failure, ventricular, left) 428.1
kidney 592.0
prostate 602.0
pulp (dental) 522.2
renal 592.0
salivary duct or gland (any) 527.5
ureter 592.1
urethra (impacted) 594.2
urinary (duct) (impacted) (passage) 592.9
bladder 594.1
diverticulum 594.0
lower tract NEC 594.9
specified site 594.8
xanthine 277.2
Stonecutters' lung 502
tuberculous (*see also* Tuberculosis) 011.4 ☑
Stonemasons'
asthma, disease, or lung 502
tuberculous (*see also* Tuberculosis) 011.4 ☑
phthisis (*see also* Tuberculosis) 011.4 ☑
Stoppage
bowel (*see also* Obstruction, intestine) 560.9
heart (*see also* Arrest, cardiac) 427.5
intestine (*see also* Obstruction, intestine) 560.9
urine NEC (*see also* Retention, urine) 788.20
Storm, thyroid (apathetic) — *see also* Thyrotoxicosis 242.9 ☑
Strabismus (alternating) (congenital) (nonparalytic) 378.9
concomitant (*see also* Heterotropia) 378.30
convergent (*see also* Esotropia) 378.00
divergent (*see also* Exotropia) 378.10
convergent (*see also* Esotropia) 378.00
divergent (*see also* Exotropia) 378.10
due to adhesions, scars — *see* Strabismus, mechanical
in neuromuscular disorder NEC 378.73
intermittent 378.20

Strabismus — *continued*
in neuromuscular disorder — *continued*
intermittent — *continued*
vertical 378.31
latent 378.40
convergent (esophoria) 378.41
divergent (exophoria) 378.42
vertical 378.43
mechanical 378.60
due to
Brown's tendon sheath syndrome 378.61
specified musculofascial disorder NEC 378.62
paralytic 378.50
third or oculomotor nerve (partial) 378.51
total 378.52
fourth or trochlear nerve 378.53
sixth or abducens nerve 378.54
specified type NEC 378.73
vertical (hypertropia) 378.31
Strain — *see also* Sprain, by site
eye NEC 368.13
heart — *see* Disease, heart
meaning gonorrhea — *see* Gonorrhea
on urination 788.65
physical NEC V62.89
postural 729.90
psychological NEC V62.89
Strands
conjunctiva 372.62
vitreous humor 379.25
Strangulation, strangulated 994.7
appendix 543.9
asphyxiation or suffocation by 994.7
bladder neck 596.0
bowel — *see* Strangulation, intestine
colon — *see* Strangulation, intestine
cord (umbilical) — *see* Compression, umbilical cord
due to birth injury 767.8
food or foreign body (*see also* Asphyxia, food) 933.1
hemorrhoids 455.8
external 455.5
internal 455.2
hernia (*see also* Hernia, by site, with obstruction)
gangrenous — *see* Hernia, by site, with gangrene
intestine (large) (small) 560.2
with hernia (*see also* Hernia, by site, with obstruction)
gangrenous — *see* Hernia, by site, with gangrene
congenital (small) 751.1
large 751.2
mesentery 560.2
mucus (*see also* Asphyxia, mucus) 933.1
newborn 770.18
omentum 560.2
organ or site, congenital NEC — *see* Atresia
ovary 620.8
due to hernia 620.4
penis 607.89
foreign body 939.3
rupture (*see also* Hernia, by site, with obstruction) 552.9
gangrenous (*see also* Hernia, by site, with gangrene) 551.9
stomach, due to hernia (*see also* Hernia, by site, with obstruction) 552.9
with gangrene (*see also* Hernia, by site, with gangrene) 551.9
umbilical cord — *see* Compression, umbilical cord
vesicourethral orifice 596.0
Strangury 788.1
Strawberry
gallbladder (*see also* Disease, gallbladder) 575.6
mark 757.32
tongue (red) (white) 529.3
Straw itch 133.8
Streak, ovarian 752.0

Strephosymbolia 315.01
secondary to organic lesion 784.69
Streptobacillary fever 026.1
Streptobacillus moniliformis 026.1
Streptococcemia 038.0
Streptococcicosis — *see* Infection, streptococcal
Streptococcus, streptococcal — *see* condition
Streptoderma 686.00
Streptomycosis — *see* Actinomycosis
Streptothricosis — *see* Actinomycosis
Streptothrix — *see* Actinomycosis
Streptotrichosis — *see* Actinomycosis
Stress 308.9
fracture — *see* Fracture, stress
polycythemia 289.0
reaction (gross) (*see also* Reaction, stress, acute) 308.9
Stretching, nerve — *see* Injury, nerve, by site
Striae (albicantes) (atrophicae) (cutis distensae) (distensae) 701.3
Striations of nails 703.8
Stricture — *see also* Stenosis 799.89
ampulla of Vater 576.2
with calculus, cholelithiasis, or stones — *see* Choledocholithiasis
anus (sphincter) 569.2
congenital 751.2
infantile 751.2
aorta (ascending) 747.22
arch 747.10
arteriosclerotic 440.0
calcified 440.0
aortic (valve) (*see also* Stenosis, aortic) 424.1
congenital 746.3
aqueduct of Sylvius (congenital) 742.3
with spina bifida (*see also* Spina bifida) 741.0 ☑
acquired 331.4
artery 447.1
basilar — *see* Narrowing, artery, basilar
carotid (common) (internal) — *see* Narrowing, artery, carotid
celiac 447.4
cerebral 437.0
congenital 747.81
due to
embolism (*see also* Embolism, brain) 434.1 ☑
thrombus (*see also* Thrombosis, brain) 434.0 ☑
congenital (peripheral) 747.60
cerebral 747.81
coronary 746.85
gastrointestinal 747.61
lower limb 747.64
renal 747.62
retinal 743.58
specified NEC 747.69
spinal 747.82
umbilical 747.5
upper limb 747.63
coronary — *see* Arteriosclerosis, coronary
congenital 746.85
precerebral — *see* Narrowing, artery, precerebral NEC
pulmonary (congenital) 747.31
acquired 417.8
renal 440.1
vertebral — *see* Narrowing, artery, vertebral
auditory canal (congenital) (external) 744.02
acquired (*see also* Stricture, ear canal, acquired) 380.50
bile duct or passage (any) (postoperative) (*see also* Obstruction, biliary) 576.2
congenital 751.61
bladder 596.89
congenital 753.6
neck 596.0
congenital 753.6
bowel (*see also* Obstruction, intestine) 560.9
brain 348.89
bronchus 519.19
syphilitic 095.8

Stricture — *see also* Stenosis — *continued*
cardia (stomach) 537.89
congenital 750.7
cardiac (*see also* Disease, heart)
orifice (stomach) 537.89
cardiovascular (*see also* Disease, cardiovascular) 429.2
carotid artery — *see* Narrowing, artery, carotid
cecum (*see also* Obstruction, intestine) 560.9
cervix, cervical (canal) 622.4
congenital 752.49
in pregnancy or childbirth 654.6 ☑
affecting fetus or newborn 763.89
causing obstructed labor 660.2 ☑
affecting fetus or newborn 763.1
colon (*see also* Obstruction, intestine) 560.9
congenital 751.2
colostomy 569.62
common bile duct (*see also* Obstruction, biliary) 576.2
congenital 751.61
coronary (artery) — *see* Arteriosclerosis, coronary
congenital 746.85
cystic duct (*see also* Obstruction, gallbladder) 575.2
congenital 751.61
cystostomy 596.83
digestive organs NEC, congenital 751.8
duodenum 537.3
congenital 751.1
ear canal (external) (congenital) 744.02
acquired 380.50
secondary to
inflammation 380.53
surgery 380.52
trauma 380.51
ejaculatory duct 608.85
enterostomy 569.62
esophagostomy 530.87
esophagus (corrosive) (peptic) 530.3
congenital 750.3
syphilitic 095.8
congenital 090.5
eustachian tube (*see also* Obstruction, Eustachian tube) 381.60
congenital 744.24
fallopian tube 628.2
gonococcal (chronic) 098.37
acute 098.17
tuberculous (*see also* Tuberculosis) 016.6 ☑
gallbladder (*see also* Obstruction, gallbladder) 575.2
congenital 751.69
glottis 478.74
heart (*see also* Disease, heart)
congenital NEC 746.89
valve (*see also* Endocarditis)
congenital NEC 746.89
aortic 746.3
mitral 746.5
pulmonary 746.02
tricuspid 746.1
hepatic duct (*see also* Obstruction, biliary) 576.2
hourglass, of stomach 537.6
hymen 623.3
hypopharynx 478.29
intestine (*see also* Obstruction, intestine) 560.9
congenital (small) 751.1
large 751.2
ischemic 557.1
lacrimal
canaliculi 375.53
congenital 743.65
punctum 375.52
congenital 743.65
sac 375.54
congenital 743.65
lacrimonasal duct 375.56
congenital 743.65
neonatal 375.55
larynx 478.79

☑ Additional Digit Required — Refer to the Tabular List for Digit Selection ⓦ Subterms under main terms may continue to next column or page

2015 ICD-9-CM ▶◀ Revised Text ● New Line ▲ Revised Code Volume 2 — 265

Stricture — *see also* Stenosis — *continued*
larynx — *continued*
    congenital 748.3
    syphilitic 095.8
       congenital 090.5
lung 518.89
meatus
    ear (congenital) 744.02
       acquired (*see also* Stricture, ear canal, acquired) 380.50
    osseous (congenital) (ear) 744.03
       acquired (*see also* Stricture, ear canal, acquired) 380.50
    urinarius (*see also* Stricture, urethra) 598.9
       congenital 753.6
mitral (valve) (*see also* Stenosis, mitral) 394.0
    congenital 746.5
    specified cause, except rheumatic 424.0
myocardium, myocardial (*see also* Degeneration, myocardial) 429.1
    hypertrophic subaortic (idiopathic) 425.11
nares (anterior) (posterior) 478.19
    congenital 748.0
nasal duct 375.56
    congenital 743.65
    neonatal 375.55
nasolacrimal duct 375.56
    congenital 743.65
    neonatal 375.55
nasopharynx 478.29
    syphilitic 095.8
nephrostomy 997.5
nose 478.19
    congenital 748.0
nostril (anterior) (posterior) 478.19
    congenital 748.0
organ or site, congenital NEC — *see* Atresia
osseous meatus (congenital) (ear) 744.03
    acquired (*see also* Stricture, ear canal, acquired) 380.50
os uteri (*see also* Stricture, cervix) 622.4
oviduct — *see* Stricture, fallopian tube
pelviureteric junction 593.3
pharynx (dilation) 478.29
prostate 602.8
pulmonary, pulmonic
    artery (congenital) 747.31
       acquired 417.8
       noncongenital 417.8
    infundibulum (congenital) 746.83
    valve (*see also* Endocarditis, pulmonary) 424.3
       congenital 746.02
    vein (congenital) 747.49
       acquired 417.8
    vessel NEC 417.8
punctum lacrimale 375.52
    congenital 743.65
pylorus (hypertrophic) 537.0
    adult 537.0
    congenital 750.5
    infantile 750.5
rectosigmoid 569.89
rectum (sphincter) 569.2
    congenital 751.2
    due to
       chemical burn 947.3
       irradiation 569.2
       lymphogranuloma venereum 099.1
    gonococcal 098.7
    inflammatory 099.1
    syphilitic 095.8
    tuberculous (*see also* Tuberculosis) 014.8 ☑
renal artery 440.1
salivary duct or gland (any) 527.8
sigmoid (flexure) (*see also* Obstruction, intestine) 560.9
spermatic cord 608.85
stoma (following) (of)
    colostomy 569.62
    cystostomy 596.83
    enterostomy 569.62
    esophagostomy 530.87

Stricture — *see also* Stenosis — *continued*
stoma — *continued*
    gastrostomy 536.42
    ileostomy 569.62
    nephrostomy 997.5
    tracheostomy 519.02
    ureterostomy 997.5
stomach 537.89
    congenital 750.7
    hourglass 537.6
subaortic 746.81
    hypertrophic (acquired) (idiopathic) 425.11
subglottic 478.74
syphilitic NEC 095.8
tendon (sheath) 727.81
trachea 519.19
    congenital 748.3
    syphilitic 095.8
    tuberculous (*see also* Tuberculosis) 012.8 ☑
tracheostomy 519.02
tricuspid (valve) (*see also* Endocarditis, tricuspid) 397.0
    congenital 746.1
    nonrheumatic 424.2
tunica vaginalis 608.85
ureter (postoperative) 593.3
    congenital 753.29
    tuberculous (*see also* Tuberculosis) 016.2 ☑
ureteropelvic junction 593.3
    congenital 753.21
ureterovesical orifice 593.3
    congenital 753.22
urethra (anterior) (meatal) (organic) (posterior) (spasmodic) 598.9
    associated with schistosomiasis (*see also* Schistosomiasis) 120.9 [598.01]
    congenital (valvular) 753.6
    due to
       infection 598.00
        syphilis 095.8 [598.01]
       trauma 598.1
    gonococcal 098.2 [598.01]
    gonorrheal 098.2 [598.01]
    infective 598.00
    late effect of injury 598.1
    postcatheterization 598.2
    postobstetric 598.1
    postoperative 598.2
    specified cause NEC 598.8
    syphilitic 095.8 [598.01]
    traumatic 598.1
    valvular, congenital 753.6
urinary meatus (*see also* Stricture, urethra) 598.9
    congenital 753.6
uterus, uterine 621.5
    os (external) (internal) — *see* Stricture, cervix
vagina (outlet) 623.2
    congenital 752.49
valve (cardiac) (heart) (*see also* Endocarditis) 424.90
    congenital (cardiac) (heart) NEC 746.89
       aortic 746.3
       mitral 746.5
       pulmonary 746.02
       tricuspid 746.1
       urethra 753.6
valvular (*see also* Endocarditis) 424.90
vascular graft or shunt 996.1
    atherosclerosis — *see* Arteriosclerosis, extremities
    embolism 996.74
    occlusion NEC 996.74
    thrombus 996.74
vas deferens 608.85
    congenital 752.89
vein 459.2
vena cava (inferior) (superior) NEC 459.2
    congenital 747.49
ventricular shunt 996.2
vesicourethral orifice 596.0
    congenital 753.6

Stricture — *see also* Stenosis — *continued*
vulva (acquired) 624.8
Stridor 786.1
    congenital (larynx) 748.3
Stridulous — *see* condition
Strippling of nails 703.8
Stroke 434.91
    apoplectic (*see also* Disease, cerebrovascular, acute) 436
    brain — *see* Infarct, brain
    embolic 434.11
    epileptic — *see* Epilepsy
    healed or old V12.54
    heart — *see* Disease, heart
    heat 992.0
    hemorrhagic — *see* Hemorrhage, brain
    iatrogenic 997.02
    in evolution 434.91
    ischemic 434.91
    late effect — *see* Late effect(s) (of) cerebrovascular disease
    lightning 994.0
    paralytic — *see* Infarct, brain
    postoperative 997.02
    progressive 435.9
    thrombotic 434.01
Stromatosis, endometrial (M8931/1) 236.0
Strong pulse 785.9
Strongyloides stercoralis infestation 127.2
Strongyloidiasis 127.2
Strongyloidosis 127.2
Strongylus (gibsoni) infestation 127.7
Strophulus (newborn) 779.89
    pruriginosus 698.2
Struck by lightning 994.0
Struma — *see also* Goiter 240.9
    fibrosa 245.3
    Hashimoto (struma lymphomatosa) 245.2
    lymphomatosa 245.2
    nodosa (simplex) 241.9
       endemic 241.9
       multinodular 241.1
       sporadic 241.9
       toxic or with hyperthyroidism 242.3 ☑
        multinodular 242.2 ☑
        uninodular 242.1 ☑
       toxicosa 242.3 ☑
        multinodular 242.2 ☑
        uninodular 242.1 ☑
       uninodular 241.0
    ovarii (M9090/0) 220
       and carcinoid (M9091/1) 236.2
       malignant (M9090/3) 183.0
    Riedel's (ligneous thyroiditis) 245.3
    scrofulous (*see also* Tuberculosis) 017.2 ☑
    tuberculous (*see also* Tuberculosis) 017.2 ☑
       abscess 017.2 ☑
       adenitis 017.2 ☑
       lymphangitis 017.2 ☑
       ulcer 017.2 ☑
Strumipriva cachexia — *see also* Hypothyroidism 244.9
Strümpell-Marie disease or spine (ankylosing spondylitis) 720.0
Strümpell-Westphal pseudosclerosis (hepatolenticular degeneration) 275.1
Stuart's disease (congenital factor X deficiency) — *see also* Defect, coagulation 286.3
Stuart-Prower factor deficiency (congenital factor X deficiency) — *see also* Defect, coagulation 286.3
Students' elbow 727.2
Stuffy nose 478.19
Stump — *see also* Amputation
    cervix, cervical (healed) 622.8
Stupor 780.09
    catatonic (*see also* Schizophrenia) 295.2 ☑
    circular (*see also* Psychosis, manic-depressive, circular) 296.7
    manic 296.89
    manic-depressive (*see also* Psychosis, affective) 296.89
    mental (anergic) (delusional) 298.9
    psychogenic 298.8
    reaction to exceptional stress (transient) 308.2

Stupor — *continued*
    traumatic NEC (*see also* Injury, intracranial)
       with spinal (cord)
        lesion — *see* Injury, spinal, by site
        shock — *see* Injury, spinal, by site
Sturge (-Weber) (-Dimitri) disease or syndrome (encephalocutaneous angiomatosis) 759.6
Sturge-Kalischer-Weber syndrome (encephalocutaneous angiomatosis) 759.6
Stuttering 315.35
    adult onset 307.0
    childhood onset 315.35
    due to late effect of cerebrovascular disease (*see also* Late effect(s) (of) cerebrovascular disease) 438.14
    in conditions classified elsewhere 784.52
Sty, stye 373.11
    external 373.11
    internal 373.12
    meibomian 373.12
Subacidity, gastric 536.8
    psychogenic 306.4
Subacute — *see* condition
Subarachnoid — *see* condition
Subclavian steal syndrome 435.2
Subcortical — *see* condition
Subcostal syndrome 098.86
    nerve compression 354.8
Subcutaneous, subcuticular — *see* condition
Subdelirium 293.1
Subdural — *see* condition
Subendocardium — *see* condition
Subependymoma (M9383/1) 237.5
Suberosis 495.3
Subglossitis — *see* Glossitis
Subhemophilia 286.0
Subinvolution (uterus) 621.1
    breast (postlactational) (postpartum) 611.89
    chronic 621.1
    puerperal, postpartum 674.8 ☑
Sublingual — *see* condition
Sublinguitis 527.2
Subluxation — *see also* Dislocation, by site
    congenital NEC (*see also* Malposition, congenital)
       hip (unilateral) 754.32
        with dislocation of other hip 754.35
        bilateral 754.33
       joint
        lower limb 755.69
        shoulder 755.59
        upper limb 755.59
       lower limb (joint) 755.69
       shoulder (joint) 755.59
       upper limb (joint) 755.59
    lens 379.32
       anterior 379.33
       posterior 379.34
    radial head 832.2
    rotary, cervical region of spine — *see* Fracture, vertebra, cervical
Submaxillary — *see* condition
Submersion (fatal) (nonfatal) 994.1
Submissiveness (undue), in child 313.0
Submucous — *see* condition
Subnormal, subnormality
    accommodation (*see also* Disorder, accommodation) 367.9
    mental (*see also* Disability, intellectual) 319
       mild 317
       moderate 318.0
       profound 318.2
       severe 318.1
    temperature (accidental) 991.6
       not associated with low environmental temperature 780.99
Subphrenic — *see* condition
Subscapular nerve — *see* condition
Subseptus uterus 752.35
Subsiding appendicitis 542
Substance abuse in family V61.42
Substernal thyroid — *see also* Goiter 240.9
    congenital 759.2
Substitution disorder 300.11
Subtentorial — *see* condition

☑ **Additional Digit Required** — Refer to the Tabular List for Digit Selection   ▽ **Subterms under main terms may continue to next column or page**

266 — Volume 2   ▶◀ Revised Text   ● New Line   ▲ Revised Code   2015 ICD-9-CM

Subtertian
- fever 084.0
- malaria (fever) 084.0

Subthyroidism (acquired) — *see also* Hypothyroidism 244.9
- congenital 243

Succenturiata placenta — *see* Placenta, abnormal

Succussion sounds, chest 786.7

Sucking thumb, child 307.9

Sudamen 705.1

Sudamina 705.1

Sudanese kala-azar 085.0

Sudden
- death, cause unknown (less than 24 hours) 798.1
  - cardiac (SCD)
    - family history of V17.41
    - personal history of, successfully resuscitated V12.53
  - during childbirth 669.9 ☑
  - infant 798.0
  - puerperal, postpartum 674.9 ☑
- hearing loss NEC 388.2
- heart failure (*see also* Failure, heart) 428.9
- infant death syndrome 798.0

Sudeck's atrophy, disease, or syndrome 733.7

SUDS (sudden unexplained death) 798.2

Suffocation — *see also* Asphyxia 799.01
- by
  - bed clothes 994.7
  - bunny bag 994.7
  - cave-in 994.7
  - constriction 994.7
  - drowning 994.1
  - inhalation
    - food or foreign body (*see also* Asphyxia, food or foreign body) 933.1
    - oil or gasoline (*see also* Asphyxia, food or foreign body) 933.1
  - overlying 994.7
  - plastic bag 994.7
  - pressure 994.7
  - strangulation 994.7
- during birth 768.1
- mechanical 994.7

Sugar
- blood
  - high 790.29
  - low 251.2
- in urine 791.5

Suicide, suicidal (attempted)
- by poisoning — *see* Table of Drugs and Chemicals
- ideation V62.84
- risk 300.9
- tendencies 300.9
- trauma NEC (*see also* nature and site of injury) 959.9

Suipestifer infection — *see also* Infection, Salmonella 003.9

Sulfatidosis 330.0

Sulfhemoglobinemia, sulphemoglobinemia (acquired) (congenital) 289.7

Sumatran mite fever 081.2

Summer — *see* condition

Sunburn 692.71
- first degree 692.71
- second degree 692.76
- third degree 692.77
- dermatitis 692.71
- due to
  - other ultraviolet radiation 692.82
  - tanning bed 692.82

SUNCT (short lasting unilateral neuralgiform headache with conjunctival injection and tearing) 339.05

Sunken
- acetabulum 718.85
- fontanels 756.0

Sunstroke 992.0

Superfecundation 651.9 ☑
- with fetal loss and retention of one or more fetus(es) 651.6 ☑
- following (elective) fetal reduction 651.7 ☑

Superfetation 651.9 ☑
- with fetal loss and retention of one or more fetus(es) 651.6 ☑
- following (elective) fetal reduction 651.7 ☑

Superinvolution uterus 621.8

Supernumerary (congenital)
- aortic cusps 746.89
- auditory ossicles 744.04
- bone 756.9
- breast 757.6
- carpal bones 755.56
- cusps, heart valve NEC 746.89
  - mitral 746.5
  - pulmonary 746.09
- digit(s) 755.00
  - finger 755.01
  - toe 755.02
- ear (lobule) 744.1
- fallopian tube 752.19
- finger 755.01
- hymen 752.49
- kidney 753.3
- lacrimal glands 743.64
- lacrimonasal duct 743.65
- lobule (ear) 744.1
- mitral cusps 746.5
- muscle 756.82
- nipples 757.6
- organ or site NEC — *see* Accessory
- ossicles, auditory 744.04
- ovary 752.0
- oviduct 752.19
- pulmonic cusps 746.09
- rib 756.3
  - cervical or first 756.2
    - syndrome 756.2
- roots (of teeth) 520.2
- spinal vertebra 756.19
- spleen 759.0
- tarsal bones 755.67
- teeth 520.1
  - causing crowding 524.31
- testis 752.89
- thumb 755.01
- toe 755.02
- uterus 752.2
- vagina 752.49
- vertebra 756.19

Supervision (of)
- contraceptive method previously prescribed V25.40
  - intrauterine device V25.42
  - oral contraceptive (pill) V25.41
  - specified type NEC V25.49
  - subdermal implantable contraceptive V25.43
- dietary (for) V65.3
  - allergy (food) V65.3
  - colitis V65.3
  - diabetes mellitus V65.3
  - food allergy intolerance V65.3
  - gastritis V65.3
  - hypercholesterolemia V65.3
  - hypoglycemia V65.3
  - intolerance (food) V65.3
  - obesity V65.3
  - specified NEC V65.3
- lactation V24.1
- newborn health
  - 8 to 28 days old V20.32
  - under 8 days old V20.31
- pregnancy — *see* Pregnancy, supervision of

Supplemental teeth 520.1
- causing crowding 524.31

Suppression
- binocular vision 368.31
- lactation 676.5 ☑
- menstruation 626.8
- ovarian secretion 256.39
- renal 586
- urinary secretion 788.5
- urine 788.5

Suppuration, suppurative — *see also* condition

Suppuration, suppurative — *see also* condition — *continued*
- accessory sinus (chronic) (*see also* Sinusitis) 473.9
- adrenal gland 255.8
- antrum (chronic) (*see also* Sinusitis, maxillary) 473.0
- bladder (*see also* Cystitis) 595.89
- bowel 569.89
- brain 324.0
  - late effect 326
- breast 611.0
  - puerperal, postpartum 675.1 ☑
- dental periosteum 526.5
- diffuse (skin) 686.00
- ear (middle) (*see also* Otitis media) 382.4
  - external (*see also* Otitis, externa) 380.10
  - internal 386.33
- ethmoidal (sinus) (chronic) (*see also* Sinusitis, ethmoidal) 473.2
- fallopian tube (*see also* Salpingo-oophoritis) 614.2
- frontal (sinus) (chronic) (*see also* Sinusitis, frontal) 473.1
- gallbladder (*see also* Cholecystitis, acute) 575.0
- gum 523.30
- hernial sac — *see* Hernia, by site
- intestine 569.89
- joint (*see also* Arthritis, suppurative) 711.0 ☑
- labyrinthine 386.33
- lung 513.0
- mammary gland 611.0
  - puerperal, postpartum 675.1 ☑
- maxilla, maxillary 526.4
  - sinus (chronic) (*see also* Sinusitis, maxillary) 473.0
- muscle 728.0
- nasal sinus (chronic) (*see also* Sinusitis) 473.9
- pancreas 577.0
- parotid gland 527.2
- pelvis, pelvic
  - female (*see also* Disease, pelvis, inflammatory) 614.4
    - acute 614.3
  - male (*see also* Peritonitis) 567.21
- pericranial (*see also* Osteomyelitis) 730.2 ☑
- salivary duct or gland (any) 527.2
- sinus (nasal) (*see also* Sinusitis) 473.9
- sphenoidal (sinus) (chronic) (*see also* Sinusitis, sphenoidal) 473.3
- thymus (gland) 254.1
- thyroid (gland) 245.0
- tonsil 474.8
- uterus (*see also* Endometritis) 615.9
- vagina 616.10
- wound (*see also* Wound, open, by site, complicated)
  - dislocation — *see* Dislocation, by site, compound
  - fracture — *see* Fracture, by site, open
  - scratch or other superficial injury — *see* Injury, superficial, by site

Supraeruption, teeth 524.34

Supraglottitis 464.50
- with obstruction 464.51

Suprapubic drainage 596.89

Suprarenal (gland) — *see* condition

Suprascapular nerve — *see* condition

Suprasellar — *see* condition

Supraspinatus syndrome 726.10

Surfer knots 919.8
- infected 919.9

Surgery
- cosmetic NEC V50.1
  - breast reconstruction following mastectomy V51.0
  - following healed injury or operation V51.8
  - hair transplant V50.0
- elective V50.9
  - breast
    - augmentation or reduction V50.1
    - reconstruction following mastectomy V51.0

Surgery — *continued*
- elective — *continued*
  - circumcision, ritual or routine (in absence of medical indication) V50.2
  - cosmetic NEC V50.1
  - ear piercing V50.3
  - face-lift V50.1
  - following healed injury or operation V51.8
  - hair transplant V50.0
- not done because of
  - contraindication V64.1
  - patient's decision V64.2
  - specified reason NEC V64.3
- plastic
  - breast
    - augmentation or reduction V50.1
    - reconstruction following mastectomy V51.0
  - cosmetic V50.1
  - face-lift V50.1
  - following healed injury or operation V51.8
  - repair of scarred tissue (following healed injury or operation) V51.8
  - specified type NEC V50.8
- previous, in pregnancy or childbirth
  - cervix 654.6 ☑
    - affecting fetus or newborn (*see also* Newborn, affected by) 760.63
    - causing obstructed labor 660.2 ☑
      - affecting fetus or newborn 763.1
  - pelvic soft tissues NEC 654.9 ☑
    - affecting fetus or newborn (*see also* Newborn, affected by) 760.63
    - causing obstructed labor 660.2 ☑
      - affecting fetus or newborn 763.1
  - perineum or vulva 654.8 ☑
  - uterus NEC 654.9 ☑
    - affecting fetus or newborn (*see also* Newborn, affected by) 760.63
    - causing obstructed labor 660.2 ☑
      - affecting fetus or newborn 763.1
    - due to previous cesarean delivery 654.2 ☑
  - vagina 654.7 ☑

Surgical
- abortion — *see* Abortion, legal
- emphysema 998.81
- kidney (*see also* Pyelitis) 590.80
- operation NEC 799.9
- procedures, complication or misadventure — *see* Complications, surgical procedure
- shock 998.00

Survey
- fetal anatomic V28.81

Susceptibility
- genetic
  - to
    - MEN (multiple endocrine neoplasia) V84.81
  - neoplasia
    - multiple endocrine (MEN) V84.81
  - neoplasm
    - malignant, of
      - breast V84.01
      - endometrium V84.04
      - other V84.09
      - ovary V84.02
      - prostate V84.03
    - specified disease V84.89

Suspected condition, ruled out — *see also* Observation, suspected V71.9
- specified condition NEC V71.89

Suspended uterus, in pregnancy or childbirth 654.4 ☑
- affecting fetus or newborn 763.89
- causing obstructed labor 660.2 ☑
  - affecting fetus or newborn 763.1

Sutton and Gull's disease (arteriolar nephrosclerosis) — *see also* Hypertension, kidney 403.90

Sutton's disease 709.09

☑ **Additional Digit Required — Refer to the Tabular List for Digit Selection**   ▽ **Subterms under main terms may continue to next column or page**

2015 ICD-9-CM   ►◄ **Revised Text**   ● **New Line**   ▲ **Revised Code**   **Volume 2 — 267**

Suture
- burst (in external operation wound) (*see also* Dehiscence) 998.32
  - internal 998.31
- inadvertently left in operation wound 998.4
- removal V58.32
- Shirodkar, in pregnancy (with or without cervical incompetence) 654.5 ☑

Swab inadvertently left in operation wound 998.4

Swallowed, swallowing
- difficulty (*see also* Dysphagia) 787.20
- foreign body NEC (*see also* Foreign body) 938

Swamp fever 100.89

Swan neck hand (intrinsic) 736.09

Sweat(s), sweating
- disease or sickness 078.2
- excessive (*see also* Hyperhidrosis) 780.8
- fetid 705.89
- fever 078.2
- gland disease 705.9
  - specified type NEC 705.89
- miliary 078.2
- night 780.8

Sweeley-Klionsky disease (angiokeratoma corporis diffusum) 272.7

Sweet's syndrome (acute febrile neutrophilic dermatosis) 695.89

Swelling 782.3
- abdominal (not referable to specific organ) 789.3 ☑
- adrenal gland, cloudy 255.8
- ankle 719.07
- anus 787.99
- arm 729.81
- breast 611.72
- Calabar 125.2
- cervical gland 785.6
- cheek 784.2
- chest 786.6
- ear 388.8
- epigastric 789.3 ☑
- extremity (lower) (upper) 729.81
- eye 379.92
- female genital organ 625.8
- finger 729.81
- foot 729.81
- glands 785.6
- gum 784.2
- hand 729.81
- head 784.2
- inflammatory — *see* Inflammation
- joint (*see also* Effusion, joint) 719.0 ☑
  - tuberculous — *see* Tuberculosis, joint
- kidney 593.89
- leg 729.81
- limb 729.81
- liver 573.8
- lung 786.6
- lymph nodes 785.6
- mediastinal 786.6
- mouth 784.2
- muscle (limb) 729.81
- neck 784.2
- nose or sinus 784.2
- palate 784.2
- pelvis 789.3 ☑
- penis 607.83
- perineum 625.8
- rectum 787.99
- scrotum 608.86
- skin 782.2
- splenic (*see also* Splenomegaly) 789.2
- substernal 786.6
- superficial, localized (skin) 782.2
- testicle 608.86
- throat 784.2
- toe 729.81
- tongue 784.2
- tubular (*see also* Disease, renal) 593.9
- umbilicus 789.3 ☑
- uterus 625.8
- vagina 625.8
- vulva 625.8

Swelling — *continued*
- wandering, due to Gnathostoma (spinigerum) 128.1
- white — *see* Tuberculosis, arthritis

Swift's disease 985.0

Swimmers'
- ear (acute) 380.12
- itch 120.3

Swimming in the head 780.4

Swollen — *see also* Swelling
- glands 785.6

Swyer-James syndrome (unilateral hyperlucent lung) 492.8

Swyer's syndrome (XY pure gonadal dysgenesis) 752.7

Sycosis 704.8
- barbae (not parasitic) 704.8
- contagiosa 110.0
- lupoid 704.8
- mycotic 110.0
- parasitic 110.0
- vulgaris 704.8

Sydenham's chorea — *see* Chorea, Sydenham's

Sylvatic yellow fever 060.0

Sylvest's disease (epidemic pleurodynia) 074.1

Symblepharon 372.63
- congenital 743.62

Symonds' syndrome 348.2

Sympathetic — *see* condition

Sympatheticotonia — *see also* Neuropathy, peripheral, autonomic 337.9

Sympathicoblastoma (M9500/3)
- specified site — *see* Neoplasm, by site, malignant
- unspecified site 194.0

Sympathicogonioma (M9500/3) — *see* Sympathicoblastoma

Sympathoblastoma (M9500/3) — *see* Sympathicoblastoma

Sympathogonioma (M9500/3) — *see* Sympathicoblastoma

Symphalangy — *see also* Syndactylism 755.10

Symptoms, specified (general) NEC 780.99
- abdomen NEC 789.9
- bone NEC 733.90
- breast NEC 611.79
- cardiac NEC 785.9
- cardiovascular NEC 785.9
- chest NEC 786.9
- cognition 799.59
- development NEC 783.9
- digestive system NEC 787.99
- emotional state NEC 799.29
- eye NEC 379.99
- gastrointestinal tract NEC 787.99
- genital organs NEC
  - female 625.9
  - male 608.9
- head and neck NEC 784.99
- heart NEC 785.9
- jaw 784.92
- joint NEC 719.60
  - ankle 719.67
  - elbow 719.62
  - foot 719.67
  - hand 719.64
  - hip 719.65
  - knee 719.66
  - multiple sites 719.69
  - pelvic region 719.65
  - shoulder (region) 719.61
  - specified site NEC 719.68
  - temporomandibular 524.69
  - wrist 719.63
- larynx NEC 784.99
- limbs NEC 729.89
- lymphatic system NEC 785.9
- maxilla 784.92
- menopausal 627.2
- metabolism NEC 783.9
- mouth NEC 528.9
- muscle NEC 728.9
- musculoskeletal NEC 781.99
  - limbs NEC 729.89
- nervous system NEC 781.99

Symptoms, specified — *continued*
- neurotic NEC 300.9
- nutrition, metabolism, and development NEC 783.9
- pelvis NEC 789.9
  - female 625.9
- peritoneum NEC 789.9
- respiratory system NEC 786.9
- skin and integument NEC 782.9
- subcutaneous tissue NEC 782.9
- throat NEC 784.99
- tonsil NEC 784.99
- urinary system NEC 788.99
- vascular NEC 785.9

Sympus 759.89

Synarthrosis 719.80
- ankle 719.87
- elbow 719.82
- foot 719.87
- hand 719.84
- hip 719.85
- knee 719.86
- multiple sites 719.89
- pelvic region 719.85
- shoulder (region) 719.81
- specified site NEC 719.88
- wrist 719.83

Syncephalus 759.4

Synchondrosis 756.9
- abnormal (congenital) 756.9
- ischiopubic (van Neck's) 732.1

Synchysis (senile) (vitreous humor) 379.21
- scintillans 379.22

Syncope (near) (pre-) 780.2
- anginosa 413.9
- bradycardia 427.89
- cardiac 780.2
- carotid sinus 337.01
- complicating delivery 669.2 ☑
- due to lumbar puncture 349.0
- fatal 798.1
- heart 780.2
- heat 992.1
- laryngeal 786.2
- tussive 786.2
- vasoconstriction 780.2
- vasodepressor 780.2
- vasomotor 780.2
- vasovagal 780.2

Syncytial infarct — *see* Placenta, abnormal

Syndactylism, syndactyly (multiple sites) 755.10
- fingers (without fusion of bone) 755.11
  - with fusion of bone 755.12
- toes (without fusion of bone) 755.13
  - with fusion of bone 755.14

Syndrome — *see also* Disease
- with 5q deletion 238.74
- 5q minus 238.74
- abdominal
  - acute 789.0 ☑
  - migraine 346.2 ☑
  - muscle deficiency 756.79
- Abercrombie's (amyloid degeneration) 277.39
- abnormal innervation 374.43
- abstinence
  - alcohol 291.81
  - drug 292.0
  - neonatal 779.5
- Abt-Letterer-Siwe (acute histiocytosis X) (M9722/3) 202.5 ☑
- Achard-Thiers (adrenogenital) 255.2
- acid pulmonary aspiration 997.39
  - obstetric (Mendelson's) 668.0 ☑
- acquired immune deficiency 042
- acquired immunodeficiency 042
- acrocephalosyndactylism 755.55
- acute abdominal 789.0 ☑
- acute chest 517.3
- acute coronary 411.1
- Adair-Dighton (brittle bones and blue sclera, deafness) 756.51
- Adams-Stokes (-Morgagni) (syncope with heart block) 426.9
- Addisonian 255.41

Syndrome — *see also* Disease — *continued*
- Adie (-Holmes) (pupil) 379.46
- adiposogenital 253.8
- adrenal
  - hemorrhage 036.3
  - meningococcic 036.3
- adrenocortical 255.3
- adrenogenital (acquired) (congenital) 255.2
  - feminizing 255.2
  - iatrogenic 760.79
  - virilism (acquired) (congenital) 255.2
- affective organic NEC 293.89
  - drug-induced 292.84
- afferent loop NEC 537.89
- African macroglobulinemia 273.3
- Ahumada-Del Castillo (nonpuerperal galactorrhea and amenorrhea) 253.1
- air blast concussion — *see* Injury, internal, by site
- Alagille 759.89
- Albright (-Martin) (pseudohypoparathyroidism) 275.49
- Albright-McCune-Sternberg (osteitis fibrosa disseminata) 756.59
- alcohol withdrawal 291.81
- Alder's (leukocyte granulation anomaly) 288.2
- Aldrich (-Wiskott) (eczema-thrombocytopenia) 279.12
- Alibert-Bazin (mycosis fungoides) (M9700/3) 202.1 ☑
- Alice in Wonderland 293.89
- alien hand 781.8
- Allen-Masters 620.6
- Alligator baby (ichthyosis congenita) 757.1
- Alport's (hereditary hematuria-nephropathy-deafness) 759.89
- Alvarez (transient cerebral ischemia) 435.9
- alveolar capillary block 516.8
- Alzheimer's 331.0
  - with dementia — *see* Alzheimer's, dementia
- amnestic (confabulatory) 294.0
  - alcohol-induced persisting 291.1
  - drug-induced 292.83
  - posttraumatic 294.0
- amotivational 292.89
- amyostatic 275.1
- amyotrophic lateral sclerosis 335.20
- androgen insensitivity 259.51
  - partial 259.52
- Angelman 759.89
- angina (*see also* Angina) 413.9
- ankyloglossia superior 750.0
- anterior
  - chest wall 786.52
  - compartment (tibial) 958.8
  - spinal artery 433.8 ☑
    - compression 721.1
  - tibial (compartment) 958.8
- antibody deficiency 279.00
  - agammaglobulinemic 279.00
  - congenital 279.04
  - hypogammaglobulinemic 279.00
- anticardiolipin antibody 289.81
- antimongolism 758.39
- antiphospholipid antibody 289.81
- Anton (-Babinski) (hemiasomatognosia) 307.9
- anxiety (*see also* Anxiety) 300.00
  - organic 293.84
- aortic
  - arch 446.7
  - bifurcation (occlusion) 444.09
  - ring 747.21
- Apert's (acrocephalosyndactyly) 755.55
- Apert-Gallais (adrenogenital) 255.2
- aphasia-apraxia-alexia 784.69
- apical ballooning 429.83
- "approximate answers" 300.16
- arcuate ligament (-celiac axis) 447.4
- arcus aortae 446.7
- arc welders' 370.24
- argentaffin, argintaffinoma 259.2
- Argonz-Del Castillo (nonpuerperal galactorrhea and amenorrhea) 253.1

☑ **Additional Digit Required** — Refer to the Tabular List for Digit Selection   ⧉ Subterms under main terms may continue to next column or page

Syndrome — *see also* Disease — *continued*
Argyll Robertson's (syphilitic) 094.89
  nonsyphilitic 379.45
Armenian 277.31
arm-shoulder (*see also* Neuropathy, peripheral, autonomic) 337.9
Arnold-Chiari (*see also* Spina bifida) 741.0 ☑
  type I 348.4
  type II 741.0 ☑
  type III 742.0
  type IV 742.2
Arrillaga-Ayerza (pulmonary artery sclerosis with pulmonary hypertension) 416.0
arteriomesenteric duodenum occlusion 537.89
arteriovenous steal 996.73
arteritis, young female (obliterative brachiocephalic) 446.7
aseptic meningitis — *see* Meningitis, aseptic
Asherman's 621.5 ☑
Asperger's 299.8 ☑
asphyctic (*see also* Anxiety) 300.00
aspiration, of newborn (massive) 770.18
  meconium 770.12
ataxia-telangiectasia 334.8
Audry's (acropachyderma) 757.39
auriculotemporal 350.8
autoimmune lymphoproliferative (ALPS) 279.41
autosomal (*see also* Abnormal, autosomes NEC)
  deletion 758.39
    5p 758.31
    22q11.2 758.32
Avellis' 344.89
Axenfeld's 743.44
Ayerza (-Arrillaga) (pulmonary artery sclerosis with pulmonary hypertension) 416.0
Baader's (erythema multiforme exudativum) 695.19
Baastrup's 721.5
Babinski (-Vaquez) (cardiovascular syphilis) 093.89
Babinski-Fröhlich (adiposogenital dystrophy) 253.8
Babinski-Nageotte 344.89
Bagratuni's (temporal arteritis) 446.5
Bakwin-Krida (craniometaphyseal dysplasia) 756.89
Balint's (psychic paralysis of visual disorientation) 368.16
Ballantyne (-Runge) (postmaturity) 766.22
ballooning posterior leaflet 424.0
Banti's — *see* Cirrhosis, liver
Bardet-Biedl (obesity, polydactyly, and intellectual disabiilties) 759.89
Bard-Pic's (carcinoma, head of pancreas) 157.0
Barlow's (mitral valve prolapse) 424.0
Barlow (-Möller) (infantile scurvy) 267
Baron Munchausen's 301.51
Barré-Guillain 357.0
Barré-Liéou (posterior cervical sympathetic) 723.2
Barrett's (chronic peptic ulcer of esophagus) 530.85
Bársony-Polgár (corkscrew esophagus) 530.5
Bársony-Teschendorf (corkscrew esophagus) 530.5
Barth 759.89
Bartter's (secondary hyperaldosteronism with juxtaglomerular hyperplasia) 255.13
basal cell nevus 759.89
Basedow's (exophthalmic goiter) 242.0 ☑
basilar artery 435.0
basofrontal 377.04
Bassen-Kornzweig (abetalipoproteinemia) 272.5
Batten-Steinert 359.21
battered
  adult 995.81
  baby or child 995.54
  spouse 995.81

Syndrome — *see also* Disease — *continued*
Baumgarten-Cruveilhier (cirrhosis of liver) 571.5
Beals 759.82
Bearn-Kunkel (-Slater) (lupoid hepatitis) 571.49
Beau's (*see also* Degeneration, myocardial) 429.1
Bechterew-Strümpell-Marie (ankylosing spondylitis) 720.0
Beck's (anterior spinal artery occlusion) 433.8 ☑
Beckwith (-Wiedemann) 759.89
Behçet's 136.1
Bekhterev-Strümpell-Marie (ankylosing spondylitis) 720.0
Benedikt's 344.89
Béquez César (-Steinbrinck-Chédiak-Higashi) (congenital gigantism of peroxidase granules) 288.2
Bernard-Horner (*see also* Neuropathy, peripheral, autonomic) 337.9
Bernard-Sergent (acute adrenocortical insufficiency) 255.41
Bernhardt-Roth 355.1
Bernheim's (*see also* Failure, heart) 428.0
Bertolotti's (sacralization of fifth lumbar vertebra) 756.15
Besnier-Boeck-Schaumann (sarcoidosis) 135
Bianchi's (aphasia-apraxia-alexia syndrome) 784.69
Biedl-Bardet (obesity, polydactyly, and intellectual disabilities) 759.89
Biemond's (obesity, polydactyly, and intellectual disabilities) 759.89
big spleen 289.4
bilateral polycystic ovarian 256.4
Bing-Horton's 339.00
Biörck (-Thorson) (malignant carcinoid) 259.2
Birt-Hogg-Dube 759.89
Blackfan-Diamond (congenital hypoplastic anemia) 284.01
black lung 500
black widow spider bite 989.5
bladder neck (*see also* Incontinence, urine) 788.30
blast (concussion) — *see* Blast, injury
blind loop (postoperative) 579.2
Bloch-Siemens (incontinentia pigmenti) 757.33
Bloch-Sulzberger (incontinentia pigmenti) 757.33
Bloom (-Machacek) (-Torre) 757.39
Blount-Barber (tibia vara) 732.4
blue
  bloater 491.20
    with
      acute bronchitis 491.22
      exacerbation (acute) 491.21
  diaper 270.0
  drum 381.02
  sclera 756.51
  toe 445.02
Boder-Sedgwick (ataxia-telangiectasia) 334.8
Boerhaave's (spontaneous esophageal rupture) 530.4
Bonnevie-Ullrich 758.6
Bonnier's 386.19
Borjeson-Forssman-Lehmann 759.89
Bouillaud's (rheumatic heart disease) 391.9
Bourneville (-Pringle) (tuberous sclerosis) 759.5
Bouveret (-Hoffmann) (paroxysmal tachycardia) 427.2
brachial plexus 353.0
Brachman-de Lange (Amsterdam dwarf, intellectual disabilities, and brachycephaly) 759.89
bradycardia-tachycardia 427.81
Brailsford-Morquio (dystrophy) (mucopolysaccharidosis IV) 277.5
brain (acute) (chronic) (nonpsychotic) (organic) (with behavioral reaction) (with neurotic reaction) 310.9

Syndrome — *see also* Disease — *continued*
brain — *continued*
  with
    presenile brain disease (*see also* Dementia, presenile) 290.10
    psychosis, psychotic reaction (*see also* Psychosis, organic) 294.9
  chronic alcoholic 291.2
  congenital (*see also* Disability, intellectual) 319
  postcontusional 310.2
  posttraumatic
    nonpsychotic 310.2
    psychotic 293.9
      acute 293.0
      chronic (*see also* Psychosis, organic) 294.8
      subacute 293.1
  psycho-organic (*see also* Syndrome, psycho-organic) 310.9
  psychotic (*see also* Psychosis, organic) 294.9
  senile (*see also* Dementia, senile) 290.0
branchial arch 744.41
Brandt's (acrodermatitis enteropathica) 686.8
Brennemann's 289.2
Briquet's 300.81
Brissaud-Meige (infantile myxedema) 244.9
broad ligament laceration 620.6
Brock's (atelectasis due to enlarged lymph nodes) 518.0
broken heart 429.83
Brown-Séquard 344.89
brown spot 756.59
Brown's (tendon sheath) 378.61
Brugada 746.89
Brugsch's (acropachyderma) 757.39
bubbly lung 770.7
Buchem's (hyperostosis corticalis) 733.3
Budd-Chiari (hepatic vein thrombosis) 453.0
Büdinger-Ludloff-Läwen 717.89
bulbar 335.22
  lateral (*see also* Disease, cerebrovascular, acute) 436
Bullis fever 082.8
bundle of Kent (anomalous atrioventricular excitation) 426.7
Bürger-Grütz (essential familial hyperlipemia) 272.3
Burke's (pancreatic insufficiency and chronic neutropenia) 577.8
Burnett's (milk-alkali) 275.42
Burnier's (hypophyseal dwarfism) 253.3
burning feet 266.2
Bywaters' 958.5
Caffey's (infantile cortical hyperostosis) 756.59
Calvé-Legg-Perthes (osteochrondrosis, femoral capital) 732.1
Caplan (-Colinet) syndrome 714.81
capsular thrombosis (*see also* Thrombosis, brain) 434.0 ☑
carbohydrate-deficient glycoprotein (CDGS) 271.8
carcinogenic thrombophlebitis 453.1
carcinoid 259.2
cardiac asthma (*see also* Failure, ventricular, left) 428.1
cardiacos negros 416.0
cardiofaciocutaneous 759.89
cardiopulmonary obesity 278.03
cardiorenal (*see also* Hypertension, cardiorenal) 404.90
cardiorespiratory distress (idiopathic), newborn 769
cardiovascular renal (*see also* Hypertension, cardiorenal) 404.90
cardiovasorenal 272.7
Carini's (ichthyosis congenita) 757.1
carotid
  artery (internal) 435.8
  body or sinus 337.01
carpal tunnel 354.0
Carpenter's 759.89

Syndrome — *see also* Disease — *continued*
Cassidy (-Scholte) (malignant carcinoid) 259.2
cat-cry 758.31
cauda equina 344.60
causalgia 355.9
  lower limb 355.71
  upper limb 354.4
cavernous sinus 437.6
celiac 579.0
  artery compression 447.4
  axis 447.4
central pain 338.0
cerebellomedullary malformation (*see also* Spina bifida) 741.0 ☑
cerebral gigantism 253.0
cerebrohepatorenal 759.89
cervical (root) (spine) NEC 723.8
  disc 722.71
  posterior, sympathetic 723.2
  rib 353.0
  sympathetic paralysis 337.09
  traumatic (acute) NEC 847.0
cervicobrachial (diffuse) 723.3
cervicocranial 723.2
cervicodorsal outlet 353.2
Céstan's 344.89
Céstan (-Raymond) 433.8 ☑
Céstan-Chenais 344.89
chancriform 114.1
Charcôt's (intermittent claudication) 443.9
  angina cruris 443.9
  due to atherosclerosis 440.21
Charcôt-Marie-Tooth 356.1
Charcôt-Weiss-Baker 337.01
CHARGE association 759.89
Cheadle (-Möller) (-Barlow) (infantile scurvy) 267
Chédiak-Higashi (-Steinbrinck) (congenital gigantism of peroxidase granules) 288.2
chest wall 786.52
Chiari's (hepatic vein thrombosis) 453.0
Chiari-Frommel 676.6 ☑
chiasmatic 368.41
Chilaiditi's (subphrenic displacement, colon) 751.4
chondroectodermal dysplasia 756.55
chorea-athetosis-agitans 275.1
Christian's (chronic histiocytosis X) 277.89
chromosome 4 short arm deletion 758.39
chronic pain 338.4
Churg-Strauss 446.4
Clarke-Hadfield (pancreatic infantilism) 577.8
Claude's 352.6
Claude Bernard-Horner (*see also* Neuropathy, peripheral, autonomic) 337.9
Clérambault's
  automatism 348.89
  erotomania 297.8
Clifford's (postmaturity) 766.22
climacteric 627.2
Clouston's (hidrotic ectodermal dysplasia) 757.31
clumsiness 315.4
Cockayne's (microencephaly and dwarfism) 759.89
Cockayne-Weber (epidermolysis bullosa) 757.39
Coffin-Lowry 759.89
Cogan's (nonsyphilitic interstitial keratitis) 370.52
cold injury (newborn) 778.2
Collet (-Sicard) 352.6
combined immunity deficiency 279.2
compartment(al) (anterior) (deep) (posterior) 958.8
  nontraumatic
    abdomen 729.73
    arm 729.71
    buttock 729.72
    fingers 729.71
    foot 729.72
    forearm 729.71
    hand 729.71

☑ Additional Digit Required — Refer to the Tabular List for Digit Selection   ▽ Subterms under main terms may continue to next column or page

2015 ICD-9-CM   ▶◀ Revised Text   ● New Line   ▲ Revised Code   Volume 2 — 269

Syndrome — *see also* Disease — *continued*
- compartment — *continued*
  - nontraumatic — *continued*
    - hip 729.72
    - leg 729.72
    - lower extremity 729.72
    - shoulder 729.71
    - specified site NEC 729.79
    - thigh 729.72
    - toes 729.72
    - upper extremity 729.71
    - wrist 729.71
  - post-surgical (*see also* Syndrome, compartment, non-traumatic) 998.89
  - traumatic 958.90
    - abdomen 958.93
    - arm 958.91
    - buttock 958.92
    - fingers 958.91
    - foot 958.92
    - forearm 958.91
    - hand 958.91
    - hip 958.92
    - leg 958.92
    - lower extremity 958.92
    - shoulder 958.91
    - specified site NEC 958.99
    - thigh 958.92
    - tibial 958.92
    - toes 958.92
    - upper extremity 958.91
    - wrist 958.91
- complex regional pain — *see also* Dystrophy, sympathetic
  - type I — *see* Dystrophy, sympathetic (posttraumatic) (reflex)
  - type II — *see* Causalgia
- compression 958.5
  - cauda equina 344.60
    - with neurogenic bladder 344.61
- concussion 310.2
- congenital
  - affecting more than one system 759.7
    - specified type NEC 759.89
  - congenital central alveolar hypoventilation 327.25
  - facial diplegia 352.6
  - muscular hypertrophy-cerebral 759.89
- congestion-fibrosis (pelvic) 625.5
- conjunctivourethrosynovial 099.3
- Conn (-Louis) (primary aldosteronism) 255.12
- Conradi (-Hünermann) (chondrodysplasia calcificans congenita) 756.59
- conus medullaris 336.8
- Cooke-Apert-Gallais (adrenogenital) 255.2
- Cornelia de Lange's (Amsterdam dwarf, intellectual disabilities, and brachycephaly) 759.8 ☑
- coronary insufficiency or intermediate 411.1
- cor pulmonale 416.9
- corticosexual 255.2
- Costen's (complex) 524.60
- costochondral junction 733.6
- costoclavicular 353.0
- costovertebral 253.0
- Cotard's (paranoia) 297.1
- Cowden 759.6
- craniovertebral 723.2
- Creutzfeldt-Jakob 046.19
  - with dementia
    - with behavioral disturbance 046.19 [294.11]
    - without behavioral disturbance 046.19 [294.10]
  - variant 046.11
    - with dementia
      - with behavioral disturbance 046.11 [294.11]
      - without behavioral disturbance 046.11 [294.10]
- crib death 798.0
- cricopharyngeal 787.20
- cri-du-chat 758.31
- Crigler-Najjar (congenital hyperbilirubinemia) 277.4

Syndrome — *see also* Disease — *continued*
- crocodile tears 351.8
- Cronkhite-Canada 211.3
- croup 464.4
- CRST (cutaneous systemic sclerosis) 710.1
- crush 958.5
- crushed lung (*see also* Injury, internal, lung) 861.20
- Cruveilhier-Baumgarten (cirrhosis of liver) 571.5
- cubital tunnel 354.2
- Cuiffini-Pancoast (M8010/3) (carcinoma, pulmonary apex) 162.3
- Curschmann (-Batten) (-Steinert) 359.21
- Cushing's (iatrogenic) (idiopathic) (pituitary basophilism) (pituitary-dependent) 255.0
  - overdose or wrong substance given or taken 962.0
- Cyriax's (slipping rib) 733.99
- cystic duct stump 576.0
- Da Costa's (neurocirculatory asthenia) 306.2
- Dameshek's (erythroblastic anemia) 282.49
- Dana-Putnam (subacute combined sclerosis with pernicious anemia) 281.0 [336.2]
- Danbolt (-Closs) (acrodermatitis enteropathica) 686.8
- Dandy-Walker (atresia, foramen of Magendie) 742.3
  - with spina bifida (*see also* Spina bifida) 741.0 ☑
- Danlos' 756.83
- Davies-Colley (slipping rib) 733.99
- dead fetus 641.3 ☑
- defeminization 255.2
- defibrination (*see also* Fibrinolysis) 286.6
- Degos' 447.8
- Deiters' nucleus 386.19
- Déjérine-Roussy 338.0
- Déjérine-Thomas 333.0
- de Lange's (Amsterdam dwarf, intellectual disabilities, and brachycephaly) (Cornelia) 759.89
- Del Castillo's (germinal aplasia) 606.0
- deletion chromosomes 758.39
- delusional
  - induced by drug 292.11
- dementia-aphonia, of childhood (*see also* Psychosis, childhood) 299.1 ☑
- demyelinating NEC 341.9
- denial visual hallucination 307.9
- depersonalization 300.6
- de Quervain's 259.51
- Dercum's (adiposis dolorosa) 272.8
- de Toni-Fanconi (-Debré) (cystinosis) 270.0
- diabetes-dwarfism-obesity (juvenile) 258.1
- diabetes mellitus-hypertension-nephrosis 250.4 ☑ [581.81]
  - due to secondary diabetes 249.4 ☑ [581.81]
- diabetes mellitus in newborn infant 775.1
- diabetes-nephrosis 250.4 ☑ [581.81]
  - due to secondary diabetes 249.4 ☑ [581.81]
- diabetic amyotrophy 250.6 ☑ [353.5]
  - due to secondary diabetes 249.6 ☑ [353.5]
- Diamond-Blackfan (congenital hypoplastic anemia) 284.01
- Diamond-Gardener (autoerythrocyte sensitization) 287.2
- DIC (diffuse or disseminated intravascular coagulopathy) (*see also* Fibrinolysis) 286.6
- diencephalohypophyseal NEC 253.8
- diffuse cervicobrachial 723.3
- diffuse obstructive pulmonary 496
- DiGeorge's (thymic hypoplasia) 279.11
- Dighton's 756.51
- Di Guglielmo's (erythremic myelosis) (M9841/3) 207.0 ☑
- disequilibrium 276.9
- disseminated platelet thrombosis 446.6
- Ditthomska 307.81
- Doan-Wisemann (primary splenic neutropenia) 289.53

Syndrome — *see also* Disease — *continued*
- Döhle body-panmyelopathic 288.2
- Donohue's (leprechaunism) 259.8
- dorsolateral medullary (*see also* Disease, cerebrovascular, acute) 436
- double athetosis 333.71
- double whammy 360.81
- Down's (mongolism) 758.0
- Dresbach's (elliptocytosis) 282.1
- Dressler's (postmyocardial infarction) 411.0
  - hemoglobinuria 283.2
  - postcardiotomy 429.4
- drug withdrawal, infant, of dependent mother 779.5
- dry skin 701.1
  - eye 375.15
- DSAP (disseminated superficial actinic porokeratosis) 692.75
- Duane's (retraction) 378.71
- Duane-Stilling-Türk (ocular retraction syndrome) 378.71
- Dubin-Johnson (constitutional hyperbilirubinemia) 277.4
- Dubin-Sprinz (constitutional hyperbilirubinemia) 277.4
- Duchenne's 335.22
- due to abnormality
  - autosomal NEC (*see also* Abnormal, autosomes NEC) 758.5
    - 13 758.1
    - 18 758.2
    - 21 or 22 758.0
    - D1 758.1
    - E3 758.2
    - G 758.0
  - chromosomal 758.89
    - sex 758.81
- dumping 564.2
  - nonsurgical 536.8
- Duplay's 726.2
- Dupré's (meningism) 781.6
- Dyke-Young (acquired macrocytic hemolytic anemia) 283.9
- dyspraxia 315.4
- dystocia, dystrophia 654.9 ☑
- Eagle-Barret 756.71
- Eales' 362.18
- Eaton-Lambert (*see also* Syndrome, Lambert-Eaton) 358.30
- Ebstein's (downward displacement, tricuspid valve into right ventricle) 746.2
- ectopic ACTH secretion 255.0
- eczema-thrombocytopenia 279.12
- Eddowes' (brittle bones and blue sclera) 756.51
- Edwards' 758.2
- efferent loop 537.89
- effort (aviators') (psychogenic) 306.2
- Ehlers-Danlos 756.83
- Eisenmenger's (ventricular septal defect) 745.4
- Ekbom's (restless legs) 333.94
- Ekman's (brittle bones and blue sclera) 756.51
- electric feet 266.2
- Elephant man 237.71
- Ellison-Zollinger (gastric hypersecretion with pancreatic islet cell tumor) 251.5
- Ellis-van Creveld (chondroectodermal dysplasia) 756.55
- embryonic fixation 270.2
- empty sella (turcica) 253.8
- endocrine-hypertensive 255.3
- Engel-von Recklinghausen (osteitis fibrosa cystica) 252.01
- enteroarticular 099.3
- entrapment — *see* Neuropathy, entrapment
- eosinophilia myalgia 710.5
- epidemic vomiting 078.82
- Epstein's — *see* Nephrosis
- Erb (-Oppenheim)-Goldflam 358.00
- Erdheim's (acromegalic macrospondylitis) 253.0
- Erdheim-Chester 277.89
- Erlacher-Blount (tibia vara) 732.4
- erythrocyte fragmentation 283.19

Syndrome — *see also* Disease — *continued*
- euthyroid sick 790.94
- Evans' (thrombocytopenic purpura) 287.32
- excess cortisol, iatrogenic 255.0
- exhaustion 300.5
- extrapyramidal 333.90
- eyelid-malar-mandible 756.0
- eye retraction 378.71
- Faber's (achlorhydric anemia) 280.9
- Fabry (-Anderson) (angiokeratoma corporis diffusum) 272.7
- facet 724.8
- Fallot's 745.2
- falx (*see also* Hemorrhage, brain) 431
- familial eczema-thrombocytopenia 279.12
- Fanconi's (anemia) (congenital pancytopenia) 284.09
- Fanconi (-de Toni) (-Debré) (cystinosis) 270.0
- Farber (-Uzman) (disseminated lipogranulomatosis) 272.8
- fatigue NEC 300.5
  - chronic 780.71
- faulty bowel habit (idiopathic megacolon) 564.7
- FDH (focal dermal hypoplasia) 757.39
- fecal reservoir 560.39
- Feil-Klippel (brevicollis) 756.16
- Felty's (rheumatoid arthritis with splenomegaly and leukopenia) 714.1
- fertile eunuch 257.2
- fetal alcohol 760.71
  - late effect 760.71
- fibrillation-flutter 427.32
- fibrositis (periarticular) 729.0
- Fiedler's (acute isolated myocarditis) 422.91
- Fiessinger-Leroy (-Reiter) 099.3
- Fiessinger-Rendu (erythema multiforme exudativum) 695.19
- first arch 756.0
- Fisher's 357.0
- fish odor 270.8
- Fitz's (acute hemorrhagic pancreatitis) 577.0
- Fitz-Hugh and Curtis 098.86
  - due to
    - Chlamydia trachomatis 099.56
    - Neisseria gonorrhoeae (gonococcal peritonitis) 098.86
- Flajani (-Basedow) (exophthalmic goiter) 242.0 ☑
- flat back
  - acquired 737.29
  - postprocedural 738.5
- floppy
  - infant 781.99
  - iris 364.81
  - valve (mitral) 424.0
- flush 259.2
- Foix-Alajouanine 336.1
- Fong's (hereditary osteo-onychodysplasia) 756.89
- foramen magnum 348.4
- Forbes-Albright (nonpuerperal amenorrhea and lactation associated with pituitary tumor) 253.1
- Foster-Kennedy 377.04
- Foville's (peduncular) 344.89
- fragile X 759.83
- Franceschetti's (mandibulofacial dysostosis) 756.0
- Fraser's 759.89
- Freeman-Sheldon 759.89
- Frey's (auriculotemporal) 705.22
- Friderichsen-Waterhouse 036.3
- Friedrich-Erb-Arnold (acropachyderma) 757.39
- Fröhlich's (adiposogenital dystrophy) 253.8
- Froin's 336.8
- Frommel-Chiari 676.6 ☑
- frontal lobe 310.0
- Fukuhara 277.87
- Fuller Albright's (osteitis fibrosa disseminata) 756.59
- functional
  - bowel 564.9
  - prepubertal castrate 752.89

☑ Additional Digit Required — Refer to the Tabular List for Digit Selection   ⚕ Subterms under main terms may continue to next column or page

Syndrome — *see also* Disease — *continued*

Gaisböck's (polycythemia hypertonica) 289.0
ganglion (basal, brain) 333.90
geniculi 351.1
Ganser's, hysterical 300.16
Gardner-Diamond (autoerythrocyte sensitization) 287.2
gastroesophageal junction 530.0
gastroesophageal laceration-hemorrhage 530.7
gastrojejunal loop obstruction 537.89
Gayet-Wernicke's (superior hemorrhagic polioencephalitis) 265.1
Gee-Herter-Heubner (nontropical sprue) 579.0
Gélineau's (*see also* Narcolepsy) 347.00
genito-anorectal 099.1
Gerhardt's (vocal cord paralysis) 478.30
Gerstmann's (finger agnosia) 784.69
Gerstmann-Sträussler-Scheinker (GSS) 046.71
Gianotti Crosti 057.8
due to known virus — *see* Infection, virus
due to unknown virus 057.8
Gilbert's 277.4
Gilford (-Hutchinson) (progeria) 259.8
Gilles de la Tourette's 307.23
Gillespie's (dysplasia oculodentodigitalis) 759.89
Glénard's (enteroptosis) 569.89
Glinski-Simmonds (pituitary cachexia) 253.2
glucuronyl transferase 277.4
glue ear 381.20
Goldberg (-Maxwell) (-Morris) (testicular feminization) 259.51
Goldenhar's (oculoauriculovertebral dysplasia) 756.0
Goldflam-Erb 358.00
Goltz-Gorlin (dermal hypoplasia) 757.39
Good's 279.06
Goodpasture's (pneumorenal) 446.21
Gopalan's (burning feet) 266.2
Gorlin's 759.89
Gorlin-Chaudhry-Moss 759.89
Gougerot-Blum (pigmented purpuric lichenoid dermatitis) 709.1
Gougerot-Carteaud (confluent reticulate papillomatosis) 701.8
Gougerot (-Houwer)-Sjögren (keratoconjunctivitis sicca) 710.2
Gouley's (constrictive pericarditis) 423.2
Gowers' (vasovagal attack) 780.2
Gowers-Paton-Kennedy 377.04
Gradenigo's 383.02
gray or grey (chloramphenicol) (newborn) 779.4
Greig's (hypertelorism) 756.0
GSS (Gerstmann-Sträussler-Scheinker) 046.71
Gubler-Millard 344.89
Guérin-Stern (arthrogryposis multiplex congenita) 754.89
Guillain-Barré (-Strohl) 357.0
Gunn's (jaw-winking syndrome) 742.8
Günther's (congenital erythropoietic porphyria) 277.1
gustatory sweating 350.8
H₃O 759.81
Hadfield-Clarke (pancreatic infantilism) 577.8
Haglund-Läwen-Fründ 717.89
hairless women 257.8
hair tourniquet (*see also* Injury, superficial, by site)
finger 915.8
infected 915.9
penis 911.8
infected 911.9
toe 917.8
infected 917.9
Hallermann-Streiff 756.0
Hallervorden-Spatz 333.0
Hamman's (spontaneous mediastinal emphysema) 518.1

Syndrome — *see also* Disease — *continued*

Hamman-Rich (diffuse interstitial pulmonary fibrosis) 516.33
hand-foot 693.0
Hand-Schüller-Christian (chronic histiocytosis X) 277.89
Hanot-Chauffard (-Troisier) (bronze diabetes) 275.01
Harada's 363.22
Hare's (M8010/3) (carcinoma, pulmonary apex) 162.3
Harkavy's 446.0
harlequin color change 779.89
Harris' (organic hyperinsulinism) 251.1
Hart's (pellagra-cerebellar ataxia-renal aminoaciduria) 270.0
Hayem-Faber (achlorhydric anemia) 280.9
Hayem-Widal (acquired hemolytic jaundice) 283.9
headache — *see* Headache, syndrome
Heberden's (angina pectoris) 413.9
Hedinger's (malignant carcinoid) 259.2
Hegglin's 288.2
Heller's (infantile psychosis) (*see also* Psychosis, childhood) 299.1 ☑
H.E.L.L.P 642.5 ☑
hemolytic-uremic (adult) (child) 283.11
hemophagocytic 288.4
infection-associated 288.4
Hench-Rosenberg (palindromic arthritis) (*see also* Rheumatism, palindromic) 719.3 ☑
Henoch-Schönlein (allergic purpura) 287.0
hepatic flexure 569.89
hepatopulmonary 573.5
hepatorenal 572.4
due to a procedure 997.49
following delivery 674.8 ☑
hepatourologic 572.4
Herrick's (hemoglobin S disease) 282.61
Herter (-Gee) (nontropical sprue) 579.0
Heubner-Herter (nontropical sprue) 579.0
Heyd's (hepatorenal) 572.4
HHHO 759.81
high grade myelodysplastic 238.73
with 5q deletion 238.73
Hilger's 337.09
histiocytic 288.4
Hoffa (-Kastert) (liposynovitis prepatellaris) 272.8
Hoffmann's 244.9 [359.5]
Hoffmann-Bouveret (paroxysmal tachycardia) 427.2
Hoffmann-Werdnig 335.0
Holländer-Simons (progressive lipodystrophy) 272.6
Holmes' (visual disorientation) 368.16
Holmes-Adie 379.46
Hoppe-Goldflam 358.00
Horner's (*see also* Neuropathy, peripheral, autonomic) 337.9
traumatic — *see* Injury, nerve, cervical sympathetic
hospital addiction 301.51
hungry bone 275.5
Hunt's (herpetic geniculate ganglionitis) 053.11
dyssynergia cerebellaris myoclonica 334.2
Hunter (-Hurler) (mucopolysaccharidosis II) 277.5
hunterian glossitis 529.4
Hurler (-Hunter) (mucopolysaccharidosis II) 277.5
Hutchinson-Boeck (sarcoidosis) 135
Hutchinson-Gilford (progeria) 259.8
Hutchinson's incisors or teeth 090.5
hydralazine
correct substance properly administered 695.4
overdose or wrong substance given or taken 972.6
hydraulic concussion (abdomen) (*see also* Injury, internal, abdomen) 868.00
hyperabduction 447.8
hyperactive bowel 564.9

Syndrome — *see also* Disease — *continued*

hyperaldosteronism with hypokalemic alkalosis (Bartter's) 255.13
hypercalcemic 275.42
hypercoagulation NEC 289.89
hypereosinophilic (idiopathic) 288.3
hyperkalemic 276.7
hyperkinetic (*see also* Hyperkinesia)
heart 429.82
hyperlipemia-hemolytic anemia-icterus 571.1
hypermobility 728.5
hypernatremia 276.0
hyperosmolarity 276.0
hyperperfusion 997.01
hypersomnia-bulimia 349.89
hypersplenic 289.4
hypersympathetic (*see also* Neuropathy, peripheral, autonomic) 337.9
hypertransfusion, newborn 776.4
hyperventilation, psychogenic 306.1
hyperviscosity (of serum) NEC 273.3
polycythemic 289.0
sclerothymic 282.8
hypoglycemic (familial) (neonatal) 251.2
functional 251.1
hypokalemic 276.8
hypophyseal 253.8
hypophyseothalamic 253.8
hypopituitarism 253.2
hypoplastic left heart 746.7
hypopotassemia 276.8
hyposmolality 276.1
hypotension, maternal 669.2 ☑
hypothenar hammer 443.89
hypotonia-hypomentia-hypogonadism-obesity 759.81
ICF (intravascular coagulation-fibrinolysis) (*see also* Fibrinolysis) 286.6
idiopathic cardiorespiratory distress, newborn 769
idiopathic nephrotic (infantile) 581.9
iliotibial band 728.89
Imerslund (-Gräsbeck) (anemia due to familial selective vitamin B₁₂ malabsorption) 281.1
immobility (paraplegic) 728.3
immune reconstitution inflammatory (IRIS) 995.90
immunity deficiency, combined 279.2
impending coronary 411.1
impingement
shoulder 726.2
vertebral bodies 724.4
inappropriate secretion of antidiuretic hormone (ADH) 253.6
incomplete
mandibulofacial 756.0
infant
death, sudden (SIDS) 798.0
Hercules 255.2
of diabetic mother 775.0
shaken 995.55
infantilism 253.3
inferior vena cava 459.2
influenza-like (*see also* Influenza) 487.1
inspissated bile, newborn 774.4
insufficient sleep 307.44
intermediate coronary (artery) 411.1
internal carotid artery (*see also* Occlusion, artery, carotid) 433.1 ☑
interspinous ligament 724.8
intestinal
carcinoid 259.2
gas 787.3
knot 560.2
intraoperative floppy iris (IFIS) 364.81
intravascular
coagulation-fibrinolysis (ICF) (*see also* Fibrinolysis) 286.6
coagulopathy (*see also* Fibrinolysis) 286.6
inverted Marfan's 759.89
IRDS (idiopathic respiratory distress, newborn) 769
irritable
bowel 564.1

Syndrome — *see also* Disease — *continued*

irritable — *continued*
heart 306.2
weakness 300.5
ischemic bowel (transient) 557.9
chronic 557.1
due to mesenteric artery insufficiency 557.1
Itsenko-Cushing (pituitary basophilism) 255.0
IVC (intravascular coagulopathy) (*see also* Fibrinolysis) 286.6
Ivemark's (asplenia with congenital heart disease) 759.0
Jaccoud's 714.4
Jackson's 344.89
Jadassohn-Lewandowski (pachyonchia congenita) 757.5
Jaffe-Lichtenstein (-Uehlinger) 252.01
Jahnke's (encephalocutaneous angiomatosis) 759.6
Jakob-Creutzfeldt 046.19
with dementia
with behavioral disturbance 046.19 [294.11]
without behavioral disturbance 046.19 [294.10]
variant 046.11
with dementia
with behavioral disturbance 046.11 [294.11]
without behavioral disturbance 046.11 [294.10]
Jaksch's (pseudoleukemia infantum) 285.8
Jaksch-Hayem (-Luzet) (pseudoleukemia infantum) 285.8
jaw-winking 742.8
jejunal 564.2
Jervell-Lange-Nielsen 426.82
jet lag 327.35
Jeune's (asphyxiating thoracic dystrophy of newborn) 756.4
Job's (chronic granulomatous disease) 288.1
Jordan's 288.2
Joseph-Diamond-Blackfan (congenital hypoplastic anemia) 284.01
Joubert 759.89
jugular foramen 352.6
Kabuki 759.89
Kahler's (multiple myeloma) (M9730/3) 203.0 ☑
Kalischer's (encephalocutaneous angiomatosis) 759.6
Kallmann's (hypogonadotropic hypogonadism with anosmia) 253.4
Kanner's (autism) (*see also* Psychosis, childhood) 299.0 ☑
Kartagener's (sinusitis, bronchiectasis, situs inversus) 759.3
Kasabach-Merritt (capillary hemangioma associated with thrombocytopenic purpura) 287.39
Kast's (dyschondroplasia with hemangiomas) 756.4
Kaznelson's (congenital hypoplastic anemia) 284.01
Kearns-Sayre 277.87
Kelly's (sideropenic dysphagia) 280.8
Kimmelstiel-Wilson (intercapillary glomerulosclerosis) 250.4 ☑ [581.81]
due to secondary diabetes 249.4 ☑ [581.81]
Klauder's (erythema multiforme exudativum) 695.19
Kleine-Levin 327.13
Klein-Waardenburg (ptosis-epicanthus) 270.2
Klinefelter's 758.7
Klippel-Feil (brevicollis) 756.16
Klippel-Trenaunay 759.89
Klumpke (-Déjérine) (injury to brachial plexus at birth) 767.6
Klüver-Bucy (-Terzian) 310.0
Köhler-Pellegrini-Stieda (calcification, knee joint) 726.62
König's 564.89

☑ **Additional Digit Required — Refer to the Tabular List for Digit Selection**   ⵣ **Subterms under main terms may continue to next column or page**

Syndrome — *see also* Disease — *continued*
Korsakoff's (nonalcoholic) 294.0
Korsakoff (-Wernicke) (nonalcoholic) 294.0
  alcoholic 291.1
  alcoholic 291.1
Kostmann's (infantile genetic agranulocytosis) 288.01
Krabbe's
  congenital muscle hypoplasia 756.89
  cutaneocerebral angioma 759.6
Kunkel (lupoid hepatitis) 571.49
labyrinthine 386.50
laceration, broad ligament 620.6
Lambert-Eaton 358.30
  in
    diseases classified elsewhere 358.39
    neoplastic disease 358.31
Landau-Kieffner 345.8 ☑
Langdon Down (mongolism) 758.0
Larsen's (flattened facies and multiple congenital dislocations) 755.8
lateral
  cutaneous nerve of thigh 355.1
  medullary (*see also* Disease, cerebrovascular acute) 436
Launois' (pituitary gigantism) 253.0
Launois-Cléret (adiposogenital dystrophy) 253.8
Laurence-Moon (-Bardet)-Biedl (obesity, polydactyly, and intellectual disabilities) 759.89
Lawford's (encephalocutaneous angiomatosis) 759.6
lazy
  leukocyte 288.09
  posture 728.3
Lederer-Brill (acquired infectious hemolytic anemia) 283.19
Legg-Calvé-Perthes (osteochondrosis capital femoral) 732.1
Lemiere 451.89
Lennox's (*see also* Epilepsy) 345.0 ☑
Lennox-Gastaut syndrome 345.0 ☑
  with tonic seizures 345.1 ☑
lenticular 275.1
Léopold-Lévi's (paroxysmal thyroid instability) 242.9 ☑
Lepore hemoglobin 282.45
Leriche's (aortic bifurcation occlusion) 444.09
Léri-Weill 756.59
Lermoyez's (*see also* Disease, Ménière's) 386.00
Lesch-Nyhan (hypoxanthine-guanine-phosphoribosyltransferase deficiency) 277.2
leukoencephalopathy, reversible, posterior 348.5
Lev's (acquired complete heart block) 426.0
Levi's (pituitary dwarfism) 253.3
Lévy-Roussy 334.3
Lichtheim's (subacute combined sclerosis with pernicious anemia) 281.0 *[336.2]*
Li-Fraumeni V84.01
Lightwood's (renal tubular acidosis) 588.89
Lignac (-de Toni) (-Fanconi) (-Debré) (cystinosis) 270.0
Likoff's (angina in menopausal women) 413.9
liver-kidney 572.4
Lloyd's 258.1
lobotomy 310.0
Löffler's (eosinophilic pneumonitis) 518.3
Löfgren's (sarcoidosis) 135
long arm 18 or 21 deletion 758.39
Looser (-Debray)-Milkman (osteomalacia with pseudofractures) 268.2
Lorain-Levi (pituitary dwarfism) 253.3
Louis-Bar (ataxia-telangiectasia) 334.8
low
  atmospheric pressure 993.2
  back 724.2
    psychogenic 306.0
  output (cardiac) (*see also* Failure, heart) 428.9
Lowe's (oculocerebrorenal dystrophy) 270.8

Syndrome — *see also* Disease — *continued*
lower radicular, newborn 767.4
Lowe-Terrey-MacLachlan (oculocerebrorenal dystrophy) 270.8
Lown (-Ganong)-Levine (short P-R interval, normal QRS complex, and supraventricular tachycardia) 426.81
Lucey-Driscoll (jaundice due to delayed conjugation) 774.30
Luetscher's (dehydration) 276.51
lumbar vertebral 724.4
Lutembacher's (atrial septal defect with mitral stenosis) 745.5
Lyell's (toxic epidermal necrolysis) 695.15
  due to drug
    correct substance properly administered 695.15
    overdose or wrong substance given or taken 977.9
      specified drug — *see* Table of Drugs and Chemicals
MacLeod's 492.8
macrogenitosomia praecox 259.8
macroglobulinemia 273.3
macrophage activation 288.4
Maffucci's (dyschondroplasia with hemangiomas) 756.4
Magenblase 306.4
magnesium-deficiency 781.7
malabsorption 579.9
  postsurgical 579.3
  spinal fluid 331.3
Mal de Debarquement 780.4
malignant carcinoid 259.2
Mallory-Weiss 530.7
mandibulofacial dysostosis 756.0
manic-depressive (*see also* Psychosis, affective) 296.80
Mankowsky's (familial dysplastic osteopathy) 731.2
maple syrup (urine) 270.3
Marable's (celiac artery compression) 447.4
Marchesani (-Weill) (brachymorphism and ectopia lentis) 759.89
Marchiafava-Bignami 341.8
Marchiafava-Micheli (paroxysmal nocturnal hemoglobinuria) 283.2
Marcus Gunn's (jaw-winking syndrome) 742.8
Marfan's (arachnodactyly) 759.82
  meaning congenital syphilis 090.49
    with luxation of lens 090.49 *[379.32]*
Marie's (acromegaly) 253.0
  primary or idiopathic (acropachyderma) 757.39
  secondary (hypertrophic pulmonary osteoarthropathy) 731.2
Markus-Adie 379.46
Maroteaux-Lamy (mucopolysaccharidosis VI) 277.5
Martin's 715.27
Martin-Albright (pseudohypoparathyroidism) 275.49
Martorell-Fabré (pulseless disease) 446.7
massive aspiration of newborn 770.18
Masters-Allen 620.6
mastocytosis 757.33
maternal hypotension 669.2 ☑
maternal obesity 646.1 ☑
May (-Hegglin) 288.2
McArdle (-Schmid) (-Pearson) (glycogenosis V) 271.0
McCune-Albright (osteitis fibrosa disseminata) 756.59
McQuarrie's (idiopathic familial hypoglycemia) 251.2
meconium
  aspiration 770.12
  plug (newborn) NEC 777.1
median arcuate ligament 447.4
mediastinal fibrosis 519.3
Meekeren-Ehlers-Danlos 756.83
Meige (blepharospasm-oromandibular dystonia) 333.82
 -Milroy (chronic hereditary edema) 757.0

Syndrome — *see also* Disease — *continued*
MELAS (mitochondrial encephalopathy, lactic acidosis and stroke-like episodes) 277.87
Melkersson (-Rosenthal) 351.8
MEN (multiple endocrine neoplasia)
  type I 258.01
  type IIA 258.02
  type IIB 258.03
Mende's (ptosis-epicanthus) 270.2
Mendelson's (resulting from a procedure) 997.32
  during labor 668.0 ☑
  obstetric 668.0 ☑
Ménétrier's (hypertrophic gastritis) 535.2 ☑
Ménière's (*see also* Disease, Ménière's) 386.00
meningo-eruptive 047.1
Menkes' 759.89
  glutamic acid 759.89
  maple syrup (urine) disease 270.3
menopause 627.2
  postartificial 627.4
menstruation 625.4
MERRF (myoclonus with epilepsy and with ragged red fibers) 277.87
mesenteric
  artery, superior 557.1
  vascular insufficiency (with gangrene) 557.1
metabolic 277.7
metastatic carcinoid 259.2
Meyenburg-Altherr-Uehlinger 733.99
Meyer-Schwickerath and Weyers (dysplasia oculodentodigitalis) 759.89
Micheli-Rietti (thalassemia minor) 282.46
Michotte's 721.5
micrognathia-glossoptosis 756.0
microphthalmos (congenital) 759.89
midbrain 348.89
middle
  lobe (lung) (right) 518.0
  radicular 353.0
Miescher's
  familial acanthosis nigricans 701.2
  granulomatosis disciformis 709.3
Mieten's 759.89
migraine 346.0 ☑
Mikity-Wilson (pulmonary dysmaturity) 770.7
Mikulicz's (dryness of mouth, absent or decreased lacrimation) 527.1
milk alkali (milk drinkers') 275.42
Milkman (-Looser) (osteomalacia with pseudofractures) 268.2
Millard-Gubler 344.89
Miller-Dieker 758.33
Miller Fisher's 357.0
Milles' (encephalocutaneous angiomatosis) 759.6
Minkowski-Chauffard (*see also* Spherocytosis) 282.0
Mirizzi's (hepatic duct stenosis) 576.2
  with calculus, cholelithiasis, or stones — *see* Choledocholithiasis
mitochondrial neurogastrointestinal encephalopathy (MNGIE) 277.87
mitral
  click (-murmur) 785.2
  valve prolapse 424.0
MNGIE (mitochondrial neurogastrointestinal encephalopathy) 277.87
Möbius'
  congenital oculofacial paralysis 352.6
  ophthalmoplegic migraine 346.2 ☑
Mohr's (types I and II) 759.89
monofixation 378.34
Moore's (*see also* Epilepsy) 345.5 ☑
Morel-Moore (hyperostosis frontalis interna) 733.3
Morel-Morgagni (hyperostosis frontalis interna) 733.3
Morgagni (-Stewart-Morel) (hyperostosis frontalis interna) 733.3
Morgagni-Adams-Stokes (syncope with heart block) 426.9

Syndrome — *see also* Disease — *continued*
Morquio (-Brailsford) (-Ullrich) (mucopolysaccharidosis IV) 277.5
Morris (testicular feminization) 259.51
Morton's (foot) (metatarsalgia) (metatarsal neuralgia) (neuralgia) (neuroma) (toe) 355.6
Moschcowitz (-Singer-Symmers) (thrombotic thrombocytopenic purpura) 446.6
Mounier-Kuhn 748.3
  with
    acute exacerbation 494.1
    bronchiectasis 494.0
      with (acute) exacerbation 494.1
  acquired 519.19
    with bronchiectasis 494.0
      with (acute) exacerbation 494.1
Mucha-Haberman (acute parapsoriasis varioliformis) 696.2
mucocutaneous lymph node (acute) (febrile) (infantile) (MCLS) 446.1
multiple
  deficiency 260
  endocrine neoplasia (MEN)
    type I 258.01
    type IIA 258.02
    type IIB 258.03
  operations 301.51
Munchausen's 301.51
Münchmeyer's (exostosis luxurians) 728.11
Murchison-Sanderson — *see* Disease, Hodgkin's
myasthenic — *see* Myasthenia, syndrome
myelodysplastic 238.75
  with 5q deletion 238.74
  high grade with 5q deletion 238.73
  lesions, low grade 238.72
  therapy-related 289.83
myeloproliferative (chronic) (M9960/1) 238.79
myofascial pain NEC 729.1
Naffziger's 353.0
Nager-de Reynier (dysostosis mandibularis) 756.0
nail-patella (hereditary osteo-onychodysplasia) 756.89
NARP (neuropathy, ataxia and retinitis pigmentosa) 277.87
Nebécourt's 253.3
Neill-Dingwall (microencephaly and dwarfism) 759.89
nephrotic (*see also* Nephrosis) 581.9
  diabetic 250.4 ☑ *[581.81]*
    due to secondary diabetes 249.4 ☑ *[581.81]*
Netherton's (ichthyosiform erythroderma) 757.1
neurocutaneous 759.6
neuroleptic malignant 333.92
Nezelof's (pure alymphocytosis) 279.13
Niemann-Pick (lipid histiocytosis) 272.7
Nonne-Milroy-Meige (chronic hereditary edema) 757.0
nonsense 300.16
Noonan's 759.89
Nothnagel's
  ophthalmoplegia-cerebellar ataxia 378.52
  vasomotor acroparesthesia 443.89
nucleus ambiguous-hypoglossal 352.6
OAV (oculoauriculovertebral dysplasia) 756.0
obesity hypoventilation 278.03
obsessional 300.3
oculocutaneous 364.24
oculomotor 378.81
oculourethroarticular 099.3
Ogilvie's (sympathicotonic colon obstruction) 560.89
ophthalmoplegia-cerebellar ataxia 378.52
Oppenheim-Urbach (necrobiosis lipoidica diabeticorum) 250.8 ☑ *[709.3]*
  due to secondary diabetes 249.8 ☑ *[709.3]*
oral-facial-digital 759.89

☑ **Additional Digit Required** — Refer to the Tabular List for Digit Selection   ▽ **Subterms under main terms may continue to next column or page**

Syndrome — *see also* Disease — *continued*
organic
  affective NEC 293.83
    drug-induced 292.84
  anxiety 293.84
  delusional 293.81
    alcohol-induced 291.5
    drug-induced 292.11
    due to or associated with
      arteriosclerosis 290.42
      presenile brain disease 290.12
      senility 290.20
  depressive 293.83
    drug-induced 292.84
    due to or associated with
      arteriosclerosis 290.43
      presenile brain disease 290.13
      senile brain disease 290.21
  hallucinosis 293.82
    drug-induced 292.84
organic affective 293.83
  induced by drug 292.84
organic personality 310.1
  induced by drug 292.89
Ormond's 593.4
orodigitofacial 759.89
orthostatic hypotensive-dysautonomic
  dyskinetic 333.0
Osler-Weber-Rendu (familial hemorrhagic
  telangiectasia) 448.0
osteodermopathic hyperostosis 757.39
osteoporosis-osteomalacia 268.2
Österreicher-Turner (hereditary osteo-onychodysplasia) 756.89
os trigonum 755.69
Ostrum-Furst 756.59
otolith 386.19
otopalatodigital 759.89
outlet (thoracic) 353.0
ovarian remnant 620.8
Owren's (*see also* Defect, coagulation) 286.3
OX 758.6
pacemaker 429.4
Paget-Schroetter (intermittent venous
  claudication) 453.89
pain (*see also* Pain)
  central 338.0
  chronic 338.4
  complex regional 355.9
    type I 337.20
      lower limb 337.22
      specified site NEC 337.29
      upper limb 337.21
    type II
      lower limb 355.71
      upper limb 354.4
  myelopathic 338.0
  thalamic (hyperesthetic) 338.0
painful
  apicocostal vertebral (M8010/3) 162.3
  arc 726.19
  bruising 287.2
  feet 266.2
Pancoast's (carcinoma, pulmonary apex)
  (M8010/3) 162.3
panhypopituitary (postpartum) 253.2
papillary muscle 429.81
  with myocardial infarction 410.8 ☑
Papillon-Léage and Psaume (orodigitofacial
  dysostosis) 759.89
parabiotic (transfusion)
  donor (twin) 772.0
  recipient (twin) 776.4
paralysis agitans 332.0
paralytic 344.9
  specified type NEC 344.89
paraneoplastic — *see* condition
Parinaud's (paralysis of conjugate upward
  gaze) 378.81
  oculoglandular 372.02
Parkes Weber and Dimitri (encephalocutaneous angiomatosis) 759.6
Parkinson's (*see also* Parkinsonism) 332.0
parkinsonian (*see also* Parkinsonism) 332.0
Parry's (exophthalmic goiter) 242.0 ☑
Parry-Romberg 349.89

Syndrome — *see also* Disease — *continued*
Parsonage-Aldren-Turner 353.5
Parsonage-Turner 353.5
Patau's (trisomy D1) 758.1
patella clunk 719.66
patellofemoral 719.46
Paterson (-Brown) (-Kelly) (sideropenic dysphagia) 280.8
Payr's (splenic flexure syndrome) 569.89
pectoral girdle 447.8
pectoralis minor 447.8
Pelger-Huët (hereditary hyposegmentation)
  288.2
pellagra-cerebellar ataxia-renal
  aminoaciduria 270.0
pellagroid 265.2
Pellegrini-Stieda 726.62
Pellizzi's (pineal) 259.8
pelvic congestion (-fibrosis) 625.5
Pendred's (familial goiter with deaf-mutism)
  243
Penfield's (*see also* Epilepsy) 345.5 ☑
Penta X 758.81
peptic ulcer — *see* Ulcer, peptic 533.9 ☑
perabduction 447.8
periodic 277.31
periurethral fibrosis 593.4
persistent fetal circulation 747.83
Petges-Cléjat (poikilodermatomyositis)
  710.3
Peutz-Jeghers 759.6
Pfeiffer (acrocephalosyndactyly) 755.55
phantom limb 353.6
pharyngeal pouch 279.11
Pick's (pericardial pseudocirrhosis of liver)
  423.2
  heart 423.2
  liver 423.2
Pick-Herxheimer (diffuse idiopathic cutaneous atrophy) 701.8
Pickwickian (cardiopulmonary obesity)
  278.03
PIE (pulmonary infiltration with eosinophilia) 518.3
Pierre Marie-Bamberger (hypertrophic pulmonary osteoarthropathy) 731.2
Pierre Mauriac's (diabetes-dwarfism-obesity)
  258.1
Pierre Robin 756.0
pigment dispersion, iris 364.53
pineal 259.8
pink puffer 492.8
pituitary 253.0
placental
  dysfunction 762.2
  insufficiency 762.2
  transfusion 762.3
plantar fascia 728.71
plateau iris (without glaucoma) 364.82
  with glaucoma 365.23
plica knee 727.83
Plummer-Vinson (sideropenic dysphagia)
  280.8
pluricarential of infancy 260
plurideficiency of infancy 260
pluriglandular (compensatory) 258.8
Poland 756.81
polycarential of infancy 260
polyglandular 258.8
polysplenia 759.0
pontine 433.8 ☑
popliteal
  artery entrapment 447.8
  web 756.89
postartificial menopause 627.4
postcardiac injury
  postcardiotomy 429.4
  postmyocardial infarction 411.0
postcardiotomy 429.4
post chemoembolization — code to associated conditions
postcholecystectomy 576.0
postcommissurotomy 429.4
postconcussional 310.2
postcontusional 310.2
postencephalitic 310.89

Syndrome — *see also* Disease — *continued*
posterior
  cervical sympathetic 723.2
  fossa compression 348.4
  inferior cerebellar artery (*see also* Dis-
    ease, cerebrovascular, acute) 436
  reversible encephalopathy (PRES) 348.39
postgastrectomy (dumping) 564.2
post-gastric surgery 564.2
posthepatitis 780.79
postherpetic (neuralgia) (zoster) 053.19
  geniculate ganglion 053.11
  ophthalmica 053.19
postimmunization — *see* Complications,
  vaccination
postinfarction 411.0
postinfluenza (asthenia) 780.79
postirradiation 990
postlaminectomy 722.80
  cervical, cervicothoracic 722.81
  lumbar, lumbosacral 722.83
  thoracic, thoracolumbar 722.82
postleukotomy 310.0
postlobotomy 310.0
postmastectomy lymphedema 457.0
postmature (of newborn) 766.22
postmyocardial infarction 411.0
postoperative NEC 998.9
  blind loop 579.2
postpartum panhypopituitary 253.2
postperfusion NEC 999.89
  bone marrow 996.85
postpericardiotomy 429.4
postphlebitic (asymptomatic) 459.10
  with
    complications NEC 459.19
    inflammation 459.12
      and ulcer 459.13
    stasis dermatitis 459.12
      with ulcer 459.13
    ulcer 459.11
      with inflammation 459.13
postpolio (myelitis) 138
postvagotomy 564.2
postvalvulotomy 429.4
postviral (asthenia) NEC 780.79
Potain's (gastrectasis with dyspepsia) 536.1
potassium intoxication 276.7
Potter's 753.0
Prader (-Labhart) -Willi (-Fanconi) 759.81
preinfarction 411.1
preleukemic 238.75
premature senility 259.8
premenstrual 625.4
premenstrual tension 625.4
pre ulcer 536.9
Prinzmetal-Massumi (anterior chest wall
  syndrome) 786.52
Profichet's 729.90
progeria 259.8
progressive pallidal degeneration 333.0
prolonged gestation 766.22
Proteus (dermal hypoplasia) 757.39
prune belly 756.71
prurigo-asthma 691.8
pseudocarpal tunnel (sublimis) 354.0
pseudohermaphroditism-virilism-hirsutism
  255.2
pseudoparalytica 358.00
pseudo-Turner's 759.89
psycho-organic 293.9
  acute 293.0
  anxiety type 293.84
  depressive type 293.83
  hallucinatory type 293.82
  nonpsychotic severity 310.1
    specified focal (partial) NEC 310.89
  paranoid type 293.81
  specified type NEC 293.89
  subacute 293.1
pterygolymphangiectasia 758.6
ptosis-epicanthus 270.2
pulmonary
  arteriosclerosis 416.0
  hypoperfusion (idiopathic) 769
  renal (hemorrhagic) 446.21

Syndrome — *see also* Disease — *continued*
pulseless 446.7
Putnam-Dana (subacute combined sclerosis
  with pernicious anemia) 281.0 [336.2]
pyloroduodenal 537.89
pyramidopallidonigral 332.0
pyriformis 355.0
QT interval prolongation 426.82
radicular NEC 729.2
  lower limbs 724.4
  upper limbs 723.4
    newborn 767.4
Raeder-Harbitz (pulseless disease) 446.7
Ramsay Hunt's
  dyssynergia cerebellaris myoclonica
    334.2
  herpetic geniculate ganglionitis 053.11
rapid time-zone change 327.35
Raymond (-Céstan) 433.8 ☑
Raynaud's (paroxysmal digital cyanosis)
  443.0
RDS (respiratory distress syndrome, newborn) 769
Refsum's (heredopathia atactica polyneuritiformis) 356.3
Reichmann's (gastrosuccorrhea) 536.8
Reifenstein's (hereditary familial hypogonadism, male) 259.52
Reilly's (*see also* Neuropathy, peripheral,
  autonomic) 337.9
Reiter's 099.3
renal glomerulohyalinosis-diabetic
  250.4 ☑ [581.81]
  due to secondary diabetes
    249.4 ☑ [581.81]
Rendu-Osler-Weber (familial hemorrhagic
  telangiectasia) 448.0
renofacial (congenital biliary fibroan-
  giomatosis) 753.0
Rénon-Delille 253.8
respiratory distress (idiopathic) (newborn)
  769
  adult (following trauma and surgery)
    518.52
  specified NEC 518.82
  type II 770.6
restless legs (RLS) 333.94
retinoblastoma (familial) 190.5
retraction (Duane's) 378.71
retroperitoneal fibrosis 593.4
retroviral seroconversion (acute) V08
Rett's 330.8
Reye's 331.81
Reye-Sheehan (postpartum pituitary
  necrosis) 253.2
Riddoch's (visual disorientation) 368.16
Ridley's (*see also* Failure, ventricular, left)
  428.1
Rieger's (mesodermal dysgenesis, anterior
  ocular segment) 743.44
Rietti-Greppi-Micheli (thalassemia minor)
  282.46
right ventricular obstruction — *see* Failure,
  heart
Riley-Day (familial dysautonomia) 742.8
Robin's 756.0
Rokitansky-Kuster-Hauser (congenital ab-
  sence, vagina) 752.45
Romano-Ward (prolonged QT interval syn-
  drome) 426.82
Romberg's 349.89
Rosen-Castleman-Liebow (pulmonary pro-
  teinosis) 516.0
rotator cuff, shoulder 726.10
Roth's 355.1
Rothmund's (congenital poikiloderma)
  757.33
Rotor's (idiopathic hyperbilirubinemia)
  277.4
Roussy-Lévy 334.3
Roy (-Jutras) (acropachyderma) 757.39
rubella (congenital) 771.0
Rubinstein-Taybi's (brachydactylia, short
  stature, and intellectual disabilities)
  759.89

☑ **Additional Digit Required — Refer to the Tabular List for Digit Selection**   ▽ **Subterms under main terms may continue to next column or page**

2015 ICD-9-CM   ►◄ **Revised Text**   ● **New Line**   ▲ **Revised Code**   **Volume 2 — 273**

Syndrome — *see also* Disease — *continued*
Rud's (mental deficiency, epilepsy, and infantilism) 759.89
Ruiter-Pompen (-Wyers) (angiokeratoma
corporis diffusum) 272.7
Runge's (postmaturity) 766.22
Russell (-Silver) (congenital hemihypertrophy and short stature) 759.89
Rytand-Lipsitch (complete atrioventricular
block) 426.0
sacralization-scoliosis-sciatica 756.15
sacroiliac 724.6
Saenger's 379.46
salt
depletion (*see also* Disease, renal) 593.9
due to heat NEC 992.8
causing heat exhaustion or prostration 992.5
low (*see also* Disease, renal) 593.9
salt-losing (*see also* Disease, renal) 593.9
Sanfilippo's (mucopolysaccharidosis III)
277.5
Scaglietti-Dagnini (acromegalic
macrospondylitis) 253.0
scalded skin 695.81
scalenus anticus (anterior) 353.0
scapulocostal 354.8
scapuloperoneal 359.1
scapulovertebral 723.4
Schaumann's (sarcoidosis) 135
Scheie's (mucopolysaccharidosis IS) 277.5
Scheuthauer-Marie-Sainton (cleidocranialis
dysostosis) 755.59
Schirmer's (encephalocutaneous angiomatosis) 759.6
schizophrenic, of childhood NEC (*see also*
Psychosis, childhood) 299.9 ☑
Schmidt's
sphallo-pharyngo-laryngeal hemiplegia
352.6
thyroid-adrenocortical insufficiency
258.1
vagoaccessory 352.6
Schneider's 047.9
Schnitzler 273.1
Scholte's (malignant carcinoid) 259.2
Scholz (-Bielschowsky-Henneberg) 330.0
Schroeder's (endocrine-hypertensive) 255.3
Schüller-Christian (chronic histiocytosis X)
277.89
Schultz's (agranulocytosis) 288.09
Schwartz (-Jampel) 359.23
Schwartz-Bartter (inappropriate secretion
of antidiuretic hormone) 253.6
Scimitar (anomalous venous drainage, right
lung to inferior vena cava) 747.49
sclerocystic ovary 256.4
sea-blue histiocyte 272.7
Seabright-Bantam (pseudohypoparathy-
roidism) 275.49
Seckel's 759.89
Secretan's (posttraumatic edema) 782.3
secretoinhibitor (keratoconjunctivitis sicca)
710.2
Seeligmann's (ichthyosis congenita) 757.1
Senear-Usher (pemphigus erythematosus)
694.4
senilism 259.8
seroconversion, retroviral (acute) V08
serotonin 333.99
serous meningitis 348.2
Sertoli cell (germinal aplasia) 606.0
sex chromosome mosaic 758.81
Sézary's (reticulosis) (M9701/3) 202.2 ☑
shaken infant 995.55
Shaver's (bauxite pneumoconiosis) 503
Sheehan's (postpartum pituitary necrosis)
253.2
shock (traumatic) 958.4
kidney 584.5
following crush injury 958.5
lung 518.82
related to trauma and surgery 518.52
neurogenic 308.9
psychic 308.9
Shone's 746.84

Syndrome — *see also* Disease — *continued*
short
bowel 579.3
P-R interval 426.81
shoulder-arm (*see also* Neuropathy, peripheral, autonomic) 337.9
shoulder-girdle 723.4
shoulder-hand (*see also* Neuropathy, peripheral, autonomic) 337.9
Shwachman's 288.02
Shy-Drager (orthostatic hypotension with
multisystem degeneration) 333.0
Sicard's 352.6
sicca (keratoconjunctivitis) 710.2
sick
cell 276.1
cilia 759.89
sinus 427.81
sideropenic 280.8
Siemens'
ectodermal dysplasia 757.31
keratosis follicularis spinulosa (decalvans) 757.39
Silfverskiöld's (osteochondrodystrophy, extremities) 756.50
Silver's (congenital hemihypertrophy and
short stature) 759.89
Silvestroni-Bianco (thalassemia minima)
282.46
Simons' (progressive lipodystrophy) 272.6
sinusitis-bronchiectasis-situs inversus 759.3
sinus tarsi 726.79
Sipple's (medullary thyroid carcinoma-
pheochromocytoma) 258.02
Sjögren (-Gougerot) (keratoconjunctivitis
sicca) 710.2
with lung involvement 710.2 [517.8]
Sjögren-Larsson (ichthyosis congenita)
757.1
SJS-TEN (Stevens-Johnson syndrome - toxic
epidermal necrolysis overlap) 695.14
Slocumb's 255.3
Sluder's 337.09
Smith-Lemli-Opitz (cerebrohepatorenal
syndrome) 759.89
Smith-Magenis 758.33
smokers' 305.1
Sneddon-Wilkinson (subcorneal pustular
dermatosis) 694.1
Sotos' (cerebral gigantism) 253.0
South African cardiomyopathy 425.2
spasmodic
upward movement, eye(s) 378.82
winking 307.20
Spens' (syncope with heart block) 426.9
spherophakia-brachymorphia 759.89
spinal cord injury (*see also* Injury, spinal, by
site)
with fracture, vertebra — *see* Fracture,
vertebra, by site, with spinal cord
injury
cervical — *see* Injury, spinal, cervical
fluid malabsorption (acquired) 331.3
splenic
agenesis 759.0
flexure 569.89
neutropenia 289.53
sequestration 289.52
Spurway's (brittle bones and blue sclera)
756.51
staphylococcal scalded skin 695.81
Stein's (polycystic ovary) 256.4
Steinbrocker's (*see also* Neuropathy, peripheral, autonomic) 337.9
Stein-Leventhal (polycystic ovary) 256.4
Stevens-Johnson (erythema multiforme
exudativum) 695.13
toxic epidermal necrolysis overlap (SJS-
TEN overlap syndrome) 695.14
Stewart-Morel (hyperostosis frontalis interna) 733.3
Stickler 759.89
stiff-baby 759.89
stiff-man 333.91
Still's (juvenile rheumatoid arthritis) 714.30

Syndrome — *see also* Disease — *continued*
Still-Felty (rheumatoid arthritis with
splenomegaly and leukopenia) 714.1
Stilling-Türk-Duane (ocular retraction syndrome) 378.71
Stojano's (subcostal) 098.86
Stokes (-Adams) (syncope with heart block)
426.9
Stokvis-Talma (enterogenous cyanosis)
289.7
stone heart (*see also* Failure, ventricular, left)
428.1
straight-back 756.19
stroke (*see also* Disease, cerebrovascular,
acute) 436
little 435.9
Sturge-Kalischer-Weber (encephalotrigeminal angiomatosis) 759.6
Sturge-Weber (-Dimitri) (encephalocutaneous angiomatosis) 759.6
subclavian-carotid obstruction (chronic)
446.7
subclavian steal 435.2
subcoracoid-pectoralis minor 447.8
subcostal 098.86
nerve compression 354.8
subperiosteal hematoma 267
subphrenic interposition 751.4
sudden infant death (SIDS) 798.0
Sudeck's 733.7
Sudeck-Leriche 733.7
superior
cerebellar artery (*see also* Disease, cerebrovascular, acute) 436
mesenteric artery 557.1
pulmonary sulcus (tumor) (M8010/3)
162.3
semi-circular canal dehiscence 386.8
vena cava 459.2
suprarenal cortical 255.3
supraspinatus 726.10
Susac 348.39
swallowed blood 777.3
sweat retention 705.1
Sweet's (acute febrile neutrophilic dermatosis) 695.89
Swyer's (XY pure gonadal dysgenesis) 752.7
Swyer-James (unilateral hyperlucent lung)
492.8
Symonds' 348.2
sympathetic
cervical paralysis 337.09
pelvic 625.5
syndactylic oxycephaly 755.55
syphilitic-cardiovascular 093.89
systemic
fibrosclerosing 710.8
inflammatory response (SIRS) 995.90
due to
infectious process 995.91
with acute organ dysfunction
995.92
non-infectious process 995.93
with acute organ dysfunction
995.94
systolic click (-murmur) 785.2
Tabagism 305.1
tachycardia-bradycardia 427.81
Takayasu (-Onishi) (pulseless disease) 446.7
Takotsubo 429.83
Tapia's 352.6
tarsal tunnel 355.5
Taussig-Bing (transposition, aorta and
overriding pulmonary artery) 745.11
Taybi's (otopalatodigital) 759.89
Taylor's 625.5
teething 520.7
tegmental 344.89
telangiectasis-pigmentation-cataract 757.33
temporal 383.02
lobectomy behavior 310.0
temporomandibular joint-pain-dysfunction
[TMJ] NEC 524.60
specified NEC 524.69
Terry's (*see also* Retinopathy of prematurity)
362.21

Syndrome — *see also* Disease — *continued*
testicular feminization 259.51
testis, nonvirilizing 257.8
tethered (spinal) cord 742.59
thalamic 338.0
Thibierge-Weissenbach (cutaneous systemic
sclerosis) 710.1
Thiele 724.6
thoracic outlet (compression) 353.0
thoracogenous rheumatic (hypertrophic
pulmonary osteoarthropathy) 731.2
Thorn's (*see also* Disease, renal) 593.9
Thorson-Biörck (malignant carcinoid) 259.2
thrombopenia-hemangioma 287.39
thyroid-adrenocortical insufficiency 258.1
Tietze's 733.6
time-zone (rapid) 327.35
Tobias' (carcinoma, pulmonary apex)
(M8010/3) 162.3
toilet seat 926.0
Tolosa-Hunt 378.55
Toni-Fanconi (cystinosis) 270.0
Touraine's (hereditary osteo-onychodysplasia) 756.89
Touraine-Solente-Golé (acropachyderma)
757.39
toxic
oil 710.5
shock 040.82
transfusion
fetal-maternal 772.0
twin
donor (infant) 772.0
recipient (infant) 776.4
transient left ventricular apical ballooning
429.83
Treacher Collins (incomplete mandibulofacial dysostosis) 756.0
trigeminal plate 259.8
triple X female 758.81
trisomy NEC 758.5
13 or D₁ 758.1
16-18 or E 758.2
18 or E₃ 758.2
20 758.5
21 or G (mongolism) 758.0
22 or G (mongolism) 758.0
G 758.0
Troisier-Hanot-Chauffard (bronze diabetes)
275.01
tropical wet feet 991.4
Trousseau's (thrombophlebitis migrans visceral cancer) 453.1
tumor lysis (following antineoplastic drug
therapy) (spontaneous) 277.88
Türk's (ocular retraction syndrome) 378.71
Turner's 758.6
Turner-Varny 758.6
Twiddler's (due to)
automatic implantable defibrillator
996.04
pacemaker 996.01
twin-to-twin transfusion 762.3
recipient twin 776.4
Uehlinger's (acropachyderma) 757.39
Ullrich (-Bonnevie) (-Turner) 758.6
Ullrich-Feichtiger 759.89
underwater blast injury (abdominal) (*see
also* Injury, internal, abdomen)
868.00
universal joint, cervix 620.6
Unverricht (-Lundborg) 345.1 ☑
Unverricht-Wagner (dermatomyositis) 710.3
upward gaze 378.81
Urbach-Oppenheim (necrobiosis lipoidica
diabeticorum) 250.8 ☑ [709.3]
due to secondary diabetes
249.8 ☑ [709.3]
Urbach-Wiethe (lipoid proteinosis) 272.8
uremia, chronic 585.9
urethral 597.81
urethro-oculoarticular 099.3
urethro-oculosynovial 099.3
urohepatic 572.4
uveocutaneous 364.24
uveomeningeal, uveomeningitis 363.22

☑ **Additional Digit Required** — Refer to the Tabular List for Digit Selection   ⩓ **Subterms under main terms may continue to next column or page**

Syndrome — *see also* Disease — *continued*
vagohypoglossal 352.6
vagovagal 780.2
van Buchem's (hyperostosis corticalis) 733.3
van der Hoeve's (brittle bones and blue sclera, deafness) 756.51
van der Hoeve-Halbertsma-Waardenburg (ptosis-epicanthus) 270.2
van der Hoeve-Waardenburg-Gualdi (ptosis-epicanthus) 270.2
vanishing twin 651.33
van Neck-Odelberg (juvenile osteochondrosis) 732.1
vascular splanchnic 557.0
vasomotor 443.9
vasovagal 780.2
VATER 759.89
Velo-cardio-facial 758.32
vena cava (inferior) (superior) (obstruction) 459.2
Verbiest's (claudicatio intermittens spinalis) 435.1
Vernet's 352.6
vertebral
artery 435.1
compression 721.1
lumbar 724.4
steal 435.1
vertebrogenic (pain) 724.5
vertiginous NEC 386.9
video display tube 723.8
Villaret's 352.6
Vinson-Plummer (sideropenic dysphagia) 280.8
virilizing adrenocortical hyperplasia, congenital 255.2
virus, viral 079.99
visceral larval migrans 128.0
visual disorientation 368.16
vitamin B_6 deficiency 266.1
vitreous touch 997.99
Vogt's (corpus striatum) 333.71
Vogt-Koyanagi 364.24
Volkmann's 958.6
von Bechterew-Strümpell (ankylosing spondylitis) 720.0
von Graefe's 378.72
von Hippel-Lindau (angiomatosis retinocerebellosa) 759.6
von Schroetter's (intermittent venous claudication) 453.89
von Willebrand (-Jürgens) (angiohemophilia) 286.4
Waardenburg-Klein (ptosis epicanthus) 270.2
Wagner (-Unverricht) (dermatomyositis) 710.3
Waldenström's (macroglobulinemia) 273.3
Waldenström-Kjellberg (sideropenic dysphagia) 280.8
Wallenberg's (posterior inferior cerebellar artery) (*see also* Disease, cerebrovascular, acute) 436
Waterhouse (-Friderichsen) 036.3
water retention 276.69
Weber's 344.89
Weber-Christian (nodular nonsuppurative panniculitis) 729.30
Weber-Cockayne (epidermolysis bullosa) 757.39
Weber-Dimitri (encephalocutaneous angiomatosis) 759.6
Weber-Gubler 344.89
Weber-Leyden 344.89
Weber-Osler (familial hemorrhagic telangiectasia) 448.0
Wegener's (necrotizing respiratory granulomatosis) 446.4
Weill-Marchesani (brachymorphism and ectopia lentis) 759.89
Weingarten's (tropical eosinophilia) 518.3
Weiss-Baker (carotid sinus syncope) 337.01
Weissenbach-Thibierge (cutaneous systemic sclerosis) 710.1
Werdnig-Hoffmann 335.0

Syndrome — *see also* Disease — *continued*
Werlhof-Wichmann (*see also* Purpura, thrombocytopenic) 287.39
Wermer's (polyendocrine adenomatosis) 258.01
Werner's (progeria adultorum) 259.8
Wernicke's (nonalcoholic) (superior hemorrhagic polioencephalitis) 265.1
Wernicke-Korsakoff (nonalcoholic) 294.0
alcoholic 291.1
Westphal-Strümpell (hepatolenticular degeneration) 275.1
wet
brain (alcoholic) 303.9 ☑
feet (maceration) (tropical) 991.4
lung
adult 518.52
newborn 770.6
whiplash 847.0
Whipple's (intestinal lipodystrophy) 040.2
"whistling face" (craniocarpotarsal dystrophy) 759.89
Widal (-Abrami) (acquired hemolytic jaundice) 283.9
Wilkie's 557.1
Wilkinson-Sneddon (subcorneal pustular dermatosis) 694.1
Willan-Plumbe (psoriasis) 696.1
Willebrand (-Jürgens) (angiohemophilia) 286.4
Willi-Prader (hypogenital dystrophy with diabetic tendency) 759.81
Wilson's (hepatolenticular degeneration) 275.1
Wilson-Mikity 770.7
Wiskott-Aldrich (eczema-thrombocytopenia) 279.12
withdrawal
alcohol 291.81
drug 292.0
infant of dependent mother 779.5
Woakes' (ethmoiditis) 471.1
Wolff-Parkinson-White (anomalous atrioventricular excitation) 426.7
Wright's (hyperabduction) 447.8
X
cardiac 413.9
dysmetabolic 277.7
xiphoidalgia 733.99
XO 758.6
XXX 758.81
XXXXY 758.81
XXY 758.7
yellow vernix (placental dysfunction) 762.2
Zahorsky's 074.0
Zellweger 277.86
Zieve's (jaundice, hyperlipemia and hemolytic anemia) 571.1
Zollinger-Ellison (gastric hypersecretion with pancreatic islet cell tumor) 251.5
Zuelzer-Ogden (nutritional megaloblastic anemia) 281.2
Synechia (iris) (pupil) 364.70
anterior 364.72
peripheral 364.73
intrauterine (traumatic) 621.5
posterior 364.71
vulvae, congenital 752.49
Synesthesia — *see also* Disturbance, sensation 782.0
Synodontia 520.2
Synophthalmus 759.89
Synorchidism 752.89
Synorchism 752.89
Synostosis (congenital) 756.59
astragaloscaphoid 755.67
radioulnar 755.53
talonavicular (bar) 755.67
tarsal 755.67
Synovial — *see* condition
Synovioma (M9040/3) — *see also* Neoplasm, connective tissue, malignant
benign (M9040/0) — *see* Neoplasm, connective tissue, benign
Synoviosarcoma (M9040/3) — *see* Neoplasm, connective tissue, malignant

Synovitis — *see also* Tenosynovitis 727.00
chronic crepitant, wrist 727.2
due to crystals — *see* Arthritis, due to crystals
gonococcal 098.51
gouty 274.00
specified NEC 727.09
syphilitic 095.7
congenital 090.0
traumatic, current — *see* Sprain, by site
tuberculous — *see* Tuberculosis, synovitis
villonodular 719.20
ankle 719.27
elbow 719.22
foot 719.27
hand 719.24
hip 719.25
knee 719.26
multiple sites 719.29
pelvic region 719.25
shoulder (region) 719.21
specified site NEC 719.28
wrist 719.23
Syphilide 091.3
congenital 090.0
newborn 090.0
tubercular 095.8
congenital 090.0
Syphilis, syphilitic (acquired) 097.9
with lung involvement 095.1
abdomen (late) 095.2
acoustic nerve 094.86
adenopathy (secondary) 091.4
adrenal (gland) 095.8
with cortical hypofunction 095.8
age under 2 years NEC (*see also* Syphilis, congenital) 090.9
acquired 097.9
alopecia (secondary) 091.82
anemia 095.8
aneurysm (artery) (ruptured) 093.89
aorta 093.0
central nervous system 094.89
congenital 090.5
anus 095.8
primary 091.1
secondary 091.3
aorta, aortic (arch) (abdominal) (insufficiency) (pulmonary) (regurgitation) (stenosis) (thoracic) 093.89
aneurysm 093.0
arachnoid (adhesive) 094.2
artery 093.89
cerebral 094.89
spinal 094.89
arthropathy (neurogenic) (tabetic) 094.0 [713.5]
asymptomatic — *see* Syphilis, latent
ataxia, locomotor (progressive) 094.0
atrophoderma maculatum 091.3
auricular fibrillation 093.89
Bell's palsy 094.89
bladder 095.8
bone 095.5
secondary 091.61
brain 094.89
breast 095.8
bronchus 095.8
bubo 091.0
bulbar palsy 094.89
bursa (late) 095.7
cardiac decompensation 093.89
cardiovascular (early) (late) (primary) (secondary) (tertiary) 093.9
specified type and site NEC 093.89
causing death under 2 years of age (*see also* Syphilis, congenital) 090.9
stated to be acquired NEC 097.9
central nervous system (any site) (early) (late) (latent) (primary) (recurrent) (relapse) (secondary) (tertiary) 094.9
with
ataxia 094.0
paralysis, general 094.1
juvenile 090.40
paresis (general) 094.1

Syphilis, syphilitic — *continued*
central nervous system — *continued*
with — *continued*
paresis — *continued*
juvenile 090.40
tabes (dorsalis) 094.0
juvenile 090.40
taboparesis 094.1
juvenile 090.40
aneurysm (ruptured) 094.87
congenital 090.40
juvenile 090.40
remission in (sustained) 094.9
serology doubtful, negative, or positive 094.9
specified nature or site NEC 094.89
vascular 094.89
cerebral 094.89
meningovascular 094.2
nerves 094.89
sclerosis 094.89
thrombosis 094.89
cerebrospinal 094.89
tabetic 094.0
cerebrovascular 094.89
cervix 095.8
chancre (multiple) 091.0
extragenital 091.2
Rollet's 091.2
Charcôt's joint 094.0 [713.5]
choked disc 094.89 [377.00]
chorioretinitis 091.51
congenital 090.0 [363.13]
late 094.83
choroiditis 091.51
congenital 090.0 [363.13]
late 094.83
prenatal 090.0 [363.13]
choroidoretinitis (secondary) 091.51
congenital 090.0 [363.13]
late 094.83
ciliary body (secondary) 091.52
late 095.8 [364.11]
colon (late) 095.8
combined sclerosis 094.89
complicating pregnancy, childbirth or puerperium 647.0 ☑
affecting fetus or newborn 760.2
condyloma (latum) 091.3
congenital 090.9
with
encephalitis 090.41
paresis (general) 090.40
tabes (dorsalis) 090.40
taboparesis 090.40
chorioretinitis, choroiditis 090.0 [363.13]
early or less than 2 years after birth NEC 090.2
with manifestations 090.0
latent (without manifestations) 090.1
negative spinal fluid test 090.1
serology, positive 090.1
symptomatic 090.0
interstitial keratitis 090.3
juvenile neurosyphilis 090.40
late or 2 years or more after birth NEC 090.7
chorioretinitis, choroiditis 090.5 [363.13]
interstitial keratitis 090.3
juvenile neurosyphilis NEC 090.40
latent (without manifestations) 090.6
negative spinal fluid test 090.6
serology, positive 090.6
symptomatic or with manifestations NEC 090.5
interstitial keratitis 090.3
conjugal 097.9
tabes 094.0
conjunctiva 095.8 [372.10]
contact V01.6
cord, bladder 094.0
cornea, late 095.8 [370.59]
coronary (artery) 093.89
sclerosis 093.89
coryza 095.8

☑ **Additional Digit Required** — Refer to the Tabular List for Digit Selection   ▽ **Subterms under main terms may continue to next column or page**

Syphilis, syphilitic — *continued*
coryza — *continued*
  congenital 090.0
cranial nerve 094.89
cutaneous — *see* Syphilis, skin
dacryocystitis 095.8
degeneration, spinal cord 094.89
d'emblée 095.8
dementia 094.1
  paralytica 094.1
    juvenilis 090.40
destruction of bone 095.5
dilatation, aorta 093.0
due to blood transfusion 097.9
dura mater 094.89
ear 095.8
  inner 095.8
    nerve (eighth) 094.86
    neurorecurrence 094.86
early NEC 091.0
  cardiovascular 093.9
  central nervous system 094.9
    paresis 094.1
    tabes 094.0
  latent (without manifestations) (less
    than 2 years after infection) 092.9
    negative spinal fluid test 092.9
    serological relapse following treat-
      ment 092.0
    serology positive 092.9
  paresis 094.1
  relapse (treated, untreated) 091.7
  skin 091.3
  symptomatic NEC 091.89
    extragenital chancre 091.2
    primary, except extragenital chancre
      091.0
    secondary (*see also* Syphilis, sec-
      ondary) 091.3
      relapse (treated, untreated) 091.7
  tabes 094.0
  ulcer 091.3
eighth nerve 094.86
endemic, nonvenereal 104.0
endocarditis 093.20
  aortic 093.22
  mitral 093.21
  pulmonary 093.24
  tricuspid 093.23
epididymis (late) 095.8
epiglottis 095.8
epiphysitis (congenital) 090.0
esophagus 095.8
Eustachian tube 095.8
exposure to V01.6
eye 095.8 *[363.13]*
  neuromuscular mechanism 094.85
eyelid 095.8 *[373.5]*
  with gumma 095.8 *[373.5]*
  ptosis 094.89
fallopian tube 095.8
fracture 095.5
gallbladder (late) 095.8
gastric 095.8
  crisis 094.0
  polyposis 095.8
general 097.9
  paralysis 094.1
    juvenile 090.40
genital (primary) 091.0
glaucoma 095.8
gumma (late) NEC 095.9
  cardiovascular system 093.9
  central nervous system 094.9
  congenital 090.5
  heart or artery 093.89
heart 093.89
  block 093.89
  decompensation 093.89
  disease 093.89
  failure 093.89
  valve (*see also* Syphilis, endocarditis)
    093.20
hemianesthesia 094.89
hemianopsia 095.8
hemiparesis 094.89

Syphilis, syphilitic — *continued*
hemiplegia 094.89
hepatic artery 093.89
hepatitis 095.3
hepatomegaly 095.3
  congenital 090.0
hereditaria tarda (*see also* Syphilis, congenital, late) 090.7
hereditary (*see also* Syphilis, congenital)
  090.9
  interstitial keratitis 090.3
Hutchinson's teeth 090.5
hyalitis 095.8
inactive — *see* Syphilis, latent
infantum NEC (*see also* Syphilis, congenital)
  090.9
inherited — *see* Syphilis, congenital
internal ear 095.8
intestine (late) 095.8
iris, iritis (secondary) 091.52
  late 095.8 *[364.11]*
joint (late) 095.8
keratitis (congenital) (early) (interstitial)
  (late) (parenchymatous) (punctata
  profunda) 090.3
kidney 095.4
lacrimal apparatus 095.8
laryngeal paralysis 095.8
larynx 095.8
late 097.0
  cardiovascular 093.9
  central nervous system 094.9
  latent or 2 years or more after infection
    (without manifestations) 096
    negative spinal fluid test 096
    serology positive 096
  paresis 094.1
  specified site NEC 095.8
  symptomatic or with symptoms 095.9
  tabes 094.0
latent 097.1
  central nervous system 094.9
  date of infection unspecified 097.1
  early or less than 2 years after infection
    092.9
  late or 2 years or more after infection 096
  serology
    doubtful
      follow-up of latent syphilis 097.1
        central nervous system 094.9
        date of infection unspecified
          097.1
        early or less than 2 years after
          infection 092.9
        late or 2 years or more after
          infection 096
      positive, only finding 097.1
        date of infection unspecified
          097.1
        early or less than 2 years after in-
          fection 097.1
        late or 2 years or more after infec-
          tion 097.1
lens 095.8
leukoderma 091.3
  late 095.8
lienis 095.8
lip 091.3
  chancre 091.2
  late 095.8
  primary 091.2
Lissauer's paralysis 094.1
liver 095.3
  secondary 091.62
locomotor ataxia 094.0
lung 095.1
lymphadenitis (secondary) 091.4
lymph gland (early) (secondary) 091.4
  late 095.8
macular atrophy of skin 091.3
  striated 095.8
maternal, affecting fetus or newborn 760.2
  manifest syphilis in newborn — *see*
    Syphilis, congenital
mediastinum (late) 095.8

Syphilis, syphilitic — *continued*
meninges (adhesive) (basilar) (brain) (spinal
  cord) 094.2
meningitis 094.2
  acute 091.81
  congenital 090.42
meningoencephalitis 094.2
meningovascular 094.2
  congenital 090.49
mesarteritis 093.89
  brain 094.89
  spine 094.89
middle ear 095.8
mitral stenosis 093.21
monoplegia 094.89
mouth (secondary) 091.3
  late 095.8
mucocutaneous 091.3
  late 095.8
mucous
  membrane 091.3
    late 095.8
  patches 091.3
    congenital 090.0
mulberry molars 090.5
muscle 095.6
myocardium 093.82
myositis 095.6
nasal sinus 095.8
neonatorum NEC (*see also* Syphilis, congenital) 090.9
nerve palsy (any cranial nerve) 094.89
nervous system, central 094.9
neuritis 095.8
  acoustic nerve 094.86
neurorecidive of retina 094.83
neuroretinitis 094.85
newborn (*see also* Syphilis, congenital) 090.9
nodular superficial 095.8
nonvenereal, endemic 104.0
nose 095.8
  saddle back deformity 090.5
  septum 095.8
    perforated 095.8
occlusive arterial disease 093.89
ophthalmic 095.8 *[363.13]*
ophthalmoplegia 094.89
optic nerve (atrophy) (neuritis) (papilla)
  094.84
orbit (late) 095.8
orchitis 095.8
organic 097.9
osseous (late) 095.5
osteochondritis (congenital) 090.0
osteoporosis 095.5
ovary 095.8
oviduct 095.8
palate 095.8
  gumma 095.8
  perforated 090.5
pancreas (late) 095.8
pancreatitis 095.8
paralysis 094.89
  general 094.1
  juvenile 090.40
paraplegia 094.89
paresis (general) 094.1
  juvenile 090.40
paresthesia 094.89
Parkinson's disease or syndrome 094.82
paroxysmal tachycardia 093.89
pemphigus (congenital) 090.0
penis 091.0
  chancre 091.0
  late 095.8
pericardium 093.81
perichondritis, larynx 095.8
periosteum 095.5
  congenital 090.0
  early 091.61
  secondary 091.61
peripheral nerve 095.8
petrous bone (late) 095.5
pharynx 095.8
  secondary 091.3
pituitary (gland) 095.8

Syphilis, syphilitic — *continued*
placenta 095.8
pleura (late) 095.8
pneumonia, white 090.0
pontine (lesion) 094.89
portal vein 093.89
primary NEC 091.2
  anal 091.1
  and secondary (*see also* Syphilis, sec-
    ondary) 091.9
  cardiovascular 093.9
  central nervous system 094.9
  extragenital chancre NEC 091.2
  fingers 091.2
  genital 091.0
  lip 091.2
  specified site NEC 091.2
  tonsils 091.2
prostate 095.8
psychosis (intracranial gumma) 094.89
ptosis (eyelid) 094.89
pulmonary (late) 095.1
  artery 093.89
pulmonum 095.1
pyelonephritis 095.4
recently acquired, symptomatic NEC 091.89
rectum 095.8
respiratory tract 095.8
retina
  late 094.83
  neurorecidive 094.83
retrobulbar neuritis 094.85
salpingitis 095.8
sclera (late) 095.0
sclerosis
  cerebral 094.89
  coronary 093.89
  multiple 094.89
  subacute 094.89
scotoma (central) 095.8
scrotum 095.8
secondary (and primary) 091.9
  adenopathy 091.4
  anus 091.3
  bone 091.61
  cardiovascular 093.9
  central nervous system 094.9
  chorioretinitis, choroiditis 091.51
  hepatitis 091.62
  liver 091.62
  lymphadenitis 091.4
  meningitis, acute 091.81
  mouth 091.3
  mucous membranes 091.3
  periosteum 091.61
  periostitis 091.61
  pharynx 091.3
  relapse (treated) (untreated) 091.7
  skin 091.3
  specified form NEC 091.89
  tonsil 091.3
  ulcer 091.3
  viscera 091.69
  vulva 091.3
seminal vesicle (late) 095.8
seronegative
  with signs or symptoms — *see* Syphilis,
    by site or stage
seropositive
  with signs or symptoms — *see* Syphilis,
    by site and stage
  follow-up of latent syphilis — *see*
    Syphilis, latent
  only finding — *see* Syphilis, latent
seventh nerve (paralysis) 094.89
sinus 095.8
sinusitis 095.8
skeletal system 095.5
skin (early) (secondary) (with ulceration)
  091.3
  late or tertiary 095.8
small intestine 095.8
spastic spinal paralysis 094.0
spermatic cord (late) 095.8
spinal (cord) 094.89

☑ **Additional Digit Required** — Refer to the Tabular List for Digit Selection   Subterms under main terms may continue to next column or page

276 — Volume 2   ▶◀ Revised Text   ● New Line   ▲ Revised Code   2015 ICD-9-CM

Syphilis, syphilitic — *continued*
- spinal — *continued*
  - with
    - paresis 094.1
    - tabes 094.0
- spleen 095.8
- splenomegaly 095.8
- spondylitis 095.5
- staphyloma 095.8
- stigmata (congenital) 090.5
- stomach 095.8
- synovium (late) 095.7
- tabes dorsalis (early) (late) 094.0
  - juvenile 090.40
- tabetic type 094.0
  - juvenile 090.40
- taboparesis 094.1
  - juvenile 090.40
- tachycardia 093.89
- tendon (late) 095.7
- tertiary 097.0
  - with symptoms 095.8
  - cardiovascular 093.9
  - central nervous system 094.9
  - multiple NEC 095.8
  - specified site NEC 095.8
- testis 095.8
- thorax 095.8
- throat 095.8
- thymus (gland) 095.8
- thyroid (late) 095.8
- tongue 095.8
- tonsil (lingual) 095.8
  - primary 091.2
  - secondary 091.3
- trachea 095.8
- tricuspid valve 093.23
- tumor, brain 094.89
- tunica vaginalis (late) 095.8
- ulcer (any site) (early) (secondary) 091.3
  - late 095.9
  - perforating 095.9
    - foot 094.0
- urethra (stricture) 095.8
- urogenital 095.8
- uterus 095.8
- uveal tract (secondary) 091.50
  - late 095.8 [363.13]
- uveitis (secondary) 091.50
  - late 095.8 [363.13]
- uvula (late) 095.8
  - perforated 095.8
- vagina 091.0
  - late 095.8
- valvulitis NEC 093.20
- vascular 093.89
  - brain or cerebral 094.89
- vein 093.89
  - cerebral 094.89
- ventriculi 095.8
- vesicae urinariae 095.8
- viscera (abdominal) 095.2
  - secondary 091.69
- vitreous (hemorrhage) (opacities) 095.8
- vulva 091.0
  - late 095.8
  - secondary 091.3
Syphiloma 095.9
- cardiovascular system 093.9
- central nervous system 094.9
- circulatory system 093.9
- congenital 090.5
Syphilophobia 300.29
Syringadenoma (M8400/0) — *see also* Neoplasm, skin, benign
- papillary (M8406/0) — *see* Neoplasm, skin, benign
Syringobulbia 336.0
Syringocarcinoma (M8400/3) — *see* Neoplasm, skin, malignant
Syringocystadenoma (M8400/0) — *see also* Neoplasm, skin, benign
- papillary (M8406/0) — *see* Neoplasm, skin, benign
Syringocystoma (M8407/0) — *see* Neoplasm, skin, benign

Syringoma (M8407/0) — *see also* Neoplasm, skin, benign
- chondroid (M8940/0) — *see* Neoplasm, by site, benign
Syringomyelia 336.0
Syringomyelitis 323.9
- late effect — *see* category 326
Syringomyelocele — *see also* Spina bifida 741.9 ☑
Syringopontia 336.0
System, systemic — *see also* condition
- disease, combined — *see* Degeneration, combined
- fibrosclerosing syndrome 710.8
- inflammatory response syndrome (SIRS) 995.90
  - due to
    - infectious process 995.91
      - with acute organ dysfunction 995.92
    - non-infectious process 995.93
      - with acute organ dysfunction 995.94
- lupus erythematosus 710.0
  - inhibitor 795.79

T

Tab — *see* Tag
Tabacism 989.84
Tabacosis 989.84
Tabardillo 080
- flea-borne 081.0
- louse-borne 080
Tabes, tabetic
- with
  - central nervous system syphilis 094.0
  - Charcôt's joint 094.0 [713.5]
  - cord bladder 094.0
  - crisis, viscera (any) 094.0
  - paralysis, general 094.1
  - paresis (general) 094.1
  - perforating ulcer 094.0
- arthropathy 094.0 [713.5]
- bladder 094.0
- bone 094.0
- cerebrospinal 094.0
- congenital 090.40
- conjugal 094.0
- dorsalis 094.0
  - neurosyphilis 094.0
- early 094.0
- juvenile 090.40
- latent 094.0
- mesenterica (*see also* Tuberculosis) 014.8 ☑
- paralysis insane, general 094.1
- peripheral (nonsyphilitic) 799.89
- spasmodic 094.0
  - not dorsal or dorsalis 343.9
- syphilis (cerebrospinal) 094.0
Taboparalysis 094.1
Taboparesis (remission) 094.1
- with
  - Charcôt's joint 094.1 [713.5]
  - cord bladder 094.1
  - perforating ulcer 094.1
- juvenile 090.40
Tache noir 923.20
Tachyalimentation 579.3
Tachyarrhythmia, tachyrhythmia — *see also* Tachycardia
- paroxysmal with sinus bradycardia 427.81
Tachycardia 785.0
- atrial 427.89
- auricular 427.89
- AV nodal re-entry (re-entrant) 427.89
- junctional ectopic 427.0
- newborn 779.82
- nodal 427.89
  - nonparoxysmal atrioventricular 426.89
  - nonparoxysmal atrioventricular (nodal) 426.89
- nonsustained 427.2
- paroxysmal 427.2
  - with sinus bradycardia 427.81
  - atrial (PAT) 427.0
    - psychogenic 316 [427.0]

Tachycardia — *continued*
- paroxysmal — *continued*
  - atrioventricular (AV) 427.0
    - psychogenic 316 [427.0]
  - essential 427.2
  - junctional 427.0
  - nodal 427.0
  - psychogenic 316 [427.2]
    - atrial 316 [427.0]
    - supraventricular 316 [427.0]
    - ventricular 316 [427.1]
  - supraventricular 427.0
    - psychogenic 316 [427.0]
  - ventricular 427.1
    - psychogenic 316 [427.1]
- postoperative 997.1
- psychogenic 306.2
- sick sinus 427.81
- sinoauricular 427.89
- sinus 427.89
- supraventricular 427.89
- sustained 427.2
  - supraventricular 427.0
  - ventricular 427.1
- ventricular (paroxysmal) 427.1
  - psychogenic 316 [427.1]
Tachygastria 536.8
Tachypnea 786.06
- hysterical 300.11
- newborn (idiopathic) (transitory) 770.6
- psychogenic 306.1
- transitory, of newborn 770.6
TACO (transfusion associated circulatory overload) 276.61
Taenia (infection) (infestation) — *see also* Infestation, taenia 123.3
- diminuta 123.6
- echinococcal infestation (*see also* Echinococcus) 122.9
- nana 123.6
- saginata infestation 123.2
- solium (intestinal form) 123.0
  - larval form 123.1
Taeniasis (intestine) — *see also* Infestation, taenia 123.3
- saginata 123.2
- solium 123.0
Taenzer's disease 757.4
Tag (hypertrophied skin) (infected) 701.9
- adenoid 474.8
- anus 455.9
- endocardial (*see also* Endocarditis) 424.90
- hemorrhoidal 455.9
- hymen 623.8
- perineal 624.8
- preauricular 744.1
- rectum 455.9
- sentinel 455.9
- skin 701.9
  - accessory 757.39
  - anus 455.9
  - congenital 757.39
  - preauricular 744.1
  - rectum 455.9
- tonsil 474.8
- urethra, urethral 599.84
- vulva 624.8
Tahyna fever 062.5
Takayasu (-Onishi) disease or syndrome (pulseless disease) 446.7
Takotsubo syndrome 429.83
Talc granuloma 728.82
- in operation wound 998.7
Talcosis 502
Talipes (congenital) 754.70
- acquired NEC 736.79
  - planus 734
- asymmetric 754.79
  - acquired 736.79
- calcaneovalgus 754.62
  - acquired 736.76
- calcaneovarus 754.59
  - acquired 736.76
- calcaneus 754.79
  - acquired 736.76
- cavovarus 754.59

Talipes — *continued*
- cavovarus — *continued*
  - acquired 736.75
- cavus 754.71
  - acquired 736.73
- equinovalgus 754.69
  - acquired 736.72
- equinovarus 754.51
  - acquired 736.71
- equinus 754.79
  - acquired, NEC 736.72
- percavus 754.71
  - acquired 736.73
- planovalgus 754.69
  - acquired 736.79
- planus (acquired) (any degree) 734
  - congenital 754.61
  - due to rickets 268.1
- valgus 754.60
  - acquired 736.79
- varus 754.50
  - acquired 736.79
Talma's disease 728.85
Talon noir 924.20
- hand 923.20
- heel 924.20
- toe 924.3
Tamponade heart (Rose's) — *see also* Pericarditis 423.3
Tanapox 059.21
Tangier disease (familial high-density lipoprotein deficiency) 272.5
Tank ear 380.12
Tantrum (childhood) — *see also* Disturbance, conduct 312.1 ☑
Tapeworm (infection) (infestation) — *see also* Infestation, tapeworm 123.9
Tapia's syndrome 352.6
Tarantism 297.8
Target-oval cell anemia 285.8
- with thalassemia — *see* Thalassemia
Tarlov's cyst 355.9
Tarral-Besnier disease (pityriasis rubra pilaris) 696.4
Tarsalgia 729.2
Tarsal tunnel syndrome 355.5
Tarsitis (eyelid) 373.00
- syphilitic 095.8 [373.00]
- tuberculous (*see also* Tuberculosis) 017.0 ☑ [373.4]
Tartar (teeth) 523.6
Tattoo (mark) 709.09
Taurodontism 520.2
Taussig-Bing defect, heart, or syndrome (transposition, aorta and overriding pulmonary artery) 745.11
Taybi's syndrome (otopalatodigital) 759.89
Tay's choroiditis 363.41
Taylor's
- disease (diffuse idiopathic cutaneous atrophy) 701.8
- syndrome 625.5
Tay-Sachs
- amaurotic familial idiocy 330.1
- disease 330.1
TBI (traumatic brain injury) — *see also* Injury, intracranial 854.0 ☑
- with skull fracture — *see* Fracture, skull, by site
Tear stone 375.57
Tear, torn (traumatic) — *see also* Wound, open, by site
- annular fibrosis 722.51
- anus, anal (sphincter) 863.89
  - with open wound in cavity 863.99
  - complicating delivery (healed) (old) 654.8 ☑
    - with mucosa 664.3 ☑
    - not associated with third-degree perineal laceration 664.6 ☑
  - nontraumatic, nonpuerperal (healed) (old) 569.43
- articular cartilage, old (*see also* Disorder, cartilage, articular) 718.0 ☑

☑ **Additional Digit Required — Refer to the Tabular List for Digit Selection**   ▽ **Subterms under main terms may continue to next column or page**

Tear, torn — *see also* Wound, open, by site — *continued*
bladder
  with
    abortion — *see* Abortion, by type, with damage to pelvic organs
    ectopic pregnancy (*see also* categories 633.0–633.9) 639.2
    molar pregnancy (*see also* categories 630–632) 639.2
  following
    abortion 639.2
    ectopic or molar pregnancy 639.2
  obstetrical trauma 665.5 ☑
bowel
  with
    abortion — *see* Abortion, by type, with damage to pelvic organs
    ectopic pregnancy (*see also* categories 633.0–633.9) 639.2
    molar pregnancy (*see also* categories 630–632) 639.2
  following
    abortion 639.2
    ectopic or molar pregnancy 639.2
  obstetrical trauma 665.5 ☑
broad ligament
  with
    abortion — *see* Abortion, by type, with damage to pelvic organs
    ectopic pregnancy (*see also* categories 633.0–633.9) 639.2
    molar pregnancy (*see also* categories 630–632) 639.2
  following
    abortion 639.2
    ectopic or molar pregnancy 639.2
  obstetrical trauma 665.6 ☑
bucket handle (knee) (meniscus) — *see* Tear, meniscus
capsule
  joint — *see* Sprain, by site
  spleen — *see* Laceration, spleen, capsule
cartilage (*see also* Sprain, by site)
  articular, old (*see also* Disorder, cartilage, articular) 718.0 ☑
  knee — *see* Tear, meniscus
  semilunar (knee) (current injury) — *see* Tear, meniscus
cervix
  with
    abortion — *see* Abortion, by type, with damage to pelvic organs
    ectopic pregnancy (*see also* categories 633.0–633.9) 639.2
    molar pregnancy (*see also* categories 630–632) 639.2
  following
    abortion 639.2
    ectopic or molar pregnancy 639.2
  obstetrical trauma (current) 665.3 ☑
  old 622.3
dural 349.31
  accidental puncture or laceration during a procedure 349.31
  incidental (inadvertent) 349.31
  nontraumatic NEC 349.39
internal organ (abdomen, chest, or pelvis) — *see* Injury, internal, by site
ligament (*see also* Sprain, by site)
  with open wound — *see* Wound, open by site
meniscus (knee) (current injury) 836.2
  bucket handle 836.0
    old 717.0
  lateral 836.1
    anterior horn 836.1
      old 717.42
    bucket handle 836.1
      old 717.41
    old 717.40
    posterior horn 836.1
      old 717.43
    specified site NEC 836.1
      old 717.49
  medial 836.0

Tear, torn — *see also* Wound, open, by site — *continued*
meniscus — *continued*
  medial — *continued*
    anterior horn 836.0
      old 717.1
    bucket handle 836.0
      old 717.0
    old 717.3
    posterior horn 836.0
      old 717.2
  old NEC 717.5
  site other than knee — *see* Sprain, by site
muscle (*see also* Sprain, by site)
  with open wound — *see* Wound, open by site
pelvic
  floor, complicating delivery 664.1 ☑
  organ NEC
    with
      abortion — *see* Abortion, by type, with damage to pelvic organs
      ectopic pregnancy (*see also* categories 633.0–633.9) 639.2
      molar pregnancy (*see also* categories 630–632) 639.2
    following
      abortion 639.2
      ectopic or molar pregnancy 639.2
    obstetrical trauma 665.5 ☑
perineum (*see also* Laceration, perineum)
  obstetrical trauma 665.5 ☑
periurethral tissue
  with
    abortion — *see* Abortion, by type, with damage to pelvic organs
    ectopic pregnancy (*see also* categories 633.0–633.9) 639.2
    molar pregnancy (*see also* categories 630–632) 639.2
  following
    abortion 639.2
    ectopic or molar pregnancy 639.2
  obstetrical trauma 664.8 ☑
rectovaginal septum — *see* Laceration, rectovaginal septum
retina, retinal (recent) (with detachment) 361.00
  without detachment 361.30
  dialysis (juvenile) (with detachment) 361.04
  giant (with detachment) 361.03
  horseshoe (without detachment) 361.32
  multiple (with detachment) 361.02
    without detachment 361.33
  old
    delimited (partial) 361.06
    partial 361.06
    total or subtotal 361.07
  partial (without detachment)
    giant 361.03
    multiple defects 361.02
    old (delimited) 361.06
    single defect 361.01
  round hole (without detachment) 361.31
  single defect (with detachment) 361.01
  total or subtotal (recent) 361.05
    old 361.07
rotator cuff (traumatic) 840.4
  current injury 840.4
  degenerative 726.10
  nontraumatic (complete) 727.61
    partial 726.13
semilunar cartilage, knee (*see also* Tear, meniscus) 836.2
  old 717.5
tendon (*see also* Sprain, by site)
  with open wound — *see* Wound, open by site
tentorial, at birth 767.0
umbilical cord
  affecting fetus or newborn 772.0
  complicating delivery 663.8 ☑

Tear, torn — *see also* Wound, open, by site — *continued*
urethra
  with
    abortion — *see* Abortion, by type, with damage to pelvic organs
    ectopic pregnancy (*see also* categories 633.0–633.9) 639.2
    molar pregnancy (*see also* categories 630–632) 639.2
  following
    abortion 639.2
    ectopic or molar pregnancy 639.2
  obstetrical trauma 665.5 ☑
uterus — *see* Injury, internal, uterus
vagina — *see* Laceration, vagina
vessel, from catheter 998.2
vulva, complicating delivery 664.0 ☑
Teething 520.7
  syndrome 520.7
Teeth, tooth — *see also* condition
  grinding 306.8
  prenatal 520.6
Tegmental syndrome 344.89
Telangiectasia, telangiectasis (verrucous) 448.9
  ataxic (cerebellar) 334.8
  familial 448.0
  hemorrhagic, hereditary (congenital) (senile) 448.0
  hereditary hemorrhagic 448.0
  retina 362.15
  spider 448.1
Telecanthus (congenital) 743.63
Telescoped bowel or intestine — *see also* Intussusception 560.0
Teletherapy, adverse effect NEC 990
Telogen effluvium 704.02
Temperature
  body, high (of unknown origin) (*see also* Pyrexia) 780.60
  cold, trauma from 991.9
    newborn 778.2
    specified effect NEC 991.8
  high
    body (of unknown origin) (*see also* Pyrexia) 780.60
    trauma from — *see* Heat
Temper tantrum (childhood) — *see also* Disturbance, conduct 312.1 ☑
Temple — *see* condition
Temporal — *see also* condition
  lobe syndrome 310.0
Temporomandibular joint-pain-dysfunction syndrome 524.60
Temporosphenoidal — *see* condition
Tendency
  bleeding (*see also* Defect, coagulation) 286.9
  homosexual, ego-dystonic 302.0
  paranoid 301.0
  suicide 300.9
Tenderness
  abdominal (generalized) (localized) 789.6 ☑
  rebound 789.6 ☑
  skin 782.0
Tendinitis, tendonitis — *see also* Tenosynovitis 726.90
  Achilles 726.71
  adhesive 726.90
    shoulder 726.0
  calcific 727.82
    shoulder 726.11
  gluteal 726.5
  patellar 726.64
  peroneal 726.79
  pes anserinus 726.61
  psoas 726.5
  tibialis (anterior) (posterior) 726.72
  trochanteric 726.5
Tendon — *see* condition
Tendosynovitis — *see* Tenosynovitis
Tendovaginitis — *see* Tenosynovitis
Tenesmus 787.99
  rectal 787.99
  vesical 788.99
Tenia — *see* Taenia

Teniasis — *see* Taeniasis
Tennis elbow 726.32
Tenonitis — *see also* Tenosynovitis
  eye (capsule) 376.04
Tenontosynovitis — *see* Tenosynovitis
Tenontothecitis — *see* Tenosynovitis
Tenophyte 727.9
Tenosynovitis (*see also* Synovitis) 727.00
  adhesive 726.90
    shoulder 726.0
  ankle 727.06
  bicipital (calcifying) 726.12
  buttock 727.09
  due to crystals — *see* Arthritis, due to crystals
  elbow 727.09
  finger 727.05
  foot 727.06
  gonococcal 098.51
  hand 727.05
  hip 727.09
  knee 727.09
  radial styloid 727.04
  shoulder 726.10
    adhesive 726.0
  specified NEC 727.09
  spine 720.1
  supraspinatus 726.10
  toe 727.06
  tuberculous — *see* Tuberculosis, tenosynovitis
  wrist 727.05
Tenovaginitis — *see* Tenosynovitis
Tension
  arterial, high (*see also* Hypertension) 401.9
    without diagnosis of hypertension 796.2
  headache 307.81
  intraocular (elevated) 365.00
  nervous 799.21
  ocular (elevated) 365.00
  pneumothorax 512.0
    iatrogenic 512.1
    postoperative 512.1
    spontaneous 512.0
  premenstrual 625.4
  state 300.9
Tentorium — *see* condition
Teratencephalus 759.89
Teratism 759.7
Teratoblastoma (malignant) (M9080/3) — *see* Neoplasm, by site, malignant
Teratocarcinoma (M9081/3) — *see also* Neoplasm, by site, malignant
  liver 155.0
Teratoma (solid) (M9080/1) — *see also* Neoplasm, by site, uncertain behavior
  adult (cystic) (M9080/0) — *see* Neoplasm, by site, benign
  and embryonal carcinoma, mixed (M9081/3) — *see* Neoplasm, by site, malignant
  benign (M9080/0) — *see* Neoplasm, by site, benign
  combined with choriocarcinoma (M9101/3) — *see* Neoplasm, by site, malignant
  cystic (adult) (M9080/0) — *see* Neoplasm, by site, benign
  differentiated type (M9080/0) — *see* Neoplasm, by site, benign
  embryonal (M9080/3) (*see also* Neoplasm, by site, malignant)
    liver 155.0
  fetal
    sacral, causing fetopelvic disproportion 653.7 ☑
  immature (M9080/3) — *see* Neoplasm, by site, malignant
  liver (M9080/3) 155.0
    adult, benign, cystic, differentiated type or mature (M9080/0) 211.5
  malignant (M9080/3) (*see also* Neoplasm, by site, malignant)
    anaplastic type (M9082/3) — *see* Neoplasm, by site, malignant
    intermediate type (M9083/3) — *see* Neoplasm, by site, malignant
    liver (M9080/3) 155.0

☑ **Additional Digit Required** — Refer to the Tabular List for Digit Selection   ▽ **Subterms under main terms may continue to next column or page**

278 — Volume 2   ▶◀ Revised Text   ● New Line   ▲ Revised Code   2015 ICD-9-CM

Teratoma — *see also* Neoplasm, by site, uncertain behavior — *continued*
  malignant (*see also* Neoplasm, by site, malignant) — *continued*
    trophoblastic (M9102/3)
      specified site — *see* Neoplasm, by site, malignant
      unspecified site 186.9
    undifferentiated type (M9082/3) — *see* Neoplasm, by site, malignant
    mature (M9080/0) — *see* Neoplasm, by site, benign
      malignant (M9080/3) — *see* Neoplasm, by site, malignant
    ovary (M9080/0) 220
      embryonal, immature, or malignant (M9080/3) 183.0
    suprasellar (M9080/3) — *see* Neoplasm, by site, malignant
    testis (M9080/3) 186.9
      adult, benign, cystic, differentiated type or mature (M9080/0) 222.0
      undescended 186.0
Terminal care V66.7
Termination
  anomalous (*see also* Malposition, congenital)
    portal vein 747.49
    right pulmonary vein 747.42
  pregnancy (legal) (therapeutic) — *see* Abortion, legal 635.9 ☑
    fetus NEC 779.6
    illegal (*see also* Abortion, illegal) 636.9 ☑
Ternidens diminutus infestation 127.7
Terrors, night (child) 307.46
Terry's syndrome (*see also* Retinopathy of prematurity) 362.21
Tertiary — *see* condition
Tessellated fundus, retina (tigroid) 362.89
Test(s)
  adequacy
    hemodialysis V56.31
    peritoneal dialysis V56.32
  AIDS virus V72.69
  allergen V72.7
  bacterial disease NEC (*see also* Screening, by name of disease) V74.9
  basal metabolic rate V72.69
  blood
    alcohol V70.4
    drug V70.4
      for therapeutic drug monitoring V58.83
      for routine general physical examination V72.62
      prior to treatment or procedure V72.63
    typing V72.86
      Rh typing V72.86
  developmental, infant or child V20.2
  Dick V74.8
  fertility V26.21
  genetic
    female V26.32
    for genetic disease carrier status
      female V26.31
      male V26.34
    male V26.39
  hearing V72.19
    following failed hearing screening V72.11
    routine, for infant and child V20.2
  HIV V72.69
  human immunodeficiency virus V72.69
  immunity status V72.61
  Kveim V82.89
  laboratory V72.60
    for medicolegal reason V70.4
    ordered as part of a routine general medical examination V72.62
    pre-operative V72.63
    pre-procedural V72.63
    specified NEC V72.69
  male partner of female with recurrent pregnancy loss V26.35
  Mantoux (for tuberculosis) V74.1

Test(s) — *continued*
  mycotic organism V75.4
  nuchal translucency V28.89
  parasitic agent NEC V75.8
  paternity V70.4
  peritoneal equilibration V56.32
  pregnancy
    negative result V72.41
    positive result V72.42
      first pregnancy V72.42
    unconfirmed V72.40
  preoperative V72.84
    cardiovascular V72.81
    respiratory V72.82
    specified NEC V72.83
  procreative management NEC V26.29
    genetic disease carrier status
      female V26.31
      male V26.34
  Rh typing V72.86
  sarcoidosis V82.89
  Schick V74.3
  Schultz-Charlton V74.8
  skin, diagnostic
    allergy V72.7
    bacterial agent NEC (*see also* Screening, by name of disease) V74.9
    Dick V74.8
    hypersensitivity V72.7
    Kveim V82.89
    Mantoux V74.1
    mycotic organism V75.4
    parasitic agent NEC V75.8
    sarcoidosis V82.89
    Schick V74.3
    Schultz-Charlton V74.8
    tuberculin V74.1
  specified type NEC V72.85
  tuberculin V74.1
  vision V72.0
    routine, for infant and child V20.2
  Wassermann
    positive (*see also* Serology for syphilis, positive) 097.1
    false 795.6
Testicle, testicular, testis — *see also* condition
  feminization (syndrome) 259.51
Tetanus, tetanic (cephalic) (convulsions) 037
  with
    abortion — *see* Abortion, by type, with sepsis
    ectopic pregnancy (*see also* categories 633.0–633.9) 639.0
    molar pregnancy — *see* categories 630–632 639.0
  following
    abortion 639.0
    ectopic or molar pregnancy 639.0
  inoculation V03.7
    reaction (due to serum) — *see* Complications, vaccination
  neonatorum 771.3
  puerperal, postpartum, childbirth 670.8 ☑
Tetany, tetanic 781.7
  alkalosis 276.3
  associated with rickets 268.0
  convulsions 781.7
    hysterical 300.11
  functional (hysterical) 300.11
  hyperkinetic 781.7
    hysterical 300.11
  hyperpnea 786.01
    hysterical 300.11
    psychogenic 306.1
  hyperventilation 786.01
    hysterical 300.11
    psychogenic 306.1
  hypocalcemic, neonatal 775.4
  hysterical 300.11
  neonatal 775.4
  parathyroid (gland) 252.1
  parathyroprival 252.1
  postoperative 252.1
  postthyroidectomy 252.1
  pseudotetany 781.7
    hysterical 300.11

Tetany, tetanic — *continued*
  psychogenic 306.1
    specified as conversion reaction 300.11
Tetralogy of Fallot 745.2
Tetraplegia — *see* Quadriplegia
Thailand hemorrhagic fever 065.4
Thalassanemia 282.40
Thalassemia (disease) 282.40
  with other hemoglobinopathy 282.49
  alpha (major) (severe) (triple gene defect) 282.43
    silent carrier 282.46
  beta (homozygous) (major) (severe) 282.44
  delta-beta (homozygous) 282.45
  dominant 282.49
  Hb-S (without crisis) 282.41
    with
      crisis 282.42
      vaso-occlusive pain 282.42
  hemoglobin
    C (Hb-C) 282.49
    D (Hb-D) 282.49
    E (Hb-E) 282.49
    E-beta 282.47
    H (Hb-H) 282.49
    I (Hb-I) 282.49
  high fetal gene (*see also* Thalassemia) 282.40
  high fetal hemoglobin (*see also* Thalassemia) 282.40
  intermedia 282.44
  major 282.44
  minor (alpha) (beta) 282.46
  mixed 282.49
  sickle-cell (without crisis) 282.41
    with
      crisis 282.42
      vaso-occlusive pain 282.42
  specified NEC 282.49
  trait (alpha) (beta) (delta-beta) 282.46
Thalassemic variants 282.49
Thaysen-Gee disease (nontropical sprue) 579.0
Thecoma (M8600/0) 220
  malignant (M8600/3) 183.0
Thelarche, precocious 259.1
Thelitis 611.0
  puerperal, postpartum 675.0 ☑
Therapeutic — *see* condition
Therapy V57.9
  blood transfusion, without reported diagnosis V58.2
  breathing V57.0
  chemotherapy, antineoplastic V58.11
    fluoride V07.31
    prophylactic NEC V07.39
  dialysis (intermittent) (treatment)
    extracorporeal V56.0
    peritoneal V56.8
    renal V56.0
    specified type NEC V56.8
  exercise NEC V57.1
    breathing V57.0
  extracorporeal dialysis (renal) V56.0
  fluoride prophylaxis V07.31
  hemodialysis V56.0
  hormone replacement (postmenopausal) V07.4
  immunotherapy antineoplastic V58.12
  long term oxygen therapy V46.2
  occupational V57.21
  orthoptic V57.4
  orthotic V57.81
  peritoneal dialysis V56.8
  physical NEC V57.1
  postmenopausal hormone replacement V07.4
  radiation V58.0
  speech (-language) V57.3
  vocational V57.22
Thermalgesia 782.0
Thermalgia 782.0
Thermanalgesia 782.0
Thermanesthesia 782.0
Thermic — *see* condition
Thermography (abnormal) 793.99
  breast 793.89

Thermoplegia 992.0
Thesaurismosis
  amyloid 277.39
  bilirubin 277.4
  calcium 275.40
  cystine 270.0
  glycogen (*see also* Disease, glycogen storage) 271.0
  kerasin 272.7
  lipoid 272.7
  melanin 255.41
  phosphatide 272.7
  urate 274.9
Thiaminic deficiency 265.1
  with beriberi 265.0
Thibierge-Weissenbach syndrome (cutaneous systemic sclerosis) 710.1
Thickened endometrium 793.5
Thickening
  bone 733.99
    extremity 733.99
  breast 611.79
  hymen 623.3
  larynx 478.79
  nail 703.8
    congenital 757.5
  periosteal 733.99
  pleura (*see also* Pleurisy) 511.0
  skin 782.8
  subepiglottic 478.79
  tongue 529.8
  valve, heart — *see* Endocarditis
Thiele syndrome 724.6
Thigh — *see* condition
Thinning vertebra — *see also* Osteoporosis 733.00
Thirst, excessive 783.5
  due to deprivation of water 994.3
Thomsen's disease 359.22
Thomson's disease (congenital poikiloderma) 757.33
Thoracic — *see also* condition
  kidney 753.3
  outlet syndrome 353.0
  stomach — *see* Hernia, diaphragm
Thoracogastroschisis (congenital) 759.89
Thoracopagus 759.4
Thoracoschisis 756.3
Thoracoscopic surgical procedure converted to open procedure V64.42
Thorax — *see* condition
Thorn's syndrome — *see also* Disease, renal 593.9
Thornwaldt's, Tornwaldt's
  bursitis (pharyngeal) 478.29
  cyst 478.26
  disease (pharyngeal bursitis) 478.29
Thorson-Biörck syndrome (malignant carcinoid) 259.2
Threadworm (infection) (infestation) 127.4
Threatened
  abortion or miscarriage 640.0 ☑
    with subsequent abortion (*see also* Abortion, spontaneous) 634.9 ☑
    affecting fetus 762.1
  labor 644.1 ☑
    affecting fetus or newborn 761.8
    premature 644.0 ☑
  miscarriage 640.0 ☑
    affecting fetus 762.1
  premature
    delivery 644.2 ☑
      affecting fetus or newborn 761.8
    labor 644.0 ☑
      before 22 completed weeks gestation 640.0 ☑
Three-day fever 066.0
Threshers' lung 495.0
Thrix annulata (congenital) 757.4
Throat — *see* condition
Thrombasthenia (Glanzmann's) (hemorrhagic) (hereditary) 287.1
Thromboangiitis 443.1
  obliterans (general) 443.1
    cerebral 437.1

☑ **Additional Digit Required** — Refer to the Tabular List for Digit Selection   ▽ **Subterms under main terms may continue to next column or page**

2015 ICD-9-CM   ▶◀ **Revised Text**   ● **New Line**   ▲ **Revised Code**   **Volume 2 — 279**

Thromboangiitis — *continued*
  obliterans — *continued*
    vessels
      brain 437.1
      spinal cord 437.1
Thromboarteritis — *see* Arteritis
Thromboasthenia (Glanzmann's) (hemorrhagic) (hereditary) 287.1
Thrombocytasthenia (Glanzmann's) 287.1
Thrombocythemia (primary) (M9962/1) 238.71
  essential 238.71
  hemorrhagic 238.71
  idiopathic (hemorrhagic) (M9962/1) 238.71
Thrombocytopathy (dystrophic) (granulopenic) 287.1
Thrombocytopenia, thrombocytopenic 287.5
  with
    absent radii (TAR) syndrome 287.33
    giant hemangioma 287.39
  amegakaryocytic, congenital 287.33
  congenital 287.33
  cyclic 287.39
  dilutional 287.49
  due to
    drugs 287.49
    extracorporeal circulation of blood 287.49
    massive blood transfusion 287.49
    platelet alloimmunization 287.49
  essential 287.30
  fetal 678.0 ☑
  heparin-induced (HIT) 289.84
  hereditary 287.33
  Kasabach-Merritt 287.39
  neonatal, transitory 776.1
    due to
      exchange transfusion 776.1
      idiopathic maternal thrombocytopenia 776.1
      isoimmunization 776.1
  primary 287.30
  puerperal, postpartum 666.3 ☑
  purpura (*see also* Purpura, thrombocytopenic) 287.30
    thrombotic 446.6
  secondary NEC 287.49
  sex-linked 287.39
Thrombocytosis 238.71
  essential 238.71
  primary 238.71
Thromboembolism — *see* Embolism
Thrombopathy (Bernard-Soulier) 287.1
  constitutional 286.4
  Willebrand-Jürgens (angiohemophilia) 286.4
Thrombopenia — *see also* Thrombocytopenia 287.5
Thrombophlebitis 451.9
  antecubital vein 451.82
  antepartum (superficial) 671.2 ☑
    affecting fetus or newborn 760.3
    deep 671.3 ☑
  arm 451.89
    deep 451.83
    superficial 451.82
  breast, superficial 451.89
  cavernous (venous) sinus — *see* Thrombophlebitis, intracranial venous sinus
  cephalic vein 451.82
  cerebral (sinus) (vein) 325
    late effect — *see* category 326
    nonpyogenic 437.6
      in pregnancy or puerperium 671.5 ☑
      late effect — *see* Late effect(s) (of) cerebrovascular disease
  due to implanted device — *see* Complications, due to (presence) of any device, implant or graft classified to 996.0–996.5 NEC
  during or resulting from a procedure NEC 997.2
  femoral 451.11
  femoropopliteal 451.19
  following infusion, perfusion, or transfusion 999.2
  hepatic (vein) 451.89
  idiopathic, recurrent 453.1

Thrombophlebitis — *continued*
  iliac vein 451.81
  iliofemoral 451.11
  intracranial venous sinus (any) 325
    late effect — *see* category 326
    nonpyogenic 437.6
      in pregnancy or puerperium 671.5 ☑
      late effect — *see* Late effect(s) (of) cerebrovascular disease
  jugular vein 451.89
  lateral (venous) sinus — *see* Thrombophlebitis, intracranial venous sinus
  leg 451.2
    deep (vessels) 451.19
      femoral vein 451.11
      specified vessel NEC 451.19
    superficial (vessels) 451.0
      femoral vein 451.11
  longitudinal (venous) sinus — *see* Thrombophlebitis, intracranial venous sinus
  lower extremity 451.2
    deep (vessels) 451.19
      femoral vein 451.11
      specified vessel NEC 451.19
    superficial (vessels) 451.0
  migrans, migrating 453.1
  pelvic
    with
      abortion — *see* Abortion, by type, with sepsis
      ectopic pregnancy (*see also* categories 633.0–633.9) 639.0
      molar pregnancy (*see also* categories 630–632) 639.0
    following
      abortion 639.0
      ectopic or molar pregnancy 639.0
    puerperal 671.4 ☑
  popliteal vein 451.19
  portal (vein) 572.1
  postoperative 997.2
  pregnancy (superficial) 671.2 ☑
    affecting fetus or newborn 760.3
    deep 671.3 ☑
  puerperal, postpartum, childbirth (extremities) (superficial) 671.2 ☑
    deep 671.4 ☑
    pelvic 671.4 ☑
    septic 670.3 ☑
    specified site NEC 671.5 ☑
  radial vein 451.83
  saphenous (greater) (lesser) 451.0
  sinus (intracranial) — *see* Thrombophlebitis, intracranial venous sinus
  specified site NEC 451.89
  tibial vein 451.19
Thrombosis, thrombotic (marantic) (multiple) (progressive) (vein) (vessel) 453.9
  with childbirth or during the puerperium — *see* Thrombosis, puerperal, postpartum
  antepartum — *see* Thrombosis, pregnancy
  aorta, aortic 444.1
    abdominal 444.09
      saddle 444.01
    bifurcation 444.09
    saddle 444.01
    terminal 444.09
    thoracic 444.1
    valve — *see* Endocarditis, aortic
  apoplexy (*see also* Thrombosis, brain) 434.0 ☑
    late effect — *see* Late effect(s) (of) cerebrovascular disease
  appendix, septic — *see* Appendicitis, acute
  arteriolar-capillary platelet, disseminated 446.6
  artery, arteries (postinfectional) 444.9
    auditory, internal 433.8 ☑
    basilar (*see also* Occlusion, artery, basilar) 433.0 ☑
    carotid (common) (internal) (*see also* Occlusion, artery, carotid) 433.1 ☑
      with other precerebral artery 433.3 ☑

Thrombosis, thrombotic — *continued*
  artery, arteries — *continued*
    cerebellar (anterior inferior) (posterior inferior) (superior) 433.8 ☑
    cerebral (*see also* Thrombosis, brain) 434.0 ☑
    choroidal (anterior) 433.8 ☑
    communicating posterior 433.8 ☑
    coronary (*see also* Infarct, myocardium) 410.9 ☑
      without myocardial infarction 411.81
      due to syphilis 093.89
      healed or specified as old 412
    extremities 444.22
      lower 444.22
      upper 444.21
    femoral 444.22
    hepatic 444.89
    hypophyseal 433.8 ☑
    meningeal, anterior or posterior 433.8 ☑
    mesenteric (with gangrene) 557.0
    ophthalmic (*see also* Occlusion, retina) 362.30
    pontine 433.8 ☑
    popliteal 444.22
    precerebral — *see* Occlusion, artery, precerebral NEC
    pulmonary 415.19
      iatrogenic 415.11
      personal history of V12.55
      postoperative 415.11
      septic 415.12
    renal 593.81
    retinal (*see also* Occlusion, retina) 362.30
    specified site NEC 444.89
    spinal, anterior or posterior 433.8 ☑
    traumatic (complication) (early) (*see also* Injury, blood vessel, by site) 904.9
    vertebral (*see also* Occlusion, artery, vertebral) 433.2 ☑
      with other precerebral artery 433.3 ☑
  atrial (endocardial) 424.90
    without endocarditis 429.89
    due to syphilis 093.89
  auricular (*see also* Infarct, myocardium) 410.9 ☑
  axillary (acute) (vein) 453.84
    chronic 453.74
    personal history of V12.51
  basilar (artery) (*see also* Occlusion, artery, basilar) 433.0 ☑
  bland NEC 453.9
  brain (artery) (stem) 434.0 ☑
    due to syphilis 094.89
    iatrogenic 997.02
    late effect — *see* Late effect(s) (of) cerebrovascular disease
    postoperative 997.02
    puerperal, postpartum, childbirth 674.0 ☑
    sinus (*see also* Thrombosis, intracranial venous sinus) 325
  capillary 448.9
    arteriolar, generalized 446.6
  cardiac (*see also* Infarct, myocardium) 410.9 ☑
    due to syphilis 093.89
    healed or specified as old 412
    valve — *see* Endocarditis
  carotid (artery) (common) (internal) (*see also* Occlusion, artery, carotid) 433.1 ☑
    with other precerebral artery 433.3 ☑
  cavernous sinus (venous) — *see* Thrombosis, intracranial venous sinus
  cerebellar artery (anterior inferior) (posterior inferior) (superior) 433.8 ☑
    late effect — *see* Late effect(s) (of) cerebrovascular disease
  cerebral (arteries) (*see also* Thrombosis, brain) 434.0 ☑
    late effect — *see* Late effect(s) (of) cerebrovascular disese
  coronary (artery) (*see also* Infarct, myocardium) 410.9 ☑

Thrombosis, thrombotic — *continued*
  coronary (*see also* Infarct, myocardium) — *continued*
    without myocardial infarction 411.81
    due to syphilis 093.89
    healed or specified as old 412
  corpus cavernosum 607.82
  cortical (*see also* Thrombosis, brain) 434.0 ☑
  due to (presence of) any device, implant, or graft classifiable to 996.0–996.5 — *see* Complications, due to (presence of) any device, implant, or graft classified to 996.0–996.5 NEC
  effort 453.89
  endocardial — *see* Infarct, myocardium
  eye (*see also* Occlusion, retina) 362.30
  femoral (vein) 453.6
    with inflammation or phlebitis 451.11
    artery 444.22
    deep 453.41
    personal history of V12.51
  genital organ, male 608.83
  heart (chamber) (*see also* Infarct, myocardium) 410.9 ☑
  hepatic (vein) 453.0
    artery 444.89
    infectional or septic 572.1
  iliac (acute) (vein) 453.41
    with inflammation or phlebitis 451.81
    artery (common) (external) (internal) 444.81
    chronic 453.51
    personal history of V12.51
  inflammation, vein — *see* Thrombophlebitis
  internal carotid artery (*see also* Occlusion, artery, carotid) 433.1 ☑
    with other precerebral artery 433.3 ☑
  intestine (with gangrene) 557.0
  intracranial (*see also* Thrombosis, brain) 434.0 ☑
    venous sinus (any) 325
      nonpyogenic origin 437.6
        in pregnancy or puerperium 671.5 ☑
  intramural (*see also* Infarct, myocardium) 410.9 ☑
    without
      cardiac condition 429.89
      coronary artery disease 429.89
      myocardial infarction 429.89
    healed or specified as old 412
  jugular (bulb)
    external (acute) 453.89
      chronic 453.79
    internal (acute) 453.86
      chronic 453.76
  kidney 593.81
    artery 593.81
  lateral sinus (venous) — *see* Thrombosis, intracranial venous sinus
  leg (*see also* Thrombosis, lower extremity) 453.6
    with inflammation or phlebitis — *see* Thrombophlebitis
    deep (vessels) 453.40
      acute 453.40
        lower distal 453.42
        upper (proximal) 453.41
      chronic 453.50
        lower (distal) 453.52
        upper (proximal) 453.51
      lower (distal) 453.42
      upper (proximal) 453.41
    personal history of V12.51
    superficial (vessels) 453.6
  liver (venous) 453.0
    artery 444.89
    infectional or septic 572.1
    portal vein 452
  longitudinal sinus (venous) — *see* Thrombosis, intracranial venous sinus
  lower extremity (superficial) 453.6
    deep vessels 453.40
      acute 453.40
        calf 453.42
        distal (lower leg) 453.42

☑ **Additional Digit Required** — Refer to the Tabular List for Digit Selection   ᵂ Subterms under main terms may continue to next column or page

280 — Volume 2   ▶◀ Revised Text   ● New Line   ▲ Revised Code   2015 ICD-9-CM

Thrombosis, thrombotic — *continued*
lower extremity — *continued*
deep vessels — *continued*
acute — *continued*
femoral 453.41
iliac 453.41
lower leg 453.42
peroneal 453.42
popliteal 453.41
proximal (upper leg) 453.41
thigh 453.41
tibial 453.42
chronic 453.50
calf 453.52
distal (lower leg) 453.52
femoral 453.51
iliac 453.51
lower leg 453.52
peroneal 453.52
popliteal 453.51
proximal (upper leg) 453.51
thigh 453.51
tibial 453.52
personal history of V12.51
saphenous (greater) (lesser) 453.6
superficial 453.6
lung 415.19
iatrogenic 415.11
personal history of V12.55
postoperative 415.11
septic 415.12
marantic, dural sinus 437.6
meninges (brain) (*see also* Thrombosis, brain) 434.0 ☑
mesenteric (artery) (with gangrene) 557.0
vein (inferior) (superior) 557.0
mitral — *see* Insufficiency, mitral
mural (heart chamber) (*see also* Infarct, myocardium) 410.9 ☑
without
cardiac condition 429.89
coronary artery disease 429.89
myocardial infarction 429.89
due to syphilis 093.89
following myocardial infarction 429.79
healed or specified as old 412
omentum (with gangrene) 557.0
ophthalmic (artery) (*see also* Occlusion, retina) 362.30
pampiniform plexus (male) 608.83
female 620.8
parietal (*see also* Infarct, myocardium) 410.9 ☑
penis, penile 607.82
peripheral arteries 444.22
lower 444.22
upper 444.21
platelet 446.6
portal 452
due to syphilis 093.89
infectional or septic 572.1
precerebral artery (*see also* Occlusion, artery, precerebral NEC)
pregnancy 671.2 ☑
deep (vein) 671.3 ☑
superficial (vein) 671.2 ☑
puerperal, postpartum, childbirth 671.2 ☑
brain (artery) 674.0 ☑
venous 671.5 ☑
cardiac 674.8 ☑
cerebral (artery) 674.0 ☑
venous 671.5 ☑
deep (vein) 671.4 ☑
intracranial sinus (nonpyogenic) (venous) 671.5 ☑
pelvic 671.4 ☑
pulmonary (artery) 673.2 ☑
specified site NEC 671.5 ☑
superficial 671.2 ☑
pulmonary (artery) (vein) 415.19
iatrogenic 415.11
personal history of V12.55
postoperative 415.11
septic 415.12
renal (artery) 593.81
vein 453.3

Thrombosis, thrombotic — *continued*
resulting from presence of shunt or other internal prosthetic device — *see* Complications, due to (presence of) any device, implant, or graft classified to 996.0–996.5 NEC
retina, retinal (artery) 362.30
arterial branch 362.32
central 362.31
partial 362.33
vein
central 362.35
tributary (branch) 362.36
saphenous vein (greater) (lesser) 453.6
scrotum 608.83
seminal vesicle 608.83
sigmoid (venous) sinus — *see* Thrombosis, intracranial venous sinus 325
silent NEC 453.9
sinus, intracranial (venous) (any) (*see also* Thrombosis, intracranial venous sinus) 325
softening, brain (*see also* Thrombosis, brain) 434.0 ☑
specified site NEC (acute) 453.89
chronic 453.79
spermatic cord 608.83
spinal cord 336.1
due to syphilis 094.89
in pregnancy or puerperium 671.5 ☑
pyogenic origin 324.1
late effect — *see* category 326
spleen, splenic 289.59
artery 444.89
testis 608.83
traumatic (complication) (early) (*see also* Injury, blood vessel, by site) 904.9
tricuspid — *see* Endocarditis, tricuspid
tumor — *see* Neoplasm, by site
tunica vaginalis 608.83
umbilical cord (vessels) 663.6 ☑
affecting fetus or newborn 762.6
upper extremity (acute) 453.83
chronic 453.73
deep 453.72
superficial 453.71
deep 453.82
superficial 453.81
vas deferens 608.83
vein
antecubital (acute) 453.81
chronic 453.71
axillary (acute) 453.84
chronic 453.74
basilic (acute) 453.81
chronic 453.71
brachial (acute) 453.82
chronic 453.72
brachiocephalic (innominate) (acute) 453.87
chronic 453.77
cephalic (acute) 453.81
chronic 453.71
deep 453.40
personal history of V12.51
internal jugular (acute) 453.86
chronic 453.76
lower extremity — *see* Thrombosis, lower extremity
personal history of V12.51
radial (acute) 453.82
chronic 453.72
saphenous (greater) (lesser) 453.6
specified site NEC (acute) 453.89
chronic 453.79
subclavian (acute) 453.85
chronic 453.75
superior vena cava (acute) 453.87
chronic 453.77
thoracic (acute) 453.87
chronic 453.77
ulnar (acute) 453.82
chronic 453.72
upper extremity — *see* Thrombosis, upper extremity

Thrombosis, thrombotic — *continued*
vena cava
inferior 453.2
personal history of V12.51
superior (acute) 453.87
chronic 453.77
Thrombus — *see* Thrombosis
Thrush 112.0
newborn 771.7
Thumb — *see also* condition
gamekeeper's 842.12
sucking (child problem) 307.9
Thygeson's superficial punctate keratitis 370.21
Thymergasia — *see also* Psychosis, affective 296.80
Thymitis 254.8
Thymoma (benign) (M8580/0) 212.6
malignant (M8580/3) 164.0
Thymus, thymic (gland) — *see* condition
Thyrocele — *see also* Goiter 240.9
Thyroglossal — *see also* condition
cyst 759.2
duct, persistent 759.2
Thyroid (body) (gland) — *see also* condition
hormone resistance 246.8
lingual 759.2
Thyroiditis 245.9
acute (pyogenic) (suppurative) 245.0
nonsuppurative 245.0
autoimmune 245.2
chronic (nonspecific) (sclerosing) 245.8
fibrous 245.3
lymphadenoid 245.2
lymphocytic 245.2
lymphoid 245.2
complicating pregnancy, childbirth, or puerperium 648.1 ☑
de Quervain's (subacute granulomatous) 245.1
fibrous (chronic) 245.3
giant (cell) (follicular) 245.1
granulomatous (de Quervain's) (subacute) 245.1
Hashimoto's (struma lymphomatosa) 245.2
iatrogenic 245.4
invasive (fibrous) 245.3
ligneous 245.3
lymphocytic (chronic) 245.2
lymphoid 245.2
lymphomatous 245.2
pseudotuberculous 245.1
pyogenic 245.0
radiation 245.4
Riedel's (ligneous) 245.3
subacute 245.1
suppurative 245.0
tuberculous (*see also* Tuberculosis) 017.5 ☑
viral 245.1
woody 245.3
Thyrolingual duct, persistent 759.2
Thyromegaly 240.9
Thyrotoxic
crisis or storm (*see also* Thyrotoxicosis) 242.9 ☑
heart failure (*see also* Thyrotoxicosis) 242.9 ☑ *[425.7]*
Thyrotoxicosis 242.9 ☑

Note — Use the following fifth-digit subclassification with category 242:

0   *without mention of thyrotoxic crisis or storm*

1   *with mention of thyrotoxic crisis or storm*

with
goiter (diffuse) 242.0 ☑
adenomatous 242.3 ☑
multinodular 242.2 ☑
uninodular 242.1 ☑
nodular 242.3 ☑
multinodular 242.2 ☑
uninodular 242.1 ☑
infiltrative
dermopathy 242.0 ☑

Thyrotoxicosis — *continued*
with — *continued*
infiltrative — *continued*
ophthalmopathy 242.0 ☑
thyroid acropachy 242.0 ☑
complicating pregnancy, childbirth, or puerperium 648.1 ☑
due to
ectopic thyroid nodule 242.4 ☑
ingestion of (excessive) thyroid material 242.8 ☑
specified cause NEC 242.8 ☑
factitia 242.8 ☑
heart 242.9 ☑ *[425.7]*
neonatal (transient) 775.3
TIA (transient ischemic attack) 435.9
with transient neurologic deficit 435.9
late effect — *see* Late effect(s) (of) cerebrovascular disease
Tibia vara 732.4
Tic 307.20
breathing 307.20
child problem 307.21
compulsive 307.22
convulsive 307.20
degenerative (generalized) (localized) 333.3
facial 351.8
douloureux (*see also* Neuralgia, trigeminal) 350.1
atypical 350.2
habit 307.20
chronic (motor or vocal) 307.22
transient (of childhood) 307.21
lid 307.20
transient (of childhood) 307.21
motor-verbal 307.23
occupational 300.89
orbicularis 307.20
transient (of childhood) 307.21
organic origin 333.3
postchoreic — *see* Chorea
psychogenic 307.20
compulsive 307.22
salaam 781.0
spasm 307.20
chronic (motor or vocal) 307.22
transient (of childhood) 307.21
Tick-bite fever NEC 066.1
African 087.1
Colorado (virus) 066.1
Rocky Mountain 082.0
Tick (-borne) fever NEC 066.1
American mountain 066.1
Colorado 066.1
hemorrhagic NEC 065.3
Crimean 065.0
Kyasanur Forest 065.2
Omsk 065.1
mountain 066.1
nonxanthematous 066.1
Tick paralysis 989.5
Tics and spasms, compulsive 307.22
Tietze's disease or syndrome 733.6
Tight, tightness
anus 564.89
chest 786.59
fascia (lata) 728.9
foreskin (congenital) 605
hymen 623.3
introitus (acquired) (congenital) 623.3
rectal sphincter 564.89
tendon 727.81
Achilles (heel) 727.81
urethral sphincter 598.9
Tilting vertebra 737.9
Timidity, child 313.21
Tinea (intersecta) (tarsi) 110.9
amiantacea 110.0
asbestina 110.0
barbae 110.0
beard 110.0
black dot 110.0
blanca 111.2
capitis 110.0
corporis 110.5
cruris 110.3

☑ **Additional Digit Required** — Refer to the Tabular List for Digit Selection   ⬇ **Subterms under main terms may continue to next column or page**

Tinea — *continued*
  decalvans 704.09
  flava 111.0
  foot 110.4
  furfuracea 111.0
  imbricata (Tokelau) 110.5
  lepothrix 039.0
  manuum 110.2
  microsporic (*see also* Dermatophytosis)
    110.9
  nigra 111.1
  nodosa 111.2
  pedis 110.4
  scalp 110.0
  specified site NEC 110.8
  sycosis 110.0
  tonsurans 110.0
  trichophytic (*see also* Dermatophytosis)
    110.9
  unguium 110.1
  versicolor 111.0
Tingling sensation — *see also* Disturbance,
  sensation 782.0
Tin-miners' lung 503
Tinnitus (aurium) 388.30
  audible 388.32
  objective 388.32
  subjective 388.31
Tipped, teeth 524.33
Tipping
  pelvis 738.6
    with disproportion (fetopelvic) 653.0 ☑
      affecting fetus or newborn 763.1
      causing obstructed labor 660.1 ☑
        affecting fetus or newborn 763.1
  teeth 524.33
Tiredness 780.79
Tissue — *see* condition
Tobacco
  abuse (affecting health) NEC (*see also* Abuse,
    drugs, nondependent) 305.1
  heart 989.84
  use disorder complicating pregnancy,
    childbirth, or the puerperium
    649.0 ☑
Tobias' syndrome (carcinoma, pulmonary
  apex) (M8010/3) 162.3
Tocopherol deficiency 269.1
Todd's
  cirrhosis — *see* Cirrhosis, biliary
  paralysis (postepileptic transitory paralysis)
    344.89
Toe — *see* condition
Toilet, artificial opening — *see also* Attention
  to, artificial, opening V55.9
Tokelau ringworm 110.5
Tollwut 071
Tolosa-Hunt syndrome 378.55
Tommaselli's disease
  correct substance properly administered
    599.70
  overdose or wrong substance given or taken
    961.4
Tongue — *see also* condition
  worms 134.1
Tongue tie 750.0
Tonic pupil 379.46
Toni-Fanconi syndrome (cystinosis) 270.0
Tonsil — *see* condition
Tonsillitis (acute) (catarrhal) (croupous) (follicular) (gangrenous) (infective) (lacunar)
  (lingual) (malignant) (membranous)
  (phlegmonous) (pneumococcal) (pseudomembranous) (purulent) (septic)
  (staphylococcal) (subacute) (suppurative) (toxic) (ulcerative) (vesicular) (viral)
  463
  with influenza, flu, or grippe (*see also* Influen-
    za) 487.1
  chronic 474.00
  diphtheritic (membranous) 032.0
  hypertrophic 474.00
  influenzal (*see also* Influenza) 487.1
  parenchymatous 475
  streptococcal 034.0
  tuberculous (*see also* Tuberculosis) 012.8 ☑

Tonsillitis — *continued*
  Vincent's 101
Tonsillopharyngitis 465.8
Toothache 525.9
Tooth, teeth — *see* condition
Topagnosis 782.0
Tophi (gouty) 274.03
  ear 274.81
  heart 274.82
  specified site NEC 274.82
TORCH infection — *see also* Infection, congenital 760.2
Torn — *see* Tear, torn
Tornwaldt's bursitis (disease) (pharyngeal
  bursitis) 478.29
  cyst 478.26
Torpid liver 573.9
Torsion
  accessory tube 620.5
  adnexa (female) 620.5
  aorta (congenital) 747.29
    acquired 447.1
  appendix
    epididymis 608.24
    testis 608.23
  bile duct 576.8
    with calculus, choledocholithiasis or
      stones — *see* Choledocholithiasis
    congenital 751.69
  bowel, colon, or intestine 560.2
  cervix — *see* Malposition, uterus
  duodenum 537.3
  dystonia — *see* Dystonia, torsion
  epididymis 608.24
    appendix 608.24
  fallopian tube 620.5
  gallbladder (*see also* Disease, gallbladder)
    575.8
    congenital 751.69
  gastric 537.89
  hydatid of Morgagni (female) 620.5
  kidney (pedicle) 593.89
  Meckel's diverticulum (congenital) 751.0
  mesentery 560.2
  omentum 560.2
  organ or site, congenital NEC — *see*
    Anomaly, specified type NEC
  ovary (pedicle) 620.5
    congenital 752.0
  oviduct 620.5
  penis 607.89
    congenital 752.69
  renal 593.89
  spasm — *see* Dystonia, torsion
  spermatic cord 608.22
    extravaginal 608.21
    intravaginal 608.22
  spleen 289.59
  testicle, testis 608.20
    appendix 608.23
  tibia 736.89
  umbilical cord — *see* Compression, umbili-
    cal cord
  uterus (*see also* Malposition, uterus) 621.6
Torticollis (intermittent) (spastic) 723.5
  congenital 754.1
    sternomastoid 754.1
  due to birth injury 767.8
  hysterical 300.11
  ocular 781.93
  psychogenic 306.0
    specified as conversion reaction 300.11
  rheumatic 723.5
  rheumatoid 714.0
  spasmodic 333.83
  traumatic, current NEC 847.0
Tortuous
  artery 447.1
  fallopian tube 752.19
  organ or site, congenital NEC — *see* Distor-
    tion
  renal vessel (congenital) 747.62
  retina vessel (congenital) 743.58
    acquired 362.17
  ureter 593.4
  urethra 599.84

Tortuous — *continued*
  vein — *see* Varicose, vein
Torula, torular (infection) 117.5
  histolytica 117.5
  lung 117.5
Torulosis 117.5
Torus
  fracture
    fibula 823.41
      with tibia 823.42
    humerus 812.49
    radius (alone) 813.45
      with ulna 813.47
    tibia 823.40
      with fibula 823.42
    ulna (alone) 813.46
      with radius 813.47
  mandibularis 526.81
  palatinus 526.81
Touch, vitreous 997.99
Touraine-Solente-Golé syndrome
  (acropachyderma) 757.39
Touraine's syndrome (hereditary osteo-onychodysplasia) 756.89
Tourette's disease (motor-verbal tic) 307.23
Tower skull 756.0
  with exophthalmos 756.0
Toxemia 799.89
  with
    abortion — *see* Abortion, by type, with
      toxemia
  bacterial — *see* Septicemia
  biliary (*see also* Disease, biliary) 576.8
  burn — *see* Burn, by site
  congenital NEC 779.89
  eclamptic 642.6 ☑
    with pre-existing hypertension 642.7 ☑
  erysipelatous (*see also* Erysipelas) 035
  fatigue 799.89
  fetus or newborn NEC 779.89
  food (*see also* Poisoning, food) 005.9
  gastric 537.89
  gastrointestinal 558.2
  intestinal 558.2
  kidney (*see also* Disease, renal) 593.9
  lung 518.89
  malarial NEC (*see also* Malaria) 084.6
  maternal (of pregnancy), affecting fetus or
    newborn 760.0
  myocardial — *see* Myocarditis, toxic
  of pregnancy (mild) (pre-eclamptic)
    642.4 ☑
    with
      convulsions 642.6 ☑
      pre-existing hypertension 642.7 ☑
    affecting fetus or newborn 760.0
    severe 642.5 ☑
  pre-eclamptic — *see* Toxemia, of pregnancy
  puerperal, postpartum — *see* Toxemia, of
    pregnancy
  pulmonary 518.89
  renal (*see also* Disease, renal) 593.9
  septic (*see also* Septicemia) 038.9
  small intestine 558.2
  staphylococcal 038.10
    aureus 038.11
    due to food 005.0
    specified organism NEC 038.19
  stasis 799.89
  stomach 537.89
  uremic (*see also* Uremia) 586
  urinary 586
Toxemica cerebropathia psychica (nonalcoholic) 294.0
  alcoholic 291.1
Toxic (poisoning) — *see also* condition
  from drug or poison — *see* Table of Drugs
    and Chemicals
  oil syndrome 710.5
  shock syndrome 040.82
  thyroid (gland) (*see also* Thyrotoxicosis)
    242.9 ☑
Toxicemia — *see* Toxemia
Toxicity
  dilantin
    asymptomatic 796.0

Toxicity — *continued*
  dilantin — *continued*
    symptomatic — *see* Table of Drugs and
      Chemicals
  drug
    asymptomatic 796.0
    symptomatic — *see* Table of Drugs and
      Chemicals
  fava bean 282.2
  from drug or poison
    asymptomatic 796.0
    symptomatic — *see* Table of Drugs and
      Chemicals
Toxicosis — *see also* Toxemia 799.89
  capillary, hemorrhagic 287.0
Toxinfection 799.89
  gastrointestinal 558.2
Toxocariasis 128.0
Toxoplasma infection, generalized 130.9
Toxoplasmosis (acquired) 130.9
  with pneumonia 130.4
  congenital, active 771.2
  disseminated (multisystemic) 130.8
  maternal
    with suspected damage to fetus affect-
      ing management of pregnancy
      655.4 ☑
    affecting fetus or newborn 760.2
      manifest toxoplasmosis in fetus or
        newborn 771.2
  multiple sites 130.8
  multisystemic disseminated 130.8
  specified site NEC 130.7
Trabeculation, bladder 596.89
Trachea — *see* condition
Tracheitis (acute) (catarrhal) (infantile) (membranous) (plastic) (pneumococcal) (septic) (suppurative) (viral) 464.10
  with
    bronchitis 490
      acute or subacute 466.0
      chronic 491.8
      tuberculosis — *see* Tuberculosis,
        pulmonary
    laryngitis (acute) 464.20
      with obstruction 464.21
      chronic 476.1
      tuberculous (*see also* Tuberculosis,
        larynx) 012.3 ☑
    obstruction 464.11
  chronic 491.8
    with
      bronchitis (chronic) 491.8
      laryngitis (chronic) 476.1
    due to external agent — *see* Condition,
      respiratory, chronic, due to
  diphtheritic (membranous) 032.3
  due to external agent — *see* Inflamma-
    tion, respiratory, upper, due to
  edematous 464.11
  influenzal (*see also* Influenza) 487.1
  streptococcal 034.0
  syphilitic 095.8
  tuberculous (*see also* Tuberculosis) 012.8 ☑
Trachelitis (nonvenereal) — *see also* Cervicitis
  616.0
  trichomonal 131.09
Tracheobronchial — *see* condition
Tracheobronchitis — *see also* Bronchitis 490
  acute or subacute 466.0
    with bronchospasm or obstruction 466.0
  chronic 491.8
  influenzal (*see also* Influenza) 487.1
  senile 491.8
Tracheobronchomegaly (congenital) 748.3
  with bronchiectasis 494.0
    with (acute) exacerbation 494.1
  acquired 519.19
    with bronchiectasis 494.0
      with (acute) exacerbation 494.1
Tracheobronchopneumonitis — *see* Pneumonia, broncho
Tracheocele (external) (internal) 519.19
  congenital 748.3
Tracheomalacia 519.19
  congenital 748.3

☑ **Additional Digit Required — Refer to the Tabular List for Digit Selection**   ▽ **Subterms under main terms may continue to next column or page**

Tracheopharyngitis (acute) 465.8
  chronic 478.9
    due to external agent — *see* Condition, respiratory, chronic, due to
    due to external agent — *see* Inflammation, respiratory, upper, due to
Tracheostenosis 519.19
  congenital 748.3
Tracheostomy
  attention to V55.0
  complication 519.00
  granuloma 519.09
  hemorrhage 519.09
  infection 519.01
  malfunctioning 519.02
  obstruction 519.09
  sepsis 519.01
  status V44.0
  stenosis 519.02
Trachoma, trachomatous 076.9
  active (stage) 076.1
  contraction of conjunctiva 076.1
  dubium 076.0
  healed or late effect 139.1
  initial (stage) 076.0
  Türck's (chronic catarrhal laryngitis) 476.0
Trachyphonia 784.49
Traction, vitreomacular 379.27
Training
  insulin pump V65.46
  orthoptic V57.4
  orthotic V57.81
Train sickness 994.6
Trait
  hemoglobin
    abnormal NEC 282.7
      with thalassemia 282.46
    C (*see also* Disease, hemoglobin, C) 282.7
      with elliptocytosis 282.7
    S (Hb-S) 282.5
    Lepore 282.49
      with other abnormal hemoglobin NEC 282.49
  paranoid 301.0
  sickle-cell 282.5
    with
      elliptocytosis 282.5
      spherocytosis 282.5
    thalassemia (alpha) (beta) (delta-beta) 282.46
Traits, paranoid 301.0
Tramp V60.0
Trance 780.09
  hysterical 300.13
Transaminasemia 790.4
Transfusion, blood
  without reported diagnosis V58.2
  donor V59.01
    stem cells V59.02
  fetal twin to twin 678.0 ☑
  incompatible (*see also* Complications, transfusion) 999.80
    ABO (*see also* Complications, transfusion) 999.60
    minor blood group 999.89
    non-ABO (*see also* Complications, transfusion) 999.75
    Rh (antigen) (C) (c) (D) (E) (e) (*see also* Complications, transfusion) 999.70
  reaction or complication — *see* Complications, transfusion
  related acute lung injury (TRALI) 518.7
  syndrome
    fetomaternal 772.0
    twin-to-twin
      blood loss (donor twin) 772.0
      recipient twin 776.4
  twin to twin fetal 678.0 ☑
Transient — *see also* condition
  alteration of awareness 780.02
  blindness 368.12
  deafness (ischemic) 388.02
  global amnesia 437.7
  hyperglycemia (post-procedural) 790.29
  hypoglycemia (post-procedural) 251.2

Transient — *see also* condition — continued
  person (homeless) NEC V60.0
Transitional, lumbosacral joint of vertebra 756.19
Translocation
  autosomes NEC 758.5
    13-15 758.1
    16-18 758.2
    21 or 22 758.0
    balanced in normal individual 758.4
    D_1 758.1
    E_3 758.2
    G 758.0
  balanced autosomal in normal individual 758.4
  chromosomes NEC 758.89
  Down's syndrome 758.0
Translucency, iris 364.53
Transmission of chemical substances through the placenta (affecting fetus or newborn) 760.70
  alcohol 760.71
  anticonvulsants 760.77
  antifungals 760.74
  anti-infective agents 760.74
  antimetabolics 760.78
  cocaine 760.75
  "crack" 760.75
  diethylstilbestrol [DES] 760.76
  hallucinogenic agents 760.73
  medicinal agents NEC 760.79
  narcotics 760.72
  obstetric anesthetic or analgesic drug 763.5
  specified agent NEC 760.79
  suspected, affecting management of pregnancy 655.5 ☑
Transplant(ed)
  bone V42.4
    marrow V42.81
  complication (*see also* Complications, due to (presence of) any device, implant, or graft classified to 996.0–996.5 NEC)
    bone marrow 996.85
    corneal graft NEC 996.79
      infection or inflammation 996.69
      reaction 996.51
      rejection 996.51
    organ (failure) (immune or nonimmune cause) (infection) (rejection) 996.80
      bone marrow 996.85
      heart 996.83
      intestines 996.87
      kidney 996.81
      liver 996.82
      lung 996.84
      pancreas 996.86
      specified NEC 996.89
    previously removed due to complication, failure, rejection or infection V45.87
    removal status V45.87
    skin NEC 996.79
      infection or inflammation 996.69
      rejection 996.52
        artificial 996.55
        decellularized allodermis 996.55
    stem cell(s) 996.88
      from
        peripheral blood 996.88
        umbilical cord 996.88
  cornea V42.5
  hair V50.0
  heart V42.1
    valve V42.2
  intestine V42.84
  kidney V42.0
  liver V42.7
  lung V42.6
  organ V42.9
    specified NEC V42.89
  pancreas V42.83
  peripheral stem cells V42.82
  skin V42.3

Transplant(ed) — continued
  stem cells, peripheral V42.82
  tissue V42.9
    specified NEC V42.89
Transplants, ovarian, endometrial 617.1
Transposed — *see* Transposition
Transposition (congenital) — *see also* Malposition, congenital
  abdominal viscera 759.3
  aorta (dextra) 745.11
  appendix 751.5
  arterial trunk 745.10
  colon 751.5
  great vessels (complete) 745.10
    both originating from right ventricle 745.11
    corrected 745.12
    double outlet right ventricle 745.11
    incomplete 745.11
    partial 745.11
    specified type NEC 745.19
  heart 746.87
    with complete transposition of viscera 759.3
  intestine (large) (small) 751.5
  pulmonary veins 747.49
  reversed jejunal (for bypass) (status) V45.3
  scrotal 752.81
  stomach 750.7
    with general transposition of viscera 759.3
  teeth, tooth 524.30
  vessels (complete) 745.10
    partial 745.11
  viscera (abdominal) (thoracic) 759.3
Trans-sexualism 302.50
  with
    asexual history 302.51
    heterosexual history 302.53
    homosexual history 302.52
Transverse — *see also* condition
  arrest (deep), in labor 660.3 ☑
    affecting fetus or newborn 763.1
  lie 652.3 ☑
    before labor, affecting fetus or newborn 761.7
    causing obstructed labor 660.0 ☑
      affecting fetus or newborn 763.1
    during labor, affecting fetus or newborn 763.1
Transvestism, transvestitism (transvestic fetishism) 302.3
Trapped placenta (with hemorrhage) 666.0 ☑
  without hemorrhage 667.0 ☑
Traumatic — *see also* condition
  brain injury (TBI) (*see also* Injury, intracranial) 854.0 ☑
    with skull fracture — *see* Fracture, skull, by site
Trauma, traumatism — *see also* Injury, by site 959.9
  birth — *see* Birth, injury NEC
  causing hemorrhage of pregnancy or delivery 641.8 ☑
  complicating
    abortion — *see* Abortion, by type, with damage to pelvic organs
    ectopic pregnancy (*see also* categories 633.0–633.9) 639.2
    molar pregnancy (*see also* categories 630–632) 639.2
  during delivery NEC 665.9 ☑
  following
    abortion 639.2
    ectopic or molar pregnancy 639.2
  maternal, during pregnancy, affecting fetus or newborn 760.5
  neuroma — *see* Injury, nerve, by site
  previous major, affecting management of pregnancy, childbirth, or puerperium V23.89
  psychic (current) (*see also* Reaction, adjustment)
    previous (history) V15.49
  psychologic, previous (affecting health) V15.49

Trauma, traumatism — *see also* Injury, by site — continued
    transient paralysis — *see* Injury, nerve, by site
Treacher Collins' syndrome (incomplete facial dysostosis) 756.0
Treitz's hernia — *see* Hernia, Treitz's
Trematode infestation NEC 121.9
Trematodiasis NEC 121.9
Trembles 988.8
Trembling paralysis — *see also* Parkinsonism 332.0
Tremor 781.0
  essential (benign) 333.1
  familial 333.1
  flapping (liver) 572.8
  hereditary 333.1
  hysterical 300.11
  intention 333.1
  medication-induced postural 333.1
  mercurial 985.0
  muscle 728.85
  Parkinson's (*see also* Parkinsonism) 332.0
  psychogenic 306.0
    specified as conversion reaction 300.11
  senilis 797
  specified type NEC 333.1
Trench
  fever 083.1
  foot 991.4
  mouth 101
  nephritis — *see* Nephritis, acute
Treponema pallidum infection — *see also* Syphilis 097.9
Treponematosis 102.9
  due to
    T. pallidum — *see* Syphilis
    T. pertenue (yaws) (*see also* Yaws) 102.9
Triad
  Kartagener's 759.3
  Reiter's (complete) (incomplete) 099.3
  Saint's (*see also* Hernia, diaphragm) 553.3
Trichiasis 704.2
  cicatricial 704.2
  eyelid 374.05
    with entropion (*see also* Entropion) 374.00
Trichinella spiralis (infection) (infestation) 124
Trichinelliasis 124
Trichinellosis 124
Trichiniasis 124
Trichinosis 124
Trichobezoar 938
  intestine 936
  stomach 935.2
Trichocephaliasis 127.3
Trichocephalosis 127.3
Trichocephalus infestation 127.3
Trichoclasis 704.2
Trichoepithelioma (M8100/0) — *see also* Neoplasm, skin, benign
  breast 217
  genital organ NEC — *see* Neoplasm, by site, benign
  malignant (M8100/3) — *see* Neoplasm, skin, malignant
Trichofolliculoma (M8101/0) — *see* Neoplasm, skin, benign
Tricholemmoma (M8102/0) — *see* Neoplasm, skin, benign
Trichomatosis 704.2
Trichomoniasis 131.9
  bladder 131.09
  cervix 131.09
  intestinal 007.3
  prostate 131.03
  seminal vesicle 131.09
  specified site NEC 131.8
  urethra 131.02
  urogenitalis 131.00
  vagina 131.01
  vulva 131.01
  vulvovaginal 131.01
Trichomycosis 039.0
  axillaris 039.0
  nodosa 111.2

☑ **Additional Digit Required** — Refer to the Tabular List for Digit Selection   ▽ **Subterms under main terms may continue to next column or page**

2015 ICD-9-CM   ▶◀ **Revised Text**   ● **New Line**   ▲ **Revised Code**   **Volume 2 — 283**

Index

Trichomycosis — Tuberculosis, tubercular, tuberculous

Trichomycosis — *continued*
  nodularis 111.2
  rubra 039.0
Trichonocardiosis (axillaris) (palmellina) 039.0
Trichonodosis 704.2
Trichophytide — *see* Dermatophytosis
Trichophytid, trichophyton infection — *see also* Dermatophytosis 110.9
Trichophytobezoar 938
  intestine 936
  stomach 935.2
Trichophytosis — *see* Dermatophytosis
Trichoptilosis 704.2
Trichorrhexis (nodosa) 704.2
Trichosporosis nodosa 111.2
Trichostasis spinulosa (congenital) 757.4
Trichostrongyliasis (small intestine) 127.6
Trichostrongylosis 127.6
Trichostrongylus (instabilis) infection 127.6
Trichotillomania 312.39
Trichromat, anomalous (congenital) 368.59
Trichromatopsia, anomalous (congenital) 368.59
Trichuriasis 127.3
Trichuris trichiuria (any site) (infection) (infestation) 127.3
Tricuspid (valve) — *see* condition
Trifid — *see also* Accessory
  kidney (pelvis) 753.3
  tongue 750.13
Trigeminal neuralgia — *see also* Neuralgia, trigeminal 350.1
Trigeminoencephaloangiomatosis 759.6
Trigeminy 427.89
  postoperative 997.1
Trigger finger (acquired) 727.03
  congenital 756.89
Trigonitis (bladder) (chronic) (pseudomembranous) 595.3
  tuberculous (*see also* Tuberculosis) 016.1 ☑
Trigonocephaly 756.0
Trihexosidosis 272.7
Trilobate placenta — *see* Placenta, abnormal
Trilocular heart 745.8
Trimethylaminuria 270.8
Tripartita placenta — *see* Placenta, abnormal
Triple — *see also* Accessory
  kidneys 753.3
  uteri 752.2
  X female 758.81
Triplegia 344.89
  congenital or infantile 343.8
Triplet
  affected by maternal complications of pregnancy 761.5
  healthy liveborn — *see* Newborn, multiple
  pregnancy (complicating delivery) NEC 651.1 ☑
    with fetal loss and retention of one or more fetus(es) 651.4 ☑
    following (elective) fetal reduction 651.7 ☑
Triplex placenta — *see* Placenta, abnormal
Triplication — *see* Accessory
Trismus 781.0
  neonatorum 771.3
  newborn 771.3
Trisomy (syndrome) NEC 758.5
  13 (partial) 758.1
  16-18 758.2
  18 (partial) 758.2
  21 (partial) 758.0
  22 758.0
  autosomes NEC 758.5
  D_1 758.1
  E_3 758.2
  G (group) 758.0
  group D_1 758.1
  group E 758.2
  group G 758.0
Tritanomaly 368.53
Tritanopia 368.53
Troisier-Hanot-Chauffard syndrome (bronze diabetes) 275.01
Trombidiosis 133.8
Trophedema (hereditary) 757.0

Trophedema — *continued*
  congenital 757.0
Trophoblastic disease — *see also* Hydatidiform mole 630
  previous, affecting management of pregnancy V23.1
Tropholymphedema 757.0
Trophoneurosis NEC 356.9
  arm NEC 354.9
  disseminated 710.1
  facial 349.89
  leg NEC 355.8
  lower extremity NEC 355.8
  upper extremity NEC 354.9
Tropical — *see also* condition
  maceration feet (syndrome) 991.4
  wet foot (syndrome) 991.4
Trouble — *see also* Disease
  bowel 569.9
  heart — *see* Disease, heart
  intestine 569.9
  kidney (*see also* Disease, renal) 593.9
  nervous 799.21
  sinus (*see also* Sinusitis) 473.9
Trousseau's syndrome (thrombophlebitis migrans) 453.1
Truancy, childhood — *see also* Disturbance, conduct
  socialized 312.2 ☑
  undersocialized, unsocialized 312.1 ☑
Truncus
  arteriosus (persistent) 745.0
  common 745.0
  communis 745.0
Trunk — *see* condition
Trychophytide — *see* Dermatophytosis
Trypanosoma infestation — *see* Trypanosomiasis
Trypanosomiasis 086.9
  with meningoencephalitis 086.9 [323.2]
  African 086.5
    due to Trypanosoma 086.5
      gambiense 086.3
      rhodesiense 086.4
  American 086.2
    with
      heart involvement 086.0
      other organ involvement 086.1
    without mention of organ involvement 086.2
  Brazilian — *see* Trypanosomiasis, American
  Chagas' — *see* Trypanosomiasis, American
  due to Trypanosoma
    cruzi — *see* Trypanosomiasis, American
    gambiense 086.3
    rhodesiense 086.4
  gambiensis, Gambian 086.3
  North American — *see* Trypanosomiasis, American
  rhodesiensis, Rhodesian 086.4
  South American — *see* Trypanosomiasis, American
T-shaped incisors 520.2
Tsutsugamushi fever 081.2
Tubercle — *see also* Tuberculosis
  brain, solitary 013.2 ☑
  Darwin's 744.29
  epithelioid noncaseating 135
  Ghon, primary infection 010.0 ☑
Tuberculid, tuberculide (indurating) (lichenoid) (miliary) (papulonecrotic) (primary) (skin) (subcutaneous) — *see also* Tuberculosis 017.0 ☑
Tuberculoma — *see also* Tuberculosis
  brain (any part) 013.2 ☑
  meninges (cerebral) (spinal) 013.1 ☑
  spinal cord 013.4 ☑

Tuberculosis, tubercular, tuberculous (calcification) (calcified) (caseous) (chromogenic acid-fast bacilli) (congenital) (degeneration) (disease) (fibrocaseous) (fistula) (gangrene) (interstitial) (isolated circumscribed lesions) (necrosis) (parenchymatous) (ulcerative) 011.9 ☑

Note — Use the following fifth-digit subclassification with categories 010–018:

0   unspecified
1   bacteriological or histological examination not done
2   bacteriological or histological examination unknown (at present)
3   tubercle bacilli found (in sputum) by microscopy
4   tubercle bacilli not found (in sputum) by microscopy, but found by bacterial culture
5   tubercle bacilli not found by bacteriological examination, but tuberculosis confirmed histologically
6   tubercle bacilli not found by bacteriological or histological examination, but tuberculosis confirmed by other methods [inoculation of animals]

For tuberculous conditions specified as late effects or sequelae, see category 137.

  abdomen 014.8 ☑
    lymph gland 014.8 ☑
  abscess 011.9 ☑
    arm 017.9 ☑
    bone (*see also* Osteomyelitis, due to, tuberculosis) 015.9 ☑ [730.8] ☑
      hip 015.1 ☑ [730.85]
      knee 015.2 ☑ [730.86]
      sacrum 015.0 ☑ [730.88]
      specified site NEC 015.7 ☑ [730.88]
      spinal 015.0 ☑ [730.88]
      vertebra 015.0 ☑ [730.88]
    brain 013.3 ☑
    breast 017.9 ☑
    Cowper's gland 016.5 ☑
    dura (mater) 013.8 ☑
      brain 013.3 ☑
      spinal cord 013.5 ☑
    epidural 013.8 ☑
      brain 013.3 ☑
      spinal cord 013.5 ☑
    frontal sinus — *see* Tuberculosis, sinus
    genital organs NEC 016.9 ☑
      female 016.7 ☑
      male 016.5 ☑
    genitourinary NEC 016.9 ☑
    gland (lymphatic) — *see* Tuberculosis, lymph gland
    hip 015.1 ☑
    iliopsoas 015.0 ☑ [730.88]
    intestine 014.8 ☑
    ischiorectal 014.8 ☑
    joint 015.9 ☑
      hip 015.1 ☑
      knee 015.2 ☑
      specified joint NEC 015.8 ☑
      vertebral 015.0 ☑ [730.88]
    kidney 016.0 ☑ [590.81]
    knee 015.2 ☑
    lumbar 015.0 ☑ [730.88]
    lung 011.2 ☑
      primary, progressive 010.8 ☑
    meninges (cerebral) (spinal) 013.0 ☑
    pelvic 016.9 ☑
      female 016.7 ☑
      male 016.5 ☑
    perianal 014.8 ☑
      fistula 014.8 ☑
    perinephritic 016.0 ☑ [590.81]

Tuberculosis, tubercular, tuberculous — *continued*
  abscess — *continued*
    perineum 017.9 ☑
    perirectal 014.8 ☑
    psoas 015.0 ☑ [730.88]
    rectum 014.8 ☑
    retropharyngeal 012.8 ☑
    sacrum 015.0 ☑ [730.88]
    scrofulous 017.2 ☑
    scrotum 016.5 ☑
    skin 017.0 ☑
      primary 017.0 ☑
    spinal cord 013.5 ☑
    spine or vertebra (column) 015.0 ☑ [730.88]
    strumous 017.2 ☑
    subdiaphragmatic 014.8 ☑
    testis 016.5 ☑
    thigh 017.9 ☑
    urinary 016.3 ☑
      kidney 016.0 ☑ [590.81]
    uterus 016.7 ☑
  accessory sinus — *see* Tuberculosis, sinus
  Addison's disease 017.6 ☑
  adenitis (*see also* Tuberculosis, lymph gland) 017.2 ☑
  adenoids 012.8 ☑
  adenopathy (*see also* Tuberculosis, lymph gland) 017.2 ☑
    tracheobronchial 012.1 ☑
      primary progressive 010.8 ☑
  adherent pericardium 017.9 ☑ [420.0]
  adnexa (uteri) 016.7 ☑
  adrenal (capsule) (gland) 017.6 ☑
  air passage NEC 012.8 ☑
  alimentary canal 014.8 ☑
  anemia 017.9 ☑
  ankle (joint) 015.8 ☑
    bone 015.5 ☑ [730.87]
  anus 014.8 ☑
  apex (*see also* Tuberculosis, pulmonary) 011.9 ☑
  apical (*see also* Tuberculosis, pulmonary) 011.9 ☑
  appendicitis 014.8 ☑
  appendix 014.8 ☑
  arachnoid 013.0 ☑
  artery 017.9 ☑
  arthritis (chronic) (synovial) 015.9 ☑ [711.40]
    ankle 015.8 ☑ [730.87]
    hip 015.1 ☑ [711.45]
    knee 015.2 ☑ [711.46]
    specified site NEC 015.8 ☑ [711.48]
    spine or vertebra (column) 015.0 ☑ [720.81]
    wrist 015.8 ☑ [730.83]
  articular — *see* Tuberculosis, joint
  ascites 014.0 ☑
  asthma (*see also* Tuberculosis, pulmonary) 011.9 ☑
  axilla, axillary 017.2 ☑
    gland 017.2 ☑
  bilateral (*see also* Tuberculosis, pulmonary) 011.9 ☑
  bladder 016.1 ☑
  bone (*see also* Osteomyelitis, due to, tuberculosis) 015.9 ☑ [730.8] ☑
    hip 015.1 ☑ [730.85]
    knee 015.2 ☑ [730.86]
    limb NEC 015.5 ☑ [730.88]
    sacrum 015.0 ☑ [730.88]
    specified site NEC 015.7 ☑ [730.88]
    spinal or vertebral column 015.0 ☑ [730.88]
  bowel 014.8 ☑
    miliary 018.9 ☑
  brain 013.2 ☑
  breast 017.9 ☑
  broad ligament 016.7 ☑
  bronchi, bronchial, bronchus 011.3 ☑
    ectasia, ectasis 011.5 ☑
    fistula 011.3 ☑

☑ **Additional Digit Required** — **Refer to the Tabular List for Digit Selection**   ▽ **Subterms under main terms may continue to next column or page**

Tuberculosis, tubercular, tuberculous — *continued*
  bronchi, bronchial, bronchus — *continued*
    fistula — *continued*
      primary, progressive 010.8 ☑
      gland 012.1 ☑
        primary, progressive 010.8 ☑
      isolated 012.2 ☑
      lymph gland or node 012.1 ☑
        primary, progressive 010.8 ☑
    bronchiectasis 011.5 ☑
    bronchitis 011.3 ☑
    bronchopleural 012.0 ☑
    bronchopneumonia, bronchopneumonic 011.6 ☑
    bronchorrhagia 011.3 ☑
    bronchotracheal 011.3 ☑
      isolated 012.2 ☑
    bronchus — *see* Tuberculosis, bronchi
  bronze disease (Addison's) 017.6 ☑
  buccal cavity 017.9 ☑
  bulbourethral gland 016.5 ☑
  bursa (*see also* Tuberculosis, joint) 015.9 ☑
  cachexia NEC (*see also* Tuberculosis, pulmonary) 011.9 ☑
  cardiomyopathy 017.9 ☑ *[425.8]*
  caries (*see also* Tuberculosis, bone) 015.9 ☑ *[730.8]*
  cartilage (*see also* Tuberculosis, bone) 015.9 ☑ *[730.8]*
    intervertebral 015.0 *[730.88]*
  catarrhal (*see also* Tuberculosis, pulmonary) 011.9 ☑
  cecum 014.8 ☑
  cellular tissue (primary) 017.0 ☑
  cellulitis (primary) 017.0 ☑
  central nervous system 013.9 ☑
    specified site NEC 013.8 ☑
  cerebellum (current) 013.2 ☑
  cerebral (current) 013.2 ☑
    meninges 013.0 ☑
  cerebrospinal 013.6 ☑
    meninges 013.0 ☑
  cerebrum (current) 013.2 ☑
  cervical 017.2 ☑
    gland 017.2 ☑
    lymph nodes 017.2 ☑
  cervicitis (uteri) 016.7 ☑
  cervix 016.7 ☑
  chest (*see also* Tuberculosis, pulmonary) 011.9 ☑
  childhood type or first infection 010.0 ☑
  choroid 017.3 ☑ *[363.13]*
  choroiditis 017.3 ☑ *[363.13]*
  ciliary body 017.3 ☑ *[364.11]*
  colitis 014.8 ☑
  colliers' 011.4 ☑
  colliquativa (primary) 017.0 ☑
  colon 014.8 ☑
    ulceration 014.8 ☑
  complex, primary 010.0 ☑
  complicating pregnancy, childbirth, or puerperium 647.3 ☑
    affecting fetus or newborn 760.2
  congenital 771.2
  conjunctiva 017.3 ☑ *[370.31]*
  connective tissue 017.9 ☑
    bone — *see* Tuberculosis, bone
  contact V01.1
  converter (tuberculin skin test) (without disease) 795.51
  cornea (ulcer) 017.3 ☑ *[370.31]*
  Cowper's gland 016.5 ☑
  coxae 015.1 ☑ *[730.85]*
  coxalgia 015.1 ☑ *[730.85]*
  cul-de-sac of Douglas 014.8 ☑
  curvature, spine 015.0 ☑ *[737.40]*
  cutis (colliquativa) (primary) 017.0 ☑
  cystitis 016.1 ☑
  cyst, ovary 016.6 ☑
  dacryocystitis 017.3 ☑ *[375.32]*
  dactylitis 015.5 ☑
  diarrhea 014.8 ☑

Tuberculosis, tubercular, tuberculous — *continued*
  diffuse (*see also* Tuberculosis, miliary) 018.9 ☑
    lung — *see* Tuberculosis, pulmonary
    meninges 013.0 ☑
  digestive tract 014.8 ☑
  disseminated (*see also* Tuberculosis, miliary) 018.9 ☑
    meninges 013.0 ☑
  duodenum 014.8 ☑
  dura (mater) 013.9 ☑
    abscess 013.8 ☑
      cerebral 013.3 ☑
      spinal 013.5 ☑
  dysentery 014.8 ☑
  ear (inner) (middle) 017.4 ☑
    bone 015.6 ☑
    external (primary) 017.0 ☑
    skin (primary) 017.0 ☑
  elbow 015.8 ☑
  emphysema — *see* Tuberculosis, pulmonary
  empyema 012.0 ☑
  encephalitis 013.6 ☑
  endarteritis 017.9 ☑
  endocarditis (any valve) 017.9 ☑ *[424.91]*
  endocardium (any valve) 017.9 ☑ *[424.91]*
  endocrine glands NEC 017.9 ☑
  endometrium 016.7 ☑
  enteric, enterica 014.8 ☑
  enteritis 014.8 ☑
  enterocolitis 014.8 ☑
  epididymis 016.4 ☑
  epididymitis 016.4 ☑
  epidural abscess 013.8 ☑
    brain 013.3 ☑
    spinal cord 013.5 ☑
  epiglottis 012.3 ☑
  episcleritis 017.3 ☑ *[379.00]*
  erythema (induratum) (nodosum) (primary) 017.1 ☑
  esophagus 017.8 ☑
  Eustachian tube 017.4 ☑
  exposure to V01.1
  exudative 012.0 ☑
    primary, progressive 010.1 ☑
  eye 017.3 ☑
  eyelid (primary) 017.0 ☑
    lupus 017.0 ☑ *[373.4]*
  fallopian tube 016.6 ☑
  fascia 017.9 ☑
  fauces 012.8 ☑
  finger 017.9 ☑
  first infection 010.0 ☑
  fistula, perirectal 014.8 ☑
  Florida 011.6 ☑
  foot 017.9 ☑
  funnel pelvis 137.3
  gallbladder 017.9 ☑
  galloping (*see also* Tuberculosis, pulmonary) 011.9 ☑
  ganglionic 015.9 ☑
  gastritis 017.9 ☑
  gastrocolic fistula 014.8 ☑
  gastroenteritis 014.8 ☑
  gastrointestinal tract 014.8 ☑
  general, generalized 018.9 ☑
    acute 018.0 ☑
    chronic 018.8 ☑
  genital organs NEC 016.9 ☑
    female 016.7 ☑
    male 016.5 ☑
  genitourinary NEC 016.9 ☑
  genu 015.2 ☑
  glandulae suprarenalis 017.6 ☑
  glandular, general 017.2 ☑
  glottis 012.3 ☑
  grinders' 011.4 ☑
  groin 017.2 ☑
  gum 017.9 ☑
  hand 017.9 ☑
  heart 017.9 ☑ *[425.8]*
  hematogenous — *see* Tuberculosis, miliary

Tuberculosis, tubercular, tuberculous — *continued*
  hemoptysis (*see also* Tuberculosis, pulmonary) 011.9 ☑
  hemorrhage NEC (*see also* Tuberculosis, pulmonary) 011.9 ☑
  hemothorax 012.0 ☑
  hepatitis 017.9 ☑
  hilar lymph nodes 012.1 ☑
    primary, progressive 010.8 ☑
  hip (disease) (joint) 015.1 ☑
    bone 015.1 ☑ *[730.85]*
  hydrocephalus 013.8 ☑
  hydropneumothorax 012.0 ☑
  hydrothorax 012.0 ☑
  hypoadrenalism 017.6 ☑
  hypopharynx 012.8 ☑
  ileocecal (hyperplastic) 014.8 ☑
  ileocolitis 014.8 ☑
  ileum 014.8 ☑
  iliac spine (superior) 015.0 ☑ *[730.88]*
  incipient NEC (*see also* Tuberculosis, pulmonary) 011.9 ☑
  indurativa (primary) 017.1 ☑
  infantile 010.0 ☑
  infection NEC 011.9 ☑
    without clinical manifestation 010.0 ☑
  infraclavicular gland 017.2 ☑
  inguinal gland 017.2 ☑
  inguinalis 017.2 ☑
  intestine (any part) 014.8 ☑
  iris 017.3 ☑ *[364.11]*
  iritis 017.3 ☑ *[364.11]*
  ischiorectal 014.8 ☑
  jaw 015.7 ☑ *[730.88]*
  jejunum 014.8 ☑
  joint 015.9 ☑
    hip 015.1 ☑
    knee 015.2 ☑
    specified site NEC 015.8 ☑
    vertebral 015.0 ☑ *[730.88]*
  keratitis 017.3 ☑ *[370.31]*
    interstitial 017.3 ☑ *[370.59]*
  keratoconjunctivitis 017.3 ☑ *[370.31]*
  kidney 016.0 ☑
  knee (joint) 015.2 ☑
  kyphoscoliosis 015.0 ☑ *[737.43]*
  kyphosis 015.0 ☑ *[737.41]*
  lacrimal apparatus, gland 017.3 ☑
  laryngitis 012.3 ☑
  larynx 012.3 ☑
  latent 795.51
  leptomeninges, leptomeningitis (cerebral) (spinal) 013.0 ☑
  lichenoides (primary) 017.0 ☑
  linguae 017.9 ☑
  lip 017.9 ☑
  liver 017.9 ☑
  lordosis 015.0 ☑ *[737.42]*
  lung — *see* Tuberculosis, pulmonary
  luposa 017.0 ☑
    eyelid 017.0 ☑ *[373.4]*
  lymphadenitis — *see* Tuberculosis, lymph gland
  lymphangitis — *see* Tuberculosis, lymph gland
  lymphatic (gland) (vessel) — *see* Tuberculosis, lymph gland
  lymph gland or node (peripheral) 017.2 ☑
    abdomen 014.8 ☑
    bronchial 012.1 ☑
      primary, progressive 010.8 ☑
    cervical 017.2 ☑
    hilar 012.1 ☑
      primary, progressive 010.8 ☑
    intrathoracic 012.1 ☑
      primary, progressive 010.8 ☑
    mediastinal 012.1 ☑
      primary, progressive 010.8 ☑
    mesenteric 014.8 ☑
    peripheral 017.2 ☑
    retroperitoneal 014.8 ☑
    tracheobronchial 012.1 ☑

Tuberculosis, tubercular, tuberculous — *continued*
  lymph gland or node — *continued*
    tracheobronchial — *continued*
      primary, progressive 010.8 ☑
  malignant NEC (*see also* Tuberculosis, pulmonary) 011.9 ☑
  mammary gland 017.9 ☑
  marasmus NEC (*see also* Tuberculosis, pulmonary) 011.9 ☑
  mastoiditis 015.6 ☑
  maternal, affecting fetus or newborn 760.2
  mediastinal (lymph) gland or node 012.1 ☑
    primary, progressive 010.8 ☑
  mediastinitis 012.8 ☑
    primary, progressive 010.8 ☑
  mediastinopericarditis 017.9 ☑ *[420.0]*
  mediastinum 012.8 ☑
    primary, progressive 010.8 ☑
  medulla 013.9 ☑
    brain 013.2 ☑
    spinal cord 013.4 ☑
  melanosis, Addisonian 017.6 ☑
  membrane, brain 013.0 ☑
  meninges (cerebral) (spinal) 013.0 ☑
  meningitis (basilar) (brain) (cerebral) (cerebrospinal) (spinal) 013.0 ☑
  meningoencephalitis 013.0 ☑
  mesentery, mesenteric 014.8 ☑
    lymph gland or node 014.8 ☑
  miliary (any site) 018.9 ☑
    acute 018.0 ☑
    chronic 018.8 ☑
    specified type NEC 018.8 ☑
  millstone makers' 011.4 ☑
  miners' 011.4 ☑
  moulders' 011.4 ☑
  mouth 017.9 ☑
  multiple 018.9 ☑
    acute 018.0 ☑
    chronic 018.8 ☑
  muscle 017.9 ☑
  myelitis 013.6 ☑
  myocarditis 017.9 ☑ *[422.0]*
  myocardium 017.9 ☑ *[422.0]*
  nasal (passage) (sinus) 012.8 ☑
  nasopharynx 012.8 ☑
  neck gland 017.2 ☑
  nephritis 016.0 ☑ *[583.81]*
  nerve 017.9 ☑
  nose (septum) 012.8 ☑
  ocular 017.3 ☑
  old NEC 137.0
    without residuals V12.01
  omentum 014.8 ☑
  oophoritis (acute) (chronic) 016.6 ☑
  optic 017.3 ☑ *[377.39]*
    nerve trunk 017.3 ☑ *[377.39]*
    papilla, papillae 017.3 ☑ *[377.39]*
  orbit 017.3 ☑
  orchitis 016.5 ☑ *[608.81]*
  organ, specified NEC 017.9 ☑
  orificialis (primary) 017.0 ☑
  osseous (*see also* Tuberculosis, bone) 015.9 ☑ *[730.8]*
  osteitis (*see also* Tuberculosis, bone) 015.9 ☑ *[730.8]*
  osteomyelitis (*see also* Tuberculosis, bone) 015.9 ☑ *[730.8]*
  otitis (media) 017.4 ☑
  ovaritis (acute) (chronic) 016.6 ☑
  ovary (acute) (chronic) 016.6 ☑
  oviducts (acute) (chronic) 016.6 ☑
  pachymeningitis 013.0 ☑
  palate (soft) 017.9 ☑
  pancreas 017.9 ☑
  papulonecrotic (primary) 017.0 ☑
  parathyroid glands 017.9 ☑
  paronychia (primary) 017.0 ☑
  parotid gland or region 017.9 ☑
  pelvic organ NEC 016.9 ☑
    female 016.7 ☑
    male 016.5 ☑

☑ Additional Digit Required — Refer to the Tabular List for Digit Selection | ▽ Subterms under main terms may continue to next column or page

Tuberculosis, tubercular, tuberculous — *continued*
pelvis (bony) 015.7 ☑ [730.85]
penis 016.5 ☑
peribronchitis 011.3 ☑
pericarditis 017.9 ☑ [420.0]
pericardium 017.9 ☑ [420.0]
perichondritis, larynx 012.3 ☑
perineum 017.9 ☑
periostitis (*see also* Tuberculosis, bone) 015.9 ☑ [730.8] ☑
periphlebitis 017.9 ☑
  eye vessel 017.3 ☑ [362.18]
  retina 017.3 ☑ [362.18]
perirectal fistula 014.8 ☑
peritoneal gland 014.8 ☑
peritoneum 014.0 ☑
peritonitis 014.0 ☑
pernicious NEC (*see also* Tuberculosis, pulmonary) 011.9 ☑
pharyngitis 012.8 ☑
pharynx 012.8 ☑
phlyctenulosis (conjunctiva) 017.3 ☑ [370.31]
phthisis NEC (*see also* Tuberculosis, pulmonary) 011.9 ☑
pituitary gland 017.9 ☑
placenta 016.7 ☑
pleura, pleural, pleurisy, pleuritis (fibrinous) (obliterative) (purulent) (simple plastic) (with effusion) 012.0 ☑
  primary, progressive 010.1 ☑
pneumonia, pneumonic 011.6 ☑
pneumothorax 011.7 ☑
polyserositis 018.9 ☑
  acute 018.0 ☑
  chronic 018.8 ☑
potters' 011.4 ☑
prepuce 016.5 ☑
primary 010.9 ☑
  complex 010.0 ☑
  complicated 010.8 ☑
    with pleurisy or effusion 010.1 ☑
  progressive 010.8 ☑
    with pleurisy or effusion 010.1 ☑
  skin 017.0 ☑
proctitis 014.8 ☑
prostate 016.5 ☑ [601.4]
prostatitis 016.5 ☑ [601.4]
pulmonaris (*see also* Tuberculosis, pulmonary) 011.9 ☑
pulmonary (artery) (incipient) (malignant) (multiple round foci) (pernicious) (reinfection stage) 011.9 ☑
  cavitated or with cavitation 011.2 ☑
    primary, progressive 010.8 ☑
  childhood type or first infection 010.0 ☑
  chromogenic acid-fast bacilli 795.39
  fibrosis or fibrotic 011.4 ☑
  infiltrative 011.0 ☑
    primary, progressive 010.9 ☑
  nodular 011.1 ☑
  specified NEC 011.8 ☑
  sputum positive only 795.39
  status following surgical collapse of lung NEC 011.9 ☑
pyelitis 016.0 ☑ [590.81]
pyelonephritis 016.0 ☑ [590.81]
pyemia — *see* Tuberculosis, miliary
pyonephrosis 016.0 ☑
pyopneumothorax 012.0 ☑
pyothorax 012.0 ☑
rectum (with abscess) 014.8 ☑
  fistula 014.8 ☑
reinfection stage (*see also* Tuberculosis, pulmonary) 011.9 ☑
renal 016.0 ☑
renis 016.0 ☑
reproductive organ 016.7 ☑
respiratory NEC (*see also* Tuberculosis, pulmonary) 011.9 ☑
  specified site NEC 012.8 ☑
retina 017.3 ☑ [363.13]

Tuberculosis, tubercular, tuberculous — *continued*
retroperitoneal (lymph gland or node) 014.8 ☑
  gland 014.8 ☑
retropharyngeal abscess 012.8 ☑
rheumatism 015.9 ☑
rhinitis 012.8 ☑
sacroiliac (joint) 015.8 ☑
sacrum 015.0 ☑ [730.88]
salivary gland 017.9 ☑
salpingitis (acute) (chronic) 016.6 ☑
sandblasters' 011.4 ☑
sclera 017.3 ☑ [379.09]
scoliosis 015.0 ☑ [737.43]
scrofulous 017.2 ☑
scrotum 016.5 ☑
seminal tract or vesicle 016.5 ☑ [608.81]
senile NEC (*see also* Tuberculosis, pulmonary) 011.9 ☑
septic NEC (*see also* Tuberculosis, miliary) 018.9 ☑
shoulder 015.8 ☑
  blade 015.7 ☑ [730.8]
sigmoid 014.8 ☑
sinus (accessory) (nasal) 012.8 ☑
  bone 015.7 ☑ [730.88]
  epididymis 016.4 ☑
skeletal NEC (*see also* Osteomyelitis, due to tuberculosis) 015.9 ☑ [730.8] ☑
skin (any site) (primary) 017.0 ☑
small intestine 014.8 ☑
soft palate 017.9 ☑
spermatic cord 016.5 ☑
spinal
  column 015.0 ☑ [730.88]
  cord 013.4 ☑
  disease 015.0 ☑ [730.88]
  medulla 013.4 ☑
  membrane 013.0 ☑
  meninges 013.0 ☑
spine 015.0 ☑ [730.88]
spleen 017.7 ☑
splenitis 017.7 ☑
spondylitis 015.0 ☑ [720.81]
spontaneous pneumothorax — *see* Tuberculosis, pulmonary
sternoclavicular joint 015.8 ☑
stomach 017.9 ☑
stonemasons' 011.4 ☑
struma 017.2 ☑
subcutaneous tissue (cellular) (primary) 017.0 ☑
subcutis (primary) 017.0 ☑
subdeltoid bursa 017.9 ☑
submaxillary 017.9 ☑
  region 017.9 ☑
supraclavicular gland 017.2 ☑
suprarenal (capsule) (gland) 017.6 ☑
swelling, joint (*see also* Tuberculosis, joint) 015.9 ☑
symphysis pubis 015.7 ☑ [730.88]
synovitis 015.9 ☑ [727.01]
  hip 015.1 ☑ [727.01]
  knee 015.2 ☑ [727.01]
  specified site NEC 015.8 ☑ [727.01]
  spine or vertebra 015.0 ☑ [727.01]
systemic — *see* Tuberculosis, miliary
tarsitis (eyelid) 017.0 ☑ [373.4]
  ankle (bone) 015.5 ☑ [730.87]
tendon (sheath) — *see* Tuberculosis, tenosynovitis
tenosynovitis 015.9 ☑ [727.01]
  hip 015.1 ☑ [727.01]
  knee 015.2 ☑ [727.01]
  specified site NEC 015.8 ☑ [727.01]
  spine or vertebra 015.0 ☑ [727.01]
testis 016.5 ☑ [608.81]
throat 012.8 ☑
thymus gland 017.9 ☑
thyroid gland 017.5 ☑
toe 017.9 ☑
tongue 017.9 ☑

Tuberculosis, tubercular, tuberculous — *continued*
tonsil (lingual) 012.8 ☑
tonsillitis 012.8 ☑
trachea, tracheal 012.8 ☑
  gland 012.1 ☑
    primary, progressive 010.8 ☑
  isolated 012.2 ☑
tracheobronchial 011.3 ☑
  glandular 012.1 ☑
    primary, progressive 010.8 ☑
  isolated 012.2 ☑
  lymph gland or node 012.1 ☑
    primary, progressive 010.8 ☑
tubal 016.6 ☑
tunica vaginalis 016.5 ☑
typhlitis 014.8 ☑
ulcer (primary) (skin) 017.0 ☑
  bowel or intestine 014.8 ☑
  specified site NEC — *see* Tuberculosis, by site
unspecified site — *see* Tuberculosis, pulmonary
ureter 016.2 ☑
urethra, urethral 016.3 ☑
urinary organ or tract 016.3 ☑
  kidney 016.0 ☑
uterus 016.7 ☑
uveal tract 017.3 ☑ [363.13]
uvula 017.9 ☑
vaccination, prophylactic (against) V03.2
vagina 016.7 ☑
vas deferens 016.5 ☑
vein 017.9 ☑
verruca (primary) 017.0 ☑
verrucosa (cutis) (primary) 017.0 ☑
vertebra (column) 015.0 ☑ [730.88]
vesiculitis 016.5 ☑ [608.81]
viscera NEC 014.8 ☑
vulva 016.7 ☑ [616.51]
wrist (joint) 015.8 ☑
  bone 015.5 ☑ [730.83]
Tuberculum
  auriculae 744.29
  occlusal 520.2
  paramolare 520.2
Tuberosity
  jaw, excessive 524.07
  maxillary, entire 524.07
Tuberous sclerosis (brain) 759.5
Tube, tubal, tubular — *see also* condition
  ligation, admission for V25.2
Tubo-ovarian — *see* condition
Tuboplasty, after previous sterilization V26.0
Tubotympanitis 381.10
Tularemia 021.9
  with
    conjunctivitis 021.3
    pneumonia 021.2
  bronchopneumonic 021.2
  conjunctivitis 021.3
  cryptogenic 021.1
  disseminated 021.8
  enteric 021.1
  generalized 021.8
  glandular 021.8
  intestinal 021.1
  oculoglandular 021.3
  ophthalmic 021.3
  pneumonia 021.2
  pulmonary 021.2
  specified NEC 021.8
  typhoidal 021.1
  ulceroglandular 021.0
  vaccination, prophylactic (against) V03.4
Tularensis conjunctivitis 021.3
Tumefaction — *see also* Swelling
  liver (*see also* Hypertrophy, liver) 789.1
Tumor (M8000/1) — *see also* Neoplasm, by site, unspecified nature
  Abrikossov's (M9580/0) (*see also* Neoplasm, connective tissue, benign)
    malignant (M9580/3) — *see* Neoplasm, connective tissue, malignant

Tumor — *see also* Neoplasm, by site, unspecified nature — *continued*
acinar cell (M8550/1) — *see* Neoplasm, by site, uncertain behavior
acinic cell (M8550/1) — *see* Neoplasm, by site, uncertain behavior
adenomatoid (M9054/0) (*see also* Neoplasm, by site, benign)
  odontogenic (M9300/0) 213.1
    upper jaw (bone) 213.0
adnexal (skin) (M8390/0) — *see* Neoplasm, skin, benign
adrenal
  cortical (benign) (M8370/0) 227.0
    malignant (M8370/3) 194.0
  rest (M8671/0) — *see* Neoplasm, by site, benign
alpha cell (M8152/0)
  malignant (M8152/3)
    pancreas 157.4
    specified site NEC — *see* Neoplasm, by site, malignant
    unspecified site 157.4
  pancreas 211.7
  specified site NEC — *see* Neoplasm, by site, benign
  unspecified site 211.7
aneurysmal (*see also* Aneurysm) 442.9
aortic body (M8691/1) 237.3
  malignant (M8691/3) 194.6
argentaffin (M8241/1) — *see* Neoplasm, by site, uncertain behavior
basal cell (M8090/1) (*see also* Neoplasm, skin, uncertain behavior)
benign (M8000/0) — *see* Neoplasm, by site, benign
beta cell (M8151/0)
  malignant (M8151/3)
    pancreas 157.4
    specified site — *see* Neoplasm, by site, malignant
    unspecified site 157.4
  pancreas 211.7
  specified site NEC — *see* Neoplasm, by site, benign
  unspecified site 211.7
blood — *see* Hematoma
Brenner (M9000/0) 220
  borderline malignancy (M9000/1) 236.2
  malignant (M9000/3) 183.0
  proliferating (M9000/1) 236.2
Brooke's (M8100/0) — *see* Neoplasm, skin, benign
brown fat (M8880/0) — *see* Lipoma, by site
Burkitt's (M9750/3) 200.2 ☑
calcifying epithelial odontogenic (M9340/0) 213.1
  upper jaw (bone) 213.0
carcinoid (M8240/1) 209.60
  benign 209.60
    appendix 209.51
    ascending colon 209.53
    bronchus 209.61
    cecum 209.52
    colon 209.50
    descending colon 209.55
    duodenum 209.41
    foregut 209.65
    hindgut 209.67
    ileum 209.43
    jejunum 209.42
    kidney 209.64
    large intestine 209.50
    lung 209.61
    midgut 209.66
    rectum 209.57
    sigmoid colon 209.56
    small intestine 209.40
    specified NEC 209.69
    stomach 209.63
    thymus 209.62
    transverse colon 209.54
  malignant (of) 209.20
    appendix 209.11
    ascending colon 209.13
    bronchus 209.21

☑ **Additional Digit Required** — Refer to the Tabular List for Digit Selection   ▽ **Subterms under main terms may continue to next column or page**

286 — Volume 2   ►◄ **Revised Text**   ● **New Line**   ▲ **Revised Code**   **2015 ICD-9-CM**

Tumor — *see also* Neoplasm, by site, unspecified nature — *continued*
carcinoid — *continued*
  malignant — *continued*
    cecum 209.12
    colon 209.10
    descending colon 209.15
    duodenum 209.01
    foregut 209.25
    hindgut 209.27
    ileum 209.03
    jejunum 209.02
    kidney 209.24
    large intestine 209.10
    lung 209.21
    midgut 209.26
    rectum 209.17
    sigmoid colon 209.16
    small intestine 209.00
    specified NEC 209.29
    stomach 209.23
    thymus 209.22
    transverse colon 209.14
    secondary — *see* Tumor, neuroendocrine, secondary
carotid body (M8692/1) 237.3
  malignant (M8692/3) 194.5
Castleman's (mediastinal lymph node hyperplasia) 785.6
cells (M8001/1) (*see also* Neoplasm, by site, unspecified nature)
  benign (M8001/0) — *see* Neoplasm, by site, benign
  malignant (M8001/3) — *see* Neoplasm, by site, malignant
  uncertain whether benign or malignant (M8001/1) — *see* Neoplasm, by site, uncertain nature
cervix
  in pregnancy or childbirth 654.6 ☑
    affecting fetus or newborn 763.89
    causing obstructed labor 660.2 ☑
      affecting fetus or newborn 763.1
chondromatous giant cell (M9230/0) — *see* Neoplasm, bone, benign
chromaffin (M8700/0) (*see also* Neoplasm, by site, benign)
  malignant (M8700/3) — *see* Neoplasm, by site, malignant
Cock's peculiar 706.2
Codman's (benign chondroblastoma) (M9230/0) — *see* Neoplasm, bone, benign
dentigerous, mixed (M9282/0) 213.1
  upper jaw (bone) 213.0
dermoid (M9084/0) — *see* Neoplasm, by site, benign
  with malignant transformation (M9084/3) 183.0
desmoid (extra-abdominal) (M8821/1) (*see also* Neoplasm, connective tissue, uncertain behavior)
  abdominal (M8822/1) — *see* Neoplasm, connective tissue, uncertain behavior
embryonal (mixed) (M9080/1) (*see also* Neoplasm, by site, uncertain behavior)
  liver (M9080/3) 155.0
endodermal sinus (M9071/3)
  specified site — *see* Neoplasm, by site, malignant
  unspecified site
    female 183.0
    male 186.9
epithelial
  benign (M8010/0) — *see* Neoplasm, by site, benign
  malignant (M8010/3) — *see* Neoplasm, by site, malignant
Ewing's (M9260/3) — *see* Neoplasm, bone, malignant
fatty — *see* Lipoma
fetal, causing disproportion 653.7 ☑
  causing obstructed labor 660.1 ☑
fibroid (M8890/0) — *see* Leiomyoma

Tumor — *see also* Neoplasm, by site, unspecified nature — *continued*
G cell (M8153/1)
  malignant (M8153/3)
    pancreas 157.4
    specified site NEC — *see* Neoplasm, by site, malignant
    unspecified site 157.4
  specified site — *see* Neoplasm, by site, uncertain behavior
  unspecified site 235.5
giant cell (type) (M8003/1) (*see also* Neoplasm, by site, unspecified nature)
  bone (M9250/1) 238.0
    malignant (M9250/3) — *see* Neoplasm, bone, malignant
  chondromatous (M9230/0) — *see* Neoplasm, bone, benign
  malignant (M8003/3) — *see* Neoplasm, by site, malignant
  peripheral (gingiva) 523.8
  soft parts (M9251/1) (*see also* Neoplasm, connective tissue, uncertain behavior)
    malignant (M9251/3) — *see* Neoplasm, connective tissue, malignant
  tendon sheath 727.02
glomus (M8711/0) (*see also* Hemangioma, by site)
  jugulare (M8690/1) 237.3
    malignant (M8690/3) 194.6
gonadal stromal (M8590/1) — *see* Neoplasm, by site, uncertain behavior
granular cell (M9580/0) (*see also* Neoplasm, connective tissue, benign)
  malignant (M9580/3) — *see* Neoplasm, connective tissue, malignant
granulosa cell (M8620/1) 236.2
  malignant (M8620/3) 183.0
granulosa cell-theca cell (M8621/1) 236.2
  malignant (M8621/3) 183.0
Grawitz's (hypernephroma) (M8312/3) 189.0
hazard-crile (M8350/3) 193
hemorrhoidal — *see* Hemorrhoids
hilar cell (M8660/0) 220
Hürthle cell (benign) (M8290/0) 226
  malignant (M8290/3) 193
hydatid (*see also* Echinococcus) 122.9
hypernephroid (M8311/1) (*see also* Neoplasm, by site, uncertain behavior)
interstitial cell (M8650/1) (*see also* Neoplasm, by site, uncertain behavior)
  benign (M8650/0) — *see* Neoplasm, by site, benign
  malignant (M8650/3) — *see* Neoplasm, by site, malignant
islet cell (M8150/0)
  malignant (M8150/3)
    pancreas 157.4
    specified site — *see* Neoplasm, by site, malignant
    unspecified site 157.4
  pancreas 211.7
  specified site NEC — *see* Neoplasm, by site, benign
  unspecified site 211.7
juxtaglomerular (M8361/1) 236.91
Krukenberg's (M8490/6) 198.6
Leydig cell (M8650/1)
  benign (M8650/0)
    specified site — *see* Neoplasm, by site, benign
    unspecified site
      female 220
      male 222.0
  malignant (M8650/3)
    specified site — *see* Neoplasm, by site, malignant
    unspecified site
      female 183.0
      male 186.9
  specified site — *see* Neoplasm, by site, uncertain behavior
  unspecified site
    female 236.2

Tumor — *see also* Neoplasm, by site, unspecified nature — *continued*
Leydig cell — *continued*
  unspecified site — *continued*
    male 236.4
lipid cell, ovary (M8670/0) 220
lipoid cell, ovary (M8670/0) 220
lymphomatous, benign (M9590/0) (*see also* Neoplasm, by site, benign)
lysis syndrome (following antineoplastic drug therapy) (spontaneous) 277.88
Malherbe's (M8110/0) — *see* Neoplasm, skin, benign
malignant (M8000/3) (*see also* Neoplasm, by site, malignant)
  fusiform cell (type) (M8004/3) — *see* Neoplasm, by site, malignant
  giant cell (type) (M8003/3) — *see* Neoplasm, by site, malignant
  mixed NEC (M8940/3) — *see* Neoplasm, by site, malignant
  small cell (type) (M8002/3) — *see* Neoplasm, by site, malignant
  spindle cell (type) (M8004/3) — *see* Neoplasm, by site, malignant
mast cell (M9740/1) 238.5
  malignant (M9740/3) 202.6 ☑
melanotic, neuroectodermal (M9363/0) — *see* Neoplasm, by site, benign
Merkel cell — *see* Carcinoma, Merkel cell
mesenchymal
  malignant (M8800/3) — *see* Neoplasm, connective tissue, malignant
  mixed (M8990/1) — *see* Neoplasm, connective tissue, uncertain behavior
mesodermal, mixed (M8951/3) (*see also* Neoplasm, by site, malignant)
  liver 155.0
mesonephric (M9110/1) (*see also* Neoplasm, by site, uncertain behavior)
  malignant (M9110/3) — *see* Neoplasm, by site, malignant
metastatic
  from specified site (M8000/3) — *see* Neoplasm, by site, malignant
  to specified site (M8000/6) — *see* Neoplasm, by site, malignant, secondary
mixed NEC (M8940/0) (*see also* Neoplasm, by site, benign)
  malignant (M8940/3) — *see* Neoplasm, by site, malignant
mucocarcinoid, malignant (M8243/3) — *see* Neoplasm, by site, malignant
mucoepidermoid (M8430/1) — *see* Neoplasm, by site, uncertain behavior
Müllerian, mixed (M8950/3) — *see* Neoplasm, by site, malignant
myoepithelial (M8982/0) — *see* Neoplasm, by site, benign
neuroendocrine 209.60
  malignant poorly differentiated 209.30
  secondary 209.70
    bone 209.73
    distant lymph nodes 209.71
    liver 209.72
    peritoneum 209.74
    site specified NEC 209.79
neurogenic olfactory (M9520/3) 160.0
nonencapsulated sclerosing (M8350/3) 193
odontogenic (M9270/1) 238.0
  adenomatoid (M9300/0) 213.1
    upper jaw (bone) 213.0
  benign (M9270/0) 213.1
    upper jaw (bone) 213.0
  calcifying epithelial (M9340/0) 213.1
    upper jaw (bone) 213.0
  malignant (M9270/3) 170.1
    upper jaw (bone) 170.0
  squamous (M9312/0) 213.1
    upper jaw (bone) 213.0
ovarian stromal (M8590/1) 236.2
ovary
  in pregnancy or childbirth 654.4 ☑
    affecting fetus or newborn 763.89

Tumor — *see also* Neoplasm, by site, unspecified nature — *continued*
ovary — *continued*
  in pregnancy or childbirth — *continued*
    causing obstructed labor 660.2 ☑
      affecting fetus or newborn 763.1
pacinian (M9507/0) — *see* Neoplasm, skin, benign
Pancoast's (M8010/3) 162.3
papillary — *see* Papilloma
pelvic, in pregnancy or childbirth 654.9 ☑
  affecting fetus or newborn 763.89
  causing obstructed labor 660.2 ☑
    affecting fetus or newborn 763.1
phantom 300.11
plasma cell (M9731/1) 238.6
  benign (M9731/0) — *see* Neoplasm, by site, benign
  malignant (M9731/3) 203.8 ☑
polyvesicular vitelline (M9071/3)
  specified site — *see* Neoplasm, by site, malignant
  unspecified site
    female 183.0
    male 186.9
Pott's puffy (*see also* Osteomyelitis) 730.2 ☑
Rathke's pouch (M9350/1) 237.0
regaud's (M8082/3) — *see* Neoplasm, nasopharynx, malignant
rete cell (M8140/0) 222.0
retinal anlage (M9363/0) — *see* Neoplasm, by site, benign
Rokitansky's 620.2
salivary gland type, mixed (M8940/0) (*see also* Neoplasm, by site, benign)
  malignant (M8940/3) — *see* Neoplasm, by site, malignant
Sampson's 617.1
Schloffer's (*see also* Peritonitis) 567.29
Schmincke (M8082/3) — *see* Neoplasm, nasopharynx, malignant
sebaceous (*see also* Cyst, sebaceous) 706.2
secondary (M8000/6) — *see* Neoplasm, by site, secondary
  carcinoid — *see* Tumor, neuroendocrine, secondary
  neuroendocrine — *see* Tumor, neuroendocrine, secondary
Sertoli cell (M8640/0)
  with lipid storage (M8641/0)
    specified site — *see* Neoplasm, by site, benign
    unspecified site
      female 220
      male 222.0
  specified site — *see* Neoplasm, by site, benign
  unspecified site
    female 220
    male 222.0
Sertoli-Leydig cell (M8631/0)
  specified site, — *see* Neoplasm, by site, benign
  unspecified site
    female 220
    male 222.0
sex cord (-stromal) (M8590/1) — *see* Neoplasm, by site, uncertain behavior
skin appendage (M8390/0) — *see* Neoplasm, skin, benign
soft tissue
  benign (M8800/0) — *see* Neoplasm, connective tissue, benign
  malignant (M8800/3) — *see* Neoplasm, connective tissue, malignant
sternomastoid 754.1
stromal
  abdomen
    benign 215.5
    malignant NEC 171.5
    uncertain behavior 238.1
  digestive system 238.1
    benign 215.5
    malignant NEC 171.5
    uncertain behavior 238.1

☑ **Additional Digit Required — Refer to the Tabular List for Digit Selection**   ⬗ **Subterms under main terms may continue to next column or page**

Tumor — *see also* Neoplasm, by site, unspecified nature — *continued*
- stromal — *continued*
  - endometrium (endometrial) 236.0
  - gastric 238.1
    - benign 215.5
    - malignant 151.9
    - uncertain behavior 238.1
  - gastrointestinal 238.1
    - benign 215.5
    - malignant NEC 171.5
    - uncertain behavior 238.1
  - intestine (small) 238.1
    - benign 215.5
    - malignant 152.9
    - uncertain behavior 238.1
  - stomach 238.1
    - benign 215.5
    - malignant 151.9
    - uncertain behavior 238.1
- superior sulcus (lung) (pulmonary) (syndrome) (M8010/3) 162.3
- suprasulcus (M8010/3) 162.3
- sweat gland (M8400/1) (*see also* Neoplasm, skin, uncertain behavior)
  - benign (M8400/0) — *see* Neoplasm, skin, benign
  - malignant (M8400/3) — *see* Neoplasm, skin, malignant
- syphilitic brain 094.89
  - congenital 090.49
- testicular stromal (M8590/1) 236.4
- theca cell (M8600/0) 220
- theca cell-granulosa cell (M8621/1) 236.2
- theca-lutein (M8610/0) 220
- turban (M8200/0) 216.4
- uterus
  - in pregnancy or childbirth 654.1 ☑
    - affecting fetus or newborn 763.89
    - causing obstructed labor 660.2 ☑
      - affecting fetus or newborn 763.1
- vagina
  - in pregnancy or childbirth 654.7 ☑
    - affecting fetus or newborn 763.89
    - causing obstructed labor 660.2 ☑
      - affecting fetus or newborn 763.1
- varicose (*see also* Varicose, vein) 454.9
- von Recklinghausen's (M9540/1) 237.71
- vulva
  - in pregnancy or childbirth 654.8 ☑
    - affecting fetus or newborn 763.89
    - causing obstructed labor 660.2 ☑
      - affecting fetus or newborn 763.1
- Warthin's (salivary gland) (M8561/0) 210.2
- white (*see also* Tuberculosis, arthritis)
- White-Darier 757.39
- Wilms' (nephroblastoma) (M8960/3) 189.0
- yolk sac (M9071/3)
  - specified site — *see* Neoplasm, by site, malignant
  - unspecified site
    - female 183.0
    - male 186.9

Tumorlet (M8040/1) — *see* Neoplasm, by site, uncertain behavior

Tungiasis 134.1

Tunica vasculosa lentis 743.39

Tunnel vision 368.45

Turban tumor (M8200/0) 216.4

Türck's trachoma (chronic catarrhal laryngitis) 476.0

Türk's syndrome (ocular retraction syndrome) 378.71

Turner's
- hypoplasia (tooth) 520.4
- syndrome 758.6
- tooth 520.4

Turner-Kieser syndrome (hereditary osteo-onychodysplasia) 756.89

Turner-Varny syndrome 758.6

Turricephaly 756.0

Tussis convulsiva — *see also* Whooping cough 033.9

Twiddler's syndrome (due to)
- automatic implantable defibrillator 996.04
- pacemaker 996.01

Twin
- affected by maternal complications of pregnancy 761.5
- conjoined 759.4
  - fetal 678.1 ☑
- healthy liveborn — *see* Newborn, twin
- pregnancy (complicating delivery) NEC 651.0 ☑
  - with fetal loss and retention of one fetus 651.3 ☑
  - conjoined 678.1 ☑
  - following (elective) fetal reduction 651.7 ☑

Twinning, teeth 520.2

Twist, twisted
- bowel, colon, or intestine 560.2
- hair (congenital) 757.4
- mesentery 560.2
- omentum 560.2
- organ or site, congenital NEC — *see* Anomaly, specified type NEC
- ovarian pedicle 620.5
  - congenital 752.0
- umbilical cord — *see* Compression, umbilical cord

Twitch 781.0

Tylosis 700
- buccalis 528.6
- gingiva 523.8
- linguae 528.6
- palmaris et plantaris 757.39

Tympanism 787.3

Tympanites (abdominal) (intestine) 787.3

Tympanitis — *see* Myringitis

Tympanosclerosis 385.00
- involving
  - combined sites NEC 385.09
    - with tympanic membrane 385.03
  - tympanic membrane 385.01
    - with ossicles 385.02
      - and middle ear 385.03

Tympanum — *see* condition

Tympany
- abdomen 787.3
- chest 786.7

Typhlitis — *see also* Appendicitis 541

Typhoenteritis 002.0

Typhogastric fever 002.0

Typhoid (abortive) (ambulant) (any site) (fever) (hemorrhagic) (infection) (intermittent) (malignant) (rheumatic) 002.0
- with pneumonia 002.0 [484.8]
- abdominal 002.0
- carrier (suspected) of V02.1
- cholecystitis (current) 002.0
- clinical (Widal and blood test negative) 002.0
- endocarditis 002.0 [421.1]
- inoculation reaction — *see* Complications, vaccination
- meningitis 002.0 [320.7]
- mesenteric lymph nodes 002.0
- myocarditis 002.0 [422.0]
- osteomyelitis (*see also* Osteomyelitis, due to, typhoid) 002.0 [730.8] ☑
- perichondritis, larynx 002.0 [478.71]
- pneumonia 002.0 [484.8]
- spine 002.0 [720.81]
- ulcer (perforating) 002.0
- vaccination, prophylactic (against) V03.1
- Widal negative 002.0

Typhomalaria (fever) — *see also* Malaria 084.6

Typhomania 002.0

Typhoperitonitis 002.0

Typhus (fever) 081.9
- abdominal, abdominalis 002.0
- African tick 082.1
- amarillic (*see also* Fever, Yellow) 060.9
- brain 081.9
- cerebral 081.9
- classical 080
- endemic (flea-borne) 081.0
- epidemic (louse-borne) 080
- exanthematicus SAI 080
  - brillii SAI 081.1
  - Mexicanus SAI 081.0

Typhus — *continued*
- exanthematicus SAI — *continued*
  - pediculo vestimenti causa 080
  - typhus murinus 081.0
- exanthematic NEC 080
- flea-borne 081.0
- Indian tick 082.1
- Kenya tick 082.1
- louse-borne 080
- Mexican 081.0
  - flea-borne 081.0
  - louse-borne 080
  - tabardillo 080
- mite-borne 081.2
- murine 081.0
- North Asian tick-borne 082.2
- petechial 081.9
- Queensland tick 082.3
- rat 081.0
- recrudescent 081.1
- recurrent (*see also* Fever, relapsing) 087.9
- São Paulo 082.0
- scrub (China) (India) (Malaya) (New Guinea) 081.2
- shop (of Malaya) 081.0
- Siberian tick 082.2
- tick-borne NEC 082.9
- tropical 081.2
- vaccination, prophylactic (against) V05.8

Tyrosinemia 270.2
- neonatal 775.89

Tyrosinosis (Medes) (Sakai) 270.2

Tyrosinuria 270.2

Tyrosyluria 270.2

U

Uehlinger's syndrome (acropachyderma) 757.39

Uhl's anomaly or disease (hypoplasia of myocardium, right ventricle) 746.84

Ulcerosa scarlatina 034.1

Ulcer, ulcerated, ulcerating, ulceration, ulcerative 707.9
- with gangrene 707.9 [785.4]
- abdomen (wall) (*see also* Ulcer, skin) 707.8
- ala, nose 478.19
- alveolar process 526.5
- amebic (intestine) 006.9
  - skin 006.6
- anastomotic — *see* Ulcer, gastrojejunal
- anorectal 569.41
- antral — *see* Ulcer, stomach
- anus (sphincter) (solitary) 569.41
  - varicose — *see* Varicose, ulcer, anus
- aorta — *see* Aneuysm
- aphthous (oral) (recurrent) 528.2
  - genital organ(s)
    - female 616.50
    - male 608.89
  - mouth 528.2
- arm (*see also* Ulcer, skin) 707.8
- arteriosclerotic plaque — *see* Arteriosclerosis, by site
- artery NEC 447.2
  - without rupture 447.8
- atrophic NEC — *see* Ulcer, skin
- Barrett's (chronic peptic ulcer of esophagus) 530.85
- bile duct 576.8
- bladder (solitary) (sphincter) 596.89
  - bilharzial (*see also* Schistosomiasis) 120.9 [595.4]
  - submucosal (*see also* Cystitis) 595.1
  - tuberculous (*see also* Tuberculosis) 016.1 ☑
- bleeding NEC — *see* Ulcer, peptic, with hemorrhage
- bone 730.9 ☑
- bowel (*see also* Ulcer, intestine) 569.82
- breast 611.0
- bronchitis 491.8
- bronchus 519.19
- buccal (cavity) (traumatic) 528.9
- burn (acute) — *see* Ulcer, duodenum
- Buruli 031.1
- buttock (*see also* Ulcer, skin) 707.8

Ulcer, ulcerated, ulcerating, ulceration, ulcerative — *continued*
- buttock (*see also* Ulcer, skin) — *continued*
  - decubitus (*see also* Ulcer, pressure) 707.00
- cancerous (M8000/3) — *see* Neoplasm, by site, malignant
- cardia — *see* Ulcer, stomach
- cardio-esophageal (peptic) 530.20
  - with bleeding 530.21
- cecum (*see also* Ulcer, intestine) 569.82
- cervix (uteri) (trophic) 622.0
  - with mention of cervicitis 616.0
- chancroidal 099.0
- chest (wall) (*see also* Ulcer, skin) 707.8
- Chiclero 085.4
- chin (pyogenic) (*see also* Ulcer, skin) 707.8
- chronic (cause unknown) (*see also* Ulcer, skin)
  - penis 607.89
- Cochin-China 085.1
- colitis — *see* Colitis, ulcerative
- colon (*see also* Ulcer, intestine) 569.82
- conjunctiva (acute) (postinfectional) 372.00
- cornea (infectional) 370.00
  - with perforation 370.06
  - annular 370.02
  - catarrhal 370.01
  - central 370.03
  - dendritic 054.42
  - marginal 370.01
  - mycotic 370.05
  - phlyctenular, tuberculous (*see also* Tuberculosis) 017.3 ☑ [370.31]
  - ring 370.02
  - rodent 370.07
  - serpent, serpiginous 370.04
  - superficial marginal 370.01
  - tuberculous (*see also* Tuberculosis) 017.3 ☑ [370.31]
- corpus cavernosum (chronic) 607.89
- crural — *see* Ulcer, lower extremity
- Curling's — *see* Ulcer, duodenum
- Cushing's — *see* Ulcer, peptic
- cystitis (interstitial) 595.1
- decubitus (unspecified site) (*see also* Ulcer, pressure) 707.00
  - with gangrene 707.00 [785.4]
  - ankle 707.06
  - back
    - lower 707.03
    - upper 707.02
  - buttock 707.05
  - coccyx 707.03
  - elbow 707.01
  - head 707.09
  - heel 707.07
  - hip 707.04
  - other site 707.09
  - sacrum 707.03
  - shoulder blades 707.02
- dendritic 054.42
- diabetes, diabetic (mellitus) 250.8 ☑ [707.9]
  - due to secondary diabetes 249.8 ☑ [707.9]
  - lower limb 250.8 ☑ [707.10]
    - ankle 250.8 ☑ [707.13]
      - due to secondary diabetes 249.8 ☑ [707.13]
    - calf 250.8 ☑ [707.12]
      - due to secondary diabetes 249.8 ☑ [707.12]
    - foot 250.8 ☑ [707.15]
      - due to secondary diabetes 249.8 ☑ [707.15]
    - heel 250.8 ☑ [707.14]
      - due to secondary diabetes 249.8 ☑ [707.14]
    - knee 250.8 ☑ [707.19]
      - due to secondary diabetes 249.8 ☑ [707.19]
    - specified site NEC 250.8 ☑ [707.19]

☑ Additional Digit Required — Refer to the Tabular List for Digit Selection ⟍ Subterms under main terms may continue to next column or page

288 — Volume 2 ▶◀ Revised Text ● New Line ▲ Revised Code 2015 ICD-9-CM

Ulcer, ulcerated, ulcerating, ulceration, ulcerative — *continued*
  diabetes, diabetic — *continued*
    lower limb — *continued*
      specified site — *continued*
        due to secondary diabetes 249.8 ☑ *[707.19]*
      thigh 250.8 ☑ *[707.11]*
        due to secondary diabetes 249.8 ☑ *[707.11]*
      toes 250.8 ☑ *[707.15]*
        due to secondary diabetes 249.8 ☑ *[707.15]*
    specified site NEC 250.8 ☑ *[707.8]*
      due to secondary diabetes 249.8 ☑ *[707.8]*
  Dieulafoy — *see* Lesion, Dieulafoy
  due to
    infection NEC — *see* Ulcer, skin
    radiation, radium — *see* Ulcer, by site
    trophic disturbance (any region) — *see* Ulcer, skin
    x-ray — *see* Ulcer, by site
  duodenum, duodenal (eroded) (peptic) 532.9 ☑

> *Note* — *Use the following fifth-digit subclassification with categories 531–534:*
> 0 *without mention of obstruction*
> 1 *with obstruction*

  with
    hemorrhage (chronic) 532.4 ☑
      and perforation 532.6 ☑
    perforation (chronic) 532.5 ☑
      and hemorrhage 532.6 ☑
  acute 532.3 ☑
    with
      hemorrhage 532.0 ☑
        and perforation 532.2 ☑
      perforation 532.1 ☑
        and hemorrhage 532.2 ☑
  bleeding (recurrent) — *see* Ulcer, duodenum, with hemorrhage
  chronic 532.7 ☑
    with
      hemorrhage 532.4 ☑
        and perforation 532.6 ☑
      perforation 532.5 ☑
        and hemorrhage 532.6 ☑
  penetrating — *see* Ulcer, duodenum, with perforation
  perforating — *see* Ulcer, duodenum, with perforation
  dysenteric NEC 009.0
  elusive 595.1
  endocarditis (any valve) (acute) (chronic) (subacute) 421.0
  enteritis — *see* Colitis, ulcerative
  enterocolitis 556.0
  epiglottis 478.79
  esophagus (peptic) 530.20
    with bleeding 530.21
    due to ingestion
      aspirin 530.20
      chemicals 530.20
      medicinal agents 530.20
    fungal 530.20
    infectional 530.20
    varicose (*see also* Varix, esophagus) 456.1
      bleeding (*see also* Varix, esophagus, bleeding) 456.0
  eyelid (region) 373.01
  eye NEC 360.00
    dendritic 054.42
  face (*see also* Ulcer, skin) 707.8
  fauces 478.29
  Fenwick (-Hunner) (solitary) (*see also* Cystitis) 595.1
  fistulous NEC — *see* Ulcer, skin
  foot (indolent) (*see also* Ulcer, lower extremity) 707.15
    perforating 707.15
      leprous 030.1
      syphilitic 094.0

Ulcer, ulcerated, ulcerating, ulceration, ulcerative — *continued*
  foot (*see also* Ulcer, lower extremity) — *continued*
    trophic 707.15
    varicose 454.0
      inflamed or infected 454.2
  frambesial, initial or primary 102.0
  gallbladder or duct 575.8
  gall duct 576.8
  gangrenous (*see also* Gangrene) 785.4
  gastric — *see* Ulcer, stomach
  gastrocolic — *see* Ulcer, gastrojejunal
  gastroduodenal — *see* Ulcer, peptic
  gastroesophageal — *see* Ulcer, stomach
  gastrohepatic — *see* Ulcer, stomach
  gastrointestinal — *see* Ulcer, gastrojejunal
  gastrojejunal (eroded) (peptic) 534.9 ☑

> *Note* — *Use the following fifth-digit subclassification with categories 531–534:*
> 0 *without mention of obstruction*
> 1 *with obstruction*

  with
    hemorrhage (chronic) 534.4 ☑
      and perforation 534.6 ☑
    perforation 534.5 ☑
      and hemorrhage 534.6 ☑
  acute 534.3 ☑
    with
      hemorrhage 534.0 ☑
        and perforation 534.2 ☑
      perforation 534.1 ☑
        and hemorrhage 534.2 ☑
  bleeding (recurrent) — *see* Ulcer, gastrojejunal, with hemorrhage
  chronic 534.7 ☑
    with
      hemorrhage 534.4 ☑
        and perforation 534.6 ☑
      perforation 534.5 ☑
        and hemorrhage 534.6 ☑
  penetrating — *see* Ulcer, gastrojejunal, with perforation
  perforating — *see* Ulcer, gastrojejunal, with perforation
  gastrojejunocolic — *see* Ulcer, gastrojejunal
  genital organ
    female 629.89
    male 608.89
  gingiva 523.8
  gingivitis 523.10
  glottis 478.79
  granuloma of pudenda 099.2
  groin (*see also* Ulcer, skin) 707.8
  gum 523.8
  gumma, due to yaws 102.4
  hand (*see also* Ulcer, skin) 707.8
  hard palate 528.9
  heel (*see also* Ulcer, lower extremity) 707.14
    decubitus (*see also* Ulcer, pressure) 707.07
  hemorrhoids 455.8
    external 455.5
    internal 455.2
  hip (*see also* Ulcer, skin) 707.8
    decubitus (*see also* Ulcer, pressure) 707.04
  Hunner's 595.1
  hypopharynx 478.29
  hypopyon (chronic) (subacute) 370.04
  hypostaticum — *see* Ulcer, varicose
  ileocolitis 556.1
  ileum (*see also* Ulcer, intestine) 569.82
  intestine, intestinal 569.82
    with perforation 569.83
    amebic 006.9
    duodenal — *see* Ulcer, duodenum
    granulocytopenic (with hemorrhage) 288.09
    marginal 569.82
    perforating 569.83
    small, primary 569.82
    stercoraceous 569.82

Ulcer, ulcerated, ulcerating, ulceration, ulcerative — *continued*
  intestine, intestinal — *continued*
    stercoral 569.82
    tuberculous (*see also* Tuberculosis) 014.8 ☑
    typhoid (fever) 002.0
    varicose 456.8
  ischemic 707.9
    lower extremity (*see also* Ulcer, lower extremity) 707.10
      ankle 707.13
      calf 707.12
      foot 707.15
      heel 707.14
      knee 707.19
      specified site NEC 707.19
      thigh 707.11
      toes 707.15
  jejunum, jejunal — *see* Ulcer, gastrojejunal
  keratitis (*see also* Ulcer, cornea) 370.00
  knee — *see* Ulcer, lower extremity
  labium (majus) (minus) 616.50
  laryngitis (*see also* Laryngitis) 464.00
    with obstruction 464.01
  larynx (aphthous) (contact) 478.79
    diphtheritic 032.3
  leg — *see* Ulcer, lower extremity
  lip 528.5
  Lipschütz's 616.50
  lower extremity (atrophic) (chronic) (neurogenic) (perforating) (pyogenic) (trophic) (tropical) 707.10
    with gangrene (*see also* Ulcer, lower extremity) 707.10 *[785.4]*
      arteriosclerotic 440.24
    ankle 707.13
    arteriosclerotic 440.23
      with gangrene 440.24
    calf 707.12
    decubitus (*see also* Ulcer, pressure) 707.00
      with gangrene 707.00 *[785.4]*
      ankle 707.06
      buttock 707.05
      heel 707.07
      hip 707.04
    foot 707.15
    heel 707.14
    knee 707.19
    specified site NEC 707.19
    thigh 707.11
    toes 707.15
    varicose 454.0
      inflamed or infected 454.2
  luetic — *see* Ulcer, syphilitic
  lung 518.89
    tuberculous (*see also* Tuberculosis) 011.2 ☑
  malignant (M8000/3) — *see* Neoplasm, by site, malignant
  marginal NEC — *see* Ulcer, gastrojejunal
  meatus (urinarius) 597.89
  Meckel's diverticulum 751.0
  Meleney's (chronic undermining) 686.09
  Mooren's (cornea) 370.07
  mouth (traumatic) 528.9
  mycobacterial (skin) 031.1
  nasopharynx 478.29
  navel cord (newborn) 771.4
  neck (*see also* Ulcer, skin) 707.8
    uterus 622.0
  neurogenic NEC — *see* Ulcer, skin
  nose, nasal (infectional) (passage) 478.19
    septum 478.19
      varicose 456.8
    skin — *see* Ulcer, skin
    spirochetal NEC 104.8
  oral mucosa (traumatic) 528.9
  palate (soft) 528.9
  penetrating NEC — *see* Ulcer, peptic, with perforation
  penis (chronic) 607.89

Ulcer, ulcerated, ulcerating, ulceration, ulcerative — *continued*
  peptic (site unspecified) 533.9 ☑

> *Note* — *Use the following fifth-digit subclassification with categories 531–534:*
> 0 *without mention of obstruction*
> 1 *with obstruction*

  with
    hemorrhage 533.4 ☑
      and perforation 533.6 ☑
    perforation (chronic) 533.5 ☑
      and hemorrhage 533.6 ☑
  acute 533.3 ☑
    with
      hemorrhage 533.0 ☑
        and perforation 533.2 ☑
      perforation 533.1 ☑
        and hemorrhage 533.2 ☑
  bleeding (recurrent) — *see* Ulcer, peptic, with hemorrhage
  chronic 533.7 ☑
    with
      hemorrhage 533.4 ☑
        and perforation 533.6 ☑
      perforation 533.5 ☑
        and hemorrhage 533.6 ☑
  penetrating — *see* Ulcer, peptic, with perforation
  perforating NEC (*see also* Ulcer, peptic, with perforation) 533.5 ☑
  skin 707.9
  perineum (*see also* Ulcer, skin) 707.8
  peritonsillar 474.8
  phagedenic (tropical) NEC — *see* Ulcer, skin
  pharynx 478.29
  phlebitis — *see* Phlebitis
  plaster (*see also* Ulcer, pressure) 707.00
  popliteal space — *see* Ulcer, lower extremity
  postpyloric — *see* Ulcer, duodenum
  prepuce 607.89
  prepyloric — *see* Ulcer, stomach
  pressure 707.00
    with
      abrasion, blister, partial thickness skin loss involving epidermis and/or dermis 707.22
      full thickness skin loss involving damage or necrosis of subcutaneous tissue 707.23
      gangrene 707.00 *[785.4]*
      necrosis of soft tissue through to underlying muscle, tendon, or bone 707.24
    ankle 707.06
    back
      lower 707.03
      upper 707.02
    buttock 707.05
    coccyx 707.03
    elbow 707.01
    head 707.09
    healed — omit code
    healing — code to Ulcer, pressure, by stage
    heel 707.07
    hip 707.04
    other site 707.09
    sacrum 707.03
    shoulder blades 707.02
    stage
      I (healing) 707.21
      II (healing) 707.22
      III (healing) 707.23
      IV (healing) 707.24
      unspecified (healing) 707.20
    unstageable 707.25
  primary of intestine 569.82
    with perforation 569.83
  proctitis 556.2
    with ulcerative sigmoiditis 556.3
  prostate 601.8
  pseudopeptic — *see* Ulcer, peptic
  pyloric — *see* Ulcer, stomach

☑ **Additional Digit Required** — Refer to the Tabular List for Digit Selection

▽ **Subterms under main terms may continue to next column or page**

Ulcer, ulcerated, ulcerating, ulceration, ulcerative — *continued*
rectosigmoid 569.82
  with perforation 569.83
rectum (sphincter) (solitary) 569.41
  stercoraceous, stercoral 569.41
  varicose — *see* Varicose, ulcer, anus
retina (*see also* Chorioretinitis) 363.20
rodent (M8090/3) (*see also* Neoplasm, skin, malignant)
  cornea 370.07
round — *see* Ulcer, stomach
sacrum (region) (*see also* Ulcer, skin) 707.8
Saemisch's 370.04
scalp (*see also* Ulcer, skin) 707.8
sclera 379.09
scrofulous (*see also* Tuberculosis) 017.2 ☑
scrotum 608.89
  tuberculous (*see also* Tuberculosis) 016.5 ☑
  varicose 456.4
seminal vesicle 608.89
sigmoid 569.82
  with perforation 569.83
skin (atrophic) (chronic) (neurogenic) (non-healing) (perforating) (pyogenic) (trophic) 707.9
  with gangrene 707.9 *[785.4]*
  amebic 006.6
  decubitus (*see also* Ulcer, pressure) 707.00
    with gangrene 707.00 *[785.4]*
  in granulocytopenia 288.09
  lower extremity (*see also* Ulcer, lower extremity) 707.10
    with gangrene 707.10 *[785.4]*
      arteriosclerotic 440.24
    ankle 707.13
    arteriosclerotic 440.23
      with gangrene 440.24
    calf 707.12
    foot 707.15
    heel 707.14
    knee 707.19
    specified site NEC 707.19
    thigh 707.11
    toes 707.15
  mycobacterial 031.1
  syphilitic (early) (secondary) 091.3
  tuberculous (primary) (*see also* Tuberculosis) 017.0 ☑
  varicose — *see* Ulcer, varicose
sloughing NEC — *see* Ulcer, skin
soft palate 528.9
solitary, anus or rectum (sphincter) 569.41
sore throat 462
  streptococcal 034.0
spermatic cord 608.89
spine (tuberculous) 015.0 ☑ *[730.88]*
stasis (leg) (venous) 454.0
  with varicose veins 454.0
  without varicose veins 459.81
  inflamed or infected 454.2
stercoral, stercoraceous 569.82
  with perforation 569.83
  anus or rectum 569.41
stoma, stomal — *see* Ulcer, gastrojejunal
stomach (eroded) (peptic) (round) 531.9 ☑

Note — *Use the following fifth-digit subclassification with categories 531–534:*

0 *without mention of obstruction*

1 *with obstruction*

  with
    hemorrhage 531.4 ☑
      and perforation 531.6 ☑
    perforation (chronic) 531.5 ☑
      and hemorrhage 531.6 ☑
  acute 531.3 ☑
    with
      hemorrhage 531.0 ☑
        and perforation 531.2 ☑
      perforation 531.1 ☑
        and hemorrhage 531.2 ☑

Ulcer, ulcerated, ulcerating, ulceration, ulcerative — *continued*
stomach — *continued*
  bleeding (recurrent) — *see* Ulcer, stomach, with hemorrhage
  chronic 531.7 ☑
    with
      hemorrhage 531.4 ☑
        and perforation 531.6 ☑
      perforation 531.5 ☑
        and hemorrhage 531.6 ☑
  penetrating — *see* Ulcer, stomach, with perforation
  perforating — *see* Ulcer, stomach, with perforation
stomatitis 528.00
stress — *see* Ulcer, peptic
strumous (tuberculous) (*see also* Tuberculosis) 017.2 ☑
submental (*see also* Ulcer, skin) 707.8
submucosal, bladder 595.1
syphilitic (any site) (early) (secondary) 091.3
  late 095.9
  perforating 095.9
    foot 094.0
testis 608.89
thigh — *see* Ulcer, lower extremity
throat 478.29
  diphtheritic 032.0
toe — *see* Ulcer, lower extremity
tongue (traumatic) 529.0
tonsil 474.8
  diphtheritic 032.0
trachea 519.19
trophic — *see* Ulcer, skin
tropical NEC (*see also* Ulcer, skin) 707.9
tuberculous — *see* Tuberculosis, ulcer
tunica vaginalis 608.89
turbinate 730.9 ☑
typhoid (fever) 002.0
  perforating 002.0
umbilicus (newborn) 771.4
unspecified site NEC — *see* Ulcer, skin
urethra (meatus) (*see also* Urethritis) 597.89
uterus 621.8
  cervix 622.0
    with mention of cervicitis 616.0
  neck 622.0
    with mention of cervicitis 616.0
vagina 616.89
valve, heart 421.0
varicose (lower extremity, any part) 454.0
  anus — *see* Varicose, ulcer, anus
  broad ligament 456.5
  esophagus (*see also* Varix, esophagus) 456.1
    bleeding (*see also* Varix, esophagus, bleeding) 456.0
  inflamed or infected 454.2
  nasal septum 456.8
  perineum 456.6
  rectum — *see* Varicose, ulcer, anus
  scrotum 456.4
  specified site NEC 456.8
  sublingual 456.3
  vulva 456.6
vas deferens 608.89
vesical (*see also* Ulcer, bladder) 596.89
vulva (acute) (infectional) 616.50
  Behçet's syndrome 136.1 *[616.51]*
  herpetic 054.12
  tuberculous 016.7 ☑ *[616.51]*
vulvobuccal, recurring 616.50
x-ray — *see* Ulcer, by site
yaws 102.4
Ulcus — *see also* Ulcer
cutis tuberculosum (*see also* Tuberculosis) 017.0 ☑
duodeni — *see* Ulcer, duodenum
durum 091.0
  extragenital 091.2
gastrojejunale — *see* Ulcer, gastrojejunal
hypostaticum — *see* Ulcer, varicose
molle (cutis) (skin) 099.0
serpens corneae (pneumococcal) 370.04
ventriculi — *see* Ulcer, stomach

Ulegyria 742.4
Ulerythema
  acneiforma 701.8
  centrifugum 695.4
  ophryogenes 757.4
Ullrich-Feichtiger syndrome 759.89
Ullrich (-Bonnevie) (-Turner) syndrome 758.6
Ulnar — *see* condition
Ulorrhagia 523.8
Ulorrhea 523.8
Umbilicus, umbilical — *see also* condition
  cord necrosis, affecting fetus or newborn 762.6
Unacceptable
  existing dental restoration
    contours 525.65
    morphology 525.65
Unavailability of medical facilities (at) V63.9
  due to
    investigation by social service agency V63.8
    lack of services at home V63.1
    remoteness from facility V63.0
    waiting list V63.2
  home V63.1
  outpatient clinic V63.0
  specified reason NEC V63.8
Uncinaria americana infestation 126.1
Uncinariasis — *see also* Ancylostomiasis 126.9
Unconscious, unconsciousness 780.09
Underdevelopment — *see also* Undeveloped
  sexual 259.0
Underfill, endodontic 526.63
Undernourishment 269.9
Undernutrition 269.9
Under observation — *see* Observation
Underweight 783.22
  for gestational age — *see* Light-for-dates
Underwood's disease (sclerema neonatorum) 778.1
Undescended — *see also* Malposition, congenital
  cecum 751.4
  colon 751.4
  testis 752.51
Undetermined diagnosis or cause 799.9
Undeveloped, undevelopment — *see also* Hypoplasia
  brain (congenital) 742.1
  cerebral (congenital) 742.1
  fetus or newborn 764.9 ☑
  heart 746.89
  lung 748.5
  testis 257.2
  uterus 259.0
Undiagnosed (disease) 799.9
Undulant fever — *see also* Brucellosis 023.9
Unemployment, anxiety concerning V62.0
Unequal leg (acquired) (length) 736.81
  congenital 755.30
Unerupted teeth, tooth 520.6
Unextracted dental root 525.3
Unguis incarnatus 703.0
Unicornis uterus 752.33
Unicornuate uterus (with or without a separate uterine horn) 752.33
Unicorporeus uterus 752.39
Uniformis uterus 752.39
Unilateral — *see also* condition
  development, breast 611.89
  organ or site, congenital NEC — *see* Agenesis
    vagina 752.49
Unilateralis uterus 752.39
Unilocular heart 745.8
Uninhibited bladder 596.54
  with cauda equina syndrome 344.61
  neurogenic — *see also* Neurogenic, bladder 596.54
Union, abnormal — *see also* Fusion
  divided tendon 727.89
  larynx and trachea 748.3
Universal
  joint, cervix 620.6
  mesentery 751.4

Unknown
  cause of death 799.9
  diagnosis 799.9
Unna's disease (seborrheic dermatitis) 690.10
Unresponsiveness, adrenocorticotropin (ACTH) 255.41
Unsatisfactory
  cytology smear
    anal 796.78
    cervical 795.08
    vaginal 795.18
  restoration, tooth (existing) 525.60
    specified NEC 525.69
Unsoundness of mind — *see also* Psychosis 298.9
Unspecified cause of death 799.9
Unstable
  back NEC 724.9
  colon 569.89
  joint — *see* Instability, joint
  lie 652.0 ☑
    affecting fetus or newborn (before labor) 761.7
    causing obstructed labor 660.0 ☑
      affecting fetus or newborn 763.1
  lumbosacral joint (congenital) 756.19
    acquired 724.6
  sacroiliac 724.6
  spine NEC 724.9
Untruthfulness, child problem — *see also* Disturbance, conduct 312.0 ☑
Unverricht (-Lundborg) disease, syndrome, or epilepsy 345.1 ☑
Unverricht-Wagner syndrome (dermatomyositis) 710.3
Upper respiratory — *see* condition
Upset
  gastric 536.8
    psychogenic 306.4
  gastrointestinal 536.8
    psychogenic 306.4
    virus (*see also* Enteritis, viral) 008.8
  intestinal (large) (small) 564.9
    psychogenic 306.4
  menstruation 626.9
  mental 300.9
  stomach 536.8
    psychogenic 306.4
Urachus — *see also* condition
  patent 753.7
  persistent 753.7
Uratic arthritis 274.00
Urbach's lipoid proteinosis 272.8
Urbach-Oppenheim disease or syndrome (necrobiosis lipoidica diabeticorum) 250.8 ☑ *[709.3]*
  due to secondary diabetes 249.8 ☑ *[709.3]*
Urbach-Wiethe disease or syndrome (lipoid proteinosis) 272.8
Urban yellow fever 060.1
Urea, blood, high — *see* Uremia
Uremia, uremic (absorption) (amaurosis) (amblyopia) (aphasia) (apoplexy) (coma) (delirium) (dementia) (dropsy) (dyspnea) (fever) (intoxication) (mania) (paralysis) (poisoning) (toxemia) (vomiting) 586
  with
    abortion — *see* Abortion, by type, with renal failure
    ectopic pregnancy (*see also* categories 633.0–633.9) 639.3
    hypertension (*see also* Hypertension, kidney) 403.91
    molar pregnancy (*see also* categories 630–632) 639.3
  chronic 585.9
  complicating
    abortion 639.3
    ectopic or molar pregnancy 639.3
    hypertension (*see also* Hypertension, kidney) 403.91
    labor and delivery 669.3 ☑
  congenital 779.89
  extrarenal 788.99
  hypertensive (chronic) (*see also* Hypertension, kidney) 403.91

☑ **Additional Digit Required** — Refer to the Tabular List for Digit Selection   ▽ **Subterms under main terms may continue to next column or page**

290 — Volume 2   ▶◀ **Revised Text**   ● **New Line**   ▲ **Revised Code**   2015 ICD-9-CM

Uremia, uremic — *continued*
 maternal NEC, affecting fetus or newborn 760.1
 neuropathy 585.9 *[357.4]*
 pericarditis 585.9 *[420.0]*
 prerenal 788.99
 pyelitic (*see also* Pyelitis) 590.80
Ureteralgia 788.0
Ureterectasis 593.89
Ureteritis 593.89
 cystica 590.3
 due to calculus 592.1
 gonococcal (acute) 098.19
  chronic or duration of 2 months or over 098.39
 nonspecific 593.89
Ureterocele (acquired) 593.89
 congenital 753.23
Ureterolith 592.1
Ureterolithiasis 592.1
Ureterostomy status V44.6
 with complication 997.5
Ureter, ureteral — *see* condition
Urethralgia 788.99
Urethra, urethral — *see* condition
Urethritis (abacterial) (acute) (allergic) (anterior) (chronic) (nonvenereal) (posterior) (recurrent) (simple) (subacute) (ulcerative) (undifferentiated) 597.80
 diplococcal (acute) 098.0
  chronic or duration of 2 months or over 098.2
 due to Trichomonas (vaginalis) 131.02
 gonococcal (acute) 098.0
  chronic or duration of 2 months or over 098.2
 nongonococcal (sexually transmitted) 099.40
  Chlamydia trachomatis 099.41
  Reiter's 099.3
  specified organism NEC 099.49
 nonspecific (sexually transmitted) (*see also* Urethritis, nongonococcal) 099.40
 not sexually transmitted 597.80
 Reiter's 099.3
 trichomonal or due to Trichomonas (vaginalis) 131.02
 tuberculous (*see also* Tuberculosis) 016.3 ☑
 venereal NEC (*see also* Urethritis, nongonococcal) 099.40
Urethrocele
 female 618.03
  with uterine prolapse 618.4
   complete 618.3
   incomplete 618.2
 male 599.5
Urethrolithiasis 594.2
Urethro-oculoarticular syndrome 099.3
Urethro-oculosynovial syndrome 099.3
Urethrorectal — *see* condition
Urethrorrhagia 599.84
Urethrorrhea 788.7
Urethrostomy status V44.6
 with complication 997.5

Urethrotrigonitis 595.3
Urethrovaginal — *see* condition
Urgency
 fecal 787.63
 hypertensive — *see* Hypertension
Urhidrosis, uridrosis 705.89
Uric acid
 diathesis 274.9
 in blood 790.6
Uricacidemia 790.6
Uricemia 790.6
Uricosuria 791.9
Urination
 frequent 788.41
 painful 788.1
 urgency 788.63
Urinemia — *see* Uremia
Urine, urinary — *see also* condition
 abnormality NEC 788.69
 blood in (*see also* Hematuria) 599.70
 discharge, excessive 788.42
 enuresis 788.30
  nonorganic origin 307.6
 extravasation 788.8
 frequency 788.41
 hesitancy 788.64
 incontinence 788.30
  active 788.30
  female 788.30
   stress 625.6
    and urge 788.33
  male 788.30
   stress 788.32
    and urge 788.33
  mixed (stress and urge) 788.33
  neurogenic 788.39
  nonorganic origin 307.6
  overflow 788.38
  stress (female) 625.6
   male NEC 788.32
 intermittent stream 788.61
 pus in 791.9
 retention or stasis NEC 788.20
  bladder, incomplete emptying 788.21
  psychogenic 306.53
  specified NEC 788.29
 secretion
  deficient 788.5
  excessive 788.42
  frequency 788.41
 strain 788.65
 stream
  intermittent 788.61
  slowing 788.62
  splitting 788.61
  weak 788.62
 urgency 788.63
Urinoma NEC 599.9
 bladder 596.89
 kidney 593.89
 renal 593.89
 ureter 593.89
 urethra 599.84
Uroarthritis, infectious 099.3

Urodialysis 788.5
Urolithiasis 592.9
Uronephrosis 593.89
Uropathy 599.9
 obstructive 599.60
Urosepsis 599.0
 meaning sepsis 995.91
 meaning urinary tract infection 599.0
Urticaria 708.9
 with angioneurotic edema 995.1
  hereditary 277.6
 allergic 708.0
 cholinergic 708.5
 chronic 708.8
 cold, familial 708.2
 dermatographic 708.3
 due to
  cold or heat 708.2
  drugs 708.0
  food 708.0
  inhalants 708.0
  plants 708.8
  serum 999.59
 factitial 708.3
 giant 995.1
  hereditary 277.6
 gigantea 995.1
  hereditary 277.6
 idiopathic 708.1
 larynx 995.1
  hereditary 277.6
 neonatorum 778.8
 nonallergic 708.1
 papulosa (Hebra) 698.2
 perstans hemorrhagica 757.39
 pigmentosa 757.33
 recurrent periodic 708.8
 serum 999.59
 solare 692.72
 specified type NEC 708.8
 thermal (cold) (heat) 708.2
 vibratory 708.4
Urticarioides acarodermatitis 133.9
Use of
 agents affecting estrogen receptors and estrogen levels NEC V07.59
 anastrozole (Arimidex) V07.52
 aromatase inhibitors V07.52
 estrogen receptor downregulators V07.59
 exemestane (Aromasin) V07.52
 fulvestrant (Faslodex) V07.59
 gonadotropin-releasing hormone (GnRH) agonist V07.59
 goserelin acetate (Zoladex) V07.59
 letrozole (Femara) V07.52
 leuprolide acetate (leuprorelin) (Lupron) V07.59
 megestrol acetate (Megace) V07.59
 methadone 304.00
 nonprescribed drugs (*see also* Abuse, drugs, nondependent) 305.9 ☑
 patent medicines (*see also* Abuse, drugs, nondependent) 305.9 ☑
 raloxifene (Evista) V07.51

Use of — *continued*
 selective estrogen receptor modulators (SERMs) V07.51
 tamoxifen (Nolvadex) V07.51
 toremifene (Fareston) V07.51
Usher-Senear disease (pemphigus erythematosus) 694.4
Uta 085.5
Uterine size-date discrepancy 649.6 ☑
Uteromegaly 621.2
Uterovaginal — *see* condition
Uterovesical — *see* condition
Uterus — *see also* condition
 with only one functioning horn 752.33
Utriculitis (utriculus prostaticus) 597.89
Uveal — *see* condition
Uveitis (anterior) — *see also* Iridocyclitis 364.3
 acute or subacute 364.00
  due to or associated with
   gonococcal infection 098.41
   herpes (simplex) 054.44
    zoster 053.22
  primary 364.01
  recurrent 364.02
  secondary (noninfectious) 364.04
   infectious 364.03
 allergic 360.11
 chronic 364.10
  due to or associated with
   sarcoidosis 135 *[364.11]*
   tuberculosis (*see also* Tuberculosis) 017.3 ☑ *[364.11]*
 due to
  operation 360.11
  toxoplasmosis (acquired) 130.2
   congenital (active) 771.2
 granulomatous 364.10
 heterochromic 364.21
 lens-induced 364.23
 nongranulomatous 364.00
 posterior 363.20
  disseminated — *see* Chorioretinitis, disseminated
  focal — *see* Chorioretinitis, focal
 recurrent 364.02
 sympathetic 360.11
 syphilitic (secondary) 091.50
  congenital 090.0 *[363.13]*
  late 095.8 *[363.13]*
 tuberculous (*see also* Tuberculosis) 017.3 ☑ *[364.11]*
Uveoencephalitis 363.22
Uveokeratitis — *see also* Iridocyclitis 364.3
Uveoparotid fever 135
Uveoparotitis 135
Uvula — *see* condition
Uvulitis (acute) (catarrhal) (chronic) (gangrenous) (membranous) (suppurative) (ulcerative) 528.3

☑ Additional Digit Required — Refer to the Tabular List for Digit Selection   ▽ Subterms under main terms may continue to next column or page

V

Vaccination
complication or reaction — *see* Complications, vaccination
delayed V64.00
not carried out V64.00
  because of
    acute illness V64.01
    allergy to vaccine or component V64.04
    caregiver refusal V64.05
    chronic illness V64.02
    guardian refusal V64.05
    immune compromised state V64.03
    parent refusal V64.05
    patient had disease being vaccinated against V64.08
    patient refusal V64.06
    reason NEC V64.09
    religious reasons V64.07
prophylactic (against) V05.9
  arthropod-borne viral
    disease NEC V05.1
    encephalitis V05.0
  chickenpox V05.4
  cholera (alone) V03.0
    with typhoid-paratyphoid (cholera + TAB) V06.0
  common cold V04.7
  diphtheria (alone) V03.5
    with
      poliomyelitis (DTP+ polio) V06.3
      tetanus V06.5
        pertussis combined (DTP) (DTaP) V06.1
        typhoid-paratyphoid (DTP + TAB) V06.2
  disease (single) NEC V05.9
    bacterial NEC V03.9
      specified type NEC V03.89
    combination NEC V06.9
      specified type NEC V06.8
    specified type NEC V05.8
  encephalitis, viral, arthropod-borne V05.0
  Hemophilus influenzae, type B [Hib] V03.81
  hepatitis, viral V05.3
  influenza V04.81
    with
      Streptococcus pneumoniae [pneumococcus] V06.6
  leishmaniasis V05.2
  measles (alone) V04.2
    with mumps-rubella (MMR) V06.4
  mumps (alone) V04.6
    with measles and rubella (MMR) V06.4
  pertussis alone V03.6
  plague V03.3
  poliomyelitis V04.0
    with diphtheria-tetanus-pertussis (DTP + polio) V06.3
  rabies V04.5
  respiratory syncytial virus (RSV) V04.82
  rubella (alone) V04.3
    with measles and mumps (MMR) V06.4
  smallpox V04.1
  Streptococcus pneumoniae [pneumococcus] V03.82
    with
      influenza V06.6
  tetanus toxoid (alone) V03.7
    with diphtheria [Td] [DT] V06.5
      with
        pertussis (DTP) (DTaP) V06.1
        with poliomyelitis (DTP+polio) V06.3
  tuberculosis (BCG) V03.2
  tularemia V03.4
  typhoid-paratyphoid (TAB) (alone) V03.1
    with diphtheria-tetanus-pertussis (TAB + DTP) V06.2
  varicella V05.4

Vaccination — *continued*
  prophylactic — *continued*
    viral
      disease NEC V04.89
      encephalitis, arthropod-borne V05.0
      hepatitis V05.3
      yellow fever V04.4
Vaccinia (generalized) 999.0
  without vaccination 051.02
  congenital 771.2
  conjunctiva 999.39
  eyelids 999.0 [373.5]
  localized 999.39
  nose 999.39
  not from vaccination 051.02
    eyelid 051.02 [373.5]
  sine vaccinatione 051.02
Vacuum
  extraction of fetus or newborn 763.3
  in sinus (accessory) (nasal) (*see also* Sinusitis) 473.9
Vagabond V60.0
Vagabondage V60.0
Vagabonds' disease 132.1
Vaginalitis (tunica) 608.4
Vagina, vaginal — *see also* condition
  high risk human papillomavirus (HPV) DNA test positive 795.15
  low risk human papillomavirus (HPV) DNA test positive 795.19
Vaginismus (reflex) 625.1
  functional 306.51
  hysterical 300.11
  psychogenic 306.51
Vaginitis (acute) (chronic) (circumscribed) (diffuse) (emphysematous) (Hemophilus vaginalis) (nonspecific) (nonvenereal) (ulcerative) 616.10
  with
    abortion — *see* Abortion, by type, with sepsis
    ectopic pregnancy (*see also* categories 633.0–633.9) 639.0
    molar pregnancy (*see also* categories 630–632) 639.0
  adhesive, congenital 752.49
  atrophic, postmenopausal 627.3
  bacterial 616.10
  blennorrhagic (acute) 098.0
    chronic or duration of 2 months or over 098.2
  candidal 112.1
  chlamydial 099.53
  complicating pregnancy or puerperium 646.6 ☑
    affecting fetus or newborn 760.8
  congenital (adhesive) 752.49
  due to
    C. albicans 112.1
    Trichomonas (vaginalis) 131.01
  following
    abortion 639.0
    ectopic or molar pregnancy 639.0
  gonococcal (acute) 098.0
    chronic or duration of 2 months or over 098.2
  granuloma 099.2
  Monilia 112.1
  mycotic 112.1
  pinworm 127.4 [616.11]
  postirradiation 616.10
  postmenopausal atrophic 627.3
  senile (atrophic) 627.3
  syphilitic (early) 091.0
    late 095.8
  trichomonal 131.01
  tuberculous (*see also* Tuberculosis) 016.7 ☑
  venereal NEC 099.8
Vaginosis — *see* Vaginitis
Vagotonia 352.3
Vagrancy V60.0
VAIN I (vaginal intraepithelial neoplasia I) 623.0
VAIN II (vaginal intraepithelial neoplasia II) 623.0
VAIN III (vaginal intraepithelial neoplasia III) 233.31

Vallecula — *see* condition
Valley fever 114.0
Valsuani's disease (progressive pernicious anemia, puerperal) 648.2 ☑
Valve, valvular (formation) — *see also* condition
  cerebral ventricle (communicating) in situ V45.2
  cervix, internal os 752.49
  colon 751.5
  congenital NEC — *see* Atresia
  formation, congenital NEC — *see* Atresia
  heart defect — *see* Anomaly, heart, valve
  ureter 753.29
    pelvic junction 753.21
    vesical orifice 753.22
  urethra 753.6
Valvulitis (chronic) — *see also* Endocarditis 424.90
  rheumatic (chronic) (inactive) (with chorea) 397.9
    active or acute (aortic) (mitral) (pulmonary) (tricuspid) 391.1
  syphilitic NEC 093.20
    aortic 093.22
    mitral 093.21
    pulmonary 093.24
    tricuspid 093.23
Valvulopathy — *see* Endocarditis
van Bogaert-Nijssen (-Peiffer) disease 330.0
van Bogaert's leukoencephalitis (sclerosing) (subacute) 046.2
van Buchem's syndrome (hyperostosis corticalis) 733.3
Vancomycin (glycopeptide)
  intermediate staphylococcus aureus (VISA/GISA) V09.8 ☑
  resistant
    enterococcus (VRE) V09.8 ☑
    staphylococcus aureus (VRSA/GRSA) V09.8 ☑
van Creveld-von Gierke disease (glycogenosis I) 271.0
van den Bergh's disease (enterogenous cyanosis) 289.7
van der Hoeve-Halbertsma-Waardenburg syndrome (ptosis-epicanthus) 270.2
van der Hoeve-Waardenburg-Gualdi syndrome (ptosis epicanthus) 270.2
van der Hoeve's syndrome (brittle bones and blue sclera, deafness) 756.51
Vanillism 692.89
Vanishing lung 492.0
Vanishing twin 651.33
van Neck (-Odelberg) disease or syndrome (juvenile osteochondrosis) 732.1
Vapor asphyxia or suffocation NEC 987.9
  specified agent — *see* Table of Drugs and Chemicals
Vaquez's disease (M9950/1) 238.4
Vaquez-Osler disease (polycythemia vera) (M9950/1) 238.4
Variance, lethal ball, prosthetic heart valve 996.02
Variants, thalassemic 282.49
Variations in hair color 704.3
Varicella 052.9
  with
    complication 052.8
      specified NEC 052.7
    pneumonia 052.1
    vaccination and inoculation (prophylactic) V05.4
  exposure to V01.71
  vaccination and inoculation (against) (prophylactic) V05.4
Varices — *see* Varix
Varicocele (scrotum) (thrombosed) 456.4
  ovary 456.5
  perineum 456.6
  spermatic cord (ulcerated) 456.4
Varicose
  aneurysm (ruptured) (*see also* Aneurysm) 442.9
  dermatitis (lower extremity) — *see* Varicose, vein, inflamed or infected

Varicose — *continued*
  eczema — *see* Varicose, vein
  phlebitis — *see* Varicose, vein, inflamed or infected
  placental vessel — *see* Placenta, abnormal
  tumor — *see* Varicose, vein
  ulcer (lower extremity, any part) 454.0
    anus 455.8
      external 455.5
      internal 455.2
    esophagus (*see also* Varix, esophagus) 456.1
      bleeding (*see also* Varix, esophagus, bleeding) 456.0
    inflamed or infected 454.2
    nasal septum 456.8
    perineum 456.6
    rectum — *see* Varicose, ulcer, anus
    scrotum 456.4
    specified site NEC 456.8
  vein (lower extremity) (ruptured) (*see also* Varix) 454.9
    with
      complications NEC 454.8
      edema 454.8
      inflammation or infection 454.1
        ulcerated 454.2
      pain 454.8
      stasis dermatitis 454.1
        with ulcer 454.2
      swelling 454.8
      ulcer 454.0
        inflamed or infected 454.2
    anus — *see* Hemorrhoids
    broad ligament 456.5
    congenital (peripheral) 747.60
      gastrointestinal 747.61
      lower limb 747.64
      renal 747.62
      specified NEC 747.69
      upper limb 747.63
    esophagus (ulcerated) (*see also* Varix, esophagus) 456.1
      bleeding (*see also* Varix, esophagus, bleeding) 456.0
    inflamed or infected 454.1
      with ulcer 454.2
    in pregnancy or puerperium 671.0 ☑
      vulva or perineum 671.1 ☑
    nasal septum (with ulcer) 456.8
    pelvis 456.5
    perineum 456.6
      in pregnancy, childbirth, or puerperium 671.1 ☑
    rectum — *see* Hemorrhoids
    scrotum (ulcerated) 456.4
    specified site NEC 456.8
    sublingual 456.3
    ulcerated 454.0
      inflamed or infected 454.2
    umbilical cord, affecting fetus or newborn 762.6
    urethra 456.8
    vulva 456.6
      in pregnancy, childbirth, or puerperium 671.1 ☑
    vessel (*see also* Varix)
      placenta — *see* Placenta, abnormal
Varicosis, varicosities, varicosity — *see also* Varix 454.9
Variola 050.9
  hemorrhagic (pustular) 050.0
  major 050.0
  minor 050.1
  modified 050.2
Varioloid 050.2
Variolosa, purpura 050.0
Varix (lower extremity) (ruptured) 454.9
  with
    complications NEC 454.8
    edema 454.8
    inflammation or infection 454.1
      with ulcer 454.2
    pain 454.8
    stasis dermatitis 454.1
      with ulcer 454.2

☑ **Additional Digit Required** — **Refer to the Tabular List for Digit Selection**   ▥ **Subterms under main terms may continue to next column or page**

2015 ICD-9-CM   ▶◀ **Revised Text**   ● **New Line**   ▲ **Revised Code**   Volume 2 — 293

Vaccination — Varix

Varix — *continued*
  with — *continued*
    swelling 454.8
    ulcer 454.0
      with inflammation or infection 454.2
  aneurysmal (*see also* Aneurysm) 442.9
  anus — *see* Hemorrhoids
  arteriovenous (congenital) (peripheral) NEC
    747.60
    gastrointestinal 747.61
    lower limb 747.64
    renal 747.62
    specified NEC 747.69
    spinal 747.82
    upper limb 747.63
  bladder 456.5
  broad ligament 456.5
  congenital (peripheral) 747.60
  esophagus (ulcerated) 456.1
    bleeding 456.0
    in
      cirrhosis of liver 571.5 *[456.20]*
      portal hypertension
        572.3 *[456.20]*
    congenital 747.69
    in
      cirrhosis of liver 571.5 *[456.21]*
        with bleeding 571.5 *[456.20]*
      portal hypertension
        572.3 *[456.21]*
        with bleeding 572.3 *[456.20]*
  gastric 456.8
  inflamed or infected 454.1
    ulcerated 454.2
  in pregnancy or puerperium 671.0 ☑
    perineum 671.1 ☑
    vulva 671.1 ☑
  labia (majora) 456.6
  orbit 456.8
    congenital 747.69
  ovary 456.5
  papillary 448.1
  pelvis 456.5
  perineum 456.6
    in pregnancy or puerperium 671.1 ☑
  pharynx 456.8
  placenta — *see* Placenta, abnormal
  prostate 456.8
  rectum — *see* Hemorrhoids
  renal papilla 456.8
  retina 362.17
  scrotum (ulcerated) 456.4
  sigmoid colon 456.8
  specified site NEC 456.8
  spinal (cord) (vessels) 456.8
  spleen, splenic (vein) (with phlebolith) 456.8
  sublingual 456.3
  ulcerated 454.0
    inflamed or infected 454.2
  umbilical cord, affecting fetus or newborn
    762.6
  uterine ligament 456.5
  vocal cord 456.8
  vulva 456.6
    in pregnancy, childbirth, or puerperium
      671.1 ☑
Vasa previa 663.5 ☑
  affecting fetus or newborn 762.6
  hemorrhage from, affecting fetus or new-
    born 772.0
Vascular — *see also* condition
  loop on papilla (optic) 743.57
  sheathing, retina 362.13
  spasm 443.9
  spider 448.1
Vascularity, pulmonary, congenital 747.39
Vascularization
  choroid 362.16
  cornea 370.60
    deep 370.63
    localized 370.61
  retina 362.16
  subretinal 362.16
Vasculitis 447.6
  allergic 287.0
  cryoglobulinemic 273.2

Vasculitis — *continued*
  disseminated 447.6
  kidney 447.8
  leukocytoclastic 446.29
  nodular 695.2
  retinal 362.18
  rheumatic — *see* Fever, rheumatic
Vasculopathy
  cardiac allograft 996.83
Vas deferens — *see* condition
Vas deferentitis 608.4
Vasectomy, admission for V25.2
Vasitis 608.4
  nodosa 608.4
  scrotum 608.4
  spermatic cord 608.4
  testis 608.4
  tuberculous (*see also* Tuberculosis) 016.5 ☑
  tunica vaginalis 608.4
  vas deferens 608.4
Vasodilation 443.9
Vasomotor — *see* condition
Vasoplasty, after previous sterilization V26.0
Vasoplegia, splanchnic — *see also* Neuropathy, peripheral, autonomic 337.9
Vasospasm 443.9
  cerebral (artery) 435.9
    with transient neurologic deficit 435.9
  coronary 413.1
  nerve
    arm NEC 354.9
    autonomic 337.9
    brachial plexus 353.0
    cervical plexus 353.2
    leg NEC 355.8
    lower extremity NEC 355.8
    peripheral NEC 355.9
    spinal NEC 355.9
    sympathetic 337.9
    upper extremity NEC 354.9
  peripheral NEC 443.9
  retina (artery) (*see also* Occlusion, retinal,
    artery) 362.30
Vasospastic — *see* condition
Vasovagal attack (paroxysmal) 780.2
  psychogenic 306.2
Vater's ampulla — *see* condition
VATER syndrome 759.89
vCJD (variant Creutzfeldt-Jakob disease) 046.11
Vegetation, vegetative
  adenoid (nasal fossa) 474.2
  consciousness (persistent) 780.03
  endocarditis (acute) (any valve) (chronic)
    (subacute) 421.0
  heart (mycotic) (valve) 421.0
  state (persistent) 780.03
Veil
  Jackson's 751.4
  over face (causing asphyxia) 768.9
Vein, venous — *see* condition
Veldt sore — *see also* Ulcer, skin 707.9
Velo-cardio-facial syndrome 758.32
Velpeau's hernia — *see* Hernia, femoral
Venereal
  balanitis NEC 099.8
  bubo 099.1
  disease 099.9
    specified nature or type NEC 099.8
  granuloma inguinale 099.2
  lymphogranuloma (Durand-Nicolas-Favre),
    any site 099.1
  salpingitis 098.37
  urethritis (*see also* Urethritis, nongonococ-
    cal) 099.40
  vaginitis NEC 099.8
  warts 078.11
Vengefulness, in child — *see also* Disturbance,
  conduct 312.0 ☑
Venofibrosis 459.89
Venom, venomous
  bite or sting (animal or insect) 989.5
  poisoning 989.5
Venous — *see* condition
Ventouse delivery NEC 669.5 ☑
  affecting fetus or newborn 763.3
Ventral — *see* condition

Ventricle, ventricular — *see also* condition
  escape 427.69
  standstill (*see also* Arrest, cardiac) 427.5
Ventriculitis, cerebral — *see also* Meningitis
  322.9
Ventriculostomy status V45.2
Verbiest's syndrome (claudicatio intermittens
  spinalis) 435.1
Vernet's syndrome 352.6
Verneuil's disease (syphilitic bursitis) 095.7
Verruca (filiformis) 078.10
  acuminata (any site) 078.11
  necrogenica (primary) (*see also* Tuberculosis)
    017.0 ☑
  peruana 088.0
  peruviana 088.0
  plana (juvenilis) 078.19
  plantaris 078.12
  seborrheica 702.19
    inflamed 702.11
  senilis 702.0
  tuberculosa (primary) (*see also* Tuberculosis)
    017.0 ☑
  venereal 078.11
  viral 078.10
    specified NEC 078.19
  vulgaris 078.10
Verrucosities — *see also* Verruca 078.10
Verrucous endocarditis (acute) (any valve)
  (chronic) (subacute) 710.0 *[424.91]*
  nonbacterial 710.0 *[424.91]*
Verruga
  peruana 088.0
  peruviana 088.0
Verse's disease (calcinosis intervertebralis)
  275.49 *[722.90]*
Version
  before labor, affecting fetus or newborn
    761.7
  cephalic (correcting previous malposition)
    652.1 ☑
    affecting fetus or newborn 763.1
  cervix — *see* Version, uterus
  uterus (postinfectional) (postpartal, old) (*see*
    also Malposition, uterus) 621.6
    forward — *see* Anteversion, uterus
    lateral — *see* Lateroversion, uterus
Vertebra, vertebral — *see* condition
Vertigo 780.4
  auditory 386.19
  aural 386.19
  benign paroxysmal positional 386.11
  central origin 386.2
  cerebral 386.2
  Dix and Hallpike (epidemic) 386.12
  endemic paralytic 078.81
  epidemic 078.81
    Dix and Hallpike 386.12
    Gerlier's 078.81
    Pedersen's 386.12
    vestibular neuronitis 386.12
  epileptic — *see* Epilepsy
  Gerlier's (epidemic) 078.81
  hysterical 300.11
  labyrinthine 386.10
  laryngeal 786.2
  malignant positional 386.2
  Ménière's (*see also* Disease, Ménière's)
    386.00
  menopausal 627.2
  otogenic 386.19
  paralytic 078.81
  paroxysmal positional, benign 386.11
  Pedersen's (epidemic) 386.12
  peripheral 386.10
    specified type NEC 386.19
  positional
    benign paroxysmal 386.11
    malignant 386.2
Verumontanitis (chronic) — *see also* Urethritis
  597.89
Vesania — *see also* Psychosis 298.9
Vesical — *see* condition
Vesicle
  cutaneous 709.8
  seminal — *see* condition

Vesicle — *continued*
  skin 709.8
Vesicocolic — *see* condition
Vesicoperineal — *see* condition
Vesicorectal — *see* condition
Vesicourethrorectal — *see* condition
Vesicovaginal — *see* condition
Vesicular — *see* condition
Vesiculitis (seminal) 608.0
  amebic 006.8
  gonorrheal (acute) 098.14
    chronic or duration of 2 months or over
      098.34
  trichomonal 131.09
  tuberculous (*see also* Tuberculosis)
    016.5 ☑ *[608.81]*
Vestibulitis (ear) — *see also* Labyrinthitis
  386.30
  nose (external) 478.19
  vulvar 625.71
Vestibulopathy, acute peripheral (recurrent)
  386.12
Vestige, vestigial — *see also* Persistence
  branchial 744.41
  structures in vitreous 743.51
Vibriosis NEC 027.9
Vidal's disease (lichen simplex chronicus)
  698.3
Video display tube syndrome 723.8
Vienna-type encephalitis 049.8
Villaret's syndrome 352.6
Villous — *see* condition
VIN I (vulvar intraepithelial neoplasia I) 624.01
VIN II (vulvar intraepithelial neoplasia II) 624.02
VIN III (vulvar intraepithelial neoplasia III)
  233.32
Vincent's
  angina 101
  bronchitis 101
  disease 101
  gingivitis 101
  infection (any site) 101
  laryngitis 101
  stomatitis 101
  tonsillitis 101
Vinson-Plummer syndrome (sideropenic
  dysphagia) 280.8
Viosterol deficiency — *see also* Deficiency,
  calciferol 268.9
Virchow's disease 733.99
Viremia 790.8
Virilism (adrenal) (female) NEC 255.2
  with
    3-beta-hydroxysteroid dehydrogenase
      defect 255.2
    11-hydroxylase defect 255.2
    21-hydroxylase defect 255.2
    adrenal
      hyperplasia 255.2
      insufficiency (congenital) 255.2
    cortical hyperfunction 255.2
Virilization (female) (suprarenal) — *see also*
  Virilism 255.2
  isosexual 256.4
Virulent bubo 099.0
Virus, viral — *see also* condition
  infection NEC (*see also* Infection, viral)
    079.99
  septicemia 079.99
  yaba monkey tumor 059.22
VISA (vancomycin intermediate staphylococcus
  aureus) V09.8 ☑
Viscera, visceral — *see* condition
Visceroptosis 569.89
Visible peristalsis 787.4
Vision, visual
  binocular, suppression 368.31
  blurred, blurring 368.8
    hysterical 300.11
  defect, defective (*see also* Impaired, vision)
    369.9
  disorientation (syndrome) 368.16
  disturbance NEC (*see also* Disturbance, vi-
    sion) 368.9
    hysterical 300.11
  examination V72.0

☑ **Additional Digit Required** — Refer to the Tabular List for Digit Selection   ▽ **Subterms under main terms may continue to next column or page**

294 — Volume 2   ▶◀ Revised Text   ● New Line   ▲ Revised Code   2015 ICD-9-CM

Vision, visual — *continued*
  field, limitation 368.40
  fusion, with defective steropsis 368.33
  hallucinations 368.16
  halos 368.16
  loss 369.9
    both eyes (*see also* Blindness, both eyes) 369.3
    complete (*see also* Blindness, both eyes) 369.00
    one eye 369.8
    sudden 368.16
  low (both eyes) 369.20
    one eye (other eye normal) (*see also* Impaired, vision) 369.70
      blindness, other eye 369.10
  perception, simultaneous without fusion 368.32
  tunnel 368.45
Vitality, lack or want of 780.79
  newborn 779.89
Vitamin deficiency NEC — *see also* Deficiency, vitamin 269.2
Vitelline duct, persistent 751.0
Vitiligo 709.01
  due to pinta (carate) 103.2
  eyelid 374.53
  vulva 624.8
Vitium cordis — *see* Disease, heart
Vitreous — *see also* condition
  touch syndrome 997.99
VLCAD (long chain/very long chain acyl CoA dehydrogenase deficiency, LCAD) 277.85
Vocal cord — *see* condition
Vocational rehabilitation V57.22
Vogt's (Cecile) disease or syndrome 333.7 ☑
Vogt-Koyanagi syndrome 364.24
Vogt-Spielmeyer disease (amaurotic familial idiocy) 330.1
Voice
  change (*see also* Dysphonia) 784.49
  loss (*see also* Aphonia) 784.41
Volhard-Fahr disease (malignant nephrosclerosis) 403.00
Volhynian fever 083.1
Volkmann's ischemic contracture or paralysis (complicating trauma) 958.6
Voluntary starvation 307.1
Volvulus (bowel) (colon) (intestine) 560.2
  with
    hernia (*see also* Hernia, by site, with obstruction)
      gangrenous — *see* Hernia, by site, with gangrene
    perforation 560.2
  congenital 751.5
  duodenum 537.3
  fallopian tube 620.5
  oviduct 620.5
  stomach (due to absence of gastrocolic ligament) 537.89
Vomiting 787.03
  with nausea 787.01
  allergic 535.4 ☑
  asphyxia 933.1
  bilious (cause unknown) 787.04
    following gastrointestinal surgery 564.3
    newborn 779.32
  blood (*see also* Hematemesis) 578.0
  causing asphyxia, choking, or suffocation (*see also* Asphyxia, food) 933.1
  cyclical 536.2
    associated with migraine 346.2 ☑
    psychogenic 306.4
  epidemic 078.82
  fecal matter 569.87
  following gastrointestinal surgery 564.3
  functional 536.8
    psychogenic 306.4
  habit 536.2
  hysterical 300.11
  nervous 306.4
  neurotic 306.4
  newborn 779.33
    bilious 779.32
  of or complicating pregnancy 643.9 ☑

Vomiting — *continued*
  of or complicating pregnancy — *continued*
    due to
      organic disease 643.8 ☑
      specific cause NEC 643.8 ☑
    early — *see* Hyperemesis, gravidarum
    late (after 22 completed weeks of gestation) 643.2 ☑
  pernicious or persistent 536.2
    complicating pregnancy — *see* Hyperemesis, gravidarum
  psychogenic 306.4
  physiological 787.03
    bilious 787.04
  psychic 306.4
  psychogenic 307.54
  stercoral 569.89
  uncontrollable 536.2
    psychogenic 306.4
  uremic — *see* Uremia
  winter 078.82
von Bechterew (-Strumpell) disease or syndrome (ankylosing spondylitis) 720.0
von Bezold's abscess 383.01
von Economo's disease (encephalitis lethargica) 049.8
von Eulenburg's disease (congenital paramyotonia) 359.29
von Gierke's disease (glycogenosis I) 271.0
von Gies' joint 095.8
von Graefe's disease or syndrome 378.72
von Hippel (-Lindau) disease or syndrome (retinocerebral angiomatosis) 759.6
von Jaksch's anemia or disease (pseudoleukemia infantum) 285.8
von Recklinghausen-Applebaum disease (hemochromatosis) — *see also* Hemochromatosis 275.03
von Recklinghausen's
  disease or syndrome (nerves) (skin) (M9540/1) 237.71
  bones (osteitis fibrosa cystica) 252.01
  tumor (M9540/1) 237.71
von Schroetter's syndrome (intermittent venous claudication) 453.89
von Willebrand (-Jürgens) (-Minot) disease or syndrome (angiohemophilia) 286.4
von Zambusch's disease (lichen sclerosus et atrophicus) 701.0
Voorhoeve's disease or dyschondroplasia 756.4
Vossius' ring 921.3
  late effect 366.21
Voyeurism 302.82
VRE (vancomycin resistant enterococcus) V09.8 ☑
Vrolik's disease (osteogenesis imperfecta) 756.51
VRSA (vancomycin resistant staphylococcus aureus) V09.8 ☑
Vulva — *see* condition
Vulvismus 625.1
Vulvitis (acute) (allergic) (chronic) (gangrenous) (hypertrophic) (intertriginous) 616.10
  with
    abortion — *see* Abortion, by type, with sepsis
    ectopic pregnancy (*see also* categories 633.0–633.9) 639.0
    molar pregnancy (*see also* categories 630–632) 639.0
  adhesive, congenital 752.49
  blennorrhagic (acute) 098.0
    chronic or duration of 2 months or over 098.2
  chlamydial 099.53
  complicating pregnancy or puerperium 646.6 ☑
  due to Ducrey's bacillus 099.0
  following
    abortion 639.0
    ectopic or molar pregnancy 639.0
  gonococcal (acute) 098.0

Vulvitis — *continued*
  gonococcal — *continued*
    chronic or duration of 2 months or over 098.2
  herpetic 054.11
  leukoplakic 624.09
  monilial 112.1
  puerperal, postpartum, childbirth 646.6 ☑
  syphilitic (early) 091.0
    late 095.8
  trichomonal 131.01
Vulvodynia 625.70
  specified NEC 625.79
Vulvorectal — *see* condition
Vulvovaginitis — *see also* Vulvitis 616.10
  amebic 006.8
  chlamydial 099.53
  gonococcal (acute) 098.0
    chronic or duration of 2 months or over 098.2
  herpetic 054.11
  monilial 112.1
  trichomonal (Trichomonas vaginalis) 131.01

W

Waardenburg-Klein syndrome (ptosis-epicanthus) 270.2
Waardenburg's syndrome 756.89
  meaning ptosis-epicanthus 270.2
Wagner's disease (colloid milium) 709.3
Wagner (-Unverricht) syndrome (dermatomyositis) 710.3
Waiting list, person on V63.2
  undergoing social agency investigation V63.8
Wakefulness disorder — *see also* Hypersomnia 780.54
  nonorganic origin 307.43
Waldenström's
  disease (osteochondrosis, capital femoral) 732.1
  hepatitis (lupoid hepatitis) 571.49
  hypergammaglobulinemia 273.0
  macroglobulinemia 273.3
  purpura, hypergammaglobulinemic 273.0
  syndrome (macroglobulinemia) 273.3
Waldenström-Kjellberg syndrome (sideropenic dysphagia) 280.8
Walking
  difficulty 719.7
    psychogenic 307.9
  sleep 307.46
    hysterical 300.13
Wall, abdominal — *see* condition
Wallenberg's syndrome (posterior inferior cerebellar artery) — *see also* Disease, cerebrovascular, acute 436
Wallgren's
  disease (obstruction of splenic vein with collateral circulation) 459.89
  meningitis (*see also* Meningitis, aseptic) 047.9
Wandering
  acetabulum 736.39
  gallbladder 751.69
  in diseases classified elsewhere V40.31
  kidney, congenital 753.3
  organ or site, congenital NEC — *see* Malposition, congenital
  pacemaker (atrial) (heart) 427.89
  spleen 289.59
Wardrop's disease (with lymphangitis) 681.9
  finger 681.02
  toe 681.11
War neurosis 300.16
Wart (digitate) (filiform) (infectious) (viral) 078.10
  common 078.19
  external genital organs (venereal) 078.11
  fig 078.19
  flat 078.19
  genital 078.11
  Hassall-Henle's (of cornea) 371.41
  Henle's (of cornea) 371.41
  juvenile 078.19
  moist 078.10

Wart — *continued*
  Peruvian 088.0
  plantar 078.12
  prosector (*see also* Tuberculosis) 017.0 ☑
  seborrheic 702.19
    inflamed 702.11
  senile 702.0
  specified NEC 078.19
  syphilitic 091.3
  tuberculous (*see also* Tuberculosis) 017.0 ☑
  venereal (female) (male) 078.11
Warthin's tumor (salivary gland) (M8561/0) 210.2
Washerwoman's itch 692.4
Wassilieff's disease (leptospiral jaundice) 100.0
Wasting
  disease 799.4
    due to malnutrition 261
  extreme (due to malnutrition) 261
  muscular NEC 728.2
  palsy, paralysis 335.21
  pelvic muscle 618.83
Water
  clefts 366.12
  deprivation of 994.3
  in joint (*see also* Effusion, joint) 719.0 ☑
  intoxication 276.69
  itch 120.3
  lack of 994.3
  loading 276.69
  on
    brain — *see* Hydrocephalus
    chest 511.89
  poisoning 276.69
Waterbrash 787.1
Water-hammer pulse — *see also* Insufficiency, aortic 424.1
Waterhouse (-Friderichsen) disease or syndrome 036.3
Water-losing nephritis 588.89
Watermelon stomach 537.82
  with hemorrhage 537.83
  without hemorrhage 537.82
Wax in ear 380.4
Waxy
  degeneration, any site 277.39
  disease 277.39
  kidney 277.39 [583.81]
  liver (large) 277.39
  spleen 277.39
Weak, weakness (generalized) 780.79
  arches (acquired) 734
    congenital 754.61
  bladder sphincter 596.59
  congenital 779.89
  eye muscle — *see* Strabismus
  facial 781.94
  foot (double) — *see* Weak, arches
  heart, cardiac (*see also* Failure, heart) 428.9
    congenital 746.9
  mind 317
  muscle (generalized) 728.87
  myocardium (*see also* Failure, heart) 428.9
  newborn 779.89
  pelvic fundus
    pubocervical tissue 618.81
    rectovaginal tissue 618.82
  pulse 785.9
  senile 797
  urinary stream 788.62
  valvular — *see* Endocarditis
Wear, worn, tooth, teeth (approximal) (hard tissues) (interproximal) (occlusal) — *see also* Attrition, teeth 521.10
Weather, weathered
  effects of
    cold NEC 991.9
      specified effect NEC 991.8
    hot (*see also* Heat) 992.9
  skin 692.74
Weber-Christian disease or syndrome (nodular nonsuppurative panniculitis) 729.30
Weber-Cockayne syndrome (epidermolysis bullosa) 757.39

☑ **Additional Digit Required** — Refer to the Tabular List for Digit Selection
▽ **Subterms under main terms may continue to next column or page**

2015 ICD-9-CM   ▶◀ **Revised Text**   ● **New Line**   ▲ **Revised Code**   **Volume 2 — 295**

Vision, visual — Weber-Cockayne syndrome

Weber-Dimitri syndrome 759.6
Weber-Gubler syndrome 344.89
Weber-Leyden syndrome 344.89
Weber-Osler syndrome (familial hemorrhagic telangiectasia) 448.0
Weber's paralysis or syndrome 344.89
Web, webbed (congenital) — see also Anomaly, specified type NEC
  canthus 743.63
  digits (see also Syndactylism) 755.10
  duodenal 751.5
  esophagus 750.3
  fingers (see also Syndactylism, fingers) 755.11
  larynx (glottic) (subglottic) 748.2
  neck (pterygium colli) 744.5
  Paterson-Kelly (sideropenic dysphagia) 280.8
  popliteal syndrome 756.89
  toes (see also Syndactylism, toes) 755.13
Wedge-shaped or wedging vertebra — see also Osteoporosis 733.00
Wegener's granulomatosis or syndrome 446.4
Wegner's disease (syphilitic osteochondritis) 090.0
Weight
  gain (abnormal) (excessive) 783.1
    during pregnancy 646.1 ☑
      insufficient 646.8 ☑
  less than 1000 grams at birth 765.0 ☑
  loss (cause unknown) 783.21
Weightlessness 994.9
Weil's disease (leptospiral jaundice) 100.0
Weill-Marchesani syndrome (brachymorphism and ectopia lentis) 759.89
Weingarten's syndrome (tropical eosinophilia) 518.3
Weir Mitchell's disease (erythromelalgia) 443.82
Weiss-Baker syndrome (carotid sinus syncope) 337.01
Weissenbach-Thibierge syndrome (cutaneous systemic sclerosis) 710.1
Wen — see also Cyst, sebaceous 706.2
Wenckebach's phenomenon, heart block (second degree) 426.13
Werdnig-Hoffmann syndrome (muscular atrophy) 335.0
Werlhof-Wichmann syndrome — see also Purpura, thrombocytopenic 287.39
Werlhof's disease — see also Purpura, thrombocytopenic 287.39
Wermer's syndrome or disease (polyendocrine adenomatosis) 258.01
Werner's disease or syndrome (progeria adultorum) 259.8
Werner-His disease (trench fever) 083.1
Werner-Schultz disease (agranulocytosis) 288.09
Wernicke's encephalopathy, disease, or syndrome (superior hemorrhagic polioencephalitis) 265.1
Wernicke-Korsakoff syndrome or psychosis (nonalcoholic) 294.0
  alcoholic 291.1
Wernicke-Posadas disease — see also Coccidioidomycosis 114.9
Wesselsbron fever 066.3
West African fever 084.8
West Nile
  encephalitis 066.41
  encephalomyelitis 066.41
  fever 066.40
    with
      cranial nerve disorders 066.42
      encephalitis 066.41
      optic neuritis 066.42
      other complications 066.49
      other neurologic manifestations 066.42
      polyradiculitis 066.42
  virus 066.40
Westphal-Strümpell syndrome (hepatolenticular degeneration) 275.1

Wet
  brain (alcoholic) (see also Alcoholism) 303.9 ☑
  feet, tropical (syndrome) (maceration) 991.4
  lung (syndrome)
    adult 518.52
    newborn 770.6
Wharton's duct — see condition
Wheal 709.8
Wheelchair confinement status V46.3
Wheezing 786.07
Whiplash injury or syndrome 847.0
Whipple's disease or syndrome (intestinal lipodystrophy) 040.2
Whipworm 127.3
"Whistling face" syndrome (craniocarpotarsal dystrophy) 759.89
White — see also condition
  kidney
    large — see Nephrosis
    small 582.9
  leg, puerperal, postpartum, childbirth 671.4 ☑
    nonpuerperal 451.19
  mouth 112.0
  patches of mouth 528.6
  sponge nevus of oral mucosa 750.26
  spot lesions, teeth 521.01
White's disease (congenital) (keratosis follicularis) 757.39
Whitehead 706.2
Whitlow (with lymphangitis) 681.01
  herpetic 054.6
Whitmore's disease or fever (melioidosis) 025
Whooping cough 033.9
  with pneumonia 033.9 [484.3]
  due to
    Bordetella
      bronchoseptica 033.8
        with pneumonia 033.8 [484.3]
      parapertussis 033.1
        with pneumonia 033.1 [484.3]
      pertussis 033.0
        with pneumonia 033.0 [484.3]
    specified organism NEC 033.8
      with pneumonia 033.8 [484.3]
  vaccination, prophylactic (against) V03.6
Wichmann's asthma (laryngismus stridulus) 478.75
Widal (-Abrami) syndrome (acquired hemolytic jaundice) 283.9
Widening aorta — see also Ectasia, aortic 447.70
  with aneurysm 441.9
  ruptured 441.5
Wilkie's disease or syndrome 557.1
Wilkinson-Sneddon disease or syndrome (subcorneal pustular dermatosis) 694.1
Willan's lepra 696.1
Willan-Plumbe syndrome (psoriasis) 696.1
Willebrand (-Jürgens) syndrome or thrombopathy (angiohemophilia) 286.4
Willi-Prader syndrome (hypogenital dystrophy with diabetic tendency) 759.81
Willis' disease (diabetes mellitus) — see also Diabetes 250.0 ☑
  due to secondary diabetes 249.0 ☑
Wilms' tumor or neoplasm (nephroblastoma) (M8960/3) 189.0
Wilson's
  disease or syndrome (hepatolenticular degeneration) 275.1
  hepatolenticular degeneration 275.1
  lichen ruber 697.0
Wilson-Brocq disease (dermatitis exfoliativa) 695.89
Wilson-Mikity syndrome 770.7
Window — see also Imperfect, closure aorticopulmonary 745.0
Winged scapula 736.89
Winter — see also condition
  vomiting disease 078.82
Wise's disease 696.2
Wiskott-Aldrich syndrome (eczema-thrombocytopenia) 279.12

Withdrawal symptoms, syndrome
  alcohol 291.81
    delirium (acute) 291.0
      chronic 291.1
    newborn 760.71
  drug or narcotic 292.0
  newborn, infant of dependent mother 779.5
  steroid NEC
    correct substance properly administered 255.41
    overdose or wrong substance given or taken 962.0
Withdrawing reaction, child or adolescent 313.22
Witts' anemia (achlorhydric anemia) 280.9
Witzelsucht 301.9
Woakes' syndrome (ethmoiditis) 471.1
Wohlfart-Kugelberg-Welander disease 335.11
Woillez's disease (acute idiopathic pulmonary congestion) 518.52
Wolff-Parkinson-White syndrome (anomalous atrioventricular excitation) 426.7
Wolhynian fever 083.1
Wolman's disease (primary familial xanthomatosis) 272.7
Wood asthma 495.8
Woolly, wooly hair (congenital) (nevus) 757.4
Wool-sorters' disease 022.1
Word
  blindness (congenital) (developmental) 315.01
    secondary to organic lesion 784.61
  deafness (secondary to organic lesion) 784.69
    developmental 315.31
Worm(s) (colic) (fever) (infection) (infestation) — see also Infestation 128.9
  guinea 125.7
  in intestine NEC 127.9
Worm-eaten soles 102.3
Worn out — see also Exhaustion 780.79
  artificial heart valve 996.02
  cardiac defibrillator (with synchronous cardiac pacemaker) V53.32
  cardiac pacemaker lead or battery V53.31
  joint prosthesis (see also Complications, mechanical, device NEC, prosthetic NEC, joint) 996.46
"Worried well" V65.5
Wound, open (by cutting or piercing instrument) (by firearms) (cut) (dissection) (incised) (laceration) (penetration) (perforating) (puncture) (with initial hemorrhage, not internal) 879.8

Note — For fracture with open wound, see Fracture.

For laceration, traumatic rupture, tear or penetrating wound of internal organs, such as heart, lung, liver, kidney, pelvic organs, etc., whether or not accompanied by open wound or fracture in the same region, see Injury, internal.

For contused wound, see Contusion. For crush injury, see Crush. For abrasion, insect bite (nonvenomous), blister, or scratch, see Injury, superficial.

Complicated includes wounds with:

  delayed healing

  delayed treatment

  foreign body

  primary infection

For late effect of open wound, see Late, effect, wound, open, by site.

  abdomen, abdominal (external) (muscle) 879.2
    complicated 879.3
    wall (anterior) 879.2
      complicated 879.3
      lateral 879.4
        complicated 879.5
  alveolar (process) 873.62

Wound, open — continued
  alveolar — continued
    complicated 873.72
  ankle 891.0
    with tendon involvement 891.2
    complicated 891.1
  anterior chamber, eye (see also Wound, open, intraocular) 871.9
  anus 863.89
  arm 884.0
    with tendon involvement 884.2
    complicated 884.1
    forearm 881.00
      with tendon involvement 881.20
      complicated 881.10
    multiple sites — see Wound, open, multiple, upper limb
    upper 880.03
      with tendon involvement 880.23
      complicated 880.13
      multiple sites (with axillary or shoulder regions) 880.09
        with tendon involvement 880.29
        complicated 880.19
  artery — see Injury, blood vessel, by site
  auditory
    canal (external) (meatus) 872.02
      complicated 872.12
    ossicles (incus) (malleus) (stapes) 872.62
      complicated 872.72
  auricle, ear 872.01
    complicated 872.11
  axilla 880.02
    with tendon involvement 880.22
    complicated 880.12
      with tendon involvement 880.29
    involving other sites of upper arm 880.09
      complicated 880.19
  back 876.0
    complicated 876.1
  bladder — see Injury, internal, bladder
  blood vessel — see Injury, blood vessel, by site
  brain — see Injury, intracranial, with intracranial wound
  breast 879.0
    complicated 879.1
  brow 873.42
    complicated 873.52
  buccal mucosa 873.61
    complicated 873.71
  buttock 877.0
    complicated 877.1
  calf 891.0
    with tendon involvement 891.2
    complicated 891.1
  canaliculus lacrimalis 870.8
    with laceration of eyelid 870.2
  canthus, eye 870.8
    laceration — see Laceration, eyelid
  cavernous sinus — see Injury, intracranial
  cerebellum — see Injury, intracranial
  cervical esophagus 874.4
    complicated 874.5
  cervix — see Injury, internal, cervix
  cheek(s) (external) 873.41
    complicated 873.51
    internal 873.61
      complicated 873.71
  chest (wall) (external) 875.0
    complicated 875.1
  chin 873.44
    complicated 873.54
  choroid 363.63
  ciliary body (eye) (see also Wound, open, intraocular) 871.9
  clitoris 878.8
    complicated 878.9
  cochlea 872.64
    complicated 872.74
  complicated 879.9
  conjunctiva — see Wound, open, intraocular
  cornea (nonpenetrating) (see also Wound, open, intraocular) 871.9
  costal region 875.0
    complicated 875.1

☑ **Additional Digit Required** — Refer to the Tabular List for Digit Selection

▼ **Subterms under main terms may continue to next column or page**

Wound, open — *continued*
   Descemet's membrane (*see also* Wound, open, intraocular) 871.9
   digit(s)
      foot 893.0
         with tendon involvement 893.2
         complicated 893.1
      hand 883.0
         with tendon involvement 883.2
         complicated 883.1
   drumhead, ear 872.61
      complicated 872.71
   ear 872.8
      canal 872.02
         complicated 872.12
      complicated 872.9
      drum 872.61
         complicated 872.71
      external 872.00
         complicated 872.10
      multiple sites 872.69
         complicated 872.79
      ossicles (incus) (malleus) (stapes) 872.62
         complicated 872.72
      specified part NEC 872.69
         complicated 872.79
   elbow 881.01
      with tendon involvement 881.21
      complicated 881.11
   epididymis 878.2
      complicated 878.3
   epigastric region 879.2
      complicated 879.3
   epiglottis 874.01
      complicated 874.11
   esophagus (cervical) 874.4
      complicated 874.5
      thoracic — *see* Injury, internal, esophagus
   Eustachian tube 872.63
      complicated 872.73
   extremity
      lower (multiple) NEC 894.0
         with tendon involvement 894.2
         complicated 894.1
      upper (multiple) NEC 884.0
         with tendon involvement 884.2
         complicated 884.1
   eye(s) (globe) — *see* Wound, open, intraocular
   eyeball NEC 871.9
      laceration (*see also* Laceration, eyeball) 871.4
      penetrating (*see also* Penetrating wound, eyeball) 871.7
   eyebrow 873.42
      complicated 873.52
   eyelid NEC 870.8
      laceration — *see* Laceration, eyelid
   face 873.40
      complicated 873.50
      multiple sites 873.49
         complicated 873.59
      specified part NEC 873.49
         complicated 873.59
   fallopian tube — *see* Injury, internal, fallopian tube
   finger(s) (nail) (subungual) 883.0
      with tendon involvement 883.2
      complicated 883.1
   flank 879.4
      complicated 879.5
   foot (any part except toe(s) alone) 892.0
      with tendon involvement 892.2
      complicated 892.1
   forearm 881.00
      with tendon involvement 881.20
      complicated 881.10
   forehead 873.42
      complicated 873.52
   genital organs (external) NEC 878.8
      complicated 878.9
      internal — *see* Injury, internal, by site
   globe (eye) (*see also* Wound, open, eyeball) 871.9
   groin 879.4

Wound, open — *continued*
   groin — *continued*
      complicated 879.5
   gum(s) 873.62
      complicated 873.72
   hand (except finger(s) alone) 882.0
      with tendon involvement 882.2
      complicated 882.1
   head NEC 873.8
      with intracranial injury — *see* Injury, intracranial
         due to or associated with skull fracture — *see* Fracture, skull
      complicated 873.9
      scalp — *see* Wound, open, scalp
   heel 892.0
      with tendon involvement 892.2
      complicated 892.1
   high-velocity (grease gun) — *see* Wound, open, complicated, by site
   hip 890.0
      with tendon involvement 890.2
      complicated 890.1
   hymen 878.6
      complicated 878.7
   hypochondrium 879.4
      complicated 879.5
   hypogastric region 879.2
      complicated 879.3
   iliac (region) 879.4
      complicated 879.5
   incidental to
      dislocation — *see* Dislocation, open, by site
      fracture — *see* Fracture, open, by site
      intracranial injury — *see* Injury, intracranial, with open intracranial wound
      nerve injury — *see* Injury, nerve, by site
   inguinal region 879.4
      complicated 879.5
   instep 892.0
      with tendon involvement 892.2
      complicated 892.1
   interscapular region 876.0
      complicated 876.1
   intracranial — *see* Injury, intracranial, with open intracranial wound
   intraocular 871.9
      with
         partial loss (of intraocular tissue) 871.2
         prolapse or exposure (of intraocular tissue) 871.1
         without prolapse (of intraocular tissue) 871.0
      laceration (*see also* Laceration, eyeball) 871.4
      penetrating 871.7
         with foreign body (nonmagnetic) 871.6
         magnetic 871.5
   iris (*see also* Wound, open, eyeball) 871.9
   jaw (fracture not involved) 873.44
      with fracture — *see* Fracture, jaw
      complicated 873.54
   knee 891.0
      with tendon involvement 891.2
      complicated 891.1
   labium (majus) (minus) 878.4
      complicated 878.5
   lacrimal apparatus, gland, or sac 870.8
      with laceration of eyelid 870.2
   larynx 874.01
      with trachea 874.00
         complicated 874.10
      complicated 874.11
   leg (multiple) 891.0
      with tendon involvement 891.2
      complicated 891.1
      lower 891.0
         with tendon involvement 891.2
         complicated 891.1
      thigh 890.0
         with tendon involvement 890.2
         complicated 890.1

Wound, open — *continued*
   leg — *continued*
      upper 890.0
         with tendon involvement 890.2
         complicated 890.1
   lens (eye) (alone) (*see also* Cataract, traumatic) 366.20
      with involvement of other eye structures — *see* Wound, open, eyeball
   limb
      lower (multiple) NEC 894.0
         with tendon involvement 894.2
         complicated 894.1
      upper (multiple) NEC 884.0
         with tendon involvement 884.2
         complicated 884.1
   lip 873.43
      complicated 873.53
   loin 876.0
      complicated 876.1
   lumbar region 876.0
      complicated 876.1
   malar region 873.41
      complicated 873.51
   mastoid region 873.49
      complicated 873.59
   mediastinum — *see* Injury, internal, mediastinum
   midthoracic region 875.0
      complicated 875.1
   mouth 873.60
      complicated 873.70
      floor 873.64
         complicated 873.74
      multiple sites 873.69
         complicated 873.79
      specified site NEC 873.69
         complicated 873.79
   multiple, unspecified site(s) 879.8

> **Note** — *Multiple open wounds of sites classifiable to the same four-digit category should be classified to that category unless they are in different limbs.*
>
> *Multiple open wounds of sites classifiable to different four-digit categories, or to different limbs, should be coded separately.*

      complicated 879.9
      lower limb(s) (one or both) (sites classifiable to more than one three-digit category in 890 to 893) 894.0
         with tendon involvement 894.2
         complicated 894.1
      upper limb(s) (one or both) (sites classifiable to more than one three-digit category in 880 to 883) 884.0
         with tendon involvement 884.2
         complicated 884.1
   muscle — *see* Sprain, by site
   nail
      finger(s) 883.0
         complicated 883.1
      thumb 883.0
         complicated 883.1
      toe(s) 893.0
         complicated 893.1
   nape (neck) 874.8
      complicated 874.9
      specified part NEC 874.8
         complicated 874.9
   nasal (*see also* Wound, open, nose)
      cavity 873.22
         complicated 873.32
      septum 873.21
         complicated 873.31
      sinuses 873.23
         complicated 873.33
   nasopharynx 873.22
      complicated 873.32
   neck 874.8
      complicated 874.9
      nape 874.8
         complicated 874.9
      specified part NEC 874.8

Wound, open — *continued*
   neck — *continued*
      specified part — *continued*
         complicated 874.9
   nerve — *see* Injury, nerve, by site
   non-healing surgical 998.83
   nose 873.20
      complicated 873.30
      multiple sites 873.29
         complicated 873.39
      septum 873.21
         complicated 873.31
      sinuses 873.23
         complicated 873.33
   occipital region — *see* Wound, open, scalp
   ocular NEC 871.9
      adnexa 870.9
         specified region NEC 870.8
      laceration (*see also* Laceration, ocular) 871.4
      muscle (extraocular) 870.3
         with foreign body 870.4
         eyelid 870.1
         intraocular — *see* Wound, open, eyeball
      penetrating (*see also* Penetrating wound, ocular) 871.7
   orbit 870.8
      penetrating 870.3
         with foreign body 870.4
   orbital region 870.9
   ovary — *see* Injury, internal, pelvic organs
   palate 873.65
      complicated 873.75
   palm 882.0
      with tendon involvement 882.2
      complicated 882.1
   parathyroid (gland) 874.2
      complicated 874.3
   parietal region — *see* Wound, open, scalp
   pelvic floor or region 879.6
      complicated 879.7
   penis 878.0
      complicated 878.1
   perineum 879.6
      complicated 879.7
   periocular area 870.8
      laceration of skin 870.0
   pharynx 874.4
      complicated 874.5
   pinna 872.01
      complicated 872.11
   popliteal space 891.0
      with tendon involvement 891.2
      complicated 891.1
   prepuce 878.0
      complicated 878.1
   pubic region 879.2
      complicated 879.3
   pudenda 878.8
      complicated 878.9
   rectovaginal septum 878.8
      complicated 878.9
   sacral region 877.0
      complicated 877.1
   sacroiliac region 877.0
      complicated 877.1
   salivary (ducts) (glands) 873.69
      complicated 873.79
   scalp 873.0
      complicated 873.1
   scalpel, fetus or newborn 767.8
   scapular region 880.01
      with tendon involvement 880.21
      complicated 880.11
      involving other sites of upper arm 880.09
         with tendon involvement 880.29
         complicated 880.19
   sclera (*see also* Wound, open, intraocular) 871.9
   scrotum 878.2
      complicated 878.3
   seminal vesicle — *see* Injury, internal, pelvic organs
   shin 891.0
      with tendon involvement 891.2

☑ Additional Digit Required — Refer to the Tabular List for Digit Selection   ⟱ Subterms under main terms may continue to next column or page

2015 ICD-9-CM   ▶◀ Revised Text   ● New Line   ▲ Revised Code   Volume 2 — 297

Wound, open — *continued*

shin — *continued*
complicated 891.1
shoulder 880.00
with tendon involvement 880.20
complicated 880.10
involving other sites of upper arm 880.09
with tendon involvement 880.29
complicated 880.19
skin NEC 879.8
complicated 879.9
skull (*see also* Injury, intracranial, with open intracranial wound)
with skull fracture — *see* Fracture, skull
spermatic cord (scrotal) 878.2
complicated 878.3
pelvic region — *see* Injury, internal, spermatic cord
spinal cord — *see* Injury, spinal
sternal region 875.0
complicated 875.1
subconjunctival — *see* Wound, open, intraocular
subcutaneous NEC 879.8
complicated 879.9
submaxillary region 873.44
complicated 873.54
submental region 873.44
complicated 873.54
subungual
finger(s) (thumb) — *see* Wound, open, finger
toe(s) — *see* Wound, open, toe
supraclavicular region 874.8
complicated 874.9
supraorbital 873.42
complicated 873.52
surgical, non-healing 998.83
temple 873.49
complicated 873.59
temporal region 873.49
complicated 873.59
testis 878.2
complicated 878.3
thigh 890.0
with tendon involvement 890.2
complicated 890.1
thorax, thoracic (external) 875.0
complicated 875.1
throat 874.8
complicated 874.9
thumb (nail) (subungual) 883.0
with tendon involvement 883.2
complicated 883.1
thyroid (gland) 874.2
complicated 874.3
toe(s) (nail) (subungual) 893.0
with tendon involvement 893.2
complicated 893.1
tongue 873.64
complicated 873.74
tonsil — *see* Wound, open, neck
trachea (cervical region) 874.02
with larynx 874.00
complicated 874.10
complicated 874.12
intrathoracic — *see* Injury, internal, trachea
trunk (multiple) NEC 879.6
complicated 879.7
specified site NEC 879.6
complicated 879.7

Wound, open — *continued*

tunica vaginalis 878.2
complicated 878.3
tympanic membrane 872.61
complicated 872.71
tympanum 872.61
complicated 872.71
umbilical region 879.2
complicated 879.3
ureter — *see* Injury, internal, ureter
urethra — *see* Injury, internal, urethra
uterus — *see* Injury, internal, uterus
uvula 873.69
complicated 873.79
vagina 878.6
complicated 878.7
vas deferens — *see* Injury, internal, vas deferens
vitreous (humor) 871.2
vulva 878.4
complicated 878.5
wrist 881.02
with tendon involvement 881.22
complicated 881.12
Wright's syndrome (hyperabduction) 447.8
pneumonia 390 [517.1]
Wringer injury — *see* Crush injury, by site
Wrinkling of skin 701.8
Wrist — *see also* condition
drop (acquired) 736.05
Wrong drug (given in error) NEC 977.9
specified drug or substance — *see* Table of Drugs and Chemicals
Wry neck — *see also* Torticollis
congenital 754.1
Wuchereria infestation 125.0
bancrofti 125.0
Brugia malayi 125.1
malayi 125.1
Wuchereriasis 125.0
Wuchereriosis 125.0
Wuchernde struma langhans (M8332/3) 193

X

Xanthelasma 272.2
eyelid 272.2 [374.51]
palpebrarum 272.2 [374.51]
Xanthelasmatosis (essential) 272.2
Xanthelasmoidea 757.33
Xanthine stones 277.2
Xanthinuria 277.2
Xanthofibroma (M8831/0) — *see* Neoplasm, connective tissue, benign
Xanthoma(s), xanthomatosis 272.2
with
hyperlipoproteinemia
type I 272.3
type III 272.2
type IV 272.1
type V 272.3
bone 272.7
craniohypophyseal 277.89
cutaneotendinous 272.7
diabeticorum 250.8 ☑ [272.2]
due to secondary diabetes 249.8 ☑ [272.2]
disseminatum 272.7
eruptive 272.2
eyelid 272.2 [374.51]
familial 272.7
hereditary 272.7

Xanthoma(s), xanthomatosis — *continued*

hypercholesterinemic 272.0
hypercholesterolemic 272.0
hyperlipemic 272.4
hyperlipidemic 272.4
infantile 272.7
joint 272.7
juvenile 272.7
multiple 272.7
multiplex 272.7
primary familial 272.7
tendon (sheath) 272.7
tuberosum 272.2
tuberous 272.2
tubo-eruptive 272.2
Xanthosis 709.09
surgical 998.81
Xenophobia 300.29
Xeroderma (congenital) 757.39
acquired 701.1
eyelid 373.33
eyelid 373.33
pigmentosum 757.33
vitamin A deficiency 264.8
Xerophthalmia 372.53
vitamin A deficiency 264.7
Xerosis
conjunctiva 372.53
with Bitôt's spot 372.53
vitamin A deficiency 264.1
vitamin A deficiency 264.0
cornea 371.40
with corneal ulceration 370.00
vitamin A deficiency 264.3
vitamin A deficiency 264.2
cutis 706.8
skin 706.8
Xerostomia 527.7
Xiphodynia 733.90
Xiphoidalgia 733.90
Xiphoiditis 733.99
Xiphopagus 759.4
XO syndrome 758.6
X-ray
effects, adverse, NEC 990
of chest
for suspected tuberculosis V71.2
routine V72.5
XXX syndrome 758.81
XXXXY syndrome 758.81
XXY syndrome 758.7
Xyloketosuria 271.8
Xylosuria 271.8
Xylulosuria 271.8
XYY syndrome 758.81

Y

Yaba monkey tumor virus 059.22
Yawning 786.09
psychogenic 306.1
Yaws 102.9
bone or joint lesions 102.6
butter 102.1
chancre 102.0
cutaneous, less than five years after infection 102.2
early (cutaneous) (macular) (maculopapular) (micropapular) (papular) 102.2
frambeside 102.2
skin lesions NEC 102.2

Yaws — *continued*

eyelid 102.9 [373.4]
ganglion 102.6
gangosis, gangosa 102.5
gumma, gummata 102.4
bone 102.6
gummatous
frambeside 102.4
osteitis 102.6
periostitis 102.6
hydrarthrosis 102.6
hyperkeratosis (early) (late) (palmar) (plantar) 102.3
initial lesions 102.0
joint lesions 102.6
juxta-articular nodules 102.7
late nodular (ulcerated) 102.4
latent (without clinical manifestations) (with positive serology) 102.8
mother 102.0
mucosal 102.7
multiple papillomata 102.1
nodular, late (ulcerated) 102.4
osteitis 102.6
papilloma, papillomata (palmar) (plantar) 102.1
periostitis (hypertrophic) 102.6
ulcers 102.4
wet crab 102.1
Yeast infection — *see also* Candidiasis 112.9
Yellow
atrophy (liver) 570
chronic 571.8
resulting from administration of blood, plasma, serum, or other biological substance (within 8 months of administration) — *see* Hepatitis, viral
fever — *see* Fever, yellow
jack (*see also* Fever, yellow) 060.9
jaundice (*see also* Jaundice) 782.4
vernix syndrome 762.2
Yersinia septica 027.8

Z

Zagari's disease (xerostomia) 527.7
Zahorsky's disease (exanthema subitum) (*see also* Exanthem subitum) 058.10
syndrome (herpangina) 074.0
Zellweger syndrome 277.86
Zenker's diverticulum (esophagus) 530.6
Ziehen-Oppenheim disease 333.6
Zieve's syndrome (jaundice, hyperlipemia, and hemolytic anemia) 571.1
Zika fever 066.3
Zollinger-Ellison syndrome (gastric hypersecretion with pancreatic islet cell tumor) 251.5
Zona — *see also* Herpes, zoster 053.9
Zoophilia (erotica) 302.1
Zoophobia 300.29
Zoster (herpes) — *see also* Herpes, zoster 053.9
Zuelzer (-Ogden) anemia or syndrome (nutritional megaloblastic anemia) 281.2
Zygodactyly — *see also* Syndactylism 755.10
Zygomycosis 117.7
Zymotic — *see* condition

☑ **Additional Digit Required — Refer to the Tabular List for Digit Selection**

ᴺᴱᶜ **Subterms under main terms may continue to next column or page**

SECTION 2

Alphabetic Index to Poisoning and External Causes of Adverse Effects of Drugs and Other Chemical Substances

TABLE OF DRUGS AND CHEMICALS

This table contains a classification of drugs and other chemical substances to identify poisoning states and external causes of adverse effects.

Each of the listed substances in the table is assigned a code according to the poisoning classification (960-989). These codes are used when there is a statement of poisoning, overdose, wrong substance given or taken, or intoxication.

The table also contains a listing of external causes of adverse effects. An adverse effect is a pathologic manifestation due to ingestion or exposure to drugs or other chemical substances (e.g., dermatitis, hypersensitivity reaction, aspirin gastritis). The adverse effect is to be identified by the appropriate code found in Section 1, Index to Diseases and Injuries. An external cause code can then be used to identify the circumstances involved. The table headings pertaining to external causes are defined below:

Accidental poisoning (E850-E869) — accidental overdose of drug, wrong substance given or taken, drug taken inadvertently, accidents in the usage of drugs and biologicals in medical and surgical procedures, and to show external causes of poisonings classifiable to 980-989.

Therapeutic use (E930-E949) — a correct substance properly administered in therapeutic or prophylactic dosage as the external cause of adverse effects.

Suicide attempt (E950-E952) — instances in which self-inflicted injuries or poisonings are involved.

Assault (E961-E962) — injury or poisoning inflicted by another person with the intent to injure or kill.

Undetermined (E980-E982) — to be used when the intent of the poisoning or injury cannot be determined whether it was intentional or accidental.

The American Hospital Formulary Service list numbers are included in the table to help classify new drugs not identified in the table by name. The AHFS list numbers are keyed to the continually revised American Hospital Formulary Service (AHFS).* These listings are found in the table under the main term **Drug**.

Excluded from the table are radium and other radioactive substances. The classification of adverse effects and complications pertaining to these substances will be found in Section 1, Index to Diseases and Injuries, and Section 3, Index to External Causes of Injuries.

Although certain substances are indexed with one or more subentries, the majority are listed according to one use or state. It is recognized that many substances may be used in various ways, in medicine and in industry, and may cause adverse effects whatever the state of the agent (solid, liquid, or fumes arising from a liquid). In cases in which the reported data indicates a use or state not in the table, or which is clearly different from the one listed, an attempt should be made to classify the substance in the form which most nearly expresses the reported facts.

*American Hospital Formulary Service, 2 vol. (Washington, D.C.: American Society of Hospital Pharmacists, 1959-)

☑ Additional Digit Required — Refer to the Tabular List for Digit Selection   ▽ Subterms under main terms may continue to next column or page

2015 ICD-9-CM   ▶◀ Revised Text   ● New Line   ▲ Revised Code   Volume 2 — 299

	Poisoning	Accident	Therapeutic Use	Suicide Attempt	Assault	Undetermined
1-propanol	980.3	E860.4	—	E950.9	E962.1	E980.9
2-propanol	980.2	E860.3	—	E950.9	E962.1	E980.9
2, 4-D (dichlorophenoxyacetic acid)	989.4	E863.5		E950.6	E962.1	E980.7
2, 4-toluene diiso-cyanate	983.0	E864.0	—	E950.7	E962.1	E980.6
2, 4, 5-T (trichlorophenoxy-acetic acid)	989.2	E863.5		E950.6	E962.1	E980.7
14-hydroxydihydromorphi-none	965.09	E850.2	E935.2	E950.0	E962.0	E980.0
ABOB	961.7	E857	E931.7	E950.4	E962.0	E980.4
Abrus (seed)	988.2	E865.3		E950.9	E962.1	E980.9
Absinthe	980.0	E860.1	—	E950.9	E962.1	E980.9
beverage	980.0	E860.0	—	E950.9	E962.1	E980.9
Acenocoumarin, aceno-coumarol	964.2	E858.2	E934.2	E950.4	E962.0	E980.4
Acepromazine	969.1	E853.0	E939.1	E950.3	E962.0	E980.3
Acetal	982.8	E862.4	—	E950.9	E962.1	E980.9
Acetaldehyde (vapor)	987.8	E869.8	—	E952.8	E962.2	E982.8
liquid	989.89	E866.8	—	E950.9	E962.1	E980.9
Acetaminophen	965.4	E850.4	E935.4	E950.0	E962.0	E980.0
Acetaminosalol	965.1	E850.3	E935.3	E950.0	E962.0	E980.0
Acetanilid(e)	965.4	E850.4	E935.4	E950.0	E962.0	E980.0
Acetarsol, acetarsone	961.1	E857	E931.1	E950.4	E962.0	E980.4
Acetazolamide	974.2	E858.5	E944.2	E950.4	E962.0	E980.4
Acetic						
acid	983.1	E864.1	—	E950.7	E962.1	E980.6
with sodium acetate (oint-ment)	976.3	E858.7	E946.3	E950.4	E962.0	E980.4
irrigating solution	974.5	E858.5	E944.5	E950.4	E962.0	E980.4
lotion	976.2	E858.7	E946.2	E950.4	E962.0	E980.4
anhydride	983.1	E864.1	—	E950.7	E962.1	E980.6
ether (vapor)	982.8	E862.4	—	E950.9	E962.1	E980.9
Acetohexamide	962.3	E858.0	E932.3	E950.4	E962.0	E980.4
Acetomenaphthone	964.3	E858.2	E934.3	E950.4	E962.0	E980.4
Acetomorphine	965.01	E850.0	E935.0	E950.0	E962.0	E980.0
Acetone (oils) (vapor)	982.8	E862.4	—	E950.9	E962.1	E980.9
Acetophenazine						
(maleate)	969.1	E853.0	E939.1	E950.3	E962.0	E980.3
Acetophenetidin	965.4	E850.4	E935.4	E950.0	E962.0	E980.0
Acetophenone	982.0	E862.4	—	E950.9	E962.1	E980.9
Acetorphine	965.09	E850.2	E935.2	E950.0	E962.0	E980.0
Acetosulfone (sodium)	961.8	E857	E931.8	E950.4	E962.0	E980.4
Acetrizoate (sodium)	977.8	E858.8	E947.8	E950.4	E962.0	E980.4
Acetylcarbromal	967.3	E852.2	E937.3	E950.2	E962.0	E980.2
Acetylcholine (chloride)	971.0	E855.3	E941.0	E950.4	E962.0	E980.4
Acetylcysteine	975.5	E858.6	E945.5	E950.4	E962.0	E980.4
Acetyldigitoxin	972.1	E858.3	E942.1	E950.4	E962.0	E980.4
Acetyldihydrocodeine	965.09	E850.2	E935.2	E950.0	E962.0	E980.0
Acetyldihydrocodeinone	965.09	E850.2	E935.2	E950.0	E962.0	E980.0
Acetylene (gas) (industri-al)	987.1	E868.1	—	E951.8	E962.2	E981.8
incomplete combustion of — see Carbon monoxide, fuel, utility						
tetrachloride (vapor)	982.3	E862.4	—	E950.9	E962.1	E980.9
Acetyliodosalicylic acid	965.1	E850.3	E935.3	E950.0	E962.0	E980.0
Acetylphenylhydrazine	965.8	E850.8	E935.8	E950.0	E962.0	E980.0
Acetylsalicylic acid	965.1	E850.3	E935.3	E950.0	E962.0	E980.0
Achromycin	960.4	E856	E930.4	E950.4	E962.0	E980.4
ophthalmic preparation	976.5	E858.7	E946.5	E950.4	E962.0	E980.4
topical NEC	976.0	E858.7	E946.0	E950.4	E962.0	E980.4
Acidifying agents	963.2	E858.1	E933.2	E950.4	E962.0	E980.4
Acids (corrosive) NEC	983.1	E864.1	—	E950.7	E962.1	E980.6
Aconite (wild)	988.2	E865.4	—	E950.9	E962.1	E980.9
Aconitine (liniment)	976.8	E858.7	E946.8	E950.4	E962.0	E980.4
Aconitum ferox	988.2	E865.4	—	E950.9	E962.1	E980.9
Acridine	983.0	E864.0	—	E950.7	E962.1	E980.6
vapor	987.8	E869.8	—	E952.8	E962.2	E982.8
Acriflavine	961.9	E857	E931.9	E950.4	E962.0	E980.4
Acrisorcin	976.0	E858.7	E946.0	E950.4	E962.0	E980.4
Acrolein (gas)	987.8	E869.8	—	E952.8	E962.2	E982.8
liquid	989.89	E866.8	—	E950.9	E962.1	E980.9
Actaea spicata	988.2	E865.4	—	E950.9	E962.1	E980.9
Acterol	961.5	E857	E931.5	E950.4	E962.0	E980.4
ACTH	962.4	E858.0	E932.4	E950.4	E962.0	E980.4
Acthar	962.4	E858.0	E932.4	E950.4	E962.0	E980.4
Actinomycin (C) (D)	960.7	E856	E930.7	E950.4	E962.0	E980.4
Adalin (acetyl)	967.3	E852.2	E937.3	E950.2	E962.0	E980.2
Adenosine (phosphate)	977.8	E858.8	E947.8	E950.4	E962.0	E980.4
ADH	962.5	E858.0	E932.5	E950.4	E962.0	E980.4
Adhesives	989.89	E866.6	—	E950.9	E962.1	E980.9

	Poisoning	Accident	Therapeutic Use	Suicide Attempt	Assault	Undetermined
Adicillin	960.0	E856	E930.0	E950.4	E962.0	E980.4
Adiphenine	975.1	E855.6	E945.1	E950.4	E962.0	E980.4
Adjunct, pharmaceutical	977.4	E858.8	E947.4	E950.4	E962.0	E980.4
Adrenal (extract, cortex or medulla) (glucocorticoids) (hormones) (mineralocorti-coids)	962.0	E858.0	E932.0	E950.4	E962.0	E980.4
ENT agent	976.6	E858.7	E946.6	E950.4	E962.0	E980.4
ophthalmic preparation	976.5	E858.7	E946.5	E950.4	E962.0	E980.4
topical NEC	976.0	E858.7	E946.0	E950.4	E962.0	E980.4
Adrenalin	971.2	E855.5	E941.2	E950.4	E962.0	E980.4
Adrenergic blocking agents	971.3	E855.6	E941.3	E950.4	E962.0	E980.4
Adrenergics	971.2	E855.5	E941.2	E950.4	E962.0	E980.4
Adrenochrome (deriva-tives)	972.8	E858.3	E942.8	E950.4	E962.0	E980.4
Adrenocorticotropic hor-mone	962.4	E858.0	E932.4	E950.4	E962.0	E980.4
Adrenocorticotropin	962.4	E858.0	E932.4	E950.4	E962.0	E980.4
Adriamycin	960.7	E856	E930.7	E950.4	E962.0	E980.4
Aerosol spray — see Sprays						
Aerosporin	960.8	E856	E930.8	E950.4	E962.0	E980.4
ENT agent	976.6	E858.7	E946.6	E950.4	E962.0	E980.4
ophthalmic preparation	976.5	E858.7	E946.5	E950.4	E962.0	E980.4
topical NEC	976.0	E858.7	E946.0	E950.4	E962.0	E980.4
Aethusa cynapium	988.2	E865.4	—	E950.9	E962.1	E980.9
Afghanistan black	969.6	E854.1	E939.6	E950.3	E962.0	E980.3
Aflatoxin	989.7	E865.9		E950.9	E962.1	E980.9
African boxwood	988.2	E865.4	—	E950.9	E962.1	E980.9
Agar (-agar)	973.3	E858.4	E943.3	E950.4	E962.0	E980.4
Agricultural agent NEC	989.89	E863.9	—	E950.6	E962.1	E980.7
Agrypnal	967.0	E851	E937.0	E950.1	E962.0	E980.1
Air contaminant(s), source or type not specified	987.9	E869.9	—	E952.9	E962.2	E982.9
specified type — see specific substance						
Akee	988.2	E865.4	—	E950.9	E962.1	E980.9
Akrinol	976.0	E858.7	E946.0	E950.4	E962.0	E980.4
Akrinon	961.6	E857	E931.6	E950.4	E962.0	E980.4
Alantolactone	961.6	E857	E931.6	E950.4	E962.0	E980.4
Albamycin	960.8	E856	E930.8	E950.4	E962.0	E980.4
Albumin (normal human serum)	964.7	E858.2	E934.7	E950.4	E962.0	E980.4
Albuterol	975.7	E858.6	E945.7	E950.4	E962.0	E980.4
Alcohol	980.9	E860.9	—	E950.9	E962.1	E980.9
absolute	980.0	E860.1	—	E950.9	E962.1	E980.9
beverage	980.0	E860.0	E947.8	E950.9	E962.1	E980.9
amyl	980.3	E860.4	—	E950.9	E962.1	E980.9
antifreeze	980.1	E860.2	—	E950.9	E962.1	E980.9
butyl	980.3	E860.4	—	E950.9	E962.1	E980.9
dehydrated	980.0	E860.1	—	E950.9	E862.1	E980.9
beverage	980.0	E860.0	E947.8	E950.9	E962.1	E980.9
denatured	980.0	E860.1	—	E950.9	E962.1	E980.9
deterrents	977.3	E858.8	E947.3	E950.4	E962.0	E980.4
diagnostic (gastric func-tion)	977.8	E858.8	E947.8	E950.4	E962.0	E980.4
ethyl	980.0	E860.1	—	E950.9	E962.1	E980.9
beverage	980.0	E860.0	E947.8	E950.9	E962.1	E980.9
grain	980.0	E860.1	—	E950.9	E962.1	E980.9
beverage	980.0	E860.0	E947.8	E950.9	E962.1	E980.9
industrial	980.9	E860.9	—	E950.9	E962.1	E980.9
isopropyl	980.2	E860.3	—	E950.9	E962.1	E980.9
methyl	980.1	E860.2	—	E950.9	E962.1	E980.9
preparation for consump-tion	980.0	E860.0	E947.8	E950.9	E962.1	E980.9
propyl	980.3	E860.4	—	E950.9	E962.1	E980.9
secondary	980.2	E860.3	—	E950.9	E962.1	E980.9
radiator	980.1	E860.2	—	E950.9	E962.1	E980.9
rubbing	980.2	E860.3	—	E950.9	E962.1	E980.9
specified type NEC	980.8	E860.8	—	E950.9	E962.1	E980.9
surgical	980.9	E860.9	—	E950.9	E962.1	E980.9
vapor (from any type of alco-hol)	987.8	E869.8	—	E952.8	E962.2	E982.8
wood	980.1	E860.2	—	E950.9	E962.1	E980.9
Alcuronium chloride	975.2	E858.6	E945.2	E950.4	E962.0	E980.4
Aldactone	974.4	E858.5	E944.4	E950.4	E962.0	E980.4
Aldicarb	989.3	E863.2	—	E950.6	E962.1	E980.7
Aldomet	972.6	E858.3	E942.6	E950.4	E962.0	E980.4
Aldosterone	962.0	E858.0	E932.0	E950.4	E962.0	E980.4
Aldrin (dust)	989.2	E863.0	—	E950.6	E962.1	E980.7
Algeldrate	973.0	E858.4	E943.0	E950.4	E962.0	E980.4
Alidase	963.4	E858.1	E933.4	E950.4	E962.0	E980.4
Aliphatic thiocyanates	989.0	E866.8	—	E950.9	E962.1	E980.9

	External Cause (E-Code)					
	Poisoning	Accident	Therapeutic Use	Suicide Attempt	Assault	Undetermined
Alkaline antiseptic solution (aromatic)	976.6	E858.7	E946.6	E950.4	E962.0	E980.4
Alkalinizing agents (medicinal)	963.3	E858.1	E933.3	E950.4	E962.0	E980.4
Alkalis, caustic	983.2	E864.2	—	E950.7	E962.1	E980.6
Alkalizing agents (medicinal)	963.3	E858.1	E933.3	E950.4	E962.0	E980.4
Alka-seltzer	965.1	E850.3	E935.3	E950.0	E962.0	E980.0
Alkavervir	972.6	E858.3	E942.6	E950.4	E962.0	E980.4
Allegron	969.05	E854.0	E939.0	E950.3	E962.0	E980.3
Alleve — Naproxen						
Allobarbital, allobarbitone	967.0	E851	E937.0	E950.1	E962.0	E980.1
Allopurinol	974.7	E858.5	E944.7	E950.4	E962.0	E980.4
Allylestrenol	962.2	E858.0	E932.2	E950.4	E962.0	E980.4
Allylisopropylacetylurea	967.8	E852.8	E937.8	E950.2	E962.0	E980.2
Allylisopropylmalonylurea	967.0	E851	E937.0	E950.1	E962.0	E980.1
Allyltribromide	967.3	E852.2	E937.3	E950.2	E962.0	E980.2
Aloe, aloes, aloin	973.1	E858.4	E943.1	E950.4	E962.0	E980.4
Alosetron	973.8	E858.4	E943.8	E950.4	E962.0	E980.4
Aloxidone	966.0	E855.0	E936.0	E950.4	E962.0	E980.4
Aloxiprin	965.1	E850.3	E935.3	E950.0	E962.0	E980.0
Alpha-1 blockers	971.3	E855.6	E941.3	E950.4	E962.0	E980.4
Alpha amylase	963.4	E858.1	E933.4	E950.4	E962.0	E980.4
Alphaprodine (hydrochloride)	965.09	E850.2	E935.2	E950.0	E962.0	E980.0
Alpha tocopherol	963.5	E858.1	E933.5	E950.4	E962.0	E980.4
Alseroxylon	972.6	E858.3	E942.6	E950.4	E962.0	E980.4
Alum (ammonium) (potassium)	983.2	E864.2	—	E950.7	E962.1	E980.6
medicinal (astringent) NEC	976.2	E858.7	E946.2	E950.4	E962.0	E980.4
Aluminium, aluminum (gel) (hydroxide)	973.0	E858.4	E943.0	E950.4	E962.0	E980.4
acetate solution	976.2	E858.7	E946.2	E950.4	E962.0	E980.4
aspirin	965.1	E850.3	E935.3	E950.0	E962.0	E980.0
carbonate	973.0	E858.4	E943.0	E950.4	E962.0	E980.4
glycinate	973.0	E858.4	E943.0	E950.4	E962.0	E980.4
nicotinate	972.2	E858.3	E942.2	E950.4	E962.0	E980.4
ointment (surgical) (topical)	976.3	E858.7	E946.3	E950.4	E962.0	E980.4
phosphate	973.0	E858.4	E943.0	E950.4	E962.0	E980.4
subacetate	976.2	E858.7	E946.2	E950.4	E962.0	E980.4
topical NEC	976.3	E858.7	E946.3	E950.4	E962.0	E980.4
Alurate	967.0	E851	E937.0	E950.1	E962.0	E980.1
Alverine (citrate)	975.1	E858.6	E945.1	E950.4	E962.0	E980.4
Alvodine	965.09	E850.2	E935.2	E950.0	E962.0	E980.0
Amanita phalloides	988.1	E865.5	—	E950.9	E962.1	E980.9
Amantadine (hydrochloride)	966.4	E855.0	E936.4	E950.4	E962.0	E980.4
Ambazone	961.9	E857	E931.9	E950.4	E962.0	E980.4
Ambenonium	971.0	E855.3	E941.0	E950.4	E962.0	E980.4
Ambutonium bromide	971.1	E855.4	E941.1	E950.4	E962.0	E980.4
Ametazole	977.8	E858.8	E947.8	E950.4	E962.0	E980.4
Amethocaine (infiltration) (topical)	968.5	E855.2	E938.5	E950.4	E962.0	E980.4
nerve block (peripheral) (plexus)	968.6	E855.2	E938.6	E950.4	E962.0	E980.4
spinal	968.7	E855.2	E938.7	E950.4	E962.0	E980.4
Amethopterin	963.1	E858.1	E933.1	E950.4	E962.0	E980.4
Amfepramone	977.0	E858.8	E947.0	E950.4	E962.0	E980.4
Amidon	965.02	E850.1	E935.1	E950.0	E962.0	E980.0
Amidopyrine	965.5	E850.5	E935.5	E950.0	E962.0	E980.0
Aminacrine	976.0	E858.7	E946.0	E950.4	E962.0	E980.4
Aminitrozole	961.5	E857	E931.5	E950.4	E962.0	E980.4
Aminoacetic acid	974.5	E858.5	E944.5	E950.4	E962.0	E980.4
Amino acids	974.5	E858.5	E944.5	E950.4	E962.0	E980.4
Aminocaproic acid	964.4	E858.2	E934.4	E950.4	E962.0	E980.4
Aminoethylisothiourium	963.8	E858.1	E933.8	E950.4	E962.0	E980.4
Aminoglutethimide	966.3	E855.0	E936.3	E950.4	E962.0	E980.4
Aminometradine	974.3	E858.5	E944.3	E950.4	E962.0	E980.4
Aminopentamide	971.1	E855.4	E941.1	E950.4	E962.0	E980.4
Aminophenazone	965.5	E850.5	E935.5	E950.0	E962.0	E980.0
Aminophenol	983.0	E864.0	—	E950.7	E962.1	E980.6
Aminophenylpyridone	969.5	E853.8	E939.5	E950.3	E962.0	E980.3
Aminophylline	975.7	E858.6	E945.7	E950.4	E962.0	E980.4
Aminopterin	963.1	E858.1	E933.1	E950.4	E962.0	E980.4
Aminopyrine	965.5	E850.5	E935.5	E950.0	E962.0	E980.0
Aminosalicylic acid	961.8	E857	E931.8	E950.4	E962.0	E980.4
Amiphenazole	970.1	E854.3	E940.1	E950.4	E962.0	E980.4
Amiquinsin	972.6	E858.3	E942.6	E950.4	E962.0	E980.4
Amisometradine	974.3	E858.5	E944.3	E950.4	E962.0	E980.4
Amitriptyline	969.05	E854.0	E939.0	E950.3	E962.0	E980.3
Ammonia (fumes) (gas) (vapor)	987.8	E869.8	—	E952.8	E962.2	E982.8
liquid (household) NEC	983.2	E861.4	—	E950.7	E962.1	E980.6
spirit, aromatic	970.89	E854.3	E940.8	E950.4	E962.0	E980.4
Ammoniated mercury	976.0	E858.7	E946.0	E950.4	E962.0	E980.4
Ammonium						
carbonate	983.2	E864.2	—	E950.7	E962.1	E980.6
chloride (acidifying agent)	963.2	E858.1	E933.2	E950.4	E962.0	E980.4
expectorant	975.5	E858.6	E945.5	E950.4	E962.0	E980.4
compounds (household) NEC	983.2	E861.4	—	E950.7	E962.1	E980.6
fumes (any usage)	987.8	E869.8	—	E952.8	E962.2	E982.8
industrial	983.2	E864.2	—	E950.7	E962.1	E980.6
ichthyosulfonate	976.4	E858.7	E946.4	E950.4	E962.0	E980.4
mandelate	961.9	E857	E931.9	E950.4	E962.0	E980.4
Amobarbital	967.0	E851	E937.0	E950.1	E962.0	E980.1
Amodiaquin(e)	961.4	E857	E931.4	E950.4	E962.0	E980.4
Amopyroquin(e)	961.4	E857	E931.4	E950.4	E962.0	E980.4
Amphenidone	969.5	E853.8	E939.5	E950.3	E962.0	E980.3
Amphetamine	969.72	E854.2	E939.7	E950.3	E962.0	E980.3
Amphomycin	960.8	E856	E930.8	E950.4	E962.0	E980.4
Amphotericin B	960.1	E856	E930.1	E950.4	E962.0	E980.4
topical	976.0	E858.7	E946.0	E950.4	E962.0	E980.4
Ampicillin	960.0	E856	E930.0	E950.4	E962.0	E980.4
Amprotropine	971.1	E855.4	E941.1	E950.4	E962.0	E980.4
Amygdalin	977.8	E858.8	E947.8	E950.4	E962.0	E980.4
Amyl						
acetate (vapor)	982.8	E862.4	—	E950.9	E962.1	E980.9
alcohol	980.3	E860.4	—	E950.9	E962.1	E980.9
nitrite (medicinal)	972.4	E858.3	E942.4	E950.4	E962.0	E980.4
Amylase (alpha)	963.4	E858.1	E933.4	E950.4	E962.0	E980.4
Amylene hydrate	980.8	E860.8	—	E950.9	E962.1	E980.9
Amylobarbitone	967.0	E851	E937.0	E950.1	E962.0	E980.1
Amylocaine	968.9	E855.2	E938.9	E950.4	E962.0	E980.4
infiltration (subcutaneous)	968.5	E855.2	E938.5	E950.4	E962.0	E980.4
nerve block (peripheral) (plexus)	968.6	E855.2	E938.6	E950.4	E962.0	E980.4
spinal	968.7	E855.2	E938.7	E950.4	E962.0	E980.4
topical (surface)	968.5	E855.2	E938.5	E950.4	E962.0	E980.4
Amytal (sodium)	967.0	E851	E937.0	E950.1	E962.0	E980.1
Analeptics	970.0	E854.3	E940.0	E950.4	E962.0	E980.4
Analgesics	965.9	E850.9	E935.9	E950.0	E962.0	E980.0
aromatic NEC	965.4	E850.4	E935.4	E950.0	E962.0	E980.0
non-narcotic NEC	965.7	E850.7	E935.7	E950.0	E962.0	E980.0
specified NEC	965.8	E850.8	E935.8	E950.0	E962.0	E980.0
Anamirta cocculus	988.2	E865.3	—	E950.9	E962.1	E980.9
Ancillin	960.0	E856	E930.0	E950.4	E962.0	E980.4
Androgens (anabolic congeners)	962.1	E858.0	E932.1	E950.4	E962.0	E980.4
Androstalone	962.1	E858.0	E932.1	E950.4	E962.0	E980.4
Androsterone	962.1	E858.0	E932.1	E950.4	E962.0	E980.4
Anemone pulsatilla	988.2	E865.4	—	E950.9	E962.1	E980.9
Anesthesia, anesthetic (general) NEC	968.4	E855.1	E938.4	E950.4	E962.0	E980.4
block (nerve) (plexus)	968.6	E855.2	E938.6	E950.4	E962.0	E980.4
gaseous NEC	968.2	E855.1	E938.2	E950.4	E962.0	E980.4
halogenated hydrocarbon derivatives NEC	968.2	E855.1	E938.2	E950.4	E962.0	E980.4
infiltration (intradermal) (subcutaneous) (submucosal)	968.5	E855.2	E938.5	E950.4	E962.0	E980.4
intravenous	968.3	E855.1	E938.3	E950.4	E962.0	E980.4
local NEC	968.9	E855.2	E938.9	E950.4	E962.0	E980.4
nerve blocking (peripheral) (plexus)	968.6	E855.2	E938.6	E950.4	E962.0	E980.4
rectal NEC	968.3	E855.1	E938.3	E950.4	E962.0	E980.4
spinal	968.7	E855.2	E938.7	E950.4	E962.0	E980.4
surface	968.5	E855.2	E938.5	E950.4	E962.0	E980.4
topical	968.5	E855.2	E938.5	E950.4	E962.0	E980.4
Aneurine	963.5	E858.1	E933.5	E950.4	E962.0	E980.4
Anginine — see Glyceryl trinitrate						
Angio-Conray	977.8	E858.8	E947.8	E950.4	E962.0	E980.4
Angiotensin	971.2	E855.5	E941.2	E950.4	E962.0	E980.4
Anhydrohydroxyprogesterone	962.2	E858.0	E932.2	E950.4	E962.0	E980.4
Anhydron	974.3	E858.5	E944.3	E950.4	E962.0	E980.4
Anileridine	965.09	E850.2	E935.2	E950.0	E962.0	E980.0

▽ Subterms under main terms may continue to next column or page

	Poisoning	Accident	Therapeutic Use	Suicide Attempt	Assault	Undetermined
Aniline (dye) (liquid)	983.0	E864.0	—	E950.7	E962.1	E980.6
analgesic	965.4	E850.4	E935.4	E950.0	E962.0	E980.0
derivatives, therapeutic NEC	965.4	E850.4	E935.4	E950.0	E962.0	E980.0
vapor	987.8	E869.8	—	E952.8	E962.2	E982.8
Aniscoropine	971.1	E855.4	E941.1	E950.4	E962.0	E980.4
Anisindione	964.2	E858.2	E934.2	E950.4	E962.0	E980.4
Anorexic agents	977.0	E858.8	E947.0	E950.4	E962.0	E980.4
Ant (bite) (sting)	—	E905.5	—	E950.9	E962.1	E980.9
Antabuse	977.3	E858.8	E947.3	E950.4	E962.0	E980.4
Antacids	973.0	E858.4	E943.0	E950.4	E962.0	E980.4
Antazoline	963.0	E858.1	E933.0	E950.4	E962.0	E980.4
Anthralin	976.4	E858.7	E946.4	E950.4	E962.0	E980.4
Anthramycin	960.7	E856	E930.7	E950.4	E962.0	E980.4
Antiadrenergics	971.3	E855.6	E941.3	E950.4	E962.0	E980.4
Antiallergic agents	963.0	E858.1	E933.0	E950.4	E962.0	E980.4
Antianemic agents NEC	964.1	E858.2	E934.1	E950.4	E962.0	E980.4
Antiaris toxicaria	988.2	E865.4	—	E950.9	E962.1	E980.9
Antiarteriosclerotic agents	972.2	E858.3	E942.2	E950.4	E962.0	E980.4
Antiasthmatics	975.7	E858.6	E945.7	E950.4	E962.0	E980.4
Antibiotics	960.9	E856	E930.9	E950.4	E962.0	E980.4
antifungal	960.1	E856	E930.1	E950.4	E962.0	E980.4
antimycobacterial	960.6	E856	E930.6	E950.4	E962.0	E980.4
antineoplastic	960.7	E856	E930.7	E950.4	E962.0	E980.4
cephalosporin (group)	960.5	E856	E930.5	E950.4	E962.0	E980.4
chloramphenicol (group)	960.2	E856	E930.2	E950.4	E962.0	E980.4
macrolides	960.3	E856	E930.3	E950.4	E962.0	E980.4
specified NEC	960.8	E856	E930.8	E950.4	E962.0	E980.4
tetracycline (group)	960.4	E856	E930.4	E950.4	E962.0	E980.4
Anticancer agents NEC	963.1	E858.1	E933.1	E950.4	E962.0	E980.4
antibiotics	960.7	E856	E930.7	E950.4	E962.0	E980.4
Anticholinergics	971.1	E855.4	E941.1	E950.4	E962.0	E980.4
Anticholinesterase (organophosphorus) (reversible)	971.0	E855.3	E941.0	E950.4	E962.0	E980.4
Anticoagulants	964.2	E858.2	E934.2	E950.4	E962.0	E980.4
antagonists	964.5	E858.2	E934.5	E950.4	E962.0	E980.4
Anti-common cold agents NEC	975.6	E858.6	E945.6	E950.4	E962.0	E980.4
Anticonvulsants NEC	966.3	E855.0	E936.3	E950.4	E962.0	E980.4
Antidepressants	969.00	E854.0	E939.0	E950.3	E962.0	E980.3
monoamine oxidase inhibitors (MAOI)	969.01	E854.0	E939.0	E950.3	E962.0	E980.3
specified type NEC	969.09	E854.0	E939.0	E950.3	E962.0	E980.3
SSNRI (selective serotonin and norepinephrine reuptake inhibitors)	969.02	E854.0	E939.0	E950.3	E962.0	E980.3
SSRI (selective serotonin reuptake inhibitors)	969.03	E854.0	E939.0	E950.3	E962.0	E980.3
tetracyclic	969.04	E854.0	E939.0	E950.3	E962.0	E980.3
tricyclic	969.05	E854.0	E939.0	E950.3	E962.0	E980.3
Antidiabetic agents	962.3	E858.0	E932.3	E950.4	E962.0	E980.4
Antidiarrheal agents	973.5	E858.4	E943.5	E950.4	E962.0	E980.4
Antidiuretic hormone	962.5	E858.0	E932.5	E950.4	E962.0	E980.4
Antidotes NEC	977.2	E858.8	E947.2	E950.4	E962.0	E980.4
Antiemetic agents	963.0	E858.1	E933.0	E950.4	E962.0	E980.4
Antiepilepsy agent NEC	966.3	E855.0	E936.3	E950.4	E962.0	E980.4
Antifertility pills	962.2	E858.0	E932.2	E950.4	E962.0	E980.4
Antiflatulents	973.8	E858.4	E943.8	E950.4	E962.0	E980.4
Antifreeze	989.89	E866.8	—	E950.9	E962.1	E980.9
alcohol	980.1	E860.2	—	E950.9	E962.1	E980.9
ethylene glycol	982.8	E862.4	—	E950.9	E962.1	E980.9
Antifungals (nonmedicinal) (sprays)	989.4	E863.6	—	E950.6	E962.1	E980.7
medicinal NEC	961.9	E857	E931.9	E950.4	E962.0	E980.4
antibiotic	960.1	E856	E930.1	E950.4	E962.0	E980.4
topical	976.0	E858.7	E946.0	E950.4	E962.0	E980.4
Antigastric secretion agents	973.0	E858.4	E943.0	E950.4	E962.0	E980.4
Antihelmintics	961.6	E857	E931.6	E950.4	E962.0	E980.4
Antihemophilic factor (human)	964.7	E858.2	E934.7	E950.4	E962.0	E980.4
Antihistamine	963.0	E858.1	E933.0	E950.4	E962.0	E980.4
Antihypertensive agents NEC	972.6	E858.3	E942.6	E950.4	E962.0	E980.4
Anti-infectives NEC	961.9	E857	E931.9	E950.4	E962.0	E980.4
antibiotics	960.9	E856	E930.9	E950.4	E962.0	E980.4
specified NEC	960.8	E856	E930.8	E950.4	E962.0	E980.4
antihelmintic	961.6	E857	E931.6	E950.4	E962.0	E980.4
antimalarial	961.4	E857	E931.4	E950.4	E962.0	E980.4
antimycobacterial NEC	961.8	E857	E931.8	E950.4	E962.0	E980.4
Anti-infectives — *continued*						
antimycobacterial — *continued*						
antibiotics	960.6	E856	E930.6	E950.4	E962.0	E980.4
antiprotozoal NEC	961.5	E857	E931.5	E950.4	E962.0	—
blood	961.4	E857	E931.4	E950.4	E962.0	E980.4
antiviral	961.7	E857	E931.7	E950.4	E962.0	E980.4
arsenical	961.1	E857	E931.1	E950.4	E962.0	E980.4
ENT agents	976.6	E858.7	E946.6	E950.4	E962.0	E980.4
heavy metals NEC	961.2	E857	E931.2	E950.4	E962.0	E980.4
local	976.0	E858.7	E946.0	E950.4	E962.0	E980.4
ophthalmic preparation	976.5	E858.7	E946.5	E950.4	E962.0	E980.4
topical NEC	976.0	E858.7	E946.0	E950.4	E962.0	E980.4
Anti-inflammatory agents (topical)	976.0	E858.7	E946.0	E950.4	E962.0	E980.4
Antiknock (tetraethyl lead)	984.1	E862.1	—	E950.9	—	E980.9
Antilipemics	972.2	E858.3	E942.2	E950.4	E962.0	E980.4
Antimalarials	961.4	E857	E931.4	E950.4	E962.0	E980.4
Antimony (compounds) (vapor) NEC	985.4	E866.2	—	E950.9	E962.1	E980.9
anti-infectives	961.2	E857	E931.2	E950.4	E962.0	E980.4
pesticides (vapor)	985.4	E863.4	—	E950.6	E962.2	E980.7
potassium tartrate	961.2	E857	E931.2	E950.4	E962.0	E980.4
tartrated	961.2	E857	E931.2	E950.4	E962.0	E980.4
Antimuscarinic agents	971.1	E855.4	E941.1	E950.4	E962.0	E980.4
Antimycobacterials NEC	961.8	E857	E931.8	E950.4	E962.0	E980.4
antibiotics	960.6	E856	E930.6	E950.4	E962.0	E980.4
Antineoplastic agents	963.1	E858.1	E933.1	E950.4	E962.0	E980.4
antibiotics	960.7	E856	E930.7	E950.4	E962.0	E980.4
Anti-Parkinsonism agents	966.4	E855.0	E936.4	E950.4	E962.0	E980.4
Antiphlogistics	965.69	E850.6	E935.6	E950.0	E962.0	E980.0
Antiprotozoals NEC	961.5	E857	E931.5	E950.4	E962.0	E980.4
blood	961.4	E857	E931.4	E950.4	E962.0	E980.4
Antipruritics (local)	976.1	E858.7	E946.1	E950.4	E962.0	E980.4
Antipsychotic agents NEC	969.3	E853.8	E939.3	E950.3	E962.0	E980.3
Antipyretics	965.9	E850.9	E935.9	E950.0	E962.0	E980.0
specified NEC	965.8	E850.8	E935.8	E950.0	E962.0	E980.0
Antipyrine	965.5	E850.5	E935.5	E950.0	E962.0	E980.0
Antirabies serum (equine)	979.9	E858.8	E949.9	E950.4	E962.0	E980.4
Antirheumatics	965.69	E850.6	E935.6	E950.0	E962.0	E980.0
Antiseborrheics	976.4	E858.7	E946.4	E950.4	E962.0	E980.4
Antiseptics (external) (medicinal)	976.0	E858.7	E946.0	E950.4	E962.0	E980.4
Antistine	963.0	E858.1	E933.0	E950.4	E962.0	E980.4
Antithyroid agents	962.8	E858.0	E932.8	E950.4	E962.0	E980.4
Antitoxin, any	979.9	E858.8	E949.9	E950.4	E962.0	E980.4
Antituberculars	961.8	E857	E931.8	E950.4	E962.0	E980.4
antibiotics	960.6	E856	E930.6	E950.4	E962.0	E980.4
Antitussives	975.4	E858.6	E945.4	E950.4	E962.0	E980.4
Antivaricose agents (sclerosing)	972.7	E858.3	E942.7	E950.4	E962.0	E980.4
Antivenin (crotaline) (spider-bite)	979.9	E858.8	E949.9	E950.4	E962.0	E980.4
Antivert	963.0	E858.1	E933.0	E950.4	E962.0	E980.4
Antivirals NEC	961.7	E857	E931.7	E950.4	E962.0	E980.4
Ant poisons — *see* Pesticides						
Antrol	989.4	E863.4	—	E950.6	E962.1	E980.7
fungicide	989.4	E863.6	—	E950.6	E962.1	E980.7
Apomorphine hydrochloride (emetic)	973.6	E858.4	E943.6	E950.4	E962.0	E980.4
Appetite depressants, central	977.0	E858.8	E947.0	E950.4	E962.0	E980.4
Apresoline	972.6	E858.3	E942.6	E950.4	E962.0	E980.4
Aprobarbital, aprobarbitone	967.0	E851	E937.0	E950.1	E962.0	E980.1
Apronalide	967.8	E852.8	E937.8	E950.2	E962.0	E980.2
Aqua fortis	983.1	E864.1	—	E950.7	E962.1	E980.6
Arachis oil (topical)	976.3	E858.7	E946.3	E950.4	E962.0	E980.4
cathartic	973.2	E858.4	E943.2	E950.4	E962.0	E980.4
Aralen	961.4	E857	E931.4	E950.4	E962.0	E980.4
Arginine salts	974.5	E858.5	E944.5	E950.4	E962.0	E980.4
Argyrol	976.0	E858.7	E946.0	E950.4	E962.0	E980.4
ENT agent	976.6	E858.7	E946.6	E950.4	E962.0	E980.4
ophthalmic preparation	976.5	E858.7	E946.5	E950.4	E962.0	E980.4
Aristocort	962.0	E858.0	E932.0	E950.4	E962.0	E980.4
ENT agent	976.6	E858.7	E946.6	E950.4	E962.0	E980.4
ophthalmic preparation	976.5	E858.7	E946.5	E950.4	E962.0	E980.4
topical NEC	976.0	E858.7	E946.0	E950.4	E962.0	E980.4

Nontherapeutic use substance

Subterms under main terms may continue to next column or page

		External Cause (E-Code)				
	Poisoning	Accident	Therapeutic Use	Suicide Attempt	Assault	Undetermined
Aromatics, corrosive	983.0	E864.0	—	E950.7	E962.1	E980.6
disinfectants	983.0	E861.4	—	E950.7	E962.1	E980.6
Arsenate of lead (insecticide)	985.1	E863.4	—	E950.8	E962.1	E980.8
herbicide	985.1	E863.5	—	E950.8	E962.1	E980.8
Arsenic, arsenicals (compounds) (dust) (fumes) (vapor) NEC	985.1	E866.3	—	E950.8	E962.1	E980.8
anti-infectives	961.1	E857	E931.1	E950.4	E962.0	E980.4
pesticide (dust) (fumes)	985.1	E863.4	—	E950.8	E962.1	E980.8
Arsine (gas)	985.1	E866.3	—	E950.8	E962.1	E980.8
Arsphenamine (silver)	961.1	E857	E931.1	E950.4	E962.0	E980.4
Arsthinol	961.1	E857	E931.1	E950.4	E962.0	E980.4
Artane	971.1	E855.4	E941.1	E950.4	E962.0	E980.4
Arthropod (venomous) NEC	989.5	E905.5	—	E950.9	E962.1	E980.9
Asbestos	989.81	E866.8	—	E950.9	E962.1	E980.9
Ascaridole	961.6	E857	E931.6	E950.4	E962.0	E980.4
Ascorbic acid	963.5	E858.1	E933.5	E950.4	E962.0	E980.4
Asiaticoside	976.0	E858.7	E946.0	E950.4	E962.0	E980.4
Aspidium (oleoresin)	961.6	E857	E931.6	E950.4	E962.0	E980.4
Aspirin	965.1	E850.3	E935.3	E950.0	E962.0	E980.0
Astringents (local)	976.2	E858.7	E946.2	E950.4	E962.0	E980.4
Atabrine	961.3	E857	E931.3	E950.4	E962.0	E980.4
Ataractics	969.5	E853.8	E939.5	E950.3	E962.0	E980.3
Atonia drug, intestinal	973.3	E858.4	E943.3	E950.4	E962.0	E980.4
Atophan	974.7	E858.5	E944.7	E950.4	E962.0	E980.4
Atropine	971.1	E855.4	E941.1	E950.4	E962.0	E980.4
Attapulgite	973.5	E858.4	E943.5	E950.4	E962.0	E980.4
Attenuvax	979.4	E858.8	E949.4	E950.4	E962.0	E980.4
Aureomycin	960.4	E856	E930.4	E950.4	E962.0	E980.4
ophthalmic preparation	976.5	E858.7	E946.5	E950.4	E962.0	E980.4
topical NEC	976.0	E858.7	E946.0	E950.4	E962.0	E980.4
Aurothioglucose	965.69	E850.6	E935.6	E950.0	E962.0	E980.0
Aurothioglycanide	965.69	E850.6	E935.6	E950.0	E962.0	E980.0
Aurothiomalate	965.69	E850.6	E935.6	E950.0	E962.0	E980.0
Automobile fuel	981	E862.1	—	E950.9	E962.1	E980.9
Autonomic nervous system agents NEC	971.9	E855.9	E941.9	E950.4	E962.0	E980.4
Avlosulfon	961.8	E857	E931.8	E950.4	E962.0	E980.4
Avomine	967.8	E852.8	E937.8	E950.2	E962.0	E980.2
Azacyclonol	969.5	E853.8	E939.5	E950.3	E962.0	E980.3
Azapetine	971.3	E855.6	E941.3	E950.4	E962.0	E980.4
Azaribine	963.1	E858.1	E933.1	E950.4	E962.0	E980.4
Azaserine	960.7	E856	E930.7	E950.4	E962.0	E980.4
Azathioprine	963.1	E858.1	E933.1	E950.4	E962.0	E980.4
Azosulfamide	961.0	E857	E931.0	E950.4	E962.0	E980.4
Azulfidine	961.0	E857	E931.0	E950.4	E962.0	E980.4
Azuresin	977.8	E858.8	E947.8	E950.4	E962.0	E980.4
Bacimycin	976.0	E858.7	E946.0	E950.4	E962.0	E980.4
ophthalmic preparation	976.5	E858.7	E946.5	E950.4	E962.0	E980.4
Bacitracin	960.8	E856	E930.8	E950.4	E962.0	E980.4
ENT agent	976.6	E858.7	E946.6	E950.4	E962.0	E980.4
ophthalmic preparation	976.5	E858.7	E946.5	E950.4	E962.0	E980.4
topical NEC	976.0	E858.7	E946.0	E950.4	E962.0	E980.4
Baking soda	963.3	E858.1	E933.3	E950.4	E962.0	E980.4
BAL	963.8	E858.1	E933.8	E950.4	E962.0	E980.4
Bamethan (sulfate)	972.5	E858.3	E942.5	E950.4	E962.0	E980.4
Bamipine	963.0	E858.1	E933.0	E950.4	E962.0	E980.4
Baneberry	988.2	E865.4	—	E950.9	E962.1	E980.9
Banewort	988.2	E865.4	—	E950.9	E962.1	E980.9
Barbenyl	967.0	E851	E937.0	E950.1	E962.0	E980.1
Barbital, barbitone	967.0	E851	E937.0	E950.1	E962.0	E980.1
Barbiturates, barbituric acid	967.0	E851	E937.0	E950.1	E962.0	E980.1
anesthetic (intravenous)	968.3	E855.1	E938.3	E950.4	E962.0	E980.4
Barium (carbonate) (chloride) (sulfate)	985.8	E866.4	—	E950.9	E962.1	E980.9
diagnostic agent	977.8	E858.8	E947.8	E950.4	E962.0	E980.4
pesticide	985.8	E863.4	—	E950.6	E962.1	E980.7
rodenticide	985.8	E863.7	—	E950.6	E962.1	E980.7
Barrier cream	976.3	E858.7	E946.3	E950.4	E962.0	E980.4
Battery acid or fluid	983.1	E864.1	—	E950.7	E962.1	E980.6
Bay rum	980.8	E860.8	—	E950.9	E962.1	E980.9
BCG vaccine	978.0	E858.8	E948.0	E950.4	E962.0	E980.4
Bearsfoot	988.2	E865.4	—	E950.9	E962.1	E980.9
Beclamide	966.3	E855.0	E936.3	E950.4	E962.0	E980.4
Bee (sting) (venom)	989.5	E905.3	—	E950.9	E962.1	E980.9
Belladonna (alkaloids)	971.1	E855.4	E941.1	E950.4	E962.0	E980.4
Bemegride	970.0	E854.3	E940.0	E950.4	E962.0	E980.4
Benactyzine	969.8	E855.8	E939.8	E950.3	E962.0	E980.3
Benadryl	963.0	E858.1	E933.0	E950.4	E962.0	E980.4
Bendrofluazide	974.3	E858.5	E944.3	E950.4	E962.0	E980.4
Bendroflumethiazide	974.3	E858.5	E944.3	E950.4	E962.0	E980.4
Benemid	974.7	E858.5	E944.7	E950.4	E962.0	E980.4
Benethamine penicillin G	960.0	E856	E930.0	E950.4	E962.0	E980.4
Benisone	976.0	E858.7	E946.0	E950.4	E962.0	E980.4
Benoquin	976.8	E858.7	E946.8	E950.4	E962.0	E980.4
Benoxinate	968.5	E855.2	E938.5	E950.4	E962.0	E980.4
Bentonite	976.3	E858.7	E946.3	E950.4	E962.0	E980.4
Benzalkonium (chloride)	976.0	E858.7	E946.0	E950.4	E962.0	E980.4
ophthalmic preparation	976.5	E858.7	E946.5	E950.4	E962.0	E980.4
Benzamidosalicylate (calcium)	961.8	E857	E931.8	E950.4	E962.0	E980.4
Benzathine penicillin	960.0	E856	E930.0	E950.4	E962.0	E980.4
Benzcarbimine	963.1	E858.1	E933.1	E950.4	E962.0	E980.4
Benzedrex	971.2	E855.5	E941.2	E950.4	E962.0	E980.4
Benzedrine (amphetamine)	969.72	E854.2	E939.7	E950.3	E962.0	E980.3
Benzene (acetyl) (dimethyl) (methyl) (solvent) (vapor)	982.0	E862.4	—	E950.9	E962.1	E980.9
hexachloride (gamma) (insecticide) (vapor)	989.2	E863.0	—	E950.6	E962.1	E980.7
Benzethonium	976.0	E858.7	E946.0	E950.4	E962.0	E980.4
Benzhexol (chloride)	966.4	E855.0	E936.4	E950.4	E962.0	E980.4
Benzilonium	971.1	E855.4	E941.1	E950.4	E962.0	E980.4
Benzin(e) — *see* Ligroin						
Benziodarone	972.4	E858.3	E942.4	E950.4	E962.0	E980.4
Benzocaine	968.5	E855.2	E938.5	E950.4	E962.0	E980.4
Benzodiapin	969.4	E853.2	E939.4	E950.3	E962.0	E980.3
Benzodiazepines (tranquilizers) NEC	969.4	E853.2	E939.4	E950.3	E962.0	E980.3
Benzoic acid (with salicylic acid) (anti-infective)	976.0	E858.7	E946.0	E950.4	E962.0	E980.4
Benzoin	976.3	E858.7	E946.3	E950.4	E962.0	E980.4
Benzol (vapor)	982.0	E862.4	—	E950.9	E962.1	E980.9
Benzomorphan	965.09	E850.2	E935.2	E950.0	E962.0	E980.0
Benzonatate	975.4	E858.6	E945.4	E950.4	E962.0	E980.4
Benzothiadiazides	974.3	E858.5	E944.3	E950.4	E962.0	E980.4
Benzoylpas	961.8	E857	E931.8	E950.4	E962.0	E980.4
Benzperidol	969.5	E853.8	E939.5	E950.3	E962.0	E980.3
Benzphetamine	977.0	E858.8	E947.0	E950.4	E962.0	E980.4
Benzpyrinium	971.0	E855.3	E941.0	E950.4	E962.0	E980.4
Benzquinamide	963.0	E858.1	E933.0	E950.4	E962.0	E980.4
Benzthiazide	974.3	E858.5	E944.3	E950.4	E962.0	E980.4
Benztropine	971.1	E855.4	E941.1	E950.4	E962.0	E980.4
Benzyl						
acetate	982.8	E862.4	—	E950.9	E962.1	E980.9
benzoate (anti-infective)	976.0	E858.7	E946.0	E950.4	E962.0	E980.4
morphine	965.09	E850.2	E935.2	E950.0	E962.0	E980.0
penicillin	960.0	E856	E930.0	E950.4	E962.0	E980.4
Bephenium hydroxynapthoate	961.6	E857	E931.6	E950.4	E962.0	E980.4
Bergamot oil	989.89	E866.8	—	E950.9	E962.1	E980.9
Berries, poisonous	988.2	E865.3	—	E950.9	E962.1	E980.9
Beryllium (compounds) (fumes)	985.3	E866.4	—	E950.9	E962.1	E980.9
Beta-carotene	976.3	E858.7	E946.3	E950.4	E962.0	E980.4
Beta-Chlor	967.1	E852.0	E937.1	E950.2	E962.0	E980.2
Betamethasone	962.0	E858.0	E932.0	E950.4	E962.0	E980.4
topical	976.0	E858.7	E946.0	E950.4	E962.0	E980.4
Betazole	977.8	E858.8	E947.8	E950.4	E962.0	E980.4
Bethanechol	971.0	E855.3	E941.0	E950.4	E962.0	E980.4
Bethanidine	972.6	E858.3	E942.6	E950.4	E962.0	E980.4
Betula oil	976.3	E858.7	E946.3	E950.4	E962.0	E980.4
Bhang	969.6	E854.1	E939.6	E950.3	E962.0	E980.3
Bialamicol	961.5	E857	E931.5	E950.4	E962.0	E980.4
Bichloride of mercury — *see* Mercury, chloride						
Bichromates (calcium) (crystals) (potassium) (sodium)	983.9	E864.3	—	E950.7	E962.1	E980.6
fumes	987.8	E869.8	—	E952.8	E962.2	E982.8
Biguanide derivatives, oral	962.3	E858.0	E932.3	E950.4	E962.0	E980.4
Biligrafin	977.8	E858.8	E947.8	E950.4	E962.0	E980.4
Bilopaque	977.8	E858.8	E947.8	E950.4	E962.0	E980.4
Bioflavonoids	972.8	E858.3	E942.8	E950.4	E962.0	E980.4
Biological substance NEC	979.9	E858.8	E949.9	E950.4	E962.0	E980.4
Biperiden	966.4	E855.0	E936.4	E950.4	E962.0	E980.4
Bisacodyl	973.1	E858.4	E943.1	E950.4	E962.0	E980.4
Bishydroxycoumarin	964.2	E858.2	E934.2	E950.4	E962.0	E980.4

Nontherapeutic use substance

Subterms under main terms may continue to next column or page

	Poisoning	Accident	Therapeutic Use	Suicide Attempt	Assault	Undetermined
Bismarsen	961.1	E857	E931.1	E950.4	E962.0	E980.4
Bismuth (compounds)						
NEC	985.8	E866.4	—	E950.9	E962.1	E980.9
anti-infectives	961.2	E857	E931.2	E950.4	E962.0	E980.4
subcarbonate	973.5	E858.4	E943.5	E950.4	E962.0	E980.4
sulfarsphenamine	961.1	E857	E931.1	E950.4	E962.0	E980.4
Bisphosphonates						
intravenous	963.1	E858.1	E933.7	E950.4	E962.0	E980.4
oral	963.1	E858.1	E933.6	E950.4	E962.0	E980.4
Bithionol	961.6	E857	E931.6	E950.4	E962.0	E980.4
Bitter almond oil	989.0	E866.8	—	E950.9	E962.1	E980.9
Bittersweet	988.2	E865.4	—	E950.9	E962.1	E930.9
Black						
flag	989.4	E863.4	—	E950.6	E962.1	E980.7
henbane	988.2	E865.4	—	E950.9	E962.1	E980.9
leaf (40)	989.4	E863.4	—	E950.6	E962.1	E980.7
widow spider (bite)	989.5	E905.1	—	E950.9	E962.1	E980.9
antivenin	979.9	E858.8	E949.9	E950.4	E962.0	E980.4
Blast furnace gas (carbon monoxide from)	986	E868.8	—	E952.1	E962.2	E982.1
Bleaching solutions	983.9	E864.3	—	E950.7	E962.1	E980.6
Bleach NEC	983.9	E864.3	—	E950.7	E962.1	E980.6
Bleomycin (sulfate)	960.7	E856	E930.7	E950.4	E962.0	E980.4
Blockain	968.9	E855.2	E938.9	E950.4	E962.0	E980.4
infiltration (subcutaneous)	968.5	E855.2	E938.5	E950.4	E962.0	E980.4
nerve block (peripheral) (plexus)	968.6	E855.2	E938.6	E950.4	E962.0	E980.4
topical (surface)	968.5	E855.2	E938.5	E950.4	E962.0	E980.4
Blood (derivatives) (natural) (plasma) (whole)	964.7	E858.2	E934.7	E950.4	E962.0	E980.4
affecting agent	964.9	E858.2	E934.9	E950.4	E962.0	E980.4
specified NEC	964.8	E858.2	E934.8	E950.4	E962.0	E980.4
substitute (macromolecular)	964.8	E858.2	E934.8	E950.4	E962.0	E980.4
Blue velvet	965.09	E850.2	E935.2	E950.0	E962.0	E980.0
Bone meal	989.89	E866.5	—	E950.9	E962.1	E980.9
Bonine	963.0	E858.1	E933.0	E950.4	E962.0	E980.4
Boracic acid	976.0	E858.7	E946.0	E950.4	E962.0	E980.4
ENT agent	976.6	E858.7	E946.6	E950.4	E962.0	E980.4
ophthalmic preparation	976.5	E858.7	E946.5	E950.4	E962.0	E980.4
Borate (cleanser) (sodium)	989.6	E861.3	—	E950.9	E962.1	E980.9
Borax (cleanser)	989.6	E861.3	—	E950.9	E962.1	E980.9
Boric acid	976.0	E858.7	E946.0	E950.4	E962.0	E980.4
ENT agent	976.6	E858.7	E946.6	E950.4	E962.0	E980.4
ophthalmic preparation	976.5	E858.7	E946.5	E950.4	E962.0	E980.4
Boron hydride NEC	989.89	E866.8	—	E950.9	E962.1	E980.9
fumes or gas	987.8	E869.8	—	E952.8	E962.2	E982.8
Botox	975.3	E858.6	E945.3	E950.4	E962.0	E980.4
Brake fluid vapor	987.8	E869.8	—	E952.8	E962.2	E982.8
Brass (compounds) (fumes)	985.8	E866.4	—	E950.9	E962.1	E980.9
Brasso	981	E861.3	—	E950.9	E962.1	
Bretylium (tosylate)	972.6	E858.3	E942.6	E950.4	E962.0	E980.4
Brevital (sodium)	968.3	E855.1	E938.3	E950.4	E962.0	E980.4
British antilewisite	963.8	E858.1	E933.8	E950.4	E962.0	E980.4
Bromal (hydrate)	967.3	E852.2	E937.3	E950.2	E962.0	E980.2
Bromelains	963.4	E858.1	E933.4	E950.4	E962.0	E980.4
Bromides NEC	967.3	E852.2	E937.3	E950.2	E962.0	E980.2
Bromine (vapor)	987.8	E869.8	—	E952.8	E962.2	E982.8
compounds (medicinal)	967.3	E852.2	E937.3	E950.2	E962.0	E980.2
Bromisovalum	967.3	E852.2	E937.3	E950.2	E962.0	E980.2
Bromobenzyl cyanide	987.5	E869.3	—	E952.8	E962.2	E982.8
Bromodiphenhydramine	963.0	E858.1	E933.0	E950.4	E962.0	E980.4
Bromoform	967.3	E852.2	E937.3	E950.2	E962.0	E980.2
Bromophenol blue reagent	977.8	E858.8	E947.8	E950.4	E962.0	E980.4
Bromosalicylhydroxamic acid	961.8	E857	E931.8	E950.4	E962.0	E980.4
Bromo-seltzer	965.4	E850.4	E935.4	E950.0	E962.0	E980.0
Brompheniramine	963.0	E858.1	E933.0	E950.4	E962.0	E980.4
Bromural	967.3	E852.2	E937.3	E950.2	E962.0	E980.2
Brown spider (bite) (venom)	989.5	E905.1	—	E950.9	E962.1	E980.9
Brucia	988.2	E865.3	—	E950.9	E962.1	E980.9
Brucine	989.1	E863.7	—	E950.6	E962.1	E980.7
Brunswick green — *see* Copper						
Bruten — *see* Ibuprofen						
Bryonia (alba) (dioica)	988.2	E865.4	—	E950.9	E962.1	E980.9
Buclizine	969.5	E853.8	E939.5	E950.3	E962.0	E980.3
Bufferin	965.1	E850.3	E935.3	E950.0	E962.0	E980.0
Bufotenine	969.6	E854.1	E939.6	E950.3	E962.0	E980.3
Buphenine	971.2	E855.5	E941.2	E950.4	E962.0	E980.4
Bupivacaine	968.9	E855.2	E938.9	E950.4	E962.0	E980.4
infiltration (subcutaneous)	968.5	E855.2	E938.5	E950.4	E962.0	E980.4
nerve block (peripheral) (plexus)	968.6	E855.2	E938.6	E950.4	E962.0	E980.4
Busulfan	963.1	E858.1	E933.1	E950.4	E962.0	E980.4
Butabarbital (sodium)	967.0	E851	E937.0	E950.1	E962.0	E980.1
Butabarbitone	967.0	E851	E937.0	E950.1	E962.0	E980.1
Butabarpal	967.0	E851	E937.0	E950.1	E962.0	E980.1
Butacaine	968.5	E855.2	E938.5	E950.4	E962.0	E980.4
Butallylonal	967.0	E851	E937.0	E950.1	E962.0	E980.1
Butane (distributed in mobile container)	987.0	E868.0	—	E951.1	E962.2	E981.1
distributed through pipes	987.0	E867		E951.0	E962.2	E981.0
incomplete combustion of — see Carbon monoxide, butane						
Butanol	980.3	E860.4	—	E950.9	E962.1	E980.9
Butanone	982.8	E862.4	—	E950.9	E962.1	E980.9
Butaperazine	969.1	E853.0	E939.1	E950.3	E962.0	E980.3
Butazolidin	965.5	E850.5	E935.5	E950.0	E962.0	E980.0
Butethal	967.0	E851	E937.0	E950.1	E962.0	E980.1
Butethamate	971.1	E855.4	E941.1	E950.4	E962.0	E980.4
Buthalitone (sodium)	968.3	E855.1	E938.3	E950.4	E962.0	E980.4
Butisol (sodium)	967.0	E851	E937.0	E950.1	E962.0	E980.1
Butobarbital, butobarbitone	967.0	E851	E937.0	E950.1	E962.0	E980.1
Butriptyline	969.05	E854.0	E939.0	E950.3	E962.0	E980.3
Buttercups	988.2	E865.4	—	E950.9	E962.1	E980.9
Butter of antimony — *see* Antimony						
Butyl						
acetate (secondary)	982.8	E862.4	—	E950.9	E962.1	E980.9
alcohol	980.3	E860.4	—	E950.9	E962.1	E980.9
carbinol	980.8	E860.8	—	E950.9	E962.1	E980.9
carbitol	982.8	E862.4	—	E950.9	E962.1	E980.9
cellosolve	982.8	E862.4	—	E950.9	E962.1	E980.9
chloral (hydrate)	967.1	E852.0	E937.1	E950.2	E962.0	E980.2
formate	982.8	E862.4	—	E950.9	E962.1	E980.9
scopolammonium bromide	971.1	E855.4	E941.1	E950.4	E962.0	E980.4
Butyn	968.5	E855.2	E938.5	E950.4	E962.0	E980.4
Butyrophenone (-based tranquilizers)	969.2	E853.1	E939.2	E950.3	E962.0	E980.3
Cacodyl, cacodylic acid — *see* Arsenic						
Cactinomycin	960.7	E856	E930.7	E950.4	E962.0	E980.4
Cade oil	976.4	E858.7	E946.4	E950.4	E962.0	E980.4
Cadmium (chloride) (compounds) (dust) (fumes) (oxide)	985.5	E866.4	—	E950.9	E962.1	E980.9
sulfide (medicinal) NEC	976.4	E858.7	E946.4	E950.4	E962.0	E980.4
Caffeine	969.71	E854.2	E939.7	E950.3	E962.0	E980.3
Calabar bean	988.2	E865.4	—	E950.9	E962.1	E980.9
Caladium seguinium	988.2	E865.4	—	E950.9	E962.1	E980.9
Calamine (liniment) (lotion)	976.3	E858.7	E946.3	E950.4	E962.0	E980.4
Calciferol	963.5	E858.1	E933.5	E950.4	E962.0	E980.4
Calcium (salts) NEC	974.5	E858.5	E944.5	E950.4	E962.0	E980.4
acetylsalicylate	965.1	E850.3	E935.3	E950.0	E962.0	E980.0
benzamidosalicylate	961.8	E857	E931.8	E950.4	E962.0	E980.4
carbaspirin	965.1	E850.3	E935.3	E950.0	E962.0	E980.0
carbimide (citrated)	977.3	E858.8	E947.3	E950.4	E962.0	E980.4
carbonate (antacid)	973.0	E858.4	E943.0	E950.4	E962.0	E980.4
cyanide (citrated)	977.3	E858.8	E947.3	E950.4	E962.0	E980.4
dioctyl sulfosuccinate	973.2	E858.4	E943.2	E950.4	E962.0	E980.4
disodium edathamil	963.8	E858.1	E933.8	E950.4	E962.0	E980.4
disodium edetate	963.8	E858.1	E933.8	E950.4	E962.0	E980.4
EDTA	963.8	E858.1	E933.8	E950.4	E962.0	E980.4
hydrate, hydroxide	983.2	E864.2	—	E950.7	E962.1	E980.6
mandelate	961.9	E857	E931.9	E950.4	E962.0	E980.4
oxide	983.2	E864.2	—	E950.7	E962.1	E980.6
Calomel — *see* Mercury, chloride						
Caloric agents NEC	974.5	E858.5	E944.5	E950.4	E962.0	E980.4
Calusterone	963.1	E858.1	E933.1	E950.4	E962.0	E980.4
Camoquin	961.4	E857	E931.4	E950.4	E962.0	E980.4
Camphor (oil)	976.1	E858.7	E946.1	E950.4	E962.0	E980.4

	External Cause (E-Code)					
	Poisoning	Accident	Therapeutic Use	Suicide Attempt	Assault	Undeter- mined
Candeptin	976.0	E858.7	E946.0	E950.4	E962.0	E980.4
Candicidin	976.0	E858.7	E946.0	E950.4	E962.0	E980.4
Cannabinols	969.6	E854.1	E939.6	E950.3	E962.0	E980.3
Cannabis (derivatives) (indica) (sativa)	969.6	E854.1	E939.6	E950.3	E962.0	E980.3
Canned heat	980.1	E860.2	—	E950.9	E962.1	E980.9
Cantharides, cantharidin, cantharis	976.8	E858.7	E946.8	E950.4	E962.0	E980.4
Capillary agents	972.8	E858.3	E942.8	E950.4	E962.0	E980.4
Capreomycin	960.6	E856	E930.6	E950.4	E962.0	E980.4
Captodiame, captodi- amine	969.5	E853.8	E939.5	E950.3	E962.0	E980.3
Caramiphen (hydrochlo- ride)	971.1	E855.4	E941.1	E950.4	E962.0	E980.4
Carbachol	971.0	E855.3	E941.0	E950.4	E962.0	E980.4
Carbacrylamine resins	974.5	E858.5	E944.5	E950.4	E962.0	E980.4
Carbamate (sedative)	967.8	E852.8	E937.8	E950.2	E962.0	E980.2
herbicide	989.3	E863.5	—	E950.6	E962.1	E980.7
insecticide	989.3	E863.2	—	E950.6	E962.1	E980.7
Carbamazepine	966.3	E855.0	E936.3	E950.4	E962.0	E980.4
Carbamic esters	967.8	E852.8	E937.8	E950.2	E962.0	E980.2
Carbamide	974.4	E858.5	E944.4	E950.4	E962.0	E980.4
topical	976.8	E858.7	E946.8	E950.4	E962.0	E980.4
Carbamylcholine chlo- ride	971.0	E855.3	E941.0	E950.4	E962.0	E980.4
Carbarsone	961.1	E857	E931.1	E950.4	E962.0	E980.4
Carbaryl	989.3	E863.2	—	E950.6	E962.1	E980.7
Carbaspirin	965.1	E850.3	E935.3	E950.0	E962.0	E980.0
Carbazochrome	972.8	E858.3	E942.8	E950.4	E962.0	E980.4
Carbenicillin	960.0	E856	E930.0	E950.4	E962.0	E980.4
Carbenoxolone	973.8	E858.4	E943.8	E950.4	E962.0	E980.4
Carbetapentane	975.4	E858.6	E945.4	E950.4	E962.0	E980.4
Carbimazole	962.8	E858.0	E932.8	E950.4	E962.0	E980.4
Carbinol	980.1	E860.2	—	E950.9	E962.1	E980.9
Carbinoxamine	963.0	E858.1	E933.0	E950.4	E962.0	E980.4
Carbitol	982.8	E862.4	—	E950.9	E962.1	E980.9
Carbocaine	968.9	E855.2	E938.9	E950.4	E962.0	E980.4
infiltration (subcuta- neous)	968.5	E855.2	E938.5	E950.4	E962.0	E980.4
nerve block (peripheral) (plexus)	968.6	E855.2	E938.6	E950.4	E962.0	E980.4
topical (surface)	968.5	E855.2	E938.5	E950.4	E962.0	E980.4
Carbol-fuchsin solution	976.0	E858.7	E946.0	E950.4	E962.0	E980.4
Carbolic acid — see also Phe- nol)	983.0	E864.0	—	E950.7	E962.1	E980.6
Carbomycin	960.8	E856	E930.8	E950.4	E962.0	E980.4
Carbon						
bisulfide (liquid) (vapor)	982.2	E862.4	—	E950.9	E962.1	E980.9
dioxide (gas)	987.8	E869.8	—	E952.8	E962.2	E982.8
disulfide (liquid) (vapor)	982.2	E862.4	—	E950.9	E962.1	E980.9
monoxide (from incomplete combustion of) (in)						
NEC	986	E868.9	—	E952.1	E962.2	E982.1
blast furnace gas	986	E868.8	—	E952.1	E962.2	E982.1
butane (distributed in mo- bile container)	986	E868.0	—	E951.1	E962.2	E981.1
distributed through pipes	986	E867	—	E951.0	E962.2	E981.0
charcoal fumes	986	E868.3	—	E952.1	E962.2	E982.1
coal						
gas (piped)	986	E867	—	E951.0	E962.2	E981.0
solid (in domestic stoves, fireplaces)	986	E868.3	—	E952.1	E962.2	E982.1
coke (in domestic stoves, fireplaces)	986	E868.3	—	E952.1	E962.2	E982.1
exhaust gas (motor) not in transit	986	E868.2	—	E952.0	E962.2	E982.0
combustion engine, any not in watercraft	986	E868.2	—	E952.0	E962.2	E982.0
farm tractor, not in tran- sit	986	E868.2	—	E952.0	E962.2	E982.0
gas engine	986	E868.2	—	E952.0	E962.2	E982.0
motor pump	986	E868.2	—	E952.0	E962.2	E982.0
motor vehicle, not in tran- sit	986	E868.2	—	E952.0	E962.2	E982.0
fuel (in domestic use)	986	E868.3	—	E952.1	E962.2	E982.1
gas (piped)	986	E867	—	E951.0	E962.2	E981.0
in mobile container	986	E868.0	—	E951.1	E962.2	E981.1
utility	986	E868.1	—	E951.8	E962.2	E981.1
in mobile container	986	E868.0	—	E951.1	E962.2	E981.1
piped (natural)	986	E867	—	E951.0	E962.2	E981.0
illuminating gas	986	E868.1	—	E951.8	E962.2	E981.8

	External Cause (E-Code)					
	Poisoning	Accident	Therapeutic Use	Suicide Attempt	Assault	Undeter- mined
Carbon — continued						
monoxide — continued						
industrial fuels or gases, any	986	E868.8	—	E952.1	E962.2	E982.1
kerosene (in domestic stoves, fireplaces)	986	E868.3	—	E952.1	E962.2	E982.1
kiln gas or vapor	986	E868.8	—	E952.1	E962.2	E982.1
motor exhaust gas, not in transit	986	E868.2	—	E952.0	E962.2	E982.0
piped gas (manufactured) (natural)	986	E867	—	E951.0	E962.2	E981.0
producer gas	986	E868.8	—	E952.1	E962.2	E982.1
propane (distributed in mo- bile container)	986	E868.0	—	E951.1	E962.2	E981.1
distributed through pipes	986	E867	—	E951.0	E962.2	E981.0
specified source NEC	986	E868.8	—	E952.1	E962.2	E982.1
stove gas	986	E868.1	—	E951.8	E962.2	E981.8
piped	986	E867	—	E951.0	E962.2	E981.0
utility gas	986	E868.1	—	E951.8	E962.2	E981.8
piped	986	E867	—	E951.0	E962.2	E981.0
water gas	986	E868.1	—	E951.8	E962.2	E981.8
wood (in domestic stoves, fireplaces)	986	E868.3	—	E952.1	E962.2	E982.1
tetrachloride (vapor) NEC	987.8	E869.4	—	E952.8	E962.2	E982.8
liquid (cleansing agent)						
NEC	982.1	E861.3	—	E950.9	E962.1	E980.9
solvent	982.1	E862.4	—	E950.9	E962.1	E980.9
Carbonic acid (gas)	987.8	E869.8	—	E952.8	E962.2	E982.8
anhydrase inhibitors	974.2	E858.5	E944.2	E950.4	E962.0	E980.4
Carbowax	976.3	E858.7	E946.3	E950.4	E962.0	E980.4
Carbrital	967.0	E851	E937.0	E950.1	E962.0	E980.1
Carbromal (derivatives)	967.3	E852.2	E937.3	E950.2	E962.0	E980.2
Cardiac						
depressants	972.0	E858.3	E942.0	E950.4	E962.0	E980.4
rhythm regulators	972.0	E858.3	E942.0	E950.4	E962.0	E980.4
Cardiografin	977.8	E858.8	E947.8	E950.4	E962.0	E980.4
Cardio-green	977.8	E858.8	E947.8	E950.4	E962.0	E980.4
Cardiotonic glycosides	972.1	E858.3	E942.1	E950.4	E962.0	E980.4
Cardiovascular agents NEC	972.9	E858.3	E942.9	E950.4	E962.0	E980.4
Cardrase	974.2	E858.5	E944.2	E950.4	E962.0	E980.4
Carfusin	976.0	E858.7	E946.0	E950.4	E962.0	E980.4
Carisoprodol	968.0	E855.1	E938.0	E950.4	E962.0	E980.4
Carmustine	963.1	E858.1	E933.1	E950.4	E962.0	E980.4
Carotene	963.5	E858.1	E933.5	E950.4	E962.0	E980.4
Carphenazine (maleate)	969.1	E853.0	E939.1	E950.3	E962.0	E980.3
Carter's Little Pills	973.1	E858.4	E943.1	E950.4	E962.0	E980.4
Cascara (sagrada)	973.1	E858.4	E943.1	E950.4	E962.0	E980.4
Cassava	988.2	E865.4	—	E950.9	E962.1	E980.9
Castellani's paint	976.0	E858.7	E946.0	E950.4	E962.0	E980.4
Castor						
bean	988.2	E865.3	—	E950.9	E962.1	E980.9
oil	973.1	E858.4	E943.1	E950.4	E962.0	E980.4
Caterpillar (sting)	989.5	E905.5	—	E950.9	E962.1	E980.9
Catha (edulis)	970.89	E854.3	E940.8	E950.4	E962.0	E980.4
Cathartics NEC	973.3	E858.4	E943.3	E950.4	E962.0	E980.4
contact	973.1	E858.4	E943.1	E950.4	E962.0	E980.4
emollient	973.2	E858.4	E943.2	E950.4	E962.0	E980.4
intestinal irritants	973.1	E858.4	E943.1	E950.4	E962.0	E980.4
saline	973.3	E858.4	E943.3	E950.4	E962.0	E980.4
Cathomycin	960.8	E856	E930.8	E950.4	E962.0	E980.4
Caustic(s)	983.9	E864.4	—	E950.7	E962.1	E980.6
alkali	983.2	E864.2	—	E950.7	E962.1	E980.6
hydroxide	983.2	E864.2	—	E950.7	E962.1	E980.6
potash	983.2	E864.2	—	E950.7	E962.1	E980.6
soda	983.2	E864.2	—	E950.7	E962.1	E980.6
specified NEC	983.9	E864.3	—	E950.7	E962.1	E980.6
Ceepryn	976.0	E858.7	E946.0	E950.4	E962.0	E980.4
ENT agent	976.6	E858.7	E946.6	E950.4	E962.0	E980.4
lozenges	976.6	E858.7	E946.6	E950.4	E962.0	E980.4
Celestone	962.0	E858.0	E932.0	E950.4	E962.0	E980.4
topical	976.0	E858.7	E946.0	E950.4	E962.0	E980.4
Cellosolve	982.8	E862.4	—	E950.9	E962.1	E980.9
Cell stimulants and prolifer- ants	976.8	E858.7	E946.8	E950.4	E962.0	E980.4
Cellulose derivatives, cathar- tic	973.3	E858.4	E943.3	E950.4	E962.0	E980.4
nitrates (topical)	976.3	E858.7	E946.3	E950.4	E962.0	E980.4
Centipede (bite)	989.5	E905.4	—	E950.9	E962.1	E980.9
Central nervous system						
depressants	968.4	E855.1	E938.4	E950.4	E962.0	E980.4

Nontherapeutic use substance

Subterms under main terms may continue to next column or page

	External Cause (E-Code)					
	Poisoning	Accident	Therapeutic Use	Suicide Attempt	Assault	Undetermined
Central nervous system — *continued*						
depressants — *continued*						
anesthetic (general)						
NEC	968.4	E855.1	E938.4	E950.4	E962.0	E980.4
gases NEC	968.2	E855.1	E938.2	E950.4	E962.0	E980.4
intravenous	968.3	E855.1	E938.3	E950.4	E962.0	E980.4
barbiturates	967.0	E851	E937.0	E950.1	E962.0	E980.1
bromides	967.3	E852.2	E937.3	E950.2	E962.0	E980.2
cannabis sativa	969.6	E854.1	E939.6	E950.3	E962.0	E980.3
chloral hydrate	967.1	E852.0	E937.1	E950.2	E962.0	E980.2
hallucinogenics	969.6	E854.1	E939.6	E950.3	E962.0	E980.3
hypnotics	967.9	E852.9	E937.9	E950.2	E962.0	E980.2
specified NEC	967.8	E852.8	E937.8	E950.2	E962.0	E980.2
muscle relaxants	968.0	E855.1	E938.0	E950.4	E962.0	E980.4
paraldehyde	967.2	E852.1	E937.2	E950.2	E962.0	E980.2
sedatives	967.9	E852.9	E937.9	E950.2	E962.0	E980.2
mixed NEC	967.6	E852.5	E937.6	E950.2	E962.0	E980.2
specified NEC	967.8	E852.8	E937.8	E950.2	E962.0	E980.2
muscle-tone depressants	968.0	E855.1	E938.0	E950.4	E962.0	E980.4
stimulants	970.9	E854.3	E940.9	E950.4	E962.0	E980.4
amphetamines	969.72	E854.2	E939.7	E950.3	E962.0	E980.3
analeptics	970.0	E854.3	E940.0	E950.4	E962.0	E980.4
antidepressants	969.00	E854.0	E939.0	E950.3	E962.0	E980.3
opiate antagonists	970.1	E854.3	E940.1	E950.4	E962.0	E980.4
specified NEC	970.89	E854.3	E940.8	E950.4	E962.0	E980.4
Cephalexin	960.5	E856	E930.5	E950.4	E962.0	E980.4
Cephaloglycin	960.5	E856	E930.5	E950.4	E962.0	E980.4
Cephaloridine	960.5	E856	E930.5	E950.4	E962.0	E980.4
Cephalosporins NEC	960.5	E856	E930.5	E950.4	E962.0	E980.4
N (adicillin)	960.0	E856	E930.0	E950.4	E962.0	E980.4
Cephalothin (sodium)	960.5	E856	E930.5	E950.4	E962.0	E980.4
Cerbera (odallam)	988.2	E865.4	—	E950.9	E962.1	E980.9
Cerberin	972.1	E858.3	E942.1	E950.4	E962.0	E980.4
Cerebral stimulants	970.9	E854.3	E940.9	E950.4	E962.0	E980.4
psychotherapeutic	969.79	E854.2	E939.7	E950.3	E962.0	E980.3
specified NEC	970.89	E854.3	E940.8	E950.4	E962.0	E980.4
Cetalkonium (chloride)	976.0	E858.7	E946.0	E950.4	E962.0	E980.4
Cetoxime	963.0	E858.1	E933.0	E950.4	E962.0	E980.4
Cetrimide	976.2	E858.7	E946.2	E950.4	E962.0	E980.4
Cetylpyridinium	976.0	E858.7	E946.0	E950.4	E962.0	E980.4
ENT agent	976.6	E858.7	E946.6	E950.4	E962.0	E980.4
lozenges	976.6	E858.7	E946.6	E950.4	E962.0	E980.4
Cevadilla — *see* Sabadilla						
Cevitamic acid	963.5	E858.1	E933.5	E950.4	E962.0	E980.4
Chalk, precipitated	973.0	E858.4	E943.0	E950.4	E962.0	E980.4
Charcoal						
fumes (carbon monoxide)	986	E868.3	—	E952.1	E962.2	E982.1
industrial	986	E868.8	—	E952.1	E962.2	E982.1
medicinal (activated)	973.0	E858.4	E943.0	E950.4	E962.0	E980.4
Chelating agents NEC	977.2	E858.8	E947.2	E950.4	E962.0	E980.4
Chelidonium majus	988.2	E865.4	—	E950.9	E962.1	E980.9
Chemical substance	989.9	E866.9	—	E950.9	E962.1	E980.9
specified NEC	989.89	E866.8	—	E950.9	E962.1	E980.9
Chemotherapy, antineoplastic	963.1	E858.1	E933.1	E950.4	E962.0	E980.4
Chenopodium (oil)	961.6	E857	E931.6	E950.4	E962.0	E980.4
Cherry laurel	988.2	E865.4	—	E950.9	E962.1	E980.9
Chiniofon	961.3	E857	E931.3	E950.4	E962.0	E980.4
Chlophedianol	975.4	E858.6	E945.4	E950.4	E962.0	E980.4
Chloral (betaine) (formamide) (hydrate)	967.1	E852.0	E937.1	E950.2	E962.0	E980.2
Chloralamide	967.1	E852.0	E937.1	E950.2	E962.0	E980.2
Chlorambucil	963.1	E858.1	E933.1	E950.4	E962.0	E980.4
Chloramphenicol	960.2	E856	E930.2	E950.4	E962.0	E980.4
ENT agent	976.6	E858.7	E946.6	E950.4	E962.0	E980.4
ophthalmic preparation	976.5	E858.7	E946.5	E950.4	E962.0	E980.4
topical NEC	976.0	E858.7	E946.0	E950.4	E962.0	E980.4
Chlorate(s) (potassium) (sodium) NEC	983.9	E864.3	—	E950.7	E962.1	E980.6
herbicides	989.4	E863.5	—	E950.6	E962.1	E980.7
Chlorcylizine	963.0	E858.1	E933.0	E950.4	E962.0	E980.4
Chlordan(e) (dust)	989.2	E863.0	—	E950.6	E962.1	E980.7
Chlordantoin	976.0	E858.7	E946.0	E950.4	E962.0	E980.4
Chlordiazepoxide	969.4	E853.2	E939.4	E950.3	E962.0	E980.3
Chloresium	976.8	E858.7	E946.8	E950.4	E962.0	E980.4
Chlorethiazol	967.1	E852.0	E937.1	E950.2	E962.0	E980.2
Chlorethyl — *see* Ethyl, chloride						
Chloretone	967.1	E852.0	E937.1	E950.2	E962.0	E980.2
Chlorex	982.3	E862.4	—	E950.9	E962.1	E980.9

	External Cause (E-Code)					
	Poisoning	Accident	Therapeutic Use	Suicide Attempt	Assault	Undetermined
Chlorhexadol	967.1	E852.0	E937.1	E950.2	E962.0	E980.2
Chlorhexidine (hydrochloride)	976.0	E858.7	E946.0	E950.4	E962.0	E980.4
Chlorhydroxyquinolin	976.0	E858.7	E946.0	E950.4	E962.0	E980.4
Chloride of lime (bleach)	983.9	E864.3	—	E950.7	E962.1	E980.6
Chlorinated						
camphene	989.2	E863.0	—	E950.6	E962.1	E980.7
diphenyl	989.89	E866.8	—	E950.9	E962.1	E980.9
hydrocarbons NEC	989.2	E863.0	—	E950.6	E962.1	E980.7
solvent	982.3	E862.4	—	E950.9	E962.1	E980.9
lime (bleach)	983.9	E864.3	—	E950.7	E962.1	E980.6
naphthalene — *see* Naphthalene						
pesticides NEC	989.2	E863.0	—	E950.6	E962.1	E980.7
soda — *see* Sodium, hypochlorite						
Chlorine (fumes) (gas)	987.6	E869.8	—	E952.8	E962.2	E982.8
bleach	983.9	E864.3	—	E950.7	E962.1	E980.6
compounds NEC	983.9	E864.3	—	E950.7	E962.1	E980.6
disinfectant	983.9	E861.4	—	E950.7	E962.1	E980.6
releasing agents NEC	983.9	E864.3	—	E950.7	E962.1	E980.6
Chlorisondamine	972.3	E858.3	E942.3	E950.4	E962.0	E980.4
Chlormadinone	962.2	E858.0	E932.2	E950.4	E962.0	E980.4
Chlormerodrin	974.0	E858.5	E944.0	E950.4	E962.0	E980.4
Chlormethiazole	967.1	E852.0	E937.1	E950.2	E962.0	E980.2
Chlormethylenecycline	960.4	E856	E930.4	E950.4	E962.0	E980.4
Chlormezanone	969.5	E853.8	E939.5	E950.3	E962.0	E980.3
Chloroacetophenone	987.5	E869.3	—	E952.8	E962.2	E982.8
Chloroaniline	983.0	E864.0	—	E950.7	E962.1	E980.6
Chlorobenzene, chlorobenzol	982.0	E862.4	—	E950.9	E962.1	E980.9
Chlorobutanol	967.1	E852.0	E937.1	E950.2	E962.0	E980.2
Chlorodinitrobenzene	983.0	E864.0	—	E950.7	E962.1	E980.6
dust or vapor	987.8	E869.8	—	E952.8	E962.2	E982.8
Chloroethane — *see* Ethyl, chloride						
Chloroform (fumes) (vapor)	987.8	E869.8	—	E952.8	E962.2	E982.8
anesthetic (gas)	968.2	E855.1	E938.2	E950.4	E962.0	E980.4
liquid NEC	968.4	E855.1	E938.4	E950.4	E962.0	E980.4
solvent	982.3	E862.4	—	E950.9	E962.1	E980.9
Chloroguanide	961.4	E857	E931.4	E950.4	E962.0	E980.4
Chloromycetin	960.2	E856	E930.2	E950.4	E962.0	E980.4
ENT agent	976.6	E858.7	E946.6	E950.4	E962.0	E980.4
ophthalmic preparation	976.5	E858.7	E946.5	E950.4	E962.0	E980.4
otic solution	976.6	E858.7	E946.6	E950.4	E962.0	E980.4
topical NEC	976.0	E858.7	E946.0	E950.4	E962.0	E980.4
Chloronitrobenzene	983.0	E864.0	—	E950.7	E962.1	E980.6
dust or vapor	987.8	E869.8	—	E952.8	E962.2	E982.8
Chlorophenol	983.0	E864.0	—	E950.7	E962.1	E980.6
Chlorophenothane	989.2	E863.0	—	E950.6	E962.1	E980.7
Chlorophyll (derivatives)	976.8	E858.7	E946.8	E950.4	E962.0	E980.4
Chloropicrin (fumes)	987.8	E869.8	—	E952.8	E962.2	E982.8
fumigant	989.4	E863.8	—	E950.6	E962.1	E980.7
fungicide	989.4	E863.6	—	E950.6	E962.1	E980.7
pesticide (fumes)	989.4	E863.4	—	E950.6	E962.1	E980.7
Chloroprocaine	968.9	E855.2	E938.9	E950.4	E962.0	E980.4
infiltration (subcutaneous)	968.5	E855.2	E938.5	E950.4	E962.0	E980.4
nerve block (peripheral) (plexus)	968.6	E855.2	E938.6	E950.4	E962.0	E980.4
Chloroptic	976.5	E858.7	E946.5	E950.4	E962.0	E980.4
Chloropurine	963.1	E858.1	E933.1	E950.4	E962.0	E980.4
Chloroquine (hydrochloride) (phosphate)	961.4	E857	E931.4	E950.4	E962.0	E980.4
Chlorothen	963.0	E858.1	E933.0	E950.4	E962.0	E980.4
Chlorothiazide	974.3	E858.5	E944.3	E950.4	E962.0	E980.4
Chlorotrianisene	962.2	E858.0	E932.2	E950.4	E962.0	E980.4
Chlorovinyldichloroarsine	985.1	E866.3	—	E950.8	E962.1	E980.8
Chloroxylenol	976.0	E858.7	E946.0	E950.4	E962.0	E980.4
Chlorphenesin (carbamate)	968.0	E855.1	E938.0	E950.4	E962.0	E980.4
topical (antifungal)	976.0	E858.7	E946.0	E950.4	E962.0	E980.4
Chlorpheniramine	963.0	E858.1	E933.0	E950.4	E962.0	E980.4
Chlorphenoxamine	966.4	E855.0	E936.4	E950.4	E962.0	E980.4
Chlorphentermine	977.0	E858.8	E947.0	E950.4	E962.0	E980.4
Chlorproguanil	961.4	E857	E931.4	E950.4	E962.0	E980.4
Chlorpromazine	969.1	E853.0	E939.1	E950.3	E962.0	E980.3
Chlorpropamide	962.3	E858.0	E932.3	E950.4	E962.0	E980.4
Chlorprothixene	969.3	E853.8	E939.3	E950.3	E962.0	E980.3
Chlorquinaldol	976.0	E858.7	E946.0	E950.4	E962.0	E980.4

	External Cause (E-Code)					
	Poisoning	Accident	Therapeutic Use	Suicide Attempt	Assault	Undetermined
Chlortetracycline	960.4	E856	E930.4	E950.4	E962.0	E980.4
Chlorthalidone	974.4	E858.5	E944.4	E950.4	E962.0	E980.4
Chlortrianisene	962.2	E858.0	E932.2	E950.4	E962.0	E980.4
Chlor-Trimeton	963.0	E858.1	E933.0	E950.4	E962.0	E980.4
Chlorzoxazone	968.0	E855.1	E938.0	E950.4	E962.0	E980.4
Choke damp	987.8	E869.8	—	E952.8	E962.2	E982.8
Cholebrine	977.8	E858.8	E947.8	E950.4	E962.0	E980.4
Cholera vaccine	978.2	E858.8	E948.2	E950.4	E962.0	E980.4
Cholesterol-lowering agents	972.2	E858.3	E942.2	E950.4	E962.0	E980.4
Cholestyramine (resin)	972.2	E858.3	E942.2	E950.4	E962.0	E980.4
Cholic acid	973.4	E858.4	E943.4	E950.4	E962.0	E980.4
Choline						
dihydrogen citrate	977.1	E858.8	E947.1	E950.4	E962.0	E980.4
salicylate	965.1	E850.3	E935.3	E950.0	E962.0	E980.0
theophyllinate	974.1	E858.5	E944.1	E950.4	E962.0	E980.4
Cholinergics	971.0	E855.3	E941.0	E950.4	E962.0	E980.4
Cholografin	977.8	E858.8	E947.8	E950.4	E962.0	E980.4
Chorionic gonadotropin	962.4	E858.0	E932.4	E950.4	E962.0	E980.4
Chromates	983.9	E864.3	—	E950.7	E962.1	E980.6
dust or mist	987.8	E869.8	—	E952.8	E962.2	E982.8
lead	984.0	E866.0	—	E950.9	E962.1	E980.9
paint	984.0	E861.5	—	E950.9	E962.1	E980.9
Chromic acid	983.9	E864.3	—	E950.7	E962.1	E980.6
dust or mist	987.8	E869.8	—	E952.8	E962.2	E982.8
Chromium	985.6	E866.4	—	E950.9	E962.1	E980.9
compounds — see Chromates						
Chromonar	972.4	E858.3	E942.4	E950.4	E962.0	E980.4
Chromyl chloride	983.9	E864.3	—	E950.7	E962.1	E980.6
Chrysarobin (ointment)	976.4	E858.7	E946.4	E950.4	E962.0	E980.4
Chrysazin	973.1	E858.4	E943.1	E950.4	E962.0	E980.4
Chymar	963.4	E858.1	E933.4	E950.4	E962.0	E980.4
ophthalmic preparation	976.5	E858.7	E946.5	E950.4	E962.0	E980.4
Chymotrypsin	963.4	E858.1	E933.4	E950.4	E962.0	E980.4
ophthalmic preparation	976.5	E858.7	E946.5	E950.4	E962.0	E980.4
Cicuta maculata or virosa	988.2	E865.4	—	E950.9	E962.1	E980.9
Cigarette lighter fluid	981	E862.1	—	E950.9	E962.1	E980.9
Cinchocaine (spinal)	968.7	E855.2	E938.7	E950.4	E962.0	E980.4
topical (surface)	968.5	E855.2	E938.5	E950.4	E962.0	E980.4
Cinchona	961.4	E857	E931.4	E950.4	E962.0	E980.4
Cinchonine alkaloids	961.4	E857	E931.4	E950.4	E962.0	E980.4
Cinchophen	974.7	E858.5	E944.7	E950.4	E962.0	E980.4
Cinnarizine	963.0	E858.1	E933.0	E950.4	E962.0	E980.4
Citanest	968.9	E855.2	E938.9	E950.4	E962.0	E980.4
infiltration (subcutaneous)	968.5	E855.2	E938.5	E950.4	E962.0	E980.4
nerve block (peripheral) (plexus)	968.6	E855.2	E938.6	E950.4	E962.0	E980.4
Citric acid	989.89	E866.8	—	E950.9	E962.1	E980.9
Citrovorum factor	964.1	E858.2	E934.1	E950.4	E962.0	E980.4
Claviceps purpurea	988.2	E865.4	—	E950.9	E962.1	E980.9
Cleaner, cleansing agent, type not specified	989.89	E861.9	—	E950.9	E962.1	E980.9
of paint or varnish	982.8	E862.9	—	E950.9	E962.1	E980.9
specified type NEC	989.89	E861.3	—	E950.9	E962.1	E980.9
Clematis vitalba	988.2	E865.4	—	E950.9	E962.1	E980.9
Clemizole	963.0	E858.1	E933.0	E950.4	E962.0	E980.4
penicillin	960.0	E856	E930.0	E950.4	E962.0	E980.4
Clidinium	971.1	E855.4	E941.1	E950.4	E962.0	E980.4
Clindamycin	960.8	E856	E930.8	E950.4	E962.0	E980.4
Cliradon	965.09	E850.2	E935.2	E950.0	E962.0	E980.0
Clocortolone	962.0	E858.0	E932.0	E950.4	E962.0	E980.4
Clofedanol	975.4	E858.6	E945.4	E950.4	E962.0	E980.4
Clofibrate	972.2	E858.3	E942.2	E950.4	E962.0	E980.4
Clomethiazole	967.1	E852.0	E937.1	E950.2	E962.0	E980.2
Clomiphene	977.8	E858.8	E947.8	E950.4	E962.0	E980.4
Clonazepam	969.4	E853.2	E939.4	E950.3	E962.0	E980.3
Clonidine	972.6	E858.3	E942.6	E950.4	E962.0	E980.4
Clopamide	974.3	E858.5	E944.3	E950.4	E962.0	E980.4
Clorazepate	969.4	E853.2	E939.4	E950.3	E962.0	E980.3
Clorexolone	974.4	E858.5	E944.4	E950.4	E962.0	E980.4
Clorox (bleach)	983.9	E864.3	—	E950.7	E962.1	E980.6
Clortermine	977.0	E858.8	E947.0	E950.4	E962.0	E980.4
Clotrimazole	976.0	E858.7	E946.0	E950.4	E962.0	E980.4
Cloxacillin	960.0	E856	E930.0	E950.4	E962.0	E980.4
Coagulants NEC	964.5	E858.2	E934.5	E950.4	E962.0	E980.4
Coal (carbon monoxide from) — see also Carbon, monoxide, coal						
oil — see Kerosene						
Coal — see also Carbon, monoxide, coal — continued						
tar NEC	983.0	E864.0	—	E950.7	E962.1	E980.6
fumes	987.8	E869.8	—	E952.8	E962.2	E982.8
medicinal (ointment)	976.4	E858.7	E946.4	E950.4	E962.0	E980.4
analgesics NEC	965.5	E850.7	E935.5	E950.0	E962.0	E980.0
naphtha (solvent)	981	E862.0	—	E950.9	E962.1	E980.9
Cobalt (fumes) (industrial)	985.8	E866.4	—	E950.9	E962.1	E980.9
Cobra (venom)	989.5	E905.0	—	E950.9	E962.1	E980.9
Coca (leaf)	970.81	E854.3	E940.8	E950.4	E962.0	E980.4
Cocaine (hydrochloride) (salt)	970.81	E854.3	E940.8	E950.4	E962.0	E980.4
topical anesthetic	968.5	E855.2	E938.5	E950.4	E962.0	E980.4
Coccidioidin	977.8	E858.8	E947.8	E950.4	E962.0	E980.4
Cocculus indicus	988.2	E865.3	—	E950.9	E962.1	E980.9
Cochineal	989.89	E866.8	—	E950.9	E962.1	E980.9
medicinal products	977.4	E858.8	E947.4	E950.4	E962.0	E980.4
Codeine	965.09	E850.2	E935.2	E950.0	E962.0	E980.0
Coffee	989.89	E866.8	—	E950.9	E962.1	E980.9
Cogentin	971.1	E855.4	E941.1	E950.4	E962.0	E980.4
Coke fumes or gas (carbon monoxide)	986	E868.3	—	E952.1	E962.2	E982.1
industrial use	986	E868.8	—	E952.1	E962.2	E982.1
Colace	973.2	E858.4	E943.2	E950.4	E962.0	E980.4
Colchicine	974.7	E858.5	E944.7	E950.4	E962.0	E980.4
Colchicum	988.2	E865.3	—	E950.9	E962.1	E980.9
Cold cream	976.3	E858.7	E946.3	E950.4	E962.0	E980.4
Colestipol	972.2	E858.3	E942.2	E950.4	E962.0	E980.4
Colistimethate	960.8	E856	E930.8	E950.4	E962.0	E980.4
Colistin	960.8	E856	E930.8	E950.4	E962.0	E980.4
Collagen	977.8	E866.8	E947.8	E950.9	E962.1	E980.9
Collagenase	976.8	E858.7	E946.8	E950.4	E962.0	E980.4
Collodion (flexible)	976.3	E858.7	E946.3	E950.4	E962.0	E980.4
Colocynth	973.1	E858.4	E943.1	E950.4	E962.0	E980.4
Coloring matter — see Dye(s)						
Combustion gas — see Carbon, monoxide						
Compazine	969.1	E853.0	E939.1	E950.3	E962.0	E980.3
Compound						
42 (warfarin)	989.4	E863.7	—	E950.6	E962.1	E980.7
269 (endrin)	989.2	E863.0	—	E950.6	E962.1	E980.7
497 (dieldrin)	989.2	E863.0	—	E950.6	E962.1	E980.7
1080 (sodium fluoroacetate)	989.4	E863.7	—	E950.6	E962.1	E980.7
3422 (parathion)	989.3	E863.1	—	E950.6	E962.1	E980.7
3911 (phorate)	989.3	E863.1	—	E950.6	E962.1	E980.7
3956 (toxaphene)	989.2	E863.0	—	E950.6	E962.1	E980.7
4049 (malathion)	989.3	E863.1	—	E950.6	E962.1	E980.7
4124 (dicapthon)	989.4	E863.4	—	E950.6	E962.1	E980.7
E (cortisone)	962.0	E858.0	E932.0	E950.4	E962.0	E980.4
F (hydrocortisone)	962.0	E858.0	E932.0	E950.4	E962.0	E980.4
Congo red	977.8	E858.8	E947.8	E950.4	E962.0	E980.4
Coniine, conine	965.7	E850.7	E935.7	E950.0	E962.0	E980.0
Conium (maculatum)	988.2	E865.4	—	E950.9	E962.1	E980.9
Conjugated estrogens (equine)	962.2	E858.0	E932.2	E950.4	E962.0	E980.4
Contac	975.6	E858.6	E945.6	E950.4	E962.0	E980.4
Contact lens solution	976.5	E858.7	E946.5	E950.4	E962.0	E980.4
Contraceptives (oral)	962.2	E858.0	E932.2	E950.4	E962.0	E980.4
vaginal	976.8	E858.7	E946.8	E950.4	E962.0	E980.4
Contrast media (roentgenographic)	977.8	E858.8	E947.8	E950.4	E962.0	E980.4
Convallaria majalis	988.2	E865.4	—	E950.9	E962.1	E980.9
Copperhead snake (bite) (venom)	989.5	E905.0	—	E950.9	E962.1	E980.9
Copper (dust) (fumes) (salts) NEC	985.8	E866.4	—	E950.9	E962.1	E980.9
arsenate, arsenite	985.1	E866.3	—	E950.8	E962.1	E980.8
insecticide	985.1	E863.4	—	E950.8	E962.1	E980.8
emetic	973.6	E858.4	E943.6	E950.4	E962.0	E980.4
fungicide	985.8	E863.6	—	E950.6	E962.1	E980.7
insecticide	985.8	E863.4	—	E950.6	E962.1	E980.7
oleate	976.0	E858.7	E946.0	E950.4	E962.0	E980.4
sulfate	983.9	E864.3	—	E950.7	E962.1	E980.6
cupric	973.6	E858.4	E943.6	E950.4	E962.0	E980.4
cuprous	983.9	E864.3	—	E950.7	E962.1	E980.6
fungicide	983.9	E863.6	—	E950.7	E962.1	E980.6
Coral (sting)	989.5	E905.6	—	E950.9	E962.1	E980.9
snake (bite) (venom)	989.5	E905.0	—	E950.9	E962.1	E980.9
Cordran	976.0	E858.7	E946.0	E950.4	E962.0	E980.4
Corn cures	976.4	E858.7	E946.4	E950.4	E962.0	E980.4
Cornhusker's lotion	976.3	E858.7	E946.3	E950.4	E962.0	E980.4

▽ Subterms under main terms may continue to next column or page

	Poisoning	Accident	Therapeutic Use	Suicide Attempt	Assault	Undeter-mined
Corn starch	976.3	E858.7	E946.3	E950.4	E962.0	E980.4
Corrosive	983.9	E864.4	—	E950.7	E962.1	E980.6
acids NEC	983.1	E864.1	—	E950.7	E962.1	E980.6
aromatics	983.0	E864.0	—	E950.7	E962.1	E980.6
disinfectant	983.0	E861.4	—	E950.7	E962.1	E980.6
fumes NEC	987.9	E869.9	—	E952.9	E962.2	E982.9
specified NEC	983.9	E864.3	—	E950.7	E962.1	E980.6
sublimate — see Mercury, chloride						
Cortate	962.0	E858.0	E932.0	E950.4	E962.0	E980.4
Cort-Dome	962.0	E858.0	E932.0	E950.4	E962.0	E980.4
ENT agent	976.6	E858.7	E946.6	E950.4	E962.0	E980.4
ophthalmic preparation	976.5	E858.7	E946.5	E950.4	E962.0	E980.4
topical NEC	976.0	E858.7	E946.0	E950.4	E962.0	E980.4
Cortef	962.0	E858.0	E932.0	E950.4	E962.0	E980.4
ENT agent	976.6	E858.7	E946.6	E950.4	E962.0	E980.4
ophthalmic preparation	976.5	E858.7	E946.5	E950.4	E962.0	E980.4
topical NEC	976.0	E858.7	E946.0	E950.4	E962.0	E980.4
Corticosteroids (fluorinat-ed)	962.0	E858.0	E932.0	E950.4	E962.0	E980.4
ENT agent	976.6	E858.7	E946.6	E950.4	E962.0	E980.4
ophthalmic preparation	976.5	E858.7	E946.5	E950.4	E962.0	E980.4
topical NEC	976.0	E858.7	E946.0	E950.4	E962.0	E980.4
Corticotropin	962.4	E858.0	E932.4	E950.4	E962.0	E980.4
Cortisol	962.0	E858.0	E932.0	E950.4	E962.0	E980.4
ENT agent	976.6	E858.7	E946.6	E950.4	E962.0	E980.4
ophthalmic preparation	976.5	E858.7	E946.5	E950.4	E962.0	E980.4
topical NEC	976.0	E858.7	E946.0	E950.4	E962.0	E980.4
Cortisone derivatives (ac-etate)	962.0	E858.0	E932.0	E950.4	E962.0	E980.4
ENT agent	976.6	E858.7	E946.6	E950.4	E962.0	E980.4
ophthalmic preparation	976.5	E858.7	E946.5	E950.4	E962.0	E980.4
topical NEC	976.0	E858.7	E946.0	E950.4	E962.0	E980.4
Cortogen	962.0	E858.0	E932.0	E950.4	E962.0	E980.4
ENT agent	976.6	E858.7	E946.6	E950.4	E962.0	E980.4
ophthalmic preparation	976.5	E858.7	E946.5	E950.4	E962.0	E980.4
Cortone	962.0	E858.0	E932.0	E950.4	E962.0	E980.4
ENT agent	976.6	E858.7	E946.6	E950.4	E962.0	E980.4
ophthalmic preparation	976.5	E858.7	E946.5	E950.4	E962.0	E980.4
Cortril	962.0	E858.0	E932.0	E950.4	E962.0	E980.4
ENT agent	976.6	E858.7	E946.6	E950.4	E962.0	E980.4
ophthalmic preparation	976.5	E858.7	E946.5	E950.4	E962.0	E980.4
topical NEC	976.0	E858.7	E946.0	E950.4	E962.0	E980.4
Cosmetics	989.89	E866.7	—	E950.9	E962.1	E980.9
Cosyntropin	977.8	E858.8	E947.8	E950.4	E962.0	E980.4
Cotarnine	964.5	E858.2	E934.5	E950.4	E962.0	E980.4
Cottonseed oil	976.3	E858.7	E946.3	E950.4	E962.0	E980.4
Cough mixtures (antitus-sives)	975.4	E858.6	E945.4	E950.4	E962.0	E980.4
containing opiates	965.09	E850.2	E935.2	E950.0	E962.0	E980.0
expectorants	975.5	E858.6	E945.5	E950.4	E962.0	E980.4
Coumadin	964.2	E858.2	E934.2	E950.4	E962.0	E980.4
rodenticide	989.4	E863.7	—	E950.6	E962.1	E980.7
Coumarin	964.2	E858.2	E934.2	E950.4	E962.0	E980.4
Coumetarol	964.2	E858.2	E934.2	E950.4	E962.0	E980.4
Cowbane	988.2	E865.4	—	E950.9	E962.1	E980.9
Cozyme	963.5	E858.1	E933.5	E950.4	E962.0	E980.4
Crack	970.81	E854.3	E940.8	E950.4	E962.0	E980.4
Creolin	983.0	E864.0	—	E950.7	E962.1	E980.6
disinfectant	983.0	E861.4	—	E950.7	E962.1	E980.6
Creosol (compound)	983.0	E864.0	—	E950.7	E962.1	E980.6
Creosote (beechwood) (coal tar)	983.0	E864.0	—	E950.7	E962.1	E980.6
medicinal (expectorant)	975.5	E858.6	E945.5	E950.4	E962.0	E980.4
syrup	975.5	E858.6	E945.5	E950.4	E962.0	E980.4
Cresol	983.0	E864.0	—	E950.7	E962.1	E980.6
disinfectant	983.0	E861.4	—	E950.7	E962.1	E980.6
Cresylic acid	983.0	E864.0	—	E950.7	E962.1	E980.6
Cropropamide	965.7	E850.7	E935.7	E950.0	E962.0	E980.0
with crotethamide	970.0	E854.3	E940.0	E950.4	E962.0	E980.4
Crotamiton	976.0	E858.7	E946.0	E950.4	E962.0	E980.4
Crotethamide	965.7	E850.7	E935.7	E950.0	E962.0	E980.0
with cropropamide	970.0	E854.3	E940.0	E950.4	E962.0	E980.4
Croton (oil)	973.1	E858.4	E943.1	E950.4	E962.0	E980.4
chloral	967.1	E852.0	E937.1	E950.2	E962.0	E980.2
Crude oil	981	E862.1	—	E950.9	E962.1	E980.9
Cryogenine	965.8	E850.8	E935.8	E950.0	E962.0	E980.0
Cryolite (pesticide)	989.4	E863.4	—	E950.6	E962.1	E980.7
Cryptenamine	972.6	E858.3	E942.6	E950.4	E962.0	E980.4
Crystal violet	976.0	E858.7	E946.0	E950.4	E962.0	E980.4
Cuckoopint	988.2	E865.4	—	E950.9	E962.1	E980.9
Cumetharol	964.2	E858.2	E934.2	E950.4	E962.0	E980.4

	Poisoning	Accident	Therapeutic Use	Suicide Attempt	Assault	Undeter-mined
Cupric sulfate	973.6	E858.4	E943.6	E950.4	E962.0	E980.4
Cuprous sulfate	983.9	E864.3	—	E950.7	E962.1	E980.6
Curare, curarine	975.2	E858.6	E945.2	E950.4	E962.0	E980.4
Cyanic acid — see Cyanide(s)						
Cyanide(s) (compounds) (hy-drogen) (potassium) (sodi-um) NEC	989.0	E866.8	—	E950.9	E962.1	E980.9
dust or gas (inhalation) NEC	987.7	E869.8	—	E952.8	E962.2	E982.8
fumigant	989.0	E863.8	—	E950.6	E962.1	E980.7
mercuric — see Mercury						
pesticide (dust) (fumes)	989.0	E863.4	—	E950.6	E962.1	E980.7
Cyanocobalamin	964.1	E858.2	E934.1	E950.4	E962.0	E980.4
Cyanogen (chloride) (gas) NEC	987.8	E869.8	—	E952.8	E962.2	E982.8
Cyclaine	968.5	E855.2	E938.5	E950.4	E962.0	E980.4
Cyclamen europaeum	988.2	E865.4	—	E950.9	E962.1	E980.9
Cyclandelate	972.5	E858.3	E942.5	E950.4	E962.0	E980.4
Cyclazocine	965.09	E850.2	E935.2	E950.0	E962.0	E980.0
Cyclizine	963.0	E858.1	E933.0	E950.4	E962.0	E980.4
Cyclobarbital, cyclobarbi-tone	967.0	E851	E937.0	E950.1	E962.0	E980.1
Cycloguanil	961.4	E857	E931.4	E950.4	E962.0	E980.4
Cyclohexane	982.0	E862.4	—	E950.9	E962.1	E980.9
Cyclohexanol	980.8	E860.8	—	E950.9	E962.1	E980.9
Cyclohexanone	982.8	E862.4	—	E950.9	E962.1	E980.9
Cyclomethycaine	968.5	E855.2	E938.5	E950.4	E962.0	E980.4
Cyclopentamine	971.2	E855.5	E941.2	E950.4	E962.0	E980.4
Cyclopenthiazide	974.3	E858.5	E944.3	E950.4	E962.0	E980.4
Cyclopentolate	971.1	E855.4	E941.1	E950.4	E962.0	E980.4
Cyclophosphamide	963.1	E858.1	E933.1	E950.4	E962.0	E980.4
Cyclopropane	968.2	E855.1	E938.2	E950.4	E962.0	E980.4
Cycloserine	960.6	E856	E930.6	E950.4	E962.0	E980.4
Cyclothiazide	974.3	E858.5	E944.3	E950.4	E962.0	E980.4
Cycrimine	966.4	E855.0	E936.4	E950.4	E962.0	E980.4
Cymarin	972.1	E858.3	E942.1	E950.4	E962.0	E980.4
Cyproheptadine	963.0	E858.1	E933.0	E950.4	E962.0	E980.4
Cyprolidol	969.09	E854.0	E939.0	E950.3	E962.0	E980.3
Cytarabine	963.1	E858.1	E933.1	E950.4	E962.0	E980.4
Cytisus						
laburnum	988.2	E865.4	—	E950.9	E962.1	E980.9
scoparius	988.2	E865.4	—	E950.9	E962.1	E980.9
Cytomel	962.7	E858.0	E932.7	E950.4	E962.0	E980.4
Cytosine (antineoplastic)	963.1	E858.1	E933.1	E950.4	E962.0	E980.4
Cytoxan	963.1	E858.1	E933.1	E950.4	E962.0	E980.4
Dacarbazine	963.1	E858.1	E933.1	E950.4	E962.0	E980.4
Dactinomycin	960.7	E856	E930.7	E950.4	E962.0	E980.4
DADPS	961.8	E857	E931.8	E950.4	E962.0	E980.4
Dakin's solution (exter-nal)	976.0	E858.7	E946.0	E950.4	E962.0	E980.4
Dalmane	969.4	E853.2	E939.4	E950.3	E962.0	E980.3
DAM	977.2	E858.8	E947.2	E950.4	E962.0	E980.4
Danilone	964.2	E858.2	E934.2	E950.4	E962.0	E980.4
Danthron	973.1	E858.4	E943.1	E950.4	E962.0	E980.4
Dantrolene	975.2	E858.6	E945.2	E950.4	E962.0	E980.4
Daphne (gnidium) (mez-ereum)	988.2	E865.4	—	E950.9	E962.1	E980.9
berry	988.2	E865.3	—	E950.9	E962.1	E980.9
Dapsone	961.8	E857	E931.8	E950.4	E962.0	E980.4
Daraprim	961.4	E857	E931.4	E950.4	E962.0	E980.4
Darnel	988.2	E865.3	—	E950.9	E962.1	E980.9
Darvon	965.8	E850.8	E935.8	E950.0	E962.0	E980.0
Daunorubicin	960.7	E856	E930.7	E950.4	E962.0	E980.4
DBI	962.3	E858.0	E932.3	E950.4	E962.0	E980.4
D-Con (rodenticide)	989.4	E863.7	—	E950.6	E962.1	E980.7
DDS	961.8	E857	E931.8	E950.4	E962.0	E980.4
DDT	989.2	E863.0	—	E950.6	E962.1	E980.7
Deadly nightshade	988.2	E865.4	—	E950.9	E962.1	E980.9
berry	988.2	E865.3	—	E950.9	E962.1	E980.9
Deanol	969.79	E854.2	E939.7	E950.3	E962.0	E980.3
Debrisoquine	972.6	E858.3	E942.6	E950.4	E962.0	E980.4
Decaborane	989.89	E866.8	—	E950.9	E962.1	E980.9
fumes	987.8	E869.8	—	E952.8	E962.2	E982.8
Decadron	962.0	E858.0	E932.0	E950.4	E962.0	E980.4
ENT agent	976.6	E858.7	E946.6	E950.4	E962.0	E980.4
ophthalmic preparation	976.5	E858.7	E946.5	E950.4	E962.0	E980.4
topical NEC	976.0	E858.7	E946.0	E950.4	E962.0	E980.4
Decahydronaphthalene	982.0	E862.4	—	E950.9	E962.1	E980.9
Decalin	982.0	E862.4	—	E950.9	E962.1	E980.9
Decamethonium	975.2	E858.6	E945.2	E950.4	E962.0	E980.4
Decholin	973.4	E858.4	E943.4	E950.4	E962.0	E980.4
sodium (diagnostic)	977.8	E858.8	E947.8	E950.4	E962.0	E980.4

	Poisoning	Accident	Therapeutic Use	Suicide Attempt	Assault	Undetermined
External Cause (E-Code)						
Declomycin	960.4	E856	E930.4	E950.4	E962.0	E980.4
Deferoxamine	963.8	E858.1	E933.8	E950.4	E962.0	E980.4
Dehydrocholic acid	973.4	E858.4	E943.4	E950.4	E962.0	E980.4
Dekalin	982.0	E862.4	—	E950.9	E962.1	E980.9
Delalutin	962.2	E858.0	E932.2	E950.4	E962.0	E980.4
Delphinium	988.2	E865.3	—	E950.9	E962.1	E980.9
Deltasone	962.0	E858.0	E932.0	E950.4	E962.0	E980.4
Deltra	962.0	E858.0	E932.0	E950.4	E962.0	E980.4
Delvinal	967.0	E851	E937.0	E950.1	E962.0	E980.1
Demecarium (bromide)	971.0	E855.3	E941.0	E950.4	E962.0	E980.4
Demeclocycline	960.4	E856	E930.4	E950.4	E962.0	E980.4
Demecolcine	963.1	E858.1	E933.1	E950.4	E962.0	E980.4
Demelanizing agents	976.8	E858.7	E946.8	E950.4	E962.0	E980.4
Demerol	965.09	E850.2	E935.2	E950.0	E962.0	E980.0
Demethylchlortetracy-cline	960.4	E856	E930.4	E950.4	E962.0	E980.4
Demethyltetracycline	960.4	E856	E930.4	E950.4	E962.0	E980.4
Demeton	989.3	E863.1	—	E950.6	E962.1	E980.7
Demulcents	976.3	E858.7	E946.3	E950.4	E962.0	E980.4
Demulen	962.2	E858.0	E932.2	E950.4	E962.0	E980.4
Denatured alcohol	980.0	E860.1	—	E950.9	E962.1	E980.9
Dendrid	976.5	E858.7	E946.5	E950.4	E962.0	E980.4
Dental agents, topical	976.7	E858.7	E946.7	E950.4	E962.0	E980.4
Deodorant spray (feminine hygiene)	976.8	E858.7	E946.8	E950.4	E962.0	E980.4
Deoxyribonuclease	963.4	E858.1	E933.4	E950.4	E962.0	E980.4
Depressants						
appetite, central	977.0	E858.8	E947.0	E950.4	E962.0	E980.4
cardiac	972.0	E858.3	E942.0	E950.4	E962.0	E980.4
central nervous system (anesthetic)	968.4	E855.1	E938.4	E950.4	E962.0	E980.4
psychotherapeutic	969.5	E853.9	E939.5	E950.3	E962.0	E980.3
Dequalinium	976.0	E858.7	E946.0	E950.4	E962.0	E980.4
Dermolate	976.2	E858.7	E946.2	E950.4	E962.0	E980.4
DES	962.2	E858.0	E932.2	E950.4	E962.0	E980.4
Desenex	976.0	E858.7	E946.0	E950.4	E962.0	E980.4
Deserpidine	972.6	E858.3	E942.6	E950.4	E962.0	E980.4
Desipramine	969.05	E854.0	E939.0	E950.3	E962.0	E980.3
Deslanoside	972.1	E858.3	E942.1	E950.4	E962.0	E980.4
Desocodeine	965.09	E850.2	E935.2	E950.0	E962.0	E980.0
Desomorphine	965.09	E850.2	E935.2	E950.0	E962.0	E980.0
Desonide	976.0	E858.7	E946.0	E950.4	E962.0	E980.4
Desoxycorticosterone derivatives	962.0	E858.0	E932.0	E950.4	E962.0	E980.4
Desoxyephedrine	969.72	E854.2	E939.7	E950.3	E962.0	E980.3
DET	969.6	E854.1	E939.6	E950.3	E962.0	E980.3
Detergents (ingested) (synthetic)	989.6	E861.0	—	E950.9	E962.1	E980.9
ENT agent	976.6	E858.7	E946.6	E950.4	E962.0	E980.4
external medication	976.2	E858.7	E946.2	E950.4	E962.0	E980.4
ophthalmic preparation	976.5	E858.7	E946.5	E950.4	E962.0	E980.4
topical NEC	976.0	E858.7	E946.0	E950.4	E962.0	E980.4
Deterrent, alcohol	977.3	E858.8	E947.3	E950.4	E962.0	E980.4
Detrothyronine	962.7	E858.0	E932.7	E950.4	E962.0	E980.4
Dettol (external medication)	976.0	E858.7	E946.0	E950.4	E962.0	E980.4
Dexamethasone	962.0	E858.0	E932.0	E950.4	E962.0	E980.4
Dexamphetamine	969.72	E854.2	E939.7	E950.3	E962.0	E980.3
Dexedrine	969.72	E854.2	E939.7	E950.3	E962.0	E980.3
Dexpanthenol	963.5	E858.1	E933.5	E950.4	E962.0	E980.4
Dextran	964.8	E858.2	E934.8	E950.4	E962.0	E980.4
Dextriferron	964.0	E858.2	E934.0	E950.4	E962.0	E980.4
Dextroamphetamine	969.72	E854.2	E939.7	E950.3	E962.0	E980.3
Dextro calcium pantothenate	963.5	E858.1	E933.5	E950.4	E962.0	E980.4
Dextromethorphan	975.4	E858.6	E945.4	E950.4	E962.0	E980.4
Dextromoramide	965.09	E850.2	E935.2	E950.0	E962.0	E980.0
Dextro pantothenyl alcohol	963.5	E858.1	E933.5	E950.4	E962.0	E980.4
topical	976.8	E858.7	E946.8	E950.4	E962.0	E980.4
Dextropropoxyphene (hydrochloride)	965.8	E850.8	E935.8	E950.0	E962.0	E980.0
Dextrorphan	965.09	E850.2	E935.2	E950.0	E962.0	E980.0
Dextrose NEC	974.5	E858.5	E944.5	E950.4	E962.0	E980.4
Dextrothyroxin	962.7	E858.0	E932.7	E950.4	E962.0	E980.4
DFP	971.0	E855.3	E941.0	E950.4	E962.0	E980.4
DHE-45	972.9	E858.3	E942.9	E950.4	E962.0	E980.4
Diabinese	962.3	E858.0	E932.3	E950.4	E962.0	E980.4
Diacetyl monoxime	977.2	E858.8	E947.2	E950.4	E962.0	E980.4
Diacetylmorphine	965.01	E850.0	E935.0	E950.0	E962.0	E980.0
Diagnostic agents	977.8	E858.8	E947.8	E950.4	E962.0	E980.4
Dial (soap)	976.2	E858.7	E946.2	E950.4	E962.0	E980.4

	Poisoning	Accident	Therapeutic Use	Suicide Attempt	Assault	Undetermined
External Cause (E-Code)						
Dial — *continued*						
sedative	967.0	E851	E937.0	E950.1	E962.0	E980.1
Diallylbarbituric acid	967.0	E851	E937.0	E950.1	E962.0	E980.1
Diaminodiphenylsulfone	961.8	E857	E931.8	E950.4	E962.0	E980.4
Diamorphine	965.01	E850.0	E935.0	E950.0	E962.0	E980.0
Diamox	974.2	E858.5	E944.2	E950.4	E962.0	E980.4
Diamthazole	976.0	E858.7	E946.0	E950.4	E962.0	E980.4
Diaphenylsulfone	961.8	E857	E931.8	E950.4	E962.0	E980.4
Diasone (sodium)	961.8	E857	E931.8	E950.4	E962.0	E980.4
Diazepam	969.4	E853.2	E939.4	E950.3	E962.0	E980.3
Diazinon	989.3	E863.1	—	E950.6	E962.1	E980.7
Diazomethane (gas)	987.8	E869.8	—	E952.8	E962.2	E982.8
Diazoxide	972.5	E858.3	E942.5	E950.4	E962.0	E980.4
Dibenamine	971.3	E855.6	E941.3	E950.4	E962.0	E980.4
Dibenzheptropine	963.0	E858.1	E933.0	E950.4	E962.0	E980.4
Dibenzyline	971.3	E855.6	E941.3	E950.4	E962.0	E980.4
Diborane (gas)	987.8	E869.8	—	E952.8	E962.2	E982.8
Dibromomannitol	963.1	E858.1	E933.1	E950.4	E962.0	E980.4
Dibucaine (spinal)	968.7	E855.2	E938.7	E950.4	E962.0	E980.4
topical (surface)	968.5	E855.2	E938.5	E950.4	E962.0	E980.4
Dibunate sodium	975.4	E858.6	E945.4	E950.4	E962.0	E980.4
Dibutoline	971.1	E855.4	E941.1	E950.4	E962.0	E980.4
Dicapthon	989.4	E863.4	—	E950.6	E962.1	E980.7
Dichloralphenazone	967.1	E852.0	E937.1	E950.2	E962.0	E980.2
Dichlorodifluoromethane	987.4	E869.2	—	E952.8	E962.2	E982.8
Dichloroethane	982.3	E862.4	—	E950.9	E962.1	E980.9
Dichloroethylene	982.3	E862.4	—	E950.9	E962.1	E980.9
Dichloroethyl sulfide	987.8	E869.8	—	E952.8	E962.2	E982.8
Dichlorohydrin	982.3	E862.4	—	E950.9	E962.1	E980.9
Dichloromethane (solvent) (vapor)	982.3	E862.4	—	E950.9	E962.1	E980.9
Dichlorophen(e)	961.6	E857	E931.6	E950.4	E962.0	E980.4
Dichlorphenamide	974.2	E858.5	E944.2	E950.4	E962.0	E980.4
Dichlorvos	989.3	E863.1	—	E950.6	E962.1	E980.7
Diclofenac sodium	965.69	E850.6	E935.6	E950.0	E962.0	E980.0
Dicoumarin, dicumarol	964.2	E858.2	E934.2	E950.4	E962.0	E980.4
Dicyanogen (gas)	987.8	E869.8	—	E952.8	E962.2	E982.8
Dicyclomine	971.1	E855.4	E941.1	E950.4	E962.0	E980.4
Dieldrin (vapor)	989.2	E863.0	—	E950.6	E962.1	E980.7
Dienestrol	962.2	E858.0	E932.2	E950.4	E962.0	E980.4
Dietetics	977.0	E858.8	E947.0	E950.4	E962.0	E980.4
Diethazine	966.4	E855.0	E936.4	E950.4	E962.0	E980.4
Diethyl						
barbituric acid	967.0	E851	E937.0	E950.1	E962.0	E980.1
carbamazine	961.6	E857	E931.6	E950.4	E962.0	E980.4
carbinol	980.8	E860.8	—	E950.9	E962.1	E980.9
carbonate	982.8	E862.4	—	E950.9	E962.1	E980.9
dioxide	982.8	E862.4	—	E950.9	E962.1	E980.9
ether (vapor) — see Ether(s)						
glycol (monoacetate) (monoethyl ether)	982.8	E862.4	—	E950.9	E962.1	E980.9
propion	977.0	E858.8	E947.0	E950.4	E962.0	E980.4
stilbestrol	962.2	E858.0	E932.2	E950.4	E962.0	E980.4
Diethylene						
dioxide	982.8	E862.4	—	E950.9	E962.1	E980.9
glycol (monoacetate) (monoethyl ether)	982.8	E862.4	—	E950.9	E962.1	E980.9
Diethylsulfone-diethylmethane	967.8	E852.8	E937.8	E950.2	E962.0	E980.2
Difencloxazine	965.09	E850.2	E935.2	E950.0	E962.0	E980.0
Diffusin	963.4	E858.1	E933.4	E950.4	E962.0	E980.4
Diflos	971.0	E855.3	E941.0	E950.4	E962.0	E980.4
Digestants	973.4	E858.4	E943.4	E950.4	E962.0	E980.4
Digitalin(e)	972.1	E858.3	E942.1	E950.4	E962.0	E980.4
Digitalis glycosides	972.1	E858.3	E942.1	E950.4	E962.0	E980.4
Digitoxin	972.1	E858.3	E942.1	E950.4	E962.0	E980.4
Digoxin	972.1	E858.3	E942.1	E950.4	E962.0	E980.4
Dihydrocodeine	965.09	E850.2	E935.2	E950.0	E962.0	E980.0
Dihydrocodeinone	965.09	E850.2	E935.2	E950.0	E962.0	E980.0
Dihydroergocristine	972.9	E858.3	E942.9	E950.4	E962.0	E980.4
Dihydroergotamine	972.9	E858.3	E942.9	E950.4	E962.0	E980.4
Dihydroergotoxine	972.9	E858.3	E942.9	E950.4	E962.0	E980.4
Dihydrohydroxycodeinone	965.09	E850.2	E935.2	E950.0	E962.0	E980.0
Dihydrohydroxymorphinone	965.09	E850.2	E935.2	E950.0	E962.0	E980.0
Dihydroisocodeine	965.09	E850.2	E935.2	E950.0	E962.0	E980.0
Dihydromorphine	965.09	E850.2	E935.2	E950.0	E962.0	E980.0
Dihydromorphinone	965.09	E850.2	E935.2	E950.0	E962.0	E980.0
Dihydrostreptomycin	960.6	E856	E930.6	E950.4	E962.0	E980.4
Dihydrotachysterol	962.6	E858.0	E932.6	E950.4	E962.0	E980.4

Nontherapeutic use substance

▽ Subterms under main terms may continue to next column or page

	Poisoning	Accident	Therapeutic Use	Suicide Attempt	Assault	Undetermined
External Cause (E-Code)						
Dihydroxyan-thraquinone	973.1	E858.4	E943.1	E950.4	E962.0	E980.4
Dihydroxycodeinone	965.09	E850.2	E935.2	E950.0	E962.0	E980.0
Diiodohydroxyquin	961.3	E857	E931.3	E950.4	E962.0	E980.4
topical	976.0	E858.7	E946.0	E950.4	E962.0	E980.4
Diiodohydroxyquinoline	961.3	E857	E931.3	E950.4	E962.0	E980.4
Dilantin	966.1	E855.0	E936.1	E950.4	E962.0	E980.4
Dilaudid	965.09	E850.2	E935.2	E950.0	E962.0	E980.0
Diloxanide	961.5	E857	E931.5	E950.4	E962.0	E980.4
Dimefline	970.0	E854.3	E940.0	E950.4	E962.0	E980.4
Dimenhydrinate	963.0	E858.1	E933.0	E950.4	E962.0	E980.4
Dimercaprol	963.8	E858.1	E933.8	E950.4	E962.0	E980.4
Dimercaptopropanol	963.8	E858.1	E933.8	E950.4	E962.0	E980.4
Dimetane	963.0	E858.1	E933.0	E950.4	E962.0	E980.4
Dimethicone	976.3	E858.7	E946.3	E950.4	E962.0	E980.4
Dimethindene	963.0	E858.1	E933.0	E950.4	E962.0	E980.4
Dimethisoquin	968.5	E855.2	E938.5	E950.4	E962.0	E980.4
Dimethisterone	962.2	E858.0	E932.2	E950.4	E962.0	E980.4
Dimethoxanate	975.4	E858.6	E945.4	E950.4	E962.0	E980.4
Dimethyl						
arsine, arsinic acid — see Arsenic						
carbinol	980.2	E860.3	—	E950.9	E962.1	E980.9
diguanide	962.3	E858.0	E932.3	E950.4	E962.0	E980.4
ketone	982.8	E862.4	—	E950.9	E962.1	E980.9
vapor	987.8	E869.8	—	E952.8	E962.2	E982.8
meperidine	965.09	E850.2	E935.2	E950.0	E962.0	E980.0
parathion	989.3	E863.1	—	E950.6	E962.1	E980.7
polysiloxane	973.8	E858.4	E943.8	E950.4	E962.0	E980.4
sulfate (fumes)	987.8	E869.8	—	E952.8	E962.2	E982.8
liquid	983.9	E864.3	—	E950.7	E962.1	E980.6
sulfoxide NEC	982.8	E862.4	—	E950.9	E962.1	E980.9
medicinal	976.4	E858.7	E946.4	E950.4	E962.0	E980.4
triptamine	969.6	E854.1	E939.6	E950.3	E962.0	E980.3
tubocurarine	975.2	E858.6	E945.2	E950.4	E962.0	E980.4
Dindevan	964.2	E858.2	E934.2	E950.4	E962.0	E980.4
Dinitrobenzene	983.0	E864.0	—	E950.7	E962.1	E980.6
vapor	987.8	E869.8	—	E952.8	E962.2	E982.8
Dinitro (-ortho-) cresol (herbicide) (spray)	989.4	E863.5	—	E950.6	E962.1	E980.7
insecticide	989.4	E863.4	—	E950.6	E962.1	E980.7
Dinitro-orthocresol (herbicide)	989.4	E863.5	—	E950.6	E962.1	E980.7
insecticide	989.4	E863.4	—	E950.6	E962.1	E980.7
Dinitrophenol (herbicide) (spray)	989.4	E863.5	—	E950.6	E962.1	E980.7
insecticide	989.4	E863.4	—	E950.6	E962.1	E980.7
Dinoprost	975.0	E858.6	E945.0	E950.4	E962.0	E980.4
Dioctyl sulfosuccinate (calcium) (sodium)	973.2	E858.4	E943.2	E950.4	E962.0	E980.4
Diodoquin	961.3	E857	E931.3	E950.4	E962.0	E980.4
Dione derivatives NEC	966.3	E855.0	E936.3	E950.4	E962.0	E980.4
Dionin	965.09	E850.2	E935.2	E950.0	E962.0	E980.0
Dioxane	982.8	E862.4		E950.9	E962.1	E980.9
Dioxin — see Herbicide						
Dioxyline	972.5	E858.3	E942.5	E950.4	E962.0	E980.4
Dipentene	982.8	E862.4	—	E950.9	E962.1	E980.9
Diphemanil	971.1	E855.4	E941.1	E950.4	E962.0	E980.4
Diphenadione	964.2	E858.2	E934.2	E950.4	E962.0	E980.4
Diphenhydramine	963.0	E858.1	E933.0	E950.4	E962.0	E980.4
Diphenidol	963.0	E858.1	E933.0	E950.4	E962.0	E980.4
Diphenoxylate	973.5	E858.4	E943.5	E950.4	E962.0	E980.4
Diphenylchloroarsine	985.1	E866.3	—	E950.8	E962.1	E980.8
Diphenylhydantoin (sodium)	966.1	E855.0	E936.1	E950.4	E962.0	E980.4
Diphenylpyraline	963.0	E858.1	E933.0	E950.4	E962.0	E980.4
Diphtheria						
antitoxin	979.9	E858.8	E949.9	E950.4	E962.0	E980.4
toxoid	978.5	E858.8	E948.5	E950.4	E962.0	E980.4
with tetanus toxoid	978.9	E858.8	E948.9	E950.4	E962.0	E980.4
with pertussis component	978.6	E858.8	E948.6	E950.4	E962.0	E980.4
vaccine	978.5	E858.8	E948.5	E950.4	E962.0	E980.4
Dipipanone	965.09	E850.2	E935.2	E950.0	E962.0	E980.0
Diplovax	979.5	E858.8	E949.5	E950.4	E962.0	E980.4
Diprophylline	975.1	E858.6	E945.1	E950.4	E962.0	E980.4
Dipyridamole	972.4	E858.3	E942.4	E950.4	E962.0	E980.4
Dipyrone	965.5	E850.5	E935.5	E950.0	E962.0	E980.0
Diquat	989.4	E863.5	—	E950.6	E962.1	E980.7
Disinfectant NEC	983.9	E861.4	—	E950.7	E962.1	E980.6
alkaline	983.2	E861.4	—	E950.7	E962.1	E980.6
aromatic	983.0	E861.4	—	E950.7	E962.1	E980.6

	Poisoning	Accident	Therapeutic Use	Suicide Attempt	Assault	Undetermined
External Cause (E-Code)						
Disipal	966.4	E855.0	E936.4	E950.4	E962.0	E980.4
Disodium edetate	963.8	E858.1	E933.8	E950.4	E962.0	E980.4
Disulfamide	974.4	E858.5	E944.4	E950.4	E962.0	E980.4
Disulfanilamide	961.0	E857	E931.0	E950.4	E962.0	E980.4
Disulfiram	977.3	E858.8	E947.3	E950.4	E962.0	E980.4
Dithiazanine	961.6	E857	E931.6	E950.4	E962.0	E980.4
Dithioglycerol	963.8	E858.1	E933.8	E950.4	E962.0	E980.4
Dithranol	976.4	E858.7	E946.4	E950.4	E962.0	E980.4
Diucardin	974.3	E858.5	E944.3	E950.4	E962.0	E980.4
Diupres	974.3	E858.5	E944.3	E950.4	E962.0	E980.4
Diuretics NEC	974.4	E858.5	E944.4	E950.4	E962.0	E980.4
carbonic acid anhydrase inhibitors	974.2	E858.5	E944.2	E950.4	E962.0	E980.4
mercurial	974.0	E858.5	E944.0	E950.4	E962.0	E980.4
osmotic	974.4	E858.5	E944.4	E950.4	E962.0	E980.4
purine derivatives	974.1	E858.5	E944.1	E950.4	E962.0	E980.4
saluretic	974.3	E858.5	E944.3	E950.4	E962.0	E980.4
Diuril	974.3	E858.5	E944.3	E950.4	E962.0	E980.4
Divinyl ether	968.2	E855.1	E938.2	E950.4	E962.0	E980.4
D-lysergic acid diethylamide	969.6	E854.1	E939.6	E950.3	E962.0	E980.3
DMCT	960.4	E856	E930.4	E950.4	E962.0	E980.4
DMSO	982.8	E862.4	—	E950.9	E962.1	E980.9
DMT	969.6	E854.1	E939.6	E950.3	E962.0	E980.3
DNOC	989.4	E863.5	—	E950.6	E962.1	E980.7
DOCA	962.0	E858.0	E932.0	E950.4	E962.0	E980.4
Dolophine	965.02	E850.1	E935.1	E950.0	E962.0	E980.0
Doloxene	965.8	E850.8	E935.8	E950.0	E962.0	E980.0
DOM	969.6	E854.1	E939.6	E950.3	E962.0	E980.3
Domestic gas — see Gas, utility						
Domiphen (bromide) (lozenges)	976.6	E858.7	E946.6	E950.4	E962.0	E980.4
Dopa (levo)	966.4	E855.0	E936.4	E950.4	E962.0	E980.4
Dopamine	971.2	E855.5	E941.2	E950.4	E962.0	E980.4
Doriden	967.5	E852.4	E937.5	E950.2	E962.0	E980.2
Dormiral	967.0	E851	E937.0	E950.1	E962.0	E980.1
Dormison	967.8	E852.8	E937.8	E950.2	E962.0	E980.2
Dornase	963.4	E858.1	E933.4	E950.4	E962.0	E980.4
Dorsacaine	968.5	E855.2	E938.5	E950.4	E962.0	E980.4
Dothiepin hydrochloride	969.05	E854.0	E939.0	E950.3	E962.0	E980.3
Doxapram	970.0	E854.3	E940.0	E950.4	E962.0	E980.4
Doxepin	969.05	E854.0	E939.0	E950.3	E962.0	E980.3
Doxorubicin	960.7	E856	E930.7	E950.4	E962.0	E980.4
Doxycycline	960.4	E856	E930.4	E950.4	E962.0	E980.4
Doxylamine	963.0	E858.1	E933.0	E950.4	E962.0	E980.4
Dramamine	963.0	E858.1	E933.0	E950.4	E962.0	E980.4
Drano (drain cleaner)	983.2	E864.2	—	E950.7	E962.1	E980.6
Dromoran	965.09	E850.2	E935.2	E950.0	E962.0	E980.0
Dromostanolone	962.1	E858.0	E932.1	E950.4	E962.0	E980.4
Droperidol	969.2	E853.1	E939.2	E950.3	E962.0	E980.3
Drotrecogin alfa	964.2	E858.2	E934.2	E950.4	E962.0	E980.4
Drug	977.9	E858.9	E947.9	E950.5	E962.0	E980.5
AHFS List						
4:00 antihistamine drugs	963.0	E858.1	E933.0	E950.4	E962.0	E980.4
8:04 amebacides	961.5	E857	E931.5	E950.4	E962.0	E980.4
arsenical anti-infectives	961.1	E857	E931.1	E950.4	E962.0	E980.4
quinoline derivatives	961.3	E857	E931.3	E950.4	E962.0	E980.4
8:08 anthelmintics	961.6	E857	E931.6	E950.4	E962.0	E980.4
quinoline derivatives	961.3	E857	E931.3	E950.4	E962.0	E980.4
8:12.04 antifungal antibiotics	960.1	E856	E930.1	E950.4	E962.0	E980.4
8:12.06 cephalosporins	960.5	E856	E930.5	E950.4	E962.0	E980.4
8:12.08 chloramphenicol	960.2	E856	E930.2	E950.4	E962.0	E980.4
8:12.12 erythromycins	960.3	E856	E930.3	E950.4	E962.0	E980.4
8:12.16 penicillins	960.0	E856	E930.0	E950.4	E962.0	E980.4
8:12.20 streptomycins	960.6	E856	E930.6	E950.4	E962.0	E980.4
8:12.24 tetracyclines	960.4	E856	E930.4	E950.4	E962.0	E980.4
8:12.28 other antibiotics	960.8	E856	E930.8	E950.4	E962.0	E980.4
antimycobacterial	960.6	E856	E930.6	E950.4	E962.0	E980.4
macrolides	960.3	E856	E930.3	E950.4	E962.0	E980.4
8:16 antituberculars	961.8	E857	E931.8	E950.4	E962.0	E980.4
antibiotics	960.6	E856	E930.6	E950.4	E962.0	E980.4
8:18 antivirals	961.7	E857	E931.7	E950.4	E962.0	E980.4
8:20 plasmodicides (antimalarials)	961.4	E857	E931.4	E950.4	E962.0	E980.4
8:24 sulfonamides	961.0	E857	E931.0	E950.4	E962.0	E980.4
8:26 sulfones	961.8	E857	E931.8	E950.4	E962.0	E980.4
8:28 treponemicides	961.2	E857	E931.2	E950.4	E962.0	E980.4
8:32 trichomonacides	961.5	E857	E931.5	E950.4	E962.0	E980.4
nitrofuran derivatives	961.9	E857	E931.9	E950.4	E962.0	E980.4
quinoline derivatives	961.3	E857	E931.3	E950.4	E962.0	E980.4

	External Cause (E-Code)					
Drug — *continued*	Poisoning	Accident	Therapeutic Use	Suicide Attempt	Assault	Undeter-mined
8:36 urinary germicides	961.9	E857	E931.9	E950.4	E962.0	E980.4
quinoline derivatives	961.3	E857	E931.3	E950.4	E962.0	E980.4
8:40 other anti-infectives	961.9	E857	E931.9	E950.4	E962.0	E980.4
10:00 antineoplastic agents	963.1	E858.1	E933.1	E950.4	E962.0	E980.4
antibiotics	960.7	E856	E930.7	E950.4	E962.0	E980.4
progestogens	962.2	E858.0	E932.2	E950.4	E962.0	E980.4
12:04 parasympathomimetic (cholinergic) agents	971.0	E855.3	E941.0	E950.4	E962.0	E980.4
12:08 parasympatholytic (cholinergic-blocking) agents	971.1	E855.4	E941.1	E950.4	E962.0	E980.4
12:12 Sympathomimetic (adrenergic) agents	971.2	E855.5	E941.2	E950.4	E962.0	E980.4
12:16 sympatholytic (adrenergic-blocking) agents	971.3	E855.6	E941.3	E950.4	E962.0	E980.4
12:20 skeletal muscle relaxants						
central nervous system muscle-tone depressants	968.0	E855.1	E938.0	E950.4	E962.0	E980.4
myoneural blocking agents	975.2	E858.6	E945.2	E950.4	E962.0	E980.4
16:00 blood derivatives	964.7	E858.2	E934.7	E950.4	E962.0	E980.4
20:04.04 iron preparations	964.0	E858.2	E934.0	E950.4	E962.0	E980.4
20:04.08 liver and stomach preparations	964.1	E858.2	E934.1	E950.4	E962.0	E980.4
20:04 antianemia drugs	964.1	E858.2	E934.1	E950.4	E962.0	E980.4
20:12.04 anticoagulants	964.2	E858.2	E934.2	E950.4	E962.0	E980.4
20:12.08 antiheparin agents	964.5	E858.2	E934.5	E950.4	E962.0	E980.4
20:12.12 coagulants	964.5	E858.2	E934.5	E950.4	E962.0	E980.4
20:12.16 hemostatics NEC	964.5	E858.2	E934.5	E950.4	E962.0	E980.4
capillary active drugs	972.8	E858.3	E942.8	E950.4	E962.0	E980.4
24:04 cardiac drugs	972.9	E858.3	E942.9	E950.4	E962.0	E980.4
cardiotonic agents	972.1	E858.3	E942.1	E950.4	E962.0	E980.4
rhythm regulators	972.0	E858.3	E942.0	E950.4	E962.0	E980.4
24:06 antilipemic agents	972.2	E858.3	E942.2	E950.4	E962.0	E980.4
thyroid derivatives	962.7	E858.0	E932.7	E950.4	E962.0	E980.4
24:08 hypotensive agents	972.6	E858.3	E942.6	E950.4	E962.0	E980.4
adrenergic blocking agents	971.3	E855.6	E941.3	E950.4	E962.0	E980.4
ganglion blocking agents	972.3	E858.3	E942.3	E950.4	E962.0	E980.4
vasodilators	972.5	E858.3	E942.5	E950.4	E962.0	E980.4
24:12 vasodilating agents NEC	972.5	E858.3	E942.5	E950.4	E962.0	E980.4
coronary	972.4	E858.3	E942.4	E950.4	E962.0	E980.4
nicotinic acid derivatives	972.2	E858.3	E942.2	E950.4	E962.0	E980.4
24:16 sclerosing agents	972.7	E858.3	E942.7	E950.4	E962.0	E980.4
28:04 general anesthetics	968.4	E855.1	E938.4	E950.4	E962.0	E980.4
gaseous anesthetics	968.2	E855.1	E938.2	E950.4	E962.0	E980.4
halothane	968.1	E855.1	E938.1	E950.4	E962.0	E980.4
intravenous anesthetics	968.3	E855.1	E938.3	E950.4	E962.0	E980.4
28:08 analgesics and antipyretics	965.9	E850.9	E935.9	E950.0	E962.0	E980.0
antirheumatics	965.69	E850.6	E935.6	E950.0	E962.0	E980.0
aromatic analgesics	965.4	E850.4	E935.4	E950.0	E962.0	E980.0
non-narcotic NEC	965.7	E850.7	E935.7	E950.0	E962.0	E980.0
opium alkaloids	965.00	E850.2	E935.2	E950.0	E962.0	E980.0
heroin	965.01	E850.0	E935.0	E950.0	E962.0	E980.0
methadone	965.02	E850.1	E935.1	E950.0	E962.0	E980.0
specified type NEC	965.09	E850.2	E935.2	E950.0	E962.0	E980.0
pyrazole derivatives	965.5	E850.5	E935.5	E950.0	E962.0	E980.0
salicylates	965.1	E850.3	E935.3	E950.0	E962.0	E980.0
specified NEC	965.8	E850.8	E935.8	E950.0	E962.0	E980.0
28:10 narcotic antagonists	970.1	E854.3	E940.1	E950.4	E962.0	E980.4
28:12 anticonvulsants	966.3	E855.0	E936.3	E950.4	E962.0	E980.4
barbiturates	967.0	E851	E937.0	E950.1	E962.0	E980.1
benzodiazepine-based tranquilizers	969.4	E853.2	E939.4	E950.3	E962.0	E980.3
bromides	967.3	E852.2	E937.3	E950.2	E962.0	E980.2
hydantoin derivatives	966.1	E855.0	E936.1	E950.4	E962.0	E980.4
oxazolidine (derivatives)	966.0	E855.0	E936.0	E950.4	E962.0	E980.4
succinimides	966.2	E855.0	E936.2	E950.4	E962.0	E980.4

	External Cause (E-Code)					
Drug — *continued*	Poisoning	Accident	Therapeutic Use	Suicide Attempt	Assault	Undeter-mined
28:16.04 antidepressants	969.00	E854.0	E939.0	E950.3	E962.0	E980.3
28:16.08 tranquilizers	969.5	E853.9	E939.5	E950.3	E962.0	E980.3
benzodiazepine-based	969.4	E853.2	E939.4	E950.3	E962.0	E980.3
butyrophenone-based	969.2	E853.1	E939.2	E950.3	E962.0	E980.3
major NEC	969.3	E853.8	E939.3	E950.3	E962.0	E980.3
phenothiazine-based	969.1	E853.0	E939.1	E950.3	E962.0	E980.3
28:16.12 other psychotherapeutic agents	969.8	E855.8	E939.8	E950.3	E962.0	E980.3
28:20 respiratory and cerebral stimulants	970.9	E854.3	E940.9	E950.4	E962.0	E980.4
analeptics	970.0	E854.3	E940.0	E950.4	E962.0	E980.4
anorexigenic agents	977.0	E858.8	E947.0	E950.4	E962.0	E980.4
psychostimulants	969.70	E854.2	E939.7	E950.3	E962.0	E980.3
specified NEC	970.89	E854.3	E940.8	E950.4	E962.0	E980.4
28:24 sedatives and hypnotics	967.9	E852.9	E937.9	E950.2	E962.0	E980.2
barbiturates	967.0	E851	E937.0	E950.1	E962.0	E980.1
benzodiazepine-based tranquilizers	969.4	E853.2	E939.4	E950.3	E962.0	E980.3
chloral hydrate (group)	967.1	E852.0	E937.1	E950.2	E962.0	E980.2
glutethamide group	967.5	E852.4	E937.5	E950.2	E962.0	E980.2
intravenous anesthetics	968.3	E855.1	E938.3	E950.4	E962.0	E980.4
methaqualone (compounds)	967.4	E852.3	E937.4	E950.2	E962.0	E980.2
paraldehyde	967.2	E852.1	E937.2	E950.2	E962.0	E980.2
phenothiazine-based tranquilizers	969.1	E853.0	E939.1	E950.3	E962.0	E980.3
specified NEC	967.8	E852.8	E937.8	E950.2	E962.0	E980.2
thiobarbiturates	968.3	E855.1	E938.3	E950.4	E962.0	E980.4
tranquilizer NEC	969.5	E853.9	E939.5	E950.3	E962.0	E980.3
36:04 to 36:88 diagnostic agents	977.8	E858.8	E947.8	E950.4	E962.0	E980.4
40:00 electrolyte, caloric, and water balance agents NEC	974.5	E858.5	E944.5	E950.4	E962.0	E980.4
40:04 acidifying agents	963.2	E858.1	E933.2	E950.4	E962.0	E980.4
40:08 alkalinizing agents	963.3	E858.1	E933.3	E950.4	E962.0	E980.4
40:10 ammonia detoxicants	974.5	E858.5	E944.5	E950.4	E962.0	E980.4
40:12 replacement solutions	974.5	E858.5	E944.5	E950.4	E962.0	E980.4
plasma expanders	964.8	E858.2	E934.8	E950.4	E962.0	E980.4
40:16 sodium-removing resins	974.5	E858.5	E944.5	E950.4	E962.0	E980.4
40:18 potassium-removing resins	974.5	E858.5	E944.5	E950.4	E962.0	E980.4
40:20 caloric agents	974.5	E858.5	E944.5	E950.4	E962.0	E980.4
40:24 salt and sugar substitutes	974.5	E858.5	E944.5	E950.4	E962.0	E980.4
40:28 diuretics NEC	974.4	E858.5	E944.4	E950.4	E962.0	E980.4
carbonic acid anhydrase inhibitors	974.2	E858.5	E944.2	E950.4	E962.0	E980.4
mercurials	974.0	E858.5	E944.0	E950.4	E962.0	E980.4
purine derivatives	974.1	E858.5	E944.1	E950.4	E962.0	E980.4
saluretics	974.3	E858.5	E944.3	E950.4	E962.0	E980.4
thiazides	974.3	E858.5	E944.3	E950.4	E962.0	E980.4
40:36 irrigating solutions	974.5	E858.5	E944.5	E950.4	E962.0	E980.4
40:40 uricosuric agents	974.7	E858.5	E944.7	E950.4	E962.0	E980.4
44:00 enzymes	963.4	E858.1	E933.4	E950.4	E962.0	E980.4
fibrinolysis-affecting agents	964.4	E858.2	E934.4	E950.4	E962.0	E980.4
gastric agents	973.4	E858.4	E943.4	E950.4	E962.0	E980.4
48:00 expectorants and cough preparations						
antihistamine agents	963.0	E858.1	E933.0	E950.4	E962.0	E980.4
antitussives	975.4	E858.6	E945.4	E950.4	E962.0	E980.4
codeine derivatives	965.09	E850.2	E935.2	E950.0	E962.0	E980.0
expectorants	975.5	E858.6	E945.5	E950.4	E962.0	E980.4
narcotic agents NEC	965.09	E850.2	E935.2	E950.0	E962.0	E980.0
52:04.04 antibiotics (EENT)						
ENT agent	976.6	E858.7	E946.6	E950.4	E962.0	E980.4
ophthalmic preparation	976.5	E858.7	E946.5	E950.4	E962.0	E980.4
52:04.06 antivirals (EENT)						
ENT agent	976.6	E858.7	E946.6	E950.4	E962.0	E980.4
ophthalmic preparation	976.5	E858.7	E946.5	E950.4	E962.0	E980.4
52:04.08 sulfonamides (EENT)						
ENT agent	976.6	E858.7	E946.6	E950.4	E962.0	E980.4
ophthalmic preparation	976.5	E858.7	E946.5	E950.4	E962.0	E980.4
52:04.12 miscellaneous anti-infectives (EENT)						
ENT agent	976.6	E858.7	E946.6	E950.4	E962.0	E980.4

Nontherapeutic use substance

▽ Subterms under main terms may continue to next column or page

Drug — Drug

	External Cause (E-Code)					
	Poisoning	Accident	Therapeutic Use	Suicide Attempt	Assault	Undeter-mined
Drug — *continued*						
52:04.12 miscellaneous anti-infectives — *continued*						
ophthalmic preparation	976.5	E858.7	E946.5	E950.4	E962.0	E980.4
52:04 anti-infectives (EENT)						
ENT agent	976.6	E858.7	E946.6	E950.4	E962.0	E980.4
ophthalmic preparation	976.5	E858.7	E946.5	E950.4	E962.0	E980.4
52:08 anti-inflammatory agents (EENT)						
ENT agent	976.6	E858.7	E946.6	E950.4	E962.0	E980.4
ophthalmic preparation	976.5	E858.7	E946.5	E950.4	E962.0	E980.4
52:10 carbonic anhydrase inhibitors	974.2	E858.5	E944.2	E950.4	E962.0	E980.4
52:12 contact lens solutions	976.5	E858.7	E946.5	E950.4	E962.0	E980.4
52:16 local anesthetics (EENT)	968.5	E855.2	E938.5	E950.4	E962.0	E980.4
52:20 miotics	971.0	E855.3	E941.0	E950.4	E962.0	E980.4
52:24 mydriatics						
adrenergics	971.2	E855.5	E941.2	E950.4	E962.0	E980.4
anticholinergics	971.1	E855.4	E941.1	E950.4	E962.0	E980.4
antimuscarinics	971.1	E855.4	E941.1	E950.4	E962.0	E980.4
parasympatholytics	971.1	E855.4	E941.1	E950.4	E962.0	E980.4
spasmolytics	971.1	E855.4	E941.1	E950.4	E962.0	E980.4
sympathomimetics	971.2	E855.5	E941.2	E950.4	E962.0	E980.4
52:28 mouth washes and gargles	976.6	E858.7	E946.6	E950.4	E962.0	E980.4
52:32 vasoconstrictors (EENT)	971.2	E855.5	E941.2	E950.4	E962.0	E980.4
52:36 unclassified agents (EENT)						
ENT agent	976.6	E858.7	E946.6	E950.4	E962.0	E980.4
ophthalmic preparation	976.5	E858.7	E946.5	E950.4	E962.0	E980.4
56:04 antacids and adsorbents	973.0	E858.4	E943.0	E950.4	E962.0	E980.4
56:08 antidiarrhea agents	973.5	E858.4	E943.5	E950.4	E962.0	E980.4
56:10 antiflatulents	973.8	E858.4	E943.8	E950.4	E962.0	E980.4
56:12 cathartics NEC	973.3	E858.4	E943.3	E950.4	E962.0	E980.4
emollients	973.2	E858.4	E943.2	E950.4	E962.0	E980.4
irritants	973.1	E858.4	E943.1	E950.4	E962.0	E980.4
56:16 digestants	973.4	E858.4	E943.4	E950.4	E962.0	E980.4
56:20 emetics and antiemetics						
antiemetics	963.0	E858.1	E933.0	E950.4	E962.0	E980.4
emetics	973.6	E858.4	E943.6	E950.4	E962.0	E980.4
56:24 lipotropic agents	977.1	E858.8	E947.1	E950.4	E962.0	E980.4
56:40 miscellaneous G.I. drugs	973.8	E858.4	E943.8	E950.4	E962.0	E980.4
60:00 gold compounds	965.69	E850.6	E935.6	E950.0	E962.0	E980.0
64:00 heavy metal antagonists	963.8	E858.1	E933.8	E950.4	E962.0	E980.4
68:04 adrenals	962.0	E858.0	E932.0	E950.4	E962.0	E980.4
68:08 androgens	962.1	E858.0	E932.1	E950.4	E962.0	E980.4
68:12 contraceptives, oral	962.2	E858.0	E932.2	E950.4	E962.0	E980.4
68:16 estrogens	962.2	E858.0	E932.2	E950.4	E962.0	E980.4
68:18 gonadotropins	962.4	E858.0	E932.4	E950.4	E962.0	E980.4
68:20.08 insulins	962.3	E858.0	E932.3	E950.4	E962.0	E980.4
68:20 insulins and antidiabetic agents	962.3	E858.0	E932.3	E950.4	E962.0	E980.4
68:24 parathyroid	962.6	E858.0	E932.6	E950.4	E962.0	E980.4
68:28 pituitary (posterior)	962.5	E858.0	E932.5	E950.4	E962.0	E980.4
anterior	962.4	E858.0	E932.4	E950.4	E962.0	E980.4
68:32 progestogens	962.2	E858.0	E932.2	E950.4	E962.0	E980.4
68:34 other corpus luteum hormones NEC	962.2	E858.0	E932.2	E950.4	E962.0	E980.4
68:36 thyroid and antithyroid						
antithyroid	962.8	E858.0	E932.8	E950.4	E962.0	E980.4
thyroid (derivatives)	962.7	E858.0	E932.7	E950.4	E962.0	E980.4
72:00 local anesthetics NEC	968.9	E855.2	E938.9	E950.4	E962.0	E980.4
infiltration (intradermal) (subcutaneous) (submucosal)	968.5	E855.2	E938.5	E950.4	E962.0	E980.4
nerve blocking (peripheral) (plexus) (regional)	968.6	E855.2	E938.6	E950.4	E962.0	E980.4
spinal	968.7	E855.2	E938.7	E950.4	E962.0	E980.4
topical (surface)	968.5	E855.2	E938.5	E950.4	E962.0	E980.4
76:00 oxytocics	975.0	E858.6	E945.0	E950.4	E962.0	E980.4
78:00 radioactive agents	990	—	—	—	—	—
80:04 serums NEC	979.9	E858.8	E949.9	E950.4	E962.0	E980.4

	External Cause (E-Code)					
	Poisoning	Accident	Therapeutic Use	Suicide Attempt	Assault	Undeter-mined
Drug — *continued*						
80:04 serums — *continued*						
immune gamma globulin (human)	964.6	E858.2	E934.6	E950.4	E962.0	E980.4
80:08 toxoids NEC	978.8	E858.8	E948.8	E950.4	E962.0	E980.4
diphtheria	978.5	E858.8	E948.5	E950.4	E962.0	E980.4
and diphtheria	978.9	E858.8	E948.9	E950.4	E962.0	E980.4
with pertussis component	978.6	E858.8	E948.6	E950.4	E962.0	E980.4
and tetanus	978.9	E858.8	E948.9	E950.4	E962.0	E980.4
with pertussis component	978.6	E858.8	E948.6	E950.4	E962.0	E980.4
tetanus	978.4	E858.8	E948.4	E950.4	E962.0	E980.4
80:12 vaccines	979.9	E858.8	E949.9	E950.4	E962.0	E980.4
bacterial NEC	978.8	E858.8	E948.8	E950.4	E962.0	E980.4
with						
other bacterial components	978.9	E858.8	E948.9	E950.4	E962.0	E980.4
pertussis component	978.6	E858.8	E948.6	E950.4	E962.0	E980.4
viral and rickettsial components	979.7	E858.8	E949.7	E950.4	E962.0	E980.4
rickettsial NEC	979.6	E858.8	E949.6	E950.4	E962.0	E980.4
with						
bacterial component	979.7	E858.8	E949.7	E950.4	E962.0	E980.4
pertussis component	978.6	E858.8	E948.6	E950.4	E962.0	E980.4
viral component	979.7	E858.8	E949.7	E950.4	E962.0	E980.4
viral NEC	979.6	E858.8	E949.6	E950.4	E962.0	E980.4
with						
bacterial component	979.7	E858.8	E949.7	E950.4	E962.0	E980.4
pertussis component	978.6	E858.8	E948.6	E950.4	E962.0	E980.4
rickettsial component	979.7	E858.8	E949.7	E950.4	E962.0	E980.4
84:04.04 antibiotics (skin and mucous membrane)	976.0	E858.7	E946.0	E950.4	E962.0	E980.4
84:04.08 fungicides (skin and mucous membrane)	976.0	E858.7	E946.0	E950.4	E962.0	E980.4
84:04.12 scabicides and pediculicides (skin and mucous membrane)	976.0	E858.7	E946.0	E950.4	E962.0	E980.4
84:04.16 miscellaneous local anti-infectives (skin and mucous membrane)	976.0	E858.7	E946.0	E950.4	E962.0	E980.4
84:06 anti-inflammatory agents (skin and mucous membrane)	976.0	E858.7	E946.0	E950.4	E962.0	E980.4
84:08 antipruritics and local anesthetics						
antipruritics	976.1	E858.7	E946.1	E950.4	E962.0	E980.4
local anesthetics	968.5	E855.2	E938.5	E950.4	E962.0	E980.4
84:12 astringents	976.2	E858.7	E946.2	E950.4	E962.0	E980.4
84:16 cell stimulants and proliferants	976.8	E858.7	E946.8	E950.4	E962.0	E980.4
84:20 detergents	976.2	E858.7	E946.2	E950.4	E962.0	E980.4
84:24 emollients, demulcents, and protectants	976.3	E858.7	E946.3	E950.4	E962.0	E980.4
84:28 keratolytic agents	976.4	E858.7	E946.4	E950.4	E962.0	E980.4
84:32 keratoplastic agents	976.4	E858.7	E946.4	E950.4	E962.0	E980.4
84:36 miscellaneous agents (skin and mucous membrane)	976.8	E858.7	E946.8	E950.4	E962.0	E980.4
86:00 spasmolytic agents	975.1	E858.6	E945.1	E950.4	E962.0	E980.4
antiasthmatics	975.7	E858.6	E945.7	E950.4	E962.0	E980.4
papaverine	972.5	E858.3	E942.5	E950.4	E962.0	E980.4
theophylline	974.1	E858.5	E944.1	E950.4	E962.0	E980.4
88:04 vitamin A	963.5	E858.1	E933.5	E950.4	E962.0	E980.4
88:08 vitamin B complex	963.5	E858.1	E933.5	E950.4	E962.0	E980.4
hematopoietic vitamin	964.1	E858.2	E934.1	E950.4	E962.0	E980.4
nicotinic acid derivatives	972.2	E858.3	E942.2	E950.4	E962.0	E980.4
88:12 vitamin C	963.5	E858.1	E933.5	E950.4	E962.0	E980.4
88:16 vitamin D	963.5	E858.1	E933.5	E950.4	E962.0	E980.4
88:20 vitamin E	963.5	E858.1	E933.5	E950.4	E962.0	E980.4
88:24 vitamin K activity	964.3	E858.2	E934.3	E950.4	E962.0	E980.4
88:28 multivitamin preparations	963.5	E858.1	E933.5	E950.4	E962.0	E980.4

Nontherapeutic use substance   ▽ Subterms under main terms may continue to next column or page

	External Cause (E-Code)					
	Poisoning	Accident	Therapeutic Use	Suicide Attempt	Assault	Undetermined
Drug — *continued*						
92:00 unclassified therapeutic agents	977.8	E858.8	E947.8	E950.4	E962.0	E980.4
specified NEC	977.8	E858.8	E947.8	E950.4	E962.0	E980.4
Duboisine	971.1	E855.4	E941.1	E950.4	E962.0	E980.4
Dulcolax	973.1	E858.4	E943.1	E950.4	E962.0	E980.4
Duponol (C) (EP)	976.2	E858.7	E946.2	E950.4	E962.0	E980.4
Durabolin	962.1	E858.0	E932.1	E950.4	E962.0	E980.4
Dyclone	968.5	E855.2	E938.5	E950.4	E962.0	E980.4
Dyclonine	968.5	E855.2	E938.5	E950.4	E962.0	E980.4
Dydrogesterone	962.2	E858.0	E932.2	E950.4	E962.0	E980.4
Dyes NEC	989.89	E866.8	—	E950.9	E962.1	E980.9
diagnostic agents	977.8	E858.8	E947.8	E950.4	E962.0	E980.4
pharmaceutical NEC	977.4	E858.8	E947.4	E950.4	E962.0	E980.4
Dyfols	971.0	E855.3	E941.0	E950.4	E962.0	E980.4
Dymelor	962.3	E858.0	E932.3	E950.4	E962.0	E980.4
Dynamite	989.89	E866.8	—	E950.9	E962.1	E980.9
fumes	987.8	E869.8	—	E952.8	E962.2	E982.8
Dyphylline	975.1	E858.6	E945.1	E950.4	E962.0	E980.4
Ear preparations	976.6	E858.7	E946.6	E950.4	E962.0	E980.4
Echothiopate, ecothiopate	971.0	E855.3	E941.0	E950.4	E962.0	E980.4
Ecstasy	969.72	E854.2	E939.7	E950.3	E962.0	E980.3
Ectylurea	967.8	E852.8	E937.8	E950.2	E962.0	E980.2
Edathamil disodium	963.8	E858.1	E933.8	E950.4	E962.0	E980.4
Edecrin	974.4	E858.5	E944.4	E950.4	E962.0	E980.4
Edetate, disodium (calcium)	963.8	E858.1	E933.8	E950.4	E962.0	E980.4
Edrophonium	971.0	E855.3	E941.0	E950.4	E962.0	E980.4
Elase	976.8	E858.7	E946.8	E950.4	E962.0	E980.4
Elaterium	973.1	E858.4	E943.1	E950.4	E962.0	E980.4
Elder	988.2	E865.4	—	E950.9	E962.1	E980.9
berry (unripe)	988.2	E865.3		E950.9	E962.1	E980.9
Electrolytes NEC	974.5	E858.5	E944.5	E950.4	E962.0	E980.4
Electrolytic agent NEC	974.5	E858.5	E944.5	E950.4	E962.0	E980.4
Embramine	963.0	E858.1	E933.0	E950.4	E962.0	E980.4
Emetics	973.6	E858.4	E943.6	E950.4	E962.0	E980.4
Emetine (hydrochloride)	961.5	E857	E931.5	E950.4	E962.0	E980.4
Emollients	976.3	E858.7	E946.3	E950.4	E962.0	E980.4
Emylcamate	969.5	E853.8	E939.5	E950.3	E962.0	E980.3
Encyprate	969.09	E854.0	E939.0	E950.3	E962.0	E980.3
Endocaine	968.5	E855.2	E938.5	E950.4	E962.0	E980.4
Endrin	989.2	E863.0	—	E950.6	E962.1	E980.7
Enflurane	968.2	E855.1	E938.2	E950.4	E962.0	E980.4
Enovid	962.2	E858.0	E932.2	E950.4	E962.0	E980.4
ENT preparations (anti-infectives)	976.6	E858.7	E946.6	E950.4	E962.0	E980.4
Enzodase	963.4	E858.1	E933.4	E950.4	E962.0	E980.4
Enzymes NEC	963.4	E858.1	E933.4	E950.4	E962.0	E980.4
Epanutin	966.1	E855.0	E936.1	E950.4	E962.0	E980.4
Ephedra (tincture)	971.2	E855.5	E941.2	E950.4	E962.0	E980.4
Ephedrine	971.2	E855.5	E941.2	E950.4	E962.0	E980.4
Epiestriol	962.2	E858.0	E932.2	E950.4	E962.0	E980.4
Epilim — see Sodium valproate						
Epinephrine	971.2	E855.5	E941.2	E950.4	E962.0	E980.4
Epsom salt	973.3	E858.4	E943.3	E950.4	E962.0	E980.4
Equanil	969.5	E853.8	E939.5	E950.3	E962.0	E980.3
Equisetum (diuretic)	974.4	E858.5	E944.4	E950.4	E962.0	E980.4
Ergometrine	975.0	E858.6	E945.0	E950.4	E962.0	E980.4
Ergonovine	975.0	E858.6	E945.0	E950.4	E962.0	E980.4
Ergotamine (tartrate) (for migraine) NEC	972.9	E858.3	E942.9	E950.4	E962.0	E980.4
Ergotrate	975.0	E858.6	E945.0	E950.4	E962.0	E980.4
Ergot NEC	988.2	E865.4	—	E950.9	E962.1	E980.9
medicinal (alkaloids)	975.0	E858.6	E945.0	E950.4	E962.0	E980.4
Erythrityl tetranitrate	972.4	E858.3	E942.4	E950.4	E962.0	E980.4
Erythrol tetranitrate	972.4	E858.3	E942.4	E950.4	E962.0	E980.4
Erythromycin	960.3	E856	E930.3	E950.4	E962.0	E980.4
ophthalmic preparation	976.5	E858.7	E946.5	E950.4	E962.0	E980.4
topical NEC	976.0	E858.7	E946.0	E950.4	E962.0	E980.4
Eserine	971.0	E855.3	E941.0	E950.4	E962.0	E980.4
Eskabarb	967.0	E851	E937.0	E950.1	E962.0	E980.1
Eskalith	969.8	E855.8	E939.8	E950.3	E962.0	E980.3
Estradiol (cypionate) (dipropionate) (valerate)	962.2	E858.0	E932.2	E950.4	E962.0	E980.4
Estriol	962.2	E858.0	E932.2	E950.4	E962.0	E980.4
Estrogens (with progestogens)	962.2	E858.0	E932.2	E950.4	E962.0	E980.4
Estrone	962.2	E858.0	E932.2	E950.4	E962.0	E980.4
Etafedrine	971.2	E855.5	E941.2	E950.4	E962.0	E980.4
Ethacrynate sodium	974.4	E858.5	E944.4	E950.4	E962.0	E980.4

	External Cause (E-Code)					
	Poisoning	Accident	Therapeutic Use	Suicide Attempt	Assault	Undetermined
Ethacrynic acid	974.4	E858.5	E944.4	E950.4	E962.0	E980.4
Ethambutol	961.8	E857	E931.8	E950.4	E962.0	E980.4
Ethamide	974.2	E858.5	E944.2	E950.4	E962.0	E980.4
Ethamivan	970.0	E854.3	E940.0	E950.4	E962.0	E980.4
Ethamsylate	964.5	E858.2	E934.5	E950.4	E962.0	E980.4
Ethanol	980.0	E860.1	—	E950.9	E962.1	E980.9
beverage	980.0	E860.0	—	E950.9	E962.1	E980.9
Ethchlorvynol	967.8	E852.8	E937.8	E950.2	E962.0	E980.2
Ethebenecid	974.7	E858.5	E944.7	E950.4	E962.0	E980.4
Ether(s) (diethyl) (ethyl) (vapor)	987.8	E869.8	—	E952.8	E962.2	E982.8
anesthetic	968.2	E855.1	E938.2	E950.4	E962.0	E980.4
petroleum — see Ligroin						
solvent	982.8	E862.4	—	E950.9	E962.1	E980.9
Ethidine chloride (vapor)	987.8	E869.8	—	E952.8	E962.2	E982.8
liquid (solvent)	982.3	E862.4	—	E950.9	E962.1	E980.9
Ethinamate	967.8	E852.8	E937.8	E950.2	E962.0	E980.2
Ethinylestradiol	962.2	E858.0	E932.2	E950.4	E962.0	E980.4
Ethionamide	961.8	E857	E931.8	E950.4	E962.0	E980.4
Ethisterone	962.2	E858.0	E932.2	E950.4	E962.0	E980.4
Ethobral	967.0	E851	E937.0	E950.1	E962.0	E980.1
Ethocaine (infiltration) (topical)	968.5	E855.2	E938.5	E950.4	E962.0	E980.4
nerve block (peripheral) (plexus)	968.6	E855.2	E938.6	E950.4	E962.0	E980.4
spinal	968.7	E855.2	E938.7	E950.4	E962.0	E980.4
Ethoheptazine (citrate)	965.7	E850.7	E935.7	E950.0	E962.0	E980.0
Ethopropazine	966.4	E855.0	E936.4	E950.4	E962.0	E980.4
Ethosuximide	966.2	E855.0	E936.2	E950.4	E962.0	E980.4
Ethotoin	966.1	E855.0	E936.1	E950.4	E962.0	E980.4
Ethoxazene	961.9	E857	E931.9	E950.4	E962.0	E980.4
Ethoxzolamide	974.2	E858.5	E944.2	E950.4	E962.0	E980.4
Ethyl						
acetate (vapor)	982.8	E862.4	—	E950.9	E962.1	E980.9
alcohol	980.0	E860.1	—	E950.9	E962.1	E980.9
beverage	980.0	E860.0	—	E950.9	E962.1	E980.9
aldehyde (vapor)	987.8	E869.8	—	E952.8	E962.2	E982.8
liquid	989.89	E866.8	—	E950.9	E962.1	E980.9
aminobenzoate	968.5	E855.2	E938.5	E950.4	E962.0	E980.4
biscoumacetate	964.2	E858.2	E934.2	E950.4	E962.0	E980.4
bromide (anesthetic)	968.2	E855.1	E938.2	E950.4	E962.0	E980.4
carbamate (antineoplastic)	963.1	E858.1	E933.1	E950.4	E962.0	E980.4
carbinol	980.3	E860.4	—	E950.9	E962.1	E980.9
chaulmoograte	961.8	E857	E931.8	E950.4	E962.0	E980.4
chloride (vapor)	987.8	E869.8	—	E952.8	E962.2	E982.8
anesthetic (local)	968.5	E855.2	E938.5	E950.4	E962.0	E980.4
inhaled	968.2	E855.1	E938.2	E950.4	E962.0	E980.4
solvent	982.3	E862.4	—	E950.9	E962.1	E980.9
estranol	962.1	E858.0	E932.1	E950.4	E962.0	E980.4
ether — see Ether(s)						
formate (solvent) NEC	982.8	E862.4	—	E950.9	E962.1	E980.9
iodoacetate	987.5	E869.3	—	E952.8	E962.2	E982.8
lactate (solvent) NEC	982.8	E862.4	—	E950.9	E962.1	E980.9
methylcarbinol	980.8	E860.8	—	E950.9	E962.1	E980.9
morphine	965.09	E850.2	E935.2	E950.0	E962.0	E980.0
Ethylene (gas)	987.1	E869.8	—	E952.8	E962.2	E982.8
anesthetic (general)	968.2	E855.1	E938.2	E950.4	E962.0	E980.4
chlorohydrin (vapor)	982.3	E862.4	—	E950.9	E962.1	E980.9
dichloride (vapor)	982.3	E862.4	—	E950.9	E962.1	E980.9
glycol(s) (any) (vapor)	982.8	E862.4	—	E950.9	E962.1	E980.9
Ethylidene						
chloride NEC	982.3	E862.4	—	E950.9	E962.1	E980.9
diethyl ether	982.8	E862.4	—	E950.9	E962.1	E980.9
Ethynodiol	962.2	E858.0	E932.2	E950.4	E962.0	E980.4
Etidocaine	968.9	E855.2	E938.9	E950.4	E962.0	E980.4
infiltration (subcutaneous)	968.5	E855.2	E938.5	E950.4	E962.0	E980.4
nerve (peripheral) (plexus)	968.6	E855.2	E938.6	E950.4	E962.0	E980.4
Etilfen	967.0	E851	E937.0	E950.1	E962.0	E980.1
Etomide	965.7	E850.7	E935.7	E950.0	E962.0	E980.0
Etorphine	965.09	E850.2	E935.2	E950.0	E962.0	E980.0
Etoval	967.0	E851	E937.0	E950.1	E962.0	E980.1
Etryptamine	969.01	E854.0	E939.0	E950.3	E962.0	E980.3
Eucaine	968.5	E855.2	E938.5	E950.4	E962.0	E980.4
Eucalyptus (oil) NEC	975.5	E858.6	E945.5	E950.4	E962.0	E980.4
Eucatropine	971.1	E855.4	E941.1	E950.4	E962.0	E980.4
Eucodal	965.09	E850.2	E935.2	E950.0	E962.0	E980.0
Euneryl	967.0	E851	E937.0	E950.1	E962.0	E980.1
Euphthalmine	971.1	E855.4	E941.1	E950.4	E962.0	E980.4
Eurax	976.0	E858.7	E946.0	E950.4	E962.0	E980.4

Nontherapeutic use substance

▶◀ Revised Text   ● New Line   ▲ Revised Code   Subterms under main terms may continue to next column or page

	Poisoning	Accident	Therapeutic Use	Suicide Attempt	Assault	Undeter-mined
Euresol	976.4	E858.7	E946.4	E950.4	E962.0	E980.4
Euthroid	962.7	E858.0	E932.7	E950.4	E962.0	E980.4
Evans blue	977.8	E858.8	E947.8	E950.4	E962.0	E980.4
Evipal	967.0	E851	E937.0	E950.1	E962.0	E980.1
sodium	968.3	E855.1	E938.3	E950.4	E962.0	E980.1
Evipan	967.0	E851	E937.0	E950.1	E962.0	E980.1
sodium	968.3	E855.1	E938.3	E950.4	E962.0	E980.4
Exalgin	965.4	E850.4	E935.4	E950.0	E962.0	E980.0
Excipients, pharmaceuti-cal	977.4	E858.8	E947.4	E950.4	E962.0	E980.4
Exhaust gas — see Carbon, monoxide						
Ex-Lax (phenolphthalein)	973.1	E858.4	E943.1	E950.4	E962.0	E980.4
Expectorants	975.5	E858.6	E945.5	E950.4	E962.0	E980.4
External medications (skin)						
(mucous membrane)	976.9	E858.7	E946.9	E950.4	E962.0	E980.4
dental agent	976.7	E858.7	E946.7	E950.4	E962.0	E980.4
ENT agent	976.6	E858.7	E946.6	E950.4	E962.0	E980.4
ophthalmic preparation	976.5	E858.7	E946.5	E950.4	E962.0	E980.4
specified NEC	976.8	E858.7	E946.8	E950.4	E962.0	E980.4
Eye agents (anti-infec-tive)	976.5	E858.7	E946.5	E950.4	E962.0	E980.4
Factor IX complex (hu-man)	964.5	E858.2	E934.5	E950.4	E962.0	E980.4
Fecal softeners	973.2	E858.4	E943.2	E950.4	E962.0	E980.4
Fenbutrazate	977.0	E858.8	E947.0	E950.4	E962.0	E980.4
Fencamfamin	970.89	E854.3	E940.8	E950.4	E962.0	E980.4
Fenfluramine	977.0	E858.8	E947.0	E950.4	E962.0	E980.4
Fenoprofen	965.61	E850.6	E935.6	E950.0	E962.0	E980.0
Fentanyl	965.09	E850.2	E935.2	E950.0	E962.0	E980.0
Fentazin	969.1	E853.0	E939.1	E950.3	E962.0	E980.3
Fenticlor, fentichlor	976.0	E858.7	E946.0	E950.4	E962.0	E980.4
Fer de lance (bite) (ven-om)	989.5	E905.0	—	E950.9	E962.1	E980.9
Ferric — see Iron						
Ferrocholinate	964.0	E858.2	E934.0	E950.4	E962.0	E980.4
Ferrous fumerate, gluconate, lactate, salt NEC, sulfate (medicinal)	964.0	E858.2	E934.0	E950.4	E962.0	E980.4
Ferrum — see Iron						
Fertilizers NEC	989.89	E866.5	—	E950.9	E962.1	E980.4
with herbicide mixture	989.4	E863.5	—	E950.6	E962.1	E980.7
Fibrinogen (human)	964.7	E858.2	E934.7	E950.4	E962.0	E980.4
Fibrinolysin	964.4	E858.2	E934.4	E950.4	E962.0	E980.4
Fibrinolysis-affecting agents	964.4	E858.2	E934.4	E950.4	E962.0	E980.4
Filix mas	961.6	E857	E931.6	E950.4	E962.0	E980.4
Fiorinal	965.1	E850.3	E935.3	E950.0	E962.0	E980.0
Fire damp	987.1	E869.8	—	E952.8	E962.2	E982.8
Fish, nonbacterial or nox-ious	988.0	E865.2	—	E950.9	E962.1	E980.9
shell	988.0	E865.1	—	E950.9	E962.1	E980.9
Flagyl	961.5	E857	E931.5	E950.4	E962.0	E980.4
Flavoxate	975.1	E858.6	E945.1	E950.4	E962.0	E980.4
Flaxedil	975.2	E858.6	E945.2	E950.4	E962.0	E980.4
Flaxseed (medicinal)	976.3	E858.7	E946.3	E950.4	E962.0	E980.4
Flomax	971.3	E855.6	E941.3	E950.4	E962.0	E980.4
Florantyrone	973.4	E858.4	E943.4	E950.4	E962.0	E980.4
Floraquin	961.3	E857	E931.3	E950.4	E962.0	E980.4
Florinef	962.0	E858.0	E932.0	E950.4	E962.0	E980.4
ENT agent	976.6	E858.7	E946.6	E950.4	E962.0	E980.4
ophthalmic preparation	976.5	E858.7	E946.5	E950.4	E962.0	E980.4
topical NEC	976.0	E858.7	E946.0	E950.4	E962.0	E980.4
Flowers of sulfur	976.4	E858.7	E946.4	E950.4	E962.0	E980.4
Floxuridine	963.1	E858.1	E933.1	E950.4	E962.0	E980.4
Flucytosine	961.9	E857	E931.9	E950.4	E962.0	E980.4
Fludrocortisone	962.0	E858.0	E932.0	E950.4	E962.0	E980.4
ENT agent	976.6	E858.7	E946.6	E950.4	E962.0	E980.4
ophthalmic preparation	976.5	E858.7	E946.5	E950.4	E962.0	E980.4
topical NEC	976.0	E858.7	E946.0	E950.4	E962.0	E980.4
Flumethasone	976.0	E858.7	E946.0	E950.4	E962.0	E980.4
Flumethiazide	974.3	E858.5	E944.3	E950.4	E962.0	E980.4
Flumidin	961.7	E857	E931.7	E950.4	E962.0	E980.4
Flunitrazepam	969.4	E853.2	E939.4	E950.3	E962.0	E980.3
Fluocinolone	976.0	E858.7	E946.0	E950.4	E962.0	E980.4
Fluocortolone	962.0	E858.0	E932.0	E950.4	E962.0	E980.4
Fluohydrocortisone	962.0	E858.0	E932.0	E950.4	E962.0	E980.4
ENT agent	976.6	E858.7	E946.6	E950.4	E962.0	E980.4
ophthalmic preparation	976.5	E858.7	E946.5	E950.4	E962.0	E980.4
topical NEC	976.0	E858.7	E946.0	E950.4	E962.0	E980.4
Fluonid	976.0	E858.7	E946.0	E950.4	E962.0	E980.4
Fluopromazine	969.1	E853.0	E939.1	E950.3	E962.0	E980.3

	Poisoning	Accident	Therapeutic Use	Suicide Attempt	Assault	Undeter-mined
Fluoracetate	989.4	E863.7	—	E950.6	E962.1	E980.7
Fluorescein (sodium)	977.8	E858.8	E947.8	E950.4	E962.0	E980.4
Fluoride(s) (pesticides) (sodi-um) NEC	989.4	E863.4	—	E950.6	E962.1	E980.7
hydrogen — see Hydrofluoric acid						
medicinal	976.7	E858.7	E946.7	E950.4	E962.0	E980.4
not pesticide NEC	983.9	E864.4	—	E950.7	E962.1	E980.6
stannous	976.7	E858.7	E946.7	E950.4	E962.0	E980.4
Fluorinated corticos-teroids	962.0	E858.0	E932.0	E950.4	E962.0	E980.4
Fluorine (compounds) (gas)	987.8	E869.8	—	E952.8	E962.2	E982.8
salt — see Fluoride(s)						
Fluoristan	976.7	E858.7	E946.7	E950.4	E962.0	E980.4
Fluoroacetate	989.4	E863.7	—	E950.6	E962.1	E980.7
Fluorodeoxyuridine	963.1	E858.1	E933.1	E950.4	E962.0	E980.4
Fluorometholone (topical) NEC	976.0	E858.7	E946.0	E950.4	E962.0	E980.4
ophthalmic preparation	976.5	E858.7	E946.5	E950.4	E962.0	E980.4
Fluorouracil	963.1	E858.1	E933.1	E950.4	E962.0	E980.4
Fluothane	968.1	E855.1	E938.1	E950.4	E962.0	E980.4
Fluoxetine hydrochlo-ride	969.03	E854.0	E939.0	E950.3	E962.0	E980.3
Fluoxymesterone	962.1	E858.0	E932.1	E950.4	E962.0	E980.4
Fluphenazine	969.1	E853.0	E939.1	E950.3	E962.0	E980.3
Fluprednisolone	962.0	E858.0	E932.0	E950.4	E962.0	E980.4
Flurandrenolide	976.0	E858.7	E946.0	E950.4	E962.0	E980.4
Flurazepam (hydrochlo-ride)	969.4	E853.2	E939.4	E950.3	E962.0	E980.3
Flurbiprofen	965.61	E850.6	E935.6	E950.0	E962.0	E980.0
Flurobate	976.0	E858.7	E946.0	E950.4	E962.0	E980.4
Flurothyl	969.8	E855.8	E939.8	E950.3	E962.0	E980.3
Fluroxene	968.2	E855.1	E938.2	E950.4	E962.0	E980.4
Folacin	964.1	E858.2	E934.1	E950.4	E962.0	E980.4
Folic acid	964.1	E858.2	E934.1	E950.4	E962.0	E980.4
Follicle stimulating hor-mone	962.4	E858.0	E932.4	E950.4	E962.0	E980.4
Food, foodstuffs, nonbacteri-al or noxious	988.9	E865.9	—	E950.9	E962.1	E980.9
berries, seeds	988.2	E865.3	—	E950.9	E962.1	E980.9
fish	988.0	E865.2	—	E950.9	E962.1	E980.9
mushrooms	988.1	E865.5	—	E950.9	E962.1	E980.9
plants	988.2	E865.9	—	E950.9	E962.1	E980.9
specified type NEC	988.2	E865.4	—	E950.9	E962.1	E980.9
shellfish	988.0	E865.1	—	E950.9	E962.1	E980.9
specified NEC	988.8	E865.8	—	E950.9	E962.1	E980.9
Fool's parsley	988.2	E865.4	—	E950.9	E962.1	E980.9
Formaldehyde (solution)	989.89	E861.4	—	E950.9	E962.1	E980.9
fungicide	989.4	E863.6	—	E950.6	E962.1	E980.7
gas or vapor	987.8	E869.8	—	E952.8	E962.2	E982.8
Formalin	989.89	E861.4	—	E950.9	E962.1	E980.9
fungicide	989.4	E863.6	—	E950.6	E962.1	E980.7
vapor	987.8	E869.8	—	E952.8	E962.2	E982.8
Formic acid	983.1	E864.1	—	E950.7	E962.1	E980.6
automobile	981	E862.1	—	E950.9	E962.1	E980.9
exhaust gas, not in tran-sit	986	E868.2	—	E952.0	E962.2	E982.0
vapor NEC	987.1	E869.8	—	E952.8	E962.2	E982.8
gas (domestic use) (see also Carbon, monoxide, fuel)						
utility	987.1	E868.1	—	E951.8	E962.2	E981.8
incomplete combustion of — see Carbon, monox-ide, fuel, utility						
in mobile container	987.0	E868.0	—	E951.1	E962.2	E981.1
piped (natural)	987.1	E867	—	E951.0	E962.2	E981.0
industrial, incomplete combus-tion	986	E868.3	—	E952.1	E962.2	E982.1
vapor	987.8	E869.8	—	E952.8	E962.2	E982.8
Fowler's solution	985.1	E866.3	—	E950.8	E962.1	E980.8
Foxglove	988.2	E865.4	—	E950.9	E962.1	E980.9
Fox green	977.8	E858.8	E947.8	E950.4	E962.0	E980.4
Framycetin	960.8	E856	E930.8	E950.4	E962.0	E980.4
Frangula (extract)	973.1	E858.4	E943.1	E950.4	E962.0	E980.4
Frei antigen	977.8	E858.8	E947.8	E950.4	E962.0	E980.4
Freons	987.4	E869.2	—	E952.8	E962.2	E982.8
Fructose	974.5	E858.5	E944.5	E950.4	E962.0	E980.4
Frusemide	974.4	E858.5	E944.4	E950.4	E962.0	E980.4
FSH	962.4	E858.0	E932.4	E950.4	E962.0	E980.4
Fuel						
Fugillin	960.8	E856	E930.8	E950.4	E962.0	E980.4

Nontherapeutic use substance

▽ Subterms under main terms may continue to next column or page

►◄ Revised Text   ● New Line   ▲ Revised Code

	Poisoning	Accident	Therapeutic Use	Suicide Attempt	Assault	Undetermined
Fulminate of mercury	985.0	E866.1	—	E950.9	E962.1	E980.9
Fulvicin	960.1	E856	E930.1	E950.4	E962.0	E980.4
Fumadil	960.8	E856	E930.8	E950.4	E962.0	E980.4
Fumagillin	960.8	E856	E930.8	E950.4	E962.0	E980.4
Fumes (from)	987.9	E869.9	—	E952.9	E962.2	E982.9
carbon monoxide — see Carbon, monoxide						
charcoal (domestic use)	986	E868.3	—	E952.1	E962.2	E982.1
chloroform — see Chloroform						
coke (in domestic stoves, fireplaces)	986	E868.3	—	E952.1	E962.2	E982.1
corrosive NEC	987.8	E869.8	—	E952.8	E962.2	E982.8
ether — see Ether(s)						
freons	987.4	E869.2	—	E952.8	E962.2	E982.8
hydrocarbons	987.1	E869.8	—	E952.8	E962.2	E982.8
petroleum (liquefied)	987.0	E868.0	—	E951.1	E962.2	E981.1
distributed through pipes (pure or mixed with air)	987.0	E867	—	E951.0	E962.2	E981.0
lead — see Lead						
metals — see specified metal						
nitrogen dioxide	987.2	E869.0	—	E952.8	E962.2	E982.8
pesticides — see Pesticides						
petroleum (liquefied)	987.0	E868.0	—	E951.1	E962.2	E981.1
distributed through pipes (pure or mixed with air)	987.0	E867	—	E951.0	E962.2	E981.0
polyester	987.8	E869.8	—	E952.8	E962.2	E982.8
specified, source other (see also substance specified)	987.8	E869.8	—	E952.8	E962.2	E982.8
sulfur dioxide	987.3	E869.1	—	E952.8	E962.2	E982.8
Fumigants	989.4	E863.8	—	E950.6	E962.1	E980.7
Fungicides — see also Antifungals	989.4	E863.6	—	E950.6	E962.1	E980.7
Fungi, noxious, used as food	988.1	E865.5	—	E950.9	E962.1	E980.9
Fungizone	960.1	E856	E930.1	E950.4	E962.0	E980.4
topical	976.0	E858.7	E946.0	E950.4	E962.0	E980.4
Furacin	976.0	E858.7	E946.0	E950.4	E962.0	E980.4
Furadantin	961.9	E857	E931.9	E950.4	E962.0	E980.4
Furadantin	961.9	E857	E931.9	E950.4	E962.0	E980.4
Furazolidone	961.9	E857	E931.9	E950.4	E962.0	E980.4
Furnace (coal burning) (domestic), gas from	986	E868.3	—	E952.1	E962.2	E982.1
industrial	986	E868.8	—	E952.1	E962.2	E982.1
Furniture polish	989.89	E861.2	—	E950.9	E962.1	E980.9
Furosemide	974.4	E858.5	E944.4	E950.4	E962.0	E980.4
Furoxone	961.9	E857	E931.9	E950.4	E962.0	E980.4
Fusel oil (amyl) (butyl) (propyl)	980.3	E860.4	—	E950.9	E962.1	E980.9
Fusidic acid	960.8	E856	E930.8	E950.4	E962.0	E980.4
Gallamine	975.2	E858.6	E945.2	E950.4	E962.0	E980.4
Gallotannic acid	976.2	E858.7	E946.2	E950.4	E962.0	E980.4
Gamboge	973.1	E858.4	E943.1	E950.4	E962.0	E980.4
Gamimune	964.6	E858.2	E934.6	E950.4	E962.0	E980.4
Gamma-benzene hexachloride (vapor)	989.2	E863.0	—	E950.6	E962.1	E980.7
Gamma globulin	964.6	E858.2	E934.6	E950.4	E962.0	E980.4
Gamma hydroxy butyrate (GHB)	968.4	E855.1	E938.4	E950.4	E962.0	E980.4
Gamulin	964.6	E858.2	E934.6	E950.4	E962.0	E980.4
Ganglionic blocking agents	972.3	E858.3	E942.3	E950.4	E962.0	E980.4
Ganja	969.6	E854.1	E939.6	E950.3	E962.0	E980.3
Garamycin	960.8	E856	E930.8	E950.4	E962.0	E980.4
ophthalmic preparation	976.5	E858.7	E946.5	E950.4	E962.0	E980.4
topical NEC	976.0	E858.7	E946.0	E950.4	E962.0	E980.4
Gardenal	967.0	E851	E937.0	E950.1	E962.0	E980.1
Gardepanyl	967.0	E851	E937.0	E950.1	E962.0	E980.1
Gas	987.9	E869.9	—	E952.9	E962.2	E982.9
acetylene	987.1	E868.1	—	E951.8	E962.2	E981.8
incomplete combustion of — see Carbon, monoxide, fuel, utility						
air contaminants, source or type not specified	987.9	E869.9	—	E952.9	E962.2	E982.9
anesthetic (general) NEC	968.2	E855.1	E938.2	E950.4	E962.0	E980.4
blast furnace	986	E868.8	—	E952.1	E962.2	E982.1
butane — see Butane						
carbon monoxide — see Carbon, monoxide						

Gas — continued	Poisoning	Accident	Therapeutic Use	Suicide Attempt	Assault	Undetermined
chlorine	987.6	E869.8	—	E952.8	E962.2	E982.8
coal — see Carbon, monoxide, coal						
cyanide	987.7	E869.8	—	E952.8	E962.2	E982.8
dicyanogen	987.8	E869.8	—	E952.8	E962.2	E982.8
domestic — see Gas, utility						
exhaust — see Carbon, monoxide, exhaust gas						
from wood- or coal-burning stove or fireplace	986	E868.3	—	E952.1	E962.2	E982.1
fuel (domestic use) (see also Carbon, monoxide, fuel)						
industrial use	986	E868.8	—	E952.1	E962.2	E982.1
utility	987.1	E868.1	—	E951.8	E962.2	E981.8
incomplete combustion of — see Carbon, monoxide, fuel, utility						
in mobile container	987.0	E868.0	—	E951.1	E962.2	E981.1
piped (natural)	987.1	E867	—	E951.0	E962.2	E981.0
garage	986	E868.2	—	E952.0	E962.2	E982.0
hydrocarbon NEC	987.1	E869.8	—	E952.8	E962.2	E982.8
incomplete combustion of — see Carbon, monoxide, fuel, utility						
liquefied (mobile container)	987.0	E868.0	—	E951.1	E962.2	E981.1
piped	987.0	E867	—	E951.0	E962.2	E981.0
hydrocyanic acid	987.7	E869.8	—	E952.8	E962.2	E982.8
illuminating — see Gas, utility						
incomplete combustion, any — see Carbon, monoxide						
kiln	986	E868.8	—	E952.1	E962.2	E982.1
lacrimogenic	987.5	E869.3	—	E952.8	E962.2	E982.8
marsh	987.1	E869.8	—	E952.8	E962.2	E982.8
motor exhaust, not in transit	986	E868.8	—	E952.1	E962.2	E982.1
mustard — see Mustard, gas						
natural	987.1	E867	—	E951.0	E962.2	E981.0
nerve (war)	987.9	E869.9	—	E952.9	E962.2	E982.9
oils	981	E862.1	—	E950.9	E962.1	E980.9
petroleum (liquefied) (distributed in mobile containers)	987.0	E868.0	—	E951.1	E962.2	E981.1
piped (pure or mixed with air)	987.0	E867	—	E951.1	E962.2	E981.1
piped (manufactured) (natural) NEC	987.1	E867	—	E951.0	E962.2	E981.0
producer	986	E868.8	—	E952.1	E962.2	E982.1
propane — see Propane						
refrigerant (freon)	987.4	E869.2	—	E952.8	E962.2	E982.8
not freon	987.9	E869.9	—	E952.9	E962.2	E982.9
sewer	987.8	E869.8	—	E952.8	E962.2	E982.8
specified source NEC (see also substance specified)	987.8	E869.8	—	E952.8	E962.2	E982.8
stove — see Gas, utility						
tear	987.5	E869.3	—	E952.8	E962.2	E982.8
utility (for cooking, heating, or lighting) (piped) NEC	987.1	E868.1	—	E951.8	E962.2	E981.8
incomplete combustion of — see Carbon, monoxide, fuel, utility						
in mobile container	987.0	E868.0	—	E951.1	E962.2	E981.1
piped (natural)	987.1	E867	—	E951.0	E962.2	E981.0
water	987.1	E868.1	—	E951.8	E962.2	E981.8
incomplete combustion of — see Carbon, monoxide, fuel, utility						
Gaseous substance — see Gas						
Gasoline, gasolene	981	E862.1	—	E950.9	E962.1	E980.9
vapor	987.1	E869.8	—	E952.8	E962.2	E982.8
Gastric enzymes	973.4	E858.4	E943.4	E950.4	E962.0	E980.4
Gastrografin	977.8	E858.8	E947.8	E950.4	E962.0	E980.4
Gastrointestinal agents	973.9	E858.4	E943.9	E950.4	E962.0	E980.4
specified NEC	973.8	E858.4	E943.8	E950.4	E962.0	E980.4
Gaultheria procumbens	988.2	E865.4	—	E950.9	E962.1	E980.9
Gelatin (intravenous)	964.8	E858.2	E934.8	E950.4	E962.0	E980.4
absorbable (sponge)	964.5	E858.2	E934.5	E950.4	E962.0	E980.4
Gelfilm	976.8	E858.7	E946.8	E950.4	E962.0	E980.4
Gelfoam	964.5	E858.2	E934.5	E950.4	E962.0	E980.4

Subterms under main terms may continue to next column or page

		External Cause (E-Code)				
	Poisoning	Accident	Therapeutic Use	Suicide Attempt	Assault	Undetermined
Gelsemine	970.89	E854.3	E940.8	E950.4	E962.0	E980.4
Gelsemium (semper-virens)	988.2	E865.4	—	E950.9	E962.1	E980.9
Gemonil	967.0	E851	E937.0	E950.1	E962.0	E980.1
Gentamicin	960.8	E856	E930.8	E950.4	E962.0	E980.4
ophthalmic preparation	976.5	E858.7	E946.5	E950.4	E962.0	E980.4
topical NEC	976.0	E858.7	E946.0	E950.4	E962.0	E980.4
Gentian violet	976.0	E858.7	E946.0	E950.4	E962.0	E980.4
Gexane	976.0	E858.7	E946.0	E950.4	E962.0	E980.4
Gila monster (venom)	989.5	E905.0	—	E950.9	E962.1	E980.9
Ginger, Jamaica	989.89	E866.8	—	E950.9	E962.1	E980.9
Gitalin	972.1	E858.3	E942.1	E950.4	E962.0	E980.4
Gitoxin	972.1	E858.3	E942.1	E950.4	E962.0	E980.4
Glandular extract (medicinal) NEC	977.9	E858.9	E947.9	E950.5	E962.0	E980.5
Glaucarubin	961.5	E857	E931.5	E950.4	E962.0	E980.4
Globin zinc insulin	962.3	E858.0	E932.3	E950.4	E962.0	E980.4
Glucagon	962.3	E858.0	E932.3	E950.4	E962.0	E980.4
Glucochloral	967.1	E852.0	E937.1	E950.2	E962.0	E980.2
Glucocorticoids	962.0	E858.0	E932.0	E950.4	E962.0	E980.4
Glucose	974.5	E858.5	E944.5	E950.4	E962.0	E980.4
oxidase reagent	977.8	E858.8	E947.8	E950.4	E962.0	E980.4
Glucosulfone sodium	961.8	E857	E931.8	E950.4	E962.0	E980.4
Glue(s)	989.89	E866.6	—	E950.9	E962.1	E980.9
Glutamic acid (hydrochloride)	973.4	E858.4	E943.4	E950.4	E962.0	E980.4
Glutaraldehyde	989.89	E861.4	—	E950.9	E962.1	E980.9
Glutathione	963.8	E858.1	E933.8	E950.4	E962.0	E980.4
Glutethimide (group)	967.5	E852.4	E937.5	E950.2	E962.0	E980.2
Glycerin (lotion)	976.3	E858.7	E946.3	E950.4	E962.0	E980.4
Glycerol (topical)	976.3	E858.7	E946.3	E950.4	E962.0	E980.4
Glyceryl						
guaiacolate	975.5	E858.6	E945.5	E950.4	E962.0	E980.4
triacetate (topical)	976.0	E858.7	E946.0	E950.4	E962.0	E980.4
trinitrate	972.4	E858.3	E942.4	E950.4	E962.0	E980.4
Glycine	974.5	E858.5	E944.5	E950.4	E962.0	E980.4
Glycobiarsol	961.1	E857	E931.1	E950.4	E962.0	E980.4
Glycols (ether)	982.8	E862.4	—	E950.9	E962.1	E980.9
Glycopyrrolate	971.1	E855.4	E941.1	E950.4	E962.0	E980.4
Glymidine	962.3	E858.0	E932.3	E950.4	E962.0	E980.4
Gold (compounds) (salts)	965.69	E850.6	E935.6	E950.0	E962.0	E980.0
Golden sulfide of antimony	985.4	E866.2	—	E950.9	E962.1	E980.9
Goldylocks	988.2	E865.4	—	E950.9	E962.1	E980.9
Gonadal tissue extract	962.9	E858.0	E932.9	E950.4	E962.0	E980.4
female	962.2	E858.0	E932.2	E950.4	E962.0	E980.4
male	962.1	E858.0	E932.1	E950.4	E962.0	E980.4
Gonadotropin	962.4	E858.0	E932.4	E950.4	E962.0	E980.4
Grain alcohol	980.0	E860.1	—	E950.9	E962.1	E980.9
beverage	980.0	E860.0	—	E950.9	E962.1	E980.9
Gramicidin	960.8	E856	E930.8	E950.4	E962.0	E980.4
Gratiola officinalis	988.2	E865.4	—	E950.9	E962.1	E980.9
Grease	989.89	E866.8	—	E950.9	E962.1	E980.9
Green hellebore	988.2	E865.4	—	E950.9	E962.1	E980.9
Green soap	976.2	E858.7	E946.2	E950.4	E962.0	E980.4
Grifulvin	960.1	E856	E930.1	E950.4	E962.0	E980.4
Griseofulvin	960.1	E856	E930.1	E950.4	E962.0	E980.4
Growth hormone	962.4	E858.0	E932.4	E950.4	E962.0	E980.4
Guaiacol	975.5	E858.6	E945.5	E950.4	E962.0	E980.4
Guaiac reagent	977.8	E858.8	E947.8	E950.4	E962.0	E980.4
Guaifenesin	975.5	E858.6	E945.5	E950.4	E962.0	E980.4
Guaiphenesin	975.5	E858.6	E945.5	E950.4	E962.0	E980.4
Guanatol	961.4	E857	E931.4	E950.4	E962.0	E980.4
Guanethidine	972.6	E858.3	E942.6	E950.4	E962.0	E980.4
Guano	989.89	E866.5	—	E950.9	E962.1	E980.9
Guanochlor	972.6	E858.3	E942.6	E950.4	E962.0	E980.4
Guanoctine	972.6	E858.3	E942.6	E950.4	E962.0	E980.4
Guanoxan	972.6	E858.3	E942.6	E950.4	E962.0	E980.4
Hair treatment agent NEC	976.4	E858.7	E946.4	E950.4	E962.0	E980.4
Halcinonide	976.0	E858.7	E946.0	E950.4	E962.0	E980.4
Halethazole	976.0	E858.7	E946.0	E950.4	E962.0	E980.4
Hallucinogens	969.6	E854.1	E939.6	E950.3	E962.0	E980.3
Haloperidol	969.2	E853.1	E939.2	E950.3	E962.0	E980.3
Haloprogin	976.0	E858.7	E946.0	E950.4	E962.0	E980.4
Halotex	976.0	E858.7	E946.0	E950.4	E962.0	E980.4
Halothane	968.1	E855.1	E938.1	E950.4	E962.0	E980.4
Halquinols	976.0	E858.7	E946.0	E950.4	E962.0	E980.4
Hand sanitizer	976.0	E858.7	E946.0	E950.4	E962.0	E980.4
Harmonyl	972.6	E858.3	E942.6	E950.4	E962.0	E980.4
Hartmann's solution	974.5	E858.5	E944.5	E950.4	E962.0	E980.4
Hashish	969.6	E854.1	E939.6	E950.3	E962.0	E980.3

		External Cause (E-Code)				
	Poisoning	Accident	Therapeutic Use	Suicide Attempt	Assault	Undetermined
Hawaiian wood rose seeds	969.6	E854.1	E939.6	E950.3	E962.0	E980.3
Headache cures, drugs, powders NEC	977.9	E858.9	E947.9	E950.5	E962.0	E980.9
Heavenly Blue (morning glory)	969.6	E854.1	E939.6	E950.3	E962.0	E980.3
Heavy metal antagonists	963.8	E858.1	E933.8	E950.4	E962.0	E980.4
anti-infectives	961.2	E857	E931.2	E950.4	E962.0	E980.4
Hedaquinium	976.0	E858.7	E946.0	E950.4	E962.0	E980.4
Hedge hyssop	988.2	E865.4	—	E950.9	E962.1	E980.9
Heet	976.8	E858.7	E946.8	E950.4	E962.0	E980.4
Helenin	961.6	E857	E931.6	E950.4	E962.0	E980.4
Hellebore (black) (green) (white)	988.2	E865.4	—	E950.9	E962.1	E980.9
Hemlock	988.2	E865.4	—	E950.9	E962.1	E980.9
Hemostatics	964.5	E858.2	E934.5	E950.4	E962.0	E980.4
capillary active drugs	972.8	E858.3	E942.8	E950.4	E962.0	E980.4
Henbane	988.2	E865.4	—	E950.9	E962.1	E980.9
Heparin (sodium)	964.2	E858.2	E934.2	E950.4	E962.0	E980.4
Heptabarbital, heptabarbitone	967.0	E851	E937.0	E950.1	E962.0	E980.1
Heptachlor	989.2	E863.0	—	E950.6	E962.1	E980.7
Heptalgin	965.09	E850.2	E935.2	E950.0	E962.0	E980.0
Herbicides	989.4	E863.5	—	E950.6	E962.1	E980.7
Heroin	965.01	E850.0	E935.0	E950.0	E962.0	E980.0
Herplex	976.5	E858.7	E946.5	E950.4	E962.0	E980.4
HES	964.8	E858.2	E934.8	E950.4	E962.0	E980.4
Hetastarch	964.8	E858.2	E934.8	E950.4	E962.0	E980.4
Hexachlorocyclohexane	989.2	E863.0	—	E950.6	E962.1	E980.7
Hexachlorophene	976.2	E858.7	E946.2	E950.4	E962.0	E980.4
Hexadimethrine (bromide)	964.5	E858.2	E934.5	E950.4	E962.0	E980.4
Hexafluorenium	975.2	E858.6	E945.2	E950.4	E962.0	E980.4
Hexa-germ	976.2	E858.7	E946.2	E950.4	E962.0	E980.4
Hexahydrophenol	980.8	E860.8	—	E950.9	E962.1	E980.9
Hexalin	980.8	E860.8	—	E950.9	E962.1	E980.9
Hexamethonium	972.3	E858.3	E942.3	E950.4	E962.0	E980.4
Hexamethyleneamine	961.9	E857	E931.9	E950.4	E962.0	E980.4
Hexamine	961.9	E857	E931.9	E950.4	E962.0	E980.4
Hexanone	982.8	E862.4	—	E950.9	E962.1	E980.9
Hexapropymate	967.8	E852.8	E937.8	E950.2	E962.0	E980.2
Hexestrol	962.2	E858.0	E932.2	E950.4	E962.0	E980.4
Hexethal (sodium)	967.0	E851	E937.0	E950.1	E962.0	E980.1
Hexetidine	976.0	E858.7	E946.0	E950.4	E962.0	E980.4
Hexobarbital, hexobarbitone	967.0	E851	E937.0	E950.1	E962.0	E980.1
sodium (anesthetic)	968.3	E855.1	E938.3	E950.4	E962.0	E980.4
soluble	968.3	E855.1	E938.3	E950.4	E962.0	E980.4
Hexocyclium	971.1	E855.4	E941.1	E950.4	E962.0	E980.4
Hexoestrol	962.2	E858.0	E932.2	E950.4	E962.0	E980.4
Hexone	982.8	E862.4	—	E950.9	E962.1	E980.9
Hexylcaine	968.5	E855.2	E938.5	E950.4	E962.0	E980.4
Hexylresorcinol	961.6	E857	E931.6	E950.4	E962.0	E980.4
Hinkle's pills	973.1	E858.4	E943.1	E950.4	E962.0	E980.4
Histalog	977.8	E858.8	E947.8	E950.4	E962.0	E980.4
Histamine (phosphate)	972.5	E858.3	E942.5	E950.4	E962.0	E980.4
Histoplasmin	977.8	E858.8	E947.8	E950.4	E962.0	E980.4
Holly berries	988.2	E865.3	—	E950.9	E962.1	E980.9
Homatropine	971.1	E855.4	E941.1	E950.4	E962.0	E980.4
Homo-tet	964.6	E858.2	E934.6	E950.4	E962.0	E980.4
Hormones (synthetic substitute) NEC	962.9	E858.0	E932.9	E950.4	E962.0	E980.4
adrenal cortical steroids	962.0	E858.0	E932.0	E950.4	E962.0	E980.4
antidiabetic agents	962.3	E858.0	E932.3	E950.4	E962.0	E980.4
follicle stimulating	962.4	E858.0	E932.4	E950.4	E962.0	E980.4
gonadotropic	962.4	E858.0	E932.4	E950.4	E962.0	E980.4
growth	962.4	E858.0	E932.4	E950.4	E962.0	E980.4
ovarian (substitutes)	962.2	E858.0	E932.2	E950.4	E962.0	E980.4
parathyroid (derivatives)	962.6	E858.0	E932.6	E950.4	E962.0	E980.4
pituitary (posterior)	962.5	E858.0	E932.5	E950.4	E962.0	E980.4
anterior	962.4	E858.0	E932.4	E950.4	E962.0	E980.4
thyroid (derivative)	962.7	E858.0	E932.7	E950.4	E962.0	E980.4
Hornet (sting)	989.5	E905.3	—	E950.9	E962.1	E980.9
Horticulture agent NEC	989.4	E863.9	—	E950.6	E962.1	E980.7
Hyaluronidase	963.4	E858.1	E933.4	E950.4	E962.0	E980.4
Hyazyme	963.4	E858.1	E933.4	E950.4	E962.0	E980.4
Hycodan	965.09	E850.2	E935.2	E950.0	E962.0	E980.0
Hydantoin derivatives	966.1	E855.0	E936.1	E950.4	E962.0	E980.4
Hydeltra	962.0	E858.0	E932.0	E950.4	E962.0	E980.4
Hydergine	971.3	E855.6	E941.3	E950.4	E962.0	E980.4
Hydrabamine penicillin	960.0	E856	E930.0	E950.4	E962.0	E980.4

Nontherapeutic use substance

▽ Subterms under main terms may continue to next column or page

	Poisoning	Accident	Therapeutic Use	Suicide Attempt	Assault	Undeter-mined
Hydralazine, hydral-lazine	972.6	E858.3	E942.6	E950.4	E962.0	E980.4
Hydrargaphen	976.0	E858.7	E946.0	E950.4	E962.0	E980.4
Hydrazine	983.9	E864.3	—	E950.7	E962.1	E980.6
Hydriodic acid	975.5	E858.6	E945.5	E950.4	E962.0	E980.4
Hydrocarbon gas	987.1	E869.8	—	E952.8	E962.2	E982.8
incomplete combustion of — see Carbon, monoxide, fuel, utility						
liquefied (mobile container)	987.0	E868.0	—	E951.1	E962.2	E981.1
piped (natural)	987.0	E867	—	E951.0	E962.2	E981.0
Hydrochloric acid (liquid)	983.1	E864.1	—	E950.7	E962.1	E980.6
medicinal	973.4	E858.4	E943.4	E950.4	E962.0	E980.4
vapor	987.8	E869.8	—	E952.8	E962.2	E982.8
Hydrochlorothiazide	974.3	E858.5	E944.3	E950.4	E962.0	E980.4
Hydrocodone	965.09	E850.2	E935.2	E950.0	E962.0	E980.0
Hydrocortisone	962.0	E858.0	E932.0	E950.4	E962.0	E980.4
ENT agent	976.6	E858.7	E946.6	E950.4	E962.0	E980.4
ophthalmic preparation	976.5	E858.7	E946.5	E950.4	E962.0	E980.4
topical NEC	976.0	E858.7	E946.0	E950.4	E962.0	E980.4
Hydrocortone	962.0	E858.0	E932.0	E950.4	E962.0	E980.4
ENT agent	976.6	E858.7	E946.6	E950.4	E962.0	E980.4
ophthalmic preparation	976.5	E858.7	E946.5	E950.4	E962.0	E980.4
topical NEC	976.0	E858.7	E946.0	E950.4	E962.0	E980.4
Hydrocyanic acid — see Cyanide(s)						
Hydroflumethiazide	974.3	E858.5	E944.3	E950.4	E962.0	E980.4
Hydrofluoric acid (liquid)	983.1	E864.1	—	E950.7	E962.1	E980.6
vapor	987.8	E869.8	—	E952.8	E962.2	E982.8
Hydrogen	987.8	E869.8	—	E952.8	E962.2	E982.8
arsenide	985.1	E866.3	—	E950.8	E962.1	E980.8
arseniureted	985.1	E866.3	—	E950.8	E962.1	E980.8
cyanide (salts)	989.0	E866.8	—	E950.9	E962.1	E980.9
gas	987.7	E869.8	—	E952.8	E962.2	E982.8
fluoride (liquid)	983.1	E864.1	—	E950.7	E962.1	E980.6
vapor	987.8	E869.8	—	E952.8	E962.2	E982.8
peroxide (solution)	976.6	E858.7	E946.6	E950.4	E962.0	E980.4
phosphureted	987.8	E869.8	—	E952.8	E962.2	E982.8
sulfide (gas)	987.8	E869.8	—	E952.8	E962.2	E982.8
arseniureted	985.1	E866.3	—	E950.8	E962.1	E980.8
sulfureted	987.8	E869.8	—	E952.8	E962.2	E982.8
Hydromorphinol	965.09	E850.2	E935.2	E950.0	E962.0	E980.0
Hydromorphinone	965.09	E850.2	E935.2	E950.0	E962.0	E980.0
Hydromorphone	965.09	E850.2	E935.2	E950.0	E962.0	E980.0
Hydromox	974.3	E858.5	E944.3	E950.4	E962.0	E980.4
Hydrophilic lotion	976.3	E858.7	E946.3	E950.4	E962.0	E980.4
Hydroquinone	983.0	E864.0	—	E950.7	E962.1	E980.6
vapor	987.8	E869.8	—	E952.8	E962.2	E982.8
Hydrosulfuric acid (gas)	987.8	E869.8	—	E952.8	E962.2	E982.8
Hydrous wool fat (lotion)	976.3	E858.7	E946.3	E950.4	E962.0	E980.4
Hydroxide, caustic	983.2	E864.2	—	E950.7	E962.1	E980.6
Hydroxocobalamin	964.1	E858.2	E934.1	E950.4	E962.0	E980.4
Hydroxyamphetamine	971.2	E855.5	E941.2	E950.4	E962.0	E980.4
Hydroxychloroquine	961.4	E857	E931.4	E950.4	E962.0	E980.4
Hydroxydihydrocodeinone	965.09	E850.2	E935.2	E950.0	E962.0	E980.0
Hydroxyethyl starch	964.8	E858.2	E934.8	E950.4	E962.0	E980.4
Hydroxyphenamate	969.5	E853.8	E939.5	E950.3	E962.0	E980.3
Hydroxyphenylbutazone	965.5	E850.5	E935.5	E950.0	E962.0	E980.0
Hydroxyprogesterone	962.2	E858.0	E932.2	E950.4	E962.0	E980.4
Hydroxyquinoline derivatives	961.3	E857	E931.3	E950.4	E962.0	E980.4
Hydroxystilbamidine	961.5	E857	E931.5	E950.4	E962.0	E980.4
Hydroxyurea	963.1	E858.1	E933.1	E950.4	E962.0	E980.4
Hydroxyzine	969.5	E853.8	E939.5	E950.3	E962.0	E980.3
Hyoscine (hydrobromide)	971.1	E855.4	E941.1	E950.4	E962.0	E980.4
Hyoscyamine	971.1	E855.4	E941.1	E950.4	E962.0	E980.4
Hyoscyamus (albus) (niger)	988.2	E865.4	—	E950.9	E962.1	E980.9
Hypaque	977.8	E858.8	E947.8	E950.4	E962.0	E980.4
Hypertussis	964.6	E858.2	E934.6	E950.4	E962.0	E980.4
Hypnotics NEC	967.9	E852.9	E937.9	E950.2	E962.0	E980.2
Hypochlorites — see Sodium, hypochlorite						
Hypotensive agents NEC	972.6	E858.3	E942.6	E950.4	E962.0	E980.4
Ibufenac	965.69	E850.6	E935.6	E950.0	E962.0	E980.0
Ibuprofen	965.61	E850.6	E935.6	E950.0	E962.0	E980.0
ICG	977.8	E858.8	E947.8	E950.4	E962.0	E980.4
Ichthammol	976.4	E858.7	E946.4	E950.4	E962.0	E980.4
Ichthyol	976.4	E858.7	E946.4	E950.4	E962.0	E980.4
Idoxuridine	976.5	E858.7	E946.5	E950.4	E962.0	E980.4

	Poisoning	Accident	Therapeutic Use	Suicide Attempt	Assault	Undeter-mined
IDU	976.5	E858.7	E946.5	E950.4	E962.0	E980.4
Iletin	962.3	E858.0	E932.3	E950.4	E962.0	E980.4
Ilex	988.2	E865.4	—	E950.9	E962.1	E980.9
Illuminating gas — see Gas, utility						
Ilopan	963.5	E858.1	E933.5	E950.4	E962.0	E980.4
Ilotycin	960.3	E856	E930.3	E950.4	E962.0	E980.4
ophthalmic preparation	976.5	E858.7	E946.5	E950.4	E962.0	E980.4
topical NEC	976.0	E858.7	E946.0	E950.4	E962.0	E980.4
Imipramine	969.05	E854.0	E939.0	E950.3	E962.0	E980.3
Immu-G	964.6	E858.2	E934.6	E950.4	E962.0	E980.4
Immuglobin	964.6	E858.2	E934.6	E950.4	E962.0	E980.4
Immune serum globulin	964.6	E858.2	E934.6	E950.4	E962.0	E980.4
Immunosuppressive agents	963.1	E858.1	E933.1	E950.4	E962.0	E980.4
Immu-tetanus	964.6	E858.2	E934.6	E950.4	E962.0	E980.4
Indandione (derivatives)	964.2	E858.2	E934.2	E950.4	E962.0	E980.4
Inderal	972.0	E858.3	E942.0	E950.4	E962.0	E980.4
Indian						
hemp	969.6	E854.1	E939.6	E950.3	E962.0	E980.3
tobacco	988.2	E865.4	—	E950.9	E962.1	E980.9
Indigo carmine	977.8	E858.8	E947.8	E950.4	E962.0	E980.4
Indocin	965.69	E850.6	E935.6	E950.0	E962.0	E980.0
Indocyanine green	977.8	E858.8	E947.8	E950.4	E962.0	E980.4
Indomethacin	965.69	E850.6	E935.6	E950.0	E962.0	E980.0
Industrial						
alcohol	980.9	E860.9	—	E950.9	E962.1	E980.9
fumes	987.8	E869.8	—	E952.8	E962.2	E982.8
solvents (fumes) (vapors)	982.8	E862.9	—	E950.9	E962.1	E980.9
Influenza vaccine	979.6	E858.8	E949.6	E950.4	E962.0	E980.4
Ingested substances NEC	989.9	E866.9	—	E950.9	E962.1	E980.9
INH (isoniazid)	961.8	E857	E931.8	E950.4	E962.0	E980.4
Inhalation, gas (noxious) — see Gas						
Ink	989.89	E866.8	—	E950.9	E962.1	E980.9
Innovar	967.6	E852.5	E937.6	E950.2	E962.0	E980.2
Inositol niacinate	972.2	E858.3	E942.2	E950.4	E962.0	E980.4
Inproquone	963.1	E858.1	E933.1	E950.4	E962.0	E980.4
Insecticides — see also Pesticides	989.4	E863.4	—	E950.6	E962.1	E980.7
chlorinated	989.2	E863.0	—	E950.6	E962.1	E980.7
mixtures	989.4	E863.3	—	E950.6	E962.1	E980.7
organochlorine (compounds)	989.2	E863.0	—	E950.6	E962.1	E980.7
organophosphorus (compounds)	989.3	E863.1	—	E950.6	E962.1	E980.7
Insect (sting), venomous	989.5	E905.5	—	E950.9	E962.1	E980.9
Insular tissue extract	962.3	E858.0	E932.3	E950.4	E962.0	E980.4
Insulin (amorphous) (globin) (isophane) (Lente) (NPH) (protamine) (Semilente) (Ultralente) (zinc)	962.3	E858.0	E932.3	E950.4	E962.0	E980.4
Intranarcon	968.3	E855.1	E938.3	E950.4	E962.0	E980.4
Inulin	977.8	E858.8	E947.8	E950.4	E962.0	E980.4
Invert sugar	974.5	E858.5	E944.5	E950.4	E962.0	E980.4
Inza — see Naproxen						
Iodide NEC — see also Iodine	976.0	E858.7	E946.0	E950.4	E962.0	E980.4
mercury (ointment)	976.0	E858.7	E946.0	E950.4	E962.0	E980.4
methylate	976.0	E858.7	E946.0	E950.4	E962.0	E980.4
potassium (expectorant) NEC	975.5	E858.6	E945.5	E950.4	E962.0	E980.4
Iodinated glycerol	975.5	E858.6	E945.5	E950.4	E962.0	E980.4
Iodine (antiseptic, external) (tincture) NEC	976.0	E858.7	E946.0	E950.4	E962.0	E980.4
diagnostic	977.8	E858.8	E947.8	E950.4	E962.0	E980.4
for thyroid conditions (antithyroid)	962.8	E858.0	E932.8	E950.4	E962.0	E980.4
vapor	987.8	E869.8	—	E952.8	E962.2	E982.8
Iodized oil	977.8	E858.8	E947.8	E950.4	E962.0	E980.4
Iodobismitol	961.2	E857	E931.2	E950.4	E962.0	E980.4
Iodochlorhydroxyquin	961.3	E857	E931.3	E950.4	E962.0	E980.4
topical	976.0	E858.7	E946.0	E950.4	E962.0	E980.4
Iodoform	976.0	E858.7	E946.0	E950.4	E962.0	E980.4
Iodopanoic acid	977.8	E858.8	E947.8	E950.4	E962.0	E980.4
Iodophthalein	977.8	E858.8	E947.8	E950.4	E962.0	E980.4
Ion exchange resins	974.5	E858.5	E944.5	E950.4	E962.0	E980.4
Iopanoic acid	977.8	E858.8	E947.8	E950.4	E962.0	E980.4
Iophendylate	977.8	E858.8	E947.8	E950.4	E962.0	E980.4
Iothiouracil	962.8	E858.0	E932.8	E950.4	E962.0	E980.4
Ipecac	973.6	E858.4	E943.6	E950.4	E962.0	E980.4
Ipecacuanha	973.6	E858.4	E943.6	E950.4	E962.0	E980.4

Nontherapeutic use substance

	External Cause (E-Code)					
	Poisoning	Accident	Therapeutic Use	Suicide Attempt	Assault	Undetermined
Ipodate	977.8	E858.8	E947.8	E950.4	E962.0	E980.4
Ipral	967.0	E851	E937.0	E950.1	E962.0	E980.1
Ipratropium	975.1	E858.6	E945.1	E950.4	E962.0	E980.4
Iproniazid	969.01	E854.0	E939.0	E950.3	E962.0	E980.3
Iron (compounds) (medicinal)						
(preparations)	964.0	E858.2	E934.0	E950.4	E962.0	E980.4
dextran	964.0	E858.2	E934.0	E950.4	E962.0	E980.4
nonmedicinal (dust) (fumes) NEC	985.8	E866.4	—	E950.9	E962.1	E980.9
Irritant drug	977.9	E858.9	E947.9	E950.5	E962.0	E980.5
Ismelin	972.6	E858.3	E942.6	E950.4	E962.0	E980.4
Isoamyl nitrite	972.4	E858.3	E942.4	E950.4	E962.0	E980.4
Isobutyl acetate	982.8	E862.4	—	E950.9	E962.1	E980.9
Isocarboxazid	969.01	E854.0	E939.0	E950.3	E962.0	E980.3
Isoephedrine	971.2	E855.5	E941.2	E950.4	E962.0	E980.4
Isoetharine	971.2	E855.5	E941.2	E950.4	E962.0	E980.4
Isofluorophate	971.0	E855.3	E941.0	E950.4	E962.0	E980.4
Isoniazid (INH)	961.8	E857	E931.8	E950.4	E962.0	E980.4
Isopentaquine	961.4	E857	E931.4	E950.4	E962.0	E980.4
Isophane insulin	962.3	E858.0	E932.3	E950.4	E962.0	E980.4
Isopregnenone	962.2	E858.0	E932.2	E950.4	E962.0	E980.4
Isoprenaline	971.2	E855.5	E941.2	E950.4	E962.0	E980.4
Isopropamide	971.1	E855.4	E941.1	E950.4	E962.0	E980.4
Isopropanol	980.2	E860.3	—	E950.9	E962.1	E980.9
topical (germicide)	976.0	E858.7	E946.0	E950.4	E962.0	E980.4
Isopropyl						
acetate	982.8	E862.4	—	E950.9	E962.1	E980.9
alcohol	980.2	E860.3	—	E950.9	E962.1	E980.9
topical (germicide)	976.0	E858.7	E946.0	E950.4	E962.0	E980.4
ether	982.8	E862.4	—	E950.9	E962.1	E980.9
Isoproterenol	971.2	E855.5	E941.2	E950.4	E962.0	E980.4
Isosorbide dinitrate	972.4	E858.3	E942.4	E950.4	E962.0	E980.4
Isothipendyl	963.0	E858.1	E933.0	E950.4	E962.0	E980.4
Isoxazolyl penicillin	960.0	E856	E930.0	E950.4	E962.0	E980.4
Isoxsuprine hydrochloride	972.5	E858.3	E942.5	E950.4	E962.0	E980.4
l-thyroxine sodium	962.7	E858.0	E932.7	E950.4	E962.0	E980.4
Jaborandi (pilocarpus) (extract)	971.0	E855.3	E941.0	E950.4	E962.0	E980.4
Jalap	973.1	E858.4	E943.1	E950.4	E962.0	E980.4
Jamaica						
dogwood (bark)	965.7	E850.7	E935.7	E950.0	E962.0	E980.0
ginger	989.89	E866.8	—	E950.9	E962.1	E980.9
Jatropha	988.2	E865.4	—	E950.9	E962.1	E980.9
curcas	988.2	E865.3	—	E950.9	E962.1	E980.9
Jectofer	964.0	E858.2	E934.0	E950.4	E962.0	E980.4
Jellyfish (sting)	989.5	E905.6	—	E950.9	E962.1	E980.9
Jequirity (bean)	988.2	E865.3	—	E950.9	E962.1	E980.9
Jimson weed	988.2	E865.4	—	E950.9	E962.1	E980.9
seeds	988.2	E865.3	—	E950.9	E962.1	E980.9
Juniper tar (oil) (ointment)	976.4	E858.7	E946.4	E950.4	E962.0	E980.4
Kallikrein	972.5	E858.3	E942.5	E950.4	E962.0	E980.4
Kanamycin	960.6	E856	E930.6	E950.4	E962.0	E980.4
Kantrex	960.6	E856	E930.6	E950.4	E962.0	E980.4
Kaolin	973.5	E858.4	E943.5	E950.4	E962.0	E980.4
Karaya (gum)	973.3	E858.4	E943.3	E950.4	E962.0	E980.4
Kemithal	968.3	E855.1	E938.3	E950.4	E962.0	E980.4
Kenacort	962.0	E858.0	E932.0	E950.4	E962.0	E980.4
Keratolytics	976.4	E858.7	E946.4	E950.4	E962.0	E980.4
Keratoplastics	976.4	E858.7	E946.4	E950.4	E962.0	E980.4
Kerosene, kerosine (fuel) (solvent) NEC	981	E862.1	—	E950.9	E962.1	E980.9
insecticide	981	E863.4	—	E950.6	E962.1	E980.7
vapor	987.1	E869.8	—	E952.8	E962.2	E982.8
Ketamine	968.3	E855.1	E938.3	E950.4	E962.0	E980.4
Ketobemidone	965.09	E850.2	E935.2	E950.0	E962.0	E980.0
Ketols	982.8	E862.4	—	E950.9	E962.1	E980.9
Ketone oils	982.8	E862.4	—	E950.9	E962.1	E980.9
Ketoprofen	965.61	E850.6	E935.6	E950.0	E962.0	E980.0
Kiln gas or vapor (carbon monoxide)	986	E868.8	—	E952.1	E962.2	E982.1
Konsyl	973.3	E858.4	E943.3	E950.4	E962.0	E980.4
Kosam seed	988.2	E865.3	—	E950.9	E962.1	E980.9
Krait (venom)	989.5	E905.0	—	E950.9	E962.1	E980.9
Kwell (insecticide)	989.2	E863.0	—	E950.6	E962.1	E980.7
anti-infective (topical)	976.0	E858.7	E946.0	E950.4	E962.0	E980.4
Laburnum (flowers) (seeds)	988.2	E865.3	—	E950.9	E962.1	E980.9
leaves	988.2	E865.4	—	E950.9	E962.1	E980.9
Lacquers	989.89	E861.6	—	E950.9	E962.1	E980.9
Lacrimogenic gas	987.5	E869.3	—	E952.8	E962.2	E982.8

	External Cause (E-Code)					
	Poisoning	Accident	Therapeutic Use	Suicide Attempt	Assault	Undetermined
Lactic acid	983.1	E864.1	—	E950.7	E962.1	E980.6
Lactobacillus acidophilus	973.5	E858.4	E943.5	E950.4	E962.0	E980.4
Lactoflavin	963.5	E858.1	E933.5	E950.4	E962.0	E980.4
Lactuca (virosa) (extract)	967.8	E852.8	E937.8	E950.2	E962.0	E980.2
Lactucarium	967.8	E852.8	E937.8	E950.2	E962.0	E980.2
Laevulose	974.5	E858.5	E944.5	E950.4	E962.0	E980.4
Lanatoside (C)	972.1	E858.3	E942.1	E950.4	E962.0	E980.4
Lanolin (lotion)	976.3	E858.7	E946.3	E950.4	E962.0	E980.4
Largactil	969.1	E853.0	E939.1	E950.3	E962.0	E980.3
Larkspur	988.2	E865.3	—	E950.9	E962.1	E980.9
Laroxyl	969.05	E854.0	E939.0	E950.3	E962.0	E980.3
Lasix	974.4	E858.5	E944.4	E950.4	E962.0	E980.4
Latex	989.82	E866.8	—	E950.9	E962.1	E980.9
Lathyrus (seed)	988.2	E865.3	—	E950.9	E962.1	E980.9
Laudanum	965.09	E850.2	E935.2	E950.0	E962.0	E980.0
Laudexium	975.2	E858.6	E945.2	E950.4	E962.0	E980.4
Laurel, black or cherry	988.2	E865.4	—	E950.9	E962.1	E980.9
Laurolinium	976.0	E858.7	E946.0	E950.4	E962.0	E980.4
Lauryl sulfoacetate	976.2	E858.7	E946.2	E950.4	E962.0	E980.4
Laxatives NEC	973.3	E858.4	E943.3	E950.4	E962.0	E980.4
emollient	973.2	E858.4	E943.2	E950.4	E962.0	E980.4
L-dopa	966.4	E855.0	E936.4	E950.4	E962.0	E980.4
Lead (dust) (fumes) (vapor)						
NEC	984.9	E866.0	—	E950.9	E962.1	E980.9
acetate (dust)	984.1	E866.0	—	E950.9	E962.1	E980.9
anti-infectives	961.2	E857	E931.2	E950.4	E962.0	E980.4
antiknock compound (tetraethyl)	984.1	E862.1	—	E950.9	E962.1	E980.9
arsenate, arsenite (dust) (insecticide) (vapor)	985.1	E863.4	—	E950.8	E962.1	E980.8
herbicide	985.1	E863.5	—	E950.8	E962.1	E980.8
carbonate	984.0	E866.0	—	E950.9	E962.1	E980.9
paint	984.0	E861.5	—	E950.9	E962.1	E980.9
chromate	984.0	E866.0	—	E950.9	E962.1	E980.9
paint	984.0	E861.5	—	E950.9	E962.1	E980.9
dioxide	984.0	E866.0	—	E950.9	E962.1	E980.9
inorganic (compound)	984.0	E866.0	—	E950.9	E962.1	E980.9
paint	984.0	E861.5	—	E950.9	E962.1	E980.9
iodide	984.0	E866.0	—	E950.9	E962.1	E980.9
pigment (paint)	984.0	E861.5	—	E950.9	E962.1	E980.9
monoxide (dust)	984.0	E866.0	—	E950.9	E962.1	E980.9
paint	984.0	E861.5	—	E950.9	E962.1	E980.9
organic	984.1	E866.0	—	E950.9	E962.1	E980.9
oxide	984.0	E866.0	—	E950.9	E962.1	E980.9
paint	984.0	E861.5	—	E950.9	E962.1	E980.9
paint	984.0	E861.5	—	E950.9	E962.1	E980.9
salts	984.0	E866.0	—	E950.9	E962.1	E980.9
specified compound NEC	984.8	E866.0	—	E950.9	E962.1	E980.9
tetra-ethyl	984.1	E862.1	—	E950.9	E962.1	E980.9
Lebanese red	969.6	E854.1	E939.6	E950.3	E962.0	E980.3
Lente Iletin (insulin)	962.3	E858.0	E932.3	E950.4	E962.0	E980.4
Leptazol	970.0	E854.3	E940.0	E950.4	E962.0	E980.4
Leritine	965.09	E850.2	E935.2	E950.0	E962.0	E980.0
Letter	962.7	E858.0	E932.7	E950.4	E962.0	E980.4
Lettuce opium	967.8	E852.8	E937.8	E950.2	E962.0	E980.2
Leucovorin (factor)	964.1	E858.2	E934.1	E950.4	E962.0	E980.4
Leukeran	963.1	E858.1	E933.1	E950.4	E962.0	E980.4
Levalbuterol	975.7	E858.6	E945.7	E950.4	E962.0	E980.4
Levallorphan	970.1	E854.3	E940.1	E950.4	E962.0	E980.4
Levanil	967.8	E852.8	E937.8	E950.2	E962.0	E980.2
Levarterenol	971.2	E855.5	E941.2	E950.4	E962.0	E980.4
Levodopa	966.4	E855.0	E936.4	E950.4	E962.0	E980.4
Levo-dromoran	965.09	E850.2	E935.2	E950.0	E962.0	E980.0
Levoid	962.7	E858.0	E932.7	E950.4	E962.0	E980.4
Levo-iso-methadone	965.02	E850.1	E935.1	E950.0	E962.0	E980.0
Levomepromazine	967.8	E852.8	E937.8	E950.2	E962.0	E980.2
Levoprome	967.8	E852.8	E937.8	E950.2	E962.0	E980.2
Levopropoxyphene	975.4	E858.6	E945.4	E950.4	E962.0	E980.4
Levorphan, levophanol	965.09	E850.2	E935.2	E950.0	E962.0	E980.0
Levothyroxine (sodium)	962.7	E858.0	E932.7	E950.4	E962.0	E980.4
Levsin	971.1	E855.4	E941.1	E950.4	E962.0	E980.4
Levulose	974.5	E858.5	E944.5	E950.4	E962.0	E980.4
Lewisite (gas)	985.1	E866.3	—	E950.8	E962.1	E980.8
Librium	969.4	E853.2	E939.4	E950.3	E962.0	E980.3
Lidex	976	E858.7	E946.0	E950.4	E962.0	E980.4
Lidocaine (infiltration) (topical)	968.5	E855.2	E938.5	E950.4	E962.0	E980.4
nerve block (peripheral) (plexus)	968.6	E855.2	E938.6	E950.4	E962.0	E980.4
spinal	968.7	E855.2	E938.7	E950.4	E962.0	E980.4
Lighter fluid	981	E862.1	—	E950.9	E962.1	E980.9

Nontherapeutic use substance

▶◀ Revised Text   ● New Line   ▲ Revised Code   Subterms under main terms may continue to next column or page

	External Cause (E-Code)					
	Poisoning	Accident	Therapeutic Use	Suicide Attempt	Assault	Undetermined
Lignocaine (infiltration) (topical)	968.5	E855.2	E938.5	E950.4	E962.0	E980.4
nerve block (peripheral) (plexus)	968.6	E855.2	E938.6	E950.4	E962.0	E980.4
spinal	968.7	E855.2	E938.7	E950.4	E962.0	E980.4
Ligroin(e) (solvent)	981	E862.0	—	E950.9	E962.1	E980.9
vapor	987.1	E869.8	—	E952.8	E962.2	E982.8
Ligustrum vulgare	988.2	E865.3	—	E950.9	E962.1	E980.9
Lily of the valley	988.2	E865.4	—	E950.9	E962.1	E980.9
Lime (chloride)	983.2	E864.2	—	E950.7	E962.1	E980.6
solution, sulferated	976.4	E858.7	E946.4	E950.4	E962.0	E980.4
Limonene	982.8	E862.4	—	E950.9	E962.1	E980.9
Lincomycin	960.8	E856	E930.8	E950.4	E962.0	E980.4
Lindane (insecticide) (vapor)	989.2	E863.0	—	E950.6	E962.1	E980.7
anti-infective (topical)	976.0	E858.7	E946.0	E950.4	E962.0	E980.4
Liniments NEC	976.9	E858.7	E946.9	E950.4	E962.0	E980.4
Linoleic acid	972.2	E858.3	E942.2	E950.4	E962.0	E980.4
Liothyronine	962.7	E858.0	E932.7	E950.4	E962.0	E980.4
Liotrix	962.7	E858.0	E932.7	E950.4	E962.0	E980.4
Lipancreatin	973.4	E858.4	E943.4	E950.4	E962.0	E980.4
Lipo-Lutin	962.2	E858.0	E932.2	E950.4	E962.0	E980.4
Lipotropic agents	977.1	E858.8	E947.1	E950.4	E962.0	E980.4
Liquefied petroleum gases	987.0	E868.0	—	E951.1	E962.2	E981.1
piped (pure or mixed with air)	987.0	E867	—	E951.0	E962.2	E981.0
Liquid petrolatum	973.2	E858.4	E943.2	E950.4	E962.0	E980.4
substance	989.9	E866.9	—	E950.9	E962.1	E980.9
specified NEC	989.89	E866.8	—	E950.9	E962.1	E980.9
Lirugen	979.4	E858.8	E949.4	E950.4	E962.0	E980.4
Lithane	969.8	E855.8	E939.8	E950.3	E962.0	E980.3
Lithium	985.8	E866.4	—	E950.9	E962.1	E980.9
carbonate	969.8	E855.8	E939.8	E950.3	E962.0	E980.3
Lithonate	969.8	E855.8	E939.8	E950.3	E962.0	E980.3
Liver (extract) (injection) (preparations)	964.1	E858.2	E934.1	E950.4	E962.0	E980.4
Lizard (bite) (venom)	989.5	E905.0	—	E950.9	E962.1	E980.9
LMD	964.8	E858.2	E934.8	E950.4	E962.0	E980.4
Lobelia	988.2	E865.4	—	E950.9	E962.1	E980.9
Lobeline	970.0	E854.3	E940.0	E950.4	E962.0	E980.4
Locorten	976.0	E858.7	E946.0	E950.4	E962.0	E980.4
Lolium temulentum	988.2	E865.3	—	E950.9	E962.1	E980.9
Lomotil	973.5	E858.4	E943.5	E950.4	E962.0	E980.4
Lomustine	963.1	E858.1	E933.1	E950.4	E962.0	E980.4
Lophophora williamsii	969.6	E854.1	E939.6	E950.3	E962.0	E980.3
Lorazepam	969.4	E853.2	E939.4	E950.3	E962.0	E980.3
Lotions NEC	976.9	E858.7	E946.9	E950.4	E962.0	E980.4
Lotronex	973.8	E858.4	E943.8	E950.4	E962.0	E980.4
Lotusate	967.0	E851	E937.0	E950.1	E962.0	E980.1
Lowila	976.2	E858.7	E946.2	E950.4	E962.0	E980.4
Loxapine	969.3	E853.8	E939.3	E950.3	E962.0	E980.3
Lozenges (throat)	976.6	E858.7	E946.6	E950.4	E962.0	E980.4
LSD (25)	969.6	E854.1	E939.6	E950.3	E962.0	E980.3
L-Tryptophan — see amino acid						
Lubricating oil NEC	981	E862.2	—	E950.9	E962.1	E980.9
Lucanthone	961.6	E857	E931.6	E950.4	E962.0	E980.4
Luminal	967.0	E851	E937.0	E950.1	E962.0	E980.1
Lung irritant (gas) NEC	987.9	E869.9	—	E952.9	E962.2	E982.9
Lutocylol	962.2	E858.0	E932.2	E950.4	E962.0	E980.4
Lutromone	962.2	E858.0	E932.2	E950.4	E962.0	E980.4
Lututrin	975.0	E858.6	E945.0	E950.4	E962.0	E980.4
Lye (concentrated)	983.2	E864.2	—	E950.7	E962.1	E980.6
Lygranum (skin test)	977.8	E858.8	E947.8	E950.4	E962.0	E980.4
Lymecycline	960.4	E856	E930.4	E950.4	E962.0	E980.4
Lymphogranuloma venereum antigen	977.8	E858.8	E947.8	E950.4	E962.0	E980.4
Lynestrenol	962.2	E858.0	E932.2	E950.4	E962.0	E980.4
Lyovac Sodium Edecrin	974.4	E858.5	E944.4	E950.4	E962.0	E980.4
Lypressin	962.5	E858.0	E932.5	E950.4	E962.0	E980.4
Lysergic acid (amide) (diethylamide)	969.6	E854.1	E939.6	E950.3	E962.0	E980.3
Lysergide	969.6	E854.1	E939.6	E950.3	E962.0	E980.3
Lysine vasopressin	962.5	E858.0	E932.5	E950.4	E962.0	E980.4
Lysol	983.0	E864.0	—	E950.7	E962.1	E980.6
Lytta (vitatta)	976.8	E858.7	E946.8	E950.4	E962.0	E980.4
Mace	987.5	E869.3	—	E952.8	E962.2	E982.8
Macrolides (antibiotics)	960.3	E856	E930.3	E950.4	E962.0	E980.4
Mafenide	976.0	E858.7	E946.0	E950.4	E962.0	E980.4
Magaldrate	973.0	E858.4	E943.0	E950.4	E962.0	E980.4
Magic mushroom	969.6	E854.1	E939.6	E950.3	E962.0	E980.3

	External Cause (E-Code)					
	Poisoning	Accident	Therapeutic Use	Suicide Attempt	Assault	Undetermined
Magnamycin	960.8	E856	E930.8	E950.4	E962.0	E980.4
Magnesia magma	973.0	E858.4	E943.0	E950.4	E962.0	E980.4
Magnesium (compounds) (fumes) NEC	985.8	E866.4	—	E950.9	E962.1	E980.9
antacid	973.0	E858.4	E943.0	E950.4	E962.0	E980.4
carbonate	973.0	E858.4	E943.0	E950.4	E962.0	E980.4
cathartic	973.3	E858.4	E943.3	E950.4	E962.0	E980.4
citrate	973.3	E858.4	E943.3	E950.4	E962.0	E980.4
hydroxide	973.0	E858.4	E943.0	E950.4	E962.0	E980.4
oxide	973.0	E858.4	E943.0	E950.4	E962.0	E980.4
sulfate (oral)	973.3	E858.4	E943.3	E950.4	E962.0	E980.4
intravenous	966.3	E855.0	E936.3	E950.4	E962.0	E980.4
trisilicate	973.0	E858.4	E943.0	E950.4	E962.0	E980.4
Malathion (insecticide)	989.3	E863.1	—	E950.6	E962.1	E980.7
Male fern (oleoresin)	961.6	E857	E931.6	E950.4	E962.0	E980.4
Mandelic acid	961.9	E857	E931.9	E950.4	E962.0	E980.4
Manganese compounds (fumes) NEC	985.2	E866.4	—	E950.9	E962.1	E980.9
Mannitol (diuretic) (medicinal) NEC	974.4	E858.5	E944.4	E950.4	E962.0	E980.4
hexanitrate	972.4	E858.3	E942.4	E950.4	E962.0	E980.4
mustard	963.1	E858.1	E933.1	E950.4	E962.0	E980.4
Mannomustine	963.1	E858.1	E933.1	E950.4	E962.0	E980.4
MAO inhibitors	969.01	E854.0	E939.0	E950.3	E962.0	E980.3
Mapharsen	961.1	E857	E931.1	E950.4	E962.0	E980.4
Marcaine	968.9	E855.2	E938.9	E950.4	E962.0	E980.4
infiltration (subcutaneous)	968.5	E855.2	E938.5	E950.4	E962.0	E980.4
nerve block (peripheral) (plexus)	968.6	E855.2	E938.6	E950.4	E962.0	E980.4
Marezine	963.0	E858.1	E933.0	E950.4	E962.0	E980.4
Marihuana, marijuana (derivatives)	969.6	E854.1	E939.6	E950.3	E962.0	E980.3
Marine animals or plants (sting)	989.5	E905.6	—	E950.9	E962.1	E980.9
Marplan	969.01	E854.0	E939.0	E950.3	E962.0	E980.3
Marsh gas	987.1	E869.8	—	E952.8	E962.2	E982.8
Marsilid	969.01	E854.0	E939.0	E950.3	E962.0	E980.3
Matulane	963.1	E858.1	E933.1	E950.4	E962.0	E980.4
Mazindol	977.0	E858.8	E947.0	E950.4	E962.0	E980.4
MDMA	969.72	E854.2	E939.7	E950.3	E962.0	E980.3
Meadow saffron	988.2	E865.3	—	E950.9	E962.1	E980.9
Measles vaccine	979.4	E858.8	E949.4	E950.4	E962.0	E980.4
Meat, noxious or nonbacterial	988.8	E865.0	—	E950.9	E962.1	E980.9
Mebanazine	969.01	E854.0	E939.0	E950.3	E962.0	E980.3
Mebaral	967.0	E851	E937.0	E950.1	E962.0	E980.1
Mebendazole	961.6	E857	E931.6	E950.4	E962.0	E980.4
Mebeverine	975.1	E858.6	E945.1	E950.4	E962.0	E980.4
Mebhydroline	963.0	E858.1	E933.0	E950.4	E962.0	E980.4
Mebrophenhydramine	963.0	E858.1	E933.0	E950.4	E962.0	E980.4
Mebutamate	969.5	E853.8	E939.5	E950.3	E962.0	E980.3
Mecamylamine (chloride)	972.3	E858.3	E942.3	E950.4	E962.0	E980.4
Mechlorethamine hydrochloride	963.1	E858.1	E933.1	E950.4	E962.0	E980.4
Meclizene (hydrochloride)	963.0	E858.1	E933.0	E950.4	E962.0	E980.4
Meclofenoxate	970.0	E854.3	E940.0	E950.4	E962.0	E980.4
Meclozine (hydrochloride)	963.0	E858.1	E933.0	E950.4	E962.0	E980.4
Medazepam	969.4	E853.2	E939.4	E950.3	E962.0	E980.3
Medicine, medicinal substance	977.9	E858.9	E947.9	E950.5	E962.0	E980.5
specified NEC	977.8	E858.8	E947.8	E950.4	E962.0	E980.4
Medinal	967.0	E851	E937.0	E950.1	E962.0	E980.1
Medomin	967.0	E851	E937.0	E950.1	E962.0	E980.1
Medroxyprogesterone	962.2	E858.0	E932.2	E950.4	E962.0	E980.4
Medrysone	976.5	E858.7	E946.5	E950.4	E962.0	E980.4
Mefenamic acid	965.7	E850.7	E935.7	E950.0	E962.0	E980.0
Megahallucinogen	969.6	E854.1	E939.6	E950.3	E962.0	E980.3
Megestrol	962.2	E858.0	E932.2	E950.4	E962.0	E980.4
Meglumine	977.8	E858.8	E947.8	E950.4	E962.0	E980.4
Meladinin	976.3	E858.7	E946.3	E950.4	E962.0	E980.4
Melanizing agents	976.3	E858.7	E946.3	E950.4	E962.0	E980.4
Melarsoprol	961.1	E857	E931.1	E950.4	E962.0	E980.4
Melia azedarach	988.2	E865.3	—	E950.9	E962.1	E980.9
Mellaril	969.1	E853.0	E939.1	E950.3	E962.0	E980.3
Meloxine	976.3	E858.7	E946.3	E950.4	E962.0	E980.4
Melphalan	963.1	E858.1	E933.1	E950.4	E962.0	E980.4
Menadiol sodium diphosphate	964.3	E858.2	E934.3	E950.4	E962.0	E980.4
Menadione (sodium bisulfite)	964.3	E858.2	E934.3	E950.4	E962.0	E980.4
Menaphthone	964.3	E858.2	E934.3	E950.4	E962.0	E980.4

	Poisoning	Accident	Therapeutic Use	Suicide Attempt	Assault	Undetermined
Meningococcal vaccine	978.8	E858.8	E948.8	E950.4	E962.0	E980.4
Menningovax-C	978.8	E858.8	E948.8	E950.4	E962.0	E980.4
Menotropins	962.4	E858.0	E932.4	E950.4	E962.0	E980.4
Menthol NEC	976.1	E858.7	E946.1	E950.4	E962.0	E980.4
Mepacrine	961.3	E857	E931.3	E950.4	E962.0	E980.4
Meparfynol	967.8	E852.8	E937.8	E950.2	E962.0	E980.2
Mepazine	969.1	E853.0	E939.1	E950.3	E962.0	E980.3
Mepenzolate	971.1	E855.4	E941.1	E950.4	E962.0	E980.4
Meperidine	965.09	E850.2	E935.2	E950.0	E962.0	E980.0
Mephenamin(e)	966.4	E855.0	E936.4	E950.4	E962.0	E980.4
Mephenesin (carbamate)	968.0	E855.1	E938.0	E950.4	E962.0	E980.4
Mephenoxalone	969.5	E853.8	E939.5	E950.3	E962.0	E980.3
Mephentermine	971.2	E855.5	E941.2	E950.4	E962.0	E980.4
Mephenytoin	966.1	E855.0	E936.1	E950.4	E962.0	E980.4
Mephobarbital	967.0	E851	E937.0	E950.1	E962.0	E980.1
Mepiperphenidol	971.1	E855.4	E941.1	E950.4	E962.0	E980.4
Mepivacaine	968.9	E855.2	E938.9	E950.4	E962.0	E980.4
infiltration (subcutaneous)	968.5	E855.2	E938.5	E950.4	E962.0	E980.4
nerve block (peripheral) (plexus)	968.6	E855.2	E938.6	E950.4	E962.0	E980.4
topical (surface)	968.5	E855.2	E938.5	E950.4	E962.0	E980.4
Meprednisone	962.0	E858.0	E932.0	E950.4	E962.0	E980.4
Meprobam	969.5	E853.8	E939.5	E950.3	E962.0	E980.3
Meprobamate	969.5	E853.8	E939.5	E950.3	E962.0	E980.3
Mepyramine (maleate)	963.0	E858.1	E933.0	E950.4	E962.0	E980.4
Meralluride	974.0	E858.5	E944.0	E950.4	E962.0	E980.4
Merbaphen	974.0	E858.5	E944.0	E950.4	E962.0	E980.4
Merbromin	976.0	E858.7	E946.0	E950.4	E962.0	E980.4
Mercaptomerin	974.0	E858.5	E944.0	E950.4	E962.0	E980.4
Mercaptopurine	963.1	E858.1	E933.1	E950.4	E962.0	E980.4
Mercumatilin	974.0	E858.5	E944.0	E950.4	E962.0	E980.4
Mercuramide	974.0	E858.5	E944.0	E950.4	E962.0	E980.4
Mercuranin	976.0	E858.7	E946.0	E950.4	E962.0	E980.4
Mercurochrome	976.0	E858.7	E946.0	E950.4	E962.0	E980.4
Mercury, mercuric, mercurous (compounds) (cyanide) (fumes) (nonmedicinal) (vapor) NEC	985.0	E866.1	—	E950.9	E962.1	E980.9
ammoniated	976.0	E858.7	E946.0	E950.4	E962.0	E980.4
anti-infective	961.2	E857	E931.2	E950.4	E962.0	E980.4
topical	976.0	E858.7	E946.0	E950.4	E962.0	E980.4
chloride (antiseptic) NEC	976.0	E858.7	E946.0	E950.4	E962.0	E980.4
fungicide	985.0	E863.6	—	E950.6	E962.1	E980.7
diuretic compounds	974.0	E858.5	E944.0	E950.4	E962.0	E980.4
fungicide	985.0	E863.6	—	E950.6	E962.1	E980.7
organic (fungicide)	985.0	E863.6	—	E950.6	E962.1	E980.7
Merethoxylline	974.0	E858.5	E944.0	E950.4	E962.0	E980.4
Mersalyl	974.0	E858.5	E944.0	E950.4	E962.0	E980.4
Merthiolate (topical)	976.0	E858.7	E946.0	E950.4	E962.0	E980.4
ophthalmic preparation	976.5	E858.7	E946.5	E950.4	E962.0	E980.4
Meruvax	979.4	E858.8	E949.4	E950.4	E962.0	E980.4
Mescal buttons	969.6	E854.1	E939.6	E950.3	E962.0	E980.3
Mescaline (salts)	969.6	E854.1	E939.6	E950.3	E962.0	E980.3
Mesoridazine besylate	969.1	E853.0	E939.1	E950.3	E962.0	E980.3
Mestanolone	962.1	E858.0	E932.1	E950.4	E962.0	E980.4
Mestranol	962.2	E858.0	E932.2	E950.4	E962.0	E980.4
Metacresylacetate	976.0	E858.7	E946.0	E950.4	E962.0	E980.4
Metaldehyde (snail killer) NEC	989.4	E863.4	—	E950.6	E962.1	E980.7
Metals (heavy) (nonmedicinal) NEC	985.9	E866.4	—	E950.9	E962.1	E980.9
dust, fumes, or vapor NEC	985.9	E866.4	—	E950.9	E962.1	E980.9
light NEC	985.9	E866.4	—	E950.9	E962.1	E980.9
dust, fumes, or vapor NEC	985.9	E866.4	—	E950.9	E962.1	E980.9
pesticides (dust) (vapor)	985.9	E863.4	—	E950.6	E962.1	E980.7
Metamucil	973.3	E858.4	E943.3	E950.4	E962.0	E980.4
Metaphen	976.0	E858.7	E946.0	E950.4	E962.0	E980.4
Metaproterenol	975.1	E858.6	E945.1	E950.4	E962.0	E980.4
Metaraminol	972.8	E858.3	E942.8	E950.4	E962.0	E980.4
Metaxalone	968.0	E855.1	E938.0	E950.4	E962.0	E980.4
Metformin	962.3	E858.0	E932.3	E950.4	E962.0	E980.4
Methacycline	960.4	E856	E930.4	E950.4	E962.0	E980.4
Methadone	965.02	E850.1	E935.1	E950.0	E962.0	E980.0
Methallenestril	962.2	E858.0	E932.2	E950.4	E962.0	E980.4
Methamphetamine	969.72	E854.2	E939.7	E950.3	E962.0	E980.3
Methandienone	962.1	E858.0	E932.1	E950.4	E962.0	E980.4
Methandriol	962.1	E858.0	E932.1	E950.4	E962.0	E980.4
Methandrostenolone	962.1	E858.0	E932.1	E950.4	E962.0	E980.4
Methane gas	987.1	E869.8	—	E952.8	E962.2	E982.8

	Poisoning	Accident	Therapeutic Use	Suicide Attempt	Assault	Undetermined
Methanol	980.1	E860.2	—	E950.9	E962.1	E980.9
vapor	987.8	E869.8	—	E952.8	E962.2	E982.8
Methantheline	971.1	E855.4	E941.1	E950.4	E962.0	E980.4
Methaphenilene	963.0	E858.1	E933.0	E950.4	E962.0	E980.4
Methapyrilene	963.0	E858.1	E933.0	E950.4	E962.0	E980.4
Methaqualone (compounds)	967.4	E852.3	E937.4	E950.2	E962.0	E980.2
Metharbital, metharbitone	967.0	E851	E937.0	E950.1	E962.0	E980.1
Methazolamide	974.2	E858.5	E944.2	E950.4	E962.0	E980.4
Methdilazine	963.0	E858.1	E933.0	E950.4	E962.0	E980.4
Methedrine	969.72	E854.2	E939.7	E950.3	E962.0	E980.3
Methenamine (mandelate)	961.9	E857	E931.9	E950.4	E962.0	E980.4
Methenolone	962.1	E858.0	E932.1	E950.4	E962.0	E980.4
Methergine	975.0	E858.6	E945.0	E950.4	E962.0	E980.4
Methiacil	962.8	E858.0	E932.8	E950.4	E962.0	E980.4
Methicillin (sodium)	960.0	E856	E930.0	E950.4	E962.0	E980.4
Methimazole	962.8	E858.0	E932.8	E950.4	E962.0	E980.4
Methionine	977.1	E858.8	E947.1	E950.4	E962.0	E980.4
Methisazone	961.7	E857	E931.7	E950.4	E962.0	E980.4
Methitural	967.0	E851	E937.0	E950.1	E962.0	E980.1
Methixene	971.1	E855.4	E941.1	E950.4	E962.0	E980.4
Methobarbital, methobarbitone	967.0	E851	E937.0	E950.1	E962.0	E980.1
Methocarbamol	968.0	E855.1	E938.0	E950.4	E962.0	E980.4
Methohexital, methohexitone (sodium)	968.3	E855.1	E938.3	E950.4	E962.0	E980.4
Methoin	966.1	E855.0	E936.1	E950.4	E962.0	E980.4
Methopholine	965.7	E850.7	E935.7	E950.0	E962.0	E980.0
Methorate	975.4	E858.6	E945.4	E950.4	E962.0	E980.4
Methoserpidine	972.6	E858.3	E942.6	E950.4	E962.0	E980.4
Methotrexate	963.1	E858.1	E933.1	E950.4	E962.0	E980.4
Methotrimeprazine	967.8	E852.8	E937.8	E950.2	E962.0	E980.2
Methoxa-Dome	976.3	E858.7	E946.3	E950.4	E962.0	E980.4
Methoxamine	971.2	E855.5	E941.2	E950.4	E962.0	E980.4
Methoxsalen	976.3	E858.7	E946.3	E950.4	E962.0	E980.4
Methoxybenzyl penicillin	960.0	E856	E930.0	E950.4	E962.0	E980.4
Methoxychlor	989.2	E863.0	—	E950.6	E962.1	E980.7
Methoxyflurane	968.2	E855.1	E938.2	E950.4	E962.0	E980.4
Methoxyphenamine	971.2	E855.5	E941.2	E950.4	E962.0	E980.4
Methoxypromazine	969.1	E853.0	E939.1	E950.3	E962.0	E980.3
Methoxypsoralen	976.3	E858.7	E946.3	E950.4	E962.0	E980.4
Methscopolamine (bromide)	971.1	E855.4	E941.1	E950.4	E962.0	E980.4
Methsuximide	966.2	E855.0	E936.2	E950.4	E962.0	E980.4
Methyclothiazide	974.3	E858.5	E944.3	E950.4	E962.0	E980.4
Methyl						
acetate	982.8	E862.4		E950.9	E962.1	E980.9
acetone	982.8	E862.4	—	E950.9	E962.1	E980.9
alcohol	980.1	E860.2	—	E950.9	E962.1	E980.9
amphetamine	969.72	E854.2	E939.7	E950.3	E962.0	E980.3
androstanolone	962.1	E858.0	E932.1	E950.4	E962.0	E980.4
atropine	971.1	E855.4	E941.1	E950.4	E962.0	E980.4
benzene	982.0	E862.4		E950.9	E962.1	E980.9
bromide (gas)	987.8	E869.8	—	E952.8	E962.2	E982.8
fumigant	987.8	E863.8		E950.6	E962.2	E980.7
butanol	980.8	E860.8	—	E950.9	E962.1	E980.9
carbinol	980.1	E860.2	—	E950.9	E962.1	E980.9
cellosolve	982.8	E862.4		E950.9	E962.1	E980.9
cellulose	973.3	E858.4	E943.3	E950.4	E962.0	E980.4
chloride (gas)	987.8	E869.8	—	E952.8	E962.2	E982.8
cyclohexane	982.8	E862.4	—	E950.9	E962.1	E980.9
cyclohexanone	982.8	E862.4		E950.9	E962.1	E980.9
dihydromorphinone	965.09	E850.2	E935.2	E950.0	E962.0	E980.0
ergometrine	975.0	E858.6	E945.0	E950.4	E962.0	E980.4
ergonovine	975.0	E858.6	E945.0	E950.4	E962.0	E980.4
ethyl ketone	982.8	E862.4	—	E950.9	E962.1	E980.9
hydrazine	983.9	E864.3	—	E950.7	E962.1	E980.6
isobutyl ketone	982.8	E862.4	—	E950.9	E962.1	E980.9
morphine NEC	965.09	E850.2	E935.2	E950.0	E962.0	E980.0
parafynol	967.8	E852.8	E937.8	E950.2	E962.0	E980.2
parathion	989.3	E863.1	—	E950.6	E962.1	E980.7
pentynol NEC	967.8	E852.8	E937.8	E950.2	E962.0	E980.2
peridol	969.2	E853.1	E939.2	E950.3	E962.0	E980.3
phenidate	969.73	E854.2	E939.7	E950.3	E962.0	E980.3
prednisolone	962.0	E858.0	E932.0	E950.4	E962.0	E980.4
ENT agent	976.6	E858.7	E946.6	E950.4	E962.0	E980.4
ophthalmic preparation	976.5	E858.7	E946.5	E950.4	E962.0	E980.4
topical NEC	976.0	E858.7	E946.0	E950.4	E962.0	E980.4
propylcarbinol	980.8	E860.8	—	E950.9	E962.1	E980.9

	Poisoning	Accident	Therapeutic Use	Suicide Attempt	Assault	Undetermined
Methyl — *continued*						
rosaniline NEC	976.0	E858.7	E946.0	E950.4	E962.0	E980.4
salicylate NEC	976.3	E858.7	E946.3	E950.4	E962.0	E980.4
sulfate (fumes)	987.8	E869.8	—	E952.8	E962.2	E982.8
liquid	983.9	E864.3	—	E950.7	E962.1	E980.6
sulfonal	967.8	E852.8	E937.8	E950.2	E962.0	E980.2
testosterone	962.1	E858.0	E932.1	E950.4	E962.0	E980.4
thiouracil	962.8	E858.0	E932.8	E950.4	E962.0	E980.4
Methylated spirit	980.0	E860.1	—	E950.9	E962.1	E980.9
Methyldopa	972.6	E858.3	E942.6	E950.4	E962.0	E980.4
Methylene						
blue	961.9	E857	E931.9	E950.4	E962.0	E980.4
chloride or dichloride (solvent) NEC	982.3	E862.4	—	E950.9	E962.1	E980.9
Methylhexabital	967.0	E851	E937.0	E950.1	E962.0	E980.1
Methylparaben (ophthalmic)	976.5	E858.7	E946.5	E950.4	E962.0	E980.4
Methyprylon	967.5	E852.4	E937.5	E950.2	E962.0	E980.2
Methysergide	971.3	E855.6	E941.3	E950.4	E962.0	E980.4
Metoclopramide	963.0	E858.1	E933.0	E950.4	E962.0	E980.4
Metofoline	965.7	E850.7	E935.7	E950.0	E962.0	E980.0
Metopon	965.09	E850.2	E935.2	E950.0	E962.0	E980.0
Metronidazole	961.5	E857	E931.5	E950.4	E962.0	E980.4
Metycaine	968.9	E855.2	E938.9	E950.4	E962.0	E980.4
infiltration (subcutaneous)	968.5	E855.2	E938.5	E950.4	E962.0	E980.4
nerve block (peripheral) (plexus)	968.6	E855.2	E938.6	E950.4	E962.0	E980.4
topical (surface)	968.5	E855.2	E938.5	E950.4	E962.0	E980.4
Metyrapone	977.8	E858.8	E947.8	E950.4	E962.0	E980.4
Mevinphos	989.3	E863.1	—	E950.6	E962.1	E980.7
Mezereon (berries)	988.2	E865.3	—	E950.9	E962.1	E980.9
Micatin	976.0	E858.7	E946.0	E950.4	E962.0	E980.4
Miconazole	976.0	E858.7	E946.0	E950.4	E962.0	E980.4
Midol	965.1	E850.3	E935.3	E950.0	E962.0	E980.0
Mifepristone	962.9	E858.0	E932.9	E950.4	E962.0	E980.4
Milk of magnesia	973.0	E858.4	E943.0	E950.4	E962.0	E980.4
Millipede (tropical) (venomous)	989.5	E905.4	—	E950.9	E962.1	E980.9
Miltown	969.5	E853.8	E939.5	E950.3	E962.0	E980.3
Mineral						
oil (medicinal)	973.2	E858.4	E943.2	E950.4	E962.0	E980.4
nonmedicinal	981	E862.1	—	E950.9	E962.1	E980.9
topical	976.3	E858.7	E946.3	E950.4	E962.0	E980.4
salts NEC	974.6	E858.5	E944.6	E950.4	E962.0	E980.4
spirits	981	E862.0	—	E950.9	E962.1	E980.9
Minocycline	960.4	E856	E930.4	E950.4	E962.0	E980.4
Mithramycin (antineoplastic)	960.7	E856	E930.7	E950.4	E962.0	E980.4
Mitobronitol	963.1	E858.1	E933.1	E950.4	E962.0	E980.4
Mitomycin (antineoplastic)	960.7	E856	E930.7	E950.4	E962.0	E980.4
Mitotane	963.1	E858.1	E933.1	E950.4	E962.0	E980.4
Moderil	972.6	E858.3	E942.6	E950.4	E962.0	E980.4
Mogadon — *see* Nitrazepam						
Molindone	969.3	E853.8	E939.3	E950.3	E962.0	E980.3
Monistat	976.0	E858.7	E946.0	E950.4	E962.0	E980.4
Monkshood	988.2	E865.4	—	E950.9	E962.1	E980.9
Monoamine oxidase inhibitors	969.01	E854.0	E939.0	E950.3	E962.0	E980.3
Monochlorobenzene	982.0	E862.4	—	E950.9	E962.1	E980.9
Monosodium glutamate	989.89	E866.8	—	E950.9	E962.1	E980.9
Monoxide, carbon — *see* Carbon, monoxide						
Moperone	969.2	E853.1	E939.2	E950.3	E962.0	E980.3
Morning glory seeds	969.6	E854.1	E939.6	E950.3	E962.0	E980.3
Moroxydine (hydrochloride)	961.7	E857	E931.7	E950.4	E962.0	E980.4
Morphazinamide	961.8	E857	E931.8	E950.4	E962.0	E980.4
Morphinans	965.09	E850.2	E935.2	E950.0	E962.0	E980.0
Morphine NEC	965.09	E850.2	E935.2	E950.0	E962.0	E980.0
antagonists	970.1	E854.3	E940.1	E950.4	E962.0	E980.4
Morpholinylethylmorphine	965.09	E850.2	E935.2	E950.0	E962.0	E980.0
Morrhuate sodium	972.7	E858.3	E942.7	E950.4	E962.0	E980.4
Moth balls — *see also* Pesticides	989.4	E863.4	—	E950.6	E962.1	E980.7
naphthalene	983.0	E863.4	—	E950.7	E962.1	E980.6
Motor exhaust gas — *see* Carbon, monoxide, exhaust gas						
Mouth wash	976.6	E858.7	E946.6	E950.4	E962.0	E980.4

	Poisoning	Accident	Therapeutic Use	Suicide Attempt	Assault	Undetermined
Mucolytic agent	975.5	E858.6	E945.5	E950.4	E962.0	E980.4
Mucomyst	975.5	E858.6	E945.5	E950.4	E962.0	E980.4
Mucous membrane agents						
(external)	976.9	E858.7	E946.9	E950.4	E962.0	E980.4
specified NEC	976.8	E858.7	E946.8	E950.4	E962.0	E980.4
Mumps						
immune globulin (human)	964.6	E858.2	E934.6	E950.4	E962.0	E980.4
skin test antigen	977.8	E858.8	E947.8	E950.4	E962.0	E980.4
vaccine	979.6	E858.8	E949.6	E950.4	E962.0	E980.4
Mumpsvax	979.6	E858.8	E949.6	E950.4	E962.0	E980.4
Muriatic acid — *see* Hydrochloric acid						
Muscarine	971.0	E855.3	E941.0	E950.4	E962.0	E980.4
Muscle affecting agents						
NEC	975.3	E858.6	E945.3	E950.4	E962.0	E980.4
oxytocic	975.0	E858.6	E945.0	E950.4	E962.0	E980.4
relaxants	975.3	E858.6	E945.3	E950.4	E962.0	E980.4
central nervous system	968.0	E855.1	E938.0	E950.4	E962.0	E980.4
skeletal	975.2	E858.6	E945.2	E950.4	E962.0	E980.4
smooth	975.1	E858.6	E945.1	E950.4	E962.0	E980.4
Mushrooms, noxious	988.1	E865.5	—	E950.9	E962.1	E980.9
Mussel, noxious	988.0	E865.1	—	E950.9	E962.1	E980.9
Mustard (emetic)	973.6	E858.4	E943.6	E950.4	E962.0	E980.4
gas	987.8	E869.8	—	E952.8	E962.2	E982.8
nitrogen	963.1	E858.1	E933.1	E950.4	E962.0	E980.4
Mustine	963.1	E858.1	E933.1	E950.4	E962.0	E980.4
M-vac	979.4	E858.8	E949.4	E950.4	E962.0	E980.4
Mycifradin	960.8	E856	E930.8	E950.4	E962.0	E980.4
topical	976.0	E858.7	E946.0	E950.4	E962.0	E980.4
Mycitracin	960.8	E856	E930.8	E950.4	E962.0	E980.4
ophthalmic preparation	976.5	E858.7	E946.5	E950.4	E962.0	E980.4
Mycostatin	960.1	E856	E930.1	E950.4	E962.0	E980.4
topical	976.0	E858.7	E946.0	E950.4	E962.0	E980.4
Mydriacyl	971.1	E855.4	E941.1	E950.4	E962.0	E980.4
Myelobromal	963.1	E858.1	E933.1	E950.4	E962.0	E980.4
Myleran	963.1	E858.1	E933.1	E950.4	E962.0	E980.4
Myochrysin(e)	965.69	E850.6	E935.6	E950.0	E962.0	E980.0
Myoneural blocking agents	975.2	E858.6	E945.2	E950.4	E962.0	E980.4
Myristica fragrans	988.2	E865.3	—	E950.9	E962.1	E980.9
Myristicin	988.2	E865.3	—	E950.9	E962.1	E980.9
Mysoline	966.3	E855.0	E936.3	E950.4	E962.0	E980.4
Nafcillin (sodium)	960.0	E856	E930.0	E950.4	E962.0	E980.4
Nail polish remover	982.8	E862.4	—	E950.9	E962.1	E908.9
Nalidixic acid	961.9	E857	E931.9	E950.4	E962.0	E980.4
Nalorphine	970.1	E854.3	E940.1	E950.4	E962.0	E980.4
Naloxone	970.1	E854.3	E940.1	E950.4	E962.0	E980.4
Nandrolone (decanoate) (phenproprioate)	962.1	E858.0	E932.1	E950.4	E962.0	E980.4
Naphazoline	971.2	E855.5	E941.2	E950.4	E962.0	E980.4
Naphtha (painter's) (petroleum)	981	E862.0	—	E950.9	E962.1	E980.9
solvent	981	E862.0	—	E950.9	E962.1	E980.9
vapor	987.1	E869.8	—	E952.8	E962.2	E982.8
Naphthalene (chlorinated)	983.0	E864.0	—	E950.7	E962.1	E980.6
insecticide or moth repellent	983.0	E863.4	—	E950.7	E962.1	E980.6
vapor	987.8	E869.8	—	E952.8	E962.2	E982.8
Naphthol	983.0	E864.0	—	E950.7	E962.1	E980.6
Naphthylamine	983.0	E864.0	—	E950.7	E962.1	E980.6
Naprosyn — *see* Naproxen						
Naproxen	965.61	E850.6	E935.6	E950.0	E962.0	E980.0
Narcotic (drug)	967.9	E852.9	E937.9	E950.2	E962.0	E980.2
analgesic NEC	965.8	E850.8	E935.8	E950.0	E962.0	E980.0
antagonist	970.1	E854.3	E940.1	E950.4	E962.0	E980.4
specified NEC	967.8	E852.8	E937.8	E950.2	E962.0	E980.2
Narcotine	975.4	E858.6	E945.4	E950.4	E962.0	E980.4
Nardil	969.01	E854.0	E939.0	E950.3	E962.0	E980.3
Natrium cyanide — *see* Cyanide(s)						
Natural						
blood (product)	964.7	E858.2	E934.7	E950.4	E962.0	E980.4
gas (piped)	987.1	E867	—	E951.0	E962.2	E981.0
incomplete combustion	986	E867	—	E951.0	E962.2	E981.0
Nealbarbital, nealbarbitone	967.0	E851	E937.0	E950.1	E962.0	E980.1
Nectadon	975.4	E858.6	E945.4	E950.4	E962.0	E980.4
Nematocyst (sting)	989.5	E905.6	—	E950.9	E962.1	E980.9
Nembutal	967.0	E851	E937.0	E950.1	E962.0	E980.1
Neoarsphenamine	961.1	E857	E931.1	E950.4	E962.0	E980.4

Subterms under main terms may continue to next column or page

	Poisoning	Accident	Therapeutic Use	Suicide Attempt	Assault	Undetermined
Neocinchophen	974.7	E858.5	E944.7	E950.4	E962.0	E980.4
Neomycin	960.8	E856	E930.8	E950.4	E962.0	E980.4
ENT agent	976.6	E858.7	E946.6	E950.4	E962.0	E980.4
ophthalmic preparation	976.5	E858.7	E946.5	E950.4	E962.0	E980.4
topical NEC	976.0	E858.7	E946.0	E950.4	E962.0	E980.4
Neonal	967.0	E851	E937.0	E950.1	E962.0	E980.1
Neoprontosil	961.0	E857	E931.0	E950.4	E962.0	E980.4
Neosalvarsan	961.1	E857	E931.1	E950.4	E962.0	E980.4
Neosilversalvarsan	961.1	E857	E931.1	E950.4	E962.0	E980.4
Neosporin	960.8	E856	E930.8	E950.4	E962.0	E980.4
ENT agent	976.6	E858.7	E946.6	E950.4	E962.0	E980.4
opthalmic preparation	976.5	E858.7	E946.5	E950.4	E962.0	E980.4
topical NEC	976.0	E858.7	E946.0	E950.4	E962.0	E980.4
Neostigmine	971.0	E855.3	E941.0	E950.4	E962.0	E980.4
Neraval	967.0	E851	E937.0	E950.1	E962.0	E980.1
Neravan	967.0	E851	E937.0	E950.1	E962.0	E980.1
Nerium oleander	988.2	E865.4	—	E950.9	E962.1	E980.9
Nerve gases (war)	987.9	E869.9	—	E952.9	E962.2	E982.9
Nesacaine	968.9	E855.2	E938.9	E950.4	E962.0	E980.4
infiltration (subcutaneous)	968.5	E855.2	E938.5	E950.4	E962.0	E980.4
nerve block (peripheral) (plexus)	968.6	E855.2	E938.6	E950.4	E962.0	E980.4
Neurobarb	967.0	E851	E937.0	E950.1	E962.0	E980.1
Neuroleptics NEC	969.3	E853.8	E939.3	E950.3	E962.0	E980.3
Neuroprotective agent	977.8	E858.8	E947.8	E950.4	E962.0	E980.4
Neutral spirits	980.0	E860.1	—	E950.9	E962.1	E980.9
beverage	980.0	E860.0	—	E950.9	E962.1	E980.9
Niacin, niacinamide	972.2	E858.3	E942.2	E950.4	E962.0	E980.4
Nialamide	969.01	E854.0	E939.0	E950.3	E962.0	E980.3
Nickle (carbonyl) (compounds) (fumes) (tetracarbonyl) (vapor)	985.8	E866.4		E950.9	E962.1	E980.9
Niclosamide	961.6	E857	E931.6	E950.4	E962.0	E980.4
Nicomorphine	965.09	E850.2	E935.2	E950.0	E962.0	E980.0
Nicotinamide	972.2	E858.3	E942.2	E950.4	E962.0	E980.4
Nicotine (insecticide) (spray) (sulfate) NEC	989.4	E863.4		E950.6	E962.1	E980.7
not insecticide	989.89	E866.8		E950.9	E962.1	E980.9
Nicotinic acid (derivatives)	972.2	E858.3	E942.2	E950.4	E962.0	E980.4
Nicotinyl alcohol	972.2	E858.3	E942.2	E950.4	E962.0	E980.4
Nicoumalone	964.2	E858.2	E934.2	E950.4	E962.0	E980.4
Nifenazone	965.5	E850.5	E935.5	E950.0	E962.0	E980.0
Nifuraldezone	961.9	E857	E931.9	E950.4	E962.0	E980.4
Nightshade (deadly)	988.2	E865.4		E950.9	E962.1	E980.9
Nikethamide	970.0	E854.3	E940.0	E950.4	E962.0	E980.4
Nilstat	960.1	E856	E930.1	E950.4	E962.0	E980.4
topical	976.0	E858.7	E946.0	E950.4	E962.0	E980.4
Nimodipine	977.8	E858.8	E947.8	E950.4	E962.0	E980.4
Niridazole	961.6	E857	E931.6	E950.4	E962.0	E980.4
Nisentil	965.09	E850.2	E935.2	E950.0	E962.0	E980.0
Nitrates	972.4	E858.3	E942.4	E950.4	E962.0	E980.4
Nitrazepam	969.4	E853.2	E939.4	E950.3	E962.0	E980.3
Nitric						
acid (liquid)	983.1	E864.1	—	E950.7	E962.1	E980.6
vapor	987.8	E869.8	—	E952.8	E962.2	E982.8
oxide (gas)	987.2	E869.0	—	E952.8	E962.2	E982.8
Nitrite, amyl (medicinal) (vapor)	972.4	E858.3	E942.4	E950.4	E962.0	E980.4
Nitroaniline	983.0	E864.0	—	E950.7	E962.1	E980.6
vapor	987.8	E869.8	—	E952.8	E962.2	E982.8
Nitrobenzene, nitrobenzol	983.0	E864.0	—	E950.7	E962.1	E980.6
vapor	987.8	E869.8	—	E952.8	E962.2	E982.8
Nitrocellulose	976.3	E858.7	E946.3	E950.4	E962.0	E980.4
Nitrofuran derivatives	961.9	E857	E931.9	E950.4	E962.0	E980.4
Nitrofurantoin	961.9	E857	E931.9	E950.4	E962.0	E980.4
Nitrofurazone	976.0	E858.7	E946.0	E950.4	E962.0	E980.4
Nitrogen (dioxide) (gas) (oxide)	987.2	E869.0	—	E952.8	E962.2	E982.8
mustard (antineoplastic)	963.1	E858.1	E933.1	E950.4	E962.0	E980.4
nonmedicinal	989.89	E866.8	—	E950.9	E962.1	E980.9
fumes	987.8	E869.8	—	E952.8	E962.2	E982.8
Nitroglycerin, nitroglycerol (medicinal)	972.4	E858.3	E942.4	E950.4	E962.0	E980.4
Nitrohydrochloric acid	983.1	E864.1	—	E950.7	E962.1	E980.6
Nitromersol	976.0	E858.7	E946.0	E950.4	E962.0	E980.4
Nitronaphthalene	983.0	E864.0	—	E950.7	E962.2	E980.6
Nitrophenol	983.0	E864.0	—	E950.7	E962.2	E980.6
Nitrothiazol	961.6	E857	E931.6	E950.4	E962.0	E980.4
Nitrotoluene, nitrotoluol	983.0	E864.0	—	E950.7	E962.1	E980.6

	Poisoning	Accident	Therapeutic Use	Suicide Attempt	Assault	Undetermined
Nitrotoluene, nitrotoluol — *continued*						
vapor	987.8	E869.8	—	E952.8	E962.2	E982.8
Nitrous	968.2	E855.1	E938.2	E950.4	E962.0	E980.4
acid (liquid)	983.1	E864.1	—	E950.7	E962.1	E980.6
fumes	987.2	E869.0	—	E952.8	E962.2	E982.8
oxide (anesthetic) NEC	968.2	E855.1	E938.2	E950.4	E962.0	E980.4
Nitrozone	976.0	E858.7	E946.0	E950.4	E962.0	E980.4
Noctec	967.1	E852.0	E937.1	E950.2	E962.0	E980.2
Noludar	967.5	E852.4	E937.5	E950.2	E962.0	E980.2
Noptil	967.0	E851	E937.0	E950.1	E962.0	E980.1
Noradrenalin	971.2	E855.5	E941.2	E950.4	E962.0	E980.4
Noramidopyrine	965.5	E850.5	E935.5	E950.0	E962.0	E980.0
Norepinephrine	971.2	E855.5	E941.2	E950.4	E962.0	E980.4
Norethandrolone	962.1	E858.0	E932.1	E950.4	E962.0	E980.4
Norethindrone	962.2	E858.0	E932.2	E950.4	E962.0	E980.4
Norethisterone	962.2	E858.0	E932.2	E950.4	E962.0	E980.4
Norethynodrel	962.2	E858.0	E932.2	E950.4	E962.0	E980.4
Norlestrin	962.2	E858.0	E932.2	E950.4	E962.0	E980.4
Norlutin	962.2	E858.0	E932.2	E950.4	E962.0	E980.4
Normison — see Benzodiazepines						
Normorphine	965.09	E850.2	E935.2	E950.0	E962.0	E980.0
Nortriptyline	969.05	E854.0	E939.0	E950.3	E962.0	E980.3
Noscapine	975.4	E858.6	E945.4	E950.4	E962.0	E980.4
Nose preparations	976.6	E858.7	E946.6	E950.4	E962.0	E980.4
Novobiocin	960.8	E856	E930.8	E950.4	E962.0	E980.4
Novocain (infiltration) (topical)	968.5	E855.2	E938.5	E950.4	E962.0	E980.4
nerve block (peripheral) (plexus)	968.6	E855.2	E938.6	E950.4	E962.0	E980.4
spinal	968.7	E855.2	E938.7	E950.4	E962.0	E980.4
Noxythiolin	961.9	E857	E931.9	E950.4	E962.0	E980.4
NPH Iletin (insulin)	962.3	E858.0	E932.3	E950.4	E962.0	E980.4
Numorphan	965.09	E850.2	E935.2	E950.0	E962.0	E980.0
Nunol	967.0	E851	E937.0	E950.1	E962.0	E980.1
Nupercaine (spinal anesthetic)	968.7	E855.2	E938.7	E950.4	E962.0	E980.4
topical (surface)	968.5	E855.2	E938.5	E950.4	E962.0	E980.4
Nutmeg oil (liniment)	976.3	E858.7	E946.3	E950.4	E962.0	E980.4
Nux vomica	989.1	E863.7	—	E950.6	E962.1	E980.7
Nydrazid	961.8	E857	E931.8	E950.4	E962.0	E980.4
Nylidrin	971.2	E855.5	E941.2	E950.4	E962.0	E980.4
Nystatin	960.1	E856	E930.1	E950.4	E962.0	E980.4
topical	976.0	E858.7	E946.0	E950.4	E962.0	E980.4
Nytol	963.0	E858.1	E933.0	E950.4	E962.0	E980.4
Oblivion	967.8	E852.8	E937.8	E950.2	E962.0	E980.2
Octyl nitrite	972.4	E858.3	E942.4	E950.4	E962.0	E980.4
Oestradiol (cypionate) (dipropionate) (valerate)	962.2	E858.0	E932.2	E950.4	E962.0	E980.4
Oestriol	962.2	E858.0	E932.2	E950.4	E962.0	E980.4
Oestrone	962.2	E858.0	E932.2	E950.4	E962.0	E980.4
Oil (of) NEC	989.89	E866.8	—	E950.9	E962.1	E980.9
bitter almond	989.0	E866.8	—	E950.9	E962.1	E980.9
camphor	976.1	E858.7	E946.1	E950.4	E962.0	E980.4
colors	989.89	E861.6	—	E950.9	E962.1	E980.9
fumes	987.8	E869.8	—	E952.8	E962.2	E982.8
lubricating	981	E862.2	—	E950.9	E962.1	E980.9
specified source, other — see substance specified						
vitriol (liquid)	983.1	E864.1	—	E950.7	E962.1	E980.6
fumes	987.8	E869.8	—	E952.8	E962.2	E982.8
wintergreen (bitter) NEC	976.3	E858.7	E946.3	E950.4	E962.0	E980.4
Ointments NEC	976.9	E858.7	E946.9	E950.4	E962.0	E980.4
Oleander	988.2	E865.4	—	E950.9	E962.1	E980.9
Oleandomycin	960.3	E856	E930.3	E950.4	E962.0	E980.4
Oleovitamin A	963.5	E858.1	E933.5	E950.4	E962.0	E980.4
Oleum ricini	973.1	E858.4	E943.1	E950.4	E962.0	E980.4
Olive oil (medicinal) NEC	973.2	E858.4	E943.2	E950.4	E962.0	E980.4
OMPA	989.3	E863.1	—	E950.6	E962.1	E980.7
Oncovin	963.1	E858.1	E933.1	E950.4	E962.0	E980.4
Ophthaine	968.5	E855.2	E938.5	E950.4	E962.0	E980.4
Ophthetic	968.5	E855.2	E938.5	E950.4	E962.0	E980.4
Opiates, opioids, opium NEC	965.00	E850.2	E935.2	E950.0	E962.0	E980.0
antagonists	970.1	E854.3	E940.1	E950.4	E962.0	E980.4
Oracon	962.2	E858.0	E932.2	E950.4	E962.0	E980.4
Oragrafin	977.8	E858.8	E947.8	E950.4	E962.0	E980.4
Oral contraceptives	962.2	E858.0	E932.2	E950.4	E962.0	E980.4
Orciprenaline	975.1	E858.6	E945.1	E950.4	E962.0	E980.4
Organidin	975.5	E858.6	E945.5	E950.4	E962.0	E980.4
Organophosphates	989.3	E863.1	—	E950.6	E962.1	E980.7

Nontherapeutic use substance

Subterms under main terms may continue to next column or page

	Poisoning	Accident	Therapeutic Use	Suicide Attempt	Assault	Undetermined
External Cause (E-Code)						

	Poisoning	Accident	Therapeutic Use	Suicide Attempt	Assault	Undetermined
Orimune	979.5	E858.8	E949.5	E950.4	E962.0	E980.4
Orinase	962.3	E858.0	E932.3	E950.4	E962.0	E980.4
Orphenadrine	966.4	E855.0	E936.4	E950.4	E962.0	E980.4
Ortal (sodium)	967.0	E851	E937.0	E950.1	E962.0	E980.1
Orthoboric acid	976.0	E858.7	E946.0	E950.4	E962.0	E980.4
ENT agent	976.6	E858.7	E946.6	E950.4	E962.0	E980.4
ophthalmic preparation	976.5	E858.7	E946.5	E950.4	E962.0	E980.4
Orthocaine	968.5	E855.2	E938.5	E950.4	E962.0	E980.4
Ortho-Novum	962.2	E858.0	E932.2	E950.4	E962.0	E980.4
Orthotolidine (reagent)	977.8	E858.8	E947.8	E950.4	E962.0	E980.4
Osmic acid (liquid)	983.1	E864.1	—	E950.7	E962.1	E980.6
fumes	987.8	E869.8	—	E952.8	E962.2	E982.8
Osmotic diuretics	974.4	E858.5	E944.4	E950.4	E962.0	E980.4
Ouabain	972.1	E858.3	E942.1	E950.4	E962.0	E980.4
Ovarian hormones (synthetic substitutes)	962.2	E858.0	E932.2	E950.4	E962.0	E980.4
Ovral	962.2	E858.0	E932.2	E950.4	E962.0	E980.4
Ovulation suppressants	962.2	E858.0	E932.2	E950.4	E962.0	E980.4
Ovulen	962.2	E858.0	E932.2	E950.4	E962.0	E980.4
Oxacillin (sodium)	960.0	E856	E930.0	E950.4	E962.0	E980.4
Oxalic acid	983.1	E864.1	—	E950.7	E962.1	E980.6
Oxanamide	969.5	E853.8	E939.5	E950.3	E962.0	E980.3
Oxandrolone	962.1	E858.0	E932.1	E950.4	E962.0	E980.4
Oxaprozin	965.61	E850.6	E935.6	E950.0	E962.0	E980.0
Oxazepam	969.4	E853.2	E939.4	E950.3	E962.0	E980.3
Oxazolidine derivatives	966.0	E855.0	E936.0	E950.4	E962.0	E980.4
Ox bile extract	973.4	E858.4	E943.4	E950.4	E962.0	E980.4
Oxedrine	971.2	E855.5	E941.2	E950.4	E962.0	E980.4
Oxeladin	975.4	E858.6	E945.4	E950.4	E962.0	E980.4
Oxethazaine NEC	968.5	E855.2	E938.5	E950.4	E962.0	E980.4
Oxidizing agents NEC	983.9	E864.3	—	E950.7	E962.1	E980.6
Oxolinic acid	961.3	E857	E931.3	E950.4	E962.0	E980.4
Oxophenarsine	961.1	E857	E931.1	E950.4	E962.0	E980.4
Oxsoralen	976.3	E858.7	E946.3	E950.4	E962.0	E980.4
Oxtriphylline	975.7	E858.6	E945.7	E950.4	E962.0	E980.4
Oxybuprocaine	968.5	E855.2	E938.5	E950.4	E962.0	E980.4
Oxybutynin	975.1	E858.6	E945.1	E950.4	E962.0	E980.4
Oxycodone	965.09	E850.2	E935.2	E950.0	E962.0	E980.0
Oxygen	987.8	E869.8	—	E952.8	E962.2	E982.8
Oxylone	976.0	E858.7	E946.0	E950.4	E962.0	E980.4
ophthalmic preparation	976.5	E858.7	E946.5	E950.4	E962.0	E980.4
Oxymesterone	962.1	E858.0	E932.1	E950.4	E962.0	E980.4
Oxymetazoline	971.2	E855.5	E941.2	E950.4	E962.0	E980.4
Oxymetholone	962.1	E858.0	E932.1	E950.4	E962.0	E980.4
Oxymorphone	965.09	E850.2	E935.2	E950.0	E962.0	E980.0
Oxypertine	969.09	E854.0	E939.0	E950.3	E962.0	E980.3
Oxyphenbutazone	965.5	E850.5	E935.5	E950.0	E962.0	E980.0
Oxyphencyclimine	971.1	E855.4	E941.1	E950.4	E962.0	E980.4
Oxyphenisatin	973.1	E858.4	E943.1	E950.4	E962.0	E980.4
Oxyphenonium	971.1	E855.4	E941.1	E950.4	E962.0	E980.4
Oxyquinoline	961.3	E857	E931.3	E950.4	E962.0	E980.4
Oxytetracycline	960.4	E856	E930.4	E950.4	E962.0	E980.4
Oxytocics	975.0	E858.6	E945.0	E950.4	E962.0	E980.4
Oxytocin	975.0	E858.6	E945.0	E950.4	E962.0	E980.4
Ozone	987.8	E869.8	—	E952.8	E962.2	E982.8
PABA	976.3	E858.7	E946.3	E950.4	E962.0	E980.4
Packed red cells	964.7	E858.2	E934.7	E950.4	E962.0	E980.4
Paint NEC	989.89	E861.6	—	E950.9	E962.1	E980.9
cleaner	982.8	E862.9	—	E950.9	E962.1	E980.9
fumes NEC	987.8	E869.8	—	E952.8	E962.1	E982.8
lead (fumes)	984.0	E861.5	—	E950.9	E962.1	E980.9
solvent NEC	982.8	E862.9	—	E950.9	E962.1	E980.9
stripper	982.8	E862.9	—	E950.9	E962.1	E980.9
Palfium	965.09	E850.2	E935.2	E950.0	E962.0	E980.0
Palivizumab	979.9	E858.8	E949.6	E950.4	E962.0	E980.4
Paludrine	961.4	E857	E931.4	E950.4	E962.0	E980.4
PAM	977.2	E855.8	E947.2	E950.4	E962.0	E980.4
Pamaquine (naphthoate)	961.4	E857	E931.4	E950.4	E962.0	E980.4
Pamprin	965.1	E850.3	E935.3	E950.0	E962.0	E980.0
Panadol	965.4	E850.4	E935.4	E950.0	E962.0	E980.0
Pancreatic dornase (mucolytic)	963.4	E858.1	E933.4	E950.4	E962.0	E980.4
Pancreatin	973.4	E858.4	E943.4	E950.4	E962.0	E980.4
Pancrelipase	973.4	E858.4	E943.4	E950.4	E962.0	E980.4
Pangamic acid	963.5	E858.1	E933.5	E950.4	E962.0	E980.4
Panthenol	963.5	E858.1	E933.5	E950.4	E962.0	E980.4
topical	976.8	E858.7	E946.8	E950.4	E962.0	E980.4
Pantopaque	977.8	E858.8	E947.8	E950.4	E962.0	E980.4
Pantopon	965.00	E850.2	E935.2	E950.0	E962.0	E980.0
Pantothenic acid	963.5	E858.1	E933.5	E950.4	E962.0	E980.4
Panwarfin	964.2	E858.2	E934.2	E950.4	E962.0	E980.4
Papain	973.4	E858.4	E943.4	E950.4	E962.0	E980.4
Papaverine	972.5	E858.3	E942.5	E950.4	E962.0	E980.4
Para-aminobenzoic acid	976.3	E858.7	E946.3	E950.4	E962.0	E980.4
Para-aminophenol derivatives	965.4	E850.4	E935.4	E950.0	E962.0	E980.0
Para-aminosalicylic acid (derivatives)	961.8	E857	E931.8	E950.4	E962.0	E980.4
Paracetaldehyde (medicinal)	967.2	E852.1	E937.2	E950.2	E962.0	E980.2
Paracetamol	965.4	E850.4	E935.4	E950.0	E962.0	E980.0
Paracodin	965.09	E850.2	E935.2	E950.0	E962.0	E980.0
Paradione	966.0	E855.0	E936.0	E950.4	E962.0	E980.4
Paraffin(s) (wax)	981	E862.3	—	E950.9	E962.1	E980.9
liquid (medicinal)	973.2	E858.4	E943.2	E950.4	E962.0	E980.4
nonmedicinal (oil)	981	E962.1	—	E950.9	—	E980.9
Paraldehyde (medicinal)	967.2	E852.1	E937.2	E950.2	E962.0	E980.2
Paramethadione	966.0	E855.0	E936.0	E950.4	E962.0	E980.4
Paramethasone	962.0	E858.0	E932.0	E950.4	E962.0	E980.4
Paraquat	989.4	E863.5	—	E950.6	E962.1	E980.7
Parasympatholytics	971.1	E855.4	E941.1	E950.4	E962.0	E980.4
Parasympathomimetics	971.0	E855.3	E941.0	E950.4	E962.0	E980.4
Parathion	989.3	E863.1	—	E950.6	E962.1	E980.7
Parathormone	962.6	E858.0	E932.6	E950.4	E962.0	E980.4
Parathyroid (derivatives)	962.6	E858.0	E932.6	E950.4	E962.0	E980.4
Paratyphoid vaccine	978.1	E858.8	E948.1	E950.4	E962.0	E980.4
Paredrine	971.2	E855.5	E941.2	E950.4	E962.0	E980.4
Paregoric	965.00	E850.2	E935.2	E950.0	E962.0	E980.0
Pargyline	972.3	E858.3	E942.3	E950.4	E962.0	E980.4
Paris green	985.1	E866.3	—	E950.8	E962.1	E980.8
insecticide	985.1	E863.4	—	E950.8	E962.1	E980.8
Parnate	969.01	E854.0	E939.0	E950.3	E962.0	E980.3
Paromomycin	960.8	E856	E930.8	E950.4	E962.0	E980.4
Paroxypropione	963.1	E858.1	E933.1	E950.4	E962.0	E980.4
Parzone	965.09	E850.2	E935.2	E950.0	E962.0	E980.0
PAS	961.8	E857	E931.8	E950.4	E962.0	E980.4
PCBs	981	E862.3	—	E950.9	E962.1	E980.9
PCP (pentachlorophenol)	989.4	E863.6	—	E950.6	E962.1	E980.7
herbicide	989.4	E863.5	—	E950.6	E962.1	E980.7
insecticide	989.4	E863.4	—	E950.6	E962.1	E980.7
phencyclidine	968.3	E855.1	E938.3	E950.4	E962.0	E980.4
Peach kernel oil (emulsion)	973.2	E858.4	E943.2	E950.4	E962.0	E980.4
Peanut oil (emulsion) NEC	973.2	E858.4	E943.2	E950.4	E962.0	E980.4
topical	976.3	E858.7	E946.3	E950.4	E962.0	E980.4
Pearly Gates (morning glory seeds)	969.6	E854.1	E939.6	E950.3	E962.0	E980.3
Pecazine	969.1	E853.0	E939.1	E950.3	E962.0	E980.3
Pecilocin	960.1	E856	E930.1	E950.4	E962.0	E980.4
Pectin (with kaolin) NEC	973.5	E858.4	E943.5	E950.4	E962.0	E980.4
Pelletierine tannate	961.6	E857	E931.6	E950.4	E962.0	E980.4
Pemoline	969.79	E854.2	E939.7	E950.3	E962.0	E980.3
Pempidine	972.3	E858.3	E942.3	E950.4	E962.0	E980.4
Penamecillin	960.0	E856	E930.0	E950.4	E962.0	E980.4
Penethamate hydriodide	960.0	E856	E930.0	E950.4	E962.0	E980.4
Penicillamine	963.8	E858.1	E933.8	E950.4	E962.0	E980.4
Penicillin (any type)	960.0	E856	E930.0	E950.4	E962.0	E980.4
Penicillinase	963.4	E858.1	E933.4	E950.4	E962.0	E980.4
Pentachlorophenol (fungicide)	989.4	E863.6	—	E950.6	E962.1	E980.7
herbicide	989.4	E863.5	—	E950.6	E962.1	E980.7
insecticide	989.4	E863.4	—	E950.6	E962.1	E980.7
Pentaerythritol	972.4	E858.3	E942.4	E950.4	E962.0	E980.4
chloral	967.1	E852.0	E937.1	E950.2	E962.0	E980.2
tetranitrate NEC	972.4	E858.3	E942.4	E950.4	E962.0	E980.4
Pentagastrin	977.8	E858.8	E947.8	E950.4	E962.0	E980.4
Pentalin	982.3	E862.4	—	E950.9	E962.1	E980.9
Pentamethonium (bromide)	972.3	E858.3	E942.3	E950.4	E962.0	E980.4
Pentamidine	961.5	E857	E931.5	E950.4	E962.0	E980.4
Pentanol	980.8	E860.8	—	E950.9	E962.1	E980.9
Pentaquine	961.4	E857	E931.4	E950.4	E962.0	E980.4
Pentazocine	965.8	E850.8	E935.8	E950.0	E962.0	E980.0
Penthienate	971.1	E855.4	E941.1	E950.4	E962.0	E980.4
Pentobarbital, pentobarbitone (sodium)	967.0	E851	E937.0	E950.1	E962.0	E980.1
Pentolinium (tartrate)	972.3	E858.3	E942.3	E950.4	E962.0	E980.4
Pentothal	968.3	E855.1	E938.3	E950.4	E962.0	E980.4
Pentylenetetrazol	970.0	E854.3	E940.0	E950.4	E962.0	E980.4
Pentylsalicylamide	961.8	E857	E931.8	E950.4	E962.0	E980.4
Pepsin	973.4	E858.4	E943.4	E950.4	E962.0	E980.4
Peptavlon	977.8	E858.8	E947.8	E950.4	E962.0	E980.4
Percaine (spinal)	968.7	E855.2	E938.7	E950.4	E962.0	E980.4

	Poisoning	Accident	Therapeutic Use	Suicide Attempt	Assault	Undetermined
Percaine — *continued*						
topical (surface)	968.5	E855.2	E938.5	E950.4	E962.0	E980.4
Perchloroethylene (vapor)	982.3	E862.4	—	E950.9	E962.1	E980.9
medicinal	961.6	E857	E931.6	E950.4	E962.0	E980.4
Percodan	965.09	E850.2	E935.2	E950.0	E962.0	E980.0
Percogesic	965.09	E850.2	E935.2	E950.0	E962.0	E980.0
Percorten	962.0	E858.0	E932.0	E950.4	E962.0	E980.4
Pergonal	962.4	E858.0	E932.4	E950.4	E962.0	E980.4
Perhexiline	972.4	E858.3	E942.4	E950.4	E962.0	E980.4
Periactin	963.0	E858.1	E933.0	E950.4	E962.0	E980.4
Periclor	967.1	E852.0	E937.1	E950.2	E962.0	E980.2
Pericyazine	969.1	E853.0	E939.1	E950.3	E962.0	E980.3
Peritrate	972.4	E858.3	E942.4	E950.4	E962.0	E980.4
Permanganates NEC	983.9	E864.3	—	E950.7	E962.1	E980.6
potassium (topical)	976.0	E858.7	E946.0	E950.4	E962.0	E980.4
Pernocton	967.0	E851	E937.0	E950.1	E962.0	E980.1
Pernoston	967.0	E851	E937.0	E950.1	E962.0	E980.1
Peronin(e)	965.09	E850.2	E935.2	E950.0	E962.0	E980.0
Perphenazine	969.1	E853.0	E939.1	E950.3	E962.0	E980.3
Pertofrane	969.05	E854.0	E939.0	E950.3	E962.0	E980.3
Pertussis						
immune serum (human)	964.6	E858.2	E934.6	E950.4	E962.0	E980.4
vaccine (with diphtheria toxoid) (with tetanus toxoid)	978.6	E858.8	E948.6	E950.4	E962.0	E980.4
Peruvian balsam	976.8	E858.7	E946.8	E950.4	E962.0	E980.4
Pesticides (dust) (fumes) (vapor)	989.4	E863.4	—	E950.6	E962.1	E980.7
arsenic	985.1	E863.4	—	E950.8	E962.1	E980.8
chlorinated	989.2	E863.0	—	E950.6	E962.1	E980.7
cyanide	989.0	E863.4	—	E950.6	E962.1	E980.7
kerosene	981	E863.4	—	E950.6	E962.1	E980.7
mixture (of compounds)	989.4	E863.3	—	E950.6	E962.1	E980.7
naphthalene	983.0	E863.4	—	E950.7	E962.1	E980.6
organochlorine (compounds)	989.2	E863.0	—	E950.6	E962.1	E980.7
petroleum (distillate) (products) NEC	981	E863.4	—	E950.6	E962.1	E980.7
specified ingredient NEC	989.4	E863.4	—	E950.6	E962.1	E980.7
strychnine	989.1	E863.4	—	E950.6	E962.1	E980.7
thallium	985.8	E863.7	—	E950.6	E962.1	E980.7
Pethidine (hydrochloride)	965.09	E850.2	E935.2	E950.0	E962.0	E980.0
Petrichloral	967.1	E852.0	E937.1	E950.2	E962.0	E980.2
Petrol	981	E862.1	—	E950.9	E962.1	E980.9
vapor	987.1	E869.8	—	E952.8	E962.2	E982.8
Petrolatum (jelly) (ointment)	976.3	E858.7	E946.3	E950.4	E962.0	E980.4
hydrophilic	976.3	E858.7	E946.3	E950.4	E962.0	E980.4
liquid	973.2	E858.4	E943.2	E950.4	E962.0	E980.4
topical	976.3	E858.7	E946.3	E950.4	E962.0	E980.4
nonmedicinal	981	E862.1	—	E950.9	E962.1	E980.9
Petroleum (cleaners) (fuels) (products) NEC	981	E862.1	—	E950.9	E962.1	E980.9
benzin(e) — see Ligroin						
ether — see Ligroin						
jelly — see Petrolatum						
naphtha — see Ligroin						
pesticide	981	E863.4	—	E950.6	E962.1	E980.7
solids	981	E862.3	—	E950.9	E962.1	E980.9
solvents	981	E862.0	—	E950.9	E962.1	E980.9
vapor	987.1	E869.8	—	E952.8	E962.2	E982.8
Peyote	969.6	E854.1	E939.6	E950.3	E962.0	E980.3
Phanodorm, phanodorn	967.0	E851	E937.0	E950.1	E962.0	E980.1
Phanquinone, phanquone	961.5	E857	E931.5	E950.4	E962.0	E980.4
Pharmaceutical excipient or adjunct	977.4	E858.8	E947.4	E950.4	E962.0	E980.4
Phenacemide	966.3	E855.0	E936.3	E950.4	E962.0	E980.4
Phenacetin	965.4	E850.4	E935.4	E950.0	E962.0	E980.0
Phenadoxone	965.09	E850.2	E935.2	E950.0	E962.0	E980.0
Phenaglycodol	969.5	E853.8	E939.5	E950.3	E962.0	E980.3
Phenantoin	966.1	E855.0	E936.1	E950.4	E962.0	E980.4
Phenaphthazine reagent	977.8	E858.8	E947.8	E950.4	E962.0	E980.4
Phenazocine	965.09	E850.2	E935.2	E950.0	E962.0	E980.0
Phenazone	965.5	E850.5	E935.5	E950.0	E962.0	E980.0
Phenazopyridine	976.1	E858.7	E946.1	E950.4	E962.0	E980.4
Phenbenicillin	960.0	E856	E930.0	E950.4	E962.0	E980.4
Phenbutrazate	977.0	E858.8	E947.0	E950.4	E962.0	E980.4
Phencyclidine	968.3	E855.1	E938.3	E950.4	E962.0	E980.4
Phendimetrazine	977.0	E858.8	E947.0	E950.4	E962.0	E980.4
Phenelzine	969.01	E854.0	E939.0	E950.3	E962.0	E980.3
Phenergan	967.8	E852.8	E937.8	E950.2	E962.0	E980.2
Phenethicillin (potassium)	960.0	E856	E930.0	E950.4	E962.0	E980.4
Phenetsal	965.1	E850.3	E935.3	E950.0	E962.0	E980.0
Pheneturide	966.3	E855.0	E936.3	E950.4	E962.0	E980.4
Phenformin	962.3	E858.0	E932.3	E950.4	E962.0	E980.4
Phenglutarimide	971.1	E855.4	E941.1	E950.4	E962.0	E980.4
Phenicarbazide	965.8	E850.8	E935.8	E950.0	E962.0	E980.0
Phenindamine (tartrate)	963.0	E858.1	E933.0	E950.4	E962.0	E980.4
Phenindione	964.2	E858.2	E934.2	E950.4	E962.0	E980.4
Pheniprazine	969.01	E854.0	E939.0	E950.3	E962.0	E980.3
Pheniramine (maleate)	963.0	E858.1	E933.0	E950.4	E962.0	E980.4
Phenmetrazine	977.0	E858.8	E947.0	E950.4	E962.0	E980.4
Phenobal	967.0	E851	E937.0	E950.1	E962.0	E980.1
Phenobarbital	967.0	E851	E937.0	E950.1	E962.0	E980.1
Phenobarbitone	967.0	E851	E937.0	E950.1	E962.0	E980.1
Phenoctide	976.0	E858.7	E946.0	E950.4	E962.0	E980.4
Phenolphthalein	973.1	E858.4	E943.1	E950.4	E962.0	E980.4
Phenolsulfonphthalein	977.8	E858.8	E947.8	E950.4	E962.0	E980.4
Phenol (derivatives) NEC	983.0	E864.0	—	E950.7	E962.1	E980.6
disinfectant	983.0	E864.0	—	E950.7	E962.1	E980.6
pesticide	989.4	E863.4	—	E950.6	E962.1	E980.7
red	977.8	E858.8	E947.8	E950.4	E962.0	E980.4
Phenomorphan	965.09	E850.2	E935.2	E950.0	E962.0	E980.0
Phenonyl	967.0	E851	E937.0	E950.1	E962.0	E980.1
Phenoperidine	965.09	E850.2	E935.2	E950.0	E962.0	E980.0
Phenoquin	974.7	E858.5	E944.7	E950.4	E962.0	E980.4
Phenothiazines (tranquilizers) NEC	969.1	E853.0	E939.1	E950.3	E962.0	E980.3
insecticide	989.3	E863.4	—	E950.6	E962.1	E980.7
Phenoxybenzamine	971.3	E855.6	E941.3	E950.4	E962.0	E980.4
Phenoxymethyl penicillin	960.0	E856	E930.0	E950.4	E962.0	E980.4
Phenprocoumon	964.2	E858.2	E934.2	E950.4	E962.0	E980.4
Phensuximide	966.2	E855.0	E936.2	E950.4	E962.0	E980.4
Phentermine	977.0	E858.8	E947.0	E950.4	E962.0	E980.4
Phentolamine	971.3	E855.6	E941.3	E950.4	E962.0	E980.4
Phenyl						
butazone	965.5	E850.5	E935.5	E950.0	E962.0	E980.0
enediamine	983.0	E864.0	—	E950.7	E962.1	E980.6
hydrazine	983.0	E864.0	—	E950.7	E962.1	E980.6
antineoplastic	963.1	E858.1	E933.1	E950.4	E962.0	E980.4
mercuric compounds — see Mercury						
salicylate	976.3	E858.7	E946.3	E950.4	E962.0	E980.4
Phenylephrine	971.2	E855.5	E941.2	E950.4	E962.0	E980.4
Phenylethylbiguanide	962.3	E858.0	E932.3	E950.4	E962.0	E980.4
Phenylpropanolamine	971.2	E855.5	E941.2	E950.4	E962.0	E980.4
Phenylsulfthion	989.3	E863.1	—	E950.6	E962.1	E980.7
Phenyramidol, phenyramidon	965.7	E850.7	E935.7	E950.0	E962.0	E980.0
Phenytoin	966.1	E855.0	E936.1	E950.4	E962.0	E980.4
pHisoHex	976.2	E858.7	E946.2	E950.4	E962.0	E980.4
Pholcodine	965.09	E850.2	E935.2	E950.0	E962.0	E980.0
Phorate	989.3	E863.1	—	E950.6	E962.1	E980.7
Phosdrin	989.3	E863.1	—	E950.6	E962.1	E980.7
Phosgene (gas)	987.8	E869.8	—	E952.8	E962.2	E982.8
Phosphate (tricresyl)	989.89	E866.8	—	E950.9	E962.1	E980.9
organic	989.3	E863.1	—	E950.6	E962.1	E980.7
solvent	982.8	E862.4	—	E950.9	E926.1	E980.9
Phosphine	987.8	E869.8	—	E952.8	E962.2	E982.8
fumigant	987.8	E863.8	—	E950.6	E962.2	E980.7
Phospholine	971.0	E855.3	E941.0	E950.4	E962.0	E980.4
Phosphoric acid	983.1	E864.1	—	E950.7	E962.1	E980.6
Phosphorus (compounds) NEC	983.9	E864.3	—	E950.7	E962.1	E980.6
rodenticide	983.9	E863.7	—	E950.7	E962.1	E980.6
Phthalimidoglutarimide	967.8	E852.8	E937.8	E950.2	E962.0	E980.2
Phthalylsulfathiazole	961.0	E857	E931.0	E950.4	E962.0	E980.4
Phylloquinone	964.3	E858.2	E934.3	E950.4	E962.0	E980.4
Physeptone	965.02	E850.1	E935.1	E950.0	E962.0	E980.0
Physostigma venenosum	988.2	E865.4	—	E950.9	E962.1	E980.9
Physostigmine	971.0	E855.3	E941.0	E950.4	E962.0	E980.4
Phytolacca decandra	988.2	E865.4	—	E950.9	E962.1	E980.9
Phytomenadione	964.3	E858.2	E934.3	E950.4	E962.0	E980.4
Phytonadione	964.3	E858.2	E934.3	E950.4	E962.0	E980.4
Picric (acid)	983.0	E864.0	—	E950.7	E962.1	E980.6
Picrotoxin	970.0	E854.3	E940.0	E950.4	E962.0	E980.4
Pilocarpine	971.0	E855.3	E941.0	E950.4	E962.0	E980.4
Pilocarpus (jaborandi) extract	971.0	E855.3	E941.0	E950.4	E962.0	E980.4

Nontherapeutic use substance

▽ Subterms under main terms may continue to next column or page

	Poisoning	Accident	Therapeutic Use	Suicide Attempt	Assault	Undetermined
Pimaricin	960.1	E856	E930.1	E950.4	E962.0	E980.4
Piminodine	965.09	E850.2	E935.2	E950.0	E962.0	E980.0
Pine oil, pinesol (disinfectant)	983.9	E861.4	—	E950.7	E962.1	E980.6
Pinkroot	961.6	E857	E931.6	E950.4	E962.0	E980.4
Pipadone	965.09	E850.2	E935.2	E950.0	E962.0	E980.0
Pipamazine	963.0	E858.1	E933.0	E950.4	E962.0	E980.4
Pipazethate	975.4	E858.6	E945.4	E950.4	E962.0	E980.4
Pipenzolate	971.1	E855.4	E941.1	E950.4	E962.0	E980.4
Piperacetazine	969.1	E853.0	E939.1	E950.3	E962.0	E980.3
Piperazine NEC	961.6	E857	E931.6	E950.4	E962.0	E980.4
estrone sulfate	962.2	E858.0	E932.2	E950.4	E962.0	E980.4
Piper cubeba	988.2	E865.4	—	E950.9	E962.1	E980.9
Piperidione	975.4	E858.6	E945.4	E950.4	E962.0	E980.4
Piperidolate	971.1	E855.4	E941.1	E950.4	E962.0	E980.4
Piperocaine	968.9	E855.2	E938.9	E950.4	E962.0	E980.4
infiltration (subcutaneous)	968.5	E855.2	E938.5	E950.4	E962.0	E980.4
nerve block (peripheral) (plexus)	968.6	E855.2	E938.6	E950.4	E962.0	E980.4
topical (surface)	968.5	E855.2	E938.5	E950.4	E962.0	E980.4
Pipobroman	963.1	E858.1	E933.1	E950.4	E962.0	E980.4
Pipradrol	970.89	E854.3	E940.8	E950.4	E962.0	E980.4
Piscidia (bark) (erythrina)	965.7	E850.7	E935.7	E950.0	E962.0	E980.0
Pitch	983.0	E864.0	—	E950.7	E962.1	E980.6
Pitkin's solution	968.7	E855.2	E938.7	E950.4	E962.0	E980.4
Pitocin	975.0	E858.6	E945.0	E950.4	E962.0	E980.4
Pitressin (tannate)	962.5	E858.0	E932.5	E950.4	E962.0	E980.4
Pituitary extracts (posterior)	962.5	E858.0	E932.5	E950.4	E962.0	E980.4
anterior	962.4	E858.0	E932.4	E950.4	E962.0	E980.4
Pituitrin	962.5	E858.0	E932.5	E950.4	E962.0	E980.4
Placental extract	962.9	E858.0	E932.9	E950.4	E962.0	E980.4
Placidyl	967.8	E852.8	E937.8	E950.2	E962.0	E980.2
Plague vaccine	978.3	E858.8	E948.3	E950.4	E962.0	E980.4
Plant foods or fertilizers NEC	989.89	E866.5	—	E950.9	E962.1	E980.9
mixed with herbicides	989.4	E863.5	—	E950.6	E962.1	E980.7
Plants, noxious, used as food	988.2	E865.9	—	E950.9	E962.1	E980.9
berries and seeds	988.2	E865.3	—	E950.9	E962.1	E980.9
specified type NEC	988.2	E865.4	—	E950.9	E962.1	E980.9
Plasma (blood)	964.7	E858.2	E934.7	E950.4	E962.0	E980.4
expanders	964.8	E858.2	E934.8	E950.4	E962.0	E980.4
Plasmanate	964.7	E858.2	E934.7	E950.4	E962.0	E980.4
Plegicil	969.1	E853.0	E939.1	E950.3	E962.0	E980.3
Podophyllin	976.4	E858.7	E946.4	E950.4	E962.0	E980.4
Podophyllum resin	976.4	E858.7	E946.4	E950.4	E962.0	E980.4
Poisonous berries	988.2	E865.3	—	E950.9	E962.1	E980.9
Poison NEC	989.9	E866.9	—	E950.9	E962.1	E980.9
Pokeweed (any part)	988.2	E865.4	—	E950.9	E962.1	E980.9
Poldine	971.1	E855.4	E941.1	E950.4	E962.0	E980.4
Poliomyelitis vaccine	979.5	E858.8	E949.5	E950.4	E962.0	E980.4
Poliovirus vaccine	979.5	E858.8	E949.5	E950.4	E962.0	E980.4
Polish (car) (floor) (furniture) (metal) (silver)	989.89	E861.2	—	E950.9	E962.1	E980.9
abrasive	989.89	E861.3	—	E950.9	E962.1	E980.9
porcelain	989.89	E861.3	—	E950.9	E962.1	E980.9
Poloxalkol	973.2	E858.4	E943.2	E950.4	E962.0	E980.4
Polyaminostyrene resins	974.5	E858.5	E944.5	E950.4	E962.0	E980.4
Polychlorinated biphenyl — see PCBs						
Polycycline	960.4	E856	E930.4	E950.4	E962.0	E980.4
Polyester resin hardener	982.8	E862.4	—	E950.9	E962.1	E980.9
fumes	987.8	E869.8	—	E952.8	E962.2	E982.8
Polyestradiol (phosphate)	962.2	E858.0	E932.2	E950.4	E962.0	E980.4
Polyethanolamine alkyl sulfate	976.2	E858.7	E946.2	E950.4	E962.0	E980.4
Polyethylene glycol	976.3	E858.7	E946.3	E950.4	E962.0	E980.4
Polyferose	964.0	E858.2	E934.0	E950.4	E962.0	E980.4
Polymyxin B	960.8	E856	E930.8	E950.4	E962.0	E980.4
ENT agent	976.6	E858.7	E946.6	E950.4	E962.0	E980.4
ophthalmic preparation	976.5	E858.7	E946.5	E950.4	E962.0	E980.4
topical NEC	976.0	E858.7	E946.0	E950.4	E962.0	E980.4
Polynoxylin(e)	976.0	E858.7	E946.0	E950.4	E962.0	E980.4
Polyoxymethyleneurea	976.0	E858.7	E946.0	E950.4	E962.0	E980.4
Polytetrafluoroethylene (inhaled)	987.8	E869.8	—	E952.8	E962.2	E982.8
Polythiazide	974.3	E858.5	E944.3	E950.4	E962.0	E980.4
Polyvinylpyrrolidone	964.8	E858.2	E934.8	E950.4	E962.0	E980.4

	Poisoning	Accident	Therapeutic Use	Suicide Attempt	Assault	Undetermined
Pontocaine (hydrochloride) (infiltration) (topical)	968.5	E855.2	E938.5	E950.4	E962.0	E980.4
nerve block (peripheral) (plexus)	968.6	E855.2	E938.6	E950.4	E962.0	E980.4
spinal	968.7	E855.2	E938.7	E950.4	E962.0	E980.4
Pot	969.6	E854.1	E939.6	E950.3	E962.0	E980.3
Potash (caustic)	983.2	E864.2	—	E950.7	E962.1	E980.6
Potassic saline injection (lactated)	974.5	E858.5	E944.5	E950.4	E962.0	E980.4
Potassium (salts) NEC	974.5	E858.5	E944.5	E950.4	E962.0	E980.4
aminosalicylate	961.8	E857	E931.8	E950.4	E962.0	E980.4
arsenite (solution)	985.1	E866.3	—	E950.8	E962.1	E980.8
bichromate	983.9	E864.3	—	E950.7	E962.1	E980.6
bisulfate	983.9	E864.3	—	E950.7	E962.1	E980.6
bromide (medicinal) NEC	967.3	E852.2	E937.3	E950.2	E962.0	E980.2
carbonate	983.2	E864.2	—	E950.7	E962.1	E980.6
chlorate NEC	983.9	E864.3	—	E950.7	E962.1	E980.6
cyanide — see Cyanide						
hydroxide	983.2	E864.2	—	E950.7	E962.1	E980.6
iodide (expectorant) NEC	975.5	E858.6	E945.5	E950.4	E962.0	E980.4
nitrate	989.89	E866.8	—	E950.9	E962.1	E980.9
oxalate	983.9	E864.3	—	E950.7	E962.1	E980.6
perchlorate NEC	977.8	E858.8	E947.8	E950.4	E962.0	E980.4
antithyroid	962.8	E858.0	E932.8	E950.4	E962.0	E980.4
permanganate	976.0	E858.7	E946.0	E950.4	E962.0	E980.4
nonmedicinal	983.9	E864.3	—	E950.7	E962.1	E980.6
Povidone-iodine (anti-infective) NEC	976.0	E858.7	E946.0	E950.4	E962.0	E980.4
Practolol	972.0	E858.3	E942.0	E950.4	E962.0	E980.4
Pralidoxime (chloride)	977.2	E858.8	E947.2	E950.4	E962.0	E980.4
Pramoxine	968.5	E855.2	E938.5	E950.4	E962.0	E980.4
Prazosin	972.6	E858.3	E942.6	E950.4	E962.0	E980.4
Prednisolone	962.0	E858.0	E932.0	E950.4	E962.0	E980.4
ENT agent	976.6	E858.7	E946.6	E950.4	E962.0	E980.4
ophthalmic preparation	976.5	E858.7	E946.5	E950.4	E962.0	E980.4
topical NEC	976.0	E858.7	E946.0	E950.4	E962.0	E980.4
Prednisone	962.0	E858.0	E932.0	E950.4	E962.0	E980.4
Pregnanediol	962.2	E858.0	E932.2	E950.4	E962.0	E980.4
Pregneninolone	962.2	E858.0	E932.2	E950.4	E962.0	E980.4
Preludin	977.0	E858.8	E947.0	E950.4	E962.0	E980.4
Premarin	962.2	E858.0	E932.2	E950.4	E962.0	E980.4
Prenylamine	972.4	E858.3	E942.4	E950.4	E962.0	E980.4
Preparation H	976.8	E858.7	E946.8	E950.4	E962.0	E980.4
Preservatives	989.89	E866.8	—	E950.9	E962.1	E980.9
Pride of China	988.2	E865.3	—	E950.9	E962.1	E980.9
Prilocaine	968.9	E855.2	E938.9	E950.4	E962.0	E980.4
infiltration (subcutaneous)	968.5	E855.2	E938.5	E950.4	E962.0	E980.4
nerve block (peripheral) (plexus)	968.6	E855.2	E938.6	E950.4	E962.0	E980.4
Primaquine	961.4	E857	E931.4	E950.4	E962.0	E980.4
Primidone	966.3	E855.0	E936.3	E950.4	E962.0	E980.4
Primula (veris)	988.2	E865.4	—	E950.9	E962.1	E980.9
Prinadol	965.09	E850.2	E935.2	E950.0	E962.0	E980.0
Priscol, Priscoline	971.3	E855.6	E941.3	E950.4	E962.0	E980.4
Privet	988.2	E865.4	—	E950.9	E962.1	E980.9
Privine	971.2	E855.5	E941.2	E950.4	E962.0	E980.4
Pro-Banthine	971.1	E855.4	E941.1	E950.4	E962.0	E980.4
Probarbital	967.0	E851	E937.0	E950.1	E962.0	E980.1
Probenecid	974.7	E858.5	E944.7	E950.4	E962.0	E980.4
Procainamide (hydrochloride)	972.0	E858.3	E942.0	E950.4	E962.0	E980.4
Procaine (hydrochloride) (infiltration) (topical)	968.5	E855.2	E938.5	E950.4	E962.0	E980.4
nerve block (peripheral) (plexus)	968.6	E855.2	E938.6	E950.4	E962.0	E980.4
penicillin G	960.0	E856	E930.0	E950.4	E962.0	E980.4
spinal	968.7	E855.2	E938.7	E950.4	E962.0	E980.4
Procalmidol	969.5	E853.8	E939.5	E950.3	E962.0	E980.3
Procarbazine	963.1	E858.1	E933.1	E950.4	E962.0	E980.4
Prochlorperazine	969.1	E853.0	E939.1	E950.3	E962.0	E980.3
Procyclidine	966.4	E855.0	E936.4	E950.4	E962.0	E980.4
Producer gas	986	E868.8	—	E952.1	E962.2	E982.1
Profenamine	966.4	E855.0	E936.4	E950.4	E962.0	E980.4
Profenil	975.1	E858.6	E945.1	E950.4	E962.0	E980.4
Progesterones	962.2	E858.0	E932.2	E950.4	E962.0	E980.4
Progestin	962.2	E858.0	E932.2	E950.4	E962.0	E980.4
Progestogens (with estrogens)	962.2	E858.0	E932.2	E950.4	E962.0	E980.4
Progestone	962.2	E858.0	E932.2	E950.4	E962.0	E980.4
Proguanil	961.4	E857	E931.4	E950.4	E962.0	E980.4
Prolactin	962.4	E858.0	E932.4	E950.4	E962.0	E980.4

Nontherapeutic use substance

Subterms under main terms may continue to next column or page

	Poisoning	Accident	Therapeutic Use	Suicide Attempt	Assault	Undetermined
Proloid	962.7	E858.0	E932.7	E950.4	E962.0	E980.4
Proluton	962.2	E858.0	E932.2	E950.4	E962.0	E980.4
Promacetin	961.8	E857	E931.8	E950.4	E962.0	E980.4
Promazine	969.1	E853.0	E939.1	E950.3	E962.0	E980.3
Promedol	965.09	E850.2	E935.2	E950.0	E962.0	E980.0
Promethazine	967.8	E852.8	E937.8	E950.2	E962.0	E980.2
Promin	961.8	E857	E931.8	E950.4	E962.0	E980.4
Pronestyl (hydrochloride)	972.0	E858.3	E942.0	E950.4	E962.0	E980.4
Pronetalol, pronethalol	972.0	E858.3	E942.0	E950.4	E962.0	E980.4
Prontosil	961.0	E857	E931.0	E950.4	E962.0	E980.4
Propamidine isethionate	961.5	E857	E931.5	E950.4	E962.0	E980.4
Propanal (medicinal)	967.8	E852.8	E937.8	E950.2	E962.0	E980.2
Propane (gas) (distributed in mobile container)	987.0	E868.0	—	E951.1	E962.2	E981.1
distributed through pipes	987.0	E867	—	E951.0	E962.2	E981.0
incomplete combustion of — see Carbon monoxide, Propane						
Propanidid	968.3	E855.1	E938.3	E950.4	E962.0	E980.4
Propanol	980.3	E860.4	—	E950.9	E962.1	E980.9
Propantheline	971.1	E855.4	E941.1	E950.4	E962.0	E980.4
Proparacaine	968.5	E855.2	E938.5	E950.4	E962.0	E980.4
Propatyl nitrate	972.4	E858.3	E942.4	E950.4	E962.0	E980.4
Propicillin	960.0	E856	E930.0	E950.4	E962.0	E980.4
Propiolactone (vapor)	987.8	E869.8	—	E952.8	E962.2	E982.8
Propiomazine	967.8	E852.8	E937.8	E950.2	E962.0	E980.2
Propionaldehyde (medicinal)	967.8	E852.8	E937.8	E950.2	E962.0	E980.2
Propionate compound	976.0	E858.7	E946.0	E950.4	E962.0	E980.4
Propion gel	976.0	E858.7	E946.0	E950.4	E962.0	E980.4
Propitocaine	968.9	E855.2	E938.9	E950.4	E962.0	E980.4
infiltration (subcutaneous)	968.5	E855.2	E938.5	E950.4	E962.0	E980.4
nerve block (peripheral) (plexus)	968.6	E855.2	E938.6	E950.4	E962.0	E980.4
Propoxur	989.3	E863.2	—	E950.6	E962.1	E980.7
Propoxycaine	968.9	E855.2	E938.9	E950.4	E962.0	E980.4
infiltration (subcutaneous)	968.5	E855.2	E938.5	E950.4	E962.0	E980.4
nerve block (peripheral) (plexus)	968.6	E855.2	E938.6	E950.4	E962.0	E980.4
topical (surface)	968.5	E855.2	E938.5	E950.4	E962.0	E980.4
Propoxyphene (hydrochloride)	965.8	E850.8	E935.8	E950.0	E962.0	E980.0
Propranolol	972.0	E858.3	E942.0	E950.4	E962.0	E980.4
Propyl						
alcohol	980.3	E860.4	—	E950.9	E962.1	E980.9
carbinol	980.3	E860.4	—	E950.9	E962.1	E980.9
hexadrine	971.2	E855.5	E941.2	E950.4	E962.0	E980.4
iodone	977.8	E858.8	E947.8	E950.4	E962.0	E980.4
thiouracil	962.8	E858.0	E932.8	E950.4	E962.0	E980.4
Propylene	987.1	E869.8	—	E952.8	E962.2	E982.8
Propylparaben (ophthalmic)	976.5	E858.7	E946.5	E950.4	E962.0	E980.4
Proscillaridin	972.1	E858.3	E942.1	E950.4	E962.0	E980.4
Prostaglandins	975.0	E858.6	E945.0	E950.4	E962.0	E980.4
Prostigmin	971.0	E855.3	E941.0	E950.4	E962.0	E980.4
Protamine (sulfate)	964.5	E858.2	E934.5	E950.4	E962.0	E980.4
zinc insulin	962.3	E858.0	E932.3	E950.4	E962.0	E980.4
Protectants (topical)	976.3	E858.7	E946.3	E950.4	E962.0	E980.4
Protein hydrolysate	974.5	E858.5	E944.5	E950.4	E962.0	E980.4
Prothiaden — see Dothiepin hydrochloride						
Prothionamide	961.8	E857	E931.8	E950.4	E962.0	E980.4
Prothipendyl	969.5	E853.8	E939.5	E950.3	E962.0	E980.3
Protokylol	971.2	E855.5	E941.2	E950.4	E962.0	E980.4
Protopam	977.2	E858.8	E947.2	E950.4	E962.0	E980.4
Protoveratrine(s) (A) (B)	972.6	E858.3	E942.6	E950.4	E962.0	E980.4
Protriptyline	969.05	E854.0	E939.0	E950.3	E962.0	E980.3
Provera	962.2	E858.0	E932.2	E950.4	E962.0	E980.4
Provitamin A	963.5	E858.1	E933.5	E950.4	E962.0	E980.4
Proxymetacaine	968.5	E855.2	E938.5	E950.4	E962.0	E980.4
Proxyphylline	975.1	E858.6	E945.1	E950.4	E962.0	E980.4
Prozac — see Fluoxetine hydrochloride						
Prunus						
laurocerasus	988.2	E865.4	—	E950.9	E962.1	E980.9
virginiana	988.2	E865.4	—	E950.9	E962.1	E980.9
Prussic acid	989.0	E866.8	—	E950.9	E962.1	E980.9
vapor	987.7	E869.8	—	E952.8	E962.2	E982.8
Pseudoephedrine	971.2	E855.5	E941.2	E950.4	E962.0	E980.4

	Poisoning	Accident	Therapeutic Use	Suicide Attempt	Assault	Undetermined
Psilocin	969.6	E854.1	E939.6	E950.3	E962.0	E980.3
Psilocybin	969.6	E854.1	E939.6	E950.3	E962.0	E980.3
PSP	977.8	E858.8	E947.8	E950.4	E962.0	E980.4
Psychedelic agents	969.6	E854.1	E939.6	E950.3	E962.0	E980.3
Psychodysleptics	969.6	E854.1	E939.6	E950.3	E962.0	E980.3
Psychostimulants	969.70	E854.2	E939.7	E950.3	E962.0	E980.3
Psychotherapeutic agents	969.9	E855.9	E939.9	E950.3	E962.0	E980.3
antidepressants	969.00	E854.0	E939.0	E950.3	E962.0	E980.3
specified NEC	969.8	E855.8	E939.8	E950.3	E962.0	E980.3
tranquilizers NEC	969.5	E853.9	E939.5	E950.3	E962.0	E980.3
Psychotomimetic agents	969.6	E854.1	E939.6	E950.3	E962.0	E980.3
Psychotropic agents	969.9	E854.8	E939.9	E950.3	E962.0	E980.3
specified NEC	969.8	E854.8	E939.8	E950.3	E962.0	E980.3
Psyllium	973.3	E858.4	E943.3	E950.4	E962.0	E980.4
Pteroylglutamic acid	964.1	E858.2	E934.1	E950.4	E962.0	E980.4
Pteroyltriglutamate	963.1	E858.1	E933.1	E950.4	E962.0	E980.4
PTFE	987.8	E869.8	—	E952.8	E962.2	E982.8
Pulsatilla	988.2	E865.4	—	E950.9	E962.1	E980.9
Purex (bleach)	983.9	E864.3	—	E950.7	E962.1	E980.6
Purine diuretics	974.1	E858.5	E944.1	E950.4	E962.0	E980.4
Purinethol	963.1	E858.1	E933.1	E950.4	E962.0	E980.4
PVP	964.8	E858.2	E934.8	E950.4	E962.0	E980.4
Pyrabital	965.7	E850.7	E935.7	E950.0	E962.0	E980.0
Pyramidon	965.5	E850.5	E935.5	E950.0	E962.0	E980.0
Pyrantel (pamoate)	961.6	E857	E931.6	E950.4	E962.0	E980.4
Pyrathiazine	963.0	E858.1	E933.0	E950.4	E962.0	E980.4
Pyrazinamide	961.8	E857	E931.8	E950.4	E962.0	E980.4
Pyrazinoic acid (amide)	961.8	E857	E931.8	E950.4	E962.0	E980.4
Pyrazole (derivatives)	965.5	E850.5	E935.5	E950.0	E962.0	E980.0
Pyrazolone (analgesics)	965.5	E850.5	E935.5	E950.0	E962.0	E980.0
Pyrethrins, pyrethrum	989.4	E863.4	—	E950.6	E962.1	E980.7
Pyribenzamine	963.0	E858.1	E933.0	E950.4	E962.0	E980.4
Pyridine (liquid) (vapor)	982.0	E862.4	—	E950.9	E962.1	E980.9
aldoxime chloride	977.2	E858.8	E947.2	E950.4	E962.0	E980.4
Pyridium	976.1	E858.7	E946.1	E950.4	E962.0	E980.4
Pyridostigmine	971.0	E855.3	E941.0	E950.4	E962.0	E980.4
Pyridoxine	963.5	E858.1	E933.5	E950.4	E962.0	E980.4
Pyrilamine	963.0	E858.1	E933.0	E950.4	E962.0	E980.4
Pyrimethamine	961.4	E857	E931.4	E950.4	E962.0	E980.4
Pyrogallic acid	983.0	E864.0	—	E950.7	E962.1	E980.6
Pyroxylin	976.3	E858.7	E946.3	E950.4	E962.0	E980.4
Pyrrobutamine	963.0	E858.1	E933.0	E950.4	E962.0	E980.4
Pyrrocitine	968.5	E855.2	E938.5	E950.4	E962.0	E980.4
Pyrvinium (pamoate)	961.6	E857	E931.6	E950.4	E962.0	E980.4
PZI	962.3	E858.0	E932.3	E950.4	E962.0	E980.4
Quaalude	967.4	E852.3	E937.4	E950.2	E962.0	E980.2
Quaternary ammonium derivatives	971.1	E855.4	E941.1	E950.4	E962.0	E980.4
Quicklime	983.2	E864.2	—	E950.7	E962.1	E980.6
Quinacrine	961.3	E857	E931.3	E950.4	E962.0	E980.4
Quinaglute	972.0	E858.3	E942.0	E950.4	E962.0	E980.4
Quinalbarbitone	967.0	E851	E937.0	E950.1	E962.0	E980.1
Quinestradiol	962.2	E858.0	E932.2	E950.4	E962.0	E980.4
Quinethazone	974.3	E858.5	E944.3	E950.4	E962.0	E980.4
Quinidine (gluconate) (polygalacturonate) (salts) (sulfate)	972.0	E858.3	E942.0	E950.4	E962.0	E980.4
Quinine	961.4	E857	E931.4	E950.4	E962.0	E980.4
Quiniobine	961.3	E857	E931.3	E950.4	E962.0	E980.4
Quinolines	961.3	E857	E931.3	E950.4	E962.0	E980.4
Quotane	968.5	E855.2	E938.5	E950.4	E962.0	E980.4
Rabies						
immune globulin (human)	964.6	E858.2	E934.6	E950.4	E962.0	E980.4
vaccine	979.1	E858.8	E949.1	E950.4	E962.0	E980.4
Racemoramide	965.09	E850.2	E935.2	E950.0	E962.0	E980.0
Racemorphan	965.09	E850.2	E935.2	E950.0	E962.0	E980.0
Radiator alcohol	980.1	E860.2	—	E950.9	E962.1	E980.9
Radio-opaque (drugs) (materials)	977.8	E858.8	E947.8	E950.4	E962.0	E980.4
Ranunculus	988.2	E865.4	—	E950.9	E962.1	E980.9
Rat poison	989.4	E863.7	—	E950.6	E962.1	E980.7
Rattlesnake (venom)	989.5	E905.0	—	E950.9	E962.1	E980.9
Raudixin	972.6	E858.3	E942.6	E950.4	E962.0	E980.4
Rautensin	972.6	E858.3	E942.6	E950.4	E962.0	E980.4
Rautina	972.6	E858.3	E942.6	E950.4	E962.0	E980.4
Rautotal	972.6	E858.3	E942.6	E950.4	E962.0	E980.4
Rauwiloid	972.6	E858.3	E942.6	E950.4	E962.0	E980.4
Rauwoldin	972.6	E858.3	E942.6	E950.4	E962.0	E980.4
Rauwolfia (alkaloids)	972.6	E858.3	E942.6	E950.4	E962.0	E980.4
Realgar	985.1	E866.3	—	E950.8	E962.1	E980.8

	Poisoning	Accident	Therapeutic Use	Suicide Attempt	Assault	Undetermined
External Cause (E-Code)						
Red cells, packed	964.7	E858.2	E934.7	E950.4	E962.0	E980.4
Reducing agents, industrial NEC	983.9	E864.3	—	E950.7	E962.1	E980.6
Refrigerant gas (freon)	987.4	E869.2	—	E952.8	E962.2	E982.8
central nervous system	968.0	E855.1	E938.0	E950.4	E962.0	E980.4
not freon	987.9	E869.9	—	E952.9	E962.2	E982.9
Regroton	974.4	E858.5	E944.4	E950.4	E962.0	E980.4
Rela	968.0	E855.1	E938.0	E950.4	E962.0	E980.4
Relaxants, skeletal muscle (autonomic)	975.2	E858.6	E945.2	E950.4	E962.0	E980.4
Renese	974.3	E858.5	E944.3	E950.4	E962.0	E980.4
Renografin	977.8	E858.8	E947.8	E950.4	E962.0	E980.4
Replacement solutions	974.5	E858.5	E944.5	E950.4	E962.0	E980.4
Rescinnamine	972.6	E858.3	E942.6	E950.4	E962.0	E980.4
Reserpine	972.6	E858.3	E942.6	E950.4	E962.0	E980.4
Resorcin, resorcinol	976.4	E858.7	E946.4	E950.4	E962.0	E980.4
Respaire	975.5	E858.6	E945.5	E950.4	E962.0	E980.4
Respiratory agents NEC	975.8	E858.6	E945.8	E950.4	E962.0	E980.4
Retinoic acid	976.8	E858.7	E946.8	E950.4	E962.0	E980.4
Retinol	963.5	E858.1	E933.5	E950.4	E962.0	E980.4
Rh (D) immune globulin (human)	964.6	E858.2	E934.6	E950.4	E962.0	E980.4
Rhodine	965.1	E850.3	E935.3	E950.0	E962.0	E980.0
RhoGAM	964.6	E858.2	E934.6	E950.4	E962.0	E980.4
Riboflavin	963.5	E858.1	E933.5	E950.4	E962.0	E980.4
Ricin	989.89	E866.8	—	E950.9	E962.1	E980.9
Ricinus communis	988.2	E865.3	—	E950.9	E962.1	E980.9
Rickettsial vaccine NEC	979.6	E858.8	E949.6	E950.4	E962.0	E980.4
with viral and bacterial vaccine	979.7	E858.8	E949.7	E950.4	E962.0	E980.4
Rifampin	960.6	E856	E930.6	E950.4	E962.0	E980.4
Rimifon	961.8	E857	E931.8	E950.4	E962.0	E980.4
Ringer's injection (lactated)	974.5	E858.5	E944.5	E950.4	E962.0	E980.4
Ristocetin	960.8	E856	E930.8	E950.4	E962.0	E980.4
Ritalin	969.73	E854.2	E939.7	E950.3	E962.0	E980.3
Roach killers — see Pesticides						
Rocky Mountain spotted fever vaccine	979.6	E858.8	E949.6	E950.4	E962.0	E980.4
Rodenticides	989.4	E863.7	—	E950.6	E962.1	E980.7
Rohypnol	969.4	E853.2	E939.4	E950.3	E962.0	E980.3
Rolaids	973.0	E858.4	E943.0	E950.4	E962.0	E980.4
Rolitetracycline	960.4	E856	E930.4	E950.4	E962.0	E980.4
Romilar	975.4	E858.6	E945.4	E950.4	E962.0	E980.4
Rose water ointment	976.3	E858.7	E946.3	E950.4	E962.0	E980.4
Rosuvastatin calcium	972.1	E858.3	E942.2	E950.4	E962.0	E980.4
Rotenone	989.4	E863.7	—	E950.6	E962.1	E980.7
Rotoxamine	963.0	E858.1	E933.0	E950.4	E962.0	E980.4
Rough-on-rats	989.4	E863.7	—	E950.6	E962.1	E980.7
RU486	962.9	E858.0	E932.9	E950.4	E962.0	E980.4
Rubbing alcohol	980.2	E860.3	—	E950.9	E962.1	E980.9
Rubella virus vaccine	979.4	E858.8	E949.4	E950.4	E962.0	E980.4
Rubelogen	979.4	E858.8	E949.4	E950.4	E962.0	E980.4
Rubeovax	979.4	E858.8	E949.4	E950.4	E962.0	E980.4
Rubidomycin	960.7	E856	E930.7	E950.4	E962.0	E980.4
Rue	988.2	E865.4	—	E950.9	E962.1	E980.9
Ruta	988.2	E865.4	—	E950.9	E962.1	E980.9
Sabadilla (medicinal)	976.0	E858.7	E946.0	E950.4	E962.0	E980.4
pesticide	989.4	E863.4	—	E950.6	E962.1	E980.7
Sabin oral vaccine	979.5	E858.8	E949.5	E950.4	E962.0	E980.4
Saccharated iron oxide	964.0	E858.2	E934.0	E950.4	E962.0	E980.4
Saccharin	974.5	E858.5	E944.5	E950.4	E962.0	E980.4
Safflower oil	972.2	E858.3	E942.2	E950.4	E962.0	E980.4
Salbutamol sulfate	975.7	E858.6	E945.7	E950.4	E962.0	E980.4
Salicylamide	965.1	E850.3	E935.3	E950.0	E962.0	E980.0
Salicylate(s)	965.1	E850.3	E935.3	E950.0	E962.0	E980.0
methyl	976.3	E858.7	E946.3	E950.4	E962.0	E980.4
theobromine calcium	974.1	E858.5	E944.1	E950.4	E962.0	E980.4
Salicylazosulfapyridine	961.0	E857	E931.0	E950.4	E962.0	E980.4
Salicylhydroxamic acid	976.0	E858.7	E946.0	E950.4	E962.0	E980.4
Salicylic acid (keratolytic) NEC	976.4	E858.7	E946.4	E950.4	E962.0	E980.4
congeners	965.1	E850.3	E935.3	E950.0	E962.0	E980.0
salts	965.1	E850.3	E935.3	E950.0	E962.0	E980.0
Saliniazid	961.8	E857	E931.8	E950.4	E962.0	E980.4
Salol	976.3	E858.7	E946.3	E950.4	E962.0	E980.4
Salt (substitute) NEC	974.5	E858.5	E944.5	E950.4	E962.0	E980.4
Saluretics	974.3	E858.5	E944.3	E950.4	E962.0	E980.4
Saluron	974.3	E858.5	E944.3	E950.4	E962.0	E980.4
Salvarsan 606 (neosilver) (silver)	961.1	E857	E931.1	E950.4	E962.0	E980.4
Sambucus canadensis	988.2	E865.4	—	E950.9	E962.1	E980.9
Sambucus canadensis — continued						
berry	988.2	E865.3	—	E950.9	E962.1	E980.9
Sandril	972.6	E858.3	E942.6	E950.4	E962.0	E980.4
Sanguinaria canadensis	988.2	E865.4	—	E950.9	E962.1	E980.9
Saniflush (cleaner)	983.9	E861.3	—	E950.7	E962.1	E980.6
Santonin	961.6	E857	E931.6	E950.4	E962.0	E980.4
Santyl	976.8	E858.7	E946.8	E950.4	E962.0	E980.4
Sarkomycin	960.7	E856	E930.7	E950.4	E962.0	E980.4
Saroten	969.05	E854.0	E939.0	E950.3	E962.0	E980.3
Saturnine — see Lead						
Savin (oil)	976.4	E858.7	E946.4	E950.4	E962.0	E980.4
Scammony	973.1	E858.4	E943.1	E950.4	E962.0	E980.4
Scarlet red	976.8	E858.7	E946.8	E950.4	E962.0	E980.4
Scheele's green	985.1	E866.3	—	E950.8	E962.1	E980.8
insecticide	985.1	E863.4	—	E950.8	E962.1	E980.8
Schradan	989.3	E863.1	—	E950.6	E962.1	E980.7
Schweinfurt(h) green	985.1	E866.3	—	E950.8	E962.1	E980.8
insecticide	985.1	E863.4	—	E950.8	E962.1	E980.8
Scilla — see Squill						
Sclerosing agents	972.7	E858.3	E942.7	E950.4	E962.0	E980.4
Scopolamine	971.1	E855.4	E941.1	E950.4	E962.0	E980.4
Scouring powder	989.89	E861.3	—	E950.9	E962.1	E980.9
Sea						
anemone (sting)	989.5	E905.6	—	E950.9	E962.1	E980.9
cucumber (sting)	989.5	E905.6	—	E950.9	E962.1	E980.9
snake (bite) (venom)	989.5	E905.0	—	E950.9	E962.1	E980.9
urchin spine (puncture)	989.5	E905.6	—	E950.9	E962.1	E980.9
Secbutabarbital	967.0	E851	E937.0	E950.1	E962.0	E980.1
Secbutabarbitone	967.0	E851	E937.0	E950.1	E962.0	E980.1
Secobarbital	967.0	E851	E937.0	E950.1	E962.0	E980.1
Seconal	967.0	E851	E937.0	E950.1	E962.0	E980.1
Secretin	977.8	E858.8	E947.8	E950.4	E962.0	E980.4
Sedatives, nonbarbiturate	967.9	E852.9	E937.9	E950.2	E962.0	E980.2
specified NEC	967.8	E852.8	E937.8	E950.2	E962.0	E980.2
Sedormid	967.8	E852.8	E937.8	E950.2	E962.0	E980.2
Seed (plant)	988.2	E865.3	—	E950.9	E962.1	E980.9
disinfectant or dressing	989.89	E866.5	—	E950.9	E962.1	E980.9
Selective serotonin and norepinephrine reuptake inhibitors (SSNRI)	969.02	E854.0	E939.0	E950.3	E962.0	E980.3
Selective serotonin reuptake inhibitors (SSRI)	969.03	E854.0	E939.0	E950.3	E962.0	E980.3
Selenium (fumes) NEC	985.8	E866.4	—	E950.9	E962.1	E980.9
disulfide or sulfide	976.4	E858.7	E946.4	E950.4	E962.0	E980.4
Selsun	976.4	E858.7	E946.4	E950.4	E962.0	E980.4
Senna	973.1	E858.4	E943.1	E950.4	E962.0	E980.4
Septisol	976.2	E858.7	E946.2	E950.4	E962.0	E980.4
Serax	969.4	E853.2	E939.4	E950.3	E962.0	E980.3
Serenesil	967.8	E852.8	E937.8	E950.2	E962.0	E980.2
Serenium (hydrochloride)	961.9	E857	E931.9	E950.4	E962.0	E980.4
Serepax — see Oxazepam						
Sernyl	968.3	E855.1	E938.3	E950.4	E962.0	E980.4
Serotonin	977.8	E858.8	E947.8	E950.4	E962.0	E980.4
Serpasil	972.6	E858.3	E942.6	E950.4	E962.0	E980.4
Sewer gas	987.8	E869.8	—	E952.8	E962.2	E982.8
Shampoo	989.6	E861.0	—	E950.9	E962.1	E980.9
Shellfish, nonbacterial or noxious	988.0	E865.1	—	E950.9	E962.1	E980.9
Silicones NEC	989.83	E866.8	E947.8	E950.9	E962.1	E980.9
Silvadene	976.0	E858.7	E946.0	E950.4	E962.0	E980.4
Silver (compound) (medicinal) NEC	976.0	E858.7	E946.0	E950.4	E962.0	E980.4
anti-infectives	976.0	E858.7	E946.0	E950.4	E962.0	E980.4
arsphenamine	961.1	E857	E931.1	E950.4	E962.0	E980.4
nitrate	976.0	E858.7	E946.0	E950.4	E962.0	E980.4
ophthalmic preparation	976.5	E858.7	E946.5	E950.4	E962.0	E980.4
toughened (keratolytic)	976.4	E858.7	E946.4	E950.4	E962.0	E980.4
nonmedicinal (dust)	985.8	E866.4	—	E950.9	E962.1	E980.9
protein (mild) (strong)	976.0	E858.7	E946.0	E950.4	E962.0	E980.4
salvarsan	961.1	E857	E931.1	E950.4	E962.0	E980.4
Simethicone	973.8	E858.4	E943.8	E950.4	E962.0	E980.4
Sinequan	969.05	E854.0	E939.0	E950.3	E962.0	E980.3
Singoserp	972.6	E858.3	E942.6	E950.4	E962.0	E980.4
Sintrom	964.2	E858.2	E934.2	E950.4	E962.0	E980.4
Sitosterols	972.2	E858.3	E942.2	E950.4	E962.0	E980.4
Skeletal muscle relaxants	975.2	E858.6	E945.2	E950.4	E962.0	E980.4
Skin						
agents (external)	976.9	E858.7	E946.9	E950.4	E962.0	E980.4
specified NEC	976.8	E858.7	E946.8	E950.4	E962.0	E980.4

Nontherapeutic use substance

▶◀ Revised Text   ● New Line   ▲ Revised Code

Subterms under main terms may continue to next column or page

	Poisoning	Accident	Therapeutic Use	Suicide Attempt	Assault	Undetermined
Skin — *continued*						
test antigen	977.8	E858.8	E947.8	E950.4	E962.0	E980.4
Sleep-eze	963.0	E858.1	E933.0	E950.4	E962.0	E980.4
Sleeping draught (drug) (pill)						
(tablet)	967.9	E852.9	E937.9	E950.2	E962.0	E980.2
Smallpox vaccine	979.0	E858.8	E949.0	E950.4	E962.0	E980.4
Smelter fumes NEC	985.9	E866.4	—	E950.9	E962.1	E980.9
Smog	987.3	E869.1	—	E952.8	E962.2	E982.8
Smoke NEC	987.9	E869.9	—	E952.9	E962.2	E982.9
Smooth muscle relaxant	975.1	E858.6	E945.1	E950.4	E962.0	E980.4
Snail killer	989.4	E863.4		E950.6	E962.1	E980.7
Snake (bite) (venom)	989.5	E905.0	—	E950.9	E962.1	E980.9
Snuff	989.89	E866.8	—	E950.9	E962.1	E980.9
Soap (powder) (product)	989.6	E861.1	—	E950.9	E962.1	E980.9
bicarb	963.3	E858.1	E933.3	E950.4	E962.0	E980.4
chlorinated — see Sodium,						
hypochlorite						
medicinal, soft	976.2	E858.7	E946.2	E950.4	E962.0	E980.4
Soda (caustic)	983.2	E864.2	—	E950.7	E962.1	E980.6
Sodium						
acetosulfone	961.8	E857	E931.8	E950.4	E962.0	E980.4
acetrizoate	977.8	E858.8	E947.8	E950.4	E962.0	E980.4
amytal	967.0	E851	E937.0	E950.1	E962.0	E980.1
arsenate — see Arsenic						
bicarbonate	963.3	E858.1	E933.3	E950.4	E962.0	E980.4
bichromate	983.9	E864.3	—	E950.7	E962.1	E980.6
biphosphate	963.2	E858.1	E933.2	E950.4	E962.0	E980.4
bisulfate	983.9	E864.3	—	E950.7	E962.1	E980.6
borate (cleanser)	989.6	E861.3	—	E950.9	E962.1	E980.9
bromide NEC	967.3	E852.2	E937.3	E950.2	E962.0	E980.2
cacodylate (nonmedicinal)						
NEC	978.8	E858.8	E948.8	E950.4	E962.0	E980.4
anti-infective	961.1	E857	E931.1	E950.4	E962.0	E980.4
herbicide	989.4	E863.5	—	E950.6	E962.1	E980.7
calcium edetate	963.8	E858.1	E933.8	E950.4	E962.0	E980.4
carbonate NEC	983.2	E864.2	—	E950.7	E962.1	E980.6
chlorate NEC	983.9	E864.3	—	E950.7	E962.1	E980.6
herbicide	983.9	E863.5	—	E950.7	E962.1	E980.6
chloride NEC	974.5	E858.5	E944.5	E950.4	E962.0	E980.4
chromate	983.9	E864.3	—	E950.7	E962.1	E980.6
citrate	963.3	E858.1	E933.3	E950.4	E962.0	E980.4
cyanide — see Cyanide(s)						
cyclamate	974.5	E858.5	E944.5	E950.4	E962.0	E980.4
diatrizoate	977.8	E858.8	E947.8	E950.4	E962.0	E980.4
dibunate	975.4	E858.6	E945.4	E950.4	E962.0	E980.4
dioctyl sulfosuccinate	973.2	E858.4	E943.2	E950.4	E962.0	E980.4
edetate	963.8	E858.1	E933.8	E950.4	E962.0	E980.4
ethacrynate	974.4	E858.5	E944.4	E950.4	E962.0	E980.4
fluoracetate (dust) (rodenti-						
cide)	989.4	E863.7	—	E950.6	E962.1	E980.7
fluoride — see Fluoride(s)						
free salt	974.5	E858.5	E944.5	E950.4	E962.0	E980.4
glucosulfone	961.8	E857	E931.8	E950.4	E962.0	E980.4
hydroxide	983.2	E864.2	—	E950.7	E962.1	E980.6
hypochlorite (bleach)						
NEC	983.9	E864.3	—	E950.7	E962.1	E980.6
disinfectant	983.9	E861.4	—	E950.7	E962.1	E980.6
medicinal (anti-infective)						
(external)	976.0	E858.7	E946.0	E950.4	E962.0	E980.4
vapor	987.8	E869.8	—	E952.8	E962.2	E982.8
hyposulfite	976.0	E858.7	E946.0	E950.4	E962.0	E980.4
indigotindisulfonate	977.8	E858.8	E947.8	E950.4	E962.0	E980.4
iodide	977.8	E858.8	E947.8	E950.4	E962.0	E980.4
iothalamate	977.8	E858.8	E947.8	E950.4	E962.0	E980.4
iron edetate	964.0	E858.2	E934.0	E950.4	E962.0	E980.4
lactate	963.3	E858.1	E933.3	E950.4	E962.0	E980.4
lauryl sulfate	976.2	E858.7	E946.2	E950.4	E962.0	E980.4
L-triiodothyronine	962.7	E858.0	E932.7	E950.4	E962.0	E980.4
metrizoate	977.8	E858.8	E947.8	E950.4	E962.0	E980.4
monofluoracetate (dust) (ro-						
denticide)	989.4	E863.7	—	E950.6	E962.1	E980.7
morrhuate	972.7	E858.3	E942.7	E950.4	E962.0	E980.4
nafcillin	960.0	E856	E930.0	E950.4	E962.0	E980.4
nitrate (oxidizing agent)	983.9	E864.3	—	E950.7	E962.1	E980.6
nitrite (medicinal)	972.4	E858.3	E942.4	E950.4	E962.0	E980.4
nitroferricyanide	972.6	E858.3	E942.6	E950.4	E962.0	E980.4
nitroprusside	972.6	E858.3	E942.6	E950.4	E962.0	E980.4
para-aminohippurate	977.8	E858.8	E947.8	E950.4	E962.0	E980.4
perborate (nonmedicinal)						
NEC	989.89	E866.8	—	E950.9	E962.1	E980.9
medicinal	976.6	E858.7	E946.6	E950.4	E962.0	E980.4
soap	989.6	E861.1	—	E950.9	E962.1	E980.9
Sodium — *continued*						
percarbonate — see Sodium,						
perborate						
phosphate	973.3	E858.4	E943.3	E950.4	E962.0	E980.4
polystyrene sulfonate	974.5	E858.5	E944.5	E950.4	E962.0	E980.4
propionate	976.0	E858.7	E946.0	E950.4	E962.0	E980.4
psylliate	972.7	E858.3	E942.7	E950.4	E962.0	E980.4
removing resins	974.5	E858.5	E944.5	E950.4	E962.0	E980.4
salicylate	965.1	E850.3	E935.3	E950.0	E962.0	E980.0
sulfate	973.3	E858.4	E943.3	E950.4	E962.0	E980.4
sulfoxone	961.8	E857	E931.8	E950.4	E962.0	E980.4
tetradecyl sulfate	972.7	E858.3	E942.7	E950.4	E962.0	E980.4
thiopental	968.3	E855.1	E938.3	E950.4	E962.0	E980.4
thiosalicylate	965.1	E850.3	E935.3	E950.0	E962.0	E980.0
thiosulfate	976.0	E858.7	E946.0	E950.4	E962.0	E980.4
tolbutamide	977.8	E858.8	E947.8	E950.4	E962.0	E980.4
tyropanoate	977.8	E858.8	E947.8	E950.4	E962.0	E980.4
valproate	966.3	E855.0	E936.3	E950.4	E962.0	E980.4
Solanine	977.8	E858.8	E947.8	E950.4	E962.0	E980.4
Solanum dulcamara	988.2	E865.4	—	E950.9	E962.1	E980.9
Solapsone	961.8	E857	E931.8	E950.4	E962.0	E980.4
Solasulfone	961.8	E857	E931.8	E950.4	E962.0	E980.4
Soldering fluid	983.1	E864.1	—	E950.7	E962.1	E980.6
Solid substance	989.9	E866.9	—	E950.9	E962.1	E980.9
specified NEC	989.9	E866.8	—	E950.9	E962.1	E980.9
Solvents, industrial	982.8	E862.9	—	E950.9	E962.1	E980.9
naphtha	981	E862.0	—	E950.9	E962.1	E980.9
petroleum	981	E862.0	—	E950.9	E962.1	E980.9
specified NEC	982.8	E862.4	—	E950.9	E962.1	E980.9
Soma	968.0	E855.1	E938.0	E950.4	E962.0	E980.4
Somatotropin	962.4	E858.0	E932.4	E950.4	E962.0	E980.4
Sominex	963.0	E858.1	E933.0	E950.4	E962.0	E980.4
Somnal	967.1	E852.0	E937.1	E950.2	E962.0	E980.2
Somnos	967.0	E851	E937.0	E950.1	E962.0	E980.1
Somonal	967.0	E851	E937.0	E950.1	E962.0	E980.1
Soneryl	967.0	E851	E937.0	E950.1	E962.0	E980.1
Soothing syrup	977.9	E858.9	E947.9	E950.5	E962.0	E980.5
Sopor	967.4	E852.3	E937.4	E950.2	E962.0	E980.2
Soporific drug	967.9	E852.9	E937.9	E950.2	E962.0	E980.2
specified type NEC	967.8	E852.8	E937.8	E950.2	E962.0	E980.2
Sorbitol NEC	977.4	E858.8	E947.4	E950.4	E962.0	E980.4
Sotradecol	972.7	E858.3	E942.7	E950.4	E962.0	E980.4
Spacoline	975.1	E858.6	E945.1	E950.4	E962.0	E980.4
Spanish fly	976.8	E858.7	E946.8	E950.4	E962.0	E980.4
Sparine	969.1	E853.0	E939.1	E950.3	E962.0	E980.3
Sparteine	975.0	E858.6	E945.0	E950.4	E962.0	E980.4
Spasmolytics	975.1	E858.6	E945.1	E950.4	E962.0	E980.4
anticholinergics	971.1	E855.4	E941.1	E950.4	E962.0	E980.4
Spectinomycin	960.8	E856	E930.8	E950.4	E962.0	E980.4
Speed	969.72	E854.2	E939.7	E950.3	E962.0	E980.3
Spermicides	976.8	E858.7	E946.8	E950.4	E962.0	E980.4
Spider (bite) (venom)	989.5	E905.1	—	E950.9	E962.1	E980.9
antivenin	979.9	E858.8	E949.9	E950.4	E962.0	E980.4
Spigelia (root)	961.6	E857	E931.6	E950.4	E962.0	E980.4
Spiperone	969.2	E853.1	E939.2	E950.3	E962.0	E980.3
Spiramycin	960.3	E856	E930.3	E950.4	E962.0	E980.4
Spirilene	969.5	E853.8	E939.5	E950.3	E962.0	E980.3
Spirit(s) (neutral) NEC	980.0	E860.1	—	E950.9	E962.1	E980.9
beverage	980.0	E860.0	—	E950.9	E962.1	E980.9
industrial	980.9	E860.9	—	E950.9	E962.1	E980.9
mineral	981	E862.0	—	E950.9	E962.1	E980.9
of salt — see Hydrochloric						
acid						
surgical	980.9	E860.9	—	E950.9	E962.1	E980.9
Spironolactone	974.4	E858.5	E944.4	E950.4	E962.0	E980.4
Sponge, absorbable						
(gelatin)	964.5	E858.2	E934.5	E950.4	E962.0	E980.4
Sporostacin	976.0	E858.7	E946.0	E950.4	E962.0	E980.4
Sprays (aerosol)	989.89	E866.8	—	E950.9	E962.1	E980.9
cosmetic	989.89	E866.7	—	E950.9	E962.1	E980.9
medicinal NEC	977.9	E858.9	E947.9	E950.5	E962.0	E980.5
pesticides — see Pesticides						
specified content — see sub-						
stance specified						
Spurge flax	988.2	E865.4	—	E950.9	E962.1	E980.9
Spurges	988.2	E865.4	—	E950.9	E962.1	E980.9
Squill (expectorant) NEC	975.5	E858.6	E945.5	E950.4	E962.0	E980.4
rat poison	989.4	E863.7	—	E950.6	E962.1	E980.7
Squirting cucumber (cathar-						
tic)	973.1	E858.4	E943.1	E950.4	E962.0	E980.4
SSNRI (selective serotonin and						
norepinephrine reuptake in-						
hibitors)	969.02	E854.0	E939.0	E950.3	E962.0	E980.3

	Poisoning	Accident	Therapeutic Use	Suicide Attempt	Assault	Undeter-mined
		External Cause (E-Code)				
SSRI (selective serotonin reuptake inhibitors)	969.03	E854.0	E939.0	E950.3	E962.0	E980.3
Stains	989.89	E866.8	—	E950.9	E962.1	E980.9
Stannous — see also Tin						
fluoride	976.7	E858.7	E946.7	E950.4	E962.0	E980.4
Stanolone	962.1	E858.0	E932.1	E950.4	E962.0	E980.4
Stanozolol	962.1	E858.0	E932.1	E950.4	E962.0	E980.4
Staphisagria or stavesacre (pediculicide)	976.0	E858.7	E946.0	E950.4	E962.0	E980.4
Stelazine	969.1	E853.0	E939.1	E950.3	E962.0	E980.3
Stemetil	969.1	E853.0	E939.1	E950.3	E962.0	E980.3
Sterculia (cathartic) (gum)	973.3	E858.4	E943.3	E950.4	E962.0	E980.4
Sternutator gas	987.8	E869.8	—	E952.8	E962.2	E982.8
Steroids NEC	962.0	E858.0	E932.0	E950.4	E962.0	E980.4
ENT agent	976.6	E858.7	E946.6	E950.4	E962.0	E980.4
ophthalmic preparation	976.5	E858.7	E946.5	E950.4	E962.0	E980.4
topical NEC	976.0	E858.7	E946.0	E950.4	E962.0	E980.4
Stibine	985.8	E866.4	—	E950.9	E962.1	E980.9
Stibophen	961.2	E857	E931.2	E950.4	E962.0	E980.4
Stilbamide, stilbamidine	961.5	E857	E931.5	E950.4	E962.0	E980.4
Stilbestrol	962.2	E858.0	E932.2	E950.4	E962.0	E980.4
Stimulants (central nervous system)	970.9	E854.3	E940.9	E950.4	E962.0	E980.4
analeptics	970.0	E854.3	E940.0	E950.4	E962.0	E980.4
opiate antagonist	970.1	E854.3	E940.1	E950.4	E962.0	E980.4
psychotherapeutic NEC	969.09	E854.0	E939.0	E950.3	E962.0	E980.3
specified NEC	970.89	E854.3	E940.8	E950.4	E962.0	E980.4
Storage batteries (acid) (cells)	983.1	E864.1	—	E950.7	E962.1	E980.6
Stovaine	968.9	E855.2	E938.9	E950.4	E962.0	E980.4
infiltration (subcutaneous)	968.5	E855.2	E938.5	E950.4	E962.0	E980.4
nerve block (peripheral) (plexus)	968.6	E855.2	E938.6	E950.4	E962.0	E980.4
spinal	968.7	E855.2	E938.7	E950.4	E962.0	E980.4
topical (surface)	968.5	E855.2	E938.5	E950.4	E962.0	E980.4
Stovarsal	961.1	E857	E931.1	E950.4	E962.0	E980.4
Stove gas — see Gas, utility						
Stoxil	976.5	E858.7	E946.5	E950.4	E962.0	E980.4
STP	969.6	E854.1	E939.6	E950.3	E962.0	E980.3
Stramonium (medicinal) NEC	971.1	E855.4	E941.1	E950.4	E962.0	E980.4
natural state	988.2	E865.4	—	E950.9	E962.1	E980.9
Streptodornase	964.4	E858.2	E934.4	E950.4	E962.0	E980.4
Streptoduocin	960.6	E856	E930.6	E950.4	E962.0	E980.4
Streptokinase	964.4	E858.2	E934.4	E950.4	E962.0	E980.4
Streptomycin	960.6	E856	E930.6	E950.4	E962.0	E980.4
Streptozocin	960.7	E856	E930.7	E950.4	E962.0	E980.4
Stripper (paint) (solvent)	982.8	E862.9	—	E950.9	E962.1	E980.9
Strobane	989.2	E863.0	—	E950.6	E962.1	E980.7
Strophanthin	972.1	E858.3	E942.1	E950.4	E962.0	E980.4
Strophanthus hispidus or kombe	988.2	E865.4	—	E950.9	E962.1	E980.9
Strychnine (rodenticide) (salts)	989.1	E863.7	—	E950.6	E962.1	E980.7
medicinal NEC	970.89	E854.3	E940.8	E950.4	E962.0	E980.4
Strychnos (ignatii) — see Strychnine						
Styramate	968.0	E855.1	E938.0	E950.4	E962.0	E980.4
Styrene	983.0	E864.0	—	E950.7	E962.1	E980.6
Succinimide (anticonvulsant)	966.2	E855.0	E936.2	E950.4	E962.0	E980.4
mercuric — see Mercury						
Succinylcholine	975.2	E858.6	E945.2	E950.4	E962.0	E980.4
Succinylsulfathiazole	961.0	E857	E931.0	E950.4	E962.0	E980.4
Sucrose	974.5	E858.5	E944.5	E950.4	E962.0	E980.4
Sulfacetamide	961.0	E857	E931.0	E950.4	E962.0	E980.4
ophthalmic preparation	976.5	E858.7	E946.5	E950.4	E962.0	E980.4
Sulfachlorpyridazine	961.0	E857	E931.0	E950.4	E962.0	E980.4
Sulfacytine	961.0	E857	E931.0	E950.4	E962.0	E980.4
Sulfadiazine	961.0	E857	E931.0	E950.4	E962.0	E980.4
silver (topical)	976.0	E858.7	E946.0	E950.4	E962.0	E980.4
Sulfadimethoxine	961.0	E857	E931.0	E950.4	E962.0	E980.4
Sulfadimidine	961.0	E857	E931.0	E950.4	E962.0	E980.4
Sulfaethidole	961.0	E857	E931.0	E950.4	E962.0	E980.4
Sulfafurazole	961.0	E857	E931.0	E950.4	E962.0	E980.4
Sulfaguanidine	961.0	E857	E931.0	E950.4	E962.0	E980.4
Sulfamerazine	961.0	E857	E931.0	E950.4	E962.0	E980.4
Sulfameter	961.0	E857	E931.0	E950.4	E962.0	E980.4
Sulfamethizole	961.0	E857	E931.0	E950.4	E962.0	E980.4
Sulfamethoxazole	961.0	E857	E931.0	E950.4	E962.0	E980.4
Sulfamethoxydiazine	961.0	E857	E931.0	E950.4	E962.0	E980.4

	Poisoning	Accident	Therapeutic Use	Suicide Attempt	Assault	Undeter-mined
		External Cause (E-Code)				
Sulfamethoxypyridazine	961.0	E857	E931.0	E950.4	E962.0	E980.4
Sulfamethylthiazole	961.0	E857	E931.0	E950.4	E962.0	E980.4
Sulfamylon	976.0	E858.7	E946.0	E950.4	E962.0	E980.4
Sulfan blue (diagnostic dye)	977.8	E858.8	E947.8	E950.4	E962.0	E980.4
Sulfanilamide	961.0	E857	E931.0	E950.4	E962.0	E980.4
Sulfanilylguanidine	961.0	E857	E931.0	E950.4	E962.0	E980.4
Sulfaphenazole	961.0	E857	E931.0	E950.4	E962.0	E980.4
Sulfaphenylthiazole	961.0	E857	E931.0	E950.4	E962.0	E980.4
Sulfaproxyline	961.0	E857	E931.0	E950.4	E962.0	E980.4
Sulfapyridine	961.0	E857	E931.0	E950.4	E962.0	E980.4
Sulfapyrimidine	961.0	E857	E931.0	E950.4	E962.0	E980.4
Sulfarsphenamine	961.1	E857	E931.1	E950.4	E962.0	E980.4
Sulfasalazine	961.0	E857	E931.0	E950.4	E962.0	E980.4
Sulfasomizole	961.0	E857	E931.0	E950.4	E962.0	E980.4
Sulfasuxidine	961.0	E857	E931.0	E950.4	E962.0	E980.4
Sulfinpyrazone	974.7	E858.5	E944.7	E950.4	E962.0	E980.4
Sulfisoxazole	961.0	E857	E931.0	E950.4	E962.0	E980.4
ophthalmic preparation	976.5	E858.7	E946.5	E950.4	E962.0	E980.4
Sulfomyxin	960.8	E856	E930.8	E950.4	E962.0	E980.4
Sulfonal	967.8	E852.8	E937.8	E950.2	E962.0	E980.2
Sulfonamides (mixtures)	961.0	E857	E931.0	E950.4	E962.0	E980.4
Sulfones	961.8	E857	E931.8	E950.4	E962.0	E980.4
Sulfonethylmethane	967.8	E852.8	E937.8	E950.2	E962.0	E980.2
Sulfonmethane	967.8	E852.8	E937.8	E950.2	E962.0	E980.2
Sulfonphthal, sulfonph-thol	977.8	E858.8	E947.8	E950.4	E962.0	E980.4
Sulfonylurea derivatives, oral	962.3	E858.0	E932.3	E950.4	E962.0	E980.4
Sulfoxone	961.8	E857	E931.8	E950.4	E962.0	E980.4
Sulfur, sulfureted, sulfuric, sulfurous, sulfuryl (compounds) NEC	989.89	E866.8	—	E950.9	E962.1	E980.9
acid	983.1	E864.1	—	E950.7	E962.1	E980.6
dioxide	987.3	E869.1	—	E952.8	E962.2	E982.8
ether — see Ether(s)						
hydrogen	987.8	E869.8	—	E952.8	E962.2	E982.8
medicinal (keratolytic) (ointment) NEC	976.4	E858.7	E946.4	E950.4	E962.0	E980.4
pesticide (vapor)	989.4	E863.4	—	E950.6	E962.1	E980.7
vapor NEC	987.8	E869.8	—	E952.8	E962.2	E982.8
Sulkowitch's reagent	977.8	E858.8	E947.8	E950.4	E962.0	E980.4
Sulphadione	961.8	E857	E931.8	E950.4	E962.0	E980.4
Sulph — see also Sulf-						
Sulthiame, sultiame	966.3	E855.0	E936.3	E950.4	E962.0	E980.4
Superinone	975.5	E858.6	E945.5	E950.4	E962.0	E980.4
Suramin	961.5	E857	E931.5	E950.4	E962.0	E980.4
Surfacaine	968.5	E855.2	E938.5	E950.4	E962.0	E980.4
Surital	968.3	E855.1	E938.3	E950.4	E962.0	E980.4
Sutilains	976.8	E858.7	E946.8	E950.4	E962.0	E980.4
Suxamethonium (bromide) (chloride) (iodide)	975.2	E858.6	E945.2	E950.4	E962.0	E980.4
Suxethonium (bromide)	975.2	E858.6	E945.2	E950.4	E962.0	E980.4
Sweet oil (birch)	976.3	E858.7	E946.3	E950.4	E962.0	E980.4
Sym-dichloroethyl ether	982.3	E862.4	—	E950.9	E962.1	E980.9
Sympatholytics	971.3	E855.6	E941.3	E950.4	E962.0	E980.4
Sympathomimetics	971.2	E855.5	E941.2	E950.4	E962.0	E980.4
Synagis	979.6	E858.8	E949.6	E950.4	E962.0	E980.4
Synalar	976.0	E858.7	E946.0	E950.4	E962.0	E980.4
Synthroid	962.7	E858.0	E932.7	E950.4	E962.0	E980.4
Syntocinon	975.0	E858.6	E945.0	E950.4	E962.0	—
Syrosingopine	972.6	E858.3	E942.6	E950.4	E962.0	E980.4
Systemic agents (primarily)	963.9	E858.1	E933.9	E950.4	E962.0	E980.4
specified NEC	963.8	E858.1	E933.8	E950.4	E962.0	E980.4
Tablets — see also specified substance	977.9	E858.9	E947.9	E950.5	E962.0	E980.5
Tace	962.2	E858.0	E932.2	E950.4	E962.0	E980.4
Tacrine	971.0	E855.3	E941.0	E950.4	E962.0	E980.4
Talbutal	967.0	E851	E937.0	E950.1	E962.0	E980.1
Talc	976.3	E858.7	E946.3	E950.4	E962.0	E980.4
Talcum	976.3	E858.7	E946.3	E950.4	E962.0	E980.4
Tamsulosin	971.3	E855.6	E941.3	E950.4	E962.0	E980.4
Tandearil, tanderil	965.5	E850.5	E935.5	E950.0	E962.0	E980.0
Tannic acid	983.1	E864.1	—	E950.7	E962.1	E980.6
medicinal (astringent)	976.2	E858.7	E946.2	E950.4	E962.0	E980.4
Tannin — see Tannic acid						
Tansy	988.2	E865.4	—	E950.9	E962.1	E980.9
TAO	960.3	E856	E930.3	E950.4	E962.0	E980.4
Tapazole	962.8	E858.0	E932.8	E950.4	E962.0	E980.4
Taractan	969.3	E853.8	E939.3	E950.3	E962.0	E980.3
Tarantula (venomous)	989.5	E905.1	—	E950.9	E962.1	E980.9

Nontherapeutic use substance

Subterms under main terms may continue to next column or page

	External Cause (E-Code)					
	Poisoning	Accident	Therapeutic Use	Suicide Attempt	Assault	Undetermined
Tartar emetic (anti-infective)	961.2	E857	E931.2	E950.4	E962.0	E980.4
Tartaric acid	983.1	E864.1	—	E950.7	E962.1	E980.6
Tartrated antimony (anti-infective)	961.2	E857	E931.2	E950.4	E962.0	E980.4
Tar NEC	983.0	E864.0	—	E950.7	E962.1	E980.6
camphor — *see* Naphthalene						
fumes	987.8	E869.8	—	E952.8	E962.2	E982.8
TCA — *see* Trichloroacetic acid						
TDI	983.0	E864.0	—	E950.7	E962.1	E980.6
vapor	987.8	E869.8	—	E952.8	E962.2	E982.8
Tear gas	987.5	E869.3		E952.8	E962.2	E982.8
Teclothiazide	974.3	E858.5	E944.3	E950.4	E962.0	E980.4
Tegretol	966.3	E855.0	E936.3	E950.4	E962.0	E980.4
Telepaque	977.8	E858.8	E947.8	E950.4	E962.0	E980.4
Tellurium	985.8	E866.4		E950.9	E962.1	E980.9
fumes	985.8	E866.4		E950.9	E962.1	E980.9
TEM	963.1	E858.1	E933.1	E950.4	E962.0	E980.4
Temazepan — *see* Benzodiazepines						
TEPA	963.1	E858.1	E933.1	E950.4	E962.0	E980.4
TEPP	989.3	E863.1	—	E950.6	E962.1	E980.7
Terbutaline	971.2	E855.5	E941.2	E950.4	E962.0	E980.4
Teroxalene	961.6	E857	E931.6	E950.4	E962.0	E980.4
Terpin hydrate	975.5	E858.6	E945.5	E950.4	E962.0	E980.4
Terramycin	960.4	E856	E930.4	E950.4	E962.0	E980.4
Tessalon	975.4	E858.6	E945.4	E950.4	E962.0	E980.4
Testosterone	962.1	E858.0	E932.1	E950.4	E962.0	E980.4
Tetanus (vaccine)	978.4	E858.8	E948.4	E950.4	E962.0	E980.4
antitoxin	979.9	E858.8	E949.9	E950.4	E962.0	E980.4
immune globulin (human)	964.6	E858.2	E934.6	E950.4	E962.0	E980.4
toxoid	978.4	E858.8	E948.4	E950.4	E962.0	E980.4
with diphtheria toxoid	978.9	E858.8	E948.9	E950.4	E962.0	E980.4
with pertussis	978.6	E858.8	E948.6	E950.4	E962.0	E980.4
Tetrabenazine	969.5	E853.8	E939.5	E950.3	E962.0	E980.3
Tetracaine (infiltration) (topical)	968.5	E855.2	E938.5	E950.4	E962.0	E980.4
nerve block (peripheral) (plexus)	968.6	E855.2	E938.6	E950.4	E962.0	E980.4
spinal	968.7	E855.2	E938.7	E950.4	E962.0	E980.4
Tetrachlorethylene — *see* Tetrachloroethylene						
Tetrachlormethiazide	974.3	E858.5	E944.3	E950.4	E962.0	E980.4
Tetrachloroethane (liquid)	982.3	E862.4	—	E950.9	E962.1	E980.9
(vapor)	982.3	E862.4	—	E950.9	E962.1	E980.9
paint or varnish	982.3	E861.6	—	E950.9	E962.1	E980.9
Tetrachloroethylene (liquid)	982.3	E862.4	—	E950.9	E962.1	E980.9
(vapor)	982.3	E862.4	—	E950.9	E962.1	E980.9
medicinal	961.6	E857	E931.6	E950.4	E962.0	E980.4
Tetrachloromethane — *see* Carbon, tetrachloride						
Tetracycline	960.4	E856	E930.4	E950.4	E962.0	E980.4
ophthalmic preparation	976.5	E858.7	E946.5	E950.4	E962.0	E980.4
topical NEC	976.0	E858.7	E946.0	E950.4	E962.0	E980.4
Tetraethylammonium chloride	972.3	E858.3	E942.3	E950.4	E962.0	E980.4
Tetraethyl lead (antiknock compound)	984.1	E862.1	—	E950.9	E962.1	E980.9
Tetraethyl pyrophosphate	989.3	E863.1	—	E950.6	E962.1	E980.7
Tetraethylthiuram disulfide	977.3	E858.8	E947.3	E950.4	E962.0	E980.4
Tetrahydroaminoacridine	971.0	E855.3	E941.0	E950.4	E962.0	E980.4
Tetrahydrocannabinol	969.6	E854.1	E939.6	E950.3	E962.0	E980.3
Tetrahydronaphthalene	982.0	E862.4	—	E950.9	E962.1	E980.9
Tetrahydrozoline	971.2	E855.5	E941.2	E950.4	E962.0	E980.4
Tetralin	982.0	E862.4	—	E950.9	E962.1	E980.9
Tetramethylthiuram (disulfide) NEC	989.4	E863.6	—	E950.6	E962.1	E980.7
medicinal	976.2	E858.7	E946.2	E950.4	E962.0	E980.4
Tetronal	967.8	E852.8	E937.8	E950.2	E962.0	E980.2
Tetryl	983.0	E864.0	—	E950.7	E962.1	E980.6
Thalidomide	967.8	E852.8	E937.8	E950.2	E962.0	E980.2
Thallium (compounds) (dust) NEC	985.8	E866.4	—	E950.9	E962.1	E980.9
pesticide (rodenticide)	985.8	E863.7	—	E950.6	E962.1	E980.7
THC	969.6	E854.1	E939.6	E950.3	E962.0	E980.3
Thebacon	965.09	E850.2	E935.2	E950.0	E962.0	E980.0
Thebaine	965.09	E850.2	E935.2	E950.0	E962.0	E980.0
Theobromine (calcium salicylate)	974.1	E858.5	E944.1	E950.4	E962.0	E980.4
Theophylline (diuretic)	974.1	E858.5	E944.1	E950.4	E962.0	E980.4
ethylenediamine	975.7	E858.6	E945.7	E950.4	E962.0	E980.4
Thiabendazole	961.6	E857	E931.6	E950.4	E962.0	E980.4
Thialbarbital, thialbarbitone	968.3	E855.1	E938.3	E950.4	E962.0	E980.4
Thiamine	963.5	E858.1	E933.5	E950.4	E962.0	E980.4
Thiamylal (sodium)	968.3	E855.1	E938.3	E950.4	E962.0	E980.4
Thiazesim	969.09	E854.0	E939.0	E950.3	E962.0	E980.3
Thiazides (diuretics)	974.3	E858.5	E944.3	E950.4	E962.0	E980.4
Thiethylperazine	963.0	E858.1	E933.0	E950.4	E962.0	E980.4
Thimerosal (topical)	976.0	E858.7	E946.0	E950.4	E962.0	E980.4
ophthalmic preparation	976.5	E858.7	E946.5	E950.4	E962.0	E980.4
Thioacetazone	961.8	E857	E931.8	E950.4	E962.0	E980.4
Thiobarbiturates	968.3	E855.1	E938.3	E950.4	E962.0	E980.4
Thiobismol	961.2	E857	E931.2	E950.4	E962.0	E980.4
Thiocarbamide	962.8	E858.0	E932.8	E950.4	E962.0	E980.4
Thiocarbarsone	961.1	E857	E931.1	E950.4	E962.0	E980.4
Thiocarlide	961.8	E857	E931.8	E950.4	E962.0	E980.4
Thioguanine	963.1	E858.1	E933.1	E950.4	E962.0	E980.4
Thiomercaptomerin	974.0	E858.5	E944.0	E950.4	E962.0	E980.4
Thiomerin	974.0	E858.5	E944.0	E950.4	E962.0	E980.4
Thiopental, thiopentone (sodium)	968.3	E855.1	E938.3	E950.4	E962.0	E980.4
Thiopropazate	969.1	E853.0	E939.1	E950.3	E962.0	E980.3
Thioproperazine	969.1	E853.0	E939.1	E950.3	E962.0	E980.3
Thioridazine	969.1	E853.0	E939.1	E950.3	E962.0	E980.3
Thio-TEPA, thiotepa	963.1	E858.1	E933.1	E950.4	E962.0	E980.4
Thiothixene	969.3	E853.8	E939.3	E950.3	E962.0	E980.3
Thiouracil	962.8	E858.0	E932.8	E950.4	E962.0	E980.4
Thiourea	962.8	E858.0	E932.8	E950.4	E962.0	E980.4
Thiphenamil	971.1	E855.4	E941.1	E950.4	E962.0	E980.4
Thiram NEC	989.4	E863.6	—	E950.6	E962.1	E980.7
medicinal	976.2	E858.7	E946.2	E950.4	E962.0	E980.4
Thonzylamine	963.0	E858.1	E933.0	E950.4	E962.0	E980.4
Thorazine	969.1	E853.0	E939.1	E950.3	E962.0	E980.3
Thornapple	988.2	E865.4	—	E950.9	E962.1	E980.9
Throat preparation (lozenges) NEC	976.6	E858.7	E946.6	E950.4	E962.0	E980.4
Thrombin	964.5	E858.2	E934.5	E950.4	E962.0	E980.4
Thrombolysin	964.4	E858.2	E934.4	E950.4	E962.0	E980.4
Thymol	983.0	E864.0	—	E950.7	E962.1	E980.6
Thymus extract	962.9	E858.0	E932.9	E950.4	E962.0	E980.4
Thyroglobulin	962.7	E858.0	E932.7	E950.4	E962.0	E980.4
Thyroid (derivatives) (extract)	962.7	E858.0	E932.7	E950.4	E962.0	E980.4
Thyrolar	962.7	E858.0	E932.7	E950.4	E962.0	E980.4
Thyrothrophin, thyrotropin	977.8	E858.8	E947.8	E950.4	E962.0	E980.4
Thyroxin(e)	962.7	E858.0	E932.7	E950.4	E962.0	E980.4
Tigan	963.0	E858.1	E933.0	E950.4	E962.0	E980.4
Tigloidine	968.0	E855.1	E938.0	E950.4	E962.0	E980.4
Tinactin	976.0	E858.7	E946.0	E950.4	E962.0	E980.4
Tincture, iodine — *see* Iodine						
Tindal	969.1	E853.0	E939.1	E950.3	E962.0	E980.3
Tin (chloride) (dust) (oxide) NEC	985.8	E866.4	—	E950.9	E962.1	E980.9
anti-infectives	961.2	E857	E931.2	E950.4	E962.0	E980.4
Titanium (compounds) (vapor)	985.8	E866.4	—	E950.9	E962.1	E980.9
ointment	976.3	E858.7	E946.3	E950.4	E962.0	E980.4
Titroid	962.7	E858.0	E932.7	E950.4	E962.0	E980.4
TMTD — *see* Tetramethylthiuram disulfide						
TNT	989.89	E866.8	—	E950.9	E962.1	E980.9
fumes	987.8	E869.8	—	E952.8	E962.2	E982.8
Toadstool	988.1	E865.5	—	E950.9	E962.1	E980.9
Tobacco NEC	989.84	E866.8	—	E950.9	E962.1	E980.9
Indian	988.2	E865.4	—	E950.9	E962.1	E980.9
smoke, second-hand	987.8	E869.4	—	—	—	—
Tocopherol	963.5	E858.1	E933.5	E950.4	E962.0	E980.4
Tocosamine	975.0	E858.6	E945.0	E950.4	E962.0	E980.4
Tofranil	969.05	E854.0	E939.0	E950.3	E962.0	E980.3
Toilet deodorizer	989.89	E866.8	—	E950.9	E962.1	E980.9
Tolazamide	962.3	E858.0	E932.3	E950.4	E962.0	E980.4
Tolazoline	971.3	E855.6	E941.3	E950.4	E962.0	E980.4
Tolbutamide	962.3	E858.0	E932.3	E950.4	E962.0	E980.4
sodium	977.8	E858.8	E947.8	E950.4	E962.0	E980.4
Tolmetin	965.69	E850.6	E935.6	E950.0	E962.0	E980.0
Tolnaftate	976.0	E858.7	E946.0	E950.4	E962.0	E980.4
Tolpropamine	976.1	E858.7	E946.1	E950.4	E962.0	E980.4

Nontherapeutic use substance

▽ Subterms under main terms may continue to next column or page

▶◀ Revised Text   ● New Line   ▲ Revised Code

Substance	Poisoning	Accident	Therapeutic Use	Suicide Attempt	Assault	Undetermined
Tolserol	968.0	E855.1	E938.0	E950.4	E962.0	E980.4
Toluene (liquid) (vapor)	982.0	E862.4	—	E950.9	E962.1	E980.9
diisocyanate	983.0	E864.0	—	E950.7	E962.1	E980.6
Toluidine	983.0	E864.0	—	E950.7	E962.1	E980.6
vapor	987.8	E869.8	—	E952.8	E962.2	E982.8
Toluol (liquid) (vapor)	982.0	E862.4	—	E950.9	E962.1	E980.9
Tolylene-2, 4-diiso-cyanate	983.0	E864.0	—	E950.7	E962.1	E980.6
Tonics, cardiac	972.1	E858.3	E942.1	E950.4	E962.0	E980.4
Toxaphene (dust) (spray)	989.2	E863.0	—	E950.6	E962.1	E980.7
Toxoids NEC	978.8	E858.8	E948.8	E950.4	E962.0	E980.4
Tractor fuel NEC	981	E862.1	—	E950.9	E962.1	E980.9
Tragacanth	973.3	E858.4	E943.3	E950.4	E962.0	E980.4
Tramazoline	971.2	E855.5	E941.2	E950.4	E962.0	E980.4
Tranquilizers	969.5	E853.9	E939.5	E950.3	E962.0	E980.3
benzodiazepine-based	969.4	E853.2	E939.4	E950.3	E962.0	E980.3
butyrophenone-based	969.2	E853.1	E939.2	E950.3	E962.0	E980.3
major NEC	969.3	E853.8	E939.3	E950.3	E962.0	E980.3
phenothiazine-based	969.1	E853.0	E939.1	E950.3	E962.0	E980.3
specified NEC	969.5	E853.8	E939.5	E950.3	E962.0	E980.3
Trantoin	961.9	E857	E931.9	E950.4	E962.0	E980.4
Tranxene	969.4	E853.2	E939.4	E950.3	E962.0	E980.3
Tranylcypromine (sul-fate)	969.01	E854.0	E939.0	E950.3	E962.0	E980.3
Trasentine	975.1	E858.6	E945.1	E950.4	E962.0	E980.4
Travert	974.5	E858.5	E944.5	E950.4	E962.0	E980.4
Trecator	961.8	E857	E931.8	E950.4	E962.0	E980.4
Tretinoin	976.8	E858.7	E946.8	E950.4	E962.0	E980.4
Triacetin	976.0	E858.7	E946.0	E950.4	E962.0	E980.4
Triacetyloleandomycin	960.3	E856	E930.3	E950.4	E962.0	E980.4
Triamcinolone	962.0	E858.0	E932.0	E950.4	E962.0	E980.4
ENT agent	976.6	E858.7	E946.6	E950.4	E962.0	E980.4
medicinal (keratolytic)	976.4	E858.7	E946.4	E950.4	E962.0	E980.4
ophthalmic preparation	976.5	E858.7	E946.5	E950.4	E962.0	E980.4
topical NEC	976.0	E858.7	E946.0	E950.4	E962.0	E980.4
Triamterene	974.4	E858.5	E944.4	E950.4	E962.0	E980.4
Triaziquone	963.1	E858.1	E933.1	E950.4	E962.0	E980.4
Tribromacetaldehyde	967.3	E852.2	E937.3	E950.2	E962.0	E980.2
Tribromoethanol	968.2	E855.1	E938.2	E950.4	E962.0	E980.4
Tribromomethane	967.3	E852.2	E937.3	E950.2	E962.0	E980.2
Trichlorethane	982.3	E862.4	—	E950.9	E962.1	E980.9
Trichlormethiazide	974.3	E858.5	E944.3	E950.4	E962.0	E980.4
Trichloroacetic acid	983.1	E864.1	—	E950.7	E962.1	E980.6
Trichloroethanol	967.1	E852.0	E937.1	E950.2	E962.0	E980.2
Trichloroethylene (liquid) (vapor)	982.3	E862.4	—	E950.9	E962.1	E980.9
anesthetic (gas)	968.2	E855.1	E938.2	E950.4	E962.0	E980.4
Trichloroethyl phos-phate	967.1	E852.0	E937.1	E950.2	E962.0	E980.2
Trichlorofluoromethane NEC	987.4	E869.2	—	E952.8	E962.2	E982.8
Trichlorotriethylamine	963.1	E858.1	E933.1	E950.4	E962.0	E980.4
Trichomonacides NEC	961.5	E857	E931.5	E950.4	E962.0	E980.4
Trichomycin	960.1	E856	E930.1	E950.4	E962.0	E980.4
Triclofos	967.1	E852.0	E937.1	E950.2	E962.0	E980.2
Tricresyl phosphate	989.89	E866.8	—	E950.9	E962.1	E980.9
solvent	982.8	E862.4	—	E950.9	E962.1	E980.9
Tricyclamol	966.4	E855.0	E936.4	E950.4	E962.0	E980.4
Tridesilon	976.0	E858.7	E946.0	E950.4	E962.0	E980.4
Tridihexethyl	971.1	E855.4	E941.1	E950.4	E962.0	E980.4
Tridione	966.0	E855.0	E936.0	E950.4	E962.0	E980.4
Triethanolamine NEC	983.2	E864.2	—	E950.7	E962.1	E980.6
detergent	983.2	E861.0	—	E950.7	E962.1	E980.6
trinitrate	972.4	E858.3	E942.4	E950.4	E962.0	E980.4
Triethanomelamine	963.1	E858.1	E933.1	E950.4	E962.0	E980.4
Triethylene melamine	963.1	E858.1	E933.1	E950.4	E962.0	E980.4
Triethylenephospho-ramide	963.1	E858.1	E933.1	E950.4	E962.0	E980.4
Triethylenethiophospho-ramide	963.1	E858.1	E933.1	E950.4	E962.0	E980.4
Trifluoperazine	969.1	E853.0	E939.1	E950.3	E962.0	E980.3
Trifluperidol	969.2	E853.1	E939.2	E950.3	E962.0	E980.3
Triflupromazine	969.1	E853.0	E939.1	E950.3	E962.0	E980.3
Trihexyphenidyl	971.1	E855.4	E941.1	E950.4	E962.0	E980.4
Triiodothyronine	962.7	E858.0	E932.7	E950.4	E962.0	E980.4
Trilene	968.2	E855.1	E938.2	E950.4	E962.0	E980.4
Trimeprazine	963.0	E858.1	E933.0	E950.4	E962.0	E980.4
Trimetazidine	972.4	E858.3	E942.4	E950.4	E962.0	E980.4
Trimethadione	966.0	E855.0	E936.0	E950.4	E962.0	E980.4
Trimethaphan	972.3	E858.3	E942.3	E950.4	E962.0	E980.4
Trimethidinium	972.3	E858.3	E942.3	E950.4	E962.0	E980.4
Trimethobenzamide	963.0	E858.1	E933.0	E950.4	E962.0	E980.4
Trimethylcarbinol	980.8	E860.8	—	E950.9	E962.1	E980.9
Trimethylpsoralen	976.3	E858.7	E946.3	E950.4	E962.0	E980.4
Trimeton	963.0	E858.1	E933.0	E950.4	E962.0	E980.4
Trimipramine	969.05	E854.0	E939.0	E950.3	E962.0	E980.3
Trimustine	963.1	E858.1	E933.1	E950.4	E962.0	E980.4
Trinitrin	972.4	E858.3	E942.4	E950.4	E962.0	E980.4
Trinitrophenol	983.0	E864.0	—	E950.7	E962.1	E980.6
Trinitrotoluene	989.89	E866.8	—	E950.9	E962.1	E980.9
fumes	987.8	E869.8	—	E952.8	E962.2	E982.8
Trional	967.8	E852.8	E937.8	E950.2	E962.0	E980.2
Trioxide of arsenic — see Arsenic						
Trioxsalen	976.3	E858.7	E946.3	E950.4	E962.0	E980.4
Tripelennamine	963.0	E858.1	E933.0	E950.4	E962.0	E980.4
Triperidol	969.2	E853.1	E939.2	E950.3	E962.0	E980.3
Triprolidine	963.0	E858.1	E933.0	E950.4	E962.0	E980.4
Trisoralen	976.3	E858.7	E946.3	E950.4	E962.0	E980.4
Troleandomycin	960.3	E856	E930.3	E950.4	E962.0	E980.4
Trolnitrate (phosphate)	972.4	E858.3	E942.4	E950.4	E962.0	E980.4
Trometamol	963.3	E858.1	E933.3	E950.4	E962.0	E980.4
Tromethamine	963.3	E858.1	E933.3	E950.4	E962.0	E980.4
Tronothane	968.5	E855.2	E938.5	E950.4	E962.0	E980.4
Tropicamide	971.1	E855.4	E941.1	E950.4	E962.0	E980.4
Troxidone	966.0	E855.0	E936.0	E950.4	E962.0	E980.4
Tryparsamide	961.1	E857	E931.1	E950.4	E962.0	E980.4
Trypsin	963.4	E858.1	E933.4	E950.4	E962.0	E980.4
Tryptizol	969.05	E854.0	E939.0	E950.3	E962.0	E980.3
Tuaminoheptane	971.2	E855.5	E941.2	E950.4	E962.0	E980.4
Tuberculin (old)	977.8	E858.8	E947.8	E950.4	E962.0	E980.4
Tubocurare	975.2	E858.6	E945.2	E950.4	E962.0	E980.4
Tubocurarine	975.2	E858.6	E945.2	E950.4	E962.0	E980.4
Turkish green	969.6	E854.1	E939.6	E950.3	E962.0	E980.3
Turpentine (spirits of) (liquid) (vapor)	982.8	E862.4	—	E950.9	E962.1	E980.9
Tybamate	969.5	E853.8	E939.5	E950.3	E962.0	E980.3
Tyloxapol	975.5	E858.6	E945.5	E950.4	E962.0	E980.4
Tymazoline	971.2	E855.5	E941.2	E950.4	E962.0	E980.4
Typhoid vaccine	978.1	E858.8	E948.1	E950.4	E962.0	E980.4
Typhus vaccine	979.2	E858.8	E949.2	E950.4	E962.0	E980.4
Tyrothricin	976.0	E858.7	E946.0	E950.4	E962.0	E980.4
ENT agent	976.6	E858.7	E946.6	E950.4	E962.0	E980.4
ophthalmic preparation	976.5	E858.7	E946.5	E950.4	E962.0	E980.4
Undecenoic acid	976.0	E858.7	E946.0	E950.4	E962.0	E980.4
Undecylenic acid	976.0	E858.7	E946.0	E950.4	E962.0	E980.4
Unna's boot	976.3	E858.7	E946.3	E950.4	E962.0	E980.4
Uracil mustard	963.1	E858.1	E933.1	E950.4	E962.0	E980.4
Uramustine	963.1	E858.1	E933.1	E950.4	E962.0	E980.4
Urari	975.2	E858.6	E945.2	E950.4	E962.0	E980.4
Urea	974.4	E858.5	E944.4	E950.4	E962.0	E980.4
topical	976.8	E858.7	E946.8	E950.4	E962.0	E980.4
Urethan(e) (antineoplastic)	963.1	E858.1	E933.1	E950.4	E962.0	E980.4
Urginea (maritima) (scilla) — see Squill						
Uric acid metabolism agents NEC	974.7	E858.5	E944.7	E950.4	E962.0	E980.4
Urokinase	964.4	E858.2	E934.4	E950.4	E962.0	E980.4
Urokon	977.8	E858.8	E947.8	E950.4	E962.0	E980.4
Urotropin	961.9	E857	E931.9	E950.4	E962.0	E980.4
Urtica	988.2	E865.4	—	E950.9	E962.1	E980.9
Utility gas — see Gas, utility						
Vaccine NEC	979.9	E858.8	E949.9	E950.4	E962.0	E980.4
bacterial NEC	978.8	E858.8	E948.8	E950.4	E962.0	E980.4
with other bacterial component	978.9	E858.8	E948.9	E950.4	E962.0	E980.4
pertussis component	978.6	E858.8	E948.6	E950.4	E962.0	E980.4
viral-rickettsial component	979.7	E858.8	E949.7	E950.4	E962.0	E980.4
mixed NEC	978.9	E858.8	E948.9	E950.4	E962.0	E980.4
BCG	978.0	E858.8	E948.0	E950.4	E962.0	E980.4
cholera	978.2	E858.8	E948.2	E950.4	E962.0	E980.4
diphtheria	978.5	E858.8	E948.5	E950.4	E962.0	E980.4
influenza	979.6	E858.8	E949.6	E950.4	E962.0	E980.4
measles	979.4	E858.8	E949.4	E950.4	E962.0	E980.4
meningococcal	978.8	E858.8	E948.8	E950.4	E962.0	E980.4
mumps	979.6	E858.8	E949.6	E950.4	E962.0	E980.4
paratyphoid	978.1	E858.8	E948.1	E950.4	E962.0	E980.4
pertussis (with diphtheria toxoid) (with tetanus toxoid)	978.6	E858.8	E948.6	E950.4	E962.0	E980.4
plague	978.3	E858.8	E948.3	E950.4	E962.0	E980.4

Subterms under main terms may continue to next column or page

	External Cause (E-Code)					
	Poisoning	Accident	Therapeutic Use	Suicide Attempt	Assault	Undetermined
Vaccine — *continued*						
poliomyelitis	979.5	E858.8	E949.5	E950.4	E962.0	E980.4
poliovirus	979.5	E858.8	E949.5	E950.4	E962.0	E980.4
rabies	979.1	E858.8	E949.1	E950.4	E962.0	E980.4
respiratory syncytial virus	979.6	E858.8	E949.6	E950.4	E962.0	E980.4
rickettsial NEC	979.6	E858.8	E949.6	E950.4	E962.0	E980.4
with						
bacterial component	979.7	E858.8	E949.7	E950.4	E962.0	E980.4
pertussis component	978.6	E858.8	E948.6	E950.4	E962.0	E980.4
viral component	979.7	E858.8	E949.7	E950.4	E962.0	E980.4
Rocky mountain spotted fever	979.6	E858.8	E949.6		E962.0	E980.4
rotavirus	979.6	E858.8	E949.6	E950.4	E962.0	E980.4
rubella virus	979.4	E858.8	E949.4	E950.4	E962.0	E980.4
sabin oral	979.5	E858.8	E949.5	E950.4	E962.0	E980.4
smallpox	979.0	E858.8	E949.0	E950.4	E962.0	E980.4
tetanus	978.4	E858.8	E948.4	E950.4	E962.0	E980.4
typhoid	978.1	E858.8	E948.1	E950.4	E962.0	E980.4
typhus	979.2	E858.8	E949.2	E950.4	E962.0	E980.4
viral NEC	979.6	E858.8	E949.6	E950.4	E962.0	E980.4
with						
bacterial component	979.7	E858.8	E949.7	E950.4	E962.0	E980.4
pertussis component	978.6	E858.8	E948.6	E950.4	E962.0	E980.4
rickettsial component	979.7	E858.8	E949.7	E950.4	E962.0	E980.4
yellow fever	979.3	E858.8	E949.3	E950.4	E962.0	E980.4
Vaccinia immune globulin (human)	964.6	E858.2	E934.6	E950.4	E962.0	E980.4
Vaginal contraceptives	976.8	E858.7	E946.8	E950.4	E962.0	E980.4
Valethamate	971.1	E855.4	E941.1	E950.4	E962.0	E980.4
Valisone	976.0	E858.7	E946.0	E950.4	E962.0	E980.4
Valium	969.4	E853.2	E939.4	E950.3	E962.0	E980.3
Valmid	967.8	E852.8	E937.8	E950.2	E962.0	E980.2
Vanadium	985.8	E866.4	—	E950.9	E962.1	E980.9
Vancomycin	960.8	E856	E930.8	E950.4	E962.0	E980.4
Vapor — *see also* Gas	987.9	E869.9	—	E952.9	E962.2	E982.9
kiln (carbon monoxide)	986	E868.8	—	E952.1	E962.2	E982.1
lead — *see* Lead						
specified source NEC (*see also* specific substance)	987.8	E869.8	—	E952.8	E962.2	E982.8
Varidase	964.4	E858.2	E934.4	E950.4	E962.0	E980.4
Varnish	989.89	E861.6	—	E950.9	E962.1	E980.9
cleaner	982.8	E862.9	—	E950.9	E962.1	E980.9
Vaseline	976.3	E858.7	E946.3	E950.4	E962.0	E980.4
Vasodilan	972.5	E858.3	E942.5	E950.4	E962.0	E980.4
Vasodilators NEC	972.5	E858.3	E942.5	E950.4	E962.0	E980.4
coronary	972.4	E858.3	E942.4	E950.4	E962.0	E980.4
Vasopressin	962.5	E858.0	E932.5	E950.4	E962.0	E980.4
Vasopressor drugs	962.5	E858.0	E932.5	E950.4	E962.0	E980.4
Venom, venomous (bite) (sting)	989.5	E905.9	—	E950.9	E962.1	E980.9
arthropod NEC	989.5	E905.5	—	E950.9	E962.1	E980.9
bee	989.5	E905.3	—	E950.9	E962.1	E980.9
centipede	989.5	E905.4	—	E950.9	E962.1	E980.9
hornet	989.5	E905.3	—	E950.9	E962.1	E980.9
lizard	989.5	E905.0	—	E950.9	E962.1	E980.9
marine animals or plants	989.5	E905.6	—	E950.9	E962.1	E980.9
millipede (tropical)	989.5	E905.4	—	E950.9	E962.1	E980.9
plant NEC	989.5	E905.7	—	E950.9	E962.1	E980.9
marine	989.5	E905.6	—	E950.9	E962.1	E980.9
scorpion	989.5	E905.2	—	E950.9	E962.1	E980.9
snake	989.5	E905.0	—	E950.9	E962.1	E980.9
specified NEC	989.5	E905.8	—	E950.9	E962.1	E980.9
spider	989.5	E905.1	—	E950.9	E962.1	E980.9
wasp	989.5	E905.3	—	E950.9	E962.1	E980.9
Ventolin — *see* Salbutamol sulfate						
Veramon	967.0	E851	E937.0	E950.1	E962.0	E980.1
Veratrum						
album	988.2	E865.4	—	E950.9	E962.1	E980.9
alkaloids	972.6	E858.3	E942.6	E950.4	E962.0	E980.4
viride	988.2	E865.4	—	E950.9	E962.1	E980.9
Verdigris — *see also* Copper	985.8	E866.4	—	E950.9	E962.1	E980.9
Veronal	967.0	E851	E937.0	E950.1	E962.0	E980.1
Veroxil	961.6	E857	E931.6	E950.4	E962.0	E980.4
Versidyne	965.7	E850.7	E935.7	E950.0	E962.0	E980.0
Viagra	972.5	E858.3	E942.5	E950.4	E962.0	E980.4
Vienna						
green	985.1	E866.3	—	E950.8	E962.1	E980.8
insecticide	985.1	E863.4	—	E950.6	E962.1	E980.7
red	989.89	E866.8	—	E950.9	E962.1	E980.9
pharmaceutical dye	977.4	E858.8	E947.4	E950.4	E962.0	E980.4

	External Cause (E-Code)					
	Poisoning	Accident	Therapeutic Use	Suicide Attempt	Assault	Undetermined
Vinbarbital, vinbarbitone	967.0	E851	E937.0	E950.1	E962.0	E980.1
Vinblastine	963.1	E858.1	E933.1	E950.4	E962.0	E980.4
Vincristine	963.1	E858.1	E933.1	E950.4	E962.0	E980.4
Vinesthene, vinethene	968.2	E855.1	E938.2	E950.4	E962.0	E980.4
Vinyl						
bital	967.0	E851	E937.0	E950.1	E962.0	E980.1
ether	968.2	E855.1	E938.2	E950.4	E962.0	E980.4
Vioform	961.3	E857	E931.3	E950.4	E962.0	E980.4
topical	976.0	E858.7	E946.0	E930.4	E962.0	E980.4
Viomycin	960.6	E856	E930.6	E950.4	E962.0	E980.4
Viosterol	963.5	E858.1	E933.5	E950.4	E962.0	E980.4
Viper (venom)	989.5	E905.0	—	E950.9	E962.1	E980.9
Viprynium (embonate)	961.6	E857	E931.6	E950.4	E962.0	E980.4
Virugon	961.7	E857	E931.7	E950.4	E962.0	E980.4
Visine	976.5	E858.7	E946.5	E950.4	E962.0	E980.4
Vitamins NEC	963.5	E858.1	E933.5	E950.4	E962.0	E980.4
B_{12}	964.1	E858.2	E934.1	E950.4	E962.0	E980.4
hematopoietic	964.1	E858.2	E934.1	E950.4	E962.0	E980.4
K	964.3	E858.2	E934.3	E950.4	E962.0	E980.4
Vleminckx's solution	976.4	E858.7	E946.4	E950.4	E962.0	E980.4
Voltaren — *see* Diclofenac sodium						
Warfarin (potassium) (sodium)	964.2	E858.2	E934.2	E950.4	E962.0	E980.4
rodenticide	989.4	E863.7	—	E950.6	E962.1	E980.7
Wasp (sting)	989.5	E905.3	—	E950.9	E962.1	E980.9
Water						
balance agents NEC	974.5	E858.5	E944.5	E950.4	E962.0	E980.4
gas	987.1	E868.1	—	E951.8	E962.2	E981.8
incomplete combustion of — *see* Carbon, monoxide, fuel, utility						
hemlock	988.2	E865.4	—	E950.9	E962.1	E980.9
moccasin (venom)	989.5	E905.0	—	E950.9	E962.1	E980.9
Wax (paraffin) (petroleum)	981	E862.3	—	E950.9	E962.1	E980.9
automobile	989.89	E861.2	—	E950.9	E962.1	E980.9
floor	981	E862.0	—	E950.9	E962.1	E980.9
Weed killers NEC	989.4	E863.5	—	E950.6	E962.1	E980.7
Welldorm	967.1	E852.0	E937.1	E950.2	E962.0	E980.2
White						
arsenic — *see* Arsenic						
hellebore	988.2	E865.4	—	E950.9	E962.1	E980.9
lotion (keratolytic)	976.4	E858.7	E946.4	E950.4	E962.0	E980.4
spirit	981	E862.0	—	E950.9	E962.1	E980.9
Whitewashes	989.89	E861.6	—	E950.9	E962.1	E980.9
Whole blood	964.7	E858.2	E934.7	E950.4	E962.0	E980.4
Wild						
black cherry	988.2	E865.4	—	E950.9	E962.1	E980.9
poisonous plants NEC	988.2	E865.4	—	E950.9	E962.1	E980.9
Window cleaning fluid	989.89	E861.3	—	E950.9	E962.1	E980.9
Wintergreen (oil)	976.3	E858.7	E946.3	E950.4	E962.0	E980.4
Witch hazel	976.2	E858.7	E946.2	E950.4	E962.0	E980.4
Wood						
alcohol	980.1	E860.2	—	E950.9	E962.1	E980.9
spirit	980.1	E860.2	—	E950.9	E962.1	E980.9
Woorali	975.2	E858.6	E945.2	E950.4	E962.0	E980.4
Wormseed, American	961.6	E857	E931.6	E950.4	E962.0	E980.4
Xanthine diuretics	974.1	E858.5	E944.1	E950.4	E962.0	E980.4
Xanthocillin	960.0	E856	E930.0	E950.4	E962.0	E980.4
Xanthotoxin	976.3	E858.7	E946.3	E950.4	E962.0	E980.4
Xigris	964.2	E858.2	E934.2	E950.4	E962.0	E980.4
Xylene (liquid) (vapor)	982.0	E862.4	—	E950.9	E962.1	E980.9
Xylocaine (infiltration) (topical)	968.5	E855.2	E938.5	E950.4	E962.0	E980.4
nerve block (peripheral) (plexus)	968.6	E855.2	E938.6	E950.4	E962.0	E980.4
spinal	968.7	E855.2	E938.7	E950.4	E962.0	E980.4
Xylol (liquid) (vapor)	982.0	E862.4	—	E950.9	E962.1	E980.9
Xylometazoline	971.2	E855.5	E941.2	E950.4	E962.0	E980.4
Yellow						
fever vaccine	979.3	E858.8	E949.3	E950.4	E962.0	E980.4
jasmine	988.2	E865.4	—	E950.9	E962.1	E980.9
Yew	988.2	E865.4	—	E950.9	E962.1	E980.9
Zactane	965.7	E850.7	E935.7	E950.0	E962.0	E980.0
Zaroxolyn	974.3	E858.5	E944.3	E950.4	E962.0	E980.4
Zephiran (topical)	976.0	E858.7	E946.0	E950.4	E962.0	E980.4
ophthalmic preparation	976.5	E858.7	E946.5	E950.4	E962.0	E980.4
Zerone	980.1	E860.2	—	E950.9	E962.1	E980.9
Zinc (compounds) (fumes) (salts) (vapor) NEC	985.8	E866.4	—	E950.9	E962.1	E980.9
anti-infectives	976.0	E858.7	E946.0	E950.4	E962.0	E980.4

Nontherapeutic use substance

Subterms under main terms may continue to next column or page

▶◀ Revised Text   ● New Line   ▲ Revised Code

		External Cause (E-Code)				
	Poisoning	Accident	Therapeutic Use	Suicide Attempt	Assault	Undeter-mined
Zinc — *continued*						
antivaricose	972.7	E858.3	E942.7	E950.4	E962.0	E980.4
bacitracin	976.0	E858.7	E946.0	E950.4	E962.0	E980.4
chloride	976.2	E858.7	E946.2	E950.4	E962.0	E980.4
gelatin	976.3	E858.7	E946.3	E950.4	E962.0	E980.4
oxide	976.3	E858.7	E946.3	E950.4	E962.0	E980.4
peroxide	976.0	E858.7	E946.0	E950.4	E962.0	E980.4
pesticides	985.8	E863.4	—	E950.6	E962.1	E980.7
phosphide (rodenticide)	985.8	E863.7	—	E950.6	E962.1	E980.7
stearate	976.3	E858.7	E946.3	E950.4	E962.0	E980.4
sulfate (antivaricose)	972.7	E858.3	E942.7	E950.4	E962.0	E980.4
ENT agent	976.6	E858.7	E946.6	E950.4	E962.0	E980.4
ophthalmic solution	976.5	E858.7	E946.5	E950.4	E962.0	E980.4
topical NEC	976.0	E858.7	E946.0	E950.4	E962.0	E980.4
undecylenate	976.0	E858.7	E946.0	E950.4	E962.0	E980.4
Zovant	964.2	E858.2	E934.2	E950.4	E962.0	E980.4
Zoxazolamine	968.0	E855.1	E938.0	E950.4	E962.0	E980.4
Zygadenus (venenosus)	988.2	E865.4	—	E950.9	E962.1	E980.9
Zyprexa	969.3	E853.8	E939.3	E950.3	E962.0	E980.3

▽ Subterms under main terms may continue to next column or page

SECTION 3

Alphabetic Index to External Causes of Injury and Poisoning (E Code)

This section contains the index to the codes which classify environmental events, circumstances, and other conditions as the cause of injury and other adverse effects. Where a code from the section Supplementary Classification of External Causes of Injury and Poisoning (E800-E999) is applicable, it is intended that the E code shall be used in addition to a code from the main body of the classification, Chapters 1 to 17.

The alphabetic index to the E codes is organized by main terms which describe the accident, circumstance, event, or specific agent which caused the injury or other adverse effect.

Note — Transport accidents (E800-E848) include accidents involving:

- *aircraft and spacecraft (E840-E845)*
- *watercraft (E830-E838)*
- *motor vehicle (E810-E825)*
- *railway (E800-E807)*
- *other road vehicles (E826-E829)*

For definitions and examples related to transport accidents — see Volume 1 code categories E800-E848.

The fourth-digit subdivisions for use with categories E800-E848 to identify the injured person are found at the end of this section.

For identifying the place in which an accident or poisoning occurred (circumstances classifiable to categories E850-E869 and E880-E928) — see the listing in this section under "Accident, occurring."

See the Table of Drugs and Chemicals (Section 2 of this volume) for identifying the specific agent involved in drug overdose or a wrong substance given or taken in error, and for intoxication or poisoning by a drug or other chemical substance.

The specific adverse effect, reaction, or localized toxic effect to a correct drug or substance properly administered in therapeutic or prophylactic dosage should be classified according to the nature of the adverse effect (e.g., allergy, dermatitis, tachycardia) listed in Section 1 of this volume.

☑ **Additional Digit Required — Refer to the Tabular List for Digit Selection** ▼ Subterms under main terms may continue to next column or page

334 — Volume 2   ▶◀ Revised Text   ● New Line   ▲ Revised Code   2015 ICD-9-CM

A

Abandonment
  causing exposure to weather conditions — see Exposure
  child, with intent to injure or kill E968.4
  helpless person, infant, newborn E904.0
    with intent to injure or kill E968.4
Abortion, criminal, injury to child E968.8
Abuse (alleged) (suspected)
  adult
    by
      child E967.4
      ex-partner E967.3
      ex-spouse E967.3
      father E967.0
      grandchild E967.7
      grandparent E967.6
      mother E967.2
      non-related caregiver E967.8
      other relative E967.7
      other specified person E967.1
      partner E967.3
      sibling E967.5
      spouse E967.3
      stepfather E967.0
      stepmother E967.2
      unspecified person E967.9
  child
    by
      boyfriend of parent or guardian E967.0
      child E967.4
      father E967.0
      female partner of parent or guardian E967.2
      girlfriend of parent or guardian E967.2
      grandchild E967.7
      grandparent E967.6
      male partner of parent or guardian E967.0
      mother E967.2
      non-related caregiver E967.8
      other relative E967.7
      other specified person(s) E967.1
      sibling E967.5
      stepfather E967.0
      stepmother E967.2
      unspecified person E967.9
Accident (to) E928.9
  aircraft (in transit) (powered) E841 ☑
    at landing, take-off E840 ☑
    due to, caused by cataclysm — see categories E908 ☑, E909 ☑
    late effect of E929.1
    unpowered (see also Collision, aircraft, unpowered) E842 ☑
    while alighting, boarding E843 ☑
  amphibious vehicle
    on
      land — see Accident, motor vehicle
      water — see Accident, watercraft
  animal-drawn vehicle NEC E827 ☑
  animal, ridden NEC E828 ☑
  balloon (see also Collision, aircraft, unpowered) E842 ☑
  caused by, due to
    abrasive wheel (metalworking) E919.3
    animal NEC E906.9
      being ridden (in sport or transport) E828 ☑
    avalanche NEC E909.2
    band saw E919.4
    bench saw E919.4
    bore, earth-drilling or mining (land) (seabed) E919.1
    bulldozer E919.7
    cataclysmic
      earth surface movement or eruption E909.9
      storm E908.9
    chain
      hoist E919.2
        agricultural operations E919.0
        mining operations E919.1

Accident (to) — continued
  caused by, due to — continued
    chain — continued
      saw E920.1
    circular saw E919.4
    cold (excessive) (see also Cold, exposure to) E901.9
    combine E919.0
    conflagration — see Conflagration
    corrosive liquid, substance NEC E924.1
    cotton gin E919.8
    crane E919.2
      agricultural operations E919.0
      mining operations E919.1
    cutting or piercing instrument (see also Cut) E920.9
    dairy equipment E919.8
    derrick E919.2
      agricultural operations E919.0
      mining operations E919.1
    drill E920.1
      earth (land) (seabed) E919.1
      hand (powered) E920.1
        not powered E920.4
      metalworking E919.3
      woodworking E919.4
    earth(-)
      drilling machine E919.1
      moving machine E919.7
      scraping machine E919.7
    electric
      current (see also Electric shock) E925.9
      motor (see also Accident, machine, by type of machine)
        current (of) — see Electric shock
    elevator (building) (grain) E919.2
      agricultural operations E919.0
      mining operations E919.1
    environmental factors NEC E928.9
    excavating machine E919.7
    explosive material (see also Explosion) E923.9
    farm machine E919.0
    firearm missile — see Shooting
    fire, flames (see also Fire)
      conflagration — see Conflagration
    forging (metalworking) machine E919.3
    forklift (truck) E919.2
      agricultural operations E919.0
      mining operations E919.1
    gas turbine E919.5
    harvester E919.0
    hay derrick, mower, or rake E919.0
    heat (excessive) (see also Heat) E900.9
    hoist (see also Accident, caused by, due to, lift) E919.2
      chain — see Accident, caused by, due to, chain
      shaft E919.1
    hot
      liquid E924.0
        caustic or corrosive E924.1
      object (not producing fire or flames) E924.8
      substance E924.9
        caustic or corrosive E924.1
        liquid (metal) NEC E924.0
        specified type NEC E924.8
    human bite E928.3
    ignition — see Ignition
    internal combustion engine E919.5
    landslide NEC E909.2
    lathe (metalworking) E919.3
      turnings E920.8
      woodworking E919.4
    lift, lifting (appliances) E919.2
      agricultural operations E919.0
      mining operations E919.1
      shaft E919.1
    lightning NEC E907
    machine, machinery (see also Accident, machine)
      drilling, metal E919.3
      manufacturing, for manufacture of beverages E919.8

Accident (to) — continued
  caused by, due to — continued
    machine, machinery (see also Accident, machine) — continued
      manufacturing, for manufacture of — continued
        clothing E919.8
        foodstuffs E919.8
        paper E919.8
        textiles E919.8
      milling, metal E919.3
      moulding E919.4
      power press, metal E919.3
      printing E919.8
      rolling mill, metal E919.3
      sawing, metal E919.3
      specified type NEC E919.8
      spinning E919.8
      weaving E919.8
    natural factor NEC E928.9
    overhead plane E919.4
    plane E920.4
      overhead E919.4
    powered
      hand tool NEC E920.1
      saw E919.4
        hand E920.1
    printing machine E919.8
    pulley (block) E919.2
      agricultural operations E919.0
      mining operations E919.1
      transmission E919.6
    radial saw E919.4
    radiation — see Radiation
    reaper E919.0
    road scraper E919.7
      when in transport under its own power — see categories E810-E825 ☑
    roller coaster E919.8
    sander E919.4
    saw E920.4
      band E919.4
      bench E919.4
      chain E920.1
      circular E919.4
      hand E920.4
        powered E920.1
      powered, except hand E919.4
      radial E919.4
    sawing machine, metal E919.3
    shaft
      hoist E919.1
      lift E919.1
      transmission E919.6
    shears E920.4
      hand E920.4
        powered E920.1
      mechanical E919.3
    shovel E920.4
      steam E919.7
    spinning machine E919.8
    steam (see also Burning, steam)
      engine E919.5
      shovel E919.7
    thresher E919.0
    thunderbolt NEC E907
    tractor E919.0
      when in transport under its own power — see categories E810-E825 ☑
    transmission belt, cable, chain, gear, pinion, pulley, shaft E919.6
    turbine (gas) (water driven) E919.5
    under-cutter E919.1
    weaving machine E919.8
    winch E919.2
      agricultural operations E919.0
      mining operations E919.1
  diving E883.0
    with insufficient air supply E913.2
  glider (hang) (see also Collision, aircraft, unpowered) E842 ☑
  hovercraft
    on
      land — see Accident, motor vehicle

Accident (to) — continued
  hovercraft — continued
    on
      water — see Accident, watercraft
  ice yacht (see also Accident, vehicle NEC) E848
  in
    medical, surgical procedure
      as, or due to misadventure — see Misadventure
      causing an abnormal reaction or later complication without mention of misadventure — see Reaction, abnormal
  kite carrying a person (see also Collision, involving aircraft, unpowered) E842 ☑
  land yacht (see also Accident, vehicle NEC) E848
  late effect of — see Late effect
  launching pad E845 ☑
  machine, machinery (see also Accident, caused by, due to, by specific type of machine) E919.9
    agricultural including animal-powered E919.0
    earth-drilling E919.1
    earth moving or scraping E919.7
    excavating E919.7
    involving transport under own power on highway or transport vehicle — see categories E810-E825 ☑, E840-E845 ☑
    lifting (appliances) E919.2
    metalworking E919.3
    mining E919.1
    prime movers, except electric motors E919.5
      electric motors — see Accident, machine, by specific type of machine
    recreational E919.8
    specified type NEC E919.8
    transmission E919.6
    watercraft (deck) (engine room) (galley) (laundry) (loading) E836 ☑
    woodworking or forming E919.4
  motor vehicle (on public highway) (traffic) E819 ☑
    due to cataclysm — see categories E908 ☑, E909 ☑
    involving
      collision (see also Collision, motor vehicle) E812 ☑
    nontraffic, not on public highway — see categories E820-E825 ☑
    not involving collision — see categories E816-E819 ☑
  nonmotor vehicle NEC E829 ☑
    nonroad — see Accident, vehicle NEC
    road, except pedal cycle, animal-drawn vehicle, or animal being ridden E829 ☑
  nonroad vehicle NEC — see Accident, vehicle NEC
  not elsewhere classifiable involving
    cable car (not on rails) E847
      on rails E829 ☑
    coal car in mine E846
    hand truck — see Accident, vehicle NEC
    logging car E846
    sled(ge), meaning snow or ice vehicle E848
    tram, mine or quarry E846
    truck
      mine or quarry E846
      self-propelled, industrial E846
      station baggage E846
    tub, mine or quarry E846
    vehicle NEC E848
      snow and ice E848
      used only on industrial premises E846
    wheelbarrow E848
  occurring (at) (in)
    apartment E849.0
    baseball field, diamond E849.4

☑ Additional Digit Required — Refer to the Tabular List for Digit Selection   ⬙ Subterms under main terms may continue to next column or page

2015 ICD-9-CM   ▶◀ Revised Text   ● New Line   ▲ Revised Code   Volume 2 — 335

Abandonment — Accident (to)

Accident (to) — *continued*
  occurring — *continued*
    construction site, any E849.3
    dock E849.8
      yard E849.3
    dormitory E849.7
    factory (building) (premises) E849.3
    farm E849.1
      buildings E849.1
      house E849.0
    football field E849.4
    forest E849.8
    garage (place of work) E849.3
      private (home) E849.0
    gravel pit E849.2
    gymnasium E849.4
    highway E849.5
    home (private) (residential) E849.0
      institutional E849.7
    hospital E849.7
    hotel E849.6
    house (private) (residential) E849.0
      movie E849.6
      public E849.6
    institution, residential E849.7
    jail E849.7
    mine E849.2
    motel E849.6
    movie house E849.6
    office (building) E849.6
    orphanage E849.7
    park (public) E849.4
      mobile home E849.8
      trailer E849.8
    parking lot or place E849.8
    place
      industrial NEC E849.3
      parking E849.8
      public E849.8
        specified place NEC E849.5
      recreational NEC E849.4
      sport NEC E849.4
    playground (park) (school) E849.4
    prison E849.6
    public building NEC E849.6
    quarry E849.2
    railway
      line NEC E849.8
      yard E849.3
    residence
      home (private) E849.0
    resort (beach) (lake) (mountain)
      (seashore) (vacation) E849.4
    restaurant E849.6
    sand pit E849.2
    school (building) (private) (public) (state)
      E849.6
      reform E849.7
      riding E849.4
    seashore E849.8
      resort E849.4
    shop (place of work) E849.3
      commercial E849.6
    skating rink E849.4
    sports palace E849.4
    stadium E849.4
    store E849.6
    street E849.5
    swimming pool (public) E849.4
      private home or garden E849.0
    tennis court, public E849.4
    theatre, theater E849.6
    trailer court E849.8
    tunnel E849.8
      under construction E849.2
    warehouse E849.3
    yard
      dock E849.3
      industrial E849.3
      private (home) E849.0
      railway E849.3
  off-road type motor vehicle (not on public
    highway) NEC E821 ☑
    on public highway — *see* categories
      E810-E819 ☑
  pedal cycle E826 ☑

Accident (to) — *continued*
  railway E807 ☑
    due to cataclysm — *see* categories
      E908 ☑, E909 ☑
    involving
      avalanche E909.2
      burning by engine, locomotive, train
        (*see also* Explosion, railway
        engine) E803 ☑
      collision (*see also* Collision, railway)
        E800 ☑
      derailment (*see also* Derailment, rail-
        way) E802 ☑
      explosion (*see also* Explosion, railway
        engine) E803 ☑
      fall (*see also* Fall, from, railway rolling
        stock) E804 ☑
      fire (*see also* Explosion, railway en-
        gine) E803 ☑
      hitting by, being struck by
        object falling in, on, from, rolling
          stock, train, vehicle
          E806 ☑
        rolling stock, train, vehicle
          E805 ☑
      overturning, railway rolling stock,
        train, vehicle (*see also* Derail-
        ment, railway) E802 ☑
      running off rails, railway (*see also*
        Derailment, railway) E802 ☑
      specified circumstances NEC E806 ☑
      train or vehicle hit by
        avalanche E909.2
        falling object (earth, rock, tree)
          E806 ☑
          due to cataclysm — *see* cate-
            gories
            E908 ☑, E909 ☑
        landslide E909.2
  roller skate E885.1
  scooter (nonmotorized) E885.0
  skateboard E885.2
  ski(ing) E885.3
    jump E884.9
    lift or tow (with chair or gondola) E847
  snowboard E885.4
  snow vehicle, motor driven (not on public
    highway) E820 ☑
    on public highway — *see* categories
      E810-E819 ☑
  spacecraft E845 ☑
  specified cause NEC E928.8
  street car E829 ☑
  traffic NEC E819 ☑
  vehicle NEC (with pedestrian) E848
    battery powered
      airport passenger vehicle E846
      truck (baggage) (mail) E846
    powered commercial or industrial (with
      other vehicle or object within
      commercial or industrial premis-
      es) E846
  watercraft E838 ☑
    with
      drowning or submersion resulting
        from
        accident other than to watercraft
          E832 ☑
        accident to watercraft E830 ☑
      injury, except drowning or submer-
        sion, resulting from
        accident other than to watercraft
          — *see* categories
          E833-E838 ☑
        accident to watercraft E831 ☑
    due to, caused by cataclysm — *see* cate-
      gories E908 ☑, E909 ☑
    machinery E836 ☑
Acid throwing E961
Acosta syndrome E902.0
Activity (involving) E030
  aerobic and step exercise (class) E009.2
  alpine skiing E003.2
  animal care NEC E019.9
  arts and handcrafts NEC E012.9

Activity — *continued*
  athletics NEC E008.9
    played
      as a team or group NEC E007.9
      individually NEC E006.9
  baking E015.2
  ballet E005.0
  barbells E010.2
  baseball E007.3
  BASE (Building, Antenna, Span, Earth)
    jumping E004.2
  basketball E007.6
  bathing (personal) E013.0
  beach volleyball E007.7
  bike riding E006.4
  boogie boarding E002.7
  bowling E006.3
  boxing E008.0
  brass instrument playing E018.3
  building and construction E016.2
  bungee jumping E004.3
  calisthenics E009.1
  canoeing (in calm and turbulent water)
    E002.5
  capture the flag E007.8
  cardiorespiratory exercise NEC E009.9
  caregiving (providing) NEC E014.9
    bathing E014.0
    lifting E014.1
  cellular
    communication device E011.1
    telephone E011.1
  challenge course E009.4
  cheerleading E005.4
  circuit training E009.3
  cleaning
    floor E013.4
  climbing NEC E004.9
    mountain E004.0
    rock E004.0
    wall climbing E004.0
  combatives E008.4
  computer
    keyboarding E011.0
    technology NEC E011.9
  confidence course E009.4
  construction (building) E016.2
  cooking and baking E015.2
  cooking and grilling NEC E015.9
  cool down exercises E009.1
  cricket E007.9
  crocheting E012.0
  cross country skiing E003.3
  dancing (all types) E005.0
  digging
    dirt E016.0
  dirt digging E016.0
  dishwashing E015.0
  diving (platform) (springboard) E002.1
    underwater E002.4
  dodge ball E007.8
  downhill skiing E003.2
  drum playing E018.1
  dumbbells E010.2
  electronic
    devices NEC E011.9
      hand held interactive E011.1
    game playing (using) (with)
      interactive device E011.1
      keyboard or other stationary device
        E011.0
  elliptical machine E009.0
  exercise(s)
    machines (primarily for)
      cardiorespiratory conditioning
        E009.0
      muscle strengthening E010.0
    muscle strengthening (non-machine)
      NEC E010.9
  external motion NEC E017.9
    roller coaster E017.0
  field hockey E007.4
  figure skating (pairs) (singles) E003.0
  flag football E007.1
  floor mopping and cleaning E013.4
  food preparation and clean up E015.0

Activity — *continued*
  football (American) NOS E007.0
    flag E007.1
    tackle E007.0
    touch E007.1
  four square E007.8
  free weights E010.2
  frisbee (ultimate) E008.3
  furniture
    building E012.2
    finishing E012.2
    repair E012.2
  game playing (electronic)
    using
      interactive device E011.1
      keyboard or other stationary device
        E011.0
  gardening E016.1
  golf E006.2
  grass drills E009.5
  grilling and smoking food E015.1
  grooming and shearing an animal E019.2
  guerilla drills E009.5
  gymnastics (rhythmic) E005.2
  handball E008.2
  handcrafts NEC E012.9
  hand held interactive electronic device
    E011.1
  hang gliding E004.4
  hiking (on level or elevated terrain) E001.0
  hockey (ice) E003.1
    field E007.4
  horseback riding E006.1
  household maintenance NEC E013.9
  ice NEC E003.9
    dancing E003.0
    hockey E003.1
    skating E003.0
  inline roller skating E006.0
  ironing E013.3
  judo E008.4
  jumping jacks E009.1
  jumping rope E006.5
  jumping (off) NEC E004.9
    BASE (Building, Antenna, Span, Earth)
      E004.2
    bungee E004.3
    jacks E009.1
    rope E006.5
  karate E008.4
  kayaking (in calm and turbulent water)
    E002.5
  keyboarding (computer) E011.0
  kickball E007.8
  knitting E012.0
  lacrosse E007.4
  land maintenance NEC E016.9
  landscaping E016.1
  laundry E013.1
  machines (exercise) primarily for cardiores-
    piratory conditioning E009.0
  maintenance
    building E016.9
    household NEC E013.9
    land E016.9
    property E016.9
  marching (on level or elevated terrain)
    E001.0
  martial arts E008.4
  microwave oven E015.2
  milking an animal E019.1
  mopping (floor) E013.4
  mountain climbing E004.0
  muscle strengthening
    exercises (non-machine) NEC E010.9
    machines E010.0
  musical keyboard (electronic) playing E018.0
  nordic skiing E003.3
  obstacle course E009.4
  oven (microwave) E015.2
  packing up and unpacking in moving to a
    new residence E013.5
  parasailing E002.9
  percussion instrument playing NEC E018.1
  personal
    bathing and showering E013.0

☑ **Additional Digit Required** — Refer to the Tabular List for Digit Selection

⬇ **Subterms under main terms may continue to next column or page**

2015 ICD-9-CM

▶◀ **Revised Text**

● **New Line**

▲ **Revised Code**

Volume 2 — 337

Bite — *continued*
  gila monster E905.0
  human being
    accidental E928.3
    assault E968.7
  insect (nonvenomous) E906.4
    venomous — *see* Sting
  krait E905.0
  late effect of — *see* Late effect
  lizard E906.2
    venomous E905.0
  mamba E905.0
  marine animal
    nonvenomous E906.3
      snake E906.2
    venomous E905.6
      snake E905.0
  millipede E906.4
    venomous E905.4
  moray eel E906.3
  rat E906.1
  rattlesnake E905.0
  rodent, except rat E906.3
  serpent — *see* Bite, snake
  shark E906.3
  snake (venomous) E905.0
    nonvenomous E906.2
    sea E905.0
  spider E905.1
    nonvenomous E906.4
  tarantula (venomous) E905.1
  venomous NEC E905.9
    by specific animal — *see category*
      E905 ☑
  viper E905.0
  water moccasin E905.0
Blast (air)
  from nuclear explosion E996 ☑
  in
    terrorism E979.2
      from nuclear explosion E979.5
      underwater E979.0
    war operations E993.9
      from nuclear explosion — *see* War
        operations, injury due to, nu-
        clear weapons
      underwater E992.9
Blizzard E908.3
Blow E928.9
  by law-enforcing agent, police (on duty)
    E975
    with blunt object (baton) (nightstick)
      (stave) (truncheon) E973
Blowing up — *see also* Explosion E923.9
Brawl (hand) (fists) (foot) E960.0
Breakage (accidental)
  cable of cable car not on rails E847
  ladder (causing fall) E881.0
  part (any) of
    animal-drawn vehicle E827 ☑
    ladder (causing fall) E881.0
    motor vehicle
      in motion (on public highway)
        E818 ☑
        not on public highway E825 ☑
    nonmotor road vehicle, except animal-
      drawn vehicle or pedal cycle
      E829 ☑
    off-road type motor vehicle (not on
      public highway) NEC E821 ☑
      on public highway E818 ☑
    pedal cycle E826 ☑
    scaffolding (causing fall) E881.1
    snow vehicle, motor-driven (not on
      public highway) E820 ☑
      on public highway E818 ☑
    vehicle NEC — *see* Accident, vehicle
Broken
  glass
    fall on E888.0
    injury by E920.8
  power line (causing electric shock) E925.1
Bumping against, into (accidentally)
  object (moving) E917.9
    caused by crowd E917.1
      with subsequent fall E917.6

Bumping against, into — *continued*
  object — *continued*
    furniture E917.3
      with subsequent fall E917.7
    in
      running water E917.2
      sports E917.0
        with subsequent fall E917.5
      stationary E917.4
        with subsequent fall E917.8
    person(s) E917.9
      with fall E886.9
        in sports E886.0
      as, or caused by, a crowd E917.1
        with subsequent fall E917.6
      in sports E917.0
        with fall E886.0
Burning, burns (accidental) (by) (from) (on)
  E899
  acid (any kind) E924.1
    swallowed — *see* Table of Drugs and
      Chemicals
  airgun E928.7
  bedclothes (*see also* Fire, specified NEC)
    E898.0
  blowlamp (*see also* Fire, specified NEC)
    E898.1
  blowtorch (*see also* Fire, specified NEC)
    E898.1
  boat, ship, watercraft — *see* categories
    E830 ☑, E831 ☑, E837 ☑
  bonfire (controlled) E897
    uncontrolled E892
  candle (*see also* Fire, specified NEC) E898.1
  caustic liquid, substance E924.1
    swallowed — *see* Table of Drugs and
      Chemicals
  chemical E924.1
    from swallowing caustic, corrosive sub-
      stance — *see* Table of Drugs and
      Chemicals
    in
      terrorism E979.7
      war operations E997.2
  cigar(s) or cigarette(s) (*see also* Fire, speci-
    fied NEC) E898.1
  clothes, clothing, nightdress — *see* Ignition,
    clothes
    with conflagration — *see* Conflagration
  conflagration — *see* Conflagration
  corrosive liquid, substance E924.1
    swallowed — *see* Table of Drugs and
      Chemicals
  electric current (*see also* Electric shock)
    E925.9
  firearm E928.7
  fire, flames (*see also* Fire) E899
  flare, Verey pistol E922.8
  heat
    from appliance (electrical) E924.8
    in local application, or packing during
      medical or surgical procedure
      E873.5
  homicide (attempt) (*see also* Assault, burn-
    ing) E968.0
  hot
    liquid E924.0
      caustic or corrosive E924.1
    object (not producing fire or flames)
      E924.8
    substance E924.9
      caustic or corrosive E924.1
      liquid (metal) NEC E924.0
      specified type NEC E924.8
    tap water E924.2
  ignition (*see also* Ignition)
    clothes, clothing, nightdress (*see also*
      Ignition, clothes)
      with conflagration — *see* Conflagra-
        tion
    highly inflammable material (benzine)
      (fat) (gasoline) (kerosene) (paraf-
      fin) (petrol) E894
  in
    terrorism E979.3
      from nuclear explosion E979.5

Burning, burns — *continued*
  in — *continued*
    terrorism — *continued*
      petrol bomb E979.3
    war operations (from fire-producing de-
      vice or conventional weapon)
      E990.9
      from nuclear explosion (*see also* War
        operations, injury due to, nu-
        clear weapons) E996.2
      incendiary bomb E990.0
      petrol bomb E990.0
  inflicted by other person
    stated as
      homicidal, intentional (*see also* As-
        sault, burning) E968.0
      undetermined whether accidental or
        intentional (*see also* Burn,
        stated as undetermined
        whether accidental or inten-
        tional) E988.1
  internal, from swallowed caustic, corrosive
    liquid, substance — *see* Table of
    Drugs and Chemicals
  lamp (*see also* Fire, specified NEC) E898.1
  late effect of NEC E929.4
  lighter (cigar) (cigarette) (*see also* Fire,
    specified NEC) E898.1
  lightning E907
  liquid (boiling) (hot) (molten) E924.0
    caustic, corrosive (external) E924.1
      swallowed — *see* Table of Drugs and
        Chemicals
  local application of externally applied sub-
    stance in medical or surgical care
    E873.5
  machinery — *see* Accident, machine
  matches (*see also* Fire, specified NEC) E898.1
  medicament, externally applied E873.5
  metal, molten E924.0
  object (hot) E924.8
    producing fire or flames — *see* Fire
  oven (electric) (gas) E924.8
  pipe (smoking) (*see also* Fire, specified NEC)
    E898.1
  radiation — *see* Radiation
  railway engine, locomotive, train (*see also*
    Explosion, railway engine) E803 ☑
  self-inflicted (unspecified whether acciden-
    tal or intentional) E988.1
    caustic or corrosive substance NEC
      E988.7
    stated as intentional, purposeful E958.1
      caustic or corrosive substance NEC
        E958.7
  stated as undetermined whether accidental
    or intentional E988.1
    caustic or corrosive substance NEC
      E988.7
  steam E924.0
    pipe E924.8
  substance (hot) E924.9
    boiling or molten E924.0
    caustic, corrosive (external) E924.1
      swallowed — *see* Table of Drugs and
        Chemicals
  suicidal (attempt) NEC E958.1
    caustic substance E958.7
    late effect of E959
  tanning bed E926.2
  therapeutic misadventure
    overdose of radiation E873.2
  torch, welding (*see also* Fire, specified NEC)
    E898.1
  trash fire (*see also* Burning, bonfire) E897
  vapor E924.0
  vitriol E924.1
  x-rays E926.3
    in medical, surgical procedure — *see*
      Misadventure, failure, in dosage,
      radiation
Butted by animal E906.8

Cachexia, lead or saturnine E866.0

Cachexia, lead or saturnine — *continued*
  from pesticide NEC (*see also* Table of Drugs
    and Chemicals) E863.4
Caisson disease E902.2
Capital punishment (any means) E978
Car sickness E903
Casualty (not due to war) NEC E928.9
  terrorism E979.8
  war (*see also* War operations) E995.9
Cat
  bite E906.3
  scratch E906.8
Cataclysmic (any injury)
  earth surface movement or eruption E909.9
    specified type NEC E909.8
  storm or flood resulting from storm E908.9
    specified type NEC E909.8
Catching fire — *see* Ignition
Caught
  between
    objects (moving) (stationary and mov-
      ing) E918
      and machinery — *see* Accident, ma-
        chine
  by cable car, not on rails E847
  in
    machinery (moving parts of) — *see*, Ac-
      cident, machine
    object E918
Cave-in (causing asphyxia, suffocation (by
  pressure)) — *see also* Suffocation, due
  to, cave-in E913.3
  with injury other than asphyxia or suffoca-
    tion E916
    with asphyxia or suffocation (*see also*
      Suffocation, due to, cave-in)
      E913.3
  struck or crushed by E916
    with asphyxia or suffocation (*see also*
      Suffocation, due to, cave-in)
      E913.3
Change(s) in air pressure — *see also* Effects
  of, air pressure
  sudden, in aircraft (ascent) (descent) (caus-
    ing aeroneurosis or aviators' disease)
    E902.1
Chilblains E901.0
  due to manmade conditions E901.1
Choking (on) (any object except food or vomitus) E912
  apple E911
  bone E911
  food, any type (regurgitated) E911
  mucus or phlegm E912
  seed E911
Civil insurrection — *see* War operations
Cloudburst E908.8
Cold, exposure to (accidental) (excessive)
  (extreme) (place) E901.9
  causing chilblains or immersion foot E901.0
  due to
    manmade conditions E901.1
    specified cause NEC E901.8
    weather (conditions) E901.0
  late effect of NEC E929.5
  self-inflicted (undetermined whether acci-
    dental or intentional) E988.3
    suicidal E958.3
  suicide E958.3
Colic, lead, painter's, or saturnine — *see*
  category E866 ☑
Collapse
  building E916
    burning (uncontrolled fire) E891.8
      in terrorism E979.3
      private E890.8
  dam E909.3
  due to heat — *see* Heat
  machinery — *see* Accident, machine or ve-
    hicle
  man-made structure E909.3
  postoperative NEC E878.9
  structure
    burning (uncontrolled fire) NEC E891.8
      in terrorism E979.3

☑ Additional Digit Required — Refer to the Tabular List for Digit Selection

▽ Subterms under main terms may continue to next column or page

Collision (accidental)

Note — In the case of collisions between different types of vehicles, persons and objects, priority in classification is in the following order:

Aircraft

Watercraft

Motor vehicle

Railway vehicle

Pedal cycle

Animal-drawn vehicle

Animal being ridden

Streetcar or other nonmotor road vehicle

Other vehicle

Pedestrian or person using pedestrian conveyance

Object (except where falling from or set in motion by vehicle etc. listed above)

In the listing below, the combinations are listed only under the vehicle etc. having priority. For definitions, see Supplementary Classification of External Causes of Injury and Poisoning (E800-E999).

aircraft (with object or vehicle) (fixed) (movable) (moving) E841 ☑
  with
    person (while landing, taking off) (without accident to aircraft) E844 ☑
    powered (in transit) (with unpowered aircraft) E841 ☑
      while landing, taking off E840 ☑
    unpowered E842 ☑
      while landing, taking off E840 ☑
animal being ridden (in sport or transport) E828 ☑
  and
    animal (being ridden) (herded) (unattended) E828 ☑
    nonmotor road vehicle, except pedal cycle or animal-drawn vehicle E828 ☑
    object (fallen) (fixed) (movable) (moving) not falling from or set in motion by vehicle of higher priority E828 ☑
    pedestrian (conveyance or vehicle) E828 ☑
animal-drawn vehicle E827 ☑
  and
    animal (being ridden) (herded) (unattended) E827 ☑
    nonmotor road vehicle, except pedal cycle E827 ☑
    object (fallen) (fixed) (movable) (moving) not falling from or set in motion by vehicle of higher priority E827 ☑
    pedestrian (conveyance or vehicle) E827 ☑
    streetcar E827 ☑
motor vehicle (on public highway) (traffic accident) E812 ☑
  after leaving, running off, public highway (without antecedent collision) (without re-entry) E816 ☑
  with antecedent collision on public highway — *see* categories E810-E815 ☑
  with re-entrance collision with another motor vehicle E811 ☑
  and
    abutment (bridge) (overpass) E815 ☑
    animal (herded) (unattended) E815 ☑

Collision — *continued*

motor vehicle — *continued*
  and — *continued*
    animal — *continued*
      carrying person, property E813 ☑
    animal-drawn vehicle E813 ☑
    another motor vehicle (abandoned) (disabled) (parked) (stalled) (stopped) E812 ☑
      with, involving re-entrance (on same roadway) (across median strip) E811 ☑
    any object, person, or vehicle off the public highway resulting from a noncollision motor vehicle nontraffic accident E816 ☑
    avalanche, fallen or not moving E815 ☑
      falling E909.2
    boundary fence E815 ☑
    culvert E815 ☑
    fallen
      stone E815 ☑
      tree E815 ☑
    guard post or guard rail E815 ☑
    inter-highway divider E815 ☑
    landslide, fallen or not moving E815 ☑
      moving E909
    machinery (road) E815 ☑
    nonmotor road vehicle NEC E813 ☑
    object (any object, person, or vehicle off the public highway resulting from a noncollision motor vehicle nontraffic accident) E815 ☑
    off, normally not on, public highway resulting from a noncollision motor vehicle traffic accident E816 ☑
    pedal cycle E813 ☑
    pedestrian (conveyance) E814 ☑
    person (using pedestrian conveyance) E814 ☑
    post or pole (lamp) (light) (signal) (telephone) (utility) E815 ☑
    railway rolling stock, train, vehicle E810 ☑
    safety island E815 ☑
    street car E813 ☑
    traffic signal, sign, or marker (temporary) E815 ☑
    tree E815 ☑
    tricycle E813 ☑
    wall of cut made for road E815 ☑
  due to cataclysm — *see* categories E908 ☑, E909 ☑
  not on public highway, nontraffic accident E822 ☑
  and
    animal (carrying person, property) (herded) (unattended) E822 ☑
    animal-drawn vehicle E822 ☑
    another motor vehicle (moving), except off-road motor vehicle E822 ☑
      stationary E823 ☑
    avalanche, fallen, not moving E823 ☑
      moving E909.2
    landslide, fallen, not moving E823 ☑
      moving E909.2
    nonmotor vehicle (moving) E822 ☑
      stationary E823 ☑
    object (fallen) (normally) (fixed) (movable but not in motion) (stationary) E823 ☑
      moving, except when falling from, set in motion by, aircraft or cataclysm E822 ☑
    pedal cycle (moving) E822 ☑

Collision — *continued*

motor vehicle — *continued*
  not on public highway, nontraffic accident — *continued*
  and — *continued*
    pedal cycle — *continued*
      stationary E823 ☑
    pedestrian (conveyance) E822 ☑
    person (using pedestrian conveyance) E822 ☑
    railway rolling stock, train, vehicle (moving) E822 ☑
      stationary E823 ☑
    road vehicle (any) (moving) E822 ☑
      stationary E823 ☑
    tricycle (moving) E822 ☑
      stationary E823 ☑
  off-road type motor vehicle (not on public highway) E821 ☑
  and
    animal (being ridden) (-drawn vehicle) E821 ☑
    another off-road motor vehicle, except snow vehicle E821 ☑
    other motor vehicle, not on public highway E821 ☑
    other object or vehicle NEC, fixed or movable, not set in motion by aircraft, motor vehicle on highway, or snow vehicle, motor driven E821 ☑
    pedal cycle E821 ☑
    pedestrian (conveyance) E821 ☑
    railway train E821 ☑
  on public highway — *see* Collision, motor vehicle
pedal cycle E826 ☑
  and
    animal (carrying person, property) (herded) (unherded) E826 ☑
    animal-drawn vehicle E826 ☑
    another pedal cycle E826 ☑
    nonmotor road vehicle E826 ☑
    object (fallen) (fixed) (movable) (moving) not falling from or set in motion by aircraft, motor vehicle, or railway train NEC E826 ☑
    pedestrian (conveyance) E826 ☑
    person (using pedestrian conveyance) E826 ☑
    street car E826 ☑
pedestrian(s) (conveyance) E917.9
  with fall E886.9
    in sports E886.0
  and
    crowd, human stampede E917.1
      with subsequent fall E917.6
    furniture E917.3
      with subsequent fall E917.7
    machinery — *see* Accident, machine
    object (fallen) (moving) not falling from NEC, fixed or set in motion by any vehicle classifiable to E800-E848 ☑, E917.9
      with subsequent fall E917.6
    caused by a crowd E917.1
      with subsequent fall E917.6
    furniture E917.3
      with subsequent fall E917.7
    in
      running water E917.2
        with drowning or submersion — *see* Submersion
      sports E917.0
        with subsequent fall E917.5
      stationary E917.4
        with subsequent fall E917.8
    vehicle, nonmotor, nonroad E848
  in
    running water E917.2

Collision — *continued*

pedestrian(s) — *continued*
  in — *continued*
    running water — *continued*
      with drowning or submersion — *see* Submersion
    sports E917.0
      with fall E886.0
  person(s) (using pedestrian conveyance) (*see also* Collision, pedestrian) E917.9
  railway (rolling stock) (train) (vehicle) (with (subsequent) derailment, explosion, fall or fire) E800 ☑
  with antecedent derailment E802 ☑
  and
    animal (carrying person) (herded) (unattended) E801 ☑
    another railway train or vehicle E800 ☑
    buffers E801 ☑
    fallen tree on railway E801 ☑
    farm machinery, nonmotor (in transport) (stationary) E801 ☑
    gates E801 ☑
    nonmotor vehicle E801 ☑
    object (fallen) (fixed) (movable) (moving) not falling from, set in motion by, aircraft or motor vehicle NEC E801 ☑
    pedal cycle E801 ☑
    pedestrian (conveyance) E805 ☑
    person (using pedestrian conveyance) E805 ☑
    platform E801 ☑
    rock on railway E801 ☑
    street car E801 ☑
  snow vehicle, motor-driven (not on public highway) E820 ☑
  and
    animal (being ridden) (-drawn vehicle) E820 ☑
    another off-road motor vehicle E820 ☑
    other motor vehicle, not on public highway E820 ☑
    other object or vehicle NEC, fixed or movable, not set in motion by aircraft or motor vehicle on highway E820 ☑
    pedal cycle E820 ☑
    pedestrian (conveyance) E820 ☑
    railway train E820 ☑
  on public highway — *see* Collision, motor vehicle
street car(s) E829 ☑
  and
    animal, herded, not being ridden, unattended E829 ☑
    nonmotor road vehicle NEC E829 ☑
    object (fallen) (fixed) (movable) (moving) not falling from or set in motion by aircraft, animal-drawn vehicle, animal being ridden, motor vehicle, pedal cycle, or railway train E829 ☑
    pedestrian (conveyance) E829 ☑
    person (using pedestrian conveyance) E829 ☑
vehicle
  animal-drawn — *see* Collision, animal-drawn vehicle
  motor — *see* Collision, motor vehicle
  nonmotor
    nonroad E848
    and
      another nonmotor, nonroad vehicle E848

Collision — Divers' disease, palsy, paralysis, squeeze

☑ **Additional Digit Required** — Refer to the Tabular List for Digit Selection

▽ **Subterms under main terms may continue to next column or page**

340 — Volume 2

▶◀ **Revised Text**   ● **New Line**   ▲ **Revised Code**

2015 ICD-9-CM

Dog bite E906.0
Dragged by
    cable car (not on rails) E847
        on rails E829 ☑
    motor vehicle (on highway) E814 ☑
        not on highway, nontraffic accident
            E825 ☑
    street car E829 ☑
Drinking poison (accidental) — *see* Table of
    Drugs and Chemicals
Drowning — *see* Submersion
Dust in eye E914

E

Earth falling (on) (with asphyxia or suffocation
    (by pressure)) — *see also* Suffocation,
    due to, cave-in E913.3
    as, or due to, a cataclysm (involving any
        transport vehicle) — *see* categories
        E908 ☑, E909 ☑
    not due to cataclysmic action E913.3
        motor vehicle (in motion) (on public
            highway) E813 ☑
            not on public highway E825 ☑
        nonmotor road vehicle NEC E829 ☑
        pedal cycle E826 ☑
        railway rolling stock, train, vehicle
            E806 ☑
        street car E829 ☑
        struck or crushed by E916
            with asphyxiation or suffocation
                E913.3
            with injury other than asphyxia, suf-
                focation E916
Earthquake (any injury) E909.0
Effect(s) (adverse) of
    air pressure E902.9
        at high altitude E902.9
            in aircraft E902.1
            residence or prolonged visit (causing
                conditions classifiable to
                E902.0) E902.0
        due to
            diving E902.2
            specified cause NEC E902.8
        in aircraft E902.1
    cold, excessive (exposure to) (*see also* Cold,
        exposure to) E901.9
    heat (excessive) (*see also* Heat) E900.9
    hot
        place — *see* Heat
        weather E900.0
    insulation — *see* Heat
    late — *see* Late effect of
    motion E903
    nuclear explosion or weapon
        in
            terrorism E979.5
            war operations (*see also* War opera-
                tions, injury due to, nuclear
                weapons) E996.9
    radiation — *see* Radiation
    terrorism, secondary E979.9
    travel E903
Electric shock, electrocution (accidental)
    (from exposed wire, faulty appliance,
    high voltage cable, live rail, open socket)
    (by) (in) E925.9
    appliance or wiring
        domestic E925.0
        factory E925.2
        farm (building) E925.8
            house E925.0
        home E925.0
        industrial (conductor) (control appara-
            tus) (transformer) E925.2
        outdoors E925.8
        public building E925.8
        residential institution E925.8
        school E925.8
        specified place NEC E925.8
    caused by other person
        stated as
            intentional, homicidal E968.8

Electric shock, electrocution — *continued*
    caused by other person — *continued*
        stated as — *continued*
            undetermined whether accidental or
                intentional E988.4
    electric power generating plant, distribution
        station E925.1
    electroshock gun (taser) (stun gun) E925.8
        caused by other person E968.8
        legal intervention E975
        stated as accidental E925.8
        stated as intentional E968.8
        due to legal intervention E975
        stated as intentional self-harm (suicidal
            attempt) E958.4
        stated as undetermined whether acciden-
            tal or intentional E988.4
        suicide (attempt) E958.4
    homicidal (attempt) E968.8
    legal execution E978
    lightning E907
    machinery E925.9
        domestic E925.0
        factory E925.2
        farm E925.8
        home E925.0
    misadventure in medical or surgical proce-
        dure
        in electroshock therapy E873.4
    self-inflicted (undetermined whether acci-
        dental or intentional) E988.4
        stated as intentional E958.4
        stated as undetermined whether accidental
            or intentional E988.4
    suicidal (attempt) E958.4
    transmission line E925.1
Electrocution — *see* Electric shock
Embolism
    air (traumatic) NEC — *see* Air, embolism
Encephalitis
    lead or saturnine E866.0
        from pesticide NEC E863.4
Entanglement
    in
        bedclothes, causing suffocation E913.0
        wheel of pedal cycle E826 ☑
Entry of foreign body, material, any — *see*
    Foreign body
Execution, legal (any method) E978
Exertion, excessive physical, from pro-
    longed activity E927.2
Exhaustion
    cold — *see* Cold, exposure to
    due to excessive exertion E927.2
    heat — *see* Heat
Explosion (accidental) (in) (of) (on) E923.9
    acetylene E923.2
    aerosol can E921.8
    aircraft (in transit) (powered) E841 ☑
        at landing, take-off E840 ☑
        in
            terrorism E979.1
            war operations
                from
                    enemy fire or explosive(s)
                        (device placed on air-
                        craft) E994.0
                  own onboard explosives
                      E994.1
        unpowered E842 ☑
    air tank (compressed) (in machinery) E921.1
    anesthetic gas in operating theatre E923.2
    automobile tire NEC E921.8
        causing transport accident — *see* cate-
            gories E810-E825 ☑
    blasting (cap) (materials) E923.1
    boiler (machinery), not on transport vehicle
        E921.0
        steamship — *see* Explosion, watercraft
    bomb E923.8
        in
            terrorism E979.2
            war operations E993.8
                after cessation of hostilities
                    E998.1

Explosion — *continued*
    bomb — *continued*
        in — *continued*
            war operations — *continued*
                atom, hydrogen or nuclear (*see*
                    also War operations, injury
                    due to, nuclear weapons)
                    E996.9
                injury by fragments from E991.9
                antipersonnel bomb E991.3
    butane E923.2
    caused by
        other person
            stated as
                intentional, homicidal — *see* As-
                    sault, explosive
                undetermined whether acciden-
                    tal or homicidal E985.5
    coal gas E923.2
    detonator E923.1
    dynamite E923.1
    explosive (material) NEC E923.9
        gas(es) E923.2
        missile E923.8
            in
                terrorism E979.2
                war operations E993.1
                    injury by fragments from
                      E991.9
                    antipersonnel bomb
                      E991.3
        used in blasting operations E923.1
    fire-damp E923.2
    fireworks E923.0
    gas E923.2
        cylinder (in machinery) E921.1
        pressure tank (in machinery) E921.1
    gasoline (fumes) (tank) not in moving motor
        vehicle E923.2
    grain store (military) (munitions) E923.8
    grenade E923.8
        in
            terrorism E979.2
            war operations E993.8
                injury by fragments from E991.4
    homicide (attempt) — *see* Assault, explosive
    hot water heater, tank (in machinery) E921.0
    in mine (of explosive gases) NEC E923.2
    late effect of NEC E929.8
    machinery (*see also* Accident, machine)
        pressure vessel — *see* Explosion, pres-
            sure vessel
    methane E923.2
    missile E923.8
        in
            terrorism E979.2
            war operations E993.1
                injury by fragments from E991.4
    motor vehicle (part of)
        in motion (on public highway) E818 ☑
        not on public highway E825 ☑
    munitions (dump) (factory) E923.8
        in
            terrorism E979.2
            war operations E993.9
    of mine E923.8
        in
            terrorism
                at sea or in harbor E979.0
                land E979.2
                marine E979.0
            war operations
                after cessation of hostilities
                    E998.0
                at sea or in harbor E992.2
                land E993.8
                  after cessation of hostilities
                    E998.0
                  injury by fragments from
                    E991.4
                marine E992.2
    own weapons
        in
            terrorism (*see also* Suicide) E979.2
            war operations E993.7
                injury by fragments from E991.9

Explosion — *continued*
    own weapons — *continued*
        in — *continued*
            war operations — *continued*
                injury by fragments from — *con-*
                  tinued
                  antipersonnel bomb E991.3
    pressure
        cooker E921.8
        gas tank (in machinery) E921.1
        vessel (in machinery) E921.9
            on transport vehicle — *see* cate-
                gories E800-E848 ☑
            specified type NEC E921.8
    propane E923.2
    railway engine, locomotive, train (boiler)
        (with subsequent collision, derail-
        ment, fall) E803 ☑
        with
            collision (antecedent) (*see also* Colli-
                sion, railway) E800 ☑
            derailment (antecedent) E802 ☑
            fire (without antecedent collision or
                derailment) E803 ☑
    secondary fire resulting from — *see* Fire
    self-inflicted (unspecified whether acciden-
        tal or intentional) E985.5
        stated as intentional, purposeful E955.5
    shell (artillery) E923.8
        in
            terrorism E979.2
            war operations E993.2
                injury by fragments from E991.4
    stated as undetermined whether caused
        accidentally or purposely inflicted
        E985.5
    steam or water lines (in machinery) E921.0
    suicide (attempted) E955.5
    terrorism — *see* Terrorism, explosion
    torpedo E923.8
        in
            terrorism E979.0
            war operations E992.0
    transport accident — *see* categories
        E800-E848 ☑
    war operations — *see* War operations, ex-
        plosion
    watercraft (boiler) E837 ☑
        causing drowning, submersion (after
            jumping from watercraft) E830 ☑
Exposure (weather) (conditions) (rain) (wind)
    E904.3
    with homicidal intent E968.4
    environmental
        to
            algae bloom E928.6
            blue-green algae bloom E928.6
            brown tide E928.6
            cyanobacteria bloom E928.6
            Florida red tide E928.6
            harmful alage
                and toxins E928.6
                bloom E928.6
            pfiesteria piscicida E928.6
            red tide E928.6
    excessive E904.3
        cold (*see also* Cold, exposure to) E901.9
            self-inflicted — *see* Cold, exposure
                to, self-inflicted
        heat (*see also* Heat) E900.9
    helpless person, infant, newborn due to
        abandonment or neglect E904.0
    noise E928.1
    prolonged in deep-freeze unit or refrigerator
        E901.1
    radiation — *see* Radiation
    resulting from transport accident — *see*
        categories E800-E848 ☑
    smoke from, due to
        fire — *see* Fire
        tobacco, second-hand E869.4
    vibration E928.2
External cause status E000.9
    child assisting in compensated work of
        other family member E000.8

☑ **Additional Digit Required — Refer to the Tabular List for Digit Selection**   ▽ **Subterms under main terms may continue to next column or page**

Index

External cause status   Index to External Causes

External cause status — Fire

External cause status — *continued*
 civilian
  done for
   financial or other compensation
    E000.0
   pay or income E000.0
  family member assisting in compensated
   work of other family member E000.8
  for income E000.0
  hobby or leisure E000.8
 military E000.1
  off duty E000.8
 off duty military E000.8
 recreation E000.8
 specified NEC E000.8
 sport not for income E000.8
 student E000.8
 volunteer E000.2

F

Fallen on by
 animal (horse) (not being ridden) E906.8
  being ridden (in sport or transport)
   E828 ☑
Fall, falling (accidental) E888.9
 building E916
  burning E891.8
   private E890.8
 down
  escalator E880.0
  ladder E881.0
   in boat, ship, watercraft E833 ☑
  staircase E880.9
  stairs, steps — *see* Fall, from, stairs
 earth (with asphyxia or suffocation (by
  pressure)) (*see also* Earth, falling)
  E913.3
 from, off
  aircraft (at landing, take-off) (in-transit)
   (while alighting, boarding)
   E843 ☑
   resulting from accident to aircraft —
    see categories E840-E842 ☑
  animal (in sport or transport) E828 ☑
  animal-drawn vehicle E827 ☑
  balcony E882
  bed E884.4
  bicycle E826 ☑
  boat, ship, watercraft (into water)
   E832 ☑
   after accident to, collision, fire on
    E830 ☑
    and subsequently struck by (part
     of) boat E831 ☑
    and subsequently struck by (part of)
     while alighting, boat E831 ☑
   burning, crushed, sinking E830 ☑
    and subsequently struck by (part
     of) boat E831 ☑
  bridge E882
  building E882
   burning (uncontrolled fire) E891.8
    in terrorism E979.3
   private E890.8
  bunk in boat, ship, watercraft E834 ☑
   due to accident to watercraft
    E831 ☑
  cable car (not on rails) E847
   on rails E829 ☑
  car — *see* Fall from motor vehicle
  chair E884.2
  cliff E884.1
  commode E884.6
  curb (sidewalk) E880.1
  elevation aboard ship E834 ☑
   due to accident to ship E831 ☑
  embankment E884.9
  escalator E880.0
  fire escape E882
  flagpole E882
  furniture NEC E884.5
  gangplank (into water) (*see also* Fall,
   from, boat) E832 ☑
   to deck, dock E834 ☑
  hammock on ship E834 ☑

Fall, falling — *continued*
 from, off — *continued*
  hammock on ship — *continued*
   due to accident to watercraft
    E831 ☑
  haystack E884.9
  heelies E885.1
  high place NEC E884.9
   stated as undetermined whether ac-
    cidental or intentional — *see*
    Jumping, from, high place
  horse (in sport or transport) E828 ☑
  in-line skates E885.1
  ladder E881.0
   in boat, ship, watercraft E833 ☑
   due to accident to watercraft
    E831 ☑
  machinery (*see also* Accident, machine)
   not in operation E884.9
  motorized
   mobility scooter E884.3
   wheelchair E884.3
  motor vehicle (in motion) (on public
   highway) E818 ☑
   not on public highway E825 ☑
    stationary, except while alighting,
     boarding, entering, leav-
     ing E884.9
    while alighting, boarding, enter-
     ing, leaving E824 ☑
   stationary, except while alighting,
    boarding, entering, leaving
    E884.9
   while alighting, boarding, entering,
    leaving, except off-road type
    motor vehicle E817 ☑
   off-road type — *see* Fall, from,
    off-road type motor vehi-
    cle
  nonmotor road vehicle (while alighting,
   boarding) NEC E829 ☑
   stationary, except while alighting,
    boarding, entering, leaving
    E884.9
  off road type motor vehicle (not on
   public highway) NEC E821 ☑
   on public highway E818 ☑
    while alighting, boarding, enter-
     ing, leaving E817 ☑
   snow vehicle — *see* Fall from snow
    vehicle, motor-driven
  one
   deck to another on ship E834 ☑
    due to accident to ship E831 ☑
   level to another NEC E884.9
    boat, ship, or watercraft E834 ☑
    due to accident to watercraft
     E831 ☑
  pedal cycle E826 ☑
  playground equipment E884.0
  railway rolling stock, train, vehicle (while
   alighting, boarding) E804 ☑
   with
    collision (*see also* Collision, rail-
     way) E800 ☑
    derailment (*see also* Derailment,
     railway) E802 ☑
    explosion (*see also* Explosion,
     railway engine) E803 ☑
  rigging (aboard ship) E834 ☑
   due to accident to watercraft
    E831 ☑
  roller skates E885.1
  scaffolding E881.1
  scooter (nonmotorized) E885.0
   motorized mobility E884.3
  sidewalk (curb) E880.1
   moving E885.9
  skateboard E885.2
  skis E885.3
  snowboard E885.4
  snow vehicle, motor-driven (not on
   public highway) E820 ☑
   on public highway E818 ☑

Fall, falling — *continued*
 from, off — *continued*
  snow vehicle, motor-driven — *continued*
   on public highway — *continued*
    while alighting, boarding, enter-
     ing, leaving E817 ☑
  stairs, steps E880.9
   boat, ship, watercraft E833 ☑
    due to accident to watercraft
     E831 ☑
   motor bus, motor vehicle — *see* Fall,
    from, motor vehicle, while
    alighting, boarding
   street car E829 ☑
  stationary vehicle NEC E884.9
  stepladder E881.0
  street car (while boarding, alighting)
   E829 ☑
   stationary, except while boarding or
    alighting E884.9
  structure NEC E882
   burning (uncontrolled fire) E891.8
    in terrorism E979.3
  table E884.9
  toilet E884.6
  tower E882
  tree E884.9
  turret E882
  vehicle NEC (*see also* Accident, vehicle
   NEC)
   stationary E884.9
  viaduct E882
  wall E882
  wheelchair (electric) (motorized) E884.3
  wheelies E885.1
  window E882
 in, on
  aircraft (at landing, take-off) (in-transit)
   E843 ☑
   resulting from accident to aircraft —
    see categories E840-E842 ☑
  boat, ship, watercraft E835 ☑
   due to accident to watercraft
    E831 ☑
   one level to another NEC E834 ☑
   on ladder, stairs E833 ☑
  cutting or piercing instrument or machine E888.0
  deck (of boat, ship, watercraft) E835 ☑
   due to accident to watercraft
    E831 ☑
  escalator E880.0
  gangplank E835 ☑
  glass, broken E888.0
  knife E888.0
  ladder E881.0
   in boat, ship, watercraft E833 ☑
   due to accident to watercraft
    E831 ☑
  object
   edged, pointed or sharp E888.0
   other E888.1
  pitchfork E888.0
  railway rolling stock, train, vehicle (while
   alighting, boarding) E804 ☑
   with
    collision (*see also* Collision, rail-
     way) E800 ☑
    derailment (*see also* Derailment,
     railway) E802 ☑
    explosion (see also Explosion,
     railway engine) E803 ☑
  scaffolding E881.1
  scissors E888.0
  staircase, stairs, steps (*see also* Fall, from,
   stairs) E880.9
  street car E829 ☑
  water transport (*see also* Fall, in, boat)
   E835 ☑
 into
  cavity E883.9
  dock E883.9
   from boat, ship, watercraft (*see also*
    Fall, from, boat) E832 ☑

Fall, falling — *continued*
 into — *continued*
  hold (of ship) E834 ☑
   due to accident to watercraft
    E831 ☑
  hole E883.9
  manhole E883.2
  moving part of machinery — *see* Accident, machine
  opening in surface NEC E883.9
  pit E883.9
  quarry E883.9
  shaft E883.9
  storm drain E883.2
  tank E883.9
  water (with drowning or submersion)
   E910.9
  well E883.1
 late effect of NEC E929.3
 object (*see also* Hit by, object, falling) E916
 other E888.8
 over
  animal E885.9
  cliff E884.1
  embankment E884.9
  small object E885.9
 overboard (*see also* Fall, from, boat) E832 ☑
 resulting in striking against object E888.1
  sharp E888.0
 rock E916
 same level NEC E888.9
  aircraft (any kind) E843 ☑
   resulting from accident to aircraft —
    see categories E840-E842 ☑
  boat, ship, watercraft E835 ☑
   due to accident to, collision, water-
    craft E831 ☑
  from
   collision, pushing, shoving, by or
    with other person(s) E886.9
    as, or caused by, a crowd E917.6
    in sports E886.0
   in-line skates E885.1
   roller skates E885.1
   scooter (nonmotorized) E885.0
   skateboard E885.2
   slipping stumbling, tripping E885 ☑
   snowboard E885.4
 snowslide E916
  as avalanche E909.2
 stone E916
 through
  hatch (on ship) E834 ☑
   due to accident to watercraft
    E831 ☑
  roof E882
  window E882
 timber E916
 while alighting from, boarding, entering,
  leaving
  aircraft (any kind) E843 ☑
  motor bus, motor vehicle — *see* Fall,
   from, motor vehicle, while
   alighting, boarding
  nonmotor road vehicle NEC E829 ☑
  railway train E804 ☑
  street car E829 ☑
Fell or jumped from high place, so stated —
 see Jumping, from, high place
Felo-de-se — *see also* Suicide E958.9
Fever
 heat — *see* Heat
 thermic — *see* Heat
Fight (hand) (fist) (foot) — *see also* Assault,
 fight E960.0
Fire (accidental) (caused by great heat from
 appliance (electrical), hot object or hot
 substance) (secondary, resulting from
 explosion) E899
 conflagration — *see* Conflagration
 controlled, normal (in brazier, fireplace,
  furnace, or stove) (charcoal) (coal)
  (coke) (electric) (gas) (wood)
  bonfire E897
  brazier, not in building or structure E897

☑ **Additional Digit Required — Refer to the Tabular List for Digit Selection**   ▽ **Subterms under main terms may continue to next column or page**

Fire, hot object or hot substance — *continued*
  controlled, normal — *continued*
    in building or structure, except private
      dwelling (barn) (church) (convalescent or residential home) (factory) (farm outbuilding) (hospital) (hotel) (institution (educational) (dormitory) (residential) (private garage) (school) (shop) (store) (theatre) E896
    in private dwelling (apartment) (boarding house) (camping place) (caravan) (farmhouse) (home (private)) (house) (lodging house) (rooming house) (tenement) E895
    not in building or structure E897
    trash E897
  forest (uncontrolled) E892
  grass (uncontrolled) E892
  hay (uncontrolled) E892
  homicide (attempt) E968.0
    late effect of E969
  in, of, on, starting in E892
    aircraft (in transit) (powered) E841 ☑
      at landing, take-off E840 ☑
      stationary E892
      unpowered (balloon) (glider) E842 ☑
    balloon E842 ☑
    boat, ship, watercraft — *see categories* E830 ☑, E831 ☑, E837 ☑
    building or structure, except private dwelling (barn) (church) (convalescent or residential home) (factory) (farm outbuilding) (hospital) (hotel) (institution (educational) (dormitory) (residential)) (school) (shop) (store) (theatre) (*see also* Conflagration, building or structure, except private dwelling) E891.9
    forest (uncontrolled) E892
    glider E842 ☑
    grass (uncontrolled) E892
    hay (uncontrolled) E892
    lumber (uncontrolled) E892
    machinery — *see* Accident, machine
    mine (uncontrolled) E892
    motor vehicle (in motion) (on public highway) E818 ☑
      not on public highway E825 ☑
      stationary E892
    prairie (uncontrolled) E892
    private dwelling (apartment) (boarding house) (camping place) (caravan) (farmhouse) (home (private)) (house) (lodging house) (private garage) (rooming house) (tenement) (*see also* Conflagration, private dwelling) E890.9
    railway rolling stock, train, vehicle (*see also* Explosion, railway engine) E803 ☑
      stationary E892
    room NEC E898.1
    street car (in motion) E829 ☑
      stationary E892
    terrorism (by fire-producing device) E979.3
      fittings or furniture (burning building) (uncontrolled fire) E979.3
      from nuclear explosion E979.5
    transport vehicle, stationary NEC E892
    tunnel (uncontrolled) E892
    war operations (by fire-producing device or conventional weapon) E990.9
      from nuclear explosion (*see also* War operations, injury due to, nuclear weapons) E996.2
      incendiary bomb E990.0
      petrol bomb E990.0
  late effect of NEC E929.4
  lumber (uncontrolled) E892
  mine (uncontrolled) E892
  prairie (uncontrolled) E892

Fire, hot object or hot substance — *continued*
  self-inflicted (unspecified whether accidental or intentional) E988.1
    stated as intentional, purposeful E958.1
  specified NEC E898.1
    with
      conflagration — *see* Conflagration
      ignition (of)
        clothing — *see* Ignition, clothes
        highly inflammable material (benzine) (fat) (gasoline) (kerosene) (paraffin) (petrol) E894
  started by other person
    stated as
      with intent to injure or kill E968.0
      undetermined whether or not with intent to injure or kill E988.1
  suicide (attempted) E958.1
    late effect of E959
  tunnel (uncontrolled) E892
Fireball effects from nuclear explosion
  in
    terrorism E979.5
    war operations (*see also* War operations, injury due to, nuclear weapons) E996.2
Fireworks (explosion) E923.0
Flash burns from explosion — *see also* Explosion E923.9
Flood (any injury) (resulting from storm) E908.2
  caused by collapse of dam or manmade structure E909.3
Forced landing (aircraft) E840 ☑
Foreign body, object or material (entrance into) (accidental)
  air passage (causing injury) E915
    with asphyxia, obstruction, suffocation E912
      food or vomitus E911
    nose (with asphyxia, obstruction, suffocation) E912
      causing injury without asphyxia, obstruction, suffocation E915
  alimentary canal (causing injury) (with obstruction) E915
    with asphyxia, obstruction respiratory passage, suffocation E912
      food E911
    mouth E915
      with asphyxia, obstruction, suffocation E912
        food E911
    pharynx E915
      with asphyxia, obstruction, suffocation E912
        food E911
  aspiration (with asphyxia, obstruction respiratory passage, suffocation) E912
    causing injury without asphyxia, obstruction respiratory passage, suffocation E915
    food (regurgitated) (vomited) E911
      causing injury without asphyxia, obstruction respiratory passage, suffocation E915
    mucus (not of newborn) E912
    phlegm E912
  bladder (causing injury or obstruction) E915
  bronchus, bronchi — *see* Foreign body, air passages
  conjunctival sac E914
  digestive system — *see* Foreign body, alimentary canal
  ear (causing injury or obstruction) E915
  esophagus (causing injury or obstruction) (*see also* Foreign body, alimentary canal) E915
  eye (any part) E914
  eyelid E914
  hairball (stomach) (with obstruction) E915
  ingestion — *see* Foreign body, alimentary canal
  inhalation — *see* Foreign body, aspiration

Foreign body, object or material — *continued*
  intestine (causing injury or obstruction) E915
  iris E914
  lacrimal apparatus E914
  larynx — *see* Foreign body, air passage
  late effect of NEC E929.8
  lung — *see* Foreign body, air passage
  mouth — *see* Foreign body, alimentary canal, mouth
  nasal passage — *see* Foreign body, air passage, nose
  nose — *see* Foreign body, air passage, nose
  ocular muscle E914
  operation wound (left in) — *see* Misadventure, foreign object
  orbit E914
  pharynx — *see* Foreign body, alimentary canal, pharynx
  rectum (causing injury or obstruction) E915
  stomach (hairball) (causing injury or obstruction) E915
  tear ducts or glands E914
  trachea — *see* Foreign body, air passage
  urethra (causing injury or obstruction) E915
  vagina (causing injury or obstruction) E915
Found dead, injured
  from exposure (to) — *see* Exposure
  on
    public highway E819 ☑
    railway right of way E807 ☑
Fracture (circumstances unknown or unspecified) E887
  due to specified external means — *see* manner of accident
  late effect of NEC E929.3
  occurring in water transport NEC E835 ☑
Freezing — *see* Cold, exposure to
Frostbite E901.0
  due to manmade conditions E901.1
Frozen — *see* Cold, exposure to

G

Garrotting, homicidal (attempted) E963
Gored E906.8
Gunshot wound — *see also* Shooting E922.9

H

Hailstones, injury by E904.3
Hairball (stomach) (with obstruction) E915
Hanged himself — *see also* Hanging, self-inflicted E983.0
Hang gliding E842 ☑
Hanging (accidental) E913.8
  caused by other person
    in accidental circumstances E913.8
    stated as
      intentional, homicidal E963
      undetermined whether accidental or intentional E983.0
  homicide (attempt) E963
  in bed or cradle E913.0
  legal execution E978
  self-inflicted (unspecified whether accidental or intentional) E983.0
    in accidental circumstances E913.8
    stated as intentional, purposeful E953.0
    stated as undetermined whether accidental or intentional E983.0
  suicidal (attempt) E953.0
Heat (apoplexy) (collapse) (cramps) (effects of) (excessive) (exhaustion) (fever) (prostration) (stroke) E900.9
  due to
    manmade conditions (as listed in E900.1, except boat, ship, watercraft) E900.1
    weather (conditions) E900.0
  from
    electric heating appartus causing burning E924.8
    nuclear explosion
      in
        terrorism E979.5

Heat — *continued*
  from — *continued*
    nuclear explosion — *continued*
      in — *continued*
        war operations (*see also* War operations, injury due to, nuclear weapons) E996.2
    generated in, boiler, engine, evaporator, fire room of boat, ship, watercraft E838
    inappropriate in local application or packing in medical or surgical procedure E873.5
  late effect of NEC E989
Hemorrhage
  delayed following medical or surgical treatment without mention of misadventure — *see* Reaction, abnormal
  during medical or surgical treatment as misadventure — *see* Misadventure, cut
High
  altitude, effects E902.9
  level of radioactivity, effects — *see* Radiation
  pressure effects (*see also* Effects of, air pressure)
    from rapid descent in water (causing caisson or divers' disease, palsy, or paralysis) E902.2
  temperature, effects — *see* Heat
Hit, hitting (accidental) by
  aircraft (propeller) (without accident to aircraft) E844 ☑
    unpowered E842 ☑
  avalanche E909.2
  being thrown against object in or part of motor vehicle (in motion) (on public highway) E818 ☑
    not on public highway E825 ☑
    nonmotor road vehicle NEC E829 ☑
    street car E829 ☑
  boat, ship, watercraft
    after fall from watercraft E838 ☑
      damaged, involved in accident E831 ☑
    while swimming, water skiing E838 ☑
  bullet (*see also* Shooting) E922.9
    from air gun E922.4
    in
      terrorism E979.4
      war operations E991.2
        rubber E991.0
  flare, Verey pistol (*see also* Shooting) E922.8
  hailstones E904.3
  landslide E909.2
  law-enforcing agent (on duty) E975
    with blunt object (baton) (night stick) (stave) (truncheon) E973
  machine — *see* Accident, machine
  missile
    firearm (*see also* Shooting) E922.9
    in
      terrorism — *see* Terrorism, missile
      war operations — *see* War operations, missile
  motor vehicle (on public highway) (traffic accident) E814 ☑
    not on public highway, nontraffic accident E822 ☑
  nonmotor road vehicle NEC E829 ☑
  object
    falling E916
      from, in, on
        aircraft E844 ☑
          due to accident to aircraft — *see categories* E840-E842
          unpowered E842 ☑
        boat, ship, watercraft E838 ☑
          due to accident to watercraft E831 ☑
        building E916
          burning (uncontrolled fire) E891.8
          in terrorism E979.3

☑ Additional Digit Required — Refer to the Tabular List for Digit Selection   ▽ Subterms under main terms may continue to next column or page

Hit, hitting by — *continued*
  object — *continued*
    falling — *continued*
      from, in, on — *continued*
        building — *continued*
          burning — *continued*
            private E890.8
        cataclysmic
          earth surface movement or
            eruption E909.9
          storm E908.9
        cave-in E916
          with asphyxiation or suffoca-
            tion (*see also* Suffoca-
            tion, due to, cave-in)
            E913.3
        earthquake E909.0
        motor vehicle (in motion) (on
          public highway) E818 ☑
          not on public highway
            E825 ☑
          stationary E916
        nonmotor road vehicle NEC
          E829 ☑
        pedal cycle E826 ☑
        railway rolling stock, train, vehicle
          E806 ☑
        street car E829 ☑
        structure, burning NEC E891.8
        vehicle, stationary E916
    moving NEC — *see* Striking against, ob-
      ject
    projected NEC — *see* Striking against,
      object
    set in motion by
      compressed air or gas, spring, strik-
        ing, throwing — *see* Striking
        against, object
      explosion — *see* Explosion
    thrown into, on, or towards
      motor vehicle (in motion) (on public
        highway) E818 ☑
        not on public highway E825 ☑
      nonmotor road vehicle NEC E829 ☑
      pedal cycle E826 ☑
      street car E829 ☑
    off-road type motor vehicle (not on public
      highway) E821 ☑
      on public highway E814 ☑
  other person(s) E917.9
    with blunt or thrown object E917.9
      in sports E917.0
        with subsequent fall E917.5
      intentionally, homicidal E968.2
    as, or caused by, a crowd E917.1
      with subsequent fall E917.6
    in sports E917.0
  pedal cycle E826 ☑
  police (on duty) E975
    with blunt object (baton) (nightstick)
      (stave) (truncheon) E973
  railway, rolling stock, train, vehicle (part of)
    E805 ☑
  shot — *see* Shooting
  snow vehicle, motor-driven (not on public
    highway) E820 ☑
    on public highway E814 ☑
    street car E829 ☑
  vehicle NEC — *see* Accident, vehicle NEC
Homicide, homicidal (attempt) (justifiable) —
  see also Assault E968.9
Hot
  liquid, object, substance, accident caused
    by (*see also* Accident, caused by, hot,
    by type of substance)
    late effect of E929.8
  place, effects — *see* Heat
  weather, effects E900.0
Humidity, causing problem E904.3
Hunger E904.1
  resulting from
    abandonment or neglect E904.0
    transport accident — *see* categories
      E800-E848 ☑
Hurricane (any injury) E908.0

Hypobarism, hypobaropathy — *see* Effects
  of, air pressure
Hypothermia — *see* Cold, exposure to

I

Ictus
  caloris — *see* Heat
  solaris E900.0
Ignition (accidental)
  anesthetic gas in operating theatre E923.2
  bedclothes
    with
      conflagration — *see* Conflagration
      ignition (of)
        clothing — *see* Ignition, clothes
        highly inflammable material
          (benzine) (fat) (gasoline)
          (kerosene) (paraffin)
          (petrol) E894
  benzine E894
  clothes, clothing (from controlled fire) (in
    building) E893.9
    with conflagration — *see* Conflagration
    from
      bonfire E893.2
      highly inflammable material E894
      sources or material as listed in E893.8
      trash fire E893.2
      uncontrolled fire — *see* Conflagra-
        tion
    in
      private dwelling E893.0
      specified building or structure, ex-
        cept private dwelling E893.1
    not in building or structure E893.2
  explosive material — *see* Explosion
  fat E894
  gasoline E894
  kerosene E894
  material
    explosive — *see* Explosion
    highly inflammable E894
      with conflagration — *see* Conflagra-
        tion
      with explosion E923.2
  nightdress — *see* Ignition, clothes
  paraffin E894
  petrol E894
Immersion — *see* Submersion
Implantation of quills of porcupine E906.8
Inanition (from) E904.9
  hunger — *see* Lack of, food
  resulting from homicidal intent E968.4
  thirst — *see* Lack of, water
Inattention after, at birth E904.0
  homicidal, infanticidal intent E968.4
Infanticide — *see also* Assault
Ingestion
  foreign body (causing injury) (with obstruc-
    tion) — *see* Foreign body, alimentary
    canal
  poisonous substance NEC — *see* Table of
    Drugs and Chemicals
Inhalation
  excessively cold substance, manmade
    E901.1
  foreign body — *see* Foreign body, aspiration
  liquid air, hydrogen, nitrogen E901.1
  mucus, not of newborn (with asphyxia, ob-
    struction respiratory passage, suffo-
    cation) E912
  phlegm (with asphyxia, obstruction respira-
    tory passage, suffocation) E912
  poisonous gas — *see* Table of Drugs and
    Chemicals
  smoke from, due to
    fire — *see* Fire
    tobacco, second-hand E869.4
  vomitus (with asphyxia, obstruction respira-
    tory passage, suffocation) E911
Injury, injured (accidental(ly)) NEC E928.9
  by, caused by, from
    air rifle (BB gun) E922.4
    animal (not being ridden) NEC E906.9
      being ridden (in sport or transport)
      E828 ☑

Injury, injured — *continued*
  by, caused by, from — *continued*
    assault (*see also* Assault) E968.9
    avalanche E909.2
    bayonet (*see also* Bayonet wound)
      E920.3
    being thrown against some part of, or
      object in
      motor vehicle (in motion) (on public
        highway) E818 ☑
        not on public highway E825 ☑
      nonmotor road vehicle NEC E829 ☑
      off-road motor vehicle NEC E821 ☑
      railway train E806 ☑
      snow vehicle, motor-driven E820 ☑
      street car E829 ☑
    bending
      due to
        repetitive movement E927.3
        sudden strenuous movement
          E927.0
    bite, human E928.3
    broken glass E920.8
    bullet — *see* Shooting
    cave-in (*see also* Suffocation, due to,
      cave-in) E913.3
      without asphyxiation or suffocation
        E916
      earth surface movement or eruption
        E909.9
      storm E908.9
    cloudburst E908.8
    component of firearm or air gun E928.7
    cutting or piercing instrument (*see also*
      Cut) E920.9
    cyclone E908.1
    earthquake E909.0
    earth surface movement or eruption
      E909.9
    electric current (*see also* Electric shock)
      E925.9
    explosion (*see also* Explosion) E923.9
      of gun part E928.7
    fire — *see* Fire
    flare, Verey pistol E922.8
    flood E908.2
    foreign body — *see* Foreign body
    gun recoil E928.7
    hailstones E904.3
    hurricane E908.0
    landslide E909.2
    law-enforcing agent, police, in course of
      legal intervention — *see* Legal
      intervention
    lightning E907
    live rail or live wire — *see* Electric shock
    machinery (*see also* Accident, machine)
      aircraft, without accident to aircraft
        E844 ☑
      boat, ship, watercraft (deck) (engine
        room) (galley) (laundry)
        (loading) E836 ☑
    mechanism of firearm or air gun E928.7
    missile
      explosive E923.8
      firearm — *see* Shooting
      in
        terrorism — *see* Terrorism, mis-
          sile
        war operations — *see* War opera-
          tions, missile
    moving part of motor vehicle (in motion)
      (on public highway) E818 ☑
      not on public highway, nontraffic
        accident E825 ☑
      while alighting, boarding, entering,
        leaving — *see* Fall, from, mo-
        tor vehicle, while alighting,
        boarding
    nail E920.8
    needle (sewing) E920.4
      hypodermic E920.5
    noise E928.1

Injury, injured — *continued*
  by, caused by, from — *continued*
    object
      fallen on
        motor vehicle (in motion) (on
          public highway) E818 ☑
        not on public highway
          E825 ☑
      falling — *see* Hit by, object, falling
    paintball gun E922.5
    radiation — *see* Radiation
    railway rolling stock, train, vehicle (part
      of) E805 ☑
      door or window E806 ☑
    recoil of firearm E928.7
    rotating propeller, aircraft E844 ☑
    rough landing of off-road type motor
      vehicle (after leaving ground or
      rough terrain) E821 ☑
      snow vehicle E820 ☑
    saber (*see also* Wound, saber) E920.3
    shot — *see* Shooting
    sound waves E928.1
    splinter or sliver, wood E920.8
    straining
      due to
        repetitive movement E927.3
        sudden strenuous movement
          E927.0
    street car (door) E829 ☑
    suicide (attempt) E958.9
    sword E920.3
    terrorism — *see* Terrorism
    third rail — *see* Electric shock
    thunderbolt E907
    tidal wave E909.4
      caused by storm E908.0
    tornado E908.1
    torrential rain E908.2
    twisting
      due to
        repetitive movement E927.3
        sudden strenuous movement
          E927.0
    vehicle NEC — *see* Accident, vehicle NEC
    vibration E928.2
    volcanic eruption E909.1
    weapon burst, in war operations E993.9
    weightlessness (in spacecraft, real or
      simulated) E928.0
    wood splinter or sliver E920.8
  due to
    civil insurrection — *see* War operations
      occurring after cessation of hostilities
        E998.9
    terrorism — *see* Terrorism
    war operations — *see* War operations
      occurring after cessation of hostilities
        E998.9
    weapon of mass destruction [WMD]
      E997.3
  homicide (*see also* Assault) E968.9
  inflicted (by)
    in course of arrest (attempted), suppres-
      sion of disturbance, maintenance
      of order, by law enforcing agents
      — *see* Legal intervention
    law-enforcing agent (on duty) — *see*
      Legal intervention
    other person
      stated as
        accidental E928.9
        homicidal, intentional — *see* As-
          sault
        undetermined whether acciden-
          tal or intentional — *see*
          Injury, stated as undeter-
          mined
    police (on duty) — *see* Legal interven-
      tion
  in, on
    civil insurrection — *see* War operations
    fight E960.0
    parachute descent (voluntary) (without
      accident to aircraft) E844 ☑

☑ Additional Digit Required — Refer to the Tabular List for Digit Selection   ▽ Subterms under main terms may continue to next column or page

344 — Volume 2   ▶◀ Revised Text   ● New Line   ▲ Revised Code   2015 ICD-9-CM

Injury, injured — *continued*
  in, on — *continued*
    parachute descent — *continued*
      with accident to aircraft — *see* categories E840-E842 ☑
      public highway E819 ☑
      railway right of way E807 ☑
      terrorism — *see* Terrorism
      war operations — *see* War operations
    late effect of E929.9
    purposely (inflicted) by other person(s) — *see* Assault
    self-inflicted (unspecified whether accidental or intentional) E988.9
      stated as
        accidental E928.9
        intentionally, purposely E958.9
  specified cause NEC E928.8
  stated as
    hanging E983.0
    knife E986
    late effect of E989
    puncture (any part of body) E986
    shooting — *see* Shooting, stated as undetermined whether accidental or intentional
    specified means NEC E988.8
    stab (any part of body) E986
    strangulation — *see* Suffocation, stated as undetermined whether accidental or intentional
    submersion E984
    suffocation — *see* Suffocation, stated as undetermined whether accidental or intentional
    undetermined whether accidentally or purposely inflicted (by) E988.9
      cut (any part of body) E986
      cutting or piercing instrument (classifiable to E920) E986
      drowning E984
      explosive(s) (missile) E985.5
      falling from high place E987.9
        manmade structure, except residential E987.1
        natural site E987.2
        residential premises E987.0
    to child due to criminal abortion E968.8
Insufficient nourishment — *see also* Lack of, food
    homicidal intent E968.4
Insulation, effects — *see* Heat
Interruption of respiration by
    food lodged in esophagus E911
    foreign body, except food, in esophagus E912
Intervention, legal — *see* Legal intervention
Intoxication, drug or poison — *see* Table of Drugs and Chemicals
Irradiation — *see* Radiation

Jammed (accidentally)
    between objects (moving) (stationary and moving) E918
    in object E918
Jumped or fell from high place, so stated — *see* Jumping, from, high place, stated as in undetermined circumstances
Jumping
    before train, vehicle or other moving object (unspecified whether accidental or intentional) E988.0
      stated as
        intentional, purposeful E958.0
        suicidal (attempt) E958.0
    from
      aircraft
        by parachute (voluntarily) (without accident to aircraft) E844
        due to accident to aircraft — *see* categories E840-E842 ☑
      boat, ship, watercraft (into water)
        after accident to, fire on, watercraft E830 ☑

Jumping — *continued*
  from — *continued*
    boat, ship, watercraft — *continued*
      after accident to, fire on, watercraft — *continued*
        and subsequently struck by (part of) boat E831 ☑
        burning, crushed, sinking E830 ☑
          and subsequently struck by (part of) boat E831 ☑
        voluntarily, without accident (to boat) with injury other than drowning or submersion E883.0
    building (*see also* Jumping, from, high place)
      burning (uncontrolled fire) E891.8
        in terrorism E979.3
        private E890.8
    cable car (not on rails) E847
      on rails E829 ☑
    high place
      in accidental circumstances or in sport — *see* categories E880-E884 ☑
      stated as
        with intent to injure self E957.9
          man-made structures NEC E957.1
          natural sites E957.2
          residential premises E957.0
        in undetermined circumstances E987.9
          man-made structures NEC E987.1
          natural sites E987.2
          residential premises E987.0
        suicidal (attempt) E957.9
          man-made structures NEC E957.1
          natural sites E957.1
          residential premises E957.0
    motor vehicle (in motion) (on public highway) — *see* Fall, from, motor vehicle
    nonmotor road vehicle NEC E829 ☑
    street car E829 ☑
    structure (*see also* Jumping, from, high place)
      burning NEC (uncontrolled fire) E891.8
        in terrorism E979.3
  into water
    with injury other than drowning or submersion E883.0
    drowning or submersion — *see* Submersion
  from, off, watercraft — *see* Jumping, from, boat
Justifiable homicide — *see* Assault

Kicked by
    animal E906.8
    person(s) (accidentally) E917.9
      with intent to injure or kill E960.0
      as, or caused by a crowd E917.1
        with subsequent fall E917.6
      in fight E960.0
      in sports E917.0
        with subsequent fall E917.5
Kicking against
    object (moving) E917.9
      in sports E917.0
        with subsequent fall E917.5
      stationary E917.4
        with subsequent fall E917.8
    person — *see* Striking against, person
Killed, killing (accidentally) NEC — *see also* Injury E928.9
    in
      action — *see* War operations
      brawl, fight (hand) (fists) (foot) E960.0
        by weapon (*see also* Assault)
          cutting, piercing E966
          firearm — *see* Shooting, homicide

Killed, killing — *see also* Injury — *continued*
  self
    stated as
      accident E928.9
      suicide — *see* Suicide
    unspecified whether accidental or suicidal E988.9
Knocked down (accidentally) (by) NEC E928.9
    animal (not being ridden) E906.8
      being ridden (in sport or transport) E828 ☑
    blast from explosion (*see also* Explosion) E923.9
    crowd, human stampede E917.6
    late effect of — *see* Late effect
    person (accidentally) E917.9
      in brawl, fight E960.0
      in sports E917.5
    transport vehicle — *see* vehicle involved under Hit by
    while boxing E917.5

Laceration NEC E928.9
Lack of
    air (refrigerator or closed place), suffocation by E913.2
    care (helpless person) (infant) (newborn) E904.0
      homicidal intent E968.4
    food except as result of transport accident E904.1
      helpless person, infant, newborn due to abandonment or neglect E904.0
    water except as result of transport accident E904.2
      helpless person, infant, newborn due to abandonment or neglect E904.0
Landslide E909.2
    falling on, hitting
      motor vehicle (any) (in motion) (on or off public highway) E909.2
      railway rolling stock, train, vehicle E909.2
Late effect of
    accident NEC (accident classifiable to E928.9) E929.9
      specified NEC (accident classifiable to E910-E928.8) E929.8
    assault E969
    fall, accidental (accident classifiable to E880-E888) E929.3
    fire, accident caused by (accident classifiable to E890-E899) E929.4
    homicide, attempt (any means) E969
    injury due to terrorism E999.1
    injury undetermined whether accidentally or purposely inflicted (injury classifiable to E980-E988) E989
    legal intervention (injury classifiable to E970-E976) E977
    medical or surgical procedure, test or therapy
      as, or resulting in, or from
        abnormal or delayed reaction or complication — *see* Reaction, abnormal
        misadventure — *see* Misadventure
    motor vehicle accident (accident classifiable to E810-E825) E929.0
    natural or environmental factor, accident due to (accident classifiable to E900-E909) E929.5
    poisoning, accidental (accident classifiable to E850-E858, E860-E869) E929.2
    suicide, attempt (any means) E959
    transport accident NEC (accident classifiable to E800-E807, E826-E838, E840-E848) E929.1
    war operations, injury due to (injury classifiable to E990-E998) E999.0
Launching pad accident E845 ☑
Legal
    execution, any method E978
    intervention (by) (injury from) E976
      baton E973

Legal — *continued*
  intervention — *continued*
    bayonet E974
    blow E975
    blunt object (baton) (nightstick) (stave) (truncheon) E973
    cutting or piercing instrument E974
    dynamite E971
    execution, any method E973
    explosive(s) (shell) E971
    firearm(s) E970
    gas (asphyxiation) (poisoning) (tear) E972
    grenade E971
    late effect of E977
    machine gun E970
    manhandling E975
    mortar bomb E971
    nightstick E973
    revolver E970
    rifle E970
    specified means NEC E975
    stabbing E974
    stave E973
    truncheon E973
Lifting, injury
    due to
      repetitive movement E927.3
      sudden strenuous movement E927.0
Lightning (shock) (stroke) (struck by) E907
Liquid (noncorrosive) in eye E914
    corrosive E924.1
Loss of control
    motor vehicle (on public highway) (without antecedent collision) E816 ☑
      with
        antecedent collision on public highway — *see* Collision, motor vehicle
        involving any object, person or vehicle not on public highway E816 ☑
        not on public highway, nontraffic accident E825 ☑
          with antecedent collision — *see* Collision, motor vehicle, not on public highway
        on public highway — *see* Collision, motor vehicle
      off-road type motor vehicle (not on public highway) E821 ☑
        on public highway — *see* Loss of control, motor vehicle
      snow vehicle, motor-driven (not on public highway) E820 ☑
        on public highway — *see* Loss of control, motor vehicle
Lost at sea E832 ☑
    with accident to watercraft E830 ☑
    in war operations E995.8
Low
    pressure, effects — *see* Effects of, air pressure
    temperature, effects — *see* Cold, exposure to
Lying before train, vehicle or other moving object (unspecified whether accidental or intentional) E988.0
    stated as intentional, purposeful, suicidal (attempt) E958.0
Lynching — *see also* Assault E968.9

Malfunction, atomic power plant in water transport E838 ☑
Mangled (accidentally) NEC E928.9
Manhandling (in brawl, fight) E960.0
    legal intervention E975
Manslaughter (nonaccidental) — *see* Assault
Marble in nose E912
Mauled by animal E906.8
Medical procedure, complication of
    delayed or as an abnormal reaction without mention of misadventure — *see* Reaction, abnormal

☑ Additional Digit Required — Refer to the Tabular List for Digit Selection
⩔ Subterms under main terms may continue to next column or page
2015 ICD-9-CM
►◄ Revised Text
● New Line
▲ Revised Code
Volume 2 — 345

Medical procedure, complication of

Medical procedure, complication of — *continued*
　due to or as a result of misadventure — *see* Misadventure
Melting of fittings and furniture in burning
　in terrorism E979.3
Minamata disease E865.2
Misadventure(s) to patient(s) during surgical or medical care E876.9
　contaminated blood, fluid, drug or biological substance (presence of agents and toxins as listed in E875) E875.9
　　administered (by) NEC E875.9
　　　infusion E875.0
　　　injection E875.1
　　　specified means NEC E875.2
　　　transfusion E875.0
　　　vaccination E875.1
　cut, cutting, puncture, perforation or hemorrhage (accidental) (inadvertent) (inappropriate) (during) E870.9
　　aspiration of fluid or tissue (by puncture or catheterization, except heart) E870.5
　　biopsy E870.8
　　　needle (aspirating) E870.5
　　blood sampling E870.5
　　catheterization E870.5
　　　heart E870.6
　　dialysis (kidney) E870.2
　　endoscopic examination E870.4
　　enema E870.7
　　infusion E870.1
　　injection E870.3
　　lumbar puncture E870.5
　　needle biopsy E870.5
　　paracentesis, abdominal E870.5
　　perfusion E870.2
　　specified procedure NEC E870.8
　　surgical operation E870.0
　　thoracentesis E870.5
　　transfusion E870.1
　　vaccination E870.3
　excessive amount of blood or other fluid during transfusion or infusion E873.0
　failure
　　in dosage E873.9
　　　electroshock therapy E873.4
　　　inappropriate temperature (too hot or too cold) in local application and packing E873.5
　　　infusion
　　　　excessive amount of fluid E873.0
　　　　incorrect dilution of fluid E873.1
　　　insulin-shock therapy E873.4
　　　nonadministration of necessary drug or medicinal E873.6
　　　overdose (*see also* Overdose)
　　　　radiation, in therapy E873.2
　　　radiation
　　　　inadvertent exposure of patient (receiving radiation for test or therapy) E873.3
　　　　not receiving radiation for test or therapy — *see* Radiation
　　　overdose E873.2
　　　specified procedure NEC E873.8
　　　transfusion
　　　　excessive amount of blood E873.0
　　mechanical, of instrument or apparatus (during procedure) E874.9
　　　aspiration of fluid or tissue (by puncture or catheterization, except of heart) E874.4
　　　biopsy E874.8
　　　　needle (aspirating) E874.4
　　　blood sampling E874.4
　　　catheterization E874.4
　　　　heart E874.5
　　　dialysis (kidney) E874.2
　　　endoscopic examination E874.3
　　　enema E874.8
　　　infusion E874.1
　　　injection E874.8
　　　lumbar puncture E874.4

Misadventure(s) to patient(s) during surgical or medical care — *continued*

failure — *continued*
　mechanical, of instrument or apparatus — *continued*
　　needle biopsy E874.4
　　paracentesis, abdominal E874.4
　　perfusion E874.2
　　specified procedure NEC E874.8
　　surgical operation E874.0
　　thoracentesis E874.4
　　transfusion E874.1
　　vaccination E874.8
　sterile precautions (during procedure) E872.9
　　aspiration of fluid or tissue (by puncture or catheterization, except heart) E872.5
　　biopsy E872.8
　　　needle (aspirating) E872.5
　　blood sampling E872.5
　　catheterization E872.5
　　　heart E872.6
　　dialysis (kidney) E872.2
　　endoscopic examination E872.4
　　enema E872.8
　　infusion E872.1
　　injection E872.3
　　lumbar puncture E872.5
　　needle biopsy E872.5
　　paracentesis, abdominal E872.5
　　perfusion E872.2
　　removal of catheter or packing E872.8
　　specified procedure NEC E872.8
　　surgical operation E872.0
　　thoracentesis E872.5
　　transfusion E872.1
　　vaccination E872.3
　suture or ligature during surgical procedure E876.2
　to introduce or to remove tube or instrument E876.4
　foreign object left in body — *see* Misadventure, foreign object
foreign object left in body (during procedure) E871.9
　aspiration of fluid or tissue (by puncture or catheterization, except heart) E871.5
　biopsy E871.8
　　needle (aspirating) E871.5
　blood sampling E871.5
　catheterization E871.5
　　heart E871.6
　dialysis (kidney) E871.2
　endoscopic examination E871.4
　enema E871.8
　infusion E871.1
　injection E871.3
　lumbar puncture E871.5
　needle biopsy E871.5
　paracentesis, abdominal E871.5
　perfusion E871.2
　removal of catheter or packing E871.7
　specified procedure NEC E871.8
　surgical operation E871.0
　thoracentesis E871.5
　transfusion E871.1
　vaccination E871.3
hemorrhage — *see* Misadventure, cut
inadvertent exposure of patient to radiation (being received for test or therapy) E873.3
inappropriate
　temperature (too hot or too cold) in local application or packing E873.5
infusion (*see also* Misadventure, by specific type, infusion)
　excessive amount of fluid E873.0
　incorrect dilution of fluid E873.1
　wrong fluid E876.1
mismatched blood in transfusion E876.0
nonadministration of necessary drug or medicinal E873.6
overdose (*see also* Overdose)

Misadventure(s) to patient(s) during surgical or medical care — *continued*

overdose (*see also* Overdose) — *continued*
　radiation, in therapy E873.2
perforation — *see* Misadventure, cut
performance of correct operation (procedure) on wrong
　body part E876.7
　side E876.7
　site E876.7
performance of operation (procedure)
　intended for another patient E876.6
　on patient not scheduled for surgery E876.6
　on wrong patient E876.6
performance of wrong operation on correct patient E876.5
puncture — *see* Misadventure, cut
specified type NEC E876.8
　failure
　　suture or ligature during surgical operation E876.2
　　to introduce or to remove tube or instrument E876.4
　　　foreign object left in body E871.9
　infusion of wrong fluid E876.1
　performance of inappropriate operation E876.5
　transfusion of mismatched blood E876.0
　wrong
　　fluid in infusion E876.1
　　placement of endotracheal tube during anesthetic procedure E876.3
transfusion (*see also* Misadventure, by specific type, transfusion)
　excessive amount of blood E873.0
　mismatched blood E876.0
wrong
　device implanted into correct surgical site E876.5
　drug given in error — *see* Table of Drugs and Chemicals
　fluid in infusion E876.1
　placement of endotracheal tube during anesthetic procedure E876.3
　procedure (operation) performed on the correct patient E876.5
Motion (effects) E903
　sickness E903
Mountain sickness E902.0
Mucus aspiration or inhalation, not of newborn (with asphyxia, obstruction respiratory passage, suffocation) E912
Mudslide of cataclysmic nature E909.2
Murder (attempt) — *see also* Assault E968.9

N

Nail, injury by E920.8
Needlestick (sewing needle) E920.4
　hypodermic E920.5
Neglect — *see also* Privation
　criminal E968.4
　homicidal intent E968.4
Noise (causing injury) (pollution) E928.1
Nuclear weapon — *see also* War operations, injury due to, nuclear weapons E996.9

O

Object
　falling
　　from, in, on, hitting
　　　aircraft E844 ☑
　　　　due to accident to aircraft — *see* categories E840–E842 ☑
　　　machinery (*see also* Accident, machine)
　　　　not in operation E916
　　　motor vehicle (in motion) (on public highway) E818 ☑
　　　　nonmotor road vehicle NEC E829 ☑
　　　　not on public highway E825 ☑
　　　　pedal cycle E826 ☑

Object — *continued*

falling — *continued*
　from, in, on, hitting — *continued*
　　motor vehicle — *continued*
　　　person E916
　　　railway rolling stock, train, vehicle E806 ☑
　　　stationary E916
　　　street car E829 ☑
　　　watercraft E838 ☑
　　　　due to accident to watercraft E831 ☑
　set in motion by
　　accidental explosion of pressure vessel — *see* category E921 ☑
　　firearm — *see* category E922 ☑
　　machine(ry) — *see* Accident, machine
　　transport vehicle — *see* categories E800–E848 ☑
　thrown from, in, on, towards
　　aircraft E844 ☑
　　cable car (not on rails) E847
　　　on rails E829 ☑
　　motor vehicle (in motion) (on public highway) E818 ☑
　　　not on public highway E825 ☑
　　nonmotor road vehicle NEC E829 ☑
　　pedal cycle E826 ☑
　　street car E829 ☑
　　vehicle NEC — *see* Accident, vehicle NEC
Obstruction
　air passages, larynx, respiratory passages by
　　external means NEC — *see* Suffocation
　　food, any type (regurgitated) (vomited) E911
　　material or object, except food E912
　　mucus E912
　　phlegm E912
　　vomitus E911
　digestive tract, except mouth or pharynx by
　　food, any type E915
　　foreign body (any) E915
　esophagus
　　without asphyxia or obstruction of respiratory passage E915
　　food E911
　　foreign body, except food E912
　mouth or pharynx by
　　food, any type E911
　　material or object, except food E912
　respiration — *see* Obstruction, air passages
Oil in eye E914
Overdose
　anesthetic (drug) — *see* Table of Drugs and Chemicals
　drug — *see* Table of Drugs and Chemicals
Overexertion E927.9
　from
　　lifting
　　　repetitive movement E927.3
　　　sudden strenuous movement E927.0
　　maintaining prolonged positions E927.1
　　　holding E927.1
　　　sitting E927.1
　　　standing E927.1
　　prolonged static position E927.1
　　pulling
　　　repetitive movement E927.3
　　　sudden strenuous movement E927.0
　　pushing
　　　repetitive movement E927.3
　　　sudden strenuous movement E927.0
　　specified NEC E927.8
　　sudden strenuous movement E927.0
Overexposure (accidental) (to)
　cold (*see also* Cold, exposure to) E901.9
　　due to manmade conditions E901.1
　heat (*see also* Heat) E900.9
　radiation — *see* Radiation
　radioactivity — *see* Radiation
　sun, except sunburn E900.0
　weather — *see* Exposure

▶◀ Revised Text　　● New Line　　▲ Revised Code

Overexposure — *continued*
  wind — *see* Exposure
Overheated — *see also* Heat E900.9
Overlaid E913.0
Overturning (accidental)
  animal-drawn vehicle E827 ☑
  boat, ship, watercraft
    causing
      drowning, submersion E830 ☑
      injury except drowning, submersion E831 ☑
  machinery — *see* Accident, machine
  motor vehicle (*see also* Loss of control, motor vehicle) E816 ☑
    with antecedent collision on public highway — *see* Collision, motor vehicle
    not on public highway, nontraffic accident E825 ☑
      with antecedent collision — *see* Collision, motor vehicle, not on public highway
  nonmotor road vehicle NEC E829 ☑
  off-road type motor vehicle — *see* Loss of control, off-road type motor vehicle
  pedal cycle E826 ☑
  railway rolling stock, train, vehicle (*see also* Derailment, railway) E802 ☑
  street car E829 ☑
  vehicle NEC — *see* Accident, vehicle NEC

P

Palsy, divers' E902.2
Parachuting (voluntary) (without accident to aircraft) E844 ☑
  due to accident to aircraft — *see* categories E840-E842 ☑
Paralysis
  divers' E902.2
  lead or saturnine E866.0
    from pesticide NEC E863.4
Pecked by bird E906.8
Performance of correct operation (procedure) **on wrong**
  body part E876.7
  side E876.7
  site E876.7
Performance of operation (procedure)
  intended for another patient E876.6
  on patient not scheduled for surgery E876.6
  on wrong patient E876.6
Performance of wrong operation on correct patient E876.5
Phlegm aspiration or inhalation (with asphyxia, obstruction respiratory passage, suffocation) E912
Piercing — *see also* Cut E920.9
  by slide trigger mechanism, scope or other part of gun E928.7
Pinched
  between objects (moving) (stationary and moving) E918
  by slide trigger mechanism, scope or other part of gun E928.7
  in object E918
Pinned under
  machine(ry) — *see* Accident, machine
Place of occurrence of accident — *see* Accident (to), occurring (at) (in)
Plumbism E866.0
  from insecticide NEC E863.4
Poisoning (accidental) (by) — *see also* Table of Drugs and Chemicals
  carbon monoxide
    generated by
      aircraft in transit E844 ☑
      motor vehicle
        in motion (on public highway) E818 ☑
        not on public highway E825 ☑
      watercraft (in transit) (not in transit) E838 ☑

Poisoning — *see also* Table of Drugs and Chemicals — *continued*
  caused by injection of poisons or toxins into or through skin by plant thorns, spines, or other mechanism E905.7
    marine or sea plants E905.6
  fumes or smoke due to
    conflagration — *see* Conflagration
    explosion or fire — *see* Fire
    ignition — *see* Ignition
  gas
    in legal intervention E972
    legal execution, by E978
    on watercraft E838 ☑
    used as anesthetic — *see* Table of Drugs and Chemicals
  in
    terrorism (chemical weapons) E979.7
    war operations E997.2
      execution E978
      intervention
        by gas E972
  late effect of — *see* Late effect
  legal
Pressure, external, causing asphyxia, suffocation — *see also* Suffocation E913.9
Privation E904.9
  food (*see also* Lack of, food) E904.1
  helpless person, infant, newborn due to abandonment or neglect E904.0
  late effect of NEC E929.5
  resulting from transport accident — *see* categories E800-E848 ☑
  water (*see also* Lack of, water) E904.2
Projected objects, striking against or struck by — *see* Striking against, object
Prolonged stay in
  high altitude (causing conditions as listed in E902.0) E902.0
  weightless environment E928.0
Prostration
  heat — *see* Heat
Pulling, injury
  due to
    repetitive movement E927.3
    sudden strenuous movement E927.0
Puncture, puncturing — *see also* Cut E920.9
  by
    plant thorns or spines E920.8
      toxic reaction E905.7
        marine or sea plants E905.6
    sea-urchin spine E905.6
Pushing (injury in) (overexertion)
  by other person(s) (accidental) E917.9
    with fall E886.9
      in sports E886.0
    as, or caused by, a crowd, human stampede E917.1
      with subsequent fall E917.6
    before moving vehicle or object
      stated as
        intentional, homicidal E968.5
        undetemined whether accidental or intentional E988.8
    from
      high place
        in accidental circum-stances — *see* categories E880-E884 ☑
        stated as
          intentional, homicidal E968.1
          undetermined whether accidental or intentional E987.9
          man-made structure, except residential E987.1
          natural site E987.2
          residential E987.0
    motor vehicle (*see also* Fall, from, motor vehicle) E818 ☑
      stated as
        intentional, homicidal E968.5
        undetermined whether accidental or intentional E988.8

Pushing — *continued*
  by other person(s) — *continued*
    in sports E917.0
      with fall E886.0
  due to
    repetitive movement E927.3
    sudden strenuous movement E927.0

R

Radiation (exposure to) E926.9
  abnormal reaction to medical test or therapy E879.2
  arc lamps E926.2
  atomic power plant (malfunction) NEC E926.9
    in water transport E838 ☑
  electromagnetic, ionizing E926.3
  gamma rays E926.3
  in
    terrorism (from or following nuclear explosion) (direct) (secondary) E979.5
      laser E979.8
    war operations (*see also* War operations, injury due to, nuclear weapons) E996.3
      laser(s) E997.0
    water transport E838 ☑
  inadvertent exposure of patient (receiving test or therapy) E873.3
  infrared (heaters and lamps) E926.1
    excessive heat E900.1
  ionized, ionizing (particles, artificially accelerated) E926.8
    electromagnetic E926.3
  isotopes, radioactive — *see* Radiation, radioactive isotopes
  laser(s) E926.4
    in
      terrorism E979.8
      war operations E997.0
    misadventure in medical care — *see* Misadventure, failure, in dosage, radiation
  late effect of NEC E929.8
    excessive heat from — *see* Heat
  light sources (visible) (ultraviolet) E926.2
  misadventure in medical or surgical procedure — *see* Misadventure, failure, in dosage, radiation
  overdose (in medical or surgical procedure) E873.2
  radar E926.0
  radioactive isotopes E926.5
    atomic power plant malfunction E926.5
      in water transport E838 ☑
    misadventure in medical or surgical treatment — *see* Misadventure, failure, in dosage, radiation
  radiobiologicals — *see* Radiation, radioactive isotopes
  radiofrequency E926.0
  radiopharmaceuticals — *see* Radiation, radioactive isotopes
  radium NEC E926.9
  sun E926.2
    excessive heat from E900.0
  tanning bed E926.2
  welding arc or torch E926.2
    excessive heat from E900.1
  x-rays (hard) (soft) E926.3
    misadventure in medical or surgical treatment — *see* Misadventure, failure, in dosage, radiation
Rape E960.1
Reaction, abnormal to or following (medical or surgical procedure) E879.9
  amputation (of limbs) E878.5
  anastomosis (arteriovenous) (blood vessel) (gastrojejunal) (skin) (tendon) (natural, artificial material, tissue) E878.2
    external stoma, creation of E878.3
  aspiration (of fluid) E879.4
    tissue E879.8
  biopsy E879.8

Reaction, abnormal to or following — *continued*
  blood
    sampling E879.7
    transfusion
      procedure E879.8
  bypass — *see* Reaction, abnormal, anastomosis
  catheterization
    cardiac E879.0
    urinary E879.6
  colostomy E878.3
  cystostomy E878.3
  dialysis (kidney) E879.1
  drugs or biologicals — *see* Table of Drugs and Chemicals
  duodenostomy E878.3
  electroshock therapy E879.3
  formation of external stoma E878.3
  gastrostomy E878.3
  graft — *see* Reaction, abnormal, anastomosis
  hypothermia E879.8
  implant, implantation (of)
    artificial
      internal device (cardiac pacemaker) (electrodes in brain) (heart valve prosthesis) (orthopedic) E878.1
    material or tissue (for anastomosis or bypass) E878.2
      with creation of external stoma E878.3
    natural tissues (for anastomosis or bypass) E878.2
      with creation of external stoma E878.3
    as transplantion — *see* Reaction, abnormal, transplant
  infusion
    procedure E879.8
  injection
    procedure E879.8
      specific type of procedure) E879.9
  insertion of gastric or duodenal sound E879.5
  insulin-shock therapy E879.3
  lumbar puncture E879.4
  perfusion E879.1
  procedures other than surgical operation (*see also* Reaction, abnormal, by specified procedure NEC E879.8
  radiological procedure or therapy E879.2
  removal of organ (partial) (total) NEC E878.6
    with
      anastomosis, bypass or graft E878.2
      formation of external stoma E878.3
      implant of artificial internal device E878.1
      transplant(ation)
        partial organ E878.4
        whole organ E878.0
  sampling
    blood E879.7
    fluid NEC E879.4
    tissue E879.8
  shock therapy E879.3
  surgical operation (*see also* Reaction, abnormal, by specified type of operation) E878.9
    restorative NEC E878.4
      with
        anastomosis, bypass or graft E878.2
        fomation of external stoma E878.3
        implant(ation) — *see* Reaction, abnormal, implant
        transplant(ation) — *see* Reaction, abnormal, transplant
    specified operation NEC E878.8
  thoracentesis E879.4
  transfusion
    procedure E879.8
  transplant, transplantation (heart) (kidney) (liver) E878.0

☑ **Additional Digit Required — Refer to the Tabular List for Digit Selection**
ᴺᴱᶜ **Subterms under main terms may continue to next column or page**

Reaction, abnormal to or following —
  continued
  transplant, transplantation — *continued*
    partial organ E878.4
    ureterostomy E878.3
    vaccination E879.8
Reduction in
  atmospheric pressure (*see also* Effects of, air
    pressure)
    while surfacing from
      deep water diving causing caisson
        or divers' disease, palsy or
        paralysis E902.2
      underground E902.8
Repetitive movements NEC E927.8
Residual (effect) — *see* Late effect
Rock falling on or hitting (accidentally)
  motor vehicle (in motion) (on public high-
    way) E818 ☑
    not on public highway E825 ☑
  nonmotor road vehicle NEC E829 ☑
  pedal cycle E826 ☑
  person E916
  railway rolling stock, train, vehicle E806 ☑
Running off, away
  animal (being ridden) (in sport or transport)
    E828 ☑
    not being ridden E906.8
  animal-drawn vehicle E827 ☑
  rails, railway (*see also* Derailment) E802 ☑
  roadway
    motor vehicle (without antecedent colli-
      sion) E816 ☑
      with
        antecedent collision — *see* Colli-
          sion motor vehicle
        subsequent collision
          involving any object, person
            or vehicle not on pub-
            lic highway E816 ☑
          on public highway E811 ☑
      nontraffic accident E825 ☑
        with antecedent collision — *see*
          Collision, motor vehicle,
          not on public highway
    nonmotor road vehicle NEC E829 ☑
    pedal cycle E826 ☑
Run over (accidentally) (by)
  animal (not being ridden) E906.8
    being ridden (in sport or transport)
      E828 ☑
  animal-drawn vehicle E827 ☑
  machinery — *see* Accident, machine
  motor vehicle (on public highway) — *see*
    Hit by, motor vehicle
  nonmotor road vehicle NEC E829 ☑
  railway train E805 ☑
  street car E829 ☑
  vehicle NEC E848

S

Saturnism E866.0
  from insecticide NEC E863.4
Scald, scalding (accidental) (by) (from) (in)
  E924.0
  acid — *see* Scald, caustic
  boiling tap water E924.2
  caustic or corrosive liquid, substance E924.1
    swallowed — *see* Table of Drugs and
      Chemicals
  homicide (attempt) — *see* Assault, burning
  inflicted by other person
    stated as
      intentional or homicidal E968.3
      undetermined whether accidental or
        intentional E988.2
  late effect of NEC E929.8
  liquid (boiling) (hot) E924.0
  local application of externally applied sub-
    stance in medical or surgical care
    E873.5
  molten metal E924.0
  self-inflicted (unspecified whether acciden-
    tal or intentional) E988.2
    stated as intentional, purposeful E958.2

Scald, scalding — *continued*
  stated as undetermined whether accidental
    or intentional E988.2
  steam E924.0
  tap water (boiling) E924.2
  transport accident — *see* categories
    E800-E848 ☑
  vapor E924.0
Scratch, cat E906.8
Sea
  sickness E903
Self-mutilation — *see* Suicide
Sequelae (of)
  in
    terrorism E999.1
    war operations E999.0
Shock
  anaphylactic (*see also* Table of Drugs and
    Chemicals) E947.9
    due to
      bite (venomous) — *see* Bite, ven-
        omous NEC
      sting — *see* Sting
  electric (*see also* Electric shock) E925.9
  from electric appliance or current (*see also*
    Electric shock) E925.9
Shooting, shot (accidental(ly)) E922.9
  air gun E922.4
  BB gun E922.4
  hand gun (pistol) (revolver) E922.0
  himself (*see also* Shooting, self-inflicted)
    E985.4
    hand gun (pistol) (revolver) E985.0
    military firearm, except hand gun E985.3
      hand gun (pistol) (revolver) E985.0
    rifle (hunting) E985.2
      military E985.3
    shotgun (automatic) E985.1
    specified firearm NEC E985.4
    Verey pistol E985.4
  homicide (attempt) E965.4
    air gun E968.6
    BB gun E968.6
    hand gun (pistol) (revolver) E965.0
    military firearm, except hand gun E965.3
      hand gun (pistol) (revolver) E965.0
    paintball gun E965.4
    rifle (hunting) E965.2
      military E965.3
    shotgun (automatic) E965.1
    specified firearm NEC E965.4
    Verey pistol E965.4
  in
    terrorism — *see* Terrorism, shooting
    war operations — *see* War operations,
      shooting
  inflicted by other person
    in accidental circumstances E922.9
      hand gun (pistol) (revolver) E922.0
      military firearm, except hand gun
        E922.3
        hand gun (pistol) (revolver)
          E922.0
      rifle (hunting) E922.2
        military E922.3
      shotgun (automatic) E922.1
      specified firearm NEC E922.8
      Verey pistol E922.8
    stated as
      intentional, homicidal E965.4
        hand gun (pistol) (revolver)
          E965.0
        military firearm, except hand gun
          E965.3
          hand gun (pistol) (revolver)
            E965.0
        paintball gun E965.4
        rifle (hunting) E965.2
          military E965.3
        shotgun (automatic) E965.1
        specified firearm E965.4
        Verey pistol E965.4
      undetermined whether accidental or
        intentional E985.4
        air gun E985.6
        BB gun E985.6

Shooting, shot — *continued*
  inflicted by other person — *continued*
    stated as
      undetermined whether accidental or
        intentional — *continued*
        hand gun (pistol) (revolver)
          E985.0
        military firearm, except hand gun
          E985.3
          hand gun (pistol) (revolver)
            E985.0
        paintball gun E985.7
        rifle (hunting) E985.2
        shotgun (automatic) E985.1
        specified firearm NEC E985.4
        Verey pistol E985.4
  legal
    execution E978
    intervention E970
  military firearm, except hand gun E922.3
    hand gun (pistol) (revolver) E922.0
  paintball gun E922.5
  rifle (hunting) E922.2
    military E922.3
  self-inflicted (unspecified whether acciden-
    tal or intentional) E985.4
    air gun E985.6
    BB gun E985.6
    hand gun (pistol) (revolver) E985.0
    military firearm, except hand gun E985.3
      hand gun (pistol) (revolver) E985.0
    paintball gun E985.7
    rifle (hunting) E985.2
      military E985.3
    shotgun (automatic) E985.1
    specified firearm NEC E985.4
    stated as
      accidental E922.9
        hand gun (pistol) (revolver)
          E922.0
        military firearm, except hand gun
          E922.3
          hand gun (pistol) (revolver)
            E922.0
        paintball gun E922.5
        rifle (hunting) E922.2
          military E922.3
        shotgun (automatic) E922.1
        specified firearm NEC E922.8
        Verey pistol E922.8
      intentional, purposeful E955.4
        hand gun (pistol) (revolver)
          E955.0
        military firearm, except hand gun
          E955.3
          hand gun (pistol) (revolver)
            E955.0
        paintball gun E955.7
        rifle (hunting) E955.2
          military E955.3
        shotgun (automatic) E955.1
        specified firearm NEC E955.4
        Verey pistol E955.4
  shotgun (automatic) E922.1
  specified firearm NEC E922.8
  stated as undetermined whether accidental
    or intentional E985.4
    hand gun (pistol) (revolver) E985.0
    military firearm, except hand gun E985.3
      hand gun (pistol) (revolver) E985.0
    paintball gun E985.7
    rifle (hunting) E985.2
      military E985.3
    shotgun (automatic) E985.1
    specified firearm NEC E985.4
    Verey pistol E985.4
  suicidal (attempt) E955.4
    air gun E955.6
    BB gun E955.6
    hand gun (pistol) (revolver) E955.0
    military firearm, except hand gun E955.3
      hand gun (pistol) (revolver) E955.0
    paintball gun E955.7
    rifle (hunting) E955.2
      military E955.3
    shotgun (automatic) E955.1

Shooting, shot — *continued*
  suicidal — *continued*
    specified firearm NEC E955.4
    Verey pistol E955.4
  Verey pistol E922.8
Shoving (accidentally) by other person — *see*
  also Pushing by other person E917.9
Sickness
  air E903
  alpine E902.0
  car E903
  motion E903
  mountain E902.0
  sea E903
  travel E903
Sinking (accidental)
  boat, ship, watercraft (causing drowning,
    submersion) E830 ☑
    causing injury except drowning, submer-
      sion E831 ☑
Siriasis E900.0
Skydiving E844 ☑
Slashed wrists — *see also* Cut, self-inflicted
  E986
Slipping (accidental)
  on
    deck (of boat, ship, watercraft) (icy) (oily)
      (wet) E835 ☑
    ice E885.9
    ladder of ship E833 ☑
      due to accident to watercraft
        E831 ☑
    mud E885.9
    oil E885.9
    snow E885.9
    stairs of ship E833 ☑
      due to accident to watercraft
        E831 ☑
    surface
      slippery E885 ☑
      wet E885 ☑
Sliver, wood, injury by E920.8
Smothering, smothered — *see also* Suffoca-
  tion E913.9
**Smouldering building or structure in terror-
ism** E979.3
Sodomy (assault) E960.1
Solid substance in eye (any part) or adnexa
  E914
Sound waves (causing injury) E928.1
Splinter, injury by E920.8
Stab, stabbing E966
  accidental — *see* Cut
Starvation E904.1
  helpless person, infant, newborn — *see* Lack
    of food
  homicidal intent E968.4
  late effect of NEC E929.5
  resulting from accident connected with
    transport — *see* categories
    E800-E848 ☑
Stepped on
  by
    animal (not being ridden) E906.8
      being ridden (in sport or transport)
        E828 ☑
    crowd E917.1
    person E917.9
      in sports E917.0
    in sports E917.0
Stepping on
  object (moving) E917.9
    in sports E917.0
      with subsequent fall E917.5
    stationary E917.4
      with subsequent fall E917.8
  person E917.9
    as, or caused by a crowd E917.1
      with subsequent fall E917.6
    in sports E917.0
Sting E905.9
  ant E905.5
  bee E905.3
  caterpillar E905.5
  coral E905.6
  hornet E905.3

☑ **Additional Digit Required** — Refer to the Tabular List for Digit Selection   ▽ **Subterms under main terms may continue to next column or page**

348 — Volume 2   ▶◀ Revised Text   ● New Line   ▲ Revised Code   2015 ICD-9-CM

Sting — *continued*
  insect NEC E905.5
  jellyfish E905.6
  marine animal or plant E905.6
  nematocysts E905.6
  scorpion E905.2
  sea anemone E905.6
  sea cucumber E905.6
  wasp E905.3
  yellow jacket E905.3
Storm E908.9
  specified type NEC E908.8
Straining, injury
  due to
    repetitive movement E927.3
    sudden strenuous movement E927.0
Strangling — *see* Suffocation
Strangulation — *see* Suffocation
Strenuous movements (in recreational or other activities) NEC E927.8
Striking against
  bottom (when jumping or diving into water) E883.0
  object (moving) E917.9
    caused by crowd E917.1
      with subsequent fall E917.6
    furniture E917.3
      with subsequent fall E917.7
    in
      running water E917.2
        with drowning or submersion — *see* Submersion
      sports E917.0
        with subsequent fall E917.5
    stationary E917.4
      with subsequent fall E917.8
  person(s) E917.9
    with fall E886.9
      in sports E886.0
    as, or caused by, a crowd E917.1
      with subsequent fall E917.6
    in sports E917.0
      with fall E886.0
Stroke
  heat — *see* Heat
  lightning E907
Struck by — *see also* Hit by
  bullet
    in
      terrorism E979.4
      war operations E991.2
        rubber E991.0
  lightning E907
  missile
    in terrorism — *see* Terrorism, missile
  object
    falling
      from, in, on
        building
          burning (uncontrolled fire) in terrorism E979.3
  thunderbolt E907
Stumbling over animal, carpet, curb, rug or (small) object (with fall) E885.9
  without fall — *see* Striking against, object
Submersion (accidental) E910.8
  boat, ship, watercraft (causing drowning, submersion) E830 ☑
    causing injury except drowning, submersion E831 ☑
  by other person
    in accidental circumstances — *see* category E910 ☑
    intentional, homicidal E964
    stated as undetermined whether accidental or intentional E984
  due to
    accident
      machinery — *see* Accident, machine
      to boat, ship, watercraft E830 ☑
      transport — *see* categories E800-E848 ☑
    avalanche E909.2
    cataclysmic
      earth surface movement or eruption E909.9

Submersion (accidental) — *continued*
  due to — *continued*
    cataclysmic — *continued*
      storm E908.9
    cloudburst E908.8
    cyclone E908.1
    fall
      from
        boat, ship, watercraft (not involved in accident) E832 ☑
          burning, crushed E830 ☑
          involved in accident, collision E830 ☑
        gangplank (into water) E832 ☑
        overboard NEC E832 ☑
    flood E908.2
    hurricane E908.0
    jumping into water E910.8
      from boat, ship, watercraft
        burning, crushed, sinking E830 ☑
        involved in accident, collision E830 ☑
        not involved in accident, for swim E910.2
      in recreational activity (without diving equipment) E910.2
        with or using diving equipment E910.1
      to rescue another person E910.3
  homicide (attempt) E964
  in
    bathtub E910.4
    specified activity, not sport, transport or recreational E910.3
    sport or recreational activity (without diving equipment) E910.2
      with or using diving equipment E910.1
      water skiing E910.0
    swimming pool NEC E910.8
    terrorism E979.8
    war operations E995.4
      intentional E995.3
    water transport E832 ☑
      due to accident to boat, ship, watercraft E830 ☑
  landslide E909.2
    overturning boat, ship, watercraft E909.2
    sinking boat, ship, watercraft E909.2
    submersion boat, ship, watercraft E909.2
    tidal wave E909.4
      caused by storm E908.0
    torrential rain E908.2
  late effect of NEC E929.8
  quenching tank E910.8
  self-inflicted (unspecified whether accidental or intentional) E984
    in accidental circumstances — *see* category E910 ☑
    stated as intentional, purposeful E954
  stated as undetermined whether accidental or intentional E984
  suicidal (attempted) E954
  while
    attempting rescue of another person E910.3
    engaged in
      marine salvage E910.3 ●
      underwater construction or repairs E910.3 ●
    fishing, not from boat E910.2
    hunting, not from boat E910.2
    ice skating E910.2
    pearl diving E910.3
    placing fishing nets E910.3
    playing in water E910.2
    scuba diving E910.1
      nonrecreational E910.3
    skin diving E910.1
    snorkel diving E910.2
    spear fishing underwater E910.1
    surfboarding E910.2
    swimming (swimming pool) E910.2
    wading (in water) E910.2
    water skiing E910.0

Sucked
  into
    jet (aircraft) E844 ☑
Suffocation (accidental) (by external means) (by pressure) (mechanical) E913.9
  caused by other person
    in accidental circumstances — *see* category E913 ☑
    stated as
      intentional, homicidal E963
      undetermined whether accidental or intentional E983.9
        by, in
          hanging E983.0
          plastic bag E983.1
          specified means NEC E983.8
  due to, by
    avalanche E909.2
    bedclothes E913.0
    bib E913.0
    blanket E913.0
    cave-in E913.3
      caused by cataclysmic earth surface movement or eruption E909.9
    conflagration — *see* Conflagration
    explosion — *see* Explosion
    falling earth, other substance E913.3
    fire — *see* Fire
    food, any type (ingestion) (inhalation) (regurgitated) (vomited) E911
    foreign body, except food (ingestion) (inhalation) E912
    ignition — *see* Ignition
    landslide E909.2
    machine(ry) — *see* Accident, machine
    material, object except food entering by nose or mouth, ingested, inhaled E912
    mucus (aspiration) (inhalation), not of newborn E912
    phlegm (aspiration) (inhalation) E912
    pillow E913.0
    plastic bag — *see* Suffocation, in, plastic bag
    sheet (plastic) E913.0
    specified means NEC E913.8
    vomitus (aspiration) (inhalation) E911
  homicidal (attempt) E963
    in war operations E995.3
  in
    airtight enclosed place E913.2
    baby carriage E913.0
    bed E913.0
    closed place E913.2
    cot, cradle E913.0
    perambulator E913.0
    plastic bag (in accidental circumstances) E913.1
      homicidal, purposely inflicted by other person E963
      self-inflicted (unspecified whether accidental or intentional) E983.1
        in accidental circumstances E913.1
        intentional, suicidal E953.1
      stated as undetermined whether accidentally or purposely inflicted E983.1
      suicidal, purposely self-inflicted E953.1
    refrigerator E913.2
    war operations E995.3
  self-inflicted (*see also* Suffocation, stated as undetermined whether accidental or intentional) E953.9
    in accidental circumstances — *see* category E913 ☑
    stated as intentional, purposeful — *see* Suicide, suffocation
  stated as undetermined whether accidental or intentional E983.9
    by, in
      hanging E983.0
      plastic bag E983.1
      specified means NEC E983.8

Suffocation — *continued*
  suicidal — *see* Suicide, suffocation
Suicide, suicidal (attempted) (by) E958.9
  burning, burns E958.1
  caustic substance E958.7
    poisoning E950.7
    swallowed E950.7
  cold, extreme E958.3
  cut (any part of body) E956
  cutting or piercing instrument (classifiable to E920) E956
  drowning E954
  electrocution E958.4
  explosive(s) (classifiable to E923) E955.5
  fire E958.1
  firearm (classifiable to E922) — *see* Shooting, suicidal
  hanging E953.0
  jumping
    before moving object, train, vehicle E958.0
    from high place — *see* Jumping, from, high place, stated as, suicidal
  knife E956
  late effect of E959
  motor vehicle, crashing of E958.5
  poisoning — *see* Table of Drugs and Chemicals
  puncture (any part of body) E956
  scald E958.2
  shooting — *see* Shooting, suicidal
  specified means NEC E958.8
  stab (any part of body) E956
  strangulation — *see* Suicide, suffocation
  submersion E954
  suffocation E953.9
    by, in
      hanging E953.0
      plastic bag E953.1
      specified means NEC E953.8
  wound NEC E958.9
Sunburn E926.2
Sunstroke E900.0
Supersonic waves (causing injury) E928.1
Surgical procedure, complication of
  delayed or as an abnormal reaction without mention of misadventure — *see* Reaction, abnormal
  due to or as a result of misadventure — *see* Misadventure
Swallowed, swallowing
  foreign body — *see* Foreign body, alimentary canal
  poison — *see* Table of Drugs and Chemicals
  substance
    caustic — *see* Table of Drugs and Chemicals
    corrosive — *see* Table of Drugs and Chemicals
    poisonous — *see* Table of Drugs and Chemicals
Swimmers cramp — *see also* category E910 E910.2
  not in recreation or sport E910.3
Syndrome, battered
  baby or child — *see* Abuse, child
  wife — *see* Assault

T

Tackle in sport E886.0
Terrorism (injury) (by) (in) E979.8
  air blast E979.2
  aircraft burned, destroyed, exploded, shot down E979.1
    used as a weapon E979.1
  anthrax E979.6
  asphyxia from
    chemical (weapons) E979.7
    fire, conflagration (caused by fire-producing device) E979.3
      from nuclear explosion E979.5
    gas or fumes E979.7
  bayonet E979.8
  biological agents E979.6
  blast (air) (effects) E979.2
    from nuclear explosion E979.5

☑ Additional Digit Required — Refer to the Tabular List for Digit Selection   ▽ Subterms under main terms may continue to next column or page

2015 ICD-9-CM   ▶◀ Revised Text   ● New Line   ▲ Revised Code   October 2014 • Volume 2 — 349

Sting — Terrorism

☑ Additional Digit Required — Refer to the Tabular List for Digit Selection   ▽ Subterms under main terms may continue to next column or page

War operations — *continued*

exposure to ionizing radiation from nuclear explosion (*see also* War operations, injury due to, nuclear weapons) E996.3

falling aircraft E994.8

fireball effects from nuclear explosion E996.2

fire or fire-producing device E990.9
flamethrower E990.1
incendiary bomb E990.0
incendiary bullet E990.2
indirectly caused from conventional weapon E990.3
petrol bomb E990.0

fragments from
antipersonnel bomb E991.3
artillery shell E991.4
bomb NEC E991.4
grenade E991.4
guided missile E991.4
land mine E991.4
rocket E991.4
shell E991.4
shrapnel E991.9

fumes E997.2

gas E997.2

grenade (explosion) E993.8
fragments, injury by E991.4

guided missile (explosion) E993.1
fragments, injury by E991.4

nuclear (*see also* War operations, injury due to, nuclear weapons) E996.9

heat from nuclear explosion E996.2

injury due to
aerial bomb E993.0
air blast E993.9
aircraft shot down E994.0
artillery shell E993.2
blast E993.9
wave E993.9
wind E993.9
bomb E993.8
but occurring after cessation of hostilities
explosion of bombs E998.1
explosion of mines E998.0
specified NEC E998.8
conventional warfare E995.9
specified form NEC E995.8
depth charge E992.1
destruction of aircraft E994.9
due to
air to air missile E994.0
collision with other aircraft E994.2
enemy fire or explosives E994.0
on board explosion (explosives) E994.1
on board fire E994.3
rocket propelled grenade [RPG] E994.0
small arms fire E994.0
surface to air missile E994.0
specified NEC E994.8
dirty bomb (*see also* War operations, injury due to, nuclear weapons) E996.9
drowning E995.4
explosion (direct pressure) (indirect pressure) (due to) E993.9
depth charge E992.1

War operations — *continued*

injury due to — *continued*
explosion — *continued*
improvised explosive device [IED]
person borne E993.3
roadside E993.5
specified NEC E993.5
transport vehicle (air) (land) (water) borne E993.4
vehicle (air) (land) (water) borne E993.4
marine mines (in harbor) (at sea) E992.2
marine weapons E992.9
specified NEC E992.8
sea based artillery shell E992.3
specified NEC E993.8
torpedo E992.0
unintentional (of own)
autocannons E993.7
automatic grenade launchers E993.7
launch device discharge E993.7
missile launchers E993.7
munitions detonation (ammunition) (artillery) (mortars) E993.6
small arms E993.7
fragments (from) E991.9
artillery E991.8
artillery shells E991.4
autocannons E991.8
automatic grenade launchers [AGL] E991.8
bombs E991.4
antipersonnel E991.3
detonation of unexploded ordnance [UXO] E991.4
grenade E991.4
guided missile E991.4
improvised explosive device [IED]
person borne E991.5
roadside E991.7
specified NEC E991.7
transport vehicle (air) (land) (water) borne E991.6
vehicle (air) (land) (water) borne E991.6
land mine E991.4
missile launchers E991.8
mortars E991.8
munitions (artillery shells) (bombs) (grenades) (rockets) (shells) E991.4
rockets E991.4
shells E991.4
small arms E991.8
specified NEC E991.9
weapons (artillery) (autocannons) (mortars) (small arms) E991.8
grenade E993.8
guided missile E993.1
hand to hand combat, unarmed E995.0
improvised explosive device [IED]
person borne E993.3
roadside E993.5
specified NEC E993.5
transport vehicle (air) (land) (water) borne E993.4
vehicle (air) (land) (water) borne E993.4
inability to surface or obtain air E995.4

War operations — *continued*

injury due to — *continued*
land mine E993.8
marine mines (in harbor) (at sea) E992.2
marine weapons E992.9
specified NEC E992.8
mortar E993.2
nuclear weapons E996.9
beta burns E996.3
blast debris E996.1
blast pressure E996.0
burns due to thermal radiation E996.2
direct blast effect E996.0
fallout exposure E996.3
fireball effect E996.2
flash burns E996.2
heat effect E996.2
indirect blast effect E996.1
nuclear radiation effects E996.3
radiation exposure (acute) E996.3
radiation sickness E996.3
secondary effects E996.3
specified effects NEC E996.8
thermal radiation effect E996.2
piercing object E995.2
restriction of airway, intentional E995.3
sea based artillery shell E992.3
shrapnel E991.9
stave E995.1
strangulation E995.3
strike by blunt object (baton) (nightstick) (stave) E995.1
submersion (accidental) (unintentional) E995.4
intentional E995.3
suffocation E995.3
accidental E995.4
torpedo E992.0
underwater blast E992.9
weapon of mass destruction [WMD] E997.3
knife E995.2
lacrimator (gas) (chemical) E997.2
land mine (explosion) E993.8
after cessation of hostilities E998.0
fragments, injury by E991.4
laser(s) E997.0
late effect of E999.0
lewisite E997.2
lung irritant (chemical) (fumes) (gas) E997.2
marine mine E992.2
mine
after cessation of hostilities E998.0
at sea E992.2
in harbor E992.2
land (explosion) E993.8
fragments, injury by E991.4
marine E992.2
missile (guided) (explosion) E993.1
fragments, injury by E991.4
marine E992.8
nuclear (*see also* War operations, injury due to, nuclear weapons) E996.9
mortar bomb (explosion) E993.2
fragments, injury by E991.4
mustard gas E997.2
nerve gas E997.2
phosgene E997.2
piercing object E995.2
poisoning (chemical) (fumes) (gas) E997.2

War operations — *continued*

radiation, ionizing from nuclear explosion (*see also* War operations, injury due to, nuclear weapons) E996.3

rocket (explosion) E993.8
fragments, injury by E991.4

saber, sabre E995.2

screening smoke E997.8

shell (aircraft) (artillery) (cannon) (land based) (explosion) E993.2
fragments, injury by E991.4
sea-based E992.3

shooting E991.2
after cessation of hostilities E998.8
bullet(s) E991.2
rubber E991.0
pellet(s) (rifle) E991.1
shrapnel E991.9
submersion E995 ☑
torpedo E992 ☑

stave E995.2

strike by blunt object (baton) (nightstick) (stave) E995.1

submersion E995.4
intentional E995.3

sword E995.2

torpedo E992.0

unconventional warfare, except by nuclear weapon E997.9
biological (warfare) E997.1
gas, fumes, chemicals E997.2
laser(s) E997.0
specified type NEC E997.8

underwater blast E992.9

vesicant (chemical) (fumes) (gas) E997.2

weapon burst E993.9

Washed
away by flood — *see* Flood
away by tidal wave — *see* Tidal wave
off road by storm (transport vehicle) E908.9
overboard E832 ☑

Weapon of mass destruction [WMD] E997.3

Weather exposure — *see also* Exposure
cold E901.0
hot E900.0

Weightlessness (causing injury) (effects of) (in spacecraft, real or simulated) E928.0

Wound (accidental) NEC — *see also* Injury E928.9
battle (*see also* War operations) E995.9
bayonet E920.3
in
legal intervention E974
war operations E995.2
gunshot — *see* Shooting
incised — *see* Cut
saber, sabre E920.3
in war operations E995.2

Wrong
body part, performance of correct operation (procedure) on E876.7
device implanted into correct surgical site E876.5
patient, performance of operation (procedure) on E876.6
procedure (operation) performed on correct patient E876.5
side, performance of correct operation (procedure) on E876.7
site, performance of correct operation (procedure) on E876.7

☑ Additional Digit Required — Refer to the Tabular List for Digit Selection ⠀⠀⠀⠀⠀ ▽ Subterms under main terms may continue to next column or page

Railway Accidents (E800-E807)

The following fourth-digit subdivisions are for use with categories E800-E807 to identify the injured person:

.0   Railway employee
Any person who by virtue of his employment in connection with a railway, whether by the railway company or not, is at increased risk of involvement in a railway accident, such as:
  catering staff on train
  postal staff on train
  driver
  railway fireman
  guard
  shunter
  porter
  sleeping car attendant

.1   Passenger on railway
Any authorized person traveling on a train, except a railway employee
> EXCLUDES   intending passenger waiting at station (.8)
>   unauthorized rider on railway vehicle (.8)

.2   Pedestrian See definition (r), E-Codes-2

.3   Pedal cyclist See definition (p), E-Codes-2

.8   Other specified person Intending passenger waiting at station
Unauthorized rider on railway vehicle

.9   Unspecified person

Motor Vehicle Traffic and Nontraffic Accidents (E810-E825)

The following fourth-digit subdivisions are for use with categories E810-E819 and E820-E825 to identify the injured person:

.0   Driver of motor vehicle other than motorcycle See definition (1), E-Codes-2

.1   Passenger in motor vehicle other than motorcycle See definition (1), E-Codes-2

.2   Motorcyclist See definition (1), E-Codes-2

.3   Passenger on motorcycle See definition (1), E-Codes-2

.4   Occupant of streetcar

.5   Rider of animal; occupant of animal-drawn vehicle

.6   Pedal cyclist See definition (p), E-Codes-2

.7   Pedestrian See definition (r), E-Codes-2

.8   Other specified person
Occupant of vehicle other than above
Person in railway train involved in accident
Unauthorized rider of motor vehicle

.9   Unspecified person

Other Road Vehicle Accidents (E826-E829)

(animal-drawn vehicle, streetcar, pedal cycle, and other nonmotor road vehicle accidents)

The following fourth-digit subdivisions are for use with categories E826-E829 to identify the injured person:

.0   Pedestrian See definition (r), E-Codes-2

.1   Pedal cyclist (does not apply to codes E827, E828, E829) See definition (p), E-Codes-2

.2   Rider of animal (does not apply to code E829)

.3   Occupant of animal-drawn vehicle (does not apply to codes E828, E829)

.4   Occupant of streetcar

.8   Other specified person

.9   Unspecified person

Water Transport Accidents (E830-E838)

The following fourth-digit subdivisions are for use with categories E830-E838 to identify the injured person:

.0   Occupant of small boat, unpowered

.1   Occupant of small boat, powered See definition (t), E-Codes-2
> EXCLUDES   water skier (.4)

.2   Occupant of other watercraft — crew
Persons:
  engaged in operation of watercraft
    providing passenger services [cabin attendants, ship's physician, catering personnel]
    working on ship during voyage in other capacity [musician in band, operators of shops and beauty parlors]

.3   Occupant of other watercraft — other than crew
Passenger
Occupant of lifeboat, other than crew, after abandoning ship

.4   Water skier

.5   Swimmer

.6   Dockers, stevedores
Longshoreman employed on the dock in loading and unloading ships

.8   Other specified person
Immigration and custom officials on board ship
Persons:
  accompanying passenger or member of crew visiting boat
Pilot (guiding ship into port)

.9   Unspecified person

Air and Space Transport Accidents (E840-E845)

The following fourth-digit subdivisions are for use with categories E840-E845 to identify the injured person:

.0   Occupant of spacecraft
  Crew
  Passenger (civilian)   in military aircraft [air force]
  (military)   [army] [national guard] [navy]
  Troops

.1   Occupant of military aircraft, any
> EXCLUDES   occupants of aircraft operated under jurisdiction of police departments (.5) parachutist (.7)

.2   Crew of commercial aircraft (powered) in surface to surface transport

.3   Other occupant of commercial aircraft (powered) in surface to surface transport
Flight personnel:
  not part of crew
  on familiarization flight Passenger on aircraft

.4   Occupant of commercial aircraft (powered) in surface to air transport
Occupant [crew] [passenger] of aircraft (powered) engaged in activities, such as:
  air drops of emergency supplies
  air drops of parachutists, except from military craft
  crop dusting
  lowering of construction material [bridge or telephone pole]
  sky writing

.5   Occupant of other powered aircraft
Occupant [crew] [passenger] of aircraft (powered) engaged in activities, such as:
  aerial spraying (crops)(fire retardants)
  aerobatic flying
  aircraft racing
  rescue operation
  storm surveillance
  traffic suveillance
Occupant of private plane NOS

.6   Occupant of unpowered aircraft, except parachutist
Occupant of aircraft classifiable to E842

.7   Parachutist (military)(other)
Person making voluntary descent
  person making descent after accident to aircraft (.1-.6)

.8   Ground crew, airline employee
Persons employed at airfields (civil)(military) or launching pads, not occupants of aircraft

.9   Other person

☑ **Additional Digit Required — Refer to the Tabular List for Digit Selection**   ▽ **Subterms under main terms may continue to next column or page**

1. Infectious and Parasitic Diseases (001-139)

NOTE Categories for "late effects" of infectious and parasitic diseases are to be found at 137-139.

INCLUDES diseases generally recognized as communicable or transmissible as well as a few diseases of unknown but possibly infectious origin

EXCLUDES acute respiratory infections (460-466)
carrier or suspected carrier of infectious organism (V02.0-V02.9)
certain localized infections
influenza (487.0-487.8, 488.01-488.19)

Intestinal Infectious Diseases (001-009)

EXCLUDES helminthiases (120.0-129)

√4ᵗʰ 001 Cholera

DEF: An acute infectious enteritis caused by a potent enterotoxin produced by *Vibrio cholerae*; changes the permeability of the mucosa of the intestines and leads to diarrhea and dehydration.

001.0 Due to Vibrio cholerae

001.1 Due to Vibrio cholerae el tor

001.9 Cholera, unspecified

√4ᵗʰ 002 Typhoid and paratyphoid fevers

DEF: Typhoid fever: an acute generalized illness caused by *Salmonella typhi*; clinical features are fever, headache, abdominal pain, cough, toxemia, leukopenia, abnormal pulse, rose spots on the skin, bacteremia, hyperplasia of intestinal lymph nodes, mesenteric lymphadenopathy, and Peyer's patches in the intestines.
DEF: Paratyphoid fever: a prolonged febrile illness, caused by salmonella serotypes other than *S. typhi*, especially *S. enteritidis* serotypes paratyphi A and B and *S. choleraesuis*.

002.0 Typhoid fever
Typhoid (fever) (infection) [any site]

002.1 Paratyphoid fever A

002.2 Paratyphoid fever B

002.3 Paratyphoid fever C

002.9 Paratyphoid fever, unspecified

√4ᵗʰ 003 Other salmonella infections

INCLUDES infection or food poisoning by Salmonella [any serotype]
DEF: Infections caused by a genus of gram-negative, anaerobic bacteria of the family *Enterobacteriaceae*; major symptoms are enteric fevers, acute gastroenteritis and septicemia.

003.0 Salmonella gastroenteritis
Salmonellosis

003.1 Salmonella septicemia

√5ᵗʰ 003.2 Localized salmonella infections

003.20 Localized salmonella infection, unspecified

003.21 Salmonella meningitis

003.22 Salmonella pneumonia

003.23 Salmonella arthritis

003.24 Salmonella osteomyelitis

003.29 Other

003.8 Other specified salmonella infections

003.9 Salmonella infection, unspecified

√4ᵗʰ 004 Shigellosis

INCLUDES bacillary dysentery
DEF: Acute infectious dysentery caused by the genus *Shigella*, of the family *Enterobacteriaceae*; affecting the colon causing blood- stained stools, tenesmus, abdominal cramps and fever.

004.0 Shigella dysenteriae
Infection by group A Shigella (Schmitz) (Shiga)

004.1 Shigella flexneri
Infection by group B Shigella

004.2 Shigella boydii
Infection by group C Shigella

004.3 Shigella sonnei
Infection by group D Shigella

004.8 Other specified Shigella infections

004.9 Shigellosis, unspecified

√4ᵗʰ 005 Other food poisoning (bacterial)

EXCLUDES salmonella infections (003.0-003.9)
toxic effect of:
food contaminants (989.7)
noxious foodstuffs (988.0-988.9)

DEF: Enteritis caused by ingesting contaminated foods and characterized by diarrhea, abdominal pain, vomiting; symptoms may be mild or life threatening.

005.0 Staphylococcal food poisoning
Staphylococcal toxemia specified as due to food

005.1 Botulism food poisoning
Botulism NOS
Food poisoning due to Clostridium botulinum
EXCLUDES infant botulism (040.41)
wound botulism (040.42)

005.2 Food poisoning due to Clostridium perfringens [C. welchii]
Enteritis necroticans

005.3 Food poisoning due to other Clostridia

005.4 Food poisoning due to Vibrio parahaemolyticus

√5ᵗʰ 005.8 Other bacterial food poisoning

EXCLUDES salmonella food poisoning (003.0-003.9)

005.81 Food poisoning due to Vibrio vulnificus

005.89 Other bacterial food poisoning
Food poisoning due to Bacillus cereus

005.9 Food poisoning, unspecified

√4ᵗʰ 006 Amebiasis

INCLUDES infection due to Entamoeba histolytica
EXCLUDES amebiasis due to organisms other than Entamoeba histolytica (007.8)

DEF: Infection of the large intestine caused by *Entamoeba histolytica*; usually asymptomatic but symptoms may range from mild diarrhea to profound life-threatening dysentery. Extraintestinal complications include hepatic abscess, which may rupture, causing life-threatening infections.

006.0 Acute amebic dysentery without mention of abscess
Acute amebiasis
DEF: Sudden, severe *Entamoeba histolytica* infection causing bloody stools.

006.1 Chronic intestinal amebiasis without mention of abscess
Chronic:
amebiasis
amebic dysentery

006.2 Amebic nondysenteric colitis
DEF: *Entamoeba histolytica* infection with inflamed colon but no dysentery.

006.3 Amebic liver abscess
Hepatic amebiasis

006.4 Amebic lung abscess
Amebic abscess of lung (and liver)

006.5 Amebic brain abscess
Amebic abscess of brain (and liver) (and lung)

006.6 Amebic skin ulceration
Cutaneous amebiasis

006.8 Amebic infection of other sites
Amebic: Ameboma
appendicitis
balanitis
EXCLUDES specific infections by free-living amebae (136.21-136.29)

006.9 Amebiasis, unspecified
Amebiasis NOS

√4ᵗʰ / √5ᵗʰ Additional Digit Required | Unspecified Code | Other Specified Code | Manifestation Code | ▶◀ Revised Text | ● New Code | ▲ Revised Code Title

2015 ICD-9-CM

Volume 1 – 1

Infectious and Parasitic Diseases

007–009.0

✓4ᵗʰ **007 Other protozoal intestinal diseases**
    INCLUDES   protozoal:
       colitis
       diarrhea
       dysentery

   007.0 Balantidiasis
      Infection by Balantidium coli

   007.1 Giardiasis
      Infection by Giardia lamblia
      Lambliasis

   007.2 Coccidiosis
      Infection by Isospora belli and Isospora hominis
      Isosporiasis

   007.3 Intestinal trichomoniasis
      DEF: Colitis, diarrhea, or dysentery caused by the protozoa *Trichomonas.*

   007.4 Cryptosporidiosis
      DEF: An intestinal infection by protozoan parasites causing intractable diarrhea in patients with AIDS and other immunosuppressed individuals.
      AHA: 4Q, '97, 30

   007.5 Cyclosporiasis
      DEF: An infection of the small intestine by the protozoal organism, *Cyclospora cayetenanesis,* spread to humans through ingestion of contaminated water or food. Symptoms include watery diarrhea, loss of appetite, increased gas, stomach cramps, nausea, vomiting, muscle aches, low grade fever, and fatigue.
      AHA: 4Q, '00, 38

   007.8 Other specified protozoal intestinal diseases
      Amebiasis due to organisms other than Entamoeba histolytica

   007.9 Unspecified protozoal intestinal disease
      Flagellate diarrhea
      Protozoal dysentery NOS

✓4ᵗʰ **008 Intestinal infections due to other organisms**
    INCLUDES   any condition classifiable to 009.0-009.3 with mention of the responsible organisms
    EXCLUDES   food poisoning by these organisms (005.0-005.9)

✓5ᵗʰ   **008.0 Escherichia coli [E. coli]**
      AHA: 4Q, '92, 17

     008.00 E. coli, unspecified
       E. coli enteritis NOS

     008.01 Enteropathogenic E. coli
       DEF: *E. coli* causing inflammation of intestines.

     008.02 Enterotoxigenic E. coli
       DEF: A toxic reaction to *E. coli* of the intestinal mucosa, causing voluminous watery secretions.

     008.03 Enteroinvasive E. coli
       DEF: *E. coli* infection penetrating intestinal mucosa.

     008.04 Enterohemorrhagic E. coli
       DEF: E. coli infection penetrating the intestinal mucosa, producing microscopic ulceration and bleeding.
       AHA: 4Q, '11, 83

     008.09 Other intestinal E. coli infections

   008.1 Arizona group of paracolon bacilli

   008.2 Aerobacter aerogenes
      Enterobacter aeogenes

   008.3 Proteus (mirabilis) (morganii)

✓5ᵗʰ   **008.4 Other specified bacteria**
      AHA: 4Q, '92, 18

     008.41 Staphylococcus
       Staphylococcal enterocolitis

     008.42 Pseudomonas
       AHA: 2Q, '89, 10

     008.43 Campylobacter

     008.44 Yersinia enterocolitica

     008.45 Clostridium difficile
       Pseudomembranous colitis
       DEF: An overgrowth of a species of bacterium that is a part of the normal colon flora in human infants and sometimes in adults; produces a toxin that causes pseudomembranous enterocolitis.; typically is seen in patients undergoing antibiotic therapy.
       A04.7 Enterocolitis due to clostridium difficile   I-10

     008.46 Other anaerobes
       Anaerobic enteritis NOS
       Bacteroides (fragilis)
       Gram-negative anaerobes

     008.47 Other gram-negative bacteria
       Gram-negative enteritis NOS
       EXCLUDES   *gram-negative anaerobes (008.46)*

     008.49 Other
       AHA: 2Q, '89, 10; 1Q, '88, 6

   008.5 Bacterial enteritis, unspecified

✓5ᵗʰ   **008.6 Enteritis due to specified virus**
      AHA: 4Q, '92, 18

     008.61 Rotavirus

     008.62 Adenovirus

     008.63 Norwalk virus
       Norovirus
       Norwalk-like agent

     008.64 Other small round viruses [SRVs]
       Small round virus NOS

     008.65 Calicivirus
       DEF: Enteritis due to a subgroup of *Picornaviruses.*

     008.66 Astrovirus

     008.67 Enterovirus NEC
       Coxsackie virus
       Echovirus
       EXCLUDES   *poliovirus (045.0-045.9)*

     008.69 Other viral enteritis
       Torovirus
       AHA: 1Q, '03, 10

   008.8 Other organism, not elsewhere classified
      Viral:
       enteritis NOS
       gastroenteritis
      EXCLUDES   *influenza with involvement of gastrointestinal tract (487.8, 488.09, 488.19)*
      A08.4 Viral intestinal infection unspecified   I-10

✓4ᵗʰ **009 Ill-defined intestinal infections**
    EXCLUDES   *diarrheal disease or intestinal infection due to specified organism (001.0-008.8)*
       diarrhea following gastrointestinal surgery (564.4)
       intestinal malabsorption (579.0-579.9)
       ischemic enteritis (557.0-557.9)
       other noninfectious gastroenteritis and colitis (558.1-558.9)
       regional enteritis (555.0-555.9)
       ulcerative colitis (556)

   009.0 Infectious colitis, enteritis, and gastroenteritis
      Colitis
      Enteritis   } septic
      Gastroenteritis
      Dysentery:
       NOS
       catarrhal
       hemorrhagic
      DEF: Colitis: An inflammation of mucous membranes of the colon.
      DEF: Enteritis: An inflammation of mucous membranes of the small intestine.
      DEF: Gastroenteritis: An inflammation of mucous membranes of stomach and intestines.
      AHA: 3Q, '99, 4
      A09 Infectious gastroenteritis and colitis unspec   I-10

   N   Newborn Age: 0   P   Pediatric Age: 0-17   M   Maternity Age: 12-55   A   Adult Age: 15-124

009.1 Colitis, enteritis, and gastroenteritis of presumed infectious origin

EXCLUDES   colitis NOS (558.9)
enteritis NOS (558.9)
gastroenteritis NOS (558.9)

AHA: 3Q, '99, 6

009.2 Infectious diarrhea

Diarrhea:
dysenteric
epidemic
Infectious diarrheal disease NOS

009.3 Diarrhea of presumed infectious origin

EXCLUDES   diarrhea NOS (787.91)

AHA: N-D, '87, 7

Tuberculosis (010-018)

INCLUDES   infection by Mycobacterium tuberculosis (human)
(bovine)

EXCLUDES   congenital tuberculosis (771.2)
late effects of tuberculosis (137.0-137.4)

The following fifth digit subclassification is for use with categories 010-018:

0 unspecified
1 bacteriological or histological examination not done
2 bacteriological or histological examination unknown (at present)
3 tubercle bacilli found (in sputum) by microscopy
4 tubercle bacilli not found (in sputum) by microscopy, but found by bacterial culture
5 tubercle bacilli not found by bacteriological examination, but tuberculosis confirmed histologically
6 tubercle bacilli not found by bacteriological or histological examination but tuberculosis confirmed by other methods [inoculation of animals]

DEF: An infection by *Mycobacterium tuberculosis* causing the formation of small, rounded nodules, called tubercles, that can disseminate throughout the body via lymph and blood vessels. Localized tuberculosis is most often seen in the lungs.

√4ᵗʰ **010 Primary tuberculous infection**

DEF: Tuberculosis of the lungs occurring when the patient is first infected.

§ √5ᵗʰ **010.0 Primary tuberculous infection**
[0-6]   EXCLUDES   nonspecific reaction to test for tuberculosis without active tuberculosis (795.51-795.52)
positive PPD (795.51)
positive tuberculin skin test without active tuberculosis (795.51)

DEF: Hilar or paratracheal lymph node enlargement in pulmonary tuberculosis.

§ √5ᵗʰ **010.1 Tuberculous pleurisy in primary progressive**
[0-6]   **tuberculosis**

DEF: Inflammation and exudation in the lining of the tubercular lung.

§ √5ᵗʰ **010.8 Other primary progressive tuberculosis**
[0-6]   EXCLUDES   tuberculous erythema nodosum (017.1)

§ √5ᵗʰ **010.9 Primary tuberculous infection, unspecified**
[0-6]

√4ᵗʰ **011 Pulmonary tuberculosis**

Use additional code to identify any associated silicosis (502)

§ √5ᵗʰ **011.0 Tuberculosis of lung, infiltrative**
[0-6]

§ √5ᵗʰ **011.1 Tuberculosis of lung, nodular**
[0-6]

§ √5ᵗʰ **011.2 Tuberculosis of lung with cavitation**
[0-6]

§ √5ᵗʰ **011.3 Tuberculosis of bronchus**
[0-6]   EXCLUDES   isolated bronchial tuberculosis (012.2)

§ √5ᵗʰ **011.4 Tuberculous fibrosis of lung**
[0-6]

§ √5ᵗʰ **011.5 Tuberculous bronchiectasis**
[0-6]

§ √5ᵗʰ **011.6 Tuberculous pneumonia [any form]**
[0-6]   DEF: Inflammatory pulmonary reaction to tuberculous cells.

§ √5ᵗʰ **011.7 Tuberculous pneumothorax**
[0-6]   DEF: Spontaneous rupture of damaged tuberculous pulmonary tissue.

§ √5ᵗʰ **011.8 Other specified pulmonary tuberculosis**
[0-6]

§ √5ᵗʰ **011.9 Pulmonary tuberculosis, unspecified**
[0-6]   Respiratory tuberculosis NOS
Tuberculosis of lung NOS

√4ᵗʰ **012 Other respiratory tuberculosis**

EXCLUDES   respiratory tuberculosis, unspecified (011.9)

§ √5ᵗʰ **012.0 Tuberculous pleurisy**
[0-6]   Tuberculosis of pleura
Tuberculous empyema
Tuberculous hydrothorax

EXCLUDES   pleurisy with effusion without mention of cause (511.9)
tuberculous pleurisy in primary progressive tuberculosis (010.1)

DEF: Inflammation and exudation in the lining of the tubercular lung.

§ √5ᵗʰ **012.1 Tuberculosis of intrathoracic lymph nodes**
[0-6]   Tuberculosis of lymph nodes:
hilar
mediastinal
tracheobronchial
Tuberculous tracheobronchial adenopathy

EXCLUDES   that specified as primary (010.0-010.9)

§ √5ᵗʰ **012.2 Isolated tracheal or bronchial tuberculosis**
[0-6]

§ √5ᵗʰ **012.3 Tuberculous laryngitis**
[0-6]   Tuberculosis of glottis

§ √5ᵗʰ **012.8 Other specified respiratory tuberculosis**
[0-6]   Tuberculosis of:
mediastinum
nasopharynx
nose (septum)
sinus [any nasal]

√4ᵗʰ **013 Tuberculosis of meninges and central nervous system**

§ √5ᵗʰ **013.0 Tuberculous meningitis**
[0-6]   Tuberculosis of meninges (cerebral) (spinal)
Tuberculous:
leptomeningitis
meningoencephalitis

EXCLUDES   tuberculoma of meninges (013.1)

§ √5ᵗʰ **013.1 Tuberculoma of meninges**
[0-6]

§ √5ᵗʰ **013.2 Tuberculoma of brain**
[0-6]   Tuberculosis of brain (current disease)

§ √5ᵗʰ **013.3 Tuberculous abscess of brain**
[0-6]

§ √5ᵗʰ **013.4 Tuberculoma of spinal cord**
[0-6]

§ √5ᵗʰ **013.5 Tuberculous abscess of spinal cord**
[0-6]

§ √5ᵗʰ **013.6 Tuberculous encephalitis or myelitis**
[0-6]

§ √5ᵗʰ **013.8 Other specified tuberculosis of central nervous system**
[0-6]

§ √5ᵗʰ **013.9 Unspecified tuberculosis of central nervous system**
[0-6]   Tuberculosis of central nervous system NOS

√4ᵗʰ **014 Tuberculosis of intestines, peritoneum, and mesenteric glands**

§ √5ᵗʰ **014.0 Tuberculous peritonitis**
[0-6]   Tuberculous ascites

DEF: Tuberculous inflammation of the membrane lining the abdomen.

---

§   Requires fifth digit. Valid digits are in [brackets] under each code. See beginning of section 010-018 for codes and definitions.

√4ᵗʰ √5ᵗʰ Additional Digit Required   Unspecified Code   Other Specified Code   Manifestation Code   ▶◀ Revised Text   ● New Code   ▲ Revised Code Title

§ ✓5ᵗʰ **014.8 Other**
[0-6]   Tuberculosis (of):
           anus
           intestine (large) (small)
           mesenteric glands
           rectum
           retroperitoneal (lymph nodes)
         Tuberculous enteritis

✓4ᵗʰ **015 Tuberculosis of bones and joints**
         Use additional code to identify manifestation, as:
         tuberculous:
           arthropathy (711.4)
           necrosis of bone (730.8)
           osteitis (730.8)
           osteomyelitis (730.8)
           synovitis (727.01)
           tenosynovitis (727.01)

§ ✓5ᵗʰ **015.0 Vertebral column**
[0-6]   Pott's disease
         Use additional code to identify manifestation, as:
           curvature of spine [Pott's] (737.4)
           kyphosis (737.4)
           spondylitis (720.81)

§ ✓5ᵗʰ **015.1 Hip**
[0-6]

§ ✓5ᵗʰ **015.2 Knee**
[0-6]

§ ✓5ᵗʰ **015.5 Limb bones**
[0-6]   Tuberculous dactylitis

§ ✓5ᵗʰ **015.6 Mastoid**
[0-6]   Tuberculous mastoiditis

§ ✓5ᵗʰ **015.7 Other specified bone**
[0-6]

§ ✓5ᵗʰ **015.8 Other specified joint**
[0-6]

§ ✓5ᵗʰ **015.9 Tuberculosis of unspecified bones and joints**
[0-6]

✓4ᵗʰ **016 Tuberculosis of genitourinary system**

§ ✓5ᵗʰ **016.0 Kidney**
[0-6]   Renal tuberculosis
         Use additional code to identify manifestation, as:
         tuberculous:
           nephropathy (583.81)
           pyelitis (590.81)
           pyelonephritis (590.81)

§ ✓5ᵗʰ **016.1 Bladder**
[0-6]

§ ✓5ᵗʰ **016.2 Ureter**
[0-6]

§ ✓5ᵗʰ **016.3 Other urinary organs**
[0-6]

§ ✓5ᵗʰ **016.4 Epididymis**   ♂
[0-6]

§ ✓5ᵗʰ **016.5 Other male genital organs**   ♂
[0-6]   Use additional code to identify manifestation, as:
         tuberculosis of:
           prostate (601.4)
           seminal vesicle (608.81)
           testis (608.81)

§ ✓5ᵗʰ **016.6 Tuberculous oophoritis and salpingitis**   ♀
[0-6]

§ ✓5ᵗʰ **016.7 Other female genital organs**   ♀
[0-6]   Tuberculous:
           cervicitis
           endometritis

§ ✓5ᵗʰ **016.9 Genitourinary tuberculosis, unspecified**
[0-6]

✓4ᵗʰ **017 Tuberculosis of other organs**

§ ✓5ᵗʰ **017.0 Skin and subcutaneous cellular tissue**
[0-6]   Lupus: Tuberculosis:
           exedens   colliquativa
           vulgaris   cutis
         Scrofuloderma   lichenoides
                               papulonecrotica
                               verrucosa cutis

         EXCLUDES *lupus erythematosus (695.4)*
                    disseminated (710.0)
                  lupus NOS (710.0)
                  nonspecific reaction to test for tuberculosis without
                       active tuberculosis (795.51-795.52)
                  positive PPD (795.51)
                  positive tuberculin skin test without active
                       tuberculosis (795.51)

§ ✓5ᵗʰ **017.1 Erythema nodosum with hypersensitivity**
[0-6]   **reaction in tuberculosis**
         Bazin's disease
         Erythema:
           induratum
           nodosum, tuberculous
         Tuberculosis indurativa

         EXCLUDES *erythema nodosum NOS (695.2)*

         DEF: Tender, inflammatory, bilateral nodules appearing on the shins
         and thought to be an allergic reaction to tuberculotoxin.

§ ✓5ᵗʰ **017.2 Peripheral lymph nodes**
[0-6]   Scrofula
         Scrofulous abscess
         Tuberculous adenitis

         EXCLUDES *tuberculosis of lymph nodes:*
                    bronchial and mediastinal (012.1)
                    mesenteric and retroperitoneal (014.8)
                  tuberculous tracheobronchial adenopathy (012.1)

         DEF: Scrofula: Old name for tuberculous cervical lymphadenitis.

§ ✓5ᵗʰ **017.3 Eye**
[0-6]   Use additional code to identify manifestation, as:
         tuberculous:
           chorioretinitis, disseminated (363.13)
           episcleritis (379.09)
           interstitial keratitis (370.59)
           iridocyclitis, chronic (364.11)
           keratoconjunctivitis (phlyctenular) (370.31)

§ ✓5ᵗʰ **017.4 Ear**
[0-6]   Tuberculosis of ear
         Tuberculous otitis media

         EXCLUDES *tuberculous mastoiditis (015.6)*

§ ✓5ᵗʰ **017.5 Thyroid gland**
[0-6]

§ ✓5ᵗʰ **017.6 Adrenal glands**
[0-6]   Addison's disease, tuberculous

§ ✓5ᵗʰ **017.7 Spleen**
[0-6]

§ ✓5ᵗʰ **017.8 Esophagus**
[0-6]

§ ✓5ᵗʰ **017.9 Other specified organs**
[0-6]   Use additional code to identify manifestation, as:
         tuberculosis of:
           endocardium [any valve] (424.91)
           myocardium (422.0)
           pericardium (420.0)

✓4ᵗʰ **018 Miliary tuberculosis**
         INCLUDES tuberculosis:
                   disseminated
                   generalized
                   miliary, whether of a single specified site, multiple sites,
                       or unspecified site
                   polyserositis

         DEF: A form of tuberculosis caused by caseous material carried through the
         bloodstream planting seedlike tubercles in various body organs.

---

§   Requires fifth digit. Valid digits are in [brackets] under each code. See beginning of section 010-018 for codes and definitions.

§ ✓5ᵗʰ **018.0 Acute miliary tuberculosis**
[0-6]

§ ✓5ᵗʰ **018.8 Other specified miliary tuberculosis**
[0-6]

§ ✓5ᵗʰ **018.9 Miliary tuberculosis, unspecified**
[0-6]

Zoonotic Bacterial Diseases (020-027)

✓4ᵗʰ **020 Plague**

INCLUDES infection by Yersinia [Pasteurella] pestis

020.0 Bubonic
DEF: Most common acute and severe form of plague characterized by lymphadenopathy (buboes), chills, fever and headache.

020.1 Cellulocutaneous
DEF: Plague characterized by inflammation and necrosis of skin.

020.2 Septicemic
DEF: Plague characterized by massive infection in the bloodstream.

020.3 Primary pneumonic
DEF: Plague characterized by massive pulmonary infection.

020.4 Secondary pneumonic
DEF: Lung infection as a secondary complication of plague.

020.5 Pneumonic, unspecified

020.8 Other specified types of plague
Abortive plague
Ambulatory plague
Pestis minor

020.9 Plague, unspecified

✓4ᵗʰ **021 Tularemia**

INCLUDES deerfly fever
infection by Francisella [Pasteurella] tularensis
rabbit fever
DEF: A febrile disease transmitted by the bites of deer flies, fleas and ticks, by inhalations of aerosolized F. tularensis or by ingestion of contaminated food or water; patients quickly develop fever, chills, weakness, headache, backache and malaise.

021.0 Ulceroglandular tularemia
DEF: Lesions occur at the site Francisella tularensis organism enters body, usually the fingers or hands.

021.1 Enteric tularemia
Tularemia:
cryptogenic
intestinal
typhoidal

021.2 Pulmonary tularemia
Bronchopneumonic tularemia

021.3 Oculoglandular tularemia
DEF: Painful conjunctival infection by Francisella tularensis organism with possible corneal, preauricular lymph, or lacrimal involvement.

021.8 Other specified tularemia
Tularemia:
generalized or disseminated
glandular

021.9 Unspecified tularemia

✓4ᵗʰ **022 Anthrax**
DEF: An bacterial disease usually transmitted by contact with infected animals or their discharges; primary routes of inoculation are cutaneous, gastrointestinal and by inhalation.
AHA: 4Q '02, 70

022.0 Cutaneous anthrax
Malignant pustule

022.1 Pulmonary anthrax
Respiratory anthrax
Wool-sorters' disease

022.2 Gastrointestinal anthrax

022.3 Anthrax septicemia

022.8 Other specified manifestations of anthrax

022.9 Anthrax, unspecified

✓4ᵗʰ **023 Brucellosis**
INCLUDES fever:
Malta
Mediterranean
undulant
DEF: An infectious disease caused by gram-negative, aerobic coccobacilli organisms transmitted to humans through contact with infected tissue or dairy products; fever, sweating, weakness and aching are symptoms.

023.0 Brucella melitensis
DEF: Infection from direct or indirect contact with infected sheep or goats.

023.1 Brucella abortus
DEF: Infection from direct or indirect contact with infected cattle.

023.2 Brucella suis
DEF: Infection from direct or indirect contact with infected swine.

023.3 Brucella canis
DEF: Infection from direct or indirect contact with infected dogs.

023.8 Other brucellosis
Infection by more than one organism

023.9 Brucellosis, unspecified

024 Glanders
Infection by:
Actinobacillus mallei
Malleomyces mallei
Pseudomonas mallei
Farcy
Malleus
DEF: Equine infection causing mucosal inflammation and skin ulcers in humans.

025 Melioidosis
Infection by:
Malleomyces pseudomallei
Pseudomonas pseudomallei
Whitmore's bacillus
Pseudoglanders
DEF: Rare infection caused by Pseudomonas pseudomallei; clinical symptoms range from localized infection to fatal septicemia.

✓4ᵗʰ **026 Rat-bite fever**

026.0 Spirillary fever
Rat-bite fever due to Spirillum minor [S. minus]
Sodoku

026.1 Streptobacillary fever
Epidemic arthritic erythema
Haverhill fever
Rat-bite fever due to Streptobacillus moniliformis

026.9 Unspecified rat-bite fever

✓4ᵗʰ **027 Other zoonotic bacterial diseases**

027.0 Listeriosis
Infection
Septicemia } by Listeria monocytogenes

Use additional code to identify manifestation, as meningitis (320.7)
EXCLUDES congenital listeriosis (771.2)

027.1 Erysipelothrix infection
Erysipeloid (of Rosenbach)
Infection } by Erysipelothrix insidiosa
Septicemia } [E. rhusiopathiae]
DEF: Usually associated with handling of fish, meat, or poultry; symptoms range from localized inflammation to septicemia.

027.2 Pasteurellosis
Pasteurella pseudotuberculosis infection
Mesenteric adenitis }
Septic infection (cat bite) } by Pasteurella multocida
(dog bite) } [P. septica]
EXCLUDES infection by:
Francisella [Pasteurella] tularensis (021.0-021.9)
Yersinia [Pasteurella] pestis (020.0-020.9)
DEF: Swelling, abscesses, or septicemia from Pasteurella multocida, commonly transmitted to humans by a dog or cat scratch.
AHA: 3Q, '12, 13

027.8 Other specified zoonotic bacterial diseases

---

§ Requires fifth digit. Valid digits are in [brackets] under each code. See beginning of section 010-018 for codes and definitions.

✓4ᵗʰ / ✓5ᵗʰ Additional Digit Required | Unspecified Code | Other Specified Code | Manifestation Code | ►◄ Revised Text | ● New Code | ▲ Revised Code Title

027.9 Unspecified zoonotic bacterial disease

Other Bacterial Diseases (030-041)

EXCLUDES   bacterial venereal diseases (098.0-099.9)
bartonellosis (088.0)

√4ᵗʰ **030 Leprosy**

INCLUDES   Hansen's disease
infection by Mycobacterium leprae

030.0 Lepromatous [type L]
Lepromatous leprosy (macular) (diffuse) (infiltrated) (nodular) (neuritic)
DEF: Infectious, disseminated leprosy bacilli with lesions and deformities.

030.1 Tuberculoid [type T]
Tuberculoid leprosy (macular) (maculoanesthetic) (major) (minor) (neuritic)
DEF: Relatively benign, self-limiting leprosy with neuralgia and scales.

030.2 Indeterminate [group I]
Indeterminate [uncharacteristic] leprosy (macular) (neuritic)
DEF: Uncharacteristic leprosy, frequently an early manifestation.

030.3 Borderline [group B]
Borderline or dimorphous leprosy (infiltrated) (neuritic)
DEF: Transitional form of leprosy, neither lepromatous nor tuberculoid.

030.8 Other specified leprosy

030.9 Leprosy, unspecified

√4ᵗʰ **031 Diseases due to other mycobacteria**

031.0 Pulmonary
Battey disease
Infection by Mycobacterium:
avium
intracellulare [Battey bacillus]
kansasii
AHA: ▶2Q, '13, 17◀

031.1 Cutaneous
Buruli ulcer
Infection by Mycobacterium:
marinum [M. balnei]
ulcerans

031.2 Disseminated
Disseminated mycobacterium avium-intracellulare complex (DMAC)
Mycobacterium avium-intracellulare complex (MAC) bacteremia
DEF: Disseminated mycobacterium avium-intracellulare complex (DMAC): A serious systemic form of MAC commonly observed in patients in the late course of AIDS.
DEF: Mycobacterium avium-intracellulare complex (MAC) bacterium: Human pulmonary disease, lymphadenitis in children and systemic disease in immunocompromised individuals caused by a slow growing, gram-positive, aerobic organism.
AHA: 4Q, '97, 31

031.8 Other specified mycobacterial diseases

031.9 Unspecified diseases due to mycobacteria
Atypical mycobacterium infection NOS

√4ᵗʰ **032 Diphtheria**

INCLUDES   infection by Corynebacterium diphtheriae

032.0 Faucial diphtheria
Membranous angina, diphtheritic
DEF: Diphtheria of the throat.

032.1 Nasopharyngeal diphtheria

032.2 Anterior nasal diphtheria

032.3 Laryngeal diphtheria
Laryngotracheitis, diphtheritic

√5ᵗʰ **032.8 Other specified diphtheria**

032.81 Conjunctival diphtheria
Pseudomembranous diphtheritic conjunctivitis

032.82 Diphtheritic myocarditis

032.83 Diphtheritic peritonitis

032.84 Diphtheritic cystitis

032.85 Cutaneous diphtheria
AHA: ▶1Q, '14, 5◀

032.89 Other

032.9 Diphtheria, unspecified

√4ᵗʰ **033 Whooping cough**

INCLUDES   pertussis

Use additional code to identify any associated pneumonia (484.3)
DEF: An acute, highly contagious respiratory tract infection caused by Bordetella pertussis and B. bronchiseptica; characteristic paroxysmal cough.

033.0 Bordetella pertussis [B. pertussis]

033.1 Bordetella parapertussis [B. parapertussis]

033.8 Whooping cough due to other specified organism
Bordetella bronchiseptica [B. bronchiseptica]

033.9 Whooping cough, unspecified organism

√4ᵗʰ **034 Streptococcal sore throat and scarlet fever**

034.0 Streptococcal sore throat

Septic:	Streptococcal:
angina	laryngitis
sore throat	pharyngitis
Streptococcal:	tonsillitis
angina	

J02.0 Streptococcal pharyngitis   I-10

034.1 Scarlet fever
Scarlatina
EXCLUDES   parascarlatina (057.8)
DEF: Streptococcal infection and fever with red rash spreading from trunk.

035 Erysipelas
EXCLUDES   postpartum or puerperal erysipelas (670.8)
DEF: An acute superficial cellulitis involving the dermal lymphatics; it is often caused by group A streptococci.

√4ᵗʰ **036 Meningococcal infection**

036.0 Meningococcal meningitis
Cerebrospinal fever (meningococcal)
Meningitis:
cerebrospinal
epidemic

036.1 Meningococcal encephalitis

036.2 Meningococcemia
Meningococcal septicemia

036.3 Waterhouse-Friderichsen syndrome, meningococcal
Meningococcal hemorrhagic adrenalitis
Meningococcic adrenal syndrome
Waterhouse-Friderichsen syndrome NOS

√5ᵗʰ **036.4 Meningococcal carditis**

036.40 Meningococcal carditis, unspecified

036.41 Meningococcal pericarditis
DEF: Meningococcal infection of the outer membrane of the heart.

036.42 Meningococcal endocarditis
DEF: Meningococcal infection of the membranes lining the cavities of the heart.

036.43 Meningococcal myocarditis
DEF: Meningococcal infection of the muscle of the heart.

√5ᵗʰ **036.8 Other specified meningococcal infections**

036.81 Meningococcal optic neuritis

036.82 Meningococcal arthropathy

036.89 Other

036.9 Meningococcal infection, unspecified
Meningococcal infection NOS

N Newborn Age: 0   P Pediatric Age: 0-17   M Maternity Age: 12-55   A Adult Age: 15-124

037 Tetanus

> EXCLUDES *tetanus:*
> *complicating:*
> *abortion (634-638 with .0, 639.0)*
> *ectopic or molar pregnancy (639.0)*
> *neonatorum (771.3)*
> *puerperal (670.8)*

DEF: An acute, often fatal, infectious disease caused by the anaerobic, spore-forming bacillus *Clostridium tetani;* the bacillus enters the body through a contaminated wound, burns, surgical wounds, or cutaneous ulcers. Symptoms: lockjaw, spasms, seizures, and paralysis.

√4ᵗʰ **038 Septicemia**

Use additional code for systemic inflammatory response syndrome (SIRS) (995.91-995.92)

> EXCLUDES *bacteremia (790.7)*
> *during labor (659.3)*
> *following ectopic or molar pregnancy (639.0)*
> *following infusion, injection, transfusion, or vaccination (999.3)*
> *postpartum, puerperal (670)*
> *septicemia (sepsis) of newborn (771.81)*
> *that complicating abortion (634-638 with .0, 639.0)*

DEF: A systemic disease associated with the presence and persistence of pathogenic microorganisms or their toxins in the blood.
AHA: 3Q, '12, 11-12; 1Q, '12, 19; 2Q, '10, 4; 2Q, '04, 16; 4Q, '88, 10; 3Q, '88, 12
TIP: When septicemia is due to a complication of care, sequence the complication code first (e.g., due to device or injury).

038.0 Streptococcal septicemia
> **AHA:** 4Q, '03, 79; 2Q, '96, 5

√5ᵗʰ **038.1 Staphylococcal septicemia**
> **AHA:** 4Q, '97, 32

    038.10 Staphylococcal septicemia, unspecified

    038.11 Methicillin susceptible Staphylococcus aureus septicemia
> MSSA septicemia
> Staphylococcus aureus septicemia NOS
> **AHA:** 4Q, '08, 69-70; 1Q, '05, 7; 2Q, '00, 5; 4Q, '98, 42
> **A41.01** Sepsis d/t Methicillin susceptible   I-10
> Staphylococcus aureus

    038.12 Methicillin resistant Staphylococcus aureus septicemia
> **AHA:** 4Q, '11,153; 3Q, '11, 15; 4Q, '08, 69-73

    038.19 Other staphylococcal septicemia
> **AHA:** 2Q, '00, 5
> **A41.1** Sepsis due to other spec Staphylococcus   I-10

038.2 Pneumococcal septicemia [Streptococcus pneumoniae septicemia]
> **AHA:** 2Q, '96, 5; 1Q, '91, 13

038.3 Septicemia due to anaerobes
> Septicemia due to bacteroides
> EXCLUDES *gas gangrene (040.0)*
> *that due to anaerobic streptococci (038.0)*
> **DEF:** Infection of blood by microorganisms that thrive without oxygen.

√5ᵗʰ **038.4 Septicemia due to other gram-negative organisms**
> **DEF:** Infection of blood by microorganisms categorized as gram-negative by Gram's method of staining for identification of bacteria.

    038.40 Gram-negative organism, unspecified
> Gram-negative septicemia NOS

    038.41 Hemophilus influenzae [H. influenzae]

    038.42 Escherichia coli [E. coli]
> **AHA:** 4Q, '03, 73
> **A41.51** Sepsis due to Escherichia coli [E coli]   I-10

    038.43 Pseudomonas

    038.44 Serratia

    038.49 Other
> **A41.59** Other Gram-negative sepsis   I-10
> **AHA:** 3Q, '12, 13

038.8 Other specified septicemias
> EXCLUDES *septicemia (due to):*
> *anthrax (022.3)*
> *gonococcal (098.89)*
> *herpetic (054.5)*
> *meningococcal (036.2)*
> *septicemic plague (020.2)*

038.9 Unspecified septicemia
> Septicemia NOS
> EXCLUDES *bacteremia NOS (790.7)*
> **AHA:** 4Q, '07, 97; 2Q, '05, 18-19; 2Q, '04, 16; 4Q, '03, 79; 2Q, '00, 3; 3Q, '99, 5, 9; 1Q, '98, 5; 3Q, '96, 16; 2Q, '96, 6
> **TIP:** Ensure that documentation includes clinical evidence of systemic infection; do not code if documentation indicates "urosepsis" only.
> **A41.9** Sepsis unspecified   I-10

√4ᵗʰ **039 Actinomycotic infections**
> INCLUDES actinomycotic mycetoma
> infection by Actinomycetales, such as species of Actinomyces, Actinomadura, Nocardia, Streptomyces
> maduromycosis (actinomycotic)
> schizomycetoma (actinomycotic)

DEF: Inflammatory lesions and abscesses at site of infection by *Actinomyces israelii.*

039.0 Cutaneous
> Erythrasma
> Trichomycosis axillaris

039.1 Pulmonary
> Thoracic actinomycosis

039.2 Abdominal

039.3 Cervicofacial

039.4 Madura foot
> EXCLUDES *madura foot due to mycotic infection (117.4)*

039.8 Of other specified sites

039.9 Of unspecified site
> Actinomycosis NOS
> Maduromycosis NOS
> Nocardiosis NOS

√4ᵗʰ **040 Other bacterial diseases**
> EXCLUDES *bacteremia NOS (790.7)*
> *bacterial infection NOS (041.9)*

040.0 Gas gangrene
> Gas bacillus infection or gangrene
> Infection by Clostridium:
> histolyticum
> oedematiens
> perfringens [welchii]
> septicum
> sordellii
> Malignant edema
> Myonecrosis, clostridial
> Myositis, clostridial
> **AHA:** 1Q, '95, 11

040.1 Rhinoscleroma
> **DEF:** Growths on the nose and nasopharynx caused by *Klebsiella rhinoscleromatis.*

040.2 Whipple's disease
> Intestinal lipodystrophy

040.3 Necrobacillosis
> **DEF:** Infection with *Fusobacterium necrophorum* causing abscess or necrosis.
> **AHA:** 4Q, '07, 85

√4ᵗʰ √5ᵗʰ Additional Digit Required   Unspecified Code   Other Specified Code   Manifestation Code   ▶◀ Revised Text   ● New Code   ▲ Revised Code Title

2015 ICD-9-CM   **Volume 1 – 7**

Infectious and Parasitic Diseases

037–040.3

√5ᵗʰ **040.4 Other specified botulism**
Non-foodborne intoxication due to toxins of Clostridium botulinum [C. botulinum]

> **EXCLUDES** *botulism NOS (005.1)*
> *food poisoning due to toxins of Clostridium botulinum (005.1)*

040.41 Infant botulism   **P**
DEF: Colonization of Clostridium botulinum spores in the large intestine; release of neurotoxins results in constipation; may progress to neuromuscular paralysis; affects infants of less than six months.
AHA: 4Q, '07, 60

040.42 Wound botulism
Non-foodborne botulism NOS
Use additional code to identify complicated open wound
AHA: 4Q, '07, 60

√5ᵗʰ **040.8 Other specified bacterial diseases**

040.81 Tropical pyomyositis

040.82 Toxic shock syndrome
Use additional code to identify the organism
DEF: Syndrome caused by staphylococcal exotoxin that may rapidly progress to severe and intractable shock; symptoms include sunburn-like rash with peeling of skin on palms and soles, sudden onset high fever, vomiting, diarrhea, myalgia, and hypotension.
AHA: ▶2Q, '13, 21;◀ 4Q, '02, 44

040.89 Other
AHA: N-D, '86, 7

√4ᵗʰ **041 Bacterial infection in conditions classified elsewhere and of unspecified site**
> **NOTE** This category is provided to be used as an additional code to identify the bacterial agent in diseases classified elsewhere. This category will also be used to classify bacterial infections of unspecified nature or site.

> **EXCLUDES** *septicemia (038.0-038.9)*
AHA: 2Q, '01, 12; J-A, '84, 19

√5ᵗʰ **041.0 Streptococcus**

041.00 Streptococcus, unspecified

041.01 Group A
AHA: 1Q, '02, 3

041.02 Group B
B95.1 Streptococcus group B cause of dz class elsewhere   **I-10**

041.03 Group C

041.04 Group D [Enterococcus]
B95.2 Enterococcus as the cause of dz class elsewhere   **I-10**

041.05 Group G

041.09 Other Streptococcus
B95.4 Oth streptococcus cause of dz class elsewhere   **I-10**

√5ᵗʰ **041.1 Staphylococcus**

041.10 Staphylococcus, unspecified
AHA: 2Q, '06, 15

041.11 Methicillin susceptible Staphylococcus aureus
MSSA
Staphylococcus aureus NOS
AHA: 4Q, '08, 69-70; 2Q, '06, 16; 4Q, '03, 104, 106; 2Q, '01, 11; 4Q, '98, 42, 54; 4Q, '97, 32
A49.01 Methicillin suscep staph infection, unsp site   **I-10**

041.12 Methicillin resistant Staphylococcus aureus
Methicillin-resistant staphylococcus aureus (MRSA)
AHA: 4Q, '09, 98; 4Q, '08, 69-70, 73
TIP: Do not assign if combination code (with localized infection) available, or if only colonization or carrier status documented.

041.19 Other Staphylococcus
AHA: 2Q, '11, 7; 2Q, '08, 3
B95.7 Other staphylococcus cause of dz class elsewhere   **I-10**

041.2 Pneumococcus

041.3 Klebsiella pneumoniae
AHA: 4Q, '08, 149

√5ᵗʰ **041.4 Escherichia coli [E. coli]**
AHA: 4Q, '11, 81-83

041.41 Shiga toxin-producing Escherichia coli [E. coli] (STEC) O157
E. coli O157:H- (nonmotile) with confirmation of Shiga toxin
E. coli O157 with confirmation of Shiga toxin when H antigen is unknown, or is not H7
O157:H7 Escherichia coli [E.coli] with or without confirmation of Shiga toxin-production
Shiga toxin-producing Escherichia coli [E.coli] O157:H7 with or without confirmation of Shiga toxin-production
STEC O157:H7 with or without confirmation of Shiga toxin-production
AHA: 4Q, '11, 83

041.42 Other specified Shiga toxin-producing Escherichia coli [E. coli] (STEC)
Non-O157 Shiga toxin-producing Escherichia coli [E.coli]
Non-O157 Shiga toxin-producing Escherichia coli [E.coli] with known O group

041.43 Shiga toxin-producing Escherichia coli [E. coli] (STEC), unspecified
Shiga toxin-producing Escherichia coli [E. coli] with unspecified O group
STEC NOS

041.49 Other and unspecified Escherichia coli [E. coli]
Escherichia coli [E. coli] NOS
Non-Shiga toxin-producing E. Coli
AHA: 4Q, '11, 155
B96.20 Unsp Escherichia coli as cause of diseases classd elswhr   **I-10**

041.5 Hemophilus influenzae [H. influenzae]

041.6 Proteus (mirabilis) (morganii)

041.7 Pseudomonas
AHA: 1Q, '10, 9; 4Q, '02, 45
B96.5 Pseudomonas as the cause of dz class elsewhere   **I-10**

√5ᵗʰ **041.8 Other specified bacterial infections**

041.81 Mycoplasma
Eaton's agent
Pleuropneumonia-like organisms [PPLO]

041.82 Bacteroides fragilis
DEF: Anaerobic gram-negative bacilli of the gastrointestinal tract; frequently implicated in intra-abdominal infection; commonly resistant to antibiotics.

041.83 Clostridium perfringens

041.84 Other anaerobes
Gram-negative anaerobes
> **EXCLUDES** *Helicobacter pylori (041.86)*

041.85 Other gram-negative organisms
Aerobacter aerogenes
Gram-negative bacteria NOS
Mima polymorpha
Serratia
> **EXCLUDES** *gram-negative anaerobes (041.84)*
AHA: 1Q, '95, 18

041.86 Helicobacter pylori [H. pylori]
AHA: 4Q, '95, 60
B96.81 Helicobacter pylori cause of dz class elsewhere   **I-10**

041.89 Other specified bacteria
AHA: 2Q, '06, 7; 2Q, '03, 7
A49.8 Other bacterial infections of unspec site   **I-10**

041.9 Bacterial infection, unspecified
AHA: 2Q, '91, 9

N Newborn Age: 0   **P** Pediatric Age: 0-17   **M** Maternity Age: 12-55   **A** Adult Age: 15-124

Human Immunodeficiency Virus (HIV) Infection (042)

042 Human immunodeficiency virus [HIV] disease
Acquired immune deficiency syndrome
Acquired immunodeficiency syndrome
AIDS
AIDS-like syndrome
AIDS-related complex
ARC
HIV infection, symptomatic

Use additional code(s) to identify all manifestations of HIV

Use additional code to identify HIV-2 infection (079.53)

EXCLUDES asymptomatic HIV infection status (V08)
exposure to HIV virus (V01.79)
nonspecific serologic evidence of HIV (795.71)

AHA: 3Q, '10, 13; 4Q, '07, 63; 3Q, '06, 15; 1Q, '05, 7; 2Q, '04, 11; 1Q, '04, 5; 1Q, '03, 15; 1Q, '99, 14; 4Q, '97, 30, 31; 1Q, '93, 21; 2Q, '92, 11; 3Q, '90, 17; J-A, '87, 8

TIP: Code only confirmed cases of HIV infection/illness; may be coded from provider's diagnostic statement.

B20 Human immunodeficiency virus [HIV] disease   I-10

Poliomyelitis and Other Non-Arthropod-Borne Viral Diseases and Prion Diseases of Central Nervous System (045-049)

045 Acute poliomyelitis

EXCLUDES late effects of acute poliomyelitis (138)

The following fifth-digit subclassification is for use with category 045:
0 poliovirus, unspecified type
1 poliovirus type I
2 poliovirus type II
3 poliovirus type III

§ **045.0 Acute paralytic poliomyelitis specified as bulbar**
[0-3] Infantile paralysis (acute) } specified as
Poliomyelitis (acute) (anterior) } bulbar
Polioencephalitis (acute) (bulbar)
Polioencephalomyelitis (acute) (anterior) (bulbar)

DEF: Acute paralytic infection occurring where the brain merges with the spinal cord; affecting breathing, swallowing, and heart rate.

§ **045.1 Acute poliomyelitis with other paralysis**
[0-3] Paralysis:
acute atrophic, spinal
infantile, paralytic
Poliomyelitis (acute) } with paralysis except
anterior } bulbar
epidemic }

DEF: Paralytic infection affecting peripheral or spinal nerves.

§ **045.2 Acute nonparalytic poliomyelitis**
[0-3] Poliomyelitis (acute) }
anterior } specified as nonparalytic
epidemic }

DEF: Nonparalytic infection causing pain, stiffness, and paresthesias.

§ **045.9 Acute poliomyelitis, unspecified**
[0-3] Infantile paralysis }
Poliomyelitis (acute) } unspecified whether
anterior } paralytic or
epidemic } nonparalytic

046 Slow virus infections and prion diseases of central nervous system

046.0 Kuru
DEF: A chronic, progressive, fatal nervous system disorder; clinical symptoms include cerebellar ataxia, trembling, spasticity and progressive dementia.

046.1 Jakob-Creutzfeldt disease
Use additional code to identify dementia:
with behavioral disturbance (294.11)
without behavioral disturbance (294.10)

046.11 Variant Creutzfeldt-Jakob disease
vCJD
AHA: 4Q, '08, 73-75

046.19 Other and unspecified Creutzfeldt-Jacob disease
CJD
Familial Creutzfeldt-Jakob disease
Iatrogenic Creutzfeldt-Jakob disease
Jakob-Creutzfeldt disease, unspecified
Sporadic Creutzfeldt-Jakob disease
Subacute spongiform encephalopathy
EXCLUDES variant Creutzfeldt-Jakob disease (vCJD) (046.11)
DEF: Communicable, progressive spongiform encephalopathy thought to be caused by an infectious particle known as a "prion" (proteinaceous infection particle); a progressive, fatal disease manifested principally by mental deterioration.
AHA: 4Q, '08, 73-75

046.2 Subacute sclerosing panencephalitis
Dawson's inclusion body encephalitis
Van Bogaert's sclerosing leukoencephalitis
DEF: Progressive viral infection causing cerebral dysfunction, blindness, dementia, and death (SSPE).

046.3 Progressive multifocal leukoencephalopathy
Multifocal leukoencephalopathy NOS
DEF: Infection affecting cerebral cortex in patients with weakened immune systems.

046.7 Other specified prion diseases of central nervous system
EXCLUDES Creutzfeldt-Jakob disease (046.11-046.19)
Jakob-Creutzfeldt disease (046.11-046.19)
kuru (046.0)
variant Creutzfeldt-Jakob disease (vCJD) (046.11)

046.71 Gerstmann-Sträussler-Scheinker syndrome
GSS syndrome
AHA: 4Q, '08, 73-75

046.72 Fatal familial insomnia
FFI
AHA: 4Q, '08, 73-75

046.79 Other and unspecified prion disease of central nervous system

046.8 Other specified slow virus infection of central nervous system

046.9 Unspecified slow virus infection of central nervous system

047 Meningitis due to enterovirus
INCLUDES meningitis:
abacterial
aseptic
viral
EXCLUDES meningitis due to:
adenovirus (049.1)
arthropod-borne virus (060.0-066.9)
leptospira (100.81)
virus of:
herpes simplex (054.72)
herpes zoster (053.0)
lymphocytic choriomeningitis (049.0)
mumps (072.1)
poliomyelitis (045.0-045.9)
any other infection specifically classified elsewhere
AHA: J-F, '87, 6

047.0 Coxsackie virus

047.1 ECHO virus
Meningo-eruptive syndrome

047.8 Other specified viral meningitis

047.9 Unspecified viral meningitis
Viral meningitis NOS
A87.9 Viral meningitis unspecified   I-10

048 Other enterovirus diseases of central nervous system
Boston exanthem

---

§ Requires fifth digit. Valid digits are in [brackets] under each code. See category 045 for codes and definitions.

Additional Digit Required **Unspecified Code** **Other Specified Code** **Manifestation Code** ►◄ Revised Text ● New Code ▲ Revised Code Title

2015 ICD-9-CM **Volume 1 – 9**

Infectious and Parasitic Diseases

049–054.2

✓4ᵗʰ **049 Other non-arthropod-borne viral diseases of central nervous system**

> EXCLUDES *late effects of viral encephalitis (139.0)*

049.0 Lymphocytic choriomeningitis
Lymphocytic:
meningitis (serous) (benign)
meningoencephalitis (serous) (benign)

049.1 Meningitis due to adenovirus
> DEF: Inflammation of lining of brain caused by Arenaviruses and usually occurring in adults in fall and winter months.

049.8 Other specified non-arthropod-borne viral diseases of central nervous system
Encephalitis: Encephalitis:
acute: lethargica
inclusion body   Rio Bravo
necrotizing   von Economo's disease
epidemic
> EXCLUDES *human herpesvirus 6 encephalitis (058.21)*
> *other human herpesvirus encephalitis (058.29)*

049.9 Unspecified non-arthropod-borne viral diseases of central nervous system
Viral encephalitis NOS

Viral Diseases Generally Accompanied by Exanthem (050-059)

> EXCLUDES *arthropod-borne viral diseases (060.0-066.9)*
> *Boston exanthem (048)*

✓4ᵗʰ **050 Smallpox**

050.0 Variola major
Hemorrhagic (pustular) smallpox
Malignant smallpox
Purpura variolosa
> DEF: Form of smallpox known for its high mortality; exists only in laboratories.

050.1 Alastrim
Variola minor
> DEF: Mild form of smallpox known for its low mortality rate.

050.2 Modified smallpox
Varioloid
> DEF: Mild form occurring in patients with history of infection or vaccination.

050.9 Smallpox, unspecified

✓4ᵗʰ **051 Cowpox and paravaccinia**

✓5ᵗʰ **051.0 Cowpox and vaccinia not from vaccination**

051.01 Cowpox
> DEF: A disease contracted by milking infected cows; vesicles usually appear on the fingers, hands and adjacent areas and usually disappear without scarring; other symptoms: local edema, lymphangitis, and regional lymphadenitis with or without fever.
> AHA: 4Q, '08, 76-77

051.02 Vaccinia not from vaccination
> EXCLUDES *vaccinia (generalized) (from vaccination) (999.0)*
> AHA: 4Q, '08, 76-77

051.1 Pseudocowpox
Milkers' node
> DEF: Hand lesions and mild fever in dairy workers caused by exposure to paravaccinia.

051.2 Contagious pustular dermatitis
Ecthyma contagiosum
Orf
> DEF: Skin eruptions caused by exposure to poxvirus-infected sheep or goats.

051.9 Paravaccinia, unspecified

✓4ᵗʰ **052 Chickenpox**
> DEF: Contagious infection by *Varicella-zoster* virus causing rash with pustules and fever.

052.0 Postvaricella encephalitis
Postchickenpox encephalitis

052.1 Varicella (hemorrhagic) pneumonitis

052.2 Postvaricella myelitis
Postchickenpox myelitis
> AHA: 4Q, '06, 58-63

052.7 With other specified complications
> AHA: 1Q, '02, 3

052.8 With unspecified complication

052.9 Varicella without mention of complication
Chickenpox NOS   Varicella NOS

✓4ᵗʰ **053 Herpes zoster**
> INCLUDES shingles
> zona
> DEF: Self-limiting infection by *Varicella-zoster* virus causing unilateral eruptions and neuralgia along affected nerves.

053.0 With meningitis
> DEF: *Varicella-zoster* virus infection causing inflammation of the lining of the brain and/or spinal cord.

✓5ᵗʰ **053.1 With other nervous system complications**

053.10 With unspecified nervous system complication

053.11 Geniculate herpes zoster
Herpetic geniculate ganglionitis
> DEF: Unilateral eruptions and neuralgia along the facial nerve geniculum affecting face and outer and middle ear.

053.12 Postherpetic trigeminal neuralgia
> DEF: Severe oral or nasal pain following a herpes zoster infection.

053.13 Postherpetic polyneuropathy
> DEF: Multiple areas of pain following a herpes zoster infection.

053.14 Herpes zoster myelitis
> AHA: 4Q, '06, 58-63

053.19 Other

✓5ᵗʰ **053.2 With ophthalmic complications**

053.20 Herpes zoster dermatitis of eyelid
Herpes zoster ophthalmicus

053.21 Herpes zoster keratoconjunctivitis

053.22 Herpes zoster iridocyclitis

053.29 Other

✓5ᵗʰ **053.7 With other specified complications**

053.71 Otitis externa due to herpes zoster

053.79 Other

053.8 With unspecified complication

053.9 Herpes zoster without mention of complication
Herpes zoster NOS
> **B02.9** Zoster without complications   I-10

✓4ᵗʰ **054 Herpes simplex**
> EXCLUDES *congenital herpes simplex (771.2)*

054.0 Eczema herpeticum
Kaposi's varicelliform eruption
> DEF: Herpes simplex virus invading site of preexisting skin inflammation.

✓5ᵗʰ **054.1 Genital herpes**
> AHA: J-F, '87, 15, 16

054.10 Genital herpes, unspecified
Herpes progenitalis
> AHA: 2Q, '10, 10
> **A60.00** Herpesviral infection urogenital system unspec   I-10

054.11 Herpetic vulvovaginitis   ♀

054.12 Herpetic ulceration of vulva   ♀

054.13 Herpetic infection of penis   ♂

054.19 Other

054.2 Herpetic gingivostomatitis

Infectious and Parasitic Diseases

054.3　Herpetic meningoencephalitis
Herpes encephalitis　Simian B disease
　　EXCLUDES　*human herpesvirus 6 encephalitis (058.21)*
　　　　　　　　other human herpesvirus encephalitis (058.29)
　　DEF: Inflammation of the brain and its lining, caused by infection of
　　herpes simplex 1 in adults and simplex 2 in newborns.

√5th **054.4　With ophthalmic complications**

　　054.40　With unspecified ophthalmic complication

　　054.41　Herpes simplex dermatitis of eyelid

　　054.42　Dendritic keratitis

　　054.43　Herpes simplex disciform keratitis

　　054.44　Herpes simplex iridocyclitis

　　054.49　Other

054.5　Herpetic septicemia
　　AHA: 2Q, '00, 5

054.6　Herpetic whitlow
Herpetic felon
　　DEF: A primary infection of the terminal segment of a finger by
　　herpes simplex; intense itching and pain start the disease, vesicles
　　form, and tissue ultimately is destroyed.

√5th **054.7　With other specified complications**

　　054.71　Visceral herpes simplex

　　054.72　Herpes simplex meningitis

　　054.73　Herpes simplex otitis externa

　　054.74　Herpes simplex myelitis
　　　　AHA: 4Q, '06, 58-63

　　054.79　Other

054.8　With unspecified complication

054.9　Herpes simplex without mention of complication
　　B00.9　Herpesviral infection unspecified　　I-10

√4th **055　Measles**
　　INCLUDES　morbilli
　　　　　　　　rubeola

055.0　Postmeasles encephalitis

055.1　Postmeasles pneumonia

055.2　Postmeasles otitis media

√5th **055.7　With other specified complications**

　　055.71　Measles keratoconjunctivitis
　　　　Measles keratitis

　　055.79　Other

055.8　With unspecified complication

055.9　Measles without mention of complication

√4th **056　Rubella**
　　INCLUDES　German measles
　　EXCLUDES　*congenital rubella (771.0)*
　　DEF: Acute but usually benign togavirus infection causing fever, sore throat,
　　and rash; associated with complications to fetus as a result of maternal
　　infection.

√5th **056.0　With neurological complications**

　　056.00　With unspecified neurological complication

　　056.01　Encephalomyelitis due to rubella
　　　　Encephalitis　　　　　　　}
　　　　Meningoencephalitis　　　} due to rubella

　　056.09　Other

√5th **056.7　With other specified complications**

　　056.71　Arthritis due to rubella

　　056.79　Other

056.8　With unspecified complications

056.9　Rubella without mention of complication

√4th **057　Other viral exanthemata**
　　DEF: Skin eruptions or rashes and fever caused by viruses, including
　　poxviruses.

057.0　Erythema infectiosum [fifth disease]
　　DEF: A moderately contagious, benign, epidemic disease, usually
　　seen in children, of probable viral etiology; a red macular rash
　　appears on face and may spread to the limbs and trunk.

057.8　Other specified viral exanthemata
Dukes (-Filatow) disease
Fourth disease
Parascarlatina
Pseudoscarlatina
　　EXCLUDES　*exanthema subitum [sixth disease] (058.10-058.12)*
　　　　　　　　roseola infantum (058.10-058.12)

057.9　Viral exanthem, unspecified

√4th **058　Other human herpesvirus**
　　EXCLUDES　*congenital herpes (771.2)*
　　　　　　　　cytomegalovirus (078.5)
　　　　　　　　Epstein-Barr virus (075)
　　　　　　　　herpes NOS (054.0-054.9)
　　　　　　　　herpes simplex (054.0-054.9)
　　　　　　　　herpes zoster (053.0-053.9)
　　　　　　　　human herpesvirus NOS (054.0-054.9)
　　　　　　　　human herpesvirus 1 (054.0-054.9)
　　　　　　　　human herpesvirus 2 (054.0-054.9)
　　　　　　　　human herpesvirus 3 (052.0-053.9)
　　　　　　　　human herpesvirus 4 (075)
　　　　　　　　human herpesvirus 5 (078.5)
　　　　　　　　varicella (052.0-052.9)
　　　　　　　　varicella-zoster virus (052.0-053.9)
　　AHA: 4Q, '07, 61

√5th **058.1　Roseola infantum**
　　Exanthema subitum [sixth disease]

　　058.10　Roseola infantum, unspecified　　P
　　　　Exanthema subitum [sixth disease], unspecified
　　　　AHA: 4Q, '07, 63

　　058.11　Roseola infantum due to human herpesvirus 6　　P
　　　　Exanthema subitum [sixth disease] due to human
　　　　herpesvirus 6

　　058.12　Roseola infantum due to human herpesvirus 7　　P
　　　　Exanthema subitum [sixth disease] due to human
　　　　herpesvirus 7

√5th **058.2　Other human herpesvirus encephalitis**
　　EXCLUDES　*herpes encephalitis NOS (054.3)*
　　　　　　　　herpes simplex encephalitis (054.3)
　　　　　　　　human herpesvirus encephalitis NOS (054.3)
　　　　　　　　simian B herpesvirus encephalitis (054.3)

　　058.21　Human herpesvirus 6 encephalitis

　　058.29　Other human herpesvirus encephalitis
　　　　Human herpesvirus 7 encephalitis

√5th **058.8　Other human herpesvirus infections**

　　058.81　Human herpesvirus 6 infection

　　058.82　Human herpesvirus 7 infection

　　058.89　Other human herpesvirus infection
　　　　Human herpesvirus 8 infection
　　　　Kaposi's sarcoma-associated herpesvirus infection
　　　　AHA: 4Q, '07, 63

√4th **059　Other poxvirus infections**
　　EXCLUDES　*contagious pustular dermatitis (051.2)*
　　　　　　　　cowpox (051.01)
　　　　　　　　ecthyma contagiosum (051.2)
　　　　　　　　milker's nodule (051.1)
　　　　　　　　orf (051.2)
　　　　　　　　paravaccinia NOS (051.9)
　　　　　　　　pseudocowpox (051.1)
　　　　　　　　smallpox (050.0-050.9)
　　　　　　　　vaccinia (generalized) (from vaccination) (999.0)
　　　　　　　　vaccinia not from vaccination (051.02)
　　AHA: 4Q, '08, 76-78

√5th **059.0　Other orthopoxvirus infections**

　　059.00　Orthopoxvirus infection, unspecified

059.01 **Monkeypox**

059.09 Other orthopoxvirus infection

☑5ᵗʰ 059.1 **Other parapoxvirus infections**

059.10 Parapoxvirus infection, unspecified

059.11 **Bovine stomatitis**

059.12 **Sealpox**

059.19 Other parapoxvirus infections

☑5ᵗʰ 059.2 **Yatapoxvirus infections**

059.20 Yatapoxvirus infection, unspecified

059.21 **Tanapox**

059.22 **Yaba monkey tumor virus**

059.8 Other poxvirus infections

059.9 Poxvirus infections, unspecified

Arthropod-borne Viral Diseases (060-066)

Use additional code to identify any associated meningitis (321.2)

EXCLUDES late effects of viral encephalitis (139.0)

☑4ᵗʰ 060 **Yellow fever**

DEF: Fever and jaundice from infection by mosquito-borne virus of genus *Flavivirus*.

060.0 **Sylvatic**

Yellow fever: Yellow fever:
  jungle   sylvan

DEF: Yellow fever transmitted from animal to man, via mosquito.

060.1 **Urban**

DEF: Yellow fever transmitted from man to man, via mosquito.

060.9 Yellow fever, unspecified

061 **Dengue**

Breakbone fever

EXCLUDES *hemorrhagic fever caused by dengue virus (065.4)*

DEF: Acute, self-limiting infection by mosquito-borne virus characterized by fever and generalized aches.

☑4ᵗʰ 062 **Mosquito-borne viral encephalitis**

062.0 **Japanese encephalitis**

Japanese B encephalitis

DEF: Flavivirus causing inflammation of the brain, with a wide range of clinical manifestations.

062.1 **Western equine encephalitis**

DEF: Alphavirus WEE infection causing inflammation of the brain, found in areas west of the Mississippi; transmitted horse to mosquito to man.

062.2 **Eastern equine encephalitis**

EXCLUDES *Venezuelan equine encephalitis (066.2)*

DEF: Alphavirus EEE causing inflammation of the brain and spinal cord, found from Canada to South America and Mexico; transmitted horse to mosquito to man.

062.3 **St. Louis encephalitis**

DEF: Epidemic form caused by Flavivirus and transmitted by mosquito, and characterized by fever, difficulty in speech, and headache.

062.4 **Australian encephalitis**

Australian arboencephalitis
Australian X disease
Murray Valley encephalitis

DEF: Flavivirus causing inflammation of the brain, occurring in Australia and New Guinea.

062.5 **California virus encephalitis**

Encephalitis: Tahyna fever
  California
  La Crosse

DEF: Bunyamwere virus causing inflammation of the brain.

062.8 Other specified mosquito-borne viral encephalitis

Encephalitis by Ilheus virus

EXCLUDES *West Nile virus (066.40-066.49)*

062.9 Mosquito-borne viral encephalitis, unspecified

☑4ᵗʰ 063 **Tick-borne viral encephalitis**

INCLUDES diphasic meningoencephalitis

063.0 **Russian spring-summer [taiga] encephalitis**

063.1 **Louping ill**

DEF: Inflammation of brain caused by virus transmitted sheep to tick to man; incidence usually limited to British Isles.

063.2 **Central European encephalitis**

DEF: Inflammation of brain caused by virus transmitted by tick; limited to central Europe and presenting with two distinct phases.

063.8 Other specified tick-borne viral encephalitis

Langat encephalitis   Powassan encephalitis

063.9 Tick-borne viral encephalitis, unspecified

064 Viral encephalitis transmitted by other and unspecified arthropods

Arthropod-borne viral encephalitis, vector unknown
Negishi virus encephalitis

EXCLUDES *viral encephalitis NOS (049.9)*

☑4ᵗʰ 065 **Arthropod-borne hemorrhagic fever**

065.0 **Crimean hemorrhagic fever [CHF Congo virus]**

Central Asian hemorrhagic fever

065.1 **Omsk hemorrhagic fever**

065.2 **Kyasanur Forest disease**

065.3 Other tick-borne hemorrhagic fever

065.4 **Mosquito-borne hemorrhagic fever**

Chikungunya hemorrhagic fever
Dengue hemorrhagic fever

EXCLUDES *Chikungunya fever (066.3)*
dengue (061)
yellow fever (060.0-060.9)

065.8 Other specified arthropod-borne hemorrhagic fever

Mite-borne hemorrhagic fever

065.9 Arthropod-borne hemorrhagic fever, unspecified

Arbovirus hemorrhagic fever NOS

☑4ᵗʰ 066 **Other arthropod-borne viral diseases**

066.0 **Phlebotomus fever**

Changuinola fever   Sandfly fever

DEF: Sandfly-borne viral infection occurring in Asia, Mideast and South America.

066.1 **Tick-borne fever**

Nairobi sheep disease   Tick fever:
Tick fever: Kemerovo
  American mountain   Quaranfil
  Colorado

066.2 **Venezuelan equine fever**

Venezuelan equine encephalitis

DEF: Alphavirus VEE infection causing inflammation of the brain, usually limited to South America, Mexico, and Florida; transmitted horse to mosquito to man.

066.3 Other mosquito-borne fever

Fever (viral):   Fever (viral):
  Bunyamwera   Oropouche
  Bwamba   Pixuna
  Chikungunya   Rift valley
  Guama   Ross river
  Mayaro   Wesselsbron
  Mucambo   Zika
  O'Nyong-Nyong

EXCLUDES *dengue (061)*
yellow fever (060.0-060.9)

☑5ᵗʰ 066.4 **West Nile fever**

AHA: 4Q, '02, 44

DEF: Mosquito-borne fever causing fatal inflammation of the brain, the lining of the brain, or of the lining of the brain and spinal cord.

066.40 West Nile fever, unspecified

West Nile fever NOS
West Nile fever without complications
West Nile virus NOS

Ⓝ Newborn Age: 0   Ⓟ Pediatric Age: 0-17   Ⓜ Maternity Age: 12-55   Ⓐ Adult Age: 15-124

Infectious and Parasitic Diseases

066.41 **West Nile fever with encephalitis**
West Nile encephalitis
West Nile encephalomyelitis
AHA: 4Q, '04, 51

066.42 **West Nile fever with other neurologic manifestation**
Use additional code to specify the neurologic manifestation
AHA: 4Q, '04, 51

066.49 **West Nile fever with other complications**
Use additional code to specify the other conditions

066.8 **Other specified arthropod-borne viral diseases**
Chandipura fever
Piry fever

066.9 **Arthropod-borne viral disease, unspecified**
Arbovirus infection NOS

Other Diseases Due to Viruses and Chlamydiae (070-079)

✓4ᵗʰ **070** **Viral hepatitis**
INCLUDES viral hepatitis (acute) (chronic)
EXCLUDES cytomegalic inclusion virus hepatitis (078.5)

The following fifth-digit subclassification is for use with categories 070.2 and 070.3:
  0 acute or unspecified, without mention of hepatitis delta
  1 acute or unspecified, with hepatitis delta
  2 chronic, without mention of hepatitis delta
  3 chronic, with hepatitis delta

DEF: Hepatitis A: HAV infection is self-limiting with flulike symptoms; transmission, fecal-oral.
DEF: Hepatitis B: HBV infection can be chronic and systemic; transmission, bodily fluids.
DEF: Hepatitis C: HCV infection can be chronic and systemic; transmission, blood transfusion and unidentified agents.
DEF: Hepatitis D (delta): HDV occurs only in the presence of hepatitis B virus.
DEF: Hepatitis E: HEV is epidemic form; transmission and nature under investigation.
AHA: 2Q,' 07, 5

070.0 **Viral hepatitis A with hepatic coma**

070.1 **Viral hepatitis A without mention of hepatic coma**
Infectious hepatitis

§ ✓5ᵗʰ **070.2** **Viral hepatitis B with hepatic coma**
[0-3]   **AHA:** 4Q, '91, 28; **For code 070.20:** 2Q, '07, 6

§ ✓5ᵗʰ **070.3** **Viral hepatitis B without mention of hepatic coma**
[0-3]   Serum hepatitis
  AHA: 1Q, '93, 28; 4Q, '91, 28
  B16.9 Acute hep B w/o delta-agent & w/o hepatic coma   **I-10**

✓5ᵗʰ **070.4** **Other specified viral hepatitis with hepatic coma**
  AHA: 4Q, '91, 28

  070.41 **Acute hepatitis C with hepatic coma**

  070.42 **Hepatitis delta without mention of active hepatitis B disease with hepatic coma**
    Hepatitis delta with hepatitis B carrier state

  070.43 **Hepatitis E with hepatic coma**

  070.44 **Chronic hepatitis C with hepatic coma**
    AHA: 2Q, '07, 5

  070.49 **Other specified viral hepatitis with hepatic coma**

✓5ᵗʰ **070.5** **Other specified viral hepatitis without mention of hepatic coma**
  AHA: 4Q, '91, 28

  070.51 **Acute hepatitis C without mention of hepatic coma**

  070.52 **Hepatitis delta without mention of active hepatititis B disease or hepatic coma**

  070.53 **Hepatitis E without mention of hepatic coma**

  070.54 **Chronic hepatitis C without mention of hepatic coma**
    AHA: 1Q, '11, 23; 4Q, '08, 120; 3Q, '07, 7; 2Q, '06, 13
    B18.2 Chronic viral hepatitis C   **I-10**

  070.59 **Other specified viral hepatitis without mention of hepatic coma**

070.6 **Unspecified viral hepatitis with hepatic coma**
  EXCLUDES unspecified viral hepatitis C with hepatic coma (070.71)

✓5ᵗʰ **070.7** **Unspecified viral hepatitis C**

  070.70 **Unspecified viral hepatitis C without hepatic coma**
    Unspecified viral hepatitis C NOS
    AHA: 4Q, '04, 52
    B19.20 Unspecified viral hepatits C w/o hepatic coma   **I-10**

  070.71 **Unspecified viral hepatitis C with hepatic coma**
    AHA: 4Q, '04, 52

070.9 **Unspecified viral hepatitis without mention of hepatic coma**
  Viral hepatitis NOS
  EXCLUDES unspecified viral hepatitis C without hepatic coma (070.70)

071 **Rabies**
Hydrophobia
Lyssa
DEF: Acute infectious disease of the CNS caused by a rhabdovirus; usually spread by bites by infected animals; progresses from fever, restlessness, and extreme excitability, to hydrophobia, seizures, confusion and death.

✓4ᵗʰ **072** **Mumps**
DEF: Acute infectious disease caused by paramyxovirus; usually seen in children less than 15 years of age; salivary glands are typically enlarged, involves other organs, such as testes, pancreas and meninges.

  072.0 **Mumps orchitis**   ♂

  072.1 **Mumps meningitis**

  072.2 **Mumps encephalitis**
    Mumps meningoencephalitis

  072.3 **Mumps pancreatitis**

✓5ᵗʰ   **072.7** **Mumps with other specified complications**

    072.71 **Mumps hepatitis**

    072.72 **Mumps polyneuropathy**

    072.79 **Other**

  072.8 **Mumps with unspecified complication**

  072.9 **Mumps without mention of complication**
    Epidemic parotitis
    Infectious parotitis

✓4ᵗʰ **073** **Ornithosis**
INCLUDES parrot fever
       psittacosis
DEF: *Chlamydia psittaci* infection often transmitted from birds to humans.

  073.0 **With pneumonia**
    Lobular pneumonitis due to ornithosis

  073.7 **With other specified complications**

  073.8 **With unspecified complication**

  073.9 **Ornithosis, unspecified**

✓4ᵗʰ **074** **Specific diseases due to Coxsackie virus**
EXCLUDES Coxsackie virus:
    infection NOS (079.2)
    meningitis (047.0)

  074.0 **Herpangina**
    Vesicular pharyngitis
    DEF: Acute infectious coxsackie virus infection causing throat lesions, fever, and vomiting; generally affects children in summer.

  074.1 **Epidemic pleurodynia**
    Bornholm disease
    Devil's grip
    Epidemic:
      myalgia
      myositis
    DEF: Paroxysmal pain in chest, accompanied by fever and usually limited to children and young adults; caused by coxsackie virus.

---

§   Requires fifth digit. Valid digits are in [brackets] under each code. See category 070 for codes and definitions.

✓4ᵗʰ
✓5ᵗʰ   Additional Digit Required   **Unspecified Code**   Other Specified Code   Manifestation Code   ►◄ Revised Text   ● New Code   ▲ Revised Code Title

2015 ICD-9-CM   **Volume 1 – 13**

√5ᵗʰ **074.2 Coxsackie carditis**

074.20 Coxsackie carditis, unspecified

074.21 Coxsackie pericarditis
DEF: Coxsackie infection of the outer lining of the heart.

074.22 Coxsackie endocarditis
DEF: Coxsackie infection within the heart's cavities.

074.23 Coxsackie myocarditis
Aseptic myocarditis of newborn
DEF: Coxsackie infection of the muscle of the heart.

074.3 Hand, foot, and mouth disease
Vesicular stomatitis and exanthem
DEF: Mild coxsackie infection causing lesions on hands, feet and oral mucosa, most commonly seen in preschool children.

074.8 Other specified diseases due to Coxsackie virus
Acute lymphonodular pharyngitis

075 Infectious mononucleosis
Glandular fever
Monocytic angina
Pfeiffer's disease
DEF: Acute infection by Epstein-Barr virus causing fever, sore throat, enlarged lymph glands and spleen, and fatigue; usually seen in teens and young adults.
AHA: 3Q, '01, 13; M-A, '87, 8

√4ᵗʰ **076 Trachoma**
EXCLUDES late effect of trachoma (139.1)
DEF: A chronic infectious disease of the cornea and conjunctiva caused by a strain of the bacteria *Chlamydia trachomatis;* the infection can cause photophobia, pain, excessive tearing and sometimes blindness.

076.0 Initial stage
Trachoma dubium

076.1 Active stage
Granular conjunctivitis (trachomatous)
Trachomatous:
follicular conjunctivitis
pannus

076.9 Trachoma, unspecified
Trachoma NOS

√4ᵗʰ **077 Other diseases of conjunctiva due to viruses and Chlamydiae**
EXCLUDES ophthalmic complications of viral diseases classified elsewhere

077.0 Inclusion conjunctivitis
Paratrachoma   Swimming pool conjunctivitis
EXCLUDES inclusion blennorrhea (neonatal) (771.6)
DEF: Pus in conjunctiva caused by *Chlamydiae trachomatis.*

077.1 Epidemic keratoconjunctivitis
Shipyard eye
DEF: Highly contagious corneal or conjunctival infection caused by adenovirus type 8; symptoms include inflammation and corneal infiltrates.

077.2 Pharyngoconjunctival fever
Viral pharyngoconjunctivitis

077.3 Other adenoviral conjunctivitis
Acute adenoviral follicular conjunctivitis

077.4 Epidemic hemorrhagic conjunctivitis
Apollo:
conjunctivitis
disease
Conjunctivitis due to enterovirus type 70
Hemorrhagic conjunctivitis (acute) (epidemic)

077.8 Other viral conjunctivitis
Newcastle conjunctivitis

√5ᵗʰ **077.9 Unspecified diseases of conjunctiva due to viruses and Chlamydiae**

077.98 Due to Chlamydiae

077.99 Due to viruses
Viral conjunctivitis NOS
B30.9 Viral conjunctivitis, unspecified   I-10

√4ᵗʰ **078 Other diseases due to viruses and Chlamydiae**
EXCLUDES viral infection NOS (079.0-079.9)
viremia NOS (790.8)

078.0 Molluscum contagiosum
DEF: Benign poxvirus infection causing small bumps on the skin or conjunctiva; transmitted by close contact.

√5ᵗʰ **078.1 Viral warts**
Viral warts due to human papilloma virus
DEF: A keratotic papilloma of the epidermis caused by the human papilloma virus; the superficial vegetative lesions last for varying durations and eventually regress spontaneously.
AHA: 2Q, '97, 9; 4Q, '93, 22

078.10 Viral warts, unspecified
Verruca:
NOS
Vulgaris
Warts (infectious)

078.11 Condyloma acuminatum
Condyloma NOS
Genital warts NOS
DEF: Clusters of mucosa or epidermal lesions on external genitalia; viral infection is sexually transmitted.

078.12 Plantar wart
Verruca plantaris
AHA: 4Q, '08, 78-79

078.19 Other specified viral warts
Common wart
Flat wart
Verruca plana

078.2 Sweating fever
Miliary fever
Sweating disease
DEF: A viral infection characterized by profuse sweating; various papular, vesicular and other eruptions cause the blockage of sweat glands.

078.3 Cat-scratch disease
Benign lymphoreticulosis (of inoculation)
Cat-scratch fever

078.4 Foot and mouth disease
Aphthous fever
Epizootic:
aphthae
stomatitis
DEF: Ulcers on oral mucosa, legs, and feet after exposure to infected animal.

078.5 Cytomegaloviral disease
Cytomegalic inclusion disease
Salivary gland virus disease
Use additional code to identify manifestation, as:
cytomegalic inclusion virus:
hepatitis (573.1)
pneumonia (484.1)
EXCLUDES congenital cytomegalovirus infection (771.1)
DEF: A herpesvirus associated with serious disease morbidity including fever, leukopenia, pneumonia, retinitis, hepatitis and organ transplant; often leads to hepatomegaly, splenomegaly and thrombocytopenia; a common post-transplant complication.
AHA: 3Q, '11, 5; 1Q, '03, 10; 3Q, '98, 4; 2Q, '93, 11; 1Q, '89, 9

078.6 Hemorrhagic nephrosonephritis
Hemorrhagic fever:
epidemic
Korean
Russian
with renal syndrome
DEF: Viral infection causing kidney dysfunction and bleeding disorders.

078.7 Arenaviral hemorrhagic fever
Hemorrhagic fever: Hemorrhagic fever:
Argentine   Junin virus
Bolivian   Machupo virus

√5ᵗʰ **078.8 Other specified diseases due to viruses and Chlamydiae**
EXCLUDES epidemic diarrhea (009.2)
lymphogranuloma venereum (099.1)

078.81 Epidemic vertigo

078.82 Epidemic vomiting syndrome
Winter vomiting disease

078.88 Other specified diseases due to Chlamydiae
AHA: 4Q, '96, 22

078.89 Other specified diseases due to viruses
Epidemic cervical myalgia
Marburg disease

√4ᵗʰ **079 Viral and chlamydial infection in conditions classified elsewhere and of unspecified site**

NOTE This category is provided to be used as an additional code to identify the viral agent in diseases classifiable elsewhere. This category will also be used to classify virus infection of unspecified nature or site.

079.0 Adenovirus

079.1 ECHO virus
DEF: An "orphan" enteric RNA virus, certain serotypes of which are associated with human disease, especially aseptic meningitis.

079.2 Coxsackie virus
DEF: A heterogenous group of viruses associated with aseptic meningitis, myocarditis, pericarditis, and acute onset juvenile diabetes.

079.3 Rhinovirus
DEF: Rhinoviruses affect primarily the upper respiratory tract. Over 100 distinct types infect humans.

079.4 Human papillomavirus
DEF: Viral infection caused by the genus *Papillomavirus* causing cutaneous and genital warts, including verruca vulgaris and condyloma acuminatum; certain types are associated with cervical dysplasia, cancer and other genital malignancies.
AHA: 2Q, '97, 9; 4Q, '93, 22
TIP: Do not assign for viral warts; see instead subcategory 078.1.

√5ᵗʰ **079.5 Retrovirus**
EXCLUDES human immunodeficiency virus, type 1 [HIV-1] (042)
human T-cell lymphotrophic virus, type III [HTLV-III] (042)
lymphadenopathy-associated virus [LAV] (042)
DEF: A large group of RNA viruses that carry reverse transcriptase and include the leukoviruses and lentiviruses.
AHA: 4Q, '93, 22, 23

079.50 Retrovirus, unspecified

079.51 Human T-cell lymphotrophic virus, type I [HTLV-I]

079.52 Human T-cell lymphotrophic virus, type II [HTLV-II]

079.53 Human immunodeficiency virus, type 2 [HIV-2]

079.59 Other specified retrovirus

079.6 Respiratory syncytial virus [RSV]
DEF: The major respiratory pathogen of young children, causing severe bronchitis and bronchopneumonia, and minor infection in adults.
AHA: 4Q, '96, 27, 28

√5ᵗʰ **079.8 Other specified viral and chlamydial infections**
AHA: 1Q, '88, 12

079.81 Hantavirus
DEF: An infection caused by the Muerto Canyon virus whose primary rodent reservoir is the deer mouse Peromyscus maniculatus; commonly characterized by fever, myalgias, headache, cough.
AHA: 4Q, '95, 60

079.82 SARS-associated coronavirus
DEF: A life-threatening respiratory disease, severe acute respiratory syndrome (SARS); etiology coronavirus; presenting symptoms may range from mild to severe forms of flu-like conditions; fever, chills, cough, headache, myalgia; diagnosis of SARS is based upon clinical, laboratory, and epidemiological criteria.
AHA: 4Q, '03, 46

079.83 Parvovirus B19
Human parvovirus   Parvovirus NOS
EXCLUDES erythema infectiosum [fifth disease] (057.0)
DEF: The only known parvovirus to cause disease in humans; manifestation is erythema infectiosum; also associated with polyarthropathy, chronic anemia, red cell aplasia, and fetal hydrops.
AHA: 4Q, '07, 64

079.88 Other specified chlamydial infection

079.89 Other specified viral infection

√5ᵗʰ **079.9 Unspecified viral and chlamydial infections**
EXCLUDES viremia NOS (790.8)

079.98 Unspecified chlamydial infection
Chlamydial infections NOS

079.99 Unspecified viral infection
Viral infections NOS
B97.89 Other viral agents cause of dz class elsewhere   I-10

Rickettsioses and Other Arthropod-borne Diseases (080-088)

EXCLUDES arthropod-borne viral diseases (060.0-066.9)

080 Louse-borne [epidemic] typhus
Typhus (fever):
classical
epidemic
exanthematic NOS
louse-borne
DEF: *Rickettsia prowazekii;* causes severe headache, rash, high fever.

√4ᵗʰ **081 Other typhus**

081.0 Murine [endemic] typhus
Typhus (fever):
endemic
flea-borne
DEF: Milder typhus caused by *Rickettsia typhi (mooseri);* transmitted by rat flea.

081.1 Brill's disease
Brill-Zinsser disease
Recrudescent typhus (fever)

081.2 Scrub typhus
Japanese river fever
Kedani fever
Mite-borne typhus
Tsutsugamushi
DEF: Typhus caused by *Rickettsia tsutsugamushi* transmitted by chigger.

081.9 Typhus, unspecified
Typhus (fever) NOS

√4ᵗʰ **082 Tick-borne rickettsioses**

082.0 Spotted fevers
Rocky mountain spotted fever
Sao Paulo fever

082.1 Boutonneuse fever
African tick typhus
India tick typhus
Kenya tick typhus
Marseilles fever
Mediterranean tick fever

082.2 North Asian tick fever
Siberian tick typhus

082.3 Queensland tick typhus

√5ᵗʰ **082.4 Ehrlichiosis**
AHA: 3Q, '06, 11; 4Q, '00, 38

082.40 Ehrlichiosis, unspecified

082.41 Ehrlichiosis chaffensis [E. chaffeensis]
DEF: A febrile illness caused by bacterial infection, also called human monocytic ehrlichiosis (HME). Causal organism is *Ehrlichia chaffensis,* transmitted by the Lone Star tick. Symptoms include fever, chills, myalgia, nausea, vomiting, diarrhea, confusion, and severe headache occurring one week after a tick bite. Clinical findings are lymphadenopathy, rash, thrombocytopenia, leukopenia, and abnormal liver function tests.

082.49 Other ehrlichiosis

082.8 Other specified tick-borne rickettsioses
Lone star fever
AHA: 4Q, '99, 19

082.9 Tick-borne rickettsiosis, unspecified
Tick-borne typhus NOS

√4ᵗʰ √5ᵗʰ Additional Digit Required   Unspecified Code   Other Specified Code   Manifestation Code   ►◄ Revised Text   ● New Code   ▲ Revised Code Title
2015 ICD-9-CM   Volume 1 – 15

078.82–082.9

✓4ᵗʰ **083 Other rickettsioses**

083.0 Q fever
   DEF: Infection of *Coxiella burnettii* usually acquired through airborne organisms.

083.1 Trench fever
   Quintan fever
   Wolhynian fever

083.2 Rickettsialpox
   Vesicular rickettsiosis
   DEF: Infection of *Rickettsia akari* usually acquired through a mite bite.

083.8 Other specified rickettsioses

083.9 Rickettsiosis, unspecified

✓4ᵗʰ **084 Malaria**
   NOTE Subcategories 084.0-084.6 exclude the listed conditions with mention of pernicious complications (084.8-084.9).
   EXCLUDES *congenital malaria (771.2)*
   DEF: Mosquito-borne disease causing high fever and prostration and cataloged by species of *Plasmodium: P. falciparum, P. malariae, P. ovale,* and *P. vivax.*

084.0 Falciparum malaria [malignant tertian]
   Malaria (fever):
     by Plasmodium falciparum
     subtertian

084.1 Vivax malaria [benign tertian]
   Malaria (fever) by Plasmodium vivax

084.2 Quartan malaria
   Malaria (fever) by Plasmodium malariae
   Malariae malaria

084.3 Ovale malaria
   Malaria (fever) by Plasmodium ovale

084.4 Other malaria
   Monkey malaria

084.5 Mixed malaria
   Malaria (fever) by more than one parasite

084.6 Malaria, unspecified
   Malaria (fever) NOS

084.7 Induced malaria
   Therapeutically induced malaria
   EXCLUDES *accidental infection from syringe, blood transfusion, etc. (084.0-084.6, above, according to parasite species)*
       transmission from mother to child during delivery (771.2)

084.8 Blackwater fever
   Hemoglobinuric:
     fever (bilious)
     malaria
   Malarial hemoglobinuria
   DEF: Severe hemic and renal complication of *Plasmodium falciparum* infection.

084.9 Other pernicious complications of malaria
   Algid malaria
   Cerebral malaria
   Use additional code to identify complication, as:
     malarial:
       hepatitis (573.2)
       nephrosis (581.81)

✓4ᵗʰ **085 Leishmaniasis**

085.0 Visceral [kala-azar]
   Dumdum fever
   Infection by Leishmania:
     donovani
     infantum
   Leishmaniasis:
     dermal, post-kala-azar
     Mediterranean
     visceral (Indian)

085.1 Cutaneous, urban
   Aleppo boil
   Baghdad boil
   Delhi boil
   Infection by Leishmania tropica (minor)
   Leishmaniasis, cutaneous:
     dry form
     late
     recurrent
     ulcerating
   Oriental sore

085.2 Cutaneous, Asian desert
   Infection by Leishmania tropica major
   Leishmaniasis, cutaneous:
     acute necrotizing
     rural
     wet form
     zoonotic form

085.3 Cutaneous, Ethiopian
   Infection by Leishmania ethiopica
   Leishmaniasis, cutaneous:
     diffuse
     lepromatous

085.4 Cutaneous, American
   Chiclero ulcer
   Infection by Leishmania mexicana
   Leishmaniasis tegumentaria diffusa

085.5 Mucocutaneous (American)
   Espundia
   Infection by Leishmania braziliensis
   Uta

085.9 Leishmaniasis, unspecified

✓4ᵗʰ **086 Trypanosomiasis**
   Use additional code to identify manifestations, as:
     trypanosomiasis:
       encephalitis (323.2)
       meningitis (321.3)

086.0 Chagas' disease with heart involvement
   American trypanosomiasis ⎱ with heart involvement
   Infection by Trypanosoma cruzi ⎰
   Any condition classifiable to 086.2 with heart involvement

086.1 Chagas' disease with other organ involvement
   American trypanosomiasis ⎱ with involvement of organ
   Infection by Trypanosoma cruzi ⎰ other than heart
   Any condition classifiable to 086.2 with involvement of organ other than heart

086.2 Chagas' disease without mention of organ involvement
   American trypanosomiasis
   Infection by Trypanosoma cruzi

086.3 Gambian trypanosomiasis
   Gambian sleeping sickness
   Infection by Trypanosoma gambiense

086.4 Rhodesian trypanosomiasis
   Infection by Trypanosoma rhodesiense
   Rhodesian sleeping sickness

086.5 African trypanosomiasis, unspecified
   Sleeping sickness NOS

086.9 Trypanosomiasis, unspecified

✓4ᵗʰ **087 Relapsing fever**
   INCLUDES recurrent fever
   DEF: Infection of *Borrelia;* symptoms are episodic and include fever and arthralgia.

087.0 Louse-borne

087.1 Tick-borne

087.9 Relapsing fever, unspecified

✓4ᵗʰ **088 Other arthropod-borne diseases**

088.0 Bartonellosis
   Carrión's disease   Verruga peruana
   Oroya fever

✓5ᵗʰ **088.8 Other specified arthropod-borne diseases**

    088.81 Lyme disease
        Erythema chronicum migrans

        DEF: A recurrent multisystem disorder caused by the spirochete *Borrelia burgdorferi* with the carrier being the tick; begins with lesions of erythema chronicum migrans; followed by arthritis of the large joints, myalgia, malaise, and neurological and cardiac manifestations.

        AHA: 4Q, '91, 15; 3Q, '90, 14; 2Q, '89, 10

        TIP: Do not assign if patient has been cured of Lyme disease but has residual chronic condition; refer instead to late-effect code 139.8.

    088.82 Babesiosis
        Babesiasis

        DEF: A tick-borne disease caused by infection of *Babesia*, characterized by fever, malaise, listlessness, severe anemia and hemoglobinuria.

        AHA: 4Q, '93, 23

    088.89 Other

    088.9 Arthropod-borne disease, unspecified

Syphilis and Other Venereal Diseases (090-099)

    EXCLUDES nonvenereal endemic syphilis (104.0)
                  urogenital trichomoniasis (131.0)

✓4ᵗʰ **090 Congenital syphilis**

    DEF: Infection by spirochete *Treponema pallidum* acquired in utero from the infected mother.

    090.0 Early congenital syphilis, symptomatic

Congenital syphilitic:	Congenital syphilitic:
choroiditis	splenomegaly
coryza (chronic)	Syphilitic (congenital):
hepatomegaly	epiphysitis
mucous patches	osteochondritis
periostitis	pemphigus

        Any congenital syphilitic condition specified as early or manifest less than two years after birth

    090.1 Early congenital syphilis, latent
        Congenital syphilis without clinical manifestations, with positive serological reaction and negative spinal fluid test, less than two years after birth

    090.2 Early congenital syphilis, unspecified
        Congenital syphilis NOS, less than two years after birth

    090.3 Syphilitic interstitial keratitis
        Syphilitic keratitis:
           parenchymatous
           punctata profunda

        EXCLUDES interstitial keratitis NOS (370.50)

✓5ᵗʰ **090.4 Juvenile neurosyphilis**

    Use additional code to identify any associated mental disorder

    DEF: *Treponema pallidum* infection involving the nervous system.

    090.40 Juvenile neurosyphilis, unspecified
        Congenital neurosyphilis
        Dementia paralytica juvenilis
        Juvenile:
           general paresis
           tabes
           taboparesis

    090.41 Congenital syphilitic encephalitis

        DEF: Congenital *Treponema pallidum* infection involving the brain.

    090.42 Congenital syphilitic meningitis

        DEF: Congenital *Treponema pallidum* infection involving the lining of the brain and/or spinal cord.

    090.49 Other

    090.5 Other late congenital syphilis, symptomatic
        Gumma due to congenital syphilis
        Hutchinson's teeth
        Syphilitic saddle nose

        Any congenital syphilitic condition specified as late or manifest two years or more after birth

    090.6 Late congenital syphilis, latent
        Congenital syphilis without clinical manifestations, with positive serological reaction and negative spinal fluid test, two years or more after birth

    090.7 Late congenital syphilis, unspecified
        Congenital syphilis NOS, two years or more after birth

    090.9 Congenital syphilis, unspecified

✓4ᵗʰ **091 Early syphilis, symptomatic**

    EXCLUDES early cardiovascular syphilis (093.0-093.9)
                  early neurosyphilis (094.0-094.9)

    091.0 Genital syphilis (primary)
        Genital chancre

        DEF: Genital lesion at the site of initial infection by *Treponema pallidum*.

    091.1 Primary anal syphilis

        DEF: Anal lesion at the site of initial infection by *Treponema pallidum*.

    091.2 Other primary syphilis

Primary syphilis of:	Primary syphilis of:
breast	lip
fingers	tonsils

        DEF: Lesion at the site of initial infection by *Treponema pallidum*.

    091.3 Secondary syphilis of skin or mucous membranes

Condyloma latum	Secondary syphilis of:
Secondary syphilis of:	skin
anus	tonsils
mouth	vulva
pharynx	

        DEF: Transitory or chronic lesions following initial syphilis infection.

    091.4 Adenopathy due to secondary syphilis
        Syphilitic adenopathy (secondary)
        Syphilitic lymphadenitis (secondary)

✓5ᵗʰ **091.5 Uveitis due to secondary syphilis**

    091.50 Syphilitic uveitis, unspecified

    091.51 Syphilitic chorioretinitis (secondary)

        DEF: Inflammation of choroid and retina as a secondary infection.

    091.52 Syphilitic iridocyclitis (secondary)

        DEF: Inflammation of iris and ciliary body as a secondary infection.

✓5ᵗʰ **091.6 Secondary syphilis of viscera and bone**

    091.61 Secondary syphilitic periostitis

        DEF: Inflammation of outer layers of bone as a secondary infection.

    091.62 Secondary syphilitic hepatitis
        Secondary syphilis of liver

    091.69 Other viscera

    091.7 Secondary syphilis, relapse
        Secondary syphilis, relapse (treated) (untreated)

        DEF: Return of symptoms of syphilis following asymptomatic period.

✓5ᵗʰ **091.8 Other forms of secondary syphilis**

    091.81 Acute syphilitic meningitis (secondary)

        DEF: Sudden, severe inflammation of the lining of the brain and/or spinal cord as a secondary infection.

    091.82 Syphilitic alopecia

        DEF: Hair loss following initial syphilis infection.

    091.89 Other

    091.9 Unspecified secondary syphilis

✓4ᵗʰ **092 Early syphilis, latent**

    INCLUDES syphilis (acquired) without clinical manifestations, with positive serological reaction and negative spinal fluid test, less than two years after infection

    092.0 Early syphilis, latent, serological relapse after treatment

    092.9 Early syphilis, latent, unspecified

✓4ᵗʰ **093 Cardiovascular syphilis**

    093.0 Aneurysm of aorta, specified as syphilitic
        Dilatation of aorta, specified as syphilitic

✓4ᵗʰ
✓5ᵗʰ   Additional Digit Required   Unspecified Code   Other Specified Code   Manifestation Code   ▶◀ Revised Text   ● New Code   ▲ Revised Code Title

2015 ICD-9-CM   **Volume 1 – 17**

Infectious and Parasitic Diseases

093.1–098.19

093.1 Syphilitic aortitis
DEF: Inflammation of the aorta — the main artery leading from the heart.

√5ᵗʰ **093.2 Syphilitic endocarditis**
DEF: Inflammation of the tissues lining the cavities of the heart.

093.20 Valve, unspecified
Syphilitic ostial coronary disease

093.21 Mitral valve

093.22 Aortic valve
Syphilitic aortic incompetence or stenosis

093.23 Tricuspid valve

093.24 Pulmonary valve

√5ᵗʰ **093.8 Other specified cardiovascular syphilis**

093.81 Syphilitic pericarditis
DEF: Inflammation of the outer lining of the heart.

093.82 Syphilitic myocarditis
DEF: Inflammation of the muscle of the heart.

093.89 Other

093.9 Cardiovascular syphilis, unspecified

√4ᵗʰ **094 Neurosyphilis**
Use additional code to identify any associated mental disorder

094.0 Tabes dorsalis
Locomotor ataxia (progressive)
Posterior spinal sclerosis (syphilitic)
Tabetic neurosyphilis
Use additional code to identify manifestation, as:
neurogenic arthropathy [Charcot's joint disease] (713.5)
DEF: Progressive degeneration of nerves associated with long-term syphilis; causing pain, wasting away, incontinence, and ataxia.
AHA: 3Q, '12, 4

094.1 General paresis
Dementia paralytica
General paralysis (of the insane) (progressive)
Paretic neurosyphilis
Taboparesis
DEF: Degeneration of brain associated with long-term syphilis, causing loss of brain function, progressive dementia, and paralysis.

094.2 Syphilitic meningitis
Meningovascular syphilis
EXCLUDES acute syphilitic meningitis (secondary) (091.81)
DEF: Inflammation of the lining of the brain and/or spinal cord.

094.3 Asymptomatic neurosyphilis

√5ᵗʰ **094.8 Other specified neurosyphilis**

094.81 Syphilitic encephalitis

094.82 Syphilitic Parkinsonism
DEF: Decreased motor function, tremors, and muscular rigidity.

094.83 Syphilitic disseminated retinochoroiditis
DEF: Inflammation of retina and choroid due to neurosyphilis.

094.84 Syphilitic optic atrophy
DEF: Degeneration of the eye and its nerves due to neurosyphilis.

094.85 Syphilitic retrobulbar neuritis
DEF: Inflammation of the posterior optic nerve due to neurosyphilis.

094.86 Syphilitic acoustic neuritis
DEF: Inflammation of acoustic nerve due to neurosyphilis.

094.87 Syphilitic ruptured cerebral aneurysm

094.89 Other

094.9 Neurosyphilis, unspecified
Gumma (syphilitic) ⎫
Syphilis (early) (late) ⎬ of central nervous system
Syphiloma ⎭   NOS

095 Other forms of late syphilis, with symptoms
INCLUDES gumma (syphilitic)
syphilis, late, tertiary, or unspecified stage

095.0 Syphilitic episcleritis

095.1 Syphilis of lung

095.2 Syphilitic peritonitis

095.3 Syphilis of liver

095.4 Syphilis of kidney

095.5 Syphilis of bone

095.6 Syphilis of muscle
Syphilitic myositis

095.7 Syphilis of synovium, tendon, and bursa
Syphilitic:
bursitis
synovitis

095.8 Other specified forms of late symptomatic syphilis
EXCLUDES cardiovascular syphilis (093.0-093.9)
neurosyphilis (094.0-094.9)

095.9 Late symptomatic syphilis, unspecified

096 Late syphilis, latent
Syphilis (acquired) without clinical manifestations, with positive serological reaction and negative spinal fluid test, two years or more after infection

√4ᵗʰ **097 Other and unspecified syphilis**

097.0 Late syphilis, unspecified

097.1 Latent syphilis, unspecified
Positive serological reaction for syphilis

097.9 Syphilis, unspecified
Syphilis (acquired) NOS
EXCLUDES syphilis NOS causing death under two years of age (090.9)

√4ᵗʰ **098 Gonococcal infections**
DEF: *Neisseria gonorrhoeae* infection generally acquired in utero or in sexual congress.

098.0 Acute, of lower genitourinary tract
Gonococcal:
Bartholinitis (acute)
urethritis (acute)
vulvovaginitis (acute)
Gonorrhea (acute):
NOS
genitourinary (tract) NOS

√5ᵗʰ **098.1 Acute, of upper genitourinary tract**

098.10 Gonococcal infection (acute) of upper genitourinary tract, site unspecified

098.11 Gonococcal cystitis (acute) upper
Gonorrhea (acute) of bladder

098.12 Gonococcal prostatitis (acute) ♂

098.13 Gonococcal epididymo-orchitis (acute) ♂
Gonococcal orchitis (acute)
DEF: Acute inflammation of the testes.

098.14 Gonococcal seminal vesiculitis (acute) ♂
Gonorrhea (acute) of seminal vesicle

098.15 Gonococcal cervicitis (acute) ♀
Gonorrhea (acute) of cervix

098.16 Gonococcal endometritis (acute) ♀
Gonorrhea (acute) of uterus

098.17 Gonococcal salpingitis, specified as acute ♀
DEF: Acute inflammation of the fallopian tubes.

098.19 Other

N Newborn Age: 0   P Pediatric Age: 0-17   M Maternity Age: 12-55   A Adult Age: 15-124

098.2 Chronic, of lower genitourinary tract

Gonoccocal:
  Bartholinitis
  urethritis   }   specified as chronic or with
  vulvovaginitis   duration of two months
Gonorrhea: or more
  NOS
  genitourinary (tract)

Any condition classifiable to 098.0 specified as chronic or with duration of two months or more

√5ᵗʰ 098.3 Chronic, of upper genitourinary tract

  INCLUDES any condition classifiable to 098.1 stated as chronic or with a duration of two months or more

  098.30 Chronic gonococcal infection of upper genitourinary tract, site unspecified

  098.31 Gonococcal cystitis, chronic
    Gonorrhea of bladder, chronic
    Any condition classifiable to 098.11, specified as chronic

  098.32 Gonococcal prostatitis, chronic   ♂
    Any condition classifiable to 098.12, specified as chronic

  098.33 Gonococcal epididymo-orchitis, chronic   ♂
    Chronic gonococcal orchitis
    Any condition classifiable to 098.13, specified as chronic
    DEF: Chronic inflammation of the testes.

  098.34 Gonococcal seminal vesiculitis, chronic   ♂
    Gonorrhea of seminal vesicle, chronic
    Any condition classifiable to 098.14, specified as chronic

  098.35 Gonococcal cervicitis, chronic   ♀
    Gonorrhea of cervix, chronic
    Any condition classifiable to 098.15, specified as chronic

  098.36 Gonococcal endometritis, chronic   ♀
    Any condition classifiable to 098.16, specified as chronic
    DEF: Chronic inflammation of the uterus.

  098.37 Gonococcal salpingitis (chronic)   ♀
    DEF: Chronic inflammation of the fallopian tubes.

  098.39 Other

√5ᵗʰ 098.4 Gonococcal infection of eye

  098.40 Gonococcal conjunctivitis (neonatorum)
    Gonococcal ophthalmia (neonatorum)
    DEF: Infection of conjunctiva present at birth.

  098.41 Gonococcal iridocyclitis
    DEF: Inflammation and infection of iris and ciliary body.

  098.42 Gonococcal endophthalmia
    DEF: Inflammation and infection of contents of eyeball.

  098.43 Gonococcal keratitis
    DEF: Inflammation and infection of the cornea.

  098.49 Other

√5ᵗʰ 098.5 Gonococcal infection of joint

  098.50 Gonococcal arthritis
    Gonococcal infection of joint NOS

  098.51 Gonococcal synovitis and tenosynovitis

  098.52 Gonococcal bursitis
    DEF: Inflammation of the sac-like cavities in a joint.

  098.53 Gonococcal spondylitis

  098.59 Other
    Gonococcal rheumatism

098.6 Gonococcal infection of pharynx

098.7 Gonococcal infection of anus and rectum
  Gonococcal proctitis

√5ᵗʰ 098.8 Gonococcal infection of other specified sites

  098.81 Gonococcal keratosis (blennorrhagica)
    DEF: Pustular skin lesions caused by *Neisseria gonorrhoeae*.

  098.82 Gonococcal meningitis
    DEF: Inflammation of lining of brain and/or spinal cord.

  098.83 Gonococcal pericarditis
    DEF: Inflammation of the outer lining of the heart.

  098.84 Gonococcal endocarditis
    DEF: Inflammation of tissues lining the cavities of heart.

  098.85 Other gonococcal heart disease

  098.86 Gonococcal peritonitis
    DEF: Inflammation of the membrane lining the abdomen.

  098.89 Other
    Gonococcemia

√4ᵗʰ 099 Other venereal diseases

099.0 Chancroid
  Bubo (inguinal):
    chancroidal
    due to Hemophilus ducreyi
  Chancre:
    Ducrey's
    simple
    soft
  Ulcus molle (cutis)(skin)
  DEF: A sexually transmitted disease caused by *Haemophilus ducreyi*; identified by a painful primary ulcer at the site of inoculation (usually external genitalia) with related lymphadenitis.

099.1 Lymphogranuloma venereum
  Climatic or tropical bubo
  (Durand-) Nicolas-Favre disease
  Esthiomene
  Lymphogranuloma inguinale
  DEF: Sexually transmitted infection of *Chlamydia trachomatis* causing skin lesions.

099.2 Granuloma inguinale
  Donovanosis
  Granuloma pudendi (ulcerating)
  Granuloma venereum
  Pudendal ulcer
  DEF: Chronic, sexually transmitted infection of *Calymmatobacterium granulomatis* causing progressive, anogenital skin ulcers.

099.3 Reiter's disease
  Reactive arthritis
  Reiter's syndrome
  Use additional code for associated:
    arthropathy (711.1)
    conjunctivitis (372.33)
  DEF: A symptom complex of unknown etiology consisting of urethritis, conjunctivitis, arthritis and myocutaneous lesions; occurs most commonly in young men and patients with HIV. Also a form of reactive arthritis.

√5ᵗʰ 099.4 Other nongonococcal urethritis [NGU]

  099.40 Unspecified
    Nonspecific urethritis

  099.41 Chlamydia trachomatis

  099.49 Other specified organism

√5ᵗʰ 099.5 Other venereal diseases due to Chlamydia trachomatis
  EXCLUDES *Chlamydia trachomatis* infection of conjunctiva (076.0-076.9, 077.0, 077.9)
    Lymphogranuloma venereum (099.1)
  DEF: Venereal diseases caused by *Chlamydia trachomatis* at other sites besides the urethra (e.g., pharynx, anus and rectum, conjunctiva and peritoneum).

  099.50 Unspecified site

  099.51 Pharynx

  099.52 Anus and rectum

√4ᵗʰ / √5ᵗʰ   Additional Digit Required   Unspecified Code   Other Specified Code   Manifestation Code   ►◄ Revised Text   ● New Code   ▲ Revised Code Title

2015 ICD-9-CM   **Volume 1 – 19**

Infectious and Parasitic Diseases

098.2–099.52

Infectious and Parasitic Diseases

099.53–104.9

099.53 Lower genitourinary sites
Use additional code to specify site of infection, such as:
bladder (595.4)
cervix (616.0)
vagina and vulva (616.11)
EXCLUDES urethra (099.41)

099.54 Other genitourinary sites
Use additional code to specify site of infection, such as:
pelvic inflammatory disease NOS (614.9)
testis and epididymis (604.91)

099.55 Unspecified genitourinary site

099.56 Peritoneum
Perihepatitis

099.59 Other specified site

099.8 Other specified venereal diseases

099.9 Venereal disease, unspecified

Other Spirochetal Diseases (100-104)

✓4th **100 Leptospirosis**
DEF: A blood infection of any spirochete of the genus Leptospire; transmitted to humans by exposure to contaminated animal tissues or water. Patients present with flulike symptoms, characteristic muscle aches involving the thighs and low back.

100.0 Leptospirosis icterohemorrhagica
Leptospiral or spirochetal jaundice (hemorrhagic)
Weil's disease

✓5th **100.8 Other specified leptospiral infections**

100.81 Leptospiral meningitis (aseptic)

100.89 Other
Fever:
Fort Bragg
pretibial
swamp
Infection by Leptospira:
australis
bataviae
pyrogenes

100.9 Leptospirosis, unspecified

101 Vincent's angina
Acute necrotizing ulcerative:
gingivitis
stomatitis
Fusospirochetal pharyngitis
Spirochetal stomatitis
Trench mouth
Vincent's:
gingivitis
infection [any site]
DEF: Painful ulceration with edema and hypermic patches of the oropharyngeal and throat membranes; it is caused by spreading of acute ulcerative gingivitis.

✓4th **102 Yaws**
INCLUDES frambesia
pian
DEF: An infectious, endemic, tropical disease caused by *Treponema pertenue*; usually affects persons 15 years old or younger; a primary cutaneous lesion develops, then a granulomatous skin eruption, and occasionally lesions that destroy skin and bone.

102.0 Initial lesions
Chancre of yaws
Frambesia, initial or primary
Initial frambesial ulcer
Mother yaw

102.1 Multiple papillomata and wet crab yaws
Butter yaws
Frambesioma
Pianoma
Plantar or palmar papilloma of yaws

102.2 Other early skin lesions
Cutaneous yaws, less than five years after infection
Early yaws (cutaneous) (macular) (papular) (maculopapular) (micropapular)
Frambeside of early yaws

102.3 Hyperkeratosis
Ghoul hand
Hyperkeratosis, palmar or plantar (early) (late) due to yaws
Worm-eaten soles
DEF: Overgrowth of skin of palm or bottoms of feet, due to yaws.

102.4 Gummata and ulcers
Gummatous frambeside
Nodular late yaws (ulcerated)
DEF: Rubbery lesions and areas of dead skin caused by yaws.

102.5 Gangosa
Rhinopharyngitis mutilans
DEF: Massive, mutilating lesions of the nose and oral cavity caused by yaws.

102.6 Bone and joint lesions
Goundou
Gumma, bone } of yaws (late)
Gummatous osteitis or periostitis

Hydrarthrosis
Osteitis } of yaws (early) (late)
Periostitis (hypertrophic)

102.7 Other manifestations
Juxta-articular nodules of yaws
Mucosal yaws

102.8 Latent yaws
Yaws without clinical manifestations, with positive serology

102.9 Yaws, unspecified

✓4th **103 Pinta**
DEF: A chronic form of treponematosis, endemic in areas of tropical America; it is identified by the presence of red, violet, blue, coffee-colored or white spots on the skin.

103.0 Primary lesions
Chancre (primary)
Papule (primary) } of pinta [carate]
Pintid

103.1 Intermediate lesions
Erythematous plaques
Hyperchronic lesions } of pinta [carate]
Hyperkeratosis

103.2 Late lesions
Cardiovascular lesions
Skin lesions:
achromic
cicatricial } of pinta [carate]
dyschromic
Vitiligo

103.3 Mixed lesions
Achromic and hyperchromic skin lesions of pinta [carate]

103.9 Pinta, unspecified

✓4th **104 Other spirochetal infection**

104.0 Nonvenereal endemic syphilis
Bejel
Njovera
DEF: *Treponema pallidum, T. pertenue*, or *T. caroteum* infection transmitted non-sexually, causing lesions on mucosa and skin.

104.8 Other specified spirochetal infections
EXCLUDES relapsing fever (087.0-087.9)
syphilis (090.0-097.9)

104.9 Spirochetal infection, unspecified

Mycoses (110-118)

Use additional code to identify manifestation as:
arthropathy (711.6)
meningitis (321.0-321.1)
otitis externa (380.15)

EXCLUDES *infection by Actinomycetales, such as species of Actinomyces, Actinomadura, Nocardia, Streptomyces (039.0-039.9)*

√4ᵗʰ **110 Dermatophytosis**

INCLUDES infection by species of Epidermophyton, Microsporum, and Trichophyton
tinea, any type except those in 111

DEF: Superficial infection of the skin caused by a parasitic fungus.

110.0 Of scalp and beard
Kerion
Sycosis, mycotic
Trichophytic tinea [black dot tinea], scalp

110.1 Of nail
Dermatophytic onychia
Onychomycosis
Tinea unguium
B35.1 Tinea unguium   I-10

110.2 Of hand
Tinea manuum

110.3 Of groin and perianal area
Dhobie itch
Eczema marginatum
Tinea cruris

110.4 Of foot
Athlete's foot
Tinea pedis

110.5 Of the body
Herpes circinatus
Tinea imbricata [Tokelau]

110.6 Deep seated dermatophytosis
Granuloma trichophyticum
Majocchi's granuloma

110.8 Of other specified sites

110.9 Of unspecified site
Favus NOS
Microsporic tinea NOS
Ringworm NOS

√4ᵗʰ **111 Dermatomycosis, other and unspecified**

111.0 Pityriasis versicolor
Infection by Malassezia [Pityrosporum] furfur
Tinea flava
Tinea versicolor

111.1 Tinea nigra
Infection by Cladosporium species
Keratomycosis nigricans
Microsporosis nigra
Pityriasis nigra
Tinea palmaris nigra

111.2 Tinea blanca
Infection by Trichosporon (beigelii) cutaneum
White piedra

111.3 Black piedra
Infection by Piedraia hortai

111.8 Other specified dermatomycoses

111.9 Dermatomycosis, unspecified

√4ᵗʰ **112 Candidiasis**

INCLUDES infection by Candida species
moniliasis

EXCLUDES *neonatal monilial infection (771.7)*

DEF: Fungal infection caused by *Candida*; usually seen in mucous membranes or skin.

112.0 Of mouth
Thrush (oral)
B37.0 Candidal stomatitis   I-10

112.1 Of vulva and vagina   ♀
Candidal vulvovaginitis
Monilial vulvovaginitis
B37.3 Candidiasis of vulva and vagina   I-10

112.2 Of other urogenital sites
Candidal balanitis
AHA: 3Q, '12, 11-12; 4Q, '03, 105; 4Q, '96, 33

112.3 Of skin and nails
Candidal intertrigo
Candidal onychia
Candidal perionyxis [paronychia]
B37.2 Candidiasis of skin and nail   I-10

112.4 Of lung
Candidal pneumonia
AHA: 2Q, '98, 7

112.5 Disseminated
Systemic candidiasis
AHA: 3Q, '12, 11-12; 2Q, '00, 5; 2Q, '89, 10
TIP: Report for candidal sepsis, followed by the appropriate subcategory 995.9 code. If due to underlying candidal UTI, code also 112.2.

√5ᵗʰ **112.8 Of other specified sites**

112.81 Candidal endocarditis

112.82 Candidal otitis externa
Otomycosis in moniliasis

112.83 Candidal meningitis

112.84 Candidal esophagitis
AHA: 4Q, '92, 19
B37.81 Candidal esophagitis   I-10

112.85 Candidal enteritis
AHA: 4Q, '92, 19

112.89 Other
AHA: 1Q, '92, 17; 3Q, '91, 20

112.9 Of unspecified site

√4ᵗʰ **114 Coccidioidomycosis**

INCLUDES infection by Coccidioides (immitis)
Posada-Wernicke disease

DEF: A fungal disease caused by inhalation of dust particles containing arthrospores of *Coccidiodes immitis*; a self-limited respiratory infection; the primary form is known as San Joaquin fever, desert fever or valley fever.
AHA: 4Q, '93, 23

114.0 Primary coccidioidomycosis (pulmonary)
Acute pulmonary coccidioidomycosis
Coccidioidomycotic pneumonitis
Desert rheumatism
Pulmonary coccidioidomycosis
San Joaquin Valley fever
DEF: Acute, self-limiting *Coccidioides immitis* infection of the lung.
B38.0 Acute pulmonary coccidioidomycosis   I-10

114.1 Primary extrapulmonary coccidioidomycosis
Chancriform syndrome
Primary cutaneous coccidioidomycosis
DEF: Acute, self-limiting *Coccidioides immitis* infection in nonpulmonary site.

114.2 Coccidioidal meningitis
DEF: *Coccidioides immitis* infection of the lining of the brain and/or spinal cord.

114.3 Other forms of progressive coccidioidomycosis
Coccidioidal granuloma
Disseminated coccidioidomycosis

114.4 Chronic pulmonary coccidioidomycosis

114.5 Pulmonary coccidioidomycosis, unspecified

114.9 Coccidioidomycosis, unspecified

√4ᵗʰ √5ᵗʰ Additional Digit Required   Unspecified Code   Other Specified Code   Manifestation Code   ►◄ Revised Text   ● New Code   ▲ Revised Code Title

Infectious and Parasitic Diseases

115–121.2

✓4ᵗʰ **115 Histoplasmosis**

> The following fifth-digit subclassification is for use with category 115:
> 0 **without mention of manifestation**
> 1 **meningitis**
> 2 **retinitis**
> 3 **pericarditis**
> 4 **endocarditis**
> 5 **pneumonia**
> 9 **other**

§ ✓5ᵗʰ **115.0 Infection by Histoplasma capsulatum**
[0-5, 9]   American histoplasmosis
       Darling's disease
       Reticuloendothelial cytomycosis
       Small form histoplasmosis
       DEF: Infection resulting from inhalation of fungal spores, causing acute pneumonia, an influenza-like illness, or a disseminated disease of the reticuloendothelial system. In immunocompromised patients it can reactivate, affecting lungs, meninges, heart, peritoneum and adrenals.

§ ✓5ᵗʰ **115.1 Infection by Histoplasma duboisii**
[0-5, 9]   African histoplasmosis
       Large form histoplasmosis

§ ✓5ᵗʰ **115.9 Histoplasmosis, unspecified**
[0-5, 9]   Histoplasmosis NOS

✓4ᵗʰ **116 Blastomycotic infection**

116.0 Blastomycosis
       Blastomycotic dermatitis
       Chicago disease
       Cutaneous blastomycosis
       Disseminated blastomycosis
       Gilchrist's disease
       Infection by Blastomyces [Ajellomyces] dermatitidis
       North American blastomycosis
       Primary pulmonary blastomycosis

116.1 Paracoccidioidomycosis
       Brazilian blastomycosis
       Infection by Paracoccidioides [Blastomyces] brasiliensis
       Lutz-Splendore-Almeida disease
       Mucocutaneous-lymphangitic paracoccidioidomycosis
       Pulmonary paracoccidioidomycosis
       South American blastomycosis
       Visceral paracoccidioidomycosis

116.2 Lobomycosis
       Infections by Loboa [Blastomyces] loboi
       Keloidal blastomycosis
       Lobo's disease

✓4ᵗʰ **117 Other mycoses**

117.0 Rhinosporidiosis
       Infection by Rhinosporidium seeberi

117.1 Sporotrichosis
       Cutaneous sporotrichosis
       Disseminated sporotrichosis
       Infection by Sporothrix [Sporotrichum] schenckii
       Lymphocutaneous sporotrichosis
       Pulmonary sporotrichosis
       Sporotrichosis of the bones

117.2 Chromoblastomycosis
       Chromomycosis
       Infection by Cladosporidium carrionii, Fonsecaea compactum, Fonsecaea pedrosoi, Phialophora verrucosa

117.3 Aspergillosis
       Infection by Aspergillus species, mainly A. fumigatus, A. flavus group, A. terreus group
       AHA: 4Q, '97, 40

117.4 Mycotic mycetomas
       Infection by various genera and species of Ascomycetes and Deuteromycetes, such as Acremonium [Cephalosporium] falciforme, Neotestudina rosatii, Madurella grisea, Madurella mycetomii, Pyrenochaeta romeroi, Zopfia [Leptosphaeria] senegalensis
       Madura foot, mycotic
       Maduromycosis, mycotic
       EXCLUDES *actinomycotic mycetomas (039.0-039.9)*

117.5 Cryptococcosis
       Busse-Buschke's disease
       European cryptococcosis
       Infection by Cryptococcus neoformans
       Pulmonary cryptococcosis
       Systemic cryptococcosis
       Torula

117.6 Allescheriosis [Petriellidosis]
       Infections by Allescheria [Petriellidium] boydii [Monosporium apiospermum]
       EXCLUDES *mycotic mycetoma (117.4)*

117.7 Zygomycosis [Phycomycosis or Mucormycosis]
       Infection by species of Absidia, Basidiobolus, Conidiobolus, Cunninghamella, Entomophthora, Mucor, Rhizopus, Saksenaea

117.8 Infection by dematiacious fungi, [Phaehyphomycosis]
       Infection by dematiacious fungi, such as Cladosporium trichoides [bantianum], Dreschlera hawaiiensis, Phialophora gougerotii, Phialophora jeanselmi

117.9 Other and unspecified mycoses

118 Opportunistic mycoses
       Infection of skin, subcutaneous tissues, and/or organs by a wide variety of fungi generally considered to be pathogenic to compromised hosts only (e.g., infection by species of Alternaria, Dreschlera, Fusarium)
       Use additional code to identify manifestation, such as:
       keratitis (370.8)

Helminthiases (120-129)

✓4ᵗʰ **120 Schistosomiasis [bilharziasis]**
       DEF: Infection caused by *Schistosoma*, a genus of flukes or trematode parasites.

120.0 Schistosoma haematobium
       Vesical schistosomiasis NOS

120.1 Schistosoma mansoni
       Intestinal schistosomiasis NOS

120.2 Schistosoma japonicum
       Asiatic schistosomiasis NOS
       Katayama disease or fever

120.3 Cutaneous
       Cercarial dermatitis
       Infection by cercariae of Schistosoma
       Schistosome dermatitis
       Swimmers' itch

120.8 Other specified schistosomiasis
       Infection by Schistosoma:
         bovis
         intercalatum
         mattheii
         spindale
       Schistosomiasis chestermani

120.9 Schistosomiasis, unspecified
       Blood flukes NOS
       Hemic distomiasis

✓4ᵗʰ **121 Other trematode infections**

121.0 Opisthorchiasis
       Infection by:
         cat liver fluke
         Opisthorchis (felineus) (tenuicollis) (viverrini)

121.1 Clonorchiasis
       Biliary cirrhosis due to clonorchiasis
       Chinese liver fluke disease
       Hepatic distomiasis due to Clonorchis sinensis
       Oriental liver fluke disease

121.2 Paragonimiasis
       Infection by Paragonimus
       Lung fluke disease (oriental)
       Pulmonary distomiasis

---

§ Requires fifth digit. Valid digits are in [brackets] under each code. See category 115 for codes and definitions.

121.3 Fascioliasis
Infection by Fasciola:
    gigantica
    hepatica
    Liver flukes NOS
    Sheep liver fluke infection

121.4 Fasciolopsiasis
Infection by Fasciolopsis (buski)
Intestinal distomiasis

121.5 Metagonimiasis
Infection by Metagonimus yokogawai

121.6 Heterophyiasis
Infection by:
    Heterophyes heterophyes
    Stellantchasmus falcatus

121.8 Other specified trematode infections
Infection by:
    Dicrocoelium dendriticum
    Echinostoma ilocanum
    Gastrodiscoides hominis

121.9 Trematode infection, unspecified
Distomiasis NOS
Fluke disease NOS

✓4th 122 Echinococcosis
INCLUDES echinococciasis
      hydatid disease
      hydatidosis
DEF: Infection caused by larval forms of tapeworms of the genus *Echinococcus.*

122.0 Echinococcus granulosus infection of liver

122.1 Echinococcus granulosus infection of lung

122.2 Echinococcus granulosus infection of thyroid

122.3 Echinococcus granulosus infection, other

122.4 Echinococcus granulosus infection, unspecified

122.5 Echinococcus multilocularis infection of liver

122.6 Echinococcus multilocularis infection, other

122.7 Echinococcus multilocularis infection, unspecified

122.8 Echinococcosis, unspecified, of liver

122.9 Echinococcosis, other and unspecified

✓4th 123 Other cestode infection

123.0 Taenia solium infection, intestinal form
Pork tapeworm (adult) (infection)

123.1 Cysticercosis
Cysticerciasis
Infection by Cysticercus cellulosae [larval form of Taenia solium]
AHA: 2Q, '97, 8

123.2 Taenia saginata infection
Beef tapeworm (infection)
Infection by Taeniarhynchus saginatus

123.3 Taeniasis, unspecified

123.4 Diphyllobothriasis, intestinal
Diphyllobothrium (adult) (latum) (pacificum) infection
Fish tapeworm (infection)

123.5 Sparganosis [larval diphyllobothriasis]
Infection by:
    Diphyllobothrium larvae
    Sparganum (mansoni) (proliferum)
    Spirometra larvae

123.6 Hymenolepiasis
Dwarf tapeworm (infection)
Hymenolepis (diminuta) (nana) infection
Rat tapeworm (infection)

123.8 Other specified cestode infection
Diplogonoporus (grandis) ⎫
Dipylidium (caninum)   ⎬ infection
Dog tapeworm (infection)

123.9 Cestode infection, unspecified
Tapeworm (infection) NOS

124 Trichinosis
Trichinella spiralis infection
Trichinellosis
Trichiniasis
DEF: Infection by *Trichinella spiralis,* the smallest of the parasitic nematodes.

✓4th 125 Filarial infection and dracontiasis

125.0 Bancroftian filariasis
Chyluria   ⎫
Elephantiasis
Infection   ⎬ due to Wuchereria bancrofti
Lymphadenitis
Lymphangitis   ⎭
Wuchereriasis

125.1 Malayan filariasis
Brugia filariasis ⎫
Chyluria
Elephantiasis
Infection   ⎬ due to Brugia [Wuchereria] malayi
Lymphadenitis
Lymphangitis ⎭

125.2 Loiasis
Eyeworm disease of Africa
Loa loa infection

125.3 Onchocerciasis
Onchocerca volvulus infection
Onchocercosis

125.4 Dipetalonemiasis
Infection by:
    Acanthocheilonema perstans
    Dipetalonema perstans

125.5 Mansonella ozzardi infection
Filariasis ozzardi

125.6 Other specified filariasis
Dirofilaria infection
Infection by:
    Acanthocheilonema streptocerca
    Dipetalonema streptocerca

125.7 Dracontiasis
Guinea-worm infection
Infection by Dracunculus medinensis

125.9 Unspecified filariasis

✓4th 126 Ancylostomiasis and necatoriasis
INCLUDES cutaneous larva migrans due to Ancylostoma
      hookworm (disease) (infection)
      uncinariasis

126.0 Ancylostoma duodenale

126.1 Necator americanus

126.2 Ancylostoma braziliense

126.3 Ancylostoma ceylanicum

126.8 Other specified Ancylostoma

126.9 Ancylostomiasis and necatoriasis, unspecified
Creeping eruption NOS
Cutaneous larva migrans NOS

✓4th 127 Other intestinal helminthiases

127.0 Ascariasis
Ascaridiasis
Infection by Ascaris lumbricoides
Roundworm infection

127.1 Anisakiasis
Infection by Anisakis larva

127.2 Strongyloidiasis
Infection by Strongyloides stercoralis
EXCLUDES trichostrongyliasis (127.6)

127.3 Trichuriasis
Infection by Trichuris trichiura
Trichocephaliasis
Whipworm (disease) (infection)

✓4th✓5th Additional Digit Required   Unspecified Code   Other Specified Code   Manifestation Code   ▶◀ Revised Text   ● New Code   ▲ Revised Code Title

2015 ICD-9-CM   **Volume 1 – 23**

Infectious and Parasitic Diseases

127.4–135

127.4 Enterobiasis
Infection by Enterobius vermicularis
Oxyuriasis
Oxyuris vermicularis infection
Pinworm (disease) (infection)
Threadworm infection

127.5 Capillariasis
Infection by Capillaria philippinensis
EXCLUDES *infection by Capillaria hepatica (128.8)*

127.6 Trichostrongyliasis
Infection by Trichostrongylus species

127.7 Other specified intestinal helminthiasis
Infection by:
Oesophagostomum apiostomum and related species
Ternidens diminutus
other specified intestinal helminth
Physalopteriasis

127.8 Mixed intestinal helminthiasis
Infection by intestinal helminths classified to more than one
of the categories 120.0-127.7
Mixed helminthiasis NOS

127.9 Intestinal helminthiasis, unspecified

√4ᵗʰ **128 Other and unspecified helminthiases**

128.0 Toxocariasis
Larva migrans visceralis
Toxocara (canis) (cati) infection
Visceral larva migrans syndrome

128.1 Gnathostomiasis
Infection by Gnathostoma spinigerum and related species

128.8 Other specified helminthiasis
Infection by:
Angiostrongylus cantonensis
Capillaria hepatica
other specified helminth

128.9 Helminth infection, unspecified
Helminthiasis NOS
Worms NOS

129 Intestinal parasitism, unspecified

Other Infectious and Parasitic Diseases (130–136)

√4ᵗʰ **130 Toxoplasmosis**
INCLUDES infection by toxoplasma gondii
toxoplasmosis (acquired)
EXCLUDES *congenital toxoplasmosis (771.2)*

130.0 Meningoencephalitis due to toxoplasmosis
Encephalitis due to acquired toxoplasmosis

130.1 Conjunctivitis due to toxoplasmosis

130.2 Chorioretinitis due to toxoplasmosis
Focal retinochoroiditis due to acquired toxoplasmosis

130.3 Myocarditis due to toxoplasmosis

130.4 Pneumonitis due to toxoplasmosis

130.5 Hepatitis due to toxoplasmosis

130.7 Toxoplasmosis of other specified sites

130.8 Multisystemic disseminated toxoplasmosis
Toxoplasmosis of multiple sites

130.9 Toxoplasmosis, unspecified

√4ᵗʰ **131 Trichomoniasis**
INCLUDES infection due to Trichomonas (vaginalis)

√5ᵗʰ **131.0 Urogenital trichomoniasis**

131.00 Urogenital trichomoniasis, unspecified
Fluor (vaginalis) ⎱ trichomonal or due to
Leukorrhea (vaginalis) ⎰ Trichomonas
(vaginalis)

DEF: *Trichomonas vaginalis* infection of reproductive and
urinary organs, transmitted through coitus.

131.01 Trichomonal vulvovaginitis   ♀
Vaginitis, trichomonal or due to Trichomonas
(vaginalis)
DEF: *Trichomonas vaginalis* infection of vulva and vagina;
often asymptomatic, transmitted through coitus.

131.02 Trichomonal urethritis
DEF: *Trichomonas vaginalis* infection of the urethra.

131.03 Trichomonal prostatitis   ♂
DEF: *Trichomonas vaginalis* infection of the prostate.

131.09 Other

131.8 Other specified sites
EXCLUDES *intestinal (007.3)*

131.9 Trichomoniasis, unspecified

√4ᵗʰ **132 Pediculosis and phthirus infestation**

132.0 Pediculus capitis [head louse]

132.1 Pediculus corporis [body louse]

132.2 Phthirus pubis [pubic louse]
Pediculus pubis

132.3 Mixed infestation
Infestation classifiable to more than one of the categories
132.0-132.2

132.9 Pediculosis, unspecified

√4ᵗʰ **133 Acariasis**

133.0 Scabies
Infestation by Sarcoptes scabiei
Norwegian scabies
Sarcoptic itch

133.8 Other acariasis
Chiggers
Infestation by:
Demodex folliculorum
Trombicula

133.9 Acariasis, unspecified
Infestation by mites NOS

√4ᵗʰ **134 Other infestation**

134.0 Myiasis
Infestation by:
Dermatobia (hominis)
fly larvae
Gasterophilus (intestinalis)
maggots
Oestrus ovis

134.1 Other arthropod infestation
Infestation by: Jigger disease
chigoe   Scarabiasis
sand flea   Tungiasis
Tunga penetrans

134.2 Hirudiniasis
Hirudiniasis (external) (internal)
Leeches (aquatic) (land)

134.8 Other specified infestations

134.9 Infestation, unspecified
Infestation (skin) NOS   Skin parasites NOS

135 Sarcoidosis
Besnier-Boeck-Schaumann disease
Lupoid (miliary) of Boeck
Lupus pernio (Besnier)
Lymphogranulomatosis, benign (Schaumann's)
Sarcoid (any site):
NOS
Boeck
Darier-Roussy
Uveoparotid fever
DEF: A chronic, granulomatous reticulosis (abnormal increase in cells),
affecting any organ or tissue; acute form has high rate of remission; chronic
form is progressive.
D86.9 Sarcoidosis unspecified   I-10

✓4ᵗʰ **136 Other and unspecified infectious and parasitic diseases**

136.0 Ainhum
Dactylolysis spontanea
DEF: A disease affecting the toes, especially the fifth digit, and the fingers, mostly seen in black adult males; characterized by a linear constriction around the affected digit leading to spontaneous amputation of the distal part of the digit.

136.1 Behçet's syndrome
DEF: A chronic inflammatory disorder of unknown etiology involving the small blood vessels; characterized by recurrent aphthous ulceration of the oral and pharyngeal mucous membranes and the genitalia, skin lesions, severe uveitis, retinal vascularitis and optic atrophy.

✓5ᵗʰ **136.2 Specific infections by free-living amebae**
AHA: 4Q, '08, 79-81

136.21 Specific infection due to acanthamoeba
Use additional code to identify manifestation, such as:
keratitis (370.8)
AHA: 4Q, '08, 81

136.29 Other specific infections by free-living amebae
Meningoencephalitis due to Naegleria

136.3 Pneumocystosis
Pneumonia due to Pneumocystis carinii
Pneumonia due to Pneumocystis jiroveci
AHA: 1Q, '05, 7; 1Q, '03, 15; N-D, '87, 5-6
DEF: *Pneumocystis carinii* fungus causing pneumonia in immunocompromised patients; a leading cause of death among AIDS patients.

136.4 Psorospermiasis

136.5 Sarcosporidiosis
Infection by Sarcocystis lindemanni
DEF: *Sarcocystis* infection causing muscle cysts of intestinal inflammation.

136.8 Other specified infectious and parasitic diseases
Candiru infestation

136.9 Unspecified infectious and parasitic diseases
Infectious disease NOS
Parasitic disease NOS
AHA: 2Q, '91, 8

Late Effects of Infectious and Parasitic Diseases (137-139)

✓4ᵗʰ **137 Late effects of tuberculosis**
NOTE This category is to be used to indicate conditions classifiable to 010-018 as the cause of late effects, which are themselves classified elsewhere. The "late effects" include those specified as such, as sequelae, or as due to old or inactive tuberculosis, without evidence of active disease.

137.0 Late effects of respiratory or unspecified tuberculosis

137.1 Late effects of central nervous system tuberculosis

137.2 Late effects of genitourinary tuberculosis

137.3 Late effects of tuberculosis of bones and joints

137.4 Late effects of tuberculosis of other specified organs

138 Late effects of acute poliomyelitis
NOTE This category is to be used to indicate conditions classifiable to 045 as the cause of late effects, which are themselves classified elsewhere. The "late effects" include conditions specified as such, or as sequelae, or as due to old or inactive poliomyelitis, without evidence of active disease.
B91 Sequelae of poliomyelitis   I-10

✓4ᵗʰ **139 Late effects of other infectious and parasitic diseases**
NOTE This category is to be used to indicate conditions classifiable to categories 001-009, 020-041, 046-136 as the cause of late effects, which are themselves classified elsewhere. The "late effects" include conditions specified as such; they also include sequela of diseases classifiable to the above categories if there is evidence that the disease itself is no longer present.

139.0 Late effects of viral encephalitis
Late effects of conditions classifiable to 049.8-049.9, 062-064

139.1 Late effects of trachoma
Late effects of conditions classifiable to 076

139.8 Late effects of other and unspecified infectious and parasitic diseases
AHA: 2Q, '06, 17; 4Q, '91, 15; 3Q, '90, 14; M-A, '87, 8

2. Neoplasms (140-239)

NOTES

1. Content

This chapter contains the following broad groups:

140-195   Malignant neoplasms, stated or presumed to be primary, of specified sites, except of lymphatic and hematopoietic tissue

196-198   Malignant neoplasms, stated or presumed to be secondary, of specified sites

199   Malignant neoplasms, without specification of site

200-208   Malignant neoplasms, stated or presumed to be primary, of lymphatic and hematopoietic tissue

209   Neuroendocrine tumors

210-229   Benign neoplasms

230-234   Carcinoma in situ

235-238   Neoplasms of uncertain behavior [see Note, above category 235]

239   Neoplasms of unspecified nature

2. Functional activity

All neoplasms are classified in this chapter, whether or not functionally active. An additional code from Chapter 3 may be used to identify such functional activity associated with any neoplasm, e.g.:

catecholamine-producing malignant pheochromocytoma of adrenal:

code 194.0, additional code 255.6

basophil adenoma of pituitary with Cushing's syndrome:

code 227.3, additional code 255.0

3. Morphology [Histology]

For those wishing to identify the histological type of neoplasms, a comprehensive coded nomenclature, which comprises the morphology rubrics of the ICD-Oncology, is given in Appendix A.

4. Malignant neoplasms overlapping site boundaries

Categories 140-195 are for the classification of primary malignant neoplasms according to their point of origin. A malignant neoplasm that overlaps two or more subcategories within a three-digit rubric and whose point of origin cannot be determined should be classified to the subcategory .8 "Other."

For example, "carcinoma involving tip and ventral surface of tongue" should be assigned to 141.8. On the other hand, "carcinoma of tip of tongue, extending to involve the ventral surface" should be coded to 141.2, as the point of origin, the tip, is known. Three subcategories (149.8, 159.8, 165.8) have been provided for malignant neoplasms that overlap the boundaries of three-digit rubrics within certain systems.

Overlapping malignant neoplasms that cannot be classified as indicated above should be assigned to the appropriate subdivision of category 195 (Malignant neoplasm of other and ill-defined sites).

DEF: An abnormal growth; morphology determines behavior, i.e., whether it will remain intact (benign) or spread to adjacent tissue (malignant). The term mass is not synonymous with neoplasm, as it is often used to describe cysts and thickenings such as those occurring with hematoma or infection. **AHA:** 2Q, '90, 7

Malignant Neoplasm of Lip, Oral Cavity, and Pharynx (140-149)

EXCLUDES   *carcinoma in situ (230.0)*

√4ᵗʰ **140   Malignant neoplasm of lip**

EXCLUDES   *malignant melanoma of skin of lip (172.0)*
malignant neoplasm of skin of lip (173.00-173.09)

140.0   Upper lip, vermilion border
Upper lip:
NOS
external
lipstick area

140.1   Lower lip, vermilion border
Lower lip:
NOS
external
lipstick area

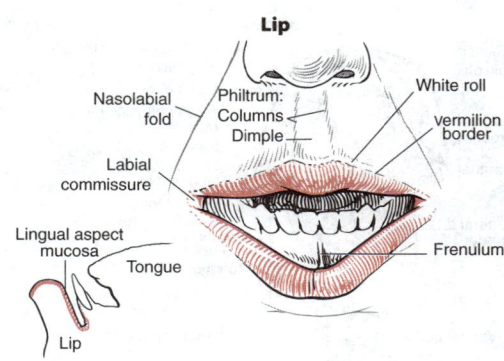

Lip

Nasolabial fold · Philtrum: Columns Dimple · White roll · vermilion border · Labial commissure · Lingual aspect mucosa · Tongue · Frenulum · Lip

140.3   Upper lip, inner aspect
Upper lip:
buccal aspect
frenulum
mucosa
oral aspect

140.4   Lower lip, inner aspect
Lower lip:
buccal aspect
frenulum
mucosa
oral aspect

140.5   Lip, unspecified, inner aspect
Lip, not specified whether upper or lower:
buccal aspect
frenulum
mucosa
oral aspect

140.6   Commissure of lip
Labial commissure

140.8   Other sites of lip
Malignant neoplasm of contiguous or overlapping sites of lip whose point of origin cannot be determined

140.9   Lip, unspecified, vermilion border
Lip, not specified as upper or lower:
NOS
external
lipstick area

√4ᵗʰ **141   Malignant neoplasm of tongue**

141.0   Base of tongue
Dorsal surface of base of tongue
Fixed part of tongue NOS
AHA: 4Q, '06, 90

141.1   Dorsal surface of tongue
Anterior two-thirds of tongue, dorsal surface
Dorsal tongue NOS
Midline of tongue
EXCLUDES   *dorsal surface of base of tongue (141.0)*

141.2   Tip and lateral border of tongue

141.3   Ventral surface of tongue
Anterior two-thirds of tongue, ventral surface
Frenulum linguae

141.4   Anterior two-thirds of tongue, part unspecified
Mobile part of tongue NOS

141.5   Junctional zone
Border of tongue at junction of fixed and mobile parts at insertion of anterior tonsillar pillar

√4ᵗʰ √5ᵗʰ Additional Digit Required   Unspecified Code   Other Specified Code   Manifestation Code   ►◄ Revised Text   ● New Code   ▲ Revised Code Title

2015 ICD-9-CM   **Volume 1 – 27**

Tongue

Main Salivary Glands

Mouth

Oropharynx

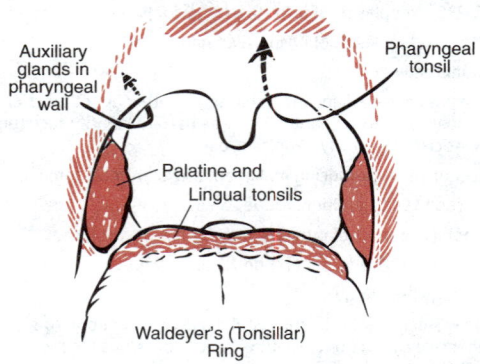

141.6 Lingual tonsil

141.8 Other sites of tongue
Malignant neoplasm of contiguous or overlapping sites of tongue whose point of origin cannot be determined

141.9 Tongue, unspecified
Tongue NOS

√4ᵗʰ 142 Malignant neoplasm of major salivary glands
INCLUDES salivary ducts
EXCLUDES *malignant neoplasm of minor salivary glands:*
NOS (145.9)
buccal mucosa (145.0)
soft palate (145.3)
tongue (141.0-141.9)
tonsil, palatine (146.0)

142.0 Parotid gland

142.1 Submandibular gland
Submaxillary gland

142.2 Sublingual gland

142.8 Other major salivary glands
Malignant neoplasm of contiguous or overlapping sites of salivary glands and ducts whose point of origin cannot be determined

142.9 Salivary gland, unspecified
Salivary gland (major) NOS

√4ᵗʰ 143 Malignant neoplasm of gum
INCLUDES alveolar (ridge) mucosa
gingiva (alveolar) (marginal)
interdental papillae
EXCLUDES *malignant odontogenic neoplasms (170.0-170.1)*

143.0 Upper gum

143.1 Lower gum

143.8 Other sites of gum
Malignant neoplasm of contiguous or overlapping sites of gum whose point of origin cannot be determined

143.9 Gum, unspecified

√4ᵗʰ 144 Malignant neoplasm of floor of mouth

144.0 Anterior portion
Anterior to the premolar-canine junction

144.1 Lateral portion

144.8 Other sites of floor of mouth
Malignant neoplasm of contiguous or overlapping sites of floor of mouth whose point of origin cannot be determined

144.9 Floor of mouth, part unspecified

√4ᵗʰ 145 Malignant neoplasm of other and unspecified parts of mouth
EXCLUDES *mucosa of lips (140.0-140.9)*

145.0 Cheek mucosa
Buccal mucosa
Cheek, inner aspect

145.1 Vestibule of mouth
Buccal sulcus (upper) (lower)
Labial sulcus (upper) (lower)

145.2 Hard palate

145.3 Soft palate
EXCLUDES *nasopharyngeal [posterior] [superior] surface of soft palate (147.3)*

145.4 Uvula

145.5 Palate, unspecified
Junction of hard and soft palate
Roof of mouth

145.6 Retromolar area

145.8 Other specified parts of mouth
Malignant neoplasm of contiguous or overlapping sites of mouth whose point of origin cannot be determined

145.9 Mouth, unspecified
Buccal cavity NOS
Minor salivary gland, unspecified site
Oral cavity NOS

N Newborn Age: 0   P Pediatric Age: 0-17   M Maternity Age: 12-55   A Adult Age: 15-124

Nasopharynx

Nasal septum
Pharyngeal tonsil
Opening of auditory tube
Pharyngeal recess (of Rosenmüller)
Soft palate

Hypopharynx

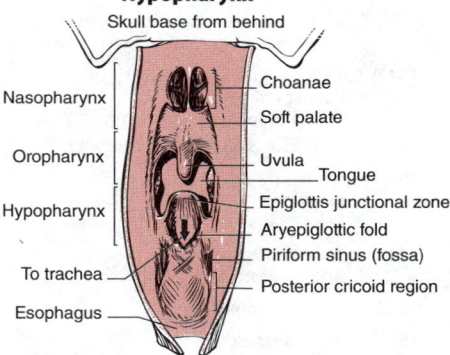

Skull base from behind

Nasopharynx
Oropharynx
Hypopharynx
To trachea
Esophagus

Choanae
Soft palate
Uvula
Tongue
Epiglottis junctional zone
Aryepiglottic fold
Piriform sinus (fossa)
Posterior cricoid region

✓4th 146 Malignant neoplasm of oropharynx

146.0 Tonsil
Tonsil:
  NOS
  faucial
  palatine
  EXCLUDES lingual tonsil (141.6)
  pharyngeal tonsil (147.1)
  AHA: S-O, '87, 8

146.1 Tonsillar fossa

146.2 Tonsillar pillars (anterior) (posterior)
Faucial pillar
Glossopalatine fold
Palatoglossal arch
Palatopharyngeal arch

146.3 Vallecula
Anterior and medial surface of the pharyngoepiglottic fold

146.4 Anterior aspect of epiglottis
Epiglottis, free border [margin]
Glossoepiglottic fold(s)
  EXCLUDES epiglottis:
  NOS (161.1)
  suprahyoid portion (161.1)

146.5 Junctional region
Junction of the free margin of the epiglottis, the aryepiglottic fold, and the pharyngoepiglottic fold

146.6 Lateral wall of oropharynx

146.7 Posterior wall of oropharynx

146.8 Other specified sites of oropharynx
Branchial cleft
Malignant neoplasm of contiguous or overlapping sites of oropharynx whose point of origin cannot be determined

146.9 Oropharynx, unspecified
  AHA: 2Q, '02, 6

✓4th 147 Malignant neoplasm of nasopharynx

147.0 Superior wall
Roof of nasopharynx

147.1 Posterior wall
Adenoid
Pharyngeal tonsil

147.2 Lateral wall
Fossa of Rosenmüller
Opening of auditory tube
Pharyngeal recess

147.3 Anterior wall
Floor of nasopharynx
Nasopharyngeal [posterior] [superior] surface of soft palate
Posterior margin of nasal septum and choanae

147.8 Other specified sites of nasopharynx
Malignant neoplasm of contiguous or overlapping sites of nasopharynx whose point of origin cannot be determined

147.9 Nasopharynx, unspecified
Nasopharyngeal wall NOS

✓4th 148 Malignant neoplasm of hypopharynx

148.0 Postcricoid region

148.1 Pyriform sinus
Pyriform fossa

148.2 Aryepiglottic fold, hypopharyngeal aspect
Aryepiglottic fold or interarytenoid fold:
  NOS
  marginal zone
  EXCLUDES aryepiglottic fold or interarytenoid fold, laryngeal aspect (161.1)

148.3 Posterior hypopharyngeal wall

148.8 Other specified sites of hypopharynx
Malignant neoplasm of contiguous or overlapping sites of hypopharynx whose point of origin cannot be determined

148.9 Hypopharynx, unspecified
Hypopharyngeal wall NOS
Hypopharynx NOS

✓4th 149 Malignant neoplasm of other and ill-defined sites within the lip, oral cavity, and pharynx

149.0 Pharynx, unspecified

149.1 Waldeyer's ring

149.8 Other
Malignant neoplasms of lip, oral cavity, and pharynx whose point of origin cannot be assigned to any one of the categories 140-148
  EXCLUDES "book leaf" neoplasm [ventral surface of tongue and floor of mouth] (145.8)

149.9 Ill-defined

Malignant Neoplasm of Digestive Organs and Peritoneum (150-159)
  EXCLUDES carcinoma in situ (230.1-230.9)

✓4th 150 Malignant neoplasm of esophagus

150.0 Cervical esophagus

150.1 Thoracic esophagus

150.2 Abdominal esophagus
  EXCLUDES adenocarcinoma (151.0)
  cardio-esophageal junction (151.0)

150.3 Upper third of esophagus
Proximal third of esophagus

150.4 Middle third of esophagus

150.5 Lower third of esophagus
Distal third of esophagus
  EXCLUDES adenocarcinoma (151.0)
  cardio-esophageal junction (151.0)

150.8 Other specified part
Malignant neoplasm of contiguous or overlapping sites of esophagus whose point of origin cannot be determined

150.9 Esophagus, unspecified

Neoplasms

151–155.2

✓4ᵗʰ 151 Malignant neoplasm of stomach

> **EXCLUDES** *benign carcinoid tumor of stomach (209.63)*
> *malignant carcinoid tumor of stomach (209.23)*

151.0 Cardia
Cardiac orifice
Cardio-esophageal junction
> **EXCLUDES** *squamous cell carcinoma (150.2, 150.5)*

151.1 Pylorus
Prepylorus
Pyloric canal

151.2 Pyloric antrum
Antrum of stomach NOS

151.3 Fundus of stomach

151.4 Body of stomach

151.5 Lesser curvature, unspecified
Lesser curvature, not classifiable to 151.1-151.4

151.6 Greater curvature, unspecified
Greater curvature, not classifiable to 151.0-151.4

151.8 Other specified sites of stomach
Anterior wall, not classifiable to 151.0-151.4
Posterior wall, not classifiable to 151.0-151.4
Malignant neoplasm of contiguous or overlapping sites of stomach whose point of origin cannot be determined

151.9 Stomach, unspecified
Carcinoma ventriculi
Gastric cancer
AHA: 2Q, '01, 17

✓4ᵗʰ 152 Malignant neoplasm of small intestine, including duodenum

> **EXCLUDES** *benign carcinoid tumor of small intestine and duodenum (209.40-209.43)*
> *malignant carcinoid tumor of small intestine and duodenum (209.00-209.03)*

152.0 Duodenum

152.1 Jejunum

152.2 Ileum
> **EXCLUDES** *ileocecal valve (153.4)*

152.3 Meckel's diverticulum

152.8 Other specified sites of small intestine
Duodenojejunal junction
Malignant neoplasm of contiguous or overlapping sites of small intestine whose point of origin cannot be determined

152.9 Small intestine, unspecified

✓4ᵗʰ 153 Malignant neoplasm of colon

> **EXCLUDES** *benign carcinoid tumor of colon (209.50-209.56)*
> *malignant carcinoid tumor of colon (209.10-209.16)*

153.0 Hepatic flexure

153.1 Transverse colon
AHA: ▶3Q, '13, 9◀

153.2 Descending colon
Left colon

153.3 Sigmoid colon
Sigmoid (flexure)
> **EXCLUDES** *rectosigmoid junction (154.0)*

153.4 Cecum
Ileocecal valve
C18.0 Malignant neoplasm of cecum   I-10

153.5 Appendix

153.6 Ascending colon
Right colon
C18.2 Malignant neoplasm of ascending colon   I-10

153.7 Splenic flexure

153.8 Other specified sites of large intestine
Malignant neoplasm of contiguous or overlapping sites of colon whose point of origin cannot be determined
> **EXCLUDES** *ileocecal valve (153.4)*
> *rectosigmoid junction (154.0)*

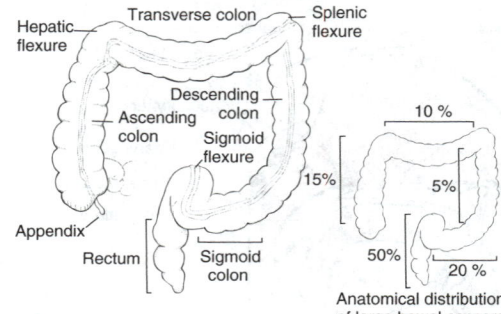

Colon

Anatomical distribution of large bowel cancers

153.9 Colon, unspecified
Large intestine NOS
AHA: 2Q, '10, 12
C18.9 Malignant neoplasm of colon unspecified   I-10

✓4ᵗʰ 154 Malignant neoplasm of rectum, rectosigmoid junction, and anus

> **EXCLUDES** *benign carcinoid tumor of rectum (209.57)*
> *malignant carcinoid tumor of rectum (209.17)*

154.0 Rectosigmoid junction
Colon with rectum
Rectosigmoid (colon)

154.1 Rectum
Rectal ampulla
C20 Malignant neoplasm of rectum   I-10

154.2 Anal canal
Anal sphincter
> **EXCLUDES** *malignant melanoma of skin of anus (172.5)*
> *malignant neoplasm of skin of anus (173.50-173.59)*

AHA: 1Q, '01, 8

154.3 Anus, unspecified
> **EXCLUDES** *malignant melanoma of:*
> *anus:*
> *margin (172.5)*
> *skin (172.5)*
> *perianal skin (172.5)*
> *malignant neoplasm of:*
> *anus:*
> *margin (173.50-173.59)*
> *skin (173.50-173.59)*
> *perianal skin (173.50-173.59)*

154.8 Other
Anorectum
Cloacogenic zone
Malignant neoplasm of contiguous or overlapping sites of rectum, rectosigmoid junction, and anus whose point of origin cannot be determined

✓4ᵗʰ 155 Malignant neoplasm of liver and intrahepatic bile ducts

155.0 Liver, primary
Carcinoma:
hepatocellular
liver cell
liver, specified as primary
Hepatoblastoma
AHA: 4Q, '08, 82
C22.0 Liver cell carcinoma   I-10

155.1 Intrahepatic bile ducts
Canaliculi biliferi
Interlobular:
bile ducts
biliary canals
Intrahepatic:
biliary passages
canaliculi
gall duct
> **EXCLUDES** *hepatic duct (156.1)*

155.2 Liver, not specified as primary or secondary

Retroperitoneum and Peritoneum

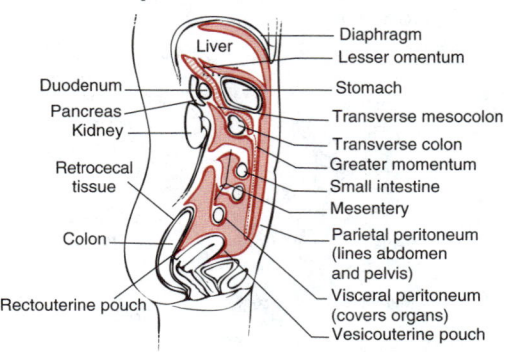

✓4ᵗʰ **156 Malignant neoplasm of gallbladder and extrahepatic bile ducts**

156.0 Gallbladder

156.1 Extrahepatic bile ducts
Biliary duct or passage NOS
Common bile duct
Cystic duct
Hepatic duct
Sphincter of Oddi

156.2 Ampulla of Vater
DEF: Malignant neoplasm in the area of dilation at the juncture of the common bile and pancreatic ducts near the opening into the lumen of the duodenum.

156.8 Other specified sites of gallbladder and extrahepatic bile ducts
Malignant neoplasm of contiguous or overlapping sites of gallbladder and extrahepatic bile ducts whose point of origin cannot be determined

156.9 Biliary tract, part unspecified
Malignant neoplasm involving both intrahepatic and extrahepatic bile ducts

✓4ᵗʰ **157 Malignant neoplasm of pancreas**
AHA: 4Q, '07, 72

157.0 Head of pancreas
AHA: 2Q, '05, 9; 4Q, '00, 40

157.1 Body of pancreas

157.2 Tail of pancreas

157.3 Pancreatic duct
Duct of:
Santorini
Wirsung

157.4 Islets of Langerhans
Islets of Langerhans, any part of pancreas
Use additional code to identify any functional activity
DEF: Malignant neoplasm within the structures of the pancreas that produce insulin, somatostatin and glucagon.

157.8 Other specified sites of pancreas
Ectopic pancreatic tissue
Malignant neoplasm of contiguous or overlapping sites of pancreas whose point of origin cannot be determined

157.9 Pancreas, part unspecified
AHA: 4Q, '89, 11
C25.9 Malignant neoplasm of pancreas unspecified   I-10

✓4ᵗʰ **158 Malignant neoplasm of retroperitoneum and peritoneum**

158.0 Retroperitoneum
Periadrenal tissue   Perirenal tissue
Perinephric tissue   Retrocecal tissue

158.8 Specified parts of peritoneum
Cul-de-sac (of Douglas)
Malignant neoplasm of contiguous or overlapping sites of retroperitoneum and peritoneum whose point of origin cannot be determined
Mesentery
Mesocolon
Omentum
Peritoneum:
parietal
pelvic
Rectouterine pouch

158.9 Peritoneum, unspecified

✓4ᵗʰ **159 Malignant neoplasm of other and ill-defined sites within the digestive organs and peritoneum**

159.0 Intestinal tract, part unspecified
Intestine NOS

159.1 Spleen, not elsewhere classified
Angiosarcoma ⎤ of spleen
Fibrosarcoma ⎦
EXCLUDES *Hodgkin's disease (201.0-201.9)*
lymphosarcoma (200.1)
reticulosarcoma (200.0)

159.8 Other sites of digestive system and intra-abdominal organs
Malignant neoplasm of digestive organs and peritoneum whose point of origin cannot be assigned to any one of the categories 150-158
EXCLUDES *anus and rectum (154.8)*
cardio-esophageal junction (151.0)
colon and rectum (154.0)

159.9 Ill-defined
Alimentary canal or tract NOS
Gastrointestinal tract NOS
EXCLUDES *abdominal NOS (195.2)*
intra-abdominal NOS (195.2)

Neoplasm of Respiratory and Intrathoracic Organs (160-165)
EXCLUDES *carcinoma in situ (231.0-231.9)*

✓4ᵗʰ **160 Malignant neoplasm of nasal cavities, middle ear, and accessory sinuses**

160.0 Nasal cavities
Cartilage of nose   Septum of nose
Conchae, nasal   Vestibule of nose
Internal nose
EXCLUDES *malignant melanoma of skin of nose (172.3)*
malignant neoplasm of skin of nose (173.30-173.39)
nasal bone (170.0)
nose NOS (195.0)
olfactory bulb (192.0)
posterior margin of septum and choanae (147.3)
turbinates (170.0)

160.1 Auditory tube, middle ear, and mastoid air cells
Antrum tympanicum
Eustachian tube
Tympanic cavity
EXCLUDES *bone of ear (meatus) (170.0)*
cartilage of ear (171.0)
malignant melanoma of:
auditory canal (external) (172.2, 173.2)
ear (external) (skin) (172.2)
malignant neoplasm of:
auditory canal (external) (173.20-173.29)
ear (external) (skin) (173.20-173.29)

160.2 Maxillary sinus
Antrum (Highmore) (maxillary)

160.3 Ethmoidal sinus

160.4 Frontal sinus

160.5 Sphenoidal sinus

160.8 Other
Malignant neoplasm of contiguous or overlapping sites of nasal cavities, middle ear, and accessory sinuses whose point of origin cannot be determined

✓4ᵗʰ
✓5ᵗʰ Additional Digit Required   Unspecified Code   Other Specified Code   Manifestation Code   ▶◀ Revised Text   ● New Code   ▲ Revised Code Title
2015 ICD-9-CM   **Volume 1 – 31**

Neoplasms

160.9   Accessory sinus, unspecified

☑4ᵗʰ **161**   **Malignant neoplasm of larynx**

     161.0   **Glottis**
         Intrinsic larynx
         Laryngeal commissure (anterior) (posterior)
         True vocal cord
         Vocal cord NOS

     161.1   **Supraglottis**
         Aryepiglottic fold or interarytenoid fold, laryngeal aspect
         Epiglottis (suprahyoid portion) NOS
         Extrinsic larynx
         False vocal cords
         Posterior (laryngeal) surface of epiglottis
         Ventricular bands
         EXCLUDES *anterior aspect of epiglottis (146.4)*
                 aryepiglottic fold or interarytenoid fold:
                 NOS (148.2)
                 hypopharyngeal aspect (148.2)
                 marginal zone (148.2)

     161.2   **Subglottis**

     161.3   **Laryngeal cartilages**
         Cartilage: Cartilage:
           arytenoid   cuneiform
           cricoid   thyroid

     161.8   **Other specified sites of larynx**
         Malignant neoplasm of contiguous or overlapping sites of larynx whose point of origin cannot be determined
         AHA: 3Q, '07, 7

     161.9   **Larynx, unspecified**

☑4ᵗʰ **162**   **Malignant neoplasm of trachea, bronchus, and lung**
     EXCLUDES *benign carcinoid tumor of bronchus (209.61)*
                 malignant carcinoid tumor of bronchus (209.21)

     162.0   **Trachea**
         Cartilage }
         Mucosa } of trachea

     162.2   **Main bronchus**
         Carina   Hilus of lung

     162.3   **Upper lobe, bronchus or lung**
         AHA: 1Q, '04, 4
         C34.10 Malig neoplasm upper lobe unspec bronchus/lung   I-10

     162.4   **Middle lobe, bronchus or lung**

     162.5   **Lower lobe, bronchus or lung**
         AHA: 3Q, '10, 3

     162.8   **Other parts of bronchus or lung**
         Malignant neoplasm of contiguous or overlapping sites of bronchus or lung whose point of origin cannot be determined
         AHA: 3Q, '06, 7

     162.9   **Bronchus and lung, unspecified**
         AHA: 2Q, '10, 14; 3Q, '06, 14-15; 2Q, '97, 3; 4Q, '96, 48
         C34.90 Malig neoplasm unsp part of unspec bronchus/lung   I-10

☑4ᵗʰ **163**   **Malignant neoplasm of pleura**

     163.0   **Parietal pleura**

     163.1   **Visceral pleura**

     163.8   **Other specified sites of pleura**
         Malignant neoplasm of contiguous or overlapping sites of pleura whose point of origin cannot be determined

     163.9   **Pleura, unspecified**

☑4ᵗʰ **164**   **Malignant neoplasm of thymus, heart, and mediastinum**

     164.0   **Thymus**
         EXCLUDES *benign carcinoid tumor of the thymus (209.62)*
                 malignant carcinoid tumor of the thymus (209.22)

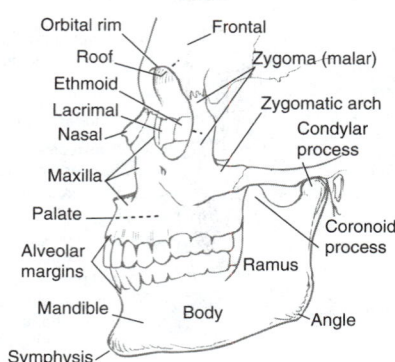

Skull

     164.1   **Heart**
         Endocardium   Myocardium
         Epicardium   Pericardium
         EXCLUDES *great vessels (171.4)*

     164.2   **Anterior mediastinum**

     164.3   **Posterior mediastinum**

     164.8   **Other**
         Malignant neoplasm of contiguous or overlapping sites of thymus, heart, and mediastinum whose point of origin cannot be determined

     164.9   **Mediastinum, part unspecified**

☑4ᵗʰ **165**   **Malignant neoplasm of other and ill-defined sites within the respiratory system and intrathoracic organs**

     165.0   **Upper respiratory tract, part unspecified**

     165.8   **Other**
         Malignant neoplasm of respiratory and intrathoracic organs whose point of origin cannot be assigned to any one of the categories 160-164

     165.9   **Ill-defined sites within the respiratory system**
         Respiratory tract NOS
         EXCLUDES *intrathoracic NOS (195.1)*
                 thoracic NOS (195.1)

Malignant Neoplasm of Bone, Connective Tissue, Skin, and Breast (170-176)

     EXCLUDES *carcinoma in situ:*
                 breast (233.0)
                 skin (232.0-232.9)

☑4ᵗʰ **170**   **Malignant neoplasm of bone and articular cartilage**
     INCLUDES cartilage (articular) (joint)
                 periosteum
     EXCLUDES *bone marrow NOS (202.9)*
                 cartilage:
                   ear (171.0)
                   eyelid (171.0)
                   larynx (161.3)
                   nose (160.0)
                 synovia (171.0-171.9)
     AHA: 4Q, '06, 103
     TIP: Do not assign for bone metastasis; see instead code 198.5.

     170.0   **Bones of skull and face, except mandible**
         Bone: Bone:
           ethmoid   sphenoid
           frontal   temporal
           malar   zygomatic
           nasal   Maxilla (superior)
           occipital   Turbinate
           orbital   Upper jaw bone
           parietal   Vomer
         EXCLUDES *carcinoma, any type except intraosseous or odontogenic:*
                 maxilla, maxillary (sinus) (160.2)
                 upper jaw bone (143.0)
                 jaw bone (lower) (170.1)

170.1 Mandible
Inferior maxilla
Jaw bone NOS
Lower jaw bone
> **EXCLUDES** carcinoma, any type except intraosseous or
> odontogenic:
> jaw bone NOS (143.9)
> lower (143.1)
> upper jaw bone (170.0)

170.2 Vertebral column, excluding sacrum and coccyx
Spinal column
Spine
Vertebra
> **EXCLUDES** sacrum and coccyx (170.6)

170.3 Ribs, sternum, and clavicle
Costal cartilage
Costovertebral joint
Xiphoid process

170.4 Scapula and long bones of upper limb
Acromion
Bones NOS of upper limb
Humerus
Radius
Ulna
AHA: 2Q, '99, 9

170.5 Short bones of upper limb
Carpal
Cuneiform, wrist
Metacarpal
Navicular, of hand
Phalanges of hand
Pisiform
Scaphoid (of hand)
Semilunar or lunate
Trapezium
Trapezoid
Unciform

170.6 Pelvic bones, sacrum, and coccyx
Coccygeal vertebra
Ilium
Ischium
Pubic bone
Sacral vertebra

170.7 Long bones of lower limb
Bones NOS of lower limb
Femur
Fibula
Tibia

170.8 Short bones of lower limb
Astragalus [talus]
Calcaneus
Cuboid
Cuneiform, ankle
Metatarsal
Navicular (of ankle)
Patella
Phalanges of foot
Tarsal

170.9 Bone and articular cartilage, site unspecified

✓4ᵗʰ 171 Malignant neoplasm of connective and other soft tissue
> **INCLUDES** blood vessel
> bursa
> fascia
> fat
> ligament, except uterine
> muscle
> peripheral, sympathetic, and parasympathetic nerves and
> ganglia
> synovia
> tendon (sheath)

> **EXCLUDES** cartilage (of):
> articular (170.0-170.9)
> larynx (161.3)
> nose (160.0)
> connective tissue:
> breast (174.0-175.9)
> internal organs — code to malignant neoplasm of the site
> [e.g., leiomyosarcoma of stomach, 151.9]
> heart (164.1)
> uterine ligament (183.4)

171.0 Head, face, and neck
Cartilage of:
ear
eyelid
AHA: 2Q, '99, 6

171.2 Upper limb, including shoulder
Arm
Finger
Forearm
Hand

171.3 Lower limb, including hip
Foot
Leg
Popliteal space
AHA: 3Q, '12, 7-8
Thigh
Toe

171.4 Thorax
Axilla
Diaphragm
Great vessels
> **EXCLUDES** heart (164.1)
> mediastinum (164.2-164.9)
> thymus (164.0)

171.5 Abdomen
Abdominal wall
Hypochondrium
> **EXCLUDES** peritoneum (158.8)
> retroperitoneum (158.0)

171.6 Pelvis
Buttock
Groin
Inguinal region
Perineum
> **EXCLUDES** pelvic peritoneum (158.8)
> retroperitoneum (158.0)
> uterine ligament, any (183.3-183.5)

171.7 Trunk, unspecified
Back NOS
Flank NOS

171.8 Other specified sites of connective and other soft tissue
Malignant neoplasm of contiguous or overlapping sites of
connective tissue whose point of origin cannot be
determined

171.9 Connective and other soft tissue, site unspecified

✓4ᵗʰ 172 Malignant melanoma of skin
> **INCLUDES** melanocarcinoma
> melanoma (skin) NOS
> melanoma in situ of skin

> **EXCLUDES** skin of genital organs (184.0-184.9, 187.1-187.9)
> sites other than skin — code to malignant neoplasm of the
> site

DEF: Malignant neoplasm of melanocytes; most common in skin, may
involve oral cavity, esophagus, anal canal, vagina, leptomeninges, or
conjunctiva.

172.0 Lip
> **EXCLUDES** vermilion border of lip (140.0-140.1, 140.9)

172.1 Eyelid, including canthus

172.2 Ear and external auditory canal
Auricle (ear)
Auricular canal, external
External [acoustic] meatus
Pinna

172.3 Other and unspecified parts of face
Cheek (external)
Chin
Eyebrow
Forehead
Nose, external
Temple

172.4 Scalp and neck

172.5 Trunk, except scrotum
Axilla
Breast
Buttock
Groin
Perianal skin
Perineum
Umbilicus
> **EXCLUDES** anal canal (154.2)
> anus NOS (154.3)
> scrotum (187.7)

| ✓4ᵗʰ ✓5ᵗʰ Additional Digit Required | Unspecified Code | Other Specified Code | Manifestation Code | ►◄ Revised Text | ● New Code | ▲ Revised Code Title |

2015 ICD-9-CM

Volume 1 – 33

172.6 Upper limb, including shoulder

Arm	Forearm
Finger	Hand

172.7 Lower limb, including hip

Ankle	Leg
Foot	Popliteal area
Heel	Thigh
Knee	Toe

172.8 Other specified sites of skin

Malignant melanoma of contiguous or overlapping sites of skin whose point of origin cannot be determined

172.9 Melanoma of skin, site unspecified

√4ᵗʰ **173 Other and unspecified malignant neoplasm of skin**

INCLUDES malignant neoplasm of:
  sebaceous glands
  sudoriferous, sudoriparous glands
  sweat glands

EXCLUDES Kaposi's sarcoma (176.0-176.9)
  malignant melanoma of skin (172.0-172.9)
  Merkel cell carcinoma of skin (209.31-209.36)
  skin of genital organs (184.0-184.9, 187.1-187.9)

AHA: 4Q, '11, 83-87; 1Q, '00, 18; 2Q, '96, 12

TIP: Do not assign for malignant neoplasm of skin documented as melanoma; see instead category 172.

√5ᵗʰ **173.0 Other and unspecified malignant neoplasm of skin of lip**

EXCLUDES vermilion border of lip (140.0-140.1, 140.9)

173.00 Unspecified malignant neoplasm of skin of lip

173.01 Basal cell carcinoma of skin of lip

173.02 Squamous cell carcinoma of skin of lip

173.09 Other specified malignant neoplasm of skin of lip

√5ᵗʰ **173.1 Other and unspecified malignant neoplasm of skin of eyelid, including canthus**

EXCLUDES cartilage of eyelid (171.0)

173.10 Unspecified malignant neoplasm of eyelid, including canthus

173.11 Basal cell carcinoma of eyelid, including canthus

173.12 Squamous cell carcinoma of eyelid, including canthus

173.19 Other specified malignant neoplasm of eyelid, including canthus

√5ᵗʰ **173.2 Other and unspecified malignant neoplasm of skin of ear and external auditory canal**

Auricle (ear)
Auricular canal, external
External meatus
Pinna

EXCLUDES cartilage of ear (171.0)

173.20 Unspecified malignant neoplasm of skin of ear and external auditory canal

173.21 Basal cell carcinoma of skin of ear and external auditory canal

173.22 Squamous cell carcinoma of skin of ear and external auditory canal

173.29 Other specified malignant neoplasm of skin of ear and external auditory canal

√5ᵗʰ **173.3 Other and unspecified malignant neoplasm of skin of other and unspecified parts of face**

Cheek, external	Forehead
Chin	Nose, external
Eyebrow	Temple

AHA: 1Q, '00, 3

173.30 Unspecified malignant neoplasm of skin of other and unspecified parts of face

173.31 Basal cell carcinoma of skin of other and unspecified parts of face

173.32 Squamous cell carcinoma of skin of other and unspecified parts of face

173.39 Other specified malignant neoplasm of skin of other and unspecified parts of face

√5ᵗʰ **173.4 Other and unspecified malignant neoplasm of scalp and skin of neck**

173.40 Unspecified malignant neoplasm of scalp and skin of neck

173.41 Basal cell carcinoma of scalp and skin of neck

173.42 Squamous cell carcinoma of scalp and skin of neck

173.49 Other specified malignant neoplasm of scalp and skin of neck

√5ᵗʰ **173.5 Other and unspecified malignant neoplasm of skin of trunk, except scrotum**

Axillary fold	Skin of:
Perianal skin	buttock
Skin of:	chest wall
abdominal wall	groin
anus	perineum
back	umbilicus
breast	

EXCLUDES anal canal (154.2)
  anus NOS (154.3)
  skin of scrotum (187.7)

AHA: 1Q, '01, 8

173.50 Unspecified malignant neoplasm of skin of trunk, except scrotum

173.51 Basal cell carcinoma of skin of trunk, except scrotum

173.52 Squamous cell carcinoma of skin of trunk, except scrotum

173.59 Other specified malignant neoplasm of skin of trunk, except scrotum

√5ᵗʰ **173.6 Other and unspecified malignant neoplasm of skin of upper limb, including shoulder**

Arm	Forearm
Finger	Hand

173.60 Unspecified malignant neoplasm of skin of upper limb, including shoulder

173.61 Basal cell carcinoma of skin of upper limb, including shoulder

173.62 Squamous cell carcinoma of skin of upper limb, including shoulder

173.69 Other specified malignant neoplasm of skin of upper limb, including shoulder

√5ᵗʰ **173.7 Other and unspecified malignant neoplasm of skin of lower limb, including hip**

Ankle	Leg
Foot	Popliteal area
Heel	Thigh
Knee	Toe

173.70 Unspecified malignant neoplasm of skin of lower limb, including hip

173.71 Basal cell carcinoma of skin of lower limb, including hip

173.72 Squamous cell carcinoma of skin of lower limb, including hip

173.79 Other specified malignant neoplasm of skin of lower limb, including hip

√5ᵗʰ **173.8 Other and unspecified malignant neoplasm of other specified sites of skin**

Malignant neoplasm of contiguous or overlapping sites of skin whose point of origin cannot be determined

173.80 Unspecified malignant neoplasm of other specified sites of skin

173.81 Basal cell carcinoma of other specified sites of skin

173.82 Squamous cell carcinoma of other specified sites of skin

173.89 Other specified malignant neoplasm of other specified sites of skin

√5ᵗʰ **173.9 Other and unspecified malignant neoplasm of skin, site unspecified**

173.90 Unspecified malignant neoplasm of skin, site unspecified

Malignant neoplasm of skin NOS

173.91 Basal cell carcinoma of skin, site unspecified

173.92 Squamous cell carcinoma of skin, site unspecified

N Newborn Age: 0   P Pediatric Age: 0-17   M Maternity Age: 12-55   A Adult Age: 15-124

173.99 Other specified malignant neoplasm of skin, site unspecified

☑4ᵗʰ 174 Malignant neoplasm of female breast

Use additional code to identify estrogen receptor status (V86.0, V86.1)

INCLUDES   breast (female)
     connective tissue
     soft parts
  Paget's disease of:
     breast
     nipple

EXCLUDES *malignant melanoma of skin of breast (172.5)*
malignant neoplasm of skin of breast (173.50-173.59)

AHA: 3Q, '97, 8; 4Q, '89, 11

TIP: For bilateral breast malignancy, do not assign two codes unless documentation indicates separate sites (i.e., different fourth digits).

174.0 Nipple and areola   ♀

174.1 Central portion   ♀

174.2 Upper-inner quadrant   ♀

174.3 Lower-inner quadrant   ♀

174.4 Upper-outer quadrant   ♀
     AHA: 4Q, '08, 155; 1Q, '04, 3; 3Q, '97, 8

174.5 Lower-outer quadrant   ♀

174.6 Axillary tail   ♀

174.8 Other specified sites of female breast   ♀
     Ectopic sites
     Inner breast
     Lower breast
     Midline of breast
     Outer breast
     Upper breast
     Malignant neoplasm of contiguous or overlapping sites of breast whose point of origin cannot be determined

174.9 Breast (female), unspecified   ♀
     AHA: 3Q, '09, 3; 3Q, '05, 11; 2Q, '94, 10; 4Q, '89, 11
     C50.911 Malig neoplasm of uns site of rt female breast   **I-10**

☑4ᵗʰ 175 Malignant neoplasm of male breast

Use additional code to identify estrogen receptor status (V86.0, V86.1)

EXCLUDES *malignant melanoma of skin of breast (172.5)*
malignant neoplasm of skin of breast (173.50-173.59)

175.0 Nipple and areola   ♂

175.9 Other and unspecified sites of male breast   ♂
     Ectopic breast tissue, male

☑4ᵗʰ 176 Kaposi's sarcoma
     AHA: 4Q, '91, 24

176.0 Skin
     AHA: 4Q, '07, 63; 4Q, '94, 29; 4Q, '91, 24

176.1 Soft tissue
     Blood vessel   Ligament
     Connective tissue   Lymphatic(s) NEC
     Fascia   Muscle
     EXCLUDES *lymph glands and nodes (176.5)*

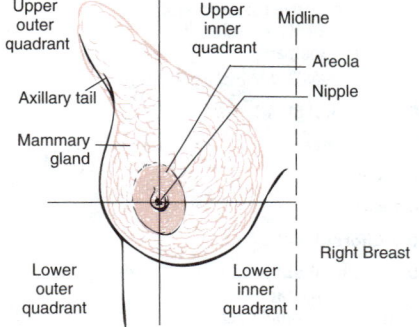

Female Breast

Upper outer quadrant
Upper inner quadrant
Midline
Areola
Nipple
Axillary tail
Mammary gland
Lower outer quadrant
Lower inner quadrant
Right Breast

176.2 Palate

176.3 Gastrointestinal sites

176.4 Lung

176.5 Lymph nodes

176.8 Other specified sites
     Oral cavity NEC

176.9 Unspecified
     Viscera NOS

Malignant Neoplasm of Genitourinary Organs (179-189)

     EXCLUDES *carcinoma in situ (233.1-233.9)*

179 Malignant neoplasm of uterus, part unspecified   ♀

☑4ᵗʰ 180 Malignant neoplasm of cervix uteri
     INCLUDES invasive malignancy [carcinoma]
     EXCLUDES *carcinoma in situ (233.1)*

180.0 Endocervix   ♀
     Cervical canal NOS
     Endocervical canal
     Endocervical gland

180.1 Exocervix   ♀

180.8 Other specified sites of cervix   ♀
     Cervical stump
     Squamocolumnar junction of cervix
     Malignant neoplasm of contiguous or overlapping sites of cervix uteri whose point of origin cannot be determined

180.9 Cervix uteri, unspecified   ♀

181 Malignant neoplasm of placenta   ♀
     Choriocarcinoma NOS
     Chorioepithelioma NOS
     EXCLUDES *chorioadenoma (destruens) (236.1)*
     hydatidiform mole (630)
        malignant (236.1)
     invasive mole (236.1)
     male choriocarcinoma NOS (186.0-186.9)

☑4ᵗʰ 182 Malignant neoplasm of body of uterus
     EXCLUDES *carcinoma in situ (233.2)*

182.0 Corpus uteri, except isthmus   ♀
     Cornu   Fundus
     Endometrium   Myometrium
     AHA: 3Q, '09, 5
     C54.9 Malignant neoplasm of corpus uteri unspecified   **I-10**

182.1 Isthmus
     Lower uterine segment

182.8 Other specified sites of body of uterus   ♀
     Malignant neoplasm of contiguous or overlapping sites of body of uterus whose point of origin cannot be determined
     EXCLUDES *uterus NOS (179)*

☑4ᵗʰ 183 Malignant neoplasm of ovary and other uterine adnexa
     EXCLUDES *Douglas' cul-de-sac (158.8)*

183.0 Ovary   ♀
     Use additional code to identify any functional activity
     AHA: 4Q, '07, 96
     C56.9 Malignant neoplasm of unspec ovary   **I-10**

183.2 Fallopian tube   ♀
     Oviduct
     Uterine tube

183.3 Broad ligament   ♀
     Mesovarium
     Parovarian region

183.4 Parametrium   ♀
     Uterine ligament NOS
     Uterosacral ligament

183.5 Round ligament   ♀
     AHA: 3Q, '99, 5

☑4ᵗʰ ☑5ᵗʰ Additional Digit Required	Unspecified Code	Other Specified Code	Manifestation Code	►◄ Revised Text	● New Code	▲ Revised Code Title

2015 ICD-9-CM   **Volume 1 – 35**

Neoplasms

183.8–190.7

183.8 Other specified sites of uterine adnexa ♀
Tubo-ovarian
Utero-ovarian
Malignant neoplasm of contiguous or overlapping sites of ovary and other uterine adnexa whose point of origin cannot be determined

183.9 Uterine adnexa, unspecified ♀

√4ᵗʰ **184 Malignant neoplasm of other and unspecified female genital organs**
EXCLUDES *carcinoma in situ (233.30-233.39)*

184.0 Vagina ♀
Gartner's duct
Vaginal vault

184.1 Labia majora ♀
Greater vestibular [Bartholin's] gland

184.2 Labia minora ♀

184.3 Clitoris ♀

184.4 Vulva, unspecified ♀
External female genitalia NOS
Pudendum

184.8 Other specified sites of female genital ♀
Malignant neoplasm of contiguous or overlapping sites of female genital organs whose point of origin cannot be determined

184.9 Female genital organ, site unspecified ♀
Female genitourinary tract NOS

185 Malignant neoplasm of prostate ♂
EXCLUDES *seminal vesicles (187.8)*
AHA: 2Q, '10, 3; 3Q, '03, 13; 3Q, '99, 5; 3Q, '92, 7
TIP: Assign as a secondary diagnosis if patient treated for BPH and incidental finding of carcinoma of the prostate is made.
C61 Malignant neoplasm of prostate   I-10

√4ᵗʰ **186 Malignant neoplasm of testis**
Use additional code to identify any functional activity

186.0 Undescended testis ♂
Ectopic testis
Retained testis

186.9 Other and unspecified testis ♂
Testis:
NOS
descended
scrotal

√4ᵗʰ **187 Malignant neoplasm of penis and other male genital organs**

187.1 Prepuce ♂
Foreskin

187.2 Glans penis ♂

187.3 Body of penis ♂
Corpus cavernosum

187.4 Penis, part unspecified ♂
Skin of penis NOS

187.5 Epididymis ♂

187.6 Spermatic cord ♂
Vas deferens

187.7 Scrotum ♂
Skin of scrotum

187.8 Other specified sites of male genital organs ♂
Seminal vesicle
Tunica vaginalis
Malignant neoplasm of contiguous or overlapping sites of penis and other male genital organs whose point of origin cannot be determined

187.9 Male genital organ, site unspecified ♂
Male genital organ or tract NOS

√4ᵗʰ **188 Malignant neoplasm of bladder**
EXCLUDES *carcinoma in situ (233.7)*

188.0 Trigone of urinary bladder

188.1 Dome of urinary bladder

188.2 Lateral wall of urinary bladder

188.3 Anterior wall of urinary bladder

188.4 Posterior wall of urinary bladder

188.5 Bladder neck
Internal urethral orifice

188.6 Ureteric orifice

188.7 Urachus

188.8 Other specified sites of bladder
Malignant neoplasm of contiguous or overlapping sites of bladder whose point of origin cannot be determined

188.9 Bladder, part unspecified
Bladder wall NOS
AHA: 1Q, '00, 5
C67.9 Malignant neoplasm of bladder unspecified   I-10

√4ᵗʰ **189 Malignant neoplasm of kidney and other and unspecified urinary organs**
EXCLUDES *benign carcinoid tumor of kidney (209.64)*
malignant carcinoid tumor of kidney (209.24)

189.0 Kidney, except pelvis
Kidney NOS
Kidney parenchyma
AHA: 2Q, '05, 4; 2Q, '04, 4
C64.9 Malig neoplasm unspec kidney no renal pelvis   I-10

189.1 Renal pelvis
Renal calyces
Ureteropelvic junction

189.2 Ureter
EXCLUDES *ureteric orifice of bladder (188.6)*

189.3 Urethra
EXCLUDES *urethral orifice of bladder (188.5)*

189.4 Paraurethral glands

189.8 Other specified sites of urinary organs
Malignant neoplasm of contiguous or overlapping sites of kidney and other urinary organs whose point of origin cannot be determined

189.9 Urinary organ, site unspecified
Urinary system NOS

Malignant Neoplasm of Other and Unspecified Sites (190-199)
EXCLUDES *carcinoma in situ (234.0-234.9)*

√4ᵗʰ **190 Malignant neoplasm of eye**
EXCLUDES *carcinoma in situ (234.0)*
dark area on retina and choroid (239.81)
cartilage (171.0)
malignant melanoma of eyelid (skin) (172.1)
malignant neoplasm of eyelid (skin) (173.10-173.19)
optic nerve (192.0)
orbital bone (170.0)
retinal freckle (239.81)

190.0 Eyeball, except conjunctiva, cornea, retina, and choroid
Ciliary body   Sclera
Crystalline lens   Uveal tract
Iris

190.1 Orbit
Connective tissue of orbit
Extraocular muscle
Retrobulbar
EXCLUDES *bone of orbit (170.0)*

190.2 Lacrimal gland

190.3 Conjunctiva

190.4 Cornea

190.5 Retina

190.6 Choroid

190.7 Lacrimal duct
Lacrimal sac
Nasolacrimal duct

Ⓝ Newborn Age: 0   Ⓟ Pediatric Age: 0-17   Ⓜ Maternity Age: 12-55   Ⓐ Adult Age: 15-124

Brain and Meninges

Fourth ventricle — Cerebrum — Corpus callosum — Thalamus — Hypothalamus — Hypophysis — Pons — Cerebellum — Medulla oblongata

Midsagittal Section (between hemispheres)

190.8 Other specified sites of eye

Malignant neoplasm of contiguous or overlapping sites of eye whose point of origin cannot be determined

190.9 Eye, part unspecified

191 Malignant neoplasm of brain

> EXCLUDES   cranial nerves (192.0)
> retrobulbar area (190.1)

AHA: 4Q, '07, 104

191.0 Cerebrum, except lobes and ventricles
Basal ganglia   Globus pallidus
Cerebral cortex   Hypothalamus
Corpus striatum   Thalamus

191.1 Frontal lobe
AHA: 4Q, '05, 118

191.2 Temporal lobe
Hippocampus
Uncus
AHA: 3Q, '09, 8; 4Q, '06, 123

191.3 Parietal lobe

191.4 Occipital lobe

191.5 Ventricles
Choroid plexus
Floor of ventricle

191.6 Cerebellum NOS
Cerebellopontine angle

191.7 Brain stem
Cerebral peduncle
Medulla oblongata
Midbrain
Pons

191.8 Other parts of brain
Corpus callosum
Tapetum
Malignant neoplasm of contiguous or overlapping sites of brain whose point of origin cannot be determined

191.9 Brain, unspecified
Cranial fossa NOS
AHA: 4Q, '09, 143

192 Malignant neoplasm of other and unspecified parts of nervous system

> EXCLUDES   peripheral, sympathetic, and parasympathetic nerves and ganglia (171.0-171.9)

192.0 Cranial nerves
Olfactory bulb

192.1 Cerebral meninges
Dura (mater)   Meninges NOS
Falx (cerebelli) (cerebri)   Tentorium

192.2 Spinal cord
Cauda equina

192.3 Spinal meninges

192.8 Other specified sites of nervous system
Malignant neoplasm of contiguous or overlapping sites of other parts of nervous system whose point of origin cannot be determined

192.9 Nervous system, part unspecified
Nervous system (central) NOS
> EXCLUDES   meninges NOS (192.1)

193 Malignant neoplasm of thyroid gland
Thyroglossal duct
Use additional code to identify any functional activity
C73 Malignant neoplasm of thyroid gland   I-10

194 Malignant neoplasm of other endocrine glands and related structures

> EXCLUDES   islets of Langerhans (157.4)
> neuroendocrine tumors (209.00-209.69)
> ovary (183.0)
> testis (186.0-186.9)
> thymus (164.0)

194.0 Adrenal gland
Adrenal cortex   Suprarenal gland
Adrenal medulla

194.1 Parathyroid gland

194.3 Pituitary gland and craniopharyngeal duct
Craniobuccal pouch   Rathke's pouch
Hypophysis   Sella turcica
AHA: J-A, '85, 9

194.4 Pineal gland

194.5 Carotid body

194.6 Aortic body and other paraganglia
Coccygeal body
Glomus jugulare
Para-aortic body

194.8 Other
Pluriglandular involvement NOS
> NOTE   If the sites of multiple involvements are known, they should be coded separately.

194.9 Endocrine gland, site unspecified

195 Malignant neoplasm of other and ill-defined sites

> INCLUDES   malignant neoplasms of contiguous sites, not elsewhere classified, whose point of origin cannot be determined

> EXCLUDES   malignant neoplasm:
> lymphatic and hematopoietic tissue (200.0-208.9)
> secondary sites (196.0-198.8)
> unspecified site (199.0-199.1)

195.0 Head, face, and neck
Cheek NOS   Nose NOS
Jaw NOS   Supraclavicular region NOS
AHA: 4Q, '03, 107

195.1 Thorax
Axilla
Chest (wall) NOS
Intrathoracic NOS

195.2 Abdomen
Intra-abdominal NOS
AHA: 2Q, '97, 3

195.3 Pelvis
Groin
Inguinal region NOS
Presacral region
Sacrococcygeal region
Sites overlapping systems within pelvis, as:
rectovaginal (septum)
rectovesical (septum)

195.4 Upper limb

195.5 Lower limb

195.8 Other specified sites
Back NOS
Flank NOS
Trunk NOS

Additional Digit Required   Unspecified Code   Other Specified Code   Manifestation Code   ►◄ Revised Text   ● New Code   ▲ Revised Code Title

2015 ICD-9-CM   **Volume 1 – 37**

190.8–195.8

Neoplasms

196–199.1

Lymph Nodes

- Head, neck, and face
- Thoracic duct empties into the left subclavian vein
- Left subclavian vein
- Intrathoracic
- Axillary and upper limb
- Intraabdominal
- Cisterna chyli
- Thoracic duct (transmits lymph through diaphragm using one-way valves)
- Nodes generally accompany large blood vessels
- Inguinal and lower limb
- Intrapelvic

✓4ᵗʰ **196 Secondary and unspecified malignant neoplasm of lymph nodes**

EXCLUDES *any malignant neoplasm of lymph nodes, specified as primary (200.0-202.9)*
Hodgkin's disease (201.0-201.9)
lymphosarcoma (200.1)
other forms of lymphoma (202.0-202.9)
reticulosarcoma (200.0)
secondary neuroendocrine tumor of (distant) lymph nodes (209.71)

AHA: 2Q, '92, 3; M-J, '85, 3

196.0 Lymph nodes of head, face, and neck
- Cervical
- Cervicofacial
- Scalene
- Supraclavicular

AHA: 3Q, '07, 7
C77.0 Sec & uns malig neo lymph nodes head face & neck   I-10

196.1 Intrathoracic lymph nodes
- Bronchopulmonary
- Intercostal
- Mediastinal
- Tracheobronchial

AHA: 3Q, '06, 7

196.2 Intra-abdominal lymph nodes
- Intestinal
- Mesenteric
- Retroperitoneal

AHA: 4Q, '03, 111
C77.2 Sec & uns malig neoplasm intra-abd lymph nodes   I-10

196.3 Lymph nodes of axilla and upper limb
- Brachial
- Epitrochlear
- Infraclavicular
- Pectoral

196.5 Lymph nodes of inguinal region and lower limb
- Femoral
- Groin
- Popliteal
- Tibial

196.6 Intrapelvic lymph nodes
- Hypogastric
- Iliac
- Obturator
- Parametrial

AHA: 2Q, '12, 9

196.8 Lymph nodes of multiple sites

196.9 Site unspecified
Lymph nodes NOS

✓4ᵗʰ **197 Secondary malignant neoplasm of respiratory and digestive systems**

EXCLUDES *lymph node metastasis (196.0-196.9)*
secondary neuroendocrine tumor of liver (209.72)
secondary neuroendocrine tumor of respiratory organs (209.79)

AHA: M-J, '85, 3

197.0 Lung
Bronchus
AHA: 3Q, '10, 3; 1Q, '06, 4; 2Q, '99, 9
C78.00 Secondary malignant neoplasm of unspec lung   I-10

197.1 Mediastinum
AHA: 3Q, '06, 7

197.2 Pleura
AHA: 1Q, '08, 16; 3Q, '07, 3; 4Q, '03, 110; 4Q, '89, 11
TIP: Do not assign for malignant pleural effusion; see instead code 511.81.
C78.2 Secondary malignant neoplasm of pleura   I-10

197.3 Other respiratory organs
Trachea

197.4 Small intestine, including duodenum

197.5 Large intestine and rectum

197.6 Retroperitoneum and peritoneum
AHA: 3Q, '10, 3;2Q, '04, 4; 4Q, '89, 11
C78.6 Sec malignant neoplasm of retroperiton & periton   I-10

197.7 Liver, specified as secondary
AHA: 3Q, '10, 3; 1Q, '06, 4; 2Q, '05, 9
C78.7 Secondary malignant neoplasm of liver   I-10

197.8 Other digestive organs and spleen
AHA: 2Q, '97, 3; 2Q, '92, 3

✓4ᵗʰ **198 Secondary malignant neoplasm of other specified sites**

EXCLUDES *lymph node metastasis (196.0-196.9)*
secondary neuroendocrine tumor of other specified sites (209.79)

AHA: M-J, '85, 3

198.0 Kidney

198.1 Other urinary organs

198.2 Skin
Skin of breast

198.3 Brain and spinal cord
AHA: 3Q, '07, 4; 3Q, '99, 7
C79.31 Secondary malignant neoplasm of brain   I-10

198.4 Other parts of nervous system
Meninges (cerebral) (spinal)
AHA: J-F, '87, 7

198.5 Bone and bone marrow
AHA: 1Q, '07, 6; 4Q, '03, 110; 3Q, '99, 5; 2Q, '92, 3; 1Q, '91, 16; 4Q, '89, 10
C79.51 Secondary malignant neoplasm of bone   I-10

198.6 Ovary   ♀

198.7 Adrenal gland
Suprarenal gland
C79.70 Sec malignant neoplasm of unspec adrenal gland   I-10

✓5ᵗʰ **198.8 Other specified sites**

198.81 Breast
EXCLUDES *skin of breast (198.2)*

198.82 Genital organs

198.89 Other
EXCLUDES *retroperitoneal lymph nodes (196.2)*
AHA: 2Q, '05, 4; 2Q, '97, 4
TIP: Assign for intra-abdominal metastasis when no further specificity of site is documented.
C79.89 Secondary malignant neoplasm of other spec sites   I-10

✓4ᵗʰ **199 Malignant neoplasm without specification of site**

EXCLUDES *malignant carcinoid tumor of unknown primary site (209.20)*
malignant (poorly differentiated) neuroendocrine carcinoma, any site (209.30)
malignant (poorly differentiated) neuroendocrine tumor, any site (209.30)
neuroendocrine carcinoma (high grade), any site (209.30)

199.0 Disseminated
Carcinomatosis
Generalized:
  cancer
  malignancy
Multiple cancer
} unspecified site (primary) (secondary)
AHA: 4Q, '89, 10

199.1 Other
Cancer
Carcinoma
Malignancy
} unspecified site (primary) (secondary)
AHA: 3Q, '06, 14-15; 1Q, '06, 4
TIP: Assign if patient is assessed for a metastatic tumor but primary site is unknown.
C80.1 Malignant neoplasm unspecified   I-10

N Newborn Age: 0   P Pediatric Age: 0-17   M Maternity Age: 12-55   A Adult Age: 15-124

199.2 Malignant neoplasm associated with transplanted organ
Code first complication of transplanted organ (996.80-996.89)
Use additional code for specific malignancy
AHA: 4Q, '08, 82-83
TIP: Assign first the appropriate code from subcategory 996.8, Complications of transplanted organ; use additional code for the specific malignancy.

Malignant Neoplasm of Lymphatic and Hematopoietic Tissue (200-208)

EXCLUDES   autoimmune lymphoproliferative syndrome (279.41)
secondary and unspecified neoplasm of lymph nodes (196.0-196.9)
secondary neoplasm of:
bone marrow (198.5)
spleen (197.8)

The following fifth-digit subclassification is for use with categories 200-202:
0 unspecified site, extranodal and solid organ sites
1 lymph nodes of head, face, and neck
2 intrathoracic lymph nodes
3 intra-abdominal lymph nodes
4 lymph nodes of axilla and upper limb
5 lymph nodes of inguinal region and lower limb
6 intrapelvic lymph nodes
7 spleen
8 lymph nodes of multiple sites

√4ᵗʰ **200 Lymphosarcoma and reticulosarcoma and other specified malignant tumors of lymphatic tissue**
AHA: 4Q, '07, 65; 2Q, '92, 3; N-D, '86, 5

§ √5ᵗʰ **200.0 Reticulosarcoma**
[0-8]   Lymphoma (malignant):   Reticulum cell sarcoma:
histiocytic (diffuse):   NOS
nodular   pleomorphic cell type
pleomorphic cell type
reticulum cell type
DEF: Malignant lymphoma of primarily histolytic cells; commonly originates in reticuloendothelium of lymph nodes.
AHA: For Code 200.03: 3Q, '01, 12; For Code 200.04: 3Q, '09, 4

§ √5ᵗʰ **200.1 Lymphosarcoma**
[0-8]   Lymphoblastoma (diffuse)
Lymphoma (malignant):
lymphoblastic (diffuse)
lymphocytic (cell type) (diffuse)
lymphosarcoma type
Lymphosarcoma:
NOS
diffuse NOS
lymphoblastic (diffuse)
lymphocytic (diffuse)
prolymphocytic
EXCLUDES   lymphosarcoma:
follicular or nodular (202.0)
mixed cell type (200.8)
lymphosarcoma cell leukemia (207.8)
DEF: Malignant lymphoma created from anaplastic lymphoid cells resembling lymphocytes or lymphoblasts.

§ √5ᵗʰ **200.2 Burkitt's tumor or lymphoma**
[0-8]   Malignant lymphoma, Burkitt's type
DEF: Large osteolytic lesion most common in jaw or as abdominal mass; usually found in central Africa but reported elsewhere.

§ √5ᵗʰ **200.3 Marginal zone lymphoma**
[0-8]   Extranodal marginal zone B-cell lymphoma
Mucosa associated lymphoid tissue [MALT]
Nodal marginal zone B-cell lymphoma
Splenic marginal zone B-cell lymphoma
AHA: 4Q, '07, 65

§ √5ᵗʰ **200.4 Mantle cell lymphoma**
[0-8]   AHA: 4Q, '07, 65

§ √5ᵗʰ **200.5 Primary central nervous system lymphoma**
[0-8]   AHA: ▶ 1Q, '13, 4;◀ 4Q, '07, 66

§ √5ᵗʰ **200.6 Anaplastic large cell lymphoma**
[0-8]   AHA: 4Q, '07, 66

§ √5ᵗʰ **200.7 Large cell lymphoma**
[0-8]   AHA: 4Q, '07, 66

§ √5ᵗʰ **200.8 Other named variants**
[0-8]   Lymphoma (malignant):
lymphoplasmacytoid type
mixed lymphocytic-histiocytic (diffuse)
Lymphosarcoma, mixed cell type (diffuse)
Reticulolymphosarcoma (diffuse)

√4ᵗʰ **201 Hodgkin's disease**
DEF: Painless, progressive enlargement of lymph nodes, spleen and general lymph tissue; symptoms include anorexia, lassitude, weight loss, fever, pruritis, night sweats, anemia.
AHA: 2Q, '92, 3; N-D, '86, 5

§ √5ᵗʰ **201.0 Hodgkin's paragranuloma**
[0-8]

§ √5ᵗʰ **201.1 Hodgkin's granuloma**
[0-8]   AHA: 2Q, '99, 7

§ √5ᵗʰ **201.2 Hodgkin's sarcoma**
[0-8]

§ √5ᵗʰ **201.4 Lymphocytic-histiocytic predominance**
[0-8]

§ √5ᵗʰ **201.5 Nodular sclerosis**
[0-8]   Hodgkin's disease, nodular sclerosis:
NOS
cellular phase

§ √5ᵗʰ **201.6 Mixed cellularity**
[0-8]

§ √5ᵗʰ **201.7 Lymphocytic depletion**
[0-8]   Hodgkin's disease, lymphocytic depletion:
NOS
diffuse fibrosis
reticular type

§ √5ᵗʰ **201.9 Hodgkin's disease, unspecified**
[0-8]   Hodgkin's: Malignant:
disease NOS   lymphogranuloma
lymphoma NOS   lymphogranulomatosis

√4ᵗʰ **202 Other malignant neoplasms of lymphoid and histiocytic tissue**
AHA: 2Q, '92, 3; N-D, '86, 5

§ √5ᵗʰ **202.0 Nodular lymphoma**
[0-8]   Brill-Symmers disease
Lymphoma:
follicular (giant) (large cell)
lymphocytic, nodular
Lymphosarcoma:
follicular (giant)
nodular
DEF: Lymphomatous cells clustered into nodules within the lymph node; usually occurs in older adults and may involve all nodes and possibly extranodal sites.
AHA: For code 202.04: 3Q, '09, 4

§ √5ᵗʰ **202.1 Mycosis fungoides**
[0-8]   EXCLUDES   peripheral T-cell lymphoma (202.7)
DEF: Type of cutaneous T-cell lymphoma; may evolve into generalized lymphoma; formerly thought to be of fungoid origin.
AHA: 2Q, '92, 4

§ √5ᵗʰ **202.2 Sézary's disease**
[0-8]   DEF: Type of cutaneous T-cell lymphoma with erythroderma, intense pruritus, peripheral lymphadenopathy, abnormal hyperchromatic mononuclear cells in skin, lymph nodes and peripheral blood.
AHA: 2Q, '99, 7

§ √5ᵗʰ **202.3 Malignant histiocytosis**
[0-8]   Histiocytic medullary reticulosis
Malignant:
reticuloendotheliosis
reticulosis

§ √5ᵗʰ **202.4 Leukemic reticuloendotheliosis**
[0-8]   Hairy-cell leukemia
DEF: Chronic leukemia with large, mononuclear cells with "hairy" appearance in marrow, spleen, liver, blood.

§   Requires fifth digit. Valid digits are in [brackets] under each code. See appropriate category for codes and definitions.

√4ᵗʰ / √5ᵗʰ Additional Digit Required   Unspecified Code   Other Specified Code   Manifestation Code   ▶◀ Revised Text   ● New Code   ▲ Revised Code Title

2015 ICD-9-CM   **October 2014 • Volume 1 – 39**

Neoplasms

202.5–206.8

§ ✓5ᵗʰ **202.5 Letterer-Siwe disease**
[0-8] Acute:
  differentiated progressive histiocytosis
  histiocytosis X (progressive)
  infantile reticuloendotheliosis
  reticulosis of infancy

  EXCLUDES *adult pulmonary Langerhans cell histiocytosis*
  (516.5)
  Hand-Schüller-Christian disease (277.89)
  histiocytosis (acute) (chronic) (277.89)
  histiocytosis X (chronic) (277.89)

  DEF: A recessive reticuloendotheliosis of early childhood, with a hemorrhagic tendency, eczema-like skin eruption, hepatosplenomegaly, lymph node enlargement, and progressive anemia; often a fatal disease with no established cause.

§ ✓5ᵗʰ **202.6 Malignant mast cell tumors**
[0-8] Malignant: Mast cell sarcoma
  mastocytoma   Systemic tissue mast
  mastocytosis   cell disease

  EXCLUDES *mast cell leukemia (207.8)*

  AHA: ►For code 202.60: 2Q, '13, 12 ◄

§ ✓5ᵗʰ **202.7 Peripheral T-cell lymphoma**
[0-8] **AHA:** 4Q, '07, 66

§ ✓5ᵗʰ **202.8 Other lymphomas**
[0-8] Lymphoma (malignant):
  NOS
  diffuse

  EXCLUDES *benign lymphoma (229.0)*

  AHA: 4Q, '06, 135; 2Q, '06, 20-21; 2Q, '92, 4; **For code 202.80:**
  4Q, '08, 83; 1Q, '08, 16; 3Q, '07, 3

  C85.80 Oth spec types non-Hodgkins lymphoma unspec site I-10

§ ✓5ᵗʰ **202.9 Other and unspecified malignant neoplasms of**
[0-8] **lymphoid and histiocytic tissue**
  Follicular dendritic cell sarcoma
  Interdigitating dendritic cell sarcoma
  Langerhans cell sarcoma
  Malignant neoplasm of bone marrow NOS

✓4ᵗʰ **203 Multiple myeloma and immunoproliferative neoplasms**
  AHA: 4Q, '08, 83-84; 4Q, '91, 26

  The following fifth-digit subclassification is for use with category 203:
   0 without mention of having achieved remission
     Failed remission
   1 in remission
   2 in relapse

§ ✓5ᵗʰ **203.0 Multiple myeloma**
[0-2] Kahler's disease   Myelomatosis

  EXCLUDES *solitary myeloma (238.6)*

  AHA: 1Q, '96, 16; 4Q, '89, 10; **For code 203.00:** 3Q, '12,16; 2Q, '10, 6; 2Q, '07, 8 **For code 203.01:** 4Q, '08, 91

  C90.00 Multiple myeloma not in remission I-10

§ ✓5ᵗʰ **203.1 Plasma cell leukemia**
[0-2] Plasmacytic leukemia
  AHA: 4Q, '91, 26; S-0, '86, 12

§ ✓5ᵗʰ **203.8 Other immunoproliferative neoplasms**
[0-2] **AHA:** 4Q, '90, 26; S-0, '86, 12

✓4ᵗʰ **204 Lymphoid leukemia**
  INCLUDES leukemia:
  lymphatic
  lymphoblastic
  lymphocytic
  lymphogenous

  AHA: 4Q, '08, 83-84; 3Q, '93, 4

  The following fifth-digit subclassification is for use with category 204:
   0 without mention of having achieved remission
     Failed remission
   1 in remission
   2 in relapse

§ ✓5ᵗʰ **204.0 Acute**
[0-2] **EXCLUDES** *acute exacerbation of chronic lymphoid leukemia*
  (204.1)

  AHA: 3Q, '99, 6; **For code 204.00:** 2Q, '11, 4; **For code 204.02:** 1Q, '12, 13

§ ✓5ᵗʰ **204.1 Chronic**
[0-2] **C91.10** Chronic lymphocytic leukemia not in remission I-10

§ ✓5ᵗʰ **204.2 Subacute**
[0-2]

§ ✓5ᵗʰ **204.8 Other lymphoid leukemia**
[0-2] Aleukemic leukemia: Aleukemic leukemia:
  lymphatic   lymphoid
  lymphocytic

  AHA: 3Q, '09, 4
  TIP: Assign for T-cell large granular lymphocytic leukemia.

§ ✓5ᵗʰ **204.9 Unspecified lymphoid leukemia**
[0-2]

✓4ᵗʰ **205 Myeloid leukemia**
  INCLUDES leukemia:
  granulocytic
  myeloblastic
  myelocytic
  myelogenous
  myelomonocytic
  myelosclerotic
  myelosis

  AHA: 4Q, '08, 83-84; 3Q, '93, 3; 4Q, '91, 26; 4Q, '90, 3; M-J, '85, 18

  The following fifth-digit subclassification is for use with category 205:
   0 without mention of having achieved remission
     Failed remission
   1 in remission
   2 in relapse

§ ✓5ᵗʰ **205.0 Acute**
[0-2] Acute promyelocytic leukemia

  EXCLUDES *acute exacerbation of chronic myeloid leukemia*
  (205.1)

  AHA: 2Q, '06, 20-2; **For code 205.00:** 4Q, '09, 79;
  For code 205.01: 2Q, '12, 16

  C92.00 Acute myeloid leukemia not in remission I-10

§ ✓5ᵗʰ **205.1 Chronic**
[0-2] Eosinophilic leukemia
  Neutrophilic leukemia

  AHA: 1Q, '00, 6; J-A, '85, 13 ; **For code 205.10:** 4Q, '08, 142

§ ✓5ᵗʰ **205.2 Subacute**
[0-2]

§ ✓5ᵗʰ **205.3 Myeloid sarcoma**
[0-2] Chloroma   Granulocytic sarcoma

§ ✓5ᵗʰ **205.8 Other myeloid leukemia**
[0-2] Aleukemic leukemia: Aleukemic leukemia:
  granulocytic   myeloid
  myelogenous   Aleukemic myelosis

§ ✓5ᵗʰ **205.9 Unspecified myeloid leukemia**
[0-2]

✓4ᵗʰ **206 Monocytic leukemia**
  INCLUDES leukemia:
  histiocytic
  monoblastic
  monocytoid

  AHA: 4Q, '08, 83-84

  The following fifth-digit subclassification is for use with category 206:
   0 without mention of having achieved remission
     Failed remission
   1 in remission
   2 in relapse

§ ✓5ᵗʰ **206.0 Acute**
[0-2] **EXCLUDES** *acute exacerbation of chronic monocytic leukemia*
  (206.1)

§ ✓5ᵗʰ **206.1 Chronic**
[0-2]

§ ✓5ᵗʰ **206.2 Subacute**
[0-2]

§ ✓5ᵗʰ **206.8 Other monocytic leukemia**
[0-2] Aleukemic:
  monocytic leukemia
  monocytoid leukemia

---

§ Requires fifth digit. Valid digits are in [brackets] under each code. See appropriate category for codes and definitions.

N Newborn Age: 0   P Pediatric Age: 0-17   M Maternity Age: 12-55   A Adult Age: 15-124

§ √5ᵗʰ **206.9 Unspecified monocytic leukemia**
[0-2]

√4ᵗʰ **207 Other specified leukemia**
EXCLUDES leukemic reticuloendotheliosis (202.4)
plasma cell leukemia (203.1)
AHA: 4Q, '08, 83-85

The following fifth-digit subclassification is for use with category 207:
  0 without mention of having achieved remission
    Failed remission
  1 in remission
  2 in relapse

§ √5ᵗʰ **207.0 Acute erythremia and erythroleukemia**
[0-2]   Acute erythremic myelosis
  Di Guglielmo's disease
  Erythremic myelosis
  DEF: Erythremia: polycythemia vera.
  DEF: Erythroleukemia: a malignant blood dyscrasia (a myeloproliferative disorder).

§ √5ᵗʰ **207.1 Chronic erythremia**
[0-2]   Heilmeyer-Schöner disease

§ √5ᵗʰ **207.2 Megakaryocytic leukemia**
[0-2]   Megakaryocytic myelosis
  Thrombocytic leukemia

§ √5ᵗʰ **207.8 Other specified leukemia**
[0-2]   Lymphosarcoma cell leukemia

√4ᵗʰ **208 Leukemia of unspecified cell type**
AHA: 4Q, '08, 83-85

The following fifth-digit subclassification is for use with category 208:
  0 without mention of having achieved remission
    Failed remission
  1 in remission
  2 in relapse

§ √5ᵗʰ **208.0 Acute**
[0-2]   Acute leukemia NOS   Stem cell leukemia
  Blast cell leukemia
  EXCLUDES acute exacerbation of chronic unspecified leukemia (208.1)

§ √5ᵗʰ **208.1 Chronic**
[0-2]   Chronic leukemia NOS

§ √5ᵗʰ **208.2 Subacute**
[0-2]   Subacute leukemia NOS

§ √5ᵗʰ **208.8 Other leukemia of unspecified cell type**
[0-2]

§ √5ᵗʰ **208.9 Unspecified leukemia**
[0-2]   Leukemia NOS
  AHA: For code 208.90: 4Q, '11, 148

Neuroendocrine Tumors (209)

√4ᵗʰ **209 Neuroendocrine tumors**
Code first any associated multiple endocrine neoplasia syndrome (258.01-258.03)
Use additional code to identify associated endocrine syndrome, such as:
  carcinoid syndrome (259.2)
EXCLUDES benign pancreatic islet cell tumors (211.7)
malignant pancreatic islet cell tumors (157.4)
AHA: 4Q, '09, 150; 4Q, '08, 85-89

√5ᵗʰ **209.0 Malignant carcinoid tumors of the small intestine**

  209.00 Malignant carcinoid tumor of the small intestine, unspecified portion

  209.01 Malignant carcinoid tumor of the duodenum

  209.02 Malignant carcinoid tumor of the jejunum

  209.03 Malignant carcinoid tumor of the ileum

√5ᵗʰ **209.1 Malignant carcinoid tumors of the appendix, large intestine, and rectum**

  209.10 Malignant carcinoid tumor of the large intestine, unspecified portion
    Malignant carcinoid tumor of the colon NOS

  209.11 Malignant carcinoid tumor of the appendix

  209.12 Malignant carcinoid tumor of the cecum

  209.13 Malignant carcinoid tumor of the ascending colon

  209.14 Malignant carcinoid tumor of the transverse colon

  209.15 Malignant carcinoid tumor of the descending colon

  209.16 Malignant carcinoid tumor of the sigmoid colon

  209.17 Malignant carcinoid tumor of the rectum

√5ᵗʰ **209.2 Malignant carcinoid tumors of other and unspecified sites**

  209.20 Malignant carcinoid tumor of unknown primary site

  209.21 Malignant carcinoid tumor of the bronchus and lung

  209.22 Malignant carcinoid tumor of the thymus

  209.23 Malignant carcinoid tumor of the stomach
    AHA: 4Q, '08, 89

  209.24 Malignant carcinoid tumor of the kidney

  209.25 Malignant carcinoid tumor of the foregut NOS

  209.26 Malignant carcinoid tumor of the midgut NOS

  209.27 Malignant carcinoid tumor of the hindgut NOS

  209.29 Malignant carcinoid tumors of other sites

√5ᵗʰ **209.3 Malignant poorly differentiated neuroendocrine tumors**
AHA: 4Q, '09, 73-74

  209.30 Malignant poorly differentiated neuroendocrine carcinoma, any site
    High grade neuroendocrine carcinoma, any site
    Malignant poorly differentiated neuroendocrine tumor NOS
    EXCLUDES Merkel cell carcinoma (209.31-209.36)
    AHA: ►1Q, '14, 5 ◄

  209.31 Merkel cell carcinoma of the face
    Merkel cell carcinoma of the ear
    Merkel cell carcinoma of the eyelid, including canthus
    Merkel cell carcinoma of the lip

  209.32 Merkel cell carcinoma of the scalp and neck

  209.33 Merkel cell carcinoma of the upper limb

  209.34 Merkel cell carcinoma of the lower limb

  209.35 Merkel cell carcinoma of the trunk

  209.36 Merkel cell carcinoma of other sites
    Merkel cell carcinoma of the buttock
    Merkel cell carcinoma of the genitals
    Merkel cell carcinoma NOS
    AHA: 4Q, '09, 74

√5ᵗʰ **209.4 Benign carcinoid tumors of the small intestine**

  209.40 Benign carcinoid tumor of the small intestine, unspecified portion

  209.41 Benign carcinoid tumor of the duodenum

  209.42 Benign carcinoid tumor of the jejunum

  209.43 Benign carcinoid tumor of the ileum

√5ᵗʰ **209.5 Benign carcinoid tumors of the appendix, large intestine, and rectum**

  209.50 Benign carcinoid tumor of the large intestine, unspecified portion
    Benign carcinoid tumor of the colon NOS

  209.51 Benign carcinoid tumor of the appendix

  209.52 Benign carcinoid tumor of the cecum

  209.53 Benign carcinoid tumor of the ascending colon

  209.54 Benign carcinoid tumor of the transverse colon

  209.55 Benign carcinoid tumor of the descending colon

  209.56 Benign carcinoid tumor of the sigmoid colon

  209.57 Benign carcinoid tumor of the rectum

§ Requires fifth digit. Valid digits are in [brackets] under each code. See appropriate category for codes and definitions.

√4ᵗʰ √5ᵗʰ Additional Digit Required   Unspecified Code   Other Specified Code   Manifestation Code   ►◄ Revised Text   ● New Code   ▲ Revised Code Title

√5ᵗʰ **209.6** **Benign carcinoid tumors of other and unspecified sites**

209.60 **Benign carcinoid tumor of unknown primary site**
Carcinoid tumor NOS
Neuroendocrine tumor NOS

209.61 **Benign carcinoid tumor of the bronchus and lung**
AHA: 4Q, '09, 151

209.62 **Benign carcinoid tumor of the thymus**

209.63 **Benign carcinoid tumor of the stomach**

209.64 **Benign carcinoid tumor of the kidney**

209.65 **Benign carcinoid tumor of the foregut NOS**

209.66 **Benign carcinoid tumor of the midgut NOS**

209.67 **Benign carcinoid tumor of the hindgut NOS**

209.69 **Benign carcinoid tumors of other sites**

√5ᵗʰ **209.7** **Secondary neuroendocrine tumors**
Secondary carcinoid tumors
AHA: 4Q, '09, 74

209.70 **Secondary neuroendocrine tumor, unspecified site**

209.71 **Secondary neuroendocrine tumor of distant lymph nodes**
AHA: ▶ 1Q, '14, 5◀

209.72 **Secondary neuroendocrine tumor of liver**

209.73 **Secondary neuroendocrine tumor of bone**

209.74 **Secondary neuroendocrine tumor of peritoneum**
Mesentery metastasis of neuroendocrine tumor
AHA: 4Q, '11, 181; 4Q, '09, 150

209.75 **Secondary Merkel cell carcinoma**
Merkel cell carcinoma nodal presentation
Merkel cell carcinoma visceral metastatic presentation
Secondary Merkel cell carcinoma, any site

209.79 **Secondary neuroendocrine tumor of other sites**
AHA: ▶ 1Q, '14, 5◀

Benign Neoplasms (210-229)

√4ᵗʰ **210** **Benign neoplasm of lip, oral cavity, and pharynx**
EXCLUDES cyst (of):
jaw (526.0-526.2, 526.89)
oral soft tissue (528.4)
radicular (522.8)

210.0 **Lip**
Frenulum labii
Lip (inner aspect) (mucosa) (vermilion border)
EXCLUDES labial commissure (210.4)
skin of lip (216.0)

210.1 **Tongue**
Lingual tonsil

210.2 **Major salivary glands**
Gland: Gland:
parotid   submandibular
sublingual
EXCLUDES benign neoplasms of minor salivary glands:
NOS (210.4)
buccal mucosa (210.4)
lips (210.0)
palate (hard) (soft) (210.4)
tongue (210.1)
tonsil, palatine (210.5)

210.3 **Floor of mouth**

210.4 **Other and unspecified parts of mouth**
Gingiva   Oral mucosa
Gum (upper) (lower)   Palate (hard) (soft)
Labial commissure   Uvula
Oral cavity NOS
EXCLUDES benign odontogenic neoplasms of bone
(213.0-213.1)
developmental odontogenic cysts (526.0)
mucosa of lips (210.0)
nasopharyngeal [posterior] [superior] surface of soft
palate (210.7)

210.5 **Tonsil**
Tonsil (faucial) (palatine)
EXCLUDES lingual tonsil (210.1)
pharyngeal tonsil (210.7)
tonsillar:
fossa (210.6)
pillars (210.6)

210.6 **Other parts of oropharynx**
Branchial cleft or vestiges
Epiglottis, anterior aspect
Fauces NOS
Mesopharynx NOS
Tonsillar:
fossa
pillars
Vallecula
EXCLUDES epiglottis:
NOS (212.1)
suprahyoid portion (212.1)

210.7 **Nasopharynx**
Adenoid tissue
Lymphadenoid tissue
Pharyngeal tonsil
Posterior nasal septum

210.8 **Hypopharynx**
Arytenoid fold   Postcricoid region
Laryngopharynx   Pyriform fossa

210.9 **Pharynx, unspecified**
Throat NOS

√4ᵗʰ **211** **Benign neoplasm of other parts of digestive system**
EXCLUDES benign stromal tumors of digestive system (215.5)

211.0 **Esophagus**

211.1 **Stomach**
Body ⎫
Cardia ⎬ of stomach
Fundus ⎭
Cardiac orifice
Pylorus
EXCLUDES benign carcinoid tumors of the stomach (209.63)
D13.1 Benign neoplasm of stomach   I-10

211.2 **Duodenum, jejunum, and ileum**
Small intestine NOS
EXCLUDES ampulla of Vater (211.5)
benign carcinoid tumors of the small intestine
(209.40-209.43)
ileocecal valve (211.3)

211.3 **Colon**
Appendix   Ileocecal valve
Cecum   Large intestine NOS
EXCLUDES benign carcinoid tumors of the large intestine
(209.50-209.56)
rectosigmoid junction (211.4)
AHA: ▶ 4Q, '13, 103, 104;◀ 2Q, '11, 9; 3Q, '05, 17; 2Q, '05, 16;
4Q, '01, 56
D12.6 Benign neoplasm of colon unspecified   I-10

211.4 **Rectum and anal canal**
Anal canal or sphincter   Rectosigmoid junction
Anus NOS
EXCLUDES anus:
margin (216.5)
skin (216.5)
benign carcinoid tumors of the rectum (209.57)
perianal skin (216.5)
AHA: 2Q, '11, 9

211.5 **Liver and biliary passages**
Ampulla of Vater   Gallbladder
Common bile duct   Hepatic duct
Cystic duct   Sphincter of Oddi

211.6 **Pancreas, except islets of Langerhans**

211.7 **Islets of Langerhans**
Islet cell tumor
Use additional code to identify any functional activity

211.8 Retroperitoneum and peritoneum
   Mesentery
   Mesocolon
   Omentum
   Retroperitoneal tissue

211.9 Other and unspecified site
   Alimentary tract NOS
   Digestive system NOS
   Gastrointestinal tract NOS
   Intestinal tract NOS
   Intestine NOS
   Spleen, not elsewhere classified

√4ᵗʰ **212   Benign neoplasm of respiratory and intrathoracic organs**

212.0 Nasal cavities, middle ear, and accessory sinuses
   Cartilage of nose
   Eustachian tube
   Nares
   Septum of nose
   Sinus:
      ethmoidal
      frontal
      maxillary
      sphenoidal

   EXCLUDES   *auditory canal (external) (216.2)*
      bone of:
         ear (213.0)
         nose [turbinates] (213.0)
      cartilage of ear (215.0)
      ear (external) (skin) (216.2)
      nose NOS (229.8)
         skin (216.3)
      olfactory bulb (225.1)
      polyp of:
         accessory sinus (471.8)
         ear (385.30-385.35)
         nasal cavity (471.0)
      posterior margin of septum and choanae (210.7)

212.1 Larynx
   Cartilage: Epiglottis (suprahyoid portion) NOS
      arytenoid   Glottis
      cricoid   Vocal cords (false)(true)
      cuneiform
      thyroid

   EXCLUDES   *epiglottis, anterior aspect (210.6)*
      polyp of vocal cord or larynx (478.4)

212.2 Trachea

212.3 Bronchus and lung
   Carina
   Hilus of lung

   EXCLUDES   *benign carcinoid tumors of bronchus and lung*
      (209.61)

212.4 Pleura

212.5 Mediastinum

212.6 Thymus

   EXCLUDES   *benign carcinoid tumors of thymus (209.62)*

212.7 Heart

   EXCLUDES   *great vessels (215.4)*

212.8 Other specified sites

212.9 Site unspecified
   Respiratory organ NOS
   Upper respiratory tract NOS

   EXCLUDES   *intrathoracic NOS (229.8)*
      thoracic NOS (229.8)

√4ᵗʰ **213   Benign neoplasm of bone and articular cartilage**

   INCLUDES   cartilage (articular) (joint)
      periosteum

   EXCLUDES   *cartilage of:*
      ear (215.0)
      eyelid (215.0))
      larynx (212.1)
      nose (212.0)
   exostosis NOS (726.91)
   synovia (215.0-215.9)

213.0 Bones of skull and face

   EXCLUDES   *lower jaw bone (213.1)*

213.1 Lower jaw bone

213.2 Vertebral column, excluding sacrum and coccyx

213.3 Ribs, sternum, and clavicle

213.4 Scapula and long bones of upper limb

213.5 Short bones of upper limb

213.6 Pelvic bones, sacrum, and coccyx

213.7 Long bones of lower limb

213.8 Short bones of lower limb

213.9 Bone and articular cartilage, site unspecified

√4ᵗʰ **214   Lipoma**

   INCLUDES   angiolipoma
      fibrolipoma
      hibernoma
      lipoma (fetal) (infiltrating) (intramuscular)
      myelolipoma
      myxolipoma

   DEF: Benign tumor frequently composed of mature fat cells; may
   occasionally be composed of fetal fat cells.

214.0 Skin and subcutaneous tissue of face

214.1 Other skin and subcutaneous tissue

214.2 Intrathoracic organs

214.3 Intra-abdominal organs

214.4 Spermatic cord   ♂

214.8 Other specified sites
   AHA: 3Q, '94, 7

214.9 Lipoma, unspecified site

√4ᵗʰ **215   Other benign neoplasm of connective and other soft tissue**

   INCLUDES   blood vessel
      bursa
      fascia
      ligament
      muscle
      peripheral, sympathetic, and parasympathetic nerves and
         ganglia
      synovia
      tendon (sheath)

   EXCLUDES   *cartilage:*
      articular (213.0-213.9)
      larynx (212.1)
      nose (212.0)
   connective tissue of:
      breast (217)
      internal organ, except lipoma and hemangioma — code
         to benign neoplasm of the site
   lipoma (214.0-214.9)

215.0 Head, face, and neck

215.2 Upper limb, including shoulder

215.3 Lower limb, including hip

215.4 Thorax

   EXCLUDES   *heart (212.7)*
      mediastinum (212.5)
      thymus (212.6)

215.5 Abdomen
   Abdominal wall
   Benign stromal tumors of abdomen
   Hypochondrium

√4ᵗʰ √5ᵗʰ Additional Digit Required   Unspecified Code   Other Specified Code   Manifestation Code   ►◄ Revised Text   ● New Code   ▲ Revised Code Title

2015 ICD-9-CM   **Volume 1 – 43**

Neoplasms

215.6 Pelvis
   Buttock
   Groin
   Inguinal region
   Perineum
   EXCLUDES *uterine:*
      leiomyoma (218.0-218.9)
      ligament, any (221.0)

215.7 **Trunk, unspecified**
   Back NOS
   Flank NOS

215.8 **Other specified sites**

215.9 **Site unspecified**

✓4ᵗʰ 216 **Benign neoplasm of skin**
   INCLUDES blue nevus
      dermatofibroma
      hydrocystoma
      pigmented nevus
      syringoadenoma
      syringoma
   EXCLUDES *skin of genital organs (221.0-222.9)*
   AHA: 1Q, '00, 21

216.0 **Skin of lip**
   EXCLUDES *vermilion border of lip (210.0)*

216.1 **Eyelid, including canthus**
   EXCLUDES *cartilage of eyelid (215.0)*

216.2 **Ear and external auditory canal**
   Auricle (ear)
   Auricular canal, external
   External meatus
   Pinna
   EXCLUDES *cartilage of ear (215.0)*

216.3 **Skin of other and unspecified parts of face**
   Cheek, external
   Eyebrow
   Nose, external
   Temple

216.4 **Scalp and skin of neck**
   AHA: 3Q, '91, 12

216.5 **Skin of trunk, except scrotum**
   Axillary fold   Skin of:
   Perianal skin   buttock
   Skin of: chest wall
      abdominal wall   groin
      anus   perineum
      back   Umbilicus
      breast
   EXCLUDES *anal canal (211.4)*
      anus NOS (211.4)
      skin of scrotum (222.4)

216.6 **Skin of upper limb, including shoulder**

216.7 **Skin of lower limb, including hip**

216.8 **Other specified sites of skin**

216.9 **Skin, site unspecified**

217 **Benign neoplasm of breast**
   Breast (male) (female):
      connective tissue
      glandular tissue
      soft parts
   EXCLUDES *adenofibrosis (610.2)*
      benign cyst of breast (610.0)
      fibrocystic disease (610.1)
      skin of breast (216.5)
   AHA: 1Q, '00, 4

Types of Uterine Fibroids

✓4ᵗʰ 218 **Uterine leiomyoma**
   INCLUDES fibroid (bleeding) (uterine)
      uterine:
         fibromyoma
         myoma
   DEF: Benign tumor primarily derived from uterine smooth muscle tissue; may contain fibrous, fatty, or epithelial tissue; also called uterine fibroid or myoma.

218.0 **Submucous leiomyoma of uterus**   ♀

218.1 **Intramural leiomyoma of uterus**   ♀
   Interstitial leiomyoma of uterus
   D25.1 Intramural leiomyoma of uterus   **I-10**

218.2 **Subserous leiomyoma of uterus**   ♀

218.9 **Leiomyoma of uterus, unspecified**   ♀
   AHA: 1Q, '03, 4
   D25.9 Leiomyoma of uterus unspecified   **I-10**

✓4ᵗʰ 219 **Other benign neoplasm of uterus**

219.0 **Cervix uteri**   ♀

219.1 **Corpus uteri**   ♀
   Endometrium
   Fundus
   Myometrium

219.8 **Other specified parts of uterus**   ♀

219.9 **Uterus, part unspecified**   ♀

220 **Benign neoplasm of ovary**   ♀
   Use additional code to identify any functional activity (256.0-256.1)
   EXCLUDES *cyst:*
      corpus albicans (620.2)
      corpus luteum (620.1)
      endometrial (617.1)
      follicular (atretic) (620.0)
      graafian follicle (620.0)
      ovarian NOS (620.2)
      retention (620.2)
   D27.9 Benign neoplasm of unspec ovary   **I-10**

✓4ᵗʰ 221 **Benign neoplasm of other female genital organs**
   INCLUDES adenomatous polyp
      benign teratoma
   EXCLUDES *cyst:*
      epoophoron (752.11)
      fimbrial (752.11)
      Gartner's duct (752.11)
      parovarian (752.11)

221.0 **Fallopian tube and uterine ligaments**   ♀
   Oviduct
   Parametruim
   Uterine ligament (broad) (round) (uterosacral)
   Uterine tube

221.1 **Vagina**   ♀

221.2 **Vulva**   ♀
   Clitoris
   External female genitalia NOS
   Greater vestibular [Bartholin's] gland
   Labia (majora) (minora)
   Pudendum
   EXCLUDES *Bartholin's (duct) (gland) cyst (616.2)*

N Newborn Age: 0   P Pediatric Age: 0-17   M Maternity Age: 12-55   A Adult Age: 15-124

Neoplasms

221.8 **Other specified sites of female genital organs** ♀

221.9 **Female genital organ, site unspecified** ♀
Female genitourinary tract NOS

✓4ᵗʰ **222 Benign neoplasm of male genital organs**

222.0 **Testis** ♂
Use additional code to identify any functional activity

222.1 **Penis** ♂
Corpus cavernosum
Glans penis
Prepuce

222.2 **Prostate** ♂
EXCLUDES *adenomatous hyperplasia of prostate*
(600.20-600.21)
prostatic:
adenoma (600.20-600.21)
enlargement (600.00-600.01)
hypertrophy (600.00-600.01)

222.3 **Epididymis** ♂

222.4 **Scrotum** ♂
Skin of scrotum

222.8 **Other specified sites of male genital organs** ♂
Seminal vesicle
Spermatic cord

222.9 **Male genital organ, site unspecified** ♂
Male genitourinary tract NOS

✓4ᵗʰ **223 Benign neoplasm of kidney and other urinary organs**

223.0 **Kidney, except pelvis**
Kidney NOS
EXCLUDES *benign carcinoid tumors of kidney (209.64)*
renal:
calyces (223.1)
pelvis (223.1)

223.1 **Renal pelvis**

223.2 **Ureter**
EXCLUDES *ureteric orifice of bladder (223.3)*

223.3 **Bladder**

✓5ᵗʰ 223.8 **Other specified sites of urinary organs**

223.81 **Urethra**
EXCLUDES *urethral orifice of bladder (223.3)*

223.89 **Other**
Paraurethral glands

223.9 **Urinary organ, site unspecified**
Urinary system NOS

✓4ᵗʰ **224 Benign neoplasm of eye**
EXCLUDES *cartilage of eyelid (215.0)*
eyelid (skin) (216.1)
optic nerve (225.1)
orbital bone (213.0)

224.0 **Eyeball, except conjunctiva, cornea, retina, and choroid**
Ciliary body
Iris
Sclera
Uveal tract

224.1 **Orbit**
EXCLUDES *bone of orbit (213.0)*

224.2 **Lacrimal gland**

224.3 **Conjunctiva**

224.4 **Cornea**

224.5 **Retina**
EXCLUDES *hemangioma of retina (228.03)*

224.6 **Choroid**

224.7 **Lacrimal duct**
Lacrimal sac
Nasolacrimal duct

224.8 **Other specified parts of eye**

Eyeball

Posterior segment
Vitreous
Optic nerve
Optic disc
Optic disc
Choroid
Sclera
Retina
Pars plana
Conjunctiva
Sclera
Lens
Cornea
Iris
Anterior chamber

224.9 **Eye, part unspecified**

✓4ᵗʰ **225 Benign neoplasm of brain and other parts of nervous system**
EXCLUDES *hemangioma (228.02)*
neurofibromatosis (237.70-237.79)
peripheral, sympathetic, and parasympathetic nerves and
ganglia (215.0-215.9)
retrobulbar (224.1)

225.0 **Brain**

225.1 **Cranial nerves**
Acoustic neuroma
AHA: 4Q, '04, 113

225.2 **Cerebral meninges**
Meninges NOS
Meningioma (cerebral)
D32.0 Benign neoplasm of cerebral meninges   I-10

225.3 **Spinal cord**
Cauda equina

225.4 **Spinal meninges**
Spinal meningioma

225.8 **Other specified sites of nervous system**

225.9 **Nervous system, part unspecified**
Nervous system (central) NOS
EXCLUDES *meninges NOS (225.2)*

226 Benign neoplasm of thyroid glands
Use additional code to identify any functional activity

✓4ᵗʰ **227 Benign neoplasm of other endocrine glands and related structures**
Use additional code to identify any functional activity
EXCLUDES *ovary (220)*
pancreas (211.6)
testis (222.0)

227.0 **Adrenal gland**
Suprarenal gland

227.1 **Parathyroid gland**

227.3 **Pituitary gland and craniopharyngeal duct (pouch)**
Craniobuccal pouch
Hypophysis
Rathke's pouch
Sella turcica

227.4 **Pineal gland**
Pineal body

227.5 **Carotid body**

227.6 **Aortic body and other paraganglia**
Coccygeal body
Glomus jugulare
Para-aortic body
AHA: N-D, '84, 17

227.8 **Other**

227.9 **Endocrine gland, site unspecified**

Neoplasms

228–232.3

✓4ᵗʰ **228 Hemangioma and lymphangioma, any site**

INCLUDES angioma (benign) (cavernous) (congenital) NOS
cavernous nevus
glomus tumor
hemangioma (benign) (congenital)

EXCLUDES benign neoplasm of spleen, except hemangioma and
lymphangioma (211.9)
glomus jugulare (227.6)
nevus:
NOS (216.0-216.9)
blue or pigmented (216.0-216.9)
vascular (757.32)

AHA: 1Q, '00, 21

✓5ᵗʰ **228.0 Hemangioma, any site**

AHA: J-F, '85, 19

DEF: A common benign tumor usually occurring in infancy;
composed of newly formed blood vessels due to malformation of
angioblastic tissue.

228.00 Of unspecified site

228.01 Of skin and subcutaneous tissue

AHA: 3Q, '10, 16

228.02 Of intracranial structures

228.03 Of retina

228.04 Of intra-abdominal structures
Peritoneum
Retroperitoneal tissue

228.09 Of other sites
Systemic angiomatosis
AHA: 3Q, '91, 20

228.1 Lymphangioma, any site
Congenital lymphangioma
Lymphatic nevus

✓4ᵗʰ **229 Benign neoplasm of other and unspecified sites**

229.0 Lymph nodes
EXCLUDES lymphangioma (228.1)

229.8 Other specified sites
Intrathoracic NOS
Thoracic NOS

229.9 Site unspecified

Carcinoma In Situ (230-234)

INCLUDES Bowen's disease
erythroplasia
Queyrat's erythroplasia

EXCLUDES leukoplakia — see Alphabetic Index

DEF: A neoplastic type; with tumor cells confined to epithelium of origin;
without further invasion.

✓4ᵗʰ **230 Carcinoma in situ of digestive organs**

230.0 Lip, oral cavity, and pharynx
Gingiva
Hypopharynx
Mouth [any part]
Nasopharynx
Oropharynx
Salivary gland or duct
Tongue

EXCLUDES aryepiglottic fold or interarytenoid fold, laryngeal
aspect (231.0)
epiglottis:
NOS (231.0)
suprahyoid portion (231.0)
skin of lip (232.0)

230.1 Esophagus

230.2 Stomach
Body ⎫
Cardia ⎬ of stomach
Fundus ⎭
Cardiac orifice
Pylorus

230.3 Colon
Appendix
Cecum
Ileocecal valve
Large intestine NOS

EXCLUDES rectosigmoid junction (230.4)

230.4 Rectum
Rectosigmoid junction

230.5 Anal canal
Anal sphincter

230.6 Anus, unspecified
EXCLUDES anus:
margin (232.5)
skin (232.5)
perianal skin (232.5)

230.7 Other and unspecified parts of intestine
Duodenum
Ileum
Jejunum
Small intestine NOS

EXCLUDES ampulla of Vater (230.8)

230.8 Liver and biliary system
Ampulla of Vater
Common bile duct
Cystic duct
Gallbladder
Hepatic duct
Sphincter of Oddi

230.9 Other and unspecified digestive organs
Digestive organ NOS
Gastrointestinal tract NOS
Pancreas
Spleen

✓4ᵗʰ **231 Carcinoma in situ of respiratory system**

231.0 Larynx
Cartilage:
arytenoid
cricoid
cuneiform
thyroid
Epiglottis:
NOS
posterior surface
suprahyoid portion
Vocal cords (false)(true)

EXCLUDES aryepiglottic fold or interarytenoid fold:
NOS (230.0)
hypopharyngeal aspect (230.0)
marginal zone (230.0)

231.1 Trachea

231.2 Bronchus and lung
Carina
Hilus of lung

231.8 Other specified parts of respiratory system
Accessory sinuses
Middle ear
Nasal cavities
Pleura

EXCLUDES ear (external) (skin) (232.2)
nose NOS (234.8)
skin (232.3)

231.9 Respiratory system, part unspecified
Respiratory organ NOS

✓4ᵗʰ **232 Carcinoma in situ of skin**
INCLUDES pigment cells
EXCLUDES melanoma in situ of skin (172.0-172.9)

232.0 Skin of lip
EXCLUDES vermilion border of lip (230.0)

232.1 Eyelid, including canthus

232.2 Ear and external auditory canal

232.3 Skin of other and unspecified parts of face

232.4 Scalp and skin of neck

232.5 Skin of trunk, except scrotum

Anus, margin	Skin of:
Axillary fold	breast
Perianal skin	buttock
Skin of:	chest wall
abdominal wall	groin
anus	perineum
back	Umbilicus

> *EXCLUDES* anal canal (230.5)
> anus NOS (230.6)
> skin of genital organs (233.30-233.39, 233.5-233.6)

232.6 Skin of upper limb, including shoulder

232.7 Skin of lower limb, including hip

232.8 Other specified sites of skin

232.9 Skin, site unspecified

√4th 233 Carcinoma in situ of breast and genitourinary system

> **TIP:** For patients with carcinoma in situ found incidentally when admitted for treatment of another condition, sequence the 233 code as a secondary condition.

233.0 Breast

> *EXCLUDES* Paget's disease (174.0-174.9)
> skin of breast (232.5)

> **TIP:** Assign for tumors specified as intraductal carcinoma.

233.1 Cervix uteri ♀
> Adenocarcinoma in situ of cervix
> Cervical intraepithelial glandular neoplasia, grade III
> Cervical intraepithelial neoplasia III [CIN III]
> Severe dysplasia of cervix

> *EXCLUDES* cervical intraepithelial neoplasia II [CIN II] (622.12)
> cytologic evidence of malignancy without histologic
>   confirmation (795.06)
> high grade squamous intraepithelial lesion (HGSIL)
>   (795.04)
> moderate dysplasia of cervix (622.12)

> **AHA:** 3Q, '92, 7; 3Q, '92, 8; 1Q, '91, 11

233.2 Other and unspecified parts of uterus ♀

√5th 233.3 Other and unspecified female genital organs
> **AHA:** 4Q, '07, 67

233.30 Unspecified female genital organ ♀

233.31 Vagina ♀
> Severe dysplasia of vagina
> Vaginal intraepithelial neoplasia III [VAIN III]

233.32 Vulva ♀
> Severe dysplasia of vulva
> Vulvar intraepithelial neoplasia III [VIN III]

233.39 Other female genital organ ♀

233.4 Prostate ♂

233.5 Penis ♂

233.6 Other and unspecified male genital organs ♂

233.7 Bladder
> **AHA:** 2Q, '12, 10

233.9 Other and unspecified urinary organs

√4th 234 Carcinoma in situ of other and unspecified sites

234.0 Eye
> *EXCLUDES* cartilage of eyelid (234.8)
> eyelid (skin) (232.1)
> optic nerve (234.8)
> orbital bone (234.8)

234.8 Other specified sites
> Endocrine gland [any]

234.9 Site unspecified
> Carcinoma in situ NOS

Neoplasms of Uncertain Behavior (235-238)

> **NOTE** Categories 235–238 classify by site certain histomorphologically well-defined neoplasms, the subsequent behavior of which cannot be predicted from the present appearance.

> **TIP:** Typically assigned for cases in which the tumor is in transition and may be undergoing malignant transformation, but continued study is required for accurate classification.

√4th 235 Neoplasm of uncertain behavior of digestive and respiratory systems

> *EXCLUDES* stromal tumors of uncertain behavior of digestive system
>   (238.1)

235.0 Major salivary glands
> Gland:
>   parotid
>   sublingual
>   submandibular

> *EXCLUDES* minor salivary glands (235.1)

235.1 Lip, oral cavity, and pharynx
> Gingiva
> Hypopharynx
> Minor salivary glands
> Mouth
> Nasopharynx
> Oropharynx
> Tongue

> *EXCLUDES* aryepiglottic fold or interarytenoid fold, laryngeal
>   aspect (235.6)
> epiglottis:
>   NOS (235.6)
>   suprahyoid portion (235.6)
> skin of lip (238.2)

235.2 Stomach, intestines, and rectum

235.3 Liver and biliary passages
> Ampulla of Vater
> Bile ducts [any]
> Gallbladder
> Liver

235.4 Retroperitoneum and peritoneum

235.5 Other and unspecified digestive organs
> Anal:
>   canal
>   sphincter
> Anus NOS
> Esophagus
> Pancreas
> Spleen

> *EXCLUDES* anus:
>   margin (238.2)
>   skin (238.2)
> perianal skin (238.2)

235.6 Larynx
> *EXCLUDES* aryepiglottic fold or interarytenoid fold:
>   NOS (235.1)
>   hypopharyngeal aspect (235.1)
>   marginal zone (235.1)

235.7 Trachea, bronchus, and lung

235.8 Pleura, thymus, and mediastinum

235.9 Other and unspecified respiratory organs
> Accessory sinuses
> Middle ear
> Nasal cavities
> Respiratory organ NOS

> *EXCLUDES* ear (external) (skin) (238.2)
> nose (238.8)
> skin (238.2)

√4th 236 Neoplasm of uncertain behavior of genitourinary organs

236.0 Uterus ♀

236.1 Placenta ♀
> Chorioadenoma (destruens)
> Invasive mole
> Malignant hydatid mole
> Malignant hydatidiform mole

√4th √5th Additional Digit Required	Unspecified Code	Other Specified Code	Manifestation Code	►◄ Revised Text	● New Code	▲ Revised Code Title

2015 ICD-9-CM   **Volume 1 – 47**

236.2 Ovary ♀

Use additional code to identify any functional activity

236.3 Other and unspecified female genital organs ♀

236.4 Testis ♂

Use additional code to identify any functional activity

236.5 Prostate ♂

236.6 Other and unspecified male genital organs ♂

236.7 Bladder

√5ᵗʰ **236.9 Other and unspecified urinary organs**

236.90 Urinary organ, unspecified

236.91 Kidney and ureter

236.99 Other

√4ᵗʰ **237 Neoplasm of uncertain behavior of endocrine glands and nervous system**

237.0 Pituitary gland and craniopharyngeal duct

Use additional code to identify any functional activity

237.1 Pineal gland

237.2 Adrenal gland

Suprarenal gland

Use additional code to identify any functional activity

237.3 Paraganglia

Aortic body   Coccygeal body
Carotid body   Glomus jugulare

AHA: N-D, '84, 17

237.4 Other and unspecified endocrine glands

Parathyroid gland
Thyroid gland

237.5 Brain and spinal cord

237.6 Meninges

Meninges:
NOS
cerebral
spinal

AHA: ▶1Q, '14, 16◀

√5ᵗʰ **237.7 Neurofibromatosis**

DEF: An inherited condition with developmental changes in the nervous system, muscles, bones and skin; multiple soft tumors (neurofibromas) distributed over the entire body.

237.70 Neurofibromatosis, unspecified

237.71 Neurofibromatosis, type 1 [von Recklinghausen's disease]

AHA: 4Q, '10, 76

237.72 Neurofibromatosis, type 2 [acoustic neurofibromatosis]

DEF: Inherited condition with cutaneous lesions, benign tumors of peripheral nerves and bilateral 8th nerve masses.

AHA: 4Q, '10, 76

237.73 Schwannomatosis

DEF: A genetic mutation (SMARCB1/INI1) causing multiple benign tumors along nerve pathways; characterized by the exception of 8th cranial nerve involvement.

AHA: 4Q, '10, 76-77

237.79 Other neurofibromatosis

AHA: 4Q, '10, 76-77

237.9 Other and unspecified parts of nervous system

Cranial nerves

EXCLUDES peripheral, sympathetic, and parasympathetic nerves and ganglia (238.1)

√4ᵗʰ **238 Neoplasm of uncertain behavior of other and unspecified sites and tissues**

238.0 Bone and articular cartilage

EXCLUDES cartilage:
ear (238.1)
eyelid (238.1)
larynx (235.6)
nose (235.9)
synovia (238.1)

AHA: 4Q, '04, 128

238.1 Connective and other soft tissue

Peripheral, sympathetic, and parasympathetic nerves and ganglia
Stromal tumors of digestive system

EXCLUDES cartilage (of):
articular (238.0)
larynx (235.6)
nose (235.9)
connective tissue of breast (238.3)

238.2 Skin

EXCLUDES anus NOS (235.5)
skin of genital organs (236.3, 236.6)
vermilion border of lip (235.1)

TIP: Assign when documentation indicates keratocanthoma only.

238.3 Breast

EXCLUDES skin of breast (238.2)

238.4 Polycythemia vera

DEF: Abnormal proliferation of all bone marrow elements, increased red cell mass and total blood volume; unknown etiology, frequently associated with splenomegaly, leukocytosis, and thrombocythemia.

D45 Polycythemia vera   I-10

238.5 Histiocytic and mast cells

Mast cell tumor NOS
Mastocytoma NOS

238.6 Plasma cells

Plasmacytoma NOS
Solitary myeloma

√5ᵗʰ **238.7 Other lymphatic and hematopoietic tissues**

EXCLUDES acute myelogenous leukemia (205.0)
chronic myelomonocytic leukemia (205.1)
myelosclerosis NOS (289.89)
myelosis:
NOS (205.9)
megakaryocytic (207.2)

AHA: 3Q, '01, 13; 1Q, '97, 5; 2Q, '89, 8

238.71 Essential thrombocythemia

Essential hemorrhagic thrombocythemia
Essential thrombocytosis
Idiopathic (hemorrhagic) thrombocythemia
Primary thrombocytosis

AHA: 4Q, '06, 63-66

D47.3 Essential (hemorrhagic) thrombocythemia   I-10

238.72 Low grade myelodysplastic syndrome lesions

Refractory anemia (RA)
Refractory anemia with excess blasts-1 (RAEB-1)
Refractory anemia with ringed sideroblasts (RARS)
Refractory cytopenia with multilineage dysplasia (RCMD)
Refractory cytopenia with multilineage dysplasia and ringed sideroblasts (RCMD-RS)

DEF: Refractory anemia (RA): Form of bone marrow disorder (myelodysplastic syndrome) that interferes with red blood cell production in the bone marrow; unresponsive to hematinics; characteristic normal or hypercellular marrow with abnormal erythrocyte development and reticulocytopenia.

AHA: 4Q, '06, 63-66

238.73 High grade myelodysplastic syndrome lesions

Refractory anemia with excess blasts-2 (RAEB-2)

AHA: 4Q, '06, 63-66

238.74 Myelodysplastic syndrome with 5q deletion

5q minus syndrome NOS

EXCLUDES constitutional 5q deletion (758.39)
high grade myelodysplastic syndrome with 5q deletion (238.73)

AHA: 4Q, '06, 63-66

238.75 Myelodysplastic syndrome, unspecified

AHA: 4Q, '06, 63-66

D46.9 Myelodysplastic syndrome unspecified   I-10

N Newborn Age: 0   P Pediatric Age: 0-17   M Maternity Age: 12-55   A Adult Age: 15-124

238.76 **Myelofibrosis with myeloid metaplasia**
Agnogenic myeloid metaplasia
Idiopathic myelofibrosis (chronic)
Myelosclerosis with myeloid metaplasia
Primary myelofibrosis

EXCLUDES   myelofibrosis NOS (289.83)
myelophthisic anemia (284.2)
myelophthisis (284.2)
secondary myelofibrosis (289.83)

AHA: 4Q, '06, 63-66

238.77 **Post-transplant lymphoproliferative disorder [PTLD]**
Code first complications of transplant (996.80-996.89)
DEF: Excessive proliferation of B-cell lymphocytes following Epstein-Barr virus infection in organ transplant patients; may progress to non-Hodgkins lymphoma.
AHA: 4Q, '08, 90-91

238.79 **Other lymphatic and hematopoietic tissues**
Lymphoproliferative disease (chronic) NOS
Megakaryocytic myelosclerosis
Myeloproliferative disease (chronic) NOS
Panmyelosis (acute)
AHA: 4Q, '06, 63-66

238.8 **Other specified sites**
Eye   Heart
EXCLUDES   eyelid (skin) (238.2)
cartilage (238.1)

238.9 **Site unspecified**

Neoplasms of Unspecified Nature (239)

√4ᵗʰ **239   Neoplasms of unspecified nature**
NOTE Category 239 classifies by site neoplasms of unspecified morphology and behavior. The term "mass," unless otherwise stated, is not to be regarded as a neoplastic growth.

INCLUDES   "growth" NOS
neoplasm NOS
new growth NOS
tumor NOS

TIP: Do not assign for inpatient cases; more information should be available.

239.0 **Digestive system**
EXCLUDES   anus:
margin (239.2)
skin (239.2)
perianal skin (239.2)

239.1 **Respiratory system**

239.2 **Bone, soft tissue, and skin**
EXCLUDES   anal canal (239.0)
anus NOS (239.0)
bone marrow (202.9)
cartilage:
larynx (239.1)
nose (239.1)
connective tissue of breast (239.3)
skin of genital organs (239.5)
vermilion border of lip (239.0)

239.3 **Breast**
EXCLUDES   skin of breast (239.2)

239.4 **Bladder**

239.5 **Other genitourinary organs**

239.6 **Brain**
EXCLUDES   cerebral meninges (239.7)
cranial nerves (239.7)

239.7 **Endocrine glands and other parts of nervous system**
EXCLUDES   peripheral, sympathetic, and parasympathetic nerves and ganglia (239.2)

√5ᵗʰ 239.8 **Other specified sites**
EXCLUDES   eyelid (skin) (239.2)
cartilage (239.2)
great vessels (239.2)
optic nerve (239.7)
AHA: 4Q, '09, 75

239.81 **Retina and choroid**
Dark area on retina
Retinal freckle
TIP: Assign for documentation of retinal "freckles" or spots that may be indicative of malignant melanoma. Histologic confirmation is not required.

239.89 **Other specified sites**

239.9 **Site unspecified**

3. Endocrine, Nutritional and Metabolic Diseases, and Immunity Disorders (240-279)

EXCLUDES *endocrine and metabolic disturbances specific to the fetus and newborn (775.0-775.9)*

NOTE All neoplasms, whether functionally active or not, are classified in Chapter 3. Codes in Chapter 3 (i.e., 242.8, 246.0, 251-253, 255-259) may be used to identify such functional activity associated with any neoplasm, or by ectopic endocrine tissue.

Disorders of Thyroid Gland (240-246)

√4ᵗʰ 240 Simple and unspecified goiter

DEF: An enlarged thyroid gland often caused by an inadequate dietary intake of iodine.

240.0 Goiter, specified as simple

Any condition classifiable to 240.9, specified as simple

240.9 Goiter, unspecified

Enlargement of thyroid
Goiter or struma:
 NOS
 diffuse colloid
 endemic
 hyperplastic
 nontoxic (diffuse)
 parenchymatous
 sporadic

EXCLUDES *congenital (dyshormonogenic) goiter (246.1)*

√4ᵗʰ 241 Nontoxic nodular goiter

EXCLUDES *adenoma of thyroid (226)*
cystadenoma of thyroid (226)

241.0 Nontoxic uninodular goiter

Thyroid nodule
Uninodular goiter (nontoxic)

DEF: Enlarged thyroid, commonly due to decreased thyroid production, with single nodule; no clinical hypothyroidism.
E04.1 Nontoxic single thyroid nodule   `I-10`

241.1 Nontoxic multinodular goiter

Multinodular goiter (nontoxic)

DEF: Enlarged thyroid, commonly due to decreased thyroid production with multiple nodules; no clinical hypothyroidism.

241.9 Unspecified nontoxic nodular goiter

Adenomatous goiter
Nodular goiter (nontoxic) NOS
Struma nodosa (simplex)

√4ᵗʰ 242 Thyrotoxicosis with or without goiter

EXCLUDES *neonatal thyrotoxicosis (775.3)*

DEF: A condition caused by excess quantities of thyroid hormones being introduced into the tissues

The following fifth-digit subclassification is for use with categories 242:
 0 without mention of thyrotoxic crisis or storm
 1 with mention of thyrotoxic crisis or storm

§ √5ᵗʰ 242.0 Toxic diffuse goiter
[0-1]

Basedow's disease
Exophthalmic or toxic goiter NOS
Graves' disease
Primary thyroid hyperplasia

DEF: Diffuse thyroid enlargement accompanied by hyperthyroidism, bulging eyes, and dermopathy.

§ √5ᵗʰ 242.1 Toxic uninodular goiter
[0-1]

Thyroid nodule ⎫
Uninodular goiter ⎭ toxic or with hyperthyroidism

DEF: Symptomatic hyperthyroidism with a single nodule on the enlarged thyroid gland. Abrupt onset of symptoms; including extreme nervousness, insomnia, weight loss, tremors, and psychosis or coma.

§ √5ᵗʰ 242.2 Toxic multinodular goiter
[0-1]

Secondary thyroid hyperplasia

DEF: Symptomatic hyperthyroidism with multiple nodules on the enlarged thyroid gland. Abrupt onset of symptoms; including extreme nervousness, insomnia, weight loss, tremors, and psychosis or coma.

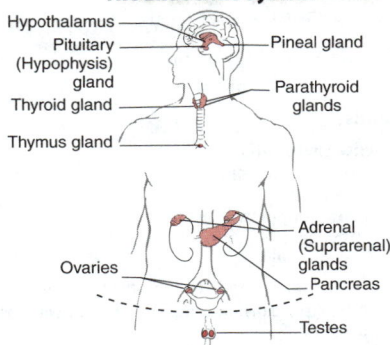

The Endocrine System

Hypothalamus
Pituitary (Hypophysis) gland
Thyroid gland
Thymus gland
Pineal gland
Parathyroid glands
Adrenal (Suprarenal) glands
Ovaries
Pancreas
Testes

§ √5ᵗʰ 242.3 Toxic nodular goiter, unspecified
[0-1]

Adenomatous goiter ⎫
Nodular goiter ⎬ toxic or with hyperthyroidism
Struma nodosa ⎭

Any condition classifiable to 241.9 specified as toxic or with hyperthyroidism

§ √5ᵗʰ 242.4 Thyrotoxicosis from ectopic thyroid nodule
[0-1]

§ √5ᵗʰ 242.8 Thyrotoxicosis of other specified origin
[0-1]

Overproduction of thyroid-stimulating hormone [TSH]
Thyrotoxicosis:
 factitia from ingestion of excessive thyroid material

Use additional E code to identify cause, if drug-induced

§ √5ᵗʰ 242.9 Thyrotoxicosis without mention of goiter or other cause
[0-1]

Hyperthyroidism NOS
Thyrotoxicosis NOS

E05.90 Thyrotoxicosis uns w/o thyrotoxic crisis or storm   `I-10`

243 Congenital hypothyroidism

Congenital thyroid insufficiency
Cretinism (athyrotic) (endemic)

Use additional code to identify associated intellectual disabilities

EXCLUDES *congenital (dyshormonogenic) goiter (246.1)*

DEF: Underproduction of thyroid hormone present from birth.

√4ᵗʰ 244 Acquired hypothyroidism

INCLUDES athyroidism (acquired)
hypothyroidism (acquired)
myxedema (adult) (juvenile)
thyroid (gland) insufficiency (acquired)

244.0 Postsurgical hypothyroidism

DEF: Underproduction of thyroid hormone due to surgical removal of all or part of the thyroid gland.
E89.0 Postprocedural hypothyroidism   `I-10`

244.1 Other postablative hypothyroidism

Hypothyroidism following therapy, such as irradiation

244.2 Iodine hypothyroidism

Hypothyroidism resulting from administration or ingestion of iodide

EXCLUDES *hypothyroidism resulting from administration of radioactive iodine (244.1)*

Use additional E code to identify drug

244.3 Other iatrogenic hypothyroidism

Hypothyroidism resulting from:
 P-aminosalicylic acid [PAS]
 Phenylbutazone
 Resorcinol
Iatrogenic hypothyroidism NOS

Use additional E code to identify drug

244.8 Other specified acquired hypothyroidism

Secondary hypothyroidism NEC

AHA: J-A, '85, 9

---

§ Requires fifth digit. Valid digits are in [brackets] under each code. See category 242 for codes and definitions.

√4ᵗʰ √5ᵗʰ Additional Digit Required   **Unspecified Code**   **Other Specified Code**   **Manifestation Code**   ▶◀ Revised Text   ● New Code   ▲ Revised Code Title

2015 ICD-9-CM   **Volume 1 – 51**

Endocrine, Nutritional and Metabolic Diseases, and Immunity

244.9–249.7

244.9 Unspecified hypothyroidism

Hypothyroidism
Myxedema   } primary or NOS

AHA: 3Q, '99, 19; 4Q, '96, 29

E03.9 Hypothyroidism unspecified   I-10

√4ᵗʰ 245 Thyroiditis

245.0 Acute thyroiditis

Abscess of thyroid
Thyroiditis:
  nonsuppurative, acute
  pyogenic
  suppurative

Use additional code to identify organism

DEF: Inflamed thyroid caused by infection, with abscess and liquid puris.

245.1 Subacute thyroiditis

Thyroiditis: Thyroiditis:
  de Quervain's   granulomatous
  giant cell   viral

DEF: Inflammation of the thyroid, characterized by fever and painful enlargement of the thyroid gland, with granulomas in the gland.

245.2 Chronic lymphocytic thyroiditis

Hashimoto's disease   Thyroiditis:
Struma lymphomatosa   autoimmune
                             lymphocytic (chronic)

DEF: Autoimmune disease of thyroid; lymphocytes infiltrate the gland and thyroid antibodies are produced; women more often affected.

245.3 Chronic fibrous thyroiditis

Struma fibrosa
Thyroiditis:
  invasive (fibrous)
  ligneous
  Riedel's

DEF: Persistent fibrosing inflammation of thyroid with adhesions to nearby structures; rare condition

245.4 Iatrogenic thyroiditis

Use additional code to identify cause

DEF: Thyroiditis resulting from treatment or intervention by physician or in a patient intervention setting.

245.8 Other and unspecified chronic thyroiditis

Chronic thyroiditis: Chronicthyroiditis:
  NOS   nonspecific

245.9 Thyroiditis, unspecified

Thyroiditis NOS

√4ᵗʰ 246 Other disorders of thyroid

246.0 Disorders of thyrocalcitonin secretion

Hypersecretion of calcitonin or thyrocalcitonin

246.1 Dyshormonogenic goiter

Congenital (dyshormonogenic) goiter
Goiter due to enzyme defect in synthesis of thyroid hormone
Goitrous cretinism (sporadic)

246.2 Cyst of thyroid

EXCLUDES cystadenoma of thyroid (226)

246.3 Hemorrhage and infarction of thyroid

246.8 Other specified disorders of thyroid

Abnormality of thyroid-binding globulin
Atrophy of thyroid
Hyper-TBG-nemia
Hypo-TBG-nemia

AHA: 2Q, '06, 5

246.9 Unspecified disorder of thyroid

E07.9 Disorder of thyroid unspecified   I-10

Diseases of Other Endocrine Glands (249-259)

√4ᵗʰ 249 Secondary diabetes mellitus

INCLUDES diabetes mellitus (due to) (in) (secondary) (with):
  drug-induced or chemical induced infection

Use additional code to identify any associated insulin use (V58.67)

EXCLUDES gestational diabetes (648.8)
hyperglycemia NOS (790.29)
neonatal diabetes mellitus (775.1)
nonclinical diabetes (790.29)
Type I diabetes — see category 250
Type II diabetes — see category 250

The following fifth-digit subclassification is for use with category 249:
  0 not stated as uncontrolled, or unspecified
  1 uncontrolled

AHA: 4Q, '08, 91-95

TIP: If the secondary DM is due to pancreatectomy, code first 251.3 Postsurgical hypoinsulinemia; also assign a code from category 249 and any manifestations, and code V88.1x Acquired absence of pancreas.

§ √5ᵗʰ 249.0 Secondary diabetes mellitus without mention of complication
[0-1]

Secondary diabetes mellitus without mention of complication or manifestation classifiable to 249.1-249.9
Secondary diabetes mellitus NOS

E09.9 Drug/chemical induced diabetes mellitus w/o comp   I-10

§ √5ᵗʰ 249.1 Secondary diabetes mellitus with ketoacidosis
[0-1]

Secondary diabetes mellitus with diabetic acidosis without mention of coma
Secondary diabetes mellitus with diabetic ketosis without mention of coma

§ √5ᵗʰ 249.2 Secondary diabetes mellitus with hyperosmolarity
[0-1]

Secondary diabetes mellitus with hyperosmolar (nonketotic) coma

§ √5ᵗʰ 249.3 Secondary diabetes mellitus with other coma
[0-1]

Secondary diabetes mellitus with diabetic coma (with ketoacidosis)
Secondary diabetes mellitus with diabetic hypoglycemic coma
Secondary diabetes mellitus with insulin coma NOS

EXCLUDES secondary diabetes mellitus with hyperosmolar coma (249.2)

§ √5ᵗʰ 249.4 Secondary diabetes mellitus with renal manifestations
[0-1]

Use additional code to identify manifestation, as:
  chronic kidney disease (585.1-585.9)
  diabetic nephropathy NOS (583.81)
  diabetic nephrosis (581.81)
  intercapillary glomerulosclerosis (581.81)
  Kimmelstiel-Wilson syndrome (581.81)

§ √5ᵗʰ 249.5 Secondary diabetes mellitus with ophthalmic manifestations
[0-1]

Use additional code to identify manifestation, as:
  diabetic blindness (369.00-369.9)
  diabetic cataract (366.41)
  diabetic glaucoma (365.44)
  diabetic macular edema (362.07)
  diabetic retinal edema (362.07)
  diabetic retinopathy (362.01-362.07)

§ √5ᵗʰ 249.6 Secondary diabetes mellitus with neurological manifestations
[0-1]

Use additional code to identify manifestation, as:
  diabetic amyotrophy (353.5)
  diabetic gastroparalysis (536.3)
  diabetic gastroparesis (536.3)
  diabetic mononeuropathy (354.0-355.9)
  diabetic neurogenic arthropathy (713.5)
  diabetic peripheral autonomic neuropathy (337.1)
  diabetic polyneuropathy (357.2)

AHA: For code 249.60: 4Q, '08, 94

§ √5ᵗʰ 249.7 Secondary diabetes mellitus with peripheral circulatory disorders
[0-1]

Use additional code to identify manifestation, as:
  diabetic gangrene (785.4)
  diabetic peripheral angiopathy (443.81)

---

§   Requires fifth digit. Valid digits are in [brackets] under each code. See category 249 for codes and definitions.

§ ✓5ᵗʰ **249.8 Secondary diabetes mellitus with other specified**
[0-1] **manifestations**
Secondary diabetic hypoglycemia in diabetes mellitus
Secondary hypoglycemic shock in diabetes mellitus

Use additional code to identify manifestation, as:
any associated ulceration (707.10-707.19, 707.8, 707.9)
diabetic bone changes (731.8)

§ ✓5ᵗʰ **249.9 Secondary diabetes mellitus with unspecified**
[0-1] **complication**

✓4ᵗʰ **250 Diabetes mellitus**

EXCLUDES gestational diabetes (648.8)
hyperglycemia NOS (790.29)
neonatal diabetes mellitus (775.1)
nonclinical diabetes (790.29)
secondary diabetes (249.0-249.9)

The following fifth-digit subclassification is for use with category 250:
0 type II or unspecified type, not state as uncontrolled
Fifth-digit 0 is for use for type II patients, even if the patient
requires insulin
Use additional code, if applicable, for associated long-term
(current) insulin use V58.67
1 type I [juvenile type], not stated as uncontrolled
2 type II or unspecified type, uncontrolled
Fifth-digit 2 is for use for type II patients, even if the patient
requires insulin
Use additional code, if applicable, for associated long-term
(current) insulin use V58.67
3 type I [juvenile type], uncontrolled

DEF: Diabetes mellitus: Inability to metabolize carbohydrates, proteins, and
fats due to insufficient secretion of insulin. Symptoms may be unremarkable,
with long-term complications, involving kidneys, nerves, blood vessels, and
eyes.
DEF: Uncontrolled diabetes: A nonspecific term indicating that the current
treatment regimen does not keep the blood sugar level of a patient within
acceptable levels.
AHA: 1Q, '11, 9; 4Q, '04, 56; 2Q, '04, 17; 2Q, '02, 13; 2Q,'01, 16; 2Q,'98, 15; 4Q,
'97, 32; 2Q, '97, 14; 3Q, '96, 5; 4Q, '93, 19; 2Q, '92, 5; 3Q, '91, 3; 2Q, '90, 22; N-D,
'85, 11
TIP: Use of insulin does not ensure type I DM; if patient is on routine insulin,
assign also V58.67 Long-term (current) use of insulin.

§ ✓5ᵗʰ **250.0 Diabetes mellitus without mention of complication**
[0-3] Diabetes mellitus without mention of complication or
manifestation classifiable to 250.1-250.9
Diabetes (mellitus) NOS
AHA: 1Q, '06, 14; 4Q, '97, 32; 3Q, '91, 3, 12; N-D, '85, 11; **For code 250.00:**
▶3Q, '13, 13;◀2Q, '12, 19; 4Q, '09, 77; 1Q, '05, 15; 4Q, '04, 55; 4Q, '03,
105, 108; 2Q, '03, 16; 1Q, '02, 7, 11; **For code 250.01:** 4Q, '04, 55; 4Q, '03,
110; 2Q, '03, 6; **For code 250.02:** 1Q, '03, 5; **For code 250.03:** ▶3Q, '13, 9 ◀
E11.9 Type 2 diabetes mellitus w/o comp   I-10

§ ✓5ᵗʰ **250.1 Diabetes with ketoacidosis**
[0-3] Diabetic:
acidosis ⎫
ketosis ⎬ without mention of coma
DEF: Diabetic hyperglycemic crisis causing ketone presence in body
fluids.
AHA: 3Q, '91, 6; **For code 250.11:** 4Q, '03, 82; **For code 250.13:** 2Q, '06,
19-20
E10.10 Type 1 diabetes mellitus w/ketoacidosis w/o coma   I-10

§ ✓5ᵗʰ **250.2 Diabetes with hyperosmolarity**
[0-3] Hyperosmolar (nonketotic) coma
AHA: 4Q, '93, 19; 3Q, '91, 7

§ ✓5ᵗʰ **250.3 Diabetes with other coma**
[0-3] Diabetic coma (with ketoacidosis)
Diabetic hypoglycemic coma
Insulin coma NOS
EXCLUDES diabetes with hyperosmolar coma (250.2)
DEF: Coma (not hyperosmolar) caused by hyperglycemia or
hypoglycemia as complication of diabetes.
AHA: 3Q, '91, 7, 12

§ ✓5ᵗʰ **250.4 Diabetes with renal manifestations**
[0-3] Use additional code to identify manifestation, as:
chronic kidney disease (585.1-585.9)
diabetic:
nephropathy NOS (583.81)
nephrosis (581.81)
intercapillary glomerulosclerosis (581.81)
Kimmelstiel-Wilson syndrome (581.81)
AHA: 3Q, '91, 8, 12; S-O, '87, 9; S-O, '84, 3; **For code 250.40:** 2Q,'12, 19;
1Q, '03, 20; **For code 250.41:** ▶2Q, '13, 6 ◀
E11.22 Type 2 diabetes mellitus w/diabetic CKD   I-10

§ ✓5ᵗʰ **250.5 Diabetes with ophthalmic manifestations**
[0-3] Use additional code to identify manifestation, as:
diabetic:
blindness (369.00-369.9)
cataract (366.41)
glaucoma (365.44)
macular edema (362.07)
retinal edema (362.07)
retinopathy (362.01-362.07)
AHA: 4Q, '05, 65; 3Q, '91, 8; S-O, '85, 11; **For code 250.50:** 4Q, '05, 67
E10.36 Type 1 diabetes mellitus with diabetic cataract   I-10

§ ✓5ᵗʰ **250.6 Diabetes with neurological manifestations**
[0-3] Use additional code to identify manifestation, as:
diabetic:
amyotrophy (353.5)
gastroparalysis (536.3)
gastroparesis (536.3)
mononeuropathy (354.0-355.9)
neurogenic arthropathy (713.5)
peripheral autonomic neuropathy (337.1)
polyneuropathy (357.2)
AHA: 4Q, '09, 151; 2Q, '09, 13, 15; 3Q, '08, 5; 2Q, '93, 6; 2Q, '92, 15; 3Q,
'91, 9; N-D, '84, 9; **For code 250.60:** 4Q, '03, 105; **For code 250.61:** 2Q, '04,
7
E11.40 Type 2 diabetes mellitus w/diab neuropathy   I-10

§ ✓5ᵗʰ **250.7 Diabetes with peripheral circulatory disorders**
[0-3] Use additional code to identify manifestation, as:
diabetic:
gangrene (785.4)
peripheral angiopathy (443.81)
DEF: Blood vessel damage or disease, usually in the feet, legs, or
hands, as a complication of diabetes.
AHA: 1Q, '96, 10; 3Q, '94, 5; 2Q, '94, 17; 3Q, '91, 10, 12; 3Q, '90, 15; **For
code 250.70:** 1Q, '04, 10
E10.51 Type 1 DM w/diab periph angiopathy w/o gangrene   I-10

§ ✓5ᵗʰ **250.8 Diabetes with other specified manifestations**
[0-3] Diabetic hypoglycemia NOS
Hypoglycemic shock NOS

Use additional code to identify manifestation, as:
any associated ulceration (707.10-707.19, 707.8, 707.9)
diabetic bone changes (731.8)
AHA: 4Q, '00, 44; 4Q, '97, 43; 2Q, '97, 16; 4Q, '93, 20; 3Q, '91, 10;
For code 250.80: 1Q, '04, 14
TIP: Assign for diabetic osteomyelitis, along with code 731.8 and the
appropriate code from category 730.
E11.618 Type 2 DM with other diabetic arthropathy   I-10

§ ✓5ᵗʰ **250.9 Diabetes with unspecified complication**
[0-3] **AHA:** 2Q, '92, 15; 3Q, '91, 7, 12
TIP: Do not assign with any other code in category 250.
E10.8 Type 1 diabetes mellitus with unspecified comp   I-10

✓4ᵗʰ **251 Other disorders of pancreatic internal secretion**

251.0 Hypoglycemic coma
Iatrogenic hyperinsulinism
Non-diabetic insulin coma
Use additional E code to identify cause, if drug-induced
EXCLUDES hypoglycemic coma in diabetes mellitus (249.3,
250.3)
DEF: Coma induced by low blood sugar in non-diabetic patient.
AHA: M-A, '85, 8

§   Requires fifth digit. Valid digits are in [brackets] under each code. See appropriate category for codes and definitions.

✓4ᵗʰ / ✓5ᵗʰ Additional Digit Required   Unspecified Code   Other Specified Code   Manifestation Code   ▶◀ Revised Text   ● New Code   ▲ Revised Code Title

2015 ICD-9-CM   **October 2014 · Volume 1 – 53**

Endocrine, Nutritional and Metabolic Diseases, and Immunity   249.8–251.0

251.1 Other specified hypoglycemia

Hyperinsulinism: Hyperplasia of pancreatic
   NOS   islet beta cells NOS
   ectopic
   functional

Use additional E code to identify cause, if drug-induced

EXCLUDES hypoglycemia:
   in diabetes mellitus (249.8, 250.8)
   in infant of diabetic mother (775.0)
   hypoglycemic coma (251.0)
   neonatal hypoglycemia (775.6)

DEF: Excessive production of insulin by the pancreas; associated with obesity and insulin-producing tumors.

AHA: ▶3Q, '13, 12;◀ 1Q, '03, 10

251.2 Hypoglycemia, unspecified

Hypoglycemia: Hypoglycemia:
   NOS   spontaneous
   reactive

EXCLUDES hypoglycemia:
   with coma (251.0)
   in diabetes mellitus (249.8, 250.8)
   leucine-induced (270.3)

AHA: M-A, '85, 8

E16.2 Hypoglycemia unspecified   I-10

251.3 Postsurgical hypoinsulinemia

Hypoinsulinemia following complete or partial
   pancreatectomy
Postpancreatectomy hyperglycemia

Use additional code to identify (any associated):
   acquired absence of pancreas (V88.11-V88.12)
   insulin use (V58.67)
   secondary diabetes mellitus (249.00-249.91)

EXCLUDES transient hyperglycemia post procedure (790.29)
   transient hypoglycemia post procedure (251.2)

AHA: 3Q, '91, 6

251.4 Abnormality of secretion of glucagon

Hyperplasia of pancreatic islet alpha cells with glucagon
   excess

DEF: Production malfunction of a pancreatic hormone secreted by cells of the islets of Langerhans.

251.5 Abnormality of secretion of gastrin

Hyperplasia of pancreatic alpha cells with gastrin excess
Zollinger-Ellison syndrome

251.8 Other specified disorders of pancreatic internal secretion

AHA: 2Q, '98, 15; 3Q, '91, 6

E16.8 Oth spec d/o of pancreatic internal secretion   I-10

251.9 Unspecified disorder of pancreatic internal secretion

Islet cell hyperplasia NOS

√4ᵗʰ **252 Disorders of parathyroid gland**

EXCLUDES hungry bone syndrome (275.5)

√5ᵗʰ **252.0 Hyperparathyroidism**

EXCLUDES ectopic hyperparathyroidism (259.3)

DEF: Abnormally high secretion of parathyroid hormones causing bone deterioration, reduced renal function, kidney stones.

252.00 Hyperparathyroidism, unspecified

E21.3 Hyperparathyroidism unspecified   I-10

Dorsal View of Parathyroid Glands

Pharynx

Thyroid gland

Parathyroid glands

Trachea

Esophagus

Parathyroid glands
↓
Parathyroid hormone (PTH)

Calcium in bones ←———→ Calcium in blood

252.01 Primary hyperparathyroidism

Hyperplasia of parathyroid

DEF: Parathyroid dysfunction commonly caused by hyperplasia of two or more glands; characteristic hypercalcemia and increased parathyroid hormone levels.

252.02 Secondary hyperparathyroidism, non-renal

EXCLUDES secondary hyperparathyroidism (of renal origin) (588.81)

DEF: Underlying disease of nonrenal origin decreases blood levels of calcium causing the parathyroid to release increased levels of parathyroid hormone; parathyroid hormone levels return to normal once underlying condition is treated and blood calcium levels are normal.

AHA: 4Q, '04, 57-59

252.08 Other hyperparathyroidism

Tertiary hyperparathyroidism

DEF: Tertiary hyperparathyroidism: chronic secondary hyperparathyroidism with adenomatous parathyroid causing irreversible abnormal production of parathyroid hormone (PTH); PTH remains high after the serum calcium levels are brought under control.

252.1 Hypoparathyroidism

Parathyroiditis (autoimmune)
Tetany:
   parathyroid
   parathyroprival

EXCLUDES pseudohypoparathyroidism (275.4)
   pseudopseudohypoparathyroidism (275.4)
   tetany NOS (781.7)
   transitory neonatal hypoparathyroidism (775.4)

DEF: Abnormally low secretion of parathyroid hormones which causes decreased calcium and increased phosphorus in the blood, resulting in muscle cramps, tetany, urinary frequency and cataracts.

252.8 Other specified disorders of parathyroid gland

Cyst
Hemorrhage   } of parathyroid

252.9 Unspecified disorder of parathyroid gland

√4ᵗʰ **253 Disorders of the pituitary gland and its hypothalamic control**

INCLUDES the listed conditions whether the disorder is in the pituitary or the hypothalamus

EXCLUDES Cushing's syndrome (255.0)

253.0 Acromegaly and gigantism

Overproduction of growth hormone

DEF: Acromegaly: chronic, middle age condition; caused by hypersecretion of the pituitary growth hormone; enlarged parts of skeleton, especially the nose, ears, jaws, fingers and toes.

DEF: Gigantism: pituitary gigantism caused by excess growth of short flat bones; men may grow 78 to 80 inches tall.

253.1 Other and unspecified anterior pituitary hyperfunction

Forbes-Albright syndrome

EXCLUDES overproduction of:
   ACTH (255.3)
   thyroid-stimulating hormone [TSH] (242.8)

DEF: Spontaneous galactorrhea-amenorrhea syndrome unrelated to pregnancy; usually related to presence of pituitary tumor.

AHA: J-A, '85, 9

253.2 Panhypopituitarism

Cachexia, pituitary   Sheehan's syndrome
Necrosis of pituitary (postpartum)   Simmonds' disease
Pituitary insufficiency NOS

EXCLUDES iatrogenic hypopituitarism (253.7)

DEF: Damage to or absence of pituitary gland leading to impaired sexual function, weight loss, fatigue, bradycardia, hypotension, pallor, depression, and impaired growth in children; called Simmonds' disease if cachexia is prominent.

253.3 Pituitary dwarfism

Isolated deficiency of (human) growth hormone [HGH]
Lorain-Levi dwarfism

DEF: Dwarfism with infantile physical characteristics due to abnormally low secretion of growth hormone and gonadotropin deficiency.

253.4 Other anterior pituitary disorders

Isolated or partial deficiency of an anterior pituitary hormone, other than growth hormone
Prolactin deficiency

AHA: J-A, '85, 9

Ⓝ Newborn Age: 0   Ⓟ Pediatric Age: 0-17   Ⓜ Maternity Age: 12-55   Ⓐ Adult Age: 15-124

253.5 Diabetes insipidus
Vasopressin deficiency

EXCLUDES   *nephrogenic diabetes insipidus (588.1)*

DEF: Metabolic disorder causing insufficient antidiuretic hormone release; symptoms include frequent urination, thirst, ravenous hunger, loss of weight, fatigue.

253.6 Other disorders of neurohypophysis
Syndrome of inappropriate secretion of antidiuretic hormone [ADH]

EXCLUDES   *ectopic antidiuretic hormone secretion (259.3)*

E22.2 Synd inappropriate secrectn antiduretic hormone   `I-10`

253.7 Iatrogenic pituitary disorders
Hypopituitarism:
   hormone-induced
   hypophysectomy-induced
   postablative
   radiotherapy-induced

Use additional E code to identify cause

DEF: Pituitary dysfunction that results from drug therapy, radiation therapy, or surgery, causing mild to severe symptoms.

253.8 Other disorders of the pituitary and other syndromes of diencephalohypophyseal origin
Abscess of pituitary   Cyst of Rathke's pouch
Adiposogenital dystrophy   Fröhlich's syndrome

EXCLUDES   *craniopharyngioma (237.0)*

253.9 Unspecified
Dyspituitarism

√4th 254 Diseases of thymus gland

EXCLUDES   *aplasia or dysplasia with immunodeficiency (279.2)*
           hypoplasia with immunodeficiency (279.2)
           myasthenia gravis (358.00-358.01)

254.0 Persistent hyperplasia of thymus
Hypertrophy of thymus

DEF: Continued abnormal growth of the twin lymphoid lobes that produce T lymphocytes.

254.1 Abscess of thymus

254.8 Other specified diseases of thymus gland
Astrophy   ⎫
Cyst   ⎬ of thymus

EXCLUDES   *thymoma (212.6)*

254.9 Unspecified disease of thymus gland

√4th 255 Disorders of adrenal glands

INCLUDES   the listed conditions whether the basic disorder is in the adrenals or is pituitary-induced

255.0 Cushing's syndrome
Adrenal hyperplasia due to excess ACTH
Cushing's syndrome:
   NOS
   iatrogenic
   idiopathic
   pituitary-dependent
Ectopic ACTH syndrome
Iatrogenic syndrome of excess cortisol
Overproduction of cortisol

Use additional E code to identify cause, if drug-induced

EXCLUDES   *congenital adrenal hyperplasia (255.2)*

DEF: Due to adrenal cortisol oversecretion or glucocorticoid medications; may cause excess fatty tissue of the face, neck and body; osteoporosis and curvature of spine, hypertension, diabetes mellitus, female genitourinary problems, male impotence, degeneration of muscle tissues, weakness.

√5th 255.1 Hyperaldosteronism
DEF: Oversecretion of aldosterone causing fluid retention, hypertension.

AHA: 4Q, '03, 48

255.10 Hyperaldosteronism, unspecified
Aldosteronism NOS
Primary aldosteronism, unspecified

EXCLUDES   *Conn's syndrome (255.12)*

255.11 Glucocorticoid-remediable aldosteronism
Familial aldosteronism type I

EXCLUDES   *Conn's syndrome (255.12)*

DEF: Rare autosomal dominant familial form of primary aldosteronism in which the secretion of aldosterone is under the influence of adrenocorticotrophic hormone (ACTH) rather than the renin-angiotensin mechanism; moderate hypersecretion of aldosterone and suppressed plasma renin activity rapidly reversed by administration of glucosteroids; symptoms include hypertension and mild hypokalemia.

255.12 Conn's syndrome
DEF: A type of primary aldosteronism caused by an adenoma of the glomerulosa cells in the adrenal cortex; presence of hypertension.

255.13 Bartter's syndrome
DEF: A cluster of symptoms caused by a defect in the ability of the kidney to reabsorb potassium; signs include alkalosis (hypokalemic alkalosis), increased aldosterone, increased plasma renin, and normal blood pressure; symptoms include muscle cramping, weakness, constipation, frequency of urination, and failure to grow; also known as urinary potassium wasting or juxtaglomerular cell hyperplasia.

255.14 Other secondary aldosteronism
AHA: 3Q, '06, 24

255.2 Adrenogenital disorders
Achard-Thiers syndrome
Adrenogenital syndromes, virilizing or feminizing, whether acquired or associated with congenital adrenal hyperplasia consequent on inborn enzyme defects in hormone synthesis
Congenital adrenal hyperplasia
Female adrenal pseudohermaphroditism
Male:
   macrogenitosomia praecox
   sexual precocity with adrenal hyperplasia
Virilization (female) (suprarenal)

EXCLUDES   *adrenal hyperplasia due to excess ACTH (255.0)*
           isosexual virilization (256.4)

255.3 Other corticoadrenal overactivity
Acquired benign adrenal androgenic overactivity
Overproduction of ACTH

√5th 255.4 Corticoadrenal insufficiency

EXCLUDES   *tuberculous Addison's disease (017.6)*

DEF: Underproduction of adrenal hormones causing low blood pressure.

AHA: 4Q, '07, 68; 3Q, '06, 24

255.41 Glucocorticoid deficiency
Addisonian crisis
Addison's disease NOS
Adrenal atrophy (autoimmune)
Adrenal calcification
Adrenal crisis
Adrenal hemorrhage
Adrenal infarction
Adrenal insufficiency NOS
Combined glucocorticoid and mineralocorticoid deficiency
Corticoadrenal insufficiency NOS

DEF: Decreased function of the adrenal cortex resulting in insufficient production of glucocorticoid, the hormone regulating carbohydrate, fat, and protein metabolism; manifestations: hyponatremia, hyperpigmentation, orthostatic hypotension, anemia, loss of appetite, and malaise.

AHA: 4Q, '07, 68, 69

E27.1 Primary adrenocortical insufficiency   `I-10`

255.42 Mineralocorticoid deficiency
Hypoaldosteronism

EXCLUDES   *combined glucocorticoid and*
           mineralocorticoid deficiency (255.41)

DEF: Decreased function of the adrenal cortex resulting in insufficient production of mineralocorticoid, which regulates electrolyte and water balance; manifestations: hyponatremia, hyperkalemia, and mild acidosis.

√4th √5th Additional Digit Required   **Unspecified Code**   Other Specified Code   Manifestation Code   ▶◀ Revised Text   ● New Code   ▲ Revised Code Title

255.5 Other adrenal hypofunction
Adrenal medullary insufficiency

EXCLUDES *Waterhouse-Friderichsen syndrome (meningococcal) (036.3)*

255.6 Medulloadrenal hyperfunction
Catecholamine secretion by pheochromocytoma

255.8 Other specified disorders of adrenal glands
Abnormality of cortisol-binding globulin

255.9 Unspecified disorder of adrenal glands

√4th 256 Ovarian dysfunction
AHA: 4Q, '00, 51

256.0 Hyperestrogenism ♀
DEF: Excess secretion of estrogen by the ovaries; characterized by ovaries containing multiple follicular cysts filled with serous fluid.

256.1 Other ovarian hyperfunction ♀
Hypersecretion of ovarian androgens
AHA: 3Q, '95, 15

256.2 Postablative ovarian failure ♀
Ovarian failure:
  iatrogenic
  postirradiation
  postsurgical

Use additional code for states associated with artificial menopause (627.4)

EXCLUDES *acquired absence of ovary (V45.77)*
asymptomatic age-related (natural) postmenopausal status (V49.81)

DEF: Failed ovarian function after medical or surgical intervention.
AHA: 2Q, '02, 12

√5th 256.3 Other ovarian failure
Use additional code for states associated with natural menopause (627.2)

EXCLUDES *asymptomatic age-related (natural) postmenopausal status (V49.81)*

AHA: 4Q, '01, 41

256.31 Premature menopause A♀
DEF: Permanent cessation of ovarian function before the age of 40 occuring naturally of unknown cause.

256.39 Other ovarian failure ♀
Delayed menarche
Ovarian hypofunction
Primary ovarian failure NOS

256.4 Polycystic ovaries ♀
Isosexual virilization
Stein-Leventhal syndrome
DEF: Multiple serous filled cysts of ovary; symptoms of infertility, hirsutism, oligomenorrhea or amenorrhea.
E28.2 Polycystic ovarian syndrome `I-10`

256.8 Other ovarian dysfunction ♀

256.9 Unspecified ovarian dysfunction ♀

√4th 257 Testicular dysfunction

257.0 Testicular hyperfunction ♂
Hypersecretion of testicular hormones

257.1 Postablative testicular hypofunction ♂
Testicular hypofunction:
  iatrogenic
  postirradiation
  postsurgical

257.2 Other testicular hypofunction
Defective biosynthesis of testicular androgen
Eunuchoidism:
  NOS
  hypogonadotropic
Failure:
  Leydig's cell, adult
  seminiferous tubule, adult
Testicular hypogonadism
EXCLUDES *azoospermia (606.0)*

257.8 Other testicular dysfunction
EXCLUDES *androgen insensitivity syndromes (259.50-259.52)*

257.9 Unspecified testicular dysfunction ♂

√4th 258 Polyglandular dysfunction and related disorders

√5th 258.0 Polyglandular activity in multiple endocrine adenomatosis
Multiple endocrine neoplasia [MEN] syndromes

Use additional codes to identify any malignancies and other conditions associated with the syndromes

AHA: 4Q, '09, 150; 4Q, '07, 70

258.01 Multiple endocrine neoplasia [MEN] type I
Wermer's syndrome
DEF: Wermer's syndrome: A rare hereditary condition characterized by the presence of adenomas or hyperplasia in more than one endocrine gland causing premature aging.
AHA: 4Q, '08, 86, 89; 4Q, '07, 70, 72

258.02 Multiple endocrine neoplasia [MEN] type IIA
Sipple's syndrome
DEF: Sipple's syndrome: A hereditary disorder caused by a defect in the RET gene causing overactivity of the thyroid, adrenal, and parathyroid glands, resulting in adrenal pheochromocytoma and thyroid medullary carcinoma.

258.03 Multiple endocrine neoplasia [MEN] type IIB

258.1 Other combinations of endocrine dysfunction
Lloyd's syndrome
Schmidt's syndrome

258.8 Other specified polyglandular dysfunction

258.9 Polyglandular dysfunction, unspecified

√4th 259 Other endocrine disorders

259.0 Delay in sexual development and puberty, not elsewhere classified
Delayed puberty

259.1 Precocious sexual development and puberty, not elsewhere classified `P`
Sexual precocity: Sexual precocity:
  NOS   cryptogenic
  constitutional   idiopathic

259.2 Carcinoid syndrome
Hormone secretion by carcinoid tumors
DEF: Presence of carcinoid tumors that spread to liver; characterized by cyanotic flushing of skin, diarrhea, bronchospasm, acquired tricuspid and pulmonary stenosis, sudden drops in blood pressure, edema, ascites.
AHA: 4Q, '08, 85-86, 89

259.3 Ectopic hormone secretion, not elsewhere classified
Ectopic:
  antidiuretic hormone secretion [ADH]
  hyperparathyroidism
EXCLUDES *ectopic ACTH syndrome (255.0)*
AHA: N-D, '85, 4

259.4 Dwarfism, not elsewhere classified
Dwarfism: Dwarfism:
  NOS   constitutional
EXCLUDES *dwarfism:*
    achondroplastic (756.4)
    intrauterine (759.7)
    nutritional (263.2)
    pituitary (253.3)
    renal (588.0)
    progeria (259.8)

√5th 259.5 Androgen insensitivity syndrome
DEF: X chromosome abnormality that prohibits the body from recognizing androgen; XY genotype with ambiguous genitalia.
AHA: 4Q, '08, 95-96; 4Q, '05, 53

259.50 Androgen insensitivity, unspecified

259.51 Androgen insensitivity syndrome
Complete androgen insensitivity
de Quervain's syndrome
Goldberg-Maxwell Syndrome

259.52 Partial androgen insensitivity
Partial androgen insensitivity syndrome
Reifenstein syndrome

259.8 Other specified endocrine disorders
Pineal gland dysfunction   Werner's syndrome
Progeria

N Newborn Age: 0   **P** Pediatric Age: 0-17   **M** Maternity Age: 12-55   **A** Adult Age: 15-124

259.9 Unspecified endocrine disorder

Disturbance:
endocrine NOS
hormone NOS
Infantilism NOS

Nutritional Deficiencies (260-269)

EXCLUDES *deficiency anemias (280.0-281.9)*

TIP: Assign first a code for the underlying condition (e.g., anorexia nervosa) if specified.

260 Kwashiorkor

Nutritional edema with dyspigmentation of skin and hair

DEF: Syndrome, particulary of children; excessive carbohydrate with inadequate protein intake, inhibited growth potential, anomalies in skin and hair pigmentation, edema and liver disease.

AHA: 3Q, '09, 6

TIP: Do not assign when documentation indicates "mild or moderate protein malnutrition" only. Kwashiorkor is a rare severe protein deficiency.

E40 Kwashiorkor   I-10

261 Nutritional marasmus

Nutritional atrophy   Severe malnutrition NOS
Severe calorie deficiency

DEF: Protein-calorie malabsorption or malnutrition in children; characterized by tissue wasting, dehydration, and subcutaneous fat depletion; may occur with infectious disease; also called infantile atrophy.

AHA: 3Q, '12, 10; 4Q, '07, 97; 3Q, '06, 14; 2Q, '06, 12

E41 Nutritional marasmus   I-10

262 Other severe, protein-calorie malnutrition

Nutritional edema without mention of dyspigmentation of skin and hair

AHA: 4Q, '92, 24; J-A, '85, 12

√4ᵗʰ 263 Other and unspecified protein-calorie malnutrition

AHA: 4Q, '92, 24

263.0 Malnutrition of moderate degree

DEF: Malnutrition characterized by biochemical changes in electrolytes, lipids, blood plasma.

AHA: 3Q, '12, 10; 3Q, '09, 6; J-A, '85, 1

263.1 Malnutrition of mild degree

AHA: J-A, '85, 1

263.2 Arrested development following protein-calorie malnutrition

Nutritional dwarfism
Physical retardation due to malnutrition

263.8 Other protein-calorie malnutrition

263.9 Unspecified protein-calorie malnutrition

Dystrophy due to malnutrition
Malnutrition (calorie) NOS

EXCLUDES *nutritional deficiency NOS (269.9)*

AHA: 3Q, '12, 9; 4Q, '03, 109; N-D, '84, 19

E46 Unspecified protein-calorie malnutrition   I-10

√4ᵗʰ 264 Vitamin A deficiency

264.0 With conjunctival xerosis

DEF: Vitamin A deficiency with conjunctival dryness.

264.1 With conjunctival xerosis and Bitot's spot

Bitot's spot in the young child

DEF: Vitamin A deficiency with conjunctival dryness, superficial spots of keratinized epithelium.

264.2 With corneal xerosis

DEF: Vitamin A deficiency with corneal dryness.

264.3 With corneal ulceration and xerosis

DEF: Vitamin A deficiency with corneal dryness, epithelial ulceration.

264.4 With keratomalacia

DEF: Vitamin A deficiency creating corneal dryness; progresses to corneal insensitivity, softness, necrosis; usually bilateral.

264.5 With night blindness

DEF: Vitamin A deficiency causing vision failure in dim light.

264.6 With xerophthalmic scars of cornea

DEF: Vitamin A deficiency with corneal scars from dryness.

264.7 Other ocular manifestations of vitamin A deficiency

Xerophthalmia due to vitamin A deficiency

264.8 Other manifestations of vitamin A deficiency

Follicular keratosis
Xeroderma   } due to vitamin A deficiency

264.9 Unspecified vitamin A deficiency

Hypovitaminosis A NOS

√4ᵗʰ 265 Thiamine and niacin deficiency states

265.0 Beriberi

DEF: Inadequate vitamin B_1 (thiamine) intake, affects heart and peripheral nerves; individual may become edematous and develop cardiac disease due to the excess fluid; affects alcoholics and people with a diet of excessive polished rice.

265.1 Other and unspecified manifestations of thiamine deficiency

Other vitamin B_1 deficiency states

265.2 Pellagra

Deficiency:
niacin (-tryptophan)
nicotinamide
nicotinic acid
vitamin PP
Pellagra (alcoholic)

DEF: Niacin deficiency causing dermatitis, inflammation of mucous membranes, diarrhea, and psychic disturbances.

√4ᵗʰ 266 Deficiency of B-complex components

266.0 Ariboflavinosis

Riboflavin [vitamin B_2] deficiency

DEF: Vitamin B_2 (riboflavin) deficiency marked by swollen lips and tongue fissures, corneal vascularization, scaling lesions, and anemia.

AHA: S-O, '86, 10

266.1 Vitamin B_6 deficiency

Deficiency:
pyridoxal
pyridoxamine
pyridoxine
Vitamin B_6 deficiency syndrome

EXCLUDES *vitamin B_6-responsive sideroblastic anemia (285.0)*

DEF: Vitamin B_6 deficiency causing skin, lip, and tongue disturbances, peripheral neuropathy; and convulsions in infants.

266.2 Other B-complex deficiencies

Deficiency:
cyanocobalamin
folic acid
vitamin B_{12}

EXCLUDES *combined system disease with anemia (281.0-281.1)*
deficiency anemias (281.0-281.9)
subacute degeneration of spinal cord with anemia (281.0-281.1)

E53.8 Deficiency of other specified B group vitamins   I-10

266.9 Unspecified vitamin B deficiency

267 Ascorbic acid deficiency

Deficiency of vitamin C
Scurvy

EXCLUDES *scorbutic anemia (281.8)*

DEF: Vitamin C deficiency causing swollen gums, myalgia, weight loss, and weakness.

√4ᵗʰ 268 Vitamin D deficiency

EXCLUDES *vitamin D-resistant:*
osteomalacia (275.3)
rickets (275.3)

268.0 Rickets, active

EXCLUDES *celiac rickets (579.0)*
renal rickets (588.0)

DEF: Inadequate vitamin D intake, usually in pediatrics, that affects bones most involved with muscular action; may cause nodules on ends and sides of bones; delayed closure of fontanels in infants; symptoms may include muscle soreness, and profuse sweating.

268.1 Rickets, late effect

Any condition specified as due to rickets and stated to be a late effect or sequela of rickets

Code first the nature of late effect

DEF: Distorted or demineralized bones as a result of vitamin D deficiency.

Endocrine, Nutritional and Metabolic Diseases, and Immunity

268.2–271.3

268.2 Osteomalacia, unspecified
DEF: Softening of bones due to decrease in calcium; marked by pain, tenderness, muscular weakness, anorexia, and weight loss.

268.9 Unspecified vitamin D deficiency
Avitaminosis D

✓4th 269 Other nutritional deficiencies

269.0 Deficiency of vitamin K
EXCLUDES deficiency of coagulation factor due to vitamin K deficiency (286.7)
vitamin K deficiency of newborn (776.0)

269.1 Deficiency of other vitamins
Deficiency:
vitamin E
vitamin P

269.2 Unspecified vitamin deficiency
Multiple vitamin deficiency NOS

269.3 Mineral deficiency, not elsewhere classified
Deficiency:
calcium, dietary
iodine
EXCLUDES deficiency:
calcium NOS (275.4)
potassium (276.8)
sodium (276.1)

269.8 Other nutritional deficiency
EXCLUDES adult failure to thrive (783.7)
failure to thrive in childhood (783.41)
feeding problems (783.3)
newborn (779.31-779.34)

269.9 Unspecified nutritional deficiency

Other Metabolic and Immunity Disorders (270-279)
Use additional code to identify any associated intellectual disabilities

✓4th 270 Disorders of amino-acid transport and metabolism
EXCLUDES abnormal findings without manifest disease (790.0-796.9)
disorders of purine and pyrimidine metabolism (277.1-277.2)
gout (274.00-274.9)

270.0 Disturbances of amino-acid transport
Cystinosis
Cystinuria
Fanconi (-de Toni) (-Debré) syndrome
Glycinuria (renal)
Hartnup disease

270.1 Phenylketonuria [PKU]
Hyperphenylalaninemia
DEF: Inherited metabolic condition causing excess phenylpyruvic and other acids in urine; results in mental retardation, neurological manifestations, including spasticity and tremors, light pigmentation, eczema, and mousy odor.

270.2 Other disturbances of aromatic amino-acid metabolism
Albinism
Alkaptonuria
Alkaptonuric ochronosis
Disturbances of metabolism of tyrosine and tryptophan
Homogentisic acid defects
Hydroxykynureninuria
Hypertyrosinemia
Indicanuria
Kynureninase defects
Oasthouse urine disease
Ochronosis
Tyrosinosis
Tyrosinuria
Waardenburg syndrome
EXCLUDES vitamin B_6-deficiency syndrome (266.1)
AHA: 3Q, '99, 20

270.3 Disturbances of branched-chain amino-acid metabolism
Disturbances of metabolism of leucine, isoleucine, and valine
Hypervalinemia
Intermittent branched-chain ketonuria
Leucine-induced hypoglycemia
Leucinosis
Maple syrup urine disease
AHA: 3Q, '00, 8

270.4 Disturbances of sulphur-bearing amino-acid metabolism
Cystathioninemia
Cystathioninuria
Disturbances of metabolism of methionine, homocystine, and cystathionine
Homocystinuria
Hypermethioninemia
Methioninemia
AHA: ▶4Q, '13, 87; ◄2Q, '07, 7;1Q, '04, 6

270.5 Disturbances of histidine metabolism
Carnosinemia
Histidinemia
Hyperhistidinemia
Imidazole aminoaciduria

270.6 Disorders of urea cycle metabolism
Argininosuccinic aciduria
Citrullinemia
Disorders of metabolism of ornithine, citrulline, argininosuccinic acid, arginine, and ammonia
Hyperammonemia
Hyperomithinemia

270.7 Other disturbances of straight-chain amino-acid metabolism
Glucoglycinuria
Glycinemia (with methyl-malonic acidemia)
Hyperglycinemia
Hyperlysinemia
Other disturbances of metabolism of glycine, threonine, serine, glutamine, and lysine
Pipecolic acidemia
Saccharopinuria
AHA: 3Q, '00, 8

270.8 Other specified disorders of amino-acid metabolism
Alaninemia	Iminoacidopathy
Ethanolaminuria	Prolinemia
Glycoprolinuria	Prolinuria
Hydroxyprolinemia	Sarcosinemia
Hyperprolinemia	

270.9 Unspecified disorder of amino-acid metabolism

✓4th 271 Disorders of carbohydrate transport and metabolism
EXCLUDES abnormality of secretion of glucagon (251.4)
diabetes mellitus (249.0-249.9, 250.0-250.9)
hypoglycemia NOS (251.2)
mucopolysaccharidosis (277.5)

271.0 Glycogenosis
Amylopectinosis
Glucose-6-phosphatase deficiency
Glycogen storage disease
McArdle's disease
Pompe's disease
von Gierke's disease
DEF: Excess glycogen storage; rare inherited trait affects liver, kidneys; causes various symptoms depending on type, though often weakness and muscle cramps.
AHA: 1Q, '98, 5

271.1 Galactosemia
Galactose-1-phosphate uridyl transferase deficiency
Galactosuria
DEF: Any of three genetic disorders due to defective galactose metabolism; symptoms include failure to thrive in infancy, jaundice, liver and spleen damage, cataracts, and mental retardation.

271.2 Hereditary fructose intolerance
Essential benign fructosuria
Fructosemia
DEF: Chromosome recessive disorder of carbohydrate metabolism; in infants, occurs after dietary sugar introduced; characterized by enlarged spleen, yellowish cast to skin, and progressive inability to thrive.

271.3 Intestinal disaccharidase deficiencies and disaccharide malabsorption
Intolerance or malabsorption (congenital) (of):
glucose-galactose
lactose
sucrose-isomaltose
E73.9 Lactose intolerance unspecified ▐I-10▌

271.4 Renal glycosuria
Renal diabetes
DEF: Persistent abnormal levels of glucose in urine, with normal blood glucose levels; caused by failure of the renal tubules to reabsorb glucose.

271.8 Other specified disorders of carbohydrate transport and metabolism
Essential benign pentosuria　　Mannosidosis
Fucosidosis　　　　　　　　　Oxalosis
Glycolic aciduria　　　　　　　Xylosuria
Hyperoxaluria (primary)　　　　Xylulosuria

271.9 Unspecified disorder of carbohydrate transport and metabolism

√4ᵗʰ 272 Disorders of lipoid metabolism
EXCLUDES *localized cerebral lipidoses (330.1)*

272.0 Pure hypercholesterolemia
Familial hypercholesterolemia
Fredrickson Type IIa hyperlipoproteinemia
Hyperbetalipoproteinemia
Hyperlipidemia, Group A
Low-density-lipoid-type [LDL] hyperlipoproteinemia
AHA: 4Q, '05, 71
E78.0 Pure hypercholesterolemia　　　　　　　　I-10

272.1 Pure hyperglyceridemia
Endogenous hyperglyceridemia
Fredrickson Type IV hyperlipoproteinemia
Hyperlipidemia, Group B
Hyperprebetalipoproteinemia
Hypertriglyceridemia, essential
Very-low-density-lipoid-type [VLDL] hyperlipoproteinemia

272.2 Mixed hyperlipidemia
Broad- or floating-betalipoproteinemia
Combined hyperlipidemia
Elevated cholesterol with elevated triglycerides NEC
Fredrickson Type IIb or III hyperlipoproteinemia
Hypercholesterolemia with endogenous hyperglyceridemia
Hyperbetalipoproteinemia with prebetalipoproteinemia
Tubo-eruptive xanthoma
Xanthoma tuberosum
DEF: Elevated levels of lipoprotein, a complex of fats and proteins, in blood due to inherited metabolic disorder.

272.3 Hyperchylomicronemia
Bürger-Grütz syndrome
Fredrickson type I or V hyperlipoproteinemia
Hyperlipidemia, Group D
Mixed hyperglyceridemia

272.4 Other and unspecified hyperlipidemia
Alpha-lipoproteinemia　　Hyperlipoproteinemia NOS
Hyperlipidemia NOS
DEF: Hyperlipoproteinemia: elevated levels of transient chylomicrons in the blood which are a form of lipoproteins that transport dietary cholesterol and triglycerides from the small intestine to the blood.
AHA: 1Q, '05, 17
E78.4 Other hyperlipidemia　　　　　　　　　　I-10

272.5 Lipoprotein deficiencies
Abetalipoproteinemia
Bassen-Kornzweig syndrome
High-density lipoid deficiency
Hypoalphalipoproteinemia
Hypobetalipoproteinemia (familial)
DEF: Abnormally low levels of lipoprotein, a complex of fats and protein, in the blood.

272.6 Lipodystrophy
Barraquer-Simons disease　　Progressive lipodystrophy
Use additional E code to identify cause, if iatrogenic
EXCLUDES *intestinal lipodystrophy (040.2)*
DEF: Disturbance of fat metabolism resulting in loss of fatty tissue in some areas of the body.

Lipid Metabolism

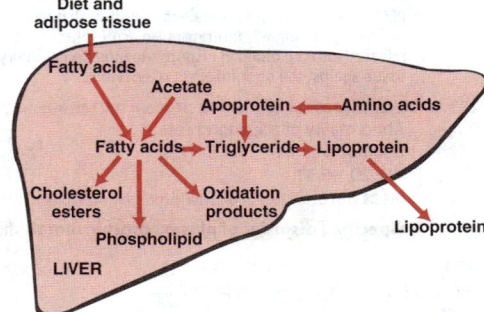

272.7 Lipidoses
Chemically-induced lipidosis
Disease:
　Anderson's
　Fabry's
　Gaucher's
　I cell [mucolipidosis I]
　lipoid storage NOS
　Niemann-Pick
　pseudo-Hurler's or mucolipdosis III
　triglyceride storage, Type I or II
　Wolman's or triglyceride storage, Type III
Mucolipidosis II
Primary familial xanthomatosis
EXCLUDES *cerebral lipidoses (330.1)*
　　　　　Tay-Sachs disease (330.1)
DEF: Lysosomal storage diseases marked by an abnormal amount of lipids in reticuloendothelial cells.

272.8 Other disorders of lipoid metabolism
Hoffa's disease or liposynovitis prepatellaris
Launois-Bensaude's lipomatosis
Lipoid dermatoarthritis

272.9 Unspecified disorder of lipoid metabolism

√4ᵗʰ 273 Disorders of plasma protein metabolism
EXCLUDES *agammaglobulinemia and hypogammaglobulinemia*
　　　　　(279.0-279.2)
　　　　　coagulation defects (286.0-286.9)
　　　　　hereditary hemolytic anemias (282.0-282.9)

273.0 Polyclonal hypergammaglobulinemia
Hypergammaglobulinemic purpura:
　benign primary
　Waldenström's
DEF: Elevated blood levels of gamma globulins, frequently found in patients with chronic infectious diseases.

273.1 Monoclonal paraproteinemia
Benign monoclonal hypergammaglobulinemia [BMH]
Monoclonal gammopathy:
　NOS
　associated with lymphoplasmacytic dyscrasias
　benign
Paraproteinemia:
　benign (familial)
　secondary to malignant or inflammatory disease

273.2 Other paraproteinemias
Cryoglobulinemic:
　purpura
　vasculitis
Mixed cryoglobulinemia
AHA: 2Q, '08, 17

273.3 Macroglobulinemia
Macroglobulinemia (idiopathic) (primary)
Waldenström's macroglobulinemia
DEF: Elevated blood levels of macroglobulins (plasma globulins of high weight); characterized by malignant neoplasms of bone marrow, spleen, liver, or lymph nodes; symptoms include weakness, fatigue, bleeding disorders, and vision problems.

Endocrine, Nutritional and Metabolic Diseases, and Immunity

273.4–276.1

273.4 Alpha-1-antitrypsin deficiency
AAT deficiency

DEF: Disorder of plasma protein metabolism that results in a deficiency of Alpha-1-antitrypsin, an acute-phase reactive protein, released into the blood in response to infection or injury to protect tissue against the harmful effect of enzymes.

273.8 Other disorders of plasma protein metabolism
Abnormality of transport protein
Bisalbuminemia
AHA: 2Q, '98, 11
E88.09 Oth disorders of plasma-protein metablolis NEC   I-10

273.9 Unspecified disorder of plasma protein metabolism

✓4ᵗʰ **274 Gout**
EXCLUDES lead gout (984.0-984.9)
DEF: Purine and pyrimidine metabolic disorders; manifested by hyperuricemia and recurrent acute inflammatory arthritis; monosodium urate or monohydrate crystals may be deposited in and around the joints, leading to joint destruction, and severe crippling.
AHA: 2Q, '95, 4

✓5ᵗʰ **274.0 Gouty arthropathy**
AHA: 4Q, '09, 76-77

274.00 Gouty arthropathy, unspecified
M10.00 Idiopathic gout unspecified site   I-10

274.01 Acute gouty arthropathy
Acute gout
Gout attack
Gout flare
Podagra

274.02 Chronic gouty arthropathy without mention of tophus (tophi)
Chronic gout

274.03 Chronic gouty arthropathy with tophus (tophi)
Chronic tophaceous gout
Gout with tophi NOS
AHA: 4Q, '09, 77

✓5ᵗʰ **274.1 Gouty nephropathy**

274.10 Gouty nephropathy, unspecified
AHA: N-D, '85, 15

274.11 Uric acid nephrolithiasis
DEF: Sodium urate stones in the kidney.

274.19 Other

✓5ᵗʰ **274.8 Gout with other specified manifestations**

274.81 Gouty tophi of ear
DEF: Chalky sodium urate deposit in the ear due to gout; produces chronic inflammation of external ear.

274.82 Gouty tophi of other sites
Gouty tophi of heart
EXCLUDES gout with tophi NOS (274.03)
gouty arthropathy with tophi (274.03)

274.89 Other
Use additional code to identify manifestations, as:
gouty:
iritis (364.11)
neuritis (357.4)

274.9 Gout, unspecified
M10.9 Gout unspecified   I-10

✓4ᵗʰ **275 Disorders of mineral metabolism**
EXCLUDES abnormal findings without manifest disease (790.0-796.9)

✓5ᵗʰ **275.0 Disorders of iron metabolism**
EXCLUDES anemia:
iron deficiency (280.0-280.9)
sideroblastic (285.0)
AHA: 4Q, '10, 77-78; 2Q, '97, 11

275.01 Hereditary hemochromatosis
Bronzed diabetes
Pigmentary cirrhosis (of liver)
Primary (hereditary) hemochromatosis
E83.110 Hereditary hemochromatosis   I-10

275.02 Hemochromatosis due to repeated red blood cell transfusions
Iron overload due to repeated red blood cell transfusions
Transfusion (red blood cell) associated hemochromatosis
AHA: 4Q, '10, 77-78
E83.111 Hemochromatosis due to repeated red blood cell transfusions   I-10

275.03 Other hemochromatosis
Hemochromatosis NOS
E83.118 Other hemochromatosis   I-10

275.09 Other disorders of iron metabolism
E83.10 Disorder of iron-metabolism unspecified   I-10

275.1 Disorders of copper metabolism
Hepatolenticular degeneration
Wilson's disease

275.2 Disorders of magnesium metabolism
HypermagnesemiaHypomagnesemia
AHA: 1Q, '10, 14; 3Q, '09, 21
E83.40 Disorders of magnesium metabolism unspec   I-10

275.3 Disorders of phosphorus metabolism
Familial hypophosphatemia
Hypophosphatasia
Vitamin D-resistant:
osteomalacia
rickets

✓5ᵗʰ **275.4 Disorders of calcium metabolism**
EXCLUDES hungry bone syndrome (275.5)
parathyroid disorders (252.00-252.9)
vitamin D deficiency (268.0-268.9)
AHA: 4Q, '97, 33

275.40 Unspecified disorder of calcium metabolism

275.41 Hypocalcemia
DEF: Abnormally decreased blood calcium level; symptoms include hyperactive deep tendon reflexes, muscle, abdominal cramps, and carpopedal spasm.
AHA: 3Q, '07, 5
E83.51 Hypocalcemia   I-10

275.42 Hypercalcemia
DEF: Abnormally increased blood calcium level; symptoms include muscle weakness, fatigue, nausea, depression, and constipation.
AHA: 3Q, '12,16; 4Q, '03, 110

275.49 Other disorders of calcium metabolism
Nephrocalcinosis
Pseudohypoparathyroidism
Pseudopseudohypoparathyroidism
DEF: Nephrocalcinosis: calcium phosphate deposits in the tubules of the kidney with resultant renal insufficiency.
DEF: Pseudohypoparathyroidism: inherited hypoparathyroidismdisorder; caused by inadequate response to parathyroid hormone, not hormonal deficiency; includes muscle cramps, tetany, urinary frequency, blurred vision due to cataracts, and dry scaly skin.
DEF: Pseudopseudohypoparathyroidism: clinical manifestations of hypoparathyroidism without affecting blood calcium levels.

275.5 Hungry bone syndrome
DEF: Marked and prolonged hypocalcemia; usually involves an extended history of elevated levels of parathyroid hormone, related bone demineralization causing the bone to sequester calcium.
AHA: 4Q, 08, 96-97

275.8 Other specified disorders of mineral metabolism

275.9 Unspecified disorder of mineral metabolism

✓4ᵗʰ **276 Disorders of fluid, electrolyte, and acid-base balance**
EXCLUDES diabetes insipidus (253.5)
familial periodic paralysis (359.3)

276.0 Hyperosmolality and/or hypernatremia
Sodium [Na] excess
Sodium [Na] overload

276.1 Hyposmolality and/or hyponatremia
Sodium [Na] deficiency
E87.1 Hypo-osmolality and hyponatremia   I-10

N Newborn Age: 0   P Pediatric Age: 0-17   M Maternity Age: 12-55   A Adult Age: 15-124

276.2 Acidosis

Acidosis:	Acidosis:
NOS	metabolic
lactic	respiratory

EXCLUDES *diabetic acidosis (249.1, 250.1)*

DEF: Disorder involves decrease of pH (hydrogen ion) concentration in blood and cellular tissues; caused by increase in acid and decrease in bicarbonate.

AHA: J-F, '87, 15

E87.2 Acidosis   I-10

276.3 Alkalosis

Alkalosis:	Alkalosis:
NOS	respiratory
metabolic	

DEF: Increased blood alkalinity (base) without relative loss of base in body fluids; caused by increased arterial plasma bicarbonate concentration or loss of carbon dioxide due to hyperventilation.

276.4 Mixed acid-base balance disorder

Hypercapnia with mixed acid-base disorder

√5ᵗʰ 276.5 Volume depletion

EXCLUDES *hypovolemic shock:*
postoperative (998.09)
traumatic (958.4)

AHA: 4Q, '05, 54; 2Q, '05, 9; 1Q, '03, 5, 22; 3Q, '02, 21; 4Q, '97, 30; 2Q, '88, 9

276.50 Volume depletion, unspecified

DEF: Depletion of total body water (dehydration) and/or contraction of total intravascular plasma (hypovolemia).

E86.9 Volume depletion unspecified   I-10

276.51 Dehydration

DEF: Depletion of total body water; blood volume may be normal while fluid is pulled from other tissues.

AHA: 1Q, '08, 10

E86.0 Dehydration   I-10

276.52 Hypovolemia

Depletion of volume of plasma

DEF: Depletion of volume plasma; depletion of total blood volume.

√5ᵗʰ 276.6 Fluid overload

EXCLUDES *ascites (789.51-789.59)*
localized edema (782.3)

AHA: 4Q, '10, 79; 3Q, '07, 9; 4Q, '06, 136

276.61 Transfusion associated circulatory overload

Fluid overload due to transfusion (blood) (blood components)

TACO

AHA: 4Q, '10, 79-80

E87.71 Transfusion associated circulatory overload   I-10

276.69 Other fluid overload

Fluid retention

E87.79 Other fluid overload   I-10

276.7 Hyperpotassemia

Hyperkalemia	Potassium [K]:
Potassium [K]:	intoxication
excess	overload

DEF: Elevated blood levels of potassium; symptoms include abnormal EKG readings, weakness; related to defective renal excretion.

AHA: 2Q, '11, 6; 1Q, '05, 9; 2Q, '01, 12

E87.5 Hyperkalemia   I-10

276.8 Hypopotassemia

Hypokalemia   Potassium [K] deficiency

DEF: Decreased blood levels of potassium; symptoms include neuromuscular disorders.

E87.6 Hypokalemia   I-10

276.9 Electrolyte and fluid disorders not elsewhere classified

Electrolyte imbalance	Hypochloremia
Hyperchloremia	

EXCLUDES *electrolyte imbalance:*
associated with hyperemesis gravidarum (643.1)
complicating labor and delivery (669.0)
following abortion and ectopic or molar pregnancy (634-638 with .4, 639.4)

AHA: J-F, '87, 15

E87.8 Oth disorders of electrolyte & fluid balance NEC   I-10

√4ᵗʰ 277 Other and unspecified disorders of metabolism

√5ᵗʰ 277.0 Cystic fibrosis

Fibrocystic disease of the pancreas
Mucoviscidosis

DEF: Genetic disorder of infants, children, and young adults marked by exocrine gland dysfunction; characterized by chronic pulmonary disease with excess mucus production, pancreatic deficiency, and high levels of electrolytes in the sweat.

AHA: 4Q, '90, 16; 3Q, '90, 18

TIP: Sequencing of CF is determined by circumstances of admission. If a patient is admitted for CF, sequence the CF first. If admitted for a complication of CF (e.g., pneumothorax, acute bronchitis, or acute cor pulmonale), sequence the complication first.

277.00 Without mention of meconium ileus

Cystic fibrosis NOS

AHA: 2Q, '03, 12

E84.9 Cystic fibrosis unspecified   I-10

277.01 With meconium ileus   N

Meconium:
ileus (of newborn)
obstruction of intestine in mucoviscidosis

277.02 With pulmonary manifestations

Cystic fibrosis with pulmonary exacerbation

Use additional code to identify any infectious organism present, such as:
pseudomonas (041.7)

277.03 With gastrointestinal manifestations

EXCLUDES *with meconium ileus (277.01)*

AHA: 4Q, '02, 45

277.09 With other manifestations

277.1 Disorders of porphyrin metabolism

Hematoporphyria	Porphyrinuria
Hematoporphyrinuria	Protocoproporphyria
Hereditary coproporphyria	Protoporphyria
Porphyria	Pyrroloporphyria

277.2 Other disorders of purine and pyrimidine metabolism

Hypoxanthine-guanine-phosphoribosyltransferase deficiency [HG-PRT deficiency]
Lesch-Nyhan syndrome
Xanthinuria

EXCLUDES *gout (274.00-274.9)*
orotic aciduric anemia (281.4)

√5ᵗʰ 277.3 Amyloidosis

DEF: Conditions of diverse etiologies characterized by the accumulation of insoluble fibrillar proteins (amyloid) in various organs and tissues of the body, compromising vital functions.

AHA: 1Q, '96, 16

277.30 Amyloidosis, unspecified

Amyloidosis NOS

AHA: 4Q, '06, 66

277.31 Familial Mediterranean fever

Benign paroxysmal peritonitis
Hereditary amyloid nephropathy
Periodic familial polyserositis
Recurrent polyserositis

DEF: Early-life onset of recurrent attacks characterized by high fevers with pain and inflammation of chest and abdominal cavities, skin and joints, also rash or vasculitis. Etiology unknown, possibly genetic, but may be precipitated by stress, trauma or exertion.

AHA: 2Q, '12, 18; 4Q, '06, 66

277.39 Other amyloidosis

Hereditary cardiac amyloidosis
Inherited systemic amyloidosis
Neuropathic (Portuguese) (Swiss) amyloidosis
Secondary amyloidosis

AHA: 1Q, '09, 9; 2Q, '08, 8; 4Q, '06, 66

√4ᵗʰ / √5ᵗʰ Additional Digit Required   Unspecified Code   Other Specified Code   Manifestation Code   ►◄ Revised Text   ● New Code   ▲ Revised Code Title

2015 ICD-9-CM   **Volume 1 – 61**

Endocrine, Nutritional and Metabolic Diseases, and Immunity

277.4–278.2

277.4 Disorders of bilirubin excretion
Hyperbilirubinemia:
   congenital
   constitutional
Syndrome:
   Crigler-Najjar
   Dubin-Johnson
   Gilbert's
   Rotor's

> **EXCLUDES** *hyperbilirubinemias specific to the perinatal period (774.0-774.7)*

AHA: ▶1Q, '14, 8◀

277.5 Mucopolysaccharidosis
Gargoylism
Hunter's syndrome
Hurler's syndrome
Lipochondrodystrophy
Maroteaux-Lamy syndrome
Morquio-Brailsford disease
Osteochondrodystrophy
Sanfilippo's syndrome
Scheie's syndrome

DEF: Metabolic disorders evidenced by excretion of various mucopolysaccharides in urine and infiltration of these substances into connective tissue, with resulting defects of bone, cartilage and connective tissue.

277.6 Other deficiencies of circulating enzymes
Hereditary angioedema
AHA: 2Q, '10, 12

277.7 Dysmetabolic syndrome X
Use additional code for associated manifestation, such as:
   cardiovascular disease (414.00-414.07)
   obesity (278.00-278.03)

DEF: A specific group of metabolic disorders that are related to the state of insulin resistance (decreased cellular response to insulin) without elevated blood sugars; often related to elevated cholesterol and triglycerides, obesity, cardiovascular disease, and high blood pressure.
AHA: 4Q, '01, 42

√5ᵗʰ 277.8 Other specified disorders of metabolism
AHA: 4Q, '03, 50; 2Q, '01, 18; S-O, '87, 9

277.81 Primary carnitine deficiency

277.82 Carnitine deficiency due to inborn errors of metabolism

277.83 Iatrogenic carnitine deficiency
Carnitine deficiency due to:
   hemodialysis
   valproic acid therapy

277.84 Other secondary carnitine deficiency

277.85 Disorders of fatty acid oxidation
Carnitine palmitoyltransferase deficiencies (CPT1, CPT2)
Glutaric aciduria type II (type IIA, IIB, IIC)
Long chain 3-hydroxyacyl CoA dehydrogenase deficiency (LCHAD)
Long chain/very long chain acyl CoA dehydrogenase deficiency (LCAD, VLCAD)
Medium chain acyl CoA dehydrogenase deficiency (MCAD)
Short chain acyl CoA dehydrogenase deficiency (SCAD)

> **EXCLUDES** *primary carnitine deficiency (277.81)*

277.86 Peroxisomal disorders
Adrenomyeloneuropathy
Neonatal adrenoleukodystrophy
Rhizomelic chrondrodysplasia punctata
X-linked adrenoleukodystrophy
Zellweger syndrome

> **EXCLUDES** *infantile Refsum disease (356.3)*

277.87 Disorders of mitochondrial metabolism
Kearns-Sayre syndrome
Mitochondrial Encephalopathy, Lactic Acidosis and Stroke-like episodes (MELAS syndrome)
Mitochondrial Neurogastrointestinal Encephalopathy syndrome (MNGIE)
Myoclonus with Epilepsy and with Ragged Red Fibers (MERRF syndrome)
Neuropathy, Ataxia and Retinitis Pigmentosa (NARP syndrome)

Use additional code for associated conditions

> **EXCLUDES** *disorders of pyruvate metabolism (271.8)*
> *Leber's optic atrophy (377.16)*
> *Leigh's subacute necrotizing encephalopathy (330.8)*
> *Reye's syndrome (331.81)*

AHA: 4Q, '04, 62

277.88 Tumor lysis syndrome
Spontaneous tumor lysis syndrome
Tumor lysis syndrome following antineoplastic drug therapy

Use additional E code to identify cause, if drug-induced

DEF: A potentially fatal metabolic complication of tumor necrosis caused by either spontaneous or treatment-related accumulation of byproducts from dying cancer cells; symptoms include hyperkalemia, hyperphosphatemia, hypocalcemia, hyperuricemia, and hyperuricosuria.
AHA: 4Q, '09, 78-79

277.89 Other specified disorders of metabolism
Hand-Schüller-Christian disease
Histiocytosis (acute) (chronic)
Histiocytosis X (chronic)

> **EXCLUDES** *histiocytosis:*
> *acute differentiated progressive (202.5)*
> *adult pulmonary Lan*
> *gerhans cell (516.5)*
> *X, acute (progressive) (202.5)*

277.9 Unspecified disorder of metabolism
Enzymopathy NOS

√4ᵗʰ 278 Overweight, obesity and other hyperalimentation
> **EXCLUDES** *hyperalimentation NOS (783.6)*
> *poisoning by vitamins NOS (963.5)*
> *polyphagia (783.6)*

√5ᵗʰ 278.0 Overweight and obesity
Use additional code to identify Body Mass Index (BMI), if known (V85.0-V85.54)

> **EXCLUDES** *adiposogenital dystrophy (253.8)*
> *obesity of endocrine origin NOS (259.9)*

AHA: 3Q, '11, 4; 4Q, '05, 97

278.00 Obesity, unspecified
Obesity NOS
DEF: BMI (body mass index) between 30.0 and 39.9.
AHA: 4Q, '01, 42; 1Q, '99, 5, 6

278.01 Morbid obesity
Severe obesity
DEF: BMI (body mass index) 40 or greater.
AHA: 4Q, '10, 81; 2Q, '09, 11; 2Q, '06, 5-6; 3Q, '03, 6-8
E66.01 Morbid (severe) obesity due to excess calories   **I-10**

278.02 Overweight
DEF: BMI (body mass index) between 25 and 29.9.
AHA: 4Q, '05, 55
E66.3 Overweight   **I-10**

278.03 Obesity hypoventilation syndrome
Pickwickian syndrome
DEF: Hypoventilation, somnolence and erythrocytosis due to excessive weight against the chest wall.
AHA: 4Q, '10, 80-81
E66.2 Morbid obesity w/alveolar hyperventilation   **I-10**

278.1 Localized adiposity
Fat pad
AHA: 2Q, '06, 10

278.2 Hypervitaminosis A

N Newborn Age: 0   **P** Pediatric Age: 0-17   **M** Maternity Age: 12-55   **A** Adult Age: 15-124

278.3 Hypercarotinemia
　　DEF: Elevated blood carotene level due to ingesting excess carotenoids or the inability to convert carotenoids to vitamin A.

278.4 Hypervitaminosis D
　　DEF: Weakness, fatigue, loss of weight, and other symptoms resulting from ingesting excessive amounts of vitamin D.

278.8 Other hyperalimentation
　　AHA: 2Q, '09, 11

√4th **279 Disorders involving the immune mechanism**
　Use additional code for associated manifestations

√5th **279.0 Deficiency of humoral immunity**
　　DEF: Inadequate immune response to bacterial infections with potential reinfection by viruses due to lack of circulating immunoglobulins (acquired antibodies).

　　279.00 Hypogammaglobulinemia, unspecified
　　　　Agammaglobulinemia NOS

　　279.01 Selective IgA immunodeficiency

　　279.02 Selective IgM immunodeficiency

　　279.03 Other selective immunoglobulin deficiencies
　　　　Selective deficiency of IgG

　　279.04 Congenital hypogammaglobulinemia
　　　　Agammaglobulinemia:
　　　　　Bruton's type
　　　　　X-linked

　　279.05 Immunodeficiency with increased IgM
　　　　Immunodeficiency with hyper-IgM:
　　　　　autosomal recessive
　　　　　X-linked

　　279.06 Common variable immunodeficiency
　　　　Dysgammaglobulinemia (acquired) (congenital) (primary)
　　　　Hypogammaglobulinemia:
　　　　　acquired primary
　　　　　congenital non-sex-linked
　　　　　sporadic

　　279.09 Other
　　　　Transient hypogammaglobulinemia of infancy

√5th **279.1 Deficiency of cell-mediated immunity**

　　279.10 Immunodeficiency with predominant T-cell defect, unspecified
　　　　AHA: S-O, '87, 10

　　279.11 DiGeorge's syndrome
　　　　Pharyngeal pouch syndrome
　　　　Thymic hypoplasia
　　　　DEF: Congenital hypoplasia or aplasia of the thymus, parathyroid glands; related heart defects, anomalies of the great vessels, esophageal atresia, and abnormalities of facial structures.

　　279.12 Wiskott-Aldrich syndrome
　　　　DEF: A disease characterized by chronic conditions, such as eczema, suppurative otitis media and anemia; results from an X-linked recessive gene and is classified as an immune deficiency syndrome.

　　279.13 Nezelof's syndrome
　　　　Cellular immunodeficiency with abnormal immunoglobulin deficiency
　　　　DEF: Immune system disorder characterized by a pathological deficiency in cellular immunity and humoral antibodies resulting in inability to fight infectious diseases.

　　279.19 Other
　　　　EXCLUDES ataxia-telangiectasia (334.8)

279.2 Combined immunity deficiency
　　Agammaglobulinemia:
　　　autosomal recessive
　　　Swiss-type
　　　x-linked recessive
　　Severe combined immunodeficiency [SCID]
　　Thymic:
　　　alymphoplasia
　　　aplasia or dysplasia with immunodeficiency
　　EXCLUDES thymic hypoplasia (279.11)
　　DEF: Agammaglobulinemia: No immunoglobulins in the blood.
　　DEF: Thymic alymphoplasia: Severe combined immunodeficiency; result of failed lymphoid tissue development.
　　AHA: 4Q, '11, 148

279.3 Unspecified immunity deficiency

√5th **279.4 Autoimmune disease, not elsewhere classified**
　　EXCLUDES transplant failure or rejection (996.80-996.89)
　　AHA: 4Q, '09, 80; 3Q, 08, 5

　　279.41 Autoimmune lymphoproliferative syndrome
　　　　ALPS
　　　　DEF: Rare genetic alteration of the *Fas* protein; impairs normal cellular apoptosis (normal cell death), causing abnormal accumulation of lymphocytes in the lymph glands, liver, and spleen; symptoms include neutropenia, anemia, and thrombocytopenia.

　　279.49 Autoimmune disease, not elsewhere classified
　　　　Autoimmune disease NOS
　　　　AHA: 3Q, '12, 8; 2Q, '11, 15
　　　　TIP: Assign for pediatric autoimmune neuropsychiatric disorder associated with streptococcal infection (PANDAS), with additional codes to report specific neurological or psychiatric manifestations.

√5th **279.5 Graft-versus-host disease**
　　Code first underlying cause, such as:
　　　complication of blood transfusion (999.89)
　　　complication of transplanted organ (996.80-996.89)
　　Use additional code to identify associated manifestations, such as:
　　　desquamative dermatitis (695.89)
　　　diarrhea (787.91)
　　　elevated bilirubin (782.4)
　　　hair loss (704.09)
　　DEF: A complication of transplantation, most commonly bone marrow; may involve skin, GI tract, liver and cause increased susceptibility to infection; results when donor cells responsible for immune response attack the cells of the transplant recipient.
　　AHA: 4Q, 08, 97-99, 154

　　279.50 Graft-versus-host disease, unspecified
　　　　AHA: 4Q, 08, 99

　　279.51 Acute graft-versus-host disease
　　　　AHA: 4Q, '11, 148; 4Q, 08, 99

　　279.52 Chronic graft-versus-host disease

　　279.53 Acute on chronic graft-versus-host disease

279.8 Other specified disorders involving the immune mechanism
　　Single complement [C_1-C_9] deficiency or dysfunction

279.9 Unspecified disorder of immune mechanism
　　AHA: 3Q, '92, 13

√4th √5th Additional Digit Required　Unspecified Code　Other Specified Code　Manifestation Code　▶◀ Revised Text　● New Code　▲ Revised Code Title

2015 ICD-9-CM　　　　　　　　　　　　　　　　　　　　　　　　　　　　　　　　　**Volume 1 – 63**

4. Diseases of the Blood and Blood-Forming Organs (280-289)

EXCLUDES anemia complicating pregnancy or the puerperium (648.2)

✓4ᵗʰ 280 Iron deficiency anemias

INCLUDES anemia:
  asiderotic
  hypochromic-microcytic
  sideropenic

EXCLUDES familial microcytic anemia (282.49)

280.0 Secondary to blood loss (chronic)
Normocytic anemia due to blood loss

EXCLUDES acute posthemorrhagic anemia (285.1)

AHA: ►3Q, '13, 4;◄ 4Q, '93, 34

280.1 Secondary to inadequate dietary iron intake

280.8 Other specified iron deficiency anemias
Paterson-Kelly syndrome
Plummer-Vinson syndrome
Sideropenic dysphagia

280.9 Iron deficiency anemia, unspecified
Anemia:
  achlorhydric
  chlorotic
Anemia:
  idiopathic hypochromic
  iron [Fe] deficiency NOS

✓4ᵗʰ 281 Other deficiency anemias

281.0 Pernicious anemia
Anemia:
  Addison's
  Biermer's
  congenital pernicious
Congenital intrinsic factor [Castle's] deficiency

EXCLUDES combined system disease without mention of anemia (266.2)
subacute degeneration of spinal cord without mention of anemia (266.2)

DEF: Chronic progressive anemia due to Vitamin B12 malabsorption; caused by lack of a secretion of intrinsic factor, which is produced by the gastric mucosa of the stomach.

AHA: N-D, '84, 1; S-O, '84, 16

281.1 Other vitamin B$_{12}$ deficiency anemia
Anemia:
  vegan's
  vitamin B$_{12}$ deficiency (dietary)
  due to selective vitamin B$_{12}$ malabsorption with proteinuria
Syndrome:
  Imerslund's
  Imerslund-Gräsbeck

EXCLUDES combined system disease without mention of anemia (266.2)
subacute degeneration of spinal cord without mention of anemia (266.2)

281.2 Folate-deficiency anemia
Congenital folate malabsorption
Folate or folic acid deficiency anemia:
  NOS
  dietary
  drug-induced
Goat's milk anemia
Nutritional megaloblastic anemia (of infancy)

Use additional E code to identify drug

DEF: Macrocytic anemia resembles pernicious anemia but without absence of hydrochloric acid secretions; responsive to folic acid therapy.

281.3 Other specified megaloblastic anemias not elsewhere classified
Combined B$_{12}$ and folate-deficiency anemia
Refractory megaloblastic anemia

DEF: Megaloblasts predominant in bone marrow with few normoblasts; rare familial type associated with proteinuria and genitourinary tract anomalies.

281.4 Protein-deficiency anemia
Amino-acid-deficiency anemia

281.8 Anemia associated with other specified nutritional deficiency
Scorbutic anemia

281.9 Unspecified deficiency anemia
Anemia:
  dimorphic
  macrocytic
  megaloblastic NOS
Anemia:
  nutritional NOS
  simple chronic

✓4ᵗʰ 282 Hereditary hemolytic anemias

DEF: Escalated rate of erythrocyte destruction; similar to all anemias, occurs when imbalance exists between blood loss and blood production.

282.0 Hereditary spherocytosis
Acholuric (familial) jaundice
Congenital hemolytic anemia (spherocytic)
Congenital spherocytosis
Minkowski-Chauffard syndrome
Spherocytosis (familial)

EXCLUDES hemolytic anemia of newborn (773.0-773.5)

DEF: Hereditary, chronic illness marked by abnormal red blood cell membrane; symptoms include enlarged spleen, jaundice; and anemia in severe cases.

282.1 Hereditary elliptocytosis
Elliptocytosis (congenital)
Ovalocytosis (congenital) (hereditary)

DEF: Genetic hemolytic anemia characterized by malformed, elliptical erythrocytes; there is increased destruction of red cells with resulting anemia.

282.2 Anemias due to disorders of glutathione metabolism
Anemia:
  6-phosphogluconic dehydrogenase deficiency
  enzyme deficiency, drug-induced
  erythrocytic glutathione deficiency
  glucose-6-phosphate dehydrogenase [G-6-PD] deficiency
  glutathione-reductase deficiency
  hemolytic nonspherocytic (hereditary), type I
Disorder of pentose phosphate pathway
Favism

282.3 Other hemolytic anemias due to enzyme deficiency
Anemia:
  hemolytic nonspherocytic (hereditary), type II
  hexokinase deficiency
  pyruvate kinase [PK] deficiency
  triosephosphate isomerase deficiency

✓5ᵗʰ 282.4 Thalassemias

EXCLUDES sickle-cell:
  disease (282.60-282.69)
  trait (282.5)

DEF: Inherited hemolytic disorders characterized by decreased production of at least one polypeptide globin chain results in defective hemoglobin synthesis; symptoms include severe anemia, expanded marrow spaces, transfusional and absorptive iron overload, impaired growth rate, thickened cranial bones, and pathologic fractures.

AHA: 4Q, '03, 51

282.40 Thalassemia, unspecified
Thalassemia NOS

AHA: 4Q, '11, 87-91

282.41 Sickle-cell thalassemia without crisis
Microdrepanocytosis
Sickle-cell thalassemia NOS
Thalassemia Hb-S disease without crisis

282.42 Sickle-cell thalassemia with crisis
Sickle-cell thalassemia with vaso-occlusive pain
Thalassemia Hb-S disease with crisis

Use additional code for type of crisis, such as:
  acute chest syndrome (517.3)
  splenic sequestration (289.52)

✓4ᵗʰ ✓5ᵗʰ Additional Digit Required Unspecified Code Other Specified Code Manifestation Code ►◄ Revised Text ● New Code ▲ Revised Code Title

2015 ICD-9-CM **October 2014 · Volume 1 – 65**

282.43 Alpha thalassemia
Alpha thalassemia major
Hemoglobin H Constant Spring
Hemoglobin H disease
Hydrops fetalis due to alpha thalassemia
Severe alpha thalassemia
Triple gene defect alpha thalassemia

EXCLUDES   *alpha thalassemia trait or minor (282.46)*
*hydrops fetalis due to isoimmunization
(773.3)*
*hydrops fetalis not due to immune hemolysis
(778.0)*

DEF: HBA1 and HBA2 genetic variant of chromosome 16
prevalent among Western African and South Asian descent;
associated with a wide spectrum of anemic presentation,
includes hemoglobin H disease subtypes.
AHA: 4Q, '11, 87-91

282.44 Beta thalassemia
Beta thalassemia major
Cooley's anemia
Homozygous beta thalassemia
Severe beta thalassemia
Thalassemia intermedia
Thalassemia major

EXCLUDES   *beta thalassemia minor (282.46)*
beta thalassemia trait (282.46)
delta-beta thalassemia (282.45)
hemoglobin E-beta thalassemia (282.47)
sickle-cell beta thalassemia (282.41, 282.42)

DEF: Diversity of mutations of HBB gene on chromosome 11
prevalent among Mediterranean and certain South Asian
descent with significant cellular damage, can result in
toxicity and increased disease severity (e.g., severe beta
thalassemia, thalassemia major).
AHA: 4Q, '11, 87-91

282.45 Delta-beta thalassemia
Homozygous delta-beta thalassemia

EXCLUDES   *delta-beta thalassemia trait (282.46)*

AHA: 4Q, '11, 87-91

282.46 Thalassemia minor
Alpha thalassemia minor
Alpha thalassemia trait
Alpha thalassemia silent carrier
Beta thalassemia minor
Beta thalassemia trait
Delta-beta thalassemia trait
Thalassemia trait NOS

EXCLUDES   *alpha thalassemia (282.43)*
beta thalassemia (282.44)
delta-beta thalassemia (282.45)
hemoglobin E-beta thalassemia (282.47)
sickle-cell trait (282.5)

DEF: Solitary abnormal gene that identifies a carrier of the
disease, yet with an absence of symptoms or a clinically
mild anemic presentation.
AHA: 4Q, '11, 87-91

282.47 Hemoglobin E-beta thalassemia

EXCLUDES   *beta thalassemia (282.44)*
beta thalassemia minor (282.46)
beta thalassemia trait (282.46)
delta-beta thalassemia (282.45)
delta-beta thalassemia trait (282.46)
hemoglobin E disease (282.7)
other hemoglobinopathies (282.7)
sickle-cell beta thalassemia (282.41, 282.42)

DEF: Clinically similar phenotype to B thalassemia major
prevalent among Southeast Asian and certain Indian
descent; results in severe transfusion-dependent anemia
when present with certain B mutations.
AHA: 4Q, '11, 87-91

282.49 Other thalassemia
Dominant thalassemia
Hemoglobin C thalassemia
Hereditary leptocytosis
Mediterranean anemia (with other
hemoglobinopathy)
Mixed thalassemia
Thalassemia with other hemoglobinopathy

EXCLUDES   *hemoglobin C disease (282.7)*
hemoglobin E disease (282.7)
other hemoglobinopathies (282.7)
sickle-cell anemias (282.60-282.69)
sickle-cell beta thalassemia (282.41-282.42)

282.5 Sickle-cell trait
Hb-AS genotype   Heterozygous:
Hemoglobin S [Hb-S] trait   hemoglobin S
                               Hb-S

EXCLUDES   *that with other hemoglobinopathy (282.60-282.69)*
that with thalassemia (282.41-282.42)

DEF: Heterozygous genetic makeup characterized by one gene for
normal hemoglobin and one for sickle-cell hemoglobin; clinical
disease rarely present.
AHA: 3Q, '12, 5
TIP: Report in addition to the appropriate code for the live birth
(V30–V39) for a newborn with sickle cell trait.
TIP: Do not assign along with another code for sickle-cell disease or
thalassemia.

√5th **282.6 Sickle-cell disease**
Sickle-cell anemia

EXCLUDES   *sickle-cell thalassemia (282.41-282.42)*
sickle-cell trait (282.5)

DEF: Inherited blood disorder; sickle-shaped red blood cells are hard
and pointed, clogging blood flow; anemia characterized by periodic
episodes of pain, acute abdominal discomfort, skin ulcerations of
the legs, increased infections.

282.60 Sickle-cell disease, unspecified
Sickle-cell anemia NOS
AHA: 2Q, '97, 11

282.61 Hb-SS disease without crisis

282.62 Hb-SS disease with crisis
Hb-SS disease with vaso-occlusive pain
Sickle-cell crisis NOS

Use additional code for type of crisis, such as:
acute chest syndrome (517.3)
splenic sequestration (289.52)

AHA: 4Q, '10, 78; 4Q, '03, 56; 2Q, '98, 8; 2Q, '91, 15

282.63 Sickle-cell/Hb-C disease without crisis
Hb-S/Hb-C disease without crisis

282.64 Sickle-cell/Hb-C disease with crisis
Hb-S/Hb-C disease with crisis
Sickle-cell/Hb-C disease with vaso-occlusive pain

Use additional code for type of crisis, such as:
acute chest syndrome (517.3)
splenic sequestration (289.52)

AHA: 4Q, '03, 51

282.68 Other sickle-cell disease without crisis
Hb-S/Hb-D
Hb-S/Hb-E   } diseases without
Sickle-cell/Hb-D   crisis
Sickle-cell/Hb-E

AHA: 4Q, '03, 51

282.69 Other sickle-cell disease with crisis
Hb-S/Hb-D
Hb-S/Hb-E   } diseases with crisis
Sickle-cell/Hb-D
Sickle-cell/Hb-E

Other sickle-cell disease with vaso-occlusive pain

Use additional code for type of crisis, such as:
acute chest syndrome (517.3)
splenic sequestration (289.52)

282.7 Other hemoglobinopathies
Abnormal hemoglobin NOS
Congenital Heinz-body anemia
Disease:
  hemoglobin C [Hb-C]
  hemoglobin D [Hb-D]
  hemoglobin E [Hb-E]
  hemoglobin Zurich [Hb-Zurich]
Hemoglobinopathy NOS
Hereditary persistence of fetal hemoglobin [HPFH]
Unstable hemoglobin hemolytic disease

EXCLUDES *familial polycythemia (289.6)*
hemoglobin E-beta thalassemia (282.47)
hemoglobin M [Hb-M] disease (289.7)
high-oxygen-affinity hemoglobin (289.0)
other hemoglobinopathies with thalassemia (282.49)

DEF: Any disorder of hemoglobin due to alteration of molecular structure; may include overt anemia.

282.8 Other specified hereditary hemolytic anemias
Stomatocytosis

282.9 Hereditary hemolytic anemia, unspecified
Hereditary hemolytic anemia NOS

√4ᵗʰ 283 Acquired hemolytic anemias
DEF: Non-hereditary anemia characterized by premature destruction of red blood cells; caused by infectious organisms, poisons, and physical agents.
AHA: N-D, '84, 1

283.0 Autoimmune hemolytic anemias
Autoimmune hemolytic disease (cold type) (warm type)
Chronic cold hemagglutinin disease
Cold agglutinin disease or hemoglobinuria
Hemolytic anemia:
  cold type (secondary) (symptomatic)
  drug-induced
  warm type (secondary) (symptomatic)
Use additional E code to identify cause, if drug-induced
EXCLUDES *Evans' syndrome (287.32)*
hemolytic disease of newborn (773.0-773.5)
AHA: 3Q, '08, 5

√5ᵗʰ 283.1 Non-autoimmune hemolytic anemias
Use additional E code to identify cause
DEF: Hemolytic anemia and thrombocytopenia with acute renal failure; relatively rare condition; 50 percent of patients require renal dialysis.
AHA: 4Q, '93, 25

283.10 Non-autoimmune hemolytic anemia, unspecified

283.11 Hemolytic-uremic syndrome
Use additional code to identify associated:
  E. coli infection (041.41-041.49)
  Pneumococcal pnemonia (481)
  Shigella dysenteriae (004.0)

283.19 Other non-autoimmune hemolytic anemias
Hemolytic anemia:
  mechanical
  microangiopathic
  toxic

283.2 Hemoglobinuria due to hemolysis from external causes
Acute intravascular hemolysis
Hemoglobinuria:
  from exertion
  march
  paroxysmal (cold) (nocturnal)
  due to other hemolysis
Marchiafava-Micheli syndrome
Use additional E code to identify cause

283.9 Acquired hemolytic anemia, unspecified
Acquired hemolytic anemia NOS
Chronic idiopathic hemolytic anemia

√4ᵗʰ 284 Aplastic anemia and other bone marrow failure syndromes
DEF: Bone marrow failure to produce the normal amount of blood components; generally non-responsive to usual therapy.
AHA: 1Q, '91, 14; N-D, '84, 1; S-0, '84, 16

√5ᵗʰ 284.0 Constitutional aplastic anemia
AHA: 1Q, '91, 14

284.01 Constitutional red blood cell aplasia
Aplasia, (pure) red cell:
  congenital
  of infants
  primary
Blackfan-Diamond syndrome
Familial hypoplastic anemia
AHA: 4Q, '06, 67-69

284.09 Other constitutional aplastic anemia
Fanconi's anemia
Pancytopenia with malformations
AHA: 4Q, '06, 67-69

√5ᵗʰ 284.1 Pancytopenia
EXCLUDES *pancytopenia (due to) (with):*
aplastic anemia NOS (284.9)
bone marrow infiltration (284.2)
constitutional red blood cell aplasia (284.01)
hairy cell leukemia (202.4)
human immunodeficiency virus disease (042)
leukoerythroblastic anemia (284.2)
malformations (284.09)
myelodysplastic syndromes (238.72-238.75)
myeloproliferative disease (238.79)
other constitutional aplastic anemia (284.09)
AHA: 4Q, '11, 91-92; 4Q, '06, 67-69

284.11 Antineoplastic chemotherapy induced pancytopenia
EXCLUDES *aplastic anemia due to antineoplastic chemotherapy (284.89)*
AHA: 4Q, '11, 92

284.12 Other drug-induced pancytopenia
EXCLUDES *aplastic anemia due to drugs (284.89)*

284.19 Other pancytopenia
AHA: ▶1Q, '14, 7◀

284.2 Myelophthisis
Leukoerythroblastic anemia
Myelophthisic anemia
Code first the underlying disorder, such as:
  malignant neoplasm of breast (174.0-174.9, 175.0-175.9)
  tuberculosis (015.0-015.9)
EXCLUDES *idiopathic myelofibrosis (238.76)*
myelofibrosis NOS (289.83)
myelofibrosis with myeloid metaplasia (238.76)
primary myelofibrosis (238.76)
secondary myelofibrosis (289.83)
DEF: A secondary disease process involving replacement of normal hematopoeitic tissue in the bone marrow with abnormal tissue, such as fibrous tissue or tumors. Occurs with advanced-stage neoplasms, granulomatous diseases such as miliary tuberculosis, and other inflammatory diseases.
AHA: 4Q, '06, 67-69

√5ᵗʰ 284.8 Other specified aplastic anemias
AHA: 4Q, '07, 72; 3Q, '05, 11; 1Q, '97, 5; 1Q, '92, 15; 1Q, '91, 14

284.81 Red cell aplasia (acquired) (adult) (with thymoma)
Red cell aplasia NOS

284.89 Other specified aplastic anemias
Aplastic anemia (due to):   Aplastic anemia (due to):
  chronic systemic disease   radiation
  drugs   toxic (paralytic)
  infection
Use additional E code to identify cause
AHA: 1Q, '11, 6; 1Q, '09, 20; 2Q, '08, 6

284.9 Aplastic anemia, unspecified
Anemia: Anemia:
  aplastic (idiopathic) NOS   nonregenerative
  aregenerative   Medullary hypoplasia
  hypoplastic NOS
EXCLUDES *refractory anemia (238.72)*

√4ᵗʰ √5ᵗʰ Additional Digit Required	Unspecified Code	Other Specified Code	Manifestation Code	▶◀ Revised Text	● New Code	▲ Revised Code Title

Diseases of the Blood and Blood-Forming Organs

285–286.3

√4ᵗʰ **285   Other and unspecified anemias**
    AHA: 1Q, '91, 14; N-D, '84, 1

285.0   Sideroblastic anemia
Anemia:
   hypochromic with iron loading
   sideroachrestic
   sideroblastic:
     acquired
     congenital
     hereditary
     primary
     secondary (drug-induced) (due to disease)
     sex-linked hypochromic
     vitamin B6-responsive
Pyridoxine-responsive (hypochromic) anemia

Use additional E code to identify cause, if drug induced

EXCLUDES *refractory sideroblastic anemia (238.72)*

DEF: Characterized by a disruption of final heme synthesis; results in iron overload of reticuloendothelial tissues.

285.1   Acute posthemorrhagic anemia
Anemia due to acute blood loss

EXCLUDES *anemia due to chronic blood loss (280.0)*
         blood loss anemia NOS (280.0)

AHA: ▶3Q, '13, 9;◀ 4Q, '11, 146; 1Q. '07, 19; 2Q, '92, 15

√5ᵗʰ ### 285.2   Anemia of chronic disease
Anemia in (due to) (with) chronic illness

AHA: 4Q, '00, 39

285.21   Anemia in chronic kidney disease
Anemia in end stage renal disease
Erythropoietin-resistant anemia (EPO resistant anemia)

TIP: Assign also a code for the chronic kidney disease (585.X).

285.22   Anemia in neoplastic disease

EXCLUDES *anemia due to antineoplastic chemotherapy (285.3)*
         aplastic anemia due to antineoplastic chemotherapy (284.89)

AHA: 4Q, '09, 81

TIP: Assign also a code for the neoplasm causing the anemia. Do not assign if anemia is caused by chemotherapy drugs, which is instead reported with 285.3.

D63.0 Anemia in neoplastic disease   I-10

285.29   Anemia of other chronic disease
Anemia in other chronic illness

285.3   Antineoplastic chemotherapy induced anemia
Anemia due to antineoplastic chemotherapy

EXCLUDES *anemia due to drug NEC — code to type of anemia*
         anemia in neoplastic disease (285.22)
         aplastic anemia due to antineoplastic chemotherapy (284.89)

DEF: Reversible adverse effect of chemotherapy, causing inhibition of bone marrow production; decrease in red blood cell production prevents adequate oxygenation of the tissues and organs causing fatigue, SOB, and exacerbation of other medical conditions.

AHA: 4Q, '09, 80-82

285.8   Other specified anemias
Anemia:
   dyserythropoietic (congenital)
   dyshematopoietic (congenital)
   von Jaksch's
Infantile pseudoleukemia

AHA: 1Q, '91, 16

285.9   Anemia, unspecified

Anemia:	Anemia:
NOS	profound
essential	progressive
normocytic, not due	secondary
to blood loss	Oligocythemia

EXCLUDES *anemia (due to):*
     blood loss:
       acute (285.1)
       chronic or unspecified (280.0)
     iron deficiency (280.0-280.9)

AHA: 1Q, '11, 16; 1Q, '09, 17, 20; 1Q. '07, 19; 1Q, '02, 14; 2Q, '92, 16; M-A, '85, 13; N-D, '84, 1

TIP: Assign for "postoperative anemia" if there is no mention of blood loss.

√4ᵗʰ **286   Coagulation defects**
    AHA: 2Q, '06, 17

286.0   Congenital factor VIII disorder
Antihemophilic globulin [AHG] deficiency
Factor VIII (functional)deficiency
Hemophilia:
   NOS
   A
   classical
   familial
   hereditary
Subhemophilia

EXCLUDES *factor VIII deficiency with vascular defect (286.4)*

DEF: Hereditary, sex-linked, results in missing antihemophilic globulin (AHG) (factor VIII); causes abnormal coagulation characterized by increased bleeding, large bruises of skin, bleeding in mouth, nose, gastrointestinal tract; hemorrhages into joints, resulting in swelling and impaired function.

286.1   Congenital factor IX disorder
Christmas disease
Deficiency:
   factor IX (functional)
   plasma thromboplastin component [PTC]
Hemophilia B

DEF: Deficiency of plasma thromboplastin component (PTC) (factor IX) and plasma thromboplastin antecedent (PTA); PTC deficiency clinically indistinguishable from classical hemophilia.

286.2   Congenital factor XI deficiency
Hemophilia C
Plasma thromboplastin antecedent [PTA] deficiency
Rosenthal's disease

286.3   Congenital deficiency of other clotting factors
Congenital afibrinogenemia
Deficiency:
   AC globulin factor:
     I [fibrinogen]
     II [prothrombin]
     V [labile]
     VII [stable]
     X [Stuart-Prower]
     XII [Hageman]
     XIII [fibrin stabilizing]
   Laki-Lorand factor
   proaccelerin
Disease:
   Owren's
   Stuart-Prower
Dysfibrinogenemia (congenital)
Dysprothrombinemia (constitutional)
Hypoproconvertinemia
Hypoprothrombinemia (hereditary)
Parahemophilia

AHA: ▶4Q, '13, 87◀

N   Newborn Age: 0   P   Pediatric Age: 0-17   M   Maternity Age: 12-55   A   Adult Age: 15-124

286.4 von Willebrand's disease
Angiohemophilia (A) (B)
Constitutional thrombopathy
Factor VIII deficiency with vascular defect
Pseudohemophilia type B
Vascular hemophilia
von Willebrand's (-Jürgens') disease

EXCLUDES *factor VIII deficiency:*
NOS (286.0)
with functional defect (286.0)
hereditary capillary fragility (287.8)

DEF: Abnormal blood coagulation caused by deficient blood Factor VII; congenital; symptoms include excess or prolonged bleeding.

√5ᵗʰ 286.5 Hemorrhagic disorder due to intrinsic circulating anticoagulants, antibodies, or inhibitors
AHA: 4Q, '11, 93-95; 3Q, '04, 7; No.5, '93, 16; 3Q, '92, 15; 3Q, '90, 14
TIP: Do not assign a code from subcategory 286.5 for Coumadin/warfarin toxicity, poisoning or adverse effect. Follow coding guidelines for poisoning and adverse reactions.

286.52 Acquired hemophilia
Autoimmune hemophilia
Autoimmune inhibitors to clotting factors
Secondary hemophilia

286.53 Antiphospholipid antibody with hemorrhagic disorder
Lupus anticoagulant [LAC] with hemorrhagic disorder
Systemic lupus erythematosus [SLE] inhibitor with hemorrhagic disorder

EXCLUDES *anti-phospholipid antibody, finding without diagnosis (795.79)*
anti-phospholipid antibody syndrome (289.81)
anti-phospholipid antibody with hypercoagulable state (289.81)
lupus anticoagulant [LAC] finding without diagnosis (795.79)
lupus anticoagulant [LAC] with hypercoagulable state (289.81)
systemic lupus erythematosus [SLE] inhibitor finding without diagnosis (795.79)
systemic lupus erythematosus [SLE] inhibitor with hypercoagulable state (289.81)

TIP: When a resulting associated hypercoagulable state is present, assign code 289.81.

286.59 Other hemorrhagic disorder due to intrinsic circulating anticoagulants, antibodies, or inhibitors
Antithrombinemia
Antithromboplastinemia
Antithromboplastinogenemia
Increase in:
anti-II (prothrombin)
anti-VIIIa
anti-IXa
anti-XIa

286.6 Defibrination syndrome
Afibrinogenemia, acquired
Consumption coagulopathy
Diffuse or disseminated intravascular coagulation [DIC syndrome]
Fibrinolytic hemorrhage, acquired
Hemorrhagic fibrinogenolysis
Pathologic fibrinolysis
Purpura:
fibrinolytic
fulminans

EXCLUDES *that complicating:*
abortion (634-638 with .1, 639.1)
pregnancy or the puerperium (641.3, 666.3)
disseminated intravascular coagulation in newborn (776.2)

DEF: Characterized by destruction of circulating fibrinogen; often precipitated by other conditions, such as injury, causing release of thromboplastic particles in blood stream.
AHA: 4Q, '93, 29

286.7 Acquired coagulation factor deficiency
Deficiency of coagulation factor due to:
liver disease
vitamin K deficiency
Hypoprothrombinemia, acquired
Use additional E code to identify cause, if drug induced

EXCLUDES *vitamin K deficiency of newborn (776.0)*
AHA: 4Q, '93, 29

286.9 Other and unspecified coagulation defects
Defective coagulation NOS   Disorder:
Deficiency, coagulation factor   coagulation
NOS   hemostasis
Delay, coagulation

EXCLUDES *abnormal coagulation profile (790.92)*
hemorrhagic disease of newborn (776.0)
that complicating:
abortion (634-638 with.1, 639.1)
pregnancy or the puerperium (641.3, 666.3)

AHA: 4Q, '99, 22; 4Q, '93, 29

√4ᵗʰ 287 Purpura and other hemorrhagic conditions
EXCLUDES *hemorrhagic thrombocythemia (238.71)*
purpura fulminans (286.6)
AHA: 1Q, '91, 14

287.0 Allergic purpura
Peliosis rheumatica   Purpura:
Purpura: rheumatica
anaphylactoid   Schönlein-Henoch
autoimmune   vascular
Henoch's   Vasculitis, allergic
nonthrombocytopenic:
hemorrhagic
idiopathic

EXCLUDES *hemorrhagic purpura (287.39)*
purpura annularis telangiectodes (709.1)

DEF: Any hemorrhagic condition, thrombocytic or nonthrombocytopenic in origin, caused by a presumed allergic reaction.

287.1 Qualitative platelet defects
Thrombasthenia (hemorrhagic) (hereditary)
Thrombocytasthenia
Thrombocytopathy (dystrophic)
Thrombopathy (Bernard-Soulier)

EXCLUDES *von Willebrand's disease (286.4)*

287.2 Other nonthrombocytopenic purpuras
Purpura: Purpura:
NOS   simplex
senile

√5ᵗʰ 287.3 Primary thrombocytopenia
EXCLUDES *thrombotic thrombocytopenic purpura (446.6)*
transient thrombocytopenia of newborn (776.1)

DEF: Decrease in number of blood platelets in circulating blood and purpural skin hemorrhages.
AHA: 4Q, '05, 56

287.30 Primary thrombocytopenia, unspecified
Megakaryocytic hypoplasia

287.31 Immune thrombocytopenic purpura
Idiopathic thrombocytopenic purpura
Tidal platelet dysgenesis

DEF: Tidal platelet dysgenesis: Platelet counts fluctuate from normal to very low within periods of 20 to 40 days and may involve autoimmune platelet destruction.
AHA: ►1Q, '14, 7;◄ 4Q, '05, 57

287.32 Evans' syndrome
DEF: Combination of immunohemolytic anemia and autoimmune hemolytic anemia, sometimes with neutropenia.

| √4ᵗʰ | Additional Digit Required | Unspecified Code | Other Specified Code | Manifestation Code | ►◄ Revised Text | ● New Code | ▲ Revised Code Title |

2015 ICD-9-CM   **October 2014 • Volume 1 – 69**

Diseases of the Blood and Blood-Forming Organs

286.4–287.32

Diseases of the Blood and Blood-Forming Organs

287.33–288.62

287.33 Congenital and hereditary thrombocytopenic purpura
Congenital and hereditary thrombocytopenia
Thrombocytopenia with absent radii (TAR) syndrome
EXCLUDES *Wiskott-Aldrich syndrome (279.12)*
DEF: Thrombocytopenia with absent radii (TAR) syndrome: autosomal recessive syndrome characterized by thrombocytopenia and bilateral radial aplasia; manifestations include skeletal, gastrointestinal, hematologic, and cardiac system abnormalities.

287.39 Other primary thrombocytopenia

√5ᵗʰ **287.4 Secondary thrombocytopenia**
Use additional E code to identify cause
EXCLUDES *heparin-induced thrombocytopenia (HIT) (289.84)*
transient thrombocytopenia of newborn (776.1)
AHA: 4Q, '10, 81-82; M-A, '85, 14

287.41 Posttransfusion purpura
Posttransfusion purpura from whole blood (fresh) or blood products
PTP
DEF: A potentially fatal transfusion complication characterized by sudden onset of severe thrombocytopenia, fever, chills, and cutaneous hemorrhaging.

287.49 Other secondary thrombocytopenia
Thrombocytopenia (due to):
dilutional
drugs
extracorporeal circulation of blood
massive blood transfusion
platelet alloimmunization
secondary NOS
DEF: Reduced number of platelets in circulating blood as consequence of an underlying disease or condition.

287.5 Thrombocytopenia, unspecified

287.8 Other specified hemorrhagic conditions
Capillary fragility (hereditary)
Vascular pseudohemophilia

287.9 Unspecified hemorrhagic conditions
Hemorrhagic diathesis (familial)

√4ᵗʰ **288 Diseases of white blood cells**
EXCLUDES *leukemia (204.0-208.9)*
AHA: 4Q, '06, 69; 1Q, '91, 14

√5ᵗʰ **288.0 Neutropenia**
Decreased absolute neutrophil count [ANC]
Use additional code for any associated:
fever (780.61)
mucositis (478.11, 528.00-528.09, 538, 616.81)
EXCLUDES *neutropenic splenomegaly (289.53)*
transitory neonatal neutropenia (776.7)
DEF: Sudden, severe condition characterized by reduced number of white blood cells; results in sores in the throat, stomach or skin; symptoms include chills, fever.
AHA: 4Q, '06, 69-73; 3Q, '05, 11; 3Q, '99, 6; 2Q, '99, 9; 3Q, '96, 16; 2Q, '96, 6

288.00 Neutropenia, unspecified
AHA: 4Q, '06, 69-73

288.01 Congenital neutropenia
Congenital agranulocytosis
Infantile genetic agranulocytosis
Kostmann's syndrome
AHA: 4Q, '06, 69-73

288.02 Cyclic neutropenia
Cyclic hematopoiesis   Periodic neutropenia
AHA: 4Q, '06, 69-73

288.03 Drug induced neutropenia
Use additional E code to identify drug
AHA: 4Q, '06, 69-73
TIP: Assign for neutropenic fever due to chemotherapy drugs, along with codes for the fever, adverse effect, and the underlying malignancy.

288.04 Neutropenia due to infection
AHA: 4Q, '06, 69-73

288.09 Other neutropenia
Agranulocytosis
Neutropenia:
immune
toxic
AHA: 4Q, '06, 69-73

288.1 Functional disorders of polymorphonuclear neutrophils
Chronic (childhood) granulomatous disease
Congenital dysphagocytosis
Job's syndrome
Lipochrome histiocytosis (familial)
Progressive septic granulomatosis

288.2 Genetic anomalies of leukocytes
Anomaly (granulation) (granulocyte) or syndrome:
Alder's (-Reilly)
Chédiak-Steinbrinck (-Higashi)
Jordan's
May-Hegglin
Pelger-Huet
Hereditary:
hypersegmentation
hyposegmentation
leukomelanopathy

288.3 Eosinophilia
Eosinophilia: Eosinophilia:
allergic   secondary
hereditary   Eosinophilic leukocytosis
idiopathic
EXCLUDES *Löffler's syndrome (518.3)*
pulmonary eosinophilia (518.3)
DEF: Elevated number of eosinophils in the blood; characteristic of allergic states and various parasitic infections.
AHA: 3Q, '00, 11

288.4 Hemophagocytic syndromes
Familial hemophagocytic lymphohistiocytosis
Familial hemophagocytic reticulosis
Hemophagocytic syndrome, infection-associated
Histiocytic syndromes
Macrophage activation syndrome
AHA: 4Q, '06, 69-73

√5ᵗʰ **288.5 Decreased white blood cell count**
EXCLUDES *neutropenia (288.01-288.09)*

288.50 Leukocytopenia, unspecified
Decreased leukocytes, unspecified
Decreased white blood cell count, unspecified
Leukopenia NOS
AHA: 4Q, '06, 69-73

288.51 Lymphocytopenia
Decreased lymphocytes
AHA: 4Q, '06, 69-73

288.59 Other decreased white blood cell count
Basophilic leukopenia
Eosinophilic leukopenia
Monocytopenia
Plasmacytopenia
AHA: 4Q, '06, 69-73

√5ᵗʰ **288.6 Elevated white blood cell count**
EXCLUDES *eosinophilia (288.3)*

288.60 Leukocytosis, unspecified
Elevated leukocytes, unspecified
Elevated white blood cell count, unspecified
AHA: 4Q, '06, 69-73

288.61 Lymphocytosis (symptomatic)
Elevated lymphocytes
AHA: 4Q, '06, 69-73

288.62 Leukemoid reaction
Basophilic leukemoid reaction
Lymphocytic leukemoid reaction
Monocytic leukemoid reaction
Myelocytic leukemoid reaction
Neutrophilic leukemoid reaction
AHA: 4Q, '06, 69-73

N Newborn Age: 0   **P** Pediatric Age: 0-17   **M** Maternity Age: 12-55   **A** Adult Age: 15-124

288.63 Monocytosis (symptomatic)
> EXCLUDES *infectious mononucleosis (075)*
> AHA: 4Q, '06, 69-73

288.64 Plasmacytosis
> AHA: 4Q, '06, 69-73

288.65 Basophilia
> AHA: 4Q, '06, 69-73

288.66 Bandemia
Bandemia without diagnosis of specific infection
> EXCLUDES *confirmed infection — code to infection*
> *leukemia (204.00-208.9)*
> DEF: Increase in early neutrophil cells, called band cells; may indicate infection.
> AHA: 4Q, '07, 73
> TIP: Do not assign based on lab values alone; physician must substantiate bandemia without evidence of corresponding infection.

288.69 Other elevated white blood cell count
> AHA: 4Q, '06, 69-73

288.8 Other specified disease of white blood cells
> EXCLUDES *decreased white blood cell counts (288.50-288.59)*
> *elevated white blood cell counts (288.60-288.69)*
> *immunity disorders (279.0-279.9)*
> AHA: M-A, '87, 12

288.9 Unspecified disease of white blood cells

√4ᵗʰ 289 Other diseases of blood and blood-forming organs

289.0 Polycythemia, secondary
High-oxygen-affinity hemoglobin
Polycythemia:
  acquired
  benign
  due to:
    fall in plasma volume
    high altitude
  emotional
  erythropoietin
  hypoxemic
  nephrogenous
  relative
  spurious
  stress
> EXCLUDES *polycythemia:*
> *neonatal (776.4)*
> *primary (238.4)*
> *vera (238.4)*
> DEF: Elevated number of red blood cells in circulating blood as result of reduced oxygen supply to the tissues.
> D75.1 Secondary polycythemia   I-10

289.1 Chronic lymphadenitis
Chronic:
  adenitis   } any lymph node, except
  lymphadenitis }   mesenteric
> EXCLUDES *acute lymphadenitis (683)*
> *mesenteric (289.2)*
> *enlarged glands NOS (785.6)*
> DEF: Persistent inflammation of lymph node tissue; origin of infection is usually elsewhere.
> I88.1 Chronic lymphadenitis except mesenteric   I-10

289.2 Nonspecific mesenteric lymphadenitis
Mesenteric lymphadenitis (acute) (chronic)
> DEF: Inflammation of the lymph nodes in peritoneal fold that encases abdominal organs; disease resembles acute appendicitis; unknown etiology.
> I88.0 Nonspecific mesenteric lymphadenitis   I-10

289.3 Lymphadenitis, unspecified, except mesenteric
> AHA: 2Q, '12, 18; 2Q, '92, 8
> I88.9 Nonspecific lymphadenitis unspecified   I-10

289.4 Hypersplenism
"Big spleen" syndrome
Dyssplenism
Hypersplenia
> EXCLUDES *primary splenic neutropenia (289.53)*
> DEF: An overactive spleen causing a deficiency of the peripheral blood components, an increase in bone marrow cells and sometimes a notable increase in the size of the spleen.
> D73.1 Hypersplenism   I-10

√5ᵗʰ 289.5 Other diseases of spleen

289.50 Disease of spleen, unspecified
> D73.9 Disease of spleen unspecified   I-10

289.51 Chronic congestive splenomegaly
> D73.2 Chronic congestive splenomegaly   I-10

289.52 Splenic sequestration
> *Code first sickle-cell disease in crisis (282.42, 282.62, 282.64, 282.69)*
> DEF: Blood is entrapped in the spleen due to vessel occlusion; most often associated with sickle-cell disease; spleen becomes enlarged and there is a sharp drop in hemoglobin.
> AHA: 4Q, '03, 51

289.53 Neutropenic splenomegaly
> AHA: 4Q, '06, 73
> D73.81 Neutropenic splenomegaly   I-10

289.59 Other
Lien migrans   Splenic:
Perisplenitis   fibrosis
Splenic: infarction
  abscess   rupture, nontraumatic
  atrophy   Splenitis
  cyst   Wandering spleen
> EXCLUDES *bilharzial splenic fibrosis (120.0-120.9)*
> *hepatolienal fibrosis (571.5)*
> *splenomegaly NOS (789.2)*
> AHA: ▶ 1Q, '14, 11◀
> D73.89 Other diseases of spleen   I-10

289.6 Familial polycythemia
Familial:
  benign polycythemia
  erythrocytosis
> DEF: Elevated number of red blood cells.

289.7 Methemoglobinemia
Congenital NADH [DPNH]-methemoglobin- reductase deficiency
Hemoglobin M [Hb-M] disease
Methemoglobinemia:
  NOS
  acquired (with sulfhemoglobinemia)
  hereditary
  toxic
Stokvis' disease
Sulfhemoglobinemia
> *Use additional E code to identify cause*
> DEF: Presence of blood methemoglobin, a chemically altered form of hemoglobin; causes cyanosis, headache, ataxia, dyspnea, tachycardia, nausea, stupor, and coma.
> D74.0 Congenital methemoglobinemia   I-10

√4ᵗʰ √5ᵗʰ Additional Digit Required	Unspecified Code	Other Specified Code	Manifestation Code	▶◀ Revised Text	● New Code	▲ Revised Code Title

Diseases of the Blood and Blood-Forming Organs

289.8–289.9

✓5ᵗʰ **289.8 Other specified diseases of blood and blood-forming organs**

DEF: Hypercoagulable states: a group of inherited or acquired abnormalities of specific proteins and anticoagulant factors; also called thromboembolic states or thrombotic disorders, result in abnormal development of blood clots.

AHA: 4Q, '03, 56; 1Q, '02, 16; 2Q, '89, 8; M-A, '87, 12

289.81 Primary hypercoagulable state

Activated protein C resistance
Antiphospholipid antibody syndrome
Antithrombin III deficiency
Factor V Leiden mutation
Lupus anticoagulant with hypercoagulable state
Protein C deficiency
Protein S deficiency
Prothrombin gene mutation
Systemic lupus erythematosus [SLE] inhibitor with hypercoagulable state

EXCLUDES *anti-phospholipid antibody, finding without diagnosis (795.79)*
anti-phospholipid antibody with hemorrhagic disorder (286.53)
lupus anticoagulant [LAC] finding without diagnosis (795.79)
lupus anticoagulant [LAC] with hemorrhagic disorder (286.53)
secondary activated protein C resistance (289.82)
secondary antiphospholipid antibody syndrome (289.82)
secondary lupus anticoagulant with hypercoagulable state (289.82)
secondary systemic lupus erythematosus [SLE] inhibitor with hypercoagulable state (289.82)
systemic lupus erythematosus [SLE] inhibitor finding without diagnosis (795.79)
systemic lupus erythematosus [SLE] inhibitor with hypercoagulable state (286.53)

DEF: Activated protein C resistance: decreased effectiveness of protein C to degrade factor V, necessary to inhibit clotting cascade; also called Factor V Leiden mutation.
DEF: Antithrombin III deficiency: deficiency in plasma antithrombin III one of six naturally occurring antithrombins that limit coagulation.
DEF: Factor V Leiden mutation: also called activated protein C resistance.
DEF: Lupus anticoagulant: autoimmune deficiency in a circulating anticoagulant that inhibits the conversion of prothrombin into thrombin; also called anti-phospholipid syndrome.
DEF: Protein C deficiency: deficiency of activated protein C which functions to bring the blood-clotting process into balance; same outcome as factor V Leiden mutation.
DEF: Protein S deficiency: similar to protein C deficiency; protein S is a vitamin K dependent cofactor in the activation of protein C.
DEF: Prothrombin gene mutation: increased levels of prothrombin, or factor II, a plasma protein that is converted to thrombin, which acts upon fibrinogen to form the fibrin.
AHA: 4Q, '11, 93

D68.59 Other primary thrombophilia   `I-10`

289.82 Secondary hypercoagulable state

EXCLUDES *heparin-induced thrombocytopenia (HIT) (289.84)*

D68.69 Other thrombophilia   `I-10`

289.83 Myelofibrosis

Myelofibrosis NOS   Secondary myelofibrosis

Code first the underlying disorder, such as:
malignant neoplasm of breast (174.0-174.9, 175.0-175.9)

Use additional code for associated therapy-related myelodysplastic syndrome, if applicable (238.72, 238.73)

Use additional external cause code if due to antineoplastic chemotherapy (E933.1)

EXCLUDES *idiopathic myelofibrosis (238.76)*
leukoerythroblastic anemia (284.2)
myelofibrosis with myeloid metaplasia (238.76)
myelophthisic anemia (284.2)
myelophthisis (284.2)
primary myelofibrosis (238.76)

DEF: A progressive bone marrow disease characterized by the replacement of bone marrow with the overgrowth of neoplastic stem cells and fibrotic tissue, also progressive anemia and enlarged spleen.
AHA: 4Q, '06, 73

D75.81 Myelofibrosis   `I-10`

289.84 Heparin-induced thrombocytopenia [HIT]

DEF: Immune-mediated reaction to heparin therapy causing an abrupt fall in platelet count and serious complications such as pulmonary embolism, stroke, AMI, or DVT.
AHA: 4Q, '08, 100-101

289.89 Other specified diseases of blood and blood-forming organs

Hypergammaglobulinemia
Pseudocholinesterase deficiency

D75.89 Oth specified dz of blood & blood-forming organs   `I-10`

289.9 Unspecified diseases of blood and blood-forming organs

Blood dyscrasia NOS   Erythroid hyperplasia

AHA: M-A, '85, 14

D75.9 Disease of blood and blood-forming organs unspecified   `I-10`

N Newborn Age: 0   **P** Pediatric Age: 0-17   **M** Maternity Age: 12-55   **A** Adult Age: 15-124

5. Mental, Behavioral and Neurodevelopmental Disorders (290-319)

Psychoses (290-299)

EXCLUDES intellectual disabilities (317-319)

Organic Psychotic Conditions (290-294)

INCLUDES psychotic organic brain syndrome

EXCLUDES nonpsychotic syndromes of organic etiology (310.0-310.9)
psychoses classifiable to 295-298 and without impairment of orientation, comprehension, calculation, learning capacity, and judgment, but associated with physical disease, injury, or condition affecting the brain [eg., following childbirth] (295.0-298.8)

✓4th **290 Dementias**

Code first the associated neurological condition

EXCLUDES dementia due to alcohol (291.0-291.2)
dementia due to drugs (292.82)
dementia not classified as senile, presenile, or arteriosclerotic (294.10-294.11)
psychoses classifiable to 295-298 occurring in the senium without dementia or delirium (295.0-298.8)
senility with mental changes of nonpsychotic severity (310.1)
transient organic psychotic conditions (293.0-293.9)

290.0 Senile dementia, uncomplicated   A
Senile dementia:
NOS
simple type
EXCLUDES mild memory disturbances, not amounting to dementia, associated with senile brain disease (310.89)
senile dementia with:
delirium or confusion (290.3)
delusional [paranoid] features (290.20)
depressive features (290.21)
AHA: 4Q, '99, 4
F03.90 Unspecif dementia w/o behavioral disturbance   I-10

✓5th **290.1 Presenile dementia**
Brain syndrome with presenile brain disease
EXCLUDES arteriosclerotic dementia (290.40-290.43)
dementia associated with other cerebral conditions (294.10-294.11)
AHA: N-D, '84, 20

290.10 Presenile dementia, uncomplicated   A
Presenile dementia:
NOS
simple type

290.11 Presenile dementia with delirium   A
Presenile dementia with acute confusional state
AHA: 1Q, '88, 3

290.12 Presenile dementia with delusional features   A
Presenile dementia, paranoid type

290.13 Presenile dementia with depressive features   A
Presenile dementia, depressed type

✓5th **290.2 Senile dementia with delusional or depressive features**
EXCLUDES senile dementia:
NOS (290.0)
with delirium and/or confusion (290.3)

290.20 Senile dementia with delusional features   A
Senile dementia, paranoid type
Senile psychosis NOS

290.21 Senile dementia with depressive features   A

290.3 Senile dementia with delirium   A
Senile dementia with acute confusional state
EXCLUDES senile:
dementia NOS (290.0)
psychosis NOS (290.20)
AHA: 3Q, '09, 11

✓5th **290.4 Vascular dementia**
Multi-infarct dementia or psychosis
Use additional code to identify cerebral atherosclerosis (437.0)
EXCLUDES suspected cases with no clear evidence of arteriosclerosis (290.9)
AHA: 1Q, '88, 3

290.40 Vascular dementia, uncomplicated   A
Arteriosclerotic dementia:
NOS
simple type
F01.50 Vascular dementia without behavioral disturbance   I-10

290.41 Vascular dementia with delirium   A
Arteriosclerotic dementia with acute confusional state

290.42 Vascular dementia with delusions   A
Arteriosclerotic dementia, paranoid type

290.43 Vascular dementia with depressed mood   A
Arteriosclerotic dementia, depressed type

290.8 Other specified senile psychotic conditions
Presbyophrenic psychosis

290.9 Unspecified senile psychotic condition   A

✓4th **291 Alcohol induced mental disorders**
EXCLUDES alcoholism without psychosis (303.0-303.9)
AHA: 1Q, '88, 3; S-O, '86, 3

291.0 Alcohol withdrawal delirium
Alcoholic delirium
Delirium tremens
EXCLUDES alcohol withdrawal (291.81)
AHA: 2Q, '91, 11
F10.921 Alcohol use unsp w/intox delirium   I-10

291.1 Alcohol induced persisting amnestic disorder
Alcoholic polyneuritic psychosis
Korsakoff's psychosis, alcoholic
Wernicke-Korsakoff syndrome (alcoholic)
DEF: Prominent and lasting reduced memory span, disordered time appreciation and confabulation, occurring in alcoholics, as sequel to acute alcoholic psychosis.
AHA: 1Q, '88, 3

291.2 Alcohol induced persisting dementia
Alcoholic dementia NOS
Alcoholism associated with dementia NOS
Chronic alcoholic brain syndrome
F10.27 Alcohol depend alcohol-induced persist dementia   I-10

291.3 Alcohol induced psychotic disorder with hallucinations
Alcoholic:
hallucinosis (acute)
psychosis with hallucinosis
EXCLUDES alcohol withdrawal with delirium (291.0)
schizophrenia (295.0-295.9) and paranoid states (297.0-297.9) taking the form of chronic hallucinosis with clear consciousness in an alcoholic
DEF: Psychosis lasting less than six months with slight or no clouding of consciousness in which auditory hallucinations predominate.
AHA: 2Q, '91, 11

291.4 Idiosyncratic alcohol intoxication
Pathologic:
alcohol intoxication
drunkenness
EXCLUDES acute alcohol intoxication (305.0)
in alcoholism (303.0)
simple drunkenness (305.0)
DEF: Unique behavioral patterns, like belligerence, after intake of relatively small amounts of alcohol; behavior not due to excess consumption.

✓4th
✓5th
Additional Digit Required   **Unspecified Code**   Other Specified Code   Manifestation Code   ►◄ Revised Text   ● New Code   ▲ Revised Code Title

2015 ICD-9-CM   **Volume 1 – 73**

291.5 Alcohol induced psychotic disorder with delusions

Alcoholic:
   paranoia
   psychosis, paranoid type
     EXCLUDES   *nonalcoholic paranoid states (297.0-297.9)*
          schizophrenia, paranoid type (295.3)

√5ᵗʰ 291.8 Other specified alcohol induced mental disorders

AHA: 3Q, '94, 13; J-A, '85, 10

291.81 Alcohol withdrawal

Alcohol:
   abstinence syndrome or symptoms
   withdrawal syndrome or symptoms
     EXCLUDES   *alcohol withdrawal:*
          delirium (291.0)
          hallucinosis (291.3)
          delirium tremens (291.0)
    AHA: 2Q, '12, 9; 4Q, '96, 28; 2Q, '91, 11
    F10.239 Alcohol dependence with withdrawal unspecified   I-10

291.82 Alcohol induced sleep disorders

Alcohol induced circadian rhythm sleep disorders
Alcohol induced hypersomnia
Alcohol induced insomnia
Alcohol induced parasomnia

291.89 Other

Alcohol induced anxiety disorder
Alcohol induced mood disorder
Alcohol induced sexual dysfunction

291.9 Unspecified alcohol induced mental disorders

Alcoholic:
   mania NOS
   psychosis NOS
Alcoholism (chronic) with psychosis
Alcohol related disorder NOS

√4ᵗʰ 292 Drug induced mental disorders

INCLUDES   organic brain syndrome associated with consumption of drugs

Use additional code for any associated drug dependence (304.0-304.9)
Use additional E code to identify drug
AHA: 3Q, '04, 8; 2Q, '91, 11; S-O, '86, 3

292.0 Drug withdrawal

Drug:
   abstinence syndrome or symptoms
   withdrawal syndrome or symptoms
    AHA: 1Q, '97, 12; 1Q, '88, 3
    TIP: Assign only for patients who suffer mental or behavioral disturbances due to drug withdrawal, regardless of the circumstances.
    F19.939 Oth psychoactive sbstnc use uns w/withdraw uns   I-10

√5ᵗʰ 292.1 Drug induced psychotic disorders

292.11 Drug induced psychotic disorder with delusions

Paranoid state induced by drugs

292.12 Drug induced psychotic disorder with hallucinations

Hallucinatory state induced by drugs
     EXCLUDES   *states following LSD or other hallucinogens, lasting only a few days or less ["bad trips"] (305.3)*

292.2 Pathological drug intoxication

Drug reaction:
   NOS   ⎫ resulting in brief psychotic
   idiosyncratic ⎬   states
   pathologic   ⎭
     EXCLUDES   *expected brief psychotic reactions to hallucinogens ["bad trips"] (305.3)*
          physiological side-effects of drugs (e.g., dystonias)

√5ᵗʰ 292.8 Other specified drug induced mental disorders

292.81 Drug induced delirium

AHA: 1Q, '88, 3
F19.921 Oth psychoactv sbstnc use uns intoxcat delirium   I-10

292.82 Drug induced persisting dementia

292.83 Drug induced persisting amnestic disorder

292.84 Drug induced mood disorder

Depressive state induced by drugs

292.85 Drug induced sleep disorders

Drug induced circadian rhythm sleep disorder
Drug induced hypersomnia
Drug induced insomnia
Drug induced parasomnia

292.89 Other

Drug induced anxiety disorder
Drug induced organic personality syndrome
Drug induced sexual dysfunction
Drug intoxication

292.9 Unspecified drug induced mental disorder

Drug related disorder NOS
Organic psychosis NOS due to or associated with drugs

√4ᵗʰ 293 Transient mental disorders due to conditions classified elsewhere

INCLUDES   transient organic mental disorders not associated with alcohol or drugs

Code first the associated physical or neurological condition
     EXCLUDES   *confusional state or delirium superimposed on senile dementia (290.3)*
          dementia due to:
          alcohol (291.0-291.9)
          arteriosclerosis (290.40-290.43)
          drugs (292.82)
          senility (290.0)

293.0 Delirium due to conditions classified elsewhere

Acute:
   confusional state
   infective psychosis
   organic reaction
   posttraumatic organic psychosis
   psycho-organic syndrome
Acute psychosis associated with endocrine, metabolic, or cerebrovascular disorder
Epileptic:
   confusional state
   twilight state
    AHA: 1Q, '88, 3
    F05 Delirium due to known physiological condition   I-10

293.1 Subacute delirium

Subacute:
   confusional state
   infective psychosis
   organic reaction
   posttraumatic organic psychosis
   psycho-organic syndrome
   psychosis associated with endocrine or metabolic disorder

√5ᵗʰ 293.8 Other specified transient mental disorders due to conditions classified elsewhere

293.81 Psychotic disorder with delusions in conditions classified elsewhere

Transient organic psychotic condition, paranoid type
AHA: 1Q, '11, 12

293.82 Psychotic disorder with hallucinations in conditions classified elsewhere

Transient organic psychotic condition, hallucinatory type

293.83 Mood disorder in conditions classified elsewhere

Transient organic psychotic condition, depressive type

293.84 Anxiety disorder in conditions classified elsewhere

AHA: 4Q, '96, 29

293.89 Other

Catatonic disorder in conditions classified elsewhere

N   Newborn Age: 0   P   Pediatric Age: 0-17   M   Maternity Age: 12-55   A   Adult Age: 15-124

293.9 Unspecified transient mental disorder in conditions classified elsewhere
Organic psychosis:
   infective NOS
   posttraumatic NOS
   transient NOS
Psycho-organic syndrome

√4ᵗʰ **294 Persistent mental disorders due to conditions classified elsewhere**
  INCLUDES   organic psychotic brain syndromes (chronic), not elsewhere classified
  AHA: M-A, '85, 12

294.0 Amnestic disorder in conditions classified elsewhere
Korsakoff's psychosis or syndrome (nonalcoholic)
Code first underlying condition
  EXCLUDES   *alcoholic:*
    amnestic syndrome (291.1)
    Korsakoff's psychosis (291.1)

√5ᵗʰ **294.1 Dementia in conditions classified elsewhere**
Dementia of the Alzheimer's type
Code first any underlying physical condition, as:
   Alzheimer's disease (331.0)
   cerebral lipidoses (330.1)
   dementia with Lewy bodies (331.82)
   dementia with Parkinsonism (331.82)
   epilepsy (345.0-345.9)
   frontal dementia (331.19)
   frontotemporal dementia (331.19)
   general paresis [syphilis] (094.1)
   hepatolenticular degeneration (275.1)
   Huntington's chorea (333.4)
   Jakob-Creutzfeldt disease (046.11-046.19)
   multiple sclerosis (340)
   Parkinson's disease (332.0)
   Pick's disease of the brain (331.11)
   polyarteritis nodosa (446.0)
   syphilis (094.1)
  EXCLUDES   *dementia:*
    arteriosclerotic (290.40-290.43)
    presenile (290.10-290.13)
    senile (290.0)
    epileptic psychosis NOS (294.8)
  AHA: 4Q, '00, 40; 1Q, '99, 14; N-D, '85, 5

294.10 Dementia in conditions classified elsewhere without behavioral disturbance
Dementia in conditions classified elsewhere NOS
F02.80 Dementia in oth dz class elsw w/o behavrl distur   I-10

294.11 Dementia in conditions classified elsewhere with behavioral disturbance
Aggressive behavior   Violent behavior
Combative behavior
Use additional code, where applicable, to identify: wandering in conditions classified elsewhere (V40.31)
  AHA: 4Q, '00, 41
  TIP: Review entire medical record for documentation of behavioral disturbance (aggressive, combative, violent behavior, wandering off); requires physician substantiation.

√5ᵗʰ **294.2 Dementia, unspecified**
  EXCLUDES   *mild memory disturbances, not amounting to dementia (310.89)*
  AHA: 4Q, '11, 95-96

294.20 Dementia, unspecified, without behavioral disturbance
Dementia NOS

294.21 Dementia, unspecified, with behavioral disturbance
Aggressive behavior
Combative behavior
Violent behavior
Use additional code, where applicable, to identify: wandering in conditions classified elsewhere (V40.31)
  AHA: 4Q, '11, 95

294.8 Other persistent mental disorders due to conditions classified elsewhere
Amnestic disorder NOS
Epileptic psychosis NOS
Mixed paranoid and affective organic psychotic states
Use additional code for associated epilepsy (345.0-345.9)
  EXCLUDES   *mild memory disturbances, not amounting to dementia (310.89)*
  AHA: 3Q, '09, 11; 3Q, '03, 14; 1Q, '88, 5
  F06.8 Oth spec mental disord d/t known physiol cond   I-10

294.9 Unspecified persistent mental disorders due to conditions classified elsewhere
Cognitive disorder NOS
Organic psychosis (chronic)
  AHA: 2Q, '07, 4

Other Psychoses (295-299)

Use additional code to identify any associated physical disease, injury, or condition affecting the brain with psychoses classifiable to 295-298

√4ᵗʰ **295 Schizophrenic disorders**
  INCLUDES   schizophrenia of the types described in 295.0-295.9 occurring in children
  EXCLUDES   *childhood type schizophrenia (299.9)*
    infantile autism (299.0)

The following fifth-digit subclassification is for use with category 295:
  0 unspecified
  1 subchronic
  2 chronic
  3 subchronic with acute exacerbation
  4 chronic with acute exacerbation
  5 in remission

DEF: Group of disorders with disturbances in thought (delusions, hallucinations), mood (blunted, flattened, inappropriate affect), sense of self; also bizarre, purposeless behavior, repetitious activity, or inactivity.

§ √5ᵗʰ **295.0 Simple type**
[0-5]   Schizophrenia simplex
  EXCLUDES   *latent schizophrenia (295.5)*

§ √5ᵗʰ **295.1 Disorganized type**
[0-5]   Hebephrenia   Hebephrenic type schizophrenia
  DEF: Inappropriate behavior; results in extreme incoherence and disorganization of time, place and sense of social appropriateness; withdrawal from routine social interaction may occur.

§ √5ᵗʰ **295.2 Catatonic type**
[0-5]   Catatonic (schizophrenia):   Schizophrenic:
   agitation   catalepsy
   excitation   catatonia
   excited type   flexibilitas cerea
   stupor
   withdrawn type
  Schizophrenic:
  DEF: Extreme changes in motor activity; one extreme is decreased response or reaction to the environment and the other is spontaneous activity.

§ √5ᵗʰ **295.3 Paranoid type**
[0-5]   Paraphrenic schizophrenia
  EXCLUDES   *involutional paranoid state (297.2)*
    paranoia (297.1)
    paraphrenia (297.2)
  DEF: Preoccupied with delusional suspicions and auditory hallucinations related to single theme; usually hostile, grandiose, overly religious, occasionally hypochondriacal.
  F20.0 Paranoid schizophrenia   I-10

§ √5ᵗʰ **295.4 Schizophreniform disorder**
[0-5]   Oneirophrenia
  Schizophreniform:
   attack
   psychosis, confusional type
  EXCLUDES   *acute forms of schizophrenia of:*
    catatonic type (295.2)
    hebephrenic type (295.1)
    paranoid type (295.3)
    simple type (295.0)
    undifferentiated type (295.8)

§ Requires fifth digit. Valid digits are in [brackets] under each code. See category 295 for codes and definitions.

√4ᵗʰ √5ᵗʰ Additional Digit Required   Unspecified Code   Other Specified Code   Manifestation Code   ►◄ Revised Text   ● New Code   ▲ Revised Code Title

Mental, Behavioral and Neurodevelopmental Disorders

295.5–296.90

§ ✓5ᵗʰ **295.5 Latent schizophrenia**
[0-5]   Latent schizophrenic reaction
Schizophrenia:
   borderline
   incipient
   prepsychotic
   prodromal
   pseudoneurotic
   pseudopsychopathic
   EXCLUDES *schizoid personality (301.20-301.22)*
AHA: For code 295.50: 1Q, '06, 10

§ ✓5ᵗʰ **295.6 Residual type**
[0-5]   Chronic undifferentiated schizophrenia
Restzustand (schizophrenic)
Schizophrenic residual state
AHA: For code 295.62: 4Q, '06, 78

§ ✓5ᵗʰ **295.7 Schizoaffective disorder**
[0-5]   Cyclic schizophrenia
Mixed schizophrenic and affective psychosis
Schizo-affective psychosis
Schizophreniform psychosis, affective type
F25.9 Schizoaffective disorder unspecified   I-10

§ ✓5ᵗʰ **295.8 Other specified types of schizophrenia**
[0-5]   Acute (undifferentiated) schizophrenia
Atypical schizophrenia
Cenesthopathic schizophrenia
   EXCLUDES *infantile autism (299.0)*

§ ✓5ᵗʰ **295.9 Unspecified schizophrenia**
[0-5]   Schizophrenia:
   NOS
   mixed NOS
   undifferentiated NOS
   undifferentiated type
Schizophrenic reaction NOS
Schizophreniform psychosis NOS
AHA: 3Q, '95, 6
F20.9 Schizophrenia unspecified   I-10

✓4ᵗʰ **296 Episodic mood disorders**
   INCLUDES episodic affective disorders
   EXCLUDES *neurotic depression (300.4)*
     reactive depressive psychosis (298.0)
     reactive excitation (298.1)

The following fifth-digit subclassification is for use with categories 296.0-296.6:
   0 unspecified
   1 mild
   2 moderate
   3 severe, without mention of psychotic behavior
   4 severe, specified as with psychotic behavior
   5 in partial or unspecified remission
   6 in full remission

AHA: M-A, '85, 14

§ ✓5ᵗʰ **296.0 Bipolar I disorder, single manic episode**
[0-6]   Hypomania (mild) NOS
Hypomanic psychosis
Mania (monopolar) NOS
Manic-depressive psychosis or reaction:
   hypomanic
   manic
     } single episode or unspecified
   EXCLUDES *circular type, if there was a previous attack of depression (296.4)*
DEF: Mood disorder identified by hyperactivity; may show extreme agitation or exaggerated excitability; speech and thought processes may be accelerated.

§ ✓5ᵗʰ **296.1 Manic disorder, recurrent episode**
[0-6]   Any condition classifiable to 296.0, stated to be recurrent
   EXCLUDES *circular type, if there was a previous attack of depression (296.4)*

§ ✓5ᵗʰ **296.2 Major depressive disorder, single episode**
[0-6]   Depressive psychosis
Endogenous depression
Involutional melancholia
Manic-depressive psychosis or reaction, depressed type
Monopolar depression
Psychotic depression
     } single episode or unspecified
   EXCLUDES *circular type, if previous attack was of manic type (296.5)*
     depression NOS (311)
     reactive depression (neurotic) (300.4)
     psychotic (298.0)
DEF: Mood disorder that produces depression; may exhibit as sadness, low self-esteem, or guilt feelings; other manifestations may be withdrawal from friends and family; interrupted sleep.
AHA: For code 296.20: 3Q, '09, 18
F32.9 Major depressive disorder single episode uns   I-10

§ ✓5ᵗʰ **296.3 Major depressive disorder, recurrent episode**
[0-6]   Any condition classifiable to 296.2, stated to be recurrent
   EXCLUDES *circular type, if previous attack was of manic type (296.5)*
     depression NOS (311)
     reactive depression (neurotic) (300.4)
     psychotic (298.0)
F33.2 Maj dprsv disord recur sev w/o psychot features   I-10

§ ✓5ᵗʰ **296.4 Bipolar I disorder, most recent episode (or current) manic**
[0-6]   Bipolar disorder, now manic
Manic-depressive psychosis, circular type but currently manic
   EXCLUDES *brief compensatory or rebound mood swings (296.99)*
F31.2 Bipolar d/o currnt epis mnic sev w/psychotc features   I-10

§ ✓5ᵗʰ **296.5 Bipolar I disorder, most recent episode (or current) depressed**
[0-6]   Bipolar disorder, now depressed
Manic-depressive psychosis, circular type but currently depressed
   EXCLUDES *brief compensatory or rebound mood swings (296.99)*
F31.30 Bipol disord currnt epis dprsd mild/mod sev uns   I-10

§ ✓5ᵗʰ **296.6 Bipolar I disorder, most recent episode (or current) mixed**
[0-6]   Manic-depressive psychosis, circular type, mixed

296.7 Bipolar I disorder, most recent episode (or current) unspecified
   Atypical bipolar affective disorder NOS
Manic-depressive psychosis, circular type, current condition not specified as either manic or depressive
DEF: Manic-depressive disorder referred to as bipolar because of the mood range from manic to depressive.

✓5ᵗʰ **296.8 Other and unspecified bipolar disorders**

296.80 Bipolar disorder, unspecified
   Bipolar disorder NOS
Manic-depressive:
   reaction NOS
   syndrome NOS
F31.9 Bipolar disorder unspecified   I-10

296.81 Atypical manic disorder

296.82 Atypical depressive disorder

296.89 Other
   Bipolar II disorder
Manic-depressive psychosis, mixed type
F31.81 Bipolar II disorder   I-10

✓5ᵗʰ **296.9 Other and unspecified episodic mood disorder**
   EXCLUDES *psychogenic affective psychoses (298.0-298.8)*

296.90 Unspecified episodic mood disorder
   Affective psychosis NOS
Melancholia NOS
Mood disorder NOS
AHA: M-A, '85, 14
F39 Unspecified mood [affective] disorder   I-10

---

§ Requires fifth digit. Valid digits are in [brackets] under each code. See appropriate category for codes and definitions

N Newborn Age: 0   **P** Pediatric Age: 0-17   **M** Maternity Age: 12-55   **A** Adult Age: 15-124

296.99 Other specified episodic mood disorder
Mood swings:
brief compensatory
rebound

✓4th **297 Delusional disorders**
INCLUDES   paranoid disorders
EXCLUDES   *acute paranoid reaction (298.3)*
alcoholic jealousy or paranoid state (291.5)
paranoid schizophrenia (295.3)

297.0 Paranoid state, simple

297.1 Delusional disorder
Chronic paranoid psychosis
Sander's disease
Systematized delusions
EXCLUDES   *paranoid personality disorder (301.0)*
F22 Delusional disorders   I-10

297.2 Paraphrenia
Involutional paranoid state
Late paraphrenia
Paraphrenia (involutional)
DEF: Paranoid schizophrenic disorder that persists over a prolonged period but does not distort personality despite persistent delusions.

297.3 Shared psychotic disorder
Folie à deux
Induced psychosis or paranoid disorder
DEF: Mental disorder two people share; first person with the delusional disorder convinces second person because of a close relationship and shared experiences to accept the delusions.

297.8 Other specified paranoid states
Paranoia querulans
Sensitiver Beziehungswahn
EXCLUDES   *acute paranoid reaction or state (298.3)*
senile paranoid state (290.20)

297.9 Unspecified paranoid state
Paranoid:
disorder NOS
psychosis NOS
reaction NOS
state NOS
AHA: J-A, '85, 9

✓4th **298 Other nonorganic psychoses**
INCLUDES   psychotic conditions due to or provoked by:
emotional stress
environmental factors as major part of etiology

298.0 Depressive type psychosis
Psychogenic depressive psychosis
Psychotic reactive depression
Reactive depressive psychosis
EXCLUDES   *manic-depressive psychosis, depressed type (296.2-296.3)*
neurotic depression (300.4)
reactive depression NOS (300.4)

298.1 Excitative type psychosis
Acute hysterical psychosis
Psychogenic excitation
Reactive excitation
EXCLUDES   *manic-depressive psychosis, manic type (296.0-296.1)*
DEF: Affective disorder similar to manic-depressive psychosis, in the manic phase, seemingly brought on by stress.

298.2 Reactive confusion
Psychogenic confusion
Psychogenic twilight state
EXCLUDES   *acute confusional state (293.0)*
DEF: Confusion, disorientation, cloudiness in consciousness; brought on by severe emotional upheaval.

298.3 Acute paranoid reaction
Acute psychogenic paranoid psychosis
Bouffée délirante
EXCLUDES   *paranoid states (297.0-297.9)*

298.4 Psychogenic paranoid psychosis
Protracted reactive paranoid psychosis

298.8 Other and unspecified reactive psychosis
Brief psychotic disorder
Brief reactive psychosis NOS
Hysterical psychosis
Psychogenic psychosis NOS
Psychogenic stupor
EXCLUDES   *acute hysterical psychosis (298.1)*

298.9 Unspecified psychosis
Atypical psychosis
Psychosis NOS
Psychotic disorder NOS
AHA: 3Q, '06, 22
F28 Oth psych d/o not d/t sbstnc/knwn physiolog cond   I-10

✓4th **299 Pervasive developmental disorders**
EXCLUDES   *adult type psychoses occurring in childhood, as:*
affective disorders (296.0-296.9)
manic-depressive disorders (296.0-296.9)
schizophrenia (295.0-295.9)

The following fifth-digit subclassification is for use with category 299:
0   current or active state
1   residual state

§ ✓5th **299.0 Autistic disorder**
[0-1]   Childhood autism
Infantile psychosis
Kanner's syndrome
EXCLUDES   *disintegrative psychosis (299.1)*
Heller's syndrome (299.1)
schizophrenic syndrome of childhood (299.9)
DEF: Severe mental disorder of children, results in impaired social behavior; abnormal development of communicative skills, appears to be unaware of the need for emotional support and little emotional response to family members.
AHA: For code 299.00: 3Q, '12, 19-20

§ ✓5th **299.1 Childhood disintegrative disorder**
[0-1]   Heller's syndrome
Use additional code to identify any associated neurological disorder
EXCLUDES   *infantile autism (299.0)*
schizophrenic syndrome of childhood (299.9)
DEF: Mental disease of children identified by impaired development of reciprocal social skills, verbal and nonverbal communication skills, imaginative play.

§ ✓5th **299.8 Other specified pervasive developmental disorders**
[0-1]   Asperger's disorder
Atypical childhood psychosis
Borderline psychosis of childhood
EXCLUDES   *simple stereotypes without psychotic disturbance (307.3)*

§ ✓5th **299.9 Unspecified pervasive developmental disorder**
[0-1]   Child psychosis NOS
Pervasive developmental disorder NOS
Schizophrenia, childhood type NOS
Schizophrenic syndrome of childhood NOS
EXCLUDES   *schizophrenia of adult type occurring in childhood (295.0-295.9)*

§   Requires fifth digit. Valid digits are in [brackets] under each code. See category 299 for codes and definitions.

✓4th
✓5th   Additional Digit Required   Unspecified Code   Other Specified Code   Manifestation Code   ►◄ Revised Text   ● New Code   ▲ Revised Code Title
2015 ICD-9-CM   **Volume 1 – 77**

Neurotic Disorders, Personality Disorders, and Other Nonpsychotic Mental Disorders (300-316)

√4ᵗʰ **300 Anxiety, dissociative and somatoform disorders**

√5ᵗʰ **300.0 Anxiety states**

> **EXCLUDES** anxiety in:
> acute stress reaction (308.0)
> transient adjustment reaction (309.24)
> neurasthenia (300.5)
> psychophysiological disorders (306.0-306.9)
> separation anxiety (309.21)

> **DEF:** Mental disorder characterized by anxiety and avoidance behavior not particularly related to any specific situation or stimulus; symptoms include emotional instability, apprehension, fatigue.

300.00 Anxiety state, unspecified

Anxiety:
   neurosis
   reaction
   state (neurotic)
Atypical anxiety disorder

AHA: 3Q, '11, 6; 2Q, '11, 5; 1Q, '02, 6

TIP: For chest pain due to anxiety, assign chest pain code first, because chest pain is not integral to the diagnosis of anxiety.

F41.9 Anxiety disorder unspecified   I-10

300.01 Panic disorder without agoraphobia

Panic:
   attack
   state

> **EXCLUDES** panic disorder with agoraphobia (300.21)

> **DEF:** Neurotic disorder characterized by recurrent panic or anxiety, apprehension, fear or terror; symptoms include shortness of breath, palpitations, dizziness, shakiness; fear of dying may persist.

F41.0 Panic d/o [epis paroxysmal anxiety] w/o agoraphobia   I-10

300.02 Generalized anxiety disorder

300.09 Other

√5ᵗʰ **300.1 Dissociative, conversion and factitious disorders**

> **EXCLUDES** adjustment reaction (309.0-309.9)
> anorexia nervosa (307.1)
> gross stress reaction (308.0-308.9)
> hysterical personality (301.50-301.59)
> psychophysiologic disorders (306.0-306.9)

300.10 Hysteria, unspecified

300.11 Conversion disorder

Astasia-abasia, hysterical
Conversion hysteria or reaction
Hysterical:
   blindness
   deafness
   paralysis

> **DEF:** Mental disorder that impairs physical functions with no physiological basis; sensory motor symptoms include seizures, paralysis, temporary blindness; increase in stress or avoidance of unpleasant responsibilities may precipitate onset of symptoms.

AHA: 2Q, '11, 5; N-D, '85, 15

300.12 Dissociative amnesia

Hysterical amnesia

300.13 Dissociative fugue

Hysterical fugue

> **DEF:** Dissociative hysteria; identified by loss of memory, flight from familiar surroundings; conscious activity is not associated with perception of surroundings, no later memory of episode.

300.14 Dissociative identity disorder

300.15 Dissociative disorder or reaction, unspecified

> **DEF:** Hysterical neurotic episode; sudden but temporary changes in perceived identity, memory, consciousness, segregated memory patterns exist separate from dominant personality.

300.16 Factitious disorder with predominantly psychological signs and symptoms

Compensation neurosis
Ganser's syndrome, hysterical

> **DEF:** A disorder characterized by the purposeful assumption of mental illness symptoms; which are acted out more often when another person is present.

300.19 Other and unspecified factitious illness

Factitious disorder (with combined psychological and physical signs and symptoms) (with predominantly physical signs and symptoms) NOS

> **EXCLUDES** multiple operations or hospital addiction syndrome (301.51)

√5ᵗʰ **300.2 Phobic disorders**

> **EXCLUDES** anxiety state not associated with a specific situation or object (300.00-300.09)
> obsessional phobias (300.3)

300.20 Phobia, unspecified

Anxiety-hysteria NOS
Phobia NOS

300.21 Agoraphobia with panic disorder

Fear of:
   open spaces ⎫
   streets   ⎬ with panic attacks
   travel   ⎭
Panic disorder with agoraphobia

> **EXCLUDES** agoraphobia without panic disorder (300.22)
> panic disorder without agoraphobia (300.01)

300.22 Agoraphobia without mention of panic attacks

Any condition classifiable to 300.21 without mention of panic attacks

300.23 Social phobia

Fear of:
   eating in public
   public speaking
   washing in public

300.29 Other isolated or specific phobias

Acrophobia   Claustrophobia
Animal phobias   Fear of crowds

300.3 Obsessive-compulsive disorders

Anancastic neurosis
Compulsive neurosis
Obsessional phobia [any]

> **EXCLUDES** obsessive-compulsive symptoms occurring in:
> endogenous depression (296.2-296.3)
> organic states (eg., encephalitis)
> schizophrenia (295.0-295.9)

300.4 Dysthymic disorder

Anxiety depression
Depression with anxiety
Depressive reaction
Neurotic depressive state
Reactive depression

> **EXCLUDES** adjustment reaction with depressive symptoms (309.0-309.1)
> depression NOS (311)
> manic-depressive psychosis, depressed type (296.2-296.3)
> reactive depressive psychosis (298.0)

> **DEF:** Depression without psychosis; less severe depression related to personal change or unexpected circumstances; also referred to as "reactional depression"

AHA: 3Q, '11, 6

F34.1 Dysthymic disorder   I-10

300.5 Neurasthenia
Fatigue neurosis
Nervous debility
Psychogenic:
  asthenia
  general fatigue
Use additional code to identify any associated physical
  disorder
EXCLUDES anxiety state (300.00-300.09)
  neurotic depression (300.4)
  psychophysiological disorders (306.0-306.9)
  specific nonpsychotic mental disorders following
    organic brain damage (310.0-310.9)
DEF: Physical and mental symptoms caused primarily by what is
known as mental exhaustion; symptoms include chronic weakness,
fatigue.

300.6 Depersonalization disorder
Derealization (neurotic)
Neurotic state with depersonalization episode
EXCLUDES depersonalization associated with:
  anxiety (300.00-300.09)
  depression (300.4)
  manic-depressive disorder or psychosis
    (296.0-296.9)
  schizophrenia (295.0-295.9)
DEF: Dissociative disorder characterized by feelings of strangeness
about self or body image; symptoms include dizziness, anxiety, fear
of insanity, loss of reality of surroundings.

300.7 Hypochondriasis
Body dysmorphic disorder
EXCLUDES hypochondriasis in:
  hysteria (300.10-300.19)
  manic-depressive psychosis, depressed type
    (296.2-296.3)
  neurasthenia (300.5)
  obsessional disorder (300.3)
  schizophrenia (295.0-295.9)

√5ᵗʰ **300.8 Somatoform disorders**

300.81 Somatization disorder
Briquet's disorder
Severe somatoform disorder

300.82 Undifferentiated somatoform disorder
Atypical somatoform disorder
Somatoform disorder NOS
DEF: Disorders in which patients have symptoms that
suggest an organic disease but no evidence of physical
disorder after repeated testing.
AHA: 4Q, '96, 29

300.89 Other somatoform disorders
Occupational neurosis, including writers' cramp
Psychasthenia
Psychasthenic neurosis

300.9 Unspecified nonpsychotic mental disorder
Psychoneurosis NOS

√4ᵗʰ **301 Personality disorders**
INCLUDES character neurosis
Use additional code to identify any associated neurosis or psychosis,
  or physical condition
EXCLUDES nonpsychotic personality disorder associated with organic
  brain syndromes (310.0-310.9)

301.0 Paranoid personality disorder
Fanatic personality
Paranoid personality (disorder)
Paranoid traits
EXCLUDES acute paranoid reaction (298.3)
  alcoholic paranoia (291.5)
  paranoid schizophrenia (295.3)
  paranoid states (297.0-297.9)
AHA: J-A, '85, 9

√5ᵗʰ **301.1 Affective personality disorder**
EXCLUDES affective psychotic disorders (296.0-296.9)
  neurasthenia (300.5)
  neurotic depression (300.4)

301.10 Affective personality disorder, unspecified

301.11 Chronic hypomanic personality disorder
Chronic hypomanic disorder
Hypomanic personality

301.12 Chronic depressive personality disorder
Chronic depressive disorder
Depressive character or personality

301.13 Cyclothymic disorder
Cycloid personality
Cyclothymia
Cyclothymic personality

√5ᵗʰ **301.2 Schizoid personality disorder**
EXCLUDES schizophrenia (295.0-295.9)

301.20 Schizoid personality disorder, unspecified

301.21 Introverted personality

301.22 Schizotypal personality disorder

301.3 Explosive personality disorder
Aggressive:
  personality
  reaction
Aggressiveness
Emotional instability (excessive)
Pathological emotionality
Quarrelsomeness
EXCLUDES dyssocial personality (301.7)
  hysterical neurosis (300.10-300.19)

301.4 Obsessive-compulsive personality disorder
Anancastic personality
Obsessional personality
EXCLUDES obsessive-compulsive disorder (300.3)
  phobic state (300.20-300.29)

√5ᵗʰ **301.5 Histrionic personality disorder**
EXCLUDES hysterical neurosis (300.10-300.19)
DEF: Extreme emotional behavior, often theatrical; often concerned
about own appeal; may demand attention, exhibit seductive
behavior.

301.50 Histrionic personality disorder, unspecified
Hysterical personality NOS

301.51 Chronic factitious illness with physical symptoms
Hospital addiction syndrome
Multiple operations syndrome
Munchausen syndrome

301.59 Other histrionic personality disorder
Personality:
  emotionally unstable
  labile
  psychoinfantile

301.6 Dependent personality disorder
Asthenic personality
Inadequate personality
Passive personality
EXCLUDES neurasthenia (300.5)
  passive-aggressive personality (301.84)
DEF: Overwhelming feeling of helplessness; fears of abandonment
may persist; difficulty in making personal decisions without
confirmation by others; low self-esteem due to irrational sensitivity
to criticism.

| √4ᵗʰ / √5ᵗʰ Additional Digit Required | Unspecified Code | Other Specified Code | Manifestation Code | ►◄ Revised Text | ● New Code | ▲ Revised Code Title |

2015 ICD-9-CM **Volume 1 – 79**

Mental, Behavioral and Neurodevelopmental Disorders

301.7–302.9

301.7 Antisocial personality disorder
Amoral personality
Asocial personality
Dyssocial personality
Personality disorder with predominantly sociopathic or asocial manifestation

EXCLUDES disturbance of conduct without specifiable personality disorder (312.0-312.9)
explosive personality (301.3)

DEF: Continuous antisocial behavior that violates rights of others; social traits include extreme aggression, total disregard for traditional social rules.

AHA: S-0, '84, 16

√5th **301.8 Other personality disorders**

301.81 Narcissistic personality disorder
DEF: Grandiose fantasy or behavior, lack of social empathy, hypersensitive to the lack of others' judgment, exploits others; need for continual admiration.

301.82 Avoidant personality disorder
DEF: Personality disorder marked by feelings of social inferiority; sensitivity to criticism, emotionally restrained due to fear of rejection.

301.83 Borderline personality disorder
DEF: Personality disorder characterized by unstable moods, self-image, and interpersonal relationships; uncontrolled anger, impulsive and self-destructive acts, fears of abandonment, feelings of emptiness and boredom, recurrent suicide threats or self-mutilation.
F60.3 Borderline personality disorder   I-10

301.84 Passive-aggressive personality
DEF: Pattern of procrastination and refusal to meet standards; introduce own obstacles to success and exploit failure.

301.89 Other
Personality: Personality:
  eccentric   masochistic
  "haltlose" type   psychoneurotic
  immature
EXCLUDES psychoinfantile personality (301.59)

301.9 Unspecified personality disorder
Pathological personality NOS
Personality disorder NOS
Psychopathic:
  constitutional state
  personality (disorder)

√4th **302 Sexual and gender identity disorders**
EXCLUDES sexual disorder manifest in:
  organic brain syndrome (290.0-294.9, 310.0-310.9)
  psychosis (295.0-298.9)

302.0 Ego-dystonic sexual orientation
Ego-dystonic lesbianism
Sexual orientation conflict disorder
EXCLUDES homosexual pedophilia (302.2)

302.1 Zoophilia
Bestiality
DEF: A sociodeviant disorder marked by engaging in sexual intercourse with animals.

302.2 Pedophilia
DEF: A sociodeviant condition of adults characterized by sexual activity with children.

302.3 Transvestic fetishism
EXCLUDES trans-sexualism (302.5)
DEF: The desire to dress in clothing of opposite sex.

302.4 Exhibitionism
DEF: Sexual deviant behavior; exposure of genitals to strangers; behavior prompted by intense sexual urges and fantasies.

√5th **302.5 Trans-sexualism**
Sex reassignment surgery status
EXCLUDES transvestism (302.3)
DEF: Gender identity disturbance; overwhelming desire to change anatomic sex, due to belief that individual is a member of the opposite sex.

302.50 With unspecified sexual history

302.51 With asexual history

302.52 With homosexual history

302.53 With heterosexual history

302.6 Gender identity disorder in children
Feminism in boys
Gender identity disorder NOS
EXCLUDES gender identity disorder in adult (302.85)
trans-sexualism (302.50-302.53)
transvestism (302.3)

√5th **302.7 Psychosexual dysfunction**
EXCLUDES impotence of organic origin (607.84)
normal transient symptoms from ruptured hymen
transient or occasional failures of erection due to fatigue, anxiety, alcohol, or drugs

302.70 Psychosexual dysfunction, unspecified
Sexual dysfunction NOS

302.71 Hypoactive sexual desire disorder
EXCLUDES decreased sexual desire NOS (799.81)

302.72 With inhibited sexual excitement
Female sexual arousal disorder
Frigidity
Impotence
Male erectile disorder

302.73 Female orgasmic disorder   ♀

302.74 Male orgasmic disorder   ♂

302.75 Premature ejaculation   ♂

302.76 Dyspareunia, psychogenic   ♀
DEF: Difficult or painful sex due to psychosomatic state.

302.79 With other specified psychosexual dysfunctions
Sexual aversion disorder

√5th **302.8 Other specified psychosexual disorders**

302.81 Fetishism
DEF: Psychosexual disorder noted for intense sexual urges and arousal precipitated by fantasies; use of inanimate objects, such as clothing, to stimulate sexual arousal, orgasm.

302.82 Voyeurism
DEF: Psychosexual disorder characterized by uncontrollable impulse to observe others, without their knowledge, who are nude or engaged in sexual activity.

302.83 Sexual masochism
DEF: Psychosexual disorder noted for need to achieve sexual gratification through humiliating or hurtful acts inflicted on self.

302.84 Sexual sadism
DEF: Psychosexual disorder noted for need to achieve sexual gratification through humiliating or hurtful acts inflicted on someone else.

302.85 Gender identity disorder in adolescents or adults
Use additional code to identify sex reassignment surgery status (302.5)
EXCLUDES gender identity disorder NOS (302.6)
gender identity disorder in children (302.6)

302.89 Other
Frotteurism
Nymphomania
Satyriasis

302.9 Unspecified psychosexual disorder
Paraphilia NOS
Pathologic sexuality NOS
Sexual deviation NOS
Sexual disorder NOS

N Newborn Age: 0   P Pediatric Age: 0-17   M Maternity Age: 12-55   A Adult Age: 15-124

√4ᵗʰ **303   Alcohol dependence syndrome**

Use additional code to identify any associated condition, as:
    alcoholic psychoses (291.0-291.9)
    drug dependence (304.0-304.9)
    physical complications of alcohol, such as:
      cerebral degeneration (331.7)
      cirrhosis of liver (571.2)
      epilepsy (345.0-345.9)
      gastritis (535.3)
      hepatitis (571.1)
      liver damage NOS (571.3)

EXCLUDES   drunkenness NOS (305.0)

The following fifth-digit subclassification is for use with category 303:
   0   unspecified
   1   continuous
   2   episodic
   3   in remission

AHA: 1Q, '10, 20-21; 3Q, '95, 6; 2Q, '91, 9; 4Q, '88, 8; S-O, '86, 3
TIP: The patient has become physically addicted to alcohol and often experiences withdrawal symptoms when not drinking. Do not assign both 303.0X and 303.9X on the same encounter.

§ √5ᵗʰ **303.0   Acute alcoholic intoxication**
[0-3]   Acute drunkenness in alcoholism

§ √5ᵗʰ **303.9   Other and unspecified   alcohol dependence**
[0-3]   Chronic alcoholism
      Dipsomania
      AHA: 2Q, '02, 4; 2Q, '89, 9; **For code 303.90:** 2Q,'12, 9; 2Q, '07, 6
      F10.20 Alcohol dependence uncomplicated   `I-10`
      F10.21 Alcohol dependence in remission   `I-10`

√4ᵗʰ **304   Drug dependence**

EXCLUDES   nondependent abuse of drugs (305.1-305.9)

The following fifth-digit subclassification is for use with category 304:
   0   unspecified
   1   continuous
   2   episodic
   3   in remission

AHA: 1Q, '10, 20-21; 2Q, '91, 10; 4Q, '88, 8; S-O, '86, 3

§ √5ᵗʰ **304.0   Opioid type dependence**
[0-3]   Heroin
      Meperidine
      Methadone
      Morphine
      Opium
      Opium alkaloids and their derivatives
      Synthetics with morphine-like effects
      AHA: 2Q, '06, 7; **For code 304.00:** ▶2Q, '13, 14;◀ 1Q, '11, 15; 2Q, '10, 13

§ √5ᵗʰ **304.1   Sedative, hypnotic or anxiolytic dependence**
[0-3]   Barbiturates
      Nonbarbiturate sedatives and tranquilizers with a similar
        effect:
         chlordiazepoxide
         diazepam
         glutethimide
         meprobamate
         methaqualone
      AHA: For code 304.10: ▶2Q, '13, 14◀

§ √5ᵗʰ **304.2   Cocaine dependence**
[0-3]   Coca leaves and derivatives
      F14.20 Cocaine dependence uncomplicated   `I-10`

§ √5ᵗʰ **304.3   Cannabis dependence**
[0-3]   Hashish
      Hemp
      Marihuana

§ √5ᵗʰ **304.4   Amphetamine and other psychostimulant dependence**
[0-3]   Methylphenidate
      Phenmetrazine

§ √5ᵗʰ **304.5   Hallucinogen dependence**
[0-3]   Dimethyltryptamine [DMT]
      Lysergic acid diethylamide [LSD] and derivatives
      Mescaline
      Psilocybin

§ √5ᵗʰ **304.6   Other specified drug dependence**
[0-3]   Absinthe addiction
      Glue sniffing
      Inhalant dependence
      Phencyclidine dependence
      EXCLUDES   tobacco dependence (305.1)

§ √5ᵗʰ **304.7   Combinations of opioid type drug with any other**
[0-3]   **AHA:** M-A, '86, 12

§ √5ᵗʰ **304.8   Combinations of drug dependence excluding opioid type drug**
[0-3]   **AHA:** M-A, '86, 12

§ √5ᵗʰ **304.9   Unspecified drug dependence**
[0-3]   Drug addiction NOS
      Drug dependence NOS
      AHA: For code 304.90: 2Q, '12, 16; 4Q, '03, 103

√4ᵗʰ **305   Nondependent abuse of drugs**

NOTE Includes cases where a person, for whom no other diagnosis is possible, has come under medical care because of the maladaptive effect of a drug on which he is not dependent and that he has taken on his own initiative to the detriment of his health or social functioning.

EXCLUDES   alcohol dependence syndrome (303.0-303.9)
       drug dependence (304.0-304.9)
       drug withdrawal syndrome (292.0)
       poisoning by drugs or medicinal substances (960.0-979.9)

The following fifth-digit subclassification is for use with codes 305.0, 305.2-305.9:
   0   unspecified
   1   continuous
   2   episodic
   3   in remission

AHA: 1Q, '10, 20-21; 2Q, '91, 10; 4Q, '88, 8; S-O, '86, 3

§ √5ᵗʰ **305.0   Alcohol abuse**
[0-3]   Drunkenness NOS
      Excessive drinking of alcohol NOS
      "Hangover" (alcohol)
      Inebriety NOS
      EXCLUDES   acute alcohol intoxication in alcoholism (303.0)
              alcoholic psychoses (291.0-291.9)
      AHA: 3Q, '96, 16; **For code 305.00:** 4Q, '09, 112
      F10.10 Alcohol abuse uncomplicated   `I-10`

305.1   Tobacco use disorder
      Tobacco dependence
      EXCLUDES   history of tobacco use (V15.82)
              smoking complicating pregnancy (649.0)
              tobacco use disorder complicating pregnancy (649.0)
      AHA: 1Q, '09, 16; 2Q, '96, 10; N-D, '84, 12
      F17.210 Nicotine dependence cigarettes uncomplicated   `I-10`

§ √5ᵗʰ **305.2   Cannabis abuse**
[0-3]   **F12.10** Cannabis abuse uncomplicated   `I-10`

§ √5ᵗʰ **305.3   Hallucinogen abuse**
[0-3]   Acute intoxication from hallucinogens ["bad trips"]
      LSD reaction

§ √5ᵗʰ **305.4   Sedative, hypnotic or anxiolytic abuse**
[0-3]

§ √5ᵗʰ **305.5   Opioid abuse**
[0-3]

§ √5ᵗʰ **305.6   Cocaine abuse**
[0-3]   **AHA:** 1Q, '93, 25; **For code 305.60:** 1Q, '05, 6
      F14.10 Cocaine abuse uncomplicated   `I-10`

§ √5ᵗʰ **305.7   Amphetamine or related acting sympathomimetic abuse**
[0-3]   **AHA: For code 305.70:** 2Q, '03, 10-11

§ √5ᵗʰ **305.8   Antidepressant type abuse**
[0-3]

---

§   Requires fifth digit. Valid digits are in [brackets] under each code. See appropriate category for codes and definitions.

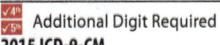

| √4ᵗʰ Additional Digit Required | Unspecified Code | Other Specified Code | Manifestation Code | ▶◀ Revised Text | ● New Code | ▲ Revised Code Title |

§ ✓5ᵗʰ **305.9 Other, mixed, or unspecified drug abuse**
[0-3]   Caffeine intoxication
      Inhalant abuse
      "Laxative habit"
      Misuse of drugs NOS
      Nonprescribed use of drugs or patent medicinals
      Phencyclidine abuse
      AHA: 3Q, '99, 20

✓4ᵗʰ **306 Physiological malfunction arising from mental factors**
   INCLUDES   psychogenic:
              physical symptoms ⎫
              physiological   ⎬ not involving tissue
              manifestations ⎭ damage

   EXCLUDES   *hysteria (300.11-300.19)*
       physical symptoms secondary to a psychiatric disorder
         classified elsewhere
       psychic factors associated with physical conditions involving
         tissue damage classified elsewhere (316)
       specific nonpsychotic mental disorders following organic
         brain damage (310.0-310.9)

   DEF: Functional disturbances or interruptions due to mental or psychological causes; no tissue damage sustained in these conditions.

306.0 Musculoskeletal
      Psychogenic paralysis   Psychogenic torticollis
   EXCLUDES   *Gilles de la Tourette's syndrome (307.23)*
       paralysis as hysterical or conversion reaction (300.11)
       tics (307.20-307.22)

306.1 Respiratory
      Psychogenic: Psychogenic:
      air hunger   hyperventilation
      cough   yawning
      hiccough
   EXCLUDES   *psychogenic asthma (316 and 493.9)*

306.2 Cardiovascular
      Cardiac neurosis
      Cardiovascular neurosis
      Neurocirculatory asthenia
      Psychogenic cardiovascular disorder
   EXCLUDES   *psychogenic paroxysmal tachycardia (316 and 427.2)*
   DEF: Neurocirculatory asthenia: functional nervous and circulatory irregularities with palpitations, dyspnea, fatigue, rapid pulse, precordial pain, fear of effort, discomfort during exercise, anxiety; also called DaCosta's syndrome, Effort syndrome, Irritable or Soldier's Heart.
   AHA: J-A, '85, 14

306.3 Skin
      Psychogenic pruritus
   EXCLUDES   *psychogenic:*
       alopecia (316 and 704.00)
       dermatitis (316 and 692.9)
       eczema (316 and 691.8 or 692.9)
       urticaria (316 and 708.0-708.9)

306.4 Gastrointestinal
      Aerophagy
      Cyclical vomiting, psychogenic
      Diarrhea, psychogenic
      Nervous gastritis
      Psychogenic dyspepsia
   EXCLUDES   *cyclical vomiting NOS (536.2)*
       associated with migraine (346.2)
       globus hystericus (300.11)
       mucous colitis (316 and 564.9)
       psychogenic:
         cardiospasm (316 and 530.0)
         duodenal ulcer (316 and 532.0-532.9)
         gastric ulcer (316 and 531.0-531.9)
         peptic ulcer NOS (316 and 533.0-533.9)
         vomiting NOS (307.54)
   DEF: Aerophagy: excess swallowing of air, usually unconscious; related to anxiety; results in distended abdomen or belching, often interpreted by the patient as a physical disorder.
   AHA: 2Q, '89, 11

306.5 Genitourinary
   EXCLUDES   *enuresis, psychogenic (307.6)*
       frigidity (302.72)
       impotence (302.72)
       psychogenic dyspareunia (302.76)

306.50 Psychogenic genitourinary malfunction, unspecified

306.51 Psychogenic vaginismus   ♀
      Functional vaginismus
   DEF: Psychogenic response resulting in painful contractions of vaginal canal muscles; can be severe enough to prevent sexual intercourse.

306.52 Psychogenic dysmenorrhea   ♀

306.53 Psychogenic dysuria

306.59 Other
   AHA: M-A, '87, 11

306.6 Endocrine

306.7 Organs of special sense
   EXCLUDES   *hysterical blindness or deafness (300.11)*
       psychophysical visual disturbances (368.16)

306.8 Other specified psychophysiological malfunction
      Bruxism
      Teeth grinding

306.9 Unspecified psychophysiological malfunction
      Psychophysiologic disorder NOS
      Psychosomatic disorder NOS

✓4ᵗʰ **307 Special symptoms or syndromes, not elsewhere classified**
   NOTE This category is intended for use if the psychopathology is manifested by a single specific symptom or group of symptoms which is not part of an organic illness or other mental disorder classifiable elsewhere.
   EXCLUDES   *those due to mental disorders classified elsewhere*
       those of organic origin

307.0 Adult onset fluency disorder
   EXCLUDES   *childhood onset fluency disorder (315.35)x*
       dysphasia (784.59)
       fluency disorder due to late effect of cerebrovascular
         accident (438.14)
       fluency disorder in conditions classified elsewhere
         (784.52)
       lisping or lalling (307.9)
       retarded development of speech (315.31-315.39)
   AHA: 4Q, '10, 83

307.1 Anorexia nervosa
   EXCLUDES   *eating disturbance NOS (307.50)*
       feeding problem (783.3)
         of nonorganic origin (307.59)
       loss of appetite (783.0)
         of nonorganic origin (307.59)
   AHA: 2Q, '06, 12; 4Q, '89, 11
   TIP: Assign an additional code for any associated malnutrition.

✓5ᵗʰ **307.2 Tics**
   EXCLUDES   *nail-biting or thumb-sucking (307.9)*
       stereotypes occurring in isolation (307.3)
       tics of organic origin (333.3)
   DEF: Involuntary muscle response usually confined to the face, shoulders.

307.20 Tic disorder, unspecified
      Tic disorder NOS

307.21 Transient tic disorder

307.22 Chronic motor or vocal tic disorder

307.23 Tourette's disorder
      Motor-verbal tic disorder
   DEF: Syndrome of facial and vocal tics in childhood; progresses to spontaneous or involuntary jerking, obscene utterances, other uncontrollable actions considered inappropriate.

---

§   Requires fifth digit. Valid digits are in [brackets] under each code. See category 305 for codes and definitions.

307.3 Stereotypic movement disorder
Body-rocking
Head banging
Spasmus nutans
Stereotypes NOS

> EXCLUDES   tics (307.20-307.23)
>   of organic origin (333.3)

√5th **307.4 Specific disorders of sleep of nonorganic origin**

> EXCLUDES   narcolepsy (347.00-347.11)
>   organic hypersomnia (327.10-327.19)
>   organic insomnia (327.00-327.09)
>   those of unspecified cause (780.50-780.59)

307.40 Nonorganic sleep disorder, unspecified

307.41 Transient disorder of initiating or maintaining sleep
Adjustment insomnia
Hyposomnia ⎫ associated with intermittent
Insomnia   ⎬ emotional reactions
Sleeplessness ⎭ or conflicts

307.42 Persistent disorder of initiating or maintaining sleep
Hyposomnia, insomnia, or sleeplessness associated
    with:
    anxiety
    conditioned arousal
    depression (major) (minor)
    psychosis
Idiopathic insomnia
Paradoxical insomnia
Primary insomnia
Psychophysiological insomnia

307.43 Transient disorder of initiating or maintaining wakefulness
Hypersomnia associated with acute or intermittent
    emotional reactions or conflicts

307.44 Persistent disorder of initiating or maintaining wakefulness
Hypersomnia associated with depression (major)
    (minor)
Insufficient sleep syndrome
Primary hypersomnia

> EXCLUDES   sleep deprivation (V69.4)

307.45 Circadian rhythm sleep disorder of nonorganic origin

307.46 Sleep arousal disorder
Night terror disorder
Night terrors
Sleep terror disorder
Sleepwalking
Somnambulism

DEF: Sleepwalking marked by extreme terror, panic,
screaming, confusion; no recall of event upon arousal; term
may refer to simply the act of sleepwalking.

307.47 Other dysfunctions of sleep stages or arousal from sleep
Nightmare disorder
Nightmares:
    NOS
    REM-sleep type
Sleep drunkenness

307.48 Repetitive intrusions of sleep
Repetitive intrusion of sleep with:
    atypical polysomnographic features
    environmental disturbances
    repeated REM-sleep interruptions

307.49 Other
"Short-sleeper"
Subjective insomnia complaint

√5th **307.5 Other and unspecified disorders of eating**

> EXCLUDES   anorexia:
>   nervosa (307.1)
>   of unspecified cause (783.0)
> overeating, of unspecified cause (783.6)
> vomiting:
>   NOS (787.03)
>   cyclical (536.2)
>   associated with migraine (346.2)
>   psychogenic (306.4)

307.50 Eating disorder, unspecified
Eating disorder NOS

307.51 Bulimia nervosa
Overeating of nonorganic origin
DEF: Mental disorder commonly characterized by binge
eating followed by self-induced vomiting; perceptions of
being fat; and fear the inability to stop eating voluntarily.
AHA: 3Q, '12, 9

307.52 Pica
Perverted appetite of nonorganic origin
DEF: Compulsive eating disorder characterized by craving
for substances other than food, such as paint chips or dirt.

307.53 Rumination disorder
Regurgitation, of nonorganic origin, of food with
    reswallowing

> EXCLUDES   obsessional rumination (300.3)

307.54 Psychogenic vomiting

307.59 Other
Feeding disorder of infancy or early childhood of
    nonorganic origin
Infantile feeding disturbances ⎫ of nonorganic
Loss of appetite   ⎬ origin

307.6 Enuresis
Enuresis (primary) (secondary) of nonorganic origin

> EXCLUDES   enuresis of unspecified cause (788.3)

DEF: Involuntary urination past age of normal control; also called
bedwetting; no trace to biological problem; focus on psychological
issues.

307.7 Encopresis
Encopresis (continuous) (discontinuous) of nonorganic origin

> EXCLUDES   encopresis of unspecified cause (787.60-787.63)

DEF: Inability to control bowel movements; cause traced to
psychological, not biological, problems.

√5th **307.8 Pain disorders related to psychological factors**

307.80 Psychogenic pain, site unspecified

307.81 Tension headache

> EXCLUDES   headache:
>   NOS (784.0)
>   migraine (346.0-346.9)
>   syndromes (339.00-339.89)
>   tension type (339.10-339.12)

AHA: 4Q, '08, 103; N-D, '85, 16

307.89 Other
Code first to type or site of pain

> EXCLUDES   pain disorder exclusively attributed to
>   psychological factors (307.80)
> psychogenic pain (307.80)

307.9 Other and unspecified special symptoms or syndromes, not elsewhere classified
Communication disorder NOS
Hair plucking
Lalling
Lisping
Masturbation
Nail-biting
Thumb-sucking

√4th
√5th   Additional Digit Required   Unspecified Code   Other Specified Code   Manifestation Code   ►◄ Revised Text   ● New Code   ▲ Revised Code Title

√4ᵗʰ **308 Acute reaction to stress**

INCLUDES   combat and operational stress reaction

EXCLUDES   *adjustment reaction or disorder (309.0-309.9)*
chronic stress reaction (309.1-309.9)

308.0 Predominant disturbance of emotions

Anxiety
Emotional crisis   }   as acute reaction to exceptional
Panic state   [gross] stress

308.1 Predominant disturbance of consciousness

Fugues as acute reaction to exceptional [gross] stress

308.2 Predominant psychomotor disturbance

Agitation states }   as acute reaction to exceptional
Stupor   [gross] stress

308.3 Other acute reactions to stress

Acute situational disturbance
Acute stress disorder

EXCLUDES   *prolonged posttraumatic emotional disturbance (309.81)*

308.4 Mixed disorders as reaction to stress

308.9 Unspecified acute reaction to stress

√4ᵗʰ **309 Adjustment reaction**

INCLUDES   adjustment disorders
reaction (adjustment) to chronic stress

EXCLUDES   *acute reaction to major stress (308.0-308.9)*
neurotic disorders (300.0-300.9)

309.0 Adjustment disorder with depressed mood

Grief reaction

EXCLUDES   *affective psychoses (296.0-296.9)*
neurotic depression (300.4)
prolonged depressive reaction (309.1)
psychogenic depressive psychosis (298.0)

AHA: ▶1Q, '14, 10◀

F43.21 Adjustment disorder with depressed mood   I-10

309.1 Prolonged depressive reaction

EXCLUDES   *affective psychoses (296.0-296.9)*
brief depressive reaction (309.0)
neurotic depression (300.4)
psychogenic depressive psychosis (298.0)

√5ᵗʰ **309.2 With predominant disturbance of other emotions**

309.21 Separation anxiety disorder

DEF: Abnormal apprehension by a child when physically separated from support environment; byproduct of abnormal symbiotic child-parent relationship.

309.22 Emancipation disorder of adolescence and early adult life

DEF: Adjustment reaction of late adolescence; conflict over independence from parental supervision; symptoms include difficulty in making decisions, increased reliance on parental advice, deliberate adoption of values in opposition of parents.

309.23 Specific academic or work inhibition

309.24 Adjustment disorder with anxiety

309.28 Adjustment disorder with mixed anxiety and depressed mood

Adjustment reaction with anxiety and depression

F43.23 Adjustment d/o w/mixed anxiety & depressed   I-10
mood

309.29 Other

Culture shock

309.3 Adjustment disorder with disturbance of conduct

Conduct disturbance }   as adjustment reaction
Destructiveness

EXCLUDES   *destructiveness in child (312.9)*
disturbance of conduct NOS (312.9)
dyssocial behavior without manifest psychiatric disorder (V71.01-V71.02)
personality disorder with predominantly sociopathic or asocial manifestations (301.7)

309.4 Adjustment disorder with mixed disturbance of emotions and conduct

√5ᵗʰ **309.8 Other specified adjustment reactions**

309.81 Posttraumatic stress disorder

Chronic posttraumatic stress disorder
Concentration camp syndrome
Posttraumatic stress disorder NOS
Post-traumatic stress disorder (PTSD)

EXCLUDES   *acute stress disorder (308.3)*
posttraumatic brain syndrome:
nonpsychotic (310.2)
psychotic (293.0-293.9)

DEF: Preoccupation with traumatic events beyond normal experience; i.e., rape, personal assault, etc,; also recurring flashbacks of trauma; symptoms include difficulty remembering, sleeping, or concentrating, and guilt feelings for surviving.

AHA: 2Q, '11, 5

309.82 Adjustment reaction with physical symptoms

309.83 Adjustment reaction with withdrawal

Elective mutism as adjustment reaction
Hospitalism (in children) NOS

309.89 Other

309.9 Unspecified adjustment reaction

Adaptation reaction NOS
Adjustment reaction NOS

√4ᵗʰ **310 Specific nonpsychotic mental disorders due to brain damage**

EXCLUDES   *neuroses, personality disorders, or other nonpsychotic conditions occurring in a form similar to that seen with functional disorders but in association with a physical condition (300.0-300.9, 301.0-301.9)*

310.0 Frontal lobe syndrome

Lobotomy syndrome
Postleucotomy syndrome [state]

EXCLUDES   *postcontusion syndrome (310.2)*

310.1 Personality change due to conditions classified elsewhere

Cognitive or personality change of other type, of nonpsychotic severity
Organic psychosyndrome of nonpsychotic severity
Presbyophrenia NOS
Senility with mental changes of nonpsychotic severity

EXCLUDES   *mild cognitive impairment (331.83)*
postconcussion syndrome (310.2)
signs and symptoms involving emotional state (799.21-799.29)

DEF: Personality disorder caused by organic factors, such as brain lesions, head trauma, or cerebrovascular accident (CVA).

AHA: 2Q, '05, 6

310.2 Postconcussion syndrome

Postcontusion syndrome or encephalopathy
Posttraumatic brain syndrome, nonpsychotic
Status postcommotio cerebri

Use additional code to identify associated post-traumatic headache, if applicable (339.20-339.22)

EXCLUDES   *any organic psychotic conditions following head injury (293.0-294.0)*
frontal lobe syndrome (310.0)
postencephalitic syndrome (310.89)

DEF: Nonpsychotic disorder due to brain trauma, causes symptoms unrelated to any disease process; symptoms include amnesia, serial headaches, rapid heartbeat, fatigue, disrupted sleep patterns, inability to concentrate.

AHA: 4Q, '90, 24

TIP: For treatment within 24 to 48 hours of the concussion, clarify with physician whether the concussion is still in the acute phase; if so, assign instead a code from 850.x subcategory.

√5ᵗʰ **310.8 Other specified nonpsychotic mental disorders following organic brain damage**

AHA: 4Q, '11, 96-97

N   Newborn Age: 0   P   Pediatric Age: 0-17   M   Maternity Age: 12-55   A   Adult Age: 15-124

310.81 Pseudobulbar affect

Involuntary emotional expression disorder

Code first underlying cause, if known, such as:
amyotrophic lateral sclerosis (335.20)
late effect of cerebrovascular accident (438.89)
late effect of traumatic brain injury (907.0)
mutiple sclerosis (340)

AHA: 4Q, '11, 97

310.89 Other specified nonpsychotic mental disorders following organic brain damage

Mild memory disturbance
Other focal (partial) organic psychosyndromes
Postencephalitic syndrome

EXCLUDES memory loss of unknown cause (780.93)

310.9 Unspecified nonpsychotic mental disorder following organic brain damage

AHA: 4Q, '03, 103

311 Depressive disorder, not elsewhere classified

Depressive disorder NOS
Depressive state NOS
Depression NOS

EXCLUDES acute reaction to major stress with depressive symptoms (308.0)
affective personality disorder (301.10-301.13)
affective psychoses (296.0-296.9)
brief depressive reaction (309.0)
depressive states associated with stressful events (309.0-309.1)
disturbance of emotions specific to childhood and adolescence, with misery and unhappiness (313.1)
mixed adjustment reaction with depressive symptoms (309.4)
neurotic depression (300.4)
prolonged depressive adjustment reaction (309.1)
psychogenic depressive psychosis (298.0)

AHA: 3Q, '11, 6;4Q, '03, 75

✓4ᵗʰ 312 Disturbance of conduct, not elsewhere classified

EXCLUDES adjustment reaction with disturbance of conduct (309.3)
drug dependence (304.0-304.9)
dyssocial behavior without manifest psychiatric disorder (V71.01-V71.02)
personality disorder with predominantly sociopathic or asocial manifestations (301.7)
sexual deviations (302.0-302.9)

The following fifth-digit subclassification is for use with categories 312.0-312.2

0 unspecified
1 mild
2 moderate
3 severe

§ ✓5ᵗʰ 312.0 Undersocialized conduct disorder, aggressive type

[0-3]   Aggressive outburst
Anger reaction
Unsocialized aggressive disorder

DEF: Mental condition identified by behaviors disrespectful of others' rights and of age-appropriate social norms or rules; symptoms include bullying, vandalism, verbal and physical abusiveness, lying, stealing, defiance.

§ ✓5ᵗʰ 312.1 Undersocialized conduct disorder, unaggressive type

[0-3]   Childhood truancy, unsocialized
Solitary stealing
Tantrums

§ ✓5ᵗʰ 312.2 Socialized conduct disorder

[0-3]   Childhood truancy, socialized
Group delinquency

EXCLUDES gang activity without manifest psychiatric disorder (V71.01)

✓5ᵗʰ 312.3 Disorders of impulse control, not elsewhere classified

312.30 Impulse control disorder, unspecified

312.31 Pathological gambling

312.32 Kleptomania

312.33 Pyromania

312.34 Intermittent explosive disorder

312.35 Isolated explosive disorder

312.39 Other

Trichotillomania

312.4 Mixed disturbance of conduct and emotions

Neurotic delinquency

EXCLUDES compulsive conduct disorder (312.3)

✓5ᵗʰ 312.8 Other specified disturbances of conduct, not elsewhere classified

312.81 Conduct disorder, childhood onset type

312.82 Conduct disorder, adolescent onset type

312.89 Other conduct disorder

Conduct disorder of unspecified onset

312.9 Unspecified disturbance of conduct

Delinquency (juvenile)
Disruptive behavior disorder NOS

AHA: 2Q, '11, 5

✓4ᵗʰ 313 Disturbance of emotions specific to childhood and adolescence

EXCLUDES adjustment reaction (309.0-309.9)
emotional disorder of neurotic type (300.0-300.9)
masturbation, nail-biting, thumbsucking, and other isolated symptoms (307.0-307.9)

313.0 Overanxious disorder

Anxiety and fearfulness ⎫ of childhood and
Overanxious disorder ⎭ adolescence

EXCLUDES abnormal separation anxiety (309.21)
anxiety states (300.00-300.09)
hospitalism in children (309.83)
phobic state (300.20-300.29)

313.1 Misery and unhappiness disorder

EXCLUDES depressive neurosis (300.4)

✓5ᵗʰ 313.2 Sensitivity, shyness, and social withdrawal disorder

EXCLUDES infantile autism (299.0)
schizoid personality (301.20-301.22)
schizophrenia (295.0-295.9)

313.21 Shyness disorder of childhood

Sensitivity reaction of childhood or adolescence

313.22 Introverted disorder of childhood

Social withdrawal ⎫ of childhood and
Withdrawal reaction ⎭ adolescence

313.23 Selective mutism

EXCLUDES elective mutism as adjustment reaction (309.83)

313.3 Relationship problems

Sibling jealousy

EXCLUDES relationship problems associated with aggression, destruction, or other forms of conduct disturbance (312.0-312.9)

✓5ᵗʰ 313.8 Other or mixed emotional disturbances of childhood or adolescence

313.81 Oppositional defiant disorder

DEF: Mental disorder of children noted for pervasive opposition, defiance of authority.

313.82 Identity disorder

Identity problem

DEF: Distress of adolescents caused by inability to form acceptable self-identity; uncertainty about career choice, sexual orientation, moral values.

313.83 Academic underachievement disorder

313.89 Other   P

Reactive attachment disorder of infancy or early childhood

---

§ Requires fifth digit. Valid digits are in [brackets] under each code. See category 312 for codes and definitions.

| ✓4ᵗʰ ✓5ᵗʰ Additional Digit Required | Unspecified Code | Other Specified Code | Manifestation Code | ▶◀ Revised Text | ● New Code | ▲ Revised Code Title |

Mental, Behavioral and Neurodevelopmental Disorders

313.9–319

313.9 Unspecified emotional disturbance of childhood or adolescence P

Mental disorder of infancy, childhood or adolescence NOS

√4th **314 Hyperkinetic syndrome of childhood**

EXCLUDES *hyperkinesis as symptom of underlying disorder — code the underlying disorder*

√5th **314.0 Attention deficit disorder**

Adult
Child

DEF: A behavioral disorder usually diagnosed at an early age; characterized by the inability to focus attention for a normal period of time.

TIP: These codes may be assigned for patients of any age.

314.00 Without mention of hyperactivity

Predominantly inattentive type

AHA: 1Q, '97, 8

314.01 With hyperactivity

Combined type
Overactivity NOS
Predominantly hyperactive/impulsive type
Simple disturbance of attention with overactivity

AHA: 3Q, '12, 19; 2Q, '11, 5; 1Q, '97, 8

F90.1 ADHD predominantly hyperactive type I-10

314.1 Hyperkinesis with developmental delay

Developmental disorder of hyperkinesis

Use additional code to identify any associated neurological disorder

314.2 Hyperkinetic conduct disorder

Hyperkinetic conduct disorder without developmental delay

EXCLUDES *hyperkinesis with significant delays in specific skills (314.1)*

314.8 Other specified manifestations of hyperkinetic syndrome

314.9 Unspecified hyperkinetic syndrome

Hyperkinetic reaction of childhood or adolescence NOS
Hyperkinetic syndrome NOS

√4th **315 Specific delays in development**

EXCLUDES *that due to a neurological disorder (320.0-389.9)*

√5th **315.0 Specific reading disorder**

315.00 Reading disorder, unspecified

315.01 Alexia

DEF: Lack of ability to understand written language; manifestation of aphasia.

315.02 Developmental dyslexia

DEF: Serious impairment of reading skills unexplained in relation to general intelligence and teaching processes.

315.09 Other

Specific spelling difficulty

315.1 Mathematics disorder

Dyscalculia

315.2 Other specific learning difficulties

Disorder of written expression

EXCLUDES *specific arithmetical disorder (315.1)*
specific reading disorder (315.00-315.09)

√5th **315.3 Developmental speech or language disorder**

315.31 Expressive language disorder

Developmental aphasia
Word deafness

EXCLUDES *acquired aphasia (784.3)*
elective mutism (309.83, 313.0, 313.23)

315.32 Mixed receptive-expressive language disorder

Central auditory processing disorder

EXCLUDES *acquired auditory processing disorder (388.45)*

315.34 Speech and language developmental delay due to hearing loss

AHA: 4Q, '07, 80, 81

315.35 Childhood onset fluency disorder

Cluttering NOS
Stuttering NOS

EXCLUDES *adult onset fluency disorder (307.0)*
fluency disorder due to late effect of cerebrovascular accident (438.14)
fluency disorder in conditions classified elsewhere (784.52)

AHA: 4Q, '10, 83-84

F80.81 Child onset fluency disorder I-10

315.39 Other

Developmental articulation disorder
Dyslalia
Phonological disorder

EXCLUDES *lisping and lalling (307.9)*

AHA: 3Q, '07, 7

315.4 Developmental coordination disorder

Clumsiness syndrome
Dyspraxia syndrome
Specific motor development disorder

315.5 Mixed development disorder

AHA: 2Q, '02, 11

315.8 Other specified delays in development

F88 Other disorders of psychological development I-10

315.9 Unspecified delay in development

Developmental disorder NOS
Learning disorder NOS

316 Psychic factors associated with diseases classified elsewhere

Psychologic factors in physical conditions classified elsewhere

Use additional code to identify the associated physical condition, as:

psychogenic:
asthma (493.9)
dermatitis (692.9)
duodenal ulcer (532.0-532.9)
eczema (691.8, 692.9)
gastric ulcer (531.0-531.9)
mucous colitis (564.9)
paroxysmal tachycardia (427.2)
ulcerative colitis (556)
urticaria (708.0-708.9)
psychosocial dwarfism (259.4)

EXCLUDES *physical symptoms and physiological malfunctions, not involving tissue damage, of mental origin (306.0-306.9)*

INTELLECTUAL DISABILITIES (317-319)

Use additional code(s) to identify any associated psychiatric or physical condition(s)

AHA: 4Q, '11, 98

317 Mild intellectual disabilities

High-grade defect
IQ 50-70
Mild mental subnormality

F70 Mild intellectual disabilities I-10

√4th **318 Other specified intellectual disabilities**

AHA: 4Q, '11, 98

318.0 Moderate intellectual disabilities

IQ 35-49
Moderate mental subnormality

318.1 Severe intellectual disabilities

IQ 20-34
Severe mental subnormality

318.2 Profound intellectual disabilities

IQ under 20
Profound mental subnormality

319 Unspecified intellectual disabilities

Mental deficiency NOS
Mental subnormality NOS

AHA: 4Q, '11, 98

F79 Unspecified intellectual disabilities I-10

6. Diseases of the Nervous System and Sense Organs (320-389)

Inflammatory Diseases of the Central Nervous System (320-326)

✓4ᵗʰ 320 Bacterial meningitis

INCLUDES
arachnoiditis
leptomeningitis
meningitis
meningoencephalitis
meningomyelitis
pachymeningitis
} bacterial

DEF: Bacterial infection causing inflammation of the lining of the brain and/or spinal cord.
AHA: J-F, '87, 6

320.0 Hemophilus meningitis
Meningitis due to Hemophilus influenzae [H. influenzae]

320.1 Pneumococcal meningitis

320.2 Streptococcal meningitis

320.3 Staphylococcal meningitis

320.7 Meningitis in other bacterial diseases classified elsewhere
Code first underlying disease, as:
actinomycosis (039.8)
listeriosis (027.0)
typhoid fever (002.0)
whooping cough (033.0-033.9)
EXCLUDES meningitis (in):
epidemic (036.0)
gonococcal (098.82)
meningococcal (036.0)
salmonellosis (003.21)
syphilis:
NOS (094.2)
congenital (090.42)
meningovascular (094.2)
secondary (091.81)
tuberculous (013.0)

✓5ᵗʰ 320.8 Meningitis due to other specified bacteria

320.81 Anaerobic meningitis
Bacteroides (fragilis)　　Gram-negative anaerobes

320.82 Meningitis due to gram-negative bacteria, not elsewhere classified
Aerobacter aerogenes　　Klebsiella
　　pneumoniae　　Proteus morganii
Escherichia coli [E. coli]　　Pseudomonas
Friedländer bacillus
EXCLUDES gram-negative anaerobes (320.81)
AHA: 4Q, '11, 155

320.89 Meningitis due to other specified bacteria
Bacillus pyocyaneus

320.9 Meningitis due to unspecified bacterium
Meningitis:　　Meningitis:
bacterial NOS　　pyogenic NOS
purulent NOS　　suppurative NOS

✓4ᵗʰ 321 Meningitis due to other organisms

INCLUDES
arachnoiditis
leptomeningitis
meningitis
pachymeningitis
} due to organisms other than bacterial

DEF: Infection causing inflammation of the lining of the brain and/or spinal cord, due to organisms other than bacteria.
AHA: J-F, '87, 6

321.0 Cryptococcal meningitis
Code first underlying disease (117.5)

321.1 Meningitis in other fungal diseases
Code first underlying disease (110.0-118)
EXCLUDES meningitis in:
candidiasis (112.83)
coccidioidomycosis (114.2)
histoplasmosis (115.01, 115.11, 115.91)

321.2 Meningitis due to viruses not elsewhere classified
Code first underlying disease, as:
meningitis due to arbovirus (060.0-066.9)
EXCLUDES meningitis (due to):
abacterial (047.0-047.9)
adenovirus (049.1)
aseptic NOS (047.9)
Coxsackie (virus)(047.0)
ECHO virus (047.1)
enterovirus (047.0-047.9)
herpes simplex virus (054.72)
herpes zoster virus (053.0)
lymphocytic choriomeningitis virus (049.0)
mumps (072.1)
viral NOS (047.9)
meningo-eruptive syndrome (047.1)
AHA: 4Q, '04, 51

321.3 Meningitis due to trypanosomiasis
Code first underlying disease (086.0-086.9)

321.4 Meningitis in sarcoidosis
Code first underlying disease (135)

321.8 Meningitis due to other nonbacterial organisms classified elsewhere
Code first underlying disease
EXCLUDES leptospiral meningitis (100.81)

✓4ᵗʰ 322 Meningitis of unspecified cause

INCLUDES
arachnoiditis
leptomeningitis
meningitis
pachymeningitis
} with no organism specified as cause

DEF: Infection causing inflammation of the lining of the brain and/or spinal cord, due to unspecified cause.
AHA: J-F, '87, 6

322.0 Nonpyogenic meningitis
Meningitis with clear cerebrospinal fluid

322.1 Eosinophilic meningitis

322.2 Chronic meningitis

322.9 Meningitis, unspecified

✓4ᵗʰ 323 Encephalitis, myelitis, and encephalomyelitis

INCLUDES
acute disseminated encephalomyelitis
meningoencephalitis, except bacterial
meningomyelitis, except bacterial
myelitis:
ascending
transverse
EXCLUDES acute transverse myelitis NOS (341.20)
acute transverse myelitis in conditions classified elsewhere (341.21)
bacterial:
meningoencephalitis (320.0-320.9)
meningomyelitis (320.0-320.9)
idiopathic transverse myelitis (341.22)

DEF: Encephalitis: inflammation of brain tissues.
DEF: Myelitis: inflammation of the spinal cord.
DEF: Encephalomyelitis: inflammation of brain and spinal cord.

✓4ᵗʰ ✓5ᵗʰ Additional Digit Required	Unspecified Code	Other Specified Code	Manifestation Code	►◄ Revised Text　● New Code　▲ Revised Code Title

Diseases of the Nervous System and Sense Organs

323.0–324.9

√5ᵗʰ **323.0 Encephalitis, myelitis, and encephalomyelitis in viral diseases classified elsewhere**

Code first underlying disease, as:
  cat-scratch disease (078.3)
  human immunodeficiency virus [HIV] disease (042)
  infectious mononucleosis (075)
  ornithosis (073.7)

323.01 *Encephalitis and encephalomyelitis in viral diseases classified elsewhere*

EXCLUDES encephalitis (in):
  arthropod-borne viral (062.0-064)
  herpes simplex (054.3)
  mumps (072.2)
  other viral diseases of central nervous system (049.8-049.9)
  poliomyelitis (045.0-045.9)
  rubella (056.01)
  slow virus infections of central nervous system (046.0-046.9)
  viral NOS (049.9)
  West Nile (066.41)

AHA: 3Q, '10, 13; 4Q, '06, 58-63

323.02 *Myelitis in viral diseases classified elsewhere*

EXCLUDES myelitis (in):
  herpes simplex (054.74)
  herpes zoster (053.14)
  poliomyelitis (045.0-045.9)
  rubella (056.01)
  other viral diseases of central nervous system (049.8-049.9)

AHA: 4Q, '06, 58-63

323.1 *Encephalitis, myelitis, and encephalomyelitis in rickettsial diseases classified elsewhere*

Code first underlying disease (080-083.9)
DEF: Inflammation of the brain caused by rickettsial disease carried by louse, tick, or mite.

323.2 *Encephalitis, myelitis, and encephalomyelitis in protozoal diseases classified elsewhere*

Code first underlying disease, as:
  malaria (084.0-084.9)
  trypanosomiasis (086.0-086.9)
DEF: Inflammation of the brain caused by protozoal disease carried by mosquitoes and flies.

√5ᵗʰ **323.4 Other encephalitis, myelitis, and encephalomyelitis due to other infections classified elsewhere**

Code first underlying disease

323.41 *Other encephalitis and encephalomyelitis due to other infections classified elsewhere*

EXCLUDES encephalitis (in):
  meningococcal (036.1)
  syphilis:
    NOS (094.81)
    congenital (090.41)
  toxoplasmosis (130.0)
  tuberculosis (013.6)
  meningoencephalitis due to free-living ameba [Naegleria] (136.29)

AHA: 4Q, '06, 58-63

323.42 *Other myelitis due to other infections classified elsewhere*

EXCLUDES myelitis (in):
  syphilis (094.89)
  tuberculosis (013.6)

AHA: 4Q, '06, 58-63

√5ᵗʰ **323.5 Encephalitis, myelitis, and encephalomyelitis following immunization procedures**

Use additional E code to identify vaccine

323.51 Encephalitis and encephalomyelitis following immunization procedures

Encephalitis postimmunization or postvaccinal
Encephalomyelitis postimmunization or postvaccinal
AHA: 4Q, '06, 58-63

323.52 Myelitis following immunization procedures

Myelitis postimmunization or postvaccinal
AHA: 4Q, '06, 58-63

√5ᵗʰ **323.6 Postinfectious encephalitis, myelitis, and encephalomyelitis**

Code first underlying disease
DEF: Infection, inflammation of brain several weeks following the outbreak of a systemic infection.

323.61 *Infectious acute disseminated encephalomyelitis [ADEM]*

Acute necrotizing hemorrhagic encephalopathy
EXCLUDES noninfectious acute disseminated encephalomyelitis (ADEM) (323.81)

AHA: 4Q, '06, 58-63

323.62 *Other postinfectious encephalitis and encephalomyelitis*

EXCLUDES encephalitis:
  postchickenpox (052.0)
  postmeasles (055.0)

AHA: 4Q, '06, 58-63

323.63 *Postinfectious myelitis*

EXCLUDES postchickenpox myelitis (052.2)
  herpes simplex myelitis (054.74)
  herpes zoster myelitis (053.14)

AHA: 4Q, '06, 58-63

√5ᵗʰ **323.7 Toxic encephalitis, myelitis, and encephalomyelitis**

Code first underlying cause, as:
  carbon tetrachloride (982.1)
  hydroxyquinoline derivatives (961.3)
  lead (984.0-984.9)
  mercury (985.0)
  thallium (985.8)
AHA: 2Q, '97, 8

323.71 *Toxic encephalitis and encephalomyelitis*
AHA: 4Q, '06, 58-63

323.72 *Toxic myelitis*
AHA: 4Q, '06, 58-63

√5ᵗʰ **323.8 Other causes of encephalitis, myelitis, and encephalomyelitis**

323.81 Other causes of encephalitis and encephalomyelitis

Noninfectious acute disseminated encephalomyelitis (ADEM)
AHA: 1Q, '11, 12; 3Q, '10, 15; 4Q, '06, 58-63

323.82 Other causes of myelitis

Transverse myelitis NOS
AHA: 4Q, '06, 58-63

323.9 Unspecified cause of encephalitis, myelitis, and encephalomyelitis

√4ᵗʰ **324 Intracranial and intraspinal abscess**

324.0 Intracranial abscess

Abscess (embolic):
  cerebellar
  cerebral
Abscess (embolic) of brain [any part]:
  epidural
  extradural
  otogenic
  subdural

EXCLUDES tuberculous (013.3)

324.1 Intraspinal abscess

Abscess (embolic) of spinal cord [any part]:
  epidural
  extradural
  subdural

EXCLUDES tuberculous (013.5)

324.9 Of unspecified site

Extradural or subdural abscess NOS

N Newborn Age: 0   P Pediatric Age: 0-17   M Maternity Age: 12-55   A Adult Age: 15-124

325 Phlebitis and thrombophlebitis of intracranial venous sinuses

Embolism
Endophlebitis
Phlebitis, septic or suppurative } of cavernous, lateral or other intracranial or unspecified intracranial venous sinus
Thrombophlebitis
Thrombosis

EXCLUDES that specified as:
  complicating pregnancy, childbirth, or the puerperium (671.5)
  of nonpyogenic origin (437.6)

DEF: Inflammation and formation of blood clot in a vein within the brain or its lining.

326 Late effects of intracranial abscess or pyogenic infection

NOTE This category is to be used to indicate conditions whose primary classification is to 320-325 [excluding 320.7, 321.0-321.8, 323.01-323.42, 323.6-323.7] as the cause of late effects, themselves classifiable elsewhere. The "late effects" include conditions specified as such, or as sequelae, which may occur at any time after the resolution of the causal condition.

Use additional code to identify condition, as:
  hydrocephalus (331.4)
  paralysis (342.0-342.9, 344.0-344.9)

Organic sleep disorders (327)

TIP: If the sleep disorder is not documented with the etiology related to an organic disease process, see instead subcategory 307.4.

√4th 327 Organic sleep disorders
  AHA: 4Q, '05, 59-64

√5th 327.0 Organic disorders of initiating and maintaining sleep [Organic insomnia]

EXCLUDES insomnia NOS (780.52)
  insomnia not due to a substance or known physiological condition (307.41-307.42)
  insomnia with sleep apnea NOS (780.51)

327.00 Organic insomnia, unspecified

327.01 Insomnia due to medical condition classified elsewhere

Code first underlying condition

EXCLUDES insomnia due to mental disorder (327.02)

327.02 Insomnia due to mental disorder

Code first mental disorder

EXCLUDES alcohol induced insomnia (291.82)
  drug induced insomnia (292.85)

327.09 Other organic insomnia

√5th 327.1 Organic disorder of excessive somnolence [Organic hypersomnia]

EXCLUDES hypersomnia NOS (780.54)
  hypersomnia not due to a substance or known physiological condition (307.43-307.44)
  hypersomnia with sleep apnea NOS (780.53)

327.10 Organic hypersomnia, unspecified

327.11 Idiopathic hypersomnia with long sleep time

327.12 Idiopathic hypersomnia without long sleep time

327.13 Recurrent hypersomnia
  Kleine-Levin syndrome
  Menstrual related hypersomnia

327.14 Hypersomnia due to medical condition classified elsewhere

Code first underlying condition

EXCLUDES hypersomnia due to mental disorder (327.15)

327.15 Hypersomnia due to mental disorder

Code first mental disorder

EXCLUDES alcohol induced hypersomnia (291.82)
  drug induced hypersomnia (292.85)

327.19 Other organic hypersomnia

√5th 327.2 Organic sleep apnea

EXCLUDES Cheyne-Stokes breathing (786.04)
  hypersomnia with sleep apnea NOS (780.53)
  insomnia with sleep apnea NOS (780.51)
  sleep apnea in newborn (770.81-770.82)
  sleep apnea NOS (780.57)

327.20 Organic sleep apnea, unspecified

327.21 Primary central sleep apnea

327.22 High altitude periodic breathing

327.23 Obstructive sleep apnea (adult) (pediatric)
  G47.33 Obstructive sleep apnea (adult) (pediatric)   I-10

327.24 Idiopathic sleep related nonobstructive alveolar hypoventilation
  Sleep related hypoxia

327.25 Congenital central alveolar hypoventilation syndrome

327.26 Sleep related hypoventilation/ hypoxemia in conditions classifiable elsewhere

Code first underlying condition

327.27 Central sleep apnea in conditions classified elsewhere

Code first underlying condition

327.29 Other organic sleep apnea

√4th 327.3 Circadian rhythm sleep disorder
  Organic disorder of sleep wake cycle
  Organic disorder of sleep wake schedule

EXCLUDES alcohol induced circadian rhythm sleep disorder (291.82)
  circadian rhythm sleep disorder of nonorganic origin (307.45)
  disruption of 24 hour sleep wake cycle NOS (780.55)
  drug induced circadian rhythm sleep disorder (292.85)

327.30 Circadian rhythm sleep disorder, unspecified

327.31 Circadian rhythm sleep disorder, delayed sleep phase type

327.32 Circadian rhythm sleep disorder, advanced sleep phase type

327.33 Circadian rhythm sleep disorder, irregular sleep-wake type

327.34 Circadian rhythm sleep disorder, free-running type

327.35 Circadian rhythm sleep disorder, jet lag type

327.36 Circadian rhythm sleep disorder, shift work type

327.37 Circadian rhythm sleep disorder in conditions classified elsewhere

Code first underlying condition

327.39 Other circadian rhythm sleep disorder

√5th 327.4 Organic parasomnia

EXCLUDES alcohol induced parasomnia (291.82)
  drug induced parasomnia (292.85)
  parasomnia not due to a known physiological condition (307.47)

327.40 Organic parasomnia, unspecified

327.41 Confusional arousals

327.42 REM sleep behavior disorder

327.43 Recurrent isolated sleep paralysis

327.44 Parasomnia in conditions classified elsewhere

Code first underlying condition

327.49 Other organic parasomnia

√5th 327.5 Organic sleep related movement disorders

EXCLUDES restless legs syndrome (333.94)
  sleep related movement disorder NOS (780.58)

327.51 Periodic limb movement disorder
  Periodic limb movement sleep disorder

327.52 Sleep related leg cramps

| √4th √5th Additional Digit Required | Unspecified Code | Other Specified Code | Manifestation Code | ►◄ Revised Text | ● New Code | ▲ Revised Code Title |

Diseases of the Nervous System and Sense Organs

327.53–331.82

327.53 Sleep related bruxism

327.59 **Other organic sleep related movement disorders**

327.8 **Other organic sleep disorders**

    AHA: 2Q, '07, 6

Hereditary and Degenerative Diseases of the Central Nervous System (330-337)

    EXCLUDES *hepatolenticular degeneration (275.1)*
    multiple sclerosis (340)
    other demyelinating diseases of central nervous system (341.0-341.9)

√4th **330** **Cerebral degenerations usually manifest in childhood**

    Use additional code to identify associated intellectual disabilities

330.0 **Leukodystrophy**

Krabbe's disease	Leukodystrophy:
Leukodystrophy:	sudanophilic
NOS	Pelizaeus-Merzbacher disease
globoid cell	Sulfatide lipidosis
metachromatic	

    DEF: Hereditary disease of arylsulfatase or cerebroside sulfatase; characterized by a diffuse loss of myelin in CNS; infantile form causes blindness, motor disturbances, rigidity, mental deterioration and, occasionally, convulsions.

330.1 **Cerebral lipidoses**

Amaurotic (familial) idiocy	Disease:
Disease:	Spielmeyer-Vogt
Batten	Tay-Sachs
Jansky-Bielschowsky	Gangliosidosis
Kufs'	

    DEF: Genetic disorder causing abnormal lipid accumulation in the reticuloendothelial cells of the brain.

330.2 *Cerebral degeneration in generalized lipidoses*

    Code first underlying disease, as:
    Fabry's disease (272.7)
    Gaucher's disease (272.7)
    Niemann-Pick disease (272.7)
    sphingolipidosis (272.7)

330.3 *Cerebral degeneration of childhood in other diseases classified elsewhere*

    Code first underlying disease, as:
    Hunter's disease (277.5)
    mucopolysaccharidosis (277.5)

330.8 **Other specified cerebral degenerations in childhood**

    Alpers' disease or gray-matter degeneration
    Infantile necrotizing encephalomyelopathy
    Leigh's disease
    Subacute necrotizing encephalopathy or
    encephalomyelopathy

    AHA: N-D, '85, 5

330.9 **Unspecified cerebral degeneration in childhood**

√4th **331** **Other cerebral degenerations**

    Use additional code, where applicable, to identify dementia:
    with behavioral disturbance (294.11)
    without behavioral disturbance (294.10)

331.0 **Alzheimer's disease**

    DEF: Diffuse atrophy of cerebral cortex; causing a progressive decline in intellectual and physical functions, including memory loss, personality changes and profound dementia.
    AHA: 4Q, '00, 41; 4Q, '99, 7; N-D, '84, 20

    G30.9 Alzheimer's disease unspecified   I-10

√5th **331.1** **Frontotemporal dementia**

    DEF: Rare, progressive degenerative brain disease, similar to Alzheimer's; cortical atrophy affects the frontal and temporal lobes.
    AHA: 4Q, '03, 57

331.11 **Pick's disease**

    DEF: A progressive frontotemporal dementia with asymmetrical atrophy of the frontal and temporal regions of the cerebral cortex, abnormal rounded brain cells called Pick cells with the presence of abnormal staining of protein (called tau); symptoms include prominent apathy, behavioral changes such as disinhibition and restlessness, echolalia, impairment of language, memory, and intellect, increased carelessness, poor personal hygiene, and decreased attention span.

331.19 **Other frontotemporal dementia**

    Frontal dementia

331.2 **Senile degeneration of brain**

    EXCLUDES *senility NOS (797)*

331.3 **Communicating hydrocephalus**

    Secondary normal pressure hydrocephalus

    EXCLUDES *congenital hydrocephalus (742.3)*
    idiopathic normal pressure hydrocephalus (331.5)
    normal pressure hydrocephalus (331.5)
    spina bifida with hydrocephalus (741.0)

    DEF: Subarachnoid hemorrhage and meningitis causing excess buildup of cerebrospinal fluid in cavities due to nonabsorption of fluid back through fluid pathways.
    AHA: S-O, '85, 12

331.4 **Obstructive hydrocephalus**

    Acquired hydrocephalus NOS

    EXCLUDES *congenital hydrocephalus (742.3)*
    idiopathic normal pressure hydrocephalus (331.5)
    normal pressure hydrocephalus (331.5)
    spina bifida with hydrocephalus (741.0)

    DEF: Obstruction of cerebrospinal fluid passage from brain into spinal canal.
    AHA: 4Q, '03, 106; 1Q, '99, 9

    G91.1 Obstructive hydrocephalus   I-10

331.5 **Idiopathic normal pressure hydrocephalus [INPH]**

    Normal pressure hydrocephalus NOS

    EXCLUDES *congenital hydrocephalus (742.3)*
    secondary normal pressure hydrocephalus (331.3)
    spina bifida with hydrocephalus (741.0)

    DEF: Abnormal increase of cerebrospinal fluid in the brain's ventricles; results in dementia, progressive mental impairment, gait disturbance, and impaired bladder control.
    AHA: 4Q, '07, 74

331.6 **Corticobasal degeneration**

    AHA: 4Q, '11, 98

331.7 *Cerebral degeneration in diseases classified elsewhere*

    Code first underlying disease, as:
    alcoholism (303.0-303.9)
    beriberi (265.0)
    cerebrovascular disease (430-438)
    congenital hydrocephalus (741.0, 742.3)
    myxedema (244.0-244.9)
    neoplastic disease (140.0-239.9)
    vitamin B12 deficiency (266.2)

    EXCLUDES *cerebral degeneration in:*
    Jakob-Creutzfeldt disease (046.11-046.19)
    progressive multifocal leukoencephalopathy (046.3)
    subacute spongiform encephalopathy (046.1)

√5th **331.8** **Other cerebral degeneration**

331.81 **Reye's syndrome**   P

    DEF: Rare childhood illness, often developed after a viral upper respiratory infection; characterized by vomiting, elevated serum transaminase, changes in liver and other viscera; brain swelling, disturbances of consciousness and seizures; can be fatal.

331.82 **Dementia with Lewy bodies**

Dementia with Parkinsonism	Lewy body disease
Lewy body dementia	

    DEF: A cerebral dementia with neurophysiologic changes, increased hippocampal volume, hypoperfusion in the occipital lobes, and beta amyloid deposits with neurofibrillary tangles, atrophy of cortex and brainstem, hallmark neuropsychologic characteristics are fluctuating cognition with pronounced variation in attention and alertness; recurrent hallucinations; and parkinsonism.
    AHA: 4Q, '03, 57

    G31.83 Dementia with Lewy bodies   I-10

N Newborn Age: 0   P Pediatric Age: 0-17   M Maternity Age: 12-55   A Adult Age: 15-124

331.83 Mild cognitive impairment, so stated

EXCLUDES *altered mental status (780.97)*
cerebral degeneration (331.0-331.9)
change in mental status (780.97)
cognitive deficits following (late effects of)
cerebral hemorrhage or infarction
(438.0)
cognitive impairment due to intracranial or
head injury (850-854, 959.01)
cognitive impairment due to late effect of
intracranial injury (907.0)
cognitive impairment due to skull fracture
(800-801, 803-804)
dementia (290.0-290.43, 294.20-294.21)
mild memory disturbance (310.89)
neurologic neglect syndrome (781.8)
personality change, nonpsychotic (310.1)

AHA: 4Q, '06, 75

331.89 Other
Cerebral ataxia

331.9 Cerebral degeneration, unspecified

√4th **332 Parkinson's disease**

EXCLUDES *dementia with Parkinsonism (331.82)*

332.0 Paralysis agitans
Parkinsonism or Parkinson's disease:
NOS
idiopathic
primary
DEF: Form of progressive parkinsonism, characterized by masklike
facial expressions, in ability to stand or walk smoothly, muscle
weakness, and involuntary trembling movement.
AHA: M-A, '87, 7
G20 Parkinson's disease   I-10

332.1 Secondary Parkinsonism
Neuroleptic-induced Parkinsonism
Parkinsonism due to drugs

Use additional E code to identify drug, if drug-induced

EXCLUDES *Parkinsonism (in):*
Huntington's disease (333.4)
progressive supranuclear palsy (333.0)
Shy-Drager syndrome (333.0)
syphilitic (094.82)

√4th **333 Other extrapyramidal disease and abnormal movement
disorders**

INCLUDES other forms of extrapyramidal, basal ganglia, or
striatopallidal disease

EXCLUDES *abnormal movements of head NOS (781.0)*
sleep related movement disorders (327.51-327.59)

333.0 Other degenerative diseases of the basal ganglia
Atrophy or degeneration:
olivopontocerebellar [Déjérine-Thomas syndrome]
pigmentary pallidal [Hallervorden-Spatz disease]
striatonigral
Parkinsonian syndrome associated with:
idiopathic orthostatic hypotension
symptomatic orthostatic hypotension
Progressive supranuclear ophthalmoplegia
Shy-Drager syndrome
AHA: 3Q, '96, 8

333.1 Essential and other specified forms of tremor
Benign essential tremor
Familial tremor
Medication-induced postural tremor

Use additional E code to identify drug, if drug-induced

EXCLUDES *tremor NOS (781.0)*

333.2 Myoclonus
Familial essential myoclonus   Palatal myoclonus

EXCLUDES *progressive myoclonic epilepsy (345.1)*
Unverricht-Lundborg disease (345.1)

Use additional E code to identify drug, if drug-induced
DEF: Spontaneous movements or contractions of muscles.
AHA: 3Q, '97, 4; M-A, '87, 12

333.3 Tics of organic origin

Use additional E code to identify drug, if drug-induced

EXCLUDES *Gilles de la Tourette's syndrome (307.23)*
habit spasm (307.22)
tic NOS (307.20)

333.4 Huntington's chorea
DEF: Genetic disease characterized by chronic progressive mental
deterioration; dementia and death within 15 years of onset.

333.5 Other choreas
Hemiballism(us)   Paroxysmal choreo-athetosis

Use additional E code to identify drug, if drug-induced

EXCLUDES *Sydenham's or rheumatic chorea (392.0-392.9)*

333.6 Genetic torsion dystonia
Dystonia:
deformans progressiva
musculorum deformans
(Schwalbe-) Ziehen-Oppenheim disease
DEF: Sustained muscular contractions, causing twisting and
repetitive movements that result in abnormal postures of trunk and
limbs; etiology unknown.

√5th **333.7 Acquired torsion dystonia**

333.71 Athetoid cerebral palsy
Double athetosis (syndrome)   Vogt's disease

EXCLUDES *infantile cerebral palsy (343.0-343.9)*

AHA: 4Q, '06, 76-78

333.72 Acute dystonia due to drugs
Acute dystonic reaction due to drugs
Neuroleptic induced acute dystonia

Use additional E code to identify drug

EXCLUDES *blepharospasm due to drugs (333.85)*
orofacial dyskinesia due to drugs (333.85)
secondary Parkinsonism (332.1)
subacute dyskinesia due to drugs (333.85)
tardive dyskinesia (333.85)

AHA: 4Q, '06, 76-78

333.79 Other acquired torsion dystonia
AHA: 4Q, '06, 76-78

√5th **333.8 Fragments of torsion dystonia**
Use additional E code to identify drug, if drug-induced

333.81 Blepharospasm

EXCLUDES *blepharospasm due to drugs (333.85)*
DEF: Uncontrolled winking or blinking due to orbicularis
oculi muscle spasm.

333.82 Orofacial dyskinesia

EXCLUDES *orofacial dyskinesia due to drugs (333.85)*
DEF: Uncontrolled movement of mouth or facial muscles.

333.83 Spasmodic torticollis

EXCLUDES *torticollis:*
NOS (723.5)
hysterical (300.11)
psychogenic (306.0)
DEF: Uncontrolled movement of head due to spasms of
neck muscle.

333.84 Organic writers' cramp

EXCLUDES *pychogenic (300.89)*

333.85 Subacute dyskinesia due to drugs
Blepharospasm due to drugs
Orofacial dyskinesia due to drugs
Tardive dyskinesia

Use additional E code to identify drug

EXCLUDES *acute dystonia due to drugs (333.72)*
acute dystonic reaction due to drugs (333.72)
secondary Parkinsonism (332.1)

AHA: 4Q, '06, 76-78

333.89 Other

√4th
√5th Additional Digit Required   Unspecified Code   Other Specified Code   Manifestation Code   ▶◀ Revised Text   ● New Code   ▲ Revised Code Title

2015 ICD-9-CM   **Volume 1 – 91**

√5ᵗʰ **333.9 Other and unspecified extrapyramidal diseases and abnormal movement disorders**

333.90 Unspecified extrapyramidal disease and abnormal movement disorder
Medication-induced movement disorders NOS

Use additional E code to identify drug, if drug-induced

333.91 Stiff-man syndrome

333.92 Neuroleptic malignant syndrome

Use additional E code to identify drug

EXCLUDES neuroleptic induced Parkinsonism (332.1)

AHA: 4Q, '94, 37

333.93 Benign shuddering attacks

AHA: 4Q, '94, 37

333.94 Restless legs syndrome [RLS]
DEF: Neurological disorder of unknown etiology with an irresistible urge to move the legs, which may temporarily relieve the symptoms, is accompanied by motor restlessness and sensations of pain, burning, prickling, or tingling.

AHA: 4Q, '06, 79

TIP: Assign an additional code if the underlying cause of the RLS is specified (e.g., iron deficiency anemia).

G25.81 Restless legs syndrome   I-10

333.99 Other
Neuroleptic-induced acute akathisia

Use additional E code to identify drug, if drug-induced

AHA: 4Q, '04, 95; 2Q, '04, 12; 4Q, '94, 37

√4ᵗʰ **334 Spinocerebellar disease**

EXCLUDES olivopontocerebellar degeneration (333.0)
peroneal muscular atrophy (356.1)

334.0 Friedreich's ataxia
DEF: Genetic recessive disease of children; sclerosis of dorsal, lateral spinal cord columns; characterized by ataxia, speech impairment, swaying and irregular movements, with muscle paralysis, especially of lower limbs.

334.1 Hereditary spastic paraplegia

334.2 Primary cerebellar degeneration
Cerebellar ataxia:
Marie's
Sanger-Brown
Dyssynergia cerebellaris myoclonica
Primary cerebellar degeneration:
NOS
hereditary
sporadic

AHA: M-A, '87, 9

334.3 Other cerebellar ataxia
Cerebellar ataxia NOS

Use additional E code to identify drug, if drug-induced

334.4 Cerebellar ataxia in diseases classified elsewhere

Code first underlying disease, as:
alcoholism (303.0-303.9)
myxedema (244.0-244.9)
neoplastic disease (140.0-239.9)

334.8 Other spinocerebellar diseases
Ataxia-telangiectasia [Louis-Bar syndrome]
Corticostriatal-spinal degeneration

334.9 Spinocerebellar disease, unspecified

√4ᵗʰ **335 Anterior horn cell disease**

335.0 Werdnig-Hoffmann disease
Infantile spinal muscular atrophy
Progressive muscular atrophy of infancy

DEF: Spinal muscle atrophy manifested in prenatal period or shortly after birth; symptoms include hypotonia, atrophy of skeletal muscle; death occurs in infancy.

√5ᵗʰ **335.1 Spinal muscular atrophy**

335.10 Spinal muscular atrophy, unspecified

335.11 Kugelberg-Welander disease
Spinal muscular atrophy:
familial
juvenile

DEF: Hereditary; juvenile muscle atrophy; appears during first two decades of life; due to lesions of anterior horns of spinal cord; includes wasting, diminution of lower body muscles and twitching.

335.19 Other
Adult spinal muscular atrophy

√5ᵗʰ **335.2 Motor neuron disease**

335.20 Amyotrophic lateral sclerosis   A
Motor neuron disease (bulbar) (mixed type)

AHA: 4Q, '95, 81

335.21 Progressive muscular atrophy
Duchenne-Aran muscular atrophy
Progressive muscular atrophy (pure)

335.22 Progressive bulbar palsy

335.23 Pseudobulbar palsy

335.24 Primary lateral sclerosis

335.29 Other

335.8 Other anterior horn cell diseases

335.9 Anterior horn cell disease, unspecified

√4ᵗʰ **336 Other diseases of spinal cord**

336.0 Syringomyelia and syringobulbia
AHA: 1Q, '89, 10

336.1 Vascular myelopathies
Acute infarction of spinal cord (embolic) (nonembolic)
Arterial thrombosis of spinal cord
Edema of spinal cord
Hematomyelia
Subacute necrotic myelopathy

336.2 Subacute combined degeneration of spinal cord in diseases classified elsewhere

Code first underlying disease, as:
pernicious anemia (281.0)
other vitamin B12 deficiency anemia (281.1)
vitamin B12 deficiency (266.2)

336.3 Myelopathy in other diseases classified elsewhere

Code first underlying disease, as:
myelopathy in neoplastic disease (140.0-239.9)

EXCLUDES myelopathy in:
intervertebral disc disorder (722.70-722.73)
spondylosis (721.1, 721.41-721.42, 721.91)

AHA: 3Q, '99, 5

336.8 Other myelopathy
Myelopathy:
drug-induced
radiation-induced

Use additonal E code to identify cause

336.9 Unspecified disease of spinal cord
Cord compression NOS
Myelopathy NOS

EXCLUDES myelitis (323.02, 323.1, 323.2, 323.42, 323.52, 323.63, 323.72, 323.82, 323.9)
spinal (canal) stenosis (723.0, 724.00-724.09)

√4ᵗʰ **337 Disorders of the autonomic nervous system**

INCLUDES disorders of peripheral autonomic, sympathetic, parasympathetic, or vegetative system

EXCLUDES familial dysautonomia [Riley-Day syndrome] (742.8)

√5ᵗʰ **337.0 Idiopathic peripheral autonomic neuropathy**

337.00 Idiopathic peripheral autonomic neuropathy, unspecified

337.01 Carotid sinus syndrome
Carotid sinus syncope

DEF: Vagal activation caused by pressure on the carotid sinus baroreceptors; sympathetic nerve impulses may cause sinus arrest or AV block.

AHA: 4Q, '08, 101-102

N Newborn Age: 0   P Pediatric Age: 0-17   M Maternity Age: 12-55   A Adult Age: 15-124

337.09 Other idiopathic peripheral autonomic neuropathy
Cervical sympathetic dystrophy or paralysis

337.1 Peripheral autonomic neuropathy in disorders classified elsewhere
Code first underlying disease, as:
amyloidosis (277.30-277.39)
diabetes (249.6, 250.6)
AHA: 2Q, '09, 13; 2Q, '93, 6; 3Q, '91, 9; N-D, '84, 9

√5ᵗʰ 337.2 Reflex sympathetic dystrophy
DEF: Disturbance of the sympathetic nervous system evidenced by sweating, pain, pallor and edema following injury to nerves or blood vessels.
AHA: 4Q, '93, 24

337.20 Reflex sympathetic dystrophy, unspecified
Complex regional pain syndrome type I, unspecified

337.21 Reflex sympathetic dystrophy of the upper limb
Complex regional pain syndrome type I of the upper limb

337.22 Reflex sympathetic dystrophy of the lower limb
Complex regional pain syndrome type I of the lower limb

337.29 Reflex sympathetic dystrophy of other specified site
Complex regional pain syndrome type I of other specified site

337.3 Autonomic dysreflexia
Use additional code to identify the cause, such as:
fecal impaction (560.32)
pressure ulcer (707.00-707.09)
urinary tract infection (599.0)
DEF: Noxious stimuli evokes paroxysmal hypertension, bradycardia, excess sweating, headache, pilomotor responses, facial flushing, and nasal congestion due to uncontrolled parasympathetic nerve response; occurs in patients with spinal cord injury above sympathetic outflow tract (T₆).
AHA: 4Q, '98, 37

337.9 Unspecified disorder of autonomic nervous system

Pain (338)

√4ᵗʰ 338 Pain, not elsewhere classified
Use additional code to identify:
pain associated with psychological factors (307.89)
EXCLUDES generalized pain (780.96)
headache syndromes (339.00-339.89)
localized pain, unspecified type — code to pain by site
migraines (346.0-346.9)
pain disorder exclusively attributed to psychological factors (307.80)
vulvar vestibulitis (625.71)
vulvodynia (625.70-625.79)
AHA: 2Q, '07, 12
TIP: Do not assign a 338 code if the pain is not specified as acute or chronic, unless post-thoracotomy, postoperative, neoplasm related or central pain syndrome.

338.0 Central pain syndrome
Déjérine-Roussy syndrome
Myelopathic pain syndrome
Thalamic pain syndrome (hyperesthetic)
AHA: 4Q, '06, 79-81

√5ᵗʰ 338.1 Acute pain

338.11 Acute pain due to trauma
AHA: 1Q, '07, 7; 4Q, '06, 79-81

338.12 Acute post-thoracotomy pain
Post-thoracotomy pain NOS
AHA: 4Q, '06, 79-81

338.18 Other acute postoperative pain
Postoperative pain NOS
AHA: 2Q, '07, 11; 4Q, '06, 79-81
G89.18 Other acute postprocedural pain   I-10

338.19 Other acute pain
EXCLUDES neoplasm related acute pain (338.3)
AHA: 2Q, '07, 11; 4Q, '06, 79-81

√5ᵗʰ 338.2 Chronic pain
EXCLUDES causalgia (355.9)
lower limb (355.71)
upper limb (354.4)
chronic pain syndrome (338.4)
myofascial pain syndrome (729.1)
neoplasm related chronic pain (338.3)
reflex sympathetic dystrophy (337.20-337.29)

338.21 Chronic pain due to trauma
AHA: 4Q, '06, 79-81

338.22 Chronic post-thoracotomy pain
AHA: 4Q, '06, 79-81

338.28 Other chronic postoperative pain
AHA: 4Q, '06, 79-81
G89.28 Other chronic postprocedural pain   I-10

338.29 Other chronic pain
AHA: 4Q, '06, 79-81

338.3 Neoplasm related pain (acute) (chronic)
Cancer associated pain
Pain due to malignancy (primary) (secondary)
Tumor associated pain
AHA: 2Q, '07, 11; 4Q, '06, 79-81
G89.3 Neoplasm related pain (acute) (chronic)   I-10

338.4 Chronic pain syndrome
Chronic pain associated with significant psychosocial dysfunction
AHA: 2Q, '07, 11; 4Q, '06, 79-81
G89.4 Chronic pain syndrome   I-10

Other Headache Syndromes (339)

√4ᵗʰ 339 Other headache syndromes
EXCLUDES headache:
NOS (784.0)
due to lumbar puncture (349.0)
migraine (346.0-346.9)
AHA: 4Q, '08, 102-105

√5ᵗʰ 339.0 Cluster headaches and other trigeminal autonomic cephalgias
TACS

339.00 Cluster headache syndrome, unspecified
Ciliary neuralgia
Cluster headache NOS
Histamine cephalgia
Lower half migraine
Migrainous neuralgia

339.01 Episodic cluster headache

339.02 Chronic cluster headache

339.03 Episodic paroxysmal hemicrania
Paroxysmal hemicrania NOS

339.04 Chronic paroxysmal hemicrania

339.05 Short lasting unilateral neuralgiform headache with conjunctival injection and tearing
SUNCT

339.09 Other trigeminal autonomic cephalgias

√5ᵗʰ 339.1 Tension type headache
EXCLUDES tension headache NOS (307.81)
tension headache related to psychological factors (307.81)
AHA: 4Q, '08, 103

339.10 Tension type headache, unspecified

339.11 Episodic tension type headache

339.12 Chronic tension type headache

√5ᵗʰ 339.2 Post-traumatic headache
TIP: Do not assign during the acute phase of the trauma (e.g., head injury). When assigning 339.2X, report also a late effect code (e.g., 907.0 for intracranial injury).

339.20 Post-traumatic headache, unspecified
AHA: 4Q, '08, 108

339.21 Acute post-traumatic headache

√4ᵗʰ √5ᵗʰ Additional Digit Required   **Unspecified Code**   Other Specified Code   Manifestation Code   ▶◀ Revised Text   ● New Code   ▲ Revised Code Title

339.22 Chronic post-traumatic headache

339.3 Drug induced headache, not elsewhere classified
Medication overuse headache
Rebound headache

√5ᵗʰ **339.4 Complicated headache syndromes**

339.41 Hemicrania continua

339.42 New daily persistent headache
NDPH

339.43 Primary thunderclap headache

339.44 Other complicated headache syndrome

√5ᵗʰ **339.8 Other specified headache syndromes**

339.81 Hypnic headache

339.82 Headache associated with sexual activity
Orgasmic headache
Preorgasmic headache

339.83 Primary cough headache

339.84 Primary exertional headache

339.85 Primary stabbing headache

339.89 Other specified headache syndromes

Other Disorders of the Central Nervous System (340-349)

340 Multiple sclerosis
Disseminated or multiple sclerosis:
NOS
brain stem
cord
generalized
G35 Multiple sclerosis   I-10

√4ᵗʰ **341 Other demyelinating diseases of central nervous system**

341.0 Neuromyelitis optica

341.1 Schilder's disease
Baló's concentric sclerosis
Encephalitis periaxialis:
concentrica [Baló's]
diffusa [Schilder's]
DEF: Chronic leukoencephalopathy of children and adolescents; symptoms include blindness, deafness, bilateral spasticity and progressive mental deterioration.

√5ᵗʰ **341.2 Acute (transverse) myelitis**
EXCLUDES *acute (transverse) myelitis (in) (due to):*
following immunization procedures (323.52)
infection classified elsewhere (323.42)
postinfectious (323.63)
protozoal diseases classified elsewhere (323.2)
rickettsial diseases classified elsewhere (323.1)
toxic (323.72)
viral diseases classified elsewhere (323.02)
transverse myelitis NOS (323.82)

341.20 Acute (transverse) myelitis NOS
AHA: 4Q, '06, 58-63

341.21 Acute (transverse) myelitis in conditions classified elsewhere
Code first underlying condition
AHA: 4Q, '06, 58-63

341.22 Idiopathic transverse myelitis
AHA: 4Q, '06, 58-63

341.8 Other demyelinating diseases of central nervous system
Central demyelination of corpus callosum
Central pontine myelinosis
Marchiafava (-Bignami) disease
AHA: N-D, '87, 6

341.9 Demyelinating disease of central nervous system, unspecified

√4ᵗʰ **342 Hemiplegia and hemiparesis**
NOTE This category is to be used when hemiplegia (complete) (incomplete) is reported without further specification, or is stated to be old or long-standing but of unspecified cause. The category is also for use in multiple coding to identify these types of hemiplegia resulting from any cause.
EXCLUDES *congenital (343.1)*
hemiplegia due to late effect of cerebrovascular accident (438.20-438.22)
infantile NOS (343.4)

The following fifth-digits are for use with codes 342.0-342.9:
0 affecting unspecified side
1 affecting dominant side
2 affecting nondominant side

AHA: 4Q, '94, 38

§ √5ᵗʰ **342.0 Flaccid hemiplegia**
[0-2]

§ √5ᵗʰ **342.1 Spastic hemiplegia**
[0-2]

§ √5ᵗʰ **342.8 Other specified hemiplegia**
[0-2]

§ √5ᵗʰ **342.9 Hemiplegia, unspecified**
[0-2]   **AHA:** 3Q, '06, 5; 4Q, '98, 87
G81.90 Hemiplegia unspecified affect unspecified side   I-10

√4ᵗʰ **343 Infantile cerebral palsy**
INCLUDES cerebral:
palsy NOS
spastic infantile paralysis
congenital spastic paralysis (cerebral)
Little's disease
paralysis (spastic) due to birth injury:
intracranial
spinal
EXCLUDES *athetoid cerebral palsy (333.71)*
hereditary cerebral paralysis, such as:
hereditary spastic paraplegia (334.1)
Vogt's disease (333.71)
spastic paralysis specified as noncongenital or noninfantile (344.0-344.9)

343.0 Diplegic
Congenital diplegia
Congenital paraplegia
DEF: Paralysis affecting both sides of the body simultaneously.

343.1 Hemiplegic
Congenital hemiplegia
EXCLUDES *infantile hemiplegia NOS (343.4)*

343.2 Quadriplegic
Tetraplegic

343.3 Monoplegic

343.4 Infantile hemiplegia
Infantile hemiplegia (postnatal) NOS

343.8 Other specified infantile cerebral palsy

343.9 Infantile cerebral palsy, unspecified
Cerebral palsy NOS
AHA: 4Q, '05, 89
G80.9 Cerebral palsy unspecified   I-10

√4ᵗʰ **344 Other paralytic syndromes**
NOTE This category is to be used when the listed conditions are reported without further specification or are stated to be old or long-standing but of unspecified cause. The category is also for use in multiple coding to identify these conditions resulting from any cause.
INCLUDES paralysis (complete) (incomplete), except as classifiable to 342 and 343
EXCLUDES *congenital or infantile cerebral palsy (343.0-343.9)*
hemiplegia (342.0-342.9)
congenital or infantile (343.1, 343.4)

√5ᵗʰ **344.0 Quadriplegia and quadriparesis**
TIP: Assign also a code from subcategory 438.5 if late effect of CVA.

---

§   Requires fifth digit. Valid digits are in [brackets] under each code. See category 342 for codes and definitions.

344.00 Quadriplegia unspecified
AHA: 4Q, '03, 103; 4Q, '98, 38
G82.50 Quadriplegia unspecified   I-10

344.01 C₁-C₄ complete

344.02 C₁-C₄ incomplete

344.03 C₅-C₇ complete

344.04 C₅-C₇ incomplete

344.09 Other
AHA: 1Q, '01, 12; 4Q, '98, 39

344.1 Paraplegia
Paralysis of both lower limbs   Paraplegia (lower)
AHA: 4Q, '03, 110; M-A, '87, 10
G82.20 Paraplegia unspecified   I-10

344.2 Diplegia of upper limbs
Diplegia (upper)   Paralysis of both upper limbs

✓5th **344.3 Monoplegia of lower limb**
Paralysis of lower limb
EXCLUDES *monoplegia of lower limb due to late effect of cerebrovascular accident (438.40-438.42)*

344.30 Affecting unspecified side

344.31 Affecting dominant side

344.32 Affecting nondominant side

✓5th **344.4 Monoplegia of upper limb**
Paralysis of upper limb
EXCLUDES *monoplegia of upper limb due to late effect of cerebrovascular accident (438.30-438.32)*

344.40 Affecting unspecified side

344.41 Affecting dominant side

344.42 Affecting nondominant side

344.5 Unspecified monoplegia

✓5th **344.6 Cauda equina syndrome**
DEF: Dull pain and paresthesias in sacrum, perineum and bladder due to compression of spinal nerve roots; pain radiates down buttocks, back of thigh, calf of leg and into foot with prickling, burning sensations.

344.60 Without mention of neurogenic bladder

344.61 With neurogenic bladder
Acontractile bladder
Autonomic hyperreflexia of bladder
Cord bladder
Detrusor hyperreflexia
AHA: M-J, '87, 12; M-A, '87, 10

✓5th **344.8 Other specified paralytic syndromes**

344.81 Locked-in state
DEF: State of consciousness where patients are paralyzed and unable to respond to environmental stimuli; patients have eye movements, and stimuli can enter the brain but patients unable to respond.
AHA: 4Q, '93, 24

344.89 Other specified paralytic syndrome
AHA: 2Q, '99, 4

344.9 Paralysis, unspecified

✓4th **345 Epilepsy and recurrent seizures**

> The following fifth-digit subclassification is for use with categories 345.0, .1, .4-.9:
> **0 without mention of intractable epilepsy**
> **1 with intractable epilepsy**
>   pharmacoresistant (pharmacologically resistant)
>   poorly controlled
>   refractory (medically)
>   treatment resistant

EXCLUDES *hippocampal sclerosis (348.81)*
mesial temporal sclerosis (348.81)
temporal sclerosis (348.81)
DEF: Brain disorder characterized by electrical-like disturbances; may include occasional impairment or loss of consciousness, abnormal motor phenomena and psychic or sensory disturbances.
AHA: 4Q, '09, 82; 1Q, '93, 24; 2Q, '92, 8; 4Q, '92, 23

§ ✓5th **345.0 Generalized nonconvulsive epilepsy**
[0-1] Absences: Pykno-epilepsy
    atonic   Seizures:
    typical   akinetic
Minor epilepsy   atonic
Petit mal
AHA: For code 345.00: 1Q, '04, 18; For code 345.01: ▶1Q, '14, 12◀

§ ✓5th **345.1 Generalized convulsive epilepsy**
[0-1] Epileptic seizures: Grand mal
    clonic   Major epilepsy
    myoclonic   Progressive myoclonic epilepsy
    tonic   Unverricht-Lundborg disease
    tonic-clonic
EXCLUDES *convulsions:*
    NOS (780.39)
    infantile (780.39)
    newborn (779.0)
    infantile spasms (345.6)
DEF: Convulsive seizures with tension of limbs (tonic) or rhythmic contractions (clonic).
AHA: 3Q, '97, 4

345.2 Petit mal status
Epileptic absence status
DEF: Minor myoclonic spasms and sudden momentary loss of consciousness in epilepsy.
AHA: ▶1Q, '14, 11◀

345.3 Grand mal status
Status epilepticus NOS
EXCLUDES *epilepsia partialis continua (345.7)*
status:
    psychomotor (345.7)
    temporal lobe (345.7)
DEF: Sudden loss of consciousness followed by generalized convulsions in epilepsy.
AHA: 3Q, '05, 12
G40.301 Gen idiopath epilep&epi syn not intractabl w/se   I-10

§ ✓5th **345.4 Localization-related (focal) (partial) epilepsy and**
[0-1] **epileptic syndromes with complex partial seizures**
Epilepsy:
    limbic system
    partial:
        secondarily generalized
        with impairment of consciousness
        with memory and ideational disturbances
    psychomotor
    psychosensory
    temporal lobe
Epileptic automatism
AHA: For code 345.41 4Q, '09, 83

§ ✓5th **345.5 Localization-related (focal) (partial) epilepsy and**
[0-1] **epileptic syndromes with simple partial seizures**
Epilepsy: Epilepsy:
    Bravais-Jacksonian NOS   somatomotor
    focal (motor) NOS   somatosensory
    Jacksonian NOS   visceral
    motor partial   visual
    partial NOS:
        without impairment of consciousness
    sensory-induced

---

§   Requires fifth digit. Valid digits are in [brackets] under each code. See category 345 for codes and definitions.

| ✓4th ✓5th Additional Digit Required | Unspecified Code | Other Specified Code | Manifestation Code | ▶◀ Revised Text | ● New Code | ▲ Revised Code Title |

§ ✓5th **345.6 Infantile spasms**
[0-1]　　Hypsarrhythmia　　　　Lightning spasms
　　　　Salaam attacks
　　　　EXCLUDES *salaam tic (781.0)*
　　　　AHA: N-D, '84, 12

§ ✓5th **345.7 Epilepsia partialis continua**
[0-1]　　Kojevnikov's epilepsy
　　　　AHA: ▶1Q, '14, 11◀
　　　　DEF: Continuous muscle contractions and relaxation; result of abnormal neural discharge.

§ ✓5th **345.8 Other forms of epilepsy and recurrent seizures**
[0-1]　　Epilepsy:
　　　　　cursive [running]
　　　　　gelastic
　　　　AHA: ▶1Q, '14, 11◀

§ ✓5th **345.9 Epilepsy, unspecified**
[0-1]　　Epileptic convulsions, fits, or seizures NOS
　　　　Seizure disorder NOS
　　　　EXCLUDES *convulsion (convulsive) disorder (780.39)*
　　　　　　　　convulsive seizure or fit NOS (780.39)
　　　　　　　　recurrent convulsions (780.39)
　　　　AHA: 1Q, '08, 17; N-D, '87, 12; **For code 345.90:** ▶4Q, '13, 86;◀ 2Q, '12, 9; 2Q, '09, 10
　　　　TIP: Code also alcohol withdrawal seizure with epileptic seizure when both conditions are documented by the provider. Assign a separate code for the alcohol dependence.
　　　　G40.909 Epilepsy uns not intractbl w/o status epilepticus　I-10

✓4th **346 Migraine**
　　　　EXCLUDES *headache:*
　　　　　　　　NOS (784.0)
　　　　　　　　syndromes (339.00-339.89)
　　　　AHA: 4Q, '08, 103, 105-107

The following fifth-digit subclassification is for use with category 346:

0 **without mention of intractable migraine without mention of status migrainosus**
　　without mention of refractory migraine without mention of status migrainosus
1 **with intractable migraine, so stated, without mention of status migrainosus**
　　with refractory migraine, so stated, without mention of status migrainosus
2 **without mention of intractable migraine with status migrainosus**
　　without mention of refractory migraine with status migrainosus
3 **with intractable migraine, so stated, with status migrainosus**
　　with refractory migraine, so stated, with status migrainosus

DEF: Benign vascular headache of extreme pain; commonly associated with irritability, nausea, vomiting and often photophobia; premonitory visual hallucination of a crescent in the visual field (scotoma).

§ ✓5th **346.0 Migraine with aura**
[0-3]　　Basilar migraine
　　　　Classic migraine
　　　　Migraine preceded or accompanied by transient focal neurological phenomena
　　　　Migraine triggered seizures
　　　　Migraine with acute-onset aura
　　　　Migraine with aura without headache (migraine equivalents)
　　　　Migraine with prolonged aura
　　　　Migraine with typical aura
　　　　Retinal migraine
　　　　EXCLUDES *persistent migraine aura (346.5, 346.6)*

§ ✓5th **346.1 Migraine without aura**
[0-3]　　Common migraine

§ ✓5th **346.2 Variants of migraine, not elsewhere classified**
[0-3]　　Abdominal migraine
　　　　Cyclical vomiting associated with migraine
　　　　Ophthalmoplegic migraine
　　　　Periodic headache syndromes in child or adolescent
　　　　EXCLUDES *cyclical vomiting NOS (536.2)*
　　　　　　　　psychogenic cyclical vomiting (306.4)

§ ✓5th **346.3 Hemiplegic migraine**
[0-3]　　Familial migraine　　　　Sporadic migraine

§ ✓5th **346.4 Menstrual migraine**　　　　　　　　　　　♀
[0-3]　　Menstrual headache　　　　Premenstrual migraine
　　　　Menstrually related migraine　Pure menstrual migraine
　　　　Premenstrual headache

§ ✓5th **346.5 Persistent migraine aura without cerebral infarction**
[0-3]　　Persistent migraine aura NOS

§ ✓5th **346.6 Persistent migraine aura with cerebral infarction**
[0-3]　　**AHA: For code 346.60:** 4Q, '08, 108
　　　　TIP: Assign also a code for the specific type of cerebral infarction.

§ ✓5th **346.7 Chronic migraine without aura**
[0-3]　　Transformed migraine without aura

§ ✓5th **346.8 Other forms of migraine**
[0-3]

§ ✓5th **346.9 Migraine, unspecified**
[0-3]　　**AHA:** N-D, '85, 16
　　　　G43.909 Migraine unspecified not intract w/o stat migran　I-10

✓4th **347 Cataplexy and narcolepsy**
　　　　DEF: Cataplexy: Sudden onset of muscle weakness with loss of tone and strength; caused by aggressive or spontaneous emotions.
　　　　DEF: Narcolepsy: Brief, recurrent, uncontrollable episodes of sound sleep.

✓5th **347.0 Narcolepsy**

　　　　347.00 Without cataplexy
　　　　　　Narcolepsy NOS

　　　　347.01 With cataplexy

✓5th **347.1 Narcolepsy in conditions classified elsewhere**
　　　　Code first underlying condition

　　　　347.10 Without cataplexy

　　　　347.11 With cataplexy

✓4th **348 Other conditions of brain**

　　348.0 Cerebral cysts
　　　　Arachnoid cyst　　　　Porencephaly, acquired
　　　　Porencephalic cyst　　Pseudoporencephaly
　　　　EXCLUDES *porencephaly (congenital) (742.4)*

　　348.1 Anoxic brain damage
　　　　Use additional E code to identify cause
　　　　EXCLUDES *that occurring in:*
　　　　　　　　abortion (634-638 with .7, 639.8)
　　　　　　　　ectopic or molar pregnancy (639.8)
　　　　　　　　labor or delivery (668.2, 669.4)
　　　　　　　　that of newborn (767.0, 768.0-768.9, 772.1-772.2)
　　　　DEF: Brain injury due to lack of oxygen, other than birth trauma.
　　　　AHA: ▶3Q, '13, 10◀
　　　　G93.1 Anoxic brain damage not elsewhere classified　I-10

　　348.2 Benign intracranial hypertension
　　　　Pseudotumor cerebri
　　　　EXCLUDES *hypertensive encephalopathy (437.2)*
　　　　DEF: Elevated pressure in brain due to fluid retention in brain cavities.

✓5th **348.3 Encephalopathy, not elsewhere classified**
　　　　AHA: 4Q, '03, 58; 3Q, '97, 4

　　　　348.30 Encephalopathy, unspecified
　　　　　　G93.40 Encephalopathy unspecified　　　I-10

　　　　348.31 Metabolic encephalopathy
　　　　　　Septic encephalopathy
　　　　　　EXCLUDES *toxic metabolic encephalopathy (349.82)*
　　　　　　TIP: Physician documentation of "acute confusional state" denotes delirium inherent to the encephalopathy. Do not report an additional code for the delirium.

　　　　348.39 Other encephalopathy
　　　　　　EXCLUDES *encephalopathy:*
　　　　　　　　　alcoholic (291.2)
　　　　　　　　　hepatic (572.2)
　　　　　　　　　hypertensive (437.2)
　　　　　　　　　toxic (349.82)

§　Requires fifth digit. Valid digits are in [brackets] under each code. See appropriate category for codes and definitions.

N Newborn Age: 0　　P Pediatric Age: 0-17　　M Maternity Age: 12-55　　A Adult Age: 15-124

348.4 Compression of brain

Compression ⎱
Herniation ⎰ brain (stem)

Posterior fossa compression syndrome

DEF: Elevated pressure in brain due to blood clot, tumor, fracture, abscess, other condition.

AHA: ▶2Q, '13, 8;◀3Q, '11, 11; 4Q, '94, 37

TIP: Assign for Arnold-Chiari syndrome, Type I. For Type II, III, or IV, refer to categories 741 and 742.

348.5 Cerebral edema

DEF: Elevated pressure in the brain due to fluid retention in brain tissues.

AHA: 4Q, '11, 99; 1Q, '10, 8; 3Q, '09, 8

G93.6 Cerebral edema   `I-10`

√5th 348.8 Other conditions of brain

AHA: S-O, '87, 9

348.81 Temporal sclerosis

Hippocampal sclerosis   Mesial temporal sclerosis

DEF: Abnormal hardening or scarring of frontal lobe tissues due to injury, tumor, congenital anomaly, or hypoxia, resulting in loss of functional neurons; commonly associated with temporal lobe epilepsy.

AHA: 4Q, '09, 83

348.82 Brain death

AHA: 4Q, '11, 99-100

348.89 Other conditions of brain

Cerebral: Cerebral:
calcification   fungus

EXCLUDES brain death (348.82)

348.9 Unspecified condition of brain

√4th 349 Other and unspecified disorders of the nervous system

AHA: 4Q, '08, 109

349.0 Reaction to spinal or lumbar puncture

Headache following lumbar puncture

AHA: 2Q, '99, 9; 3Q, '90, 18

G97.1 Other reaction to spinal and lumbar puncture   `I-10`

349.1 Nervous system complications from surgically implanted device

EXCLUDES immediate postoperative complications (997.00-997.09)

mechanical complications of nervous system device (996.2)

349.2 Disorders of meninges, not elsewhere classified

Adhesions, meningeal (cerebral) (spinal)
Cyst, spinal meninges
Meningocele, acquired
Pseudomeningocele, acquired

AHA: 1Q, '06, 15; 2Q, '98, 18; 3Q, '94, 4

√5th 349.3 Dural tear

349.31 Accidental puncture or laceration of dura during a procedure

Incidental (inadvertent) durotomy

AHA: 4Q, '08, 109-110

TIP: Do not assign code 998.2 Accidental puncture or laceration during a procedure, for an incidental dural tear.

349.39 Other dural tear

√5th 349.8 Other specified disorders of nervous system

349.81 Cerebrospinal fluid rhinorrhea

EXCLUDES cerebrospinal fluid otorrhea (388.61)

DEF: Cerebrospinal fluid discharging from the nose; caused by fracture of frontal bone with tearing of dura mater and arachnoid.

349.82 Toxic encephalopathy

Toxic metabolic encephalopathy

Use additional E code to identify cause

DEF: Brain tissue degeneration due to toxic substance.

AHA: 4Q, '93, 29

G92 Toxic encephalopathy   `I-10`

349.89 Other

349.9 Unspecified disorders of nervous system

Disorder of nervous system (central) NOS

AHA: 3Q, '12, 4

Cranial Nerves

Pons

- Olfactory bulb (I)
- Optic nerve (II)
- Oculomotor nerve (III)
- Trochlear nerve (IV)
- Trigeminal nerve (V)
- Abducens nerve (VI)
- Facial nerve (VII)
- Vestibulocochlear nerve (VIII)
- Glossopharyngeal nerve (IX)
- Vagus nerve (X)
- Accessory nerve (XI)
- Hypoglossal nerve (XII)

Trigeminal and Facial Nerve Branches

Temporal branches
Zygomatic branches
Buccal branches
Mandibular branch
Cervical branch
Branches of Facial Nerve (above)
Maxillary (V2)

Divisions of Trigeminal Nerve (below)
Ophthalmic (V1)
Trigeminal nerve (CN V)
Mandibulary (V3)

Disorders of the Peripheral Nervous System (350-359)

EXCLUDES diseases of:
acoustic [8th] nerve (388.5)
oculomotor [3rd, 4th, 6th] nerves (378.0-378.9)
optic [2nd] nerve (377.0-377.9)
peripheral autonomic nerves (337.0-337.9)

neuralgia ⎱
neuritis ⎰ NOS or "rheumatic" (729.2)
radiculitis

peripheral neuritis in pregnancy (646.4)

√4th 350 Trigeminal nerve disorders

INCLUDES disorders of 5th cranial nerve

350.1 Trigeminal neuralgia

Tic douloureux   Trigeminal neuralgia NOS
Trifacial neuralgia

EXCLUDES postherpetic (053.12)

G50.0 Trigeminal neuralgia   `I-10`

350.2 Atypical face pain

350.8 Other specified trigeminal nerve disorders

350.9 Trigeminal nerve disorder, unspecified

√4th 351 Facial nerve disorders

INCLUDES disorders of 7th cranial nerve

EXCLUDES that in newborn (767.5)

351.0 Bell's palsy

Facial palsy

DEF: Unilateral paralysis of face due to lesion on facial nerve; produces facial distortion.

G51.0 Bell's palsy   `I-10`

351.1 Geniculate ganglionitis

Geniculate ganglionitis NOS

EXCLUDES herpetic (053.11)

DEF: Inflammation of tissue at bend in facial nerve.

351.8 Other facial nerve disorders

Facial myokymia
Melkersson's syndrome

AHA: 3Q, '02, 13

351.9 Facial nerve disorder, unspecified

√4th
√5th Additional Digit Required   **Unspecified Code**   Other Specified Code   Manifestation Code   ▶◀ Revised Text   ● New Code   ▲ Revised Code Title

2015 ICD-9-CM   **October 2014 · Volume 1 – 97**

Diseases of the Nervous System and Sense Organs

352–355.4

✓4th 352 Disorders of other cranial nerves

352.0 Disorders of olfactory [lst] nerve

352.1 Glossopharyngeal neuralgia
DEF: Pain between throat and ear along petrosal and jugular ganglia.
AHA: 2Q, '02, 8

352.2 Other disorders of glossopharyngeal [9th] nerve

352.3 Disorders of pneumogastric [10th] nerve
Disorders of vagal nerve
EXCLUDES paralysis of vocal cords or larynx (478.30-478.34)
DEF: Nerve disorder affecting ear, tongue, pharynx, larynx, esophagus, viscera and thorax.

352.4 Disorders of accessory [11th] nerve
DEF: Nerve disorder affecting palate, pharynx, larynx, thoracic viscera, sternocleidomastoid and trapezius muscles.

352.5 Disorders of hypoglossal [12th] nerve
DEF: Nerve disorder affecting tongue muscles.

352.6 Multiple cranial nerve palsies
Collet-Sicard syndrome
Polyneuritis cranialis

352.9 Unspecified disorder of cranial nerves

✓4th 353 Nerve root and plexus disorders
EXCLUDES conditions due to:
intervertebral disc disorders (722.0-722.9)
spondylosis (720.0-721.9)
vertebrogenic disorders (723.0-724.9)

353.0 Brachial plexus lesions
Cervical rib syndrome   Scalenus anticus syndrome
Costoclavicular syndrome   Thoracic outlet syndrome
EXCLUDES brachial neuritis or radiculitis NOS (723.4)
that in newborn (767.6)
DEF: Acquired disorder in tissue along nerves in shoulder; causes corresponding motor and sensory dysfunction.
AHA: 3Q, '06, 12

353.1 Lumbosacral plexus lesions
DEF: Acquired disorder in tissue along nerves in lower back; causes corresponding motor and sensory dysfunction.

353.2 Cervical root lesions, not elsewhere classified

353.3 Thoracic root lesions, not elsewhere classified

353.4 Lumbosacral root lesions, not elsewhere classified

353.5 Neuralgic amyotrophy
Parsonage-Aldren-Turner syndrome
Code first any associated underlying disease, such as:
diabetes mellitus (249.6, 250.6)

353.6 Phantom limb (syndrome)
DEF: Abnormal tingling or a burning sensation, transient aches, and intermittent or continuous pain perceived as originating in the absent limb.

353.8 Other nerve root and plexus disorders

353.9 Unspecified nerve root and plexus disorder

✓4th 354 Mononeuritis of upper limb and mononeuritis multiplex
DEF: Inflammation of a single nerve; known as mononeuritis multiplex when several nerves in unrelated body areas are affected.

354.0 Carpal tunnel syndrome
Median nerve entrapment
Partial thenar atrophy
DEF: Compression of median nerve by tendons; causes pain, tingling, numbness and burning sensation in hand.
G56.00 Carpal tunnel syndrome unspec upper limb   I-10

354.1 Other lesion of median nerve
Median nerve neuritis

354.2 Lesion of ulnar nerve
Cubital tunnel syndrome   Tardy ulnar nerve palsy

354.3 Lesion of radial nerve
Acute radial nerve palsy
AHA: N-D, '87, 6

354.4 Causalgia of upper limb
Complex regional pain syndrome type II of the upper limb
EXCLUDES causalgia:
NOS (355.9)
lower limb (355.71)
complex regional pain syndrome type II of the lower limb (355.71)
DEF: Peripheral nerve damage, upper limb; usually due to injury; causes burning sensation and trophic skin changes.

354.5 Mononeuritis multiplex
Combinations of single conditions classifiable to 354 or 355

354.8 Other mononeuritis of upper limb

354.9 Mononeuritis of upper limb, unspecified

✓4th 355 Mononeuritis of lower limb

355.0 Lesion of sciatic nerve
EXCLUDES sciatica NOS (724.3)
DEF: Acquired disorder of sciatic nerve; causes motor and sensory dysfunction in back, buttock and leg.
AHA: 2Q, '89, 12

355.1 Meralgia paresthetica
Lateral cutaneous femoral nerve of thigh compression or syndrome
DEF: Inguinal ligament entraps lateral femoral cutaneous nerve; causes tingling, pain and numbness along outer thigh.

355.2 Other lesion of femoral nerve

355.3 Lesion of lateral popliteal nerve
Lesion of common peroneal nerve

355.4 Lesion of medial popliteal nerve

Peripheral Nervous System

Brain
Spinal cord
Brachial plexus
Musculocutaneous
Radial
Median
Deep branch of radial
Superficial branch of radial
Ulnar
Femoral
Common peroneal
Deep peroneal
Superficial peroneal
Intercostal
Subcostal
Lumbar plexus
Sacral plexus
Sciatic
Muscular branches of femoral
Saphenous
Tibial

355.5 Tarsal tunnel syndrome
  DEF: Compressed, entrapped posterior tibial nerve; causes tingling, pain and numbness in sole of foot.

355.6 Lesion of plantar nerve
  Morton's metatarsalgia, neuralgia, or neuroma

✓5ᵗʰ **355.7 Other mononeuritis of lower limb**

  355.71 Causalgia of lower limb
    EXCLUDES causalgia:
      NOS (355.9)
      upper limb (354.4)
      complex regional pain syndrome type II of upper limb (354.4)
    DEF: Dysfunction of lower limb peripheral nerve, usually due to injury; causes burning pain and trophic skin changes.

  355.79 Other mononeuritis of lower limb

355.8 Mononeuritis of lower limb, unspecified

355.9 Mononeuritis of unspecified site
  Causalgia NOS   Complex regional pain syndrome NOS
  EXCLUDES causalgia:
    lower limb (355.71)
    upper limb (354.4)
    complex regional pain syndrome:
    lower limb (355.71)
    upper limb (354.4)
  G58.9 Mononeuropathy unspecified   I-10

✓4ᵗʰ **356 Hereditary and idiopathic peripheral neuropathy**

  356.0 Hereditary peripheral neuropathy
    Déjérine-Sottas disease

  356.1 Peroneal muscular atrophy
    Charcôt-Marie-Tooth disease
    Neuropathic muscular atrophy
    DEF: Genetic disorder, in muscles innervated by peroneal nerves; symptoms include muscle wasting in lower limbs and locomotor difficulties.

  356.2 Hereditary sensory neuropathy
    DEF: Inherited disorder in dorsal root ganglia, optic nerve, and cerebellum, causing sensory losses, shooting pains, and foot ulcers.

  356.3 Refsum's disease
    Heredopathia atactica polyneuritiformis
    DEF: Genetic disorder of lipid metabolism; causes persistent, painful inflammation of nerves and retinitis pigmentosa.

  356.4 Idiopathic progressive polyneuropathy

  356.8 Other specified idiopathic peripheral neuropathy
    Supranuclear paralysis

  356.9 Unspecified
    AHA: ▶1Q, '13, 3◀
    G60.9 Hereditary & idiopathic neuropathy unspecified   I-10

✓4ᵗʰ **357 Inflammatory and toxic neuropathy**

  357.0 Acute infective polyneuritis
    Guillain-Barré syndrome   Postinfectious polyneuritis
    DEF: Guillain-Barré syndrome: acute demyelinating polyneuropathy preceded by viral illness (i.e., herpes, cytomegalovirus [CMV], Epstein-Barr virus [EBV]) or a bacterial illness; areflexic motor paralysis with mild sensory disturbance and acellular rise in spinal fluid protein.
    AHA: 2Q, '98, 12

  357.1 Polyneuropathy in collagen vascular disease
    Code first underlying disease, as:
      disseminated lupus erythematosus (710.0)
      polyarteritis nodosa (446.0)
      rheumatoid arthritis (714.0)

  357.2 Polyneuropathy in diabetes
    Code first underlying disease (249.6, 250.6)
    AHA: 4Q, '09, 151; 2Q, '09, 13, 15; 3Q, '08, 5; 4Q, '03, 105; 2Q, '92, 15; 3Q, '91, 9

  357.3 Polyneuropathy in malignant disease
    Code first underlying disease (140.0-208.9)

357.4 Polyneuropathy in other diseases classified elsewhere
  Code first underlying disease, as:
    amyloidosis (277.30-277.39)
    beriberi (265.0)
    chronic uremia (585.9)
    deficiency of B vitamins (266.0-266.9)
    diphtheria (032.0-032.9)
    hypoglycemia (251.2)
    pellagra (265.2)
    porphyria (277.1)
    sarcoidosis (135)
    uremia NOS (586)
    EXCLUDES polyneuropathy in:
      herpes zoster (053.13)
      mumps (072.72)
    AHA: 2Q, '08, 8; 2Q, '98, 15
    G63 Polyneuropathy in diseases classified elsewhere   I-10

357.5 Alcoholic polyneuropathy

357.6 Polyneuropathy due to drugs
  Use additional E code to identify drug

357.7 Polyneuropathy due to other toxic agents
  Use additional E code to identify toxic agent

✓5ᵗʰ **357.8 Other**
  AHA: 4Q, '02, 47; 2Q, '98, 12

  357.81 Chronic inflammatory demyelinating polyneuritis
    DEF: Inflammation of peripheral nerves resulting in destruction of myelin sheath; associated with diabetes mellitus, dysproteinemia, renal failure and malnutrition; symptoms include tingling, numbness, burning pain, diminished tendon reflexes, weakness of lower extremities.

  357.82 Critical illness polyneuropathy
    Acute motor neuropathy
    DEF: An acute axonal neuropathy, both sensory and motor, that is associated with Systemic Inflammatory Response Syndrome (SIRS).
    AHA: 4Q, '03, 111

  357.89 Other inflammatory and toxic neuropathy
    AHA: ▶1Q, '14, 10; 1Q, '13, 3◀

357.9 Unspecified

✓4ᵗʰ **358 Myoneural disorders**

✓5ᵗʰ **358.0 Myasthenia gravis**
    DEF: Autoimmune disorder of acetylcholine at neuromuscular junction; causing fatigue of voluntary muscles.
    AHA: 4Q, '03, 59

  358.00 Myasthenia gravis without (acute) exacerbation
    Myasthenia gravis NOS
    G70.00 Myasthenia gravis w/o (acute) exacerbation   I-10

  358.01 Myasthenia gravis with (acute) exacerbation
    Myasthenia gravis in crisis
    AHA: 4Q, '07, 109; 1Q, '05, 4; 4Q, '04, 139

358.1 Myasthenic syndromes in diseases classified elsewhere
  Code first underlying disease, as:
    botulism (005.1, 040.41-040.42)
    hypothyroidism (244.0-244.9)
    malignant neoplasm (140.0-208.9)
    pernicious anemia (281.0)
    thyrotoxicosis (242.0-242.9)

358.2 Toxic myoneural disorders
  Use additional E code to identify toxic agent

✓5ᵗʰ **358.3 Lambert-Eaton syndrome**
    Eaton-Lambert syndrome
    AHA: 4Q, '11, 100-101

  358.30 Lambert-Eaton syndrome, unspecified
    Lambert-Eaton syndrome NOS
    AHA: 4Q, '11, 101

  358.31 Lambert-Eaton syndrome in neoplastic disease
    Code first the underlying neoplastic disease

  358.39 Lambert-Eaton syndrome in other diseases classified elsewhere
    Code first the underlying condition

✓4ᵗʰ/✓5ᵗʰ Additional Digit Required   Unspecified Code   Other Specified Code   Manifestation Code   ▶◀ Revised Text   ● New Code   ▲ Revised Code Title

Diseases of the Nervous System and Sense Organs

358.8–360.03

358.8 Other specified myoneural disorders

358.9 Myoneural disorders, unspecified
>AHA: 2Q, '02, 16

√4th 359 Muscular dystrophies and other myopathies
>EXCLUDES idiopathic polymyositis (710.4)

359.0 Congenital hereditary muscular dystrophy
>Benign congenital myopathy
>Central core disease
>Centronuclear myopathy
>Myotubular myopathy
>Nemaline body disease
>
>EXCLUDES arthrogryposis multiplex congenita (754.89)
>
>DEF: Genetic disorder; causing progressive or nonprogressive muscle weakness.

359.1 Hereditary progressive muscular dystrophy
>Muscular dystrophy:
> NOS
> distal
> Duchenne
> Erb's
> fascioscapulohumeral
>Muscular dystrophy:
> Gower's
> Landouzy-Déjérine
> limb-girdle
> ocular
> oculopharyngeal
>
>DEF: Genetic degenerative, muscle disease; causes progressive weakness, wasting of muscle with no nerve involvement.

√5th 359.2 Myotonic disorders
>EXCLUDES periodic paralysis (359.3)
>
>DEF: Impaired movement due to spasmatic, rigid muscles.
>
>AHA: 4Q, '07, 75

359.21 Myotonic muscular dystrophy
>Dystrophia myotonica
>Myotonia atrophica
>Myotonic dystrophy
>Proximal myotonic myopathy [PROMM]
>Steinert's disease

359.22 Myotonia congenita
>Acetazolamide responsive myotonia congenita
>Dominant form [Thomsen's disease]
>Myotonia levior
>Recessive form [Becker's disease]

359.23 Myotonic chondrodystrophy
>Congenital myotonic chondrodystrophy
>Schwartz-Jampel disease

359.24 Drug induced myotonia
>Use additional E code to identify drug

359.29 Other specified myotonic disorder
>Myotonia fluctuans
>Myotonia permanens
>Paramyotonia congenita (of von Eulenburg)

359.3 Periodic paralysis
>Familial periodic paralysis
>Hypokalemic familial periodic paralysis
>Hyperkalemic periodic paralysis
>Hypokalemic periodic paralysis
>Potassium sensitive periodic paralysis
>
>EXCLUDES paramyotonia congenita (of von Eulenburg) (359.29)
>
>DEF: Genetic disorder; characterized by rapidly progressive flaccid paralysis; attacks often occur after exercise or exposure to cold or dietary changes.

359.4 Toxic myopathy
>Use additional E code to identify toxic agent
>
>DEF: Muscle disorder caused by toxic agent.
>
>AHA: 1Q, '88, 5

359.5 Myopathy in endocrine diseases classified elsewhere
>Code first underlying disease, as:
> Addison's disease (255.41)
> Cushing's syndrome (255.0)
> hypopituitarism (253.2)
> myxedema (244.0-244.9)
> thyrotoxicosis (242.0-242.9)
>
>DEF: Muscle disorder secondary to dysfunction in hormone secretion.

Eye

Globe (Eyeball)

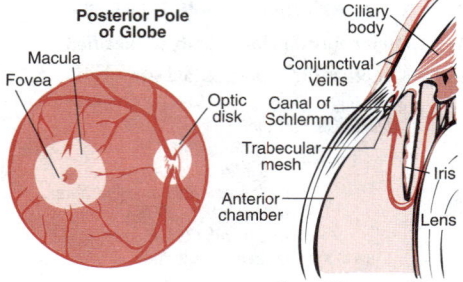

Posterior Pole of Globe

Flow of Aqueous Humor

359.6 Symptomatic inflammatory myopathy in diseases classified elsewhere
>Code first underlying disease, as:
> amyloidosis (277.30-277.39)
> disseminated lupus erythematosus (710.0)
> malignant neoplasm (140.0-208.9)
> polyarteritis nodosa (446.0)
> rheumatoid arthritis (714.0)
> sarcoidosis (135)
> scleroderma (710.1)
> Sjögren's disease (710.2)

√5th 359.7 Inflammatory and immune myopathies, NEC

359.71 Inclusion body myositis
>IBM
>
>DEF: Progressive, debilitating inflammatory muscle disease characterized by dysphagia, chronic muscle swelling, weakness, and atrophy (wasting); impairs fine motor functions.
>
>AHA: 4Q, '09, 84

359.79 Other inflammatory and immune myopathies, NEC
>Inflammatory myopathy NOS

√5th 359.8 Other myopathies
>AHA: 4Q, '02, 47; 3Q, '90, 17

359.81 Critical illness myopathy
>Acute necrotizing myopathy
>Acute quadriplegic myopathy
>Intensive care (ICU) myopathy
>Myopathy of critical illness

359.89 Other myopathies

359.9 Myopathy, unspecified

Disorders of the Eye and Adnexa (360-379)

Use additional external cause code, if applicable, to identify the cause of the eye condition

√4th 360 Disorders of the globe
>INCLUDES disorders affecting multiple structures of eye

√5th 360.0 Purulent endophthalmitis
>EXCLUDES bleb associated endophthalmitis (379.63)

360.00 Purulent endophthalmitis, unspecified

360.01 Acute endophthalmitis

360.02 Panophthalmitis

360.03 Chronic endophthalmitis

Adnexa

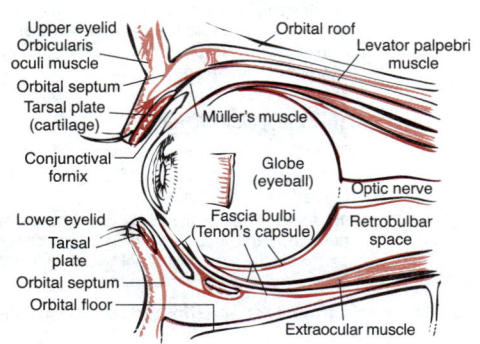

Upper eyelid
Orbicularis oculi muscle
Orbital septum
Tarsal plate (cartilage)
Conjunctival fornix
Lower eyelid
Tarsal plate
Orbital septum
Orbital floor
Orbital roof
Levator palpebri muscle
Müller's muscle
Globe (eyeball)
Optic nerve
Fascia bulbi (Tenon's capsule)
Retrobulbar space
Extraocular muscle

360.04 Vitreous abscess

✓5ᵗʰ **360.1 Other endophthalmitis**
> **EXCLUDES** bleb associated endophthalmitis (379.63)

360.11 Sympathetic uveitis
> **DEF:** Inflammation of vascular layer of uninjured eye; follows injury to other eye.

360.12 Panuveitis
> **DEF:** Inflammation of entire vascular layer of eye, including choroid, iris and ciliary body.

360.13 Parasitic endophthalmitis NOS
> **DEF:** Parasitic infection causing inflammation of the entire eye.

360.14 Ophthalmia nodosa
> **DEF:** Conjunctival inflammation caused by embedded hairs.

360.19 Other
> Phacoanaphylactic endophthalmitis

✓5ᵗʰ **360.2 Degenerative disorders of globe**
> **AHA:** 3Q, '91, 3

360.20 Degenerative disorder of globe, unspecified

360.21 Progressive high (degenerative) myopia
> Malignant myopia
> **DEF:** Severe, progressive nearsightedness in adults, complicated by serious disease of the choroid; leads to retinal detachment and blindness.

360.23 Siderosis
> **DEF:** Iron pigment deposits within tissue of eyeball; caused by high iron content of blood.

360.24 Other metallosis
> Chalcosis
> **DEF:** Metal deposits, other than iron, within eyeball tissues.

360.29 Other
> **EXCLUDES** xerophthalmia (264.7)

✓5ᵗʰ **360.3 Hypotony of eye**

360.30 Hypotony, unspecified
> **DEF:** Low osmotic pressure causing lack of tone, tension and strength.

360.31 Primary hypotony

360.32 Ocular fistula causing hypotony
> **DEF:** Low intraocular pressure due to leak through abnormal passage.

360.33 Hypotony associated with other ocular disorders

360.34 Flat anterior chamber
> **DEF:** Low pressure behind cornea, causing compression.

✓5ᵗʰ **360.4 Degenerated conditions of globe**

360.40 Degenerated globe or eye, unspecified

360.41 Blind hypotensive eye
> Atrophy of globe　　Phthisis bulbi
> **DEF:** Vision loss due to extremely low intraocular pressure.

360.42 Blind hypertensive eye
> Absolute glaucoma
> **DEF:** Vision loss due to painful, high intraocular pressure.

360.43 Hemophthalmos, except current injury
> **EXCLUDES** traumatic (871.0-871.9, 921.0-921.9)
> **DEF:** Pool of blood within eyeball, not from current injury.

360.44 Leucocoria
> **DEF:** Whitish mass or reflex in the pupil behind lens; also called cat's eye reflex; often indicative of retinoblastoma.

✓5ᵗʰ **360.5 Retained (old) intraocular foreign body, magnetic**
> Use additional code to identify foreign body (V90.11)
> **EXCLUDES** current penetrating injury with magnetic foreign body (871.5)
> retained (old) foreign body of orbit (376.6)

360.50 Foreign body, magnetic, intraocular, unspecified

360.51 Foreign body, magnetic, in anterior chamber

360.52 Foreign body, magnetic, in iris or ciliary body

360.53 Foreign body, magnetic, in lens

360.54 Foreign body, magnetic, in vitreous

360.55 Foreign body, magnetic, in posterior wall

360.59 Foreign body, magnetic, in other or multiple sites

✓5ᵗʰ **360.6 Retained (old) intraocular foreign body, nonmagnetic**
> Retained (old) foreign body:
> NOS
> nonmagnetic
> Use additional code to identify foreign body (V90.01-V90.10, V90.12, V90.2-V90.9)
> **EXCLUDES** current penetrating injury with (nonmagnetic) foreign body (871.6)
> retained (old) foreign body in orbit (376.6)

360.60 Foreign body, intraocular, unspecified

360.61 Foreign body in anterior chamber

360.62 Foreign body in iris or ciliary body

360.63 Foreign body in lens

360.64 Foreign body in vitreous

360.65 Foreign body in posterior wall

360.69 Foreign body in other or multiple sites

✓5ᵗʰ **360.8 Other disorders of globe**

360.81 Luxation of globe
> **DEF:** Displacement of eyeball.

360.89 Other

360.9 Unspecified disorder of globe

✓4ᵗʰ **361 Retinal detachments and defects**
> **DEF:** Disorders of light-sensitive layer at back of eye, which separates from blood supply, disrupting vision.

✓5ᵗʰ **361.0 Retinal detachment with retinal defect**
> Rhegmatogenous retinal detachment
> **EXCLUDES** detachment of retinal pigment epithelium (362.42-362.43)
> retinal detachment (serous) (without defect) (361.2)

361.00 Retinal detachment with retinal defect, unspecified

361.01 Recent detachment, partial, with single defect

361.02 Recent detachment, partial, with multiple defects

361.03 Recent detachment, partial, with giant tear

361.04 Recent detachment, partial, with retinal dialysis
> Dialysis (juvenile) of retina (with detachment)

361.05 Recent detachment, total or subtotal

361.06 Old detachment, partial
> Delimited old retinal detachment

361.07 Old detachment, total or subtotal

Diseases of the Nervous System and Sense Organs

361.1–362.33

✓5ᵗʰ **361.1 Retinoschisis and retinal cysts**

> **EXCLUDES**   *juvenile retinoschisis (362.73)*
> *microcystoid degeneration of retina (362.62)*
> *parasitic cyst of retina (360.13)*

361.10 Retinoschisis, unspecified

> **DEF:** Separation of retina due to degenerative process of aging; should not be confused with acute retinal detachment.

361.11 Flat retinoschisis

> **DEF:** Slow, progressive split of retinal sensory layers.

361.12 Bullous retinoschisis

> **DEF:** Fluid retention between split retinal sensory layers.

361.13 Primary retinal cysts

361.14 Secondary retinal cysts

361.19 Other

> Pseudocyst of retina

361.2 Serous retinal detachment

> Retinal detachment without retinal defect
>
> **EXCLUDES**   *central serous retinopathy (362.41)*
> *retinal pigment epithelium detachment (362.42-362.43)*

✓5ᵗʰ **361.3 Retinal defects without detachment**

> **EXCLUDES**   *chorioretinal scars after surgery for detachment (363.30-363.35)*
> *peripheral retinal degeneration without defect (362.60-362.66)*

361.30 Retinal defect, unspecified

> Retinal break(s) NOS

361.31 Round hole of retina without detachment

361.32 Horseshoe tear of retina without detachment

> Operculum of retina without mention of detachment

361.33 Multiple defects of retina without detachment

✓5ᵗʰ **361.8 Other forms of retinal detachment**

361.81 Traction detachment of retina

> Traction detachment with vitreoretinal organization

361.89 Other

> **AHA:** 3Q, '99, 12

361.9 Unspecified retinal detachment

> **AHA:** N-D, '87, 10

✓4ᵗʰ **362 Other retinal disorders**

> **EXCLUDES**   *chorioretinal scars (363.30-363.35)*
> *chorioretinitis (363.0-363.2)*

✓5ᵗʰ **362.0 Diabetic retinopathy**

> *Code first diabetes (249.5, 250.5)*
>
> **DEF:** Retinal changes in diabetes of long duration; causes hemorrhages, microaneurysms, waxy deposits and proliferative noninflammatory degenerative disease of retina.
> **AHA:** 4Q, '05, 65; 3Q, '91, 8

362.01 Background diabetic retinopathy

> Diabetic retinal microaneurysms
> Diabetic retinopathy NOS

362.02 Proliferative diabetic retinopathy

> **DEF:** Occurrence of the ischemic effects of vessel blockages result in neovascularization; new blood vessels begin to form to compensate for restricted blood flow; multiple areas of the retina and inner vitreous may be affected.
> **AHA:** 3Q, '96, 5

362.03 Nonproliferative diabetic retinopathy NOS

362.04 Mild nonproliferative diabetic retinopathy

> **DEF:** Early stages of degenerative condition of the retina due to diabetes; microaneurysm formation; small balloon-like swelling of the retinal vessels.

362.05 Moderate nonproliferative diabetic retinopathy

> **DEF:** Stage of degenerative condition of the retina due to diabetes with pronounced microaneurysms; vessel blockages can occur.

362.06 Severe nonproliferative diabetic retinopathy

> **DEF:** Stage of degenerative condition of the retina due to diabetes in which vascular breakdown in the retina results in multiple vascular blockages, or "beadings," with intraretinal hemorrhages.
> **AHA:** 4Q, '05, 67

362.07 Diabetic macular edema

> **NOTE** Code 362.07 must be used with a code for diabetic retinopathy (362.01-362.06)
> Diabetic retinal edema
>
> **DEF:** Leakage from retinal blood vessels causes swelling of the macula and impaired vision; exudates or plaques may develop in the posterior pole of the retina due to the breakdown of retinal vasculature.

✓5ᵗʰ **362.1 Other background retinopathy and retinal vascular changes**

362.10 Background retinopathy, unspecified

> **AHA:** 1Q, '06, 12

362.11 Hypertensive retinopathy

> **DEF:** Retinal irregularities caused by systemic hypertension.
> **AHA:** 3Q, '90, 3

362.12 Exudative retinopathy

> Coats' syndrome
> **AHA:** 3Q, '99, 12

362.13 Changes in vascular appearance

> Vascular sheathing of retina
> Use additional code for any associated atherosclerosis (440.8)

362.14 Retinal microaneurysms NOS

> **DEF:** Microscopic dilation of retinal vessels in nondiabetic.

362.15 Retinal telangiectasia

> **DEF:** Dilation of blood vessels of the retina.

362.16 Retinal neovascularization NOS

> Neovascularization: Neovascularization:
> choroidal   subretinal
> **DEF:** New and abnormal vascular growth in the retina.

362.17 Other intraretinal microvascular abnormalities

> Retinal sclerosis
> Retinal varices

362.18 Retinal vasculitis

> Eales' disease   Retinal:
> Retinal: perivasculitis
> arteritis   phlebitis
> endarteritis
> **DEF:** Inflammation of retinal blood vessels.

✓5ᵗʰ **362.2 Other proliferative retinopathy**

> **AHA:** 4Q, '08, 110-111

362.20 Retinopathy of prematurity, unspecified

> Retinopathy of prematurity NOS

362.21 Retrolental fibroplasia

> Cicatricial retinopathy of prematurity
> **DEF:** Fibrous tissue in vitreous, from retina to lens, causing blindness; associated with premature infants requiring high amounts of oxygen.

362.22 Retinopathy of prematurity, stage 0

362.23 Retinopathy of prematurity, stage 1

362.24 Retinopathy of prematurity, stage 2

362.25 Retinopathy of prematurity, stage 3

362.26 Retinopathy of prematurity, stage 4

362.27 Retinopathy of prematurity, stage 5

362.29 Other nondiabetic proliferative retinopathy

> **AHA:** 3Q, '96, 5

✓5ᵗʰ **362.3 Retinal vascular occlusion**

> **DEF:** Obstructed blood flow to and from retina.

362.30 Retinal vascular occlusion, unspecified

362.31 Central retinal artery occlusion

362.32 Arterial branch occlusion

362.33 Partial arterial occlusion

> Hollenhorst plaque   Retinal microembolism

N Newborn Age: 0   P Pediatric Age: 0-17   M Maternity Age: 12-55   A Adult Age: 15-124

362.34 Transient arterial occlusion
Amaurosis fugax
AHA: 1Q, '00, 16

362.35 Central retinal vein occlusion
AHA: 2Q, '93, 6

362.36 Venous tributary (branch) occlusion

362.37 Venous engorgement
Occlusion:
incipient
partial } of retinal vein

√5ᵗʰ **362.4 Separation of retinal layers**
EXCLUDES retinal detachment (serous) (361.2)
rhegmatogenous (361.00-361.07)

362.40 Retinal layer separation, unspecified

362.41 Central serous retinopathy
DEF: Serous-filled blister causing detachment of retina from pigment epithelium.

362.42 Serous detachment of retinal pigment epithelium
Exudative detachment of retinal pigment epithelium
DEF: Blister of fatty fluid causing detachment of retina from pigment epithelium.

362.43 Hemorrhagic detachment of retinal pigment epithelium
DEF: Blood-filled blister causing detachment of retina from pigment epithelium.

√5ᵗʰ **362.5 Degeneration of macula and posterior pole**
EXCLUDES degeneration of optic disc (377.21-377.24)
hereditary retinal degeneration [dystrophy] (362.70-362.77)

362.50 Macular degeneration (senile), unspecified

362.51 Nonexudative senile macular degeneration
Senile macular degeneration:
atrophic
dry

362.52 Exudative senile macular degeneration
Kuhnt-Junius degeneration
Senile macular degeneration:
disciform
wet
DEF: Leakage in macular blood vessels with loss of visual acuity.

362.53 Cystoid macular degeneration
Cystoid macular edema
DEF: Retinal swelling and cyst formation in macula.

362.54 Macular cyst, hole, or pseudohole
AHA: 4Q, '11, 106

362.55 Toxic maculopathy
Use additional E code to identify drug, if drug induced

362.56 Macular puckering
Preretinal fibrosis

362.57 Drusen (degenerative)
DEF: White, hyaline deposits on Bruch's membrane (lamina basalis choroideae).

√5ᵗʰ **362.6 Peripheral retinal degenerations**
EXCLUDES hereditary retinal degeneration [dystrophy] (362.70-362.77)
retinal degeneration with retinal defect (361.00-361.07)

362.60 Peripheral retinal degeneration, unspecified

362.61 Paving stone degeneration
DEF: Degeneration of peripheral retina; causes thinning through which choroid is visible.

362.62 Microcystoid degeneration
Blessig's cysts Iwanoff's cysts

362.63 Lattice degeneration
Palisade degeneration of retina
DEF: Degeneration of retina; often bilateral, usually benign; characterized by lines intersecting at irregular intervals in peripheral retina; retinal thinning and retinal holes may occur.

362.64 Senile reticular degeneration
DEF: Net-like appearance of retina; sign of degeneration.

362.65 Secondary pigmentary degeneration
Pseudoretinitis pigmentosa

362.66 Secondary vitreoretinal degenerations

√5ᵗʰ **362.7 Hereditary retinal dystrophies**
DEF: Genetically induced progressive changes in retina.

362.70 Hereditary retinal dystrophy, unspecified

362.71 Retinal dystrophy in systemic or cerebroretinal lipidoses
Code first underlying disease, as:
cerebroretinal lipidoses (330.1)
systemic lipidoses (272.7)

362.72 Retinal dystrophy in other systemic disorders and syndromes
Code first underlying disease, as:
Bassen-Kornzweig syndrome (272.5)
Refsum's disease (356.3)

362.73 Vitreoretinal dystrophies
Juvenile retinoschisis

362.74 Pigmentary retinal dystrophy
Retinal dystrophy, albipunctate
Retinitis pigmentosa

362.75 Other dystrophies primarily involving the sensory retina
Progressive cone(-rod) dystrophy
Stargardt's disease

362.76 Dystrophies primarily involving the retinal pigment epithelium
Fundus flavimaculatus   Vitelliform dystrophy

362.77 Dystrophies primarily involving Bruch's membrane
Dystrophy:
hyaline
pseudoinflammatory foveal
Hereditary drusen

√5ᵗʰ **362.8 Other retinal disorders**
EXCLUDES chorioretinal inflammations (363.0-363.2)
chorioretinal scars (363.30-363.35)

362.81 Retinal hemorrhage
Hemorrhage: Hemorrhage:
preretinal   subretinal
retinal (deep) (superficial)
AHA: 4Q, '96, 43

362.82 Retinal exudates and deposits

362.83 Retinal edema
Retinal:
cotton wool spots
edema (localized) (macular) (peripheral)
DEF: Retinal swelling due to fluid accumulation.

362.84 Retinal ischemia
DEF: Reduced retinal blood supply.

362.85 Retinal nerve fiber bundle defects

362.89 Other retinal disorders

362.9 Unspecified retinal disorder

√4ᵗʰ **363 Chorioretinal inflammations, scars, and other disorders of choroid**

√5ᵗʰ **363.0 Focal chorioretinitis and focal retinochoroiditis**
EXCLUDES focal chorioretinitis or retinochoroiditis in:
histoplasmosis (115.02, 115.12, 115.92)
toxoplasmosis (130.2)
congenital infection (771.2)

363.00 Focal chorioretinitis, unspecified
Focal:
choroiditis or chorioretinitis NOS
retinitis or retinochoroiditis NOS

363.01 Focal choroiditis and chorioretinitis, juxtapapillary

363.03 Focal choroiditis and chorioretinitis of other posterior pole

√4ᵗʰ √5ᵗʰ Additional Digit Required	Unspecified Code	Other Specified Code	Manifestation Code	►◄ Revised Text	● New Code	▲ Revised Code Title

363.04 Focal choroiditis and chorioretinitis, peripheral

363.05 Focal retinitis and retinochoroiditis, juxtapapillary
Neuroretinitis

363.06 Focal retinitis and retinochoroiditis, macular or paramacular

363.07 Focal retinitis and retinochoroiditis of other posterior pole

363.08 Focal retinitis and retinochoroiditis, peripheral

√5th **363.1 Disseminated chorioretinitis and disseminated retinochoroiditis**

> EXCLUDES   *disseminated choroiditis or chorioretinitis in secondary syphilis (091.51)*
> *neurosyphilitic disseminated retinitis or retinochoroiditis (094.83)*
> *retinal (peri)vasculitis (362.18)*

363.10 Disseminated chorioretinitis, unspecified
Disseminated:
choroiditis or chorioretinitis NOS
retinitis or retinochoroiditis NOS

363.11 Disseminated choroiditis and, chorioretinitis posterior pole

363.12 Disseminated choroiditis and chorioretinitis, peripheral

363.13 Disseminated choroiditis and chorioretinitis, generalized
> Code first any underlying disease, as:
> tuberculosis (017.3)

363.14 Disseminated retinitis and retinochoroiditis, metastatic

363.15 Disseminated retinitis and retinochoroiditis, pigment epitheliopathy
Acute posterior multifocal placoid pigment epitheliopathy
> DEF: Widespread inflammation of retina and choroid; characterized by pigmented epithelium involvement.

√5th **363.2 Other and unspecified forms of chorioretinitis and retinochoroiditis**

> EXCLUDES   *panophthalmitis (360.02)*
> *sympathetic uveitis (360.11)*
> *uveitis NOS (364.3)*

363.20 Chorioretinitis, unspecified
Choroiditis NOS   Uveitis, posterior NOS
Retinitis NOS

363.21 Pars planitis
Posterior cyclitis
> DEF: Inflammation of peripheral retina and ciliary body; characterized by bands of white cells.

363.22 Harada's disease
> DEF: Retinal detachment and bilateral widespread exudative choroiditis; symptoms include headache, vomiting, increased lymphocytes in cerebrospinal fluid; with temporary or permanent deafness.

√5th **363.3 Chorioretinal scars**
Scar (postinflammatory) (postsurgical) (posttraumatic):
choroid
retina

363.30 Chorioretinal scar, unspecified

363.31 Solar retinopathy
> DEF: Retinal scarring caused by solar radiation.

363.32 Other macular scars

363.33 Other scars of posterior pole

363.34 Peripheral scars

363.35 Disseminated scars

√5th **363.4 Choroidal degenerations**

363.40 Choroidal degeneration, unspecified
Choroidal sclerosis NOS

363.41 Senile atrophy of choroid
> DEF: Wasting away of choroid; due to aging.

363.42 Diffuse secondary atrophy of choroid
> DEF: Wasting away of choroid in systemic disease.

363.43 Angioid streaks of choroid
> DEF: Degeneration of choroid; characterized by dark brown streaks radiating from optic disc; occurs with pseudoxanthoma, elasticum or Paget's disease.

√5th **363.5 Hereditary choroidal dystrophies**
Hereditary choroidal atrophy:
partial [choriocapillaris]
total [all vessels]

363.50 Hereditary choroidal dystrophy or atrophy, unspecified

363.51 Circumpapillary dystrophy of choroid, partial

363.52 Circumpapillary dystrophy of choroid, total
Helicoid dystrophy of choroid

363.53 Central dystrophy of choroid, partial
Dystrophy, choroidal: Dystrophy, choroidal:
central areolar   circinate

363.54 Central choroidal atrophy, total
Dystrophy, choroidal: Dystrophy, choroidal:
central gyrate   serpiginous

363.55 Choroideremia
> DEF: Hereditary choroid degeneration, occurs in first decade; characterized by constricted visual field and ultimately blindness in males; less debilitating in females.

363.56 Other diffuse or generalized dystrophy, partial
Diffuse choroidal sclerosis

363.57 Other diffuse or generalized dystrophy, total
Generalized gyrate atrophy, choroid

√5th **363.6 Choroidal hemorrhage and rupture**

363.61 Choroidal hemorrhage, unspecified

363.62 Expulsive choroidal hemorrhage

363.63 Choroidal rupture

√5th **363.7 Choroidal detachment**

363.70 Choroidal detachment, unspecified

363.71 Serous choroidal detachment
> DEF: Detachment of choroid from sclera; due to blister of serous fluid.

363.72 Hemorrhagic choroidal detachment
> DEF: Detachment of choroid from sclera; due to blood-filled blister.

363.8 Other disorders of choroid

363.9 Unspecified disorder of choroid

√4th **364 Disorders of iris and ciliary body**

√5th **364.0 Acute and subacute iridocyclitis**
Anterior uveitis
Cylitis   } acute, subacute
Iridocyclitis
Iritis

> EXCLUDES   *gonococcal (098.41)*
> *herpes simplex (054.44)*
> *herpes zoster (053.22)*

364.00 Acute and subacute iridocyclitis, unspecified

364.01 Primary iridocyclitis

364.02 Recurrent iridocyclitis

364.03 Secondary iridocyclitis, infectious

364.04 Secondary iridocyclitis, noninfectious
Aqueous: Aqueous:
cells   flare
fibrin

364.05 Hypopyon
> DEF: Accumulation of white blood cells between cornea and lens.

√5th **364.1 Chronic iridocyclitis**
> EXCLUDES   *posterior cyclitis (363.21)*

364.10 Chronic iridocyclitis, unspecified

N   Newborn Age: 0   P   Pediatric Age: 0-17   M   Maternity Age: 12-55   A   Adult Age: 15-124

364.11 Chronic iridocyclitis in diseases classified elsewhere

> Code first underlying disease, as:
> sarcoidosis (135)
> tuberculosis (017.3)

EXCLUDES syphilitic iridocyclitis (091.52)

DEF: Persistent inflammation of iris and ciliary body; due to underlying disease or condition.

√5ᵗʰ **364.2 Certain types of iridocyclitis**

EXCLUDES posterior cyclitis (363.21)
sympathetic uveitis (360.11)

364.21 Fuchs' heterochromic cyclitis

DEF: Chronic cyclitis characterized by differences in the color of the two irises; the lighter iris appears in the inflamed eye.

364.22 Glaucomatocyclitic crises

DEF: An uncommon inflammatory unilateral eye condition, characteristic recurrent episodes of high intraocular pressure accompanied by mild inflammation.

364.23 Lens-induced iridocyclitis

DEF: Inflammation of iris; due to immune reaction to proteins in lens following trauma or other lens abnormality.

364.24 Vogt-Koyanagi syndrome

DEF: Uveomeningitis with exudative iridocyclitis and choroiditis; causes depigmentation of hair and skin, detached retina; tinnitus and loss of hearing.

364.3 Unspecified iridocyclitis

Uveitis NOS

√5ᵗʰ **364.4 Vascular disorders of iris and ciliary body**

364.41 Hyphema

Hemorrhage of iris or ciliary body

DEF: Hemorrhage in anterior chamber; also called hyphemia or "blood shot" eyes.

364.42 Rubeosis iridis

Neovascularization of iris or ciliary body

DEF: Blood vessel and connective tissue formation on surface of iris; symptomatic of diabetic retinopathy, central retinal vein occlusion and retinal detachment.

√5ᵗʰ **364.5 Degenerations of iris and ciliary body**

364.51 Essential or progressive iris atrophy

364.52 Iridoschisis

DEF: Splitting of the iris into two layers.

364.53 Pigmentary iris degeneration

Acquired heterochromia
Pigment dispersion syndrome } of iris
Translucency

364.54 Degeneration of pupillary margin

Atrophy of sphincter
Ectropion of pigment epithelium } of iris

364.55 Miotic cysts of pupillary margin

DEF: Serous-filled sacs in pupillary margin of iris.

364.56 Degenerative changes of chamber angle

364.57 Degenerative changes of ciliary body

364.59 Other iris atrophy

Iris atrophy (generalized) (sector shaped)

√5ᵗʰ **364.6 Cysts of iris, ciliary body, and anterior chamber**

EXCLUDES miotic pupillary cyst (364.55)
parasitic cyst (360.13)

364.60 Idiopathic cysts

DEF: Fluid-filled sacs in iris or ciliary body; unknown etiology.

364.61 Implantation cysts

Epithelial down-growth, anterior chamber
Implantation cysts (surgical) (traumatic)

364.62 Exudative cysts of iris or anterior chamber

364.63 Primary cyst of pars plana

DEF: Fluid-filled sacs of outermost ciliary ring.

364.64 Exudative cyst of pars plana

DEF: Protein, fatty-filled sacs of outermost ciliary ring; due to fluid leak from blood vessels.

√5ᵗʰ **364.7 Adhesions and disruptions of iris and ciliary body**

EXCLUDES flat anterior chamber (360.34)

364.70 Adhesions of iris, unspecified

Synechiae (iris) NOS

364.71 Posterior synechiae

DEF: Adhesion binding iris to lens.

364.72 Anterior synechiae

DEF: Adhesion binding the iris to cornea.

364.73 Goniosynechiae

Peripheral anterior synechiae

DEF: Adhesion binding the iris to cornea at the angle of the anterior chamber.

364.74 Pupillary membranes

Iris bombé   Pupillary:
Pupillary: seclusion
  occlusion

DEF: Membrane traversing the pupil and blocking vision.

364.75 Pupillary abnormalities

Deformed pupil   Rupture of sphincter, pupil
Ectopic pupil

364.76 Iridodialysis

DEF: Separation of the iris from the ciliary body base; due to trauma or surgical accident.

364.77 Recession of chamber angle

DEF: Receding of anterior chamber angle of the eye; restricts vision.

√5ᵗʰ **364.8 Other disorders of iris and ciliary body**

AHA: 2Q, '07, 9

364.81 Floppy iris syndrome

Intraoperative floppy iris syndrome [IFIS]

Use additional E code to identify cause, such as:
sympatholytics [antiadrenergics] causing adverse effect in therapeutic use (E941.3)

DEF: Condition complicating cataract surgery for patients who have received alpha blocker treatment for urinary retention problems; iris dilator muscle fails to dilate, and the iris may billow or flap.

AHA: 4Q, '07, 77, 79

364.82 Plateau iris syndrome

DEF: A postoperative chronic angle-closure glaucoma characterized by closing of the anterior chamber angle secondary to a large or anteriorly positioned ciliary body that impairs the normal flow of aqueous fluid.

AHA: 4Q, '08, 112

364.89 Other disorders of iris and ciliary body

Prolapse of iris NOS

EXCLUDES prolapse of iris in recent wound (871.1)

364.9 Unspecified disorder of iris and ciliary body

√4ᵗʰ **365 Glaucoma**

EXCLUDES blind hypertensive eye [absolute glaucoma] (360.42)
congenital glaucoma (743.20-743.22)

DEF: Rise in intraocular pressure restricting blood flow; multiple causes.

√5ᵗʰ **365.0 Borderline glaucoma [glaucoma suspect]**

AHA: 1Q, '90, 8

365.00 Preglaucoma, unspecified

365.01 Open angle with borderline findings, low risk

Open angle, low risk

DEF: Minor block of aqueous outflow from eye

AHA: 4Q, '11, 102

365.02 Anatomical narrow angle

Primary angle closure suspect

365.03 Steroid responders

365.04 Ocular hypertension

DEF: High fluid pressure within eye; no clear cause.

365.05 Open angle with borderline findings, high risk

Open angle, high risk

AHA: 4Q, '11, 102-103

| √4ᵗʰ √5ᵗʰ Additional Digit Required | Unspecified Code | Other Specified Code | Manifestation Code | ►◄ Revised Text | ● New Code | ▲ Revised Code Title |

Plateau Iris Syndrome

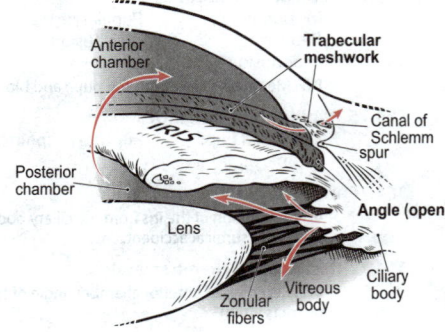

Normal Aqueous Flow

365.06 Primary angle closure without glaucoma damage
AHA: 4Q, '11, 102-103

√5ᵗʰ **365.1 Open-angle glaucoma**

365.10 Open-angle glaucoma, unspecified
Wide-angle glaucoma NOS
Use additional code to identify glaucoma stage
(365.70-365.74)

365.11 Primary open angle glaucoma
Chronic simple glaucoma
Use additional code to identify glaucoma stage
(365.70-365.74)
DEF: High intraocular pressure, despite free flow of aqueous.

365.12 Low tension glaucoma
Use additional code to identify glaucoma stage
(365.70-365.74)

365.13 Pigmentary glaucoma
Use additional code to identify glaucoma stage
(365.70-365.74)
DEF: High intraocular pressure; due to iris pigment granules blocking aqueous flow.

365.14 Glaucoma of childhood
Infantile or juvenile glaucoma

365.15 Residual stage of open angle glaucoma

√5ᵗʰ **365.2 Primary angle-closure glaucoma**
DEF: Glaucoma caused by a shift in the position of the iris of the eye that blocks the surface of the trabecular meshwork causing impairment of the normal flow of aqueous fluid.

365.20 Primary angle-closure glaucoma, unspecified
Use additional code to identify glaucoma stage
(365.70-365.74)

365.21 Intermittent angle-closure glaucoma
Angle-closure glaucoma:
  interval
  subacute
DEF: Recurring attacks of high intraocular pressure; due to blocked aqueous flow.

365.22 Acute angle-closure glaucoma
Acute angle-closure glaucoma attack
Acute angle-closure glaucoma crisis
DEF: Sudden, severe rise in intraocular pressure due to blockage in aqueous drainage.

Angle Closure Glaucoma

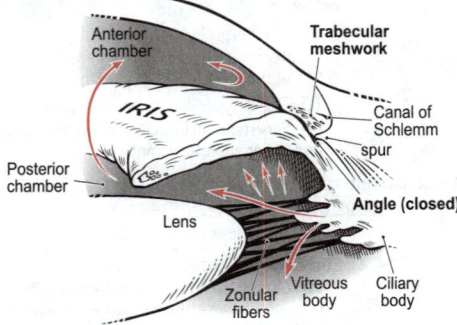

365.23 Chronic angle-closure glaucoma
Chronic primary angle closure glaucoma
Use additional code to identify glaucoma stage
(365.70-365.74)
AHA: 2Q, '98, 16

365.24 Residual stage of angle-closure glaucoma

√5ᵗʰ **365.3 Corticosteroid-induced glaucoma**
DEF: Elevated intraocular pressure; due to long-term corticosteroid therapy.

365.31 Glaucomatous stage
Use additional code to identify glaucoma stage
(365.70-365.74)

365.32 Residual stage

√5ᵗʰ **365.4 Glaucoma associated with congenital anomalies, dystrophies, and systemic syndromes**

365.41 Glaucoma associated with chamber angle anomalies

365.42 Glaucoma associated with anomalies of iris

365.43 Glaucoma associated with other anterior segment anomalies

365.44 *Glaucoma associated with systemic syndromes*
Code first associated disease, as
  neurofibromatosis (237.70-237.79)
  Sturge-Weber (-Dimitri) syndrome (759.6)

√5ᵗʰ **365.5 Glaucoma associated with disorders of the lens**

365.51 Phacolytic glaucoma
DEF: Elevated intraocular pressure; due to lens protein blocking aqueous flow.

365.52 Pseudoexfoliation glaucoma
Use additional code to identify glaucoma stage
(365.70-365.74)
DEF: Glaucoma characterized by small grayish particles deposited on the lens.

365.59 Glaucoma associated with other lens disorders

√5ᵗʰ **365.6 Glaucoma associated with other ocular disorders**

365.60 Glaucoma associated with unspecified ocular disorder

365.61 Glaucoma associated with pupillary block
DEF: Acute, open-angle glaucoma caused by mature cataract; aqueous flow is blocked by lens material and macrophages.

365.62 Glaucoma associated with ocular inflammations
Use additional code to identify glaucoma stage
(365.70-365.74)

365.63 Glaucoma associated with vascular disorders
Use additional code to identify glaucoma stage
(365.70-365.74)

365.64 Glaucoma associated with tumors or cysts

365.65 Glaucoma associated with ocular trauma
Use additional code to identify glaucoma stage
(365.70-365.74)

N Newborn Age: 0   P Pediatric Age: 0-17   M Maternity Age: 12-55   A Adult Age: 15-124

✓5ᵗʰ 365.7 Glaucoma stage

Code first associated type of glaucoma (365.10-365.13,
365.20, 365.23, 365.31, 365.52, 365.62-365.63, 365.65)

AHA: 4Q, '11, 102-105

TIP: If a patient has bilateral glaucoma with different stages or the
stage evolves during the encounter from one stage to another,
assign one code for the highest stage documented.

365.70 Glaucoma stage, unspecified
Glaucoma stage NOS

365.71 Mild stage glaucoma
Early stage glaucoma

365.72 Moderate stage glaucoma

365.73 Severe stage glaucoma
Advanced stage glaucoma　　End-stage glaucoma

365.74 Indeterminate stage glaucoma

✓5ᵗʰ 365.8 Other specified forms of glaucoma

365.81 Hypersecretion glaucoma

**365.82 Glaucoma with increased episcleral venous
pressure**

365.83 Aqueous misdirection
Malignant glaucoma

DEF: A form of secondary angle-closure glaucoma that
occurs when aqueous humor flows into the posterior
chamber of the eye (vitreous) rather than through the
normal recycling channels.
AHA: 4Q, '02, 48

365.89 Other specified glaucoma
AHA: 2Q, '98, 16

365.9 Unspecified glaucoma
AHA: 3Q, '03, 14; 2Q, '01, 16
H40.9 Unspecified glaucoma　　　　**I-10**

✓4ᵗʰ 366 Cataract

EXCLUDES congenital cataract (743.30-743.34)

DEF: A variety of conditions that create a cloudy, or calcified lens that
obstructs vision.

✓5ᵗʰ 366.0 Infantile, juvenile, and presenile cataract

366.00 Nonsenile cataract, unspecified

366.01 Anterior subcapsular polar cataract
DEF: Defect within the front, center lens surface.

366.02 Posterior subcapsular polar cataract
DEF: Defect within the rear, center lens surface.

366.03 Cortical, lamellar, or zonular cataract
DEF: Opacities radiating from center to edge of lens; appear
as thin, concentric layers of lens.

366.04 Nuclear cataract

366.09 Other and combined forms of nonsenile cataract

✓5ᵗʰ 366.1 Senile cataract
AHA: 3Q, '91, 9; S-0, '85, 10

366.10 Senile cataract, unspecified　　**A**
AHA: 1Q, '03, 5

366.11 Pseudoexfoliation of lens capsule　　**A**

366.12 Incipient cataract　　**A**
Cataract:　　　　Cataract:
coronary　　　　punctate
immature NOS　　Water clefts
DEF: Minor disorders of lens not affecting vision; due to
aging.

366.13 Anterior subcapsular polar senile cataract　　**A**

366.14 Posterior subcapsular polar senile cataract　　**A**

366.15 Cortical senile cataract　　**A**

366.16 Nuclear sclerosis　　**A**
Cataracta brunescens　　　Nuclear cataract
AHA: 4Q, '07, 79

366.17 Total or mature cataract　　**A**

366.18 Hypermature cataract　　**A**
Morgagni cataract

366.19 Other and combined forms of senile cataract　　**A**

Cataract

Sclera
Trebeculae
Ciliary suspensory fibers
Lens
Posterior polar cataract
Cornea
Cortical cataract
Iris
Anterior polar cataract

✓5ᵗʰ 366.2 Traumatic cataract

366.20 Traumatic cataract, unspecified

366.21 Localized traumatic opacities
Vossius' ring

366.22 Total traumatic cataract

366.23 Partially resolved traumatic cataract

✓5ᵗʰ 366.3 Cataract secondary to ocular disorders

366.30 Cataracta complicata, unspecified

366.31 Glaucomatous flecks (subcapsular)
Code first underlying glaucoma (365.0-365.9)

366.32 Cataract in inflammatory disorders
Code first underlying condition, as:
chronic choroiditis (363.0-363.2)

366.33 Cataract with neovascularization
Code first underlying condition, as:
chronic iridocyclitis (364.10)

366.34 Cataract in degenerative disorders
Sunflower cataract
Code first underlying condition, as:
chalcosis (360.24)
degenerative myopia (360.21)
pigmentary retinal dystrophy (362.74)

✓5ᵗʰ 366.4 Cataract associated with other disorders

366.41 Diabetic cataract
Code first diabetes (249.5, 250.5)
AHA: 3Q, '91, 9; S-0, '85, 11

366.42 Tetanic cataract
Code first underlying disease, as:
calcinosis (275.4)
hypoparathyroidism (252.1)

366.43 Myotonic cataract
Code first underlying disorder (359.21, 359.23)

366.44 Cataract associated with other syndromes
Code first underlying condition, as:
craniofacial dysostosis (756.0)
galactosemia (271.1)

366.45 Toxic cataract
Drug-induced cataract
Use additional E code to identify drug or other toxic
substance

**366.46 Cataract associated with radiation and
other physical influences**
Use additional E code to identify cause

✓5ᵗʰ 366.5 After-cataract

366.50 After-cataract, unspecified
Secondary cataract NOS

366.51 Soemmering's ring
DEF: A donut-shaped lens remnant and a capsule behind
the pupil as a result of cataract surgery or trauma.

366.52 Other after-cataract, not obscuring vision

366.53 After-cataract, obscuring vision

366.8 Other cataract
Calcification of lens

✓4ᵗʰ **✓5ᵗʰ** Additional Digit Required	Unspecified Code	Other Specified Code	Manifestation Code	►◄ Revised Text	● New Code	▲ Revised Code Title

366.9 **Unspecified cataract**
AHA: 4Q, '09, 131
H26.9 Unspecified cataract   I-10

√4ᵗʰ **367 Disorders of refraction and accommodation**

367.0 **Hypermetropia**
Far-sightedness   Hyperopia
DEF: Refraction error, called also hyperopia, focal point is posterior to retina; abnormally short anteroposterior diameter or subnormal refractive power; causes farsightedness.

367.1 **Myopia**
Near-sightedness
DEF: Refraction error, focal point is anterior to retina; causes near-sightedness.

√5ᵗʰ 367.2 **Astigmatism**

367.20 **Astigmatism, unspecified**

367.21 **Regular astigmatism**

367.22 **Irregular astigmatism**

√5ᵗʰ 367.3 **Anisometropia and aniseikonia**

367.31 **Anisometropia**
DEF: Eyes with refractive powers that differ by at least one diopter.

367.32 **Aniseikonia**
DEF: Eyes with unequal retinal imaging; usually due to refractive error.

367.4 **Presbyopia**
DEF: Loss of crystalline lens elasticity; causes errors of accommodation; due to aging.

√5ᵗʰ 367.5 **Disorders of accommodation**

367.51 **Paresis of accommodation**
Cycloplegia
DEF: Partial paralysis of ciliary muscle, causing focus problems.

367.52 **Total or complete internal ophthalmoplegia**
DEF: Total paralysis of ciliary muscle; large pupil incapable of focus.

367.53 **Spasm of accommodation**
DEF: Abnormal contraction of ciliary muscle; causes focus problems.

√5ᵗʰ 367.8 **Other disorders of refraction and accommodation**

367.81 **Transient refractive change**

367.89 **Other**
Drug-induced ⎫ disorders of refraction and
Toxic   ⎭ accommodation

367.9 **Unspecified disorder of refraction and accommodation**

√4ᵗʰ **368 Visual disturbances**
EXCLUDES electrophysiological disturbances (794.11-794.14)

√5ᵗʰ 368.0 **Amblyopia ex anopsia**
DEF: Vision impaired due to disuse; esotropia often cause.

368.00 **Amblyopia, unspecified**

368.01 **Strabismic amblyopia**
Suppression amblyopia

368.02 **Deprivation amblyopia**
DEF: Decreased vision associated with suppressed retinal image of one eye.

368.03 **Refractive amblyopia**

√5ᵗʰ 368.1 **Subjective visual disturbances**

368.10 **Subjective visual disturbance, unspecified**

368.11 **Sudden visual loss**

368.12 **Transient visual loss**
Concentric fading   Scintillating scotoma

368.13 **Visual discomfort**
Asthenopia   Photophobia
Eye strain

368.14 **Visual distortions of shape and size**
Macropsia   Micropsia
Metamorphopsia

368.15 **Other visual distortions and entoptic phenomena**
Photopsia   Refractive:
Refractive: polyopia
diplopia   Visual halos

368.16 **Psychophysical visual disturbances**
Prosopagnosia   Visual:
Visual: hallucinations
agnosia   object agnosia
disorientation syndrome

368.2 **Diplopia**
Double vision
H53.2 Diplopia   I-10

√5ᵗʰ 368.3 **Other disorders of binocular vision**

368.30 **Binocular vision disorder, unspecified**

368.31 **Suppression of binocular vision**

368.32 **Simultaneous visual perception without fusion**

368.33 **Fusion with defective stereopsis**
DEF: Faulty depth perception though normal ability to focus.

368.34 **Abnormal retinal correspondence**

√5ᵗʰ 368.4 **Visual field defects**

368.40 **Visual field defect, unspecified**

368.41 **Scotoma involving central area**
Scotoma: Scotoma:
central   paracentral
centrocecal
DEF: Vision loss (blind spot) in central five degrees of visual field.

368.42 **Scotoma of blind spot area**
Enlarged: Paracecal scotoma
angioscotoma
blind spot

368.43 **Sector or arcuate defects**
Scotoma: Scotoma:
arcuate   Seidel
Bjerrum
DEF: Arc-shaped blind spot caused by retinal nerve damage.

368.44 **Other localized visual field defect**
Scotoma: Visual field defect:
NOS   nasal step
ring   peripheral

368.45 **Generalized contraction or constriction**

368.46 **Homonymous bilateral field defects**
Hemianopsia (altitudinal) (homonymous)
Quadrant anopia
DEF: Disorders found in the corresponding vertical halves of the visual fields of both eyes.

368.47 **Heteronymous bilateral field defects**
Hemianopsia: Hemianopsia:
binasal   bitemporal
DEF: Disorders in the opposite halves of the visual fields of both eyes.

√5ᵗʰ 368.5 **Color vision deficiencies**
Color blindness

368.51 **Protan defect**
Protanomaly   Protanopia
DEF: Mild difficulty distinguishing green and red hues with shortened spectrum; sex-linked affecting one percent of males.

368.52 **Deutan defect**
Deuteranomaly   Deuteranopia
DEF: Male-only disorder; difficulty in distinguishing green and red, no shortened spectrum.

368.53 **Tritan defect**
Tritanomaly   Tritanopia
DEF: Difficulty in distinguishing blue and yellow; occurs often due to drugs, retinal detachment and central nervous system diseases.

368.54 Achromatopsia
Monochromatism (cone) (rod)
DEF: Complete color blindness; caused by disease, injury to retina, optic nerve or pathway.

368.55 Acquired color vision deficiencies

368.59 Other color vision deficiencies

√5ᵗʰ **368.6 Night blindness**
Nyctalopia
DEF: Nyctalopia: disorder of vision in dim light or night blindness.

368.60 Night blindness, unspecified

368.61 Congenital night blindness
Hereditary night blindness   Oguchi's disease

368.62 Acquired night blindness
EXCLUDES that due to vitamin A deficiency (264.5)

368.63 Abnormal dark adaptation curve
Abnormal threshold ⎫
Delayed adaptation ⎬ of cones or rods

368.69 Other night blindness

368.8 Other specified visual disturbances
Blurred vision NOS
AHA: 4Q, '02, 56

368.9 Unspecified visual disturbance
AHA: 3Q, '06, 22; 1Q, '04, 15

√4ᵗʰ **369 Blindness and low vision**
NOTE Visual impairment refers to a functional limitation of the eye (e.g., limited visual acuity or visual field). It should be distinguished from visual disability, indicating a limitation of the abilities of the individual (e.g., limited reading skills, vocational skills), and from visual handicap, indicating a limitation of personal and socioeconomic independence (e.g., limited mobility, limited employability).

The levels of impairment defined in the table on the next page are based on the recommendations of the WHO Study Group on Prevention of Blindness (Geneva, November 6-10, 1972; WHO Technical Report Series 518), and of the International Council of Ophthalmology (1976).

Note that definitions of blindness vary in different settings.

For international reporting WHO defines blindness as profound impairment. This definition can be applied to blindness of one eye (369.1, 369.6) and to blindness of the individual (369.0).

For determination of benefits in the U.S.A., the definition of legal blindness as severe impairment is often used. This definition applies to blindness of the individual only.

EXCLUDES correctable impaired vision due to refractive errors (367.0-367.9)

√5ᵗʰ **369.0 Profound impairment, both eyes**

369.00 Impairment level not further specified
Blindness:
    NOS according to WHO definition
    both eyes

369.01 Better eye: total impairment; lesser eye: total impairment

369.02 Better eye: near-total impairment; lesser eye: not further specified

369.03 Better eye: near-total impairment; lesser eye: total impairment

369.04 Better eye: near-total impairment; lesser eye: near-total impairment

369.05 Better eye: profound impairment; lesser eye: not further specified

369.06 Better eye: profound impairment; lesser eye: total impairment

369.07 Better eye: profound impairment; lesser eye: near-total impairment

369.08 Better eye: profound impairment; lesser eye: profound impairment

√4ᵗʰ **369.1 Moderate or severe impairment, better eye, profound impairment lesser eye**

369.10 Impairment level not further specified
Blindness, one eye, low vision other eye

369.11 Better eye: severe impairment; lesser eye: blind, not further specified

369.12 Better eye: severe impairment; lesser eye: total impairment

369.13 Better eye: severe impairment; lesser eye: near-total impairment

369.14 Better eye: severe impairment; lesser eye: profound impairment

369.15 Better eye: moderate impairment; lesser eye: blind, not further specified

369.16 Better eye: moderate impairment; lesser eye: total impairment

369.17 Better eye: moderate impairment; lesser eye: near-total impairment

369.18 Better eye: moderate impairment; lesser eye: profound impairment

√5ᵗʰ **369.2 Moderate or severe impairment, both eyes**

369.20 Impairment level not further specified
Low vision, both eyes NOS

369.21 Better eye: severe impairment; lesser eye: not further specified

369.22 Better eye: severe impairment; lesser eye: severe impairment

369.23 Better eye: moderate impairment; lesser eye: not further specified

369.24 Better eye: moderate impairment; lesser eye: severe impairment

369.25 Better eye: moderate impairment; lesser eye: moderate impairment

369.3 Unqualified visual loss, both eyes
EXCLUDES blindness NOS:
    legal [U.S.A. definition] (369.4)
    WHO definition (369.00)

369.4 Legal blindness, as defined in U.S.A.
Blindness NOS according to U.S.A. definition
EXCLUDES legal blindness with specification of impairment level (369.01-369.08, 369.11-369.14, 369.21-369.22)
H54.8 Legal blindness as defined in USA   I-10

√5ᵗʰ **369.6 Profound impairment, one eye**

369.60 Impairment level not further specified
Blindness, one eye

369.61 One eye: total impairment; other eye: not specified

369.62 One eye: total impairment; other eye: near normal vision

369.63 One eye: total impairment; other eye: normal vision

369.64 One eye: near-total impairment; other eye: not specified

369.65 One eye: near-total impairment; other eye: near-normal vision

369.66 One eye: near-total impairment; other eye: normal vision

369.67 One eye: profound impairment; other eye: not specified

369.68 One eye: profound impairment; other eye: near-normal vision

369.69 One eye: profound impairment; other eye: normal vision

√5ᵗʰ **369.7 Moderate or severe impairment, one eye**

369.70 Impairment level not further specified
Low vision, one eye

Diseases of the Nervous System and Sense Organs

369.71–370.60

Classification		LEVELS OF VISUAL IMPAIRMENT	Additional descriptors which may be encountered
"legal"	WHO	Visual acuity and/or visual field limitation (whichever is worse)	
	(NEAR-) NORMAL VISION	RANGE OF NORMAL VISION 20/10 20/13 20/16 20/20 20/25 2.0 1.6 1.25 1.0 0.8	
		NEAR-NORMAL VISION 20/30 20/40 20/50 20/60 0.7 0.6 0.5 0.4 0.3	
LOW VISION	LOW VISION	MODERATE VISUAL IMPAIRMENT 20/70 20/80 20/100 20/125 20/160 0.25 0.20 0.16 0.12	Moderate low vision
		SEVERE VISUAL IMPAIRMENT 20/200 20/250 20/320 20/400 0.10 0.08 0.06 0.05 Visual field: 20 degrees or less	Severe low vision, "Legal" blindness
LEGAL BLINDNESS (U.S.A.) both eyes	BLINDNESS (WHO) one or both eyes	PROFOUND VISUAL IMPAIRMENT 20/500 20/630 20/800 20/1000 0.04 0.03 0.025 0.02 Count fingers at: less than 3m (10 ft.) Visual field: 10 degrees or less	Profound low vision, Moderate blindness
		NEAR-TOTAL VISUAL IMPAIRMENT Visual acuity: less than 0.02 (20/1000) Count fingers at: 1m (3 ft.) or less Hand movements: 5m (15 ft.) or less Light projection, light perception Visual field: 5 degrees or less	Severe blindness Near-total blindness
		TOTAL VISUAL IMPAIRMENT No light perception (NLP)	Total blindness

Visual acuity refers to best achievable acuity with correction.
Non-listed Snellen fractions may be classified by converting to the nearest decimal equivalent, e.g. 10/200 = 0.05, 6/30 = 0.20.
CF (count fingers) without designation of distance, may be classified to profound impairment.
HM (hand motion) without designation of distance, may be classified to near-total impairment.
Visual field measurements refer to the largest field diameter for a 1/100 white test object.

369.71 One eye: severe impairment; other eye: not specified

369.72 One eye: severe impairment; other eye: near-normal vision

369.73 One eye: severe impairment; other eye: normal vision

369.74 One eye: moderate impairment; other eye: not specified

369.75 One eye: moderate impairment; other eye: near-normal vision

369.76 One eye: moderate impairment; other eye: normal vision

369.8 Unqualified visual loss, one eye

369.9 Unspecified visual loss
    AHA: 4Q, '02, 114; 3Q, '02, 20

✓4ᵗʰ **370 Keratitis**

✓5ᵗʰ **370.0 Corneal ulcer**
    EXCLUDES *that due to vitamin A deficiency (264.3)*

370.00 Corneal ulcer, unspecified

370.01 Marginal corneal ulcer

370.02 Ring corneal ulcer

370.03 Central corneal ulcer

370.04 Hypopyon ulcer
    Serpiginous ulcer
    DEF: Corneal ulcer with an accumulation of pus in the eye's anterior chamber.

370.05 Mycotic corneal ulcer
    DEF: Fungal infection causing corneal tissue loss.

370.06 Perforated corneal ulcer
    DEF: Tissue loss through all layers of cornea.

370.07 Mooren's ulcer
    DEF: Tissue loss, with chronic inflammation, at junction of cornea and sclera; seen in elderly.

✓5ᵗʰ **370.2 Superficial keratitis without conjunctivitis**
    EXCLUDES *dendritic [herpes simplex] keratitis (054.42)*

370.20 Superficial keratitis, unspecified

370.21 Punctate keratitis
    Thygeson's superficial punctate keratitis
    DEF: Formation of cellular and fibrinous deposits (keratic precipitates) on posterior surface; deposits develop after injury or iridocyclitis.

370.22 Macular keratitis
    Keratitis: Keratitis:
      areolar   stellate
      nummular   striate

370.23 Filamentary keratitis
    DEF: Keratitis characterized by twisted filaments of mucoid material on the cornea's surface.

370.24 Photokeratitis
    Snow blindness   Welders' keratitis
    DEF: Painful, inflamed cornea; due to extended exposure to ultraviolet light.
    AHA: 3Q, '96, 6

✓5ᵗʰ **370.3 Certain types of keratoconjunctivitis**

370.31 Phlyctenular keratoconjunctivitis
    Phlyctenulosis
    Use additional code for any associated tuberculosis (017.3)
    DEF: Miniature blister on conjunctiva or cornea; associated with tuberculosis and malnutrition disorders.

370.32 Limbar and corneal involvement in vernal conjunctivitis
    Use additional code for vernal conjunctivitis (372.13)
    DEF: Corneal itching and inflammation in conjunctivitis; often limited to lining of eyelids.

370.33 Keratoconjunctivitis sicca, not specified as Sjögren's
    EXCLUDES *Sjögren's syndrome (710.2)*
    DEF: Inflammation of conjunctiva and cornea; characterized by "horny" looking tissue and excess blood in these areas; decreased flow of lacrimal (tear) is a contributing factor.

370.34 Exposure keratoconjunctivitis
    DEF: Incomplete closure of eyelid causing dry, inflamed eye.

370.35 Neurotrophic keratoconjunctivitis

✓5ᵗʰ **370.4 Other and unspecified keratoconjunctivitis**

370.40 Keratoconjunctivitis, unspecified
    Superficial keratitis with conjunctivitis NOS

370.44 Keratitis or keratoconjunctivitis in exanthema
    Code first underlying condition (050.0-052.9)
    EXCLUDES *herpes simplex (054.43)*
            herpes zoster (053.21)
            measles (055.71)

370.49 Other
    EXCLUDES *epidemic keratoconjunctivitis (077.1)*

✓5ᵗʰ **370.5 Interstitial and deep keratitis**

370.50 Interstitial keratitis, unspecified

370.52 Diffuse interstitial keratitis
    Cogan's syndrome
    DEF: Inflammation of cornea; with deposits in middle corneal layers; may obscure vision.

370.54 Sclerosing keratitis
    DEF: Chronic corneal inflammation leading to opaque scarring.

370.55 Corneal abscess
    DEF: Pocket of pus and inflammation on the cornea.

370.59 Other
    EXCLUDES *disciform herpes simplex keratitis (054.43)*
            syphilitic keratitis (090.3)

✓5ᵗʰ **370.6 Corneal neovascularization**

370.60 Corneal neovascularization, unspecified

370.61 Localized vascularization of cornea
DEF: Limited infiltration of cornea by new blood vessels.

370.62 Pannus (corneal)
DEF: Buildup of superficial vascularization and granulated tissue under epithelium of cornea.
AHA: 3Q, '02, 20

370.63 Deep vascularization of cornea
DEF: Deep infiltration of cornea by new blood vessels.

370.64 Ghost vessels (corneal)

370.8 Other forms of keratitis
Code first underlying condition, such as:
Acanthamoeba (136.21)
Fusarium (118)
AHA: 4Q, '08, 80-81; 3Q, '94, 5

370.9 Unspecified keratitis

√4ᵗʰ **371 Corneal opacity and other disorders of cornea**

√5ᵗʰ **371.0 Corneal scars and opacities**
EXCLUDES that due to vitamin A deficiency (264.6)

371.00 Corneal opacity, unspecified
Corneal scar NOS

371.01 Minor opacity of cornea
Corneal nebula

371.02 Peripheral opacity of cornea
Corneal macula not interfering with central vision

371.03 Central opacity of cornea
Corneal:
leucoma
macula } interfering with central vision

371.04 Adherent leucoma
DEF: Dense, opaque corneal growth adhering to the iris; also spelled as leukoma.

371.05 Phthisical cornea
Code first underlying tuberculosis (017.3)

√5ᵗʰ **371.1 Corneal pigmentations and deposits**

371.10 Corneal deposit, unspecified

371.11 Anterior pigmentations
Stähli's lines

371.12 Stromal pigmentations
Hematocornea

371.13 Posterior pigmentations
Krukenberg spindle

371.14 Kayser-Fleischer ring
DEF: Copper deposits forming ring at outer edge of cornea; seen in Wilson's disease and other liver disorders.

371.15 Other deposits associated with metabolic disorders

371.16 Argentous deposits
DEF: Silver deposits in cornea.

√5ᵗʰ **371.2 Corneal edema**

371.20 Corneal edema, unspecified

371.21 Idiopathic corneal edema
DEF: Corneal swelling and fluid retention of unknown cause.

371.22 Secondary corneal edema
DEF: Corneal swelling and fluid retention caused by an underlying disease, injury, or condition.

371.23 Bullous keratopathy
DEF: Corneal degeneration; characterized by recurring, rupturing epithelial "blisters;" ruptured blebs expose corneal nerves; occurs in glaucoma, iridocyclitis and Fuchs' epithelial dystrophy.

371.24 Corneal edema due to wearing of contact lenses

√5ᵗʰ **371.3 Changes of corneal membranes**

371.30 Corneal membrane change, unspecified

371.31 Folds and rupture of Bowman's membrane

371.32 Folds in Descemet's membrane

371.33 Rupture in Descemet's membrane

√5ᵗʰ **371.4 Corneal degenerations**

371.40 Corneal degeneration, unspecified

371.41 Senile corneal changes
Arcus senilis   Hassall-Henle bodies

371.42 Recurrent erosion of cornea
EXCLUDES Mooren's ulcer (370.07)

371.43 Band-shaped keratopathy
DEF: Horizontal bands of superficial corneal calcium deposits.

371.44 Other calcerous degenerations of cornea

371.45 Keratomalacia NOS
EXCLUDES that due to vitamin A deficiency (264.4)
DEF: Destruction of the cornea by keratinization of the epithelium with ulceration and perforation of the cornea; seen in cases of vitamin A deficiency.

371.46 Nodular degeneration of cornea
Salzmann's nodular dystrophy

371.48 Peripheral degenerations of cornea
Marginal degeneration of cornea [Terrien's]

371.49 Other
Discrete colliquative keratopathy

√5ᵗʰ **371.5 Hereditary corneal dystrophies**
DEF: Genetic disorder; leads to opacities, edema or lesions of cornea.

371.50 Corneal dystrophy, unspecified

371.51 Juvenile epithelial corneal dystrophy

371.52 Other anterior corneal dystrophies
Corneal dystrophy: Corneal dystrophy:
microscopic cystic   ring-like

371.53 Granular corneal dystrophy

371.54 Lattice corneal dystrophy

371.55 Macular corneal dystrophy

371.56 Other stromal corneal dystrophies
Crystalline corneal dystrophy

371.57 Endothelial corneal dystrophy
Combined corneal dystrophy
Cornea guttata
Fuchs' endothelial dystrophy

371.58 Other posterior corneal dystrophies
Polymorphous corneal dystrophy

√5ᵗʰ **371.6 Keratoconus**
DEF: Bilateral bulging protrusion of anterior cornea; often due to noninflammatory thinning.

371.60 Keratoconus, unspecified

371.61 Keratoconus, stable condition

371.62 Keratoconus, acute hydrops

√5ᵗʰ **371.7 Other corneal deformities**

371.70 Corneal deformity, unspecified

371.71 Corneal ectasia
DEF: Bulging protrusion of thinned, scarred cornea.

371.72 Descemetocele
DEF: Protrusion of Descemet's membrane into cornea.

371.73 Corneal staphyloma
DEF: Protrusion of cornea into adjacent tissue.

√5ᵗʰ **371.8 Other corneal disorders**

371.81 Corneal anesthesia and hypoesthesia
DEF: Decreased or absent sensitivity of cornea.

371.82 Corneal disorder due to contact lens
EXCLUDES corneal edema due to contact lens (371.24)
DEF: Contact lens wear causing cornea disorder, excluding swelling.

371.89 Other
AHA: 3Q, '99, 12

371.9 Unspecified corneal disorder

Diseases of the Nervous System and Sense Organs

372–372.75

✓4ᵗʰ **372 Disorders of conjunctiva**
> EXCLUDES *keratoconjunctivitis (370.3-370.4)*

✓5ᵗʰ **372.0 Acute conjunctivitis**

372.00 Acute conjunctivitis, unspecified

372.01 Serous conjunctivitis, except viral
> EXCLUDES *viral conjunctivitis NOS (077.9)*
> AHA: 3Q, '08, 6

372.02 Acute follicular conjunctivitis
Conjunctival folliculosis NOS
> EXCLUDES *conjunctivitis:*
> *adenoviral (acute follicular) (077.3)*
> *epidemic hemorrhagic (077.4)*
> *inclusion (077.0)*
> *Newcastle (077.8)*
> *epidemic keratoconjunctivitis (077.1)*
> *pharyngoconjunctival fever (077.2)*
> DEF: Severe conjunctival inflammation with dense
> infiltrations of lymphoid tissues of inner eyelids; may be
> traced to a viral or chlamydial etiology.

372.03 Other mucopurulent conjunctivitis
Catarrhal conjunctivitis
> EXCLUDES *blennorrhea neonatorum (gonococcal)*
> *(098.40)*
> *neonatal conjunctivitis(771.6)*
> *ophthalmia neonatorum NOS (771.6)*

372.04 Pseudomembranous conjunctivitis
Membranous conjunctivitis
> EXCLUDES *diphtheritic conjunctivitis (032.81)*
> DEF: Severe inflammation of conjunctiva; false membrane
> develops on inner surface of eyelid; membrane can be
> removed without harming epithelium, due to bacterial
> infections, toxic and allergic factors, and viral infections.

372.05 Acute atopic conjunctivitis
> DEF: Sudden, severe conjunctivitis due to allergens.

372.06 Acute chemical conjunctivitis
Acute toxic conjunctivitis
> Use additional E code to identify the chemical or toxic
> agent
> EXCLUDES *burn of eye and adnexa (940.0-940.9)*
> *chemical corrosion injury of eye*
> *(940.2-940.3)*
> AHA: 4Q, '09, 85

✓5ᵗʰ **372.1 Chronic conjunctivitis**

372.10 Chronic conjunctivitis, unspecified

372.11 Simple chronic conjunctivitis

372.12 Chronic follicular conjunctivitis
> DEF: Persistent conjunctival inflammation with dense,
> localized infiltrations of lymphoid tissues of inner eyelids.

372.13 Vernal conjunctivitis
> AHA: 3Q, '96, 8

372.14 Other chronic allergic conjunctivitis
> AHA: 3Q, '96, 8

372.15 Parasitic conjunctivitis
> *Code first underlying disease, as:*
> *filariasis (125.0-125.9)*
> *mucocutaneous leishmaniasis (085.5)*

✓5ᵗʰ **372.2 Blepharoconjunctivitis**

372.20 Blepharoconjunctivitis, unspecified

372.21 Angular blepharoconjunctivitis
> DEF: Inflammation at junction of upper and lower eyelids;
> may block lacrimal secretions.

372.22 Contact blepharoconjunctivitis

✓5ᵗʰ **372.3 Other and unspecified conjunctivitis**

372.30 Conjunctivitis, unspecified
> H10.9 Unspecified conjunctivitis   I-10

372.31 Rosacea conjunctivitis
> *Code first underlying rosacea dermatitis (695.3)*

372.33 Conjunctivitis in mucocutaneous disease
> *Code first underlying disease, as:*
> *erythema multiforme (695.10-695.19)*
> *Reiter's disease (099.3)*
> EXCLUDES *ocular pemphigoid (694.61)*

372.34 Pingueculitis
> EXCLUDES *pinguecula (372.51)*
> AHA: 4Q, '08, 112-113

372.39 Other
> AHA: 2Q, '07, 9

✓5ᵗʰ **372.4 Pterygium**
> EXCLUDES *pseudopterygium (372.52)*
> DEF: Wedge-shaped, conjunctival thickening that advances from the
> inner corner of the eye toward the cornea.

372.40 Pterygium, unspecified

372.41 Peripheral pterygium, stationary

372.42 Peripheral pterygium, progressive

372.43 Central pterygium

372.44 Double pterygium

372.45 Recurrent pterygium

✓5ᵗʰ **372.5 Conjunctival degenerations and deposits**

372.50 Conjunctival degeneration, unspecified

372.51 Pinguecula
> EXCLUDES *pingueculitis (372.34)*
> DEF: Proliferative spot on the bulbar conjunctiva located
> near the sclerocorneal junction, usually on the nasal side; it
> is seen in elderly people.

372.52 Pseudopterygium
> DEF: Conjunctival scar joined to the cornea; it looks like a
> pterygium but is not attached to the tissue.

372.53 Conjunctival xerosis
> EXCLUDES *conjunctival xerosis due to vitamin A*
> *deficiency (264.0, 264.1, 264.7)*
> DEF: Dry conjunctiva due to vitamin A deficiency; related to
> Bitot's spots; may develop into xerophthalmia and
> keratomalacia.

372.54 Conjunctival concretions
> DEF: Calculus or deposit on conjunctiva.

372.55 Conjunctival pigmentations
Conjunctival argyrosis
> DEF: Color deposits in conjunctiva.

372.56 Conjunctival deposits

✓5ᵗʰ **372.6 Conjunctival scars**

372.61 Granuloma of conjunctiva

372.62 Localized adhesions and strands of conjunctiva
> DEF: Abnormal fibrous connections in conjunctiva.

372.63 Symblepharon
Extensive adhesions of conjunctiva
> DEF: Adhesion of the eyelids to the eyeball.

372.64 Scarring of conjunctiva
Contraction of eye socket (after enucleation)

✓5ᵗʰ **372.7 Conjunctival vascular disorders and cysts**

372.71 Hyperemia of conjunctiva
> DEF: Conjunctival blood vessel congestion causing eye
> redness.

372.72 Conjunctival hemorrhage
Hyposphagma   Subconjunctival hemorrhage

372.73 Conjunctival edema
Chemosis of conjunctiva   Subconjunctival edema
> DEF: Fluid retention and swelling in conjunctival tissue.

372.74 Vascular abnormalities of conjunctiva
Aneurysm(ata) of conjunctiva

372.75 Conjunctival cysts
> DEF: Abnormal sacs of fluid in conjunctiva.

N Newborn Age: 0   P Pediatric Age: 0-17   M Maternity Age: 12-55   A Adult Age: 15-124

√5ᵗʰ **372.8 Other disorders of conjunctiva**

   372.81 Conjunctivochalasis
     DEF: Bilateral condition of redundant conjunctival tissue between globe and lower eyelid margin; may cover lower punctum, interfering with normal tearing.
     AHA: 4Q, '00, 41

   372.89 Other disorders of conjunctiva

372.9 Unspecified disorder of conjunctiva

√4ᵗʰ **373 Inflammation of eyelids**

√5ᵗʰ **373.0 Blepharitis**
   EXCLUDES *blepharoconjunctivitis (372.20-372.22)*

   373.00 Blepharitis, unspecified

   373.01 Ulcerative blepharitis

   373.02 Squamous blepharitis

√5ᵗʰ **373.1 Hordeolum and other deep inflammation of eyelid**
   DEF: Purulent, localized, staphylococcal infection in sebaceous glands of eyelids.

   373.11 Hordeolum externum
     Hordeolum NOS   Stye
     DEF: Infection of the oil glands in the eyelash follicles.

   373.12 Hordeolum internum
     Infection of meibomian gland
     DEF: Infection of the oil gland of the eyelid margin.

   373.13 Abscess of eyelid
     Furuncle of eyelid
     DEF: Inflamed pocket of pus on the eyelid.

373.2 Chalazion
   Meibomian (gland) cyst
   EXCLUDES *infected meibomian gland (373.12)*
   DEF: Chronic inflammation of the meibomian gland, causing an eyelid mass.

√5ᵗʰ **373.3 Noninfectious dermatoses of eyelid**

   373.31 Eczematous dermatitis of eyelid

   373.32 Contact and allergic dermatitis of eyelid

   373.33 Xeroderma of eyelid

   373.34 Discoid lupus erythematosus of eyelid

373.4 Infective dermatitis of eyelid of types resulting in deformity
   Code first underlying disease, as:
     leprosy (030.0-030.9)
     lupus vulgaris (tuberculous) (017.0)
     yaws (102.0-102.9)

373.5 Other infective dermatitis of eyelid
   Code first underlying disease, as:
     actinomycosis (039.3)
     impetigo (684)
     mycotic dermatitis (110.0-111.9)
     vaccinia (051.0)
     postvaccination (999.0)
   EXCLUDES *herpes:*
     simplex (054.41)
     zoster (053.20)

373.6 Parasitic infestation of eyelid
   Code first underlying disease, as:
     leishmaniasis (085.0-085.9)
     loiasis (125.2)
     onchocerciasis (125.3)
     pediculosis (132.0)

373.8 Other inflammations of eyelids

373.9 Unspecified inflammation of eyelid

√4ᵗʰ **374 Other disorders of eyelids**

√5ᵗʰ **374.0 Entropion and trichiasis of eyelid**
   DEF: Entropion: turning inward of eyelid edge toward eyeball.
   DEF: Trichiasis: ingrowing eyelashes marked by irritation with possible distortion of sight.

   374.00 Entropion, unspecified

   374.01 Senile entropion   A

Entropion and Ectropion

Normal eyelashes   Entropion   Ectropion

   374.02 Mechanical entropion

   374.03 Spastic entropion

   374.04 Cicatricial entropion

   374.05 Trichiasis without entropion

√5ᵗʰ **374.1 Ectropion**
   DEF: Turning outward (eversion) of eyelid edge; exposes palpebral conjunctiva; dryness irritation result.

   374.10 Ectropion, unspecified

   374.11 Senile ectropion   A

   374.12 Mechanical ectropion

   374.13 Spastic ectropion

   374.14 Cicatricial ectropion

√5ᵗʰ **374.2 Lagophthalmos**
   DEF: Incomplete closure of eyes; causes dry eye and other complications.

   374.20 Lagophthalmos, unspecified

   374.21 Paralytic lagophthalmos

   374.22 Mechanical lagophthalmos

   374.23 Cicatricial lagophthalmos

√5ᵗʰ **374.3 Ptosis of eyelid**

   374.30 Ptosis of eyelid, unspecified
     AHA: 2Q, '96, 11

   374.31 Paralytic ptosis
     DEF: Drooping of upper eyelid due to nerve disorder.

   374.32 Myogenic ptosis
     DEF: Drooping of upper eyelid due to muscle disorder.

   374.33 Mechanical ptosis
     DEF: Outside force causes drooping of upper eyelid.

   374.34 Blepharochalasis
     Pseudoptosis
     DEF: Loss of elasticity, thickened or indurated skin of eyelids associated with recurrent episodes of idiopathic edema causing intracellular tissue atrophy.

√5ᵗʰ **374.4 Other disorders affecting eyelid function**
   EXCLUDES *blepharoclonus (333.81)*
     blepharospasm (333.81)
     facial nerve palsy (351.0)
     third nerve palsy or paralysis (378.51-378.52)
     tic (psychogenic) (307.20-307.23)
     organic (333.3)

   374.41 Lid retraction or lag

   374.43 Abnormal innervation syndrome
     Jaw-blinking   Paradoxical facial movements

   374.44 Sensory disorders

   374.45 Other sensorimotor disorders
     Deficient blink reflex

   374.46 Blepharophimosis
     Ankyloblepharon
     DEF: Narrowing of palpebral fissure horizontally; caused by laterally displaced inner canthi; either acquired or congenital.

√5ᵗʰ **374.5 Degenerative disorders of eyelid and periocular area**

   374.50 Degenerative disorder of eyelid, unspecified

√4ᵗʰ / √5ᵗʰ Additional Digit Required   Unspecified Code   Other Specified Code   Manifestation Code   ▶◀ Revised Text   ● New Code   ▲ Revised Code Title

2015 ICD-9-CM   **Volume 1 – 113**

Diseases of the Nervous System and Sense Organs

374.51–376.11

374.51 Xanthelasma
Xanthoma (planum) (tuberosum) of eyelid
Code first underlying condition (272.0-272.9)
DEF: Fatty tumors of the eyelid linked to high fat content of blood.

374.52 Hyperpigmentation of eyelid
Chloasma   Dyspigmentation
DEF: Excess pigment of eyelid.

374.53 Hypopigmentation of eyelid
Vitiligo of eyelid
DEF: Lack of color pigment of the eyelid.

374.54 Hypertrichosis of eyelid
DEF: Excessive eyelash growth.

374.55 Hypotrichosis of eyelid
Madarosis of eyelid
DEF: Less than normal, or absent, eyelashes.

374.56 Other degenerative disorders of skin affecting eyelid

√5ᵗʰ **374.8 Other disorders of eyelid**

374.81 Hemorrhage of eyelid
EXCLUDES *black eye (921.0)*

374.82 Edema of eyelid
Hyperemia of eyelid
DEF: Swelling and fluid retention in eyelid.
AHA: 4Q, '08, 131

374.83 Elephantiasis of eyelid
DEF: Filarial disease causing dermatitis and enlargement of eyelid.

374.84 Cysts of eyelids
Sebaceous cyst of eyelid

374.85 Vascular anomalies of eyelid

374.86 Retained foreign body of eyelid
Use additional code to identify foreign body (V90.01-V90.9)

374.87 Dermatochalasis
DEF: Acquired form of connective tissue disorder associated with decreased elastic tissue and abnormal elastin formation resulting in loss of elasticity of the skin of the eyelid, generally associated with aging.

374.89 Other disorders of eyelid

374.9 Unspecified disorder of eyelid

√4ᵗʰ **375 Disorders of lacrimal system**

√5ᵗʰ **375.0 Dacryoadenitis**

375.00 Dacryoadenitis, unspecified

375.01 Acute dacryoadenitis
DEF: Severe, sudden inflammation of the lacrimal gland.

375.02 Chronic dacryoadenitis
DEF: Persistent inflammation of the lacrimal gland.

375.03 Chronic enlargement of lacrimal gland

√5ᵗʰ **375.1 Other disorders of lacrimal gland**

375.11 Dacryops
DEF: Overproduction and constant flow of tears; may cause distended lacrimal duct.

375.12 Other lacrimal cysts and cystic degeneration

375.13 Primary lacrimal atrophy

375.14 Secondary lacrimal atrophy
DEF: Wasting away of the lacrimal gland due to another disease.

375.15 Tear film insufficiency, unspecified
Dry eye syndrome
AHA: 3Q, '96, 6
DEF: Eye dryness and irritation from insufficient tear production.

375.16 Dislocation of lacrimal gland

√5ᵗʰ **375.2 Epiphora**
DEF: Abnormal development of tears due to stricture of lacrimal passages.

375.20 Epiphora, unspecified as to cause

375.21 Epiphora due to excess lacrimation
DEF: Tear overflow due to overproduction.

375.22 Epiphora due to insufficient drainage
DEF: Tear overflow due to blocked drainage.

√5ᵗʰ **375.3 Acute and unspecified inflammation of lacrimal passages**
EXCLUDES *neonatal dacryocystitis (771.6)*

375.30 Dacryocystitis, unspecified

375.31 Acute canaliculitis, lacrimal

375.32 Acute dacryocystitis
Acute peridacryocystitis

375.33 Phlegmonous dacryocystitis
DEF: Infection of the tear sac with pockets of pus.

√5ᵗʰ **375.4 Chronic inflammation of lacrimal passages**

375.41 Chronic canaliculitis

375.42 Chronic dacryocystitis

375.43 Lacrimal mucocele

√5ᵗʰ **375.5 Stenosis and insufficiency of lacrimal passages**

375.51 Eversion of lacrimal punctum
DEF: Abnormal turning outward of the tear duct.

375.52 Stenosis of lacrimal punctum
DEF: Abnormal narrowing of the tear duct.

375.53 Stenosis of lacrimal canaliculi

375.54 Stenosis of lacrimal sac
DEF: Abnormal narrowing of the tear sac.

375.55 Obstruction of nasolacrimal duct, neonatal
EXCLUDES *congenital anomaly of nasola- crimal duct (743.65)*
DEF: Acquired, abnormal obstruction of tear drainage system from the eye to the nose; in an infant.

375.56 Stenosis of nasolacrimal duct, acquired

375.57 Dacryolith
DEF: Concretion or stone anywhere in lacrimal system.

√5ᵗʰ **375.6 Other changes of lacrimal passages**

375.61 Lacrimal fistula
DEF: Abnormal communication from the lacrimal system.

375.69 Other

√5ᵗʰ **375.8 Other disorders of lacrimal system**

375.81 Granuloma of lacrimal passages
DEF: Abnormal nodules within lacrimal system.

375.89 Other

375.9 Unspecified disorder of lacrimal system

√4ᵗʰ **376 Disorders of the orbit**

√5ᵗʰ **376.0 Acute inflammation of orbit**

376.00 Acute inflammation of orbit, unspecified

376.01 Orbital cellulitis
Abscess of orbit
DEF: Infection of tissue between the orbital bone and eyeball.

376.02 Orbital periostitis
DEF: Inflammation of connective tissue covering the orbital bone.

376.03 Orbital osteomyelitis
DEF: Inflammation of the orbital bone.

376.04 Tenonitis

√5ᵗʰ **376.1 Chronic inflammatory disorders of orbit**

376.10 Chronic inflammation of orbit, unspecified

376.11 Orbital granuloma
Pseudotumor (inflammatory) of orbit
DEF: Abnormal nodule between orbital bone and eyeball.

N Newborn Age: 0	**P** Pediatric Age: 0-17	**M** Maternity Age: 12-55	**A** Adult Age: 15-124

Lacrimal System

Superior and inferior lobes of lacrimal gland

Medial angle

Lacrimal ducts

Lacrimal canaliculi

Nasolacrimal sac

Lacrimal caruncle

Superior, inferior lacrimal puncta

Left eye

376.12 Orbital myositis
DEF: Painful inflammation of the muscles of the eye.

376.13 Parasitic infestation of orbit
Code first underlying disease, as:
hydatid infestation of orbit (122.3, 122.6, 122.9)
myiasis of orbit (134.0)

√5ᵗʰ **376.2 Endocrine exophthalmos**
Code first underlying thyroid disorder (242.0-242.9)

376.21 Thyrotoxic exophthalmos
DEF: Painful inflammation of eye muscles.

376.22 Exophthalmic ophthalmoplegia
DEF: Inability to rotate eye as a result of bulging eyes.

√5ᵗʰ **376.3 Other exophthalmic conditions**

376.30 Exophthalmos, unspecified
DEF: Abnormal protrusion of eyeball.

376.31 Constant exophthalmos
DEF: Continuous, abnormal protrusion or bulging of eyeball.

376.32 Orbital hemorrhage
DEF: Bleeding behind the eyeball, causing it to bulge forward.

376.33 Orbital edema or congestion
DEF: Fluid retention behind eyeball, causing forward bulge.

376.34 Intermittent exophthalmos

376.35 Pulsating exophthalmos
DEF: Bulge or protrusion; associated with a carotid-cavernous fistula.

376.36 Lateral displacement of globe
DEF: Abnormal displacement of the eyeball away from nose, toward temple.

√5ᵗʰ **376.4 Deformity of orbit**

376.40 Deformity of orbit, unspecified

376.41 Hypertelorism of orbit
DEF: Abnormal increase in interorbital distance; associated with congenital facial deformities; may be accompanied by mental deficiency.

376.42 Exostosis of orbit
DEF: Abnormal bony growth of orbit.

376.43 Local deformities due to bone disease
DEF: Acquired abnormalities of orbit; due to bone disease.

376.44 Orbital deformities associated with craniofacial deformities

376.45 Atrophy of orbit
DEF: Wasting away of bone tissue of orbit.

376.46 Enlargement of orbit

376.47 Deformity due to trauma or surgery

√5ᵗʰ **376.5 Enophthalmos**
DEF: Recession of eyeball deep into eye socket.

376.50 Enophthalmos, unspecified as to cause

376.51 Enophthalmos due to atrophy of orbital tissue

376.52 Enophthalmos due to trauma or surgery

376.6 Retained (old) foreign body following penetrating wound of orbit
Retrobulbar foreign body
Use additional code to identify foreign body (V90.01-V90.9)

√5ᵗʰ **376.8 Other orbital disorders**

376.81 Orbital cysts
Encephalocele of orbit
AHA: 3Q, '99, 13

376.82 Myopathy of extraocular muscles
DEF: Disease in the muscles that control eyeball movement.

376.89 Other

376.9 Unspecified disorder of orbit

√4ᵗʰ **377 Disorders of optic nerve and visual pathways**

√5ᵗʰ **377.0 Papilledema**

377.00 Papilledema, unspecified

377.01 Papilledema associated with increased intracranial pressure

377.02 Papilledema associated with decreased ocular pressure

377.03 Papilledema associated with retinal disorder

377.04 Foster-Kennedy syndrome
DEF: Retrobulbar optic neuritis, central scotoma and optic atrophy; caused by tumors in frontal lobe of brain that press downward.

√5ᵗʰ **377.1 Optic atrophy**

377.10 Optic atrophy, unspecified

377.11 Primary optic atrophy
EXCLUDES neurosyphilitic optic atrophy (094.84)

377.12 Postinflammatory optic atrophy
DEF: Adverse effect of inflammation causing wasting away of eye.

377.13 Optic atrophy associated with retinal dystrophies
DEF: Progressive changes in retinal tissue due to metabolic disorder causing wasting away of eye.

377.14 Glaucomatous atrophy [cupping] of optic disc

377.15 Partial optic atrophy
Temporal pallor of optic disc

377.16 Hereditary optic atrophy
Optic atrophy: Optic atrophy:
dominant hereditary   Leber's

√5ᵗʰ **377.2 Other disorders of optic disc**

377.21 Drusen of optic disc

377.22 Crater-like holes of optic disc

377.23 Coloboma of optic disc
DEF: Ocular malformation caused by the failure of fetal fissure of optic stalk to close.

377.24 Pseudopapilledema

√5ᵗʰ **377.3 Optic neuritis**
EXCLUDES meningococcal optic neuritis (036.81)

377.30 Optic neuritis, unspecified

377.31 Optic papillitis
DEF: Swelling and inflammation of the optic disc.

377.32 Retrobulbar neuritis (acute)
EXCLUDES syphilitic retrobulbar neuritis (094.85)
DEF: Inflammation of optic nerve immediately behind the eyeball.

377.33 Nutritional optic neuropathy
DEF: Malnutrition causing optic nerve disorder.

377.34 Toxic optic neuropathy
Toxic amblyopia
DEF: Toxic substance causing optic nerve disorder.

377.39 Other
EXCLUDES ischemic optic neuropathy (377.41)

√5ᵗʰ **377.4 Other disorders of optic nerve**

377.41 Ischemic optic neuropathy
DEF: Decreased blood flow affecting optic nerve.

377.42 Hemorrhage in optic nerve sheaths
DEF: Bleeding in meningeal lining of optic nerve.

377.43 Optic nerve hypoplasia
AHA: 4Q, '06, 81

377.49 Other
Compression of optic nerve

√5ᵗʰ **377.5 Disorders of optic chiasm**

377.51 Associated with pituitary neoplasms and disorders
DEF: Abnormal pituitary growth causing disruption in nerve chain from retina to brain.

377.52 Associated with other neoplasms
DEF: Abnormal growth, other than pituitary, causing disruption in nerve chain from retina to brain.

377.53 Associated with vascular disorders
DEF: Vascular disorder causing disruption in nerve chain from retina to brain.

377.54 Associated with inflammatory disorders
DEF: Inflammatory disease causing disruption in nerve chain from retina to brain.

√5ᵗʰ **377.6 Disorders of other visual pathways**

377.61 Associated with neoplasms

377.62 Associated with vascular disorders

377.63 Associated with inflammatory disorders

√5ᵗʰ **377.7 Disorders of visual cortex**
EXCLUDES visual:
agnosia (368.16)
hallucinations (368.16)
halos (368.15)

377.71 Associated with neoplasms

377.72 Associated with vascular disorders

377.73 Associated with inflammatory

377.75 Cortical blindness
DEF: Blindness due to brain disorder, rather than eye disorder.

377.9 Unspecified disorder of optic nerve and visual pathways

√4ᵗʰ **378 Strabismus and other disorders of binocular eye movements**
EXCLUDES nystagmus and other irregular eye movements (379.50-379.59)
DEF: Misalignment of the eyes due to imbalance in extraocular muscles.

√5ᵗʰ **378.0 Esotropia**
Convergent concomitant strabismus
EXCLUDES intermittent esotropia (378.20-378.22)
DEF: Visual axis deviation created by one eye fixing upon an image and the other eye deviating inward.

378.00 Esotropia, unspecified

378.01 Monocular esotropia

378.02 Monocular esotropia with A pattern

378.03 Monocular esotropia with V pattern

378.04 Monocular esotropia with other noncomitancies
Monocular esotropia with X or Y pattern

378.05 Alternating esotropia

378.06 Alternating esotropia with A pattern

378.07 Alternating esotropia with V pattern

378.08 Alternating esotropia with other noncomitancies
Alternating esotropia with X or Y pattern

√5ᵗʰ **378.1 Exotropia**
Divergent concomitant strabismus
EXCLUDES intermittent exotropia (378.20, 378.23-378.24)
DEF: Visual axis deviation created by one eye fixing upon an image and the other eye deviating outward.

378.10 Exotropia, unspecified

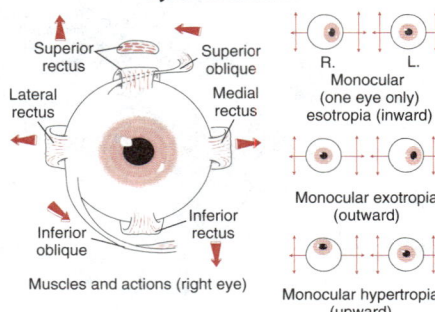

Eye Musculature

Superior rectus
Superior oblique
Lateral rectus
Medial rectus
Inferior oblique
Inferior rectus

Muscles and actions (right eye)

R.   L.
Monocular (one eye only) esotropia (inward)

Monocular exotropia (outward)

Monocular hypertropia (upward)

378.11 Monocular exotropia

378.12 Monocular exotropia with A pattern

378.13 Monocular exotropia with V pattern

378.14 Monocular exotropia with other noncomitancies
Monocular exotropia with X or Y pattern

378.15 Alternating exotropia

378.16 Alternating exotropia with A pattern

378.17 Alternating exotropia with V pattern

378.18 Alternating exotropia with other noncomitancies
Alternating exotropia with X or Y pattern

√5ᵗʰ **378.2 Intermittent heterotropia**
EXCLUDES vertical heterotropia (intermittent) (378.31)
DEF: Deviation of eyes seen only at intervals; it is also called strabismus.

378.20 Intermittent heterotropia, unspecified
Intermittent: Intermittent:
esotropia NOS   exotropia NOS

378.21 Intermittent esotropia, monocular

378.22 Intermittent esotropia, alternating

378.23 Intermittent exotropia, monocular

378.24 Intermittent exotropia, alternating

√5ᵗʰ **378.3 Other and unspecified heterotropia**

378.30 Heterotropia, unspecified

378.31 Hypertropia
Vertical heterotropia (constant) (intermittent)

378.32 Hypotropia

378.33 Cyclotropia

378.34 Monofixation syndrome
Microtropia

378.35 Accommodative component in esotropia

√5ᵗʰ **378.4 Heterophoria**
DEF: Deviation occurring only when the other eye is covered.

378.40 Heterophoria, unspecified

378.41 Esophoria

378.42 Exophoria

378.43 Vertical heterophoria

378.44 Cyclophoria

378.45 Alternating hyperphoria

√5ᵗʰ **378.5 Paralytic strabismus**
DEF: Deviation of the eye due to nerve paralysis affecting muscle.

378.50 Paralytic strabismus, unspecified

378.51 Third or oculomotor nerve palsy, partial
AHA: 3Q, '91, 9

378.52 Third or oculomotor nerve palsy, total
AHA: 2Q, '89, 12

378.53 Fourth or trochlear nerve palsy
AHA: 2Q, '01, 21

378.54 Sixth or abducens nerve palsy
AHA: 2Q, '89, 12

N Newborn Age: 0   **P** Pediatric Age: 0-17   **M** Maternity Age: 12-55   **A** Adult Age: 15-124

378.55 External ophthalmoplegia

378.56 Total ophthalmoplegia

√5ᵗʰ 378.6 Mechanical strabismus
> **DEF:** Deviation of the eye due to an outside force upon the extraocular muscles.

378.60 Mechanical strabismus, unspecified

378.61 Brown's (tendon) sheath syndrome
> **DEF:** Congenital or acquired shortening of the anterior sheath of superior oblique muscle; eye is unable to move upward and inward; usually unilateral.

378.62 Mechanical strabismus from other musculofascial disorders

378.63 Limited duction associated with other conditions

√5ᵗʰ 378.7 Other specified strabismus

378.71 Duane's syndrome
> **DEF:** Congenital; affects one eye; due to abnormal fibrous bands attached to rectus muscle; inability to abduct affected eye with retraction of globe.

378.72 Progressive external ophthalmoplegia
> **DEF:** Paralysis progressing from one eye muscle to another.

378.73 Strabismus in other neuromuscular disorders

√5ᵗʰ 378.8 Other disorders of binocular eye movements
> **EXCLUDES** *nystagmus (379.50-379.56)*

378.81 Palsy of conjugate gaze
> **DEF:** Paralysis progressing from one eye muscle to another.

378.82 Spasm of conjugate gaze
> **DEF:** Muscle contractions impairing parallel movement of eye.

378.83 Convergence insufficiency or palsy

378.84 Convergence excess or spasm

378.85 Anomalies of divergence

378.86 Internuclear ophthalmoplegia
> **DEF:** Eye movement anomaly due to brainstem lesion.

378.87 Other dissociated deviation of eye movements
> Skew deviation

378.9 Unspecified disorder of eye movements
> Ophthalmoplegia NOS   Strabismus NOS
> **AHA:** 2Q, '01, 21

√4ᵗʰ 379 Other disorders of eye

√5ᵗʰ 379.0 Scleritis and episcleritis
> **EXCLUDES** *syphilitic episcleritis (095.0)*

379.00 Scleritis, unspecified
> Episcleritis NOS

379.01 Episcleritis periodica fugax
> **DEF:** Hyperemia (engorgement) of the sclera and overlying conjunctiva characterized by a sudden onset and short duration.

379.02 Nodular episcleritis
> **DEF:** Inflammation of the outermost layer of the sclera, with formation of nodules.

379.03 Anterior scleritis

379.04 Scleromalacia perforans
> **DEF:** Scleral thinning, softening and degeneration; seen with rheumatoid arthritis.

379.05 Scleritis with corneal involvement
> Scleroperikeratitis

379.06 Brawny scleritis
> **DEF:** Severe scleral inflammation with thickening corneal margins.

379.07 Posterior scleritis
> Sclerotenonitis

379.09 Other
> Scleral abscess

√5ᵗʰ 379.1 Other disorders of sclera
> **EXCLUDES** *blue sclera (743.47)*

379.11 Scleral ectasia
> Scleral staphyloma NOS
> **DEF:** Protrusion of the contents of the eyeball where the sclera has thinned.

379.12 Staphyloma posticum
> **DEF:** Ring-shaped protrusion or bulging of sclera and uveal tissue at posterior pole of eye.

379.13 Equatorial staphyloma
> **DEF:** Ring-shaped protrusion or bulging of sclera and uveal tissue midway between front and back of eye.

379.14 Anterior staphyloma, localized

379.15 Ring staphyloma

379.16 Other degenerative disorders of sclera

379.19 Other

√5ᵗʰ 379.2 Disorders of vitreous body
> **DEF:** Disorder of clear gel that fills space between retina and lens.

379.21 Vitreous degeneration
> Vitreous: Vitreous:
>   cavitation   liquefaction
>   detachment

379.22 Crystalline deposits in vitreous
> Asteroid hyalitis   Synchysis scintillans

379.23 Vitreous hemorrhage
> **AHA:** 3Q, '91, 15

379.24 Other vitreous opacities
> Vitreous floaters

379.25 Vitreous membranes and strands

379.26 Vitreous prolapse
> **DEF:** Slipping of vitreous from normal position.

379.27 Vitreomacular adhesion   **A**
> Vitreomacular traction
> **EXCLUDES** *traction detachment with vitreoretinal organization (361.81)*
> **AHA:** 4Q, '11, 105-106

379.29 Other disorders of vitreous
> **EXCLUDES** *vitreous abscess (360.04)*
> **AHA:** 1Q, '99, 11

√5ᵗʰ 379.3 Aphakia and other disorders of lens
> **EXCLUDES** *after-cataract (366.50-366.53)*

379.31 Aphakia
> **EXCLUDES** *cataract extraction status (V45.61)*
> **DEF:** Absence of eye's crystalline lens.

379.32 Subluxation of lens

379.33 Anterior dislocation of lens
> **DEF:** Lens displaced toward iris.

379.34 Posterior dislocation of lens
> **DEF:** Lens displaced backward toward vitreous.

379.39 Other disorders of lens

√5ᵗʰ 379.4 Anomalies of pupillary function

379.40 Abnormal pupillary function, unspecified

379.41 Anisocoria
> **DEF:** Unequal pupil diameter.

379.42 Miosis (persistent), not due to miotics
> **DEF:** Abnormal contraction of pupil less than 2 mil.

379.43 Mydriasis (persistent), not due to mydriatics
> **DEF:** Morbid dilation of pupil.

379.45 Argyll Robertson pupil, atypical
> Argyll Robertson phenomenon or pupil, nonsyphilitic
> **EXCLUDES** *Argyll Robertson pupil (syphilitic) (094.89)*
> **DEF:** Failure of pupil to respond to light; affects both eyes; may be caused by diseases such as syphilis of the central nervous system or miosis.

379.46 Tonic pupillary reaction
> Adie's pupil or syndrome

√4ᵗʰ √5ᵗʰ Additional Digit Required   Unspecified Code   Other Specified Code   Manifestation Code   ▶◀ Revised Text   ● New Code   ▲ Revised Code Title

2015 ICD-9-CM   **Volume 1 – 117**

Diseases of the Nervous System and Sense Organs

379.49–380.50

379.49 Other
Hippus   Pupillary paralysis

√5ᵗʰ **379.5 Nystagmus and other irregular eye movements**

379.50 Nystagmus, unspecified
DEF: Involuntary, rapid, rhythmic movement of eyeball; vertical, horizontal, rotatory or mixed; cause may be congenital, acquired, physiological, neurological, myopathic, or due to ocular diseases.
AHA: 4Q, '02, 68; 2Q, '01, 21

379.51 Congenital nystagmus

379.52 Latent nystagmus

379.53 Visual deprivation nystagmus

379.54 Nystagmus associated with disorders of the vestibular system

379.55 Dissociated nystagmus

379.56 Other forms of nystagmus

379.57 Deficiencies of saccadic eye movements
Abnormal optokinetic response
DEF: Saccadic eye movements; small, rapid, involuntary movements by both eyes simultaneously, due to changing point of fixation on visualized object.

379.58 Deficiencies of smooth pursuit movements

379.59 Other irregularities of eye movements
Opsoclonus

√5ᵗʰ **379.6 Inflammation (infection) of postprocedural bleb**
Postprocedural blebitis

379.60 Inflammation (infection) of postprocedural bleb, unspecified
AHA: 4Q, '06, 82

379.61 Inflammation (infection) of postprocedural bleb, stage 1
AHA: 4Q, '06, 82

379.62 Inflammation (infection) of postprocedural bleb, stage 2
AHA: 4Q, '06, 82

379.63 Inflammation (infection) of postprocedural bleb, stage 3
Bleb associated endophthalmitis
AHA: 4Q, '06, 82

379.8 Other specified disorders of eye and adnexa

√5ᵗʰ **379.9 Unspecified disorder of eye and adnexa**

379.90 Disorder of eye, unspecified

379.91 Pain in or around eye

379.92 Swelling or mass of eye

379.93 Redness or discharge of eye

379.99 Other ill-defined disorders of eye
EXCLUDES blurred vision NOS (368.8)

Diseases of the Ear and Mastoid Process (380-389)

Use additional external cause code, if applicable, to identify the cause of the ear condition

√4ᵗʰ **380 Disorders of external ear**

√5ᵗʰ **380.0 Perichondritis and chondritis of pinna**
Chondritis of auricle   Perichondritis of auricle

380.00 Perichondritis of pinna, unspecified

380.01 Acute perichondritis of pinna

380.02 Chronic perichondritis of pinna

380.03 Chondritis of pinna
DEF: Infection that has progressed into the cartilage; presents as indurated and edematous skin over the pinna; vascular compromise occurs with tissue necrosis and deformity.
AHA: 4Q, '04, 76

Ear and Mastoid Process

√5ᵗʰ **380.1 Infective otitis externa**

380.10 Infective otitis externa, unspecified
Otitis externa (acute):   Otitis externa (acute):
NOS   hemorrhagica
circumscribed   infective NOS
diffuse

380.11 Acute infection of pinna
EXCLUDES furuncular otitis externa (680.0)

380.12 Acute swimmers' ear
Beach ear   Tank ear
DEF: Otitis externa due to swimming.

380.13 Other acute infections of external ear
Code first underlying disease, as:
erysipelas (035)
impetigo (684)
seborrheic dermatitis (690.10-690.18)
EXCLUDES herpes simplex (054.73)
herpes zoster (053.71)

380.14 Malignant otitis externa
DEF: Severe necrotic otitis externa; due to bacteria.

380.15 Chronic mycotic otitis externa
Code first underlying disease, as:
aspergillosis (117.3)
otomycosis NOS (111.9)
EXCLUDES candidal otitis externa (112.82)

380.16 Other chronic infective otitis externa
Chronic infective otitis externa NOS

√5ᵗʰ **380.2 Other otitis externa**

380.21 Cholesteatoma of external ear
Keratosis obturans of external ear (canal)
EXCLUDES cholesteatoma NOS (385.30-385.35)
postmastoidectomy (383.32)
DEF: Cystlike mass filled with debris, including cholesterol; rare, congenital condition.

380.22 Other acute otitis externa
Acute otitis externa: Acute otitis externa:
actinic   eczematoid
chemical   reactive
contact

380.23 Other chronic otitis externa
Chronic otitis externa NOS

√5ᵗʰ **380.3 Noninfectious disorders of pinna**

380.30 Disorder of pinna, unspecified

380.31 Hematoma of auricle or pinna

380.32 Acquired deformities of auricle or pinna
EXCLUDES cauliflower ear (738.7)
AHA: 3Q, '03, 12

380.39 Other
EXCLUDES gouty tophi of ear (274.81)

380.4 Impacted cerumen
Wax in ear

√5ᵗʰ **380.5 Acquired stenosis of external ear canal**
Collapse of external ear canal

380.50 Acquired stenosis of external ear canal, unspecified as to cause

N Newborn Age: 0   P Pediatric Age: 0-17   M Maternity Age: 12-55   A Adult Age: 15-124

380.51 Secondary to trauma
DEF: Narrowing of the external ear canal; due to trauma.

380.52 Secondary to surgery
DEF: Postsurgical narrowing of the external ear canal.

380.53 Secondary to inflammation
DEF: Narrowing of the external ear canal; due to chronic inflammation.

√5ᵗʰ **380.8 Other disorders of external ear**

380.81 Exostosis of external ear canal

380.89 Other

380.9 Unspecified disorder of external ear

√4ᵗʰ **381 Nonsuppurative otitis media and Eustachian tube disorders**

√5ᵗʰ **381.0 Acute nonsuppurative otitis media**
Acute tubotympanic catarrh
Otitis media, acute or subacute:
catarrhal
exudative
transudative
with effusion
EXCLUDES *otitic barotrauma (993.0)*

381.00 Acute nonsuppurative otitis media, unspecified

381.01 Acute serous otitis media
Acute or subacute secretory otitis media
DEF: Sudden, severe infection of the middle ear.

381.02 Acute mucoid otitis media
Acute or subacute seromucinous otitis media
Blue drum syndrome
DEF: Sudden, severe infection of the middle ear, with mucous.

381.03 Acute sanguinous otitis media
DEF: Sudden, severe infection of the middle ear, with blood.

381.04 Acute allergic serous otitis media

381.05 Acute allergic mucoid otitis media

381.06 Acute allergic sanguinous otitis media

√5ᵗʰ **381.1 Chronic serous otitis media**
Chronic tubotympanic catarrh

381.10 Chronic serous otitis media, simple or unspecified
DEF: Persistent infection of the middle ear, without pus.

381.19 Other
Serosanguinous chronic otitis media

√5ᵗʰ **381.2 Chronic mucoid otitis media**
Glue ear
EXCLUDES *adhesive middle ear disease (385.10-385.19)*
DEF: Chronic condition; characterized by viscous fluid in middle ear; due to obstructed Eustachian tube.

381.20 Chronic mucoid otitis media, simple or unspecified

381.29 Other
Mucosanguinous chronic otitis media

381.3 Other and unspecified chronic nonsuppurative otitis media
Otitis media, chronic:
allergic
exudative
secretory
Otitis media, chronic:
seromucinous
transudative
with effusion

381.4 Nonsuppurative otitis media, not specified as acute or chronic
Otitis media:
allergic
catarrhal
exudative
mucoid
Otitis media:
secretory
seromucinous
serous
transudative
with effusion

√5ᵗʰ **381.5 Eustachian salpingitis**

381.50 Eustachian salpingitis, unspecified

381.51 Acute Eustachian salpingitis
DEF: Sudden, severe inflammation of the Eustachian tube.

381.52 Chronic Eustachian salpingitis
DEF: Persistent inflammation of the Eustachian tube.

√5ᵗʰ **381.6 Obstruction of Eustachian tube**
Stenosis
Stricture } of Eustachian tube

381.60 Obstruction of Eustachian tube, unspecified

381.61 Osseous obstruction of Eustachian tube
Obstruction of Eustachian tube from cholesteatoma, polyp, or other osseous lesion

381.62 Intrinsic cartilaginous obstruction of Eustachian tube
DEF: Blockage of Eustachian tube; due to cartilage overgrowth.

381.63 Extrinsic cartilaginous obstruction of Eustachian tube
Compression of Eustachian tube

381.7 Patulous Eustachian tube
DEF: Distended, oversized Eustachian tube.

√5ᵗʰ **381.8 Other disorders of Eustachian tube**

381.81 Dysfunction of Eustachian tube

381.89 Other

381.9 Unspecified Eustachian tube disorder

√4ᵗʰ **382 Suppurative and unspecified otitis media**

√5ᵗʰ **382.0 Acute suppurative otitis media**
Otitis media, acute:
necrotizing NOS
Otitis media, acute
purulent

382.00 Acute suppurative otitis media without spontaneous rupture of ear drum
DEF: Sudden, severe inflammation of middle ear, with pus.

382.01 Acute suppurative otitis media with spontaneous rupture of ear drum
DEF: Sudden, severe inflammation of middle ear, with pressure tearing ear drum tissue.

382.02 Acute suppurative otitis media in diseases classified elsewhere
Code first underlying disease, as:
influenza (487.8, 488.09, 488.19)
scarlet fever (034.1)
EXCLUDES *postmeasles otitis (055.2)*

382.1 Chronic tubotympanic suppurative otitis media
Benign chronic suppurative
ottis media
Chronic tubotympanic disease } (with anterior perforation of ear drum)
DEF: Inflammation of tympanic cavity and auditory tube; with pus formation.

382.2 Chronic atticoantral suppurative otitis media
Chronic atticoantral disease
Persistent mucosal disease } (with posterior or superior maginal perforation of ear drum)
DEF: Inflammation of upper tympanic membrane and mastoid antrum with pus formation.

382.3 Unspecified chronic suppurative otitis media
Chronic purulent otitis media
EXCLUDES *tuberculous otitis media (017.4)*

382.4 Unspecified suppurative otitis media
Purulent otitis media NOS

382.9 Unspecified otitis media
Otitis media:
NOS
acute NOS
Otitis media:
chronic NOS
AHA: N-D, '84, 16
H66.93 Otitis media unspecified bilateral   I-10

√4ᵗʰ **383 Mastoiditis and related conditions**

√5ᵗʰ **383.0 Acute mastoiditis**
Abscess of mastoid   Empyema of mastoid

383.00 Acute mastoiditis without complications
DEF: Sudden, severe inflammation of mastoid air cells.

√4ᵗʰ √5ᵗʰ Additional Digit Required	Unspecified Code	Other Specified Code	Manifestation Code	►◄ Revised Text	● New Code	▲ Revised Code Title

2015 ICD-9-CM   **Volume 1 – 119**

Diseases of the Nervous System and Sense Organs

383.01–385.24

383.01 Subperiosteal abscess of mastoid
DEF: Pocket of pus within the mastoid bone.

383.02 Acute mastoiditis with other complications
Gradenigo's syndrome

383.1 Chronic mastoiditis
Caries of mastoid   Fistula of mastoid
EXCLUDES *tuberculous mastoiditis (015.6)*
DEF: Persistent inflammation of the mastoid air cells.

√5th **383.2 Petrositis**
Coalescing osteitis
Inflammation } of petrous bone
Osteomyelitis

383.20 Petrositis, unspecified

383.21 Acute petrositis
DEF: Sudden, severe inflammation of dense bone behind the ear.

383.22 Chronic petrositis
DEF: Persistent inflammation of dense bone behind the ear.

√5th **383.3 Complications following mastoidectomy**

383.30 Postmastoidectomy complication, unspecified

383.31 Mucosal cyst of postmastoidectomy cavity
DEF: Mucous-lined cyst cavity following removal of mastoid bone.

383.32 Recurrent cholesteatoma of postmastoidectomy cavity
DEF: Cystlike mass of cell debris in cavity following removal of mastoid bone.

383.33 Granulations of postmastoidectomy cavity
Chronic inflammation of postmastoidectomy cavity
DEF: Granular tissue in cavity following removal of mastoid bone.

√5th **383.8 Other disorders of mastoid**

383.81 Postauricular fistula
DEF: Abnormal passage behind mastoid cavity.

383.89 Other

383.9 Unspecified mastoiditis

√4th **384 Other disorders of tympanic membrane**

√5th **384.0 Acute myringitis without mention of otitis media**

384.00 Acute myringitis, unspecified
Acute tympanitis NOS
DEF: Sudden, severe inflammation of ear drum.

384.01 Bullous myringitis
Myringitis bullosa hemorrhagica
DEF: Type of viral otitis media characterized by the appearance of serous or hemorrhagic blebs on the tympanic membrane.

384.09 Other

384.1 Chronic myringitis without mention of otitis media
Chronic tympanitis
DEF: Persistent inflammation of ear drum; with no evidence of middle ear infection.

Middle and Inner Ear

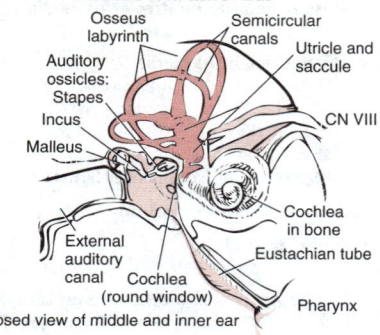

Osseus labyrinth
Semicircular canals
Utricle and saccule
Auditory ossicles: Stapes
Incus
Malleus
CN VIII
Cochlea in bone
External auditory canal
Cochlea (round window)
Eustachian tube
Pharynx
Exposed view of middle and inner ear

√5th **384.2 Perforation of tympanic membrane**
Perforation of ear drum: Perforation of ear drum:
NOS   postinflammatory
persistent posttraumatic
EXCLUDES *otitis media with perforation of tympanic membrane (382.00-382.9)*
traumatic perforation [current injury] (872.61)

384.20 Perforation of tympanic membrane, unspecified

384.21 Central perforation of tympanic membrane

384.22 Attic perforation of tympanic membrane
Pars flaccida

384.23 Other marginal perforation of tympanic membrane

384.24 Multiple perforations of tympanic membrane

384.25 Total perforation of tympanic membrane

√5th **384.8 Other specified disorders of tympanic membrane**

384.81 Atrophic flaccid tympanic membrane
Healed perforation of ear drum

384.82 Atrophic nonflaccid tympanic membrane

384.9 Unspecified disorder of tympanic membrane

√4th **385 Other disorders of middle ear and mastoid**
EXCLUDES *mastoiditis (383.0-383.9)*

√5th **385.0 Tympanosclerosis**

385.00 Tympanosclerosis, unspecified as to involvement

385.01 Tympanosclerosis involving tympanic membrane only
DEF: Tough, fibrous tissue impeding functions of ear drum.

385.02 Tympanosclerosis involving tympanic membrane and ear ossicles
DEF: Tough, fibrous tissue impeding functions of middle ear bones (stapes, malleus, incus).

385.03 Tympanosclerosis involving tympanic membrane, ear ossicles, and middle ear
DEF: Tough, fibrous tissue impeding functions of ear drum, middle ear bones and middle ear canal.

385.09 Tympanosclerosis involving other combination of structures

√5th **385.1 Adhesive middle ear disease**
Adhesive otitis   Otitis media:
Otitis media: fibrotic
chronic adhesive
EXCLUDES *glue ear (381.20-381.29)*
DEF: Adhesions of middle ear structures.

385.10 Adhesive middle ear disease, unspecified as to involvement

385.11 Adhesions of drum head to incus

385.12 Adhesions of drum head to stapes

385.13 Adhesions of drum head to promontorium

385.19 Other adhesions and combinations

√5th **385.2 Other acquired abnormality of ear ossicles**

385.21 Impaired mobility of malleus
Ankylosis of malleus

385.22 Impaired mobility of other ear ossicles
Ankylosis of ear ossicles, except malleus

385.23 Discontinuity or dislocation of ear ossicles
DEF: Disruption in auditory chain; created by malleus, incus and stapes.

385.24 Partial loss or necrosis of ear ossicles
DEF: Tissue loss in malleus, incus and stapes.

Cholesteatoma

Middle ear chamber

Cholesteatoma sac   Ear drum

√5ᵗʰ 385.3 Cholesteatoma of middle ear and mastoid

Cholesterosis
Epidermosis
Keratosis
Polyp
} of (middle) ear

EXCLUDES cholesteatoma:
    external ear canal (380.21)
    recurrent of postmastoidectomy cavity (383.32)

DEF: Cystlike mass of middle ear and mastoid antrum filled with debris, including cholesterol.

385.30 Cholesteatoma, unspecified

385.31 Cholesteatoma of attic

385.32 Cholesteatoma of middle ear

385.33 Cholesteatoma of middle ear and mastoid

DEF: Cystlike mass of cell debris in middle ear and mastoid air cells behind ear.
AHA: 3Q, '00, 10

385.35 Diffuse cholesteatosis

√5ᵗʰ 385.8 Other disorders of middle ear and mastoid

385.82 Cholesterin granuloma

DEF: Granuloma formed of fibrotic tissue; contains cholesterol crystals surrounded by foreign-body cells; found in the middle ear and mastoid area.

385.83 Retained foreign body of middle ear

Use additional code to identify foreign body (V90.01-V90.9)
AHA: 3Q, '94, 7; N-D, '87, 9

385.89 Other

385.9 Unspecified disorder of middle ear and mastoid

√4ᵗʰ 386 Vertiginous syndromes and other disorders of vestibular system

EXCLUDES vertigo NOS (780.4)
AHA: M-A, '85, 12

√5ᵗʰ 386.0 Ménière's disease

Endolymphatic hydrops   Ménière's syndrome or vertigo
Lermoyez's syndrome

DEF: Distended membranous labyrinth of middle ear from endolymphatic hydrops; causes ischemia, failure of nerve function; hearing and balance dysfunction; symptoms include fluctuating deafness, ringing in ears and dizziness.

386.00 Ménière's disease, unspecified

Ménière's disease (active)
H81.03 Ménière's disease bilateral   **I-10**

386.01 Active Ménière's disease, cochleovestibular

386.02 Active Ménière's disease, cochlear

386.03 Active Ménière's disease, vestibular

386.04 Inactive Ménière's disease

Ménière's disease in remission

√5ᵗʰ 386.1 Other and unspecified peripheral vertigo

EXCLUDES epidemic vertigo (078.81)

386.10 Peripheral vertigo, unspecified

386.11 Benign paroxysmal positional vertigo

Benign paroxysmal positional nystagmus

386.12 Vestibular neuronitis

Acute (and recurrent) peripheral vestibulopathy
DEF: Transient benign vertigo, unknown cause; characterized by response to caloric stimulation on one side, nystagmus with rhythmic movement of eyes; normal auditory function present.

386.19 Other

Aural vertigo   Otogenic vertigo

386.2 Vertigo of central origin

Central positional nystagmus   Malignant positional vertigo

√5ᵗʰ 386.3 Labyrinthitis

386.30 Labyrinthitis, unspecified

386.31 Serous labyrinthitis

Diffuse labyrinthitis
DEF: Inflammation of labyrinth; with fluid buildup.

386.32 Circumscribed labyrinthitis

Focal labyrinthitis

386.33 Suppurative labyrinthitis

Purulent labyrinthitis
DEF: Inflammation of labyrinth; with pus.

386.34 Toxic labyrinthitis

DEF: Inflammation of labyrinth; due to toxic reaction.

386.35 Viral labyrinthitis

√5ᵗʰ 386.4 Labyrinthine fistula

386.40 Labyrinthine fistula, unspecified

386.41 Round window fistula

386.42 Oval window fistula

386.43 Semicircular canal fistula

386.48 Labyrinthine fistula of combined sites

√5ᵗʰ 386.5 Labyrinthine dysfunction

386.50 Labyrinthine dysfunction, unspecified

386.51 Hyperactive labyrinth, unilateral

DEF: Abnormal increased sensitivity of labyrinth to stimuli such as sound, pressure or gravitational change, affecting one ear.

386.52 Hyperactive labyrinth, bilateral

DEF: Abnormal increased sensitivity of labyrinth to stimuli such as sound, pressure or gravitational change, affecting both ears.

386.53 Hypoactive labyrinth, unilateral

DEF: Abnormal decreased sensitivity of labyrinth to stimuli such as sound, pressure or gravitational change, affecting one ear.

386.54 Hypoactive labyrinth, bilateral

DEF: Abnormal decreased sensitivity of labyrinth to stimuli such as sound, pressure or gravitational change, affecting both ears.

386.55 Loss of labyrinthine reactivity, unilateral

DEF: Decreased function of the labyrinth sensors, affecting one ear

386.56 Loss of labyrinthine reactivity, bilateral

DEF: Decreased function of the labyrinth sensors, affecting both ears

386.58 Other forms and combinations

386.8 Other disorders of labyrinth

AHA: 1Q, '11, 6

386.9 Unspecified vertiginous syndromes and labyrinthine disorders

√4ᵗʰ 387 Otosclerosis

INCLUDES otospongiosis
DEF: Synonym for otospongiosis, spongy bone formation in the labyrinth bones of the ear; it causes progressive hearing impairment.

387.0 Otosclerosis involving oval window, nonobliterative

DEF: Tough, fibrous tissue impeding functions of oval window.

387.1 Otosclerosis involving oval window, obliterative

DEF: Tough, fibrous tissue blocking oval window.

√4ᵗʰ √5ᵗʰ Additional Digit Required   **Unspecified Code**   Other Specified Code   Manifestation Code   ►◄ Revised Text   ● New Code   ▲ Revised Code Title

2015 ICD-9-CM   **Volume 1 – 121**

Diseases of the Nervous System and Sense Organs

387.2–389.9

387.2 Cochlear otosclerosis
Otosclerosis involving: Otosclerosis involving:
  otic capsule   round window
DEF: Tough, fibrous tissue impeding functions of cochlea.

387.8 Other otosclerosis

387.9 Otosclerosis, unspecified

✓4ᵗʰ **388 Other disorders of ear**

  ✓5ᵗʰ **388.0 Degenerative and vascular disorders of ear**

    388.00 Degenerative and vascular disorders, unspecified

    388.01 Presbyacusis
      DEF: Progressive, bilateral perceptive hearing loss caused by advancing age; it is also known as presbycusis.

    388.02 Transient ischemic deafness
      DEF: Restricted blood flow to auditory organs causing temporary hearing loss.

  ✓5ᵗʰ **388.1 Noise effects on inner ear**

    388.10 Noise effects on inner ear, unspecified

    388.11 Acoustic trauma (explosive) to ear
      Otitic blast injury

    388.12 Noise-induced hearing loss

  388.2 Sudden hearing loss, unspecified

  ✓5ᵗʰ **388.3 Tinnitus**
    DEF: Abnormal noises in ear; may be heard by others beside the affected individual; noises include ringing, clicking, roaring and buzzing.

    388.30 Tinnitus, unspecified

    388.31 Subjective tinnitus

    388.32 Objective tinnitus

  ✓5ᵗʰ **388.4 Other abnormal auditory perception**

    388.40 Abnormal auditory perception, unspecified

    388.41 Diplacusis
      DEF: Perception of a single auditory sound as two sounds at two different levels of intensity.

    388.42 Hyperacusis
      DEF: Exceptionally acute sense of hearing caused by such conditions as Bell's palsy; this term may also refer to painful sensitivity to sounds.

    388.43 Impairment of auditory discrimination
      DEF: Impaired ability to distinguish tone of sound.

    388.44 Recruitment
      DEF: Perception of abnormally increased loudness caused by a slight increase in sound intensity; it is a term used in audiology.

    388.45 Acquired auditory processing disorder
      Auditory processing disorder NOS
      EXCLUDES central auditory processing disorder (315.32)
      DEF: Difficulty in recognizing and interpreting sounds; a failure of the brain to process auditory information; due to neurological problems due to injury, infection, and degenerative conditions.
      AHA: 4Q, '07, 79

  388.5 Disorders of acoustic nerve
    Acoustic neuritis
    Degeneration
    Disorder   } of acoustic or eighth nerve
    EXCLUDES acoustic neuroma (225.1)
                 syphilitic acoustic neuritis (094.86)
    AHA: M-A, '87, 8

  ✓5ᵗʰ **388.6 Otorrhea**

    388.60 Otorrhea, unspecified
      Discharging ear NOS

    388.61 Cerebrospinal fluid otorrhea
      EXCLUDES cerebrospinal fluid rhinorrhea (349.81)
      DEF: Spinal fluid leakage from ear.
      AHA: ▶2Q, '13, 8◄

    388.69 Other
      Otorrhagia

✓5ᵗʰ **388.7 Otalgia**

  388.70 Otalgia, unspecified
    Earache NOS

  388.71 Otogenic pain

  388.72 Referred pain

388.8 Other disorders of ear

388.9 Unspecified disorder of ear

✓4ᵗʰ **389 Hearing loss**

  ✓5ᵗʰ **389.0 Conductive hearing loss**
    Conductive deafness
    EXCLUDES mixed conductive and sensorineural hearing loss (389.20-389.22)
    DEF: Dysfunction in sound-conducting structures of external or middle ear causing hearing loss.
    AHA: 4Q, '07, 80; 4Q, '89, 5

    389.00 Conductive hearing loss, unspecified
      AHA: ▶2Q, '13, 8◄

    389.01 Conductive hearing loss, external ear

    389.02 Conductive hearing loss, tympanic membrane

    389.03 Conductive hearing loss, middle ear

    389.04 Conductive hearing loss, inner ear

    389.05 Conductive hearing loss, unilateral

    389.06 Conductive hearing loss, bilateral
      AHA: 4Q, '07, 81

    389.08 Conductive hearing loss of combined types

  ✓5ᵗʰ **389.1 Sensorineural hearing loss**
    Perceptive hearing loss or deafness
    EXCLUDES abnormal auditory perception (388.40-388.44)
            mixed conductive and sensorineural hearing loss (389.20-389.22)
            psychogenic deafness (306.7)
    DEF: Nerve conduction causing hearing loss.
    AHA: 4Q, '07, 80; 4Q, '89, 5

    389.10 Sensorineural hearing loss, unspecified
      AHA: 1Q, '93, 29

    389.11 Sensory hearing loss, bilateral

    389.12 Neural hearing loss, bilateral

    389.13 Neural hearing loss, unilateral

    389.14 Central hearing loss

    389.15 Sensorineural hearing loss, unilateral
      AHA: 4Q, '06, 84

    389.16 Sensorineural hearing loss, asymmetrical
      AHA: 4Q, '06, 84

    389.17 Sensory hearing loss, unilateral

    389.18 Sensorineural hearing loss, bilateral
      AHA: 4Q, '06, 84

  ✓5ᵗʰ **389.2 Mixed conductive and sensorineural hearing loss**
    Deafness or hearing loss of type classifiable to 389.00-389.08 with type classifiable to 389.10-389.18
    AHA: 4Q, '07, 80

    389.20 Mixed hearing loss, unspecified

    389.21 Mixed hearing loss, unilateral

    389.22 Mixed hearing loss, bilateral

  389.7 Deaf, non-speaking, not elsewhere classifiable

  389.8 Other specified forms of hearing loss

  389.9 Unspecified hearing loss
    Deafness NOS
    AHA: 1Q, '04, 15
    H91.93 Unspecified hearing loss bilateral   I-10

N Newborn Age: 0   P Pediatric Age: 0-17   M Maternity Age: 12-55   A Adult Age: 15-124

7. Diseases of the Circulatory System (390-459)

Acute Rheumatic Fever (390-392)

DEF: Febrile disease occurs mainly in children or young adults following throat infection by group A streptococci; symptoms include fever, joint pain, lesions of heart, blood vessels and joint connective tissue, abdominal pain, skin changes, and chorea.

390   Rheumatic fever without mention of heart involvement

Arthritis, rheumatic, acute or subacute
Rheumatic fever (active) (acute)
Rheumatism, articular, acute or subacute
EXCLUDES   *that with heart involvement (391.0-391.9)*

✓4th 391   Rheumatic fever with heart involvement

EXCLUDES   *chronic heart diseases of rheumatic origin (393-398.99)*
       unless rheumatic fever is also present or there is
       evidence of recrudescence or activity of the rheumatic
       process

391.0   Acute rheumatic pericarditis
Rheumatic:
    fever (active) (acute) with pericarditis
    pericarditis (acute)
Any condition classifiable to 390 with pericarditis
EXCLUDES   *that not specified as rheumatic (420.0-420.9)*
DEF: Sudden, severe inflammation of heart lining due to rheumatic fever.

391.1   Acute rheumatic endocarditis
Rheumatic:
    endocarditis, acute
    fever (active) (acute) with endocarditis or valvulitis
    valvulitis acute
Any condition classifiable to 390 with endocarditis or valvulitis
DEF: Sudden, severe inflammation of heart cavities due to rheumatic fever.

391.2   Acute rheumatic myocarditis
Rheumatic fever (active) (acute) with myocarditis
Any condition classifiable to 390 with myocarditis
DEF: Sudden, severe inflammation of heart muscles due to rheumatic fever.

391.8   Other acute rheumatic heart disease
Rheumatic:
    fever (active) (acute) with other or multiple types of heart
        involvement
    pancarditis, acute
Any condition classifiable to 390 with other or multiple types
    of heart involvement

391.9   Acute rheumatic heart disease, unspecified
Rheumatic:
    carditis, acute
    fever (active) (acute) with unspecified type of heart
        involvement
    heart disease, active or acute
Any condition classifiable to 390 with unspecified type of
    heart involvement

Sections of Heart Muscle

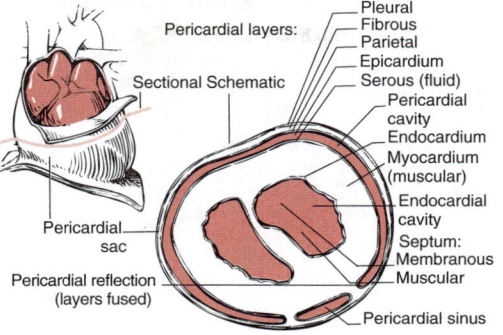

Pericardial layers:
Pleural
Fibrous
Parietal
Epicardium
Serous (fluid)
Pericardial cavity
Endocardium
Myocardium (muscular)
Endocardial cavity
Septum:
Membranous
Muscular

Sectional Schematic

Pericardial sac
Pericardial reflection (layers fused)
Pericardial sinus

✓4th 392   Rheumatic chorea

INCLUDES   Sydenham's chorea
EXCLUDES   *chorea:*
       NOS (333.5)
       Huntington's (333.4)
DEF: Childhood disease linked with rheumatic fever and streptococcal infections; symptoms include spasmodic, involuntary movements of limbs or facial muscles, psychic symptoms, and irritability.

392.0   With heart involvement
Rheumatic chorea with heart involvement of any type classifiable to 391

392.9   Without mention of heart involvement

Chronic Rheumatic Heart Disease (393-398)

393   Chronic rheumatic pericarditis

Adherent pericardium, rheumatic
Chronic rheumatic:
    mediastinopericarditis
    myopericarditis
EXCLUDES   *pericarditis NOS or not specified as rheumatic (423.0-423.9)*
DEF: Persistent inflammation of heart lining due to rheumatic heart disease.

✓4th 394   Diseases of mitral valve

EXCLUDES   *that with aortic valve involvement (396.0-396.9)*

394.0   Mitral stenosis
Mitral (valve):
    obstruction (rheumatic)
    stenosis NOS
DEF: Narrowing, of mitral valve between left atrium and left ventricle; due to rheumatic heart disease.
TIP: Assign when documentation indicates mitral valve stenosis or obstruction with no further specification of cause.

394.1   Rheumatic mitral insufficiency
Rheumatic mitral:
    incompetence
    regurgitation
EXCLUDES   *that not specified as rheumatic (424.0)*
DEF: Malfunction of mitral valve between left atrium and left ventricle; due to rheumatic heart disease.
AHA: 2Q, '05, 14

394.2   Mitral stenosis with insufficiency
Mitral stenosis with incompetence or regurgitation
DEF: A narrowing or stricture of the mitral valve situated between the left atrium and left ventricle; valve does not completely close, is insufficient (inadequate)in preventing regurgitation into the atrium; also called incompetence.
AHA: 1Q, '07, 11

394.9   Other and unspecified mitral valve diseases
Mitral (valve):
    disease (chronic)
    failure

✓4th 395   Diseases of aortic valve

EXCLUDES   *that not specified as rheumatic (424.1)*
       that with mitral valve involvement (396.0-396.9)

395.0   Rheumatic aortic stenosis
Rheumatic aortic (valve) obstruction
DEF: Narrowing of the aortic valve; results in backflow into ventricle; due to rheumatic heart disease.
AHA: 4Q, '88, 8

395.1   Rheumatic aortic insufficiency
Rheumatic aortic:
    incompetence
    regurgitation
DEF: Malfunction of the aortic valve; results in backflow into left ventricle; due to rheumatic heart disease.

395.2   Rheumatic aortic stenosis with insufficiency
Rheumatic aortic stenosis with incompetence or regurgitation
DEF: Malfunction and narrowing, of the aortic valve; results in backflow into left ventricle; due to rheumatic heart disease.

395.9   Other and unspecified rheumatic aortic diseases
Rheumatic aortic (valve) disease

✓4th ✓5th Additional Digit Required   Unspecified Code   Other Specified Code   Manifestation Code   ►◄ Revised Text   ● New Code   ▲ Revised Code Title

2015 ICD-9-CM   **Volume 1 – 123**

✓4th **396 Diseases of mitral and aortic valves**

> INCLUDES involvement of both mitral and aortic valves, whether specified as rheumatic or not

> AHA: N-D, '87, 8

396.0 Mitral valve stenosis and aortic valve stenosis
Atypical aortic (valve) stenosis
Mitral and aortic (valve) obstruction (rheumatic)

396.1 Mitral valve stenosis and aortic valve insufficiency

396.2 Mitral valve insufficiency and aortic valve stenosis
> AHA: 2Q, '09, 17; 1Q, '09, 18; 2Q, '00, 16

396.3 Mitral valve insufficiency and aortic valve insufficiency
Mitral and aortic (valve):
    incompetence
    regurgitation
I08.0 Rheumatic d/o of both mitral & aortic valves   I-10

396.8 Multiple involvement of mitral and aortic valves
Stenosis and insufficiency of mitral or aortic valve with stenosis or insufficiency, or both, of the other valve

396.9 Mitral and aortic valve diseases, unspecified

✓4th **397 Diseases of other endocardial structures**

397.0 Diseases of tricuspid valve
Tricuspid (valve) (rheumatic):
    disease
    insufficiency
    obstruction
    regurgitation
    stenosis
> DEF: Malfunction of the valve between right atrium and right ventricle; due to rheumatic heart disease.
> AHA: 3Q, '06, 7; 2Q, '00, 16
I07.2 Rheumatic tricuspid stenosis and insufficiency   I-10

397.1 Rheumatic diseases of pulmonary valve
> EXCLUDES that not specified as rheumatic (424.3)

397.9 Rheumatic diseases of endocardium, valve unspecified
Rheumatic:
    endocarditis (chronic)
    valvulitis (chronic)
> EXCLUDES that not specified as rheumatic (424.90-424.99)

✓4th **398 Other rheumatic heart disease**

398.0 Rheumatic myocarditis
Rheumatic degeneration of myocardium
> EXCLUDES myocarditis not specified as rheumatic (429.0)
> DEF: Chronic inflammation of heart muscle; due to rheumatic heart disease.

✓5th **398.9 Other and unspecified rheumatic heart diseases**

398.90 Rheumatic heart disease, unspecified
Rheumatic:
    carditis
    heart disease NOS
> EXCLUDES carditis not specified as rheumatic (429.89)
> heart disease NOS not specified as rheumatic (429.9)

398.91 Rheumatic heart failure (congestive)
Rheumatic left ventricular failure
> DEF: Decreased cardiac output, edema and hypertension; due to rheumatic heart disease.
> AHA: 2Q, '05, 14; 1Q, '95, 6; 3Q, '88, 3
I09.81 Rheumatic heart failure   I-10

398.99 Other

Hypertensive Disease (401-405)

> EXCLUDES that complicating pregnancy, childbirth, or the puerperium (642.0-642.9)
> that involving coronary vessels (410.00-414.9)
> AHA: 3Q, '90, 3; 2Q, '89, 12; S-O, '87, 9; J-A, '84, 11

✓4th **401 Essential hypertension**

> INCLUDES high blood pressure
> hyperpiesia
> hyperpiesis
> hypertension (arterial) (essential) (primary) (systemic)
> hypertensive vascular:
>   degeneration
>   disease

> EXCLUDES elevated blood pressure without diagnosis of hypertension (796.2)
> pulmonary hypertension (416.0-416.9)
> that involving vessels of:
>   brain (430-438)
>   eye (362.11)

> DEF: Hypertension that occurs without apparent organic cause; idiopathic.
> AHA: 2Q, '92, 5

401.0 Malignant
> DEF: Severe high arterial blood pressure; results in necrosis in kidney, retina, etc.; hemorrhages occur and death commonly due to uremia or rupture of cerebral vessel.
> AHA: M-J, '85, 19

401.1 Benign
> DEF: Mildly elevated arterial blood pressure.

401.9 Unspecified
> AHA: 1Q, '12, 14; 4Q, '10,124,125, 135; 4Q, '09, 77, 129; 1Q, '09, 18; 2Q, '08, 16; 4Q, '05, 71; 3Q, '05, 8; 4Q, '04, 78; 4Q, '03, 105, 108, 111; 3Q, '03, 14; 2Q, '03, 16; 4Q, '97, 37
I10 Essential (primary) hypertension   I-10

✓4th **402 Hypertensive heart disease**

> INCLUDES hypertensive:
>   cardiomegaly
>   cardiopathy
>   cardiovascular disease
>   heart (disease) (failure)
> any condition classifiable to 429.0-429.3, 429.8, 429.9 due to hypertension

Use additional code to specify type of heart failure (428.0-428.43), if known

> AHA: 4Q, '02, 49; 2Q, '93, 9; N-D, '84, 18
> TIP: Assign when a cardiac condition is stated (due to hypertension) or implied (hypertensive).

✓5th **402.0 Malignant**

402.00 Without heart failure

402.01 With heart failure
> AHA: 4Q, '08, 180

✓5th **402.1 Benign**

402.10 Without heart failure

402.11 With heart failure

✓5th **402.9 Unspecified**

402.90 Without heart failure
I11.9 Hypertensive heart disease without heart failure   I-10

402.91 With heart failure
> AHA: 4Q, '02, 52; 1Q, '93, 19; 2Q, '89, 12

N Newborn Age: 0   P Pediatric Age: 0-17   M Maternity Age: 12-55   A Adult Age: 15-124

Diseases of the Circulatory System

403–410.2

✓4ᵗʰ 403 Hypertensive chronic kidney disease

INCLUDES arteriolar nephritis
arteriosclerosis of:
    kidney
    renal arterioles
arteriosclerotic nephritis (chronic) (interstitial)
hypertensive:
    nephropathy
    renal failure
    uremia (chronic)
nephrosclerosis
renal sclerosis with hypertension
any condition classifiable to 585 and 587 with any condition classifiable to 401

EXCLUDES *acute kidney failure (584.5-584.9)*
renal disease stated as not due to hypertension
renovascular hypertension (405.0-405.9 with
    fifth-digit 1)

The following fifth-digit subclassification is for use with category 403:
  0 with chronic kidney disease stage I through stage IV, or unspecified
     Use additional code to identify the stage of chronic kidney disease (585.1-585.4, 585.9)
  1 with chronic kidney disease stage V or end stage renal disease
     Use additional code to identify the stage of chronic kidney disease (585.5, 585.6)

AHA: 4Q, '06, 84-86; 4Q, '05, 68; 4Q, '92, 22; 2Q, '92, 5
TIP: Assign whenever a patient has both chronic kidney disease and hypertension (presumed cause-and-effect relationship).

§ ✓5ᵗʰ **403.0 Malignant**
[0-1]

§ ✓5ᵗʰ **403.1 Benign**
[0-1]   AHA: For code 403.11: 3Q, '10, 12

§ ✓5ᵗʰ **403.9 Unspecified**
[0-1]   AHA: For code 403.90: 4Q, '10, 137; 1Q, '08, 10 ;2Q, '07, 3; 4Q, '06, 86; For code 403.91: 4Q, '10, 137; 1Q ,'08, 7; 4Q, '05, 69; 1Q, '04, 14; 1Q, '03, 20; 2Q, '01, 11; 3Q, '91, 8
    I12.9 HTN CKD w/stage I thru IV CKD/UNS CKD I-10

✓4ᵗʰ 404 Hypertensive heart and chronic kidney disease

INCLUDES disease:
    cardiorenal
    cardiovascular renal
any condition classifiable to 402 with any condition classifiable to 403

Use additional code to specify type of heart failure (428.0-428.43), if known

The following fifth-digit subclassification is for use with category 404:
  0 without heart failure and with chronic kidney disease stage I through stage IV, or unspecified
     Use additional code to identify the stage of chronic kidney disease (585.1-585.4, 585.9)
  1 with heart failure and with chronic kidney disease stage I through stage IV, or unspecified
     Use additional code to identify the stage of chronic kidney disease (585.1-585.4, 585.9)
  2 without heart failure and with chronic kidney disease stage V or end stage renal disease
     Use additional code to identify the stage of chronic kidney disease (585.5, 585.6)
  3 with heart failure and chronic kidney disease stage V or end stage renal disease
     Use additional code to identify the stage of chronic kidney disease (585.5, 585.6)

AHA: 4Q, '06, 84-86; 4Q, '05, 68; 4Q, '02, 49; 3Q, '90, 3; J-A, '84, 14

§ ✓5ᵗʰ **404.0 Malignant**
[0-3]

§ ✓5ᵗʰ **404.1 Benign**
[0-3]

§ ✓5ᵗʰ **404.9 Unspecified**
[0-3]   **I13.0 HTN heart & CKD HF & stage I thru IV CKD/UNS CKD** I-10

✓4ᵗʰ 405 Secondary hypertension

DEF: High arterial blood pressure due to or with a variety of primary diseases, such as renal disorders, CNS disorders, endocrine, and vascular diseases.
AHA: 3Q, '90, 3; S-O, '87, 9, 11; J-A, '84, 14

✓5ᵗʰ **405.0 Malignant**

    405.01 Renovascular

    405.09 Other

✓5ᵗʰ **405.1 Benign**

    405.11 Renovascular

    405.19 Other

✓5ᵗʰ **405.9 Unspecified**

    405.91 Renovascular

    405.99 Other
      AHA: 3Q, '00, 4

Ischemic Heart Disease (410-414)

INCLUDES that with mention of hypertension

Use additional code to identify presence of hypertension (401.0-405.9)

AHA: 3Q, '91, 10; J-A, '84, 5

✓4ᵗʰ 410 Acute myocardial infarction

INCLUDES cardiac infarction
coronary (artery):
    embolism
    occlusion
    rupture
    thrombosis
infarction of heart, myocardium, or ventricle
rupture of heart, myocardium, or ventricle
ST elevation (STEMI) and non-ST elevation (NSTEMI) myocardial infarction
any condition classifiable to 414.1-414.9 specified as acute or with a stated duration of 8 weeks or less

The following fifth-digit subclassification is for use with category 410:
  0 episode of care unspecified
     Use when the source document does not contain sufficient information for the assigment of fifth-digit 1 or 2.
  1 initial episode of care
     Use fifth-digit 1 to designate the first episode of care (regardless of facility site) for a newly diagnosed myocardial infarction. The fifth-digit 1 is assigned regardless of the number of times a patient may be transferred during the initial episode of care.
  2 subsequent episode of care
     Use fifth-digit 2 to designate an episode of care following the initial episode when the patient is admitted for further observation, evaluation or treatment for a myocardial infarction that has received initial treatment, but is still less than 8 weeks old.

DEF: A sudden insufficiency of blood supply to an area of the heart muscle; usually due to a coronary artery occlusion.
AHA: 1Q, '12, 7; 2Q, '06, 9; 4Q, '05, 69; 3Q, '01, 21; 3Q, '98, 15; 4Q, '97, 37; 3Q, '95, 9; 4Q, 92, 24; 1Q, '92, 10; 3Q, '91, 18; 1Q, '91, 14; 3Q, '89, 3
TIP: Assign an acute MI code with a fifth digit of "1," initial episode of care, for all care provided before the AMI has resolved, regardless of type or number of transfers between facilities.

§ ✓5ᵗʰ **410.0 Of anterolateral wall**
[0-2]   ST elevation myocardial infarction (STEMI) of anterolateral wall
     AHA: For code 410.01: 4Q, '09, 129; 4Q, '08, 72

§ ✓5ᵗʰ **410.1 Of other anterior wall**
[0-2]   Infarction:
     anterior (wall) NOS ⎫ (with contiguous portion of
     anteroapical   ⎬   intraventricular
     anteroseptal   ⎭   septum)
    ST elevation myocardial infarction (STEMI) of other anterior wall
     AHA: For code 410.11: 3Q, '03, 10

§ ✓5ᵗʰ **410.2 Of inferolateral wall**
[0-2]   ST elevation myocardial infarction (STEMI) of inferolateral wall

---

§ Requires fifth digit. Valid digits are in [brackets] under each code. See appropriate category for codes and definitions.

✓4ᵗʰ ✓5ᵗʰ Additional Digit Required   Unspecified Code   Other Specified Code   Manifestation Code   ►◄ Revised Text   ● New Code   ▲ Revised Code Title

2015 ICD-9-CM   Volume 1 – 125

Diseases of the Circulatory System

410.3–413.9

Acute Myocardial Infarction

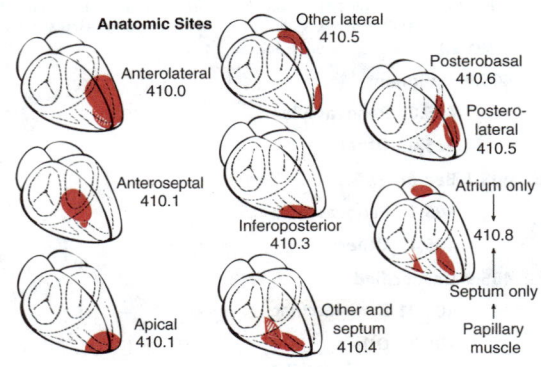

Anatomic Sites

Anterolateral 410.0

Other lateral 410.5

Posterobasal 410.6

Postero-lateral 410.5

Anteroseptal 410.1

Inferoposterior 410.3

Atrium only 410.8

Apical 410.1

Other and septum 410.4

Septum only

Papillary muscle

§ ✓5ᵗʰ **410.3 Of inferoposterior wall**
[0-2]   ST elevation myocardial infarction (STEMI) of inferoposterior wall

§ ✓5ᵗʰ **410.4 Of other inferior wall**
[0-2]   Infarction:
         diaphragmatic wall NOS ⎫ (with contiguous portion of
         inferior (wall) NOS   ⎭   intraventricular septum)
         ST elevation myocardial infarction (STEMI) of other inferior wall
         AHA: 1Q, '00, 7, 26; 4Q, '99, 9; 3Q, '97, 10; **For code 410.41:** 3Q, '09, 10; 2Q, '01, 8, 9
         I21.19 STEMI invlv oth coronary artery of inferior wall   **I-10**

§ ✓5ᵗʰ **410.5 Of other lateral wall**
[0-2]   Infarction:
         apical-lateral
         basal-lateral
         high lateral
         posterolateral
         ST elevation myocardial infarction (STEMI) of other lateral wall
         AHA: For code 410.51: 3Q, '09, 9

§ ✓5ᵗʰ **410.6 True posterior wall infarction**
[0-2]   Infarction:
         posterobasal
         strictly posterior
         ST elevation myocardial infarction (STEMI) of true posterior wall

§ ✓5ᵗʰ **410.7 Subendocardial infarction**
[0-2]   Non-ST elevation myocardial infarction (NSTEMI)
         Nontransmural infarction
         AHA: 1Q, '00, 7; **For code 410.71:** 2Q, '10, 8-9; 4Q, '05, 71; 2Q, '05, 19
         I21.4 Non-ST elevation (NSTEMI) myocardial infarction   **I-10**

§ ✓5ᵗʰ **410.8 Of other specified sites**
[0-2]   Infarction of:
         atrium
         papillary muscle
         septum alone
         ST elevation myocardial infarction (STEMI) of other specified sites

§ ✓5ᵗʰ **410.9 Unspecified site**
[0-2]   Acute myocardial infarction NOS
         Coronary occlusion NOS
         Myocardial infarction NOS
         AHA: 1Q, '96, 17; 1Q, '92, 9; **For code 410.91:** 2Q, '05, 18; 3Q, '02, 5
         I21.3 ST elevation myocardial infarction of uns site   **I-10**

✓4ᵗʰ **411 Other acute and subacute forms of ischemic heart disease**
     AHA: 4Q, '94, 55; 3Q, '91, 24

     411.0 Postmyocardial infarction syndrome
             Dressler's syndrome
             DEF: Complication developing several days/weeks after myocardial infarction; symptoms include fever, leukocytosis, chest pain, pericarditis, pleurisy, and pneumonitis; tendency to recur.

411.1 Intermediate coronary syndrome
        Impending infarction   Preinfarction syndrome
        Preinfarction angina   Unstable angina
        EXCLUDES *angina (pectoris) (413.9)*
                    decubitus (413.0)
        DEF: A condition representing an intermediate stage between angina of effort and acute myocardial infarction. It is often documented by the physician as "unstable angina."
        AHA: 3Q, '07, 9; 4Q, '05, 105; 2Q, '04, 3; 1Q, '03, 12; 3Q, '01, 15; 2Q, '01, 7, 9; 4Q, '98, 86; 2Q, '96, 10; 3Q, '91, 24; 1Q, '91, 14; 3Q, '90, 6; 4Q, '89, 10
        TIP: Do not assign code 411.1 on the same episode of care as an acute myocardial infarction (category 410). Assign 411.1 for accelerated angina.
        I20.0 Unstable angina   **I-10**

✓5ᵗʰ **411.8 Other**
     AHA: 3Q, '91, 18; 3Q, '89, 4

     411.81 Acute coronary occlusion without myocardial infarction
             Acute coronary (artery):
                embolism   ⎫ without or not resulting
                obstruction   ⎬   in myocardial
                occlusion   ⎪   infarction
                thrombosis   ⎭
             EXCLUDES *obstruction without infarction due to atherosclerosis (414.00-414.07)*
                         occlusion without infarction due to atherosclerosis (414.00-414.07)
             DEF: Interrupted blood flow to a portion of the heart; without tissue death.
             AHA: 3Q, '91, 24; 1Q, '91, 14

     411.89 Other
             Coronary insufficiency (acute)
             Subendocardial ischemia
             AHA: 3Q, '01, 14; 1Q, '92, 9

412 Old myocardial infarction
     Healed myocardial infarction
     Past myocardial infarction diagnosed on ECG [EKG] or other special investigation, but currently presenting no symptoms
     AHA: 2Q, '03, 10; 2Q, '01, 9; 3Q, '98, 15; 2Q, '91, 22; 3Q, '90, 7
     TIP: Assign for any acute myocardial infarction stated to be older than 8 weeks.
     I25.2 Old myocardial infarction   **I-10**

✓4ᵗʰ **413 Angina pectoris**
     DEF: Severe constricting pain in the chest, often radiating from the precordium to the left shoulder and down the arm, due to ischemia of the heart muscle; usually caused by coronary disease; pain is often precipitated by effort or excitement.

     413.0 Angina decubitus
             Nocturnal angina
             DEF: Angina occurring only in the recumbent position.

     413.1 Prinzmetal angina
             Variant angina pectoris
             DEF: Angina occurring when patient is recumbent; associated with ST-segment elevations.
             AHA: 3Q, '06, 23

     413.9 Other and unspecified angina pectoris
             Angina: Anginal syndrome
                NOS   Status anginosus
                cardiac   Stenocardia
                equivalent   Syncope anginosa
                of effort
             Use additional code(s) for symptoms associated with angina equivalent
             EXCLUDES *preinfarction angina (411.1)*
             AHA: 2Q, '08, 16; 3Q, '02, 4; 3Q, '91, 16; 3Q, '90, 6
             TIP: For patients with both angina and coronary artery disease, sequence the CAD (subcategory 414.0) code first.
             I20.9 Angina pectoris unspecified   **I-10**

---

§   Requires fifth digit. Valid digits are in [brackets] under each code. See category 410 for codes and definitions.

N Newborn Age: 0   **P** Pediatric Age: 0-17   **M** Maternity Age: 12-55   **A** Adult Age: 15-124

☑4ᵗʰ **414 Other forms of chronic ischemic heart disease**

EXCLUDES *arteriosclerotic cardiovascular disease [ASCVD] (429.2)*
cardiovascular:
arteriosclerosis or sclerosis (429.2)
degeneration or disease (429.2)

☑5ᵗʰ **414.0 Coronary atherosclerosis**

Arteriosclerotic heart disease [ASHD] Coronary (artery):
Atherosclerotic heart disease arteritis or endarteritis
Coronary (artery): atheroma
arteriosclerosis sclerosis
  stricture

Use additional code, if applicable, to identify chronic total occlusion of coronary artery (414.2)

EXCLUDES *embolism of graft (996.72)*
occlusion NOS of graft (996.72)
thrombus of graft (996.72)

DEF: A chronic condition marked by thickening and loss of elasticity of the coronary artery; caused by deposits of plaque containing cholesterol, lipoid material and lipophages.

AHA: 2Q, '97, 13; 2Q, '95, 17; 4Q, '94, 49; 2Q, '94, 13; 1Q, '94, 6; 3Q, '90, 7

414.00 Of unspecified type of vessel, native or graft Ⓐ
AHA: 1Q, '04, 24; 2Q, '03, 16; 3Q, '01, 15; 4Q, '99, 4; 3Q, '97, 15; 4Q, '96, 31

414.01 Of native coronary artery Ⓐ
DEF: Plaque deposits in natural heart vessels.
AHA: 3Q, '12, 17; 3Q, '09, 9, 10; 3Q, '08, 10; 2Q, '08, 16; 3Q, '06, 25; 4Q, '05, 71; 2Q, '04, 3; 4Q, '03, 108; 3Q, '03, 9, 14; 3Q, '02, 4-9; 3Q, '01, 15; 2Q, '01, 8, 9; 3Q, '97, 15; 2Q, '96, 10; 4Q, '96, 31
TIP: Assign for documentation of CAD NOS in a patient with no history of coronary artery bypass procedure.
I25.10 ASHD of native cor artery w/o angina pectoris I-10

414.02 Of autologous vein bypass graft Ⓐ
AHA: 2Q, '10, 8-9
DEF: Plaque deposit in grafted vein originating within patient.

414.03 Of nonautologous biological bypass graft Ⓐ
DEF: Plaque deposits in grafted vessel originating outside patient.

414.04 Of artery bypass graft Ⓐ
Internal mammary artery
DEF: Plaque deposits in grafted artery originating within patient.
AHA: 4Q, '96, 31

414.05 Of unspecified type of bypass graft Ⓐ
Bypass graft NOS
AHA: 3Q, '97, 15; 4Q, '96, 31

414.06 Of native coronary artery of transplanted heart
AHA: 4Q, '03, 60; 4Q, '02, 53

414.07 Of bypass graft (artery) (vein) of transplanted heart Ⓐ

☑5ᵗʰ **414.1 Aneurysm and dissection of heart**
AHA: 4Q, '02, 54

414.10 Aneurysm of heart (wall)
Aneurysm (arteriovenous):
mural
ventricular

Arteries of the Heart

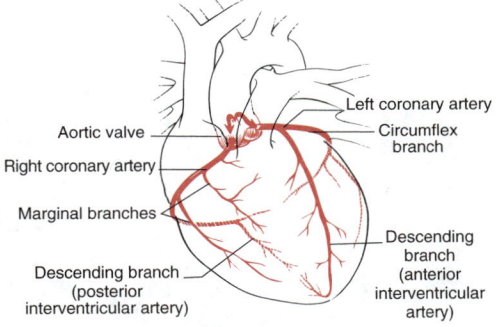

Aortic valve
Right coronary artery
Marginal branches
Descending branch (posterior interventricular artery)
Left coronary artery
Circumflex branch
Descending branch (anterior interventricular artery)

414.11 Aneurysm of coronary vessels
Aneurysm (arteriovenous) of coronary vessels
DEF: Dilatation of all three-vessel wall layers forming a sac filled with blood.
AHA: 2Q, '10, 8-9; 3Q, '03, 10; 1Q, '99, 17

414.12 Dissection of coronary artery
DEF: A tear in the intimal arterial wall of a coronary artery resulting in the sudden intrusion of blood within the layers of the wall.
AHA: 1Q, '11, 3-4

414.19 Other aneurysm of heart
Arteriovenous fistula, acquired, of heart

414.2 Chronic total occlusion of coronary artery
Complete occlusion of coronary artery
Total occlusion of coronary artery
Code first coronary atherosclerosis (414.00-414.07)
EXCLUDES *acute coronary occlusion with myo- cardial infarction (410.00-410.92)*
acute coronary occlusion without myocardial infarction (411.81)
DEF: Complete blockage of coronary artery due to plaque accumulation over an extended period of time; results in substantial reduction of blood flow.
AHA: 4Q, '07, 82

414.3 Coronary atherosclerosis due to lipid rich plaque Ⓐ
Code first coronary atherosclerosis (414.00-414.07)
AHA: 4Q, '08, 113

414.4 Coronary atherosclerosis due to calcified coronary lesion
Coronary atherosclerosis due to severely calcified coronary lesion
Code first coronary atherosclerosis (414.00-414.07)
AHA: 4Q, '11, 107

414.8 Other specified forms of chronic ischemic heart disease
Chronic coronary insufficiency
Ischemia, myocardial (chronic)
Any condition classifiable to 410 specified as chronic, or presenting with symptoms after 8 weeks from date of infarction
EXCLUDES *coronary insufficiency (acute) (411.89)*
AHA: ►4Q, '13, 102;◄ 3Q, '01, 15; 1Q, '92, 10; 3Q, '90, 7, 15; 2Q, '90, 19
I25.89 Other forms of chronic ischemic heart disease I-10

414.9 Chronic ischemic heart disease, unspecified
Ischemic heart disease NOS

Diseases of Pulmonary Circulation (415-417)

☑4ᵗʰ **415 Acute pulmonary heart disease**

415.0 Acute cor pulmonale
EXCLUDES *cor pulmonale NOS (416.9)*
DEF: A heart-lung disease marked by dilation and failure of the right side of heart; due to pulmonary embolism; ventilatory function is impaired and pulmonary hypertension results.

☑5ᵗʰ **415.1 Pulmonary embolism and infarction**
Pulmonary (artery) (vein): Pulmonary (artery) (vein):
apoplexy infarction (hemorrhagic)
embolism thrombosis
EXCLUDES *chronic pulmonary embolism (416.2)*
personal history of pulmonary embolism (V12.55)
that complicating:
abortion (634-638 with .6, 639.6)
ectopic or molar pregnancy (639.6)
pregnancy, childbirth, or the puerperium (673.0-673.8)
DEF: Embolism: Closure of the pulmonary artery or branch; due to thrombosis (blood clot).
DEF: Infarction: Necrosis of lung tissue; due to obstructed arterial blood supply, most often by pulmonary embolism.
AHA: 4Q, '90, 25

415.11 Iatrogenic pulmonary embolism and infarction
Use additional code for associated septic pulmonary embolism, if applicable, 415.12
AHA: 4Q, '95, 58
TIP: Do not report code 997.39 Other respiratory complications, with code 415.11.

☑4ᵗʰ
☑5ᵗʰ Additional Digit Required Unspecified Code Other Specified Code Manifestation Code ►◄ Revised Text ● New Code ▲ Revised Code Title

2015 ICD-9-CM **October 2014 • Volume 1 – 127**

415.12 Septic pulmonary embolism
Septic embolism NOS

Code first underlying infection, such as:
septicemia (038.0-038.9)

EXCLUDES *septic arterial embolism (449)*

AHA: 4Q, '07, 84-86

415.13 Saddle embolus of pulmonary artery

AHA: 4Q, '11, 107-108

415.19 Other

AHA: 3Q, '10, 10; 4Q, '09, 86

I26.99 Other pulmonary embolism w/o acute cor pulmonale ▐I-10▌

√4ᵗʰ **416 Chronic pulmonary heart disease**

416.0 Primary pulmonary hypertension
Idiopathic pulmonary arteriosclerosis
Pulmonary hypertension (essential) (idiopathic) (primary)

EXCLUDES *pulmonary hypertension NOS (416.8)*
secondary pulmonary hypertension (416.8)

DEF: A rare increase in pulmonary circulation, often resulting in right ventricular failure or fatal syncope.

I27.0 Primary pulmonary hypertension ▐I-10▌

416.1 Kyphoscoliotic heart disease

DEF: High blood pressure within the lungs as a result of curvature of the spine.

416.2 Chronic pulmonary embolism

Use additional code, if applicable, for associated long-term (current) use of anticoagulants (V58.61)

EXCLUDES *personal history of pulmonary embolism (V12.55)*

DEF: A long-standing condition commonly associated with pulmonary hypertension in which small blood clots travel to the lungs repeatedly over many weeks, months, or years, requiring continuation of established anticoagulant or thrombolytic therapy.

AHA: 4Q, '09, 85-86

416.8 Other chronic pulmonary heart diseases
Pulmonary hypertension NOS
Pulmonary hypertension, secondary

AHA: 1Q, '12, 17; 1Q, '11, 10; 3Q, '10, 12; 2Q, '10, 10

I27.89 Other specified pulmonary heart diseases ▐I-10▌

416.9 Chronic pulmonary heart disease, unspecified
Chronic cardiopulmonary disease
Cor pulmonale (chronic) NOS

√4ᵗʰ **417 Other diseases of pulmonary circulation**

417.0 Arteriovenous fistula of pulmonary vessels

EXCLUDES *congenital arteriovenous fistula (747.32)*

DEF: Abnormal communication between blood vessels within lung.

417.1 Aneurysm of pulmonary artery

EXCLUDES *congenital aneurysm (747.39)*
congenital arteriovenous aneurysm (747.32)

417.8 Other specified diseases of pulmonary circulation
Pulmonary:
arteritis
endarteritis
Rupture } of pulmonary vessel
Stricture

417.9 Unspecified disease of pulmonary circulation

Anatomy

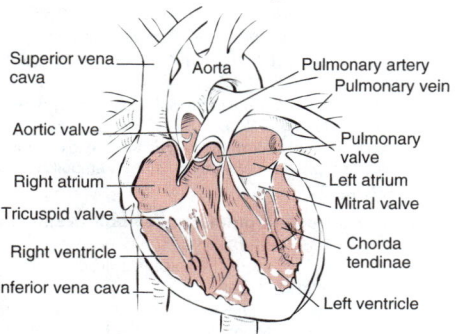

Superior vena cava
Aorta
Pulmonary artery
Pulmonary vein
Aortic valve
Pulmonary valve
Right atrium
Left atrium
Tricuspid valve
Mitral valve
Right ventricle
Chorda tendinae
Inferior vena cava
Left ventricle

Blood Flow

Other Forms of Heart Disease (420-429)

√4ᵗʰ **420 Acute pericarditis**

INCLUDES acute:
mediastinopericarditis
myopericarditis
pericardial effusion
pleuropericarditis
pneumopericarditis

EXCLUDES *acute rheumatic pericarditis (391.0)*
postmyocardial infarction syndrome [Dressler's] (411.0)

DEF: Inflammation of the pericardium (heart sac); pericardial friction rub results from this inflammation and is heard as a scratchy or leathery sound.

420.0 Acute pericarditis in diseases classified elsewhere

Code first underlying disease, as:
actinomycosis (039.8)
amebiasis (006.8)
chronic uremia (585.9)
nocardiosis (039.8)
tuberculosis (017.9)
uremia NOS (586)

EXCLUDES *pericarditis (acute) (in):*
Coxsackie (virus) (074.21)
gonococcal (098.83)
histoplasmosis (115.0-115.9 with fifth-digit 3)
meningococcal infection (036.41)
syphilitic (093.81)

√5ᵗʰ **420.9 Other and unspecified acute pericarditis**

420.90 Acute pericarditis, unspecified
Pericarditis (acute):   Periocarditis (acute):
NOS   sicca
infective NOS

AHA: 2Q, '89, 12

420.91 Acute idiopathic pericarditis
Pericarditis, acute: Periocarditis (acute):
benign   viral
nonspecific

420.99 Other
Pericarditis (acute):   Pericarditis (acute):
pneumococcal   suppurative
purulent   Pneumopyopericardium
staphylococcal   Pyopericardium
streptococcal

EXCLUDES *pericarditis in diseases classified elsewhere (420.0)*

√4th **421 Acute and subacute endocarditis**
> **DEF:** Bacterial inflammation of the endocardium (intracardiac area); major symptoms include fever, fatigue, heart murmurs, splenomegaly, embolic episodes and areas of infarction.

421.0 Acute and subacute bacterial endocarditis
Endocarditis (acute)(chronic) (subacute):
> bacterial
> infective NOS
> lenta
> malignant
> purulent
> septic
> ulcerative
> vegetative

Infective aneurysm
Subacute bacterial endocarditis [SBE]

Use additional code to identify infectious organism [e.g., Streptococcus 041.0, Staphylococcus 041.1]

AHA: 4Q, '08, 73; 1Q, '99, 12; 1Q, '91, 15

I33.0 Acute and subacute infective endocarditis   I-10

421.1 **Acute and subacute infective endocarditis in diseases classified elsewhere**
> *Code first underlying disease, as:*
> blastomycosis (116.0)
> Q fever (083.0)
> typhoid (fever) (002.0)

EXCLUDES *endocarditis (in):*
> *Coxsackie (virus) (074.22)*
> *gonococcal (098.84)*
> *histoplasmosis (115.0-115.9 with fifth-digit 4)*
> *meningococcal infection (036.42)*
> *monilial (112.81)*

421.9 Acute endocarditis, unspecified
Endocarditis
Myoendocarditis } acute or subacute
Periendocarditis

EXCLUDES *acute rheumatic endocarditis (391.1)*

√4th **422 Acute myocarditis**
> **EXCLUDES** *acute rheumatic myocarditis (391.2)*
> **DEF:** Acute inflammation of the muscular walls of the heart (myocardium).

422.0 **Acute myocarditis in diseases classified elsewhere**
> *Code first underlying disease, as:*
> myocarditis (acute):
> influenzal (487.8, 488.09, 488.19)
> tuberculous (017.9)

EXCLUDES *myocarditis (acute) (due to):*
> *aseptic, of newborn (074.23)*
> *Coxsackie (virus) (074.23)*
> *diphtheritic (032.82)*
> *meningococcal infection (036.43)*
> *syphilitic (093.82)*
> *toxoplasmosis (130.3)*

√5th **422.9 Other and unspecified acute myocarditis**

422.90 Acute myocarditis, unspecified
Acute or subacute (interstitial) myocarditis

422.91 Idiopathic myocarditis
Myocarditis (acute or subacute):
> Fiedler's
> giant cell
> isolated (diffuse) (granulomatous)
> nonspecific granulomatous

422.92 Septic myocarditis
Myocarditis, acute or subacute:
> pneumococcal
> staphylococcal

Use additional code to identify infectious organism [e.g., Staphylococcus 041.1]

EXCLUDES *myocarditis, acute or subacute:*
> *in bacterial diseases classified elsewhere (422.0)*
> *streptococcal (391.2)*

Cardiac Tamponade

Normal   Cardiac Tamponade

422.93 Toxic myocarditis
> **DEF:** Inflammation of the heart muscle due to an adverse reaction to certain drugs or chemicals reaching the heart through the bloodstream.

422.99 Other

√4th **423 Other diseases of pericardium**
> **EXCLUDES** *that specified as rheumatic (393)*

423.0 Hemopericardium
> **DEF:** Blood in the pericardial sac (pericardium).

423.1 Adhesive pericarditis
Adherent pericardium   Pericarditis:
Fibrosis of pericardium   adhesive
Milk spots   obliterative
                   Soldiers' patches

> **DEF:** Two layers of serous pericardium adhere to each other by fibrous adhesions.

423.2 Constrictive pericarditis
Concato's disease
Pick's disease of heart (and liver)
> **DEF:** Inflammation identified by a rigid, thickened and sometimes calcified pericardium; ventricles of the heart not adequately filled; congestive heart failure may result.

423.3 Cardiac tamponade
> Code first the underlying cause
> **DEF:** Life-threatening condition in which fluid or blood accumulates between the muscle of the heart (myocardium) and the outer sac (pericardium), resulting in compression of the heart, which decreases cardiac output.
> **AHA:** 4Q, '07, 86, 87

423.8 Other specified diseases of pericardium
Calcification
Fistula } of pericardium
AHA: 2Q, '89, 12

423.9 Unspecified disease of pericardium
AHA: 1Q, '07, 11

√4th **424 Other diseases of endocardium**
> **EXCLUDES** *bacterial endocarditis (421.0-421.9)*
> *rheumatic endocarditis (391.1, 394.0-397.9)*
> *syphilitic endocarditis (093.20-093.24)*

424.0 Mitral valve disorders
Mitral (valve):
> incompetence
> insufficiency } NOS of specified cause, except rheumatic
> regurgitation

EXCLUDES *mitral (valve):*
> *disease (394.9)*
> *failure (394.9)*
> *stenosis (394.0)*
> *the listed conditions:*
> *specified as rheumatic (394.1)*
> *unspecified as to cause but with mention of:*
> *diseases of aortic valve (396.0-396.9)*
> *mitral stenosis or obstruction (394.2)*

AHA: 3Q, '06, 7; 2Q, '00, 16; 3Q, '98, 11; N-D, '87, 8; N-D, '84, 8

I34.8 Other nonrheumatic mitral valve disorders   I-10

√4th √5th Additional Digit Required   Unspecified Code   Other Specified Code   Manifestation Code   ►◄ Revised Text   ● New Code   ▲ Revised Code Title

2015 ICD-9-CM   **Volume 1 – 129**

Diseases of the Circulatory System

424.1–426.10

Heart Valve Disorders

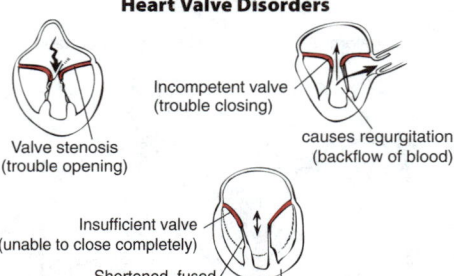

Normal Heart Valve Function

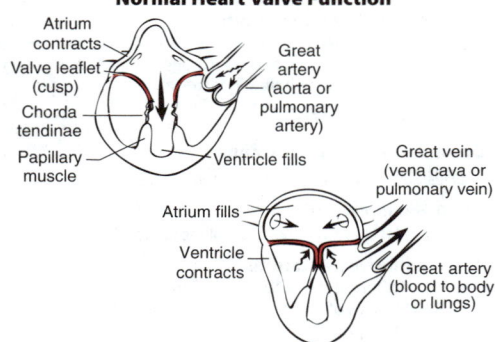

424.1 Aortic valve disorders
Aortic (valve):
  incompetence
  insufficiency   } NOS of specified cause,
  regurgitation   except rheumatic
  stenosis

EXCLUDES *hypertrophic subaortic stenosis (425.11)*
that specified as rheumatic (395.0-395.9)
that of unspecified cause but with mention of diseases of mitral valve (396.0-396.9)
AHA: 4Q, '11, 152; 4Q, '08, 179; 4Q, '88, 8; N-D, '87, 8

424.2 Tricuspid valve disorders, specified as nonrheumatic
Tricuspid valve:
  incompetence
  insufficiency   } of specified cause, except
  regurgitation   rheumatic
  stenosis

EXCLUDES *rheumatic or of unspecified cause (397.0)*

424.3 Pulmonary valve disorders
Pulmonic: Pulmonic:
  incompetence NOS   regurgitation NOS
  insufficiency NOS   stenosis NOS

EXCLUDES *that specified as rheumatic (397.1)*

√5ᵗʰ **424.9 Endocarditis, valve unspecified**

424.90 Endocarditis, valve unspecified, unspecified cause
Endocarditis (chronic):
  NOS
  nonbacterial thrombotic
Valvular:
  incompetence
  insufficiency   } of unspecified valve,
  regurgitation   unspecified cause
  stenosis
Valvulitis (chronic)
I38 Endocarditis valve unspecified   I-10

424.91 Endocarditis in diseases classified elsewhere
Code first underlying disease as:
  atypical verrucous endocarditis [Libman-Sacks] (710.0)
  disseminated lupus erythematosus (710.0)
  tuberculosis (017.9)
EXCLUDES *syphilitic (093.20-093.24)*

424.99 Other
Any condition classifiable to 424.90 with specified cause, except rheumatic
EXCLUDES *endocardial fibroelastosis (425.3)*
that specified as rheumatic (397.9)

√4ᵗʰ **425 Cardiomyopathy**
INCLUDES myocardiopathy
AHA: J-A, '85, 15

425.0 Endomyocardial fibrosis

√5ᵗʰ **425.1 Hypertrophic cardiomyopathy**
EXCLUDES *ventricular hypertrophy (429.3)*
AHA: 4Q, '11, 109-110

425.11 Hypertrophic obstructive cardiomyopathy
Hypertrophic subaortic stenosis (idiopathic)
DEF: Cardiomyopathy marked by left ventricle hypertrophy, enlarged septum; results in obstructed blood flow.
AHA: ▶3Q, '13, 10◀

425.18 Other hypertrophic cardiomyopathy
Nonobstructive hypertrophic cardiomyopathy

425.2 Obscure cardiomyopathy of Africa
Becker's disease
Idiopathic mural endomyocardial disease

425.3 Endocardial fibroelastosis
Elastomyofibrosis
DEF: A condition marked by left ventricle hypertrophy and conversion of the endocardium into a thick fibroelastic coat; capacity of the ventricle may be reduced, but is often increased.

425.4 Other primary cardiomyopathies
Cardiomyopathy: Cardiomyopathy:
  NOS   idiopathic
  congestive   obstructive
  constrictive   restrictive
  familial   Cardiovascular collagenosis
AHA: 4Q, '11, 109-110; 4Q, '09, 141; 1Q, '07, 20; 2Q, '05, 14; 1Q, '00, 22; 4Q, '97, 55; 2Q, '90, 19
TIP: For congestive cardiomyopathy, assign first a code for the CHF (category 428) if the treatment is directed toward the CHF.
I42.8 Other cardiomyopathies   I-10

425.5 Alcoholic cardiomyopathy
DEF: Heart disease as result of excess alcohol consumption.
AHA: S-O, '85, 15

425.7 *Nutritional and metabolic cardiomyopathy*
Code first underlying disease, as:
  amyloidosis (277.30-277.39)
  beriberi (265.0)
  cardiac glycogenosis (271.0)
  mucopolysaccharidosis (277.5)
  thyrotoxicosis (242.0-242.9)
EXCLUDES *gouty tophi of heart (274.82)*

425.8 *Cardiomyopathy in other diseases classified elsewhere*
Code first underlying disease, as:
  Friedreich's ataxia (334.0)
  myotonia atrophica (359.21)
  progressive muscular dystrophy (359.1)
  sarcoidosis (135)
EXCLUDES *cardiomyopathy in Chagas' disease (086.0)*
AHA: 2Q, '93, 9
I43 Cardiomyopathy in diseases classified elsewhere   I-10

425.9 Secondary cardiomyopathy, unspecified

√4ᵗʰ **426 Conduction disorders**
DEF: Disruption or disturbance in the electrical impulses that regulate heartbeats.

426.0 Atrioventricular block, complete
Third degree atrioventricular block
AHA: 2Q, '06, 14
TIP: Assign if documentation indicates intermittent complete heart block.

√5ᵗʰ **426.1 Atrioventricular block, other and unspecified**
AHA: 2Q, '06, 14
TIP: Assign separate codes for each type of AV block documented.

426.10 Atrioventricular block, unspecified
Atrioventricular [AV] block (incomplete) (partial)

Nerve Conduction of the Heart

Normal and Long QT Electrocardiogram

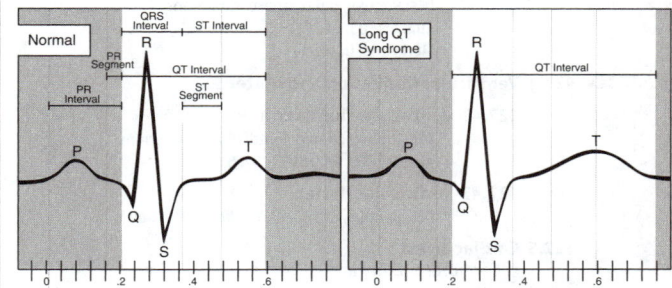

426.11 First degree atrioventricular block
Incomplete atrioventricular block, first degree
Prolonged P-R interval NOS
AHA: 2Q, '06, 14
I44.0 Atrioventricular block first degree [I-10]

426.12 Mobitz (type) II atrioventricular block
Incomplete atrioventricular block:
Mobitz (type) II
second degree, Mobitz (type) II
DEF: Impaired conduction of excitatory impulse from cardiac atrium to ventricle through AV node.
AHA: 2Q, '06, 14

426.13 Other second degree atrioventricular block
Incomplete atrioventricular block:
Mobitz (type) I [Wenckebach's]
second degree:
NOS
Mobitz (type) I
with 2:1 atrioventricular response [block]
Wenckebach's phenomenon
DEF: Wenckebach's phenomenon: impulses generated at constant rate to sinus node, P-R interval lengthens; results in cycle of ventricular inadequacy and shortened P-R interval; second-degree A-V block commonly called "Mobitz type 1."

426.2 Left bundle branch hemiblock
Block: Block:
left anterior fascicular   left posterior fascicular

426.3 Other left bundle branch block
Left bundle branch block:
NOS
anterior fascicular with posterior fascicular
complete
main stem
I44.7 Left bundle-branch block unspecified [I-10]

426.4 Right bundle branch block
AHA: 3Q, '00, 3
I45.10 Unspecified right bundle-branch block [I-10]

√5ᵗʰ 426.5 Bundle branch block, other and unspecified

426.50 Bundle branch block, unspecified

426.51 Right bundle branch block and left posterior fascicular block

426.52 Right bundle branch block and left anterior fascicular block

426.53 Other bilateral bundle branch block
Bifascicular block NOS
Bilateral bundle branch block NOS
Right bundle branch with left bundle branch block (incomplete) (main stem)

426.54 Trifascicular block

426.6 Other heart block
Intraventricular block:
NOS
diffuse
myofibrillar
Sinoatrial block
Sinoauricular block

426.7 Anomalous atrioventricular excitation
Atrioventricular   Ventricular pre-excitation accelerated
conduction: Wolff-Parkinson-White syndrome
accessory
pre-excitation
DEF: Wolff-Parkinson-White: normal conduction pathway is bypassed; results in short P-R interval on EKG; tendency to supraventricular tachycardia.

√5ᵗʰ 426.8 Other specified conduction disorders

426.81 Lown-Ganong-Levine syndrome
Syndrome of short P-R interval, normal QRS complexes, and supraventricular tachycardias

426.82 Long QT syndrome
DEF: Condition characterized by recurrent syncope, malignant arrhythmias, and sudden death; characteristic prolonged Q-T interval on electrocardiogram.
AHA: 4Q, '05, 72

426.89 Other
Dissociation: Nonparoxysmal AV
atrioventricular [AV]   nodal tachycardia
interference
isorhythmic
AHA: ▶2Q, '13, 25◀

426.9 Conduction disorder, unspecified
Heart block NOS   Stokes-Adams syndrome

√4ᵗʰ 427 Cardiac dysrhythmias
EXCLUDES that complicating:
abortion (634-638 with .7, 639.8)
ectopic or molar pregnancy (639.8)
labor or delivery (668.1, 669.4)
DEF: Disruption or disturbance in the rhythm of heartbeats.
AHA: J-A, '85, 15

427.0 Paroxysmal supraventricular tachycardia
Paroxysmal tachycardia: Paroxysmal tachycardia:
atrial [PAT]   junctional
atrioventricular [AV]   nodal
DEF: Rapid atrial rhythm.

427.1 Paroxysmal ventricular tachycardia
Ventricular tachycardia (paroxysmal)
DEF: Rapid ventricular rhythm.
AHA: ▶3Q, '13, 6; 1Q, '13, 10;◀2Q, '09, 14; 1Q, '08, 14; 2Q, '06, 15-16; 3Q, '95, 9; M-A, '86, 11
TIP: If a ventricular tachycardia is documented as sustained or nonsustained but is induced during an EP study, assign 427.1.
I47.2 Ventricular tachycardia [I-10]

427.2 Paroxysmal tachycardia, unspecified
Bouveret-Hoffmann syndrome
Paroxysmal tachycardia:
NOS
essential

√5ᵗʰ 427.3 Atrial fibrillation and flutter
TIP: Assign V58.61 Long-term (current) use of anticoagulants, as a secondary diagnosis if the patient is maintained on Coumadin.

427.31 Atrial fibrillation
DEF: Irregular, rapid atrial contractions.
AHA: ▶4Q, '13, 98, 101;◀1Q, '12, 7; 4Q, '08, 135; 3Q, '05, 8; 4Q, '04, 78, 121; 3Q, '04, 7; 4Q, '03, 95, 105; 1Q, '03, 8; 2Q, '99, 17; 3Q, '95, 8
I48.0 Atrial fibrillation [I-10]

Diseases of the Circulatory System

427.32–428.43

427.32 Atrial flutter
DEF: Regular, rapid atrial contractions.
AHA: 4Q, '03, 94
I48.1 Atrial flutter I-10

√5ᵗʰ **427.4 Ventricular fibrillation and flutter**

427.41 Ventricular fibrillation
DEF: Irregular, rapid ventricular contractions.
AHA: 2Q, '09, 14-15; 3Q, '02, 5

427.42 Ventricular flutter
DEF: Regular, rapid, ventricular contractions.

427.5 Cardiac arrest
Cardiorespiratory arrest
AHA: ▶1Q, '13, 9-11;◀ 3Q, '02, 5; 2Q, '00, 12; 3Q, '95, 8; 2Q, '88, 8
I46.9 Cardiac arrest cause unspecified I-10

√5ᵗʰ **427.6 Premature beats**

427.60 Premature beats, unspecified
Ectopic beats
Extrasystoles
Extrasystolic arrhythmia
Premature contractions or systoles NOS

427.61 Supraventricular premature beats
Atrial premature beats, contractions, or systoles

427.69 Other
Ventricular premature beats, contractions, or systoles
AHA: 4Q, '93, 42

√5ᵗʰ **427.8 Other specified cardiac dysrhythmias**

427.81 Sinoatrial node dysfunction
Sinus bradycardia: Syndrome:
  persistent   sick sinus
  severe   tachycardia-bradycardia
EXCLUDES sinus bradycardia NOS (427.89)
DEF: Complex cardiac arrhythmia; appears as severe sinus bradycardia, sinus bradycardia with tachycardia, or sinus bradycardia with atrioventricular block.
AHA: 4Q, '11, 168; 3Q, '10, 9; 3Q, '00, 8
I49.5 Sick sinus syndrome I-10

427.89 Other
Rhythm disorder:
  coronary sinus
  ectopic
  nodal
Wandering (atrial) pacemaker
EXCLUDES carotid sinus syncope (337.0)
  neonatal bradycardia (779.81)
  neonatal tachycardia (779.82)
  reflex bradycardia (337.0)
  tachycardia NOS (785.0)
AHA: 3Q, '12, 9
I49.8 Other specified cardiac arrhythmias I-10

427.9 Cardiac dysrhythmia, unspecified
Arrhythmia (cardiac) NOS
AHA: 2Q, '89, 10

Echocardiography of Heart Failure

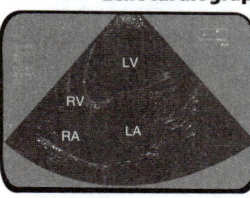
Systolic dysfunction with dilated LV

Diastolic dysfunction with LV hypertrophy

Four-chamber echocardiograms, two-dimensional views.
LV: Left ventricle
RV: Right ventricle
RA: Right atrium
LA: Left atrium

√4ᵗʰ **428 Heart failure**
Code, if applicable, heart failure due to hypertension first (402.0-402.9, with fifth-digit 1 or 404.0-404.9 with fifth-digit 1 or 3)
EXCLUDES following cardiac surgery (429.4)
  rheumatic (398.91)
  that complicating:
    abortion (634-638 with .7, 639.8)
    ectopic or molar pregnancy (639.8)
    labor or delivery (668.1, 669.4)
AHA: 4Q, '02, 49; 3Q, '98, 5; 2Q, '90, 16; 2Q, '90, 19; 2Q, '89, 10; 3Q, '88, 3

428.0 Congestive heart failure, unspecified
Congestive heart disease
Right heart failure (secondary to left heart failure)
EXCLUDES fluid overload NOS (276.69)
DEF: Mechanical inadequacy; caused by inability of heart to pump and circulate blood; results in fluid collection in lungs, hypertension, congestion and edema of tissue.
AHA: 3Q, '12, 9; 4Q, '09, 141; 1Q, '09, 8, 18; 4Q, '08, 72, 180, 182; 3Q, '08, 12; 3Q, '07, 9; 1Q, 07, 20; 3Q, '06, 7; 4Q, '05, 120; 3Q, '05, 8; 1Q, '05, 5, 9; 1Q, '05, 5, 9; 4Q, '04, 140; 3Q, '04, 7;4Q, '03, 109; 1Q, '03, 9; 4Q, '02, 52; 2Q, '01, 13; 4Q, '00, 48; 2Q, '00, 16; 1Q, '00, 22; 4Q, '99, 4; 1Q, '99, 11; 4Q, '97, 55; 3Q, '97, 10; 3Q, '96, 9; 3Q, '91, 18; 3Q, '91, 19; 2Q, '89, 12
TIP: Assign additional code(s) from subcategory 428.2, 428.3, or 428.4 to specify the type of heart failure.
I50.9 Heart failure unspecified I-10

428.1 Left heart failure
Acute edema of lung   } with heart disease NOS or
Acute pulmonary edema }   heart failure
Cardiac asthma
Left ventricular failure
DEF: Mechanical inadequacy of left ventricle; causing fluid in lungs.

√5ᵗʰ **428.2 Systolic heart failure**
EXCLUDES combined systolic and diastolic heart failure (428.40-428.43)
DEF: Heart failure due to a defect in expulsion of blood caused by an abnormality in systolic function, or ventricular contractile dysfunction.

428.20 Unspecified
I50.20 Unspecified systolic congestive heart failure I-10

428.21 Acute
I50.21 Acute systolic congestive heart failure I-10

428.22 Chronic
AHA: 4Q, '05, 120

428.23 Acute on chronic
AHA: 1Q, '09, 8, 18;1Q, '03, 9

√5ᵗʰ **428.3 Diastolic heart failure**
EXCLUDES combined systolic and diastolic heart failure (428.40-428.43)
DEF: Heart failure due to resistance to ventricular filling caused by an abnormality in the diastolic function.
AHA: 1Q, '12, 7

428.30 Unspecified
AHA: 4Q, '02, 52
I50.30 Unspecified diastolic congestive heart failure I-10

428.31 Acute

428.32 Chronic
AHA: 3Q, '08, 12
I50.32 Chronic diastolic congestive heart failure I-10

428.33 Acute on chronic
AHA: 4Q, '09, 141; 3Q, '08, 12; 1Q, '07, 20
I50.33 Acute on chronic diastolic heart failure I-10

√5ᵗʰ **428.4 Combined systolic and diastolic heart failure**

428.40 Unspecified

428.41 Acute
AHA: 4Q, '04, 140

428.42 Chronic

428.43 Acute on chronic
AHA: 3Q, '06, 7; 4Q, '02, 52

N Newborn Age: 0   P Pediatric Age: 0-17   M Maternity Age: 12-55   A Adult Age: 15-124

428.9 Heart failure, unspecified
Cardiac failure NOS   Myocardial failure NOS
Heart failure NOS   Weak heart
AHA: 2Q, '89, 10; N-D, '85, 14

√4ᵗʰ **429 Ill-defined descriptions and complications of heart disease**

429.0 Myocarditis, unspecified
Myocarditis
 NOS
 chronic (interstitial)   ⎱ (with mention of
 fibroid   ⎰ arteriosclerosis)
 senile

Use additional code to identify presence of arteriosclerosis

EXCLUDES   acute or subacute (422.0-422.9)
           rheumatic (398.0)
            acute (391.2)
           that due to hypertension (402.0-402.9)

429.1 Myocardial degeneration
Degeneration of heart or
 myocardium:
 fatty
 mural   ⎱ (with mention of
 muscular   ⎰ arteriosclerosis)
Myocardial:
 degeneration
 disease

Use additional code to identify presence of arteriosclerosis

EXCLUDES   that due to hypertension (402.0-402.9)

429.2 Cardiovascular disease, unspecified
Arteriosclerotic cardiovascular disease [ASCVD]
Cardiovascular arteriosclerosis
Cardiovascular:
 degeneration   ⎱ (with mention of
 disease   ⎰ arteriosclerosis)
 sclerosis

Use additional code to identify presence of arteriosclerosis

EXCLUDES   that due to hypertension (402.0-402.9)
AHA: 3Q, '12, 17

429.3 Cardiomegaly
Cardiac: Ventricular dilatation
 dilatation
 hypertrophy

EXCLUDES   that due to hypertension (402.0-402.9)
I51.7 Cardiomegaly   I-10

429.4 Functional disturbances following cardiac surgery
Cardiac insufficiency ⎱ following cardiac surgery or
Heart failure   ⎰ due to prosthesis
Postcardiotomy syndrome
Postvalvulotomy syndrome

EXCLUDES   cardiac failure in the immediate postoperative period
           (997.1)
AHA: 2Q, '02, 12; N-D, '85, 6

429.5 Rupture of chordae tendineae
DEF: Torn tissue, between heart valves and papillary muscles.

429.6 Rupture of papillary muscle
DEF: Torn muscle, between chordae tendineae and heart wall.

√5ᵗʰ **429.7 Certain sequelae of myocardial infarction, not elsewhere classified**
Use additional code to identify the associated myocardial
 infarction:
 with onset of 8 weeks or less (410.00-410.92)
 with onset of more than 8 weeks (414.8)

EXCLUDES   congenital defects of heart (745, 746)
           coronary aneurysm (414.11)
           disorders of papillary muscle (429.6, 429.81)
           postmyocardial infarction syndrome (411.0)
           rupture of chordae tendineae (429.5)
AHA: 3Q, '89, 5

429.71 Acquired cardiac septal defect   A
EXCLUDES   acute septal infarction (410.00-410.92)
DEF: Abnormal communication, between opposite heart
 chambers; due to defect of septum; not present at birth.

429.79 Other   A
Mural thrombus (atrial) (ventricular), acquired,
 following myocardial infarction
AHA: 1Q, '92, 10

√5ᵗʰ **429.8 Other ill-defined heart diseases**

429.81 Other disorders of papillary muscle
Papillary muscle: Papillary muscle:
 atrophy   incompetence
 degeneration   incoordination
 dysfunction   scarring

429.82 Hyperkinetic heart disease
DEF: Condition of unknown origin in young adults; marked
 by increased cardiac output at rest, increased rate of
 ventricular ejection; may lead to heart failure.

429.83 Takotsubo syndrome
Broken heart syndrome
Reversible left ventricular dysfunction following
 sudden emotional stress
Stress induced cardiomyopathy
Transient left ventricular apical ballooning syndrome
AHA: 4Q, '06, 87

429.89 Other
Carditis
EXCLUDES   that due to hypertension (402.0-402.9)
AHA: 2Q, '06, 18; 3Q, '05, 14; 1Q, '92, 10

429.9 Heart disease, unspecified
Heart disease (organic) NOS   Morbus cordis NOS
EXCLUDES   that due to hypertension (402.0-402.9)
AHA: 1Q, '09, 7; 1Q, '93, 19
I51.9 Heart disease unspecified   I-10

Cerebrovascular Disease (430-438)

INCLUDES   with mention of hypertension (conditions classifiable to
           401-405)

Use additional code to identify presence of hypertension

EXCLUDES   any condition classifiable to 430-434, 436, 437 occurring
           during pregnancy, childbirth, or the puerperium, or
           specified as puerperal (674.0)
           iatrogenic cerebrovascular infarction or hemorrhage
           (997.02)
AHA: 1Q, '93, 27; 3Q, '91, 10; 3Q, '90, 3; 2Q, '89, 8; M-A, '85, 6

430 Subarachnoid hemorrhage
Meningeal hemorrhage   Ruptured:
Ruptured: (congenital) cerebral aneurysm NOS
 berry aneurysm

EXCLUDES   berry aneurysm, nonruptured (437.3)
           syphilitic ruptured cerebral aneurysm (094.87)
AHA: 4Q, '04, 77
DEF: Bleeding in space between brain and lining.

431 Intracerebral hemorrhage
Hemorrhage (of):   Hemorrhage (of):
 basilar   internal capsule
 bulbar   intrapontine
 cerebellar   pontine
 cerebral   subcortical
 cerebromeningeal   ventricular
 corticalRupture of blood vessel in brain
DEF: Bleeding within the brain.
AHA: ▶2Q, '13, 10;◄ 1Q, '12, 14; 3Q, '10, 5-6; 1Q, '10, 8; 3Q, '07, 4; 4Q, '04, 77
I61.9 Nontraumatic intracerebral hemorrhage unspec   I-10

Berry Aneurysms

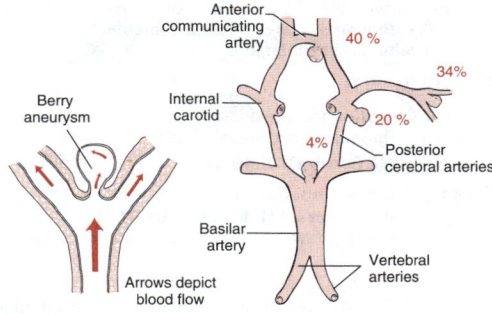

Anterior
communicating
artery
40 %
34%
20 %
4%
Berry
aneurysm
Internal
carotid
Posterior
cerebral arteries
Basilar
artery
Vertebral
arteries
Arrows depict
blood flow

Diseases of the Circulatory System

432–437.4

Cerebrovascular Arteries

Posterior parietal
Parietal-occipital
Calcarine
Posterior cerebral
Anterior inferior cerebellar
Posterior inferior cerebellar
Basilar
Vertebral

Callosal-marginal
Pericallosal
Anterior cerebral
Anterior communicating
Middle cerebral
Ophthalmic
Posterior communicating
External carotid
Internal carotid
Aorta

✓4ᵗʰ **432 Other and unspecified intracranial hemorrhage**
     AHA: 4Q, '04, 7

     432.0 Nontraumatic extradural hemorrhage
         Nontraumatic epidural hemorrhage
         DEF: Bleeding, nontraumatic, between skull and brain lining.

     432.1 Subdural hemorrhage
         Subdural hematoma, nontraumatic
         DEF: Bleeding, between outermost and other layers of brain lining.

     432.9 Unspecified intracranial hemorrhage
         Intracranial hemorrhage NOS

✓4ᵗʰ **433 Occlusion and stenosis of precerebral arteries**
     INCLUDES embolism
         narrowing   of basilar, carotid, and vertebral
         obstruction   arteries
         thrombosis

     Use additional code, if applicable, to identify status post administration of tPA (rtPA) in a different facility within the last 24 hours prior to admission to current facility (V45.88)

     EXCLUDES insufficiency NOS of precerebral arteries (435.0-435.9)

     The following fifth-digit subclassification is for use with category 433:
       0 without mention of cerebral infarction
       1 with cerebral infarction

     DEF: Blockage, stricture, arteries branching into brain.
     AHA: 2Q, '95, 14; 3Q, '90, 16

§ ✓5ᵗʰ **433.0 Basilar artery**
     [0-1]

§ ✓5ᵗʰ **433.1 Carotid artery**
     [0-1]   AHA: 1Q, '00, 16; **For code 433.10:** 1Q, '06, 17; 1Q, '02, 7, 10
         I65.29 Occlusion and stenosis of unspec carotid artery   I-10
         I63.239 Cerbral infarct d/t usp occ/stenosis of uns carotid art   I-10

§ ✓5ᵗʰ **433.2 Vertebral artery**
     [0-1]

§ ✓5ᵗʰ **433.3 Multiple and bilateral**
     [0-1]   AHA: 2Q, '02, 19

§ ✓5ᵗʰ **433.8 Other specified precerebral artery**
     [0-1]

§ ✓5ᵗʰ **433.9 Unspecified precerebral artery**
     [0-1]   Precerebral artery NOS

✓4ᵗʰ **434 Occlusion of cerebral arteries**
     Use additional code, if applicable, to identify status post administration of tPA (rtPA) in a different facility within the last 24 hours prior to admission to current facility (V45.88)

     The following fifth-digit subclassification is for use with category 434:
       0 without mention of cerebral infarction
       1 with cerebral infarction

     AHA: 2Q, '95, 14

§ ✓5ᵗʰ **434.0 Cerebral thrombosis**
     [0-1]   Thrombosis of cerebral arteries
         AHA: **For code 434.01:** 4Q, '04, 77

§ ✓5ᵗʰ **434.1 Cerebral embolism**
     [0-1]   AHA: **For code 434.11:** 4Q, '04, 77; 3Q, '97, 11
         I63.449 Cerbral infarct d/t embo of uns cerebellar art   I-10

---

§ ✓5ᵗʰ **434.9 Cerebral artery occlusion, unspecified**
     [0-1]   AHA: **For code 434.91:** ▶2Q, '13, 10;◀ 3Q, '10, 5-6; 4Q, '08, 108; 3Q, '07, 9; 1Q, '07, 23; 4Q, '04, 77-78; 4Q, '98, 87

✓4ᵗʰ **435 Transient cerebral ischemia**
     INCLUDES cerebrovascular insufficiency (acute) with transient focal neurological signs and symptoms
         insufficiency of basilar, carotid, and vertebral arteries
         spasm of cerebral arteries

     EXCLUDES acute cerebrovascular insufficiency NOS (437.1)
         that due to any condition classifiable to 433 (433.0-433.9)

     DEF: Temporary restriction of blood flow to arteries branching into brain.

     435.0 Basilar artery syndrome

     435.1 Vertebral artery syndrome

     435.2 Subclavian steal syndrome
         DEF: Cerebrovascular insufficiency, due to occluded subclavian artery; symptoms include pain in mastoid and posterior head regions, flaccid paralysis of arm and diminished or absent radial pulse on affected side.

     435.3 Vertebrobasilar artery syndrome
         DEF: Transient ischemic attack; due to brainstem dysfunction; symptoms include confusion, vertigo, binocular blindness, diplopia, unilateral or bilateral weakness and paresthesis of extremities.
         AHA: 4Q, '95, 60

     435.8 Other specified transient cerebral ischemias

     435.9 Unspecified transient cerebral ischemia
         Impending cerebrovascular accident
         Intermittent cerebral ischemia
         Transient ischemic attack [TIA]
         AHA: N-D, '85, 12
         G45.9 Transient cerebral ischemic attack unspecified   I-10

436 Acute, but ill-defined, cerebrovascular disease
     Apoplexy, apoplectic: Apoplexy, apoplectic:
       NOS   seizure
       attack   Cerebral seizure
       cerebral

     EXCLUDES any condition classifiable to categories 430-435
         cerebrovascular accident (434.91)
         CVA (ischemic) (434.91)
             embolic (434.11)
             hemorrhagic (430, 431, 432.0-432.9)
             thrombotic (434.01)
         postoperative cerebrovascular accident (997.02)
         stroke (ischemic) (434.91)
             embolic (434.11)
             hemorrhagic (430, 431, 432.0-432.9)
             thrombotic (434.01)

     AHA: 4Q, '04, 77; 4Q, '99, 3

     TIP: Do not assign when documentation indicates "CVA, stroke, or cerebral infarction." See instead default code 434.91.

✓4ᵗʰ **437 Other and ill-defined cerebrovascular disease**

     437.0 Cerebral atherosclerosis   **A**
         Atheroma of cerebral arteries
         Cerebral arteriosclerosis
         AHA: 3Q, '10, 15
         I67.2 Cerebral atherosclerosis   I-10

     437.1 Other generalized ischemic cerebrovascular disease
         Acute cerebrovascular insufficiency NOS
         Cerebral ischemia (chronic)
         AHA: 1Q, '09, 8

     437.2 Hypertensive encephalopathy
         DEF: Cerebral manifestations (such as visual disturbances and headache) due to high blood pressure.
         AHA: J-A, '84, 14

     437.3 Cerebral aneurysm, nonruptured
         Internal carotid artery, intracranial portion
         Internal carotid artery NOS
         EXCLUDES congenital cerebral aneurysm, nonruptured (747.81)
             internal carotid artery, extracranial portion (442.81)
         AHA: ▶4Q, '13, 92;◀ 2Q, '09, 12

     437.4 Cerebral arteritis
         DEF: Inflammation of a cerebral artery or arteries.
         AHA: 4Q, '99, 21

---

§   Requires fifth digit. Valid digits are in [brackets] under each code. See appropriate category for codes and definitions.

N Newborn Age: 0   **P** Pediatric Age: 0-17   **M** Maternity Age: 12-55   **A** Adult Age: 15-124

437.5 Moyamoya disease

DEF: Cerebrovascular ischemia; vessels occlude and rupture causing tiny hemorrhages at base of brain; predominantly affects Japanese.

437.6 Nonpyogenic thrombosis of intracranial venous sinus

EXCLUDES pyogenic (325)

437.7 Transient global amnesia

DEF: Episode of short-term memory loss, not often recurrent; pathogenesis unknown; with no signs or symptoms of neurological disorder.
AHA: 4Q, '92, 20

437.8 Other

AHA: ▶2Q, '13, 10◀

437.9 Unspecified

Cerebrovascular disease or lesion NOS
AHA: 1Q, '09, 9

√4ᵗʰ **438 Late effects of cerebrovascular disease**

NOTE This category is to be used to indicate conditions in 430-437 as the cause of late effects. The "late effects" include conditions specified as such, as sequelae, which may occur at any time after the onset of the causal condition.

EXCLUDES personal history of:
cerebral infarction without residual deficits (V12.54)
PRIND [Prolonged reversible ischemic neurologic deficit] (V12.54)
RIND [Reversible ischemic neurological deficit] (V12.54)
transient ischemic attack [TIA] (V12.54)

AHA: 3Q, '06, 3-4, 6; 4Q, '99, 4, 6, 7; 4Q, '98, 39, 88; 4Q, '97, 35, 37; 4Q, '92, 21;N-D,'86, 12; M-A, '86, 7

TIP: Assign instead code V12.54 TIA and cerebral infarction without residual effects, if no residual deficits are present.

438.0 Cognitive deficits

√5ᵗʰ **438.1 Speech and language deficits**

438.10 Speech and language deficit, unspecified

438.11 Aphasia

DEF: Impairment or absence of the ability to communicate by speech, writing or signs or to comprehend the spoken or written language due to disease or injury to the brain.
AHA: 4Q, '03, 105; 4Q, '97, 36

438.12 Dysphasia

DEF: Impaired speech; marked by inability to sequence language.
AHA: 4Q, '99, 3, 9

438.13 Dysarthria

DEF: Speech disorder caused by paralysis, spasticity, or other nerve damage resulting in difficulty expressing words or sounds; characterized by slurring, interrupted rhythm of speech, or distorted vowel sounds.
AHA: 4Q, '09, 87-88

TIP: If dysarthria or other speech disturbances are not due to underlying cerebrovascular disease, see subcategory 784.5 codes.

438.14 Fluency disorder

Stuttering due to late effect of cerebrovascular accident
DEF: Interruption in the flow of speech that significantly interferes with communication; characterized by primary sound and syllable repetitions, articulatory fixations, and abnormal prolongation of speech sounds.
AHA: 4Q, '10, 83; 4Q, '09, 87-88

438.19 Other speech and language deficits

√5ᵗʰ **438.2 Hemiplegia/hemiparesis**

DEF: Paralysis of one side of the body.
AHA: 1Q, '10, 5

438.20 Hemiplegia affecting unspecified side

AHA: 4Q, '07, 94; 4Q, '03, 105; 4Q, '99, 3, 9
I69.959 Hempl & hemiparesis flw uns CVD affect uns side [I-10]

438.21 Hemiplegia affecting dominant side

438.22 Hemiplegia affecting nondominant side

AHA: 4Q, '03, 105; 1Q, '02, 16

√5ᵗʰ **438.3 Monoplegia of upper limb**

DEF: Paralysis of one limb or one muscle group.

438.30 Monoplegia of upper limb affecting unspecified side

438.31 Monoplegia of upper limb affecting dominant side

438.32 Monoplegia of upper limb affecting nondominant side

√5ᵗʰ **438.4 Monoplegia of lower limb**

438.40 Monoplegia of lower limb affecting unspecified side

438.41 Monoplegia of lower limb affecting dominant side

438.42 Monoplegia of lower limb affecting nondominant side

√5ᵗʰ **438.5 Other paralytic syndrome**

Use additional code to identify type of paralytic syndrome, such as:
locked-in state (344.81)
quadriplegia (344.00-344.09)

EXCLUDES late effects of cerebrovascular accident with:
hemiplegia/hemiparesis (438.20-438.22)
monoplegia of lower limb (438.40-438.42)
monoplegia of upper limb (438.30-438.32)

438.50 Other paralytic syndrome affecting unspecified side

438.51 Other paralytic syndrome affecting dominant side

438.52 Other paralytic syndrome affecting nondominant side

438.53 Other paralytic syndrome, bilateral

AHA: 4Q, '98, 39

438.6 Alterations of sensations

Use additional code to identify the altered sensation

438.7 Disturbances of vision

Use additional code to identify the visual disturbance
AHA: 4Q, '02, 56

√5ᵗʰ **438.8 Other late effects of cerebrovascular disease**

438.81 Apraxia

DEF: Inability to activate learned movements; no known sensory or motor impairment.

438.82 Dysphagia

Use additional code to identify the type of dysphagia, if known (787.20-787.29)
DEF: Inability or difficulty in swallowing.
AHA: 4Q, '07, 94
I69.991 Dysphagia following uns cerebrovascular dis [I-10]

438.83 Facial weakness

Facial droop

438.84 Ataxia

AHA: 4Q, '02, 56

438.85 Vertigo

438.89 Other late effects of cerebrovascular disease

Use additional code to identify the late effect
AHA: 2Q, '09, 10; 1Q, '05, 13; 4Q, '98, 39
TIP: Assign 438.89 and 728.87 Muscle weakness, for residual weakness secondary to late effect of CVA.
I69.998 Other sequelae flw uns cerebrovascular disease [I-10]

438.9 Unspecified late effects of cerebrovascular disease

√4ᵗʰ √5ᵗʰ Additional Digit Required   Unspecified Code   Other Specified Code   Manifestation Code   ▶◄ Revised Text   ● New Code   ▲ Revised Code Title

Map of Major Arteries

Branches of Abdominal Aorta

Diseases of Arteries, Arterioles, and Capillaries (440-449)

✓4ᵗʰ 440 Atherosclerosis

    INCLUDES arteriolosclerosis
                 arteriosclerosis (obliterans) (senile)
                 arteriosclerotic vascular disease
                 atheroma
                 degeneration:
                    arterial
                    arteriovascular
                    vascular
                 endarteritis deformans or obliterans
                 senile:
                    arteritis
                    endarteritis

    EXCLUDES atheroembolism (445.01-445.89)
                 atherosclerosis of bypass graft of the extremities
                    (440.30-440.32)

    DEF: Stricture and reduced elasticity of artery; due to plaque deposits.

440.0 Of aorta   **A**
    AHA: 2Q, '93, 7; 2Q, '93, 8; 4Q, '88, 8

440.1 Of renal artery   **A**
    EXCLUDES atherosclerosis of renal arterioles (403.00-403.91)

✓5ᵗʰ 440.2 Of native arteries of the extremities

Use additional code, if applicable, to identify chronic total occlusion of artery of the extremities (440.4)

    EXCLUDES atherosclerosis of bypass graft of the extremities
                    (440.30-440.32)

AHA: 4Q, '94, 49; 4Q, '93, 27; 4Q, '92, 25; 3Q, '90, 15; M-A, '87, 6

TIP: Codes are listed in order of increasing severity; all patients who have gangrene (regardless of whether ulceration, rest pain, and/or intermittent claudication are present) are coded to 440.24. Patients without gangrene, but with ulceration (regardless of whether they also suffer from rest pain or intermittent claudication) are coded to 440.23.

440.20 Atherosclerosis of the extremities, unspecified   **A**

    I70.209 Uns atherosclero natv art of extrem uns extrem   **I-10**

440.21 Atherosclerosis of the extremities with intermittent claudication   **A**

    DEF: Atherosclerosis; marked by pain, tension and weakness after walking; no symptoms while at rest.

    I70.219 Atherosclerosis native arteries ext interm claud uns ext   **I-10**

440.22 Atherosclerosis of the extremities with rest pain   **A**

    INCLUDES any condition classifiable to 440.21

    DEF: Atherosclerosis, marked by pain, tension and weakness while at rest.

N Newborn Age: 0   **P** Pediatric Age: 0-17   **M** Maternity Age: 12-55   **A** Adult Age: 15-124

440.23 Atherosclerosis of the extremities with ulceration [A]

INCLUDES any condition classifiable to 440.21 and 440.22

Use additional code for any associated ulceration (707.10-707.19, 707.8, 707.9)

AHA: 4Q, '00, 44

I70.249 Atherosclero natv art lt leg ulceration uns site [I-10]

440.24 Atherosclerosis of the extremities with gangrene

INCLUDES any condition classifiable to 440.21, 440.22, and 440.23 with ischemic gangrene 785.4

Use additional code for any associated ulceration (707.10-707.19, 707.8, 707.9)

EXCLUDES gas gangrene (040.0)

AHA: 4Q, '03, 109; 3Q, '03, 14; 4Q, '95, 54; 1Q, '95, 11

440.29 Other [A]

√5ᵗʰ **440.3 Of bypass graft of extremities**

EXCLUDES atherosclerosis of native arteries of the extremities (440.21-440.24)
embolism [occlusion NOS] [thrombus] of graft (996.74)

AHA: 4Q, '94, 49

440.30 Of unspecified graft [A]

440.31 Of autologous vein bypass graft [A]

440.32 Of nonautologous biological bypass graft [A]

440.4 Chronic total occlusion of artery of the extremities
Complete occlusion of artery of the extremities
Total occlusion of artery of the extremities

Code first atherosclerosis of arteries of the extremities (440.20-440.29, 440.30-440.32)

EXCLUDES acute occlusion of artery of extremity (444.21-444.22)

AHA: 4Q, '07, 82

440.8 Of other specified arteries [A]

EXCLUDES basilar (433.0)
carotid (433.1)
cerebral (437.0)
coronary (414.00-414.07)
mesenteric (557.1)
precerebral (433.0-433.9)
pulmonary (416.0)
vertebral (433.2)

AHA: 3Q, '09, 9

TIP: Assign for arteriosclerosis of the iliac artery.

440.9 Generalized and unspecified atherosclerosis [A]
Arteriosclerotic vascular disease NOS

EXCLUDES arteriosclerotic cardiovascular disease [ASCVD] (429.2)

I70.91 Generalized atherosclerosis [I-10]

√4ᵗʰ **441 Aortic aneurysm and dissection**

EXCLUDES aortic ectasia (447.70-447.73)
syphilitic aortic aneurysm (093.0)
traumatic aortic aneurysm (901.0, 902.0)

√5ᵗʰ **441.0 Dissection of aorta**
DEF: Dissection or splitting of wall of the aorta; due to blood entering through intimal tear or interstitial hemorrhage.
AHA: 4Q, '89, 10

441.00 Unspecified site

441.01 Thoracic
AHA: ▶4Q, '13, 92;◀ 1Q, '09, 16; 4Q, '07, 87

441.02 Abdominal

441.03 Thoracoabdominal

441.1 Thoracic aneurysm, ruptured

441.2 Thoracic aneurysm without mention of rupture
AHA: 3Q, '92, 10
I71.2 Thoracic aortic aneurysm without rupture [I-10]

441.3 Abdominal aneurysm, ruptured
I71.3 Abdominal aortic aneurysm, ruptured [I-10]

Thoracic and Abdominal Aortic Aneurysm

Thoracic aneurysm
Abdominal aneurysm
Aorta

441.4 Abdominal aneurysm without mention of rupture
AHA: 4Q, '00, 64; 1Q, '99, 15, 16, 17; 3Q, '92, 10
I71.4 Abdominal aortic aneurysm without rupture [I-10]

441.5 Aortic aneurysm of unspecified site, ruptured
Rupture of aorta NOS

441.6 Thoracoabdominal aneurysm, ruptured

441.7 Thoracoabdominal aneurysm, without mention of rupture
AHA: 2Q, '06, 16

441.9 Aortic aneurysm of unspecified site without mention of rupture
Aneurysm
Dilatation
Hyaline necrosis } of aorta

AHA: 4Q, '10, 84

√4ᵗʰ **442 Other aneurysm**

INCLUDES aneurysm (ruptured) (cirsoid) (false) (varicose)
aneurysmal varix

EXCLUDES arteriovenous aneurysm or fistula:
acquired (447.0)
congenital (747.60-747.69)
traumatic (900.0-904.9)

DEF: Dissection or splitting of arterial wall; due to blood entering through intimal tear or interstitial hemorrhage.

442.0 Of artery of upper extremity

442.1 Of renal artery

442.2 Of iliac artery
AHA: 1Q, '99, 16, 17

442.3 Of artery of lower extremity
Aneurysm: 　　　　 Aneurysm:
femoral artery 　　 popliteal artery
AHA: 2Q, '08, 13; 3Q, '02, 24-26; 1Q, '99, 16

√5ᵗʰ **442.8 Of other specified artery**

442.81 Artery of neck
Aneurysm of carotid artery (common) (external) (internal, extracranial portion)

EXCLUDES internal carotid artery, intra- cranial portion (437.3)

442.82 Subclavian artery

442.83 Splenic artery

442.84 Other visceral artery
Aneurysm:
celiac
gastroduodenal
gastroepiploic
hepatic } artery
pancreaticoduodenal
superior mesenteric

√4ᵗʰ / √5ᵗʰ Additional Digit Required　　Unspecified Code　　Other Specified Code　　Manifestation Code　　▶◀ Revised Text　　● New Code　　▲ Revised Code Title

Diseases of the Circulatory System

442.89–445.02

442.89 Other

Aneurysm:
  mediastinal artery
  spinal artery

EXCLUDES *cerebral (nonruptured) (437.3)*
     congenital (747.81)
     ruptured (430)
    coronary (414.11)
    heart (414.10)
    pulmonary (417.1)

442.9 Of unspecified site

√4ᵗʰ **443 Other peripheral vascular disease**

443.0 Raynaud's syndrome

Raynaud's:
  disease
  phenomenon (secondary)

Use additional code to identify gangrene (785.4)

DEF: Constriction of the arteries, due to cold or stress; bilateral ischemic attacks of fingers, toes, nose or ears; symptoms include pallor, paresthesia and pain.

I73.00 Raynaud's syndrome without gangrene   `I-10`

443.1 Thromboangiitis obliterans [Buerger's disease]

Presenile gangrene

DEF: Inflammatory disease of extremity blood vessels, mainly the lower; occurs primarily in young men and leads to tissue ischemia and gangrene.

√5ᵗʰ **443.2 Other arterial dissection**

EXCLUDES *dissection of aorta (441.00-441.03)*
    dissection of coronary arteries (414.12)

AHA: 4Q, '02, 54

443.21 Dissection of carotid artery

  AHA: ▶4Q, '13, 92◀

443.22 Dissection of iliac artery

443.23 Dissection of renal artery

443.24 Dissection of vertebral artery

443.29 Dissection of other artery

√5ᵗʰ **443.8 Other specified peripheral vascular diseases**

443.81 *Peripheral angiopathy in diseases classified elsewhere*

Code first underlying disease, as:
  diabetes mellitus (249.7, 250.7)

AHA: 1Q, '04, 14; 3Q, '91, 10

I79.8 Oth d/o art arterioles & cap in dz clas elsw   `I-10`

443.82 Erythromelalgia

DEF: Rare syndrome of paroxysmal vasodilation; maldistribution of blood flow causes redness, pain, increased skin temperature, and burning sensations in various parts of the body.

AHA: 4Q, '05, 73

443.89 Other

Acrocyanosis   Erythrocyanosis
Acroparesthesia:
  simple [Schultze's type]
  vasomotor [Nothnagel's type]

EXCLUDES *chilblains (991.5)*
    frostbite (991.0-991.3)
    immersion foot (991.4)

AHA: 4Q, '07, 124

I73.89 Other specified peripheral vascular dz   `I-10`

443.9 Peripheral vascular disease, unspecified

Intermittent claudication NOS
Peripheral:
  angiopathy NOS
  vascular disease NOS
Spasm of artery

EXCLUDES *atherosclerosis of the arteries of the extremities (440.20-440.22)*
    spasm of cerebral artery (435.0-435.9)

AHA: 4Q, '92, 25; 3Q, '91, 10

I73.9 Peripheral vascular disease unspecified   `I-10`

Arterial Diseases and Disorders

Lipids
Calcium deposits

Atherosclerosis narrowing lumen   Thrombus (clot) forming in lumen

Intimal proliferation   Organization of thrombus and recanalization

Aneurysm bypasses lumen or...

Embolus (from elsewhere) occluding lumen   ...bulges from arterial wall   Arteriovenous fistula

√4ᵗʰ **444 Arterial embolism and thrombosis**

INCLUDES infarction:
  embolic
  thrombotic
occlusion

EXCLUDES *atheroembolism (445.01-445.89)*
  that complicating:
    abortion (634-638 with .6, 639.6)
    ectopic or molar pregnancy (639.6)
    pregnancy, childbirth, or the pueperium (673.0-673.8)
  septic arterial embolism (449)

AHA: 2Q, '92, 11; 4Q, '90, 27

√5ᵗʰ **444.0 Of abdominal aorta**

  AHA: 4Q, '11, 107-109; 2Q, '93, 7; 4Q, '90, 27

444.01 Saddle embolus of abdominal aorta

  AHA: 4Q, '11, 108

444.09 Other arterial embolism and thrombosis of abdominal aorta

Aortic bifurcation syndrome   Leriche's syndrome
Aortoiliac obstruction

444.1 Of thoracic aorta

Embolism or thrombosis of aorta (thoracic)

√5ᵗʰ **444.2 Of arteries of the extremities**

  AHA: M-A, '87, 6

444.21 Upper extremity

444.22 Lower extremity

Arterial embolism or thrombosis:
  femoral
  peripheral NOS
  popliteal

EXCLUDES *iliofemoral (444.81)*

AHA: 2Q, '11, 8; 4Q, '07, 85; 3Q, '03, 10; 1Q, '03, 17; 3Q, '90, 16

I74.3 Embo & thromb of arteries of the low extremities   `I-10`

√5ᵗʰ **444.8 Of other specified artery**

444.81 Iliac artery

  AHA: 1Q, '03, 16

444.89 Other

EXCLUDES *basilar (433.0)*
  carotid (433.1)
  cerebral (434.0-434.9)
  coronary (410.00-410.92)
  mesenteric (557.0)
  ophthalmic (362.30-362.34)
  precerebral (433.0-433.9)
  pulmonary (415.11-415.19)
  renal (593.81)
  retinal (362.30-362.34)
  vertebral (433.2)

444.9 Of unspecified artery

√4ᵗʰ **445 Atheroembolism**

INCLUDES atherothrombotic microembolism
cholesterol embolism

AHA: 4Q, '02, 57

√5ᵗʰ **445.0 Of extremities**

445.01 Upper extremity

445.02 Lower extremity

N Newborn Age: 0   **P** Pediatric Age: 0-17   **M** Maternity Age: 12-55   **A** Adult Age: 15-124

✓5ᵗʰ 445.8 Of other sites

445.81 Kidney

Use additional code for any associated acute kidney failure or chronic kidney disease (584, 585)

445.89 Other site

✓4ᵗʰ 446 Polyarteritis nodosa and allied conditions

446.0 Polyarteritis nodosa

Disseminated necrotizing periarteritis
Necrotizing angiitis
Panarteritis (nodosa)
Periarteritis (nodosa)

DEF: Inflammation of small and mid-size arteries; symptoms related to involved arteries in kidneys, muscles, gastrointestinal tract and heart; results in tissue death.

446.1 Acute febrile mucocutaneous lymph node syndrome [MCLS]

Kawasaki disease

DEF: Acute febrile disease of children; marked by erythema of conjunctiva and mucous membranes of upper respiratory tract, skin eruptions and edema.

✓5ᵗʰ 446.2 Hypersensitivity angiitis

EXCLUDES antiglomerular basement membrane disease without pulmonary hemorrhage (583.89)

446.20 Hypersensitivity angiitis, unspecified

446.21 Goodpasture's syndrome

Antiglomerular basement membrane antibody-mediated nephritis with pulmonary hemorrhage

Use additional code to identify renal disease (583.81)

DEF: Glomerulonephritis associated with hematuria, progresses rapidly; results in death from renal failure.

446.29 Other specified hypersensitivity angiitis

AHA: 1Q, '95, 3

446.3 Lethal midline granuloma

Malignant granuloma of face

DEF: Granulomatous lesion; in nose or paranasal sinuses; often fatal; occurs chiefly in males.

AHA: 3Q, '00, 11

446.4 Wegener's granulomatosis

Necrotizing respiratory granulomatosis
Wegener's syndrome

DEF: A disease occurring mainly in men; marked by necrotizing granulomas and ulceration of the upper respiratory tract; cause is a vasculitis affecting small vessels due to an immune disorder.

AHA: 3Q, '00, 11

446.5 Giant cell arteritis

Bagratuni's syndrome
Cranial arteritis
Horton's disease
Temporal arteritis

DEF: Inflammation of arteries; due to giant cells affecting carotid artery branches, resulting in occlusion; symptoms include fever, headache and neurological problems.

M31.6 Other giant cell arteritis   I-10

446.6 Thrombotic microangiopathy

Moschcowitz's syndrome
Thrombotic thrombocytopenic purpura

DEF: Blockage of small blood vessels; due to hyaline deposits; symptoms include purpura, CNS disorders; results in protracted disease or rapid death.

446.7 Takayasu's disease

Aortic arch arteritis   Pulseless disease

DEF: Progressive obliterative arteritis of brachiocephalic trunk, left subclavian, and left common carotid arteries above aortic arch; results in ischemia in brain, heart and arm.

✓4ᵗʰ 447 Other disorders of arteries and arterioles

447.0 Arteriovenous fistula, acquired

Arteriovenous aneurysm, acquired

EXCLUDES cerebrovascular (437.3)
coronary (414.19)
pulmonary (417.0)
surgically created arteriovenous shunt or fistula:
complication (996.1, 996.61-996.62)
status or presence (V45.11)
traumatic (900.0-904.9)

DEF: Communication between an artery and vein caused by error in healing.

447.1 Stricture of artery

AHA: 2Q, '93, 8; M-A, '87, 6

I77.1 Stricture of artery   I-10

447.2 Rupture of artery

Erosion
Fistula, except arteriovenous
Ulcer
} of artery

EXCLUDES traumatic rupture of artery (900.0-904.9)

447.3 Hyperplasia of renal artery

Fibromuscular hyperplasia of renal artery

DEF: Overgrowth of cells in muscular lining of renal artery.

447.4 Celiac artery compression syndrome

Celiac axis syndrome   Marable's syndrome

447.5 Necrosis of artery

447.6 Arteritis, unspecified

Aortitis NOS   Endarteritis NOS

EXCLUDES arteritis, endarteritis:
aortic arch (446.7)
cerebral (437.4)
coronary (414.00-414.07)
deformans (440.0-440.9)
obliterans (440.0-440.9)
pulmonary (417.8)
senile (440.0-440.9)
polyarteritis NOS (446.0)
syphilitic aortitis (093.1)

AHA: 1Q, '95, 3

✓5ᵗʰ 447.7 Aortic ectasia

Ectasis aorta

EXCLUDES aortic aneurysm and dissection (441.00-441.9)

DEF: A diffuse, irregular dilation of the aorta less than 3 cm in diameter; increases the patient's risk of developing an aortic aneurysm.

AHA: 4Q, '10, 84-85

447.70 Aortic ectasia, unspecified site

447.71 Thoracic aortic ectasia

447.72 Abdominal aortic ectasia

447.73 Thoracoabdominal aortic ectasia

447.8 Other specified disorders of arteries and arterioles

Fibromuscular hyperplasia of arteries, except renal

447.9 Unspecified disorders of arteries and arterioles

✓4ᵗʰ 448 Disease of capillaries

448.0 Hereditary hemorrhagic telangiectasia

Rendu-Osler-Weber disease

DEF: Genetic disease with onset after puberty; results in multiple telangiectases, dilated venules on skin and mucous membranes; recurrent bleeding may occur.

448.1 Nevus, non-neoplastic

Nevus:
araneus
senile
Nevus:
spider
stellar

EXCLUDES neoplastic (216.0-216.9)
port wine (757.32)
strawberry (757.32)

DEF: Enlarged or malformed blood vessels of skin; results in reddish swelling, skin patch, or birthmark.

448.9 Other and unspecified capillary diseases

Capillary:
hemorrhage
hyperpermeability
Capillary:
thrombosis

EXCLUDES capillary fragility (hereditary) (287.8)

449 Septic arterial embolism

Code first underlying infection, such as:
infective endocarditis (421.0)
lung abscess (513.0)

Use additional code to identify the site of the embolism (433.0-433.9, 444.01-444.9)

EXCLUDES septic pulmonary embolism (415.12)

AHA: 4Q, '07, 84-85

| ✓4ᵗʰ ✓5ᵗʰ Additional Digit Required | Unspecified Code | Other Specified Code | Manifestation Code | ►◄ Revised Text | ● New Code | ▲ Revised Code Title |

Diseases of the Circulatory System

451–453.6

Diseases of Veins and Lymphatics, and Other Diseases of Circulatory System (451-459)

☑4ᵗʰ 451 Phlebitis and thrombophlebitis

> INCLUDES   endophlebitis
> inflammation, vein
> periphlebitis
> suppurative phlebitis

Use additional E code to identify drug, if drug-induced

> EXCLUDES   that complicating:
> abortion (634-638 with .7, 639.8)
> ectopic or molar pregnancy (639.8)
> pregnancy, childbirth, or the puerperium (671.0-671.9)
> that due to or following:
> implant or catheter device (996.61-996.62)
> infusion, perfusion, or transfusion (999.2)

DEF: Inflammation of a vein (phlebitis) with formation of a thrombus (thrombophlebitis).

AHA: ▶2Q, '13, 3;◀ 1Q, '11, 19; 1Q, '92, 16

TIP: Assign an additional code from category 453 for thrombosis; if both conditions are present, assign codes from both categories 451 and 453.

451.0 Of superficial vessels of lower extremities
Saphenous vein (greater) (lesser)
AHA: 3Q, '91, 16

☑5ᵗʰ 451.1 Of deep vessels of lower extremities
AHA: 3Q, '91, 16

   451.11 Femoral vein (deep) (superficial)

   451.19 Other
      Femoropopliteal vein   Tibial vein
      Popliteal vein

451.2 Of lower extremities, unspecified
AHA: 4Q, '04, 80

☑5ᵗʰ 451.8 Of other sites
> EXCLUDES   intracranial venous sinus (325)
> nonpyogenic (437.6)
> portal (vein) (572.1)

   451.81 Iliac vein

   451.82 Of superficial veins of upper extremities
      Antecubital vein   Cephalic vein
      Basilic vein

   451.83 Of deep veins of upper extremities
      Brachial vein   Ulnar vein
      Radial vein

   451.84 Of upper extremities, unspecified

   451.89 Other
      Axillary vein
      Jugular vein
      Subclavian vein
      Thrombophlebitis of breast (Mondor's disease)

451.9 Of unspecified site

452 Portal vein thrombosis
Portal (vein) obstruction
> EXCLUDES   hepatic vein thrombosis (453.0)
> phlebitis of portal vein (572.1)

DEF: Formation of a blood clot in main vein of liver.

☑4ᵗʰ 453 Other venous embolism and thrombosis
> EXCLUDES   that complicating:
> abortion (634-638 with .7, 639.8)
> ectopic or molar pregnancy (639.8)
> pregnancy, childbirth, or the puerperium (671.0-671.9)

AHA: 1Q, '11, 19-21; 1Q, '92, 16

453.0 Budd-Chiari syndrome
Hepatic vein thrombosis
DEF: Thrombosis or other obstruction of hepatic vein; symptoms include enlarged liver, extensive collateral vessels, intractable ascites and severe portal hypertension.

453.1 Thrombophlebitis migrans
DEF: Slow, advancing thrombophlebitis; appearing first in one vein then another.

453.2 Of inferior vena cava

453.3 Of renal vein

☑5ᵗʰ 453.4 Acute venous embolism and thrombosis of deep vessels of lower extremity
AHA: 4Q, '09, 88-92; 3Q, '08,16

   453.40 Acute venous embolism and thrombosis of unspecified deep vessels of lower extremity
      Deep vein thrombosis NOS
      DVT NOS
      AHA: 1Q, '12, 18
      TIP: Assign as the default code for "deep vein thrombosis," whether documented as acute or subacute.
      I82.409 Ac embo & thrombo of uns deep veins of unsp lower ext   I-10

   453.41 Acute venous embolism and thrombosis of deep vessels of proximal lower extremity
      Femoral   Thigh
      Iliac   Upper leg NOS
      Popliteal
      AHA: 4Q, '04, 79

   453.42 Acute venous embolism and thrombosis of deep vessels of distal lower extremity
      Calf   Peroneal
      Lower leg NOS   Tibial

☑5ᵗʰ 453.5 Chronic venous embolism and thrombosis of deep vessels of lower extremity
Use additional code, if applicable, for associated long-term (current) use of anticoagulants (V58.61)
> EXCLUDES   personal history of venous thrombosis and embolism (V12.51)

AHA: 4Q, '09, 88-92

   453.50 Chronic venous embolism and thrombosis of unspecified deep vessels of lower

   453.51 Chronic venous embolism and thrombosis of deep vessels of proximal lower extremity
      Femoral   Thigh
      Iliac   Upper leg NOS
      Popliteal

   453.52 Chronic venous embolism and thrombosis of deep vessels of distal lower extremity
      Calf   Peroneal
      Lower leg NOS   Tibial

453.6 Venous embolism and thrombosis of superficial vessels of lower extremity
Saphenous vein (greater) (lesser)
Use additional code, if applicable, for associated long-term (current) use of anticoagulants (V58.61)
AHA: 4Q, '09, 88-92

Veins of Head and Neck

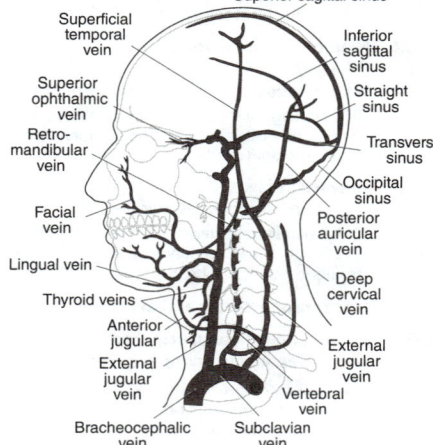

Map of Major Veins

√5ᵗʰ 453.7 Chronic venous embolism and thrombosis of other specified vessels

Use additional code, if applicable, for associated long-term (current) use of anticoagulants (V58.61)

EXCLUDES *personal history of venous thrombosis and embolism (V12.51)*

AHA: 4Q, '09, 88-92

453.71 Chronic venous embolism and thrombosis of superficial veins of upper extremity
Antecubital vein   Cephalic vein
Basilic vein

453.72 Chronic venous embolism and thrombosis of deep veins of upper extremity
Brachial vein   Ulnar vein
Radial vein

453.73 Chronic venous embolism and thrombosis of upper extremity, unspecified

453.74 Chronic venous embolism and thrombosis of axillary veins

453.75 Chronic venous embolism and thrombosis of subclavian veins

453.76 Chronic venous embolism and thrombosis of internal jugular veins

453.77 Chronic venous embolism and thrombosis of other thoracic veins
Brachiocephalic (innominate)
Superior vena cava

453.79 Chronic venous embolism and thrombosis of other specified veins

√5ᵗʰ 453.8 Acute venous embolism and thrombosis of other specified veins

EXCLUDES *cerebral (434.0-434.9)*
coronary (410.00-410.92)
intracranial venous sinus (325)
nonpyogenic (437.6)
mesenteric (557.0)
portal (452)
precerebral (433.0-433.9)
pulmonary (415.19)

AHA: 4Q, '09, 88-92; 3Q, '91, 16; M-A, '87, 6

453.81 Acute venous embolism and thrombosis of superficial veins of upper extremity
Antecubital vein
Basilic vein
Cephalic vein

453.82 Acute venous embolism and thrombosis of deep veins of upper extremity
Brachial vein   Ulnar vein
Radial vein

453.83 Acute venous embolism and thrombosis of upper extremity, unspecified

453.84 Acute venous embolism and thrombosis of axillary veins

453.85 Acute venous embolism and thrombosis of subclavian veins

453.86 Acute venous embolism and thrombosis of internal jugular veins

√4ᵗʰ / √5ᵗʰ Additional Digit Required | **Unspecified Code** | Other Specified Code | **Manifestation Code** | ►◄ Revised Text | ● New Code | ▲ Revised Code Title

2015 ICD-9-CM | **Volume 1 – 141**

Diseases of the Circulatory System

453.87–457.0

453.87 Acute venous embolism and thrombosis of other thoracic veins
Brachiocephalic (innominate)
Superior vena cava

453.89 Acute venous embolism and thrombosis of other specified veins
I82.890 Ac embolism and thrombosis of other spec veins   I-10

453.9 Of unspecified site
Embolism of vein
Thrombosis (vein)
AHA: 1Q, '12, 18

√4ᵗʰ 454 Varicose veins of lower extremities
EXCLUDES   that complicating pregnancy, childbirth, or the puerperium (671.0)
DEF: Dilated leg veins; due to incompetent vein valves that allow reversed blood flow and cause tissue erosion or weakness of wall; may be painful.
AHA: 2Q, '91, 20

454.0 With ulcer   A
Varicose ulcer (lower extremity, any part)
Varicose veins with ulcer of lower extremity [any part] or of unspecified site
Any condition classifiable to 454.9 with ulcer or specified as ulcerated
AHA: 4Q, '99, 18

454.1 With inflammation   A
Stasis dermatitis
Varicose veins with inflammation of lower extremity [any part] or of unspecified site
Any condition classifiable to 454.9 with inflammation or specified as inflamed

454.2 With ulcer and inflammation   A
Varicose veins with ulcer and inflammation of lower extremity [any part] or of unspecified site
Any condition classifiable to 454.9 with ulcer and inflammation

454.8 With other complications
Edema   Swelling
Pain
AHA: 4Q, '02, 58

454.9 Asymptomatic varicose veins   A
Phlebectasia }
Varicose veins } of lower extremity [any part]
Varix } or of unspecified site
Varicose veins NOS
AHA: 4Q, '02, 58
TIP: Do not assign if patient seen for surgical treatment of varicose veins; query physician for specific symptom (inflammation, pain, edema, swelling).

√4ᵗʰ 455 Hemorrhoids
INCLUDES   hemorrhoids (anus) (rectum)
piles
varicose veins, anus or rectum
EXCLUDES   that complicating pregnancy, childbirth, or the puerperium (671.8)
DEF: Varicose condition of external hemorrhoidal veins causing painful swellings at the anus.

455.0 Internal hemorrhoids without mention of complication
AHA: 3Q, '05, 17
K64.0 First degree hemorrhoids   I-10

455.1 Internal thrombosed hemorrhoids

455.2 Internal hemorrhoids with other complication
Internal hemorrhoids: Internal hemorrhoids:
   bleeding   strangulated
   prolapsed   ulcerated
AHA: 3Q, '05, 17; 1Q, '03, 8
K64.2 Third degree hemorrhoid   I-10

455.3 External hemorrhoids without mention of complication
AHA: 1Q, '07, 13; 3Q, '05, 17
K64.4 Residual hemorrhoidal skin tags   I-10

455.4 External thrombosed hemorrhoids

455.5 External hemorrhoids with other complication
External hemorrhoids: External hemorrhoids:
   bleeding   strangulated
   prolapsed   ulcerated
AHA: 3Q, '05, 17; 1Q, '03, 8

455.6 Unspecified hemorrhoids without mention of complication
Hemorrhoids NOS

455.7 Unspecified thrombosed hemorrhoids
Thrombosed hemorrhoids, unspecified whether internal or external

455.8 Unspecified hemorrhoids with other complication
Hemorrhoids, unspecified whether internal or external:
   bleeding
   prolapsed
   strangulated
   ulcerated

455.9 Residual hemorrhoidal skin tags
Skin tags, anus or rectum

√4ᵗʰ 456 Varicose veins of other sites

456.0 Esophageal varices with bleeding
DEF: Distended, tortuous, veins of lower esophagus, usually due to portal hypertension.

456.1 Esophageal varices without mention of bleeding

√5ᵗʰ 456.2 Esophageal varices in diseases classified elsewhere
Code first underlying cause, as:
   cirrhosis of liver (571.0-571.9)
   portal hypertension (572.3)

   456.20 With bleeding
     AHA: N-D, '85, 14
     I85.11 Secondary esophageal varices with bleeding   I-10

   456.21 Without mention of bleeding
     AHA: 3Q, '05, 15; 2Q, '02, 4

456.3 Sublingual varices
DEF: Distended, tortuous veins beneath tongue.

456.4 Scrotal varices   ♂
Varicocele

456.5 Pelvic varices
Varices of broad ligament

456.6 Vulval varices   ♀
Varices of perineum
EXCLUDES   that complicating pregnancy, childbirth, or the puerperium (671.1)

456.8 Varices of other sites
Varicose veins of nasal septum (with ulcer)
EXCLUDES   placental varices (656.7)
     retinal varices (362.17)
     varicose ulcer of unspecified site (454.0)
     varicose veins of unspecified site (454.9)
AHA: 2Q, '02, 4

√4ᵗʰ 457 Noninfectious disorders of lymphatic channels

457.0 Postmastectomy lymphedema syndrome   A
Elephantiasis }
Obliteration of lymphatic } due to mastectomy
   vessel }
DEF: Reduced lymphatic circulation following mastectomy; symptoms include swelling of the arm on the operative side.
AHA: 2Q, '02, 12

N Newborn Age: 0   P Pediatric Age: 0-17   M Maternity Age: 12-55   A Adult Age: 15-124

457.1 Other lymphedema

Elephantiasis (nonfilarial) NOS
Lymphangiectasis
Lymphedema:
   acquired (chronic)
   praecox

Lymphedema:
   secondary
Obliteration, lymphatic
   vessel

> **EXCLUDES** *elephantiasis (nonfilarial):*
>   *congenital (757.0)*
>   *eyelid (374.83)*
>   *vulva (624.8)*

DEF: Fluid retention due to reduced lymphatic circulation; due to other than mastectomy.
AHA: 3Q, '04, 5
I89.0 Lymphedema not elsewhere classified   **I-10**

457.2 Lymphangitis

Lymphangitis:
   NOS
   chronic

Lymphangitis:
   subacute

> **EXCLUDES** *acute lymphangitis (682.0-682.9)*

457.8 Other noninfectious disorders of lymphatic channels

Chylocele (nonfilarial)
Chylous:
   ascites
   cyst
Lymph node or vessel:
   fistula
   infarction
   rupture

> **EXCLUDES** *chylocele:*
>   *filarial (125.0-125.9)*
>   *tunica vaginalis (nonfilarial) (608.84)*

AHA: 1Q, '04, 5; 3Q, '03, 17

457.9 Unspecified noninfectious disorder of lymphatic channels

458 Hypotension

> **INCLUDES** hypopiesis
> **EXCLUDES** *cardiovascular collapse (785.50)*
>   *maternal hypotension syndrome (669.2)*
>   *shock (785.50-785.59)*
>   *Shy-Drager syndrome (333.0)*

458.0 Orthostatic hypotension

Hypotension:
   orthostatic (chronic)

Hypotension:
   postural

DEF: Low blood pressure; occurs when standing.
AHA: 3Q, '00, 8; 3Q, '91, 9
I95.1 Orthostatic hypotension   **I-10**

458.1 Chronic hypotension

Permanent idiopathic hypotension
DEF: Persistent low blood pressure.

458.2 Iatrogenic hypotension

DEF: Abnormally low blood pressure; due to medical treatment.
AHA: 4Q, '03, 60; 3Q, '02, 12; 4Q, '95, 57

458.21 Hypotension of hemodialysis

Intra-dialytic hypotension
AHA: 4Q, '03, 61

458.29 Other iatrogenic hypotension

Postoperative hypotension
I95.81 Postprocedural hypotension   **I-10**

458.8 Other specified hypotension

AHA: 4Q, '97, 37

458.9 Hypotension, unspecified

Hypotension (arterial) NOS
I95.9 Hypotension unspecified   **I-10**

459 Other disorders of circulatory system

459.0 Hemorrhage, unspecified

Rupture of blood vessel NOS
Spontaneous hemorrhage NEC

> **EXCLUDES** *hemorrhage:*
>   *gastrointestinal NOS (578.9)*
>   *in newborn NOS (772.9)*
>   *secondary or recurrent following trauma (958.2)*
>   *traumatic rupture of blood vessel (900.0-904.9)*
>   *nontraumatic hematoma of soft tissue (729.92)*

AHA: 4Q, '90, 26
R58 Hemorrhage not elsewhere classified   **I-10**

459.1 Postphlebitic syndrome

Chronic venous hypertension due to deep vein thrombosis

> **EXCLUDES** *chronic venous hypertension without deep vein thrombosis (459.30-459.39)*

DEF: Various conditions following deep vein thrombosis; including edema, pain, stasis dermatitis, cellulitis, varicose veins and ulceration of the lower leg.
AHA: 4Q, '02, 58; 2Q, '91, 20

459.10 Postphlebitic syndrome without complications

Asymptomatic postphlebitic syndrome
Postphlebitic syndrome NOS

459.11 Postphlebitic syndrome with ulcer

459.12 Postphlebitic syndrome with inflammation

459.13 Postphlebitic syndrome with ulcer and inflammation

459.19 Postphlebitic syndrome with other complication

459.2 Compression of vein

Stricture of vein
Vena cava syndrome (inferior) (superior)

459.3 Chronic venous hypertension (idiopathic)

Stasis edema

> **EXCLUDES** *chronic venous hypertension due to deep vein thrombosis (459.10-459.9)*
>   *varicose veins (454.0-454.9)*

AHA: 4Q, '02, 59

459.30 Chronic venous hypertension without complications

Asymptomatic chronic venous hypertension
Chronic venous hypertension NOS

459.31 Chronic venous hypertension with ulcer

AHA: 4Q, '02, 43

459.32 Chronic venous hypertension with inflammation

459.33 Chronic venous hypertension with ulcer and inflammation

459.39 Chronic venous hypertension with other complication

459.8 Other specified disorders of circulatory system

459.81 Venous (peripheral) insufficiency, unspecified

Chronic venous insufficiency NOS
Use additional code for any associated ulceration (707.10-707.19, 707.8, 707.9)
DEF: Insufficient drainage, venous blood, any part of body, results in edema or dermatosis.
AHA: 3Q, '04, 5; 2Q, '91, 20; M-A, '87, 6
TIP: Assign for stasis dermatitis without varicose veins or past DVT.
I87.2 Venous insufficiency (chronic) (peripheral)   **I-10**

459.89 Other

Collateral circulation (venous), any site
Phlebosclerosis
Venofibrosis

459.9 Unspecified circulatory system disorder

AHA: ▶1Q, '13, 7◀

✓4ᵗʰ / ✓5ᵗʰ   Additional Digit Required   Unspecified Code   Other Specified Code   Manifestation Code   ▶◀ Revised Text   ● New Code   ▲ Revised Code Title

2015 ICD-9-CM   October 2014 • Volume 1 – 143

8. Diseases of the Respiratory System (460-519)

Use additional code to identify infectious organism

Acute Respiratory Infections (460-466)

> **EXCLUDES** pneumonia and influenza (480.0-488.19)

460 Acute nasopharyngitis [common cold]

Coryza (acute)   Rhinitis:
Nasal catarrh, acute   acute
Nasopharyngitis: infective
  NOS
  acute
  infective NOS

> **EXCLUDES** nasopharyngitis, chronic (472.2)
>   pharyngitis:
>   acute or unspecified (462)
>   chronic (472.1)
>   rhinitis:
>   allergic (477.0-477.9)
>   chronic or unspecified (472.0)
>   sore throat:
>   acute or unspecified (462)
>   chronic (472.1)

DEF: Acute inflammation of mucous membranes; extends from nares to pharynx.
AHA: 1Q, '88, 12

√4ᵗʰ 461 Acute sinusitis

> **INCLUDES** abscess
> empyema
> infection   acute, of sinus
> inflammation   (accessory) (nasal)
> suppuration

> **EXCLUDES** chronic or unspecified sinusitis (473.0-473.9)

461.0 Maxillary
Acute antritis

461.1 Frontal

461.2 Ethmoidal

461.3 Sphenoidal

461.8 Other acute sinusitis
Acute pansinusitis

461.9 Acute sinusitis, unspecified
Acute sinusitis NOS
J01.90 Acute sinusitis unspecified   I-10

462 Acute pharyngitis
Acute sore throat NOS
Pharyngitis (acute):
  NOS
  gangrenous
  infective
  phlegmonous
  pneumococcal
  staphylococcal
  suppurative
  ulcerative
Sore throat (viral) NOS
Viral pharyngitis

> **EXCLUDES** abscess:
>   peritonsillar [quinsy] (475)
>   pharyngeal NOS (478.29)
>   retropharyngeal (478.24)
>   chronic pharyngitis (472.1)
>   infectious mononucleosis (075)
>   that specified as (due to):
>   Coxsackie (virus) (074.0)
>   gonococcus (098.6)
>   herpes simplex (054.79)
>   influenza (487.1, 488.02, 488.12)
>   septic (034.0)
>   streptococcal (034.0)

AHA: 2Q, '12, 18; 4Q, '99, 26; S-O, '85, 8
J02.9 Acute pharyngitis unspecified   I-10

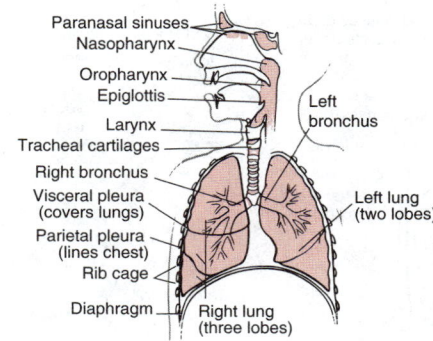

Respiratory System

Paranasal sinuses
Nasopharynx
Oropharynx
Epiglottis
Larynx
Tracheal cartilages
Right bronchus
Visceral pleura (covers lungs)
Parietal pleura (lines chest)
Rib cage
Diaphragm
Left bronchus
Left lung (two lobes)
Right lung (three lobes)

463 Acute tonsillitis

Tonsillitis (acute):   Tonsillitis (acute):
  NOS   septic
  follicular   staphylococcal
  gangrenous   suppurative
  infective   ulcerative
  pneumococcal   viral

> **EXCLUDES** chronic tonsillitis (474.0)
>   hypertrophy of tonsils (474.1)
>   peritonsillar abscess [quinsy] (475)
>   sore throat:
>   acute or NOS (462)
>   septic (034.0)
>   streptococcal tonsillitis (034.0)

AHA: N-D, '84, 16

√4ᵗʰ 464 Acute laryngitis and tracheitis

> **EXCLUDES** that associated with influenza (487.1, 488.02, 488.12)
>   that due to Streptococcus (034.0)

√5ᵗʰ 464.0 Acute laryngitis
Laryngitis (acute):
  NOS
  edematous
  Hemophilus influenzae [H. influenzae]
  pneumococcal
  septic
  suppurative
  ulcerative

> **EXCLUDES** chronic laryngitis (476.0-476.1)
>   influenzal laryngitis (487.1, 488.02, 488.12)

AHA: 4Q, '01, 42

464.00 Without mention of obstruction

464.01 With obstruction

√5ᵗʰ 464.1 Acute tracheitis
Tracheitis (acute):
  NOS
  catarrhal
  viral

> **EXCLUDES** chronic tracheitis (491.8)

464.10 Without mention of obstruction

464.11 With obstruction

√5ᵗʰ 464.2 Acute laryngotracheitis
Laryngotracheitis (acute)
Tracheitis (acute) with laryngitis (acute)

> **EXCLUDES** chronic laryngotracheitis (476.1)

464.20 Without mention of obstruction

464.21 With obstruction

√5ᵗʰ 464.3 Acute epiglottitis
Viral epiglottitis

> **EXCLUDES** epiglottitis, chronic (476.1)

464.30 Without mention of obstruction

464.31 With obstruction

√4ᵗʰ
√5ᵗʰ Additional Digit Required   Unspecified Code   Other Specified Code   Manifestation Code   ▶◀ Revised Text   ● New Code   ▲ Revised Code Title

Diseases of the Respiratory System

464.4–473.9

Upper Respiratory System

464.4 Croup
Croup syndrome
DEF: Acute laryngeal obstruction due to allergy, foreign body or infection; symptoms include barking cough, hoarseness and harsh, persistent high-pitched respiratory sound.
J05.0 Acute obstructive laryngitis [croup] `I-10`

✓5ᵗʰ 464.5 Supraglottitis, unspecified
DEF: A rapidly advancing generalized upper respiratory infection of the lingual tonsillar area, epiglottic folds, false vocal cords, and the epiglottis.
AHA: 4Q, '01, 42

464.50 Without mention of obstruction
AHA: 4Q, '01, 43

464.51 With obstruction

✓4ᵗʰ 465 Acute upper respiratory infections of multiple or unspecified sites
EXCLUDES   upper respiratory infection due to:
     influenza (487.1, 488.02, 488.12)
     Streptococcus (034.0)

465.0 Acute laryngopharyngitis
DEF: Acute infection of the vocal cords and pharynx.

465.8 Other multiple sites
Multiple URI
AHA: 4Q, '07, 85

465.9 Unspecified site
Acute URI NOS
Upper respiratory infection (acute)
J06.9 Acute upper respiratory infection unspecified `I-10`

✓4ᵗʰ 466 Acute bronchitis and bronchiolitis
INCLUDES   that with:
     bronchospasm
     obstruction

466.0 Acute bronchitis
Bronchitis, acute or subacute:
     fibrinous
     membranous
     pneumococcal
     purulent
     septic
     viral
     with tracheitis
Croupous bronchitis
Tracheobronchitis, acute
EXCLUDES   acute bronchitis with chronic obstructive pulmonary disease (491.22)
DEF: Acute inflammation of main branches of bronchial tree due to infectious or irritant agents; symptoms include cough with a varied production of sputum, fever, substernal soreness, and lung rales.
AHA: 4Q, '04, 137; 1Q, '04, 3; 4Q, '02, 46; 4Q, '96, 28; 4Q, '91, 24; 1Q, '88, 12
TIP: If documented with COPD, assign only 491.22 Obstructive chronic bronchitis with acute bronchitis.
J20.9 Acute bronchitis unspecified `I-10`

✓5ᵗʰ 466.1 Acute bronchiolitis
Bronchiolitis (acute)   Capillary pneumonia
EXCLUDES   respiratory bronchiolitis interstitial lung disease (516.34)
DEF: Acute inflammation of the smallest branches of bronchial tree due to infectious or irritant agents; symptoms include cough, tachycardia, labored breathing, and lung crackles.

466.11 Acute bronchiolitis due to respiratory syncytial virus (RSV)
AHA: 1Q, '05, 10; 4Q, '96, 27
J21.0 Acute bronchiolitis d/t resp syncytial virus `I-10`

466.19 Acute bronchiolitis due to other infectious organisms
Use additional code to identify organism
J21.8 Acute bronchiolitis d/t oth specified organisms `I-10`

Other Diseases of the Upper Respiratory Tract (470-478)

470 Deviated nasal septum
Deflected septum (nasal) (acquired)
EXCLUDES   congenital (754.0)

✓4ᵗʰ 471 Nasal polyps
EXCLUDES   adenomatous polyps (212.0)

471.0 Polyp of nasal cavity
Polyp: Polyp:
   choanal   nasopharyngeal

471.1 Polypoid sinus degeneration
Woakes' syndrome or ethmoiditis

471.8 Other polyp of sinus
Polyp of sinus: Polyp of sinus:
   accessory   maxillary
   ethmoidal   sphenoidal

471.9 Unspecified nasal polyp
Nasal polyp NOS

✓4ᵗʰ 472 Chronic pharyngitis and nasopharyngitis

472.0 Chronic rhinitis
Ozena   Rhinitis:
Rhinitis: hypertrophic
   NOS   obstructive
   atrophic   purulent
   granulomatous   ulcerative
EXCLUDES   allergic rhinitis (477.0-477.9)
DEF: Persistent inflammation of mucous membranes of nose.

472.1 Chronic pharyngitis
Chronic sore throat   Pharyngitis:
Pharyngitis: granular (chronic)
   atrophic   hypertrophic

472.2 Chronic nasopharyngitis
EXCLUDES   acute or unspecified nasopharyngitis (460)
DEF: Persistent inflammation of mucous membranes extending from nares to pharynx.

✓4ᵗʰ 473 Chronic sinusitis
INCLUDES   abscess
     empyema
     infection   (chronic) of sinus (accessory) (nasal)
     suppuration
EXCLUDES   acute sinusitis (461.0-461.9)

473.0 Maxillary
Antritis (chronic)
J32.0 Chronic maxillary sinusitis `I-10`

473.1 Frontal

473.2 Ethmoidal
EXCLUDES   Woakes' ethmoiditis (471.1)

473.3 Sphenoidal

473.8 Other chronic sinusitis
Pansinusitis (chronic)

473.9 Unspecified sinusitis (chronic)
Sinusitis (chronic) NOS
J32.9 Chronic sinusitis unspecified `I-10`

Diseases of the Respiratory System

474–478.4

Paranasal Sinuses

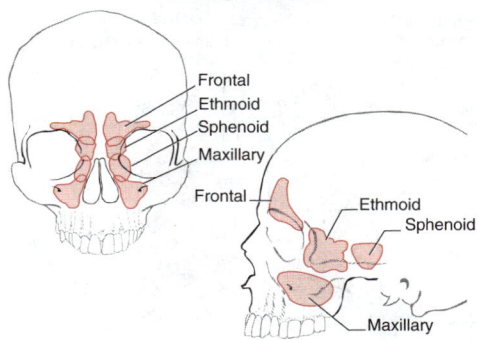

Frontal
Ethmoid
Sphenoid
Maxillary

Frontal

Ethmoid
Sphenoid

Maxillary

474 Chronic disease of tonsils and adenoids

474.0 Chronic tonsillitis and adenoiditis
> **EXCLUDES** *acute or unspecified tonsillitis (463)*
> **AHA:** 4Q, '97, 38

474.00 Chronic tonsillitis

474.01 Chronic adenoiditis

474.02 Chronic tonsillitis and adenoiditis

474.1 Hypertrophy of tonsils and adenoids
> Enlargement
> Hyperplasia } of tonsils or adenoids
> Hypertrophy
>
> **EXCLUDES** *that with:*
> *adenoiditis (474.01)*
> *adenoiditis and tonsillitis (474.02)*
> *tonsillitis (474.00)*

474.10 Tonsils with adenoids
> **AHA:** 2Q, '05, 16

474.11 Tonsils alone

474.12 Adenoids alone

474.2 Adenoid vegetations
> **DEF:** Fungus-like growth of lymph tissue between the nares and pharynx.

474.8 Other chronic disease of tonsils and adenoids
> Amygdalolith
> Calculus, tonsil
> Cicatrix of tonsil (and adenoid)
> Tonsillar tag
> Ulcer, tonsil

474.9 Unspecified chronic disease of tonsils and adenoids
> Disease (chronic) of tonsils (and adenoids)

475 Peritonsillar abscess
> Abscess of tonsil
> Peritonsillar cellulitis
> Quinsy
> **EXCLUDES** *tonsillitis:*
> *acute or NOS (463)*
> *chronic (474.0)*
> **J36** Peritonsillar abscess   `I-10`

476 Chronic laryngitis and laryngotracheitis

476.0 Chronic laryngitis
> Laryngitis: Laryngitis:
> catarrhal   sicca
> hypertrophic

476.1 Chronic laryngotracheitis
> Laryngitis, chronic, with tracheitis (chronic)
> Tracheitis, chronic, with laryngitis
> **EXCLUDES** *chronic tracheitis (491.8)*
> *laryngitis and tracheitis, acute or unspecified*
> *(464.00-464.51)*

477 Allergic rhinitis
> **INCLUDES** allergic rhinitis (nonseasonal) (seasonal)
> hay fever
> spasmodic rhinorrhea
> **EXCLUDES** *allergic rhinitis with asthma (bronchial) (493.0)*
> **DEF:** True immunoglobulin E (IgE)-mediated allergic reaction of nasal mucosa; seasonal (typical hay fever) or perennial (year-round allergens: dust, food, dander).

477.0 Due to pollen
> Pollinosis

477.1 Due to food
> **AHA:** 4Q, '00, 42

477.2 Due to animal (cat) (dog) hair and dander

477.8 Due to other allergen

477.9 Cause unspecified
> **AHA:** 2Q, '97, 9
> **J30.9** Allergic rhinitis unspecified   `I-10`

478 Other diseases of upper respiratory tract

478.0 Hypertrophy of nasal turbinates
> **DEF:** Overgrowth, enlargement of shell-shaped bones in nasal cavity.

478.1 Other diseases of nasal cavity and sinuses
> **EXCLUDES** *varicose ulcer of nasal septum (456.8)*

478.11 Nasal mucositis (ulcerative)
> Use additional E code to identify adverse effects of therapy, such as:
> antineoplastic and immunosuppressive drugs (E930.7, E933.1)
> radiation therapy (E879.2)
> **AHA:** 4Q, '06, 88-90

478.19 Other diseases of nasal cavity and sinuses
> Abscess
> Necrosis } of nose (septum)
> Ulcer
> Cyst or mucocele of sinus (nasal)
> Rhinolith
> **AHA:** 4Q, '06, 88-90
> **J34.1** Cyst and mucocele of nose and nasal sinus   `I-10`

478.2 Other diseases of pharynx, not elsewhere classified

478.20 Unspecified disease of pharynx

478.21 Cellulitis of pharynx or nasopharynx

478.22 Parapharyngeal abscess

478.24 Retropharyngeal abscess
> **DEF:** Purulent infection, behind pharynx and front of precerebral fascia.

478.25 Edema of pharynx or nasopharynx

478.26 Cyst of pharynx or nasopharynx

478.29 Other
> Abscess of pharynx or nasopharynx
> **EXCLUDES** *ulcerative pharyngitis (462)*

478.3 Paralysis of vocal cords or larynx
> **DEF:** Loss of motor ability of vocal cords or larynx; due to nerve or muscle damage.

478.30 Paralysis, unspecified
> Laryngoplegia   Paralysis of glottis

478.31 Unilateral, partial

478.32 Unilateral, complete

478.33 Bilateral, partial

478.34 Bilateral, complete

478.4 Polyp of vocal cord or larynx
> **EXCLUDES** *adenomatous polyps (212.1)*

`Additional Digit Required`   `Unspecified Code`   `Other Specified Code`   `Manifestation Code`   ►◄ Revised Text   ● New Code   ▲ Revised Code Title

2015 ICD-9-CM   **Volume 1 – 147**

478.5 Other diseases of vocal cords

Abscess
Cellulitis
Granuloma   } of vocal cords
Leukoplakia

Chorditis (fibrinous) (nodosa) (tuberosa)
Singers' nodes

478.6 Edema of larynx

Edema (of):   Edema (of):
  glottis   supraglottic
  subglottic

✓5ᵗʰ 478.7 Other diseases of larynx, not elsewhere classified

478.70 Unspecified disease of larynx

478.71 Cellulitis and perichondritis of larynx
DEF: Inflammation of deep soft tissues or lining of bone of the larynx.

478.74 Stenosis of larynx

478.75 Laryngeal spasm
Laryngismus (stridulus)
DEF: Involuntary muscle contraction of the larynx.

478.79 Other
Abscess
Necrosis
Obstruction   } of larynx
Pachyderma
Ulcer
EXCLUDES ulcerative laryngitis (464.00-464.01)
AHA: 3Q, '91, 20

478.8 Upper respiratory tract hypersensitivity reaction, site unspecified
EXCLUDES hypersensitivity reaction of lower respiratory tract, as:
    extrinsic allergic alveolitis (495.0-495.9)
    pneumoconiosis (500-505)

478.9 Other and unspecified diseases of upper respiratory tract
Abscess   } of trachea
Cicatrix

Pneumonia and Influenza (480-488)

EXCLUDES pneumonia:
  allergic or eosinophilic (518.3)
  aspiration:
    NOS (507.0)
    newborn (770.18)
    solids and liquids (507.0-507.8)
  congenital (770.0)
  lipoid (507.1)
  passive (514)
  rheumatic (390)
  ventilator-associated (997.31)

✓4ᵗʰ 480 Viral pneumonia

480.0 Pneumonia due to adenovirus

480.1 Pneumonia due to respiratory syncytial virus
AHA: 4Q, '10, 98; 4Q, '96, 28; 1Q, '88, 12

480.2 Pneumonia due to parainfluenza virus

480.3 Pneumonia due to SARS-associated coronavirus
DEF: A severe adult respiratory syndrome caused by the coronavirus, specified as inflammation of the lungs with consolidation.
AHA: 4Q, '03, 46-47

480.8 Pneumonia due to other virus not elsewhere classified
EXCLUDES congenital rubella pneumonitis (771.0)
    pneumonia complicating viral diseases classified elsewhere (484.1-484.8)

480.9 Viral pneumonia, unspecified
AHA: 3Q, '98, 5

481 Pneumococcal pneumonia [Streptococcus pneumoniae pneumonia]
Lobar pneumonia, organism unspecified
AHA: 2Q, '98, 7; 4Q, '92, 19; 1Q, '92, 18; 1Q, '91, 13; 1Q, '88, 13; M-A, '85, 6

Lungs

Right Lung (Three Lobes) — Trachea — Left Lung (Two Lobes)
Bronchopulmonary segments: — S1 S3 — Primary bronchus — Secondary bronchus
Upper lobe — S2 — S1,2 — S3 S4 S5 Upper lobe
Middle lobe — S5 — S6
S4 — S7,8 Lower lobe
Lower lobe — S8 — S9
Diaphragm — S9 S10 — S7 S10

✓4ᵗʰ 482 Other bacterial pneumonia
AHA: 4Q, '93, 39

482.0 Pneumonia due to Klebsiella pneumoniae

482.1 Pneumonia due to Pseudomonas

482.2 Pneumonia due to Hemophilus influenzae [H. influenzae]
AHA: 2Q, '05, 19

✓5ᵗʰ 482.3 Pneumonia due to Streptococcus
EXCLUDES Streptococcus pneumoniae (481)
AHA: 1Q, '88, 13

482.30 Streptococcus, unspecified

482.31 Group A

482.32 Group B

482.39 Other Streptococcus

✓5ᵗʰ 482.4 Pneumonia due to Staphylococcus
AHA: 3Q, '91, 16

482.40 Pneumonia due to Staphylococcus, unspecified

482.41 Methicillin susceptible pneumonia due to Staphylococcus aureus
MSSA pneumonia
Pneumonia due to Staphylococcus aureus NOS
J15.211 Pneumonia d/t methicillin suscep staph   I-10

482.42 Methicillin resistant pneumonia due to Staphylococcus aureus
AHA: 4Q, '08, 69, 71, 72

482.49 Other Staphylococcus pneumonia
AHA: ▶2Q, '13, 21◀

✓5ᵗʰ 482.8 Pneumonia due to other specified bacteria
EXCLUDES pneumonia, complicating infectious disease classified elsewhere (484.1-484.8)
AHA: 3Q, '88, 11

482.81 Anaerobes
Bacteroides (melaninogenicus)
Gram-negative anaerobes

482.82 Escherichia coli [E. coli]

482.83 Other gram-negative bacteria
Gram-negative pneumonia NOS
Proteus
Serratia marcescens
EXCLUDES gram-negative anaerobes (482.81)
    Legionnaires' disease (482.84)
AHA: 2Q, '98, 5; 3Q, '94, 9
TIP: Do not assign based solely on laboratory findings of gram-negative bacteria on gram-stain. Physician substantiation is required.
J15.6 Pneumonia d/t oth aerobic Gram-negative bacteria   I-10

482.84 Legionnaires' disease
DEF: Severe and often fatal infection by Legionella pneumophila; symptoms include high fever, gastrointestinal pain, headache, myalgia, dry cough, and pneumonia; usually transmitted airborne via air conditioning systems.
AHA: 4Q, '97, 38

N Newborn Age: 0   **P** Pediatric Age: 0-17   **M** Maternity Age: 12-55   **A** Adult Age: 15-124

482.89 Other specified bacteria
AHA: ▶2Q, '13, 17;◀ 2Q, '97, 6
TIP: Do not assign based on documentation of "mixed bacterial pneumonia" or "gram-positive pneumonia." See instead 482.9.

482.9 Bacterial pneumonia unspecified
AHA: 2Q, '98, 6; 2Q, '97, 6; 1Q, '94, 17
J15.9 Unspecified bacterial pneumonia `I-10`

✓4th **483 Pneumonia due to other specified organism**
AHA: N-D, '87, 5
TIP: Do not assign if pneumonia due to candidiasis; see code 112.4.

483.0 Mycoplasma pneumoniae
Eaton's agent   Pleuropneumonia-like organism [PPLO]

483.1 Chlamydia
AHA: 4Q, '96, 31

483.8 Other specified organism

✓4th **484 Pneumonia in infectious diseases classified elsewhere**

484.1 Pneumonia in cytomegalic inclusion disease
Code first underlying disease (078.5)

484.3 Pneumonia in whooping cough
Code first underlying disease (033.0-033.9)

484.5 Pneumonia in anthrax
Code first underlying disease (022.1)

484.6 Pneumonia in aspergillosis
Code first underlying disease (117.3)
AHA: 4Q, '97, 40

484.7 Pneumonia in other systemic mycoses
Code first underlying disease
EXCLUDES pneumonia in:
candidiasis (112.4)
coccidioidomycosis (114.0)
histoplasmosis (115.0-115.9 with fifth-digit 5)

484.8 Pneumonia in other infectious diseases classified elsewhere
Code first underlying disease, as:
Q fever (083.0)
typhoid fever (002.0)
EXCLUDES pneumonia in:
actinomycosis (039.1)
measles (055.1)
nocardiosis (039.1)
ornithosis (073.0)
Pneumocystis carinii (136.3)
salmonellosis (003.22)
toxoplasmosis (130.4)
tuberculosis (011.6)
tularemia (021.2)
varicella (052.1)

485 Bronchopneumonia, organism unspecified
Bronchopneumonia: Pneumonia:
hemorrhagic   lobular
terminal   segmental
Pleurobronchopneumonia
EXCLUDES bronchiolitis (acute) (466.11-466.19)
chronic (491.8)
lipoid pneumonia (507.1)

486 Pneumonia, organism unspecified
EXCLUDES hypostatic or passive pneumonia (514)
inhalation or aspiration pneumonia due to foreign materials (507.0-507.8)
pneumonitis due to fumes and vapors (506.0)
AHA: 4Q, '10, 135; 1Q, '10, 3, 12; 3Q, '09, 16; 4Q, '08, 142; 4Q, '99, 6; 3Q, '99, 9; 3Q, '98, 7; 2Q, '98, 4, 5; 1Q, '98, 8; 3Q, '97, 9; 3Q, '94, 10; 3Q, '88, 11
TIP: Never assume a causal organism based on laboratory or radiology findings alone.
J18.9 Pneumonia unspecified organism `I-10`

✓4th **487 Influenza**
Influenza caused by unspecified influenza virus
EXCLUDES Hemophilus influenzae [H. influenzae]:
infection NOS (041.5)
influenza due to identified avian influenza virus (488.01-488.09)
influenza due to 2009 H1N1 [swine] influenza virus (488.11-488.19)
influenza due to identified (novel) 2009 H1N1 influenza virus (488.11-488.19)
laryngitis (464.00-464.01)
meningitis (320.0)

487.0 With pneumonia
Influenza with pneumonia, any form   Influenzal:
Influenzal: pneumonia
bronchopneumonia
Use additional code to identify the type of pneumonia (480.0-480.9, 481, 482.0-482.9, 483.0-483.8, 485)
AHA: 1Q, '06, 18; 2Q, '05, 18
TIP: Selection of the principal diagnosis will be dependent on the circumstances of admission

487.1 With other respiratory manifestations
Influenza NEC   Influenzal:
Influenza NOS   pharyngitis
Influenzal: respiratory infection (upper) (acute)
laryngitis
AHA: 4Q, '11, 114; 1Q, '10, 4; 1Q, '06, 18; 2Q, '05, 18; 4Q, '99, 26
J10.1 Influenza d/t oth influenza virus w/resp manifst `I-10`

487.8 With other manifestations
Encephalopathy due to influenza
Influenza with involvement of gastrointestinal tract
EXCLUDES "intestinal flu" [viral gastroenteritis] (008.8)

✓4th **488 Influenza due to certain identified influenza viruses**
EXCLUDES influenza caused by unspecified or seasonal influenza viruses (487.0-487.8)
AHA: 4Q, '09, 92-93
TIP: Do not assign a code from this category unless the specified influenza virus is confirmed.

✓5th **488.0 Influenza due to identified avian influenza virus**
Avian influenza
Bird flu
Influenza A/H5N1
DEF: Infection caused by contact with bird influenza viruses; results in flu-like symptoms that may progress to other severe and life-threatening complications.
AHA: 4Q, '10, 85-87; 4Q, '07, 87

488.01 Influenza due to identified avian influenza virus with pneumonia
Avian influenzal:
bronchopneumonia
pneumonia
Influenza due to identified avian influenza virus with pneumonia, any form
Use additional code to identify the type of pneumonia (480.0- 480.9, 481, 482.0-482.9, 483.0-483.8, 485)
J09.X1 Influenza d/t ident novel influenza A virus w/pneumonia `I-10`

488.02 Influenza due to identified avian influenza virus with other respiratory manifestations
Avian influenzal: Identified avian influenza NOS
laryngitis
pharyngitis
respiratory infection (acute) (upper)
J09.X2 Flu d/t ident novel influenza A virus w/oth resp manifest `I-10`

488.09 Influenza due to identified avian influenza virus with other manifestations
Avian influenza with involvement of gastrointestinal tract
Encephalopathy due to identified avian influenza
EXCLUDES "intestinal flu" [viral gastroenteritis] (008.8)

✓4th ✓5th Additional Digit Required | Unspecified Code | Other Specified Code | Manifestation Code | ▶◀ Revised Text | ● New Code | ▲ Revised Code Title

Bronchioli and Alveoli

To trachea
Pulmonary arteriole
Terminal bronchiolus
Elastic fibers
Capillary network over all alveoli
Alveoli
Alveolus

✓5ᵗʰ 488.1 Influenza due to identified 2009 H1N1 influenza virus
2009 H1N1 swine influenza virus   Novel H1N1 influenza
(Novel) 2009 influenza H1N1   Novel influenza A/H1N1

   EXCLUDES *bird influenza virus infection (488.01-488.09)*
     influenza A/H5N1 (488.01-488.09)
     other human infection with influenza virus of animal
       origin (488.81-488.89)
     swine influenza virus infection (488.81-488.89)

   AHA: 4Q, '11, 110-112, 114; 4Q, '10, 85-87; 1Q, '10, 3-4

488.11 Influenza due to identified 2009 H1N1 influenza virus with pneumonia
Influenza due to identified (novel) 2009 H1N1 with pneumonia, any form
(Novel) 2009 H1N1 influenzal:
   bronchopneumonia
   pneumonia
Use additional code to identify the type of pneumonia (480.0- 480.9, 481, 482.0-482.9, 483.0-483.8, 485)

   J10.08 Influenza d/t oth ident influenza virus w/oth pneumonia   **I-10**

488.12 Influenza due to identified 2009 H1N1 influenza virus with other respiratory manifestations
(Novel) 2009 H1N1 influenza NOS
(Novel) 2009 H1N1 influenzal:
   laryngitis
   pharyngitis
   respiratory infection (acute) (upper)

   J10.1 Flu d/t oth ident influenza virus w/oth resp manifest   **I-10**

488.19 Influenza due to identified 2009 H1N1 influenza virus with other manifestations
Encephalopathy due to identified (novel) 2009 H1N1 influenza
(Novel) 2009 H1N1 influenza with involvement of gastrointestinal tract

   EXCLUDES *"intestinal flu" [viral gastroenteritis] (008.8)*

✓5ᵗʰ 488.8 Influenza due to novel influenza A
Influenza due to animal origin influenza virus
Infection with influenza viruses occurring in pigs or other animals
Other novel influenza A viruses not previously found in humans

   EXCLUDES *bird influenza virus infection (488.01-488.09)*
     influenza A/H5N1 (488.01-488.09)
     influenza due to identified 2009 H1N1 influenza virus
       (488.11- 488.19)

   AHA: 4Q, '11, 110-114

488.81 Influenza due to identified novel influenza A virus with pneumonia
Influenza due to animal origin influenza virus with pneumonia, any form
Novel influenza A:
   bronchopneumonia
   pneumonia
Use additional code to identify the type of pneumonia (480.0-480.9, 481, 482.0-482.9, 483.0-483.8, 485)

488.82 Influenza due to identified novel influenza A virus with other respiratory manifestations
Influenza due to animal origin influenza A virus with other respiratory manifestations
Novel influenza A:
   laryngitis
   pharyngitis
   respiratory infection (acute) (upper)

488.89 Influenza due to identified novel influenza A virus with other manifestations
Encephalopathy due to novel influenza A
Influenza due to animal origin influenza virus with encephalopathy
Influenza due to animal origin influenza virus with involvement of gastrointestinal tract
Novel influenza A with involvement of gastrointestinal tract

   EXCLUDES *"intestinal flu" [viral gastroenteritis] (008.8)*

Chronic Obstructive Pulmonary Disease and Allied Conditions (490-496)

AHA: 3Q, '88, 5

TIP: Due to the overlapping nature of conditions that make up COPD, it's essential that the coder review all instructional notes carefully.

490 Bronchitis, not specified as acute or chronic
Bronchitis NOS: Tracheobronchitis NOS
   catarrhal
   with tracheitis NOS

   EXCLUDES *bronchitis:*
     allergic NOS (493.9)
     asthmatic NOS (493.9)
     due to fumes and vapors (506.0)

   J40 Bronchitis not specified as acute or chronic   **I-10**

✓4ᵗʰ 491 Chronic bronchitis
   EXCLUDES *chronic obstructive asthma (493.2)*

491.0 Simple chronic bronchitis
Catarrhal bronchitis, chronic   Smokers' cough

   J41.0 Simple chronic bronchitis   **I-10**

491.1 Mucopurulent chronic bronchitis
Bronchitis (chronic) (recurrent):
   fetid
   mucopurulent
   purulent

   DEF: Chronic bronchial infection characterized by both mucus and pus secretions in the bronchial tree; recurs after asymptomatic periods; signs are coughing, expectoration and secondary changes in the lung.

   AHA: 3Q, '88, 12

✓5ᵗʰ 491.2 Obstructive chronic bronchitis
Bronchitis: Bronchitis with:
   emphysematous   chronic airway obstruction
   obstructive (chronic)   emphysema
   (diffuse)

   EXCLUDES *asthmatic bronchitis (acute) NOS (493.9)*
     chronic obstructive asthma (493.2)

   AHA: 3Q, '97, 9; 4Q, '91, 25; 2Q, '91, 21

491.20 Without exacerbation
Emphysema with chronic bronchitis

   AHA: 3Q, '97, 9

   J44.9 Chronic obst pulmonary disease, unspecified   **I-10**

Interrelationship Between Chronic Airway Obstruction, Chronic Bronchitis, and Emphysema

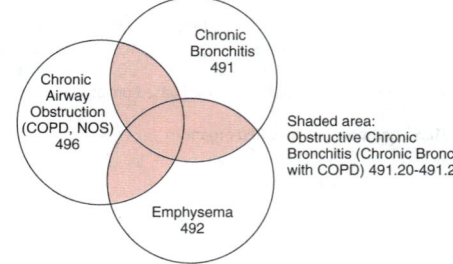

Chronic Bronchitis 491
Chronic Airway Obstruction (COPD, NOS) 496
Emphysema 492
Shaded area: Obstructive Chronic Bronchitis (Chronic Bronchitis with COPD) 491.20-491.21

491.21 With (acute) exacerbation
Acute exacerbation of chronic obstructive pulmonary disease [COPD]
Decompensated chronic obstructive pulmonary disease [COPD]
Decompensated chronic obstructive pulmonary disease [COPD] with exacerbation
EXCLUDES *chronic obstructive asthma with acute exacerbation (493.22)*
AHA: 1Q, '10, 12; 1Q, '04, 3; 3Q, '02, 18, 19; 4Q, '01, 43; 2Q, '96, 10
J44.1 Chronic obst pulmonary disease with exacerbation   **I-10**

491.22 With acute bronchitis
AHA: 3Q, '06, 20; 4Q, '04, 82
J44.0 Chronic obst pulmonary disease w/exacerbation   **I-10**

491.8 Other chronic bronchitis
Chronic: Chronic:
  tracheitis   tracheobronchitis

491.9 Unspecified chronic bronchitis
J42 Unspecified chronic bronchitis   **I-10**

492 Emphysema
AHA: 2Q, '91, 21

492.0 Emphysematous bleb
Giant bullous emphysema
Ruptured emphysematous bleb
Tension pneumatocele
Vanishing lung
DEF: Formation of vesicle or bulla in emphysematous lung, more than one millimeter; contains serum or blood.
AHA: 2Q, '93, 3

492.8 Other emphysema
Emphysema (lung or pulmonary):
  NOS
  centriacinar
  centrilobular
  obstructive
  panacinar
  panlobular
  unilateral
  vesicular
MacLeod's syndrome
Swyer-James syndrome
Unilateral hyperlucent lung
EXCLUDES *emphysema:*
    with chronic bronchitis (491.20-491.22)
    compensatory (518.2)
    due to fumes and vapors (506.4)
    interstitial (518.1)
      newborn (770.2)
    mediastinal (518.1)
    surgical (subcutaneous) (998.81)
    traumatic (958.7)
AHA: 4Q, '08, 175; 1Q, '05, 4; 4Q, '93, 41; J-A, '84, 17
J43.9 Emphysema unspecified   **I-10**

493 Asthma
EXCLUDES *wheezing NOS (786.07)*

The following fifth-digit subclassification is for use with codes 493.0-493.2, 493.9:
  0 unspecified
  1 with status asthmaticus
  2 with (acute) exacerbation

DEF: Status asthmaticus: severe, intractable episode of asthma unresponsive to normal therapeutic measures.
AHA: 4Q, '04, 137; 4Q, '03, 62; 4Q, '01, 43; 4Q, '00, 42; 1Q, '91, 13; 3Q, '88, 9; J-A, '85, 8; N-D, '84, 17
TIP: If documentation indicates both exacerbation and status asthmaticus, assign only the code for status asthmaticus.

§ √5th 493.0 Extrinsic asthma
[0-2]   Asthma:
        allergic with stated cause
        atopic
        childhood
        hay
        platinum
      Hay fever with asthma
      EXCLUDES *asthma:*
        allergic NOS (493.9)
        detergent (507.8)
        miners' (500)
        wood (495.8)
      DEF: Transient stricture of airway diameters of bronchi; due to environmental factor; also called allergic (bronchial) asthma.
      J45.20 Mild intermittent asthma uncomplicated   **I-10**

§ √5th 493.1 Intrinsic asthma
[0-2]   Late-onset asthma
      DEF: Transient stricture of airway diameters of bronchi; due to pathophysiological disturbances.
      AHA: 3Q, '88, 9; M-A, '85, 7

§ √5th 493.2 Chronic obstructive asthma
[0-2]   Asthma with chronic obstructive pulmonary disease [COPD]
      Chronic asthmatic bronchitis
      EXCLUDES *acute bronchitis (466.0)*
        chronic obstructive bronchitis (491.20-491.22)
      DEF: Persistent narrowing of airway diameters in the bronchial tree, restricting airflow and causing constant labored breathing.
      AHA: 2Q, '91, 21; 2Q, '90, 20; **For code 493.20:** 4Q, '03, 108; **For code 493.22:** 1Q, '09, 17; 3Q, '06, 20

√5th 493.8 Other forms of asthma
      AHA: 4Q, '03, 62

493.81 Exercise induced bronchospasm

493.82 Cough variant asthma

§ √5th 493.9 Asthma, unspecified
[0-2]   Asthma (bronchial) (allergic NOS)
      Bronchitis:
        allergic
        asthmatic
      AHA: 4Q, '97, 40, **For code 493.90:** 4Q, '04, 137; 4Q, '03, 108; 4Q, '99, 25; 1Q, '97, 7; **For code 493.91:** 1Q, '05, 5; **For code 493.92:** 1Q, '03, 9
      J45.909 Unspecified asthma uncomplicated   **I-10**
      J45.901 Unspecified asthma with acute exacerbation   **I-10**

494 Bronchiectasis
Bronchiectasis (fusiform) (postinfectious) (recurrent)
Bronchiolectasis
EXCLUDES *congenital (748.61)*
    tuberculous bronchiectasis (current disease) (011.5)
DEF: Dilation of bronchi; due to infection or chronic conditions; causes decreased lung capacity and recurrent infections of lungs.
AHA: 4Q, '00, 42

494.0 Bronchiectasis without acute exacerbation
J47.9 Bronchiectasis uncomplicated   **I-10**

494.1 Bronchiectasis with acute exacerbation

---

§ Requires fifth digit. Valid digits are in [brackets] under each code. See category 493 for codes and definitions.

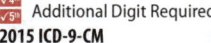
  Additional Digit Required   Unspecified Code   Other Specified Code   Manifestation Code   ►◄ Revised Text   ● New Code   ▲ Revised Code Title

2015 ICD-9-CM   **Volume 1 – 151**

Diseases of the Respiratory System

495–507.0

✓4ᵗʰ **495 Extrinsic allergic alveolitis**

INCLUDES allergic alveolitis and pneumonitis due to inhaled organic dust particles of fungal, thermophilic actinomycete, or other origin

DEF: Pneumonitis due to particles inhaled into lung, often at workplace; symptoms include cough, chills, fever, increased heart and respiratory rates; develops within hours of exposure.

495.0 Farmers' lung

495.1 Bagassosis

495.2 Bird-fanciers' lung
  Budgerigar-fanciers' disease or lung
  Pigeon-fanciers' disease or lung

495.3 Suberosis
  Cork-handlers' disease or lung

495.4 Malt workers' lung
  Alveolitis due to Aspergillus clavatus

495.5 Mushroom workers' lung

495.6 Maple bark-strippers' lung
  Alveolitis due to Cryptostroma corticale

495.7 "Ventilation" pneumonitis
  Allergic alveolitis due to fungal, thermophilic actinomycete, and other organisms growing in ventilation [air conditioning] systems

495.8 Other specified allergic alveolitis and pneumonitis
  Cheese-washers' lung   Grain-handlers' disease or lung
  Coffee workers' lung   Pituitary snuff-takers' disease
  Fish-meal workers' lung   Sequoiosis or red-cedar asthma
  Furriers' lung   Wood asthma

495.9 Unspecified allergic alveolitis and pneumonitis
  Alveolitis, allergic (extrinsic)   Hypersensitivity pneumonitis

496 Chronic airway obstruction, not elsewhere classified

NOTE This code is not to be used with any code from categories 491-493

Chronic:
  nonspecific lung disease
  obstructive lung disease
  obstructive pulmonary disease [COPD] NOS

EXCLUDES chronic obstructive lung disease [COPD] specified (as) (with):
  allergic alveolitis (495.0-495.9)
  asthma (493.20-493.22)
  bronchiectasis (494.0-494.1)
  bronchitis (491.20-491.22)
    with emphysema (491.20-491.22)
    decompensated (491.21)
  emphysema (492.0-492.8)

AHA: 1Q, '10, 5, 18; 1Q, '09, 16; 3Q, '07, 10; 4Q, '03, 109; 2Q, '00, 15; 2Q, '92, 16; 2Q, '91, 21; 3Q, '88, 56

TIP: COPD is a nonspecific term that encompasses many different respiratory conditions; review medical record and query physician for more specific documentation of emphysema, bronchitis, asthma, etc.

J44.9 Chronic obstructive pulmonary disease unspec   I-10

Pneumoconioses and Other Lung Diseases Due to External Agents (500-508)

DEF: Permanent deposits of particulate matter, within lungs; due to occupational or environmental exposure; results in chronic induration and fibrosis. (See specific listings in 500-508 code range).

500 Coal workers' pneumoconiosis   A
  Anthracosilicosis   Coal workers' lung
  Anthracosis   Miner's asthma
  Black lung disease

501 Asbestosis   A

502 Pneumoconiosis due to other silica or silicates
  Pneumoconiosis due to talc
  Silicotic fibrosis (massive) of lung
  Silicosis (simple) (complicated)

503 Pneumoconiosis due to other inorganic dust
  Aluminosis (of lung)   Graphite fibrosis (of lung)
  Baritosis   Siderosis
  Bauxite fibrosis (of lung)   Stannosis
  Berylliosis

504 Pneumonopathy due to inhalation of other dust
  Byssinosis   Flax-dressers' disease
  Cannabinosis

EXCLUDES allergic alveolitis (495.0-495.9)
  asbestosis (501)
  bagassosis (495.1)
  farmers' lung (495.0)

505 Pneumoconiosis, unspecified

✓4ᵗʰ **506 Respiratory conditions due to chemical fumes and vapors**

Use additional code to identify associated respiratory conditions, such as:
acute respiratory failure (518.81)

506.0 Bronchitis and pneumonitis due to fumes and vapors
  Chemical bronchitis (acute)
  AHA: 3Q. '10, 19; 3Q, '08, 7

506.1 Acute pulmonary edema due to fumes and vapors
  Chemical pulmonary edema (acute)
  EXCLUDES acute pulmonary edema NOS (518.4)
    chronic or unspecified pulmonary edema (514)
  AHA: 3Q, '88, 4

506.2 Upper respiratory inflammation due to fumes and vapors
  AHA: 3Q, '05, 10

506.3 Other acute and subacute respiratory conditions due to fumes and vapors
  AHA: 3Q, '10, 19

506.4 Chronic respiratory conditions due to fumes and vapors
  Emphysema (diffuse) (chronic) ⎫ due to inhalation
  Obliterative bronchiolitis ⎪ of chemical
    (chronic) (subacute) ⎬ fumes and
  Pulmonary fibrosis (chronic) ⎭ vapors

506.9 Unspecified respiratory conditions due to fumes and vapors
  Silo-fillers' disease

✓4ᵗʰ **507 Pneumonitis due to solids and liquids**

EXCLUDES fetal aspiration pneumonitis (770.18)
  postprocedural pneumonitis (997.32)
  AHA: 3Q, '91, 16

507.0 Due to inhalation of food or vomitus
  Aspiration pneumonia (due to):
    NOS
    food (regurgitated)
    gastric secretions
    milk
    saliva
    vomitus
  AHA: 4Q, '11, 150; 1Q, '11, 16; 1Q, '08, 18; 1Q, '89,10
  TIP: If postprocedural or postoperative aspiration pneumonia is specified, assign instead 997.32.
  J69.0 Pneumonitis due to inhalation of food and vomit   I-10

N Newborn Age: 0   P Pediatric Age: 0-17   M Maternity Age: 12-55   A Adult Age: 15-124

507.1 Due to inhalation of oils and essences
Lipoid pneumonia (exogenous)
EXCLUDES *endogenous lipoid pneumonia (516.8)*

507.8 Due to other solids and liquids
Detergent asthma

✓4ᵗʰ **508 Respiratory conditions due to other and unspecified external agents**
Use additional code to identify associated respiratory conditions, such as:
acute respiratory failure (518.81)

508.0 Acute pulmonary manifestations due to radiation
Radiation pneumonitis
AHA: 2Q, '88, 4

508.1 Chronic and other pulmonary manifestations due to radiation
Fibrosis of lung following radiation

508.2 Respiratory conditions due to smoke inhalation
Smoke inhalation NOS
EXCLUDES *smoke inhalation due to chemical fumes and vapors (506.9)*
AHA: 4Q, '11, 114-115
TIP: Assign for smoke inhalation, along with the appropriate E code describing the source of the smoke and fumes.

508.8 Respiratory conditions due to other specified external agents

508.9 Respiratory conditions due to unspecified external agent

Other Diseases of Respiratory System (510-519)

✓4ᵗʰ **510 Empyema**
Use additional code to identify infectious organism (041.0-041.9)
EXCLUDES *abscess of lung (513.0)*
DEF: Purulent infection within pleural space.

510.0 With fistula
Fistula:	Fistula:
bronchocutaneous	mediastinal
bronchopleural	pleural
hepatopleural	thoracic

Any condition classifiable to 510.9 with fistula
DEF: Purulent infection of respiratory cavity, with communication from cavity to another structure.

510.9 Without mention of fistula
Abscess:	Pleurisy:
pleura	purulent
thorax	septic
Empyema (chest) (lung)	seropurulent
(pleura)	suppurative
Fibrinopurulent pleurisy	Pyopneumothorax
	Pyothorax

AHA: 4Q, '07, 113; 3Q, '94, 6
J86.9 Pyothorax without fistula [I-10]

✓4ᵗʰ **511 Pleurisy**
EXCLUDES *pleurisy with mention of tuberculosis, current disease (012.0)*
DEF: Inflammation of serous membrane of lungs and lining of thoracic cavity; causes exudation in cavity or membrane surface.

511.0 Without mention of effusion or current tuberculosis
Adhesion, lung or pleura	Pleurisy:
Calcification of pleura	NOS
Pleurisy (acute) (sterile):	pneumococcal
diaphragmatic	staphylococcal
fibrinous	streptococcal
interlobar	Thickening of pleura

AHA: 3Q, '94, 5

511.1 With effusion, with mention of a bacterial cause other than tuberculosis
Pleurisy with effusion (exudative) (serous):
pneumococcal
staphylococcal
streptococcal
other specified nontuberculous bacterial cause

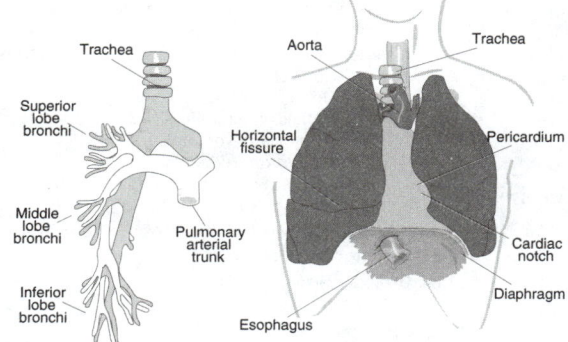
Lower Respiratory System

Trachea, Aorta, Trachea, Superior lobe bronchi, Horizontal fissure, Pericardium, Middle lobe bronchi, Pulmonary arterial trunk, Cardiac notch, Inferior lobe bronchi, Diaphragm, Esophagus

✓5ᵗʰ **511.8 Other specified forms of effusion, except tuberculous**
EXCLUDES *traumatic (860.2-860.5, 862.29, 862.39)*
AHA: 4Q, '08, 113-114; 1Q, '97, 10

511.81 Malignant pleural effusion
Code first malignant neoplasm, if known
J91.0 Malignant pleural effusion [I-10]

511.89 Other specified forms of effusion, except tuberculous
Encysted pleurisy	Hydropneumothorax
Hemopneumothorax	Hydrothorax
Hemothorax	

511.9 Unspecified pleural effusion
Pleural effusion NOS	Pleurisy:
Pleurisy:	serous
exudative	with effusion NOS
serofibrinous	

AHA: 2Q, '03, 7; 3Q, '91, 19; 4Q, '89, 11
TIP: Do not assign when the pleural effusion is a symptom of CHF and no therapeutic treatment (e.g., thoracentesis) is directed towards the pleural effusion.
J90 Pleural effusion not elsewhere classified [I-10]

✓4ᵗʰ **512 Pneumothorax and air leak**
DEF: Collapsed lung; due to gas or air in pleural space.
AHA: 4Q, '11, 115-116

512.0 Spontaneous tension pneumothorax
DEF: Leaking air from lung into lining causing collapse.
AHA: 3Q, '94, 5

512.1 Iatrogenic pneumothorax
Postoperative pneumothorax
DEF: Air trapped in the lining of the lung following surgery.
AHA: 1Q, '11, 14; 4Q, '94, 40
TIP: Pneumothorax is a known risk associated with most thoracic surgery; do not assign based on radiology findings alone, without physician substantiation.
J95.811 Postprocedural pneumothorax [I-10]

512.2 Postoperative air leak
AHA: 4Q, '11, 115-117

✓5ᵗʰ **512.8 Other pneumothorax and air leak**
Pneumothorax:	Pneumothorax:
NOS	chronic
acute	

EXCLUDES *pneumothorax:*
congenital (770.2)
traumatic (860.0-860.1, 860.4-860.5)
tuberculous, current disease (011.7)
AHA: 4Q, '11, 115-117; 2Q, '93, 3

512.81 Primary spontaneous pneumothorax
J93.11 Primary spontaneous pneumothorax [I-10]

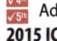

Diseases of the Respiratory System

512.82–517.3

512.82 Secondary spontaneous pneumothorax
Code first underlying condition, such as:
cancer metastatic to lung (197.0)
catamenial pneumothorax due to endometriosis (617.8)
cystic fibrosis (277.02)
eosinophilic pneumonia (518.3)
lymphangioleiomyomatosis (516.4)
Marfan syndrome (759.82)
pneumocystis carinii pneumonia (136.3)
primary lung cancer (162.3-162.9)
spontaneous rupture of the esophagus (530.4)

512.83 Chronic pneumothorax

512.84 Other air leak
Persistent air leak

512.89 Other pneumothorax
Acute pneumothorax
Spontaneous pneumothorax NOS
Pneumothorax NOS
J93.9 Pneumothorax unspecified   `I-10`

✓4ᵗʰ 513 Abscess of lung and mediastinum

513.0 Abscess of lung
Abscess (multiple) of lung
Gangrenous or necrotic pneumonia
Pulmonary gangrene or necrosis
AHA: 4Q, '07, 85; 2Q '98, 7

513.1 Abscess of mediastinum

514 Pulmonary congestion and hypostasis
Hypostatic: Pulmonary edema:
   bronchopneumonia   NOS
   pneumonia   chronic
Passive pneumonia
Pulmonary congestion (chronic) (passive)
EXCLUDES acute pulmonary edema:
NOS (518.4)
with mention of heart disease or failure (428.1)
hypostatic pneumonia due to or specified as a specific type of pneumonia— code to the type of pneumonia (480.0-480.9, 481, 482.0-482.9, 483.0-483.8, 487.0, 488.01, 488.11)
DEF: Excessive retention of interstitial fluid in the lungs and pulmonary vessels; due to poor circulation.
AHA: 2Q, '98, 6; 3Q, '88, 5
J81.1 Chronic pulmonary edema   `I-10`

515 Postinflammatory pulmonary fibrosis
Cirrhosis of lung
Fibrosis of lung (atrophic) (confluent) (massive) (perialveolar) (peribronchial) } chronic or unspecified
Induration of lung
DEF: Fibrosis and scarring of the lungs due to inflammatory reaction.
J84.10 Pulmonary fibrosis, unspecified   `I-10`

✓4ᵗʰ 516 Other alveolar and parietoalveolar pneumonopathy

516.0 Pulmonary alveolar proteinosis
DEF: Reduced ventilation; due to proteinaceous deposits on alveoli; symptoms include dyspnea, cough, chest pain, weakness, weight loss, and hemoptysis.

516.1 Idiopathic pulmonary hemosiderosis
Code first underlying disease (275.01-275.09)
Essential brown induration of lung
EXCLUDES acute idiopathic pulmonary hemorrhage in infants [AIPHI] (786.31)
DEF: Fibrosis of alveolar walls; marked by abnormal amounts hemosiderin in lungs; primarily affects children; symptoms include anemia, fluid in lungs, and blood in sputum; etiology unknown.

516.2 Pulmonary alveolar microlithiasis
DEF: Small calculi in pulmonary alveoli resembling sand-like particles on x-ray.

✓5ᵗʰ 516.3 Idiopathic interstitial pneumonia
AHA: 4Q, '11, 117-119

516.30 Idiopathic interstitial pneumonia, not otherwise specified
Idiopathic fibrosing alveolitis

516.31 Idiopathic pulmonary fibrosis
Cryptogenic fibrosing alveolitis
DEF: Chronic disease of unknown causation characterized by scarring and thickening of the lungs affecting males over 50

516.32 Idiopathic non-specific interstitial pneumonitis
EXCLUDES non-specific interstitial pneumonia NOS, or due to known underlying cause (516.8)

516.33 Acute interstitial pneumonitis
Hamman Rich syndrome
EXCLUDES pneumocystis pneumonia (136.3)

516.34 Respiratory bronchiolitis interstitial lung disease

516.35 Idiopathic lymphoid interstitial pneumonia
Idiopathic lymphocytic interstitial pneumonitis
EXCLUDES lymphoid interstitial pneumonia NOS, or due to known underlying cause (516.8)
pneumocystis pneumonia (136.3)

516.36 Cryptogenic organizing pneumonia
EXCLUDES organizing pneumonia NOS, or due to known underlying cause (516.8)

516.37 Desquamative interstitial pneumonia

516.4 Lymphangioleiomyomatosis   ♀
Lymphangiomyomatosis
AHA: 4Q, '11, 119

516.5 Adult pulmonary Langerhans cell histiocytosis   `A`
Adult PLCH
AHA: 4Q, '11, 119

✓5ᵗʰ 516.6 Interstitial lung diseases of childhood
AHA: 4Q, '11, 120-123

516.61 Neuroendocrine cell hyperplasia of infancy

516.62 Pulmonary interstitial glycogenosis

516.63 Surfactant mutations of the lung
DEF: Genetic disorders resulting in insufficient secretion of a complex mixture of phospholipids and proteins that reduce surface tension in the alveoli following the onset of breathing to facilitate lung expansion in the newborn; leading indication for pediatric lung transplantation.

516.64 Alveolar capillary dysplasia with vein misalignment

516.69 Other interstitial lung diseases of childhood

516.8 Other specified alveolar and parietoalveolar pneumonopathies
Endogenous lipoid pneumonia
Interstitial pneumonia
Lymphoid interstitial pneumonia due to known underlying cause
Lymphoid interstitial pneumonia NOS
Non-specific interstitial pneumonia due to known underlying cause
Non-specific interstitial pneumonia NOS
Organizing pneumonia due to known underlying cause
Organizing pneumonia NOS
Code first, if applicable, underlying cause of pneumonopathy, if known
Use additional E code, if applicable, for drug-induced or toxic pneumonopathy
EXCLUDES cryptogenic organizing pneumonia (516.36)
idiopathic lymphoid interstitial pneumonia (516.35)
idiopathic non-specific interstitial pneumonitis (516.32)
lipoid pneumonia, exogenous or unspecified (507.1)
AHA: 1Q, '11, 16; 1Q, '10, 6; 2Q, '06, 20; 1Q, '92, 12

516.9 Unspecified alveolar and parietoalveolar pneumonopathy

✓4ᵗʰ 517 Lung involvement in conditions classified elsewhere
EXCLUDES rheumatoid lung (714.81)

517.1 Rheumatic pneumonia
Code first underlying disease (390)

517.2 Lung involvement in systemic sclerosis
Code first underlying disease (710.1)

517.3 Acute chest syndrome
Code first sickle-cell disease in crisis (282.42, 282.62, 282.64, 282.69)
AHA: 4Q, '03, 51, 56

`N` Newborn Age: 0   `P` Pediatric Age: 0-17   `M` Maternity Age: 12-55   `A` Adult Age: 15-124

Diseases of the Respiratory System

517.8 — 518.84

517.8 Lung involvement in other diseases classified elsewhere

Code first underlying disease, as:
amyloidosis (277.30-277.39)
polymyositis (710.4)
sarcoidosis (135)
Sjögren's disease (710.2)
systemic lupus erythematosus (710.0)

EXCLUDES syphilis (095.1)

AHA: 2Q, '03, 7

518 Other diseases of lung

518.0 Pulmonary collapse

Atelectasis   Middle lobe syndrome
Collapse of lung

EXCLUDES atelectasis:
congenital (partial) (770.5)
primary (770.4)
tuberculous, current disease (011.8)

AHA: 4Q, '90, 25

J98.11 Atelectasis   I-10

518.1 Interstitial emphysema

Mediastinal emphysema

EXCLUDES surgical (subcutaneous) emphysema (998.81)
that in fetus or newborn (770.2)
traumatic emphysema (958.7)

DEF: Escaped air from the alveoli trapped in the interstices of the lung; trauma or cough may cause the disease.

518.2 Compensatory emphysema

DEF: Distention of all or part of the lung caused by disease processes or surgical intervention that decreased volume in another part of the lung; overcompensation reaction to the loss of capacity in another part of the lung.

518.3 Pulmonary eosinophilia

Eosinophilic asthma   Pneumonia:
Löffler's syndrome   eosinophilic
Pneumonia: Tropical eosinophilia
    allergic

EXCLUDES pulmonary infiltrate NOS (793.19)

DEF: Infiltration, into pulmonary parenchyma of eosinophils; results in cough, fever, and dyspnea.

AHA: 4Q, '11, 139

518.4 Acute edema of lung, unspecified

Acute pulmonary edema NOS
Pulmonary edema, postoperative

EXCLUDES pulmonary edema:
acute, with mention of heart disease or failure (428.1)
chronic or unspecified (514)
due to external agents (506.0-508.9)

DEF: Severe, sudden fluid retention within lung tissues.

TIP: Do not assign separately if associated with CHF or heart disease; it is incorporated into those codes.

518.5 Pulmonary insufficiency following trauma and surgery

EXCLUDES adult respiratory distress syndrome associated with other conditions (518.82)
pneumonia:
aspiration (507.0)
hypostatic (514)
respiratory failure in other conditions (518.81, 518.83-518.84)

AHA: 4Q, '11, 123-125; 3Q, '10, 19; 4Q, '04, 139; 3Q, '88, 3; 3Q, '88, 7; S-O, '87, 1

518.51 Acute respiratory failure following trauma and surgery

Respiratory failure, not otherwise specified, following trauma and surgery

EXCLUDES acute respiratory failure in other conditions (518.81)

J95.821 Acute postprocedural respiratory failure   I-10

518.52 Other pulmonary insufficiency, not elsewhere classified, following trauma and surgery

Adult respiratory distress syndrome
Pulmonary insufficiency following surgery
Pulmonary insufficiency following trauma
Shock lung related to trauma and surgery

EXCLUDES adult respiratory distress syndrome associated with other conditions (518.82)
aspiration pneumonia (507.0)
hypostatic pneumonia (514)
shock lung, not related to trauma or surgery (518.82)

518.53 Acute and chronic respiratory failure following trauma and surgery

EXCLUDES acute and chronic respiratory failure in other conditions (518.84)

518.6 Allergic bronchopulmonary aspergillosis

DEF: Noninvasive hypersensitive reaction; due to allergic reaction to Aspergillus fumigatus (mold).

AHA: 4Q, '97, 39

518.7 Transfusion related acute lung injury [TRALI]

DEF: A relatively rare, but serious pulmonary complication of blood transfusion, with acute respiratory distress, noncardiogenic pulmonary edema, cyanosis, hypoxemia, hypotension, fever and chills.

AHA: 4Q, '06, 91

518.8 Other diseases of lung

518.81 Acute respiratory failure

Respiratory failure NOS

EXCLUDES acute and chronic respiratory failure (518.84)
acute respiratory distress (518.82)
acute respiratory failure following trauma and surgery (518.51)
chronic respiratory failure (518.83)
respiratory arrest (799.1)
respiratory failure, newborn (770.84)

AHA: 3Q, '12, 21-22; 4Q, '10, 80; 1Q, '10, 18-19; 3Q, '09, 14; 2Q, '09, 11; 1Q, '08, 18; 3Q, '07, 6; 2Q, '06, 25; 4Q, '05, 96; 2Q, '05, 19; 1Q, '05, 3-8; 1Q, '05, 3-8; 4Q, '04, 139; 1Q, '03, 15; 4Q, '98, 41; 3Q, '91, 14; 2Q, '91, 3; 4Q, '90, 25; 2Q, '90, 20; 3Q, '88, 7; 3Q, '88, 10; S-O, '87, 1

TIP: If both respiratory failure and another acute condition are equally responsible for admission, either may be sequenced as principal diagnosis in the absence of chapter-specific guidelines to the contrary.

J96.01 Acute respiratory failure with hypoxia   I-10

518.82 Other pulmonary insufficiency, not elsewhere classified

Acute respiratory distress
Acute respiratory insufficiency
Adult respiratory distress syndrome NEC

EXCLUDES acute interstitial pneumonitis (516.33)
adult respiratory distress syndrome associated with trauma or surgery (518.52)
pulmonary insufficiency following trauma or surgery (518.52)
respiratory distress:
NOS (786.09)
newborn (770.89)
syndrome, newborn (769)

AHA: 4Q, '03, 105; 2Q, '91, 21; 3Q, '88, 7

J80 Acute respiratory distress syndrome   I-10

518.83 Chronic respiratory failure

AHA: 4Q, '05, 96; 4Q, '03, 103, 111

J96.10 Chronic respiratory failure, unsp w/ hypox or hypercap   I-10

518.84 Acute and chronic respiratory failure

Acute on chronic respiratory failure

EXCLUDES acute and chronic respiratory failure following trauma or surgery (518.53)

AHA: 2Q, '11, 7

J96.20 Ac & chr resp failure unsp w/hypox or hypercap   I-10

Additional Digit Required   **Unspecified Code**   Other Specified Code   Manifestation Code   ►◄ Revised Text   ● New Code   ▲ Revised Code Title

2015 ICD-9-CM   **Volume 1 – 155**

Diseases of the Respiratory System

518.89 Other diseases of lung, not elsewhere classified
Broncholithiasis   Lung disease NOS
Calcification of lung   Pulmolithiasis
DEF: Broncholithiasis: calculi in lumen of transbronchial tree.
DEF: Pulmolithiasis: calculi in lung.
AHA: 3Q, '90, 18; 4Q, '88, 6
TIP: Do not assign for solitary lung nodule; see instead code 793.11.
J98.4 Other disorders of lung   `I-10`

✓4ᵗʰ **519 Other diseases of respiratory system**

✓5ᵗʰ **519.0 Tracheostomy complications**

519.00 Tracheostomy complication, unspecified

519.01 Infection of tracheostomy
Use additional code to identify type of infection, such as:
abscess or cellulitis of neck (682.1)
septicemia (038.0-038.9)
Use additional code to identify organism (041.00-041.9)
AHA: 4Q, '98, 41

519.02 Mechanical complication of tracheostomy
Tracheal stenosis due to tracheostomy

519.09 Other tracheostomy complications
Hemorrhage due to tracheostomy
Tracheoesophageal fistula due to tracheostomy

✓5ᵗʰ **519.1 Other diseases of trachea and bronchus, not elsewhere classified**
AHA: 3Q, '02, 18; 3Q, '88, 6

519.11 Acute bronchospasm
Bronchospasm NOS
EXCLUDES *acute bronchitis with bronchospasm (466.0)*
asthma (493.00-493.92)
exercise induced bronchospasm (493.81)
AHA: 4Q, '06, 92

519.19 Other diseases of trachea and bronchus
Calcification
Stenosis } of bronchus or trachea
Ulcer
AHA: 4Q, '06, 92

519.2 Mediastinitis
DEF: Inflammation of tissue between organs behind sternum.

519.3 Other diseases of mediastinum, not elsewhere classified
Fibrosis
Hernia } of mediastinum
Retraction

519.4 Disorders of diaphragm
Diaphragmitis   Relaxation of diaphragm
Paralysis of diaphragm
EXCLUDES *congenital defect of diaphragm (756.6)*
diaphragmatic hernia (551-553 with .3)
congenital (756.6)

519.8 Other diseases of respiratory system, not elsewhere classified
AHA: 4Q, '89, 12

519.9 Unspecified disease of respiratory system
Respiratory disease (chronic) NOS

9. Diseases of the Digestive System (520-579)

Diseases of Oral Cavity, Salivary Glands, and Jaws (520-529)

√4ᵗʰ **520 Disorders of tooth development and eruption**

520.0 Anodontia
Absence of teeth (complete) (congenital) (partial)
Hypodontia
Oligodontia
EXCLUDES *acquired absence of teeth (525.10-525.19)*

520.1 Supernumerary teeth
Distomolar
Fourth molar
Mesiodens
Paramolar
Supplemental teeth
EXCLUDES *supernumerary roots (520.2)*

520.2 Abnormalities of size and form
Concrescence ⎱
Fusion   ⎰ of teeth
Gemination

Dens evaginatus
Dens in dente
Dens invaginatus
Enamel pearls
Macrodontia
Microdontia
Peg-shaped [conical] teeth
Supernumerary roots
Taurodontism
Tuberculum paramolare
EXCLUDES *that due to congenital syphilis (090.5)*
tuberculum Carabelli, which is regarded as a normal variation

520.3 Mottled teeth
Mottling of enamel
Dental fluorosis
Nonfluoride enamel opacities

Digestive System

The Oral Cavity

Teeth

Maxillary view

Mandibulary view

520.4 Disturbances of tooth formation
Aplasia and hypoplasia of cementum
Dilaceration of tooth
Enamel hypoplasia (neonatal) (postnatal) (prenatal)
Horner's teeth
Hypocalcification of teeth
Regional odontodysplasia
Turner's tooth
EXCLUDES *Hutchinson's teeth and mulberry molars in congenital syphilis (090.5)*
mottled teeth (520.3)

520.5 Hereditary disturbances in tooth structure, not elsewhere classified
Amelogensis ⎫
Dentinogenesis ⎬ imperfecta
Odontogenesis ⎭

Dentinal dysplasia
Shell teeth

520.6 Disturbances in tooth eruption
Teeth:
  embedded
  impacted
  natal
  neonatal
  prenatal
  primary [deciduous]:
    persistent
    shedding, premature
Tooth eruption:
  late
  obstructed
  premature
EXCLUDES *exfoliation of teeth (attributable to disease of surrounding tissues) (525.0-525.19)*
AHA: 1Q, '06, 18; 2Q, '05, 15

520.7 Teething syndrome

520.8 Other specified disorders of tooth development and eruption
Color changes during tooth formation
Pre-eruptive color changes
EXCLUDES *posteruptive color changes (521.7)*

520.9 Unspecified disorder of tooth development and eruption

Diseases of the Digestive System

521–522.8

✓4th **521**   **Diseases of hard tissues of teeth**

✓5th   **521.0 Dental caries**
> **AHA:** 4Q, '01, 44

> **521.00** Dental caries, unspecified

> **521.01** **Dental caries limited to enamel**
> > Initial caries
> > White spot lesion

> **521.02** **Dental caries extending into dentine**

> **521.03** **Dental caries extending into pulp**

> **521.04** **Arrested dental caries**

> **521.05** **Odontoclasia**
> > Infantile melanodontia
> > Melanodontoclasia
> > **EXCLUDES**   *internal and external resorption of teeth (521.40-521.49)*
> > **DEF:** A pathological dental condition described as stained areas, loss of tooth substance, and hypoplasia linked to nutritional deficiencies during tooth development and to cariogenic oral conditions.

> **521.06** **Dental caries pit and fissure**
> > Primary dental caries, pit and fissure origin

> **521.07** **Dental caries of smooth surface**
> > Primary dental caries, smooth surface origin

> **521.08** **Dental caries of root surface**
> > Primary dental caries, root surface

> **521.09** Other dental caries
> > **AHA:** 3Q, '02, 14

✓5th   **521.1 Excessive attrition (approximal wear) (occlusal wear)**

> **521.10** Excessive attrition, unspecified

> **521.11** **Excessive attrition, limited to enamel**

> **521.12** **Excessive attrition, extending into dentine**

> **521.13** **Excessive attrition, extending into pulp**

> **521.14** **Excessive attrition, localized**

> **521.15** **Excessive attrition, generalized**

✓5th   **521.2 Abrasion**
> Abrasion:
> > dentifrice
> > habitual
> > occupational   } of teeth
> > ritual
> > traditional
> > Wedge defect NOS

> **521.20** Abrasion, unspecified

> **521.21** **Abrasion, limited to enamel**

> **521.22** **Abrasion, extending into dentine**

> **521.23** **Abrasion, extending into pulp**

> **521.24** **Abrasion, localized**

> **521.25** **Abrasion, generalized**

✓5th   **521.3 Erosion**
> Erosion of teeth:
> > NOS
> > due to:
> > > medicine
> > > persistent vomiting
> > idiopathic
> > occupational

> **521.30** Erosion, unspecified

> **521.31** **Erosion, limited to enamel**

> **521.32** **Erosion, extending into dentine**

> **521.33** **Erosion, extending into pulp**

> **521.34** **Erosion, localized**

> **521.35** **Erosion, generalized**

✓5th **521.4 Pathological resorption**
> **DEF:** Loss of dentin and cementum due to disease process.

> **521.40** Pathological resorption, unspecified

> **521.41** **Pathological resorption, internal**

> **521.42** **Pathological resorption, external**

> **521.49** Other pathological resorption
> > Internal granuloma of pulp

521.5 Hypercementosis
> Cementation hyperplasia
> **DEF:** Excess deposits of cementum, on tooth root.

521.6 Ankylosis of teeth
> **DEF:** Adhesion of tooth to surrounding bone.

521.7 Intrinsic posteruptive color changes
> Staining [discoloration] of teeth:
> > NOS
> > due to:
> > > drugs
> > > metals
> > > pulpal bleeding
> > **EXCLUDES**   *accretions [deposits] on teeth (523.6)*
> > > *extrinsic color changes (523.6)*
> > > *pre-eruptive color changes (520.8)*

✓5th **521.8 Other specified diseases of hard tissues of teeth**

> **521.81** **Cracked tooth**
> > **EXCLUDES**   *asymptomatic craze lines in enamel — omit code*
> > > *broken tooth due to trauma (873.63, 873.73)*
> > > *fractured tooth due to trauma (873.63, 873.73)*

> **521.89** Other specified diseases of hard tissues of teeth
> > Irradiated enamel
> > Sensitive dentin

521.9 Unspecified disease of hard tissues of teeth

✓4th **522**   **Diseases of pulp and periapical tissues**

522.0 Pulpitis
> Pulpal: Pulpitis:
> > abscess   acute
> > polyp   chronic (hyperplastic) (ulcerative)
> >   suppurative

522.1 Necrosis of the pulp
> Pulp gangrene
> **DEF:** Death of pulp tissue.

522.2 Pulp degeneration
> Denticles   Pulp stones
> Pulp calcifications

522.3 Abnormal hard tissue formation in pulp
> Secondary or irregular dentin

522.4 Acute apical periodontitis of pulpal origin
> **DEF:** Severe inflammation of periodontal ligament due to pulpal inflammation or necrosis.

522.5 Periapical abscess without sinus
> Abscess:
> > dental
> > dentoalveolar
> > **EXCLUDES**   *periapical abscess with sinus (522.7)*

522.6 Chronic apical periodontitis
> Apical or periapical granuloma
> Apical periodontitis NOS

522.7 Periapical abscess with sinus
> Fistula:
> > alveolar process
> > dental

522.8 Radicular cyst
> Cyst:
> > apical (periodontal)
> > periapical
> > radiculodental
> > residual radicular
> > **DEF:** Cyst in tissue around tooth apex due to chronic infection of granuloma around root.

N Newborn Age: 0   **P** Pediatric Age: 0-17   **M** Maternity Age: 12-55   **A** Adult Age: 15-124

522.9 Other and unspecified diseases of pulp and periapical tissues

√4ᵗʰ **523 Gingival and periodontal diseases**

√5ᵗʰ **523.0 Acute gingivitis**
> EXCLUDES *acute necrotizing ulcerative gingivitis (101)*
> *herpetic gingivostomatitis (054.2)*

> **523.00 Acute gingivitis, plaque induced**
> Acute gingivitis NOS

> **523.01 Acute gingivitis, non-plaque induced**

√5ᵗʰ **523.1 Chronic gingivitis**
> Gingivitis (chronic):
> desquamative
> hyperplastic
> simple marginal
> ulcerative
> EXCLUDES *herpetic gingivostomatitis (054.2)*

> **523.10 Chronic gingivitis, plaque induced**
> Chronic gingivitis NOS
> Gingivitis NOS

> **523.11 Chronic gingivitis, non-plaque induced**

√5ᵗʰ **523.2 Gingival recession**
> Gingival recession (postinfective) (postoperative)

> **523.20 Gingival recession, unspecified**

> **523.21 Gingival recession, minimal**

> **523.22 Gingival recession, moderate**

> **523.23 Gingival recession, severe**

> **523.24 Gingival recession, localized**

> **523.25 Gingival recession, generalized**

√5ᵗʰ **523.3 Aggressive and acute periodontitis**
> Acute:
> pericementitis
> pericoronitis
> EXCLUDES *acute apical periodontitis (522.4)*
> *periapical abscess (522.5, 522.7)*
> DEF: Severe inflammation of tissues supporting teeth.

> **523.30 Aggressive periodontitis, unspecified**

> **523.31 Aggressive periodontitis, localized**
> Periodontal abscess

> **523.32 Aggressive periodontitis, generalized**

> **523.33 Acute periodontitis**

√5ᵗʰ **523.4 Chronic periodontitis**
> Chronic pericoronitis
> Pericementitis (chronic)
> Periodontitis:
> NOS
> complex
> simplex
> EXCLUDES *chronic apical periodontitis (522.6)*

> **523.40 Chronic periodontitis, unspecified**

> **523.41 Chronic periodontitis, localized**

> **523.42 Chronic periodontitis, generalized**

523.5 Periodontosis

523.6 Accretions on teeth
> Dental calculus:
> subgingival
> supragingival
> Deposits on teeth:
> betel
> materia alba
> soft
> tartar
> tobacco
> Extrinsic discoloration of teeth
> EXCLUDES *intrinsic discoloration of teeth (521.7)*
> DEF: Foreign material on tooth surface, usually plaque or calculus.

523.8 Other specified periodontal diseases
> Giant cell:
> epulis
> peripheral granuloma
> Gingival:
> cysts
> enlargement NOS
> fibromatosis
> Gingival polyp
> Periodontal lesions due to traumatic occlusion
> Peripheral giant cell granuloma
> EXCLUDES *leukoplakia of gingiva (528.6)*

523.9 Unspecified gingival and periodontal disease
> AHA: 3Q ,'02, 14

√4ᵗʰ **524 Dentofacial anomalies, including malocclusion**

√5ᵗʰ **524.0 Major anomalies of jaw size**
> EXCLUDES *hemifacial atrophy or hypertrophy (754.0)*
> *unilateral condylar hyperplasia or hypoplasia of mandible (526.89)*

> **524.00 Unspecified anomaly**
> DEF: Unspecified deformity of jaw size.

> **524.01 Maxillary hyperplasia**
> DEF: Overgrowth or over development of upper jaw bone.

> **524.02 Mandibular hyperplasia**
> DEF: Overgrowth or over development of lower jaw bone.

> **524.03 Maxillary hypoplasia**
> DEF: Incomplete or underdeveloped upper jaw bone.

> **524.04 Mandibular hypoplasia**
> DEF: Incomplete or underdeveloped lower jaw bone.
> AHA: 2Q, '12, 17

> **524.05 Macrogenia**
> DEF: Enlarged jaw, especially chin; affects bone, soft tissue, or both.

> **524.06 Microgenia**
> DEF: Underdeveloped mandible, characterized by an extremely small chin.

> **524.07 Excessive tuberosity of jaw**
> Entire maxillary tuberosity

> **524.09 Other specified anomaly**

√5ᵗʰ **524.1 Anomalies of relationship of jaw to cranial base**

> **524.10 Unspecified anomaly**
> Prognathism
> Retrognathism
> DEF: Prognathism: protrusion of lower jaw.
> DEF: Retrognathism: jaw is located posteriorly to a normally positioned jaw; backward position of mandible.

> **524.11 Maxillary asymmetry**
> DEF: Absence of symmetry of maxilla.

> **524.12 Other jaw asymmetry**

> **524.19 Other specified anomaly**

Angle's Classification of Malocclusion

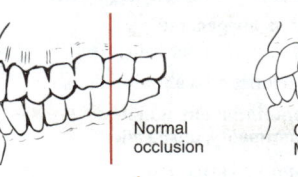

Normal occlusion   Class I Malocclusion

Class II Malocclusion   Class III Malocclusion

√4ᵗʰ √5ᵗʰ Additional Digit Required   Unspecified Code   Other Specified Code   Manifestation Code   ▶◀ Revised Text   ● New Code   ▲ Revised Code Title

2015 ICD-9-CM   **Volume 1 – 159**

Diseases of the Digestive System

524.2–525.19

√5th **524.2 Anomalies of dental arch relationship**
Anomaly of dental arch
EXCLUDES *hemifacial atrophy or hypertrophy (754.0)*
soft tissue impingement (524.81-524.82)
unilateral condylar hyperplasia or hypoplasia of
mandible (526.89)

524.20 Unspecified anomaly of dental arch relationship

524.21 Malocclusion, Angle's class I
Neutro-occlusion

524.22 Malocclusion, Angle's class II
Disto-occlusion Division I
Disto-occlusion Division II

524.23 Malocclusion, Angle's class III
Mesio-occlusion

524.24 Open anterior occlusal relationship
Anterior open bite

524.25 Open posterior occlusal relationship
Posterior open bite

524.26 Excessive horizontal overlap
Excessive horizontal overjet

524.27 Reverse articulation
Anterior articulation
Crossbite
Posterior articulation

524.28 Anomalies of interarch distance
Excessive interarch distance
Inadequate interarch distance

524.29 Other anomalies of dental arch relationship
Other anomalies of dental arch

√5th **524.3 Anomalies of tooth position of fully erupted teeth**
EXCLUDES *impacted or embedded teeth with abnormal position*
of such teeth or adjacent teeth (520.6)

524.30 Unspecified anomaly of tooth position
Diastema of teeth NOS
Displacement of teeth NOS
Transposition of teeth NOS

524.31 Crowding of teeth

524.32 Excessive spacing of teeth

524.33 Horizontal displacement of teeth
Tipped teeth
Tipping of teeth

524.34 Vertical displacement of teeth
Extruded tooth
Infraeruption of teeth
Intruded tooth
Supraeruption of teeth

524.35 Rotation of tooth/teeth

524.36 Insufficient interocclusal distance of teeth (ridge)
Lack of adequate intermaxillary vertical dimension

524.37 Excessive interocclusal distance of teeth
Excessive intermaxillary vertical dimension
Loss of occlusal vertical dimension

524.39 Other anomalies of tooth position

524.4 Malocclusion, unspecified
DEF: Malposition of top and bottom teeth; interferes with chewing.

√5th **524.5 Dentofacial functional abnormalities**

524.50 Dentofacial functional abnormality, unspecified

524.51 Abnormal jaw closure

524.52 Limited mandibular range of motion

524.53 Deviation in opening and closing of the mandible

524.54 Insufficient anterior guidance
Insufficient anterior occlusal guidance

524.55 Centric occlusion maximum intercuspation discrepancy
Centric occlusion of teeth discrepancy

524.56 Non-working side interference
Balancing side interference

524.57 Lack of posterior occlusal support

524.59 Other dentofacial functional abnormalities
Abnormal swallowing'   Sleep postures
Mouth breathing   Tongue, lip, or finger habits

√5th **524.6 Temporomandibular joint disorders**
EXCLUDES *current temporomandibular joint:*
dislocation (830.0-830.1)
strain (848.1)

524.60 Temporomandibular joint disorders, unspecified
Temporomandibular joint-pain-dysfunction syndrome [TMJ]

524.61 Adhesions and ankylosis (bony or fibrous)
DEF: Stiffening or union of temporomandibular joint due to bony or fibrous union across joint.

524.62 Arthralgia of temporomandibular joint
DEF: Pain in temporomandibular joint; not inflammatory in nature.

524.63 Articular disc disorder (reducing or non-reducing)

524.64 Temporomandibular joint sounds on opening and/or closing the jaw

524.69 Other specified temporomandibular joint disorders

√5th **524.7 Dental alveolar anomalies**

524.70 Unspecified alveolar anomaly

524.71 Alveolar maxillary hyperplasia
DEF: Excessive tissue formation in the dental alveoli of upper jaw.

524.72 Alveolar mandibular hyperplasia
DEF: Excessive tissue formation in the dental alveoli of lower jaw.

524.73 Alveolar maxillary hypoplasia
DEF: Incomplete or underdeveloped alveolar tissue of upper jaw.

524.74 Alveolar mandibular hypoplasia
DEF: Incomplete or underdeveloped alveolar tissue of lower jaw.

524.75 Vertical displacement of alveolus and teeth
Extrusion of alveolus and teeth

524.76 Occlusal plane deviation

524.79 Other specified alveolar anomaly

√5th **524.8 Other specified dentofacial anomalies**

524.81 Anterior soft tissue impingement

524.82 Posterior soft tissue impingement

524.89 Other specified dentofacial anomalies

524.9 Unspecified dentofacial anomalies

√4th **525 Other diseases and conditions of the teeth and supporting structures**

525.0 Exfoliation of teeth due to systemic causes
DEF: Deterioration of teeth and surrounding structures due to systemic disease.

√5th **525.1 Loss of teeth due to trauma, extraction, or periodontal disease**
Code first class of edentulism (525.40-525.44, 525.50-525.54)
AHA: 4Q, '05, 74; 4Q, '01, 44

525.10 Acquired absence of teeth, unspecified
Tooth extraction status, NOS

525.11 Loss of teeth due to trauma

525.12 Loss of teeth due to periodontal disease

525.13 Loss of teeth due to caries

525.19 Other loss of teeth

√5ᵗʰ **525.2 Atrophy of edentulous alveolar ridge**

    525.20 Unspecified atrophy of edentulous alveolar ridge
        Atrophy of the mandible NOS
        Atrophy of the maxilla NOS

    525.21 Minimal atrophy of the mandible

    525.22 Moderate atrophy of the mandible

    525.23 Severe atrophy of the mandible

    525.24 Minimal atrophy of the maxilla

    525.25 Moderate atrophy of the maxilla

    525.26 Severe atrophy of the maxilla

525.3 Retained dental root

√5ᵗʰ **525.4 Complete edentulism**
    Use additional code to identify cause of edentulism (525.10-525.19)
    AHA: 4Q, '05, 74

    525.40 Complete edentulism, unspecified
        Edentulism NOS

    525.41 Complete edentulism, class I

    525.42 Complete edentulism, class II

    525.43 Complete edentulism, class III

    525.44 Complete edentulism, class IV

√5ᵗʰ **525.5 Partial edentulism**
    Use additional code to identify cause of edentulism (525.10-525.19)
    AHA: 4Q, '05, 74

    525.50 Partial edentulism, unspecified

    525.51 Partial edentulism, class I

    525.52 Partial edentulism, class II

    525.53 Partial edentulism, class III

    525.54 Partial edentulism, class IV

√5ᵗʰ **525.6 Unsatisfactory restoration of tooth**
    Defective bridge, crown, fillings
    Defective dental restoration
    EXCLUDES *dental restoration status (V45.84)*
        unsatisfactory endodontic treatment (526.61-526.69)

    525.60 Unspecified unsatisfactory restoration of tooth
        Unspecified defective dental restoration

    525.61 Open restoration margins
        Dental restoration failure of marginal integrity
        Open margin on tooth restoration

    525.62 Unrepairable overhanging of dental restorative materials
        Overhanging of tooth restoration

    525.63 Fractured dental restorative material without loss of material
        EXCLUDES *cracked tooth (521.81)*
            fractured tooth (873.63, 873.73)

    525.64 Fractured dental restorative material with loss of material
        EXCLUDES *cracked tooth (521.81)*
            fractured tooth (873.63, 873.73)

    525.65 Contour of existing restoration of tooth biologically incompatible with oral health
        Dental restoration failure of periodontal anatomical integrity
        Unacceptable contours of existing restoration
        Unacceptable morphology of existing restoration

    525.66 Allergy to existing dental restorative material
        Use additional code to identify the specific type of allergy

    525.67 Poor aesthetics of existing restoration
        Dental restoration aesthetically inadequate or displeasing

    525.69 Other unsatisfactory restoration of existing tooth

√5ᵗʰ **525.7 Endosseous dental implant failure**

    525.71 Osseointegration failure of dental implant
        Failure of dental implant due to infection
        Failure of dental implant due to unintentional loading
        Failure of dental implant osseointegration due to premature loading
        Failure of dental implant to osseointegrate prior to intentional prosthetic loading
        Hemorrhagic complications of dental implant placement
        Iatrogenic osseointegration failure of dental implant
        Osseointegration failure of dental implant due to complications of systemic disease
        Osseointegration failure of dental implant due to poor bone quality
        Pre-integration failure of dental implant NOS
        Pre-osseointegration failure of dental implant

    525.72 Post-osseointegration biological failure of dental implant
        Failure of dental implant due to lack of attached gingiva
        Failure of dental implant due to occlusal trauma (caused by poor prosthetic design)
        Failure of dental implant due to parafunctional habits
        Failure of dental implant due to periodontal infection (peri-implantitis)
        Failure of dental implant due to poor oral hygiene
        Failure of dental implant to osseointegrate following intentional prosthetic loading
        Iatrogenic post-osseointegration failure of dental implant
        Post-osseointegration failure of dental implant due to complications of systemic disease

    525.73 Post-osseointegration mechanic failure of dental implant
        Failure of dental prosthesis causing loss of dental implant
        Fracture of dental implant
        Mechanical failure of dental implant NOS
        EXCLUDES *cracked tooth (521.81)*
            fractured dental restorative material with loss of material (525.64)
            fractured dental restorative material without loss of material (525.63)
            fractured tooth (873.63, 873.73)

    525.79 Other endosseous dental implant failure
        Dental implant failure NOS

525.8 Other specified disorders of the teeth and supporting structures
    Enlargement of alveolar ridge NOS
    Irregular alveolar process

525.9 Unspecified disorder of the teeth and supporting structures

√4ᵗʰ **526 Diseases of the jaws**

526.0 Developmental odontogenic cysts
    Cyst: Cyst:
      dentigerous   lateral periodontal
      eruption   primordial
      follicular   Keratocyst
      lateral developmental
    EXCLUDES *radicular cyst (522.8)*

526.1 Fissural cysts of jaw
    Cyst: Cyst:
      globulomaxillary   median palatal
      incisor canal   nasopalatine
      median anterior maxillary   palatine of papilla
    EXCLUDES *cysts of oral soft tissues (528.4)*

526.2 Other cysts of jaws
    Cyst of jaw: Cyst of jaw:
      NOS   hemorrhagic
      aneurysmal   traumatic

526.3 Central giant cell (reparative) granuloma
    EXCLUDES *peripheral giant cell granuloma (523.8)*

√4ᵗʰ√5ᵗʰ Additional Digit Required   Unspecified Code   Other Specified Code   Manifestation Code   ►◄ Revised Text   ● New Code   ▲ Revised Code Title

526.4 Inflammatory conditions

Abscess
Osteitis   } of jaw (acute) (chronic)
Osteomyelitis (neonatal)   (suppurative)
Periostitis

Sequestrum of jaw bone

EXCLUDES   *alveolar osteitis (526.5)*
osteonecrosis of jaw (733.45)

526.5 Alveolitis of jaw

Alveolar osteitis   Dry socket

DEF: Inflammation of alveoli or tooth socket.

✓5th **526.6 Periradicular pathology associated with previous endodontic treatment**

526.61 Perforation of root canal space

526.62 Endodontic overfill

526.63 Endodontic underfill

526.69 Other periradicular pathology associated with previous endodontic treatment

✓5th **526.8 Other specified diseases of the jaws**

526.81 Exostosis of jaw

Torus mandibularis   Torus palatinus

DEF: Spur or bony outgrowth on the jaw.

526.89 Other

Cherubism
Fibrous dysplasia   } of jaw(s)
Latent bone cyst
Osteoradionecrosis

Unilateral condylar hyperplasia or hypoplasia of mandible

526.9 Unspecified disease of the jaws

AHA: 4Q, '10, 93-94

✓4th **527 Diseases of the salivary glands**

527.0 Atrophy

DEF: Wasting away, necrosis of salivary gland tissue.

527.1 Hypertrophy

DEF: Overgrowth or overdeveloped salivary gland tissue.

527.2 Sialoadenitis

Parotitis: Sialoangitis
   NOS   Sialodochitis
   allergic
   toxic

EXCLUDES   *epidemic or infectious parotitis (072.0-072.9)*
uveoparotid fever (135)

DEF: Inflammation of salivary gland.

527.3 Abscess

527.4 Fistula

EXCLUDES   *congenital fistula of salivary gland (750.24)*

527.5 Sialolithiasis

Calculus   } of salivary gland or duct
Stone

Sialodocholithiasis

527.6 Mucocele

Mucous:
   extravasation cyst of salivary gland
   retention cyst of salivary gland
Ranula

DEF: Dilated salivary gland cavity filled with mucous.

527.7 Disturbance of salivary secretion

Hyposecretion   Sialorrhea
Ptyalism   Xerostomia

527.8 Other specified diseases of the salivary glands

Benign lymphoepithelial lesion of salivary gland
Sialectasia
Sialosis
Stenosis   } of salivary duct
Stricture

527.9 Unspecified disease of the salivary glands

✓4th **528 Diseases of the oral soft tissues, excluding lesions specific for gingiva and tongue**

✓5th **528.0 Stomatitis and mucositis (ulcerative)**

EXCLUDES   *cellulitis and abscess of mouth (528.3)*
diphtheritic stomatitis (032.0)
epizootic stomatitis (078.4)
gingivitis (523.0-523.1)
oral thrush (112.0)
Stevens-Johnson syndrome (695.13)
stomatitis:
   acute necrotizing ulcerative (101)
   aphthous (528.2)
   gangrenous (528.1)
   herpetic (054.2)
   Vincent's (101)

DEF: Stomatitis: Inflammation of oral mucosa; labial and buccal mucosa, tongue, palate, floor of the mouth, and gingivae.

AHA: 2Q, '99, 9

TIP: Do not assign if documented as fungal oral thrush, or as due to candidiasis. See instead 112.0.

528.00 Stomatitis and mucositis, unspecified

Mucositis NOS
Ulcerative mucositis NOS
Ulcerative stomatitis NOS
Vesicular stomatitis NOS

AHA: 4Q, '06, 88-90

528.01 Mucositis (ulcerative) due to antineoplastic therapy

Use additional E code to identify adverse effects of therapy, such as:
   antineoplastic and immunosuppressive drugs (E930.7, E933.1)
   radiation therapy (E879.2)

AHA: 4Q, '06, 88-90

528.02 Mucositis (ulcerative) due to other drugs

Use additional E code to identify drug

AHA: 4Q, '06, 88-90

528.09 Other stomatitis and mucositis (ulcerative)

AHA: 4Q, '06, 88-90

528.1 Cancrum oris

Gangrenous stomatitis
Noma

DEF: A severely gangrenous lesion of mouth due to fusospirochetal infection; destroys buccal, labial and facial tissues; can be fatal; found primarily in debilitated and malnourished children.

528.2 Oral aphthae

Aphthous stomatitis
Canker sore
Periadenitis mucosa necrotica recurrens
Recurrent aphthous ulcer
Stomatitis herpetiformis

EXCLUDES   *herpetic stomatitis (054.2)*

DEF: Small oval or round ulcers of the mouth marked by a grayish exudate and a red halo effect.

AHA: 2Q, '12, 18

528.3 Cellulitis and abscess

Cellulitis of mouth (floor)
Ludwig's angina
Oral fistula

EXCLUDES   *abscess of tongue (529.0)*
cellulitis or abscess of lip (528.5)
fistula (of):
   dental (522.7)
   lip (528.5)
gingivitis (523.00-523.11)

528.4 Cysts

Dermoid cyst
Epidermoid cyst
Epstein's pearl   } of mouth
Lymphoepithelial cyst
Nasoalveolar cyst
Nasolabial cyst

EXCLUDES   *cyst:*
   gingiva (523.8)
   tongue (529.8)

528.5 Diseases of lips

Abscess
Cellulitis
Fistula   } of lips
Hypertrophy

Cheilitis:
    NOS
    angular
Cheilodynia
Cheilosis

> **EXCLUDES** *actinic cheilitis (692.79)*
> *congenital fistula of lip (750.25)*
> *leukoplakia of lips (528.6)*

> **AHA:** S-O, '86, 10

528.6 Leukoplakia of oral mucosa, including tongue

Leukokeratosis of oral mucosa
Leukoplakia of:
    gingiva
    lips
    tongue

> **EXCLUDES** *carcinoma in situ (230.0, 232.0)*
> *leukokeratosis nicotina palati (528.79)*

> **DEF:** Thickened white patches of epithelium on mucous membranes of mouth.

✓5ᵗʰ 528.7 Other disturbances of oral epithelium, including tongue

> **EXCLUDES** *carcinoma in situ (230.0, 232.0)*
> *leukokeratosis NOS (702.8)*

528.71 Minimal keratinized residual ridge mucosa
Minimal keratinization of alveolar ridge mucosa

528.72 Excessive keratinized residual ridge mucosa
Excessive keratinization of alveolar ridge mucosa

528.79 Other disturbances of oral epithelium, including tongue
Erythroplakia of mouth or tongue
Focal epithelial hyperplasia of mouth or tongue
Leukoedema of mouth or tongue
Leukokeratosis nicotina palate
Other oral epithelium disturbances

528.8 Oral submucosal fibrosis, including of tongue

528.9 Other and unspecified diseases of the oral soft tissues
Cheek and lip biting
Denture sore mouth
Denture stomatitis
Melanoplakia
Papillary hyperplasia of palate

Eosinophilic granuloma
Irritative hyperplasisa   } of oral mucosa
Pyogenic granuloma
Ulcer (traumatic)

✓4ᵗʰ 529 Diseases and other conditions of the tongue

529.0 Glossitis

Abscess   } of tongue
Ulceration (traumatic)

> **EXCLUDES** *glossitis:*
> *benign migratory (529.1)*
> *Hunter's (529.4)*
> *median rhomboid (529.2)*
> *Moeller's (529.4)*

529.1 Geographic tongue
Benign migratory glossitis
Glossitis areata exfoliativa

> **DEF:** Chronic glossitis; marked by filiform papillae atrophy and inflammation; no known etiology.

529.2 Median rhomboid glossitis

> **DEF:** A noninflammatory, congenital disease characterized by rhomboid-like lesions at the middle third of the tongue's dorsal surface.

529.3 Hypertrophy of tongue papillae
Black hairy tongue
Coated tongue
Hypertrophy of foliate papillae
Lingua villosa nigra

529.4 Atrophy of tongue papillae
Bald tongue
Glazed tongue
Glossitis:
    Hunter's
    Moeller's
Glossodynia exfoliativa
Smooth atrophic tongue

529.5 Plicated tongue
Fissured
Furrowed   } tongue
Scrotal

> **EXCLUDES** *fissure of tongue, congenital (750.13)*
> **DEF:** Cracks, fissures or furrows, on dorsal surface of tongue.

529.6 Glossodynia
Glossopyrosis
Painful tongue

> **EXCLUDES** *glossodynia exfoliativa (529.4)*

529.8 Other specified conditions of the tongue
Atrophy
Crenated
Enlargement   } (of) tongue
Hypertrophy

Glossocele
Glossoptosis

> **EXCLUDES** *erythroplasia of tongue (528.79)*
> *leukoplakia of tongue (528.6)*
> *macroglossia (congenital) (750.15)*
> *microglossia (congenital) (750.16)*
> *oral submucosal fibrosis (528.8)*

529.9 Unspecified condition of the tongue

Diseases of Esophagus, Stomach, and Duodenum (530-539)

✓4ᵗʰ 530 Diseases of esophagus

> **EXCLUDES** *esophageal varices (456.0-456.2)*

530.0 Achalasia and cardiospasm
Achalasia (of cardia)
Aperistalsis of esophagus
Megaesophagus

> **EXCLUDES** *congenital cardiospasm (750.7)*
> **DEF:** Failure of smooth muscle fibers to relax at gastrointestinal junctures, such as esophagogastric sphincter when swallowing.

✓5ᵗʰ 530.1 Esophagitis

Esophagitis: Esphagitis:
   chemical   postoperative
   peptic   regurgitant

> Use additional E code to identify cause, if induced by chemical
> **EXCLUDES** *tuberculous esophagitis (017.8)*
> **AHA:** 4Q, '93, 27; 1Q, '92, 17; 3Q, '91, 20
> **TIP:** Do not assign if esophagitis due to candidiasis; see instead code 112.84.

530.10 Esophagitis, unspecified
Esophagitis NOS

> **AHA:** 3Q, '05, 17

Esophagus

Pharyngeal constrictors
Front view
Epiglottis
Cricoid cartilage
Trachea
C6
Pharyngoesophageal sphincter
Side view
Gastroesophageal sphincter
Diaphragm
Stomach

| ✓4ᵗʰ ✓5ᵗʰ | Additional Digit Required | Unspecified Code | Other Specified Code | Manifestation Code | ►◄ Revised Text | ● New Code | ▲ Revised Code Title |

2015 ICD-9-CM   **Volume 1 – 163**

Diseases of the Digestive System

530.11–531.4

530.11 Reflux esophagitis
DEF: Inflammation of lower esophagus; due to regurgitated gastric acid.
AHA: 4Q, '95, 82
K21.0 Gastro-esophageal reflux disease w/esophagitis ▮I-10▮

530.12 Acute esophagitis
DEF: An acute inflammation of the mucous lining or submucosal coat of the esophagus.
AHA: 4Q, '01, 45

530.13 Eosinophilic esophagitis
AHA: 4Q, '08, 115-116

530.19 Other esophagitis
Abscess of esophagus
AHA: 3Q, '01, 10
K20.8 Other esophagitis ▮I-10▮

✓5th **530.2 Ulcer of esophagus**
Ulcer of esophagus:
  fungal
  peptic
Ulcer of esophagus due to ingestion of:
  aspirin
  chemicals
  medicines
Use additional E code to identify cause, if induced by chemical or drug
AHA: 4Q, '03, 63

530.20 Ulcer of esophagus without bleeding
Ulcer of esophagus NOS

530.21 Ulcer of esophagus with bleeding
EXCLUDES bleeding esophageal varices (456.0, 456.20)

530.3 Stricture and stenosis of esophagus
Compression of esophagus
Obstruction of esophagus
EXCLUDES congenital stricture of esophagus (750.3)
AHA: 1Q, '12, 15; 2Q, '01, 4; 2Q, '97, 3; 1Q, '88, 13
TIP: If esophageal obstruction is due to impacted foreign body, such as meat or other substance, assign instead code 935.1.
K22.2 Esophageal obstruction ▮I-10▮

530.4 Perforation of esophagus
Rupture of esophagus
EXCLUDES traumatic perforation of esophagus (862.22, 862.32, 874.4-874.5)

530.5 Dyskinesia of esophagus
Corkscrew esophagus
Curling esophagus
Esophagospasm
Spasm of esophagus
EXCLUDES cardiospasm (530.0)
DEF: Difficulty performing voluntary esophageal movements.
AHA: 1Q, '88, 13; N-D, '84, 19

530.6 Diverticulum of esophagus, acquired
Diverticulum, acquired:
  epiphrenic
  pharyngoesophageal
  pulsion
  subdiaphragmatic
  traction
  Zenker's (hypopharyngeal)
Esophageal pouch, acquired
Esophagocele, acquired
EXCLUDES congenital diverticulum of esophagus (750.4)
AHA: J-F, '85, 3

530.7 Gastroesophageal laceration-hemorrhage syndrome
Mallory-Weiss syndrome
DEF: Laceration of distal esophagus and proximal stomach due to vomiting, hiccups or other sustained activity.

✓5th **530.8 Other specified disorders of esophagus**

530.81 Esophageal reflux
Gastroesophageal reflux
EXCLUDES reflux esophagitis (530.11)
DEF: Regurgitation of the gastric contents into esophagus and possibly pharynx.
AHA: 4Q, '10, 97; 2Q, '01, 4; 1Q, '95, 7; 4Q, '92, 27
K21.9 Gastro-esophageal reflux dz w/o esophagitis ▮I-10▮

530.82 Esophageal hemorrhage
EXCLUDES hemorrhage due to esophageal varices (456.0-456.2)
AHA: 1Q, '05, 17

530.83 Esophageal leukoplakia

530.84 Tracheoesophageal fistula
EXCLUDES congenital tracheoesophageal fistula (750.3)

530.85 Barrett's esophagus
DEF: A metaplastic disorder in which specialized columnar epithelial cells replace the normal squamous epithelial cells; secondary to chronic gastroesophageal reflux damage to the mucosa; increases risk of developing adenocarcinoma.
AHA: 4Q, '03, 63
K22.70 Barrett's esophagus w/o dysphagia ▮I-10▮

530.86 Infection of esophagostomy
Use additional code to specify infection

530.87 Mechanical complication of esophagostomy
Malfunction of esophagostomy

530.89 Other
EXCLUDES Paterson-Kelly syndrome (280.8)

530.9 Unspecified disorder of esophagus

✓4th **531 Gastric ulcer**
INCLUDES ulcer (peptic):
  prepyloric
  pylorus
  stomach
Use additional E code to identify drug, if drug-induced
EXCLUDES peptic ulcer NOS (533.0-533.9)

The following fifth-digit subclassification is for use with category 531:
  0 without mention of obstruction
  1 with obstruction

DEF: Destruction of tissue in lumen of stomach due to action of gastric acid and pepsin on gastric mucosa decreasing resistance to ulcers.
AHA: 1Q, '91, 15; 4Q, '90, 27

§ ✓5th **531.0 Acute with hemorrhage**
[0-1]   **AHA:** N-D, '84, 15

§ ✓5th **531.1 Acute with perforation**
[0-1]

§ ✓5th **531.2 Acute with hemorrhage and perforation**
[0-1]

§ ✓5th **531.3 Acute without mention of hemorrhage or perforation**
[0-1]

§ ✓5th **531.4 Chronic or unspecified with hemorrhage**
[0-1]   **AHA:** 4Q, '90, 22
K25.4 Chronic/unspec gastric ulcer w/hemorrhage ▮I-10▮

Stomach

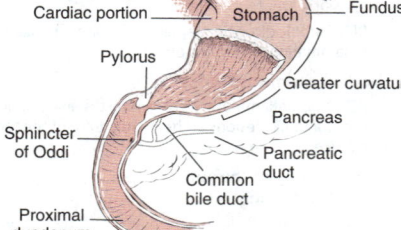

§   Requires fifth digit. Valid digits are in [brackets] under each code. See category 531 for codes and definitions.

N Newborn Age: 0   **P** Pediatric Age: 0-17   **M** Maternity Age: 12-55   **A** Adult Age: 15-124

Diseases of the Digestive System

531.5–535.4

§ ✓5ᵗʰ **531.5 Chronic or unspecified with perforation**
[0-1]

§ ✓5ᵗʰ **531.6 Chronic or unspecified with hemorrhage and perforation**
[0-1]

§ ✓5ᵗʰ **531.7 Chronic without mention of hemorrhage or perforation**
[0-1]

§ ✓5ᵗʰ **531.9 Unspecified as acute or chronic, without mention of hemorrhage or perforation**
[0-1]
     K25.9 Gastric ulcer uns acute/chronic w/o hem/perf   I-10

✓4ᵗʰ **532 Duodenal ulcer**
INCLUDES erosion (acute) of duodenum
     ulcer (peptic):
       duodenum
       postpyloric
Use additional E code to identify drug, if drug-induced
EXCLUDES peptic ulcer NOS (533.0-533.9)

The following fifth-digit subclassification is for use with category 532:
  0 without mention of obstruction
  1 with obstruction

DEF: Ulcers in duodenum due to action of gastric acid and pepsin on mucosa decreasing resistance to ulcers.
AHA: 4Q, '90, 27; 1Q, '91, 15

§ ✓5ᵗʰ **532.0 Acute with hemorrhage**
[0-1]   **AHA:** 4Q, '90, 22

§ ✓5ᵗʰ **532.1 Acute with perforation**
[0-1]

§ ✓5ᵗʰ **532.2 Acute with hemorrhage and perforation**
[0-1]

§ ✓5ᵗʰ **532.3 Acute without mention of hemorrhage or perforation**
[0-1]

§ ✓5ᵗʰ **532.4 Chronic or unspecified with hemorrhage**
[0-1]   K26.4 Chronic/unspecified duodenal ulcer w/hemorrhage   I-10

§ ✓5ᵗʰ **532.5 Chronic or unspecified with perforation**
[0-1]

§ ✓5ᵗʰ **532.6 Chronic or unspecified with hemorrhage and perforation**
[0-1]

§ ✓5ᵗʰ **532.7 Chronic without mention of hemorrhage or perforation**
[0-1]

§ ✓5ᵗʰ **532.9 Unspecified as acute or chronic, without mention of hemorrhage or perfortaion**
[0-1]   K26.9 Duodenal ulcer uns acute/chronic w/o hem/perf   I-10

✓4ᵗʰ **533 Peptic ulcer, site unspecified**
INCLUDES gastroduodenal ulcer NOS
     peptic ulcer NOS
     stress ulcer NOS
Use additional E code to identify drug, if drug-induced
EXCLUDES peptic ulcer:
     duodenal (532.0-532.9)
     gastric (531.0-531.9)

The following fifth-digit subclassification is for use with category 533:
  0 without mention of obstruction
  1 with obstruction

DEF: Ulcer of mucous membrane of esophagus, stomach or duodenum due to gastric acid secretion.
AHA: 1Q, '91, 15; 4Q, '90, 27

§ ✓5ᵗʰ **533.0 Acute with hemorrhage**
[0-1]

§ ✓5ᵗʰ **533.1 Acute with perforation**
[0-1]

§ ✓5ᵗʰ **533.2 Acute with hemorrhage and perforation**
[0-1]

§ ✓5ᵗʰ **533.3 Acute without mention of hemorrhage and perforation**
[0-1]

§ ✓5ᵗʰ **533.4 Chronic or unspecified with hemorrhage**
[0-1]

§ ✓5ᵗʰ **533.5 Chronic or unspecified with perforation**
[0-1]

§ ✓5ᵗʰ **533.6 Chronic or unspecified with hemorrhage and perforation**
[0-1]

§ ✓5ᵗʰ **533.7 Chronic without mention of hemorrhage or perforation**
[0-1]   **AHA:** 2Q, '89, 16

§ ✓5ᵗʰ **533.9 Unspecified as acute or chronic, without mention of hemorrhage or perforation**
[0-1]

✓4ᵗʰ **534 Gastrojejunal ulcer**
INCLUDES ulcer (peptic) or erosion:
     anastomotic
     gastrocolic
     gastrointestinal
     gastrojejunal
     jejunal
     marginal
     stomal
EXCLUDES primary ulcer of small intestine (569.82)

The following fifth-digit subclassification is for use with category 534:
  0 without mention of obstruction
  1 with obstruction

AHA: 1Q, '91, 15; 4Q, '90, 27

§ ✓5ᵗʰ **534.0 Acute with hemorrhage**
[0-1]

§ ✓5ᵗʰ **534.1 Acute with perforation**
[0-1]

§ ✓5ᵗʰ **534.2 Acute with hemorrhage and perforation**
[0-1]

§ ✓5ᵗʰ **534.3 Acute without mention of hemorrhage or perforation**
[0-1]

§ ✓5ᵗʰ **534.4 Chronic or unspecified with hemorrhage**
[0-1]

§ ✓5ᵗʰ **534.5 Chronic or unspecified with perforation**
[0-1]

§ ✓5ᵗʰ **534.6 Chronic or unspecified with hemorrhage and perforation**
[0-1]

§ ✓5ᵗʰ **534.7 Chronic without mention of hemorrhage or perforation**
[0-1]

§ ✓5ᵗʰ **534.9 Unspecified as acute or chronic, without mention of hemorrhage or perforation**
[0-1]

✓4ᵗʰ **535 Gastritis and duodenitis**
The following fifth-digit subclassification is for use with category 535:
  0 without mention of hemorrhage
  1 with hemorrhage

AHA: 2Q, '92, 9; 4Q, '91, 25

§ ✓5ᵗʰ **535.0 Acute gastritis**
[0-1]   **AHA:** 2Q, '92, 8; N-D, '86, 9

§ ✓5ᵗʰ **535.1 Atrophic gastritis**
[0-1] Gastritis:
     atrophic-hyperplastic
     chronic (atrophic)
  DEF: Inflammation of stomach, with mucous membrane atrophy and peptic gland destruction.
  AHA: 1Q, '94, 18
  K29.50 Unspecified chronic gastritis without bleeding   I-10

§ ✓5ᵗʰ **535.2 Gastric mucosal hypertrophy**
[0-1] Hypertrophic gastritis

§ ✓5ᵗʰ **535.3 Alcoholic gastritis**
[0-1]

§ ✓5ᵗʰ **535.4 Other specified gastritis**
[0-1] Gastritis: Gastritis:
     allergic   superficial
     bile induced   toxic
     irritant
  EXCLUDES eosinophilic gastritis (535.7)
  AHA: 4Q, '90, 27

---

§ Requires fifth digit. Valid digits are in [brackets] under each code. See appropriate category for codes and definitions.

✓4ᵗʰ Additional Digit Required   Unspecified Code   Other Specified Code   Manifestation Code   ►◄ Revised Text   ● New Code   ▲ Revised Code Title

Diseases of the Digestive System

535.5–537.9

§ ✓5ᵗʰ **535.5 Unspecified gastritis and gastroduodenitis**
[0-1]   **AHA: For code 535.50:** 3Q, '05, 17; 4Q, '99, 25

§ ✓5ᵗʰ **535.6 Duodenitis**
[0-1]   **DEF:** Inflammation of intestine, between pylorus and jejunum.
     AHA: For code 535.60: 3Q, '05, 17
     K29.80 Duodenitis without bleeding   `I-10`

§ ✓5ᵗʰ **535.7 Eosinophilic gastritis**
[0-1]   **AHA:** 4Q, '08, 115-116

✓4ᵗʰ **536 Disorders of function of stomach**
     EXCLUDES *functional disorders of stomach specified as psychogenic (306.4)*

536.0 Achlorhydria
     DEF: Absence of gastric acid due to gastric mucosa atrophy; unresponsive to histamines; also known as gastric anacidity.

536.1 Acute dilatation of stomach
     Acute distention of stomach

536.2 Persistent vomiting
     Cyclical vomiting
     Habit vomiting
     Persistent vomiting [not of pregnancy]
     Uncontrollable vomiting
     EXCLUDES *bilious emesis (vomiting) (787.04)*
         excessive vomiting in pregnancy (643.0-643.9)
         vomiting NOS (787.03)
           cyclical, associated with migraine (346.2)
         vomiting of fecal matter (569.87)

536.3 Gastroparesis
     Gastroparalysis
     Code first underlying disease, if known, such as:
       diabetes mellitus (249.6, 250.6)
     DEF: Slight degree of paralysis within muscular coat of stomach.
     AHA: 4Q, '08, 94; 2Q, '04, 7; 2Q, '01, 4; 4Q, '94, 42

✓5ᵗʰ **536.4 Gastrostomy complications**
     AHA: 4Q, '98, 42
     TIP: Do not assign code 997.4 Digestive system complications, for any gastrostomy complications.

536.40 Gastrostomy complication, unspecified

536.41 Infection of gastrostomy
     Use additional code to identify organism (041.00-041.9)
     Use additional code to specify type of infection, such as:
     abscess or cellulitis of abdomen (682.2)
     septicemia (038.0-038.9)
     AHA: 4Q, '98, 42

536.42 Mechanical complication of gastrostomy

536.49 Other gastrostomy complications
     AHA: 4Q, '98, 42

536.8 Dyspepsia and other specified disorders of function of stomach
     Achylia gastrica   Hypochlorhydria
     Hourglass contraction of stomach   Indigestion
     Hyperacidity   Tachygastria
     Hyperchlorhydria
     EXCLUDES *achlorhydria (536.0)*
         heartburn (787.1)
     AHA: 2Q, '93, 6; 2Q, '89, 16; N-D, '84, 9
     K30 Functional dyspepsia   `I-10`

536.9 Unspecified functional disorder of stomach
     Functional gastrointestinal:
       disorder
       disturbance
       irritation

✓4ᵗʰ **537 Other disorders of stomach and duodenum**

537.0 Acquired hypertrophic pyloric stenosis
     Constriction
     Obstruction } of pylorus, acquired or adult
     Stricture
     EXCLUDES *congenital or infantile pyloric stenosis (750.5)*
     AHA: 2Q, '01, 4; J-F, '85, 14

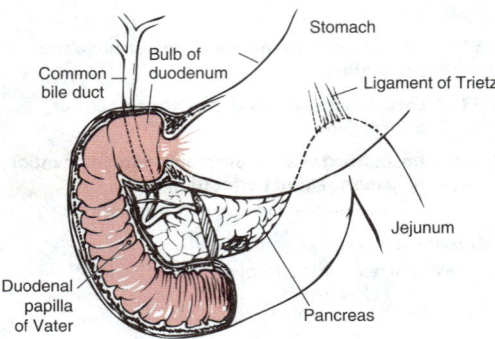

Duodenum

Stomach
Bulb of duodenum
Ligament of Trietz
Common bile duct
Jejunum
Pancreas
Duodenal papilla of Vater

537.1 Gastric diverticulum
     EXCLUDES *congenital diverticulum of stomach (750.7)*
     DEF: Herniated sac or pouch within stomach or duodenum.
     AHA: J-F, '85, 4

537.2 Chronic duodenal ileus
     DEF: Persistent obstruction between pylorus and jejunum.

537.3 Other obstruction of duodenum
     Cicatrix
     Stenosis } of duodenum
     Stricture
     Volvulus
     EXCLUDES *congenital obstruction of duodenum (751.1)*

537.4 Fistula of stomach or duodenum
     Gastrocolic fistula
     Gastrojejunocolic fistula
     AHA: 1Q, '12, 10
     TIP: Assign when a previous G-tube site has failed to spontaneously close and requires further treatment.

537.5 Gastroptosis
     DEF: Downward displacement of stomach.

537.6 Hourglass stricture or stenosis of stomach
     Cascade stomach
     EXCLUDES *congenital hourglass stomach (750.7)*
         hourglass contraction of stomach (536.8)

✓5ᵗʰ **537.8 Other specified disorders of stomach and duodenum**
     AHA: 4Q, '91, 25

537.81 Pylorospasm
     EXCLUDES *congenital pylorospasm (750.5)*
     DEF: Spasm of the pyloric sphincter.

537.82 Angiodysplasia of stomach and duodenum (without mention of hemorrhage)
     AHA: 2Q, '07, 7; 3Q, '96, 10; 4Q, '90, 4

537.83 Angiodysplasia of stomach and duodenum with hemorrhage
     DEF: Bleeding of stomach and duodenum due to vascular abnormalities.
     AHA: 2Q, '07, 7

537.84 Dieulafoy lesion (hemorrhagic) of stomach and duodenum
     DEF: An abnormally large and convoluted submucosal artery protruding through a defect in the mucosa in the stomach or intestines that can erode the epithelium causing hemorrhaging.
     AHA: 4Q, '02, 60

537.89 Other
     Gastric or duodenal:
       prolapse
       rupture
     Intestinal metaplasia of gastric mucosa
     Passive congestion of stomach
     EXCLUDES *diverticula of duodenum (562.00-562.01)*
         gastrointestinal hemorrhage (578.0-578.9)
     AHA: 1Q, '11, 10-11; 3Q, '05, 15; N-D, '84, 7
     TIP: Assign for congestive portal gastropathy or portal hypertensive gastropathy.

537.9 Unspecified disorder of stomach and duodenum

N Newborn Age: 0   P Pediatric Age: 0-17   M Maternity Age: 12-55   A Adult Age: 15-124

538 Gastrointestinal mucositis (ulcerative)

Use additional E code to identify adverse effects of therapy, such as: antineoplastic and immunosuppressive drugs (E930.7, E933.1) radiation therapy (E879.2)

EXCLUDES *mucositis (ulcerative) of mouth and oral soft tissue (528.00-528.09)*

AHA: 4Q, '06, 88-90

√4th **539 Complications of bariatric procedures**

TIP: If associated dumping syndrome is documented, assign also code 564.2.

√5th **539.0 Complications of gastric band procedure**

AHA: 4Q, '11, 125-127

539.01 Infection due to gastric band procedure

Use additional code to specify type of infection, such as:
abscess or cellulitis of abdomen (682.2)
septicemia (038.0-038.9)
Use additional code to identify organism (041.00-041.9)

AHA: 4Q, '11, 127

539.09 Other complications of gastric band procedure

Use additional code(s) to further specify the complication

√5th **539.8 Complications of other bariatric procedure**

EXCLUDES *complications of gastric band procedure (539.01-539.09)*

AHA: 4Q, '11, 125-127

539.81 Infection due to other bariatric procedure

Use additional code to specify type of infection, such as:
abscess or cellulitis of abdomen (682.2)
septicemia (038.0-038.9)
Use additional code to identify organism (041.00-041.9)

539.89 Other complications of other bariatric procedure

Use additional code(s) to further specify the complication

AHA: ▶3Q, '13, 12◀

Appendicitis (540-543)

√4th **540 Acute appendicitis**

DEF: Inflammation of vermiform appendix due to fecal obstruction, neoplasm or foreign body of appendiceal lumen; causes infection, edema and infarction of appendiceal wall; may result in mural necrosis, and perforation.

AHA: N-D, '84, 19

540.0 With generalized peritonitis

Appendicitis ⎱ perforation ⎰ fulminating
(acute) ⎰ peritonitis (generalized) ⎰ gangrenous
with: ⎰ rupture ⎰ obstructive

Cecitis (acute) with perforation, peritonitis (generalized), rupture

Rupture of appendix

EXCLUDES *acute appendicitis with peritoneal abscess (540.1)*

K35.2 Acute appendicitis w/generalized peritonitis   I-10

540.1 With peritoneal abscess

Abscess of appendix   With generalized peritonitis

AHA: N-D, '84, 19

Appendix

Appendicular artery
Mesoappendix
Cecum
Vermiform appendix

Inguinal Hernias

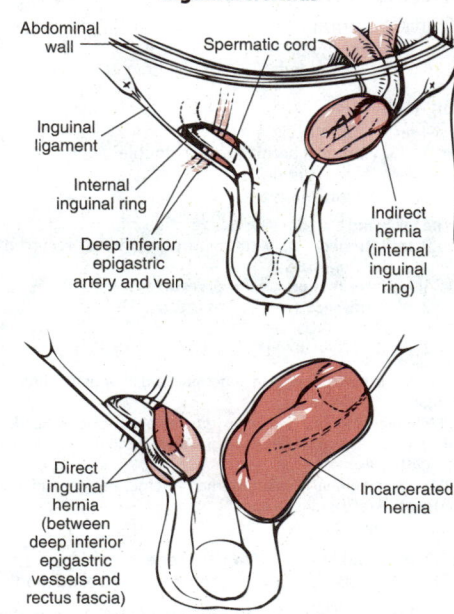

Abdominal wall
Spermatic cord
Inguinal ligament
Internal inguinal ring
Deep inferior epigastric artery and vein
Indirect hernia (internal inguinal ring)
Direct inguinal hernia (between deep inferior epigastric vessels and rectus fascia)
Incarcerated hernia

540.9 Without mention of peritonitis

Acute appendicitis without mention of perforation, peritonitis, or rupture:
fulminating
gangrenous
inflamed
obstructive

Acute cecitis without mention of perforation, peritonitis, or rupture

AHA: ▶2Q, '13, 7;◀ 1Q, '01, 15; 4Q, '97, 52

K35.80 Unspecified acute appendicitis   I-10

541 Appendicitis, unqualified

AHA: 2Q, '90, 26

TIP: Do not assign for normal appendix found at appendectomy. Assign instead symptom code (e.g., abdominal pain).

542 Other appendicitis

Appendicitis: Appendicitis:
chronic   relapsing
recurrent   subacute

EXCLUDES *hyperplasia (lymphoid) of appendix (543.0)*

AHA: 1Q, '01, 15

√4th **543 Other diseases of appendix**

543.0 Hyperplasia of appendix (lymphoid)

DEF: Proliferation of cells in appendix tissue.

543.9 Other and unspecified diseases of appendix

Appendicular or appendiceal:
colic
concretion
fistula
Diverticulum
Fecalith ⎱
Intussusception ⎰ of appendix
Mucocele
Stercolith

√4th
√5th Additional Digit Required   Unspecified Code   Other Specified Code   Manifestation Code   ▶◀ Revised Text   ● New Code   ▲ Revised Code Title

2015 ICD-9-CM   **October 2014 • Volume 1 – 167**

Diseases of the Digestive System

550–552.9

Hernia of Abdominal Cavity (550-553)

INCLUDES   hernia:
     acquired
     congenital, except diaphragmatic or hiatal

✓4th **550 Inguinal hernia**

INCLUDES   bubonocele
     inguinal hernia (direct) (double) (indirect) (oblique)
        (sliding)
     scrotal hernia

> The following fifth-digit subclassification is for use with category 550:
> **0 unilateral or unspecified (not specified as recurrent)**
>   Unilateral NOS
> **1 unilateral or unspecified, recurrent**
> **2 bilateral (not specified as recurrent)**
>   Bilateral NOS
> **3 bilateral, recurrent**

DEF: Hernia protrusion of an abdominal organ or tissue through inguinal canal.
DEF: Indirect inguinal hernia: (external or oblique) leaves abdomen through deep inguinal ring, passes through inguinal canal lateral to the inferior epigastric artery.
DEF: Direct inguinal hernia: (internal) emerges between inferior epigastric artery and rectus muscle edge.
AHA: N-D, '85, 12

§   ✓5th **550.0 Inguinal hernia, with gangrene**
   [0-3]   Inguinal hernia with gangrene (and obstruction)

§   ✓5th **550.1 Inguinal hernia, with obstruction, without mention**
   [0-3]   **of gangrene**
       Inguinal hernia with mention of incarceration, irreducibility, or strangulation

§   ✓5th **550.9 Inguinal hernia, without mention of obstruction**
   [0-3]   **or gangrene**
       Inguinal hernia NOS
       AHA: For code 550.91: 3Q, '03, 10; 1Q, '03, 4
       K40.90 Uni ingin hernia w/o obst/gangrene not spec recur   `I-10`

✓4th **551 Other hernia of abdominal cavity, with gangrene**
INCLUDES   *that with gangrene (and obstruction)*

✓5th **551.0 Femoral hernia with gangrene**

     551.00 Unilateral or unspecified (not specified as recurrent)
        Femoral hernia NOS with gangrene

     551.01 Unilateral or unspecified, recurrent

     551.02 Bilateral (not specified as recurrent)

     551.03 Bilateral, recurrent

   551.1 Umbilical hernia with gangrene
     Parumbilical hernia specified as gangrenous

✓5th **551.2 Ventral hernia with gangrene**

     551.20 Ventral, unspecified, with gangrene

     551.21 Incisional, with gangrene
       Hernia:
       postoperative   } specified as
       recurrent, ventral   gangrenous

     551.29 Other
       Epigastric hernia specified as gangrenous

Hernias of Abdominal Cavity

Hiatal hernia
Diaphragm
Epigastric hernia
Incisional hernia
Umbilical hernia
Inguinal hernia

Femoral Hernia

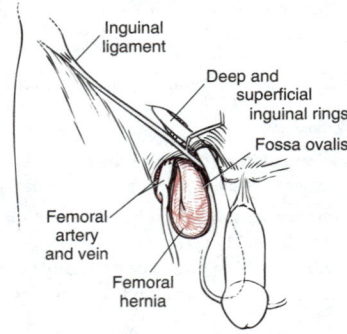

Inguinal ligament
Deep and superficial inguinal rings
Fossa ovalis
Femoral artery and vein
Femoral hernia

551.3 Diaphragmatic hernia with gangrene
   Hernia:
     hiatal (esophageal) (sliding) } specified as
     paraesophageal   gangrenous
     Thoracic stomach
     EXCLUDES *congenital diaphragmatic hernia (756.6)*

551.8 Hernia of other specified sites, with gangrene
   Any condition classifiable to 553.8 if specified as gangrenous

551.9 Hernia of unspecified site, with gangrene
   Any condition classifiable to 553.9 if specified as gangrenous

✓4th **552 Other hernia of abdominal cavity, with obstruction, but without mention of gangrene**
EXCLUDES *that with mention of gangrene (551.0-551.9)*

✓5th **552.0 Femoral hernia with obstruction**
   Femoral hernia specified as incarcerated, irreducible, strangulated, or causing obstruction

     552.00 Unilateral or unspecified (not specified as recurrent)

     552.01 Unilateral or unspecified, recurrent

     552.02 Bilateral (not specified as recurrent)

     552.03 Bilateral, recurrent

   552.1 Umbilical hernia with obstruction
     Parumbilical hernia specified as incarcerated, irreducible, strangulated, or causing obstruction

✓5th **552.2 Ventral hernia with obstruction**
   Ventral hernia specified as incarcerated, irreducible, strangulated, or causing obstruction

     552.20 Ventral, unspecified, with obstruction
       AHA: 2Q, '11, 18

     552.21 Incisional, with obstruction
       Hernia:
       postoperative } specified as incarcerated,
       recurrent,   irreducible, strangulated,
       ventral   or causing obstruction
       AHA: 1Q, '12, 8; 3Q, '03, 11

     552.29 Other
       Epigastric hernia specified as incarcerated, irreducible, strangulated, or causing obstruction

   552.3 Diaphragmatic hernia with obstruction
     Hernia:
     hiatal (esophageal) } specified as caracerated,
     (sliding)   irreducible,
     paraesophageal   strangulated, or
     Thoracic stomach   causing obstruction
     EXCLUDES *congenital diaphragmatic hernia (756.6)*

552.8 Hernia of other specified sites, with obstruction
   Any condition classifiable to 553.8 if specified as incarcerated, irreducible, strangulated, or causing obstruction
   AHA: 1Q, '04, 10

552.9 Hernia of unspecified site, with obstruction
   Any condition classifiable to 553.9 if specified as incarcerated, irreducible, strangulated, or causing obstruction

---

§   Requires fifth digit. Valid digits are in [brackets] under each code. See category 550 for codes and definitions.

Diseases of the Digestive System

553–556.9

Diaphragmatic Hernias

Esophagus

Gastroesophageal junction (remains in place)

Stomach

Diaphragm

Gastroesophageal junction (slides up and down)

Paraesophageal Hiatal Hernia

Sliding Hiatal Hernia

☑4ᵗʰ 553 Other hernia of abdominal cavity without mention of obstruction or gangrene

> **EXCLUDES** *the listed conditions with mention of:*
> *gangrene (and obstruction) (551.0-551.9)*
> *obstruction (552.0-552.9)*

☑5ᵗʰ 553.0 Femoral hernia

    553.00 Unilateral or unspecified (not specified as recurrent)
        Femoral hernia NOS

    553.01 Unilateral or unspecified, recurrent

    553.02 Bilateral (not specified as recurrent)

    553.03 Bilateral, recurrent

553.1 Umbilical hernia
    Parumbilical hernia
    K42.9 Umbilical hernia without obstruction/gangrene   `I-10`

☑5ᵗʰ 553.2 Ventral hernia

    553.20 Ventral, unspecified
        AHA: 2Q, '06, 10; 3Q, '03, 6

    553.21 Incisional
        Hernia:
          postoperative
          recurrent, ventral
        AHA: 3Q, '03, 6
        K43.2 Incisional hernia w/o obstruction or gangrene   `I-10`

    553.29 Other
        Hernia:
          epigastric
          spigelian

553.3 Diaphragmatic hernia
    Hernia:
      hiatal (esophageal) (sliding)
      paraesophageal
    Thoracic stomach
> **EXCLUDES** *congenital:*
> *diaphragmatic hernia (756.6)*
> *hiatal hernia (750.6)*
> *esophagocele (530.6)*

    AHA: 2Q, '01, 6; 1Q, '00, 6
    K44.9 Diaphragmatic hernia w/o obstruction/gangrene   `I-10`

553.8 Hernia of other specified sites
    Hernia:
      ischiatic
      ischiorectal
      lumbar
      obturator
      pudendal
      retroperitoneal
      sciatic
    Other abdominal hernia of specified site
> **EXCLUDES** *vaginal enterocele (618.6)*

553.9 Hernia of unspecified site
    Enterocele   Hernia:
    Epiplocele   intestinal
    Hernia: intra-abdominal
      NOS   Rupture (nontraumatic)
      interstitial   Sarcoepiplocele

Noninfectious Enteritis and Colitis (555-558)

☑4ᵗʰ 555 Regional enteritis

> **INCLUDES** Crohn's disease
> Granulomatous enteritis
> **EXCLUDES** *ulcerative colitis (556)*

DEF: Inflammation of intestine; classified to site.
TIP: Assign separate code for fistula, if present. Sequence 555 code as first-listed/principal diagnosis (if underlying cause of fistula).

555.0 Small intestine
    Ileitis: Regional enteritis or Crohn's disease of:
      regional   duodenum
      segmental   ileum
      terminal   jejunum

555.1 Large intestine
    Colitis:
      granulmatous
      regional
      transmural
    Regional enteritis or Crohn's disease of:
      colon
      large bowel
      rectum
    AHA: 3Q, '99, 8

555.2 Small intestine with large intestine
    Regional ileocolitis
    AHA: 1Q, '03, 18

555.9 Unspecified site
    Crohn's disease NOS
    Regional enteritis NOS
    AHA: 1Q, '09, 5; 2Q, '05, 11; 3Q, '99, 8; 4Q, '97, 42; 2Q, '97, 3
    K50.90 Crohns disease unspecified w/o complications   `I-10`

☑4ᵗʰ 556 Ulcerative colitis

DEF: Chronic inflammation of mucosal lining of intestinal tract; may be single area or entire colon.
AHA: 3Q, '99, 8

556.0 Ulcerative (chronic) enterocolitis

556.1 Ulcerative (chronic) ileocolitis

556.2 Ulcerative (chronic) proctitis

556.3 Ulcerative (chronic) proctosigmoiditis

556.4 Pseudopolyposis of colon

556.5 Left-sided ulcerative (chronic) colitis

556.6 Universal ulcerative (chronic) colitis
    Pancolitis

556.8 Other ulcerative colitis

556.9 Ulcerative colitis, unspecified
    Ulcerative enteritis NOS
    AHA: 1Q, '03, 10
    K51.90 Ulcerative colitis unspecified w/o complications   `I-10`

Large Intestine

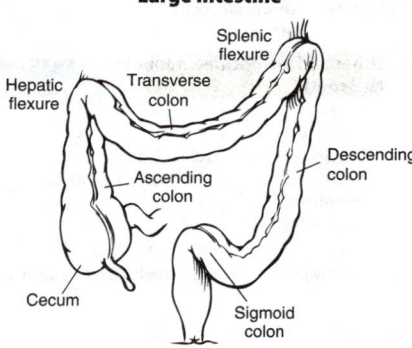

Splenic flexure

Hepatic flexure

Transverse colon

Descending colon

Ascending colon

Cecum

Sigmoid colon

☑4ᵗʰ ☑5ᵗʰ Additional Digit Required   **Unspecified Code**   Other Specified Code   Manifestation Code   ►◄ Revised Text   ● New Code   ▲ Revised Code Title

2015 ICD-9-CM   **Volume 1 – 169**

Diseases of the Digestive System

557–560.39

☑4ᵗʰ 557 Vascular insufficiency of intestine

> **EXCLUDES** *necrotizing enterocolitis of the newborn (777.50-777.53)*
> **DEF:** Inadequacy of intestinal vessels.

557.0 Acute vascular insufficiency of intestine
Acute:
  hemorrhagic enterocolitis
  ischemic colitis, enteritis, or enterocolitis
  massive necrosis of intestine
Bowel infarction
Embolism of mesenteric artery
Fulminant enterocolitis
Hemorrhagic necrosis of intestine
Infarction of appendices epiploicae
Intestinal gangrene
Intestinal infarction (acute) (agnogenic) (hemorrhagic)
  (nonocclusive)
Mesenteric infarction (embolic) (thrombotic)
Necrosis of intestine
Terminal hemorrhagic enteropathy
Thrombosis of mesenteric artery
AHA: 3Q, '11, 11; 2Q, '08, 15; 4Q, '01, 53
TIP: Do not assign an additional code for GI bleeding; it is inherent in 557.0.
K55.0 Acute vascular disorders of intestine   `I-10`

557.1 Chronic vascular insufficiency of intestine
Angina, abdominal
Chronic ischemic colitis, enteritis, or enterocolitis
Ischemic stricture of intestine
Mesenteric:
  angina
  artery syndrome (superior)
  vascular insufficiency
AHA: 3Q, '96, 9; 4Q, '90, 4; N-D, '86, 11; N-D, '84, 7

557.9 Unspecified vascular insufficiency of intestine
Alimentary pain due to vascular insufficiency
Ischemic colitis, enteritis, or enterocolitis NOS
K55.9 Vascular disorder of intestine unspecified   `I-10`

☑4ᵗʰ 558 Other and unspecified noninfectious gastroenteritis and colitis

> **EXCLUDES** *infectious:*
>   *colitis, enteritis, or gastroenteritis (009.0-009.1)*
>   *diarrhea (009.2-009.3)*

558.1 Gastroenteritis and colitis due to radiation
Radiation enterocolitis

558.2 Toxic gastroenteritis and colitis
Use additional E code to identify cause

558.3 Allergic gastroenteritis and colitis
Use additional code to identify type of food allergy
  (V15.01-V15.05)
DEF: True immunoglobulin E (IgE)-mediated allergic reaction of the lining of the stomach, intestines, or colon to food proteins; causes nausea, vomiting, diarrhea, and abdominal cramping.
AHA: 4Q, '08, 116; 1Q, '03, 12; 4Q, '00, 42

☑5ᵗʰ 558.4 Eosinophilic gastroenteritis and colitis
AHA: 4Q, '08, 116

558.41 Eosinophilic gastroenteritis
Eosinophilic enteritis
AHA: 4Q, '08, 116

558.42 Eosinophilic colitis
AHA: 4Q, '08, 115-116

558.9 Other and unspecified noninfectious gastroenteritis and colitis
Colitis ⎫
Enteritis ⎪
Gastroenteritis ⎬ NOS, dietetic, or
Ileitis ⎪ noninfectious
Jejunitis ⎪
Sigmoiditis ⎭
AHA: 3Q, '11, 11; 2Q, '08, 10; 1Q, '08, 10; 3Q, '99, 4, 6; N-D, '87, 7
K52.9 Noninfective gastroenteritis & colitis unspec   `I-10`

Other Diseases of Intestines and Peritoneum (560-569)

☑4ᵗʰ 560 Intestinal obstruction without mention of hernia

> **EXCLUDES** *duodenum (537.2-537.3)*
>   *inguinal hernia with obstruction (550.1)*
>   *intestinal obstruction complicating hernia (552.0-552.9)*
>   *mesenteric:*
>   *embolism (557.0)*
>   *infarction (557.0)*
>   *thrombosis (557.0)*
>   *neonatal intestinal obstruction (277.01, 777.1-777.2, 777.4)*

TIP: If intestinal obstruction is due to abdominal carcinomatosis or Crohn's disease, sequence that condition first.

560.0 Intussusception
Intussusception (colon) (intestine) (rectum)
Invagination of intestine or colon
> **EXCLUDES** *intussusception of appendix (543.9)*
DEF: Prolapse of a bowel section into adjacent section; occurs primarily in children; symptoms include paroxysmal pain, vomiting, presence of blood, and mucous passage from rectum.
AHA: 4Q, '98, 82

560.1 Paralytic ileus
Adynamic ileus
Ileus (of intestine) (of bowel) (of colon)
Paralysis of intestine or colon
> **EXCLUDES** *gallstone ileus (560.31)*
DEF: Obstruction of ileus due to inhibited bowel motility.
AHA: 1Q, '12, 6; J-F, '87, 13
K56.0 Paralytic ileus   `I-10`

560.2 Volvulus
Knotting ⎫
Strangulation ⎬ if intestine, bowel, or colon
Torsion ⎪
Twist ⎭
DEF: Entanglement of bowel; causes obstruction; may compromise bowel circulation.

☑5ᵗʰ 560.3 Impaction of intestine

560.30 Impaction of intestine, unspecified
Impaction of colon

560.31 Gallstone ileus
Obstruction of intestine by gallstone

560.32 Fecal impaction
> **EXCLUDES** *constipation (564.00-564.09)*
>   *incomplete defecation (787.61)*
AHA: 4Q, '10, 87-89
K56.41 Fecal impaction   `I-10`

560.39 Other
Concretion of intestine
Enterolith
AHA: 4Q, '98, 38
K56.49 Other impaction of intestine   `I-10`

Volvulus and Diverticulitis

Knotted intestine (volvulus)

Diverticulum

☒ **N** Newborn Age: 0   ☐ **P** Pediatric Age: 0-17   ☐ **M** Maternity Age: 12-55   ☐ **A** Adult Age: 15-124

☑5ᵗʰ 560.8 Other specified intestinal obstruction

    560.81 Intestinal or peritoneal adhesions with obstruction (postoperative) (postinfection)

        EXCLUDES *adhesions without obstruction (568.0)*

        DEF: Obstruction of peritoneum or intestine due to abnormal union of tissues.

        AHA: 1Q, '10, 11; 4Q, '95, 55; 3Q, '95, 6; N-D, '87, 9

        TIP: Do not assign additional code from subcategory 997.4 Digestive system complications.

        K56.5 Intestinal adhes [bands] w/obst (postproc) (postinfec)   `I-10`

    560.89 Other

        Acute pseudo-obstruction of intestine

        Mural thickening causing obstruction

        EXCLUDES *ischemic stricture of intestine (557.1)*

        AHA: 2Q, '97, 3; 1Q, '88, 6

560.9 Unspecified intestinal obstruction

    Enterostenosis

    Obstruction

    Occlusion   } of intestine or colon

    Stenosis

    Stricture

    EXCLUDES *congenital stricture or stenosis of intestine (751.1-751.2)*

    K56.60 Unspecified intestinal obstruction   `I-10`

☑4ᵗʰ 562 Diverticula of intestine

    Use additional code to identify any associated:

    peritonitis (567.0-567.9)

    EXCLUDES *congenital diverticulum of colon (751.5)*

        diverticulum of appendix (543.9)

        Meckel's diverticulum (751.0)

    AHA: 4Q, '91, 25; J-F, '85, 1

☑5ᵗʰ 562.0 Small intestine

    562.00 Diverticulosis of small intestine (without mention of hemorrhage)

        Diverticulosis:

          duodenum

          ileum   } without mention of diverticulitis

          jejunum

        DEF: Saclike herniations of mucous lining of small intestine.

    562.01 Diverticulitis of small intestine (without mention of hemorrhage)

        Diverticulitis (with diverticulosis):

          duodenum

          ileum

          jejunum

          small intestine

        DEF: Inflamed saclike herniations of mucous lining of small intestine

    562.02 Diverticulosis of small intestine with hemorrhage

    562.03 Diverticulitis of small intestine with hemorrhage

☑5ᵗʰ 562.1 Colon

    562.10 Diverticulosis of colon (without mention of hemorrhage)

        Diverticulosis:

          NOS

          intestine (large)   } without metion of diverticulitis

          Diverticular disease (colon)

        DEF: Saclike herniations of mucous lining of large intestine.

        AHA: 3Q, '05, 17; 3Q, '02, 15; 4Q, '90, 21; J-F, '85, 5

        K57.30 Divrticulos lg intest uns w/o perf/absc w/o bldg   `I-10`

    562.11 Diverticulitis of colon (without mention of hemorrhage)

        Diverticulitis (with diverticulosis):

          NOS

          colon

          intestine (large)

        DEF: Inflamed saclike herniations of mucosal lining of large intestine.

        AHA: 1Q, '96, 14; J-F, '85, 5

        K57.32 Divrticulit lg intest uns w/o perf/absc w/o bldg   `I-10`

    562.12 Diverticulosis of colon with hemorrhage

    562.13 Diverticulitis of colon with hemorrhage

☑4ᵗʰ 564 Functional digestive disorders, not elsewhere classified

    EXCLUDES *functional disorders of stomach (536.0-536.9)*

        those specified as psychogenic (306.4)

☑5ᵗʰ 564.0 Constipation

    EXCLUDES *fecal impaction (560.32)*

        incomplete defecation (787.61)

    AHA: 4Q, '01, 45

    564.00 Constipation, unspecified

        K59.00 Constipation unspecified   `I-10`

    564.01 Slow transit constipation

        DEF: Delay in the transit of fecal material through the colon secondary to smooth muscle dysfunction or decreased peristaltic contractions along the colon: also called colonic inertia or delayed transit.

    564.02 Outlet dysfunction constipation

        DEF: Failure to relax the paradoxical contractions of the striated pelvic floor muscles during the attempted defecation.

    564.09 Other constipation

564.1 Irritable bowel syndrome

    Irritable colon   Spastic colon

    DEF: Functional gastrointestinal disorder (FGID); symptoms include diarrhea, constipation, abdominal pain, gas, distended abdomen, nausea, vomiting, emotional distress, and depression.

    AHA: 1Q, '88, 6

    K58.9 Irritable bowel syndrome without diarrhea   `I-10`

564.2 Postgastric surgery syndromes

    Dumping syndrome   Postgastrectomy syndrome

    Jejunal syndrome   Postvagotomy syndrome

    EXCLUDES *malnutrition following gastrointestinal surgery (579.3)*

        postgastrojejunostomy ulcer (534.0-534.9)

    AHA: 1Q, '95, 11

564.3 Vomiting following gastrointestinal surgery

    Vomiting (bilious) following gastrointestinal surgery

564.4 Other postoperative functional disorders

    Diarrhea following gastrointestinal surgery

    EXCLUDES *colostomy and enterostomy complications (569.60-569.69)*

564.5 Functional diarrhea

    EXCLUDES *diarrhea:*

        NOS (787.91)

        psychogenic (306.4)

    DEF: Diarrhea with no detectable organic cause.

564.6 Anal spasm

    Proctalgia fugax

564.7 Megacolon, other than Hirschsprung's

    Dilatation of colon

    EXCLUDES *megacolon:*

        congenital [Hirschsprung's] (751.3)

        toxic (556)

    DEF: Enlarged colon; congenital or acquired; can occur acutely or become chronic.

☑5ᵗʰ 564.8 Other specified functional disorders of intestine

    EXCLUDES *malabsorption (579.0-579.9)*

    AHA: 1Q, '88, 6

    564.81 Neurogenic bowel

        DEF: Disorder of bowel due to spinal cord lesion above conus medullaris; symptoms include precipitous micturition, nocturia, headache, sweating, nasal obstruction and spastic contractions.

        AHA: 1Q, '01, 12; 4Q, '98, 45

    564.89 Other functional disorders of intestine

        Atony of colon

        DEF: Absence of normal bowel tone or strength.

        AHA: 3Q, '12, 22

        TIP: Assign for visceral hypersensitivity; an overstimulation response causing extreme pain.

564.9 Unspecified functional disorder of intestine

☑4ᵗʰ ☑5ᵗʰ Additional Digit Required	Unspecified Code	Other Specified Code	Manifestation Code	►◄ Revised Text	● New Code	▲ Revised Code Title

2015 ICD-9-CM   **Volume 1 – 171**

Diseases of the Digestive System

565–567.9

Anal Fistula and Abscess

Urethra
Fistula
Bladder
Abscess
Rectum

Psoas Muscle Abscess

Psoas minor muscle
Psoas major muscle
Small intestine (ilium)
Peritoneal cavity
Small intestine (jejunum)
Ascending colon
Abscess
Ascending colon
Psoas major muscle
Pelvic bone
Psoas major muscle
Spinous process of L4
Erector spinae muscles

✓4ᵗʰ **565 Anal fissure and fistula**

  565.0 Anal fissure

    EXCLUDES *anal sphincter tear (healed) (non-traumatic) (old) (569.43)*
    traumatic (863.89, 863.99)

    DEF: Ulceration of cleft at anal mucosa; causes pain, itching, bleeding, infection, and sphincter spasm; may occur with hemorrhoids.

  565.1 Anal fistula

    Fistula:
      anorectal
      rectal
      rectum to skin

    EXCLUDES *fistula of rectum to internal organs — see Alphabetic Index*
    ischiorectal fistula (566)
    rectovaginal fistula (619.1)

    DEF: Abnormal opening on cutaneous surface near anus; may lack connection with rectum.
    AHA: 1Q, '07, 13

566 Abscess of anal and rectal regions

  Abscess: Cellulitis:
    ischiorectal   anal
    perianal   perirectal
    perirectal   rectal
                     Ischiorectal fistula

✓4ᵗʰ **567 Peritonitis and retroperitoneal infections**

    EXCLUDES *peritonitis:*
    benign paroxysmal (277.31)
    pelvic, female (614.5, 614.7)
    periodic familial (277.31)
    puerperal (670.8)
    with or following:
      abortion (634-638 with .0, 639.0)
      appendicitis (540.0-540.1)
      ectopic or molar pregnancy (639.0)

    DEF: Inflammation of the peritoneal cavity.

  567.0 Peritonitis in infectious diseases classified elsewhere

    Code first underlying disease

    EXCLUDES *peritonitis:*
    gonococcal (098.86)
    syphilitic (095.2)
    tuberculous (014.0)

  567.1 Pneumococcal peritonitis

✓5ᵗʰ **567.2 Other suppurative peritonitis**
    AHA: 4Q, '05, 74; 2Q, '01, 11, 12; 3Q, '99, 9; 2Q, '98, 19

    567.21 Peritonitis (acute) generalized
      Pelvic peritonitis, male
      TIP: For pelvic peritonitis in a female patient, refer to code 614.5.

    567.22 Peritoneal abscess
      Abscess (of):
        abdominopelvic
        mesenteric
        omentum
        peritoneum
        retrocecal
        subdiaphragmatic
        subhepatic
        subphrenic
      K65.1 Peritoneal abscess   I-10

    567.23 Spontaneous bacterial peritonitis
      EXCLUDES *bacterial peritonitis NOS (567.29)*

    567.29 Other suppurative peritonitis
      Subphrenic peritonitis
      AHA: 2Q, '10, 4

✓5ᵗʰ **567.3 Retroperitoneal infections**
    AHA: 4Q, '05, 74

    567.31 Psoas muscle abscess
      DEF: Infection that extends into or around the psoas muscle that connects the lumbar vertebrae to the femur.

    567.38 Other retroperitoneal abscess
      AHA: 4Q, '05, 77

    567.39 Other retroperitoneal infections

✓5ᵗʰ **567.8 Other specified peritonitis**
    AHA: 4Q, '05, 74

    567.81 Choleperitonitis
      Peritonitis due to bile
      DEF: Inflammation or infection due to presence of bile in the peritoneum resulting from rupture of the bile passages or gallbladder.

    567.82 Sclerosing mesenteritis
      Fat necrosis of peritoneum
      (Idiopathic) sclerosing mesenteric fibrosis
      Mesenteric lipodystrophy
      Mesenteric panniculitis
      Retractile mesenteritis
      DEF: Inflammatory processes involving the mesenteric fat; progresses to fibrosis and necrosis of tissue.
      AHA: 4Q, '05, 77

    567.89 Other specified peritonitis
      Chronic proliferative peritonitis
      Mesenteric saponification
      Peritonitis due to urine

  567.9 Unspecified peritonitis
    Peritonitis NOS
    Peritonitis of unspecified cause
    AHA: ▶2Q, '13, 3;◀ 1Q, '04, 10

N Newborn Age: 0   P Pediatric Age: 0-17   M Maternity Age: 12-55   A Adult Age: 15-124

√4ᵗʰ 568 Other disorders of peritoneum

568.0 Peritoneal adhesions (postoperative) (postinfection)

Adhesions (of):
- abdominal (wall)
- diaphragm
- intestine
- male pelvis
- mesenteric
- omentum
- stomach

Adhesive bands

> **EXCLUDES** adhesions:
>> pelvic, female (614.6)
>> with obstruction:
>>> duodenum (537.3)
>>> intestine (560.81)

DEF: Abnormal union of tissues in peritoneum.

AHA: 1Q, '12, 8; 2Q, '11, 18; 3Q, '03, 7, 11; 4Q, '95, 55; 3Q, '95, 7; S-O, '85, 11

TIP: Do not assign additional code from subcategory 997.4 Digestive system complications.

K66.0 Peritoneal adhesns (postprocedural) (postinfection)   I-10

√5ᵗʰ 568.8 Other specified disorders of peritoneum

568.81 Hemoperitoneum (nontraumatic)

568.82 Peritoneal effusion (chronic)

> **EXCLUDES** ascites NOS (789.51-789.59)

DEF: Persistent leakage of fluid within peritoneal cavity.

568.89 Other

Peritoneal:
- cyst
- granuloma

568.9 Unspecified disorder of peritoneum

√4ᵗʰ 569 Other disorders of intestine

569.0 Anal and rectal polyp

Anal and rectal polyp NOS

> **EXCLUDES** adenomatous anal and rectal polyp (211.4)

569.1 Rectal prolapse

Procidentia:	Prolapse:
anus (sphincter)	anal canal
rectum (sphincter)	rectal mucosa
Proctoptosis	

> **EXCLUDES** prolapsed hemorrhoids (455.2, 455.5)

569.2 Stenosis of rectum and anus

Stricture of anus (sphincter)

569.3 Hemorrhage of rectum and anus

> **EXCLUDES** gastrointestinal bleeding NOS (578.9)
>> melena (578.1)

AHA: 3Q, '05, 17

K62.5 Hemorrhage of anus and rectum   I-10

√5ᵗʰ 569.4 Other specified disorders of rectum and anus

569.41 Ulcer of anus and rectum

Solitary ulcer ⎱ of anus (sphincter) or
Stercoral ulcer ⎰   rectum (sphincter)

569.42 Anal or rectal pain

AHA: 1Q, '03, 8; 1Q, '96, 13

Rectum and Anus

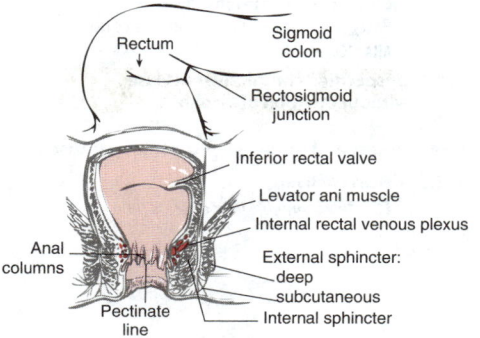

569.43 Anal sphincter tear (healed) (old)

Tear of anus, nontraumatic

Use additional code for any associated fecal incontinence (787.60-787.63)

> **EXCLUDES** anal fissure (565.0)
>> anal sphincter tear (healed) (old) complicating delivery (654.8)

AHA: 4Q, '07, 88

569.44 Dysplasia of anus

Anal intraepithelial neoplasia I and II (AIN I and II) (histologically confirmed)

Dysplasia of anus NOS

Mild and moderate dysplasia of anus (histologically confirmed)

> **EXCLUDES** abnormal results from anal cytologic examination without histologic confirmation (796.70-796.79)
>> anal intraepithelial neoplasia III (230.5, 230.6)
>> carcinoma in situ of anus (230.5, 230.6)
>> HGSIL of anus (796.74)
>> severe dysplasia of anus (230.5, 230.6)

AHA: 4Q, '08, 117

569.49 Other

Granuloma ⎱ of rectum (sphincter)
Rupture ⎰

Hypertrophy of anal papillae

Proctitis NOS

Use additional code for any associated fecal incontinence (787.60-787.63)

> **EXCLUDES** fistula of rectum to:
>> internal organs — see Alphabetic Index
>> skin (565.1)
>> hemorrhoids (455.0-455.9)

569.5 Abscess of intestine

> **EXCLUDES** appendiceal abscess (540.1)

K63.0 Abscess of intestine   I-10

√5ᵗʰ 569.6 Colostomy and enterostomy complications

DEF: Complication in a surgically created opening, from intestine to surface skin.

AHA: 4Q, '95, 58

TIP: Do not assign additional code from subcategory 997.4 Digestive system complications.

569.60 Colostomy and enterostomy complication, unspecified

569.61 Infection of colostomy or enterostomy

Use additional code to identify organism (041.00-041.9)

Use additional code to specify type of infection, such as:

abscess or cellulitis of abdomen (682.2)
septicemia (038.0-038.9)

569.62 Mechanical complication of colostomy and enterostomy

Malfunction of colostomy and enterostomy

AHA: 2Q, '05, 11 ; 1Q, '03, 10; 4Q, '98, 44

569.69 Other complication

Fistula	Prolapse
Hernia	

AHA: 3Q, '98, 16

√5ᵗʰ 569.7 Complications of intestinal pouch

TIP: Do not assign code from subcategory 997.4 Digestive system complications in addition to a code from this subcategory.

569.71 Pouchitis

Inflammation of internal ileoanal pouch

DEF: Inflammatory complication of an existing surgically created ileoanal pouch, resulting in multiple GI complaints, including diarrhea, abdominal pain, rectal bleeding, fecal urgency, or incontinence.

AHA: 4Q, '09, 94

569.79 Other complications of intestinal pouch

√4ᵗʰ √5ᵗʰ Additional Digit Required	Unspecified Code	Other Specified Code	Manifestation Code	►◄ Revised Text	● New Code	▲ Revised Code Title

√5ᵗʰ **569.8 Other specified disorders of intestine**
    AHA: 4Q, '91, 25

569.81 Fistula of intestine, excluding rectum and anus
    Fistula: Fistula:
     abdominal wall   enteroenteric
     enterocolic   ileorectal
    EXCLUDES *fistula of intestine to internal organs — see Alphabetic Index*
              persistent postoperative fistula (998.6)
    AHA: 3Q, '99, 8

569.82 Ulceration of intestine
    Primary ulcer of intestine
    Ulceration of colon
    EXCLUDES *that with perforation (569.83)*

569.83 Perforation of intestine
    AHA: 2Q, '12, 5

569.84 Angiodysplasia of intestine (without mention of hemorrhage)
    DEF: Small vascular abnormalities of the intestinal tract without bleeding problems.
    AHA: 3Q, '96, 10; 4Q, '90, 4; 4Q, '90, 21
    TIP: Assign code 569.84 or 569.85 for documentation of either intestinal arteriovenous (AV) malformation or angiodysplasia.

569.85 Angiodysplasia of intestine with hemorrhage
    DEF: Small vascular abnormalities of the intestinal tract with bleeding problems.
    AHA: 3Q, '96, 9

569.86 Dieulafoy lesion (hemorrhagic) of intestine
    AHA: 4Q, '02, 60-61

569.87 Vomiting of fecal matter
    DEF: Spasmodic expulsion of partially digested substance with similar odor to fecal matter; often suggestive of bowel obstruction or other underlying causal pathology.
    AHA: 4Q, '09, 105

569.89 Other
    Enteroptosis
    Granuloma   ⎫
    Prolapse   ⎬ of intestine
    Pericolitis
    Perisigmoiditis
    Visceroptosis
    EXCLUDES *gangrene of intestine, mesentery, or omentum (557.0)*
             hemorrhage of intestine NOS (578.9)
             obstruction of intestine (560.0-560.9)
    AHA: ▶2Q, '13, 3;◀ 3Q, '96, 9

569.9 Unspecified disorder of intestine

Other Diseases of Digestive System (570-579)

570 Acute and subacute necrosis of liver
    Acute hepatic failure
    Acute or subacute hepatitis, not specified as infective
    Necrosis of liver (acute) (diffuse) (massive) (subacute)
    Parenchymatous degeneration of liver
    Yellow atrophy (liver) (acute) (subacute)
    EXCLUDES *icterus gravis of newborn (773.0-773.2)*
             serum hepatitis (070.2-070.3)
             that with:
                 abortion (634-638 with .7, 639.8)
                 ectopic or molar pregnancy (639.8)
                 pregnancy, childbirth, or the puerperium (646.7)
             viral hepatitis (070.0-070.9)
    AHA: 2Q, '05, 9; 1Q, '00, 22
    K72.00 Acute and subacute hepatic failure without coma   I-10

√4ᵗʰ **571 Chronic liver disease and cirrhosis**

571.0 Alcoholic fatty liver   A

571.1 Acute alcoholic hepatitis   A
    Acute alcoholic liver disease
    AHA: 2Q, '02, 4

Liver

Inferior vena cava — Hepatic veins
Diaphragm — Caudate lobe
Gallbladder — Portal vein
Common bile duct — Medial segment — Lateral segment
Right lobe — Left lobe

571.2 Alcoholic cirrhosis of liver   A
    Florid cirrhosis
    Laennec's cirrhosis (alcoholic)
    DEF: Fibrosis and dysfunction of liver due to alcoholic liver disease.
    AHA: 1Q, '11, 23; 3Q, '07, 7; 2Q, '07, 6; 2Q, '02, 4; 1Q, '02, 3; N-D, '85, 14
    TIP: For a patient admitted for bleeding esophageal varices due to alcoholic liver cirrhosis, sequence the liver cirrhosis first.
    K70.30 Alcoholic cirrhosis of liver without ascites   I-10

571.3 Alcoholic liver damage, unspecified   A

√5ᵗʰ **571.4 Chronic hepatitis**
    EXCLUDES *viral hepatitis (acute) (chronic) (070.0-070.9)*

571.40 Chronic hepatitis, unspecified

571.41 Chronic persistent hepatitis

571.42 Autoimmune hepatitis
    AHA: 4Q, '08, 120

571.49 Other
    Chronic hepatitis:
     active
     aggressive
    Recurrent hepatitis
    AHA: 3Q, '99, 19; N-D, '85, 14

571.5 Cirrhosis of liver without mention of alcohol
    Cirrhosis of liver:
     NOS
     cryptogenic
     macronodular
     micronodular
     posthepatitic
     postnecrotic
    Healed yellow atrophy (liver)
    Portal cirrhosis
    Code first, if applicable, viral hepatitis (acute) (chronic) (070.0-070.9)
    DEF: Fibrosis and dysfunction of liver; not alcohol related.
    AHA: 1Q, '11, 23; 3Q, '07, 7; 2Q, '07, 5
    TIP: For a patient admitted for bleeding esophageal varices due to liver cirrhosis, sequence the liver cirrhosis first.

571.6 Biliary cirrhosis
    Chronic nonsuppurative destructive cholangitis
    Cirrhosis:
     cholangitic
     cholestatic

571.8 Other chronic nonalcoholic liver disease
    Chronic yellow atrophy (liver)
    Fatty liver, without mention of alcohol
    AHA: 2Q, '96, 12

571.9 Unspecified chronic liver disease without mention of alcohol

√4ᵗʰ **572 Liver abscess and sequelae of chronic liver disease**

572.0 Abscess of liver
    EXCLUDES *amebic liver abscess (006.3)*

572.1 Portal pyemia

Phlebitis of portal vein   Pylephlebitis
Portal thrombophlebitis   Pylethrombophlebitis

DEF: Inflammation of portal vein or branches; may be due to intestinal disease; symptoms include fever, chills, jaundice, sweating, and abscess in various body parts.

572.2 Hepatic encephalopathy

Hepatic coma
Hepatocerebral intoxication
Portal-systemic encephalopathy

EXCLUDES *hepatic coma associated with viral hepatitis — see category 070*

AHA: 2Q, '07, 5; 2Q, '05, 9; 1Q, '02, 3; 3Q, '95, 14

TIP: Do not assign if hepatic coma is documented with viral hepatitis; see category 070 with fourth digit indicating hepatic coma.

K72.91 Hepatic failure unspecified with coma   `I-10`

572.3 Portal hypertension

Use additional code for any associated complications, such as:
portal hypertensive gastropathy (537.89)

DEF: Abnormally high blood pressure in the portal vein.

AHA: 3Q, '05, 15

K76.6 Portal hypertension   `I-10`

572.4 Hepatorenal syndrome

EXCLUDES *that following delivery (674.8)*

DEF: Hepatic and renal failure characterized by cirrhosis with ascites or obstructive jaundice, oliguria, and low sodium concentration.

AHA: 3Q, '93, 15

572.8 Other sequelae of chronic liver disease

EXCLUDES *hepatopulmonary syndrome (573.5)*

✓4ᵗʰ 573 Other disorders of liver

EXCLUDES *amyloid or lardaceous degeneration of liver (277.39)*
congenital cystic disease of liver (751.62)
glycogen infiltration of liver (271.0)
hepatomegaly NOS (789.1)
portal vein obstruction (452)

573.0 Chronic passive congestion of liver

DEF: Blood accumulation in liver tissue.

573.1 Hepatitis in viral diseases classified elsewhere

Code first underlying disease as:
Coxsackie virus disease (074.8)
cytomegalic inclusion virus disease (078.5)
infectious mononucleosis (075)

EXCLUDES *hepatitis (in):*
mumps (072.71)
viral (070.0-070.9)
yellow fever (060.0-060.9)

573.2 Hepatitis in other infectious diseases classified elsewhere

Code first underlying disease, as:
malaria (084.9)

EXCLUDES *hepatitis in:*
late syphilis (095.3)
secondary syphilis (091.62)
toxoplasmosis (130.5)

Hepatic portal veins

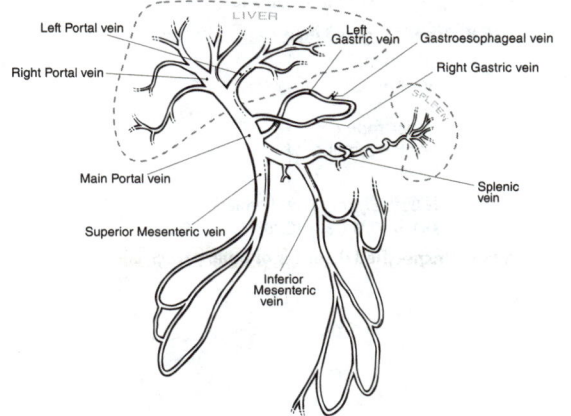

Gallbladder and Bile Ducts

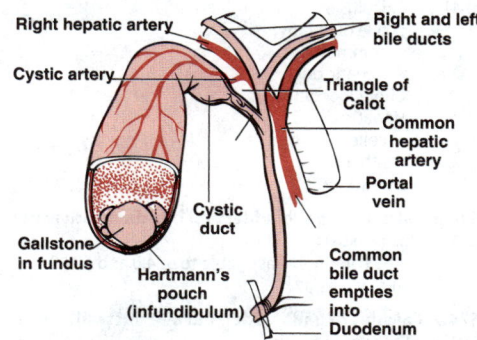

573.3 Hepatitis, unspecified

Toxic (noninfectious) hepatitis

Use additional E code to identify cause

AHA: 3Q, '98, 3, 4; 4Q, '90, 26

K75.9 Inflammatory liver disease unspecified   `I-10`

573.4 Hepatic infarction

573.5 Hepatopulmonary syndrome

Code first underlying liver disease, such as:
alcoholic cirrhosis of liver (571.2)
cirrhosis of liver without mention of alcohol (571.5)

AHA: 4Q, '11, 127-128

573.8 Other specified disorders of liver

Hepatoptosis

AHA: ▶1Q, '14, 8◀

573.9 Unspecified disorder of liver

✓4ᵗʰ 574 Cholelithiasis

The following fifth-digit subclassification is for use with category 574:
0 without mention of obstruction
1 with obstruction

EXCLUDES *retained cholelithiasis following cholecystectomy (997.41)*

§ ✓5ᵗʰ 574.0 Calculus of gallbladder with acute cholecystitis
[0-1]

Biliary calculus
Calculus of cystic duct   } with acute cholecystitis
Cholelithiasis

Any condition classifiable to 574.2 with acute cholecystitis

AHA: 4Q, '96, 32

K80.00 Calculus of GB w/acute cholecystitis w/o obst   `I-10`

§ ✓5ᵗʰ 574.1 Calculus of gallbladder with other cholecystitis
[0-1]

Biliary calculus
Calculus of cystic duct   } with cholecystitis
Cholelithiasis

Cholecystitis with cholelithiasis NOS

Any condition classifiable to 574.2 with cholecystitis (chronic)

AHA: 3Q, '99, 9; 4Q, '96, 32, 69; 2Q, '96, 13; **For code 574.10:** 1Q, '03, 5

K80.10 Calculus of GB w/chronic cholecystitis w/o obst   `I-10`

§ ✓5ᵗʰ 574.2 Calculus of gallbladder without mention of cholecystitis
[0-1]

Biliary:
calculus NOS
colic NOS
Calculus of cystic duct
Cholelithiasis NOS
Colic (recurrent) of gallbladder
Gallstone (impacted)

AHA: For code 574.20: 1Q, '88, 14

K80.20 Calculus of GB w/o cholecystitis w/o obst   `I-10`

§ ✓5ᵗʰ 574.3 Calculus of bile duct with acute cholecystitis
[0-1]

Calculus of bile duct (any)   } with acute cholecystitis
Choledocholithiasis

Any condition classifiable to 574.5 with acute cholecystitis

§ ✓5ᵗʰ 574.4 Calculus of bile duct with other cholecystitis
[0-1]

Calculus of bile duct
(any)   } with cholecystitis (chronic)
Choledocholithiasis

Any condition classifiable to 574.5 with cholecystitis (chronic)

---

§   Requires fifth digit. Valid digits are in [brackets] under each code. See category 574 for codes and definitions.

| ✓4ᵗʰ ✓5ᵗʰ Additional Digit Required | Unspecified Code | Other Specified Code | Manifestation Code | ▶◀ Revised Text | ● New Code | ▲ Revised Code Title |

2015 ICD-9-CM   **October 2014 • Volume 1 – 175**

Diseases of the Digestive System

574.5–576.9

§ ✓5ᵗʰ **574.5 Calculus of bile duct without mention of cholecystitis**
　[0-1]　Calculus of:
　　　　　　bile duct [any]
　　　　　　common duct
　　　　　　hepatic duct
　　　　　Choledocholithiasis
　　　　　Hepatic:
　　　　　　colic (recurrent)
　　　　　　lithiasis
　　　　　AHA: 3Q, '94, 11

§ ✓5ᵗʰ **574.6 Calculus of gallbladder and bile duct with acute**
　[0-1]　**cholecystitis**
　　　　　Any condition classifiable to 574.0 and 574.3
　　　　　AHA: 4Q, '96, 32

§ ✓5ᵗʰ **574.7 Calculus of gallbladder and bile duct with**
　[0-1]　**other cholecytitis**
　　　　　Any condition classifiable to 574.1 and 574.4
　　　　　AHA: 4Q, '96, 32

§ ✓5ᵗʰ **574.8 Calculus of gallbladder and bile duct with acute**
　[0-1]　**and chronic cholcystitis**
　　　　　Any condition classifiable to 574.6 and 574.7
　　　　　AHA: 4Q, '96, 32

§ ✓5ᵗʰ **574.9 Calculus of gallbladder and bile duct without cholecystitis**
　[0-1]　Any condition classifiable to 574.2 and 574.5
　　　　　AHA: 4Q, '96, 32

✓4ᵗʰ **575 Other disorders of gallbladder**

　　575.0 Acute cholecystitis
　　　　　Abscess of gallbladder ⎤
　　　　　Angiocholecystitis ⎟
　　　　　Cholecystitis: ⎟
　　　　　　emphysematous (acute) ⎬ without mention of
　　　　　　gangrenous ⎟ 　　calculus
　　　　　　suppurative ⎟
　　　　　Empyema of gallbladder ⎟
　　　　　Gangrene of gallbladder ⎦

　　　　　EXCLUDES that with:
　　　　　　　acute and chronic cholecystitis (575.12)
　　　　　　　choledocholithiasis (574.3)
　　　　　　　choledocholithiasis and cholelithiasis (574.6)
　　　　　　　cholelithiasis (574.0)
　　　　　AHA: 3Q, '91, 17
　　　　　TIP: Do not assign a separate cholecystitis code from category 575 with a code from category 574.
　　　　　K81.0 Acute cholecystitis　　　　　　　　　　I-10

✓5ᵗʰ **575.1 Other cholecystitis**
　　　　　Cholecystitis: ⎤
　　　　　　NOS ⎬ without mention of calculus
　　　　　　chronic ⎦

　　　　　EXCLUDES that with:
　　　　　　　choledocholithiasis (574.4)
　　　　　　　choledocholithiasis and cholelithiasis (574.8)
　　　　　　　cholelithiasis (574.1)
　　　　　AHA: 4Q, '96, 32

　　575.10 Cholecystitis, unspecified
　　　　　Cholecystitis NOS

　　575.11 Chronic cholecystitis
　　　　　K81.1 Chronic cholecystitis　　　　　　　　I-10

　　575.12 Acute and chronic cholecystitis
　　　　　AHA: 4Q, '97, 52; 4Q, '96, 32

　　575.2 Obstruction of gallbladder
　　　　　Occlusion ⎤
　　　　　Stenosis ⎬ of cystic duct or gallbladder without
　　　　　Stricture ⎦ 　　mention of calculus

　　　　　EXCLUDES that with calculus (574.0-574.2 with
　　　　　　　fifth-digit 1)

　　575.3 Hydrops of gallbladder
　　　　　Mucocele of gallbladder
　　　　　DEF: Serous fluid accumulation in bladder.
　　　　　AHA: 2Q, '89, 13

　　575.4 Perforation of gallbladder
　　　　　Rupture of cystic duct or gallbladder

　　575.5 Fistula of gallbladder
　　　　　Fistula:
　　　　　　cholecystoduodenal
　　　　　　cholecystoenteric

　　575.6 Cholesterolosis of gallbladder
　　　　　Strawberry gallbladder
　　　　　DEF: Cholesterol deposits in gallbladder tissue.
　　　　　AHA: 4Q, '90, 17

　　575.8 Other specified disorders of gallbladder
　　　　　Adhesions ⎤
　　　　　Atrophy ⎟
　　　　　Cyst ⎟
　　　　　Hypertrophy ⎬ of cystic duct or gallbladder
　　　　　Nonfunctioning ⎟
　　　　　Ulcer ⎦

　　　　　Biliary dyskinesia
　　　　　EXCLUDES Hartmann's pouch of intestine (V44.3)
　　　　　　　nonvisualization of gallbladder (793.3)
　　　　　AHA: 4Q, '90, 26; 2Q, '89, 13

　　575.9 Unspecified disorder of gallbladder

✓4ᵗʰ **576 Other disorders of biliary tract**
　　　　　EXCLUDES that involving the:
　　　　　　　cystic duct (575.0-575.9)
　　　　　　　gallbladder (575.0-575.9)

　　576.0 Postcholecystectomy syndrome
　　　　　DEF: Jaundice or abdominal pain following cholecystectomy.
　　　　　AHA: 1Q, '88, 10
　　　　　TIP: Do not assign additional code from subcategory 997.4 Digestive system complications.

　　576.1 Cholangitis
　　　　　Cholangitis:　　　Cholangitis:
　　　　　　NOS　　　　　　recurrent
　　　　　　acute　　　　　sclerosing
　　　　　　ascending　　　secondary
　　　　　　chronic　　　　stenosing
　　　　　　primary　　　　suppurative
　　　　　AHA: 2Q, '99, 13
　　　　　K83.0 Cholangitis　　　　　　　　　　　I-10

　　576.2 Obstruction of bile duct
　　　　　Occlusion ⎤
　　　　　Stenosis ⎬ of bile duct, except cystic duct, without
　　　　　Stricture ⎦ 　　mention of calculus

　　　　　EXCLUDES congenital (751.61)
　　　　　　　that with calculus (574.3-574.5 with
　　　　　　　　fifth-digit 1)
　　　　　AHA: 3Q, '03, 17-18; 1Q, '01, 8; 2Q, '99, 13
　　　　　K83.1 Obstruction of bile duct　　　　　I-10

　　576.3 Perforation of bile duct
　　　　　Rupture of bile duct, except cystic duct

　　576.4 Fistula of bile duct
　　　　　Choledochoduodenal fistula

　　576.5 Spasm of sphincter of Oddi

　　576.8 Other specified disorders of biliary tract
　　　　　Adhesions ⎤
　　　　　Atrophy ⎟
　　　　　Cyst ⎟
　　　　　Hypertrophy ⎬ of bile duct (any)
　　　　　Nonfunctioning ⎟
　　　　　Ulcer ⎦

　　　　　EXCLUDES congenital choledochal cyst (751.69)
　　　　　AHA: ▶1Q, '14, 8;◀ 3Q, '03, 17; 2Q, '99, 14

　　576.9 Unspecified disorder of biliary tract

---

§　Requires fifth digit. Valid digits are in [brackets] under each code. See category 574 for codes and definitions.

Pancreas

✓4ᵗʰ **577 Diseases of pancreas**

577.0 Acute pancreatitis
Abscess of pancreas
Necrosis of pancreas:
acute
infective
Pancreatitis:
NOS
acute (recurrent)
apoplectic
hemorrhagic
subacute
suppurative
EXCLUDES *mumps pancreatitis (072.3)*
AHA: 3Q, '99, 9; 2Q, '98, 19; 2Q, '96, 13; 2Q, '89, 9
K85.0 Idiopathic acute pancreatitis   I-10

577.1 Chronic pancreatitis
Chronic pancreatitis:
NOS
infectious
interstitial
Pancreatitis:
painless
recurrent
relapsing
AHA: 1Q, '01, 8; 2Q, '96, 13; 3Q, '94, 11
K86.1 Other chronic pancreatitis   I-10

577.2 Cyst and pseudocyst of pancreas
K86.2 Cyst of pancreas   I-10

577.8 Other specified diseases of pancreas
Atrophy ⎫
Calculus ⎬ of pancreas
Cirrhosis ⎪
Fibrosis ⎭
Pancreatic:
infantilism
necrosis:
NOS
aseptic
fat
Pancreatolithiasis
EXCLUDES *fibrocystic disease of pancreas (277.00-277.09)*
islet cell tumor of pancreas (211.7)
pancreatic steatorrhea (579.4)
AHA: 1Q, '01, 8

577.9 Unspecified disease of pancreas

✓4ᵗʰ **578 Gastrointestinal hemorrhage**
EXCLUDES *that with mention of:*
angiodysplasia of stomach and duodenum (537.83)
angiodysplasia of intestine (569.85)
diverticulitis, intestine:
large (562.13)
small (562.03)
diverticulosis, intestine:
large (562.12)
small (562.02)
gastritis and duodenitis (535.0-535.6)
ulcer:
*duodenal, gastric, gastrojejuunal or peptic
(531.00-534.91)*
AHA: 2Q, '92, 9; 4Q, '90, 20

578.0 Hematemesis
Vomiting of blood
AHA: 2Q, '02, 4

578.1 Blood in stool
Melena
EXCLUDES *melena of the newborn (772.4, 777.3)*
occult blood (792.1)
AHA: ▶4Q, '13, 83; 3Q, '13, 9;◀ 2Q, '06, 17; 2Q, '92, 8
K92.1 Melena   I-10

578.9 Hemorrhage of gastrointestinal tract, unspecified
Gastric hemorrhage
Intestinal hemorrhage
AHA: 4Q, '06, 91; 3Q, '05, 17; N-D, '86, 9
TIP: Assign 578.9 if the physician does not establish a causal link between GI bleeding and any possible causes found on endoscopy.
K92.2 Gastrointestinal hemorrhage unspecified   I-10

✓4ᵗʰ **579 Intestinal malabsorption**

579.0 Celiac disease
Celiac: Gee (-Herter) disease
crisis   Gluten enteropathy
infantilism   Idiopathic steatorrhea
rickets   Nontropical sprue
DEF: Malabsorption syndrome due to gluten consumption; symptoms include fetid, bulky, frothy, oily stools, distended abdomen, gas, asthenia, electrolyte depletion and vitamin B, D and K deficiency.

579.1 Tropical sprue
Sprue:
NOS
tropical
Tropical steatorrhea
DEF: Diarrhea, occurs in tropics; may be due to enteric infection and malnutrition.

579.2 Blind loop syndrome
Postoperative blind loop syndrome
DEF: Obstruction or impaired passage in small intestine due to alterations, from strictures or surgery; causes stasis, abnormal bacterial flora, diarrhea, weight loss, multiple vitamin deficiency, and megaloblastic anemia.
TIP: Do not assign additional code from subcategory 997.4 Digestive system complications.

579.3 Other and unspecified postsurgical nonabsorption
Hypoglycemia ⎫ following gastrointestinal
Malnutrition ⎬ surgery
AHA: 4Q, '03, 104

579.4 Pancreatic steatorrhea
DEF: Excess fat in feces due to absence of pancreatic secretions in intestine.

579.8 Other specified intestinal malabsorption
Enteropathy:
exudative
protein-losing
Steatorrhea (chronic)
AHA: 1Q, '88, 6

579.9 Unspecified intestinal malabsorption
Malabsorption syndrome NOS
AHA: 2Q, '11, 15; 4Q, '04, 59

577-579.9

✓4ᵗʰ ✓5ᵗʰ Additional Digit Required   Unspecified Code   Other Specified Code   Manifestation Code   ▶◀ Revised Text   ● New Code   ▲ Revised Code Title
2015 ICD-9-CM   **October 2014 • Volume 1 – 177**

10. Diseases of the Genitourinary System (580-629)

Nephritis, Nephrotic Syndrome, and Nephrosis (580-589)

EXCLUDES hypertensive chronic kidney disease (403.00-403.91, 404.00-404.93)

✓4th 580 Acute glomerulonephritis

INCLUDES acute nephritis

DEF: Acute, severe inflammation in tuft of capillaries that filter the kidneys.

580.0 With lesion of proliferative glomerulonephritis
Acute (diffuse) proliferative glomerulonephritis
Acute poststreptococcal glomerulonephritis

580.4 With lesion of rapidly progressive glomerulonephritis
Acute nephritis with lesion of necrotizing glomerulitis
DEF: Acute glomerulonephritis; progresses to ESRD with diffuse epithelial proliferation.

✓5th 580.8 With other specified pathological lesion in kidney

580.81 Acute glomerulonephritis in diseases classified elsewhere

Code first underlying disease, as:
infectious hepatitis (070.0-070.9)
mumps (072.79)
subacute bacterial endocarditis (421.0)
typhoid fever (002.0)

580.89 Other
Glomerulonephritis, acute, with lesion of:
exudative nephritis
interstitial (diffuse) (focal) nephritis

580.9 Acute glomerulonephritis with unspecified pathological lesion in kidney

Glomerulonephritis
  NOS
  hemorrhagic   } specified as acute
Nephritis
Nephropathy

✓4th 581 Nephrotic syndrome

DEF: Disease process marked by symptoms such as extensive edema, notable proteinuria, hypoalbuminemia, and susceptibility to intercurrent infections.

581.0 With lesion of proliferative glomerulonephritis

581.1 With lesion of membranous glomerulonephritis
Epimembranous nephritis
Idiopathic membranous glomerular disease
Nephrotic syndrome with lesion of:
  focal glomerulosclerosis
  sclerosing membranous glomerulonephritis
  segmental hyalinosis

581.2 With lesion of membranoproliferative glomerulonephritis
Nephrotic syndrome with lesion (of):
  endothelial
  hypocomplementemic persistent
  lobular
  mesangiocapillary
  mixed membranous and
  proliferative   } glomerulonephritis

DEF: Glomerulonephritis combined with clinical features of nephrotic syndrome; characterized by uneven thickening of glomerular capillary walls and mesangial cell increase; slowly progresses to ESRD.

581.3 With lesion of minimal change glomerulonephritis
Foot process disease
Lipoid nephrosis
Minimal change:
  glomerular disease
  glomerulitis
  nephrotic syndrome
AHA: 1Q, '07, 23

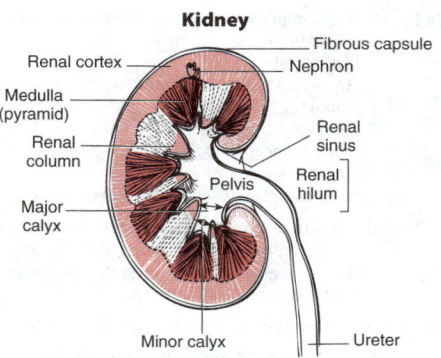

Kidney

Renal cortex — Fibrous capsule
— Nephron
Medulla (pyramid)
Renal column — Renal sinus
— Renal hilum
Pelvis
Major calyx
Minor calyx — Ureter

✓5th 581.8 With other specified pathological lesion in kidney

581.81 Nephrotic syndrome in diseases classified elsewhere

Code first underlying disease, as:
amyloidosis (277.30-277.39)
diabetes mellitus (249.4, 250.4)
tes mellitus (250.4)
malaria (084.9)
polyarteritis (446.0)
systemic lupus erythematosus (710.0)
EXCLUDES nephrosis in epidemic hemorrhagic fever (078.6)
AHA: 3Q, '91, 8, 12; S-O, '85, 3

581.89 Other
Glomerulonephritis with edema and lesion of:
exudative nephritis
interstitial (diffuse) (focal) nephritis

581.9 Nephrotic syndrome with unspecified pathological lesion in kidney
Glomerulonephritis with edema NOS
Nephritis:
  nephrotic NOS
  with edema NOS
Nephrosis NOS
Renal disease with edema NOS

✓4th 582 Chronic glomerulonephritis

INCLUDES chronic nephritis

DEF: Slow progressive type of nephritis characterized by inflammation of the capillary loops in the glomeruli of the kidney, which leads to renal failure.

582.0 With lesion of proliferative glomerulonephritis
Chronic (diffuse) proliferative glomerulonephritis

582.1 With lesion of membranous glomerulonephritis
Chronic glomerulonephritis:
  membranous
  sclerosing
Focal glomerulosclerosis
Segmental hyalinosis
AHA: S-O, '84, 16

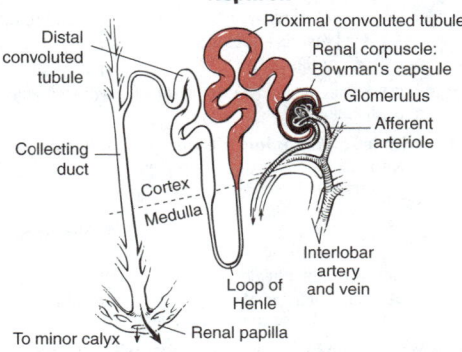

Nephron

Distal convoluted tubule — Proximal convoluted tubule
Renal corpuscle: Bowman's capsule
Collecting duct
Cortex
Medulla
Glomerulus
Afferent arteriole
Loop of Henle
Interlobar artery and vein
To minor calyx — Renal papilla

✓4th ✓5th Additional Digit Required   **Unspecified Code**   Other Specified Code   Manifestation Code   ►◄ Revised Text   ● New Code   ▲ Revised Code Title

2015 ICD-9-CM   **Volume 1 – 179**

582.2 With lesion of membranoproliferative glomerulonephritis

Chronic glomerulonephritis:
endothelial
hypocomplementemic persistent
lobular
membranoproliferative
mesangiocapillary
mixed membranous and proliferative

DEF: Chronic glomerulonephritis with mesangial cell proliferation.

582.4 With lesion of rapidly progressive glomerulonephritis

Chronic nephritis with lesion of necrotizing glomerulitis

DEF: Chronic glomerulonephritis rapidly progresses to ESRD; marked by diffuse epithelial proliferation.

√5ᵗʰ **582.8 With other specified pathological lesion in kidney**

582.81 **Chronic glomerulonephritis in diseases classified elsewhere**

Code first underlying disease, as:
amyloidosis (277.30-277.39)
systemic lupus erythematosus (710.0)

582.89 Other

Chronic glomerulonephritis with lesion of:
exudative nephritis
interstitial (diffuse) (focal) nephritis

582.9 Chronic glomerulonephritis with unspecified pathological lesion in kidney

Glomerulonephritis:
  NOS
  hemorrhagic   ⎤
Nephritis   ⎬ specified as chronic
Nephropathy   ⎦

AHA: 2Q, '01, 12

√4ᵗʰ **583 Nephritis and nephropathy, not specified as acute or chronic**

INCLUDES "renal disease" so stated, not specified as acute or chronic but with stated pathology or cause

583.0 With lesion of proliferative glomerulonephritis

Proliferative:
glomerulonephritis (diffuse) NOS
nephritis NOS
nephropathy NOS

583.1 With lesion of membranous glomerulonephritis

Membranous:
glomerulonephritis NOS
nephritis NOS
Membranous nephropathy NOS

DEF: Kidney inflammation or dysfunction with deposits on glomerular capillary basement membranes.

N05.2 Uns nephritic syndr w/ diffuse membranous gln   I-10

583.2 With lesion of membranoproliferative glomerulonephritis

Membranoproliferative:
glomerulonephritis NOS
nephritis NOS
nephropathy NOS
Nephritis NOS, with lesion of:
  hypocomplementemic persistent ⎤
  lobular   ⎬ glomerulonephritis
  mesangiocapillary   ⎪
  mixed membranous and   ⎦
    proliferative

DEF: Kidney inflammation or dysfunction with mesangial cell proliferation.

583.4 With lesion of rapidly progressive glomerulonephritis

Necrotizing or rapidly progressive:
glomerulitis NOS
glomerulonephritis NOS
nephritis NOS
nephropathy NOS
Nephritis, unspecified, with lesion of necrotizing glomerulitis

DEF: Kidney inflammation or dysfunction; rapidly progresses to ESRD marked by diffuse epithelial proliferation.

583.6 With lesion of renal cortical necrosis

Nephritis, NOS   ⎤
Nephropathy NOS ⎬ with (renal) cortical necrosis
               ⎦
Renal cortical necrosis NOS

583.7 With lesion of renal medullary necrosis

Nephritis, NOS   ⎤ with (renal) medullary
Nephropathy NOS ⎬ [papillary] necrosis
               ⎦

√5ᵗʰ **583.8 With other specified pathological lesion in kidney**

583.81 **Nephritis and nephropathy, not specified as acute or chronic, in diseases classified elsewhere**

Code first underlying disease, as:
amyloidosis (277.30-277.39)
diabetes mellitus (249.4, 250.4)
gonococcal infection (098.19)
Goodpasture's syndrome (446.21)
systemic lupus erythematosus (710.0)
tuberculosis (016.0)

EXCLUDES gouty nephropathy (274.10)
syphilitic nephritis (095.4)

AHA: ▶2Q, '13, 6;◀ 2Q, '12, 19; 2Q, '03, 7; 3Q, '91, 8; S-O, '85, 3

583.89 Other

Glomerulitis   ⎤
Glomerulonephritis ⎪ with lesions of:
Nephritis   ⎬ exudative nephritis
Nephropathy   ⎪ interstitial nephritis
Renal disease   ⎦

583.9 With unspecified pathological lesion in kidney

Glomerulitis   ⎤
Glomerulonephritis ⎬ NOS
Nephritis   ⎪
Nephropathy   ⎦

EXCLUDES nephropathy complicating pregnancy, labor, or the puerperium (642.0-642.9, 646.2)
renal disease NOS with no stated cause (593.9)

√4ᵗʰ **584 Acute kidney failure**

INCLUDES acute renal failure

EXCLUDES following labor and delivery (669.3)
posttraumatic (958.5)
that complicating:
  abortion (634-638 with .3, 639.3)
  ectopic or molar pregnancy (639.3)

DEF: State resulting from increasing urea and related substances from the blood (azotemia), often with urine output of less than 500 ml per day.

AHA: 2Q, '11, 15; 3Q, '10, 15; 1Q, '93, 18; 2Q, '92, 5; 4Q, '92, 22

TIP: Report acute renal failure separately when documented in addition to or in association with hypertensive renal disease..

584.5 Acute kidney failure with lesion of tubular necrosis

Lower nephron nephrosis
Renal failure with (acute) tubular necrosis
Tubular necrosis:
  NOS
  acute

DEF: Acute decline in kidney efficiency with destruction of tubules.

N17.0 Acute renal failure with tubular necrosis   I-10

584.6 Acute kidney failure with lesion of renal cortical necrosis

DEF: Acute decline in kidney efficiency with destruction of renal tissues that filter blood.

584.7 Acute kidney failure with lesion of renal medullary [papillary] necrosis

Necrotizing renal papillitis

DEF: Acute decline in kidney efficiency with destruction of renal tissues that collect urine.

584.8 Acute kidney failure with other specified pathological lesion in kidney

AHA: 3Q, '11, 16-17; N-D, '85, 1

584.9 Acute kidney failure, unspecified

Acute kidney injury (nontraumatic)

EXCLUDES traumatic kidney injury (866.00-866.13)

AHA: 3Q, '11, 16-17; 4Q, '09, 98; 4Q, '08, 192; 4Q, '07, 97; 2Q, '05, 18; 2Q, '03, 7; 1Q, '03, 22; 3Q, '02, 21, 28; 2Q, '01, 14; 1Q, '00, 22; 3Q, '96, 9; 4Q, '88, 1

N17.9 Acute renal failure unspecified   I-10

N Newborn Age: 0   **P** Pediatric Age: 0-17   **M** Maternity Age: 12-55   **A** Adult Age: 15-124

Diseases of the Genitourinary System

585–590.2

✓4th **585 Chronic kidney disease [CKD]**
Chronic uremia

Code first hypertensive chronic kidney disease, if applicable, (403.00-403.91, 404.00-404.93)

Use additional code to identify kidney transplant status, if applicable (V42.0)

Use additional code to identify manifestation as:
uremic:
neuropathy (357.4)
pericarditis (420.0)

AHA: 4Q, '06, 84-86; 4Q, '05, 68, 77; 1Q, '04, 5; 4Q, '03, 61, 111; 2Q, '03, 7; 2Q, '01, 12, 13; 1Q, '01, 3; 4Q, '98, 55; 3Q, '98, 6, 7; 2Q, '98, 20; 3Q, '96, 9; 1Q, '93, 18; 3Q, '91, 8; 4Q, '89, 1; N-D, '85, 15; S-O, '84, 3

585.1 Chronic kidney disease, Stage I
DEF: Some kidney damage; normal or slightly increased GFR (> 90).

585.2 Chronic kidney disease, Stage II (mild)
DEF: Kidney damage with mild decrease in GFR (60–89).

585.3 Chronic kidney disease, Stage III (moderate)
AHA: ▶2Q, '13, 13;◀ 4Q, '05, 69
DEF: Kidney damage with moderate decrease in GFR (30–59).
N18.3 Chronic kidney disease stage 3 (moderate) I-10

585.4 Chronic kidney disease, Stage IV (severe)
DEF: Kidney damage with severe decrease in GFR (15–29).
N18.4 Chronic kidney disease stage 4 (severe) I-10

585.5 Chronic kidney disease, Stage V
EXCLUDES chronic kidney disease, stage V requiring chronic dialysis (585.6)
DEF: Kidney failure with GFR value of less than 15.
AHA: ▶2Q, '13, 6;◀ 4Q, '10, 137

585.6 End stage renal disease
Chronic kidney disease requiring chronic dialysis
DEF: Federal government indicator of a stage V CKD patient undergoing treatment by dialysis or transplantation.
AHA: ▶2Q, '13, 5;◀ 3Q, '11,15; 2Q, '11, 6; 3Q, '10, 12, 15; 4Q, '08, 193; 1Q, '08, 7; 4Q, '07, 86; 3Q, '07, 5, 9; 4Q, '06, 136; 4Q, '05, 79
N18.6 End stage renal disease I-10

585.9 Chronic kidney disease, unspecified
Chronic renal disease   Chronic renal insufficiency
Chronic renal failure NOS
AHA: 1Q, '08, 10; 2Q, '07, 3; 4Q, '06, 86; 4Q, '05, 79
N18.9 Chronic kidney disease unspecified I-10

586 Renal failure, unspecified
Uremia NOS
EXCLUDES following labor and delivery (669.3)
posttraumatic renal failure (958.5)
that complicating:
abortion (634-638 with .3, 639.3)
ectopic or molar pregnancy (639.3)
uremia:
extrarenal (788.9)
prerenal (788.9)
DEF: Renal failure: kidney functions cease; malfunction may be due to inability to excrete metabolized substances or retain level of electrolytes.
DEF: Uremia: excess urea, creatinine and other nitrogenous products of protein and amino acid metabolism in blood due to reduced excretory function in bilateral kidney disease; also called azotemia.
AHA: 3Q, '98, 6; 1Q, '93, 18; 1Q, '88, 3
N19 Unspecified renal failure I-10

Genitourinary System

Inferior vena cava
Right kidney
Anterior division of internal iliac artery
Superior and Inferior vesicular arteries
Ureteral orifice
Urethra
Aorta
Left kidney
Ureter
Ovarian or testicular artery and vein
Urinary bladder
Urogenital diaphragm

587 Renal sclerosis, unspecified
Atrophy of kidney
Contracted kidney
Renal:
cirrhosis
fibrosis
AHA: 4Q, '10, 137

✓4th **588 Disorders resulting from impaired renal function**

588.0 Renal osteodystrophy
Azotemic osteodystrophy
Phosphate-losing tubular disorders
Renal:
dwarfism
infantilism
rickets
DEF: Condition resulting from chronic renal failure results in osteomalacia, osteoporosis or osteosclerosis; an abnormal level of phosphorus in the blood and impaired stimulation of the parathyroid.

588.1 Nephrogenic diabetes insipidus
EXCLUDES diabetes insipidus NOS (253.5)
DEF: Type of diabetes due to renal tubules inability to reabsorb water; not responsive to vasopressin; may develop into chronic renal insufficiency.

✓5th **588.8 Other specified disorders resulting from impaired renal function**
EXCLUDES secondary hypertension (405.0-405.9)

588.81 Secondary hyperparathyroidism (of renal origin)
Secondary hyperparathyroidism NOS
DEF: Parathyroid dysfunction caused by chronic renal failure; phosphate clearance is impaired, phosphate is released from bone, vitamin D is not produced, intestinal calcium absorption is low, and blood levels of calcium are lowered causing excessive production of parathyroid hormone.
AHA: 4Q, '04, 58-59
N25.81 Secondary hyperparathyroidism of renal origin I-10

588.89 Other specified disorders resulting from impaired renal function
Hypokalemic nephropathy

588.9 Unspecified disorder resulting from impaired renal function

✓4th **589 Small kidney of unknown cause**

589.0 Unilateral small kidney

589.1 Bilateral small kidneys

589.9 Small kidney, unspecified

Other Diseases of Urinary System (590-599)

✓4th **590 Infections of kidney**
Use additional code to identify organism, such as Escherichia coli [E. coli] (041.41-041.49)

✓5th **590.0 Chronic pyelonephritis**
Chronic pyelitis
Chronic pyonephrosis
Code if applicable, any casual condition first

590.00 Without lesion of renal medullary necrosis

590.01 With lesion of renal medullary necrosis

✓5th **590.1 Acute pyelonephritis**
Acute pyelitis
Acute pyonephrosis

590.10 Without lesion of renal medullary necrosis

590.11 With lesion of renal medullary necrosis

590.2 Renal and perinephric abscess
Abscess:
kidney
nephritic
perirenal
Carbuncle of kidney

✓4th ✓5th Additional Digit Required   **Unspecified Code**   Other Specified Code   Manifestation Code   ▶◀ Revised Text   ● New Code   ▲ Revised Code Title

Diseases of the Genitourinary System

585–590.2

Diseases of the Genitourinary System

590.3–594.9

590.3 Pyeloureteritis cystica
Infection of renal pelvis and ureter
Ureteritis cystica
DEF: Inflammation and formation of submucosal cysts in the kidney, pelvis, and ureter.

√5ᵗʰ **590.8 Other pyelonephritis or pyonephrosis, not specified as acute or chronic**

590.80 Pyelonephritis, unspecified
Pyelitis NOS
Pyelonephritis NOS
AHA: 1Q, '98, 10; 4Q, '97, 40
N11.9 Chronic tubulo-interstitial nephritis uns   I-10

590.81 Pyelitis or pyelonephritis in diseases classified elsewhere
Code first underlying disease, as:
tuberculosis (016.0)

590.9 Infection of kidney, unspecified
EXCLUDES urinary tract infection NOS (599.0)

591 Hydronephrosis
Hydrocalycosis
Hydronephrosis
Hydroureteronephrosis
EXCLUDES congenital hydronephrosis (753.29)
hydroureter (593.5)
DEF: Distention of kidney and pelvis, with urine build-up due to ureteral obstruction; pyonephrosis may result.
AHA: 3Q, '12, 11-12; 2Q, '98, 9
TIP: Hydronephrosis is not inherent in urinary obstructions and should be coded separately.
N13.30 Unspecified hydronephrosis   I-10

√4ᵗʰ **592 Calculus of kidney and ureter**
EXCLUDES nephrocalcinosis (275.4)

592.0 Calculus of kidney
Nephrolithiasis NOS
Renal calculus or stone
Staghorn calculus
Stone in kidney
EXCLUDES uric acid nephrolithiasis (274.11)
AHA: 3Q, '12, 11-12; 1Q, '00, 4
N20.0 Calculus of kidney   I-10

592.1 Calculus of ureter
Ureteric stone
Ureterolithiasis
AHA: 2Q, '98, 9; 1Q, '98, 10; 1Q, '91, 11
N20.1 Calculus of ureter   I-10

592.9 Urinary calculus, unspecified
AHA: 1Q, '98, 10; 4Q, '97, 40

√4ᵗʰ **593 Other disorders of kidney and ureter**

593.0 Nephroptosis
Floating kidney
Mobile kidney

593.1 Hypertrophy of kidney

593.2 Cyst of kidney, acquired
Cyst (multiple) (solitary) of kidney, not congenital
Peripelvic (lymphatic) cyst
EXCLUDES calyceal or pyelogenic cyst of kidney (591)
congenital cyst of kidney (753.1)
polycystic (disease of) kidney (753.1)
DEF: Abnormal, fluid-filled sac in the kidney, not present at birth.
AHA: 4Q, '90, 3
N28.1 Cyst of kidney acquired   I-10

593.3 Stricture or kinking of ureter
Angulation ⎫
Constriction ⎬ of ureter (post-operative)
Stricture of pelviureteric junction
DEF: Stricture or knot in tube connecting kidney to bladder.
AHA: 2Q, '98, 9

593.4 Other ureteric obstruction
Idiopathic retroperitoneal fibrosis
Occlusion NOS of ureter
EXCLUDES that due to calculus (592.1)
AHA: 1Q, '10, 9; 2Q, '97, 4

593.5 Hydroureter
EXCLUDES congenital hydroureter (753.22)
hydroureteronephrosis (591)

593.6 Postural proteinuria
Benign postural proteinuria
Orthostatic proteinuria
EXCLUDES proteinuria NOS (791.0)
DEF: Excessive amounts of serum protein in the urine caused by the body position, e.g., orthostatic and lordotic.

√5ᵗʰ **593.7 Vesicoureteral reflux**
DEF: Backflow of urine, from bladder into ureter due to obstructed bladder neck.
AHA: 4Q, '94, 42

593.70 Unspecified or without reflux nephropathy

593.71 With reflux nephropathy, unilateral

593.72 With reflux nephropathy, bilateral

593.73 With reflux nephropathy NOS

√5ᵗʰ **593.8 Other specified disorders of kidney and ureter**

593.81 Vascular disorders of kidney
Renal (artery):
embolism
hemorrhage
thrombosis
Renal infarction

593.82 Ureteral fistula
Intestinoureteral fistula
EXCLUDES fistula between ureter and female genital tract (619.0)
DEF: Abnormal communication, between tube connecting kidney to bladder and another structure.

593.89 Other
Adhesions, kidney or ureter
Periureteritis
Polyp of ureter
Pyelectasia
Ureterocele
EXCLUDES tuberculosis of ureter (016.2)
ureteritis cystica (590.3)

593.9 Unspecified disorder of kidney and ureter
Acute renal disease
Acute renal insufficiency
Renal disease NOS
Salt-losing nephritis or syndrome
EXCLUDES chronic renal insufficiency (585.9)
cystic kidney disease (753.1)
nephropathy, so stated (583.0-583.9)
renal disease:
arising in pregnancy or the puerperium
(642.1-642.2, 642.4-642.7, 646.2)
not specified as acute or chronic, but with stated
pathology or cause (583.0-583.9)
AHA: 4Q, '05, 79; 1Q, '93, 17
N28.9 Disorder of kidney and ureter unspecified   I-10

√4ᵗʰ **594 Calculus of lower urinary tract**

594.0 Calculus in diverticulum of bladder
DEF: Stone or mineral deposit in abnormal sac on the bladder wall.

594.1 Other calculus in bladder
Urinary bladder stone
EXCLUDES staghorn calculus (592.0)
DEF: Stone or mineral deposit in bladder.

594.2 Calculus in urethra
DEF: Stone or mineral deposit in tube that empties urine from bladder.

594.8 Other lower urinary tract calculus
AHA: J-F, '85, 16

594.9 Calculus of lower urinary tract, unspecified
EXCLUDES calculus of urinary tract NOS (592.9)

Bladder

Anterior View

Fundus
Left ureter
Right ureter
Lateral wall
Ureteral orifice
Trigone
Uvula of bladder
Urethra

Lateral View

Urachus
Left ureter
Peritoneum
Pubic bone
Urogenital diaphragm

✓4ᵗʰ 595 Cystitis

EXCLUDES *prostatocystitis (601.3)*

Use additional code to identify organism, such as Escherichia coli [E. coli] (041.41-041.49)

595.0 Acute cystitis

EXCLUDES *trigonitis (595.3)*

DEF: Acute inflammation of bladder.

AHA: 2Q, '99, 15

N30.00 Acute cystitis without hematuria I-10

595.1 Chronic interstitial cystitis

Hunner's ulcer
Panmural fibrosis of bladder
Submucous cystitis

DEF: Inflamed lesion affecting bladder wall; symptoms include urinary frequency, pain on bladder filling, nocturia, and distended bladder.

595.2 Other chronic cystitis

Chronic cystitis NOS
Subacute cystitis

EXCLUDES *trigonitis (595.3)*

DEF: Persistent inflammation of bladder.

595.3 Trigonitis

Follicular cystitis
Trigonitis (acute) (chronic)
Urethrotrigonitis

DEF: Inflammation of the triangular area of the bladder called the trigonum vesicae.

595.4 Cystitis in diseases classified elsewhere

Code first underlying disease, as:
actinomycosis (039.8)
amebiasis (006.8)
bilharziasis (120.0-120.9)
Echinococcus infestation (122.3, 122.6)

EXCLUDES *cystitis:*
diphtheritic (032.84)
gonococcal (098.11, 098.31)
monilial (112.2)
trichomonal (131.09)
tuberculous (016.1)

✓5ᵗʰ 595.8 Other specified types of cystitis

595.81 Cystitis cystica

DEF: Inflammation of the bladder characterized by formation of multiple cysts.

595.82 Irradiation cystitis

Use additional E code to identify cause

DEF: Inflammation of the bladder due to effects of radiation.

595.89 Other

Abscess of bladder:
Cystitis:
bullous
emphysematous
glandularis

595.9 Cystitis, unspecified

✓4ᵗʰ 596 Other disorders of bladder

Use additional code to identify urinary incontinence (625.6, 788.30-788.39)

AHA: M-A, '87, 10

596.0 Bladder neck obstruction

Contracture (acquired) } of bladder neck or
Obstruction (acquired) } vesicourethral
Stenosis (acquired) } orifice

EXCLUDES *congenital (753.6)*

DEF: Bladder outlet and vesicourethral obstruction; occurs as a consequence of benign prostatic hypertrophy or prostatic cancer; may also occur in either sex due to strictures, following radiation, cystoscopy, catheterization, injury, infection, blood clots, bladder cancer, impaction or disease compressing bladder neck.

AHA: 3Q, '02, 28; 2Q, '01, 14; N-D, '86, 10

N32.0 Bladder-neck obstruction I-10

596.1 Intestinovesical fistula

Fistula:
enterovesical
vesicocolic
vesicoenteric
vesicorectal

DEF: Abnormal communication, between intestine and bladder.

596.2 Vesical fistula, not elsewhere classified

Fistula:
bladder NOS
urethrovesical
vesicocutaneous
vesicoperineal

EXCLUDES *fistula between bladder and female genital tract (619.0)*

DEF: Abnormal communication between bladder and another structure.

596.3 Diverticulum of bladder

Diverticulitis } of bladder
Diverticulum (acquired) (false) }

EXCLUDES *that with calculus in diverticulum of bladder (594.0)*

DEF: Abnormal pouch in bladder wall.

596.4 Atony of bladder

High compliance bladder
Hypotonicity } of bladder
Inertia }

EXCLUDES *neurogenic bladder (596.54)*

DEF: Distended, bladder with loss of expulsive force; linked to CNS disease.

✓5ᵗʰ 596.5 Other functional disorders of bladder

EXCLUDES *cauda equina syndrome with neurogenic bladder (344.61)*

596.51 Hypertonicity of bladder

Hyperactivity
Overactive bladder

DEF: Abnormal tension of muscular wall of bladder; may appear after surgery of voluntary nerve.

N32.81 Overactive bladder I-10

596.52 Low bladder compliance

DEF: Low bladder capacity; causes increased pressure and frequent urination.

596.53 Paralysis of bladder

DEF: Impaired bladder motor function due to nerve or muscle damage.

596.54 Neurogenic bladder NOS

DEF: Unspecified dysfunctional bladder due to lesion of central, peripheral nervous system; may result in incontinence, residual urine retention, urinary infection, stones and renal failure.

AHA: 1Q, '01, 12

N31.9 Neuromuscular dysfunction of bladder unspecified I-10

✓4ᵗʰ ✓5ᵗʰ Additional Digit Required | **Unspecified Code** | Other Specified Code | Manifestation Code | ►◄ Revised Text | ● New Code | ▲ Revised Code Title

Diseases of the Genitourinary System

596.55–599.72

596.55 Detrusor sphincter dyssynergia
DEF: Instability of the urinary bladder sphincter muscle associated with urinary incontinence.

596.59 Other functional disorder of bladder
Detrusor instability
DEF: Detrusor instability: instability of bladder; marked by uninhibited contractions often leading to incontinence.

596.6 Rupture of bladder, nontraumatic

596.7 Hemorrhage into bladder wall
Hyperemia of bladder
EXCLUDES *acute hemorrhagic cystitis (595.0)*

√5th **596.8 Other specified disorders of bladder**
EXCLUDES *cystocele, female (618.01-618.02, 618.09, 618.2-618.4)*
hernia or prolapse of bladder, female (618.01-618.02, 618.09, 618.2-618.4)
AHA: 4Q, '11, 128-129; J-F, '85, 8

596.81 Infection of cystostomy
Use additional code to specify type of infection, such as:
abscess or cellulitis of abdomen (682.2)
septicemia (038.0-038.9)
Use additional code to identify organism (041.00-041.9)
AHA: 4Q, '11, 129

596.82 Mechanical complication of cystostomy
Malfunction of cystostomy

596.83 Other complication of cystostomy
Fistula
Hernia
Prolapse

596.89 Other specified disorders of bladder
Bladder hemorrhage
Bladder hypertrophy
Calcified bladder
Contracted bladder
AHA: ▶1Q, '13, 5◀

596.9 Unspecified disorder of bladder
AHA: J-F, '85, 8

√4th **597 Urethritis, not sexually transmitted, and urethral syndrome**
EXCLUDES *nonspecific urethritis, so stated (099.4)*

597.0 Urethral abscess
Abscess: Abscess of:
  periurethral   Cowper's gland
  urethral (gland)   Littré's gland
Abscess of: Periurethral cellulitis
  bulbourethral gland
EXCLUDES *urethral caruncle (599.3)*
DEF: Pocket of pus in tube that empties urine from the bladder.

√5th **597.8 Other urethritis**

597.80 Urethritis, unspecified

597.81 Urethral syndrome NOS

597.89 Other
Adenitis, Skene's glands
Cowperitis
Meatitis, urethral
Ulcer, urethra (meatus)
Verumontanitis
EXCLUDES *trichomonal (131.02)*

√4th **598 Urethral stricture**
Use additional code to identify urinary incontinence (625.6, 788.30-788.39)
INCLUDES pinhole meatus
stricture of urinary meatus
EXCLUDES *congenital stricture of urethra and urinary meatus (753.6)*
DEF: Narrowing of tube that empties urine from bladder.

√5th **598.0 Urethral stricture due to infection**

598.00 Due to unspecified infection

598.01 Due to infective diseases classified elsewhere
Code first underlying disease, as:
gonococcal infection (098.2)
schistosomiasis (120.0-120.9)
syphilis (095.8)

598.1 Traumatic urethral stricture
Stricture of urethra:
late effect of injury
postobstetric
EXCLUDES *postoperative following surgery on genitourinary tract (598.2)*

598.2 Postoperative urethral stricture
Postcatheterization stricture of urethra
AHA: 3Q, '97, 6

598.8 Other specified causes of urethral stricture
AHA: N-D, '84, 9

598.9 Urethral stricture, unspecified

√4th **599 Other disorders of urethra and urinary tract**

599.0 Urinary tract infection, site not specified
EXCLUDES *candidiasis of urinary tract (112.2)*
urinary tract infection of newborn (771.82)
Use additional code to identify organism, such as Escherichia coli [E. coli] (041.41-041.49)
AHA: 2Q, '12, 20; 1Q, '12, 11; 4Q, '11, 129; 1Q, '10, 9; 3Q, '09, 10-11; 3Q, '05, 12; 2Q, '04, 13; 4Q, '03, 79; 4Q, '99, 6; 2Q, '99, 15; 1Q, '98, 5; 2Q, '96, 7; 4Q, '96, 33; 2Q, '95, 7; 1Q, '92, 13
N39.0 Urinary tract infection site not specified   I-10

599.1 Urethral fistula
Fistula: Urinary fistula NOS
  urethroperineal
  urethrorectal
EXCLUDES *fistula:*
urethroscrotal (608.89)
urethrovaginal (619.0)
urethrovesicovaginal (619.0)
AHA: 2Q, '11, 13; 3Q, '97, 6

599.2 Urethral diverticulum
DEF: Abnormal pouch in urethral wall.

599.3 Urethral caruncle
Polyp of urethra

599.4 Urethral false passage
DEF: Abnormal opening in urethra due to surgery; trauma or disease.

599.5 Prolapsed urethral mucosa
Prolapse of urethra   Urethrocele
EXCLUDES *urethrocele, female (618.03, 618.09, 618.2-618.4)*

√5th **599.6 Urinary obstruction**
Use additional code to identify urinary incontinence (625.6, 788.30-788.39)
EXCLUDES *obstructive nephropathy NOS (593.89)*
AHA: 4Q, '05, 80

599.60 Urinary obstruction, unspecified
Obstructive uropathy NOS
Urinary (tract) obstruction NOS
N13.9 Obstructive and reflux uropathy unspec   I-10

599.69 Urinary obstruction, not elsewhere classified
Code, if applicable, any causal condition first, such as:
hyperplasia of prostate (600.0-600.9 with fifth-digit 1)
AHA: 4Q, '06, 93

√5th **599.7 Hematuria**
Hematuria (benign) (essential)
EXCLUDES *hemoglobinuria (791.2)*
AHA: 4Q, '08, 121; 1Q, '00, 5; 3Q, '95, 8

599.70 Hematuria, unspecified
R31.9 Hematuria unspecified   I-10

599.71 Gross hematuria
AHA: 2Q, '10, 3; 2Q, '10, 3

599.72 Microscopic hematuria

N Newborn Age: 0   P Pediatric Age: 0-17   M Maternity Age: 12-55   A Adult Age: 15-124

✓5ᵗʰ **599.8 Other specified disorders of urethra and urinary tract**

Use additional code to identify urinary incontinence (625.6, 788.30-788.39), if present

EXCLUDES symptoms and other conditions classifiable to 788.0-788.2, 788.4-788.9, 791.0-791.9

599.81 Urethral hypermobility
DEF: Hyperactive urethra.

599.82 Intrinsic (urethral) sphincter deficiency [ISD]
DEF: Malfunctioning urethral sphincter.
AHA: 2Q, '96, 15

599.83 Urethral instability
DEF: Inconsistent functioning of urethra.

599.84 Other specified disorders of urethra
Rupture of urethra (nontraumatic)
Urethral:
    cyst
    granuloma
DEF: Rupture of urethra due to herniation or breaking down of tissue; not due to trauma.
DEF: Urethral cyst: abnormal sac in urethra; usually fluid filled.
DEF: Granuloma: inflammatory cells forming small nodules in urethra.
AHA: 1Q, '09, 15

599.89 Other specified disorders of urinary tract

599.9 Unspecified disorder of urethra and urinary tract

Diseases of Male Genital Organs (600-608)

✓4ᵗʰ **600 Hyperplasia of prostate**
INCLUDES enlarged prostate
DEF: Fibrostromal proliferation in periurethral glands, causes blood in urine; etiology unknown.
AHA: 3Q, '05, 20; 4Q, '00, 43; 3Q, '94, 12; 3Q, '92, 7; N-D, '86, 10

✓5ᵗʰ **600.0 Hypertrophy (benign) of prostate**
Benign prostatic hypertrophy   Soft enlarged prostate
Enlargement of prostate
Smooth enlarged prostate
AHA: 4Q, '06, 93-95; 3Q, '05, 20; 4Q, '03, 63; 1Q, '03, 6; 3Q, '02, 28; 2Q, '01, 14

600.00 Hypertrophy (benign) of prostate without urinary obstruction and other lower urinary tract symptoms [LUTS]   A ♂
Hypertrophy (benign) of prostate NOS
N40.0 Enlarged prostate without LUTS   I-10

600.01 Hypertrophy (benign) of prostate with urinary obstruction and other lower urinary tract symptoms [LUTS]   A ♂
Hypertrophy (benign) of prostate with urinary retention

Use additional code to identify symptoms:
    incomplete bladder emptying (788.21)
    nocturia (788.43)
    straining on urination (788.65)
    urinary frequency (788.41)
    urinary hesitancy (788.64)
    urinary incontinence (788.30-788.39)
    urinary obstruction (599.69)
    urinary retention (788.20)
    urinary urgency (788.63)
    weak urinary stream (788.62)
AHA: 4Q, '06, 93-95; 4Q, '03, 64

✓5ᵗʰ **600.1 Nodular prostate**
Hard, firm prostate
Multinodular prostate
EXCLUDES malignant neoplasm of prostate (185)
DEF: Hard, firm nodule in prostate.
AHA: 4Q, '03, 63

600.10 Nodular prostate without urinary obstruction   A ♂
Nodular prostate NOS

600.11 Nodular prostate with urinary obstruction   A ♂
Nodular prostate with urinary retention

Male Pelvic Organs

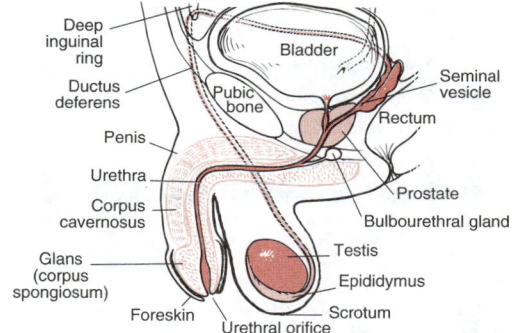

✓5ᵗʰ **600.2 Benign localized hyperplasia of prostate**
Adenofibromatous hypertrophy of prostate
Adenoma of prostate
Fibroadenoma of prostate
Fibroma of prostate
Myoma of prostate
Polyp of prostate
EXCLUDES benign neoplasms of prostate (222.2)
    hypertrophy of prostate (600.00-600.01)
    malignant neoplasm of prostate (185)
DEF: Benign localized hyperplasia clearly defined epithelial tumor.
AHA: 4Q, '06, 93-95; 4Q, '03, 63

600.20 Benign localized hyperplasia of prostate without urinary obstruction and other lower urinary tract symptoms [LUTS]   A ♂
Benign localized hyperplasia of prostate NOS

600.21 Benign localized hyperplasia of prostate with urinary obstruction and other lower urinary tract symptoms [LUTS]   A ♂
Benign localized hyperplasia of prostate with urinary retention

Use additional code to identify symptoms:
    incomplete bladder emptying (788.21)
    nocturia (788.43)
    straining on urination (788.65)
    urinary frequency (788.41)
    urinary hesitancy (788.64)
    urinary incontinence (788.30-788.39)
    urinary obstruction (599.69)
    urinary retention (788.20)
    urinary urgency (788.63)
    weak urinary stream (788.62)

600.3 Cyst of prostate   A ♂
DEF: Sacs of fluid, which differentiate this from either nodular or adenomatous tumors.

✓5ᵗʰ **600.9 Hyperplasia of prostate, unspecified**
Median bar
Prostatic obstruction NOS
AHA: 4Q, '06, 93-95; 4Q, '03, 63

600.90 Hyperplasia of prostate, unspecified, without urinary obstruction and other lower urinary tract symptoms [LUTS]   A ♂
Hyperplasia of prostate NOS

600.91 Hyperplasia of prostate, unspecified with urinary obstruction and other lower urinary tract symptoms [LUTS]   A ♂
Hyperplasia of prostate, unspecified, with urinary retention
Use additional code to identify symptoms:
    incomplete bladder emptying (788.21)
    nocturia (788.43)
    straining on urination (788.65)
    urinary frequency (788.41)
    urinary hesitancy (788.64)
    urinary incontinence (788.30-788.39)
    urinary obstruction (599.69)
    urinary retention (788.20)
    urinary urgency (788.63)
    weak urinary stream (788.62)

Diseases of the Genitourinary System

601–606.9

✓4ᵗʰ **601 Inflammatory diseases of prostate**

Use additional code to identify organism, such as Staphylococcus (041.1), or Streptococcus (041.0)

601.0 Acute prostatitis   A ♂

601.1 Chronic prostatitis   A ♂

601.2 Abscess of prostate   A ♂

601.3 Prostatocystitis   A ♂

601.4 Prostatitis in diseases classified elsewhere   A ♂

Code first underlying disease, as:
actinomycosis (039.8)
blastomycosis (116.0)
syphilis (095.8)
tuberculosis (016.5)

EXCLUDES *prostatitis:*
gonococcal (098.12, 098.32)
monilial (112.2)
trichomonal (131.03)

601.8 Other specified inflammatory diseases of prostate   A ♂
Prostatitis:
cavitary
diverticular
granulomatous

601.9 Prostatitis, unspecified   A ♂
Prostatitis NOS

✓4ᵗʰ **602 Other disorders of prostate**

602.0 Calculus of prostate   A ♂
Prostatic stone
DEF: Stone or mineral deposit in prostate.

602.1 Congestion or hemorrhage of prostate   A ♂
DEF: Bleeding or fluid collection in prostate.

602.2 Atrophy of prostate   A ♂

602.3 Dysplasia of prostate   ♂
Prostatic intraepithelial neoplasia I (PIN I)
Prostatic intraepithelial neoplasia II (PIN II)
EXCLUDES *prostatic intraepithelial neoplasia III (PIN III) (233.4)*
DEF: Abnormality of shape and size of the intraepithelial tissues of the prostate; premalignant condition characterized by stalks and absence of a basilar cell layer; synonyms are intraductal dysplasia, large acinar atypical hyperplasia, atypical primary hyperplasia, hyperplasia with malignant changes, marked atypia, or duct-acinar dysplasia.
AHA: 4Q, '01, 46

602.8 Other specified disorders of prostate   A ♂
Fistula
Infarction } of prostate
Stricture
Periprostatic adhesions

602.9 Unspecified disorder of prostate   A ♂

✓4ᵗʰ **603 Hydrocele**

INCLUDES hydrocele of spermatic cord, testis or tunica vaginalis
EXCLUDES *congenital (778.6)*
DEF: Circumscribed collection of fluid in tunica vaginalis, spermatic cord or testis.

603.0 Encysted hydrocele   ♂

603.1 Infected hydrocele   ♂
Use additional code to identify organism

603.8 Other specified types of hydrocele   ♂

603.9 Hydrocele, unspecified   ♂

Common Inguinal Canal Anomalies

✓4ᵗʰ **604 Orchitis and epididymitis**

Use additional code to identify organism, such as:
Escherichia coli [E. coli] (041.41-041.49)
Staphylococcus (041.10-041.19)
Streptococcus (041.00-041.09)

604.0 Orchitis, epididymitis, and epididymo-orchitis, with abscess   ♂
Abscess of epididymis or testis

✓5ᵗʰ **604.9 Other orchitis, epididymitis, and epididymo-orchitis, without mention of abscess**

604.90 Orchitis and epididymitis, unspecified   ♂

604.91 Orchitis and epididymitis in diseases classified elsewhere   ♂

Code first underlying disease, as:
diphtheria (032.89)
filariasis (125.0-125.9)
syphilis (095.8)

EXCLUDES *orchitis:*
gonococcal (098.13, 098.33)
mumps (072.0)
tuberculous (016.5)
tuberculous epididymitis (016.4)

604.99 Other   ♂

605 Redundant prepuce and phimosis   ♂
Adherent prepuce
Paraphimosis
Phimosis (congenital)
Tight foreskin
DEF: Constriction of preputial orifice causing inability of the prepuce to be drawn back over the glans; it may be congenital or caused by infection.
AHA: 3Q, '08, 9

✓4ᵗʰ **606 Infertility, male**
AHA: 2Q, '96, 9

606.0 Azoospermia   A ♂
Absolute infertility
Infertility due to:
germinal (cell) aplasia
spermatogenic arrest (complete)
DEF: Absence of spermatozoa in the semen or inability to produce spermatozoa.

606.1 Oligospermia   A ♂
Infertility due to:
germinal cell desquamation
hypospermatogenesis
incomplete spermatogenic arrest
DEF: Insufficient number of sperm in semen.

606.8 Infertility due to extratesticular causes   A ♂
Infertility due to:
drug therapy
infection
obstruction of efferent ducts
radiation
systemic disease

606.9 Male infertility, unspecified   A ♂

N Newborn Age: 0   **P** Pediatric Age: 0-17   **M** Maternity Age: 12-55   **A** Adult Age: 15-124

√4ᵗʰ **607 Disorders of penis**
> *EXCLUDES* phimosis (605)

607.0 Leukoplakia of penis ♂
> Kraurosis of penis
> *EXCLUDES* carcinoma in situ of penis (233.5)
> erythroplasia of Queyrat (233.5)
> **DEF:** White, thickened patches on glans penis.

607.1 Balanoposthitis ♂
> Balanitis
> Use additional code to identify organism
> **DEF:** Inflammation of glans penis and prepuce.

607.2 Other inflammatory disorders of penis ♂
> Abscess
> Boil ⎫ of corpus cavernosum or
> Carbuncle ⎬ penis
> Cellulitis ⎭
> Cavernitis (penis)
> Use additional code to identify organism
> *EXCLUDES* herpetic infection (054.13)

607.3 Priapism ♂
> Painful erection
> **DEF:** Prolonged penile erection without sexual stimulation.

√5ᵗʰ **607.8 Other specified disorders of penis**

607.81 Balanitis xerotica obliterans ♂
> Induratio penis plastica
> **DEF:** Inflammation of the glans penis, caused by stricture of the opening of the prepuce.

607.82 Vascular disorders of penis ♂
> Embolisim
> Hematoma ⎫ of corpus
> (nontraumatic) ⎬ cavernosum
> Hemorrhage ⎬ or penis
> Thrombosis ⎭

607.83 Edema of penis ♂
> **DEF:** Fluid retention within penile tissues.

607.84 Impotence of organic origin Ⓐ ♂
> *EXCLUDES* nonorganic (302.72)
> **DEF:** Physiological cause interfering with erection.
> **AHA:** 3Q, '91, 11
> **TIP:** If impotence is a result of previous radical prostatectomy, report code 997.99 first.

607.85 Peyronie's disease ♂
> **DEF:** A severe curvature of the erect penis due to fibrosis of the cavernous sheaths.
> **AHA:** 4Q, '03, 64

607.89 Other ♂
> Atrophy
> Fibrosis ⎫ of corpus cavernosum or
> Hypertrophy ⎬ penis
> Ulcer (chronic) ⎭

607.9 Unspecified disorder of penis ♂

√4ᵗʰ **608 Other disorders of male genital organs**

608.0 Seminal vesiculitis ♂
> Abscess ⎫ of seminal vesicle
> Cellulitis ⎬
> Vesiculitis (seminal)
> Use additional code to identify organism
> *EXCLUDES* gonococcal infection (098.14, 098.34)
> **DEF:** Inflammation of seminal vesicle.

608.1 Spermatocele ♂
> **DEF:** Cystic enlargement of the epididymis or the testis; the cysts contain spermatozoa.

√5ᵗʰ **608.2 Torsion of testis**
> **DEF:** Twisted or rotated testis; may compromise blood flow.

608.20 Torsion of testis, unspecified ♂
> **AHA:** 4Q, '06, 95

Torsion of the Testis

Appendix testis · Appendix epididymis · Epididymis · Spermatic cord · Torsion of appendix epididymis · Extravaginal torsion · Intravaginal torsion · Testicle · Torsion of appendix testis · Tunica vaginalis · Tunica vaginalis

608.21 Extravaginal torsion of spermatic cord ♂
> **DEF:** Torsion of the spermatic cord just below the tunica vaginalis attachments.
> **AHA:** 4Q, '06, 95

608.22 Intravaginal torsion of spermatic cord ♂
> Torsion of spermatic cord NOS
> **DEF:** Torsion within the tunica vaginalis also called the "bell-clapper" anomaly. It usually occurs in older children.
> **AHA:** 4Q, '06, 95

608.23 Torsion of appendix testis ♂
> **DEF:** Torsion of small solid projection of tissue on the upper outer surface of the testis (hydatid of Morgagni); a remnant of the embryologic Müllerian duct.
> **AHA:** 4Q, '06, 95

608.24 Torsion of appendix epididymis ♂
> **DEF:** Torsion of small stalked appendage of the head of the epididymis (pedunculated hydatid); a detached embryologic efferent duct.
> **AHA:** 4Q, '06, 95

608.3 Atrophy of testis ♂

608.4 Other inflammatory disorders of male genital organs ♂
> Abscess ⎫ of scrotum, spermatic cord, testis
> Boil ⎬ [except abscess], tunica
> Carbuncle ⎬ vaginalis, or vas deferens
> Cellulitis ⎭
> Vasitis
> Use additional code to identify organism
> *EXCLUDES* abscess of testis (604.0)

√5ᵗʰ **608.8 Other specified disorders of male genital organs**

608.81 Disorders of male genital organs in diseases classified elsewhere ♂
> *Code first underlying disease, as:*
> *filariasis (125.0-125.9)*
> *tuberculosis (016.5)*

608.82 Hematospermia ♂
> **DEF:** Presence of blood in the ejaculate; relatively common, affecting men of any age after puberty; cause is often the result of a viral or bacterial infection and inflammation.
> **AHA:** 4Q, '01, 46

608.83 Vascular disorders ♂
> Hematoma (non- ⎫ of seminal vessel, spermatic
> traumatic) ⎬ cord, testis, scrotum,
> Hemorrhage ⎬ tunica vaginalis, or vas
> Thrombosis ⎭ deferens
> Hematocele NOS, male
> **AHA:** 4Q, '03, 110
> **TIP:** Assign for Fournier's gangrene, which is a result of an infection in the genital area.

608.84 Chylocele of tunica vaginalis ♂
> **DEF:** Chylous effusion into tunica vaginalis; due to infusion of lymphatic fluids.

608.85 Stricture ♂
> Stricture of:
> spermatic cord
> tunica vaginalis
> vas deferens

608.86 Edema ♂

√4ᵗʰ / √5ᵗʰ Additional Digit Required   **Unspecified Code**   **Other Specified Code**   **Manifestation Code**   ►◄ Revised Text   ● New Code   ▲ Revised Code Title

2015 ICD-9-CM   **Volume 1 – 187**

Diseases of the Genitourinary System

608.87–612.1

608.87 Retrograde ejaculation   ♂
DEF: Condition where the semen travels to the bladder rather than out through the urethra due to damaged nerves causing the bladder neck to remain open during ejaculation.
AHA: 4Q, '01, 46

608.89 Other   ♂
Atrophy ⎱ of seminal vessel, spermatic
Fibrosis   cord, testis, scrotum,
Hypertrophy ⎰ tunica vaginalis, or vas
Ulcer   deferens
EXCLUDES atrophy of testis (608.3)

608.9 Unspecified disorder of male genital organs   ♂

Disorders of Breast (610-612)

✓4ᵗʰ 610 Benign mammary dysplasias

610.0 Solitary cyst of breast
Cyst (solitary) of breast

610.1 Diffuse cystic mastopathy   A
Chronic cystic mastitis
Cystic breast
Fibrocystic disease of
breast
DEF: Extensive formation of nodular cysts in breast tissue; symptoms include tenderness, change in size and hyperplasia of ductal epithelium.
AHA: 2Q, '06, 10
TIP: Assign in addition to screening mammography V code; is a normal variant, commonly found in normal breasts and not a pathological condition.

610.2 Fibroadenosis of breast
Fibroadenosis of breast:
NOS
chronic
cystic
diffuse
periodic
segmental
DEF: Non-neoplastic nodular condition of breast.

610.3 Fibrosclerosis of breast
DEF: Fibrous tissue in breast.

610.4 Mammary duct ectasia
Comedomastitis
Duct ectasia
Mastitis:
periductal
plasma cell
DEF: Atrophy of duct epithelium; causes distended collecting ducts of mammary gland, drying up of breast secretion, intraductal inflammation and periductal and interstitial chronic inflammatory reaction.

610.8 Other specified benign mammary dysplasias
Mazoplasia
Sebaceous cyst of breast
AHA: 2Q, '09, 9

610.9 Benign mammary dysplasia, unspecified

✓4ᵗʰ 611 Other disorders of breast
EXCLUDES that associated with lactation or the puerperium (675.0-676.9)

611.0 Inflammatory disease of breast
Abscess (acute) (chronic) (nonpuerperal) of:
areola
breast
Mammillary fistula
Mastitis (acute) (subacute) (nonpuerperal):
NOS
infective
retromammary
submammary
EXCLUDES carbuncle of breast (680.2)
chronic cystic mastitis (610.1)
neonatal infective mastitis (771.5)
thrombophlebitis of breast [Mondor's disease] (451.89)
AHA: ▶2Q, '13, 23◀

611.1 Hypertrophy of breast
Gynecomastia
Hypertrophy of breast:
NOS
massive pubertal
EXCLUDES breast engorgement in newborn (778.7)
disproportion of reconstructed breast (612.1)

611.2 Fissure of nipple

611.3 Fat necrosis of breast
Fat necrosis (segmental) of breast
Code first breast necrosis due to breast graft (996.79)
DEF: Splitting of neutral fats in adipose tissue cells as a result of trauma; a firm circumscribed mass is then formed in the breast.

611.4 Atrophy of breast

611.5 Galactocele
DEF: Milk-filled cyst in breast due to blocked duct.

611.6 Galactorrhea not associated with childbirth
DEF: Flow of milk not associated with childbirth or pregnancy.

✓5ᵗʰ 611.7 Signs and symptoms in breast

611.71 Mastodynia
Pain in breast

611.72 Lump or mass in breast
AHA: 4Q, '09, 106; 2Q, '03, 4-5
TIP: Do not assign if the underlying cause of the breast lump or mass is determined and documented during the episode of care.

611.79 Other
Induration of breast
Inversion of nipple
Nipple discharge
Retraction of nipple

✓5ᵗʰ 611.8 Other specified disorders of breast
AHA: 4Q, '08, 121-122

611.81 Ptosis of breast   A
EXCLUDES ptosis of native breast in relation to reconstructed breast (612.1)

611.82 Hypoplasia of breast   A
Micromastia
EXCLUDES congenital absence of breast (757.6)
hypoplasia of native breast in relation to reconstructed breast (612.1)

611.83 Capsular contracture of breast implant   A
TIP: Do not assign additional code from category 996 Complications peculiar to certain specified procedures.

611.89 Other specified disorders of breast
Hematoma (nontraumatic) of breast
Infarction of breast
Occlusion of breast duct
Subinvolution of breast (postlactational) (postpartum)

611.9 Unspecified breast disorder

✓4ᵗʰ 612 Deformity and disproportion of reconstructed breast
AHA: 4Q, '08, 123

612.0 Deformity of reconstructed breast   A
Contour irregularity in reconstructed breast
Excess tissue in reconstructed breast
Misshapen reconstructed breast

612.1 Disproportion of reconstructed breast   A
Breast asymmetry between native breast and reconstructed breast
Disproportion between native breast and reconstructed breast

N Newborn Age: 0   **P** Pediatric Age: 0-17   **M** Maternity Age: 12-55   **A** Adult Age: 15-124

Inflammatory Disease of Female Pelvic Organs (614-616)

Use additional code to identify organism, such as Staphylococcus (041.1), or Streptococcus (041.0)

> **EXCLUDES** *that associated with pregnancy, abortion, childbirth, or the puerperium (630-676.9)*

√4ᵗʰ 614 Inflammatory disease of ovary, fallopian tube, pelvic cellular tissue, and peritoneum

> **EXCLUDES** *endometritis (615.0-615.9)*
> *major infection following delivery (670.0-670.8)*
> *that complicating:*
> *abortion (634-638 with .0, 639.0)*
> *ectopic or molar pregnancy (639.0)*
> *pregnancy or labor (646.6)*

614.0 Acute salpingitis and oophoritis ♀
Any condition classifiable to 614.2, specified as acute or subacute
DEF: Acute inflammation of ovary and fallopian tube.

614.1 Chronic salpingitis and oophoritis ♀
Hydrosalpinx
Salpingitis:
 follicularis
 isthmica nodosa
Any condition classifiable to 614.2, specified as chronic
DEF: Persistent inflammation of ovary and fallopian tube.

614.2 Salpingitis and oophoritis not specified as acute, subacute, or chronic ♀
Abscess (of):
 fallopian tube
 ovary
 tubo-ovarian
Oophoritis
Perioophoritis
Perisalpingitis
Pyosalpinx
Salpingitis
Salpingo-oophoritis
Tubo-ovarian inflammatory disease

> **EXCLUDES** *gonococcal infection (chronic) (098.37)*
> *acute (098.17)*
> *tuberculous (016.6)*

AHA: 2Q, '91, 5

614.3 Acute parametritis and pelvic cellulitis ♀
Acute inflammatory pelvic disease
Any condition classifiable to 614.4, specified as acute
DEF: Parametritis: inflammation of the parametrium; pelvic cellulitis is a synonym for parametritis.

614.4 Chronic or unspecified parametritis and pelvic cellulitis ♀
Abscess (of):
 broad ligament ⎫
 parametrium ⎬ chronic or NOS
 pelvis, femal ⎪
 pouch of Douglas ⎭
Chronic inflammatory pelvic disease
Pelvic cellulitis, female

> **EXCLUDES** *tuberculous (016.7)*

614.5 Acute or unspecified pelvic peritonitis, female ♀
AHA: 4Q, '05, 74
TIP: For pelvic peritonitis in a male patient, refer to code 567.21.

614.6 Pelvic peritoneal adhesions, female (postoperative) (postinfection) ♀
Adhesions:
 peritubal
 tubo-ovarian

Use additional code to identify any associated infertility (628.2)
DEF: Fibrous scarring abnormally joining structures within abdomen.
AHA: 2Q, '11, 19; 3Q, '03, 6; 1Q, '03, 4; 3Q, '95, 7; 3Q, '94, 12
N73.6 Female pelvic peritoneal adhesions (postinfective) `I-10`

614.7 Other chronic pelvic peritonitis, female ♀
> **EXCLUDES** *tuberculous (016.7)*

614.8 Other specified inflammatory disease of female pelvic organs and tissues ♀

614.9 Unspecified inflammatory disease of female pelvic organs and tissues ♀
Pelvic infection or inflammation, female NOS
Pelvic inflammatory disease [PID]

√4ᵗʰ 615 Inflammatory diseases of uterus, except cervix

> **EXCLUDES** *following delivery (670.0-670.8)*
> *hyperplastic endometritis (621.30-621.35)*
> *that complicating:*
> *abortion (634-638 with .0, 639.0)*
> *ectopic or molar pregnancy (639.0)*
> *pregnancy or labor (646.6)*

615.0 Acute ♀
Any condition classifiable to 615.9, specified as acute or subacute

615.1 Chronic ♀
Any condition classifiable to 615.9, specified as chronic

615.9 Unspecified inflammatory disease of uterus ♀
Endometritis   Myometritis
Endomyometritis   Perimetritis
Intrauterine infection Pyometra
Metritis   Uterine abscess
N71.9 Inflammatory disease of uterus unspecified `I-10`

√4ᵗʰ 616 Inflammatory disease of cervix, vagina, and vulva

> **EXCLUDES** *that complicating:*
> *abortion (634-638 with .0, 639.0)*
> *ectopic or molar pregnancy (639.0)*
> *pregnancy, childbirth, or the puerperium (646.6)*

616.0 Cervicitis and endocervicitis ♀
Cervicitis ⎫ with or without mention of
Endocervicitis ⎬ erosion or ectropion
Nabothian (gland) cyst or follicle

> **EXCLUDES** *erosion or ectropion without mention of cervicitis (622.0)*

N72 Inflammatory disease of cervix uteri `I-10`

√5ᵗʰ 616.1 Vaginitis and vulvovaginitis

> **EXCLUDES** *vulvar vestibulitis (625.71)*

DEF: Inflammation or infection of vagina or external female genitalia.

616.10 Vaginitis and vulvovaginitis, unspecified ♀
Vaginitis:
 NOS
 postirradiation
Vulvitis NOS
Vulvovaginitis NOS

Use additional code to identify organism, such as:
 Escherichia coli [E. coli] (041.41-041.49)
 Staphylococcus (041.10-041.19)
 Streptococcus (041.00-041.09)

> **EXCLUDES** *noninfective leukorrhea (623.5)*
> *postmenopausal or senile vaginitis (627.3)*

616.11 Vaginitis and vulvovaginitis in diseases classified elsewhere ♀

Code first underlying disease, as:
 pinworm vaginitis (127.4)

> **EXCLUDES** *herpetic vulvovaginitis (054.11)*
> *monilial vulvovaginitis (112.1)*
> *trichomonal vaginitis or vulvovaginitis (131.01)*

616.2 Cyst of Bartholin's gland ♀
Bartholin's duct cyst
DEF: Fluid-filled sac within gland of vaginal orifice.

616.3 Abscess of Bartholin's gland ♀
Vulvovaginal gland abscess

616.4 Other abscess of vulva ♀
Abscess ⎫
Carbuncle ⎬ of vulva
Furuncle ⎭

Diseases of the Genitourinary System

616.5–618.09

✓5ᵗʰ **616.5 Ulceration of vulva**

     616.50 Ulceration of vulva, unspecified ♀
       Ulcer NOS of vulva

     616.51 *Ulceration of vulva in diseases classified elsewhere* ♀

       Code first underlying disease, as:
         Behçet's syndrome (136.1)
         tuberculosis (016.7)

       EXCLUDES *vulvar ulcer (in):*
          gonococcal (098.0)
          herpes simplex (054.12)
          syphilitic (091.0)

✓5ᵗʰ **616.8 Other specified inflammatory diseases of cervix, vagina, and vulva**

       EXCLUDES *noninflammatory disorders of:*
          cervix (622.0-622.9)
          vagina (623.0-623.9)
          vulva (624.0-624.9)

     616.81 Mucositis (ulcerative) of cervix, vagina, and vulva ♀

       Use additional E code to identify adverse effects of therapy, such as:
         antineoplastic and immunosuppressive drugs (E930.7, E933.1)
         radiation therapy (E879.2)
       AHA: 4Q, '06, 88-90

     616.89 Other inflammatory disease of cervix, vagina and vulva ♀
       Caruncle, vagina or labium
       Ulcer, vagina
       AHA: 4Q, '06, 88-90

     616.9 Unspecified inflammatory disease of cervix, vagina, and vulva ♀

Other Disorders of Female Genital Tract (617-629)

✓4ᵗʰ **617 Endometriosis**

     617.0 Endometriosis of uterus ♀
       Adenomyosis
       Endometriosis:
         cervix
         internal
         myometrium
       EXCLUDES *stromal endometriosis (236.0)*
       DEF: Aberrant uterine mucosal tissue; creating products of menses and inflamed uterine tissues.
       AHA: 3Q, '92, 7
       N80.0 Endometriosis of uterus   `I-10`

     617.1 Endometriosis of ovary ♀
       Chocolate cyst of ovary
       Endometrial cystoma of ovary
       DEF: Aberrant uterine tissue; creating products of menses and inflamed ovarian tissues.
       N80.1 Endometriosis of ovary   `I-10`

     617.2 Endometriosis of fallopian tube ♀
       DEF: Aberrant uterine tissue; creating products of menses and inflamed tissues of fallopian tubes.

     617.3 Endometriosis of pelvic peritoneum ♀
       Endometriosis:
         broad ligament
         cul-de-sac (Douglas')
         parametrium
         round ligament
       DEF: Aberrant uterine tissue; creating products of menses and inflamed peritoneum tissues.

     617.4 Endometriosis of rectovaginal septum and vagina ♀
       DEF: Aberrant uterine tissue; creating products of menses and inflamed tissues in and behind vagina.

     617.5 Endometriosis of intestine ♀
       Endometriosis: Endometriosis:
         appendix   rectum
         colon
       DEF: Aberrant uterine tissue; creating products of menses and inflamed intestinal tissues.

Female Genitourinary System

Uterine (fallopian) tube — Ovary — Rectouterine pouch (of Douglas) — Uterus (fundus) — Cervix — Bladder — Rectum — Pubic bone — Clitoris — Urogenital diaphragm — Anus — Urethral orifice (meatus) — Labia minora — Labia majora — Vaginal canal

Common Sites of Endometriosis

Common sites of endometriosis, in descending order of frequency:
(1) ovary
(2) cul de sac
(3) uterosacral ligaments
(4) broad ligaments
(5) fallopian tube
(6) uterovesical fold
(7) round ligament
(8) vermiform appendix
(9) vagina
(10) rectovaginal septum

     617.6 Endometriosis in scar of skin ♀

     617.8 Endometriosis of other specified sites ♀
       Endometriosis: Endometriosis:
         bladder   umbilicus
         lung   vulva

     617.9 Endometriosis, site unspecified ♀

✓4ᵗʰ **618 Genital prolapse**

     Use additional code to identify urinary incontinence (625.6, 788.31, 788.33-788.39)

       EXCLUDES *that complicating pregnancy, labor, or delivery (654.4)*

✓5ᵗʰ **618.0 Prolapse of vaginal walls without mention of uterine prolapse**

       EXCLUDES *that with uterine prolapse (618.2-618.4)*
         enterocele (618.6)
         vaginal vault prolapse following hysterectomy (618.5)

     618.00 Unspecified prolapse of vaginal walls ♀
       Vaginal prolapse NOS

     618.01 Cystocele, midline ♀
       Cystocele NOS
       DEF: Defect in the pubocervical fascia, the supportive layer of the bladder, causing bladder drop and herniated into the vagina along the midline.
       N81.11 Cystocele midline   `I-10`

     618.02 Cystocele, lateral ♀
       Paravaginal
       DEF: Loss of support of the lateral attachment of the vagina at the arcus tendinous results in bladder drop; bladder herniates into the vagina laterally.

     618.03 Urethrocele ♀

     618.04 Rectocele ♀
       Proctocele
       Use additional code for any associated fecal incontinence (787.60-787.63)
       N81.6 Rectocele   `I-10`

     618.05 Perineocele ♀

     618.09 Other prolapse of vaginal walls without mention of uterine prolapse ♀
       Cystourethrocele

   N Newborn Age: 0   **P** Pediatric Age: 0-17   **M** Maternity Age: 12-55   **A** Adult Age: 15-124

Vaginal Midline Cystocele

Vaginal Lateral Cystocele

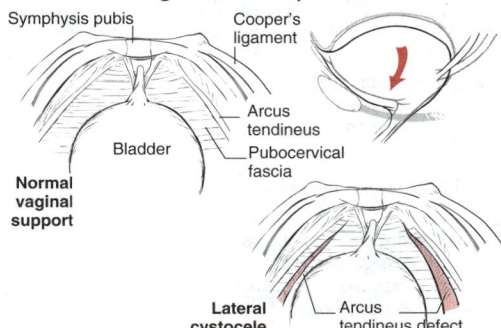

Types of Vaginal Hernias

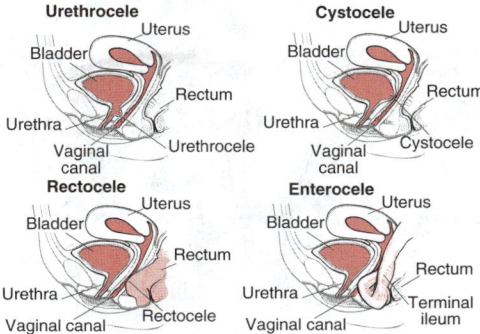

618.1 Uterine prolapse without mention of vaginal wall prolapse ♀

Descensus uteri

Uterine prolapse:
  NOS
  complete

Uterine prolapse:
  first degree
  second degree
  third degree

EXCLUDES *that with mention of cystocele, urethrocele, or rectocele (618.2-618.4)*

618.2 Uterovaginal prolapse, incomplete ♀
  DEF: Downward displacement of uterus downward into vagina.
  N81.2 Incomplete uterovaginal prolapse `I-10`

618.3 Uterovaginal prolapse, complete ♀
  DEF: Downward displacement of uterus exposed within external genitalia.

618.4 Uterovaginal prolapse, unspecified ♀
  N81.4 Uterovaginal prolapse unspecified `I-10`

618.5 Prolapse of vaginal vault after hysterectomy ♀
  N99.3 Prolapse of vaginal vault after hysterectomy `I-10`

618.6 Vaginal enterocele, congenital or acquired ♀
  Pelvic enterocele, congenital or acquired
  DEF: Vaginal vault hernia formed by the loop of the small intestine protruding into the rectal vaginal pouch; can also accompany uterine prolapse or follow hysterectomy.
  N81.5 Vaginal enterocele `I-10`

618.7 Old laceration of muscles of pelvic floor ♀

√5ᵗʰ **618.8 Other specified genital prolapse**

  618.81 Incompetence or weakening of pubocervical tissue ♀

  618.82 Incompetence or weakening of rectovaginal tissue ♀

  618.83 Pelvic muscle wasting ♀
    Disuse atrophy of pelvic muscles and anal sphincter

  618.84 Cervical stump prolapse ♀
    AHA: 4Q, '06, 97

  618.89 Other specified genital prolapse ♀

618.9 Unspecified genital prolapse ♀

√4ᵗʰ **619 Fistula involving female genital tract**
  EXCLUDES *vesicorectal and intestinovesical fistula (596.1)*

619.0 Urinary-genital tract fistula, female ♀
  Fistula:
    cervicovesical
    ureterovaginal
    urethrovaginal
    urethrovesicovaginal
  Fistula:
    uteroureteric
    uterovesical
    vesicocervicovaginal
    vesicovaginal

619.1 Digestive-genital tract fistula, female ♀
  Fistula:
    intestinouterine
    intestinovaginal
    rectovaginal
  Fistula:
    rectovulval
    sigmoidovaginal
    uterorectal

619.2 Genital tract-skin fistula, female ♀
  Fistula:
    uterus to abdominal wall
    vaginoperineal

619.8 Other specified fistulas involving female genital tract ♀
  Fistula:
    cervix
    cul-de-sac (Douglas')
    uterus
    vagina
  DEF: Abnormal communication between female reproductive tract and skin.

619.9 Unspecified fistula involving female genital tract ♀

√4ᵗʰ **620 Noninflammatory disorders of ovary, fallopian tube, and broad ligament**
  EXCLUDES *hydrosalpinx (614.1)*

620.0 Follicular cyst of ovary ♀
  Cyst of graafian follicle
  DEF: Fluid-filled, encapsulated cyst due to occluded follicle duct that secretes hormones into ovaries.
  N83.0 Follicular cyst of ovary `I-10`

620.1 Corpus luteum cyst or hematoma ♀
  Corpus luteum hemorrhage or rupture
  Lutein cyst
  DEF: Fluid-filled cyst due to serous developing from corpus luteum or clotted blood.
  N83.1 Corpus luteum cyst `I-10`

620.2 Other and unspecified ovarian cyst ♀
  Cyst:
    NOS
    corpus albicans
    retention NOS ⎫ of ovary
    serous
    theca-lutein
  Simple cystoma of ovary
  EXCLUDES *cystadenoma (benign) (serous) (220)*
    developmental cysts (752.0)
    neoplastic cysts (220)
    polycystic ovaries (256.4)
    Stein-Leventhal syndrome (256.4)
  N83.20 Unspecified ovarian cysts `I-10`

620.3 Acquired atrophy of ovary and fallopian tube ♀
  Senile involution of ovary

√4ᵗʰ √5ᵗʰ Additional Digit Required   Unspecified Code   Other Specified Code   Manifestation Code   ►◄ Revised Text   ● New Code   ▲ Revised Code Title

2015 ICD-9-CM   **Volume 1 – 191**

Diseases of the Genitourinary System

620.4–622.11

Uterus and Ovaries

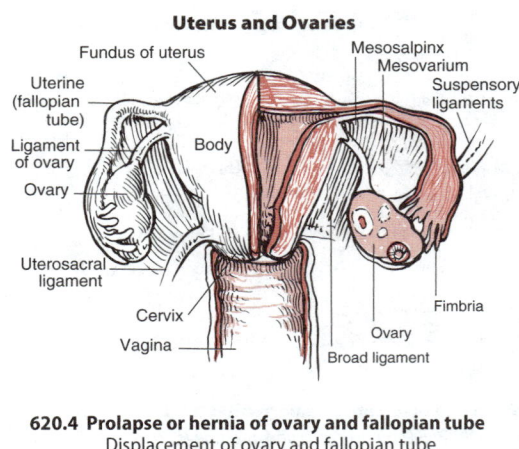

620.4 Prolapse or hernia of ovary and fallopian tube ♀
Displacement of ovary and fallopian tube
Salpingocele

620.5 Torsion of ovary, ovarian pedicle, or fallopian tube ♀
Torsion:
accessory tube
hydatid of Morgagni

620.6 Broad ligament laceration syndrome ♀
Masters-Allen syndrome

620.7 Hematoma of broad ligament ♀
Hematocele, broad ligament
DEF: Blood within peritoneal fold that supports uterus.

620.8 Other noninflammatory disorders of ovary, fallopian tube, and broad ligament ♀
Cyst / of broad ligament or
Polyp / fallopian tube

Infarction / of ovary or fallopian tube
Rupture
Hematosalpinx
EXCLUDES *hematosalpinx in ectopic pregnancy (639.2)*
peritubal adhesions (614.6)
torsion of ovary, ovarian pedicle, or fallopian tube (620.5)

620.9 Unspecified noninflammatory disorder of ovary, fallopian tube, and broad ligament ♀

✓4ᵗʰ 621 Disorders of uterus, not elsewhere classified

621.0 Polyp of corpus uteri ♀
Polyp:
endometrium
uterus NOS
EXCLUDES *cervical polyp NOS (622.7)*
N84.0 Polyp of corpus uteri **I-10**

621.1 Chronic subinvolution of uterus ♀
EXCLUDES *puerperal (674.8)*
DEF: Abnormal size of uterus after delivery; the uterus does not return to its normal size after the birth of a child.
AHA: 1Q, '91, 11

621.2 Hypertrophy of uterus ♀
Bulky or enlarged uterus
EXCLUDES *puerperal (674.8)*

✓5ᵗʰ 621.3 Endometrial hyperplasia
DEF: Abnormal cystic overgrowth of endometrial tissue.

621.30 Endometrial hyperplasia, unspecified ♀
Endometrial hyperplasia NOS
Hyperplasia (adenomatous) (cystic) (glandular) of endometrium
Hyperplastic endometritis

621.31 Simple endometrial hyperplasia without atypia ♀
EXCLUDES *benign endometrial hyperplasia (621.34)*

621.32 Complex endometrial hyperplasia without atypia ♀
EXCLUDES *benign endometrial hyperplasia (621.34)*

621.33 Endometrial hyperplasia with atypia ♀
EXCLUDES *endometrial intraepithelial neoplasia [EIN] (621.35)*

621.34 Benign endometrial hyperplasia
DEF: Excessive cell growth of the endometrium due to primary hormonal changes (menopause) that result in secondary effects to the endometrial stroma and associated structures.
AHA: 4Q, '09, 95-96

621.35 Endometrial intraepithelial neoplasia [EIN] ♀
EXCLUDES *malignant neoplasm of endometrium with endometrial intraepithelial neoplasia [EIN] (182.0)*
DEF: Abnormal premalignant neoplastic changes of the endometrial glands prone to malignant transformation.
AHA: 4Q, '09, 95-96
TIP: Do not confuse (EIN) with unrelated serous intraepithelial carcinoma (serous EIC), which is an early phase of (Type II) papillary serous adenocarcinoma of the endometrium.

621.4 Hematometra ♀
Hemometra
EXCLUDES *that in congenital anomaly (752.2-752.39)*
DEF: Accumulated blood in uterus.

621.5 Intrauterine synechiae ♀
Adhesions of uterus   Band(s) of uterus

621.6 Malposition of uterus ♀
Anteversion
Retroflexion / of uterus
Retroversion
EXCLUDES *malposition complicating pregnancy, labor, or delivery (654.3-654.4)*
prolapse of uterus (618.1-618.4)

621.7 Chronic inversion of uterus ♀
EXCLUDES *current obstetrical trauma (665.2)*
prolapse of uterus (618.1-618.4)

621.8 Other specified disorders of uterus, not elsewhere classified ♀
Atrophy, acquired
Cyst
Fibrosis NOS / of uterus
Old laceration (postpartum)
Ulcer
EXCLUDES *bilharzial fibrosis (120.0-120.9)*
endometriosis (617.0)
fistulas (619.0-619.8)
inflammatory diseases (615.0-615.9)

621.9 Unspecified disorder of uterus ♀

✓4ᵗʰ 622 Noninflammatory disorders of cervix
EXCLUDES *abnormality of cervix complicating pregnancy, labor, or delivery (654.5-654.6)*
fistula (619.0-619.8)

622.0 Erosion and ectropion of cervix ♀
Eversion / of cervix
Ulcer
EXCLUDES *that in chronic cervicitis (616.0)*
DEF: Ulceration or turning outward of uterine cervix.

✓5ᵗʰ 622.1 Dysplasia of cervix (uteri)
EXCLUDES *abnormal results from cervical cytologic examination without histologic confirmation (795.00-795.09)*
carcinoma in situ of cervix (233.1)
cervical intraepithelial neoplasia III [CIN III] (233.1)
HGSIL of cervix (795.04)
DEF: Abnormal cell structures in portal between uterus and vagina.
AHA: 1Q, '91, 11

622.10 Dysplasia of cervix, unspecified ♀
Anaplasia of cervix   Cervical dysplasia NOS
Cervical atypism

622.11 Mild dysplasia of cervix ♀
Cervical intraepithelial neoplasia I [CIN I]

622.12 Moderate dysplasia of cervix ♀
Cervical intraepithelial neoplasia II [CIN II]
EXCLUDES *carcinoma in situ of cervix (233.1)*
cervical intraepithelial neoplasia III [CIN III] (233.1)
severe dysplasia (233.1)

622.2 Leukoplakia of cervix (uteri) ♀
EXCLUDES *carcinoma in situ of cervix (233.1)*
DEF: Thickened, white patches on portal between uterus and vagina.

622.3 Old laceration of cervix ♀
Adhesions
Band(s)   } of cervix
Cicatrix (postpartum)
EXCLUDES *current obstetrical trauma (665.3)*
DEF: Scarring or other evidence of old wound on cervix.

622.4 Stricture and stenosis of cervix ♀
Atresia (acquired)
Contracture   } of cervix
Occlusion
Pinpoint os uteri
EXCLUDES *congenital (752.49)*
that complicating labor (654.6)

622.5 Incompetence of cervix ♀
EXCLUDES *complicating pregnancy (654.5)*
that affecting fetus or newborn (761.0)
DEF: Inadequate functioning of cervix; marked by abnormal widening during pregnancy; causing miscarriage.

622.6 Hypertrophic elongation of cervix ♀
DEF: Overgrowth of cervix tissues extending down into vagina.

622.7 Mucous polyp of cervix ♀
Polyp NOS of cervix
EXCLUDES *adenomatous polyp of cervix (219.0)*

622.8 Other specified noninflammatory disorders of cervix ♀
Atrophy (senile)
Cyst   } of cervix
Fibrosis
Hemorrhage
EXCLUDES *endometriosis (617.0)*
fistula (619.0-619.8)
inflammatory diseases (616.0)

622.9 Unspecified noninflammatory disorder of cervix ♀

✓4ᵗʰ **623 Noninflammatory disorders of vagina**
EXCLUDES *abnormality of vagina complicating pregnancy, labor, or delivery (654.7)*
congenital absence of vagina (752.49)
congenital diaphragm or bands (752.49)
fistulas involving vagina (619.0-619.8)

623.0 Dysplasia of vagina ♀
Mild and moderate dysplasia of vagina
Vaginal intraepithelial neoplasia I and II [VAIN I and II]
EXCLUDES *abnormal results from vaginal cytological examination without histologic confirmation (795.10-795.19)*
carcinoma in situ of vagina (233.31)
HGSIL of vagina (795.14)
severe dysplasia of vagina (233.31)
vaginal intraepithelial neoplasia III [VAIN III] (233.31)

623.1 Leukoplakia of vagina ♀
DEF: Thickened white patches on vaginal canal.

623.2 Stricture or atresia of vagina ♀
Adhesions (postoperative) (postradiation) of vagina
Occlusion of vagina
Stenosis, vagina
Use additional E code to identify any external cause
EXCLUDES *congenital atresia or stricture (752.49)*

623.3 Tight hymenal ring ♀
Rigid hymen
Tight hymenal ring   } acquired or congenital
Tight introitus
EXCLUDES *imperforate hymen (752.42)*

623.4 Old vaginal laceration ♀
EXCLUDES *old laceration involving muscles of pelvic floor (618.7)*
DEF: Scarring or other evidence of old wound on vagina.

623.5 Leukorrhea, not specified as infective ♀
Leukorrhea NOS of vagina
Vaginal discharge NOS
EXCLUDES *trichomonal (131.00)*
DEF: Viscid whitish discharge from vagina.

623.6 Vaginal hematoma ♀
EXCLUDES *current obstetrical trauma (665.7)*

623.7 Polyp of vagina ♀

623.8 Other specified noninflammatory disorders of vagina ♀
Cyst   } of vagina
Hemorrhage

623.9 Unspecified noninflammatory disorder of vagina ♀

✓4ᵗʰ **624 Noninflammatory disorders of vulva and perineum**
EXCLUDES *abnormality of vulva and perineum complicating pregnancy, labor, or delivery (654.8)*
condyloma acuminatum (078.11)
fistulas involving:
perineum — see Alphabetic Index
vulva (619.0-619.8)
vulval varices (456.6)
vulvar involvement in skin conditions (690-709.9)

✓5ᵗʰ **624.0 Dystrophy of vulva**
EXCLUDES *carcinoma in situ of vulva (233.32)*
severe dysplasia of vulva (233.32)
vulvar intraepithelial neoplasia III [VIN III] (233.32)
AHA: 4Q, '07, 90

624.01 Vulvar intraepithelial neoplasia I [VIN I] ♀
Mild dysplasia of vulva

624.02 Vulvar intraepithelial neoplasia II [VIN II] ♀
Moderate dysplasia of vulva
AHA: 4Q, '07, 91

624.09 Other dystrophy of vulva ♀
Kraurosis of vulva
Leukoplakia of vulva

624.1 Atrophy of vulva ♀

624.2 Hypertrophy of clitoris ♀
EXCLUDES *that in endocrine disorders (255.2, 256.1)*

624.3 Hypertrophy of labia ♀
Hypertrophy of vulva NOS
DEF: Overgrowth of fleshy folds on either side of vagina.

624.4 Old laceration or scarring of vulva ♀
DEF: Scarring or other evidence of old wound on external female genitalia.

624.5 Hematoma of vulva ♀
EXCLUDES *that complicating delivery (664.5)*
DEF: Blood in tissue of external genitalia.

624.6 Polyp of labia and vulva ♀

624.8 Other specified noninflammatory disorders of vulva and perineum ♀
Cyst
Edema   } of vulva
Stricture
AHA: 1Q, '03, 13; 1Q, '95, 8

624.9 Unspecified noninflammatory disorder of vulva and perineum ♀

✓4ᵗʰ **625 Pain and other symptoms associated with female genital organs**

625.0 Dyspareunia ♀
EXCLUDES *psychogenic dyspareunia (302.76)*
DEF: Difficult or painful sexual intercourse.

625.1 Vaginismus ♀
Colpospasm
Vulvismus
EXCLUDES *psychogenic vaginismus (306.51)*
DEF: Vaginal spasms; due to involuntary contraction of musculature; prevents intercourse.

Diseases of the Genitourinary System

625.2–628.3

625.2 Mittelschmerz ♀
Intermenstrual pain
Ovulation pain
DEF: Pain occurring between menstrual periods.

625.3 Dysmenorrhea ♀
Painful menstruation
EXCLUDES psychogenic dysmenorrhea (306.52)
AHA: 2Q, '94, 12
N94.6 Dysmenorrhea unspecified   `I-10`

625.4 Premenstrual tension syndromes ♀
Menstrual molimen
Premenstrual dysphoric disorder
Premenstrual syndrome
Premenstrual tension NOS
EXCLUDES menstrual migraine (346.4)
AHA: 4Q, '03, 116

625.5 Pelvic congestion syndrome ♀
Congestion-fibrosis syndrome
Taylor's syndrome
DEF: Excessive accumulation of blood in vessels of pelvis; may occur after orgasm; causes abnormal menstruation, lower back pain and vaginal discharge.

625.6 Stress incontinence, female ♀
EXCLUDES mixed incontinence (788.33)
     stress incontinence, male (788.32)
DEF: Involuntary leakage of urine due to insufficient sphincter control; occurs upon sneezing, laughing, coughing, sudden movement or lifting.
N39.3 Stress incontinence(female) (male)   `I-10`

`✓5ᵗʰ` **625.7 Vulvodynia**
DEF: Vulvar pain without an identifiable cause that persists for three months or longer.
AHA: 4Q, '08, 124

     625.70 Vulvodynia, unspecified ♀
         Vulvodynia NOS

     625.71 Vulvar vestibulitis ♀

     625.79 Other vulvodynia ♀

625.8 Other specified symptoms associated with female genital organs ♀
AHA: N-D, '85, 16

625.9 Unspecified symptom associated with female genital organs ♀
AHA: 4Q, '06, 110
R10.2 Pelvic and perineal pain   `I-10`

`✓4ᵗʰ` **626 Disorders of menstruation and other abnormal bleeding from female genital tract**
EXCLUDES menopausal and premenopausal bleeding (627.0)
     pain and other symptoms associated with menstrual cycle (625.2–625.4)
     postmenopausal bleeding (627.1)
     precocious puberty (259.1)

626.0 Absence of menstruation ♀
Amenorrhea (primary) (secondary)

626.1 Scanty or infrequent menstruation ♀
Hypomenorrhea   Oligomenorrhea

626.2 Excessive or frequent menstruation ♀
Heavy periods   Menorrhagia
Menometrorrhagia   Plymenorrhea
EXCLUDES premenopausal (627.0)
     that in puberty (626.3)
AHA: 4Q, '11, 146
N92.0 Excess & frequent menstruation w/regular cycle   `I-10`

626.3 Puberty bleeding ♀
Excessive bleeding associated with onset of menstrual periods
Pubertal menorrhagia

626.4 Irregular menstrual cycle ♀
Irregular: Irregular:
   bleeding NOS   periods
   menstruation

626.5 Ovulation bleeding ♀
Regular intermenstrual bleeding

626.6 Metrorrhagia ♀
Bleeding unrelated to menstrual cycle
Irregular intermenstrual bleeding

626.7 Postcoital bleeding
DEF: Bleeding from vagina after sexual intercourse.

626.8 Other ♀
Dysfunctional or functional uterine hemorrhage NOS
Menstruation:
   retained
   suppression of
N92.5 Other specified irregular menstruation   `I-10`

626.9 Unspecified ♀

`✓4ᵗʰ` **627 Menopausal and postmenopausal disorders**
EXCLUDES asymptomatic age-related (natural) postmenopausal status (V49.81)

627.0 Premenopausal menorrhagia ♀
Excessive bleeding associated with onset of menopause
Menorrhagia:
   climacteric
   menopausal
   preclimacteric

627.1 Postmenopausal bleeding ♀
N95.0 Postmenopausal bleeding   `I-10`

627.2 Symptomatic menopausal or female climacteric states ♀
Symptoms, such as flushing, sleeplessness, headache, lack of concentration, associated with the menopause

627.3 Postmenopausal atrophic vaginitis ♀
Senile (atrophic) vaginitis

627.4 Symptomatic states associated with artificial menopause ♀
Postartificial menopause syndromes
Any condition classifiable to 627.1, 627.2, or 627.3 which follows induced menopause
DEF: Conditions arising after hysterectomy.

627.8 Other specified menopausal and postmenopausal disorders ♀
EXCLUDES premature menopause NOS (256.31)

627.9 Unspecified menopausal and postmenopausal disorder ♀

`✓4ᵗʰ` **628 Infertility, female**
INCLUDES primary and secondary sterility
DEF: Infertility: inability to conceive for at least one year with regular intercourse.
DEF: Primary infertility: occurring in patients who have never conceived.
DEF: Secondary infertility: occurring in patients who have previously conceived.
AHA: 2Q, '96, 9; 1Q, '95, 7

628.0 Associated with anovulation ♀
Anovulatory cycle
Use additional code for any associated Stein-Leventhal syndrome (256.4)

628.1 Of pituitary-hypothalamic origin ♀
Code first underlying cause, as:
   adiposogenital dystrophy (253.8)
   anterior pituitary disorder (253.0-253.4)

628.2 Of tubal origin ♀
Infertility associated with congenital anomaly of tube
Tubal:
   block
   occlusion
   stenosis
Use additional code for any associated peritubal adhesions (614.6)

628.3 Of uterine origin ♀
Infertility associated with congenital anomaly of uterus
Nonimplantation
Use additional code for any associated tuberculous endometritis (016.7)

`N` Newborn Age: 0   `P` Pediatric Age: 0-17   `M` Maternity Age: 12-55   `A` Adult Age: 15-124

628.4 Of cervical or vaginal origin ♀
Infertility associated with:
anomaly of cervical mucus
congenital structural anomaly
dysmucorrhea

628.8 Of other specified origin ♀

628.9 Of unspecified origin ♀

✓4ᵗʰ **629 Other disorders of female genital organs**

629.0 Hematocele, female, not elsewhere classified ♀
EXCLUDES *hematocele or hematoma:*
broad ligament (620.7)
fallopian tube (620.8)
that associated with ectopic pregnancy
(633.00-633.91)
uterus (621.4)
vagina (623.6)
vulva (624.5)

629.1 Hydrocele, canal of Nuck ♀
Cyst of canal of Nuck (acquired)
EXCLUDES *congenital (752.41)*

✓5ᵗʰ **629.2 Female genital mutilation status** ♀
Female circumcision status
Female genital cutting
AHA: 4Q, '04, 88

629.20 Female genital mutilation status, unspecified ♀
Female genital cutting status, unspecified
Female genital mutilation status NOS

629.21 Female genital mutilation Type I status ♀
Clitorectomy status
Female genital cutting Type I status
DEF: Female genital mutilation involving clitorectomy, with part or all of the clitoris removed.

629.22 Female genital mutilation Type II status ♀
Clitorectomy with excision of labia minora status
Female genital cutting Type II status
DEF: Female genital mutilation involving clitoris and the labia minora amputation.
AHA: 4Q, '04, 90

629.23 Female genital mutilation Type III status ♀
Female genital cutting Type III status
Infibulation status
DEF: Female genital mutilation involving removal, most or all of the labia minora excised, labia majora incised which is then made into a hood of skin over the urethral and vaginal opening.
AHA: 4Q, '04, 90

629.29 Other female genital mutilation status ♀
Female genital cutting Type IV status
Female genital mutilation Type IV status
Other female genital cutting status
AHA: 4Q, '06, 97

✓5ᵗʰ **629.3 Complication of implanted vaginal mesh and other prosthetic materials**
AHA: 4Q, '11, 130-131

629.31 Erosion of implanted vaginal mesh and other prosthetic materials to surrounding organ or tissue ♀
Erosion of implanted vaginal mesh and other prosthetic materials into pelvic floor muscles

629.32 Exposure of implanted vaginal mesh and other prosthetic materials into vagina ♀
Exposure of vaginal mesh and other prosthetic materials through vaginal wall

✓5ᵗʰ **629.8 Other specified disorders of female genital organs**

629.81 Recurrent pregnancy loss without current pregnancy ♀
EXCLUDES *recurrent pregnancy loss with current pregnancy (646.3)*
AHA: 4Q, '06, 98

629.89 Other specified disorders of female genital organs ♀
AHA: 4Q, '06, 98

629.9 Unspecified disorder of female genital organs ♀

11. Complications of Pregnancy, Childbirth, and the Puerperium (630-679)

Ectopic and Molar Pregnancy (630-633)

Use additional code from category 639 to identify any complications

630 Hydatidiform mole Ⓜ♀
Trophoblastic disease NOS
Vesicular mole

> **EXCLUDES** *chorioadenoma (destruens) (236.1)*
> *chorionepithelioma (181)*
> *malignant hydatidiform mole (236.1)*

DEF: Abnormal product of pregnancy; marked by mass of cysts resembling bunch of grapes due to chorionic villi proliferation, and dissolution; must be surgically removed.

√4th **631 Other abnormal product of conception**
AHA: 4Q, '11, 131-132

631.0 Inappropriate change in quantitative human chorionic gonadotropin (hCG) in early pregnancy Ⓜ♀
Biochemical pregnancy
Chemical pregnancy
Inappropriate level of quantitative human chorionic gonadotropin (hCG) for gestational age in early pregnancy

> **EXCLUDES** *blighted ovum (631.8)*
> *molar pregnancy (631.8)*

631.8 Other abnormal products of conception Ⓜ♀
Blighted ovum

632 Missed abortion Ⓜ♀
Early fetal death before completion of 22 weeks' gestation with retention of dead fetus
Retained products of conception, not following spontaneous or induced abortion or delivery

> **EXCLUDES** *failed induced abortion (638.0-638.9)*
> *fetal death (intrauterine) (late) (656.4)*
> *missed delivery (656.4)*
> *that with hydatidiform mole (630)*
> *that with other abnormal products of conception (631.8)*

AHA: 1Q, '01, 5
002.1 Missed abortion   I-10

√4th **633 Ectopic pregnancy**
INCLUDES ruptured ectopic pregnancy
DEF: Fertilized egg develops outside uterus.
AHA: 4Q, '02, 61

√5th **633.0 Abdominal pregnancy**
Intraperitoneal pregnancy

633.00 Abdominal pregnancy without intrauterine pregnancy Ⓜ♀

633.01 Abdominal pregnancy with intrauterine pregnancy Ⓜ♀

√5th **633.1 Tubal pregnancy**
Fallopian pregnancy
Rupture of (fallopian) tube due to pregnancy
Tubal abortion
AHA: 2Q, '90, 27

633.10 Tubal pregnancy without intrauterine pregnancy Ⓜ♀
000.1 Tubal pregnancy   I-10

633.11 Tubal pregnancy with intrauterine pregnancy Ⓜ♀

√5th **633.2 Ovarian pregnancy**

633.20 Ovarian pregnancy without intrauterine pregnancy Ⓜ♀

633.21 Ovarian pregnancy with intrauterine pregnancy Ⓜ♀

√5th **633.8 Other ectopic pregnancy**
Pregnancy:
cervical
combined
cornual
intraligamentous
mesometric
mural

633.80 Other ectopic pregnancy without intrauterine pregnancy Ⓜ♀

633.81 Other ectopic pregnancy with intrauterine pregnancy Ⓜ♀

√5th **633.9 Unspecified ectopic pregnancy**

633.90 Unspecified ectopic pregnancy without intrauterine pregnancy Ⓜ♀

633.91 Unspecified ectopic pregnancy with intrauterine pregnancy Ⓜ♀

Other Pregnancy with Abortive Outcome (634-639)

The following fourth-digit subdivisions are for use with categories 634-638:
.0 Complicated by genital tract and pelvic infection
Endometritis
Salpingo-oophoritis
Sepsis NOS
Septicemia NOS
Any condition classifiable to 639.0 with condition classifiable to 634-638
> **EXCLUDES** *urinary tract infection (634-638 with .7)*

.1 Complicated by delayed or excessive hemorrhage
Afibrinogenemia
Defibrination syndrome
Intravascular hemolysis
Any condition classifiable to 639.1 with condition classifiable to 634-638

.2 Complicated by damage to pelvic organs and tissues
Laceration, perforation, or tear of:
bladder
uterus
Any condition classifiable to 639.2 with condition classifiable to 634-638

.3 Complicated by renal failure
Oliguria
Uremia
Any condition classifiable to 639.3, with condition classifiable to 634-638

.4 Complicated by metabolic disorder
Electrolyte imbalance with conditions classfiable to 634-638

.5 Complicated by shock
Circulatory collapse
Shock (postoperative) (septic)
Any condition classifiable to 639.5 with condition classifiable to 634-638

.6 Complicated by embolism
Embolism:
NOS
amniotic fluid
pulmonary
Any condition classifiable to 639.6, with condition classifiable to 634-638

.7 With other specified complications
Cardiac arrest or failure
Urinary tract infection
Any condition classiable to 639.8 with condition classifiable to 634-638

.8 With unspecified complication
.9 Without mention of complication

§ √4th **634 Spontaneous abortion**

> Requires fifth-digit to identify stage:
> 0   unspecified
> 1   incomplete
> 2   complete

> **INCLUDES** miscarriage
> spontaneous abortion

DEF: Spontaneous premature expulsion of the products of conception from the uterus.
AHA: 4Q, '11, 181; 2Q, '91, 16

§§ √5th **634.0 Complicated by genital tract and pelvic infection** Ⓜ♀
[0-2]

§§ √5th **634.1 Complicated by delayed or excessive hemorrhage** Ⓜ♀
[0-2]   AHA: For Code 634.11: 1Q, '03, 6

---

§   See beginning of section 634-639 for fourth-digit definitions.
§§   Requires fifth digit. Valid digits are in [brackets] under each code. See appropriate category for codes and definitions.

√4th √5th Additional Digit Required   **Unspecified Code**   Other Specified Code   Manifestation Code   ▶◀ Revised Text   ● New Code   ▲ Revised Code Title

Complications of Pregnancy, Childbirth, and the Puerperium

634.2–638

Ectopic Pregnancy Sites

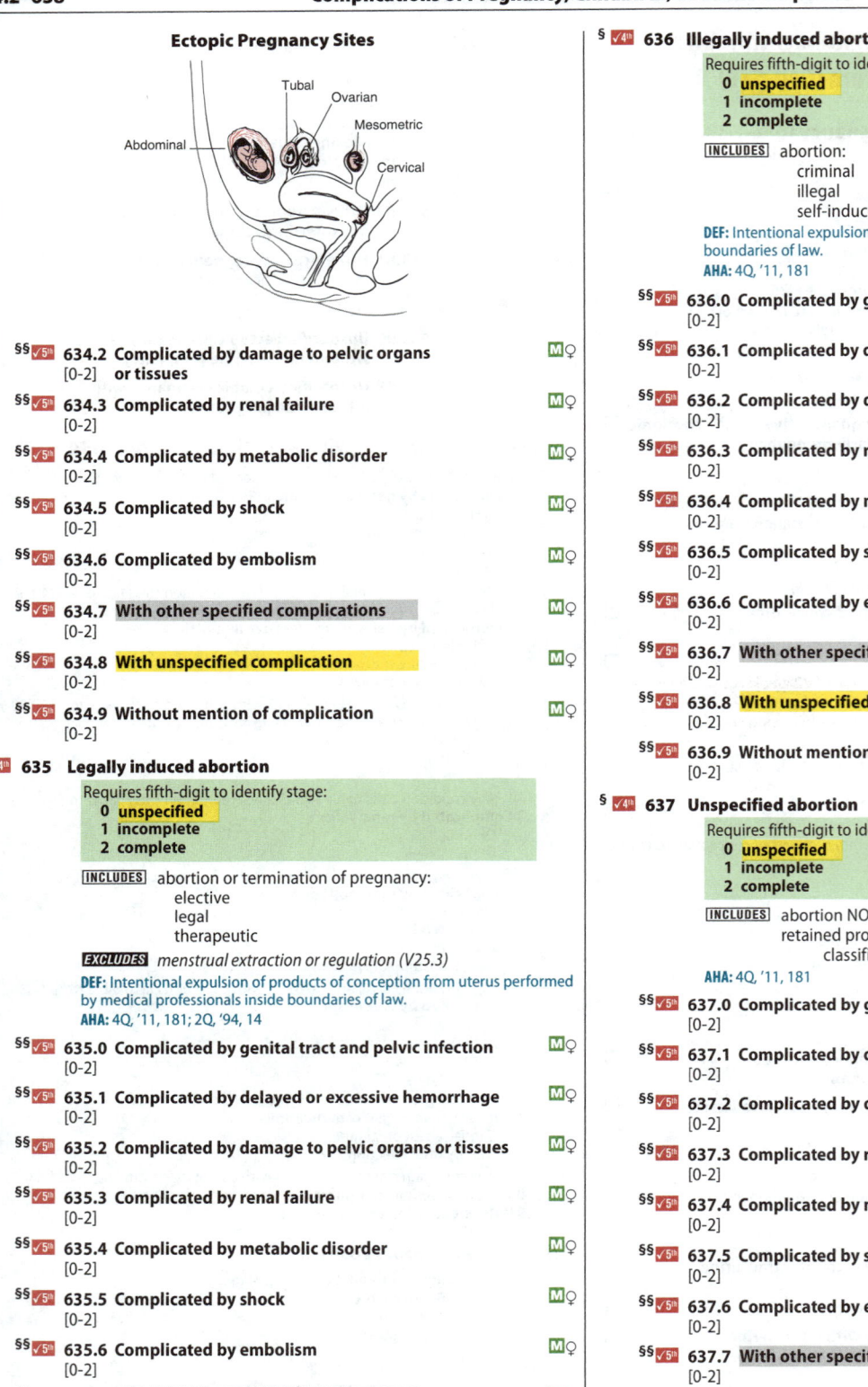

§§ √5th **634.2 Complicated by damage to pelvic organs or tissues** [0-2] M♀

§§ √5th **634.3 Complicated by renal failure** [0-2] M♀

§§ √5th **634.4 Complicated by metabolic disorder** [0-2] M♀

§§ √5th **634.5 Complicated by shock** [0-2] M♀

§§ √5th **634.6 Complicated by embolism** [0-2] M♀

§§ √5th **634.7 With other specified complications** [0-2] M♀

§§ √5th **634.8 With unspecified complication** [0-2] M♀

§§ √5th **634.9 Without mention of complication** [0-2] M♀

§ √4th **635 Legally induced abortion**

Requires fifth-digit to identify stage:
0 unspecified
1 incomplete
2 complete

INCLUDES abortion or termination of pregnancy:
elective
legal
therapeutic

EXCLUDES *menstrual extraction or regulation (V25.3)*

DEF: Intentional expulsion of products of conception from uterus performed by medical professionals inside boundaries of law.
AHA: 4Q, '11, 181; 2Q, '94, 14

§§ √5th **635.0 Complicated by genital tract and pelvic infection** [0-2] M♀

§§ √5th **635.1 Complicated by delayed or excessive hemorrhage** [0-2] M♀

§§ √5th **635.2 Complicated by damage to pelvic organs or tissues** [0-2] M♀

§§ √5th **635.3 Complicated by renal failure** [0-2] M♀

§§ √5th **635.4 Complicated by metabolic disorder** [0-2] M♀

§§ √5th **635.5 Complicated by shock** [0-2] M♀

§§ √5th **635.6 Complicated by embolism** [0-2] M♀

§§ √5th **635.7 With other specified complications** [0-2] M♀

§§ √5th **635.8 With unspecified complication** [0-2] M♀

§§ √5th **635.9 Without mention of complication** [0-2] M♀
AHA: For code 635.92: 2Q, '10, 6-7; 2Q, '94, 14

§ √4th **636 Illegally induced abortion**

Requires fifth-digit to identify stage:
0 unspecified
1 incomplete
2 complete

INCLUDES abortion:
criminal
illegal
self-induced

DEF: Intentional expulsion of products of conception from uterus; outside boundaries of law.
AHA: 4Q, '11, 181

§§ √5th **636.0 Complicated by genital tract and pelvic infection** [0-2] M♀

§§ √5th **636.1 Complicated by delayed or excessive hemorrhage** [0-2] M♀

§§ √5th **636.2 Complicated by damage to pelvic organs or tissues** [0-2] M♀

§§ √5th **636.3 Complicated by renal failure** [0-2] M♀

§§ √5th **636.4 Complicated by metabolic disorder** [0-2] M♀

§§ √5th **636.5 Complicated by shock** [0-2] M♀

§§ √5th **636.6 Complicated by embolism** [0-2] M♀

§§ √5th **636.7 With other specified complications** [0-2] M♀

§§ √5th **636.8 With unspecified complication** [0-2] M♀

§§ √5th **636.9 Without mention of complication** [0-2] M♀

§ √4th **637 Unspecified abortion**

Requires fifth-digit to identify stage:
0 unspecified
1 incomplete
2 complete

INCLUDES abortion NOS
retained products of conception following abortion, not classifiable elsewhere

AHA: 4Q, '11, 181

§§ √5th **637.0 Complicated by genital tract and pelvic infection** [0-2] M♀

§§ √5th **637.1 Complicated by delayed or excessive hemorrhage** [0-2] M♀

§§ √5th **637.2 Complicated by damage to pelvic organs or tissues** [0-2] M♀

§§ √5th **637.3 Complicated by renal failure** [0-2] M♀

§§ √5th **637.4 Complicated by metabolic disorder** [0-2] M♀

§§ √5th **637.5 Complicated by shock** [0-2] M♀

§§ √5th **637.6 Complicated by embolism** [0-2] M♀

§§ √5th **637.7 With other specified complications** [0-2] M♀

§§ √5th **637.8 With unspecified complication** [0-2] M♀

§§ √5th **637.9 Without mention of complication** [0-2] M♀

§ √4th **638 Failed attempted abortion**

INCLUDES failure of attempted induction of (legal) abortion

EXCLUDES *incomplete abortion (634.0-637.9)*

DEF: Continued pregnancy despite an attempted legal abortion.

§ See beginning of section 634-639 for fourth-digit definitions.
§§ Requires fifth digit. Valid digits are in [brackets] under each code. See appropriate category for codes and definitions.

N Newborn Age: 0   P Pediatric Age: 0-17   M Maternity Age: 12-55   A Adult Age: 15-124

638.0 Complicated by genital tract and pelvic infection ♂♀

638.1 Complicated by delayed or excessive hemorrhage ♂♀

638.2 Complicated by damage to pelvic organs or tissues ♂♀

638.3 Complicated by renal failure ♂♀

638.4 Complicated by metabolic disorder ♂♀

638.5 Complicated by shock ♂♀

638.6 Complicated by embolism ♂♀

638.7 With other specified complications ♂♀

638.8 With unspecified complication ♂♀

638.9 Without mention of complication ♂♀

✓4th **639 Complications following abortion and ectopic and molar pregnancies**

NOTE This category is provided for use when it is required to classify separately the complications classifiable to the fourth-digit level in categories 634-638; for example:

a) when the complication itself was responsible for an episode of medical care, the abortion, ectopic or molar pregnancy itself having been dealt with at a previous episode

b) when these conditions are immediate complications of ectopic or molar pregnancies classifiable to 630-633 where they cannot be identified at fourth-digit level.

639.0 Genital tract and pelvic infection ♂♀

Endometritis
Parametritis
Pelvic peritonitis
Salpingitis   } following conditions classifiable to 630-638
Salpingo-oophoritis
Sepsis NOS
Septicemia NOS

EXCLUDES urinary tract infection (639.8)

639.1 Delayed or excessive hemorrhage ♂♀

Afibrinogenemia
Defibrination syndrome   } following conditions classfiable to 630-638
Intravascular

639.2 Damage to pelvic organs and tissues ♂♀

Laceration, perforation, or tear of:

bladder
bowel
broad ligament   } following conditions classifiable to 630-638
cervix
periurethral tissue
uterus
vagina

639.3 Kidney failure ♀

Oliguria
Renal (kidney):
  failure (acute)   } following conditions classifiable to 630-638
  shutdown
  tubular necrosis
Uremia

639.4 Metabolic disorders ♀

Electrolyte imbalance following conditions classifiable to 630-638

639.5 Shock ♂♀

Circulatory collapse
Shock (postoperative)   } following conditions classifiable to 630-638
(septic)

639.6 Embolism ♂♀

Embolism:

NOS
air
amniotic fluid
blood-clot
fat   } following conditions classifiable to 630-638
pulmonary
pyemic
septic
soap

639.8 **Other specified complications following abortion or ectopic and molar pregnancy** ♂♀

Acute yellow atrophy
  or necrosis of
  liver   } following conditons classifiable to 630-638
Cardiac arrest or failure
Cerebral anoxia
Urinary tract infection

639.9 **Unspecified complication following abortion or ectopic and molar pregnancy** ♂♀

Complication(s) not further specified following conditions classifiable to 630-638

Complications Mainly Related to Pregnancy (640-649)

INCLUDES the listed conditions even if they arose or were present during labor, delivery, or the puerperium

AHA: 2Q, '90, 11

The following fifth-digit subclassification is for use with categories 640-649 to denote the current episode of care. Valid fifth-digits are in [brackets] under each code.

0 unspecified as to episode of care or not applicable
1 delivered, with or without mention of antepartum condition
  Antepartum condition with delivery
  Delivery NOS (with mention of antepartum complication during current episode of care)
  Intrapartum obstetric condition (with mention of antepartum complication during current episode of care)
  Pregnancy, delivered (with mention of antepartum complication during current episode of care)
2 delivered, with mention of postpartum complication
  Delivery with mention of puerperal complication during current episode of care
3 antepartum condition or complication
  Antepartum obstetric condtion, not delivered during the current episode of care
4 postpartum condition or complication
  Postpartum or puerperal obstetric condition or complication following delivery that occurred:
  during previous episode of care
  outside hospital, with subsequent admission for observation or care

✓4th **640 Hemorrhage in early pregnancy**

INCLUDES hemorrhage before completion of 22 weeks' gestation

§ ✓5th **640.0 Threatened abortion** ♂♀
[0,1,3]   DEF: Bloody discharge during pregnancy; cervix may be dilated and pregnancy is threatened, but the pregnancy is not terminated.

§ ✓5th **640.8 Other specified hemorrhage in early pregnancy** ♂♀
[0,1,3]

§ ✓5th **640.9 Unspecified hemorrhage in early pregnancy** ♂♀
[0,1,3]

✓4th **641 Antepartum hemorrhage, abruptio placentae, and placenta previa**

§ ✓5th **641.0 Placenta previa without hemorrhage** ♂♀
[0,1,3]   Low impantation of placenta
  Placenta previa noted:
   during pregnancy   } without hemorrhage
   before labor (and delivered by caesarean delivery

DEF: Placenta implanted in lower segment of uterus; commonly causes hemorrhage in the last trimester of pregnancy.

Placenta Previa

| Low (marginal) implantation | Partial placenta previa | Total placenta previa |

§ Requires fifth digit. Valid digits are in [brackets] under each code. See beginning of section 640-649 for codes and definitions.

✓4th
✓5th Additional Digit Required   **Unspecified Code**   Other Specified Code   Manifestation Code   ►◄ Revised Text   ● New Code   ▲ Revised Code Title

2015 ICD-9-CM   **Volume 1 – 199**

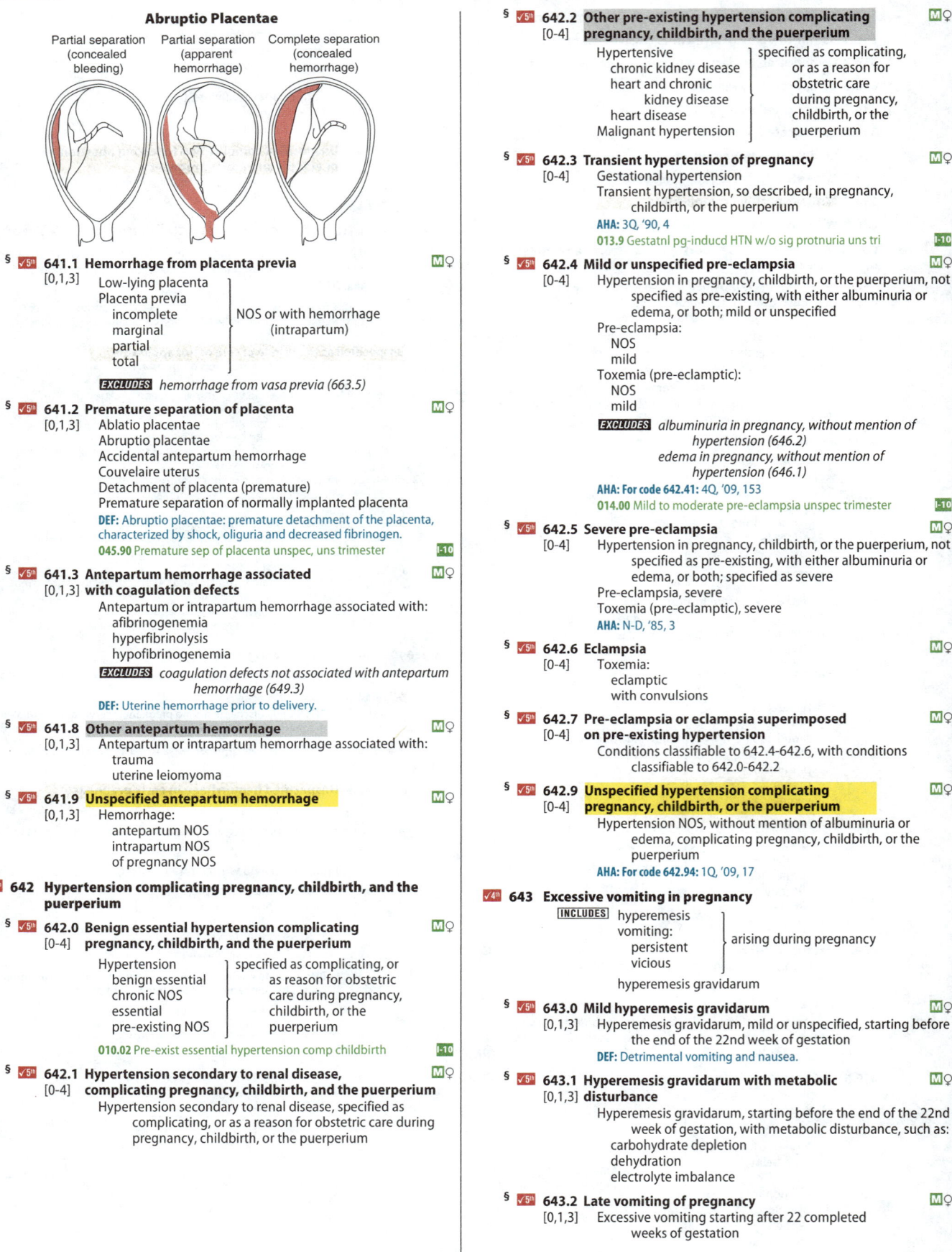

Abruptio Placentae

Partial separation (concealed bleeding)   Partial separation (apparent hemorrhage)   Complete separation (concealed hemorrhage)

§ ✓5ᵗʰ **641.1 Hemorrhage from placenta previa** Ⓜ♀
[0,1,3]
Low-lying placenta
Placenta previa
  incomplete   ⎱ NOS or with hemorrhage
  marginal   ⎰ (intrapartum)
  partial
  total

EXCLUDES *hemorrhage from vasa previa (663.5)*

§ ✓5ᵗʰ **641.2 Premature separation of placenta** Ⓜ♀
[0,1,3]
Ablatio placentae
Abruptio placentae
Accidental antepartum hemorrhage
Couvelaire uterus
Detachment of placenta (premature)
Premature separation of normally implanted placenta
DEF: Abruptio placentae: premature detachment of the placenta, characterized by shock, oliguria and decreased fibrinogen.
045.90 Premature sep of placenta unspec, uns trimester   [I-10]

§ ✓5ᵗʰ **641.3 Antepartum hemorrhage associated** Ⓜ♀
[0,1,3] **with coagulation defects**
Antepartum or intrapartum hemorrhage associated with:
  afibrinogenemia
  hyperfibrinolysis
  hypofibrinogenemia
EXCLUDES *coagulation defects not associated with antepartum hemorrhage (649.3)*
DEF: Uterine hemorrhage prior to delivery.

§ ✓5ᵗʰ **641.8 Other antepartum hemorrhage** Ⓜ♀
[0,1,3] Antepartum or intrapartum hemorrhage associated with:
  trauma
  uterine leiomyoma

§ ✓5ᵗʰ **641.9 Unspecified antepartum hemorrhage** Ⓜ♀
[0,1,3] Hemorrhage:
  antepartum NOS
  intrapartum NOS
  of pregnancy NOS

✓4ᵗʰ **642 Hypertension complicating pregnancy, childbirth, and the puerperium**

§ ✓5ᵗʰ **642.0 Benign essential hypertension complicating** Ⓜ♀
[0-4] **pregnancy, childbirth, and the puerperium**
Hypertension   ⎱ specified as complicating, or
  benign essential ⎰ as reason for obstetric
  chronic NOS   care during pregnancy,
  essential   childbirth, or the
  pre-existing NOS   puerperium
010.02 Pre-exist essential hypertension comp childbirth   [I-10]

§ ✓5ᵗʰ **642.1 Hypertension secondary to renal disease,** Ⓜ♀
[0-4] **complicating pregnancy, childbirth, and the puerperium**
Hypertension secondary to renal disease, specified as complicating, or as a reason for obstetric care during pregnancy, childbirth, or the puerperium

§ ✓5ᵗʰ **642.2 Other pre-existing hypertension complicating** Ⓜ♀
[0-4] **pregnancy, childbirth, and the puerperium**
Hypertensive   ⎱ specified as complicating,
  chronic kidney disease ⎰ or as a reason for
  heart and chronic   obstetric care
    kidney disease   during pregnancy,
  heart disease   childbirth, or the
Malignant hypertension   puerperium

§ ✓5ᵗʰ **642.3 Transient hypertension of pregnancy** Ⓜ♀
[0-4]
Gestational hypertension
Transient hypertension, so described, in pregnancy, childbirth, or the puerperium
AHA: 3Q, '90, 4
013.9 Gestatnl pg-inducd HTN w/o sig protnuria uns tri   [I-10]

§ ✓5ᵗʰ **642.4 Mild or unspecified pre-eclampsia** Ⓜ♀
[0-4]
Hypertension in pregnancy, childbirth, or the puerperium, not specified as pre-existing, with either albuminuria or edema, or both; mild or unspecified
Pre-eclampsia:
  NOS
  mild
Toxemia (pre-eclamptic):
  NOS
  mild
EXCLUDES *albuminuria in pregnancy, without mention of hypertension (646.2)*
edema in pregnancy, without mention of hypertension (646.1)
AHA: For code 642.41: 4Q, '09, 153
014.00 Mild to moderate pre-eclampsia unspec trimester   [I-10]

§ ✓5ᵗʰ **642.5 Severe pre-eclampsia** Ⓜ♀
[0-4]
Hypertension in pregnancy, childbirth, or the puerperium, not specified as pre-existing, with either albuminuria or edema, or both; specified as severe
Pre-eclampsia, severe
Toxemia (pre-eclamptic), severe
AHA: N-D, '85, 3

§ ✓5ᵗʰ **642.6 Eclampsia** Ⓜ♀
[0-4] Toxemia:
  eclamptic
  with convulsions

§ ✓5ᵗʰ **642.7 Pre-eclampsia or eclampsia superimposed** Ⓜ♀
[0-4] **on pre-existing hypertension**
Conditions classifiable to 642.4-642.6, with conditions classifiable to 642.0-642.2

§ ✓5ᵗʰ **642.9 Unspecified hypertension complicating** Ⓜ♀
[0-4] **pregnancy, childbirth, or the puerperium**
Hypertension NOS, without mention of albuminuria or edema, complicating pregnancy, childbirth, or the puerperium
AHA: For code 642.94: 1Q, '09, 17

✓4ᵗʰ **643 Excessive vomiting in pregnancy**
INCLUDES hyperemesis
  vomiting: ⎱ arising during pregnancy
    persistent   ⎰
    vicious
  hyperemesis gravidarum

§ ✓5ᵗʰ **643.0 Mild hyperemesis gravidarum** Ⓜ♀
[0,1,3] Hyperemesis gravidarum, mild or unspecified, starting before the end of the 22nd week of gestation
DEF: Detrimental vomiting and nausea.

§ ✓5ᵗʰ **643.1 Hyperemesis gravidarum with metabolic** Ⓜ♀
[0,1,3] **disturbance**
Hyperemesis gravidarum, starting before the end of the 22nd week of gestation, with metabolic disturbance, such as:
  carbohydrate depletion
  dehydration
  electrolyte imbalance

§ ✓5ᵗʰ **643.2 Late vomiting of pregnancy** Ⓜ♀
[0,1,3] Excessive vomiting starting after 22 completed weeks of gestation

---

§   Requires fifth digit. Valid digits are in [brackets] under each code. See beginning of section 640-649 for codes and definitions.

Ⓝ Newborn Age: 0   Ⓟ Pediatric Age: 0-17   Ⓜ Maternity Age: 12-55   Ⓐ Adult Age: 15-124

§ ✓5ᵗʰ **643.8 Other vomiting complicating pregnancy** Ⓜ♀
[0,1,3]   Vomiting due to organic disease or other cause, specified as complicating pregnancy, or as a reason for obstetric care during pregnancy

   Use additional code to specify cause

§ ✓5ᵗʰ **643.9 Unspecified vomiting of pregnancy** Ⓜ♀
[0,1,3]   Vomiting as a reason for care during pregnancy, length of gestation unspecified

✓4ᵗʰ **644 Early or threatened labor**

§ ✓5ᵗʰ **644.0 Threatened premature labor** Ⓜ♀
[0,3]   Premature labor after 22 weeks, but before 37 completed weeks of gestation without delivery

   EXCLUDES that occurring before 22 completed weeks of gestation (640.0)

   060.00 Preterm labor without delivery unspec trimester �Ⅰ-10

§ ✓5ᵗʰ **644.1 Other threatened labor** Ⓜ♀
[0,3]   False labor:
      NOS
      after 37 completed weeks
         of gestation   } without delivery
      Threatened labor NOS

§ ✓5ᵗʰ **644.2 Early onset of delivery** Ⓜ♀
[0,1]   Onset (spontaneous) of delivery } before 37 completed
      Premature labor with onset of } weeks of
      delivery   } gestation

   AHA: ▶1Q, '14, 19; 2Q, '13, 27;◀ 2Q, '91, 16; For code 644.21: 3Q, '11, 3
   TIP: Assign if an attempted termination of pregnancy results in a liveborn fetus.
   060.14x0 Pt labor 3rd tri w/pt del 3rd tri not applic/uns �Ⅰ-10

✓4ᵗʰ **645 Late pregnancy**
   AHA: 4Q, '00, 43; 4Q, '91, 26

§ ✓5ᵗʰ **645.1 Post term pregnancy** Ⓜ♀
[0,1,3]   Pregnancy over 40 completed weeks to 42 completed weeks gestation

   048.0 Post-term pregnancy �Ⅰ-10

§ ✓5ᵗʰ **645.2 Prolonged pregnancy** Ⓜ♀
[0,1,3]   Pregnancy which has advanced beyond 42 completed weeks gestation

✓4ᵗʰ **646 Other complications of pregnancy, not elsewhere classified**
   Use additional code(s) to further specify complication
   AHA: 4Q, '95, 59

§ ✓5ᵗʰ **646.0 Papyraceous fetus** Ⓜ♀
[0,1,3]   DEF: Fetus that dies in the second trimester of pregnancy and is retained in the uterus, with subsequent atrophy and mummification; commonly occurs in twin pregnancy, nonviable fetus becomes compressed by growth of living twin.

§ ✓5ᵗʰ **646.1 Edema or excessive weight gain in** Ⓜ♀
[0-4]   **pregnancy, without mention of hypertension**
      Gestational edema
      Maternal obesity syndrome

   EXCLUDES that with mention of hypertension (642.0-642.9)

§ ✓5ᵗʰ **646.2 Unspecified renal disease in pregnancy,** Ⓜ♀
[0-4]   **without mention of hypertension**

      Albuminuria   } in pregnancy or the
      Nephropathy NOS } puerperium, without
      Renal disease NOS } mention of
      Uremia   } hypertension

      Gestational proteinuria
   EXCLUDES that with mention of hypertension (642.0-642.9)

§ ✓5ᵗʰ **646.3 Recurrent pregnancy loss** Ⓜ♀
[0,1,3]   *EXCLUDES with current abortion (634.0-634.9)*
             without current pregnancy (629.81)
      DEF: Three or more consecutive spontaneous abortions.

§ ✓5ᵗʰ **646.4 Peripheral neuritis in pregnancy** Ⓜ♀
[0-4]

§ ✓5ᵗʰ **646.5 Asymptomatic bacteriuria in pregnancy** Ⓜ♀
[0-4]

§ ✓5ᵗʰ **646.6 Infections of genitourinary tract in pregnancy** Ⓜ♀
[0-4]   Conditions classifiable to 590, 595, 597, 599.0, 616 complicating pregnancy, childbirth, or the puerperium
      Conditions classifiable to 614.0-614.5, 614.7-614.9, 615 complicating pregnancy or labor

   EXCLUDES major puerperal infection (670.0-670.8)
   AHA: For code 646.63: 4Q, '04, 90
   023.90 Unspec GU tract infection in pregnancy uns tri Ⅰ-10

§ ✓5ᵗʰ **646.7 Liver and biliary tract disorders in pregnancy** Ⓜ♀
[0,1,3]   Acute yellow atrophy of liver }
            (obstetric) (true)   } of pregnancy
         Icterus gravis   }
         Necrosis of liver   }

   EXCLUDES hepatorenal syndrome following delivery (674.8)
            viral hepatitis (647.6)

§ ✓5ᵗʰ **646.8 Other specified complications of pregnancy** Ⓜ♀
[0-4]   Fatigue during pregnancy
      Herpes gestationis
      Insufficient weight gain of pregnancy
   AHA: 3Q, '98, 16; J-F, '85, 15

§ ✓5ᵗʰ **646.9 Unspecified complication of pregnancy** Ⓜ♀
[0,1,3]

✓4ᵗʰ **647 Infectious and parasitic conditions in the mother classifiable elsewhere, but complicating pregnancy, childbirth, or the puerperium**
   INCLUDES the listed conditions when complicating the pregnant state, aggravated by the pregnancy, or when a main reason for obstetric care

   Use additional code(s) to further specify complication
   EXCLUDES those conditions in the mother known or suspected to have affected the fetus (655.0-655.9)

§ ✓5ᵗʰ **647.0 Syphilis** Ⓜ♀
[0-4]   Conditions classifiable to 090-097

§ ✓5ᵗʰ **647.1 Gonorrhea** Ⓜ♀
[0-4]   Conditions classifiable to 098

§ ✓5ᵗʰ **647.2 Other venereal diseases** Ⓜ♀
[0-4]   Conditions classifiable to 099

§ ✓5ᵗʰ **647.3 Tuberculosis** Ⓜ♀
[0-4]   Conditions classifiable to 010-018

§ ✓5ᵗʰ **647.4 Malaria** Ⓜ♀
[0-4]   Conditions classifiable to 084

§ ✓5ᵗʰ **647.5 Rubella** Ⓜ♀
[0-4]   Conditions classifiable to 056

§ ✓5ᵗʰ **647.6 Other viral diseases** Ⓜ♀
[0-4]   Conditions classifiable to 042, 050-055, 057-079, 795.05, 795.15, 796.75

   AHA: J-F, '85, 15; For code 647.61: 2Q, '10, 10
   TIP: Assign when pregnant patient has any HIV-related condition or is stated to have an asymptomatic HIV infection.
   098.52 Other viral diseases complicating childbirth Ⅰ-10

§ ✓5ᵗʰ **647.8 Other specified infectious and parasitic** Ⓜ♀
[0-4]   **diseases**

§ ✓5ᵗʰ **647.9 Unspecified infection or infestation** Ⓜ♀
[0-4]

✓4ᵗʰ **648 Other current conditions in the mother classifiable elsewhere, but complicating pregnancy, childbirth, or the puerperium**
   INCLUDES the listed conditions when complicating the pregnant state, aggravated by the pregnancy, or when a main reason for obstetric care

   Use additional code(s) to identify the condition
   EXCLUDES those conditions in the mother known or suspected to have affected the fetus (655.0-655.9)

§ ✓5ᵗʰ **648.0 Diabetes mellitus** Ⓜ♀
[0-4]   Conditions classifiable to 249, 250
      EXCLUDES gestational diabetes (648.8)
   AHA: 3Q, '91, 5, 11
   024.32 Uns pre-existing diabetes mellitus in childbirth Ⅰ-10

---

§ Requires fifth digit. Valid digits are in [brackets] under each code. See beginning of section 640-649 for codes and definitions.

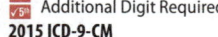

✓4ᵗʰ/✓5ᵗʰ Additional Digit Required | **Unspecified Code** | Other Specified Code | **Manifestation Code** | ▶◀ Revised Text | ● New Code | ▲ Revised Code Title

Complications of Pregnancy, Childbirth, and the Puerperium

648.1–650

§ ✓5ᵗʰ **648.1 Thyroid dysfunction**   Ⓜ♀
[0-4]   Conditions classifiable to 240-246

§ ✓5ᵗʰ **648.2 Anemia**   Ⓜ♀
[0-4]   Conditions classifiable to 280-285
    AHA: For Code 648.22: 1Q, '02, 14; **For code 648.24:** 1Q, '09, 17
    TIP: Assign with fifth digit 2 for postpartum anemia.
    099.013 Anemia complicating pregnancy third trimester   I-10

§ ✓5ᵗʰ **648.3 Drug dependence**   Ⓜ♀
[0-4]   Conditions classifiable to 304
    AHA: 2Q, '98, 13; 4Q, '88, 8

§ ✓5ᵗʰ **648.4 Mental disorders**   Ⓜ♀
[0-4]   Conditions classifiable to 290-303, 305.0, 305.2-305.9,
      306-316, 317-319
    AHA: 2Q, '98, 13; 4Q, '95, 63
    099.314 Alcohol use complicating childbirth   I-10

§ ✓5ᵗʰ **648.5 Congenital cardiovascular disorders**   Ⓜ♀
[0-4]   Conditions classifiable to 745-747

§ ✓5ᵗʰ **648.6 Other cardiovascular diseases**   Ⓜ♀
[0-4]   Conditions classifiable to 390-398, 410-429
    EXCLUDES *cerebrovascular disorders in the puerperium (674.0)*
         peripartum cardiomyopathy (674.5)
         venous complications (671.0-671.9)
    AHA: 3Q, '98, 11; **For code 648.64:** ▶3Q, '12, 9◀

§ ✓5ᵗʰ **648.7 Bone and joint disorders of back, pelvis, and**   Ⓜ♀
[0-4]   **lower limbs**
    Conditions classifiable to 720-724, and those classifiable to
      711-719 or 725-738, specified as affecting the lower
      limbs

§ ✓5ᵗʰ **648.8 Abnormal glucose tolerance**   Ⓜ♀
[0-4]   Conditions classifiable to 790.21-790.29
    Gestational diabetes
    Use additional code, if applicable, for associated long-term
      (current) insulin use (V58.67)
    DEF: Glucose intolerance arising in pregnancy, resolving at end of
    pregnancy.
    AHA: 3Q, '91, 5; **For code 648.83:** 4Q, '04, 56
    TIP: Do not assign if patient was diabetic before becoming pregnant;
    should never be assigned in combination with code 648.0X.
    024.429 Gestational diab mellitus childbirth uns cntrl   I-10

§ ✓5ᵗʰ **648.9 Other current conditions classifiable elsewhere**   Ⓜ♀
[0-4]   Conditions classifiable to 440-459, 795.01-795.04, 795.06,
      795.10-795.14, 795.16, 796.70-796.74, 796.76
    Nutritional deficiencies [conditions classifiable to 260-269]
    AHA: 3Q, '06, 14; 4Q, '04, 88; N-D, '87, 10; **For code 648.91:** 1Q, '02, 14;
    For code 648.93: 4Q, '04, 90; **For code 648.94:** 1Q, '09, 17
    TIP: Assign for group B streptococcus carrier patients, along with
    code V02.51 Carrier or suspected carrier of infectious diseases.

✓4ᵗʰ **649 Other conditions or status of the mother complicating**
    pregnancy, childbirth, or the puerperium
    AHA: 4Q, '06, 99

§ ✓5ᵗʰ **649.0 Tobacco use disorder complicating pregnancy,**   Ⓜ♀
[0-4]   **childbirth, or the puerperium**
    Smoking complicating pregnancy, childbirth, or the
      puerperium
    AHA: 4Q, '06, 99
    099.334 Smoking tobacco complicating childbirth   I-10

§ ✓5ᵗʰ **649.1 Obesity complicating pregnancy, childbirth,**   Ⓜ♀
[0-4]   **or the puerperium**
    Use additional code to identify the obesity (278.00- 278.03)
    AHA: 4Q, '06, 99
    099.214 Obesity complicating childbirth   I-10

§ ✓5ᵗʰ **649.2 Bariatric surgery status complicating**   Ⓜ♀
[0-4]   **pregnancy, childbirth, or the puerperium**
    Gastric banding status complicating pregnancy, childbirth, or
      the puerperium
    Gastric bypass status for obesity complicating pregnancy,
      childbirth, or the puerperium
    Obesity surgery status complicating pregnancy, childbirth, or
      the puerperium
    AHA: 4Q, '06, 99, 118

§ ✓5ᵗʰ **649.3 Coagulation defects complicating pregnancy,**   Ⓜ♀
[0-4]   **childbirth, or the puerperium**
    Conditions classifiable to 286, 287, 289
    Use additional code to identify the specific coagulation defect
      (286.0-286.9, 287.0-287.9, 289.0-289.9)
    EXCLUDES *coagulation defects causing antepartum*
         hemorrhage (641.3)
         postpartum coagulation defects (666.3)
    AHA: 4Q, '06, 99

§ ✓5ᵗʰ **649.4 Epilepsy complicating pregnancy, childbirth,**   Ⓜ♀
[0-4]   **or the puerperium**
    Conditions classifiable to 345
    Use additional code to identify the specific type of epilepsy
      (345.00-345.91)
    EXCLUDES *eclampsia (642.6)*
    AHA: 4Q, '06, 99

§ ✓5ᵗʰ **649.5 Spotting complicating pregnancy**   Ⓜ♀
[0,1,3]   **EXCLUDES** *antepartum hemorrhage (641.0-641.9)*
         hemorrhage in early pregnancy (640.0-640.9)
    AHA: 4Q, '06, 99

§ ✓5ᵗʰ **649.6 Uterine size date discrepancy**   Ⓜ♀
[0-4]   **EXCLUDES** *suspected problem with fetal growth not found*
         (V89.04)
    AHA: 4Q, '06, 99

§ ✓5ᵗʰ **649.7 Cervical shortening**   Ⓜ♀
[0,1,3]   **EXCLUDES** *suspected cervical shortening not found (V89.05)*
    DEF: A cervix that has shortened to < 25 mm in length by the 16th
    week of pregnancy; warning sign for impending premature delivery;
    treated by cervical cerclage placement or progesterone.
    AHA: 4Q, '08, 124-125; **For code 649.73:** 4Q, '08, 125

§ ✓5ᵗʰ **649.8 Onset (spontaneous) of labor after 37 completed**   Ⓜ♀
[1,2]   **weeks of gestation but before 39 completed weeks**
    gestation, with delivery by (planned) cesarean section
    Delivery by (planned) cesarean section occurring after 37
      completed weeks of gestation but before 39 completed
      weeks gestation due to (spontaneous) onset of labor
    Use additional code to specify reason for planned cesarean
      section such as:
      cephalopelvic disproportion (normally formed fetus)
      (653.4)
      previous cesarean delivery (654.2)
    AHA: 4Q, '11, 132-133; **For code 649.81:** 4Q, '11, 133

Normal Delivery, and Other Indications for Care in Pregnancy, Labor, and Delivery (650-659)

The following fifth-digit subclassification is for use with categories 651-659 to denote the current episode of care. Valid fifth-digits are in [brackets] under each code.

0   unspecified as to episode of care or not applicable
1   delivered, with or without mention of antepartum condition
2   delivered, with mention of postpartum complication
3   antepartum condition or complication
4   postpartum condition or complication

650 Normal delivery   Ⓜ♀
    NOTE Delivery requiring minimal or no assistance, with or without
    episiotomy, without fetal manipulation [e.g., rotation version]
    or instrumentation [forceps] of spontaneous, cephalic, vaginal,
    full-term, single, live-born infant. This code is for use as a single
    diagnosis code and is not to be used with any other code in the
    range 630-676.
    Use additional code to indicate outcome of delivery (V27.0)
    EXCLUDES *breech delivery (assisted) (spontaneous) NOS (652.2)*
         delivery by vacuum extractor, forceps, cesarean section, or
         breech extraction, without specified complication
         (669.5-669.7)
    AHA: 2Q, '02, 10; 3Q, '01, 12; 3Q, '00, 5; 4Q, '95, 28, 59
    TIP: Code 650 is to be assigned only for the episode of care during which the
    patient delivers and may be assigned if the patient is admitted for induction
    of labor.
    080 Encounter for full-term uncomplicated delivery   I-10

---

§   Requires fifth digit. Valid digits are in [brackets] under each code. See beginning of section 640-649 for codes and definitions.

Ⓝ Newborn Age: 0   Ⓟ Pediatric Age: 0-17   Ⓜ Maternity Age: 12-55   Ⓐ Adult Age: 15-124

Malposition and Malpresentation

Breech

Shoulder (arm prolapse)

Mother's pelvis

Face (mentum)

Compound (extremity together with head)

Oblique

Cephalopelvic Disproportion

Pubic symphysis

Cephalopelvic disproportion due to: Contraction of pelvic inlet, or large fetus, or hydrocephalus

Ischial tuberosity

Contraction of pelvic outlet (from below)

Pubic symphysis

Pelvic inlet from above

Complications of Pregnancy, Childbirth, and the Puerperium

651–653.9

✓4ᵗʰ **651 Multiple gestation**
Use additional code to specify placenta status (V91.00-V91.99)

§ ✓5ᵗʰ **651.0 Twin pregnancy**   M♀
[0,1,3]
   EXCLUDES *fetal conjoined twins (678.1)*
   AHA: 3Q, '06, 16
   030.009 Twin preg unspec numb of placenta & unspec numb   I-10
   amniotic sacs unspec tri

§ ✓5ᵗʰ **651.1 Triplet pregnancy**   M♀
[0,1,3]

§ ✓5ᵗʰ **651.2 Quadruplet pregnancy**   M♀
[0,1,3]

§ ✓5ᵗʰ **651.3 Twin pregnancy with fetal loss and retention of one**   M♀
[0,1,3] **fetus**
   Vanishing twin syndrome (651.33)

§ ✓5ᵗʰ **651.4 Triplet pregnancy with fetal loss and retention of one**   M♀
[0,1,3] **or more fetus(es)**

§ ✓5ᵗʰ **651.5 Quadruplet pregnancy with fetal loss and retention**   M♀
[0,1,3] **of one or more fetus(es)**

§ ✓5ᵗʰ **651.6 Other multiple pregnancy with fetal loss and**   M♀
[0,1,3] **retention of one or more fetus(es)**

§ ✓5ᵗʰ **651.7 Multiple gestation following (elective)**   M♀
[0,1,3] **fetal reduction**
   Fetal reduction of multiple fetuses reduced to single fetus
   AHA: 3Q, '06, 18; **For code 651.71:** 4Q, '05, 81

§ ✓5ᵗʰ **651.8 Other specified multiple gestation**   M♀
[0,1,3]

§ ✓5ᵗʰ **651.9 Unspecified multiple gestation**   M♀
[0,1,3]

✓4ᵗʰ **652 Malposition and malpresentation of fetus**
Code first any associated obstructed labor (660.0)

§ ✓5ᵗʰ **652.0 Unstable lie**   M♀
[0,1,3]   **DEF:** Changing fetal position.

§ ✓5ᵗʰ **652.1 Breech or other malpresentation successfully**   M♀
[0,1,3] **converted to cephalic presentation**
   Cephalic version NOS

§ ✓5ᵗʰ **652.2 Breech presentation without mention of version**   M♀
[0,1,3] Breech delivery (assisted) (spontaneous) NOS
   Buttocks presentation
   Complete breech
   Frank breech
   EXCLUDES *footling presentation (652.8)*
     incomplete breech (652.8)
   DEF: Fetal presentation of buttocks or feet at birth canal.
   AHA: **For code 652.21:** ▶3Q, '13, 7◀
   032.1xx0 Maternal care breech presentation not applic/uns   I-10

§ ✓5ᵗʰ **652.3 Transverse or oblique presentation**   M♀
[0,1,3] Oblique lie   Transverse lie
   EXCLUDES *transverse arrest of fetal head (660.3)*
   DEF: Delivery of fetus, shoulder first.

§ ✓5ᵗʰ **652.4 Face or brow presentation**   M♀
[0,1,3] Mentum presentation

---

§ ✓5ᵗʰ **652.5 High head at term**   M♀
[0,1,3] Failure of head to enter pelvic brim
   AHA: For code 652.51: ▶3Q, '13, 8◀
   032.4xx0 Maternal care high head at term not applic/uns   I-10

§ ✓5ᵗʰ **652.6 Multiple gestation with malpresentation**   M♀
[0,1,3] **of one fetus or more**

§ ✓5ᵗʰ **652.7 Prolapsed arm**   M♀
[0,1,3]

§ ✓5ᵗʰ **652.8 Other specified malposition or malpresentation**   M♀
[0,1,3] Compound presentation

§ ✓5ᵗʰ **652.9 Unspecified malposition or malpresentation**   M♀
[0,1,3]

✓4ᵗʰ **653 Disproportion**
Code first any associated obstructed labor (660.1)

§ ✓5ᵗʰ **653.0 Major abnormality of bony pelvis, not**   M♀
[0,1,3] **further specified**
   Pelvic deformity NOS

§ ✓5ᵗʰ **653.1 Generally contracted pelvis**   M♀
[0,1,3] Contracted pelvis NOS

§ ✓5ᵗʰ **653.2 Inlet contraction of pelvis**   M♀
[0,1,3] Inlet contraction (pelvis)

§ ✓5ᵗʰ **653.3 Outlet contraction of pelvis**   M♀
[0,1,3] Outlet contraction (pelvis)

§ ✓5ᵗʰ **653.4 Fetopelvic disproportion**   M♀
[0,1,3] Cephalopelvic disproportion NOS
   Disproportion of mixed maternal and fetal origin, with
     normally formed fetus
   033.4xx0 Mtrn care dispropor mtrn & fetal orig not applic   I-10

§ ✓5ᵗʰ **653.5 Unusually large fetus causing disproportion**   M♀
[0,1,3] Disproportion of fetal origin with normally formed fetus
   Fetal disproportion NOS
   EXCLUDES *that when the reason for medical care was concern*
     for the fetus (656.6)

§ ✓5ᵗʰ **653.6 Hydrocephalic fetus causing disproportion**   M♀
[0,1,3]   **EXCLUDES** *that when the reason for medical care was concern*
     for the fetus (655.0)

§ ✓5ᵗʰ **653.7 Other fetal abnormality causing disproportion**   M♀
[0,1,3] Fetal:
   ascites
   hydrops
   myelomeningocele
   sacral teratoma
   tumor
   EXCLUDES *conjoined twins causing disproportion (678.1)*

§ ✓5ᵗʰ **653.8 Disproportion of other origin**   M♀
[0,1,3]   **EXCLUDES** *shoulder (girdle) dystocia (660.4)*

§ ✓5ᵗʰ **653.9 Unspecified disproportion**   M♀
[0,1,3]

---

§   Requires fifth digit. Valid digits are in [brackets] under each code. See beginning of section 640-649 for codes and definitions.

✓4ᵗʰ / ✓5ᵗʰ Additional Digit Required   **Unspecified Code**   Other Specified Code   Manifestation Code   ▶◀ Revised Text   ● New Code   ▲ Revised Code Title

Complications of Pregnancy, Childbirth, and the Puerperium

654–656.5

✓4ᵗʰ **654 Abnormality of organs and soft tissues of pelvis**
   INCLUDES the listed conditions during pregnancy, childbirth, or the puerperium
   Code first any associated obstructed labor (660.2)
   EXCLUDES trauma to perineum and vulva complicating current delivery (664.0-664.9)

§ ✓5ᵗʰ **654.0 Congenital abnormalities of uterus**   M♀
 [0-4]   Double uterus
         Uterus bicornis

§ ✓5ᵗʰ **654.1 Tumors of body of uterus**   M♀
 [0-4]   Uterine fibroids

§ ✓5ᵗʰ **654.2 Previous cesarean delivery**   M♀
 [0,1,3]   Uterine scar from previous cesarean delivery
         AHA: 1Q, '92, 8; **For code 654.21:** ▶3Q, '13, 6;◀ 4Q, '11, 133
         O34.21 Maternal care for scar from prev cesarean del   I-10

§ ✓5ᵗʰ **654.3 Retroverted and incarcerated gravid uterus**   ♀
 [0-4]   **DEF:** Retroverted: tilted back uterus; no change in angle of longitudinal axis.
         DEF: Incarcerated: immobile, fixed uterus.

§ ✓5ᵗʰ **654.4 Other abnormalities in shape or position of gravid uterus and of neighboring structures**   ♀
 [0-4]   Cystocele
         Pelvic floor repair
         Pendulous abdomen
         Prolapse of gravid uterus
         Rectocele
         Rigid pelvic floor

§ ✓5ᵗʰ **654.5 Cervical incompetence**   M♀
 [0-4]   Presence of Shirodkar suture with or without mention of cervical incompetence
         DEF: Abnormal cervix; tendency to dilate in second trimester; causes premature fetal expulsion.
         DEF: Shirodkar suture: purse-string suture used to artificially close incompetent cervix.

§ ✓5ᵗʰ **654.6 Other congenital or acquired abnormality of cervix**   M♀
 [0-4]   Cicatricial cervix
         Polyp of cervix
         Previous surgery to cervix
         Rigid cervix (uteri)
         Stenosis or stricture of cervix
         Tumor of cervix

§ ✓5ᵗʰ **654.7 Congenital or acquired abnormality of vagina**   M♀
 [0-4]   Previous surgery to vagina
         Septate vagina
         Stenosis of vagina (acquired) (congenital)
         Stricture of vagina
         Tumor of vagina

§ ✓5ᵗʰ **654.8 Congenital or acquired abnormality of vulva**   M♀
 [0-4]   Anal sphincter tear (healed) (old) complicating delivery
         Fibrosis of perineum
         Persistent hymen
         Previous surgery to perineum or vulva
         Rigid perineum
         Tumor of vulva
         EXCLUDES anal sphincter tear (healed) (old) not associated with delivery (569.43)
              varicose veins of vulva (671.1)
         AHA: 1Q, '03, 14

§ ✓5ᵗʰ **654.9 Other and unspecified**   M♀
 [0-4]   Uterine scar NEC

✓4ᵗʰ **655 Known or suspected fetal abnormality affecting management of mother**
   INCLUDES the listed conditions in the fetus as a reason for observation or obstetrical care of the mother, or for termination of pregnancy
   AHA: 3Q, '90, 4
   TIP: Only assign when the fetal condition affects the management of the mother. Assign on mother's chart when in utero procedures are performed on the fetus.

§ ✓5ᵗʰ **655.0 Central nervous system malformation in fetus**   M♀
 [0,1,3]   Fetal or suspected fetal:
         anencephaly
         hydrocephalus
         spina bifida (with myelomeningocele)

§ ✓5ᵗʰ **655.1 Chromosomal abnormality in fetus**   M♀
 [0,1,3]

§ ✓5ᵗʰ **655.2 Hereditary disease in family possibly affecting fetus**   M♀
 [0,1,3]

§ ✓5ᵗʰ **655.3 Suspected damage to fetus from viral disease in the mother**   M♀
 [0,1,3]   Suspected damage to fetus from maternal rubella

§ ✓5ᵗʰ **655.4 Suspected damage to fetus from other disease in the mother**   M♀
 [0,1,3]   Suspected damage to fetus from maternal:
         alcohol addiction
         listeriosis
         toxoplasmosis

§ ✓5ᵗʰ **655.5 Suspected damage to fetus from drugs**   M♀
 [0,1,3]

§ ✓5ᵗʰ **655.6 Suspected damage to fetus from radiation**   M♀
 [0,1,3]

§ ✓5ᵗʰ **655.7 Decreased fetal movements**   M♀
 [0,1,3]   **AHA:** 4Q, '97, 41

§ ✓5ᵗʰ **655.8 Other known or suspected fetal abnormality, not elsewhere classified**   M♀
 [0,1,3]   Suspected damage to fetus from:
         environmental toxins
         intrauterine contraceptive device
         AHA: 3Q, '06, 16, 18

§ ✓5ᵗʰ **655.9 Unspecified**   M♀
 [0,1,3]   **AHA: For code 655.93:** 2Q, '10, 6-7

✓4ᵗʰ **656 Other known or suspected fetal and placental problems affecting management of mother**
   EXCLUDES fetal hematologic conditions (678.0)
           suspected placental problems not found (V89.02)

§ ✓5ᵗʰ **656.0 Fetal-maternal hemorrhage**   M♀
 [0,1,3]   Leakage (microscopic) of fetal blood into maternal circulation

§ ✓5ᵗʰ **656.1 Rhesus isoimmunization**   M♀
 [0,1,3]   Anti-D [Rh] antibodies
         Rh incompatibility
         DEF: Antibodies developing against Rh factor; mother with Rh negative develops antibodies against Rh positive fetus.
         O36.0190 Mtrn care anti-D Rh antibods uns tri not applic   I-10

§ ✓5ᵗʰ **656.2 Isoimmunization from other and unspecified blood-group incompatibility**   M♀
 [0,1,3]   ABO isoimmunization
         AHA: 4Q, '06, 135

§ ✓5ᵗʰ **656.3 Fetal distress**   M♀
 [0,1,3]   Fetal metabolic acidemia
         EXCLUDES abnormal fetal acid-base balance (656.8)
              abnormality in fetal heart rate or rhythm (659.7)
              fetal bradycardia (659.7)
              fetal tachycardia (659.7)
              meconium in liquor (656.8)
         DEF: Life-threatening disorder; fetal anoxia, hemolytic disease and other miscellaneous diseases cause fetal distress.
         AHA: N-D, '86, 4

§ ✓5ᵗʰ **656.4 Intrauterine death**   M♀
 [0,1,3]   Fetal death:
         NOS
         after completion of 22 weeks' gestation
         late
         Missed delivery
         EXCLUDES missed abortion (632)

§ ✓5ᵗʰ **656.5 Poor fetal growth**   M♀
 [0,1,3]   "Light-for-dates"
         "Placental insufficiency"
         "Small-for-dates"
         O36.5190 Mtrn care known/spct placental insuff uns tri   I-10

§   Requires fifth digit. Valid digits are in [brackets] under each code. See beginning of section 640-649 for codes and definitions.

N Newborn Age: 0   P Pediatric Age: 0-17   M Maternity Age: 12-55   A Adult Age: 15-124

§ √5ᵗʰ **656.6 Excessive fetal growth**   Ⓜ♀
[0,1,3]   "Large-for-dates"
    036.60x0 Mtrn care excess fetl grwth uns tri not applic   I-10

§ √5ᵗʰ **656.7 Other placental conditions**   Ⓜ♀
[0,1,3]   Abnormal placenta
    Placental infarct
    EXCLUDES *placental polyp (674.4)*
               placentitis (658.4)

§ √5ᵗʰ **656.8 Other specified fetal and placental problems**   Ⓜ♀
[0,1,3]   Abnormal acid-base balance
    Intrauterine acidosis
    Lithopedian
    Meconium in liquor
    Subchorionic hematoma
    DEF: Lithopedian: Calcified fetus; not expelled by mother.
    036.20x0 Mtrn care hydrops fetalis uns tri not applic/uns   I-10

§ √5ᵗʰ **656.9 Unspecified fetal and placental problem**   Ⓜ♀
[0,1,3]

√4ᵗʰ **657 Polyhydramnios**   Ⓜ♀
[0,1,3]

§ √5ᵗʰ **Use 0 as fourth-digit for this category**

    Hydramnios
    EXCLUDES *suspected polyhydramnios not found (V89.01)*
    DEF: Excess amniotic fluid.
    AHA: 3Q, '06, 16; 4Q, '91, 26
    040.9xx0 Polyhydramnios uns trimester not applicable/uns   I-10

√4ᵗʰ **658 Other problems associated with amniotic cavity and membranes**
    EXCLUDES *amniotic fluid embolism (673.1)*
               suspected problems with amniotic cavity and membranes not found (V89.01)

§ √5ᵗʰ **658.0 Oligohydramnios**   Ⓜ♀
[0,1,3]   Oligohydramnios without mention of rupture of membranes
    DEF: Deficient amount of amniotic fluid.
    AHA: 3Q, '06, 16
    041.00x0 Oligohydramnios uns trimester not applicable/uns   I-10

§ √5ᵗʰ **658.1 Premature rupture of membranes**   Ⓜ♀
[0,1,3]   Rupture of amniotic sac less than 24 hours prior to the onset of labor
    AHA: For code 658.13: 1Q, '01, 5; 4Q, '98, 77
    042.00 Prmat rom ool w/in 24 hrs of rup uns wks gestatn   I-10

§ √5ᵗʰ **658.2 Delayed delivery after spontaneous or**
[0,1,3] **unspecified rupture of membranes**
    Prolonged rupture of membranes NOS
    Rupture of amniotic sac 24 hours or more prior to the onset of labor
    AHA: For code 658.21: ▶1Q, '14, 19◀

§ √5ᵗʰ **658.3 Delayed delivery after artificial rupture**   Ⓜ♀
[0,1,3] **of membranes**

§ √5ᵗʰ **658.4 Infection of amniotic cavity**   Ⓜ♀
[0,1,3]   Amnionitis   Membranitis
    Chorioamnionitis   Placentitis
    041.1090 Inf amniotic sac & memb uns, uns tri not applic/uns   I-10

§ √5ᵗʰ **658.8 Other**   Ⓜ♀
[0,1,3]   Amnion nodosum
    Amniotic cyst

§ √5ᵗʰ **658.9 Unspecified**   Ⓜ♀
[0,1,3]

√4ᵗʰ **659 Other indications for care or intervention related to labor and delivery, not elsewhere classified**

§ √5ᵗʰ **659.0 Failed mechanical induction**   Ⓜ♀
[0,1,3]   Failure of induction of labor by surgical or other instrumental methods

§ √5ᵗʰ **659.1 Failed medical or unspecified induction**   Ⓜ♀
[0,1,3]   Failed induction NOS
    Failure of induction of labor by medical methods, such as oxytocic drugs
    061.9 Failed induction of labor unspecified   I-10

§ √5ᵗʰ **659.2 Maternal pyrexia during labor, unspecified**   Ⓜ♀
[0,1,3]   **DEF:** Fever during labor.
    075.2 Pyrexia during labor not elsewhere classified   I-10

§ √5ᵗʰ **659.3 Generalized infection during labor**   Ⓜ♀
[0,1,3]   Septicemia during labor

§ √5ᵗʰ **659.4 Grand multiparity**   Ⓜ♀
    EXCLUDES *supervision only, in pregnancy (V23.3)*
               without current pregnancy (V61.5)
    DEF: Having borne six or more children previously.

§ √5ᵗʰ **659.5 Elderly primigravida**   Ⓜ♀
[0,1,3]   First pregnancy in a woman who will be 35 years of age or older at expected date of delivery
    EXCLUDES *supervision only, in pregnancy (V23.81)*
    AHA: 3Q, '01, 12
    009.519 Supervisn of elderly primigravida uns trimester   I-10

§ √5ᵗʰ **659.6 Elderly multigravida**   Ⓜ♀
[0,1,3]   Second or more pregnancy in a woman who will be 35 years of age or older at expected date of delivery
    EXCLUDES *elderly primigravida 659.5*
               supervision only, in pregnancy (V23.82)
    AHA: 3Q, '01, 12
    009.529 Supervisn of elderly multigravida uns trimester   I-10

§ √5ᵗʰ **659.7 Abnormality in fetal heart rate or rhythm**   Ⓜ♀
[0,1,3]   Depressed fetal heart tones
    Fetal:
      bradycardia
      tachycardia
    Fetal heart rate decelerations
    Non-reassuring fetal heart rate or rhythm
    AHA: 4Q, '98, 48; **For code 659.71:** ▶1Q, '14, 14◀
    076 Abn in fetal heart rate & rhythm comp L&D   I-10

§ √5ᵗʰ **659.8 Other specified indications for care or**   Ⓜ♀
[0,1,3] **intervention related to labor and delivery**
    Pregnancy in a female less than 16 years old at expected date of delivery
    Very young maternal age
    AHA: 3Q, '01, 12

§ √5ᵗʰ **659.9 Unspecified indication for care or intervention**   Ⓜ♀
[0,1,3] **related to labor and delivery**

Complications Occurring Mainly in the Course of Labor and Delivery (660–669)

The following fifth-digit subclassification is for use with categories 660-669 to denote the current episode of care. Valid fifth-digits are in [brackets] under each code.

0 unspecified as to episode of care or not applicable
1 delivered, with or without mention of antepartum condition
2 delivered, with mention of postpartum complication
3 antepartum condition or complication
4 postpartum condition or complication

√4ᵗʰ **660 Obstructed labor**
    AHA: 3Q, '95, 10

§ √5ᵗʰ **660.0 Obstruction caused by malposition of fetus at**   Ⓜ♀
[0,1,3] **onset of labor**
    Any condition classifiable to 652, causing obstruction during labor
    Use additional code from 652.0-652.9 to identify condition
    AHA: For code 660.01: ▶3Q, '13, 7, 8◀

§ √5ᵗʰ **660.1 Obstruction by bony pelvis**   Ⓜ♀
[0,1,3]   Any condition classifiable to 653, causing obstruction during labor
    Use additional code from 653.0-653.9 to identify condition

§ √5ᵗʰ **660.2 Obstruction by abnormal pelvic soft tissues**   Ⓜ♀
[0,1,3]   Prolapse of anterior lip of cervix
    Any condition classifiable to 654, causing obstruction during labor
    Use additional code from 654.0-654.9 to identify condition

§ √5ᵗʰ **660.3 Deep transverse arrest and persistent**   Ⓜ♀
[0,1,3] **occipitoposterior position**
    064.0xx0 Obst labor incpl rotat of fetal head not applic   I-10

§ Requires fifth digit. Valid digits are in [brackets] under each code. See beginning of section 640-649 for codes and definitions.

√4ᵗʰ/√5ᵗʰ Additional Digit Required   **Unspecified Code**   Other Specified Code   Manifestation Code   ▶◀ Revised Text   ● New Code   ▲ Revised Code Title

2015 ICD-9-CM   **October 2014 · Volume 1 – 205**

Complications of Pregnancy, Childbirth, and the Puerperium

660.4–664.4

§ √5th **660.4 Shoulder (girdle) dystocia**   M♀
[0,1,3]   Impacted shoulders
DEF: Obstructed labor due to impacted fetal shoulders.
066.0 Obstructed labor due to shoulder dystocia   I-10

§ √5th **660.5 Locked twins**   M♀
[0,1,3]

§ √5th **660.6 Failed trial of labor, unspecified**   M♀
[0,1,3]   Failed trial of labor, without mention of
condition or suspected condition

§ √5th **660.7 Failed forceps or vacuum extractor,**   M♀
[0,1,3] **unspecified**
Application of ventouse or forceps, without mention of
condition

§ √5th **660.8 Other causes of obstructed labor**   M♀
[0,1,3]   Use additional code to identify condition
AHA: 4Q, '04, 88

§ √5th **660.9 Unspecified obstructed labor**   M♀
[0,1,3]   Dystocia:
NOS
fetal NOS
maternal NOS

√4th **661 Abnormality of forces of labor**

§ √5th **661.0 Primary uterine inertia**   M♀
[0,1,3]   Failure of cervical dilation
Hypotonic uterine dysfunction, primary
Prolonged latent phase of labor
DEF: Lack of efficient contractions during labor causing prolonged labor.
062.0 Primary inadequate contractions   I-10

§ √5th **661.1 Secondary uterine inertia**   M♀
[0,1,3]   Arrested active phase of labor
Hypotonic uterine dysfunction, secondary
062.1 Secondary uterine inertia   I-10

§ √5th **661.2 Other and unspecified uterine inertia**   M♀
[0,1,3]   Atony of uterus without hemorrhage
Desultory labor
Irregular labor
Poor contractions
Slow slope active phase of labor
EXCLUDES atony of uterus with hemorrhage (666.1)
postpartum atony of uterus without hemorrhage
(669.8)

§ √5th **661.3 Precipitate labor**   M♀
[0,1,3]   **DEF:** Rapid labor and delivery.

§ √5th **661.4 Hypertonic, incoordinate, or prolonged**   M♀
[0,1,3] **uterine contractions**
Cervical spasm
Contraction ring (dystocia)
Dyscoordinate labor
Hourglass contraction of uterus
Hypertonic uterine dysfunction
Incoordinate uterine action
Retraction ring (Bandl's) (pathological)
Tetanic contractions
Uterine dystocia NOS
Uterine spasm

§ √5th **661.9 Unspecified abnormality of labor**   M♀
[0,1,3]

√4th **662 Long labor**

§ √5th **662.0 Prolonged first stage**   M♀
[0,1,3]

§ √5th **662.1 Prolonged labor, unspecified**   M♀
[0,1,3]

§ √5th **662.2 Prolonged second stage**   M♀
[0,1,3]

§ √5th **662.3 Delayed delivery of second twin, triplet, etc.**   M♀
[0,1,3]

√4th **663 Umbilical cord complications**

§ √5th **663.0 Prolapse of cord**   M♀
[0,1,3]   Presentation of cord
DEF: Abnormal presentation of fetus; marked by protruding umbilical
cord during labor; can cause fetal death.

§ √5th **663.1 Cord around neck, with compression**   M♀
[0,1,3]   Cord tightly around neck
069.1xx0 L&D comp by cord arnd neck with comprs   I-10
not applic/uns

§ √5th **663.2 Other and unspecified cord entanglement,**   M♀
[0,1,3] **with compression**
Entanglement of cords of twins in mono-amniotic sac
Knot in cord (with compression)

§ √5th **663.3 Other and unspecified cord entanglement,**   M♀
[0,1,3] **without mention of compression**
AHA: For code 663.31: 2Q, '03, 9
069.82x0 L&D comp by oth cord entanglement   I-10
w/o comprs unsp. fetus

§ √5th **663.4 Short cord**   M♀
[0,1,3]

§ √5th **663.5 Vasa previa**   M♀
[0,1,3]   **DEF:** Abnormal presentation of fetus marked by blood vessels of
umbilical cord in front of fetal head.

§ √5th **663.6 Vascular lesions of cord**   M♀
[0,1,3]   Bruising of cord
Hematoma of cord
Thrombosis of vessels of cord

§ √5th **663.8 Other umbilical cord complications**   M♀
[0,1,3]   Velamentous insertion of umbilical cord

§ √5th **663.9 Unspecified umbilical cord complication**   M♀
[0,1,3]

√4th **664 Trauma to perineum and vulva during delivery**
INCLUDES damage from instruments
that from extension of episiotomy
AHA: 1Q, '92, 11; N-D, '84, 10

§ √5th **664.0 First-degree perineal laceration**   M♀
[0,1,4]   Perineal laceration, rupture, or tear involving:
fourchette
hymen
labia
skin
vagina
vulva
070.0 First degree perineal laceration during delivery   I-10

§ √5th **664.1 Second-degree perineal laceration**   M♀
[0,1,4]   Perineal laceration, rupture, or tear (following episiotomy)
involving:
pelvic floor
perineal muscles
vaginal muscles
EXCLUDES that involving anal sphincter (664.2)
AHA: For code 664.11: 4Q, '08, 192
070.1 Second degree perineal laceration dur delivery   I-10

§ √5th **664.2 Third-degree perineal laceration**   M♀
[0,1,4]   Perineal laceration, rupture, or tear
(following episiotomy) involving:
anal sphincter
rectovaginal septum
sphincter NOS
EXCLUDES anal sphincter tear during delivery not associated
with third-degree perineal laceration (664.6)
that with anal or rectal mucosal laceration (664.3)
070.2 Third degree perineal laceration during delivery   I-10

§ √5th **664.3 Fourth-degree perineal laceration**   M♀
[0,1,4]   Perineal laceration, rupture, or tear as
classifiable to 664.2 and involving also:
anal mucosa
rectal mucosa

§ √5th **664.4 Unspecified perineal laceration**   M♀
[0,1,4]   Central laceration
AHA: 1Q, '92, 8

N Newborn Age: 0   P Pediatric Age: 0–17   M Maternity Age: 12–55   A Adult Age: 15–124

Perineal Lacerations

First degree

Second degree

Anus

Third degree

Fourth degree

§ √5ʰ **664.5 Vulval and perineal hematoma**   Ⓜ♀
[0,1,4]   AHA: N-D, '84, 10

§ √5ʰ **664.6 Anal sphincter tear complicating delivery,**   Ⓜ♀
[0,1,4] **not associated with third-degree perineal laceration**
    EXCLUDES *third-degree perineal laceration (664.2)*
    AHA: For code 664.61: 4Q, '07, 88, 90

§ √5ʰ **664.8 Other specified trauma to perineum and vulva**   Ⓜ♀
[0,1,4]   Periurethral trauma
    AHA: For code 664.81: 4Q, '07, 125
    TIP: Assign when documentation indicates periurethral laceration only.

§ √5ʰ **664.9 Unspecified trauma to perineum and vulva**   Ⓜ♀
[0,1,4]

√4ʰ **665 Other obstetrical trauma**
    INCLUDES damage from instruments

§ √5ʰ **665.0 Rupture of uterus before onset of labor**   Ⓜ♀
[0,1,3]

§ √5ʰ **665.1 Rupture of uterus during labor**   Ⓜ♀
[0,1]   Rupture of uterus NOS

§ √5ʰ **665.2 Inversion of uterus**   Ⓜ♀
[0,2,4]

§ √5ʰ **665.3 Laceration of cervix**   Ⓜ♀
[0,1,4]

§ √5ʰ **665.4 High vaginal laceration**   Ⓜ♀
[0,1,4]   Laceration of vaginal wall or sulcus without mention of perineal laceration
    071.4 Obstetric high vaginal laceration alone   I-10

§ √5ʰ **665.5 Other injury to pelvic organs**   Ⓜ♀
[0,1,4]   EXCLUDES *periurethral trauma (664.8)*
    Injury to:
      bladder
      urethra
    AHA: M-A, '87, 10
    071.5 Other obstetric injury to pelvic organs   I-10

§ √5ʰ **665.6 Damage to pelvic joints and ligaments**   Ⓜ♀
[0,1,4]   Avulsion of inner symphyseal cartilage
    Damage to coccyx
    Separation of symphysis (pubis)
    AHA: N-D, '84, 12

§ √5ʰ **665.7 Pelvic hematoma**   Ⓜ♀
[0,1,2,4]   Hematoma of vagina

§ √5ʰ **665.8 Other specified obstetrical trauma**   Ⓜ♀
[0-4]

§ √5ʰ **665.9 Unspecified obstetrical trauma**   Ⓜ♀
[0-4]

√4ʰ **666 Postpartum hemorrhage**
    AHA: 1Q, '88, 14

§ √5ʰ **666.0 Third-stage hemorrhage**   Ⓜ♀
[0,2,4]   Hemorrhage associated with retained, trapped, or adherent placenta
    Retained placenta NOS

§ √5ʰ **666.1 Other immediate postpartum hemorrhage**   Ⓜ♀
[0,2,4]   Atony of uterus with hemorrhage
    Hemorrhage within the first 24 hours following delivery of placenta
    Postpartum atony of uterus with hemorrhage
    Postpartum hemorrhage (atonic) NOS
    EXCLUDES *atony of uterus without hemorrhage (661.2)*
      postpartum atony of uterus without hemorrhage (669.8)
    072.1 Other immediate postpartum hemorrhage   I-10

§ √5ʰ **666.2 Delayed and secondary postpartum hemorrhage**   Ⓜ♀
[0,2,4]   Hemorrhage:
      after the first 24 hours following delivery
      associated with retained portions of placenta or membranes
    Postpartum hemorrhage specified as delayed or secondary
    Retained products of conception NOS, following delivery

§ √5ʰ **666.3 Postpartum coagulation defects**   Ⓜ♀
[0,2,4]   Postpartum:
      afibrinogenemia
      fibrinolysis

√4ʰ **667 Retained placenta or membranes, without hemorrhage**
    NOTE Requires fifth digit; valid digits are in [brackets] under each code. See beginning of section 660-669 for definitions.
    DEF: Postpartum condition resulting from failure to expel placental membrane tissues due to failed contractions of uterine wall.
    AHA: 1Q, '88, 14
    TIP: A retained placenta is one that has not separated or been expelled within one hour after completion of the second stage of labor (birth of the fetus).

§ √5ʰ **667.0 Retained placenta without hemorrhage**   Ⓜ♀
[0,2,4]   Placenta accreta
    Retained
      placenta: } without hemorrhage
    NOS
    total
    073.0 Retained placenta without hemorrhage   I-10

§ √5ʰ **667.1 Retained portions of placenta or**   Ⓜ♀
[0,2,4] **membranes, without hemorrhage**
    Retained products of conception following delivery, without hemorrhage

√4ʰ **668 Complications of the administration of anesthetic or other sedation in labor and delivery**
    INCLUDES complications arising from the administration of a general or local anesthetic, analgesic, or other sedation in labor and delivery
    EXCLUDES *reaction to spinal or lumbar puncture (349.0)*
      spinal headache (349.0)
    Use additional code(s) to further specify complication

§ √5ʰ **668.0 Pulmonary complications**   Ⓜ♀
[0-4]   Inhalation (aspiration) of
      stomach contents or   } following anesthesia or
      secretions   other sedation in
    Mendelson's syndrome   labor or delivery
    Pressure collapse of lung

§ √5ʰ **668.1 Cardiac complications**   Ⓜ♀
[0-4]   Cardiac arrest or failure following anesthesia or other sedation in labor and delivery

§ √5ʰ **668.2 Central nervous system complications**   Ⓜ♀
[0-4]   Cerebral anoxia following anesthesia or other sedation in labor and delivery

§ √5ʰ **668.8 Other complications of anesthesia or**   Ⓜ♀
[0-4] **other sedation in labor and delivery**
    AHA: 2Q, '99, 9

§ √5ʰ **668.9 Unspecified complication of anesthesia**   Ⓜ♀
[0-4] **and other sedation**

√4ʰ **669 Other complications of labor and delivery, not elsewhere classified**

§ √5ʰ **669.0 Maternal distress**   Ⓜ♀
[0-4]   Metabolic disturbance in labor and delivery

---

§   Requires fifth digit. Valid digits are in [brackets] under each code. See beginning of section 640-649 for codes and definitions.

√4ʰ √5ʰ Additional Digit Required   Unspecified Code   Other Specified Code   Manifestation Code   ►◄ Revised Text   ● New Code   ▲ Revised Code Title

2015 ICD-9-CM   **Volume 1 – 207**

Complications of Pregnancy, Childbirth, and the Puerperium

669.1–673.2

§ ✓5ᵗʰ **669.1 Shock during or following labor and delivery** Ⓜ♀
[0-4]   Obstetric shock

§ ✓5ᵗʰ **669.2 Maternal hypotension syndrome** Ⓜ♀
[0-4]   **DEF:** Low arterial blood pressure in mother during labor and delivery.

§ ✓5ᵗʰ **669.3 Acute kidney failure following labor and delivery** Ⓜ♀
[0,2,4]

§ ✓5ᵗʰ **669.4 Other complications of obstetrical surgery** Ⓜ♀
[0-4]   **and procedures**
     Cardiac:
       arrest   following cesarean or other obstetrical
       failure   surgery or procedure, including
     Cerebral anoxia   delivery NOS
      EXCLUDES *complications of obstetrical surgical wounds (674.1-674.3)*
      AHA: For code 669.42: ▶1Q, '14, 14◀

§ ✓5ᵗʰ **669.5 Forceps or vacuum extractor delivery** Ⓜ♀
[0,1]   **without mention of indication**
     Delivery by ventouse, without mention of indication

§ ✓5ᵗʰ **669.6 Breech extraction, without mention of** Ⓜ♀
[0,1]   **indication**
      EXCLUDES *breech delivery NOS (652.2)*

§ ✓5ᵗʰ **669.7 Cesarean delivery, without mention of indication** Ⓜ♀
[0,1]   **AHA: For code 669.71:** 1Q, '01, 11
     082 Encounter for cesarean delivery w/o indication   I-10

§ ✓5ᵗʰ **669.8 Other complications of labor and delivery** Ⓜ♀
[0-4]   **AHA:** 4Q, '06, 135

§ ✓5ᵗʰ **669.9 Unspecified complication of labor and delivery** Ⓜ♀
[0-4]

Complications of the Puerperium (670-677)

NOTE Categories 671 and 673-676 include the listed conditions even if they occur during pregnancy or childbirth.

The following fifth-digit subclassification is for use with categories 670-676 to denote the current episode of care. Valid fifth-digits are in [brackets] under each code.
0 unspecified as to episode of care or not applicable
1 delivered, with or without mention of antepartum condition
2 delivered, with mention of postpartum complication
3 antepartum condition or complication
4 postpartum condition or complication

✓4ᵗʰ **670 Major puerperal infection**
      EXCLUDES *infection following abortion (639.0)*
              minor genital tract infection following delivery (646.6)
              puerperal pyrexia NOS (672)
              puerperal fever NOS (672)
              puerperal pyrexia of unknown origin (672)
              urinary tract infection following delivery (646.6)
      DEF: Infection and inflammation following childbirth.
      AHA: 4Q, '91, 26; 2Q, '91, 7

§ ✓5ᵗʰ **670.0 Major puerperal infection, unspecified** Ⓜ♀
[0,2,4]   **AHA: For code 670.02:** 3Q, '07, 8

§ ✓5ᵗʰ **670.1 Puerperal endometritis** Ⓜ♀
[0,2,4]

§ ✓5ᵗʰ **670.2 Puerperal sepsis** Ⓜ♀
[0,2,4]   Puerperal pyemia
     Use additional code to identify severe sepsis (995.92) and any associated acute organ dysfunction, if applicable
     AHA: For code 670.24: 4Q, '09, 98
     TIP: Do not assign a code from category 038 or 995.91 Sepsis, along with a code from this subcategory. If applicable, assign additional codes to indicate severe sepsis (995.92), and any associated acute organ dysfunction.

§ ✓5ᵗʰ **670.3 Puerperal septic thrombophlebitis** Ⓜ♀
[0,2,4]

§ ✓5ᵗʰ **670.8 Other major puerperal infection** Ⓜ♀
[0,2,4]   Puerperal: Puerperal:
     pelvic cellulitis   salpingitis
     peritonitis

✓4ᵗʰ **671 Venous complications in pregnancy and the puerperium**
      EXCLUDES *personal history of venous complications prior to pregnancy, such as:*
              thrombophlebitis (V12.52)
              thrombosis and embolism (V12.51)

§ ✓5ᵗʰ **671.0 Varicose veins of legs** Ⓜ♀
[0-4]   Varicose veins NOS
     DEF: Distended, tortuous veins on legs associated with pregnancy.

§ ✓5ᵗʰ **671.1 Varicose veins of vulva and perineum** Ⓜ♀
[0-4]   **DEF:** Distended, tortuous veins on external female genitalia associated with pregnancy.

§ ✓5ᵗʰ **671.2 Superficial thrombophlebitis** Ⓜ♀
[0-4]   Phlebitis NOS
     Thrombophlebitis (superficial)
     Thrombosis NOS
     Use additional code to identify the superficial thrombophlebitis (453.6, 453.71, 453.81)

§ ✓5ᵗʰ **671.3 Deep phlebothrombosis, antepartum** Ⓜ♀
[0,1,3]   Deep vein thrombosis antepartum
     Use additional code to identify the deep vein thrombosis (453.40-453.42, 453.50-453.52, 453.72-453.79, 453.82-453.89)
     Use additional code for long term (current) use of anticoagulants, if applicable (V58.61)

§ ✓5ᵗʰ **671.4 Deep phlebothrombosis, postpartum** Ⓜ♀
[0,2,4]   Deep-vein thrombosis, postpartum
     Pelvic thrombophlebitis, postpartum
     Phlegmasia alba dolens (puerperal)
     Use additional code to identify the deep vein thrombosis (453.40-453.42, 453.50-453.52, 453.72-453.79, 453.82-453.89)
     Use additional code for long term (current) use of anticoagulants, if applicable (V58.61)

§ ✓5ᵗʰ **671.5 Other phlebitis and thrombosis** Ⓜ♀
[0-4]   Cerebral venous thrombosis
     Thrombosis of intracranial venous sinus

§ ✓5ᵗʰ **671.8 Other venous complications** Ⓜ♀
[0-4]   Hemorrhoids

§ ✓5ᵗʰ **671.9 Unspecified venous complication** Ⓜ♀
[0-4]

✓4ᵗʰ **672 Pyrexia of unknown origin during the puerperium** Ⓜ♀
[0,2,4]

§ ✓5ᵗʰ   **Use 0 as fourth-digit for this category**
     Postpartum fever NOS
     Puerperal fever NOS
     Puerperal pyrexia NOS
     DEF: Fever of unknown origin experienced by the mother after childbirth.
     AHA: 4Q, '91, 26
     086.4 Pyrexia of unknown origin following delivery   I-10

✓4ᵗʰ **673 Obstetrical pulmonary embolism**
      INCLUDES *pulmonary emboli in pregnancy, childbirth, or the puerperium, or specified as puerperal*
      EXCLUDES *embolism following abortion (639.6)*

§ ✓5ᵗʰ **673.0 Obstetrical air embolism** Ⓜ♀
[0-4]   **DEF:** Sudden blocking of pulmonary artery with air or nitrogen bubbles during puerperium.

§ ✓5ᵗʰ **673.1 Amniotic fluid embolism** Ⓜ♀
[0-4]   **DEF:** Sudden onset of pulmonary artery blockage from amniotic fluid entering the mother's circulation near the end of pregnancy due to strong uterine contractions.

§ ✓5ᵗʰ **673.2 Obstetrical blood-clot embolism** Ⓜ♀
[0-4]   Puerperal pulmonary embolism NOS
     AHA: For code 673.24: 1Q, '05, 6
     DEF: Blood clot blocking artery in the lung; associated with pregnancy.
     TIP: If a pregnant or postpartum patient develops a pulmonary embolism that progresses to acute respiratory failure, the code for the pregnancy/delivery complication (673.2X) should be sequenced first.

---

§   Requires fifth digit. Valid digits are in [brackets] under each code. See beginning of section 640-649 for codes and definitions.

Ⓝ Newborn Age: 0   Ⓟ Pediatric Age: 0-17   Ⓜ Maternity Age: 12-55   Ⓐ Adult Age: 15-124

§ ✓5ᵗʰ **673.3 Obstetrical pyemic and septic embolism**   Ⓜ♀
[0-4]

§ ✓5ᵗʰ **673.8 Other pulmonary embolism**   Ⓜ♀
[0-4]   Fat embolism

✓4ᵗʰ **674 Other and unspecified complications of the puerperium, not elsewhere classified**

§ ✓5ᵗʰ **674.0 Cerebrovascular disorders in the puerperium**   Ⓜ♀
[0-4]   Any condition classifiable to 430-434, 436-437 occurring during pregnancy, childbirth, or the puerperium, or specified as puerperal
EXCLUDES *intracranial venous sinus thrombosis (671.5)*

§ ✓5ᵗʰ **674.1 Disruption of cesarean wound**   Ⓜ♀
[0,2,4]   Dehiscence or disruption of uterine wound
EXCLUDES *uterine rupture before onset of labor (665.0)*
uterine rupture during labor (665.1)
AHA: ▶3Q, '13, 6◀

§ ✓5ᵗʰ **674.2 Disruption of perineal wound**   Ⓜ♀
[0,2,4]   Breakdown of perineum
Disruption of wound of:
episiotomy
perineal laceration
Secondary perineal tear
AHA: For code 674.24: 1Q, '97, 9

§ ✓5ᵗʰ **674.3 Other complications of obstetrical surgical**   Ⓜ♀
[0,2,4] **wounds**
Hematoma }
Hemorrhage } of cesarean section or
Infection } perineal wound
EXCLUDES *damage from instruments in delivery (664.0-665.9)*
AHA: For code 674.32: 2Q, '91, 7; **For code 674.34:** 4Q, '09, 98

§ ✓5ᵗʰ **674.4 Placental polyp**   Ⓜ♀
[0,2,4]

§ ✓5ᵗʰ **674.5 Peripartum cardiomyopathy**   Ⓜ♀
[0-4]   Postpartum cardiomyopathy
DEF: Any structural or functional abnormality of the ventricular myocardium, non-inflammatory disease of obscure or unknown etiology with onset during the postpartum period.
AHA: 4Q, '03, 65; **For code 674.54:** 3Q, '12, 9

§ ✓5ᵗʰ **674.8 Other**   Ⓜ♀
[0,2,4]   Hepatorenal syndrome, following delivery
Postpartum:
subinvolution of uterus
uterine hypertrophy
AHA: 3Q, '98, 16

§ ✓5ᵗʰ **674.9 Unspecified**   Ⓜ♀
[0,2,4]   Sudden death of unknown cause during the puerperium

✓4ᵗʰ **675 Infections of the breast and nipple associated with childbirth**
INCLUDES the listed conditions during pregnancy, childbirth, or the puerperium

§ ✓5ᵗʰ **675.0 Infections of nipple**   Ⓜ♀
[0-4]   Abscess of nipple

§ ✓5ᵗʰ **675.1 Abscess of breast**   Ⓜ♀
[0-4]   Abscess: Abscess:
mammary   purulent
subareolar   retromammary
submammary   submammary

§ ✓5ᵗʰ **675.2 Nonpurulent mastitis**   Ⓜ♀
[0-4]   Lymphangitis of breast
Mastitis:
NOS
interstitial
parenchymatous

§ ✓5ᵗʰ **675.8 Other specified infections of the breast and**   Ⓜ♀
[0-4] **nipple**

§ ✓5ᵗʰ **675.9 Unspecified infection of the breast and nipple**   Ⓜ♀
[0-4]

Lactation Process: Ejection Reflex Arc

✓4ᵗʰ **676 Other disorders of the breast associated with childbirth and disorders of lactation**
INCLUDES the listed conditions during pregnancy, the puerperium, or lactation

§ ✓5ᵗʰ **676.0 Retracted nipple**   Ⓜ♀
[0-4]

§ ✓5ᵗʰ **676.1 Cracked nipple**   Ⓜ♀
[0-4]   Fissure of nipple

§ ✓5ᵗʰ **676.2 Engorgement of breasts**   Ⓜ♀
[0-4]   **DEF:** Abnormal accumulation of milk in ducts of breast.

§ ✓5ᵗʰ **676.3 Other and unspecified disorder of breast**   Ⓜ♀
[0-4]

§ ✓5ᵗʰ **676.4 Failure of lactation**   Ⓜ♀
[0-4]   Agalactia
DEF: Abrupt ceasing of milk secretion by breast.

§ ✓5ᵗʰ **676.5 Suppressed lactation**   Ⓜ♀
[0-4]

§ ✓5ᵗʰ **676.6 Galactorrhea**   Ⓜ♀
[0-4]   **EXCLUDES** *galactorrhea not associated with childbirth (611.6)*
DEF: Excessive or persistent milk secretion by breast; may be in absence of nursing.

§ ✓5ᵗʰ **676.8 Other disorders of lactation**   Ⓜ♀
[0-4]   Galactocele
DEF: Galactocele: Obstructed mammary gland, creating retention cyst, results in milk-filled cysts enlarging mammary gland.
AHA: 3Q, '12, 7

§ ✓5ᵗʰ **676.9 Unspecified disorder of lactation**   Ⓜ♀
[0-4]

677 Late effect of complication of pregnancy, childbirth, and the puerperium   ♀
NOTE This category is to be used to indicate conditions in 632-648.9 and 651-676.9 as the cause of the late effect, themselves classifiable elsewhere. The "late effects" include conditions specified as such, or as sequelae, which may occur at any time after puerperium.
Code first any sequelae
AHA: ▶3Q, '13, 6;◀ 1Q, '97, 9; 4Q, '94, 42
TIP: Sequence as a secondary diagnosis, after the code for the late effect complication. May be assigned at any time after the initial postpartum period (six weeks following delivery).

---

§ Requires fifth digit. Valid digits are in [brackets] under each code. See beginning of section 640-649 for codes and definitions.

| ✓4ᵗʰ ✓5ᵗʰ Additional Digit Required | Unspecified Code | Other Specified Code | Manifestation Code | ▶◀ Revised Text | ● New Code | ▲ Revised Code Title |

Other Maternal and Fetal Complications (678-679)

The following fifth-digit subclassification is for use with categories 678-679 to denote the current episode of care. Valid fifth-digits are in [brackets] under each code.

0 **unspecified as to episode of care or not applicable**
1 **delivered, with or without mention of antepartum condition**
2 **delivered, with mention of postpartum complication**
3 **antepartum condition or complication**
4 **postpartum condition or complication**

√4ᵗʰ **678**   **Other fetal conditions**

§ √5ᵗʰ   **678.0 Fetal hematologic conditions**   M ♀
    [0,1,3]   Fetal anemia
           Fetal thrombocytopenia
           Fetal twin to twin transfusion

         EXCLUDES *fetal and neonatal hemorrhage (772.0-772.9)*
                  fetal hematologic disorders affecting newborn (776.0-776.9)
                  fetal-maternal hemorrhage (656.00-656.03)
                  isoimmunization incompatibility (656.10-656.13, 656.20-656.23)

         AHA: 4Q, '08, 125-127

§ √5ᵗʰ   **678.1 Fetal conjoined twins**   M ♀
    [0,1,3]   **AHA:** 4Q, '08, 125-127

√4ᵗʰ **679**   **Complications of in utero procedures**
      AHA: 4Q, '08, 127-128, 158

§ √5ᵗʰ   **679.0 Maternal complications from in utero procedure**   M ♀
    [0-4]   **EXCLUDES** *maternal history of in utero procedure during previous pregnancy (V23.86)*

§ √5ᵗʰ   **679.1 Fetal complications from in utero procedure**   M ♀
    [0-4]   Fetal complications from amniocentesis
         EXCLUDES *newborn affected by in utero procedure (760.61-760.64)*

         TIP: Assign only on the mother's record. Although there is a fetal complication, it affects the mother's pregnancy.

---

§   Requires fifth digit. Valid digits are in [brackets] under each code. See beginning of section 640-649 for codes and definitions.

N Newborn Age: 0   **P** Pediatric Age: 0-17   **M** Maternity Age: 12-55   **A** Adult Age: 15-124

12. Diseases of the Skin and Subcutaneous Tissue (680-709)

Infections of Skin and Subcutaneous Tissue (680-686)

EXCLUDES *certain infections of skin classified under "Infectious and Parasitic Diseases," such as:*
erysipelas (035)
erysipeloid of Rosenbach (027.1)
herpes:
simplex (054.0-054.9)
zoster (053.0-053.9)
molluscum contagiosum (078.0)
viral warts (078.10-078.19)

✓4ᵗʰ 680 Carbuncle and furuncle

INCLUDES boil
furunculosis

DEF: Carbuncle: necrotic boils in skin and subcutaneous tissue of neck or back mainly due to staphylococcal infection.
DEF: Furuncle: circumscribed inflammation of corium and subcutaneous tissue due to staphylococcal infection.

680.0 Face
Ear [any part]
Face [any part, except eye]
Nose (septum)
Temple (region)
EXCLUDES *eyelid (373.13)*
lacrimal apparatus (375.31)
orbit (376.01)

680.1 Neck

680.2 Trunk
Abdominal wall
Back [any part, except buttocks]
Breast
Chest wall
Flank
Groin
Pectoral region
Perineum
Umbilicus
EXCLUDES *buttocks (680.5)*
external genital organs:
female (616.4)
male (607.2, 608.4)

680.3 Upper arm and forearm
Arm [any part, except hand]
Axilla
Shoulder

680.4 Hand
Finger [any]
Thumb
Wrist

680.5 Buttock
Anus
Gluteal region

680.6 Leg, except foot
Ankle
Hip
Knee
Thigh

680.7 Foot
Heel
Toe

680.8 Other specified sites
Head [any part, except face]
Scalp
EXCLUDES *external genital organs:*
female (616.4)
male (607.2, 608.4)

680.9 Unspecified site
Boil NOS
Carbuncle NOS
Furuncle NOS

Skin and Subcutaneous Layer

Hair follicle
Epidermis
Dermis
Hypodermis (subcutaneous layer)
Bulb
Sebaceous gland
Arrector pili muscle
Thick-skin epidermis
Hair shaft
Pacinian corpuscle
Hair matrix
Sweat (eccrine gland)
Sensory nerve
Blood vessels

✓4ᵗʰ 681 Cellulitis and abscess of finger and toe

INCLUDES that with lymphangitis

Use additional code to identify organism, such as Staphylococcus (041.1)

DEF: Acute suppurative inflammation and edema in subcutaneous tissue or muscle of finger or toe.
AHA: 2Q, '91, 5; J-F, '87, 12
TIP: Coding of cellulitis due to superficial injury, burn, or frostbite requires two codes, one for the injury and one for the cellulitis. Sequencing depends on the circumstances of the admission.

✓5ᵗʰ 681.0 Finger

681.00 Cellulitis and abscess, unspecified
L03.019 Cellulitis of unspecified finger `I-10`

681.01 Felon
Pulp abscess   Whitlow
EXCLUDES *herpetic whitlow (054.6)*
DEF: Painful abscess of fingertips caused by infection in the closed space of terminal phalanx.

681.02 Onychia and paronychia of finger
Panaritium
Perionychia } of finger
DEF: Onychia: inflammation of nail matrix; causes nail loss.
DEF: Paronychia: inflammation of tissue folds around nail.

✓5ᵗʰ 681.1 Toe

681.10 Cellulitis and abscess, unspecified
AHA: 1Q, '05, 14
L03.039 Cellulitis of unspecified toe `I-10`

681.11 Onychia and paronychia of toe
Panaritium
Perionychia } of toe

681.9 Cellulitis and abscess of unspecified digit
Infection of nail NOS

✓4ᵗʰ 682 Other cellulitis and abscess

INCLUDES abscess (acute
cellulitis (diffuse)
lymphangitis, acute } (with lymphangitis) except of finger or toe

Use additional code to identify organism, such as Staphylococcus (041.1)

EXCLUDES *lymphangitis (chronic) (subacute) (457.2)*
DEF: Cellulitis: Acute suppurative inflammation of deep subcutaneous tissue and sometimes muscle due to infection of wound, burn or other lesion.
AHA: 2Q, '91, 5; J-F, '87, 12; S-O, '85, 10
TIP: Coding of cellulitis due to superficial injury, burn, or frostbite requires two codes, one for the injury and one for the cellulitis. Sequencing depends on the circumstances of the admission.

682.0 Face
Cheek, external   Nose, external
Chin   Submandibular
Forehead   Temple (region)
EXCLUDES *ear [any part] (380.10-380.16)*
eyelid (373.13)
lacrimal apparatus (375.31)
lip (528.5)
mouth (528.3)
nose (internal) (478.1)
orbit (376.01)
AHA: ▶4Q, '13, 98◀
L03.211 Cellulitis of face `I-10`

| ✓4ᵗʰ ✓5ᵗʰ Additional Digit Required | Unspecified Code | Other Specified Code | Manifestation Code | ▶◀ Revised Text | ● New Code | ▲ Revised Code Title |

Diseases of the Skin and Subcutaneous Tissue

682.1–686.1

682.1 Neck
L03.221 Cellulitis of neck   I-10

682.2 Trunk
Abdominal wall
Back [any part, except buttock]
Chest wall
Flank
Groin
Pectoral region
Perineum
Umbilicus, except newborn

EXCLUDES   anal and rectal regions (566)
breast:
NOS (611.0)
puerperal (675.1)
external genital organs:
female (616.3-616.4)
male (604.0, 607.2, 608.4)
umbilicus, newborn (771.4)

AHA: 4Q, '98, 42
L03.319 Cellulitis of trunk unspecified   I-10

682.3 Upper arm and forearm
Arm [any part, except hand]
Axilla
Shoulder

EXCLUDES   hand (682.4)

AHA: 2Q, '03, 7
L03.113 Cellulitis of right upper limb   I-10

682.4 Hand, except fingers and thumb
Wrist

EXCLUDES   finger and thumb (681.00-681.02)

682.5 Buttock
Gluteal region

EXCLUDES   anal and rectal regions (566)
L03.317 Cellulitis of buttock   I-10

682.6 Leg, except foot
Ankle
Hip
Knee
Thigh

AHA: 3Q, '12, 13; 1Q, '09, 10; 3Q, '04, 5; 4Q, '03, 108
L03.115 Cellulitis of right lower limb   I-10

682.7 Foot, except toes
Heel

EXCLUDES   toe (681.10-681.11)

682.8 Other specified sites
Head [except face]
Scalp

EXCLUDES   face (682.0)

682.9 Unspecified site
Abscess NOS
Cellulitis NOS
Lymphangitis, acute NOS

EXCLUDES   lymphangitis NOS (457.2)

683 Acute lymphadenitis
Abscess (acute)
Adenitis, acute   } lymph gland or node, except mesenteric
Lymphadenitis, acute

Use additional code to identify organism, such as Staphylococcus (041.1)

EXCLUDES   enlarged glands NOS (785.6)
lymphadenitis:
chronic or subacute, except mesenteric (289.1)
mesenteric (acute) (chronic) (subacute) (289.2)
unspecified (289.3)

DEF: Acute inflammation of lymph nodes due to primary infection located elsewhere in the body.

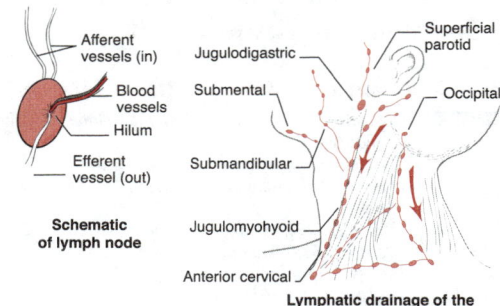

Lymphatic System of Head and Neck

Afferent vessels (in)
Blood vessels
Hilum
Efferent vessel (out)
Schematic of lymph node
Jugulodigastric
Submental
Submandibular
Jugulomyohyoid
Anterior cervical
Superficial parotid
Occipital

Lymphatic drainage of the head, neck, and face

684 Impetigo
Impetiginization of other dermatoses
Impetigo (contagiosa) [any site] [any organism]:
bullous
circinate
neonatorum
simplex
Pemphigus neonatorum

EXCLUDES   impetigo herpetiformis (694.3)

DEF: Infectious skin disease commonly occurring in children; caused by group A streptococci or *Staphylococcus aureus;* skin lesions usually appear on the face and consist of subcorneal vesicles and bullae that burst and form yellow crusts.

✓4th **685 Pilonidal cyst**
INCLUDES   fistula   } coccygeal or pilonidal
              sinus

DEF: Hair-containing cyst or sinus in the tissues of the sacrococcygeal area; often drains through opening at the postanal dimple.

685.0 With abscess

685.1 Without mention of abscess
AHA: 3Q, '11, 9

✓4th **686 Other local infections of skin and subcutaneous tissue**
Use additional code to identify any infectious organism (041.0-041.8)

✓5th **686.0 Pyoderma**
Dermatitis: Dermatitis:
purulent   suppurative
septic

DEF: Nonspecific purulent skin disease related most to furuncles, pustules, or possibly carbuncles.

686.00 Pyoderma, unspecified

686.01 Pyoderma gangrenosum
DEF: Persistent debilitating skin disease characterized by irregular, boggy, blue-red ulcerations, with central healing and undermined edges.
AHA: 4Q, '97, 42

686.09 Other pyoderma

686.1 Pyogenic granuloma
Granuloma: Granuloma:
septic   telangiectaticum
suppurative

EXCLUDES   pyogenic granuloma of oral mucosa (528.9)

DEF: Solitary polypoid capillary hemangioma often associated with local irritation, trauma, and superimposed inflammation; located on the skin and gingival or oral mucosa.

Stages of Pilonidal Disease

Normal follicle
Stretched follicle
Infected follicle
Acute abscess
Chronic abscess
Epithelial tube

686.8 Other specified local infections of skin and subcutaneous tissue
Bacterid (pustular)
Dermatitis vegetans
Ecthyma
Perlèche
> *EXCLUDES* *dermatitis infectiosa eczematoides (690.8)*
> *panniculitis (729.30-729.39)*

686.9 Unspecified local infection of skin and subcutaneous tissue
Fistula of skin NOS
Skin infection NOS
> *EXCLUDES* *fistula to skin from internal organs — see Alphabetic Index*

Other Inflammatory Conditions of Skin and Subcutaneous Tissue (690-698)

> *EXCLUDES* *panniculitis (729.30-729.39)*

690 Erythematosquamous dermatosis
> *EXCLUDES* *eczematous dermatitis of eyelid (373.31)*
> *parakeratosis variegata (696.2)*
> *psoriasis (696.0-696.1)*
> *seborrheic keratosis (702.11-702.19)*

690.1 Seborrheic dermatitis
AHA: 4Q, '95, 58

690.10 Seborrheic dermatitis, unspecified
Seborrheic dermatitis NOS
L21.9 Seborrheic dermatitis unspecified   I-10

690.11 Seborrhea capitis   P
Cradle cap

690.12 Seborrheic infantile dermatitis   P

690.18 Other seborrheic dermatitis

690.8 Other erythematosquamous dermatosis

691 Atopic dermatitis and related conditions
DEF: Atopic dermatitis: chronic, pruritic, inflammatory skin disorder found on the face and antecubital and popliteal fossae; often accompanied by allergic rhinitis, hay fever, asthma, and extreme itching; also called allergic dermatitis, or disseminated neurodermatitis.

691.0 Diaper or napkin rash
Ammonia dermatitis
Diaper or napkin:
   dermatitis
   erythema
   rash
Psoriasiform napkin eruption

691.8 Other atopic dermatitis and related conditions
Atopic dermatitis
Besnier's prurigo
Eczema:
   atopic
   flexural
   intrinsic (allergic)
Neurodermatitis:
   atopic
   diffuse (of Brocq)

692 Contact dermatitis and other eczema
> INCLUDES dermatitis:
>   NOS
>   contact
>   occupational
>   venenata
> eczema (acute) (chronic):
>   NOS
>   allergic
>   erythematous
>   occupational
> *EXCLUDES* *allergy NOS (995.3)*
> *contact dermatitis of eyelids (373.32)*
> *dermatitis due to substances taken internally (693.0-693.9)*
> *eczema of external ear (380.22)*
> *perioral dermatitis (695.3)*
> *urticarial reactions (708.0-708.9, 995.1)*

DEF: Contact dermatitis: acute or chronic dermatitis caused by initial irritant effect of a substance, or by prior sensitization to a substance coming once again in contact with skin.

692.0 Due to detergents

692.1 Due to oils and greases

692.2 Due to solvents
Dermatitis due to solvents of:
   chlorocompound ⎫
   cyclohexane |
   ester   ⎬ group
   glycol |
   hydrocarbon |
   ketone   ⎭

692.3 Due to drugs and medicines in contact with skin
Dermatitis (allergic) (contact) due to:
   arnica
   fungicides
   iodine
   keratolytics
   mercurials
   neomycin
   pediculocides
   phenols
   scabicides
   any drug applied to skin
Dermatitis medicamentosa due to drug applied to skin
Use additional E code to identify drug
> *EXCLUDES* *allergy NOS due to drugs (995.27)*
> *dermatitis due to ingested drugs (693.0)*
> *dermatitis medicamentosa NOS (693.0)*

692.4 Due to other chemical products
Dermatitis due to:
   acids
   adhesive plaster
   alkalis
   caustics
   dichromate
   insecticide
   nylon
   plastic
   rubber
AHA: 3Q, '08, 6-7; 2Q, '89, 16

692.5 Due to food in contact with skin
Dermatitis, contact, due to:
   cereals
   fish
   flour
   fruit
   meat
   milk
> *EXCLUDES* *dermatitis due to:*
> *dyes (692.89)*
> *ingested foods (693.1)*
> *preservatives (692.89)*

√4ᵗʰ √5ᵗʰ Additional Digit Required   Unspecified Code   Other Specified Code   Manifestation Code   ►◄ Revised Text   ● New Code   ▲ Revised Code Title

2015 ICD-9-CM   **Volume 1 – 213**

692.6 Due to plants [except food]
Dermatitis due to:
lacquer tree [Rhus verniciflua]
poison:
ivy [Rhus toxicodendron]
oak [Rhus diversiloba]
sumac [Rhus venenata]
vine [Rhus radicans]
primrose [Primula]
ragweed [Senecio jacobae]
other plants in contact with the skin

> EXCLUDES   *allergy NOS due to pollen (477.0)*
>   *nettle rash (708.8)*

√5ᵗʰ **692.7 Due to solar radiation**

> EXCLUDES   *sunburn due to other ultraviolet radiation exposure*
>   *(692.82)*

692.70 Unspecified dermatitis due to sun

692.71 Sunburn
First degree sunburn
Sunburn NOS
AHA: 4Q, '01, 47
TIP: Do not assign if sunburn is due to tanning bed use; see instead code 692.82.

692.72 Acute dermatitis due to solar radiation
Acute solar skin damage NOS
Berloque dermatitis
Photoallergic response
Phototoxic response
Polymorphus light eruption
Use additional E code to identify drug, if drug induced

> EXCLUDES   *sunburn (692.71, 692.76-692.77)*

DEF: Berloque dermatitis: Phytophotodermatitis due to sun exposure after use of a product containing bergamot oil; causes red patches, that turn brown.
DEF: Photoallergic response: Dermatitis due to hypersensitivity to the sun; causes papulovesicular, eczematous or exudative eruptions.
DEF: Phototoxic response: Chemically induced sensitivity to sun causes burn-like reaction, occasionally vesiculation and subsequent hyperpigmentation.
DEF: Polymorphous light eruption: Inflammatory skin eruptions due to sunlight exposure; eruptions differ in size and shape.
DEF: Acute solar skin damage (NOS): Rapid, unspecified injury to skin from sun.

692.73 Actinic reticuloid and actinic granuloma
DEF: Actinic reticuloid: Dermatosis aggravated by light, causes chronic eczema-like eruption on exposed skin which extends to other unexposed surfaces; occurs in the elderly.
DEF: Actinic granuloma: Inflammatory response of skin to sun causing small nodule of microphages.

692.74 Other chronic dermatitis due to solar radiation
Chronic solar skin damage NOS
Solar elastosis

> EXCLUDES   *actinic [solar] keratosis (702.0)*

DEF: Solar elastosis: Premature aging of skin of light-skinned people; causes inelasticity, thinning or thickening, wrinkling, dryness, scaling and hyperpigmentation.
DEF: Chronic solar skin damage (NOS): Chronic skin impairment due to exposure to the sun, not otherwise specified.

692.75 Disseminated superficial actinic porokeratosis [DSAP]
DEF: Autosomal dominant skin condition occurring in skin that has been overexposed to the sun; characterized by superficial annular, keratotic, brownish-red spots or thickenings with depressed centers and sharp, ridged borders, may evolve into squamous cell carcinoma.
AHA: 4Q, '00, 43

692.76 Sunburn of second degree
AHA: 4Q, '01, 47
TIP: Do not assign if sunburn is due to tanning bed use; see instead code 692.82.

692.77 Sunburn of third degree
AHA: 4Q, '01, 47
TIP: Do not assign if sunburn is due to tanning bed use; see instead code 692.82.

692.79 Other dermatitis due to solar radiation
Hydroa aestivale
Photodermatitis   }
Photosensitiveness } (due to sun)
Solar skin damage NOS

√5ᵗʰ **692.8 Due to other specified agents**

692.81 Dermatitis due to cosmetics

692.82 Dermatitis due to other radiation
Infrared rays
Light, except from sun
Radiation NOS
Tanning bed
Ultraviolet rays, except from sun
X-rays

> EXCLUDES   *solar radiation (692.70-692.79)*

AHA: 4Q, '01, 47; 3Q, '00, 5

692.83 Dermatitis due to metals
Jewelry

692.84 Due to animal (cat) (dog) dander
Due to animal (cat) (dog) hair

692.89 Other
Dermatitis due to:
cold weather
dyes
hot weather
preservatives

> EXCLUDES   *allergy (NOS) (rhinitis) due to animal hair or*
>   *dander (477.2)*
>   *allergy to dust (477.8)*
>   *sunburn (692.71, 692.76-692.77)*

692.9 Unspecified cause
Dermatitis:
NOS
contact NOS
venenata NOS
Eczema NOS
L23.9 Allergic contact dermatitis unspecified cause   I-10

√4ᵗʰ **693 Dermatitis due to substances taken internally**

> EXCLUDES   *adverse effect NOS of drugs and medicines (995.20)*
>   *allergy NOS (995.3)*
>   *contact dermatitis (692.0-692.9)*
>   *urticarial reactions (708.0-708.9, 995.1)*

DEF: Inflammation of skin due to ingested substance.

693.0 Due to drugs and medicines
Dermatitis medicamentosa NOS
Use additional E code to identify drug

> EXCLUDES   *that due to drugs in contact with skin (692.3)*

AHA: 2Q, '07, 8
TIP: Assign for palmar plantar erythrodysesthesia (PPE) or hand-foot syndrome due to chemotherapy drugs.
L27.0 Gen skin eruption d/t Rx & med taken internally   I-10

693.1 Due to food

693.8 Due to other specified substances taken internally

693.9 Due to unspecified substance taken internally

> EXCLUDES   *dermatitis NOS (692.9)*

✓4ᵗʰ 694 Bullous dermatoses

694.0 Dermatitis herpetiformis
Dermatosis herpetiformis
Duhring's disease
Hydroa herpetiformis

EXCLUDES *herpes gestationis (646.8)*
dermatitis herpetiformis:
juvenile (694.2)
senile (694.5)

DEF: Chronic, multisystem disease manifested most in the cutaneous system; seen as an extremely pruritic eruption of various lesions that frequently heal leaving hyperpigmentation or hypopigmentation and occasionally scarring; usually associated with an asymptomatic gluten-sensitive enteropathy, and immunogenic factors.

694.1 Subcorneal pustular dermatosis
Sneddon-Wilkinson disease or syndrome

DEF: Chronic relapses of sterile pustular blebs beneath the horny skin layer of the trunk and skin folds; resembles dermatitis herpetiformis.

694.2 Juvenile dermatitis herpetiformis
Juvenile pemphigoid

694.3 Impetigo herpetiformis

DEF: Rare dermatosis associated with pregnancy; marked by itching pustules in third trimester, hypocalcemia, tetany, fever and lethargy; may result in maternal or fetal death.

694.4 Pemphigus
Pemphigus:
NOS
erythematosus
foliaceus
malignant
vegetans
vulgaris

EXCLUDES *pemphigus neonatorum (684)*

DEF: Chronic, relapsing, sometimes fatal skin diseases; causes vesicles, bullae; autoantibodies against intracellular connections cause acantholysis.

694.5 Pemphigoid
Benign pemphigus NOS
Bullous pemphigoid
Herpes circinatus bullosus
Senile dermatitis herpetiformis

✓5ᵗʰ 694.6 Benign mucous membrane pemphigoid
Cicatricial pemphigoid
Mucosynechial atrophic bullous dermatitis

694.60 Without mention of ocular involvement

694.61 With ocular involvement
Ocular pemphigus

DEF: Mild self-limiting, subepidermal blistering of mucosa including the conjunctiva, seen predominantly in the elderly, produces adhesions and scarring.

694.8 Other specified bullous dermatoses

EXCLUDES *herpes gestationis (646.8)*

694.9 Unspecified bullous dermatoses

✓4ᵗʰ 695 Erythematous conditions

695.0 Toxic erythema
Erythema venenatum

✓5ᵗʰ 695.1 Erythema multiforme
Use additional code to identify associated manifestations, such as:
arthropathy associated with dermatological disorders (713.3)
conjunctival edema (372.73)
conjunctivitis (372.04, 372.33)
corneal scars and opacities (371.00-371.05)
corneal ulcer (370.00-370.07)
edema of eyelid (374.82)
inflammation of eyelid (373.8)
keratoconjunctivitis sicca (370.33)
mechanical lagophthalmos (374.22)
mucositis (478.11, 528.00, 538, 616.81)
stomatitis (528.00)
symblepharon (372.63)
Use additional E code to identify drug, if drug-induced
Use additional code to identify percentage of skin exfoliation (695.50-695.59)

EXCLUDES *(Staphylococcal) scalded skin syndrome (695.81)*

DEF: Symptom complex with varied skin eruption pattern of macular, bullous, papular, nodose, or vesicular lesions on the neck, face, and legs; gastritis and rheumatic pains; secondary to number of factors, including infections, ingestants, physical agents, malignancy and pregnancy.
AHA: 4Q, '08, 128-130

695.10 Erythema multiforme, unspecified
Erythema iris
Herpes iris

695.11 Erythema multiforme minor

695.12 Erythema multiforme major

695.13 Stevens-Johnson syndrome

695.14 Stevens-Johnson syndrome-toxic epidermal necrolysis overlap syndrome
SJS-TEN overlap syndrome
AHA: 4Q, '08, 131

695.15 Toxic epidermal necrolysis
Lyell's syndrome

695.19 Other erythema multiforme

695.2 Erythema nodosum

EXCLUDES *tuberculous erythema nodosum (017.1)*

DEF: Panniculitis (an inflammatory reaction of the subcutaneous fat) of women, usually seen as a hypersensitivity reaction to infections, drugs, sarcoidosis, and specific enteropathies; the acute stage associated with fever, malaise, and arthralgia; the lesions are pink to blue in color as tender nodules and are found on the front of the legs below the knees.

695.3 Rosacea
Acne:
erythematosa
rosacea
Perioral dermatitis
Rhinophyma

DEF: Chronic skin disease, usually of the face, characterized by persistent erythema and telangiectasis with acute episodes of edema, engorgement papules, and pustules.

695.4 Lupus erythematosus
Lupus:
erythematodes (discoid)
erythematosus (discoid), not disseminated

EXCLUDES *lupus (vulgaris) NOS (017.0)*
systemic [disseminated] lupus erythematosus (710.0)

DEF: Group of connective tissue disorders occurring as various cutaneous diseases of unknown origin; it primarily affects women between the ages of 20 and 40.

Diseases of the Skin and Subcutaneous Tissue

695.5–698.2

✓5ᵗʰ **695.5 Exfoliation due to erythematous conditions according to extent of body surface involved**

Code first erythematous condition causing exfoliation, such as:
Ritter's disease (695.81)
(Staphylococcal) scalded skin syndrome (695.81)
Stevens-Johnson syndrome (695.13)
Stevens-Johnson syndrome-toxic epidermal necrolysis overlap syndrome (695.14)
toxic epidermal necrolysis (695.15)
AHA: 4Q, '08, 128-131

695.50 Exfoliation due to erythematous condition involving less than 10 percent of body surface
Exfoliation due to erythematous condition NOS

695.51 Exfoliation due to erythematous condition involving 10-19 percent of body surface

695.52 Exfoliation due to erythematous condition involving 20-29 percent of body surface

695.53 Exfoliation due to erythematous condition involving 30-39 percent of body surface
AHA: 4Q, '08, 131

695.54 Exfoliation due to erythematous condition involving 40-49 percent of body surface

695.55 Exfoliation due to erythematous condition involving 50-59 percent of body surface

695.56 Exfoliation due to erythematous condition involving 60-69 percent of body surface

695.57 Exfoliation due to erythematous condition involving 70-79 percent of body surface

695.58 Exfoliation due to erythematous condition involving 80-89 percent of body surface

695.59 Exfoliation due to erythematous condition involving 90 percent or more of body surface

✓5ᵗʰ **695.8 Other specified erythematous conditions**

695.81 Ritter's disease
Dermatitis exfoliativa neonatorum
(Staphylococcal) Scalded skin syndrome
Use additional code to identify percentage of skin exfoliation (695.50-695.59)
DEF: Infectious skin disease of young children marked by eruptions ranging from a localized bullous to widespread of easily ruptured fine vesicles and bullae; results in exfoliation of large planes of skin and leaves raw areas.

695.89 Other
Erythema intertrigo
Intertrigo
Pityriasis rubra (Hebra)
EXCLUDES mycotic intertrigo (111.0-111.9)
AHA: S-O, '86, 10

695.9 Unspecified erythematous condition
Erythema NOS
Erythroderma (secondary)

✓4ᵗʰ **696 Psoriasis and similar disorders**

696.0 Psoriatic arthropathy
DEF: Psoriasis associated with inflammatory arthritis; often involves interphalangeal joints.

696.1 Other psoriasis
Acrodermatitis continua
Dermatitis repens
Psoriasis:
NOS
any type, except arthropathic
EXCLUDES psoriatic arthropathy (696.0)
L40.9 Psoriasis unspecified   I-10

696.2 Parapsoriasis
Parakeratosis variegata
Parapsoriasis lichenoides chronica
Pityriasis lichenoides et varioliformis
DEF: Erythrodermas similar to lichen, planus and psoriasis; symptoms include redness and itching; resistant to treatment.

696.3 Pityriasis rosea
Pityriasis circinata (et maculata)
DEF: Common, self-limited rash of unknown etiology marked by a solitary erythematous, salmon or fawn-colored herald plaque on the trunk, arms or thighs; followed by development of papular or macular lesions that tend to peel and form a scaly collarette.

696.4 Pityriasis rubra pilaris
Devergie's disease
Lichen ruber acuminatus
EXCLUDES pityriasis rubra (Hebra) (695.89)
DEF: Inflammatory disease of hair follicles; marked by firm, red lesions topped by horny plugs; may form patches; occurs on fingers elbows, knees.

696.5 Other and unspecified pityriasis
Pityriasis:
NOS
alba
streptogenes
EXCLUDES pityriasis:
simplex (690.18)
versicolor (111.0)

696.8 Other

✓4ᵗʰ **697 Lichen**
EXCLUDES lichen:
obtusus corneus (698.3)
pilaris (congenital) (757.39)
ruber acuminatus (696.4)
sclerosus et atrophicus (701.0)
scrofulosus (017.0)
simplex chronicus (698.3)
spinulosus (congenital) (757.39)
urticatus (698.2)

697.0 Lichen planus
Lichen: Lichen:
planopilaris   ruber planus
DEF: Inflammatory, pruritic skin disease; marked by angular, flat-top, violet-colored papules; may be acute and widespread or chronic and localized.

697.1 Lichen nitidus
Pinkus' disease
DEF: Chronic, inflammatory, asymptomatic skin disorder, characterized by numerous glistening, flat-topped, discrete, skin-colored micropapules most often on penis, lower abdomen, inner thighs, wrists, forearms, breasts and buttocks.

697.8 Other lichen, not elsewhere classified
Lichen:
ruber moniliforme
striata

697.9 Lichen, unspecified

✓4ᵗʰ **698 Pruritus and related conditions**
EXCLUDES pruritus specified as psychogenic (306.3)
DEF: Pruritus: Intense, persistent itching due to irritation of sensory nerve endings from organic or psychogenic causes.

698.0 Pruritus ani
Perianal itch

698.1 Pruritus of genital organs

698.2 Prurigo
Lichen urticatus
Prurigo:
NOS
Hebra's
mitis
simplex
Urticaria papulosa (Hebra)
EXCLUDES prurigo nodularis (698.3)

698.3 Lichenification and lichen simplex chronicus
Hyde's disease
Neurodermatitis (circumscripta) (local)
Prurigo nodularis

EXCLUDES *neurodermatitis, diffuse (of Brocq) (691.8)*

DEF: Lichenification: thickening of skin due to prolonged rubbing or scratching.

DEF: Lichen simplex chronicus: eczematous dermatitis, of face, neck, extremities, scrotum, vulva, and perianal region due to repeated itching, rubbing and scratching; spontaneous or evolves with other dermatoses.

698.4 Dermatitis factitia [artefacta]
Dermatitis ficta
Neurotic excoriation

Use additional code to identify any associated mental disorder

DEF: Various types of self-inflicted skin lesions characterized in appearance as an erythema to a gangrene.

698.8 Other specified pruritic conditions
Pruritus:
　hiemalis
　senilis
Winter itch

698.9 Unspecified pruritic disorder
Itch NOS
Pruritus NOS

L29.9 Pruritus unspecified 　　　　　　　　　　**I-10**

Other Diseases of Skin and Subcutaneous Tissue (700-709)

EXCLUDES *conditions confined to eyelids (373.0-374.9)*
congenital conditions of skin, hair, and nails (757.0-757.9)

700　Corns and callosities
Callus
Clavus

DEF: Corns: Conical or horny thickening of skin on toes, due to friction, pressure from shoes and hosiery; pain and inflammation may develop.

DEF: Callosities: Localized overgrowth (hyperplasia) of the horny epidermal layer due to pressure or friction.

√4ᵗʰ 701　Other hypertrophic and atrophic conditions of skin

EXCLUDES *dermatomyositis (710.3)*
hereditary edema of legs (757.0)
scleroderma (generalized) (710.1)

701.0 Circumscribed scleroderma
Addison's keloid
Dermatosclerosis, localized
Lichen sclerosus et atrophicus
Morphea
Scleroderma, circumscribed or localized

DEF: Thickened, hardened, skin and subcutaneous tissue; may involve musculoskeletal system.

701.1 Keratoderma, acquired
Acquired:
　ichthyosis
　keratoderma palmaris et plantaris
Elastosis perforans serpiginosa
Hyperkeratosis:
　NOS
　follicularis in cutem penetrans
　palmoplantaris climacterica
Keratoderma:
　climactericum
　tylodes, progressive
Keratosis (blennorrhagica)

EXCLUDES *Darier's disease [keratosis follicularis] (congenital) (757.39)*
keratosis:
*　arsenical (692.4)*
*　gonococcal (098.81)*

AHA: 4Q, '94, 48

701.2 Acquired acanthosis nigricans
Keratosis nigricans

DEF: Diffuse velvety hyperplasia of the spinous skin layer of the axilla and other body folds marked by gray, brown, or black pigmentation; in adult form often associated with malignant acanthosis nigricans in a benign, nevoid form relatively generalized.

701.3 Striae atrophicae
Atrophic spots of skin
Atrophoderma maculatum
Atrophy blanche (of Milian)
Degenerative colloid atrophy
Senile degenerative atrophy
Striae distensae

DEF: Bands of atrophic, depressed, wrinkled skin associated with stretching of skin from pregnancy, obesity, or rapid growth during puberty.

701.4 Keloid scar
Cheloid
Hypertrophic scar
Keloid

DEF: Overgrowth of scar tissue due to excess amounts of collagen during connective tissue repair; occurs mainly on upper trunk, face.

701.5 Other abnormal granulation tissue
Excessive granulation

701.8 Other specified hypertrophic and atrophic conditions of skin
Acrodermatitis atrophicans chronica
Atrophia cutis senilis
Atrophoderma neuriticum
Confluent and reticulate papillomatosis
Cutis laxa senilis
Elastosis senilis
Folliculitis ulerythematosa reticulata
Gougerot-Carteaud syndrome or disease

AHA: 1Q, '08, 7

TIP: Assign for nephrogenic fibrosing dermopathy (NFD) or nephrogenic systemic dermopathy (NSD), a systemic condition occurring only in patients with kidney disease.

701.9 Unspecified hypertrophic and atrophic conditions of skin
Atrophoderma
Skin tag

√4ᵗʰ 702　Other dermatoses

EXCLUDES *carcinoma in situ (232.0-232.9)*

702.0 Actinic keratosis
DEF: Wart-like growth, red or skin-colored; may form a cutaneous horn.
AHA: 1Q, '92, 18

√5ᵗʰ 702.1 Seborrheic keratosis
DEF: Common, benign, lightly pigmented, warty growth composed of basaloid cells.

702.11 Inflamed seborrheic keratosis
AHA: 4Q, '94, 48

702.19 Other seborrheic keratosis
Seborrheic keratosis NOS

702.8 Other specified dermatoses

√4ᵗʰ 703　Diseases of nail

EXCLUDES *congenital anomalies (757.5)*
onychia and paronychia (681.02, 681.11)

703.0 Ingrowing nail
Ingrowing nail with infection
Unguis incarnatus

EXCLUDES *infection, nail NOS (681.9)*

703.8 Other specified diseases of nail
Dystrophia unguium
Hypertrophy of nail
Koilonychia
Leukonychia (punctata) (striata)
Onychauxis
Onychogryposis
Onycholysis

703.9 Unspecified disease of nail

Diseases of the Skin and Subcutaneous Tissue

704–706.1

✓4th **704 Diseases of hair and hair follicles**
> **EXCLUDES** *congenital anomalies (757.4)*

✓5th **704.0 Alopecia**
> **EXCLUDES** *madarosis (374.55)*
> *syphilitic alopecia (091.82)*
> **DEF:** Lack of hair, especially on scalp; often called baldness; may be partial or total; occurs at any age.

704.00 Alopecia, unspecified
Baldness   Loss of hair

704.01 Alopecia areata
Ophiasis
DEF: Alopecia areata: usually reversible, inflammatory, patchy hair loss found in beard or scalp.
DEF: Ophiasis: alopecia areata of children; marked by band around temporal and occipital scalp margins.

704.02 Telogen effluvium
DEF: Shedding of hair from premature telogen development in follicles due to stress, including shock, childbirth, surgery, drugs or weight loss.

704.09 Other
Folliculitis decalvans
Hypotrichosis:
   NOS
   postinfectional NOS
Pseudopelade

704.1 Hirsutism
Hypertrichosis: Polytrichia
   NOS
   lanuginosa, acquired
> **EXCLUDES** *hypertrichosis of eyelid (374.54)*
> **DEF:** Excess hair growth; often in unexpected places and amounts.

704.2 Abnormalities of the hair
Atrophic hair
Clastothrix
Fragilitas crinium
Trichiasis:
   NOS
   cicatrical
Trichorrhexis (nodosa)
> **EXCLUDES** *trichiasis of eyelid (374.05)*

704.3 Variations in hair color
Canities (premature)
Grayness, hair (premature)
Heterochromia of hair
Poliosis:
   NOS
   circumscripta, acquired

✓5th **704.4 Pilar and trichilemmal cysts**
AHA: 4Q, '11, 134-135

704.41 Pilar cyst

704.42 Trichilemmal cyst
Trichilemmal proliferating cyst
AHA: 4Q, '11, 135

704.8 Other specified diseases of hair and hair follicles
Folliculitis:
   NOS
   abscedens et suffodiens
   pustular
Perifolliculitis:
   NOS
   capitis abscedens et suffodiens
   scalp
Sycosis:
   NOS
   barbae [not parasitic]
   lupoid
   vulgaris
AHA: 1Q, '11, 8

704.9 Unspecified disease of hair and hair follicles

✓4th **705 Disorders of sweat glands**

705.0 Anhidrosis
Hypohidrosis   Oligohidrosis
DEF: Lack or deficiency of ability to sweat.

705.1 Prickly heat
Heat rash
Miliaria rubra (tropicalis)
Sudamina

✓5th **705.2 Focal hyperhidrosis**
> **EXCLUDES** *generalized (secondary) hyperhidrosis (780.8)*

705.21 Primary focal hyperhidrosis
Focal hyperhidrosis NOS
Hyperhidrosis NOS
Hyperhidrosis of:
   axilla
   face
   palms
   soles
DEF: A rare disorder of the sweat glands resulting in excessive production of sweat; occurs in the absence of any underlying condition, almost always focal, confined to one or more specific areas of the body.
AHA: 4Q, '04, 91

705.22 Secondary focal hyperhidrosis
Frey's syndrome
DEF: Secondary focal hyperhidrosis: a symptom of an underlying disease process resulting in excessive sweating beyond what the body requires to maintain thermal control, confined to one or more specific areas of the body.
DEF: Frey's syndrome: an auriculotemporal syndrome due to lesion on the parotid gland; characteristic redness and excessive sweating on the cheek in connection with eating.
AHA: 4Q, '04, 91

✓5th **705.8 Other specified disorders of sweat glands**

705.81 Dyshidrosis
Cheiropompholyx
Pompholyx
DEF: Vesicular eruption, on hands, feet causing itching and burning.

705.82 Fox-Fordyce disease
DEF: Chronic, usually pruritic disease evidenced by small follicular papular eruptions, especially in the axillary and pubic areas; develops from the closure and rupture of the affected apocrine glands' intraepidermal portion of the ducts.

705.83 Hidradenitis
Hidradenitis suppurativa
DEF: Inflamed sweat glands.

705.89 Other
Bromhidrosis
Chromhidrosis
Granulosis rubra nasi
Urhidrosis
> **EXCLUDES** *generalized hyperhidrosis (780.8)*
> *hidrocystoma (216.0-216.9)*
DEF: Bromhidrosis: foul-smelling axillary sweat due to decomposed bacteria.
DEF: Chromhidrosis: secretion of colored sweat.
DEF: Granulosis rubra nasi: idiopathic condition of children; causes redness, sweating around nose, face and chin; tends to end by puberty.
DEF: Urhidrosis: urinous substance, such as uric acid, in sweat; occurs in uremia.

705.9 Unspecified disorder of sweat glands
Disorder of sweat glands NOS

✓4th **706 Diseases of sebaceous glands**

706.0 Acne varioliformis
Acne:
   frontalis
   necrotica
DEF: Rare form of acne characterized by persistent brown papulo-pustules usually on the brow and temporoparietal part of the scalp.

706.1 Other acne
Acne: Acne:
   NOS   vulgaris
   conglobata   Blackhead
   cystic   Comedo
   pustular
> **EXCLUDES** *acne rosacea (695.3)*

N Newborn Age: 0	**P** Pediatric Age: 0-17	**M** Maternity Age: 12-55	**A** Adult Age: 15-124	

706.2 Sebaceous cyst
Atheroma, skin
Keratin cyst
Wen

EXCLUDES pilar cyst (704.41)
trichilemmal (proliferating) cyst (704.42)
DEF: Benign epidermal cyst, contains sebum and keratin; presents as firm, circumscribed nodule.

706.3 Seborrhea
EXCLUDES seborrhea:
capitis (690.11)
sicca (690.18)
seborrheic
dermatitis (690.10)
keratosis (702.11-702.19)
DEF: Seborrheic dermatitis marked by excessive secretion of sebum; the sebum forms an oily coating, crusts, or scales on the skin; it is also called hypersteatosis.

706.8 Other specified diseases of sebaceous glands
Asteatosis (cutis)
Xerosis cutis

706.9 Unspecified disease of sebaceous glands

707 Chronic ulcer of skin
INCLUDES non-infected sinus of skin
non-healing ulcer
EXCLUDES varicose ulcer (454.0, 454.2)
AHA: 4Q, '04, 92

707.0 Pressure ulcer
Bed sore
Decubitus ulcer
Plaster ulcer

Use additional code to identify pressure ulcer stage (707.20-707.25)
AHA: 4Q, '08, 132-133; 1Q, '04, 14; 4Q, '03, 110; 4Q, '99, 20; 1Q, '96, 15; 3Q, '90, 15; N-D, '87, 9

707.00 Unspecified site

707.01 Elbow

707.02 Upper back
Shoulder blades

707.03 Lower back
Coccyx
Sacrum
AHA: 3Q, '08, 17; 1Q, '05, 16
L89.159 Pressure ulcer of sacral region uns stage **I-10**

707.04 Hip
L89.209 Pressure ulcer of unspecified hip uns stage **I-10**

707.05 Buttock
AHA: 2Q, '12, 3
L89.309 Pressure ulcer of unspecified buttock uns stage **I-10**

707.06 Ankle

707.07 Heel
AHA: 4Q, '09, 150; 1Q, '05, 16
L89.609 Pressure ulcer of unspecified heel uns stage **I-10**

707.09 Other site
Head
L89.899 Pressure ulcer of other site unspecified stage **I-10**

Four Stages of Pressure Ulcers

Epidermis
Dermis
Subcutaneous tissue

First Stage
Persistent focal erythema

Second Stage
Partial thickness skin loss involving epidermis, dermis, or both

Superficial fascia
Muscle
Bone
Deep fascia

Third Stage
Full thickness skin loss extending through subcutaneous tissue

Fourth Stage
Necrosis of soft tissue extending to muscle and bone

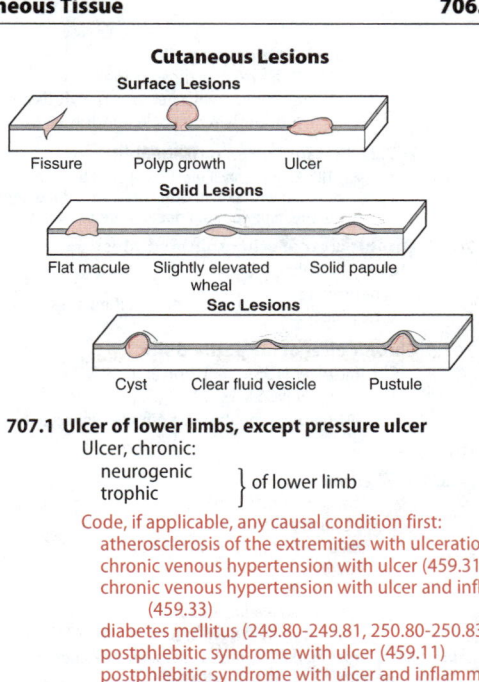

Cutaneous Lesions

Surface Lesions

Fissure   Polyp growth   Ulcer

Solid Lesions

Flat macule   Slightly elevated wheal   Solid papule

Sac Lesions

Cyst   Clear fluid vesicle   Pustule

707.1 Ulcer of lower limbs, except pressure ulcer
Ulcer, chronic:
neurogenic
trophic } of lower limb

Code, if applicable, any causal condition first:
atherosclerosis of the extremities with ulceration (440.23)
chronic venous hypertension with ulcer (459.31)
chronic venous hypertension with ulcer and inflammation (459.33)
diabetes mellitus (249.80-249.81, 250.80-250.83)
postphlebitic syndrome with ulcer (459.11)
postphlebitic syndrome with ulcer and inflammation (459.13)
AHA: 4Q, '00, 44; 4Q, '99, 15

707.10 Ulcer of lower limb, unspecified
AHA: 3Q, '04, 5; 4Q, '02, 43
L97.901 Non-prss chr ulcr uns part uns lw leg brkdwn skn **I-10**

707.11 Ulcer of thigh

707.12 Ulcer of calf
L97.229 Non-press chronic ulcer left calf w/uns severity **I-10**

707.13 Ulcer of ankle
L97.309 Non-press chronic ulcer uns ankle uns severity **I-10**

707.14 Ulcer of heel and midfoot
Plantar surface of midfoot
L97.409 Non-press chr ulcer uns heel & midft uns sevrity **I-10**

707.15 Ulcer of other part of foot
Toes
L97.509 Non-press chr ulcer oth part uns ft uns severity **I-10**

707.19 Ulcer of other part of lower limb
L97.819 Non-press chr ulcer oth part rt low leg uns sevr **I-10**

707.2 Pressure ulcer stages
Code first site of pressure ulcer (707.00-707.09)
AHA: 4Q, '08, 132-134
TIP: If a pressure ulcer progresses during an admission from one stage to another, assign only the code for the higher stage.

707.20 Pressure ulcer, unspecified stage
Healing pressure ulcer NOS
Healing pressure ulcer, unspecified stage

707.21 Pressure ulcer stage I
Healing pressure ulcer, stage I
Pressure pre-ulcer skin changes limited to persistent focal erythema

707.22 Pressure ulcer stage II
Healing pressure ulcer, stage II
Pressure ulcer with abrasion, blister, partial thickness skin loss involving epidermis and/or dermis
AHA: 2Q, '12, 3

707.23 Pressure ulcer stage III
Healing pressure ulcer, stage III
Pressure ulcer with full thickness skin loss involving damage or necrosis of subcutaneous tissue
AHA: 4Q, '09, 150

| Additional Digit Required | Unspecified Code | Other Specified Code | Manifestation Code | ▶◀ Revised Text | ● New Code | ▲ Revised Code Title |

707.24 Pressure ulcer stage IV
Healing pressure ulcer, stage IV
Pressure ulcer with necrosis of soft tissues through to underlying muscle, tendon, or bone

707.25 Pressure ulcer, unstageable
TIP: Assign only if ulcer is covered by eschar, has been treated with skin or other graft, or is documented as a deep tissue injury but not documented as due to trauma.

707.8 Chronic ulcer of other specified sites
Ulcer, chronic:
  neurogenic } of other specified sites
  trophic

707.9 Chronic ulcer of unspecified site
Chronic ulcer NOS   Tropical ulcer NOS
Trophic ulcer NOS   Ulcer of skin NOS
L98.499 Non-press chr ulcer skin oth sites uns severity   `I-10`

√4ᵗʰ 708 Urticaria
EXCLUDES *edema:*
  angioneurotic (995.1)
  Quincke's (995.1)
  hereditary angioedema (277.6)
  urticaria:
  giant (995.1)
  papulosa (Hebra) (698.2)
  pigmentosa (juvenile) (congenital) (757.33)
DEF: Skin disorder marked by raised edematous patches of skin or mucous membrane with intense itching; also called hives.

708.0 Allergic urticaria

708.1 Idiopathic urticaria

708.2 Urticaria due to cold and heat
Thermal urticaria

708.3 Dermatographic urticaria
Dermatographia
Factitial urticaria

708.4 Vibratory urticaria

708.5 Cholinergic urticaria

708.8 Other specified urticaria
Nettle rash
Urticaria:
  chronic
  recurrent periodic

708.9 Urticaria, unspecified
Hives NOS

√4ᵗʰ 709 Other disorders of skin and subcutaneous tissue

√5ᵗʰ 709.0 Dyschromia
EXCLUDES *albinism (270.2)*
  pigmented nevus (216.0-216.9)
  that of eyelid (374.52-374.53)
DEF: Pigment disorder of skin or hair.

709.00 Dyschromia, unspecified

709.01 Vitiligo
DEF: Persistent, progressive development of nonpigmented white patches on otherwise normal skin.

709.09 Other

709.1 Vascular disorders of skin
Angioma serpiginosum
Purpura (primary)annularis telangiectodes

709.2 Scar conditions and fibrosis of skin
Adherent scar (skin)
Cicatrix
Disfigurement (due to scar)
Fibrosis, skin NOS
Scar NOS
EXCLUDES *keloid scar (701.4)*
AHA: N-D, '84, 19

709.3 Degenerative skin disorders
Calcinosis: Degeneration, skin
  circumscripta   Deposits, skin
  cutis   Senile dermatosis NOS
Colloid milium   Subcutaneous calcification

709.4 Foreign body granuloma of skin and subcutaneous tissue
Use additional code to identify foreign body (V90.01-V90.9)
EXCLUDES *residual foreign body without granuloma of skin and subcutaneous tissue (729.6)*
  that of muscle (728.82)

709.8 Other specified disorders of skin
Epithelial hyperplasia
Menstrual dermatosis
Vesicular eruption
DEF: Epithelial hyperplasia: increased number of epithelial cells.
DEF: Vesicular eruption: liquid-filled structures appearing through skin.
AHA: ▶2Q, '13, 9;◄ 4Q, '08, 99; N-D, '87, 6
L98.8 Other spec disorders skin & subcutaneous tissue   `I-10`

709.9 Unspecified disorder of skin and subcutaneous tissue
Dermatosis NOS

N Newborn Age: 0   **P** Pediatric Age: 0-17   **M** Maternity Age: 12-55   **A** Adult Age: 15-124

13. Diseases of the Musculoskeletal System and Connective Tissue (710-739)

Use additional external cause code, if applicable, to identify the cause of the musculoskeletal condition

The following fifth-digit subclassification is for use with categories 711-712, 715-716, 718-719, and 730:

0 site unspecified

1 shoulder region
Acromioclavicular joint(s)
Clavicle
Glenohumeral joint(s)
Scapula
Sternoclavicular joint(s)

2 upper arm
Elbow joint
Humerus

3 forearm
Radius
Ulna
Wrist joint

4 hand
Carpus
Metacarpus
Phalanges [fingers]

5 pelvic region and thigh
Buttock
Femur
Hip (joint)

6 lower leg
Fibula
Knee joint
Patella
Tibia

7 ankle and foot
Ankle joint
Digits [toes]
Metatarsus
Phalanges, foot
Tarsus
Other joints in foot

8 other specified sites
Head
Neck
Ribs
Skull
Trunk
Vertebral column

9 multiple sites

Arthropathies and Related Disorders (710-719)

> **EXCLUDES** *disorders of spine (720.0-724.9)*

✓4ᵗʰ 710 Diffuse diseases of connective tissue

> **INCLUDES** all collagen diseases whose effects are not mainly confined to a single system

> **EXCLUDES** *those affecting mainly the cardiovascular system, i.e., polyarteritis nodosa and allied conditions (446.0-446.7)*

710.0 Systemic lupus erythematosus
Disseminated lupus erythematosus
Libman-Sacks disease

Use additional code to identify manifestation, as:
endocarditis (424.91)
nephritis (583.81)
chronic (582.81)
nephrotic syndrome (581.81)

> **EXCLUDES** *lupus erythematosus (discoid) NOS (695.4)*

DEF: A chronic multisystemic inflammatory disease affecting connective tissue; marked by anemia, leukopenia, muscle and joint pains, fever, rash of a butterfly pattern around cheeks and forehead area; of unknown etiology.
AHA: 2Q, '03, 7-8; 2Q, '97, 8
M32.9 Systemic lupus erythematosus unspecified   I-10

710.1 Systemic sclerosis
Acrosclerosis
CRST syndrome
Progressive systemic sclerosis
Scleroderma

Use additional code to identify manifestation, as:
lung involvement (517.2)
myopathy (359.6)

> **EXCLUDES** *circumscribed scleroderma (701.0)*

DEF: Systemic disease, involving excess fibrotic collagen build-up; symptoms include thickened skin, fibrotic degenerative changes in various organs, and vascular abnormalities; condition occurs more often in females.
AHA: 1Q, '88, 6

710.2 Sicca syndrome
Keratoconjunctivitis sicca
Sjögren's disease

DEF: Autoimmune disease; associated with keratoconjunctivitis, laryngopharyngitis, rhinitis, dry mouth, enlarged parotid gland, and chronic polyarthritis.

710.3 Dermatomyositis
Poikilodermatomyositis
Polymyositis with skin involvement

DEF: Polymyositis characterized by flat-top purple papules on knuckles; upper eyelid rash, edema of eyelids and orbit area, red rash on forehead, neck, shoulders, trunk and arms; symptoms include fever, weight loss, aching muscles; visceral cancer.

710.4 Polymyositis

DEF: Chronic, progressive, inflammatory skeletal muscle disease; causes weakness of limb girdles, neck, pharynx; may precede or follow scleroderma, Sjogren's disease, systemic lupus erythematosus, arthritis, or malignancy.

710.5 Eosinophilia myalgia syndrome
Toxic oil syndrome

Use additional E code to identify drug, if drug induced

DEF: Eosinophilia myalgia syndrome (EMS): inflammatory, multisystem fibrosis; associated with ingesting elementary L-tryptophan; symptoms include myalgia, weak limbs and bulbar muscles, distal sensory loss, areflexia, arthralgia, cough, fever, fatigue, skin rashes, myopathy, and eosinophil counts greater than 1000/microliter.
DEF: Toxic oil syndrome: syndrome similar to EMS due to ingesting contaminated cooking oil.
AHA: 4Q, '92, 21

710.8 Other specified diffuse diseases of connective tissue
Multifocal fibrosclerosis (idiopathic) NEC
Systemic fibrosclerosing syndrome
AHA: M-A, '87, 12

710.9 Unspecified diffuse connective tissue disease
Collagen disease NOS

✓4ᵗʰ 711 Arthropathy associated with infections

> **INCLUDES** arthritis
> arthropathy   associated with conditions
> polyarthritis   classifiable below
> polyarthropathy

> **EXCLUDES** *rheumatic fever (390)*

The following fifth-digit subclassification is for use with category 711; valid digits are in [brackets] under each code. See list at beginning of chapter for definitions.

0 site unspecified
1 shoulder region
2 upper arm
3 forearm
4 hand
5 pelvic region and thigh
6 lower leg
7 ankle and foot
8 other specified sites
9 multiple sites

AHA: 1Q, '92, 17

§ ✓5ᵗʰ 711.0 Pyogenic arthritis
[0-9]
Arthritis or polyarthritis (due to):
coliform [Escherichia coli]
Hemophilus influenzae [H. influenzae]
pneumococcal
Pseudomonas
staphylococcal
streptococcal
Pyarthrosis

Use additional code to identify infectious organism (041.0-041.8)

DEF: Infectious arthritis caused by various bacteria; marked by inflamed synovial membranes, and purulent effusion in joints.
AHA: 1Q, '92, 16; 1Q, '91, 15
M00.869 Arthritis due to other bacteria unspecified knee   I-10

§ ✓5ᵗʰ 711.1 Arthropathy associated with Reiter's disease and nonspecific urethritis
[0-9]

Code first underlying disease as:
nonspecific urethritis (099.4)
Reiter's disease (099.3)

DEF: Reiter's disease: joint disease marked by diarrhea, urethritis, conjunctivitis, keratosis and arthritis; of unknown etiology; affects young males.
DEF: Urethritis: inflamed urethra.

---

§ Requires fifth digit. Valid digits are in [brackets] under each code. See beginning of section 710-739 for codes and defintions.

Joint Structures

Muscle
Periosteum (covers bone)
Cortical bone
Medullary bone
Fascia over Muscle
Sesamoid bone
Bursa (with synovial fluid)
Tendon (muscle to bone)
Muscle insertion into bone (crosses one or more joints)
Retinaculum
Tendon sheath around Tendon
Synovium lines Joint capsule around Synovial cavity (with fluid)
Articular cartilage
Ligament (bone to bone)
Bursa
Bone covered with periosteum

§ √5th **711.2 Arthropathy in Behçet's syndrome**
[0-9]   *Code first underlying disease (136.1)*
    DEF: Behçet's syndrome: Chronic inflammatory disorder, of unknown etiology; affects small blood vessels; causes ulcers of oral and pharyngeal mucous membranes and genitalia, skin lesions, retinal vasculitis, optic atrophy and severe uveitis.

§ √5th **711.3 Postdysenteric arthropathy**
[0-9]   *Code first underlying disease as:*
    dysentery (009.0)
    enteritis, infectious (008.0-009.3)
    paratyphoid fever (002.1-002.9)
    typhoid fever (002.0)
    EXCLUDES *salmonella arthritis (003.23)*

§ √5th **711.4 Arthropathy associated with other bacterial diseases**
[0-9]   *Code first underlying disease as:*
    diseases classifiable to 010-040, 090-099, except as in 711.1, 711.3, and 713.5
    leprosy (030.0-030.9)
    tuberculosis (015.0-015.9)
    EXCLUDES *gonococcal arthritis (098.50)*
          meningococcal arthritis (036.82)

§ √5th **711.5 Arthropathy associated with other viral diseases**
[0-9]   *Code first underlying disease as:*
    diseases classifiable to 045-049, 050-079, 480, 487
    O'nyong nyong (066.3)
    EXCLUDES *that due to rubella (056.71)*

§ √5th **711.6 Arthropathy associated with mycoses**
[0-9]   *Code first underlying disease (110.0-118)*

§ √5th **711.7 Arthropathy associated with helminthiasis**
[0-9]   *Code first underlying disease as:*
    filariasis (125.0-125.9)

§ √5th **711.8 Arthropathy associated with other infectious and parasitic diseases**
    Code first underlying disease as:
    diseases classifiable to 080-088, 100-104, 130-136
    EXCLUDES *arthropathy associated with sarcoidosis (713.7)*
    AHA: 4Q, '91, 15; 3Q, '90, 14

§ √5th **711.9 Unspecified infective arthritis**
[0-9]   Infective arthritis or polyarthritis (acute) (chronic) (subacute) NOS

√4th **712 Crystal arthropathies**
    INCLUDES crystal-induced arthritis and synovitis
    EXCLUDES *gouty arthropathy (274.00-274.03)*
    DEF: Joint disease due to urate crystal deposit in joints or synovial membranes.

The following fifth-digit subclassification is for use with category 712; valid digits are in [brackets] under each code. See list at beginning of chapter for definitions.
    0 site unspecified
    1 shoulder region
    2 upper arm
    3 forearm
    4 hand
    5 pelvic region and thigh
    6 lower leg
    7 ankle and foot
    8 other specified sites
    9 multiple sites

§ √5th **712.1 Chondrocalcinosis due to dicalcium phosphate crystals**
[0-9]   Chondrocalcinosis due to dicalcium phosphate crystals (with other crystals)
    Code first underlying disease (275.4)

§ √5th **712.2 Chondrocalcinosis due to pyrophosphate crystals**
[0-9]   *Code first underlying disease (275.4)*

§ √5th **712.3 Chondrocalcinosis, unspecified**
[0-9]   *Code first underlying disease (275.4)*

§ √5th **712.8 Other specified crystal arthropathies**
[0-9]

§ √5th **712.9 Unspecified crystal arthropathy**
[0-9]

√4th **713 Arthropathy associated with other disorders classified elsewhere**
    INCLUDES arthritis
           arthropathy   } associated with
           polyarthritis   conditions
           polyarthropathy   classifiable below

713.0 Arthropathy associated with other endocrine and metabolic disorders
    Code first underlying disease as:
    acromegaly (253.0)
    hemochromatosis (275.01-275.09)
    hyperparathyroidism (252.00-252.08)
    hypogammaglobulinemia (279.00-279.09)
    hypothyroidism (243-244.9)
    lipoid metabolism disorder (272.0-272.9)
    ochronosis (270.2)
    EXCLUDES *arthropathy associated with:*
          amyloidosis (713.7)
          crystal deposition disorders, except gout (712.1-712.9)
          diabetic neuropathy (713.5)
          gout (274.00-274.03)

713.1 Arthropathy associated with gastrointestinal conditions other than infections
    Code first underlying disease as:
    regional enteritis (555.0-555.9)
    ulcerative colitis (556)

713.2 Arthropathy associated with hematological disorders
    Code first underlying disease as:
    hemoglobinopathy (282.4-282.7)
    hemophilia (286.0-286.2)
    leukemia (204.0-208.9)
    malignant reticulosis (202.3)
    multiple myelomatosis (203.0)
    EXCLUDES *arthropathy associated with Henoch-Schönlein purpura (713.6)*

713.3 Arthropathy associated with dermatological disorders
    Code first underlying disease as:
    erythema multiforme (695.10-695.19)
    erythema nodosum (695.2)
    EXCLUDES *psoriatic arthropathy (696.0)*

---

§   Requires fifth digit. Valid digits are in [brackets] under each code. See beginning of section 710-739 for codes and defintions.

N Newborn Age: 0   **P** Pediatric Age: 0-17   **M** Maternity Age: 12-55   **A** Adult Age: 15-124

713.4 Arthropathy associated with respiratory disorders

Code first underlying disease as:
diseases classifiable to 490-519

EXCLUDES *arthropathy associated with respiratory infections (711.0, 711.4-711.8)*

713.5 Arthropathy associated with neurological disorders

Charcôt's arthropathy   } associated with diseases
Neuropathic arthritis   } classifiable elsewhere

Code first underlying disease as:
neuropathic joint disease [Charcôt's joints]:
    NOS (094.0)
    diabetic (249.6, 250.6)
    syringomyelic (336.0)
    tabetic [syphilitic] (094.0)

AHA: 3Q, '12, 4

713.6 Arthropathy associated with hypersensitivity reaction

Code first underlying disease as:
Henoch (-Schönlein) purpura (287.0)
serum sickness (999.51-999.59)

EXCLUDES *allergic arthritis NOS (716.2)*

713.7 Other general diseases with articular involvement

Code first underlying disease as:
amyloidosis (277.30-277.39)
familial Mediterranean fever (277.31)
sarcoidosis (135)

AHA: 2Q, '97, 12

713.8 Arthropathy associated with other condition classifiable elsewhere

Code first underlying disease as:
conditions classifiable elsewhere except as in 711.1-711.8, 712, and 713.0-713.7

√4ᵗʰ 714 Rheumatoid arthritis and other inflammatory polyarthropathies

EXCLUDES *rheumatic fever (390)*
rheumatoid arthritis of spine NOS (720.0)

AHA: 2Q, '95, 3

714.0 Rheumatoid arthritis
Arthritis or polyarthritis:
    atrophic
    rheumatic (chronic)

Use additional code to identify manifestation, as:
myopathy (359.6)
polyneuropathy (357.1)

EXCLUDES *juvenile rheumatoid arthritis NOS (714.30)*

DEF: Chronic systemic disease principally of joints, manifested by inflammatory changes in articular structures and synovial membranes, atrophy, and loss in bone density.

AHA: 2Q, '06, 20; 1Q, '90, 5

M06.9 Rheumatoid arthritis unspecified   I-10

714.1 Felty's syndrome
Rheumatoid arthritis with splenoadenomegaly and leukopenia

DEF: Syndrome marked by rheumatoid arthritis, splenomegaly, leukopenia, pigmented spots on lower extremity skin, anemia, and thrombocytopenia.

714.2 Other rheumatoid arthritis with visceral or systemic involvement
Rheumatoid carditis

√5ᵗʰ 714.3 Juvenile chronic polyarthritis

DEF: Rheumatoid arthritis of more than one joint; lasts longer than six weeks in age 17 or younger; symptoms include fever, erythematous rash, weight loss, lymphadenopathy, hepatosplenomegaly and pericarditis.

714.30 Polyarticular juvenile rheumatoid arthritis, chronic or unspecified
Juvenile rheumatoid arthritis NOS
Still's disease

714.31 Polyarticular juvenile rheumatoid arthritis, acute

714.32 Pauciarticular juvenile rheumatoid arthritis

714.33 Monoarticular juvenile rheumatoid arthritis

714.4 Chronic postrheumatic arthropathy
Chronic rheumatoid nodular fibrositis
Jaccoud's syndrome

DEF: Persistent joint disorder; follows previous rheumatic infection.

√5ᵗʰ 714.8 Other specified inflammatory polyarthropathies

714.81 Rheumatoid lung
Caplan's syndrome
Diffuse interstitial rheumatoid disease of lung
Fibrosing alveolitis, rheumatoid

DEF: Lung disorders associated with rheumatoid arthritis.

714.89 Other

714.9 Unspecified inflammatory polyarthropathy
Inflammatory polyarthropathy or polyarthritis NOS

EXCLUDES *polyarthropathy NOS (716.5)*

√4ᵗʰ 715 Osteoarthrosis and allied disorders

NOTE Localized, in the subcategories below, includes bilateral involvement of the same site.

INCLUDES arthritis or polyarthritis:
    degenerative
    hypertrophic
degenerative joint disease
osteoarthritis

EXCLUDES *Marie-Strümpell spondylitis (720.0)*
osteoarthrosis [osteoarthritis] of spine (721.0-721.9)

The following fifth-digit subclassification is for use with category 715; valid digits are in [brackets] under each code. See list at beginning of chapter for definitions.

  0 site unspecified
  1 shoulder region
  2 upper arm
  3 forearm
  4 hand
  5 pelvic region and thigh
  6 lower leg
  7 ankle and foot
  8 other specified sites
  9 multiple sites

§ √5ᵗʰ 715.0 Osteoarthrosis, generalized
[0,4,9] Degenerative joint disease, involving multiple joints
Primary generalized hypertrophic osteoarthrosis

DEF: Chronic noninflammatory arthritis; marked by degenerated articular cartilage and enlarged bone; symptoms include pain and stiffness with activity.

§ √5ᵗʰ 715.1 Osteoarthrosis, localized, primary
[0-8] Localized osteoarthropathy, idiopathic

M17.0 Bilateral primary osteoarthritis of knee   I-10

§ √5ᵗʰ 715.2 Osteoarthrosis, localized, secondary
[0-8] Coxae malum senilis

§ √5ᵗʰ 715.3 Osteoarthrosis, localized, not specified whether
[0-8] **primary or secondary**
Otto's pelvis

AHA: For code 715.35: 3Q, '04, 12; 2Q, '04, 15; **For code 715.36:** 4Q, '03, 118; 2Q, '95, 5

M16.9 Osteoarthritis of hip unspecified   I-10

§ √5ᵗʰ 715.8 Osteoarthrosis involving, or with mention of
[0,9] **more than one site, but not specified as generalized**

§ √5ᵗʰ 715.9 Osteoarthrosis, unspecified whether
[0-8] **generalized or localized**

AHA: For code 715.90: 2Q, '97, 12

M19.90 Unspecified osteoarthritis unspecified site   I-10
M17.9 Osteoarthritis of knee unspecified   I-10

---

§   Requires fifth digit. Valid digits are in [brackets] under each code. See beginning of section 710-739 for codes and definitions.

√4ᵗʰ √5ᵗʰ Additional Digit Required   <mark>Unspecified Code</mark>   Other Specified Code   Manifestation Code   ▶◀ Revised Text   ● New Code   ▲ Revised Code Title

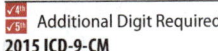

✓4ᵗʰ **716 Other and unspecified arthropathies**

EXCLUDES cricoarytenoid arthropathy (478.79)

The following fifth-digit subclassification is for use with category 716; valid digits are in [brackets] under each code. See list at beginning of chapter for definitions.

    0 **site unspecified**
    1 **shoulder region**
    2 **upper arm**
    3 **forearm**
    4 **hand**
    5 **pelvic region and thigh**
    6 **lower leg**
    7 **ankle and foot**
    8 **other specified sites**
    9 **multiple sites**

AHA: 2Q, '95, 3

§ ✓5ᵗʰ **716.0 Kaschin-Beck disease**
[0-9]   Endemic polyarthritis
DEF: Chronic degenerative disease of spine and peripheral joints; occurs in eastern Siberian, northern Chinese, and Korean youth; may be a mycotoxicosis caused by eating cereals infected with fungus.

§ ✓5ᵗʰ **716.1 Traumatic arthropathy**
[0-9]   **AHA:** For Code 716.11: 1Q, '02, 9; For code 716.15: 2Q, '09, 11

§ ✓5ᵗʰ **716.2 Allergic arthritis**
[0-9]   **EXCLUDES** arthritis associated with Henoch-Schönlein purpura or serum sickness (713.6)

§ ✓5ᵗʰ **716.3 Climacteric arthritis**   ♀
[0-9]   Menopausal arthritis
DEF: Ovarian hormone deficiency; causes pain in small joints, shoulders, elbows or knees; affects females at menopause; also called arthropathia ovaripriva.

§ ✓5ᵗʰ **716.4 Transient arthropathy**
[0-9]   **EXCLUDES** palindromic rheumatism (719.3)

§ ✓5ᵗʰ **716.5 Unspecified polyarthropathy or polyarthritis**
[0-9]

§ ✓5ᵗʰ **716.6 Unspecified monoarthritis**
[0-8]   Coxitis

§ ✓5ᵗʰ **716.8 Other specified arthropathy**
[0-9]

§ ✓5ᵗʰ **716.9 Arthropathy, unspecified**
[0-9]   Arthritis ⎫
    Arthropathy ⎬ (acute) (chronic) (subacute)
    Articular rheumatism (chronic)
    Inflammation of joint NOS
    M12.9 Arthropathy unspecified   I-10

✓4ᵗʰ **717 Internal derangement of knee**
INCLUDES degeneration ⎫
    rupture, old   ⎬ of articular cartilage or
    tear, old ⎭ meniscus of knee

EXCLUDES acute derangement of knee (836.0-836.6)
    ankylosis (718.5)
    contracture (718.4)
    current injury (836.0-836.6)
    deformity (736.4-736.6)
    recurrent dislocation (718.3)

717.0 Old bucket handle tear of medial meniscus
    Old bucket handle tear of unspecified cartilage

717.1 Derangement of anterior horn of medial meniscus

717.2 Derangement of posterior horn of medial meniscus

717.3 Other and unspecified derangement of medial meniscus
    Degeneration of internal semilunar cartilage

Disruption and Tears of Meniscus

Bucket-handle   Flap-type   Peripheral   Radial

Horizontal cleavage   Vertical   Congenital discoid meniscus

Internal Derangements of Knee

Disruptions of Cruciate Ligament   Chondromalacia of Patella

Anterior   Posterior   "Kissing" lesion of femur

✓5ᵗʰ **717.4 Derangement of lateral meniscus**

    717.40 Derangement of lateral meniscus, unspecified

    717.41 Bucket handle tear of lateral meniscus

    717.42 Derangement of anterior horn of lateral meniscus

    717.43 Derangement of posterior horn of lateral meniscus

    717.49 Other

717.5 Derangement of meniscus, not elsewhere classified
    Congenital discoid meniscus
    Cyst of semilunar cartilage
    Derangement of semilunar cartilage NOS

717.6 Loose body in knee
    Joint mice, knee
    Rice bodies, knee (joint)
DEF: The presence in the joint synovial area of a small, frequently calcified, loose body created from synovial membrane, organized fibrin fragments of articular cartilage or arthritis osteophytes.

717.7 Chondromalacia of patella
    Chondromalacia patellae
    Degeneration [softening] of articular cartilage of patella
DEF: Softened patella cartilage.
AHA: M-A, '85, 14; N-D, '84, 9

✓5ᵗʰ **717.8 Other internal derangement of knee**

    717.81 Old disruption of lateral collateral ligament

    717.82 Old disruption of medial collateral ligament

    717.83 Old disruption of anterior cruciate ligament

    717.84 Old disruption of posterior cruciate ligament

    717.85 Old disruption of other ligaments of knee
      Capsular ligament of knee

    717.89 Other
      Old disruption of ligaments NOS

717.9 Unspecified internal derangement of knee
    Derangement NOS of knee

---

§   Requires fifth digit. Valid digits are in [brackets] under each code. See beginning of section 710-739 for codes and defintions.

718 Other derangement of joint

EXCLUDES   current injury (830.0-848.9)
         jaw (524.60-524.69)

The following fifth-digit subclassification is for use with category 718; valid digits are in [brackets] under each code. See list at beginning of chapter for definitions.

   0   site unspecified
   1   shoulder region
   2   upper arm
   3   forearm
   4   hand
   5   pelvic region and thigh
   6   lower leg
   7   ankle and foot
   8   other specified sites
   9   multiple sites

§ **718.0 Articular cartilage disorder**

[0-5,7-9] Meniscus:
       disorder
       rupture, old
       tear, old
       Old rupture of ligament(s) of joint NOS

EXCLUDES   articular cartilage disorder:
         in ochronosis (270.2)
         knee (717.0-717.9)
         chondrocalcinosis (275.4)
         metastatic calcification (275.4)

§ **718.1 Loose body in joint**

[0-5,7-9] Joint mice

EXCLUDES   knee (717.6)

DEF: Calcified loose bodies in synovial fluid; due to arthritic osteophytes.

AHA: For code 718.17: 2Q, '01, 15

§ **718.2 Pathological dislocation**

[0-9] Dislocation or displacement of joint, not recurrent and not current injury
Spontaneous dislocation (joint)

§ **718.3 Recurrent dislocation of joint**

[0-9] AHA: N-D, '87, 7

§ **718.4 Contracture of joint**

[0-9] AHA: 4Q, '98, 40

TIP: Assign an additional code from category 438 if the contracture is a result of a CVA.

§ **718.5 Ankylosis of joint**

[0-9] Ankylosis of joint (fibrous) (osseous)

EXCLUDES   spine (724.9)
         stiffness of joint without mention of ankylosis (719.5)

DEF: Immobility and solidification of joint; due to disease, injury or surgical procedure.

§ **718.6 Unspecified intrapelvic protrusion of acetabulum**

[5] Protrusio acetabuli, unspecified

DEF: Sinking of the floor of acetabulum, causing femoral head to protrude, limits hip movement; of unknown etiology.

§ **718.7 Developmental dislocation of joint**

[0-9] EXCLUDES   congenital dislocation of joint (754.0-755.8)
            traumatic dislocation of joint (830-839)

AHA: 4Q, '01, 48

Joint Derangements and Disorders

Loose body in joint   Dislocation of joint

Joint contracture   Ankylosis of joint   Synovial effusion (fluid)   Hemarthrosis (blood)

---

§ **718.8 Other joint derangement, not elsewhere classified**

[0-9] Flail joint (paralytic)   Instability of joint

EXCLUDES   deformities classifiable to 736 (736.0-736.9)

AHA: For code 718.81: 2Q, '00, 14

TIP: Assign 718.81 for multidirectional shoulder instability.

§ **718.9 Unspecified derangement of joint**

[0-5,7-9] EXCLUDES   knee (717.9)

719 Other and unspecified disorders of joint

EXCLUDES   jaw (524.60-524.69)

The following fifth-digit subclassification is for use with codes 719.0-719.6, 719.8-719.9; valid digits are in [brackets] under each code. See list at beginning of chapter for definitions.

   0   site unspecified
   1   shoulder region
   2   upper arm
   3   forearm
   4   hand
   5   pelvic region and thigh
   6   lower leg
   7   ankle and foot
   8   other specified sites
   9   multiple sites

§ **719.0 Effusion of joint**

[0-9] Hydrarthrosis
Swelling of joint, with or without pain

EXCLUDES   intermittent hydrarthrosis (719.3)

M25.469 Effusion unspecified knee   I-10

§ **719.1 Hemarthrosis**

[0-9] EXCLUDES   current injury (840.0-848.9)

§ **719.2 Villonodular synovitis**

[0-9] DEF: Overgrowth of synovial tissue, especially at knee joint; due to macrophage infiltration of giant cells in synovial villi and fibrous nodules.

§ **719.3 Palindromic rheumatism**

[0-9] Hench-Rosenberg syndrome
Intermittent hydrarthrosis

DEF: Recurrent episodes of afebrile arthritis and periarthritis marked by their complete disappearance after a few days or hours; causes swelling, redness, and disability usually affecting only one joint; no known cause.

§ **719.4 Pain in joint**

[0-9] Arthralgia

AHA: For code 719.46: 1Q, '01, 3

TIP: Assign 719.46 for patellofemoral syndrome, a chronic knee pain common among athletes.

M25.519 Pain in unspecified shoulder   I-10
M25.552 Pain in left hip   I-10

§ **719.5 Stiffness of joint, not elsewhere classified**

[0-9]

§ **719.6 Other symptoms referable to joint**

[0-9] Joint crepitus
Snapping hip

AHA: 1Q, '94, 15; For code 719.66: 2Q, '07, 6

TIP: Assign 719.66 for patellar clunk syndrome, which is a fibrous reaction caused by chronic pressure on the patella, S/P knee replacement surgery.

719.7 Difficulty in walking

EXCLUDES   abnormality of gait (781.2)

AHA: 2Q, '04, 15; 4Q, '03, 66

R26.2 Difficulty in walking not elsewhere classified   I-10

§ **719.8 Other specified disorders of joint**

[0-9] Calcification of joint
Fistula of joint

EXCLUDES   temporomandibular joint-pain-dysfunction syndrome [Costen's syndrome] (524.60)

§ **719.9 Unspecified disorder of joint**

[0-9]

---

§ Requires fifth digit. Valid digits are in [brackets] under each code. See beginning of section 710-739 for codes and defintions.

| ✓4th ✓5th Additional Digit Required | Unspecified Code | Other Specified Code | Manifestation Code | ▶◀ Revised Text | ● New Code | ▲ Revised Code Title |

Diseases of the Musculoskeletal System and Connective Tissue

720–722.39

Dorsopathies (720-724)

EXCLUDES   curvature of spine (737.0-737.9)
     osteochondrosis of spine (juvenile) (732.0)
       adult (732.8)

✓4ᵗʰ **720 Ankylosing spondylitis and other inflammatory spondylopathies**

     720.0 Ankylosing spondylitis
       Rheumatoid arthritis of spine NOS
       Spondylitis:
         Marie-Strümpell
         rheumatoid
       DEF: Rheumatoid arthritis of spine and sacroiliac joints; fusion and deformity in spine follows; affects mainly males; cause unknown.

     720.1 Spinal enthesopathy
       Disorder of peripheral ligamentous or muscular attachments of spine
       Romanus lesion
       DEF: Tendinous or muscular vertebral bone attachment abnormality.

     720.2 Sacroiliitis, not elsewhere classified
       Inflammation of sacroiliac joint NOS
       DEF: Pain due to inflammation in joint, at juncture of sacrum and hip.

   ✓5ᵗʰ **720.8 Other inflammatory spondylopathies**

       720.81 Inflammatory spondylopathies in diseases classified elsewhere
         Code first underlying disease as:
           tuberculosis (015.0)

       720.89 Other

     720.9 Unspecified inflammatory spondylopathy
       Spondylitis NOS

✓4ᵗʰ **721 Spondylosis and allied disorders**
     DEF: Degenerative changes in spinal joint.
     AHA: 2Q, '89, 14

     721.0 Cervical spondylosis without myelopathy
       Cervical or cervicodorsal:
         arthritis
         osteoarthritis
         spondylarthritis

     721.1 Cervical spondylosis with myelopathy
       Anterior spinal artery compression syndrome
       Spondylogenic compression of cervical spinal cord
       Vertebral artery compression syndrome
       M47.12 Other spondylosis w/myelopathy cervical region   ‖-10

     721.2 Thoracic spondylosis without myelopathy
       Thoracic:
         arthritis
         osteoarthritis
         spondylarthritis

     721.3 Lumbosacral spondylosis without myelopathy
       Lumbar or lumbosacral:
         arthritis
         osteoarthritis
         spondylarthritis
       AHA: 4Q, '02, 107
       M47.817 Spondylosis w/o myelopath/radiculopath lumboscrl   ‖-10

   ✓5ᵗʰ **721.4 Thoracic or lumbar spondylosis with myelopathy**

       721.41 Thoracic region
         Spondylogenic compression of thoracic spinal cord

       721.42 Lumbar region

     721.5 Kissing spine
       Baastrup's syndrome
       DEF: Compression of spinous processes of adjacent vertebrae; due to mutual contact.

     721.6 Ankylosing vertebral hyperostosis

     721.7 Traumatic spondylopathy
       Kümmell's disease or spondylitis

     721.8 Other allied disorders of spine

   ✓5ᵗʰ **721.9 Spondylosis of unspecified site**

       721.90 Without mention of myelopathy
         Spinal:
           arthritis (deformans) (degenerative) (hypertrophic)
           osteoarthritis NOS
         Spondylarthrosis NOS

       721.91 With myelopathy
         Spondylogenic compression of spinal cord NOS

✓4ᵗʰ **722 Intervertebral disc disorders**
     AHA: 1Q, '88, 10

     722.0 Displacement of cervical intervertebral disc without myelopathy
       Neuritis (brachial) or radiculitis due to displacement or rupture of cervical intervertebral disc
       Any condition classifiable to 722.2 of the cervical or cervicothoracic intervertebral disc
       M50.20 Other cerv disc displacement uns cerv region   ‖-10

   ✓5ᵗʰ **722.1 Displacement of thoracic or lumbar intervertebral disc without myelopathy**

       722.10 Lumbar intervertebral disc without myelopathy
         Lumbago or sciatica due to displacement of intervertebral disc
         Neuritis or radiculitis due to displacement or rupture of lumbar intervertebral disc
         Any condition classifiable to 722.2 of the lumbar or lumbosacral intervertebral disc
         AHA: 4Q, '08, 184; 1Q, '07, 9; 3Q, '03, 12; 1Q, '03, 7; 4Q, '02, 107
         M51.26 Oth intervertebral disc displcmnt lumbar region   ‖-10

       722.11 Thoracic intervertebral disc without myelopathy
         Any condition classifiable to 722.2 of thoracic intervertebral disc

     722.2 Displacement of intervertebral disc, site unspecified, without myelopathy
       Discogenic syndrome NOS
       Herniation of nucleus pulposus NOS
       Intervertebral disc NOS:
         extrusion
         prolapse
         protrusion
         rupture
       Neuritis or radiculitis due to displacement or rupture of intervertebral disc

   ✓5ᵗʰ **722.3 Schmorl's nodes**
       DEF: Irregular bone defect in the margin of the vertebral body; causes herniation into end plate of vertebral body.

       722.30 Unspecified region

       722.31 Thoracic region

       722.32 Lumbar region

       722.39 Other

Normal Anatomy of Vertebral Disc

Lamina · Ligamentum flavum · Spinal canal · Spinal cord in dural sac · Intervertebral disk · Annulus · Nucleus pulposus · Vertebral body · Spinal nerve · Lamina · Disk annulus · Nucleus pulposus · **Normal Top View** · **Normal Side View**

Derangement of Vertebral Disc

Nucleus pulposus
Herniates through Annulus
Spinal cord
Spinal nerve
Spinal stenosis
Schmorl's nodule
Osteophyte
Folded or thickened ligamentum flavum
Collapsed disk
Laminectomy and/or diskectomy decompresses spinal canal

Stenosis in Cervical Region

Spinal cord in fluid-filled
Dural sac
Old displacement/ dislocation of C₁ on C₂
Posterior longitudinal ligament
Spinal cord
Vertebral body
Spinal canal
Torticollis

722.4 Degeneration of cervical intervertebral disc
Degeneration of cervicothoracic intervertebral disc
M50.30 Other cerv disc degeneration uns cerv region [I-10]

✓5ᵗʰ **722.5 Degeneration of thoracic or lumbar intervertebral disc**

722.51 Thoracic or thoracolumbar intervertebral disc
AHA: 2Q, '11, 8

722.52 Lumbar or lumbosacral intervertebral disc
AHA: 2Q, '06, 18; 4Q, '04, 133
M51.37 Oth intervertebral disc degen lumbosacral region [I-10]

722.6 Degeneration of intervertebral disc, site unspecified
Degenerative disc disease NOS
Narrowing of intervertebral disc or space NOS

✓5ᵗʰ **722.7 Intervertebral disc disorder with myelopathy**

722.70 Unspecified region

722.71 Cervical region

722.72 Thoracic region

722.73 Lumbar region

✓5ᵗʰ **722.8 Postlaminectomy syndrome**
DEF: Spinal disorder due to spinal laminectomy surgery.
AHA: J-F, '87, 7
TIP: Assign if documentation indicates that pain is due to scar tissue formation following disc surgery.

722.80 Unspecified region

722.81 Cervical region

722.82 Thoracic region

722.83 Lumbar region
AHA: 2Q, '97, 15
M96.1 Postlaminectomy syndrome NEC [I-10]

✓5ᵗʰ **722.9 Other and unspecified disc disorder**
Calcification of intervertebral cartilage or disc
Discitis

722.90 Unspecified region
AHA: N-D, '84, 19

722.91 Cervical region

722.92 Thoracic region

722.93 Lumbar region
M51.86 Other intervertebral disc disorder lumbar region [I-10]

✓4ᵗʰ **723 Other disorders of cervical region**
EXCLUDES conditions due to:
intervertebral disc disorders (722.0-722.9)
spondylosis (721.0-721.9)
AHA: 3Q, '94, 14; 2Q, '89, 14

723.0 Spinal stenosis in cervical region
AHA: 4Q, '03, 101
M48.02 Spinal stenosis cervical region [I-10]

723.1 Cervicalgia
Pain in neck
DEF: Pain in cervical spine or neck region.
M54.2 Cervicalgia [I-10]

723.2 Cervicocranial syndrome
Barré-Liéou syndrome
Posterior cervical sympathetic syndrome
DEF: Neurologic disorder of upper cervical spine and nerve roots.

723.3 Cervicobrachial syndrome (diffuse)
DEF: Complex of symptoms due to scalenus anterior muscle compressing the brachial plexus; pain radiates from shoulder to arm or back of neck.
AHA: N-D, '85, 12

723.4 Brachial neuritis or radiculitis NOS
Cervical radiculitis   Radicular syndrome of upper limbs

723.5 Torticollis, unspecified
Contracture of neck
EXCLUDES congenital (754.1)
due to birth injury (767.8)
hysterical (300.11)
ocular torticollis (781.93)
psychogenic (306.0)
spasmodic (333.83)
traumatic, current (847.0)
DEF: Abnormally positioned neck relative to head due to cervical muscle or fascia contractions; also called wryneck.
AHA: 2Q, '01, 21; 1Q, '95, 7

723.6 Panniculitis specified as affecting neck
DEF: Inflammation of the panniculus adiposus (subcutaneous fat) in the neck.

723.7 Ossification of posterior longitudinal ligament in cervical region

723.8 Other syndromes affecting cervical region
Cervical syndrome NEC   Occipital neuralgia
Klippel's disease
AHA: 1Q, '00, 7

723.9 Unspecified musculoskeletal disorders and symptoms referable to neck
Cervical (region) disorder NOS

✓4ᵗʰ **724 Other and unspecified disorders of back**
EXCLUDES collapsed vertebra (code to cause, e.g., osteoporosis, 733.00-733.09)
conditions due to:
intervertebral disc disorders (722.0-722.9)
spondylosis (721.0-721.9)
AHA: 2Q, '89, 14

✓5ᵗʰ **724.0 Spinal stenosis, other than cervical**

724.00 Spinal stenosis, unspecified region
M48.00 Spinal stenosis site unspecified [I-10]

724.01 Thoracic region

724.02 Lumbar region, without neurogenic claudication
Lumbar region NOS
AHA: 4Q, '08, 109; 4Q, '07, 120; 1Q, '07, 10, 20; 4Q, '99, 13
M48.06 Spinal stenosis lumbar region [I-10]

724.03 Lumbar region, with neurogenic claudication
DEF: Spinal canal narrowing with nerve root compression causing muscle pain, fatigue, and weakness during extension of the lumbar spine; pain is relieved by sitting or bending.
AHA: 2Q, '11, 10; 4Q, '10, 89

724.09 Other

724.1 Pain in thoracic spine

724.2 Lumbago
Low back pain
Low back syndrome
Lumbalgia
AHA: 2Q, '07, 11; N-D, '85, 12
M54.5 Low back pain [I-10]

724.3 Sciatica
Neuralgia or neuritis of sciatic nerve
EXCLUDES specified lesion of sciatic nerve (355.0)
AHA: 2Q, '89, 12
M54.30 Sciatica unspecified side [I-10]

724.4 Thoracic or lumbosacral neuritis or radiculitis, unspecified
Radicular syndrome of lower limbs
AHA: 2Q, '99, 3
M51.14 Intervertebral disc d/o w/radiculopathy thoracic [I-10]

724.5 Backache, unspecified
Vertebrogenic (pain) syndrome NOS
M54.9 Dorsalgia unspecified [I-10]

724.6 Disorders of sacrum
Ankylosis ⎤
Instability ⎦ lumbosacral or sacroiliac (joint)

√5th 724.7 Disorders of coccyx

724.70 Unspecified disorder of coccyx

724.71 Hypermobility of coccyx

724.79 Other
Coccygodynia

724.8 Other symptoms referable to back
Ossification of posterior longitudinal ligament NOS
Panniculitis specified as sacral or affecting back

724.9 Other unspecified back disorders
Ankylosis of spine NOS
Compression of spinal nerve root NEC
Spinal disorder NOS
EXCLUDES sacroiliitis (720.2)

Rheumatism, Excluding the Back (725-729)

INCLUDES disorders of muscles and tendons and their attachments, and of other soft tissues

725 Polymyalgia rheumatica
DEF: Joint and muscle pain, pelvis, and shoulder girdle stiffness, high sedimentation rate and temporal arteritis; occurs in elderly.
M35.3 Polymyalgia rheumatica [I-10]

√4th 726 Peripheral enthesopathies and allied syndromes
NOTE Enthesopathies are disorders of peripheral ligamentous or muscular attachments.
EXCLUDES spinal enthesopathy (720.1)

726.0 Adhesive capsulitis of shoulder

√5th 726.1 Rotator cuff syndrome of shoulder and allied disorders

726.10 Disorders of bursae and tendons in shoulder region, unspecified
Rotator cuff syndrome NOS
Supraspinatus syndrome NOS
AHA: 2Q, '01, 11
M75.50 Bursitis of unspecified shoulder [I-10]

726.11 Calcifying tendinitis of shoulder

726.12 Bicipital tenosynovitis

726.13 Partial tear of rotator cuff
EXCLUDES complete rupture of rotator cuff, nontraumatic (727.61)
AHA: 4Q, '11, 135-136

726.19 Other specified disorders
EXCLUDES complete rupture of rotator cuff, nontraumatic (727.61)

726.2 Other affections of shoulder region, not elsewhere classified
Periarthritis of shoulder
Scapulohumeral fibrositis

√5th 726.3 Enthesopathy of elbow region

726.30 Enthesopathy of elbow, unspecified

726.31 Medial epicondylitis

726.32 Lateral epicondylitis
Epicondylitis NOS
Golfers' elbow
Tennis elbow

726.33 Olecranon bursitis
Bursitis of elbow

726.39 Other

726.4 Enthesopathy of wrist and carpus
Bursitis of hand or wrist
Periarthritis of wrist

726.5 Enthesopathy of hip region
Bursitis of hip
Gluteal tendinitis
Iliac crest spur
Psoas tendinitis
Trochanteric tendinitis

√5th 726.6 Enthesopathy of knee

726.60 Enthesopathy of knee, unspecified
Bursitis of knee NOS

726.61 Pes anserinus tendinitis or bursitis
DEF: Inflamed tendons of sartorius, gracilis and semitendinosus muscles of medial aspect of knee.

726.62 Tibial collateral ligament bursitis
Pellegrini-Stieda syndrome

726.63 Fibular collateral ligament bursitis

726.64 Patellar tendinitis

726.65 Prepatellar bursitis
AHA: 2Q, '06, 15

726.69 Other
Bursitis:
infrapatellar
subpatellar

√5th 726.7 Enthesopathy of ankle and tarsus

726.70 Enthesopathy of ankle and tarsus, unspecified
Metatarsalgia NOS
EXCLUDES Morton's metatarsalgia (355.6)

726.71 Achilles bursitis or tendinitis

726.72 Tibialis tendinitis
Tibialis (anterior) (posterior) tendinitis

726.73 Calcaneal spur
DEF: Overgrowth of calcaneus bone; causes pain on walking; due to chronic avulsion injury of plantar fascia from calcaneus.

726.79 Other
Peroneal tendinitis

726.8 Other peripheral enthesopathies

√5th 726.9 Unspecified enthesopathy

726.90 Enthesopathy of unspecified site
Capsulitis NOS
Periarthritis NOS
Tendinitis NOS

726.91 Exostosis of unspecified site
Bone spur NOS
AHA: 2Q, '01, 15

√4th 727 Other disorders of synovium, tendon, and bursa

√5th 727.0 Synovitis and tenosynovitis

727.00 Synovitis and tenosynovitis, unspecified
Synovitis NOS
Tenosynovitis NOS
M65.9 Synovitis and tenosynovitis unspecified [I-10]

N ⬤ Newborn Age: 0   P ⬛ Pediatric Age: 0-17   M ⬛ Maternity Age: 12-55   A ⬛ Adult Age: 15-124

727.01 Synovitis and tenosynovitis in diseases classified elsewhere

Code first underlying disease as:
tuberculosis (015.0-015.9)

EXCLUDES crystal-induced (275.4)
gonococcal (098.51)
gout (274.00-274.03)
syphilitic (095.7)

727.02 Giant cell tumor of tendon sheath

727.03 Trigger finger (acquired)

DEF: Stenosing tenosynovitis or nodule in flexor tendon; cessation of flexion or extension movement in finger, followed by snapping into place.

727.04 Radial styloid tenosynovitis
de Quervain's disease

727.05 Other tenosynovitis of hand and wrist

727.06 Tenosynovitis of foot and ankle

727.09 Other

727.1 Bunion

DEF: Enlarged first metatarsal head due to inflamed bursa; results in laterally displaced great toe.

727.2 Specific bursitides often of occupational origin

Beat: Chronic crepitant synovitis of wrist
elbow   Miners':
hand   elbow
knee   knee

727.3 Other bursitis
Bursitis NOS

EXCLUDES bursitis:
gonococcal (098.52)
subacromial (726.19)
subcoracoid (726.19)
subdeltoid (726.19)
syphilitic (095.7)
"frozen shoulder" (726.0)

√5ᵗʰ 727.4 Ganglion and cyst of synovium, tendon, and bursa

727.40 Synovial cyst, unspecified

EXCLUDES that of popliteal space (727.51)
AHA: 2Q, '97, 6

727.41 Ganglion of joint

727.42 Ganglion of tendon sheath

Bunion

Normal
metatarsophalangeal
joint

Exostosis

Ganglia

Extensor
tendon
sheaths

Ganglion of wrist
(fluid-filled sac)

Baker's cyst
connected to
knee joint
synovial cavity

727.43 Ganglion, unspecified

727.49 Other
Cyst of bursa

√5ᵗʰ 727.5 Rupture of synovium

727.50 Rupture of synovium, unspecified

727.51 Synovial cyst of popliteal space
Baker's cyst (knee)

727.59 Other

√5ᵗʰ 727.6 Rupture of tendon, nontraumatic

727.60 Nontraumatic rupture of unspecified tendon

727.61 Complete rupture of rotator cuff

EXCLUDES partial tear of rotator cuff (726.13)
AHA: 4Q, '11, 136

727.62 Tendons of biceps (long head)

727.63 Extensor tendons of hand and wrist

727.64 Flexor tendons of hand and wrist

727.65 Quadriceps tendon

727.66 Patellar tendon

727.67 Achilles tendon

727.68 Other tendons of foot and ankle

727.69 Other

√5ᵗʰ 727.8 Other disorders of synovium, tendon, and bursa

727.81 Contracture of tendon (sheath)
Short Achilles tendon (acquired)

727.82 Calcium deposits in tendon and bursa
Calcification of tendon NOS
Calcific tendinitis NOS

EXCLUDES peripheral ligamentous or muscular attachments (726.0-726.9)

727.83 Plica syndrome
Plica knee

DEF: A fold in the synovial tissue formed before birth, creating a septum between two pockets of synovial tissue; most common are the medial patellar plica and the suprapatellar plica. Plica syndrome, or plica knee, refers to symptomatic plica.
AHA: 4Q, '00, 44

727.89 Other
Abscess of bursa or tendon

EXCLUDES xanthomatosis localized to tendons (272.7)
AHA: 2Q, '89, 15

727.9 Unspecified disorder of synovium, tendon, and bursa

√4ᵗʰ 728 Disorders of muscle, ligament, and fascia

EXCLUDES enthesopathies (726.0-726.9)
muscular dystrophies (359.0-359.1)
myoneural disorders (358.00-358.9)
myopathies (359.2-359.9)
nontraumatic hematoma of muscle (729.92)
old disruption of ligaments of knee (717.81-717.89)

728.0 Infective myositis
Myositis:
purulent
suppurative

EXCLUDES myositis:
epidemic (074.1)
interstitial (728.81)
syphilitic (095.6)
tropical (040.81)

DEF: Inflamed connective septal tissue of muscle.

√5ᵗʰ 728.1 Muscular calcification and ossification

728.10 Calcification and ossification, unspecified
Massive calcification (paraplegic)

728.11 Progressive myositis ossificans

DEF: Progressive myositic disease; marked by bony tissue formed by voluntary muscle; occurs among very young.

Diseases of the Musculoskeletal System and Connective Tissue   727.01–728.11

728.12 Traumatic myositis ossificans
Myositis ossificans (circumscripta)

728.13 Postoperative heterotopic calcification
DEF: Abnormal formation of calcium deposits in muscular tissue after surgery, marked by a corresponding loss of muscle tone and tension.

728.19 Other
Polymyositis ossificans

728.2 Muscular wasting and disuse atrophy, not elsewhere classified
Amyotrophia NOS
Myofibrosis
EXCLUDES *neuralgic amyotrophy (353.5)*
pelvic muscle wasting and disuse atrophy (618.83)
progressive muscular atrophy (335.0-335.9)

728.3 Other specific muscle disorders
Arthrogryposis
Immobility syndrome (paraplegic)
EXCLUDES *arthrogryposis multiplex congenita (754.89)*
stiff-man syndrome (333.91)

728.4 Laxity of ligament

728.5 Hypermobility syndrome

728.6 Contracture of palmar fascia   **A**
Dupuytren's contracture
DEF: Dupuytren's contracture: flexion deformity of finger, due to shortened, thickened fibrosing of palmar fascia; cause unknown; associated with long-standing epilepsy.

√5ᵗʰ **728.7 Other fibromatoses**

728.71 Plantar fascial fibromatosis
Contracture of plantar fascia
Plantar fasciitis (traumatic)
DEF: Plantar fascia fibromatosis; causes nodular swelling and pain; not associated with contractures.

728.79 Other
Garrod's or knuckle pads
Nodular fasciitis
Pseudosarcomatous fibromatosis (proliferative) (subcutaneous)
DEF: Knuckle pads: Pea-size nodules on dorsal surface of interphalangeal joints; new growth of fibrous tissue with thickened dermis and epidermis.

√5ᵗʰ **728.8 Other disorders of muscle, ligament, and fascia**

728.81 Interstitial myositis
DEF: Inflammation of septal connective parts of muscle tissue.

728.82 Foreign body granuloma of muscle
Talc granuloma of muscle
Use additional code to identify foreign body (V90.01-V90.9)

728.83 Rupture of muscle, nontraumatic

728.84 Diastasis of muscle
Diastasis recti (abdomen)
EXCLUDES *diastasis recti complicating pregnancy, labor, and delivery (665.8)*
DEF: Muscle separation, such as recti abdominis after repeated pregnancies.

728.85 Spasm of muscle
M62.838 Other muscle spasm   **I-10**

728.86 Necrotizing fasciitis
Use additional code to identify:
gangrene (785.4), if applicable
infectious organism (041.00-041.89)
DEF: Fulminating infection begins with extensive cellulitis, spreads to superficial and deep fascia; causes thrombosis of subcutaneous vessels, and gangrene of underlying tissue.
AHA: 4Q, '95, 54

728.87 Muscle weakness (generalized)
EXCLUDES *generalized weakness (780.79)*
AHA: 1Q, '05, 13; 4Q, '03, 66
TIP: Assign an additional code from category 438 if the weakness is a result of a CVA.

728.88 Rhabdomyolysis
DEF: A disintegration or destruction of muscle; an acute disease characterized by the excretion of myoglobin into the urine.
AHA: 4Q, '03, 66

728.89 Other
Eosinophilic fasciitis
Use additional E code to identify drug, if drug induced
DEF: Eosinophilic fasciitis: inflammation of fascia of extremities associated with eosinophilia, edema, and swelling; occurs alone or as part of myalgia syndrome.
AHA: 3Q, '06, 13; 3Q, '02, 28; 2Q, '01, 14, 15

728.9 Unspecified disorder of muscle, ligament, and fascia

√4ᵗʰ **729 Other disorders of soft tissues**
EXCLUDES *acroparesthesia (443.89)*
carpal tunnel syndrome (354.0)
disorders of the back (720.0-724.9)
entrapment syndromes (354.0-355.9)
palindromic rheumatism (719.3)
periarthritis (726.0-726.9)
psychogenic rheumatism (306.0)

729.0 Rheumatism, unspecified and fibrositis
DEF: General term describes diseases of muscle, tendon, nerve, joint, or bone; symptoms include pain and stiffness.

729.1 Myalgia and myositis, unspecified
Fibromyositis NOS
DEF: Myalgia: muscle pain.
DEF: Myositis: inflamed voluntary muscle.
DEF: Fibromyositis: inflamed fibromuscular tissue.
M79.1 Myalgia   **I-10**

729.2 Neuralgia, neuritis, and radiculitis, unspecified
EXCLUDES *brachial radiculitis (723.4)*
cervical radiculitis (723.4)
lumbosacral radiculitis (724.4)
mononeuritis (354.0-355.9)
radiculitis due to intervertebral disc involvement (722.0-722.2, 722.7)
sciatica (724.3)
DEF: Neuralgia: paroxysmal pain along nerve; symptoms include brief pain and tenderness at point nerve exits.
DEF: Neuritis: inflamed nerve, symptoms include paresthesia, paralysis and loss of reflexes at nerve site.
DEF: Radiculitis: inflamed nerve root.

√5ᵗʰ **729.3 Panniculitis, unspecified**
DEF: Inflammatory reaction of subcutaneous fat; causes nodules; often develops in abdominal region.

729.30 Panniculitis, unspecified site
Weber-Christian disease
DEF: Febrile, nodular, nonsuppurative, relapsing inflammation of subcutaneous fat.

729.31 Hypertrophy of fat pad, knee
Hypertrophy of infrapatellar fat pad

729.39 Other site
EXCLUDES *panniculitis specified as (affecting):*
back (724.8)
neck (723.6)
sacral (724.8)
AHA: 2Q, '11, 3

729.4 Fasciitis, unspecified
EXCLUDES *necrotizing fasciitis (728.86)*
nodular fasciitis (728.79)
AHA: 2Q, '94, 13

729.5 Pain in limb
AHA: 2Q, '07, 11
M79.609 Pain in unspecified limb   **I-10**

729.6 Residual foreign body in soft tissue
Use additional code to identify foreign body (V90.01-V90.9)
EXCLUDES *foreign body granuloma:*
muscle (728.82)
skin and subcutaneous tissue (709.4)

N Newborn Age: 0   **P** Pediatric Age: 0-17   **M** Maternity Age: 12-55   **A** Adult Age: 15-124

✓5ᵗʰ **729.7 Nontraumatic compartment syndrome**

Code first, if applicable, postprocedural complication (998.89)

EXCLUDES compartment syndrome NOS (958.90)
traumatic compartment syndrome (958.90-958.99)

DEF: Compression of nerves and blood vessels within an enclosed space, leading to impaired blood flow and muscle and nerve damage.

729.71 Nontraumatic compartment syndrome of upper extremity

Nontraumatic compartment syndrome of shoulder, arm, forearm, wrist, hand, and fingers

AHA: 4Q, '06, 100-102

729.72 Nontraumatic compartment syndrome of lower extremity

Nontraumatic compartment syndrome of hip, buttock, thigh, leg, foot, and toes

AHA: 4Q, '06, 100-102

729.73 Nontraumatic compartment syndrome of abdomen

AHA: 4Q, '06, 100-102

729.79 Nontraumatic compartment syndrome of other sites

AHA: 4Q, '06, 100-102

✓5ᵗʰ **729.8 Other musculoskeletal symptoms referable to limbs**

TIP: Assign for pseudothrombophlebitis, which involves painful swelling of the lower extremity and mimics deep vein thrombosis (DVT).

729.81 Swelling of limb

AHA: 4Q, '88, 6

TIP: Assign for hyperalgesic pseudothrombophlebitis, which involves painful swelling of the lower extremity and mimics deep vein thrombosis (DVT).

729.82 Cramp

729.89 Other

EXCLUDES abnormality of gait (781.2)
tetany (781.7)
transient paralysis of limb (781.4)

AHA: 4Q, '88, 12

R29.898 Oth symptoms & signs involv musculo sys   I-10

✓5ᵗʰ **729.9 Other and unspecified disorders of soft tissue**

AHA: 4Q, '08, 134-136

729.90 Disorders of soft tissue, unspecified

729.91 Post-traumatic seroma

EXCLUDES seroma complicating a procedure (998.13)

729.92 Nontraumatic hematoma of soft tissue

Nontraumatic hematoma of muscle

AHA: ▶2Q, '13, 8;◀ 4Q, '08, 135

TIP: Assign an additional E code for a drug adverse effect if caused by Coumadin or other anticoagulants.

729.99 Other disorders of soft tissue

Polyalgia

Osteopathies, Chondropathies, and Acquired Musculoskeletal Deformities (730-739)

✓4ᵗʰ **730 Osteomyelitis, periostitis, and other infections involving bone**

EXCLUDES jaw (526.4-526.5)
petrous bone (383.2)

Use additional code to identify organism, such as Staphylococcus (041.1)

The following fifth-digit subclassification is for use with category 730; valid digits are in [brackets] under each code. See list at beginning of chapter for definitions.

  0 **site unspecified**
  1 **shoulder region**
  2 **upper arm**
  3 **forearm**
  4 **hand**
  5 **pelvic region and thigh**
  6 **lower leg**
  7 **ankle and foot**
  8 **other specified sites**
  9 **multiple sites**

DEF: Osteomyelitis: bacterial inflammation of bone tissue and marrow.
DEF: Periostitis: inflammation of specialized connective tissue; causes swelling of bone and aching pain.

AHA: 4Q, '97, 43

§ ✓5ᵗʰ **730.0 Acute osteomyelitis**
[0-9]

Abscess of any bone except accessory sinus, jaw, or mastoid
Acute or subacute osteomyelitis, with or without mention of periostitis

Use additional code to identify major osseous defect, if applicable (731.3)

AHA: 4Q, '06, 103; **For code 730.06:** 1Q, '02, 4; **For code 730.07:** 1Q, '04, 14

§ ✓5ᵗʰ **730.1 Chronic osteomyelitis**
[0-9]

Brodie's abscess
Chronic or old osteomyelitis, with or without mention of periostitis
Sclerosing osteomyelitis of Garré
Sequestrum of bone

Use additional code to identify major osseous defect, if applicable (731.3)

EXCLUDES aseptic necrosis of bone (733.40-733.49)

AHA: 4Q, '06, 103; **For code 730.17:** 3Q, '11, 15; 3Q, '00, 4

§ ✓5ᵗʰ **730.2 Unspecified osteomyelitis**
[0-9]

Osteitis or osteomyelitis NOS, with or without mention of periostitis

Use additional code to identify major osseous defect, if applicable (731.3)

AHA: 4Q, '06, 103

M86.9 Osteomyelitis unspecified   I-10

§ ✓5ᵗʰ **730.3 Periostitis without mention of osteomyelitis**
[0-9]

Abscess of periosteum   ⎱ without mention of
Periostosis   ⎰ osteomyelitis

EXCLUDES that in secondary syphilis (091.61)

§ ✓5ᵗʰ **730.7 Osteopathy resulting from poliomyelitis**
[0-9]

Code first underlying disease (045.0-045.9)

§ ✓5ᵗʰ **730.8 Other infections involving bone in diseases classified elsewhere**
[0-9]

Code first underlying disease as:
tuberculosis (015.0-015.9)
typhoid fever (002.0)

EXCLUDES syphilis of bone NOS (095.5)

AHA: 2Q, '97, 16; 3Q, '91, 10

§ ✓5ᵗʰ **730.9 Unspecified infection of bone**
[0-9]

| ✓4ᵗʰ ✓5ᵗʰ Additional Digit Required | Unspecified Code | Other Specified Code | Manifestation Code | ►◄ Revised Text | ● New Code | ▲ Revised Code Title |

☑4ᵗʰ **731 Osteitis deformans and osteopathies associated with other disorders classified elsewhere**

DEF: Osteitis deformans: Bone disease marked by episodes of increased bone loss, excessive repair attempts; causes weakened, deformed bones with increased mass, bowed long bones, deformed flat bones, pain and pathological fractures; may be fatal if associated with congestive heart failure, giant cell tumors or bone sarcoma; also called Paget's disease.

731.0 Osteitis deformans without mention of bone tumor
  Paget's disease of bone

731.1 Osteitis deformans in diseases classified elsewhere

  Code first underlying disease as:
    malignant neoplasm of bone (170.0-170.9)

731.2 Hypertrophic pulmonary osteoarthropathy
  Bamberger-Marie disease
  DEF: Clubbing of fingers and toes; related to enlarged ends of long bones, due to chronic lung and heart disease.

731.3 Major osseous defects
  Code first underlying disease, if known, such as:
    aseptic necrosis (733.40-733.49)
    malignant neoplasm of bone (170.0-170.9)
    osteomyelitis (730.00-730.29)
    osteoporosis (733.00-733.09)
    peri-prosthetic osteolysis (996.45)
  AHA: 4Q, '06, 103

731.8 Other bone involvement in diseases classified elsewhere

  Code first underlying disease as:
    diabetes mellitus (249.8, 250.8)

  Use additional code to specify bone condition, such as:
    acute osteomyelitis (730.00-730.09)
  AHA: 2Q, '10, 6; 1Q, '04, 14; 4Q, '97, 43; 2Q, '97, 16
  TIP: For diabetic osteomyelitis, assign a total of three codes: 250.8X, 731.8, and a code from category 730.
  M90.89 Osteopathy dz classified elsewhere multiple site   I-10

☑4ᵗʰ **732 Osteochondropathies**

  DEF: Conditions related to both bone and cartilage, or conditions in which cartilage is converted to bone (enchondral ossification).

732.0 Juvenile osteochondrosis of spine
  Juvenile osteochondrosis (of):
    marginal or vertebral epiphysis (of Scheuermann)
    spine NOS
  Vertebral epiphysitis
    EXCLUDES *adolescent postural kyphosis (737.0)*

732.1 Juvenile osteochondrosis of hip and pelvis
  Coxa plana
  Ischiopubic synchondrosis (of van Neck)
  Osteochondrosis (juvenile) of:
    acetabulum
    head of femur (of Legg-Calvé-Perthes)
    iliac crest (of Buchanan)
    symphysis pubis (of Pierson)
  Pseudocoxalgia

732.2 Nontraumatic slipped upper femoral epiphysis
  Slipped upper femoral epiphysis NOS

732.3 Juvenile osteochondrosis of upper extremity
  Osteochondrosis (juvenile) of:
    capitulum of humerus (of Panner)
    carpal lunate (of Kienbock)
    hand NOS
    head of humerus (of Haas)
    heads of metacarpals (of Mauclaire)
    lower ulna (of Burns)
    radial head (of Brailsford)
    upper extremity NOS

732.4 Juvenile osteochondrosis of lower extremity, excluding foot
  Osteochondrosis (juvenile) of:
    lower extremity NOS
    primary patellar center (of Köhler)
    proximal tibia (of Blount)
    secondary patellar center (of Sinding-Larsen)
    tibial tubercle (of Osgood-Schlatter)
  Tibia vara

Slipped Femoral Epiphysis

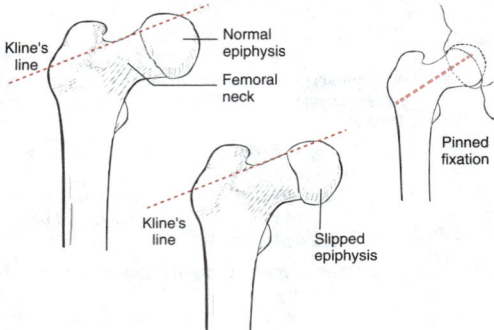

732.5 Juvenile osteochondrosis of foot
  Calcaneal apophysitis
  Epiphysitis, os calcis
  Osteochondrosis (juvenile) of:
    astragalus (of Diaz)
    calcaneum (of Sever)
    foot NOS
    metatarsal
      second (of Freiberg)
      fifth (of Iselin)
    os tibiale externum (of Haglund)
    tarsal navicular (of Köhler)

732.6 Other juvenile osteochondrosis
  Apophysitis
  Epiphysitis   ⎱ specified as juvenile, of other
  Osteochondritis ⎰ site, or site NOS
  Osteochondrosis

732.7 Osteochondritis dissecans

732.8 Other specified forms of osteochondropathy
  Adult osteochondrosis of spine

732.9 Unspecified osteochondropathy
  Apophysitis
  Epiphysitis   ⎱ NOS
  Osteochondritis ⎰ not specified as adult or juvenile, of
  Osteochondrosis   unspecified site

☑4ᵗʰ **733 Other disorders of bone and cartilage**

  EXCLUDES *bone spur (726.91)*
    cartilage of, or loose body in, joint (717.0-717.9, 718.0-718.9)
    giant cell granuloma of jaw (526.3)
    osteitis fibrosa cystica generalisata (252.01)
    osteomalacia (268.2)
    polyostotic fibrous dysplasia of bone (756.54)
    prognathism, retrognathism (524.1)
    xanthomatosis localized to bone (272.7)

☑5ᵗʰ **733.0 Osteoporosis**
  Use additional code to identify major osseous defect, if applicable (731.3)
  Use additional code to identify personal history of pathologic (healed) fracture (V13.51)
  DEF: Bone mass reduction that ultimately results in fractures after minimal trauma; dorsal kyphosis or loss of height often occur.
  AHA: 4Q, '06, 103

  733.00 Osteoporosis, unspecified
    Wedging of vertebra NOS
    AHA: 4Q, '07, 92;1Q, '07, 22; 3Q, '01, 19; 2Q, '98, 12
    M81.0 Age-related osteoporosis w/o curr path fx   I-10

  733.01 Senile osteoporosis
    Postmenopausal osteoporosis
    AHA: 1Q, '07, 5, 6
    M81.0 Age-related osteoporosis without current   I-10
    pathological fracture

  733.02 Idiopathic osteoporosis
    M81.8 Other osteoporosis w/o current pathological fx   I-10

  733.03 Disuse osteoporosis

733.09 Other
Drug-induced osteoporosis
Use additional E code to identify drug
AHA: 4Q, '03, 108
M81.6 Localized osteoporosis [Lequesne] `I-10`

√5ᵗʰ **733.1 Pathologic fracture**
Chronic fracture
Spontaneous fracture
EXCLUDES stress fracture (733.93-733.95)
traumatic fracture (800-829)
DEF: Fracture due to bone structure weakening by pathological processes (e.g., osteoporosis, neoplasms and osteomalacia).
AHA: 4Q, '08, 158; 1Q, '07, 3-4; 4Q, '93, 25; N-D, '86, 10; N-D, '85, 16
TIP: Assign only for newly diagnosed fractures; refer to V code aftercare categories if patient is receiving routine care during healing or recovery phase.

733.10 Pathologic fracture, unspecified site

733.11 Pathologic fracture of humerus
AHA: 2Q, '10, 6

733.12 Pathologic fracture of distal radius and ulna
Wrist NOS

733.13 Pathologic fracture of vertebrae
Collapse of vertebra NOS
AHA: 3Q, '08, 4; 1Q, '07, 5, 6, 22; 3Q, '99, 5
TIP: Assign for a chronic vertebral pathological fracture for which the patient is receiving medication.
M48.53xA Collasped vertebra NEC cervicothorac `I-10`
initial enc

733.14 Pathologic fracture of neck of femur
Femur NOS
Hip NOS
AHA: 1Q, '01, 1; 1Q, '96, 16

733.15 Pathologic fracture of other specified part of femur
AHA: 2Q, '98, 12
M84.453A Pathological fracture, unspec femur, `I-10`
initial encounter for fx

733.16 Pathologic fracture of tibia or fibula
Ankle NOS

733.19 Pathologic fracture of other specified site

√5ᵗʰ **733.2 Cyst of bone**

733.20 Cyst of bone (localized), unspecified

733.21 Solitary bone cyst
Unicameral bone cyst

733.22 Aneurysmal bone cyst
DEF: Solitary bone lesion, bulges into periosteum; marked by calcified rim.

733.29 Other
Fibrous dysplasia (monostotic)
EXCLUDES cyst of jaw (526.0-526.2, 526.89)
osteitis fibrosa cystica (252.01)
polyostotic fibrousdysplasia of bone (756.54)

733.3 Hyperostosis of skull
Hyperostosis interna frontalis
Leontiasis ossium
DEF: Abnormal bone growth on inner aspect of cranial bones.

√5ᵗʰ **733.4 Aseptic necrosis of bone**
Use additional code to identify major osseous defect, if applicable (731.3)
EXCLUDES osteochondropathies (732.0-732.9)
DEF: Infarction of bone tissue due to a noninfectious etiology, such as a fracture, ischemic disorder or administration of immunosuppressive drugs; leads to degenerative joint disease or nonunion of fractures.
AHA: 4Q, '06, 103

733.40 Aseptic necrosis of bone, site unspecified

733.41 Head of humerus

733.42 Head and neck of femur
Femur NOS
EXCLUDES Legg-Calvé-Perthes disease (732.1)
M87.256 Osteonecrosis due to previous `I-10`
trauma uns femur

733.43 Medial femoral condyle

733.44 Talus

733.45 Jaw
Use additional E code to identify drug, if drug-induced
EXCLUDES osteoradionecrosis of jaw (526.89)
AHA: 4Q, '07, 91

733.49 Other

733.5 Osteitis condensans
Piriform sclerosis of ilium
DEF: Idiopathic condition marked by low back pain; associated with oval or triangular sclerotic, opaque bone next to sacroiliac joints in the ileum.

733.6 Tietze's disease
Costochondral junction syndrome
Costochondritis
DEF: Painful, idiopathic, nonsuppurative, swollen costal cartilage sometimes confused with cardiac symptoms because the anterior chest pain resembles that of coronary artery disease.
M94.0 Chondrocostal junction syndrome (Tietze dz) `I-10`

733.7 Algoneurodystrophy
Disuse atrophy of bone
Sudeck's atrophy
DEF: Painful, idiopathic complex reflex sympathetic dystrophy, a chronic progressive disease characterized by severe pain, swelling, and changes in the skin.

√5ᵗʰ **733.8 Malunion and nonunion of fracture**
AHA: 2Q, '94, 5

733.81 Malunion of fracture

733.82 Nonunion of fracture
Pseudoarthrosis (bone)

√5ᵗʰ **733.9 Other unspecified disorders of bone and cartilage**
AHA: 4Q, '08, 136-137

733.90 Disorder of bone and cartilage unspecified
M89.9 Disorder of bone, unspecified `I-10`

733.91 Arrest of bone development or growth
Epiphyseal arrest

733.92 Chondromalacia
Chondromalacia:
NOS
localized, except patella
systemic
tibial plateau
EXCLUDES chondromalacia of patella (717.7)
DEF: Articular cartilage softening.

733.93 Stress fracture of tibia or fibula
Stress reaction of tibia or fibula
Use additional external cause code(s) to identify the cause of the stress fracture
AHA: 4Q, '08, 158; 4Q, '01, 48

733.94 Stress fracture of the metatarsals
Stress reaction of metatarsals
Use additional external cause code(s) to identify the cause of the stress fracture
AHA: 4Q, '08, 158; 4Q, '01, 48

733.95 Stress fracture of other bone
Stress reaction of other bone
Use additional external cause code(s) to identify the cause of the stress fracture
EXCLUDES stress fracture of:
femoral neck (733.96)
fibula (733.93)
metatarsals (733.94)
pelvis (733.98)
shaft of femur (733.97)
tibia (733.93)
AHA: 4Q, '08, 158; 4Q, '01, 48

√4ᵗʰ √5ᵗʰ Additional Digit Required   Unspecified Code   Other Specified Code   Manifestation Code   ▶◀ Revised Text   ● New Code   ▲ Revised Code Title

733.96 Stress fracture of femoral neck
Stress reaction of femoral neck

Use additional external cause code(s) to identify the cause of the stress fracture

AHA: 4Q, '08, 158

733.97 Stress fracture of shaft of femur
Stress reaction of shaft of femur

Use additional external cause code(s) to identify the cause of the stress fracture

AHA: 4Q, '08, 158

733.98 Stress fracture of pelvis
Stress reaction of pelvis

Use additional external cause code(s) to identify the cause of the stress fracture

AHA: 4Q, '08, 158

733.99 Other
Diaphysitis
Hypertrophy of bone
Relapsing polychondritis

AHA: 1Q, '11, 6; J-F, '87, 14

734 Flat foot
Pes planus (acquired)
Talipes planus (acquired)

EXCLUDES congenital (754.61)
rigid flat foot (754.61)
spastic (everted) flat foot (754.61)

✓4ᵗʰ **735 Acquired deformities of toe**

EXCLUDES congenital (754.60-754.69, 755.65-755.66)

735.0 Hallux valgus (acquired)
DEF: Angled displacement of the great toe, causing it to ride over or under other toes.

735.1 Hallux varus (acquired)
DEF: Angled displacement of the great toe toward the body midline, away from the other toes.

735.2 Hallux rigidus
DEF: Limited flexion movement at metatarsophalangeal joint of great toe; due to degenerative joint disease.

735.3 Hallux malleus
DEF: Extended proximal phalanx, flexed distal phalanges of great toe; foot resembles claw or hammer.

735.4 Other hammer toe (acquired)

735.5 Claw toe (acquired)
DEF: Hyperextended proximal phalanges, flexed middle and distal phalanges.

735.8 Other acquired deformities of toe
AHA: 4Q, '07, 123
TIP: Assign for hallux limitus, a deformity of the first metatarsophalangeal joint, which restricts the range of motion and can lead to stiffness and pain in the joint.

735.9 Unspecified acquired deformity of toe

✓4ᵗʰ **736 Other acquired deformities of limbs**

EXCLUDES congenital (754.3-755.9)

✓5ᵗʰ **736.0 Acquired deformities of forearm, excluding fingers**

736.00 Unspecified deformity
Deformity of elbow, forearm, hand, or wrist (acquired) NOS

736.01 Cubitus valgus (acquired)
DEF: Deviation of the elbow away from the body midline upon extension; it occurs when the palm is turning outward.

736.02 Cubitus varus (acquired)
DEF: Elbow joint displacement angled laterally; when the forearm is extended, it is deviated toward the midline of the body; also called "gun stock" deformity.

736.03 Valgus deformity of wrist (acquired)
DEF: Abnormal angulation away from the body midline.

736.04 Varus deformity of wrist (acquired)
DEF: Abnormal angulation toward the body midline.

Acquired Deformities of Toe

Hallux valgus

Hallux varus

Hallux malleus
(hammer of big toe)

Hammertoe

Acquired Deformities of Forearm

Varus deformity of wrist

Valgus deformity of wrist

Cubitus valgus

Cubitus varus

Claw hand

Wrist drop

Club hand

736.05 Wrist drop (acquired)
DEF: Inability to extend the hand at the wrist due to extensor muscle paralysis.

736.06 Claw hand (acquired)
DEF: Flexion and atrophy of the hand and fingers; found in ulnar nerve lesions, syringomyelia, and leprosy.

736.07 Club hand, acquired
DEF: Twisting of the hand out of shape or position; caused by the congenital absence of the ulna or radius.

736.09 Other

736.1 Mallet finger
DEF: Permanently flexed distal phalanx.

✓5ᵗʰ **736.2 Other acquired deformities of finger**

736.20 Unspecified deformity
Deformity of finger (acquired) NOS

736.21 Boutonniere deformity
DEF: A deformity of the finger caused by flexion of the proximal interphalangeal joint and hyperextension of the distal joint; also called buttonhole deformity.

736.22 Swan-neck deformity
DEF: Flexed distal and hyperextended proximal interphalangeal joint.

736.29 Other
EXCLUDES trigger finger (727.03)
AHA: 2Q, '05, 7; 2Q, '89, 13

✓5ᵗʰ **736.3 Acquired deformities of hip**

736.30 Unspecified deformity
Deformity of hip (acquired) NOS

736.31 Coxa valga (acquired)
DEF: Increase of at least 140 degrees in the angle formed by the axis of the head and the neck of the femur, and the axis of its shaft.

736.32 Coxa vara (acquired)
DEF: The bending downward of the neck of the femur, causing difficulty in movement; a right angle or less may be formed by the axis of the head and neck of the femur, and the axis of its shaft.

736.39 Other
AHA: 4Q, '11, 156; 2Q, '08, 4; 2Q, '91, 18
TIP: Do not assign as principal diagnosis for patient encounters for joint replacement following previous explantation of joint prosthesis, assign code V54.82 instead.

Deformities of Lower Limb

Cavus
deformity

Equinovarus   Cavovarus

Axis of Deformity
(may be multiple)

Dorsal

Valgus   Varus

Genu recurvatum

Plantar   Equinus Calcaneus

Kyphosis and Lordosis

Kyphosis
(hump)

Lordosis
(concave)

√5ᵗʰ **736.4 Genu valgum or varum (acquired)**

736.41 Genu valgum (acquired)
DEF: Abnormally close together and an abnormally large
space between the ankles; also called "knock-knees."

736.42 Genu varum (acquired)
DEF: Abnormally separated knees and the inward bowing of
the legs; it is also called "bowlegs."

736.5 Genu recurvatum (acquired)
DEF: Hyperextended knees; also called "backknee."

736.6 Other acquired deformities of knee
Deformity of knee (acquired) NOS

√5ᵗʰ **736.7 Other acquired deformities of ankle and foot**
EXCLUDES deformities of toe (acquired) (735.0-735.9)
pes planus (acquired) (734)

736.70 Unspecified deformity of ankle
and foot, acquired

736.71 Acquired equinovarus deformity
Clubfoot, acquired
EXCLUDES clubfoot not specified as acquired
(754.5-754.7)

736.72 Equinus deformity of foot, acquired
DEF: A plantar flexion deformity that forces people to walk
on their toes.

736.73 Cavus deformity of foot
EXCLUDES that with claw foot (736.74)
DEF: Abnormally high longitudinal arch of the foot.

736.74 Claw foot, acquired
DEF: High foot arch with hyperextended toes at
metatarsophalangeal joint and flexed toes at distal joints;
also called "main en griffe."

736.75 Cavovarus deformity of foot, acquired
DEF: Inward turning of the heel from the midline of the leg
and an abnormally high longitudinal arch.

736.76 Other calcaneus deformity

736.79 Other
Acquired:
pes
talipes } not elsewhere classified

√5ᵗʰ **736.8 Acquired deformities of other parts of limbs**

736.81 Unequal leg length (acquired)

736.89 Other
Deformity (acquired):
arm or leg, not elsewhere classified
shoulder
AHA: 4Q, '11, 156; 2Q, '08, 5
TIP: Do not assign as principal diagnosis for patient
encounters for joint replacement following previous
explantation of joint prosthesis, assign code V54.82
instead.

736.9 Acquired deformity of limb, site unspecified

√4ᵗʰ **737 Curvature of spine**
EXCLUDES congenital (754.2)

737.0 Adolescent postural kyphosis
EXCLUDES osteochondrosis of spine (juvenile) (732.0)
adult (732.8)

√5ᵗʰ **737.1 Kyphosis (acquired)**

737.10 Kyphosis (acquired) (postural)
M40.05 Postural kyphosis thoracolumbar region   I-10

737.11 Kyphosis due to radiation

737.12 Kyphosis, postlaminectomy
AHA: J-F, '87, 7
M96.3 Postlaminectomy kyphosis   I-10

737.19 Other
EXCLUDES that associated with conditions classifiable
elsewhere (737.41)
AHA: 1Q, '07, 20

√5ᵗʰ **737.2 Lordosis (acquired)**
DEF: Swayback appearance created by an abnormally increased
spinal curvature; it is also referred to as "hollow back" or "saddle
back."

737.20 Lordosis (acquired) (postural)

737.21 Lordosis, postlaminectomy

737.22 Other postsurgical lordosis

737.29 Other
EXCLUDES that associated with conditions classifiable
elsewhere (737.42)

√5ᵗʰ **737.3 Kyphoscoliosis and scoliosis**
DEF: Kyphoscoliosis: backward and lateral curvature of the spinal
column; it is found in vertebral osteochondrosis.
DEF: Scoliosis: an abnormal deviation of the spine to the left or right
of the midline.

737.30 Scoliosis [and kyphoscoliosis], idiopathic
AHA: 3Q, '03, 19
M41.115 Juvenile idiopathic scoliosis thoracolumbar   I-10
region

737.31 Resolving infantile idiopathic scoliosis

737.32 Progressive infantile idiopathic scoliosis
AHA: 3Q, '02, 12

Scoliosis and Kyphoscoliosis

Scoliosis   Kyphoscoliosis

√4ᵗʰ
√5ᵗʰ Additional Digit Required   Unspecified Code   Other Specified Code   Manifestation Code   ►◄ Revised Text   ● New Code   ▲ Revised Code Title

737.33 Scoliosis due to radiation

737.34 Thoracogenic scoliosis

737.39 Other

> EXCLUDES *that associated with conditions classifiable elsewhere (737.43)*
> *that in kyphoscoliotic heart disease (416.1)*

AHA: 2Q, '02, 16

√5th **737.4 Curvature of spine associated with other conditions**

Code first associated condition as:
Charcôt-Marie-Tooth disease (356.1)
mucopolysaccharidosis (277.5)
neurofibromatosis (237.70-237.79)
osteitis deformans (731.0)
osteitis fibrosa cystica (252.01)
osteoporosis (733.00-733.09)
poliomyelitis (138)
tuberculosis [Pott's curvature] (015.0)

737.40 Curvature of spine, unspecified

737.41 Kyphosis

737.42 Lordosis

737.43 Scoliosis

737.8 Other curvatures of spine

737.9 Unspecified curvature of spine

Curvature of spine (acquired) (idiopathic) NOS
Hunchback, acquired

> EXCLUDES *deformity of spine NOS (738.5)*

√4th **738 Other acquired deformity**

> EXCLUDES *congenital (754.0-756.9, 758.0-759.9)*
> *dentofacial anomalies (524.0-524.9)*

738.0 Acquired deformity of nose

Deformity of nose (acquired)
Overdevelopment of nasal bones

> EXCLUDES *deflected or deviated nasal septum (470)*

√5th **738.1 Other acquired deformity of head**

738.10 Unspecified deformity

738.11 Zygomatic hyperplasia

DEF: Abnormal enlargement of the zygoma (processus zygomaticus temporalis).

738.12 Zygomatic hypoplasia

DEF: Underdevelopment of the zygoma (processus zygomaticus temporalis).

738.19 Other specified deformity

AHA: 1Q, '06, 8; 2Q, '03, 13

738.2 Acquired deformity of neck

738.3 Acquired deformity of chest and rib

Deformity:
chest (acquired)
rib (acquired)
Pectus:
carinatum, acquired
excavatum, acquired

738.4 Acquired spondylolisthesis

Degenerative spondylolisthesis
Spondylolysis, acquired

> EXCLUDES *congenital (756.12)*

DEF: Vertebra displaced forward over another; due to bilateral defect in vertebral arch, eroded articular surface of posterior facets and elongated pedicle between fifth lumbar vertebra and sacrum.
AHA: 4Q, '07, 120; 1Q, '07, 10

M43.10 Spondylolisthesis site unspecified   I-10

738.5 Other acquired deformity of back or spine

Deformity of spine NOS

> EXCLUDES *curvature of spine (737.0-737.9)*

AHA: 1Q, '08, 11
TIP: Assign for post procedural flat back syndrome, which may be the result of a previous spinal fusion surgery. Do not assign a surgical complication code.

738.6 Acquired deformity of pelvis

Pelvic obliquity

> EXCLUDES *intrapelvic protrusion of acetabulum (718.6)*
> *that in relation to labor and delivery (653.0-653.4, 653.8-653.9)*

DEF: Pelvic obliquity: slanting or inclination of the pelvis at an angle between 55 and 60 degrees between the plane of the pelvis and the horizontal plane.

738.7 Cauliflower ear

DEF: Abnormal external ear; due to injury, subsequent perichondritis.

738.8 Acquired deformity of other specified site

Deformity of clavicle

AHA: 2Q, '01, 15

738.9 Acquired deformity of unspecified site

√4th **739 Nonallopathic lesions, not elsewhere classified**

> INCLUDES segmental dysfunction
> somatic dysfunction

DEF: Disability, loss of function or abnormality of a body part that is neither classifiable to a particular system nor brought about therapeutically to counteract another disease.

739.0 Head region

Occipitocervical region

739.1 Cervical region

Cervicothoracic region

739.2 Thoracic region

Thoracolumbar region

739.3 Lumbar region

Lumbosacral region

739.4 Sacral region

Sacrococcygeal region
Sacroiliac region

739.5 Pelvic region

Hip region
Pubic region

739.6 Lower extremities

739.7 Upper extremities

Acromioclavicular region
Sternoclavicular region

739.8 Rib cage

Costochondral region
Costovertebral region
Sternochondral region

739.9 Abdomen and other

AHA: 2Q, '89, 14

N   Newborn Age: 0   P   Pediatric Age: 0-17   M   Maternity Age: 12-55   A   Adult Age: 15-124

14. Congenital Anomalies (740-759)

AHA: 2Q, '12, 17

TIP: Codes from chapter 14 may be assigned throughout the life of the patient, whenever the congenital anomaly is diagnosed.

√4ᵗʰ 740 Anencephalus and similar anomalies

740.0 Anencephalus
Acrania
Amyelencephalus
Hemicephaly
Hemianencephaly
DEF: Fetus without cerebrum, cerebellum and flat bones of skull.

740.1 Craniorachischisis
DEF: Congenital slit in cranium and vertebral column.

740.2 Iniencephaly
DEF: Spinal cord passes through enlarged occipital bone (foramen magnum); absent vertebral bone layer and spinal processes; resulting in both reduction in number and proper fusion of the vertebrae.

√4ᵗʰ 741 Spina bifida
EXCLUDES spina bifida occulta (756.17)

The following fifth-digit subclassification is for use with category 741:
0 **unspecified region**
1 **cervical region**
2 **dorsal [thoracic] region**
3 **lumbar region**

DEF: Lack of closure of spinal cord's bony encasement; marked by cord protrusion into lumbosacral area; evident by elevated alpha-fetoprotein of amniotic fluid.
AHA: 3Q, '94, 7
TIP: For Arnold-Chiari syndrome, Type I, refer to code 348.4.

§ √5ᵗʰ 741.0 With hydrocephalus
[0-3] Arnold-Chiari syndrome, type II
Chiari malformation, type II
Any condition classifiable to 741.9 with any condition classifiable to 742.3
AHA: 4Q, '97, 51; 4Q, '94, 37; S-O, '87, 10
Q05.4 Unspecified spina bifida with hydrocephalus [I-10]

§ √5ᵗʰ 741.9 Without mention of hydrocephalus
[0-3] Hydromeningocele (spinal)
Hydromyelocele
Meningocele (spinal)
Meningomyelocele
Myelocele
Myelocystocele
Rachischisis
Spina bifida (aperta)
Syringomyelocele
Q05.8 Sacral spina bifida without hydrocephalus [I-10]

√4ᵗʰ 742 Other congenital anomalies of nervous system
EXCLUDES congenital central alveolar hypoventilation syndrome (327.25)

742.0 Encephalocele
Encephalocystocele
Encephalomyelocele
Hydroencephalocele
Hydromeningocele, cranial
Meningocele, cerebral
Meningoencephalocele
DEF: Brain tissue protrudes through skull defect.
AHA: 4Q, '94, 37

742.1 Microcephalus
Hydromicrocephaly
Micrencephaly
DEF: Extremely small head or brain.

Spina Bifida

Normal spinal cord
Cerebrospinal fluid space
Skin

Spinal cord (placode) in section
Cerebrospinal fluid
Skin
Unfused posterior vertebral bone

742.2 Reduction deformities of brain
Absence
Agenesis } of part of brain
Aplasia
Hypoplasia

Agyria
Arhinencephaly
Holoprosencephaly
Microgyria
AHA: 3Q, '03, 15; 4Q, '94, 37
TIP: Assign for septo-optic dysplasia.

742.3 Congenital hydrocephalus
Aqueduct of Sylvius:
anomaly
obstruction, congenital
stenosis
Atresia of foramina of Magendie and Luschka
Hydrocephalus in newborn
EXCLUDES hydrocephalus:
acquired (331.3-331.4)
due to congenital toxoplasmosis (771.2)
with any condition classifiable to 741.9 (741.0)
DEF: Fluid accumulation within the skull; involves subarachnoid (external) or ventricular (internal) brain spaces.
AHA: 4Q, '05, 83
Q03.9 Congenital hydrocephalus unspecified [I-10]

742.4 Other specified anomalies of brain
Congenital cerebral cyst | Multiple anomalies of brain NOS
Macroencephaly | Porencephaly
Macrogyria | Ulegyria
Megalencephaly
AHA: 1Q, '99, 9; 3Q, '92, 12

Normal Ventricles and Hydrocephalus

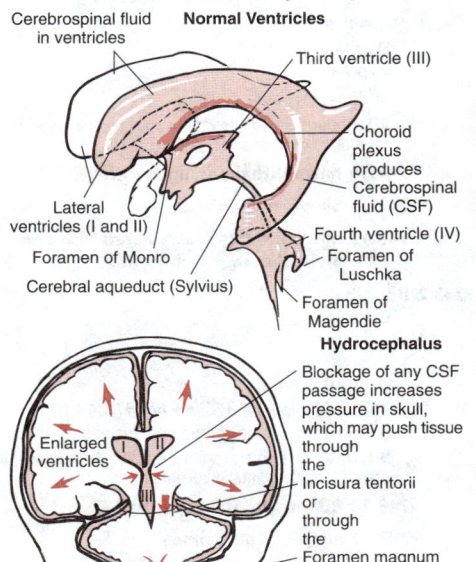

Cerebrospinal fluid in ventricles
Normal Ventricles
Third ventricle (III)
Choroid plexus produces Cerebrospinal fluid (CSF)
Lateral ventricles (I and II)
Foramen of Monro
Cerebral aqueduct (Sylvius)
Fourth ventricle (IV)
Foramen of Luschka
Foramen of Magendie

Hydrocephalus
Enlarged ventricles
Blockage of any CSF passage increases pressure in skull, which may push tissue through the Incisura tentorii or through the Foramen magnum

---

§ Requires fifth digit. Valid digits are in [brackets] under each code. See category 741 for codes and definitions.

√5th **742.5 Other specified anomalies of spinal cord**

742.51 Diastematomyelia
DEF: Congenital anomaly often associated with spina bifida; the spinal cord is separated into halves by a bony tissue resembling a "spike" (a spicule), each half surrounded by a dural sac.

742.53 Hydromyelia
Hydrorhachis
DEF: Dilated central spinal cord canal; characterized by increased fluid accumulation.

742.59 Other
Amyelia
Atelomyelia
Congenital anomaly of spinal meninges
Defective development of cauda equina
Hypoplasia of spinal cord
Myelatelia
Myelodysplasia
AHA: 2Q, '91, 14; 1Q, '89, 10
TIP: Assign for tethered spinal cord syndrome, regardless of when it is diagnosed.

742.8 Other specified anomalies of nervous system
Agenesis of nerve
Displacement of brachial plexus
Familial dysautonomia
Jaw-winking syndrome
Marcus-Gunn syndrome
Riley-Day syndrome
EXCLUDES neurofibromatosis (237.70-237.79)

742.9 Unspecified anomaly of brain, spinal cord, and nervous system
Anomaly
Congenital: ⎫   ⎧ brain
  disease   ⎬ of: ⎨ nervous system
  lesion   ⎭   ⎩ spinal cord
Deformity

√4th **743 Congenital anomalies of eye**

√5th **743.0 Anophthalmos**
DEF: Complete absence of the eyes or the presence of vestigial eyes.

743.00 Clinical anophthalmos, unspecified
Agenesis   ⎫
Cogenital absence ⎬ of eye
Anophthalmos NOS ⎭

743.03 Cystic eyeball, congenital

743.06 Cryptophthalmos
DEF: Skin is continuous over eyeball, results in apparent absence of eyelids.

√5th **743.1 Microphthalmos**
Dysplasia ⎫
Hypoplasia ⎬ of eye
Rudimentary eye
DEF: Abnormally small eyeballs, may be opacities of cornea and lens, scarring of choroid and retina.

743.10 Microphthalmos, unspecified

743.11 Simple microphthalmos

743.12 Microphthalmos associated with other anomalies of eye and adnexa

√5th **743.2 Buphthalmos**
Glaucoma:
  congenital
  newborn
Hydrophthalmos
EXCLUDES glaucoma of childhood (365.14)
  traumatic glaucoma due to birth injury (767.8)
DEF: Distended, enlarged fibrous coats of eye; due to intraocular pressure of congenital glaucoma.

743.20 Buphthalmos, unspecified

743.21 Simple buphthalmos

743.22 Buphthalmos associated with other ocular anomalies
Keratoglobus,   ⎫
  cogenital   ⎬ associated with
Megalocornea   ⎭ buphthalmos

√5th **743.3 Congenital cataract and lens anomalies**
EXCLUDES infantile cataract (366.00-366.09)
DEF: Opaque eye lens.

743.30 Congenital cataract, unspecified

743.31 Capsular and subcapsular cataract

743.32 Cortical and zonular cataract

743.33 Nuclear cataract

743.34 Total and subtotal cataract, congenital

743.35 Congenital aphakia
Congenital absence of lens

743.36 Anomalies of lens shape
Microphakia
Spherophakia

743.37 Congenital ectopic lens

743.39 Other

√5th **743.4 Coloboma and other anomalies of anterior segment**
DEF: Coloboma: ocular tissue defect associated with defect of ocular fetal intraocular fissure; may cause small pit on optic disk, major defects of iris, ciliary body, choroid, and retina.

743.41 Anomalies of corneal size and shape
Microcornea
EXCLUDES that associated with buphthalmos (743.22)

743.42 Corneal opacities, interfering with vision, congenital

743.43 Other corneal opacities, congenital

743.44 Specified anomalies of anterior chamber, chamber angle, and related structures
Anomaly:
  Axenfeld's
  Peters'
  Rieger's

743.45 Aniridia
DEF: Incompletely formed or absent iris; affects both eyes; dominant trait; also called congenital absence of iris.
AHA: 2Q, '10, 4-5; 3Q, '02, 20

743.46 Other specified anomalies of iris and ciliary body
Anisocoria, congenital
Atresia of pupil
Coloboma of iris
Corectopia

743.47 Specified anomalies of sclera

743.48 Multiple and combined anomalies of anterior segment

743.49 Other

√5th **743.5 Congenital anomalies of posterior segment**

743.51 Vitreous anomalies
Congenital vitreous opacity

743.52 Fundus coloboma
DEF: Absent retinal and choroidal tissue; occurs in lower fundus; a bright white ectatic zone of exposed sclera extends into and changes the optic disk.

743.53 Chorioretinal degeneration, congenital

743.54 Congenital folds and cysts of posterior segment

743.55 Congenital macular changes

743.56 Other retinal changes, congenital
AHA: 3Q, '99, 12

743.57 Specified anomalies of optic disc
Coloboma of optic disc (congenital)

743.58 Vascular anomalies
Congenital retinal aneurysm

743.59 Other

N Newborn Age: 0   P Pediatric Age: 0-17   M Maternity Age: 12-55   A Adult Age: 15-124

☑5ʰ **743.6 Congenital anomalies of eyelids, lacrimal system, and orbit**

　　743.61 Congenital ptosis
　　　　DEF: Drooping of eyelid.

　　743.62 Congenital deformities of eyelids
　　　　Ablepharon
　　　　Absence of eyelid
　　　　Accessory eyelid
　　　　Congenital:
　　　　　ectropion
　　　　　entropion
　　　　AHA: 1Q, '00, 22
　　　　TIP: Assign for epiblepharon, in which a redundant horizontal skin fold under the eyelid causes an abnormal vertical orientation of the eyelashes; may result in the eyelashes touching the eyeball.

　　743.63 Other specified congenital anomalies of eyelid
　　　　Absence, agenesis, of cilia

　　743.64 Specified congenital anomalies of lacrimal gland

　　743.65 Specified congenital anomalies of lacrimal passages
　　　　Absence, agenesis of:
　　　　　lacrimal apparatus
　　　　　punctum lacrimale
　　　　Accessory lacrimal canal

　　743.66 Specified congenital anomalies of orbit

　　743.69 Other
　　　　Accessory eye muscles

　743.8 Other specified anomalies of eye
　　　EXCLUDES *congenital nystagmus (379.51)*
　　　　　　　　ocular albinism (270.2)
　　　　　　　　optic nerve hypoplasia (377.43)
　　　　　　　　retinitis pigmentosa (362.74)

　743.9 Unspecified anomaly of eye
　　　Congenital:
　　　　anomaly NOS　⎫ of eye (any part)
　　　　deformity NOS ⎭

☑4ʰ **744 Congenital anomalies of ear, face, and neck**
　　EXCLUDES *anomaly of:*
　　　　　　　cervical spine (754.2, 756.10-756.19)
　　　　　　　larynx (748.2-748.3)
　　　　　　　nose (748.0-748.1)
　　　　　　　parathyroid gland (759.2)
　　　　　　　thyroid gland (759.2)
　　　　　　　cleft lip (749.10-749.25)

☑5ʰ **744.0 Anomalies of ear causing impairment of hearing**
　　　EXCLUDES *congenital deafness without mention of cause (389.0-389.9)*

　　744.00 Unspecified anomaly of ear with impairment of hearing

　　744.01 Absence of external ear
　　　　Absence of:
　　　　　auditory canal (external)
　　　　　auricle (ear) (with stenosis or atresia of auditory canal)

　　744.02 Other anomalies of external ear with impairment of hearing
　　　　Atresia or stricture of auditory canal (external)

　　744.03 Anomaly of middle ear, except ossicles
　　　　Atresia or stricture of osseous meatus (ear)

　　744.04 Anomalies of ear ossicles
　　　　Fusion of ear ossicles

　　744.05 Anomalies of inner ear
　　　　Congenital anomaly of:
　　　　　membranous labyrinth
　　　　　organ of Corti

　　744.09 Other
　　　　Absence of ear, congenital

744.1 Accessory auricle
　　Accessory tragus　　　　Supernumerary:
　　Polyotia　　　　　　　　　ear
　　Preauricular appendage　　lobule
　　DEF: Redundant tissue or structures of ear.

☑5ʰ **744.2 Other specified anomalies of ear**
　　EXCLUDES *that with impairment of hearing (744.00-744.09)*

　　744.21 Absence of ear lobe, congenital

　　744.22 Macrotia
　　　　DEF: Abnormally large pinna of ear.

　　744.23 Microtia
　　　　DEF: Hypoplasia of pinna; associated with absent or closed auditory canal.

　　744.24 Specified anomalies of Eustachian tube
　　　　Absence of Eustachian tube

　　744.29 Other
　　　　Bat ear
　　　　Darwin's tubercle
　　　　Pointed ear
　　　　Prominence of auricle
　　　　Ridge ear
　　　　EXCLUDES *preauricular sinus (744.46)*

744.3 Unspecified anomaly of ear
　　Congenital:
　　　anomaly NOS　⎫ of ear, not elsewhere
　　　deformity NOS ⎭　　classified

☑5ʰ **744.4 Branchial cleft cyst or fistula; preauricular sinus**

　　744.41 Branchial cleft sinus or fistula
　　　　Branchial:
　　　　　sinus (external) (internal)
　　　　　vestige
　　　　DEF: Cyst due to failed closure of embryonic branchial cleft.

　　744.42 Branchial cleft cyst

　　744.43 Cervical auricle

　　744.46 Preauricular sinus or fistula

　　744.47 Preauricular cyst

　　744.49 Other
　　　　Fistula (of):
　　　　　auricle, congenital
　　　　　cervicoaural

744.5 Webbing of neck
　　Pterygium colli
　　DEF: Thick, triangular skinfold, stretches from lateral side of neck across shoulder; associated with Turner's and Noonan's syndromes.

☑5ʰ **744.8 Other specified anomalies of face and neck**

　　744.81 Macrocheilia
　　　　Hypertrophy of lip, congenital
　　　　DEF: Abnormally large lips.

　　744.82 Microcheilia
　　　　DEF: Abnormally small lips.

　　744.83 Macrostomia
　　　　DEF: Bilateral or unilateral anomaly of mouth due to malformed maxillary and mandibular processes; results in mouth extending toward ear.

　　744.84 Microstomia
　　　　DEF: Abnormally small mouth.

　　744.89 Other
　　　　EXCLUDES *congenital fistula of lip (750.25)*
　　　　　　　　musculoskeletal anomalies (754.0-754.1, 756.0)

744.9 Unspecified anomalies of face and neck
　　Congenital:
　　　anomaly NOS　⎫ of face [any part] or neck [any
　　　deformity NOS ⎭　　part]

☑4ʰ ☑5ʰ Additional Digit Required　　Unspecified Code　　　Other Specified Code　　　Manifestation Code　　　▶◀ Revised Text　　　● New Code　　　▲ Revised Code Title

Congenital Anomalies

743.6 – 744.9

✓4th **745 Bulbus cordis anomalies and anomalies of cardiac septal closure**

745.0 Common truncus

Absent septum }
Communication (abnormal) } between aorta and pulmonary artery

Aortic septal defect
Common aortopulmonary trunk
Persistent truncus arteriosus

✓5th **745.1 Transposition of great vessels**

745.10 Complete transposition of great vessels

Transposition of great vessels:
NOS
classical

745.11 Double outlet right ventricle

Dextratransposition of aorta
Incomplete transposition of great vessels
Origin of both great vessels from right ventricle
Taussig-Bing syndrome or defect

745.12 Corrected transposition of great vessels

745.19 Other

745.2 Tetralogy of Fallot

Fallot's pentalogy
Ventricular septal defect with pulmonary stenosis or atresia, dextraposition of aorta, and hypertrophy of right ventricle

EXCLUDES *Fallot's triad (746.09)*

DEF: Obstructed cardiac outflow causes pulmonary stenosis, interventricular septal defect and right ventricular hypertrophy.

745.3 Common ventricle

Cor triloculare biatriatum
Single ventricle

745.4 Ventricular septal defect

Eisenmenger's defect or complex
Gerbo dedefect
Interventricular septal defect
Left ventricular-right atrial communication
Roger's disease

EXCLUDES *common atrioventricular canal type (745.69)*
single ventricle (745.3)

Q21.0 Ventricular septal defect I-10

745.5 Ostium secundum type atrial septal defect

Defect:
  atrium secundum
  fossa ovalis
Patent or persistent:
  foramen ovale
  ostium secundum
Lutembacher's syndrome

DEF: Opening in atrial septum due to failure of the septum secundum and the endocardial cushions to fuse; there is a rim of septum surrounding the defect.

AHA: 2Q, '12, 3; 3Q, '09, 17; 3Q, '09, 17

Q21.1 Atrial septal defect I-10

✓5th **745.6 Endocardial cushion defects**

DEF: Atrial and/or ventricular septal defects causing abnormal fusion of cushions in atrioventricular canal.

745.60 Endocardial cushion defect, unspecified type

DEF: Septal defect due to imperfect fusion of endocardial cushions.

Heart Defects

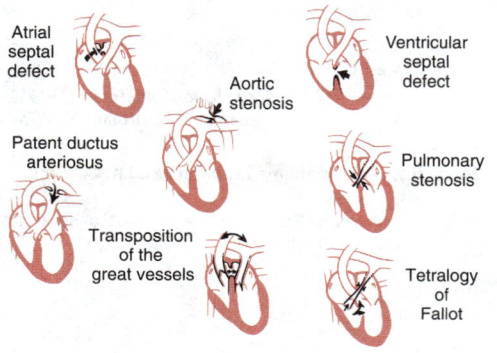

Atrial septal defect

Ventricular septal defect

Aortic stenosis

Patent ductus arteriosus

Pulmonary stenosis

Transposition of the great vessels

Tetralogy of Fallot

745.61 Ostium primum defect

Persistent ostium primum

DEF: Opening in low, posterior septum primum; causes cleft in basal portion of atrial septum; associated with cleft mitral valve.

745.69 Other

Absence of atrial septum
Atrioventricular canal type ventricular septal defect
Common atrioventricular canal
Common atrium

745.7 Cor biloculare

Absence of atrial and ventricular septa

DEF: Atrial and ventricular septal defect; marked by heart with two cardiac chambers (one atrium, one ventricle), and one atrioventricular valve.

745.8 Other

745.9 Unspecified defect of septal closure

Septal defect NOS

✓4th **746 Other congenital anomalies of heart**

EXCLUDES *endocardial fibroelastosis (425.3)*

✓5th **746.0 Anomalies of pulmonary valve**

EXCLUDES *infundibular or subvalvular pulmonic stenosis (746.83)*
tetralogy of Fallot (745.2)

746.00 Pulmonary valve anomaly, unspecified

746.01 Atresia, congenital

Congenital absence of pulmonary valve

746.02 Stenosis, congenital

DEF: Stenosis of opening between pulmonary artery and right ventricle; causes obstructed blood outflow from right ventricle.

746.09 Other

Congenital insufficiency of pulmonary valve
Fallot's triad or trilogy

746.1 Tricuspid atresia and stenosis, congenital

Absence of tricuspid valve

746.2 Ebstein's anomaly

DEF: Malformation of the tricuspid valve characterized by septal and posterior leaflets attaching to the wall of the right ventricle; causing the right ventricle to fuse with the atrium into a large right atrium and a small ventricle; causes heart failure and abnormal cardiac rhythm.

746.3 Congenital stenosis of aortic valve

Congenital aortic stenosis

EXCLUDES *congenital:*
subaortic stenosis (746.81)
supravalvular aortic stenosis (747.22)

DEF: Stenosis of orifice of aortic valve; obstructs blood outflow from left ventricle.

AHA: 4Q, '88, 8

746.4 Congenital insufficiency of aortic valve

Bicuspid aortic valve
Congenital aortic insufficiency

DEF: Impaired functioning of aortic valve due to incomplete closure; causes backflow (regurgitation) of blood from aorta to left ventricle.

Q23.1 Congenital insufficiency of aortic valve I-10

746.5 Congenital mitral stenosis

Fused commissure }
Parachute deformity } of mitral valve
Supernumerary cusps }

DEF: Stenosis of left atrioventricular orifice.

AHA: 3Q, '07, 3

746.6 Congenital mitral insufficiency

DEF: Impaired functioning of mitral valve due to incomplete closure; causes backflow of blood from left ventricle to left atrium.

746.7 Hypoplastic left heart syndrome

Atresia, or marked hypoplasia, of aortic orifice or valve, with hypoplasia of ascending aorta and defective development of left ventricle (with mitral valve atresia)

N Newborn Age: 0 **P** Pediatric Age: 0-17 **M** Maternity Age: 12-55 **A** Adult Age: 15-124

✓5ᵗʰ **746.8 Other specified anomalies of heart**

746.81 Subaortic stenosis

DEF: Stenosis, of left ventricular outflow tract due to fibrous tissue ring or septal hypertrophy below aortic valve.

AHA: 3Q, '07, 3

746.82 Cor triatriatum

DEF: Transverse septum divides left atrium due to failed resorption of embryonic common pulmonary vein; results in three atrial chambers.

746.83 Infundibular pulmonic stenosis

Subvalvular pulmonic stenosis

DEF: Stenosis of right ventricle outflow tract within infundibulum due to fibrous diaphragm below valve or long, narrow fibromuscular channel.

746.84 Obstructive anomalies of heart, not elsewhere classified

Shone's syndrome
Uhl's disease

Use additional code for associated anomalies, such as:
coarctation of aorta (747.10)
congenital mitral stenosis (746.5)
subaortic stenosis (746.81)

AHA: 2Q, '12, 3

746.85 Coronary artery anomaly

Anomalous origin or communication of coronary artery
Arteriovenous malformation of coronary artery
Coronary artery:
absence
arising from aorta or pulmonary trunk
single

AHA: N-D, '85, 3

746.86 Congenital heart block

Complete or incomplete atrioventricular [AV] block

DEF: Impaired conduction of electrical impulses; due to maldeveloped junctional tissue.

746.87 Malposition of heart and cardiac apex

Abdominal heart
Dextrocardia
Ectopia cordis
Levocardia (isolated)
Mesocardia

EXCLUDES dextrocardia with complete transposition of viscera (759.3)

746.89 Other

Atresia ⎱
Hypoplasia ⎰ of cardiac vein

Congenital:
cardiomegaly
diverticulum, left ventricle
pericardial defect

AHA: 3Q, '00, 3; 1Q, '99, 11; J-F, '85, 3

TIP: Assign for Brugada syndrome. Additional codes may be required.

Q24.8 Oth specified congenital malformations of heart I-10

746.9 Unspecified anomaly of heart

Congenital:
anomaly of heart NOS
heart disease NOS

✓4ᵗʰ **747 Other congenital anomalies of circulatory system**

747.0 Patent ductus arteriosus

Patent ductus Botalli
Persistent ductus arteriosus

DEF: Open lumen in ductus arteriosus causes arterial blood recirculation in lungs; inhibits blood supply to aorta; symptoms such as shortness of breath more noticeable upon activity.

AHA: 3Q, '09, 17

Q25.0 Patent ductus arteriosus I-10

✓5ᵗʰ **747.1 Coarctation of aorta**

DEF: Localized deformity of aortic media seen as a severe constriction of the vessel lumen; major symptom is high blood pressure in the arms and low pressure in the legs; may result in a CVA, rupture of the aorta, bacterial endocarditis or congestive heart failure.

747.10 Coarctation of aorta (preductal) (postductal)

Hypoplasia of aortic arch

AHA: 3Q, '07, 3; 1Q, '99, 11; 4Q, '88, 8

747.11 Interruption of aortic arch

✓5ᵗʰ **747.2 Other anomalies of aorta**

747.20 Anomaly of aorta, unspecified

747.21 Anomalies of aortic arch

Anomalous origin, right subclavian artery
Dextraposition of aorta
Double aortic arch
Kommerell's diverticulum
Overriding aorta
Persistent:
convolutions, aortic arch
right aortic arch
Vascular ring

EXCLUDES hypoplasia of aortic arch (747.10)

AHA: 1Q, '03, 15

747.22 Atresia and stenosis of aorta

Absence ⎫
Aplasia ⎬ of aorta
Hypoplasia ⎪
Stricture ⎭

Supra (valvular)-aortic stenosis

EXCLUDES congenital aortic (valvular) stenosis or stricture, so stated (746.3)
hypoplasia of aorta in hypoplastic left heart syndrome (746.7)

747.29 Other

Aneurysm of sinus of Valsalva
Congenital:
aneurysm ⎱ of aorta
dilation ⎰

✓5ᵗʰ **747.3 Anomalies of pulmonary artery**

AHA: 4Q, '11, 137-138

747.31 Pulmonary artery coarctation and atresia

Agenesis of pulmonary artery
Atresia of pulmonary artery
Coarctation of pulmonary artery
Hypoplasia of pulmonary artery
Stenosis of pulmonary artery

AHA: 2Q, '12, 3

747.32 Pulmonary arteriovenous malformation

Pulmonary arteriovenous aneurysm

EXCLUDES acquired pulmonary arteriovenous fistula (417.0)

AHA: 4Q, '11, 138

747.39 Other anomalies of pulmonary artery and pulmonary circulation

Anomaly of pulmonary artery

✓5ᵗʰ **747.4 Anomalies of great veins**

747.40 Anomaly of great veins, unspecified

Anomaly NOS of:
pulmonary veins
vena cava

747.41 Total anomalous pulmonary venous connection

Total anomalous pulmonary venous return [TAPVR]:
subdiaphragmatic
supradiaphragmatic

747.42 Partial anomalous pulmonary venous connection

Partial anomalous pulmonary venous return

747.49 Other anomalies of great veins

Absence ⎫
Congenital ⎬ of vena cava (inferior)
stenosis ⎭ (superior)

Persistent:
left posterior cardinal vein
left superior vena cava
Scimitar syndrome
Transposition of pulmonary veins NOS

747.5 Absence or hypoplasia of umbilical artery

Single umbilical artery

✓4ᵗʰ ✓5ᵗʰ Additional Digit Required   **Unspecified Code**   Other Specified Code   Manifestation Code   ◄► Revised Text   ● New Code   ▲ Revised Code Title

2015 ICD-9-CM   **Volume 1 – 241**

Congenital Anomalies

747.6–748.4

√5ᵗʰ **747.6 Other anomalies of peripheral vascular system**

Absence
Anomaly } of artery or vein, NEC
Atresia

Arteriovenous aneurysm (peripheral)
Arteriovenous malformation of the peripheral vascular system
Congenital:
  aneurysm (peripheral)
  phlebectasia
  stricture, artery
  varix
Multiple renal arteries

EXCLUDES *anomalies of:*
  cerebral vessels (747.81)
  pulmonary artery (747.39)
  congenital retinal aneurysm (743.58)
  hemangioma (228.00-228.09)
  lymphangioma (228.1)

747.60 Anomaly of the peripheral vascular system, unspecified site

747.61 Gastrointestinal vessel anomaly
AHA: 3Q, '96, 10
TIP: Do not assign for gastric or intestinal AV malformation or angiodysplasia not stated to be congenital. See instead code 537.82, 537.83, 569.84, or 569.85.

747.62 Renal vessel anomaly

747.63 Upper limb vessel anomaly

747.64 Lower limb vessel anomaly

747.69 Anomalies of other specified sites of peripheral vascular system

√5ᵗʰ **747.8 Other specified anomalies of circulatory system**

747.81 Anomalies of cerebrovascular system
Arteriovenous malformation of brain
Cerebral arteriovenous aneurysm, congenital
Congenital anomalies of cerebral vessels
EXCLUDES *ruptured cerebral (arteriovenous) aneurysm (430)*
Q28.3 Other malformations of cerebral vessels   I-10

747.82 Spinal vessel anomaly
Arteriovenous malformation of spinal vessel
AHA: 3Q, '95, 5

747.83 Persistent fetal circulation   N
Persistent pulmonary hypertension
Primary pulmonary hypertension of newborn
DEF: A return to fetal circulation due to constriction of pulmonary arterioles and opening of the ductus arteriosus and foramen ovale, right-to-left shunting, oxygenation of the blood does not occur, and the lungs remain constricted after birth; is seen in term or post-term infants; causes include asphyxiation, meconium aspiration syndrome, acidosis, sepsis, and developmental immaturity.
AHA: 4Q, '02, 62

Persistent Fetal Circulation

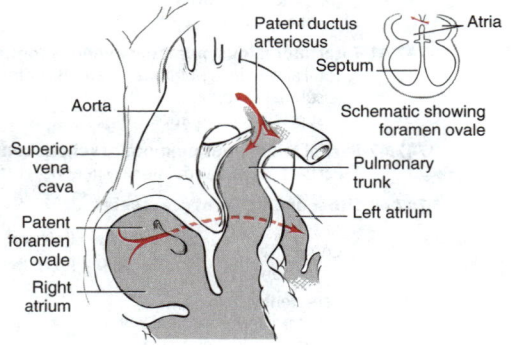

747.89 Other
Aneurysm, congenital, specified site not elsewhere classified
EXCLUDES *congenital aneurysm:*
  coronary (746.85)
  peripheral (747.6)
  pulmonary (747.39)
    arteriovenous (747.32)
  retinal (743.58)
AHA: 4Q, '02, 63

747.9 Unspecified anomaly of circulatory system

√4ᵗʰ **748 Congenital anomalies of respiratory system**
EXCLUDES *congenital central alveolar hypoventilation syndrome (327.25)*
  congenital defect of diaphragm (756.6)

748.0 Choanal atresia
Atresia
Congenital stenosis } of nares (anterior) (posterior)
DEF: Occluded posterior nares (choana), bony or membranous due to failure of embryonic bucconasal membrane to rupture.

748.1 Other anomalies of nose
Absent nose
Accessory nose
Cleft nose
Congenital:
  deformity of nose
  notching of tip of nose
  perforation of wall of nasal sinus
Deformity of wall of nasal sinus
EXCLUDES *congenital deviation of nasal septum (754.0)*

748.2 Web of larynx
Web of larynx:
  NOS
  glottic
  subglottic
DEF: Malformed larynx; marked by thin, translucent, or thick, fibrotic spread between vocal folds; affects speech.

748.3 Other anomalies of larynx, trachea, and bronchus
Absence or agenesis of:
  bronchus
  larynx
  trachea
Anomaly (of):
  cricoid cartilage
  epiglottis
  thyroid cartilage
  tracheal cartilage
Atresia (of):
  epiglottis
  glottis
  larynx
  trachea
Cleft thyroid, cartilage, congenital
Congenital:
  dilation, trachea
  stenosis:
    larynx
    trachea
  tracheocele
Diverticulum:
  bronchus
  trachea
Fissure of epiglottis
Laryngocele
Posterior cleft of cricoid cartilage (congenital)
Rudimentary tracheal bronchus
Stridor, laryngeal, congenital
AHA: 1Q, '99, 14
Q32.4 Other congenital malformations of bronchus   I-10

748.4 Congenital cystic lung
Disease, lung:
  cystic, congenital
  polycystic, congenital
Honeycomb lung, congenital
EXCLUDES *acquired or unspecified cystic lung (518.89)*
DEF: Enlarged air spaces of lung parenchyma.

N Newborn Age: 0   P Pediatric Age: 0-17   M Maternity Age: 12-55   A Adult Age: 15-124

748.5 Agenesis, hypoplasia, and dysplasia of lung
Absence of lung (fissures) (lobe) (lobe)
Aplasia of lung
Hypoplasia of lung
Sequestration of lung

√5ᵗʰ **748.6 Other anomalies of lung**

748.60 Anomaly of lung, unspecified

748.61 Congenital bronchiectasis

748.69 Other
Accessory lung (lobe)
Azygos lobe (fissure), lung

748.8 Other specified anomalies of respiratory system
Abnormal communication between pericardial and pleural sacs
Anomaly, pleural folds
Atresia of nasopharynx
Congenital cyst of mediastinum

748.9 Unspecified anomaly of respiratory system
Anomaly of respiratory system NOS

√4ᵗʰ **749 Cleft palate and cleft lip**
AHA: 2Q, '12, 17

√5ᵗʰ **749.0 Cleft palate**

749.00 Cleft palate, unspecified

749.01 Unilateral, complete

749.02 Unilateral, incomplete
Cleft uvula

749.03 Bilateral, complete

749.04 Bilateral, incomplete

√5ᵗʰ **749.1 Cleft lip**
Cheiloschisis   Harelip
Congenital fissure of lip   Labium leporinum

749.10 Cleft lip, unspecified

749.11 Unilateral, complete

749.12 Unilateral, incomplete

749.13 Bilateral, complete

749.14 Bilateral, incomplete

√5ᵗʰ **749.2 Cleft palate with cleft lip**
Cheilopalatoschisis

749.20 Cleft palate with cleft lip, unspecified

749.21 Unilateral, complete

749.22 Unilateral, incomplete

Cleft Lip and Palate

Unilateral cleft lip

No cleft palate

Cleft lip with cleft alveolar ridge

No cleft palate

Unilateral cleft lip and cleft palate
Alveolar ridge
Cleft palate

Prolabium
Bilateral cleft lip and cleft palate

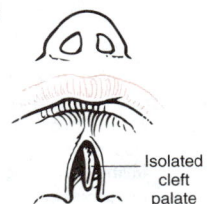
Isolated cleft palate

749.23 Bilateral, complete
AHA: 1Q, '96, 14

749.24 Bilateral, incomplete

749.25 Other combinations

√4ᵗʰ **750 Other congenital anomalies of upper alimentary tract**
EXCLUDES dentofacial anomalies (524.0-524.9)

750.0 Tongue tie
Ankyloglossia
DEF: Restricted tongue movement due to lingual frenum extending toward tip of tongue. Tongue may be fused to mouth floor affecting speech.

√5ᵗʰ **750.1 Other anomalies of tongue**

750.10 Anomaly of tongue, unspecified

750.11 Aglossia
DEF: Absence of tongue.

750.12 Congenital adhesions of tongue

750.13 Fissure of tongue
Bifid tongue
Double tongue

750.15 Macroglossia
Congenital hypertrophy of tongue

750.16 Microglossia
Hypoplasia of tongue

750.19 Other

√5ᵗʰ **750.2 Other specified anomalies of mouth and pharynx**

750.21 Absence of salivary gland

750.22 Accessory salivary gland

750.23 Atresia, salivary duct
Imperforate salivary duct

750.24 Congenital fistula of salivary gland

750.25 Congenital fistula of lip
Congenital (mucus) lip pits

750.26 Other specified anomalies of mouth
Absence of uvula

750.27 Diverticulum of pharynx
Pharyngeal pouch

750.29 Other specified anomalies of pharynx
Imperforate pharynx

750.3 Tracheoesophageal fistula, esophageal atresia and stenosis
Absent esophagus
Atresia of esophagus
Congenital:
    esophageal ring
    stenosis of esophagus
    stricture of esophagus
Congenital fistula:
    esophagobronchial
    esophagotracheal
Imperforate esophagus
Webbed esophagus
AHA: 1Q, '12, 15

750.4 Other specified anomalies of esophagus
Dilatation, congenital
Displacement, congenital
Diverticulum   } (of) esophagus
Duplication
Giant

Esophageal pouch
EXCLUDES congenital hiatus hernia (750.6)
AHA: J-F, '85, 3

√4ᵗʰ / √5ᵗʰ Additional Digit Required   Unspecified Code   Other Specified Code   Manifestation Code   ◄► Revised Text   ● New Code   ▲ Revised Code Title

Congenital Anomalies

750.5–751.8

750.5 Congenital hypertrophic pyloric stenosis
Congenital or infantile:
   constriction ⎫
   hypertrophy ⎪
   spasm   ⎬ of pylorus
   stenosis   ⎪
   stricture   ⎭

DEF: Obstructed pylorus due to overgrowth of pyloric muscle.
Q40.0 Congenital hypertrophic pyloric stenosis   **I-10**

750.6 Congenital hiatus hernia
Displacement of cardia through esophageal hiatus
EXCLUDES *congenital diaphragmatic hernia (756.6)*

750.7 Other specified anomalies of stomach
Congenital:
   cardiospasm
   hourglass stomach
Displacement of stomach
Diverticulum of stomach, congenital
Duplication of stomach
Megalogastria
Microgastria
Transposition of stomach

750.8 Other specified anomalies of upper alimentary tract

750.9 Unspecified anomaly of upper alimentary tract
Congenital:
   anomaly NOS ⎫ of upper alimentary tract [any
   deformity NOS ⎬   part, except tongue]

√4ᵗʰ 751 Other congenital anomalies of digestive system

751.0 Meckel's diverticulum
Meckel's diverticulum (displaced) (hypertrophic)
Persistent:
   omphalomesenteric duct
   vitelline duct

DEF: Malformed sacs or appendages of ileum of small intestine; can cause strangulation, volvulus and intussusception.
AHA: 1Q, '04, 10
TIP: Assign for mesodiverticular band, a fibrous band connecting the tip of the diverticulum to the mesentery; can cause small bowel herniation and obstruction.

751.1 Atresia and stenosis of small intestine
Atresia of:
   duodenum
   ileum
   intestine NOS
Congenital:
   absence   ⎫
   obstruction ⎬ of small intestine or intestine
   stenosis   ⎪   NOS
   stricture   ⎭
Imperforate jejunum

751.2 Atresia and stenosis of large intestine rectum, and anal canal
Absence:
   anus (congenital)
   appendix, congenital
   large intestine, congenital
   rectum
Atresia of:
   anus
   colon
   rectum
Congenital or infantile:
   obstruction of large intestine
   occlusion of anus
   stricture of anus
Imperforate:
   anus
   rectum
Stricture of rectum, congenital
AHA: 2Q, '11, 13; 2Q, '98, 16

751.3 Hirschsprung's disease and other congenital functional disorders of colon
Aganglionosis   Congenital megacolon
Congenital dilation of colon   Macrocolon
DEF: Hirschsprung's disease: enlarged or dilated colon (megacolon), with absence of ganglion cells in the narrowed wall distally; causes inability to defecate.

751.4 Anomalies of intestinal fixation
Congenital adhesions: Rotation of cecum or colon:
   omental, anomalous   failure of
   peritoneal   incomplete
Jackson's membrane   insufficient
Malrotation of colon   Universal mesentery

751.5 Other anomalies of intestine
Congenital diverticulum, colon   Megaloappendix
Dolichocolon   Megaloduodenum
Duplication of: Microcolon
   anus   Persistent cloaca
   appendix   Transposition of:
   cecum   appendix
   intestine   colon
Ectopic anus   intestine
AHA: ▶2Q, '13, 3; ◀2Q, '10, 12; 3Q, '02, 11; 3Q, '01, 8
Q43.9 Congenital malformation of intestine unspecified   **I-10**

√5ᵗʰ 751.6 Anomalies of gallbladder, bile ducts, and liver

751.60 Unspecified anomaly of gallbladder, bile ducts, and liver

751.61 Biliary atresia
Congenital:
   absence   ⎫
   hypoplasia ⎬ of bile duct
   obstruction ⎪ (common) of
   stricture   ⎭ passage
AHA: S-O, '87, 8

751.62 Congenital cystic disease of liver
Congenital polycystic disease of liver
Fibrocystic disease of liver

751.69 Other anomalies of gallbladder, bile ducts, and liver
Absence of:
   gallbladder, congenital
   liver (lobe)
Accessory:
   hepatic ducts
   liver
Congenital:
   choledochal cyst
   hepatomegaly
Duplication of:
   biliary duct
   cystic duct
   gallbladder
   liver
Floating:
   gallbladder
   liver
Intrahepatic gallbladder
AHA: S-O, '87, 8

751.7 Anomalies of pancreas
Absence   ⎫
Accessory   ⎪
Agenesis   ⎬ (of) pancreas
Annular   ⎪
Hypoplasia ⎭
Ectopic pancreatic tissue
Pancreatic heterotopia
EXCLUDES *diabetes mellitus (249.0-249.9, 250.0-250.9)*
             fibrocystic disease of pancreas
                 (277.00-277.09)
             neonatal diabetes mellitus (775.1)

751.8 Other specified anomalies of digestive system
Absence (complete) (partial) of alimentary tract NOS
Duplication   ⎫
Malposition, congenital ⎬ of digestive organs NOS
EXCLUDES *congenital diaphragmatic hernia (756.6)*
             congenital hiatus hernia (750.6)

N Newborn Age: 0   **P** Pediatric Age: 0-17   **M** Maternity Age: 12-55   **A** Adult Age: 15-124

751.9 Unspecified anomaly of digestive system
Congenital:
anomaly NOS
deformity NOS } of digestive system NOS

√4th 752 Congenital anomalies of genital organs
EXCLUDES syndromes associated with anomalies in the number and form of chromosomes (758.0-758.9)

752.0 Anomalies of ovaries ♀
Absence, congenital
Accessory
Ectopic
Streak } (of) ovary

√5th 752.1 Anomalies of fallopian tubes and broad ligaments

752.10 Unspecified anomaly of fallopian tubes and broad ligaments ♀

752.11 Embryonic cyst of fallopian tubes and broad ligaments ♀
Cyst: Cyst:
epoophoron   parovarian
fimbrial
AHA: S-O, '85, 13

752.19 Other ♀
Absence
Accessory
Atresia } (of) fallopian tube or broad ligament

752.2 Doubling of uterus ♀
Didelphic uterus
Doubling of uterus [any degree] (associated with doubling of cervix and vagina)

√5th 752.3 Other anomalies of uterus
AHA: 4Q, '10, 90-91; 3Q, '06, 18

752.31 Agenesis of uterus ♀
Congenital absence of uterus
Q51.0 Congenital absence of uterus **I-10**

752.32 Hypoplasia of uterus ♀
Q51.811 Hypoplasia of uterus **I-10**

752.33 Unicornuate uterus ♀
Unicornuate uterus with or without a separate uterine horn
Uterus with only one functioning horn
Q51.4 Unicornuate uterus **I-10**

752.34 Bicornuate uterus ♀
Bicornuate uterus, complete or partial
Q51.3 Bicornuate uterus **I-10**

752.35 Septate uterus ♀
Septate uterus, complete or partial

752.36 Arcuate uterus ♀
Q51.810 Arcuate uterus **I-10**

752.39 Other anomalies of uterus ♀
Aplasia of uterus NOS
Müllerian anomaly of the uterus, NEC
EXCLUDES anomaly of uterus due to exposure to diethylstilbestrol [DES] in utero (760.76)
didelphic uterus (752.2)
doubling of uterus (752.2)
DEF: Müllerian anomalies: The failure or disruption of female embryonic Müllerian ducts to transform into the upper vagina, cervix uterus, and oviducts, resulting in anomalous organ development.

√5th 752.4 Anomalies of cervix, vagina, and external female genitalia

752.40 Unspecified anomaly of cervix, vagina, and external female genitalia ♀

752.41 Embryonic cyst of cervix, vagina, and external female genitalia ♀
Cyst of:
canal of Nuck, congenital
Gartner's duct
vagina, embryonal
vulva, congenital
DEF: Embryonic fluid-filled cysts of cervix, vagina or external female genitalia.

Hypospadias and Epispadias

Hypospadias (ventral view) — Glans penis, Glandular hypospadias, Penile hypospadias, Scrotal hypospadias, Scrotum, Scrotal raphe, Penile raphe

Epispadias (dorsal view) — Normal external urethral orifice, Glans penis, Foreskin (retracted), Epispadias

752.42 Imperforate hymen ♀
DEF: Complete closure of membranous fold around external opening of vagina.

752.43 Cervical agenesis ♀
Cervical hypoplasia
AHA: 4Q, '10, 90-92
Q51.5 Agenesis and aplasia of cervix **I-10**

752.44 Cervical duplication ♀
AHA: 4Q, '10, 90-92

752.45 Vaginal agenesis ♀
Agenesis of vagina, total or partial
AHA: 4Q, '10, 90-92
Q52.0 Congenital absence of vagina **I-10**

752.46 Transverse vaginal septum ♀
AHA: 4Q, '10, 90-92

752.47 Longitudinal vaginal septum ♀
Longitudinal vaginal septum with or without obstruction
AHA: 4Q, '10, 90-92

752.49 Other anomalies of cervix, vagina, and external female genitalia ♀
Absence of clitoris or vulva
Agenesis of clitoris or vulva
Anomalies of cervix, NEC
Anomalies of hymen, NEC
Congenital stenosis or stricture of:
cervical canal
vagina
Müllerian anomalies of the cervix and vagina, NEC
EXCLUDES double vagina associated with total duplication (752.2)
AHA: 3Q, '06, 18

√5th 752.5 Undescended and retractile testicle
AHA: 4Q, '96, 33

752.51 Undescended testis ♂
Cryptorchism   Ectopic testis
Q53.20 Undescended testicle unspecified bilateral **I-10**

752.52 Retractile testis ♂

√5th 752.6 Hypospadias and epispadias and other penile anomalies
AHA: 4Q, '96, 34, 35

752.61 Hypospadias ♂
DEF: Abnormal opening of urethra on the ventral surface of the penis or perineum.
AHA: 4Q, '03, 67-68; 3Q, '97, 6
Q54.1 Hypospadias penile **I-10**

752.62 Epispadias ♂
Anaspadias
DEF: Urethra opening on dorsal surface of penis.

752.63 Congenital chordee ♂
DEF: Ventral bowing of penis due to fibrous band along corpus spongiosum; occurs with hypospadias.

752.64 Micropenis ♂

752.65 Hidden penis ♂

752.69 Other penile anomalies ♂

√4th √5th Additional Digit Required   Unspecified Code   Other Specified Code   Manifestation Code   ►◄ Revised Text   ● New Code   ▲ Revised Code Title

Congenital Anomalies

752.7–753.9

752.7 Indeterminate sex and pseudohermaphroditism
Gynandrism
Hermaphroditism
Ovotestis
Pseudohermaphroditism (male) (female)
Pure gonadal dysgenesis

EXCLUDES androgen insensitivity (259.50-259.52)
pseudohermaphroditism:
female, with adrenocortical disorder (255.2)
male, with gonadal disorder (257.8)
with specified chromosomal anomaly
(758.0-758.9)
testicular feminization syndrome (259.50-259.52)

DEF: Pseudohermaphroditism: presence of gonads of one sex and external genitalia of other sex.

✓5ᵗʰ 752.8 Other specified anomalies of genital organs
EXCLUDES congenital hydrocele (778.6)
penile anomalies (752.61-752.69)
phimosis or paraphimosis (605)

752.81 Scrotal transposition ♂
AHA: 4Q, '03, 67-68

752.89 Other specified anomalies of genital organs
Absence of: Atresia of:
prostate   ejaculatory duct
spermatic cord   vas deferens
vas deferens   Fusion of testes
Anorchism   Hypoplasia of testis
Aplasia (congenital) of: Monorchism
prostate   Polyorchism
round ligament
testicle

752.9 Unspecified anomaly of genital organs
Congenital:
anomaly NOS ⎱ of genital organ, not
deformity NOS ⎰ elsewhere classified

✓4ᵗʰ 753 Congenital anomalies of urinary system

753.0 Renal agenesis and dysgenesis
Atrophy of kidney: Congenital absence of kidney(s)
congenital   Hypoplasia of kidney(s)
infantile
Q60.2 Renal agenesis unspecified   I-10

✓5ᵗʰ 753.1 Cystic kidney disease
EXCLUDES acquired cyst of kidney (593.2)
AHA: 4Q, '90, 3

753.10 Cystic kidney disease, unspecified
Q61.9 Cystic kidney disease unspecified   I-10

753.11 Congenital single renal cyst

753.12 Polycystic kidney, unspecified type
AHA: ▶3Q, '13, 6◀
Q61.3 Polycystic kidney unspecified   I-10

753.13 Polycystic kidney, autosomal dominant
DEF: Slow progressive disease characterized by bilateral cysts causing increased kidney size and impaired function.

753.14 Polycystic kidney, autosomal recessive
DEF: Rare disease characterized by multiple cysts involving kidneys and liver, producing renal and hepatic failure in childhood or adolescence.

753.15 Renal dysplasia

753.16 Medullary cystic kidney
Nephronopthisis
DEF: Diffuse kidney disease results in uremia onset prior to age 20.

753.17 Medullary sponge kidney
DEF: Dilated collecting tubules; usually asymptomatic but calcinosis in tubules may cause renal insufficiency.

753.19 Other specified cystic kidney disease
Multicystic kidney

✓5ᵗʰ 753.2 Obstructive defects of renal pelvis and ureter
AHA: 4Q, '96, 35

753.20 Unspecified obstructive defect of renal pelvis and ureter

753.21 Congenital obstruction of ureteropelvic junction
DEF: Stricture at junction of ureter and renal pelvis.

753.22 Congenital obstruction of ureterovesical junction
Adynamic ureter
Congenital hydroureter
DEF: Stricture at junction of ureter and bladder.

753.23 Congenital ureterocele

753.29 Other
Q62.11 Congen occlusion of ureteropelvic junct   I-10

753.3 Other specified anomalies of kidney
Accessory kidney   Fusion of kidneys
Congenital: Giant kidney
calculus of kidney   Horseshoe kidney
displaced kidney   Hyperplasia of kidney
Discoid kidney   Lobulation of kidney
Double kidney with   Malrotation of kidney
double pelvis   Trifid kidney (pelvis)
Ectopic kidney
AHA: 1Q, '07, 23
TIP: Assign for Finnish-type congenital nephrosis, along with code 581.3 Nephrotic syndrome.
Q63.8 Oth specified congenital malformations of kidney   I-10

753.4 Other specified anomalies of ureter
Absent ureter
Accessory ureter
Deviation of ureter
Displaced ureteric orifice
Double ureter
Ectopic ureter
Implantation, anomalous of ureter

753.5 Exstrophy of urinary bladder
Ectopia vesicae
Extroversion of bladder
DEF: Absence of lower abdominal and anterior bladder walls with posterior bladder wall protrusion.

753.6 Atresia and stenosis of urethra and bladder neck
Congenital obstruction:
bladder neck
urethra
Congenital stricture of:
urethra (valvular)
urinary meatus
vesicourethral orifice
Imperforate urinary meatus
Impervious urethra
Urethral valve formation

753.7 Anomalies of urachus
Cyst ⎱
Fistula ⎰ (of) urachussinus
Patent
Persistent umbilical sinus

753.8 Other specified anomalies of bladder and urethra
Absence, congenital of:
bladder
urethra
Accessory:
bladder
urethra
Congenital:
diverticulum of bladder
hernia of bladder
prolapse of:
bladder (mucosa)
urethra
urethrorectal fistula
Double:
urethra
urinary meatus

753.9 Unspecified anomaly of urinary system
Congenital:
anomaly NOS ⎱ of urinary system [any part,
deformity NOS ⎰ except urachus]
AHA: 2Q, '11, 6

N Newborn Age: 0   **P** Pediatric Age: 0-17   **M** Maternity Age: 12-55   **A** Adult Age: 15-124

754   Certain congenital musculoskeletal deformities

INCLUDES   nonteratogenic deformities which are considered to be due to intrauterine malposition and pressure

754.0   Of skull, face, and jaw
Asymmetry of face
Compression facies
Depressions in skull
Deviation of nasal septum, congenital
Dolichocephaly
Plagiocephaly
Potter's facies
Squashed or bent nose, congenital

EXCLUDES   dentofacial anomalies (524.0-524.9)
syphilitic saddle nose (090.5)

754.1   Of sternocleidomastoid muscle
Congenital sternomastoid torticollis
Congenital wryneck
Contracture of sternocleidomastoid (muscle)
Sternomastoid tumor

754.2   Of spine
Congenital postural:
lordosis
scoliosis

754.3   Congenital dislocation of hip

754.30   Congenital dislocation of hip, unilateral
Congenital dislocation of hip NOS

754.31   Congenital dislocation of hip, bilateral

754.32   Congenital subluxation of hip, unilateral
Congenital flexion deformity, hip or thigh
Predislocation status of hip at birth
Preluxation of hip, congenital

754.33   Congenital subluxation of hip, bilateral

754.35   Congenital dislocation of one hip with subluxation of other hip

754.4   Congenital genu recurvatum and bowing of long bones of leg

754.40   Genu recurvatum
DEF: Backward curving of knee joint.

754.41   Congenital dislocation of knee (with genu recurvatum)

754.42   Congenital bowing of femur

754.43   Congenital bowing of tibia and fibula

754.44   Congenital bowing of unspecified long bones of leg

754.5   Varus deformities of feet
EXCLUDES   acquired (736.71, 736.75, 736.79)

754.50   Talipes varus
Congenital varus deformity of foot, unspecified
Pes varus
DEF: Inverted foot marked by outer sole resting on ground.

754.51   Talipes equinovarus
Equinovarus (congenital)
DEF: Elevated, outward rotation of heel; also called clubfoot.

754.52   Metatarsus primus varus
DEF: Malformed first metatarsal bone, with bone angled toward body.

754.53   Metatarsus varus

754.59   Other
Talipes calcaneovarus

754.6   Valgus deformities of feet
EXCLUDES   valgus deformity of foot (acquired) (736.79)

754.60   Talipes valgus
Congenital valgus deformity of foot, unspecified

754.61   Congenital pes planus
Congenital rocker bottom flat foot
Flat foot, congenital
EXCLUDES   pes planus (acquired) (734)

754.62   Talipes calcaneovalgus

754.69   Other
Talipes:
equinovalgus
planovalgus

754.7   Other deformities of feet
EXCLUDES   acquired (736.70-736.79)

754.70   Talipes, unspecified
Congenital deformity of foot NOS

754.71   Talipes cavus
Cavus foot (congenital)

754.79   Other
Asymmetric talipes
Talipes:
calcaneus
equinus

754.8   Other specified nonteratogenic anomalies

754.81   Pectus excavatum
Congenital funnel chest

754.82   Pectus carinatum
Congenital pigeon chest [breast]

754.89   Other
Club hand (congenital)
Congenital:
deformity of chest wall
dislocation of elbow
Generalized flexion contractures of lower limb joints, congenital
Spade-like hand (congenital)

755   Other congenital anomalies of limbs
EXCLUDES   those deformities classifiable to 754.0-754.8

755.0   Polydactyly

755.00   Polydactyly, unspecified digits
Supernumerary digits

755.01   Of fingers
Accessory fingers

755.02   Of toes
Accessory toes

755.1   Syndactyly
Symphalangy
Webbing of digits

755.10   Of multiple and unspecified sites

755.11   Of fingers without fusion of bone

755.12   Of fingers with fusion of bone

755.13   Of toes without fusion of bone

755.14   Of toes with fusion of bone

755.2   Reduction deformities of upper limb

755.20   Unspecified reduction deformity of upper limb
Ectromelia NOS ⎱
Hemimelia NOS ⎰ of upper limb

Shortening of arm, congenital

755.21   Transverse deficiency of upper limb
Amelia of upper limb
Congenital absence of:
fingers, all (complete or partial)
forearm, including hand and fingers
upper limb, complete
Congenital amputation of upper limb
Transverse hemimelia of upper limb

755.22   Longitudinal deficiency of upper limb, not elsewhere classified
Phocomelia NOS of upper limb
Rudimentary arm

755.23   Longitudinal deficiency, combined, involving humerus, radius, and ulna (complete or incomplete)
Congenital absence of arm and forearm (complete or incomplete) with or without metacarpal deficiency and/or phalangeal deficiency, incomplete
Phocomelia, complete, of upper limb

| ✓4th ✓5th | Additional Digit Required | Unspecified Code | Other Specified Code | Manifestation Code | ►◄ Revised Text | ● New Code | ▲ Revised Code Title |

2015 ICD-9-CM   **Volume 1 – 247**

Congenital Anomalies

754–755.23

Congenital Anomalies

755.24–755.64

755.24 Longitudinal deficiency, humeral, complete or partial (with or without distal deficiencies, incomplete)
Congenital absence of humerus (with or without absence of some [but not all] distal elements)
Proximal phocomelia of upper limb

755.25 Longitudinal deficiency, radioulnar, complete or partial (with or without distal deficiencies, incomplete)
Congenital absence of radius and ulna (with or without absence of some [but not all] distal elements)
Distal phocomelia of upper limb

755.26 Longitudinal deficiency, radial, complete or partial (with or without distal deficiencies, incomplete)
Agenesis of radius
Congenital absence of radius (with or without absence of some [but not all] distal elements)

755.27 Longitudinal deficiency, ulnar, complete or partial (with or without distal deficiencies, incomplete)
Agenesis of ulna
Congenital absence of ulna (with or without absence of some [but not all] distal elements)

755.28 Longitudinal deficiency, carpals or metacarpals, complete or partial (with or without incomplete phalangeal deficiency)

755.29 Longitudinal deficiency, phalanges, complete or partial
Absence of finger, congenital
Aphalangia of upper limb, terminal, complete or partial
EXCLUDES *terminal deficiency of all five digits (755.21)*
transverse deficiency of phalanges (755.21)

√5ᵗʰ **755.3 Reduction deformities of lower limb**

755.30 Unspecified reduction deformity of lower limb
Ectromelia NOS ⎫
Hemimelia NOS ⎬ of lower limb
Shortening of leg, congenital

755.31 Transverse deficiency of lower limb
Amelia of lower limb
Congenital absence of:
  foot
  leg, including foot and toes
  lower limb, complete
  toes, all, complete
Transverse hemimelia of lower limb

755.32 Longitudinal deficiency of lower limb, not elsewhere classified
Phocomelia NOS of lower limb

755.33 Longitudinal deficiency, combined, involving femur, tibia, and fibula (complete or incomplete)
Congenital absence of thigh and (lower) leg (complete or incomplete) with or without metacarpal deficiency and/or phalangeal deficiency, incomplete
Phocomelia, complete, of lower limb

755.34 Longitudinal deficiency, femoral, complete or partial (with or without distal deficiencies, incomplete)
Congenital absence of femur (with or without absence of some [but not all] distal elements)
Proximal phocomelia of lower limb

755.35 Longitudinal deficiency, tibiofibular, complete or partial (with or without distal deficiencies, incomplete)
Congenital absence of tibia and fibula (with or without absence of some [but not all] distal elements)
Distal phocomelia of lower limb

755.36 Longitudinal deficiency, tibia, complete or partial (with or without distal deficiencies, incomplete)
Agenesis of tibia
Congenital absence of tibia (with or without absence of some [but not all] distal elements)

755.37 Longitudinal deficiency, fibular, complete or partial (with or without distal deficiencies, incomplete)
Agenesis of fibula
Congenital absence of fibula (with or without absence of some [but not all] distal elements)

755.38 Longitudinal deficiency, tarsals or metatarsals, complete or partial (with or without incomplete phalangeal deficiency)

755.39 Longitudinal deficiency, phalanges, complete or partial
Absence of toe, congenital
Aphalangia of lower limb, terminal, complete or partial
EXCLUDES *terminal deficiency of all five digits (755.31)*
transverse deficiency of phalanges (755.31)

755.4 Reduction deformities, unspecified limb
Absence, congenital (complete or partial) of limb NOS
Amelia ⎫
Ectromelia ⎬ of unspecified limb
Hemimelia ⎬
Phocomelia ⎭

√5ᵗʰ **755.5 Other anomalies of upper limb, including shoulder girdle**

755.50 Unspecified anomaly of upper limb

755.51 Congenital deformity of clavicle

755.52 Congenital elevation of scapula
Sprengel's deformity

755.53 Radioulnar synostosis
DEF: Osseous adhesion of radius and ulna.

755.54 Madelung's deformity
DEF: Distal ulnar overgrowth or radial shortening; also called carpus curvus.

755.55 Acrocephalosyndactyly
Apert's syndrome
DEF: Premature cranial suture fusion (craniostenosis); marked by cone-shaped or pointed (acrocephaly) head and webbing of the fingers (syndactyly); similar to craniofacial dysostosis.

755.56 Accessory carpal bones

755.57 Macrodactylia (fingers)
DEF: Abnormally large fingers, toes.

755.58 Cleft hand, congenital
Lobster-claw hand
DEF: Extended separation between fingers into metacarpus; also may refer to large fingers and absent middle fingers of hand.

755.59 Other
Cleidocranial dysostosis
Cubitus:
  valgus, congenital
  varus, congenital
EXCLUDES *club hand (congenital) (754.89)*
congenital dislocation of elbow (754.89)

√5ᵗʰ **755.6 Other anomalies of lower limb, including pelvic girdle**

755.60 Unspecified anomaly of lower limb

755.61 Coxa valga, congenital
DEF: Abnormally wide angle between the neck and shaft of the femur.

755.62 Coxa vara, congenital
DEF: Diminished angle between neck and shaft of femur.

755.63 Other congenital deformity of hip (joint)
Congenital anteversion of femur (neck)
EXCLUDES *congenital dislocation of hip (754.30-754.35)*
AHA: 1Q, '94, 15; S-O, '84, 15
Q65.9 Congenital deformity of hip unspecified **I-10**

755.64 Congenital deformity of knee (joint)
Congenital:
  absence of patella
  genu valgum [knock-knee]
  genu varum [bowleg]
Rudimentary patella

N Newborn Age: 0   **P** Pediatric Age: 0-17   **M** Maternity Age: 12-55   **A** Adult Age: 15-124

755.65 Macrodactylia of toes
DEF: Abnormally large toes.

755.66 Other anomalies of toes
Congenital:
hallux valgus
hallux varus
hammer toe

755.67 Anomalies of foot, not elsewhere classified
Astragaloscaphoid synostosis
Calcaneonavicular bar
Coalition of calcaneus
Talonavicular synostosis
Tarsal coalitions

755.69 Other
Congenital:
angulation of tibia
deformity (of):
ankle (joint)
sacroiliac (joint)
fusion of sacroiliac joint

755.8 Other specified anomalies of unspecified limb

755.9 Unspecified anomaly of unspecified limb
Congenital:
anomaly NOS } of unspecified limb
deformity NOS
EXCLUDES reduction deformity of unspecified limb (755.4)

✔4th **756 Other congenital musculoskeletal anomalies**
EXCLUDES congenital myotonic chondrodystrophy (359.23)
those deformities classifiable to 754.0-754.8

756.0 Anomalies of skull and face bones
Absence of skull bones
Acrocephaly
Congenital deformity of forehead
Craniosynostosis
Crouzon's disease
Hypertelorism
Imperfect fusion of skull
Oxycephaly
Platybasia
Premature closure of cranial sutures
Tower skull
Trigonocephaly
EXCLUDES acrocephalosyndactyly [Apert's syndrome] (755.55)
dentofacial anomalies (524.0-524.9)
skull defects associated with brain anomalies, such
as:
anencephalus (740.0)
encephalocele (742.0)
hydrocephalus (742.3)
microcephalus (742.1)
AHA: 2Q, '12, 17; 3Q, '98, 9; 3Q, '96, 15
TIP: Assign for Nager syndrome (preaxial acrofacial dysostosis), along
with codes for any additional features that are not captured in the
code.
Q75.8 Other spec cong malformations skull & face bones   I-10

✔5th **756.1 Anomalies of spine**

756.10 Anomaly of spine, unspecified

756.11 Spondylolysis, lumbosacral region
Prespondylolisthesis (lumbosacral)
DEF: Bilateral or unilateral defect through the pars
interarticularis of a vertebra causes spondylolisthesis.

756.12 Spondylolisthesis
DEF: Downward slipping of lumbar vertebra over next
vertebra; usually related to pelvic deformity.
Q76.2 Congenital spondylolisthesis   I-10

756.13 Absence of vertebra, congenital

756.14 Hemivertebra
DEF: Incomplete development of one side of a vertebra.

756.15 Fusion of spine [vertebra], congenital

756.16 Klippel-Feil syndrome
DEF: Short, wide neck; limits range of motion due to
abnormal number of cervical vertebra or fused
hemivertebrae.

756.17 Spina bifida occulta
EXCLUDES spina bifida (aperta) (741.0-741.9)
DEF: Spina bifida marked by a bony spinal canal defect
without a protrusion of the cord or meninges; it is
diagnosed by radiography and has no symptoms.

756.19 Other
Platyspondylia
Supernumerary vertebra

756.2 Cervical rib
Supernumerary rib in the cervical region
DEF: Costa cervicalis: extra rib attached to cervical vertebra.

756.3 Other anomalies of ribs and sternum
Congenital absence of:
rib
sternum
Congenital:
fissure of sternum
fusion of ribs
Sternum bifidum
EXCLUDES nonteratogenic deformity of chest wall
(754.81-754.89)

756.4 Chondrodystrophy
Achondroplasia   Enchondromatosis
Chondrodystrophia (fetalis)   Ollier's disease
Dyschondroplasia
EXCLUDES congenital myotonic chondrodystrophy (359.23)
lipochondrodystrophy [Hurler's syndrome] (277.5)
Morquio's disease (277.5)
DEF: Abnormal development of cartilage.
AHA: 2Q, '02, 16; S-O, '87, 10
TIP: Assign for Jeune's syndrome, and also for cartilage-hair
syndrome (cartilage-hair hypoplasia).

✔5th **756.5 Osteodystrophies**

756.50 Osteodystrophy, unspecified

756.51 Osteogenesis imperfecta
Fragilitas ossium
Osteopsathyrosis
DEF: A collagen disorder commonly characterized by brittle,
osteoporotic, easily fractured bones, hypermobility of
joints, blue sclerae, and a tendency to hemorrhage.

756.52 Osteopetrosis
DEF: Abnormally dense bone, optic atrophy,
hepatosplenomegaly, deafness; sclerosing depletes bone
marrow and nerve foramina of skull; often fatal.

756.53 Osteopoikilosis
DEF: Multiple sclerotic foci on ends of long bones, stippling
in round, flat bones; identified by x-ray.

756.54 Polyostotic fibrous dysplasia of bone
DEF: Fibrous tissue displaces bone results in segmented
ragged-edge café-au-lait spots; occurs in girls of early
puberty.

756.55 Chondroectodermal dysplasia
Ellis-van Creveld syndrome
DEF: Inadequate enchondral bone formation; impaired
development of hair and teeth, polydactyly, and cardiac
septum defects.

756.56 Multiple epiphyseal dysplasia

756.59 Other
Albright (-McCune)-Sternberg syndrome

Congenital Anomalies

756.6–757.6

Omphalocele

756.6 Anomalies of diaphragm
Absence of diaphragm
Congenital hernia:
  diaphragmatic
  foramen of Morgagni
Eventration of diaphragm
> **EXCLUDES** *congenital hiatus hernia (750.6)*

✓5ᵗʰ 756.7 Anomalies of abdominal wall

  756.70 Anomaly of abdominal wall, unspecified

  756.71 Prune belly syndrome
    Eagle-Barrett syndrome
    Prolapse of bladder mucosa
    DEF: Prune belly syndrome: absence of lower rectus abdominis muscle and lower and medial oblique muscles; results in dilated bladder and ureters, dysplastic kidneys and hydronephrosis; common in male infants with undescended testicles.
    AHA: 4Q, '97, 44

  756.72 Omphalocele
    Exomphalos
    DEF: Exomphalos: umbilical hernia prominent navel.
    DEF: Omphalocele: hernia of umbilicus due to impaired abdominal wall; results in membrane-covered intestine protruding through peritoneum and amnion.
    AHA: 4Q, '09, 98-99

  756.73 Gastroschisis
    DEF: Fissure of abdominal wall, results in protruding small or large intestine.
    AHA: 4Q, '09, 98-99

  756.79 Other congenital anomalies of abdominal wall
    > **EXCLUDES** *umbilical hernia (551-553 with .1)*

✓5ᵗʰ 756.8 Other specified anomalies of muscle, tendon, fascia, and connective tissue

  756.81 Absence of muscle and tendon
    Absence of muscle (pectoral)
    AHA: 1Q, '10, 13

  756.82 Accessory muscle

  756.83 Ehlers-Danlos syndrome
    DEF: Danlos syndrome: connective tissue disorder causes hyperextended skin and joints; results in fragile blood vessels with bleeding, poor wound healing and subcutaneous pseudotumors.

Gastroschisis

756.89 Other
Amyotrophia congenita
Congenital shortening of tendon
AHA: 3Q, '99, 16
TIP: Assign for Stickler's syndrome, a hereditary progressive arthro-ophthalmopathy, along with codes for the specific manifestations.

756.9 Other and unspecified anomalies of musculoskeletal system
Congenital:
  anomaly NOS   ⎱ of musculoskeletal system, not
  deformity NOS ⎰   elsewhere classified

✓4ᵗʰ 757 Congenital anomalies of the integument
> **INCLUDES** anomalies of skin, subcutaneous tissue, hair, nails, and breast
> **EXCLUDES** *hemangioma (228.00-228.09)*
> *pigmented nevus (216.0-216.9)*

757.0 Hereditary edema of legs
Congenital lymphedema   Milroy's disease
Hereditary trophedema

757.1 Ichthyosis congenita
Congenital ichthyosis   Ichthyosiform erythroderma
Harlequin fetus
DEF: Overproduction of skin cells causes scaling of skin; may result in stillborn fetus or death soon after birth.

757.2 Dermatoglyphic anomalies
Abnormal palmar creases
DEF: Abnormal skin-line patterns of fingers, palms, toes and soles; initial finding of possible chromosomal abnormalities.

✓5ᵗʰ 757.3 Other specified anomalies of skin

  757.31 Congenital ectodermal dysplasia
    DEF: Tissues and structures originate in embryonic ectoderm; includes anhidrotic and hidrotic ectodermal dysplasia and EEC syndrome.

  757.32 Vascular hamartomas
    Birthmarks   Strawberry nevus   Port-wine stain
    DEF: Benign tumor of blood vessels; due to malformed angioblastic tissues.
    AHA: 2Q, '12, 7
    TIP: Assign for nevus flammeus, which may be associated with increased risk for seizure or glaucoma. Further testing may be required.
    Q82.5 Congenital non-neoplastic nevus   I-10

  757.33 Congenital pigmentary anomalies of skin
    Congenital poikiloderma   Xeroderma pigmentosum
    Urticaria pigmentosa
    > **EXCLUDES** *albinism (270.2)*
    AHA: ▶1Q, '13, 14◀
    Q82.2 Mastocytosis   I-10

  757.39 Other
    Accessory skin tags, congenital
    Congenital scar
    Epidermolysis bullosa
    Keratoderma (congenital)
    > **EXCLUDES** *pilonidal cyst (685.0-685.1)*
    AHA: ▶1Q, '13, 15◀
    Q82.8 Other specified congenital malformations of skin   I-10

757.4 Specified anomalies of hair
Congenital: Congenital:
  alopecia   hypertrichosis
  atrichosis   monilethrix
  beaded hair   Persistent lanugo

757.5 Specified anomalies of nails
Anonychia   Congenital:
Congenital: leukonychia
  clubnail   onychauxis
  koilonychia   pachyonychia

757.6 Specified congenital anomalies of breast
Accessory   ⎱
Congenital absent ⎰ breast or nipple
Supernumerary
> **EXCLUDES** *absence of pectoral muscle (756.81)*
> *hypoplasia of breast (611.82)*
> *micromastia (611.82)*

N Newborn Age: 0   **P** Pediatric Age: 0-17   **M** Maternity Age: 12-55   **A** Adult Age: 15-124

757.8 Other specified anomalies of the integument

757.9 Unspecified anomaly of the integument
Congenital:
anomaly NOS
deformity NOS } of integument

√4ᵗʰ 758 Chromosomal anomalies
INCLUDES syndromes associated with anomalies in the number and form of chromosomes
Use additional codes for conditions associated with the chromosomal anomalies

758.0 Down syndrome
Mongolism
Translocation Down syndrome
Trisomy:
21 or 22
G
Q90.9 Down syndrome unspecified   I-10

758.1 Patau's syndrome
Trisomy:
13
D_1
DEF: Trisomy of 13th chromosome; characteristic failure to thrive, severe mental impairment, seizures, abnormal eyes, low-set ears and sloped forehead.

758.2 Edwards' syndrome
Trisomy:
18
E_3
DEF: Trisomy of 18th chromosome; characteristic mental and physical impairments; mainly affects females.

√5ᵗʰ 758.3 Autosomal deletion syndromes

758.31 Cri-du-chat syndrome
Deletion 5p
DEF: Hereditary congenital syndrome caused by a microdeletion of short arm of chromosome 5; characterized by catlike cry in newborn, microencephaly, severe mental deficiency, and hypertelorism.

758.32 Velo-cardio-facial syndrome
Deletion 22q11.2
DEF: Microdeletion syndrome affecting multiple organs; characteristic cleft palate, heart defects, elongated face with almond-shaped eyes, wide nose, small ears, weak immune systems, weak musculature, hypothyroidism, short stature, and scoliosis; deletion at q11.2 on the long arm of the chromosome 22.

758.33 Other microdeletions
Miller-Dieker syndrome
Smith-Magenis syndrome
DEF: Miller-Dieker syndrome: deletion from the short arm of chromosome 17; characteristic mental retardation, speech and motor development delays, neurological complications, and multiple abnormalities affecting the kidneys, heart, gastrointestinal tract; death in infancy or early childhood.
DEF: Smith-Magenis syndrome: deletion in a certain area of chromosome 17 that results in craniofacial changes, speech delay, hoarse voice, hearing loss and behavioral problems, such as self-destructive head banging, wrist biting, and tearing at nails.

758.39 Other autosomal deletions

758.4 Balanced autosomal translocation in normal individual

758.5 Other conditions due to autosomal anomalies
Accessory autosomes NEC

758.6 Gonadal dysgenesis
Ovarian dysgenesis   XO syndrome
Turner's syndrome
EXCLUDES *pure gonadal dysgenesis (752.7)*

758.7 Klinefelter's syndrome   ♂
XXY syndrome
DEF: Impaired embryonic development of seminiferous tubes; results in small testes, azoospermia, infertility and enlarged mammary glands.

√5ᵗʰ 758.8 Other conditions due to chromosome anomalies

758.81 Other conditions due to sex chromosome anomalies

758.89 Other
Q99.8 Other specified chromosome abnormalities   I-10

758.9 Conditions due to anomaly of unspecified chromosome

√4ᵗʰ 759 Other and unspecified congenital anomalies

759.0 Anomalies of spleen
Aberrant
Absent } spleen
Accessory
Congenital splenomegaly
Ectopic spleen
Lobulation of spleen

759.1 Anomalies of adrenal gland
Aberrant
Absent } adrenal gland
Accessory
EXCLUDES *adrenogenital disorders (255.2)*
congenital disorders of steroid metabolism (255.2)

759.2 Anomalies of other endocrine glands
Absent parathyroid gland
Accessory thyroid gland
Persistent thyroglossal or thyrolingual duct
Thyroglossal (duct) cyst
EXCLUDES *congenital:*
goiter (246.1)
hypothyroidism (243)

759.3 Situs inversus
Situs inversus or transversus:
abdominalis
thoracis
Transposition of viscera:
abdominal
thoracic
EXCLUDES *dextrocardia without mention of complete transposition (746.87)*
DEF: Laterally transposed thoracic and abdominal viscera.

759.4 Conjoined twins
Craniopagus   Thoracopagus
Dicephalus   Xiphopagus
Pygopagus

759.5 Tuberous sclerosis
Bourneville's disease
Epiloia
DEF: Hamartomas of brain, retina and viscera, impaired mental ability, seizures and adenoma sebaceum.

759.6 Other hamartoses, not elsewhere classified
Syndrome:
Peutz-Jeghers
Sturge-Weber (-Dimitri)
von Hippel-Lindau
EXCLUDES *neurofibromatosis (237.70-237.79)*
DEF: Peutz-Jeghers: hereditary syndrome characterized by hamartomas of small intestine.
DEF: Sturge-Weber: congenital syndrome characterized by unilateral port-wine stain over trigeminal nerve, underlying meninges and cerebral cortex.
DEF: von Hipple-Lindau: hereditary syndrome of congenital angiomatosis of the retina and cerebellum.
AHA: 3Q, '92, 12

759.7 Multiple congenital anomalies, so described
Congenital:
anomaly, multiple NOS
deformity, multiple NOS

√5ᵗʰ 759.8 Other specified anomalies
AHA: S-O, '87, 9; S-O, '85, 11

759.81 Prader-Willi syndrome

759.82 Marfan syndrome
AHA: 3Q, '93, 11

| √4ᵗʰ √5ᵗʰ Additional Digit Required | Unspecified Code | Other Specified Code | Manifestation Code | ►◄ Revised Text | ● New Code | ▲ Revised Code Title |

759.83 Fragile X syndrome
AHA: 4Q, '94, 41

759.89 Other
Congenital malformation syndromes affecting
multiple systems, not elsewhere classified
Laurence-Moon-Biedl syndrome
AHA: ▶4Q, '13, 92; ◀2Q, '12, 3; 3Q, '08, 3; 3Q, '06, 21; 2Q, '05,
17; 2Q, '04, 12; 1Q, '01, 3; 3Q, '99, 17, 18; 3Q, '98, 8
TIP: Assign for the following syndromes:
Alagille s.
Alport's s.
Antley-Bixler s.
branchio-oto-renal ((BOR) s.
Borjeson-Forsmann-Lehmann s.
cardiofaciocutaneous (CFC) s.
Costello s.
fasciocutaneoskeletal (FCS)s.
mutliple pterygium s.
Noonan's s.
Startle s.
Williams s.
Assign additional codes for any documented
manifestations.

759.9 Congenital anomaly, unspecified

15. Certain Conditions Originating in the Perinatal Period (760-779)

INCLUDES conditions which have their origin in the perinatal period, before birth through the first 28 days after birth, even though death or morbidity occurs later

Use additional code(s) to further specify condition

Maternal Causes of Perinatal Morbidity and Mortality (760-763)

AHA: 2Q, '89, 14; 3Q, '90, 5

TIP: A newborn condition is clinically significant when it has implications for the newborn's *future* health care. This is an exception to the UHDDS guidelines.

√4th **760 Fetus or newborn affected by maternal conditions which may be unrelated to present pregnancy**

INCLUDES the listed maternal conditions only when specified as a cause of mortality or morbidity of the fetus or newborn

EXCLUDES *maternal endocrine and metabolic disorders affecting fetus or newborn (775.0-775.9)*

AHA: 1Q, '94, 8; 2Q, '92, 12; N-D, '84, 11

TIP: Do not assign unless the mother's condition has actually affected the fetus or newborn.

760.0 Maternal hypertensive disorders
Fetus or newborn affected by maternal conditions classifiable to 642

760.1 Maternal renal and urinary tract diseases
Fetus or newborn affected by maternal conditions classifiable to 580-599

760.2 Maternal infections
Fetus or newborn affected by maternal infectious disease classifiable to 001-136 and 487, but fetus or newborn not manifesting that disease
EXCLUDES *congenital infectious diseases (771.0-771.8)*
maternal genital tract and other localized infections (760.8)

760.3 Other chronic maternal circulatory and respiratory diseases
Fetus or newborn affected by chronic maternal conditions classifiable to 390-459, 490-519, 745-748

760.4 Maternal nutritional disorders
Fetus or newborn affected by:
maternal disorders classifiable to 260-269
maternal malnutrition NOS
EXCLUDES *fetal malnutrition (764.10-764.29)*

760.5 Maternal injury
Fetus or newborn affected by maternal conditions classifiable to 800-995

√5th **760.6 Surgical operation on mother and fetus**
EXCLUDES *cesarean section for present delivery (763.4)*
damage to placenta from amniocentesis, cesarean section, or surgical induction (762.1)
AHA: 4Q, '08, 137-138
TIP: These codes include existing conditions present at the time of birth that are related to procedures performed before the time of delivery.

760.61 Newborn affected by amniocentesis
EXCLUDES *fetal complications from amniocentesis (679.1)*

760.62 Newborn affected by other in utero procedure
EXCLUDES *fetal complications of in utero procedure (679.1)*

760.63 Newborn affected by other surgical operations on mother during pregnancy
EXCLUDES *newborn affected by previous surgical procedure on mother not associated with pregnancy (760.64)*

760.64 Newborn affected by previous surgical procedure on mother not associated with pregnancy

√5th **760.7 Noxious influences affecting fetus or newborn via placenta or breast milk**
Fetus or newborn affected by noxious substance transmitted via placenta or breast milk
EXCLUDES *anesthetic and analgesic drugs administered during labor and delivery (763.5)*
drug withdrawal syndrome in newborn (779.5)
AHA: 3Q, '91, 21

760.70 Unspecified noxious substance
Fetus or newborn affected by:
Drug NEC

760.71 Alcohol
Fetal alcohol syndrome

760.72 Narcotics

760.73 Hallucinogenic agents

760.74 Anti-infectives
Antibiotics   Antifungals

760.75 Cocaine
AHA: 3Q, '94, 6; 2Q, '92, 12; 4Q, '91, 26
TIP: If documentation indicates drug withdrawal in the newborn, also assign code 779.5 Drug withdrawal syndrome in newborn.

760.76 Diethylstilbestrol [DES]
AHA: 4Q, '94, 45

760.77 Anticonvulsants   N
Carbamazepine   Phenytoin
Phenobarbital   Valproic acid
AHA: 4Q, '05, 82

760.78 Antimetabolic agents   N
Methotrexate
Retinoic acid
Statins
AHA: 4Q, '05, 82-83

760.79 Other
Fetus or newborn affected by:
immune sera   } transmitted via
medicinal agents NEC   placenta
toxic substance NEC   or breast
AHA: 1Q, '10, 14; 3Q, '09, 21
P04.8 Newborn (suspected) affected by oth maternl noxious subst   I-10

760.8 Other specified maternal conditions affecting fetus or newborn
Maternal genital tract and other localized infection affecting fetus or newborn, but fetus or newborn not manifesting that disease
EXCLUDES *maternal urinary tract infection affecting fetus or newborn (760.1)*

760.9 Unspecified maternal condition affecting fetus or newborn

√4th **761 Fetus or newborn affected by maternal complications of pregnancy**
INCLUDES the listed maternal conditions only when specified as a cause of mortality or morbidity of the fetus or newborn

761.0 Incompetent cervix
DEF: Inadequate functioning of uterine cervix.

761.1 Premature rupture of membranes

761.2 Oligohydramnios
EXCLUDES *that due to premature rupture of membranes (761.1)*
DEF: Deficient amniotic fluid.

761.3 Polyhydramnios
Hydramnios (acute) (chronic)
DEF: Excess amniotic fluid.

761.4 Ectopic pregnancy
Pregnancy:
abdominal
intraperitoneal
tubal

761.5 Multiple pregnancy
Triplet (pregnancy)   Twin (pregnancy)

√4th √5th Additional Digit Required   Unspecified Code   Other Specified Code   Manifestation Code   ►◄ Revised Text   ● New Code   ▲ Revised Code Title

Certain Conditions Originating in the Perinatal Period

761.6–763.9

761.6 Maternal death

761.7 Malpresentation before labor
Breech presentation
External version
Oblique lie } before labor
Transverse lie
Unstable lie

761.8 Other specified maternal complications of pregnancy affecting fetus or newborn
Spontaneous abortion, fetus

761.9 Unspecified maternal complication of pregnancy affecting fetus or newborn

√4ᵗʰ **762 Fetus or newborn affected by complications of placenta, cord, and membranes**
INCLUDES the listed maternal conditions only when specified as a cause of mortality or morbidity in the fetus or newborn
AHA: 1Q, '94, 8

762.0 Placenta previa   N
DEF: Placenta developed in lower segment of uterus; causes hemorrhaging in last trimester.

762.1 Other forms of placental separation and hemorrhage   N
Abruptio placentae
Antepartum hemorrhage
Damage to placenta from amniocentesis, cesarean section, or surgical induction
Maternal blood loss
Premature separation of placenta
Rupture of marginal sinus

762.2 Other and unspecified morphological and functional abnormalities of placenta   N
Placental:
dysfunction
infarction
insufficiency

762.3 Placental transfusion syndromes   N
Placental and cord abnormality resulting in twin-to-twin or other transplacental transfusion
Use additional code to indicate resultant condition in newborn:
fetal blood loss (772.0)
polycythemia neonatorum (776.4)

762.4 Prolapsed cord   N
Cord presentation

762.5 Other compression of umbilical cord   N
Cord around neck
Entanglement of cord
Knot in cord
Torsion of cord
AHA: 2Q, '03, 9
TIP: Assign only if the cord compression or entanglement was documented as having affected the fetus/newborn.
P02.5 Newborn (suspected) affected by oth compression umb cord   I-10

762.6 Other and unspecified conditions of umbilical cord   N
Short cord
Thrombosis
Varices } of umbilical cord
Velamentous insertion
Vasa previa
EXCLUDES infection of umbilical cord (771.4)
single umbilical artery (747.5)
P02.69 Newborn (suspected) affected by oth cond umbil cord   I-10

762.7 Chorioamnionitis   N
Amnionitis   Placentitis
Membranitis
DEF: Inflamed fetal membrane.

762.8 Other specified abnormalities of chorion and amnion   N

762.9 Unspecified abnormality of chorion and amnion   N

√4ᵗʰ **763 Fetus or newborn affected by other complications of labor and delivery**
INCLUDES the listed conditions only when specified as a cause of mortality or morbidity in the fetus or newborn
EXCLUDES newborn affected by surgical procedures on mother (760.61-760.64)
AHA: 1Q, '94, 8

763.0 Breech delivery and extraction   N

763.1 Other malpresentation, malposition, and disproportion during labor and delivery   N
Fetus or newborn affected by:
abnormality of bony pelvis
contracted pelvis
persistent occipitoposterior position
shoulder presentation
transverse lie
Fetus or newborn affected by conditions classifiable to 652, 653, and 660

763.2 Forceps delivery   N
Fetus or newborn affected by forceps extraction

763.3 Delivery by vacuum extractor   N

763.4 Cesarean delivery   N
EXCLUDES placental separation or hemorrhage from cesarean section (762.1)

763.5 Maternal anesthesia and analgesia   N
Reactions and intoxications from maternal opiates and tranquilizers during labor and delivery
EXCLUDES drug withdrawal syndrome in newborn (779.5)

763.6 Precipitate delivery   N
Rapid second stage

763.7 Abnormal uterine contractions   N
Fetus or newborn affected by:
contraction ring
hypertonic labor
hypotonic uterine dysfunction
uterine inertia or dysfunction
Fetus or newborn affected by conditions classifiable to 661, except 661.3

√5ᵗʰ **763.8 Other specified complications of labor and delivery affecting fetus or newborn**
AHA: 4Q, '98, 46

763.81 Abnormality in fetal heart rate or rhythm before the onset of labor   N

763.82 Abnormality in fetal heart rate or rhythm during labor   N
AHA: 4Q, '98, 46

763.83 Abnormality in fetal heart rate or rhythm, unspecified as to time of onset   N

763.84 Meconium passage during delivery   N
EXCLUDES meconium aspiration (770.11, 770.12)
meconium staining (779.84)
DEF: Fetal intestinal activity that increases in response to a distressed state during delivery; anal sphincter relaxes, and meconium is passed into the amniotic fluid.
AHA: ▶4Q, '13, 94, 95;◀ 4Q, '05, 83
TIP: If the meconium was documented as aspirated or had any effect on the newborn, see codes 770.11 and 770.12.

763.89 Other specified complications of labor and delivery affecting fetus or newborn   N
Fetus or newborn affected by:
abnormality of maternal soft tissues
destructive operation on live fetus to facilitate delivery
induction of labor (medical)
other procedures used in labor and delivery
Fetus or newborn affected by other conditions classifiable to 650-669

763.9 Unspecified complication of labor and delivery affecting fetus or newborn   N

N Newborn Age: 0   P Pediatric Age: 0-17   M Maternity Age: 12-55   A Adult Age: 15-124

Other Conditions Originating in the Perinatal Period (764-779)

The following fifth-digit subclassification is for use with category 764 and codes 765.0-765.1 to denote birthweight:

0 unspecified [weight]
1 less than 500 grams
2 500-749 grams
3 750-999 grams
4 1,000-1,249 grams
5 1,250-1,499 grams
6 1,500-1,749 grams
7 1,750-1,999 grams
8 2,000-2,499 grams
9 2,500 grams and over

√4ᵗʰ 764 Slow fetal growth and fetal malnutrition
AHA: 1Q, '09, 13; 3Q, '04, 4; 4Q, '02, 63; 1Q, '94, 8; 2Q, '91, 19; 2Q, '89, 15

§ √5ᵗʰ **764.0 "Light-for-dates" without mention of fetal malnutrition** N
[0-9] Infants underweight for gestational age
"Small-for-dates"
P05.00 Newborn light for gest age unsp weight I-10

§ √5ᵗʰ **764.1 "Light-for-dates" with signs of fetal malnutrition** N
[0-9] Infants "light-for-dates" classifiable to 764.0, who in addition show signs of fetal malnutrition, such as dry peeling skin and loss of subcutaneous tissue

§ √5ᵗʰ **764.2 Fetal malnutrition without mention of "light-for-dates"** N
[0-9] Infants, not underweight for gestational age, showing signs of fetal malnutrition, such as dry peeling skin and loss of subcutaneous tissue
Intrauterine malnutrition

§ √5ᵗʰ **764.9 Fetal growth retardation, unspecified** N
[0-9] Intrauterine growth retardation
AHA: For code 764.97: 1Q, '97, 6

√4ᵗʰ 765 Disorders relating to short gestation and low birthweight
INCLUDES the listed conditions, without further specification, as causes of mortality, morbidity, or additional care, in fetus or newborn
AHA: 1Q, '97, 6; 1Q, '94, 8; 2Q, '91, 19; 2Q, '89, 15

§ √5ᵗʰ **765.0 Extreme immaturity** N
[0-9] NOTE Usually implies a birthweight of less than 1000 grams.
Use additional code for weeks of gestation (765.20-765.29)
AHA: 1Q, '09, 13; 3Q, '04, 4; 4Q, '02, 63; For code 765.01:▶ 1Q, '14, 16;◀
For code 765.03: 4Q, '01, 51

§ √5ᵗʰ **765.1 Other preterm infants** N
[0-9] NOTE Usually implies a birthweight of 1000-2499 grams.
Prematurity NOS
Prematurity or small size, not classifiable to 765.0 or as "light-for-dates" in 764
Use additional code for weeks of gestation (765.20-765.29)
AHA: 1Q, '09, 13; 3Q, '04, 4; 4Q, '02, 63; For code 765.10: 1Q, '09, 15; 1Q, '94, 14; For code 765.17: 4Q, '08, 139; 1Q, '97, 6;
For code 765.18: 4Q, '02, 64
P07.10 Other low birth weight newborn uns weight I-10

√5ᵗʰ **765.2 Weeks of gestation**
AHA: 3Q, '04, 4; 4Q, '02, 63
TIP: Assign as an additional code with category 764 and codes from 765.0 and 765.1, as documented by the provider.

765.20 Unspecified weeks of gestation N

765.21 Less than 24 completed weeks of gestation N
AHA: ▶1Q, '14, 16◀

765.22 24 completed weeks of gestation N

765.23 25-26 completed weeks of gestation N
AHA: 1Q, '09, 14

765.24 27-28 completed weeks of gestation N

765.25 29-30 completed weeks of gestation N
P07.32 Preterm newborn, gestl age 29 compl wks I-10

765.26 31-32 completed weeks of gestation N
AHA: 1Q, '09, 14; 4Q, '08, 139

765.27 33-34 completed weeks of gestation N
AHA: 4Q, '10, 97

765.28 35-36 completed weeks of gestation N
AHA: 4Q, '02, 64
P07.38 Preterm newborn, gestl age 35 compl wks I-10

765.29 37 or more completed weeks of gestation N

√4ᵗʰ 766 Disorders relating to long gestation and high birthweight
INCLUDES the listed conditions, without further specification, as causes of mortality, morbidity, or additional care, in fetus or newborn

766.0 Exceptionally large baby N
NOTE Usually implies a birthweight of 4500 grams or more.

766.1 Other "heavy-for-dates" infants N
Other fetus or infant "heavy-" or "large-for-dates" regardless of period of gestation
P08.1 Other heavy for gestational age newborn I-10

√5ᵗʰ **766.2 Late infant, not "heavy-for-dates"**
AHA: 2Q, '06, 12; 4Q, '03, 69
TIP: May be assigned based on gestational age alone, without documentation of any related specific condition or disorder.

766.21 Post-term infant N
Infant with gestation period over 40 completed weeks to 42 completed weeks
AHA: 1Q, '09, 12;
P08.21 Post-term newborn I-10

766.22 Prolonged gestation of infant N
Infant with gestation period over 42 completed weeks
Postmaturity NOS
AHA: 1Q, '09, 12

√4ᵗʰ 767 Birth trauma

767.0 Subdural and cerebral hemorrhage N
Subdural and cerebral hemorrhage, whether described as due to birth trauma or to intrapartum anoxia or hypoxia
Subdural hematoma (localized)
Tentorial tear
Use additional code to identify cause
EXCLUDES intraventricular hemorrhage (772.10-772.14)
subarachnoid hemorrhage (772.2)

√5ᵗʰ **767.1 Injuries to scalp**
AHA: 4Q, '03, 69

767.11 Epicranial subaponeurotic hemorrhage (massive) N
Subgaleal hemorrhage
DEF: A hemorrhage that occurs within the space between the galea aponeurotica, or epicranial aponeurosis, a thin tendinous structure that is attached to the skull laterally, and the periosteum of the skull.

767.19 Other injuries to scalp N
Caput succedaneum
Cephalhematoma
Chignon (from vacuum extraction)
P12.89 Other birth injuries to scalp I-10

767.2 Fracture of clavicle N

767.3 Other injuries to skeleton N
Fracture of: Fracture of:
long bones   skull
EXCLUDES congenital dislocation of hip (754.30-754.35)
fracture of spine, congenital (767.4)

767.4 Injury to spine and spinal cord N
Dislocation
Fracture   } of spine or spinal cord due to
Laceration   birth trauma
Rupture

767.5 Facial nerve injury N
Facial palsy

767.6 Injury to brachial plexus N
Palsy or paralysis: Palsy or paralysis:
brachial   Klumpke (-Déjérine)
Erb (-Duchenne)

767.7 Other cranial and peripheral nerve injuries N
Phrenic nerve paralysis

---

§ Requires fifth digit. Valid digits are in [brackets] under each code. See beginning of section 764-779 for codes and definitions.

√4ᵗʰ √5ᵗʰ Additional Digit Required | Unspecified Code | Other Specified Code | Manifestation Code | ►◄ Revised Text | ● New Code | ▲ Revised Code Title

Certain Conditions Originating in the Perinatal Period

767.8–770.18

Epicranial Aponeurosis

767.8 **Other specified birth trauma**

Eye damage	Rupture of:
Hematoma of:	liver
liver (subcapsular)	spleen
testes	Scalpel wound
vulva	Traumatic glaucoma

     EXCLUDES *hemorrhage classifiable to 772.0-772.9*

767.9 **Birth trauma, unspecified**
     Birth injury NOS

768 **Intrauterine hypoxia and birth asphyxia**
     NOTE Use only when associated with newborn morbidity classifiable elsewhere
     EXCLUDES *acidemia NOS of newborn (775.81)*
         acidosis NOS of newborn (775.81)
         cerebral ischemia NOS (779.2)
         hypoxia NOS of newborn (770.88)
         mixed metabolic and respiratory acidosis of newborn (775.81)
         respiratory arrest of newborn (770.87)
     DEF: Oxygen intake insufficiency due to interrupted placental circulation or premature separation of placenta.
     AHA: 4Q, '92, 20

768.0 **Fetal death from asphyxia or anoxia before onset of labor or at unspecified time**

768.1 **Fetal death from asphyxia or anoxia during labor**

768.2 **Fetal distress before onset of labor, in liveborn infant**
     Fetal metabolic acidemia before onset of labor, in liveborn infant

768.3 **Fetal distress first noted during labor and delivery, in liveborn infant**
     Fetal metabolic acidemia first noted during labor and delivery, in liveborn infant

768.4 **Fetal distress, unspecified as to time of onset, in liveborn infant**
     Fetal metabolic acidemia unspecified as to time of onset, in liveborn infant
     AHA: N-D, '86, 10

768.5 **Severe birth asphyxia**
     Birth asphyxia with neurologic involvement
     EXCLUDES *hypoxic-ischemic encephalopathy [HIE] (768.70-768.73)*
     AHA: N-D, '86, 3

768.6 **Mild or moderate birth asphyxia**
     Other specified birth asphyxia (without mention of neurologic involvement)
     EXCLUDES *hypoxic-ischemic encephalopathy [HIE] (768.70-768.73)*
     AHA: N-D, '86, 3

768.7 **Hypoxic-ischemic encephalopathy [HIE]**
     AHA: 4Q, '09, 99-101; 4Q, '06, 104

     768.70 **Hypoxic-ischemic encephalopathy, unspecified**
     768.71 **Mild hypoxic-ischemic encephalopathy**
     768.72 **Moderate hypoxic-ischemic encephalopathy**
         AHA: 4Q, '09, 101
     768.73 **Severe hypoxic-ischemic encephalopathy**

768.9 **Unspecified birth asphyxia in liveborn infant**
     Anoxia   } NOS, in liveborn infant
     Asphyxia

769 **Respiratory distress syndrome**
     Cardiorespiratory distress syndrome of newborn
     Hyaline membrane disease (pulmonary)
     Idiopathic respiratory distress syndrome [IRDS or RDS] of newborn
     Pulmonary hypoperfusion syndrome
     EXCLUDES *transient tachypnea of newborn (770.6)*
     DEF: Severe chest contractions upon air intake and expiratory grunting; infant appears blue due to oxygen deficiency and has rapid respiratory rate; formerly called hyaline membrane disease.
     AHA: 1Q, '89, 10; N-D, '86, 6
     TIP: Do not assign if documentation specifies Type II respiratory distress syndrome, which usually resolves within six to 24 hours after birth; see instead 770.6.
     P22.0 Respiratory distress syndrome of newborn   **I-10**

770 **Other respiratory conditions of fetus and newborn**

     770.0 **Congenital pneumonia**
     Infective pneumonia acquired prenatally
     EXCLUDES *pneumonia from infection acquired after birth (480.0-486)*
     AHA: 1Q, '05, 10

     770.1 **Fetal and newborn aspiration**
     EXCLUDES *aspiration of postnatal stomach contents (770.85, 770.86)*
         meconium passage during delivery (763.84)
         meconium staining (779.84)
     AHA: 4Q, '05, 83

         770.10 **Fetal and newborn aspiration, unspecified**

         770.11 **Meconium aspiration without respiratory symptoms**
         Meconium aspiration NOS

         770.12 **Meconium aspiration with respiratory symptoms**
         Meconium aspiration pneumonia
         Meconium aspiration pneumonitis
         Meconium aspiration syndrome NOS
         Use additional code to identify any secondary pulmonary hypertension (416.8), if applicable
         DEF: Meconium aspiration syndrome: aspiration of fetal intestinal material during or prior to delivery, usually a complication of placental insufficiency, causing pneumonitis and bronchial obstruction (inflammatory reaction of lungs).

         770.13 **Aspiration of clear amniotic fluid without respiratory symptoms**
         Aspiration of clear amniotic fluid NOS

         770.14 **Aspiration of clear amniotic fluid with respiratory symptoms**
         Aspiration of clear amniotic fluid with pneumonia
         Aspiration of clear amniotic fluid with pneumonitis
         Use additional code to identify any secondary pulmonary hypertension (416.8), if applicable

         770.15 **Aspiration of blood without respiratory symptoms**
         Aspiration of blood NOS

         770.16 **Aspiration of blood with respiratory symptoms**
         Aspiration of blood with pneumonia
         Aspiration of blood with pneumonitis
         Use additional code to identify any secondary pulmonary hypertension (416.8), if applicable

         770.17 **Other fetal and newborn aspiration without respiratory symptoms**

         770.18 **Other fetal and newborn aspiration with respiratory symptoms**
         Other aspiration pneumonia
         Other aspiration pneumonitis
         Use additional code to identify any secondary pulmonary hypertension (416.8), if applicable

---

770.2 Interstitial emphysema and related conditions   N
Pneumomediastinum
Pneumopericardium   } originating in the perinatal
Pneumothorax   period

P25.0 Interstitial emphysema origin perinatal period   I-10

770.3 Pulmonary hemorrhage   N
Hemorrhage:
alveolar (lung)
intra-alveolar (lung)   } originating in the
massive pulmonary   perinatal period

770.4 Primary atelectasis   N
Pulmonary immaturity NOS
DEF: Alveoli fail to expand causing insufficient air intake by newborn.

770.5 Other and unspecified atelectasis   N
Atelectasis:
NOS
partial   } originating in the perinatal
secondary   period
Pulmonary collapse

770.6 Transitory tachypnea of newborn   N
Idiopathic tachypnea of newborn
Wet lung syndrome
EXCLUDES respiratory distress syndrome (769)
DEF: Quick, shallow breathing of newborn; short-term problem.
AHA: 4Q, '95, 4; 1Q, '94, 12; 3Q, '93, 7; 1Q, '89, 10; N-D, '86, 6
P22.1 Transient tachypnea of newborn   I-10

770.7 Chronic respiratory disease arising in the perinatal period
Bronchopulmonary dysplasia
Interstitial pulmonary fibrosis of prematurity
Wilson-Mikity syndrome
AHA: 1Q, '11, 16; 2Q, '91, 19; N-D, '86, 11
P27.8 Other chronic resp dz origin perinatal period   I-10

√5ʰ 770.8 Other respiratory problems after birth
EXCLUDES mixed metabolic and respiratory acidosis of newborn
(775.81)
AHA: 4Q, '02, 65; 2Q, '98, 10; 2Q, '96, 10

770.81 Primary apnea of newborn   N
Apneic spells of newborn NOS
Essential apnea of newborn
Sleep apnea of newborn
DEF: Cessation of breathing when a neonate makes no
respiratory effort for 15 seconds, resulting in cyanosis and
bradycardia.
P28.3 Primary sleep apnea of newborn   I-10

770.82 Other apnea of newborn   N
Obstructive apnea of newborn

770.83 Cyanotic attacks of newborn   N

770.84 Respiratory failure of newborn   N
EXCLUDES respiratory distress syndrome (769)
AHA: 4Q, '08, 99

**770.85 Aspiration of postnatal stomach
contents without respiratory symptoms**   N
Aspiration of postnatal stomach contents NOS
AHA: 4Q, '05, 83

**770.86 Aspiration of postnatal stomach
contents with respiratory symptoms**   N
Aspiration of postnatal stomach contents with
pneumonia
Aspiration of postnatal stomach contents with
pneumonitis
Use additional code to identify any secondary
pulmonary hypertension (416.8), if applicable
AHA: 4Q, '05, 83

770.87 Respiratory arrest of newborn   N
AHA: 4Q, '06, 104-106

770.88 Hypoxemia of newborn   N
Hypoxia NOS of newborn
AHA: 4Q, '06, 104-106

770.89 Other respiratory problems after birth   N
AHA: 3Q, '09, 20
P28.89 Oth specified respiratory conditions   I-10
of newborn

**770.9 Unspecified respiratory condition of fetus
and newborn**   N

√4ʰ 771 Infections specific to the perinatal period
INCLUDES infections acquired before or during birth or via the
umbilicus or during the first 28 days after birth
EXCLUDES congenital pneumonia (770.0)
congenital syphilis (090.0-090.9)
infant botulism (040.41)
maternal infectious disease as a cause of mortality or
morbidity in fetus or newborn, but fetus or newborn
not manifesting the disease (760.2)
ophthalmia neonatorum due to gonococcus (098.40)
other infections not specifically classified to this category
AHA: N-D, '85, 4

771.0 Congenital rubella   N
Congenital rubella pneumonitis

771.1 Congenital cytomegalovirus infection   N
Congenital cytomegalic inclusion disease

771.2 Other congenital infections   N
Congenital: Congenital:
herpes simplex   toxoplasmosis
listeriosis   tuberculosis
malaria

771.3 Tetanus neonatorum   N
Tetanus omphalitis
EXCLUDES hypocalcemic tetany (775.4)
DEF: Severe infection of central nervous system; due to exotoxin of
tetanus bacillus from navel infection prompted by nonsterile
technique during umbilical ligation.

771.4 Omphalitis of the newborn   N
Infection:
navel cord
umbilical stump
EXCLUDES tetanus omphalitis (771.3)
DEF: Inflamed umbilicus.
AHA: 4Q, '09, 102

771.5 Neonatal infective mastitis   N
EXCLUDES noninfective neonatal mastitis (778.7)

771.6 Neonatal conjunctivitis and dacryocystitis   N
Ophthalmia neonatorum NOS
EXCLUDES ophthalmia neonatorum due to gonococcus (098.40)

771.7 Neonatal Candida infection   N
Neonatal moniliasis
Thrush in newborn

√5ʰ 771.8 Other infection specific to the perinatal period
Use additional code to identify organism or specific infection
AHA: 4Q, '02, 66

771.81 Septicemia [sepsis] of newborn   N
Use additional codes to identify severe sepsis (995.92)
and any associated acute organ dysfunction, if
applicable
AHA: 4Q, '08, 99
TIP: Assign instead of 038 or 995.91.
P36.9 Bacterial sepsis newborn unspecified   I-10

771.82 Urinary tract infection of newborn   N

771.83 Bacteremia of newborn   N

**771.89 Other infections specific to the
perinatal period**   N
Intra-amniotic infection of fetus NOS
Infection of newborn NOS

√4ʰ
√5ʰ Additional Digit Required   Unspecified Code   Other Specified Code   Manifestation Code   ▶◀ Revised Text   ● New Code   ▲ Revised Code Title

2015 ICD-9-CM   **Volume 1 – 257**

Certain Conditions Originating in the Perinatal Period

772–774.6

✓4th **772   Fetal and neonatal hemorrhage**

> EXCLUDES   fetal hematologic conditions complicating pregnancy (678.0)
> hematological disorders of fetus and newborn (776.0-776.9)

772.0   Fetal blood loss affecting newborn   N

Fetal blood loss from:
- cut end of co-twin's cord
- placenta
- ruptured cord
- vasa previa

Fetal exsanguination

Fetal hemorrhage into:
- co-twin
- mother's circulation

✓5th **772.1   Intraventricular hemorrhage**

Intraventricular hemorrhage from any perinatal cause

AHA: 4Q, '01, 49; 3Q, '92, 8; 4Q, '88, 8

772.10   Unspecified grade   N

772.11   Grade I   N
Bleeding into germinal matrix

772.12   Grade II   N
Bleeding into ventricle

772.13   Grade III   N
Bleeding with enlargement of ventricle
AHA: 4Q, '01, 51

772.14   Grade IV   N
Bleeding into cerebral cortex

772.2   Subarachnoid hemorrhage   N
Subarachnoid hemorrhage from any perinatal cause
> EXCLUDES   subdural and cerebral hemorrhage (767.0)

772.3   Umbilical hemorrhage after birth   N
Slipped umbilical ligature

772.4   Gastrointestinal hemorrhage   N
> EXCLUDES   swallowed maternal blood (777.3)

772.5   Adrenal hemorrhage   N

772.6   Cutaneous hemorrhage   N
- Bruising
- Ecchymoses   } in fetus or newborn
- Petechiae
- Superficial hematoma
P54.5 Neonatal cutaneous hemorrhage   I-10

772.8   Other specified hemorrhage of fetus or newborn   N
> EXCLUDES   hemorrhagic disease of newborn (776.0)
> pulmonary hemorrhage (770.3)

772.9   Unspecified hemorrhage of newborn   N

✓4th **773   Hemolytic disease of fetus or newborn, due to isoimmunization**

DEF: Hemolytic anemia of fetus or newborn due to maternal antibody formation against fetal erythrocytes; infant blood contains nonmaternal antigen.

TIP: Do not assign unless the physician substantiates confirmation by a positive Coomb's (direct antibody or direct antiglobulin) test.

773.0   Hemolytic disease due to Rh isoimmunization   N

- Anemia
- Erythroblastosis (fetalis)   } due to RH:
- Hemolytic disease (fetus)   antibodies
- (newborn)   isoimmunization
- Jaundice   maternal/fetal incompatibility

Rh hemolytic disease
Rh isoimmunization

773.1   Hemolytic disease due to ABO isoimmunization   N
ABO hemolytic disease
ABO isoimmunization
- Anemia   due to ABO:
- Erythroblastosis (fetalis)   antibodies
- Hemolytic disease (fetus)   isoimmunization
- (newborn)   maternal/fetal
- Jaundice   incompatibility

DEF: Incompatible Rh fetal-maternal blood grouping; prematurely destroys red blood cells; detected by Coombs test.
AHA: 3Q, '92, 8
P55.1 ABO isoimmunization of newborn   I-10

773.2   Hemolytic disease due to other and unspecified isoimmunization   N
Erythroblastosis (fetalis) (neonatorum) NOS
Hemolytic disease (fetus) (newborn) NOS
Jaundice or anemia due to other and unspecified blood-group incompatibility
AHA: 1Q, '94, 13
P55.9 Hemolytic disease of newborn unspecified   I-10

773.3   Hydrops fetalis due to isoimmunization   N
Use additional code to identify type of isoimmunization (773.0-773.2)
DEF: Massive edema of entire body and severe anemia; may result in fetal death or stillbirth.

773.4   Kernicterus due to isoimmunization   N
Use additional code to identify type of isoimmunization (773.0-773.2)
DEF: Complication of erythroblastosis fetalis associated with severe neural symptoms, high blood bilirubin levels and nerve cell destruction; results in bilirubin-pigmented gray matter of central nervous system.

773.5   Late anemia due to isoimmunization   N

✓4th **774   Other perinatal jaundice**

774.0   Perinatal jaundice from hereditary hemolytic anemias   N
Code first underlying disease (282.0-282.9)

774.1   Perinatal jaundice from other excessive hemolysis   N
Fetal or neonatal jaundice from:
- bruising
- drugs or toxins transmitted from mother
- infection
- polycythemia
- swallowed maternal blood
Use additional code to identify cause
> EXCLUDES   jaundice due to isoimmunization (773.0-773.2)

774.2   Neonatal jaundice associated with preterm delivery   N
Hyperbilirubinemia of prematurity
Jaundice due to delayed conjugation associated with preterm delivery
AHA: 3Q, '91, 21
P59.0 Neonatal jaundice associated w/preterm delivery   I-10

✓5th **774.3   Neonatal jaundice due to delayed conjugation from other causes**

774.30   Neonatal jaundice due to delayed conjugation, cause unspecified   N
DEF: Jaundice of newborn with abnormal bilirubin metabolism; causes excess accumulated unconjugated bilirubin in blood.

774.31   Neonatal jaundice due to delayed conjugation in diseases classified elsewhere   N
Code first underlying diseases as:
- congenital hypothyroidism (243)
- Crigler-Najjar syndrome (277.4)
- Gilbert's syndrome (277.4)

774.39   Other   N
Jaundice due to delayed conjugation from causes, such as:
- breast milk inhibitors
- delayed development of conjugating system

774.4   Perinatal jaundice due to hepatocellular damage   N
Fetal or neonatal hepatitis
Giant cell hepatitis
Inspissated bile syndrome

774.5   Perinatal jaundice from other causes   N
Code first underlying cause as:
- congenital obstruction of bile duct (751.61)
- galactosemia (271.1)
- mucoviscidosis (277.00-277.09)

774.6   Unspecified fetal and neonatal jaundice   N
Icterus neonatorum
Neonatal hyperbilirubinemia (transient)
Physiologic jaundice NOS in newborn
> EXCLUDES   that in preterm infants (774.2)
AHA: 1Q, '94, 13; 2Q, '89, 15
P59.9 Neonatal jaundice unspecified   I-10

N Newborn Age: 0   P Pediatric Age: 0-17   M Maternity Age: 12-55   A Adult Age: 15-124

774.7 Kernicterus not due to isoimmunization N
Bilirubin encephalopathy
Kernicterus of newborn NOS
> **EXCLUDES** *kernicterus due to isoimmunization (773.4)*

√4th **775 Endocrine and metabolic disturbances specific to the fetus and newborn**
> **INCLUDES** transitory endocrine and metabolic disturbances caused by the infant's response to maternal endocrine and metabolic factors, its removal from them, or its adjustment to extrauterine existence

775.0 Syndrome of "infant of a diabetic mother" N
Maternal diabetes mellitus affecting fetus or newborn (with hypoglycemia)
> **AHA:** 1Q, '04, 7-8; 3Q, '91, 5
> **TIP:** Do not assign if the infant has no manifestations or symptoms of the syndrome; refer instead to code V18.0 Family history, diabetes mellitus.
> **P70.1** Syndrome of infant of diabetic mother   I-10

775.1 Neonatal diabetes mellitus N
Diabetes mellitus syndrome in newborn infant
> **AHA:** 3Q, '91, 6

775.2 Neonatal myasthenia gravis N

775.3 Neonatal thyrotoxicosis N
Neonatal hyperthyroidism (transient)

775.4 Hypocalcemia and hypomagnesemia of newborn N
Cow's milk hypocalcemia
Hypocalcemic tetany, neonatal
Neonatal hypoparathyroidism
Phosphate-loading hypocalcemia

775.5 Other transitory neonatal electrolyte disturbances N
Dehydration, neonatal
> **AHA:** 1Q, '10, 14; 3Q, '09, 21; 1Q, '05, 9
> **TIP:** If the patient has neonatal hyperkalemia, assign also code 276.7 Hyperpotassemia.
> **P74.1** Dehydration of newborn   I-10

775.6 Neonatal hypoglycemia N
> **EXCLUDES** *infant of mother with diabetes mellitus (775.0)*
> **AHA:** 1Q '94, 8
> **P70.4** Other neonatal hypoglycemia   I-10

775.7 Late metabolic acidosis of newborn N

√5th **775.8 Other neonatal endocrine and metabolic disturbances**

  775.81 Other acidosis of newborn N
  Acidemia NOS of newborn
  Acidosis of newborn NOS
  Mixed metabolic and respiratory acidosis of newborn
>   **AHA:** 4Q, '06, 104-106

  775.89 Other neonatal endocrine and metabolic disturbances N
  Amino-acid metabolic disorders described as transitory
>   **AHA:** 4Q, '06, 104-106

775.9 Unspecified endocrine and metabolic disturbances specific to the fetus and newborn N

√4th **776 Hematological disorders of newborn**
> **INCLUDES** disorders specific to the newborn though possibly originating in utero
> **EXCLUDES** *fetal hematologic conditions (678.0)*

776.0 Hemorrhagic disease of newborn N
Hemorrhagic diathesis of newborn
Vitamin K deficiency of newborn
> **EXCLUDES** *fetal or neonatal hemorrhage (772.0-772.9)*

776.1 Transient neonatal thrombocytopenia N
Neonatal thrombocytopenia due to:
  exchange transfusion
  idiopathic maternal thrombocytopenia
  isoimmunization
> **DEF:** Temporary decrease in blood platelets of newborn.
> **P61.0** Transient neonatal thrombocytopenia   I-10

776.2 Disseminated intravascular coagulation in newborn N
> **DEF:** Disseminated intravascular coagulation of newborn: clotting disorder due to excess thromboplastic agents in blood as a result of disease or trauma; causes blood clotting within vessels and reduces available elements necessary for blood coagulation.

776.3 Other transient neonatal disorders of coagulation N
Transient coagulation defect, newborn

776.4 Polycythemia neonatorum N
Plethora of newborn
Polycythemia due to:
  donor twin transfusion
  maternal-fetal transfusion
> **DEF:** Abnormal increase of total red blood cells of newborn.

776.5 Congenital anemia N
Anemia following fetal blood loss
> **EXCLUDES** *anemia due to isoimmunization (773.0-773.2, 773.5)*
> *hereditary hemolytic anemias (282.0-282.9)*

776.6 Anemia of prematurity N
> **P61.2** Anemia of prematurity   I-10

776.7 Transient neonatal neutropenia N
Isoimmune neutropenia   Maternal transfer neutropenia
> **EXCLUDES** *congenital neutropenia (nontransient) (288.01)*
> **DEF:** Decreased neutrophilic leukocytes in blood of newborn.

776.8 Other specified transient hematological disorders N

776.9 Unspecified hematological disorder specific to newborn N

√4th **777 Perinatal disorders of digestive system**
> **INCLUDES** disorders specific to the fetus and newborn
> **EXCLUDES** *intestinal obstruction classifiable to 560.0-560.9*

777.1 Meconium obstruction N
Congenital fecaliths
Delayed passage of meconium
Meconium ileus NOS
Meconium plug syndrome
> **EXCLUDES** *meconium ileus in cystic fibrosis (277.01)*
> **DEF:** Meconium blocked digestive tract of newborn.

777.2 Intestinal obstruction due to inspissated milk N

777.3 Hematemesis and melena due to swallowed maternal blood N
Swallowed blood syndrome in newborn
> **EXCLUDES** *that not due to swallowed maternal blood (772.4)*

777.4 Transitory ileus of newborn N
> **EXCLUDES** *Hirschsprung's disease (751.3)*

√5th **777.5 Necrotizing enterocolitis in newborn**
> **DEF:** Serious intestinal infection and inflammation in preterm infants; severity is measured by stages and may progress to life-threatening perforation or peritonitis; resection surgical treatment may be necessary.
> **AHA:** 4Q, '08, 138-140

  777.50 Necrotizing enterocolitis in newborn, unspecified N
  Necrotizing enterocolitis in newborn, NOS

  777.51 Stage I necrotizing enterocolitis in newborn N
  Necrotizing enterocolitis without pneumatosis, without perforation
>   **DEF:** Broad-spectrum symptoms with non-specific signs including feeding intolerance, sepsis, gastroenteritis, ileus, metabolic abnormalities.

  777.52 Stage II necrotizing enterocolitis in newborn N
  Necrotizing enterocolitis with pneumatosis, without perforation
>   **DEF:** Radiographic confirmation of necrotizing enterocolitis showing intestinal dilatation, fixed loops of bowels, pneumatosis intestinalis, metabolic acidosis, and thrombocytopenia.

  777.53 Stage III necrotizing enterocolitis in newborn N
  Necrotizing enterocolitis with perforation
  Necrotizing enterocolitis with pneumatosis and perforation
>   **DEF:** Advanced stage in which infant demonstrates signs of bowel perforation, septic shock, metabolic acidosis, ascites, disseminated intravascular coagulopathy, neutropenia.
>   **AHA:** 4Q, '08, 139

√4th √5th Additional Digit Required   Unspecified Code   Other Specified Code   Manifestation Code   ▶◀ Revised Text   ● New Code   ▲ Revised Code Title

777.6 Perinatal intestinal perforation　　　N
　　Meconium peritonitis

777.8 Other specified perinatal disorders of digestive system　　　N
　　AHA: 4Q, '10, 97

777.9 Unspecified perinatal disorder of digestive system　　　N

√4ᵗʰ **778 Conditions involving the integument and temperature regulation of fetus and newborn**

778.0 Hydrops fetalis not due to isoimmunization　　　N
　　Idiopathic hydrops
　　EXCLUDES hydrops fetalis due to isoimmunization (773.3)
　　DEF: Edema of entire body, unrelated to immune response.

778.1 Sclerema neonatorum　　　N
　　Subcutaneous fat necrosis
　　DEF: Diffuse, rapidly progressing white, waxy, nonpitting hardening of tissue, usually of legs and feet, life-threatening; found in preterm or debilitated infants; unknown etiology.

778.2 Cold injury syndrome of newborn　　　N

778.3 Other hypothermia of newborn　　　N

778.4 Other disturbances of temperature regulation of newborn　　　N
　　Dehydration fever in newborn
　　Environmentally-induced pyrexia
　　Hyperthermia in newborn
　　Transitory fever of newborn
　　P81.9 Disturbance of temp regulation newborn uns　　I-10

778.5 Other and unspecified edema of newborn　　　N
　　Edema neonatorum

778.6 Congenital hydrocele
　　Congenital hydrocele of tunica vaginalis
　　P83.5 Congenital hydrocele　　I-10

778.7 Breast engorgement in newborn　　　N
　　Noninfective mastitis of newborn
　　EXCLUDES infective mastitis of newborn (771.5)

778.8 Other specified conditions involving the integument of fetus and newborn　　　N
　　Urticaria neonatorum
　　EXCLUDES impetigo neonatorum (684)
　　　　　　pemphigus neonatorum (684)
　　P83.8 Oth spec conditions integument specific to newborn　　I-10

778.9 Unspecified condition involving the integument and temperature regulation of fetus and newborn　　　N

√4ᵗʰ **779 Other and ill-defined conditions originating in the perinatal period**

779.0 Convulsions in newborn　　　N
　　Fits ⎫
　　Seizures ⎬ in newborn
　　AHA: N-D, '84, 11
　　TIP: Clarify with the physician that convulsions are not actually infantile spasms; if so, refer to subcategory 345.6.

779.1 Other and unspecified cerebral irritability in newborn　　　N

779.2 Cerebral depression, coma, and other abnormal cerebral signs　　　N
　　Cerebral ischemia NOS of newborn
　　CNS dysfunction in newborn NOS
　　EXCLUDES cerebral ischemia due to birth trauma (767.0)
　　　　　　intrauterine cerebral ischemia (768.2-768.9)
　　　　　　intraventricular hemorrhage (772.10-772.14)

√5ᵗʰ **779.3 Disorder of stomach function and feeding problems in newborn**
　　AHA: 2Q, '89, 15

　　779.31 Feeding problems in newborn　　　N
　　　　Slow feeding in newborn
　　　　EXCLUDES feeding problem in child over 28 days old (783.3)
　　　　AHA: 4Q, '09, 102
　　　　P92.9 Feeding problem of newborn unspecified　　I-10

779.32 Bilious vomiting in newborn　　　N
　　EXCLUDES bilious vomiting in child over 28 days old (787.04)

779.33 Other vomiting in newborn
　　Regurgitation of food in newborn
　　EXCLUDES vomiting in child over 28 days old (536.2, 787.01-787.04)

779.34 Failure to thrive in newborn　　　N
　　EXCLUDES failure to thrive in child over 28 days old (783.41)

779.4 Drug reactions and intoxications specific to newborn　　　N
　　Gray syndrome from chloramphenicol administration in newborn
　　EXCLUDES fetal alcohol syndrome (760.71)
　　　　　　reactions and intoxications from maternal opiates and tranquilizers (763.5)

779.5 Drug withdrawal syndrome in newborn　　　N
　　Drug withdrawal syndrome in infant of dependent mother
　　EXCLUDES fetal alcohol syndrome (760.71)
　　AHA: 3Q, '94, 6
　　TIP: If the infant is asymptomatic but has a positive drug screen (e.g., for cocaine), assign instead 760.75.

779.6 Termination of pregnancy (fetus)　　　N
　　Fetal death due to:
　　　induced abortion
　　　termination of pregnancy
　　EXCLUDES spontaneous abortion (fetus) (761.8)

779.7 Periventricular leukomalacia
　　DEF: Necrosis of white matter adjacent to lateral ventricles with the formation of cysts; cause of PVL has not been firmly established, but thought to be related to inadequate blood flow in certain areas of the brain.
　　AHA: 4Q, '01, 50, 51

√5ᵗʰ **779.8 Other specified conditions originating in the perinatal period**
　　AHA: 4Q, '02, 67; 1Q, '94, 15

　　779.81 Neonatal bradycardia　　　N
　　　　EXCLUDES abnormality in fetal heart rate or rhythm complicating labor and delivery (763.81-763.83)
　　　　　　　bradycardia due to birth asphyxia (768.5-768.9)
　　　　P29.12 Neonatal bradycardia　　I-10

　　779.82 Neonatal tachycardia　　　N
　　　　EXCLUDES abnormality in fetal heart rate or rhythm complicating labor and delivery (763.81-763.83)

　　779.83 Delayed separation of umbilical cord　　　N
　　　　AHA: 4Q, '03, 71

　　779.84 Meconium staining　　　N
　　　　EXCLUDES meconium aspiration (770.11, 770.12)
　　　　　　　meconium passage during delivery (763.84)
　　　　AHA: ▶4Q, '13, 95;◄ 4Q, '05, 83, 88
　　　　P96.83 Meconium staining　　I-10

　　779.85 Cardiac arrest of newborn　　　N
　　　　AHA: 4Q, '06, 104-106

　　779.89 Other specified conditions originating in the perinatal period　　　N
　　　　Use additional code to specify condition
　　　　AHA: 3Q, '12, 5; 3Q, '11, 3-4; 2Q, '11, 13; 1Q, '06, 18; 2Q, '05, 15; 1Q, '05, 9
　　　　P96.89 Oth spec conditions originating perinatal period　　I-10

779.9 Unspecified condition originating in the perinatal period　　　N
　　Congenital debility NOS
　　Stillbirth NEC

---

16. Symptoms, Signs, and Ill-Defined Conditions (780-799)

This section includes symptoms, signs, abnormal results of laboratory or other investigative procedures, and ill-defined conditions regarding which no diagnosis classifiable elsewhere is recorded.

Signs and symptoms that point rather definitely to a given diagnosis are assigned to some category in the preceding part of the classification. In general, categories 780-796 include the more ill-defined conditions and symptoms that point with perhaps equal suspicion to two or more diseases or to two or more systems of the body, and without the necessary study of the case to make a final diagnosis. Practically all categories in this group could be designated as "not otherwise specified," or as "unknown etiology," or as "transient." The Alphabetic Index should be consulted to determine which symptoms and signs are to be allocated here and which to more specific sections of the classification; the residual subcategories numbered .9 are provided for other relevant symptoms which cannot be allocated elsewhere in the classification.

The conditions and signs or symptoms included in categories 780-796 consist of: (a) cases for which no more specific diagnosis can be made even after all facts bearing on the case have been investigated; (b) signs or symptoms existing at the time of initial encounter that proved to be transient and whose causes could not be determined; (c) provisional diagnoses in a patient who failed to return for further investigation or care; (d) cases referred elsewhere for investigation or treatment before the diagnosis was made; (e) cases in which a more precise diagnosis was not available for any other reason; (f) certain symptoms which represent important problems in medical care and which it might be desired to classify in addition to a known cause.

AHA: 3Q, '11, 12

Symptoms (780-789)

AHA: 1Q, '91, 12; 2Q, '90, 3; 2Q, '90, 5; 2Q, '90, 15; M-A, '85, 3

√4th 780 General symptoms

√5th 780.0 Alteration of consciousness

EXCLUDES alteration of consciousness due to:
intracranial injuries (850.0-854.19)
skull fractures (800.00-801.99, 803.00-804.99)
coma:
diabetic (249.2-249.3, 250.2-250.3)
hepatic (572.2)
originating in the perinatal period (779.2)

AHA: 4Q, '92, 20

780.01 Coma

DEF: State of unconsciousness from which the patient cannot be awakened.
AHA: ▶3Q, '13, 10;◄ 1Q, '12, 14; 3Q, '96, 16
TIP: Although found in the symptoms and signs chapter, coma is not inherent in other conditions and should be reported whenever appropriately documented.

780.02 Transient alteration of awareness

DEF: Temporary, recurring spells of reduced consciousness.

780.03 Persistent vegetative state

DEF: Persistent wakefulness without consciousness due to nonfunctioning cerebral cortex.

780.09 Other

Drowsiness
Semicoma
Somnolence
Stupor
Unconsciousness
R40.1 Stupor   I-10

780.1 Hallucinations

Hallucinations:
NOS
auditory
gustatory
olfactory
tactile

EXCLUDES those associated with mental disorders, as functional psychoses (295.0-298.9)
organic brain syndromes (290.0-294.9, 310.0-310.9)
visual hallucinations (368.16)

DEF: Perception of external stimulus in absence of stimulus; inability to distinguish between real and imagined.

780.2 Syncope and collapse

Blackout
Fainting
(Near) (Pre) syncope
Vasovagal attack

EXCLUDES carotid sinus syncope (337.0)
heat syncope (992.1)
neurocirculatory asthenia (306.2)
orthostatic hypotension (458.0)
shock NOS (785.50)

DEF: Sudden unconsciousness due to reduced blood flow to brain.
AHA: 1Q, '02, 6; 3Q, '00, 12; 4Q, '95, 42; 3Q, '95, 14; N-D, '85, 12
R55 Syncope and collapse   I-10

√5th 780.3 Convulsions

EXCLUDES convulsions:
epileptic (345.10-345.91)
in newborn (779.0)

DEF: Sudden, involuntary contractions of the muscles.
AHA: 2Q, '12, 9; 2Q, '97, 8; 1Q, '97, 12; 3Q, '94, 9; 1Q, '93, 24; 4Q, '92, 23; N-D, '87, 12

780.31 Febrile convulsions (simple), unspecified

Febrile seizure NOS
AHA: 4Q, '97, 45

780.32 Complex febrile convulsions

Febrile seizure:
atypical
complex
complicated

EXCLUDES status epilepticus (345.3)
AHA: 4Q, '06, 106

780.33 Post traumatic seizures

EXCLUDES post traumatic epilepsy (345.00-345.91)
AHA: ▶4Q, '13, 86;◄ 4Q, '10, 92-93

780.39 Other convulsions

Convulsive disorder NOS
Fit NOS
Recurrent convulsions NOS
Seizure NOS

AHA: ▶4Q, '13, 89;◄ 2Q, '12, 9; 2Q, '11, 5; 1Q, '08, 17; 3Q, '06, 22; 4Q, '04, 51; 1Q, '03, 7; 2Q, '99, 17; 4Q, '98, 39
R56.9 Unspecified convulsions   I-10

780.4 Dizziness and giddiness

Light-headedness
Vertigo NOS

EXCLUDES Ménière's disease and other specified vertiginous syndromes (386.0-386.9)

DEF: Whirling sensations in head with feeling of falling.
AHA: 2Q, '03, 11; 3Q, '00, 12; 2Q, '97, 9; 2Q, '91, 17
R42 Dizziness and giddiness   I-10

√5th 780.5 Sleep disturbances

EXCLUDES circadian rhythm sleep disorders (327.30-327.39)
organic hypersomnia (327.10-327.19)
organic insomnia (327.00-327.09)
organic sleep apnea (327.20-327.29)
organic sleep related movement disorders (327.51-327.59)
parasomnias (327.40-327.49)
that of nonorganic origin (307.40-307.49)

AHA: 4Q, '05, 59

780.50 Sleep disturbance, unspecified

780.51 Insomnia with sleep apnea, unspecified

DEF: Transient cessation of breathing disturbing sleep.

780.52 Insomnia, unspecified

DEF: Inability to maintain adequate sleep cycle.
G47.00 Insomnia unspecified   I-10

780.53 Hypersomnia with sleep apnea, unspecified

DEF: Autonomic response inhibited during sleep; causes insufficient oxygen intake, acidosis and pulmonary hypertension.
AHA: 1Q, '93, 28; N-D, '85, 4

780.54 Hypersomnia, unspecified

DEF: Prolonged sleep cycle.

780.55 Disruptions of 24 hour sleep wake cycle, unspecified

√4th √5th Additional Digit Required   **Unspecified Code**   Other Specified Code   Manifestation Code   ►◄ Revised Text   ● New Code   ▲ Revised Code Title

2015 ICD-9-CM   **October 2014 • Volume 1 – 261**

780.56 Dysfunctions associated with sleep stages or arousal from sleep

780.57 Unspecified sleep apnea

AHA: 1Q, '01, 6 ; 1Q, '97, 5; 1Q, '93, 28

G47.30 Sleep apnea unspecified   I-10

780.58 Sleep related movement disorder, unspecified

EXCLUDES restless legs syndrome (333.94)

AHA: 4Q, '04, 95

780.59 Other

780.6 Fever and other physiologic disturbances of temperature regulation

EXCLUDES effects of reduced environmental temperature (991.0-991.9)
effects of heat and light (992.0-992.9)
fever, chills or hypothermia associated with confirmed infection — code to infection

AHA: 4Q, '08,140-142; 3Q, '05, 16; 3Q, '00,13; 4Q, '99, 26; 2Q, '91, 8

780.60 Fever, unspecified

Chills with fever
Fever NOS
Fever of unknown origin (FUO)
Hyperpyrexia NOS
Pyrexia NOS
Pyrexia of unknown origin

EXCLUDES chills without fever (780.64)
neonatal fever (778.4)
pyrexia of unknown origin (during):
in newborn (778.4)
labor (659.2)
the puerperium (672)

R50.9 Fever unspecified   I-10

780.61 Fever presenting with conditions classified elsewhere

Code first underlying condition when associated fever is present, such as with:
leukemia (conditions classifiable to 204-208)
neutropenia (288.00-288.09)
sickle-cell disease (282.60-282.69)

AHA: 2Q, '12, 18; 4Q, '08, 142

780.62 Postprocedural fever

EXCLUDES posttransfusion fever (780.66)
postvaccination fever (780.63)

TIP: Do not assign a code from category 998 for post-procedural fever.

780.63 Postvaccination fever

Postimmunization fever

780.64 Chills (without fever)

Chills NOS

EXCLUDES chills with fever (780.60)

780.65 Hypothermia not associated with low environmental temperature

EXCLUDES hypothermia:
associated with low environmental temperature (991.6)
due to anesthesia (995.89)
of newborn (778.2, 778.3)

780.66 Febrile nonhemolytic transfusion reaction

FNHTR
Posttransfusion fever

AHA: 4Q, '10, 99-100

780.7 Malaise and fatigue

EXCLUDES debility, unspecified (799.3)
fatigue (during):
combat (308.0-308.9)
heat (992.6)
pregnancy (646.8)
neurasthenia (300.5)
senile asthenia (797)

AHA: 4Q, '88, 12; M-A, '87, 8

780.71 Chronic fatigue syndrome

DEF: Persistent fatigue, symptoms include weak muscles, sore throat, lymphadenitis, headache, depression and mild fever; no known cause; also called chronic mononucleosis, benign myalgic encephalomyelitis, Iceland disease and neurosthenia.

AHA: 4Q, '98, 48

780.72 Functional quadriplegia

Complete immobility due to severe physical disability or frailty

EXCLUDES hysterical paralysis (300.11)
immobility syndrome (728.3)
neurologic quadriplegia (344.00-344.09)
quadriplegia NOS (344.00)

DEF: Inability to move due to another condition such as dementia, severe contractures, or arthritis, not a physiologic one; no mental ability to move independently; typically found in severely demented patients.

AHA: 4Q, '08, 143

TIP: The functional quadriplegic patient typically has severe dementia and the quadriplegia will be due to a nonneurologic condition.

780.79 Other malaise and fatigue

Asthenia NOS   Postviral (asthenic) syndrome
Lethargy   Tiredness

DEF: Asthenia: Any weakness, lack of strength or loss of energy, especially neuromuscular.
DEF: Lethargy: Listlessness, drowsiness, stupor and apathy.
DEF: Malaise: Vague feeling of debility or lack of good health.
DEF: Postviral (asthenic) syndrome: Listlessness, drowsiness, stupor and apathy; follows acute viral infection.
DEF: Tiredness: General exhaustion or fatigue.

AHA: 4Q, '04, 78; 1Q, '00, 6; 4Q, '99, 26

R53.83 Other fatigue   I-10

780.8 Generalized hyperhidrosis

Diaphoresis   Secondary hyperhidrosis
Excessive sweating

EXCLUDES focal (localized) (primary) (secondary) hyperhidrosis (705.21-705.22)
Frey's syndrome (705.22)

DEF: Excessive sweating, appears as droplets on skin; general or localized.

780.9 Other general symptoms

EXCLUDES hypothermia:
NOS (accidental) (991.6)
due to anesthesia (995.89)
of newborn (778.2-778.3)
memory disturbance as part of a pattern of mental disorder

AHA: 4Q, '02, 67; 4Q, '99, 10; 3Q, '93, 11; N-D, '85, 12

780.91 Fussy infant (baby)   P

780.92 Excessive crying of infant (baby)   N

EXCLUDES excessive crying of child, adolescent or adult (780.95)

780.93 Memory loss

Amnesia (retrograde)
Memory loss NOS

EXCLUDES memory loss due to:
intracranial injuries (850.0-854.19)
skull fractures (800.00-801.99, 803.00-804.99)
mild memory disturbance due to organic brain damage (310.89)
transient global amnesia (437.7)

AHA: 4Q, '03, 71

780.94 Early satiety
DEF: The premature feeling of being full; mechanism of satiety is multifactorial.
AHA: 4Q, '03, 72

780.95 Excessive crying of child, adolescent, or adult
EXCLUDES   excessive crying of infant (baby) (780.92)
AHA: 4Q, '05, 89

780.96 Generalized pain
Pain NOS
AHA: 4Q, '06, 79-81
TIP: For pain syndromes, refer to category 338; if site is specified, refer to index.

780.97 Altered mental status
Change in mental status
EXCLUDES   altered level of consciousness (780.01-780.09)
     altered mental status due to known condition — code to condition
     delirium NOS (780.09)
AHA: 4Q, '06, 107
R41.82 Altered mental status unspecified   I-10

780.99 Other general symptoms
AHA: 4Q, '03, 103

√4ᵗʰ **781 Symptoms involving nervous and musculoskeletal systems**
EXCLUDES   depression NOS (311)
     disorders specifically relating to:
       back (724.0-724.9)
       hearing (388.0-389.9)
       joint (718.0-719.9)
       limb (729.0-729.9)
       neck (723.0-723.9)
       vision (368.0-369.9)
     pain in limb (729.5)

781.0 Abnormal involuntary movements
Abnormal head movements   Spasms NOS
Fasciculation   Tremor NOS
EXCLUDES   abnormal reflex (796.1)
     chorea NOS (333.5)
     infantile spasms (345.60-345.61)
     spastic paralysis (342.1, 343.0-344.9)
     specified movement disorders classifiable to 333 (333.0-333.9)
     that of nonorganic origin (307.2-307.3)
R25.9 Unspecified abnormal involuntary movements   I-10

781.1 Disturbances of sensation of smell and taste
Anosmia   Parosmia
Parageusia
DEF: Anosmia: loss of sense of smell due to organic factors, including loss of olfactory nerve conductivity, cerebral disease, nasal fossae formation and peripheral olfactory nerve diseases; can also be psychological disorder.
DEF: Parageusia: distorted sense of taste, or bad taste in mouth.
DEF: Parosmia: distorted sense of smell.

781.2 Abnormality of gait
Gait: Gait:
   ataxic   spastic
   paralytic   staggering
EXCLUDES   ataxia:
     NOS (781.3)
     locomotor (progressive) (094.0)
     difficulty in walking (719.7)
DEF: Abnormal, asymmetric gait.
AHA: 1Q, '11, 9; 2Q, '05, 6; 2Q, '04, 15
TIP: If the patient's gait abnormality is due to a joint problem, refer to code 719.7 Difficulty in walking.
R26.9 Unspecified abnormalities of gait and mobility   I-10

781.3 Lack of coordination
Ataxia NOS
Muscular incoordination
EXCLUDES   ataxic gait (781.2)
     cerebellar ataxia (334.0-334.9)
     difficulty in walking (719.7)
     vertigo NOS (780.4)
AHA: 4Q, '04, 51; 3Q, '97, 12

781.4 Transient paralysis of limb
Monoplegia, transient NOS
EXCLUDES   paralysis (342.0-344.9)

781.5 Clubbing of fingers
DEF: Enlarged soft tissue of distal fingers.

781.6 Meningismus
Dupré's syndrome
Meningism
DEF: Condition with signs and symptoms that resemble meningeal irritation; it is associated with febrile illness and dehydration with no evidence of infection.
AHA: 3Q, '00,13; J-F, '87, 7

781.7 Tetany
Carpopedal spasm
EXCLUDES   tetanus neonatorum (771.3)
     tetany:
       hysterical (300.11)
       newborn (hypocalcemic) (775.4)
       parathyroid (252.1)
       psychogenic (306.0)
DEF: Nerve and muscle hyperexcitability; symptoms include muscle spasms, twitching, cramps, laryngospasm with inspiratory stridor, hyperreflexia and choreiform movements.

781.8 Neurologic neglect syndrome
Asomatognosia   Left-sided neglect
Hemi-akinesia   Sensory extinction
Hemi-inattention   Sensory neglect
Hemispatial neglect   Visuospatial neglect
EXCLUDES   visuospatial deficit (799.53)
AHA: 4Q, '94, 37
TIP: If documented as sequelae of a CVA, assign also a code from category 438.

√5ᵗʰ **781.9 Other symptoms involving nervous and musculoskeletal systems**
AHA: 4Q, '00, 45

781.91 Loss of height
EXCLUDES   osteoporosis (733.00-733.09)

781.92 Abnormal posture

781.93 Ocular torticollis
DEF: Abnormal head posture as a result of a contracted state of cervical muscles to correct a visual disturbance; either double vision or a visual field defect.
AHA: 4Q, '02, 68

781.94 Facial weakness
Facial droop
EXCLUDES   facial weakness due to late effect of cerebrovascular accident (438.83)
AHA: 4Q, '03, 72
TIP: Do not assign if facial droop or weakness is due to Bell's palsy; see instead code 351.0.
R29.810 Facial weakness   I-10

781.99 Other symptoms involving nervous and musculoskeletal systems

√4ᵗʰ **782 Symptoms involving skin and other integumentary tissue**
EXCLUDES   symptoms relating to breast (611.71-611.79)

782.0 Disturbance of skin sensation
Anesthesia of skin   Hypoesthesia
Burning or prickling   Numbness
   sensation   Paresthesia
Hyperesthesia   Tingling
R20.9 Unspecified disturbances of skin sensation   I-10

782.1 Rash and other nonspecific skin eruption
Exanthem
EXCLUDES   vesicular eruption (709.8)
AHA: 4Q, '08, 99

782.2 Localized superficial swelling, mass, or lump
Subcutaneous nodules
EXCLUDES   localized adiposity (278.1)

√4ᵗʰ
√5ᵗʰ
Additional Digit Required   Unspecified Code   Other Specified Code   Manifestation Code   ▶◀ Revised Text   ● New Code   ▲ Revised Code Title

2015 ICD-9-CM   **Volume 1 – 263**

Symptoms, Signs, and Ill-Defined Conditions

782.3–784.2

782.3 Edema
Anasarca   Localized edema NOS
Dropsy
     EXCLUDES   *ascites (789.51-789.59)*
               edema of:
                  newborn NOS (778.5)
                  pregnancy (642.0-642.9, 646.1)
                fluid retention (276.69)
                hydrops fetalis (773.3, 778.0)
                hydrothorax (511.81-511.89)
                nutritional edema (260, 262)
     DEF: Edema: excess fluid in intercellular body tissue.
     DEF: Anasarca: massive edema in all body tissues.
     DEF: Dropsy: serous fluid accumulated in body cavity or cellular tissue.
     DEF: Localized edema: edema in specific body areas.
     AHA: 2Q, '00, 18
     R60.9 Edema unspecified   `I-10`

782.4 Jaundice, unspecified, not of newborn
Cholemia NOS
Icterus NOS
     EXCLUDES   *jaundice in newborn (774.0-774.7)*
                due to isoimmunization (773.0-773.2, 773.4)
     DEF: Bilirubin deposits of skin, causing yellow cast.
     R17 Unspecified jaundice   `I-10`

782.5 Cyanosis
     EXCLUDES   *newborn (770.83)*
     DEF: Deficient oxygen of blood; causes blue cast to skin.

✓5ᵗʰ 782.6 Pallor and flushing

782.61 Pallor

782.62 Flushing
Excessive blushing

782.7 Spontaneous ecchymoses
Petechiae
     EXCLUDES   *ecchymosis in fetus or newborn (772.6)*
                purpura (287.0-287.9)
     DEF: Hemorrhagic spots of skin; resemble freckles.

782.8 Changes in skin texture
Induration   } of skin
Thickening

782.9 Other symptoms involving skin and integumentary tissues

✓4ᵗʰ 783 Symptoms concerning nutrition, metabolism, and development

783.0 Anorexia
Loss of appetite
     EXCLUDES   *anorexia nervosa (307.1)*
                loss of appetite of nonorganic origin (307.59)
     R63.0 Anorexia   `I-10`

783.1 Abnormal weight gain
     EXCLUDES   *excessive weight gain in pregnancy (646.1)*
                obesity (278.00)
                morbid (278.01)

✓5ᵗʰ 783.2 Abnormal loss of weight and underweight
Use additional code to identify Body Mass Index (BMI), if known (V85.0-V85.54)
     AHA: 4Q, '00, 45

783.21 Loss of weight
     AHA: 4Q, '05, 96
     R63.4 Abnormal weight loss   `I-10`

783.22 Underweight
     AHA: 4Q, '05, 96

783.3 Feeding difficulties and mismanagement
Feeding problem (elderly) (infant)
     EXCLUDES   *feeding disturbance or problems:*
                in newborn (779.31-779.34)
                of nonorganic origin (307.50-307.59
     AHA: 3Q, '97, 12

✓5ᵗʰ 783.4 Lack of expected normal physiological development in childhood
     EXCLUDES   *delay in sexual development and puberty (259.0)*
                gonadal dysgenesis (758.6)
                pituitary dwarfism (253.3)
                slow fetal growth and fetal malnutrition (764.00-764.99)
                specific delays in mental development (315.0-315.9)
     AHA: 4Q, '00, 45; 3Q, '97, 4

783.40 Lack of normal physiological development, unspecified
Inadequate development
Lack of development

783.41 Failure to thrive   `P`
Failure to gain weight
     EXCLUDES   *failure to thrive in newborn (779.34)*
     DEF: Organic failure to thrive: acute or chronic illness that interferes with nutritional intake, absorption, metabolism excretion and energy requirements. Nonorganic FTT is symptom of neglect or abuse.
     AHA: 1Q, '03, 12

783.42 Delayed milestones   `P`
Late talker
Late walker

783.43 Short stature
Growth failure   Lack of growth
Growth retardation   Physical retardation
     DEF: Constitutional short stature: stature inconsistent with chronological age. Genetic short stature is when skeletal maturation matches chronological age.

783.5 Polydipsia
Excessive thirst

783.6 Polyphagia
Excessive eating
Hyperalimentation NOS
     EXCLUDES   *disorders of eating of nonorganic origin (307.50-307.59)*

783.7 Adult failure to thrive   `A`
     R62.7 Adult failure to thrive   `I-10`

783.9 Other symptoms concerning nutrition, metabolism, and development
Hypometabolism
     EXCLUDES   *abnormal basal metabolic rate (794.7)*
                dehydration (276.51)
                other disorders of fluid, electrolyte, and acid-base balance (276.0-276.9)
     AHA: 2Q, '04, 3

✓4ᵗʰ 784 Symptoms involving head and neck
     EXCLUDES   *encephalopathy NOS (348.30)*
                specific symptoms involving neck classifiable to 723 (723.0-723.9)

784.0 Headache
Facial pain
Pain in head NOS
     EXCLUDES   *atypical face pain (350.2)*
                migraine (346.0-346.9)
                tension headache (307.81)
     AHA: 3Q, '06, 22; 2Q, '06, 17; 3Q, '00, 13; 1Q, '90, 4; 3Q, '92, 14
     TIP: Do not assign if headache syndrome has been diagnosed, refer to category 339.
     R51 Headache   `I-10`

784.1 Throat pain
     EXCLUDES   *dysphagia (787.20-787.29)*
                neck pain (723.1)
                sore throat (462)
                chronic (472.1)

784.2 Swelling, mass, or lump in head and neck
Space-occupying lesion, intracranial NOS
     AHA: 1Q, '03, 8

N Newborn Age: 0   **P** Pediatric Age: 0-17   **M** Maternity Age: 12-55   **A** Adult Age: 15-124

784.3 Aphasia

    EXCLUDES *aphasia due to late effects of cerebrovascular disease (438.11)*
        developmental aphasia (315.31)

    DEF: Inability to communicate through speech, written word, or sign language.

    AHA: 3Q, '10, 5; 4Q, '04, 78; 4Q, '98, 87; 3Q, '97, 12

    R47.01 Aphasia   **I-10**

✓5th 784.4 Voice and resonance disorders

    AHA: 4Q, '09, 102-103

    784.40 Voice and resonance disorder, unspecified

    784.41 Aphonia
        Loss of voice

    784.42 Dysphonia
        Hoarseness

    784.43 Hypernasality

    784.44 Hyponasality

    784.49 Other voice and resonance disorders
        Change in voice

✓5th 784.5 Other speech disturbance

    EXCLUDES *speech disorder due to late effect of cerebrovascular accident (438.10-438.19)*
        stuttering (315.35)

    AHA: 4Q, '09, 87-88

    784.51 Dysarthria

        EXCLUDES *dysarthria due to late effect of cerebrovascular accident (438.13)*

    784.52 *Fluency disorder in conditions classified elsewhere*
        Stuttering in conditions classified elsewhere

        Code first underlying disease or condition, such as:
        Parkinson's disease (332.0)

        EXCLUDES *adult onset fluency disorder (307.0)*
            childhood onset fluency disorder (315.35)
            fluency disorder due to late effect of cerebrovascular accident (438.14)

        AHA: 4Q, '10, 83-84

    784.59 Other speech disturbance
        Dysphasia
        Slurred speech
        Speech disturbance NOS
        R47.89 Other speech disturbances   **I-10**

✓5th 784.6 Other symbolic dysfunction

    EXCLUDES *developmental learning delays (315.0-315.9)*

    784.60 Symbolic dysfunction, unspecified

    784.61 Alexia and dyslexia
        Alexia (with agraphia)
        DEF: Alexia: Inability to understand written word due to central brain lesion.
        DEF: Dyslexia: Ability to recognize letters but inability to read, spell, and write words; genetic.

    784.69 Other
        Acalculia   Agraphia NOS
        Agnosia   Apraxia

784.7 Epistaxis
    Hemorrhage from nose
    Nosebleed
    AHA: 3Q, '04, 7
    R04.0 Epistaxis   **I-10**

784.8 Hemorrhage from throat
    EXCLUDES *hemoptysis (786.30-786.39)*

✓5th 784.9 Other symptoms involving head and neck

    784.91 Postnasal drip
        AHA: 4Q, '06, 108

    784.92 Jaw pain
        Mandibular pain
        Maxilla pain
        EXCLUDES *temporomandibular joint arthralgia (524.62)*
        AHA: 4Q, '10, 93-94
        R68.84 Jaw pain

784.99 Other symptoms involving head and neck
    Choking sensation
    Feeling of foreign body in throat
    Halitosis
    Mouth breathing
    Sneezing
    EXCLUDES *foreign body in throat (933.0)*
    AHA: 4Q, '06, 108

✓4th 785 Symptoms involving cardiovascular system

    EXCLUDES *heart failure NOS (428.9)*

    785.0 Tachycardia, unspecified
        Rapid heart beat
        EXCLUDES *neonatal tachycardia (779.82)*
            paroxysmal tachycardia (427.0-427.2)
        DEF: Excessively rapid heart rate.
        AHA: 2Q, '03, 11
        R00.0 Tachycardia unspecified   **I-10**

    785.1 Palpitations
        Awareness of heart beat
        EXCLUDES *specified dysrhythmias (427.0-427.9)*
        R00.2 Palpitations   **I-10**

    785.2 Undiagnosed cardiac murmurs
        Heart murmurs NOS
        AHA: 4Q, '92, 16
        R01.1 Cardiac murmur unspecified   **I-10**

    785.3 Other abnormal heart sounds
        Cardiac dullness, increased or decreased
        Friction fremitus, cardiac
        Precordial friction

    785.4 Gangrene
        Gangrene: Gangrenous cellulitis
          NOS   Phagedena
          spreading cutaneous
        Code first any associated underlying condition
        EXCLUDES *gangrene of certain sites — see Alphabetic Index*
            gangrene with atherosclerosis of the extremities (440.24)
            gas gangrene (040.0)
        DEF: Gangrene: necrosis of skin tissue due to bacterial infection, diabetes, embolus and vascular supply loss.
        DEF: Gangrenous cellulitis: group A streptococcal infection; begins with severe cellulitis, spreads to superficial and deep fascia; produces gangrene of underlying tissues.
        AHA: ▶4Q, '13, 83;◀ 1Q, '04, 14; 3Q, '91, 12; 3Q, '90, 15; M-A, '86, 12
        I96 Gangrene not elsewhere classified   **I-10**

    ✓5th 785.5 Shock without mention of trauma

        785.50 Shock, unspecified
            Failure of peripheral circulation
            DEF: Peripheral circulatory failure due to heart insufficiencies.
            AHA: 2Q, '96, 10

        785.51 Cardiogenic shock
            DEF: Shock syndrome: associated with myocardial infarction, cardiac tamponade and massive pulmonary embolism; symptoms include mental confusion, reduced blood pressure, tachycardia, pallor and cold, clammy skin.
            AHA: 4Q, '08, 182; 3Q, '05, 14
            R57.0 Cardiogenic shock   **I-10**

        785.52 *Septic shock*
            Shock:
              endotoxic
              gram-negative
            Code first underlying infection
            Use additional code, if applicable, to identify systemic inflammatory response syndrome due to infectious process with organ dysfunction (995.92)
            AHA: ▶2Q, '13, 21;◀ 2Q, '10, 4; 4Q, '08, 99; 4Q, '06, 113; 2Q, '05, 18-19; 4Q, '03, 73, 79
            TIP: The diagnosis of septic shock indicates the presence of severe sepsis; code 785.52 should not be assigned without first assigning code 995.92.

| ✓4th ✓5th Additional Digit Required | Unspecified Code | Other Specified Code | Manifestation Code | ▶◀ Revised Text | ● New Code | ▲ Revised Code Title |

2015 ICD-9-CM   **October 2014 • Volume 1 – 265**

Symptoms, Signs, and Ill-Defined Conditions

785.59–786.9

785.59 Other
Shock:
hypovolemic
EXCLUDES   *shock (due to):*
anesthetic (995.4)
anaphylactic (995.0)
due to serum (999.41-999.49)
electric (994.8)
following abortion (639.5)
lightning (994.0)
obstetrical (669.1)
postoperative (998.00-998.09)
traumatic (958.4)
AHA: 2Q, '00, 3

785.6 Enlargement of lymph nodes
Lymphadenopathy
"Swollen glands"
EXCLUDES   *lymphadenitis (chronic) (289.1-289.3)*
acute (683)
R59.9 Enlarged lymph nodes unspecified   `I-10`

785.9 Other symptoms involving cardiovascular system
Bruit (arterial)
Weak pulse

√4ᵗʰ **786 Symptoms involving respiratory system and other chest symptoms**

√5ᵗʰ **786.0 Dyspnea and respiratory abnormalities**

786.00 Respiratory abnormality, unspecified

786.01 Hyperventilation
EXCLUDES   *hyperventilation, psychogenic (306.1)*
DEF: Rapid breathing causes carbon dioxide loss from blood.

786.02 Orthopnea
DEF: Difficulty breathing except in upright position.

786.03 Apnea
EXCLUDES   *apnea of newborn (770.81, 770.82)*
sleep apnea (780.51, 780.53, 780.57)
DEF: Cessation of breathing.
AHA: 4Q, '98, 50

786.04 Cheyne-Stokes respiration
DEF: Rhythmic increase of depth and frequency of breathing with apnea; occurs in frontal lobe and diencephalic dysfunction.
AHA: 4Q, '98, 50

786.05 Shortness of breath
DEF: Inability to take in sufficient oxygen.
AHA: 4Q, '99, 25; 1Q, '99, 6; 4Q, '98, 50
R06.02 Shortness of breath   `I-10`

786.06 Tachypnea
EXCLUDES   *transitory tachypnea of newborn (770.6)*
DEF: Abnormal rapid respiratory rate; called hyperventilation.
AHA: 1Q, '11, 16-17; 4Q, '98, 50

786.07 Wheezing
EXCLUDES   *asthma (493.00-493.92)*
DEF: Stenosis of respiratory passageway; causes whistling sound; due to asthma, coryza, croup, emphysema, hay fever, edema, and pleural effusion.
AHA: 4Q, '98, 50

786.09 Other
Respiratory:
distress
insufficiency
EXCLUDES   *respiratory distress:*
following trauma and surgery (518.52)
newborn (770.89)
syndrome (newborn) (769)
adult (518.52)
respiratory failure (518.81, 518.83-518.84)
newborn (770.84)
AHA: 4Q, '05, 90; 2Q, '98, 10; 1Q, '97, 7; 1Q, '90, 9
R06.00 Dyspnea, unspecified   `I-10`

786.1 Stridor
EXCLUDES   *congenital laryngeal stridor (748.3)*
DEF: Obstructed airway causes harsh sound.

786.2 Cough
EXCLUDES   *cough:*
psychogenic (306.1)
smokers' (491.0)
with hemorrhage (786.39)
AHA: 4Q, '99, 26
R05 Cough   `I-10`

√5ᵗʰ **786.3 Hemoptysis**
DEF: Coughing up blood or blood-stained sputum.
AHA: 3Q, '11, 12; 4Q, '10, 94-95; 2Q, '06, 17; 4Q, '90, 26

786.30 Hemoptysis, unspecified
Pulmonary hemorrhage NOS
AHA: ▶4Q, '13, 83◀
R04.2 Hemoptysis   `I-10`

786.31 Acute idiopathic pulmonary hemorrhage in infants [AIPHI]   `P`
Acute idiopathic pulmonary hemorrhage in infant over 28 days old
EXCLUDES   *pulmonary hemorrhage of newborn under 28 days old (770.3)*
von Willebrand's disease (286.4)
DEF: An abrupt onset of bleeding or blood in the airway with acute respiratory distress or failure in a patient with no prior history of an identifiable causal condition.
R04.81 Acute idiopathic pulmonary hemorrhage in infants

786.39 Other hemoptysis
Cough with hemorrhage
R04.89 Hemorrhage from othr site in resp passages   `I-10`

786.4 Abnormal sputum
Abnormal:
amount
color   } (of) sputum
odor
Excessive

√5ᵗʰ **786.5 Chest pain**

786.50 Chest pain, unspecified
AHA: 1Q, '07, 19; 2Q, '06, 7; 1Q, '03, 6; 1Q, '02, 4; 4Q, '99, 25
R07.9 Chest pain unspecified   `I-10`

786.51 Precordial pain
DEF: Chest pain over heart and lower thorax.

786.52 Painful respiration
Pain: Pleurodynia
anterior chest wall
pleuritic
EXCLUDES   *epidemic pleurodynia (074.1)*
AHA: N-D, '84, 17
R07.1 Chest pain on breathing   `I-10`

786.59 Other
Discomfort
Pressure   } in chest
Tightness
EXCLUDES   *pain in breast (611.71)*
AHA: 1Q, '02, 6
TIP: Assign for chest pain due to anxiety, along with an additional code for anxiety. Chest pain is not integral to the diagnosis of anxiety.
R07.89 Other chest pain   `I-10`

786.6 Swelling, mass, or lump in chest
EXCLUDES   *lump in breast (611.72)*
R22.2 Localized swelling, mass, lump, trunk   `I-10`

786.7 Abnormal chest sounds
Abnormal percussion, chest   Rales
Friction sounds, chest   Tympany, chest
EXCLUDES   *wheezing (786.07)*

786.8 Hiccough
EXCLUDES   *psychogenic hiccough (306.1)*

786.9 Other symptoms involving respiratory system and chest
Breath-holding spell

`N` Newborn Age: 0   `P` Pediatric Age: 0-17   `M` Maternity Age: 12-55   `A` Adult Age: 15-124

☑️4ᵗʰ **787 Symptoms involving digestive system**
EXCLUDES constipation (564.00-564.09)
pylorospasm (537.81)
congenital (750.5)

☑️5ᵗʰ **787.0 Nausea and vomiting**
Emesis
EXCLUDES hematemesis NOS (578.0)
vomiting:
bilious, following gastrointestinal surgery (564.3)
cyclical (536.2)
associated with migraine (346.2)
psychogenic (306.4)
excessive, in pregnancy (643.0-643.9)
fecal matter (569.87)
habit (536.2)
of newborn (779.32, 779.33)
persistent (536.2)
psychogenic NOS (307.54)
AHA: M-A, '85, 11

787.01 Nausea with vomiting
AHA: 1Q, '03, 5
R11.2 Nausea with vomiting, unspecified I-10

787.02 Nausea alone
AHA: 3Q, '00, 12; 2Q, '97, 9
R11.0 Nausea alone I-10

787.03 Vomiting alone
787.04 Bilious emesis
Bilious vomiting
EXCLUDES bilious emesis (vomiting) in newborn (779.32)
AHA: 4Q, '09, 103-104

787.1 Heartburn
Pyrosis Waterbrash
EXCLUDES dyspepsia or indigestion (536.8)
AHA: 2Q, '01, 6

☑️5ᵗʰ **787.2 Dysphagia**
Code first, if applicable, dysphagia due to late effect of cerebrovascular accident (438.82)
AHA: 4Q, '07, 92-94; 3Q, '07, 7; 4Q, '03, 103, 109; 2Q, '01, 4

787.20 Dysphagia, unspecified
Difficulty in swallowing NOS

787.21 Dysphagia, oral phase
787.22 Dysphagia, oropharyngeal phase
AHA: 4Q, '07, 94

787.23 Dysphagia, pharyngeal phase
787.24 Dysphagia, pharyngoesophageal phase
787.29 Other dysphagia
Cervical dysphagia
Neurogenic dysphagia
R13.19 Other dysphagia I-10

Phases of Swallowing

Oral phase

Oropharyngeal phase

Pharyngeal phase

Pharyngeoesophageal phase

787.3 Flatulence, eructation, and gas pain
Abdominal distention (gaseous)
Bloating
Tympanites (abdominal) (intestinal)
EXCLUDES aerophagy (306.4)
DEF: Flatulence: excess air or gas in intestine or stomach,
DEF: Eructation: belching, expelling gas through mouth.
DEF: Gas pain: gaseous pressure affecting gastrointestinal system.

787.4 Visible peristalsis
Hyperperistalsis
DEF: Increase in involuntary movements of intestines.

787.5 Abnormal bowel sounds
Absent bowel sounds
Hyperactive bowel sounds

☑️5ᵗʰ **787.6 Incontinence of feces**
Encopresis NOS
Incontinence of sphincter ani
EXCLUDES that of nonorganic origin (307.7)
AHA: 4Q, '10, 87-89; 1Q, '97, 9

787.60 Full incontinence of feces
Fecal incontinence NOS
R15.9 Full incontinence of feces I-10

787.61 Incomplete defecation
EXCLUDES constipation (564.00-564.09)
fecal impaction (560.32)

787.62 Fecal smearing
Fecal soiling

787.63 Fecal urgency
R15.2 Fecal urgency

787.7 Abnormal feces
Bulky stools
EXCLUDES abnormal stool content (792.1)
melena:
NOS (578.1)
newborn (772.4, 777.3)

☑️5ᵗʰ **787.9 Other symptoms involving digestive system**
EXCLUDES gastrointestinal hemorrhage (578.0-578.9)
intestinal obstruction (560.0-560.9)
specific functional digestive disorders:
esophagus (530.0-530.9)
stomach and duodenum (536.0-536.9)
those not elsewhere classified (564.00-564.9)

787.91 Diarrhea
Diarrhea NOS
AHA: 2Q, '10, 12; 4Q, '08, 99; 4Q, '95, 54
R19.7 Diarrhea unspecified I-10

787.99 Other
Change in bowel habits
Tenesmus (rectal)
DEF: Tenesmus: Painful, ineffective straining at the rectum with limited passage of fecal matter.

☑️4ᵗʰ **788 Symptoms involving urinary system**
EXCLUDES hematuria (599.70-599.72)
nonspecific findings on examination of the urine (791.0-791.9)
small kidney of unknown cause (589.0-589.9)
uremia NOS (586)
urinary obstruction (599.60, 599.69)

788.0 Renal colic
Colic (recurrent) of:
kidney
ureter
DEF: Kidney pain.
AHA: 3Q, '04, 8
TIP: Do not assign if renal colic is due to calculus; see category 592.

788.1 Dysuria
Painful urination
Strangury

Symptoms, Signs, and Ill-Defined Conditions

787–788.1

√5ᵗʰ **788.2 Retention of urine**

Code, if applicable, any causal condition first, such as:
   hyperplasia of prostate (600.0-600.9 with fifth-digit 1)
DEF: Accumulation of urine in the bladder due to inability to void.

788.20 Retention of urine, unspecified
   AHA: ▶ 1Q, '13, 5;◀ 4Q, '06, 93, 95; 2Q, '04, 18; 3Q, '03, 12-13;
   1Q, '03, 6; 3Q, '96, 10
   R33.9 Retention of urine unspecified   I-10

788.21 Incomplete bladder emptying
   AHA: 4Q, '06, 93

788.29 Other specified retention of urine

√5ᵗʰ **788.3 Urinary incontinence**

Code, if applicable, any causal condition first, such as:
   congenital ureterocele (753.23)
   genital prolapse (618.00-618.9)
   hyperplasia of prostate (600.0-600.9 with fifth-digit 1)
EXCLUDES functional urinary incontinence (788.91)
   that of nonorganic origin (307.6)
   urinary incontinence associated with cognitive
   impairment (788.91)
   AHA: 4Q, '06, 93; 4Q, '92, 22

788.30 Urinary incontinence, unspecified
   Enuresis NOS
   AHA: 1Q, '09, 15
   R32 Unspecified urinary incontinence   I-10

788.31 Urge incontinence
   DEF: Inability to control urination, upon urge to urinate.
   AHA: 1Q, '00, 19

788.32 Stress incontinence, male   ♂
   EXCLUDES stress incontinence, female (625.6)
   DEF: Inability to control urination associated with weak
   sphincter in males.

788.33 Mixed incontinence, (male) (female)
   Urge and stress
   DEF: Urge, stress incontinence: involuntary discharge of
   urine due to anatomic displacement.

788.34 Incontinence without sensory awareness
   DEF: Involuntary discharge of urine without sensory
   warning.

788.35 Post-void dribbling
   DEF: Involuntary discharge of residual urine after voiding.

788.36 Nocturnal enuresis
   DEF: Involuntary discharge of urine during the night.

788.37 Continuous leakage
   DEF: Continuous, involuntary urine seepage.

788.38 Overflow incontinence
   DEF: Leakage caused by pressure of retained urine in the
   bladder after the bladder has fully contracted due to
   weakened bladder muscles or an obstruction of the
   urethra.

788.39 Other urinary incontinence

√5ᵗʰ **788.4 Frequency of urination and polyuria**

Code, if applicable, any causal condition first, such as:
   hyperplasia of prostate (600.0-600.9 with fifth-digit 1)

788.41 Urinary frequency
   Frequency of micturition
   AHA: 4Q, '06, 93

788.42 Polyuria
   DEF: Excessive urination.

788.43 Nocturia
   DEF: Urination affecting sleep patterns.
   AHA: 4Q, '06, 93

788.5 Oliguria and anuria
   Deficient secretion of urine
   Suppression of urinary secretion
   EXCLUDES that complicating:
      abortion (634-638 with .3, 639.3)
      ectopic or molar pregnancy (639.3)
      pregnancy, childbirth, or the puerperium
         (642.0-642.9, 646.2)
   DEF: Oliguria: diminished urinary secretion related to fluid intake.
   DEF: Anuria: lack of urinary secretion due to renal failure or
   obstructed urinary tract.

√5ᵗʰ **788.6 Other abnormality of urination**

Code, if applicable, any causal condition first, such as:
   hyperplasia of prostate (600.0-600.9 with fifth-digit 1)

788.61 Splitting of urinary stream
   Intermittent urinary stream

788.62 Slowing of urinary stream
   Weak stream
   AHA: 4Q, '06, 93

788.63 Urgency of urination
   EXCLUDES urge incontinence (788.31, 788.33)
   DEF: Feeling of intense need to urinate; abrupt sensation of
   imminent urination.
   AHA: 4Q, '06, 93; 4Q, '03, 74

788.64 Urinary hesitancy
   AHA: 4Q, '06, 93, 109

788.65 Straining on urination
   AHA: 4Q, '06, 93, 109

788.69 Other

788.7 Urethral discharge
   Penile discharge
   Urethrorrhea

788.8 Extravasation of urine
   DEF: Leaking or infiltration of urine into tissues.

√5ᵗʰ **788.9 Other symptoms involving urinary system**
   AHA: 1Q, '05, 12; 4Q, '88, 1

788.91 Functional urinary incontinence
   Urinary incontinence due to cognitive impairment, or
   severe physical disability or immobility
   EXCLUDES urinary incontinence due to physiologic
   condition (788.30-788.39)
   AHA: 4Q, '08, 144-145

788.99 Other symptoms involving urinary system
   Extrarenal uremia
   Vesical:
      pain
      tenesmus

√4ᵗʰ **789 Other symptoms involving abdomen and pelvis**
   EXCLUDES symptoms referable to genital organs:
      female (625.0-625.9)
      male (607.0-608.9)
      psychogenic (302.70-302.79)

The following fifth-digit subclassification is to be used for codes 789.0,
789.3, 789.4, 789.6:
   0 unspecified site
   1 right upper quadrant
   2 left upper quadrant
   3 right lower quadrant
   4 left lower quadrant
   5 periumbilic
   6 epigastric
   7 generalized
   9 other specified site
      Multiple sites

§ √5ᵗʰ **789.0 Abdominal pain**
   [0-7, 9]   Cramps, abdominal
   AHA: 1Q, '95, 3; **For code 789.06:** 1Q, '02, 5
   R10.9 Unspecified abdominal pain   I-10
   R10.31 Right lower quadrant pain   I-10
   R10.13 Epigastric pain   I-10
   R10.84 Generalized abdominal pain   I-10

§ Requires fifth digit. Valid digits are in [brackets] under each code. See category 789 for codes and definitions.

789.1 Hepatomegaly
Enlargement of liver

789.2 Splenomegaly
Enlargement of spleen

§ ✓5ᵗʰ **789.3 Abdominal or pelvic swelling, mass, or lump**
[0-7, 9]   Diffuse or generalized swelling or mass:
     abdominal NOS
     umbilical
     EXCLUDES   *abdominal distention (gaseous) (787.3)*
              ascites (789.51-789.59)

§ ✓5ᵗʰ **789.4 Abdominal rigidity**
[0-7, 9]

✓5ᵗʰ **789.5 Ascites**
Fluid in peritoneal cavity
DEF: Serous fluid effusion and accumulation in abdominal cavity.
AHA: 4Q, '07, 95; 2Q, '05, 8; 4Q, '89, 11

     789.51 Malignant ascites
         Code first malignancy, such as:
            malignant neoplasm of ovary (183.0)
            secondary malignant neoplasm of retroperitoneum
               and peritoneum (197.6)
         AHA: 4Q, '07, 96
         R18.0 Malignant ascities   I-10

     789.59 Other ascites
         AHA: 4Q, '08, 99
         R18.8 Other ascites   I-10

§ ✓5ᵗʰ **789.6 Abdominal tenderness**
[0-7, 9]   Rebound tenderness

     789.7 Colic   P
         Colic NOS   Infantile colic
         EXCLUDES   *colic in adult and child over 12 months old (789.0)*
               renal colic (788.0)
         DEF: Inconsolable crying in an otherwise well-fed and healthy infant
         for more than three hours in a day, three days a week, for more than
         three weeks.
         AHA: 4Q, '09, 104-105

     789.9 Other symtoms involving abdomen and pelvis
         Umbilical:
            bleeding
            discharge

Nonspecific Abnormal Findings (790-796)

     AHA: 3Q, '11, 4; 2Q, '90, 16

✓4ᵗʰ **790 Nonspecific findings on examination of blood**
     EXCLUDES   *abnormality of:*
         platelets (287.0-287.9)
         thrombocytes (287.0-287.9)
         white blood cells (288.00-288.9)

✓5ᵗʰ **790.0 Abnormality of red blood cells**
     EXCLUDES   *anemia:*
         congenital (776.5)
         newborn, due to isoimmunization (773.0-773.2,
            773.5)
         of premature infant (776.6)
         other specified types (280.0-285.9)
         hemoglobin disorders (282.5-282.7)
         polycythemia:
         familial (289.6)
         neonatorum (776.4)
         secondary (289.0)
         vera (238.4)
     AHA: 4Q, '00, 46

     790.01 Precipitous drop in hematocrit
         Drop in hematocritDrop in hemoglobin
         TIP: Typically reported as a reason for encounter at a dialysis
         center.

     790.09 Other abnormality of red blood cells
         Abnormal red cell morphology NOS
         Abnormal red cell volume NOS
         Anisocytosis
         Poikilocytosis

790.1 Elevated sedimentation rate

✓5ᵗʰ **790.2 Abnormal glucose**
     EXCLUDES   *diabetes mellitus (249.00-249.91, 250.00-250.93)*
         dysmetabolic syndrome X (277.7)
         gestational diabetes (648.8)
         glycosuria (791.5)
         hypoglycemia (251.2)
         that complicating pregnancy, childbirth, or
            puerperium (648.8)
     AHA: 1Q, '11, 9; 4Q, '03, 74; 3Q, '91, 5
     TIP: These codes are typically assigned on encounters before a
     patient is diagnosed with diabetes mellitus.

     790.21 Impaired fasting glucose
         Elevated fasting glucose

     790.22 Impaired glucose tolerance test (oral)
         Elevated glucose tolerance test

     790.29 Other abnormal glucose
         Abnormal glucose NOS
         Abnormal non-fasting glucose
         Hyperglycemia NOS
         Pre-diabetes NOS
         AHA: 1Q, '12, 17; 3Q, '09, 5; 2Q, '05, 21
         TIP: Assign for any stress hyperglycemia for which no causal
         condition is determined including postoperative
         hyperglycemia that is not specifically documented as a
         complication of the procedure.
         R73.09 Other abnormal glucose   I-10

790.3 Excessive blood level of alcohol
Elevated blood-alcohol
AHA: S-O, '86, 3

790.4 Nonspecific elevation of levels of transaminase or lactic acid dehydrogenase [LDH]
R74.0 Nonspecific elevation levels transaminase & LDH   I-10

790.5 Other nonspecific abnormal serum enzyme levels
Abnormal serum level of:
   acid phosphatase
   alkaline phosphatase
   amylase
   lipase
EXCLUDES   *deficiency of circulating enzymes (277.6)*
R74.8 Abnormal levels of other serum enzymes   I-10

790.6 Other abnormal blood chemistry
Abnormal blood level of:
   cobalt
   copper
   iron
   lead
   lithium
   magnesium
   mineral
   zinc
EXCLUDES   *abnormality of electrolyte or acid-base balance*
         (276.0-276.9)
       hypoglycemia NOS (251.2)
       lead poisoning (984.0-984.9)
       specific finding indicating abnormality of:
         amino-acid transport and metabolism
           (270.0-270.9)
         carbohydrate transport and metabolism
           (271.0-271.9)
         lipid metabolism (272.0-272.9)
       uremia NOS (586)
AHA: ▶2Q, '13, 13;◀ 4Q, '88, 1
TIP: If only azotemia is documented (indexed to 790.6), clarify with
physician; if due to uremia or renal failure, code to those conditions
instead.
R78.89 Finding oth spec substances not norm found blood   I-10

---

§   Requires fifth digit. Valid digits are in [brackets] under each code. See category 789 for codes and definitions.

✓4ᵗʰ / ✓5ᵗʰ   Additional Digit Required   **Unspecified Code**   Other Specified Code   Manifestation Code   ▶◀ Revised Text   ● New Code   ▲ Revised Code Title

2015 ICD-9-CM   **October 2014 • Volume 1 – 269**

790.7 Bacteremia

> **EXCLUDES** *bacteremia of newborn (771.83)*
> *septicemia (038)*

> **Use additional code to identify organism (041)**

> **DEF:** Laboratory finding of bacteria in the blood in the absence of two or more signs of sepsis; transient in nature, progresses to septicemia with severe infectious process.
> **AHA:** ▶1Q, '14, 18;◀ 2Q, '11, 7; 2Q, '03, 7; 4Q, '93, 29; 3Q, '88, 12
> **TIP:** If clinical signs or symptoms indicating systemic disease exist, query physician for the presence of sepsis; code to category 038 if documented.

790.8 Viremia, unspecified

> **DEF:** Presence of a virus in the blood stream.
> **AHA:** 4Q, '88, 10

√5ᵗʰ 790.9 Other nonspecific findings on examination of blood

> **AHA:** 4Q, '93, 29

790.91 Abnormal arterial blood gases

790.92 Abnormal coagulation profile

> Abnormal or prolonged:
> bleeding time
> coagulation time
> partial thromboplastin time [PTT]
> prothrombin time [PT]

> **EXCLUDES** *coagulation (hemorrhagic) disorders (286.0-286.9)*

> **R79.1** Abnormal coagulaton profile   **I-10**

790.93 Elevated prostate specific antigen, [PSA]   **A♂**

790.94 Euthyroid sick syndrome

> **DEF:** Transient alteration of thyroid hormone metabolism due to nonthyroid illness or stress.
> **AHA:** 4Q, '97, 45

790.95 Elevated C-reactive protein [CRP]

> **DEF:** Inflammation in an arterial wall results in elevated C-reactive protein (CRP) in the blood; CRP is a recognized risk factor in cardiovascular disease.

790.99 Other

> **AHA:** 3Q, '12, 18; 3Q, '11, 4; 2Q, '03, 14
> **TIP:** Assign for documentation of secondary thrombocytosis as clinically significant but without other reportable underlying cause.

√4ᵗʰ 791 Nonspecific findings on examination of urine

> **EXCLUDES** *hematuria NOS (599.70-599.72)*
> *specific findings indicating abnormality of:*
> *amino-acid transport and metabolism (270.0-270.9)*
> *carbohydrate transport and metabolism (271.0-271.9)*

791.0 Proteinuria

> Albuminuria
> Bence-Jones proteinuria

> **EXCLUDES** *postural proteinuria (593.6)*
> *that arising during pregnancy or the puerperium (642.0-642.9, 646.2)*

> **DEF:** Excess protein in urine.
> **AHA:** 2Q, '12, 19; 3Q, '91, 8

791.1 Chyluria

> **EXCLUDES** *filarial (125.0-125.9)*

> **DEF:** Excess chyle in urine.

791.2 Hemoglobinuria

> **DEF:** Free hemoglobin in blood due to rapid hemolysis of red blood cells.

791.3 Myoglobinuria

> **DEF:** Myoglobin (oxygen-transporting pigment) in urine.

791.4 Biliuria

> **DEF:** Bile pigments in urine.

791.5 Glycosuria

> **EXCLUDES** *renal glycosuria (271.4)*

> **DEF:** Sugar in urine.

791.6 Acetonuria

> Ketonuria

> **DEF:** Excess acetone in urine.

791.7 Other cells and casts in urine

791.9 Other nonspecific findings on examination of urine

> Crystalluria
> Elevated urine levels of:
> 17-ketosteroids
> catecholamines
> indolacetic acid
> vanillylmandelic acid [VMA]
> Melanuria
> **AHA:** 1Q, '05, 12

√4ᵗʰ 792 Nonspecific abnormal findings in other body substances

> **EXCLUDES** *that in chromosomal analysis (795.2)*

792.0 Cerebrospinal fluid

792.1 Stool contents

> Abnormal stool color   Occult stool
> Fat in stool   Pus in stool
> Mucus in stool

> **EXCLUDES** *blood in stool [melena] (578.1)*
> *newborn (772.4, 777.3)*

> **AHA:** 2Q, '92, 9

792.2 Semen   ♂

> Abnormal spermatozoa

> **EXCLUDES** *azoospermia (606.0)*
> *oligospermia (606.1)*

792.3 Amniotic fluid   **M♀**

> **DEF:** Nonspecific abnormal findings in amniotic fluid.
> **AHA:** N-D, '86, 4

792.4 Saliva

> **EXCLUDES** *that in chromosomal analysis (795.2)*

792.5 Cloudy (hemodialysis) (peritoneal) dialysis effluent

> **AHA:** 4Q, '00, 46

792.9 Other nonspecific abnormal findings in body substances

> Peritoneal fluid
> Pleural fluid
> Synovial fluid
> Vaginal fluids

√4ᵗʰ 793 Nonspecific (abnormal) findings on radiological and other examination of body structure

> **INCLUDES** nonspecific abnormal findings of:
> thermography
> ultrasound examination [echogram]
> x-ray examination

> **EXCLUDES** *abnormal results of function studies and radioisotope scans (794.0-794.9)*

793.0 Skull and head

> **EXCLUDES** *nonspecific abnormal echoencephalogram (794.01)*

> **AHA:** 3Q, '06, 22

√5ᵗʰ 793.1 Lung field

> **AHA:** 4Q, '11, 138-139

793.11 Solitary pulmonary nodule

> Coin lesion lung
> Solitary pulmonary nodule, subsegmental branch of the bronchial tree

793.19 Other nonspecific abnormal finding of lung field

> Pulmonary infiltrate NOS
> Shadow, lung
> **AHA:** 4Q, '11, 139

793.2 Other intrathoracic organ

> Abnormal:
> echocardiogram
> heart shadow
> ultrasound cardiogram
> Mediastinal shift
> **AHA:** 1Q, '12, 17

793.3 Biliary tract

> Nonvisualization of gallbladder

793.4 Gastrointestinal tract

793.5 Genitourinary organs

> Filling defect:
> bladder
> kidney
> ureter

N Newborn Age: 0   **P** Pediatric Age: 0-17   **M** Maternity Age: 12-55   **A** Adult Age: 15-124

793.6 Abdominal area, including retroperitoneum

793.7 Musculoskeletal system

√5ᵗʰ **793.8 Breast**

    AHA: 4Q, '01, 51

    793.80 Abnormal mammogram, unspecified

    793.81 Mammographic microcalcification

        EXCLUDES *mammographic calcification (793.89)*
            mammographic calculus (793.89)

        DEF: Calcium and cellular debris deposits in the breast that cannot be felt but can be detected on a mammogram; can be a sign of cancer, benign conditions, or changes in the breast tissue as a result of inflammation, injury, or obstructed duct.

    793.82 Inconclusive mammogram
        Dense breasts NOS
        Inconclusive mammogram NEC
        Inconclusive mammography due to dense breasts
        Inconclusive mammography NEC
        AHA: 4Q, '09, 105-106

    793.89 Other (abnormal) findings on radiological examination of breast
        Mammographic calcification
        Mammographic calculus

√5ᵗʰ **793.9 Other**

    EXCLUDES *abnormal finding by radioisotope localization of placenta (794.9)*

    TIP: Sequence a code for the sign or symptom that was the reason for the imaging or radiological test first.

    793.91 Image test inconclusive due to excess body fat
        Use additional code to identify Body Mass Index (BMI), if known (V85.0-V85.54)
        AHA: 4Q, '06, 109

    793.99 Other nonspecific (abnormal) findings on radiological and other examinations of body structure
        Abnormal:
           placental finding by x-ray or ultrasound method
           radiological findings in skin and subcutaneous tissue
        AHA: 4Q, '06, 109

√4ᵗʰ **794 Nonspecific abnormal results of function studies**

    INCLUDES radioisotope:
        scans
        uptake studies
        scintiphotography

√5ᵗʰ **794.0 Brain and central nervous system**

    794.00 Abnormal function study, unspecified

    794.01 Abnormal echoencephalogram

    794.02 Abnormal electroencephalogram [EEG]

    794.09 Other
        Abnormal brain scan

√5ᵗʰ **794.1 Peripheral nervous system and special senses**

    794.10 Abnormal response to nerve stimulation, unspecified

    794.11 Abnormal retinal function studies
        Abnormal electroretinogram [ERG]

    794.12 Abnormal electro-oculogram [EOG]

    794.13 Abnormal visually evoked potential

    794.14 Abnormal oculomotor studies

    794.15 Abnormal auditory function studies
        AHA: 1Q, '04, 15-16
        TIP: If the reason for the encounter was for a hearing examination, sequence a code from subcategory V72.1 first. When nonspecific hearing loss is documented, assign 389.9 instead of 794.15.

    794.16 Abnormal vestibular function studies

    794.17 Abnormal electromyogram [EMG]
        EXCLUDES *that of eye (794.14)*

    794.19 Other

794.2 Pulmonary
    Abnormal lung scan
    Reduced:
        ventilatory capacity
        vital capacity

√5ᵗʰ **794.3 Cardiovascular**

    794.30 Abnormal function study, unspecified

    794.31 Abnormal electrocardiogram [ECG] [EKG]
        EXCLUDES *long QT syndrome (426.82)*
        R94.31 Abnormal electrocardiogram [ECG] [EKG]   I-10

    794.39 Other
        Abnormal:
           ballistocardiogram
           phonocardiogram
           vectorcardiogram
        R94.39 Abnormal result oth cardiovasculr function study   I-10

794.4 Kidney
    Abnormal renal function test

794.5 Thyroid
    Abnormal thyroid:
        scan
        uptake

794.6 Other endocrine function study

794.7 Basal metabolism
    Abnormal basal metabolic rate [BMR]

794.8 Liver
    Abnormal liver scan
    R94.5 Abnormal results of liver function studies   I-10

794.9 Other
    Bladder   Placenta
    Pancreas   Spleen

√4ᵗʰ **795 Other and nonspecific abnormal cytological, histological, immunological and DNA test findings**

    EXCLUDES *abnormal cytologic smear of anus and anal HPV (796.70-796.79)*
        nonspecific abnormalities of red blood cells (790.01-790.09)

√5ᵗʰ **795.0 Abnormal Papanicolaou smear of cervix and cervical HPV**
    Abnormal thin preparation smear of cervix
    Abnormal cervical cytology
    EXCLUDES *abnormal cytologic smear of vagina and vaginal HPV (795.10-795.19)*
        carcinoma in situ of cervix (233.1)
        cervical intraepithelial neoplasia I (CIN I) (622.11)
        cervical intraepithelial neoplasia II (CIN II) (622.12)
        cervical intraepithelial neoplasia III (CIN III) (233.1)
        dysplasia (histologically confirmed) of cervix (uteri) NOS (622.10)
        mild cervical dysplasia (histologically confirmed) (622.11)
        moderate cervical dysplasia (histologically confirmed) (622.12)
        severe cervical dysplasia (histologically confirmed) (233.1)
    AHA: 4Q, '08, 145-146; 4Q, '02, 69

    795.00 Abnormal glandular Papanicolaou smear of cervix   ♀
        Atypical endocervical cells NOS
        Atypical endometrial cells NOS
        Atypical cervical glandular cells NOS

    795.01 Papanicolaou smear of cervix with atypical squamous cells of undetermined significance [ASC-US]   ♀
        AHA: 2Q, '06, 4

    795.02 Papanicolaou smear of cervix with atypical squamous cells cannot exclude high grade squamous intraepithelial lesion [ASC-H]   ♀

    795.03 Papanicolaou smear of cervix with low grade squamous intraepithelial lesion [LGSIL]   ♀

    795.04 Papanicolaou smear of cervix with high grade squamous intraepithelial lesion [HGSIL]   ♀

√4ᵗʰ / √5ᵗʰ Additional Digit Required   Unspecified Code   Other Specified Code   Manifestation Code   ▶◀ Revised Text   ● New Code   ▲ Revised Code Title

Symptoms, Signs, and Ill-Defined Conditions

795.05–795.71

795.05 Cervical high risk human papillomavirus [HPV] DNA test positive ♀

795.06 Papanicolaou smear of cervix with cytologic evidence of malignancy ♀
AHA: 4Q, '06, 110

795.07 Satisfactory cervical smear but lacking transformation zone ♀

795.08 Unsatisfactory cervical cytology smear ♀
Inadequate cervical cytology sample
AHA: 2Q, '06, 4

795.09 Other abnormal Papanicolaou smear of cervix and cervical HPV ♀
Cervical low risk human papillomavirus (HPV) DNA test positive

Use additional code for associated human papillomavirus (079.4)

EXCLUDES encounter for Papanicolaou cervical smear to confirm findings of recent normal smear following initial abnormal smear (V72.32)

√5ᵗʰ **795.1 Abnormal Papanicolaou smear of vagina and vaginal HPV**
Abnormal thin preparation smear of vagina NOS
Abnormal vaginal cytology NOS

Use additional code to identify acquired absence of uterus and cervix, if applicable (V88.01-V88.03)

EXCLUDES abnormal cytologic smear of cervix and cervical HPV (795.00-795.09)
carcinoma in situ of vagina (233.31)
carcinoma in situ of vulva (233.32)
dysplasia (histologically confirmed) of vagina NOS (623.0, 233.31)
dysplasia (histologically confirmed) of vulva NOS (624.01, 624.02, 233.32)
mild vaginal dysplasia (histologically confirmed) (623.0)
mild vulvar dysplasia (histologically confirmed) (624.01)
moderate vaginal dysplasia (histologically confirmed) (623.0)
moderate vulvar dysplasia (histologically confirmed) (624.02)
severe vaginal dysplasia (histologically confirmed) (233.31)
severe vulvar dysplasia (histologically confirmed) (233.32)
vaginal intraepithelial neoplasia I (VAIN I) (623.0)
vaginal intraepithelial neoplasia II (VAIN II) (623.0)
vaginal intraepithelial neoplasia III (VAIN III) (233.31)
vulvar intraepithelial neoplasia I (VIN I) (624.01)
vulvar intraepithelial neoplasia II (VIN II) (624.02)
vulvar intraepithelial neoplasia III (VIN III) (233.32)
AHA: 4Q, '08, 145-148

795.10 Abnormal glandular Papanicolaou smear of vagina ♀
Atypical vaginal glandular cells NOS

795.11 Papanicolaou smear of vagina with atypical squamous cells of undetermined significance [ASC-US] ♀

795.12 Papanicolaou smear of vagina with atypical squamous cells cannot exclude high grade squamous intraepithelial lesion [ASC-H] ♀

795.13 Papanicolaou smear of vagina with low grade squamous intraepithelial lesion [LGSIL] ♀

795.14 Papanicolaou smear of vagina with high grade squamous intraepithelial lesion [HGSIL] ♀

795.15 Vaginal high risk human papillomavirus [HPV] DNA test positive ♀
EXCLUDES condyloma acuminatum (078.11)
genital warts (078.11)

795.16 Papanicolaou smear of vagina with cytologic evidence of malignancy ♀

795.18 Unsatisfactory vaginal cytology smear ♀
Inadequate vaginal cytology sample

795.19 Other abnormal Papanicolaou smear of vagina and vaginal HPV ♀
Vaginal low risk human papillomavirus (HPV) DNA test positive

Use additional code for associated human papillomavirus (079.4)

795.2 Nonspecific abnormal findings on chromosomal analysis
Abnormal karyotype

√5ᵗʰ **795.3 Nonspecific positive culture findings**
Positive culture findings in:
nose   sputum
throat   wound
EXCLUDES that of:
blood (790.7-790.8)
urine (791.9)

795.31 Nonspecific positive findings for anthrax
Positive findings by nasal swab
AHA: 4Q, '02, 70
TIP: If the patient has been exposed only to anthrax, assign instead V01.81. If a patient has not been exposed but fears anthrax and tests negative, assign instead V71.82.

795.39 Other nonspecific positive culture findings
EXCLUDES colonization status (V02.0-V02.9)

795.4 Other nonspecific abnormal histological findings

√5ᵗʰ **795.5 Nonspecific reaction to test for tuberculosis**
AHA: 4Q, '11, 140-141

795.51 Nonspecific reaction to tuberculin skin test without active tuberculosis
Abnormal result of Mantoux test
PPD positive
Tuberculin (skin test) positive
Tuberculin (skin test) reactor
EXCLUDES nonspecific reaction to cell mediated immunity measurement of gamma interferon antigen response without active tuberculosis (795.52)
AHA: 4Q, '11, 182
TIP: Assign when documentation indicates "latent tuberculosis."

795.52 Nonspecific reaction to cell mediated immunity measurement of gamma interferon antigen response without active tuberculosis
Nonspecific reaction to QuantiFERON-TB test (QFT) without active tuberculosis
EXCLUDES nonspecific reaction to tuberculin skin test without active tuberculosis (795.51)
positive tuberculin skin test (795.51)

795.6 False positive serological test for syphilis
False positive Wassermann reaction

√5ᵗʰ **795.7 Other nonspecific immunological findings**
EXCLUDES abnormal tumor markers (795.81-795.89)
elevated prostate specific antigen [PSA] (790.93)
elevated tumor associated antigens (795.81-795.89)
isoimmunization, in pregnancy (656.1-656.2)
affecting fetus or newborn (773.0-773.2)
AHA: 2Q, '93, 6

795.71 Nonspecific serologic evidence of human immunodeficiency virus [HIV]
Inclusive human immunodeficiency [HIV] test (adult) (infant)
NOTE This code is **only** to be used when a test finding is reported as nonspecific. Asymptomatic positive findings are coded to V08. If any HIV infection symptom or condition is present, see code 042. Negative findings are not coded.
EXCLUDES acquired immunodeficiency syndrome [AIDS] (042)
asymptomatic human immunodeficiency virus, [HIV] infection status (V08)
HIV infection, symptomatic (042)
human immunodeficiency virus [HIV] disease (042)
positive (status) NOS (V08)
AHA: 2Q, '04, 11; 1Q, '93, 21; 1Q, '93, 22; 2Q, '92, 11; J-A, '87, 24

N Newborn Age: 0   P Pediatric Age: 0-17   M Maternity Age: 12-55   A Adult Age: 15-124

795.79 Other and unspecified nonspecific immunological findings
Raised antibody titer
Raised level of immunoglobulins
AHA: 4Q, '11, 93

√5ᵗʰ **795.8 Abnormal tumor markers**
Elevated tumor associated antigens [TAA]
Elevated tumor specific antigens [TSA]
EXCLUDES elevated prostate specific antigen [PSA] (790.93)

795.81 Elevated carcinoembryonic antigen [CEA]
AHA: 4Q, '06, 111

795.82 Elevated cancer antigen 125 [CA 125]   ♀
AHA: 4Q, '06, 111

795.89 Other abnormal tumor markers
AHA: 4Q, '06, 111

√4ᵗʰ **796 Other nonspecific abnormal findings**

796.0 Nonspecific abnormal toxicological findings
Abnormal levels of heavy metals or drugs in blood, urine, or other tissue
Use additional code for retained foreign body, if applicable, (V90.01-V90.9)
EXCLUDES excessive blood level of alcohol (790.3)
AHA: 1Q, '97, 16

796.1 Abnormal reflex

796.2 Elevated blood pressure reading without diagnosis of hypertension
NOTE This category is to be used to record an episode of elevated blood pressure in a patient in whom no formal diagnosis of hypertension has been made, or as an incidental finding.
AHA: 2Q, '03, 11; 3Q, '90, 4; J-A, '84, 12
TIP: Assign an additional E code for poisoning or adverse effect of a drug if the documentation indicates it's the underlying cause of the elevated blood pressure.
R03.0 Elevated blood-pressure reading without dx HTN   I-10

796.3 Nonspecific low blood pressure reading

796.4 Other abnormal clinical findings
AHA: 1Q, '97, 16

796.5 Abnormal finding on antenatal screening   M ♀
AHA: 4Q, '97, 46

796.6 Abnormal findings on neonatal screening   N
EXCLUDES nonspecific serologic evidence of human immunodeficiency virus [HIV] (795.71)
AHA: 4Q, '04, 99

√5ᵗʰ **796.7 Abnormal cytologic smear of anus and anal HPV**
EXCLUDES abnormal cytologic smear of cervix and cervical HPV (795.00-795.09)
abnormal cytologic smear of vagina and vaginal HPV (795.10-795.19)
anal intraepithelial neoplasia I (AIN I) (569.44)
anal intraepithelial neoplasia II (AIN II) (569.44)
anal intraepithelial neoplasia III (AIN III) (230.5, 230.6)
carcinoma in situ of anus (230.5, 230.6)
dysplasia (histologically confirmed) of anus NOS (569.44)
mild anal dysplasia (histologically confirmed) (569.44)
moderate anal dysplasia (histologically confirmed) (569.44)
severe anal dysplasia (histologically confirmed) (230.5, 230.6)
AHA: 4Q, '08, 117-119

796.70 Abnormal glandular Papanicolaou smear of anus
Atypical anal glandular cells NOS

796.71 Papanicolaou smear of anus with atypical squamous cells of undetermined significance [ASC-US]

796.72 Papanicolaou smear of anus with atypical squamous cells cannot exclude high grade squamous intraepithelial lesion [ASC-H]

796.73 Papanicolaou smear of anus with low grade squamous intraepithelial lesion [LGSIL]

796.74 Papanicolaou smear of anus with high grade squamous intraepithelial lesion [HGSIL]

796.75 Anal high risk human papillomavirus [HPV] DNA test positive

796.76 Papanicolaou smear of anus with cytologic evidence of malignancy

796.77 Satisfactory anal smear but lacking transformation zone

796.78 Unsatisfactory anal cytology smear
Inadequate anal cytology sample

796.79 Other abnormal Papanicolaou smear of anus and anal HPV
Anal low risk human papillomavirus (HPV) DNA test positive
Use additional code for associated human papillomavirus (079.4)

796.9 Other

Ill-Defined and Unknown Causes of Morbidity and Mortality (797-799)

797 Senility without mention of psychosis
Frailty   Senile asthenia
Old age   Senile:
Senescence   debility
                      exhaustion
EXCLUDES senile psychoses (290.0-290.9)

√4ᵗʰ **798 Sudden death, cause unknown**

798.0 Sudden infant death syndrome   P
Cot death
Crib death
Sudden death of nonspecific cause in infancy
DEF: Death of infant under age one due to nonspecific cause.

798.1 Instantaneous death

798.2 Death occurring in less than 24 hours from onset of symptoms, not otherwise explained
Death known not to be violent or instantaneous, for which no cause could be discovered
Died without sign of disease

798.9 Unattended death
Death in circumstances where the body of the deceased was found and no cause could be discovered
Found dead

√4ᵗʰ **799 Other ill-defined and unknown causes of morbidity and mortality**

√5ᵗʰ **799.0 Asphyxia and hypoxemia**
EXCLUDES asphyxia and hypoxemia (due to):
carbon monoxide (986)
hypercapnia (786.09)
inhalation of food or foreign body (932-934.9)
newborn (768.0-768.9)
traumatic (994.7)

799.01 Asphyxia
DEF: Lack of oxygen in inspired air, causing a deficiency of oxygen in tissues (hypoxia) and elevated levels of arterial carbon dioxide (hypercapnia).
AHA: 4Q, '05, 90

799.02 Hypoxemia
DEF: Deficient oxygenation of the blood.
AHA: 3Q, '09, 20; 2Q, '06, 24, 25; 4Q, '05, 90
TIP: Hypoxia is not inherent in COPD (496) and may be assigned in addition, if applicable.
R09.02 Hypoxemia   I-10

Symptoms, Signs, and Ill-Defined Conditions

799.1–799.9

799.1 Respiratory arrest
Cardiorespiratory failure
> **EXCLUDES**   cardiac arrest (427.5)
> failure of peripheral circulation (785.50)
> respiratory distress:
>> NOS (786.09)
>> acute (518.82)
>> following trauma and surgery (518.52)
>> newborn (770.89)
>> syndrome (newborn) (769)
>>> adult (following trauma and surgery) (518.52)
>> other (518.82)
> respiratory failure (518.81, 518.83-518.84)
>> newborn (770.84)
> respiratory insufficiency (786.09)
>> acute (518.82)

√5ᵗʰ 799.2 Signs and symptoms involving emotional state
> **EXCLUDES**   anxiety (293.84, 300.00-300.09)
> depression (311)

AHA: 4Q, '09,107

TIP: If associated with underlying history of traumatic brain injury (TBI), assign in addition to a code for the late effect of TBI (e.g., 905.0 or 907.0).

799.21 Nervousness
Nervous
AHA: 4Q, '09,108

799.22 Irritability
Irritable
AHA: 4Q, '09,108

799.23 Impulsiveness
Impulsive
> **EXCLUDES**   impulsive neurosis (300.3)

799.24 Emotional lability

799.25 Demoralization and apathy
Apathetic

799.29 Other signs and symptoms involving emotional state

799.3 Debility, unspecified
> **EXCLUDES**   asthenia (780.79)
> nervous debility (300.5)
> neurasthenia (300.5)
> senile asthenia (797)

799.4 Cachexia
Wasting disease
Code first underlying condition, if known
DEF: General ill health and poor nutrition.
AHA: ▶1Q, '13, 13;◀ 3Q, '06, 14, 15; 3Q, '90, 17
TIP: Assign an additional code for any associated malnutrition, if documented.
R64 Cachexia   **I-10**

√5ᵗʰ 799.5 Signs and symptoms involving cognition
> **EXCLUDES**   amnesia (780.93)
> amnestic syndrome (294.0)
> attention deficit disorder (314.00-314.01)
> late effects of cerebrovascular disease (438.0)
> memory loss (780.93)
> mild cognitive impairment, so stated (331.83)
> specific problems in developmental delay
>> (315.00-315.9)
> transient global amnesia (437.7)
> visuospatial neglect (781.8)

AHA: 3Q, '12, 19-20; 4Q, '10, 95-96

TIP: Report as additional diagnoses not integral to a known condition to describe the nature or type of deficit due to unknown or unrelated cause.

799.51 Attention or concentration deficit
AHA: 3Q, '12, 20

799.52 Cognitive communication deficit
AHA: 3Q, '12, 19-21

799.53 Visuospatial deficit

799.54 Psychomotor deficit
AHA: 4Q, '10, 95-97

799.55 Frontal lobe and executive function deficit
AHA: 3Q, '12, 20

799.59 Other signs and symptoms involving cognition

√5ᵗʰ 799.8 Other ill-defined conditions

799.81 Decreased libido   **A**
Decreased sexual desire
> **EXCLUDES**   psychosexual dysfunction with inhibited
>> sexual desire (302.71)

AHA: 4Q, '03, 75

799.82 Apparent life threatening event in infant   **P**
ALTE
Apparent life threatening event in newborn and infant

Code first confirmed diagnosis, if known

Use additional code(s) for associated signs and symptoms if no confirmed diagnosis established, or if signs and symptoms are not associated routinely with confirmed diagnosis, or provide additional information for cause of ALTE

AHA: 4Q, '10, 97-98; 4Q, '09, 109

799.89 Other ill-defined conditions

799.9 Other unknown and unspecified cause
Undiagnosed disease, not specified as to site or system involved
Unknown cause of morbidity or mortality
AHA: 1Q, '98,.4; 1Q, '90, 20

N Newborn Age: 0   **P** Pediatric Age: 0-17   **M** Maternity Age: 12-55   **A** Adult Age: 15-124

17. Injury and Poisoning (800-999)

Use additional code for retained foreign body, if applicable, (V90.01-V90.9)

Use E code(s) to identify the cause and intent of the injury or poisoning (E800-E999)

NOTE

1. The principle of multiple coding of injuries should be followed wherever possible. Combination categories for multiple injuries are provided for use when there is insufficient detail as to the nature of the individual conditions, or for primary tabulation purposes when it is more convenient to record a single code; otherwise, the component injuries should be coded separately.

   Where multiple sites of injury are specified in the titles, the word "with" indicates involvement of both sites, and the word "and" indicates involvement of either or both sites. The word "finger" includes thumb.

2. Categories for "late effect" of injuries are to be found at 905-909.

FRACTURES (800-829)

EXCLUDES malunion (733.81)
nonunion (733.82)
pathological or spontaneous fracture (733.10-733.19)
stress fractures (733.93-733.95)

NOTE The terms "condyle," "coronoid process," "ramus," and "symphysis" indicate the portion of the bone fractured, not the name of the bone involved.

The descriptions "closed" and "open" used in the fourth-digit subdivisions include the following terms:

closed (with or without delayed healing):
comminuted	impacted
depressed	linear
elevated	simple
fissured	slipped epiphysis
fracture NOS	spiral
greenstick	

open (with or without delayed healing):
compound	puncture
infected	with foreign body
missile	

NOTE A fracture not indicated as closed or open should be classified as closed.

AHA: 4Q, '08, 158; 1Q, '07, 3-4; 4Q, '90, 26; 3Q, '90, 5; 3Q, '90, 13; 2Q, '90, 7; 2Q, '89, 15, S-O, '85, 3

TIP: Assign the acute fracture codes only while the patient is receiving active treatment for the fracture, such as during surgical care, an ED encounter, or evaluation and treatment by a new physician. Otherwise, refer to aftercare category V54.

Fracture of Skull (800-804)

INCLUDES traumatic brain injury due to fracture of skull

The following fifth-digit subclassification is for use with the appropriate codes in category 800, 801, 803, and 804:

0 unspecified state of consciousness
1 with no loss of consciousness
2 with brief [less than one hour] loss of consciousness
3 with moderate [1-24 hours] loss of consciousness
4 with prolonged [more than 24 hours] loss of consciousness and return to pre-existing conscious level
5 with prolonged [more than 24 hours] loss of consciousness, without return to pre-existing conscious level
　Use fifth-digit 5 to designate when a patient is unconscious and dies before regaining consciousness, regardless of the duration of the loss of consciousness
6 with loss of consciousness of unspecified duration
9 with concussion, unspecified

√4ᵗʰ 800 Fracture of vault of skull

INCLUDES frontal bone
parietal bone

DEF: Fracture of bone that forms skull dome and protects brain.
AHA: 4Q,'96, 36

§ **√5ᵗʰ 800.0 Closed without mention of intracranial injury**
[0-6, 9]

§ **√5ᵗʰ 800.1 Closed with cerebral laceration and contusion**
[0-6, 9]

Skull

§ **√5ᵗʰ 800.2 Closed with subarachnoid, subdural, and extradural**
[0-6, 9] hemorrhage

§ **√5ᵗʰ 800.3 Closed with other and unspecified intracranial**
[0-6, 9] hemorrhage

§ **√5ᵗʰ 800.4 Closed with intracranial injury of other and**
[0-6, 9] unspecified nature

§ **√5ᵗʰ 800.5 Open without mention of intracranial injury**
[0-6, 9]

§ **√5ᵗʰ 800.6 Open with cerebral laceration and contusion**
[0-6, 9]

§ **√5ᵗʰ 800.7 Open with subarachnoid, subdural, and**
[0-6, 9] extradural hemorrhage

§ **√5ᵗʰ 800.8 Open with other and unspecified intracranial**
[0-6, 9] hemorrhage

§ **√5ᵗʰ 800.9 Open with intracranial injury of other and**
[0-6, 9] unspecified nature

√4ᵗʰ 801 Fracture of base of skull

INCLUDES fossa:
anterior
middle
posterior
occiput bone
orbital roof
sinus:
ethmoid
frontal
sphenoid bone
temporal bone

DEF: Fracture of bone that forms skull floor.
AHA: 4Q, '96, 36

§ **√5ᵗʰ 801.0 Closed without mention of intracranial injury**
[0-6, 9]

§ **√5ᵗʰ 801.1 Closed with cerebral laceration and contusion**
[0-6, 9]　**AHA: For code 801.15:** 4Q, '96, 36

§ **√5ᵗʰ 801.2 Closed with subarachnoid, subdural, and**
[0-6, 9] extradural hemorrhage

§ **√5ᵗʰ 801.3 Closed with other and unspecified intracranial**
[0-6, 9] hemorrhage

§ **√5ᵗʰ 801.4 Closed with intracranial injury of other and**
[0-6, 9] unspecified nature

§ **√5ᵗʰ 801.5 Open without mention of intracranial injury**
[0-6, 9]

§ **√5ᵗʰ 801.6 Open with cerebral laceration and contusion**
[0-6, 9]

§ **√5ᵗʰ 801.7 Open with subarachnoid, subdural, and**
[0-6, 9] extradural hemorrhage

§ **√5ᵗʰ 801.8 Open with other and unspecified intracranial**
[0-6, 9] hemorrhage

§ **√5ᵗʰ 801.9 Open with intracranial injury of other and**
[0-6, 9] unspecified nature

---

§　Requires fifth digit. Valid digits are in [brackets] under each code. See beginning of section 800-804 for codes and definitions.

| √4ᵗʰ √5ᵗʰ Additional Digit Required | Unspecified Code | Other Specified Code | Manifestation Code | ►◄ Revised Text | ● New Code | ▲ Revised Code Title |

2015 ICD-9-CM　　　　　　　　　　　　　　　　　　　　　　　　　　**Volume 1 – 275**

Injury and Poisoning

802–804.9

Fractures

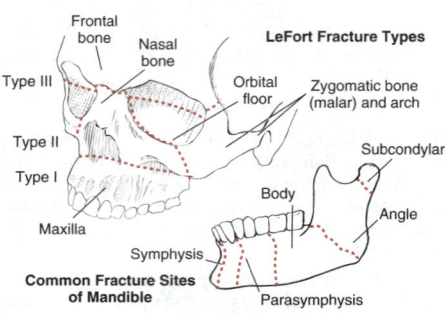

Facial Fracture

802.9 Other facial bones, open

☑4th **802 Fracture of face bones**
AHA: 4Q, '96, 36

802.0 Nasal bones, closed
S02.2xxA Fracture nasal bones initial encounter closed fx   I-10

802.1 Nasal bones, open

☑5th **802.2 Mandible, closed**
Inferior maxilla   Lower jaw (bone)

   802.20 Unspecified site

   802.21 Condylar process

   802.22 Subcondylar

   802.23 Coronoid process

   802.24 Ramus, unspecified

   802.25 Angle of jaw

   802.26 Symphysis of body

   802.27 Alveolar border of body

   802.28 Body, other and unspecified

   802.29 Multiple sites

☑5th **802.3 Mandible, open**

   802.30 Unspecified site

   802.31 Condylar process

   802.32 Subcondylar

   802.33 Coronoid process

   802.34 Ramus, unspecified

   802.35 Angle of jaw

   802.36 Symphysis of body

   802.37 Alveolar border of body

   802.38 Body, other and unspecified

   802.39 Multiple sites

802.4 Malar and maxillary bones, closed
Superior maxilla   Zygoma
Upper jaw (bone)   Zygomatic arch
S02.400A Malar fx uns initial enc closed fx   I-10
S02.401A Maxillary fx uns initial enc closed fx   I-10
S02.402A Zygomatic fx uns initial enc closed fx   I-10

802.5 Malar and maxillary bones, open

802.6 Orbital floor (blow-out), closed
S02.3xxA Fracture orbital floor initial encounter clos fx   I-10

802.7 Orbital floor (blow-out), open

802.8 Other facial bones, closed
Alveolus
Orbit:
   NOS
   part other than roof or floor
Palate
EXCLUDES *orbital:*
    floor (802.6)
    roof (801.0-801.9)
S02.42xA Fx of alveolus of maxilla initial enc closed fx   I-10

☑4th **803 Other and unqualified skull fractures**
INCLUDES   skull NOS
         skull multiple NOS
AHA: 4Q, '96, 36

§ ☑5th **803.0 Closed without mention of intracranial injury**
[0-6, 9]

§ ☑5th **803.1 Closed with cerebral laceration and contusion**
[0-6, 9]

§ ☑5th **803.2 Closed with subarachnoid, subdural, and**
[0-6, 9] **extradural hemorrhage**

§ ☑5th **803.3 Closed with other and unspecified intracranial**
[0-6, 9] **hemorrhage**

§ ☑5th **803.4 Closed with intracranial injury of other and**
[0-6, 9] **unspecified nature**

§ ☑5th **803.5 Open without mention of intracranial injury**
[0-6, 9]

§ ☑5th **803.6 Open with cerebral laceration and contusion**
[0-6, 9]

§ ☑5th **803.7 Open with subarachnoid, subdural, and**
[0-6, 9] **extradural hemorrhage**

§ ☑5th **803.8 Open with other and unspecified intracranial**
[0-6, 9] **hemorrhage**

§ ☑5th **803.9 Open with intracranial injury of other and**
[0-6, 9] **unspecified nature**

☑4th **804 Multiple fractures involving skull or face with other bones**
AHA: 4Q, '96, 36

§ ☑5th **804.0 Closed without mention of intracranial injury**
[0-6, 9]

§ ☑5th **804.1 Closed with cerebral laceration and contusion**
[0-6, 9]   AHA: For code 804.10: 1Q, '06, 6

§ ☑5th **804.2 Closed with subarachnoid, subdural, and**
[0-6, 9] **extradural hemorrhage**

§ ☑5th **804.3 Closed with other and unspecified intracranial**
[0-6, 9] **hemorrhage**

§ ☑5th **804.4 Closed with intracranial injury of other and**
[0-6, 9] **unspecified nature**

§ ☑5th **804.5 Open without mention of intracranial injury**
[0-6, 9]

§ ☑5th **804.6 Open with cerebral laceration and contusion**
[0-6, 9]

§ ☑5th **804.7 Open with subarachnoid, subdural, and**
[0-6, 9] **extradural hemorrage**

§ ☑5th **804.8 Open with other and unspecified intracranial**
[0-6, 9] **hemorrhage**

§ ☑5th **804.9 Open with intracranial injury of other and**
[0-6, 9] **unspecified nature**

---

§   Requires fifth digit. Valid digits are in [brackets] under each code. See beginning of section 800-804 for codes and definitions.

N Newborn Age: 0   P Pediatric Age: 0-17   M Maternity Age: 12-55   A Adult Age: 15-124

Fracture of Neck and Trunk (805-809)

✓4ᵗʰ **805 Fracture of vertebral column without mention of spinal cord injury**

INCLUDES   neural arch
spine
spinous process
transverse process
vertebra

The following fifth-digit subclassification is for use with codes 805.0-805.1:

   0 cervical vertebra, unspecified level
   1 first cervical vertebra
   2 second cervical vertebra
   3 third cervical vertebra
   4 fourth cervical vertebra
   5 fifth cervical vertebra
   6 sixth cervical vertebra
   7 seventh cervical vertebra
   8 multiple cervical vertebrae

§ ✓5ᵗʰ **805.0 Cervical, closed**
[0-8]   Atlas
        Axis
        S12.101A Uns nondisplcd fx 2nd cerv vert initial enc   I-10
        closed fx

§ ✓5ᵗʰ **805.1 Cervical, open**
[0-8]

805.2 Dorsal [thoracic], closed
     S22.008A Oth fx uns thoracic vertebra initial enc clos fx   I-10

805.3 Dorsal [thoracic], open

805.4 Lumbar, closed
     AHA: 1Q, '07, 7; 4Q, '99, 12
     S32.008A Oth fx uns lumbar vertebra initial enc closed fx   I-10

805.5 Lumbar, open

805.6 Sacrum and coccyx, closed
     S32.19xA Other fx of sacrum initial encounter closed fx   I-10

805.7 Sacrum and coccyx, open

805.8 Unspecified, closed

805.9 Unspecified, open

Vertebral Column

Articular facets · Odontoid process · Atlas (C-1) · Axis (C-2) · Spinous process · Skull · Side view · C1 · C2 · Atlas · Axis · Odontoid process · C-1—C-4 · C-5—C-7 · T-1—T-12 · L-1—L-5 · Sacrum (fused) · Coccyx · Spinous process · Body · Pedicle · Facet · Nerve foramen · Nerve root · Vertebral body · Pedicle Transverse process · Facet · Lamina · Spinal cord

✓4ᵗʰ **806 Fracture of vertebral column with spinal cord injury**

INCLUDES   any condition classifiable to 805 with:
     complete or incomplete transverse lesion (of cord)
     hematomyelia
     injury to:
       cauda equina
       nerve
     paralysis
     paraplegia
     quadriplegia
     spinal concussion

✓5ᵗʰ **806.0 Cervical, closed**

806.00 C_1-C_4 level with unspecified spinal cord injury
     Cervical region NOS with spinal cord injury NOS

806.01 C_1-C_4 level with complete lesion of cord

806.02 C_1-C_4 level with anterior cord syndrome

806.03 C_1-C_4 level with central cord syndrome

806.04 C_1-C_4 level with other specified spinal cord injury
     C_1-C_4 level with:
       incomplete spinal cord lesion NOS
       posterior cord syndrome

806.05 C_5-C_7 level with unspecified spinal cord injury

806.06 C_5-C_7 level with complete lesion of cord

806.07 C_5-C_7 level with anterior cord syndrome

806.08 C_5-C_7 level with central cord syndrome

806.09 C_5-C_7 level with other specified spinal cord injury
     C_5-C_7 level with:
       incomplete spinal cord lesion NOS
       posterior cord syndrome

✓5ᵗʰ **806.1 Cervical, open**

806.10 C_1-C_4 level with unspecified spinal cord injury

806.11 C_1-C_4 level with complete lesion of cord

806.12 C_1-C_4 level with anterior cord syndrome

806.13 C_1-C_4 level with central cord syndrome

806.14 C_1-C_4 level with other specified spinal cord injury
     C_1-C_4 level with:
       incomplete spinal cord lesion NOS
       posterior cord syndrome

806.15 C_5-C_7 level with unspecified spinal cord injury

806.16 C_5-C_7 level with complete lesion of cord

806.17 C_5-C_7 level with anterior cord syndrome

806.18 C_5-C_7 level with central cord syndrome

806.19 C_5-C_7 level with other specified spinal cord injury
     C_5-C_7 level with:
       incomplete spinal cord lesion NOS
       posterior cord syndrome

✓5ᵗʰ **806.2 Dorsal [thoracic], closed**

806.20 T_1-T_6 level with unspecified spinal cord injury
     Thoracic region NOS with spinal cord injury NOS

806.21 T_1-T_6 level with complete lesion of cord

806.22 T_1-T_6 level with anterior cord syndrome

806.23 T_1-T_6 level with central cord syndrome

806.24 T_1-T_6 level with other specified spinal cord injury
     T_1-T_6 level with:
       incomplete spinal cord lesion NOS
       posterior cord syndrome

806.25 T_7-T_{12} level with unspecified spinal cord injury

806.26 T_7-T_{12} level with complete lesion of cord

806.27 T_7-T_{12} level with anterior cord syndrome

806.28 T_7-T_{12} level with central cord syndrome

806.29 T_7-T_{12} level with other specified spinal cord injury
     T_7-T_{12} level with:
       incomplete spinal cord lesion NOS
       posterior cord syndrome

---

§   Requires fifth digit. Valid digits are in [brackets] under each code. See category 805 for codes and definitions.

✓4ᵗʰ
✓5ᵗʰ   Additional Digit Required   **Unspecified Code**   Other Specified Code   Manifestation Code   ►◄ Revised Text   ● New Code   ▲ Revised Code Title

√5th **806.3 Dorsal [thoracic], open**

806.30 T_1-T_6 level with unspecified spinal cord injury

806.31 T_1-T_6 level with complete lesion of cord

806.32 T_1-T_6 level with anterior cord syndrome

806.33 T_1-T_6 level with central cord syndrome

806.34 T_1-T_6 level with other specified spinal cord injury
T_1-T_6 level with:
incomplete spinal cord lesion NOS
posterior cord syndrome

806.35 T_7-T_{12} level with unspecified spinal cord injury

806.36 T_7-T_{12} level with complete lesion of cord

806.37 T_7-T_{12} level with anterior cord syndrome

806.38 T_7-T_{12} level with central cord syndrome

806.39 T_7-T_{12} level with other specified spinal cord injury
T_7-T_{12} level with:
incomplete spinal cord lesion NOS
posterior cord syndrome

806.4 Lumbar, closed
AHA: 4Q, '99, 11, 13

806.5 Lumbar, open

√5th **806.6 Sacrum and coccyx, closed**

806.60 With unspecified spinal cord injury

806.61 With complete cauda equina lesion

806.62 With other cauda equina injury

806.69 With other spinal cord injury

√5th **806.7 Sacrum and coccyx, open**

806.70 With unspecified spinal cord injury

806.71 With complete cauda equina lesion

806.72 With other cauda equina injury

806.79 With other spinal cord injury

806.8 Unspecified, closed

806.9 Unspecified, open

√4th **807 Fracture of rib(s), sternum, larynx, and trachea**

The following fifth-digit subclassification is for use with codes 807.0-807.1:
  0 rib(s) unspecifed
  1 one rib
  2 two ribs
  3 three ribs
  4 four ribs
  5 five ribs
  6 six ribs
  7 seven ribs
  8 eight or more ribs
  9 multiple ribs, unspecified

§ √5th **807.0 Rib(s), closed**
[0-9]
AHA: For codes 807.00-807.02: ▶1Q, '13, 15◀
S22.31xA Fracture one rib right side, initial encounter closed fx   I-10
S22.43xG Mx fx ribs bilat subseqnt enc fx delayed healing   I-10

§ √5th **807.1 Rib(s), open**
[0-9]

Ribs, Sternum, Larynx, and Trachea

Hyoid bone
Laryngeal cartilage
Clavicle
Mandible
Cricoid cartilage
Trachea
Manubrium of sternum
Sternum
Rib cage
Xiphoid process
Costal cartilages

807.2 Sternum, closed
DEF: Break in flat bone (breast bone) in anterior thorax.

807.3 Sternum, open
DEF: Break, with open wound, in flat bone in mid anterior thorax.

807.4 Flail chest

807.5 Larynx and trachea, closed
Hyoid bone
Thyroid cartilage
Trachea

807.6 Larynx and trachea, open

√4th **808 Fracture of pelvis**

808.0 Acetabulum, closed

808.1 Acetabulum, open

808.2 Pubis, closed
AHA: 1Q, '08, 9
S32.509A Unspec fx unspec pubis initial encounter closed fx   I-10

808.3 Pubis, open

√5th **808.4 Other specified part, closed**

808.41 Ilium

808.42 Ischium

808.43 Multiple closed pelvic fractures with disruption of pelvic circle
Multiple closed pelvic fractures with disruption of pelvic ring
AHA: 1Q, '08, 9
TIP: To assign, documentation must indicate multiple pelvic fractures with complete disruption of the pelvic circle.

808.44 Multiple closed pelvic fractures without disruption of pelvic circle
Multiple closed pelvic fractures without disruption of pelvic ring
AHA: 4Q, '11, 141-142

808.49 Other
Innominate bone
Pelvic rim

√5th **808.5 Other specified part, open**

808.51 Ilium

808.52 Ischium

808.53 Multiple open pelvic fractures with disruption of pelvic circle
Multiple open pelvic fractures with disruption of pelvic ring

808.54 Multiple open pelvic fractures without disruption of pelvic circle
Multiple open pelvic fractures without disruption of pelvic ring
AHA: 4Q, '11, 141-142

808.59 Other

808.8 Unspecified, closed

808.9 Unspecified, open

√4th **809 Ill-defined fractures of bones of trunk**

INCLUDES bones of trunk with other bones except those of skull and face
multiple bones of trunk

EXCLUDES multiple fractures of:
pelvic bones alone (808.0-808.9)
ribs alone (807.0-807.1, 807.4)
ribs or sternum with limb bones (819.0-819.1, 828.0-828.1)
skull or face with other bones (804.0-804.9)

809.0 Fracture of bones of trunk, closed

809.1 Fracture of bones of trunk, open

§ Requires fifth digit. Valid digits are in [brackets] under each code. See category 807 for codes and definitions.

N Newborn Age: 0   P Pediatric Age: 0-17   M Maternity Age: 12-55   A Adult Age: 15-124

Pelvis and Pelvic Fractures

Right Clavicle and Scapula, Anterior View

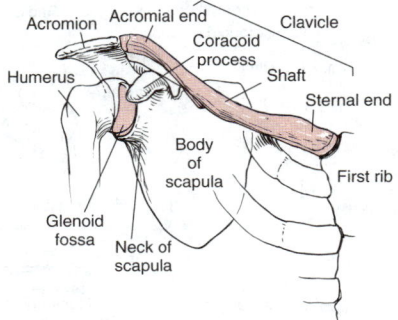

Fracture of Upper Limb (810-819)

✓4th 810 Fracture of clavicle

INCLUDES collar bone
interligamentous part of clavicle

The following fifth-digit subclassification is for use with category 810:
  0 unspecified part
     Clavicle NOS
  1 sternal end of clavicle
  2 shaft of clavicle
  3 acromial end of clavicle

§ ✓5th 810.0 Closed
[0-3]

§ ✓5th 810.1 Open
[0-3]

✓4th 811 Fracture of scapula

INCLUDES shoulder blade

The following fifth-digit subclassification is for use with category 811:
  0 unspecified part
  1 acromial process
     Acromion (process)
  2 coracoid process
  3 glenoid cavity and neck of scapula
  9 other

§ ✓5th 811.0 Closed
[0-3, 9]

§ ✓5th 811.1 Open
[0-3, 9]

✓4th 812 Fracture of humerus

✓5th 812.0 Upper end, closed

812.00 Upper end, unspecified part
Proximal end   Shoulder

812.01 Surgical neck
Neck of humerus NOS
S42.214A Uns nondsplcd fx surg neck rt   I-10
humerus inital enc closed fx

812.02 Anatomical neck

812.03 Greater tuberosity

812.09 Other
Head   Upper epiphysis
Lesser tuberosity
S42.294A Oth nondsplcd fx up end rt humerus   I-10
initial enc clos fx

✓5th 812.1 Upper end, open

812.10 Upper end, unspecified part

812.11 Surgical neck

812.12 Anatomical neck

812.13 Greater tuberosity

812.19 Other

Right Humerus, Anterior View

✓5th 812.2 Shaft or unspecified part, closed

812.20 Unspecified part of humerus
Humerus NOS   Upper arm NOS

812.21 Shaft of humerus
AHA: 4Q, '05, 129; 3Q, '99, 14

✓5th 812.3 Shaft or unspecified part, open

812.30 Unspecified part of humerus

812.31 Shaft of humerus

✓5th 812.4 Lower end, closed
Distal end of humerus   Elbow

812.40 Lower end, unspecified part

812.41 Supracondylar fracture of humerus

812.42 Lateral condyle
External condyle

812.43 Medial condyle
Internal epicondyle

812.44 Condyle(s), unspecified
Articular process NOS   Lower epiphysis NOS

812.49 Other
Multiple fractures of lower end   Trochlea

✓5th 812.5 Lower end, open

812.50 Lower end, unspecified part

812.51 Supracondylar fracture of humerus

812.52 Lateral condyle

812.53 Medial condyle

812.54 Condyle(s), unspecified

812.59 Other

✓4th 813 Fracture of radius and ulna

✓5th 813.0 Upper end, closed
Proximal end

813.00 Upper end of forearm, unspecified

813.01 Olecranon process of ulna

813.02 Coronoid process of ulna

---

§   Requires fifth digit. Valid digits are in [brackets] under each code. See appropriate category for codes and definitions.

| ✓4th ✓5th Additional Digit Required | Unspecified Code | Other Specified Code | Manifestation Code | ▶◀ Revised Text | ● New Code | ▲ Revised Code Title |

Right Radius and Ulna, Anterior View

813.03 Monteggia's fracture
> **DEF:** Fracture near the head of the ulnar shaft, causing dislocation of the radial head.

813.04 Other and unspecified fractures of proximal end of ulna (alone)
> Multiple fractures of ulna, upper end

813.05 Head of radius

813.06 Neck of radius

813.07 Other and unspecified fractures of proximal end of radius (alone)
> Multiple fractures of radius, upper end

813.08 Radius with ulna, upper end [any part]

√5th **813.1 Upper end, open**

813.10 Upper end of forearm, unspecified

813.11 Olecranon process of ulna

813.12 Coronoid process of ulna

813.13 Monteggia's fracture

813.14 Other and unspecified fractures of proximal end of ulna (alone)

813.15 Head of radius

813.16 Neck of radius

813.17 Other and unspecified fractures of proximal end of radius (alone)

813.18 Radius with ulna, upper end [any part]

√5th **813.2 Shaft, closed**

813.20 Shaft, unspecified

813.21 Radius (alone)

813.22 Ulna (alone)

813.23 Radius with ulna
> AHA: 4Q, '09, 120

√5th **813.3 Shaft, open**

813.30 Shaft, unspecified

813.31 Radius (alone)

813.32 Ulna (alone)

813.33 Radius with ulna

√5th **813.4 Lower end, closed**
> Distal end

813.40 Lower end of forearm, unspecified

813.41 Colles' fracture
> Smith's fracture
> **DEF:** Break of lower end of radius; associated with backward movement of the radius lower section.

813.42 Other fractures of distal end of radius (alone)
> Dupuytren's fracture, radius   Radius, lower end
> **DEF:** Dupuytren's fracture: fracture and dislocation of the forearm; the fracture is of the radius above the wrist, and the dislocation is of the ulna at the lower end.
> **S52.501A** Uns fx lower end rt radius initial enc closed fx   I-10

813.43 Distal end of ulna (alone)
> Ulna: Ulna:
> head   lower epiphysis
> lower end   styloid process

813.44 Radius with ulna, lower end
> AHA: 1Q, '07, 7

813.45 Torus fracture of radius (alone)
> **EXCLUDES** torus fracture of radius and ulna (813.47)
> AHA: 4Q, '02, 70

813.46 Torus fracture of ulna (alone)
> **EXCLUDES** torus fracture of radius and ulna (813.47)
> AHA: 4Q, '09, 110

813.47 Torus fracture of radius and ulna
> AHA: 4Q, '09, 110

√5th **813.5 Lower end, open**

813.50 Lower end of forearm, unspecified

813.51 Colles' fracture

813.52 Other fractures of distal end of radius (alone)

813.53 Distal end of ulna (alone)

813.54 Radius with ulna, lower end

√5th **813.8 Unspecified part, closed**

813.80 Forearm, unspecified

813.81 Radius (alone)
> AHA: 2Q, '98, 19

813.82 Ulna (alone)

813.83 Radius with ulna

√5th **813.9 Unspecified part, open**

813.90 Forearm, unspecified

813.91 Radius (alone)

813.92 Ulna (alone)

813.93 Radius with ulna

√4th **814 Fracture of carpal bone(s)**

> The following fifth-digit subclassification is for use with category 814:
> 0 carpal bone, unspecified
>   Wrist NOS
> 1 navicular [scaphoid] of wrist
> 2 lunate [semilunar] bone of wrist
> 3 triquetral [cuneiform] bone of wrist
> 4 pisiform
> 5 trapezium bone [larger multangular]
> 6 trapezoid bone [smaller multangular]
> 7 capitate bone [os magnum]
> 8 hamate [unciform] bone
> 9 other

§ √5th **814.0 Closed**
> [0-9]

§ √5th **814.1 Open**
> [0-9]

Hand Fractures

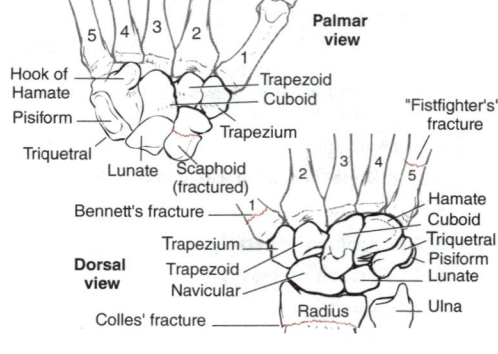

§ Requires fifth digit. Valid digits are in [brackets] under each code. See category 814 for codes and definitions.

√4th **815** **Fracture of metacarpal bone(s)**

INCLUDES hand [except finger]
metacarpus

The following fifth-digit subclassification is for use with category 815:
0 **metacarpal bone(s), site unspecified**
1 **base of thumb [first] metacarpal**
Bennett's fracture
2 **base of other metacarpal bone(s)**
3 **shaft of metacarpal bone(s)**
4 **neck of metacarpal bone(s)**
9 **multiple sites of metacarpus**

§ √5th **815.0 Closed**
[0-4, 9]

§ √5th **815.1 Open**
[0-4, 9]

√4th **816** **Fracture of one or more phalanges of hand**

INCLUDES finger(s)
thumb

The following fifth-digit subclassification is for use with category 816:
0 **phalanx or phalanges, unspecified**
1 **middle or proximal phalanx or phalanges**
2 **distal phalanx or phalanges**
3 **multiple sites**

TIP: If phalangeal fracture(s) are due to crushing injury, sequence that code (927.3) first.

§ √5th **816.0 Closed**
[0-3]

§ √5th **816.1 Open**
[0-3] AHA: For code 816.12: 4Q, '03, 77

√4th **817** **Multiple fractures of hand bones**

INCLUDES metacarpal bone(s) with phalanx or phalanges of same hand

817.0 Closed

817.1 Open

√4th **818** **Ill-defined fractures of upper limb**

INCLUDES arm NOS
multiple bones of same upper limb

EXCLUDES multiple fractures of:
metacarpal bone(s) with phalanx or phalanges (817.0-817.1)
phalanges of hand alone (816.0-816.1)
radius with ulna (813.0-813.9)

818.0 Closed

818.1 Open

√4th **819** **Multiple fractures involving both upper limbs, and upper limb with rib(s) and sternum**

INCLUDES arm(s) with rib(s) or sternum
both arms [any bones]

819.0 Closed

819.1 Open

Fracture of Lower Limb (820-829)

√4th **820** **Fracture of neck of femur**

√5th **820.0 Transcervical fracture, closed**

820.00 Intracapsular section, unspecified

820.01 Epiphysis (separation) (upper)
Transepiphyseal

820.02 Midcervical section
Transcervical NOS
AHA: 3Q, '03, 12

820.03 Base of neck
Cervicotrochanteric section

820.09 Other
Head of femur   Subcapital
S72.064A Nondsplcd art fx head rt femur   I-10
initial enc closed fx

√5th **820.1 Transcervical fracture, open**

820.10 Intracapsular section, unspecified

820.11 Epiphysis (separation) (upper)

820.12 Midcervical section

820.13 Base of neck

820.19 Other

√5th **820.2 Pertrochanteric fracture, closed**

820.20 Trochanteric section, unspecified
Trochanter:
NOS
greater
lesser

820.21 Intertrochanteric section

820.22 Subtrochanteric section
S72.25xA Nondsplcd subtrochant fx lt femur   I-10
inital enc closed fx

√5th **820.3 Pertrochanteric fracture, open**

820.30 Trochanteric section, unspecified

820.31 Intertrochanteric section

820.32 Subtrochanteric section

820.8 Unspecified part of neck of femur, closed
Hip NOS   Neck of femur NOS
S72.002A Fx uns part neck left femur initial enc clos fx   I-10

820.9 Unspecified part of neck of femur, open

√4th **821** **Fracture of other and unspecified parts of femur**

√5th **821.0 Shaft or unspecified part, closed**

821.00 Unspecified part of femur
Thigh   Upper leg
EXCLUDES hip NOS (820.8)

821.01 Shaft
AHA: 1Q, '07, 4; 1Q, '99, 5
S72.331A Displaced obl fx shaft rt femur initial   I-10
enc clos fx

√5th **821.1 Shaft or unspecified part, open**

821.10 Unspecified part of femur

821.11 Shaft

√5th **821.2 Lower end, closed**
Distal end

821.20 Lower end, unspecified part

821.21 Condyle, femoral

821.22 Epiphysis, lower (separation)

821.23 Supracondylar fracture of femur

821.29 Other
Multiple fractures of lower end

√5th **821.3 Lower end, open**

821.30 Lower end, unspecified part

821.31 Condyle, femoral

821.32 Epiphysis, lower (separation)

821.33 Supracondylar fracture of femur

821.39 Other

√4th **822** **Fracture of patella**

822.0 Closed
S82.001A Uns fx right patella initial encounter closed fx   I-10

822.1 Open

---

§ Requires fifth digit. Valid digits are in [brackets] under each code. See appropriate category for codes and definitions.

√4th
√5th Additional Digit Required   Unspecified Code   Other Specified Code   Manifestation Code   ►◄ Revised Text   ● New Code   ▲ Revised Code Title

Injury and Poisoning

823–825.29

Right Femur, Anterior View

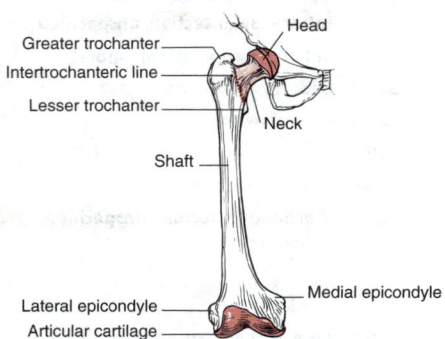

Right Tibia and Fibula, Anterior View

Torus Fracture

Anterior views of torus compression fracture

✓4th **823 Fracture of tibia and fibula**

> EXCLUDES Dupuytren's fracture (824.4-824.5)
> ankle (824.4-824.5)
> radius (813.42, 813.52)
> Pott's fracture (824.4-824.5)
> that involving ankle (824.0-824.9)

> The following fifth-digit subclassification is for use with category 823:
>   **0 tibia alone**
>   **1 fibula alone**
>   **2 fibula with tibia**

§ ✓5th **823.0 Upper end, closed**
[0-2]   Head
     Proximal end
     Tibia:
       condyles
       tuberosity
     S82.121A Displcd fx lat condyle rt tibia initial enc clos fx   I-10

§ ✓5th **823.1 Upper end, open**
[0-2]

§ ✓5th **823.2 Shaft, closed**
[0-2]

§ ✓5th **823.3 Shaft, open**
[0-2]

§ ✓5th **823.4 Torus fracture**
[0-2]   **DEF:** A bone deformity in children, occurring commonly in the tibia and fibula, in which the bone bends and buckles but does not fracture.
     AHA: 4Q, '02, 70

§ ✓5th **823.8 Unspecified part, closed**
[0-2]   Lower leg NOS
     AHA: For code 823.82: 1Q, '97, 8

§ ✓5th **823.9 Unspecified part, open**
[0-2]

✓4th **824 Fracture of ankle**

> **TIP:** If ankle fracture also includes syndesmotic injury, assign also code 845.03 Sprains and strains of tibiofibular (ligament), distal.

   824.0 Medial malleolus, closed
     Tibia involving:
       ankle
       malleolus
     AHA: 1Q, '04, 9

   824.1 Medial malleolus, open

   824.2 Lateral malleolus, closed
     Fibula involving:
       ankle
       malleolus
     AHA: 2Q, '02, 3

   824.3 Lateral malleolus, open

   824.4 Bimalleolar, closed
     Dupuytren's fracture, fibula   Pott's fracture
     DEF: Bimalleolar, closed: Breaking of both nodules (malleoli) on either side of ankle joint, without an open wound.
     DEF: Dupuytren's fracture (Pott's fracture): The breaking of the farthest end of the lower leg bone (fibula), with injury to the farthest end joint of the other lower leg bone (tibia).
     AHA: 2Q, '12, 11
     S82.841A Displcd bimalleolar fx rt lw leg initl enc clos fx   I-10

   824.5 Bimalleolar, open

   824.6 Trimalleolar, closed
     Lateral and medial malleolus with anterior or posterior lip of tibia
     S82.855A Nondispl trimalleolar fx of left lower leg, init   I-10

   824.7 Trimalleolar, open

   824.8 Unspecified, closed
     Ankle NOS
     AHA: 3Q, '00, 12
     S89.302A Uns physeal fx low end lt fibula initial enc clo fx   I-10

   824.9 Unspecified, open

✓4th **825 Fracture of one or more tarsal and metatarsal bones**

   825.0 Fracture of calcaneus, closed
     Heel bone   Os calcis

   825.1 Fracture of calcaneus, open

✓5th **825.2 Fracture of other tarsal and metatarsal bones, closed**

     825.20 Unspecified bone(s) of foot [except toes]
       Instep

     825.21 Astragalus
       Talus

     825.22 Navicular [scaphoid], foot

     825.23 Cuboid

     825.24 Cuneiform, foot

     825.25 Metatarsal bone(s)

     825.29 Other
       Tarsal with metatarsal bone(s) only
       EXCLUDES calcaneus (825.0)

---

§   Requires fifth digit. Valid digits are in [brackets] under each code. See category 823 for codes and definitions.

Right Foot, Dorsal

√5ᵗʰ **825.3 Fracture of other tarsal and metatarsal bones, open**

825.30 Unspecified bone(s) of foot [except toes]

825.31 Astragalus

825.32 Navicular [scaphoid], foot

825.33 Cuboid

825.34 Cuneiform, foot

825.35 Metatarsal bone(s)

825.39 Other

√4ᵗʰ **826 Fracture of one or more phalanges of foot**
   INCLUDES   toe(s)

826.0 Closed

826.1 Open

√4ᵗʰ **827 Other, multiple, and ill-defined fractures of lower limb**
   INCLUDES   leg NOS
              multiple bones of same lower limb
   EXCLUDES   multiple fractures of:
              ankle bones alone (824.4-824.9)
              phalanges of foot alone (826.0-826.1)
              tarsal with metatarsal bones (825.29, 825.39)
              tibia with fibula (823.0-823.9 with fifth-digit 2)

827.0 Closed

827.1 Open

√4ᵗʰ **828 Multiple fractures involving both lower limbs, lower with upper limb, and lower limb(s) with rib(s) and sternum**
   INCLUDES   arm(s) with leg(s) [any bones]
              both legs [any bones]
              leg(s) with rib(s) or sternum

828.0 Closed

828.1 Open

√4ᵗʰ **829 Fracture of unspecified bones**

829.0 Unspecified bone, closed

829.1 Unspecified bone, open

Dislocation (830-839)

   INCLUDES   displacement
              subluxation
   EXCLUDES   congenital dislocation (754.0-755.8)
              pathological dislocation (718.2)
              recurrent dislocation (718.3)

   NOTE   The descriptions "closed" and "open," used in the fourth-digit subdivisions, include the following terms:

closed:	open:
complete	compound
dislocation NOS	infected
partial	with foreign body
simple	
uncomplicated	

   A dislocation not indicated as closed or open should be classified as closed.
   AHA: 3Q, '90, 12
   TIP: Do not assign if documentation indicates developmental dislocation; see instead subcategory 718.7.

√4ᵗʰ **830 Dislocation of jaw**
   INCLUDES   jaw (cartilage) (meniscus)
              mandible
              maxilla (inferior)
              temporomandibular (joint)

830.0 Closed dislocation

830.1 Open dislocation

√4ᵗʰ **831 Dislocation of shoulder**
   EXCLUDES   sternoclavicular joint (839.61, 839.71)
              sternum (839.61, 839.71)

   The following fifth-digit subclassification is for use with category 831:
   0 shoulder, unspecified
       Humerus NOS
   1 anterior dislocation of humerus
   2 posterior dislocation of humerus
   3 inferior dislocation of humerus
   4 acromioclavicular (joint)
       Clavicle
   9 other
       Scapula

   TIP: Do not assign if documentation indicates recurrent shoulder dislocation; see instead code 718.31.

§ √5ᵗʰ **831.0 Closed dislocation**
   [0-4, 9]

§ √5ᵗʰ **831.1 Open dislocation**
   [0-4, 9]

√4ᵗʰ **832 Dislocation of elbow**

   The following fifth-digit subclassification is for use with subcategories 832.0 and 832.1:
   0 elbow, unspecified
   1 anterior dislocation of elbow
   2 posterior dislocation of elbow
   3 medial dislocation of elbow
   4 lateral dislocation of elbow
   9 other

§ √5ᵗʰ **832.0 Closed dislocation**
   [0-4, 9]

§ √5ᵗʰ **832.1 Open dislocation**
   [0-4, 9]

832.2 Nursemaid's elbow
   Subluxation of radial head
   AHA: 4Q, '09, 110-111

√4ᵗʰ **833 Dislocation of wrist**

   The following fifth-digit subclassification is for use with category 833:
   0 wrist unspecified part
       Carpal (bone)
       Radius, distal end
   1 radioulnar (joint), distal
   2 radiocarpal (joint)
   3 midcarpal (joint)
   4 carpometacarpal (joint)
   5 metacarpal (bone), proximal end
   9 other
       Ulna, distal end

§ √5ᵗʰ **833.0 Closed dislocation**
   [0-5, 9]

§ √5ᵗʰ **833.1 Open dislocation**
   [0-5, 9]

√4ᵗʰ **834 Dislocation of finger**
   INCLUDES   finger(s)
              phalanx of hand
              thumb

   The following fifth-digit subclassification is for use with category 834:
   0 finger unspecified part
   1 metacarpophalangeal (joint)
       Metacarpal (bone), distal end
   2 interphalangeal (joint), hand

§ √5ᵗʰ **834.0 Closed dislocation**
   [0-2]

§ √5ᵗʰ **834.1 Open dislocation**
   [0-2]

---

§   Requires fifth digit. Valid digits are in [brackets] under each code. See appropriate category for codes and definitions.

√4ᵗʰ / √5ᵗʰ   Additional Digit Required   Unspecified Code   Other Specified Code   Manifestation Code   ▶◀ Revised Text   ● New Code   ▲ Revised Code Title

2015 ICD-9-CM   **Volume 1 – 283**

Injury and Poisoning

835–839.59

√4th **835 Dislocation of hip**

The following fifth-digit subclassification is for use with category 835:
0 dislocation of hip, unspecified
1 posterior dislocation
2 obturator dislocation
3 other anterior dislocation

§ √5th **835.0 Closed dislocation**
[0-3]

§ √5th **835.1 Open dislocation**
[0-3]

√4th **836 Dislocation of knee**

EXCLUDES   *dislocation of knee:*
old or pathological (718.2)
recurrent (718.3)
internal derangement of knee joint (717.0-717.5,
717.8-717.9)
old tear of cartilage or meniscus of knee (717.0-717.5,
717.8-717.9)

836.0 Tear of medial cartilage or meniscus of knee, current
Bucket handle tear:
NOS   } current injury
medial meniscus

836.1 Tear of lateral cartilage or meniscus of knee, current

836.2 Other tear of cartilage or meniscus of knee, current
Tear of:
cartilage
(semilunar)   } current injury, not specified as
meniscus   medial or lateral

836.3 Dislocation of patella, closed

836.4 Dislocation of patella, open

√5th **836.5 Other dislocation of knee, closed**

     836.50 Dislocation of knee, unspecified

     836.51 Anterior dislocation of tibia, proximal end
Posterior dislocation of femur, distal end, closed

     836.52 Posterior dislocation of tibia, proximal end
Anterior dislocation of femur, distal end, closed

     836.53 Medial dislocation of tibia, proximal end

     836.54 Lateral dislocation of tibia, proximal end

     836.59 Other

√5th **836.6 Other dislocation of knee, open**

     836.60 Dislocation of knee, unspecified

     836.61 Anterior dislocation of tibia, proximal end
Posterior dislocation of femur, distal end, open

     836.62 Posterior dislocation of tibia, proximal end
Anterior dislocation of femur, distal end, open

     836.63 Medial dislocation of tibia, proximal end

     836.64 Lateral dislocation of tibia, proximal end

     836.69 Other

√4th **837 Dislocation of ankle**

INCLUDES   astragalus
fibula, distal end
navicular, foot
scaphoid, foot
tibia, distal end

837.0 Closed dislocation

837.1 Open dislocation

√4th **838 Dislocation of foot**

The following fifth-digit subclassification is for use with category 838:
0 foot unspecified
1 tarsal (bone), joint unspecified
2 midtarsal (joint)
3 tarsometatarsal (joint)
4 metatarsal (bone), joint unspecified
5 metatarsophalangeal (joint)
6 interphalangeal (joint), foot
9 other
Phalanx of foot
Toe(s)

§ √5th **838.0 Closed dislocation**
[0-6, 9]

§ √5th **838.1 Open dislocation**
[0-6, 9]

√4th **839 Other, multiple, and ill-defined dislocations**

√5th **839.0 Cervical vertebra, closed**
Cervical spine
Neck

     839.00 Cervical vertebra, unspecified

     839.01 First cervical vertebra

     839.02 Second cervical vertebra

     839.03 Third cervical vertebra

     839.04 Fourth cervical vertebra

     839.05 Fifth cervical vertebra

     839.06 Sixth cervical vertebra

     839.07 Seventh cervical vertebra

     839.08 Multiple cervical vertebrae

√5th **839.1 Cervical vertebra, open**

     839.10 Cervical vertebra, unspecified

     839.11 First cervical vertebra

     839.12 Second cervical vertebra

     839.13 Third cervical vertebra

     839.14 Fourth cervical vertebra

     839.15 Fifth cervical vertebra

     839.16 Sixth cervical vertebra

     839.17 Seventh cervical vertebra

     839.18 Multiple cervical vertebrae

√5th **839.2 Thoracic and lumbar vertebra, closed**

     839.20 Lumbar vertebra

     839.21 Thoracic vertebra
Dorsal [thoracic] vertebra

√5th **839.3 Thoracic and lumbar vertebra, open**

     839.30 Lumbar vertebra

     839.31 Thoracic vertebra

√5th **839.4 Other vertebra, closed**

     839.40 Vertebra, unspecified site
Spine NOS

     839.41 Coccyx

     839.42 Sacrum
Sacroiliac (joint)

     839.49 Other

√5th **839.5 Other vertebra, open**

     839.50 Vertebra, unspecified site

     839.51 Coccyx

     839.52 Sacrum

     839.59 Other

§   Requires fifth digit. Valid digits are in [brackets] under each code. See appropriate category for codes and definitions.

N Newborn Age: 0   P Pediatric Age: 0-17   M Maternity Age: 12-55   A Adult Age: 15-124

√5th **839.6 Other location, closed**

839.61 Sternum
Sternoclavicular joint

839.69 Other
Pelvis

√5th **839.7 Other location, open**

839.71 Sternum

839.79 Other

839.8 Multiple and ill-defined, closed
Arm
Back
Hand
Multiple locations, except fingers or toes alone
Other ill-defined locations
Unspecified location

839.9 Multiple and ill-defined, open

Sprains and Strains of Joints and Adjacent Muscles (840-848)

INCLUDES
avulsion
hemarthrosis
laceration   of:
rupture   joint capsule
sprain   ligament
strain   muscle
tear   tendon

EXCLUDES laceration of tendon in open wounds (880-884 and 890-894 with .2)

√4th **840 Sprains and strains of shoulder and upper arm**

840.0 Acromioclavicular (joint) (ligament)

840.1 Coracoclavicular (ligament)

840.2 Coracohumeral (ligament)

840.3 Infraspinatus (muscle) (tendon)

840.4 Rotator cuff (capsule)
EXCLUDES complete rupture of rotator cuff, nontraumatic (727.61)

840.5 Subscapularis (muscle)

840.6 Supraspinatus (muscle) (tendon)

840.7 Superior glenoid labrum lesion
SLAP lesion
AHA: 2Q, '12, 15; 4Q,'01, 52
DEF: Detachment injury of the superior aspect of the glenoid labrum which is the ring of fibrocartilage attached to the rim of the glenoid cavity of the scapula.

840.8 Other specified sites of shoulder and upper arm

840.9 Unspecified site of shoulder and upper arm
Arm NOS
Shoulder NOS

√4th **841 Sprains and strains of elbow and forearm**

841.0 Radial collateral ligament

841.1 Ulnar collateral ligament

841.2 Radiohumeral (joint)

841.3 Ulnohumeral (joint)

841.8 Other specified sites of elbow and forearm

841.9 Unspecified site of elbow and forearm
Elbow NOS

√4th **842 Sprains and strains of wrist and hand**

√5th **842.0 Wrist**

842.00 Unspecified site

842.01 Carpal (joint)

842.02 Radiocarpal (joint) (ligament)

842.09 Other
Radioulnar joint, distal

√5th **842.1 Hand**

842.10 Unspecified site

842.11 Carpometacarpal (joint)

842.12 Metacarpophalangeal (joint)

842.13 Interphalangeal (joint)

842.19 Other
Midcarpal (joint)

√4th **843 Sprains and strains of hip and thigh**

843.0 Iliofemoral (ligament)

843.1 Ischiocapsular (ligament)

843.8 Other specified sites of hip and thigh

843.9 Unspecified site of hip and thigh
Hip NOS   Thigh NOS

√4th **844 Sprains and strains of knee and leg**

844.0 Lateral collateral ligament of knee

844.1 Medial collateral ligament of knee

844.2 Cruciate ligament of knee

844.3 Tibiofibular (joint) (ligament), superior

844.8 Other specified sites of knee and leg

844.9 Unspecified site of knee and leg
Knee NOS   Leg NOS

√4th **845 Sprains and strains of ankle and foot**

√5th **845.0 Ankle**

845.00 Unspecified site
AHA: 2Q, '02, 3

845.01 Deltoid (ligament), ankle
Internal collateral (ligament), ankle

845.02 Calcaneofibular (ligament)

845.03 Tibiofibular (ligament), distal
AHA: 1Q, '04, 9

845.09 Other
Achilles tendon

√5th **845.1 Foot**

845.10 Unspecified site

845.11 Tarsometatarsal (joint) (ligament)

845.12 Metatarsophalangeal (joint)

845.13 Interphalangeal (joint), toe

845.19 Other

√4th **846 Sprains and strains of sacroiliac region**

846.0 Lumbosacral (joint) (ligament)

846.1 Sacroiliac ligament

846.2 Sacrospinatus (ligament)

846.3 Sacrotuberous (ligament)

846.8 Other specified sites of sacroiliac region

846.9 Unspecified site of sacroiliac region

√4th **847 Sprains and strains of other and unspecified parts of back**
EXCLUDES lumbosacral (846.0)

847.0 Neck
Anterior longitudinal (ligament), cervical
Atlanto-axial (joints)
Atlanto-occipital (joints)
Whiplash injury
EXCLUDES neck injury NOS (959.0)
thyroid region (848.2)
S13.4xxA Sprain ligaments cervical spine initial encounter I-10

847.1 Thoracic

847.2 Lumbar

847.3 Sacrum
Sacrococcygeal (ligament)

847.4 Coccyx

847.9 Unspecified site of back
Back NOS

Injury and Poisoning

848–852.5

☑4ᵗʰ **848 Other and ill-defined sprains and strains**

848.0 Septal cartilage of nose

848.1 Jaw
    Temporomandibular (joint) (ligament)

848.2 Thyroid region
    Cricoarytenoid (joint) (ligament)   Thyroid cartilage
    Cricothyroid (joint) (ligament)

848.3 Ribs
    Chondrocostal (joint)   } without mention of injury
    Costal cartilage   } to sternum

☑5ᵗʰ **848.4 Sternum**

848.40 Unspecified site

848.41 Sternoclavicular (joint) (ligament)

848.42 Chondrosternal (joint)

848.49 Other
    Xiphoid cartilage

848.5 Pelvis
    Symphysis pubis
    EXCLUDES *that in childbirth (665.6)*

848.8 Other specified sites of sprains and strains

848.9 Unspecified site of sprain and strain

Intracranial Injury, Excluding those with Skull Fracture (850-854)

INCLUDES   traumatic brain injury without skull fracture
EXCLUDES   *intracranial injury with skull fracture (800-801 and 803-804, except .0 and .5)*
    open wound of head without intracranial injury (870.0-873.9)
    skull fracture alone (800-801 and 803-804 with .0, .5)

NOTE   The description "with open intracranial wound," used in the fourth-digit subdivisions, includes those specified as open or with mention of infection or foreign body.

The following fifth-digit subclassification is for use with categories 851-854:
  0 unspecified state of consciousness
  1 with no loss of consciousness
  2 with brief [less than one hour] loss of consciousness
  3 with moderate [1-24 hours] loss of consciousness
  4 with prolonged [more than 24 hours] loss of consciousness and return to pre-existing conscious level
  5 with prolonged [more than 24 hours] loss of consciousness without return to pre-existing conscious level
    Use fifth-digit 5 to designate when a patient is unconscious and dies before regaining consciousness, regardless of the duration of the loss of consciousness
  6 with loss of consciousness of unspecified duration
  9 with concussion, unspecified

AHA: 1Q, '93, 22
TIP: If documentation specifies only "head injury," with no further specificity, and is self-limiting, assign instead code 959.01 Head injury, unspecified.

☑4ᵗʰ **850 Concussion**

INCLUDES   commotio cerebri
EXCLUDES   *concussion with:*
    cerebral laceration or contusion (851.0-851.9)
    cerebral hemorrhage (852-853)
    head injury NOS (959.01)

AHA: 2Q, '96, 6; 4Q, '90, 24
TIP: When a patient is treated for symptoms within 24 to 48 hours of the concussion, clarify with the physician whether the concussion is still in the acute phase or is a postconcussion syndrome; if so, assign instead code 310.2.

850.0 With no loss of consciousness
    Concussion with mental confusion or disorientation, without loss of consciousness

☑5ᵗʰ **850.1 With brief loss of consciousness**
    Loss of consciousness for less than one hour
    AHA: 4Q, '03, 76; 1Q, '99, 10; 2Q, '92, 5

850.11 With loss of consciousness of 30 minutes or less
    S06.0x1A Concussion w/loc 30 min/less initial encounter I-10

850.12 With loss of consciousness from 31 to 59 minutes
    AHA: 4Q, '10, 111

850.2 With moderate loss of consciousness
    Loss of consciousness for 1-24 hours

850.3 With prolonged loss of consciousness and return to pre-existing conscious level
    Loss of consciousness for more than 24 hours with complete recovery

850.4 With prolonged loss of consciousness, without return to pre-existing conscious level

850.5 With loss of consciousness of unspecified duration
    S06.0x9A Concussion w/loc uns duration initial encounter   I-10

850.9 Concussion, unspecified

☑4ᵗʰ **851 Cerebral laceration and contusion**
    AHA: 4Q, '96, 36; 1Q, '93, 22; 4Q, '90, 24

§ ☑5ᵗʰ **851.0 Cortex (cerebral) contusion without mention of**
  [0-6, 9]**open intracranial wound**
    AHA: For code 851.00: 4Q, '10, 93

§ ☑5ᵗʰ **851.1 Cortex (cerebral) contusion with open**
  [0-6, 9]**intracranial wound**
    AHA: 1Q, '92, 9

§ ☑5ᵗʰ **851.2 Cortex (cerebral) laceration without mention of**
  [0-6, 9]**open intracranial wound**
    S06.330A Contus/lac cereb, w/o loss of consciousness, init   I-10

§ ☑5ᵗʰ **851.3 Cortex (cerebral) laceration with open intracranial wound**
  [0-6, 9]

§ ☑5ᵗʰ **851.4 Cerebellar or brain stem contusion without mention of**
  [0-6, 9]**open intracranial wound**

§ ☑5ᵗʰ **851.5 Cerebellar or brain stem contusion with open**
  [0-6, 9]**intracranial wound**

§ ☑5ᵗʰ **851.6 Cerebellar or brain stem laceration without**
  [0-6, 9]**mention of open intracranial wound**

§ ☑5ᵗʰ **851.7 Cerebellar or brain stem laceration with open**
  [0-6, 9]**intracranial wound**

§ ☑5ᵗʰ **851.8 Other and unspecified cerebral laceration and**
  [0-6, 9]**contusion, without mention of open intracranial wound**
    Brain (membrane) NOS
    AHA: 4Q, '96, 37

§ ☑5ᵗʰ **851.9 Other and unspecified cerebral laceration and**
  [0-6, 9]**contusion, with open intracranial wound**

☑4ᵗʰ **852 Subarachnoid, subdural, and extradural hemorrhage, following injury**
    EXCLUDES   *cerebral contusion or laceration (with hemorrhage) (851.0-851.9)*
    DEF: Bleeding from lining of brain; due to injury.

§ ☑5ᵗʰ **852.0 Subarachnoid hemorrhage following injury**
  [0-6, 9]**without mention of open intracranial wound**
    Middle meningeal hemorrhage following injury

§ ☑5ᵗʰ **852.1 Subarachnoid hemorrhage following injury with**
  [0-6, 9]**open intracranial wound**

§ ☑5ᵗʰ **852.2 Subdural hemorrhage following injury without**
  [0-6, 9]**mention of open intracranial wound**
    AHA: For code 852.25: 4Q, '11, 99; 4Q, '96, 43; For codes 852.21-852.29: 4Q, '07, 107

§ ☑5ᵗʰ **852.3 Subdural hemorrhage following injury with**
  [0-6, 9]**open intracranial wound**

§ ☑5ᵗʰ **852.4 Extradural hemorrhage following injury without**
  [0-6, 9]**mention of open intracranial wound**
    Epidural hematoma following injury

§ ☑5ᵗʰ **852.5 Extradural hemorrhage following injury with**
  [0-6, 9]**open intracranial wound**

---

§   Requires fifth digit. Valid digits are in [brackets] under each code. See beginning of section 850-854 for codes and definitions.

N Newborn Age: 0   P Pediatric Age: 0-17   M Maternity Age: 12-55   A Adult Age: 15-124

Brain

853 ✓4th **Other and unspecified intracranial hemorrhage following injury**

§ ✓5th **853.0 Without mention of open intracranial wound**
[0-6, 9]   Cerebral compression due to injury
Intracranial hematoma following injury
Traumatic cerebral hemorrhage
AHA: 3Q, '90, 14

§ ✓5th **853.1 With open intracranial wound**
[0-6, 9]

854 ✓4th **Intracranial injury of other and unspecified nature**
INCLUDES injury:
brain NOS
cavernous sinus
intracranial
traumatic brain NOS
EXCLUDES any condition classifiable to 850-853
head injury NOS (959.01)
AHA: 1Q, '99, 10; 2Q, '92, 6
TIP: Assign a code from category 854 for traumatic brain injury (TBI) with diffuse axonal injury (DAI), also known as a shear injury.

§ ✓5th **854.0 Without mention of open intracranial wound**
[0-6, 9]   **AHA: For code 854.00:** 4Q, '09, 108; 2Q, '05, 6

§ ✓5th **854.1 With open intracranial wound**
[0-6, 9]

Internal Injury of Thorax, Abdomen, and Pelvis (860-869)

INCLUDES   blast injuries
blunt trauma
bruise
concussion injuries (except cerebral)   } of internal
crushing   organs
hematoma
laceration
puncture
tear
traumatic rupture

EXCLUDES concussion NOS (850.0-850.9)
flail chest (807.4)
foreign body entering through orifice (930.0-939.9)
injury to blood vessels (901.0-902.9)

NOTE The description "with open wound," used in the fourth-digit
subdivisions, includes those with mention of infection or
foreign body.

860 ✓4th **Traumatic pneumothorax and hemothorax**
DEF: Traumatic pneumothorax: air or gas leaking into pleural space of lung due to trauma.
DEF: Traumatic hemothorax: blood buildup in pleural space of lung due to trauma.
AHA: 2Q, '93, 4
TIP: If there's no mention of trauma associated with pneumothorax, see instead category 512.

860.0 Pneumothorax without mention of open wound into thorax
S27.0xxA Traumatic pneumothorax initial encounter   I-10

860.1 Pneumothorax with open wound into thorax

860.2 Hemothorax without mention of open wound into thorax

860.3 Hemothorax with open wound into thorax

860.4 Pneumohemothorax without mention of open wound into thorax

860.5 Pneumohemothorax with open wound into thorax

861 ✓4th **Injury to heart and lung**
EXCLUDES injury to blood vessels of thorax (901.0-901.9)

✓5th **861.0 Heart, without mention of open wound into thorax**
AHA: 1Q, '92, 9

861.00 Unspecified injury

861.01 Contusion
Cardiac contusion
Myocardial contusion
DEF: Bruising within the pericardium with no mention of open wound.

861.02 Laceration without penetration of heart chambers
DEF: Tearing injury of heart tissue, without penetration of chambers; no open wound.

861.03 Laceration with penetration of heart chambers

✓5th **861.1 Heart, with open wound into thorax**

861.10 Unspecified injury

861.11 Contusion

861.12 Laceration without penetration of heart chambers

861.13 Laceration with penetration of heart chambers

✓5th **861.2 Lung, without mention of open wound into thorax**

861.20 Unspecified injury

861.21 Contusion
DEF: Bruising of lung without mention of open wound.
S27.321A Contusion of lung unilateral initial encounter   I-10

861.22 Laceration

✓5th **861.3 Lung, with open wound into thorax**

861.30 Unspecified injury

861.31 Contusion

861.32 Laceration

862 ✓4th **Injury to other and unspecified intrathoracic organs**
EXCLUDES injury to blood vessels of thorax (901.0-901.9)

862.0 Diaphragm, without mention of open wound into cavity

862.1 Diaphragm, with open wound into cavity

✓5th **862.2 Other specified intrathoracic organs, without mention of open wound into cavity**

862.21 Bronchus

862.22 Esophagus

862.29 Other
Pleura
Thymus gland

✓5th **862.3 Other specified intrathoracic organs, with open wound into cavity**

862.31 Bronchus

862.32 Esophagus

862.39 Other

§   Requires fifth digit. Valid digits are in [brackets] under each code. See beginning of section 850-854 for codes and definitions.

| ✓4th ✓5th Additional Digit Required | Unspecified Code | Other Specified Code | Manifestation Code | ►◄ Revised Text | ● New Code | ▲ Revised Code Title |

Injury and Poisoning

862.8–867.7

862.8 Multiple and unspecified intrathoracic organs, without mention of open wound into cavity
Crushed chest   Multiple intrathoracic organs

862.9 Multiple and unspecified intrathoracic organs, with open wound into cavity

√4th **863 Injury to gastrointestinal tract**
EXCLUDES *anal sphincter laceration during delivery (664.2)*
bile duct (868.0-868.1 with fifth-digit 2)
gallbladder (868.0-868.1 with fifth-digit 2)

863.0 Stomach, without mention of open wound into cavity

863.1 Stomach, with open wound into cavity

√5th **863.2 Small intestine, without mention of open wound into cavity**

     863.20 Small intestine, unspecified site

     863.21 Duodenum

     863.29 Other

√5th **863.3 Small intestine, with open wound into cavity**

     863.30 Small intestine, unspecified site

     863.31 Duodenum

     863.39 Other

√5th **863.4 Colon or rectum, without mention of open wound into cavity**

     863.40 Colon, unspecified site

     863.41 Ascending [right] colon

     863.42 Transverse colon

     863.43 Descending [left] colon

     863.44 Sigmoid colon

     863.45 Rectum

     863.46 Multiple sites in colon and rectum

     863.49 Other

√5th **863.5 Colon or rectum, with open wound into cavity**

     863.50 Colon, unspecified site

     863.51 Ascending [right] colon

     863.52 Transverse colon

     863.53 Descending [left] colon

     863.54 Sigmoid colon

     863.55 Rectum

     863.56 Multiple sites in colon and rectum

     863.59 Other

√5th **863.8 Other and unspecified gastrointestinal sites, without mention of open wound into cavity**

     863.80 Gastrointestinal tract, unspecified site

     863.81 Pancreas, head

     863.82 Pancreas, body

     863.83 Pancreas, tail

     863.84 Pancreas, multiple and unspecified sites

     863.85 Appendix

     863.89 Other
         Intestine NOS

√5th **863.9 Other and unspecified gastrointestinal sites, with open wound into cavity**

     863.90 Gastrointestinal tract, unspecified site

     863.91 Pancreas, head

     863.92 Pancreas, body

     863.93 Pancreas, tail

     863.94 Pancreas, multiple and unspecified sites

     863.95 Appendix

863.99 Other

√4th **864 Injury to liver**
The following fifth-digit subclassification is for use with category 864:
   0   unspecified injury
   1   hematoma and contusion
   2   laceration, minor
       Laceration involving capsule only, or without significant involvement of hepatic parenchyma [i.e., less than 1 cm deep]
   3   laceration, moderate
       Laceration involving parenchyma but without major disruption of parenchyma [i.e., less than 10 cm long and less than 3 cm deep]
   4   laceration, major
       Laceration with significant disruption of hepatic parenchyma [i.e., 10 cm long and 3 cm deep]
       Multiple moderate lacerations, with or without hematoma
       Stellate lacerations of liver
   5   laceration, unspecified
   9   other

§ √5th **864.0 Without mention of open wound into cavity**
[0-5, 9]

§ √5th **864.1 With open wound into cavity**
[0-5, 9]

√4th **865 Injury to spleen**
The following fifth-digit subclassification is for use with category 865:
   0   unspecified injury
   1   hematoma without rupture of capsule
   2   capsular tears, without major disruption of parenchyma
   3   laceration extending into parenchyma
   4   massive parenchymal disruption
   9   other

§ √5th **865.0 Without mention of wound into cavity**
[0-4, 9]

§ √5th **865.1 With open wound into cavity**
[0-4, 9]

√4th **866 Injury to kidney**
EXCLUDES *acute kidney injury (nontraumatic) (584.9)*
The following fifth-digit subclassification is for use with category 866:
   0   unspecified injury
   1   hematoma without rupture of capsule
   2   laceration
   3   complete disruption of kidney parenchyma
AHA: 4Q, '08, 192

§ √5th **866.0 Without mention of open wound into cavity**
[0-3]

§ √5th **866.1 With open wound into cavity**
[0-3]

√4th **867 Injury to pelvic organs**
EXCLUDES *injury during delivery (664.0-665.9)*

867.0 Bladder and urethra, without mention of open wound into cavity
     AHA: ▶1Q, '14, 12;◀ N-D, '85, 15
     TIP: Assign for urethral injury due to patient's pulling out indwelling urinary catheter.
     S37.20xA Unspecified injury of bladder initial encounter   I-10

867.1 Bladder and urethra, with open wound into cavity

867.2 Ureter, without mention of open wound into cavity

867.3 Ureter, with open wound into cavity

867.4 Uterus, without mention of open wound into cavity   ♀

867.5 Uterus, with open wound into cavity   ♀

867.6 Other specified pelvic organs, without mention of open wound into cavity
     Fallopian tube   Seminal vesicle
     Ovary   Vas deferens
     Prostate

867.7 Other specified pelvic organs, with open wound into cavity

---

§ Requires fifth digit. Valid digits are in [brackets] under each code. See appropriate category for codes and definitions.

N Newborn Age: 0   P Pediatric Age: 0-17   M Maternity Age: 12-55   A Adult Age: 15-124

867.8 Unspecified pelvic organ, without mention of open wound into cavity

867.9 Unspecified pelvic organ, with open wound into cavity

√4th **868 Injury to other intra-abdominal organs**

The following fifth-digit subclassification is for use with category 868:

> 0 unspecified intra-abdominal organ
> 1 adrenal gland
> 2 bile duct and gallbladder
> 3 peritoneum
> 4 retroperitoneum
> 9 other and multiple intra-abdominal organs

§ √5th **868.0 Without mention of open wound into cavity**
[0-4, 9]

§ √5th **868.1 With open wound into cavity**
[0-4, 9]

√4th **869 Internal injury to unspecified or ill-defined organs**

INCLUDES internal injury NOS
multiple internal injury NOS

869.0 Without mention of open wound into cavity

869.1 With open wound into cavity
AHA: 2Q, '89, 15

Open Wound (870-897)

INCLUDES animal bite
avulsion
cut
laceration
puncture wound
traumatic amputation

EXCLUDES burn (940.0-949.5)
crushing (925-929.9)
puncture of internal organs (860.0-869.1)
superficial injury (910.0-919.9)
that incidental to:
dislocation (830.0-839.9)
fracture (800.0-829.1)
internal injury (860.0-869.1)
intracranial injury (851.0-854.1)

NOTE The description "complicated" used in the fourth-digit subdivisions includes those with mention of delayed healing, delayed treatment, foreign body, or infection.

AHA: 4Q, '01, 52

TIP: Do not assign a code designated as "complicated" based only on physician documentation of complicated. For coding purposes, there must be indications of delayed healing, delayed treatment, infection, or foreign body.

Open Wound of Head, Neck, and Trunk (870-879)

√4th **870 Open wound of ocular adnexa**

870.0 Laceration of skin of eyelid and periocular area

870.1 Laceration of eyelid, full-thickness, not involving lacrimal passages

870.2 Laceration of eyelid involving lacrimal passages

870.3 Penetrating wound of orbit, without mention of foreign body

870.4 Penetrating wound of orbit with foreign body
EXCLUDES retained (old) foreign body in orbit (376.6)

870.8 Other specified open wounds of ocular adnexa

870.9 Unspecified open wound of ocular adnexa

√4th **871 Open wound of eyeball**

EXCLUDES 2nd cranial nerve [optic] injury (950.0-950.9)
3rd cranial nerve [oculomotor] injury (951.0)

871.0 Ocular laceration without prolapse of intraocular tissue
DEF: Tear in ocular tissue without displacing structures.
AHA: 3Q, '96, 7

871.1 Ocular laceration with prolapse or exposure of intraocular tissue

871.2 Rupture of eye with partial loss of intraocular tissue
DEF: Forcible tearing of eyeball, with tissue loss.

871.3 Avulsion of eye
Traumatic enucleation
DEF: Traumatic extraction of eyeball from socket.

871.4 Unspecified laceration of eye

871.5 Penetration of eyeball with magnetic foreign body
EXCLUDES retained (old) magnetic foreign body in globe (360.50-360.59)

871.6 Penetration of eyeball with (nonmagnetic) foreign body
EXCLUDES retained (old) (nonmagnetic) foreign body in globe (360.60-360.69)

871.7 Unspecified ocular penetration

871.9 Unspecified open wound of eyeball

√4th **872 Open wound of ear**

√5th **872.0 External ear, without mention of complication**

872.00 External ear, unspecified site

872.01 Auricle, ear
Pinna
DEF: Open wound of fleshy, outer ear.

872.02 Auditory canal
DEF: Open wound of passage from external ear to eardrum.

√5th **872.1 External ear, complicated**

872.10 External ear, unspecified site

872.11 Auricle, ear

872.12 Auditory canal

√5th **872.6 Other specified parts of ear, without mention of complication**

872.61 Ear drum
Drumhead   Tympanic membrane

872.62 Ossicles

872.63 Eustachian tube
DEF: Open wound of channel between nasopharynx and tympanic cavity.

872.64 Cochlea
DEF: Open wound of snail shell shaped tube of inner ear.

872.69 Other and multiple sites

√5th **872.7 Other specified parts of ear, complicated**

872.71 Ear drum

872.72 Ossicles

872.73 Eustachian tube

872.74 Cochlea

872.79 Other and multiple sites

872.8 Ear, part unspecified, without mention of complication
Ear NOS

872.9 Ear, part unspecified, complicated

√4th **873 Other open wound of head**

873.0 Scalp, without mention of complication
S01.01xA Laceration w/o foreign body scalp initial enc   I-10

873.1 Scalp, complicated

√5th **873.2 Nose, without mention of complication**

873.20 Nose, unspecified site

873.21 Nasal septum
DEF: Open wound between nasal passages.

873.22 Nasal cavity
DEF: Open wound of nostrils.

873.23 Nasal sinus
DEF: Open wound of mucous-lined respiratory cavities.

873.29 Multiple sites

√5th **873.3 Nose, complicated**

873.30 Nose, unspecified site

§ Requires fifth digit. Valid digits are in [brackets] under each code. See category 868 for codes and definitions.

873.31 **Nasal septum**

873.32 **Nasal cavity**

873.33 **Nasal sinus**

873.39 **Multiple sites**

√5ᵗʰ 873.4 **Face, without mention of complication**

     873.40 **Face, unspecified site**

     873.41 **Cheek**

     873.42 **Forehead**
        Eyebrow
        AHA: 4Q, '96, 43
        S01.81xA Laceration w/o FB other part head   I-10
        initial enc

     873.43 **Lip**

     873.44 **Jaw**

     873.49 **Other and multiple sites**

√5ᵗʰ 873.5 **Face, complicated**

     873.50 **Face, unspecified site**

     873.51 **Cheek**

     873.52 **Forehead**

     873.53 **Lip**

     873.54 **Jaw**

     873.59 **Other and multiple sites**

√5ᵗʰ 873.6 **Internal structures of mouth, without mention of complication**

     873.60 **Mouth, unspecified site**

     873.61 **Buccal mucosa**
        DEF: Open wound of inside of cheek.

     873.62 **Gum (alveolar process)**

     873.63 **Tooth (broken) (fractured) (due to trauma)**
        EXCLUDES *cracked tooth (521.81)*
        AHA: 1Q, '04, 17

     873.64 **Tongue and floor of mouth**

     873.65 **Palate**
        DEF: Open wound of roof of mouth.

     873.69 **Other and multiple sites**

√5ᵗʰ 873.7 **Internal structures of mouth, complicated**

     873.70 **Mouth, unspecified site**

     873.71 **Buccal mucosa**

     873.72 **Gum (alveolar process)**

     873.73 **Tooth (broken) (fractured) (due to trauma)**
        EXCLUDES *cracked tooth (521.81)*
        AHA: 1Q, '04, 17

     873.74 **Tongue and floor of mouth**

     873.75 **Palate**

     873.79 **Other and multiple sites**

873.8 **Other and unspecified open wound of head without mention of complication**
     Head NOS

873.9 **Other and unspecified complicated open wound of head**

√4ᵗʰ 874 **Open wound of neck**

√5ᵗʰ 874.0 **Larynx and trachea, without mention of complication**

     874.00 **Larynx with trachea**

     874.01 **Larynx**

     874.02 **Trachea**

√5ᵗʰ 874.1 **Larynx and trachea, complicated**

     874.10 **Larynx with trachea**

     874.11 **Larynx**

     874.12 **Trachea**

874.2 **Thyroid gland, without mention of complication**

874.3 **Thyroid gland, complicated**

874.4 **Pharynx, without mention of complication**
     Cervical esophagus

874.5 **Pharynx, complicated**

874.8 **Other and unspecified parts, without mention of complication**
     Nape of neck
     Supraclavicular region
     Throat NOS

874.9 **Other and unspecified parts, complicated**

√4ᵗʰ 875 **Open wound of chest (wall)**
     EXCLUDES *open wound into thoracic cavity (860.0-862.9)*
              traumatic pneumothorax and hemothorax (860.1, 860.3, 860.5)
     AHA: 3Q, '95, 17; 3Q, '93, 17

875.0 **Without mention of complication**

875.1 **Complicated**

√4ᵗʰ 876 **Open wound of back**
     INCLUDES loin
               lumbar region
     EXCLUDES *open wound into thoracic cavity (860.0-862.9)*
              traumatic pneumothorax and hemothorax (860.1, 860.3, 860.5)

876.0 **Without mention of complication**

876.1 **Complicated**

√4ᵗʰ 877 **Open wound of buttock**
     INCLUDES sacroiliac region

877.0 **Without mention of complication**

877.1 **Complicated**

√4ᵗʰ 878 **Open wound of genital organs (external), including traumatic amputation**
     EXCLUDES *injury during delivery (664.0-665.9)*
              internal genital organs (867.0-867.9)

878.0 **Penis, without mention of complication**   ♂

878.1 **Penis, complicated**   ♂

878.2 **Scrotum and testes, without mention of complication**   ♂

878.3 **Scrotum and testes, complicated**   ♂

878.4 **Vulva, without mention of complication**   ♀
     Labium (majus) (minus)

878.5 **Vulva, complicated**   ♀

878.6 **Vagina, without mention of complication**   ♀

878.7 **Vagina, complicated**   ♀

878.8 **Other and unspecified parts, without mention of complication**

878.9 **Other and unspecified parts, complicated**

√4ᵗʰ 879 **Open wound of other and unspecified sites, except limbs**

879.0 **Breast, without mention of complication**

879.1 **Breast, complicated**

879.2 **Abdominal wall, anterior, without mention of complication**
     Abdominal wall NOS   Pubic region
     Epigastric region   Umbilical region
     Hypogastric region
     AHA: 2Q, '91, 22; 3Q, '90, 5
     TIP: If the abdominal wall open wound results in aortic rupture, sequence code 902.0 first.

879.3 **Abdominal wall, anterior, complicated**

879.4 **Abdominal wall, lateral, without mention of complication**
     Flank   Iliac (region)
     Groin   Inguinal region
     Hypochondrium

879.5 **Abdominal wall, lateral, complicated**

N Newborn Age: 0   P Pediatric Age: 0-17   M Maternity Age: 12-55   A Adult Age: 15-124

879.6 Other and unspecified parts of trunk, without mention of complication
Pelvic region   Trunk NOS
Perineum

879.7 Other and unspecified parts of trunk, complicated

879.8 Open wound(s) (multiple) of unspecified site(s) without mention of complication
Multiple open wounds NOS   Open wound NOS

879.9 Open wound(s) (multiple) of unspecified site(s), complicated

Open Wound of Upper Limb (880-887)

AHA: N-D, '85, 5
TIP: For degloving injuries, assign code for open wound of the specified site, most often involving extremities.

√4th 880 Open wound of shoulder and upper arm

The following fifth-digit subclassification is for use with category 880:
   0 shoulder region
   1 scapular region
   2 axillary region
   3 upper arm
   9 multiple sites

§ √5th **880.0 Without mention of complication**
[0-3, 9]

§ √5th **880.1 Complicated**
[0-3, 9]   **AHA: For code 880.13:** 2Q, '06, 7

§ √5th **880.2 With tendon involvement**
[0-3, 9]

√4th 881 Open wound of elbow, forearm, and wrist

The following fifth-digit subclassification is for use with category 881:
   0 forearm
   1 elbow
   2 wrist

§ √5th **881.0 Without mention of complication**
[0-2]

§ √5th **881.1 Complicated**
[0-2]

§ √5th **881.2 With tendon involvement**
[0-2]

√4th 882 Open wound of hand except finger(s) alone

882.0 Without mention of complication

882.1 Complicated
     AHA: 4Q, '08, 152

882.2 With tendon involvement

√4th 883 Open wound of finger(s)
INCLUDES   fingernail
           thumb (nail)

883.0 Without mention of complication

883.1 Complicated

883.2 With tendon involvement

√4th 884 Multiple and unspecified open wound of upper limb
INCLUDES   arm NOS
           multiple sites of one upper limb
           upper limb NOS

884.0 Without mention of complication

884.1 Complicated

884.2 With tendon involvement

√4th 885 Traumatic amputation of thumb (complete) (partial)
INCLUDES   thumb(s) (with finger(s) of either hand)

885.0 Without mention of complication
     AHA: 1Q, '03, 7

885.1 Complicated

√4th 886 Traumatic amputation of other finger(s) (complete) (partial)
INCLUDES   finger(s) of one or both hands, without mention of thumb(s)

886.0 Without mention of complication

886.1 Complicated

√4th 887 Traumatic amputation of arm and hand (complete) (partial)

887.0 Unilateral, below elbow, without mention of complication

887.1 Unilateral, below elbow, complicated

887.2 Unilateral, at or above elbow, without mention of complication

887.3 Unilateral, at or above elbow, complicated

887.4 Unilateral, level not specified, without mention of complication

887.5 Unilateral, level not specified, complicated

887.6 Bilateral [any level], without mention of complication
One hand and other arm

887.7 Bilateral [any level], complicated

Open Wound of Lower Limb (890-897)

AHA: N-D, '85, 5

√4th 890 Open wound of hip and thigh

890.0 Without mention of complication

890.1 Complicated

890.2 With tendon involvement

√4th 891 Open wound of knee, leg [except thigh], and ankle
INCLUDES   leg NOS
           multiple sites of leg, except thigh
EXCLUDES   that of thigh (890.0-890.2)
           with multiple sites of lower limb (894.0-894.2)

891.0 Without mention of complication
     S81.031A Puncture wound w/o FB rt knee initial   I-10
     encounter

891.1 Complicated

891.2 With tendon involvement

√4th 892 Open wound of foot except toe(s) alone
INCLUDES   heel

892.0 Without mention of complication

892.1 Complicated

892.2 With tendon involvement

√4th 893 Open wound of toe(s)
INCLUDES   toenail

893.0 Without mention of complication

893.1 Complicated
     AHA: 4Q, '08, 73

893.2 With tendon involvement

√4th 894 Multiple and unspecified open wound of lower limb
INCLUDES   lower limb NOS
           multiple sites of one lower limb, with thigh

894.0 Without mention of complication

894.1 Complicated

894.2 With tendon involvement

√4th 895 Traumatic amputation of toe(s) (complete) (partial)
INCLUDES   toe(s) of one or both feet

895.0 Without mention of complication

895.1 Complicated

√4th 896 Traumatic amputation of foot (complete) (partial)

896.0 Unilateral, without mention of complication

896.1 Unilateral, complicated

---

§ Requires fifth digit. Valid digits are in [brackets] under each code. See appropriate category for codes and definitions.

Injury and Poisoning

896.2 Bilateral, without mention of complication
> EXCLUDES *one foot and other leg (897.6-897.7)*

896.3 Bilateral, complicated

✓4ᵗʰ **897 Traumatic amputation of leg(s) (complete) (partial)**

897.0 Unilateral, below knee, without mention of complication

897.1 Unilateral, below knee, complicated

897.2 Unilateral, at or above knee, without mention of complication

897.3 Unilateral, at or above knee, complicated

897.4 Unilateral, level not specified, without mention of complication

897.5 Unilateral, level not specified, complicated

897.6 Bilateral [any level], without mention of complication
> One foot and other leg

897.7 Bilateral [any level], complicated
> AHA: 3Q, '90, 5

Injury to Blood Vessels (900-904)

INCLUDES
arterial hematoma
avulsion
cut
laceration
rupture
traumatic aneurysm or fistula (arteriovenous)
} of blood vessel secondary to other injuries, e.g.; fracture or open wound

EXCLUDES *accidental puncture or laceration during medical procedure (998.2)*
intracranial hemorrhage following injury (851.0-854.1)
> AHA: 3Q, '90, 5

✓4ᵗʰ **900 Injury to blood vessels of head and neck**

✓5ᵗʰ **900.0 Carotid artery**

900.00 Carotid artery, unspecified
> AHA: ▶1Q, '14, 20; 4Q, '13, 92◀

900.01 Common carotid artery

900.02 External carotid artery

900.03 Internal carotid artery
> AHA: ▶1Q, '14, 20◀

900.1 Internal jugular vein

✓5ᵗʰ **900.8 Other specified blood vessels of head and neck**

900.81 External jugular vein
> Jugular vein NOS

900.82 Multiple blood vessels of head and neck

900.89 Other

900.9 Unspecified blood vessel of head and neck

✓4ᵗʰ **901 Injury to blood vessels of thorax**
> EXCLUDES *traumatic hemothorax (860.2-860.5)*

901.0 Thoracic aorta
> AHA: ▶4Q, '13, 92◀

901.1 Innominate and subclavian arteries

901.2 Superior vena cava

901.3 Innominate and subclavian veins

✓5ᵗʰ **901.4 Pulmonary blood vessels**

901.40 Pulmonary vessel(s), unspecified

901.41 Pulmonary artery

901.42 Pulmonary vein

✓5ᵗʰ **901.8 Other specified blood vessels of thorax**

901.81 Intercostal artery or vein

901.82 Internal mammary artery or vein

901.83 Multiple blood vessels of thorax

901.89 Other
> Azygos vein   Hemiazygos vein

901.9 Unspecified blood vessel of thorax

✓4ᵗʰ **902 Injury to blood vessels of abdomen and pelvis**

902.0 Abdominal aorta

✓5ᵗʰ **902.1 Inferior vena cava**

902.10 Inferior vena cava, unspecified

902.11 Hepatic veins

902.19 Other

✓5ᵗʰ **902.2 Celiac and mesenteric arteries**

902.20 Celiac and mesenteric arteries, unspecified

902.21 Gastric artery

902.22 Hepatic artery

902.23 Splenic artery

902.24 Other specified branches of celiac axis

902.25 Superior mesenteric artery (trunk)

902.26 Primary branches of superior mesenteric artery
> Ileocolic artery

902.27 Inferior mesenteric artery

902.29 Other

✓5ᵗʰ **902.3 Portal and splenic veins**

902.31 Superior mesenteric vein and primary subdivisions
> Ileocolic vein

902.32 Inferior mesenteric vein

902.33 Portal vein

902.34 Splenic vein

902.39 Other
> Cystic vein   Gastric vein

✓5ᵗʰ **902.4 Renal blood vessels**

902.40 Renal vessel(s), unspecified

902.41 Renal artery

902.42 Renal vein

902.49 Other
> Suprarenal arteries

✓5ᵗʰ **902.5 Iliac blood vessels**

902.50 Iliac vessel(s), unspecified

902.51 Hypogastric artery

902.52 Hypogastric vein

902.53 Iliac artery

902.54 Iliac vein

902.55 Uterine artery ♀

902.56 Uterine vein ♀

902.59 Other

✓5ᵗʰ **902.8 Other specified blood vessels of abdomen and pelvis**

902.81 Ovarian artery ♀

902.82 Ovarian vein ♀

902.87 Multiple blood vessels of abdomen and pelvis

902.89 Other

902.9 Unspecified blood vessel of abdomen and pelvis

✓4ᵗʰ **903 Injury to blood vessels of upper extremity**

✓5ᵗʰ **903.0 Axillary blood vessels**

903.00 Axillary vessel(s), unspecified

903.01 Axillary artery

903.02 Axillary vein

903.1 Brachial blood vessels

903.2 Radial blood vessels

903.3 Ulnar blood vessels

903.4 Palmar artery

903.5 Digital blood vessels

N Newborn Age: 0   P Pediatric Age: 0-17   M Maternity Age: 12-55   A Adult Age: 15-124

903.8 Other specified blood vessels of upper extremity
Multiple blood vessels of upper extremity

903.9 Unspecified blood vessel of upper extremity

✓4th **904 Injury to blood vessels of lower extremity and unspecified sites**

904.0 Common femoral artery
Femoral artery above profunda origin

904.1 Superficial femoral artery

904.2 Femoral veins

904.3 Saphenous veins
Saphenous vein (greater) (lesser)

✓5th **904.4 Popliteal blood vessels**

904.40 Popliteal vessel(s), unspecified

904.41 Popliteal artery

904.42 Popliteal vein

✓5th **904.5 Tibial blood vessels**

904.50 Tibial vessel(s), unspecified

904.51 Anterior tibial artery

904.52 Anterior tibial vein

904.53 Posterior tibial artery

904.54 Posterior tibial vein

904.6 Deep plantar blood vessels

904.7 Other specified blood vessels of lower extremity
Multiple blood vessels of lower extremity

904.8 Unspecified blood vessel of lower extremity

904.9 Unspecified site
Injury to blood vessel NOS

Late Effects of Injuries, Poisonings, Toxic Effects, and Other External Causes (905-909)

NOTE These categories are to be used to indicate conditions classifiable to 800-999 as the cause of late effects, which are themselves classified elsewhere. The "late effects" include those specified as such, or as sequelae, which may occur at any time after the acute injury.

✓4th **905 Late effects of musculoskeletal and connective tissue injuries**
AHA: 1Q, '95, 10; 2Q, '94, 3

905.0 Late effect of fracture of skull and face bones
Late effect of injury classifiable to 800-804
AHA: ▶2Q, '13, 8;◄ 3Q, '97, 12

905.1 Late effect of fracture of spine and trunk without mention of spinal cord lesion
Late effect of injury classifiable to 805, 807-809
AHA: 1Q, '07, 20

905.2 Late effect of fracture of upper extremities
Late effect of injury classifiable to 810-819

905.3 Late effect of fracture of neck of femur
Late effect of injury classifiable to 820

905.4 Late effect of fracture of lower extremities
Late effect of injury classifiable to 821-827
S79.001S Uns physeal fx upper end right femur sequela `I-10`

905.5 Late effect of fracture of multiple and unspecified bones
Late effect of injury classifiable to 828-829

905.6 Late effect of dislocation
Late effect of injury classifiable to 830-839

905.7 Late effect of sprain and strain without mention of tendon injury
Late effect of injury classifiable to 840-848, except tendon injury

905.8 Late effect of tendon injury
Late effect of tendon injury due to:
open wound [injury classifiable to 880-884 with .2, 890-894 with .2]
sprain and strain [injury classifiable to 840-848]
AHA: 2Q, '89, 13; 2Q, '89, 15

905.9 Late effect of traumatic amputation
Late effect of injury classifiable to 885-887, 895-897
EXCLUDES late amputation stump complication (997.60-997.69)

✓4th **906 Late effects of injuries to skin and subcutaneous tissues**

906.0 Late effect of open wound of head, neck, and trunk
Late effect of injury classifiable to 870-879

906.1 Late effect of open wound of extremities without mention of tendon injury
Late effect of injury classifiable to 880-884, 890-894 except .2

906.2 Late effect of superficial injury
Late effect of injury classifiable to 910-919

906.3 Late effect of contusion
Late effect of injury classifiable to 920-924

906.4 Late effect of crushing
Late effect of injury classifiable to 925-929

906.5 Late effect of burn of eye, face, head, and neck
Late effect of injury classifiable to 940-941
AHA: 4Q, '04, 76

906.6 Late effect of burn of wrist and hand
Late effect of injury classifiable to 944
AHA: 4Q, '94, 22

906.7 Late effect of burn of other extremities
Late effect of injury classifiable to 943 or 945
AHA: 4Q, '94, 22

906.8 Late effect of burns of other specified sites
Late effect of injury classifiable to 942, 946-947
AHA: 4Q, '94, 22

906.9 Late effect of burn of unspecified site
Late effect of injury classifiable to 948-949
AHA: 4Q, '94, 22

✓4th **907 Late effects of injuries to the nervous system**

907.0 Late effect of intracranial injury without mention of skull fracture
Late effect of injury classifiable to 850-854
AHA: ▶4Q, '13, 86;◄ 3Q, '12, 20; 4Q, '11, 97; 4Q, '10, 96; 4Q, '09, 108; 4Q, '08, 108; 4Q, '03, 103; 3Q, '90, 14
S06.2x1S Diffuse traumatic brain inj loc 30 min/less sequela `I-10`

907.1 Late effect of injury to cranial nerve
Late effect of injury classifiable to 950-951

907.2 Late effect of spinal cord injury
Late effect of injury classifiable to 806, 952
AHA: 4Q, '03, 103; 4Q, '98, 38
S34.114S Complete lesion L4 of lumbar spinal cord sequela `I-10`

907.3 Late effect of injury to nerve root(s), spinal plexus(es), and other nerves of trunk
Late effect of injury classifiable to 953-954
AHA: 2Q, '07, 11

907.4 Late effect of injury to peripheral nerve of shoulder girdle and upper limb
Late effect of injury classifiable to 955

907.5 Late effect of injury to peripheral nerve of pelvic girdle and lower limb
Late effect of injury classifiable to 956

907.9 Late effect of injury to other and unspecified nerve
Late effect of injury classifiable to 957

✓4th **908 Late effects of other and unspecified injuries**

908.0 Late effect of internal injury to chest
Late effect of injury classifiable to 860-862

908.1 Late effect of internal injury to intra-abdominal organs
Late effect of injury classifiable to 863-866, 868

908.2 Late effect of internal injury to other internal organs
Late effect of injury classifiable to 867 or 869

908.3 Late effect of injury to blood vessel of head, neck, and extremities
Late effect of injury classifiable to 900, 903-904

908.4 Late effect of injury to blood vessel of thorax, abdomen, and pelvis
Late effect of injury classifiable to 901-902

| ✓4th ✓5th Additional Digit Required | Unspecified Code | Other Specified Code | Manifestation Code | ▶◄ Revised Text | ● New Code | ▲ Revised Code Title |

Injury and Poisoning

908.5–914.3

908.5 **Late effect of foreign body in orifice**
Late effect of injury classifiable to 930-939

908.6 **Late effect of certain complications of trauma**
Late effect of complications classifiable to 958

908.9 **Late effect of unspecified injury**
Late effect of injury classifiable to 959
AHA: 3Q, '00, 4

✓4th **909 Late effects of other and unspecified external causes**

909.0 **Late effect of poisoning due to drug, medicinal or biological substance**
Late effect of conditions classifiable to 960-979
EXCLUDES late effect of adverse effect of drug, medicinal or biological substance (909.5)
AHA: 4Q, '03, 103

909.1 **Late effect of toxic effects of nonmedical substances**
Late effect of conditions classifiable to 980-989

909.2 **Late effect of radiation**
Late effect of conditions classifiable to 990

909.3 **Late effect of complications of surgical and medical care**
Late effect of conditions classifiable to 996-999
AHA: 1Q, '93, 29

909.4 **Late effect of certain other external causes**
Late effect of conditions classifiable to 991-994

909.5 **Late effect of adverse effect of drug, medical or biological substance**
EXCLUDES late effect of poisoning due to drug, medicinal or biological substance (909.0)
AHA: 4Q, '94, 48

909.9 **Late effect of other and unspecified external causes**

Superficial Injury (910-919)

EXCLUDES burn (blisters) (940.0-949.5)
contusion (920-924.9)
foreign body:
granuloma (728.82)
inadvertently left in operative wound (998.4)
residual in soft tissue (729.6)
insect bite, venomous (989.5)
open wound with incidental foreign body (870.0-897.7)
AHA: 2Q, '89, 15
TIP: Do not code separately when associated with more severe injuries of the same site.

✓4th **910 Superficial injury of face, neck, and scalp except eye**
INCLUDES cheek
ear
gum
lip
nose
throat
EXCLUDES eye and adnexa (918.0-918.9)

910.0 **Abrasion or friction burn without mention of infection**
S00.01xA Abrasion of scalp initial encounter   **I-10**

910.1 **Abrasion or friction burn, infected**

910.2 **Blister without mention of infection**

910.3 **Blister, infected**

910.4 **Insect bite, nonvenomous, without mention of infection**

910.5 **Insect bite, nonvenomous, infected**

910.6 **Superficial foreign body (splinter) without major open wound and without mention of infection**

910.7 **Superficial foreign body (splinter) without major open wound, infected**

910.8 **Other and unspecified superficial injury of face, neck, and scalp without mention of infection**

910.9 **Other and unspecified superficial injury of face, neck, and scalp, infected**

✓4th **911 Superficial injury of trunk**
INCLUDES abdominal wall   interscapular region
anus   labium (majus) (minus)
back   penis
breast   perineum
buttock   scrotum
chest wall   testis
flank   vagina
groin   vulva
EXCLUDES hip (916.0-916.9)
scapular region (912.0-912.9)

911.0 **Abrasion or friction burn without mention of infection**
AHA: 3Q, '01, 10

911.1 **Abrasion or friction burn, infected**

911.2 **Blister without mention of infection**

911.3 **Blister, infected**

911.4 **Insect bite, nonvenomous, without mention of infection**

911.5 **Insect bite, nonvenomous, infected**

911.6 **Superficial foreign body (splinter) without major open wound and without mention of infection**

911.7 **Superficial foreign body (splinter) without major open wound, infected**

911.8 **Other and unspecified superficial injury of trunk without mention of infection**

911.9 **Other and unspecified superficial injury of trunk, infected**

✓4th **912 Superficial injury of shoulder and upper arm**
INCLUDES axilla
scapular region

912.0 **Abrasion or friction burn without mention of infection**

912.1 **Abrasion or friction burn, infected**

912.2 **Blister without mention of infection**

912.3 **Blister, infected**

912.4 **Insect bite, nonvenomous, without mention of infection**

912.5 **Insect bite, nonvenomous, infected**

912.6 **Superficial foreign body (splinter) without major open wound and without mention of infection**

912.7 **Superficial foreign body (splinter) without major open wound, infected**

912.8 **Other and unspecified superficial injury of shoulder and upper arm without mention of infection**

912.9 **Other and unspecified superficial injury of shoulder and upper arm infected**

✓4th **913 Superficial injury of elbow, forearm, and wrist**

913.0 **Abrasion or friction burn without mention of infection**

913.1 **Abrasion or friction burn, infected**

913.2 **Blister without mention of infection**

913.3 **Blister, infected**

913.4 **Insect bite, nonvenomous, without mention of infection**

913.5 **Insect bite, nonvenomous, infected**

913.6 **Superficial foreign body (splinter) without major open wound and without mention of infection**

913.7 **Superficial foreign body (splinter) without major open wound, infected**

913.8 **Other and unspecified superficial injury of elbow, forearm, and wrist without mention of infection**

913.9 **Other and unspecified superficial injury of elbow, forearm, and wrist, infected**

✓4th **914 Superficial injury of hand(s) except finger(s) alone**

914.0 **Abrasion or friction burn without mention of infection**

914.1 **Abrasion or friction burn, infected**

914.2 **Blister without mention of infection**

914.3 **Blister, infected**

914.4 Insect bite, nonvenomous, without mention of infection

914.5 Insect bite, nonvenomous, infected

914.6 Superficial foreign body (splinter) without major open wound and without mention of infection

914.7 Superficial foreign body (splinter) without major open wound, infected

914.8 Other and unspecified superficial injury of hand without mention of infection

914.9 Other and unspecified superficial injury of hand, infected

√4ᵗʰ 915 Superficial injury of finger(s)

INCLUDES fingernail
thumb (nail)

915.0 Abrasion or friction burn without mention of infection

915.1 Abrasion or friction burn, infected

915.2 Blister without mention of infection

915.3 Blister, infected

915.4 Insect bite, nonvenomous, without mention of infection

915.5 Insect bite, nonvenomous, infected

915.6 Superficial foreign body (splinter) without major open wound and without mention of infection

915.7 Superficial foreign body (splinter) without major open wound, infected

915.8 Other and unspecified superficial injury of fingers without mention of infection

AHA: 3Q, '01, 10

915.9 Other and unspecified superficial injury of fingers, infected

√4ᵗʰ 916 Superficial injury of hip, thigh, leg, and ankle

916.0 Abrasion or friction burn without mention of infection

S80.812A Abrasion left lower leg initial encounter   I-10

916.1 Abrasion or friction burn, infected

916.2 Blister without mention of infection

916.3 Blister, infected

916.4 Insect bite, nonvenomous, without mention of infection

916.5 Insect bite, nonvenomous, infected

916.6 Superficial foreign body (splinter) without major open wound and without mention of infection

916.7 Superficial foreign body (splinter) without major open wound, infected

916.8 Other and unspecified superficial injury of hip, thigh, leg, and ankle without mention of infection

916.9 Other and unspecified superficial injury of hip, thigh, leg, and ankle, infected

√4ᵗʰ 917 Superficial injury of foot and toe(s)

INCLUDES heel
toenail

917.0 Abrasion or friction burn without mention of infection

917.1 Abrasion or friction burn, infected

917.2 Blister without mention of infection

917.3 Blister, infected

917.4 Insect bite, nonvenomous, without mention of infection

917.5 Insect bite, nonvenomous, infected

917.6 Superficial foreign body (splinter) without major open wound and without mention of infection

917.7 Superficial foreign body (splinter) without major open wound, infected

917.8 Other and unspecified superficial injury of foot and toes without mention of infection

AHA: 1Q, '03, 13

917.9 Other and unspecified superficial injury of foot and toes infected

AHA: 1Q, '03, 13
TIP: Assign for hair strangulation of toe, with infection.

√4ᵗʰ 918 Superficial injury of eye and adnexa

EXCLUDES burn (940.0-940.9)
foreign body on external eye (930.0-930.9)

918.0 Eyelids and periocular area
Abrasion
Insect bite
Superficial foreign body (splinter)

918.1 Cornea
Corneal abrasion   Superficial laceration
EXCLUDES corneal injury due to contact lens (371.82)

918.2 Conjunctiva

918.9 Other and unspecified superficial injuries of eye
Eye (ball) NOS

√4ᵗʰ 919 Superficial injury of other, multiple, and unspecified sites

EXCLUDES multiple sites classifiable to the same three-digit category (910.0-918.9)

919.0 Abrasion or friction burn without mention of infection

919.1 Abrasion or friction burn, infected

919.2 Blister without mention of infection

919.3 Blister, infected

919.4 Insect bite, nonvenomous, without mention of infection

919.5 Insect bite, nonvenomous, infected

919.6 Superficial foreign body (splinter) without major open wound and without mention of infection

919.7 Superficial foreign body (splinter) without major open wound, infected

919.8 Other and unspecified superficial injuries without mention of infection

919.9 Other and unspecified superficial injury, infected

Contusion with Intact Skin Surface (920-924)

INCLUDES bruise   } without fracture or open
hematoma   }   wound

EXCLUDES concussion (850.0-850.9)
hemarthrosis (840.0-848.9)
internal organs (860.0-869.1)
that incidental to:
crushing injury (925-929.9)
dislocation (830.0-839.9)
fracture (800.0-829.1)
internal injury (860.0-869.1)
intracranial injury (850.0-854.1)
nerve injury (950.0-957.9)
open wound (870.0-897.7)

920 Contusion of face, scalp, and neck except eye(s)

Cheek   Mandibular joint area
Ear (auricle)   Nose
Gum   Throat
Lip

S00.33xA Contusion of nose initial encounter   I-10

√4ᵗʰ 921 Contusion of eye and adnexa

921.0 Black eye, not otherwise specified

921.1 Contusion of eyelids and periocular area

921.2 Contusion of orbital tissues

921.3 Contusion of eyeball
TIP: If iridodialysis (rupture of the root of the iris) is present and is due to the eyeball contusion, assign also code 364.76.

921.9 Unspecified contusion of eye
Injury of eye NOS

√4ᵗʰ 922 Contusion of trunk

922.0 Breast

922.1 Chest wall
S20.212A Contusion left front wall thorax initial enc   I-10

√4ᵗʰ
√5ᵗʰ Additional Digit Required   Unspecified Code   Other Specified Code   Manifestation Code   ►◄ Revised Text   ● New Code   ▲ Revised Code Title

922.2 Abdominal wall
　　Flank　　　　　Groin

✓5ᵗʰ **922.3 Back**
　　AHA: 4Q, '96, 39

　922.31 Back
　　　EXCLUDES *interscapular region (922.33)*
　　　AHA: 3Q, '99, 14

　922.32 Buttock

　922.33 Interscapular region

922.4 Genital organs
　　Labium (majus) (minus)
　　Penis
　　Perineum
　　Scrotum
　　Testis
　　Vagina
　　Vulva

922.8 Multiple sites of trunk

922.9 Unspecified part
　　Trunk NOS

✓4ᵗʰ **923 Contusion of upper limb**

✓5ᵗʰ **923.0 Shoulder and upper arm**

　923.00 Shoulder region

　923.01 Scapular region

　923.02 Axillary region

　923.03 Upper arm

　923.09 Multiple sites

✓5ᵗʰ **923.1 Elbow and forearm**

　923.10 Forearm

　923.11 Elbow

✓5ᵗʰ **923.2 Wrist and hand(s), except finger(s) alone**

　923.20 Hand(s)

　923.21 Wrist

923.3 Finger
　　Fingernail　　　　Thumb (nail)

923.8 Multiple sites of upper limb

923.9 Unspecified part of upper limb
　　Arm NOS

✓4ᵗʰ **924 Contusion of lower limb and of other and unspecified sites**

✓5ᵗʰ **924.0 Hip and thigh**

　924.00 Thigh
　　　AHA: 1Q, '09, 10

　924.01 Hip
　　　S70.02xA Contusion of left hip initial encounter　　I-10

✓5ᵗʰ **924.1 Knee and lower leg**

　924.10 Lower leg

　924.11 Knee

✓5ᵗʰ **924.2 Ankle and foot, excluding toe(s)**

　924.20 Foot
　　　Heel

　924.21 Ankle

924.3 Toe
　　Toenail

924.4 Multiple sites of lower limb

924.5 Unspecified part of lower limb
　　Leg NOS

924.8 Multiple sites, not elsewhere classified
　　AHA: 1Q, '03, 7
　　S70.10xA Contusion of unspecified thigh initial encounter　　I-10

924.9 Unspecified site

Crushing Injury (925-929)

Use additional code to identify any associated injuries, such as:
　fractures (800-829)
　internal injuries (860.0-869.1)
　intracranial injuries (850.0-854.1)
AHA: 4Q, '03, 77; 2Q, '93, 7

✓4ᵗʰ **925 Crushing injury of face, scalp, and neck**
　　Cheek　　　　　Pharynx
　　Ear　　　　　　Throat
　　Larynx

　925.1 Crushing injury of face and scalp
　　　Cheek　　　　Ear

　925.2 Crushing injury of neck
　　　Larynx
　　　Pharynx
　　　Throat

✓4ᵗʰ **926 Crushing injury of trunk**

　926.0 External genitalia
　　　Labium (majus) (minus)
　　　Penis
　　　Scrotum
　　　Testis
　　　Vulva

✓5ᵗʰ **926.1 Other specified sites**

　926.11 Back

　926.12 Buttock

　926.19 Other
　　　Breast

　926.8 Multiple sites of trunk

　926.9 Unspecified site
　　　Trunk NOS

✓4ᵗʰ **927 Crushing injury of upper limb**

✓5ᵗʰ **927.0 Shoulder and upper arm**

　927.00 Shoulder region

　927.01 Scapular region

　927.02 Axillary region

　927.03 Upper arm

　927.09 Multiple sites

✓5ᵗʰ **927.1 Elbow and forearm**

　927.10 Forearm

　927.11 Elbow

✓5ᵗʰ **927.2 Wrist and hand(s), except finger(s) alone**

　927.20 Hand(s)

　927.21 Wrist

927.3 Finger(s)
　　AHA: 4Q, '03, 77

927.8 Multiple sites of upper limb

927.9 Unspecified site
　　Arm NOS

✓4ᵗʰ **928 Crushing injury of lower limb**

✓5ᵗʰ **928.0 Hip and thigh**

　928.00 Thigh

　928.01 Hip

✓5ᵗʰ **928.1 Knee and lower leg**

　928.10 Lower leg

　928.11 Knee

✓5ᵗʰ **928.2 Ankle and foot, excluding toe(s) alone**

　928.20 Foot
　　　Heel

　928.21 Ankle

928.3 Toe(s)

Ⓝ Newborn Age: 0　　　Ⓟ Pediatric Age: 0-17　　　Ⓜ Maternity Age: 12-55　　　Ⓐ Adult Age: 15-124

928.8 **Multiple sites of lower limb**

928.9 **Unspecified site**
　　Leg NOS

✓4ᵗʰ 929 **Crushing injury of multiple and unspecified sites**

929.0 **Multiple sites, not elsewhere classified**

929.9 **Unspecified site**

Effects Of Foreign Body Entering Through Orifice (930-939)

EXCLUDES *foreign body:*
　　granuloma (728.82)
　　inadvertently left in operative wound (998.4, 998.7)
　　in open wound (800-839, 851-897)
　　residual in soft tissues (729.6)
　　superficial without major open wound (910-919
　　　　with .6 or .7)

✓4ᵗʰ 930 **Foreign body on external eye**
EXCLUDES *foreign body in penetrating wound of:*
　　eyeball (871.5-871.6)
　　　　retained (old) (360.5-360.6)
　　ocular adnexa (870.4)
　　　　retained (old) (376.6)

930.0 **Corneal foreign body**

930.1 **Foreign body in conjunctival sac**

930.2 **Foreign body in lacrimal punctum**

930.8 **Other and combined sites**

930.9 **Unspecified site**
　　External eye NOS

931 **Foreign body in ear**
　　Auditory canal　　　　Auricle

932 **Foreign body in nose**
　　Nasal sinus　　　　Nostril

✓4ᵗʰ 933 **Foreign body in pharynx and larynx**

933.0 **Pharynx**
　　Nasopharynx　　　　Throat NOS

933.1 **Larynx**
　　Asphyxia due to foreign body
　　Choking due to:
　　　food (regurgitated)
　　　phlegm
　　TIP: Assign for mucous plug causing asphyxia; otherwise, for tracheobronchial, refer to code 519.19 Other diseases of trachea and bronchus.

✓4ᵗʰ 934 **Foreign body in trachea, bronchus, and lung**

934.0 **Trachea**

934.1 **Main bronchus**
　　AHA: 3Q, '02, 18

934.8 **Other specified parts**
　　Bronchioles
　　Lung

934.9 **Respiratory tree, unspecified**
　　Inhalation of liquid or vomitus, lower respiratory tract NOS

✓4ᵗʰ 935 **Foreign body in mouth, esophagus, and stomach**

935.0 **Mouth**

935.1 **Esophagus**
　　AHA: 1Q, '88, 13
　　TIP: If esophageal obstruction is due to stenosis, caustic stricture (e.g., lye ingestion), or tumor, assign instead code 530.3.

935.2 **Stomach**

936 **Foreign body in intestine and colon**

937 **Foreign body in anus and rectum**
　　Rectosigmoid (junction)

938 **Foreign body in digestive system, unspecified**
　　Alimentary tract NOS
　　Swallowed foreign body

✓4ᵗʰ 939 **Foreign body in genitourinary tract**

939.0 **Bladder and urethra**

939.1 **Uterus, any part**   ♀
EXCLUDES *intrauterine contraceptive device:*
　　complications from (996.32, 996.65)
　　presence of (V45.51)

939.2 **Vulva and vagina**   ♀

939.3 **Penis**   ♂

939.9 **Unspecified site**

Burns (940-949)

INCLUDES burns from:
　　electrical heating appliance
　　electricity
　　flame
　　hot object
　　lightning
　　radiation
　　chemical burns (external) (internal)
　　scalds
EXCLUDES *friction burns (910-919 with .0, .1)*
　　sunburn (692.71, 692.76-692.77)
AHA: 4Q, 94, 22; 2Q, '90, 7; 4Q, '88, 3; M-A, '86, 9
TIP: Nonhealing burns are coded as acute burns, as is necrosis of burned skin. Assign code 958.3 for any documented infected burn site.

✓4ᵗʰ 940 **Burn confined to eye and adnexa**

940.0 **Chemical burn of eyelids and periocular area**

940.1 **Other burns of eyelids and periocular area**

940.2 **Alkaline chemical burn of cornea and conjunctival sac**

940.3 **Acid chemical burn of cornea and conjunctival sac**

940.4 **Other burn of cornea and conjunctival sac**

940.5 **Burn with resulting rupture and destruction of eyeball**

940.9 **Unspecified burn of eye and adnexa**

✓4ᵗʰ 941 **Burn of face, head, and neck**
EXCLUDES *mouth (947.0)*

The following fifth-digit subclassification is for use with category 941:
　0 **face and head, unspecified site**
　1 **ear [any part]**
　2 **eye (with other parts of face, head, and neck)**
　3 **lip(s)**
　4 **chin**
　5 **nose (septum)**
　6 **scalp [any part]**
　　Temple (region)
　7 **forehead and cheek**
　8 **neck**
　9 **multiple sites [except with eye] of face, head and neck**

AHA: 4Q, '94, 22; M-A, '86, 9

§ ✓5ᵗʰ 941.0 **Unspecified degree**
　[0-9]

§ ✓5ᵗʰ 941.1 **Erythema [first degree]**
　[0-9]   **AHA: For code 941.11:** 3Q, '10, 19; **For code 941.19:** 3Q, '05, 10

§ ✓5ᵗʰ 941.2 **Blisters, epidermal loss [second degree]**
　[0-9]

§ ✓5ᵗʰ 941.3 **Full-thickness skin loss [third degree NOS]**
　[0-9]

§ ✓5ᵗʰ 941.4 **Deep necrosis of underlying tissues [deep third degree] without mention of loss of a body part**
　[0-9]

§ ✓5ᵗʰ 941.5 **Deep necrosis of underlying tissues [deep third degree] with loss of a body part**
　[0-9]

---

§　Requires fifth digit. Valid digits are in [brackets] under each code. See category 941 for codes and definitions.

| ✓4ᵗʰ ✓5ᵗʰ Additional Digit Required | Unspecified Code | Other Specified Code | Manifestation Code | ►◄ Revised Text | ● New Code | ▲ Revised Code Title |

Injury and Poisoning

942–947.9

√4ᵗʰ **942 Burn of trunk**

> EXCLUDES *scapular region (943.0-943.5 with fifth-digit 6)*

> The following fifth-digit subclassificaiton is for use with category 942:
> 0 **trunk, unspecified site**
> 1 **breast**
> 2 **chest wall, excluding breast and nipple**
> 3 **abdominal wall**
> > Flank
> > Groin
> 4 **back [any part]**
> > Buttock
> > Interscapular region
> 5 **genitalia**
> > Labium (majus) (minus)
> > Penis
> > Perineum
> > Scrotum
> > Testis
> > Vulva
> 9 **other and multiple sites of trunk**

> AHA: 4Q, '94, 22; M-A, '86, 9

§ √5ᵗʰ **942.0 Unspecified degree**
[0-5, 9]

§ √5ᵗʰ **942.1 Erythema [first degree]**
[0-5, 9]

§ √5ᵗʰ **942.2 Blisters, epidermal loss [second degree]**
[0-5, 9]

§ √5ᵗʰ **942.3 Full-thickness skin loss [third degree NOS]**
[0-5, 9]

§ √5ᵗʰ **942.4 Deep necrosis of underlying tissues [deep third**
[0-5, 9] **degree] without mention of loss of a body part**

§ √5ᵗʰ **942.5 Deep necrosis of underlying tissues [deep third**
[0-5, 9] **degree] with loss of a body part**

√4ᵗʰ **943 Burn of upper limb, except wrist and hand**

> The following fifth-digit subclassificaiton is for use with category 943:
> 0 **upper limb, unspecified site**
> 1 **forearm**
> 2 **elbow**
> 3 **upper arm**
> 4 **axilla**
> 5 **shoulder**
> 6 **scapular region**
> 9 **multiple sites of upper limb, except wrist and hand**

> AHA: 4Q, '94, 22; M-A, '86, 9

§ √5ᵗʰ **943.0 Unspecified degree**
[0-6, 9]   AHA: For code 943.00: 3Q, '10, 19

§ √5ᵗʰ **943.1 Erythema [first degree]**
[0-6, 9]

§ √5ᵗʰ **943.2 Blisters, epidermal loss [second degree]**
[0-6, 9]

§ √5ᵗʰ **943.3 Full-thickness skin loss [third degree NOS]**
[0-6, 9]

§ √5ᵗʰ **943.4 Deep necrosis of underlying tissues [deep third**
[0-6, 9] **degree] without mention of loss of a body part**

§ √5ᵗʰ **943.5 Deep necrosis of underlying tissues [deep third**
[0-6, 9] **degree] with loss of a body part**

√4ᵗʰ **944 Burn of wrist(s) and hand(s)**

> The following fifth-digit subclassification is for use with category 944:
> 0 **hand, unspecified site**
> 1 **single digit [finger (nail)] other than thumb**
> 2 **thumb (nail)**
> 3 **two or more digits, not including thumb**
> 4 **two or more digits including thumb**
> 5 **palm**
> 6 **back of hand**
> 7 **wrist**
> 8 **multiple sites of wrist(s) and hand(s)**

§ √5ᵗʰ **944.0 Unspecified degree**
[0-8]

§ √5ᵗʰ **944.1 Erythema [first degree]**
[0-8]

§ √5ᵗʰ **944.2 Blisters, epidermal loss [second degree]**
[0-8]

§ √5ᵗʰ **944.3 Full-thickness skin loss [third degree NOS]**
[0-8]

§ √5ᵗʰ **944.4 Deep necrosis of underlying tissues [deep third**
[0-8] **degree] without mention of loss of a body part**

§ √5ᵗʰ **944.5 Deep necrosis of underlying tissues [deep third**
[0-8] **degree] with loss of a body part**

√4ᵗʰ **945 Burn of lower limb(s)**

> The following fifth-digit subclassification is for use with category 945:
> 0 **lower limb [leg], unspecified site**
> 1 **toe(s) (nail)**
> 2 **foot**
> 3 **ankle**
> 4 **lower leg**
> 5 **knee**
> 6 **thigh [any part]**
> 9 **multiple sites of lower limb(s)**

> AHA: 4Q, '94, 22; M-A, '86, 9

§ √5ᵗʰ **945.0 Unspecified degree**
[0-6, 9]

§ √5ᵗʰ **945.1 Erythema [first degree]**
[0-6, 9]

§ √5ᵗʰ **945.2 Blisters, epidermal loss [second degree]**
[0-6, 9]

§ √5ᵗʰ **945.3 Full-thickness skin loss [third degree NOS]**
[0-6, 9]

§ √5ᵗʰ **945.4 Deep necrosis of underlying tissues [deep third**
[0-6, 9] **degree] without mention of loss of a body part**

§ √5ᵗʰ **945.5 Deep necrosis of underlying tissues [deep third**
[0-6, 9] **degree] with loss of a body part**

√4ᵗʰ **946 Burns of multiple specified sites**

> INCLUDES burns of sites classifiable to more than one three-digit category in 940-945

> EXCLUDES *multiple burns NOS (949.0-949.5)*

> AHA: 4Q, '94, 22; M-A, '86, 9

> TIP: Only assign if the specific sites of the multiple burns are not specified.

946.0 Unspecified degree

946.1 Erythema [first degree]

946.2 Blisters, epidermal loss [second degree]

946.3 Full-thickness skin loss [third degree NOS]

946.4 Deep necrosis of underlying tissues [deep third degree] without mention of loss of a body part

946.5 Deep necrosis of underlying tissues [deep third degree] with loss of a body part

√4ᵗʰ **947 Burn of internal organs**

> INCLUDES burns from chemical agents (ingested)

> AHA: 4Q, '94, 22; M-A, '86, 9

947.0 Mouth and pharynx
> Gum   Tongue

947.1 Larynx, trachea, and lung

947.2 Esophagus

947.3 Gastrointestinal tract
> Colon   Small intestine
> Rectum   Stomach
> AHA: 2Q, '12, 8

947.4 Vagina and uterus   ♀

947.8 Other specified sites

947.9 Unspecified site

---

§ Requires fifth digit. Valid digits are in [brackets] under each code. See appropriate category for codes and definitions.

Burns
Degrees of Burns

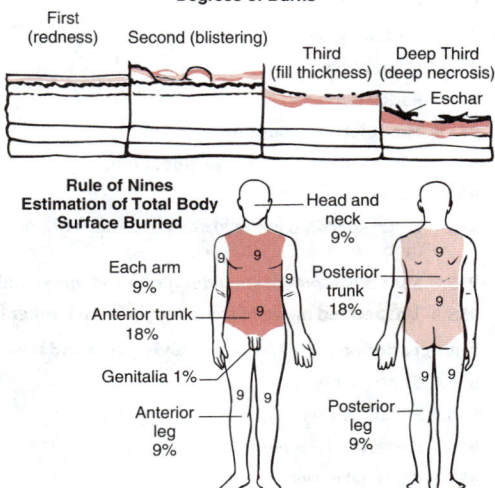

First (redness) — Second (blistering) — Third (fill thickness) — Deep Third (deep necrosis) — Eschar

Rule of Nines Estimation of Total Body Surface Burned

Head and neck 9%
Each arm 9%
Anterior trunk 18%
Posterior trunk 18%
Genitalia 1%
Anterior leg 9%
Posterior leg 9%

✓4ᵗʰ **948 Burns classified according to extent of body surface involved**

> **NOTE** This category is to be used when the site of the burn is unspecified, or with categories 940-947 when the site is specified.

> **EXCLUDES** sunburn (692.71, 692.76-692.77)

The following fifth-digit subclassification is for use with category 948 to indicate the percent of body surface with third degree burn; valid digits are in [brackets] under each code:

- 0 less than 10 percent or unspecified
- 1 10-19%
- 2 20-29%
- 3 30-39%
- 4 40-49%
- 5 50-59%
- 6 60-69%
- 7 70-79%
- 8 80-89%
- 9 90% or more of body surface

AHA: 4Q, '94, 22; 4Q, '88, 3; M-A, '86, 9; N-D, '84, 13

§ ✓5ᵗʰ **948.0 Burn [any degree] involving less than 10 percent of body surface**
[0]
    T31.0 Burns involving less than 10% of body surface   I-10

§ ✓5ᵗʰ **948.1 10-19 percent of body surface**
[0-1]

§ ✓5ᵗʰ **948.2 20-29 percent of body surface**
[0-2]

§ ✓5ᵗʰ **948.3 30-39 percent of body surface**
[0-3]

§ ✓5ᵗʰ **948.4 40-49 percent of body surface**
[0-4]

§ ✓5ᵗʰ **948.5 50-59 percent of body surface**
[0-5]

§ ✓5ᵗʰ **948.6 60-69 percent of body surface**
[0-6]

§ ✓5ᵗʰ **948.7 70-79 percent of body surface**
[0-7]

§ ✓5ᵗʰ **948.8 80-89 percent of body surface**
[0-8]

§ ✓5ᵗʰ **948.9 90 percent or more of body surface**
[0-9]

✓4ᵗʰ **949 Burn, unspecified**

> **INCLUDES** burn NOS
> multiple burns NOS

> **EXCLUDES** burn of unspecified site but with statement of the extent of body surface involved (948.0-948.9)

AHA: 4Q, '94, 22; M-A, '86, 9

    949.0 Unspecified degree

949.1 Erythema [first degree]

949.2 Blisters, epidermal loss [second degree]

949.3 Full-thickness skin loss [third degree NOS]

949.4 Deep necrosis of underlying tissues [deep third degree] without mention of loss of a body part

949.5 Deep necrosis of underlying tissues [deep third degree] with loss of a body part

Injury to Nerves and Spinal Cord (950-957)

> **INCLUDES** division of nerve
> lesion in continuity   } (with open
> traumatic neuroma   wound)
> traumatic transient paralysis

> **EXCLUDES** accidental puncture or laceration during medical procedure (998.2)

✓4ᵗʰ **950 Injury to optic nerve and pathways**

    950.0 Optic nerve injury
        Second cranial nerve

    950.1 Injury to optic chiasm

    950.2 Injury to optic pathways

    950.3 Injury to visual cortex

    950.9 Unspecified
        Traumatic blindness NOS

✓4ᵗʰ **951 Injury to other cranial nerve(s)**

    951.0 Injury to oculomotor nerve
        Third cranial nerve

    951.1 Injury to trochlear nerve
        Fourth cranial nerve

    951.2 Injury to trigeminal nerve
        Fifth cranial nerve

    951.3 Injury to abducens nerve
        Sixth cranial nerve

    951.4 Injury to facial nerve
        Seventh cranial nerve

    951.5 Injury to acoustic nerve
        Auditory nerve
        Eighth cranial nerve
        Traumatic deafness NOS

    951.6 Injury to accessory nerve
        Eleventh cranial nerve

    951.7 Injury to hypoglossal nerve
        Twelfth cranial nerve

    951.8 Injury to other specified cranial nerves
        Glossopharyngeal [9th cranial] nerve
        Olfactory [1st cranial] nerve
        Pneumogastric [10th cranial] nerve
        Traumatic anosmia NOS
        Vagus [10th cranial] nerve

    951.9 Injury to unspecified cranial nerve

✓4ᵗʰ **952 Spinal cord injury without evidence of spinal bone injury**

  ✓5ᵗʰ **952.0 Cervical**

    952.00 C_1-C_4 level with unspecified spinal cord injury
        Spinal cord injury, cervical region NOS

    952.01 C_1-C_4 level with complete lesion of spinal cord

    952.02 C_1-C_4 level with anterior cord syndrome

    952.03 C_1-C_4 level with central cord syndrome

    952.04 C_1-C_4 level with other specified spinal cord injury
        Incomplete spinal cord lesion at C_1-C_4 level:
          NOS
          with posterior cord syndrome

    952.05 C_5-C_7 level with unspecified spinal cord injury

    952.06 C_5-C_7 level with complete lesion of spinal cord

    952.07 C_5-C_7 level with anterior cord syndrome

---

§   Requires fifth digit. Valid digits are in [brackets] under each code. See category 948 for codes and definitions.

✓4ᵗʰ ✓5ᵗʰ Additional Digit Required   Unspecified Code   Other Specified Code   Manifestation Code   ▶◀ Revised Text   ● New Code   ▲ Revised Code Title

2015 ICD-9-CM   **Volume 1 – 299**

Injury and Poisoning

952.08–958.3

Spinal Nerve Roots

952.08 C_5-C_7 level with central cord syndrome

952.09 C_5-C_7 level with other specified spinal cord injury
Incomplete spinal cord lesion at C_5-C_7 level:
NOS
with posterior cord syndrome

√5ᵗʰ **952.1 Dorsal [thoracic]**

952.10 T_1-T_6 level with unspecified spinal cord injury
Spinal cord injury, thoracic region NOS

952.11 T_1-T_6 level with complete lesion of spinal cord

952.12 T_1-T_6 level with anterior cord syndrome

952.13 T_1-T_6 level with central cord syndrome

952.14 T_1-T_6 level with other specified spinal cord injury
Incomplete spinal cord lesion at T_1-T_6 level:
NOS
with posterior cord syndrome

952.15 T_7-T_{12} level with unspecified spinal cord injury

952.16 T_7-T_{12} level with complete lesion of spinal cord

952.17 T_7-T_{12} level with anterior cord syndrome

952.18 T_7-T_{12} level with central cord syndrome

952.19 T_7-T_{12} level with other specified spinal cord injury
Incomplete spinal cord lesion at T_7-T_{12} level:
NOS
with posterior cord syndrome

952.2 Lumbar

952.3 Sacral

952.4 Cauda equina

952.8 Multiple sites of spinal cord

952.9 Unspecified site of spinal cord

√4ᵗʰ **953 Injury to nerve roots and spinal plexus**

953.0 Cervical root

953.1 Dorsal root

953.2 Lumbar root

953.3 Sacral root

953.4 Brachial plexus

953.5 Lumbosacral plexus

953.8 Multiple sites

953.9 Unspecified site

√4ᵗʰ **954 Injury to other nerve(s) of trunk, excluding shoulder and pelvic girdles**

954.0 Cervical sympathetic

954.1 Other sympathetic
Celiac ganglion or plexus
Inferior mesenteric plexus
Splanchnic nerve(s)
Stellate ganglion

954.8 Other specified nerve(s) of trunk

954.9 Unspecified nerve of trunk

√4ᵗʰ **955 Injury to peripheral nerve(s) of shoulder girdle and upper limb**

955.0 Axillary nerve

955.1 Median nerve

955.2 Ulnar nerve

955.3 Radial nerve

955.4 Musculocutaneous nerve

955.5 Cutaneous sensory nerve, upper limb

955.6 Digital nerve

955.7 Other specified nerve(s) of shoulder girdle and upper limb

955.8 Multiple nerves of shoulder girdle and upper limb

955.9 Unspecified nerve of shoulder girdle and upper limb

√4ᵗʰ **956 Injury to peripheral nerve(s) of pelvic girdle and lower limb**

956.0 Sciatic nerve

956.1 Femoral nerve

956.2 Posterior tibial nerve

956.3 Peroneal nerve

956.4 Cutaneous sensory nerve, lower limb

956.5 Other specified nerve(s) of pelvic girdle and lower limb

956.8 Multiple nerves of pelvic girdle and lower limb

956.9 Unspecified nerve of pelvic girdle and lower limb

√4ᵗʰ **957 Injury to other and unspecified nerves**

957.0 Superficial nerves of head and neck

957.1 Other specified nerve(s)

957.8 Multiple nerves in several parts
Multiple nerve injury NOS

957.9 Unspecified site
Nerve injury NOS

Certain Traumatic Complications and Unspecified Injuries (958-959)

√4ᵗʰ **958 Certain early complications of trauma**
EXCLUDES *adult respiratory distress syndrome (518.52)*
flail chest (807.4)
post-traumatic seroma (729.91)
shock lung related to trauma and surgery (518.52)
that occurring during or following medical procedures (996.0-999.9)

958.0 Air embolism
Pneumathemia
EXCLUDES *that complicating:*
abortion (634-638 with .6, 639.6)
ectopic or molar pregnancy (639.6)
pregnancy, childbirth, or the puerperium (673.0)
DEF: Arterial obstruction due to introduction of air bubbles into the veins following surgery or trauma.

958.1 Fat embolism
EXCLUDES *that complicating:*
abortion (634-638 with .6, 639.6)
pregnancy, childbirth, or the puerperium (673.8)
DEF: Arterial blockage due to the entrance of fat in circulatory system, after fracture of large bones or administration of corticosteroids.

958.2 Secondary and recurrent hemorrhage

958.3 Posttraumatic wound infection, not elsewhere classified
EXCLUDES *infected open wounds — code to complicated open wound of site*
AHA: 4Q, '01, 53; S-O, '85, 10
TIP: Do not assign if the infection is documented as due to cellulitis; see instead categories 681 and 682 and complicated wound codes.

958.4 Traumatic shock
Shock (immediate) (delayed) following injury
EXCLUDES shock:
    anaphylactic (995.0)
      due to serum (999.41-999.49)
    anesthetic (995.4)
    electric (994.8)
    following abortion (639.5)
    lightning (994.0)
    nontraumatic NOS (785.50)
    obstetric (669.1)
    postoperative (998.00-998.09)
DEF: Shock, immediate or delayed following injury.

958.5 Traumatic anuria
Crush syndrome   Renal failure following crushing
EXCLUDES that due to a medical procedure (997.5)
DEF: Complete suppression of urinary secretion by kidneys due to trauma.

958.6 Volkmann's ischemic contracture
Posttraumatic muscle contracture
DEF: Muscle deterioration due to loss of blood supply from injury or tourniquet; causes muscle contraction and results in inability to extend the muscles fully.

958.7 Traumatic subcutaneous emphysema
EXCLUDES subcutaneous emphysema resulting from a procedure (998.81)

958.8 Other early complications of trauma
AHA: 2Q, '92, 13

√5th **958.9 Traumatic compartment syndrome**
EXCLUDES nontraumatic compartment syndrome (729.71-729.79)
DEF: Compression of nerves and blood vessels within an enclosed space due to previous trauma, which leads to impaired blood flow and muscle and nerve damage.
TIP: If the compartment syndrome is specified as chronic or exercise-induced, see instead subcategory 729.7.

    958.90 Compartment syndrome, unspecified
      AHA: 4Q, '06, 100-102

    958.91 Traumatic compartment syndrome of upper extremity
      Traumatic compartment syndrome of shoulder, arm, forearm, wrist, hand, and fingers
      AHA: 4Q, '06, 100-102

    958.92 Traumatic compartment syndrome of lower extremity
      Traumatic compartment syndrome of hip, buttock, thigh, leg, foot, and toes
      AHA: 4Q, '06, 100-102

    958.93 Traumatic compartment syndrome of abdomen
      AHA: 4Q, '06, 100-102

    958.99 Traumatic compartment syndrome of other sites
      AHA: 4Q, '06, 100-102

√4th **959 Injury, other and unspecified**
INCLUDES injury NOS
EXCLUDES injury NOS of:
    blood vessels (900.0-904.9)
    eye (921.0-921.9)
    internal organs (860.0-869.1)
    intracranial sites (854.0-854.1)
    nerves (950.0-951.9, 953.0-957.9)
    spinal cord (952.0-952.9)

√5th **959.0 Head, face and neck**

    959.01 Head injury, unspecified
      EXCLUDES concussion (850.1-850.9)
        with head injury NOS (850.1-850.9)
        head injury NOS with loss of consciousness (850.1-850.5)
        specified head injuries (850.0-854.1)
      AHA: 4Q, '08, 108; 4Q, '97, 46
      S09.90xA Unspecified injury of head initial encounter   I-10

    959.09 Injury of face and neck
      Cheek   Mouth
      Ear   Nose
      Eyebrow   Throat
      Lip
      AHA: 4Q, '97, 46

√5th **959.1 Trunk**
EXCLUDES scapular region (959.2)
AHA: 4Q, '03, 78; 1Q, '99, 10

    959.11 Other injury of chest wall

    959.12 Other injury of abdomen

    959.13 Fracture of corpus cavernosum penis   ♂

    959.14 Other injury of external genitals

    959.19 Other injury of other sites of trunk
      Injury of trunk NOS

959.2 Shoulder and upper arm
Axilla   Scapular region

959.3 Elbow, forearm, and wrist
AHA: 1Q, '97, 8

959.4 Hand, except finger

959.5 Finger
Fingernail   Thumb (nail)

959.6 Hip and thigh
Upper leg

959.7 Knee, leg, ankle, and foot

959.8 Other specified sites, including multiple
EXCLUDES multiple sites classifiable to the same four-digit category (959.0-959.7)

959.9 Unspecified site

Poisoning by Drugs, Medicinal and Biological Substances (960-979)

INCLUDES overdose of these substances
wrong substance given or taken in error
Use additional code to specify the effects of the poisoning
EXCLUDES adverse effects ["hypersensitivity," "reaction," etc.] of correct substance properly administered. Such cases are to be classified according to the nature of the adverse effect, such as:
    adverse effect NOS (995.20)
    allergic lymphadenitis (289.3)
    aspirin gastritis (535.4)
    blood disorders (280.0-289.9)
    dermatitis:
      contact (692.0-692.9)
      due to ingestion (693.0-693.9)
    nephropathy (583.9)
    [The drug giving rise to the adverse effect may be identified by use of categories E930-E949.]
    drug dependence (304.0-304.9)
    drug reaction and poisoning affecting the newborn (760.0-779.9)
    nondependent abuse of drugs (305.0-305.9)
    pathological drug intoxication (292.2)
AHA: 2Q, '90, 11
TIP: Assign a poisoning code for interaction between prescribed drug and alcohol or prescribed drug and other nonprescribed drug or medicinal agent. Sequence poisoning code first, then code for manifestation of poisoning.
If respiratory failure is due to a poisoning, the poisoning code must be sequenced first.

√4th **960 Poisoning by antibiotics**
EXCLUDES antibiotics:
    ear, nose, and throat (976.6)
    eye (976.5)
    local (976.0)

960.0 Penicillins
Ampicillin
Carbenicillin
Cloxacillin
Penicillin G

Injury and Poisoning

960.1–963.0

960.1 Antifungal antibiotics
Amphotericin B
Griseofulvin
Nystatin
Trichomycin
EXCLUDES *preparations intended for topical use (976.0-976.9)*

960.2 Chloramphenicol group
Chloramphenicol
Thiamphenicol

960.3 Erythromycin and other macrolides
Oleandomycin
Spiramycin

960.4 Tetracycline group
Doxycycline
Minocycline
Oxytetracycline

960.5 Cephalosporin group
Cephalexin
Cephaloglycin
Cephaloridine
Cephalothin

960.6 Antimycobacterial antibiotics
Cycloserine
Kanamycin
Rifampin
Streptomycin

960.7 Antineoplastic antibiotics
Actinomycin such as:
Bleomycin
Cactinomycin
Dactinomycin
Daunorubicin
Mitomycin

960.8 Other specified antibiotics

960.9 Unspecified antibiotic

√4ᵗʰ **961 Poisoning by other anti-infectives**
EXCLUDES *anti-infectives:*
ear, nose, and throat (976.6)
eye (976.5)
local (976.0)

961.0 Sulfonamides
Sulfadiazine
Sulfafurazole
Sulfamethoxazole

961.1 Arsenical anti-infectives

961.2 Heavy metal anti-infectives
Compounds of:
antimony
bismuth
lead
mercury
EXCLUDES *mercurial diuretics (974.0)*

961.3 Quinoline and hydroxyquinoline derivatives
Chiniofon
Diiodohydroxyquin
EXCLUDES *antimalarial drugs (961.4)*

961.4 Antimalarials and drugs acting on other blood protozoa
Chloroquine
Cycloguanil
Primaquine
Proguanil [chloroguanide]
Pyrimethamine
Quinine

961.5 Other antiprotozoal drugs
Emetine

961.6 Anthelmintics
Hexylresorcinol
Piperazine
Thiabendazole

961.7 Antiviral drugs
Methisazone
EXCLUDES *amantadine (966.4)*
cytarabine (963.1)
idoxuridine (976.5)

961.8 Other antimycobacterial drugs
Ethambutol
Ethionamide
Isoniazid
Para-aminosalicylic acid derivatives
Sulfones

961.9 Other and unspecified anti-infectives
Flucytosine
Nitrofuran derivatives

√4ᵗʰ **962 Poisoning by hormones and synthetic substitutes**
EXCLUDES *oxytocic hormones (975.0)*

962.0 Adrenal cortical steroids
Cortisone derivatives
Desoxycorticosterone derivatives
Fluorinated corticosteroids

962.1 Androgens and anabolic congeners
Methandriol
Nandrolone
Oxymetholone
Testosterone

962.2 Ovarian hormones and synthetic substitutes
Contraceptives, oral
Estrogens
Estrogens and progestogens, combined
Progestogens

962.3 Insulins and antidiabetic agents
Acetohexamide
Biguanide derivatives, oral
Chlorpropamide
Glucagon
Insulin
Phenformin
Sulfonylurea derivatives, oral
Tolbutamide
AHA: 4Q, '93, 19; M-A, '85, 8
TIP: Assign only if documentation indicates overdose of insulin; if due to diabetic adjusting dosage, assign instead 250.8X or 249.8X and E932.3 for adverse reaction to insulin, if applicable.

962.4 Anterior pituitary hormones
Corticotropin
Gonadotropin
Somatotropin [growth hormone]

962.5 Posterior pituitary hormones
Vasopressin
EXCLUDES *oxytocic hormones (975.0)*

962.6 Parathyroid and parathyroid derivatives

962.7 Thyroid and thyroid derivatives
Dextrothyroxin
Levothyroxine sodium
Liothyronine
Thyroglobulin

962.8 Antithyroid agents
Iodides
Thiouracil
Thiourea

962.9 Other and unspecified hormones and synthetic substitutes

√4ᵗʰ **963 Poisoning by primarily systemic agents**
963.0 Antiallergic and antiemetic drugs
Antihistamines
Chlorpheniramine
Diphenhydramine
Diphenylpyraline
Thonzylamine
Tripelennamine
EXCLUDES *phenothiazine-based tranquilizers (969.1)*

963.1 Antineoplastic and immunosuppressive drugs
     Azathioprine
     Busulfan
     Chlorambucil
     Cyclophosphamide
     Cytarabine
     Fluorouracil
     Mercaptopurine
     thio-TEPA
     EXCLUDES *antineoplastic antibiotics (960.7)*

963.2 Acidifying agents

963.3 Alkalizing agents

963.4 Enzymes, not elsewhere classified
     Penicillinase

963.5 Vitamins, not elsewhere classified
     Vitamin A
     Vitamin D
     EXCLUDES *nicotinic acid (972.2)*
                   vitamin K (964.3)

963.8 Other specified systemic agents
     Heavy metal antagonists

963.9 Unspecified systemic agent

✓4ᵗʰ 964 Poisoning by agents primarily affecting blood constituents

964.0 Iron and its compounds
     Ferric salts
     Ferrous sulfate and other ferrous salts

964.1 Liver preparations and other antianemic agents
     Folic acid

964.2 Anticoagulants
     Coumarin
     Heparin
     Phenindione
     Warfarin sodium
     AHA: 1Q, '94, 22
     TIP: If documentation indicates an adverse reaction to Coumadin, assign instead manifestation (e.g., hematuria or epistaxis), code 790.92 if abnormal coagulation profile is documented, and E934.2.

964.3 Vitamin K [phytonadione]

964.4 Fibrinolysis-affecting drugs
     Aminocaproic acid
     Streptodornase
     Streptokinase
     Urokinase

964.5 Anticoagulant antagonists and other coagulants
     Hexadimethrine
     Protamine sulfate

964.6 Gamma globulin

964.7 Natural blood and blood products
     Blood plasma
     Human fibrinogen
     Packed red cells
     Whole blood
     EXCLUDES *transfusion reactions (999.41-999.8)*

964.8 Other specified agents affecting blood constituents
     Macromolecular blood substitutes
     Plasma expanders

964.9 Unspecified agent affecting blood constituents

✓4ᵗʰ 965 Poisoning by analgesics, antipyretics, and antirheumatics
     EXCLUDES *drug dependence (304.0-304.9)*
                   nondependent abuse (305.0-305.9)

✓5ᵗʰ 965.0 Opiates and related narcotics

     965.00 Opium (alkaloids), unspecified
         AHA: 3Q, '07, 6

     965.01 Heroin
         Diacetylmorphine

     965.02 Methadone

     965.09 Other
         Codeine [methylmorphine]
         Meperidine [pethidine]
         Morphine
         AHA: 3Q, '07, 6
         T40.4x1A Poisoning oth synthetic narc accidnt initial enc **I-10**

965.1 Salicylates
     Acetylsalicylic acid [aspirin]
     Salicylic acid salts
     AHA: N-D, '94, 15

965.4 Aromatic analgesics, not elsewhere classified
     Acetanilid
     Paracetamol [acetaminophen]
     Phenacetin [acetophenetidin]

965.5 Pyrazole derivatives
     Aminophenazone [aminopyrine]
     Phenylbutazone

✓5ᵗʰ 965.6 Antirheumatics [antiphlogistics]
     EXCLUDES *salicylates (965.1)*
                   steroids (962.0-962.9)
     AHA: 4Q, '98, 50

     965.61 Propionic acid derivatives
         Fenoprofen
         Flurbiprofen
         Ibuprofen
         Ketoprofen
         Naproxen
         Oxaprozin
         AHA: 4Q, '98, 50

     965.69 Other antirheumatics
         Gold salts
         Indomethacin

965.7 Other non-narcotic analgesics
     Pyrabital

965.8 Other specified analgesics and antipyretics
     Pentazocine

965.9 Unspecified analgesic and antipyretic

✓4ᵗʰ 966 Poisoning by anticonvulsants and anti-Parkinsonism drugs

966.0 Oxazolidine derivatives
     Paramethadione
     Trimethadione

966.1 Hydantoin derivatives
     Phenytoin

966.2 Succinimides
     Ethosuximide
     Phensuximide

966.3 Other and unspecified anticonvulsants
     Primidone
     EXCLUDES *barbiturates (967.0)*
                   sulfonamides (961.0)

966.4 Anti-Parkinsonism drugs
     Amantadine
     Ethopropazine [profenamine]
     Levodopa [L-dopa]

✓4ᵗʰ 967 Poisoning by sedatives and hypnotics
     EXCLUDES *drug dependence (304.0-304.9)*
                   nondependent abuse (305.0-305.9)

967.0 Barbiturates
     Amobarbital [amylobarbitone]
     Barbital [barbitone]
     Butabarbital [butabarbitone]
     Pentobarbital [pentobarbitone]
     Phenobarbital [phenobarbitone]
     Secobarbital [quinalbarbitone]
     EXCLUDES *thiobarbiturate anesthetics (968.3)*

967.1 Chloral hydrate group

967.2 Paraldehyde

967.3 Bromine compounds
     Bromide
     Carbromal (derivatives)

✓4ᵗʰ ✓5ᵗʰ Additional Digit Required	Unspecified Code	Other Specified Code	Manifestation Code	►◄ Revised Text	● New Code	▲ Revised Code Title

967.4 Methaqualone compounds

967.5 Glutethimide group

967.6 Mixed sedatives, not elsewhere classified

967.8 Other sedatives and hypnotics

967.9 Unspecified sedative or hypnotic
     Sleeping:
         drug
         pill   } NOS
         tablet

√4ᵗʰ **968 Poisoning by other central nervous system depressants and anesthetics**
     EXCLUDES drug dependence (304.0-304.9)
                nondependent abuse (305.0-305.9)

968.0 Central nervous system muscle-tone depressants
     Chlorphenesin (carbamate)
     Mephenesin
     Methocarbamol

968.1 Halothane

968.2 Other gaseous anesthetics
     Ether
     Halogenated hydrocarbon derivatives, except halothane
     Nitrous oxide

968.3 Intravenous anesthetics
     Ketamine
     Methohexital [methohexitone]
     Thiobarbiturates, such as thiopental sodium

968.4 Other and unspecified general anesthetics

968.5 Surface (topical) and infiltration anesthetics
     Cocaine (topical)
     Lidocaine (lignocaine)
     Procaine
     Tetracaine
     EXCLUDES poisoning by cocaine used as a central nervous system stimulant (970.81)
     AHA: 1Q, '93, 25

968.6 Peripheral nerve- and plexus-blocking anesthetics

968.7 Spinal anesthetics

968.9 Other and unspecified local anesthetics
     T41.44xA Poisoning uns anesthetic undetermind initial enc   **I-10**

√4ᵗʰ **969 Poisoning by psychotropic agents**
     EXCLUDES drug dependence (304.0-304.9)
                nondependent abuse (305.0-305.9)

√5ᵗʰ **969.0 Antidepressants**
     AHA: 4Q, '09, 111-112

     969.00 Antidepressant, unspecified
         AHA: 3Q, '07, 6; #5, '94, 9; 3Q, '91, 14; N-D, '84, 14

     969.01 Monoamine oxidase inhibitors
         MAOI

     969.02 Selective serotonin and norepinephrine reuptake inhibitors
         SSNRI antidepressants
         TIP: Assign for serotonin syndrome due to poisoning, along with 333.99 and E854.0, for accidental poisoning.

     969.03 Selective serotonin reuptake inhibitors
         SSRI antidepressants
         TIP: Assign for serotonin syndrome due to poisoning, along with 333.99 and E854.0, for accidental poisoning.

     969.04 Tetracyclic antidepressants

     969.05 Tricyclic antidepressants
         AHA: 4Q, '09, 112

     969.09 Other antidepressants

969.1 Phenothiazine-based tranquilizers
     Chlorpromazine
     Fluphenazine
     Prochlorperazine
     Promazine

969.2 Butyrophenone-based tranquilizers
     Haloperidol
     Spiperone
     Trifluperidol

969.3 Other antipsychotics, neuroleptics, and major tranquilizers

969.4 Benzodiazepine-based tranquilizers
     Chlordiazepoxide   Lorazepam
     Diazepam   Medazepam
     Flurazepam   Nitrazepam
     AHA: 4Q, '09, 112
         T42.4X1A Poisoning by benzodiazepines, accidental, init   **I-10**

969.5 Other tranquilizers
     Hydroxyzine
     Meprobamate

969.6 Psychodysleptics [hallucinogens]
     Cannabis (derivatives)
     Lysergide [LSD]
     Marihuana (derivatives)
     Mescaline
     Psilocin
     Psilocybin
     AHA: ▶2Q, '13, 16◀

√5ᵗʰ **969.7 Psychostimulants**
     EXCLUDES central appetite depressants (977.0)
     AHA: 4Q, '09, 113-114

     969.70 Psychostimulant, unspecified
         AHA: 2Q, '03, 11

     969.71 Caffeine

     969.72 Amphetamines
         Methamphetamines
         TIP: Assign for overdose and poisoning by the club drug ecstasy.

     969.73 Methylphenidate

     969.79 Other psychostimulants

969.8 Other specified psychotropic agents

969.9 Unspecified psychotropic agent

√4ᵗʰ **970 Poisoning by central nervous system stimulants**

970.0 Analeptics
     Lobeline
     Nikethamide

970.1 Opiate antagonists
     Levallorphan
     Nalorphine
     Naloxone

√5ᵗʰ **970.8 Other specified central nervous system stimulants**
     AHA: 4Q, '10, 98-99; 1Q, '05, 6

     970.81 Cocaine
         Crack

     970.89 Other central nervous system stimulants
         AHA: ▶2Q, '13, 15◀

970.9 Unspecified central nervous system stimulant

√4ᵗʰ **971 Poisoning by drugs primarily affecting the autonomic nervous system**

971.0 Parasympathomimetics [cholinergics]
     Acetylcholine
     Anticholinesterase:
         organophosphorus
         reversible
     Pilocarpine

971.1 Parasympatholytics [anticholinergics and antimuscarinics] and spasmolytics
     Atropine
     Homatropine
     Hyoscine [scopolamine]
     Quaternary ammonium derivatives
     EXCLUDES papaverine (972.5)

971.2 Sympathomimetics [adrenergics]
     Epinephrine [adrenalin]
     Levarterenol [noradrenalin]

971.3 Sympatholytics [antiadrenergics]
     Phenoxybenzamine
     Tolazoline hydrochloride

N Newborn Age: 0   **P** Pediatric Age: 0-17   **M** Maternity Age: 12-55   **A** Adult Age: 15-124

971.9 Unspecified drug primarily affecting autonomic nervous system

☑4ᵗʰ **972 Poisoning by agents primarily affecting the cardiovascular system**

972.0 Cardiac rhythm regulators
Practolol
Procainamide
Propranolol
Quinidine
EXCLUDES *lidocaine (968.5)*

972.1 Cardiotonic glycosides and drugs of similar action
Digitalis glycosides
Digoxin
Strophanthins

972.2 Antilipemic and antiarteriosclerotic drugs
Clofibrate
Nicotinic acid derivatives

972.3 Ganglion-blocking agents
Pentamethonium bromide

972.4 Coronary vasodilators
Dipyridamole
Nitrates [nitroglycerin]
Nitrites

972.5 Other vasodilators
Cyclandelate
Diazoxide
Papaverine
EXCLUDES *nicotinic acid (972.2)*

972.6 Other antihypertensive agents
Clonidine
Guanethidine
Rauwolfia alkaloids
Reserpine

972.7 Antivaricose drugs, including sclerosing agents
Sodium morrhuate
Zinc salts

972.8 Capillary-active drugs
Adrenochrome derivatives
Metaraminol

972.9 Other and unspecified agents primarily affecting the cardiovascular system

☑4ᵗʰ **973 Poisoning by agents primarily affecting the gastrointestinal system**

973.0 Antacids and antigastric secretion drugs
Aluminum hydroxide
Magnesium trisilicate
AHA: 1Q, '03, 19

973.1 Irritant cathartics
Bisacodyl
Castor oil
Phenolphthalein

973.2 Emollient cathartics
Dioctyl sulfosuccinates

973.3 Other cathartics, including intestinal atonia drugs
Magnesium sulfate

973.4 Digestants
Pancreatin
Papain
Pepsin

973.5 Antidiarrheal drugs
Kaolin
Pectin
EXCLUDES *anti-infectives (960.0-961.9)*

973.6 Emetics

973.8 Other specified agents primarily affecting the gastrointestinal system

973.9 Unspecified agent primarily affecting the gastrointestinal system

☑4ᵗʰ **974 Poisoning by water, mineral, and uric acid metabolism drugs**

974.0 Mercurial diuretics
Chlormerodrin
Mercaptomerin
Mersalyl

974.1 Purine derivative diuretics
Theobromine
Theophylline
EXCLUDES *aminophylline [theophylline ethylenediamine] (975.7)*
caffeine (969.71)

974.2 Carbonic acid anhydrase inhibitors
Acetazolamide

974.3 Saluretics
Benzothiadiazides
Chlorothiazide group

974.4 Other diuretics
Ethacrynic acid
Furosemide

974.5 Electrolytic, caloric, and water-balance agents

974.6 Other mineral salts, not elsewhere classified

974.7 Uric acid metabolism drugs
Allopurinol
Colchicine
Probenecid

☑4ᵗʰ **975 Poisoning by agents primarily acting on the smooth and skeletal muscles and respiratory system**

975.0 Oxytocic agents
Ergot alkaloids
Oxytocin
Prostaglandins

975.1 Smooth muscle relaxants
Adiphenine
Metaproterenol [orciprenaline]
EXCLUDES *papaverine (972.5)*

975.2 Skeletal muscle relaxants

975.3 Other and unspecified drugs acting on muscles

975.4 Antitussives
Dextromethorphan
Pipazethate

975.5 Expectorants
Acetylcysteine
Guaifenesin
Terpin hydrate

975.6 Anti-common cold drugs

975.7 Antiasthmatics
Aminophylline [theophylline ethylenediamine]

975.8 Other and unspecified respiratory drugs

☑4ᵗʰ **976 Poisoning by agents primarily affecting skin and mucous membrane, ophthalmological, otorhinolaryngological, and dental drugs**

976.0 Local anti-infectives and anti-inflammatory drugs

976.1 Antipruritics

976.2 Local astringents and local detergents

976.3 Emollients, demulcents, and protectants

976.4 Keratolytics, keratoplastics, other hair treatment drugs and preparations

976.5 Eye anti-infectives and other eye drugs
Idoxuridine

976.6 Anti-infectives and other drugs and preparations for ear, nose, and throat

976.7 Dental drugs topically applied
EXCLUDES *anti-infectives (976.0)*
local anesthetics (968.5)

976.8 Other agents primarily affecting skin and mucous membrane
Spermicides [vaginal contraceptives]

Injury and Poisoning

976.9–985.5

976.9 Unspecified agent primarily affecting skin and mucous membrane

✓4ᵗʰ **977 Poisoning by other and unspecified drugs and medicinal substances**

977.0 Dietetics
Central appetite depressants

977.1 Lipotropic drugs

977.2 Antidotes and chelating agents, not elsewhere classified

977.3 Alcohol deterrents

977.4 Pharmaceutical excipients
Pharmaceutical adjuncts

977.8 Other specified drugs and medicinal substances
Contrast media used for diagnostic x-ray procedures
Diagnostic agents and kits

977.9 Unspecified drug or medicinal substance

✓4ᵗʰ **978 Poisoning by bacterial vaccines**

978.0 BCG

978.1 Typhoid and paratyphoid

978.2 Cholera

978.3 Plague

978.4 Tetanus

978.5 Diphtheria

978.6 Pertussis vaccine, including combinations with a pertussis component

978.8 Other and unspecified bacterial vaccines

978.9 Mixed bacterial vaccines, except combinations with a pertussis component

✓4ᵗʰ **979 Poisoning by other vaccines and biological substances**
EXCLUDES gamma globulin (964.6)

979.0 Smallpox vaccine

979.1 Rabies vaccine

979.2 Typhus vaccine

979.3 Yellow fever vaccine

979.4 Measles vaccine

979.5 Poliomyelitis vaccine

979.6 Other and unspecified viral and rickettsial vaccines
Mumps vaccine

979.7 Mixed viral-rickettsial and bacterial vaccines, except combinations with a pertussis component
EXCLUDES combinations with a pertussis component (978.6)

979.9 Other and unspecified vaccines and biological substances

Toxic Effects of Substances Chiefly Nonmedicinal as to Source (980-989)

Use additional code to identify:
personal history of retained foreign body fully removed (V15.53)
retained foreign body status, if applicable, (V90.01-V90.9)
Use additional code to specify the nature of the toxic effect
EXCLUDES burns from chemical agents (ingested) (947.0-947.9)
localized toxic effects indexed elsewhere (001.0-799.9)
respiratory conditions due to external agents (506.0-508.9)
respiratory conditions due to smoke inhalation NOS (508.2)
AHA: 3Q, '10, 19

✓4ᵗʰ **980 Toxic effect of alcohol**

980.0 Ethyl alcohol
Denatured alcohol   Grain alcohol
Ethanol
Use additional code to identify any associated:
acute alcohol intoxication (305.0)
in alcoholism (303.0)
drunkenness (simple) (305.0)
pathological (291.4)
AHA: 4Q, '09, 112; 3Q, '96, 16
T51.0x1A Toxic effect ethanol accidental initial encountr   I-10

980.1 Methyl alcohol
Methanol
Wood alcohol

980.2 Isopropyl alcohol
Dimethyl carbinol
Isopropanol
Rubbing alcohol

980.3 Fusel oil
Alcohol:
amyl
butyl
propyl

980.8 Other specified alcohols

980.9 Unspecified alcohol

981 Toxic effect of petroleum products
Benzine   Petroleum:
Gasoline   ether
Kerosene   naphtha
Paraffin wax   spirit

✓4ᵗʰ **982 Toxic effect of solvents other than petroleum-based**

982.0 Benzene and homologues

982.1 Carbon tetrachloride

982.2 Carbon disulfide
Carbon bisulfide

982.3 Other chlorinated hydrocarbon solvents
Tetrachloroethylene
Trichloroethylene
EXCLUDES chlorinated hydrocarbon preparations other than solvents (989.2)
AHA: 3Q, '08, 6-7

982.4 Nitroglycol

982.8 Other nonpetroleum-based solvents
Acetone

✓4ᵗʰ **983 Toxic effect of corrosive aromatics, acids, and caustic alkalis**

983.0 Corrosive aromatics
Carbolic acid or phenol
Cresol

983.1 Acids
Acid:
hydrochloric
nitric
sulfuric

983.2 Caustic alkalis
Lye
Potassium hydroxide
Sodium hydroxide

983.9 Caustic, unspecified

✓4ᵗʰ **984 Toxic effect of lead and its compounds (including fumes)**
INCLUDES that from all sources except medicinal substances

984.0 Inorganic lead compounds
Lead dioxide
Lead salts

984.1 Organic lead compounds
Lead acetate
Tetraethyl lead

984.8 Other lead compounds

984.9 Unspecified lead compound

✓4ᵗʰ **985 Toxic effect of other metals**
INCLUDES that from all sources except medicinal substances

985.0 Mercury and its compounds
Minamata disease

985.1 Arsenic and its compounds

985.2 Manganese and its compounds

985.3 Beryllium and its compounds

985.4 Antimony and its compounds

985.5 Cadmium and its compounds

N Newborn Age: 0   P Pediatric Age: 0-17   M Maternity Age: 12-55   A Adult Age: 15-124

985.6 Chromium

985.8 Other specified metals
     Brass fumes
     Copper salts
     Iron compounds
     Nickel compounds
     AHA: 1Q, '88, 5
     TIP: Assign for aluminum overloading or excessive concentration of aluminum in the body, along with E879.1 if due to renal dialysis and E879.8 if due to total parenteral nutrition.

985.9 Unspecified metal

986 Toxic effect of carbon monoxide
     Carbon monoxide from any source

✓4ᵗʰ 987 Toxic effect of other gases, fumes, or vapors

987.0 Liquefied petroleum gases
     Butane
     Propane

987.1 Other hydrocarbon gas

987.2 Nitrogen oxides
     Nitrogen dioxide
     Nitrous fumes

987.3 Sulfur dioxide

987.4 Freon
     Dichloromonofluoromethane

987.5 Lacrimogenic gas
     Bromobenzyl cyanide
     Chloroacetophenone
     Ethyliodoacetate

987.6 Chlorine gas

987.7 Hydrocyanic acid gas

987.8 Other specified gases, fumes, or vapors
     Phosgene
     Polyester fumes

987.9 Unspecified gas, fume, or vapor
     AHA: 4Q, '11, 114; 3Q, '05, 10
     TIP: Do not assign for conditions due to smoke inhalation; assign instead code 508.2.

988 Toxic effect of noxious substances eaten as food
     EXCLUDES allergic reaction to food, such as:
         gastroenteritis (558.3)
         rash (692.5, 693.1)
         food poisoning (bacterial) (005.0-005.9)
         toxic effects of food contaminants, such as:
             aflatoxin and other mycotoxin (989.7)
             mercury (985.0)

988.0 Fish and shellfish

988.1 Mushrooms

988.2 Berries and other plants

988.8 Other specified noxious substances eaten as food

988.9 Unspecified noxious substance eaten as food

✓4ᵗʰ 989 Toxic effect of other substances, chiefly nonmedicinal as to source

989.0 Hydrocyanic acid and cyanides
     Potassium cyanide
     Sodium cyanide
     EXCLUDES gas and fumes (987.7)

989.1 Strychnine and salts

989.2 Chlorinated hydrocarbons
     Aldrin
     Chlordane
     DDT
     Dieldrin
     EXCLUDES chlorinated hydrocarbon solvents (982.0-982.3)

989.3 Organophosphate and carbamate
     Carbaryl
     Dichlorvos
     Malathion
     Parathion
     Phorate
     Phosdrin

989.4 Other pesticides, not elsewhere classified
     Mixtures of insecticides

989.5 Venom
     Bites of venomous snakes, lizards, and spiders
     Tick paralysis

989.6 Soaps and detergents

989.7 Aflatoxin and other mycotoxin [food contaminants]

✓5ᵗʰ 989.8 Other substances, chiefly nonmedicinal as to source
     AHA: 4Q, '95, 60

     989.81 Asbestos
         EXCLUDES asbestosis (501)
                  exposure to asbestos (V15.84)

     989.82 Latex

     989.83 Silicone
         EXCLUDES silicone used in medical devices, implants and grafts (996.00-996.79)

     989.84 Tobacco

     989.89 Other

989.9 Unspecified substance, chiefly nonmedicinal as to source

Other and Unspecified Effects of External Causes (990-995)

990 Effects of radiation, unspecified
     Complication of:
         phototherapy
         radiation therapy
     Radiation sickness
     [The type of radiation giving rise to the adverse effect may be identified by use of the E codes.]
     EXCLUDES specified adverse effects of radiation. Such conditions are to be classified according to the nature of the adverse effect, as:
         burns (940.0-949.5)
         dermatitis (692.7-692.8)
         leukemia (204.0-208.9)
         pneumonia (508.0)
         sunburn (692.71, 692.76-692.77)

✓4ᵗʰ 991 Effects of reduced temperature

991.0 Frostbite of face

991.1 Frostbite of hand

991.2 Frostbite of foot

991.3 Frostbite of other and unspecified sites

991.4 Immersion foot
     Trench foot
     DEF: Paresthesia, edema, blotchy cyanosis of foot, the skin is soft (macerated), pale and wrinkled, and the sole is swollen with surface ridging and following sustained immersion in water.

991.5 Chilblains
     Erythema pernio
     Perniosis
     DEF: Red, swollen, itchy skin; follows damp cold exposure; also associated with pruritus and a burning feeling in hands, feet, ears, and face in children, legs and toes in women, and hands and fingers in men.

991.6 Hypothermia
     Hypothermia (accidental)
     EXCLUDES hypothermia following anesthesia (995.89)
                  hypothermia not associated with low environmental temperature (780.65)
     DEF: Reduced body temperature due to low environmental temperatures.

991.8 Other specified effects of reduced temperature

✓4ᵗʰ
✓5ᵗʰ Additional Digit Required   **Unspecified Code**   Other Specified Code   **Manifestation Code**   ►◄ Revised Text   ● New Code   ▲ Revised Code Title

2015 ICD-9-CM   **Volume 1 – 307**

991.9　Unspecified effect of reduced temperature
Effects of freezing or excessive cold NOS

√4th　**992　Effects of heat and light**
　　EXCLUDES　burns (940.0-949.5)
　　　　　　diseases of sweat glands due to heat (705.0-705.9)
　　　　　　malignant hyperpyrexia following anesthesia (995.86)
　　　　　　sunburn (692.71, 692.76-692.77)

992.0　Heat stroke and sunstroke
　　Heat apoplexy　　　Siriasis
　　Heat pyrexia　　　Thermoplegia
　　Ictus solaris
　　Use additional code(s) to identify any associated complication
　　　　of heat stroke, such as:
　　　　alterations of consciousness (780.01-780.09)
　　　　systemic inflammatory response syndrome (995.93-995.94)
　　DEF: Headache, vertigo, cramps and elevated body temperature due
　　　to high environmental temperatures.

992.1　Heat syncope
　　Heat collapse

992.2　Heat cramps

992.3　Heat exhaustion, anhydrotic
　　Heat prostration due to water depletion
　　EXCLUDES　that associated with salt depletion (992.4)

992.4　Heat exhaustion due to salt depletion
　　Heat prostration due to salt (and water) depletion

992.5　Heat exhaustion, unspecified
　　Heat prostration NOS

992.6　Heat fatigue, transient

992.7　Heat edema
　　DEF: Fluid retention due to high environmental temperatures.

992.8　Other specified heat effects

992.9　Unspecified

√4th　**993　Effects of air pressure**

993.0　Barotrauma, otitic
　　Aero-otitis media
　　Effects of high altitude on ears
　　DEF: Ringing ears, deafness, pain and vertigo due to air pressure
　　　changes.

993.1　Barotrauma, sinus
　　Aerosinusitis
　　Effects of high altitude on sinuses

993.2　Other and unspecified effects of high altitude
　　Alpine sickness　　　　Hypobaropathy
　　Andes disease　　　　Mountain sickness
　　Anoxia due to high altitude
　　AHA: 3Q, '88, 4

993.3　Caisson disease
　　Bends
　　Compressed-air disease
　　Decompression sickness
　　Divers' palsy or paralysis
　　DEF: Rapid reduction in air pressure while breathing compressed air;
　　　symptoms include skin lesions, joint pains, respiratory and
　　　neurological problems.

993.4　Effects of air pressure caused by explosion

993.8　Other specified effects of air pressure

993.9　Unspecified effect of air pressure

√4th　**994　Effects of other external causes**
　　EXCLUDES　certain adverse effects not elsewhere classified (995.0-995.8)

994.0　Effects of lightning
　　Shock from lightning
　　Struck by lightning NOS
　　EXCLUDES　burns (940.0-949.5)

994.1　Drowning and nonfatal submersion
　　Bathing cramp
　　Immersion
　　AHA: ▶3Q, '13, 10;◀ 3Q, '09, 14; 3Q, '88, 4
　　TIP: When near-drowning results in acute respiratory edema, assign
　　　also code 518.5 Post-traumatic pulmonary insufficiency.

994.2　Effects of hunger
　　Deprivation of food
　　Starvation

994.3　Effects of thirst
　　Deprivation of water

994.4　Exhaustion due to exposure

994.5　Exhaustion due to excessive exertion
　　Exhaustion due to overexertion

994.6　Motion sickness
　　Air sickness　　　　Travel sickness
　　Seasickness

994.7　Asphyxiation and strangulation
　　Suffocation (by):　　Suffocation (by):
　　　bedclothes　　　　plastic bag
　　　cave-in　　　　　pressure
　　　constriction　　　strangulation
　　　mechanical
　　EXCLUDES　asphyxia from:
　　　　　　carbon monoxide (986)
　　　　　　inhalation of food or foreign body (932-934.9)
　　　　　　other gases, fumes, and vapors (987.0-987.9)

994.8　Electrocution and nonfatal effects of electric current
　　Shock from electric current
　　Shock from electroshock gun (taser)
　　EXCLUDES　electric burns (940.0-949.5)

994.9　Other effects of external causes
　　Effects of:
　　　abnormal gravitational [G] forces or states
　　　weightlessness

√4th　**995　Certain adverse effects not elsewhere classified**
　　EXCLUDES　complications of surgical and medical care (996.0-999.9)

995.0　Other anaphylactic reaction
　　Allergic shock
　　Anaphylactic reaction
　　Anaphylactic shock NOS or due to adverse effect of correct
　　　medicinal substance properly administered
　　Anaphylactoid reaction, NOS
　　Anaphylaxis
　　Use additional E code to identify external cause, such as:
　　　adverse effects of correct medicinal substance properly
　　　administered [E930-E949]
　　EXCLUDES　anaphylactic reaction to serum (999.41-999.49)
　　　　　　anaphylactic shock or reaction due to adverse food
　　　　　　reaction (995.60-995.69)
　　DEF: Immediate sensitivity response after exposure to specific
　　　antigen; results in life-threatening respiratory distress; usually
　　　followed by vascular collapse, shock, urticaria, angioedema and
　　　pruritus.
　　AHA: ▶2Q, '13, 12;◀ 4Q, '93, 30

995.1　Angioneurotic edema
　　Allergic angioedema
　　Giant urticaria
　　EXCLUDES　urticaria:
　　　　　　due to serum (999.51-999.59)
　　　　　　other specified (698.2, 708.0-708.9, 757.33)
　　DEF: Circulatory response of deep dermis, subcutaneous or
　　　submucosal tissues; causes localized edema and wheals.

√5th　**995.2　Other and unspecified adverse effect of drug, medicinal
　　and biological substance**
　　EXCLUDES　pathological drug intoxication (292.2)
　　AHA: 2Q, '97, 12; 3Q, '95, 13; 3Q, '92, 16
　　TIP: Codes from this subcategory should not be assigned for
　　　inpatient cases; their use is limited to certain outpatient cases in
　　　which there is no documentation of specific symptoms associated
　　　with the adverse effect.

**995.20　Unspecified adverse effect of unspecified
　　drug, medicinal and biological substance**
　　Unspecified adverse effect of unspecified medicinal
　　　substance properly administered
　　AHA: 4Q, '06, 112

995.21　Arthus phenomenon
　　Arthus reaction
　　AHA: 4Q, '06, 112

N　Newborn Age: 0　　　P　Pediatric Age: 0-17　　　M　Maternity Age: 12-55　　　A　Adult Age: 15-124

995.22 Unspecified adverse effect of anesthesia

　　AHA: 4Q, '06, 112

995.23 Unspecified adverse effect of insulin

　　AHA: 4Q, '06, 112

995.24 Failed moderate sedation during procedure

　　Failed conscious sedation during procedure

　　AHA: 4Q, '09, 114

　　TIP: If documentation indicates a personal history of failed moderate sedation, assign instead code V15.80 History of failed moderate sedation.

995.27 Other drug allergy

　　Allergic reaction NEC (due) to correct medical
　　　　substance properly administered
　　Drug allergy NOS
　　Drug hypersensitivity NOS
　　Hypersensitivity (due) to correct medical substance
　　　　properly administered

　　AHA: 4Q, '06, 112

995.29 Unspecified adverse effect of other drug, medicinal and biological substance

　　Unspecified adverse effect of medicinal substance
　　　　NEC properly administered

　　AHA: 4Q, '06, 112

995.3 Allergy, unspecified

　　Allergic reaction NOS　　　Idiosyncrasy NOS
　　Hypersensitivity NOS

　　EXCLUDES *allergic reaction NOS to correct medicinal substance*
　　　　　　properly administered (995.27)
　　　　　allergy to existing dental restorative materials
　　　　　　(525.66)
　　　　　specific types of allergic reaction, such as:
　　　　　　allergic diarrhea (558.3)
　　　　　　dermatitis (691.0-693.9)
　　　　　　hayfever (477.0-477.9)

995.4 Shock due to anesthesia

　　Shock due to anesthesia in which the correct substance was
　　　　properly administered

　　EXCLUDES *complications of anesthesia in labor or delivery*
　　　　　　(668.0-668.9)
　　　　　overdose or wrong substance given (968.0-969.9)
　　　　　postoperative shock NOS (998.00)
　　　　　specified adverse effects of anesthesia classified
　　　　　　elsewhere, such as:
　　　　　　anoxic brain damage (348.1)
　　　　　　hepatitis (070.0-070.9), etc.
　　　　　unspecified adverse effect of anesthesia (995.22)

√5ᵗʰ **995.5** Child maltreatment syndrome

　　Use additional code(s), if applicable, to identify any associated
　　　　injuries

　　Use additional E code to identify:
　　　nature of abuse (E960-E968)
　　　perpetrator (E967.0-E967.9)

　　AHA: 2Q, '12, 12; 1Q, '98, 11

　　TIP: Although separate codes for any associated injuries should be
　　assigned, codes from this subcategory may be assigned alone if
　　there are no documented injuries or associated conditions.

995.50 Child abuse, unspecified　　**P**

995.51 Child emotional/psychological abuse　　**P**

　　AHA: 4Q, '96, 38, 40

995.52 Child neglect (nutritional)　　**P**

　　AHA: 4Q, '96, 38, 40

995.53 Child sexual abuse　　**P**

　　AHA: 4Q, '96, 39, 40

995.54 Child physical abuse　　**P**

　　Battered baby or child syndrome

　　EXCLUDES *shaken infant syndrome (995.55)*

　　AHA: 3Q, '99, 14; 4Q, '96, 39, 40

995.55 Shaken infant syndrome　　**P**

　　Use additional code(s) to identify any associated
　　　　injuries

　　AHA: 4Q, '96, 40, 43

995.59 Other child abuse and neglect　　**P**

　　Multiple forms of abuse

√5ᵗʰ **995.6** Anaphylactic reaction due to food

　　Anaphylactic reaction due to adverse food reaction
　　Anaphylactic shock or reaction due to nonpoisonous foods
　　Anaphylactoid reaction due to food

　　AHA: 4Q, '11, 142-145; 4Q, '93, 30

　　TIP: Codes from this subcategory may be assigned not only for
　　anaphylactic shock, but also for any documentation of anaphylactic
　　reaction to food.

995.60 Anaphylactic reaction due to unspecified food

995.61 Anaphylactic reaction due to peanuts

995.62 Anaphylactic reaction due to crustaceans

995.63 Anaphylactic reaction due to fruits and vegetables

995.64 Anaphylactic reaction due to tree nuts and seeds

　　AHA: 1Q, '08, 12

995.65 Anaphylactic reaction due to fish

995.66 Anaphylactic reaction due to food additives

995.67 Anaphylactic reaction due to milk products

995.68 Anaphylactic reaction due to eggs

995.69 Anaphylactic reaction due to other specified food

995.7 Other adverse food reactions, not elsewhere classified

　　Use additional code to identify the type of reaction,
　　　　such as:
　　hives (708.0)
　　wheezing (786.07)

　　EXCLUDES *anaphylactic reaction or shock due to adverse food*
　　　　　　reaction (995.60-995.69)
　　　　　asthma (493.0, 493.9)
　　　　　dermatitis due to food (693.1)
　　　　　　in contact with skin (692.5)
　　　　　gastroenteritis and colitis due to food (558.3)
　　　　　rhinitis due to food (477.1)

√5ᵗʰ **995.8** Other specified adverse effects, not elsewhere classified

995.80 Adult maltreatment, unspecified　　**A**

　　Abused person NOS

　　Use additional code to identify:
　　　any associated injury
　　　perpetrator (E967.0-E967.9)

　　AHA: 2Q, '12, 12; 4Q, '96, 41, 43

995.81 Adult physical abuse　　**A**

　　Battered:　　　　　　　　　　Battered:
　　　person syndrome NEC　　　spouse
　　　man　　　　　　　　　　　woman

　　Use additional code to identify:
　　　any association injury
　　　nature of abuse (E960-E968)
　　　perpetrator (E967.0-E967.9)

　　AHA: 2Q, '12, 12; 4Q, '96, 42, 43

995.82 Adult emotional/psychological abuse　　**A**

　　Use additional E code to identify perpetrator
　　　(E967.0-E967.9)

　　AHA: 2Q, '12, 12

995.83 Adult sexual abuse　　**A**

　　Use additional code(s) to identify:
　　　any associated injury
　　　perpetrator (E967.0-E967.9)

　　AHA: 2Q, '12, 12

995.84 Adult neglect (nutritional)　　**A**

　　Use additional code(s) to identify:
　　　intent of neglect (E904.0, E968.4)
　　　perpetrator (E967.0-E967.9)

　　AHA: 2Q, '12, 12

Continuum of Illness Due to Infection

Bacteremia ➡ Septicemia ➡ Sepsis

Severe Sepsis ⬅ Severe Sepsis
with Septic Shock

MODS
(Multiple Organ
Dysfunction Syndrome)　　➡　　Death

√4ᵗʰ √5ᵗʰ Additional Digit Required　　Unspecified Code　　Other Specified Code　　Manifestation Code　　►◄ Revised Text　　● New Code　　▲ Revised Code Title

2015 ICD-9-CM　　　　　　　　　　　　　　　　　　　　　　　　　　　　　　**Volume 1 – 309**

Injury and Poisoning

995.85–996

995.85 Other adult abuse and neglect [A]
Multiple forms of abuse and neglect

Use additional code(s) to identify
  any associated injury
  intent of neglect (E904.0, E968.4)
  nature of abuse (E960-E968)
  perpetrator (E967.0-E967.9)

AHA: 2Q, '12, 12

995.86 Malignant hyperthermia
Malignant hyperpyrexia due to anesthesia

AHA: 4Q, '98, 51

995.89 Other
Hypothermia due to anesthesia

AHA: 2Q, '04, 18; 3Q, '03, 12

√5ᵗʰ 995.9 Systemic inflammatory response syndrome (SIRS)
DEF: Clinical response to infection or trauma that can trigger an acute inflammatory reaction and progresses to coagulation, impaired fibrinolysis, and organ failure; manifested by two or more of the following symptoms: fever, tachycardia, tachypnea, leukocytosis or leukopenia.

AHA: 4Q, '06, 113-116; 2Q, '04, 16; 4Q, '02, 71

TIP: Coding these conditions requires a minimum of two codes: the underlying cause (e.g., Infection or trauma) is sequenced first, followed by a code from subcategory 995.9.

995.90 Systemic inflammatory response syndrome, unspecified
SIRS NOS

995.91 Sepsis
Systemic inflammatory response syndrome due to infectious process without acute organ dysfunction

Code first underlying infection

EXCLUDES sepsis with acute organ dysfunction (995.92)
    sepsis with multiple organ dysfunction (995.92)
    severe sepsis (995.92)

AHA: 3Q, '12, 11,13; 2Q,'12, 21; 3Q, '11, 15; 4Q, '08, 72; 4Q, '07, 86; 4Q, '06, 113-116; 2Q, '04, 16; 4Q, '03, 79

995.92 Severe sepsis
Sepsis with acute organ dysfunction
Sepsis with multiple organ dysfunction (MOD)
Systemic inflammatory response syndrome due to infectious process with acute organ dysfunction

Code first underlying infection

Use additional code to specify acute organ
  dysfunction, such as:
  acute kidney failure (584.5-584.9)
  acute respiratory failure (518.81)
  critical illness myopathy (359.81)
  critical illness polyneuropathy (357.82)
  disseminated intravascular coagulopathy [DIC]
    (286.6)
  encephalopathy (348.31)
  hepatic failure (570)
  septic shock (785.52)

AHA: ▶2Q, '13, 21;◀ 3Q, '12, 11; 4Q, '11, 153; 2Q, '10, 4; 4Q, '09, 98; 4Q, '08, 99; 4Q, '07, 97; 4Q, '06, 113-116; 2Q, '05, 18-19; 1Q, '05, 7; 1Q, '05, 7; 2Q, '04, 16; 4Q, '03, 73, 79

R65.21 Severe sepsis with septic shock   [I-10]

995.93 Systemic inflammatory response syndrome due to noninfectious process without acute organ dysfunction
Code first underlying conditions, such as:
  acute pancreatitis (577.0)
  trauma

EXCLUDES systemic inflammatory response syndrome
    due to noninfectious process with
    acute organ dysfunction (995.94)

AHA: 1Q, '11, 22; 1Q, '10, 10-11; 4Q, '06, 113-116

995.94 Systemic inflammatory response syndrome due to noninfectious process with acute organ dysfunction
Code first underlying conditions, such as:
  acute pancreatitis (577.0)
  heat stroke (992.0)
  trauma

Use additional code to specify acute organ
  dysfunction, such as:
  acute kidney failure (584.5-584.9)
  acute respiratory failure (518.81)
  critical illness myopathy (359.81)
  critical illness polyneuropathy (357.82)
  disseminated intravascular coagulopathy [DIC]
    syndrome (286.6)
  encephalopathy (348.31)
  hepatic failure (570)

EXCLUDES severe sepsis (995.92)

AHA: 1Q, '10, 10; 4Q, '06, 113-116; 4Q, '03, 79

Complications of Surgical and Medical Care, Not Elsewhere Classified (996-999)

EXCLUDES adverse effects of medicinal agents (001.0-799.9,
    995.0-995.8)
burns from local applications and irradiation (940.0-949.5)
complications of:
  conditions for which the procedure was performed
  surgical procedures during abortion, labor, and delivery
    (630-676.9)
poisoning and toxic effects of drugs and chemicals
  (960.0-989.9)
postoperative conditions in which no complications are
  present, such as:
  artificial opening status (V44.0-V44.9)
  closure of external stoma (V55.0-V55.9)
  fitting of prosthetic device (V52.0-V52.9)
specified complications classified elsewhere
  anesthetic shock (995.4)
  electrolyte imbalance (276.0-276.9)
  postlaminectomy syndrome (722.80-722.83)
  postmastectomy lymphedema syndrome (457.0)
  postoperative psychosis (293.0-293.9)
  any other condition classified elsewhere in the Alphabetic
    Index when described as due to a procedure

AHA: 2Q, '12, 5, 8

TIP: Assign additional codes to further specify the nature of the complication unless the complication code provides a complete description of the condition.

√4ᵗʰ 996 Complications peculiar to certain specified procedures

INCLUDES complications, not elsewhere classified, in the use of
    artificial substitutes [e.g., Dacron, metal, Silastic,
    Teflon] or natural sources [e.g., bone] involving:
anastomosis (internal)
graft (bypass) (patch)
implant
internal device:
  catheter
  electronic
  fixation
  prosthetic
reimplant
transplant

EXCLUDES accidental puncture or laceration during procedure (998.2)
capsular contracture of breast implant (611.83)
complications of internal anastomosis of:
  gastrointestinal tract (997.49)
  urinary tract (997.5)
endosseous dental implant failures (525.71-525.79)
intraoperative floppy iris syndrome [IFIS] (364.81)
mechanical complication of respirator (V46.14)
other specified complications classified elsewhere, such as:
  hemolytic anemia (283.1)
  functional cardiac disturbances (429.4)
  serum hepatitis (070.2-070.3)

AHA: 1Q, '94, 3

N Newborn Age: 0   P Pediatric Age: 0-17   M Maternity Age: 12-55   A Adult Age: 15-124

✓5ᵗʰ 996.0 Mechanical complication of cardiac device, implant, and graft

Breakdown (mechanical)   Obstruction, mechanical
Displacement   Perforation
Leakage   Protrusion

AHA: 2Q, '08, 9; 2Q, '93, 9

TIP: If the documentation indicates that the cardiac device (e.g., pacemaker, heart valve prosthesis) has reached its normally occurring end of life, do not assign a complication code; see instead subcategory V53.3.

996.00 Unspecified device, implant, and graft

996.01 Due to cardiac pacemaker (electrode)
     AHA: 2Q, '06, 15; 2Q, '99, 11
     T82.120A Displacement cardiac electrode initial encounter   `I-10`

996.02 Due to heart valve prosthesis

996.03 Due to coronary bypass graft
     EXCLUDES *atherosclerosis of graft (414.02, 414.03)*
          embolism [occlusion NOS] [thrombus] of graft (996.72)
     AHA: 2Q, '95, 17; N-D, '86, 5

996.04 Due to automatic implantable cardiac defibrillator
     AHA: 2Q, '05, 3

996.09 Other
     AHA: ►1Q, '13, 4;◄ 2Q, '93, 9

996.1 Mechanical complication of other vascular device, implant, and graft

Mechanical complications involving:
   aortic (bifurcation) graft (replacement)
   arteriovenous:

     dialysis catheter
     fistula   } surgically created
     shunt

   balloon (counterpulsation) device, intra-aortic
   carotid artery bypass graft
   femoral-popliteal bypass graft
   umbrella device, vena cava

     EXCLUDES *atherosclerosis of biological graft (440.30-440.32)*
          embolism [occlusion NOS] [thrombus] of (biological) (synthetic) graft (996.74)
          peritoneal dialysis catheter (996.56)

     AHA: 1Q, '12, 18; 1Q, '11, 5; 1Q, '06, 10; 2Q, '05, 8; 1Q, '02, 13; 1Q, '95, 3

     TIP: Assign for a nonmaturing AV fistula and also for postprocedural reduction in transjugular intrahepatic portosystemic shunt flow in a patient with a TIPS catheter.

     T82.330A Leakage aortic bifurcation graft initial enc   `I-10`

996.2 Mechanical complication of nervous system device, implant, and graft

Mechanical complications involving:
   dorsal column stimulator
   electrodes implanted in brain [brain "pacemaker"]
   peripheral nerve graft
   ventricular (communicating) shunt

     AHA: 2Q, '99, 4; S-O, '87, 10

✓5ᵗʰ 996.3 Mechanical complication of genitourinary device, implant, and graft
     AHA: 3Q, '01, 13; S-O, '85, 3

996.30 Unspecified device, implant, and graft

996.31 Due to urethral [indwelling] catheter

996.32 Due to intrauterine contraceptive device   ♀

996.39 Other
     Prosthetic reconstruction of vas deferens
     Repair (graft) of ureter without mention of resection
     EXCLUDES *complications due to:*
          external stoma of urinary tract (596.81-596.83)
          internal anastomosis of urinary tract (997.5)

✓5ᵗʰ 996.4 Mechanical complication of internal orthopedic device, implant, and graft

Mechanical complications involving:
   external (fixation) device utilizing internal screw(s), pin(s) or other methods of fixation
   grafts of bone, cartilage, muscle, or tendon
   internal (fixation) device such as nail, plate, rod, etc.

Use additional code to identify prosthetic joint with mechanical complication (V43.60-V43.69)

     EXCLUDES *complications of external orthopedic device, such as: pressure ulcer due to cast (707.00-707.09)*

     AHA: 4Q, '05, 91; 2Q, '99, 10; 2Q, '98, 19; 2Q, '96, 11; 3Q, '95, 16; N-D, '85, 11

     TIP: Since these codes may be used for any joint device complications, assign an additional code from subcategory V43.6 to specify the joint involved.

996.40 Unspecified mechanical complication of internal orthopedic device, implant, and graft

996.41 Mechanical loosening of prosthetic joint
     Aseptic loosening
     AHA: 4Q, '05, 112
     T84.031A Mech loosening int lt hip prosth jnt initial enc   `I-10`

996.42 Dislocation of prosthetic joint
     Instability of prosthetic joint
     Subluxation of prosthetic joint
     T84.020A Disloc of internal rt hip prosthesis, init encntr   `I-10`

996.43 Broken prosthetic joint implant
     Breakage (fracture) of prosthetic joint

996.44 Peri-prosthetic fracture around prosthetic joint
     AHA: 4Q, '05, 93

996.45 Peri-prosthetic osteolysis
     Use additional code to identify major osseous defect, if applicable (731.3)
     AHA: 4Q, '06, 103

996.46 Articular bearing surface wear of prosthetic joint

996.47 Other mechanical complication of prosthetic joint implant
     Mechanical complication of prosthetic joint NOS
     Prosthetic joint implant failure NOS

996.49 Other mechanical complication of other internal orthopedic device, implant, and graft
     Breakage of internal fixation device in bone
     Dislocation of internal fixation device in bone
     EXCLUDES *mechanical complication of prosthetic joint implant (996.41-996.47)*
     AHA: ►2Q, '13, 22;◄ 1Q, '10, 7

✓5ᵗʰ 996.5 Mechanical complication of other specified prosthetic device, implant, and graft

Mechanical complications involving:
   nonabsorbable surgical material NOS
   other graft, implant, and internal device, not elsewhere classified
   prosthetic implant in:
     bile duct   chin
     breast   orbit of eye

     AHA: 1Q, '98, 11

996.51 Due to corneal graft
     AHA: 2Q, '10, 4-5

996.52 Due to graft of other tissue, not elsewhere classified
     Skin graft failure or rejection
     EXCLUDES *failure of artificial skin graft (996.55)*
          failure of decellularized allodermis (996.55)
          sloughing of temporary skin allografts or xenografts (pigskin) — omit code
     AHA: 3Q, '12, 6; 1Q, '96, 10
     TIP: Assign for failure of living biological wound care materials used to treat nonhealing wounds recalcitrant to conventional therapy (e.g., Apligraft, CelTx, Dermagraft).

996.53 Due to ocular lens prosthesis
     EXCLUDES *contact lenses — code to condition*
     AHA: 1Q, '00, 9

Injury and Poisoning

996.0–996.53

✓4ᵗʰ ✓5ᵗʰ Additional Digit Required   Unspecified Code   Other Specified Code   Manifestation Code   ►◄ Revised Text   ● New Code   ▲ Revised Code Title

2015 ICD-9-CM   **October 2014 · Volume 1 – 311**

Injury and Poisoning

996.54–996.73

996.54 Due to breast prosthesis
Breast capsule (prosthesis)
Mammary implant
AHA: 2Q, '98, 14; 3Q, '92, 4
TIP: If documentation indicates capsular contracture of breast implant, see instead code 611.83.

996.55 Due to artificial skin graft and decellularized allodermis
Dislodgement
Displacement
Failure
Non-adherence
Poor incorporation
Shearing
AHA: 4Q, '98, 52

996.56 Due to peritoneal dialysis catheter
EXCLUDES *mechanical complication of arteriovenous dialysis catheter (996.1)*
AHA: 4Q, '98, 54

996.57 Due to insulin pump
AHA: 4Q, '03, 81-82

996.59 Due to other implant and internal device, not elsewhere classified
Nonabsorbable surgical material NOS
Prosthetic implant in:
    bile duct
    chin
    orbit of eye
AHA: ▶2Q, '13, 11;◀ 1Q, '11, 10-11; 2Q, '99, 13; 3Q, '94, 7
TIP: Assign for clogged biliary stent and also for nonfunctioning pressure equalization (PE) tubes.

√5ᵗʰ **996.6 Infection and inflammatory reaction due to internal prosthetic device, implant, and graft**
Infection (causing ⎫ due to (presence of) any device,
  obstruction)   ⎬   implant, and graft
Inflammation   ⎭   classifiable to 996.0-996.5
Use additional code to identify specified infections
AHA: 2Q, '89, 16; J-F, '87, 14

996.60 Due to unspecified device, implant, and graft

996.61 Due to cardiac device, implant, and graft
Cardiac pacemaker or defibrillator:
    electrode(s), lead(s)
    pulse generator
    subcutaneous pocket
Coronary artery bypass graft
Heart valve prosthesis

996.62 Due to other vascular device, implant, and graft
Arterial graft
Arteriovenous fistula or shunt
Infusion pump
Vascular catheter (arterial) (dialysis) (peripheral venous)
EXCLUDES *infection due to:*
    central venous catheter (999.31-999.32)
    Hickman catheter (999.31-999.32)
    peripherally inserted central catheter [PICC] (999.31-999.32)
    portacath (port-a-cath) (999.31-999.32)
    triple lumen catheter (999.31-999.32)
    umbilical venous catheter (999.31-999.32)
AHA: 2Q, '10, 8; 4Q, '07, 86; 2Q, '04, 16; 1Q, '04, 5; 4Q, '03, 107, 111; 2Q, '03, 7; 2Q, '94, 13
T82.7xxA Inf & inflam react oth card vasc dev   I-10
gft initial enc

996.63 Due to nervous system device, implant, and graft
Electrodes implanted in brain
Peripheral nerve graft
Spinal canal catheter
Ventricular (communicating) shunt (catheter)

996.64 Due to indwelling urinary catheter
Use additional code to identify specified infections, such as:
  cystitis (595.0-595.9)
  sepsis (038.0-038.9)
EXCLUDES *complications due to:*
    external stoma of urinary tract (596.81-596.83)
AHA: 2Q, '12, 20; 1Q, '12, 11; 3Q, '09, 10-11; 3Q, '93, 6
TIP: Assign for documented infection due to the presence of an indwelling urinary catheter, whether Foley, suprapubic, or other type.
T83.51XA Infect/inflm reaction d/t indwell   I-10
urinary catheter, init

996.65 Due to other genitourinary device implant, and graft
Intrauterine contraceptive device
AHA: 1Q, '00, 15

996.66 Due to internal joint prosthesis
Use additional code to identify infected prosthetic joint (V43.60-V43.69)
AHA: ▶1Q, '14, 5;◀ 4Q, '11, 156; 2Q, '08, 3-5; 2Q, '07, 7; 4Q, '05, 91, 113; 2Q, '91, 18
TIP: Do not assign as principal diagnosis for patient encounters for joint replacement following previous explantation of joint prosthesis, assign code V54.82 instead.
T84.51xA Inf & inflam reaction int rt hip pros   I-10
initial enc

996.67 Due to other internal orthopedic device, implant, and graft
Bone growth stimulator (electrode)
Internal fixation device (pin) (rod) (screw)

996.68 Due to peritoneal dialysis catheter
Exit-site infection or inflammation
AHA: 4Q, '98, 54

996.69 Due to other internal prosthetic device, implant, and graft
Breast prosthesis
Ocular lens prosthesis
Prosthetic orbital implant
AHA: 1Q, '11, 10; 2Q, '08, 11; 4Q, '03, 108; 4Q, '98, 52

√5ᵗʰ **996.7 Other complications of internal (biological) (synthetic) prosthetic device, implant, and graft**
Complication NOS ⎫
Occlusion NOS   ⎪
Embolism   ⎪ due to (presence of) any device,
Fibrosis   ⎬   implant, and graft
Hemorrhage   ⎪   classifiable to 996.0-996.5
Pain   ⎪
Stenosis   ⎪
Thrombus   ⎭
Use additional code to identify complication, such as:
  pain due to presence of device, implant or graft (338.18-338.19, 338.28-338.29)
  venous embolism and thrombosis (453.2-453.9)
EXCLUDES *disruption (dehiscence) of internal suture material (998.31)*
    transplant rejection (996.80-996.89)
AHA: 2Q,'12, 5; 2Q, '07, 12; 4Q, '05, 94; 1Q, '89, 9; N-D, '86, 5

996.70 Due to unspecified device, implant, and graft

996.71 Due to heart valve prosthesis

996.72 Due to other cardiac device, implant, and graft
Cardiac pacemaker or defibrillator:
    electrode(s), lead(s)
    subcutaneous pocket
Coronary artery bypass (graft)
EXCLUDES *occlusion due to atherosclerosis (414.02-414.06)*
AHA: 2Q, '10, 8-9; 3Q, '08, 10; 3Q, '06, 8, 25; 3Q, '01, 20
TIP: Assign for in-stent stenosis of previously placed coronary artery stent.
T82.847A Pain cardiac prosth devc impl graft initial enc   I-10

996.73 Due to renal dialysis device, implant, and graft
AHA: 2Q, '91, 18
T82.858A Stenosis vasc prosth devc impl graft initial enc   I-10

996.74 Due to other vascular device, implant, and graft

> **EXCLUDES** occlusion of biological graft due to atherosclerosis (440.30-440.32)

> **AHA:** ▶2Q, '13, 3;◀ 1Q, '12, 18; 2Q, '11, 8;1Q, '03, 16, 17
> **TIP:** Assign for clotted peripherally inserted central catheter (PICC) line.

996.75 Due to nervous system device, implant, and graft

996.76 Due to genitourinary device, implant, and graft

> **EXCLUDES** complications of implanted vaginal mesh (629.31-629.32)

> **AHA:** 1Q, '09, 15; 1Q, '00, 15
> **T83.83xA** Hemorrhage GU prosth devc impl graft initial enc **I-10**

996.77 Due to internal joint prosthesis

> Use additional code to identify prosthetic joint (V43.60-V43.69)

> **AHA:** 4Q, '05, 91
> **T84.84xA** Pain int ortho prosth devc impl gft initial enc **I-10**

996.78 Due to other internal orthopedic device, implant, and graft

> **AHA:** 2Q, '03, 14

996.79 Due to other internal prosthetic device, implant, and graft

> **AHA:** 2Q, '04, 7; 1Q,'01, 8; 3Q, '95, 14; 3Q, '92, 4

√5ᵗʰ 996.8 Complications of transplanted organ

Transplant failure or rejection

Use additional code to identify nature of complication, such as:
cytomegalovirus (CMV) infection (078.5)
graft-versus-host disease (279.50-279.53)
malignancy associated with organ transplant (199.2)
post-transplant lymphoproliferative disorder (PTLD) (238.77)

> **AHA:** 4Q, '08, 82-83; 3Q, '01, 12; 3Q, '93, 3, 4; 2Q, '93, 11; 1Q, '93, 24
> **TIP:** Assign only if the complication affects the function of the transplanted organ. Assign also a code for the specific complication.

996.80 Transplanted organ, unspecified

996.81 Kidney

> **AHA:** 2Q, '12, 6; 2Q, '11, 6; 1Q, '10, 9; 4Q, '08, 83; 3Q, '03, 16; 3Q, '98, 6, 7; 3Q, '94, 8; 2Q, '94, 9; 1Q, '93, 24
> **TIP:** Do not assign for chronic kidney disease (CKD) status following kidney transplant. The provider must indicate transplant failure, rejection, or other complication to support assignment of this code.
> **T86.11** Kidney transplant rejection **I-10**

996.82 Liver

> **AHA:** 4Q, '08, 82, 99; 3Q, '03, 17; 3Q, '98, 3, 4

996.83 Heart

> **AHA:** 3Q, '03, 16; 4Q, '02, 53; 3Q, '98, 5

996.84 Lung

> **AHA:** 2Q, '03, 12; 3Q, '98, 5

996.85 Bone marrow

> **AHA:** 1Q, '12, 13; 4Q, '08, 91; 4Q, '90, 4
> **TIP:** Do not assign for recurrence or relapse of hematopoietic or lymphatic malignancy following bone marrow/stem cell transplant.

996.86 Pancreas

996.87 Intestine

996.88 Stem cell

Complications from stem cells from:
peripheral blood
umbilical cord

> **AHA:** 4Q, '11, 147-148

996.89 Other specified transplanted organ

> **AHA:** 1Q, '11, 8; 3Q, '94, 5

√5ᵗʰ 996.9 Complications of reattached extremity or body part

996.90 Unspecified extremity

996.91 Forearm

996.92 Hand

996.93 Finger(s)

996.94 Upper extremity, other and unspecified

996.95 Foot and toe(s)

996.96 Lower extremity, other and unspecified

996.99 Other specified body part

√4ᵗʰ 997 Complications affecting specified body systems, not elsewhere classified

Use additional code to identify complications

> **EXCLUDES** the listed conditions when specified as:
> causing shock (998.00-998.09)
> complications of:
> anesthesia:
> adverse effect (001.0-799.9, 995.0-995.8)
> in labor or delivery (668.0-668.9)
> poisoning (968.0-969.9)
> implanted device or graft (996.0-996.9)
> obstetrical procedures (669.0-669.4)
> reattached extremity (996.90-996.96)
> transplanted organ (996.80-996.89)

> **AHA:** 1Q, '94, 4; 1Q, '93, 26

√5ᵗʰ 997.0 Nervous system complications

997.00 Nervous system complication, unspecified

997.01 Central nervous system complication

Anoxic brain damage
Cerebral hypoxia

> **EXCLUDES** cerebrovascular hemorrhage or infarction (997.02)

> **AHA:** 1Q, '07, 22; 1Q, '06, 15
> **TIP:** Assign for hyperperfusion syndrome, a complication of carotid endarterectomy.

997.02 Iatrogenic cerebrovascular infarction or hemorrhage

Postoperative stroke

> **AHA:** 3Q, '10, 5; 3Q, '06, 6; 2Q, '04, 8; 4Q, '95, 57
> **TIP:** Assign an additional code to specify the type of postoperative stroke involved.
> **I97.810** Intraop cerebrvascular infarct during card surg **I-10**

997.09 Other nervous system complications

> **G97.0** Cerebrospinal fluid leak from spinal puncture **I-10**

997.1 Cardiac complications

Cardiac:
arrest
insufficiency
Cardiorespiratory failure
Heart failure } during or resulting from a procedure

> **EXCLUDES** the listed conditions as long-term effects of cardiac surgery or due to the presence of cardiac prosthetic device (429.4)

> **AHA:** ▶4Q, '13, 98; 1Q, '13, 11;◀ 1Q, '11, 3-4; 4Q, '08, 179; 2Q, '02, 12
> **I97.711** Intraoperative cardiac arrest during oth surgery **I-10**

997.2 Peripheral vascular complications

Phlebitis or thrombophlebitis during or resulting from a procedure

> **EXCLUDES** the listed conditions due to:
> implant or catheter device (996.62)
> infusion, perfusion, or transfusion (999.2)
> complications affecting blood vessels (997.71-997.79)

> **AHA:** 1Q, '03, 6; 3Q, '02, 24-26
> **T81.72xA** Complication of vein following a procedure NEC init. enc **I-10**

Injury and Poisoning

996.74–997.2

Injury and Poisoning

997.3–997.99

✓5ᵗʰ 997.3 Respiratory complications

EXCLUDES *iatrogenic [postoperative] pneumothorax (512.1)*
iatrogenic pulmonary embolism (415.11)
specified complications classified elsewhere, such as:
adult respiratory distress syndrome (518.52)
pulmonary edema, postoperative (518.4)
respiratory insufficiency, acute, postoperative (518.52)
shock lung related to trauma and surgery (518.52)
tracheostomy complications (519.00-519.09)
transfusion related acute lung injury [TRALI] (518.7)

AHA: 4Q, '11, 148-150; 1Q, '97, 10; 2Q, '93, 3; 2Q, '93, 9; 4Q, '90, 25

997.31 Ventilator associated pneumonia
Ventilator associated pneumonitis

Use additional code to identify organism

AHA: 4Q, '08, 148-149

TIP: Do not assign unless the provider has documented the relationship between the pneumonia and ventilation status.

997.32 Postprocedural aspiration pneumonia
Chemical pneumonitis resulting from a procedure
Mendelson's syndrome resulting from a procedure

EXCLUDES *aspiration pneumonia during labor and delivery (668.0)*

DEF: Mendelson's syndrome: acid pneumonitis due to aspiration of gastric acids, may occur after anesthesia or sedation.

AHA: 4Q, '11, 150

TIP: Do not assign code 507.0 in addition to 997.32; aspiration pneumonia due to a procedure is fully captured with this code.

997.39 Other respiratory complications

AHA: 1Q, '11, 16

J95.4 Chem pneumonitis d/t anesthesia [Mendelson syndrm]   **I-10**

✓5ᵗʰ 997.4 Digestive system complications

Complications of:
intestinal (internal) anastomosis and bypass, not elsewhere classified, except that involving urinary tract
Hepatic failure ⎫
Hepatorenal syndrome ⎬ specified as due to a
Intestinal obstruction NOS ⎭ procedure

EXCLUDES *complications of gastric band procedure (539.01-539.09)*
complications of other bariatric procedure (539.81-539.89)
gastrostomy complications (536.40-536.49)
specified gastrointestinal complications classified elsewhere, such as:
blind loop syndrome (579.2)
colostomy and enterostomy complications (569.60-569.69)
complications of intestinal pouch (569.71-569.79)
gastrojejunal ulcer (534.0-534.9)
infection of esophagostomy (530.86)
infection of external stoma (569.61)
mechanical complication of esophagostomy (530.87)
pelvic peritoneal adhesions, female (614.6)
peritoneal adhesions (568.0)
peritoneal adhesions with obstruction (560.81)
postcholecystectomy syndrome (576.0)
postgastric surgery syndromes (564.2)
pouchitis (569.71)
vomiting following gastrointestinal surgery (564.3)

AHA: 4Q, '11, 125, 148-150; 2Q, '01, 4-6; 3Q, '99, 4; 2Q, '99, 14; 3Q, '97, 7; 1Q, '97, 11; 2Q, '95, 7; 1Q, '93, 26; 3Q, '92, 15; 2Q, '89, 15; 1Q, '88, 14

997.41 Retained cholelithiasis following cholecystectomy

997.49 Other digestive system complications

AHA: 1Q, '12, 6

TIP: Assign for ileus following gastrointestinal surgery; physician documentation of the cause-and-effect relationship is not required.

K91.89 Oth postproc comp & disorder of digest syst   **I-10**

997.5 Urinary complications

Complications of:
internal anastomosis and bypass of urinary tract, including that involving intestinal tract
Oliguria or anuria ⎫
Renal (kidney): ⎪
failure (acute) ⎬ specified as due to
insufficiency (acute) ⎪ procedure
Tubular necrosis (acute) ⎭

EXCLUDES *complications of cystostomy (596.81-596.83)*
complications of external stoma of urinary tract (596.81-596.83)
specified complications classified elsewhere, such as:
postoperative stricture of:
ureter (593.3)
urethra (598.2)

AHA: ▶1Q, '14, 12;◀ 1Q '12, 11; 3Q, '03, 13; 3Q, '96, 10, 15; 4Q, '95, 73; 1Q, '92, 13; 2Q, '89, 16; M-A, '87, 10; S-O, '85, 3

TIP: Assign for a urostomy-associated urinary tract infection with poor self-catheterization technique/hygiene.

N99.0 Postprocedural (acute) (chronic) renal failure   **I-10**

✓5ᵗʰ 997.6 Amputation stump complication

EXCLUDES *admission for treatment for a current traumatic amputation — code to complicated traumatic amputation*
phantom limb (syndrome) (353.6)

AHA: 4Q, '95, 82

997.60 Unspecified complication

997.61 Neuroma of amputation stump
DEF: Hyperplasia generated nerve cell mass following amputation.

997.62 Infection (chronic)
Use additional code to identify the organism

AHA: 1Q, '05, 15 4Q, '96, 46

TIP: If cellulitis is specified as a manifestation of the infection, assign an additional code from category 681 or 682.

T87.43 Infection amputation stump right lower extremity   **I-10**

997.69 Other
AHA: 1Q, '05, 15

✓5ᵗʰ 997.7 Vascular complications of other vessels

EXCLUDES *peripheral vascular complications (997.2)*

997.71 Vascular complications of mesenteric artery
AHA: 4Q, '01, 53

TIP: For postoperative mesenteric artery embolism, assign also code 557.0 Acute vascular insufficiency of intestine.

997.72 Vascular complications of renal artery

997.79 Vascular complications of other vessels

✓5ᵗʰ 997.9 Complications affecting other specified body systems, not elsewhere classified

EXCLUDES *specified complications classified elsewhere, such as:*
broad ligament laceration syndrome (620.6)
postartificial menopause syndrome (627.4)
postoperative stricture of vagina (623.2)

997.91 Hypertension
EXCLUDES *essential hypertension (401.0-401.9)*

AHA: 4Q, '95, 57

997.99 Other
Vitreous touch syndrome

DEF: Vitreous touch syndrome: vitreous protruding through pupil and attaches to corneal epithelium; causes aqueous fluid in vitreous body; marked by corneal edema, loss of lucidity; complication of cataract surgery.

AHA: 2Q, '94, 12; 1Q, '94, 17

N Newborn Age: 0   **P** Pediatric Age: 0-17   **M** Maternity Age: 12-55   **A** Adult Age: 15-124

☑4ᵗʰ **998 Other complications of procedures, not elsewhere classified**

     EXCLUDES   *fluid overload due to transfusion (blood) (276.61)*
                     TACO (276.61)
                     transfusion associated circulatory overload (276.61)

     AHA: 1Q, '94, 4

☑5ᵗʰ **998.0 Postoperative shock**

     Shock during or resulting from a surgical procedure

     EXCLUDES   *shock:*
                     anaphylactic due to serum (999.41-999.49)
                     anesthetic (995.4)
                     electric (994.8)
                     following abortion (639.5)
                     obstetric (669.1)
                     traumatic (958.4)

     AHA: 4Q, '11, 150-153

     998.00 Postoperative shock, unspecified
            Collapse, not otherwise specified, during or resulting from a surgical procedure
            Failure of peripheral circulation, postoperative

     998.01 Postoperative shock, cardiogenic
            AHA: 4Q, '11, 152

     998.02 Postoperative shock, septic
            Postoperative endotoxic shock
            Postoperative gram-negative shock
            Code first underlying infection
            Use additional code, to identify severe sepsis (995.92) and any associated acute organ dysfunction, if applicable
            AHA: 4Q, '11, 153

     998.09 Postoperative shock, other
            Postoperative hypovolemic shock

☑5ᵗʰ **998.1 Hemorrhage or hematoma or seroma complicating a procedure**

     EXCLUDES   *hemorrhage, hematoma, or seroma:*
                     complicating cesarean section or puerperal perineal wound (674.3)
                     due to implanted device or graft (996.70-996.79)

     998.11 Hemorrhage complicating a procedure
            AHA: 1Q, '11, 13; 3Q '03, 13; 1Q, '03, 4; 4Q, '97, 52; 1Q, '97, 10
            I97.410 Intraop hemorrhage circ sys organ comp card cath   I-10

     998.12 Hematoma complicating a procedure
            AHA: 1Q, '11, 13; 3Q '06, 12; 1Q, '03, 6; 3Q '02, 24, 26

     998.13 Seroma complicating a procedure
            AHA: 4Q, '96, 46; 1Q, '93, 26; 2Q, '92, 15; S-O, '87, 8

998.2 Accidental puncture or laceration during a procedure

     Accidental perforation by catheter or other instrument during a procedure on:
       blood vessel   nerve   organ

     EXCLUDES   *iatrogenic [postoperative] pneumothorax (512.1)*
                     puncture or laceration caused by implanted device intentionally left in operation wound (996.0-996.5)
                     specified complications classified elsewhere, such as:
                     broad ligament laceration syndrome (620.6)
                     dural tear (349.31)
                     incidental durotomy (349.31)
                     trauma from instruments during delivery (664.0-665.9)

     AHA: 2Q, '12, 5; 1Q, '10, 8, 11; 2Q, '07, 9; 1Q, '06, 15; 3Q, '02, 24, 26; 3Q, '94, 6; 3Q, '90, 17; 3Q, '90, 18

     TIP: Assign an additional code to describe the nature or site (e.g., organ) of the perforation.

     I97.51 Accidentl punct lac circ sys organ dur circ proc   I-10

☑5ᵗʰ **998.3 Disruption of wound**

     Dehiscence ⎫
     Rupture   ⎬ of operation wound
     Disruption of any suture materials or other closure method

     EXCLUDES   *disruption of:*
                     cesarean wound (674.1)
                     perineal wound, puerperal (674.2)

     AHA: 4Q, '08, 149-152; 4Q, '02, 73; 1Q, '93, 19

     998.30 Disruption of wound, unspecified
            Disruption of wound NOS

     998.31 Disruption of internal operation (surgical) wound
            Disruption or dehiscence of closure of:
                fascia, superficial or muscular
                internal organ
                muscle or muscle flap
                ribs or rib cage
                skull or craniotomy
                sternum or sternotomy
                tendon or ligament
            Deep disruption or dehiscence of operation wound NOS

            EXCLUDES   *complications of internal anastomosis of:*
                              gastrointestinal tract (997.49)
                              urinary tract (997.5)

            AHA: 4Q, '10,131

     998.32 Disruption of external operation (surgical) wound
            Disruption of operation wound NOS
            Disruption or dehiscence of closure of:
                cornea
                mucosa
                skin
                subcutaneous tissue
            Full-thickness skin disruption or dehiscence
            Superficial disruption or dehiscence of operation wound

            AHA: ▶1Q, '14, 5;◀ 1Q, '06, 8; 1Q, '05, 11; 4Q, '03, 104, 106
            T81.31xA Disruption ext operation wound NEC initial enc   I-10

     998.33 Disruption of traumatic injury wound repair
            Disruption or dehiscence of closure of traumatic laceration (external) (internal)
            AHA: 4Q, '08, 151, 152

998.4 Foreign body accidentally left during a procedure

     Adhesions   ⎫ due to foreign body accidentally left in
     Obstruction   ⎬ operative wound or body cavity
     Perforation   ⎭ during a procedure

     EXCLUDES   *obstruction or perforation caused by implanted device intentionally left in body (996.0-996.5)*

     AHA: ▶1Q, '14, 14;◀ 1Q, '12, 12; 1Q, '11, 5-6; 1Q, '09,18; 1Q, '89, 9
     TIP: Report for an unintended retention of a foreign object following any type of procedure, in any type of setting..

☑5ᵗʰ **998.5 Postoperative infection**

     EXCLUDES   *bleb associated endophthalmitis (379.63)*
                     infection due to:
                     implanted device (996.60-996.69)
                     infusion, perfusion, or transfusion (999.31-999.39)
                     postoperative obstetrical wound infection (674.3)

     998.51 Infected postoperative seroma
            Use additional code to identify organism
            AHA: 4Q, '96, 46

     998.59 Other postoperative infection
            Abscess:
                intra-abdominal ⎫
                stitch   ⎬ postoperative
                subphrenic   ⎪
                wound   ⎭
            Septicemia
            Use additional code to identify infection
            AHA: 4Q, '11, 153; 2Q, '06, 23; 4Q, '04, 76; 4Q, '03, 104, 106-107; 3Q, '98, 3; 3Q, '95, 5; 2Q, '95, 7; 3Q, '94, 6; 1Q, '93, 19; J-F, '87, 14
            TIP: Do not assign if the infection is related to an internal prosthetic device, implant, or graft; see instead subcategory 996.6.
            T81.4xxA Infection following procedure initl encounter   I-10

998.6 Persistent postoperative fistula
     AHA: J-F, '87, 14
     T81.83XA Persistent postprocedural fistula, init encntr   I-10

998.7 Acute reaction to foreign substance accidentally left during a procedure
     Peritonitis:
       aseptic
       chemical

☑4ᵗʰ / ☑5ᵗʰ Additional Digit Required   **Unspecified Code**   Other Specified Code   Manifestation Code   ▶◀ Revised Text   ● New Code   ▲ Revised Code Title

Injury and Poisoning

998.8–999.39

√5ᵗʰ **998.8 Other specified complications of procedures, not elsewhere classified**
  AHA: 4Q, '94, 46; 1Q, '89, 9

  998.81 Emphysema (subcutaneous) (surgical) resulting from a procedure

  998.82 Cataract fragments in eye following cataract surgery

  998.83 Non-healing surgical wound
    AHA: 4Q, '96, 47

  998.89 Other specified complications
    AHA: ▶4Q, '13, 90;◀ 2Q, '12, 8; 2Q, '09, 11; 3Q, '06, 9;
    3Q, '05, 16; 3Q, '99, 13; 2Q, '98, 16
    TIP: Assign for cases in which a procedure is performed on the wrong body site (e.g., right leg versus left leg), along with E876.5-E876.7.
    T81.89xA Other complications of procedures NEC, init enc   I-10

998.9 Unspecified complication of procedure, not elsewhere classified
  Postoperative complication NOS
    EXCLUDES complication NOS of obstetrical, surgery or procedure (669.4)
  AHA: 4Q, '93, 37

√4ᵗʰ **999 Complications of medical care, not elsewhere classified**
  INCLUDES complications, not elsewhere classified, of:
    dialysis (hemodialysis) (peritoneal) (renal)
    extracorporeal circulation
    hyperalimentation therapy
    immunization
    infusion
    inhalation therapy
    injection
    inoculation
    perfusion
    transfusion
    vaccination
    ventilation therapy

  Use additional code, where applicable, to identify specific complication
    EXCLUDES specified complications classified elsewhere such as:
      complications of implanted device (996.0-996.9)
      contact dermatitis due to drugs (692.3)
      dementia dialysis (294.8)
      transient (293.9)
      dialysis disequilibrium syndrome (276.0-276.9)
      poisoning and toxic effects of drugs and chemicals (960.0-989.9)
      postvaccinal encephalitis (323.51)
      water and electrolyte imbalance (276.0-276.9)

  999.0 Generalized vaccinia
    EXCLUDES vaccinia not from vaccine (051.02)
    DEF: Skin eruption, self-limiting; follows vaccination; due to transient viremia with virus localized in skin.

  999.1 Air embolism
    Air embolism to any site following infusion, perfusion, or transfusion
    EXCLUDES embolism specified as:
      complicating:
        abortion (634-638 with .6, 639.6)
        ectopic or molar pregnancy (639.6)
        pregnancy, childbirth, or the puerperium (673.0)
      due to implanted device (996.7)
      traumatic (958.0)

999.2 Other vascular complications
  Phlebitis ⎫
  Thromboembolism ⎬ following infusion, perfusion, or transfusion
  Thrombophlebitis ⎭
    EXCLUDES extravasation of vesicant drugs (999.81, 999.82)
      the listed conditions when specified as:
        due to implanted device (996.61-996.62.
          996.72-996.74)
        postoperative NOS (997.2, 997.71-997.79)
  AHA: 2Q, '97, 5
  TIP: Do not assign for IV infiltration; if the infiltration is severe enough to cause other complications, a code for the specific complication should be assigned. For chemotherapy extravasation, see code 999.81.
  T80.1xxA Vasc comp follw inf transfusn tx inj initial enc   I-10

√5ᵗʰ **999.3 Other infection**
  Infection ⎫
  Sepsis ⎬ following infusion, injection, transfusion, or vaccination
  Septicemia ⎭
  Use additional code to identify the specified infection, such as:
    septicemia (038.0-038.9)
    EXCLUDES the listed conditions when specified as:
      due to implanted device (996.60-996.69)
      postoperative NOS (998.51-998.59)
  AHA: 4Q, '07, 96; 2Q, '01, 11, 12; 2Q, '97, 5; J-F, '87, 14

  999.31 Other and unspecified infection due to central venous catheter
    Central line-associated infection
    Infection due to:
      central venous catheter NOS
      Hickman catheter
      peripherally inserted central catheter (PICC)
      triple lumen catheter
      umbilical venous catheter
    EXCLUDES infection due to:
      arterial catheter (996.62)
      catheter NOS (996.69)
      peripheral venous catheter (996.62)
      urinary catheter (996.64)
    AHA: ▶1Q, '14, 18;◀ 2Q, '12, 16; 2Q, '11, 7; 4Q, '08, 72, 193;
    4Q, '07, 97

  999.32 Bloodstream infection due to central venous catheter
    Bloodstream infection due to:
      Hickman catheter
      peripherally inserted central catheter (PICC)
      portacath (port-a-cath)
      triple lumen catheter
      umbilical venous catheter
    Catheter-related bloodstream infection (CRBSI) NOS
    Central line-associated bloodstream infection (CLABSI)
    AHA: ▶1Q, '14, 18;◀ 4Q, '11, 153-155

  999.33 Local infection due to central venous catheter
    Exit or insertion site infection
    Local infection due to:
      Hickman catheter
      peripherally inserted central catheter (PICC)
      portacath (port-a-cath)
      triple lumen catheter
      umbilical venous catheter
    Port or reservoir infection
    Tunnel infection
    AHA: 4Q, '11, 153-155

  999.34 Acute infection following transfusion, infusion, or injection of blood and blood products
    AHA: 4Q, '11, 153-155
    TIP: If the acute infection transmitted via transfusion, infusion, or injection is HIV, sequence code 042 first.

  999.39 Infection following other infusion, injection, transfusion, or vaccination
    AHA: 4Q, '08, 99

√5ᵗʰ **999.4 Anaphylactic reaction due to serum**
Allergic shock
Anaphylactic shock due to serum
Anaphylactoid reaction due to serum
Anaphylaxis

EXCLUDES *ABO incompatibility reaction due to transfusion of*
blood or blood products (999.60-999.69)
reaction:
allergic NOS (995.0)
anaphylactic:
NOS (995.0)
due to drugs and chemicals (995.0)
other serum (999.51-999.59)
shock:
allergic NOS (995.0)
anaphylactic:
NOS (995.0)
due to drugs and chemicals (995.0)

DEF: Life-threatening hypersensitivity to foreign serum; causes
respiratory distress, vascular collapse, and shock.
AHA: 4Q, '11, 142-147

999.41 Anaphylactic reaction due to administration of
blood and blood products
AHA: 4Q, '11, 146

999.42 Anaphylactic reaction due to vaccination

999.49 Anaphylactic reaction due to other serum

√5ᵗʰ **999.5 Other serum reaction**
Intoxication by serum
Protein sickness
Serum rash
Serum sickness
Urticaria due to serum

EXCLUDES *serum hepatitis (070.2-070.3)*
DEF: Serum sickness: Hypersensitivity to foreign serum; causes fever,
hives, swelling, and lymphadenopathy.
AHA: 4Q, '11, 142-146

999.51 Other serum reaction due to administration
of blood and blood products

999.52 Other serum reaction due to vaccination

999.59 Other serum reaction

√5ᵗʰ **999.6 ABO incompatibility reaction due to transfusion of blood or**
blood products

EXCLUDES *minor blood group antigens reactions (Duffy) (E)*
(K(ell)) (Kidd) (Lewis) (M) (N) (P) (S)
(999.75-999.79)

AHA: 4Q, '10, 99-102

999.60 ABO incompatibility reaction, unspecified
ABO incompatible blood transfusion NOS
Reaction to ABO incompatibility from transfusion
NOS

999.61 ABO incompatibility with hemolytic
transfusion reaction not specified as acute or
delayed
ABO incompatibility with hemolytic transfusion
reaction at unspecified time after transfusion
Hemolytic transfusion reaction (HTR) due to ABO
incompatibility

999.62 ABO incompatibility with acute hemolytic
transfusion reaction
ABO incompatibility with hemolytic transfusion
reaction less than 24 hours after transfusion
Acute hemolytic transfusion reaction (AHTR) due to
ABO incompatibility

999.63 ABO incompatibility with delayed hemolytic
transfusion reaction
ABO incompatibility with hemolytic transfusion
reaction 24 hours or more after transfusion
Delayed hemolytic transfusion reaction (DHTR) due to
ABO incompatibility

999.69 Other ABO incompatibility reaction
Delayed serologic transfusion reaction (DSTR) from
ABO incompatibility
Other ABO incompatible blood transfusion
Other reaction to ABO incompatibility from
transfusion

√5ᵗʰ **999.7 Rh and other non-ABO incompatibility reaction due to**
transfusion of blood or blood products
Elevation of Rh titer
AHA: 4Q, '10, 99-100,102-105

999.70 Rh incompatibility reaction, unspecified
Reaction due to Rh factor in transfusion NOS
Rh incompatible blood transfusion NOS
Unspecified reaction due to incompatibility related to
Rh antigens (C) (c) (D) (E) (e)
Unspecified reaction to Rh incompatibility

999.71 Rh incompatibility with hemolytic transfusion
reaction not specified as acute or delayed
Hemolytic transfusion reaction (HTR) due to Rh
incompatibility
HTR due to incompatibility related to Rh antigens (C)
(c) (D) (E) (e), not specified as acute or delayed
Rh incompatibility with hemolytic transfusion
reaction at unspecified time after transfusion

999.72 Rh incompatibility with acute hemolytic
transfusion reaction
Acute hemolytic transfusion reaction (AHTR) due to
Rh incompatibility
AHTR due to incompatibility related to Rh antigens
(C) (c) (D) (E) (e)
Rh incompatibility with hemolytic transfusion
reaction less than 24 hours after transfusion

999.73 Rh incompatibility with delayed hemolytic
transfusion reaction
Delayed hemolytic transfusion reaction (DHTR) due to
Rh incompatibility
DHTR due to incompatibility related to Rh antigens
(C) (c) (D) (E) (e)
Rh incompatibility with hemolytic transfusion
reaction 24 hours or more after transfusion

999.74 Other Rh incompatibility reaction
Delayed serologic transfusion reaction (DSTR) from
Rh incompatibility
Other reaction due to incompatibility related to Rh
antigens (C) (c) (D) (E) (e)
Other reaction to Rh incompatible blood transfusion

999.75 Non-ABO incompatibility reaction, unspecified
Non-ABO incompatible blood transfusion NOS
Reaction to non-ABO antigen incompatibility from
transfusion NOS
Unspecified reaction due to incompatibility related to
minor antigens (Duffy) (Kell) (Kidd) (Lewis) (M)
(N) (P) (S)

999.76 Non-ABO incompatibility with hemolytic
transfusion reaction not specified as acute or
delayed
Hemolytic transfusion reaction (HTR) due to non-ABO
incompatibility
HTR from incompatibility related to minor antigens
(Duffy) (Kell) (Kidd) (Lewis) (M) (N) (P) (S)
Non-ABO incompatibility with hemolytic transfusion
reaction at unspecified time after transfusion

999.77 Non-ABO incompatibility with acute hemolytic
transfusion reaction
Acute hemolytic transfusion reaction (AHTR) due to
non-ABO incompatibility
AHTR from incompatibility related to minor antigens
(Duffy) (Kell) (Kidd) (Lewis) (M) (N) (P) (S)
Non-ABO incompatibility with hemolytic transfusion
reaction less than 24 hours after transfusion

999.78 Non-ABO incompatibility with delayed
hemolytic transfusion reaction
Delayed hemolytic transfusion reaction (DHTR) due to
non-ABO incompatibility
DHTR from incompatibility related to minor antigens
(Duffy) (Kell) (Kidd) (Lewis) (M) (N) (P) (S)
Non-ABO incompatibility with hemolytic transfusion
reaction 24 hours or more after transfusion

Injury and Poisoning

999.4–999.78

√4ᵗʰ √5ᵗʰ Additional Digit Required   **Unspecified Code**   **Other Specified Code**   **Manifestation Code**   ▶◀ Revised Text   ● New Code   ▲ Revised Code Title

2015 ICD-9-CM   **Volume 1 – 317**

Injury and Poisoning

999.79–999.9

999.79 Other non-ABO incompatibility reaction
Delayed serologic transfusion reaction (DSTR) from non-ABO incompatibility
Other non-ABO incompatible blood transfusion
Other reaction due to incompatibility related to minor antigens (Duffy) (Kell) (Kidd) (Lewis) (M) (N) (P) (S)
Other reaction to non-ABO incompatibility from transfusion

√5ᵗʰ **999.8 Other and unspecified infusion and transfusion reaction**
EXCLUDES   *ABO incompatibility reactions (999.60-999.69)*
febrile nonhemolytic transfusion reaction (FNHTR) (780.66)
hemochromatosis due to repeated red blood cell transfusions (275.02)
non-ABO incompatibility reactions (999.70-999.79)
postoperative shock (998.00-998.09)
posttransfusion purpura (287.41)
Rh incompatibility reactions (999.70-999.74)
transfusion associated circulatory overload (TACO) (276.61)
transfusion related acute lung injury [TRALI] (518.7)
AHA: 4Q, '08, 152-155; 3Q, '00, 9

999.80 Transfusion reaction, unspecified
Incompatible blood transfusion NOS
Reaction to blood group incompatibility in infusion or transfusion NOS
AHA: 4Q, '10, 99-100, 106-107

999.81 Extravasation of vesicant chemotherapy
Infiltration of vesicant chemotherapy
AHA: 4Q, '08, 155

999.82 Extravasation of other vesicant agent
Infiltration of other vesicant agent

999.83 Hemolytic transfusion reaction, incompatibility unspecified
Hemolytic transfusion reaction (HTR) with antigen incompatibility unspecified, not specified as acute or delayed
HTR with incompatibility unspecified at unspecified time after transfusion
AHA: 4Q, '10, 99-100, 106-107

999.84 Acute hemolytic transfusion reaction, incompatibility unspecified
Acute hemolytic transfusion reaction (AHTR) with antigen incompatibility unspecified
AHTR, incompatibility unspecified
AHA: 4Q, '10, 99-100, 106-107

999.85 Delayed hemolytic transfusion reaction, incompatibility unspecified
Delayed hemolytic transfusion reaction (DHTR) with antigen incompatibility unspecified
DHTR, incompatibility unspecified
AHA: 4Q, '10, 99-100, 106-107

999.88 Other infusion reaction

999.89 Other transfusion reaction
Delayed serologic transfusion reaction (DSTR), incompatibility unspecified
Use additional code to identify graft-versus-host reaction (279.5)
AHA: 4Q, '08, 99, 154

999.9 Other and unspecified complications of medical care, not elsewhere classified
Complications, not elsewhere classified, of:
electroshock
inhalation
ultrasound   } therapy
ventilation
Unspecified misadventure of medical care
EXCLUDES   *unspecified complication of:*
phototherapy (990)
radiation therapy (999)
ventilator associated pneumonia (997.31)
AHA: 3Q, '06, 25; 1Q, '03, 19; 2Q, '97, 5

N   Newborn Age: 0   P   Pediatric Age: 0-17   M   Maternity Age: 12-55   A   Adult Age: 15-124

Supplementary Classification of Factors Influencing Health Status and Contact with Health Services (V01-V91)

This classification is provided to deal with occasions when circumstances other than a disease or injury classifiable to categories 001-999 (the main part of ICD) are recorded as "diagnoses" or "problems." This can arise mainly in three ways:

a) When a person who is not currently sick encounters the health services for some specific purpose, such as to act as a donor of an organ or tissue, to receive prophylactic vaccination, or to discuss a problem which is in itself not a disease or injury. This will be a fairly rare occurrence among hospital inpatients, but will be relatively more common among hospital outpatients and patients of family practitioners, health clinics, etc.

b) When a person with a known disease or injury, whether it is current or resolving, encounters the health care system for a specific treatment of that disease or injury (e.g., dialysis for renal disease; chemotherapy for malignancy; cast change).

c) When some circumstance or problem is present which influences the person's health status but is not in itself a current illness or injury. Such factors may be elicited during population surveys, when the person may or may not be currently sick, or be recorded as an additional factor to be borne in mind when the person is receiving care for some current illness or injury classifiable to categories 001-999.

In the latter circumstances the V code should be used only as a supplementary code and should not be the one selected for use in primary, single cause tabulations. Examples of these circumstances are a personal history of certain diseases, or a person with an artificial heart valve in situ.

> **AHA:** J-F, '87, 8

Persons with Potential Health Hazards Related to Communicable Diseases (V01-V06)

> **EXCLUDES** *family history of infectious and parasitic diseases (V18.8)*
> *personal history of infectious and parasitic diseases (V12.0)*

√4ᵗʰ **V01 Contact with or exposure to communicable diseases**
> **TIP:** Do not assign if the patient shows signs or symptoms of the disease to which he or she was exposed.

V01.0 Cholera
Conditions classifiable to 001

V01.1 Tuberculosis
Conditions classifiable to 010-018

V01.2 Poliomyelitis
Conditions classifiable to 045

V01.3 Smallpox
Conditions classifiable to 050

V01.4 Rubella
Conditions classifiable to 056

V01.5 Rabies
Conditions classifiable to 071

V01.6 Venereal diseases
Conditions classifiable to 090-099
> **AHA:** 4Q, '07, 125

√5ᵗʰ **V01.7 Other viral diseases**
Conditions classifiable to 042-078 and V08, except as above
> **AHA:** 2Q, '92, 11

V01.71 Varicella

V01.79 Other viral diseases

√5ᵗʰ **V01.8 Other communicable diseases**
Conditions classifiable to 001-136, except as above
> **AHA:** J-A, '87, 24

V01.81 Anthrax
> **AHA:** 4Q, '02, 70, 78

V01.82 Exposure to SARS-associated coronavirus
> **AHA:** 4Q, '03, 46-47

V01.83 Escherichia coli (E. coli)

V01.84 Meningococcus
> **Z20.811** Contact with and exposure to meningococcus   I-10

V01.89 Other communicable diseases

V01.9 Unspecified communicable diseases

√4ᵗʰ **V02 Carrier or suspected carrier of infectious diseases**
> **INCLUDES** colonization status
> **AHA:** 3Q, '95, 18; 3Q, '94, 4

V02.0 Cholera

V02.1 Typhoid

V02.2 Amebiasis

V02.3 Other gastrointestinal pathogens

V02.4 Diphtheria

√5ᵗʰ **V02.5 Other specified bacterial diseases**

V02.51 Group B streptococcus
> **AHA:** 3Q, '06, 14; 1Q, '02, 14; 4Q, '98, 56

V02.52 Other streptococcus

V02.53 Methicillin susceptible Staphylococcus aureus
MSSA colonization
> **AHA:** 4Q, '08, 69, 71, 156

V02.54 Methicillin resistant Staphylococcus aureus
MRSA colonization
> **AHA:** 4Q, '08, 69, 71, 72, 156

V02.59 Other specified bacterial diseases
Meningococcal
Staphylococcal

√5ᵗʰ **V02.6 Viral hepatitis**
Hepatitis Australian-antigen [HAA] [SH] carrier
Serum hepatitis carrier

V02.60 Viral hepatitis carrier, unspecified
> **AHA:** 4Q, '97, 47

V02.61 Hepatitis B carrier
> **AHA:** 4Q, '97, 47
> **Z22.51** Carrier of viral hepatitis B   I-10

V02.62 Hepatitis C carrier
> **AHA:** 4Q, '97, 47

V02.69 Other viral hepatitis carrier
> **AHA:** 4Q, '97, 47

V02.7 Gonorrhea

V02.8 Other venereal diseases

V02.9 Other specified infectious organism
> **AHA:** 3Q, '95, 18; 1Q, '93, 22; J-A, '87, 24

√4ᵗʰ **V03 Need for prophylactic vaccination and inoculation against bacterial diseases**
> **EXCLUDES** *vaccination not carried out (V64.00-V64.09)*
> *vaccines against combinations of diseases (V06.0-V06.9)*

V03.0 Cholera alone

V03.1 Typhoid-paratyphoid alone [TAB]

V03.2 Tuberculosis [BCG]

V03.3 Plague

V03.4 Tularemia

V03.5 Diphtheria alone

V03.6 Pertussis alone

V03.7 Tetanus toxoid alone

√5ᵗʰ **V03.8 Other specified vaccinations against single bacterial diseases**

V03.81 Hemophilus influenza, type B [Hib]

V03.82 Streptococcus pneumoniae [pneumococcus]

V03.89 Other specified vaccination
> **AHA:** 2Q, '00, 9
> **TIP:** Assign for vaccination against Lyme disease.

V03.9 Unspecified single bacterial disease

√4ᵗʰ **V04 Need for prophylactic vaccination and inoculation against certain viral diseases**
> **EXCLUDES** *vaccines against combinations of diseases (V06.0-V06.9)*

V04.0 Poliomyelitis

V04.1 Smallpox

√4ᵗʰ √5ᵗʰ Additional Digit Required   Unspecified Code   Other Specified Code   Manifestation Code   ►◄ Revised Text   ● New Code   ▲ Revised Code Title

V04.2 Measles alone

V04.3 Rubella alone

V04.4 Yellow fever

V04.5 Rabies

V04.6 Mumps alone

V04.7 Common cold

✓5ᵗʰ **V04.8 Other viral diseases**
AHA: 4Q, '03, 83

V04.81 Influenza

V04.82 Respiratory syncytial virus (RSV)
AHA: 1Q, '09, 14

V04.89 Other viral diseases
AHA: 2Q, '07, 9
TIP: Assign for vaccination against human papilloma virus (HPV).

✓4ᵗʰ **V05 Need for other prophylactic vaccination and inoculation against single diseases**
EXCLUDES vaccines against combinations of diseases (V06.0-V06.9)

V05.0 Athropod-borne viral encephalitis

V05.1 Other arthropod-borne viral diseases

V05.2 Leshmaniasis

V05.3 Viral hepatitis

V05.4 Varicella
Chickenpox

V05.8 Other specified disease
AHA: 1Q, '01, 4; 3Q, '91, 20

V05.9 Unspecified single disease

✓4ᵗʰ **V06 Need for prophylactic vaccination and inoculation against combinations of diseases**
NOTE Use additional single vaccination codes from categories V03-V05 to identify any vaccinations not included in a combination code.

V06.0 Cholera with typhoid-paratyphoid [cholera+TAB]

V06.1 Diphtheia-tetanus-pertussis, combined [DTP] [DTaP]
AHA: 4Q, '03, 83; 3Q, '98, 13

V06.2 Diphtheria-tetanus-pertussis with typhoid-paratyphoid [DTP+TAB]

V06.3 Diphtheria-tetanus-pertussis with poliomyelitis [DTP+polio]

V06.4 Measles-mumps-rubella [MMR]

V06.5 Tetanus-diphtheria [Td] [DT]
AHA: 4Q, '03, 83

V06.6 Streptococcus pneumoniae [pneumococcus] and influenza

V06.8 Other combinations
EXCLUDES multiple single vaccination codes (V03.0-V05.9)
AHA: 1Q, '12, 11; 1Q, '94, 19

V06.9 Unspecified combined vaccine

Persons with Need for Isolation, Other Potential Health Hazards and Prophylactic Measures (V07-V09)

✓4ᵗʰ **V07 Need for isolation and other prophylactic or treatment measures**
EXCLUDES long-term (current) (prophylactic) use of certain specific drugs (V58.61-V58.69)
prophylactic organ removal (V50.41-V50.49)

V07.0 Isolation
Admission to protect the individual from his surroundings or for isolation of individual after contact with infectious diseases

V07.1 Desensitization to allergens

V07.2 Prophylactic immunotherapy
Administration of:
antivenin
immune sera [gamma globulin]
RhoGAM
tetanus antitoxin

✓5ᵗʰ **V07.3 Other prophylactic chemotherapy**

V07.31 Prophylactic fluoride administration

V07.39 Other prophylactic chemotherapy
EXCLUDES maintenance chemotherapy following disease (V58.11)

V07.4 Hormone replacement therapy (postmenopausal) ♀
Z79.890 Hormone replacement therapy postmenopausal   I-10

✓5ᵗʰ **V07.5 Use of agents affecting estrogen receptors and estrogen levels**
Code first, if applicable:
malignant neoplasm of breast (174.0-174.9, 175.0-175.9)
malignant neoplasm of prostate (185)
Use additional code, if applicable, to identify:
estrogen receptor positive status (V86.0)
family history of breast cancer (V16.3)
genetic susceptibility to cancer (V84.01-V84.09)
personal history of breast cancer (V10.3)
personal history of prostate cancer (V10.46)
postmenopausal status (V49.81)
EXCLUDES hormone replacement therapy (postmenopausal) (V07.4)
AHA: 4Q, '10, 108; 4Q, '08, 156

V07.51 Use of selective estrogen receptor modulators [SERMs]
Use of:
raloxifene (Evista)
tamoxifen (Nolvadex)
toremifene (Fareston)
Z79.810 Lng term sel estrogen receptor modulators SERMS   I-10

V07.52 Use of aromatase inhibitors
Use of:
anastrozole (Arimidex)
exemestane (Aromasin)
letrozole (Femara)

V07.59 Use of other agents affecting estrogen receptors and estrogen levels
Use of:
estrogen receptor downregulators
fulvestrant (Faslodex)
gonadotropin-releasing hormone (GnRH) agonist
goserelin acetate (Zoladex)
leuprolide acetate (leuprorelin) (Lupron)
megestrol acetate (Megace)

V07.8 Other specified prophylactic or treatment measure
AHA: ▶1Q, '13, 8;◄ 2Q, '10, 6, 14; 1Q, '92, 11
TIP: Assign for patients having prophylactic breast removal because of a strong family history of breast cancer, along with code V16.3 Family history of breast cancer.

V07.9 Unspecified prophylactic or treatment measure

V08 Asymptomatic human immunodeficiency virus [HIV] infection status
HIV positive NOS
NOTE This code is only to be used when no HIV infection symptoms or conditions are present. If any HIV infection symptoms or conditions are present, see code 042.
EXCLUDES AIDS (042)
human immunodeficiency virus [HIV] disease (042)
exposure to HIV (V01.79)
nonspecific serologic evidence of HIV (795.71)
symptomatic human immunodeficiency virus [HIV] infection (042)
AHA: 2Q, '04, 11; 2Q, '99, 8; 3Q, '95, 18
Z21 Asymptomatic HIV infection status   I-10

✓4th V09 Infection with drug-resistant microorganisms

> NOTE This category is intended for use as an additional code for infectious conditions classified elsewhere to indicate the presence of drug-resistance of the infectious organism.
>
> AHA: 3Q, '94, 4; 4Q, '93, 22

V09.0 Infection with microorganisms resistant to penicillins

> AHA: 2Q, '06, 16; 4Q, '03, 104, 106

V09.1 Infection with microorganisms resistant to cephalosporins and other B-lactam antibiotics

V09.2 Infection with microorganisms resistant to macrolides

V09.3 Infection with microorganisms resistant to tetracyclines

V09.4 Infection with microorganisms resistant to aminoglycosides

✓5th V09.5 Infection with microorganisms resistant to quinolones and fluoroquinolones

> **V09.50 Without mention of resistance to multiple quinolones and fluoroquinoles**
>
> **V09.51 With resistance to multiple quinolones and fluoroquinoles**

V09.6 Infection with microorganisms resistant to sulfonamides

✓5th V09.7 Infection with microorganisms resistant to other specified antimycobacterial agents

> EXCLUDES Amikacin (V09.4)
> Kanamycin (V09.4)
> Streptomycin [SM] (V09.4)
>
> **V09.70 Without mention of resistance to multiple antimycobacterial agents**
>
> **V09.71 With resistance to multiple antimycobacterial agents**

✓5th V09.8 Infection with microorganisms resistant to other specified drugs

> Vancomycin (glycopeptide) intermediate staphylococcus aureus (VISA/GISA)
> Vancomycin (glycopeptide) resistant enterococcus (VRE)
> Vancomycin (glycopeptide) resistant staphylococcus aureus (VRSA/GRSA)
>
> **V09.80 Without mention of resistance to multiple drugs**
>
> **V09.81 With resistance to multiple drugs**

✓5th V09.9 Infection with drug-resistant microorganisms, unspecified

> Drug resistance, NOS
>
> **V09.90 Without mention of multiple drug resistance**
>
> > Z16.30 Resist to unspec antimicrobial drugs **I-10**
>
> **V09.91 With multiple drug resistance**
>
> > Multiple drug resistance NOS

Persons with Potential Health Hazards Related to Personal and Family History (V10-V19)

> EXCLUDES obstetric patients where the possibility that the fetus might be affected is the reason for observation or management during pregnancy (655.0-655.9)
>
> AHA: J-F, '87, 1

✓4th V10 Personal history of malignant neoplasm

> AHA: 4Q, '02, 80; 4Q, '98, 69; 1Q, '95, 4; 3Q, '92, 5; M-J, '85, 10; 2Q, '90, 9
> TIP: Assign the codes in this category only for a personal history of primary malignancy (not metastatic malignancies).

✓5th V10.0 Gastrointestinal tract

> History of conditions classifiable to 140-159
>
> EXCLUDES personal history of malignant carcinoid tumor (V10.91)
> personal history of malignant neuroendocrine tumor (V10.91)
>
> **V10.00 Gastrointestinal tract, unspecified**
>
> **V10.01 Tongue**
>
> **V10.02 Other and unspecified oral cavity and pharynx**
>
> **V10.03 Esophagus**
>
> **V10.04 Stomach**

V10.05 Large intestine

> AHA: 3Q, '99, 7; 1Q, '95, 4
> Z85.038 Personal hx othr malig neoplasm large intestine **I-10**

V10.06 Rectum, rectosigmoid junction, and anus

V10.07 Liver

V10.09 Other

> AHA: 4Q, '03, 111

✓5th V10.1 Trachea, bronchus, and lung

> History of conditions classifiable to 162
>
> EXCLUDES personal history of malignant carcinoid tumor (V10.91)
> personal history of malignant neuroendocrine tumor (V10.91)
>
> **V10.11 Bronchus and lung**
>
> > AHA: ▶1Q, '13, 8◀
>
> **V10.12 Trachea**

✓5th V10.2 Other respiratory and intrathoracic organs

> History of conditions classifiable to 160, 161, 163-165
>
> **V10.20 Respiratory organ, unspecified**
>
> **V10.21 Larynx**
>
> > AHA: 4Q, '03, 108, 110
>
> **V10.22 Nasal cavities, middle ear, and accessory sinuses**
>
> **V10.29 Other**

V10.3 Breast

> History of conditions classifiable to 174 and 175
> AHA: 1Q, '12, 11; 2Q, '11, 12; 3Q, '07, 4; 1Q, '07, 6; 2Q, '03, 5; 4Q, '01, 66; 4Q, '98, 65; 4Q, '97, 50; 1Q, '91, 16; 1Q, '90, 21
> TIP: Do not assign for personal history of ductal carcinoma in situ (DCIS); assign code V13.89.
> Z85.3 Personal history primary malig neoplasm breast **I-10**

✓5th V10.4 Genital organs

> History of conditions classifiable to 179-187
>
> **V10.40 Female genital organ, unspecfied** ♀
>
> **V10.41 Cervix uteri** ♀
>
> > AHA: 4Q, '07, 99
>
> **V10.42 Other parts of uterus** ♀
>
> **V10.43 Ovary** ♀
>
> **V10.44 Other female genital organs** ♀
>
> **V10.45 Male genital organ, unspecfied** ♂
>
> **V10.46 Prostate** ♂
>
> > AHA: 1Q, '09, 15
>
> **V10.47 Testis** ♂
>
> > Z85.47 Personal history primary malig neoplasm testis **I-10**
>
> **V10.48 Epididymis** ♂
>
> **V10.49 Other male genital organs** ♂

✓5th V10.5 Urinary organs

> History of conditions classifiable to 188 and 189
>
> EXCLUDES personal history of malignant carcinoid tumor (V10.91)
> personal history of malignant neuroendocrine tumor (V10.91)
>
> **V10.50 Urinary organ, unspecified**
>
> **V10.51 Bladder**
>
> **V10.52 Kidney**
>
> > EXCLUDES renal pelvis (V10.53)
> > AHA: 2Q, '04, 4
>
> **V10.53 Renal pelvis**
>
> > AHA: 4Q, '01, 55
>
> **V10.59 Other**

✓5th V10.6 Leukemia

> Conditions classifiable to 204-208
>
> EXCLUDES leukemia in remission (204-208)
> AHA: 2Q, '92, 13; 4Q, '91, 26; 4Q, '90, 3
>
> **V10.60 Leukemia, unspecified**

| ✓4th ✓5th Additional Digit Required | Unspecified Code | Other Specified Code | Manifestation Code | ▶◀ Revised Text | ● New Code | ▲ Revised Code Title |

V10.61 Lymphoid leukemia

V10.62 Myeloid leukemia

V10.63 Monocytic leukemia

V10.69 Other

√5th **V10.7 Other lymphatic and hematopoietic neoplasms**
Conditions classifiable to 200-203
EXCLUDES listed conditions in 200-203 in remission
AHA: M-J, '85, 18

V10.71 Lymphosarcoma and reticulosarcoma

V10.72 Hodgkin's disease

V10.79 Other

√5th **V10.8 Personal history of malignant neoplasm of other sites**
History of conditions classifiable to 170-173, 190-195
EXCLUDES personal history of malignant carcinoid tumor (V10.91)
personal history of malignant neuroendocrine tumor (V10.91)

V10.81 Bone
AHA: 2Q, '03, 13

V10.82 Malignant melanoma of skin

V10.83 Other malignant neoplasm of skin

V10.84 Eye

V10.85 Brain
AHA: 1Q, '01, 6

V10.86 Other parts of the nervous system
EXCLUDES peripheral sympathetic, and parasympathetic nerves (V10.89)

V10.87 Thyroid

V10.88 Other endocrine glands and related structures

V10.89 Other

√5th **V10.9 Other and unspecified personal history of malignant neoplasm**
AHA: 4Q, '09, 115

V10.90 Personal history of unspecified malignant neoplasm
Personal history of malignant neoplasm NOS
EXCLUDES personal history of malignant carcinoid tumor (V10.91)
personal history of malignant neuroendocrine tumor (V10.91)
personal history of Merkel cell carcinoma (V10.91)

V10.91 Personal history of malignant neuroendocrine tumor
Personal history of malignant carcinoid tumor NOS
Personal history of malignant neuroendocrine tumor NOS
Personal history of Merkel cell carcinoma NOS
Code first any continuing functional activity, such as: carcinoid syndrome (259.2)

√4th **V11 Personal history of mental disorder**

V11.0 Schizophrenia
EXCLUDES that in remission (295.0-295.9 with fifth-digit 5)

V11.1 Affective disorders
Personal history of manic-depressive psychosis
EXCLUDES that in remission (296.0-296.6 with fifth-digit 5, 6)

V11.2 Neurosis

V11.3 Alcoholism

V11.4 Combat and operational stress reaction **A**
AHA: 4Q, '10, 108

V11.8 Other mental disorders

V11.9 Unspecified mental disorder

√4th **V12 Personal history of certain other diseases**
AHA: 3Q, '92, 11

√5th **V12.0 Infectious and parasitic diseases**
EXCLUDES personal history of infectious diseases specific to a body system

V12.00 Unspecified infectious and parasitic disease

V12.01 Tuberculosis

V12.02 Poliomyelitis
Z86.12 Personal history of poliomyelitis   I-10

V12.03 Malaria

V12.04 Methicillin resistant Staphylococcus aureus
MRSA
AHA: 4Q, '08, 69, 71

V12.09 Other

V12.1 Nutritional deficiency

√5th **V12.2 Endocrine, metabolic, and immunity disorders**
AHA: 4Q, '11, 156

V12.21 Gestational diabetes ♀

V12.29 Other endocrine, metabolic, and immunity disorders

V12.3 Diseases of blood and blood-forming organs

√5th **V12.4 Disorders of nervous system and sense organs**

V12.40 Unspecified disorder of nervous system and sense organs

V12.41 Benign neoplasm of the brain
AHA: 4Q, '97, 48
TIP: Benign neoplasms of the brain are tracked separately because, besides being potentially life-threatening, they often recur and can be difficult to treat.

V12.42 Infections of the central nervous system
Encephalitis   Meningitis
AHA: 4Q, '05, 95

V12.49 Other disorders of nervous system and sense organs
AHA: 4Q, '98, 59

√5th **V12.5 Diseases of circulatory system**
EXCLUDES history of anaphylactic shock (V13.81)
old myocardial infarction (412)
postmyocardial infarction syndrome (411.0)
AHA: 4Q, '95, 61

V12.50 Unspecified circulatory disease

V12.51 Venous thrombosis and embolism
EXCLUDES pulmonary embolism (V12.55)
AHA: 1Q, '11, 20; 3Q, '06, 12; 4Q, '03, 108; 1Q, '02, 15

V12.52 Thrombophlebitis

V12.53 Sudden cardiac arrest
Sudden cardiac death successfully resuscitated
AHA: 4Q, '07, 98

V12.54 Transient ischemic attack [TIA], and cerebral infarction without residual deficits
Prolonged reversible ischemic neurological deficit [PRIND]
Reversible ischemic neurologic deficit [RIND]
Stroke NOS without residual deficits
EXCLUDES history of traumatic brain injury (V15.52)
late effects of cerebrovascular disease (438.0-438.9)
AHA: 4Q, '07, 98
TIP: Assign for old CVA for which the patient has no residual deficits; if deficits are present, see category 438.
Z86.73 Personal hx TIA & cerebral infarct w/o deficits   I-10

V12.55 Pulmonary embolism
AHA: ►4Q, '13, 83;◄ 4Q, '11, 156

V12.59 Other
AHA: ►4Q, '13, 101;◄ 2Q, '07, 3; 4Q, '99, 4; 4Q, '98, 88; 4Q, '97, 37

N Newborn Age: 0   **P** Pediatric Age: 0-17   **M** Maternity Age: 12-55   **A** Adult Age: 15-124   **PDx** Primary Diagnosis

322 – Volume 1 • October 2014   2015 ICD-9-CM

√5th **V12.6 Diseases of respiratory system**
> **EXCLUDES** *tuberculosis (V12.01)*

V12.60 Unspecified disease of respiratory system

V12.61 Pneumonia (recurrent)
> AHA: 4Q, '05, 95

V12.69 Other diseases of respiratory system

√5th **V12.7 Diseases of digestive system**
> AHA: 1Q, '95, 3; 2Q, '89, 16

V12.70 Unspecified digestive disease

V12.71 Peptic ulcer disease

V12.72 Colonic polyps
> AHA: ▶4Q, '13, 104, 105;◀ 3Q, '02, 15
> Z86.010 Personal history of colonic polyps   I-10

V12.79 Other

√4th **V13 Personal history of other diseases**

√5th **V13.0 Disorders of urinary system**

V13.00 Unspecified urinary disorder

V13.01 Urinary calculi

V13.02 Urinary (tract) infection
> AHA: 4Q, '05, 95

V13.03 Nephrotic syndrome
> AHA: 4Q, '05, 95

V13.09 Other

V13.1 Trophoblastic disease ♀
> **EXCLUDES** *supervision during a current pregnancy (V23.1)*

√5th **V13.2 Other genital system and obstetric disorders**
> **EXCLUDES** *recurrent pregnancy loss (646.3)*
> *without current pregnancy (629.81)*
> *supervision during a current pregnancy of a woman*
> *with poor obstetric history (V23.0-V23.9)*

V13.21 Personal history of pre-term labor ♀
> **EXCLUDES** *current pregnancy with history of pre-term*
> *labor (V23.41)*
> AHA: 4Q, '02, 78

V13.22 Personal history of cervical dysplasia ♀
> Personal history of conditions classifiable to
> 622.10-622.12
> **EXCLUDES** *personal history of malignant neoplasm of*
> *cervix uteri (V10.41)*
> AHA: 4Q, '07, 98

V13.23 Personal history of vaginal dysplasia ♀
> Personal history of conditions classifiable to 623.0
> **EXCLUDES** *personal history of malignant neoplasm of*
> *vagina (V10.44)*
> AHA: 4Q, '10, 108

V13.24 Personal history of vulvar dysplasia ♀
> Personal history of conditions classifiable to
> 624.01-624.02
> **EXCLUDES** *personal history of malignant neoplasm of*
> *vulva (V10.44)*
> AHA: 4Q, '10, 108

V13.29 Other genital system and obstetric disorders ♀

V13.3 Diseases of skin and subcutaneous tissue

V13.4 Arthritis

√5th **V13.5 Other musculoskeletal disorders**
> AHA: 4Q, '08, 158
> TIP: Personal histories of pathological, stress, or traumatic fractures
> are separately classified because a patient with such a history is at
> much higher risk of refracture of the same site.

V13.51 Pathologic fracture
> Healed pathologic fracture
> **EXCLUDES** *personal history of traumatic fracture*
> *(V15.51)*

V13.52 Stress fracture
> Healed stress fracture
> **EXCLUDES** *personal history of traumatic fracture*
> *(V15.51)*

V13.59 Other musculoskeletal disorders

√5th **V13.6 Congenital (corrected) malformations**
> AHA: 4Q, '10, 108, 136; 4Q, '98, 63

V13.61 Personal history of (corrected) hypospadias ♂

V13.62 Personal history of other (corrected) congenital malformations of genitourinary system

V13.63 Personal history of (corrected) congenital malformations of nervous system

V13.64 Personal history of (corrected) congenital malformations of eye, ear, face and neck
> Corrected cleft lip and palate

V13.65 Personal history of (corrected) congenital malformations of heart and circulatory system

V13.66 Personal history of (corrected) congenital malformations of respiratory system

V13.67 Personal history of (corrected) congenital malformations of digestive system

V13.68 Personal history of (corrected) congenital malformations of integument, limbs, and musculoskeletal systems

V13.69 Personal history of other (corrected) congenital malformations
> AHA: 4Q, '10, 108; 1Q, '04, 16

V13.7 Perinatal problems
> **EXCLUDES** *low birth weight status (V21.30-V21.35)*

√5th **V13.8 Other specified diseases**
> AHA: 4Q, '11, 156

V13.81 Anaphylaxis

V13.89 Other specified diseases
> AHA: 1Q, '12, 11

V13.9 Unspecified disease
> AHA: 4Q, '06, 117

√4th **V14 Personal history of allergy to medicinal agents**

V14.0 Penicillin
> Z88.0 Allergy status to penicillin   I-10

V14.1 Other antibiotic agent

V14.2 Sulfonamides

V14.3 Other anti-infective agent

V14.4 Anesthetic agent

V14.5 Narcotic agent

V14.6 Analgesic agent

V14.7 Serum or vaccine

V14.8 Other specified medicinal agents

V14.9 Unspecified medicinal agent

√4th **V15 Other personal history presenting hazards to health**
> **EXCLUDES** *personal history of drug therapy (V87.41-V87.49)*

√5th **V15.0 Allergy, other than to medicinal agents**
> **EXCLUDES** *allergy to food substance used as base for medicinal*
> *agent (V14.0-V14.9)*
> AHA: 4Q, '00, 42, 49
> TIP: A person who has had an allergic episode to a substance in the
> past should always be considered allergic to the substance.

V15.01 Allergy to peanuts
> Z91.010 Allergy to peanuts   I-10

V15.02 Allergy to milk products
> **EXCLUDES** *lactose intolerance (271.3)*
> AHA: 1Q, '03, 12

V15.03 Allergy to eggs

V15.04 Allergy to seafood
> Seafood (octopus) (squid) ink   Shellfish

V15.05 Allergy to other foods
> Food additives   Nuts other than peanuts

| √4th √5th Additional Digit Required | Unspecified Code | Other Specified Code | Manifestation Code | ▶◀ Revised Text | ● New Code | ▲ Revised Code Title |

2015 ICD-9-CM   **October 2014 • Volume 1 – 323**

V Codes

V15.06–V16.59

V15.06 Allergy to insects and arachnids
Bugs   Spiders
Insect bites and stings

V15.07 Allergy to latex
Latex sensitivity

V15.08 Allergy to radiographic dye
Contrast media used for diagnostic x-ray procedures

V15.09 Other allergy, other than to medicinal agents

V15.1 Surgery to heart and great vessels
EXCLUDES replacement by transplant or other means (V42.1-V42.2, V43.2-V43.4)
AHA: 1Q, '04, 16

√5ᵗʰ V15.2 Surgery to other organs
EXCLUDES replacement by transplant or other means (V42.0-V43.8)
AHA: 4Q, '08, 158

V15.21 Personal history of undergoing in utero procedure during pregnancy ♀
AHA: 4Q, '08, 158

V15.22 Personal history of undergoing in utero procedure while a fetus
AHA: 4Q, '08, 158

V15.29 Surgery to other organs

V15.3 Irradiation
Previous exposure to therapeutic or other ionizing radiation
AHA: 2Q, '11, 12;

√5ᵗʰ V15.4 Psychological trauma
EXCLUDES history of condition classifiable to 290-316 (V11.0-V11.9)

V15.41 History of physical abuse
Rape
AHA: 3Q, '99, 15

V15.42 History of emotional abuse
Neglect
AHA: 3Q, '99, 15

V15.49 Other
AHA: 3Q, '99, 15

√5ᵗʰ V15.5 Injury
AHA: 4Q, '08, 158

V15.51 Traumatic fracture
Healed traumatic fracture
EXCLUDES personal history of pathologic and stress fracture (V13.51, V13.52)
TIP: Personal histories of pathological, stress, or traumatic fractures are separately classified because a patient with such a history is at much higher risk of refracture of the same site.

V15.52 History of traumatic brain injury
EXCLUDES personal history of cerebrovascular accident (cerebral infarction) without residual deficits (V12.54)
AHA: 4Q, '09, 115

V15.53 Personal history of retained foreign body fully removed
AHA: 4Q, '10, 108

V15.59 Other injury

V15.6 Poisoning

V15.7 Contraception
EXCLUDES current contraceptive management (V25.0-V25.4)
presence of intrauterine contraceptive device as incidental finding (V45.5)

√5ᵗʰ V15.8 Other specified personal history presenting hazards to health
EXCLUDES contact with and (suspected) exposure to:
aromatic compounds and dyes (V87.11-V87.19)
arsenic and other metals (V87.01-V87.09)
molds (V87.31)
AHA: 4Q, '95, 62

V15.80 History of failed moderate sedation
History of failed conscious sedation
AHA: 4Q, '09, 115

V15.81 Noncompliance with medical treatment
EXCLUDES noncompliance with renal dialysis (V45.12)
AHA: 2Q,'12, 16; 3Q, '07, 9; 4Q, '06, 136; 2Q, '03, 7; 2Q, '01, 11, 12, 13; 2Q, '99, 17; 2Q, '97, 11; 1Q, '97, 12; 3Q, '96, 9

V15.82 History of tobacco use
EXCLUDES tobacco dependence (305.1)
AHA: 1Q, '09, 17
Z87.891 Personal history of nicotine dependence   I-10

V15.83 Underimmunization status
Delinquent immunization status
Lapsed immunization schedule status
AHA: 4Q, '09, 115

V15.84 Contact with and (suspected) exposure to asbestos
AHA: 4Q, '09, 116

V15.85 Contact with and (suspected) exposure to potentially hazardous body fluids
AHA: 4Q, '09, 116

V15.86 Contact with and (suspected) exposure to lead
AHA: 4Q, '09, 116

V15.87 History of extracorporeal membrane oxygenation [ECMO]
AHA: 4Q, '03, 84

V15.88 History of fall
At risk for falling
AHA: 4Q, '05, 95
Z91.81 History of falling   I-10

V15.89 Other
EXCLUDES contact with and (suspected) exposure to other potentially hazardous:
chemicals (V87.2)
substances (V87.39)
AHA: 3Q, '08, 7; 3Q, '07, 5; 1Q, '90, 21; N-D, '84, 12

V15.9 Unspecified personal history presenting hazards to health

√4ᵗʰ V16 Family history of malignant neoplasm

V16.0 Gastrointestinal tract
Family history of condition classifiable to 140-159
AHA: 1Q, '99, 4
TIP: Family history of colon cancer is a condition that meets the criteria of "high risk" for a screening colonoscopy.

V16.1 Trachea, bronchus, and lung
Family history of condition classifiable to 162

V16.2 Other respiratory and intrathoracic organs
Family history of condition classifiable to 160-161, 163-165

V16.3 Breast
Family history of condition classifiable to 174
AHA: 4Q, '04, 107; 2Q, '03, 4; 2Q, '00, 8; 1Q, '92, 11
Z80.3 Family history of malignant neoplasm of breast   I-10

√5ᵗʰ V16.4 Genital organs
Family history of condition classifiable to 179-187
AHA: 4Q, '97, 48

V16.40 Genital organ, unspecified

V16.41 Ovary
AHA: 3Q, '09, 5

V16.42 Prostate
Z80.42 Family history of malignant neoplasm of prostate   I-10

V16.43 Testis

V16.49 Other
AHA: 2Q, '06, 2

√5ᵗʰ V16.5 Urinary organs
Family history of condition classifiable to 188-189

V16.51 Kidney

V16.52 Bladder
AHA: 4Q, '07, 98

V16.59 Other

V16.6 Leukemia
    Family history of condition classifiable to 204-208

V16.7 Other lymphatic and hematopoietic neoplasms
    Family history of condition classifiable to 200-203

V16.8 Other specified malignant neoplasm
    Family history of other condition classifiable to 140-199

V16.9 Unspecified malignant neoplasm

✓4ᵗʰ **V17 Family history of certain chronic disabling diseases**

V17.0 Psychiatric condition
    EXCLUDES *family history of intellectual disabilities (V18.4)*

V17.1 Stroke (cerebrovascular)
    Z82.3 Family history of stroke   I-10

V17.2 Other neurological diseases
    Epilepsy
    Huntington's chorea

V17.3 Ischemic heart disease

✓5ᵗʰ **V17.4 Other cardiovascular diseases**
    AHA: 1Q, '04, 6

    V17.41 Family history of sudden cardiac death [SCD]
        EXCLUDES *family history of ischemic heart disease (V17.3)*
        family history of myocardial infarction (V17.3)
        AHA: 4Q, '07, 98

    V17.49 Family history of other cardiovascular diseases
        Family history of cardiovascular disease NOS

V17.5 Asthma

V17.6 Other chronic respiratory conditions

V17.7 Arthritis

✓5ᵗʰ **V17.8 Other musculoskeletal diseases**

    V17.81 Osteoporosis
        AHA: 4Q, '05, 95

    V17.89 Other musculoskeletal diseases

✓4ᵗʰ **V18 Family history of certain other specific conditions**

V18.0 Diabetes mellitus
    AHA: 1Q, '04, 8
    TIP: Assign for a normal infant born to a diabetic mother who presents with no manifestations of the syndrome.

✓5ᵗʰ **V18.1 Other endocrine and metabolic diseases**

    V18.11 Multiple endocrine neoplasia [MEN] syndrome
        AHA: 4Q, '07, 98, 100

    V18.19 Other endocrine and metabolic diseases

V18.2 Anemia

V18.3 Other blood disorders

V18.4 Intellectual disabilities

✓5ᵗʰ **V18.5 Digestive disorders**

    V18.51 Colonic polyps
        EXCLUDES *family history of malignant neoplasm of gastrointestinal tract (V16.0)*
        AHA: 4Q, '06, 117
        Z83.71 Family history of colonic polyps   I-10

    V18.59 Other digestive disorders

✓5ᵗʰ **V18.6 Kidney diseases**

    V18.61 Polycystic kidney

    V18.69 Other kidney diseases

V18.7 Other genitourinary diseases

V18.8 Infectious and parasitic diseases

V18.9 Genetic disease carrier
    AHA: 4Q, '05, 95

✓4ᵗʰ **V19 Family history of other conditions**

V19.0 Blindness or visual loss

✓5ᵗʰ **V19.1 Other eye disorders**
    AHA: 4Q, '11, 156

    V19.11 Glaucoma

    V19.19 Other specified eye disorder

V19.2 Deafness or hearing loss

V19.3 Other ear disorders

V19.4 Skin conditions

V19.5 Congenital anomalies

V19.6 Allergic disorders

V19.7 Consanguinity

V19.8 Other condition

Persons Encountering Health Services in Circumstances Related to Reproduction and Development (V20-V29)

✓4ᵗʰ **V20 Health supervision of infant or child**

V20.0 Foundling   PDx P

V20.1 Other healthy infant or child receiving care   PDx P
    Medical or nursing care supervision of healthy infant in cases of:
        maternal illness, physical or psychiatric
        socioeconomic adverse condition at home
        too many children at home preventing or interfering with normal care
    AHA: 1Q, '00, 25; 3Q, '89, 14

V20.2 Routine infant or child health check   PDx P
    Developmental testing of infant or child
    Health check for child over 28 days old
    Immunizations appropriate for age
    Routine vision and hearing testing
    Use additional code(s) to identify:
        special screening examination(s) performed (V73.0-V82.9)
    EXCLUDES *health check for child under 29 days old (V20.31-V20.32)*
        newborn health supervision (V20.31-V20.32)
        special screening for developmental handicaps (V79.3)
    AHA: 4Q, '09, 115; 1Q, '09, 15; 1Q, '04, 15

✓5ᵗʰ **V20.3 Newborn health supervision**
    Health check for child under 29 days old
    EXCLUDES *health check for child over 28 days old (V20.2)*
    AHA: 4Q, '09, 117

    V20.31 Health supervision for newborn under 8 days old   PDx N
        Health check for newborn under 8 days old

    V20.32 Health supervision for newborn 8 to 28 days old   PDx N
        Health check for newborn 8 to 28 days old
        Newborn weight check
        AHA: 4Q, '09, 102,117

✓4ᵗʰ **V21 Constitutional states in development**

V21.0 Period of rapid growth in childhood

V21.1 Puberty

V21.2 Other adolescence

✓5ᵗʰ **V21.3 Low birth weight status**
    EXCLUDES *history of perinatal problems*
    AHA: 4Q, '00, 51
    TIP: There are no age restrictions on these V codes after the perinatal period; assign for patients without the initial condition who may continue to manifest the consequences of it.

    V21.30 Low birth weight status, unspecified

    V21.31 Low birth weight status, less than 500 grams

    V21.32 Low birth weight status, 500-999 grams

    V21.33 Low birth weight status, 1000-1499 grams

    V21.34 Low birth weight status, 1500-1999 grams

    V21.35 Low birth weight status, 2000-2500 grams

V21.8 Other specified constitutional states in development

V21.9 Unspecified constitutional state in development

✓4ᵗʰ ✓5ᵗʰ Additional Digit Required   Unspecified Code   Other Specified Code   Manifestation Code   ►◄ Revised Text   ● New Code   ▲ Revised Code Title

2015 ICD-9-CM   **Volume 1 – 325**

V16.6–V21.9

V Codes

V22–V25.41

✓4th **V22 Normal pregnancy**

> **EXCLUDES** *pregnancy examination or test, pregnancy unconfirmed (V72.40)*

> **AHA:** 1Q, '12, 10; 4Q, '07, 125

> **TIP:** Do not assign with any code from chapter 11, "Complications of Pregnancy, Childbirth, and the Puerperium."

V22.0 Supervision of normal first pregnancy [PDx] ♀

> **AHA:** 3Q, '99, 16

> **Z34.00** Encounter suprvisn norm 1 pregnancy uns trimestr [I-10]

V22.1 Supervision of other normal pregnancy [PDx] ♀

> **AHA:** 3Q, '99, 16

V22.2 Pregnant state, incidental ♀
> Pregnant state NOS

✓4th **V23 Supervision of high-risk pregnancy**

> **AHA:** 1Q, '12, 10; 1Q, '90, 10

V23.0 Pregnancy with history of infertility [M] ♀

V23.1 Pregnancy with history of trophoblastic disease [M] ♀
> Pregnancy with history of:
> hydatidiform mole
> vesicular mole

> **EXCLUDES** *that without current pregnancy (V13.1)*

V23.2 Pregnancy with history of abortion [M] ♀
> Pregnancy with history of conditions classifiable to 634-638

> **EXCLUDES** *recurrent pregnancy loss:*
> *care during pregnancy (646.3)*
> *that without current pregnancy (629.81)*

V23.3 Grand multiparity [M] ♀

> **EXCLUDES** *care in relation to labor and delivery (659.4)*
> *that without current pregnancy (V61.5)*

✓5th **V23.4 Pregnancy with other poor obstetric history**
> Pregnancy with history of other conditions classifiable to 630-676

V23.41 Pregnancy with history of labor pre-term [M] ♀
> **AHA:** 4Q, '02, 79

V23.42 Pregnancy with history of ectopic pregnancy [M] ♀
> **AHA:** 4Q, '11, 157

V23.49 Pregnancy with other poor obstetric history [M] ♀

V23.5 Pregnancy with other poor reproductive history [M] ♀
> Pregnancy with history of stillbirth or neonatal death

V23.7 Insufficient prenatal care [M] ♀
> History of little or no prenatal care

✓5th **V23.8 Other high-risk pregnancy**
> **AHA:** 4Q, '08, 158; 4Q, '98, 56, 63

V23.81 Elderly primigravida [M] ♀
> First pregnancy in a woman who will be 35 years of age or older at expected date of delivery

> **EXCLUDES** *elderly primigravida complicating pregnancy (659.5)*

V23.82 Elderly multigravida [M] ♀
> Second or more pregnancy in a woman who will be 35 years of age or older at expected date of delivery

> **EXCLUDES** *elderly multigravida complicating pregnancy (659.6)*

> **AHA:** 4Q, '11, 133

V23.83 Young primigravida [M] ♀
> First pregnancy in a female less than 16 years old at expected date of delivery

> **EXCLUDES** *young primigravida complicating pregnancy (659.8)*

V23.84 Young multigravida [M] ♀
> Second or more pregnancy in a female less than 16 years old at expected date of delivery

> **EXCLUDES** *young multigravida complicating pregnancy (659.8)*

V23.85 Pregnancy resulting from assisted reproductive technology [A] ♀
> Pregnancy resulting from in vitro fertilization

> **AHA:** 4Q, '08, 160

V23.86 Pregnancy with history of in utero procedure during previous pregnancy [M] ♀

> **EXCLUDES** *management of pregnancy affected by in utero procedure during current pregnancy (679.0-679.1)*

> **AHA:** 4Q, '08, 158, 160

V23.87 Pregnancy with inconclusive fetal viability [M] ♀
> Encounter to determine fetal viability of pregnancy

> **AHA:** 4Q, '11, 157

V23.89 Other high-risk pregnancy [M] ♀
> **AHA:** 3Q, '06, 14

V23.9 Unspecified high-risk pregnancy [M] ♀

✓4th **V24 Postpartum care and examination**

V24.0 Immediately after delivery [PDx] [M] ♀
> Care and observation in uncomplicated cases

> **AHA:** 3Q, '06, 11

V24.1 Lactating mother [PDx] ♀
> Supervision of lactation

> **AHA:** 3Q, '12, 7

V24.2 Routine postpartum follow-up [PDx] ♀

✓4th **V25 Encounter for contraceptive management**
> **AHA:** 4Q, '92, 24

✓5th **V25.0 General counseling and advice**

V25.01 Prescription of oral contraceptives ♀

V25.02 Initiation of other contraceptive measures
> Fitting of diaphragm
> Prescription of foams, creams, or other agents

> **AHA:** 3Q, '97, 7

V25.03 Encounter for emergency contraceptive counseling and prescription
> Encounter for postcoital contraceptive counseling and prescription

> **AHA:** 4Q, '03, 84

V25.04 Counseling and instruction in natural family planning to avoid pregnancy
> **AHA:** 4Q, '07, 99

> **Z30.02** Counsel & instruct natural family plan avoid pg [I-10]

V25.09 Other
> Family planning advice

✓5th **V25.1 Encounter for insertion or removal of intrauterine contraceptive device**

> **EXCLUDES** *encounter for routine checking of intrauterine contraceptive device (V25.42)*

> **AHA:** 4Q, '10, 109

V25.11 Encounter for insertion of intrauterine contraceptive device ♀

V25.12 Encounter for removal of intrauterine contraceptive device ♀

V25.13 Encounter for removal and reinsertion of intrauterine contraceptive device ♀
> Encounter for replacement of intrauterine contraceptive device

V25.2 Sterilization
> Admission for interruption of fallopian tubes or vas deferens

V25.3 Menstrual extraction ♀
> Menstrual regulation

✓5th **V25.4 Surveillance of previously prescribed contraceptive methods**
> Checking, reinsertion, or removal of contraceptive device
> Repeat prescription for contraceptive method
> Routine examination in connection with contraceptive maintenance

V25.40 Contraceptive surveillance, unspecified

V25.41 Contraceptive pill ♀

[N] Newborn Age: 0   [P] Pediatric Age: 0-17   [M] Maternity Age: 12-55   [A] Adult Age: 15-124   [PDx] Primary Diagnosis

V25.42 Intrauterine contraceptive device ♀
  Checking of intrauterine device
  EXCLUDES *insertion or removal of intrauterine contraceptive device (V25.11-V25.13)*
  presence of intrauterine contraceptive device as incidental finding (V45.51)
  AHA: 4Q, '10, 109-110

V25.43 Implantable subdermal contraceptive ♀

V25.49 Other contraceptive method
  AHA: 3Q, '97, 7

V25.5 Insertion of implantable subdermal contraceptive ♀
  AHA: 3Q, '92, 9

V25.8 Other specified contraceptive management
  Postvasectomy sperm count
  EXCLUDES *sperm count following sterilization reversal (V26.22)*
  sperm count for fertility testing (V26.21)
  AHA: 3Q, '96, 9

V25.9 Unspecified contraceptive management

✓⁴ᵗʰ **V26 Procreative management**

V26.0 Tuboplasty or vasoplasty after previous sterilization
  AHA: 2Q, '95, 10
  TIP: Assign for encounters for tubal ligation or vasectomy reversal procedures.

V26.1 Artificial insemination ♀

✓⁵ᵗʰ **V26.2 Investigation and testing**
  EXCLUDES *postvasectomy sperm count (V25.8)*
  AHA: 4Q, '00, 56

V26.21 Fertility testing
  Fallopian insufflation
  Sperm count for fertility testing
  EXCLUDES *genetic counseling and testing (V26.31-V26.39)*

V26.22 Aftercare following sterilization reversal
  Fallopian insufflation following sterilization reversal
  Sperm count following sterilization reversal

V26.29 Other investigation and testing
  AHA: 2Q, '96, 9; N-D, '85, 15

✓⁵ᵗʰ **V26.3 Genetic counseling and testing**
  EXCLUDES *fertility testing (V26.21)*
  nonprocreative genetic screening (V82.71, V82.79)
  AHA: 4Q, '05, 96

V26.31 Testing of female for genetic disease carrier status ♀
  AHA: 4Q, '06, 117

V26.32 Other genetic testing of female ♀
  Use additional code to identify recurrent pregnancy loss (629.81, 646.3)
  AHA: 4Q, '06, 117
  Z31.438 Encounter oth genetic test female procreative mngmnt   I-10

V26.33 Genetic counseling

V26.34 Testing of male for genetic disease carrier status ♂
  AHA: 4Q, '06, 117

V26.35 Encounter for testing of male partner of female with recurrent pregnancy loss ♂
  AHA: 4Q, '06, 117

V26.39 Other genetic testing of male ♂
  AHA: 4Q, '06, 117

✓⁵ᵗʰ **V26.4 General counseling and advice**

V26.41 Procreative counseling and advice using natural family planning
  AHA: 4Q, '07, 99

V26.42 Encounter for fertility preservation counseling
  Encounter for fertility preservation counseling prior to cancer therapy
  Encounter for fertility preservation counseling prior to surgical removal of gonads
  AHA: 4Q, '09, 117

V26.49 Other procreative management, counseling and advice

✓⁵ᵗʰ **V26.5 Sterilization status**

V26.51 Tubal ligation status ♀
  EXCLUDES *infertility not due to previous tubal ligation (628.0-628.9)*
  Z98.51 Tubal ligation status   I-10

V26.52 Vasectomy status ♂

✓⁵ᵗʰ **V26.8 Other specified procreative management**

V26.81 Encounter for assisted reproductive fertility procedure cycle PDx ♀
  Patient undergoing in vitro fertilization cycle
  Use additional code to identify the type of infertility
  EXCLUDES *pre-cycle diagnosis and testing — code to reason for encounter*
  AHA: 4Q, '07, 99

V26.82 Encounter for fertility preservation procedure PDx
  Encounter for fertility preservation procedure prior to cancer therapy
  Encounter for fertility preservation procedure prior to surgical removal of gonads
  AHA: 4Q, '09, 117

V26.89 Other specified procreative management

V26.9 Unspecified procreative management

✓⁴ᵗʰ **V27 Outcome of delivery**
  NOTE This category is intended for the coding of the outcome of delivery on the mother's record.
  AHA: 2Q, '91, 16
  TIP: Assign on the maternal chart for every admission during which a delivery occurs.

V27.0 Single liveborn M ♀
  AHA: ▶1Q, '14, 14;◄ 4Q, '11, 133; 4Q, '08, 192; 4Q, '05, 81; 2Q, '03, 9; 2Q, '02, 10; 1Q, '01, 10; 3Q, '00, 5; 4Q, '98, 77; 4Q, '95, 59; 1Q, '92, 9
  Z37.0 Single live birth   I-10

V27.1 Single stillborn M ♀

V27.2 Twins, both liveborn M ♀
  Z37.2 Twins both liveborn   I-10

V27.3 Twins, one liveborn and one stillborn M ♀

V27.4 Twins, both stillborn M ♀

V27.5 Other multiple birth, all liveborn M ♀

V27.6 Other multiple birth, some liveborn M ♀

V27.7 Other multiple birth, all stillborn M ♀

V27.9 Unspecified outcome of delivery M ♀
  Single birth ⎫
  Multiple birth ⎬ outcome to infant unspecified

✓⁴ᵗʰ **V28 Encounter for antenatal screening of mother**
  EXCLUDES *abnormal findings on screening — code to findings*
  routine prenatal care (V22.0-V23.9)
  suspected fetal conditions affecting management of pregnancy (655.00-655.93, 656.00- 656.93, 657.00-657.03, 658.00, 658.93)
  suspected fetal conditions not found (V89.01-V89.09)
  AHA: 4Q, '06, 117; 1Q, '04, 11

V28.0 Screening for chromosomal anomalies by amniocentesis M ♀

V28.1 Screening for raised alpha-fetoprotein levels in amniotic fluid M ♀

V28.2 Other screening based on amniocentesis M ♀

V28.3 Encounter for routine screening for malformation using ultrasonics ♀
  Encounter for routine fetal ultrasound NOS
  EXCLUDES *encounter for fetal anatomic survey (V28.81)*
  genetic counseling and testing (V26.31-V26.39)

V28.4 Screening for fetal growth retardation using ultrasonics ♀

V28.5 Screening for isoimmunization ♀

✓⁴ᵗʰ ✓⁵ᵗʰ Additional Digit Required   Unspecified Code   Other Specified Code   Manifestation Code   ▶◄ Revised Text   ● New Code   ▲ Revised Code Title

2015 ICD-9-CM   **October 2014 • Volume 1 – 327**

V25.42–V28.5

V28.6 Screening for Streptococcus B   M ♀
  AHA: 4Q, '97, 46

√5ᵗʰ **V28.8 Other specified antenatal screening**
  AHA: 4Q, '08, 159; 3Q, '99, 16

     V28.81 Encounter for fetal anatomic survey   M ♀

     V28.82 Encounter for screening for risk of pre-term labor   M ♀

     V28.89 Other specified antenatal screening   M ♀
        Chorionic villus sampling
        Genomic screening
        Nuchal translucency testing
        Proteomic screening

V28.9 Unspecified antenatal screening   ♀

√4ᵗʰ **V29 Observation and evaluation of newborns and infants for suspected condition not found**
  NOTE This category is to be used for newborns, within the neonatal period, (the first 28 days of life) who are suspected of having an abnormal condition resulting from exposure from the mother or the birth process, but without signs or symptoms, and, which after examination and observation, is found not to exist.
  EXCLUDES suspected fetal conditions not found (V89.01-V89.09)
  AHA: 1Q, '00, 25; 4Q, '94, 47; 1Q, '94, 9; 4Q, '92, 21
  TIP: Do not assign if the infant shows any signs or symptoms.

[1] **V29.0 Observation for suspected infectious condition**   N
  AHA: 1Q, '01, 10

[1] **V29.1 Observation for suspected neurological condition**   N

[1] **V29.2 Observation for suspected respiratory condition**   N

[1] **V29.3 Observation for suspected genetic or metabolic condition**   N
  AHA: 2Q, '05, 21; 4Q, '98, 59, 68

[1] **V29.8 Observation for other specified suspected condition**   N
  AHA: 2Q, '03, 15

[1] **V29.9 Observation for unspecified suspected condition**   N
  AHA: 1Q, '02, 6

Liveborn Infants According to Type of Birth (V30-V39)

  NOTE These categories are intended for the coding of liveborn infants who are consuming health care [e.g., crib or bassinet occupancy].

  The following fourth-digit subdivisions are for use with categories V30-V39:
  √5ᵗʰ   0   Born in hospital   N
       1   Born before admission to hospital   N
       2   Born outside hospital and not hospitalized
  The following two fifth-digits are for use with the fourth-digit .0, Born in hospital:
       0   delivered without mention of cesarean delivery
       1   delivered by cesarean delivery

  AHA: 1Q, '01, 10

§ √4ᵗʰ **V30 Single liveborn**   PDx
  AHA: 3Q, '12, 5; 2Q, '03, 9; 4Q, '98, 46, 59; 1Q, '94, 9; **For code V30.00:** 2Q, '12, 17; 1Q, '04, 8, 16; 4Q, '03, 68; **For code V30.01:** 4Q, '09, 101; 4Q, '05, 88; **For code V30.10:** 3Q, '06, 10
  Z38.00 Single liveborn infant delivered vaginally   I-10

§ √4ᵗʰ **V31 Twin, mate liveborn**   PDx
  AHA: 3Q, '92, 10
  Z38.31 Twin liveborn infant delivered by cesarean   I-10

§ √4ᵗʰ **V32 Twin, mate stillborn**   PDx

§ √4ᵗʰ **V33 Twin, unspecified**   PDx

§ √4ᵗʰ **V34 Other multiple, mates all liveborn**   PDx

§ √4ᵗʰ **V35 Other multiple, mates all stillborn**   PDx

§ √4ᵗʰ **V36 Other multiple, mates live and stillborn**   PDx

§ √4ᵗʰ **V37 Other multiple, unspecified**   PDx

§ √4ᵗʰ **V39 Unspecified**   PDx

Persons with a Condition Influencing their Health Status (V40-V49)

  NOTE These categories are intended for use when these conditions are recorded as "diagnoses" or "problems."
  TIP: Includes patients with a carrier status or who have sequelae or residual of a past condition or disease, which may affect current or future treatment.

√4ᵗʰ **V40 Mental and behavioral problems**

V40.0 Problems with learning

V40.1 Problems with communication [including speech]

V40.2 Other mental problems

√5ᵗʰ **V40.3 Other behavioral problems**
  AHA: 4Q, '11, 158

     V40.31 Wandering in diseases classified elsewhere
  Code first underlying disorder such as:
     Alzheimer's disease (331.0)
     autism or pervasive developmental disorder (299.0-299.9)
     dementia, unspecified, with behavioral disturbance (294.21)
     intellectual disabilities (317-319)

     V40.39 Other specified behavioral problem

V40.9 Unspecified mental or behavioral problem

√4ᵗʰ **V41 Problems with special senses and other special functions**

V41.0 Problems with sight

V41.1 Other eye problems

V41.2 Problems with hearing

V41.3 Other ear problems

V41.4 Problems with voice production

V41.5 Problems with smell and taste

V41.6 Problems with swallowing and mastication

V41.7 Problems with sexual function
  EXCLUDES marital problems (V61.10)
       psychosexual disorders (302.0-302.9)

V41.8 Other problems with special functions

V41.9 Unspecified problem with special functions

√4ᵗʰ **V42 Organ or tissue replaced by transplant**
  INCLUDES homologous or heterologous (animal) (human) transplant organ status
  AHA: 3Q, '11, 5; 3Q, '98, 3, 4
  TIP: Do not assign if the patient has a complication of the transplanted organ; the code from subcategory 996.8 provides the information.

V42.0 Kidney
  AHA: ▶3Q, '13, 6;◀1Q, '08, 10; 1Q, '03, 10; 3Q, '01, 12
  Z94.0 Kidney transplant status   I-10

V42.1 Heart
  AHA: 3Q, '03, 16; 3Q, '01, 13

V42.2 Heart valve

V42.3 Skin

V42.4 Bone

V42.5 Cornea

V42.6 Lung

V42.7 Liver
  AHA: 3Q, '11, 5
  Z94.4 Liver transplant status   I-10

√5ᵗʰ **V42.8 Other specified organ or tissue**
  AHA: 4Q, '98, 64; 4Q, '97, 49

     V42.81 Bone marrow
  AHA: 1Q, '12, 13

     V42.82 Peripheral stem cells

     V42.83 Pancreas
  AHA: 1Q, '03, 10; 2Q, '01, 16

---

[1]   V29 observation codes are to be used as first-listed/principal Dx only, except when the first-listed/principal Dx is required to be a code from the V30.
§   Require fourth and fifth digits. See beginning of section V30-V39 for codes and definitions.

V42.84 Intestines
   AHA: 4Q, '00, 48, 50

V42.89 Other

V42.9 Unspecified organ or tissue

☑4th **V43 Organ or tissue replaced by other means**
   INCLUDES organ or tissue assisted by other means
   replacement of organ by:
      artificial device
      mechanical device
      prosthesis
   EXCLUDES cardiac pacemaker in situ (V45.01)
   fitting and adjustment of prosthetic device (V52.0-V52.9)
   renal dialysis status (V45.11)

V43.0 Eye globe

V43.1 Lens
   Pseudophakos
   AHA: 4Q, '98, 65

☑5th **V43.2 Heart**
   Fully implantable artificial heart
   Heart assist device
   AHA: 4Q, '03, 85

   V43.21 Heart assist device

   V43.22 Fully implantable artificial heart

V43.3 Heart valve
   AHA: 3Q, '06, 7; 3Q, '02, 13, 14
   TIP: If the status post heart valve replacement information includes
   "porcine" or mention of other homologous or heterologous tissue,
   assign instead V42.2.
   Z95.2 Presence of prosthetic heart valve   I-10

V43.4 Blood vessel

V43.5 Bladder

☑5th **V43.6 Joint**
   AHA: 4Q, '05, 91

   V43.60 Unspecified joint

   V43.61 Shoulder

   V43.62 Elbow

   V43.63 Wrist

   V43.64 Hip
      AHA: 1Q, '09, 6; 2Q, '08, 3-5; 3Q, '06, 4, 5; 4Q, '05, 93, 112; 2Q,
      '04, 15
      Z96.641 Presence of right artificial hip joint   I-10

   V43.65 Knee
      AHA: ▶1Q, '14, 5;◀ 3Q, '06, 5

   V43.66 Ankle

   V43.69 Other

V43.7 Limb

☑5th **V43.8 Other organ or tissue**

   V43.81 Larynx
      AHA: 4Q, '95, 55

   V43.82 Breast
      AHA: 4Q, '95, 55
      Z98.82 Breast implant status   I-10

   V43.83 Artificial skin

   V43.89 Other

☑4th **V44 Artificial opening status**
   EXCLUDES artificial openings requiring attention or
   management (V55.0-V55.9)
   TIP: Do not assign if the patient has a complication of the artificial opening,
   such as infection or obstruction; assign only the complication code.

V44.0 Tracheostomy
   AHA: 4Q, '03, 103, 107, 111; 1Q, '01, 6

V44.1 Gastrostomy
   AHA: 4Q, '03, 103, 107-108, 110; 1Q, '01, 12; 3Q, '97, 12; 1Q, '93, 26

V44.2 Ileostomy

V44.3 Colostomy
   AHA: 4Q, '03, 110
   Z93.3 Colostomy status   I-10

V44.4 Other artificial opening of gastrointestinal tract

☑5th **V44.5 Cystostomy**

   V44.50 Cystostomy, unspecified

   V44.51 Cutaneous-vesicostomy

   V44.52 Appendico-vesicostomy

   V44.59 Other cystostomy

V44.6 Other artificial opening of urinary tract
   Nephrostomy   Ureterostomy   Urethrostomy
   AHA: 3Q, '12, 11-12

V44.7 Artificial vagina

V44.8 Other artificial opening status

V44.9 Unspecified artificial opening status

☑4th **V45 Other postprocedural states**
   EXCLUDES aftercare management (V51-V58.9)
   malfunction or other complication — code to condition
   AHA: 4Q, '03, 85

☑5th **V45.0 Cardiac device in situ**
   EXCLUDES artificial heart (V43.22)
   heart assist device (V43.21)

   V45.00 Unspecified cardiac device

   V45.01 Cardiac pacemaker
      EXCLUDES cardiac defibrillator with synchronous
      cardiac pacemaker (V45.02)

   V45.02 Automatic implantable cardiac defibrillator
      With synchronous cardiac pacemaker
      Z95.810 Presence auto implantable cardiac   I-10
      defibrillator

   V45.09 Other specified cardiac device
      Carotid sinus pacemaker in situ

☑5th **V45.1 Renal dialysis status**
   EXCLUDES admission for dialysis treatment or session (V56.0)
   AHA: 4Q, '08, 157; 1Q, '08, 7; 4Q, '07, 86; 3Q, '07, 9; 4Q, '06, 136; 4Q, '05,
   96; 2Q, '03, 7; 2Q, '01, 12, 13

   V45.11 Renal dialysis status
      Hemodialysis status
      Patient requiring intermittent renal dialysis
      Peritoneal dialysis status
      Presence of arterial-venous shunt (for dialysis)
      AHA: 3Q, '11, 15; 4Q, '08, 157, 193
      Z99.2 Dependence on renal dialysis   I-10

   V45.12 Noncompliance with renal dialysis

V45.2 Presence of cerebrospinal fluid drainage device
   Cerebral ventricle (communicating) shunt, valve, or device in
   situ
   EXCLUDES malfunction (996.2)
   AHA: 4Q, '03, 106

V45.3 Intestinal bypass or anastomosis status
   EXCLUDES bariatric surgery status (V45.86)
   gastric bypass status (V45.86)
   obesity surgery status (V45.86)

V45.4 Arthrodesis status
   AHA: ▶2Q, '13, 22;◀ N-D, '84, 18
   TIP: If there is a complication of the fusion graft site that requires
   refusion or revision, assign instead a code from subcategory 996.4.

☑5th **V45.5 Presence of contraceptive device**

   V45.51 Intrauterine contraceptive device   ♀
      EXCLUDES checking of device (V25.42)
      complication from device (996.32)
      insertion and removal of device
      (V25.11-V25.13)
      Z97.5 Presence of intrauterine contraceptive   I-10
      device

   V45.52 Subdermal contraceptive implant

   V45.59 Other

√5th **V45.6 States following surgery of eye and adnexa**

Cataract extraction } state following eye
Filtering bleb } surgery
Surgical eyelid adhesion

EXCLUDES *aphakia (379.31)*
artificial eye globe (V43.0)

AHA: 4Q, '98, 65; 4Q, '97, 49

V45.61 Cataract extraction status
Use additional code for associated artificial
lens status (V43.1)

**V45.69 Other states following surgery of eye
and adnexa**
AHA: 2Q, '01, 16; 1Q, '98, 10; 4Q, '97, 19

√5th **V45.7 Acquired absence of organ**
AHA: 4Q, '98, 65; 4Q, '97, 50

V45.71 Acquired absence of breast and nipple
EXCLUDES *congenital absence of breast and nipple
(757.6)*
AHA: 4Q, '08, 159; 4Q, '01, 66

V45.72 Acquired absence of intestine (large)(small)

V45.73 Acquired absence of kidney

V45.74 Other parts of urinary tract
Bladder
AHA: 4Q, '00, 51

V45.75 Stomach
AHA: 4Q, '00, 51

V45.76 Lung
AHA: 4Q, '00, 51

V45.77 Genital organs
EXCLUDES *acquired absence of cervix and uterus
(V88.01-V88.03)*
*female genital mutilation status
(629.20-629.29)*
AHA: 1Q, '03, 13, 14; 4Q, '00, 51

V45.78 Eye
AHA: 4Q, '00, 51

V45.79 Other acquired absence of organ
EXCLUDES *acquired absence of pancreas
(V88.11-V88.12)*
AHA: 4Q, '00, 51

√5th **V45.8 Other postprocedural status**

V45.81 Aortocoronary bypass status
AHA: 4Q, '11, 153; 4Q, '10, 131; 4Q, '03, 105; 3Q, '01, 15; 3Q,
'97, 16

**V45.82 Percutaneous transluminal coronary angioplasty
status**

V45.83 Breast implant removal status
AHA: 4Q, '95, 55

V45.84 Dental restoration status
Dental crowns status   Dental fillings status
AHA: 4Q, '01, 54

V45.85 Insulin pump status

V45.86 Bariatric surgery status
Gastric banding status
Gastric bypass status for obesity
Obesity surgery status
EXCLUDES *bariatric surgery status complicating
pregnancy, childbirth or the
puerperium (649.2)*
*intestinal bypass or anastomosis status
(V45.3)*
AHA: 2Q, '09, 10; 4Q, '06, 118
Z98.84 Bariatric surgery status   I-10

V45.87 Transplanted organ removal status
Transplanted organ previously removed due to
complication, failure, rejection or infection
EXCLUDES *encounter for removal of transplanted organ
— code to complication of
transplanted organ (996.80-996.89)*
AHA: 4Q, '08, 157

**V45.88 Status post administration of tPA (rtPA) in a
different facility within the last 24 hours prior to
admission to current facility**
Code first condition requiring tPA administration,
such as:
acute cerebral infarction (433.0-433.9
with fifth-digit 1, 434.0-434.9 with fifth
digit 1)
acute myocardial infarction (410.00-410.92)
AHA: ▶4Q, '13, 99;◀ 4Q, '08, 157
TIP: Assign only on receiving facility record; assign even if
the patient is still receiving tPA at the time of transfer.

V45.89 Other
Presence of neuropacemaker or other electronic
device
EXCLUDES *artificial heart valve in situ (V43.3)*
vascular prosthesis in situ (V43.4)
AHA: 1Q, '95, 11

√4th **V46 Other dependence on machines and devices**

V46.0 Aspirator

√5th **V46.1 Respirator [Ventilator]**
Iron lung
AHA: 4Q, '05, 96; 4Q, '03, 103; 1Q, '01, 12; J-F, '87, 7 3

V46.11 Dependence on respirator, status
AHA: ▶2Q, '13, 25;◀ 4Q, '04, 100
Z99.11 Dependence on respirator ventilator status   I-10

**V46.12 Encounter for respirator dependence
during power failure**   PDx
AHA: 4Q, '04, 100

**V46.13 Encounter for weaning from respirator
[ventilator]**   PDx

V46.14 Mechanical complication of respirator [ventilator]
Mechanical failure of respirator [ventilator]

V46.2 Supplemental oxygen
Long-term oxygen therapy
AHA: 4Q, '03, 108; 4Q, '02, 79

V46.3 Wheelchair dependence
Wheelchair confinement status
Code first cause of dependence, such as:
muscular dystrophy (359.1)
obesity (278.00-278.03)
AHA: 4Q, '08, 157

V46.8 Other enabling machines
Hyperbaric chamber
Possum [Patient-Operated-Selector-Mechanism]
EXCLUDES *cardiac pacemaker (V45.0)*
kidney dialysis machine (V45.11)

V46.9 Unspecified machine dependence
AHA: 4Q, '06, 117

√4th **V47 Other problems with internal organs**

V47.0 Deficiencies of internal organs

V47.1 Mechanical and motor problems with internal organs

V47.2 Other cardiorespiratory problems
Cardiovascular exercise intolerance with pain (with):
at rest
less than ordinary activity
ordinary activity

V47.3 Other digestive problems

V47.4 Other urinary problems

V47.5 Other genital problems

V47.9 Unspecified

√4th **V48 Problems with head, neck, and trunk**

V48.0 Deficiencies of head
EXCLUDES *deficiencies of ears, eyelids, and nose (V48.8)*

V48.1 Deficiencies of neck and trunk

V48.2 Mechanical and motor problems with head

V48.3 Mechanical and motor problems with neck and trunk

V48.4 Sensory problem with head

V48.5 Sensory problem with neck and trunk

V48.6 Disfigurements of head

V48.7 Disfigurements of neck and trunk

V48.8 Other problems with head, neck, and trunk

V48.9 Unspecified problem with head, neck, or trunk

✓4ᵗʰ **V49 Other conditions influencing health status**

V49.0 Deficiencies of limbs

V49.1 Mechanical problems with limbs

V49.2 Motor problems with limbs

V49.3 Sensory problems with limbs

V49.4 Disfigurements of limbs

V49.5 Other problems of limbs

✓5ᵗʰ **V49.6 Upper limb amputation status**
AHA: 4Q, '05, 94; 4Q, '98, 42; 4Q, '94, 39

V49.60 Unspecified level
Z89.201 Acquired absence of right upper limb uns level   I-10

V49.61 Thumb

V49.62 Other finger(s)
AHA: 2Q, '05, 7

V49.63 Hand

V49.64 Wrist
Disarticulation of wrist

V49.65 Below elbow

V49.66 Above elbow
Disarticulation of elbow

V49.67 Shoulder
Disarticulation of shoulder

✓5ᵗʰ **V49.7 Lower limb amputation status**
AHA: 3Q, '06, 5; 4Q, '05, 94; 4Q, '98, 42; 4Q, '94, 39

V49.70 Unspecified level

V49.71 Great toe

V49.72 Other toe(s)

V49.73 Foot

V49.74 Ankle
Disarticulation of ankle

V49.75 Below knee
Z89.512 Acq absence of lt leg below knee   I-10

V49.76 Above knee
Disarticulation of knee

V49.77 Hip
Disarticulation of hip

✓5ᵗʰ **V49.8 Other specified conditions influencing health status**
AHA: 4Q, '00, 51

V49.81 Asymptomatic postmenopausal status (age-related) (natural)   A ♀
EXCLUDES menopausal and premenopausal disorder (627.0-627.9)
postsurgical menopause (256.2)
premature menopause (256.31)
symptomatic menopause (627.0-627.9)
AHA: 4Q, '09, 106; 4Q, '02, 79; 4Q, '00, 54

V49.82 Dental sealant status
AHA: 4Q, '01, 54

V49.83 Awaiting organ transplant status

V49.84 Bed confinement status
AHA: 4Q, '05, 96

V49.85 Dual sensory impairment
Blindness with deafness
Combined visual hearing impairment
Code first:
hearing impairment (389.00-389.9)
visual impairment (369.00-369.9)
AHA: 4Q, '07, 100

V49.86 Do not resuscitate status
AHA: 1Q, '12, 14; 4Q, '10, 108
Z66 Do not resuscitate   I-10

V49.87 Physical restraints status
EXCLUDES restraint due to a procedure – omit code
AHA: 4Q, '10, 108-109

V49.89 Other specified conditions influencing health status
AHA: 4Q, '05, 94

V49.9 Unspecified

Persons Encountering Health Services for Specific Procedures and Aftercare (V50-V59)

NOTE Categories V51-V59 are intended for use to indicate a reason for care in patients who may have already been treated for some disease or injury not now present, or who are receiving care to consolidate the treatment, to deal with residual states, or to prevent recurrence.
EXCLUDES follow-up examination for medical surveillance following treatment (V67.0-V67.9)

✓4ᵗʰ **V50 Elective surgery for purposes other than remedying health states**

V50.0 Hair transplant

V50.1 Other plastic surgery for unacceptable cosmetic appearance
Breast augmentation or reduction
Face-lift
EXCLUDES encounter for breast reduction (611.1)
plastic surgery following healed injury or operation (V51.0-V51.8)

V50.2 Routine or ritual circumcision   ♂
Circumcision in the absence of significant medical indication

V50.3 Ear piercing

✓5ᵗʰ **V50.4 Prophylactic organ removal**
EXCLUDES organ donations (V59.0-V59.9)
therapeutic organ removal — code to condition
AHA: 4Q, '94, 44
TIP: Assign an additional code, such as one from category V16 Family history of malignant neoplasm, to indicate the reason for the prophylactic organ removal.

V50.41 Breast
AHA: 2Q, '11, 12; 4Q, '04, 107

V50.42 Ovary   ♀
AHA: 3Q, '09, 5

V50.49 Other
AHA: 3Q, '09, 5

V50.8 Other
Z40.8 Encounter for other prophylactic surgery   I-10

V50.9 Unspecified

✓4ᵗʰ **V51 Aftercare involving the use of plastic surgery**
Plastic surgery following healed injury or operation
EXCLUDES cosmetic plastic surgery (V50.2)
plastic surgery as treatment for current condition or injury — code to condition or injury
repair of scarred tissue — code to scar
AHA: 4Q, '08, 159

V51.0 Encounter for breast reconstruction following mastectomy   PDx A
EXCLUDES deformity and disproportion of reconstructed breast (612.0-612.1)
AHA: 4Q, '08, 159-160

V51.8 Other aftercare involving the use of plastic surgery

✓4ᵗʰ **V52 Fitting and adjustment of prosthetic device and implant**
INCLUDES removal of device
EXCLUDES malfunction or complication of prosthetic device (996.0-996.7)
status only, without need for care (V43.0-V43.8)
AHA: 4Q, '05, 94; 4Q, '95, 55 ; 1Q, '90, 7

V52.0 Artificial arm (complete) (partial)

✓4ᵗʰ ✓5ᵗʰ Additional Digit Required   Unspecified Code   Other Specified Code   Manifestation Code   ►◄ Revised Text   ● New Code   ▲ Revised Code Title

2015 ICD-9-CM   Volume 1 – 331

V Codes

V52.1–V54.19

V52.1 Artificial leg (complete) (partial)

V52.2 Artificial eye

V52.3 Dental prosthetic device

V52.4 Breast prosthesis and implant ♀
Elective implant exchange (different material) (different size)
Removal of tissue expander without synchronous insertion of permanent implant
> **EXCLUDES** admission for initial breast implant insertion for breast augmentation (V50.1)
> complications of breast implant (996.54, 996.69, 996.79)
> encounter for breast reconstruction following mastectomy (V51.0)
> **AHA:** 4Q, '95, 80, 81

V52.8 Other specified prosthetic device
> **AHA:** 2Q, '02, 12, 16

V52.9 Unspecified prosthetic device

✓4ᵗʰ **V53 Fitting and adjustment of other device**
> **INCLUDES** removal of device
> replacement of device
> **EXCLUDES** status only, without need for care (V45.0-V45.8)

✓5ᵗʰ **V53.0 Devices related to nervous system and special senses**
> **AHA:** 4Q, '98, 66; 4Q, '97, 51

> **V53.01 Fitting and adjustment of cerebral ventricular (communicating) shunt**
> > **AHA:** 4Q, '97, 51

> **V53.02 Neuropacemaker (brain) (peripheral nerve) (spinal cord)**

> **V53.09 Fitting and adjustment of other devices related to nervous system and special senses**
> Auditory substitution device
> Visual substitution device
> > **AHA:** 2Q, '99, 4

V53.1 Spectacles and contact lenses

V53.2 Hearing aid

✓5ᵗʰ **V53.3 Cardiac device**
> Reprogramming
> **AHA:** 3Q, '92, 3; 1Q, '90, 7; M-J, '87, 8; N-D, '84, 18
> **TIP:** Assign for cardiac device replacement when the device has reached normal end-of-life parameters.

> **V53.31 Cardiac pacemaker**
> > **EXCLUDES** automatic implantable cardiac defibrillator with synchronous cardiac pacemaker (V53.32)
> > mechanical complication of cardiac pacemaker (996.01)
> > **AHA:** 3Q, '10, 9; 1Q, '02, 3

> **V53.32 Automatic implantable cardiac defibrillator**
> With synchronous cardiac pacemaker
> > **AHA:** 3Q, '05, 8

> **V53.39 Other cardiac device**
> > **AHA:** 4Q, '10, 124,125; 2Q, '08, 9; 1Q, '07, 20

V53.4 Orthodontic devices

✓5ᵗʰ **V53.5 Other gastrointestinal appliance and device**
> **EXCLUDES** colostomy (V55.3)
> ileostomy (V55.2)
> other artificial opening of digestive tract (V55.4)
> **AHA:** 4Q, '09, 116

> **V53.50 Fitting and adjustment of intestinal appliance and device**

> **V53.51 Fitting and adjustment of gastric lap band**

> **V53.59 Fitting and adjustment of other gastrointestinal appliance and device**

V53.6 Urinary devices
Urinary catheter
> **EXCLUDES** cystostomy (V55.5)
> nephrostomy (V55.6)
> ureterostomy (V55.6)
> urethrostomy (V55.6)

V53.7 Orthopedic devices
Orthopedic: Orthopedic:
brace   corset
cast   shoes
> **EXCLUDES** other orthopedic aftercare (V54)
> **AHA:** ▶4Q, '13, 101◀

V53.8 Wheelchair

✓5ᵗʰ **V53.9 Other and unspecified device**
> **AHA:** 2Q, '03, 6

> **V53.90 Unspecified device**

> **V53.91 Fitting and adjustment of insulin pump**
> Insulin pump titration

> **V53.99 Other device**
> > **AHA:** 2Q, '09, 10

✓4ᵗʰ **V54 Other orthopedic aftercare**
> **EXCLUDES** fitting and adjustment of orthopedic devices (V53.7)
> malfunction of internal orthopedic device (996.40-996.49)
> other complication of nonmechanical nature (996.60-996.79)
> **AHA:** 4Q, '08, 158; 1Q, '07, 3-4; 3Q, '95, 3

✓5ᵗʰ **V54.0 Aftercare involving internal fixation device**
> **EXCLUDES** malfunction of internal orthopedic device (996.40-996.49)
> other complication of nonmechanical nature (996.60-996.79)
> removal of external fixation device (V54.89)
> **AHA:** 4Q, '03, 87

> **V54.01 Encounter for removal of internal fixation device**

> **V54.02 Encounter for lengthening/adjustment of growth rod**

> **V54.09 Other aftercare involving internal fixation device**

✓5ᵗʰ **V54.1 Aftercare for healing traumatic fracture**
> **EXCLUDES** aftercare following joint replacement (V54.81)
> aftercare for amputation stump (V54.89)
> **AHA:** 4Q, '02, 80
> **TIP:** Assign for follow-up and treatment during the healing phase of the fracture; an aftercare code should be used for all subsequent encounters after the initial encounter for care of a fracture.

> **V54.10 Aftercare for healing traumatic fracture of arm, unspecified**

> **V54.11 Aftercare for healing traumatic fracture of upper arm**

> **V54.12 Aftercare for healing traumatic fracture of lower arm**
> > **AHA:** 1Q, '07, 7

> **V54.13 Aftercare for healing traumatic fracture of hip**
> > **AHA:** 1Q, '09, 6; 4Q, '03, 103, 105; 2Q, '03, 16

> **V54.14 Aftercare for healing traumatic fracture of leg, unspecified**

> **V54.15 Aftercare for healing traumatic fracture of upper leg**
> > **EXCLUDES** aftercare for healing traumatic fracture of hip (V54.13)
> > **AHA:** 3Q, '06, 6

> **V54.16 Aftercare for healing traumatic fracture of lower leg**

> **V54.17 Aftercare for healing traumatic fracture of vertebrae**

> **V54.19 Aftercare for healing traumatic fracture of other bone**
> > **AHA:** 1Q, '05, 13; 4Q, '02, 80

N Newborn Age: 0   **P** Pediatric Age: 0-17   **M** Maternity Age: 12-55   **A** Adult Age: 15-124   **PDx** Primary Diagnosis

332 – Volume 1 · October 2014   **2015 ICD-9-CM**

V Codes

☑5ᵗʰ **V54.2 Aftercare for healing pathologic fracture**
> EXCLUDES *aftercare following joint replacement (V54.81)*
> AHA: 4Q, '02, 80

V54.20 Aftercare for healing pathologic fracture of arm, unspecified

V54.21 Aftercare for healing pathologic fracture of upper arm

V54.22 Aftercare for healing pathologic fracture of lower arm

V54.23 Aftercare for healing pathologic fracture of hip

V54.24 Aftercare for healing pathologic fracture of leg, unspecified

V54.25 Aftercare for healing pathologic fracture of upper leg
> EXCLUDES *aftercare for healing pathologic fracture of hip (V54.23)*

V54.26 Aftercare for healing pathologic fracture of lower leg

V54.27 Aftercare for healing pathologic fracture of vertebrae
> AHA: 1Q, '07, 6; 4Q, '03, 108

V54.29 Aftercare for healing pathologic fracture of other bone
> AHA: 4Q, '02, 80

☑5ᵗʰ **V54.8 Other orthopedic aftercare**
> AHA: 3Q, '01, 19; 4Q, '99, 5

V54.81 Aftercare following joint replacement
> Use additional code to identify joint replacement site (V43.60-V43.69)
> AHA: 1Q, '11, 9; 1Q, '09, 6; 3Q, '06, 4; 2Q, '04, 15; 4Q, '02, 80

V54.82 Aftercare following explantation of joint prosthesis
> Aftercare following explantation of joint prosthesis, staged procedure
> Encounter for joint prosthesis insertion following prior explantation of joint prosthesis
> AHA: 4Q, '11, 156
> TIP: Assign also a code from subcategory V88.2 to identify the specific joint.

V54.89 Other orthopedic aftercare
> Aftercare for healing fracture NOS

V54.9 Unspecified orthopedic aftercare

☑4ᵗʰ **V55 Attention to artificial openings**
> INCLUDES adjustment or repositioning of catheter
> closure
> passage of sounds or bougies
> reforming
> removal or replacement of catheter
> toilet or cleansing
> EXCLUDES *complications of external stoma (519.00-519.09, 569.60-569.69, 596.81-596.83, 997.49)*
> *status only, without need for care (V44.0-V44.9)*

V55.0 Tracheostomy

V55.1 Gastrostomy
> AHA: 4Q, '99, 9; 3Q, '97, 7, 8; 1Q, '96, 14; 3Q, '95, 13
> TIP: Assign for gastrostomy or PEG tube that has been dislodged or clogged, for which simple irrigation or replacement is performed.

V55.2 Ileostomy

V55.3 Colostomy
> AHA: 1Q, '09, 5; 2Q, '05, 4; 3Q, '97, 9
> Z43.3 Encounter for attention to colostomy   I-10

V55.4 Other artificial opening of digestive tract
> AHA: 2Q, '05, 14; 1Q, '03, 10

V55.5 Cystostomy

V55.6 Other artificial opening of urinary tract
> Nephrostomy   Urethrostomy
> Ureterostomy

V55.7 Artificial vagina

V55.8 Other specified artificial opening

V55.9 Unspecified artificial opening

☑4ᵗʰ **V56 Encounter for dialysis and dialysis catheter care**
> Use additional code to identify the associated condition
> EXCLUDES *dialysis preparation — code to condition*
> AHA: 4Q, '98, 66; 1Q, '93, 29

V56.0 Extracorporeal dialysis   PDx
> Dialysis (renal) NOS
> EXCLUDES *dialysis status (V45.11)*
> AHA: 4Q, '05, 79; 1Q, '04, 23; 4Q, '00, 40; 3Q, '98, 6; 2Q, '98, 20

V56.1 Fitting and adjustment of extracorporeal dialysis catheter
> Removal or replacement of catheter
> Toilet or cleansing
> Use additional code for any concurrent extracorporeal dialysis (V56.0)
> AHA: 2Q, '98, 20

V56.2 Fitting and adjustment of peritoneal dialysis catheter
> Use additional code for any concurrent peritoneal dialysis (V56.8)
> AHA: 4Q, '98, 55

☑5ᵗʰ **V56.3 Encounter for adequacy testing for dialysis**
> AHA: 4Q, '00, 55

V56.31 Encounter for adequacy testing for hemodialysis

V56.32 Encounter for adequacy testing for peritoneal dialysis
> Peritoneal equilibration test

V56.8 Other dialysis
> Peritoneal dialysis
> AHA: 4Q, '98, 55

☑4ᵗʰ **V57 Care involving use of rehabilitation procedures**
> Use additional code to identify underlying condition
> AHA: 3Q, '06, 3; 1Q, '02, 19; 3Q, '97, 12; 1Q, '90, 6; S-O, '86, 3
> TIP: Assign codes from this category for episodes of care related to rehabilitation.

V57.0 Breathing exercises   PDx

V57.1 Other physical therapy   PDx
> Therapeutic and remedial exercises, except breathing
> AHA: 3Q, '06, 4; 2Q, '04, 15; 4Q, '02, 56; 4Q, '99, 5

☑5ᵗʰ **V57.2 Occupational therapy and vocational rehabilitation**

V57.21 Encounter for occupational therapy   PDx
> AHA: 4Q, '99, 7

V57.22 Encounter for vocational therapy   PDx

V57.3 Speech-language therapy   PDx
> AHA: 4Q, '97, 36

V57.4 Orthoptic training   PDx

☑5ᵗʰ **V57.8 Other specified rehabilitation procedure**

V57.81 Orthotic training   PDx
> Gait training in the use of artificial limbs

V57.89 Other   PDx
> Multiple training or therapy
> AHA: 4Q, '07, 94; 3Q, '06, 6; 4Q, '03, 105-106, 108; 2Q, '03, 16; 1Q '02, 16; 3Q, '01, 21; 3Q, '97, 11, 12; S-O, '86, 4

V57.9 Unspecified rehabilitation procedure   PDx

☑4ᵗʰ **V58 Encounter for other and unspecified procedures and aftercare**
> EXCLUDES *convalescence and palliative care (V66)*
> TIP: If a patient is admitted for both radiation therapy and chemotherapy, either code V58.0 or V58.11 may be sequenced as the principal diagnosis.

V58.0 Radiotherapy   PDx
> Encounter or admission for radiotherapy
> EXCLUDES *encounter for radioactive implant — code to condition*
> *radioactive iodine therapy — code to condition*
> AHA: ►1Q, '13, 8;◄ 3Q, '92, 5; 2Q, '90, 7; J-F, '87, 13
> Z51.0 Encounter for antineoplastic radiation therapy   I-10

☑4ᵗʰ / ☑5ᵗʰ Additional Digit Required   Unspecified Code   Other Specified Code   Manifestation Code   ►◄ Revised Text   ● New Code   ▲ Revised Code Title

2015 ICD-9-CM   **October 2014 • Volume 1 – 333**

V Codes

V58.1–V58.74

√5th **V58.1 Encounter for antineoplastic chemotherapy and immunotherapy**
Encounter or admission for chemotherapy
EXCLUDES *chemotherapy and immunotherapy for nonneoplastic conditions — code to condition*
AHA: 1Q, '04, 13; 2Q, '03, 16; 3Q, '93, 4; 2Q, '92, 6; 2Q, '91, 17; 2Q, '90, 7; S-O, '84, 5

V58.11 Encounter for antineoplastic chemotherapy PDx
AHA: 1Q, '12, 13; 2Q, '11, 4; 4Q, '09, 79; 4Q, '08, 82, 155; 4Q, '07, 104; 2Q, '06, 20-21; 4Q, '05, 98
Z51.11 Encounter for antineoplastic chemotherapy I-10

V58.12 Encounter for antineoplastic immunotherapy PDx
AHA: 4Q, '05, 98

V58.2 Blood transfusion, without reported diagnosis

√5th **V58.3 Attention to dressings and sutures**
Change or removal of wound packing
EXCLUDES *attention to drains (V58.49)*
planned postoperative wound closure (V58.41)
AHA: 2Q, '05, 14

V58.30 Encounter for change or removal of nonsurgical wound dressing
Encounter for change or removal of wound dressing NOS
AHA: 4Q, '09, 150; 4Q, '06, 117

V58.31 Encounter for change or removal of surgical wound dressing
AHA: 4Q, '06, 117
Z48.01 Encounter change/removal surgical wound dressing I-10

V58.32 Encounter for removal of sutures
Encounter for removal of staples
AHA: 4Q, '06, 117
Z48.02 Encounter for removal of sutures I-10

√5th **V58.4 Other aftercare following surgery**
NOTE Codes from this subcategory should be used in conjunction with other aftercare codes to fully identify the reason for the aftercare encounter
EXCLUDES *aftercare following sterilization reversal surgery (V26.22)*
attention to artificial openings (V55.0-V55.9)
orthopedic aftercare (V54.0-V54.9)
AHA: 4Q, '99, 9; N-D, '87, 9

V58.41 Encounter for planned postoperative wound closure
EXCLUDES *disruption of operative wound (998.31-998.32)*
encounter for dressings and suture aftercare (V58.30-V58.32)
AHA: 4Q, '99, 15

V58.42 Aftercare following surgery for neoplasm
Conditions classifiable to 140-239
AHA: 4Q, '02, 80

V58.43 Aftercare following surgery for injury and trauma
Conditions classifiable to 800-999
EXCLUDES *aftercare for healing traumatic fracture (V54.10-V54.19)*
AHA: 4Q, '02, 80

V58.44 Aftercare following organ transplant
Use additional code to identify the organ transplanted (V42.0-V42.9)
AHA: 3Q, '11, 5; 4Q, '04, 101

V58.49 Other specified aftercare following surgery
Change or removal of drains
AHA: 1Q, '96, 8, 9

V58.5 Orthodontics
EXCLUDES *fitting and adjustment of orthodontic device (V53.4)*

√5th **V58.6 Long-term (current) drug use**
Long-term (current) prophylactic drug use
EXCLUDES *drug abuse and dependence complicating pregnancy (648.3-648.4)*
drug abuse (305.00-305.93)
drug dependence (304.00-304.93)
hormone replacement therapy (postmenopausal) (V07.4)
use of agents affecting estrogen receptors and estrogen levels (V07.51-V07.59)
AHA: 1Q, '11, 15; 4Q, '08, 159; 4Q, '03, 85; 4Q, '02, 84; 3Q, '02, 15; 4Q, '95, 61
TIP: Do not assign for patients on detoxification drugs or maintenance programs to prevent withdrawal symptoms related to drug dependence; assign instead drug dependence code(s).

V58.61 Long-term (current) use of anticoagulants
EXCLUDES *long-term (current) use of aspirin (V58.66)*
AHA: ▶4Q, '13, 101;◀ 4Q, '08, 135; 3Q, '06, 13; 3Q, '04, 7; 4Q, '03, 108; 3Q, '02, 13-16; 1Q, '02, 15, 16
Z79.01 Long term (current) use of anticoagulants I-10

V58.62 Long-term (current) use of antibiotics
AHA: 4Q, '98, 59

V58.63 Long-term (current) use of antiplatelets/ antithrombotics
EXCLUDES *long-term (current) use of aspirin (V58.66)*

V58.64 Long-term (current) use of non-steroidal anti-inflammatories (NSAID)
EXCLUDES *long-term (current) use of aspirin (V58.66)*

V58.65 Long-term (current) use of steroids
Z79.52 Long term (current) use of systemic steroids I-10

V58.66 Long-term (current) use of aspirin
AHA: 4Q, '04, 102

V58.67 Long-term (current) use of insulin
AHA: ▶3Q, '13, 9;◀ 4Q, '04, 55-56, 103
Z79.4 Long term (current) use of insulin I-10

V58.68 Long term (current) use of bisphosphonates
AHA: 4Q, '11, 157

V58.69 Long-term (current) use of other medications
Other high-risk medications
Long term current use of methadone for pain control
Long term current use of opiate analgesic
EXCLUDES *methadone maintenance NOS (304.00)*
methadone use NOS (304.00)
AHA: ▶2Q, '13, 13, 14;◀ 2Q, '11, 7; 2Q, '10, 10, 13; 4Q, '09, 83; 3Q, '09, 3; 4Q, '08, 156; 2Q, '04, 10; 1Q, '04, 13; 1Q, '03, 11; 2Q, '00, 8; 3Q, '99, 13; 2Q, '99, 17; 1Q, '97, 12; 2Q, '96, 7

√5th **V58.7 Aftercare following surgery to specified body systems, not elsewhere classified**
NOTE Codes from this subcategory should be used in conjunction with other aftercare codes to fully identify the reason for the aftercare encounter
EXCLUDES *aftercare following organ transplant (V58.44)*
aftercare following surgery for neoplasm (V58.42)
AHA: 4Q, '03, 104; 4Q, '02, 80

V58.71 Aftercare following surgery of the sense organs, NEC
Conditions classifiable to 360-379, 380-389
AHA: ▶2Q, '13, 11◀

V58.72 Aftercare following surgery of the nervous system, NEC
Conditions classifiable to 320-359
EXCLUDES *aftercare following surgery of the sense organs, NEC (V58.71)*

V58.73 Aftercare following surgery of the circulatory system, NEC
Conditions classifiable to 390-459
AHA: 2Q, '09, 12; 4Q, '03, 105

V58.74 Aftercare following surgery of the respiratory system, NEC
Conditions classifiable to 460-519

V58.75 Aftercare following surgery of the teeth, oral cavity and digestive system, NEC
Conditions classifiable to 520-579
AHA: 2Q, '05, 14

V58.76 Aftercare following surgery of the genitourinary system, NEC
Conditions classifiable to 580-629
EXCLUDES   *aftercare following sterilization reversal (V26.22)*
AHA: 1Q, '05, 11-12

V58.77 Aftercare following surgery of the skin and subcutaneous tissue, NEC
Conditions classifiable to 680-709

V58.78 Aftercare following surgery of the musculoskeletal system, NEC
Conditions classifiable to 710-739
EXCLUDES   *orthopedic aftercare (V54.01-V54.9)*

√5ᵗʰ **V58.8 Other specified procedures and aftercare**
AHA: 4Q, '94, 45; 2Q, '94, 8

V58.81 Fitting and adjustment of vascular catheter
Removal or replacement of catheter
Toilet or cleansing
EXCLUDES   *complication of renal dialysis (996.73)*
complication of vascular catheter (996.74)
dialysis preparation — code to condition
encounter for dialysis (V56.0-V56.8)
fitting and adjustment of dialysis catheter (V56.1)
AHA: 2Q, '11, 4

V58.82 Fitting and adjustment of nonvascular catheter, NEC
Removal or replacement of catheter
Toilet or cleansing
EXCLUDES   *fitting and adjustment of peritoneal dialysis catheter (V56.2)*
fitting and adjustment of urinary catheter (V53.6)

V58.83 Encounter for therapeutic drug monitoring
Use additional code for any associated long- term (current) drug use (V58.61-V58.69)
EXCLUDES   *blood-drug testing for medico- legal reasons (V70.4)*
DEF: Drug monitoring: Measurement of the level of a specific drug in the body or measurement of a specific function to assess effectiveness of a drug.
AHA: 4Q, '08, 156; 2Q, '04, 10; 1Q, '04, 13;4Q, '03, 85; 4Q, '02, 84; 3Q, '02, 13-16

V58.89 Other specified aftercare
AHA: 4Q, '98, 59

V58.9 Unspecified aftercare

√4ᵗʰ **V59 Donors**
EXCLUDES   *examination of potential donor (V70.8)*
self-donation of organ or tissue — code to condition
AHA: 4Q, '95, 62; 1Q, '90, 10; N-D, '84,
TIP: Assign only for living donations to other individuals, not for self-donation or for cadaveric donations.

√5ᵗʰ **V59.0 Blood**

   V59.01 Whole blood   PDx

   V59.02 Stem cells   PDx

   V59.09 Other   PDx

V59.1 Skin   PDx

V59.2 Bone   PDx

V59.3 Bone marrow   PDx

V59.4 Kidney   PDx

V59.5 Cornea   PDx

V59.6 Liver   PDx

√5ᵗʰ **V59.7 Egg (oocyte) (ovum)**
AHA: 4Q, '05, 99

   V59.70 Egg (oocyte) (ovum) donor, unspecified   PDx ♀

   V59.71 Egg (oocyte) (ovum) donor, under age 35, anonymous recipient   PDx ♀
Egg donor, under age 35 NOS

   V59.72 Egg (oocyte) (ovum) donor, under age 35, designated recipient   PDx ♀

   V59.73 Egg (oocyte) (ovum) donor, age 35 and over, anonymous recipient   PDx ♀
Egg donor, age 35 and over NOS

   V59.74 Egg (oocyte) (ovum) donor, age 35 and over, designated recipient   PDx ♀

V59.8 Other specified organ or tissue   PDx
AHA: 3Q, '02, 20

V59.9 Unspecified organ or tissue   PDx

Persons Encountering Health Services in Other Circumstances (V60-V69)

√4ᵗʰ **V60 Housing, household, and economic circumstances**

V60.0 Lack of housing
Hobos   Transients
Social migrants   Vagabonds
Tramps

V60.1 Inadequate housing
Lack of heating
Restriction of space
Technical defects in home preventing adequate care

V60.2 Inadequate material resources
Economic problem   Poverty NOS

V60.3 Person living alone

V60.4 No other household member able to render care
Person requiring care (has) (is):
family member too handicapped, ill, or otherwise unsuited to render care
partner temporarily away from home
temporarily away from usual place of abode
EXCLUDES   *holiday relief care (V60.5)*

V60.5 Holiday relief care
Provision of health care facilities to a person normally cared for at home, to enable relatives to take a vacation

V60.6 Person living in residential institution
Boarding school resident

√5ᵗʰ **V60.8 Other specified housing or economic circumstances**
AHA: 4Q, '09, 118

   V60.81 Foster care (status)

   V60.89 Other specified housing or economic circumstances

V60.9 Unspecified housing or economic circumstance

√4ᵗʰ **V61 Other family circumstances**
INCLUDES   when these circumstances or fear of them, affecting the person directly involved or others, are mentioned as the reason, justified or not, for seeking or receiving medical advice or care
AHA: 1Q, '90, 9

√5ᵗʰ **V61.0 Family disruption**
AHA: 4Q, '08, 160

   V61.01 Family disruption due to family member on military deployment
Individual or family affected by other family member being on deployment
EXCLUDES   *family disruption due to family member on non-military extended absence from home (V61.08)*

   V61.02 Family disruption due to return of family member from military deployment
Individual or family affected by other family member having returned from deployment (current or past conflict)

   V61.03 Family disruption due to divorce or legal separation

---

√4ᵗʰ √5ᵗʰ Additional Digit Required   Unspecified Code   Other Specified Code   Manifestation Code   ►◄ Revised Text   ● New Code   ▲ Revised Code Title

V Codes

V61.04–V62.84

V61.04 Family disruption due to parent-child estrangement
> **EXCLUDES** *other family estrangement (V61.09)*

V61.05 Family disruption due to child in welfare custody

V61.06 Family disruption due to child in foster care or in care of non-parental family member

V61.07 Family disruption due to death of family member
> **EXCLUDES** *bereavement (V62.82)*
> **AHA:** 4Q, '09, 117

V61.08 Family disruption due to other extended absence of family member
> **EXCLUDES** *family disruption due to family member on military deployment (V61.01)*
> **AHA:** 4Q, '09, 117

V61.09 Other family disruption
> Family estrangement NOS

✓5ᵗʰ V61.1 Counseling for marital and partner problems
> **EXCLUDES** *problems related to:*
> *psychosexual disorders (302.0-302.9)*
> *sexual function (V41.7)*

V61.10 Counseling for marital and partner problems, unspecified
> Marital conflict
> Marital relationship problem
> Partner conflict
> Partner relationship problem

V61.11 Counseling for victim of spousal and partner abuse
> **EXCLUDES** *encounter for treatment of current injuries due to abuse (995.80-995.85)*

V61.12 Counseling for perpetrator of spousal and partner abuse

✓5ᵗʰ V61.2 Parent-child problems

V61.20 Counseling for parent-child problem, unspecified
> Concern about behavior of child
> Parent-child conflict
> Parent-child relationship problem

V61.21 Counseling for victim of child abuse
> Child battering   Child neglect
> **EXCLUDES** *current injuries due to abuse (995.50-995.59)*

V61.22 Counseling for perpetrator of parental child abuse
> **EXCLUDES** *counseling for non-parental abuser (V62.83)*

V61.23 Counseling for parent-biological child problem
> Concern about behavior of biological child
> Parent-biological child conflict
> Parent-biological child relationship problem
> **AHA:** 4Q, '09, 117

V61.24 Counseling for parent-adopted child problem
> Concern about behavior of adopted child
> Parent-adopted child conflict
> Parent-adopted child relationship problem
> **AHA:** 4Q, '09, 117

V61.25 Counseling for parent (guardian)-foster child problem
> Concern about behavior of foster child
> Parent (guardian)-foster child conflict
> Parent (guardian)-foster child relationship problem
> **AHA:** 4Q, '09, 117

V61.29 Other parent-child problems
> **AHA:** 3Q, '99, 16

V61.3 Problems with aged parents or in-laws

✓5ᵗʰ V61.4 Health problems within family

V61.41 Alcoholism in family

V61.42 Substance abuse in family
> **AHA:** 4Q, '09, 117

V61.49 Other
> Care of   } sick or handicapped person
> Presence of }   in family or household

V61.5 Multiparity

V61.6 Illegitimacy or illegitimate pregnancy Ⓜ ♀

V61.7 Other unwanted pregnancy Ⓜ ♀

V61.8 Other specified family circumstances
> Problems with family members NEC
> Sibling relationship problem

V61.9 Unspecified family circumstance

✓4ᵗʰ V62 Other psychosocial circumstances
> **INCLUDES** *those circumstances or fear of them, affecting the person directly involved or others, mentioned as the reason, justified or not, for seeking or receiving medical advice or care*
> **EXCLUDES** *previous psychological trauma (V15.41-V15.49)*

V62.0 Unemployment
> **EXCLUDES** *circumstances when main problem is economic inadequacy or poverty (V60.2)*

V62.1 Adverse effects of work environment

✓5ᵗʰ V62.2 Other occupational circumstances or maladjustment
> **AHA:** 4Q, '08, 160

V62.21 Personal current military deployment status Ⓐ
> Individual (civilian or military) currently deployed in theater or in support of military war, peacekeeping and humanitarian operations

V62.22 Personal history of return from military deployment Ⓐ
> Individual (civilian or military) with past history of military war, peacekeeping and humanitarian deployment (current or past conflict)

V62.29 Other occupational circumstances or maladjustment Ⓐ
> Career choice problem
> Dissatisfaction with employment
> Occupational problem

V62.3 Educational circumstances
> Academic problem
> Dissatisfaction with school environment
> Educational handicap

V62.4 Social maladjustment
> Acculturation problem
> Cultural deprivation
> Political, religious, or sex discrimination
> Social:
>   isolation
>   persecution

V62.5 Legal circumstances
> Imprisonment   Litigation
> Legal investigation   Prosecution

V62.6 Refusal of treatment for reasons of religion or conscience

✓5ᵗʰ V62.8 Other psychological or physical stress, not elsewhere classified

V62.81 Interpersonal problems, not elsewhere classified
> Relational problem NOS

V62.82 Bereavement, uncomplicated
> **EXCLUDES** *bereavement as adjustment reaction (309.0)*
> *family disruption due to death of family member (V61.07)*

V62.83 Counseling for perpetrator of physical/sexual abuse
> **EXCLUDES** *counseling for perpetrator of parental child abuse (V61.22)*
> *counseling for perpetrator of spousal and partner abuse (V61.12)*

V62.84 Suicidal ideation
> **EXCLUDES** *suicidal tendencies (300.9)*
> **DEF:** Thoughts of committing suicide; no actual attempt of suicide has been made.
> **AHA:** 4Q, '05, 96
> **TIP:** Assign for patients who have not attempted suicide, and who may not be considered a suicide risk, but who have indicated thoughts about suicide.
> **R45.851** Suicidal ideations   I-10

V62.85 Homicidal ideation
AHA: 4Q, '10, 110
R45.850 Homicidal ideations

V62.89 Other
Borderline intellectual functioning
Life circumstance problems
Phase of life problems
Religious or spiritual problem

V62.9 Unspecified psychosocial circumstance

✓4ᵗʰ **V63 Unavailability of other medical facilities for care**
AHA: 1Q, '91, 21

V63.0 Residence remote from hospital or other health care facility

V63.1 Medical services in home not available
EXCLUDES no other household member able to render care
(V60.4)
AHA: 4Q, '01, 67; 1Q, '01, 12

V63.2 Person awaiting admission to adequate facility elsewhere

V63.8 Other specified reasons for unavailability of medical facilities
Person on waiting list undergoing social agency investigation

V63.9 Unspecified reason for unavailability of medical facilities

✓4ᵗʰ **V64 Persons encountering health services for specific procedures, not carried out**

✓5ᵗʰ **V64.0 Vaccination not carried out**
AHA: 4Q, '05, 99

V64.00 Vaccination not carried out, unspecified reason

V64.01 Vaccination not carried out because of acute illness

V64.02 Vaccination not carried out because of chronic illness or condition

V64.03 Vaccination not carried out because of immune compromised state

V64.04 Vaccination not carried out because of allergy to vaccine or component
Z28.04 Immunization not carried out pt allergy vaccine I-10

V64.05 Vaccination not carried out because of caregiver refusal
Guardian refusal   Parent refusal
EXCLUDES vaccination not carried out because of caregiver refusal for religious reasons (V64.07)
AHA: ▶3Q, '13, 4;◀ 4Q, '09, 115; 1Q, '07, 12

V64.06 Vaccination not carried out because of patient refusal

V64.07 Vaccination not carried out for religious reasons

V64.08 Vaccination not carried out because patient had disease being vaccinated against

V64.09 Vaccination not carried out for other reason

V64.1 Surgical or other procedure not carried out because of contraindication
TIP: Assign an additional code to indicate the contraindication (reason the surgery or other procedure was canceled).

V64.2 Surgical or other procedure not carried out because of patient's decision
AHA: 2Q, '01, 8

V64.3 Procedure not carried out for other reasons

✓5ᵗʰ **V64.4 Closed surgical procedure converted to open procedure**
AHA: 4Q, '03, 87; 4Q, '98, 68; 4Q, '97, 52

V64.41 Laparoscopic surgical procedure converted to open procedure
AHA: 1Q, '11, 14-15

V64.42 Thoracoscopic surgical procedure converted to open procedure

V64.43 Arthroscopic surgical procedure converted to open procedure

✓4ᵗʰ **V65 Other persons seeking consultation**

V65.0 Healthy person accompanying sick person
Boarder

✓5ᵗʰ **V65.1 Person consulting on behalf of another person**
Advice or treatment for nonattending third party
EXCLUDES concern (normal) about sick person in family (V61.41-V61.49)
AHA: 4Q, '03, 84

V65.11 Pediatric pre-birth visit for expectant parent(s)
Pre-adoption visit for adoptive parent(s)

V65.19 Other person consulting on behalf of another person

V65.2 Person feigning illness
Malingerer   Peregrinating patient
AHA: 3Q, '99, 20
TIP: Assign for patients engaged in what is documented as "drug-seeking behavior."

V65.3 Dietary surveillance and counseling
Dietary surveillance and counseling (in):
NOS
colitis
diabetes mellitus
food allergies or intolerance
gastritis
hypercholesterolemia
hypoglycemia
obesity
Use additional code to identify Body Mass Index (BMI), if known (V85.0-V85.54)
AHA: 4Q, '05, 96

✓5ᵗʰ **V65.4 Other counseling, not elsewhere classified**
Health:
advice
education
instruction
EXCLUDES counseling (for):
contraception (V25.40-V25.49)
genetic (V26.31-V26.39)
on behalf of third party (V65.11-V65.19)
procreative management (V26.41-V26.49)

V65.40 Counseling NOS

V65.41 Exercise counseling

V65.42 Counseling on substance use and abuse
Z71.6 Tobacco abuse counseling I-10

V65.43 Counseling on injury prevention

V65.44 Human immunodeficiency virus [HIV] counseling

V65.45 Counseling on other sexually transmitted diseases

V65.46 Encounter for insulin pump training
Z46.81 Encounter for fitting & adjustment insulin pump I-10

V65.49 Other specified counseling
AHA: 4Q, '08, 156; 2Q, '00, 8

V65.5 Person with feared complaint in whom no diagnosis was made
Feared condition not demonstrated
Problem was normal state
"Worried well"

V65.8 Other reasons for seeking consultation
EXCLUDES specified symptoms
AHA: 3Q, '92, 4

V65.9 Unspecified reason for consultation

✓4ᵗʰ **V66 Convalescence and palliative care**

V66.0 Following surgery PDx

V66.1 Following radiotherapy PDx

V66.2 Following chemotherapy PDx

V66.3 Following psychotherapy and other treatment for mental disorder PDx

---

✓4ᵗʰ
✓5ᵗʰ Additional Digit Required   Unspecified Code   Other Specified Code   Manifestation Code   ▶◀ Revised Text   ● New Code   ▲ Revised Code Title
2015 ICD-9-CM   October 2014 · Volume 1 – 337

V Codes

V66.4–V70.2

V66.4 Following treatment of fracture `PDx`

V66.5 Following other treatment `PDx`

V66.6 Following combined treatment `PDx`

V66.7 Encounter for palliative care
End of life care
Hospice care
Terminal care
Code first underlying disease
AHA: 3Q, '12, 16; 1Q, '12, 14; 3Q, '10, 18; 3Q, '08, 13; 2Q, '05, 9; 4Q, '03, 107; 1Q, '98, 11; 4Q, '96, 47, 48
TIP: Assign as secondary diagnosis when treatment is focused on management of pain and symptoms in a patient with an incurable disease.
Z51.5 Encounter for palliative care `I-10`

V66.9 Unspecified convalescence `PDx`
AHA: 4Q, '99, 8

✓4ᵗʰ **V67 Follow-up examination**
INCLUDES surveillance only following completed treatment
EXCLUDES surveillance of contraception (V25.40-V25.49)
AHA: 4Q, '08, 157; 2Q, '03, 5; 4Q, '94, 98

✓5ᵗʰ **V67.0 Following surgery**
AHA: 4Q, '00, 56; 4Q, '98, 69; 4Q, '97, 50; 2Q, '95, 8;1Q, '95, 4; 3Q, '92, 11

V67.00 Following surgery, unspecified

V67.01 Follow-up vaginal pap smear ♀
Vaginal pap-smear, status-post hysterectomy for malignant condition
Use additional code to identify:
acquired absence of uterus (V88.01-V88.03)
personal history of malignant neoplasm (V10.40-V10.44)
EXCLUDES vaginal pap smear status-post hysterectomy for non-malignant condition (V76.47)
AHA: 4Q, '08, 157

V67.09 Following other surgery
EXCLUDES sperm count following sterilization reversal (V26.22)
sperm count for fertility testing (V26.21)
AHA: ▶4Q, '13, 105;◄ 3Q, '08, 6; 3Q, '03, 16; 3Q, '02, 15

V67.1 Following radiotherapy

V67.2 Following chemotherapy
Cancer chemotherapy follow-up

V67.3 Following psychotherapy and other treatment for mental disorder

V67.4 Following treatment of healed fracture
EXCLUDES current (healing) fracture aftercare (V54.0-V54.9)
AHA: 1Q, '09, 6; 1Q, '90, 7

✓5ᵗʰ **V67.5 Following other treatment**

V67.51 Following completed treatment with high-risk medications, not elsewhere classified
EXCLUDES long-term (current) drug use (V58.61-V58.69)
AHA: 1Q, '99, 5, 6;4Q, '95, 61 ; 1Q, '90, 18

V67.59 Other

V67.6 Following combined treatment

V67.9 Unspecified follow-up examination

✓4ᵗʰ **V68 Encounters for administrative purposes**

✓5ᵗʰ **V68.0 Issue of medical certificates**
EXCLUDES encounter for general medical examination (V70.0-V70.9)

V68.01 Disability examination `PDx`
Use additional code(s) to identify specific examination(s), screening and testing performed (V72.0-V82.9)
AHA: 4Q, '07, 101

V68.09 Other issue of medical certificates `PDx`

V68.1 Issue of repeat prescriptions `PDx`
Issue of repeat prescription for:
appliance
glasses
medications
EXCLUDES repeat prescription for contraceptives (V25.41-V25.49)

V68.2 Request for expert evidence `PDx`

✓5ᵗʰ **V68.8 Other specified administrative purpose**

V68.81 Referral of patient without examination or treatment `PDx`

V68.89 Other `PDx`

V68.9 Unspecified administrative purpose `PDx`

✓4ᵗʰ **V69 Problems related to lifestyle**
AHA: 4Q, '94, 48

V69.0 Lack of physical exercise

V69.1 Inappropriate diet and eating habits
EXCLUDES anorexia nervosa (307.1)
bulimia (783.6)
malnutrition and other nutritional deficiencies (260-269.9)
other and unspecified eating disorders (307.50-307.59)

V69.2 High-risk sexual behavior

V69.3 Gambling and betting
EXCLUDES pathological gambling (312.31)

V69.4 Lack of adequate sleep
Sleep deprivation
EXCLUDES insomnia (780.52)

V69.5 Behavioral insomnia of childhood `P`
DEF: Behaviors on the part of the child or caregivers that cause negative compliance with a child's sleep schedule; results in lack of adequate sleep.
AHA: 4Q, '05, 99

V69.8 Other problems related to lifestyle
Self-damaging behavior

V69.9 Problem related to lifestyle, unspecified

Persons without Reported Diagnosis Encountered During Examination and Investigation of Individuals and Populations (V70-V82)

NOTE Nonspecific abnormal findings disclosed at the time of these examinations are classifiable to categories 790-796.

✓4ᵗʰ **V70 General medical examination**
Use additional code(s) to identify any special screening examination(s) performed (V73.0-V82.9)

V70.0 Routine general medical examination at a health care facility `PDx`
Health checkup
EXCLUDES health checkup of infant or child over 28 days old (V20.2)
health supervision of newborn 8 to 28 days old (V20.32)
health supervision of newborn under 8 days old (V20.31)
pre-procedural general physical examination (V72.83)
AHA: ▶4Q, '13, 101◄

V70.1 General psychiatric examination, requested by the authority `PDx`

V70.2 General psychiatric examination, other and unspecified `PDx`

V70.3 Other medical examination for administrative purposes `PDx`

General medical examination for:
admission to old age home
adoption
camp
driving license
immigration and naturalization
insurance certification
marriage
prison
school admission
sports competition

EXCLUDES *attendance for issue of medical certificates (V68.0)*
pre-employment screening (V70.5)

AHA: 3Q, '08, 6; 1Q, '90, 6
Z02.6 Encounter for exam for insurance purposes `I-10`

V70.4 Examination for medicolegal reasons `PDx`

Blood-alcohol tests   Paternity testing
Blood-drug tests

EXCLUDES *examination and observation following:*
accidents (V71.3, V71.4)
assault (V71.6)
rape (V71.5)

V70.5 Health examination of defined subpopulations

Armed forces personnel
Inhabitants of institutions
Occupational healthexaminations
Pre-employment screening
Preschool children
Prisoners
Prostitutes
Refugees
School children
Students

V70.6 Health examination in population surveys `PDx`

EXCLUDES *special screening (V73.0-V82.9)*

V70.7 Examination of participant in clinical trial

Examination of participant or control in clinical research

AHA: 2Q, '06, 5-6; 4Q, '01, 55

V70.8 Other specified general medical examinations `PDx`

Examination of potential donor of organ or tissue

V70.9 Unspecified general medical examination `PDx`

`√4th` **V71 Observation and evaluation for suspected conditions not found**

INCLUDES This category is to be used when persons without a diagnosis are suspected of having an abnormal condition, without signs or symptoms, which requires study, but after examination and observation, is found not to exist. This category is also for use for administrative and legal observation status.

EXCLUDES *suspected maternal and fetal conditions not found (V89.01-V89.09)*

AHA: 4Q, '94, 47; 2Q, '90, 5; M-A, '87, 1
TIP: Assign observation codes only as principal/first-listed diagnosis and only if there is no documentation of any signs or symptoms.

`√5th` **V71.0 Observation for suspected mental condition**

V71.01 Adult antisocial behavior `A` `PDx`

Dyssocial behavior or gang activity in adult without manifest psychiatric disorder

V71.02 Childhood or adolescent antisocial behavior `PDx`

Dyssocial behavior or gang activity in child or adolescent without manifest psychiatric disorder

V71.09 Other suspected mental condition `PDx`

V71.1 Observation for suspected malignant neoplasm `PDx`

V71.2 Observation for suspected tuberculosis `PDx`

V71.3 Observation following accident at work `PDx`

V71.4 Observation following other accident `PDx`

Examination of individual involved in motor vehicle traffic accident

AHA: 1Q, '06, 9

V71.5 Observation following alleged rape or seduction `PDx`

Examination of victim or culprit

V71.6 Observation following other inflicted injury `PDx`

Examination of victim or culprit

V71.7 Observation for suspected cardiovascular disease `PDx`

AHA: 1Q, '04, 6; 3Q, '90, 10; S-O, '87, 10

`√5th` **V71.8 Observation and evaluation for other specified suspected conditions**

EXCLUDES *contact with and (suspected) exposure to (potentially) hazardous substances (V15.84-V15.86, V87.0-V87.31)*

AHA: 4Q, '00, 54 ; 1Q, '90, 19

V71.81 Abuse and neglect `PDx`

EXCLUDES *adult abuse and neglect (995.80-995.85)*
child abuse and neglect (995.50-995.59)

AHA: 4Q, '00, 55

V71.82 Observation and evaluation for suspected exposure to anthrax `PDx`

AHA: 4Q, '02, 70, 85

V71.83 Observation and evaluation for suspected exposure to other biological agent `PDx`

AHA: 4Q, '03, 47

V71.89 Other specified suspected conditions `PDx`

AHA: 2Q, '11, 4; 3Q, '08, 7; 2Q, '03, 15

V71.9 Observation for unspecified suspected condition `PDx`

AHA: 1Q, '02, 6

`√4th` **V72 Special investigations and examinations**

INCLUDES routine examination of specific system

Use additional code(s) to identify any special screening examination(s) performed (V73.0-V82.9)

EXCLUDES *general medical examination (V70.0-V70.4)*
general screening examination of defined population groups (V70.5, V70.6, V70.7)
health supervision of newborn 8 to 28 days old (V20.32)
health supervision of newborn under 8 days old (V20.31)
routine examination of infant or child over 28 days old (V20.2)

V72.0 Examination of eyes and vision

AHA: 1Q, '04, 15

`√5th` **V72.1 Examination of ears and hearing**

AHA: 1Q, '04, 15

V72.11 Encounter for hearing examination following failed hearing screening

AHA: 3Q, '11, 3; 4Q, '06, 118
Z01.110 Encounter hearing exam follow failed hearing scr `I-10`

V72.12 Encounter for hearing conservation and treatment

AHA: 4Q, '07, 100

V72.19 Other examination of ears and hearing

V72.2 Dental examination

`√5th` **V72.3 Gynecological examination**

EXCLUDES *cervical Papanicolaou smear without general gynecological examination (V76.2)*
routine examination in contraceptive management (V25.40-V25.49)

V72.31 Routine gynecological examination ♀

General gynecological examination with or without Papanicolaou cervical smear
Pelvic examination (annual) (periodic)

Use additional code to identify:
human papillomavirus (HPV) screening (V73.81)
routine vaginal Papanicolaou smear (V76.47)

AHA: 2Q, '06, 2-3; 4Q, '05, 98

`√4th` `√5th` Additional Digit Required   Unspecified Code   Other Specified Code   Manifestation Code   ►◄ Revised Text   ● New Code   ▲ Revised Code Title

V Codes

V72.32–V76.10

V72.32 Encounter for Papanicolaou cervical smear to confirm findings of recent normal smear following initial abnormal smear ♀
AHA: 2Q, '06, 4

✓5th **V72.4 Pregnancy examination or test**
AHA: 4Q, '05, 98

V72.40 Pregnancy examination or test, pregnancy unconfirmed ♀
Possible pregnancy, not (yet) confirmed

V72.41 Pregnancy examination or test, negative result ♀

V72.42 Pregnancy examination or test, positive result ♀ M

V72.5 Radiological examination, not elsewhere classified
Routine chest x-ray
EXCLUDES *radiologic examinations as part of pre-procedural testing (V72.81-V72.84)*
AHA: 1Q, '90, 19

✓5th **V72.6 Laboratory examination**
Encounters for blood and urine testing
AHA: 4Q, '09, 117-118; 2Q, '06, 4; 1Q, '90, 22

V72.60 Laboratory examination, unspecified

V72.61 Antibody response examination
Immunity status testing
EXCLUDES *encounter for allergy testing (V72.7)*

V72.62 Laboratory examination ordered as part of a routine general medical examination
Blood tests for routine general physical examination

V72.63 Pre-procedural laboratory examination
Blood tests prior to treatment or procedure
Pre-operative laboratory examination

V72.69 Other laboratory examination

V72.7 Diagnostic skin and sensitization tests
Allergy tests
Skin tests for hypersensitivity
EXCLUDES *diagnostic skin tests for bacterial diseases (V74.0-V74.9)*

✓5th **V72.8 Other specified examinations**
EXCLUDES *pre-procedural laboratory examinations (V72.63)*

V72.81 Pre-operative cardiovascular examination
Pre-procedural cardiovascular examination
Z01.810 Encounter for preprocedural cardiovascular exam   I-10

V72.82 Pre-operative respiratory examination
Pre-procedural respiratory examination
AHA: 3Q, '96, 14

V72.83 Other specified pre-operative examination
Examination prior to chemotherapy
Other pre-procedural examination
Pre-procedural general physical examination
EXCLUDES *routine general medical examination (V70.0)*
AHA: ▶2Q, '13, 11;◀ 3Q, '96, 14

V72.84 Pre-operative examination, unspecified
Pre-procedural examination, unspecified

V72.85 Other specified examination
AHA: 1Q, '12, 10; 4Q, '05, 96; 1Q, '04, 12

V72.86 Encounter for blood typing

V72.9 Unspecified examination
AHA: 4Q, '06, 117

✓4th **V73 Special screening examination for viral and chlamydial diseases**
AHA: 1Q, '04, 11

V73.0 Poliomyelitis

V73.1 Smallpox

V73.2 Measles

V73.3 Rubella

V73.4 Yellow fever

V73.5 Other arthropod-borne viral diseases
Dengue fever
Hemorrhagic fever
Viral encephalitis:
mosquito-borne
tick-borne

V73.6 Trachoma

✓5th **V73.8 Other specified viral and chlamydial diseases**

V73.81 Human papillomavirus [HPV]
AHA: 4Q, '07, 100

V73.88 Other specified chlamydial diseases
AHA: 4Q, '07, 124

V73.89 Other specified viral diseases

✓5th **V73.9 Unspecified viral and chlamydial disease**

V73.98 Unspecified chlamydial disease

V73.99 Unspecified viral disease

✓4th **V74 Special screening examination for bacterial and spirochetal diseases**
INCLUDES diagnostic skin tests for these diseases
AHA: 1Q, '04, 11

V74.0 Cholera

V74.1 Pulmonary tuberculosis

V74.2 Leprosy [Hansen's disease]

V74.3 Diphtheria

V74.4 Bacterial conjunctivitis

V74.5 Venereal disease
Screening for bacterial and spirochetal sexually transmitted diseases
Screening for sexually transmitted diseases NOS
EXCLUDES *special screening for nonbacterial sexually transmitted diseases (V73.81-V73.89, V75.4, V75.8)*
AHA: 4Q, '07, 124

V74.6 Yaws

V74.8 Other specified bacterial and spirochetal diseases
Brucellosis
Leptospirosis
Plague
Tetanus
Whooping cough

V74.9 Unspecified bacterial and spirochetal disease

✓4th **V75 Special screening examination for other infectious diseases**
AHA: 1Q, '04, 11

V75.0 Rickettsial diseases

V75.1 Malaria

V75.2 Leishmaniasis

V75.3 Trypanosomiasis
Chagas' disease
Sleeping sickness

V75.4 Mycotic infections

V75.5 Schistosomiasis

V75.6 Filariasis

V75.7 Intestinal helminthiasis

V75.8 Other specified parasitic infections

V75.9 Unspecified infectious disease

✓4th **V76 Special screening for malignant neoplasms**
AHA: 1Q, '04, 11
TIP: Whenever a screening examination is performed, the screening code is the first-listed code, regardless of the findings or any procedure that is performed as a result of the findings.

V76.0 Respiratory organs

✓5th **V76.1 Breast**
AHA: 4Q, '98, 67

V76.10 Breast screening, unspecified

V76.11 Screening mammogram for high-risk patient ♀
　　AHA: 2Q, '03, 4

V76.12 Other screening mammogram
　　AHA: 4Q, '09, 106; 2Q, '06, 10; 2Q, '03, 3-4

V76.19 Other screening breast examination

V76.2 Cervix ♀
　　Routine cervical Papanicolaou smear
　　EXCLUDES special screening for human papillomavirus (V73.81)
　　　　that as part of a general gynecological examination
　　　　(V72.31)

V76.3 Bladder

√5ᵗʰ **V76.4 Other sites**

V76.41 Rectum

V76.42 Oral cavity

V76.43 Skin

V76.44 Prostate ♂
　　Z12.5 Encounter screening malignant neoplasm　I-10
　　prostate

V76.45 Testis ♂

V76.46 Ovary ♀
　　AHA: 4Q, '00, 52

V76.47 Vagina ♀
　　Vaginal pap smear status-post hysterectomy for
　　　non-malignant condition
　　Use additional code to identify acquired absence of
　　uterus (V88.01-V88.03)
　　EXCLUDES vaginal pap smear status-post hysterectomy
　　　　for malignant condition (V67.01)
　　AHA: 4Q, '08, 157; 4Q, '00, 52

V76.49 Other sites
　　AHA: 1Q, '99, 4

√5ᵗʰ **V76.5 Intestine**
　　AHA: 4Q, '00, 52

V76.50 Intestine, unspecified

V76.51 Colon
　　Screening colonoscopy NOS
　　EXCLUDES rectum (V76.41)
　　AHA: ▶4Q, '13, 103, 104;◀4Q, '01, 56
　　Z12.11 Encounter screening malignant neoplasm　I-10
　　of colon

V76.52 Small intestine

√5ᵗʰ **V76.8 Other neoplasm**
　　AHA: 4Q, '00, 52

V76.81 Nervous system

V76.89 Other neoplasm

V76.9 Unspecified

√4ᵗʰ **V77 Special screening for endocrine, nutritional, metabolic, and
immunity disorders**
　　AHA: 1Q, '04, 11

V77.0 Thyroid disorders

V77.1 Diabetes mellitus

V77.2 Malnutrition

V77.3 Phenylketonuria [PKU]

V77.4 Galactosemia

V77.5 Gout

V77.6 Cystic fibrosis
　　Screening for mucoviscidosis

V77.7 Other inborn errors of metabolism

V77.8 Obesity

√5ᵗʰ **V77.9 Other and unspecified endocrine, nutritional, metabolic,
and immunity disorders**
　　AHA: 4Q, '00, 53

V77.91 Screening for lipoid disorders
　　Screening for cholesterol level
　　Screening for hypercholesterolemia
　　Screening for hyperlipidemia

**V77.99 Other and unspecified endocrine nutritional
metabolic and immunity disorders**

√4ᵗʰ **V78 Special screening for disorders of blood and blood-forming
organs**
　　AHA: 1Q, '04, 11

V78.0 Iron deficiency anemia

V78.1 Other and unspecified deficiency anemia

V78.2 Sickle cell disease or trait

V78.3 Other hemoglobinopathies

V78.8 Other disorders of blood and blood-forming organs

V78.9 Unspecified disorder of blood and blood-forming organs

√4ᵗʰ **V79 Special screening for mental disorders and developmental
handicaps**
　　AHA: 1Q, '04, 11

V79.0 Depression

V79.1 Alcoholism

V79.2 Intellectual disabilities

V79.3 Developmental handicaps in early childhood

**V79.8 Other specified mental disorders and
developmental handicaps**

**V79.9 Unspecified mental disorder and
developmental handicap**

√4ᵗʰ **V80 Special screening for neurological, eye, and ear diseases**
　　AHA: 1Q, '04, 11

√5ᵗʰ **V80.0 Neurological conditions**
　　AHA: 4Q, '09, 116

V80.01 Traumatic brain injury
V80.09 Other neurological conditions

V80.1 Glaucoma

V80.2 Other eye conditions
　　Screening for:
　　　cataract
　　　congenital anomaly of eye
　　　senile macular lesions
　　EXCLUDES general vision examination (V72.0)

V80.3 Ear diseases
　　EXCLUDES general hearing examination (V72.11-V72.19)

√4ᵗʰ **V81 Special screening for cardiovascular, respiratory, and
genitourinary diseases**
　　AHA: 1Q, '04, 11

V81.0 Ischemic heart disease

V81.1 Hypertension

V81.2 Other and unspecified cardiovascular conditions

V81.3 Chronic bronchitis and emphysema

V81.4 Other and unspecified respiratory conditions
　　EXCLUDES screening for:
　　　lung neoplasm (V76.0)
　　　pulmonary tuberculosis (V74.1)

V81.5 Nephropathy
　　Screening for asymptomatic bacteriuria

V81.6 Other and unspecified genitourinary conditions

√4ᵗʰ **V82 Special screening for other conditions**
　　AHA: 1Q, '04, 11

V82.0 Skin conditions

V82.1 Rheumatoid arthritis

V82.2 Other rheumatic disorders

√4ᵗʰ √5ᵗʰ Additional Digit Required　　Unspecified Code　　Other Specified Code　　Manifestation Code　　▶◀ Revised Text　　● New Code　　▲ Revised Code Title

V Codes

V82.3 Congenital dislocation of hip

V82.4 Maternal postnatal screening for chromosomal anomalies ♀

> EXCLUDES *antenatal screening by amniocentesis (V28.0)*

V82.5 Chemical poisoning and other contamination
Screening for:
heavy metal poisoning
ingestion of radioactive substance
poisoning from contaminated water supply
radiation exposure

V82.6 Multiphasic screening

✓5ᵗʰ **V82.7 Genetic screening**

> EXCLUDES *genetic testing for procreative management (V26.31-V26.39)*

V82.71 Screening for genetic disease carrier status
AHA: 4Q, '06, 118

V82.79 Other genetic screening
AHA: 4Q, '06, 118

✓5ᵗʰ **V82.8 Other specified conditions**
AHA: 4Q, '00, 53

V82.81 Osteoporosis
Use additional code to identify:
hormone replacement therapy (postmenopausal) status (V07.4)
postmenopausal (age-related) (natural) status (V49.81)
AHA: 4Q, '00, 54

V82.89 Other specified conditions

V82.9 Unspecified condition

Genetics (V83-V84)

✓4ᵗʰ **V83 Genetic carrier status**
AHA: 4Q, '02, 79; 4Q, '01, 54
TIP: The patient does not have the disease or carry a risk of developing it, but may genetically pass it to offspring who then may develop it.

✓5ᵗʰ **V83.0 Hemophilia A carrier**

V83.01 Asymptomatic hemophilia A carrier

V83.02 Symptomatic hemophilia A carrier

✓5ᵗʰ **V83.8 Other genetic carrier status**

V83.81 Cystic fibrosis gene carrier

V83.89 Other genetic carrier status

✓4ᵗʰ **V84 Genetic susceptibility to disease**

> INCLUDES confirmed abnormal gene
> EXCLUDES *chromosomal anomalies (758.0-758.9)*

Use additional code, if applicable, for any associated family history of the disease (V16-V19)
AHA: 4Q, '04, 106
TIP: The patient has a gene that increases the risk of developing a specific disease; assign only as a secondary condition.

✓5ᵗʰ **V84.0 Genetic susceptibility to malignant neoplasm**
Code first, if applicable, any current malignant neoplasms (140.0-195.8, 200.0-208.9, 230.0-234.9)
Use additional code, if applicable, for any personal history of malignant neoplasm (V10.0-V10.9)

V84.01 Genetic susceptibility to malignant neoplasm of breast
AHA: 2Q, '11, 12; 4Q, '04, 107
Z15.01 Genetic susceptibility malignant neoplasm breast I-10

V84.02 Genetic susceptibility to malignant neoplasm of ovary ♀

V84.03 Genetic susceptibility to malignant neoplasm of prostate ♂

V84.04 Genetic susceptibility to malignant neoplasm of endometrium ♀

V84.09 Genetic susceptibility to other malignant neoplasm
AHA: ▶2Q, '13, 15◀

✓5ᵗʰ **V84.8 Genetic susceptibility to other disease**

V84.81 Genetic susceptibility to multiple endocrine neoplasia [MEN]

> EXCLUDES *multiple endocrine neoplasia [MEN] syndromes (258.01-258.03)*

AHA: 4Q, '07, 100

V84.89 Genetic susceptibility to other disease
AHA: ▶4Q, '13, 87◀

Body Mass Index (V85)

✓4ᵗʰ **V85 Body Mass Index [BMI]**
Kilograms per meters squared
NOTE BMI adult codes are for use for persons over 20 years old
AHA: 3Q, '11, 4-5; 2Q, '10, 15; 4Q, '08, 191; 4Q, '05, 97
TIP: While BMI may be coded from dietician or other caregiver documentation, the diagnosis of being overweight or obese must be coded from physician documentation.

V85.0 Body Mass Index less than 19, adult A

V85.1 Body Mass Index between 19-24, adult A

✓5ᵗʰ **V85.2 Body Mass Index between 25-29, adult**

V85.21 Body Mass Index 25.0-25.9, adult A

V85.22 Body Mass Index 26.0-26.9, adult A

V85.23 Body Mass Index 27.0-27.9, adult A

V85.24 Body Mass Index 28.0-28.9, adult A

V85.25 Body Mass Index 29.0-29.9, adult A

✓5ᵗʰ **V85.3 Body Mass Index between 30-39, adult**

V85.30 Body Mass Index 30.0-30.9, adult A

V85.31 Body Mass Index 31.0-31.9, adult A

V85.32 Body Mass Index 32.0-32.9, adult A

V85.33 Body Mass Index 33.0-33.9, adult A

V85.34 Body Mass Index 34.0-34.9, adult A

V85.35 Body Mass Index 35.0-35.9, adult A

V85.36 Body Mass Index 36.0-36.9, adult A

V85.37 Body Mass Index 37.0-37.9, adult A

V85.38 Body Mass Index 38.0-38.9, adult A

V85.39 Body Mass Index 39.0-39.9, adult A

✓5ᵗʰ **V85.4 Body Mass Index 40 and over, adult**
AHA: 4Q, '10, 81, 109

V85.41 Body Mass Index 40.0-44.9, adult A
AHA: 4Q, '10, 109

V85.42 Body Mass Index 45.0-49.9, adult A

V85.43 Body Mass Index 50.0-59.9, adult A

V85.44 Body Mass Index 60.0-69.9, adult A

V85.45 Body Mass Index 70 and over, adult A

✓5ᵗʰ **V85.5 Body Mass Index, pediatric**
NOTE BMI pediatric codes are for use for persons age 2-20 years old. These percentiles are based on the growth charts published by the Centers for Disease Control and Prevention (CDC)
AHA: 4Q, '06, 118

V85.51 Body Mass Index, pediatric, less than 5th percentile for age P

V85.52 Body Mass Index, pediatric, 5th percentile to less than 85th percentile for age P

V85.53 Body Mass Index, pediatric, 85th percentile to less than 95th percentile for age P

V85.54 Body Mass Index, pediatric, greater than or equal to 95th percentile for age P
Z68.54 Body mass index (BMI) ≥ 95% for age I-10

N Newborn Age: 0   P Pediatric Age: 0-17   M Maternity Age: 12-55   A Adult Age: 15-124   PDx Primary Diagnosis

Estrogen Receptor Status (V86)

√4ᵗʰ **V86 Estrogen receptor status**
Code first malignant neoplasm of breast (174.0-174.9, 175.0-175.9)
AHA: 4Q, '06, 118

V86.0 Estrogen receptor positive status [ER+]

V86.1 Estrogen receptor negative status [ER-]

Other Specified Personal Exposures and History Presenting Hazards to Health (V87)

√4ᵗʰ **V87 Other specified personal exposures and history presenting hazards to health**

√5ᵗʰ **V87.0 Contact with and (suspected) exposure to hazardous metals**
EXCLUDES exposure to lead (V15.86)
toxic effect of metals (984.0-985.9)
AHA: 4Q, '08, 158

V87.01 Arsenic

V87.02 Contact with and (suspected) exposure to uranium
EXCLUDES retained depleted uranium fragments (V90.01)
AHA: 4Q, '11, 156

V87.09 Other hazardous metals
Chromium compounds   Nickel dust

√5ᵗʰ **V87.1 Contact with and (suspected) exposure to hazardous aromatic compounds**
EXCLUDES toxic effects of aromatic compounds (982.0, 983.0)
AHA: 4Q, '08, 158

V87.11 Aromatic amines

V87.12 Benzene

V87.19 Other hazardous aromatic compounds
Aromatic dyes NOS
Polycyclic aromatic hydrocarbons

V87.2 Contact with and (suspected) exposure to other potentially hazardous chemicals
Dyes NOS
EXCLUDES exposure to asbestos (V15.84)
toxic effect of chemicals (980-989)
AHA: 4Q, '08, 158

√5ᵗʰ **V87.3 Contact with and (suspected) exposure to other potentially hazardous substances**
EXCLUDES contact with and (suspected) exposure to potentially hazardous body fluids (V15.85)
personal history of retained foreign body fully removed (V15.53)
toxic effect of substances (980-989)

V87.31 Exposure to mold

V87.32 Contact with and (suspected) exposure to algae bloom
AHA: 4Q, '09, 116

V87.39 Contact with and (suspected) exposure to other potentially hazardous substances

√5ᵗʰ **V87.4 Personal history of drug therapy**
EXCLUDES long-term (current) drug use (V58.61-V58.69)
AHA: 4Q, '09, 116; 4Q, '08, 159

V87.41 Personal history of antineoplastic chemotherapy
Z92.21 Personal hx antineoplastic chemotherapy   I-10

V87.42 Personal history of monoclonal drug therapy

V87.43 Personal history of estrogen therapy

V87.44 Personal history of inhaled steroid therapy

V87.45 Personal history of systemic steroid therapy
Personal history of steroid therapy NOS

V87.46 Personal history of immunosuppression therapy
EXCLUDES personal history of steroid therapy (V87.44, V87.45)

V87.49 Personal history of other drug therapy

Acquired Absence of Other Organs and Tissue (V88)

√4ᵗʰ **V88 Acquired absence of other organs and tissue**

√5ᵗʰ **V88.0 Acquired absence of cervix and uterus**
AHA: 4Q, '08, 157

V88.01 Acquired absence of both cervix and uterus   ♀
Acquired absence of uterus NOS
Status post total hysterectomy

V88.02 Acquired absence of uterus with remaining cervical stump   ♀
Status post partial hysterectomy with remaining cervical stump

V88.03 Acquired absence of cervix with remaining uterus   ♀

√5ᵗʰ **V88.1 Acquired absence of pancreas**
Use additional code to identify any associated:
insulin use (V58.67)
secondary diabetes mellitus (249.00-249.91)
AHA: 4Q, '10, 109

V88.11 Acquired total absence of pancreas
Acquired absence of pancreas NOS

V88.12 Acquired partial absence of pancreas

√5ᵗʰ **V88.2 Acquired absence of joint**
Acquired absence of joint following prior explantation of joint prosthesis
Joint prosthesis explantation status
AHA: 4Q, '11, 156-157

V88.21 Acquired absence of hip joint
Acquired absence of hip joint following explantation of joint prosthesis, with or without presence of antibiotic-impregnated cement spacer

V88.22 Acquired absence of knee joint
Acquired absence of knee joint following explantation of joint prosthesis, with or without presence of antibiotic-impregnated cement spacer

V88.29 Acquired absence of other joint
Acquired absence of other joint following explantation of joint prosthesis, with or without presence of antibiotic-impregnated cement spacer

Other Suspected Conditions Not Found (V89)

√4ᵗʰ **V89 Other suspected conditions not found**

√5ᵗʰ **V89.0 Suspected maternal and fetal conditions not found**
EXCLUDES known or suspected fetal anomalies affecting management of mother, not ruled out (655.00, 655.93, 656.00-656.93, 657.00-657.03, 658.00-658.93)
newborn and perinatal conditions — code to condition
AHA: 4Q, '08, 159
TIP: These investigations are performed while the fetus is in utero; the codes should be assigned only on the mother's medical record.

V89.01 Suspected problem with amniotic cavity and membrane not found   M♀
Suspected oligohydramnios not found
Suspected polyhydramnios not found

V89.02 Suspected placental problem not found   M♀

V89.03 Suspected fetal anomaly not found   M♀

V89.04 Suspected problem with fetal growth not found   M♀

V89.05 Suspected cervical shortening not found   M♀

V89.09 Other suspected maternal and fetal condition not found   M♀

√4ᵗʰ
√5ᵗʰ Additional Digit Required   **Unspecified Code**   Other Specified Code   Manifestation Code   ►◄ Revised Text   ● New Code   ▲ Revised Code Title

Retained Foreign Body (V90)

✓4ᵗʰ **V90 Retained foreign body**

Embedded fragment (status)

Embedded splinter (status)

Retained foreign body status

> EXCLUDES   *artificial joint prosthesis status (V43.60-V43.69)*
> *foreign body accidentally left during a procedure (998.4)*
> *foreign body entering through orifice (930.0-939.9)*
> *in situ cardiac devices (V45.00-V45.09)*
> *organ or tissue replaced by other means (V43.0-V43.89)*
> *organ or tissue replaced by transplant (V42.0-V42.9)*
> *personal history of retained foreign body removed (V15.53)*
> *superficial foreign body (splinter) (categories 910-917 and 919 with 4ᵗʰ character 6 or 7, 918.0)*

AHA: 4Q, '10, 109

✓5ᵗʰ **V90.0 Retained radioactive fragment**

    V90.01 Retained depleted uranium fragments

    V90.09 Other retained radioactive fragments

        Other retained depleted isotope fragments

        Retained nontherapeutic radioactive fragments

✓5ᵗʰ **V90.1 Retained metal fragments**

> EXCLUDES   *retained radioactive metal fragments (V90.01-V90.09)*

    V90.10 Retained metal fragments, unspecified

        Retained metal fragment NOS

    V90.11 Retained magnetic metal fragments

    V90.12 Retained nonmagnetic metal fragments

V90.2 Retained plastic fragments

    Acrylics fragments

    Diethylhexylphthalates fragments

    Isocyanate fragments

✓5ᵗʰ **V90.3 Retained organic fragments**

    V90.31 Retained animal quills or spines

    V90.32 Retained tooth

    V90.33 Retained wood fragments

    V90.39 Other retained organic fragments

✓5ᵗʰ **V90.8 Other specified retained foreign body**

    V90.81 Retained glass fragments

    V90.83 Retained stone or crystalline fragments

        Retained concrete or cement fragments

    V90.89 Other specified retained foreign body

V90.9 Retained foreign body, unspecified material

Multiple Gestation Placenta Status (V91)

✓4ᵗʰ **V91 Multiple gestation placenta status**

Code first multiple gestation (651.0-651.9)

AHA: 4Q, '10, 110

✓5ᵗʰ **V91.0 Twin gestation placenta status**

    V91.00 Twin gestation, unspecified number of placenta, unspecified number of amniotic sacs   M♀

    V91.01 Twin gestation, monochorionic/monoamniotic (one placenta, one amniotic sac)   M♀

    V91.02 Twin gestation, monochorionic/diamniotic (one placenta, two amniotic sacs)   M♀

    V91.03 Twin gestation, dichorionic/diamniotic (two placentae, two amniotic sacs)   M♀

    V91.09 Twin gestation, unable to determine number of placenta and number of amniotic sacs   M♀

✓5ᵗʰ **V91.1 Triplet gestation placenta status**

    V91.10 Triplet gestation, unspecified number of placenta and unspecified number of amniotic sacs   M♀

    V91.11 Triplet gestation, with two or more monochorionic fetuses   M♀

    V91.12 Triplet gestation, with two or more monoamniotic fetuses   M♀

    V91.19 Triplet gestation, unable to determine number of placenta and number of amniotic sacs   M♀

✓5ᵗʰ **V91.2 Quadruplet gestation placenta status**

    V91.20 Quadruplet gestation, unspecified number of placenta and unspecified number of amniotic sacs   M♀

    V91.21 Quadruplet gestation, with two or more monochorionic fetuses   M♀

    V91.22 Quadruplet gestation, with two or more monoamniotic fetuses   M♀

    V91.29 Quadruplet gestation, unable to determine number of placenta and number of amniotic sacs   M♀

✓5ᵗʰ **V91.9 Other specified multiple gestation placenta status**

Placenta status for multiple gestations greater than quadruplets

    V91.90 Other specified multiple gestation, unspecified number of placenta and unspecified number of amniotic sacs   M♀

    V91.91 Other specified multiple gestation, with two or more monochorionic fetuses   M♀

    V91.92 Other specified multiple gestation, with two or more monoamniotic fetuses   M♀

    V91.99 Other specified multiple gestation, unable to determine number of placenta and number of amniotic sacs   M♀

Supplementary Classification of External Causes of Injury and Poisoning (E000-E999)

This section is provided to permit the classification of environmental events, circumstances, and conditions as the cause of injury, poisoning, and other adverse effects. Where a code from this section is applicable, it is intended that it shall be used in addition to a code from one of the main chapters of ICD-9-CM, indicating the nature of the condition. Certain other conditions which may be stated to be due to external causes are classified in Chapters 1 to 16 of ICD-9-CM. For these, the "E" code classification should be used as an additional code for more detailed analysis.

Machinery accidents [other than those connected with transport] are classifiable to category E919, in which the fourth digit allows a broad classification of the type of machinery involved.

Categories for "late effects" of accidents and other external causes are to be found at E929, E959, E969, E977, E989, and E999.

External Cause Status (E000)

NOTE A code from category E000 may be used in conjunction with the external cause code(s) assigned to a record to indicate the status of the person at the time the event occurred. A single code from category E000 should be assigned for an encounter.

√4th E000 External cause status

E000.0 Civilian activity done for income or pay
Civilian activity done for financial or other compensation
EXCLUDES *military activity (E000.1)*

E000.2 Volunteer activity
EXCLUDES *activity of child or other family member assisting in compensated work of other family member (E000.8)*

E000.1 Military activity
EXCLUDES *activity of off-duty military personnel (E000.8)*

E000.8 Other external cause status
Activity of child or other family member assisting in compensated work of other family member
Activity NEC
Hobby not done for income
Leisure activity
Off-duty activity of military personnel
Recreation or sport not for income or while a student
Student activity
EXCLUDES *civilian activity done for income or compensation (E000.0)*
military activity (E000.1)

E000.9 Unspecified external cause status

Activity (E001-E030)

NOTE Categories E001 to E030 are provided for use to indicate the activity of the person seeking healthcare for an injury or health condition, such as a heart attack while shoveling snow, which resulted from, or was contributed to, by the activity. These codes are appropriate for use for both acute injuries, such as those from chapter 17, and conditions that are due to the long-term, cumulative affects of an activity, such as those from chapter 13. They are also appropriate for use with external cause codes for cause and intent if identifying the activity provides additional information on the event.

These codes should be used in conjunction with other external cause codes for external cause status (E000) and place of occurrence (E849).

This section contains the following broad activity categories:

E001 Activities involving walking and running
E002 Activities involving water and water craft
E003 Activities involving ice and snow
E004 Activities involving climbing, rappelling, and jumping off
E005 Activities involving dancing and other rhythmic movement
E006 Activities involving other sports and athletics played individually
E007 Activities involving other sports and athletics played as a team or group
E008 Activities involving other specified sports and athletics
E009 Activity involving other cardiorespiratory exercise
E010 Activity involving other muscle strengthening exercises
E011 Activities involving computer technology and electronic devices
E012 Activities involving arts and handcrafts
E013 Activities involving personal hygiene and household maintenance
E014 Activities involving person providing caregiving
E015 Activities involving food preparation, cooking and grilling
E016 Activities involving property and land maintenance, building and construction
E017 Activities involving roller coasters and other types of external motion
E018 Activities involving playing musical instrument
E019 Activities involving animal care
E029 Other activity
E030 Unspecified activity

√4th E001 Activities involving walking and running
EXCLUDES *walking an animal (E019.0)*
walking or running on a treadmill (E009.0)

E001.0 Walking, marching and hiking
Walking, marching and hiking on level or elevated terrain
EXCLUDES *mountain climbing (E004.0)*

E001.1 Running

√4th E002 Activities involving water and water craft
EXCLUDES *activities involving ice (E003.0-E003.9)*
boating and other watercraft transport accidents (E830-E838)

E002.0 Swimming

E002.1 Springboard and platform diving

E002.2 Water polo

E002.3 Water aerobics and water exercise

E002.4 Underwater diving and snorkeling
SCUBA diving

E002.5 Rowing, canoeing, kayaking, rafting and tubing
Canoeing, kayaking, rafting and tubing in calm and turbulent water

E002.6 Water skiing and wake boarding

E002.7 Surfing, windsurfing and boogie boarding

E002.8 Water sliding

E002.9 Other activity involving water and watercraft
Activity involving water NOS
Parasailing
Water survival training and testing

√4th E003 Activities involving ice and snow
EXCLUDES *shoveling ice and snow (E016.0)*

E003.0 Ice skating
Figure skating (singles) (pairs)
Ice dancing
EXCLUDES *ice hockey (E003.1)*

E003.1 Ice hockey

E003.2 Snow (alpine) (downhill) skiing, snow boarding, sledding, tobogganing and snow tubing
EXCLUDES *cross country skiing (E003.3)*

E003.3 Cross country skiing
Nordic skiing

E003.9 Other activity involving ice and snow
Activity involving ice and snow NOS

√4th E004 Activities involving climbing, rappelling, and jumping off
EXCLUDES *hiking on level or elevated terrain (E001.0)*
jumping rope (E006.5)
sky diving (E840-E844)
trampoline jumping (E005.3)

E004.0 Mountain climbing, rock climbing and wall climbing

E004.1 Rappelling

E004.2 BASE jumping
Building, Antenna, Span, Earth jumping

E004.3 Bungee jumping

E004.4 Hang gliding

E004.9 Other activity involving climbing, rappelling and jumping off

☑4ᵗʰ **E005 Activities involving dancing and other rhythmic movement**
    EXCLUDES *martial arts (E008.4)*

E005.0 Dancing

E005.1 Yoga

E005.2 Gymnastics
    Rhythmic gymnastics
    EXCLUDES *trampoline (E005.3)*

E005.3 Trampoline

E005.4 Cheerleading

E005.9 Other activity involving dancing and other rhythmic movements

☑4ᵗʰ **E006 Activities involving other sports and athletics played individually**
    EXCLUDES *dancing (E005.0)*
          gymnastic (E005.2)
          trampoline (E005.3)
          yoga (E005.1)

E006.0 Roller skating (inline) and skateboarding

E006.1 Horseback riding

E006.2 Golf

E006.3 Bowling

E006.4 Bike riding
    EXCLUDES *transport accident involving bike riding (E800-E829)*

E006.5 Jumping rope

E006.6 Non-running track and field events
    EXCLUDES *running (any form) (E001.1)*

E006.9 Other activity involving other sports and athletics played individually
    EXCLUDES *activities involving climbing, rappelling, and jumping (E004.0-E004.9)*
          activities involving ice and snow (E003.0-E003.9)
          activities involving walking and running (E001.0-E001.9)
          activities involving water and watercraft (E002.0-E002.9)

☑4ᵗʰ **E007 Activities involving other sports and athletics played as a team or group**
    EXCLUDES *ice hockey (E003.1)*
          water polo (E002.2)

E007.0 American tackle football
    Football NOS

E007.1 American flag or touch football

E007.2 Rugby

E007.3 Baseball
    Softball

E007.4 Lacrosse and field hockey

E007.5 Soccer

E007.6 Basketball

E007.7 Volleyball (beach) (court)

E007.8 Physical games generally associated with school recess, summer camp and children
    Capture the flag   Four square
    Dodge ball   Kickball

E007.9 Other activity involving other sports and athletics played as a team or group
    Cricket

☑4ᵗʰ **E008 Activities involving other specified sports and athletics**

E008.0 Boxing

E008.1 Wrestling

E008.2 Racquet and hand sports
    Handball   Squash
    Racquetball   Tennis

E008.3 Frisbee
    Ultimate frisbee

E008.4 Martial arts
    Combatives

E008.9 Other specified sports and athletics activity
    EXCLUDES *sports and athletics activities specified in categories E001-E007*

☑4ᵗʰ **E009 Activity involving other cardiorespiratory exercise**
    Activity involving physical training

E009.0 Exercise machines primarily for cardiorespiratory conditioning
    Elliptical and stepper machines
    Stationary bike
    Treadmill

E009.1 Calisthenics
    Jumping jacks   Warm up and cool down

E009.2 Aerobic and step exercise

E009.3 Circuit training

E009.4 Obstacle course
    Challenge course   Confidence course

E009.5 Grass drills
    Guerilla drills

E009.9 Other activity involving cardiorespiratory exercise
    EXCLUDES *activities involving cardiorespiratory exercise specified in categories E001-E008*

☑4ᵗʰ **E010 Activity involving other muscle strengthening exercises**

E010.0 Exercise machines primarily for muscle strengthening

E010.1 Push-ups, pull-ups, sit-ups

E010.2 Free weights
    Barbells
    Dumbbells

E010.3 Pilates

E010.9 Other activity involving other muscle strengthening exercises
    EXCLUDES *activities involving muscle strengthening specified in categories E001-E009*

☑4ᵗʰ **E011 Activities involving computer technology and electronic devices**
    EXCLUDES *electronic musical keyboard or instruments (E018.0)*

E011.0 Computer keyboarding
    Electronic game playing using keyboard or other stationary device

E011.1 Hand held interactive electronic device
    Cellular telephone and communication device
    Electronic game playing using interactive device
    EXCLUDES *electronic game playing using keyboard or other stationary device (E011.0)*

E011.9 Other activity involving computer technology and electronic devices

☑4ᵗʰ **E012 Activities involving arts and handcrafts**
    EXCLUDES *activities involving playing musical instrument (E018.0-E018.3)*

E012.0 Knitting and crocheting

E012.1 Sewing

E012.2 Furniture building and finishing
    Furniture repair

E012.9 Activity involving other arts and handcrafts

☑4ᵗʰ **E013 Activities involving personal hygiene and household maintenance**
    EXCLUDES *activities involving cooking and grilling (E015.0-E015.9)*
          activities involving property and land maintenance, building and construction (E016.0-E016.9)
          activity involving persons providing caregiving (E014.0-E014.9)
          dishwashing (E015.0)
          food preparation (E015.0)
          gardening (E016.1)

E013.0 Personal bathing and showering

☑4ᵗʰ Fourth-digit Required   ▶◀ Revised Text   ● New Code   ▲ Revised Code Title

✓4ᵗʰ **E014** **Activities involving person providing caregiving**

E013.1 Laundry

E013.2 Vacuuming

E013.3 Ironing

E013.4 Floor mopping and cleaning

E013.5 Residential relocation
   Packing up and unpacking involved in moving to a new residence

E013.8 Other personal hygiene activity

E013.9 Other household maintenance

✓4ᵗʰ **E014** **Activities involving person providing caregiving**

E014.0 Caregiving involving bathing

E014.1 Caregiving involving lifting

E014.9 Other activity involving person providing caregiving

✓4ᵗʰ **E015** **Activities involving food preparation, cooking and grilling**

E015.0 Food preparation and clean up
   Dishwasing

E015.1 Grilling and smoking food

E015.2 Cooking and baking
   Use of stove, oven and microwave oven

E015.9 Other activity involving cooking and grilling

✓4ᵗʰ **E016** **Activities involving property and land maintenance, building and construction**

E016.0 Digging, shoveling and raking
   Dirt digging
   Raking leaves
   Snow shoveling

E016.1 Gardening and landscaping
   Pruning, trimming shrubs, weeding

E016.2 Building and construction

E016.9 Other activity involving property and land maintenance, building and construction

✓4ᵗʰ **E017** **Activities involving roller coasters and other types of external motion**

E017.0 Roller coaster riding

E017.9 Other activity involving external motion

✓4ᵗʰ **E018** **Activities involving playing musical instrument**
   Activity involving playing electric musical instrument

E018.0 Piano playing
   Musical keyboard (electronic) playing

E018.1 Drum and other percussion instrument playing

E018.2 String instrument playing

E018.3 Wind and brass instrument playing

✓4ᵗʰ **E019** **Activities involving animal care**
   EXCLUDES horseback riding (E006.1)

E019.0 Walking an animal

E019.1 Milking an animal

E019.2 Grooming and shearing an animal

E019.9 Other activity involving animal care

✓4ᵗʰ **E029** **Other activity**

E029.0 Refereeing a sports activity

E029.1 Spectator at an event

E029.2 Rough housing and horseplay

E029.9 Other activity

E030 **Unspecified activity**

Transport Accidents (E800-E848)

Definitions and Examples Related to Transport Accidents

(a) A **transport accident** (E800-E848) is any accident involving a device designed primarily for, or being used at the time primarily for, conveying persons or goods from one place to another.

INCLUDES accidents involving:
   aircraft and spacecraft (E840-E845)
   watercraft (E830-E838)
   motor vehicle (E810-E825)
   railway (E800-E807)
   other road vehicles (E826-E829)

In classifying accidents which involve more than one kind of transport, the above order of precedence of transport accidents should be used.

Accidents involving agricultural and construction machines, such as tractors, cranes, and bulldozers, are regarded as transport accidents only when these vehicles are under their own power on a highway [otherwise the vehicles are regarded as machinery]. Vehicles which can travel on land or water, such as hovercraft and other amphibious vehicles, are regarded as watercraft when on the water, as motor vehicles when on the highway, and as off-road motor vehicles when on land, but off the highway.

EXCLUDES accidents:
   in sports which involve the use of transport but where the transport vehicle itself was not involved in the accident
   involving vehicles which are part of industrial equipment used entirely on industrial premises
   occurring during transportation but unrelated to the hazards associated with the means of transportation [e.g., injuries received in a fight on board ship; transport vehicle involved in a cataclysm such as an earthquake]
   to persons engaged in the maintenance or repair of transport equipment or vehicle not in motion, unlesss injured by another vehicle in motion

(b) A **railway accident** is a transport accident involving a railway train or other railway vehicle operated on rails, whether in motion or not.

EXCLUDES accidents:
   in repair shops
   in roundhouse or on turntable
   on railway premises but not involving a train or other railway vehicle

(c) A **railway train** or **railway vehicle** is any device with or without cars coupled to it, desiged for traffic on a railway.

INCLUDES interurban:
   electric car   } (operated chiefly on its own
   street car   right-of-way, not open to
                         other traffic)
   railway train, any power [diesel] [electric] [steam]:
   funicular
   monorail or two-rail
   subterranean or elevated
   other vehicle designed to run on a railway track

EXCLUDES interurban electric cars [streetcars] specified to be operating on a right-of-way that forms part of the public street or highway [definition (h)]

(d) A **railway** or **railroad** is a right-of-way designed for traffic on rails, which is used by carriages or wagons transporting passengers or freight, and by other rolling stock, and which is not open to other public vehicular traffic.

(e) A **motor vehicle accident** is a transport accident involving a motor vehicle. It is defined as a motor vehicle traffic accident or as a motor vehicle nontraffic accident according to whether the accident occurs on a public highway or elsewhere.

EXCLUDES injury or damage due to cataclysm
   injury or damage while a motor vehicle, not under its own power, is being loaded on, or unloaded from, another conveyance

(f) A **motor vehicle traffic accident** is any motor vehicle accident occurring on a public highway [i.e., originating, terminating, or involving a vehicle partially on the highway]. A motor vehicle accident is assumed to have occurred on the highway unless another place is specified, except in the case of accidents involving only off-road motor vehicles which are classified as nontraffic accidents unless the contrary is stated.

(g) A **motor vehicle nontraffic accident** is any motor vehicle accident which occurs entirely in any place other than a public highway.

(h) A **public highway [trafficway]** or **street** is the entire width between property lines [or other boundary lines] of every way or place, of which any part is open to the use of the public for purposes of vehicular traffic as a matter of right or custom. A **roadway** is that part of the public highway designed, improved, and ordinarily used, for vehicular travel.

INCLUDES   approaches (public) to:
- docks
- public building
- station

EXCLUDES   *driveway (private)*
parking lot
ramp
roads in:
- *airfield*
- *farm*
- *industrial premises*
- *mine*
- *private grounds*
- *quarry*

(i) A **motor vehicle** is any mechanically or electrically powered device, not operated on rails, upon which any person or property may be transported or drawn upon a highway. Any object such as a trailer, coaster, sled, or wagon being towed by a motor vehicle is considered a part of the motor vehicle.

INCLUDES   automobile [any type]
bus
construction machinery, farm and industrial machinery, steam roller, tractor, army tank, highway grader, or similar vehicle on wheels or treads, while in transport under own power
fire engine (motorized)
motorcycle
motorized bicycle [moped] or scooter
trolley bus not operating on rails
truck
van

EXCLUDES   *devices used solely to move persons or materials within the confines of a building and its premises, such as:*
- *building elevator*
- *coal car in mine*
- *electric baggage or mail truck used solely within a railroad station*
- *electric truck used solely within an industrial plant*
- *moving overhead crane*

(j) A **motorcycle** is a two-wheeled motor vehicle having one or two riding saddles and sometimes having a third wheel for the support of a sidecar. The sidecar is considered part of the motorcycle.

INCLUDES   motorized:
- bicycle [moped]
- scooter
- tricycle

(k) An **off-road motor vehicle** is a motor vehicle of special design, to enable it to negotiate rough or soft terrain or snow. Examples of special design are high construction, special wheels and tires, driven by treads, or support on a cushion of air.

INCLUDES   all terrain vehicle [ATV]
army tank
hovercraft, on land or swamp
snowmobile

(l) A **driver** of a motor vehicle is the occupant of the motor vehicle operating it or intending to operate it. A **motorcyclist** is the driver of a motorcycle. Other authorized occupants of a motor vehicle are **passengers**.

(m) An **other road vehicle** is any device, except a motor vehicle, in, on, or by which any person or property may be transported on a highway.

INCLUDES   animal carrying a person or goods
animal-drawn vehicles
animal harnessed to conveyance
bicycle [pedal cycle]
streetcar
tricycle (pedal)

EXCLUDES   *pedestrian conveyance [definition (q)]*

(n) A **streetcar** is a device designed and used primarily for transporting persons within a municipality, running on rails, usually subject to normal traffic control signals, and operated principally on a right-of-way that forms part of the traffic way. A trailer being towed by a streetcar is considered a part of the streetcar.

INCLUDES   interurban or intraurban electric or streetcar, when specified to be operating on a street or public highway
tram (car)
trolley (car)

(o) A **pedal cycle** is any road transport vehicle operated solely by pedals.

INCLUDES   bicycle
pedal cycle
tricycle

EXCLUDES   *motorized bicycle [definition (j)]*

(p) A **pedal cyclist** is any person riding on a pedal cycle or in a sidecar attached to such a vehicle.

(q) A **pedestrian conveyance** is any human powered device by which a pedestrian may move other than by walking or by which a walking person may move another pedestrian.

INCLUDES   baby carriage
coaster wagon
heelies, wheelies
ice skates
motorized mobility scooter
perambulator
pushcart
pushchair
roller skates
scooter
skateboard
skis
sled
wheelchair (electric)

(r) A **pedestrian** is any person involved in an accident who was not at the time of the accident riding in or on a motor vehicle, railroad train, streetcar, animal-drawn or other vehicle, or on a bicycle or animal.

INCLUDES   person:
- changing tire of vehicle
- in or operating a pedestrian conveyance
- making adjustment to motor of vehicle
- on foot

(s) A **watercraft** is any device for transporting passengers or goods on the water.

(t) A **small boat** is any watercraft propelled by paddle, oars, or small motor, with a passenger capacity of less than ten.

INCLUDES   boat NOS
canoe
coble
dinghy
punt
raft
rowboat
rowing shell
scull
skiff
small motorboat

EXCLUDES   *barge*
lifeboat (used after abandoning ship)
raft (anchored) being used as a diving platform
yacht

(u) An **aircraft** is any device for transporting passengers or goods in the air.

INCLUDES   airplane [any type]
balloon
bomber
dirigible
glider (hang)
military aircraft
parachute

(v) A **commercial transport aircraft** is any device for collective passenger or freight transportation by air, whether run on commercial lines for profit or by government authorities, with the exception of military craft.

Railway Accidents (E800-E807)

NOTE For definitions of railway accident and related terms see definitions (a) to (d).

EXCLUDES *accidents involving railway train and:*
aircraft (E840.0-E845.9)
motor vehicle (E810.0-E825.9)
watercraft (E830.0-E838.9)

The following fourth digit subdivisions are for use with categories E800-E807 to identify the injured person:

.0 Railway employee
Any person who by virtue of his employment in connection with a railway, whether by the railway company or not, is at increased risk of involvement in a railway accident, such as:
catering staff of train
driver
guard
porter
postal staff on train
railway fireman
shunter
sleeping car attendant

.1 Passenger on railway
Any authorized person traveling on a train, except a railway employee.
EXCLUDES *intending passenger waiting at station (.8)*
unauthorized rider on railway vehicle (.8)

.2 Pedestrian
See definition (r)

.3 Pedal cyclist
See definition (p)

.8 Other specified person
Intending passenger or bystander waiting at station
Unauthorized rider on railway vehicle

.9 Unspecified person

§ ✓4ᵗʰ **E800   Railway accident involving collision with rolling stock**
INCLUDES collision between railway trains or railway vehicles, any kind
collision NOS on railway
derailment with antecedent collision with rolling stock or NOS

§ ✓4ᵗʰ **E801   Railway accident involving collision with other object**
INCLUDES collision of railway train with:
buffers
fallen tree on railway
gates
platform
rock on railway
streetcar
other nonmotor vehicle
other object
EXCLUDES *collision with:*
aircraft (E840.0-E842.9)
motor vehicle (E810.0-E810.9, E820.0-E822.9)

§ ✓4ᵗʰ **E802   Railway accident involving derailment without antecedent collision**

§ ✓4ᵗʰ **E803   Railway accident involving explosion, fire, or burning**
EXCLUDES *explosion or fire, with antecedent derailment (E802.0-E802.9)*
explosion or fire, with mention of antecedent collision (E800.0-E801.9)

§ ✓4ᵗʰ **E804   Fall in, on, or from railway train**
INCLUDES fall while alighting from or boarding railway train
EXCLUDES *fall related to collision, derailment, or explosion of railway train (E800.0-E803.9)*

§ ✓4ᵗʰ **E805   Hit by rolling stock**
INCLUDES crushed
injured
killed   } by railway train or part
knocked down
run over
EXCLUDES *pedestrian hit by object set in motion by railway train (E806.0-E806.9)*

§ ✓4ᵗʰ **E806   Other specified railway accident**
INCLUDES hit by object falling in railway train
injured by door or window on railway train
nonmotor road vehicle or pedestrian hit by object set in motion by railway train
railway train hit by falling:
earth NOS
rock
tree
other object
EXCLUDES *railway accident due to cataclysm (E908-E909)*

§ ✓4ᵗʰ **E807   Railway accident of unspecified nature**
INCLUDES found dead
injured   } on railway right-of-way NOS
railway accident NOS

Motor Vehicle Traffic Accidents (E810-E819)

NOTE For definitions of motor vehicle traffic accident, and related terms, see definitions (e) to (k).

EXCLUDES *accidents involving motor vehicle and aircraft (E840.0-E845.9)*

The following fourth digit subdivisions are for use with categories E810-E819 to identify the injured person:

.0 Driver of motor vehicle other than motorcycle
See definition (l)
.1 Passenger in motor vehicle other than motorcycle
See definition (l)
.2 Motorcyclist
See definition (l)
.3 Passenger on motorcycle
See definition (l)
.4 Occupant of streetcar
.5 Rider of animal; occupant of animal-drawn vehicle
.6 Pedal cyclist
See definition (p)
.7 Pedestrian
See definition (r)
.8 Other specified person
Occupant of vehicle other than above
Person in railway train involved in accident
Unauthorized rider of motor vehicle
.9 Unspecified person

§ ✓4ᵗʰ **E810   Motor vehicle traffic accident involving collision with train**
EXCLUDES *motor vehicle collision with object set in motion by railway train (E815.0-E815.9)*
railway train hit by object set in motion by motor vehicle (E818.0-E818.9)

§ ✓4ᵗʰ **E811   Motor vehicle traffic accident involving re-entrant collision with another motor vehicle**
INCLUDES collision between motor vehicle which accidentally leaves the roadway then re-enters the same roadway, or the opposite roadway on a divided highway, and another motor vehicle
EXCLUDES *collision on the same roadway when none of the motor vehicles involved have left and re-entered the highway (E812.0-E812.9)*

§ ✓4ᵗʰ **E812   Other motor vehicle traffic accident involving collision with motor vehicle**
INCLUDES collision with another motor vehicle parked, stopped, stalled, disabled, or abandoned on the highway
motor vehicle collision NOS
EXCLUDES *collision with object set in motion by another motor vehicle (E815.0-E815.9)*
re-entrant collision with another motor vehicle (E811.0-E811.9)

E800–E812

---

§ Requires fourth digit. See beginning of appropriate section for codes and definitions.

✓4ᵗʰ Fourth-digit Required   ►◄ Revised Text   ● New Code   ▲ Revised Code Title

§ ✓4ᵗʰ **E813 Motor vehicle traffic accident involving collision with other vehicle**

    INCLUDES collision between motor vehicle, any kind, and:
        other road (nonmotor transport) vehicle, such as:
           animal carrying a person
           animal-drawn vehicle
           pedal cycle
           streetcar

    EXCLUDES *collision with:*
        object set in motion by nonmotor road vehicle (E815.0-E815.9)
        pedestrian (E814.0-E814.9)
        nonmotor road vehicle hit by object set in motion by motor vehicle (E818.0-E818.9)

§ ✓4ᵗʰ **E814 Motor vehicle traffic accident involving collision with pedestrian**

    INCLUDES collision between motor vehicle, any kind, and:
        pedestrian
        pedestrian dragged, hit, or run over by motor vehicle, any kind

    EXCLUDES *pedestrian hit by object set in motion by motor vehicle (E818.0-E818.9)*

§ ✓4ᵗʰ **E815 Other motor vehicle traffic accident involving collision on the highway**

    INCLUDES collision (due to loss of control) (on highway) between motor vehicle, any kind, and:
        abutment (bridge) (overpass)
        animal (herded) (unattended)
        fallen stone, traffic sign, tree, utility pole
        guard rail or boundary fence
        interhighway divider
        landslide (not moving)
        object set in motion by railway train or road vehicle (motor) (nonmotor)
        object thrown in front of motor vehicle
        other object, fixed, movable, or moving
        safety island
        temporary traffic sign or marker
        wall of cut made for road

    EXCLUDES *collision with:*
        any object off the highway (resulting from loss of control) (E816.0-E816.9)
        any object which normally would have been off the highway and is not stated to have been on it (E816.0-E816.9)
        motor vehicle parked, stopped, stalled, disabled, or abandoned on highway (E812.0-E812.9)
        moving landslide (E909)
        motor vehicle hit by object:
          set in motion by railway train or road vehicle (motor) (nonmotor) (E818.0-E818.9)
          thrown into or on vehicle (E818.0-E818.9)

§ ✓4ᵗʰ **E816 Motor vehicle traffic accident due to loss of control, without collision on the highway**

    INCLUDES motor vehicle:
        failing to make curve
        going out of control (due to):   and:
          blowout   coliding with object off the highway
          burst tire   overturning
          driver falling asleep   stopping abruptly off the highway
          drive inattention
          excessive speed
          failure of mechanical part

    EXCLUDES *collision on highway following loss of control (E810.0-E815.9)*
        loss of control of motor vehicle following collision on the highway (E810.0-E815.9)

§ ✓4ᵗʰ **E817 Noncollision motor vehicle traffic accident while boarding or alighting**

    INCLUDES fall down stairs of motor bus
        fall from car in street
        injured by moving part of the vehicle   } while boarding or alighting
        trapped by door of motor bus

§ ✓4ᵗʰ **E818 Other noncollision motor vehicle traffic accident**

    INCLUDES accidental poisoning from exhaust gas generated by
        breakage of any part of
        explosion of any part of
        fall, jump, or being accidentally pushed from
        fire starting in   } motor vehicle while in motion
        hit by object thrown into or on
        injured by being thrown against some part of, or object in
        injury from moving part of
        object falling in or on
        object thrown on

        collision of railway train or road vehicle except motor vehicle, with object set in motion by motor vehicle
        motor vehicle hit by object set in motion by railway train or road vehicle (motor) (nonmotor)
        pedestrian, railway train, or road vehicle (motor) (nonmotor) hit by object set in motion by motor vehicle

    EXCLUDES *collision between motor vehicle and:*
        object set in motion by railway train or road vehicle (motor) (nonmotor) (E815.0-E815.9)
        object thrown towards the motor vehicle (E815.0-E815.9)
        person overcome by carbon monoxide generated by stationary motor vehicle off the roadway with motor running (E868.2)

§ ✓4ᵗʰ **E819 Motor vehicle traffic accident of unspecified nature**

    INCLUDES motor vehicle traffic accident NOS
        traffic accident NOS

Motor Vehicle Nontraffic Accidents (E820-E825)

  NOTE For definitions of motor vehicle nontraffic accident and related terms see definition (a) to (k).

  INCLUDES accidents involving motor vehicles being used in recreational or sporting activities off the highway
      collision and noncollision motor vehicle accidents occurring entirely off the highway

  EXCLUDES *accidents involving motor vehicle and:*
      aircraft (E840.0-E845.9)
      watercraft (E830.0-E838.9)
      accidents, not on the public highway, involving agricultural and construction machinery but not involving another motor vehicle (E919.0, E919.2, E919.7)

The following fourth digit subdivisions are for use with categories E820-E825 to identify the injured person:

  .0 Driver of motor vehicle other than motorcycle
    See definition (l)
  .1 Passenger in motor vehicle other than motorcycle
    See definition (l)
  .2 Motorcyclist
    See definition (l)
  .3 Passenger on motorcycle
    See definition (l)
  .4 Occupant of streetcar
  .5 Rider of animal; occupant of animal-drawn vehicle
  .6 Pedal cyclist
    See definition (p)
  .7 Pedestrian
    See definition (r)
  .8 Other specified person
    Occupant of vehicle other than above
    Person in railway train involved in accident
    Unauthorized rider of motor vehicle
  .9 Unspecified person

---

§   Requires fourth digit. See beginning of appropriate section for codes and definitions.

§ ✓4ᵗʰ **E820 Nontraffic accident involving motor-driven snow vehicle**

INCLUDES breakage of part of ⎫
fall from   ⎬ motor-driven snow
hit by   ⎪ vehicle (not on
overturning of   ⎪ public highway)
run over or dragged by ⎭

collision of motor-driven snow vehicle with:
  animal (being ridden) (-drawn vehicle)
  another off-road motor vehicle
  other motor vehicle, not on public highway
  railway train
  other object, fixed or movable
injury caused by rough landing of motor-driven snow
  vehicle (after leaving ground on rough terrain)

EXCLUDES *accident on the public highway involving motor driven
snow vehicle (E810.0-E819.9)*

§ ✓4ᵗʰ **E821 Nontraffic accident involving other off-road motor vehicle**

INCLUDES breakage of part of ⎫
fall from   ⎪
hit by   ⎬ off-road motorvehicle
overturning of   ⎪ except snow
run over or dragged by ⎪ vehicle (not on
thrown against some part ⎪ public highway
  of or object in   ⎭

collision with:
  animal (being ridden) (-drawn vehicle)
  another off-road motor vehicle, except snow vehicle
  other motor vehicle, not on public highway
  other object, fixed or movable

EXCLUDES *accident on public highway involving off-road motor
vehicle (E810.0-E819.9)*
*collision between motor driven snow vehicle and other
off-road motor vehicle (E820.0-E820.9)*
hovercraft accident on water (E830.0-E838.9)

§ ✓4ᵗʰ **E822 Other motor vehicle nontraffic accident involving collision
with moving object**

INCLUDES collision, not on public highway, between motor vehicle,
  except off-road motor vehicle and:
  animal
  nonmotor vehicle
  other motor vehicle, except off-road motor vehicle
  pedestrian
  railway train
  other moving object

EXCLUDES *collision with:*
  motor-driven snow vehicle (E820.0-E820.9)
  other off-road motor vehicle (E821.0-E821.9)

§ ✓4ᵗʰ **E823 Other motor vehicle nontraffic accident involving collision
with stationary object**

INCLUDES collision, not on public highway, between motor vehicle,
  except off-road motor vehicle, and any object,
  fixed or movable, but not in motion

§ ✓4ᵗʰ **E824 Other motor vehicle nontraffic accident while boarding and
alighting**

INCLUDES fall   ⎫
injury from oving part ⎪ while boarding or alighting
  of motor   ⎬ from motor vehicle,
  vehicle   ⎪ except off-road motor
trapped by door of ⎪ vehicle, not on public
  motor vehhicle ⎭ highway

§ ✓4ᵗʰ **E825 Other motor vehicle nontraffic accident of other and
unspecified nature**

INCLUDES accidental poisoning from carbon ⎫
  monoxide generated by ⎪
breakage of any part of ⎪
explosion of any part of ⎪
fall, jump, or being accidentally ⎪
  pushed from ⎬ motor vehicle
fire starting in ⎪ while in
hit by object thrown into, towards, ⎪ motion, not
  or on ⎪ on public
injured by being thrown against ⎪ highway
  some part of, or object in ⎪
injury from moving part of ⎪
object falling in or on ⎭
motor vehicle nontraffic accident NOS

EXCLUDES *fall from or in stationary motor vehicle (E884.9, E885.9)*
*overcome by carbon monoxide or exhaust gas generated by
stationary motor vehicle off the roadway with motor
running (E868.2)*
*struck by falling object from or in stationary motor vehicle
(E916)*

Other Road Vehicle Accidents (E826-E829)

NOTE Other road vehicle accidents are transport accidents involving road
vehicles other than motor vehicles. For definitions of other road
vehicle and related terms see definitions (m) to (o).

INCLUDES accidents involving other road vehicles being used in recreational
or sporting activities

EXCLUDES *collision of other road vehicle [any] with:*
  aircraft (E840.0-E845.9)
  motor vehicle (E813.0-E813.9, E820.0-E822.9)
  railway train (E801.0-E801.9))

The following fourth digit subdivisions are for use with categories E826-E829
to identify the injured person:
.0 Pedestrian
  See definition (r)
.1 Pedal cyclist
  See definition (p)
.2 Rider of animal
.3 Occupant of animal-drawn vehicle
.4 Occupant of streetcar
.8 Other specified person
.9 Unspecified person

§ ✓4ᵗʰ **E826 Pedal cycle accident**

[0-9] INCLUDES breakage of any part of pedal cycle
collision between pedal cycle and:
  animal (being ridden) (herded) (unattended)
  another pedal cycle
  any pedestrian
  nonmotor road vehicle
  other object, fixed, movable, or moving, not set in
    motion by motor vehicle, railway train, or aircraft
entanglement in wheel of pedal cycle
fall from pedal cycle
hit by object falling or thrown on the pedal cycle
pedal cycle accident NOS
pedal cycle overturned

§ ✓4ᵗʰ **E827 Animal-drawn vehicle accident**

[0,2,4,8,9] INCLUDES breakage of any part of vehicle
collision between animal-drawn vehicle and:
  animal (being ridden) (herded) (unattended)
  nonmotor road vehicle, except pedal cycle
  pedestrian, pedestrian conveyance, or pedestrian
    vehicle
  other object, fixed, movable, or moving, not set in
    motion by motor vehicle, railway train, or aircraft

fall from   ⎫
knocked down by ⎪
overturning of   ⎬ animal drawn vehicle
running over by ⎪
thrown from   ⎭

EXCLUDES *collision of animal-drawn vehicle with pedal cycle
(E826.0-E826.9)*

---

§ Requires fourth digit. See beginning of appropriate section for codes and definitions.

§ ✓4ᵗʰ **E828 Accident involving animal being ridden**

[0,2,4,8,9] INCLUDES collision between animal being ridden and:
  another animal
  nonmotor road vehicle, except pedal cycle, and
    animal-drawn vehicle
  pedestrian, pedestrian conveyance, or pedestrian
    vehicle
  other object, fixed, movable, or moving, not set in
    motion by motor vehicle, railway train, or aircraft

fall from
knocked down by   } animal being ridden
thrown from
trampled by

ridden animal stumbled and fell

EXCLUDES *collision of animal being ridden with:*
  animal-drawn vehicle (E827.0-E827.9)
  pedal cycle (E826.0-E826.9)

§ ✓4ᵗʰ **E829 Other road vehicle accidents**

[0,4,8,9] INCLUDES accident while boarding
  or alighting from
blow from object in   streetcar
breakage of any part of   nonmotor road vehicle
caught in door of   not classifiable to
derailment of   E826-E828
fall in, on, or from
fire in

collision between streetcar or nonmotor road vehicle,
  except as in E826-E828, and:
  animal (not being ridden)
  another nonmotor road vehicle not classifiable to
    E826-E828
  pedestrian
  other object, fixed, movable, or moving, not set in
    motion by motor vehicle, railway train, or aircraft
nonmotor road vehicle accident NOS
streetcar accident NOS

EXCLUDES *collision with:*
  animal being ridden (E828.0-E828.9)
  animal-drawn vehicle (E827.0-E827.9)
  pedal cycle (E826.0-E826.9)

Water Transport Accidents (E830-E838)

NOTE For definitions of water transport accident and related terms see
  definitions (a), (s), and (t).

INCLUDES watercraft accidents in the course of recreational activities

EXCLUDES *accidents involving both aircraft, including objects set in motion by*
  aircraft, and watercraft (E840.0-E845.9)

The following fourth digit subdivisions are for use with categories E830-E838
to identify the injured person:
.0 Occupant of small boat, unpowered
.1 Occupant of small boat, powered
  See definition (t)
  EXCLUDES *water skier (.4)*
.2 Occupant of other watercraft — crew
  Persons:
    engaged in operation of watercraft
    providing passenger services [cabin attendants, ship's physician,
      catering personnel]
    working on ship during voyage in other capacity [musician in
      band, operators of shops and beauty parlors]
.3 Occupant of other watercraft — other than crew
  Passenger
  Occupant of lifeboat, other than crew, after abandoning ship
.4 Water skier
.5 Swimmer
.6 Dockers, stevedores
  Longshoreman employed on the dock in loading and unloading ships
.7 Occupant of military watercraft, any type
.8 Other specified person
  Immigration and custom officials on board ship
  Person:
    accompanying passenger or member of crew visiting boat
  Pilot (guiding ship into port)
.9 Unspecified person

§ ✓4ᵗʰ **E830 Accident to watercraft causing submersion**

INCLUDES submersion and drowning due to:
  boat overturning
  boat submerging
  falling or jumping from burning ship
  falling or jumping from crushed watercraft
  ship sinking
  other accident to watercraft

§ ✓4ᵗʰ **E831 Accident to watercraft causing other injury**

INCLUDES any injury, except submersion and drowning, as a result
    of an accident to watercraft
  burned while ship on fire
  crushed between ships in collision
  crushed by lifeboat after abandoning ship
  fall due to collision or other accident to watercraft
  hit by falling object due to accident to watercraft
  injured in watercraft accident involving collision
  struck by boat or part thereof after fall or jump from
    damaged boat

EXCLUDES *burns from localized fire or explosion on board ship*
  (E837.0-E837.9)

§ ✓4ᵗʰ **E832 Other accidental submersion or drowning in water transport
  accident**

INCLUDES submersion or drowning as a result of an accident other
    than accident to the watercraft, such as:
  fall:
    from gangplank
    from ship
    overboard
  thrown overboard by motion of ship
  washed overboard

EXCLUDES *submersion or drowning of swimmer or diver who*
  voluntarily jumps from boat not involved in an
  accident (E910.0-E910.9)

§ ✓4ᵗʰ **E833 Fall on stairs or ladders in water transport**

EXCLUDES *fall due to accident to watercraft (E831.0-E831.9)*

§ ✓4ᵗʰ **E834 Other fall from one level to another in water transport**

EXCLUDES *fall due to accident to watercraft (E831.0-E831.9)*

§ ✓4ᵗʰ **E835 Other and unspecified fall in water transport**

EXCLUDES *fall due to accident to watercraft (E831.0-E831.9)*

§ ✓4ᵗʰ **E836 Machinery accident in water transport**

INCLUDES injuries in water transport caused by:
  deck
  engine room
  galley   } machinery
  laundry
  loading

§ ✓4ᵗʰ **E837 Explosion, fire, or burning in watercraft**

INCLUDES explosion of boiler on steamship
  localized fire on ship

EXCLUDES *burning ship (due to collision or explosion) resulting in:*
  submersion or drowning (E830.0-E830.9)
  other injury (E831.0-E831.9)

§ ✓4ᵗʰ **E838 Other and unspecified water transport accident**

INCLUDES accidental poisoning by gases or fumes on ship
  atomic power plant malfunction in watercraft
  crushed between ship and stationary object [wharf]
  crushed between ships without accident to watercraft
  crushed by falling object on ship or while loading or
    unloading
  hit by boat while water skiing
  struck by boat or part thereof (after fall from boat)
  watercraft accident NOS

---

§ Requires fourth digit. Valid digits are in [brackets] under each code. See beginning of appropriate section for codes and definitions.

✓4ᵗʰ Fourth-digit Required   ▶◀ Revised Text   ● New Code   ▲ Revised Code Title

Air and Space Transport Accidents (E840-E845)

NOTE For definition of aircraft and related terms see definitions (u) and (v).

The following fourth digit subdivisions are for use with categories E840-E845 to identify the injured person. Valid fourth digits are in [brackets] under codes E842-E845:

.0 Occupant of spacecraft
.1 Occupant of military aircraft, any
  Crew in military aircraft [air force] [army] [national guard] [navy]
  Passenger (civilian) (military) in military aircraft [air force] [army] [national guard] [navy]
  Troops in military aircraft [air force] [army] [national guard] [navy]
    EXCLUDES occupants of aircraft operated under jurisdiction of police departments (.5)
                    parachutist (.7)
.2 Crew of commercial aircraft (powered) in surface to surface transport
.3 Other occupant of commercial aircraft (powered) in surface to surface transport
  Flight personnel:
    not part of crew
    on familiarization flight
  Passenger on aircraft (powered) NOS
.4 Occupant of commercial aircraft (powered) in surface to air transport
  Occupant [crew] [passenger] of aircraft (powered) engaged in activities, such as:
    aerial spraying (crops) (fire retardants)
    air drops of emergency supplies
    air drops of parachutists, except from military craft
    crop dusting
    lowering of construction material [bridge or telephone pole]
    sky writing
.5 Occupant of other powered aircraft
  Occupant [crew] [passenger] of aircraft (powered) engaged in activities, such as:
    aerobatic flying
    aircraft racing
    rescue operation
    storm surveillance
    traffic surveillance
  Occupant of private plane NOS
.6 Occupant of unpowered aircraft, except parachutist
  Occupant of aircraft classifiable to E842
.7 Parachutist (military) (other)
  Person making voluntary descent
    EXCLUDES person making descent after accident to aircraft (.1-.6)
.8 Ground crew, airline employee
  Persons employed at airfields (civil) (military) or launching pads, not occupants of aircraft
.9 Other person

§ ✓4ᵗʰ **E840 Accident to powered aircraft at takeoff or landing**
  INCLUDES collision of aircraft with any object, fixed, movable, or moving
            crash
            explosion on aircraft   while taking off or landing
            fire on aircraft
            forced landing

§ ✓4ᵗʰ **E841 Accident to powered aircraft, other and unspecified**
  INCLUDES aircraft accident NOS
            aircraft crash or wreck NOS
            any accident to powered aircraft while in transit or when not specified whether in transit, taking off, or landing
            collision of aircraft with another aircraft, bird, or any object, while in transit
            explosion on aircraft while in transit
            fire on aircraft while in transit

§ ✓4ᵗʰ **E842 Accident to unpowered aircraft**
  [6-9]   INCLUDES any accident, except collision with powered aircraft, to:
                    balloon
                    glider
                    hang glider
                    kite carrying a person
                  hit by object falling from unpowered aircraft

§ ✓4ᵗʰ **E843 Fall in, on, or from aircraft**
  [0-9]   INCLUDES accident in boarding or alighting from aircraft, any kind
                    fall in, on, or from aircraft [any kind], while in transit, taking off, or landing, except when as a result of an accident to aircraft

§ ✓4ᵗʰ **E844 Other specified air transport accidents**
  [0-9]   INCLUDES hit by:
                    aircraft
                    object falling from aircraft
                  injury by or from:
                    machinery of aircraft   without
                    rotating propellar   accident
                    voluntary parachute descent to aircraft
                  poisoning by carbon monoxide from aircraft while in transit
                  sucked into jet
                  any accident involving other transport vehicle (motor) (nonmotor) due to being hit by object set in motion by aircraft (powered)
    EXCLUDES air sickness (E903)
              effects of:
                high altitude (E902.0-E902.1)
                pressure change (E902.0-E902.1)
              injury in parachute descent due to accident to aircraft (E840.0-E842-9)

§ ✓4ᵗʰ **E845 Accident involving spacecraft**
  [0,8,9] INCLUDES launching pad accident
           EXCLUDES effects of weightlessness in spacecraft (E928.0)

Vehicle Accidents Not Elsewhere Classifiable (E846-E848)

E846 Accidents involving powered vehicles used solely within the buildings and premises of industrial or commercial establishment
  Accident to, on, or involving:
    battery powered airport passenger vehicle
    battery powered trucks (baggage) (mail)
    coal car in mine
    logging car
    self propelled truck, industrial
    station baggage truck (powered)
    tram, truck, or tub (powered) in mine or quarry
  Collision with:
    pedestrian
    other vehicle or object within premises
  Explosion of
  Fall from   powered vehicle, industrial or commercial
  Overturning of
  Struck by
    EXCLUDES accidental poisoning by exhaust gas from vehicle not elsewhere classifiable (E868.2)
              injury by crane, lift (fork), or elevator (E919.2)

E847 Accidents involving cable cars not running on rails
  Accident to, on, or involving:
    cable car, not on rails
    ski chair-lift
    ski-lift with gondola
    téléférique
  Breakage of cable
  Caught or dragged by
  Fall or jump from   cable car, not on rails
  Object thrown from or in

E848 Accidents involving other vehicles, not elsewhere classifiable
  Accident to, on, or involving:
    ice yacht
    land yacht
    nonmotor, nonroad vehicle NOS

---

§ Requires fourth digit. See beginning of appropriate section for codes and definitions.

✓4ᵗʰ Fourth-digit Required   ▶◀ Revised Text   ● New Code   ▲ Revised Code Title

E Codes

E849–E851

Place of Occurrence (E849)

☑4th **E849 Place of Occurrence**

NOTE The following category is for use to denote the place where the injury or poisoning occurred.

E849.0 Home

Apartment
Boarding house
Farm house
Home premises
House (residential)
Noninstitutional place
  of residence
Private:
  driveway

Private:
  garage
  garden
  home
  walk
Swimming pool in private
  house or garden
Yard of home

EXCLUDES home under construction but not yet occupied
  (E849.3)
institutional place of residence (E849.7)

E849.1 Farm

Farm:
  buildings
  land under cultivation

EXCLUDES farm house and home premises of farm (E849.0)

E849.2 Mine and quarry

Gravel pit
Sand pit

Tunnel under construction

E849.3 Industrial place and premises

Building under construction
Dockyard
Dry dock
Factory
  building
  premises
Garage (place of work)

Industrial yard
Loading platform (factory)
  (store)
Plant, industrial
Railway yard
Shop (place of work)
Warehouse
Workhouse

E849.4 Place for recreation and sport

Amusement park
Baseball field
Basketball court
Beach resort
Cricket ground
Fives court
Football field
Golf course
Gymnasium
Hockey field
Holiday camp
Ice palace
Lake resort
Mountain resort

Playground, including school
  playground
Public park
Racecourse
Resort NOS
Riding school
Rifle range
Seashore resort
Skating rink
Sports palace
Stadium
Swimming pool, public
Tennis court
Vacation resort

EXCLUDES that in private house or garden (E849.0)

E849.5 Street and highway

E849.6 Public building

Building (including adjacent grounds) used by the general
  public or by a particular group of the public, such as:

airport
bank
café
casino
church
cinema
clubhouse
courthouse
dance hall
garage building
  (for car storage)
hotel
market (grocery or
  other commodity)
movie house

music hall
nightclub
office
office building
opera house
post office
public hall
radio broadcasting station
restaurant
school (state) (public) (private)
shop, commercial
station (bus) (railway)
store
theater

EXCLUDES home garage (E849.0)
industrial building or workplace (E849.3)

E849.7 Residential institution

Children's home
Dormitory
Hospital
Jail

Old people's home
Orphanage
Prison
Reform school

E849.8 Other specified places

Beach NOS
Canal
Caravan site NOS
Derelict house
Desert
Dock
Forest
Harbor
Hill
Lake NOS
Mountain
Parking lot
Parking place

Pond or pool (natural)
Prairie
Public place NOS
Railway line
Reservoir
River
Sea
Seashore NOS
Stream
Swamp
Trailer court
Woods

E849.9 Unspecified place

Accidental Poisoning by Drugs, Medicinal Substances, and Biologicals (E850-E858)

INCLUDES accidental overdose of drug, wrong drug given or taken
  in error, and drug taken inadvertently
accidents in the use of drugs and biologicals in medical
  and surgical procedures

EXCLUDES administration with suicidal or homicidal intent or intent to
  harm, or in circumstances classifiable to E980-E989
  (E950.0-E950.5, E962.0, E980.0-E980.5)
correct drug properly administered in therapeutic or
  prophylactic dosage, as the cause of adverse effect
  (E930.0-E949.9)

NOTE See Alphabetic Index for more complete list of specific drugs
  to be classified under the fourth digit subdivisions. The
  American Hospital Formulary numbers can be used to
  classify new drugs listed by the American Hospital
  Formulary Service (AHFS). See Appendix C.

☑4th **E850 Accidental poisoning by analgesics, antipyretics, and
  antirheumatics**

E850.0 Heroin
  Diacetylmorphine

E850.1 Methadone

E850.2 Other opiates and related narcotics
  Codeine [methylmorphine]
  Meperidine [pethidine]
  Morphine
  Opium (alkaloids)

E850.3 Salicylates
  Acetylsalicylic acid [aspirin]
  Amino derivatives of salicylic acid
  Salicylic acid salts

E850.4 Aromatic analgesics, not elsewhere classified
  Acetanilid
  Paracetamol [acetaminophen]
  Phenacetin [acetophenetidin]

E850.5 Pyrazole derivatives
  Aminophenazone [amidopyrine]
  Phenylbutazone

E850.6 Antirheumatics [antiphlogistics]
  Gold salts
  Indomethacin
  EXCLUDES salicylates (E850.3)
    steroids (E858.0)

E850.7 Other non-narcotic analgesics
  Pyrabital

E850.8 Other specified analgesics and antipyretics
  Pentazocine

E850.9 Unspecified analgesic or antipyretic

E851 Accidental poisoning by barbiturates
  Amobarbital [amylobarbitone]
  Barbital [barbitone]
  Butabarbital [butabarbitone]
  Pentobarbital [pentobarbitone]
  Phenobarbital [phenobarbitone]
  Secobarbital [quinalbarbitone]
  EXCLUDES thiobarbiturates (E855.1)

✓4ᵗʰ **E852 Accidental poisoning by other sedatives and hypnotics**

E852.0 Chloral hydrate group

E852.1 Paraldehyde

E852.2 Bromine compounds
Bromides
Carbromal (derivatives)

E852.3 Methaqualone compounds

E852.4 Glutethimide group

E852.5 Mixed sedatives, not elsewhere classified

E852.8 Other specified sedatives and hypnotics

E852.9 Unspecified sedative or hypnotic
Sleeping:
drug
pill } NOS
tablet

✓4ᵗʰ **E853 Accidental poisoning by tranquilizers**

E853.0 Phenothiazine-based tranquilizers
Chlorpromazine   Prochlorperazine
Fluphenazine   Promazine

E853.1 Butyrophenone-based tranquilizers
Haloperidol   Trifluperidol
Spiperone

E853.2 Benzodiazepine-based tranquilizers
Chlordiazepoxide   Lorazepam
Diazepam   Medazepam
Flurazepam   Nitrazepam

E853.8 Other specified tranquilizers
Hydroxyzine   Meprobamate

E853.9 Unspecified tranquilizer

✓4ᵗʰ **E854 Accidental poisoning by other psychotropic agents**

E854.0 Antidepressants
Amitriptyline
Imipramine
Monoamine oxidase [MAO] inhibitors

E854.1 Psychodysleptics [hallucinogens]
Cannabis derivatives   Mescaline
Lysergide [LSD]   Psilocin
Marihuana (derivatives) Psilocybin

E854.2 Psychostimulants
Amphetamine
Caffeine
EXCLUDES *central appetite depressants (E858.8)*

E854.3 Central nervous system stimulants
Analeptics
Opiate antagonists

E854.8 Other psychotropic agents

✓4ᵗʰ **E855 Accidental poisoning by other drugs acting on central and autonomic nervous system**

E855.0 Anticonvulsant and anti-Parkinsonism drugs
Amantadine
Hydantoin derivatives
Levodopa [L-dopa]
Oxazolidine derivatives [paramethadione] [trimethadione]
Succinimides

E855.1 Other central nervous system depressants
Ether
Gaseous anesthetics
Halogenated hydrocarbon derivatives
Intravenous anesthetics
Thiobarbiturates, such as thiopental sodium

E855.2 Local anesthetics
Cocaine   Procaine
Lidocaine [lignocaine] Tetracaine

E855.3 Parasympathomimetics [cholinergics]
Acetylcholine   Anticholinesterase:
Anticholinesterase: reversible
organophosphorus   Pilocarpine

E855.4 Parasympatholytics [anticholinergics and antimuscarinics] and spasmolytics
Atropine   Hyoscine [scopolamine]
Homatropine   Quaternary ammonium derivatives

E855.5 Sympathomimetics [adrenergics]
Epinephrine [adrenalin]
Levarterenol [noradrenalin]

E855.6 Sympatholytics [antiadrenergics]
Phenoxybenzamine
Tolazoline hydrochloride

E855.8 Other specified drugs acting on central and autonomic nervous systems

E855.9 Unspecified drug acting on central and autonomic nervous systems

E856 Accidental poisoning by antibiotics

E857 Accidental poisoning by other anti-infectives

✓4ᵗʰ **E858 Accidental poisoning by other drugs**

E858.0 Hormones and synthetic substitutes

E858.1 Primarily systemic agents

E858.2 Agents primarily affecting blood constituents

E858.3 Agents primarily affecting cardiovascular system

E858.4 Agents primarily affecting gastrointestinal system

E858.5 Water, mineral, and uric acid metabolism drugs

E858.6 Agents primarily acting on the smooth and skeletal muscles and respiratory system

E858.7 Agents primarily affecting skin and mucous membrane, ophthalmological, otorhinolaryngological, and dental drugs

E858.8 Other specified drugs
Central appetite depressants

E858.9 Unspecified drug

Accidental Poisoning by Other Solid and Liquid Substances, Gases, and Vapors (E860-E869)

NOTE Categories in this section are intended primarily to indicate the external cause of poisoning states classifiable to 980-989. They may also be used to indicate external causes of localized effects classifiable to 001-799.

✓4ᵗʰ **E860 Accidental poisoning by alcohol, not elsewhere classified**

E860.0 Alcoholic beverages
Alcohol in preparations intended for consumption

E860.1 Other and unspecified ethyl alcohol and its products
Denatured alcohol   Grain alcohol NOS
Ethanol NOS   Methylated spirit

E860.2 Methyl alcohol
Methanol   Wood alcohol

E860.3 Isopropyl alcohol
Dimethyl carbinol   Rubbing alcohol subsitute
Isopropanol   Secondary propyl alcohol

E860.4 Fusel oil
Alcohol: Alcohol:
amyl   propyl
butyl

E860.8 Other specified alcohols

E860.9 Unspecified alcohol

✓4ᵗʰ **E861 Accidental poisoning by cleansing and polishing agents, disinfectants, paints, and varnishes**

E861.0 Synthetic detergents and shampoos

E861.1 Soap products

E861.2 Polishes

E861.3 Other cleansing and polishing agents
Scouring powders

E861.4 Disinfectants
Household and other disinfectants not ordinarily used on the person
EXCLUDES carbolic acid or phenol (E864.0)

E861.5 Lead paints

E861.6 Other paints and varnishes
Lacquers   Paints, other than lead
Oil colors   White washes

E861.9 Unspecified

√4ᵗʰ **E862 Accidental poisoning by petroleum products, other solvents and their vapors, not elsewhere classified**

E862.0 Petroleum solvents
Petroleum: Petroleum:
  ether   naphtha
  benzine

E862.1 Petroleum fuels and cleaners
Antiknock additives to petroleum fuels
Gas oils
Gasoline or petrol
Kerosene
EXCLUDES kerosene insecticides (E863.4)

E862.2 Lubricating oils

E862.3 Petroleum solids
Paraffin wax

E862.4 Other specified solvents
Benzene

E862.9 Unspecified solvent

√4ᵗʰ **E863 Accidental poisoning by agricultural and horticultural chemical and pharmaceutical preparations other than plant foods and fertilizers**
EXCLUDES plant foods and fertilizers (E866.5)

E863.0 Insecticides of organochlorine compounds
Benzene hexachloride   Dieldrin
Chlordane   Endrine
DDT   Toxaphene

E863.1 Insecticides of organophosphorus compounds
Demeton   Parathion
Diazinon   Phenylsulphthion
Dichlorvos   Phorate
Malathion   Phosdrin
Methyl parathion

E863.2 Carbamates
Aldicarb   Propoxur
Carbaryl

E863.3 Mixtures of insecticides

E863.4 Other and unspecified insecticides
Kerosene insecticides

E863.5 Herbicides
2, 4-Dichlorophenoxyacetic acid [2, 4-D]
2, 4, 5-Trichlorophenoxyacetic acid [2, 4, 5-T]
Chlorates
Diquat
Mixtures of plant foods and fertilizers with herbicides
Paraquat

E863.6 Fungicides
Organic mercurials (used in seed dressing)
Pentachlorophenols

E863.7 Rodenticides
Fluoroacetates   Warfarin
Squill and derivatives   Zinc phosphide
Thallium

E863.8 Fumigants
Cyanides   Phosphine
Methyl bromide

E863.9 Other and unspecified

√4ᵗʰ **E864 Accidental poisoning by corrosives and caustics, not elsewhere classified**
EXCLUDES those as components of disinfectants (E861.4)

E864.0 Corrosive aromatics
Carbolic acid or phenol

E864.1 Acids
Acid:
  hydrochloric
  nitric
  sulfuric

E864.2 Caustic alkalis
Lye

E864.3 Other specified corrosives and caustics

E864.4 Unspecified corrosives and caustics

√4ᵗʰ **E865 Accidental poisoning from poisonous foodstuffs and poisonous plants**
INCLUDES any meat, fish, or shellfish
plants, berries, and fungi eaten as, or in mistake for, food, or by a child
EXCLUDES anaphylactic shock due to adverse food reaction (995.60-995.69)
food poisoning (bacterial) (005.0-005.9)
poisoning and toxic reactions to venomous plants (E905.6-E905.7)

E865.0 Meat

E865.1 Shellfish

E865.2 Other fish

E865.3 Berries and seeds

E865.4 Other specified plants

E865.5 Mushrooms and other fungi

E865.8 Other specified foods

E865.9 Unspecified foodstuff or poisonous plant

√4ᵗʰ **E866 Accidental poisoning by other and unspecified solid and liquid substances**
EXCLUDES these substances as a component of:
medicines (E850.0-E858.9)
paints (E861.5-E861.6)
pesticides (E863.0-E863.9)
petroleum fuels (E862.1)

E866.0 Lead and its compounds and fumes

E866.1 Mercury and its compounds and fumes

E866.2 Antimony and its compounds and fumes

E866.3 Arsenic and its compounds and fumes

E866.4 Other metals and their compounds and fumes
Beryllium (compounds)   Iron (compounds)
Brass fumes   Manganese (compounds)
Cadmium (compounds)   Nickel (compounds)
Copper salts   Thallium (compounds)

E866.5 Plant foods and fertilizers
EXCLUDES mixtures with herbicides (E863.5)

E866.6 Glues and adhesives

E866.7 Cosmetics

E866.8 Other specified solid or liquid substances

E866.9 Unspecified solid or liquid substance

E867 Accidental poisoning by gas distributed by pipeline
Carbon monoxide from incomplete combustion of piped gas
Coal gas NOS
Liquefied petroleum gas distributed through pipes (pure or mixed with air)
Piped gas (natural) (manufactured)

√4ᵗʰ Fourth-digit Required   ▶◀ Revised Text   ● New Code   ▲ Revised Code Title

√4ᵗʰ **E868 Accidental poisoning by other utility gas and other carbon monoxide**

  E868.0 Liquefied petroleum gas distributed in mobile containers

    Butane
    Liquefied hydrocarbon gas NOS
    Propane
      } or carbon monoxide from incomplete combustion of these gases

  E868.1 Other and unspecified utility gas

    Acetylene
    Gas NOS used for lighting, heating, or cooking
    Water gas
      } or carbon monoxide from incomplete combustion of these gases

  E868.2 Motor vehicle exhaust gas

    Exhaust gas from:
      any type of combustion engine not in watercraft
      farm tractor, not in transit
      gas engine
      motor pump
      motor vehicle, not in transit

    EXCLUDES poisoning by carbon monoxide from:
      aircraft while in transit (E844.0-E844.9)
      motor vehicle while in transit (E818.0-E818.9)
      watercraft whether or not in transit (E838.0-E838.9)

  E868.3 Carbon monoxide from incomplete combustion of other domestic fuels

    Carbon monoxide from incomplete combustion of:
      coal
      coke
      kerosene
      wood
      } in domestic stove or fireplace

    EXCLUDES carbon monoxide from smoke and fumes due to conflagration (E890.0-E893.9)

  E868.8 Carbon monoxide from other sources

    Carbon monoxide from:
      blast furnace gas
      incomplete combustion of fuels in industrial use
      kiln vapor

  E868.9 Unspecified carbon monoxide

√4ᵗʰ **E869 Accidental poisoning by other gases and vapors**

  EXCLUDES effects of gases used as anesthetics (E855.1, E938.2)
    fumes from heavy metals (E866.0-E866.4)
    smoke and fumes due to conflagration or explosion (E890.0-E899)

  E869.0 Nitrogen oxides

  E869.1 Sulfur dioxide

  E869.2 Freon

  E869.3 Lacrimogenic gas [tear gas]

    Bromobenzyl cyanide
    Chloroacetophenone
    Ethyliodoacetate

  E869.4 Second-hand tobacco smoke

  E869.8 Other specified gases and vapors

    Chlorine
    Hydrocyanic acid gas

  E869.9 Unspecified gases and vapors

Misadventures to Patients During Surgical and Medical Care (E870-E876)

  EXCLUDES accidental overdose of drug and wrong drug given in error (E850.0-E858.9)
    surgical and medical procedures as the cause of abnormal reaction by the patient, without mention of misadventure at the time of procedure (E878.0-E879.9)

√4ᵗʰ **E870 Accidental cut, puncture, perforation, or hemorrhage during medical care**

  E870.0 Surgical operation

  E870.1 Infusion or transfusion

  E870.2 Kidney dialysis or other perfusion

  E870.3 Injection or vaccination

  E870.4 Endoscopic examination

  E870.5 Aspiration of fluid or tissue, puncture, and catheterization

    Abdominal paracentesis
    Aspirating needle biopsy
    Blood sampling
    Lumbar puncture
    Thoracentesis
      EXCLUDES heart catheterization (E870.6)

  E870.6 Heart catheterization

  E870.7 Administration of enema

  E870.8 Other specified medical care

  E870.9 Unspecified medical care

√4ᵗʰ **E871 Foreign object left in body during procedure**

  E871.0 Surgical operation

  E871.1 Infusion or transfusion

  E871.2 Kidney dialysis or other perfusion

  E871.3 Injection or vaccination

  E871.4 Endoscopic examination

  E871.5 Aspiration of fluid or tissue, puncture, and catheterization

    Abdominal paracentesis
    Aspiration needle biopsy
    Blood sampling
    Lumbar puncture
    Thoracentesis
      EXCLUDES heart catheterization (E871.6)

  E871.6 Heart catheterization

  E871.7 Removal of catheter or packing

  E871.8 Other specified procedures

  E871.9 Unspecified procedure

√4ᵗʰ **E872 Failure of sterile precautions during procedure**

  E872.0 Surgical operation

  E872.1 Infusion or transfusion

  E872.2 Kidney dialysis and other perfusion

  E872.3 Injection or vaccination

  E872.4 Endoscopic examination

  E872.5 Aspiration of fluid or tissue, puncture, and catheterization

    Abdominal paracentesis   Lumbar puncture
    Aspiration needle biopsy   Thoracentesis
    Blood sampling
      EXCLUDES heart catheterization (E872.6)

  E872.6 Heart catheterization

  E872.8 Other specified procedures

  E872.9 Unspecified procedure

√4ᵗʰ **E873 Failure in dosage**

  EXCLUDES accidental overdose of drug, medicinal or biological substance (E850.0-E858.9)

  E873.0 Excessive amount of blood or other fluid during transfusion or infusion

  E873.1 Incorrect dilution of fluid during infusion

  E873.2 Overdose of radiation in therapy

  E873.3 Inadvertent exposure of patient to radiation during medical care

  E873.4 Failure in dosage in electroshock or insulin-shock therapy

  E873.5 Inappropriate [too hot or too cold] temperature in local application and packing

  E873.6 Nonadministration of necessary drug or medicinal substance

  E873.8 Other specified failure in dosage

  E873.9 Unspecified failure in dosage

√4ᵗʰ Fourth-digit Required   ►◄ Revised Text   ● New Code   ▲ Revised Code Title

☑4ᵗʰ **E874 Mechanical failure of instrument or apparatus during procedure**

E874.0 Surgical operation

E874.1 Infusion and transfusion
Air in system

E874.2 Kidney dialysis and other perfusion

E874.3 Endoscopic examination

E874.4 Aspiration of fluid or tissue, puncture, and catheterization
Abdominal paracentesis   Lumbar puncture
Aspiration needle biopsy   Thoracentesis
Blood sampling
EXCLUDES   *heart catheterization (E874.5)*

E874.5 Heart catheterization

E874.8 Other specified procedures

E874.9 Unspecified procedure

☑4ᵗʰ **E875 Contaminated or infected blood, other fluid, drug, or biological substance**
INCLUDES   presence of:
bacterial pyrogens
endotoxin-producing bacteria
serum hepatitis-producing agent

E875.0 Contaminated substance transfused or infused

E875.1 Contaminated substance injected or used for vaccination

E875.2 Contaminated drug or biological substance administered by other means

E875.8 Other

E875.9 Unspecified

☑4ᵗʰ **E876 Other and unspecified misadventures during medical care**

E876.0 Mismatched blood in transfusion

E876.1 Wrong fluid in infusion

E876.2 Failure in suture and ligature during surgical operation

E876.3 Endotracheal tube wrongly placed during anesthetic procedure

E876.4 Failure to introduce or to remove other tube or instrument
EXCLUDES   *foreign object left in body during procedure (E871.0-E871.9)*

* **E876.5 Performance of wrong operation (procedure) on correct patient**
Wrong device implanted into correct surgical site
EXCLUDES   *correct operation (procedure) performed on wrong body part (E876.7)*

* **E876.6 Performance of operation (procedure) on patient not scheduled for surgery**
Performance of operation (procedure) intended for another patient
Performance of operation (procedure) on wrong patient

* **E876.7 Performance of correct operation (procedure) on wrong side/body part**
Performance of correct operation (procedure) on wrong side
Performance of correct operation (procedure) on wrong site

E876.8 Other specified misadventures during medical care
Performance of inappropriate treatment NEC

E876.9 Unspecified misadventure during medical care

Surgical and Medical Procedures as the Cause of Abnormal Reaction of Patient or Later Complication, Without Mention of Misadventure at the Time of Procedure (E878-E879)

INCLUDES   procedures as the cause of abnormal reaction, such as:
displacement or malfunction of prosthetic device
hepatorenal failure, postoperative
malfunction of external stoma
postoperative intestinal obstruction
rejection of transplanted organ

EXCLUDES   *anesthetic management properly carried out as the cause of adverse effect (E937.0-E938.9)*
infusion and transfusion, without mention of misadventure in the technique of procedure (E930.0-E949.9)

☑4ᵗʰ **E878 Surgical operation and other surgical procedures as the cause of abnormal reaction of patient, or of later complication, without mention of misadventure at the time of operation**

E878.0 Surgical operation with transplant of whole organ
Transplantation of:
heart
kidney
liver

E878.1 Surgical operation with implant of artificial internal device
Cardiac pacemaker
Electrodes implanted in brain
Heart valve prosthesis
Internal orthopedic device

E878.2 Surgical operation with anastomosis, bypass, or graft, with natural or artificial tissues used as implant
Anastomosis:
arteriovenous
gastrojejunal
Graft of blood vessel, tendon, or skin
EXCLUDES   *external stoma (E878.3)*

E878.3 Surgical operation with formation of external stoma
Colostomy   Gastrostomy
Cystostomy   Ureterostomy
Duodenostomy

E878.4 Other restorative surgery

E878.5 Amputation of limb(s)

E878.6 Removal of other organ (partial) (total)

E878.8 Other specified surgical operations and procedures

E878.9 Unspecified surgical operations and procedures

☑4ᵗʰ **E879 Other procedures, without mention of misadventure at the time of procedure, as the cause of abnormal reaction of patient, or of later complication**

E879.0 Cardiac catheterization

E879.1 Kidney dialysis

E879.2 Radiological procedure and radiotherapy
EXCLUDES   *radio-opaque dyes for diagnostic x-ray procedures (E947.8)*

E879.3 Shock therapy
Electroshock therapy
Insulin-shock therapy

E879.4 Aspiration of fluid
Lumbar puncture
Thoracentesis

E879.5 Insertion of gastric or duodenal sound

E879.6 Urinary catheterization

E879.7 Blood sampling

E879.8 Other specified procedures
Blood transfusion

E879.9 Unspecified procedure

---

*   Wrong surgery (MCE) edit applies.

Accidental Falls (E880-E888)

EXCLUDES falls (in or from):
  burning building (E890.8, E891.8)
  into fire (E890.0-E899)
  into water (with submersion or drowning)
    (E910.0-E910.9)
  machinery (in operation) (E919.0-E919.9)
  on edged, pointed, or sharp object (E920.0-E920.9)
  transport vehicle (E800.0-E845.9)
  vehicle not elsewhere classifiable (E846-E848)

✓4ᵗʰ E880 Fall on or from stairs or steps

E880.0 Escalator

E880.1 Fall on or from sidewalk curb
  EXCLUDES fall from moving sidewalk (E885.9)

E880.9 Other stairs or steps

✓4ᵗʰ E881 Fall on or from ladders or scaffolding

E881.0 Fall from ladder

E881.1 Fall from scaffolding

E882 Fall from or out of building or other structure

Fall from: Fall from:
  balcony   turret
  bridge   viaduct
  building   wall
  flagpole   window
  tower   Fall through roof

  EXCLUDES collapse of a building or structure (E916)
    fall or jump from burning building (E890.8, E891.8)

✓4ᵗʰ E883 Fall into hole or other opening in surface

  INCLUDES fall into: fall into:
    cavity   shaft
    dock   swimming pool
    hole   tank
    pit   well
    quarry

  EXCLUDES fall into water NOS (E910.9)
    that resulting in drowning or submersion without mention
      of injury (E910.0-E910.9)

E883.0 Accident from diving or jumping into water [swimming pool]
  Strike or hit:
    against bottom when jumping or diving into water
    wall or board of swimming pool
    water surface
  EXCLUDES diving with insufficient air supply (E913.2)
    effects of air pressure from diving (E902.2)

E883.1 Accidental fall into well

E883.2 Accidental fall into storm drain or manhole

E883.9 Fall into other hole or other opening in surface

✓4ᵗʰ E884 Other fall from one level to another

E884.0 Fall from playground equipment
  EXCLUDES recreational machinery (E919.8)

E884.1 Fall from cliff

E884.2 Fall from chair

E884.3 Fall from wheelchair
  Fall from motorized mobility scooter
  Fall from motorized wheelchair

E884.4 Fall from bed

E884.5 Fall from other furniture

E884.6 Fall from commode
  Toilet

E884.9 Other fall from one level to another
  Fall from: Fall from:
    embankment   stationary vehicle
    haystack   tree

✓4ᵗʰ E885 Fall on same level from slipping, tripping, or stumbling

E885.0 Fall from (nonmotorized) scooter
  EXCLUDES fall from motorized mobility scooter (E884.3)

E885.1 Fall from roller skates
  Heelies   Wheelies
  In-line skates

E885.2 Fall from skateboard

E885.3 Fall from skis

E885.4 Fall from snowboard

E885.9 Fall from other slipping, tripping, or stumbling
  Fall on moving sidewalk

✓4ᵗʰ E886 Fall on same level from collision, pushing, or shoving, by or with other person
  EXCLUDES crushed or pushed by a crowd or human stampede (E917.1, E917.6)

E886.0 In sports
  Tackles in sports
  EXCLUDES kicked, stepped on, struck by object, in sports (E917.0, E917.5)

E886.9 Other and unspecified
  Fall from collision of pedestrian (conveyance) with another pedestrian (conveyance)

E887 Fracture, cause unspecified

✓4ᵗʰ E888 Other and unspecified fall
  Accidental fall NOS
  Fall on same level NOS

E888.0 Fall resulting in striking against sharp object
  Use additional external cause code to identify object (E920)

E888.1 Fall resulting in striking against other object

E888.8 Other fall

E888.9 Unspecified fall
  Fall NOS

Accidents Caused by Fire and Flames (E890-E899)

  INCLUDES asphyxia or poisoning due to conflagration or ignition
    burning by fire
    secondary fires resulting from explosion

  EXCLUDES arson (E968.0)
    fire in or on:
      machinery (in operation) (E919.0-E919.9)
      transport vehicle other than stationary vehicle
        (E800.0-E845.9)
      vehicle not elsewhere classifiable (E846-E848)

✓4ᵗʰ E890 Conflagration in private dwelling
  INCLUDES conflagration in:
    apartment
    boarding house
    camping place
    caravan
    farmhouse
    house
    lodging house
    mobile home
    private garage
    rooming house
    tenement
  conflagration originating from sources classifiable to
    E893-E898 in the above buildings

E890.0 Explosion caused by conflagration

E890.1 Fumes from combustion of polyvinylchloride [PVC] and similar material in conflagration

E890.2 Other smoke and fumes from conflagration
  Carbon monoxide ⎫
  Fumes NOS   ⎬ from conflagration in private building
  Smoke NOS   ⎭

E890.3 Burning caused by conflagration

E890.8 Other accident resulting from conflagration
  Collapse of   ⎫
  Fall from   ⎬ burning private building
  Hit by object falling from
  Jump from   ⎭

E890.9 Unspecified accident resulting from conflagration in private dwelling

E Codes

E891–E899

✓4ᵗʰ **E891 Conflagration in other and unspecified building or structure**

Conflagration in:

    barn
    church
    convalescent and other residential home
    dormitory of educational institution
    factory
    farm outbuildings
    hospital
    hotel
    school
    store
    theater

Conflagration originating from sources classifiable to E893-E898, in the above buildings

E891.0 Explosion caused by conflagration

E891.1 Fumes from combustion of polyvinylchloride [PVC] and similar material in conflagration

E891.2 Other smoke and fumes from conflagration

Carbon monoxide ⎫
Fumes NOS   ⎬ from conflagration in private
Smoke NOS   ⎭ building or structure

E891.3 Burning caused by conflagration

E891.8 Other accident resulting from conflagration

Collapse of   ⎫
Fall from   ⎬ burning private
Hit by object falling from ⎬ building or
Jump from   ⎭ structure

E891.9 Unspecified accident resulting from conflagration of other and unspecified building or structure

E892 Conflagration not in building or structure

Fire (uncontrolled) (in) (of):   Fire (uncontrolled) (in) (of):
    forest   prairie
    grass   transport vehicle [any],
    hay   except while in transit
    lumber   tunnel
    mine

✓4ᵗʰ **E893 Accident caused by ignition of clothing**

EXCLUDES *ignition of clothing:*
    from highly inflammable material (E894)
    with conflagration (E890.0-E892)

E893.0 From controlled fire in private dwelling

Ignition of clothing from:

    normal fire (charcoal) (coal) ⎫
        (electric) (gas) (wood) in: ⎬ in private dwelling
    brazier   ⎬ (as listed in
    fireplace   ⎬ E890)
    furnace   ⎬
    stove   ⎭

E893.1 From controlled fire in other building or structure

Ignition of clothing from:

    normal fire (charcoal) (coal) ⎫
        (electric) (gas) (wood) in: ⎬ in other building or
    brazier   ⎬ structure (as
    fireplace   ⎬ listed in E891)
    furnace   ⎬
    stove   ⎭

E893.2 From controlled fire not in building or structure

Ignition of clothing from:

    bonfire (controlled)
    brazier fire (controlled), not in building or structure
    trash fire (controlled)

EXCLUDES *conflagration not in building (E892)*
    trash fire out of control (E892)

E893.8 From other specified sources

Ignition of clothing from: Ignition of clothing from:
    blowlamp   cigarette
    blowtorch   lighter
    burning bedspread   matches
    candle   pipe
    cigar   welding torch

E893.9 Unspecified source

Ignition of clothing (from controlled fire NOS) (in building NOS) NOS

E894 Ignition of highly inflammable material

Ignition of:

    benzine   ⎫
    gasoline   ⎬
    fat   ⎬ (with ignition of clothing)
    kerosene   ⎬
    paraffin   ⎬
    petrol   ⎭

EXCLUDES *ignition of highly inflammable material with:*
    conflagration (E890.0-E892)
    explosion (E923.0-E923.9)

E895 Accident caused by controlled fire in private dwelling

Burning by (flame of) normal fire (charcoal) (coal) (electric) (gas) (wood) in:

    brazier   ⎫
    fireplace ⎬ in private dwelling (as listed in E890)
    furnace   ⎬
    stove   ⎭

EXCLUDES *burning by hot objects not producing fire or flames (E924.0-E924.9)*
    ignition of clothing from these sources (E893.0)
    poisoning by carbon monoxide from incomplete combustion of fuel (E867-E868.9)
    that with conflagration (E890.0-E890.9)

E896 Accident caused by controlled fire in other and unspecified building or structure

Burning by (flame of) normal fire (charcoal) (coal)(electric)(gas)(wood) in:

    brazier   ⎫
    fireplace ⎬ in other building or structure (as
    furnace   ⎬ listed in E891)
    stove   ⎭

EXCLUDES *burning by hot objects not producing fire or flames (E924.0-E924.9)*
    ignition of clothing from these sources (E893.1)
    poisoning by carbon monoxide from incomplete combustion of fuel (E867-E868.9)
    that with conflagration (E891.0-E891.9)

E897 Accident caused by controlled fire not in building or structure

Burns from flame of:

    bonfire   ⎫
    brazier fire, not in building or structure ⎬ controlled
    trash fire   ⎭

EXCLUDES *ignition of clothing from these sources (E893.2)*
    trash fire out of control (E892)
    that with conflagration (E892)

✓4ᵗʰ **E898 Accident caused by other specified fire and flames**

EXCLUDES *conflagration (E890.0-E892)*
    that with ignition of:
      clothing (E893.0-E893.9)
      highly inflammable material (E894)

E898.0 Burning bedclothes

Bed set on fire NOS

E898.1 Other

Burning by: Burning by:
    blowlamp   lamp
    blowtorch   lighter
    candle   matches
    cigar   pipe
    cigarette   welding torch
    fire in room NOS

E899 Accident caused by unspecified fire

Burning NOS

Accidents Due to Natural and Environmental Factors (E900-E909)

✓4ᵗʰ **E900 Excessive heat**

E900.0 Due to weather conditions
Excessive heat as the external cause of:
ictus solaris
siriasis
sunstroke

E900.1 Of man-made origin

Heat (in):	Heat (in):
boiler room	furnace room
drying room	generated in transport vehicle
factory	kitchen

E900.9 Of unspecified origin

✓4ᵗʰ **E901 Excessive cold**

E901.0 Due to weather conditions
Excessive cold as the cause of:
chilblains NOS
immersion foot

E901.1 Of man-made origin

Contact with or inhalation of:	Prolonged exposure in:
dry ice	deep freeze unit
liquid air	refrigerator
liquid hydrogen	
liquid nitrogen	

E901.8 Other specified origin

E901.9 Of unspecified origin

✓4ᵗʰ **E902 High and low air pressure and changes in air pressure**

E902.0 Residence or prolonged visit at high altitude
Residence or prolonged visit at high altitude as the cause of:
Acosta syndrome
Alpine sickness
altitude sickness
Andes disease
anoxia, hypoxia
barotitis, barodontalgia, barosinusitis, otitic barotrauma
hypobarism, hypobaropathy
mountain sickness
range disease

E902.1 In aircraft
Sudden change in air pressure in aircraft during ascent or descent as the cause of:
aeroneurosis
aviators' disease

E902.2 Due to diving
High air pressure from rapid descent in water
Reduction in atmospheric pressure while surfacing from deep water diving
} as the cause of:
caisson disease
divers' disease
divers' palsy or paralysis

E902.8 Due to other specified causes
Reduction in atmospheric pressure while surfacing from underground

E902.9 Unspecified cause

E903 Travel and motion

✓4ᵗʰ **E904 Hunger, thirst, exposure, and neglect**
EXCLUDES   any condition resulting from homicidal intent (E968.0-E968.9)
hunger, thirst, and exposure resulting from accidents connected with transport (E800.0-E848)

E904.0 Abandonment or neglect of infants and helpless persons
Exposure to weather conditions
Hunger or thirst
} resulting from abandonment or neglect
Desertion of newborn
Inattention at or after birth
Lack of care (helpless person) (infant)
EXCLUDES   criminal [purposeful] neglect (E968.4)

E904.1 Lack of food
Lack of food as the cause of:
inanition
insufficient nourishment
starvation
EXCLUDES   hunger resulting from abandonment or neglect (E904.0)

E904.2 Lack of water
Lack of water as the cause of:
dehydration
inanition
EXCLUDES   dehydration due to acute fluid loss (276.51)

E904.3 Exposure (to weather conditions), not elsewhere classifiable

Exposure NOS	Struck by hailstones
Humidity	

EXCLUDES   struck by lightning (E907)

E904.9 Privation, unqualified
Destitution

✓4ᵗʰ **E905 Venomous animals and plants as the cause of poisoning and toxic reactions**
INCLUDES   chemical released by animal
insects
release of venom through fangs, hairs, spines, tentacles, and other venom apparatus
EXCLUDES   eating of poisonous animals or plants (E865.0-E865.9)

E905.0 Venomous snakes and lizards

Cobra	Mamba
Copperhead snake	Rattlesnake
Coral snake	Sea snake
Fer de lance	Snake (venomous)
Gila monster	Viper
Krait	Water moccasin

EXCLUDES   bites of snakes and lizards known to be nonvenomous (E906.2)

E905.1 Venomous spiders

Black widow spider	Tarantula (venomous)
Brown spider	

E905.2 Scorpion

E905.3 Hornets, wasps, and bees
Yellow jacket

E905.4 Centipede and venomous millipede (tropical)

E905.5 Other venomous arthropods
Sting of:
ant
caterpillar

E905.6 Venomous marine animals and plants

Puncture by sea urchin spine	Sting of:
Sting of:	sea anemone
coral	sea cucumber
jelly fish	other marine animal
nematocysts	or plant

EXCLUDES   bites and other injuries caused by nonvenomous marine animal (E906.2-E906.8)
bite of sea snake (venomous) (E905.0)

E905.7 Poisoning and toxic reactions caused by other plants
Injection of poisons or toxins into or through skin by plant thorns, spines, or other mechanisms
EXCLUDES   puncture wound NOS by plant thorns or spines (E920.8)

E905.8 Other specified

E905.9 Unspecified
Sting NOS
Venomous bite NOS

✓4ᵗʰ **E906 Other injury caused by animals**
EXCLUDES   poisoning and toxic reactions caused by venomous animals and insects (E905.0-E905.9)
road vehicle accident involving animals (E827.0-E828.9)
tripping or falling over an animal (E885.9)

E906.0 Dog bite

E906.1 Rat bite

E906.2 Bite of nonvenomous snakes and lizards

E906.3 Bite of other animal except arthropod
Cats   Rodents, except rats
Moray eel   Shark

E906.4 Bite of nonvenomous arthropod
Insect bite NOS

E906.5 Bite by unspecified animal
Animal bite NOS

E906.8 Other specified injury caused by animal
Butted by animal
Fallen on by horse or other animal, not being ridden
Gored by animal
Implantation of quills of porcupine
Pecked by bird
Run over by animal, not being ridden
Stepped on by animal, not being ridden
EXCLUDES   *injury by animal being ridden (E828.0-E828.9)*

E906.9 Unspecified injury caused by animal

E907 Lightning
EXCLUDES   *injury from:*
fall of tree or other object caused by lightning (E916)
fire caused by lightning (E890.0-E892)

✓4ᵗʰ **E908 Cataclysmic storms, and floods resulting from storms**
EXCLUDES   *collapse of dam or man-made structure causing flood (E909.3)*

E908.0 Hurricane
Storm surge
"Tidal wave" caused by storm action
Typhoon

E908.1 Tornado
Cyclone
Twisters

E908.2 Floods
Torrential rainfall
Flash flood
EXCLUDES   *collapse of dam or man-made structure causing flood (E909.3)*

E908.3 Blizzard (snow)(ice)

E908.4 Dust storm

E908.8 Other cataclysmic storms
Cloudburst

E908.9 Unspecified cataclysmic storms, and floods resulting from storms
Storm NOS

✓4ᵗʰ **E909 Cataclysmic earth surface movements and eruptions**

E909.0 Earthquakes

E909.1 Volcanic eruptions
Burns from lava
Ash inhalation

E909.2 Avalanche, landslide, or mudslide

E909.3 Collapse of dam or man-made structure

E909.4 Tidalwave caused by earthquake
Tidalwave NOS
Tsunami
EXCLUDES   *tidalwave caused by tropical storm (E908.0)*

E909.8 Other cataclysmic earth surface movements and eruptions

E909.9 Unspecified cataclysmic earth surface movements and eruptions

Accidents Caused by Submersion, Suffocation, and Foreign Bodies (E910-E915)

✓4ᵗʰ **E910 Accidental drowning and submersion**
INCLUDES   immersion
swimmers' cramp
EXCLUDES   *diving accident (NOS) (resulting in injury except drowning) (E883.0)*
diving with insufficient air supply (E913.2)
drowning and submersion due to:
cataclysm (E908-E909)
machinery accident (E919.0-E919.9)
transport accident (E800.0-E845.9)
effect of high and low air pressure (E902.2)
injury from striking against objects while in running water (E917.2)

E910.0 While water-skiing
Fall from water skis with submersion or drowning
EXCLUDES   *accident to water-skier involving a watercraft and resulting in submersion or other injury (E830.4, E831.4)*

E910.1 While engaged in other sport or recreational activity with diving equipment
Scuba diving NOS
Skin diving NOS
Underwater spear fishing NOS

E910.2 While engaged in other sport or recreational activity without diving equipment
Fishing or hunting, except from boat or with diving equipment
Ice skating
Playing in water
Surfboarding
Swimming NOS
Voluntarily jumping from boat, not involved in accident, for swim NOS
Wading in water
EXCLUDES   *jumping into water to rescue another person (E910.3)*

E910.3 While swimming or diving for purposes other than recreation or sport
Marine salvage
Pearl diving
Placement of fishing nets   (with diving
Rescue (attempt) of another   equipment)
person
Underwater construction or
repairs

E910.4 In bathtub

E910.8 Other accidental drowning or submersion
Drowning in:
quenching tank
swimming pool

E910.9 Unspecified accidental drowning or submersion
Accidental fall into water NOS
Drowning NOS

E911 Inhalation and ingestion of food causing obstruction of respiratory tract or suffocation
Aspiration and inhalation of food [any] (into respiratory tract) NOS
Asphyxia by   food [including bone, seed in food,
Choked on   regurgitated food]
Suffocation by

Compression of trachea   by food lodged in
Interruption of respiration   esophagus
Obstruction of respiration

Obstruction of pharynx by food (bolus)
EXCLUDES   *injury, except asphyxia and obstruction of respiratory passage, caused by food (E915)*
obstruction of esophagus by food without mention of asphyxia or obstruction of respiratory passage (E915)

E912 Inhalation and ingestion of other object causing obstruction of respiratory tract or suffocation

Aspiration and inhalation of foreign body except food (into respiratory tract) NOS

Foreign object [bean] [marble] in nose

Obstruction of pharynx by foreign body

Compression

Interruption of respiration   } by foreign body in

Obstruction of respiration   esophagus

EXCLUDES *injury, except asphyxia and obstruction of respiratory passage, caused by foreign body (E915)*

obstruction of esophagus by foreign body without mention of asphyxia or obstruction in respiratory passage (E915)

√4ᵗʰ E913 Accidental mechanical suffocation

EXCLUDES *mechanical suffocation from or by:*

accidental inhalation or ingestion of:

food (E911)

foreign object (E912)

cataclysm (E908-E909)

explosion (E921.0-E921.9, E923.0-E923.9)

machinery accident (E919.0-E919.9)

E913.0 In bed or cradle

EXCLUDES *suffocation by plastic bag (E913.1)*

E913.1 By plastic bag

E913.2 Due to lack of air (in closed place)

Accidentally closed up in refrigerator or other airtight enclosed space

Diving with insufficient air supply

EXCLUDES *suffocation by plastic bag (E913.1)*

E913.3 By falling earth or other substance

Cave-in NOS

EXCLUDES *cave-in caused by cataclysmic earth surface movements and eruptions (E909)*

struck by cave-in without asphyxiation or suffocation (E916)

E913.8 Other specified means

Accidental hanging, except in bed or cradle

E913.9 Unspecified means

Asphyxia, mechanical NOS

Strangulation NOS

Suffocation NOS

E914 Foreign body accidentally entering eye and adnexa

EXCLUDES *corrosive liquid (E924.1)*

E915 Foreign body accidentally entering other orifice

EXCLUDES *aspiration and inhalation of foreign body, any, (into respiratory tract) NOS (E911-E912)*

Other Accidents (E916-E928)

E916 Struck accidentally by falling object

Collapse of building, except on fire

Falling:

rock

snowslide NOS

stone

tree

Object falling from:

machine, not in operation

stationary vehicle

Code first:

collapse of building on fire (E890.0-E891.9)

falling object in:

cataclysm (E908-E909)

machinery accidents (E919.0-E919.9)

transport accidents (E800.0-E845.9)

vehicle accidents not elsewhere classifiable (E846-E848)

object set in motion by:

explosion (E921.0-E921.9, E923.0-E923.9)

firearm (E922.0-E922.9)

projected object (E917.0-E917.9)

√4ᵗʰ E917 Striking against or struck accidentally by objects or persons

INCLUDES bumping into or against

colliding with

kicking against

stepping on

struck by

} object (moving) (projected) (stationary)

pedestrian conveyance

person

EXCLUDES *fall from:*

collision with another person, except when caused by a crowd (E886.0-E886.9)

stumbling over object (E885.9)

fall resulting in striking against object (E888.0, E888.1)

injury caused by:

assault (E960.0-E960.1, E967.0-E967.9)

cutting or piercing instrument (E920.0-E920.9)

explosion (E921.0-E921.9, E923.0-E923.9)

firearm (E922.0-E922.9)

machinery (E919.0-E919.9)

transport vehicle (E800.0-E845.9)

vehicle not elsewhere classifiable (E846-E848)

E917.0 In sports without subsequent fall

Kicked or stepped on during game (football) (rugby)

Struck by hit or thrown ball

Struck by hockey stick or puck

E917.1 Caused by a crowd, by collective fear or panic without subsequent fall

Crushed

Pushed   } by crowd or human

Stepped on   stampede

E917.2 In running water without subsequent fall

EXCLUDES *drowning or submersion (E910.0-E910.9)*

that in sports (E917.0, E917.5)

E917.3 Furniture without subsequent fall

EXCLUDES *fall from furniture (E884.2, E884.4-E884.5)*

E917.4 Other stationary object without subsequent fall

Bath tub

Fence

Lamp-post

E917.5 Object in sports with subsequent fall

Knocked down while boxing

E917.6 Caused by a crowd, by collective fear or panic with subsequent fall

E917.7 Furniture with subsequent fall

EXCLUDES *fall from furniture (E884.2, E884.4-E884.5)*

E917.8 Other stationary object with subsequent fall

Bath tub

Fence

Lamp-post

E917.9 Other striking against with or without subsequent fall

E918 Caught accidentally in or between objects

Caught, crushed, jammed, or pinched in or between moving or stationary objects, such as:

escalator

folding object

hand tools, appliances, or implements

sliding door and door frame

under packing crate

washing machine wringer

EXCLUDES *injury caused by:*

cutting or piercing instrument (E920.0-E920.9)

machinery (E919.0-E919.9)

mechanism or component of firearm and air gun (E928.7)

transport vehicle (E800.0-E845.9)

vehicle not elsewhere classifiable (E846-E848)

struck accidentally by:

falling object (E916)

object (moving) (projected) (E917.0-E917.9)

✓4ᵗʰ **E919 Accidents caused by machinery**

INCLUDES   burned by
caught in (moving parts of)
collapse of
crushed by
cut or pierced by
drowning or submersion caused by
explosion of, on, in
fall from or into moving part of
fire starting in or on   machinery
mechanical suffocation caused by   (accident)
object falling from, on, in motion
    by
overturning of
pinned under
run over by
struck by
thrown from

caught between machinery and other object
machinery accident NOS

EXCLUDES   accidents involving machinery, not in operation (E884.9,
     E916-E918)
injury caused by:
     electric current in connection with machinery
         (E925.0-E925.9)
     escalator (E880.0, E918)
     explosion of pressure vessel in connection with
         machinery (E921.0-E921.9)
     mechanism or component of firearm and air gun
         (E928.7)
     moving sidewalk (E885.9)
     powered hand tools, appliances, and implements
         (E916-E918, E920.0-E921.9, E923.0-E926.9)
     transport vehicle accidents involving machinery
         (E800.0-E848)
     poisoning by carbon monoxide generated by machine
         (E868.8)

E919.0 Agricultural machines

Animal-powered   Farm tractor
   agricultural machine   Harvester
Combine   Hay mower or rake
Derrick, hay   Reaper
Farm machinery NOS   Thresher

EXCLUDES   that in transport under own power on the highway
     (E810.0-E819.9)
that being towed by another vehicle on the
     highway (E810.0-E819.9, E827.0-E827.9,
     E829.0-E829.9)
that involved in accident classifiable to E820-E829
     (E820.0-E829.9)

E919.1 Mining and earth-drilling machinery

Bore or drill (land) (seabed)
Shaft hoist
Shaft lift
Under-cutter

EXCLUDES   coal car, tram, truck, and tub in mine (E846)

E919.2 Lifting machines and appliances

Chain hoist
Crane
Derrick
Elevator (building) (grain)   except in agricultural
Forklift truck   or mining
Lift   operations
Pulley block
Winch

EXCLUDES   that being towed by another vehicle on the
     highway (E810.0-E819.9, E827.0-E827.9,
     E829.0-829.9)
that in transport under own power on the highway
     (E810.0-E819.9)
that involved in accident classifiable to E820-E829
     (E820.0-E829.9)

E919.3 Metalworking machines

Abrasive wheel   Metal:
Forging machine   milling machine
Lathe   power press
Mechanical shears   rolling-mill
Metal: sawing machine
   drilling machine

E919.4 Woodworking and forming machines

Band saw   Overhead plane
Bench saw   Powered saw
Circular saw   Radial saw
Molding machine   Sander

EXCLUDES   *hand saw (E920.1)*

E919.5 Prime movers, except electrical motors

Gas turbine
Internal combustion engine
Steam engine
Water driven turbine

EXCLUDES   *that being towed by other vehicle on the highway*
     (E810.0-E819.9, E827.0-E827.9,
     E829.0-E829.9)
that in transport under own power on the highway
     (E810.0-E819.9)

E919.6 Transmission machinery

Transmission: Transmission:
  belt   pinion
  cable   pulley
  chain   shaft
  gear

E919.7 Earth moving, scraping, and other excavating machines

Bulldozer   Steam shovel
Road scraper

EXCLUDES   *that being towed by other vehicle on the highway*
     (E810.0-E819.9, E827.0-E827.9,
     E829.0-E829.9)
that in transport under own power on the highway
     (E810.0-E819.9)

E919.8 Other specified machinery

Machines for manufacture of:
   clothing
   foodstuffs and beverages
   paper
Printing machine
Recreational machinery
Spinning, weaving, and textile machines

E919.9 Unspecified machinery

✓4ᵗʰ **E920 Accidents caused by cutting and piercing instruments or objects**

INCLUDES   edged
     accidental injury (by) object   pointed
                     sharp

EXCLUDES   *injury caused by mechanism or component of firearm and*
     air gun (E928.7)

E920.0 Powered lawn mower

E920.1 Other powered hand tools

Any powered hand tool [compressed air] [electric]
     [explosive cartridge] [hydraulic power], such as:
   drill
   hand saw
   hedge clipper
   rivet gun
   snow blower
   staple gun

EXCLUDES   *band saw (E919.4)*
           bench saw (E919.4)

E920.2 Powered household appliances and implements

Blender   Electric:
Electric: knife
  beater or mixer   sewing machine
  can opener   Garbage disposal appliance
  fan

E920.3 Knives, swords, and daggers

E920.4 Other hand tools and implements

Axe	Paper cutter
Can opener NOS	Pitchfork
Chisel	Rake
Fork	Scissors
Hand saw	Screwdriver
Hoe	Sewing machine, not powered
Ice pick	Shovel
Needle (sewing)	

E920.5 Hypodermic needle
Contaminated needle
Needle stick

E920.8 Other specified cutting and piercing instruments or objects

Arrow	Nail
Broken glass	Plant thorn
Dart	Splinter
Edge of stiff paper	Tin can lid
Lathe turnings	

EXCLUDES *animal spines or quills (E906.8)*
flying glass due to explosion (E921.0-E923.9)

E920.9 Unspecified cutting and piercing instrument or object

☑4ᵗʰ **E921 Accident caused by explosion of pressure vessel**

INCLUDES accidental explosion of pressure vessels, whether or not part of machinery

EXCLUDES *explosion of pressure vessel on transport vehicle (E800.0-E845.9)*

E921.0 Boilers

E921.1 Gas cylinders
Air tank   Pressure gas tank

E921.8 Other specified pressure vessels
Aerosol can   Tin can lid
Automobile tire

E921.9 Unspecified pressure vessel

☑4ᵗʰ **E922 Accident caused by firearm, and air gun missile**

EXCLUDES *injury caused by mechanism or component of firearm and air gun (E928.7)*

E922.0 Handgun
Pistol   Revolver
EXCLUDES *Verey pistol (E922.8)*

E922.1 Shotgun (automatic)

E922.2 Hunting rifle

E922.3 Military firearms
Army rifle   Machine gun

E922.4 Air gun
BB gun   Pellet gun

E922.5 Paintball gun

E922.8 Other specified firearm missile
Verey pistol [flare]

E922.9 Unspecified firearm missile
Gunshot wound NOS
Shot NOS

☑4ᵗʰ **E923 Accident caused by explosive material**

INCLUDES flash burns and other injuries resulting from explosion of explosive material
ignition of highly explosive material with explosion

EXCLUDES *explosion:*
in or on machinery (E919.0-E919.9)
on any transport vehicle, except stationary motor vehicle (E800.0-E848)
with conflagration (E890.0, E891.0,E892)
injury caused by mechanism or component of firearm and air gun (E928.7)
secondary fires resulting from explosion (E890.0-E899)

E923.0 Fireworks

E923.1 Blasting materials
Blasting cap   Dynamite
Detonator   Explosive [any] used in blasting operations

E923.2 Explosive gases

Acetylene	Fire damp
Butane	Gasoline fumes
Coal gas	Methane
Explosion in mine NOS	Propane

E923.8 Other explosive materials

Bomb	Torpedo
Explosive missile	Explosion in munitions:
Grenade	dump
Mine	factory
Shell	

E923.9 Unspecified explosive material
Explosion NOS

☑4ᵗʰ **E924 Accident caused by hot substance or object, caustic or corrosive material, and steam**

EXCLUDES *burning NOS (E899)*
chemical burn resulting from swallowing a corrosive substance (E860.0-E864.4)
fire caused by these substances and objects (E890.0-E894)
radiation burns (E926.0-E926.9)
therapeutic misadventures (E870.0-E876.9)

E924.0 Hot liquids and vapors, including steam
Burning or scalding by:
boiling water
hot or boiling liquids not primarily caustic or corrosive
liquid metal
steam
other hot vapor
EXCLUDES *hot (boiling) tap water (E924.2)*

E924.1 Caustic and corrosive substances
Burning by:
acid [any kind]
ammonia
caustic oven cleaner or other substance
corrosive substance
lye
vitriol

E924.2 Hot (boiling) tap water

E924.8 Other
Burning by:
heat from electric heating appliance
hot object NOS
light bulb
steam pipe

E924.9 Unspecified

☑4ᵗʰ **E925 Accident caused by electric current**

INCLUDES electric current from exposed wire, faulty appliance, high voltage cable, live rail, or open electric socket as the cause of:
burn
cardiac fibrillation
convulsion
electric shock
electrocution
puncture wound
respiratory paralysis

EXCLUDES *burn by heat from electrical appliance (E924.8)*
lightning (E907)

E925.0 Domestic wiring and appliances

E925.1 Electric power generating plants, distribution stations, transmission lines
Broken power line

E925.2 Industrial wiring, appliances, and electrical machinery
Conductors
Control apparatus
Electrical equipment and machinery
Transformers

E925.8 Other electric current
Wiring and appliances in or on:
farm [not farmhouse]
outdoors
public building
residential institutions
schools

E925.9 Unspecified electric current
Burns or other injury from electric current NOS
Electric shock NOS
Electrocution NOS

☑4ᵗʰ **E926 Exposure to radiation**
EXCLUDES *abnormal reaction to or complication of treatment without*
mention of misadventure (E879.2)
atomic power plant malfunction in water transport
(E838.0-E838.9)
misadventure to patient in surgical and medical procedures
(E873.2-E873.3)
use of radiation in war operations (E996-E997.9)

E926.0 Radiofrequency radiation

Overexposure to:	from:
microwave radiation	high-powered radio and
radar radiation	television transmitters
radiofrequency	industrial radiofrequency
radiofrequency	induction heaters
radiation [any]	radar installations

E926.1 Infrared heaters and lamps
Exposure to infrared radiation from heaters and lamps as
the cause of:
blistering
burning
charring
inflammatory change
EXCLUDES *physical contact with heater or lamp (E924.8)*

E926.2 Visible and ultraviolet light sources
Arc lamps
Black light sources
Electrical welding arc
Oxygas welding torch
Sun rays
Tanning bed
EXCLUDES *excessive heat from these sources (E900.1-E900.9)*

E926.3 X-rays and other electromagnetic ionizing radiation
Gamma rays
X-rays (hard) (soft)

E926.4 Lasers

E926.5 Radioactive isotopes
Radiobiologicals
Radiopharmaceuticals

E926.8 Other specified radiation
Artificially accelerated beams of ionized particles generated
by:
betatrons
synchrotrons

E926.9 Unspecified radiation
Radiation NOS

☑4ᵗʰ **E927 Overexertion and strenuous and repetitive movements or
loads**
Use additional code to identify activity (E001-E030)

E927.0 Overexertion from sudden strenuous movement
Sudden trauma from strenuous movement

E927.1 Overexertion from prolonged static position
Overexertion from maintaining prolonged positions, such
as:
holding
sitting
standing

E927.2 Excessive physical exertion from prolonged activity

E927.3 Cumulative trauma from repetitive motion
Cumulative trauma from repetitive movements

E927.4 Cumulative trauma from repetitive impact

**E927.8 Other overexertion and strenuous and repetitive
movements or loads**

**E927.9 Unspecified overexertion and strenuous and repetitive
movements or loads**

☑4ᵗʰ **E928 Other and unspecified environmental and accidental causes**
E928.0 Prolonged stay in weightless environment
Weightlessness in spacecraft (simulator)

E928.1 Exposure to noise
Noise (pollution)
Sound waves
Supersonic waves

E928.2 Vibration

E928.3 Human bite

E928.4 External constriction caused by hair

E928.5 External constriction caused by other object

E928.6 Environmental exposure to harmful algae and toxins

Algae bloom NOS	Florida red tide
Blue-green algae bloom	Harmful algae bloom
Brown tide	Pfiesteria piscicida
Cyanobacteria bloom	Red tide

E928.7 Mechanism or component of firearm and air gun
Injury due to:
explosion of gun parts
recoil
Pierced, cut, crushed, or pinched by slide, trigger
mechanism, scope, or other gun part
Powder burn from firearm or air gun
EXCLUDES *accident caused by firearm and air gun missile*
(E922.0-E922.9)

E928.8 Other

E928.9 Unspecified accident

Accident NOS	
Blow NOS	stated as accidentally
Casualty (not due to war)	inflicted
Decapitation	

Knocked down	
Killed	stated as accidentally
Injury [any part of body, or	inflicted, but not
unspecified]	otherwise
Mangled	specified
Wound	

EXCLUDES *fracture, cause unspecified (E887)*
injuries undetermined whether accidentally or
purposely inflicted (E980.0-E989)

Late Effects Of Accidental Injury (E929)

NOTE This category is to be used to indicate accidental injury as the cause of
death or disability from late effects, which are themselves classifiable
elsewhere. The "late effects" include conditions reported as such, or as
sequelae which may occur at any time after the attempted suicide or
self-inflicted injury.

☑4ᵗʰ **E929 Late effects of accidental injury**
EXCLUDES *late effects of:*
surgical and medical procedures (E870.0-E879.9)
therapeutic use of drugs and medicines (E930.0-E949.9)

E929.0 Late effects of motor vehicle accident
Late effects of accidents classifiable to E810-E825

E929.1 Late effects of other transport accident
Late effects of accidents classifiable to E800-E807,
E826-E838, E840-E848

E929.2 Late effects of accidental poisoning
Late effects of accidents classifiable to E850-E858,
E860-E869

E929.3 Late effects of accidental fall
Late effects of accidents classifiable to E880-E888

E929.4 Late effects of accident caused by fire
Late effects of accidents classifiable to E890-E899

**E929.5 Late effects of accident due to natural and environmental
factors**
Late effects of accidents classifiable to E900-E909

E929.8 Late effects of other accidents
Late effects of accidents classifiable to E910-E928.8

E929.9 Late effects of unspecified accident
Late effects of accidents classifiable to E928.9

Drugs, Medicinal And Biological Substances Causing Adverse Effects In Therapeutic Use (E930-E949)

INCLUDES correct drug properly administered in therapeutic or prophylactic dosage, as the cause of any adverse effect including allergic or hypersensitivity reactions

EXCLUDES *accidental overdose of drug and wrong drug given or taken in error (E850.0-E858.9)*

accidents in the technique of administration of drug or biological substance, such as accidental puncture during injection, or contamination of drug (E870.0-E876.9)

administration with suicidal or homicidal intent or intent to harm, or in circumstances classifiable to E950.0-E950.5, E962.0, E980.0-E980.5

NOTE See Alphabetic Index for more complete list of specific drugs to be classified under the fourth digit subdivisions. The American Hospital Formulary numbers can be used to classify new drugs listed by the American Hospital Formulary Service (AHFS). See Appendix C.

✔4ᵗʰ E930　Antibiotics

EXCLUDES *that used as eye, ear, nose, and throat [ENT], and local anti-infectives (E946.0-E946.9)*

E930.0　Penicillins
Natural　　　　　　　　Semisynthetic, such as:
Synthetic　　　　　　　　cloxacillin
Semisynthetic, such as:　　nafcillin
　ampicillin　　　　　　　oxacillin

E930.1　Antifungal antibiotics
Amphotericin B　　　　Hachimycin [trichomycin]
Griseofulvin　　　　　　Nystatin

E930.2　Chloramphenicol group
Chloramphenicol　　　　Thiamphenicol

E930.3　Erythromycin and other macrolides
Oleandomycin　　　　　Spiramycin

E930.4　Tetracycline group
Doxycycline　　　　　　Oxytetracycline
Minocycline

E930.5　Cephalosporin group
Cephalexin　　　　　　Cephaloridine
Cephaloglycin　　　　　Cephalothin

E930.6　Antimycobacterial antibiotics
Cycloserine　　　　　　Rifampin
Kanamycin　　　　　　Streptomycin

E930.7　Antineoplastic antibiotics
Actinomycins, such as:　Actinomycins, such as:
　Bleomycin　　　　　　Daunorubicin
　Cactinomycin　　　　　Mitomycin
　Dactinomycin

EXCLUDES *other antineoplastic drugs (E933.1)*

E930.8　Other specified antibiotics

E930.9　Unspecified antibiotic

✔4ᵗʰ E931　Other anti-infectives

EXCLUDES *ENT, and local anti-infectives (E946.0-E946.9)*

E931.0　Sulfonamides
Sulfadiazine　　　　　Sulfamethoxazole
Sulfafurazole

E931.1　Arsenical anti-infectives

E931.2　Heavy metal anti-infectives
Compounds of:　　Compounds of:
　antimony　　　　　lead
　bismuth　　　　　mercury

EXCLUDES *mercurial diuretics (E944.0)*

E931.3　Quinoline and hydroxyquinoline derivatives
Chiniofon
Diiodohydroxyquin

EXCLUDES *antimalarial drugs (E931.4)*

E931.4　Antimalarials and drugs acting on other blood protozoa
Chloroquine phosphate　Proguanil [chloroguanide]
Cycloguanil　　　　　Pyrimethamine
Primaquine　　　　　Quinine (sulphate)

E931.5　Other antiprotozoal drugs
Emetine

E931.6　Anthelmintics
Hexylresorcinol　　　　Piperazine
Male fern oleoresin　　Thiabendazole

E931.7　Antiviral drugs
Methisazone

EXCLUDES *amantadine (E936.4)*
cytarabine (E933.1)
idoxuridine (E946.5)

E931.8　Other antimycobacterial drugs
Ethambutol　　　　Para-aminosalicylic acid derivatives
Ethionamide　　　　Sulfones
Isoniazid

E931.9　Other and unspecified anti-infectives
Flucytosine　　　　Nitrofuranderivatives

✔4ᵗʰ E932　Hormones and synthetic substitutes

E932.0　Adrenal cortical steroids
Cortisone derivatives
Desoxycorticosterone derivatives
Fluorinated corticosteroid

E932.1　Androgens and anabolic congeners
Nandrolone phenpropionate
Oxymetholone
Testosterone and preparations

E932.2　Ovarian hormones and synthetic substitutes
Contraceptives, oral
Estrogens
Estrogens and progestogens combined
Progestogens

E932.3　Insulins and antidiabetic agents
Acetohexamide　　　　Insulin
Biguanide derivatives, oral　Phenformin
Chlorpropamide　　　　Sulfonylurea derivatives, oral
Glucagon　　　　　　Tolbutamide

EXCLUDES *adverse effect of insulin administered for shock therapy (E879.3)*

E932.4　Anterior pituitary hormones
Corticotropin　　　Somatotropin [growth hormone]
Gonadotropin

E932.5　Posterior pituitary hormones
Vasopressin

EXCLUDES *oxytocic agents (E945.0)*

E932.6　Parathyroid and parathyroid derivatives

E932.7　Thyroid and thyroid derivatives
Dextrothyroxine　　　Liothyronine
Levothyroxine sodium　Thyroglobulin

E932.8　Antithyroid agents
Iodides　　　　　　Thiourea
Thiouracil

E932.9　Other and unspecified hormones and synthetic substitutes

✔4ᵗʰ E933　Primarily systemic agents

E933.0　Antiallergic and antiemetic drugs
Antihistamines　　　Diphenylpyraline
Chlorpheniramine　　Thonzylamine
Diphenhydramine　　Tripelennamine

EXCLUDES *phenothiazine-based tranquilizers (E939.1)*

E933.1　Antineoplastic and immunosuppressive drugs
Azathioprine　　　Mechlorethamine hydrochloride
Busulfan　　　　　Mercaptopurine
Chlorambucil　　　Triethylenethiophosphoramide
Cyclophosphamide　　[thio-TEPA]
Cytarabine
Fluorouracil

EXCLUDES *antineoplastic antibiotics (E930.7)*

E933.2　Acidifying agents

E933.3　Alkalizing agents

E933.4　Enzymes, not elsewhere classified
Penicillinase

✔4ᵗʰ Fourth-digit Required　　　▶◀ Revised Text　　　● New Code　　　▲ Revised Code Title

E Codes

E933.5–E939.2

E933.5 Vitamins, not elsewhere classified
Vitamin A
Vitamin D
EXCLUDES nicotinic acid (E942.2)
vitamin K (E934.3)

E933.6 Oral bisphosphonates

E933.7 Intravenous bisphosphonates

E933.8 Other systemic agents, not elsewhere classified
Heavy metal antagonists

E933.9 Unspecified systemic agent

✓4th E934 Agents primarily affecting blood constituents

E934.0 Iron and its compounds
Ferric salts
Ferrous sulphate and other ferrous salts

E934.1 Liver preparations and other antianemic agents
Folic acid

E934.2 Anticoagulants
Coumarin   Prothrombin synthesis inhibitor
Heparin   Warfarin sodium
Phenindione

E934.3 Vitamin K [phytonadione]

E934.4 Fibrinolysis-affecting drugs
Aminocaproic acid   Streptokinase
Streptodornase   Urokinase

E934.5 Anticoagulant antagonists and other coagulants
Hexadimethrine bromide
Protamine sulfate

E934.6 Gamma globulin

E934.7 Natural blood and blood products
Blood plasma   Packed red cells
Human fibrinogen   Whole blood

E934.8 Other agents affecting blood constituents
Macromolecular blood substitutes

E934.9 Unspecified agent affecting blood constituents

✓4th E935 Analgesics, antipyretics, and antirheumatics

E935.0 Heroin
Diacetylmorphine

E935.1 Methadone

E935.2 Other opiates and related narcotics
Codeine [methylmorphine]
Meperidine [pethidine]
Morphine
Opium (alkaloids)

E935.3 Salicylates
Acetylsalicylic acid [aspirin]
Amino derivatives of salicylic acid
Salicylic acid salts

E935.4 Aromatic analgesics, not elsewhere classified
Acetanilid
Paracetamol [acetaminophen]
Phenacetin [acetophenetidin]

E935.5 Pyrazole derivatives
Aminophenazone [aminopyrine]
Phenylbutazone

E935.6 Antirheumatics [antiphlogistics]
Gold salts   Indomethacin
EXCLUDES salicylates (E935.3)
steroids (E932.0)

E935.7 Other non-narcotic analgesics
Pyrabital

E935.8 Other specified analgesics and antipyretics
Pentazocine

E935.9 Unspecified analgesic and antipyretic

✓4th E936 Anticonvulsants and anti-Parkinsonism drugs

E936.0 Oxazolidine derivatives
Paramethadione   Trimethadione

E936.1 Hydantoin derivatives
Phenytoin

E936.2 Succinimides
Ethosuximide   Phensuximide

E936.3 Other and unspecified anticonvulsants
Beclamide
Primidone

E936.4 Anti-Parkinsonism drugs
Amantadine
Ethopropazine [profenamine]
Levodopa [L-dopa]

✓4th E937 Sedatives and hypnotics

E937.0 Barbiturates
Amobarbital [amylobarbitone]
Barbital [barbitone]
Butabarbital [butabarbitone]
Pentobarbital [pentobarbitone]
Phenobarbital [phenobarbitone]
Secobarbital [quinalbarbitone]
EXCLUDES thiobarbiturates (E938.3)

E937.1 Chloral hydrate group

E937.2 Paraldehyde

E937.3 Bromine compounds
Bromide
Carbromal (derivatives)

E937.4 Methaqualone compounds

E937.5 Glutethimide group

E937.6 Mixed sedatives, not elsewhere classified

E937.8 Other sedatives and hypnotics

E937.9 Unspecified
Sleeping:
drug
pill   } NOS
tablet

✓4th E938 Other central nervous system depressants and anesthetics

E938.0 Central nervous system muscle-tone depressants
Chlorphenesin (carbamate)
Mephenesin
Methocarbamol

E938.1 Halothane

E938.2 Other gaseous anesthetics
Ether
Halogenated hydrocarbon derivatives, except halothane
Nitrous oxide

E938.3 Intravenous anesthetics
Ketamine
Methohexital [methohexitone]
Thiobarbiturates, such as thiopental sodium

E938.4 Other and unspecified general anesthetics

E938.5 Surface and infiltration anesthetics
Cocaine
Lidocaine [lignocaine]
Procaine
Tetracaine

E938.6 Peripheral nerve- and plexus-blocking anesthetics

E938.7 Spinal anesthetics

E938.9 Other and unspecified local anesthetics

✓4th E939 Psychotropic agents

E939.0 Antidepressants
Amitriptyline   Monoamine oxidase
Imipramine   [MAO] inhibitors

E939.1 Phenothiazine-based tranquilizers
Chlorpromazine   Prochlorperazine
Fluphenazine   Promazine
Phenothiazine

E939.2 Butyrophenone-based tranquilizers
Haloperidol   Trifluperidol
Spiperone

✓4th Fourth-digit Required   ▶◀ Revised Text   ● New Code   ▲ Revised Code Title

E939.3 Other antipsychotics, neuroleptics, and major tranquilizers

E939.4 Benzodiazepine-based tranquilizers
Chlordiazepoxide	Lorazepam
Diazepam	Medazepam
Flurazepam	Nitrazepam

E939.5 Other tranquilizers
Hydroxyzine	Meprobamate

E939.6 Psychodysleptics [hallucinogens]
Cannabis (derivatives)	Mescaline
Lysergide [LSD]	Psilocin
Marihuana (derivatives)	Psilocybin

E939.7 Psychostimulants
Amphetamine	Caffeine

EXCLUDES *central appetite depressants (E947.0)*

E939.8 Other psychotropic agents

E939.9 Unspecified psychotropic agent

√4ᵗʰ **E940 Central nervous system stimulants**

E940.0 Analeptics
Lobeline	Nikethamide

E940.1 Opiate antagonists
Levallorphan	Naloxone
Nalorphine	

E940.8 Other specified central nervous system stimulants

E940.9 Unspecified central nervous system stimulant

√4ᵗʰ **E941 Drugs primarily affecting the autonomic nervous system**

E941.0 Parasympathomimetics [cholinergics]
Acetylcholine
Anticholinesterase:
　organophosphorus
　reversible
Pilocarpine

E941.1 Parasympatholytics [anticholinergics and antimuscarinics] and spasmolytics
Atropine	Hyoscine [scopamine]
Homatropine	Quaternary ammonium derivatives

EXCLUDES *papaverine (E942.5)*

E941.2 Sympathomimetics [adrenergics]
Epinephrine [adrenalin]
Levarterenol [noradrenalin]

E941.3 Sympatholytics [antiadrenergics]
Phenoxybenzamine
Tolazolinehydrochloride

E941.9 Unspecified drug primarily affecting the autonomic nervous system

√4ᵗʰ **E942 Agents primarily affecting the cardiovascular system**

E942.0 Cardiac rhythm regulators
Practolol	Propranolol
Procainamide	Quinidine

E942.1 Cardiotonic glycosides and drugs of similar action
Digitalis glycosides	Strophanthins
Digoxin	

E942.2 Antilipemic and antiarteriosclerotic drugs
Cholestyramine	Nicotinic acid derivatives
Clofibrate	Sitosterols

EXCLUDES *dextrothyroxine (E932.7)*

E942.3 Ganglion-blocking agents
Pentamethonium bromide

E942.4 Coronary vasodilators
Dipyridamole	Nitrites
Nitrates [nitroglycerin]	Prenylamine

E942.5 Other vasodilators
Cyclandelate	Hydralazine
Diazoxide	Papaverine

E942.6 Other antihypertensive agents
Clonidine	Rauwolfia alkaloids
Guanethidine	Reserpine

E942.7 Antivaricose drugs, including sclerosing agents
Monoethanolamine	Zinc salts

E942.8 Capillary-active drugs
Adrenochrome derivatives	Metaraminol
Bioflavonoids	

E942.9 Other and unspecified agents primarily affecting the cardiovascular system

√4ᵗʰ **E943 Agents primarily affecting gastrointestinal system**

E943.0 Antacids and antigastric secretion drugs
Aluminum hydroxide	Magnesium trisilicate

E943.1 Irritant cathartics
Bisacodyl	Phenolphthalein
Castor oil	

E943.2 Emollient cathartics
Sodium dioctyl sulfosuccinate

E943.3 Other cathartics, including intestinal atonia drugs
Magnesium sulfate

E943.4 Digestants
Pancreatin	Pepsin
Papain	

E943.5 Antidiarrheal drugs
Bismuth subcarbonate	Kaolin
Pectin	

EXCLUDES *anti-infectives (E930.0-E931.9)*

E943.6 Emetics

E943.8 Other specified agents primarily affecting the gastrointestinal system

E943.9 Unspecified agent primarily affecting the gastrointestinal system

√4ᵗʰ **E944 Water, mineral, and uric acid metabolism drugs**

E944.0 Mercurial diuretics
Chlormerodrin	Mercurophylline
Mercaptomerin	Mersalyl

E944.1 Purine derivative diuretics
Theobromine
Theophylline

EXCLUDES *aminophylline [theophylline ethylenediamine] (E945.7)*

E944.2 Carbonic acid anhydrase inhibitors
Acetazolamide

E944.3 Saluretics
Benzothiadiazides	Chlorothiazide group

E944.4 Other diuretics
Ethacrynic acid	Furosemide

E944.5 Electrolytic, caloric, and water-balance agents

E944.6 Other mineral salts, not elsewhere classified

E944.7 Uric acid metabolism drugs
Cinchophen and congeners	Phenoquin
Colchicine	Probenecid

√4ᵗʰ **E945 Agents primarily acting on the smooth and skeletal muscles and respiratory system**

E945.0 Oxytocic agents
Ergot alkaloids	Prostaglandins

E945.1 Smooth muscle relaxants
Adiphenine
Metaproterenol [orciprenaline]

EXCLUDES *papaverine (E942.5)*

E945.2 Skeletal muscle relaxants
Alcuronium chloride
Suxamethonium chloride

E945.3 Other and unspecified drugs acting on muscles

E945.4 Antitussives
Dextromethorphan
Pipazethate hydrochloride

E Codes

E945.5–E957.0

E945.5 Expectorants
Acetylcysteine
Cocillana
Guaifenesin [glyceryl guaiacolate]
Ipecacuanha
Terpin hydrate

E945.6 Anti-common cold drugs

E945.7 Antiasthmatics
Aminophylline [theophylline ethylenediamine]

E945.8 Other and unspecified respiratory drugs

✓4th **E946 Agents primarily affecting skin and mucous membrane, ophthalmological, otorhinolaryngological, and dental drugs**

E946.0 Local anti-infectives and anti-inflammatory drugs

E946.1 Antipruritics

E946.2 Local astringents and local detergents

E946.3 Emollients, demulcents, and protectants

E946.4 Keratolytics, kerstoplastics, other hair treatment drugs and preparations

E946.5 Eye anti-infectives and other eye drugs
Idoxuridine

E946.6 Anti-infectives and other drugs and preparations for ear, nose, and throat

E946.7 Dental drugs topically applied

E946.8 Other agents primarily affecting skin and mucous membrane
Spermicides

E946.9 Unspecified agent primarily affecting skin and mucous membrane

✓4th **E947 Other and unspecified drugs and medicinal substances**

E947.0 Dietetics

E947.1 Lipotropic drugs

E947.2 Antidotes and chelating agents, not elsewhere classified

E947.3 Alcohol deterrents

E947.4 Pharmaceutical excipients

E947.8 Other drugs and medicinal substances
Contrast media used for diagnostic x-ray procedures
Diagnostic agents and kits

E947.9 Unspecified drug or medicinal substance

✓4th **E948 Bacterial vaccines**

E948.0 BCG vaccine

E948.1 Typhoid and paratyphoid

E948.2 Cholera

E948.3 Plague

E948.4 Tetanus

E948.5 Diphtheria

E948.6 Pertussis vaccine, including combinations with a pertussis component

E948.8 Other and unspecified bacterial vaccines

E948.9 Mixed bacterial vaccines, except combinations with a pertussis component

✓4th **E949 Other vaccines and biological substances**
EXCLUDES *gamma globulin (E934.6)*

E949.0 Smallpox vaccine

E949.1 Rabies vaccine

E949.2 Typhus vaccine

E949.3 Yellow fever vaccine

E949.4 Measles vaccine

E949.5 Poliomyelitis vaccine

E949.6 Other and unspecified viral and rickettsial vaccines
Mumps vaccine

E949.7 Mixed viral-rickettsial and bacterial vaccines, except combinations with a pertussis component
EXCLUDES *combinations with a pertussis component (E948.6)*

E949.9 Other and unspecified vaccines and biological substances

Suicide and Self-inflicted Injury (E950-E959)

INCLUDES injuries in suicide and attempted suicide
self-inflicted injuries specified as intentional

✓4th **E950 Suicide and self-inflicted poisoning by solid or liquid substances**

E950.0 Analgesics, antipyretics, and antirheumatics

E950.1 Barbiturates

E950.2 Other sedatives and hypnotics

E950.3 Tranquilizers and other psychotropic agents

E950.4 Other specified drugs and medicinal substances

E950.5 Unspecified drug or medicinal substance

E950.6 Agricultural and horticultural chemical and pharmaceutical preparations other than plant foods and fertilizers

E950.7 Corrosive and caustic substances
Suicide and self-inflicted poisoning by substances classifiable to E864

E950.8 Arsenic and its compounds

E950.9 Other and unspecified solid and liquid substances

✓4th **E951 Suicide and self-inflicted poisoning by gases in domestic use**

E951.0 Gas distributed by pipeline

E951.1 Liquefied petroleum gas distributed in mobile containers

E951.8 Other utility gas

✓4th **E952 Suicide and self-inflicted poisoning by other gases and vapors**

E952.0 Motor vehicle exhaust gas

E952.1 Other carbon monoxide

E952.8 Other specified gases and vapors

E952.9 Unspecified gases and vapors

✓4th **E953 Suicide and self-inflicted injury by hanging, strangulation, and suffocation**

E953.0 Hanging

E953.1 Suffocation by plastic bag

E953.8 Other specified means

E953.9 Unspecified means

E954 Suicide and self-inflicted injury by submersion [drowning]

✓4th **E955 Suicide and self-inflicted injury by firearms, air guns and explosives**

E955.0 Handgun

E955.1 Shotgun

E955.2 Hunting rifle

E955.3 Military firearms

E955.4 Other and unspecified firearm
Gunshot NOS
Shot NOS

E955.5 Explosives

E955.6 Air gun
BB gun
Pellet gun

E955.7 Paintball gun

E955.9 Unspecified

E956 Suicide and self-inflicted injury by cutting and piercing instrument

✓4th **E957 Suicide and self-inflicted injuries by jumping from high place**

E957.0 Residential premises

✓4th Fourth-digit Required   ▶◀ Revised Text   ● New Code   ▲ Revised Code Title

E957.1 **Other man-made structures**

E957.2 **Natural sites**

E957.9 **Unspecified**

✓4ᵗʰ **E958 Suicide and self-inflicted injury by other and unspecified means**

E958.0 **Jumping or lying before moving object**

E958.1 **Burns, fire**

E958.2 **Scald**

E958.3 **Extremes of cold**

E958.4 **Electrocution**

E958.5 **Crashing of motor vehicle**

E958.6 **Crashing of aircraft**

E958.7 **Caustic substances, except poisoning**

> EXCLUDES *poisoning by caustic substance (E950.7)*

E958.8 **Other specified means**

E958.9 **Unspecified means**

E959 Late effects of self-inflicted injury

> NOTE This category is to be used to indicate circumstances classifiable to E950-E958 as the cause of death or disability from late effects, which are themselves classifiable elsewhere. The "late effects" include conditions reported as such, or as sequelae which may occur at any time after the attempted suicide or self-inflicted injury.

Homicide and Injury Purposely Inflicted by Other Persons (E960-E969)

> INCLUDES injuries inflicted by another person with intent to injure or kill, by any means

> EXCLUDES injuries due to:
> *legal intervention (E970-E978)*
> *operations of war (E990-E999)*
> *terrorism (E979)*

✓4ᵗʰ **E960 Fight, brawl, rape**

E960.0 **Unarmed fight or brawl**
Beatings NOS
Brawl or fight with hands, fists, feet
Injured or killed in fight NOS

> EXCLUDES *homicidal:*
> *injury by weapons (E965.0-E966, E969)*
> *strangulation (E963)*
> *submersion (E964)*

E960.1 **Rape**

E961 Assault by corrosive or caustic substance, except poisoning
Injury or death purposely caused by corrosive or caustic substance, such as:
acid [any]
corrosive substance
vitriol

> EXCLUDES *burns from hot liquid (E968.3)*
> *chemical burns from swallowing a corrosive substance (E962.0-E962.9)*

✓4ᵗʰ **E962 Assault by poisoning**

E962.0 **Drugs and medicinal substances**
Homicidal poisoning by any drug or medicinal substance

E962.1 **Other solid and liquid substances**

E962.2 **Other gases and vapors**

E962.9 **Unspecified poisoning**

E963 Assault by hanging and strangulation
Homicidal (attempt):   Homicidal (attempt):
garrotting or ligature   strangulation
hanging   suffocation

E964 Assault by submersion [drowning]

✓4ᵗʰ **E965 Assault by firearms and explosives**

E965.0 **Handgun**
Pistol   Revolver

E965.1 **Shotgun**

E965.2 **Hunting rifle**

E965.3 **Military firearms**

E965.4 **Other and unspecified firearm**

E965.5 **Antipersonnel bomb**

E965.6 **Gasoline bomb**

E965.7 **Letter bomb**

E965.8 **Other specified explosive**
Bomb NOS (placed in):
car
house
Dynamite

E965.9 **Unspecified explosive**

E966 Assault by cutting and piercing instrument
Assassination (attempt), homicide (attempt) by any instrument classifiable under E920
Homicidal:
cut
puncture } any part of the body
stab
Stabbed any part of the body

✓4ᵗʰ **E967 Perpetrator of child and adult abuse**

> NOTE Selection of the correct perpetrator code is based on the relationship between the perpetrator and the victim

E967.0 **By father, stepfather, or boyfriend**
Male partner of child's parent or guardian

E967.1 **By other specified person**

E967.2 **By mother, stepmother, or girlfriend**
Female partner of child's parent or guardian

E967.3 **By spouse or partner**
Abuse of spouse or partner by ex-spouse or ex-partner

E967.4 **By child**

E967.5 **By sibling**

E967.6 **By grandparent**

E967.7 **By other relative**

E967.8 **By non-related caregiver**

E967.9 **By unspecified person**

✓4ᵗʰ **E968 Assault by other and unspecified means**

E968.0 **Fire**
Arson   Homicidal burns NOS

> EXCLUDES *burns from hot liquid (E968.3)*

E968.1 **Pushing from a high place**

E968.2 **Striking by blunt or thrown object**

E968.3 **Hot liquid**
Homicidal burns by scalding

E968.4 **Criminal neglect**
Abandonment of child, infant, or other helpless person with intent to injure or kill

E968.5 **Transport vehicle**
Being struck by other vehicle or run down with intent to injure
Pushed in front of, thrown from, or dragged by moving vehicle with intent to injure

E968.6 **Air gun**
BB gun
Pellet gun

E968.7 **Human bite**

E968.8 **Other specified means**

E968.9 **Unspecified means**
Assassination (attempt) NOS
Homicidal (attempt):
injury NOS
wound NOS
Manslaughter (nonaccidental)
Murder (attempt) NOS
Violence, non-accidental

E969 Late effects of injury purposely inflicted by other person

NOTE This category is to be used to indicate circumstances classifiable to E960-E968 as the cause of death or disability from late effects, which are themselves classifiable elsewhere. The "late effects" include conditions reported as such, or as sequelae which may occur at any time after injury purposely inflicted by another person.

Legal Intervention (E970-E978)

INCLUDES injuries inflicted by the police or other law-enforcing agents, including military on duty, in the course of arresting or attempting to arrest lawbreakers, suppressing disturbances, maintaining order, and other legal action
legal execution

EXCLUDES injuries caused by civil insurrections (E990.0-E999)

E970 Injury due to legal intervention by firearms

Gunshot wound	Injury by:
Injury by:	rifle pellet or rubber bullet
machine gun	shot NOS
revolver	

E971 Injury due to legal intervention by explosives

Injury by:	Injury by:
dynamite	grenade
explosive shell	mortar bomb

E972 Injury due to legal intervention by gas

Asphyxiation by gas	Poisoning by gas
Injury by tear gas	

E973 Injury due to legal intervention by blunt object

Hit, struck by:	Hit, struck by:
baton (nightstick)	stave
blunt object	

E974 Injury due to legal intervention by cutting and piercing instrument

Cut	Injured by bayonet
Incised wound	Stab wound

E975 Injury due to legal intervention by other specified means

Blow	Manhandling

E976 Injury due to legal intervention by unspecified means

E977 Late effects of injuries due to legal intervention

NOTE This category is to be used to indicate circumstances classifiable to E970-E976 as the cause of death or disability from late effects, which are themselves classifiable elsewhere. The "late effects" include conditions reported as such, or as sequelae, which may occur at any time after the injury due to legal intervention.

E978 Legal execution

All executions performed at the behest of the judiciary or ruling authority [whether permanent or temporary] as:

asphyxiation by gas
beheading, decapitation (by guillotine)
capital punishment
electrocution
hanging
poisoning
shooting
other specified means

Terrorism (E979)

✓4ᵗʰ **E979 Terrorism**

Injuries resulting from the unlawful use of force or violence against persons or property to intimidate or coerce a Government, the civilian population, or any segment thereof, in furtherance of political or social objective

E979.0 Terrorism involving explosion of marine weapons

Depth-charge	Sea-based artillery shell
Marine mine	Torpedo
Mine NOS, at sea or in harbour	Underwater blast

E979.1 Terrorism involving destruction of aircraft

Aircraft used as a weapon	Aircraft:
Aircraft:	shot down
burned	Crushed by falling aircraft
exploded	

E979.2 Terrorism involving other explosions and fragments

Antipersonnel bomb (fragments)	Fragments from: artillery shell
Blast NOS	bomb
Explosion (of):	grenade
artillery shell	guided missile
breech-block	land-mine
cannon block	rocket
mortar bomb	shell
munitions being used in terrorism	shrapnel
NOS	Mine NOS

E979.3 Terrorism involving fires, conflagration and hot substances

Burning building or structure:	Fire (causing): NOS
collapse of	Other injury
fall from	Melting of fittings and
hit by falling object in	furniture in burning
jump from	Petrol bomb
Conflagration NOS	Smouldering building
Fire (causing):	or structure
Asphyxia	
Burns	

E979.4 Terrorism involving firearms

Bullet:	Bullet:
carbine	rifle
machine gun	rubber (rifle)
pistol	Pellets (shotgun)

E979.5 Terrorism involving nuclear weapons

Blast effects
Exposure to ionizing radiation from nuclear weapon
Fireball effects
Heat from nuclear weapon
Other direct and secondary effects of nuclear weapons

E979.6 Terrorism involving biological weapons

Anthrax	Smallpox
Cholera	

E979.7 Terrorism involving chemical weapons

Gases, fumes, chemicals	Phosgene
Hydrogen cyanide	Sarin

E979.8 Terrorism involving other means

Drowning and submersion
Lasers
Piercing or stabbing instruments
Terrorism NOS

E979.9 Terrorism, secondary effects

NOTE This code is for use to identify conditions occurring subsequent to a terrorist attack not those that are due to the initial terrorist act

EXCLUDES late effect of terrorist attack (E999.1)

Injury Undetermined Whether Accidentally or Purposely Inflicted (E980-E989)

NOTE Categories E980-E989 are for use when it is unspecified or it cannot be determined whether the injuries are accidental (unintentional), suicide (attempted), or assault.

✓4ᵗʰ **E980 Poisoning by solid or liquid substances, undetermined whether accidentally or purposely inflicted**

E980.0 Analgesics, antipyretics, and antirheumatics

E980.1 Barbiturates

E980.2 Other sedatives and hypnotics

E980.3 Tranquilizers and other psychotropic agents

E980.4 Other specified drugs and medicinal substances

E980.5 Unspecified drug or medicinal substance

E980.6 Corrosive and caustic substances

Poisoning, undetermined whether accidental or purposeful, by substances classifiable to E864

E980.7 Agricultural and horticultural chemical and pharmaceutical preparations other than plant foods and fertilizers

E980.8 Arsenic and its compounds

E980.9 **Other and unspecified solid and liquid substances**

✓4ᵗʰ E981 **Poisoning by gases in domestic use, undetermined whether accidentally or purposely inflicted**

E981.0 **Gas distributed by pipeline**

E981.1 **Liquefied petroleum gas distributed in mobile containers**

E981.8 **Other utility gas**

✓4ᵗʰ E982 **Poisoning by other gases, undetermined whether accidentally or purposely inflicted**

E982.0 **Motor vehicle exhaust gas**

E982.1 **Other carbon monoxide**

E982.8 **Other specified gases and vapors**

E982.9 **Unspecified gases and vapors**

✓4ᵗʰ E983 **Hanging, strangulation, or suffocation, undetermined whether accidentally or purposely inflicted**

E983.0 **Hanging**

E983.1 **Suffocation by plastic bag**

E983.8 **Other specified means**

E983.9 **Unspecified means**

E984 **Submersion [drowning], undetermined whether accidentally or purposely inflicted**

✓4ᵗʰ E985 **Injury by firearms, air guns and explosives, undetermined whether accidentally or purposely inflicted**

E985.0 **Handgun**

E985.1 **Shotgun**

E985.2 **Hunting rifle**

E985.3 **Military firearms**

E985.4 **Other and unspecified firearm**

E985.5 **Explosives**

E985.6 **Air gun**
BB gun   Pellet gun

E985.7 **Paintball gun**

E986 **Injury by cutting and piercing instruments, undetermined whether accidentally or purposely inflicted**

✓4ᵗʰ E987 **Falling from high place, undetermined whether accidentally or purposely inflicted**

E987.0 **Residential premises**

E987.1 **Other man-made structures**

E987.2 **Natural sites**

E987.9 **Unspecified site**

✓4ᵗʰ E988 **Injury by other and unspecified means, undetermined whether accidentally or purposely inflicted**

E988.0 **Jumping or lying before moving object**

E988.1 **Burns, fire**

E988.2 **Scald**

E988.3 **Extremes of cold**

E988.4 **Electrocution**

E988.5 **Crashing of motor vehicle**

E988.6 **Crashing of aircraft**

E988.7 **Caustic substances, except poisoning**

E988.8 **Other specified means**

E988.9 **Unspecified means**

E989 **Late effects of injury, undetermined whether accidentally or purposely inflicted**

NOTE This category is to be used to indicate circumstances classifiable to E980-E988 as the cause of death or disability from late effects, which are themselves classifiable elsewhere. The "late effects" include conditions reported as such, or as sequelae, which may occur at any time after injury, undetermined whether accidentally or purposely inflicted.

Injury Resulting from Operations of War (E990-E999)

INCLUDES injuries to military personnel and civilians caused by war and civil insurrections and occurring during the time of war and insurrection, and peacekeeping missions

EXCLUDES accidents during training of military personnel manufacture of war material and transport, unless attributable to enemy action

✓4ᵗʰ E990 **Injury due to war operations by fires and conflagrations**

INCLUDES asphyxia, burns, or other injury originating from fire caused by a fire-producing device or indirectly by any conventional weapon

E990.0 **From gasoline bomb**
Incendiary bomb

E990.1 **From flamethrower**

E990.2 **From incendiary bullet**

E990.3 **From fire caused indirectly from conventional weapon**
EXCLUDES fire aboard military aircraft (E994.3)

E990.9 **From other and unspecified source**

✓4ᵗʰ E991 **Injury due to war operations by bullets and fragments**

EXCLUDES injury due to bullets and fragments due to war operations, but occurring after cessation of hostilities (E998.0)
injury due to explosion of artillery shells and mortars (E993.2)
injury due to explosion of improvised explosive device [IED] (E993.3-E993.5)
injury due to sea-based artillery shell (E992.3)

E991.0 **Rubber bullets (rifle)**

E991.1 **Pellets (rifle)**

E991.2 **Other bullets**
Bullet [any, except rubber bullets and pellets]:
carbine
machine gun
pistol
rifle
shotgun

E991.3 **Antipersonnel bomb (fragments)**

E991.4 **Fragments from munitions**
Fragments from: Fragments from:
artillery shell   guided missile
bombs, except antipersonnel land mine
detonation of unexploded   rockets
    ordnance [UXO]   shell
grenade

E991.5 **Fragments from person-borne improvised explosive device [IED]**

E991.6 **Fragments from vehicle-borne improvised explosive device [IED]**
IED borne by land, air, or water transport vehicle

E991.7 **Fragments from other improvised explosive device [IED]**
Roadside IED

E991.8 **Fragments from weapons**
Fragments from: Fragments from:
artillery   missile launchers
autocannons   mortars
automatic grenade launchers small arms

E991.9 **Other and unspecified fragments**
Shrapnel NOS

✓4ᵗʰ E992 **Injury due to war operations by explosion of marine weapons**

E992.0 **Torpedo**

E992.1 **Depth charge**

E992.2 **Marine mines**
Marine mines at sea or in harbor

E992.3 **Sea-based artillery shell**

E992.8 **Other marine weapons**

E992.9 **Unspecified marine weapon**
Underwater blast NOS

✓4ᵗʰ Fourth-digit Required   ►◄ Revised Text   ● New Code   ▲ Revised Code Title

✓4ᵗʰ **E993 Injury due to war operations by other explosion**

Injuries due to direct or indirect pressure or air blast of an explosion occurring during war operations

EXCLUDES *injury due to fragments resulting from an explosion (E991.0-E991.9)*
injury due to detonation of unexploded ordnance but occurring after cessation of hostilities (E998.0-E998.9)
injury due to nuclear weapons (E996.0-E996.9)

E993.0 Aerial bomb

E993.1 Guided missile

E993.2 Mortar
Artillery shell

E993.3 Person-borne improvised explosive device [IED]

E993.4 Vehicle-borne improvised explosive device [IED]
IED borne by land, air, or water transport vehicle

E993.5 Other improvised explosive device [IED]
Roadside IED

E993.6 Unintentional detonation of own munitions
Unintentional detonation of own ammunition (artillery) (mortars)

E993.7 Unintentional discharge of own munitions launch device
Unintentional explosion of own:
autocannons
automatic grenade launchers
missile launchers
small arms

E993.8 Other specified explosion
Bomb   Land mine
Grenade

E993.9 Unspecified explosion
Air blast NOS   Blast wind NOS
Blast NOS   Explosion NOS
Blast wave NOS

✓4ᵗʰ **E994 Injury due to war operations by destruction of aircraft**

E994.0 Destruction of aircraft due to enemy fire or explosives
Air to air missile   Rocket propelled grenade [RPG]
Explosive device placed   Small arms fire
  on aircraft   Surface to air missile

E994.1 Unintentional destruction of aircraft due to own onboard explosives

E994.2 Destruction of aircraft due to collision with other aircraft

E994.3 Destruction of aircraft due to onboard fire

E994.8 Other destruction of aircraft

E994.9 Unspecified destruction of aircraft

✓4ᵗʰ **E995 Injury due to war operations by other and unspecified forms of conventional warfare**

E995.0 Unarmed hand-to-hand combat
EXCLUDES *intentional restriction of airway (E995.3)*

E995.1 Struck by blunt object
Baton (nightstick)
Stave

E995.2 Piercing object
Bayonet
Knife
Sword

E995.3 Intentional restriction of air and airway
Intentional submersion
Strangulation
Suffocation

E995.4 Unintentional drowning due to inability to surface or obtain air
Submersion

E995.8 Other forms of conventional warfare

E995.9 Unspecified form of conventional warfare

✓4ᵗʰ **E996 Injury due to war operations by nuclear weapons**
Dirty bomb NOS

EXCLUDES *late effects of injury due to nuclear weapons (E999.0, E999.1)*

E996.0 Direct blast effect of nuclear weapon
Injury to bodily organs due to blast pressure

E996.1 Indirect blast effect of nuclear weapon
Injury due to being thrown by blast
Injury due to being struck or crushed by blast debris

E996.2 Thermal radiation effect of nuclear weapon
Burns due to thermal radiation
Fireball effects
Flash burns
Heat effects

E996.3 Nuclear radiation effects
Acute radiation exposure
Beta burns
Fallout exposure
Radiation sickness
Secondary effects of nuclear weapons

E996.8 Other effects of nuclear weapons

E996.9 Unspecified effect of nuclear weapon

✓4ᵗʰ **E997 Injury due to war operations by other forms of unconventional warfare**

E997.0 Lasers

E997.1 Biological warfare

E997.2 Gases, fumes, and chemicals

E997.3 Weapon of mass destruction [WMD], unspecified

E997.8 Other specified forms of unconventional warfare

E997.9 Unspecified form of unconventional warfare

✓4ᵗʰ **E998 Injury due to war operations but occurring after cessation of hostilities**

Injuries due to operations of war but occurring after cessation of hostilities by any means classifiable under E990-E997
Injuries by explosion of bombs or mines placed in the course of operations of war, if the explosion occurred after cessation of hostilities

E998.0 Explosion of mines

E998.1 Explosion of bombs

E998.8 Injury due to other war operations but occurring after cessation of hostilities

E998.9 Injury due to unspecified war operations but occurring after cessation of hostilities

✓4ᵗʰ **E999 Late effect of injury due to war operations and terrorism**

NOTE This category is to be used to indicate circumstances classifiable to E979, E990-E998 as the cause of death or disability from late effects, which are themselves classifiable elsewhere. The "late effects" include conditions reported as such, or as sequelae, which may occur at any time after the injury, resulting from operations of war or terrorism

E999.0 Late effect of injury due to war operations

E999.1 Late effect of injury due to terrorism

Official ICD-9-CM Government Appendixes

Appendix A: Morphology of Neoplasms

The World Health Organization has published an adaptation of the International Classification of Diseases for oncology (ICD-O). It contains a coded nomenclature for the morphology of neoplasms, which is reproduced here for those who wish to use it in conjunction with Chapter 2 of the International Classification of Diseases, 9th Revision, Clinical Modification.

The morphology code numbers consist of five digits; the first four identify the histological type of the neoplasm and the fifth indicates its behavior. The one-digit behavior code is as follows:

/0 Benign
/1 Uncertain whether benign or malignant
    Borderline malignancy
/2 Carcinoma in situ
    Intraepithelial
    Noninfiltrating
    Noninvasive
/3 Malignant, primary site
/6 Malignant, metastatic site
    Secondary site
/9 Malignant, uncertain whether primary or metastatic site

In the nomenclature below, the morphology code numbers include the behavior code appropriate to the histological type of neoplasm, but this behavior code should be changed if other reported information makes this necessary. For example, "chordoma (M9370/3)" is assumed to be malignant; the term "benign chordoma" should be coded M9370/0. Similarly, "superficial spreading adenocarcinoma (M8143/3)" described as "noninvasive" should be coded M8143/2 and "melanoma (M8720/3)" described as "secondary" should be coded M8720/6.

The following table shows the correspondence between the morphology code and the different sections of Chapter 2:

Morphology Code Histology/Behavior		ICD-9-CM Chapter 2	
Any	0	210-229	Benign neoplasms
M8000-M8004	1	239	Neoplasms of unspecified nature
M8010+	1	235-238	Neoplasms of uncertain behavior
Any	2	230-234	Carcinoma in situ
Any	3	140-195 200-208	Malignant neoplasms, stated or presumed to be primary
Any	6	196-198	Malignant neoplasms, stated or presumed to be secondary

The ICD-O behavior digit /9 is inapplicable in an ICD context, since all malignant neoplasms are presumed to be primary (/3) or secondary (/6) according to other information on the medical record. Only the first-listed term of the full ICD-O morphology nomenclature appears against each code number in the list below. The ICD-9-CM Alphabetical Index (Volume 2), however, includes all the ICD-O synonyms as well as a number of other morphological names still likely to be encountered on medical records but omitted from ICD-O as outdated or otherwise undesirable.

A coding difficulty sometimes arises where a morphological diagnosis contains two qualifying adjectives that have different code numbers. An example is "transitional cell epidermoid carcinoma." "Transitional cell carcinoma NOS" is M8120/3 and "epidermoid carcinoma NOS" is M8070/3. In such circumstances, the higher number (M8120/3 in this example) should be used, as it is usually more specific.

Coded Nomenclature for Morphology of Neoplasms

M800	**Neoplasms NOS**
M8000/0	Neoplasm, benign
M8000/1	Neoplasm, uncertain whether benign or malignant
M8000/3	Neoplasm, malignant
M8000/6	Neoplasm, metastatic
M8000/9	Neoplasm, malignant, uncertain whether primary or metastatic
M8001/0	Tumor cells, benign
M8001/1	Tumor cells, uncertain whether benign or malignant
M8001/3	Tumor cells, malignant
M8002/3	Malignant tumor, small cell type
M8003/3	Malignant tumor, giant cell type
M8004/3	Malignant tumor, fusiform cell type
M801-M804	**Epithelial neoplasms NOS**
M8010/0	Epithelial tumor, benign
M8010/2	Carcinoma in situ NOS
M8010/3	Carcinoma NOS
M8010/6	Carcinoma, metastatic NOS
M8010/9	Carcinomatosis
M8011/0	Epithelioma, benign
M8011/3	Epithelioma, malignant
M8012/3	Large cell carcinoma NOS
M8020/3	Carcinoma, undifferentiated type NOS
M8021/3	Carcinoma, anaplastic type NOS
M8022/3	Pleomorphic carcinoma
M8030/3	Giant cell and spindle cell carcinoma
M8031/3	Giant cell carcinoma
M8032/3	Spindle cell carcinoma
M8033/3	Pseudosarcomatous carcinoma
M8034/3	Polygonal cell carcinoma
M8035/3	Spheroidal cell carcinoma
M8040/1	Tumorlet
M8041/3	Small cell carcinoma NOS
M8042/3	Oat cell carcinoma
M8043/3	Small cell carcinoma, fusiform cell type
M805-M808	**Papillary and squamous cell neoplasms**
M8050/0	Papilloma NOS (except Papilloma of urinary bladder M8120/1)
M8050/2	Papillary carcinoma in situ
M8050/3	Papillary carcinoma NOS
M8051/0	Verrucous papilloma
M8051/3	Verrucous carcinoma NOS
M8052/0	Squamous cell papilloma
M8052/3	Papillary squamous cell carcinoma
M8053/0	Inverted papilloma
M8060/0	Papillomatosis NOS
M8070/2	Squamous cell carcinoma in situ NOS
M8070/3	Squamous cell carcinoma NOS
M8070/6	Squamous cell carcinoma, metastatic NOS
M8071/3	Squamous cell carcinoma, keratinizing type NOS
M8072/3	Squamous cell carcinoma, large cell, nonkeratinizing type
M8073/3	Squamous cell carcinoma, small cell, nonkeratinizing type
M8074/3	Squamous cell carcinoma, spindle cell type
M8075/3	Adenoid squamous cell carcinoma
M8076/2	Squamous cell carcinoma in situ with questionable stromal invasion
M8076/3	Squamous cell carcinoma, microinvasive
M8080/2	Queyrat's erythroplasia
M8081/2	Bowen's disease
M8082/3	Lymphoepithelial carcinoma
M809-M811	**Basal cell neoplasms**
M8090/1	Basal cell tumor
M8090/3	Basal cell carcinoma NOS
M8091/3	Multicentric basal cell carcinoma
M8092/3	Basal cell carcinoma, morphea type
M8093/3	Basal cell carcinoma, fibroepithelial type
M8094/3	Basosquamous carcinoma
M8095/3	Metatypical carcinoma
M8096/0	Intraepidermal epithelioma of Jadassohn
M8100/0	Trichoepithelioma
M8101/0	Trichofolliculoma
M8102/0	Tricholemmoma
M8110/0	Pilomatrixoma
M812-M813	**Transitional cell papillomas and carcinomas**
M8120/0	Transitional cell papilloma NOS
M8120/1	Urothelial papilloma
M8120/2	Transitional cell carcinoma in situ
M8120/3	Transitional cell carcinoma NOS
M8121/0	Schneiderian papilloma
M8121/1	Transitional cell papilloma, inverted type
M8121/3	Schneiderian carcinoma
M8122/3	Transitional cell carcinoma, spindle cell type
M8123/3	Basaloid carcinoma
M8124/3	Cloacogenic carcinoma
M8130/3	Papillary transitional cell carcinoma
M814-M838	**Adenomas and adenocarcinomas**
M8140/0	Adenoma NOS
M8140/1	Bronchial adenoma NOS
M8140/2	Adenocarcinoma in situ
M8140/3	Adenocarcinoma NOS
M8140/6	Adenocarcinoma, metastatic NOS
M8141/3	Scirrhous adenocarcinoma
M8142/3	Linitis plastica
M8143/3	Superficial spreading adenocarcinoma
M8144/3	Adenocarcinoma, intestinal type
M8145/3	Carcinoma, diffuse type
M8146/0	Monomorphic adenoma
M8147/0	Basal cell adenoma
M8150/0	Islet cell adenoma
M8150/3	Islet cell carcinoma
M8151/0	Insulinoma NOS
M8151/3	Insulinoma, malignant
M8152/0	Glucagonoma NOS
M8152/3	Glucagonoma, malignant
M8153/1	Gastrinoma NOS
M8153/3	Gastrinoma, malignant
M8154/3	Mixed islet cell and exocrine adenocarcinoma
M8160/0	Bile duct adenoma
M8160/3	Cholangiocarcinoma

M8161/0	Bile duct cystadenoma	
M8161/3	Bile duct cystadenocarcinoma	
M8170/0	Liver cell adenoma	
M8170/3	Hepatocellular carcinoma NOS	
M8180/0	Hepatocholangioma, benign	
M8180/3	Combined hepatocellular carcinoma and cholangiocarcinoma	
M8190/0	Trabecular adenoma	
M8190/3	Trabecular adenocarcinoma	
M8191/0	Embryonal adenoma	
M8200/0	Eccrine dermal cylindroma	
M8200/3	Adenoid cystic carcinoma	
M8201/3	Cribriform carcinoma	
M8210/0	Adenomatous polyp NOS	
M8210/3	Adenocarcinoma in adenomatous polyp	
M8211/0	Tubular adenoma NOS	
M8211/3	Tubular adenocarcinoma	
M8220/0	Adenomatous polyposis coli	
M8220/3	Adenocarcinoma in adenomatous polyposis coli	
M8221/0	Multiple adenomatous polyps	
M8230/3	Solid carcinoma NOS	
M8231/3	Carcinoma simplex	
M8240/1	Carcinoid tumor NOS	
M8240/3	Carcinoid tumor, malignant	
M8241/1	Carcinoid tumor, argentaffin NOS	
M8241/3	Carcinoid tumor, argentaffin, malignant	
M8242/1	Carcinoid tumor, nonargentaffin NOS	
M8242/3	Carcinoid tumor, nonargentaffin, malignant	
M8243/3	Mucocarcinoid tumor, malignant	
M8244/3	Composite carcinoid	
M8250/1	Pulmonary adenomatosis	
M8250/3	Bronchiolo-alveolar adenocarcinoma	
M8251/0	Alveolar adenoma	
M8251/3	Alveolar adenocarcinoma	
M8260/0	Papillary adenoma NOS	
M8260/3	Papillary adenocarcinoma NOS	
M8261/1	Villous adenoma NOS	
M8261/3	Adenocarcinoma in villous adenoma	
M8262/3	Villous adenocarcinoma	
M8263/0	Tubulovillous adenoma	
M8270/0	Chromophobe adenoma	
M8270/3	Chromophobe carcinoma	
M8280/0	Acidophil adenoma	
M8280/3	Acidophil carcinoma	
M8281/0	Mixed acidophil-basophil adenoma	
M8281/3	Mixed acidophil-basophil carcinoma	
M8290/0	Oxyphilic adenoma	
M8290/3	Oxyphilic adenocarcinoma	
M8300/0	Basophil adenoma	
M8300/3	Basophil carcinoma	
M8310/0	Clear cell adenoma	
M8310/3	Clear cell adenocarcinoma NOS	
M8311/1	Hypernephroid tumor	
M8312/3	Renal cell carcinoma	
M8313/0	Clear cell adenofibroma	
M8320/3	Granular cell carcinoma	
M8321/0	Chief cell adenoma	
M8322/0	Water-clear cell adenoma	
M8322/3	Water-clear cell adenocarcinoma	
M8323/0	Mixed cell adenoma	
M8323/3	Mixed cell adenocarcinoma	
M8324/0	Lipoadenoma	
M8330/0	Follicular adenoma	
M8330/3	Follicular adenocarcinoma NOS	
M8331/3	Follicular adenocarcinoma, well differentiated type	
M8332/3	Follicular adenocarcinoma, trabecular type	

M8333/0	Microfollicular adenoma
M8334/0	Macrofollicular adenoma
M8340/3	Papillary and follicular adenocarcinoma
M8350/3	Nonencapsulated sclerosing carcinoma
M8360/1	Multiple endocrine adenomas
M8361/1	Juxtaglomerular tumor
M8370/0	Adrenal cortical adenoma NOS
M8370/3	Adrenal cortical carcinoma
M8371/0	Adrenal cortical adenoma, compact cell type
M8372/0	Adrenal cortical adenoma, heavily pigmented variant
M8373/0	Adrenal cortical adenoma, clear cell type
M8374/0	Adrenal cortical adenoma, glomerulosa cell type
M8375/0	Adrenal cortical adenoma, mixed cell type
M8380/0	Endometrioid adenoma NOS
M8380/1	Endometrioid adenoma, borderline malignancy
M8380/3	Endometrioid carcinoma
M8381/0	Endometrioid adenofibroma NOS
M8381/1	Endometrioid adenofibroma, borderline malignancy
M8381/3	Endometrioid adenofibroma, malignant

M839-M842   Adnexal and skin appendage neoplasms

M8390/0	Skin appendage adenoma
M8390/3	Skin appendage carcinoma
M8400/0	Sweat gland adenoma
M8400/1	Sweat gland tumor NOS
M8400/3	Sweat gland adenocarcinoma
M8401/0	Apocrine adenoma
M8401/3	Apocrine adenocarcinoma
M8402/0	Eccrine acrospiroma
M8403/0	Eccrine spiradenoma
M8404/0	Hidrocystoma
M8405/0	Papillary hydradenoma
M8406/0	Papillary syringadenoma
M8407/0	Syringoma NOS
M8410/0	Sebaceous adenoma
M8410/3	Sebaceous adenocarcinoma
M8420/0	Ceruminous adenoma
M8420/3	Ceruminous adenocarcinoma

M843   Mucoepidermoid neoplasms

M8430/1	Mucoepidermoid tumor
M8430/3	Mucoepidermoid carcinoma

M844-M849   Cystic, mucinous, and serous neoplasms

M8440/0	Cystadenoma NOS
M8440/3	Cystadenocarcinoma NOS
M8441/0	Serous cystadenoma NOS
M8441/1	Serous cystadenoma, borderline malignancy
M8441/3	Serous cystadenocarcinoma NOS
M8450/0	Papillary cystadenoma NOS
M8450/1	Papillary cystadenoma, borderline malignancy
M8450/3	Papillary cystadenocarcinoma NOS
M8460/0	Papillary serous cystadenoma NOS
M8460/1	Papillary serous cystadenoma, borderline malignancy
M8460/3	Papillary serous cystadenocarcinoma
M8461/0	Serous surface papilloma NOS
M8461/1	Serous surface papilloma, borderline malignancy
M8461/3	Serous surface papillary carcinoma
M8470/0	Mucinous cystadenoma NOS
M8470/1	Mucinous cystadenoma, borderline malignancy

M8470/3	Mucinous cystadenocarcinoma NOS
M8471/0	Papillary mucinous cystadenoma NOS
M8471/1	Papillary mucinous cystadenoma, borderline malignancy
M8471/3	Papillary mucinous cystadenocarcinoma
M8480/0	Mucinous adenoma
M8480/3	Mucinous adenocarcinoma
M8480/6	Pseudomyxoma peritonei
M8481/3	Mucin-producing adenocarcinoma
M8490/3	Signet ring cell carcinoma
M8490/6	Metastatic signet ring cell carcinoma

M850-M854   Ductal, lobular, and medullary neoplasms

M8500/2	Intraductal carcinoma, noninfiltrating NOS
M8500/3	Infiltrating duct carcinoma
M8501/2	Comedocarcinoma, noninfiltrating
M8501/3	Comedocarcinoma NOS
M8502/3	Juvenile carcinoma of the breast
M8503/0	Intraductal papilloma
M8503/2	Noninfiltrating intraductal papillary adenocarcinoma
M8504/0	Intracystic papillary adenoma
M8504/2	Noninfiltrating intracystic carcinoma
M8505/0	Intraductal papillomatosis NOS
M8506/0	Subareolar duct papillomatosis
M8510/3	Medullary carcinoma NOS
M8511/3	Medullary carcinoma with amyloid stroma
M8512/3	Medullary carcinoma with lymphoid stroma
M8520/2	Lobular carcinoma in situ
M8520/3	Lobular carcinoma NOS
M8521/3	Infiltrating ductular carcinoma
M8530/3	Inflammatory carcinoma
M8540/3	Paget's disease, mammary
M8541/3	Paget's disease and infiltrating duct carcinoma of breast
M8542/3	Paget's disease, extramammary (except Paget's disease of bone)

M855   Acinar cell neoplasms

M8550/0	Acinar cell adenoma
M8550/1	Acinar cell tumor
M8550/3	Acinar cell carcinoma

M856-M858   Complex epithelial neoplasms

M8560/3	Adenosquamous carcinoma
M8561/0	Adenolymphoma
M8570/3	Adenocarcinoma with squamous metaplasia
M8571/3	Adenocarcinoma with cartilaginous and osseous metaplasia
M8572/3	Adenocarcinoma with spindle cell metaplasia
M8573/3	Adenocarcinoma with apocrine metaplasia
M8580/0	Thymoma, benign
M8580/3	Thymoma, malignant

M859-M867   Specialized gonadal neoplasms

M8590/1	Sex cord-stromal tumor
M8600/0	Thecoma NOS
M8600/3	Theca cell carcinoma
M8610/0	Luteoma NOS
M8620/1	Granulosa cell tumor NOS
M8620/3	Granulosa cell tumor, malignant
M8621/1	Granulosa cell-theca cell tumor
M8630/0	Androblastoma, benign
M8630/1	Androblastoma NOS
M8630/3	Androblastoma, malignant
M8631/0	Sertoli-Leydig cell tumor

M8632/1	Gynandroblastoma
M8640/0	Tubular androblastoma NOS
M8640/3	Sertoli cell carcinoma
M8641/0	Tubular androblastoma with lipid storage
M8650/0	Leydig cell tumor, benign
M8650/1	Leydig cell tumor NOS
M8650/3	Leydig cell tumor, malignant
M8660/0	Hilar cell tumor
M8670/0	Lipid cell tumor of ovary
M8671/0	Adrenal rest tumor

M868-M871 Paragangliomas and glomus tumors

M8680/1	Paraganglioma NOS
M8680/3	Paraganglioma, malignant
M8681/1	Sympathetic paraganglioma
M8682/1	Parasympathetic paraganglioma
M8690/1	Glomus jugulare tumor
M8691/1	Aortic body tumor
M8692/1	Carotid body tumor
M8693/1	Extra-adrenal paraganglioma NOS
M8693/3	Extra-adrenal paraganglioma, malignant
M8700/0	Pheochromocytoma NOS
M8700/3	Pheochromocytoma, malignant
M8710/3	Glomangiosarcoma
M8711/0	Glomus tumor
M8712/0	Glomangioma

M872-M879 Nevi and melanomas

M8720/0	Pigmented nevus NOS
M8720/3	Malignant melanoma NOS
M8721/3	Nodular melanoma
M8722/0	Balloon cell nevus
M8722/3	Balloon cell melanoma
M8723/0	Halo nevus
M8724/0	Fibrous papule of the nose
M8725/0	Neuronevus
M8726/0	Magnocellular nevus
M8730/0	Nonpigmented nevus
M8730/3	Amelanotic melanoma
M8740/0	Junctional nevus
M8740/3	Malignant melanoma in junctional nevus
M8741/2	Precancerous melanosis NOS
M8741/3	Malignant melanoma in precancerous melanosis
M8742/2	Hutchinson's melanotic freckle
M8742/3	Malignant melanoma in Hutchinson's melanotic freckle
M8743/3	Superficial spreading melanoma
M8750/0	Intradermal nevus
M8760/0	Compound nevus
M8761/1	Giant pigmented nevus
M8761/3	Malignant melanoma in giant pigmented nevus
M8770/0	Epithelioid and spindle cell nevus
M8771/3	Epithelioid cell melanoma
M8772/3	Spindle cell melanoma NOS
M8773/3	Spindle cell melanoma, type A
M8774/3	Spindle cell melanoma, type B
M8775/3	Mixed epithelioid and spindle cell melanoma
M8780/0	Blue nevus NOS
M8780/3	Blue nevus, malignant
M8790/0	Cellular blue nevus

M880 Soft tissue tumors and sarcomas NOS

M8800/0	Soft tissue tumor, benign
M8800/3	Sarcoma NOS
M8800/9	Sarcomatosis NOS
M8801/3	Spindle cell sarcoma
M8802/3	Giant cell sarcoma (except of bone M9250/3)

M8803/3	Small cell sarcoma
M8804/3	Epithelioid cell sarcoma

M881-M883 Fibromatous neoplasms

M8810/0	Fibroma NOS
M8810/3	Fibrosarcoma NOS
M8811/0	Fibromyxoma
M8811/3	Fibromyxosarcoma
M8812/0	Periosteal fibroma
M8812/3	Periosteal fibrosarcoma
M8813/0	Fascial fibroma
M8813/3	Fascial fibrosarcoma
M8814/3	Infantile fibrosarcoma
M8820/0	Elastofibroma
M8821/1	Aggressive fibromatosis
M8822/1	Abdominal fibromatosis
M8823/1	Desmoplastic fibroma
M8830/0	Fibrous histiocytoma NOS
M8830/1	Atypical fibrous histiocytoma
M8830/3	Fibrous histiocytoma, malignant
M8831/0	Fibroxanthoma NOS
M8831/1	Atypical fibroxanthoma
M8831/3	Fibroxanthoma, malignant
M8832/0	Dermatofibroma NOS
M8832/1	Dermatofibroma protuberans
M8832/3	Dermatofibrosarcoma NOS

M884 Myxomatous neoplasms

M8840/0	Myxoma NOS
M8840/3	Myxosarcoma

M885-M888 Lipomatous neoplasms

M8850/0	Lipoma NOS
M8850/3	Liposarcoma NOS
M8851/0	Fibrolipoma
M8851/3	Liposarcoma, well differentiated type
M8852/0	Fibromyxolipoma
M8852/3	Myxoid liposarcoma
M8853/3	Round cell liposarcoma
M8854/3	Pleomorphic liposarcoma
M8855/3	Mixed type liposarcoma
M8856/0	Intramuscular lipoma
M8857/0	Spindle cell lipoma
M8860/0	Angiomyolipoma
M8860/3	Angiomyoliposarcoma
M8861/0	Angiolipoma NOS
M8861/1	Angiolipoma, infiltrating
M8870/0	Myelolipoma
M8880/0	Hibernoma
M8881/0	Lipoblastomatosis

M889-M892 Myomatous neoplasms

M8890/0	Leiomyoma NOS
M8890/1	Intravascular leiomyomatosis
M8890/3	Leiomyosarcoma NOS
M8891/1	Epithelioid leiomyoma
M8891/3	Epithelioid leiomyosarcoma
M8892/1	Cellular leiomyoma
M8893/0	Bizarre leiomyoma
M8894/0	Angiomyoma
M8894/3	Angiomyosarcoma
M8895/0	Myoma
M8895/3	Myosarcoma
M8900/0	Rhabdomyoma NOS
M8900/3	Rhabdomyosarcoma NOS
M8901/3	Pleomorphic rhabdomyosarcoma
M8902/3	Mixed type rhabdomyosarcoma
M8903/0	Fetal rhabdomyoma
M8904/0	Adult rhabdomyoma
M8910/3	Embryonal rhabdomyosarcoma
M8920/3	Alveolar rhabdomyosarcoma

M893-M899 Complex mixed and stromal neoplasms

M8930/3	Endometrial stromal sarcoma
M8931/1	Endolymphatic stromal myosis
M8932/0	Adenomyoma
M8940/0	Pleomorphic adenoma
M8940/3	Mixed tumor, malignant NOS
M8950/3	Mullerian mixed tumor
M8951/3	Mesodermal mixed tumor
M8960/1	Mesoblastic nephroma
M8960/3	Nephroblastoma NOS
M8961/3	Epithelial nephroblastoma
M8962/3	Mesenchymal nephroblastoma
M8970/3	Hepatoblastoma
M8980/3	Carcinosarcoma NOS
M8981/3	Carcinosarcoma, embryonal type
M8982/0	Myoepithelioma
M8990/0	Mesenchymoma, benign
M8990/1	Mesenchymoma NOS
M8990/3	Mesenchymoma, malignant
M8991/3	Embryonal sarcoma

M900-M903 Fibroepithelial neoplasms

M9000/0	Brenner tumor NOS
M9000/1	Brenner tumor, borderline malignancy
M9000/3	Brenner tumor, malignant
M9010/0	Fibroadenoma NOS
M9011/0	Intracanalicular fibroadenoma NOS
M9012/0	Pericanalicular fibroadenoma
M9013/0	Adenofibroma NOS
M9014/0	Serous adenofibroma
M9015/0	Mucinous adenofibroma
M9020/0	Cellular intracanalicular fibroadenoma
M9020/1	Cystosarcoma phyllodes NOS
M9020/3	Cystosarcoma phyllodes, malignant
M9030/0	Juvenile fibroadenoma

M904 Synovial neoplasms

M9040/0	Synovioma, benign
M9040/3	Synovial sarcoma NOS
M9041/3	Synovial sarcoma, spindle cell type
M9042/3	Synovial sarcoma, epithelioid cell type
M9043/3	Synovial sarcoma, biphasic type
M9044/3	Clear cell sarcoma of tendons and aponeuroses

M905 Mesothelial neoplasms

M9050/0	Mesothelioma, benign
M9050/3	Mesothelioma, malignant
M9051/0	Fibrous mesothelioma, benign
M9051/3	Fibrous mesothelioma, malignant
M9052/0	Epithelioid mesothelioma, benign
M9052/3	Epithelioid mesothelioma, malignant
M9053/0	Mesothelioma, biphasic type, benign
M9053/3	Mesothelioma, biphasic type, malignant
M9054/0	Adenomatoid tumor NOS

M906-M909 Germ cell neoplasms

M9060/3	Dysgerminoma
M9061/3	Seminoma NOS
M9062/3	Seminoma, anaplastic type
M9063/3	Spermatocytic seminoma
M9064/3	Germinoma
M9070/3	Embryonal carcinoma NOS
M9071/3	Endodermal sinus tumor
M9072/3	Polyembryoma
M9073/1	Gonadoblastoma
M9080/0	Teratoma, benign
M9080/1	Teratoma NOS
M9080/3	Teratoma, malignant NOS
M9081/3	Teratocarcinoma

Appendix A: Morphology of Neoplasms

M9082/3	Malignant teratoma, undifferentiated type
M9083/3	Malignant teratoma, intermediate type
M9084/0	Dermoid cyst
M9084/3	Dermoid cyst with malignant transformation
M9090/0	Struma ovarii NOS
M9090/3	Struma ovarii, malignant
M9091/1	Strumal carcinoid

M910   **Trophoblastic neoplasms**

M9100/0	Hydatidiform mole NOS
M9100/1	Invasive hydatidiform mole
M9100/3	Choriocarcinoma
M9101/3	Choriocarcinoma combined with teratoma
M9102/3	Malignant teratoma, trophoblastic

M911   **Mesonephromas**

M9110/0	Mesonephroma, benign
M9110/1	Mesonephric tumor
M9110/3	Mesonephroma, malignant
M9111/1	Endosalpingioma

M912-M916   **Blood vessel tumors**

M9120/0	Hemangioma NOS
M9120/3	Hemangiosarcoma
M9121/0	Cavernous hemangioma
M9122/0	Venous hemangioma
M9123/0	Racemose hemangioma
M9124/3	Kupffer cell sarcoma
M9130/0	Hemangioendothelioma, benign
M9130/1	Hemangioendothelioma NOS
M9130/3	Hemangioendothelioma, malignant
M9131/0	Capillary hemangioma
M9132/0	Intramuscular hemangioma
M9140/3	Kaposi's sarcoma
M9141/0	Angiokeratoma
M9142/0	Verrucous keratotic hemangioma
M9150/0	Hemangiopericytoma, benign
M9150/1	Hemangiopericytoma NOS
M9150/3	Hemangiopericytoma, malignant
M9160/0	Angiofibroma NOS
M9161/1	Hemangioblastoma

M917   **Lymphatic vessel tumors**

M9170/0	Lymphangioma NOS
M9170/3	Lymphangiosarcoma
M9171/0	Capillary lymphangioma
M9172/0	Cavernous lymphangioma
M9173/0	Cystic lymphangioma
M9174/0	Lymphangiomyoma
M9174/1	Lymphangiomyomatosis
M9175/0	Hemolymphangioma

M918-M920   **Osteomas and osteosarcomas**

M9180/0	Osteoma NOS
M9180/3	Osteosarcoma NOS
M9181/3	Chondroblastic osteosarcoma
M9182/3	Fibroblastic osteosarcoma
M9183/3	Telangiectatic osteosarcoma
M9184/3	Osteosarcoma in Paget's disease of bone
M9190/3	Juxtacortical osteosarcoma
M9191/0	Osteoid osteoma NOS
M9200/0	Osteoblastoma

M921-M924   **Chondromatous neoplasms**

M9210/0	Osteochondroma
M9210/1	Osteochondromatosis NOS
M9220/0	Chondroma NOS
M9220/1	Chondromatosis NOS
M9220/3	Chondrosarcoma NOS
M9221/0	Juxtacortical chondroma
M9221/3	Juxtacortical chondrosarcoma
M9230/0	Chondroblastoma NOS
M9230/3	Chondroblastoma, malignant
M9240/3	Mesenchymal chondrosarcoma
M9241/0	Chondromyxoid fibroma

M925   **Giant cell tumors**

M9250/1	Giant cell tumor of bone NOS
M9250/3	Giant cell tumor of bone, malignant
M9251/1	Giant cell tumor of soft parts NOS
M9251/3	Malignant giant cell tumor of soft parts

M926   **Miscellaneous bone tumors**

M9260/3	Ewing's sarcoma
M9261/3	Adamantinoma of long bones
M9262/0	Ossifying fibroma

M927-M934   **Odontogenic tumors**

M9270/0	Odontogenic tumor, benign
M9270/1	Odontogenic tumor NOS
M9270/3	Odontogenic tumor, malignant
M9271/0	Dentinoma
M9272/0	Cementoma NOS
M9273/0	Cementoblastoma, benign
M9274/0	Cementifying fibroma
M9275/0	Gigantiform cementoma
M9280/0	Odontoma NOS
M9281/0	Compound odontoma
M9282/0	Complex odontoma
M9290/0	Ameloblastic fibro-odontoma
M9290/3	Ameloblastic odontosarcoma
M9300/0	Adenomatoid odontogenic tumor
M9301/0	Calcifying odontogenic cyst
M9310/0	Ameloblastoma NOS
M9310/3	Ameloblastoma, malignant
M9311/0	Odontoameloblastoma
M9312/0	Squamous odontogenic tumor
M9320/0	Odontogenic myxoma
M9321/0	Odontogenic fibroma NOS
M9330/0	Ameloblastic fibroma
M9330/3	Ameloblastic fibrosarcoma
M9340/0	Calcifying epithelial odontogenic tumor

M935-M937   **Miscellaneous tumors**

M9350/1	Craniopharyngioma
M9360/1	Pinealoma
M9361/1	Pineocytoma
M9362/3	Pineoblastoma
M9363/0	Melanotic neuroectodermal tumor
M9370/3	Chordoma

M938-M948   **Gliomas**

M9380/3	Glioma, malignant
M9381/3	Gliomatosis cerebri
M9382/3	Mixed glioma
M9383/1	Subependymal glioma
M9384/1	Subependymal giant cell astrocytoma
M9390/0	Choroid plexus papilloma NOS
M9390/3	Choroid plexus papilloma, malignant
M9391/3	Ependymoma NOS
M9392/3	Ependymoma, anaplastic type
M9393/1	Papillary ependymoma
M9394/1	Myxopapillary ependymoma
M9400/3	Astrocytoma NOS
M9401/3	Astrocytoma, anaplastic type
M9410/3	Protoplasmic astrocytoma
M9411/3	Gemistocytic astrocytoma
M9420/3	Fibrillary astrocytoma
M9421/3	Pilocytic astrocytoma
M9422/3	Spongioblastoma NOS
M9423/3	Spongioblastoma polare
M9430/3	Astroblastoma

M9440/3	Glioblastoma NOS
M9441/3	Giant cell glioblastoma
M9442/3	Glioblastoma with sarcomatous component
M9443/3	Primitive polar spongioblastoma
M9450/3	Oligodendroglioma NOS
M9451/3	Oligodendroglioma, anaplastic type
M9460/3	Oligodendroblastoma
M9470/3	Medulloblastoma NOS
M9471/3	Desmoplastic medulloblastoma
M9472/3	Medullomyoblastoma
M9480/3	Cerebellar sarcoma NOS
M9481/3	Monstrocellular sarcoma

M949-M952   **Neuroepitheliomatous neoplasms**

M9490/0	Ganglioneuroma
M9490/3	Ganglioneuroblastoma
M9491/0	Ganglioneuromatosis
M9500/3	Neuroblastoma NOS
M9501/3	Medulloepithelioma NOS
M9502/3	Teratoid medulloepithelioma
M9503/3	Neuroepithelioma NOS
M9504/3	Spongioneuroblastoma
M9505/1	Ganglioglioma
M9506/0	Neurocytoma
M9507/0	Pacinian tumor
M9510/3	Retinoblastoma NOS
M9511/3	Retinoblastoma, differentiated type
M9512/3	Retinoblastoma, undifferentiated type
M9520/3	Olfactory neurogenic tumor
M9521/3	Esthesioneurocytoma
M9522/3	Esthesioneuroblastoma
M9523/3	Esthesioneuroepithelioma

M953   **Meningiomas**

M9530/0	Meningioma NOS
M9530/1	Meningiomatosis NOS
M9530/3	Meningioma, malignant
M9531/0	Meningotheliomatous meningioma
M9532/0	Fibrous meningioma
M9533/0	Psammomatous meningioma
M9534/0	Angiomatous meningioma
M9535/0	Hemangioblastic meningioma
M9536/0	Hemangiopericytic meningioma
M9537/0	Transitional meningioma
M9538/1	Papillary meningioma
M9539/3	Meningeal sarcomatosis

M954-M957   **Nerve sheath tumor**

M9540/0	Neurofibroma NOS
M9540/1	Neurofibromatosis NOS
M9540/3	Neurofibrosarcoma
M9541/0	Melanotic neurofibroma
M9550/0	Plexiform neurofibroma
M9560/0	Neurilemmoma NOS
M9560/1	Neurinomatosis
M9560/3	Neurilemmoma, malignant
M9570/0	Neuroma NOS

M958   **Granular cell tumors and alveolar soft part sarcoma**

M9580/0	Granular cell tumor NOS
M9580/3	Granular cell tumor, malignant
M9581/3	Alveolar soft part sarcoma

M959-M963   **Lymphomas, NOS or diffuse**

M9590/0	Lymphomatous tumor, benign
M9590/3	Malignant lymphoma NOS
M9591/3	Malignant lymphoma, non Hodgkin's type
M9600/3	Malignant lymphoma, undifferentiated cell type NOS
M9601/3	Malignant lymphoma, stem cell type

M9602/3	Malignant lymphoma, convoluted cell type NOS
M9610/3	Lymphosarcoma NOS
M9611/3	Malignant lymphoma, lymphoplasmacytoid type
M9612/3	Malignant lymphoma, immunoblastic type
M9613/3	Malignant lymphoma, mixed lymphocytic-histiocytic NOS
M9614/3	Malignant lymphoma, centroblastic-centrocytic, diffuse
M9615/3	Malignant lymphoma, follicular center cell NOS
M9620/3	Malignant lymphoma, lymphocytic, well differentiated NOS
M9621/3	Malignant lymphoma, lymphocytic, intermediate differentiation NOS
M9622/3	Malignant lymphoma, centrocytic
M9623/3	Malignant lymphoma, follicular center cell, cleaved NOS
M9630/3	Malignant lymphoma, lymphocytic, poorly differentiated NOS
M9631/3	Prolymphocytic lymphosarcoma
M9632/3	Malignant lymphoma, centroblastic type NOS
M9633/3	Malignant lymphoma, follicular center cell, noncleaved NOS

M964   *Reticulosarcomas*

M9640/3	Reticulosarcoma NOS
M9641/3	Reticulosarcoma, pleomorphic cell type
M9642/3	Reticulosarcoma, nodular

M965-M966   *Hodgkin's disease*

M9650/3	Hodgkin's disease NOS
M9651/3	Hodgkin's disease, lymphocytic predominance
M9652/3	Hodgkin's disease, mixed cellularity
M9653/3	Hodgkin's disease, lymphocytic depletion NOS
M9654/3	Hodgkin's disease, lymphocytic depletion, diffuse fibrosis
M9655/3	Hodgkin's disease, lymphocytic depletion, reticular type
M9656/3	Hodgkin's disease, nodular sclerosis NOS
M9657/3	Hodgkin's disease, nodular sclerosis, cellular phase
M9660/3	Hodgkin's paragranuloma
M9661/3	Hodgkin's granuloma
M9662/3	Hodgkin's sarcoma

M969   **Lymphomas, nodular or follicular**

M9690/3	Malignant lymphoma, nodular NOS

M9691/3	Malignant lymphoma, mixed lymphocytic-histiocytic, nodular
M9692/3	Malignant lymphoma, centroblastic-centrocytic, follicular
M9693/3	Malignant lymphoma, lymphocytic, well differentiated, nodular
M9694/3	Malignant lymphoma, lymphocytic, intermediate differentiation, nodular
M9695/3	Malignant lymphoma, follicular center cell, cleaved, follicular
M9696/3	Malignant lymphoma, lymphocytic, poorly differentiated, nodular
M9697/3	Malignant lymphoma, centroblastic type, follicular
M9698/3	Malignant lymphoma, follicular center cell, noncleaved, follicular

M970   **Mycosis fungoides**

M9700/3	Mycosis fungoides
M9701/3	Sezary's disease

M971-M972   **Miscellaneous reticuloendothelial neoplasms**

M9710/3	Microglioma
M9720/3	Malignant histiocytosis
M9721/3	Histiocytic medullary reticulosis
M9722/3	Letterer-Siwe's disease

M973   **Plasma cell tumors**

M9730/3	Plasma cell myeloma
M9731/0	Plasma cell tumor, benign
M9731/1	Plasmacytoma NOS
M9731/3	Plasma cell tumor, malignant

M974   **Mast cell tumors**

M9740/1	Mastocytoma NOS
M9740/3	Mast cell sarcoma
M9741/3	Malignant mastocytosis

M975   **Burkitt's tumor**

M9750/3	Burkitt's tumor

M980-M994   **Leukemias NOS**

M9800/3	Leukemias NOS
M9800/3	Leukemia NOS
M9801/3	Acute leukemia NOS
M9802/3	Subacute leukemia NOS
M9803/3	Chronic leukemia NOS
M9804/3	Aleukemic leukemia NOS

M981   **Compound leukemias**

M9810/3	Compound leukemia

M982   **Lymphoid leukemias**

M9820/3	Lymphoid leukemia NOS

M9821/3	Acute lymphoid leukemia
M9822/3	Subacute lymphoid leukemia
M9823/3	Chronic lymphoid leukemia
M9824/3	Aleukemic lymphoid leukemia
M9825/3	Prolymphocytic leukemia

M983   **Plasma cell leukemias**

M9830/3	Plasma cell leukemia

M984   **Erythroleukemias**

M9840/3	Erythroleukemia
M9841/3	Acute erythremia
M9842/3	Chronic erythremia

M985   **Lymphosarcoma cell leukemias**

M9850/3	Lymphosarcoma cell leukemia

M986   **Myeloid leukemias**

M9860/3	Myeloid leukemia NOS
M9861/3	Acute myeloid leukemia
M9862/3	Subacute myeloid leukemia
M9863/3	Chronic myeloid leukemia
M9864/3	Aleukemic myeloid leukemia
M9865/3	Neutrophilic leukemia
M9866/3	Acute promyelocytic leukemia

M987   **Basophilic leukemias**

M9870/3	Basophilic leukemia

M988   **Eosinophilic leukemias**

M9880/3	Eosinophilic leukemia

M989   **Monocytic leukemias**

M9890/3	Monocytic leukemia NOS
M9891/3	Acute monocytic leukemia
M9892/3	Subacute monocytic leukemia
M9893/3	Chronic monocytic leukemia
M9894/3	Aleukemic monocytic leukemia

M990-M994   **Miscellaneous leukemias**

M9900/3	Mast cell leukemia
M9910/3	Megakaryocytic leukemia
M9920/3	Megakaryocytic myelosis
M9930/3	Myeloid sarcoma
M9940/3	Hairy cell leukemia

M995-M997   **Miscellaneous myeloproliferative and lymphoproliferative disorders**

M9950/1	Polycythemia vera
M9951/1	Acute panmyelosis
M9960/1	Chronic myeloproliferative disease
M9961/1	Myelosclerosis with myeloid metaplasia
M9962/1	Idiopathic thrombocythemia
M9970/1	Chronic lymphoproliferative disease

Appendix B: Glossary of Mental Disorders

was officially deleted October 1, 2004

Appendix C: Classification of Drugs by American Hospital Formulary Service List Number and Their ICD-9-CM Equivalents

The coding of adverse effects of drugs is keyed to the continually revised Hospital Formulary of the American Hospital Formulary Service (AHFS) published under the direction of the American Society of Hospital Pharmacists.

The following section gives the ICD-9-CM diagnosis code for each AHFS list.

AHFS* List	ICD-9-CM Dx Code
4:00 ANTIHISTAMINE DRUGS	963.0
8:00 ANTI-INFECTIVE AGENTS	
8:04 Amebacides	961.5
hydroxyquinoline derivatives	961.3
arsenical anti-infectives	961.1
quinoline derivatives	961.3
8:12.04 Antifungal Antibiotics	960.1
nonantibiotics	961.9
8:12.06 Cephalosporins	960.5
8:12.08 Chloramphenicol	960.2
8:12.12 The Erythromycins	960.3
8:12.16 The Penicillins	960.0
8:12.20 The Streptomycins	960.6
8:12.24 The Tetracyclines	960.4
8:12.28 Other Antibiotics	960.8
antimycobacterial antibiotics	960.6
macrolides	960.3
8:16 Antituberculars	961.8
antibiotics	960.6
8:18 Antivirals	961.7
8:20 Plasmodicides (antimalarials)	961.4
8:24 Sulfonamides	961.0
8:26 The Sulfones	961.8
8:28 Treponemicides	961.2
8:32 Trichomonacides	961.5
hydroxyquinoline derivatives	961.3
nitrofuran derivatives	961.9
8:36 Urinary Germicides	961.9
quinoline derivatives	961.3
8:40 Other Anti-Infectives	961.9
10:00 ANTINEOPLASTIC AGENTS	963.1
antibiotics	960.7
progestogens	962.2
12:00 AUTONOMIC DRUGS	
12:04 Parasympathomimetic (Cholinergic) Agents	971.0
12:08 Parasympatholytic (Cholinergic Blocking Agents	971.1
12:12 Sympathomimetic (Adrenergic) Agents	971.2
12:16 Sympatholytic (Adrenergic Blocking) Agents	971.3
12:20 Skeletal Muscle Relaxants	975.2
central nervous system	
muscle-tone depressants	968.0
16:00 BLOOD DERIVATIVES	964.7
20:00 BLOOD FORMATION AND COAGULATION	
20:04 Antianemia Drugs	964.1
20:04.04 Iron Preparations	964.0
20:04.08 Liver and Stomach Preparations	964.1
20:12.04 Anticoagulants	964.2
20:12.08 Antiheparin Agents	964.5
20:12.12 Coagulants	964.5
20:12.16 Hemostatics	964.5
capillary-active drugs	972.8
fibrinolysis-affecting agents	964.4
natural products	964.7
24:00 CARDIOVASCULAR DRUGS	
24:04 Cardiac Drugs	972.9
cardiotonic agents	972.1
rhythm regulators	972.0
24:06 Antilipemic Agents	972.2
thyroid derivatives	962.7

AHFS* List	ICD-9-CM Dx Code
24:08 Hypotensive Agents	972.6
adrenergic blocking agents	971.3
ganglion-blocking agents	972.3
vasodilators	972.5
24:12 Vasodilating Agents	972.5
coronary	972.4
nicotinic acid derivatives	972.2
24:16 Sclerosing Agents	972.7
28:00 CENTRAL NERVOUS SYSTEM DRUGS	
28:04 General Anesthetics	968.4
gaseous anesthetics	968.2
halothane	968.1
intravenous anesthetics	968.3
28:08 Analgesics and Antipyretics	965.9
antirheumatics	965.61-965.69
aromatic analgesics	965.4
non-narcotics NEC	965.7
opium alkaloids	965.00
heroin	965.01
methadone	965.02
specified type NEC	965.09
pyrazole derivatives	965.5
salicylates	965.1
specified type NEC	965.8
28:10 Narcotic Antagonists	970.1
28:12 Anticonvulsants	966.3
barbiturates	967.0
benzodiazepine-based tranquilizers	969.4
bromides	967.3
hydantoin derivatives	966.1
oxazolidine derivative	966.0
succinimides	966.2
28:16.04 Antidepressants	969.00-969.09
28:16.08 Tranquilizers	969.5
benzodiazepine-based	969.4
butyrophenone-based	969.2
major NEC	969.3
phenothiazine-based	969.1
28:16.12 Other Psychotherapeutic Agents	969.8
28:20 Respiratory and Cerebral Stimulants	970.9
analeptics	970.0
anorexigenic agents	977.0
psychostimulants	969.70-969.79
specified type NEC	970.81-970.89
28:24 Sedatives and Hypnotics	967.9
barbiturates	967.0
benzodiazepine-based tranquilizers	969.4
chloral hydrate group	967.1
glutethamide group	967.5
intravenous anesthetics	968.3
methaqualone	967.4
paraldehyde	967.2
phenothiazine-based tranquilizers	969.1
specified type NEC	967.8
thiobarbiturates	968.3
tranquilizer NEC	969.5
36:00 DIAGNOSTIC AGENTS	977.8
40:00 ELECTROLYTE, CALORIC, AND WATER BALANCE AGENTS NEC	974.5
40:04 Acidifying Agents	963.2
40:08 Alkalinizing Agents	963.3
40:10 Ammonia Detoxicants	974.5
40:12 Replacement Solutions NEC	974.5
plasma volume expanders	964.8
40:16 Sodium-Removing Resins	974.5
40:18 Potassium-Removing Resins	974.5
40:20 Caloric Agents	974.5
40:24 Salt and Sugar Substitutes	974.5
40:28 Diuretics NEC	974.4
carbonic acid anhydrase inhibitors	974.2
mercurials	974.0
purine derivatives	974.1
saluretics	974.3

	AHFS* List	ICD-9-CM Dx Code
40:36	Irrigating Solutions	974.5
40:40	Uricosuric Agents	974.7
44:00	ENZYMES NEC	963.4
	fibrinolysis-affecting agents	964.4
	gastric agents	973.4
48:00	EXPECTORANTS AND COUGH PREPARATIONS	
	antihistamine agents	963.0
	antitussives	975.4
	codeine derivatives	965.09
	expectorants	975.5
	narcotic agents NEC	965.09
52:00	EYE, EAR, NOSE, AND THROAT PREPARATIONS	
52:04	Anti-Infectives	
	ENT	976.6
	ophthalmic	976.5
52:04.04	Antibiotics	
	ENT	976.6
	ophthalmic	976.5
52:04.06	Antivirals	
	ENT	976.6
	ophthalmic	976.5
52:04.08	Sulfonamides	
	ENT	976.6
	ophthalmic	976.5
52:04.12	Miscellaneous Anti-Infectives	
	ENT	976.6
	ophthalmic	976.5
52:08	Anti-Inflammatory Agents	
	ENT	976.6
	ophthalmic	976.5
52:10	Carbonic Anhydrase Inhibitors	974.2
52:12	Contact Lens Solutions	976.5
52:16	Local Anesthetics	968.5
52:20	Miotics	971.0
52:24	Mydriatics	
	adrenergics	971.2
	anticholinergics	971.1
	antimuscarinics	971.1
	parasympatholytics	971.1
	spasmolytics	971.1
	sympathomimetics	971.2
52:28	Mouth Washes and Gargles	976.6
52:32	Vasoconstrictors	971.2
52:36	Unclassified Agents	
	ENT	976.6
	ophthalmic	976.5
56:00	GASTROINTESTINAL DRUGS	
56:04	Antacids and Absorbents	973.0
56:08	Anti-Diarrhea Agents	973.5
56:10	Antiflatulents	973.8
56:12	Cathartics NEC	973.3
	emollients	973.2
	irritants	973.1
56:16	Digestants	973.4
56:20	Emetics and Antiemetics	
	antiemetics	963.0
	emetics	973.6
56:24	Lipotropic Agents	977.1
60:00	GOLD COMPOUNDS	965.69
64:00	HEAVY METAL ANTAGONISTS	963.8
68:00	HORMONES AND SYNTHETIC SUBSTITUTES	
68:04	Adrenals	962.0
68:08	Androgens	962.1
68:12	Contraceptives	962.2
68:16	Estrogens	962.2
68:18	Gonadotropins	962.4
68:20	Insulins and Antidiabetic Agents	962.3
68:20.08	Insulins	962.3
68:24	Parathyroid	962.6
68:28	Pituitary	
	anterior	962.4
	posterior	962.5
68:32	Progestogens	962.2

	AHFS* List	ICD-9-CM Dx Code
68:34	Other Corpus Luteum Hormones	962.2
68:36	Thyroid and Antithyroid	
	antithyroid	962.8
	thyroid	962.7
72:00	LOCAL ANESTHETICS NEC	968.9
	topical (surface) agents	968.5
	infiltrating agents (intradermal) (subcutaneous) (submucosal)	968.5
	nerve blocking agents (peripheral) (plexus) (regional)	968.6
	spinal	968.7
76:00	OXYTOCICS	975.0
78:00	RADIOACTIVE AGENTS	990
80:00	SERUMS, TOXOIDS, AND VACCINES	
80:04	Serums	979.9
	immune globulin (gamma) (human)	964.6
80:08	Toxoids NEC	978.8
	diphtheria	978.5
	and tetanus	978.9
	with pertussis component	978.6
	tetanus	978.4
	and diphtheria	978.9
	with pertussis component	978.6
80:12	Vaccines NEC	979.9
	bacterial NEC	978.8
	with other bacterial component	978.9
	pertussis component	978.6
	viral and rickettsial component	979.7
	rickettsial NEC	979.6
	with bacterial component	979.7
	pertussis component	978.6
	viral component	979.7
	viral NEC	979.6
	with bacterial component	979.7
	pertussis component	978.6
	rickettsial component	979.7
84:00	SKIN AND MUCOUS MEMBRANE PREPARATIONS	
84:04	Anti-Infectives	976.0
84:04.04	Antibiotics	976.0
84:04.08	Fungicides	976.0
84:04.12	Scabicides and Pediculicides	976.0
84:04.16	Miscellaneous Local Anti-Infectives	976.0
84:06	Anti-Inflammatory Agents	976.0
84:08	Antipruritics and Local Anesthetics	
	antipruritics	976.1
	local anesthetics	968.5
84:12	Astringents	976.2
84:16	Cell Stimulants and Proliferants	976.8
84:20	Detergents	976.2
84:24	Emollients, Demulcents, and Protectants	976.3
84:28	Keratolytic Agents	976.4
84:32	Keratoplastic Agents	976.4
84:36	Miscellaneous Agents	976.8
86:00	SPASMOLYTIC AGENTS	975.1
	antiasthmatics	975.7
	papaverine	972.5
	theophyllin	974.1
88:00	VITAMINS	
88:04	Vitamin A	963.5
88:08	Vitamin B Complex	963.5
	hematopoietic vitamin	964.1
	nicotinic acid derivatives	972.2
88:12	Vitamin C	963.5
88:16	Vitamin D	963.5
88:20	Vitamin E	963.5
88:24	Vitamin K Activity	964.3
88:28	Multivitamin Preparations	963.5
92:00	UNCLASSIFIED THERAPEUTIC AGENTS	977.8

* American Hospital Formulary Service

Appendix D: Classification of Industrial Accidents According to Agency

Annex B to the Resolution concerning Statistics of Employment Injuries adopted by the Tenth International Conference of Labor Statisticians on 12 October 1962

1 Machines

11	Prime-Movers, except Electrical Motors
111	Steam engines
112	Internal combustion engines
119	Others
12	Transmission Machinery
121	Transmission shafts
122	Transmission belts, cables, pulleys, pinions, chains, gears
129	Others
13	Metalworking Machines
131	Power presses
132	Lathes
133	Milling machines
134	Abrasive wheels
135	Mechanical shears
136	Forging machines
137	Rolling-mills
139	Others
14	Wood and Assimilated Machines
141	Circular saws
142	Other saws
143	Molding machines
144	Overhand planes
149	Others
15	Agricultural Machines
151	Reapers (including combine reapers)
152	Threshers
159	Others
16	Mining Machinery
161	Under-cutters
169	Others
19	Other Machines Not Elsewhere Classified
191	Earth-moving machines, excavating and scraping machines, except means of transport
192	Spinning, weaving and other textile machines
193	Machines for the manufacture of food- stuffs and beverages
194	Machines for the manufacture of paper
195	Printing machines
199	Others

2 Means of Transport and Lifting Equipment

21	Lifting Machines and Appliances
211	Cranes
212	Lifts and elevators
213	Winches
214	Pulley blocks
219	Others
22	Means of Rail Transport
221	Inter-urban railways
222	Rail transport in mines, tunnels, quarries, industrial establishments, docks, etc.
229	Others
23	Other Wheeled Means of Transport, Excluding Rail Transport
231	Tractors
232	Lorries
233	Trucks
234	Motor vehicles, not elsewhere classified
235	Animal-drawn vehicles
236	Hand-drawn vehicles
239	Others
24	Means of Air Transport
25	Means of Water Transport
251	Motorized means of water transport
252	Non-motorized means of water transport
26	Other Means of Transport
261	Cable-cars
262	Mechanical conveyors, except cable-cars
269	Others

3 Other Equipment

31	Pressure Vessels
311	Boilers
312	Pressurized containers
313	Pressurized piping and accessories
314	Gas cylinders
315	Caissons, diving equipment
319	Others
32	Furnaces, Ovens, Kilns
321	Blast furnaces
322	Refining furnaces
323	Other furnaces
324	Kilns
325	Ovens
33	Refrigerating Plants
34	Electrical Installations, Including Electric Motors, but Excluding Electric Hand Tools
341	Rotating machines
342	Conductors
343	Transformers
344	Control apparatus
349	Others
35	Electric Hand Tools
36	Tools, Implements, and Appliances, Except Electric Hand Tools
361	Power-driven hand tools, except electrichand tools
362	Hand tools, not power-driven
369	Others
37	Ladders, Mobile Ramps
38	Scaffolding
39	Other Equipment, Not Elsewhere Classified

4 Materials, Substances and Radiations

41	Explosives
42	Dusts, Gases, Liquids and Chemicals, Excluding Explosives
421	Dusts
422	Gases, vapors, fumes
423	Liquids, not elsewhere classified
424	Chemicals, not elsewhere classified
43	Flying Fragments
44	Radiations
441	Ionizing radiations
449	Others
49	Other Materials and Substances Not Elsewhere Classified

5 Working Environment

51	Outdoor
511	Weather
512	Traffic and working surfaces
513	Water
519	Others
52	Indoor
521	Floors
522	Confined quarters
523	Stairs
524	Other traffic and working surfaces
525	Floor openings and wall openings
526	Environmental factors (lighting, ventilation, temperature, noise, etc.)
529	Others
53	Underground
531	Roofs and faces of mine roads and tunnels, etc.
532	Floors of mine roads and tunnels, etc.
533	Working-faces of mines, tunnels, etc.
534	Mine shafts
535	Fire
536	Water
539	Others

6 Other Agencies, Not Elsewhere Classified

61	Animals
611	Live animals
612	Animal products
69	Other Agencies, Not Elsewhere Classified

7 Agencies Not Classified for Lack of Sufficient Data

Appendix E: List of Three-digit Categories

1. Infectious and Parasitic Diseases

Intestinal infectious diseases (001-009)
001 Cholera
002 Typhoid and paratyphoid fevers
003 Other salmonella infections
004 Shigellosis
005 Other food poisoning (bacterial)
006 Amebiasis
007 Other protozoal intestinal diseases
008 Intestinal infections due to other organisms
009 Ill-defined intestinal infections

Tuberculosis (010-018)
010 Primary tuberculous infection
011 Pulmonary tuberculosis
012 Other respiratory tuberculosis
013 Tuberculosis of meninges and central nervous system
014 Tuberculosis of intestines, peritoneum, and mesenteric glands
015 Tuberculosis of bones and joints
016 Tuberculosis of genitourinary system
017 Tuberculosis of other organs
018 Miliary tuberculosis

Zoonotic bacterial diseases (020-027)
020 Plague
021 Tularemia
022 Anthrax
023 Brucellosis
024 Glanders
025 Melioidosis
026 Rat-bite fever
027 Other zoonotic bacterial diseases

Other bacterial diseases (030-041)
030 Leprosy
031 Diseases due to other mycobacteria
032 Diphtheria
033 Whooping cough
034 Streptococcal sore throat and scarlet fever
035 Erysipelas
036 Meningococcal infection
037 Tetanus
038 Septicemia
039 Actinomycotic infections
040 Other bacterial diseases
041 Bacterial infection in conditions classified elsewhere and of unspecified site

Human immunodeficiency virus (042)
042 Human immunodeficiency virus [HIV] disease

Poliomyelitis and other non-arthropod-borne viral diseases and prion diseases of central nervous system (045-049)
045 Acute poliomyelitis
046 Slow virus infections and prion diseases of central nervous system
047 Meningitis due to enterovirus
048 Other enterovirus diseases of central nervous system
049 Other non-arthropod-borne viral diseases of central nervous system

Viral diseases generally accompanied by exanthem (050-059)
050 Smallpox
051 Cowpox and paravaccinia
052 Chickenpox
053 Herpes zoster
054 Herpes simplex
055 Measles
056 Rubella
057 Other viral exanthemata
058 Other human herpesvirus
059 Other poxvirus infections

Arthropod-borne viral diseases (060-066)
060 Yellow fever
061 Dengue
062 Mosquito-borne viral encephalitis
063 Tick-borne viral encephalitis
064 Viral encephalitis transmitted by other and unspecified arthropods
065 Arthropod-borne hemorrhagic fever
066 Other arthropod-borne viral diseases

Other diseases due to viruses and Chlamydiae (070-079)
070 Viral hepatitis
071 Rabies
072 Mumps
073 Ornithosis
074 Specific diseases due to Coxsackie virus
075 Infectious mononucleosis
076 Trachoma
077 Other diseases of conjunctiva due to viruses and Chlamydiae
078 Other diseases due to viruses and Chlamydiae
079 Viral and chlamydial infection in conditions classified elsewhere and of unspecified site

Rickettsioses and other arthropod-borne diseases (080-088)
080 Louse-borne [epidemic] typhus
081 Other typhus
082 Tick-borne rickettsioses
083 Other rickettsioses
084 Malaria
085 Leishmaniasis
086 Trypanosomiasis
087 Relapsing fever
088 Other arthropod-borne diseases

Syphilis and other venereal diseases (090-099)
090 Congenital syphilis
091 Early syphilis, symptomatic
092 Early syphilis, latent
093 Cardiovascular syphilis
094 Neurosyphilis
095 Other forms of late syphilis, with symptoms
096 Late syphilis, latent
097 Other and unspecified syphilis
098 Gonococcal infections
099 Other venereal diseases

Other spirochetal diseases (100-104)
100 Leptospirosis
101 Vincent's angina
102 Yaws
103 Pinta
104 Other spirochetal infection

Mycoses (110-118)
110 Dermatophytosis
111 Dermatomycosis, other and unspecified
112 Candidiasis
114 Coccidioidomycosis
115 Histoplasmosis
116 Blastomycotic infection
117 Other mycoses
118 Opportunistic mycoses

Helminthiases (120-129)
120 Schistosomiasis [bilharziasis]
121 Other trematode infections
122 Echinococcosis
123 Other cestode infection
124 Trichinosis
125 Filarial infection and dracontiasis
126 Ancylostomiasis and necatoriasis
127 Other intestinal helminthiases
128 Other and unspecified helminthiases
129 Intestinal parasitism, unspecified

Other infectious and parasitic diseases (130-136)
130 Toxoplasmosis
131 Trichomoniasis
132 Pediculosis and phthirus infestation
133 Acariasis
134 Other infestation
135 Sarcoidosis
136 Other and unspecified infectious and parasitic diseases

Late effects of infectious and parasitic diseases (137-139)
137 Late effects of tuberculosis
138 Late effects of acute poliomyelitis
139 Late effects of other infectious and parasitic diseases

2. Neoplasms

Malignant neoplasm of lip, oral cavity, and pharynx (140-149)
140 Malignant neoplasm of lip
141 Malignant neoplasm of tongue
142 Malignant neoplasm of major salivary glands
143 Malignant neoplasm of gum
144 Malignant neoplasm of floor of mouth
145 Malignant neoplasm of other and unspecified parts of mouth
146 Malignant neoplasm of oropharynx
147 Malignant neoplasm of nasopharynx
148 Malignant neoplasm of hypopharynx
149 Malignant neoplasm of other and ill-defined sites within the lip, oral cavity, and pharynx

Malignant neoplasm of digestive organs and peritoneum (150-159)
150 Malignant neoplasm of esophagus
151 Malignant neoplasm of stomach
152 Malignant neoplasm of small intestine, including duodenum
153 Malignant neoplasm of colon
154 Malignant neoplasm of rectum, rectosigmoid junction, and anus
155 Malignant neoplasm of liver and intrahepatic bile ducts
156 Malignant neoplasm of gallbladder and extrahepatic bile ducts
157 Malignant neoplasm of pancreas
158 Malignant neoplasm of retroperitoneum and peritoneum
159 Malignant neoplasm of other and ill-defined sites within the digestive organs and peritoneum

Malignant neoplasm of respiratory and intrathoracic organs (160-165)
160 Malignant neoplasm of nasal cavities, middle ear, and accessory sinuses
161 Malignant neoplasm of larynx
162 Malignant neoplasm of trachea, bronchus, and lung
163 Malignant neoplasm of pleura
164 Malignant neoplasm of thymus, heart, and mediastinum
165 Malignant neoplasm of other and ill-defined sites within the respiratory system and intrathoracic organs

Malignant neoplasm of bone, connective tissue, skin, and breast (170-176)
170 Malignant neoplasm of bone and articular cartilage
171 Malignant neoplasm of connective and other soft tissue
172 Malignant melanoma of skin
173 Other and unspecified malignant neoplasm of skin
174 Malignant neoplasm of female breast
175 Malignant neoplasm of male breast
176 Kaposi's sarcoma

Malignant neoplasm of genitourinary organs (179-189)
179 Malignant neoplasm of uterus, part unspecified
180 Malignant neoplasm of cervix uteri
181 Malignant neoplasm of placenta
182 Malignant neoplasm of body of uterus
183 Malignant neoplasm of ovary and other uterine adnexa
184 Malignant neoplasm of other and unspecified female genital organs
185 Malignant neoplasm of prostate
186 Malignant neoplasm of testis
187 Malignant neoplasm of penis and other male genital organs
188 Malignant neoplasm of bladder
189 Malignant neoplasm of kidney and other unspecified urinary organs

Malignant neoplasm of other and unspecified sites (190-199)
190 Malignant neoplasm of eye
191 Malignant neoplasm of brain
192 Malignant neoplasm of other and unspecified parts of nervous system
193 Malignant neoplasm of thyroid gland
194 Malignant neoplasm of other endocrine glands and related structures
195 Malignant neoplasm of other and ill-defined sites
196 Secondary and unspecified malignant neoplasm of lymph nodes
197 Secondary malignant neoplasm of respiratory and digestive systems
198 Secondary malignant neoplasm of other specified sites
199 Malignant neoplasm without specification of site

Malignant neoplasm of lymphatic and hematopoietic tissue (200-208)
200 Lymphosarcoma and reticulosarcoma and other specified malignant tumors of lymphatic tissue
201 Hodgkin's disease
202 Other malignant neoplasm of lymphoid and histiocytic tissue
203 Multiple myeloma and immunoproliferative neoplasms
204 Lymphoid leukemia
205 Myeloid leukemia
206 Monocytic leukemia
207 Other specified leukemia
208 Leukemia of unspecified cell type

Neuroendocrine tumors (209)
209 Neuroendocrine tumors

Benign neoplasms (210-229)
210 Benign neoplasm of lip, oral cavity, and pharynx
211 Benign neoplasm of other parts of digestive system
212 Benign neoplasm of respiratory and intrathoracic organs
213 Benign neoplasm of bone and articular cartilage
214 Lipoma
215 Other benign neoplasm of connective and other soft tissue
216 Benign neoplasm of skin
217 Benign neoplasm of breast
218 Uterine leiomyoma
219 Other benign neoplasm of uterus
220 Benign neoplasm of ovary
221 Benign neoplasm of other female genital organs
222 Benign neoplasm of male genital organs
223 Benign neoplasm of kidney and other urinary organs
224 Benign neoplasm of eye
225 Benign neoplasm of brain and other parts of nervous system
226 Benign neoplasm of thyroid gland

227 Benign neoplasm of other endocrine glands and related structures
228 Hemangioma and lymphangioma, any site
229 Benign neoplasm of other and unspecified sites

Carcinoma in situ (230-234)
230 Carcinoma in situ of digestive organs
231 Carcinoma in situ of respiratory system
232 Carcinoma in situ of skin
233 Carcinoma in situ of breast and genitourinary system
234 Carcinoma in situ of other and unspecified sites

Neoplasms of uncertain behavior (235-238)
235 Neoplasm of uncertain behavior of digestive and respiratory systems
236 Neoplasm of uncertain behavior of genitourinary organs
237 Neoplasm of uncertain behavior of endocrine glands and nervous system
238 Neoplasm of uncertain behavior of other and unspecified sites and tissues

Neoplasms of unspecified nature (239)
239 Neoplasm of unspecified nature

3. Endocrine, Nutritional and Metabolic Diseases, and Immunity Disorders

Disorders of thyroid gland (240-246)
240 Simple and unspecified goiter
241 Nontoxic nodular goiter
242 Thyrotoxicosis with or without goiter
243 Congenital hypothyroidism
244 Acquired hypothyroidism
245 Thyroiditis
246 Other disorders of thyroid

Diseases of other endocrine glands (249-259)
249 Secondary diabetes mellitus
250 Diabetes mellitus
251 Other disorders of pancreatic internal secretion
252 Disorders of parathyroid gland
253 Disorders of the pituitary gland and its hypothalamic control
254 Diseases of thymus gland
255 Disorders of adrenal glands
256 Ovarian dysfunction
257 Testicular dysfunction
258 Polyglandular dysfunction and related disorders
259 Other endocrine disorders

Nutritional deficiencies (260-269)
260 Kwashiorkor
261 Nutritional marasmus
262 Other severe protein-calorie malnutrition
263 Other and unspecified protein-calorie malnutrition
264 Vitamin A deficiency
265 Thiamine and niacin deficiency states
266 Deficiency of B-complex components
267 Ascorbic acid deficiency
268 Vitamin D deficiency
269 Other nutritional deficiencies

Other metabolic disorders and immnity disorders (270-279)
270 Disorders of amino-acid transport and metabolism
271 Disorders of carbohydrate transport and metabolism
272 Disorders of lipoid metabolism
273 Disorders of plasma protein metabolism
274 Gout
275 Disorders of mineral metabolism
276 Disorders of fluid, electrolyte, and acid-base balance
277 Other and unspecified disorders of metabolism

278 Overweight, obesity and other hyperalimentation
279 Disorders involving the immune mechanism

4. Diseases of Blood and Blood-forming Organs (280-289)
280 Iron deficiency anemias
281 Other deficiency anemias
282 Hereditary hemolytic anemias
283 Acquired hemolytic anemias
284 Aplastic anemia and other bone marrow failure syndromes
285 Other and unspecified anemias
286 Coagulation defects
287 Purpura and other hemorrhagic conditions
288 Diseases of white blood cells
289 Other diseases of blood and blood-forming organs

5. Mental, Behavioral and Neurodevelopmental Disorders

Organic psychotic conditions (290-294)
290 Dementias
291 Alcoholic induced mental disorders
292 Drug induced mental disorders
293 Transient mental disorders due to conditions classified elsewhere
294 Persistent mental disorders due to conditions classified elsewhere

Other psychoses (295-299)
295 Schizophrenic disorders
296 Episodic mood disorders
297 Delusional disorders
298 Other nonorganic psychoses
299 Pervasive developmental disorders

Neurotic disorders, personality disorders, and other nonpsychotic mental disorders (300-316)
300 Anxiety, dissociative and somatoform disorders
301 Personality disorders
302 Sexual and gender identity disorders
303 Alcohol dependence syndrome
304 Drug dependence
305 Nondependent abuse of drugs
306 Physiological malfunction arising from mental factors
307 Special symptoms or syndromes, not elsewhere classified
308 Acute reaction to stress
309 Adjustment reaction
310 Specific nonpsychotic mental disorders due to brain damage
311 Depressive disorder, not elsewhere classified
312 Disturbance of conduct, not elsewhere classified
313 Disturbance of emotions specific to childhood and adolescence
314 Hyperkinetic syndrome of childhood
315 Specific delays in development
316 Psychic factors associated with diseases classified elsewhere

Intellectual Disabilities (317-319)
317 Mild intellectual disabilities
318 Other specified intellectual disabilities
319 Unspecified intellectual disabilities

6. Diseases of the Nervous System and Sense Organs

Inflammatory diseases of the central nervous system (320-326)
320 Bacterial meningitis
321 Meningitis due to other organisms
322 Meningitis of unspecified cause
323 Encephalitis, myelitis, and encephalomyelitis

324 Intracranial and intraspinal abscess
325 Phlebitis and thrombophlebitis of intracranial venous sinuses
326 Late effects of intracranial abscess or pyogenic infection

Organic Sleep Disorders (327)
327 Organic sleep disorders

Hereditary and degenerative diseases of the central nervous system (330-337)
330 Cerebral degenerations usually manifest in childhood
331 Other cerebral degenerations
332 Parkinson's disease
333 Other extrapyramidal diseases and abnormal movement disorders
334 Spinocerebellar disease
335 Anterior horn cell disease
336 Other diseases of spinal cord
337 Disorders of the autonomic nervous system

Pain (338)
338 Pain, not elsewhere classified

Other headache syndromes (339)
339 Other headache syndromes

Other disorders of the central nervous system (340-349)
340 Multiple sclerosis
341 Other demyelinating diseases of central nervous system
342 Hemiplegia and hemiparesis
343 Infantile cerebral palsy
344 Other paralytic syndromes
345 Epilepsy and recurrent seizures
346 Migraine
347 Cataplexy and narcolepsy
348 Other conditions of brain
349 Other and unspecified disorders of the nervous system

Disorders of the peripheral nervous system (350-359)
350 Trigeminal nerve disorders
351 Facial nerve disorders
352 Disorders of other cranial nerves
353 Nerve root and plexus disorders
354 Mononeuritis of upper limb and mononeuritis multiplex
355 Mononeuritis of lower limb
356 Hereditary and idiopathic peripheral neuropathy
357 Inflammatory and toxic neuropathy
358 Myoneural disorders
359 Muscular dystrophies and other myopathies

Disorders of the eye and adnexa (360-379)
360 Disorders of the globe
361 Retinal detachments and defects
362 Other retinal disorders
363 Chorioretinal inflammations and scars and other disorders of choroid
364 Disorders of iris and ciliary body
365 Glaucoma
366 Cataract
367 Disorders of refraction and accommodation
368 Visual disturbances
369 Blindness and low vision
370 Keratitis
371 Corneal opacity and other disorders of cornea
372 Disorders of conjunctiva
373 Inflammation of eyelids
374 Other disorders of eyelids
375 Disorders of lacrimal system
376 Disorders of the orbit
377 Disorders of optic nerve and visual pathways
378 Strabismus and other disorders of binocular eye movements
379 Other disorders of eye

Diseases of the ear and mastoid process (380-389)
380 Disorders of external ear
381 Nonsuppurative otitis media and Eustachian tube disorders
382 Suppurative and unspecified otitis media
383 Mastoiditis and related conditions
384 Other disorders of tympanic membrane
385 Other disorders of middle ear and mastoid
386 Vertiginous syndromes and other disorders of vestibular system
387 Otosclerosis
388 Other disorders of ear
389 Hearing loss

7. Diseases of the Circulatory System

Acute rheumatic fever (390-392)
390 Rheumatic fever without mention of heart involvement
391 Rheumatic fever with heart involvement
392 Rheumatic chorea

Chronic rheumatic heart disease (393-398)
393 Chronic rheumatic pericarditis
394 Diseases of mitral valve
395 Diseases of aortic valve
396 Diseases of mitral and aortic valves
397 Diseases of other endocardial structures
398 Other rheumatic heart disease

Hypertensive disease (401-405)
401 Essential hypertension
402 Hypertensive heart disease
403 Hypertensive chronic kidney disease
404 Hypertensive heart and chronic kidney disease
405 Secondary hypertension

Ischemic heart disease (410-414)
410 Acute myocardial infarction
411 Other acute and subacute forms of ischemic heart disease
412 Old myocardial infarction
413 Angina pectoris
414 Other forms of chronic ischemic heart disease

Diseases of pulmonary circulation (415-417)
415 Acute pulmonary heart disease
416 Chronic pulmonary heart disease
417 Other diseases of pulmonary circulation

Other forms of heart disease (420-429)
420 Acute pericarditis
421 Acute and subacute endocarditis
422 Acute myocarditis
423 Other diseases of pericardium
424 Other diseases of endocardium
425 Cardiomyopathy
426 Conduction disorders
427 Cardiac dysrhythmias
428 Heart failure
429 Ill-defined descriptions and complications of heart disease

Cerebrovascular disease (430-438)
430 Subarachnoid hemorrhage
431 Intracerebral hemorrhage
432 Other and unspecified intracranial hemorrhage
433 Occlusion and stenosis of precerebral arteries
434 Occlusion of cerebral arteries
435 Transient cerebral ischemia
436 Acute, but ill-defined, cerebrovascular disease
437 Other and ill-defined cerebrovascular disease
438 Late effects of cerebrovascular disease

Diseases of arteries, arterioles, and capillaries (440-449)
440 Atherosclerosis
441 Aortic aneurysm and dissection
442 Other aneurysm
443 Other peripheral vascular disease
444 Arterial embolism and thrombosis
445 Atheroembolism
446 Polyarteritis nodosa and allied conditions
447 Other disorders of arteries and arterioles
448 Diseases of capillaries
449 Septic arterial embolism

Diseases of veins and lymphatics, and other diseases of circulatory system (451-459)
451 Phlebitis and thrombophlebitis
452 Portal vein thrombosis
453 Other venous embolism and thrombosis
454 Varicose veins of lower extremities
455 Hemorrhoids
456 Varicose veins of other sites
457 Noninfectious disorders of lymphatic channels
458 Hypotension
459 Other disorders of circulatory system

8. Diseases of the Respiratory System

Acute respiratory infections (460-466)
460 Acute nasopharyngitis [common cold]
461 Acute sinusitis
462 Acute pharyngitis
463 Acute tonsillitis
464 Acute laryngitis and tracheitis
465 Acute upper respiratory infections of multiple or unspecified sites
466 Acute bronchitis and bronchiolitis

Other diseases of upper respiratory tract (470-478)
470 Deviated nasal septum
471 Nasal polyps
472 Chronic pharyngitis and nasopharyngitis
473 Chronic sinusitis
474 Chronic disease of tonsils and adenoids
475 Peritonsillar abscess
476 Chronic laryngitis and laryngotracheitis
477 Allergic rhinitis
478 Other diseases of upper respiratory tract

Pneumonia and influenza (480-488)
480 Viral pneumonia
481 Pneumococcal pneumonia [Streptococcus pneumoniae pneumonia]
482 Other bacterial pneumonia
483 Pneumonia due to other specified organism
484 Pneumonia in infectious diseases classified elsewhere
485 Bronchopneumonia, organism unspecified
486 Pneumonia, organism unspecified
487 Influenza
488 Influenza due to certain identified influenza viruses

Chronic obstructive pulmonary disease and allied conditions (490-496)
490 Bronchitis, not specified as acute or chronic
491 Chronic bronchitis
492 Emphysema
493 Asthma
494 Bronchiectasis
495 Extrinsic allergic alveolitis
496 Chronic airways obstruction, not elsewhere classified

Pneumoconioses and other lung diseases due to external agents (500-508)
500 Coal workers' pneumoconiosis
501 Asbestosis
502 Pneumoconiosis due to other silica or silicates
503 Pneumoconiosis due to other inorganic dust
504 Pneumopathy due to inhalation of other dust
505 Pneumoconiosis, unspecified
506 Respiratory conditions due to chemical fumes and vapors
507 Pneumonitis due to solids and liquids
508 Respiratory conditions due to other and unspecified external agents

Other diseases of respiratory system (510-519)
510　Empyema
511　Pleurisy
512　Pneumothorax and air leak
513　Abscess of lung and mediastinum
514　Pulmonary congestion and hypostasis
515　Postinflammatory pulmonary fibrosis
516　Other alveolar and parietoalveolar pneumopathy
517　Lung involvement in conditions classified elsewhere
518　Other diseases of lung
519　Other diseases of respiratory system

9. Diseases of the Digestive System

Diseases of oral cavity, salivary glands, and jaws (520-529)
520　Disorders of tooth development and eruption
521　Diseases of hard tissues of teeth
522　Diseases of pulp and periapical tissues
523　Gingival and periodontal diseases
524　Dentofacial anomalies, including malocclusion
525　Other diseases and conditions of the teeth and supporting structures
526　Diseases of the jaws
527　Diseases of the salivary glands
528　Diseases of the oral soft tissues, excluding lesions specific for gingiva and tongue
529　Diseases and other conditions of the tongue

Diseases of esophagus, stomach, and duodenum (530-539)
530　Diseases of esophagus
531　Gastric ulcer
532　Duodenal ulcer
533　Peptic ulcer, site unspecified
534　Gastrojejunal ulcer
535　Gastritis and duodenitis
536　Disorders of function of stomach
537　Other disorders of stomach and duodenum
538　Gastrointestinal mucositis (ulcerative)
539　Complications of bariatric procedures

Appendicitis (540-543)
540　Acute appendicitis
541　Appendicitis, unqualified
542　Other appendicitis
543　Other diseases of appendix

Hernia of abdominal cavity (550-553)
550　Inguinal hernia
551　Other hernia of abdominal cavity, with gangrene
552　Other hernia of abdominal cavity, with obstruction, but without mention of gangrene
553　Other hernia of abdominal cavity without mention of obstruction or gangrene

Noninfective enteritis and colitis (555-558)
555　Regional enteritis
556　Ulcerative colitis
557　Vascular insufficiency of intestine
558　Other noninfective gastroenteritis and colitis

Other diseases of intestines and peritoneum (560-569)
560　Intestinal obstruction without mention of hernia
562　Diverticula of intestine
564　Functional digestive disorders, not elsewhere classified
565　Anal fissure and fistula
566　Abscess of anal and rectal regions
567　Peritonitis and retroperitoneal infections
568　Other disorders of peritoneum
569　Other disorders of intestine

Other diseases of digestive system (570-579)
570　Acute and subacute necrosis of liver
571　Chronic liver disease and cirrhosis
572　Liver abscess and sequelae of chronic liver disease
573　Other disorders of liver
574　Cholelithiasis
575　Other disorders of gallbladder
576　Other disorders of biliary tract
577　Diseases of pancreas
578　Gastrointestinal hemorrhage
579　Intestinal Malabsorption

10. Diseases of the Genitourinary System

Nephritis, nephrotic syndrome, and nephrosis (580-589)
580　Acute gloerulonephritis
581　Nephrotic syndrome
582　Chronic glomerulonephritis
583　Nephritis and nephropathy, not specified as acute or chronic
584　Acute kidney failure
585　Chronic kidney disease (CKD)
586　Renal failure, unspecified
587　Renal sclerosis, unspecified
588　Disorders resulting from impaired renal function
589　Small kidney of unknown cause

Other diseases of urinary system (590-599)
590　Infections of kidney
591　Hydronephrosis
592　Calculus of kidney and ureter
593　Other disorders of kidney and ureter
594　Calculus of lower urinary tract
595　Cystitis
596　Other disorders of bladder
597　Urethritis, not sexually transmitted, and urethral syndrome
598　Urethral stricture
599　Other disorders of urethra and urinary tract

Diseases of male genital organs (600-608)
600　Hyperplasia of prostate
601　Inflammatory diseases of prostate
602　Other disorders of prostate
603　Hydrocele
604　Orchitis and epididymitis
605　Redundant prepuce and phimosis
606　Infertility, male
607　Disorders of penis
608　Other disorders of male genital organs

Disorders of breast (610-612)
610　Benign mammary dysplasias
611　Other disorders of breast
612　Deformity and disproportion of reconstructed breast

Inflammatory disease of female pelvic organs (614-616)
614　Inflammatory disease of ovary, fallopian tube, pelvic cellular tissue, and peritoneum
615　Inflammatory diseases of uterus, except cervix
616　Inflammatory disease of cervix, vagina, and vulva

Other disorders of female genital tract (617-629)
617　Endometriosis
618　Genital prolapse
619　Fistula involving female genital tract
620　Noninflammatory disorders of ovary, fallopian tube, and broad ligament
621　Disorders of uterus, not elsewhere classified
622　Noninflammatory disorders of cervix
623　Noninflammatory disorders of vagina
624　Noninflammatory disorders of vulva and perineum
625　Pain and other symptoms associated with female genital organs
626　Disorders of menstruation and other abnormal bleeding from female genital tract
627　Menopausal and postmenopausal disorders
628　Infertility, female
629　Other disorders of female genital organs

11. Complications of Pregnancy, Childbirth and the Puerperium

Ectopic and molar pregnancy (630-633)
630　Hydatidiform mole
631　Other abnormal product of conception
632　Missed abortion
633　Ectopic pregnancy

Other pregnancy with abortive outcome (634-639)
634　Spontaneous abortion
635　Legally induced abortion
636　Illegally induced abortion
637　Unspecified abortion
638　Failed attempted abortion
639　Complications following abortion and ectopic and molar pregnancies

Complications mainly related to pregnancy (640-649)
640　Hemorrhage in early pregnancy
641　Antepartum hemorrhage, abruptio placentae, and placenta previa
642　Hypertension complicating pregnancy, childbirth, and the puerperium
643　Excessive vomiting in pregnancy
644　Early or threatened labor
645　Late pregnancy
646　Other complications of pregnancy, not elsewhere classified
647　Infectious and parasitic conditions in the mother classifiable elsewhere, but complicating pregnancy, childbirth, and the puerperium
648　Other current conditions in the mother classifiable elsewhere, but complicating pregnancy, childbirth, and the puerperium
649　Other conditions or status of the mother complicating pregnancy, childbirth, or the puerperium

Normal delivery, and other indications for care in pregnancy, labor, and delivery (650-659)
650　Normal delivery
651　Multiple gestation
652　Malposition and malpresentation of fetus
653　Disproportion
654　Abnormality of organs and soft tissues of pelvis
655　Known or suspected fetal abnormality affecting management of mother
656　Other known or suspected fetal and placental problems affecting management of mother
657　Polyhydramnios
658　Other problems associated with amniotic cavity and membranes
659　Other indications for care or intervention related to labor and delivery, not elsewhere classified

Complications occurring mainly in the course of labor and delivery (660-669)
660　Obstructed labor
661　Abnormality of forces of labor
662　Long labor
663　Umbilical cord complications
664　Trauma to perineum and vulva during delivery
665　Other obstetrical trauma
666　Postpartum hemorrhage
667　Retained placenta or membranes, without hemorrhage
668　Complications of the administration of anesthetic or other sedation in labor and delivery
669　Other complications of labor and delivery, not elsewhere classified

Complications of the puerperium (670-677)
670　Major puerperal infection

671 Venous complications in pregnancy and the puerperium
672 Pyrexia of unknown origin during the puerperium
673 Obstetrical pulmonary embolism
674 Other and unspecified complications of the puerperium, not elsewhere classified
675 Infections of the breast and nipple associated with childbirth
676 Other disorders of the breast associated with childbirth, and disorders of lactation
677 Late effect of complication of pregnancy, childbirth, and the puerperium

Other maternal and fetal complications (678-679)
678 Other fetal conditions
679 Complications of in utero procedures

12. Diseases of the Skin and Subcutaneous Tissue

Infections of skin and subcutaneous tissue (680-686)
680 Carbuncle and furuncle
681 Cellulitis and abscess of finger and toe
682 Other cellulitis and abscess
683 Acute lymphadenitis
684 Impetigo
685 Pilonidal cyst
686 Other local infections of skin and subcutaneous tissue

Other inflammatory conditions of skin and subcutaneous tissue (690-698)
690 Erythematosquamous dermatosis
691 Atopic dermatitis and related conditions
692 Contact dermatitis and other eczema
693 Dermatitis due to substances taken internally
694 Bullous dermatoses
695 Erythematous conditions
696 Psoriasis and similar disorders
697 Lichen
698 Pruritus and related conditions

Other diseases of skin and subcutaneous tissue (700-709)
700 Corns and callosities
701 Other hypertrophic and atrophic conditions of skin
702 Other dermatoses
703 Diseases of nail
704 Diseases of hair and hair follicles
705 Disorders of sweat glands
706 Diseases of sebaceous glands
707 Chronic ulcer of skin
708 Urticaria
709 Other disorders of skin and subcutaneous tissue

13. Diseases of the Musculoskeletal System and Connective Tissue

Arthropathies and related disorders (710-719)
710 Diffuse diseases of connective tissue
711 Arthropathy associated with infections
712 Crystal arthropathies
713 Arthropathy associated with other disorders classified elsewhere
714 Rheumatoid arthritis and other inflammatory polyarthropathies
715 Osteoarthrosis and allied disorders
716 Other and unspecified arthropathies
717 Internal derangement of knee
718 Other derangement of joint
719 Other and unspecified disorder of joint

Dorsopathies (720-724)
720 Ankylosing spondylitis and other inflammatory spondylopathies
721 Spondylosis and allied disorders
722 Intervertebral disc disorders
723 Other disorders of cervical region
724 Other and unspecified disorders of back

Rheumatism, excluding the back (725-729)
725 Polymyalgia rheumatica
726 Peripheral enthesopathies and allied syndromes
727 Other disorders of synovium, tendon, and bursa
728 Disorders of muscle, ligament, and fascia
729 Other disorders of soft tissues

Osteopathies, chondropathies, and acquired musculoskeletal deformities (730-739)
730 Osteomyelitis, periostitis, and other infections involving bone
731 Osteitis deformans and osteopathies associated with other disorders classified elsewhere
732 Osteochondropathies
733 Other disorders of bone and cartilage
734 Flat foot
735 Acquired deformities of toe
736 Other acquired deformities of limbs
737 Curvature of spine
738 Other acquired deformity
739 Nonallopathic lesions, not elsewhere classified

14. Congenital Anomalies

740 Anencephalus and similar anomalies
741 Spina bifida
742 Other congenital anomalies of nervous system
743 Congenital anomalies of eye
744 Congenital anomalies of ear, face, and neck
745 Bulbus cordis anomalies and anomalies of cardiac septal closure
746 Other congenital anomalies of heart
747 Other congenital anomalies of circulatory system
748 Congenital anomalies of respiratory system
749 Cleft palate and cleft lip
750 Other congenital anomalies of upper alimentary tract
751 Other congenital anomalies of digestive system
752 Congenital anomalies of genital organs
753 Congenital anomalies of urinary system
754 Certain congenital musculoskeletal deformities
755 Other congenital anomalies of limbs
756 Other congenital musculoskeletal anomalies
757 Congenital anomalies of the integument
758 Chromosomal anomalies
759 Other and unspecified congenital anomalies

15. Certain Conditions Originating in the Perinatal Period

Maternal causes of perinatal morbidity and mortality (760-763)
760 Fetus or newborn affected by maternal conditions which may be unrelated to present pregnancy
761 Fetus or newborn affected by maternal complications of pregnancy
762 Fetus or newborn affected by complications of placenta, cord, and membranes
763 Fetus or newborn affected by other complications of labor and delivery

Other conditions originating in the perinatal period (764-779)
764 Slow fetal growth and fetal malnutrition
765 Disorders relating to short gestation and unspecified low birthweight
766 Disorders relating to long gestation and high birthweight
767 Birth trauma
768 Intrauterine hypoxia and birth asphyxia
769 Respiratory distress syndrome
770 Other respiratory conditions of fetus and newborn
771 Infections specific to the perinatal period
772 Fetal and neonatal hemorrhage
773 Hemolytic disease of fetus or newborn, due to isoimmunization
774 Other perinatal jaundice
775 Endocrine and metabolic disturbances specific to the fetus and newborn
776 Hematological disorders of newborn
777 Perinatal disorders of digestive system
778 Conditions involving the integument and temperature regulation of fetus and newborn
779 Other and ill-defined conditions originating in the perinatal period

16. Symptoms, Signs, and Ill-defined Conditions

Symptoms (780-789)
780 General symptoms
781 Symptoms involving nervous and musculoskeletal systems
782 Symptoms involving skin and other integumentary tissue
783 Symptoms concerning nutrition, metabolism, and development
784 Symptoms involving head and neck
785 Symptoms involving cardiovascular system
786 Symptoms involving respiratory system and other chest symptoms
787 Symptoms involving digestive system
788 Symptoms involving urinary system
789 Other symptoms involving abdomen and pelvis

Nonspecific abnormal findings (790-796)
790 Nonspecific findings on examination of blood
791 Nonspecific findings on examination of urine
792 Nonspecific abnormal findings in other body substances
793 Nonspecific (abnormal) findings on radiological and other examination of body structure
794 Nonspecific abnormal results of function studies
795 Other and nonspecific abnormal cystological, histological, immunological and DNA test findings
796 Other nonspecific abnormal findings

Ill-defined and unknown causes of morbidity and mortality (797-799)
797 Senility without mention of psychosis
798 Sudden death, cause unknown
799 Other ill-defined and unknown causes of morbidity and mortality

17. Injury and Poisoning

Fracture of skull (800-804)
800 Fracture of vault of skull
801 Fracture of base of skull
802 Fracture of face bones
803 Other and unqualified skull fractures
804 Multiple fractures involving skull or face with other bones

Fracture of spine and trunk (805-809)
805 Fracture of vertebral column without mention of spinal cord injury
806 Fracture of vertebral column with spinal cord injury
807 Fracture of rib(s), sternum, larynx, and trachea
808 Fracture of pelvis
809 Ill-defined fractures of bones of trunk

Fracture of upper limb (810-819)
810 Fracture of clavicle
811 Fracture of scapula
812 Fracture of humerus
813 Fracture of radius and ulna
814 Fracture of carpal bone(s)
815 Fracture of metacarpal bone(s)

816	Fracture of one or more phalanges of hand
817	Multiple fractures of hand bones
818	Ill-defined fractures of upper limb
819	Multiple fractures involving both upper limbs, and upper limb with rib(s) and sternum

Fracture of lower limb (820-829)

820	Fracture of neck of femur
821	Fracture of other and unspecified parts of femur
822	Fracture of patella
823	Fracture of tibia and fibula
824	Fracture of ankle
825	Fracture of one or more tarsal and metatarsal bones
826	Fracture of one or more phalanges of foot
827	Other, multiple, and ill-defined fractures of lower limb
828	Multiple fractures involving both lower limbs, lower with upper limb, and lower limb(s) with rib(s) and sternum
829	Fracture of unspecified bones

Dislocation (830-839)

830	Dislocation of jaw
831	Dislocation of shoulder
832	Dislocation of elbow
833	Dislocation of wrist
834	Dislocation of finger
835	Dislocation of hip
836	Dislocation of knee
837	Dislocation of ankle
838	Dislocation of foot
839	Other, multiple, and ill-defined dislocations

Sprains and strains of joints and adjacent muscles (840-848)

840	Sprains and strains of shoulder and upper arm
841	Sprains and strains of elbow and forearm
842	Sprains and strains of wrist and hand
843	Sprains and strains of hip and thigh
844	Sprains and strains of knee and leg
845	Sprains and strains of ankle and foot
846	Sprains and strains of sacroiliac region
847	Sprains and strains of other and unspecified parts of back
848	Other and ill-defined sprains and strains

Intracranial injury, excluding those with skull fracture (850-854)

850	Concussion
851	Cerebral laceration and contusion
852	Subarachnoid, subdural, and extradural hemorrhage, following injury
853	Other and unspecified intracranial hemorrhage following injury
854	Intracranial injury of other and unspecified nature

Internal injury of thorax, abdomen, and pelvis (860-869)

860	Traumatic pneumothorax and hemothorax
861	Injury to heart and lung
862	Injury to other and unspecified intrathoracic organs
863	Injury to gastrointestinal tract
864	Injury to liver
865	Injury to spleen
866	Injury to kidney
867	Injury to pelvic organs
868	Injury to other intra-abdominal organs
869	Internal injury to unspecified or ill-defined organs

Open wound of head, neck, and trunk (870-879)

870	Open wound of ocular adnexa
871	Open wound of eyeball
872	Open wound of ear
873	Other open wound of head
874	Open wound of neck
875	Open wound of chest (wall)
876	Open wound of back
877	Open wound of buttock
878	Open wound of genital organs (external), including traumatic amputation
879	Open wound of other and unspecified sites, except limbs

Open wound of upper limb (880-887)

880	Open wound of shoulder and upper arm
881	Open wound of elbow, forearm, and wrist
882	Open wound of hand except finger(s) alone
883	Open wound of finger(s)
884	Multiple and unspecified open wound of upper limb
885	Traumatic amputation of thumb (complete) (partial)
886	Traumatic amputation of other finger(s) (complete) (partial)
887	Traumatic amputation of arm and hand (complete) (partial)

Open wound of lower limb (890-897)

890	Open wound of hip and thigh
891	Open wound of knee, leg [except thigh], and ankle
892	Open wound of foot except toe(s) alone
893	Open wound of toe(s)
894	Multiple and unspecified open wound of lower limb
895	Traumatic amputation of toe(s) (complete) (partial)
896	Traumatic amputation of foot (complete) (partial)
897	Traumatic amputation of leg(s) (complete) (partial)

Injury to blood vessels (900-904)

900	Injury to blood vessels of head and neck
901	Injury to blood vessels of thorax
902	Injury to blood vessels of abdomen and pelvis
903	Injury to blood vessels of upper extremity
904	Injury to blood vessels of lower extremity and unspecified sites

Late effects of injuries, poisonings, toxic effects, and other external causes (905-909)

905	Late effects of musculoskeletal and connective tissue injuries
906	Late effects of injuries to skin and subcutaneous tissues
907	Late effects of injuries to the nervous system
908	Late effects of other and unspecified injuries
909	Late effects of other and unspecified external causes

Superficial injury (910-919)

910	Superficial injury of face, neck, and scalp except eye
911	Superficial injury of trunk
912	Superficial injury of shoulder and upper arm
913	Superficial injury of elbow, forearm, and wrist
914	Superficial injury of hand(s) except finger(s) alone
915	Superficial injury of finger(s)
916	Superficial injury of hip, thigh, leg, and ankle
917	Superficial injury of foot and toe(s)
918	Superficial injury of eye and adnexa
919	Superficial injury of other, multiple, and unspecified sites

Contusion with intact skin surface (920-924)

920	Contusion of face, scalp, and neck except eye(s)
921	Contusion of eye and adnexa
922	Contusion of trunk
923	Contusion of upper limb
924	Contusion of lower limb and of other and unspecified sites

Crushing injury (925-929)

925	Crushing injury of face, scalp, and neck
926	Crushing injury of trunk
927	Crushing injury of upper limb
928	Crushing injury of lower limb
929	Crushing injury of multiple and unspecified sites

Effects of foreign body entering through orifice (930-939)

930	Foreign body on external eye
931	Foreign body in ear
932	Foreign body in nose
933	Foreign body in pharynx and larynx
934	Foreign body in trachea, bronchus, and lung
935	Foreign body in mouth, esophagus, and stomach
936	Foreign body in intestine and colon
937	Foreign body in anus and rectum
938	Foreign body in digestive system, unspecified
939	Foreign body in genitourinary tract

Burns (940-949)

940	Burn confined to eye and adnexa
941	Burn of face, head, and neck
942	Burn of trunk
943	Burn of upper limb, except wrist and hand
944	Burn of wrist(s) and hand(s)
945	Burn of lower limb(s)
946	Burns of multiple specified sites
947	Burn of internal organs
948	Burns classified according to extent of body surface involved
949	Burn, unspecified

Injury to nerves and spinal cord (950-957)

950	Injury to optic nerve and pathways
951	Injury to other cranial nerve(s)
952	Spinal cord injury without evidence of spinal bone injury
953	Injury to nerve roots and spinal plexus
954	Injury to other nerve(s) of trunk excluding shoulder and pelvic girdles
955	Injury to peripheral nerve(s) of shoulder girdle and upper limb
956	Injury to peripheral nerve(s) of pelvic girdle and lower limb
957	Injury to other and unspecified nerves

Certain traumatic complications and unspecified injuries (958-959)

958	Certain early complications of trauma
959	Injury, other and unspecified

Poisoning by drugs, medicinals and biological substances (960-979)

960	Poisoning by antibiotics
961	Poisoning by other anti-infectives
962	Poisoning by hormones and synthetic substitutes
963	Poisoning by primarily systemic agents
964	Poisoning by agents primarily affecting blood constituents
965	Poisoning by analgesics, antipyretics, and antirheumatics
966	Poisoning by anticonvulsants and anti-Parkinsonism drugs
967	Poisoning by sedatives and hypnotics
968	Poisoning by other central nervous system depressants and anesthetics
969	Poisoning by psychotropic agents
970	Poisoning by central nervous system stimulants
971	Poisoning by drugs primarily affecting the autonomic nervous system
972	Poisoning by agents primarily affecting the cardiovascular system
973	Poisoning by agents primarily affecting the gastrointestinal system
974	Poisoning by water, mineral, and uric acid metabolism drugs
975	Poisoning by agents primarily acting on the smooth and skeletal muscles and respiratory system

976   Poisoning by agents primarily affecting skin and mucous membrane, ophthalmological, otorhinolaryngological, and dental drugs
977   Poisoning by other and unspecified drugs and medicinals
978   Poisoning by bacterial vaccines
979   Poisoning by other vaccines and biological substances

Toxic effects of substances chiefly nonmedicinal as to source (980-989)

980   Toxic effect of alcohol
981   Toxic effect of petroleum products
982   Toxic effect of solvents other than petroleum-based
983   Toxic effect of corrosive aromatics, acids, and caustic alkalis
984   Toxic effect of lead and its compounds (including fumes)
985   Toxic effect of other metals
986   Toxic effect of carbon monoxide
987   Toxic effect of other gases, fumes, or vapors
988   Effect of noxious substances eaten as food
989   Toxic effect of other substances, chiefly nonmedicinal as to source

Other and unspecified effects of external causes (990-995)

990   Effects of radiation, unspecified
991   Effects of reduced temperature
992   Effects of heat and light
993   Effects of air pressure
994   Effects of other external causes
995   Certain adverse effects, not elsewhere classified

Complications of surgical and medical care, not elsewhere classified (996-999)

996   Complications peculiar to certain specified procedures
997   Complications affecting specified body systems, not elsewhere classified
998   Other complications of procedures, not elsewhere classified
999   Complications of medical care, not elsewhere classified

Supplementary Classification of Factors Influencing Health Status and Contact With Health Services

Persons with potential health hazards related to communicable diseases (V01-V06)

V01   Contact with or exposure to communicable diseases
V02   Carrier or suspected carrier of infectious diseases
V03   Need for prophylactic vaccination and inoculation against bacterial diseases
V04   Need for prophylactic vaccination and inoculation against certain viral diseases
V05   Need for other prophylactic vaccination and inoculation against single diseases
V06   Need for prophylactic vaccination and inoculation against combinations of diseases

Persons with need for isolation, other potential health hazards, and prophylactic measures (V07-V09)

V07   Need for isolation and other prophylactic or treatment measures
V08   Asymptomatic human immunodeficiency virus [HIV] infection status
V09   Infection with drug-resistant microorganisms

Persons with potential health hazards related to personal and family history (V10-V19)

V10   Personal history of malignant neoplasm
V11   Personal history of mental disorder
V12   Personal history of certain other diseases

V13   Personal history of other diseases
V14   Personal history of allergy to medicinal agents
V15   Other personal history presenting hazards to health
V16   Family history of malignant neoplasm
V17   Family history of certain chronic disabling diseases
V18   Family history of certain other specific conditions
V19   Family history of other conditions

Persons encountering health services in circumstances related to reproduction and development (V20-V29)

V20   Health supervision of infant or child
V21   Constitutional states in development
V22   Normal pregnancy
V23   Supervision of high-risk pregnancy
V24   Postpartum care and examination
V25   Encounter for contraceptive management
V26   Procreative management
V27   Outcome of delivery
V28   Encounter for antenatal screening of mother
V29   Observation and evaluation of newborns and infants for suspected condition not found

Liveborn infants according to type of birth (V30-V39)

V30   Single liveborn
V31   Twin, mate liveborn
V32   Twin, mate stillborn
V33   Twin, unspecified
V34   Other multiple, mates all liveborn
V35   Other multiple, mates all stillborn
V36   Other multiple, mates live and stillborn
V37   Other multiple, unspecified
V39   Unspecified

Persons with a condition influencing their health status (V40-V49)

V40   Mental and behavioral problems
V41   Problems with special senses and other special functions
V42   Organ or tissue replaced by transplant
V43   Organ or tissue replaced by other means
V44   Artificial opening status
V45   Other postprocedural states
V46   Other dependence on machines and devices
V47   Other problems with internal organs
V48   Problems with head, neck, and trunk
V49   Other conditions influencing health status

Persons encountering health services for specific procedures and aftercare (V50-V59)

V50   Elective surgery for purposes other than remedying health states
V51   Aftercare involving the use of plastic surgery
V52   Fitting and adjustment of prosthetic device and implant
V53   Fitting and adjustment of other device
V54   Other orthopedic aftercare
V55   Attention to artificial openings
V56   Encounter for dialysis and dialysis catheter care
V57   Care involving use of rehabilitation procedures
V58   Encounter for other and unspecified procedures and aftercare
V59   Donors

Persons encountering health services in other circumstances (V60-V69)

V60   Housing, household, and economic circumstances
V61   Other family circumstances
V62   Other psychosocial circumstances
V63   Unavailability of other medical facilities for care
V64   Persons encountering health services for specific procedures, not carried out
V65   Other persons seeking consultation
V66   Convalescence and palliative care
V67   Follow-up examination

V68   Encounters for administrative purposes
V69   Problems related to lifestyle

Persons without reported diagnosis encountered during examination and investigation of individuals and populations (V70-V82)

V70   General medical examination
V71   Observation and evaluation for suspected conditions not found
V72   Special investigations and examinations
V73   Special screening examination for viral and chlamydial diseases
V74   Special screening examination for bacterial and spirochetal diseases
V75   Special screening examination for other infectious diseases
V76   Special screening for malignant neoplasms
V77   Special screening for endocrine, nutritional, metabolic, and immunity disorders
V78   Special screening for disorders of blood and blood-forming organs
V79   Special screening for mental disorders and developmental handicaps
V80   Special screening for neurological, eye, and ear diseases
V81   Special screening for cardiovascular, respiratory, and genitourinary diseases
V82   Special screening for other conditions

Genetics (V83-V84)

V83   Genetic carrier status
V84   Genetic susceptibility to disease

Body mass index (V85)

V85   Body Mass Index [BMI]

Estrogen receptor status (V86)

V86   Estrogen receptor status

Other specified personal exposures and history presenting hazards to health (V87)

V87   Other specified personal exposures and history presenting hazards to health

Acquired absence of other organs and tissue (V88)

V88   Acquired absence of other organs and tissue

Other suspected conditions not found (V89)

V89   Other suspected conditions not found

Retained Foreign Body (V90)

V90   Retained foreign body

Multiple Gestation Placenta Status (V91)

V91   Multiple gestation placenta status

Supplementary Classification of External Causes of Injury and Poisoning

External Cause Status (E000)

E000   External cause status

Activity (E001-E030)

E001   Activities involving walking and running
E002   Activities involving water and water craft
E003   Activities involving ice and snow
E004   Activities involving climbing, rappelling, and jumping off
E005   Activities involving dancing and other rhythmic movement
E006   Activities involving other sports and athletics played individually
E007   Activities involving other sports and athletics played as a team or group
E008   Activities involving other specified sports and athletics
E009   Activity involving other cardiorespiratory exercise
E010   Activity involving other muscle strengthening exercises

E011   Activities involving computer technology and electronic devices
E012   Activities involving arts and handcrafts
E013   Activities involving personal hygiene and household maintenance
E014   Activities involving person providing caregiving
E015   Activities involving food preparation, cooking and grilling
E016   Activities involving property and land maintenance, building and construction
E017   Activities involving roller coasters and other types of external motion
E018   Activities involving playing musical instrument
E019   Activities involving animal care
E029   Other activity
E030   Unspecified activity

Transport Accidents (E800-E848)

Railway accidents (E800-E807)
E800   Railway accident involving collision with roling stock
E801   Railway accident involving collision with other object
E802   Railway accident involving derailment without antecedent collision
E803   Railway accident involving explosion, fire, or burning
E804   Fall in, on, or from railway train
E805   Hit by rolling stock
E806   Other specified railway accident
E807   Railway accident of unspecified nature

Motor vehicle traffic accidents (E810-E819)
E810   Motor vehicle traffic accident involving collision with train
E811   Motor vehicle traffic accident involving re-entrant collision with another motor vehicle
E812   Other motor vehicle traffic accident involving collision with another motor vehicle
E813   Motor vehicle traffic accident involving collision with other vehicle
E814   Motor vehicle traffic accident involving collision with pedestrian
E815   Other motor vehicle traffic accident involving collision on the highway
E816   Motor vehicle traffic accident due to loss of control, without collision on the highway
E817   Noncollision motor vehicle traffic accident while boarding or alighting
E818   Other noncollision motor vehicle traffic accident
E819   Motor vehicle traffic accident of unspecified nature

Motor vehicle nontraffic accidents (E820-E825)
E820   Nontraffic accident involving motor-driven snow vehicle
E821   Nontraffic accident involving other off-road motor vehicle
E822   Other motor vehicle nontraffic accident involving collision with moving object
E823   Other motor vehicle nontraffic accident involving collision with stationary object
E824   Other motor vehicle nontraffic accident while boarding and alighting
E825   Other motor vehicle nontraffic accident of other and unspecified nature

Other road vehicle accidents (E826-E829)
E826   Pedal cycle accident
E827   Animal-drawn vehicle accident
E828   Accident involving animal being ridden
E829   Other road vehicle accidents

Water transport accidents (E830-E838)
E830   Accident to watercraft causing submersion
E831   Accident to watercraft causing other injury
E832   Other accidental submersion or drowning in water transport accident
E833   Fall on stairs or ladders in water transport
E834   Other fall from one level to another in water transport
E835   Other and unspecified fall in water transport
E836   Machinery accident in water transport
E837   Explosion, fire, or burning in watercraft
E838   Other and unspecified water transport accident

Air and space transport accidents (E840-E845)
E840   Accident to powered aircraft at takeoff or landing
E841   Accident to powered aircraft, other and unspecified
E842   Accident to unpowered aircraft
E843   Fall in, on, or from aircraft
E844   Other specified air transport accidents
E845   Accident involving spacecraft

Vehicle accidents, not elsewhere classfiable (E846-E849)
E846   Accidents involving powered vehicles used solely within the buildings and premises of an industrial or commercial establishment
E847   Accidents involving cable cars not running on rails
E848   Accidents involving other vehicles, not elsewhere classifiable
E849   Place of occurrence

Accidental poisoning by drugs, medicinal substances, and biologicals (E850-E858)
E850   Accidental poisoning by analgesics, antipyretics, and antirheumatics
E851   Accidental poisoning by barbiturates
E852   Accidental poisoning by other sedatives and hypnotics
E853   Accidental poisoning by tranquilizers
E854   Accidental poisoning by other psychotropic agents
E855   Accidental poisoning by other drugs acting on central and autonomic nervous systems
E856   Accidental poisoning by antibiotics
E857   Accidental poisoning by anti-infectives
E858   Accidental poisoning by other drugs

Accidental poisoning by other solid and liquid substances, gases, and vapors (E860-E869)
E860   Accidental poisoning by alcohol, not elsewhere classified
E861   Accidental poisoning by cleansing and polishing agents, disinfectants, paints, and varnishes
E862   Accidental poisoning by petroleum products, other solvents and their vapors, not elsewhere classified
E863   Accidental poisoning by agricultural and horticultural chemical and pharmaceutical preparations other than plant foods and fertilizers
E864   Accidental poisoning by corrosives and caustics, not elsewhere classified
E865   Accidental poisoning from poisonous foodstuffs and poisonous plants
E866   Accidental poisoning by other and unspecified solid and liquid substances
E867   Accidental poisoning by gas distributed by pipeline
E868   Accidental poisoning by other utility gas and other carbon monoxide
E869   Accidental poisoning by other gases and vapors

Misadventures to patients during surgical and medical care (E870-E876)
E870   Accidental cut, puncture, perforation, or hemorrhage during medical care
E871   Foreign object left in body during procedure
E872   Failure of sterile precautions during procedure
E873   Failure in dosage
E874   Mechanical failure of instrument or apparatus during procedure
E875   Contaminated or infected blood, other fluid, drug, or biological substance
E876   Other and unspecified misadventures during medical care

Surgical and medical procedures as the cause of abnormal reaction of patient or later complication, without mention of misadventure at the time of procedure (E878-E879)
E878   Surgical operation and other surgical procedures as the cause of abnormal reaction of patient, or of later complication, without mention of misadventure at the time of operation
E879   Other procedures, without mention of misadventure at the time of procedure, as the cause of abnormal reaction of patient, or of later complication

Accidental falls (E880-E888)
E880   Fall on or from stairs or steps
E881   Fall on or from ladders or scaffolding
E882   Fall from or out of building or other structure
E883   Fall into hole or other opening in surface
E884   Other fall from one level to another
E885   Fall on same level from slipping, tripping, or stumbling
E886   Fall on same level from collision, pushing or shoving, by or with other person
E887   Fracture, cause unspecified
E888   Other and unspecified fall

Accidents caused by fire and flames (E890-E899)
E890   Conflagration in private dwelling
E891   Conflagration in other and unspecified building or structure
E892   Conflagration not in building or structure
E893   Accident caused by ignition of clothing
E894   Ignition of highly inflammable material
E895   Accident caused by controlled fire in private dwelling
E896   Accident caused by controlled fire in other and unspecified building or structure
E897   Accident caused by controlled fire not in building or structure
E898   Accident caused by other specified fire and flames
E899   Accident caused by unspecified fire

Accidents due to natural and environmental factors (E900-E909)
E900   Excessive heat
E901   Excessive cold
E902   High and low air pressure and changes in air pressure
E903   Travel and motion
E904   Hunger, thirst, exposure, and neglect
E905   Venomous animals and plants as the cause of poisoning and toxic reactions
E906   Other injury caused by animals
E907   Lightning
E908   Cataclysmic storms, and floods resulting from storms
E909   Cataclysmic earth surface movements and eruptions

Accidents caused by submersion, suffocation, and foreign bodies (E910-E915)
E910   Accidental drowning and submersion
E911   Inhalation and ingestion of food causing obstruction of respiratory tract or suffocation
E912   Inhalation and ingestion of other object causing obstruction of respiratory tract or suffocation
E913   Accidental mechanical suffocation
E914   Foreign body accidentally entering eye and adnexa
E915   Foreign body accidentally entering other orifice

Other accidents (E916-E928)
E916   Struck accidentally by falling object

Appendix E: List of Three-digit Categories

E917   Striking against or struck accidentally by objects or persons
E918   Caught accidentally in or between objects
E919   Accidents caused by machinery
E920   Accidents caused by cutting and piercing instruments or objects
E921   Accident caused by explosion of pressure vessel
E922   Accident caused by firearm and air gun missile
E923   Accident caused by explosive material
E924   Accident caused by hot substance or object, caustic or corrosive material, and steam
E925   Accident caused by electric current
E926   Exposure to radiation
E927   Overexertion and strenuous and repetitive movements or loads
E928   Other and unspecified environmental and accidental causes

Late effects of accidental injury (E929)
E929   Late effects of accidental injury

Drugs, medicinal and biological substances causing adverse effects in therapeutic use (E930-E949)
E930   Antibiotics
E931   Other anti-infectives
E932   Hormones and synthetic substitutes
E933   Primarily systemic agents
E934   Agents primarily affecting blood constituents
E935   Analgesics, antipyretics, and antirheumatics
E936   Anticonvulsants and anti-Parkinsonism drugs
E937   Sedatives and hypnotics
E938   Other central nervous system depressants and anesthetics
E939   Psychotropic agents
E940   Central nervous system stimulants
E941   Drugs primarily affecting the autonomic nervous system
E942   Agents primarily affecting the cardiovascular system
E943   Agents primarily affecting gastrointestinal system
E944   Water, mineral, and uric acid metabolism drugs
E945   Agents primarily acting on the smooth and skeletal muscles and respiratory system
E946   Agents primarily affecting skin and mucous membrane, ophthalmological, otorhinolaryngological, and dental drugs
E947   Other and unspecified drugs and medicinal substances
E948   Bacterial vaccines
E949   Other vaccines and biological substances

Suicide and self-inflicted injury (E950-E959)
E950   Suicide and self-inflicted poisoning by solid or liquid substances
E951   Suicide and self-inflicted poisoning by gases in domestic use
E952   Suicide and self-inflicted poisoning by other gases and vapors
E953   Suicide and self-inflicted injury by hanging, strangulation, and suffocation
E954   Suicide and self-inflicted injury by submersion [drowning]
E955   Suicide and self-inflicted injury by firearms, air guns and explosives
E956   Suicide and self-inflicted injury by cutting and piercing instruments
E957   Suicide and self-inflicted injuries by jumping from high place
E958   Suicide and self-inflicted injury by other and unspecified means
E959   Late effects of self-inflicted injury

Homicide and injury purposely inflicted by other persons (E960-E969)
E960   Fight, brawl, and rape
E961   Assault by corrosive or caustic substance, except poisoning
E962   Assault by poisoning
E963   Assault by hanging and strangulation
E964   Assault by submersion [drowning]
E965   Assault by firearms and explosives
E966   Assault by cutting and piercing instrument
E967   Perpetrator of child and adult abuse
E968   Assault by other and unspecified means
E969   Late effects of injury purposely inflicted by other person

Legal intervention (E970-E978)
E970   Injury due to legal intervention by firearms
E971   Injury due to legal intervention by explosives
E972   Injury due to legal intervention by gas
E973   Injury due to legal intervention by blunt object
E974   Injury due to legal intervention by cutting and piercing instruments
E975   Injury due to legal intervention by other specified means
E976   Injury due to legal intervention by unspecified means
E977   Late effects of injuries due to legal intervention
E978   Legal execution

Terrorism (E979)
E979   Terrorism

Injury undetermined whether accidentally or purposely inflicted (E980-E989)
E980   Poisoning by solid or liquid substances, undetermined whether accidentally or purposely inflicted
E981   Poisoning by gases in domestic use, undetermined whether accidentally or purposely inflicted
E982   Poisoning by other gases, undetermined whether accidentally or purposely inflicted
E983   Hanging, strangulation, or suffocation, undetermined whether accidentally or purposely inflicted
E984   Submersion [drowning], undetermined whether accidentally or purposely inflicted
E985   Injury by firearms and explosives, undetermined whether accidentally or purposely inflicted
E986   Injury by cutting and piercing instruments, undetermined whether accidentally or purposely inflicted
E987   Falling from high place, undetermined whether accidentally or purposely inflicted
E988   Injury by other and unspecified means, undetermined whether accidentally or purposely inflicted
E989   Late effects of injury, undetermined whether accidentally or purposely inflicted

Injury resulting from operations of war (E990-E999)
E990   Injury due to war operations by fires and conflagrations
E991   Injury due to war operations by bullets and fragments
E992   Injury due to war operations by explosion of marine weapons
E993   Injury due to war operations by other explosion
E994   Injury due to war operations by destruction of aircraft
E995   Injury due to war operations by other and unspecified forms of conventional warfare
E996   Injury due to war operations by nuclear weapons
E997   Injury due to war operations by other forms of unconventional warfare
E998   Injury due to war operations but occurring after cessation of hostilities
E999   Late effects of injury due to war operations and terrorism

10 Steps to Correct Coding

To code accurately, it is necessary to have a working knowledge of medical terminology and to understand the characteristics, terminology and conventions of ICD-9-CM. Transforming descriptions of diseases, injuries, conditions and procedures into numerical designations (coding) is a complex activity and should not be undertaken without proper training.

Originally, coding allowed retrieval of medical information by diagnoses and operations for medical research, education and administration. Coding today is used to describe the medical necessity of a procedure and facilitate payment of health services, to evaluate utilization patterns and to study the appropriateness of health care costs. Coding provides the basis for epidemiological studies and research into the quality of health care. Incorrect or inaccurate coding can lead to investigations of fraud and abuse. Therefore, coding must be performed correctly and consistently to produce meaningful statistics to aid in planning for the health needs of the nation.

Follow the 10 steps below to correctly code encounters for healthcare services.

Step 1: Identify the reason for the visit or encounter (i.e., a sign, symptom, diagnosis and/or condition).

The medical record documentation should accurately reflect the patient's condition, using terminology that includes specific diagnoses and symptoms, or clearly states the reasons for the encounter.

Choosing the main term that best describes the reason chiefly responsible for the service provided is the most important step in coding. If symptoms are present and documented, but a definitive diagnosis has not yet been determined, code the symptoms. **Do not code conditions that are referred to as "rule out," "suspected," "probable" or "questionable."** Diagnoses often are not established at the time of the initial encounter/visit. Two or more visits may be necessary to establish the diagnosis. Code only what is documented in the available records and only to the highest degree of certainty known at the time of the patient's visit.

Step 2: After selecting the reason for the encounter, always consult the Alphabetic Index, Volume 2, before verifying code selection in the Tabular section.

The most critical rule is to begin the code selection process in the *Alphabetic Index*. Never turn first to the Tabular List (Volume 1). The Index provides cross references, essential and non-essential modifiers, and inclusion terms not found in the Tabular List. To prevent coding errors, always use both the Alphabetic Index and the Tabular List when locating and assigning a code. Always verify the code found in the Alphabetic Index in the Tabular List. First, the Index does not include the important instructional notes found in the Tabular. Second, the advantage of a classification system is that like items are grouped together. A quick scan of the Tabular might provide coding options for the coder that would have been missed.

Step 3: Locate the main term entry.

The Alphabetic Index is a listing of conditions. Conditions may be expressed as nouns or eponyms, with critical use of adjectives. Some conditions have multiple entries under synonyms. Reasons for encounters may be located under general terms such as admission, encounter, and examination. Other general terms such as history of or status post are used to locate factors influencing health.

Step 4: Read and interpret any notes listed with the main term or the subterm.

Notes such as common fifth-digit references and cross references are identified by italicized type. Always check any cross-references to ensure that all alternative terms are researched.

Step 5: Review entries for modifiers.

Nonessential modifiers are the terms located within parentheses following the main term entry. These parenthetical terms are supplementary words or explanatory information that may either be present or absent in the diagnostic statement and do not affect code selection. The subterms listed under the main term are essential modifiers that do affect coding assignment. Each line of indent represents a more specific code entry.

Step 6: Interpret abbreviations, cross-references, fifth digits, and brackets.

The cross-references used are "see," "see category" and "see also" which indicate alternative term choices for code searches. The abbreviation NEC may follow main terms or subterms. NEC (not elsewhere classified) indicates that there is no specific code for the condition even though the medical documentation may be very specific. Is a fifth digit required? You MUST refer to the Tabular List to discover the correct code. Italicized brackets *[ ]* enclose a second code that must be used along with the code immediately preceding it, with the bracketed code sequenced as the secondary code. This is a mandatory multiple code situation. Both the underlying condition and the manifestation (code in the slanted bracket) must be reported.

Step 7: Choose a potential code and locate it in the Tabular List.

The coder must follow any Includes, Excludes notes, and other instructional notes, such as "Code first" and "Use additional code," listed in the Tabular for the chapter, category, subcategory, and subclassification level of code selection which direct the coder to use a different or additional code.

Any codes in the Tabular range, 001.0 through 999.9, may be used to identify the diagnostic reason for the encounter. The Tabular encompasses many codes describing disease and injury classifications (e.g., infectious and parasitic diseases, neoplasms, symptoms, signs and ill-defined conditions, etc.).

Codes that describe symptoms and signs, as opposed to definitive diagnoses, should be used for reporting purposes when an established diagnosis has not been made (confirmed) by the physician. Chapter 16 of the ICD-9-CM code book, "Symptoms, Signs, and Ill-Defined Conditions" (codes 780.01-799.9) contains many, but not all, codes for symptoms.

ICD-9-CM classifies encounters with health care providers for circumstances other than a disease or injury using codes in the Supplementary Classification of Factors Influencing Health Status and Contact with Health Services (V01.0-V91.99). There are many occasions when circumstances other than a disease or injury are recorded as chiefly responsible for the encounter.

Step 8: Determine whether the code is at the highest level of specificity.

A code is invalid if it has not been coded to the full number of digits (greatest level of specificity) required. A three-digit code is to be used only if the category is not further subdivided. Assign four-digit codes (subcategory codes) only if there are no five-digit codes for that category. Assign five-digit codes (fifth-digit subclassification codes) for those categories mandating the use of five digits.

Step 9: Assign the code.

Having reviewed all relevant information concerning the possible code choices, assign the code that most completely describes the condition.

Repeat steps one through nine for all additional documented conditions that meet the following criteria:

- Conditions that currently exist at the time of the visit.

- Conditions that require or affect patient care, treatment or management.

Step 10: Sequence codes correctly.

Sequencing is defined as the order in which the codes are listed on the claim. List first the ICD-9-CM code for the diagnosis, condition, problem or other reason for the encounter/visit, which is shown in the medical record to be chiefly responsible for the services provided. List additional codes that describe any coexisting conditions. Follow the official coding guidelines (See Section IV Diagnostic Coding and Reporting Guidelines for Outpatient Services) concerning proper sequencing of codes.

Coding Examples

Diagnosis: Anorexia
- Step 1: The reason for the encounter was the condition, anorexia.
- Step 2. Consult the Index to Diseases.
- Step 3: Locate the main term "Anorexia."
- Step 4: There are no italicized instructional notes to interpret.
- Step 5: Note that there are two possible subterms (essential modifiers), "hysterical" and "nervosa," neither of which is documented in this instance and therefore cannot be used in code selection. The code listed next to the main term is called the default code selection.
- Step 6: There are no abbreviations, cross-references, fifth-digit notations, or brackets.

- Step 7: Turn to code 783.0 in the Tabular List and read the instructional notes. In this case the "Excludes" note indicates that anorexia determined to be of non-organic origin should be coded to Chapter 5. The diagnostic statement does not indicate non-organic origin.

- Step 8: There is no further division of the category past the fourth digit subcategory. Therefore, the subcategory code level is the highest level of specificity.

- Step 9: The default code, 783.0 is the correct code selection.

- Step 10: Since anorexia is listed as the chief reason for the healthcare encounter, the first-listed or principal diagnosis is 783.0.

Diagnosis: Acute bronchitis
- Step 1: The reason for the encounter was the condition, acute bronchitis.

- Step 2. Consult the Index to Diseases.

- Step 3: Locate the main term "Bronchitis."

- Step 4: There are no italicized instructional notes to interpret.

- Step 5: Review entries for modifiers. Since "acute" is not listed as a nonessential modifier, read past the "with" modifier until you find the subterm "acute or subacute" with code 466.0.

- Step 6: There are no abbreviations, cross-references, fifth digit notations, or brackets.

- Step 7: Since there are no more appropriate subterms, turn to code 466.0 in the Tabular List. The Includes note under category 466.0 does refer to possible infective organism, and other alternative terms for acute bronchitis. Note that inclusion term list is not exhaustive, but is only a representative selection of diagnoses that are included in the subcategory. At the beginning of chapter 8, "Diseases of the Respiratory System," you will notice the "use additional code" note that tells you to assign a code to identify the infectious organism. This instructional note applies to the entire chapter.

- Step 8: There is no further division of the category past the fourth- digit subcategory. Therefore, the subcategory code level is the highest level of specificity.

- Step 9: Assign code 466.0.

- Step 10: Repeat steps 1-9 for any additional code assignments.

Diagnosis: Acute bronchitis due to staphylococcus
- Step 1: The reason for the encounter was the condition, acute bronchitis due to staphylococcus.

- Step 2: Follow the steps listed in the above example for the diagnosis of acute bronchitis. You will now start the search for code identifying the underlying infectious organism, which in this case is staphylococcus.

- Step 3. Consult the Index to Diseases.

- Step 4: Locate the main term Staphylococcus, staphylococcal.

- Step 5: The italicized instructional notes states see condition. Locate the main term "Infection, infected, infective".

- Step 6: Review entries for modifiers. Locate the subterm "staphylococcal NEC," where you will find code 041.10 referenced. The abbreviation NEC indicates that a review of the medical record may be necessary to determine if there is documentation concerning the specific type of staphylococcus.

- Step 7: Verify code 041.10 in the Tabular List. The code title is Staphylococcus, unspecified. If there is additional information identifying the organism as aureus or other, assign the appropriate code; 041.11–041.19. Otherwise, assign code 041.10, Staphylococcus, unspecified, as an additional code.

- Step 8: There is no further division of the category past the fifth-digit subclassification level. Therefore, the subclassification code level is the highest level of specificity. The final code assignment would be 041.10.

- Step 9: Assign code 041.10.

- Step 10: Sequence codes as directed by the instructional note for category 466. Code first 466.0 and assign code 041.10 as an additional condition.

Diagnosis: Traveler's diarrhea
- Step 1: The reason for the encounter was the condition, Traveler's diarrhea.

- Step 2. Consult the Index to Diseases.

- Step 3: Locate the main term "Diarrhea" in the Alphabetic Index.

- Step 4: There are no italicized instructional notes to interpret.

- Step 5: Review entries for modifiers. Note that the nonessential modifiers (in parentheses) after the main term do not include the term "Traveler's," which means that the coder should search the subterms for the term "Traveler's." The subterm "Traveler's" has a possible code selection, 009.2, and suggests the subterm "due to specified organism NEC 008.8." The diagnostic statement does not include the infectious agent; therefore, code 008.8 does not apply.

- Step 6: There are no abbreviations, cross-references, fifth-digit notations, or brackets.

- Step 7: Locate code 009.2 in the Tabular List and read all instructional notes under the main category and subcategories. The Includes notes does not list the term "Traveler's" under code 009.2. As instructed by the Alphabetic Index, you should code the condition to 009.2. The ICD-9-CM code book implies that "Traveler's diarrhea" is the same as infectious diarrhea when it is not attributed to any specified infectious agent.

- Step 8: There is no further division of the category past the fourth-digit subcategory level. Therefore, the subcategory code level is the highest level of specificity. The final code assignment would be 009.2.

- Step 9: Assign code 009.2.

- Step 10: Since infectious diarrhea is listed as the chief reason for the healthcare encounter, the first-listed or principal diagnosis is 009.2.

Diagnosis: Ingrown toenail, infected
- Step 1: The reason for the encounter was the condition, infected ingrown toenail.

- Step 2. Consult the Index to Diseases.

- Step 3: First you must decide what the searchable main term should be. Reminder: search for condition, not anatomical site. The Alphabetic Index helps you determine the main term. Refer to "toenail" in the Alphabetic Index; the closest match is "Toe," which includes the instruction "see condition." Locate the main term "Infection" in the Alphabetic Index. The subterm toe has a subterm "nail" which refers the coder to category 681, Cellulitis and abscess of finger and toe. This does not indicate the condition ingrown toenail. The main term, therefore, is "Ingrown." A review of the Alphabetic Index takes you to "Ingrowing."

- Step 4: There are no italicized instructional notes to interpret.

- Step 5: Review the subterms. The subterm "nail" appears and lists nonessential modifiers (in parentheses) as "finger," "toe" and "infected." These nonessential modifiers complete the diagnostic statement.

- Step 6: There are no abbreviations, cross-references, fifth-digit notations, or brackets.

- Step 7: Verify code 703.0 in the Tabular List Before assigning the code, review all instructional notes under category 703 and under code 703.0. The note, "Excludes: infection, nail NOS (681.9)," can be ignored because the diagnostic statement specifies the infection is due to the ingrowing nail.

- Step 8: Therefore, the subcategory code level is the highest level of specificity. The final code assignment would be 703.0.

- Step 9: The correct code choice is 703.0, Ingrowing nail with infection.

- Step 10: Since infectious infected ingrown toenail is listed as the chief reason for the healthcare encounter, the first-listed or principal diagnosis is 703.0.

Valid Three-digit ICD-9-CM Codes

Three-digit ICD-9-CM codes are used to identify a condition or disease only when a fourth or fifth digit is not available. The following are the only ICD-9-CM codes that are valid without further specificity.

024	Glanders
025	Melioidosis
035	Erysipelas
037	Tetanus
042	Human immunodeficiency virus (HIV) disease
048	Other enterovirus diseases of central nervous system
061	Dengue
064	Viral encephalitis transmitted by other and unspecified arthropods
071	Rabies
075	Infectious mononucleosis
080	Louse-borne [epidemic] typhus
096	Late syphilis, latent
101	Vincent's angina
118	Opportunistic mycoses
124	Trichinosis
129	Intestinal parasitism, unspecified
135	Sarcoidosis
138	Late effects of acute poliomyelitis
179	Malignant neoplasm of uterus, part unspecified
181	Malignant neoplasm of placenta
185	Malignant neoplasm of prostate
193	Malignant neoplasm of thyroid gland
217	Benign neoplasm of breast
220	Benign neoplasm of ovary
226	Benign neoplasm of thyroid glands
243	Congenital hypothyroidism
260	Kwashiorkor
261	Nutritional marasmus
262	Other severe, protein-calorie malnutrition
267	Ascorbic acid deficiency
311	Depressive disorder, not elsewhere classified

316	Psychic factors associated with diseases classified elsewhere
317	Mild intellectual disabilities
319	Unspecified intellectual disabilities
325	Phlebitis and thrombophlebitis of intracranial venous sinuses
326	Late effects of intracranial abscess or pyogenic infection
340	Multiple sclerosis
390	Rheumatic fever without mention of heart involvement
393	Chronic rheumatic pericarditis
412	Old myocardial infarction
430	Subarachnoid hemorrhage
431	Intracerebral hemorrhage
436	Acute, but ill-defined, cerebrovascular disease
449	Septic arterial embolism
452	Portal vein thrombosis
460	Acute nasopharyngitis [common cold]
462	Acute pharyngitis
463	Acute tonsillitis
470	Deviated nasal septum
475	Peritonsillar abscess
481	Pneumococcal pneumonia [Streptococcus pneumoniae pneumonia]
485	Bronchopneumonia, organism unspecified
486	Pneumonia, organism unspecified
490	Bronchitis, not specified as acute or chronic
496	Chronic airway obstruction, not elsewhere classified
500	Coal workers' pneumoconiosis
501	Asbestosis
502	Pneumoconiosis due to other silica or silicates
503	Pneumoconiosis due to other inorganic dust
504	Pneumonopathy due to inhalation of other dust

505	Pneumoconiosis, unspecified
514	Pulmonary congestion and hypostasis
515	Postinflammatory pulmonary fibrosis
538	Gastrointestinal mucostitis (ulcerative)
541	Appendicitis, unqualified
542	Other appendicitis
566	Abscess of anal and rectal regions
570	Acute and subacute necrosis of liver
586	Renal failure, unspecified
587	Renal sclerosis, unspecified
591	Hydronephrosis
605	Redundant prepuce and phimosis
630	Hydatidiform mole
632	Missed abortion
650	Normal delivery
677	Late effect of complication of pregnancy, childbirth, and the puerperium
683	Acute lymphadenitis
684	Impetigo
700	Corns and callosities
725	Polymyalgia rheumatica
734	Flat foot
769	Respiratory distress syndrome
797	Senility without mention of psychosis
920	Contusion of face, scalp, and neck except eye(s)
931	Foreign body in ear
932	Foreign body in nose
936	Foreign body in intestine and colon
937	Foreign body in anus and rectum
938	Foreign body in digestive system, unspecified
981	Toxic effect of petroleum products
986	Toxic effect of carbon monoxide
990	Effects of radiation, unspecified
V08	Asymptomatic HIV infection status

Coding Tables

Abortion—Spontaneous/Legally Induced	Spontaneous Abortion (accidental) (early) (late) (miscarriage) (recurrent)				Legal Abortion (legal indication) (medical indication)(under medical supervision)			
	Incomplete (part of the products of conception are retained)	Complete (all of the products of conception are expelled)	Unspecified	Complication following abortion (separate episode of care)	Incomplete (part of the products of conception are retained)	Complete (all of the products of conception are expelled)	Unspecified	Complication following abortion (separate episode of care)
Without complication	634.91	634.92	634.90		635.91	635.92	635.90	
With complication of:								
Afibrinogenemia						635.12	635.10	639.1
Atrophy, acute yellow	634.71	634.72	634.70	639.8	635.71	635.72	635.70	639.8
Cardiac arrest	634.71	634.72	634.70	639.8	635.71	635.72	635.70	639.8
Cardiac failure	634.71	634.72	634.70	639.8	635.71	635.72	635.70	639.8
Cerebral anoxia	634.71	634.72	634.70	639.8	635.71	635.72	635.70	639.8
Circulatory collapse	634.51	634.52	634.50	639.5	635.51	635.52	635.50	639.5
Defibrination syndrome	634.11	634.12	634.10	639.1	635.11	635.12	635.10	639.1
Electrolyte imbalance	634.41	634.42	634.40	639.4	635.41	635.42	635.40	639.4
Embolism (any type)	634.61	634.62	634.60	639.6	635.61	635.62	635.60	639.6
Endometritis	634.01	634.02	634.00	639.0	635.01	635.02	635.00	639.0
Genital tract infection	634.01	634.02	634.00	639.0	635.01	635.02	635.00	639.0
Hemorrhage, delayed or excessive	634.11	634.12	634.10	639.1	635.11	635.12	635.10	639.1
Intravascular hemolysis	634.11	634.12	634.10	639.1	635.11	635.12	635.10	639.1
Kidney failure (acute)	634.31	634.32	634.30	639.3	635.31	635.32	635.30	639.3
Laceration of:								
pelvic organs	634.21	634.22	634.20	639.2	635.21	635.22	635.20	639.2
Metabolic disorder	634.41	634.42	634.40	639.4	635.41	635.42	635.40	639.4
Necrosis of liver	634.71	634.72	634.70	639.8	635.71	635.72	635.70	639.8
Oliguria	634.31	634.32	634.30	639.3	635.31	635.32	635.30	639.3
Other specified complication	634.71	634.72	634.70	639.8	635.71	635.72	635.70	639.8
Parametritis	634.01	634.02	634.00	639.0	635.01	635.02	635.00	639.0
Pelvic infection	634.01	634.02	634.00	639.0	635.01	635.02	635.00	639.0
Pelvic peritonitis	634.01	634.02	634.00	639.0	635.01	635.02	635.00	639.0
Perforation — *see* Abortion, by type, laceration								
Renal shutdown	634.31	634.32	634.30	639.3	635.31	635.32	635.30	639.3
Renal tubular necrosis	634.31	634.32	634.30	639.3	635.31	635.32	635.30	639.3
Salpingitis	634.01	634.02	634.00	639.0	635.01	635.02	635.00	639.0
Salpingo-oophoritis	634.01	634.02	634.00	639.0	635.01	635.02	635.00	639.0
Sepsis NOS	634.01	634.02	634.00	639.0	635.01	635.02	635.00	639.0
Septicemia NOS	634.01	634.02	634.00	639.0	635.01	635.02	635.00	639.0
Shock (postoperative)(septic)	634.51	634.52	634.50	639.5	635.51	635.52	635.50	639.5
Tear — *see* Abortion, by type, laceration								
Unspecified complications	634.81	634.82	634.80	639.9	635.81	635.82	635.80	639.9
Uremia	634.31	634.32	634.30	639.3	635.31	635.32	635.30	639.3
Urinary tract infection	634.71	634.72	634.70	639.8	635.71	635.72	635.70	639.8
UTI (urinary tract infection)	634.71	634.72	634.70	639.8	635.71	635.72	635.70	639.8

Abortion—Illegally Induced/Unspecified	Illegally Induced Abortion (criminal) (homicidal) (self-induced)				Unspecified Abortion — Retained products of conception following abortion, not classifiable elsewhere or not otherwise specified			
	Incomplete (part of the products of conception are retained)	Complete (all of the products of conception are expelled)	Unspecified	Complication following abortion (separate episode of care)	Incomplete (part of the products of conception are retained)	Complete (all of the products of conception are expelled)	Unspecified	Complication following abortion (separate episode of care)
Without complication	636.91	636.92	636.90		637.91	637.92	637.90	
With complication of:								
Afibrinogenemia	636.11	636.12	636.10	639.1	637.11	637.12	637.10	639.1
Atrophy, acute yellow	636.71	636.72	636.70	639.8	637.71	637.72	637.70	639.8
Cardiac arrest	636.71	636.72	636.70	639.8	637.71	637.72	637.70	639.8
Cardiac failure	636.71	636.72	636.70	639.8	637.71	637.72	637.70	639.8
Cerebral anoxia	636.71	636.72	636.70	639.8	637.71	637.72	637.70	639.8
Circulatory collapse	636.51	636.52	636.50	639.5	637.51	637.52	637.50	639.5
Defibrination syndrome	636.11	636.12	636.10	639.1	637.11	637.12	637.10	639.1
Electrolyte imbalance	636.41	636.42	636.40	639.4	637.41	637.42	637.40	639.4
Embolism (any type)	636.61	636.62	636.60	639.6	637.61	637.62	637.60	639.6
Endometritis	636.01	636.02	636.00	639.0	637.01	637.02	637.00	639.0

Abortion—Illegally Induced/Unspecified

	Illegally Induced Abortion (criminal) (homicidal) (self-induced)				Unspecified Abortion — Retained products of conception following abortion, not classifiable elsewhere or not otherwise specified			
	Incomplete (part of the products of conception are retained)	Complete (all of the products of conception are expelled)	Unspecified	Complication following abortion (separate episode of care)	Incomplete (part of the products of conception are retained)	Complete (all of the products of conception are expelled)	Unspecified	Complication following abortion (separate episode of care)
With complication of: — *continued*								
Genital tract infection	636.01	636.02	636.00	639.0	637.01	637.02	637.00	639.0
Hemorrhage, delayed or excessive	636.11	636.12	636.10	639.1	637.11	637.12	637.10	639.1
Intravascular hemolysis	636.11	636.12	636.10	639.1	637.11	637.12	637.10	639.1
Kidney failure (acute)	636.31	636.32	636.30	639.3	637.31	637.32	637.30	639.3
Laceration of:								
pelvic organs	636.21	636.22	636.20	639.2	637.21	637.22	637.20	639.2
Metabolic disorder	636.41	636.42	636.40	639.4	637.41	637.42	637.40	639.4
Necrosis of liver	636.71	636.72	636.70	639.8	637.71	637.72	637.70	639.8
Oliguria	636.31	636.32	636.30	639.3	637.31	637.32	637.30	639.3
Other specified complication	636.71	636.72	636.70	639.8	637.71	637.72	637.70	639.8
Parametritis	636.01	636.02	636.00	639.0	637.01	637.02	637.00	639.0
Pelvic infection	636.01	636.02	636.00	639.0	637.01	637.02	637.00	639.0
Pelvic peritonitis	636.01	636.02	636.00	639.0	637.01	637.02	637.00	639.0
Perforation — *see* Abortion, by type, laceration								
Renal shutdown	636.31	636.32	636.30	639.3	637.31	637.32	637.30	639.3
Renal tubular necrosis	636.31	636.32	636.30	639.3	637.31	637.32	637.30	639.3
Salpingitis	636.01	636.02	636.00	639.0	637.01	637.02	637.00	639.0
Salpingo-oophoritis	636.01	636.02	636.00	639.0	637.01	637.02	637.00	639.0
Sepsis NOS	636.01	636.02	636.00	639.0	637.01	637.02	637.00	639.0
Septicemia NOS	636.01	636.02	636.00	639.0	637.01	637.02	637.00	639.0
Shock (postoperative) (septic)	636.51	636.52	636.50	639.5	637.51	637.52	637.50	639.5
Specified complication NEC	636.71	636.72	636.70	639.8	637.71	637.72	637.70	639.8
Tear — *see* Abortion, by type, laceration								
Unspecified complications	636.81	636.82	636.80	639.9	637.81	637.82	637.80	639.9
Uremia	636.31	636.32	636.30	639.3	637.31	637.32	637.30	639.3
Urinary tract infection	636.71	636.72	636.70	639.8	637.71	637.72	637.70	639.8
UTI (urinary tract infection)	636.71	636.72	636.70	639.8	637.71	637.72	637.70	639.8

Abortion—Other Specified

	Failed Attempted Abortion / Hydatidiform Mole / Missed Abortion / Other Abnormal Product of Conception			
	Failed Attempted Abortion	Hydatidiform Mole	Missed Abortion (all products of conception retained)	Other abnormal product of conception (blighted ovum, chemical, fleshy mole, stone mole, carneous mole, mole NOS)
Without complication	638.9	630	632	
inappropriate level of hCG (chemical, false positive)				631.0
other abnormal products of conception				631.8
With complication of:				
Afibrinogenemia	638.1	639.1	639.1	639.1
Atrophy, acute yellow	638.7	639.8	639.8	639.8
Cardiac arrest	638.7	639.8	639.8	639.8
Cardiac failure	638.7	639.8	639.8	639.8
Cerebral anoxia	638.7	639.8	639.8	639.8
Circulatory collapse	638.5	639.5	639.5	639.5
Defibrination syndrome	638.1	639.1	639.1	639.1
Electrolyte imbalance	638.4	639.4	639.4	639.4
Embolism (any type)	638.6	639.6	639.6	639.6
Endometritis	638.0	639.0	639.0	639.0
Genital tract infection	638.0	639.0	639.0	639.0
Hemorrhage, delayed or excessive	638.1	639.1	639.1	639.1
Intravascular hemolysis	638.1	639.1	639.1	639.1
Kidney failure (acute)	638.3	639.3	639.3	639.3
Laceration of:				
pelvic organs	638.2	639.2	639.2	639.2
Metabolic disorder	638.4	639.4	639.4	639.4
Necrosis of liver	638.7	639.8	639.8	639.8
Oliguria	638.3	639.3	639.3	639.3

Abortion—Other Specified

With complication of: — *continued*	Failed Attempted Abortion	Hydatidiform Mole	Missed Abortion (all products of conception retained)	Other abnormal product of conception (blighted ovum, chemical, fleshy mole, stone mole, carneous mole, mole NOS)
Other specified complications	638.7	639.8	639.8	639.8
Parametritis	638.0	639.0	639.0	639.0
Pelvic infection	638.0	639.0	639.0	639.0
Pelvic peritonitis	638.0	639.0	639.0	639.0
Perforation — *see* Abortion, by type, laceration				
Renal shutdown	638.3	639.3	639.3	639.3
Renal tubular necrosis	638.3	639.3	639.3	639.3
Salpingitis	638.0	639.0	639.0	639.0
Salpingo-oophoritis	638.0	639.0	639.0	639.0
Sepsis NOS	638.0	639.0	639.0	639.0
Septicemia NOS	638.0	639.0	639.0	639.0
Shock (postoperative) (septic)	638.5	639.5	639.5	639.5
Tear — *see* Abortion, by type, laceration				
Unspecified complications	638.8	639.9	639.9	639.9
Urinary tract infection	638.7	639.8	639.8	639.8
UTI (urinary tract infection)	638.7	639.8	639.8	639.8

Burn

Burn (acid) (cathode ray) (caustic) (chemical) (electric heating appliance) (electricity) (fire) (flame) (hot liquid or object) (irradiation) (lime) (radiation) (steam) (thermal) (x-ray)	Unspecified Degree	First Degree [erythema]	Second Degree [blisters, epidermal loss]	Third Degree NOS [full-thickness skin loss]	Deep Third Degree [without mention of loss of body part]	Deep Third Degree [with loss of a body part]
Abdomen, abdominal (wall) (muscle)	942.03	942.13	942.23	942.33	942.43	942.53
with trunk	942.09	942.19	942.29	942.39	942.49	942.59
Ankle	945.03	945.13	945.23	945.33	945.43	945.53
with lower limb	945.09	945.19	945.29	945.39	945.49	945.59
Anus	942.09	942.19	942.29	942.39	942.49	942.59
Arm(s)	943.00	943.10	943.20	943.30	943.40	943.50
lower	943.01	943.11	943.21	943.31	943.41	943.51
multiple sites, except hand(s) or wrist(s)	943.09	943.19	943.29	943.39	943.49	943.59
upper	943.03	943.13	943.23	943.33	943.43	943.53
Auditory canal (external)	941.01	941.11	941.21	941.31	941.41	941.51
with face or head	941.09	941.19	941.29	941.39	941.49	941.59
Auricle (ear)	941.01	941.11	941.21	941.31	941.41	941.51
with face or head	941.09	941.19	941.29	941.39	941.49	941.59
Axilla	943.04	943.14	943.24	943.34	943.44	943.54
with upper limb, except hand(s) or wrist(s)	943.09	943.19	943.29	943.39	943.49	943.59
Back	942.04	942.14	942.24	942.34	942.44	942.54
with trunk	942.09	942.19	942.29	942.39	942.49	942.59
Biceps						
brachii	943.03	943.13	943.23	943.33	943.43	943.53
femoris	945.06	945.16	945.26	945.36	945.46	945.56
Breast(s)	942.01	942.11	942.21	942.31	942.41	942.51
with trunk	942.09	942.19	942.29	942.39	942.49	942.59
Brow	941.07	941.17	941.27	941.37	941.47	941.57
Buttock(s)	942.04	942.14	942.24	942.34	942.44	942.54
Cheek (cutaneous)	941.07	941.17	941.27	941.37	941.47	941.57
with face or head	941.09	941.19	941.29	941.39	941.49	941.59
Chest wall (anterior)	942.02	942.12	942.22	942.32	942.42	942.52
with trunk	942.09	942.19	942.29	942.39	942.49	942.59
Chin	941.04	941.14	941.24	941.34	941.44	941.54
with face or head	941.09	941.19	941.29	941.39	941.49	941.59
Clitoris	942.05	942.15	942.25	942.35	942.45	942.55
Ear (drum) (external)	941.01	941.11	941.21	941.31	941.41	941.51
with face or head	941.09	941.19	941.29	941.39	941.49	941.59
Elbow	943.02	943.12	943.22	943.32	943.42	943.52
with hand(s) and wrist(s)	946.0	946.1	946.2	946.3	946.4	946.5
with upper limb, except hand(s) or wrist(s)	943.09	943.19	943.29	943.39	943.49	943.59
Entire body	946.0	946.1	946.2	946.3	946.4	946.5
Epididymis	942.05	942.15	942.25	942.35	942.45	942.55
Epigastric region	942.03	942.13	942.23	942.33	942.43	942.53

Burn (acid) (cathode ray) (caustic) (chemical) (electric heating appliance) (electricity) (fire) (flame) (hot liquid or object) (irradiation) (lime) (radiation) (steam) (thermal) (x-ray)	Unspecified Degree	First Degree [erythema]	Second Degree [blisters, epidermal loss]	Third Degree NOS [full-thickness skin loss]	Deep Third Degree [without mention of loss of body part]	Deep Third Degree [with loss of a body part]
Extremity						
arm	943.00	943.10	943.20	943.30	943.40	943.50
lower	943.01	943.11	943.21	943.31	943.41	943.51
multiple sites	943.09	943.19	943.29	943.39	943.49	943.59
upper	943.03	943.13	943.23	943.33	943.43	943.53
leg	945.00	945.10	945.20	945.30	945.40	945.50
lower	945.04	945.14	945.24	945.34	945.44	945.54
multiple sites	945.09	945.19	945.29	945.39	945.49	945.59
upper	945.06	945.16	945.26	945.36	945.46	945.56
Eye(s), only — *see* Eye, eyeball, burn						
with						
face, head or neck	941.02	941.12	941.22	941.32	941.42	941.52
other sites	946.0	946.1	946.2	946.3	946.4	946.5
Face	941.00	941.10	941.20	941.30	941.40	941.50
multiple sites	941.09	941.19	941.29	941.39	941.49	941.59
with eye(s)	941.02	941.12	941.22	941.32	941.42	941.52
Finger (nail) (subungual)	944.01	944.11	944.21	944.31	944.41	944.41
with						
hand(s)	944.08	944.18	944.28	944.38	944.48	944.58
other sites	946.0	946.1	946.2	946.3	946.4	946.5
thumb	944.04	944.14	944.24	944.34	944.44	944.54
multiple digits	944.03	944.13	944.23	944.33	944.43	944.53
with thumb	944.04	944.14	944.24	944.34	944.44	944.54
Foot	945.02	945.12	945.22	945.32	945.42	945.52
with lower limb	945.09	945.19	945.29	945.39	945.49	945.59
Forearm(s)	943.01	943.11	943.21	943.31	943.41	943.51
with upper limb, except hand(s) or wrist(s)	943.09	943.19	943.29	943.39	943.49	943.59
Forehead	941.07	941.17	941.27	941.37	941.47	941.57
with face or head	941.09	941.19	941.29	941.39	941.49	941.59
Genitourinary organ(s)						
external	942.05	942.15	942.25	942.35	942.45	942.55
internal—*see* specific organ or site, burn						
Groin	942.03	942.13	942.23	942.33	942.43	942.53
Hand(s) (and wrist)	944.00	944.10	944.20	944.30	944.40	944.50
back (doral surface)	944.06	944.16	944.26	944.36	944.46	944.56
multiple sites	944.08	944.18	944.28	944.38	944.48	944.58
Head (and face)	941.00	941.10	941.20	941.30	941.40	941.50
multiple sites	941.09	941.19	941.29	941.39	941.49	941.59
Heel	945.02	945.12	945.22	945.32	945.42	945.52
Hip	942.09	942.19	942.29	942.39	942.49	942.59
Internal organ(s) — *see* specific organ or site, burn						
Knee	945.05	945.15	945.25	945.35	945.45	945.55
with lower limb	945.09	945.19	945.29	945.39	945.49	945.59
Labium (majus) (minus)	942.05	942.15	942.25	942.35	942.45	942.55
Leg	945.00	945.10	945.20	945.30	945.40	945.50
lower, unspecified site	945.04	945.14	945.24	945.34	945.44	945.54
multiple sites	945.09	945.19	945.29	945.39	945.49	945.59
upper (thigh) (any part)	945.06	945.16	945.26	945.36	945.46	945.56
Lip(s)	941.03	941.13	941.23	941.33	941.43	941.53
with face or head	941.09	941.19	941.29	941.39	941.49	941.59
Lumbar region	942.04	942.14	942.24	942.34	942.44	942.54
Malar region	941.07	941.17	941.27	941.37	941.47	941.57
Mastoid region	941.06	941.16	941.26	941.36	941.46	941.56
Membrane, tympanic	941.01	941.11	941.21	941.31	941.41	941.51
Multiple, specified sites, classifiable to more than one category in 940–945	946.0	946.1	946.2	946.3	946.4	946.5
Nasal (septum)	941.05	941.15	941.25	941.35	941.45	941.55
Neck	941.08	941.18	941.28	941.38	941.48	941.58
with face or head	941.09	941.19	941.29	941.39	941.49	941.59
Nose	941.05	941.15	941.25	941.35	941.45	941.55
with face or head	941.09	941.19	941.29	941.39	941.49	941.59
Palm(s)	944.05	944.15	944.25	944.35	944.45	944.55
with hand(s) or wrist(s)	944.08	944.18	944.28	944.38	944.48	944.58
Penis	942.05	942.15	942.25	942.35	942.45	942.55
Perineum	942.05	942.15	942.25	942.35	942.45	942.55
Pubic region	942.05	942.15	942.25	942.35	942.45	942.55

Burn (acid) (cathode ray) (caustic) (chemical) (electric heating appliance) (electricity) (fire) (flame) (hot liquid or object) (irradiation) (lime) (radiation) (steam) (thermal) (x-ray)	Unspecified Degree	First Degree [erythema]	Second Degree [blisters, epidermal loss]	Third Degree NOS [full-thickness skin loss]	Deep Third Degree [without mention of loss of body part]	Deep Third Degree [with loss of a body part]
Sacral region	942.04	942.14	942.24	942.34	942.44	942.54
Scalp	941.06	941.16	941.26	941.36	941.46	941.56
with face or head	941.09	941.19	941.29	941.39	941.49	941.59
Scapular region	943.06	943.16	943.26	943.36	943.46	943.56
with upper limb, except hand(s) or wrist(s)	943.09	943.19	943.29	943.39	943.49	943.59
Scrotum	942.05	942.15	942.25	942.35	942.45	942.55
Shoulder(s)	943.05	943.15	943.25	943.35	943.45	943.55
with						
hand(s) and wrist(s)	946.0	946.1	946.2	946.3	946.4	946.5
upper limb, except hand(s) or wrist(s)	943.09	943.19	943.29	943.39	943.49	943.59
Skin, unspecified site	949.0	949.1	949.2	949.3	949.4	949.5
Skull	941.00	941.10	941.20	941.30	941.40	941.50
Submental region	941.04	941.14	941.24	941.34	941.44	941.54
Supraclavicular fossa	941.08	941.18	941.28	941.38	941.48	941.58
Temple	941.06	941.16	941.26	941.36	941.46	941.56
Testicle	942.05	942.15	942.25	942.35	942.45	942.55
Thigh	945.06	945.16	945.26	945.36	945.46	945.56
with lower limb	945.09	945.19	945.29	945.39	945.49	945.59
Thumb(s) (nail)	944.02	944.12	944.22	944.32	944.42	944.52
with finger(s)	944.04	944.14	944.24	944.34	944.44	944.54
with hand(s) or wrist(s)	944.08	944.18	944.28	944.38	944.48	944.58
Toe (nail)	945.01	945.11	945.21	945.31	945.41	945.51
with lower limb	945.09	945.19	945.29	945.39	945.49	945.59
Trunk	942.00	942.10	942.20	942.30	942.40	942.50
multiple sites	942.09	942.19	942.29	942.39	942.49	942.59
specified site, NEC	942.09	942.19	942.29	942.39	942.49	942.59
Tunica vaginalis	942.05	942.15	942.25	942.35	942.45	942.55
Unspecified site	949.0	949.1	949.2	949.3	949.4	949.5
Vulva	942.05	942.15	942.25	942.35	942.45	942.55
Wrist(s)	944.07	944.17	944.27	944.37	944.47	944.57
with hand(s)	944.08	944.18	944.28	944.38	944.48	944.58

Complications due to

Complications due to (presence of)	Mechanical	Infection/inflammatory reaction	Other
Aortocoronary bypass graft	996.03	996.61	996.72
Arteriovenous			
fistula	996.1	996.62	996.74
shunt	996.1	996.62	996.74
Artificial heart	996.09	996.61	996.72
Artificial skin graft	996.55	996.69	996.79
Bariatric procedure			
gastric band		539.01	539.09
other		539.81	539.89
Bile duct	996.59	996.69	996.79
Blood vessel graft	996.1	996.62	996.74
Bone growth stimulator	996.40	996.67	996.78
Bone marrow transplant	996.85	996.85	996.85
Breast implant	996.54	996.69	996.79
Bypass graft			
aortocoronary	996.03	996.61	996.72
blood vessel	996.1	996.62	996.74
carotid artery	996.1	996.62	996.74
coronary artery	996.03	996.61	996.72
femoral-popliteal	996.1	996.62	996.74
Cardiac			
defibrillator	996.04	996.61	996.72
pulse generator	996.04	996.61	996.72
subcutaneous pocket	996.04	996.61	996.72
pacemaker		996.61	996.72
pulse generator	996.09	996.61	996.72
subcutaneous pocket	996.09	996.61	996.72
valve prosthesis	996.02	996.61	996.71
Carotid artery bypass graft	996.1	996.62	996.74
Catheter			
central venous	996.1	999.31	996.74
cystostomy	596.82	996.65	996.76

Complications due to (presence of)	Mechanical	Infection/inflammatory reaction	Other
Catheter — *continued*			
dialysis (hemodialysis)	996.1	996.62	996.73
peritoneal	996.56	996.68	996.73
Hickman	996.1	999.31	996.74
PICC	996.1	999.31	996.74
spinal	996.2	996.63	996.75
urinary, indwelling	996.31	996.64	996.76
triple lumen	996.1	999.31	996.74
vascular (peripheral)	996.1	996.62	996.74
Chin implant	996.59	996.69	996.79
Contraceptive device (intrauterine)	996.32	996.65	996.76
Corneal graft	996.51	996.69	996.79
retroprosthetic membrane	996.51		
Coronary artery bypass graft	996.03	996.61	996.72
Cystostomy	596.82	596.81	596.83
Decellularized alodermis	996.55	996.69	996.79
Dialysis catheter (hemodialysis)	996.1	996.62	996.73
peritoneal	996.56	996.68	996.73
Dorsal column stimulator	996.2	996.63	996.75
Electrodes			
brain	996.2	996.63	996.75
heart	996.01	996.61	996.72
Esophagostomy	530.87	530.86	
External fixator device	996.40	996.67	996.78
Genitourinary device	996.39	996.65	996.76
unspecified	996.30	996.65	996.70
Graft			
artificial skin	996.52	996.69	996.79
blood vessel	996.1	996.62	996.74
bone	996.40	996.67	996.78
cartilage	996.40	996.67	996.78
carotid artery	996.1	996.62	996.74
corneal	996.51	996.69	996.79
retroprosthetic membrane	996.51		
coronary artery	996.03	996.61	996.72
femoral-popliteal	996.1	996.62	996.74
muscle	996.40	996.67	996.78
peripheral nerve	996.2	996.62	996.75
skin	996.52	996.69	996.79
tendon	996.40	996.67	996.78
ureter	996.39	996.65	996.76
Heart assist device	996.09	996.61	996.72
Heart transplant	996.83	996.83	996.83
Infusion pump	996.59	996.62	996.74
Insulin pump	996.57	996.69	996.57
Internal fixator device			
nail	996.40	996.67	996.78
plate	996.40	996.67	996.78
rod	996.40	996.67	996.78
screw	996.40	996.67	996.78
Intraaortic balloon	996.1	996.62	996.74
Joint prosthesis, internal			
Articular bearing surface wear	996.46	996.66	996.77
Aseptic loosening	996.41	996.66	996.77
Breakage (fracture) of prosthetic joint	996.43	996.66	996.77
Dislocation of prosthetic joint	996.42	996.66	996.77
Failure of prosthetic joint implant	996.47	996.66	996.77
Instability of prosthetic joint	996.42	996.66	996.77
Loosening of prosthetic joint	996.41	996.66	996.77
Peri-prosthetic fracture	996.44	996.66	996.77
Peri-prosthetic osteolysis	996.45	996.66	996.77
Subluxation of prosthetic joint	996.42	996.66	996.77
Liver transplant	996.82	996.82	996.82
Lung transplant	996.84	996.84	996.84
Mammary implant	996.54	996.69	996.79
Nervous system device	996.2	996.63	996.75
Nonabsorbable surgical material NOS	996.59	996.69	996.79
Other vascular device	996.1	996.62	996.74

Complications due to (presence of)	Mechanical	Infection/inflammatory reaction	Other
Pancreas transplant	996.86	996.86	996.86
Prosthetic implant			
bile duct	996.59	996.69	996.79
breast	996.54	996.69	996.79
chin	996.59	996.69	996.79
ocular lens	996.53	996.69	996.79
orbit of eye	996.59	996.69	996.79
vaginal mesh			
erosion			629.31
exposure			629.32
vas deferens	996.39	996.65	996.76
Shunt			
arteriovenous	996.1	996.62	996.74
ventricular	996.2	996.63	996.75
Transfusion			
anaphylactic reaction			999.41
febrile			780.66
hemochromatosis			275.02
hemolytic reaction			999.83
acute			999.84
delayed			999.85
incompatibility reaction			
ABO			999.60
with HTR			999.61
acute			999.62
delayed			999.63
non-specified			999.61
specified type NEC			999.69
non-ABO			
with HTR			999.76
acute			999.77
delayed			999.78
non-specified			999.75
specified type NEC			999.79
Rh			
with HTR			999.71
acute			999.72
delayed			999.73
non-specified			999.70
specified type NEC			999.74
overload			
circulatory (TACO)			276.61
fluid			276.61
iron			275.02
purpura			287.41
serum reaction			999.51
specified reaction NEC			999.89
Transplanted organ			
bone marrow	996.85	996.85	996.85
heart	996.83	996.83	996.83
liver	996.82	996.82	996.82
lung	996.84	996.84	996.84
other specified organ	996.89	996.89	996.89
pancreas	996.86	996.86	996.86
stem cell	996.88	996.88	996.88
unspecified organ	996.80	996.80	996.80
Umbrella device, vena cava	996.1	996.62	996.74
Unspecified cardiac device	996.00	996.60	996.72
Vascular catheter (peripheral)	996.1	996.62	996.74
Ventricular shunt	996.2	996.63	996.75

Coding Tables

Diabetes

Diabetes (brittle) (congenital) (familial) (mellitus) (severe) (slight)	**TYPE I**		**TYPE II or unspecified type. The codes found in these columns are for use even if the patient requires insulin.**			**Additional Code Required**
	Controlled or not stated as uncontrolled	Uncontrolled	Controlled or not stated as uncontrolled	Uncontrolled	Other metabolic disorders or conditions	List these codes after the diabetes code
Without complication or manifestation	250.01	250.03	250.00	250.02		
With complication or manifestation						
coma (ketoacidosis)	250.31	250.33	250.30	250.32		
hyperosmolar (nonketotic)	250.21	250.23	250.20	250.22		
complication NOS	250.91	250.93	250.90	250.92		
specified NEC	250.81	250.83	250.80	250.82		
gangrene	250.71	250.73	250.70	250.72		785.4
hyperosmolarity	250.21	250.23	250.20	250.22		
ketosis, ketoacidosis	250.11	250.13	250.10	250.12		
osteomyelitis	250.81	250.83	250.80	250.82		731.8
specified manifestations NEC	250.81	250.83	250.80	250.82		
Abnormal glucose NOS						
NOS					790.29	
non-fasting					790.29	
fasting					790.21	
tolerance test					790.22	
Abnormal glucose tolerance test (GTT), **elevated glucose tolerance test**					790.22	
Acetonemia	250.11	250.13	250.10	250.12		
Acidosis	250.11	250.13	250.10	250.12		
Amyotrophy	250.61	250.63	250.60	250.62		353.1
Angiopathia, angiopathy (peripheral)	250.71	250.73	250.70	250.72		443.81
retinalis (juvenilis)	250.51	250.53	250.50	250.52		362.01
Arthritis, arthropathy	250.61	250.63	250.60	250.62		713.5
Charcôt's	250.61	250.63	250.60	250.62		713.5
neuropathic (Charcôt's)	250.61	250.63	250.60	250.62		713.5
Asymptomatic elevated (abnormal glucose)					790.29	
Ataxia, ataxy, ataxic, locomotor (progressive)	250.61	250.63	250.60	250.62		337.1
Autonomic neuropathy (peripheral)	250.61	250.63	250.60	250.62		337.1
Bone change	250.81	250.83	250.80	250.82		731.8
Bronze, bronzed					275.01	
Cataract diabetic	250.51	250.53	250.50	250.52		366.41
senile (non diabetic)	250.01	250.03	250.00	250.02		366.17
snowflake	250.51	250.53	250.50	250.52		366.41
Charcôt's joint (disease)	250.61	250.63	250.60	250.62		713.5
Chemical					790.29	
Coma (with ketoacidosis)	250.31	250.33	250.30	250.32		
hyperglycemic	250.31	250.33	250.30	250.32		
hyperosmolar (nonketotic)	250.21	250.23	250.20	250.22		
hypoglycemic	250.31	250.33	250.30	250.32		
nondiabetic					251.0	
insulin	250.31	250.33	250.30	250.32		
nondiabetic					251.0	
Kussmaul's	250.31	250.33	250.30	250.32		
prediabetic	250.21	250.23	250.20	250.22		
Complication NOS	250.91	250.93	250.90	250.92		
specified NEC	250.81	250.83	250.80	250.82		
Dermopathy	250.81	250.83	250.80	250.82		709.8
Dietary supervision					V65.3	
Ebstein's disease	250.41	250.43	250.40	250.42		581.81
Edema (macula) (retina)	250.51	250.53	250.50	250.52		362.01
Family History					V18.0	
Gangrene	250.71	250.73	250.70	250.72		785.4
Gastroparalysis/Gastroparesis	250.61	250.63	250.60	250.62		536.3
Gestational diabetes						
antepartum					648.83	
delivered w/o antepartum condition					648.81	
postpartum					648.84	
unspecified. episode. of care					648.80	
with antepartum condition					648.82	
with long term (current) insulin use						V58.67
Glaucoma	250.51	250.53	250.50	250.52		365.44
Glomerulohyalinosis — diabetic syndrome	250.41	250.43	250.40	250.42		581.81

Diabetes (brittle) (congenital) (familial) (mellitus) (severe) (slight)	TYPE I		TYPE II or unspecified type. The codes found in these columns are for use even if the patient requires insulin.			Additional Code Required
	Controlled or not stated as uncontrolled	Uncontrolled	Controlled or not stated as uncontrolled	Uncontrolled	Other metabolic disorders or conditions	List these codes after the diabetes code
Glomerulonephritis, chronic	250.41	250.43	250.40	250.42		583.81
with nephrotic syndrome	250.41	250.43	250.40	250.42		581.81
Glomerulosclerosis (intercapillary)	250.41	250.43	250.40	250.42		581.81
Glucose Intolerance					790.22	
Glycogenosis, secondary	250.81	250.83	250.80	250.82		259.8
Hemochromatosis						
hereditary	275.01					
primary	275.01					
specified type	275.03					
transfusion associated (red cell)	275.02					
Hirschfeld's disease	250.01	250.01	250.00	250.02		
Hyperglycemia						
with coma	250.31	250.33	250.30	250.32		
diabetic	250.11	250.13	250.10	250.12		
neonatal (transient)					775.1	
nondiabetic					790.6	
postpancreatectomy					251.3	
Hyperosmolar coma	250.21	250.23	250.20	250.22		
Hyperosmolarity	250.21	250.23	250.20	250.22		
Hypertension nephrosis syndrome	250.41	250.43	250.40	250.42		581.81
Hypoglycemia (diabetic) without coma	250.81	250.83	250.80	250.82		
with coma	250.31	250.33	250.30	250.32		
neonatal, transient					775.0	
nondiabetic						
with coma					251.0	
without coma					251.1	
NOS (spontaneous)					251.2	
Hypoglycemic shock	250.81	250.83	250.80	250.82		
Hypoinsulinemia, postsurgical					251.3	
Impaired fasting glucose					790.21	
Impotence	250.61	250.63	250.60	250.62		607.84
Insipidus					253.5	
nephrogenic					588.1	
pituitary					253.5	
vasopressin-resistant					588.1	
Insulin, long term (current) use						V58.67
Insulin overdose	250.x1	250.x3	250.x0	250.x2	962.3	
Insulin underdose (code to diabetes only)						
Intercapillary glomerulosclerosis	250.41	250.43	250.40	250.42		581.81
Iridis rubeosis/Iritis	250.51	250.53	250.50	250.53		364.42
Ketosis, ketoacidosis	250.11	250.13	250.10	250.12		
Kidney disease, chronic	250.41	250.43	250.40	250.42		585.9
End Stage	250.41	250.43	250.40	250.42		585.6
Stage I	250.41	250.43	250.40	250.42		585.1
Stage II	250.41	250.43	250.40	250.42		585.2
Stage III	250.41	250.43	250.40	250.42		585.3
Stage IV	250.41	250.43	250.40	250.42		585.4
Stage V	250.41	250.43	250.40	250.42		585.5
Kimmelstiel (-Wilson) disease or syndrome	250.41	250.43	250.40	250.42		581.81
Kussmaul's coma	250.31	250.33	250.30	250.32		
Lancereaux's (diabetes mellitus with marked emaciation)	250.81	250.83	250.80	250.82		261
Latent (chemical)					790.29	
Lipoidosis	250.81	250.83	250.80	250.82		272.7
Macular edema	250.51	250.53	250.50	250.52		362.01
Microangiopathy (peripheral)	250.71	250.73	250.70	250.72		443.81
Mononeuropathy, mononeuritis, unspecified site	250.61	250.63	250.60	250.62		355.9
lower limb, unspecified	250.61	250.63	250.60	250.62		355.8
upper limb, unspecified	250.61	250.63	250.60	250.62		354.9
Myelopathy	250.61	250.63	250.60	250.62		336.3
Necrobiosis lipoidica	250.81	250.83	250.80	250.82		709.3
Neonatal, transient hyperglycemia					775.1	
hypoglycemia					775.0	
Nephritis, chronic	250.41	250.43	250.40	250.42		583.81
with nephrotic syndrome	250.41	250.43	250.40	250.42		581.81

Coding Tables

Diabetes

Diabetes (brittle) (congenital) (familial) (mellitus) (severe) (slight)	TYPE I		TYPE II or unspecified type. The codes found in these columns are for use even if the patient requires insulin.			Additional Code Required
	Controlled or not stated as uncontrolled	Uncontrolled	Controlled or not stated as uncontrolled	Uncontrolled	Other metabolic disorders or conditions	List these codes after the diabetes code
Nephropathy	250.41	250.43	250.40	250.42		583.81
Nephrosis (Ebsteins) (syndrome)	250.41	250.43	250.40	250.42		581.81
Neuralgia	250.61	250.63	250.60	250.62		357.2
Neuritis	250.61	250.63	250.60	250.62		357.2
Neurogenic arthropathy	250.61	250.63	250.60	250.62		713.5
Neuropathic arthritis	250.61	250.63	250.60	250.62	713.5	
Neuropathy	250.61	250.63	250.60	250.62		357.2
autonomic (peripheral)	250.61	250.63	250.60	250.62		337.1
Neurophthisis	250.61	250.63	250.60	250.62		357.2
Nonclinical					790.29	
Ophthalmoplegia	250.51	250.53	250.50	250.52		378.86
Osteomyelitis	250.81	250.83	250.80	250.82		731.8
Peripheral angiopathy	250.71	250.73	250.70	250.72		443.81
Peripheral autonomic neuropathy	250.61	250.63	250.60	250.62		337.1
Peripheral vascular disease (occlusive)	250.71	250.73	250.70	250.72		443.81
Pre-diabetes NOS					790.29	
Phosphate					275.3	
Polyneuropathy, polyneuritis	250.61	250.63	250.60	250.62		357.2
Postpancreatectomy					251.3	
Postsurgical (hypoinsulinemia)					251.3	
Prediabetes					790.29	
Pseudotabes	250.61	250.63	250.60	250.62		337.1
Renal glycosuria (true)					271.4	
Retinal						
edema	250.51	250.53	250.50	250.52		362.07
hemorrhage	250.51	250.53	250.50	250.52		362.01
Retinitis	250.51	250.53	250.50	250.52		362.01
Retinopathy	250.51	250.53	250.50	250.52		362.01
background (simple)	250.51	250.53	250.50	250.52		362.01
nonproliferative, NOS	250.51	250.53	250.50	250.52		362.03
nonproliferative, mild	250.51	250.53	250.50	250.52		362.04
nonproliferative, moderate	250.51	250.53	250.50	250.52		362.05
nonproliferative, severe	250.51	250.53	250.50	250.52		362.06
proliferative	250.51	250.53	250.50	250.52		362.02
Rubeosis iridis	250.51	250.53	250.50	250.52		364.42
Secondary						
postsurgical					251.3	
steroid induced					251.8	E932.0
Skin						
dermopathy	250.81	250.83	250.80	250.82		709.8
necrobiosis lipoidica diabeticorum	250.81	250.83	250.80	250.82		709.3
Screening					V77.1	
Steroid induced						
correct substance properly administered					251.8	E932.0
overdose or wrong substance given or taken					962.0	
Stress					790.29	
Subclinical					790.29	
Subliminal					790.29	
Syndrome						
diabetes-dwarfism-obesity (juvenile)					258.1	
diabetes mellitus in newborn infant					775.1	
diabetes-nephrosis	250.41	250.43	250.40	250.42		581.81
diabetic amyotrophy	250.61	250.63	250.60	250.62		353.1
Hanot-Chauffard (-Troisier) (bronze diabetes)					275.01	
nephrotic	250.41	250.43	250.40	250.42		581.81
Oppenheim-Urbach (necrobiosis lipoidica diabeticorum)	250.81	250.83	250.80	250.82		709.3
Pierre Mauriac's (diabetes-dwarfism-obesity)					258.1	
renal glomerulohyalinosis-diabetic	250.41	250.43	250.40	250.42		581.81
Troisier-Hanot-Chauffard (bronze diabetes)					275.01	
Urbach-Oppenheim (necrobiosis lipoidica diabeticorum)	250.81	250.83	250.80	250.82		709.3

Diabetes (brittle) (congenital) (familial) (mellitus) (severe) (slight)	TYPE I		TYPE II or unspecified type. The codes found in these columns are for use even if the patient requires insulin.			Additional Code Required
	Controlled or not stated as uncontrolled	Uncontrolled	Controlled or not stated as uncontrolled	Uncontrolled	Other metabolic disorders or conditions	List these codes after the diabetes code
Ulcer (skin), except pressure, unspecified site	250.81	250.83	250.80	250.82		707.9
lower extremity, unspecified	250.81	250.83	250.80	250.82		707.19
lower extremity, ankle	250.81	250.83	250.80	250.82		707.13
lower extremity, calf	250.81	250.83	250.80	250.82		707.12
lower extremity, heel and midfoot	250.81	250.83	250.80	250.82		707.14
lower extremity, thigh	250.81	250.83	250.80	250.82		707.11
lower extremity, toes	250.81	250.83	250.80	250.82		707.15
specified site NEC	250.81	250.83	250.80	250.82		707.8
unspecified complication	250.91	250.93	250.90	250.92		
Willis' disease	250.01	250.03	250.00	250.02		
Xanthoma diabeticorum, xanthomatosis	250.81	250.83	250.80	250.82		272.2

Site of Hernia	Without Obstruction	With Obstruction	Gangrene (with or without obstruction)
Abdomen (wall)	553.20	552.20	551.20
recurrent	553.21	552.21	551.21
Abdominal, specified site NEC	553.8	552.8	551.8
Appendix	553.8	552.8	551.8
Bilateral — see Hernia, by site			
Bladder (sphincter)			
congenital (female) (male)	756.71		
female			
lateral	618.02		
midline	618.01		
male		596.89	
Brain (acquired) (stem)	348.4		
congenital	742.0		
Broad ligament	553.8		
Bubonocele — see Hernia, inguinal			
Cecocele — see also Hernia, by site	553.9	552.9	551.9
Cerebral (acquired)	348.4		
congenital (endaural)	742.0		
Ciliary body (acquired)	364.89		
traumatic	871.1		
Colic	553.9	552.9	551.9
Colon	553.9	552.9	551.9
Colostomy	569.69		
Cooper's	553.8	552.8	551.8
Crural — see Hernia, femoral			
Diaphragm(atic)	553.3	552.3	551.3
congenital (gross defect)	756.6		
traumatic	862.0		
with open wound	862.1		
Direct — see Hernia, inguinal			
Disc, intervertebral — see Displacement, intervertebral disc			
Diverticulum (intestine)	553.9	552.9	551.9
Double — see Hernia, inguinal			
Duodenojejunal	553.8	552.8	551.8
Encysted — see Hernia, inguinal			
En glissade — see Hernia, inguinal			
Enterocele – see also Hernia, by site	553.9	552.9	551.9
Enterostomy	569.69		
Epigastric	553.29	552.29	551.29
recurrent	553.21	552.21	551.21
Epigastrocele	553.29	552.29	551.29
recurrent	553.21	552.21	551.21
Epiplocele	553.9	552.9	551.9
Epiplosarcomphalocele	553.1	552.1	551.1
Esophageal (hiatal)	553.3	552.3	551.3
congenital	750.6		
Eventration (chest to colon)	553.3	552.3	551.3
congenital (gross defect)	756.6		
External — see Hernia, inguinal			

Site of Hernia

Site of Hernia	Without Obstruction	With Obstruction	Gangrene (with or without obstruction)
Fallopian tube	620.4		
Fascia	728.89		
Fat (pad)	729.30		
eye, eyelid	374.34		
knee		729.31	
orbit		374.34	
retro-orbital	374.34		
retropatellar	729.31		
specified site NEC	729.39		
Female			
complete	618.3		
cystocele			
lateral	618.02		
midline	618.01		
with prolapse	618.4		
incomplete	618.2		
fallopian tube	620.4		
ovary, oviduct	620.4		
rectovaginal	618.6		
uterus	621.8		
vaginal	618.6		
vesical			
congenital	756.71		
lateral	618.02		
midline	618.01		
Femoral (unilateral)	553.00	552.00	551.00
bilateral	553.02	552.02	551.02
recurrent	553.03	552.03	551.03
recurrent (unilateral)	553.01	552.01	551.01
Foramen			
Bochdale (acquired)	553.3	552.3	551.3
congenital	756.6		
magnum	348.4		
Morgagni (an) (acquired)	553.3	552.3	551.3
congenital	756.6		
Furnicular (umbilical)	553.1	552.1	551.1
spermatic cord—*see* Hernia, inguinal			
Gastric mucosa	537.89		
Gastrointestinal tract	553.9	552.9	551.9
Gluteal — *see* Hernia, femoral			
Gruber's	553.8	552.8	551.8
Hesselbach's	553.8	552.8	551.8
Hiatal (esophageal) (sliding)	553.3	552.3	551.3
Holthouse's — *see* Hernia, inguinal			
Incarcerated — *see* Hernia, by site, with obstruction			
Incisional	553.21	552.21	551.21
lumbar	553.8	552.8	551.8
Indirect — *see* Hernia, inguinal			
Infantile — *see* Hernia, inguinal			
Infrapatellar fat pad	729.31		
Inguinal (unilateral) (direct) (double) ((encysted) (external) (furnicular) (indirect) (infantile) (internal) (interstial) (oblique) (scrotal) (sliding)	550.90	550.10	550.00
bilateral	550.92	550.12	550.02
recurrent	550.93	550.13	550.03
recurrent (unilateral)	550.91	550.11	550.01
Internal	553.8	552.8	551.8
Interstitial	553.9	552.9	551.9
Intervertebral cartilage — *see* Displacement, intervertebral disc			
Intestine(al)	553.9	552.9	551.9
Intra-abdominal	553.9	552.9	551.9
Intraparietal	553.9	552.9	551.9
Iris (acquired)	364.89		
traumatic	871.1		
Irreducible — *see* Hernia, by site, with obstruction			
Ischiatic	553.8	552.8	551.8

Site of Hernia	Without Obstruction	With Obstruction	Gangrene (with or without obstruction)
Lens (acquired)	379.32		
traumatic	871.1		
Linea alba	553.29	552.29	551.29
recurrent	553.21	552.21	551.21
Linea semilunaris	553.29	552.29	551.29
Littre's	553.9	552.9	551.9
Lumbar	553.8	552.8	551.8
intervertebral disc	722.10		
Lung (acquired)	518.89		
congenital	748.69		
Male			
chylocele	608.84		
cystocele	596.89		
scrotal - *see* Hernia, inguinal			
spermatocele	608.1		
congenital	752.8		
testis	550.90	550.10	550.00
bilateral	550.92	550.12	550.02
recurrent	550.93	550.13	550.03
recurrent (unilateral)	550.91	550.11	550.01
vesical	596.89		
congenital	756.71		
Mediastinum	519.3		
Merocele — *see* Hernia, femoral			
Mesenteric (internal)	553.8	552.8	551.8
Mesocolon	553.8	552.8	551.8
Muscle (sheath)	728.89		
Nucleus polpous — *see* Displacement, intervertebral disc			
Oblique — *see* Hernia, inguinal			
Obstructive — *see* Hernia, by site with obstruction			
Orbturator	553.8	552.8	551.8
Omental	553.8	552.8	551.8
Omentocele	553.8	552.8	551.8
Orbital fat pad	374.34		
Ovary, oviduct	620.4		
Paracolostomy	569.69		
Paraduodenal	553.8	552.8	551.8
Paraesophageal	553.8	552.8	551.8
congenital	750.6		
Parahiatal	553.8	552.8	551.8
Paraumbilical	553.1	552.1	551.1
Parietal	553.9	552.9	551.9
Perineal	553.8	552.8	551.8
Peritoneal sac, lesser	553.8	552.8	551.8
Petit's	553.8	552.8	551.8
intervertebral disc	722.10		
Popliteal fat pad	729.31		
Postoperative	553.21	552.21	551.21
Prevesical	596.89		
Properitoneal	553.8	552.8	551.8
Pudendal	553.8	552.8	551.8
Rectovaginal	618.6		
Retroperitoneal	553.8	552.8	551.8
Richter's	553.9	552.9	551.9
Rieux's, Reix's	553.8	552.8	551.8
Saint's, triad — *see* Hernia, Diaphragm			
Sarcopiplocele	553.9	552.9	551.9
Sarcoepiplomphalocele	553.9	552.9	551.9
Sciatic	553.8	552.8	551.8
Scrotum, scrotal — *see* Hernia, inguinal			
Sliding			
hiatal	553.3	552.3	551.3
congenital	750.6		
inguinal — *see* Hernia, inguinal			
Spermatocele	608.1		
congenital	752.8		
Spigelian	553.29	552.29	551.29
Spinal — *see* Spina Bifida			

Coding Tables

Site of Hernia

Coding Tables

Site of Hernia	Without Obstruction	With Obstruction	Gangrene (with or without obstruction)
Strangulated — *see* Hernia, by site, wth obstruction			
Supraumbilicus	553.29	552.29	551.29
recurrent	553.21	552.21	551.21
Tendon	727.9		
Testis (nontraumatic)	550.90	550.10	550.00
bilateral	550.92	550.12	550.02
recurrent	550.93	550.13	550.03
recurrent (unilateral)	550.91	550.11	550.01
Thoracic stomach	553.8	552.8	551.8
Treitz's	553.8	552.8	551.8
Triad, Saint's — *see* Hernia, diaphragm			
Umbilical, umbilicus	553.1	552.1	551.1
Unspecified site NEC	553.9	552.9	551.9
Ureter	593.89	593.4	
Uterus NOS	621.8		
pregnant — *see* herniation of uterus—pregnancy table			
Vaginal	618.6		
Velpeau's — *see* Hernia, femoral			
Ventral	553.20	552.20	551.20
incisional	553.21	552.21	551.21
recurrent	553.21	552.21	551.21
Vertebral cartilage — *see* Displacement, intervertebral disc			
Vesical			
congenital (female) (male)	756.71		
female			
lateral	618.02		
midline	618.01		
male		596.89	
Vitreous (acquired)	379.21		
traumatic	871.1		

Ectopic Pregnancy	Abdominal pregnancy (Intraperitoneal pregnancy)	Tubal pregnancy (Fallopian pregnancy, rupture of fallopian tube due to pregnancy, tubal abortion)	Ovarian pregnancy	Other ectopic pregnancy (Includes the following pregnancy(s): cervical, cornual mural mesometric intraligamentous)	Unspecified ectopic pregnancy
Without complication					
with intrauterine pregnancy	633.01	633.11	633.21	633.81	633.91
without intrauterine pregnancy	633.00	633.10	633.20	633.80	633.90
With complication of:					
Afibrinogenemia	639.1	639.1	639.1	639.1	639.1
Atrophy, acute yellow	639.8	639.8	639.8	639.8	639.8
Cardiac arrest	639.8	639.8	639.8	639.8	639.8
Cardiac failure	639.8	639.8	639.8	639.8	639.8
Cerebral anoxia	639.8	639.8	639.8	639.8	639.8
Circulatory collapse	639.5	639.5	639.5	639.5	639.5
Defibrination syndrome	639.1	639.1	639.1	639.1	639.1
Electrolyte imbalance	639.4	639.4	639.4	639.4	639.4
Embolism (any type)	639.6	639.6	639.6	639.6	639.6
Endometritis	639.0	639.0	639.0	639.0	639.0
Genital tract infection	639.0	639.0	639.0	639.0	639.0
Hemorrhage, delayed or excessive	639.1	639.1	639.1	639.1	639.1
Intravascular hemolysis	639.1	639.1	639.1	639.1	639.1
Kidney failure (acute)	639.3	639.3	639.3	639.3	639.3
Laceration of:					
pelvic organs	639.2	639.2	639.2	639.2	639.2
Metabolic disorder	639.4	639.4	639.4	639.4	639.4
Necrosis of liver	639.8	639.8	639.8	639.8	639.8
Oliguria	639.3	639.3	639.3	639.3	639.3
Other specified complication	639.8	639.8	639.8	639.8	639.8
Parametritis	639.0	639.0	639.0	639.0	639.0
Pelvic infection	639.0	639.0	639.0	639.0	639.0
Pelvic peritonitis	639.0	639.0	639.0	639.0	639.0
Renal shutdown	639.3	639.3	639.3	639.3	639.3
Renal tubular necrosis	639.3	639.3	639.3	639.3	639.3
Salpingitis	639.0	639.0	639.0	639.0	639.0
Salpingo-oophoritis	639.0	639.0	639.0	639.0	639.0

Ectopic Pregnancy

Ectopic Pregnancy	Abdominal pregnancy (Intraperitoneal pregnancy)	Tubal pregnancy (Fallopian pregnancy, rupture of fallopian tube due to pregnancy, tubal abortion)	Ovarian pregnancy	Other ectopic pregnancy (Includes the following pregnancy(s): cervical, cornual mural mesometric intraligamentous)	Unspecified ectopic pregnancy
With complication of: — *continued*					
Sepsis NOS	639.0	639.0	639.0	639.0	639.0
Septicemia NOS	639.0	639.0	639.0	639.0	639.0
Shock (postoperative)(septic)	639.5	639.5	639.5	639.5	639.5
Unspecified complications	639.9	639.9	639.9	639.9	639.9
Urinary tract infection (UTI)	639.8	639.8	639.8	639.8	639.8

Normal Pregnancy

Pregnancy/Delivery, current (Normal) (Single) (Uterine) (without Sickness)	Code	Special Notes
Assisted reproductive technology	V23.85	
Counseling (for)		
illegitimate	V61.6	
multiparity	V61.5	
unwanted pregnancy, NEC	V61.7	
Examination (pregnancy test)		
negative results	V72.41	
positive results	V72.42	
unconfirmed	V72.40	
Normal delivery	650	This code is always a primary diagnosis.
Normal pregnancy		
with other condition not affecting the pregnancy	V22.2	V22.2 should be used in place of any other pregnancy codes and listed second on the claim form. The condition, which does not affect the pregnancy, must be listed first.
first pregnancy	V22.0	Codes V22.0 and V22.1 should never be used in conjunction with any codes from cataegories 640-648 and 651-676.
second or other normal pregnancy	V22.1	Meaning 2nd, 3rd, 4th etc. pregnancy
Postpartum care and examination		
immediately after delivery	V24.0	Normal uncomplicated cases
lactating mother	V24.1	Supervision of lactating mother
routine postpartum follow-up	V24.2	Care within 6 weeks after delivery
Previous (not affecting current pregnancy)		These codes may be used in conjunction with chapter 11 codes. A thorough review of any pertinent excludes notes (found in the tabular list) is necessary to be certain that these V codes are being used properly.
abortion	V23.2	Excludes recurrent pregnancy loss (646.3x)
difficult delivery	V23.49	
ectopic pregnancy	V23.42	
forceps delivery	V23.49	
hemorrhage, antepartum or postpartum	V23.49	
hydatidiform mole	V23.1	
infertility	V23.0	
in utero procedure	V23.86	Current pregnancy with history of in utero procedure during a prior pregnancy. Report a history of in utero procedure in a nongravid uterus with code V15.21
malignancy NEC	V23.89	
neonatal death	V23.5	
nonobstetrical conditions	V23.89	
premature delivery	V23.41	
pre-term labor	V23.41	
specified NEC	V23.89	
stillbirth	V23.5	
trophoblastic disease	V23.1	
unspecified condition	V23.9	
vesicular mole	V23.1	
Screening, prenatal (for)		If the abnormal finding is known—code the screening and the findings as additional codes
by		
amniocentesis		
chromosomal anomalies	V28.0	
raised alpha-fetoprotein levels (amniotic fluid)	V28.1	
specified, NEC	V28.2	
fetal anatomic survey	V28.81	
ultrasound		
fetal growth retardation	V28.4	
malformation	V28.3	

Coding Tables *(left margin)*

Antepartum Pregnancy *(left margin)*

Normal Pregnancy

Pregnancy/Delivery, current (Normal) (Single) (Uterine) (without Sickness)	Code	Special Notes
Screening, prenatal (for) — *continued*		
isoimmunization	V28.5	
other specified screening	V28.89	
Streptococcus B	V28.6	
unspecified, screening	V28.9	
Supervision (of) (for)		These codes may be used in conjunction with chapter 11 codes. A thorough review of any pertinent excludes notes (found in the tabular list) is necessary to be certain that these V codes are being used properly.
high-risk, NOS	V23.9	
insufficient prenatal care	V23.7	
specified problem NEC	V23.89	
inconclusive fetal viability	V23.87	
multigravida		Second or more pregnancy
elderly	V23.82	35 years of age or older at expected date of delivery
young	V23.84	Younger than 16 years of age at expected date of delivery
multiparity	V23.3	
normal NEC	V22.1	
first pregnancy	V22.0	
poor		
obstetric history	V23.49	
reproductive history	V23.5	
primigravida		First pregnancy
elderly	V23.81	35 years of age or older at expected date of delivery
young	V23.83	Younger than 16 years of age at expected date of delivery
unconfirmed	V72.40	
undelivered (no other diagnosis)	V22.2	
with false labor	644.1	
high risk	V23.9	
specified problems NEC	V23.89	
Suspected problem not found		
amniotic cavity and membrane	V89.01	
cervical shortening	V89.05	
fetal anomaly	V89.03	
fetal growth	V89.04	
placental	V89.02	

Antepartum Pregnancy Condition or Complication; affecting management of mother	Antepartum condition or complication	Delivered, with or without mention of antepartum condition	Unspecified episode of care	Assign additional code to describe the…	Affecting fetus (coded on the newborn chart only)
Ablatio placentae	641.23	641.21	641.20		762.1
Abnormal, NEC	646.93	646.91	646.90		761.8
amnion	658.93	658.91	658.90		762.9
cervix	654.63	654.61	654.60		763.89
causing obstructed labor	660.23	660.21	660.20	cause	763.1
change in	631.0				
quantitative human chorionic gonadotropin (hCG) in early pregnancy					
chorion	658.93	658.91	658.90		762.9
cord (umbilical)	663.93	663.91	663.90		762.6
fetal chromosomes (suspected)	655.13	655.11	655.10		758.89
fetal					
heart rate	659.73	659.71	659.70		763.83
before onset of labor	659.73	659.71	659.70		763.81
during labor	659.73	659.71	659.70		763.82
heart rhythm	659.73	659.71	659.70		763.8
before onset of labor	659.73	659.71	659.70		763.81
during labor	659.73	659.71	659.70		763.82
fetus, fetal (suspected) NEC	655.93	655.91	655.90		779.9
acid-base balance	656.83	656.81	656.80		768.4
causing disproportion	653.73	653.71	653.70		763.1
causing obstructed labor	660.13	660.11	660.10	cause	763.1
specified NEC	655.83	655.81	655.80		779.8

Antepartum Pregnancy Condition or Complication; affecting management of mother	Antepartum condition or complication	Delivered, with or without mention of antepartum condition	Unspecified episode of care	Assign additional code to describe the…	Affecting fetus (coded on the newborn chart only)
Abnormal, NEC — *continued*					
findings, nonspecific (a code from 640-648 should be used first when the management of the mother is affected by the abnormal findings)	796.5				
glucose tolerance test	648.83	648.81	648.80	condition	775.0
labor (forces of) NEC	661.93	661.91	661.90	condition	763.7
pelvic organs or tissues NEC	654.93	654.91	654.90		763.89
causing obstructed labor	660.23	660.21	660.20	cause	763.1
pelvis (bony)	653.03	653.01	653.00		763.1
causing obstructed labor	660.13	660.11	660.10	cause	763.1
perineum or vulva	654.83	654.81	654.80		763.89
causing obstructed labor	660.23	660.21	660.20	cause	763.1
placenta, placental (vessel)	656.73	656.71	656.70		762.2
with hemorrhage	641.83	641.81	641.80		762.1
position					
cervix	654.43	654.41	654.40		763.89
causing obstructed labor	660.23	660.21	660.20	cause	763.1
fetus	652.93	652.91	652.90		763.1
causing obstructed labor	660.03	660.01	660.00	cause	763.1
placenta (low implantation) (previa)	641.03	641.01	641.00		762.0
with hemorrhage	641.13	641.11	641.10		762.1
uterus	654.43	654.41	654.40		763.89
causing obstructed labor	660.23	660.21	660.20	cause	763.1
product(s) of conception NEC	631.8				
quality of milk	676.83	676.81	676.80		
shape of uterus	654.43	654.41	654.40		763.89
causing obstructed labor	660.23	660.21	660.20	cause	763.1
size of fetus	653.53	653.51	653.50		763.1
causing obstructed labor	660.13	660.11	660.10	cause	763.1
umbilical cord NEC	663.83	663.81	663.80		762.6
uterus (congenital)	654.03	654.01	654.00		763.89
causing obstructed labor	660.23	660.21	660.20	cause	763.1
vagina	654.73	654.71	654.70		763.89
causing obstructed labor	660.23	660.21	660.20	cause	763.1
vulva (acquired) (congenital)	654.83	654.81	654.80		763.89
causing obstructed labor	660.23	660.21	660.20	cause	763.1
weight gain	646.13	646.11	646.10	condition	761.8
with					
hypertension (mild) (pre-eclamptic)	642.43	642.41	642.40		760.0
convulsions	642.63	642.61	642.60		760.0
pre-existing hypertension	642.73	642.71	642.70		760.0
severe hypertension	642.53	642.51	642.50		760.0
Aborter, recurrent	646.33	646.31	646.30	condition	761.8
Abruption of placenta	641.23	641.21	641.20		762.1
Abscess					
areola (acute) (chronic)	675.13	675.11	675.10		
Bartholin's gland	646.63	646.61	646.60	condition	760.8
bladder	646.63	646.61	646.60	condition	760.1
breast (acute) (chronic)	675.13	675.11	675.10		
kidney	646.63	646.61	646.60	condition	760.1
labium (majus) (minus)	646.63	646.61	646.60	condition	760.8
milk	675.13	675.11	675.10		
nipple	675.03	675.01	675.00		
subareolar	675.13	675.11	675.10		
urethra	646.63	646.61	646.60	condition	760.1
vulva	646.63	646.61	646.60	condition	760.8
Absorption (of) (through placenta)					
suspected damage to fetus					
chemical	655.53	655.51	655.50		760.70
drug	655.53	655.51	655.50		760.70
Acidosis (fetal) (intrauterine)	656.83	656.81	656.80		768.4
Addiction					
alcoholic	648.43	648.41	648.40	condition	760.71
suspected fetal damage	655.43	655.41	655.40		760.71

Coding Tables *(side margin)*

Antepartum Pregnancy *(side margin)*

Antepartum Pregnancy Condition or Complication; affecting management of mother	Antepartum condition or complication	Delivered, with or without mention of antepartum condition	Unspecified episode of care	Assign additional code to describe the…	Affecting fetus (coded on the newborn chart only)
Adhesion(s), adhesive					
amnion to fetus	658.83	658.81	658.80		762.8
uterus to abdominal wall	654.43	654.41	654.40		763.89
causing obstructed labor	660.23	660.21	660.20	cause	763.1
Advanced maternal age (multigravida)	659.63	659.61	659.60		761.8
primigravida	659.53	659.51	659.50		761.8
Aerocele	673.03	673.01	673.00		
AFP (screening for raised levels in amniotic fluid)	V28.1				
Agalactia	676.43	676.41	676.40		
Air embolism	673.03	673.01	673.00		
Age					
elderly (35 years of age or older at expected date of delivery)					
multigravida (second or more pregnancy)	659.63	659.61	659.60		
primigravida (first pregnancy)	659.53	659.51	659.50		
young (less than 16 years old at expected date of delivery)	659.83	659.81	659.80		
Albuminuria (gravidarum)	646.23	646.21	646.20	condition	760.1
with hypertension (and edema)					760.1
mild	642.43	642.41	642.40		760.0
severe	642.53	642.51	642.50		760.0
gestational	646.23	646.21	646.20	condition	760.1
pre-eclamptic (mild)	642.23	642.21	642.20		760.0
severe	642.53	642.51	642.50		760.0
Alcohol, alcoholic					
addiction (maternal)	648.43	648.41	648.40	condition	760.71
with suspected fetal damage	655.43	655.41	655.40		760.71
Alphafetoprotein (screening for raised levels in amniotic fluid)	V28.1				
Amnion (nodosum)	658.83	658.81	658.80		762.9
Amnionitis	658.43	658.41	658.40		762.7
Amniotic fluid embolism	673.13	673.11	673.10		
Amputation of cervix	654.63	654.61	654.60		763.89
causing obstructed labor	660.23	660.21	660.20	cause	763.1
Android pelvis					
with disproportion (fetopelvic)	653.33	653.31	653.30		763.1
causing obstructed labor	660.13	660.11	660.10	cause	763.1
Anemia	648.23	648.21	648.20	condition	760.8
aplastic	648.23	648.21	648.20	condition	760.8
iron (Fe) deficiency	648.23	648.21	648.20	condition	760.8
macrocytic	648.23	648.21	648.20	condition	760.8
megaloblastic	648.23	648.21	648.20	condition	760.8
pernicious	648.23	648.21	648.20	condition	760.8
postpartum	648.23	648.21	648.20	condition	
Anencephalus, anencephaly (fetal)	655.03	655.01	655.00		
Anesthesia, anesthetic					
complications NEC	668.83	668.81	668.80	condition	
cardiac	668.13	668.11	668.10	condition	763.5
central nervous system	668.23	668.21	668.20	condition	763.5
pulmonary	668.03	668.01	668.00	condition	763.5
death (from) during delivery	668.93	668.91	668.90	condition	761.6
Anomaly, anomalous (congenital)					
cardiovascular system	648.53	648.51	648.50	condition	
cervix	654.63	654.61	654.60		763.89
causing obstructed labor	660.23	660.21	660.20	cause	763.1
pelvis (bony)	653.03	653.01	653.00		763.1
causing obstructed labor	660.13	660.11	660.10	cause	763.1
uterus	654.03	654.01	654.00		763.89
causing obstructed labor	660.23	660.21	660.20	cause	763.1
Anoxia cerebral					
complicating delivery (cesarean) (instrumental)	669.43	669.41	669.40		
due to obstetric anesthesia or sedation	668.23	668.21	668.20	complication	
Anteversion					
uterus, uterine (cervix)	654.43	654.41	654.40		763.89
causing obstructed labor	660.23	660.21	660.20	cause	763.1

Antepartum Pregnancy
Condition or Complication; affecting management of mother

	Antepartum condition or complication	Delivered, with or without mention of antepartum condition	Unspecified episode of care	Assign additional code to describe the…	Affecting fetus (coded on the newborn chart only)
Anthropoid pelvis					
with disproportion (fetopelvic)	653.23	653.21	653.20		763.1
causing obstructed labor	660.13	660.11	660.10	cause	763.1
Antibodies (incompatibility)					
ABO	656.23	656.21	656.20		773.2
anti-C	656.13	656.11	656.10		773.0
anti-D, cord blood	656.13	656.11	656.10		773.0
anti-E	656.13	656.11	656.10		773.0
blood group (ABO)	656.23	656.21	656.20		773.1
Rh (blood group) (factor)	656.13	656.11	656.10		773.0
Apoplexia, apoplexy, apoplectic					
placenta	641.23	641.21	641.20		762.1
uteroplacental	641.23	641.21	641.20		762.1
Arrest, arrested					
active phase of labor	661.13	661.11	661.10		763.7
any plane in pelvis complicating delivery	660.13	660.11	660.10	cause	763.1
cardiac					
anesthesia, complicating	668.13	668.11	668.10		
delivery (cesarean) (instrumental)	669.43	669.41	669.40		
deep transverse	660.33	660.31	660.30	cause	763.1
development or growth of fetus	656.53	656.51	656.50		764.90
transverse (deep)	660.33	660.31	660.30	cause	763.1
Ascites					
fetal, causing fetopelvic disproportion	653.73	653.71	653.70		763.1
causing obstructed labor	660.13	660.11	660.10	cause	763.1
Aspiration					
acid-pulmonary (syndrome)	668.03	668.01	668.00	complication	
pneumonitis	668.03	668.01	668.00	complication	
Assimilation, pelvis					
with disproportion	653.23	653.21	653.20		763.1
causing obstructed labor	660.13	660.11	660.10	cause	763.1
Asymmetry					
pelvis with disproportion	653.03	653.01	653.00		763.1
causing obstructed labor	660.13	660.11	660.10	cause	763.1
Atonia, atony, atonic (intrapartum)					
w/o hemmorage	661.23	661.21	661.20		
Atresia, atretic					
cervix	654.63	654.61	654.60		763.89
causing obstructed labor	660.23	660.21	660.20	cause	763.1
Atrophy, atrophic					
breast	676.33	676.31	676.30		
liver (acute) (subacute) (yellow)	646.73	646.71	646.70	complication	
Avulsion (traumatic)					
symphyseal cartilage (inner)		665.61	665.60		
Bacilluria, asymptomatic	646.53	646.51	646.50	complication	
Bacteremia					
during labor	659.33	659.31	659.30		
during pregnancy	647.83	647.81	647.80	condition	
Bacteriuria, asymptomatic	646.53	646.51	646.50	complication	760.1
Band(s), **amniotic**	658.83	658.81	658.80		762.8
Bandl's ring (contraction)	661.43	661.41	661.40		763.7
Bariatric surgery	649.23	649.21	649.20		
Bicornis or Bicornuate uterus	654.03	654.01	654.00		763.89
causing obstructed labor	660.23	660.21	660.20	cause	763.1
Bleeding	641.93	641.91	641.90		
accidental	641.23	641.21	641.20		762.1
before 22 completed weeks gestation NEC	640.93	640.91	640.90		
cerebrovascular	674.03	674.01	674.00		
due to					
afibrinogenemia or other coagulation defect	641.33	641.31	641.30		
fibroids	641.83	641.81	641.80		762.1
marginal sinus (rupture)	641.23	641.21	641.20		762.1
premature separation, placenta	641.23	641.21	641.20		762.1
trauma	641.83	641.81	641.80		
early (before 22 completed weeks gestation)	640.93	640.91	640.90		
threatened abortion	640.03	640.01	640.00		

Coding Tables

Antepartum Pregnancy

Antepartum Pregnancy Condition or Complication; affecting management of mother	Antepartum condition or complication	Delivered, with or without mention of antepartum condition	Unspecified episode of care	Assign additional code to describe the…	Affecting fetus (coded on the newborn chart only)
Bleeding — *continued*					
unavoidable	641.13	641.11	641.10		
Bone disorders	648.73	648.71	648.70	condition	
Borderline pelvis	653.13	653.11	653.10		763.1
with obstruction during labor	660.13	660.11	660.10	cause	763.1
Braxton Hicks contractions	644.13		644.10		
Breech presentation (buttocks) (complete) (frank)	652.23	652.21	652.20		761.7
with successful version	652.13	652.11	652.10		763.1
before labor	652.23	652.21	652.20		761.7
during labor	652.23	652.21	652.20		763.0
Brow presentation					
complicating delivery	652.43	652.41	652.40		763.1
Bruise					
umbilical cord	663.63	663.61	663.60		762.6
Caked breast	676.23	676.21	676.20		
Cardiomyopathy	674.53	674.51	674.50		
Cardiovascular disease	648.63	648.61	648.60	condition	
congenital	648.53	648.51	648.50	condition	
Cellulitis, breast	675.13	675.11	675.10		
Cephalopelvic disproportion NOS	653.43	653.41	653.40		763.1
with obstruction during labor	660.13	660.11	660.10	cause	763.1
Cerebrovascular disorders	674.03	674.01	674.00	condition	
Cervical Shortening	649.73	649.71	649.70		
Cervicitis	646.63	646.61	646.60	condition	760.8
Cervix					
adhesions	654.63	654.61	654.60		
anaplasia	654.63	654.61	654.60		
atypism	654.63	654.61	654.60		
bands	654.63	654.61	654.60		
with obstruction during labor	660.23	660.21	660.20	cause	763.1
cervicitis	654.63	654.61	654.60		
cicatrix	654.63	654.61	654.60		
cyst		654.61	654.60		
dysplasia	654.63	654.61	654.60		
ectropion	654.63	654.61	654.60		
endocervicitis	654.63	654.61	654.60		
erosion	654.63	654.61	654.60		
hypertrophic elongation	654.63	654.61	654.60		
incompetence	654.53	654.51	654.50		761.0
leukoplakia	654.63	654.61	654.60		
Nabothian (gland) cyst or follicle	654.63	654.61	654.60		
polyp		654.61	654.60		
stricture and stenosis	654.63	654.61	654.60		
ulcer		654.61	654.60		
Cesarean delivery, section NEC		669.71	669.70		763.4
post mortem		669.71	669.70		761.6
previous	654.23	654.21	654.20		
causing obstructed labor	660.23	660.21	660.20	cause	763.1
Chiari-Frommel syndrome	676.63	676.61	676.60		
Chloasma (gravidarum)	646.83	646.81	646.80	condition	
Chorioamnionitis	658.43	658.41	658.40		762.7
Cicatrix					
cervix	654.63	654.61	654.60		
causing obstructed labor	660.23	660.21	660.20	cause	763.1
vagina	654.73	654.71	654.70		
causing obstructed labor	660.23	660.21	660.20	cause	763.1
Coagulation defects	649.33	649.31	649.30	286.0-286.9, 287.0-287.9, 289.0-289.9	
Collapse (during or after labor and delivery)					
circulatory (peripheral)	669.13	669.11	669.10		779.8
lung		668.01	668.00		
vascular (peripheral)	669.13	669.11	669.10		
Colporrhexis		665.41	665.40		
Complications NEC	646.93	646.91	646.90	condition	761.9
delivery	669.93	669.91	669.90		

Antepartum Pregnancy
Condition or Complication; affecting management of mother

	Antepartum condition or complication	Delivered, with or without mention of antepartum condition	Unspecified episode of care	Assign additional code to describe the…	Affecting fetus (coded on the newborn chart only)
Complications NEC — *continued*					
labor and delivery					
procedure (instrumental) (manual) (surgical)	669.43	669.41	669.40		
specified type NEC	669.83	669.81	669.80		
umbilical cord	663.93	663.91	663.90		762.6
specified type NEC	663.83	663.81	663.80		762.6
in utero procedure					
fetal	679.13	679.11	679.10		
maternal	679.03	679.01	679.00		
intrauterine contraceptive device (IUD)	655.83	655.81	655.80		
labor and delivery	669.93	669.91	669.90		
anesthesia (sedation)	668.93	668.91	668.90		763.5
cardiac	668.13	668.11	668.10		
central nervous system	668.23	668.21	668.20		
pulmonary	668.03	668.01	668.00		
specified type NEC	668.83	668.81	668.80		
specified condition NEC	669.83	669.81	669.80		
Compound presentation					
complicating delivery	652.83	652.81	652.80		763.1
causing obstructed labor	660.03	660.01	660.00	cause	763.1
Compression, umbilical cord					
complicating delivery	663.23	663.21	663.20		762.5
cord around neck	663.13	663.11	663.10		762.5
cord prolapsed	663.03	663.01	663.00		762.4
Conjoined twins	678.10	678.11	678.10		
causing disproportion (fetopelvic)	653.73	653.71	653.70		763.1
with obstruction during labor	660.13	661.00	660.10	cause	763.1
Constriction					
ring (uterus)	661.43	661.41	661.40		763.7
Contractions					
before 37 weeks	644.03		644.00		
Braxton Hicks	644.13		644.10		
Hicks'	644.13		644.10		
hourglass uterus	661.43	661.41	661.40		763.7
pelvis, complicating delivery	653.13	653.11	653.10		763.1
causing obstructed labor	660.13	660.11	660.10	cause	763.1
generally contracted	653.13	653.11	653.10		763.1
causing obstructed labor	660.13	660.11	660.10	cause	763.1
inlet	653.23	653.21	653.20		763.1
causing obstructed labor	660.13	660.11	660.10	cause	763.1
midpelvic	653.83	653.81	653.80		763.1
causing obstructed labor	660.13	660.11	660.10	cause	763.1
midplane	653.83	653.81	653.80		763.1
causing obstructed labor	660.13	660.11	660.10	cause	763.1
outlet	653.33	653.31	653.30		763.1
causing obstructed labor	660.13	660.11	660.10	cause	763.1
ring (Bandl's)	661.43	661.41	661.40		763.7
uterus					
abnormal	661.93	661.91	661.90		763.7
clonic, hourglass or tetanic	661.43	661.41	661.40		763.7
dyscoordinate	661.43	661.41	661.40		763.7
hourglass	661.43	661.41	661.40		763.7
incoordinate	661.43	661.41	661.40		763.7
inefficient or poor	661.23	661.21	661.20		763.7
irregular	661.23	661.21	661.20		763.7
tetanic	661.43	661.41	661.40		763.7
Convulsions (eclamptic) (uremic)	642.63	642.61	642.60		760.0
with pre-existing hypertension	642.73	642.71	642.70		760.0
Cord, complicating delivery					
around neck (tightly) (with compression)	663.13	663.11	663.10		762.5
without compression	663.33	663.31	663.30		762.6
prolapse, complicating delivery	663.03	663.01	663.00		762.4
Cornual — *see* Ectopic pregnancy					761.4
CPD	653.43	653.41	653.40		763.1
causing obstructed labor	653.43	653.41	653.40		763.1
Cracked nipple	676.13	676.11	676.10		

Antepartum Pregnancy Condition or Complication; affecting management of mother	Antepartum condition or complication	Delivered, with or without mention of antepartum condition	Unspecified episode of care	Assign additional code to describe the…	Affecting fetus (coded on the newborn chart only)
Cretin, pelvis (with disproportion) (fetopelvic)	653.13	653.11	653.10		763.1
causing obstructed labor	660.13	660.11	660.10	cause	763.1
Cross birth (of fetus) **complicating delivery**	652.33	652.31	652.30		763.1
with successful version	652.13	652.11	652.10		763.1
causing obstructed labor	660.03	660.01	660.00	cause	763.1
Cyst					
amnion, amniotic	658.83	658.81	658.80		763.89
chorion	658.83	658.81	658.80		763.89
ovary	654.43	654.41	654.40		763.89
causing obstructed labor	660.23	660.21	660.20	cause	763.1
pelvic	654.43	654.41	654.40		763.89
causing obstructed labor	660.23	660.21	660.20	cause	763.1
Cystitis	646.63	646.61	646.60	condition	760.1
Cystocele	654.43	654.41	654.40		763.89
causing obstructed labor	660.23	660.21	660.20	cause	763.1
Damage					
coccyx, complicating delivery		665.61	665.60		763.89
pelvic (during delivery)					
joint or ligament		665.61	665.60		763.89
organ		665.51	665.50		
Dates vs uterine size discrepancy	646.83	646.81	646.80		
Dead, fetus					
retained in utero (after 22 completed weeks' gestation)	656.43	656.41	656.40		779.9
before 22 weeks — *see* Abortion, missed					
syndrome	641.33	641.31	641.30		779.9
Death					
fetal NEC	646.93	646.91	646.90	condition	779.9
early before 22 weeks gestation — *see* Abortion, missed					
near term	656.43	656.41	656.40		779.9
maternal, NEC	646.93	646.91	646.90	condition	761.6
during delivery	668.93	668.91	668.90		
sudden, during delivery	669.93	669.91	669.90		761.6
under anesthesia NEC	668.93	668.91	668.90		761.6
Deciduitis	646.63	646.61	646.60		760.8
Decreased fetal movements	655.73	655.71	655.70		
Defect, defective					
coagulation (factor)	641.33	641.31	641.30		762.1
causing hemorrhage of pregnancy or delivery	641.33	641.31	641.30		762.1
Deficiency, deficient					
coagulation (factor)	641.33	641.31	641.30		762.1
causing hemorrhage of pregnancy or delivery	641.33	641.31	641.30		762.1
Deformity					
fetal					
with fetopelvic disproportion	653.73	653.71	653.70		763.1
causing obstructed labor	660.13	660.11	660.10		763.1
known or suspected	655.93	655.91	655.90		763.89
pelvic, pelvis					
with disproportion (fetopelvic)	653.03	653.01	653.00		763.1
causing obstructed labor	660.13	660.11	660.10	cause	763.1
soft part, organs or tissues NEC	654.93	654.91	654.90	cause	763.89
causing obstructed labor	660.23	660.21	660.20	cause	763.1
Delay, delayed					
any plane in pelvis, complicating delivery	660.13	660.11	660.10	cause	763.1
birth or delivery NEC	662.13	662.11	662.10		763.89
second twin, triplet, or multiple mate	662.33	662.31	662.30		763.89
Dependence, maternal					
alcohol, with suspected fetal damage	655.43	655.41	655.40		779.5
drug	648.33	648.31	648.30	condition	779.5
suspected damage to fetus	655.53	655.51	655.50		779.5
Depression	648.43	648.41	648.40	condition	
Dermatitis, gestationis	646.83	646.81	646.80	condition	
Detachment					
cervix, annular		665.31	665.30		763.89

Antepartum Pregnancy Condition or Complication; affecting management of mother	Antepartum condition or complication	Delivered, with or without mention of antepartum condition	Unspecified episode of care	Assign additional code to describe the…	Affecting fetus (coded on the newborn chart only)
Development					
incomplete (fetus or newborn)	656.53	656.51	656.50		763.89
Diabetes					
condition present before pregnancy	648.03	648.01	648.00	condition	775.0
gestational (chemical) (latent)	648.83	648.81	648.80	condition	775.0
with long term (current) insulin use				V58.67	775.0
Diastasis, recti (abdomen) **complicating delivery**	665.83	665.81	665.80		763.89
Difficult delivery NEC	669.93	669.91	669.90		763.89
Dilatation					
bladder (sphincter)	654.43	654.41	654.40		763.89
causing obstructed labor	660.23	660.21	660.20	cause	763.1
cervix, complicating delivery	654.63	654.61	654.60		763.89
incomplete, poor, slow	661.03	661.01	661.00		763.7
Discrepancy-uterine size to dates	646.83	646.81	646.80		
Disease, diseased NEC	646.93	646.91	646.90	condition	
breast NEC	676.33	676.31	676.30		
cerebrovascular, NEC	674.03	674.01	674.00		
Frommel's	676.63	676.61	676.60		
heart					
placenta	656.73	656.71	656.70		762.2
renal NEC	646.23	646.21	646.20	condition	760.1
Valsuani's (progressive pernicious anemia, puerperal)	648.23	648.21	648.20	condition	
venereal NEC	647.23	647.21	647.20	condition	
virus NEC	647.63	647.61	647.60	condition	
with fetal damage	655.33	655.31	655.30		763.89
Disorders					
breast	676.33	676.31	676.30		
genital tract or organ	646.63	646.61	646.60	condition	760.8
lactation	676.93	676.91	676.90		
liver	646.73	646.71	646.70	condition	760.8
mental	648.43	648.41	648.40	condition	
metabolism NEC (in labor and delivery)	669.03	669.01	669.00		763.89
Displacement, uterus NEC	654.43	654.41	654.40		763.89
causing obstructed labor	660.23	660.21	660.20	cause	763.1
Disproportion	653.93	653.91	653.90		763.1
caused by					
conjoined twins	653.73	653.71	653.70		763.1
contraction, pelvis (general)	653.13	653.11	653.10		763.1
inlet	653.23	653.21	653.20		763.1
midpelvic	653.83	653.81	653.80		763.1
midplane	653.83	653.81	653.80		763.1
outlet	653.33	653.31	653.30		763.1
fetal NEC	653.53	653.51	653.50		763.1
ascites	653.73	653.71	653.70		763.1
hydrocephalus	653.63	653.61	653.60		763.1
hydrops	653.73	653.71	653.70		763.1
meningomyelocele	653.73	653.71	653.70		763.1
sacral teratoma	653.73	653.71	653.70		763.1
tumor	653.73	653.71	653.70		763.1
hydrocephalic fetus	653.63	653.61	653.60		763.1
pelvis, pelvic, abnormality (bony) NEC	653.03	653.01	653.00		763.1
unusually large fetus	653.53	653.51	653.50		763.1
causing obstructed labor	660.13	660.11	660.10	cause	763.1
cephalopelvic, normally formed fetus	653.43	653.41	653.40		763.1
fetopelvic, normally formed fetus	653.43	653.41	653.40		763.1
causing obstructed labor	660.13	660.11	660.10	cause	763.1
pelvis, pelvic (bony) NEC	653.13	653.11	653.10		763.1
causing obstructed labor	660.13	660.11	660.10	cause	763.1
specified type NEC	653.83	653.81	653.80		763.1
Distortion					
lumbar spine					
with disproportion (fetopelvic)	653.03	653.01	653.00		763.1
causing obstructed labor	660.13	660.11	660.10	cause	763.1
maternal	669.03	669.01	669.00		
Distress (fetal)	656.83	656.81	656.80		763.89

Coding Tables

Antepartum Pregnancy

Antepartum Pregnancy Condition or Complication; affecting management of mother	Antepartum condition or complication	Delivered, with or without mention of antepartum condition	Unspecified episode of care	Assign additional code to describe the…	Affecting fetus (coded on the newborn chart only)
Double uterus	654.03	654.01	654.00		763.89
causing obstructed labor	660.23	660.21	660.20	cause	763.1
Dropsy, amnion	657.03	657.01	657.00		761.3
Drug dependence	648.33	648.31	648.30	condition	
Dyscrasia, blood					
with antepartum hemorrhage	641.33	641.31	641.30		762.1
Dysfunction					
thyroid	648.13	648.11	648.10	condition	
uterus, complicating delivery	661.93	661.91	661.90		763.7
hypertonic	661.43	661.41	661.40		763.7
hypotonic, primary	661.03	661.01	661.00		763.7
secondary	661.13	661.11	661.10		763.7
Dysplasia of cervix	654.63	654.61	654.60		763.89
causing obstructed labor	660.23	660.21	660.20	cause	763.1
Dystocia	660.93	660.91	660.90	cause	763.1
cervical	661.23	661.21	661.20		763.7
contraction ring	661.43	661.41	661.40		763.7
fetal	660.93	660.91	660.90	cause	763.1
abnormal size	653.53	653.51	653.50		763.1
causing obstructed labor	660.13	660.11	660.10	cause	763.1
deformity	653.73	653.71	653.70		763.1
causing obstructed labor	660.13	660.11	660.10	cause	763.1
maternal	660.93	660.91	660.90		763.1
positional	660.03	660.01	660.00	cause	763.1
shoulder (girdle)	660.43	660.41	660.40	cause	763.1
uterine NEC	661.43	661.41	661.40		763.7
Early onset of delivery (spontaneous)		644.21	644.20		
Preterm neonate birthweight					
Extreme immaturity (code also weeks of gestation, codes 765.20-765.29)					
unspecified (weight)					765.00
< 500 gms					765.11
500-749 gms					765.02
750-999 gms					765.03
1,000-1,249 gms					765.04
1,250-1,499 gms					765.05
1,500-1,749 gms					765.06
1,750-1,999 gms					765.07
2,000-2,499 gms					765.08
≥ 2,500 gms					765.09
Other preterm (code also weeks of gestation, codes 765.20-765.29)					
unspecified (weight)					765.10
< 500 gms					765.11
500-749 gms					765.12
750-999 gms					765.13
1,000-1,249 gms					765.14
1,250-1,499 gms					765.15
1,500-1,749 gms					765.16
1,750-1,999 gms					765.17
2,000-2,499 gms					765.18
≥ 2,500 gms					765.19
Preterm neonate weeks of gestation (code in addition to birthweight, subcategory codes 765.0 and 765.1)					
unspecified weeks of gestation					765.20
< 24 completed weeks of gestation					765.21
24 completed weeks of gestation					765.22
25-26 completed weeks of gestation					765.23
27-28 completed weeks of gestation					765.24
29-30 completed weeks of gestation					765.25
31-32 completed weeks of gestation					765.26
33-34 completed weeks of gestation					765.27
35-36 completed weeks of gestation					765.28
≥ 37 completed weeks of gestation					765.29

Antepartum Pregnancy Condition or Complication; affecting management of mother	Antepartum condition or complication	Delivered, with or without mention of antepartum condition	Unspecified episode of care	Assign additional code to describe the…	Affecting fetus (coded on the newborn chart only)
Eclampsia, eclamptic (coma) (convulsions) (delirium)	642.63	642.61	642.60		760.0
with pre-existing hypertension	642.73	642.71	642.70		760.0
Edema	646.13	646.11	646.10	condition	
with hypertension — *see* Pregnancy, toxemia					
Effect, adverse					
anesthetic (in labor and delivery) NEC	668.93	668.91	668.90		763.5
radiation (suspected damage to fetus)	655.63	655.61	655.60	condition	
Effusion, amniotic fluid	658.13	658.11	658.10		761.1
delayed delivery following	658.23	658.21	658.20		761.1
Electrolyte imbalance with hyperemesis gravidarum (before 22 completed weeks' gestation)	643.13	643.11	643.10		761.8
Embolism					
air (pulmonary)	673.03	673.01	673.00		
amniotic fluid	673.13	673.11	673.10		
blood clot	673.23	673.21	673.20		
brain	674.03	674.01	674.00		
cerebral	674.03	674.01	674.00		
fat (cerebral) (pulmonary) (systemic)	673.83	673.81	673.80		
intracranial (venous sinus) (nonpyogenic)	671.53	671.51	671.50		
pulmonary NEC	673.23	673.21	673.20		
pyemic	673.33	673.31	673.30		
septic	673.33	673.31	673.30		
Emesis (gravidarum) — *see* Pregnancy, vomiting					
Endometritis	646.63	646.61	646.60	condition	760.8
decidual	646.63	646.61	646.60	condition	760.8
Engorgement, breast	676.23	676.21	676.20		
Entanglement, umbilical cord(s)	663.33	663.31	663.30		762.5
with compression	663.23	663.21	663.20		762.5
around neck with compression	663.13	663.11	663.10		762.5
twins in monoamniotic sac	663.23	663.21	663.20		762.5
Epilepsy	649.43	649.41	649.40	345.00-345.91	
Excessive					
large (fetus)	656.63	656.61	656.60		766.0
with obstructed labor	660.13	660.11	660.10	cause	763.1
causing disproportion	653.53	653.51	653.50		763.1
causing obstructed labor	660.13	660.11	660.10	cause	763.1
milk secretion	676.63	676.61	676.60		
weight gain	646.13	646.11	646.10	condition	
Exhaustion (complicating delivery)	669.83	669.81	669.80		763.89
Extraction					
breech NEC		669.61	669.60		763.0
manual NEC	669.83	669.81	669.80		763.89
Face presentation	652.43	652.41	652.40		763.1
causing obstructed labor	660.03	660.01	660.00	cause	763.1
Failure, failed					
cervical dilation in labor	661.03	661.01	661.00		763.7
descent of head (at term)	652.53	652.51	652.50		763.1
in labor	660.03	660.01	660.00	cause	763.1
engagement of head NEC	652.53	652.51	652.50		763.1
in labor	660.03	660.01	660.00	cause	763.1
fetal head to enter pelvic brim	652.53	652.51	652.50		763.1
in labor	660.03	660.01	660.00	cause	763.1
forceps NEC	660.73	660.71	660.70	cause	763.1
heart, complicating					
delivery (cesarean) (instrumental)	669.43	669.41	669.40		
obstetric anesthesia or sedation	668.13	668.11	668.10		
induction (of labor)	659.13	659.11	659.10		763.89
by oxytocic drugs (Pitocin)	659.13	659.11	659.10		763.89
instrumental	659.03	659.01	659.00		763.89
mechanical	659.03	659.01	659.00		763.89
medical	659.13	659.11	659.10		763.89
surgical	659.03	659.01	659.00		763.89
lactation	676.43	676.41	676.40		
to progress	661.23	661.21	661.20		763.89
trial of labor NOS	660.63	660.61	660.60	cause	763.1

Coding Tables

Antepartum Pregnancy

Antepartum Pregnancy Condition or Complication; affecting management of mother	Antepartum condition or complication	Delivered, with or without mention of antepartum condition	Unspecified episode of care	Assign additional code to describe the…	Affecting fetus (coded on the newborn chart only)
Failure, failed — *continued*					
vacuum extraction delivery NOS	660.73	660.71	660.70	cause	763.1
ventouse NOS	660.73	660.71	660.70	cause	763.1
False labor (pains)	644.13		644.10		
False positive pregnancy	631.0				
Fatigue	646.83	646.81	646.80	condition	
Fatty metamorphosis of liver	646.73	646.71	646.70	condition	760.8
Female genital mutilation	648.93	648.91	648.90	629.20-629	
Fetal					
acidosis	656.33	656.31	656.30		763.89
anemia	678.03	678.01	678.00		
following blood loss (affecting newborn)					776.5
bradycardia	659.73	659.71	659.70		763.83
before onset of labor	659.73	659.71	659.70		763.81
during labor	659.73	659.71	659.70		763.82
complication from in utero procedure	679.13	679.11	679.10		
decreased movements	655.73	655.71	655.70		763.89
demise (near term)	656.43	656.41	656.40	cause	
early (before 22 weeks completed gestation)	632				761.8
deformity	653.73	653.71	653.70		763.1
causing obstructed labor	660.13	660.11	660.10	cause	763.1
distress	656.83	656.81	656.80		
heart rate, abnormal	659.73	659.71	659.70		763.83
before onset of labor	659.73	659.71	659.70		763.81
during labor	659.73	659.71	659.70		763.82
heart rhythm, abnormal	659.73	659.71	659.70		763.83
before onset of labor	659.73	659.71	659.70		763.81
during labor	659.73	659.71	659.70		763.82
hematologic conditions	678.03	678.01	678.00		
movements, decreased	655.73	655.71	655.70		
thrombocytopenia	678.03	678.01	678.00		
twin to twin transfusion	678.03	678.01	678.00		
Fetomaternal hemorrhage	656.03	656.01	656.00		772.0
Fibrinolysis	641.33	641.31	641.30		762.1
Fibroid tumor(s)	654.13	654.11	654.10		763.89
causing obstructed labor	660.23	660.21	660.20	cause	763.1
Fibromyoma (uterus)	654.13	654.11	654.10		763.89
causing obstructed labor	660.23	660.21	660.20	cause	763.1
Fibrosis, fibrotic					
amnion	658.83	658.81	658.80		
chorion	658.83	658.81	658.80		
perineum	654.83	654.81	654.80		763.8
causing obstructed labor	660.23	660.21	660.20	cause	763.1
Fissure, nipple	676.13	676.11	676.10		
Fistula					
breast	675.13	675.11	675.10		
mammary gland	675.13	675.11	675.10		
Flat, pelvis					
with disproportion (fetopelvic)	653.23	653.21	653.20		763.1
causing obstructed labor	660.13	660.11	660.10	cause	763.1
Footling presentation	652.83	652.81	652.80		
with successful version	652.13	652.11	652.10		
Forced birth or delivery NEC		669.81	669.80		763.89
Forceps delivery NEC		669.51	669.50		763.2
Fractured coccyx complicating delivery		665.61	665.60		
Frommel's disease	676.63	676.61	676.60		
Frommel-Chiari syndrome	676.63	676.61	676.60		
Funnel pelvis with disproportion (fetopelvic)	653.33	653.31	653.30		763.1
causing obstructed labor	660.13	660.11	660.10	cause	763.1
Fusion, hymeno-urethral					
causing obstructed labor	660.13	660.11	660.10	cause	763.1
Galactocele (breast)	676.83	676.81	676.80		
Galactorrhea	676.63	676.61	676.60		
Genital (female) **mutilation**	648.93	648.91	648.90	629.20-629.29	
Goiter	648.13	648.11	648.10	condition	
Gonococcal infection	647.13	647.11	647.10	condition	760.2

Antepartum Pregnancy Condition or Complication; affecting management of mother	Antepartum condition or complication	Delivered, with or without mention of antepartum condition	Unspecified episode of care	Assign additional code to describe the…	Affecting fetus (coded on the newborn chart only)
Gonorrhea	647.13	647.11	647.10	condition	760.2
Grand multiparity, affecting labor and delivery	659.43	659.41	659.40		
Growth fetal (poor)	656.53	656.51	656.50		764.90
Heart (fetal)					
abnormal					
rate	659.73	659.71	659.70		763.81
before onset of labor	659.73	659.71	659.70		763.81
during labor	659.73	659.71	659.70		763.82
rhythm	659.73	659.71	659.70		763.83
before onset of labor	659.73	659.71	659.70		763.81
during labor	659.73	659.71	659.70		763.82
HELLP (Hemolysis, Elevated Liver function and Low Platelets)	642.53	642.51	642.50		
Hematoma					
amnion	658.83	658.81	658.80		
broad ligament		665.71	665.70		
complicating delivery (perineum) (vulva)		664.51	664.50		
pelvic		665.71	665.70	665.71	
vagina		665.71	665.70		
pelvis, complicating delivery		665.71	665.70		
perineal wound complicating delivery		664.51	664.50		
umbilical cord	663.63	663.61	663.60		762.6
vagina		665.71	665.70		
vulva, complicating delivery		664.51	664.50		767.8
Hemolysis, intravascular	641.33	641.31	641.30		762.1
Hemolysis, elevated liver function, low platelets syndrome (HELLP)	642.53	642.51	642.50		
Hemorrhage					
accidental	641.23	641.21	641.20		762.1
before 22 completed weeks gestation NEC	640.93	640.91	640.90		
brain	674.03	674.01	674.00		
cerebrovascular	674.03	674.01	674.00		
complicating delivery	641.93	641.91	641.90		762.1
associated with					
afibrinogenemia	641.33	641.31	641.30		763.89
coagulation defect	641.33	641.31	641.30		763.89
hyperfibrinolysis	641.33	641.31	641.30		763.89
hypofibrinogenemia	641.33	641.31	641.30		763.89
concealed	641.93	641.91	641.90		762.1
due to					
afibrinogenemia or other coagulation defect	641.33	641.31	641.30	condition	763.89
fibroids	641.83	641.81	641.80		763.89
low-lying placenta	641.13	641.11	641.10		762.0
marginal sinus (rupture)	641.23	641.21	641.20		762.1
placenta previa	641.13	641.11	641.10		762.0
premature separation, placenta	641.23	641.21	641.20		762.1
trauma	641.83	641.81	641.80		763.89
umbilicus, umbilical cord	663.83	663.81	663.80		772.0
due to					
afibrinogenemia or other coagulation defect	641.33	641.31	641.30	condition	762.1
fibroids	641.83	641.81	641.80		762.1
low-lying placenta	641.13	641.11	641.10		762.1
marginal sinus					
(rupture)	641.23	641.21	641.20		762.1
placenta previa	641.13	641.11	641.10		762.0
premature separation, placenta	641.23	641.21	641.20		762.1
trauma	641.83	641.81	641.80		763.89
umbilicus, umbilical cord	663.83	663.81	663.80		772.0
early (before 22 completed weeks gestation)	640.93	640.91	640.90		762.1
fetomaternal	656.03	656.01	656.00		772.0
funis (complicating delivery)	663.83	663.81	663.80		772.0
intracranial	674.03	674.01	674.00		
marginal sinus	641.23	641.21	641.20		762.1
placenta NEC	641.93	641.91	641.90		762.1
from surgical or instrumental damage	641.83	641.81	641.80		762.1
previa	641.13	641.11	641.10		762.0

Coding Tables

Antepartum Pregnancy

Antepartum Pregnancy Condition or Complication; affecting management of mother	Antepartum condition or complication	Delivered, with or without mention of antepartum condition	Unspecified episode of care	Assign additional code to describe the…	Affecting fetus (coded on the newborn chart only)
Hemorrhage — *continued*					
retroplacental	641.23	641.21	641.20		762.1
subarachnoid	674.03	674.01	674.00		
subdural	674.03	674.01	674.00		
threatened abortion	640.03	640.01	640.00		
umbilicus, umbilical cord (complicating delivery)	663.83	663.81	663.80		772.0
unavoidable	641.13	641.11	641.10		762.0
vasa previa	663.53	663.51	663.50		772.0
Hemorrhoids	671.83	671.81	671.80		
Hepatitis	646.73	646.71	646.70	condition	
viral	647.63	647.61	647.60	condition	
Herniation of uterus	654.43	654.41	654.40		
causing obstructed labor	660.23	660.21	660.20	cause	763.1
Herpes, herpetic	647.63	647.61	647.60	condition	
gestationis	646.83	646.81	646.80	condition	
High head at term	652.43	652.41	652.40		763.1
HIV	647.63	647.61	647.60	042	
asymptomatic	647.63	647.61	647.60	V08	
Hourglass uterus	661.43	661.41	661.40		763.7
Hydatidiform mole	630				
previous pregnancy, affecting management of current pregnancy	V23.1	V23.1	V23.1		
Hydramnios	657.03	657.01	657.00		761.3
Hydroa gestationis	646.83	646.81	646.80	condition	
Hydrocephalic fetus	655.03	655.01	655.00		763.1
causing disproportion	653.63	653.61	653.60		763.1
with obstructed labor	660.13	660.11	660.10	cause	763.1
Hydrops amnii	657.03	657.01	657.00		
Hydrorrhea	658.13	658.11	658.10		
Hyperemesis					
before 22 completed weeks of gestation	643.03	643.01	643.00		761.8
with					
carbohydrate depletion	643.13	643.11	643.10		761.8
dehydration	643.13	643.11	643.10		761.8
electrolyte imbalance	643.13	643.11	643.10		761.8
metabolic disturbance	643.13	643.11	643.10		761.8
mild	643.03	643.01	643.00		761.8
severe with metabolic disturbance	643.13	643.11	643.10		761.8
late (starting 23rd week of gestation)	643.23	643.21	643.20		761.8
Hypersecretion of milk	676.63	676.61	676.60		
Hypertension	642.93	642.91	642.90		760.0
with					
albuminuria (and edema) (mild)	642.43	642.41	642.40		760.0
severe	642.53	642.51	642.50		760.0
edema (mild)	642.43	642.41	642.40		760.0
severe	642.53	642.51	642.50		760.0
heart disease	642.23	642.21	642.20		760.0
and renal disease	642.23	642.21	642.20		760.0
pre-eclampsia or eclampsia	642.73	642.71	642.70		760.0
renal disease	642.23	642.21	642.20		760.0
and heart disease	642.23	642.21	642.20		760.0
benign	642.03	642.01	642.00		760.0
chronic	642.03	642.01	642.00		760.0
pre-existing	642.03	642.01	642.00		760.0
chronic	642.03	642.01	642.00		760.0
essential	642.03	642.01	642.00		760.0
with pre-eclampsia or eclampsia	642.73	642.71	642.70		760.0
gestational	642.33	642.31	642.30		
malignant	642.23	642.21	642.20		760.0
chronic	642.23	642.21	642.20		760.0
with pre-eclampsia or eclampsia	642.73	642.71	642.70		760.0
pre-existing	642.23	642.21	642.20		760.0
pre-existing	642.03	642.01	642.00		
secondary to renal disease	642.13	642.11	642.10		760.0
with pre-eclampsia or eclampsia	642.73	642.71	642.70		760.0
transient	642.33	642.31	642.30		

Antepartum Pregnancy

Condition or Complication; affecting management of mother	Antepartum condition or complication	Delivered, with or without mention of antepartum condition	Unspecified episode of care	Assign additional code to describe the…	Affecting fetus (coded on the newborn chart only)
Hypertensive					
heart and renal disease	642.23	642.21	642.20		760.0
heart disease	642.23	642.21	642.20		760.0
renal disease	642.23	642.21	642.20		760.0
Hyperthyroidism	648.13	648.11	648.10	condition	
Hypertonicity	648.13	648.11	648.10	condition	763.7
Hypertrophy					
breast	676.33	676.31	676.30		
Hypotension (following labor and delivery)	669.23	669.21	669.20		
Hypothyroidism	648.13	648.11	648.10	condition	
Hysteralgia	646.83	646.81	646.80	condition	
Icterus gravis	646.73	646.71	646.70	condition	760.8
Illegitimate	V61.6	V61.6	V61.6		
Imbalance					
electrolyte with hyperemesis gravidarum (before 22 completed weeks' gestation)	643.13	643.11	643.10		
Immunization					
ABO	656.23	656.21	656.20		773.1
Rh factor	656.13	656.11	656.10		773.0
Immunodeficiency to Rh factor	656.13	656.11	656.10		773.0
Impacted shoulder	660.43	660.41	660.40	cause	763.1
Inadequate development of fetus	656.53	656.51	656.50		764.90
Incarceration, uterus	654.33	654.31	654.30		763.1
causing obstructed labor	660.23	660.21	660.20	cause	763.1
Incompatibility, blood groups (ABO)					
ABO	656.23	656.21	656.20		773.1
Blood (group) (Duffy) (E) (K(ell)) (Kidd) (Lewis) (M) (N) (P) (S) NEC	656.23	656.21	656.20		773.2
Rh(esus) (blood group) (factor)	656.13	656.11	656.10		773.0
Incompetent cervix (os)	654.53	654.51	654.50		761.0
causing obstructed labor	660.23	660.21	660.20	cause	763.1
Incoordinate uterus (action) (contractions)	661.43	661.41	661.40		763.7
In double uterus	654.03	654.01	654.00		
causing obstructed labor	660.23	660.21	660.20	cause	763.1
Induced					
failed by method of					
drugs	659.13	659.11	659.10		
mechanical	659.03	659.01	659.00		
successful — assign code to indicate the reason for the induction					763.89
Indurated breast	676.33	676.31	676.30		
Inertia, uterus NEC					
primary	661.03	661.01	661.00		763.7
secondary	661.13	661.11	661.10		763.7
Infantile					
genitalia, genitals	654.43	654.41	654.40		763.89
causing obstructed labor	660.23	660.21	660.20	cause	763.1
pelvis	653.13	653.11	653.10		763.1
causing obstructed labor	660.13	660.11	660.10	cause	763.1
Infarct, infarction					
amnion	658.83	658.81	658.80		
brain (stem)	674.03	674.01	674.00		
chorion	658.83	658.81	658.80		
lung — see Pregnancy, embolism					
placenta	656.73	656.71	656.70		762.2
Infection	647.93	647.91	647.90	condition	760.2
amniotic fluid	658.43	658.41	658.40	condition	762.7
bladder	646.63	646.61	646.60	condition	
breast (mammary gland)	675.23	675.21	675.20		
with nipple	675.93	675.91	675.90		
specified type NEC	675.83	675.81	675.80		
nonpurulent	675.23	675.21	675.20		
purulent	675.13	675.11	675.10		
chorionic plate	658.83	658.81	658.80		
genital organs	646.63	646.61	646.60	condition	760.8
minor or localized	646.63	646.61	646.60	condition	760.8

Coding Tables (side margin)

Antepartum Pregnancy (side margin)

Antepartum Pregnancy Condition or Complication; affecting management of mother	Antepartum condition or complication	Delivered, with or without mention of antepartum condition	Unspecified episode of care	Assign additional code to describe the…	Affecting fetus (coded on the newborn chart only)
Infection — *continued*					
intrauterine, complicating delivery	646.63	646.61	646.60	condition	
kidney	646.63	646.61	646.60	condition	760.1
nipple	675.03	675.01	675.00		
with breast	675.93	675.91	675.90		
specified type NEC	675.83	675.81	675.80		
perineal wound minor	646.63	646.61	646.60	condition	760.1
urinary (tract)	646.63	646.61	646.60	condition	760.1
asymptomatic	646.53	646.51	646.50	condition	760.1
UTI	646.63	646.61	646.60	condition	760.1
asymptomatic	646.53	646.51	646.50	condition	760.1
Infective and parasitic diseases NEC	647.83	647.81	647.80	complication	
Infestation	647.93	647.91	647.90	condition	760.8
Inflammation					
areola	675.03	675.01	675.00		
bladder	646.63	646.61	646.60	condition	760.8
breast (mammary gland)	675.23	675.21	675.20		
fetal membranes (acute)	658.43	658.41	658.40		762.7
genital organ	646.63	646.61	646.60	condition	760.8
urinary tract NEC	646.63	646.61	646.60	condition	760.8
Inhalation of stomach contents or secretions in labor and delivery	668.03	668.01	668.00		
Injury	648.93	648.91	648.90	condition	
birth canal NEC	665.93	665.91	665.90		763.89
coccyx, complicating delivery		665.61	665.60		
genital organs, obstetrical					
trauma NEC	665.93	665.91	665.90		763.89
instrumental, obstetrical NEC	665.93	665.91	665.90		763.89
bladder		665.51	665.50		763.89
cervix		665.31	665.30		763.89
high vaginal		665.41	665.40		763.89
perineal NEC		664.91	664.90		763.89
urethra		665.51	665.50		763.89
uterus		665.51	665.50		763.89
obstetrical NEC	665.93	665.91	665.90		763.89
floor		664.11	664.10		763.89
joint or ligament		665.61	665.60		763.89
organs		665.51	665.50		763.89
periurethral tissue, complicating delivery		665.51	665.50		763.89
symphysis pubis, complicating delivery		665.61	665.60		763.89
Insertion of umbilical cord, lateral or velamentous	663.53	663.51	663.50		762.6
Insufficient					
prenatal care	V23.7				
weight gain	646.83	646.81	646.80	condition	
Interstitial — *see* Ectopic pregnancy	633.8x				
Intoxication					
chemical via placenta or breast milk, suspected	655.53	655.51	655.50		760.70
drug					
obstetric anesthetic or sedation	668.93	668.91	668.90		763.5
via placenta or breast milk, suspected	655.53	655.51	655.50		760.70
septic					
during labor	659.33	659.31	659.30		
Intraligamentous — *see* Ectopic pregnancy	633.8x				
Intramural — *see* Ectopic pregnancy	633.8x				
Intraperitoneal — *see* Ectopic pregnancy	633.0x				
Intrauterine fetal death					
early (before 22 completed weeks of gestation)	632				
near term NEC	656.43	656.41	656.40		
In utero procedure					
fetal complication	679.13	679.11	679.10		
maternal complication	679.03	679.01	679.00		
Inversion					
nipple	676.33	676.31	676.30		
Ischemia, cerebral	674.03	674.01	674.00		
Isoimmunization (ABO)	656.23	656.21	656.20		
Rh(esus)	656.13	656.11	656.10		

Antepartum Pregnancy Condition or Complication; affecting management of mother	Antepartum condition or complication	Delivered, with or without mention of antepartum condition	Unspecified episode of care	Assign additional code to describe the…	Affecting fetus (coded on the newborn chart only)
Isthmian (with rupture) — *see* Ectopic Pregnancy	633.1x				
Joint disorders	648.73	648.71	648.70	condition	
Kidney					
disease or failure NEC	646.23	646.21	646.20	condition	
with secondary hypertension	642.13	642.11	642.10		
hypertensive	642.23	642.21	642.20		
Knot, umbilical cord (true)	663.23	663.21	663.20		762.5
Labor					
abnormal NEC	661.93	661.91	661.90		763.7
arrested active phase	661.13	661.11	661.10		763.7
desultory	661.23	661.21	661.20		763.7
dyscoordinate	661.43	661.41	661.40		763.7
early onset (22-36 weeks gestation)		644.21	644.20		763.7
failed					763.7
induction	659.13	659.11	659.10		763.89
mechanical	659.03	659.01	659.00		763.89
medical (drug)	659.13	659.11	659.10		763.89
surgical	659.03	659.01	659.00		763.89
trial (vaginal delivery)	660.63	660.61	660.60	cause	763.1
false	644.13		644.10		
hypertonic	661.43	661.41	661.40		763.7
hypotonic, primary	661.03	661.01	661.00		763.7
secondary	661.13	661.11	661.10		763.7
incoordinate	661.43	661.41	661.40		763.7
irregular	661.23	661.21	661.20		763.7
long	662.13	662.11	662.10		763.89
first stage	662.03	662.01	662.00		763.89
second stage	662.23	662.21	662.20		763.89
missed (at or near term)	656.43	656.41	656.40		
obstructed NEC	660.93	660.91	660.90	cause	763.1
specified cause NEC	660.83	660.81	660.80	cause	763.1
onset (spontaneous) after 37 completed weeks of gestation but before 39 completed weeks of gestation, with delivery by (planned) cesarean section		649.81			
pains, spurious	644.13		644.10		
precipitate	661.33	661.31	661.30		763.6
premature		644.21	644.20		
threatened	644.03		644.00		
prolonged or protracted	662.13	662.11	662.10		763.89
first stage	662.03	662.01	662.00		763.89
second stage	662.23	662.21	662.20		763.89
threatened NEC	644.13		644.10		
undelivered	644.13		644.10		
Laceration (obstetrical trauma)					
Anus, anal (sphincter)complicating delivery					
with third degree perineal laceration		664.21	664.20		763.89
w/mucosa		664.31	664.30		763.89
w/o third degree perineal laceration		664.61	664.60		763.89
old (healed)		654.81	654.80		763.89
bladder		665.51	665.50		
bowel		665.51	665.50		
broad ligament		665.61	665.60		
central, complicating delivery		664.41	664.40		
cervix (uteri)		665.31	665.30		
fourchette, complicating delivery		664.01	664.00		
labia, complicating delivery		664.01	664.00		
pelvic (complicating delivery)					
floor (muscles)		664.11	664.10		
organ NEC (obstetrical trauma)		665.51	665.50		763.89
perineum, complicating delivery		664.41	664.40		
first degree		664.01	664.00		
second degree		664.11	664.10		
third degree		664.21	664.20		
fourth degree		664.31	664.30		

Coding Tables *(left margin)*

Antepartum Pregnancy *(left margin)*

Antepartum Pregnancy Condition or Complication; affecting management of mother	Antepartum condition or complication	Delivered, with or without mention of antepartum condition	Unspecified episode of care	Assign additional code to describe the…	Affecting fetus (coded on the newborn chart only)
Laceration (obstetrical trauma) — *continued*					
perineum, complicating delivery — *continued*					
involving					
anal sphincter		664.21	664.20		
fourchette		664.01	664.00		
hymen		664.01	664.00		
labia		664.01	664.00		
pelvic floor		664.11	664.10		
perineal muscles		664.11	664.10		
rectovaginal with septum		664.21	664.20		
with anal mucosa		664.31	664.30		
skin		664.01	664.00		
sphincter (anal)		664.21	664.20		
with anal mucosa		664.31	664.30		
vagina		664.01	664.00		
vaginal muscles		664.11	664.10		
vulva		664.01	664.00		
peritoneum (obstetrical trauma)		665.51	665.50		
periurethral tissue (obstetrical trauma)		665.51	665.50		
rectovaginal septum		665.41	665.40		
with perineum		664.21	664.20		
involving anal or rectal mucosa		664.31	664.30		
urethra (obstetrical trauma)		665.51	665.50		
uterus (obstetrical trauma NEC)		665.11	665.10		
vagina (complicating delivery)		665.41	665.40		
with perineal involvement		664.01	664.00		
first degree		664.01	664.00		
second degree		664.11	664.10		
third degree		664.21	664.20		
fourth degree		664.31	664.30		
high		664.41	664.40		
muscles		664.11	664.10		
sulcus		665.41	665.40		
wall		665.41	665.40		
vulva (complicating delivery)		664.01	664.00		
Lactation, lactating (breast)					
defective	676.43	676.41	676.40		
disorder	676.93	676.91	676.90		
specified type NEC	676.83	676.81	676.80		
examination and/or care of mother	V24.1	V24.1	V24.1		
excessive	676.63	676.61	676.60		
failed	676.43	676.41	676.40		
mastitis NEC	675.23	675.21	675.20		
suppressed	676.53	676.51	676.50		
Large					
fetus causing disproportion	653.53	653.51	653.50		763.1
with obstructed labor	660.13	660.11	660.10	cause	763.1
for-dates (fetus)	656.63	656.61	656.60		766.1
exceptionally (weight of 4500 grams or more)	656.63	656.61	656.60		766.0
childbirth complication(s)	677	677	677	condition	
Late effect(s) (of)					
complication(s) of					
childbirth	677	677	677	condition	
delivery	677	677	677	condition	
postpartum	677	677	677	condition	
pregnancy	677	677	677	condition	
puerperium	677	677	677	condition	
Lateroversion, uterus	654.43	654.41	654.40		763.89
causing obstructed labor	660.23	660.21	660.20	cause	763.1
Leakage					
amniotic fluid	658.13	658.11	658.10		761.1
with delayed delivery	658.23	658.21	658.20		761.1
blood (microscopic), fetal, into maternal circulation	656.03	656.01	656.00		
Lesion, vascular of umbilical cord	663.63	663.61	663.60		762.6
Light-for-dates	656.53	656.51	656.50		764.00
with signs of fetal malnutrition	656.53	656.51	656.50		764.10

Coding Tables

Antepartum Pregnancy

Antepartum Pregnancy Condition or Complication; affecting management of mother	Antepartum condition or complication	Delivered, with or without mention of antepartum condition	Unspecified episode of care	Assign additional code to describe the…	Affecting fetus (coded on the newborn chart only)
Listeriosis, suspected fetal damage	655.43	655.41	655.40		771.2
Lithopedion	656.83	656.81	656.80		
Locked twins	660.53	660.51	660.50	cause	763.1
Lymphadenitis, breast	675.23	675.21	675.20		
breast	675.23	675.21	675.20		
Malaria	647.43	647.41	647.40	condition	
Male type pelvis with disproportion (fetopelvic)	653.23	653.21	653.20		763.1
causing obstructed labor	660.13	660.11	660.10	cause	763.1
Malformation					
pelvic organs or tissues	654.93	654.91	654.90		763.89
causing obstructed labor	660.23	660.21	660.20	cause	763.1
placenta	656.73	656.71	656.70		
umbilical cord (complicating delivery)	663.93	663.91	663.90		762.6
uterus (congenital)	654.03	654.01	654.00		
causing obstructed labor	660.23	660.21	660.20	cause	763.1
Malnutrition	648.93	648.91	648.90	condition	
Fetal malnutrition					
Without mention of "light-for dates"					
unspecified (weight)					764.20
< 500 gms					764.21
500-749 gms					764.22
750-999 gms					764.23
1,000-1,249 gms					764.24
1,250-1,499 gms					764.25
1,500-1,749 gms					764.26
1,750-1,999 gms					764.27
2,000-2,499 gms					764.28
≥ 2,500 gms					764.29
With mention of "light-for dates" unspecified (weight)					764.10
< 500 gms					764.11
500-749 gms					764.12
750-999 gms					764.13
1,000-1,249 gms					764.14
1,250-1,499 gms					764.15
1,500-1,749 gms					764.16
1,750-1,999 gms					764.17
2,000-2,499 gms					764.18
≥ 2,500 gms					764.19
Malposition					
fetal NEC	652.93	652.91	652.90		763.1
with successful version	652.13	652.11	652.10		763.1
before labor	652.93	652.91	652.90		763.1
in multiple gestation	652.63	652.61	652.60		763.1
with locking	660.53	660.51	660.50	cause	763.1
causing obstructed labor	660.03	660.01	660.00	cause	763.1
pelvic organs or tissues	654.43	654.41	654.40		763.89
causing obstructed labor	660.23	660.21	660.20	cause	763.1
specified type NEC	652.83	652.81	652.80		763.1
causing obstructed labor	660.03	660.01	660.00	cause	763.1
uterus or cervix	654.43	654.41	654.40		763.89
causing obstructed labor	660.23	660.21	660.20	cause	763.1
Malpresentation					
fetal	652.93	652.91	652.90		763.1
with successful version	652.13	652.11	652.10		763.1
in multiple gestation	652.63	652.61	652.60		763.1
specified type NEC	652.83	652.81	652.80		763.1
causing obstructed labor	660.03	660.01	660.00	cause	763.1
uterus or cervix	654.43	654.41	654.40		
causing obstructed labor	660.03	660.01	660.00	cause	763.1
Mammillitis, puerperal	675.23	675.21	675.20		
Mammitis, puerperal	675.23	675.21	675.20		
Marginal sinus hemorrhage or rupture	641.23	641.21	641.20		762.1
Mastitis					
lactational	675.23	675.21	675.20		

Coding Tables

Antepartum Pregnancy

Antepartum Pregnancy Condition or Complication; affecting management of mother	**Antepartum condition or complication**	**Delivered, with or without mention of antepartum condition**	**Unspecified episode of care**	**Assign additional code to describe the...**	**Affecting fetus (coded on the newborn chart only)**
Mastitis — *continued*					
puerperal, (interstitial) (nonpurulent) (parenchymatous)	675.23	675.21	675.20		
purulent	675.13	675.11	675.10		
stagnation	675.23	675.21	675.20		
puerperalis	675.23	675.21	675.20		
retromammary	675.13	675.11	675.10		
submammary	675.13	675.11	675.10		
Maternal obesity syndrome	646.13	646.11	646.10	condition	
Meconium in liquor (staining)	656.83	656.81	656.80		
Membranitis, fetal	658.43	658.41	658.40		762.7
Mendelson's syndrome	668.03	668.01	668.00		
Menstruation during pregnancy	640.83	640.81	640.80		
Mental disorders	648.43	648.41	648.40	condition	
Mentum presentation	652.43	652.41	652.40		763.1
causing obstructed labor	660.03	660.01	660.00	cause	763.1
Metaplasia squamous cell amnion	658.83	658.81	658.80		763.89
Milk					
excess secretion	676.63	676.61	676.60		
Milk leg (deep vessels)	671.33	671.31	671.30		
Missed					
delivery (at or near term)	656.43	656.41	656.40		763.89
labor (at or near term)	656.43	656.41	656.40		763.89
Morning sickness	643.03	643.01	643.00		
Multiparity (grand)	659.43	659.41	659.40		763.89
Myelomeningocele fetal, causing fetopelvic disproportion	653.73	653.71	653.70		763.1
causing obstructed labor	660.13	660.11	660.10	cause	763.1
Myoma uterus (cervix) (corpus)	654.13	654.11	654.10		763.89
causing obstructed labor	660.23	660.21	660.20	cause	763.1
Nägele's pelvis with disproportion (fetopelvic)	653.03	653.01	653.00		763.1
causing obstructed labor	660.13	660.11	660.10	cause	763.1
Necrosis					
genital organ or tract	646.63	646.61	646.60	condition	760.8
kidney, cortical (acute)	646.23	646.21	646.20	condition	760.1
tubular	646.23	646.21	646.20	condition	760.1
liver	646.73	646.71	646.70	condition	760.8
placenta	656.73	656.71	656.70		762.2
renal, cortical	646.23	646.21	646.20	condition	760.1
Nephritis, nephrosis	646.23	646.21	646.20	condition	760.1
with hypertension	642.13	642.11	642.10		760.0
Nephropathy NEC	646.23	646.21	646.20	condition	
Neuritis (peripheral)	646.43	646.41	646.40	condition	
Nonengagement of head NEC	652.53	652.51	652.50		763.1
in labor	660.03	660.01	660.00	cause	763.1
Noxious substances transmitted through placenta or breast milk, suspected, unspecified	655.53	655.51	655.50		760.70
Nuchal hitch (arm)	652.83	652.81	652.80		763.1
causing obstructed labor	660.03	660.01	660.00	cause	763.1
Nutritional deficiency	648.93	648.91	648.90	condition	
Obesity					
excessive weight gain during pregnancy	646.13	646.11	646.10	complication	
morbid	649.13	649.11	649.10	278.00, 278.01-278.03, V85.30-V85.45	
Oblique lie or presentation	652.33	652.31	652.30		763.1
with successful version	652.13	652.11	652.10		763.1
causing obstructed labor	660.03	660.01	660.00	cause	763.1
Obstetrical trauma NEC (complicating delivery)	665.93	665.91	665.90		763.89
Obstruction, obstructed, obstructive					
labor	660.93	660.91	660.90	cause	763.1
borderline pelvis	660.13	660.11	660.10	cause	763.1
by					
bony pelvis	660.13	660.11	660.10	cause	763.1
deep transverse arrest	660.33	660.31	660.30	cause	763.1
impacted shoulder	660.43	660.41	660.40	cause	763.1

Antepartum Pregnancy Condition or Complication; affecting management of mother	Antepartum condition or complication	Delivered, with or without mention of antepartum condition	Unspecified episode of care	Assign additional code to describe the…	Affecting fetus (coded on the newborn chart only)
Obstruction, obstructed, obstructive — *continued*					
locked twins	660.53	660.51	660.50	cause	763.1
malposition (fetus)	660.03	660.01	660.00	cause	763.1
head during labor	660.33	660.31	660.30	cause	763.1
persistent occipitoposterior position	660.33	660.31	660.30	cause	763.1
soft tissue, pelvic	660.23	660.21	660.20	cause	763.1
Occlusion, precerebral artery NEC	674.03	674.01	674.00	condition	
Oligohydramnios NEC	658.03	658.01	658.00		761.2
due to premature rupture of membranes	658.13	658.11	658.10		761.2
Oliguria	646.23	646.21	646.20	condition	
with hypertension — *see* Pregnancy, toxemia					
Oophoritis	646.63	646.61	646.60	condition	
Oversize fetus (weight of 4500 grams or more)	656.63	656.61	656.60		766.0
causing disproportion	653.53	653.51	653.50		763.1
with obstructed labor	660.13	660.11	660.10	cause	763.1
Pain(s)	646.83	646.81	646.80	condition	
false labor	644.13		644.10		
Papyraceous fetus	646.03	646.01	646.00	condition	779.8
Paralysis, bladder		665.51	665.50		
Patent cervix	654.53	654.51	654.50		761.0
causing obstructed labor	660.23	660.21	660.20	cause	763.1
Pendulous	654.43	654.41	654.40		763.89
causing obstructed labor	660.23	660.21	660.20	cause	763.1
complication of delivery		665.11	665.10		763.89
Perforation					
bladder		665.51	665.50		
bowel		665.51	665.50		
broad ligament		665.61	665.60		
cervix		665.31	665.30		
instrumental (complicating delivery)	665.93	665.91	665.90		
pelvic (floor)		664.11	664.10		
organ		665.51	665.50		763.89
urethral		665.51	665.50		763.89
uterus		665.51	665.50		763.89
Persistence					
hymen (tag)	654.83	654.81	654.80		
causing obstructed labor	660.23	660.21	660.20	cause	763.1
occiput (anterior or posterior)	660.33	660.31	660.30	cause	763.1
Phlebitis	671.93	671.91	671.90		760.3
deep	671.33	671.31	671.30	DVT code, anticoag use (V58.61)	760.3
intracranial	671.53	671.51	671.50		
lower extremities	671.23	671.21	671.20	453.6, 453.71, 453.81	760.3
specified site NEC	671.53	671.51	671.50		
superficial	671.23	671.21	671.20	453.6, 453.71, 453.81	760.3
Phlegmasia	671.33	671.31	671.30	DVT code, anticoag use (V58.61)	760.3
PID	646.63	646.61	646.60	condition	
Pithecoid pelvis (fetopelvic)	653.23	653.21	653.20		763.1
obstructed labor	660.13	660.11	660.10	cause	763.1
Placenta, placental					
abnormal	656.73	656.71	656.70		762.2
with hemorrhage	641.83	641.81	641.80		762.1
abruptio or ablatio	641.23	641.21	641.20		762.1
absorption (suspected) of					
chemical	655.53	655.51	655.50		760.79
drug (NEC)	655.53	655.51	655.50		760.79
accessory lobe	656.73	656.71	656.70		762.2
with hemorrhage	641.83	641.81	641.80		762.1
apoplexy	641.23	641.21	641.20		762.1
battledore	656.73	656.71	656.70		762.2
with hemorrhage	641.83	641.81	641.80		762.1
bilobate	656.73	656.71	656.70		762.2
with hemorrhage	641.83	641.81	641.80		762.1
bipartita	656.73	656.71	656.70		762.2
with hemorrhage	641.83	641.81	641.80		762.1

Antepartum Pregnancy Condition or Complication; affecting management of mother	Antepartum condition or complication	Delivered, with or without mention of antepartum condition	Unspecified episode of care	Assign additional code to describe the…	Affecting fetus (coded on the newborn chart only)
Placenta, placental — *continued*					
centralis	641.03	641.01	641.00		762.0
with hemorrhage	641.13	641.11	641.10		762.1
circumvallata	656.73	656.71	656.70		762.2
with hemorrhage	641.83	641.81	641.80		762.1
cyst (amniotic)	656.73	656.71	656.70		762.2
with hemorrhage	641.83	641.81	641.80		762.1
deficiency	656.53	656.51	656.50		762.2
degeneration	656.53	656.51	656.50		762.2
detachment	641.23	641.21	641.20		762.1
dimidiata	656.73	656.71	656.70		762.2
with hemorrhage	641.83	641.81	641.80		762.1
disease	656.73	656.71	656.70		762.2
with hemorrhage	641.83	641.81	641.80		762.1
duplex	656.73	656.71	656.70		762.2
with hemorrhage	641.83	641.81	641.80		762.1
dysfunction	656.53	656.51	656.50		762.2
fenestrata	656.73	656.71	656.70		762.2
with hemorrhage	641.83	641.81	641.80		762.1
fibrosis	656.73	656.71	656.70		762.2
with hemorrhage	641.83	641.81	641.80		762.1
hematoma	656.73	656.71	656.70		762.2
with hemorrhage	641.83	641.81	641.80		762.1
hemorrhage	641.23	641.21	641.20		762.1
hormone disturbance	656.73	656.71	656.70		762.2
with hemorrhage	641.83	641.81	641.80		762.1
hyperplasia	656.73	656.71	656.70		762.2
with hemorrhage	641.83	641.81	641.80		762.1
infarct	656.73	656.71	656.70		762.2
with hemorrhage	641.83	641.81	641.80		762.1
insertion, vicious	641.03	641.01	641.00		762.0
with hemorrhage	641.13	641.11	641.10		762.1
insufficiency	656.53	656.51	656.50		762.2
lateral	641.03	641.01	641.00		762.0
with hemorrhage	641.13	641.11	641.10		762.1
low implantation	641.03	641.01	641.00		762.0
with hemorrhage	641.13	641.11	641.10		762.1
low lying	641.03	641.01	641.00		762.0
with hemorrhage	641.13	641.11	641.10		762.1
malformation	656.73	656.71	656.70		762.2
with hemorrhage	641.83	641.81	641.80		762.1
malposition	641.03	641.01	641.00		762.2
with hemorrhage	641.13	641.11	641.10		762.1
marginalis, marginata	641.03	641.01	641.00		762.0
with hemorrhage	641.13	641.11	641.10		762.1
marginal sinus (hemorrhage)	641.23	641.21	641.20		762.1
membranacea	656.73	656.71	656.70		762.2
with hemorrhage	641.83	641.81	641.80		762.1
multiload	656.73	656.71	656.70		762.2
with hemorrhage	641.83	641.81	641.80		762.1
necrosis	656.73	656.71	656.70		762.2
with hemorrhage	641.83	641.81	641.80		762.1
previa	641.03	641.01	641.00		762.0
with hemorrhage	641.13	641.11	641.10		762.1
separation (premature) (undelivered)	641.23	641.21	641.20		762.1
septuplex	656.73	656.71	656.70		762.2
with hemorrhage	641.83	641.81	641.80		762.1
small	656.53	656.51	656.50		762.2
softening	656.73	656.71	656.70		762.2
with hemorrhage	641.83	641.81	641.80		762.1
spuria	656.73	656.71	656.70		762.2
with hemorrhage	641.83	641.81	641.80		762.1
succenturiata	656.73	656.71	656.70		762.2
with hemorrhage	641.83	641.81	641.80		762.1
syphilitic	647.03	647.01	647.00	condition	760.2
manifest syphilis in the infant or fetus	647.03	647.01	647.00	condition	090.0

Antepartum Pregnancy
Condition or Complication; affecting management of mother

	Antepartum condition or complication	Delivered, with or without mention of antepartum condition	Unspecified episode of care	Assign additional code to describe the…	Affecting fetus (coded on the newborn chart only)
Placenta, placental — *continued*					
transfusion syndromes (fetus)					762.3
transmission of chemical substance (suspected, affecting pregnancy)	655.53	655.51	655.50		760.70
trilobate	656.73	656.71	656.70		762.2
with hemorrhage	641.83	641.81	641.80		762.1
triplex	656.73	656.71	656.70		762.2
with hemorrhage	641.83	641.81	641.80		762.1
varicose vessel	656.73	656.71	656.70		762.2
with hemorrhage	641.83	641.81	641.80		762.1
vicious insertion	641.03	641.01	641.00		
with hemorrhage	641.13	641.11	641.10		762.0
Placentitis	658.43	658.41	658.40		762.7
Platypelloid pelvis (disproportion)	653.23	653.21	653.20		763.1
obstructed labor	660.13	660.11	660.10	cause	763.1
Pneumonitis					
aspiration	668.03	668.01	668.00	condition	770.18
postanesthetic	668.03	668.01	668.00	condition	
postoperative	668.03	668.01	668.00		
Polygalactia	676.63	676.61	676.60		
Polyhydramnios	657.03	657.01	657.00		761.3
Polyp					
cervix	654.63	654.61	654.60		763.89
obstructed labor	660.23	660.21	660.20	cause	763.1
uterus	654.13	654.11	654.10		763.89
obstructed labor	660.23	660.21	660.20	cause	763.1
Poor					
contractions labor	661.23	661.21	661.20		763.7
fetal growth, affecting management	656.53	656.51	656.50		
Fetal growth retardation					
unspecified (weight)					764.90
< 500 gms					764.91
500-749 gms					764.92
750-999 gms					764.93
1,000-1,249 gms					764.94
1,250-1,499 gms					764.95
1,500-1,749 gms					764.96
1,750-1,999 gms					764.97
2,000-2,499 gms					764.98
≥ 2,500 gms					764.99
obstetrical history	V23.4				
Position – *see* also Presentation, fetal	652.93	652.91	652.90		763.1
causing obstructed labor	660.03	660.01	660.00	cause	763.1
Post-term (over 40 to 42 completed weeks)	645.13	645.11	645.10		766.21
Prediabetes	648.83	648.81	648.80	condition	
Prolonged (over 42 completed weeks)	645.23	645.21	645.20		766.22
Pre-eclampsia (mild)	642.43	642.41	642.40		760.0
with convulsions	642.63	642.61	642.60		760.0
severe	642.53	642.51	642.50		760.0
superimposed on pre-existing hypertensive disease	642.73	642.71	642.70		760.0
Pre-existing condition (prior to pregnancy) **affecting current pregnancy**					
abnormal glucose tolerance	648.83	648.81	648.80	condition	
anemia	648.23	648.21	648.20	condition	
bone and joint (lower limb)	648.73	648.71	648.70	condition	
cardiovascular	648.63	648.61	648.60	condition	
congenital	648.53	648.51	648.50	condition	
cerebrovascular	674.03	674.01	674.00		
diabetic	648.03	648.01	648.00	condition	
drug dependence	648.33	648.31	648.30	condition	
genital organ or tract	646.63	646.61	646.60	condition	
gonorrheal	647.13	647.11	647.10	condition	
hypertensive	642.23	642.21	642.20		
renal	642.13	642.11	642.10		
infectious	647.93	647.91	647.90	condition	
specified type NEC	647.83	647.81	647.80	condition	

Antepartum Pregnancy
Condition or Complication; affecting management of mother

	Antepartum condition or complication	Delivered, with or without mention of antepartum condition	Unspecified episode of care	Assign additional code to describe the…	Affecting fetus (coded on the newborn chart only)
Pre-existing condition (prior to pregnancy) **affecting current pregnancy** — *continued*					
liver	646.73	646.71	646.70	condition	
malarial	647.43	647.41	647.40	condition	
nutritional deficiency	648.93	648.91	648.90	condition	
parasitic NEC	647.83	647.81	647.80	condition	
renal	646.23	646.21	646.20	condition	
hypertensive	642.13	642.11	642.10		
rubella	647.53	647.51	647.50	condition	
specified condition NEC	648.93	648.91	648.90	condition	
syphilitic	647.03	647.01	647.00	condition	
thyroid	648.13	648.11	648.10	condition	
tuberculous	647.33	647.31	647.30	condition	
urinary	646.63	646.61	646.60	condition	
venereal	647.23	647.21	647.20	condition	
viral NEC	647.63	647.61	647.60	condition	
Premature					
labor		644.21	644.20		
threatened	644.03		644.00		
rupture of membranes or amnion	658.13	658.11	658.10		761.1
with delayed delivery	658.23	658.21	658.20		
Presentation, fetal					
abnormal	652.93	652.91	652.90		763.1
with successful version	652.13	652.11	652.10		761.7
causing obstructed labor	660.03	660.01	660.00	cause	763.1
in multiple gestation (one or more)	652.63	652.61	652.60		763.1
causing obstructed labor	660.03	660.01	660.00	cause	763.1
specified NEC	652.83	652.81	652.80		763.1
causing obstructed labor	660.03	660.01	660.00	cause	763.1
arm	652.73	652.71	652.70		763.1
causing obstructed labor	660.03	660.01	660.00	cause	763.1
breech	652.23	652.21	652.20		761.7
with successful version	652.13	652.11	652.10		761.7
causing obstructed labor	660.03	660.01	660.00	cause	763.0
brow	652.43	652.41	652.40		763.1
causing obstructed labor	660.03	660.01	660.00	cause	763.1
cord	663.03	663.01	663.00		762.5
extended head	652.43	652.41	652.40		763.1
causing obstructed labor	660.03	660.01	660.00	cause	763.1
face	652.43	652.41	652.40		763.1
causing obstructed labor	660.03	660.01	660.00	cause	763.1
to pubes	652.83	652.81	652.80		763.1
causing obstructed labor	660.33	660.31	660.30	cause	763.1
hand, leg, or foot NEC	652.83	652.81	652.80		763.1
causing obstructed labor	660.03	660.01	660.00	cause	763.1
mentum	652.43	652.41	652.40		763.1
causing obstructed labor	660.03	660.01	660.00	cause	763.1
multiple gestation (one fetus or more)	652.63	652.61	652.60		763.1
causing obstructed labor	660.03	660.01	660.00	cause	763.1
oblique	652.33	652.31	652.30		763.1
with successful version	652.13	652.11	652.10		763.1
causing obstructed labor	660.03	660.01	660.00	cause	763.1
shoulder	652.83	652.81	652.80		763.1
causing obstructed labor	660.03	660.01	660.00	cause	763.1
transverse	652.33	652.31	652.30		763.1
with successful version	652.13	652.11	652.10		763.1
causing obstructed labor	660.03	660.01	660.00	cause	763.1
umbilical cord	663.03	663.01	663.00		
unstable	652.03	652.01	652.00		763.1
causing obstructed labor	660.03	660.01	660.00	cause	763.1
Previous					
abortion	V23.2				
infertility	V23.0				
nonobstetric condition	V23.89				
poor obstetrical history	V23.49				
premature delivery	V23.41				

Antepartum Pregnancy
Condition or Complication; affecting management of mother

	Antepartum condition or complication	Delivered, with or without mention of antepartum condition	Unspecified episode of care	Assign additional code to describe the…	Affecting fetus (coded on the newborn chart only)
Previous — *continued*					
recurrent pregnancy loss	646.33	646.31	646.30		
trophoblastic disease	V23.1				
Primigravida, elderly	659.53	659.51	659.50		763.89
Primipara, old	659.53	659.51	659.50		763.89
Problem (with)					
fetus NOS	656.93	656.91	656.90		779.9
specified type NEC	656.83	656.81	656.80		779.8
placenta NOS	656.93	656.91	656.90		762.2
specified type NEC	656.83	656.81	656.80		762.2
Prolapse, prolapsed					
arm or hand, complicating delivery	652.73	652.71	652.70		763.1
causing obstructed labor	660.03	660.01	660.00	cause	763.1
cervix, anterior lip (obstructing labor)	660.23	660.21	660.20	cause	763.1
fetal extremity, complicating delivery	652.83	652.81	652.80		763.1
causing obstructed labor	660.03	660.01	660.00	cause	763.1
leg, complicating delivery	652.83	652.81	652.80		763.1
causing obstructed labor	660.03	660.01	660.00	cause	763.1
umbilical cord, complicating delivery	663.03	663.01	663.00		762.4
causing obstructed labor	660.23	660.21	660.20	cause	763.1
Prolonged					
labor	662.13	662.11	662.10		
first stage	662.03	662.01	662.00		763.89
second stage	662.23	662.21	662.20		763.89
pregnancy over 40 completed weeks to 42 completed weeks	645.13	645.11	645.10		766.21
pregnancy over 42 completed weeks	645.23	645.21	645.20		766.22
rupture of membranes (24 hours or more prior to onset of labor)	658.23	658.21	658.20		761.8
uterine contractions in labor	661.43	661.41	661.40		763.7
PROM	658.13	658.11	658.10		761.1
with delayed delivery	658.23	658.21	658.20		761.8
Prominence, ischial spine or sacral promontory					
with disproportion (fetopelvic)	653.33	653.31	653.30		763.1
causing obstructed labor	660.13	660.11	660.10	cause	763.1
Proteinuria (gestational)	646.23	646.21	646.20	condition	
with toxemia (mild) (pre-eclamptic)	642.43	642.41	642.40		760.0
convulsions	642.63	642.61	642.60		760.0
pre-existing hypertension	642.73	642.71	642.70		760.0
severe	642.53	642.51	642.50		760.0
Pruritus, pruritic	646.83	646.81	646.80	condition	
Psychosis or psychoneurosis	648.43	648.41	648.40	condition	
Ptyalism	646.83	646.81	646.80	condition	
Pyelitis	646.63	646.61	646.60	condition	760.1
Pyrexia (of unknown origin) (PUO), **during labor**	659.23	659.21	659.20		
Quadruplet NEC	651.23	651.21	651.20	V91.20-V91.29	761.5
with fetal loss and retention of one or more fetus(es)	651.53	651.51	651.50	V91.20-V91.29	
reduction, multiple gestation (elective)	651.73	651.71	651.70	V91.20-V91.29	
Quintuplet NEC	651.83	651.81	651.80	V91.90-V91.99	761.5
with fetal loss and retention of one or more fetus(es)	651.63	651.61	651.60	V91.90-V91.99	
reduction, multiple gestation (elective)	651.73	651.71	651.70	V91.90-V91.99	
Rachitic with disproportion (fetopelvic)	653.23	653.21	653.20		763.1
causing obstructed labor	660.13	660.11	660.10	cause	763.1
Rapid second stage (delivery)	661.33	661.31	661.30		763.6
Reaction obstetric anesthetic or analgesic NEC	668.93	668.91	668.90		763.5
Rectocele	654.43	654.41	654.40		763.1
causing obstructed labor	660.23	660.21	660.20	cause	763.1
Recurrent pregnancy loss	646.33	646.31	646.30		
Reduction, multiple gestation (elective)	651.73	651.71	651.70	placenta status	
Repair of pelvic floor, previous	654.43	654.41	654.40		763.89
causing obstructed labor	660.23	660.21	660.20	cause	763.1
Retardation fetal growth (intrauterine)	656.53	656.51	656.50		764.90
Retention, retained					
dead					
fetus (after 22 completed weeks gestation)	656.43	656.41	656.40		cause

Coding Tables

Antepartum Pregnancy

Antepartum Pregnancy Condition or Complication; affecting management of mother	Antepartum condition or complication	Delivered, with or without mention of antepartum condition	Unspecified episode of care	Assign additional code to describe the...	Affecting fetus (coded on the newborn chart only)
Retention, retained — *continued*					
early fetal death (before 22 completed weeks gestation)	632				
ovum		631.8			
Retinitis	646.83	646.81	646.80	condition	
Retraction					
nipple	676.03	676.01	676.00		
ring, uterus (Bandl's) (pathological)	661.43	661.41	661.40		763.7
Retroversion, uterus	654.33	654.31	654.30		763.89
causing obstructed labor	660.23	660.21	660.20	cause	763.1
Rh immunization, incompatibility, or sensitization	656.13	656.11	656.10		773.0
Rigid, rigidity					
cervix	654.63	654.61	654.60		763.89
causing obstructed labor	660.23	660.21	660.20	cause	763.1
pelvic floor	654.43	654.41	654.40		763.89
causing obstructed labor	660.23	660.21	660.20	cause	763.1
Ring(s), complicating delivery					
perineum or vulva	654.83	654.81	654.80		763.89
causing obstructed labor	660.23	660.21	660.20	cause	763.1
vagina	654.73	654.71	654.70		763.89
causing obstructed labor	660.23	660.21	660.20	cause	763.1
Bandl's	661.43	661.41	661.40		763.7
contraction	661.43	661.41	661.40		763.7
retraction, uterus, pathological	661.43	661.41	661.40		763.7
Robert's pelvis with disproportion (fetopelvic)	653.03	653.01	653.00		763.1
causing obstructed labor	660.13	660.11	660.10	cause	763.1
Rubella (German measles)	647.53	647.51	647.50	condition	760.2
with suspected fetal damage	655.33	655.31	655.30		771.0
Rupture					
abdominal viscera (obstetrical trauma)		665.51	665.50		
amnion (premature)	658.13	658.11	658.10		763.89
with delayed delivery	658.23	658.21	658.20		763.89
bladder (sphincter), obstetrical trauma		665.51	665.50		
cervix (uteri), obstetrical trauma		665.31	665.30		
marginal sinus (hemorrhage)	641.23	641.21	641.20		762.1
membranes (premature)	658.13	658.11	658.10		761.1
with delayed delivery	658.23	658.21	658.20		761.1
artificial with delayed delivery following	658.33	658.31	658.30		761.1
pelvic floor, complicating delivery		664.11	664.10		
perineum during delivery		664.41	664.40		
umbilical cord	663.83	663.81	663.80		772.0
urethra (obstetrical trauma)		665.51	665.50		
uterus					
before onset of labor	665.03	665.01	665.00		763.89
during labor		665.11	665.10		763.89
vulva, complicating delivery		664.01	664.00		
Sacculation, complicating delivery	654.43	654.41	654.40		763.1
causing obstructed labor	660.23	660.21	660.20	cause	763.1
Salivation (excessive)	646.83	646.81	646.80	condition	
Salpingitis	646.63	646.61	646.60	condition	760.8
Salpingo-oophoritis	646.63	646.61	646.60	condition	760.8
Scar, scarring					
cervix	654.63	654.61	654.60		763.89
causing obstructed labor	660.23	660.21	660.20	cause	763.1
uterus NEC	654.93	654.91	654.90		763.89
from previous cesarean delivery	654.23	654.21	654.20		763.89
causing obstructed labor	660.23	660.21	660.20	cause	763.1
Scoliotic pelvis with disproportion (fetopelvic)	653.03	653.01	653.00		763.1
causing obstructed labor	660.13	660.11	660.10	cause	763.1
Screening, prenatal (for)					
If the abnormal finding is known — code the findings					
by					
amniocentesis					
chromosomal anomalies	V28.0				

Antepartum Pregnancy

Condition or Complication; affecting management of mother	Antepartum condition or complication	Delivered, with or without mention of antepartum condition	Unspecified episode of care	Assign additional code to describe the...	Affecting fetus (coded on the newborn chart only)
Screening, prenatal (for) — *continued*					
If the abnormal finding is known — code the findings — *continued*					
by — *continued*					
amniocentesis — *continued*					
raised alpha-fetoprotein levels (amniotic fluid)	V28.1				
specified, NEC	V28.2				
ultrasound					
fetal growth retardation	V28.4				
malformation	V28.3				
isoimmunization	V28.5				
other specified screening	V28.89				
Streptococcus B	V28.6				
unspecified, screening	V28.9				
Separation (obstetrical trauma)					
pubic bone		665.61	665.60		
symphysis pubis		665.61	665.60		
Sepsis, complicating labor	659.33	659.31	659.30		
Septicemia	647.83	647.81	647.80	condition	
Septum, vagina	654.73	654.71	654.70		763.89
causing obstructed labor	660.23	660.21	660.20	cause	763.1
Sextuplet NEC	651.83	651.81	651.80	V91.90-V91.99	761.5
with fetal loss and retention of one or more fetus(es)	651.63	651.61	651.60	V91.90-V91.99	
reduction, multiple gestation (elective)	651.73	651.71	651.70	V91.90-V91.99	
Shirodkar suture	654.53	654.51	654.50		
causing obstructed labor	660.23	660.21	660.20	cause	763.1
Shock					
complicating labor and delivery	669.13	669.11	669.10		
following labor and delivery	669.13	669.11	669.10		
Short, shortening, shortness	663.43	663.41	663.40		762.6
cervix	649.73	649.71	649.70	complication	
umbilical cord	663.43	663.41	663.40		762.6
Sinus, marginal, rupture or bleeding	641.23	641.21	641.20		762.1
Slow fetal growth	656.53	656.51	656.50		764.90
Small					
for-dates fetus	656.53	656.51	656.50		764.00
pelvis					
with disproportion (fetopelvic)	653.13	653.11	653.10		763.1
causing obstructed labor	660.13	660.11	660.10	cause	763.1
Spasms					
cervix, complicating delivery	661.43	661.41	661.40		763.7
uterus	646.83	646.81	646.80	condition	
complicating delivery	661.43	661.41	661.40		763.7
complicating labor	661.43	661.41	661.40		763.7
Specified condition NEC	646.83	646.81	646.80	condition	
Spina bifida (aperta)**, suspected fetal**	655.03	655.01	655.00		
Spondylolisthesis with disproportion (fetopelvic)	653.33	653.31	653.30		763.1
causing obstructed labor	660.13	660.11	660.10	cause	763.1
Spondylolysis with disproportion (fetopelvic)	653.33	653.31	653.30		763.1
causing obstructed labor	660.13	660.11	660.10	cause	763.1
Spondylosis with disproportion (fetopelvic)	653.33	653.31	653.30		763.1
causing obstructed labor	660.13	660.11	660.10	cause	763.1
Spotting					
antepartum hemorrhage	641.93	641.91	641.90		
spotting	649.53	649.51	649.50		
Spurious labor pains	644.13		644.10		
Stenosis (cicatricial)					
cervix, cervical (canal)	654.63	654.61	654.60		763.89
causing obstructed labor	660.23	660.21	660.20	cause	763.1
vagina	654.73	654.71	654.70		763.89
causing obstructed labor	660.23	660.21	660.20	cause	763.1
Stricture, cervix (canal)	654.63	654.61	654.60		763.89
causing obstructed labor	660.23	660.21	660.20	cause	763.1
Sudden death					
during childbirth	669.93	669.91	669.90		

Coding Tables

Antepartum Pregnancy

Coding Tables

Antepartum Pregnancy

Antepartum Pregnancy Condition or Complication; affecting management of mother	Antepartum condition or complication	Delivered, with or without mention of antepartum condition	Unspecified episode of care	Assign additional code to describe the…	Affecting fetus (coded on the newborn chart only)
Supervision (of) (for)					
high-risk	V23.9				
insufficient prenatal care	V23.7				
specified problem NEC	V23.89				
multiparity	V23.3				
normal NEC	V22.1				
first pregnancy	V22.0				
poor					
obstetric history	V23.49				
reproductive history	V23.5				
Suppression of lactation	676.53	676.51	676.50		
Suppurative, breast, mammary gland	675.13	675.11	675.10		
Surgery, previous					
cervix	654.63	654.61	654.60		763.89
causing obstructed labor	660.23	660.21	660.20	cause	763.1
pelvic soft tissues NEC	654.93	654.91	654.90		763.89
causing obstructed labor	660.23	660.21	660.20	cause	763.1
perineum or vulva	654.83	654.81	654.80		
uterus NEC	654.93	654.91	654.90		763.89
causing obstructed labor	660.23	660.21	660.20	cause	763.1
from previous cesarean delivery	654.23	654.21	654.20		
causing obstructed labor	660.23	660.21	660.20	cause	763.1
vagina	654.73	654.71	654.70		
causing obstructed labor	660.23	660.21	660.20	cause	763.1
Suspended uterus	654.43	654.41	654.40		763.89
causing obstructed labor	660.23	660.21	660.20	cause	763.1
Suture, Shirodkar (with or without cervical incompetence)	654.53	654.51	654.50		
causing obstructed labor	660.23	660.21	660.20	cause	763.1
Syncope complicating delivery	669.23	669.21	669.20		
Syndrome					
acid pulmonary aspiration (Mendelson's)	668.03	668.01	668.00		
Chiari-Frommel	676.63	676.61	676.60		
dead fetus	641.33	641.31	641.30		
dystocia, dystrophia	654.93	654.91	654.90		
causing obstructed labor	660.23	660.21	660.20	cause	763.1
Frommel-Chiari	676.63	676.61	676.60		
H.E.L.L.P (Hemolysis, Elevated Liver function and Low Platelets)	642.53	642.51	642.50		
hypotension, maternal	669.23	669.21	669.20		
maternal hypotension	669.23	669.21	669.20		
Mendelson's (during labor) (obstetric)	668.03	668.01	668.00		
vanishing twin	651.33			V91.00-V91.09 condition	
Syphilis	647.03	647.01	647.00		760.2
Tear, torn					
Anus, anal (sphincter)complicating delivery					
with third degree perineal laceration		664.21	664.20		763.89
w/mucosa		664.31	664.30		763.89
w/o third degree perineal laceration		664.61	664.60		763.89
old (healed)		654.81	654.80		763.89
bladder, obstetrical trauma		665.51	665.50		763.89
bowel, obstetrical trauma		665.51	665.50		763.89
broad ligament, obstetrical trauma		665.51	665.50		763.89
cervix, obstetrical trauma		665.31	665.30		763.89
pelvic					
floor, complicating delivery		664.11	664.10		763.89
organ NEC, obstetrical trauma		665.51	665.50		763.89
perineum, obstetrical trauma		665.51	665.50		763.89
periurethral, obstetrical trauma		664.81	664.80		763.89
umbilical cord, complicating delivery	663.83	663.81	663.80		772.0
urethra, obstetrical trauma		665.51	665.50		
vulva, complicating delivery		664.01	664.00		763.89
Teratoma, fetal sacral, causing fetopelvic disproportion	653.73	653.71	653.70		763.1
causing obstructed labor	660.23	660.21	660.20	cause	763.1
Thelitis	675.03	675.01	675.00		

Antepartum Pregnancy

Antepartum Pregnancy
Condition or Complication; affecting management of mother

Antepartum Pregnancy	Antepartum condition or complication	Delivered, with or without mention of antepartum condition	Unspecified episode of care	Assign additional code to describe the…	Affecting fetus (coded on the newborn chart only)
Threatened					
abortion or miscarriage	640.03	640.01	640.00		762.1
labor	644.13		644.10		761.8
before 22 completed weeks gestation	640.03	640.01	640.00		762.1
premature delivery		644.21	644.20		761.8
premature labor	644.03		644.00		761.8
Thrombophlebitis	671.23	671.21	671.20	453.6, 453.71, 453.81	760.3
cerebral (sinus) (vein), nonpyogenic	671.53	671.51	671.50		760.3
deep	671.33	671.31	671.30	DVT code, anticoag use (V58.61)	760.3
intracranial venous sinus, nonpyogenic	671.53	671.51	671.50		760.3
specified site NEC	671.53	671.51	671.50		760.3
superficial	671.23	671.21	671.20	453.6, 453.71, 453.81	760.3
Thrombosis	671.93	671.91	671.90		
brain (artery) (stem)	674.03	674.01	674.00		
intracranial, venous sinus (nonpyogenic origin)	671.53	671.51	671.50		
deep	671.33	671.31	671.30	DVT code, anticoag use (V58.61)	760.3
spinal cord	671.53	671.51	671.50		
superficial	671.23	671.21	671.20	453.6, 453.71, 453.81	
umbilical cord (vessels)	663.63	663.61	663.60		762.6
venous (superficial)	671.23	671.21	671.20	453.6, 453.71, 453.81	
Thyroid dysfunction	648.13	648.11	648.10	condition	
Thyroiditis	648.13	648.11	648.10	condition	
Thyrotoxicosis	648.13	648.11	648.10	condition	
Tipping pelvis with disproportion (fetopelvic)	653.03	653.01	653.00		763.1
causing obstructed labor	660.13	660.11	660.10	cause	763.1
Tobacco use disorder	649.03	649.01	649.00		
Torsion of uterus	654.43	654.41	654.40		
causing obstructed labor	660.23	660.21	660.20	cause	763.1
Toxemia (mild) (pre-eclamptic)	642.43	642.41	642.40		760.0
with					760.0
convulsions	642.63	642.61	642.60		760.0
pre-existing hypertension	642.73	642.71	642.70		760.0
Toxemia (mild) (pre-eclamptic)	642.43	642.41	642.40		760.0
eclamptic	642.63	642.61	642.60		760.0
with pre-existing hypertension	642.73	642.71	642.70		760.0
severe	642.53	642.51	642.50		760.0
Transmission of chemical substances through the placenta, suspected	655.53	655.51	655.50		760.70
Transverse					
arrest (deep), in labor	660.33	660.31	660.30	cause	763.1
lie or presentation	652.33	652.31	652.30		761.7
with successful version	652.13	652.11	652.10		763.1
causing obstructed labor	660.03	660.01	660.00	cause	763.1
Trauma	648.93	648.91	648.90	condition	
causing hemorrhage	641.83	641.81	641.80		760.5
during delivery NEC	665.93	665.91	665.90		760.5
obstetrical	665.93	665.91	665.90		760.5
previous pregnancy (major), affecting management of current pregnancy, childbirth or puerperium	V23.89	V23.89	V23.89		
Triplet NEC	651.13	651.11	651.10	V91.10-V91.19	761.5
with fetal loss and retention of one or more fetus(es)	651.43	651.41	651.40	V91.10-V91.19	761.5
reduction, multiple gestation (elective)	651.73	651.71	651.70	V91.10-V91.19	
Trophoblastic disease	630				
previous pregnancy, affecting management of current pregnancy	V23.1	V23.1	V23.1		
Tubal (with rupture)					761.4
w/ intrauterine pregnancy	633.11				
w/o intrauterine pregnancy	633.10				
Tuberculosis	647.33	647.31	647.30	condition	760.2
Tumor					
cervix	654.63	654.61	654.60		763.89
causing obstructed labor	660.23	660.21	660.20	cause	763.1
fetal, causing disproportion	653.73	653.71	653.70		763.1
causing obstructed labor	660.13	660.11	660.10	cause	763.1

Antepartum Pregnancy Condition or Complication; affecting management of mother	Antepartum condition or complication	Delivered, with or without mention of antepartum condition	Unspecified episode of care	Assign additional code to describe the...	Affecting fetus (coded on the newborn chart only)
Tumor — *continued*					
ovary	654.43	654.41	654.40		763.89
causing obstructed labor	660.23	660.21	660.20	cause	763.1
pelvic	654.93	654.91	654.90		763.89
causing obstructed labor	660.23	660.21	660.20	cause	763.1
pelvic organs or tissue NEC	654.43	654.41	654.40		763.89
causing obstructed labor	660.23	660.21	660.20	cause	763.1
uterus	654.13	654.11	654.10		763.89
causing obstructed labor	660.23	660.21	660.20	cause	763.1
vagina	654.73	654.71	654.70		763.89
causing obstructed labor	660.23	660.21	660.20	cause	763.1
vulva	654.83	654.81	654.80		763.89
causing obstructed labor	660.23	660.21	660.20	cause	763.1
Twin NEC	651.03	651.01	651.00	V91.00-V91.09	761.5
with fetal loss and retention of one or more fetus(es)	651.33	651.31	651.30	V91.00-V91.09	761.5
reduction, multiple gestation (elective)	651.73	651.71	651.70	V91.00-V91.09	
conjoined (siamese)	678.13	678.11	678.10		759.4
Unstable lie	652.03	652.01	652.00		761.7
causing obstructed labor	660.03	660.01	660.00	cause	763.1
Unwanted NEC	V61.7				
Uremia (renal disease or failure) **NEC**	646.23	646.21	646.20	condition	760.1
with secondary hypertension	642.13	642.11	642.10		760.0
hypertensive	642.23	642.21	642.20		760.0
Urethritis	646.63	646.61	646.60	condition	760.1
Uterine size date discrepancy	649.63	649.61	649.60		
UTI	646.63	646.61	646.60	condition	760.1
Vaginitis or vulvitis	646.63	646.61	646.60	condition	760.8
Valsuani's disease	648.23	648.21	648.20	condition	
Vanishing twin	651.33			V91.00-V91.09	
Varicose					
placental vessels	656.73	656.71	656.70		
veins (legs)	671.03	671.01	671.00		
perineum	671.13	671.11	671.10		
vulva	671.13	671.11	671.10		
Varicosity, labia or vulva	671.13	671.11	671.10		
Varix (lower extremity)	671.03	671.01	671.00		
perineum	671.13	671.11	671.10		
Vulva	671.13	671.11	671.10		
Vasa previa	663.53	663.51	663.50		762.6
hemorrhage	663.53	663.51	663.50		772.0
Venereal disease NEC	647.23	647.21	647.20	disease	
Venous, unspecified	671.93	671.91	671.90		
Ventouse delivery NEC		669.51	669.50		763.3
Version					
before labor	652.13	652.11	652.10		761.7
causing obstructed labor	660.03	660.01	660.00	cause	763.1
cephalic (correcting previous malposition)	652.13	652.11	652.10		763.1
causing obstructed labor	660.03	660.01	660.00	cause	763.1
Viral disease NEC	647.63	647.61	647.60	disease	
Vomiting	643.93	643.91	643.90		761.8
due to					
organic disease or other cause	643.83	643.81	643.80		761.8
specific cause NEC	643.83	643.81	643.80		761.8
early (mild) (before 22 completed weeks gestation)	643.03	643.01	643.00		761.8
with					761.8
carbohydrate depletion	643.13	643.11	643.10		761.8
dehydration	643.13	643.11	643.10		761.8
electrolyte imbalance	643.13	643.11	643.10		761.8
late (after 22 completed weeks gestation)	643.23	643.21	643.20		761.8
severe (with metabolic disturbance)	643.13	643.11	643.10		761.8
Vulvitis	646.63	646.61	646.60	condition	760.8
Weight gain	646.13	646.11	646.10	condition	
insufficient	646.83	646.81	646.80	condition	
Young maternal age	659.83	659.81	659.80		

Postpartum Pregnancy Condition or Complication; affecting management of mother	**Postpartum condition or complication**	**Delivered with mention of postpartum complication**	**Unspecified episode of care**	**Assign additional code to describe the…**	**Affecting newborn (coded on the newborn chart only)**
Abnormal NEC					
cervix	654.64	654.62	654.60		763.89
glucose tolerance test	648.84	648.82	648.80	condition	775.0
pelvic organs or tissues NEC	654.94	654.92	654.90		763.89
perineum or vulva	654.84	654.82	654.80		763.89
position					
cervix	654.44	654.42	654.40		763.89
uterus	654.44	654.42	654.40		763.89
quality of milk	676.84	676.82	676.80		
shape of uterus	654.44	654.42	654.40		
uterus (congenital)	654.04	654.02	654.00		763.89
vagina	654.74	654.72	654.70		763.89
vulva (acquired) (congenital)	654.84	654.82	654.80		763.89
weight gain	646.14	646.12	646.10	condition	761.8
with hypertension (mild) (pre-eclamptic)	642.44	642.42	642.40		760.0
with					
convulsions	642.64	642.62	642.60		760.0
pre-existing hypertension	642.74	642.72	642.70		760.0
with severe hypertension	642.54	642.52	642.50		760.0
Abscess					
areola (acute) (chronic)	675.14	675.12	675.10		
Bartholin's gland	646.64	646.62	646.60	condition	760.8
bladder	646.64	646.62	646.60	condition	760.1
breast (acute) (chronic)	675.14	675.12	675.10		
cervix (uteri)	670.84	670.82	670.80		
fallopian tube	670.84	670.82	670.80		
genital organ or tract NEC (postpartum)	670.84	670.82	670.80		
kidney	646.64	646.62	646.60	condition	760.1
labium (majus) (minus)	646.64	646.62	646.60	condition	760.8
mesosalpinx	670.84	670.82	670.80		
milk	675.14	675.12	675.10		
nabothian	646.64	646.62	646.60	condition	
nipple	675.04	675.02	675.00		
ovary	670.84	670.82	670.80		
oviduct	670.84	670.82	670.80		
para-uterine	670.84	670.82	670.80		
pelvic	670.84	670.82	670.80		
perimetric	670.84	670.82	670.80		
peritoneum, peritoneal (perforated) (ruptured) postpartum	670.84	670.82	670.80		
periuterine	670.84	670.82	670.80		
retro-uterine	670.84	670.82	670.80		
subareolar postpartum	675.14	675.12	675.10		
suprapelvic	670.84	670.82	670.80		
tubal (ruptured)	670.84	670.82	670.80		
tubo-ovarian	67084	670.82	670.80		
urethra	646.64	646.62	646.60	condition	760.1
urinary tract NEC	646.64	646.62	646.60	condition	
uterine, uterus	670.84	670.82	670.80		
vagina (wall)	646.64	646.62	646.60	condition	
vaginorectal	646.64	646.62	646.60	condition	
vulva	646.64	646.62	646.60	condition	
vulvovaginal gland	646.64	646.62	646.60	condition	760.8
Accreta placenta	667.04	667.02	667.00		
with hemorrhage	666.04	666.02	666.00		
Accident	674.94	674.92	674.90		
Addiction					
alcoholic	648.44	648.42	648.40	condition	760.71
Adherent placenta	667.04	667.02	667.00		
with hemorrhage	666.04	666.02	666.00		
Adhesion(s), adhesive					
cervicovaginal (postpartum)	674.84	674.82	674.80		
uterus to abdominal wall	654.44	654.42	654.40		763.89
Adnexitis	670.84	670.82	670.80		
Aerocele	673.04	673.02	673.00		

Coding Tables

Postpartum Pregnancy

Condition or Complication; affecting management of mother	Postpartum condition or complication	Delivered with mention of postpartum complication	Unspecified episode of care	Assign additional code to describe the...	Affecting newborn (coded on the newborn chart only)
Afibrinogenemia (postpartum)	666.34	666.32	666.30		
AFP (screening for raised levels in amniotic fluid)	V28.1				
	676.44	676.42	676.40		
Agalactia	673.04	673.02	673.00		
Air embolism	646.24	646.22	646.20	condition	760.1
Albuminuria (gravidarum)					760.1
with hypertension (and edema)					760.0
mild	642.44	642.42	642.40		760.0
severe	642.54	642.52	642.50		760.1
gestational	646.24	646.22	646.20	condition	760.0
pre-eclamptic (mild)	642.24	642.22	642.20		760.0
severe	642.54	642.52	642.50		
Alcohol, alcoholic				condition	760.71
addiction (maternal)	648.44	648.42	648.40		
Alphafetoprotein (screening for raised levels in amniotic fluid)	V28.1				
	673.14	673.12	673.10		
Amniotic fluid embolism	654.64	654.62	654.60		763.8
Amputation of cervix	648.24	648.22	648.20	condition	760.8
Anemia	648.24	648.22	648.20	condition	760.8
aplastic	648.24	648.22	648.20	condition	760.8
iron (Fe) deficiency	648.24	648.22	648.20	condition	760.8
macrocytic	648.24	648.22	648.20	condition	760.8
megaloblastic	648.24	648.22	648.20	condition	760.8
pernicious	648.24	648.22	648.20	condition	
postpartum	648.24	648.22	648.20	condition	
Anesthesia, anesthetic	668.84	668.82	668.80	condition	763.5
complications NEC	668.14	668.12	668.10	condition	763.5
cardiac	668.24	668.22	668.20	condition	763.5
central nervous system	668.04	668.02	668.00	condition	763.5
pulmonary	668.94	668.92	668.90	condition	761.6
death (from) during delivery					
Anomaly, anomalous (congenital)				condition	
cardiovascular system	648.54	648.52	648.50		
cervix	654.64	654.62	654.60		763.89
uterus	654.04	654.02	654.00		763.89
Anoxia cerebral					
complicating delivery (cesarean) (instrumental)	669.44	669.42	669.40		
due to obstetric anesthesia or sedation	668.24	668.22	668.20	complication	
Anteversion					763.89
uterus, uterine (cervix)	654.44	654.42	654.40		
Anuria, postpartum	669.34	669.32	669.30		
Apoplexy	674.04	674.02	674.00		
Arrest, arrested					
cardiac					
anesthesia, complicating delivery (cesarean)	668.14	668.12	668.10		
(instrumental)	669.44	669.42	669.40		
Aspiration					
acid-pulmonary (syndrome)	668.04	668.02	668.00	complication	
pneumonitis	668.04	668.02	668.00	complication	
Atonia, atony, atonic					
w/hemorrhage	666.14	666.12	666.10		
w/o hemorrhage	669.84	669.82	669.80		
Atresia, atretic					
cervix	654.64	654.62	654.60		763.89
Atrophy, atrophic					
breast, postpartum	676.34	676.32	676.30		
postpartum	674.84	674.82	674.80		
Avulsion (traumatic)					
symphyseal cartilage (inner)	665.64		665.60		
Bacilluria, asymptomatic	646.54	646.52	646.50	complication	760.1
Bacteremia	647.84	647.82	647.80	condition	
Bacteriuria, asymptomatic	646.54	646.52	646.50	complication	760.1
Bariatric surgery	649.24	649.22	649.20		
Bicornis or Bicornuate uterus	654.04	654.02	654.00		763.89
Bleeding					
atonic, following delivery	666.14	666.12	666.10		
cerebrovascular	674.04	674.02	674.00		

Postpartum Pregnancy
Condition or Complication; affecting management of mother

	Postpartum condition or complication	Delivered with mention of postpartum complication	Unspecified episode of care	Assign additional code to describe the...	Affecting newborn (coded on the newborn chart only)
Bleeding — *continued*					
due to					
subinvolution, postpartum	666.24	666.22	666.20		
Blood, dyscrasia (postpartum)	666.34	666.32	666.30		
Bone disorders	648.74	648.72	648.70	condition	
Breakdown, perineum	674.24	674.22	674.20		
Breastfeeding difficulties	676.84	676.82	676.80		
Caked breast (postpartum)	676.24	676.22	676.20		
Cardiomyopathy	674.54	674.52	674.50		
Cardiovascular disease	648.64	648.62	648.60	condition	
congenital	648.54	648.52	648.50	condition	
Cellulitis (postpartum)					
breast	675.14	675.12	675.10		
pelvis	670.84	670.82	670.80		
Cerebrovascular disorders	674.04	674.02	674.00	condition	
Cervical shortening		649.70			
Cervicitis	646.64	646.62	646.60	condition	760.8
Cervix					
adhesions	654.64	654.62	654.60		
anaplasia	654.64	654.62	654.60		
atypism	654.64	654.62	654.60		
bands	654.64	654.62	654.60		
cervicitis	654.64	654.62	654.60		
cicatrix	654.64	654.62	654.60		
cyst	654.64	654.62	654.60		
dysplasia	654.64	654.62	654.60		
ectropion	654.64	654.62	654.60		
endocervicitis	654.64	654.62	654.60		
erosion	654.64	654.62	654.60		
hypertrophic elongation	654.64	654.62	654.60		
incompetence	654.54	654.52	654.50		
leukoplakia	654.64	654.62	654.60		761.0
Nabothian (gland) cyst or follicle	654.64	654.62	654.60		
old laceration	654.64	654.62	654.60		
polyp	654.64	654.62	654.60		
stricture and stenosis	654.64	654.62	654.60		
ulcer	654.64	654.62	654.60		
Chiari-Frommel syndrome	676.64	676.62	676.60		
Childbed fever	670.24	670.22	670.20	Sepsis, 995.92, organ failure, condition	
Chloasma (gravidarum)	646.84	646.82	646.80		
Cicatrix					
cervix	654.64	654.62	654.60		
vagina	654.74	654.72	654.70		
Circulating anticoagulants	666.34	666.32	666.30		
Coagulation defects	649.34	649.32	649.30	286.0-286.9	
Collapse (during or after labor and delivery)					
circulatory (peripheral)	669.14	669.12	669.10		779.8
lung	668.04	668.02	668.00		
vascular (peripheral)	669.14	669.12	669.10		
Colporrhexis	665.44		665.40		
Complications NEC					
cesarean section wound	674.34	674.32	674.30		
delivery	669.94	669.92	669.90		
procedure (instrumental) (manual) (surgical)	669.44	669.42	669.40		
specified type NEC	669.84	669.82	669.80		
fetal	679.13	679.11	679.10		
labor and delivery	669.94	669.92	669.90		
anesthesia (sedation)	668.94	668.92	668.90		763.5
cardiac	668.14	668.12	668.10		
central nervous system	668.24	668.22	668.20		
pulmonary	668.04	668.02	668.00		
specified type NEC	668.84	668.82	668.80		
specified condition NEC	669.84	669.82	669.80		
maternal	679.03	679.01	679.00		
perineal repair	674.34	674.32	674.30		

Postpartum Pregnancy Condition or Complication; affecting management of mother	Postpartum condition or complication	Delivered with mention of postpartum complication	Unspecified episode of care	Assign additional code to describe the…	Affecting newborn (coded on the newborn chart only)
Complications NEC — *continued*					
perineal repair — *continued*					
disruption	674.24	674.22	674.20		
postpartum NEC	674.94	674.92	674.90		
surgical wound	674.34	674.32	674.30		
Convulsions (eclamptic) (uremic)	642.64	642.62	642.60		760.0
with pre-existing hypertension	642.74	642.72	642.70		760.0
Cracked nipple (postpartum)	676.14	676.12	676.10		
Cyst					
ovary	654.44	654.42	654.40		763.89
pelvic	654.44	654.42	654.40		763.89
Cystitis	646.64	646.62	646.60	condition	760.1
Cystocele	654.44	654.42	654.40		763.89
Damage					
coccyx, complicating delivery	665.64		665.60		763.89
pelvic (during delivery)					
joint or ligament	665.64		665.60		763.89
organ	665.54		665.50		763.89
Death, maternal, NEC					
during delivery	668.94	668.92	668.90		761.6
postpartum (cause not stated) (sudden)	674.94	674.92	674.90		
under anesthesia NEC	668.94	668.92	668.90		761.6
Deciduitis	646.64	646.62	646.60		760.8
postpartum	670.84	670.82	670.80		
Defect, defective coagulation (factor)					
postpartum	666.34	666.32	666.30		
Deficiency, deficient coagulation (factor)					
postpartum	666.34	666.32	666.30		
Deformity					
pelvic, pelvis					
soft part, organs or tissues NEC	654.94	654.92	654.90	cause	763.89
Dehiscence (postpartum)					
cesarean wound	674.14	674.12	674.10		
episiotomy	674.24	674.22	674.20		
perineal wound	674.24	674.22	674.20		
uterine wound	674.14	674.12	674.10		
Dependence, maternal					
drug	648.34	648.32	648.30	condition	779.5
Depression, postpartum	648.44	648.42	648.40	condition	
Dermatitis, gestationis	646.84	646.82	646.80	condition	
Detachment					
cervix, annular	665.34		665.30		763.89
Diabetes					
with long term (current) insulin use				V58.67	775.0
condition present before pregnancy	648.04	648.02	648.00	condition	775.0
gestational (chemical) (latent)	648.84	648.82	648.80	condition	775.0
Diastasis, recti (abdomen) **complicating delivery**	665.84	665.82	665.80		763.89
Difficult delivery NEC	669.94	669.92	669.90		763.89
Difficulty with breast feeding	676.84	676.82	676.80		
Dilatation					
bladder (sphincter)	654.44	654.42	654.40		763.89
Disease, NEC (postpartum)	674.94	674.92	674.90		
breast NEC	676.34	676.32	676.30		
cerebrovascular, NEC	674.04	674.02	674.00		
Frommel's	676.64	676.62	676.60		
heart	648.64	648.62	648.60	condition	760.8
postpartum	674.84	674.82	674.80		
renal NEC	646.24	646.22	646.20	condition	760.1
Valsuani's (progressive pernicious anemia, puerperal)	648.24	648.22	648.20	condition	
venereal NEC	647.24	647.22	647.20	condition	
virus NEC	647.64	647.62	647.60	condition	
Disorders					
breast, postpartum	676.34	676.32	676.30		
genital tract or organ	646.64	646.62	646.60	condition	760.8
lactation	676.94	676.92	676.90		
mental	648.44	648.42	648.40	condition	

Postpartum Pregnancy
Condition or Complication; affecting management of mother

	Postpartum condition or complication	Delivered with mention of postpartum complication	Unspecified episode of care	Assign additional code to describe the…	Affecting newborn (coded on the newborn chart only)
Disorders — *continued*					
metabolism NEC (in labor and delivery)	669.04	669.02	669.00		
specified type NEC	676.84	676.82	676.80		763.8
Displacement, uterus NEC	654.44	654.42	654.40		
Disruption, wound					763.8
cesarean operation	674.14	674.12	674.10		
episiotomy	674.24	674.22	674.20		
perineal (obstetric)	674.24	674.22	674.20		
uterine	674.14	674.12	674.10		
Distortion					
maternal	669.04	669.02	669.00		
Double uterus	654.04	654.02	654.00		
Drug dependence	648.34	648.32	648.30	condition	763.89
Dyscrasia, blood					
postpartum	666.34	666.32	666.30		
Dysfunction					
thyroid	648.14	648.12	648.10	condition	
Dysplasia of cervix	654.64	654.62	654.60		
Eclampsia, eclamptic	642.64	642.62	642.60		763.89
with pre-existing hypertension	642.74	642.72	642.70		760.0
Edema	646.14	646.12	646.10	condition	760.0
with hypertension — *see* Pregnancy, toxemia					
cervix (postpartum)	674.84	674.82	674.80		
Effect, adverse					
anesthetic (in labor and delivery) NEC	668.94	668.92	668.90		763.5
Embolism					
air (pulmonary)	673.04	673.02	673.00		
amniotic fluid	673.14	673.12	673.10		
blood clot	673.24	673.22	673.20		
brain (postpartum)	674.04	674.02	674.00		
cerebral (postpartum)	674.04	674.02	674.00		
fat (cerebral) (pulmonary) (systemic)	673.84	673.82	673.80		
heart	674.84	674.82	674.80		
intracranial (venous sinus) (nonpyogenic)	671.54	671.52	671.50		
pulmonary NEC	673.24	673.22	673.20		
pyemic	673.34	673.32	673.30		
septic	673.34	673.32	673.30		
specified NEC	674.84	674.82	674.80		
spinal cord	671.54	671.52	671.50		
Emesis (gravidarum) — *see* Pregnancy, vomiting					
Endometritis	670.14	670.12	670.10	condition	760.8
decidual	670.14	670.12	670.10	condition	760.8
postpartum	670.14	670.12	670.10		
puerperal	670.14	670.12	670.10		
Engorgement, breast (postpartum)	676.24	676.22	676.20		
Epilepsy	649.44	649.42	649.40	345.00-345.91	
Erysipelas (postpartum, childbirth)	670.84	670.82	670.80		
Eversion, uterus					
complicating delivery	665.24	665.22	665.20		763.89
postpartum	674.84	674.82	674.80		
Excessive					
milk secretion	676.64	676.62	676.60		
weight gain	646.14	646.12	646.10	condition	
Exhaustion (complicating delivery)	669.84	669.82	669.80		763.89
Extraction					
manual NEC	669.84	669.82	669.80		763.89
Extroversion, uterus (complicating delivery)	665.24	665.22	665.20		763.89
Failure, failed					
heart, complicating					
delivery (cesarean) (instrumental)	669.44	669.42	669.40		
obstetric anesthesia or sedation	668.14	668.12	668.10		
lactation	676.44	676.42	676.40		
renal following labor and delivery (acute)	669.34	669.32	669.30		
Fatigue	646.84	646.82	646.80	condition	
Febris puerperalis	672.04	672.02	672.00		
Female genital mutilation	648.94	648.92	648.90	629.20-629.29	

Coding Tables

Postpartum Pregnancy

Postpartum Pregnancy Condition or Complication; affecting management of mother	Postpartum condition or complication	Delivered with mention of postpartum complication	Unspecified episode of care	Assign additional code to describe the…	Affecting newborn (coded on the newborn chart only)
Fever	672.04	672.02	672.00		
childbed	670.24	670.22	670.20	Sepsis, 995.92, organ failure	
milk	672.04	672.02	672.00		
sepsis	670.24	670.22	670.20	Sepsis, 995.92, organ failure	
Fibrinolysis postpartum	666.34	666.32	666.30		
Fibroid tumor(s)	654.14	654.12	654.10		763.89
Fibromyoma (uterus)	654.14	654.12	654.10		763.89
Fibrosis, fibrotic					
perineum	654.84	654.82	654.80		763.89
Fissure, nipple (postpartum)	676.14	676.12	676.10		
Fistula (postpartum)					
breast, mammary gland	675.14	675.12	675.10		
nipple	675.04	675.02	675.00		
Forced birth or delivery NEC	669.84	669.82	669.80		763.89
Fractured coccyx complicating delivery	665.64		665.60		
Frommel's disease	676.64	676.62	676.60		
Frommel-Chiari syndrome	676.64	676.62	676.60		
Galactocele (breast)**, postpartum**	676.84	676.82	676.80		
Galactorrhea	676.64	676.62	676.60		
Gangrene					
gas (bacillus) postpartum, childbirth	670.84	670.82	670.80		
Genital (female) **mutilation**	648.94	648.92	648.90	629.20-629.29 condition	
Goiter	648.14	648.12	648.10	condition	760.2
Gonococcal infection	647.14	647.12	647.10	condition	760.2
Gonorrhea	647.14	647.12	647.10	condition	760.2
HELLP	642.54	642.52	642.50		
Hematoma					
broad ligament	665.74	665.72	665.70		
cesarean section wound	674.34	674.32	674.30		
complicating delivery (perineum) (vulva)	664.54		664.50		
pelvic	665.74	665.72	665.70		
vagina	665.74	665.72	665.70		
episiotomy	674.34	674.32	674.30		
obstetrical surgical wound	674.34	674.32	674.30		
pelvis, complicating delivery	665.74	665.72	665.70		
perineal wound	674.34	674.32	674.30		
complicating delivery	664.54		664.50		
vagina	665.74	665.72	665.70		
vulva, complicating delivery	664.54		664.50		767.8
Hematosalpinx, infectional	670.84	670.82	670.80		
Hemiplegia, cerebral	674.04	674.02	674.00		
Hemolysis, liver dysfunction, low platelets syndrome	642.54	642.52	642.50		
Hemorrhage					
brain (postpartum, childbirth)	674.04	674.02	674.00		
bulbar	674.04	674.02	674.00		
cerebrovascular	674.04	674.02	674.00		
cesarean section wound	674.34	674.32	674.30		
retained					
placenta	666.04	666.02	666.00		
secundines	666.24	666.22	666.20		
delayed, postpartum	666.24	666.22	666.20		
due to					
episiotomy	674.34	674.32	674.30		
extradural	674.04	674.02	674.00		
internal capsule	674.04	674.02	674.00		
intracranial, postpartum, childbirth	674.04	674.02	674.00		
intrapontine	674.04	674.02	674.00		
obstetrical surgical wound	674.34	674.32	674.30		
perineal wound	674.34	674.32	674.30		
postpartum (atonic) (following delivery of placenta)	666.14	666.12	666.10		
pontine	674.04	674.02	674.00		
subarachnoid	674.04	674.02	674.00		
subcortical	674.04	674.02	674.00		

Coding Tables

Postpartum Pregnancy

Postpartum Pregnancy Condition or Complication; affecting management of mother	Postpartum condition or complication	Delivered with mention of postpartum complication	Unspecified episode of care	Assign additional code to describe the…	Affecting newborn (coded on the newborn chart only)
Hemorrhage — *continued*					
subdural	674.04	674.02	674.00		
delayed or secondary (after 24 hours)	666.24	666.22	666.20		
retained placenta	666.04	666.02	666.00		
third stage	666.04	666.02	666.00		
subarachnoid, postpartum, childbirth	674.04	674.02	674.00		
subdural, postpartum, childbirth	674.04	674.02	674.00		
third stage	666.04	666.02	666.00		
uterine, delayed	666.24	666.22	666.20		
ventricular	674.04	674.02	674.00		
Hemorrhoids	671.84	671.82	671.80		
Hepatitis, viral	647.64	647.62	647.60	condition	
Hepatorenal syndrome	674.84	674.82	674.80		
Herniation of uterus	654.44	654.42	654.40		
Herpes, herpetic	647.64	647.62	647.60	condition	
gestationis	646.84	646.82	646.80	condition	
Hydroa gestationis	646.84	646.82	646.80	condition	
Hypersecretion of milk	676.64	676.62	676.60		
Hypertension	642.94	642.92	642.90		760.0
with					
albuminuria (and edema) (mild)	642.44	642.42	642.40		760.0
severe	642.54	642.52	642.50		760.0
edema (mild)	642.44	642.42	642.40		760.0
severe	642.54	642.52	642.50		760.0
heart disease	642.24	642.22	642.20		760.0
and renal disease	642.24	642.22	642.20		760.0
pre-eclampsia or eclampsia	642.74	642.72	642.70		760.0
renal disease	642.24	642.22	642.20		760.0
and heart disease	642.24	642.22	642.20		760.0
benign	642.04	642.02	642.00		760.0
chronic	642.04	642.02	642.00		760.0
pre-existing	642.04	642.02	642.00		760.0
chronic	642.04	642.02	642.00		760.0
essential	642.04	642.02	642.00		760.0
with pre-eclampsia or eclampsia	642.74	642.72	642.70		760.0
gestational	642.34	642.32	642.30		
malignant	642.24	642.22	642.20		
chronic	642.24	642.22	642.20		760.0
with pre-eclampsia or eclampsia	642.74	642.72	642.70		760.0
pre-existing	642.24	642.22	642.20		760.0
pre-existing	642.04	642.02	642.00		
secondary to renal disease	642.14	642.12	642.10		760.0
with pre-eclampsia or eclampsia	642.74	642.72	642.70		760.0
transient	642.34	642.32	642.30		
Hypertensive					
heart and renal disease	642.24	642.22	642.20		760.0
heart disease	642.24	642.22	642.20		760.0
renal disease	642.24	642.22	642.20		760.0
Hyperthyroidism	648.14	648.12	648.10	condition	
Hypotonic uterus	666.14	666.12	666.10		
Hypertonicity	648.14	648.12	648.10	condition	763.7
Hypertrophy					
breast (postpartum)	676.34	676.32	676.30		
uterus (postpartum)	674.84	674.82	674.80		
Hypotension (following labor and delivery)	669.24	669.22	669.20		
Hypothyroidism	648.14	648.12	648.10	condition	
Hysteralgia	646.84	646.82	646.80	condition	
Incarceration, uterus	654.34	654.32	654.30		
Incompetent cervix (os)	654.54	654.52	654.50		763.1
Increased anticoagulants (postpartum)	666.34	666.32	666.30		761.0
In double uterus	654.04	654.02	654.00		
Indurated breast (postpartum)	676.34	676.32	676.30		763.89
Inertia of uterus	666.14	666.12	666.10		
Infantile					
genitalia, genitals	654.44	654.42	654.40		763.89

Postpartum Pregnancy Condition or Complication; affecting management of mother	Postpartum condition or complication	Delivered with mention of postpartum complication	Unspecified episode of care	Assign additional code to describe the...	Affecting newborn (coded on the newborn chart only)
Infarct, infarction	674.04	674.02	674.00		
brain (stem), postpartum, childbirth	647.94	647.92	647.90	condition	760.2
Infection	646.64	646.62	646.60	condition	
Bartholin's gland	646.64	646.62	646.60	condition	
bladder	675.24	675.22	675.20		
breast (mammary gland), postpartum	675.94	675.92	675.90		
with nipple	675.84	675.82	675.80		
specified type NEC	675.24	675.22	675.20		
nonpurulent	675.14	675.12	675.10		
purulent	646.64	646.62	646.60	condition	
cervix (uteri)	674.34	674.32	674.30		
cesarean section wound	646.64	646.62	646.60	condition	
endocervix	674.34	674.32	674.30		
episiotomy	670.84	670.82	670.80		
fallopian tube	670.04	670.02	670.00		
generalized	646.64	646.62	646.60	condition	760.8
genital organs	670.04	670.02	670.00		760.8
postpartum, childbirth	670.04	670.02	670.00		760.8
major (unspec.)	646.64	646.62	646.60	condition	760.8
minor or localized	646.64	646.62	646.60	condition	
intrauterine, complicating delivery	646.64	646.62	646.60	condition	760.1
kidney	675.04	675.02	675.00		
nipple	675.94	675.92	675.90		
with breast	675.84	675.82	675.80		
specified type NEC	670.84	670.82	670.80		
ovary	670.84	670.82	670.80		
pelvic	674.34	674.32	674.30		
perineal wound (obstetrical)	670.04	670.02	670.00		
postpartum (major) (unspec.)	646.64	646.62	646.60	condition	
minor	670.84	670.82	670.80		
other	670.04	670.02	670.00		
puerperal (major) (unspec.)	646.64	646.62	646.60	condition	
renal	670.84	670.82	670.80		
tubo-ovarian	646.64	646.62	646.60	condition	760.1
urinary (tract)	646.54	646.52	646.50	condition	760.1
asymptomatic	646.64	646.62	646.60	condition	760.1
UTI	646.54	646.52	646.50	condition	760.1
asymptomatic	646.64	646.62	646.60	condition	
vagina	647.84	647.82	647.80	complication	
Infective and parasitic diseases NEC	647.94	647.92	647.90	condition	760.8
Infestation					
Inflammation	675.04	675.02	675.00		
areola, postpartum	646.64	646.62	646.60	condition	
Bartholin's gland	646.64	646.62	646.60	condition	760.8
bladder	675.24	675.22	675.20		
breast (mammary gland), postpartum	646.64	646.62	646.60	condition	
cervix (uteri)	670.84	670.82	670.80		
fallopian tube	646.64	646.62	646.60	condition	760.8
genital organ	646.64	646.62	646.60	condition	760.8
urinary tract NEC	668.04	668.02	668.00		
Inhalation of stomach contents or secretions in labor and delivery	648.94	648.92	648.90	condition	
Injury	665.94	665.92	665.90		763.89
birth canal NEC	665.64		665.60		
coccyx, complicating delivery	665.94	665.92	665.90		763.89
genital organs, obstetrical trauma NEC	665.94	665.92	665.90		763.89
instrumental, obstetrical NEC	665.54		665.50		763.89
bladder	665.34		665.30		763.89
cervix	665.44		665.40		763.89
high vaginal	664.94		664.90		763.89
perineal NEC	664.84		664.80		763.89
periurethral	665.54		665.50		763.89
urethra	665.54		665.50		763.89
uterus	665.94	665.92	665.90		763.89
obstetrical NEC					

Postpartum Pregnancy Condition or Complication; affecting management of mother	Postpartum condition or complication	Delivered with mention of postpartum complication	Unspecified episode of care	Assign additional code to describe the…	Affecting newborn (coded on the newborn chart only)
Injury — *continued*	648.94	648.92	648.90	condition	
pelvic, complicating delivery					
floor	664.14		664.10		
joint or ligament	665.64		665.60		763.89
organs	665.54		665.50		763.89
periurethral tissue, complicating delivery	664.84		664.80		763.89
symphysis pubis, complicating delivery	665.64		665.60		763.89
Insufficient					763.89
prenatal care	V23.7				
weight gain	646.84	646.82	646.80	condition	
Newborn "light-for-dates" without mention of fetal malnutrition					
unspecified (weight)					
< 500 gms					764.00
500-749 gms					764.01
750-999 gms					764.02
1,000-1,249 gms					764.03
1,250-1,499 gms					764.04
1,500-1,749 gms					764.05
1,750-1,999 gms					764.06
2,000-2,499 gms					764.07
≥ 2,500 gms					764.08
					764.09
Intoxication					
drug					
obstetric anesthetic or sedation	668.94	668.92	668.90		763.5
septic, postpartum, childbirth	670.24	670.22	670.20	Sepsis, 995.92, organ failure	
Inversion					
nipple, postpartum	676.34	676.32	676.30		
uterus, complicating delivery	665.24	665.22	665.20		763.89
Ischemia, cerebral (postpartum, childbirth)	674.04	674.02	674.00		
Joint disorders	648.74	648.72	648.70	condition	
Labor		649.82			
onset (spontaneous) after 37 completed weeks of gestation but before 39 completed weeks of gestation, with delivery by (planned) cesarean section					
Laceration (obstetrical trauma)					
Anus, anal (sphincter)complicating delivery					
with third degree perineal laceration	664.24		664.20		
w/mucosa	664.34		664.30		
w/o third degree perineal laceration	664.64		664.60		
old (healed)	654.84		654.80		
bladder	665.54		665.50		
bowel	665.54		665.50		
broad ligament	665.64		665.60		
central	664.44		664.40		
cervix (uteri)	665.34		665.30		
fourchette	664.04		664.00		
labia	664.04		664.00		
pelvic					
floor (muscles)	664.14		664.10		
organ NEC	665.54		665.50		
perineum	664.44		664.40		
first degree	664.04		664.00		
second degree	664.14		664.10		
third degree	664.24		664.20		
fourth degree	664.34		664.30		
central	664.44		664.40		
involving					
anal sphincter	664.24		664.20		
fourchette	664.04		664.00		
hymen	664.04		664.00		
labia	664.04		664.00		
pelvic floor	664.14		664.10		
perineal muscles	664.14		664.10		

Coding Tables

Postpartum Pregnancy

Postpartum Pregnancy Condition or Complication; affecting management of mother	Postpartum condition or complication	Delivered with mention of postpartum complication	Unspecified episode of care	Assign additional code to describe the…	Affecting newborn (coded on the newborn chart only)
Laceration — *continued*					
perineum — *continued*					
involving — *continued*					
rectovaginal with septum	664.24		664.20		
with anal mucosa	664.34		664.30		
skin	664.04		664.00		
sphincter (anal)	664.24		664.20		
with anal mucosa	664.34		664.30		
vagina	664.04		664.00		
vaginal muscles	664.14		664.10		
vulva	664.04		664.00		
secondary	674.24	674.22	674.20		
peritoneum (obstetrical trauma)	665.54		665.50		
periurethral tissue (obstetrical trauma)	664.84		664.80		
rectovaginal septum	665.44		665.40		
with perineum	664.24		664.20		
involving anal or rectal mucosa	664.34		664.30		
urethra (obstetrical trauma)	665.54		665.50		
vagina (complicating delivery)	665.44		665.40		
with perineal involvement	664.04		664.00		
first degree	664.04		664.00		
second degree	664.14		664.10		
third degree	664.24		664.20		
fourth degree	664.34		664.30		
high	664.44		664.40		
muscles	664.14		664.10		
sulcus	665.44		665.40		
wall	665.44		665.40		
vulva (complicating delivery)	664.04		664.00		
Lactation, lactating (breast) (postpartum)					
defective	676.44	676.42	676.40		
disorder	676.94	676.92	676.90		
specified type NEC	676.84	676.82	676.80		
examination and/or care of mother	V24.1	V24.1	V24.1		
excessive	676.64	676.62	676.60		
failed	676.44	676.42	676.40		
mastitis NEC	675.24	675.22	675.20		
suppressed	676.54	676.52	676.50		
Late effect(s) (of)					
childbirth complication(s)	677	677	677	condition	
complication(s) of					
childbirth	677	677	677	condition	
delivery	677	677	677	condition	
postpartum	677	677	677	condition	
pregnancy	677	677	677	condition	
puerperium	677	677	677	condition	
Lateroversion, uterus	654.44	654.42	654.40		763.89
Lymphadenitis, breast postpartum	675.24	675.22	675.20		
Lymphangitis (postpartum)	670.84	670.82	670.80		
breast	675.24	675.22	675.20		
Malaria	647.44	647.42	647.40	condition	
Malformation					
pelvic organs or tissues	654.94	654.92	654.90		763.89
uterus (congenital)	654.04	654.02	654.00		
Malnutrition	648.94	648.92	648.90	condition	
Malposition					
pelvic organs or tissues	654.44	654.42	654.40		763.89
uterus or cervix	654.44	654.42	654.40		763.89
Malpresentation					
uterus or cervix	654.44	654.42	654.40		
Mammillitis, puerperal, postpartum	675.24	675.22	675.20		
Mammitis, puerperal, postpartum	675.24	675.22	675.20		
Mastitis					
lactational	675.24	675.22	675.20		
puerperal, postpartum, (interstitial) (nonpurulent) (parenchymatous)	675.24	675.22	675.20		

Postpartum Pregnancy

Condition or Complication; affecting management of mother	Postpartum condition or complication	Delivered with mention of postpartum complication	Unspecified episode of care	Assign additional code to describe the…	Affecting newborn (coded on the newborn chart only)
Mastitis — *continued*					
puerperal, postpartum, (interstitial) (nonpurulent) (parenchymatous) — *continued*					
purulent	675.14	675.12	675.10		
stagnation	675.24	675.22	675.20		
puerperalis	675.24	675.22	675.20		
retromammary (puerperal, postpartum)	675.14	675.12	675.10		
submammary (puerperal, postpartum)	675.14	675.12	675.10		
Maternal obesity syndrome	646.14	646.12	646.10	condition	
Membrane, retained (complicating delivery) (with hemorrhage)	666.24	666.22	666.20		
without hemorrhage	667.14	667.12	667.10		
Mendelson's syndrome	668.04	668.02	668.00		
Mental disorders	648.44	648.42	648.40	condition	
Metritis (puerperal, postpartum, childbirth)	670.14	670.12	670.10		
Metroperitonitis	670.84	670.82	670.80		
Metrorrhagia	666.24	666.22	666.20		
Metrorrhagia, postpartum	666.24	666.22	666.20		
Metrosalpingitis	670.84	670.82	670.80		
Metrovaginitis	670.84	670.82	670.80		
Milk					
excess secretion	676.64	676.62	676.60		
fever	672.04	672.02	672.00		
retention	672.04	672.02	672.00		
Milk leg (deep vessels)	671.44	671.42	671.40		
Monoplegia, cerebral	674.04	674.02	674.00		
Myocardiopathy (postpartum)	674.84	674.82	674.80		
Myoma uterus (cervix) (corpus)	654.14	654.12	654.10		763.89
Myxedema (postpartum)	674.84	674.82	674.80		
Necrosis					
genital organ or tract	646.64	646.62	646.60	condition	
kidney, cortical (acute)	646.24	646.22	646.20	condition	760.8
following labor and delivery	669.34	669.32	669.30		760.1
liver, puerperal, postpartum	674.84	674.82	674.80		
ovary	670.84	670.82	670.80		
renal, cortical	646.24	646.22	646.20	condition	760.1
tubular	646.24	646.22	646.20	condition	760.1
following labor and delivery	669.34	669.32	669.30		
Nephritis, nephrosis	646.24	646.22	646.20	condition	760.1
with hypertension	642.14	642.12	642.10		760.0
Nephropathy NEC	646.24	646.22	646.20	condition	
Neuritis (peripheral)	646.44	646.42	646.40	condition	
puerperal, postpartum	646.44	646.42	646.40	condition	
Nutritional deficiency	648.94	648.92	648.90	condition	
Obesity					
excessive weight gain during pregnancy	646.14	646.12	646.10	complication	
morbid	649.14	649.12	649.10	278.00, 278.01, 278.03, V85.39-V85.45	
Obstetrical trauma NEC (complicating delivery)	665.94	665.92	665.90		763.89
Occlusion, precerebral artery NEC (puerperal, postpartum, childbirth)	674.04	674.02	674.00	condition	
Oliguria	646.24	646.22	646.20	condition	
with hypertension — *see* Pregnancy, toxemia					
following labor and delivery (postpartum)	669.34	669.32	669.30		
Oophoritis	646.64	646.62	646.60	condition	
Pain(s),	646.84	646.82	646.80	condition	
Paralysis, bladder	665.54		665.50		
Paralytic stroke	674.04	674.02	674.00		
Parametritis	670.84	670.82	670.80		
Paravaginitis	646.64	646.62	646.60	condition	
Patent cervix	654.54	654.52	654.50		761.0
Pelvic inflammatory disease	646.64	646.62	646.60	condition	
Pelviperitonitis	670.84	670.82	670.80		
Pendulous abdomen	654.44	654.42	654.40		763.89

Coding Tables *(left margin)*

Postpartum Pregnancy *(left margin)*

Postpartum Pregnancy Condition or Complication; affecting management of mother	Postpartum condition or complication	Delivered with mention of postpartum complication	Unspecified episode of care	Assign additional code to describe the…	Affecting newborn (coded on the newborn chart only)
Perforation					
bladder	665.54		665.50		
bowel	665.54		665.50		
broad ligament	665.64		665.60		
cervix	665.34		665.30		
instrumental (complicating delivery)	665.94	665.92	665.90		
pelvic (floor)	664.14		664.10		763.89
organ	665.54		665.50		763.89
urethral	665.54		665.50		763.89
uterus	665.54		665.50		
Perimetritis	670.14	670.12	670.10		
Perimetrosalpingitis	670.84	670.82	670.80		
Perinephritis	646.64	646.62	646.60	condition	
Perioophoritis	670.84	670.82	670.80		
Perisalpingitis	670.84	670.82	670.80		
Peritoneal infection	670.84	670.82	670.80		
Peritonitis	670.84	670.82	670.80		
Perivaginitis	670.84	670.82	670.80	condition	
Persistence					
hymen (tag)	654.84	654.82	654.80		
Phlebitis	671.94	671.92	671.90		760.3
deep, postpartum	671.44	671.42	671.40		
intracranial	671.54	671.52	671.50		
lower extremities	671.24	671.22	671.20	453.6, 453.71, 453.81	760.3
specified site NEC	671.54	671.52	671.50		
superficial	671.24	671.22	671.20	453.6, 453.71, 453.81	760.3
Phlegmasia alba dolens	671.44	671.42	671.40		
PID	646.64	646.62	646.60	condition	
Placenta, placental					
accreta	667.04	667.02	667.00		
with hemorrhage	666.04	666.02	666.00		
adherent	667.04	667.02	667.00		
with hemorrhage	666.04	666.02	666.00		
increta	667.04	667.02	667.00		
with hemorrhage	666.04	666.02	666.00		
percreta	667.04	667.02	667.00		
with hemorrhage	666.04	666.02	666.00		
polyp	674.44	674.42	674.40		
retention (without hemorrhage)	667.04	667.02	667.00		
fragments (delayed hemorrhage)	666.24	666.22	666.20		
without hemorrhage	667.14	667.12	667.10		
hemorrhage	666.04	666.02	666.00		
postpartum	666.24	666.22	666.20		
syphilitic	647.04	647.02	647.00	condition	760.2
manifest syphilis in the infant or fetus	647.04	647.02	647.00	condition	090.0
trapped	667.04	667.02	667.00		
with hemorrhage	666.04	666.02	666.00		
Pneumonitis					
aspiration	668.04	668.02	668.00	condition	770.18
postanesthetic	668.04	668.02	668.00	condition	
postoperative	668.04	668.02	668.00		
Polygalactia	676.64	676.62	676.60		
Polyp					
cervix	654.64	654.62	654.60		763.89
placenta	674.44	674.42	674.40		
uterus	654.14	654.12	654.10		763.89
Pyelocystitis	646.64	646.62	646.60	condition	
Pyelohydronephrosis	646.64	646.62	646.60	condition	
Pyelonephritis	646.64	646.62	646.60	condition	
Pyelonephrosis	646.64	646.62	646.60	condition	
Pyemia	670.24	670.22	670.20	Sepsis, 995.92, organ failure	
Pyocystitis	670.84	670.82	670.80	condition	
Pyohemia	670.04	670.02	670.00		
Pyometra	670.04	670.02	670.00		
Pyonephritis	670.84	670.82	670.80	condition	

Postpartum Pregnancy Condition or Complication; affecting management of mother	Postpartum condition or complication	Delivered with mention of postpartum complication	Unspecified episode of care	Assign additional code to describe the…	Affecting newborn (coded on the newborn chart only)
Pyonephrosis	670.84	670.82	670.80	condition	
Pyo-oophoritis	670.84	670.82	670.80		
Pyosalpingitis	670.84	670.82	670.80		
Pyosalpinx	670.84	670.82	670.80		
Prediabetes	648.84	648.82	648.80	condition	
Pre-eclampsia (mild)	642.44	642.42	642.40		760.0
with convulsions	642.64	642.62	642.60		760.0
severe	642.54	642.52	642.50		760.0
superimposed on pre-existing hypertensive disease	642.74	642.72	642.70		760.0
Pre-existing condition (prior to pregnancy) affecting current pregnancy					
abnormal glucose tolerance	648.84	648.82	648.80	condition	
anemia	648.24	648.22	648.20	condition	
bone and joint (lower limb)	648.74	648.72	648.70	condition	
cardiovascular	648.64	648.62	648.60	condition	
congenital	648.54	648.52	648.50	condition	
cerebrovascular	674.04	674.02	674.00		
diabetic	648.04	648.02	648.00	condition	
drug dependence	648.34	648.32	648.30	condition	
genital organ or tract	646.64	646.62	646.60	condition	
gonorrheal	647.14	647.12	647.10	condition	
hypertensive	642.24	642.22	642.20		
renal	642.14	642.12	642.10		
infectious	647.94	647.92	647.90	condition	
specified type NEC	647.84	647.82	647.80	condition	
malarial	647.44	647.42	647.40	condition	
nutritional deficiency	648.94	648.92	648.90	condition	
parasitic NEC	647.84	647.82	647.80	condition	
renal	646.24	646.22	646.20	condition	
hypertensive	642.14	642.12	642.10		
rubella	647.54	647.52	647.50	condition	
specified condition NEC	648.94	648.92	648.90	condition	
syphilitic	647.04	647.02	647.00	condition	
thyroid	648.14	648.12	648.10	condition	
tuberculous	647.34	647.32	647.30	condition	
urinary	646.64	646.62	646.60	condition	
venereal	647.24	647.22	647.20	condition	
viral NEC	647.64	647.62	647.60	condition	
Proteinuria (gestational)	646.24	646.22	646.20	condition	
with toxemia (mild) (pre-eclamptic)	642.44	642.42	642.40		760.0
with convulsion	642.64	642.62	642.60		760.0
with pre-existing hypertension	642.74	642.72	642.70		760.0
severe	642.54	642.52	642.50		760.0
Pruritus, pruritic	646.84	646.82	646.80	condition	
Psychosis or psychoneurosis	648.44	648.42	648.40	condition	
Ptyalism	646.84	646.82	646.80	condition	
Pyelitis	646.64	646.62	646.60	condition	
Pyrexia (of unknown origin) (PUO)					760.1
postpartum	672.04	672.02	672.00		
Reaction obstetric anesthetic or analgesic NEC	668.94	668.92	668.90		763.5
Rectocele	654.44	654.42	654.40		763.1
Renal					
disease or failure NEC	646.24	646.22	646.20	condition	
with secondary hypertension	642.14	642.12	642.10		
hypertensive	642.24	642.22	642.20		
shutdown following labor and delivery	669.34	669.32	669.30		
Repair of pelvic floor, previous	654.44	654.42	654.40		763.89
Retention, retained					
decidua (following delivery) (fragments)	667.14	667.12	667.10		
with hemorrhage	666.24	666.22	666.20		
membranes (following delivery)	667.14	667.12	667.10		
with hemorrhage	666.24	666.22	666.20		
milk (postpartum)	676.24	676.22	676.20		
placenta (total) (without hemorrhage)	667.04	667.02	667.00		
with hemorrhage	666.04	666.02	666.00		

Postpartum Pregnancy Condition or Complication; affecting management of mother	Postpartum condition or complication	Delivered with mention of postpartum complication	Unspecified episode of care	Assign additional code to describe the…	Affecting newborn (coded on the newborn chart only)
Retention, retained — *continued*					
portions or fragments	667.14	667.12	667.10		
with hemorrhage	666.24	666.22	666.20		
secundines (following delivery)	667.14	667.12	667.10		
with hemorrhage	666.24	666.22	666.20		
complicating puerperium (delayed hemorrhage)	666.24	666.22	666.20		
Retinitis	646.84	646.82	646.80	condition	
Retraction					
nipple (postpartum)	676.04	676.02	676.00		
Retroversion, uterus	654.34	654.32	654.30		763.89
Rigid, rigidity					
cervix	654.64	654.62	654.60		763.89
pelvic floor	654.44	654.42	654.40		763.89
perineum or vulva	654.84	654.82	654.80		763.89
vagina	654.74	654.72	654.70		763.89
Rubella (German measles)	647.54	647.52	647.50	condition	760.2
Rupture					
abdominal viscera	665.54		665.50		
bladder (sphincter)	665.54		665.50		
cervix (uteri	665.34		665.30		
pelvic floor	664.14		664.10		
perineum	664.44		664.40		
urethra	665.54		665.50		
vulva	664.04		664.00		
Sacculation	654.44	654.42	654.40		763.1
Salivation (excessive)	646.84	646.82	646.80	condition	
Salpingitis	646.64	646.62	646.60	condition	760.8
postpartum	670.84	670.82	670.80		
Salpingo-oophoritis	646.64	646.62	646.60	condition	760.8
postpartum	670.84	670.82	670.80		
Scar, scarring					
cervix	654.64	654.62	654.60		763.89
uterus NEC	654.94	654.92	654.90		763.89
Separation (obstetrical trauma)					
pubic bone	665.64		665.60		
symphysis pubis	665.64		665.60		
Sepsis					
postpartum	670.24	670.22	670.20	Sepsis, 995.92, organ failure	
puerperal	670.24	670.22	670.20	Sepsis, 995.92, organ failure	
Septicemia	647.84	647.82	647.80	condition	771.81
postpartum	670.24	670.22	670.20	Sepsis, 995.92, organ failure	
Septum, vagina	654.74	654.72	654.70		763.89
Shirodkar suture	654.54	654.52	654.50		
Shock					
complicating labor and delivery	669.14	669.12	669.10		
following labor and delivery	669.14	669.12	669.10		
Spasms					
uterus	646.84	646.82	646.80	condition	
Specified condition NEC	646.84	646.82	646.80	condition	
Stenosis (cicatricial)					
cervix, cervical (canal)	654.64	654.62	654.60		763.89
vagina	654.74	654.72	654.70		763.89
Stricture, cervix (canal)	654.64	654.62	654.60		763.89
Subinvolution of uterus (postpartum)	674.84	674.82	674.80		
Sudden death					
during childbirth	669.94	669.92	669.90		
postpartum	674.94	674.92	674.90		
Suppression of lactation	676.54	676.52	676.50		
Suppuration, suppurative of breast or mammary gland (postpartum)	675.14	675.12	675.10		
Surgery, previous					
cervix	654.64	654.62	654.60		763.89

Postpartum Pregnancy
Condition or Complication; affecting management of mother

	Postpartum condition or complication	Delivered with mention of postpartum complication	Unspecified episode of care	Assign additional code to describe the…	Affecting newborn (coded on the newborn chart only)
Surgery, previous — *continued*					
pelvic soft tissues NEC	654.94	654.92	654.90		763.89
perineum or vulva	654.84	654.82	654.80		
uterus NEC	654.94	654.92	654.90		763.89
vagina	654.74	654.72	654.70		
Suspended uterus	654.44	654.42	654.40		763.89
Suture, Shirodkar (with or without cervical incompetence)	654.54	654.52	654.50		
Syncope complicating delivery	669.24	669.22	669.20		
Syndrome					
acid pulmonary aspiration (Mendelson's)	668.04	668.02	668.00		
Chiari-Frommel	676.64	676.62	676.60		
dystocia, dystrophia	654.94	654.92	654.90		
Frommel-Chiari	676.64	676.62	676.60		
H.E.L.L.P (Hemolysis, Elevated Liver function and Low Platelets)	642.54	642.52	642.50		
hepatorenal following delivery	674.84	674.82	674.80		
hypotension, maternal	669.24	669.22	669.20		
maternal hypotension	669.24	669.22	669.20		
Mendelson's (during labor) (obstetric)	668.04	668.02	668.00		
Syphilis	647.04	647.02	647.00	condition	760.2
Tear, torn					
Anus, anal (sphincter)					
with third degree perineal laceration	664.24		664.20		
w/mucosa	664.34		664.30		
w/o third degree perineal laceration	664.64		664.60		
old (healed)	654.84		654.80		
bladder	665.54		665.50		763.89
bowel	665.54		665.50		763.89
broad ligament	665.54		665.50		763.89
cervix	665.34		665.30		763.89
pelvic					
floor	664.14		664.10		763.89
organ NEC	665.54		665.50		763.89
perineum	665.54		665.50		763.89
periurethral	664.84		664.80		763.89
urethra	665.54		665.50		
vulva	664.04		664.00		763.89
Tetanus, tetanic (puerperal, postpartum, childbirth)	670.84	670.82	670.80		
Thelitis (puerperal, postpartum)	675.04	675.02	675.00		
Thrombocytopenia (postpartum)	666.34	666.32	666.30		
Thrombophlebitis	671.24	671.22	671.20	453.6, 453.71, 453.81	760.3
cerebral (sinus) (vein), nonpyogenic	671.54	671.52	671.50		760.3
intracranial venous sinus, nonpyogenic	671.54	671.52	671.50		760.3
pelvic, postpartum	671.44	671.42	671.40		
septic (puerperal)	670.34	670.32	670..30		
specified site NEC	671.54	671.52	671.50		760.3
superficial	671.24	671.22	671.20	453.6, 453.71, 453.81	760.3
Thrombosis	671.94	671.92	671.90		
brain (artery) (stem)	674.04	674.02	674.00		
intracranial, venous sinus (nonpyogenic origin)	671.54	671.52	671.50		
pelvic	671.44	671.42	671.40		
postpartum	671.94	671.92	671.90		
brain (artery) (stem)	674.04	674.02	674.00		
venous	671.54	671.52	671.50		760.3
cardiac	674.84	674.82	674.80		
cerebral (artery)	674.04	674.02	674.00		
venous	671.54	671.52	671.50		760.3
deep (vein)	671.44	671.42	671.40		
intracranial sinus (nonpyogenic) (venous)	671.54	671.52	671.50		760.3
pulmonary (artery)	673.24	673.22	673.20		
specified site NEC	671.54	671.52	671.50		
superficial	671.24	671.22	671.20	453.6, 453.71, 453.81	
spinal cord	671.54	671.52	671.50		
superficial	671.24	671.22	671.20	453.6, 453.71, 453.81	

Postpartum Pregnancy Condition or Complication; affecting management of mother	Postpartum condition or complication	Delivered with mention of postpartum complication	Unspecified episode of care	Assign additional code to describe the…	Affecting newborn (coded on the newborn chart only)
Thrombosis — *continued*					
venous (superficial)	671.24	671.22	671.20	453.6, 453.71, 453.81	
Thyroid dysfunction	648.14	648.12	648.10	condition	
Thyroiditis	648.14	648.12	648.10	condition	
Thyrotoxicosis	648.14	648.12	648.10	condition	
Tobacco use disorder	649.04	649.02	649.00		
Torsion of uterus	654.44	654.42	654.40		
Toxemia (mild) (pre-eclamptic)	642.44	642.42	642.40		760.0
with					760.0
convulsions	642.64	642.62	642.60		760.0
pre-existing hypertension	642.74	642.72	642.70		760.0
eclamptic	642.64	642.62	642.60		
with pre-existing hypertension	642.74	642.72	642.70		760.0
severe	642.54	642.52	642.50		760.0
Trapped placenta (without hemorrhage)	666.04	666.02	666.00		
with hemorrhage	667.04	667.02	667.00		
Trauma	648.94	648.92	648.90	condition	
during delivery NEC	665.94	665.92	665.90		760.5
obstetrical	665.94	665.92	665.90		760.5
previous pregnancy (major), affecting childbirth or postpartum management	V23.89	V23.89	V23.89		
Tuberculosis	647.34	647.32	647.30	condition	760.2
Tumor					
cervix	654.64	654.62	654.60		763.89
ovary	654.44	654.42	654.40		763.89
pelvic	654.94	654.92	654.90		763.89
pelvic organs or tissue NEC	654.44	654.42	654.40		763.89
uterus	654.14	654.12	654.10		763.89
vagina	654.74	654.72	654.70		763.89
vulva	654.84	654.82	654.80		763.89
Uremia (renal disease or failure) **NEC**	646.24	646.22	646.20	condition	760.1
with secondary hypertension	642.14	642.12	642.10		760.0
complicating labor and delivery	669.34	669.32	669.30		
hypertensive	642.24	642.22	642.20		760.0
Urethritis	646.64	646.62	646.60	condition	760.1
Urinary Tract Infection	646.64	646.62	646.60	condition	760.1
Uterine size date discrepancy	649.64	649.62	649.60		
UTI	646.64	646.62	646.60	condition	760.1
Vaginitis or vulvitis	646.64	646.62	646.60	condition	760.8
Valsuani's disease (progressive pernicious anemia, puerperal)	648.24	648.22	648.20	condition	
Varicose					
veins (legs)	671.04	671.02	671.00		
perineum	671.14	671.12	671.10		
vulva	671.14	671.12	671.10		
Varicosity, labia or vulva	671.14	671.12	671.10		
Varix (lower extremity)	671.04	671.02	671.00		
perineum	671.14	671.12	671.10		
vulva	671.14	671.12	671.10		
Venereal disease NEC	647.24	647.22	647.20	disease	
Viral disease NEC	647.64	647.62	647.60	disease	
Vulvitis	646.64	646.62	646.60	condition	760.8
Weight gain	646.14	646.12	646.10	condition	
insufficient	646.84	646.82	646.80	condition	
White leg, postpartum, childbirth	671.44	671.42	671.40		

Personal and Family History	Personal	Family	Notes
Abuse			
emotional	V15.42		Subcategory VI5.4 excludes history of conditions classifiable to 290-316 (see V11.0-V11.9)
neglect	V15.42		Subcategory VI5.4 excludes history of conditions classifiable to 290-316 (see V11.0-V11.9)
physical	V15.41		Subcategory VI5.4 excludes history of conditions classifiable to 290-316 (see V11.0-V11.9)

Personal and Family History

Personal and Family History	Personal	Family	Notes
Abuse — *continued*			
sexual	V15.41		Subcategory VI5.4 excludes history of conditions classifiable to 290-316 (see V11.0-V11.9)
Affective psychosis	V11.1	V17.0	V11.1 includes personal history of manic-depressive psychosis
			V17.0 excludes family history of mental retardation (see code V18.4)
Alcoholism	V11.3	V61.41	V17.0 excludes family history of mental retardation (see code V18.4)
Allergy to			
analgesic agent NEC	V14.6	V19.6	
anesthetic NEC	V14.4	V19.6	
antibiotic agent NEC	V14.1	V19.6	
anti-infective agent NEC	V14.3	V19.6	
arachnid bite	V15.06	V19.6	
diathesis	V15.09	V19.6	
drug allergy	V14.9	V19.6	
drug allergy, specified type NEC	V14.8	V19.6	
eggs	V15.03	V19.6	
food additives	V15.05	V19.6	
insect bite	V15.06	V19.6	
latex	V15.07	V19.6	
medicinal agents	V14.9	V19.6	
medicinal agents, specified type NEC	V14.8	V19.6	
milk products	V15.02	V19.6	
narcotic agent NEC	V14.5	V19.6	
nuts	V15.05	V19.6	
peanuts	V15.01	V19.6	
penicillin	V14.0	V19.6	
radiographic dye	V15.08	V19.6	
seafood	V15.04	V19.6	
serum	V14.7	V19.6	
specified food NEC	V15.05	V19.6	
specified nonmedicinal agents NEC	V15.09	V19.6	
spider bite	V15.06	V19.6	
sulfa	V14.2	V19.6	
sulfonamides	V14.2	V19.6	
therapeutic agent	V15.09	V19.6	
vaccine	V14.7	V19.6	
Anaphylactic shock	V15.09		
Anaphylaxis	V13.81	V19.6	
Anemia	V12.3	V18.2	For family history of other blood disorders, see code V18.3
Anomaly (corrected)			
circulatory system	V13.65	V19.5	
cleft lip, palate	V13.64	V19.5	V13.64 also includes malformations (corrected) of eye, ear, face and neck
digestive system	V13.67	V19.5	
genitourinary system	V13.62	V19.5	
musculoskeletal system	V13.68	V19.5	V13.68 includes malformations of integument and limbs
nervous system	V13.63	V19.5	
respiratory system	V13.66	V19.5	
Arrest, sudden cardiac	V12.53	V17.41	V12.5 excludes old myocardial infarction (412) and postmyocardial infarction syndrome (411.0)
			V12.53 includes successfully resuscitated sudden cardiac death
Arteriosclerosis (cardiovascular)	code to condition	V17.49	
Arthritis	V13.4	V17.7	
Asthma	code to condition	V17.5	
attack, transient ischemic (TIA)	V12.54	V17.1	V12.54 includes unspecified stroke without residual deficits
Benign neoplasm of brain	V12.41		
Blindness	code to condition	V19.0	
Blood disease	V12.3	V18.3	
Calculi, urinary	V13.01	V18.7	
Cardiovascular disease	V12.50	V17.49	
myocardial infarction	412	V17.3	
Carrier, genetic disease	V83.01-V83.89	V18.9	See category V84 for Genetic susceptibility to disease
Chemotherapy, antineoplastic	V87.41		V87.41 excludes long-term current drug use(see codes V58.61-V58.69)
Child abuse	V15.41		
Chronic respiratory condition NEC	V12.60	V17.6	
Cigarette smoking	V15.82		V15.82 excludes tobacco dependence (see code 305.1)
Circulatory system disease	V12.50	V17.3	V12.5 excludes old myocardial infarction (412) and postmyocardial infarction syndrome (411.0)
myocardial infarction	412	V17.3	

Personal and Family History	Personal	Family	Notes
Colonic polyps	V12.72	V18.51	
Combat and operational stress reaction	V11.4		
Congenital (corrected) **malformation**	V13.69	V19.5	
circulatory system	V13.65	V19.5	
digestive system	V13.67	V19.5	
ear	V13.64	V19.5	
eye	V13.64	V19.5	
face	V13.64	V19.5	
genitourinary system	V13.62	V19.5	
heart	V13.65	V19.5	
hypospadias	V13.61	V19.5	
integument (skin)	V13.68	V19.5	
limbs	V13.68	V19.5	
lip (cleft)	V13.64	V19.5	
musculsoskeletal	V13.68	V19.59	
nervous system	V13.63	V19.5	
palate (cleft)	V13.64	V19.5	
respiratory system	V13.66	V19.5	
specified type	V13.69	V19.5	
Consanguinity		V19.7	
Contact (exposure) (suspected)			
asbestos	V15.84		
bodily fluids, potentially hazardous	V15.85		
lead	V15.86		
Contraception	V15.7		
Coronary artery disease	V12.50	V17.3	V12.5 excludes old myocardial infarction (412) and postmyocardial infarction syndrome (411.0)
Cystic fibrosis	V12.69	V18.19	
Deafness	code to condition	V19.2	
Death, sudden, successfully resuscitated	V12.53	V17.41	V12.5 excludes old myocardial infarction (412) and postmyocardial infarction syndrome (411.0)
Deficit			
prolonged reversible ischemic neurologic (PRIND)	V12.54	V17.1, V17.2	V12.54 includes unspecified stroke without residual deficits
reversible ischemic neurologic (RIND)	V12.54	V17.1, V17.2	V12.54 includes unspecified stroke without residual deficits
Diabetes mellitus	code to condition	V18.0	
gestational	V12.21	V18.0	
Diathesis, allergic	V15.09	V19.6	
Digestive system disease	V12.70	V18.59	
peptic ulcer	V12.71	V18.59	
polyps, colonic	V12.72	V18.51	For family history of malignant neoplasm of gastrointestinal tract see code V16.0
specified NEC	V12.79	V18.59	
Disease (of)	V13.9	V19.8	
blood	V12.3	V18.3	
blood-forming organs	V12.3	V18.3	
cardiovascular system	V12.50	V17.49	
cerebrovascular system	V12.59	V17.2	
circulatory system	V12.50	V17.1, V17.3	
circulatory, specified NEC	V12.59	V17.1	
coronary artery	V12.50	V17.3	V12.5 excludes old myocardial infarction (412) and postmyocardial infarction syndrome (411.0)
digestive system	V12.70	V18.59	
peptic ulcer	V12.71	V18.59	
polyps, colonic	V12.72	V18.51	For family history of malignant neoplasm of gastrointestinal tract see code V16.0
digestive, specified NEC	V12.79	V18.59	
ear NEC	V12.49	V19.3	
eye NEC	V12.49	V19.19	
glaucoma	code to condition	V19.11	
hypertensive	V12.59	V17.49	
infectious	V12.00	V18.8	
malaria	V12.03	V18.8	
methicillin resistant Staphylococcus aureus (MRSA) V12.04	V12.04	V18.8	
MRSA (methicillin resistant Staphylococcus aureus) V12.04	V12.04	V18.8	
poliomyelitis	V12.02	V18.8	

Personal and Family History	Personal	Family	Notes
Disease (of) — *continued*			
infectious — *continued*			
specified NEC	V12.09	V18.8	
tuberculosis	V12.01	V18.8	
ischemic heart	V12.59	V17.3	
parasitic	V12.00	V18.8	V18.8Infectious and parasitic diseases
infectious/parasitic, specified NEC V12.09	V12.09	V18.8	V18.8Infectious and parasitic diseases
respiratory system	V12.60	V17.6	AHA CC Q2 1992 History of COPD is coded to 496, Chronic airway obstruction, not elsewhere classified.
pneumonia	V12.61	V18.8	
respiratory, specified NEC	V12.69	V17.6	
skin	V13.3	V19.4	
other, specified site NEC	V13.89	V19.8	
subcutaneous tissue	V13.3	V19.8	
trophoblastic	V13.1	V19.8	
affecting management of pregnancy	V23.1		
vaginal dysplasia	V13.23		
vulvar dysplasia	V13.24		
Disorder (of)	V13.9		
endocrine	V12.29	V18.19	
diabetes mellitus	code to condition	V18.0	
gestational diabetes	V12.21		
multiple neoplasia [MEN] syndrome	V12.29	V18.11	
genital system	V13.29	V18.7	
vaginal dysplasia	V13.23		
vulvar dysplasia	V13.24		
hematological	V12.3	V18.3	
immunity	V12.29	V19.8	V12.29 Personal history of endocrine, metabolic, and immunity disorders
kidney	code to condition	V18.69	
polycystic	code to condition	V18.61	
mental	V11.9	V17.0	V17.0 excludes family history of mental retardation (see code V18.4)
affective type	V11.1	V17.0	V11.1 includes a personal history of manic-depressive psychosis V17.0 excludes family history of mental retardation (see code V18.4)
combat and operational stress reaction	V11.4		
manic-depressive	V11.1	V17.0	V11.1 includes a personal history of manic-depressive psychosis V17.0 excludes family history of mental retardation (see code V18.4)
neurosis	V11.2	V17.0	V17.0 excludes family history of mental retardation (see code V18.4)
schizophrenia	V11.0	V17.0	V17.0 excludes family history of mental retardation (see code V18.4)
mental, specified type NEC	V11.8	V17.0	
metabolic	V12.29	V18.19	
musculoskeletal NEC	V13.59	V17.89	
osteoporosis	code to condition	V17.81	
nervous system	V12.40	V17.2	
nervous, specified type NEC	V12.49	V17.2	
obstetric	V13.29		
affecting management of current pregnancy	V23.49		
pre-term labor	V23.41		
pre-term labor	V13.21		
psychiatric condition	V11.9	V17.0	
sense organs	V12.40	V19.0-V19.4	
sense organs, specified type NEC	V12.49	V19.0-V19.4	
other, specified site NEC	V13.89	V19.8	
urinary system	V13.00	V18.61, V18.69, V18.7	
calculi	V13.01	V18.69, V18.7	
infection	V13.02	V18.69, V18.7	
nephrotic syndrome	V13.03	V18.69	
urinary, specified NEC	V13.09	V18.61, V18.69, V18.7	
Drug therapy			See code 305.9 for patent, nonprescribed (see also Abuse, drugs, nondependent)
antineoplastic chemotherapy	V87.41		
estrogen therapy	V87.43		
immunosuppression therapy	V87.46		
monoclonal drug therapy	V87.42		
other drug therapy	V87.49		
steroid therapy NOS	V87.45		
inhaled	V87.44		

Coding Tables

Personal and Family History

Personal and Family History	Personal	Family	Notes
Drug therapy — *continued*			
steroid therapy NOS — *continued*			
systemic	V87.45		
Dysplasia			V13.22 includes conditions in subcategories 622.10-622.12
cervical	V13.22	V18.7	Personal history of conditions classifiable to 623.0
vaginal	V13.23		Personal history of conditions classifiable to 624.01-624.02
vulvar	V13.24		
Effect NEC of external cause	V15.89	V19.8	
Embolism (pulmonary)	V12.55	V19.8	
Emotional abuse	V15.42		
Encephalitis	V12.42	V18.8	
Endocrine disorder	V12.29	V18.19	
multiple neoplasia [MEN] syndrome	V12.29	V18.11	
Epilepsy	code to condition	V17.2	
Extracorporeal membrane oxygenation (ECMO)	V15.87		
Failed conscious/moderate sedation	V15.80		
Falling	V15.88		Code V15.88 can be reported as either 1st-listed or secondary.
Foreign body, retained, fully removed	V15.53		
Fracture, healed			
pathologic	V13.51	V17.89	
stress	V13.52	V17.89	
traumatic	V15.51	V17.89	
Genetic disease carrier	V83.01-V83.89	V18.9	
Genital system disorder	V13.29	V18.7	
pre-term labor	V13.21		
Glaucoma	code to condition	V19.11	
Glomerulonephritis	code to condition	V18.69	
Gout	V12.29	V18.19	
Hay fever	V12.69	V17.6	
Health hazard	V15.9		
falling	V15.88		
specified cause NEC	V15.89		
Hearing loss	code to condition	V19.2	
Hematopoietic neoplasia	V10.79	V16.7	
Hepatitis, B or C	V12.09	V18.8	
Hodgkin's disease	V10.72	V16.7	
Huntington's chorea	code to condition	V17.2	
Hydrocephalus	code to condition	V19.5	
Hypertension	V12.59	V17.49	
Hypospadias (corrected)	V13.61	V19.5	
Immunity disorder	V12.29	V19.8	
Infarction, cerebral, without residual deficits	V12.54	V17.1	
Infarction, myocardial	412	V17.3	
Infection			
central nervous system	V12.42	V18.8	
urinary (tract)	V13.02	V18.7, V18.8	
Infectious disease	V12.00	V18.8	
malaria	V12.03	V18.8	
methicillin resistant Staphylococcus aureus (MRSA)	V12.04	V18.8	
MRSA (methicillin resistant Staphylococcus aureus)	V12.04	V18.8	
poliomyelitis	V12.02	V18.8	
specified NEC	V12.09	V18.8	
tuberculosis	V12.01	V18.8	
Injury NEC	V15.59		
fracture, healed			
pathologic	V13.51	V17.89	
stress	V13.52	V17.89	
traumatic	V15.51	V17.89	
traumatic brain	V15.52		
Insufficient prenatal care	V23.7		
In utero procedure			
during pregnancy	V15.21		
while a fetus	V15.22		
Irradiation	V15.3		
Ischemic heart disease	V12.59	V17.3	

Coding Tables

Personal and Family History

Personal and Family History	Personal	Family	Notes
Kidney disease	code to condition	V18.69	
polycystic	code to condition	V18.61	
Leukemia	V10.60	V16.6	
lymphoid	V10.61	V16.6	
monocytic	V10.63	V16.6	
myeloid	V10.62	V16.6	
specified type NEC	V10.69	V16.6	
Little or no prenatal care	V23.7		
Low birth weight	V21.30		Also see Status, low birth weight
Lymphatic malignant neoplasia NEC	V10.79	V16.7	
Lymphosarcoma	V10.71	V16.7	V10.7 includes conditions in categories 200-203 except those in remission
			V16.7 includes family history of conditons in categories 200-203
Malaria	V12.03	V18.8	V12.0 excludes personal history of specific body system infectious diseases
Malformations (corrected)			
circulatory system	V13.65		
cleft lip, palate	V13.64		V13.64 also includes malformations (corrected) of eye, ear, face and neck
digestive system	V13.67		
genitourinary system	V13.62		
musculoskeletal system	V13.68		V13.68 includes malformations of integument and limbs
nervous system	V13.63		
respiratory system	V13.66		
Malignant neoplasm (of)	V10.90	V16.9	
accessory sinus	V10.22	V16.2	
adrenal	V10.88	V16.7	V10.8 includes history of conditions in categories 170-173, 190-195
			V16.7 includes family history of conditons in categories 200-203
anorectal	V10.06	V16.0	
anus	V10.06	V16.0	V16.0 includes family history of conditions in categories 140-159
appendix	V10.09	V16.0	
bile duct	V10.09		V10.0 includes history of conditions in categories 140-159
bladder	V10.51	V16.52	V16.5 incudes family history of condition in categories 160-161, 163-165
bone	V10.81	V16.8	V16.8 includes family history of conditons in categories 140-199
brain	V10.85	V16.8	
breast	V10.3	V16.3	
male	V10.3	V16.8	
bronchus	V10.11	V16.1	V10.1 includes history of conditions in category 162
carcinoid tumor	V10.91	V16.8	Code V10.91 secondary to any continuing functional activity (e.g., 259.2)
cecum	V10.05	V16.0	
cervix uteri	V10.41	V16.49	
colon	V10.05	V16.0	
connective tissue NEC	V10.89	V16.8	
corpus uteri	V10.42	V16.49	
digestive system	V10.00	V16.0	
digestive, specified part NEC	V10.09	V16.0	
duodenum	V10.09	V16.0	
endocrine gland NEC	V10.88	V16.8	
epididymis	V10.48	V16.49	
esophagus	V10.03	V16.0	
eye	V10.84	V16.8	
fallopian tube	V10.44	V16.49	
female genital organ	V10.40	V16.40	
female genital, specified site NEC	V10.44	V16.49	
gallbladder	V10.09	V16.0	
gastrointestinal tract	V10.00	V16.0	
genital organs	V10.40, V10.45	V16.40	
gum	V10.02	V16.0	
hematopoietic NEC	V10.79	V16.7	
hypopharynx	V10.02	V16.0	
ileum	V10.09	V16.0	
ilium	V10.81	V16.8	
intestine	V10.05, V10.06	V16.0	
intrathoracic organs NEC	V10.20	V16.2	
jejunum	V10.09	V16.0	
kidney	V10.52	V16.51	
large intestine	V10.05	V16.0	
larynx	V10.21	V16.2	
lip	V10.02	V16.0	
liver	V10.07	V16.0	
lung	V10.11	V16.1	V10.1 includes history of conditions in category 162

Personal and Family History

Personal and Family History	Personal	Family	Notes
Malignant neoplasm (of) — *continued*			
lymph glands or nodes NEC	V10.79	V16.7	
lymphatic NEC	V10.79	V16.7	
male genital organ	V10.45	V16.40	
male genital, specified site NEC	V10.49	V16.49	
mediastinum	V10.29	V16.2	
melanoma (of skin)	V10.82	V16.8	
Merkel cell carcinoma	V10.91	V16.8	Code V10.91 secondary to any continuing functional activity (e.g., 259.2)
middle ear	V10.22	V16.2	
mouth	V10.02	V16.0	
mouth, specified part NEC	V10.02	V16.0	
nasal cavities	V10.22	V16.2	
nasopharynx	V10.02	V16.2	
nervous system NEC	V10.86	V16.8	
neuroendocrine tumor	V10.91	V16.8	Code V10.91 secondary to any continuing functional activity (e.g., 259.2)
nose	V10.22	V16.2	
oropharynx	V10.02	V16.0	
ovary	V10.43	V16.41	
oviduct	V10.44	V16.41	
pancreas	V10.09	V16.0	
parathyroid	V10.88	V16.8	
penis	V10.49	V16.49	
pharynx	V10.02	V16.0	
pineal	V10.88	V16.8	
pituitary	V10.88	V16.8	
placenta	V10.44	V16.49	
pleura	V10.29	V16.2	
prostate	V10.46	V16.42	
rectosigmoid junction	V10.06	V16.0	
rectum	V10.06	V16.0	
renal pelvis	V10.53	V16.59	
respiratory organs NEC	V10.20	V16.2	
salivary gland	V10.02	V16.0	
skin	V10.83	V16.8	
melanoma	V10.82	V16.8	
small intestine NEC	V10.09	V16.0	
soft tissue NEC	V10.89	V16.8	
specified site NEC	V10.89	V16.8	
stomach	V10.04	V16.0	
testis	V10.47	V16.43	
thymus	V10.29	V16.2	
thyroid	V10.87	V16.8	
tongue	V10.01	V16.0	
trachea	V10.12	V16.1	V10.1 includes history of conditions in category 162
ureter	V10.59	V16.59	
urethra	V10.59	V16.59	
urinary organ	V10.50	V16.59	
uterine adnexa	V10.44	V16.49	
uterus	V10.42	V16.49	
vagina	V10.44	V16.49	
vulva	V10.44	V16.49	
Manic-depressive psychosis	V11.1	V17.0	V17.0 excludes family history of mental retardation (see code V18.4)
Meningitis	V12.42	V18.8	
Mental disorder	V11.9	V17.0	V17.0 excludes family history of mental retardation (see code V18.4)
affective type	V11.1	V17.0	V17.0 excludes family history of mental retardation (see code V18.4)
combat and operational stress reaction	V11.4		
manic-depressive	V11.1	V17.0	V17.0 excludes family history of mental retardation (see code V18.4)
neurosis	V11.2	V17.0	V17.0 excludes family history of mental retardation (see code V18.4)
schizophrenia	V11.0	V17.0	V17.0 excludes family history of mental retardation (see code V18.4)
specified type NEC	V11.8	V17.0	V17.0 excludes family history of mental retardation (see code V18.4)
Mental retardation	code to condition	V18.4	
Merkel cell carcinoma	V10.91	V16.8	Code V10.91 secondary to any continuing functional activity (e.g., 259.2)
Metabolic disorder	V12.29	V18.19	
Methicillin resistant Staphylococcus aureus (MRSA)	V12.04	V18.8	
Mongolism	code to condition	V19.5	
Monoclonal drug therapy	V87.42		

Personal and Family History

Personal and Family History	Personal	Family	Notes
MRSA (methicillin resistant Staphylococcus aureus)	V12.04	V18.8	
Multiple endocrine neoplasia [MEN] syndrome	V12.29	V18.11	
Musculoskeletal disorder NEC	V13.59	V17.89	
osteoporosis	code to condition	V17.81	
Myeloma	V10.79	V16.7	
Myocardial infarction	412	V17.3	
Neglect (emotional)	V15.42		
Nephritis	V13.03	V18.69	
Nephrosis	V13.09	V18.69	
Nephrotic syndrome	V13.03	V18.69	
Nervous system disorder	V12.40	V17.2	
Nervous, specified type NEC	V12.49	V17.2	
Neurosis	V11.2	V17.0	V17.0 excludes family history of mental retardation (see code V18.4)
Noncompliance with medical treatment	V15.81		
Nutritional deficiency	V12.1		
Obstetric disorder	V13.89		
affecting management of current pregnancy	V23.49		
history of pre-term labor	V13.21		
pregnancy with history of ectopic pregnancy	V23.42		
pregnancy with history of pre-term labor	V23.41		
pregnancy with inconclusive fetal viability	V23.87		
Osteoporosis	code to condition	V17.81	
Parasitic disease	V12.00	V18.8	
parasitic/infectious, specified NEC	V12.09	V18.8	
Perinatal problems	V13.7		
low birth weight	V12.30		For V21.30 low birth weight see also Status, low birth weight
Physical abuse	V15.41		
Poisoning	V15.6		
Poliomyelitis	V12.02	V18.8	
Polycystic kidney disease	code to condition	V18.61	
Polyps, colonic	V12.72	V18.51	
Poor obstetric	V13.29		
affecting management of current pregnancy	V23.49		
history of pre-term labor	V13.21		
pregnancy with history of ectopic pregnancy	V23.42		
pregnancy with history of pre-term labor	V23.41		
pregnancy with inconclusive fetal viability	V23.87		
Prolonged reversible ischemic neurologic deficit (PRIND)	V12.54	V17.1, V17.2	
Psychiatric disorder	V11.9	V17.0	V17.0 excludes family history of mental retardation (see code V18.4)
affective type	V11.1	V17.0	V17.0 excludes family history of mental retardation (see code V18.4)
manic-depressive	V11.1	V17.0	V17.0 excludes family history of mental retardation (see code V18.4)
neurosis	V11.2	V17.0	V17.0 excludes family history of mental retardation (see code V18.4)
schizophrenia	V11.0	V17.0	V17.0 excludes family history of mental retardation (see code V18.4)
psychiatric, specified type NEC	V11.8	V17.0	V17.0 excludes family history of mental retardation (see code V18.4)
Psychological trauma	V15.49		
emotional abuse	V15.42		
neglect	V15.42		
physical abuse	V15.41		
rape	V15.41		
stress, combat and operational	V11.4		
Psychoneurosis	V11.2	V17.0	V17.0 excludes family history of mental retardation (see code V18.4)
Radiation therapy	V15.3		
Rape	V15.41		
Respiratory system disease	V12.60	V17.5, V17.6	
pneumonia	V12.61	V18.8	
respiratory, specified NEC	V12.69	V17.5, V17.6	
Retardation, mental	code to condition	V18.4	
Reticulosarcoma	V10.71	V16.7	V16.7 includes family history of conditions in cateogries 200-203
Retinitis pigmentosa	V12.49	V19.19	
Return from military deployment	V62.22		
Reversible ischemic neurologic deficit (RIND)	V12.54	V17.1, V17.2	
Schizophrenia	V11.0	V17.0	V17.0 excludes family history of mental retardation (see code V18.4)
Skin disease	V13.3	V19.4	
Smoking (tobacco)	V15.82		V15.82 excludes tobacco dependence (see code 305.1)

Coding Tables

Personal and Family History

Personal and Family History	Personal	Family	Notes
Stress, combat and operational	V11.4		
Status, low birth weight			
> 500 grams	V21.31		
500-999 grams	V21.32		
1000-1499 grams	V21.33		
1500-1999 grams	V21.34		
2000-2500	V21.35		
unspecified	V21.30		
Stroke without residual deficits	V12.54	V17.1	
Subcutaneous tissue disease	V13.3	V19.8	
Sudden			
cardiac arrest	V12.53	V17.41	V17.41 excludes family history of ischemic heart disease and myocardial infarction (see V17.3)
cardiac death (successfully resuscitated)	V12.53	V17.41	
Surgery to			
surgery, great vessels	V15.1		
surgery, heart	V15.1		
surgery, during pregnancy	V15.21		
surgery, while a fetus	V15.22		
surgery, organs NEC	V15.29		
Syndrome, nephrotic	V13.03	V18.69	
Therapy			
antineoplastic drug	V87.41		
drug NEC	V87.49		
estrogen	V87.43		
immunosuppression	V87.46		
monoclonal drug	V87.42		
steroid therapy NOS	V87.45		
inhaled	V87.44		
systemic	V87.45		
Thrombophlebitis	V12.52	V18.3	
Thrombosis	V12.51	V18.3	
Tobacco use	V15.82		V15.82 excludes tobacco dependence (see code 305.1)
Traumatic brain injury	V15.52		
Trophoblastic disease	V13.1	V19.8	
trophoblastic, affecting management of pregnancy	V23.1		
Tuberculosis	V12.01	V18.8	
Ulcer, peptic	V12.71	V18.59	
Underimmunization	V15.83		
Urinary system disorder	V13.00	V18.7	
calculi	V13.01	V18.7	
infection	V13.02	V18.7, V18.8	
nephrotic syndrome	V13.03	V18.69	
specified NEC	V13.09	V18.7	
Vaginal dysplasia	V13.23		
Visual loss	code to condition	V19.0	
Vulvar dysplasia	V13.24		